CARDIAC SURGERY

CARDIAC SURGERY

MORPHOLOGY, DIAGNOSTIC CRITERIA, NATURAL HISTORY, TECHNIQUES, RESULTS, AND INDICATIONS

JOHN W. KIRKLIN, MD

Professor and Surgeon
Cardiothoracic Division
Department of Surgery
University of Alabama at Birmingham
    Medical Center
Birmingham, Alabama
formerly
Professor and Surgeon (1950–1967)
Chairman, Department of Surgery (1964–1966)
Mayo Clinic and Mayo Foundation
Rochester, Minnesota
Chairman, Department of Surgery (1967–1982)
Director, Division of Cardiothoracic Surgery
    (1967–1985)
University of Alabama at Birmingham Medical
    Center
Birmingham, Alabama

BRIAN G. BARRATT-BOYES, KBE, MB, ChM

Surgeon-in-Charge
Cardiothoracic Surgical Unit
Green Lane Hospital
Surgeon to Mater Misericordiae Hospital
Professor of Surgery (Hon.)
University of Auckland
Auckland, New Zealand

Illustrations by John W. Desley

A WILEY MEDICAL PUBLICATION
JOHN WILEY & SONS
New York • Chichester • Brisbane • Toronto • Singapore

Copyright © 1986 by John Wiley & Sons, Inc.

Library of Congress Cataloging in Publication Data:

Kirklin, John W. (John Webster)
  Cardiac surgery.

  (A Wiley medical publication)
  Includes bibliographies and index.
  1. Heart—Surgery. I. Barratt-Boyes, Brian G.
II. Title. III. Series. [DNLM: 1. Heart Surgery.
WG 169 K59c]

RD598.K555 1986   617'.412   85-16938
ISBN 0-471-01416-8

Printed in the United States of America

10 9 8 7 6 5 4 3 2 1

FOREWORD

Perhaps you are like me in having fancied at one time or another the possibility of someday being able to encompass the entire body of essential information of a selected specialty and then "wrap it up" into a skillfully coordinated, comprehensive, concise compendium. Increasingly rare are the occasions when that fantasy can be transformed into reality. Indeed, for cardiac surgery, such an accomplishment may never again occur after this book. This is especially true if an aspiring author is also required to be a principal contributor to essentially every frontier of progress in the entire specialty. Thus, from its very inception, this book has been unique.

There was a time when I would have experienced an unwelcome sense of jealousy at encountering a remarkable volume such as this one—similar to the irrational frustration I typically experienced as a youth when listening to a virtuoso pianist. Why couldn't I play as well? But now, in maturity, I can enjoy such a performance without feeling the pain of my own inadequacies. So also can the outstanding accomplishments of this text now be appreciated. One can absorb its facts, benefit from its teaching, marvel at the skill of its authors, and still rigorously control one's envy. But it isn't easy!

It would be expected that my background of clinical experience as well as service as the editor of a journal of our specialty would assure reasonable familiarity with what is known in cardiac surgery. Nevertheless, as I have read through the various chapters of this book in a comprehensive manner, I have experienced afresh the thrill of discovering new knowledge, of setting straight some confusing and annoying misunderstandings regarding certain principles, and of filling in various lingering gaps in my knowledge. The entire expanse of cardiac surgery seems to be here, laid out in the same crisp, logical, fully documented style that we have all come to recognize and respect in the many other reports, lectures, and publications provided by these particular authors. Furthermore, not only does the book address the needs of those experienced in the subtleties of cardiac surgery, but it should serve equally well as an introduction for those just beginning the journey.

It is no exaggeration to suggest that Drs. Kirklin and Barratt-Boyes are well known by medical professionals throughout the world and are deeply and legitimately respected and admired by all of them. Though for the bulk of their careers they have worked at nearly diametrically opposite points on our globe, earlier they were associated for a time, when Brian Barratt-Boyes was a resident in cardiothoracic surgery at Mayo and John Kirklin was just embarking on his unique pioneering experience with the world's first continuous series of clinical cardiac operations using a pump oxygenator. Their subsequent collaboration through the years, culminating now in the production of this book, is evidence of their mutual respect. This tradition of cooperation between them has often resulted in a cross-fertilization of ideas and publication of analyses of their combined clinical experiences. It has also provided evidence of the shrunken dimensions of our modern world and strengthens the hope that one day such collaboration will be possible even among politicians, economists, ethicists, and every segment of society all over the world.

The temptation is great to proceed with documentation of the unexcelled qualifications of the authors of this text. A long listing of their accomplishments, honors, and awards could easily be provided to support this claim for their preeminence. Perhaps we must be content to note only that both are widely in demand by patients and referring physicians to assume responsibility for the detailed care of great numbers of patients with all types of cardiac pathology, and to note at the other end of the spectrum of acclaim that Sir Brian was knighted several years ago and that John Kirklin was recently extended the prestigious Gifted Teacher Award by the American College of Cardiology. And they have been recipients of most of the possible recognitions in between.

Whether a text is more valuable if each of its various chapters is written by a highly selected authority on the subject, or more valuable if written entirely by one or a handful of authors, with consequent advantages of consistency of style and integration of presentation, is debatable. But the question has become largely moot in modern times, particularly for the whole expanse of cardiac surgery, because the body of knowledge has become so vast that anything other than multiple authorship is increasingly impractical. The question is specifically irrelevant with respect to this book since, though it has only two authors, each chapter reflects their combined outstanding authority on that subject. Thus this text retains the advantages of both approaches. One wonders if this phenomenon can ever again be possible.

We live in an age unique for the rapid revelation of complexity and intricacy in the universe about us. So marvelous is the view that one is almost overwhelmed by fascination and excitement. In its particular way this book adds to that fascination. And even apart from the factual information and the technical descriptions that pack its pages, the book serves also as an example of artistic beauty. And I speak not only of the superb drawings of John Desley; the precise, comprehensive, compact presentation of its materials gives the work true literary status. If scientific literature can ever be regarded as subject to admiration in an artistic sense, this book can.

One enigma remains after studying the manuscript. How is something like this humanly possible for a pair of authors to accomplish, each carrying burdensome administrative, investigative, teaching, and clinical care loads, as well as coping with all of the multitudinous responsibilities and distractions imposed upon anyone who is an important leader in an extremely demanding specialty? It seems superhuman. I must accept this enigma as something inexplicable—another instance of the limitless capacity for human achievement. I come away from my reading of this book intellectually stimulated, freshly inspired, rededicated toward scientific ideals, and even newly reassured about the ultimate fulfillment of humanity's loftiest hopes. I think you will do likewise.

DWIGHT C. McGOON, MD
Professor of Surgery
Thoracic and Cardiovascular Surgery
Mayo Medical School
Mayo Clinic
Rochester, Minnesota

PREFACE

This book on cardiac surgery is designed to provide the information that is relevant to the surgical treatment of the various types of heart disease. It is based on our personal experiences, gathered during 70 combined man-years in cardiac surgery, during which approximately 50,000 open heart operations and 5,000 closed heart operations have been performed by our colleagues and us on cardiac surgical services that we have directed. This is stressed only to indicate the extent of the experience upon which the book is based.

The entire book (except Chapter 4) has been written and rewritten by both of us, not one chapter by one of us, another by the other, and so on. This has forced us to clarify our thoughts and reconcile our differences, much to the betterment of the result. The extensive contributions of surgeons, clinicians, and scientists from all over the world, as recorded in the medical and scientific literature, have been used throughout in an attempt to provide a complete and authoritative account.

A determined effort has been made to document all aspects of the text and, as part of that documentation, to present as completely as possible the early and late results of all the surgical procedures described. The surgical procedures are presented in complete detail and with illustrations to clarify the anatomy and the technical details of the operation. We have had personal experience with all the operations described under "Technique of Operation." Since the knowledge of the morphology of a condition is basic to its surgical treatment, the morphology is described in detail for each of the conditions. The surgeon should be able to evaluate the clinical features and diagnostic criteria in the patients for whom he or she accepts surgical responsibility, and these are presented in each instance. The indications for operation depend on a comparison of the results of surgical treatment with the natural history and with the results of nonsurgical treatment, and, therefore, the indications are presented near the end of each chapter or section. The indications will require continuous modification in the future as both medical and surgical treatment change. For the interest of the reader, historical notes are included in all but some of the first six chapters. This historical material is rendered reasonably accurate by the fact that we participated in and lived through the development of much of cardiac surgery. Unless it is recorded now, this history will be difficult to recapture in later years.

Part I discusses basic aspects of cardiac surgery, including a detailed discussion, in Chapter 6, of the methodology of making the comparisons that, among other things, underlie the determination of the indications for operation. The remainder of the book deals with the multitude of cardiac surgical problems that occur in ischemic heart disease (Part II), valvular heart disease (Part III), congenital heart disease (Part IV), cardiac rhythm disturbances (Part V), other cardiac conditions (Part VI), and thoracic and thoracoabdominal aortic diseases (Part VII). Since, in our opinion, there are important interrelations among these various aspects of cardiac surgery, they are presented together in one volume.

We have developed this knowledge and prepared this book with the intense collaboration of many people in various disciplines, most but not all of whom are in the institutions in which we work. Details of this are to be found in Acknowledgments. We know that there must be errors and omissions in the text, and for these we apologize. But we hope that the book represents reasonably well the current status of all aspects of cardiac surgery and can serve as a comprehensive and yet cohesive source book for surgeons, cardiologists, cardiac radiologists, pathologists, and others interested in heart disease. We hope also that, as refinements and improvements appear in the future, this book will help prevent the loss of old truths and knowledge as the new develop.

Some explanations of the conventions used in the text are in order. We believe the reader will want to know—and we want the reader to know—the source of unpublished data, photographs of specimens, cineangiograms, and who favors what when alternative methods or ideas are presented. Since one of us, Kirklin, currently works at the Medical Center of the University of Alabama at Birmingham (UAB) and the other, Barratt-Boyes, at Green Lane Hospital (GLH) in Auckland, New Zealand, the abbreviations UAB and GLH are used to indicate the origin of a particular table or statement. However, this is not to say that all of our institutional colleagues would support the details of the point of view or technique being put forth. The bibliographic references are characterized by the first letter of the last name of the first author and a number (such as [1.4]) rather than simply a number. This convention combines the convenience, simplicity, and brevity of a reference symbol in the text with the usefulness to the reader of being able easily to find the reference to a given author's paper in the chapter references, which are primarily arranged alphabetically. The secondary, numerical arrangement has no logic, and new references within each alphabetic subheading were simply added to the end of the list in that subheading without the need for renumbering all subsequent references. This method greatly simplified the preparation of the book and is recommended to others. The abbreviation CL is used throughout to denote 70% confidence limits around the point estimate. The reasons for presenting 70%, rather than 95% or 50% confidence limits, are described in Chapter 6. The drawings of surgical procedures are, with few exceptions, oriented as the field is seen from the position of the surgeon. In the case of open operations, this is from the patient's right side.

JOHN W. KIRKLIN
BRIAN G. BARRATT-BOYES

ACKNOWLEDGMENTS

Obviously, many of our colleagues participated in producing the experience, gathering the data, and generating the ideas expressed in this book. However, two people, Dr. Eugene H. Blackstone, professor of cardiovascular surgical research at the University of Alabama at Birmingham, and Dr. Louise Calder, pediatric cardiologist and morphologist at Green Lane Hospital in Auckland, New Zealand, played important roles in the development of every aspect of the book, and we extend our heartfelt thanks for their friendship, support, and contributions throughout the period of preparation.

Our surgical colleagues at the Mayo Clinic, Drs. F. Henry Ellis, Jr., Dwight C. McGoon, and Robert B. Wallace, played an important role in producing the results and generating the ideas from that early era (1950–1967). The current faculty cardiovascular surgeons at UAB, Drs. Albert D. Pacifico, George L. Zorn, Richard B. Shepard, James K. Kirklin, and David C. McGiffin, helped in a major way in producing the experiences (1967–1985) on which this book is based, and together we have developed a consistent but ever evolving approach to cardiac surgery. Drs. Robert B. Karp and Nicholas T. Kouchoukos were also important participants when they were part of the UAB experience. Dr. William Lell and his colleagues (UAB) provided superb cardiovascular anesthesia and were highly valued colleagues. Jarman Baxley directed the perfusionists (UAB) and was responsible for the excellence of their performance. Drs. Ricardo Ceballos and Jack Geer (UAB) gave expert support in cardiac pathology.

Throughout the GLH years (1956–1985), our surgical colleagues, Drs. Alan Kerr, Ken Graham, and David Hill, played an important role in the development of our knowledge, as did Drs. David Cole and Peter Clarke in an early part of that experience. Our anesthesia colleagues (GLH), Drs. Eve Seelye and Carl Moller, provided superb support and cooperation.

Drs. Patricia Clarkson, John Neutze, and James Lowe at GLH helped with many medical aspects throughout this text, as did Drs. L. M. Bargeron, Jr., William Rogers, and Vance Plumb at UAB. The cineangiograms from GLH were supplied and interpreted by Dr. Peter Brandt, and those from UAB by Drs. L. M. Bargeron, Jr., and Beningo Soto. Dr. Ceballos provided advice on the Morphology sections. The biomedical statistics (GLH) were supplied by Dr. R. M. L. Whitlock, with the expert assistance of Drs. Alastair Scott, Chris Wild, and John Pemberton of the Department of Mathematics, University of Auckland. The data analysis (UAB) was one of the results of the intimate collaboration of Dr. Blackstone throughout the preparation of the book. The preparation and photographs of anatomic specimens (GLH) were made possible by the generous and expert help of Dr. Louise Calder and Darren Brown.

The drawings of operations were made by John Desley of Rochester, Minnesota. Mr. Desley worked skillfully, long, and hard with his special expertise to capture anatomic details and operative steps with accuracy and clarity. He patiently redrew figures several times when they did not properly convey the sense of the operation or the anatomy and on a number of occasions provided original illustrative interpretations to clarify difficult subjects.

The manuscripts of the various chapters were prepared by our skillful co-workers Nancy Ferguson and Debbie Nuby, and earlier Sandy O'Brien, at UAB; and Doreen Gibson at GLH. The compilation of these chapters into a cohesive whole and the completion of the thousands of details that go into the making of a book were done expertly and cheerfully by Ms. Nuby and Ms. Ferguson. The patient cooperation initially of Ray Moloney and Linda Turner, and during the editing and actual production of the book of Rosalind Straley and Margery Carazzone at John Wiley & Sons, made our relations with the publisher a great joy.

The initial preparation of many of the chapters has been aided by a number of individuals. Some were at that time residents or registrars in cardiothoracic surgery, including Warren W. Bailey (UAB), Thomas J. Berger (UAB), Vincent R. Conti (UAB), Richard J. Cyrus (UAB), Larry S. Fox (UAB), Jacob Goldstein (GLH), Allan Hilless (GLH), Richard A. Jones (GLH), Nevin M. Katz (UAB), Garth McDonald (GLH), Lynn B. McGrath (UAB), John Pigott (UAB), Peter Raudkivi (GLH), Clive Robinson (GLH), Richard G. Rouse (UAB), Johan Steyn (GLH), and Robert W. Stewart (UAB). Others were special fellows in cardiothoracic surgery (UAB), including Azai Appelbaum, Enrique G. Bertranou, K. M. Cherian, John G. Coles, Joseph Defauw, Harold D. Head, F. Sallis Hill, Jean-Marc Jarry, Claude Labrosse, Yves Leclerc, Fernando Lucchese, Roxanne McKay, Carlos A. Nojek, Richard R. Reynolds, Ismail Sallam, Guglielmo Stefanelli, Carlo Valfre, Stephen Westaby, and Frederick E. Wideman. Some were faculty or consultant staff, including Trevor Agnew (GLH), Edwin L. Bradley (UAB), Peter Brandt (GLH), L. P. Elliott (UAB),

Ed Harris (GLH), Thomas N. James (UAB), James K. Kirklin (UAB), Carl Moller (GLH), David C. Naftel (UAB), Vance J. Plumb (UAB), Harry Rea (GLH), A. H. G. Roche (GLH), William J. Rogers (UAB), John Rutherford (GLH), Eve Seelye (GLH), Warren Smith (GLH), Richard B. Shepard (UAB), Malcolm E. Turner, Jr. (UAB), and Harvey White (GLH).

JOHN W. KIRKLIN
BRIAN G. BARRATT-BOYES

CONTENTS

CARDIAC SURGERY

GENERAL CONSIDERATIONS

PART I

ANATOMY AND TERMINOLOGY

CARDIAC CHAMBERS AND MAJOR VESSELS

The accurate diagnosis of complex congenital heart defects depends on identification of the chambers and great vessels of the heart by their morphology, regardless of their spatial positions.

Right Atrium

The right atrium (Fig. 1-1) is that chamber of the heart which normally receives systemic venous drainage from the inferior and superior vena cavae. It also normally receives the major portion of coronary venous drainage from the coronary sinus. Morphologic characteristics important for identification of the right atrium are the presence of the limbus of the fossa ovalis, which surrounds the valve of the fossa ovalis (septum primum) superiorly, anteriorly, and posteriorly; a wide-based, blunt-ended atrial appendage; the eustachian valve at the orifice of the inferior vena cava and the thebesian valve at the orifice of the coronary sinus; and the crista terminalis, which separates the trabeculated from the nontrabeculated portion of the atrium.

Clinically, the definitive morphologic features of the right atrium may be difficult to recognize.[B1] Occasionally, the atrial septum is seen well enough in profile angiocardiographically to delineate the limbus of the fossa ovalis, and sometimes the right atrial appendage is outlined sufficiently to differentiate its shape from that of the left atrial appendage. The fact that the hepatic portion of the inferior vena cava usually drains into the right atrium often makes it possible to determine the location of the right atrium by passage of a catheter from the inferior vena cava to the heart. In complex situations, various factors must be considered in determining the atrial situs: the morphologic features of the atria, the venous drainage, and the situs indicated by the pulmonary artery and bronchial anatomy.[P1,S1,V1,V2] In most cases, the wide-based blunt-ended right atrial appendage is the most secure indicator that the atrium is morphologically a right atrium.

Left Atrium

The left atrium (Fig. 1-2) is that cardiac chamber which normally receives the pulmonary venous drainage from the four pulmonary veins. The septal surface of the left atrium is

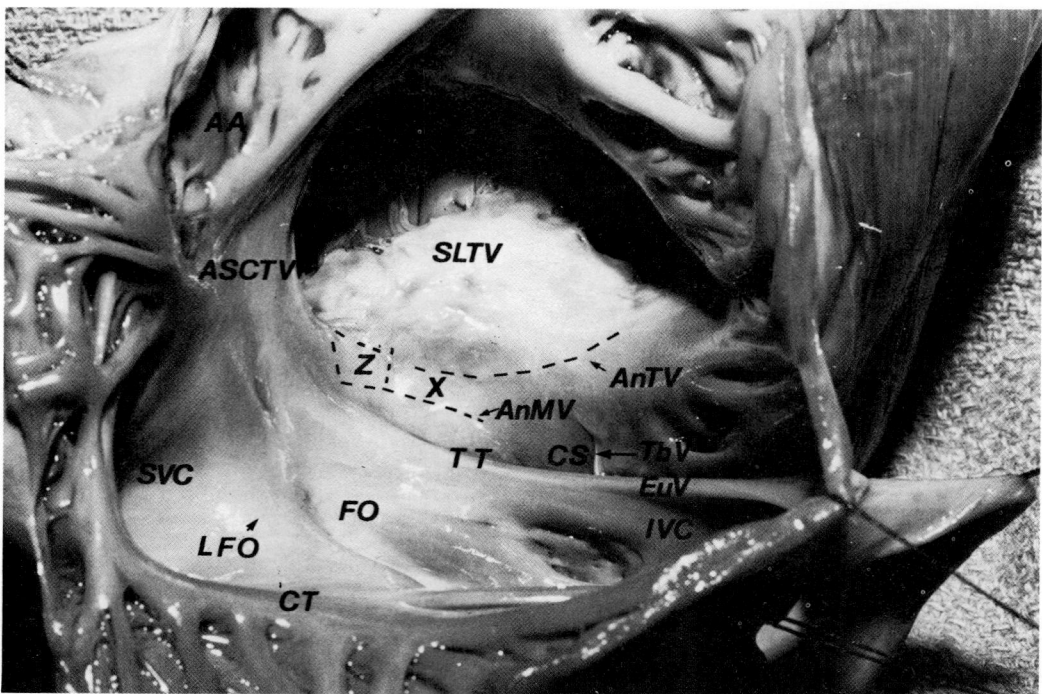

Figure 1-1 The interior of the normal right atrium, viewed from the right side at operation (UAB). AA, atrial appendage; AnMV, position of mitral valve anulus on the other side of the septum, indicated by the dotted line; AnTV, anulus of tricuspid valve, indicated by the dotted line; ASCTV, anteroseptal commissure of tricuspid valve; CS, orifice of coronary sinus; CT, crista terminalis (the inside of the sulcus terminalis); EuV, eustachian valve; FO, fossa ovalis; IVC, orifice of inferior vena cava; LFO, limbus of fossa ovalis (this is C-shaped and extends anteriorly and posteriorly to enclose the fossa ovalis); SLTV, septal leaflet of tricuspid valve; SVC, orifice of superior vena cava; ThV, thebesian valve; TT, tendon of Todaro; X, muscular portion of the atrioventricular septum; Z, membranous portion of the atrioventricular septum.

characterized by the flap valve of the septum primum, in contrast to the limbus of the fossa ovalis, present on the right atrial septal surface. The left atrial appendage is long and narrow in shape, in contrast to the bluntness of the right atrial appendage, and is the best indicator that the atrium is morphologically a left atrium. There is no crista terminalis at the base of the left atrial appendage, as there is in the right atrium; the appendage is the only trabeculated structure in the left atrium.

In general, at cardiac catheterization the location of the left atrium is determined indirectly by defining the position of the right atrium as described above. With normal pulmonary venous connection, the left atrium may be well opacified after a right ventricular or pulmonary artery injection.

Right Ventricle

The right ventricle has a large sinus portion, such surrounds and supports a tricuspid atrioventricular (AV) valve and includes the apex, and a smaller *infundibulum,* or outlet portion, which gives attachment to a semilunar valve. The inlet and outlet valves of the right ventricle are thus widely separated. The entire sinus portion of the right ventricle and most of the infundibulum (both free wall and septum) are coarsely trabeculated.

The septal surface of the right ventricle is divided into a *posterior* (basal) portion, a *middle* portion, an *apical* (anterior) portion, and an *infundibular* (conal) portion (GLH) (Fig. 1-3). Alternatively, the right ventricle's septal surface may be divided into an *inlet* portion, an *apical trabecular* portion, and an *infundibular,* or outlet, portion (UAB)[1] (Fig. 1-4).[S12] In this terminology, the inlet portion of the ventricular septum surrounds and supports the tricuspid valve. The apical trabecular portion is that portion with the coarse trabecular pattern typical of the right ventricle (Fig. 1-4). The smooth, prominent *infundibular septum*[A1] (or conal or *outlet septum*) separates the pulmonary from the aortic and tricuspid valves. Only part of the infundibular septum is interventricular (Fig. 1-4), and in some malformations, such as double-outlet right ventricle, none of it may be.

Laterally to the right, the infundibular (conal) septum imperceptibly merges with the free right ventricular wall immediately beyond its attachment to the membranous septum

---

[1]The phrase *inlet septum* is in some ways undesirable because the term has developmental implications,[A5] and the large inlet septum on the right ventricular side is not duplicated on the left side. The use of the term *trabecular* to describe a portion of the sinus septum is also undesirable in some ways, as part of the infundibular septum is also trabeculated (Fig. 1-4).

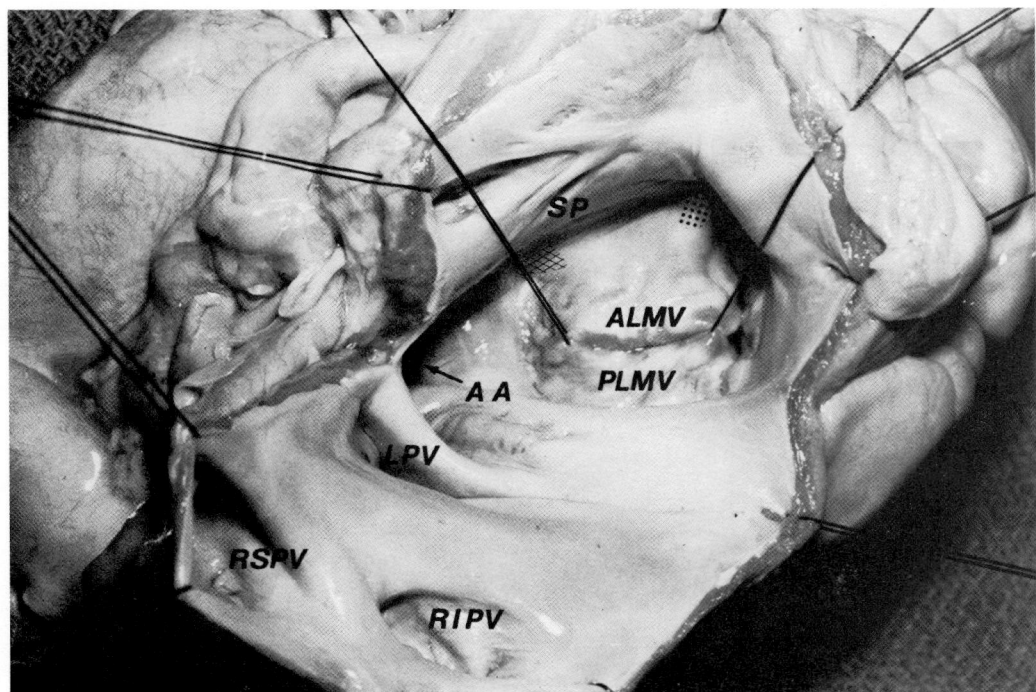

Figure 1-2 The interior of the normal left atrium, viewed from the right side at operation, as, for example, during mitral valve operations (UAB). The stippled area indicates the position of the right trigone, which contains the bundle of His. The crosshatching marks the left trigone, the area of greatest risk to the aortic valve during mitral replacement.

AA, base of atrial appendage; ALMV, anterior leaflet of mitral valve; LPV, orifices of left pulmonary veins; PLMV, posterior leaflet of mitral valve; RIPV, orifice of right inferior pulmonary vein; RSPV, orifice of right superior pulmonary vein; SP, septum primum.

and can at that point be called the *parietal extension* (band). The parietal band lies anterior to the right aortic sinus (Fig. 1-3) and partially overlies that portion of the free wall of the right ventricle termed the *ventriculo-infundibular fold.* Many surgeons call the infundibular septum and the parietal band the *crista superventricularis.* Medially and to the left, the infundibular septum merges with the ventricular septum between the limbs of a particularly prominent smooth, Y-shaped muscle bundle called the *septal band,* or *trabecula septomarginalis* (TSM) (Fig. 1-5).[A1,T1] The septal band extends apically to become continuous with the *moderator band,* a prominent trabeculation running from septum to free wall.

It should be noted that the most distal cephalad portion of the infundibular septum is not, strictly speaking, part of the ventricular septum, for in the normal heart the pulmonary valve arises from the apex of a cone of muscle and does not have a septal attachment. The anterior limb of the TSM and a high anterior trabeculated portion of septum, which becomes continuous with the trabeculated free wall, also form part of the septal surface of the infundibulum.

The junction between the infundibulum and sinus portions of the right ventricle is clearly demarcated only along the lower margin of the infundibular septum. The incomplete muscular ridge formed by the infundibular septum and the parietal band together with the septal and moderator bands

forms a natural line of division between the posteroinferior sinus portion and the anterosuperior infundibular portion of the ventricle.[V3]

The papillary muscle arrangement supporting the three leaflets of the tricuspid valve is different from that of the mitral valve in the left ventricle. In the case of the tricuspid valve, in addition to a single large anterior papillary muscle that is attached to the anterior free wall and fuses with the moderator band, there are multiple smaller posterior papillary muscles attached partly to the posterior (inferior) free wall and partly to the septum, and a group of small septal papillary muscles. The lowermost of these small septal muscles attaches posterior to the trabecula septomarginalis (septal band) (Fig. 1-4), and the uppermost, called the medial (conal) papillary muscle (muscle of Lancisi, or muscle of Lushka), to the posterior limb of the septal band.

Left Ventricle

The left ventricle consists of a larger *sinus* portion, which supports a bicuspid (mitral) atrioventricular valve and includes the apex, and a much smaller *outlet* (outflow) portion beneath a semilunar valve. The inlet and outlet valves of the left ventricle lie juxtaposed within its base, and inflow and outflow portions are separated by the anterior mitral leaflet (Fig. 1-6).

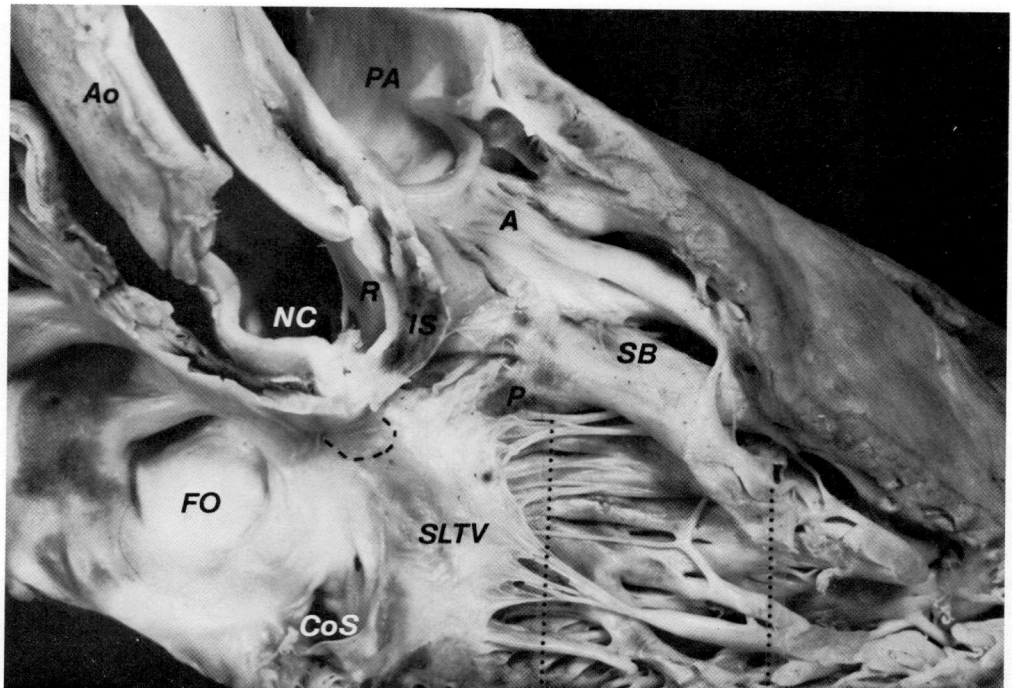

Figure 1-3 The right ventricular side of the septa after the right atrium, right ventricle, and pulmonary artery have been exposed by removing their anterior walls and the rightward portion of aorta and parietal band (or parietal extension of the infundibular septum) (GLH). The entire right ventricular septum is displayed, together with the relationship of the infundibular septum to the aortic root. In this heart, the infundibular septum is less prominent than in some. The dashed line defines the atrioventricular portion of the membranous septum. The dotted lines define the arbitrary division of the sinus septum into posterior (beneath septal tricuspid leaflet), middle, and apical portions (GLH). The specimen corresponds to a right anterior oblique projection in cineangiography.

A, left anterior division septal band; Ao, aorta; CoS, coronary sinus; FO, fossa ovalis; IS, cut end of infundibular septum; NC, noncoronary aortic sinus; P, right posterior division septal band; PA, pulmonary artery; R, right coronary aortic sinus; SB, septal band (trabecula septomarginalis); SLTV, septal tricuspid leaflet.

The entire free wall of the left ventricle and the apical half to two-thirds of the septum are trabeculated (Figs. 1-6, 1-7), but the trabeculations are characteristically fine compared to those in the right ventricle.[B1] The septal surface of the left ventricle may be considered to have a *sinus* portion, most of which is trabeculated, and a smooth *outlet* (outflow) portion (GLH) (Fig. 1-7). The part of the *sinus* portion of the septum immediately beneath the mitral valve may be termed the *inlet septum*, and the rest of the sinus portion the *trabecular septum* (UAB) (Fig. 1-8). The outlet (outflow) portion lies in front and to the right of the anterior mitral leaflet, corresponds to the inlet portion on the right ventricular side of the septum, and includes the atrioventricular septum (Fig. 1-9). In contrast to the right ventricular side, where the septal tricuspid leaflet is the only valvular attachment to the septum, on the left ventricular side the rightward half of the anterior mitral valve leaflet attaches to the septum posteriorly, and the right and part of the noncoronary aortic cusps attach to it anteriorly (Fig. 1-8). The leftward half of the anterior mitral leaflet is in fibrous continuity with the aortic valve in an area termed the *aortic-mitral anulus* (Figs. 1-8, 1-9). The anteriorly placed right ventricular infundibular

(conal) septum lies opposite the aortic valve (Fig. 1-10). It may occasionally be displaced into the left ventricular outflow beneath the aortic valve, and occasionally muscle may also extend between aortic and mitral valves, forming a true infundibulum to the left ventricle. The papillary muscle pattern of the mitral valve is distinctive. Two large papillary muscles attach to the free wall (anterolateral and posteromedial) (Fig. 1-6). No papillary muscles attach to the left side of the ventricular septum.

Aorta

The aorta is that great artery arising from the base of the heart which normally gives rise to the systemic and coronary arteries. The identity of the aorta is established by recognizing it as the vessel of origin of the brachiocephalic arteries, which never arise from the pulmonary artery. It is not so definitively the vessel of origin of the coronary arteries, as occasionally one, or very rarely both, coronary arteries may arise from the pulmonary artery.[O1]

The *main pulmonary artery* (trunk) is that great artery which normally gives rise to the pulmonary arterial system.

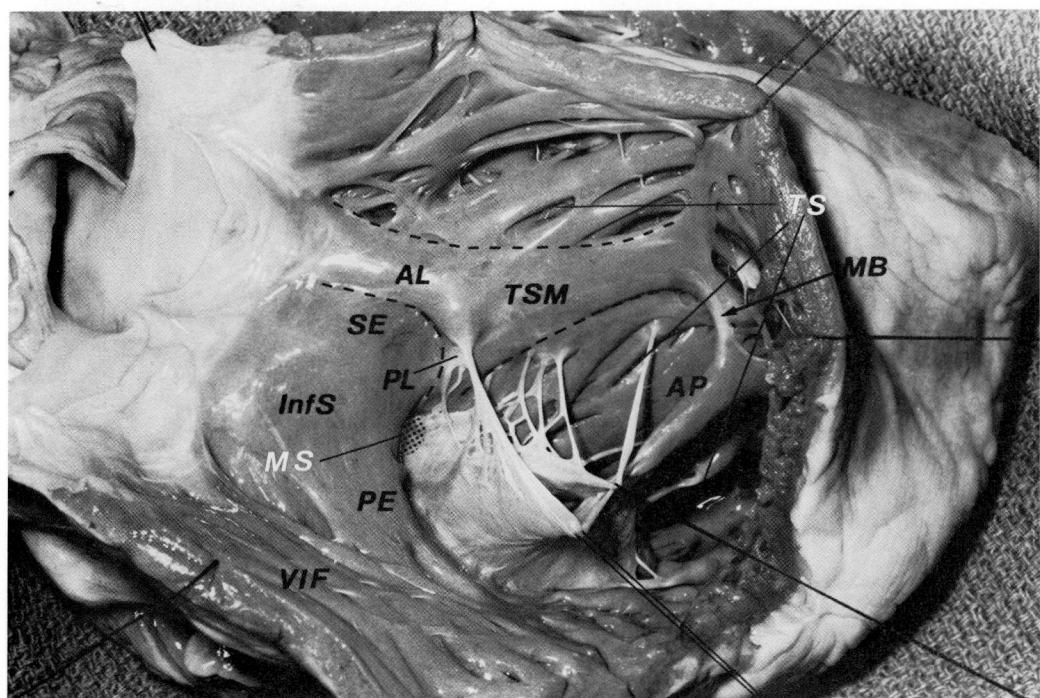

Figure 1-4 The interior of the normal right ventricle, particularly the apical trabecular and infundibular portions, oriented as at operation (UAB). As this figure and Figure 1-3 show, the infundibular (conal) septum separates the pulmonary from the tricuspid valve, and only its rightward portion and the inferior part of its central portion form part of the interventricular septum (these portions can be called the *septal extension* of the infundibular septum). The entire interventricular septum of the infundibulum is composed of the septal extension of the infundibular septum, the anterior limb of the septal band (TSM), and, in front of that, a heavily trabeculated portion of septum.

AL, anterior limb of TSM; AP, anterior papillary muscle; InfS, Infundibular (conal) septum; MB, moderator band; MS, position of membranous septum; PE, parietal extension of infundibular septum (parietal band); PL, posterior limb of TSM, giving origin to the medial papillary muscle; SE, septal extension of infundibular septum; TS, trabeculated portion of septum, part of which lies in the infundibulum and the remainder in the sinus portion of the ventricle; TSM, trabecula septomarginalis (septal band); VIF, ventriculoinfundibular fold.

As noted above, the main pulmonary trunk characteristically has no brachiocephalic vessels arising from it. At angiography, the differentiation between pulmonary trunk and aorta may require careful study, as the brachiocephalic vessels may opacify with the pulmonary trunk by filling through a patent ductus arteriosus. The pulmonary valve is normally anterior, and the aortic valve posterior and to the right in individuals with visceral and atrial situs solitus.

THE ATRIAL SEPTUM

See "Right Atrium" and "Left Atrium."

THE VENTRICULAR SEPTUM

The right and left ventricular septal surfaces are asymmetric, due mainly to the presence of an infundibulum in the right ventricle only. In addition, the higher pressure in the left ventricle makes the sinus septal surface concave on the left

side and convex on the right (Fig. 1-10), a feature that is accentuated during ventricular systole. The axes of the right and left ventricular outflow tracts differ. That of the right ventricle is almost vertically oriented, while that of the left ventricle angles sharply to the right (Fig. 1-11), a feature profiled cineangiographically in the left anterior oblique (LAO) view.[B1,B2]

Muscular Septum

See "Right Ventricle" and "Left Ventricle."

Membranous Septum

The membranous septum (pars membranacea) is the fibrous part of the cardiac septum separating the left ventricular outflow tract from, in part, the right ventricle and, in part, the right atrium. The line of division between these components is determined by the attachment of the tricuspid valve anulus to the septum (Figs. 1-9, 1-12). On the right ventricular side of this attachment is the *interventricular component*,

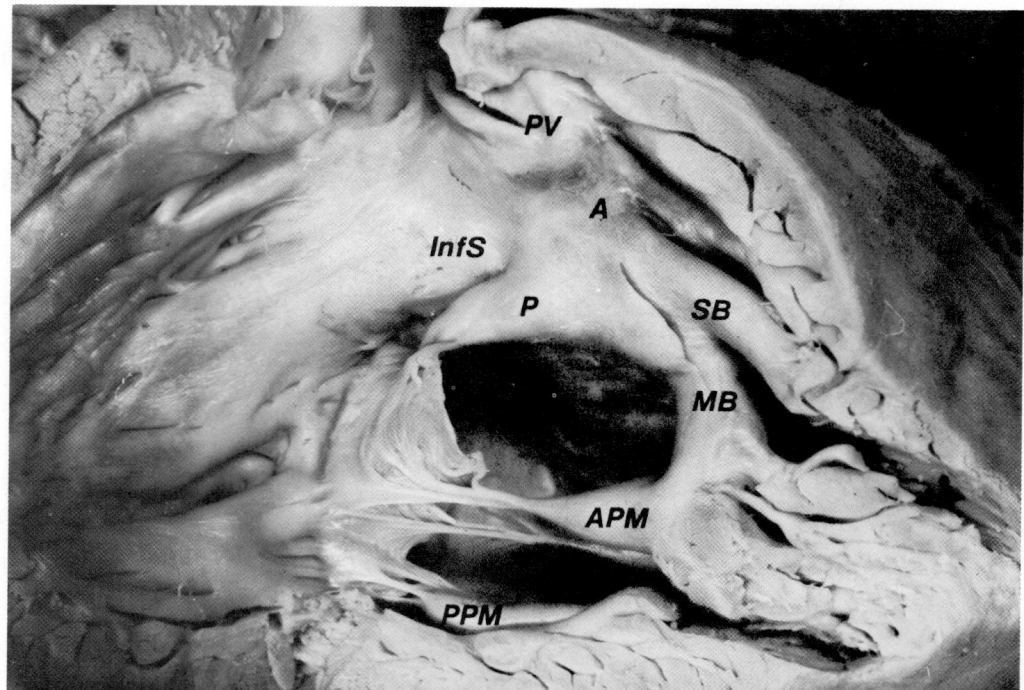

Figure 1-5 The interior of the right ventricle after it has been opened close to the anterior septal margin and along its acute margin inferiorly, and the anterior wall hinged to the right (GLH). The specimen is oriented anatomically with the aorta and pulmonary artery at the top. The pulmonary artery has also been opened. The attachments of the septal band (trabecula septomarginalis) are clearly demonstrated.

A, left anterior division of septal band; APM, anterior papillary muscle; InfS, infundibular (conal) septum; MB, moderator band; P, right posterior division of septal band, giving origin to the medial papillary muscle; PPM, posterior papillary muscle; PV, pulmonary valve; SB, septal band (trabecula septomarginalis).

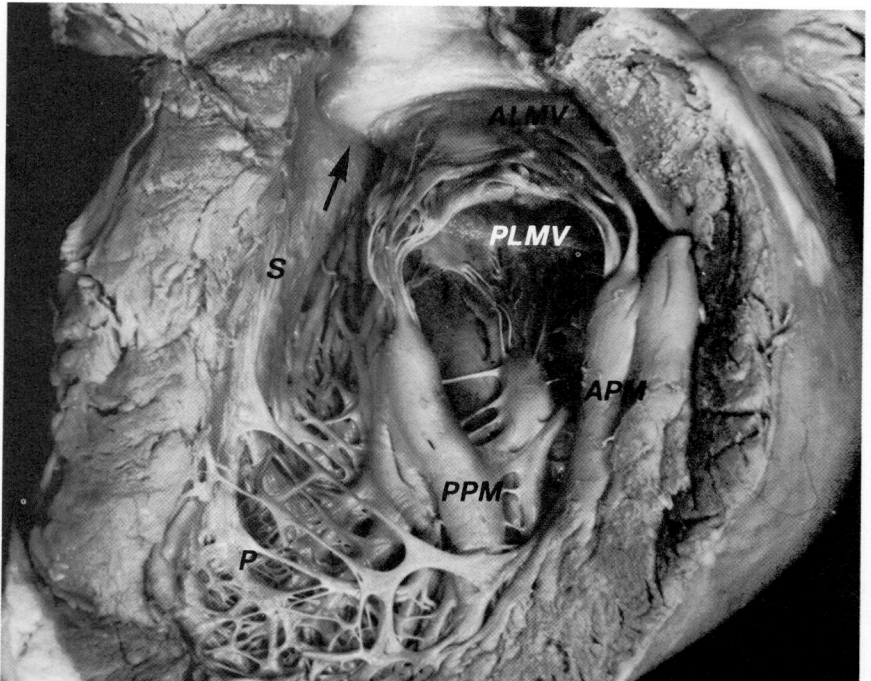

Figure 1-6 The interior of the left ventricle after the anterior ventricular and aortic walls have been excised, leaving the obtuse margin, posterior free wall, and septum intact (GLH). The specimen is anatomically oriented. The posterior (mural) leaflet of the mitral valve lies against the posterior free wall, while the anterior mitral leaflet hinges in part from the aortic ring and in part from the septum and separates the outflow portion of the ventricle from the remaining sinus portion. The arrow indicates the left ventricular outflow.

APM, anterior papillary muscle; ALMV, anterior leaflet mitral valve; PLMV, posterior leaflet mitral valve; PPM, posterior papillary muscle; S, septal surface.

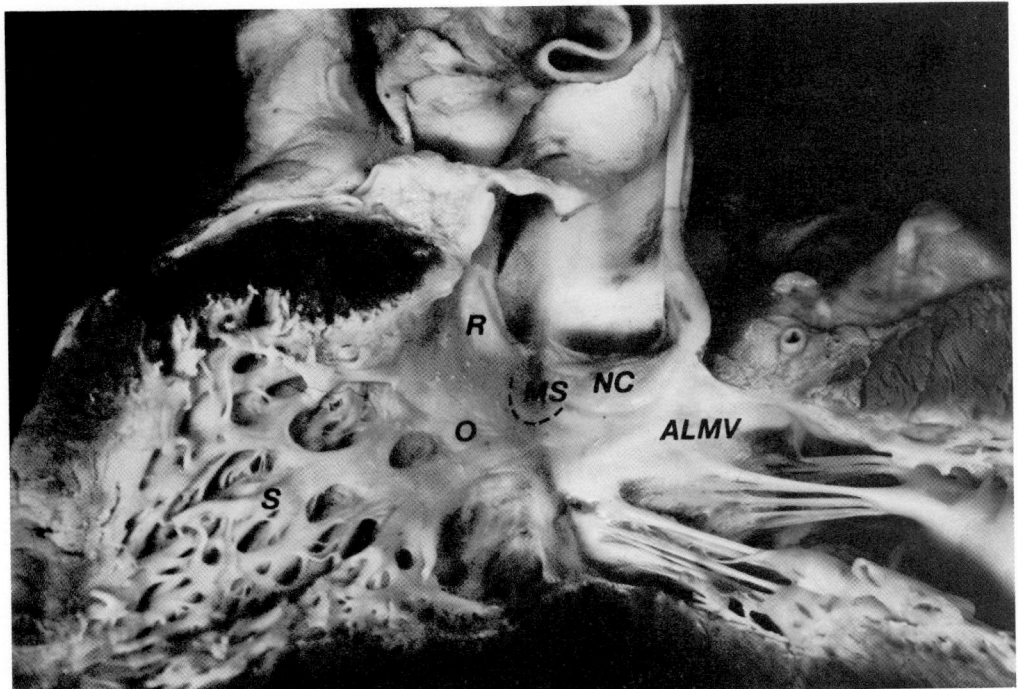

Figure 1-7 The interior of the left ventricle after the free wall, including the mitral valve apparatus, has been swung to the observer's right and away from the septal surface by a fish-mouth incision into the left ventricle and aorta (GLH). The smooth portion of the septum is much less extensive in this heart than in that in Figure 1-10.

ALMV, anterior leaflet mitral valve; MS, membranous septum; NC, noncoronary aortic cusp; O, outlet septum; R, right coronary aortic leaflet; S, sinus septum.

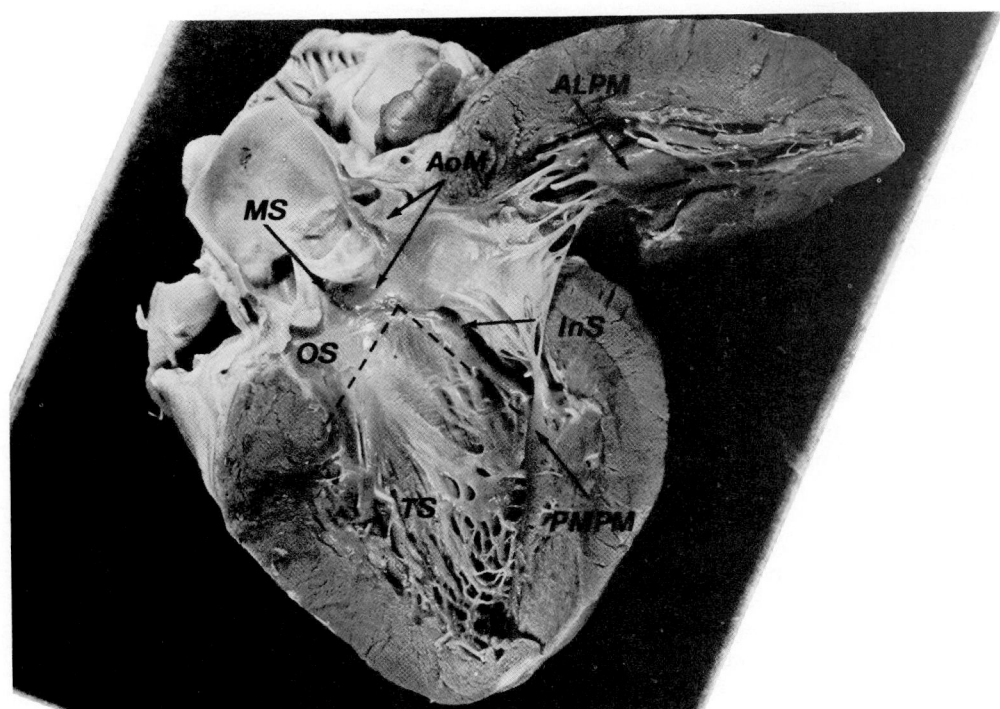

Figure 1-8 The interior of the normal left ventricle, viewed from a slightly different perspective than that of Figure 1-7 (UAB).

ALPM, anterolateral papillary muscle; AoM, aortic-mitral anulus (continuity); InS, inlet septum; MS, membranous septum; OS, outlet septum; PMPM, posteromedial papillary muscle; TS, trabecular septum.

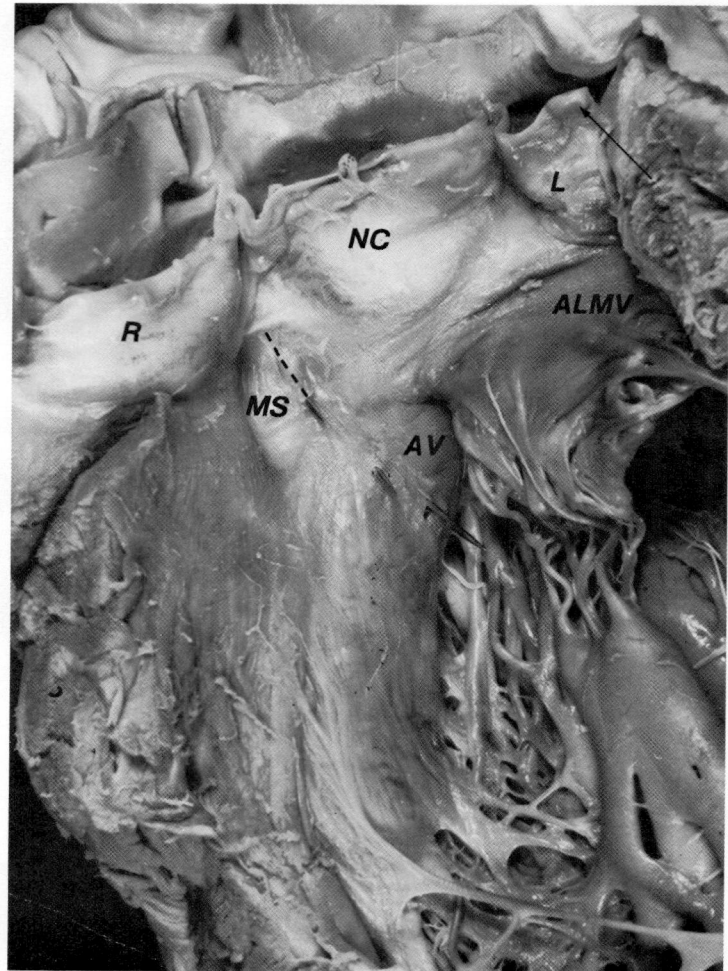

Figure 1-9   A view of the left ventricular septum, displaying the relationship between the outflow portion of the left ventricular septum and the aortic and mitral valves (GLH). The pins protrude along the line of attachment of the tricuspid septal leaflet to the right septal surface. Septal tissue inferior to this and the dashed line corresponds to the right ventricular inflow and septal tissue superior to it to the atrioventricular septum. The arrow indicates a nodulus Aranti. (In this specimen, also shown in Fig. 1-7, the right coronary artery ostium is eccentrically located near the R-NC commissure.)

ALMV, anterior leaflet mitral valve; AV, atrioventricular septum (muscular portion); L, left aortic cusp; MS, membranous septum, with the atrioventricular portion superior to the dashed line and the interventricular portion inferior to it; NC, noncoronary aortic cusp; R, right aortic cusp.

while on the right atrial side it forms the membranous portion of the atrioventricular septum.

Atrioventricular Septum

The atrioventricular septum is that portion of the cardiac septum which lies between the right atrium and the left ventricle. It consists of a superior membranous portion and an inferior muscular portion. The atrioventricular septum exists because the septal attachment of the tricuspid valve is more apical than the septal attachment of the anterior leaflet of the mitral valve (Figs. 1-10, 1-12). Viewed from the left ventricular side, the muscular component forms part of the outlet septum (Fig. 1-10). The AV node lies in the atrial septum adjacent to the junction between the membranous and mus-

cular portions of the atrioventricular septum, and the bundle of His passes toward the right trigone between these two components (Fig. 1-12).

THE CONDUCTION SYSTEM

The following description is based on studies of hearts without congenital defects.[B6] Abnormalities of the conduction system are associated with certain congenital cardiac malformations and are determined primarily by the alignment between atrial and ventricular septal structures and the pattern of ventricular architecture.[A8,A10] Such abnormalities are described in the chapters relating to these malformations (Chapters 42, 43, and 44).

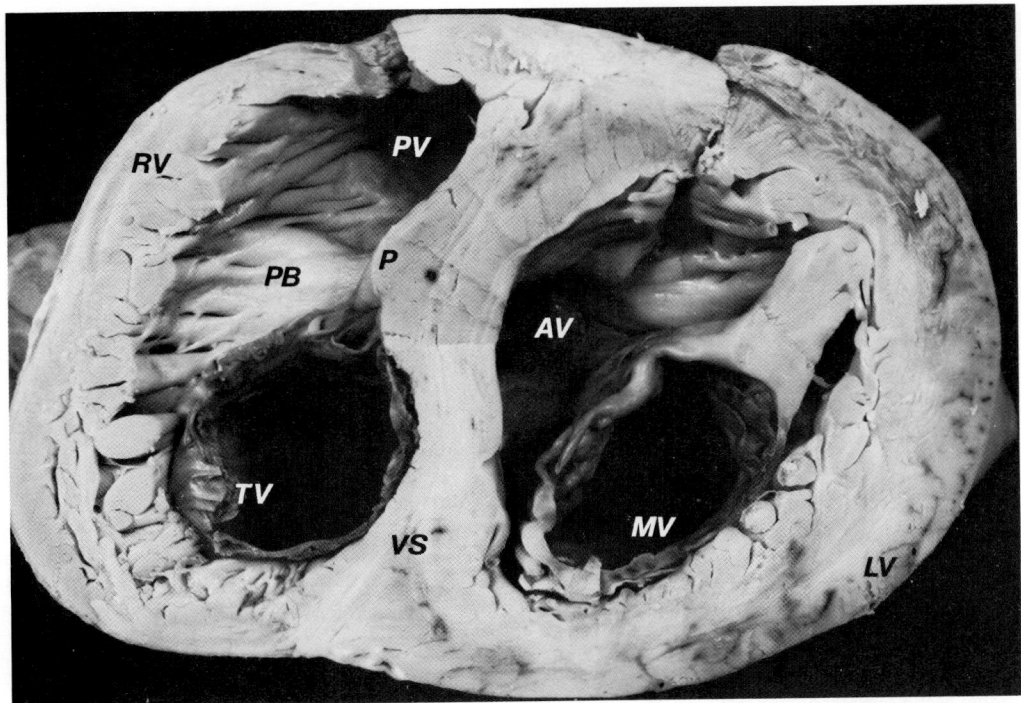

Figure 1-10 Transverse section of the heart at the level of the medial papillary muscle of the tricuspid valve to show the curvature of the septum and the manner in which the right ventricular infundibulum lies superior and anterior to the aortic valve (GLH). (This specimen is from a 9-month-old patient with a patent ductus arteriosus and pulmonary hypertension.)

AV, aortic valve; LV, left ventricle; MV, mitral valve; P, posterior division of the septal band (trabecula septomarginalis) and medial papillary muscle; PB, parietal band (parietal extension of infundibular septum); PV, pulmonary valve; RV, right ventricle; TV, tricuspid valve; VS, ventricular septum.

Sinus Node

The sinus node is located along the anterolateral aspect of the junction between the superior vena cava and the right atrial appendage (Fig. 1-13).[H1,J1,T2] In rare cases, it extends medially across the crest of the caval-atrial junction. The node is superficial, lying just beneath the epicardial surface in the sulcus terminalis, and is approximately 15 by 5 by 1.5 mm.[J1] It is pierced by the relatively large sinus node artery. (For details of the blood supply, see "Coronary Arteries.")

Internodal Pathways

The spread of activation between sinus node and atrioventricular node occurs preferentially through the muscle bundles delimited by the orifices of the right atrium.[S2,S3] Considerable histologic and electrophysiologic investigation has been carried out to determine if pathways of specialized conduction tissue exist within these broad muscle bundles and connect the sinoatrial (SA) and atrioventricular nodes. Investigators have not found discrete internodal tracts composed of homogeneous cells or fibers, although some have identified Purkinje-like cells in the major muscle bundles of adult hearts.[J2,J3,L1,T3] Controversy continues as to whether these pale cells seen in the atrial myocardium are Purkinje-type cells and whether they form the preferential conduction pathways.

Atrioventricular Node

The AV node lies directly on the right atrial side of the central fibrous body (right trigone) in the muscular portion of the atrioventricular septum, just anterosuperior to the ostium of the coronary sinus.[J4,T2] At times, its posterior margin has been found to lie directly against the coronary sinus ostium.[J4] It has a flattened oblong shape, with an average dimension in adults of 1 by 3 by 6 mm. Its left surface lies against the mitral anulus. Viewed from the right atrium, the AV node can be localized within a triangle described by Koch (Fig. 1-14) formed by the tricuspid anulus, the tendon of Todaro (the continuation of the eustachian valve that runs to the central fibrous body), and the coronary sinus ostium.

Bundle of His and Bundle Branches

The common AV bundle (bundle of His) is a direct continuation of the AV node. The bundle passes through the rightward part of the right trigone of the central fibrous body to reach the posteroinferior margin of the membranous ventricular septum. This area is just inferior to the commissure between the tricuspid valve's septal and anterior leaflets (Fig. 1-14c). Its diameter in the region of the central fibrous body is about 1 mm.[J4] The bundle courses along the posteroinferior border of the membranous septum and the crest of the muscular ventricular septum, giving off fibers that form

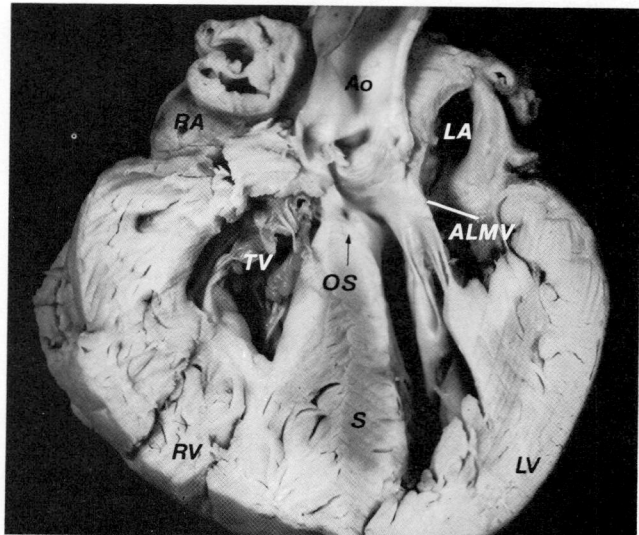

Figure 1-11 Oblique section of a heart from which the superior portion of both ventricles has been removed, including the entire right ventricular infundibulum and pulmonary artery and the front half of the aorta (GLH). The sharp rightward angulation of the outflow portion of the LV septum is well seen, as is the manner in which the anterior leaflet of the mitral valve contributes one boundary to the left ventricular outflow.

ALMV, anterior leaflet of mitral valve; Ao, aorta; LA, left atrium; LV, left ventricle; OS, LV outflow septum; RA, right atrium; RV, right ventricle; S, septum; TV, tricuspid valve.

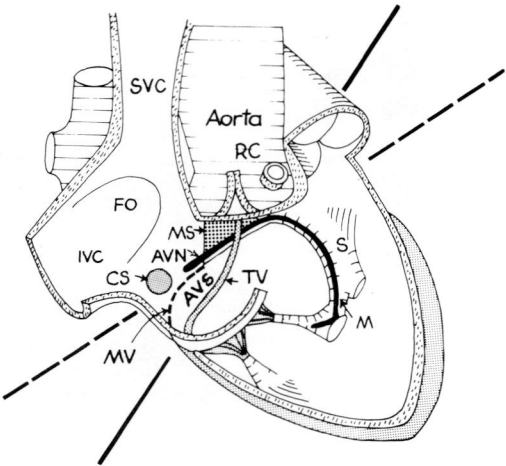

Figure 1-12 Diagram of the right heart, the aortic root, and the conduction tissue (at approximately 65° right anterior oblique [RAO] projection). The plane of the mitral valve attachment (dashed line) corresponds to the atrial edge of the muscular atrioventricular septum and the inferior edge of the membranous septum and differs from the plane of the tricuspid valve (solid line). The muscular portion of the atrioventricular septum is frequently smaller than depicted.

AVS, muscular atrioventricular septum; AVN, atrioventricular node extending into the bundle of His and the right bundle branch; CS, coronary sinus; FO, fossa ovalis; IVC, inferior vena cava; M, moderator band; MS, membranous septum, crossed by the attachment of the tricuspid valve; MV, mitral valve ring; RC, right coronary artery; S, portion of septal band (trabecula septomarginalis); SVC, superior vena cava; TV, tricuspid valve.

Modified from McAlpine.[M4]

the left bundle branch. This branching occurs beneath the commissure between the right and noncoronary cusps in close proximity to the aortic valve, over a distance of 6.5–20 mm, after which the remaining fibers form the right bundle branch (Fig. 1-15). The bundle of His lies on the left side of the ventricular septal crest in about 75%–80% percent of human hearts and on the right side of the crest in the remainder.[M1] In the latter situation, the His bundle connects to the left bundle by a relatively narrow stem.[M2]

The left bundle branch fans out over the left ventricular septal surface, gradually forming two or three main radiations.[D1,S4,T2] It is not uncommon for the anterior and posterior subdivisions to be accompanied by a central, third radiation that originates from the His bundle or from both of the former subdivisions. The anterior radiation travels toward the base of the anterolateral papillary muscle of the left ventricle. The wider posterior subdivision courses toward the base of the posteromedial papillary muscle. Multiple peripheral anastomoses occur among the subdivisions of the left bundle branch system as it distributes to the left ventricle.[D1]

The right bundle branch originates from the bundle of His in the region of the anteroinferior margin of the membranous septum and courses along the right ventricular septal surface, passing just below the medial papillary muscle and along the inferior margin of the septal band and the moderator band[L1] to the base of the anterior papillary muscle. The fibers then fan out to supply the walls of the right ventricle. Proximally, the right bundle averages about 1 mm in

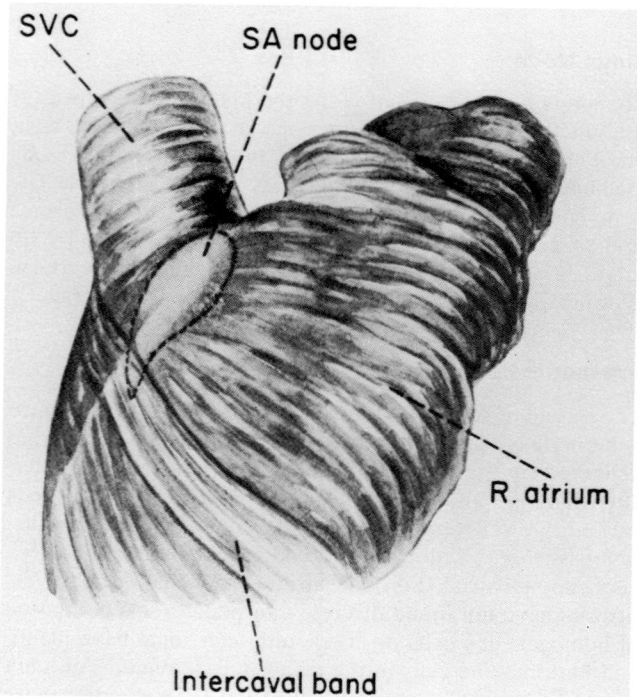

Figure 1-13 Usual location of the sinus node.

RA, right atrium; SN, sinus node; SVC, superior vena cava.

Reproduced with permission from Lev et al.[L6]

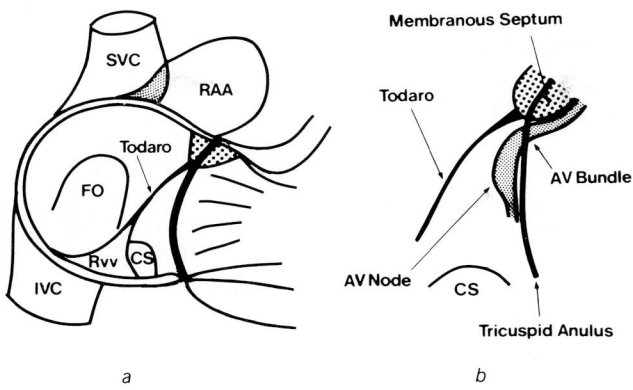

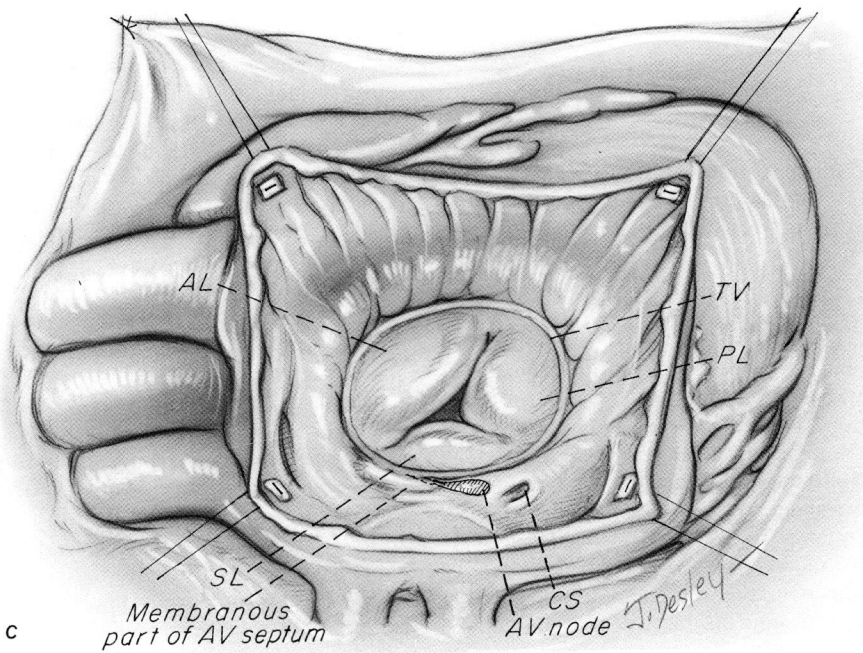

Figure 1-14 Anatomic and surgical aspects of the conduction system.

(a) Diagram of the triangle of Koch within the right atrium. The triangle is defined by the tendon of Todaro, the orifice of the coronary sinus, and the tricuspid anulus.

(b) Diagram showing the relationship of the AV node and AV bundle (His bundle) to the triangle of Koch. The AV node lies within the triangle, and the AV bundle is located at the apex of the triangle.

(c) Interior of the right atrium, as seen at operation. The membranous portion of the AV septum is easily visualized, particularly when cold cardioplegia is used. The AV node is unseen by the surgeon, but its position in the muscular portion of the AV septum is easily conceptualized at operation from the visible landmarks. This drawing should be correlated with the anatomic specimen shown in Figure 1-1.

AO, aorta; AV, atrioventricular; CS, coronary sinus; PA, pulmonary artery; SVC, superior vena cava; TV, tricuspid valve.

Parts a, b reproduced with permission from Anderson et al.[A3]

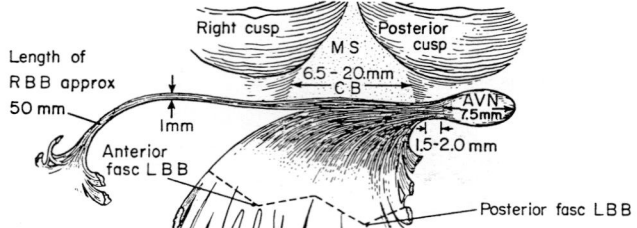

Figure 1-15 Diagram of the atrioventricular conduction system and its relationship to the membranous septum and the aortic valve, viewed from the left ventricular side. The atrioventricular node (AVN) is in the atrioventricular septum on the right atrial side of the right trigone, which is beneath the nadir of the posterior cusp of the aortic valve. The common AV bundle courses along the postero-inferior margin of the membranous septum, giving off fibers that form the left bundle branch. This region lies beneath the commissure of the right and noncoronary (posterior) aortic cusps. The right bundle branch originates from the common AV bundle in the region of the anteroinferior border of the membranous septum.

AVN, atrioventricular node; CB, branching portion of common AV bundle; fasc, fascicle; LBB, left bundle branch; MS, membranous septum; RBB, right bundle branch.

Reproduced with permission from Titus.[T2]

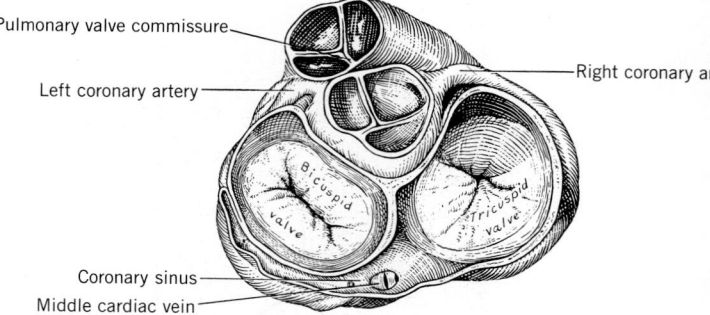

Figure 1-16 Drawing of the normal interrelationships among the heart valves. The aortic valve is centrally located and wedged between the mitral and tricuspid valves. The pulmonary valve is anterior and slightly to the left of the aortic valve.

Reproduced with permission from Gray.[G1]

diameter.[T2] It is usually subendocardial in its proximal portion, intramyocardial in its middle portion, and again subendocardial near the base of the anterior papillary muscle.[T2]

CARDIAC VALVES

The interrelationships among the heart valves in normally formed hearts are remarkably uniform.[M3] The aortic valve occupies a central position, wedged between the mitral and tricuspid valves, while the pulmonary valve is situated anterior, superior, and slightly to the left of the aortic valve (Fig. 1-16). The anuli of these valves merge with each other and with the membranous septum to form the fibrous skeleton of the heart.[G1] The core of the skeleton is the central fibrous body, with its two extensions, the right and left fibrous trigones. The right fibrous trigone forms a dense junction between the mitral, tricuspid, and aortic anuli (noncoronary cusp) and the membranous septum and is pierced by the bundle of His. The left fibrous trigone, situated more anteriorly and to the left, lies between the aortic (left cusp) and mitral anuli. The tendon of the infundibulum is a fibrous band joining the more superiorly placed pulmonary valve to the central cardiac skeleton. The tendon of Todaro also joins the central fibrous body (see ''Atrioventricular Node'').

By virtue of similarities in morphology and function, the heart valves naturally fall into two groups: the atrioventricular (mitral and tricuspid) valves, and the semilunar (aortic and pulmonary) valves.

Mitral Valve

The atrioventricular valve of the left ventricle, the mitral valve, is bicuspid, with an anterior (aortic, or septal) leaflet and a posterior (mural, or ventricular) leaflet[2] (Fig. 1-17). Tissue that could be called *commissural leaflets* is usually present at the commissures between these two leaflets. The combined area of the two mitral leaflets is twice that of the mitral orifice, resulting in a large area of coaptation.[P2,S5] When this large area of coaptation is lost because of malalignment of the leaflets, undue stress is placed on the chordae tendineae, and they may rupture. Though there has been some controversy as to the definition of commissural areas, particularly in regard to clefts in the posterior leaflet, Silver and colleagues have described chordae tendineae, which define the limits of the septal (anterior) and posterior leaflets.[L2,R1] Rusted and associates found the depth of commissures in the normal mitral valve to average 0.7–0.8 cm and never more than 1.3 cm in the 50 hearts they studied.[R2]

The larger *septal* (anterior, or aortic) *leaflet* is roughly triangular in shape, with the base of the triangle inserting on about one-third of the anulus. The septal leaflet has a relatively smooth free margin with few or no indentations. There is a distinct ridge separating the region of closure (rough zone) from the remaining leaflet (clear zone).[R1] The clear zone is devoid of direct chordal insertions. The septal (anterior) leaflet is in fibrous continuity with the aortic valve through the aortic-mitral anulus and forms a boundary of the left ventricular outflow tract.[W1] This region of continuity occupies about one-quarter of the mitral anulus and corresponds to the region beneath half the left coronary cusp and half the noncoronary cusp of the aortic valve. The limits of this attachment are demarcated by the right and left fibrous trigones (Fig. 1-18). These points do not correspond to the commissures of the mitral valve (Fig. 1-2). The AV node and bundle are at risk of surgical damage adjacent to the right trigone.

The smaller *posterior leaflet* inserts into about two-thirds of the anulus and typically has a scalloped appearance. Ranganathan and associates found the posterior leaflet to be divided into three segments in 46 of the 50 normal mitral valves

---

[2] From a surgeon's viewpoint, the terms *septal leaflet* and *posterior leaflet* seem best.

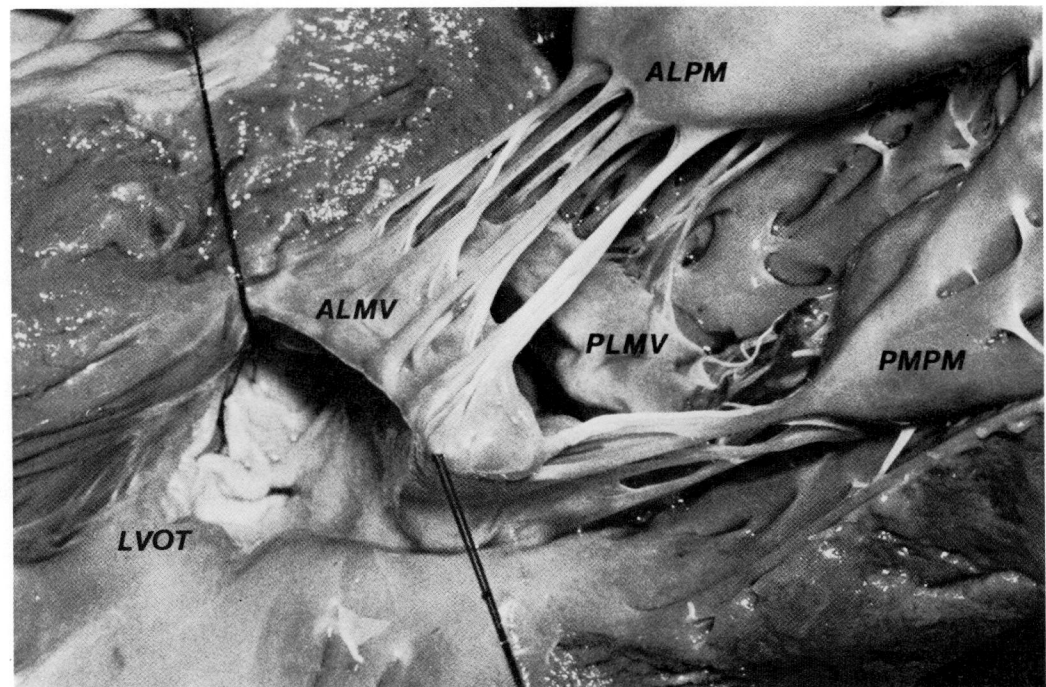

Figure 1-17 The normal mitral valve, viewed from the surgical exposure afforded by an antero-lateral left ventriculotomy (UAB). For this figure, the anterolateral left ventricular wall is held forward and to the observer's right.

ALMV, anterior leaflet; ALPM, anterolateral papillary muscle; LVOT, left ventricular outflow tract; PLMV, posterior leaflet; PMPM, posteromedial papillary muscle.

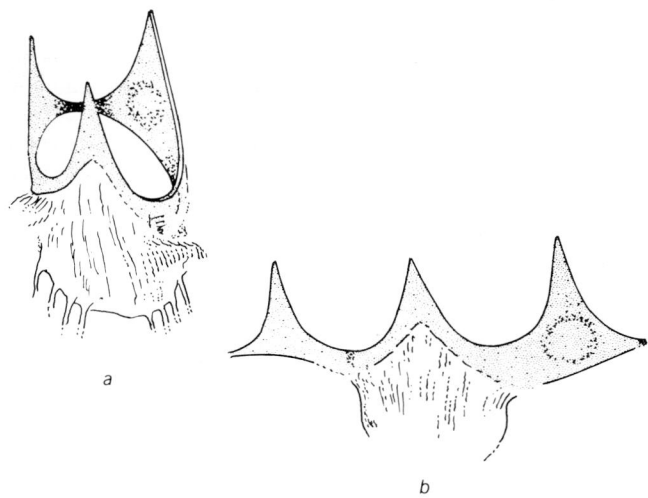

Figure 1-18

(a) Diagram of the fibrous, crownlike skeleton of the aortic valve, viewed from the direction of the mitral valve. The skeleton is in continuity with the membranous septum and the anterior (septal) leaflet of the mitral valve. The subaortic curtain is the aortic-mitral anulus.

(b) The skeleton flattened out, illustrating the U-shaped components of the aortic valve.

Reproduced from Zimmerman.[Z1]

they studied.[R1] The posterior leaflet has rough and clear zones corresponding to those of the anterior leaflet, as well as a basal zone close to the anulus, which receives chordae directly from left ventricular trabeculae.[L2,R1]

The majority of *chordae tendineae* to the mitral valve originate from the two large papillary muscles of the left ventricle, the anterolateral and posteromedial papillary muscles. Each leaflet receives chordae from both papillary muscles, and the majority insert on the free leaflet edge.[R2] Tandler defined three orders of chordae. Those of the first order insert on the free margin of the leaflet; the second order chordae insert a few to several millimeters back from the free edge; and third order chordae insert at the base of the leaflet (applicable only to the posterior leaflet).[T1] Lam and associates have reclassified chordae into rough zone (including strut chordae), cleft, basal, and commissural chordae.[L2] They suggest that this classification provides a clear definition of mitral valve leaflets and should be useful in studying mitral valve function.

Tricuspid Valve

The atrioventricular valve of the right ventricle, or tricuspid valve, has three leaflets (Fig. 1-19). Its orifice is roughly triangular in shape and is larger than the mitral orifice. The anulus is relatively indistinct, especially in the septal region.

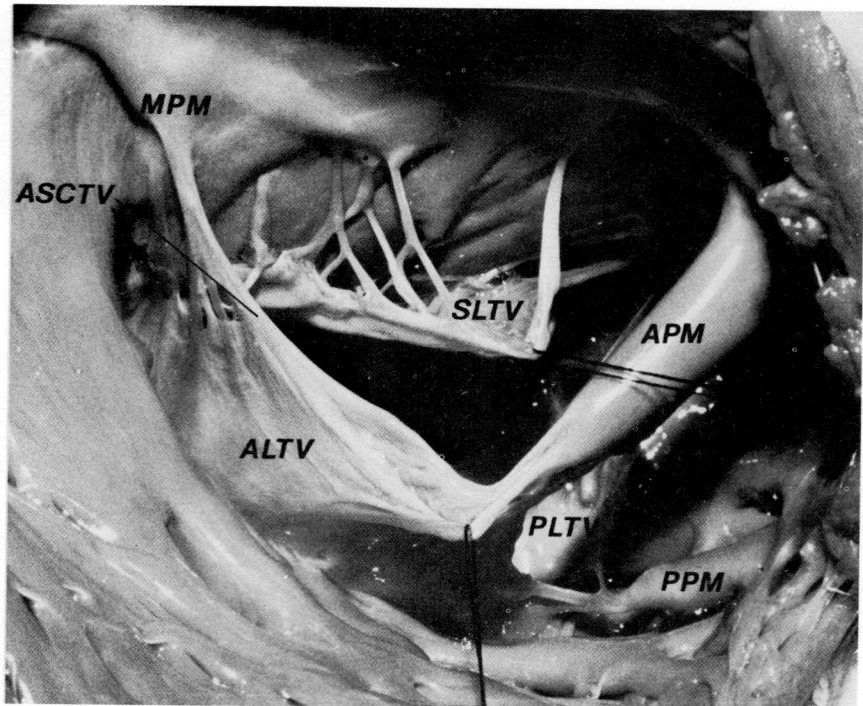

Figure 1-19 The normal open tricuspid valve, viewed from in front through the right ventricular cavity (UAB).

ALTV, anterior leaflet; APM, anterior papillary muscle; ASCTV, anteroseptal commissure; MPM, medial papillary muscle; PLTV, posterior leaflet; PPM, posterior papillary muscle; SLTV, septal leaflet.

The leaflets and chordae tendineae are thinner than those of the mitral valve.[B3,G2]

The *anterior leaflet* (actually anterosuperior in position) is the largest of the three leaflets and may have notches creating subdivisions. Silver and associates found a notch close to the anteroseptal commissure in 47 of the 50 anterior leaflets they examined.[S6] This notch was occasionally as deep as a commissure but could be differentiated from a true commissure by the type of chordal attachments. The chordae attaching to the anterior leaflet arise from the anterior and medial papillary muscles.

The *posterior leaflet* (actually inferior in position) is usually the smallest and commonly is scalloped. Its chordae originate from the posterior and anterior papillary muscle.

The *septal leaflet* is usually slightly larger than the posterior leaflet. Its chordae arise from the posterior and septal papillary muscles. Most of this leaflet attaches to the membranous and muscular portions of the ventricular septum, though part may attach to the posterior wall of the right ventricle. The transition between the attachments to posterior wall and septum is associated with a fold in the leaflet.[S6]

Of major surgical importance is the proximity of the conduction system to the septal leaflet and its anteroseptal commissure. The membranous septum usually lies beneath the septal leaflet inferior to the anteroseptal commissure, but the attachments at the septal and anterior leaflets are variable so that parts of either may attach to the membranous septum. The bundle of His penetrates the right trigone beneath the interventricular component of the membranous septum (usually about 5 mm inferior to the commissure) to run along the crest of the muscular septum (see "The Conduction System"). That portion of the septal leaflet between the membranous septum and the commissure extends around the tricuspid anulus, away from the septum, to the right ventricular free wall (Fig. 1-1). According to Sherman, this portion of the tricuspid valve may form a flap over some ventricular septal defects (VSDs).[S7]

Aortic Valve

The aortic valve is normally tricuspid and is composed of three basic components: a fibrous skeleton, delicate cusps, and sinuses of Valsalva.[Z1] These components form three cuplike structures that constitute the entire valve mechanism.

The crownlike skeleton of the valve is a composite of three U-shaped solid collagenous structures (Fig. 1-18) and is in fibrous continuity with the anterior leaflet of the mitral valve and with the membranous septum.

The three delicate fibrous cusps insert into the scalloped outline of the valve skeleton. The free edge of each cusp is of tougher consistency than the remainder of the cusp. At the midpoint of each free edge is a fibrous *nodulus Aranti*. On either side of each nodulus is an extremely thin, crescent-shaped portion of the cusp termed the *lunula* (Fig. 1-9). The lunulae are occasionally fenestrated near the commissures.

These regions form the area of coaptation during valve closure.

The aortic sinuses (sinuses of Valsalva) are dilated pockets of the aortic root that form the outer component of the three cuplike closing structures of the aortic valve. The coronary arteries arise from two of the aortic sinuses. The walls of the sinuses are considerably thinner than the wall of the aorta proper,[Z1] an important consideration in the design of proximal aortotomies.

The origins of the coronary arteries are the basis of a nomenclature for the sinuses and cusps. The ostia of the right and left coronary arteries identify the right and left sinuses and cusps. The sinus and cusp without an associated coronary artery are termed *noncoronary*. Several other nomenclatures for the cusps and sinuses have been described.[B3,G2,K1]

Pulmonary Valve

The structure of the pulmonary valve is similar to that of the aortic valve.[G2] The pulmonary valve normally has three cusps, with a nodule at the midpoint of each free edge and lunulae and thin crescent-shaped coaptive surfaces on either side of the nodules. The pocket behind each cusp is the sinus. The major differences from the aortic valve are (1) the lighter construction of the pulmonary valve cusps,[G1,G2] (2) the normal absence of coronary artery origins, (3) the normal lack of fibrous continuity with the anterior tricuspid valve leaflet, and (4) the lack of a fibrous ring or skeleton joining the bases of all three cusps, which are attached to muscle instead.

The pulmonary valve cusps have been described by several terminologies[B3,G2,K1] but are usually named by their relationships to the aortic valve. They are thus termed *right, left,* and *anterior* (nonseptal). Kerr and Goss found that a commissure of the pulmonary valve was adjacent to a commissure of the aortic valve in 199 of the 200 specimens they studied.[K1] They suggested that the cusps of each arterial valve should be termed *right adjacent, left adjacent,* and *opposite* (or, as suggested by Anderson, right facing, left facing, and nonfacing) in relation to the adjacent commissure of each valve.

CORONARY ARTERIES

From an anatomical point of view, the coronary artery system divides naturally into two distributions, left and right. From the standpoint of the surgeon, the coronary artery system is divided into four parts: the left main coronary artery, the left anterior descending coronary artery and its branches, the left circumflex coronary artery and its branches, the right coronary artery and its branches. The branches of each of the last three vessels must also be familiar to the surgeon.

The major coronary arteries form a circle and a loop about the heart (Fig. 1-20).[D2,S8] The circle is formed by the right coronary and left circumflex arteries as they traverse the atrioventricular sulci. The loop between the ventricles and at right angles to the circle is formed by the left anterior descending coronary artery anteriorly and the posterior descending coronary artery posteriorly as they encircle the septum. The blood supply to the back of the left ventricle streams down as a series of parallel obtuse marginal arteries coming from the posterior half of the circle, formed on the left by the left circumflex artery and on the right (in hearts with a dominant right coronary circulation) by the extension across the crux cordis[3] of the right coronary artery termed the *right posterolateral segment*. This latter segment supplies inferior surface (marginal) branches to the inferior (diaphragmatic) surface of the left ventricle. A right dominant artery does not necessarily supply branches to the inferior surface of the left ventricle, however, as it may terminate only as the posterior descending artery. The blood supply to the anterior portion of the left ventricle comes from the diagonal branches of this portion of the loop, the left anterior descending coronary artery. That to the lateral part of the anterior portion comes from the first branches of both the left anterior descending and circumflex arteries. The ventricular septum receives its blood supply from the loop that encircles it, formed by the left anterior descending artery in front and the posterior descending artery behind.

Variability in the origin of the posterior descending artery is expressed by the term *dominance*. A right dominant coronary circulation is one in which the posterior descending coronary artery is a terminal branch of the right coronary artery. A left dominant circulation, which occurs in about 10%–15% of hearts, is one in which the posterior descending coronary artery is a branch, usually the last one, of the left circumflex coronary artery. Left dominance occurs more frequently in males than in females. This distinction as to whether the right or left coronary artery supplies the posterior descending artery is important in evaluating patients with coronary artery disease and in the planning of coronary artery bypass grafting.

The following is a general description of coronary artery anatomy in hearts that are otherwise normal.[B4,F1,G3,J5,M4,S8,V4] As with the conduction system, some congenital cardiac malformations are associated with abnormalities of the coronary arteries (see Chapters 42 and 43). The nomenclature is based on the United States National Heart, Lung and Blood Institute's *Proposal and Manual of Operations for Collaborative Studies in Coronary Artery Surgery*[N1] (Fig. 1-21) and the American Heart Association (AHA) Coronary Artery Disease Reporting System.[A2] Both systems include rules for defining the various segments of the major coronary arteries. Figure 1-21 should be studied along with the brief descriptions that follow.

Left Main Coronary Artery

The left main coronary artery extends from the ostium in the left sinus of Valsalva to its bifurcation into the left anterior descending and left circumflex branches. Its usual length is 10–20 mm, with a range of 0–40 mm. It normally courses

---

[3]The crux cordis is an area along the posterior aspect of the atrioventricular groove where the atrial and ventricular septa meet.

between the pulmonary artery and the left atrial appendage to reach the left atrioventricular groove. Occasionally, additional vessels originate from the left main coronary artery and course parallel to the diagonal branches of the left anterior descending branch.[15] Such an additional artery (formerly called a *ramus intermedius*) is termed the *first diagonal branch* of the left anterior descending artery. Rarely (in 1% of persons), the left main coronary artery is absent, the left

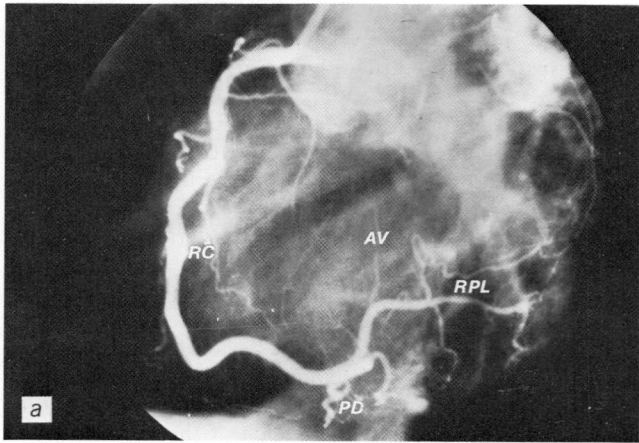

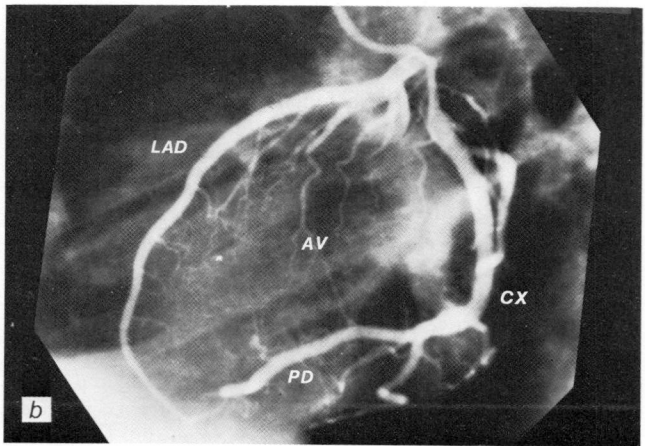

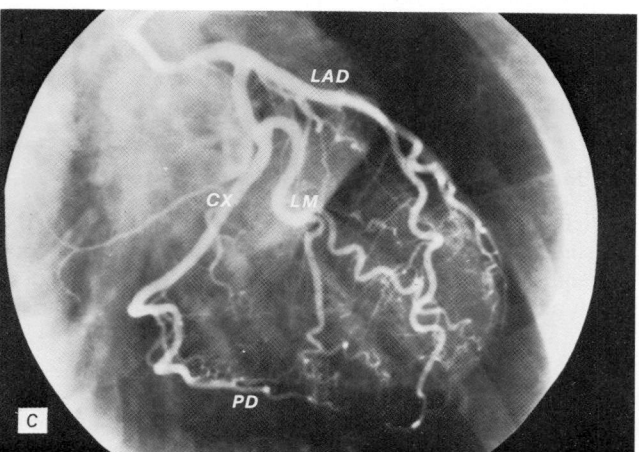

anterior descending and left circumflex coronary arteries originating directly from the aorta via two separate ostia.

Left Anterior Descending Coronary Artery

Beginning as a continuation of the left main coronary artery, the left anterior descending coronary artery courses along the anterior interventricular sulcus to the apex of the heart. Part of it may be buried in muscle. In most cases, this artery extends around the apex into the posterior interventricular sulcus, supplying the apical portion of both right and left ventricles.[15] This vessel supplies branches to the right ventricular free wall (usually small), to the septum, and to the left ventricular free wall. One or more branches to the right ventricle connect with infundibular branches from the proximal right coronary artery. This important route for collateral flow is the *loop of Vieussens*. The *septal arteries* arise almost perpendicularly from the left anterior descending coronary artery, a characteristic that is sometimes helpful in the angiographic identification of the anterior descending artery. A variable number of *diagonal arteries* course obliquely between the anterior descending and left circumflex artery and supply the left ventricular free wall anteriorly and laterally.

Variations in the left anterior descending artery are infrequent, although in about 4% of hearts, it exists as two parallel vessels of about equal size. It may terminate before the apex or extend as far as the posterior atrioventricular groove.

Left Circumflex Coronary Artery

The left circumflex artery originates from the left main coronary artery at about a 90° angle, with its initial few centimeters lying medial to the base of the left atrial appendage. The sinus node artery occasionally originates from the first few millimeters of the left circumflex artery. Rarely, the circumflex artery may terminate before the obtuse margin. A large branch originating from the proximal left circumflex artery and coursing around the left atrium near the atrioventricular groove is termed the *atrial circumflex artery*. The

Figure 1-20 Coronary arteriograms, demonstrating the circle-loop concept of coronary artery anatomy (UAB). The circle is formed by the right coronary and left circumflex arteries and is displayed in the LAO projection. The loop is formed by the left anterior descending and posterior descending arteries and is demonstrated in the RAO projection.
(a) Right coronary injection in the LAO projection. The circulation is right dominant. The right coronary artery, which forms the right component of the circle, is visualized.
(b) Left coronary injection in the LAO projection. Note that this is a left dominant circulation. The left circumflex artery, which forms the left component of the circle, is visualized.
(c) Left coronary injection in the RAO projection. The left dominant circulation allows demonstration of both components of the loop: left anterior descending and posterior descending arteries.
AV, AV node artery; CX, left circumflex artery; LAD, left anterior descending artery; LM, left marginal artery; PD, posterior descending artery; RC, right coronary artery; RPL, right posterolateral artery.

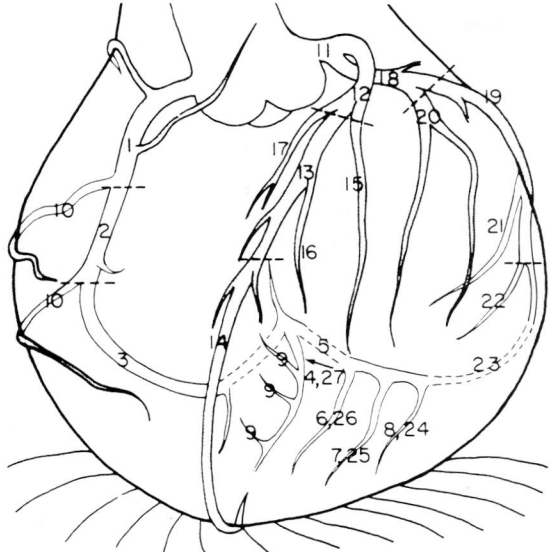

Figure 1-21 Diagram of the anatomic segments of the coronary arteries for use in locating lesions in individual patients. (1, 2, 3) Proximal, mid-, and distal portions of the right coronary artery. (4, 27) Posterior descending coronary artery, which, as the dotted segments proximal to it indicate, may arise from the right (4) or left (27) system. (5) Right posterolateral segment, an extension of the right coronary artery in association with right dominant systems. (6, 7, 8) From it come several inferior surface (marginal) branches, called right posterolateral arteries, to the back of the left ventricle. Left dominant systems have a comparable left posterolateral segment, leading to the posterior descending artery. (9) Inferior septal branches of the posterior descending artery. (10) Acute marginal branches of the coronary artery. (11) Left main coronary artery. (12, 13, 14) Proximal, mid-, and distal portions of the left anterior descending coronary artery. (15, 16) First and second diagonal branches. The first diagonal may originate almost from the bifurcation of the left main coronary artery, and was formerly called a ramus intermedius. Additional diagonal branches may be present. (17) First septal branch of the anterior descending artery. (18, 19) The proximal and distal portions of the left circumflex coronary artery. (20, 21, 22) The first, second, and third obtuse marginal branches of the circumflex artery, the first usually being a large vessel. (23) An extension of the circumflex artery, called the left AV artery, present only in patients with a left dominant system. In such patients, this vessel gives off further inferior surface ("marginal") branches to the back of the left ventricle, now called left posterolateral arteries (24, 25, 26), before terminating in the left posterior descending coronary artery (27).

Reproduced with permission from The National Heart, Lung, and Blood Institute Coronary Artery Surgery Study (CASS),[C1] and the American Heart Association, Inc.

ventricular branches of the circumflex artery, the *obtuse marginal arteries*, supply the obtuse margin of the heart and may be embedded in the muscle. Often, their position can then be identified at operation by the altered (reddish or light tan) color of the overlying thin muscle layer compared to that of the remainder of the ventricular wall. Those branches supplying the inferior surface of the left ventricle in a heart with a left dominant system (or in one with a codominant system where the right coronary artery gives rise only to a posterior descending artery) are termed *left posterolateral*

(marginal) *arteries*. In hearts with a left dominant system, the left circumflex coronary artery gives rise to the *posterior descending artery* at or usually before the crux. Variations in the origin and length of the left circumflex artery, and in the number and size of its marginal branches, are common.

Right Coronary Artery

The right coronary artery usually is a single large artery, and it courses down the right atrioventricular groove. Branches supplying the anterior right ventricular free wall exit from the atrioventricular sulcus in a looping fashion because of the depth of the right coronary artery in the sulcus. In this same area the anterior right atrial artery arises, and this branch often gives origin to the sinus node artery. More distally a lateral right atrial artery usually arises,[B9] and this artery is frequently severed when an oblique right atriotomy is made. In the region of the acute margin of the heart, a relatively constant long branch of the right coronary artery arises, the *acute marginal artery*, which courses most of the way to the apex of the heart. The right coronary artery in most hearts crosses the crux, where it takes a characteristic deep U-turn, giving off the *atrioventricular node artery* at the apex of the turn. The right coronary artery then terminates by bifurcating into the *right posterior descending coronary artery* and the *right posterolateral segment artery*. The *posterior descending coronary artery* descends in the posterior interventricular sulcus for a variable distance, giving rise to septal, right ventricular, and left ventricular branches. Variations in its anatomy are numerous, and it frequently arises before the crux. The right posterolateral segment of the right coronary artery gives origin to marginal branches to the inferior surface of the left ventricle in most hearts with a right dominant system.

Variations in the right coronary artery are common. It may have a dual origin from the right sinus of Valsalva. In about 10% of hearts, it bifurcates within a few millimeters of the aortic ostium, forming two diverging trunks of equal size. In half of the cases, the artery supplying the infundibulum of the right ventricle arises separately from the aortic sinus and is then termed the *conus artery*.[J5,S9] The *sinus node artery* originates from the second or third centimeter of the right coronary artery in many hearts (see "Coronary Arterial Supply to Specialized Areas of the Heart").[J5]

Coronary Arterial Supply to Specialized Areas of the Heart

The predominant blood supply to the ventricular septum is from the left anterior descending coronary artery via four to six large septal arteries 70–80 mm in length.[J6,J7] In contrast, the septal arteries from the posterior descending coronary artery (with the exception of the atrioventricular node artery) are rarely more than 15 mm in length (Fig. 1-22). They supply only a small zone of the ventricular septum near the posterior interventricular sulcus and in the region of the atrioventricular node. The septal arteries from the posterior descending artery may, however, serve as an important source of collateral circulation. Until their final terminations, the septal arteries from both anterior and posterior descend-

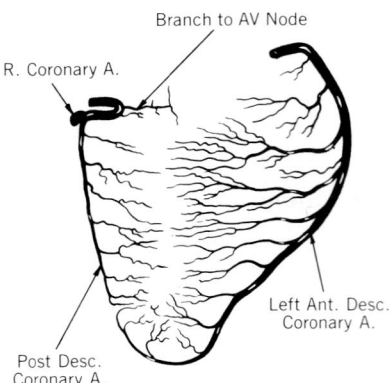

Figure 1-22 Drawing of the blood supply of the ventricular septum. Most of the septum is supplied by the left anterior descending coronary artery via large septal arteries. The septal arteries from the posterior descending artery are relatively small. In this right dominant circulation, note the origin of the AV node artery from the characteristic U-turn of the right coronary artery.

Reproduced with permission from James et al.,[J6] and the American Heart Association, Inc.

ing arteries course along the right ventricular side of the septum, where pressure is lower than on the left side.[J6] It is to be noted that in the 10% of hearts with a left dominant circulation, the entire blood supply is from the left coronary artery.

The sinus node artery arises from the right coronary artery in about 55% of hearts and from the left circumflex or main left coronary artery in the remainder. When it arises from the right coronary artery, it courses posteriorly and superiorly over the anterior wall of the right atrium beneath the right atrial appendage to the base of the superior vena cava. The sinus node artery may penetrate the interatrial septum in its course to the superior vena cava. It then encircles the cava clockwise or counterclockwise, or bifurcates and encircles it in both directions. If the sinus node artery arises from the left circumflex artery, it courses over the left atrial wall, variably penetrates the interatrial septum, and ascends to the base of the superior vena cava, encircling that vessel as when it originates from the right coronary artery (Fig. 1-23).

The atrioventricular node artery arises from the characteristic U-turn of the right coronary artery as it crosses the crux

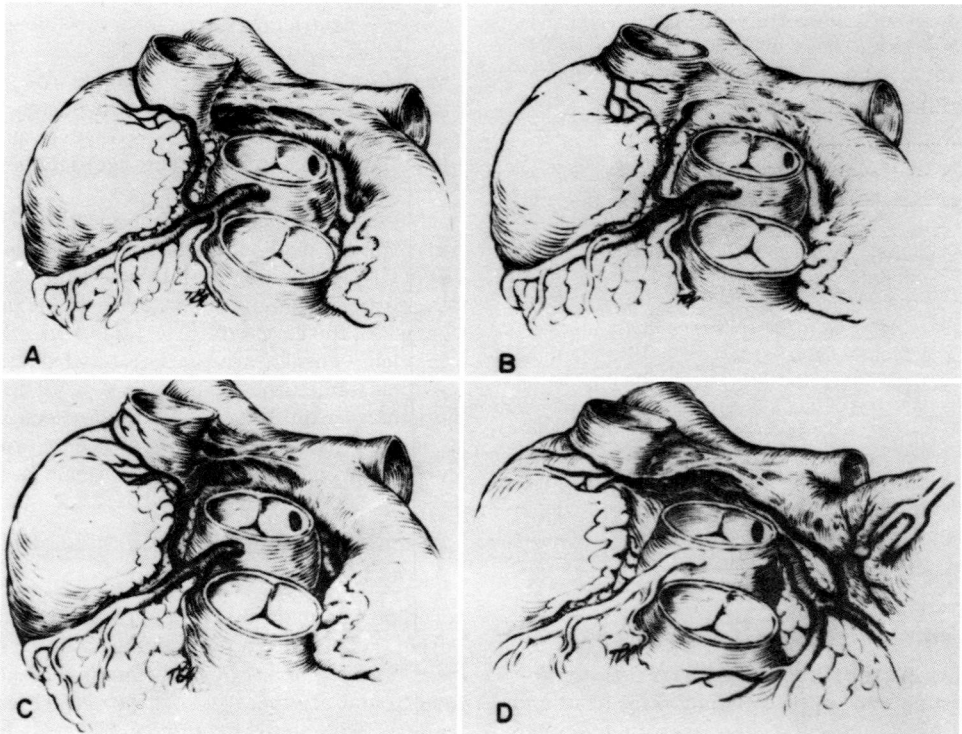

Figure 1-23 Origin and distribution of the sinus node artery. The sinus node artery may arise from the right coronary artery and encircle the base of the superior vena cava in (*a*) a clockwise direction or (*b*) a counterclockwise direction or (*c*) bifurcate and encircle it in both directions. The sinus node artery may arise from (*d*) the left circumflex artery and encircle the base of the superior vena cava as in *a*, *b*, or *c*.

Reproduced with permission from Lewis et al.[L7]

of the heart. The atrioventricular node is usually supplied by the dominant coronary artery. The atrioventricular node artery courses superiorly and anteriorly and terminates with a distinctive angulation.[S8] An important accessory blood supply to the atrioventricular node is *Kugel's artery*, which originates from the proximal segment of either the right coronary artery or the left circumflex artery and courses through the interatrial septum to the crux of the heart to anastomose with the atrioventricular node artery. In the atrial septum, Kugel's artery anastomoses with branches of the sinus node artery.[J5]

The bundle of His and the proximal few millimeters of the main bundle branches are supplied by the atrioventricular node artery. The remainder of the bundle branches and the Purkinje arborization within the septum are supplied by the septal arteries originating from the left anterior descending artery.

The anterolateral papillary muscle of the right ventricle, located near the junction of apical septum and free wall, is supplied by branches from the left anterior descending artery. The anterolateral papillary muscle of the left ventricle is supplied primarily by one or more branches from the left anterior descending coronary artery but may also be supplied by circumflex marginal branches. The arterial supply of the posteromedial papillary muscle of the left ventricle is from terminal branches of the right or circumflex arteries, depending upon the distribution of these arteries to the inferior surface of the left ventricle.

TERMINOLOGY AND CLASSIFICATION OF HEART DISEASE

Understanding the morphology of heart disease is fundamental to its surgical treatment. The morphology of heart disease could be fully described and understood using any one of a number of systems of terminology and classification. However, appropriate and accurate terminology and classification are important because they greatly facilitate the understanding and teaching of cardiac morphology, diagnosis, and surgical treatment. Also, they determine the method of categorization of cases, a procedure that is essential to the study of groups of patients.

The terminology and classification used at GLH and UAB have evolved over a period of about 25 years to a considerable extent in response to clinical, and particularly surgical, needs. It was based originally on the teaching of Edwards and his pupil, Becu, has been profoundly influenced and modified on numerous occasions by the work of Van Praagh, has benefited through the years from the work of Van Mierop and of Lev and recently his colleague, Bharati, and more recently by the concepts of Anderson.

Following the ideas of Lev, terminology based on the somewhat shifting sands of embryology has been avoided as much as possible. Any terms that have embryological implications are used only because they have become conventional. This is not to deny the importance of the science of embryology, but, rather, to emphasize the importance of precise description of morphology.

In the complete description of a cardiac anomaly in a patient, the following are tabulated:[B1,K2,K3,S10,V6]

Situs of the thoracic viscera and atria

Situs of the ventricles

Dominance of the ventricles
    Balanced ventricles
    Right ventricular (left hypoplasia)
    Left ventricular (right hypoplasia)

Cardiac connections
    Atrioventricular
    Ventriculoarterial

Cardiac and arterial position
    Heart
    Atria
    Ventricles
    Great arteries

Defects or malformations

Conventional diagnosis (when available)

Situs of the Thoracic Viscera and Atria

The possible situs of the thoracic viscera and atria are (1) situs solitus, (2) situs inversus, (3) situs ambiguus. *Situs solitus* means that the right-left relations of the asymmetric viscera and the atria are usual. That is to say, the right (eparterial) and left (hyparterial) main stem bronchi are normally positioned, the right atrium is to the right of the left atrium, and the left atrium is to the left. *Situs inversus* indicates that the right-left relations are the opposite of usual. In chemical language, these are isomers. With rare exceptions, atrial and thoracic visceral situs are concordant. *Situs ambiguus* is the absence of lateralization in the thoracic organs and atrial chambers;[V1,V2] in the case of the latter, this condition is termed *atrial isomerism* (see Chapter 46). It is usually, but not invariably, associated with the lack of abdominal lateralization, that is, asplenia or polysplenia.

In *asplenia* and *polysplenia*, the usually asymmetric structures tend to be symmetric. In both, in contrast to normal, the length of the right and left main stem bronchi are the same as is the relation of each bronchus to its pulmonary artery and the configuration of the artery.[L3,P1,V2] People with *asplenia* tend to have bilateral right-sidedness (right atriopulmonary isomerism), a condition best identified[S10,S11] by finding the right-type configuration of main stem bronchus and its pulmonary artery on both left and right sides (the bronchus is relatively short and posterior and superior to the pulmonary artery, which bifurcates into an upper and lower trunk).[B5,L3,S11] Patients with *polysplenia* tend to have bilateral left-sidedness[M5] (left atriopulmonary isomerism), with the left-type configuration of the main stem bronchus and its pulmonary artery on both sides (the bronchus is anterior and inferior to the pulmonary artery, which gives off individual branches, rather than a discrete trunk, to the upper lobe). A determination of situs can sometimes be made by study of the plain chest roentgenogram.[S1] When there is situs ambiguus, a common atrium is often present, and only the morphology of the atrial appendages indicates whether there is right or left atrial isomerism (see Chapter 46). Complex forms of congenital heart disease tend to occur in patients with atrial isomerism,[L4,L5,M5,S11] although, rarely, the heart is normal.

Situs of the Ventricles

In situs solitus, the ventricles are said to have normal (usual, concordant) situs when the morphologically right ventricle is anterior and to the right of the morphologic left ventricle, which is posterior and to the left. Van Praagh's term *D-loop*[V6,V9,V10] may be used to describe this ventricular situs, or isomer, as may his term *right-handedness*,[V13,V14] also used by Anderson.[A9] *D-loop* indicates that the *sinus portion* of the morphologic right ventricle is to the right vis-à-vis that of the left. In hearts with D-loop (as described by Van Praagh[V7]), the direction of blood flow in the right ventricle is from right to left through the right-sided tricuspid valve and inflow (sinus) portion to the usually left-sided outflow portion (infundibulum). D-loop, or right-handedness, can also be defined as existing when the palmar surface of the right hand can be placed on the septal surface of the right ventricle in such a way that the thumb is in the inlet (tricuspid valve), the wrist in the apical trabecular component, and the fingers in the outlet (pulmonary valve).

In situs solitus, the ventricles are said to be *inverted* when the morphologically right ventricle is more or less posterior and to the left of the morphologically left ventricle. Van Praagh's term *L-loop* applies here, as does the term *left-handedness*. In L-loop, the sinus (inlet) portion of the morphologically right ventricle is to the left vis-à-vis that of left; that is, the internal organization is the opposite of that in D-loop, and the direction of blood flow is from the left-sided tricuspid valve to the right-sided infundibulum. L-loop, or left-handedness, can also be defined as existing when the left hand can be placed with its palm on the septal surface of the right ventricle such that the thumb is in the inlet, the wrist in the apical trabecular component, and the fingers in the outlet. Bargeron (personal communication) has suggested that, looking through the right ventricle's AV valve toward its apex, in D-loop the septal structures are to the left and in L-loop they are to the right.

In atrial situs inversus, L-loop is the normal (usual, concordant) situs, and D-loop is the inverted situs. The definitions of the loop, or handedness, are independent of atrial or visceral situs and are thus the same as just described. Since there are two possible ventricular situs (D-loop and L-loop) in either thoracic and atrial situs solitus or inversus, there are four basic hearts, an idea expressed many years ago by Stanger, Edwards, and colleagues.[S12] (see Appendix 1A)

When the thoracic and atrial situs are ambiguus, only the ventricular situs can be described, and its relation to thoracic and atrial situs is "ambiguus."

Dominance of the Ventricles

Normally, the size (area on biplane cineangiogram) of the two ventricles is similar, and they can be said to be *balanced*. In many kinds of cardiac conditions, one ventricle is larger, or dominant, and the other is smaller and can be severely hypoplastic. The dominance may be mild, moderate, or severe. Indeed, in rare cases, only one ventricle exists (see Chapter 44).

Cardiac Connections

Information about the cardiac connections is fundamental in describing any malformed heart and requires elucidation at both atrioventricular and ventriculoarterial levels. The *atrioventricular connection* may be *concordant* (the right atrium[4] connects to the right ventricle; the left atrium connects to the left ventricle), *discordant* (the right atrium connects to the left ventricle, the left atrium to the right ventricle), *univentricular* (the atria connect to only one ventricle; see Chapter 44 for more details of this subset), or *ambiguus* (situs ambiguus of atria). When an AV valve is straddling, it is considered connected to the ventricle into which more than 50% of the valve orifice faces. As Bharati and colleagues have pointed out, it is pertinent to distinguish between straddling of the *valve anulus* across the septum and of the *chordal attachments* into an inappropriate ventricle.[B8] Milo and colleagues have suggested that the term *overriding* should be used when referring to the anulus, and *straddling* when referring to chordal attachments.[M6]

The *ventriculoarterial connection* may be concordant (the left ventricle connects wholly or nearly so to the aorta, the right ventricle to the pulmonary artery) or discordant (the right ventricle connects to the aorta, the left ventricle to the pulmonary artery; commonly called transposition of the great artery[V8]). As with the atrioventricular connections, when a semilunar valve is overriding a ventricular septal defect, it is considered connected to the ventricle from which over 50% of the valve area arises. The connection may also be *double outlet* (the great arteries arise wholly or for the most part from one ventricle).

The ventriculoarterial connection may be considered *single outlet* when there is a common arterial trunk (truncus arteriosus communis) or only a single artery, usually the aorta, connected to a ventricle. In the latter case there is usually pulmonary atresia, and categorization as single outlet ventriculoarterial connection, although morphologically precise, considerably complicates the presentation of information in many types of congenital heart disease. Alternatively, the ventriculoarterial connections can be termed concordant, discordant, or double outlet by identifying the connection, although atretic, of the pulmonary artery to a ventricle. Even when there is a ventriculo-pulmonary artery discontinuity, this is often possible. For example, when the morphology is typical for tetralogy of Fallot except that there is only a single ventricular outlet because of pulmonary atresia, the condition is called tetralogy of Fallot with pulmonary atresia (see Chapter 23).

---

[4] The adjectives left and right used to modify atrium or ventricle always mean "morphologically right" or "morphologically left." The position of the chamber is referred to as "right-sided" or "left-sided."

Cardiac and Arterial Positions

Normally, the cardiac apex points to the left, a situation called *levocardia*. The term *dextrocardia* applies when the cardiac apex points to the right; and *mesocardia,* when it is in the midline. There is merit to using the term *dextroversion* to denote dextrocardia with situs solitus of the viscera and atria, and *levoversion* to denote levocardia with situs inversus. Dextroversion and levoversion alter the geometry and position of all the cardiac chambers. Thus, the position of the heart is important surgically, but it is not a basic abnormality, such as D- or L-loop.

The left atrium is generally to the left and the right atrium to the right in situs solitus, and opposite to it in situ inversus.

The position of the ventricles is determined primarily, but not exclusively, by the ventricular situs (loop). The morphologically right ventricle is usually anterior and to the right in D-loop, and the left ventricle posterior and to the left. Generally, with L-loop (inverted ventricles), the morphologically left ventricle is anterior and to the right, and the morphologically right ventricle posterior and to the left. However, the ventricles may be side-by-side or directly anteroposterior to one another, with either ventricle in either position. Recent interest has focused on the superoinferior (over-and-under) position of the ventricles, which occurs most commonly with L-loop but can occur with D-loop.[V7] This, and probably other positional anomalies, are most clearly seen by angiocardiographic study and, indeed, may be entirely overlooked by autopsy studies. These positional interrelations are not basic pathologic entities but are best thought of as rotational anomalies producing various patterns from the four basic hearts.

The possible positions of the origins of the great arteries are nearly infinite around the 360° of a circle but may be simplified as (1) normal, with aorta to the right (in visceroatrial situs solitus) or left (in inversus) and somewhat posterior to the pulmonary artery; (2) aorta anterior to the pulmonary artery, either directly or somewhat to the right (D-malposition[V8]); (3) aorta to the left of the pulmonary artery (L-malposition); and (4) aorta posterior to the pulmonary artery.

Normally, the great arteries tend to cross rather than to run parallel. In contrast, when the great arteries are malposed, their first portions are usually parallel.[D3]

As indicated, these are all positional arterial abnormalities and are not basic parts of a malformation. However, certain probabilities exist. For example, the inflow portion of the right ventricle is usually on the side of the aortic origin.

Crisscross Atrioventricular Flow Pathways

In normal hearts, the atrioventricular flow pathways are more or less parallel. In cases of crisscross atrioventricular flow pathways, they cross over each other. The term *crisscross hearts* was introduced by Ando et al.[A6] and by Anderson et al.[A4] in 1974, but the condition had been described earlier by Lev, in 1961.[L8]

The phrase *crisscross* has caused confusion and controversy. One point of view is that in some abnormal hearts the pathways cross when viewed on cineangiography (UAB). Another point of view is that this is an illusion (GLH).[V11] In any event, *crisscross* has no implications with regard to internal ventricular architecture or atrioventricular connections. The crisscross of the flow pathways is produced by positional abnormalities of the ventricles (often resulting in their being in a superior-inferior, or two-storied, position). Hypoplasia of the inflow or sinus of the right ventricle often contributes to crisscross. In most cases of crisscross, there is ventriculoarterial discordance and either discordant ventriculoarterial connections or double-outlet right ventricle.

Defects and Abnormalities

Defects involving the heart chambers and valves are more common when there are connection and rotational anomalies. Such defects must be described separately for each heart, along with that heart's segmental situs, connections, and positions. Possible defects include atrial septal defect, atrioventricular canal, anomalous systemic and pulmonary venous connections, congenital valvar and subvalvar lesions, straddling AV valves, and abnormalities of septal morphology, including conal infundibular development.

Conventional Diagnoses

As a summarizing convenience, certain old and more or less widely used phrases that are in themselves not anatomically specific but that are well-understood by most surgeons continue to be useful. In each instance, the morphology denoted by a given phrase must be defined, in part because others may use the same phrase (such as *transposition of the great arteries*) differently. Such phrases include *AV canal* (Chapter 19), *tetralogy of Fallot* (Chapter 23), *Taussig-Bing heart* (Chapter 40), *complete transposition of the great arteries* (Chapter 39), *double-outlet ventricle* (Chapters 40 and 41), *corrected transposition of the great arteries* (Chapter 42), *isolated ventricular inversion* (Chapter 43), and *anatomically corrected malposition of the great arteries* (Chapter 45). In the interest of readability, the text does not use quotation marks for these phrases, but it would be more correct to do so, since, once defined, they are used primarily for convenience.

Symbolic Convention of Van Praagh

Van Praagh's symbolic convention for the heart, for example, S,D,D heart, is widely used and is a convenient and concise way of expressing certain features of the heart.[V5] The first symbol refers to the situs (isomerism) of thoracic viscera and atria (S for solitus, I for inversus). The second symbol indicates the situs (isomerism) of the ventricles in terms of D-loop and L-loop (see "Situs of the Ventricles"). When taken with the first symbol, it is of fundamental significance in designating which of the four basic hearts, or isomeric combinations, is present. The third symbol refers to the position of the aortic origin (D for right-sided, L for left-sided).

APPENDIX

APPENDIX **1A**

ILLUSTRATIVE MODELS OF CONGENITAL HEART DISEASE

The concepts of the Van Praagh symbolic representation may be combined with those of atrioventricular and ventricular arterial connections as shown in the figures (GLH).

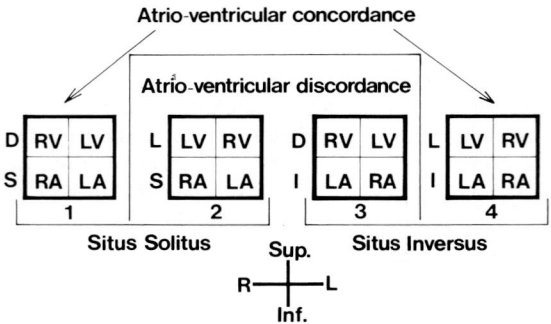

Figure 1A-1   A model of the atrioventricular connections of the four basic hearts, excluding situs ambiguus (GLH). The arrangement of boxes and the abbreviations are identical in all similar models presented here.

D, D ventricular loop; I, situs inversus; L, L ventricular loop; S, situs solitus; RV, right ventricle; LV, left ventricle; RA, right atrium; LA, left atrium.

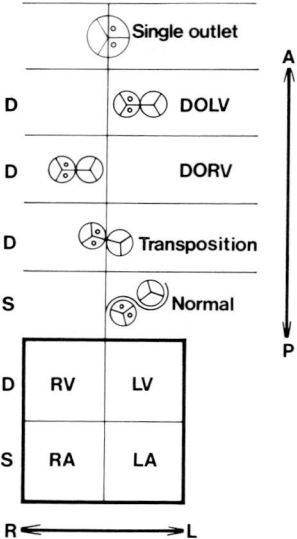

Figure 1A-3   A model of the varieties of ventriculoarterial connection (GLH). The aortic origin in transposition of the great arteries and the double-outlet ventricles (DORV, DOLV) is indicated by D when it lies to the right of the pulmonary artery origin and L when it lies to the left. When the aortic origin is anterior, it is almost always also superior to the pulmonary artery; when side by side, both origins are usually at the same level. The vertical line above the box represents the position of the ventricular septum.

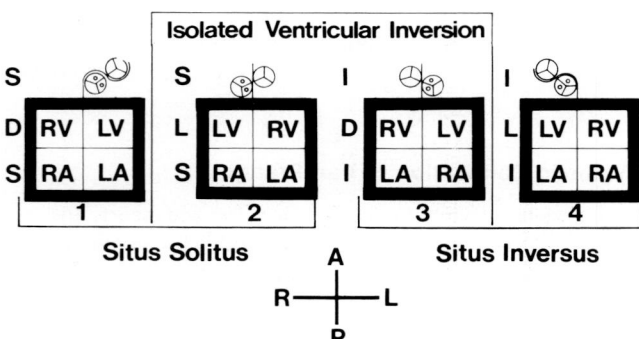

Figure 1A-2   A model of the four so-called normal hearts, that is, hearts with atrioventricular and ventriculoarterial concordance (GLH). In the Van Praagh convention, the first letter (S or I) refers to the atrial position (solitus or inversus); the second letter (D or L) to the ventricular loop; and the third letter to the position of the origin of the aorta (recognized by its two coronary ostia) in relation to the origin of the pulmonary artery.[V12] Note that in situs inversus the aortic origin lies to the left of the pulmonary artery origin.

REFERENCES

A

1. Anderson RH, Becker AE, Van Mierop LHS: What should we call the "crista"? *Br Heart J* 39:856, 1977.

2. Ad Hoc Committee for Grading of Coronary Artery Disease, Council on Cardiovascular Surgery, American Heart Association: American Heart Association committee report: A reporting system on patients evaluated for coronary artery disease. *Circulation* 51:5, 1975.

3. Anderson RH, Becker AE, Wenink ACG: The development of the conducting tissues, in NK Roberts, H Gelband (eds): *Cardiac Arrhythmias in the Neonate, Infant, and Child.* New York: Appleton-Century-Crofts, 1977, p 1.

4. Anderson RH, Shinebourne EA, Gerlis LN: Criss-cross atrioventricular relationships producing paradoxical atrioventricular concordance or discordance: Their significance to nomenclature of congenital heart disease. *Circulation* 50:176, 1974.

5. Anderson RH: Embryology of the ventricular septum, in RH Anderson, EA Shinebourne (eds): *Pediatric Cardiology 1977.* Edinburgh: Churchill Livingstone, 1978, p 103.

6. Ando M, Takao A, Cho E: Criss-cross heart by abnormal rotation of ventricular loop: Diagnostic considerations for complex cardiac anomaly. *Proc Pediatr Circ Soc* 4, 1974.

7. Anderson RH, Becker AE, in *Cardiac Anatomy.* Edinburgh, London: Churchill Livingstone, 1980.

8. Anderson RH, Ho SY, Becker AE: The surgical anatomy of the conduction tissues. *Thorax* 38:408, 1983.

9. Anderson RH: Criss-cross hearts revisited: A question of definition. *Pediatr Cardiol* 3:305, 1982.

10. Anderson RH, Ho SY, Becker AE: The clinical anatomy of the cardiac conduction system, in DJ Rowlands (ed): *Recent Advances in Cardiology.* Edinburgh: Churchill Livingstone, 1984.

B

1. Brandt PWT, Calder AL: Cardiac connections: The segmental approach to radiologic diagnosis in congenital heart disease, in *Current Problems in Diagnostic Radiology.* Chicago: Year Book Medical, 1977.

2. Bargeron LM Jr, Elliott LP, Soto B, Bream PR, Curry G: Axial cineangiography in congenital heart disease. I. Concept, Technical and Anatomic Considerations. *Circulation* 56:1075, 1977.

3. Barry A, Patten BM: The structure of the adult heart, in SE Gould (ed): *Pathology of the Heart and Blood Vessels* (ed 3). Springfield, Ill: Charles C Thomas, 1968, p 91.

4. Baltaxe HA, Amplatz K, Levin DC: *Coronary Angiography.* Springfield, Ill: Charles C Thomas, 1973.

5. Brandt HM, Liebow AA: Right pulmonary isomerism associated with venous, splenic, and other abnormalities. *Lab Invest* 7:469, 1958.

6. Bharati S, Lev M, Kirklin JW: *Cardiac Surgery and the Conduction System.* New York: John Wiley & Sons, 1983.

7. Brandt PWT, Partridge JB, Wattie WJ: Coronary arteriography: A method of presentation of the arteriogram report and a scoring system. *Clin Radiol* 28:361, 1977.

8. Bharati S, McAllister HA Jr, Lev M: Straddling and displaced atrioventricular orifice valves. *Circulation* 60:673, 1979.

9. Busquet J, Fontan F, Anderson RH, Ho SY, Davies MJ: The surgical significance of the atrial branches of the coronary arteries. *Int J Cardiol* 6:223, 1984.

C

1. Principal investigators of CASS and their associates: The National Heart, Lung, and Blood Institute Coronary Artery Surgery Study (CASS). *Circulation* 63 (Suppl 1):1 June 1981.

D

1. Demoulin JC, Kulbertus HE: Histopathological examination of concept of left hemiblock. *Br Heart J* 34:807, 1972.

2. Daves ML: Cardiac roentgenology: The loop and circle approach. *Radiology* 95:157, 1970.

3. De la Cruz MV, Berrazueta JR, Arteaga M, Attie F, Soni J: Rules for diagnosis of arterioventricular discordances and spatial identification of ventricles: Crossed great arteries and transposition of the great arteries. *Br Heart J* 38:341, 1976.

F

1. Fulton WFM: *The Coronary Arteries.* Springfield, Ill: Charles C Thomas, 1965.

G

1. Gray H, in CM Goss (ed): *Anatomy of the Human Body* (ed 29). Philadelphia: Lea & Febiger, 1973, p 543.

2. Gross L, Kugel MA: Topographic anatomy and histology of the valves in the human heart. *Am J Pathol* 7:445, 1931.

3. Gensini GG: *Coronary Arteriography.* Mount Kisco, NY: Futura, 1975.

H

1. Hudson REB: The human pacemaker and its pathology. *Br Heart J* 22:153, 1960.

J

1. James TN: Anatomy of the human sinus node. *Anat Rec* 141:109, 1961.

2. James TN: The connecting pathways between the sinus node and the AV node and between the right and left atrium in the human heart. *Am Heart J* 66:498, 1963.

3. Janse MJ, Anderson RH: Specialized internodal atrial pathways: Fact or fiction? *Eur J Cardiol* 2:117, 1974.

4. James TN: Morphology of the human atrioventricular node, with remarks pertinent to its electrophysiology. *Am Heart J* 62:756, 1961.

5. James TN: *Anatomy of the Coronary Arteries.* New York: Hoeber, 1961.

6. James TN, Burch GE: The blood supply of the human interventricular septum. *Circulation* 17:391, 1958.

7. James TN: Anatomy of the coronary arteries in health and disease. *Circulation* 32:1020, 1965.

K

1. Kerr A Jr, Goss CM: Retention of embryonic relationship of aortic and pulmonary valve cusps and a suggested nomenclature. *Anat Rec* 125:777, 1956.

2. Kirklin JW: Introduction, in JW Kirklin (ed): *Advances in Cardiovascular Surgery.* New York: Grune & Stratton, 1973, pp 3–7.

3. Kirklin JW, Pacifico AD, Bargeron LM Jr, Soto B: Cardiac repair in anatomically corrected malposition of the great arteries. *Circulation* 48:153, 1973.

L

1. Lev M, Bharati S: Anatomy of the conduction system in normal and congenitally abnormal hearts, in NK Roberts, H Gelband (eds): *Cardiac Arrhythmias in the Neonate, Infant, and Child.* New York: Appleton-Century-Crofts, 1977, p 29.
2. Lam JHC, Ranganathan N, Wigle ED, Silver MD: Morphology of the human mitral valve. I. Chordae tendineae: A new classification. *Circulation* 41:449, 1970.
3. Landing BH, Lawrence TK, Payne VC, Wells TR: Bronchial anatomy in syndromes with abnormal visceral situs, abnormal spleen, and congenital heart disease. *Am J Cardiol* 128:456, 1971.
4. Lev M, Liberthson RR, Golden JG, Eckner FAO, Arcilla RA: The pathologic anatomy of mesocardia. *Am J Cardiol* 28:428, 1971.
5. Liberthson RR, Hastreiter AR, Sinha SN, Bharati S, Novak GM, Lev M: Levocardia with visceral heterotaxy-isolated levocardia: Pathologic anatomy and its clinical implication. *Am Heart J* 85:40, 1973.
6. Lev M: The conduction system, in SE Gould (ed): *Pathology of the Heart and Blood Vessels* (ed 3). Springfield, Ill: Charles C Thomas, 1968, p 183.
7. Lewis AB, Lindesmith GG, Takahashi M, Stanton RE, Tucker BL, Stiles QR, Meyer BW: Cardiac rhythm following the mustard procedure for transposition of the great vessels. *J Thorac Cardiovasc Surg* 73:919, 1977.
8. Lev M, Rowlatt UF: The pathological anatomy of mixed levocardia: A review of 13 cases of atrial or ventricular inversion with or without corrected transposition. *Am J Cardiol* 9:216, 1961.

M

1. Massing GK, Liebman J, James TN: Cardiac conduction pathways in the infant and child, in M. A. Engle (ed): *Pediatric Cardiology.* FA Davis, 1974, p 27.
2. Massing GK, James TN: Anatomical configuration of the His bundle and proximal bundle branches in the human heart. *Circulation* 43,44(suppl II):II-64, 1971 (abstr).
3. Merkin RJ: Position and orientation of the heart valves. *Am J Anat* 125:375, 1969.
4. McAlpine WA: *Heart and Coronary Arteries.* Berlin: Springer-Verlag, 1975.
5. Moller JH, Nakib A, Anderson RC, Edwards JE: Congenital cardiac disease associated with polysplenia: A developmental complex of bilateral 'left-sideness.' *Circulation* 36:789, 1967.
6. Milo S, Ho SY, Macartney FJ, Wilkinson JL, Becker AE, Wenink ACG, Gittenberger de Grott AC, Anderson RH: Straddling and over-riding atrio-ventricular valves: Morphology and classification. *Am J Cardiol* 44:1122, 1979.

N

1. National Heart, Lung and Blood Institute: Proposal and Manual of Operations for Collaborative Studies in Coronary Artery Surgery. Contract no. 1-HV-32973, National Heart, Lung and Blood Institute, 1975.

O

1. Ogden JA: Congenital anomalies of the coronary arteries. *Am J Cardiol* 25:474, 1970.

P

1. Partridge JB, Scott O, Deverall PB, Macartney FJ: Visualization and measurement of the main bronchi by tomography as an objective indicator of thoracic situs in congenital heart disease. *Circulation* 51:188, 1975.
2. Perloff JK, Roberts WC: The mitral apparatus: Functional anatomy of mitral regurgitation. *Circulation* 46:227, 1972.

R

1. Ranganathan N, Lam JHC, Wigle ED, Silver MD: Morphology of the human mitral valve. II. The valve leaflets. *Circulation* 41:459, 1970.
2. Rusted IE, Scheifley CH, Edwards JE: Studies of the mitral valve. I. Anatomic features of the normal mitral valve and associated structures. *Circulation* 6:825, 1952.

S

1. Soto B, Pacifico AD, Souza AS, Bargeron LM Jr, Ermocilla R, Tonkin IL: Identification of thoracic isomerism from the plain chest roentgenogram. *Am J Roentgenol* 131:995, 1978.
2. Spach MS, King TD, Barr RC, Boaz DE, Morrow MN, Herman-Giddens S: Electrical potential distribution surrounding the atria during depolarization and repolarization in the dog. *Circ Res* 24:857, 1969.
3. Spach MS, Lieberman M, Scott JC, Barr RC, Johnson EA, Kootsey JM: Excitation sequences of the atrial septum and AV node in isolated hearts of the dog and rabbit. *Circ Res* 29:156, 1971.
4. Spach MS, Huang S, Armstrong SI, Canent RV Jr: Demonstration of peripheral conduction system in human hearts. *Circulation* 28:333, 1963.
5. Silverman ME, Hurst JW: The mitral complex. *Am Heart J* 76:399, 1968.
6. Silver MD, Lam JHC, Ranganathan N, Wigle ED: Morphology of the human tricuspid valve. *Circulation* 43:333, 1971.
7. Sherman FE: Ventricular septal defect, in FE Sherman (ed): *An Atlas of Congenital Heart Disease.* Philadelphia: Lea & Febiger, 1963, p 170.
8. Soto B, Russell RO Jr, Moraski RE: *Radiographic Anatomy of the Coronary Arteries: An Atlas.* Mt. Kisco, NY: Futura, 1976.
9. Schlesinger MJ, Zoll PM, Wessler S: The conus artery: A third coronary artery. *Am Heart J* 38:823, 1949.
10. Shinebourne EA, Macartney FJ, Anderson RH: Sequential chamber localization-logical approach to diagnosis in congenital heart disease. *Br Heart J* 38:327, 1976.
11. Stanger P, Rudolph AM, Edwards JE: Cardiac malpositions. *Circulation* 56:159, 1977.
12. Stanger P, Benassi RC, Korns ME, Jue KL, Edwards JE: Diagrammatic portrayal of variations in cardiac structure, reference to transposition, dextrocardia and the concept of four normal heart. *Circulation* 37(suppl IV):IV-1, 1968.

T

1. Tandler J: *Anatomie des Herzens: Handbuch des Anatomie des Mensihen,* vol 3, part 1. Jena: Gustav Fischer, 1913, p 84.

2. Titus JL: Normal anatomy of the human cardiac conduction system. *Mayo Clin Proc* 48:24, 1973.

3. Truex RC: The sinoatrial node and its connections with the atrial tissues, in HJJ Wellens, KI Lie, MJ Janse (eds): *The Conduction System of the Heart*. Philadelphia: Lea & Febiger, 1976, p 209.

V

1. Van Mierop LHS, Wiglesworth FW: Isomerism of the cardiac atria in the asplenia syndrome. *Lab Invest* 11:1303, 1962.

2. Van Mierop LHS, Eisen S, Schiebler GL: The radiographic appearance of the tracheobronchial tree as an indicator of visceral situs. *Am J Cardiol* 26:432, 1970.

3. Van Mierop LHS: Anatomy and embryology of the right ventricle, in JE Edwards, M Lev, MR Abell (eds): *The Heart*. Baltimore: Williams & Wilkins, 1974.

4. Vlodaver Z, Amplatz K, Burchell HB, Edwards JE: *Coronary Heart Disease: Clinical Angiographic and Pathologic Profiles*. New York: Springer-Verlag, 1976.

5. Van Praagh R: The segmental approach to diagnosis in congenital heart disease: Birth defects. *Original Article Series* 8:4, 1972.

6. Van Praagh R, Ongley PA, Swan HJC: Anatomic types of single or common ventricle in man. *Am J Cardiol* 13:367, 1964.

7. Van Praagh S, LaCorte M, Fellows KE, Bossina K, Busch HJ, Keck EW, Weinberg PM, Van Praagh R: Superior-inferior ventricles: Anatomic and angiocardiographic findings in 10 postmortem cases, in *Etiology and Morphogenesis of Congenital Heart Disease*. Futura, Mt. Kisco, NY: 1980, p 317.

8. Van Praagh R, Van Praagh S: Isolated ventricular inversion: A consideration of the morphogenesis, definition and diagnosis of non-transposed and transposed great arteries. *Am J Cardiol* 17:395, 1966.

9. Van Praagh R, Van Praagh S, Vlad P, Keith JD: Anatomic types of congenital dextrocardia: Diagnostic and embryologic implications. *Am J Cardiol* 13:510, 1964.

10. Van Praagh R, Plett JA, Van Praagh S: Single ventricle: Pathology, embryology, terminology, and classification. *Herz* 4:113, 1979.

11. Van Praagh R, Weinberg PM, Van Praagh S: Malposition of the heart, in AJ Moss, FH Adams, GC Emmanouilides (eds): *Heart Disease in Infants, Children and Adolescents*. Baltimore: Williams & Wilkins, 1977, p 395.

12. Van Praagh R: Terminology of congenital heart disease: Glossary and commentary. *Circulation* 56:139, 1977.

13. Van Praagh R, David I, Gordon D, Wright B, Van Praagh S: Ventricular diagnosis and designation, in MJ Godman (ed): *Pediatric Cardiology*, vol 4. London: Churchill Livingstone, 1981, p 153.

14. Van Praagh S, La Corte M, Fellows KE, Bossina K, Busch JH, Beck EW, Weinberg P, Van Praagh R: Superior-inferior ventricles: Anatomic and angiocardiographic findings in ten postmortem cases, in R Van Praagh (ed): *Etiology and Morphology of Congenital Heart Disease*. Mt Kisco, New York: Futura, 1980, p 317.

W

1. Walmsley R, Watson H: The outflow tract of the left ventricle. *Br Heart J* 28:435, 1966.

Z

1. Zimmerman J: The functional and surgical anatomy of the aortic valve. *Isr J Med Sci* 5:862, 1969.

2

HYPOTHERMIA, CIRCULATORY ARREST, AND CARDIOPULMONARY BYPASS

SECTION **1**

HYPOTHERMIA AND TOTAL CIRCULATORY ARREST

HISTORICAL NOTE

Bigelow, with his publication in 1950[B1,B2] on experimental hypothermia produced by surface cooling, introduced the idea that whole body hypothermia might be useful in cardiac surgery. Boerema in 1951[B3] reported experimental studies indicating that when animals were cooled by a femoral-femoral shunt through a cooling coil, up to 15 minutes of total circulatory arrest (produced by inflow stasis) were tolerated without apparent ill effect. Bigelow, later in 1950,[B4] reported cooling dogs to 20°C by surface cooling, with recovery after 15 minutes of total circulatory arrest. In 1953, Lewis and Taufic[L1] reported successful repair of an atrial septal defect in a 5-year-old girl with surface cooling, and Swan at about the same time reported successful results[S1] in a number of patients treated by the same technique. In 1958, Sealy, Brown, and Young reported successful clinical cases[S2] in which hypothermia was combined with cardiopulmonary bypass (CPB). In 1959, Drew[D1] reported experimental studies in which CPB (using the subject's own lungs as the oxygenator) was used to cool and rewarm the subject, and operations done during profound hypothermia (to 15°C) and total circulatory arrest. In 1960, Dubost and colleagues reported the use of profound hypothermia and total circulatory arrest for cardiac surgery.[W1] In 1961, we[K1] reported from the Mayo Clinic the results of operation with profound hypothermia and total circulatory arrest in 52 patients, using Drew's technique in 23 patients and a pump-oxygenator in 29. In 1963, Horiuchi and colleagues,[H1] from Tohoku University, in Japan, reported 16 survivors of repair of VSD in 18 infants under 1 year of age, using surface cooling to 25°C and total circulatory arrest. Dillard and colleagues modified this technique to permit surface cooling to profoundly hypothermic temperatures of 17–20°C and extension of the circulatory arrest time to 60 minutes. In 1967, they reported successful repair of total anomalous pulmonary venous connection in four infants by this method of surface cooling and rewarming.[D2] Also in 1967, Hikasa and colleagues, from Kyoto University, reported[H2] good results in the repair of a number of malformations, using the technique of surface-cooling patients to 20°C and performing the procedure during total circulatory arrest lasting 15–75 minutes with CPB rewarming. Wakusawa, at Iwate University, reported a similar experience in 1968.[W2] In 1970, we[B5] reported from GLH the repair of a variety of malformations during total circulatory arrest in 34 infants weighing less than 10 kg, using surface cooling to 22–27°C, followed by a brief period of CPB to reduce the temperature further, and rewarming with limited CPB. Hamilton, in 1973, reported[H3] operations with profound hypothermia and total circulatory arrest in 18 infants, using only CPB for cooling (core cooling).

HYPOTHESES AND ASSUMPTIONS

The hypothesis underlying the use of total circulatory arrest for cardiac surgery is that there is a "safe" duration of this state, the length of which is inversely related to the temperature of the organism during the arrest period. A "safe" period of total circulatory arrest is characterized by absence of detectable functional or structural organ derangements in the early or late postoperative period. Structural derangements without apparent functional derangement must be of concern because of the implied loss of reserve, which may be of importance to the individual in later life.

The temperature of the organism is not so easily defined. In normal humans, the temperature gradients at rest are small,[B6] so a single numerical representation of inner body temperature is acceptable. When hypothermia is produced by surface cooling, internal temperature gradients are relatively small.[C1] Of course, the skin and muscles become cooler than the inner organs, and rectal temperature is significantly lower than nasopharyngeal temperature. During cooling by hypothermic perfusion with CPB (core cooling), the relationship of rectal to nasopharyngeal temperature is reversed, and organ and regional differences in temperature are considerable, although they can be lessened by prolonging the cooling period.[C1] Thus, particularly when this technique is used wholly or in part for profound hypothermia, the specific site of temperature measurement must be noted as well as the limitations in interpretation of the measurements themselves.

The assumption is that hypothermia, without itself producing damage, reduces metabolic activity to the extent that the available energy stores in the various organs maintain cell viability throughout the ischemic period of total circulatory arrest and thus allow normal structure and function to return after recovery from the arrest period. It is also assumed that the magnitude of the reduction of oxygen consumption is directly related to the "safe" duration of total circulatory arrest.

OXYGEN CONSUMPTION DURING HYPOTHERMIA

Oxygen consumption is considered a measure of metabolic activity. Therefore, the magnitude of its decrease by hypothermia (in the anesthetized subject, in whom shivering is prevented) has been taken as an index of the degree of reduction of metabolic activity. The use of oxygen consumption as such a marker is reasonable, because for all practical purposes tissue and cellular stores of oxygen do not exist. Thus, the body is dependent upon the circulation to bring oxygen to tissues in amounts determined by the oxygen consumption.

Relationship between Oxygen Consumption and Body Temperature

The energy requirements of the body, reflected in part by oxygen consumption ($\dot{V}o_2$), are reduced during hypothermia, reflecting the dependence of the rate of biochemical reactions upon temperature.[F1] The quantitative interrelations have been expressed mathematically in various ways. Some have used a linear model. Others, including Harris, at GLH,[H4] have used a model based on Arrhenius' theory, which states that the logarithm of the rate of a chemical reaction is inversely proportional to the reciprocal of the absolute temperature. This curve describing this relationship is S-shaped (similar to the familiar oxygen dissociation curve) such that at very high temperatures the reaction rate ceases increasing with temperature (reaches an asymptote). However, at physiologic temperatures, biochemical systems operate only on the upswing of the curve. Thus, particularly when the range of temperature is relatively small, this relationship finds numerical expression in van't Hoff's law, which relates the logarithm of a chemical reaction rate directly to temperature. Conveniently, according to this equation, the reaction rate increases by two to three times for an increase of temperature of 10°C. Chemists use the symbol Q_{10} for this multiple.

Since oxygen uptake is the expression of all oxidative reactions, both direct and indirect, the logarithm of $\dot{V}o_2$ might be expected to be directly proportional to temperature. In general, this appears to be so. Whether the observed fall in $\dot{V}o_2$ during clinical hypothermia can be accounted for entirely on this physicochemical basis is doubtful, however (see "Oxygen Consumption during Hypothermia in Tissue Slices and Isolated Organs").

Total Body Oxygen Consumption after Surface Cooling

As already noted, when hypothermia is induced by cooling the surface of an anesthetized human or an experimental animal, cooling is rather uniform throughout the body and the temperatures of internal organs and regions differ by less than 2°C.[C1] Therefore, the values for whole body oxygen consumption at various body temperatures are probably useful, and the relative magnitude of reduction can be assumed to be similar throughout the body.

Good data in this area are available from the animal experiments of Ross,[R1] Bigelow,[B2] and Penrod.[P1] Data for surface cooling in humans are sparse, though Harris, at GLH,[H5] estimated Q_{10} to lie between 1.9 and 4.2 in 10 surface-cooled infants. The experimental animal data have been (UAB) reanalyzed using (1) a linear equation, (2) Arrhenius' equation, and (3) van't Hoff's law. The latter best explained this combined set of data (Fig. 2-1).[R1,B2,P1]

Oxygen Consumption during Hypothermia in Tissue Slices and Isolated Organs

Data from the studies described above could lead to an underestimation of true oxygen demand, since only areas in which perfusion of the microcirculation continues can participate in oxygen consumption (tissue and cellular stores of oxygen being trivial). In theory at least, a considerable part of the reduction in oxygen consumption from surface cooling could be from the shutting down of the microcirculation of portions of the body or from arteriovenous shunting.

Studies in tissue slices at various temperatures show that oxygen consumption is in fact reduced by hypothermia.[F2,F3,F4] These studies and those of isolated organs suggest that Q_{10}, though differing from tissue to tissue, is on the average about 2 (for references and a table of Q_{10} values, see the paper by Harris et al.[H6]). Measurement of human $\dot{V}o_2$ before and after heating, rather than cooling, indicate a Q_{10} in this same range, of about 1.9.[S3] The vasodilatation due to heating presumably ensures access of oxygen to the tissues, and this Q_{10} probably represents true tissue O_2 requirement. A Q_{10} greater than 1.9 due to cooling may therefore indicate that O_2 delivery has been compromised. Fuhrman and associates have spent many years investigating this possibility. They showed that in general there was a close agreement between resting $\dot{V}o_2$ at 37°C and tissue slice respiration.[F4,M1] However, rats cooled by immersion to 18°C exhibit a 33% lower $\dot{V}o_2$ than would be expected from studies of tissue slice respiration at this temperature.[F3] The discrepancy was not accounted for by either inhomogeneities in whole body temperature or by the known changes in Q_{10} exhibited by some tissues with temperature (in part related to altered function at reduced temperatures). The exact mechanism remains unknown. It could be due to arteriovenous shunting or to shutting down of perfusion to some areas of the body. Microvascular physiologists have referred to the latter as a decrease in the *effective capillary density*. This may result not only from reduced cardiac output and vasoconstriction but also from changes in blood viscosity, geometry and com-

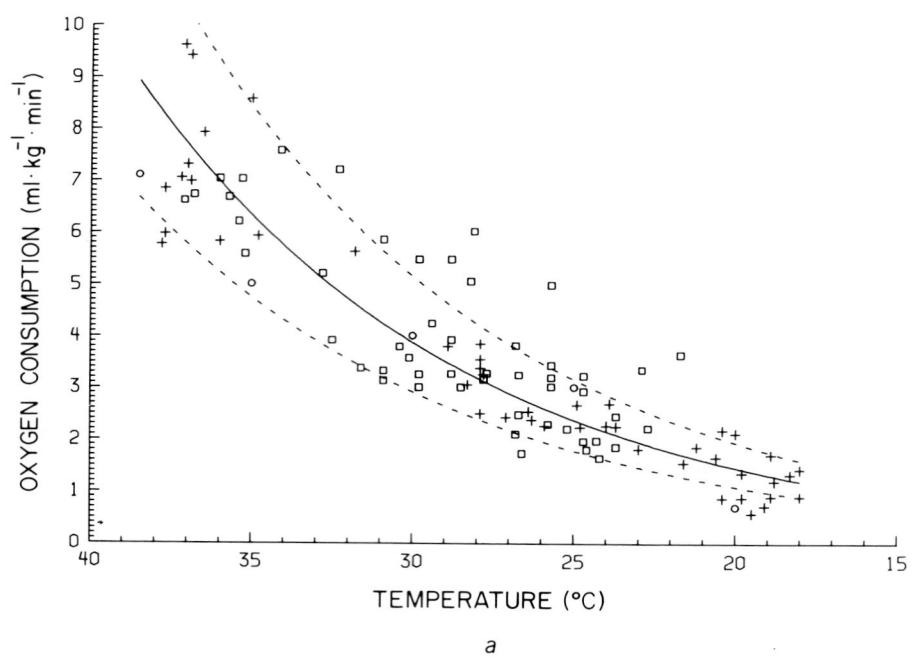

a

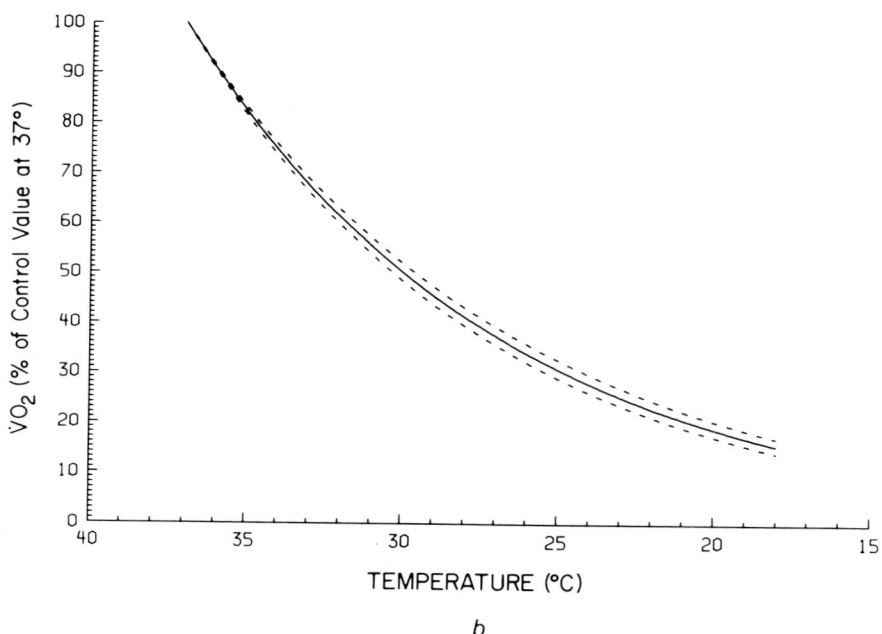

b

Figure 2-1

(*a*) Whole body oxygen consumption (V̇O₂) as a function of body temperature in dogs made hypothermic by surface cooling. The regression line for the equation (see Appendix 2A, equation 2A-1) is represented by the solid line, and the dashed lines enclose the 70% confidence limits. The slope indicates a Q_{10} of 2.7. (Crosses are data points from Ross,[R1] circles from Bigelow,[B2] and squares from Penrod.[P1])

(*b*) Nomogram of the equation derived from the data in *a*, with the oxygen consumption expressed as percent of control value at 37°C. The dotted lines surround the 70% confidence limits.

Table 2-1 Oxygen consumption ($\dot{V}O_2$) expressed as ml · hr^{-1} · gm^{-1} wet weight ± SD. Data have been rearranged and recalculated to allow for comparisons.

Organ	Tissue Slices (Rats)[F2]			Isolated, In Situ Organs (Dogs)[H19] (Cooling Coil Shunt)			Isolated, In Situ Organs (Dogs)[R10] (Surface Cooling)		
	37°C	25°C	% $\dot{V}O_2$ Reduction	37°C	25°C	% $\dot{V}O_2$ Reduction	37°C	25°C	% $\dot{V}O_2$ Reduction
Brain	1.98 ± 0.31	0.73 ± 0.139	63%	5.16 ± 0.90	3.54 ± 0.90	31%	4.31 ± 0.64	1.46 ± 0.30	66%
Kidney	3.87[a]	1.63[a]	58%	5.58 ± 1.98	0.96 ± 0.36	83%			
Muscle	0.76	0.36	53%	0.90 ± 0.30	0.30 ± 0.12	67%			

[a] Kidney cortex.

pliance of red cells, plasma "skimming," clumping of formed blood elements, and so forth.

However, some studies of tissue slices and isolated, perfused organs show a relative reduction of organ consumption at any degree of hypothermia to be *greater* than in those of the body as a whole (Table 2-1). This may be related to known species differences in tissue respiration,[M1] to suboptimal conditions for tissue respiration in the studies with tissue slices, or to increased oxygen consumption during whole body perfusion due, for example, to catecholamine release.

The striking fact from both whole body and tissue and organ studies is that oxygen consumption is not reduced to near zero even at very low temperatures.[H19,R10] Metabolic activity is therefore continuing, and the time limits of safe total circulatory arrest must be finite. Further, this continuing metabolic activity causes a tendency for organs and systems to rewarm during the arrest period. Donald and Kerr[K3] showed in dog brains cooled to 1–2°C that a rise in temperature occurred during a 30-minute period of total circulatory arrest and that this was in part related to the gradient between brain and room temperature but in part to continuing metabolic activity in the brain.

Total Body Oxygen Consumption during Cardiopulmonary Bypass and Hypothermia

Total body oxygen consumption during CPB at normothermia (37°C) theoretically should be that of an intact human under anesthesia if all parts of the microcirculation are being perfused. While at the Mayo Clinic, we determined in two studies in humans that $\dot{V}O_2$ during normothermic CPB at flows of 1.8–2.4 l · min^{-1} · m^{-2} was highly variable. Values between 74 and 162 ml · min^{-1} · m^{-2} were found in one of the studies,[M2] and in the other study of 12 patients, $\dot{V}O_2$ was 131 ± 20 (SD) l · min^{-1} · m^{-2}.[L2]

A combined analysis of experimental studies in animals during normothermic CPB indicates a best-fit hyperbolic relationship between the perfusion flow rate and $\dot{V}O_2$ (Fig. 2-2). This relationship also fits the data of Cheng et al.[C2]

The data for the combined analysis was chosen from studies expressing flow during CPB in l · min^{-1} · m^{-2} (the units in which cardiac output is commonly expressed). These units were not used in the excellent study of Andersen and Senning, nor could the data be recalculated in these terms, and therefore they could not be included.[A1] These authors, too, found increasing oxygen consumption with increasing ex-

tracorporeal flow rate and derived a linear regression equation from the data:

$$\dot{V}O_2 = 0.4437 \cdot (\dot{Q} - 62.7) + 71.6 \qquad \textbf{(2-1)}$$

Correlation coefficient = 0.83

where $\dot{V}O_2$ is oxygen consumption, expressed as percent of measured control value before bypass, and $\dot{Q}$ is flow from the pump-oxygenator expressed as ml · kg^{-1} · min^{-1}. Anderson and Senning noted, however, that flow and oxygen consumption must meet at zero and that the control value for $\dot{V}O_2$ was usually reached at high flows (100–125 ml · kg^{-1} · m^{-1}). Visual observation of their scattergram suggests that the hyperbolic model derived (UAB) fits their data and ideas well.

The temperature of the patient also affects $\dot{V}O_2$ during CPB, as it does in intact, anesthetized, nonshivering subjects. Harris, Seelye, and Squire at GLH, were the first to express mathematically the interrelationship between perfusion flow rate, temperature, and $\dot{V}O_2$,[H4] but these data covered only a narrow range of temperature. Complete data of the type desired are not available. Using the experimental data at 37°C just described and the relationship of $\dot{V}O_2$ to flow at 20°C measured during CPB in humans,[F5] an equation and a nomogram have been developed (Fig. 2-3) portraying the relations of $\dot{V}O_2$ to flow at various temperatures.

Kent[K2] has studied $\dot{V}O_2$ in experimental animals during hypothermia produced by combined surface and core cooling. His data are similar to those obtained from surface cooling alone.

OTHER PHENOMENA DURING HYPOTHERMIA AND CIRCULATORY ARREST

No-Reflow Phenomenon

It is only an assumption that a numerical relationship exists between oxygen consumption and "safe" total circulatory *arrest time* at any given temperature. In fact, the existence of a necessary and close relationship between the two over wide ranges of temperatures would be surprising, in view of other phenomena that occur during total circulatory arrest. One of these is regional vascular occlusion in the brain, leading to the no-reflow phenomenon.[A2] This phenomenon is an obstructive lesion of the microcirculation occurring in many areas of the brain, which prevents reperfusion and produces additional damage after circulatory arrest. The no-reflow phenomenon could, at least theoretically, damage the brain

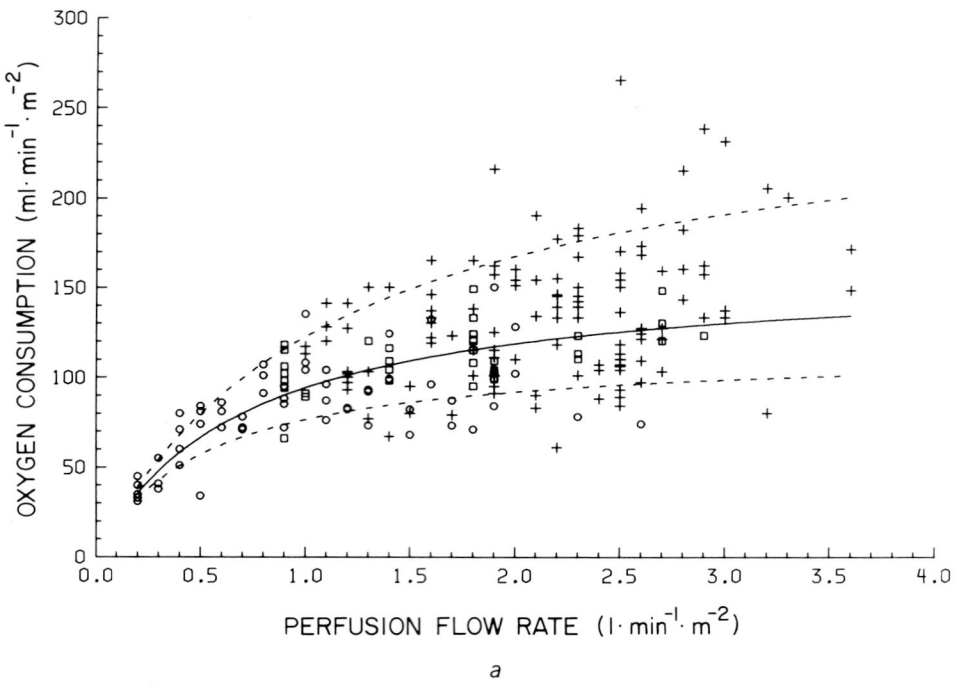

a

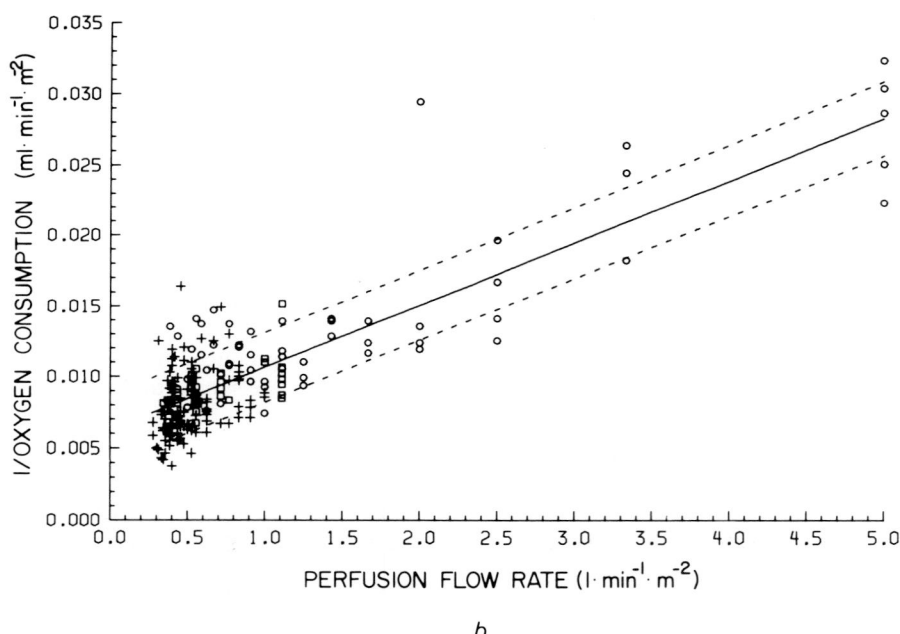

b

Figure 2-2 Relationship of total body oxygen consumption ($\dot{V}o_2$) to perfusion flow rate ($\dot{Q}$) at normothermia during nonpulsatile cardiopulmonary bypass.

(*a*) Scattergram of data from animal experiments (*n* = 213) performed at about 37°C by Cheng and colleagues[C2] (*n* = 33), Paneth and colleagues[P8] (*n* = 60), and Starr[S17] (*n* = 120). Note that scatter of the data increases as flow increases. The solid line is the nomogram of the hyperbolic equation (see Appendix 2A, equation 2A-2), with its 70% confidence limits.

(*b*) Nomogram of the transformation of data to hyperbolic model. The vertical axis is 1 over the oxygen consumption in ml · min^{-1} · m^{-2}.

Part *a* reproduced with permission from Fox et al.[F5]

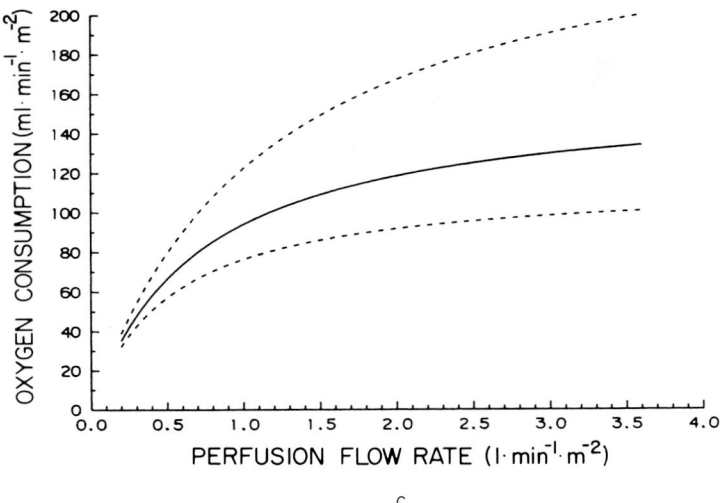

c

Figure 2-2 *(continued)*

(c) Another nomogram of equation 2A-2, with a different vertical scale. The asymptote (derived by inverting the intercept term of the hyperbolic regression equation) is 160 ml · min⁻¹ · m⁻². The dashed lines surround the 70% confidence limits.

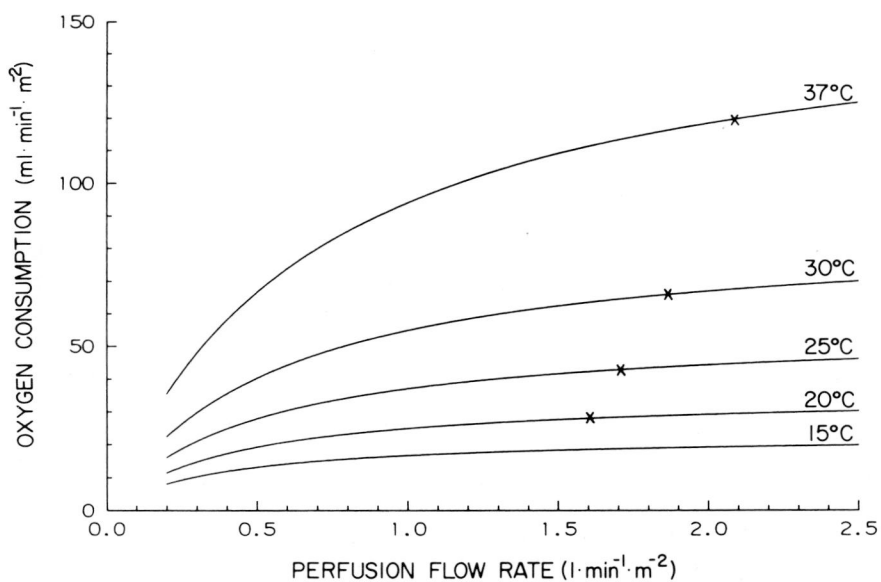

Figure 2-3 Nomogram of an equation expressing the relationship of oxygen consumption ($\dot{V}O_2$) to perfusion flow rate ($\dot{Q}$) and temperature (T). The small *x*'s have been added to represent the perfusion flow rates used clinically at these temperatures (UAB, GLH) (see Appendix 2A, equation 2A-3).

after profound hypothermia and total circulatory arrest. However, Norwood and colleagues have shown experimentally that this phenomenon develops as a result of severe hypoxia or anoxia, not of circulatory arrest per se.[N1] They have also shown that hypothermia to 20°C prevents the no-reflow phenomenon with 90 minutes of anoxia produced by continuing perfusion at an arterial PaO_2 of about 10 mmHg.

Changes in Plasma Volume

Cooling of the patient itself causes other widespread changes. Chen and colleagues have shown progressive hemoconcentration and decrease in plasma volume during surface cooling of infants to 25°C,[C14] an observation that supports their own and previous[D15] experimental studies. This may represent a sequestration of plasma in portions of the vascular bed and/or a leakage in plasma into the interstitial fluid compartment.

THE DAMAGING EFFECTS OF TOTAL CIRCULATORY ARREST DURING HYPOTHERMIA

It is generally agreed that the brain has the shortest "safe" circulatory arrest time of any organ or region of the body, although occasionally the kidney seems to be damaged by a period of total circulatory arrest when the brain is not. Although the other organs and regions can be severely damaged by long periods of total circulatory arrest, their "safe" circulatory arrest times are generally longer than those of the brain.

Brain Function and Structure

Experimental Studies
Animal experiments indicate that, when the brain itself is cooled to 15°C, 30 minutes of total circulatory arrest are accepted without evidence of functional or structural damage. Folkerth, Angell, and colleagues[F6] showed no functional or structural brain abnormalities in dogs subjected to 30 minutes of total circulatory arrest after being surface-cooled to 28°C and then taken to 20°C (site of temperature measurement not stated) by CPB.

That 30 minutes of total circulatory arrest to the brain has a high probability of being safe is also suggested by studies in dogs by Kramer and colleagues.[K3] They showed a steady decline of adenosine triphosphate (ATP) concentrations in brain to 35% of control values after 30 minutes of total circulatory arrest at an esophageal temperature of 4–5°C and a cerebral cortical temperature of 13°C produced by 50 minutes of cooling by CPB; the concentrations rapidly returned to normal after restoration of circulation. The studies of Fisk and colleagues also suggest that, with the brain cooled to 20°C, 30 minutes of total circulatory arrest is "safe," with a high probability that no functional or structural abnormality will result.[F7,F8] Studies of cerebral structure and function after cerebral circulatory arrest in gerbils at 18°C by Treasure and colleagues also support the idea that 30 minutes is a safe circulatory arrest time at these temperatures.[T15] Wolin, Massopust, White, and colleagues[W3] showed no intellectual

deterioration in trained rhesus monkeys after the brain had been cooled to 15°C and the circulation arrested for 30 minutes.

The studies by Treasure and colleagues suggest that, in the gerbil at least, circulatory arrest periods longer than 45 minutes, at 18–20°C, result in a considerable probability of structural and functional brain damage, with the probability increasing as the arrest time lengthens.[T15] Animals undergoing 45–60 minutes of total circulatory arrest in the study by Folkerth and colleagues sometimes survived without functional abnormality, but all had histologic evidence of anoxic brain damage. Kramer and colleagues state that when circulatory arrest was prolonged to 60 minutes, only two of four dogs showed recovery of brain ATP levels, again indicating the risks of the longer arrest period. One dog subjected to 90 minutes of arrest did not recover.

Experiments in infant pigs by Fisk and colleagues[F7,F8] showed histopathologic evidence of brain damage in all animals subjected to profound hypothermia produced by core cooling to an esophageal temperature of 20°C and total circulatory arrest for 60 minutes. However, studies in dogs by Molina and colleagues showed no increase in evidences of brain damage at 18°C when there was total circulatory arrest for 60 minutes compared with continuing nonpulsatile or pulsatile perfusion from the pump-oxygenator.[M11]

In summary, these experimental studies indicate that a 30-minute period of total circulatory arrest at 18–20°C is nearly uniformly safe and results in little structural or functional brain damage. The data are somewhat conflicting regarding these matters when the total circulatory arrest time is extended to 45–60 minutes. Most studies, however, indicate that, with these longer arrest times, there is a considerable probability of brain damage, both in structure and function.

Related to this question is evidence that perfusion temperatures of 15°C are not, per se, damaging to the brain. Wolin and colleagues showed in trained rhesus monkeys that continuous cold perfusion for 30 minutes (blood at 10–15°C) of brains already at 15°C does not result in intellectual deterioration.[W3]

Also of note is the suggestion of some experiments that very rapid cooling by CPB may fail to provide safe total circulatory arrest. Thus, experiments in dogs undergoing profound hypothermia and total circulatory arrest for 30 minutes by Almond and associates[A3] were interpreted by them to indicate structural and functional brain damage when the cooling by CPB was done with the perfusation 20°C colder than the patient; and they believed that this did not occur with gradients of 4–6°C. However, the damage might have been related to the short period of cooling with the very cold blood, producing very uneven whole body and brain cooling.[Z1] The longer period of cooling required with the blood only 4–6°C colder than the subject must have produced more even cooling.

Studies in Humans
The functional state of the human brain during and very early after profound hypothermia and total circulatory arrest has been studied only by electroencephalographic evidence of brain function. Generally, such evidence is related to nasopharyngeal or tympanic membrane temperature, which

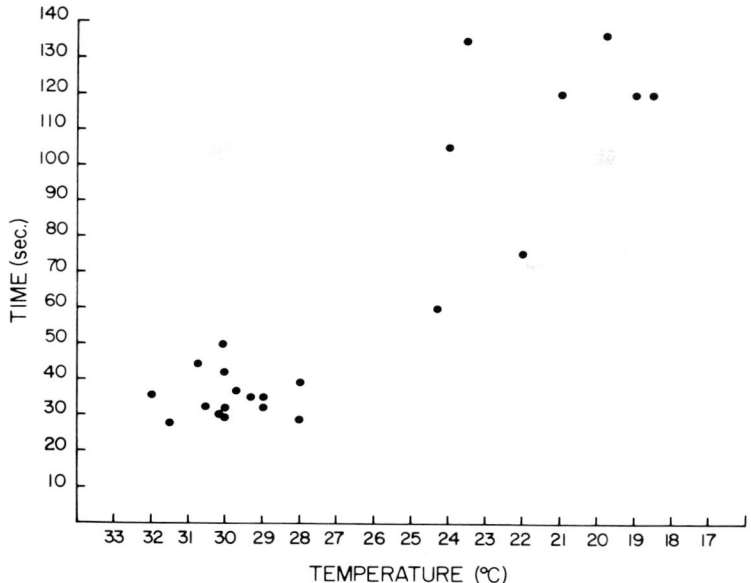

Figure 2-4 Length of time (in seconds) between the beginning of total circulatory arrest and the appearance of electroencephalographic quiescence, related to nasopharyngeal temperature at the time of circulatory arrest.

Redrawn from Harden et al.[H7]

have been shown in humans to be very similar to the temperature of the cerebral cortex.[G1,W1] The brain does, however, tend to cool unevenly,[Z1] leaving some areas more susceptible to ischemic damage than others. This can be minimized by using surface cooling or by strict adherence to a proper protocol of perfusion flow, temperature gradient between perfusate and patient, and duration of cooling during core cooling.

During core cooling in humans to 18.5°C, continuous phasic activity in the electroencephalogram (EEG) persists throughout, according to the studies of Harden and colleagues.[H7] Cohen, Olszowka, and Subramanian;[C3] Setiey and colleagues;[S4] and Weiss and colleagues[W4] reported similar findings, using surface cooling and limited CPB, and then total circulatory arrest. During the cooling, there is a gradual disappearance of fast components and an increase in slow components. Occasionally, repetitive fast discharges occur. When circulatory arrest is established, electroencephalographic activity disappears within an average time of 109 seconds (compared with 21 seconds in the dog[K3]). The time required for disappearance of EEG activity was, in the experience of Harden, Pampiglione, and Waterston,[H7] inversely related to temperature at the time of arrest (Fig. 2-4). When CPB is resumed after circulatory arrest, EEG activity is absent initially and then gradually returns as rewarming proceeds.[C3] In general, after 20–30 minutes of rewarming, the EEG has returned approximately to its control condition.[C3] This latent period, between the resumption of whole body perfusion and rewarming and the time of return of reasonably normal EEG activity, is believed by Weiss and colleagues[W4] to be related to the important metabolic (oxygen) debt that has developed during the arrest period, this in turn being influenced by brain temperature during arrest and by

the duration of the arrest. Weiss and colleagues[W4] made the observation that when circulatory arrest was less than 37–40 minutes, EEG activity always reappeared in less than 20 minutes, whereas longer periods of circulatory arrest were followed by longer and more varied latent periods. This agrees with the experimental data on the tolerance of the brain to circulatory arrest during profound hypothermia.

Weiss and colleagues[W4] also note that the persisting EEG activity during circulatory arrest reported by Reilly and associates[R2] probably reflected activity in the white matter structure and cerebellum. This is of interest because of the occasional postoperative occurrence of choreoathetoid movements in humans and high-stepping gait in experimental animals. Such results may be at least in part due to uneven brain cooling secondary to regional differences in flow during cooling.

Choreoathetosis has occurred early postoperatively in some patients with the technique of profound hypothermia and total circulatory arrest. Two instances (2.7%; CL 0.9%–6.5%) occurred among 72 patients operated on in the first 2 years of the GLH experience with this technique.[C4] Brunberg, Reilly, and Doty[B7] reported choreoathetosis in 4 (19%; CL 10%–32%) of 21 infants; Bergouignan, Fontan, and colleagues[B8] in 4 (15%; CL 8%–25%) of 27 patients; and Stewart et al., at UAB, in 5 (2.3%; CL 1.3%–3.9%) of 219 infants and young children operated on by this technique.[S5] When it occurs, choreoathetosis usually develops 2 to 6 days postoperatively. As time passes, the movements usually lessen in severity. If mild, they disappear completely, but if severe, they or hypotonia may persist to a greater or lesser degree. Brunberg and colleagues found no correlation between the circulatory arrest time or the depth of cooling (between 16 and 20°C) and the development of choreoathetosis.[B7] In toto, these reports suggest that this specific complication occurs in 1%–12% of patients and that its residual effects are permanent in some patients. Choreoathetosis seems to occur only when total circulatory arrest exceeds 30–45 minutes and is particularly likely to occur when it exceeds 60 minutes.[S5] We and others have seen this complication rarely after hypothermic CPB without circulatory arrest, but the incidence with this technique is not known.

The cause of the choreoathetosis is not clear. Profound hypothermia per se may cause damage. Egerton and colleagues report that continuous hypothermic perfusion at 10–12°C produced moderate or severe brain damage, including choreoathetosis, in 10 (63%; CL 46%–77%) of 16 patients.[E1] Air or particulate embolization to the brain may be implicated. When circulatory arrest is used, the choreoathetosis may be related to the uneven brain cooling, leading to the continuing metabolic and EEG activity over the white matter and cerebellum observed by Reilly and associates,[R2] and perhaps uneven brain reperfusion related to the vascular changes implicated in the no-reflow phenomenon.[H8,H9,C5,O1,G2] The latter is one rationale for using hemodilution during cooling, for absence of red cells in the perfusion used just before total circulatory arrest to the brain eliminates the no-reflow phenomenon.[A2]

Brunberg, Reilly, and Doty[B7] suggest that increased tissue glucose, such as is usually present at the beginning of the arrest period, may allow excessive glycolysis during the arrest period, possibly resulting in tissue damage from lactic acid accumulation. Preexisting developmental delay or other neurologic abnormalities, present in some of these patients,[B7,C4] may also increase the likelihood of postoperative choreoathetosis.

Seizures have occurred in the early postoperative period in 5%–10% of patients in whom the technique of profound hypothermia and total circulatory arrest has been used. Because the seizures are usually transient and followed by uneventful convalescence, they are not considered major neurologic events. Uncommonly, they are followed by severe brain dysfunction. Four (7%; CL 4%–12%) of 57 infants undergoing repair of ventricular septal defects at GLH during profound hypothermia and total circulatory arrest developed seizures transiently in the postoperative period and then recovered completely,[B9] and among a different group of 72 long-term survivors, 4 (5%; CL 3%–10%) had seizures early postoperatively.[C4] Brunberg, Reilly, and Doty[B7] reported generalized seizures in 2 (9%; CL 3%–20%) of 22 patients operated on under similar circumstances. Venugopal, Subramanian, and coworkers reported seizures in 6 (4.6%; CL 2.7%–7.4%) of 130 such patients.[V1] Belsey and colleagues reported 6 patients (35%; CL 22%–51%) with seizures among 17 having intracardiac operations during profound hypothermia and total circulatory arrest and without CO_2 in the ventilatory mixture during cooling, and 9 (3.6%; CL 2.4%–5.3%) among 248 patients in whom CO_2 was included.[B10]

The comments made concerning possible causes of the choreoathetosis are also applicable to seizures. However, it is well known that infants are highly susceptible to seizures from disturbances of thermoregulation and fluid balance, as well as from metabolic disorders, especially those related to glucose and calcium, and that many of these factors are operative in these patients.

More severe and gross evidences of brain damage have uncommonly occurred after profound hypothermia and total circulatory arrest, including either coma dating from surgery or developing some hours later, followed by death or lasting impairment. At UAB, 3 (1.4%; CL 0.6%–2.7%) such instances have occurred among 218 young patients undergoing repair of the common types of congenital heart disease with profound hypothermia and total circulatory arrest.[S5] Along with these 3, the 5 patients who developed choreoathetosis represent the total who developed major neurologic events early after these operations. All such events occurred in the group of patients in whom core cooling alone was used (Table 2-2). None occurred in patients in whom the duration of total circulatory arrest was less than 45 minutes, and the probability of developing major neurologic events increased as total circulatory arrest times increased beyond this (Fig. 2-5).

The effect of this form of cardiac surgery on late postoperative intellectual capacity and behavior has been difficult to study. The problems in testing small infants preoperatively so that each may serve as his or her own control contribute to the difficulty of firmly resolving the problem. Associated congenital developmental disorders, the possible effects before operation of severe congenital heart disease, and the effects of other perioperative events complicate the interpretation of the data. In general, late postoperative studies suggest that when total circulatory arrest is less than 60 minutes at nasopharyngeal temperatures of about 20°C, intellectual capacity and development are not adversely affected. When arrest is longer than 60 minutes, intellectual development may be adversely affected.

The intellectual development in 72 of the first 76 consecutive long-term survivors of profoundly hypothermic total circulatory arrest (GLH), using mainly the technique of surface cooling and core rewarming, has been reviewed.[C4] Sixty-nine children who also had taken the Stanford-Binet IQ test at an average age of 57 months and who were Caucasian singletons born after 38–42 weeks gestation, weighing

Table 2-2 Major neurologic events of patients after profound hypothermia and total circulatory arrest (UAB, January 1972 to July 1, 1979).[S5]

Method	No. of Patients	Circulating Arrest (min)	Major Neurologic Events[a]		
			No.	%	CL
Surface cooling to 28°C, then core cooling	80	42.5 (± SD 13.57)	0	0%	0–2%
Core cooling only	138	42.8 (± SD 15.35)	8	6%	4–9%
Total	218[b]				
P					.03

KEY: CL, 70% confidence limits.

[a] Excludes only seizures followed by uneventful convalescence.

[b] Repair of VSD, tetralogy of Fallot, transposition of the great arteries, and AV canal defects. Mean temperature during arrest for both groups was 19.7°C ± 1.76 (SD).

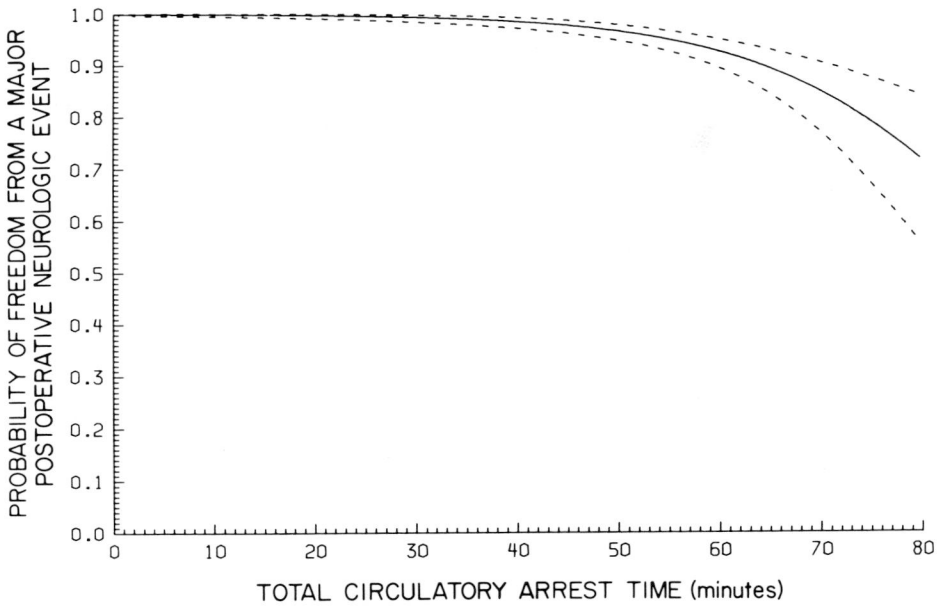

Figure 2-5 Relationship between the probability of the occurrence of a major neurologic event postoperatively and the total circulatory arrest time in 219 patients (eight events) undergoing open intracardiac operations (UAB).[S5] (See Appendix 2A, equation 2A-5.)

3,000 to 4,000 g at birth, and without evidence of congenital malformation, neonatal illness, or other adverse features. The mean IQ of the 72 patients was 92.9 (SD ± 16.5), compared with 106.2 (SD ± 11.6) for the control group (P = .0001). However, the 25 patients who met all the criteria of the control group (except that they had congenital heart disease) had a mean IQ of 101.4 (SD ± 15.0), which was not different from that of the control group (P = .21). Sixty-two patients had no important neurologic problems preoperatively and had normal birth weight for gestational age, and their mean IQ was 95.5 (SD ± 14.4) lower than that of the control group (P = .001) but higher than the mean IQ of 76.5 (± 20.0) of 10 patients with low birth weight or important neurologic problems preoperatively (P = .001) (Fig. 2-6*a*). The relation of the Stanford-Binet scores of the 72 patients to the duration of total circulatory arrest is shown in Figure 2-6*b*. Patients who had circulatory arrest of 50–60 minutes had IQs similar to those who had circulatory arrest for 35 minutes or less. There were too few patients with circulatory arrest times exceeding 60 minutes to show any significant difference, if such exists. There was no relation between nasopharyngeal temperature at the time of circulatory arrest and IQ late postoperatively (Fig. 2-6*c*). The mean nasopharyngeal temperature during arrest for these initial 72 patients was 22.2°C (± 1.6). (For at least the last 8 years, the prearrest temperature has been stabilized between 17°C and 19°C).

Subramanian and colleagues,[S6] in a study of 36 children operated upon with profound hypothermia (cooled mainly by surface means) and total circulatory arrest, found 89% (CL 81%–94%) of psychometric test scores to fall within the normal or above normal range. Four children were in the defective range. Three of the latter patients had preoperative morbidity (stroke, cardiorespiratory arrest). Dickinson and

Sambrooks[D4] (core cooling) considered the possibility that this technique may have contributed to a low IQ in 4 of 38 patients tested. They found no difference in the IQ of patients arrested for 30–39 minutes (n = 7) of those arrested for 60–69 minutes (n = 8). Haka-Ikse, Blackwood, and Steward[H10] concluded optimistically that the technique of profound hypothermia (using mainly core cooling) and total circulatory arrest can be used "without fear of retarding psychomotor development." However, the "development quotient" of their 17 patients late postoperatively was slightly but significantly (P < .05) lower than that of the patients' siblings. The duration of total circulatory arrest varied from 17 to 72 minutes, with a mean value of 44.2 ± 3.0 (SE) minutes. As in most clinical studies, they found no apparent effect of the duration of total circulatory arrest on the developmental quotient late postoperatively. Messmer and colleagues gathered data by psychomotor testing of 11 patients an average of 7 years after cardiac surgery using profound hypothermia and total circulatory arrest. In their view, there was no adverse effect of the procedure.[M3] Noteworthy are the facts that, in their patients, total circulatory arrest times varied between 8 and 43 minutes, with a mean of 23.5 ± 4.9 (SE) minutes; that temperature was 22.8°C ± 0.6 (SE); and that surface cooling without CPB was used. Stevenson, Stone, Dillard, and Morgan also studied intellectual performance late postoperatively in 32 patients undergoing intracardiac surgery during total circulatory arrest at 20°C following surface cooling and surface rewarming.[S7] Although some children had performance below the range of normal, the etiology was difficult to determine because of other factors, such as cardiac arrest or severe renal failure early postoperatively. Wright and colleagues, in a nonrandomized study in infants, compared intellectual development late (1–6 years) after intracardiac repair using

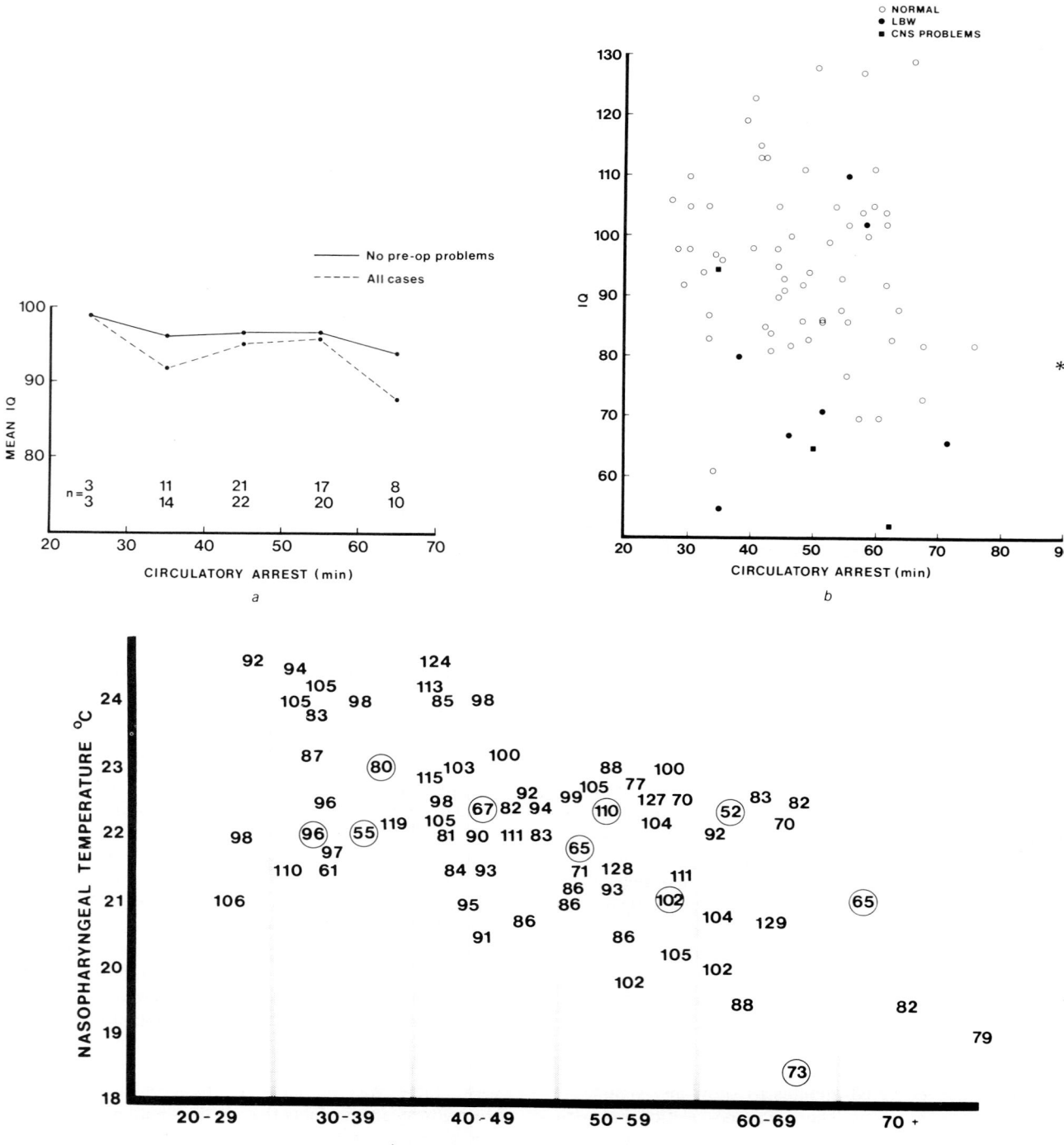

Figure 2-6

(a) Results of IQ (Stanford Binet) testing years after intracardiac repair in infancy, using profound hypothermia and total circulatory arrest.

(b) Open circles represent patients who were normal preoperatively except for heart disease; solid circles, those with low birth weight for gestational age; solid squares, those with preoperative neurologic problems. The asterisk represents a patient who sustained a cardiopulmonary arrest postoperatively.

(c) The numbers in the scattergram are the IQs at late study, distributed according to circulatory arrest time and nasopharyngeal temperature during arrest. The circled numbers represent patients with preoperative problems.

Reproduced with permission from Clarkson et al.,[C4] and the American Heart Association, Inc.

Table 2-3 The results of intelligence testing of patients some years after surgery performed in infancy utilizing profound hypothermia–circulatory arrest techniques.

	No. of Patients Tested	IQ ≤ 80			
		"Explained" by:		Unexplained	Total
		Preoperative Events	Postoperative Events		
Subramanian[S7]	36	3	0	1	4 (11%)
Dickinson[D3]	38	3	1	3	7 (18%)
Clarkson[C4]	72	6	1	5	12 (16%)
Total	146	12 (8%; CL 6%–11%)	2 (1.4%; CL 0.5%–3.2%)	9 (6.2%; CL 4.1%–9.0%)	23 (16%; CL 13%–19%)

KEY: CL, 70% confidence limits; IQ = intelligence quotient.

continuous CPB with that after profound hypothermia (15–20°C) and total circulatory arrest.[W5] Three (20%; CL 9%–36%) of 15 operated on with CPB were intellectually slow or had serious defects, according to their parents; 8 (47%; CL 32%–62%) of 17 operated on with total circulatory arrest (21–67 minutes) were slow or had serious defects. However, the study of Wright and colleagues suffers from the criticism that no data on formal psychometric testing are presented and that the criteria they used are not specific for mental development.

The results of psychomotor testing in 146 children undergoing cardiac surgery during profound hypothermia and total circulatory arrest, obtained by combining the three largest reported series, are summarized in Table 2-3. Twenty-three (16%; CL 13%–19%) of the 146 had an IQ ≤ 80, more than one standard deviation below the test mean. In approximately half the patients, preoperative events were considered likely to account for the low scores. In the remainder, an occasional child had suffered an adverse perioperative event, but the low scores were unexplained in nine (6.2%; CL 4.1%–9.0%) patients.

Wells, Lincoln, and colleagues obtained data on intellectual and psychological development in children that caused them to question the idea that 60 minutes of total circulatory arrest at 18°C is safe.[W17] They found that the intelligence quotient of patients with an arrest time of 50 minutes or greater was significantly lower late postoperatively than that of those with an arrest time of less than 50 minutes. Also, they found an inverse relationship between arrest time and intelligence quotient late postoperatively.

In summary, the data from patients are somewhat conflicting. There is considerable agreement that arrest times of longer than 60 minutes at 18–20°C are not safe, and some of the data suggest the probability that arrest periods of longer than 45 minutes may not be safe. It must be remembered that at present there are no data on late intellectual development following the use in infancy of profound hypothermia with continuous full-flow or low-flow perfusion rather than circulatory arrest.

Renal Function and Structure

Experimental Studies

At normothermia, at least in rats, 20 minutes of total circulatory arrest to the kidney produces no histochemical evidence of cell death, while 30 minutes produces extensive cell death in the distal portion of the proximal convoluted tubules, with scattered areas of cell death being seen at 25 minutes.[V2] Vogt and Farber[V2] identified the progressive accumulation of lactic acid during ischemia and the rapid fall of ATP to 20% of control values as major factors in the evolution of cell death.

Hypothermia prolongs the "safe" circulatory arrest time for the kidney in the intact dog. Ninety minutes of total circulatory arrest after surface cooling to 18–20°C produces no late morphologic changes in the kidney.[R3] However, the precise relationships among temperatures, time of total circulatory arrest, and morphologic and functional renal damage are not clear. The work of Gowing and Dexter[G3] suggests that minimal morphologic changes evolve in the kidney after 60 minutes of circulatory arrest at 21°C. It is apparent, however, that at any temperature the "safe" circulatory arrest time for the kidney is longer than it is for the brain and shorter than it is for the liver. In addition, a scattered loss of cells through cell death probably results in no detectable loss of renal function, whereas this may not be true in the brain.

As with other organs, the question of the damaging effects of hypothermia itself is not fully resolved. Ward[W6] found that the morphologic and functional derangements of the kidney after 90 minutes of total circulatory arrest were less at an arrest temperature of 15°C than when the temperatures were lower or higher. This suggests that temperatures below 15°C may themselves damage the kidney.

Studies in Humans

Important oliguria beginning about 12 hours postoperatively occasionally complicates the recovery of infants operated on with profound hypothermia and total circulatory arrest for less than 60 minutes. For example, Venugopal and colleagues reported 4 (3%; CL 2%–6%) deaths from renal failure among 130 patients operated on in this way.[V1] Renal failure was the cause of death in 14% of the patients who failed to survive.

Usually, the primary cause of the renal failure seems to be low cardiac output after repair. However, in at least some cases, the severe oliguria develops when the hemodynamic state of the patient seems by other criteria quite satisfactory. In view of the finding in experimental studies that morphologic and functional damage to the kidney does not occur

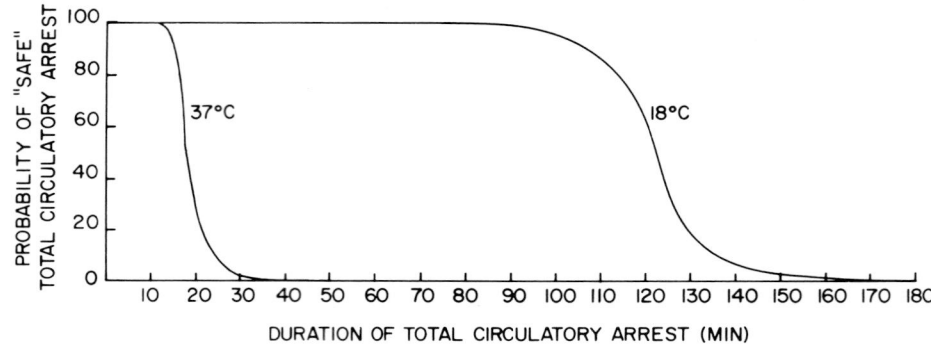

Figure 2-7 Freehand nomogram of our estimate of the relations in the kidney between the probability of "safe" total circulatory arrest and the duration of the total circulatory arrest at two temperatures. The normothermic relationship is based on the work of Vogt and Farber,[V2] and the hypothermic one, on data presented in the text.

after 60 minutes of total circulatory arrest at temperatures of 18–20°C (Fig. 2-7), damaging effects from CPB and cardiac surgery must be implicated. In part, this may be low cardiac output preceding and following the total circulatory arrest. In part, it may be damage to the kidneys by free hemoglobin, and circulating toxins that appear during CPB (see Section 2). Hemoglobin has been found in the renal tubules of some of these patients at autopsy.

Liver Function

The normothermic liver of humans resumes normal function after its complete isolation from the circulation for 35 to 40 minutes.[H11] Studies in dogs suggest that complete hepatic circulatory arrest for 45 minutes or more at 37°C is followed by serious functional derangements.[A4,B11] During profound hypothermia to 20–22°C, 60 minutes of complete circulatory arrest does not produce structural or functional abnormalities in the liver.[R3]

"SAFE" DURATION OF TOTAL CIRCULATORY ARREST

The preceding information does not allow the formulation of a table or a rigorously derived equation relating "safe" duration of total circulatory arrest to various temperatures based on rigorously derived rules. Knowledge of biological systems in general indicates that, were adequate information available, the relationships should be expressed as the probability of no functional or structural damage (i.e., the probability of "safe" circulatory arrest) at a given temperature, rather than as an absolute value.

In addition to the data already presented, a few additional comments are indicated. Our initial experiences at the Mayo Clinic[K1] suggested that 45 minutes was the maximum "safe" duration even when the nasopharyngeal temperature was reduced to 20°C. At GLH,[S8] we calculated the oxygen debt from measurements of O_2 consumption in 10 infants after a mean of 55 minutes of circulatory arrest at 23°C and con-

cluded that the total energy stores had probably been drawn upon during that interval.

As a guide to the use of total circulatory arrest, Figure 2-8 shows three curves relating the probability of "safe" total circulatory arrest to the arrest time at three temperatures: 37, 28, and 18°C. These estimates are based on currently available information and, because of lack of data, have not been rigorously derived. To emphasize that each curve would have a degree of uncertainty even were considerable data available, the 70% confidence limits around the continuous point estimate for 18°C, suggested by the little information that is available, *are* shown in Figure 2-8*b*. The preceding pages indicate that histologic changes in the central nervous system, without functional abnormalities, are the most sensitive indicators of lack of complete safety of the arrest period used. The portrayal at 18°C of essentially complete safety of 30 minutes of total circulatory arrest is consistent with all available information. The portrayal of essentially complete safety of arrest for at least 70% of subjects of 45 minutes is also consistent with the facts, and the damage produced within this time period is likely to be structural and without functional sequelae. Most patients will have some structural evidence of damage from 60 minutes of arrest, but only 10% of these patients will have evident functional damage, and in many of these the manifestations will be transient.

Other support systems, such as continuous CPB at normothermia or with moderate or profound hypothermia with or without very low perfusion flow rates, have their own potential for damage, particularly in infants. A large body of rigorously derived information about these is also lacking. Further, the heart disease being treated itself has great potential for producing damage. An inaccurate repair can produce damage, and inaccuracies are more likely to result when surgical exposure is poor. The surgical team weighs the relative risks and imponderables of these and other factors in deciding in an individual patient whether total circulatory arrest should be used and, if it is to be used, its duration and patient temperature during it (see Section 3 for further details).

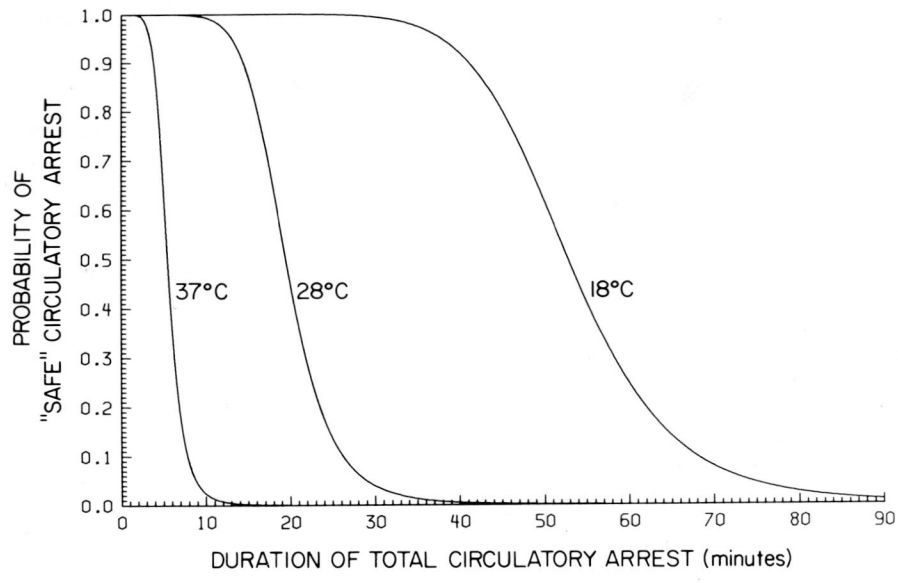

a

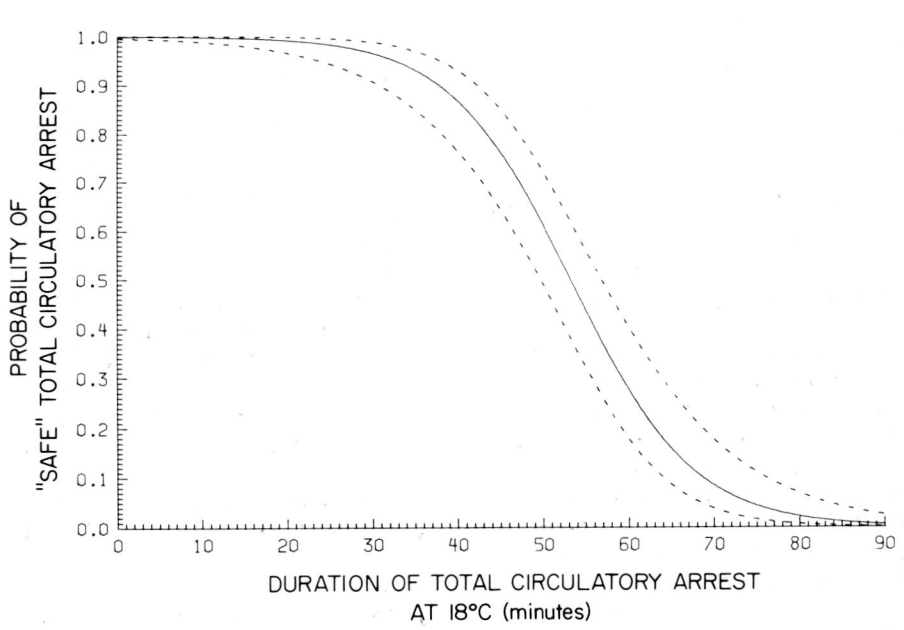

b

Figure 2-8

(*a*) Nomogram of an estimate (not rigorously derived) of the probability of "safe" total circulatory arrest (absence of structural or functional damage) according to the arrest time, at nasopharyngeal temperatures of 37, 28, and 18°C.

(*b*) Nomogram of an estimate with 70% confidence limits (dashed line) at 18°C. The number of experiments in the literature at 18°C nasopharyngeal temperature at 40 minutes of circulatory arrest are estimated at 20 as a basis for calculating these confidence limits. Note that at 30 minutes "safe" arrest is highly likely and that at 45 minutes it is probable. Other data suggest that at 45 minutes the damage will probably be only structural and without evident functional sequelae (see Fig. 2-5).

WHOLE BODY PERFUSION DURING CARDIOPULMONARY BYPASS

HISTORICAL NOTE

The historical aspects of cardiopulmonary bypass for cardiac surgery are not easily described, for it is almost impossible to know who first had the idea of diverting the circulation to an oxygenator outside the body and pumping it back to the patient's arterial system in order to allow surgery within the heart. References to extracorporeal gas exchange in blood go back to the last part of the nineteenth century. For example, Frey and Gruber worked with an "oxygenator" in 1885.[F9] Subsequently, scores of laboratory studies with oxygenators and pumps were reported. However, serious consideration of the use of pump-oxygenators for cardiac surgery had to await the development of modern anesthesia, modern surgical methods, and, particularly, scientific developments such as the discovery and use of heparin, plastic material, and the like. Without doubt, Gibbon, with his pioneering experimental work at the Massachusetts General Hospital in Boston in the late 1930s,[G4] was a major contributor to the development of CPB and its advancement to the stage of successful clinical application. Gibbon's work was interrupted by World War II, but when he came to Jefferson Medical School in Philadelphia after military service he resumed work with CPB, its pathophysiology, and the equipment required for it. Most of the medical and surgical world took little note of his work, and in fact considered it unlikely to lead to any useful knowledge. However, he persevered. As a result, the first successful operation in which the patient was totally supported by CPB was done by Gibbon, when he repaired an atrial septal defect in a young woman using a pump-oxygenator in 1953.[G5] Unfortunately, his subsequent four patients died from a variety of problems, and he became discouraged with the method.[G6]

Meantime, a few others began to work with pump-oxygenators for CPB in the late 1940s. Among these were Dennis,[D5] at the University of Minnesota. His laboratory studies led him to make what may have been the first attempt to use a pump-oxygenator for clinical cardiac surgery, in 1951.[D5] He and Varco operated on a patient thought to have an atrial septal defect and felt they had done a satisfactory repair, but the patient died. Autopsy showed that the lesion was in fact a partial AV canal defect and misinterpretation of the anatomy was a major factor in the patient's death. In Stockholm, Sweden, Bjork,[B12] and Senning[S9] also worked in the late 1940s and early 1950s with CPB. Related to this is Crafoord's early use of this method for removal of an atrial myxoma.[C6]

After Dennis' unsuccessful effort, Lillehei and colleagues, at the University of Minnesota, began working in the laboratory with controlled cross-circulation, using another intact subject as the "oxygenator."[C7] Their experimental studies led them to adopt the "azygos flow principle,"[A5] which was that only very small perfusion flow rates were needed. In April 1954, they began a spectacular series of operations for congenital heart disease using "controlled cross-circulation" and the mother (or father) as the "oxygenator."[W7] Although this particular technique was soon abandoned, the work of Lillehei and colleagues brought into being the modern era of open heart surgery.

We began experimental work at the Mayo Clinic in Rochester, Minnesota, in the early 1950s[J1,D6] with pump-oxygenators, which led to our first use of CBP with a pump-oxgenator, in March 1955, in successfully repairing a ventricular septal defect. We then began the world's first series of intracardiac operations using a pump-oxygenator.[K4] Quickly, the field of intracardiac surgery using a pump-oxygenator for CPB began to expand, and today is widely practiced. We began our work in this area at GLH in 1958.

UNIQUE FEATURES

The human being whose arterial blood flow is temporarily provided by means of a pump-oxygenator is in an abnormal situation that affects most if not all of the body's physiologic processes. When essentially all systemic venous blood returns to the pump-oxygenator instead of the heart, the situation is termed *total cardiopulmonary bypass*. When some systemic venous blood returns to the heart and is ejected into the aorta, the situation is termed *partial cardiopulmonary bypass*.

In contrast to the situation in intact humans, a number of physiologic variables are directly under external control during CPB. These include total systemic blood flow ("cardiac output"); input pressure wave form; systemic venous pressure; pulmonary venous pressure; hematocrit of the initial perfusate and its chemical composition; arterial oxygen, carbon dioxide, and nitrogen levels; and temperature of the perfusate and patients. Decisions should therefore be made by the surgeon concerning all of these matters.

Another group of variables is determined in part by the externally controlled variables but in part by the patient. These include systemic vascular resistance, total body oxygen consumption, mixed venous oxygen levels, lactic acidemia and pH, regional and organ blood flow, and regional and organ function.

A number of undesirable damaging effects occur to a greater or lesser degree with CPB. These include blood coagulation abnormalities, changes in red blood cells and plasma proteins produced by their passage through the extracorporeal system, gaseous and particulate emboli, and liberation or production of a wide variety of *vasoactive* and otherwise biologically active substances by contact of blood with foreign surfaces.

EXTERNALLY CONTROLLED VARIABLES
Total Systemic Blood Flow

During total CPB, the systemic blood flow, which is virtually the same as the perfusion flow rate, is under the control of the perfusionist. This can be set at an arbitrary level or may be kept equal to the venous return from the patient. The most rational approach is to set it at an arbitrary level.

The optimal flow rate during CPB is still being debated. A few facts are clear. Acidosis with increased lactic acid production, low oxygen consumption, and the other features of cardiogenic shock, result from normothermic CPB at flows of less than about 1.6 l · min^{-1} · m^{-2} (or less than about 50 ml · kg^{-1} · min^{-1}).[C16,D7] Animal experiments (see Fig. 2-2) and our clinical data[L2,M2] and experience indicate that, at normothermia, flows over about 1.8 l · min^{-1} · m^{-2} are quite acceptable as regards total body oxygen consumption but that flows of 2.2–2.5 l · min^{-1} · m^{-2} are more securely adequate. During hypothermic perfusions, "adequate," or "acceptable," flow rates are somewhat lower (see "Total Body Oxygen Consumption during Cardiopulmonary Bypass").

The best criterion of acceptability, or adequacy, of flow rate at any temperature is the survival of the subject without structural or functional evidence of organ or system damage. Just as in total circulatory arrest, this is no doubt a probability phenomenon, with no precise predictors or criteria of adequacy other than this. It is rational to believe that survival without damage is most likely to occur when the entire microcirculation is perfused at flows that maintain near normal tissue oxygen levels. In humans on bypass, this probably applies when whole body oxygen consumption is near ($>$ 85% of) the asymptote of the temperature-specific curve relating flow to $\dot{V}_{O_2}$ (represented by the x's in Fig. 2-3).

Mixed-venous O_2 pressure or saturation[1] have been widely used as indexes of adequate perfusion (for references, see Harris and colleagues[H12]), the assumption being that these values reflect average cellular P_{O_2}. If flow rate is high and the entire microcirculation perfused, this is true. However, it has been shown at GLH[H12] that during CPB, with perfusion within the conventional range, mixed-venous oxygenation is inversely related to $\dot{V}_{O_2}$. This might have been predicted from the Fick equation:

$$\dot{V}_{O_2} = \dot{Q}(CaO_2 - CvO_2) \qquad (2-3)$$

If $\dot{V}_{O_2}$ and CaO_2 are fixed, CvO_2 rises with $\dot{Q}$. If, instead, $\dot{Q}$ and CaO_2 are fixed, CvO_2 rises as $\dot{V}_{O_2}$ falls, and $\dot{V}_{O_2}$ may fall, despite a perfectly "adequate" total perfusion, if the capillary bed is not evenly perfused. In this case, the distance between perfused capillaries and many tissue cells increases, and these cells do not obtain their oxygen requirement. In effect, this amounts to a shunt of arterial blood into the venous system, and this effective shunt may at times amount to half the total $\dot{Q}$. Rudy, Heymann, and Edmunds,[R4] using microspheres in normothermic rhesus monkeys during CPB, found that shunting was only 1.4% of the total flow rate. This is quite consistent with the GLH data if the effective shunt is dominantly at capillary level.

A high PvO_2 or SvO_2 does not, therefore, mean that cellu-

lar oxygenation is satisfactory, whatever the total flow rate. A $\dot{V}_{O_2}$ at or near the whole body requirement does. The $\dot{V}_{O_2}$ is not difficult to measure during CPB; the problem is, rather, to decide what the oxygen requirement is in a given case.[H4,H12] Moreover, as Figures 2-2 and 2-3 suggest, if $\dot{V}_{O_2}$ is below the usual levels at conventional $\dot{Q}$, increasing $\dot{Q}$ probably will not increase it. The fault is not in $\dot{Q}$ but in the capillary bed or at a cellular level.

As might be expected, high flow is achieved at the expense of some loss of safety and convenience in other variables. Blood trauma in the oxygenator is probably greater when high blood flows pass through it, and with a bubble oxygenator the risks of gaseous emboli are also greater. The pressure gradients across the arterial cannula are greater at high flows. This increases cavitation, blood trauma, and the risk of bubbles forming as blood emerges from the cannula.

In clinical practice, at UAB and GLH when body temperature is at 28°C or above a flow of 2.5 l · min^{-1} · min^{-2} is chosen for infants and children under about 4 years of age, and one of 2.2 l · min^{-1} · m^{-2} for older patients. For very large adults with a body surface area of 2.0 m^2 or more, a flow of 1.8 to 2.0 l · min^{-1} · m^{-2} is chosen in order to avoid the disadvantage of high flows through the oxygenator. Lower flows may be chosen when body temperature is lower (see Fig. 2-3).

Temperature of the Perfusate and Patient

Since the introduction by Brown of an efficient heat exchanger for extracorporeal circulation,[B13] the temperature of the perfusate and secondarily of the patient has been under the control of the perfusionist. This has come to be one of the most important decisions to be made about CPB for each patient. The potential surgical flexibility of CPB is achieved only when it is combined with hypothermia.

In deciding on the temperature of the patient during CPB, several facts need to be considered. Somewhat lower CPB flow rates can be used at low temperatures (see Fig. 2-3). Because of the coronary collateral circulation, some of the perfusate reaches the heart and affects its temperature, even when the aorta is cross-clamped (see Chapter 3). Thus, the heart after cold cardioplegia has a tendency to return to the temperature of the body around it, although this can be effectively combated by the use of external cardiac cooling (see Chapter 3). The patient's body temperature is related to the "safe" total circulatory arrest time that is available (see Section 1). If the nasopharyngeal temperature is, for example, 28°C, 10–15 minutes of circulatory arrest are available for repair of a split arterial pump tube or electrical or mechanical pump-oxygenator failure, or to improve surgical exposure. Another fact to be considered is that longer rewarming times are required when hypothermia is profound.

A temperature of about 25°C is used in most cases (UAB, GLH). This is partly for reasons of myocardial protection (see Chapter 3) and partly for the flexibility of hypothermia as to low flow and total circulatory arrest. A nasopharyngeal temperature of 18–20°C is usually chosen when the operation is to be done during total circulatory arrest. The suggestion that long periods of perfusion at a nasopharyngeal temperature below about 15°C may produce brain damage (see

---

[1] Of course, mixed venous oxygen saturation (SvO_2); mixed venous oxygen tension, or pressure (PvO_2); and mixed venous oxygen content (CvO_2) may all be used to express mixed venous oxygen levels. The equation is

$$CvO_2 = 1.38 \cdot SvO_2 \cdot HgbConc + PvO_2 \cdot 0.003 \qquad (2-2)$$

where CvO_2 is in ml · dl^{-1}, Hg is in g · dl^{-1}, SvO_2 is a decimal fraction, and PvO_2 is in mmHg.

Section 1) implies that nasopharyngeal temperature should rarely if ever be taken below this.

During core cooling, the blood entering the patient's aorta is generally not lowered more than 10–14°C below nasopharyngeal temperature (GLH) in order to minimize the tendency for gas to come out of solution when the cold blood is warmed by the patient. This is a conservative recommendation, as some groups (UAB and others) use as cold a perfusate temperature as can be obtained once CPB is commenced.

Because blood is damaged by temperatures of 42°C and above and the boundary layer of blood next to the wall of the heat-exchanging tube probably reaches the temperature of the water, the water temperature should not exceed 42°C. The blood temperature should not exceed 39.5°C during rewarming. During cooling, the water temperature does not fall below about 5°C for operational reasons, and it is apparently safe to allow the boundary layer of blood to reach this temperature. The solubility of gas in blood is decreased when blood is warmed, but during rewarming, this is not a potential problem when the heat exchanger is upstream to the oxygenator. When it is downstream to the oxygenator, it is potentially a problem during rewarming, and this is one reason a bubble trap is used in the arterial line downstream to both at UAB. During cooling the heat exchanger is, of course, safer downstream to the oxygenator.

Arterial Input Pressure Wave Form

The most commonly used type of arterial pump is the roller pump (originally used by DeBakey for blood transfusion[D8]). It generates a relatively nonpulsatile flow, and the relatively narrow orifice of the arterial cannula tends to depulse the inflow still further. At both GLH and UAB, this type of arterial input is used.

A pulsatile arterial input can be achieved in several ways. When the atrial pressures and thus ventricular filling pressures are increased by increasing the patient's blood volume (with no tapes around the caval cannulae, arterial inflow to the patient is temporarily increased over venous return from the patient; or venous return is temporarily reduced below arterial input by partially occluding the venous line), and cardiac function is good, left ventricular ejection augments systemic blood flow and produces a pusatile arterial blood flow; in other words, pulsation is achieved by substituting partial CPB. This mechanism is used during cooling and rewarming whenever possible. A pulsatile wave form can also be produced by using intra-aortic balloon pulsation during bypass.[P2] A third method is the use of a pulsatile type of arterial pump. The effect on the organism of using a system that results in a pulsatile (versus a nonpulsatile) arterial wave form during CPB has been controversial since clinical CPB began (see ''Altered Arterial Blood Flow Patterns'').

Systemic Venous Pressure

In the patient during CPB, systemic venous pressure is determined by the methods used,[K5] since

$$Pv_{sys} = f \frac{\dot{Q}, \text{ viscosity, venous line suction}}{\text{cannula size, venous line size}} \quad (2\text{-}4)$$

where Pv_{sys} is mean systemic venous pressure and $\dot{Q}$ the systemic blood flow. The cross-sectional area of the single or multiple venous cannulae and their length, and to a lesser extent (because it usually has a large diameter) that of the venous line to the pump-oxygenator, are the fixed factors determining venous pressure during total CPB. For this reason, the largest venous cannulae compatible with the clinical situation are used. A table has been empirically derived, giving the optimum sizes of venous cannulae appropriate for various flows (Table 2-4). When smaller cannulae must be used, the other variables in equation 2-4 can be manipulated (for example, the systemic blood flow may be reduced) to assure an acceptable venous pressure.

Table 2-4 Venous cannulae for various flows.

Total Flow (liters/min) ≤	<	Single Tygon	Single USCI[bc]	Two Tygon	Two Ryggs[d]	Two USCI[b]	Pacifico Angled Metal SVC	IVC
	0.9	3/16″ (4.75)	20 FR (4.7)		4 mm	16 FR (3.18)	16 FR (3.8 mm)	20 FR (5.3 mm)
0.9 --- 1.75		4/16″ (6.35)	24 FR (5.26)	3/16″ (4.75)	5 mm			
0.9 --- 1.2						20 FR (4.17)	20 FR (5.3 mm)	20 FR (5.3 mm)
1.2 --- 1.6						22 FR (4.88)	20 FR (5.3 mm)	24 FR (6.5 mm)
1.6 --- 1.75						24 FR (5.26)	24 FR (6.5 mm)	24 FR (6.5 mm)
1.7 --- 2.2		4/16″ (6.35)	28 FR (6.60)	4/16″ (6.35)	6 mm	28 FR (6.60)	24 FR (6.5 mm)	28 FR (7.45mm)
2.2 --- 2.8		5/16″ (7.95)		4/16″ (6.35)	6 mm	30 FR (7.24)	28 FR (7.45 mm)	28 FR (7.45mm)
2.8 --- 3.2		5/16″ (7.95)		5/16″ (7.95)	6 mm	32 FR (8.05)	28 FR (7.45 mm)	28 FR (7.45mm)
3.2 --- 3.7		6/16″ (9.52)		5/16″ (7.95)	7 mm	34 FR (8.74)	28 FR (7.45 mm)	32 FR (8 mm)
3.7		8/16″ (12.69)		6/16″ (9.52)	7 mm	36 FR (9.19)	32 FR (8 mm)	32 FR (8 mm)

KEY: FR, French; IVC, inferior vena cava; SVC, superior vena cava.

[a] Outer diameter; internal diameter in mm in parentheses.

[b] United States Catheter and Instrument, a division of CR Bard, Inc., Box 666, Billerica, Mass., 01821.

[c] In adults, at UAB, USCI ''two-stage'' single cannula is used (46 FR, 11.84 mm internal diameter, tapering to 34 FR, 8.74 mm internal diameter).

[d] Ryggs venous catheters by Polystand (North America) Inc., 925 South Curry Pike, Box 1308, Bloomington, Ind. 47401.

There is no apparent physiologic advantage in having a central venous pressure above zero during CPB. Raising the venous pressure requires more intravascular volume and often an additional priming volume. The venous pressure should, therefore, be kept close to zero, and certainly not above 10 mmHg, in order to minimize increases in extracellular fluid.

Pulmonary Venous Pressure

Ideally, pulmonary venous pressure should be at zero during total CPB, and certainly not above 10 mmHg. Undue elevations are dangerous because they tend to produce increased extravascular lung water and eventually pulmonary edema, according to Starling's law of transcapillary fluid exchange:[2]

$$P_c - P_t = \pi_c - \pi_t \qquad (2\text{-}5)$$

where P_c is "effective" blood pressure within the capillary, P_t is "tissue turgor pressure" (interstitial fluid pressure), π_c is osmotic pressure of the plasma (colloid) inside the capillary, and π_t is osmotic pressure of the extracellular fluid (tissue colloid osmotic pressure). The increase in extracellular lung water is related to the duration of elevation of pulmonary venous or pulmonary capillary pressure, other things being equal.

Hemoglobin of the Mixed Patient and Pump-Oxygenator Blood Volume

The composition and amounts of blood and fluids infused before and during CPB, the blood loss, and the amount and composition of the initial (priming) volume of the pump-oxygenator determine the hemoglobin (Hb) (hematocrit [Hct][3]) of the mixed patient and pump-oxgenator blood. The hemoglobin is also affected by patient interactions, primarily transcapillary movement of fluid from the intravascular to the interstitial space and into urine volume, as discussed below.

In intact humans at 37°C, the normal hematocrit of 0.40–0.50 is optimal for oxygen transport[C8] (assuming normal red cell hemoglobin concentration). This provides sufficient oxygen delivery to maintain normal mitochondrial Po_2 levels of about 0.05–1.0 mmHg and average intracellular Po_2 levels of about 5 mmHg, these being reflected in normal oxygen levels (PvO_2) of about 40, (SvO_2 of about 75%) in mixed venous blood. The normal hematocrit is optimal rheologically in intact man as well.[C8] When the hematocrit is abnormally high, oxygen content is high but the increased viscosity tends to decrease blood flow. Thus, the rate of oxygen transport varies directly with hematocrit (because oxygen content varies directly with hematocrit, assuming normal red cell hemoglobin concentrations and adequate oxygenation) and inversely with blood's (apparent) viscosity (which is also determined primarily by hematocrit). Hypothermia increases blood's (apparent) viscosity, so at low temperatures a lower hematocrit is more appropriate than at 37°C.

A hematocrit less than normal appears desirable during hypothermic CPB, because of its lower apparent viscosity, low shear rates, and, thus, presumably better perfusion of the microcirculation. Thus, a hematocrit of about 0.25 is desirable during moderately hypothermic perfusions, and one of about 0.20 during profound hypothermic CPB. During rewarming, a higher (≥ 0.30) hematocrit is desirable because of the increased oxygen demands, and the higher apparent viscosity at these higher hematocrits is quite appropriate during normothermia.

In fact, the body's autoregulatory mechanisms, including its capacity to recover from transient abnormalities in oxygen delivery, are so well developed that a considerable range (± 0.05) of hematocrits around the desirable point is quite acceptable. This is fortunate, for otherwise the need for homologous blood in the priming volume, with its own economic and medical disadvantages, would be increased. Since essentially all CPB procedures are done with moderate or profound hypothermia (20–25°C), an initial hematocrit of 0.2–0.25 is accepted. Thus, a calculation is made of the mixed patient-machine hematocrit that will result if the pump-oxgenator is primed with an asanguineous solution, using these equations:

$$\text{Hct p} \cdot \text{m} = \frac{\text{patient red cell volume (ml)} + \text{machine red blood cell volume (ml)}}{\text{patient BV} + \text{machine BV (ml)}}$$

(2-6)

where Hct p · m is the hematocrit of combined patient-machine blood volume, and BV is blood volume. So, when no blood is in the priming volume,

$$\text{Hct p} \cdot \text{m} = \frac{[\text{body weight (kg)} \cdot f \cdot 1{,}000]\,[\text{Hct}_p]}{[\text{body weight (kg)} \cdot f \cdot 1{,}000] + \text{machine BV}}$$

(2-7)

where $f = .08$ in infants and children (≤ 12 years) and $f = .065$ when for patients over age 12.[4] If the calculated hematocrit is in the desired range, the clear prime is used. About 20% of the prime is 5% glucose and 80% balanced salt solution with enough concentrated human albumin added to make it colloidally iso-osmotic. If the calculated hematocrit is too low, an appropriate amount of blood (or packed red blood cells) is added.

"Banked blood" less than about 48 hours old is used, but older blood is accepted for adults when necessary. Packed red blood cells should be less than 5 days old. (See Section 4 for practices at GLH in infants). The blood has, of course, been rendered Ca^{2+} free by the anticoagulant solution and is acidotic, so additions of heparin, calcium, and buffer are made (Table 2-5).

---

[2] This classic equation is an oversimplification that neglects lymph flow.

[3] Although *hemoglobin* and *hematocrit* are not synonymous, in practice in this situation either may be used.

---

[4] These are average values and provide a method of estimating blood volume. More complex regression equations are available for more precise estimates.

Table 2-5 Additives to a unit of CPD blood for the pump-oxygenator.

Substance	Amount	
CPD blood	500 ml	
Heparin	3 ml	(3,000 units; 6 units · ml⁻¹ blood)
NaHCO₃ (8.4%)	10 ml	
CaCl₂ (10%)	5 ml	(added last)
Total	568 ml	

Albumin Concentration in the Mixed Patient–Pump-Oxygenator Blood Volume

The concentration of albumin in the mixed patient–pump-oxygenator blood volume is also affected by the amount of hemodilution. Theoretically, according to equation 2-5, a reduction of albumin and thus of the colloidal osmotic pressure of the plasma accentuates movement of fluid out of the vascular space into the interstitial space. That this does occur is indicated by Cohn and colleagues' data showing that the extracellular fluid volume increases more rapidly when hemodilution is used than when it is not.[C9] During long periods of CPB with hemodilution, more volume additions are required (UAB) when albumin is not added to produce more or less normal colloidal osmotic pressure than when it is. This is presumably the result of transcapillary fluid loss (and to some extent urinary losses). However, the adaptiveness of the organism allows these transient abnormalities to be well tolerated by most patients.

Albumin may not (GLH) be added routinely, in part because of restricted availability and its cost. It should, however, be added when volume additions in excess of 2 liters are required during CPB or when there is an excessive diuresis during CPB.

Glucose Concentration

When no mannitol is used in the prime, the glucose concentration (350 mg · dl⁻¹) is deliberately raised to promote osmotic diuresis during and for a few hours after operation and to provide a source of energy.

Ionic Composition of Perfusate

The perfusate should have an ionic composition similar to that of plasma. Thus, the vehicle for hemodilution is a balanced salt solution with a relatively normal pH.

Arterial Oxygen Levels

With present-day bubble and membrane oxygenators, maintenance of arterial oxygen pressure (PaO_2) of about 250 mmHg is easily accomplished and can be considered optimal. Higher PaO_2 is unnecessary and theoretically subjects the patient to the risk of oxygen toxicity and bubble formation. Oxygen pressures lower than about 85 mmHg result in a declining arterial oxygen content (according to the oxygen dissociation curve of blood) and a corresponding reduction of tissue and mixed-venous oxygen levels. Shepard showed,

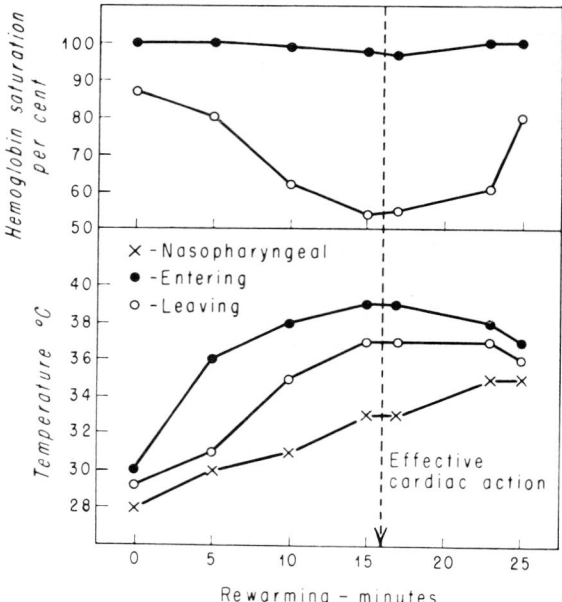

Figure 2-9 Hemoglobin saturations and temperatures during rewarming. Note the sharp fall in the mixed venous oxygen saturation, shown by the open circles in the upper panel, as rewarming proceeds. The "entering" temperatures are those in the arterial line entering the patient, and the "leaving" temperatures, those in the venous return line.

Reproduced with permission from Theye and Kirklin.[T1]

in dogs undergoing normothermic CPB, that when arterial oxygen saturation fell below 65%, total body oxygen consumption fell.[S10] This indicates hypoxic cell damage.

The temperature of the patient, related as it is to whole body oxygen consumption ($\dot{V}O_2$) (see Figs. 2-1 and 2-3), affects arterial oxygen levels with any given oxygenator at any given blood and gas flow rate. A reduction of the patient's body temperature reduces $\dot{V}O_2$ and increases PvO_2, both resulting, in this setting, in increased PaO_2. During rewarming by perfusion from the pump-oxygenator, increasing $\dot{V}O_2$, due presumably in part to the oxygen debt that has accumulated, results in relatively low mixed-venous oxygen levels and relatively high $\dot{V}O_2$ (Fig. 2-9).[T1,T2,T3] This period, then, makes maximal demands on the oxygenator as regards oxygen transfer capacity for any given patient.[L2,T2,T3]

Arterial Carbon Dioxide Pressure

A $PaCO_2$ between 30 and 40 mmHg (measured at 37°C) is desirable during CPB. As in the lungs of intact humans, this is determined by the ratio of gas flow to blood flow in the oxygenator,[H13] higher ratios resulting in lower $PaCO_2$. Present-day bubble and membrane oxygenators ventilated appropriately give a $PaCO_2$ within this range.

Optimal $PaCO_2$ during profound hypothermia is controversial, in part because of the effect of $PaCO_2$ on arterial pH. Reeves,[R5,R6] Rahn and colleagues,[R7] and Swan[S11] have emphasized that at low temperatures neutrality is associated with a higher pH than at normothermia because of the change in the dissociation constant of water. They argue that during CPB, when the perfusate and patient nasopharyngeal temperature are 20°C, $PaCO_2$ measured at 37°C should be 30–40 mmHg, which indicates a $PaCO_2$ of about 14 to 20 mmHg at 20°C (by the Reeves correction[R5,R6]), and that pH (measured at 37°C) should be about 7.38, which indicates a pH at 20°C of about 7.6 (by the Rosenthal correction[R8]). When during cooling for profound hypothermia CO_2 has been added to the ventilatory mixture (in the belief that brain cooling would be more rapid because of the assumed increase in cerebral blood flow) too acidotic a milieu develops, according to this concept. Rahn, Reeves, and Howell[R7] believe that *relative* hyperventilation should be practiced during hypothermic CPB, so that $PaCO_2$ will be below 40 mmHg and the milieu alkalotic. This can be accomplished by maintaining the ratio of gas flow to blood flow constant during cooling and *not* adding CO_2 to the ventilatory mixture. Carbon dioxide production falls as the patient cools, and relative hyperventilation results. These principles are now followed at both UAB and GLH, although measurements of $PaCO_2$ and pH during cooling may indicate the need for some change in these ratios.

PATIENT RESPONSES TO CARDIOPULMONARY BYPASS

The patient response to CPB involves the entire organism, is complex, and defies complete description because of gaps in our knowledge. Part of this response is to the damaging effects of CPB (see "The Damaging Effects of Cardiopulmonary Bypass"). Part of the response becomes apparent only in the postoperative period and is described in Chapter 5. Here are described some of the easily categorized responses during operation.

Systemic Vascular Resistance

At the onset of normothermic or moderately hypothermic CPB, systemic vascular resistance usually falls abruptly. After that it gradually rises toward normal throughout the period of CPB[C17,M10] and may become higher than normal. Considerable variation exists from patient to patient in the systemic vascular resistance and thus in the systemic arterial blood pressure during perfusion. Patients with coronary artery disease tend particularly to develop a high systemic vascular resistance during CPB.[W8] When profound hypothermia is produced during CPB, systemic vascular resistance usually falls more than during normothermic or moderately hypothermic bypass.

The advisability of pharmacologically manipulating the systemic vascular resistance during CPB has been extensively debated. Some evidence indicates that cerebral blood flow is lower than is desirable when mean arterial blood pressure during normothermic or moderately hypothermic CPB falls below about 55 mmHg. Therefore, when during rewarming it is lower than that for more than a few minutes, it is rational pharmacologically to increase systemic vascular resistance (see Chapter 4) and thus arterial blood pressure. This in turn provides more adequate coronary blood flow.

Increasing the perfusion flow rate above the usual values during rewarming is quite ineffective in increasing arterial pressure. When, during this phase of CPB, systemic vascular resistance becomes so high that mean arterial blood pressure rises above 100 mmHg mean, it is prudent to reduce it pharmacologically below that level (see Chapter 4).

Venous Tone

The veins constrict during CPB. Thus, venous tone increases during CPB, and remains high for some hours afterwards.[G11,R12]

Total Body Oxygen Consumption

Although $\dot{V}O_2$ is to a great extent determined by the perfusion flow rate (see Figs. 2-2 and 2-3) and the patient's temperature (see Figs. 2-1 and 2-3) during CPB, the patient's biological response is also a factor. The details of this response have not been completely determined.

Mixed Venous Oxygen Levels

Although mixed venous oxygen levels are related to the controlled variables of perfusion flow rate, the hemoglobin concentration of the perfusate, and the arterial oxygen tension as expressed by the Fick equation (see equation 2-3), they are also related to the patient's response in terms of $\dot{V}O_2$ and thus to some partially controllable variables that affect $\dot{V}O_2$, such as 2,3-diphosphoglyceric acid levels in the red blood cells and pH.

When most of the microcirculation is known to be perfused, mixed venous oxygen levels reflect the mean value for tissue oxygen levels. Thus, the assumption can be made that when mixed-venous oxygen levels during CPB are relatively normal (PvO_2, 30–40 mmHg; SvO_2, 60%–70%) and total body oxygen consumption is relatively normal, tissue oxygen levels are relatively normal and the whole body perfusion is meeting the patient's metabolic demands (see "Total Systemic Blood Flow: Perfusion Flow Rate").

Metabolic Acidosis

Metabolic acidosis, primarily from lactic acidemia, is well-known to complicate many situations characterized by acute reductions of systemic blood flow rate, including CPB. There is a steady and significant increase in blood lactate concentration during an operation with CPB, but when the recommended criteria are followed in setting perfusion flow rates, this concentration does not exceed 5 mmol $\cdot$ 1^{-1}.[H6]

Catecholamine Response

The response of circulating epinephrine (released primarily from the adrenal medulla) and norepinephrine (which overflows into the blood stream from generalized sympathetic nervous system discharge), has been studied by many groups, with somewhat conflicting results.[H5,H14,P3,T4,T5] However, it is now clear that CPB is associated with a massive catecholamine release, greater than from nearly any other form of stress. With the onset of CPB, plasma epinephrine levels increase in all patients, and begin to decline after bypass (Fig. 2-10a).[W8] Persisting elevation one hour after operation occurs only in patients with postoperative hypertension.

Norepinephrine levels do not rise in patients who remain normotensive postoperatively, but in those with postoperative hypertension it increases at the start of the operation and reaches a peak at the start of CPB (Fig. 2-10b). It re-

mains elevated at one hour postoperatively in this group. These patients show blood pressure responses typical for patients undergoing CPB, with a striking fall at the onset of CPB from reduced systemic arteriolar resistance (Fig. 2-10c). Mean blood pressure one hour after operation correlated positively and significantly with both plasma epinephrine and norepinephrine levels.

The sympathetic-adrenal system discharge during, and in some patients after, CPB is presumably related to the

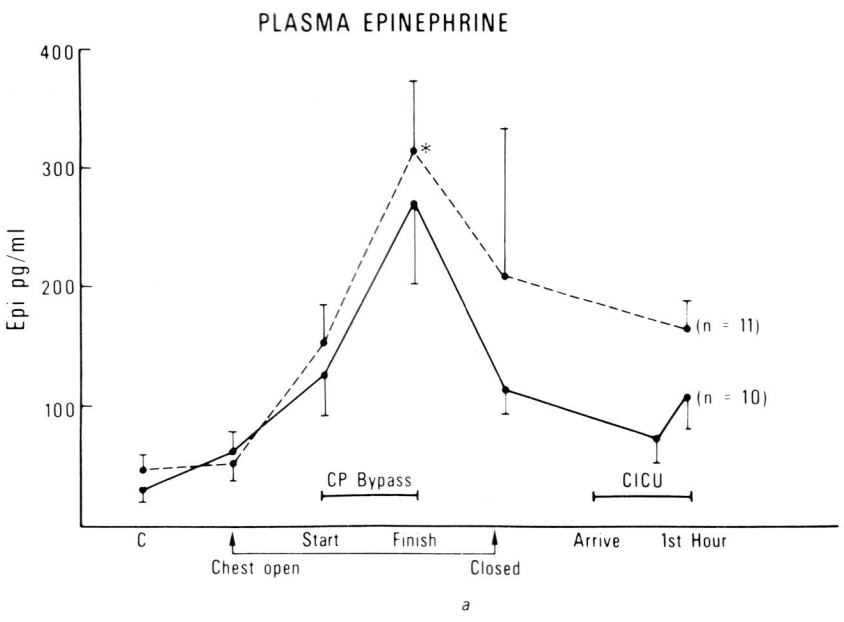

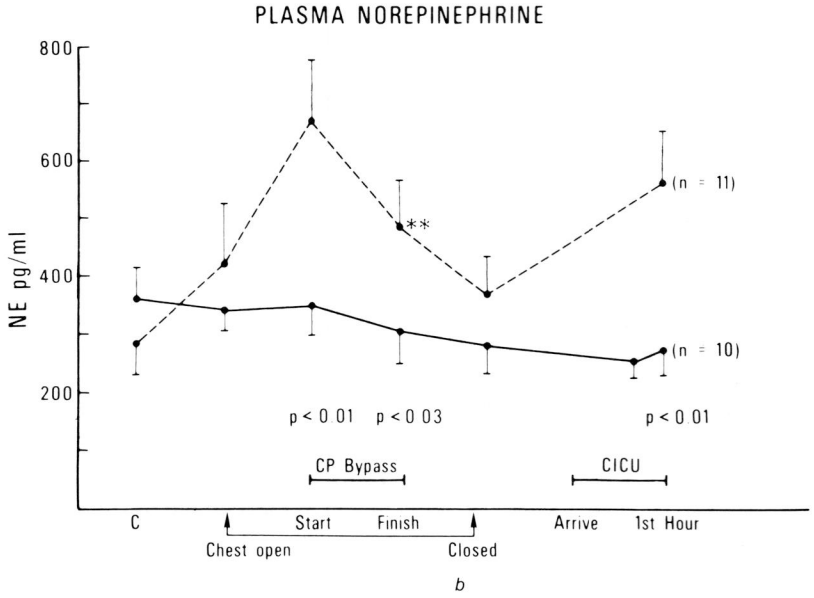

Figure 2-10 Studies in patients undergoing CPB for coronary artery bypass grafting at various stages of the operation and early postoperative period.
(a) Plasma epinephrine levels (mean ± standard error) in patients who were normotensive early postoperatively (solid line) and those who were hypertensive (dashed line).
(b) Plasma norepinephrine levels.

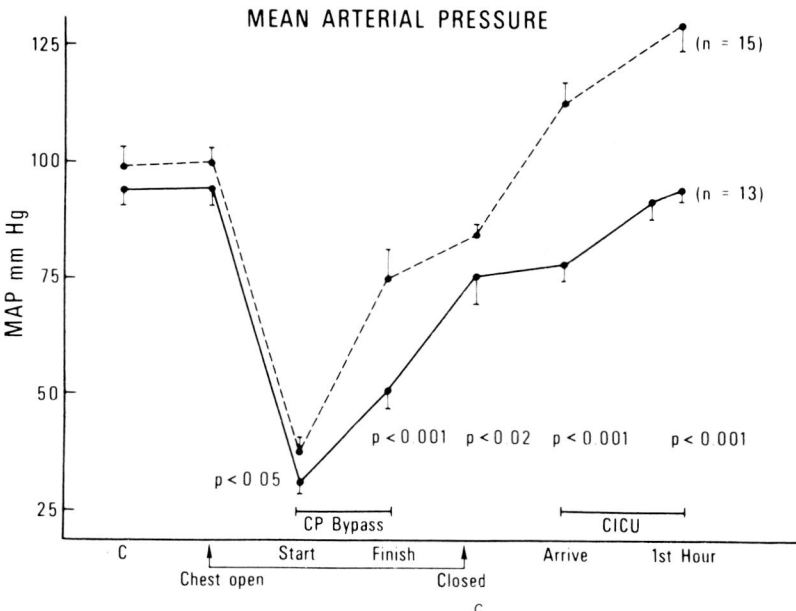

Figure 2-10 *(continued)*
(c) Mean arterial blood pressure.
CICU, Cardiac Intensive Care Unit.
Reproduced with permission from Wallach et al.[W8]

damaging effects of CPB (see "The Damaging Effects of Cardiopulmonary Bypass"). Part of the catecholamine increase, particularly the norepinephrine, is due to the fact that during CPB blood does not pass through the lungs, where the norepinephrine is largely inactivated.[R14]

Body Composition

After CPB, extracellular fluid volume is increased.[B22,C18] The increase is in the interstitial fluid compartment, as is shown by the increase in interstitial fluid pressure that is present during CPB.[C18,R13] Plasma volume tends to be decreased.[C18] The magnitude of the increase in extracellular fluid volume is directly related to the duration of the CPB (Fig. 2-11) and is greater when hemodilution is used.[C9] The large thoracic duct lymph flow that occurs during CPB is related to this tendency of the interstitial fluid to increase.[B21] Also, exchangeable sodium is increased after CPB, while total exchangeable potassium is decreased.[P9] The amount and concentration of intracellular potassium is decreased.[P9]

These acute changes are probably in part at least the result of some of the damaging effects of CPB. The "whole body inflammatory reaction" (see Section 3) includes increases in capillary permeability, which probably facilitate these changes in body composition. The neurohumoral results of a period of relatively nonpulsatile flow may also contribute to them.

Thermal Balance during and after Hypothermic Bypass

Heat is lost by the patient during CPB. A study of six adult patients cooled to 30°C during bypass lasting 130 minutes showed a mean net loss of 1,000 kJ of heat (1 kilocalorie = 4.2 kJ) by the end of hypothermia.[D9] Loss to the heat exchanger and pump circuit was 840 kJ; evaporative and convective loss amounted to 380 kJ; and the patient's own metabolism supplied 220 kJ during this period. During rewarming to a nasopharyngeal temperature of 37°C, the pump returned 670 kJ to the patient. Loss of heat during the period of anesthesia preceding bypass was not accounted for. The patients therefore left the operating room with a deficit of at least 330 kJ, equivalent to more than 1.5 hours of basal energy production. This deficit has to be made up in the early postoperative period, and the extra metabolism necessary to do this places a strain on the circulation that is at times, no doubt, important. When more profound hypothermia is used, the problem is magnified, because muscle rewarms even more slowly and total heat loss during operation is greater. It is necessary to bear in mind that the temperature of the muscles and body fat remains considerably lower than that of the nasopharynx after a short period of rewarming.

THE DAMAGING EFFECTS OF CARDIOPULMONARY BYPASS

Safe CPB is characterized by the absence of structural or functional damage after the perfusion. Most patients have no apparent ill effects from CPB, but few specific studies of organ function have been made. Walker and colleagues showed no change in the intelligence quotient and intellectual performance tests before and one week after coronary artery bypass grafting using CPB.[W16]

In general, however, the conclusion that CPB is "safe"

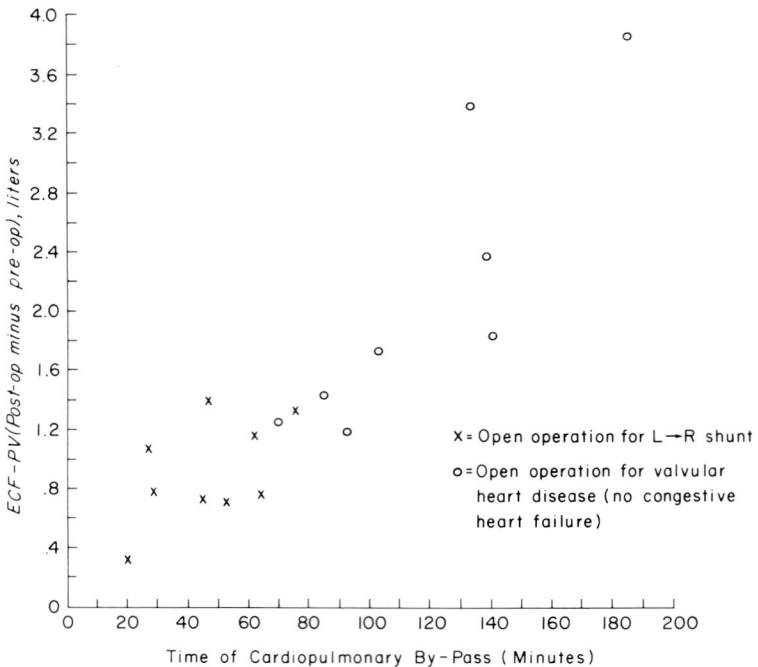

Figure 2-11   Relationship between time of cardiopulmonary bypass and increment in ECF-PV soon after operation (patients with congestive heart failure are not included).
Reproduced with permission from Cleland et al.[C18]

has not been rigorously supported. In fact, some damage is manifested in most patients. These manifestations include an abnormal tendency to bleed externally and into tissues; a diffuse or whole body "inflammatory reaction," characterized by increased capillary permeability with consequent transcapillary plasma loss, increased interstitial fluid, leukocytosis, and fever; renal dysfunction; peripheral and perhaps central vasoconstriction that persists a variable time after CPB and results in both hemodynamic and metabolic abnormalities; and breakdown of red blood cells resulting in hemoglobinemia, hemoglobinuria, and anemia, and perhaps increased susceptibility to infection. This results in variable organ dysfunction and has been referred to as a *postperfusion syndrome* or *postpump syndrome.* The fact that most patients convalesce normally after CPB only attests to the organism's ability to compensate for these damaging effects and not to their absence. The uncommon occurrence of such changes as severe pulmonary edema without elevated left atrial pressure, severe bleeding diatheses, and transient subtle neurologic changes occasionally bring these abnormalities of CPB forcefully to attention. Much of the current residual morbidity and mortality from open heart operations is secondary to these poorly understood changes.

There are some incremental risk factors for clinical manifestations of the damaging effects of CPB (Table 2-6).[K10] One is the duration of perfusion (Fig. 2-12). In infants 1 year of age, this becomes evident[5] after 80 minutes of CPB. Another

such risk factor is the age of the patient (Fig. 2-13). The incremental risk effect of young age becomes evident at age 4 years and increases further in still younger patients. Increased levels of C3a (an anaphylatoxin resulting from activation of the complement cascade, discussed further below) increase the possibility of morbidity from the damaging effects of CPB (Fig. 2-14). The interrelated effects of the three variables are such that, when CPB time is increased from 60 to 120 minutes, there is an evident difference in the probability of morbidity at all ages and all C3a levels.

Possibly, the cardiac defect being treated has an effect, in that preoperatively cyanotic patients seem more susceptible to the damaging effects of CPB. Other possible factors include the perfusion flow rate, the composition of the perfusate, the oxygenating surface, and the temperature of the patient.

The most obvious mechanisms for damage during CPB are exposure of blood to an abnormal environment, and altered

---

[5] For a definition of evident differences, see Chapter 6, "Proportions and Confidence Limits."

Table 2-6   Incremental risk factors for morbidity after CPB (UAB, $n = 116$; 26 patient events[K10]).

Variable (Incremental Risk Factor)	Logistic Coefficient ± SD	P value
(Higher) C3a levels (ng · ml⁻¹) 3 hr after CPB	.0006 ± .00033	.07
(Longer) Elapsed time of CPB (min)	.017 ± .0048	.0004
(Younger) Age at Operation (ln yr)	−.71 ± .131	< .0001
Intercept	2.0 ± .60	

KEY: CPB, cardiopulmonary bypass; ln, logarithm; SD, standard deviation.

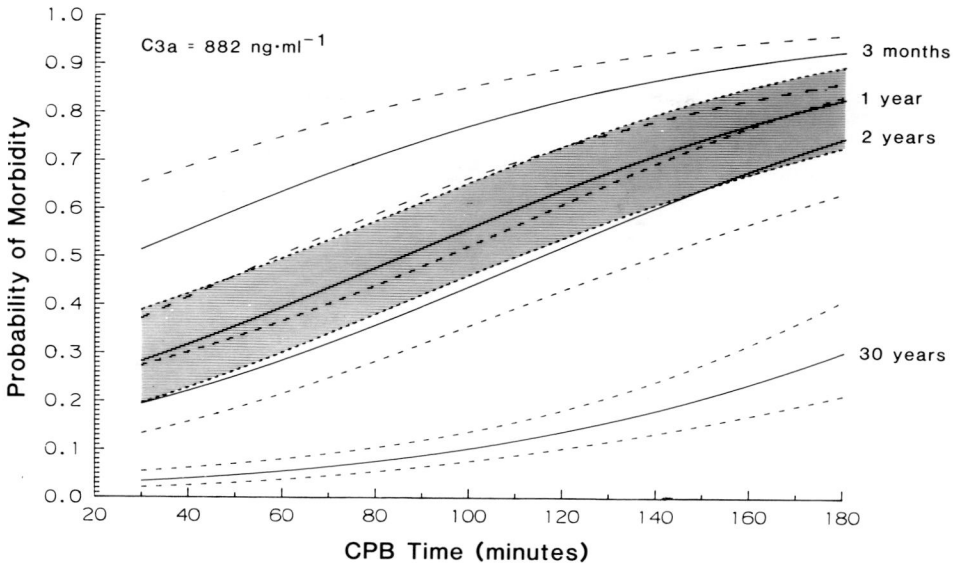

Figure 2-12 Nomogram from a multivariate analysis (Table 2-6) of the probability of morbidity (cardiac, pulmonary, renal, and coagulation dysfunction) after CPB. The presentation shows CPB time along the horizontal axis, and the relationships are shown for four age groups at a C3a level of 882 ng · ml^{-1} (the median value in the study).

Reproduced with permission from Kirklin et al.[K10]

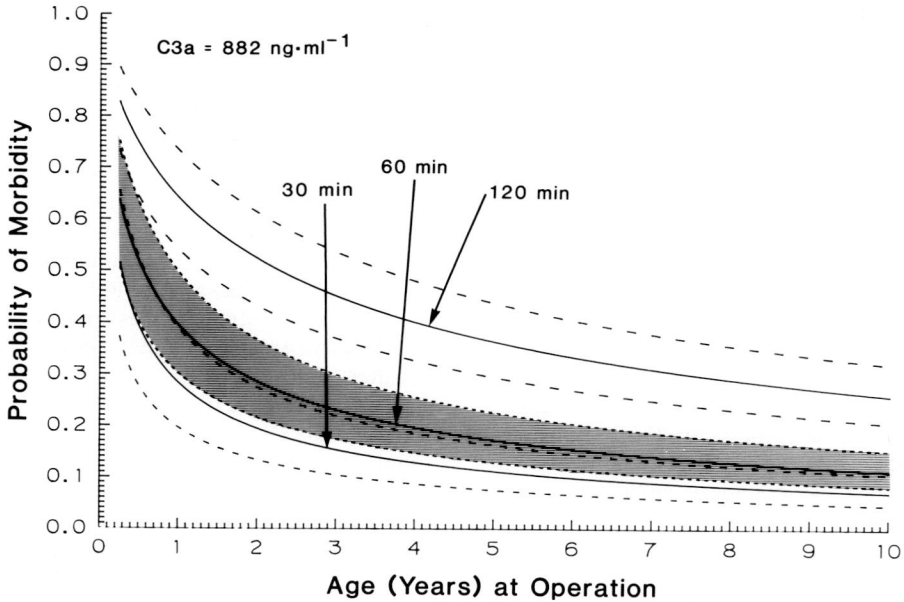

Figure 2-13 Nomogram from a multivariate analysis of probability of morbidity after CPB. The presentation is as in Figure 2-12, but here morbidity is shown as a function of age at operation, with three different cardiopulmonary bypass times.

Reproduced with permission from Kirklin et al.[K10]

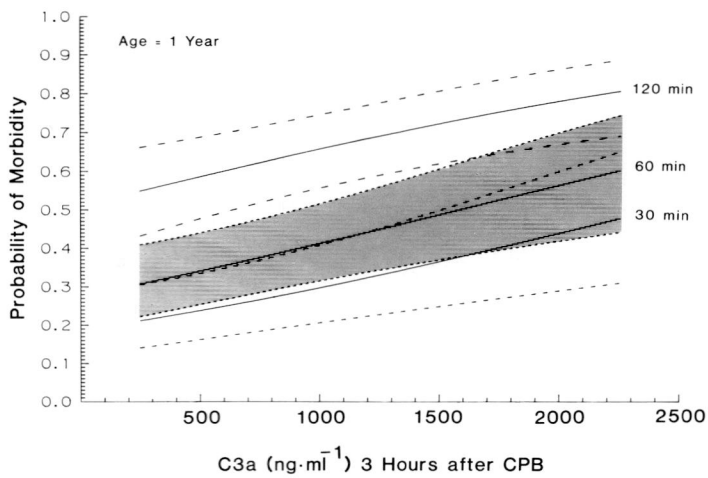

Figure 2-14 Nomogram of probability of morbidity after CPB, with the level of C3a along the horizontal axis and showing relationships for three different CPB times in a patient 1 year of age. Reproduced with permission from Kirklin et al.[K10]

arterial blood flow patterns. While both interact, the former is believed to have the more powerful detrimental effect.

Exposure of Blood to Abnormal Events

Blood is a complex substance with formed elements (red blood cells, white blood cells, and platelets) and unformed elements. Among the latter, the plasma proteins are particularly vulnerable. They can be divided into those with primarily osmotic effects (albumin), those that are carrier vehicles for other blood-borne substances (such as albumin, lipoproteins, and immunoglobulins), and those that are part of the humoral amplification systems[6] (coagulation, fibrinolytic, complement, or kallikrein-kinin).

The nonphysiologic effects on blood during CPB include exposure to nonendothelial surfaces, exposure to shear stresses, and incorporation of abnormal substances, such as bubbles, fibrin particles, and aggregates of platelets. Again, these are interacting in their effects (Fig. 2-15).

Exposure to Nonendothelial Surfaces

Other things being equal, the damage produced by contact of blood with a nonendothelial surface increases with the proportion of blood in the boundary layer where surface effects occur. Thus, the most critical surfaces are those of the oxygenator, where a relatively large proportion of blood is deliberately maneuvered into the boundary layer for gas exchange. In bubble, disk, and screen oxygenators, the

unphysiologic surface is gas (generally 100% O_2). In membrane oxygenators, the surface is generally the membrane. However, recent studies have shown[W9] that microbubbles of air have a strong tendency to cling to the membrane surface; thus, the unphysiologic surface is more complex than expected. Next largest are the surfaces of the heat exchanger, where a large proportion of blood is present in the boundary layer for heat exchange. Probably next are those of the various defoaming, debubbling, and filtering devices. The proportion of blood in the boundary layer is quite small in the reservoirs, tubes, and cannula, and thus these surfaces are the least critical.

The unphysiologic surfaces have direct and indirect effects on platelets, which result in platelet clumps, which may embolize; a reduction in the number of platelets; and a reduction simultaneously in their important adhesive and aggregating properties (as measured by their response to adenosine diphosphate [ADP], epinephrine, or collagen). Platelet aggregates have been demonstrated in membrane oxygenators after CPB by Edmunds and colleagues[E2] and in the defoaming mesh of bubble oxygenators by Hope and colleagues.[H24] Many studies have documented the reduction in the number of circulating platelets after CPB. For example Kalter and colleagues,[K6] using a bubble oxygenator, observed a decrease from a mean preoxygenator platelet count of 222,100 cells · mm^{-3} to one of 85,000 cells · mm^{-3} at the end. Han and colleagues report a platelet count of 210,950 cells · mm^{-3} before bypass and one of 138,000 cells · mm^{-3} after bypass.[H15] The decrease did not correlate with the duration of CPB. These and other workers[A6,F10,H22] have shown a significant deterioration in function in the platelets that remain, as shown by a decrease in platelet aggregation in response to ADP.[B14]

Platelets are apparently not reduced in either number or function by shear stresses per se.[A7,S12,T6] Indeed, there is no evidence that platelets are destroyed in any important quantity during CPB. Rather, the decrease in their number is due to clumping on the foreign surfaces in response to the inva-

---

[6] Humoral amplification systems are those in which a small stimulus results in a self-perpetuating and ever-widening response in the system. Generally, in intact humans these are triggered and are active in a localized area, such as a burn, an area of peritonitis, or a wound. CPB is perhaps the only situation in which the whole body is exposed directly to the results of activation of these substances. In hemodialysis, in which the blood is returned to a large vein, the heart and lungs only are exposed directly.

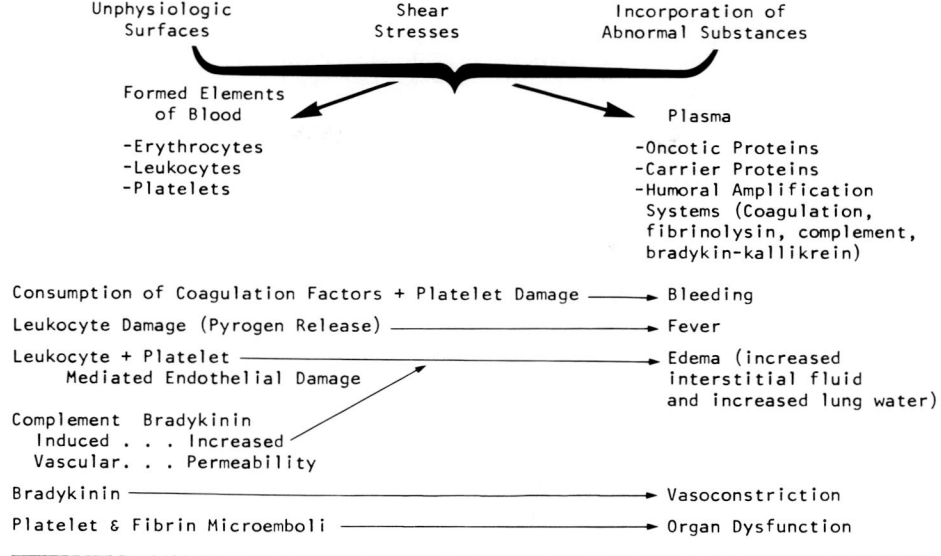

Figure 2-15 Schematic representation of a current concept of the damaging effects of CPB related to the exposure of blood to abnormal events.

sion of the organism's integrity, and to the finite number of replacement platelets available. This unwanted stimulation of clumping on foreign surfaces apparently also depletes granular-stored aggregating protein in the surviving platelets, which also adversely affects their adhesiveness.[A8] The severe reduction in the number of normally functioning platelets is probably the most important factor in the postoperative bleeding diathesis produced by CPB.

Prevention of platelet damage and depletion could theoretically be accomplished by reducing the platelet-stimulating properties of the nonbiological surface or by making the platelets reversibly nonfunctional during CPB so that they do not adhere and aggregate. Addonizio and colleagues have shown that the former can to some extent be accomplished by "coating" the membrane oxygenator surfaces with albumin.[A7] They and others have also conducted investigations suggesting the feasibility and usefulness of rendering the platelets reversibly nonfunctional by infusing prostaglandins (prostaglandin E₁ and prostacyclins) during CPB.[A6,A7,A9,A10] Jacobs and colleagues have shown that methylprednisolone given in pharmacologic doses (30 mg · kg⁻¹ body weight) just before the insult, almost completely prevents the granulocyte aggregation in vitro that C5a oridinarily induces (see below).[H20,J5]

Exposure of the blood to nonphysiologic surfaces has some effect on leukocytes, but shear stresses probably have the most important effect (see below). Damage to erythrocytes, either from direct cell fragmentation or from alterations of the cellular membrane and later cell fragmentation, results in liberation of hemoglobin into the plasma. This is generally estimated by measuring serum hemoglobin levels. The damage is produced mainly by shear forces (see below), but also to some extent from exposure of blood in the boundary layer to nonbiological surfaces.[S12]

The carrier proteins are significantly damaged by blood exposure to nonbiological surfaces. Lee and colleagues[L3] showed many years ago that protein denaturation occurred in oxygenators, the lipoproteins liberating free fat in the process. Fat microemboli result. During CPB, the large globules of free fat seen on the surface of the intracardiac or intrapericardial blood pool result from this change. Because of protein denaturation, plasma viscosity is increased, which no doubt has other widespread effects. The denatured proteins are also believed to increase the clumping of red cells, which makes them more likely to be traumatized by shear forces.

The carrier gamma globulins are denatured at the foreign interface, especially when it is a blood-gas interphase.[P4,S13] The magnitude of this is related to the proportion of the plasma in the boundary layer and also the concentration of gamma globulin. The latter argues for hemodilution during CPB. This denaturation seems to be less in the presence of albumin. In addition to the mechanical effects, denaturation of gamma globulins may contribute to the humoral and cellular immune defects that seem to be present after CPB.

Damage to the proteins that are part of the humoral amplification systems has more complex and widespread results involving all four components of this system. No doubt, the protein called *Hageman factor* (factor XII) is activated (denatured, or uncoiled) almost immediately after the start of CPB by the massive contact of blood in the boundary layers with nonbiological surfaces.[F11,V3] (Most of the evidence for this is indirect. It includes the demonstration of fibrinopeptide A,[D10] a product of fibrinogen activation, and of bradykinin and plasmin during CPB, both byproducts of the activation of Hageman factor.) This initiates the cascade of the coagulation humoral amplification system and may initiate the cascades of the other three amplification systems. Thus, even in the presence of adequate heparin levels during CPB, microcoagulation is continuing, generating fibrin, and consuming the coagulation factors to a varying degree.[K6,K10] The demonstrated reduction of essentially all of these (except the Hageman factor) is believed to be a result of this consumption, rather than of denaturation at contact with nonendothelial surfaces. The relative degree to which various nonbiological surfaces, including an air-blood interphase, activate these cascades has not been determined in detail. This microcoagulation and consumption of coagulation factors is further aggravated by the previously described platelet adhesion, aggregation, and granule release.

The fibrinolytic cascade, a second humoral amplification system, is probably activated to some degree in all operations in which CPB is used (and perhaps in many in which it is not). Thus, many studies have shown an important incidence of fibrinolysis following CPB. For example, hyperfibrinolysis has been shown to be present in 159 (20%) of 774 patients undergoing coronary artery bypass grafting.[L4] Naturally occurring plasminogen (which normally is incorporated within thrombi) can be transformed into the active fibrinolytic agent plasmin, and measurable blood plasmin levels have been demonstrated in patients shortly after initiation of CPB.[B15] This is believed to be in response to the disseminated microcoagulation mentioned above. Since the conversion of plasminogen to plasmin is facilitated by kallikrein, which also results from the activation of Hageman factor, the fibrinolytic cascade may be initiated also by the activation of factor. Further, since plasmin also serves as an activator of complement, prekallikrein, and possibly Hageman factor, the widespread activation of plasminogen into plasmin (which in intact humans is usually a circumscribed and localized phenomenon) may initiate the cascades of all the humoral amplification systems. Again, as an example of the possibly powerful effects of the systemic occurrence of events that in intact humans are localized ones, breakdown products of fibrinogen (produced by the coagulation cascade), when acted upon by plasmin, have been shown experimentally to produce important pulmonary dysfunction.

A third humoral amplification system involves complement, a group of circulating glycoproteins that function as a part of the body's response to various kinds of injury, such as traumatic, immunologic, or foreign body insult. The final product of complement activation is a complex of glycoproteins (called C5-9) that forms on antibody at immunoglobulin-coated membranes and aids in membrane lysis and phagocytosis. The complement cascade, once activated, also results in the production of powerful anaphylatoxins[H16] (called C3a and C5a), which increase vascular permeability, cause smooth muscle contraction, mediate leukocyte chemotaxis, and facilitate leukocyte aggregation and enzyme release (see below).[G7,G8] The usefulness of all this as a response to localized injury is obvious, but the problems of a *whole body response* to the generalized injury of CPB are also obvious. Complement activation occurs either via the classical pathway or via the so-called alternative pathway. The complement system can be activated upon contact of blood with nonbiological surfaces, perhaps by way of Hageman factor, but other substances, such as thrombin and plasmin, can also activate it.

Complement activation during CPB was reported by Hairston;[H17] by Parker and colleagues,[P5] from UAB; and by Hammerschmidt and colleagues.[H21] Complement consumption during cardiopulmonary bypass has also been demonstrated by Chiu and colleagues.[C19] Chenoweth, Stewart, and colleagues[C10] at UAB have demonstrated C3a, a complement breakdown product, in blood shortly after commencing CPB for cardiac surgery, with the continuing production of this breakdown product of complement being directly related to body temperature and perfusion flow rate. This results in over 50% of patients having serum C3a levels above $1,000 \text{ ng} \cdot \text{ml}^{-1}$ at the end of operation with cardiopulmonary bypass (Fig. 2-16). Complement activation has also been demonstrated to occur during hemodialysis,[C11,C12] seeming to result from exposure of blood to the cellophane dialysis membrane.[A11] Complement activation in this setting is via the alternative pathway, with depletion of C3 but not C1.[C11,C12] During CPB, activation is via the alternative pathway.[C13,K11] Further complement activation by the classical pathway occurs after the administration of protamine at the end of CPB,[K11] and this adds to the whole body inflammatory reaction in some patients.[L3,N5]

The adverse effects of complement activation are twofold: the depletion of a component (complement) necessary for normal immune response, and the adverse effects of the intravascular production of the anaphylatoxins (C5a and C3a). Hairston showed a decreased ability of postbypass serum to inhibit the growth of certain bacteria and related this in part to complement depletion.[H17] The adverse effects of the anaphylatoxins were described in general above. In this regard, pulmonary sequestration of polymorphonuclear leukocytes and neutropenia have been shown to develop during hemodialysis and to be temporarily related to complement activation.[C11] Similar observations have been made during CPB.[S5,W10] That these changes are functionally significant is evident from the increased alveoloarterial oxygen difference that develops during hemodialysis.[C12] This all suggests that leukocyte-mediated pulmonary endothelial injury (see below) and increased lung vascular permeability, perhaps mediated also by reactive oxygen metabolites,[P10] may contribute to the adverse effects of CPB on pulmonary function. Similar sequestrations may take place in other organs during CPB.

That important complement activation is dependent upon a large proportion of blood in the boundary layer (such as in an oxygenator or hemodialysis coil) is evident from the demonstration by Birek and colleagues[B16] in sheep that venovenous bypass produced no adverse effects on white blood cells, platelets, or pulmonary arterial pressure. Adding an oxygenator to the circuit resulted in a decrease in circulating white blood cells and in platelets (presumably from pulmonary sequestration), and a marked rise in pulmonary artery pressure. Fountain showed that infusion of complement-activated plasma produced the same result.[F12]

As discussed below, the shear stresses of CPB are quite damaging to leukocytes; already mentioned was the fact that the exposure to nonphysiologic surfaces has profound effects on platelets. Complement activation can be hypothesized to interact with these effects and compound them. The anaphylatoxin C5a is a stimulus to polymorphonuclear aggregation, which, with the shear stress damage, results in pulmonary sequestration of leukocytes. These

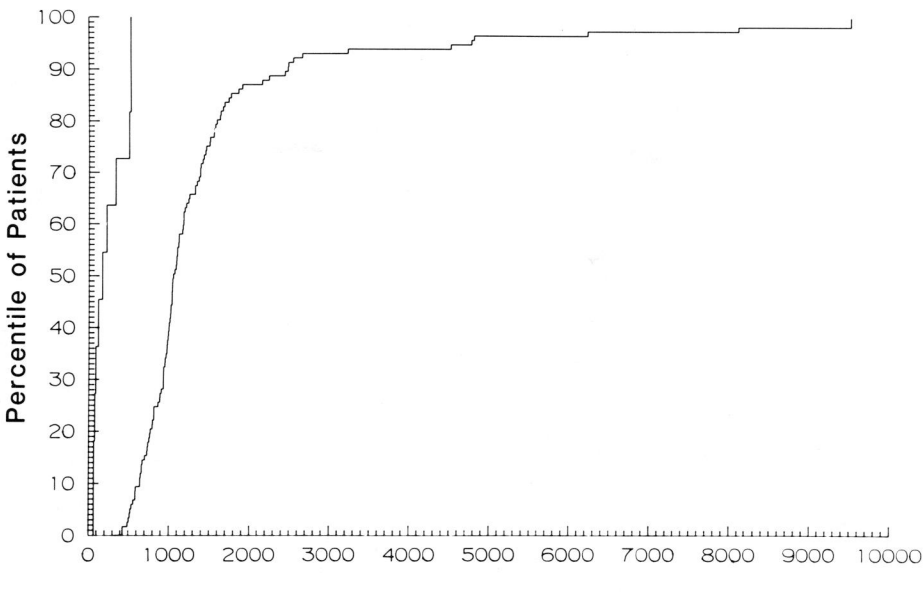

Figure 2-16 C3a levels at the end of cardiopulmonary bypass, expressed in a cumulative percentile plot. The steep vertical line on the left represents closed cases, 100% of whom had near normal or normal levels. The curve on the right represents open cases, virtually all of whom had increased levels. Fifty percent of patients had levels above 1,000 ng · ml^{-1}, and 25% had levels above 1,600. Reproduced with permission from Kirklin JK, et al.[K10]

shear-stressed and damaged leukocytes have unstable lysosomes,[M4] and the release of these against the pulmonary basement membrane and endothelial cells can be presumed to be damaging. Wilson has demonstrated in biopsy specimens of human lung taken after CPB increased numbers of polymorphonuclear leukocytes adherent to pulmonary endothelium.[W10] These granulocytes have lucent cytoplasmic areas consistent with loss of lysosomal contents. Adjacent to these leukocytes are areas of endothelial and alveolar cell swelling. This, as well as relative pulmonary ischemia, may result in a decrease of pulmonary surfactant and a strong tendency to atelectasis.[P6] Tsiao[T7] has reported similar findings in the lung and in heart and skeletal muscle.

Regarding the interactions affecting platelets, the injury of platelets at surfaces causes them to aggregate and release vasoactive substances, a trend that is aggravated by activated complement. Aggregates of activated platelets in the lungs also give rise to pulmonary endothelial injury,[J2] which is expected to result in increased pulmonary artery pressure and pulmonary dysfunction.

A fourth humoral amplification system involves kallikrein and bradykinin. Contact activation of the Hageman factor initiates the kallikrein-bradykinin cascade resulting in the production of bradykinin. Bradykinin increases vascular permeability, dilates arterioles, initiates smooth muscle contraction, and elicits pain. Kallikrein activates Hageman factor and activates plasminogen to form plasmin, demonstrating again the complex interactions between the various reactions of blood to a nonphysiologic experience.

Several studies using appropriate methodology have shown important amounts of bradykinin to be present during CPB.[E3,F13,P7] Hypothermia itself apparently results in bradykinin production. Apparently, immaturity, such as is present in young infants, results in less effective means of bradykinin elimination.[F13] Exclusion of the pulmonary circulation probably also reduces the organism's ability to cope with circulating bradykinin, since the lungs are the main site of bradykinin elimination.

Nagaoka demonstrated a reduction in peripheral resistance and in fluid requirement during CPB accompanied by the administration of Trasylol.[N2] This agent is known to neutralize the kallikrein-bradykinin system.

Shear Stresses

Shear stresses are generated by the blood pumps, by suction systems, by abrupt acceleration and deceleration of blood, and by cavitation around the end of the arterial cannula. They are an important abnormal event during CPB as regards the leukocyte. This is in part because they are the largest formed blood element and perhaps also because leukocytes are normally exposed to nonendothelialized surfaces, since they are capable of exiting from the vascular space by diapedesis and of migrating via chemotactic gradients. They are also capable of phagocytosis and, because of their proteolytic and enzymatic substances, of digesting almost any biological material. Martin has demonstrated that shear stresses not only increase leukocyte disruption but also increase degranulation and adherence and decrease aggregation, chemotactic migration, and phagocytosis in nondisrupted leukocytes.[M4]

During CPB, an initial leukopenia develops, which returns to baseline values after about 2 hours of CPB.[K7] Similar changes occur without an oxygenator in the system[K8] and are in part the result of active movement of leukocytes out of the vascular spaces. Immediately after CPB, a leukocytosis is present, consisting primarily of stab forms of polymorphonuclear leukocytes,[R9] which lasts for several days. Lymphocytes (both T and B) are decreased after CPB,[R9] and T-cell function is decreased.

Chenoweth, Stewart, and colleagues, at UAB and the Scripps Institute, have shown that pulmonary sequestration of polymorphonuclear leukocytes occurs during CPB.[C10] As indicated above, an inflammatory response follows their disruption and release of proteolytic and vasoactive substances.

Erythrocytes are damaged during CPB primarily by shear stresses. This damage results in either immediate lysis, with release of free hemoglobin or shortened life span and delayed hemolysis. The amount of hemolysis and liberated free Hb increase linearly with increased shear rates.[S12] In CPB systems, hemolysis is much less without the oxygenator in the system,[M5] and bubble oxygenators have been shown to produce more hemolysis than membrane oxygenators.[A12,C13] The interaction of the damaging effects is again demonstrated by the fact that the critical shear stress for erthrocytes is lowered by the presence of an unphysiologic surface.[M6] The intracardiac sucker systems are particularly damaging to erythrocytes, not only because of high shear stresses and deceleration injury but also because negative pressures are more damaging to erythrocytes than are positive ones.[M6]

Serum Hb levels during clinical CPB do not accurately reflect the amount of hemolysis, because Hb either bound to haptoglobins or free when haptoglobin binding sites are saturated, is continuously removed from the circulating blood by the reticuloendothelial system[D11] and in the urine. However, representative values are those reported by Han and colleagues,[H15] who found serum Hb levels to be 8.3 ± 1.3 mg $\cdot$ dl^{-1} before CPB, 33.3 ± 3.6 mg $\cdot$ dl^{-1} 10 minutes after the start of CPB and 90.7 ± 8.4 mg $\cdot$ dl^{-1} after CPB. The patient's plasma Hb level may be still higher several hours after CPB, probably because of continuing destruction of erythrocytes damaged but not destroyed during CPB. When the plasma Hb level exceeds about 40 mg $\cdot$ dl^{-1}, Hb casts may form in the tubules. There is little likelihood of renal shutdown unless the plasma Hb level exceeds 100 mg $\cdot$ dl^{-1}.

The shortened survival time of erythrocytes produced by the extracorporeal circulation of blood through the pump-oxygenator results also in a progressive loss of red cell mass in the first 3 or 4 postoperative days. Anemia may result.

Incorporation of Abnormal Substances

Normally, blood circulates in an endothelial-lined closed system, protected against abnormal intrusions. During intracardiac operations with CPB, air bubbles, fibrin and tissue debris, defoaming agents, and so forth inadvertently become incorporated in the blood as micro- and macro-emboli. Shed blood that has made contact with injured tissues contains thromboplastinogen, a coagulation activator, and its aspiration by the pump-oxygenator sucker system must contribute to intravascular coagulation and the formation of thrombin and platelet emboli.

Microembolization is greatest during the first 10–15 minutes of CPB,[C15] probably because some of the microemboli are particulate matter in the oxygenator left after its manufacture.[R11] There is some suggestion, from the work of Clark and colleagues and Donald and colleagues,[D14] that large gradients between the water bath and the blood in the heat exchanger (that is, rapid cooling and rewarming) are accompanied by showering of microemboli.

Altered Arterial Blood Flow Patterns

Most CPB for cardiac surgery is conducted with roller pumps, and during total CPB with the heart empty or not beating, the arterial blood flow is nearly linear (nonpulsatile), and the arterial pressure pulse is very small. This is an alteration from the normal state, in which the arterial blood flow is pulsatile and the arterial pulse pressure is about one-third the systolic blood pressure.

Intuitively, pulsatile flow seems advantageous over nonpulsatile flow. Several physiologic studies strongly support this idea, showing that with steady rather than pulsatile flow vascular resistance increases, red cells aggregate, renal function is impaired, renin is released, and cellular hypoxia leads to metabolic acidosis.[G9,G10,M7,W11] However, whether pulsatile flow during CPB results in fewer functional derangements than does nonpulsatile flow has been a controversial subject for many years. A number of studies have concluded that pulsatile perfusion leads to significant benefit,[D12,H18, J3,M8,N3,T8–T12] but not all of them present convincing evidence. Several studies find little or no benefit from pulsatile compared to nonpulsatile flow.[B17,N4,S14,S15,W12,W13] An extensive review of these matters was presented by Mavroudis in 1978.[M9]

At GLH, a randomized clinical study investigated pulsatile versus nonpulsatile flow during hypothermic (25–30°C) CPB.[S14] No significant differences between the two were found in whole body oxygen consumption, blood lactate concentration, systemic vascular resistance, urine flow, or thermal gradients. Thus, no suggestion was found that pulsatile flow improved the perfusion of the microcirculation during clinical CPB.

It is possible that pulsatile flow would result in fewer functional derangements at lower flows than were used in the GLH study.[D12,O3,S10] In this regard, it is interesting that Bixler and colleagues found that nonpulsatile perfusion at a mean pressure of 50 mmHg of the hypertrophied fibrillating dog's heart resulted in subendocardial ischemia, whereas pulsatile flow did not.[B18] When the mean perfusion pressure was 80 mmHg, neither pulsatile nor nonpulsatile flow resulted in subendocardial ischemia. It is also possible but not proved that pulsatile flow may have an advantage over nonpulsatile flow in infants. Williams and colleagues have drawn this conclusion from a clinical study in which they found more rapid cooling and rewarming and greater urine flow with pulsatile flow.[W14] The results of this study however are difficult to interpret. Finally, pulsatile flow could prove beneficial in patients who come to operation desperately ill with end-stage disease (with low cardiac output, acidosis, renal failure, and so on).

Thus, there is insufficient evidence to conclude that pulsatile flow from the pump-oxygenator significantly reduces the ill effects of the relatively short periods of CPB required for cardiac surgery in the great majority of patients.

SECTION **3**
CLINICAL METHODOLOGY OF CARDIOPULMONARY BYPASS

GENERAL COMMENTS AND STRATEGY

The technique of cardiopulmonary bypass as described in this section is used by some surgeons for all cardiac operations. Alternatively, it may be used routinely except for some operations in infants less than 2.5 kg in weight and for a very few special operations in older patients (UAB); or CPB may be used for all operations except those in infants less than 8 kg in weight, in which profoundly hypothermic total circulatory arrest (see Section 4) is used as a routine (GLH).

Cardiopulmonary bypass should be used as a flexible clinical tool, recognizing its physiological limitations, risks, and damaging effects. CPB is combined with at least some degree of hypothermia in essentially all situations, for the reasons given in the previous sections (GLH, UAB). The operation is planned so that the repair is being completed during the rewarming phase. An important advantage of hypothermia is that it allows a safe period of very low perfusion flow rate (about $0.5 \, 1 \cdot \min^{-1} \cdot m^{-2}$) or total circulatory arrest, when needed. Cerebral oxygen consumption is preserved during low flows by autoregulation.[F14]

The size of arterial (Table 2-7) and venous cannulae (Table 2-4) is determined primarily by the total perfusion flow rate. The total perfusion flow rate, even at normothermia, is not an absolute but a range of "acceptable" values. Thus, if the surgical situation compels the use of smaller cannulae, the total perfusion flow rate is set at a smaller value. Two venous cannulae may be used as a routine (GLH); or routinely only

for operations for congenital heart disease including those in small infants, and in operations for tricuspid valve surgery or other operations in the right atrium (UAB). A single large cavoatrial venous cannula, with additional holes which come to lie in the right atrium while the tip is in the inferior vena cava, may be (UAB) used for coronary artery bypass grafting, aortic valve operations, mitral valve operations, and combinations of these. Such a cannula has been shown experimentally to decompress the right heart efficiently.[B23] On occasions (UAB) a single venous cannula may also be used with conventional CPB and without aortic cross-clamping for a simple operation such as replacement of a valved extracardiac conduit.

The method of cannulation, the use of left atrial and left ventricular vents, monitoring lines, and indeed all aspects of clinical CPB must be flexible within certain limits. The combined knowledge and experience of the surgeon, anesthesiologist, and perfusionist should allow them to adapt the method to the surgical situation while assuring the greatest possible safety for the patient.

POSITIONING THE MONITORING DEVICES

ECG monitoring limb leads should be in position before inducing the anesthetic. Later, they can be changed for laterally placed chest leads or a posterior chest pad. Immediately after anesthetic induction, a 20 gauge plastic cannula is inserted into the radial artery (preferably the left) percutaneously by the anesthesiologist or a member of the surgical team.[D13,O2] If this is not successful, the radial artery is exposed by the surgeon through a small transverse skin incision, which is sited 3.5 cm (two finger breadths) proximal to the wrist skin crease to avoid the fibrous flexor retinaculum and is proximal therefore to the site of the failed percutaneous arterial puncture. When the failed arterial puncture has entered the artery, a tourniquet (blood pressure cuff pressurized to 300 mmHg) is helpful during the cut-down. The plastic cannula is inserted under vision elevating the artery with a loop ligature that may be removed so that the artery is not tied off distally. The skin incision is loosely approximated and the cannula secured to the skin with a stitch. Alternatively, the artery may be ligated distally, and a tie also placed around the proximal artery containing the plastic needle. This prevents occasional bleeding, and has not been detrimental. Also, all cut-down wounds may be (UAB) left unsutured and a synthetic absorbable suture (Dexon) used for ligatures. The cosmetic results are the same as when the skin is sutured and this practice has assured good healing without infection.

A three-way stopcock is attached to the cannula to provide a proximal arterial sampling site and to allow indicator dilution cardiac output measurements when desired. The cannula is connected to a strain gauge for continuous pressure monitoring. An arm board is carefully padded and securely taped onto the back of the forearm and hand with the wrist and hand in a position of function. The venous and arterial lines are taped in such a way that they are absolutely secure for as long as needed, but also so that the arterial three-way stopcock and entry port to the venous line are

Table 2-7 Arterial cannula pressure gradient (mmHg).

	Flow (liters/min)							
Cannula Size[a]	0.5	1.0	1.5	2.0	2.5	3.0	3.5	4.0
10 (1.70)	60	175	350					
12 (2.31)	40	100	225	325				
14 (2.77)	25	60	140	240	350			
16 (3.18)		25	50	90	150	200	260	
18 (3.76)		20	40	60	80	120	150	200
20 (4.17)			25	40	60	80	100	120
22 (4.88)			25	40	50	60	75	90
24 (5.26)				40	50	60	70	80

[a] Outer diameter in French scale; internal diameter in mm in parentheses.

accessible postoperatively. Properly inserted and cared for, the arterial cannula should function well for 2–3 weeks if necessary.

In infants less than about 6 weeks of age, the radial artery is usually too small to admit easily the 20-gauge needle. While a smaller needle is satisfactory for pressure measurements, repeated sampling from it may cause problems, and its use as a sampling site for indicator-dilution curves is not always feasible. Therefore, in such infants the brachial artery may be (UAB) used, approaching it through the same transverse incision used for a venous cut-down on the cephalic vein in the antecubital fossa. It is dissected and the arterial needle inserted through a purse-string of 6-0 prolene. The needle must be securely positioned to prevent bleeding postoperatively. The brachial artery is also often used in infants and young children with Down's syndrome because the radial artery may be unusually small. However, if the radial artery has been unsuccessfully tried, or is not available because of having been ligated on a previous occasion, the brachial artery must *not* be used. These are the only circumstances under which hand or arm ischemia has been seen after use of the brachial artery.

The femoral artery may also be used for arterial monitoring when the upper extremity arteries have been used previously or cannot be cannulated. The femoral arteries may be exposed surgically and an 18 gauge plastic cannula inserted into the *superficial* femoral arteries (GLH). This allows forward flow in the common and profunda femoral arteries. The transverse skin incision is made at least 3 cm distal to the groin skin crease. The artery is not ligated distally and purse-string stitches are not used. Alternatively a percutaneous method may be employed (UAB). In this, as well as in other arterial cannulations, the guidewire technique is useful.

An intravenous plastic cannula is inserted percutaneously into the cephalic vein in the forearm or more proximally in the antecubital fossa for intravenous infusion. This may be (UAB) accomplished with a small incision over the vein, so that the vein can be tied securely around the cannula. A second plastic cannula is inserted percutaneously into the external or internal jugular vein. Central venous pressure monitoring during CPB may be (GLH) accomplished via a fine catheter fused to the inside of the inferior vena caval cannula (Fig. 2-17) and via directly inserted right atrial catheter at the conclusion.

Routinely devices are inserted after the induction of anesthesia. Occasionally, in particularly ill adults, the anesthesiologist and the surgeon may decide that the arterial and venous cannulae should be inserted before beginning the anesthetic. This is then done under local anesthesia.

POSITIONING THE PATIENT

The surgeon or a senior member of the surgical team should be with the anesthesiologist to position the patient correctly for the operation, as an improperly positioned patient can make the operation much more difficult. Both arms may be placed at the side to make optimal access for the surgical

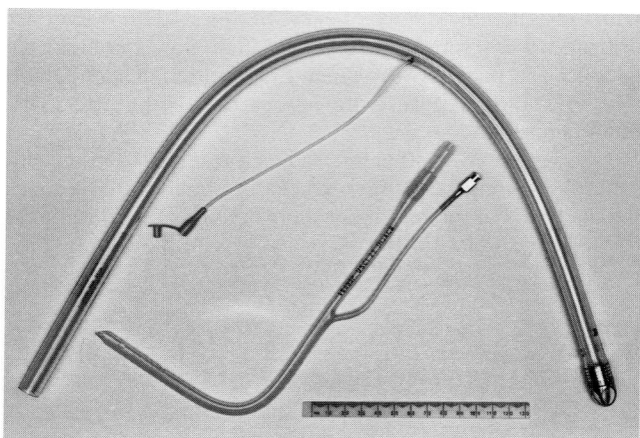

Figure 2-17 The smaller-angled left ventricular vent catheter (size, 22 FR, 5 mm internal diameter) when inserted through the base of the right superior pulmonary vein is easily manipulated so that its tip passes through the mitral valve and into the left ventricle (GLH). The pressure-monitoring side tube extends to the tip of the cannula. (The Sarns angled catheter has a similar shape.) A larger, similar catheter (8 mm internal diameter) may be used to cannulate the inferior vena cava and is representative of the venous lines (of varying diameters) used. It has a metal basket tip, side holes in the plastic proximal to the tip, and a similar pressure-monitoring side tube.

team and to avoid traction on the brachial plexus during the operation (UAB). Alternatively, a carefully positioned arm board is used for the left arm (containing the venous and arterial line) so that these can be observed by the anesthesiologist (GLH). Particularly in infants, a pad is placed behind the chest to throw this forward and extend the neck. The patient's trunk must not be rotated, and the arm at the side must be secured to prevent compression of the ulnar nerve at the elbow. The cautery pad is placed under the buttocks. A draping framework is placed over the head of the patient and extended to either side to screen effectively the patient's head and the anesthesiologist from the sterile field. A urethral catheter is inserted into the bladder. A thermistor probe is positioned in the nasopharynx.

PREPARING THE SURGICAL FIELD

The skin of the anterior thorax and abdomen is prepared with an antiseptic solution after mechanically cleansing the skin. In most patients, both groins should be prepared as well and draped into the surgical field so that the femoral vessels can be cannulated when necessary. Both legs must be surgically prepared in their entirety for individuals undergoing coronary artery bypass grafting.

Appropriate sterile drapes are then applied. The surgeon must work out a method that gives flawless aseptic protection, in spite of the large number of tubes and devices that must pass out from the surgical field to the pump-oxygenator and to the various monitoring devices. The draping must effectively shield the surgical field from the anesthesiologist, while at the same time allowing the anesthesiologist an unobstructed view into the field.

The preparation of the surgical field must of course include proper sterile garb for members of the surgical team. Overhead caps should entirely cover the hair, and separate gown backs over the usual operating gown should be worn.

The surgical field is finally covered by an impervious adhesive plastic sheet, in part to prevent the side drapes from falling away from the skin. It also prevents the drapes in the vicinity of the wound from becoming wet and thus losing their sterility.

The pump lines are passed from the operating table to the perfusionist who completes the CPB circuit, while the surgeon fixes the on-table portion of the lines securely to the drapes. The lines for myocardial temperature measurement (GLH) and cardioplegia infusion, pericardial irrigation and suction are also positioned.

THE OPERATING ROOM TEAM

The surgeon stands on the patient's right side, at the level of the median sternotomy incision. For the patient to receive the best care, the surgeon must be not only a competent surgeon in general, but also a specialist in all aspects of cardiovascular surgery. The first assistant stands exactly across from the surgeon and should face the table squarely. If the first assistant allows him- or herself to drift a little toward the foot of the table, the assistant's left shoulder and arm also drift forward and encroach upon the space over the patient's abdomen across which the surgeon and the surgical nurse must work together. The first assistant should be a resident surgeon with experience in a cardiovascular surgical team. In some cases, the option exists of using a licensed surgeon's assistant who is fully trained to assist in cardiovascular surgical procedures (UAB). A second assistant is not necessary for most operations, but if one is available, he or she is positioned to the first assistant's right or sometimes on the surgeon's left. The surgical nurse stands to the surgeon's right, for in this position the nurse can, when necessary, act as a surgical assistant as well as performing his or her usual duties. The nurse and a circulating nurse must be efficient specialists in cardiovascular operating room nursing.

The anesthesiologist and his or her assistants must not be hidden from the surgical field by the drapes because continuous communication and coordination between anesthesiologist and surgeon is vitally important. Potentially dangerous situations can be handled more quickly and effectively when these two most experienced members of the team act in unison. For the anesthesiologist to reach his or her potential and for the patient to receive the best care, the anesthesiologist should be a specialist in cardiovascular anesthesia and supportive treatment.

When CPB is used, the pump-oxygenator may be behind (UAB) the first assistant or, alternatively (GLH), behind the surgeon. The perfusionist plays a highly responsible role in the management of the patient and must be well-trained and experienced.

THE INCISION

Primary Median Sternotomy

A straight vertical midline skin incision may be used in all patients undergoing CPB through a medial sternotomy incision (UAB). The vertical skin incision commences one finger breadth below the suprasternal notch and extends to a point one to three cm below the tip of the xyphoid. The lower part of the incision is carried through the linea alba.

Alternatively, an exception may be made in pre-pubertal girls in whom a bilateral submammary skin incision is made which follows the fourth intercostal space (GLH). A flap of skin and subcutaneous tissue is raised superiorly and inferiorly to expose the full length of the sternum for a vertical sternotomy.

The exact midline over the sternum is scored with the cautery. A sharp cat's-paw retractor elevates the upper angle of the verticle skin incision, placing the underlying tissues on tension. The soft tissue is separated off the superior surface of the manubrium, and a right-angled clamp is passed over the denuded manubrium into the space behind, hugging the bone. The clamp is spread to create a space for the toe of the sternal saw. The suprasternal ligament is cut with the cautery.

The blade of an electric or air-driven saw is introduced into the space of Burns and the toe of the saw is held snugly against the posterior surface of the manubrium with the cutting edge against the superior manubrial surface. Activating the saw, the manubrium and first 2 cm of the sternum are cut, staying precisely in the midline. The saw tip is kept elevated so that the toe hugs the back of the sternum. During sawing the anesthesiologist stops ventilating and has no pressure on the lungs so that the soft tissue and pleura fall away from the sternum. After the upper third of the sternun is cut, the saw is stopped, and retracted so that the toe disengages from any soft tissue in the retrosternal area. It is then slid back into position, and another 3 cm or so of sternum split in similar fashion. This process is repeated until the whole sternum is divided in the midline. Drifting away from the midline is a serious error because the sternum will not then spread evenly and its later closure is more difficult. When the incision is made in this manner, the pleural spaces are rarely entered. A thin layer of bone wax is spread over the marrow, but excessive wax is avoided lest it result in infection and nonunion. When the sternum is fragile, as in old people, it may be better to avoid wax altogether. The bleeding points in the cut edge of the anterior and posterior sternal periosteum are cauterized and the rib spreader is inserted and opened just enough to allow dissection to begin. After a few minutes of dissection, it is opened a little more and then a few minutes later a little more and so on. When the procedure is done in this manner and if the sternum has been split in the midline, the sternum can be widely spread without fracturing.

The dissection continues by incising the fascia enveloping the thymus gland (Fig. 2-18). The right and left lobes of the thymus are separated up to the innominate vein. In infants and children the thymus may be subtotally resected, leaving only the cervical portion cephalad to the innominate vein lest

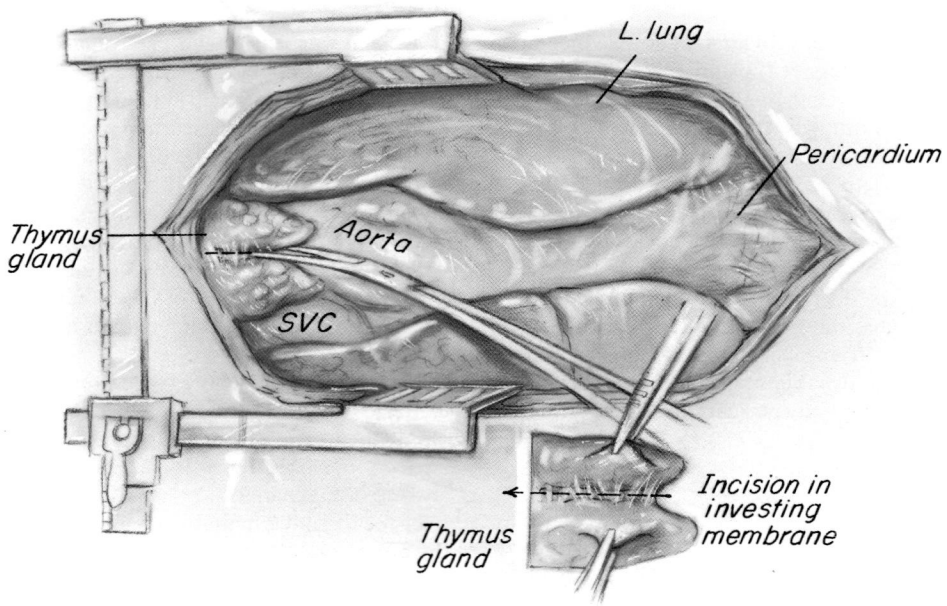

Figure 2-18   Dissection after the median sternotomy incision has been made. (In infants and young children, the rib spreader is less obstructive when the ratchet end is over the abdomen.) Note that the investing membrane over the thymus gland is divided and then the right and left lobes are separated from each other as far up as the innominate vein. In infants and children, both lobes of the thymus gland are subtotally resected as the incision is being made, since otherwise they become filled with hematoma.

expanding hematomas develop and cause postoperative bleeding (UAB).

The pericardium is then opened longitudinally in the midline from the innominate vein above to the diaphragm below. When the incision meets the diaphragm, care is taken not to open the peritoneal cavity lest considerable amounts of blood enter it during the cardiac operation. If entry is made, the opening is promptly sutured. The pericardium is cut back at right angles to the longitudinal incision at its diaphragmmatic end, further on the left than the right, after carefully pushing back the pleura to avoid entering it. Pericardial stay sutures are then applied.

Secondary Median Sternotomy

When a previous sternotomy incision has been made, an oscillating saw is used as a routine. Properly used, this saw allows the sternum to be split without damage to underlying tissues. Once the sternum is divided, a sharp cat's-paw retractor is inserted to elevate the lower left sternal fragment. The dissection is commenced just beneath the xiphisternum, dividing the tissues *just* behind the sternum. Working from below upward, the surgeon frees the left sternal edge in this manner to the suprasternal notch. An exactly similar maneuver is repeated on the right side. Returning to the left sternal edge, the surgeon fully elevates it with two retractors and carries the dissection leftward, keeping fairly close to the sternum until the divided edge of the pericardium is

identified (when the pericardium has not been sutured at the first operation, it retracts well away from the midline). The left edge of the pericardium is separated from the underlying ventricle with scissors. This plane is usually easily developed inferiorly above the diaphragm. This limited left-sided dissection is carried superiorly also, over the main pulmonary artery, avoiding damage to the tip of the left atrial appendage. Often, this part can be completed with the finger.

Only now is the rib spreader inserted and opened. The right-sided structures usually must be completely dissected. The plane of the dissection for this is also most easily developed inferiorly above the diaphragm. It is often best accomplished partly from below and partly from above where the anterior and lateral edge of the aorta is identified. It is most important, during the dissection of the aorta, to keep outside its adventitial layer. Then the outer edge of the superior vena cava is dissected. The inferior and superior dissections are frequently easily connected by blunt dissection with the finger posteriorly, just in front of the right pulmonary veins and left atrium. Finally, the lateral right atrium is freed with care, leaving a piece of pericardium attached to the atrium if it is too densely adherent. This is often at the site of previously placed purse-string sutures. The aorta requires further dissection, particularly posteriorly in front of the right pulmonary artery, to allow later cross-clamping.

Further dissection should be avoided unless it is necessary for proper exposure. Operations in which more extensive dissection may be necessary include redo coronary artery

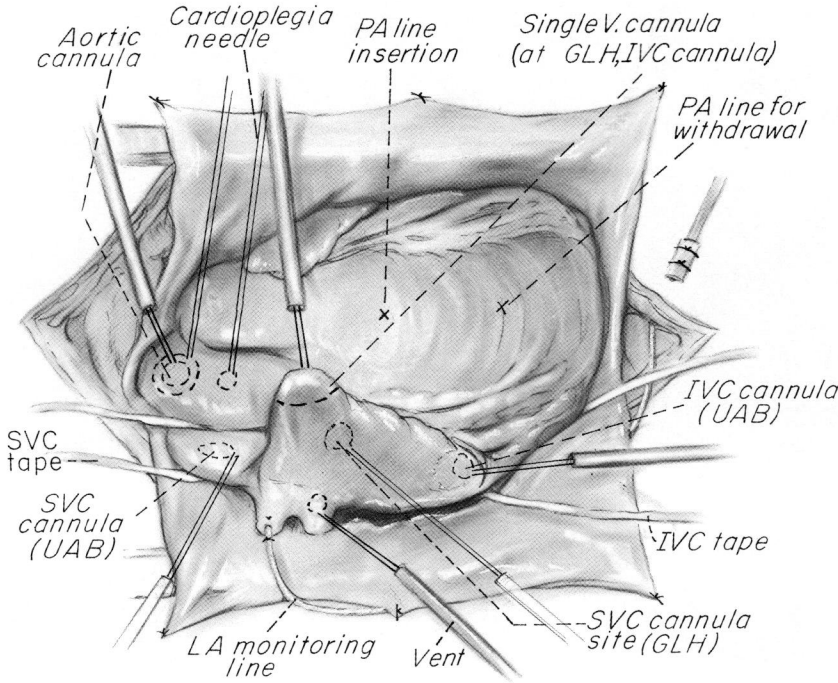

Figure 2-19 Schematic representation showing the positions of all possible cannulae and lines. As indicated in the text, not all are used in each patient.
IVC, inferior vena cava; LA, left atrium; PA, pulmonary artery; SVC, superior vena cava.

bypass grafting operations, mitral valve reoperations, and repairs inside the right or left ventricle. When further mobilization is necessary it is usually deferred until CPB has been started. The heart can then be emptied, and the dissection performed more precisely, with no hemodynamic insults. However, the perfusion at this stage should be normothermic to prevent ventricular fibrillation and overdistention of the heart. If the heart is incompletely mobilized, the left pleural space may be entered and opened widely as this allows cardiac defibrillation and the usual de-airing maneuvers at the end of operation.

PREPARATION FOR CARDIOPULMONARY BYPASS

Once the pericardial stay sutures are inserted, left atrial pressure is estimated for the anesthesiologist (from palpation of the wall tension in the main pulmonary artery, unless pulmonary vascular disease is present). The size and any pathology of the cardiac chambers are noted, anomalies of systemic venous return (especially a persistent left superior vena cava) or pulmonary venous return are sought, and the heart is palpated for evidences of mitral, tricuspid, or aortic valve incompetence. A left atrial monitoring line may be routinely inserted at this time (UAB), or it may be inserted later (GLH). For this, a 3-0 silk purse-string stitch is placed on the right superior pulmonary vein just behind the right atrium (Fig. 2-19). A fine polyvinyl catheter is threaded into

a 16 gauge Tuohy needle, the needle inserted into left atrium through the purse-string, the catheter advanced about 2 cm, the needle withdrawn, and the purse-string tied. A 5-0 silk stitch is placed and tied just snugly around the catheter, very near the purse-string. The other end of the catheter is brought through the skin (Fig. 2-19), and an attachment is made to a strain gauge manometer. This simple and inexpensive method of measuring left atrial pressure makes Swan-Ganz catheters unnecessary in most patients.

Siting and Purse-string Sutures for Arterial Cannulation

The site for aortic cannulation should whenever possible be within the pericardial reflection onto the aorta, because the aorta with this reflection fused onto the anterior surface is tougher and better for cannulation than is that part outside (beyond and downstream to) the reflection. In this location, the cannulation site is proximal (upstream) to the origin of the innominate artery. The site should be a little to the left side (to the right side in patients with right aortic arch) as an added precaution against the cannula tip entering the innominate artery. At times in infants, in children with a previously constructed Waterston anastomosis or with truncus arteriosus, in adults with short ascending aortas or ascending aortic aneurysms, and in those about to undergo coronary artery bypass grafting, this cannulation site would not leave a sufficient length of free ascending aorta more proximally

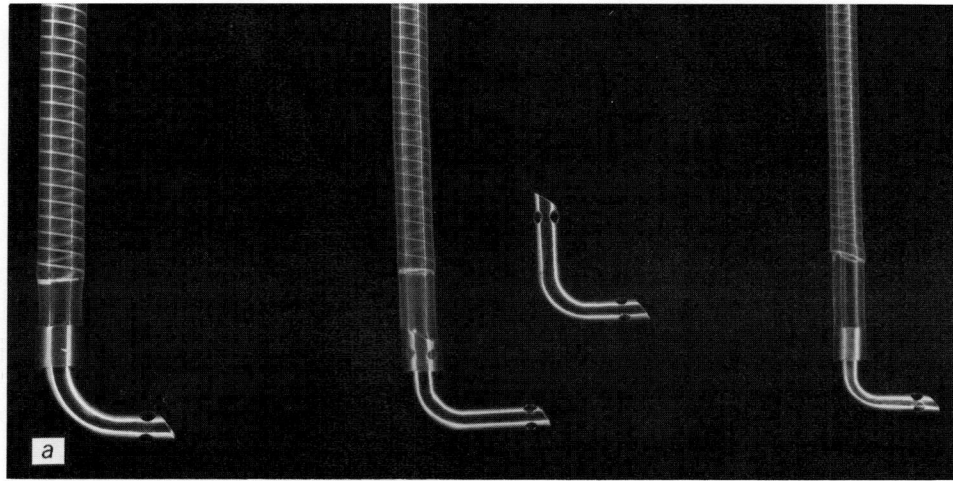

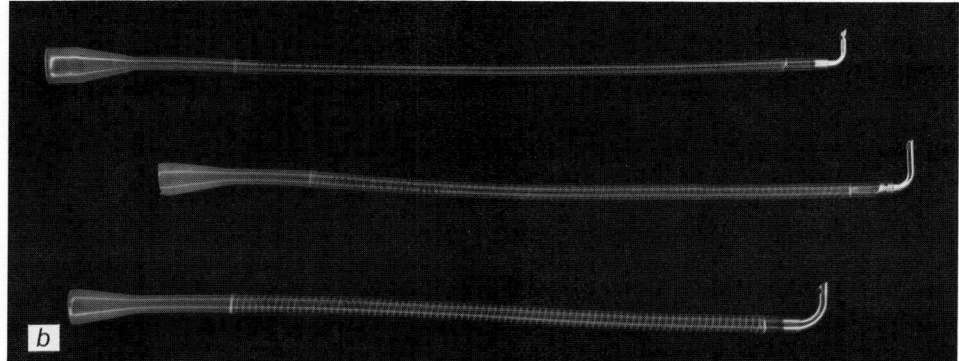

Figure 2-20 Special thin-walled, right-angled metal cannula for direct superior and inferior vena caval cannulation. These were designed by Pacifico and are similar to those used by Trusler and colleagues at Toronto Sick Children's Hospital. They are made in multiple sizes and fit in unmodified, open-ended USCI venous cannula.
(*a*) Close-up of metal cannulae.
(*b*) Metal USCI cannula assembly.
USCI, United States Catheter and Instrument, a Division of CR Bard, Inc., Box 666, Billerica, Mass., 01821.

for the aortic cross-clamp, the cardioplegic needle and other operative manipulations. In such situations, the pericardial reflection over the cephalad end of ascending aorta is incised and dissected off the aorta, the aorta retracted down, and the purse-string sutures placed on the left side of the anterior aortic wall, if necessary, distal (downstream) to the orifice of the innominate artery. In such situations, care is taken that the aortic cross-clamp is proximal (upstream) to the orifice of the innominate artery.

In infants and small children, only a single purse-string stitch of 3-0 silk is used while in older children and adults, two concentric purse-string sutures of 2-0 silk are placed. When the aorta is scarred from a previous operation, a single pledgetted 3-0 polypropylene box stitch may be used at the cannulation site. The purse-string stitch catches just adventitia and must not penetrate into the lumen. A purse-string stitch (usually pledgetted) is now placed for the cardioplegic needle (see Fig. 2-19).

Siting and Purse-string Sutures for Venous Cannulation

Generally, the purse-string sutures for venous cannulation are placed before heparinization and aortic cannulation, but they may be placed after this. The details of these depend upon the perfusion technique to be used. When a single venous cannula is used, only a right atrial appendage purse-string suture on a snare is needed.

When two venous cannulae are used, the superior vena cava (SVC) and inferior vena cava (IVC) are cannulated directly (UAB). This approach is an old one, but has been refined for use by the availability of ideal cannulae (Fig. 2-20). With this method, exposure within the atria and ventricles is excellent, even in small babies. An oval-shaped purse-string is placed on the presenting surface of the SVC (Fig. 2-19), and a tape placed around the SVC. For this, an incision is made in the pericardial reflection over the right pulmonary artery just on the medial side of the SVC and again just lateral to the SVC. These allow a right-angled clamp to be passed easily around SVC, grasp the tape, and pull it through. The tape is placed in a rubber "keeper." To pass a tape around the IVC, the pericardial reflection posterior to inferior vena cava and just inferior to the right inferior pulmonary vein is cut. This simple maneuver clearly delineates the inferior border of the right inferior pulmonary vein and left atrium; establishes a free communication between the two pericardial spaces, which allows better circulation of the external cooling fluid; and provides a place for the inferior vena caval tape now to be placed. Alternatively, the inferior vena cava is mobilized by first passing the fingers medial to and behind the cava, breaking down the pericardial reflection posteriorly by blunt dissection. The hand is then removed and a right angled forcep or Semb forcep substituted. The tip of this instrument is exposed by retracting the lateral right atrial wall forward and medially. Usually, the forcep slides through lateral to the inferior vena cava without further dissection; occasionally, tissue must be divided with scissors working lateral to the right atrium and below the inferior pulmonary vein. The surgeon alone, with DeBakey tissue forceps, retracts the right atrium superiorly to expose the presenting surface of the IVC, which may require limited dissection from the diaphragm. A purse-string stitch is placed at the right atrial caval junction or on the IVC itself, in a transverse oval shape (Fig. 2-19).

Both caval cannulae may be introduced into a single opening in the right atrial appendage, unless this is too small, using a loose strong silk ligature around the appendage and placed on a Rummel tourniquet (GLH). Otherwise, one cannula is introduced here in similar fashion (for advancement into the inferior vena cava) and the other into the lateral right atrial wall about 1 cm below the SVC junction (well clear of the sinus node) using a purse-string stitch (Fig. 2-19). Excluding clamps are used, and for greater accuracy the excluded portion of atrium is opened before the purse-string is inserted.

The line for introducing the external cardiac cooling fluid is slipped into the left side of the pericardial space, a thermistor for measuring myocardial temperature is placed into the anterior portion of the ventricular septum (GLH) (see Chapter 3), and the suction line for aspirating the pericardial cooling fluid is stitched into place over the diaphragm (GLH).

Arterial Cannulation

The patient is now heparinized (see Chapter 4) and an arterial cannula of appropriate size is selected (Table 2-6). The adventitia over the innermost area within the purse-string is excised. With the aorta stabilized by clamps on the adventitia and held by the assistant or a gauze sponge under the surgeon's left index finger, a digitally controlled stab wound of sufficient length is made within the purse-string. The aortic cannula can then be slipped into the aorta easily and almost bloodlessly. Alternatively, the sharp-pointed knife is kept in the small stab-wound, and the arterial cannula is slid down the blade into the aorta. Care is taken to adjust the cannula so that 5 to 10 mm projects into the aorta, and its obliquely cut open end faces distally *into the aortic arch.*

The "keeper" on the inner purse-string is snugged down and secured, and the cannula tied to it. The arterial cannula is now connected to the arterial line from the pump-oxygenator and carefully de-aired.

This same technique may be used in infants and adults (UAB). Alternatively, in infants and small children, an excluding (Cooley) clamp is used (GLH). All layers of the aorta, including the adventitia, are thicker in these small patients, and an excluding clamp will not damage the intima. The excluded portion of aorta is opened longitudinally with a knife, the purse-string stitch then positioned, the cannula tip positioned in the opening and the clamp released as the cannula is inserted.

Venous Cannulation

For venous cannulation when a single venous cannula is to be used, a suitable clamp is placed across the appendage, the appendage is opened, clamps are placed on either edge, the surgeon's index finger inserted to palpate the tricuspid valve, and then the venous cannula inserted into the right atrium. A single "two-stage" venous cannula with an internal diameter of $^8/_{16}$ inches (see Table 2-4) may be used in adults for the operations of coronary artery bypass grafting, aortic valve replacement, or mitral valve replacement. This completely diverts all venous return to the pump-oxygenator when properly positioned with the tip in the inferior vena cava and the side holes in the mid-right atrium. In children and infants in whom a single venous cannula is to be used, a similar cannula is fashioned from a piece of Tygon tubing.

When two venous cannulae and caval taping are to be used, a clamp is placed across the right atrial appendage, the appendage opened, and one and then the other venous cannula inserted through this opening (GLH). One is guided into the SVC and one into the IVC. Alternatively, direct caval cannulation is used (UAB). The right atrium adjacent to the IVC is retracted by the surgeon with tissue forceps, a stab wound made in the center of the IVC purse-string, and the right angled metal cannula inserted with an intracardiac sucker in the pericardium to pick up any shed blood. A similar stab wound is made in the center of the purse-string on the SVC, and this venous cannula is inserted. CPB is then established.

COMMENCING CARDIOPULMONARY BYPASS AND LEFT HEART VENTING

On command from the surgeon, the perfusionist commences CPB, and immediately the surgeon removes the arterial (if present) and venous line clamps. The perfusion flow is gradually increased to about 2.2 $1 \cdot min^{-1} \cdot m^{-2}$, and after the proper flow rate has been obtained, perfusion cooling is begun by dropping the water temperature in the heat exchanger to 4°C.

For operations in the right ventricle in which increased pulmonary venous return is anticipated, venting of the left heart is done with a left atrial vent inserted through a stab wound (GLH) (Fig. 2-19). Alternatively, when two venous cannulae are being used for operations in the right ventricle or right atrium, the caval tapes are snugged after cooling has been started and the heart has become ineffective, and the right atrium opened through a small oblique atriotomy (UAB). If a patent foramen ovale or atrial septal defect is present, a sump sucker is placed partially across this and into the left atrium. If one is not present, a stab wound is made in the fossa ovalis just beneath the superior limbus. The right atrium remains open during the repair, and external cardiac cooling is not used. If the operation is to be done through the right atrium, pulmonary venous return is picked up by a sucker or similar arrangement.

For aortic or mitral valve surgery, a vent is inserted from the right side directly into left atrium through a purse-string stitch positioned in the base of the right superior or inferior pulmonary vein. The stitch should pick up atrial wall, and not only adventitia, and should not be large enough to compromise the pulmonary vein orifice when tied down. To avoid the entrance of air into the left heart, the venous pressure is raised to 5 mmHg, a stab made within the purse-string, and the vent catheter introduced, either before connecting the catheter to the machine line or, if connected, with gentle pump suction. When the catheter tip is to lie through the mitral valve, an angled vent is used, and the line may incorporate a side arm for pressure monitoring (GLH) (Fig. 2-17).

CARDIOPULMONARY BYPASS DURING THE OPERATION AND REWARMING

The perfusate temperature is reduced as much as possible, and when the myocardial temperature reaches about 27°C, the aorta is cross-clamped and the cold cardioplegic solution injected (see Chapter 3). When both cavae have been cannulated and taped, the cardioplegic solution is aspirated from the right atrium and discarded (GLH). It may be allowed to enter the CPB circuit, except in infants and small children, in whom it is aspirated by a high vacuum sucker as it emerges from the coronary sinus and is discarded (UAB) (see Chapter 3). Cooling by the perfusate is continued until the nasopharyngeal temperature reaches 25°C, and then the perfusate temperature is stabilized at the desired level. Flows can be safely reduced to about $1.6 \ l \cdot min^{-1} \cdot m^{-2}$ at this temperature, and brief periods of low flow may be used.

At 25°C, a short period (up to 5 minutes) of total circulatory arrest may be used once or twice, but if a formal period of total circulatory arrest is contemplated, the temperature should be reduced to 20°C.

In using total circulatory arrest, it is important that the arterial line is clamped before turning off the arterial pump, so that the arterial line to the patient is pressurized to some degree, and the venous line is also clamped. Although blood will run out of the aorta during the arrest period, this clamp on the arterial line prevents the exertion of any inadvertent gravity suction on the arterial cannula and thus eliminates the possibility that air will be sucked into the aorta around the cannula. Likewise, in reestablishing CPB, the arterial line from the pump-oxygenator is pressured to 40 or 50 mmHg by turning on the arterial pump slowly, and only then is the clamp on the arterial line removed.

After completing most of the repair, rewarming is begun about 5 minutes (or, alternatively, up to 20 minutes [GLH]) before removing the aortic cross-clamp. The exact timing depends on myocardial temperature and the time elapsed from the last infusion of cardioplegic solution, for core rewarming also rewarms the heart more rapidly. This tendency is minimized by continuing the external cardiac cooling as long as the aortic clamp is in place. For rewarming, the water in the heat exchanger is raised to 42°C, and the arterial line blood temperature should not exceed 39°C. It is advantageous, but not routine, to have the nasopharyngeal temperature at 37°C for about 10 minutes before stopping CPB, lest there be an excessive downward drift of temperature post-CPB, and to have myocardial temperature normal and the myocardium contracting forcefully for about the same length of time.

DE-AIRING THE HEART

After completing the repair and as the cardiac chambers are closed, the heart must be freed of air as much as is possible *before* it begins to beat, but further maneuvers are necessary after cardiac action begins. The exact steps and sequences vary from surgeon to surgeon, but the principles are well established. These are (1) the filling of the heart with fluid before closing it, to minimize air entrapment; (2) aspiration of residual air from the heart before allowing it to eject; (3) intermittent ventilation of the lungs to express air from the pulmonary veins; and (4) continuous suction on a needle vent in the ascending aorta (or a freely bleeding stab wound) as the heart commences ejecting blood, to retrieve any air that may have remained in the heart or pulmonary veins.[H23]

One sequence that is used is best illustrated by the procedure following aortic valve replacement (GLH):

1. About 10 minutes before aortic closure is completed, suction on the left atrial vent is turned off, and the caval tapes are released, to allow the left heart to fill slowly with blood. Should blood not be escaping freely from the most anterior portion of the aortotomy prior to completing this suture line, fluid (saline or Ringer's lactate) is added via the left atrial vent line (the pressure monitoring side line incorporated in the left atrial vent is used for this) until it is flowing freely from the aorta. The anesthesiologist should *gently* inflate the lungs to remove any air from the pulmonary veins into the left atrium. Vigorous inflation is not advisable, as, when the lungs collapse, air is drawn back into the left ventricle through the still opened aorta.

2. With a 20-ml syringe and large-bore needle, the left atrium is aspirated through the base of the right superior pulmonary vein. Air is almost invariably obtained. The maneuver is repeated and combined with gentle ventilation on two or three occasions until no further air appears. A large left atrial appendage should also be aspirated (a small one can be gently pushed backward) to evacuate air.

3. The heart is gently pulled forward and to the right without dislocating it, and needle aspiration is performed through

the front of the left ventricular apex. This is a simple and effective way of removing the pocket of air that is almost always present at this site. The maneuver is repeated two or three times.

4. The operating table is tilted head down. The central venous pressure is kept near zero.

5. Perfusion flow is temporarily reduced as the aortic cross-clamp is slowly released. The aortic incision is allowed to bleed freely anteriorly initially, and then the aortic vent needle (16 gauge) is inserted and suction sufficient to aspirate 250 ml/min (the suction pump is calibrated) applied to it. A higher suction can produce cavitation with little extra flow. If runoff into the ventricle is suspected (this will occur, for example, with a cloth-covered Starr-Edwards valve and with a Bjork-Shiley valve), left ventricular overdistention must be prevented. The left ventricular diastolic pressure is monitored through the left atrial line pressure side arm (as this catheter tip still lies in the ventricle) and is not allowed to rise above 15 mmHg. The ventricle is also palpated to assess its state. Alternatively, the left atrial vent can be disconnected from the CPB line and allowed to bleed back under close observation. Should the heart beat spontaneously at this time, the open end of the left atrial vent may need to be occluded with the finger in case air is sucked through it with a vigorous beat.

6. The left atrial vent is clamped, and the heart is electrically defibrillated if not already beating. The front of the heart is vigorously vibrated with the hand several times.

7. Central venous (right atrial) pressure is *slowly* raised by the perfusionist. The heart will now begin to eject. Air may now appear in the aortic vent suction line. When the central venous pressure has been raised to 10 mmHg and the heart has ejected for several minutes, CPB flows are slowly reduced. The ventricle is again vibrated.

8. The left atrial vent is withdrawn back from the ventricle into the atrium almost to the purse-string site so that its side holes will bleed and temporarily vent the atrium. (It is mandatory that the left atrial pressure be at least 5 mmHg.) This maneuver is repeated two or three times.

9. The table is leveled. Suction on the aortic needle is stopped, the needle is removed, and the stitch is tied. These maneuvers should not be hurried. The longer the aortic vent needle is in use, the better, and it must never be withdrawn until the heart has been ejecting well for some time.

An alternative procedure for de-airing (UAB), after aortic valve replacement for example, is

1. The intracardiac vent, if present, is turned off, and with a syringe, the heart is filled with saline before aortotomy closure is completed.

2. Once the heart is closed and before the aortic clamp is released, the venous line is temporarily occluded so as to drive venous blood through the right heart and the lungs, and generate a little pressure in the left ventricle. The heart is gently elevated so that the apex of the left ventricle is the highest point, an open large bore needle (no. 13)

is inserted, and the lungs are inflated intermittently as the left ventricle is gently compressed and vibrated by the surgeon. A pocket of air is always evacuated by this maneuver, and some air is removed from the pulmonary veins and left atrium as well.

3. The left atrial vent may be removed at this time or left in place on no suction.

4. Suction is placed on the large bore cardioplegic needle in the ascending aorta as the aortic clamp is released. This is continued until the heart is beating well, and in the interim the surgeon may be placing epicardial wires and recording catheters.

5. When the heart is beating well, and with blood in the patient to produce a good left ventricular ejection, the anesthesiologist repeatedly places strong positive pressure on the lung. This facilitates the movement of blood and air out of the pulmonary veins, into the cardiac chambers, and out the suction vent. This procedure is repeated until no air escapes from the vent.

6. The left atrial appendage is compressed a few times (except in operations on the mitral valve where it may be filled with thrombi) while the anesthesiologist repeats the positive pressure maneuvers. The back of the left atrium is balloted, or vibrated, while the positive pressure maneuvers are repeated. When no further air is removed by this procedure, the surgeon intermittently squeezes and vibrates the left ventricle, particularly the apex.

7. With enough blood in the patient to allow the left ventricle to eject well, as evidenced by a normal arterial pulse pressure, the perfusionist reduces the flow rate to $0.5 \, l \cdot min^{-1} \cdot m^{-2}$, with the heart sustaining an essentially normal arterial blood pressure. The same sequences are then repeated until no further air is obtained.

8. The flow is increased to about $1 \, l \cdot min^{-1} \cdot m^{-2}$ and all blood removed from the patient by opening the venous line widely. The heart collapses, and with the repetition of these same maneuvers, at times a little additional air is removed.

9. Once this de-airing procedure is completed, full perfusion flow is reestablished, and the venting needle is removed. Rewarming continues at full CPB flows and with enough blood in the patient that the heart ejects well and maintains a normally pulsatile flow.

COMPLETING CARDIOPULMONARY BYPASS

The patient is rewarmed to a nasopharyngeal temperature of about 37°C. To accomplish this, the water going through the heat exchanger is set at 42°C. This gradually brings the arterial line temperature to about 39°C. In patients in whom the flow is relatively small because of their small size, the temperature of the water entering the heat exchanger may have to be reduced a little to prevent the arterial line temperature rising above 39.5°C.

During rewarming and after de-airing, the vent if present is removed. A polyvinyl catheter may be placed in the pulmonary artery by way of the right ventricle for pressure monitoring if desired. Pulmonary artery diastolic pressure can be measured through the pulmonary artery catheter, which reflects mean left atrial pressure reasonably well when pulmonary vascular disease is not present. After removal of the venous cannula, another catheter in the right atrium is brought out through the right atrial appendage. The left atrial pressure monitoring line may (GLH) now be inserted through the stab wound and a purse-string used for the left atrial vent, which is not, therefore, tied down securely until this is done. If a left atrial vent has not been used, the catheter is inserted through its own purse-string at this same site. This is most conveniently done using a 16-gauge Tuohy needle that will accept a plastic catheter of adequate diameter. Generally, two right atrial myocardial electrodes are positioned.[W15] To do this, a 5-0 silk stitch is used to place two bites in the right atrial epicardium, the bared end of the shielded wire electrode is caught in the loop, and the suture is tied.[W15] In most patients, a right ventricular myocardial wire is similarly placed. Drainage tubes are placed through epigastric extraperitoneal stab wounds. One is left between the diaphragm and the diaphragmatic surface of the heart to the left of the inferior vena cava, and the other to the right of the right atrium posteriorly. Of course, if either pleural space has been opened, catheters are placed therein.

When the patient has rewarmed to 37°C, CPB is discontinued with appropriate right and left atrial pressures (see Chapter 4). The venous cannulae are removed and the purse-strings tied. Similarly, the arterial cannula is removed. Protamine is administered slowly, using the ACT method for controlling dosage (see Chapter 4).

COMPLETING THE OPERATION

After stopping CPB, the surgeon's main task is obtaining hemostasis. This is best accomplished in an orderly way. All cardiac suture lines and purse-strings are inspected to be certain that they are not bleeding at all. Either fine adventitial stitches or pledgeted 4-0 or 5-0 polypropylene sutures are used to control any bleeding areas on the heart. Generally, the electrocautery suffices to control bleeding from the mediastinal tissues and around the sternum. Troublesome bleeding from the sternum itself is best managed by tying heavy encircling absorbable sutures around the sternum. The wound should be closed only after hemostasis is secure.

The pericardium is left open after operations with CPB through a median sternotomy incision. A few stitches may, however, be placed at the upper end to partially cover a particularly prominent aorta. Reoperations have not posed a problem with this technique. The advantages of leaving the pericardium open are (1) good drainage into the pericardium (and then out through the drainage tubes) of retrosternal and mediastinal bleeding, thus preventing hematomas from developing in that area; and (2) minimizing (but not eliminating) the tendency of retained blood to produce a positive intrapericardial pressure and thus reduced ventricular transmural pressure (tamponade).

Secure closure of the sternum is critically important. Stainless steel wire sutures are used, with the cephalad one or two placed through the manubrium, the next three or four

Table 2-8 Guide for use of stainless steel wire in sternal closure.

Patient's Weight (kg)		Stainless Steel Wire for Sternal Closure		
≤ <	No.	is the same size as	No.
5	28		00
5---10	26		0
10---25	25		1
25---40	22		4
40---60	20		5
60	19		6

around the sternum close to the bone, and the most inferior one again through the sternum itself. Appropriate sizes of stainless steel sutures are available to match the patient's size (Table 2-8). The wires are twisted, not tied, to bring the sternum together, and in adults are further twisted with an instrument to assure that the sternal fragments are well approximated. Completely absorbable sutures (Dexon) are used for closing the muscles over the sternum and the linea alba. The skin is closed with a subcuticular Dexon suture.

THE PUMP-OXYGENATOR

The available apparatus for CPB changes continually, but some general points are important.

A venous reservoir is generally used and is positioned to provide adequate siphonage from gravity.[P8] Such a reservoir allows escape of any air returning with the venous blood, and for the storage of excess volume. Bubble oxygenators can act as a venous reservoir. A venous pump, instead of gravity drainage, can be used to move blood directly from the cavae into the oxygenator, but such a system requires precise control.

Bubble oxygenators are the most commonly used. They have an in built medium-porosity mesh filter. Membrane oxygenators probably reduce blood trauma, and should not produce emboli. They make control of Pa_{O_2} and Pa_{CO_2} during hypothermia easier. However, in the past no clear advantage of membrane over bubble oxygenators has been demonstrated, even in children.[S16] However, the new hollow fiber membrane oxygenators have been shown experimentally to preserve blood cells and platelet function well[E4] and they may become clinically advantageous in some circumstances.

An efficient heat exchanger is necessary. These may be integral within the oxygenator or freestanding. The former tend to be less efficient.

The arterial pump is most commonly a roller pump. It should be adjusted before each perfusion so as to be slightly nonocclusive. The pump tubing should be silastic or latex, which do not become stiff at low temperatures. Other plastic tubing stiffens at low temperatures, and the recoil and thus the stroke volume of the pump and perfusion flow rate become less during hypothermia. The arterial pump should be calibrated at frequent intervals so that the flow rate can be accurately established.

The arterial line pressure in the pump-oxygenator must be continuously monitored. When this pressure becomes greater than 250–300 mmHg, the risk of disruption of the arterial line and of cavitation in the region of the arterial cannula increases. These risks are prevented by a properly positioned, adequately sized cannula (see Table 2-7).

An arterial bubble trap may be used as a safety device to remove air that has inadvertently entered the arterial line.

A low-porosity arterial filter can be used. A randomized study by Walker and colleagues[W16] at UAB failed to show any beneficial effects from such a filter.

The CPB circuit should contain at least two cardiotomy suction lines, for return of blood from the opened heart, except as described in Section 4. This blood contains particulate matter and air, and must be passed through a low-porosity filter and defoamed in a separate chamber open to air before it is returned to the circuit. During the perfusion, blood may be promptly aspirated from the pericardium with these suckers, provided that it has not become mixed with fluid used for external cardiac cooling. Blood left too long in the pericardium before being aspirated is a potent source of hemolysis. This part of the extracorporeal apparatus is the most damaging to blood. Ideally, these lines should be activated by a continuously and rapidly variable high capacity vacuum system, but this has proved impractical and roller pumps are therefore used. With this system, when the end of the line is blocked, the suction rapidly increases, which may damage either the tissue or the blood. This necessitates constant supervision of the open heart roller pump rates.

The pump-oxygenator should be designed to *minimize priming volume*. This is most critical in infants, in whom the primary volume can greatly exceed the patient's blood volume. Virtually all infant circuits are less than optimal in this regard.[T13] These considerations were paramount in the design of the GLH infant circuit (see Section 4).

SPECIAL SITUATIONS AND CONTROVERSIES

Right Anterolateral Thoracotomy for Cardiopulmonary Bypass

A right anterolateral thoracotomy through the fifth interspace may be (GLH) used for cosmetic reasons in young women with breast development for mitral valve surgery and atrial septal defect repair. This approach provides excellent access to left and right atria, although the field is relatively restricted and cannulation of the ascending aorta can be taxing. When the aorta is inaccessible, arterial cannulation is achieved via the right external iliac artery.

For a right anterolateral thoracotomy, the patient is positioned with the right side elevated 45°, using sandbags beneath the chest and hip. The patient's position is secured with adhesive strapping across the right thigh onto the side of the operating table. The tape must not prevent easy access to the right iliac fossa. The right arm is flexed at the elbow and suspended from the frame at the table top by the wrist. The left arm lies at the side. The skin incision follows the fifth intercostal space. Anteriorly, it crosses onto the center of the sternum, while laterally it finishes opposite and two

finger-breadths below the angle of the scapula. The muscles are divided over the fifth interspace, which is then entered. The internal mammary artery is preserved anteriorly by dividing the fifth costal cartilage transversely with a knife just lateral to this artery. The interspace is opened posteriorly well beyond the limits of the skin incision and the rib spreader inserted. The pericardium is opened 2 cm in front and parallel to the phrenic nerve. Superiorly, the thymus is dissected off (it seldom needs division) and the pericardium opened to the apex of the chest. A single (10-mm) venous cannula is inserted through the right atrial appendage. With this approach, minimal forward retraction of the heart is required, and caval compression never occurs. The aorta is cannulated on its right anterolateral aspect if accessible; otherwise, the right external iliac artery is exposed *retroperitoneally* through a transverse skin incision opposite the anterior iliac crest (as for appendectomy) and cannulated. In other respects, the procedure is similar to a median sternotomy approach.

Left Superior Vena Cava

A left superior vena cava (LSVC) presents no problems in situations in which a single venous cannula is chosen. When other techniques for venous cannulation are needed, several options exist. The simplest and most common method is to use two caval cannulae and to pick up the LSVC flow by the sump sucker that is partially across the atrial septum (see "Commencing Cardiopulmonary Bypass and Left Heart Venting") or in the coronary sinus ostium (UAB, GLH). The LSVC may be taped so that the cava can be occluded completely for short periods when atrial exposure may be critical (GLH).

A pressure-monitoring needle may be inserted into the LSVC, or the pressure on the left jugular vein may be monitored. As a test, the LSVC may be clamped below the needle (downstream). If the monitored pressure does not rise, the vein can be safely occluded during CPB (GLH).

Uncommonly an additional (third) cannula is inserted into the LSVC either via the right atrium and coronary sinus ostium or directly via a purse-string where the vein enters the pericardium lateral to the left atrial appendage (GLH, UAB). The latter is most easily done after CPB has been established but before the right atrium is opened, and the venous cannula is less in the surgeon's way if it is brought from the LSVC behind the heart en route to the venous connector. When three cannulae are in use, two Y connectors are required to connect the venous return to the single venous pump line.

Left Atrial Pressure Monitoring

Knowledge of left atrial pressure intra- and postoperatively is important. The most direct way of obtaining this is to insert a fine polyvinyl catheter into the left atrium. There is danger of accidental introduction of air into the left atrial line and of cerebral embolization from a tiny thrombus on its tip, but these complications have not been identified at UAB or GLH. The only complication has been the occasional occurrence of bleeding when the catheter is removed. This may be significant enough in small infants to require immediate blood replacement and, rarely, reoperation.

As an alternative, a catheter may be introduced into the pulmonary artery for intra- and postoperative monitoring (as discussed above). Unless pulmonary vascular disease is present, the pulmonary artery diastolic pressure is similar to mean left atrial pressure.

SECTION 4
CLINICAL METHODOLOGY OF PROFOUNDLY HYPOTHERMIC TOTAL CIRCULATORY ARREST

GENERAL COMMENTS AND STRATEGY

As indicated earlier, the use of this may be limited to a few special operations and to most operations in infants less than 2.5 kg (UAB) or, alternatively, it may be used as a routine in infants less than 8 kg in weight (GLH). Initial surface cooling is used, to a nasopharyngeal temperature of 20–22°C (GLH) or to 28–30°C (UAB).

The technique may be very similar to that described for operations during cardiopulmonary bypass (CPB), except that the head and body are surrounded with ice bags during the placement of devices and beginning of anesthesia (UAB). When convenient, two venous cannulae may be employed (UAB), but in very small infants a single venous cannula is used and removed during the intracardiac repair.

Alternatively, a special technique is used in which surface cooling is provided by a water bed and ice bags, with a 5-minute period of core cooling often required to complete the cooling process or, in the cyanotic group, to oxygenate fully the tissues prior to circulatory arrest (GLH). Core rewarming requires a 20–30-minute period of bypass and is assisted by circulating water at 40°C through the water bed. On theoretical grounds, this method is superior to other techniques because hypothermia produced by surface cooling is more even than that by core cooling (see Section 1), the liver functions for a longer time, and the heart continues to beat and provide a pulsatile flow. Core rewarming rapidly rewarms these central organs so that the heart can eject and again provide pulsatile flow and the liver can again begin to metabolize lactate.[B19] The period of CPB is also reduced to a minimum. The remainder of Section 4 describes this alternative of profound hypothermia with limited CPB and total circulatory arrest (GLH).

INITIAL SURFACE COOLING

The premedicated naked infant is placed supine on the cold water bed, from which the infant is partly insulated at this stage by a dry towel (Fig. 2-21). The water bed is constructed of heavyweight plastic, supported in a low profile wooden frame that fits the tabletop. Water at 1°C is rapidly circulated through the bed using a specially designed circuit (Fig. 2-21). To allow as much as possible of the infant to come into direct

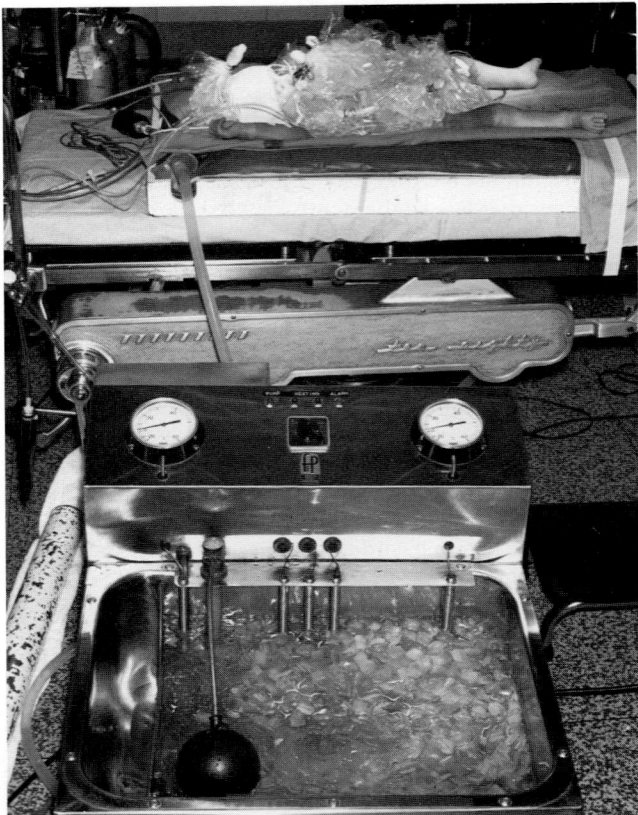

Figure 2-21   An infant anesthetized and intubated is shown on a water bed, with the control apparatus for the bed. Thorax, abdomen, and head have been surrounded by ice bags.
Reproduced with permission from Barratt-Boyes.[B20]

contact with the bed, it is not permitted to overfill. In small infants (less than 4 kg), the nasopharyngeal temperature falls 1°C in 5 minutes with this system (Fig. 2-22). The rate is slowed by 1 minute per degree for each additional kilogram of body weight. The dry towel is removed after induction of the anesthetic (see Chapter 4, Section 1 for details) and replaced by a single layer of linen cloth to ensure more direct heat transference. Ice bags are placed over the chest and flanks.

The water bed is also used to aid rewarming. Its temperature is altered more rapidly by emptying out the cold water before refilling it with warm. When the bed is empty, the infant sinks toward the tabletop, and the zero level of the pressure transducers must be adjusted accordingly.

Operating on a water bed has the theoretical disadvantage that the infant is not completely stable. In practice, the surgeon is unaware of this and is not inconvenienced.

Induction and insertion of monitoring devices usually take 40–45 minutes, by which time the nasopharyngeal temperature has already fallen significantly (Fig. 2-18). Further ice bags are positioned to cover the abdomen, protecting the genital area and avoiding contact with peripheral parts.

Surface cooling is continued until the nasopharyngeal tem-

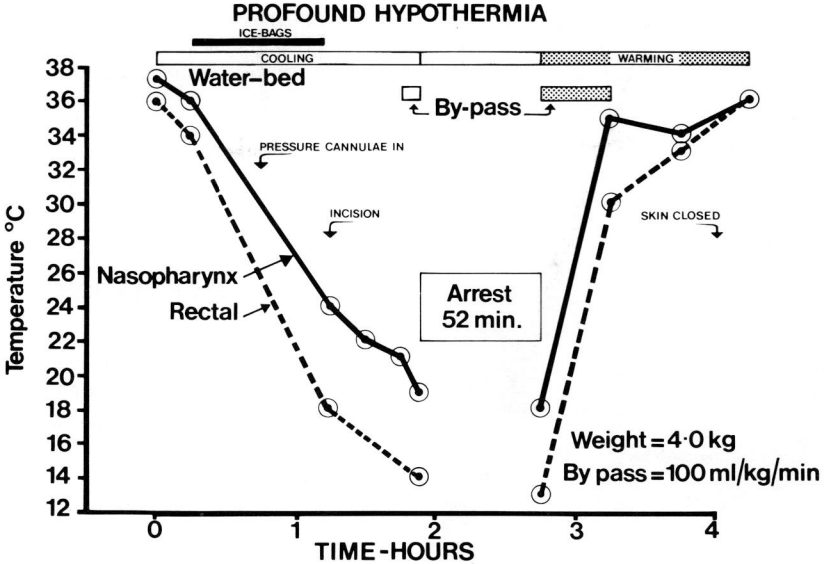

Figure 2-22 The temperature course of a 4-kg infant operated on with profound hypothermia, limited cardiopulmonary bypass, and total circulatory arrest. Note the more rapid fall of rectal than of nasopharyngeal temperature. Notice also that surface cooling is readily accomplished with a combination of ice bags and water bed.

Reproduced with permission from Barratt-Boyes.[B20]

perature reaches 24°C. Halothane inhalation is stopped at lower temperatures if the arterial blood pressure falls consistently below 30 mmHg. Sinus bradycardia is not corrected.

STERNOTOMY

The ice bags are removed, and the skin painted and draped. A median sternotomy is made, and the pericardium opened vertically. When needed for the intracardiac repair, an appropriate piece of pericardium is removed. The patient is heparinized (300 units · kg^{-1}).

The vena cavae are taped using an aneurysm needle to encircle the inferior vena cava as this avoids any manipulation of the heart that can induce ventricular fibrillation. If the latter occurs, the heart is electrically defibrillated. If defibrillation is not achieved—and this is rare—cannulation is completed without undue haste with the heart arrested.

A single right atrial cannula (4–6 mm internal diameter) is inserted through the appendage. The arterial cannula is inserted into the ascending aorta close to the valve, using a size 10 FR–14 FR Argyl arterial cannula (Fig. 2-23). The tip of the cannula is cut obliquely, about 3 mm from the shoulder on the cannula to limit its depth of insertion into the ascending aorta to this amount.

CARDIOPULMONARY BYPASS

The venous and arterial lines are connected to the primed perfusion circuit, incorporating a two-way tap in the arterial connector (Fig. 2-23), partly for use later to aspirate air from the ventricle. The arterial line is clamped on the machine side of the connector. Two milliequivalents of potassium chloride, 5 mEq of sodium bicarbonate, and 500 mg of ascorbic acid are added to the machine prime, the latter for its effect in lowering blood viscosity.[T14] Iced water has continued to circulate through the water bed during these maneuvers, and the nasopharyngeal temperature will have dropped a further 2–3°C to approximately 21°C.

Cooling perfusion is now commenced at a flow rate of 100 ml · kg^{-1} · min^{-1}. The pump-oxygenator system is shown in Figure 2-24. The temperature of the blood leaving the heat exchanger is maintained at 10°C lower than the nasopharyngeal temperature. To oxygenate the tissues as fully as possible, a minimum 3-minute perfusion time is allowed. At the desired nasopharyngeal temperature of 18°C,

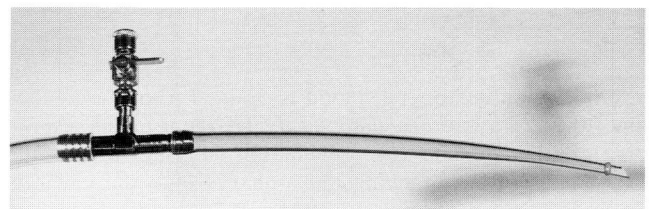

Figure 2-23 Arterial cannula assembly (Argyle Co.) for infant use (GLH). Note that the cannula tip extends for only 3–4 mm beyond the plastic O ring, which snugs against the outside of the aortic wall. This allows the aorta to be cross-clamped downstream to the cannulation site.

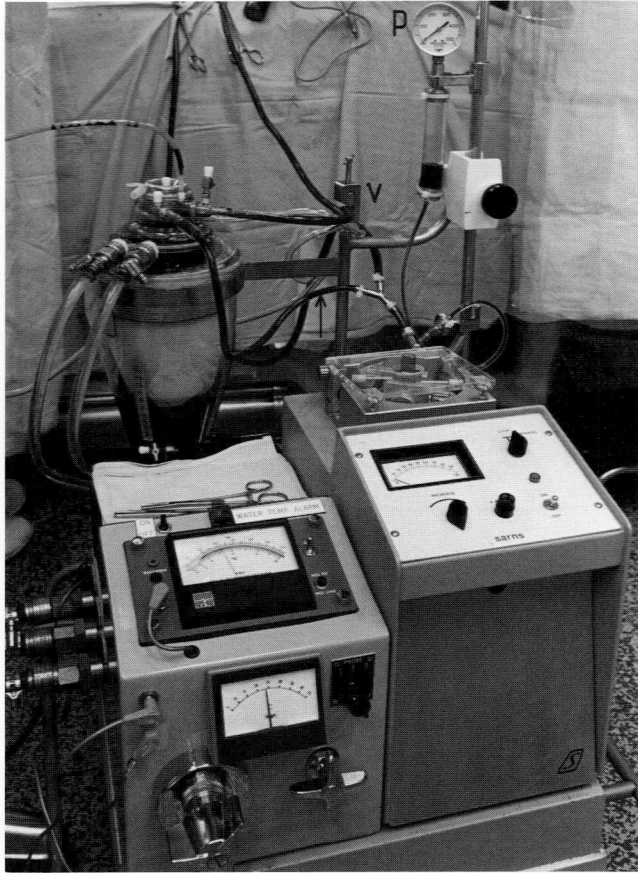

Figure 2-24 The simplified infant cardiopulmonary bypass circuit used at GLH in most profound hypothermia-circulatory arrest procedures. The single pump is for arterial return. The heat exchanger is incorporated in the hard-case infant bubble oxygenator. A recirculation line is provided (arrow) to allow the blood to be warmed to 10°C above the circulatory arrest temperature during the arrest period. This increases the speed for rewarming. The module to the left of the pump unit contains the water mixing valves and temperature monitors. In straightforward procedures in which the arrest time will not exceed 45 minutes, no open heart return pumps are provided. For more complex conditions, under which the operating time within the heart may be longer than this, two open heart return pumps with a debubbling chamber are added so that more conventional CPB is possible. Venous and arterial lines are 5/16 inches ID (7.5 mm), and the circuit priming volume is 800 ml.

V, venous line occluder; P, arterial pressure gauge.

the perfusion is stopped, blood is drained from the venous line, the aorta is cross-clamped *downstream* of the arterial line connection site (to prevent air entering around the purse-string from reaching the arch vessels), the cavae is occluded, and both lines are clamped.

Cardioplegia is not currently employed in infants operated on using this technique. It has been abandoned because the St. Thomas' solution then in use, which contained 0.98 mmol of procaine hydrochloride and did not contain albumin, appeared to be associated with impaired myocardial contractil-

ity postoperatively in these infants (see Chapter 3). It is to be noted that, using the circulatory arrest technique, the cardioplegic solution is not washed out from the coronary vascular bed but remains in contact with it in full concentration throughout the arrest period. Myocardial temperature without cardioplegia is 10°C at the time of cross-clamping and does not rise above 16°C during the arrest period.

THE CARDIAC OPERATION

The right atrial cannula is completely removed from the heart. The heart is opened where appropriate and the repair is carried out. The right atrium is always opened to close any atrial communication, including a patent foramen ovale and blood is injected by syringe through any atrial defect to flush air from the atrium into the ventricle. With the intracardiac repair completed, the cardiotomy is closed.

During circulatory arrest, the water bed temperature is raised to 15°C, and an oxygen flow of $1.5 \, l \cdot min^{-1}$ is maintained through the bubble oxygenator to ensure that the gas vent holes are not occluded by dried blood. The lungs are kept slightly inflated but are not ventilated.

DE-AIRING THE HEART

A small catheter is introduced through a stab wound in the apex of the left ventricle and controlled with a purse-string stitch. Blood that has been aspirated from the oxygenator into two or three 50-ml syringes via the Luer tap on the arterial line connector before the arrest period is syringed through the left ventricular catheter and aspirated into a dry syringe connected to the arterial Luer tap, gently massaging the heart and ventilating the lungs. The solution passes through any Teflon patch used for ventricular septal defect repair into the right ventricle. Air in the right heart is therefore readily evacuated by inserting a fine forcep between the right ventriculotomy closure sutures and also passing these upward through the pulmonary valve to render it temporarily incompetent. The catheter is not removed from the ventricle until CPB has been re-established.

CARDIOPULMONARY BYPASS FOR REWARMING

Rewarming CPB is begun, adding 2 mEq of potassium chloride, 10 mEq of sodium bicarbonate, and a further 500 mg of ascorbic acid to the perfusate. The first return from the arterial line is allowed to distend the ascending aorta momentarily and flush the coronaries before the aortic cross-clamp is released. Flow is kept at $100 \, ml \cdot kg^{-1} \cdot min^{-1}$ and mean right atrial pressure at 5 to 10 mmHg. The heart usually returns to a coordinated beat spontaneously within minutes of beginning perfusion, but if not, it is electrically defibrillated. The raised filling pressure allows it to eject and contribute a normal arterial pulse contour. In case air remains inside the ventricle, the ascending aorta is needled proximal to the arterial cannula and allowed to bleed. The left ventricle is also dislocated and suction applied to the catheter in the apex of the ventricle with the syringe, following which the catheter is removed and the stab wound closed.

As the heart is contributing to the circulation, the lungs are ventilated. If the heart rate is slow due to heart block—and this is common early in the rewarming phase—the heart is paced at an adequate rate.

The temperature of the blood leaving the heat exchanger is initially 10°C above the arrest temperature and is raised to 37°C within 5 minutes. At the start of the rewarming period, the water bed is recirculated with water at 40°C, and this is continued until the chest is closed.

During rewarming, a left atrial pressure line is inserted either through the base of the right superior pulmonary vein or through the left atrial appendage. If pacemaker wires are not already in position, they are now inserted.

Rewarming perfusion is stopped after 20–30 minutes when the nasopharyngeal temperature reaches 35°C and the rectal temperature 28°C or more, because rewarming is completed by the water bed, which is at 40°C. The heart is decannulated. Heparin is reversed with protamine sulphate (6 mg/kg) given slowly intravenously over 5 minutes. The sternum is closed over two drainage catheters.

SPECIAL SITUATIONS AND CONTROVERSIES

Complex Situations Requiring Prolonged Intracardiac Repair Time

In the past, circulatory arrest times of 60–65 minutes at 18°C nasopharyngeal have been regarded as safe at GLH.[C4] Currently circulatory arrest time is limited to no more than 45 minutes (see " 'Safe' Duration of Total Circulatory Arrest"). This is sufficient for most repairs but, in more complex situations, the repair is planned so that the most difficult portions are accomplished during a 45-minute arrest period. A few minutes are then spent in cannulating both cavae from within the opened right atrium and connecting these lines by a Y connector to the venous pump line. CPB is then commenced with the temperature at 10°C, flushing blood initially from the arterial line through the frustrated aortic valve and then releasing the aortic clamp. The aortic clamp is reapplied proximal (upstream) to the arterial cannulae after the myocardium has been perfused for about 5 minutes at this temperature and the temperature is stabilized at 15°C at a lower perfusion flow rate (approximately 50 ml · kg^{-1} · min^{-1}).

Associated Patent Ductus Arteriosus

Regardless of its size, patent ductus arteriosus can be closed without difficulty from the anterior approach. The low blood pressure at the end of surface cooling makes exposure simple, and, if necessary, the caval snares can be tightened to empty the heart completely while the ductus is dissected and ligated. Ligation only has been practiced in these infants using the anterior approach, but two ligatures are required when the ductus is large.

Reoperations

The heart is more irritable at low temperature, and while no important arrhythmia has occurred before opening the chest even at a temperature as low as 20°C, ventricular fibrillation does occur occasionally with manipulation of the heart. Accordingly, when pericardial adhesions are expected, the chest is opened at about 27°C rather than 24°C and cooling subsequently completed by a longer period of cooling CPB.

Cardiopulmonary Bypass Prime

To prime the infant circuit, 850 ml of blood are required. Fresh heparinized blood is used, obtained on the morning of operation. Each unit contains 50 ml of 5% dextrose as diluent and has a hemoglobin content of approximately 13 g · dl^{-1}.[C9] The hemoglobin is further lowered to 11 by adding an appropriate amount of 4.3% dextrose solution in 0.18% sodium chloride (assuming that the infant's blood volume is 80 ml · kg^{-1}). Citrated blood is avoided, in part because it increases the sodium load (both from the citrate itself and the additional bicarbonate necessary to reconstitute the blood and return the pH to near normal), a factor that could be detrimental in neonates, many of whom present for surgery with severe congestive heart failure.

It is relevant to note that the prime provides a considerable glucose load, which has a diuretic effect.

Potassium and Base

The amounts of potassium chloride and sodium bicarbonate added to the machine prime before cooling perfusion and again before rewarming perfusion are empirical and should, strictly speaking, be varied depending on the infant's weight. The metabolic data would also suggest that rather more base could be added during rewarming (Fig. 2-25) to correct the acid shift. However, the rapid correction of acidosis with resumption of a natural circulation at the end of rewarming perfusion indicates that additional base is seldom necessary, and it is deliberately kept to a minimum to reduce the sodium load.

Flow Rates

Rates of 100 ml/kg/min are used during both cooling and rewarming perfusion. At the low temperature already prevailing when the short period of cooling perfusion is begun, this flow is considered adequate; and during rewarming perfusion, the pump flow is deliberately kept below the expected cardiac output to allow the contracting heart to contribute a pulsatile arterial flow.

Carbon Dioxide Gas Concentration

Carbon dioxide is no longer added to the ventilatory mixture for the patient at temperatures below 30°C, for the aim is to

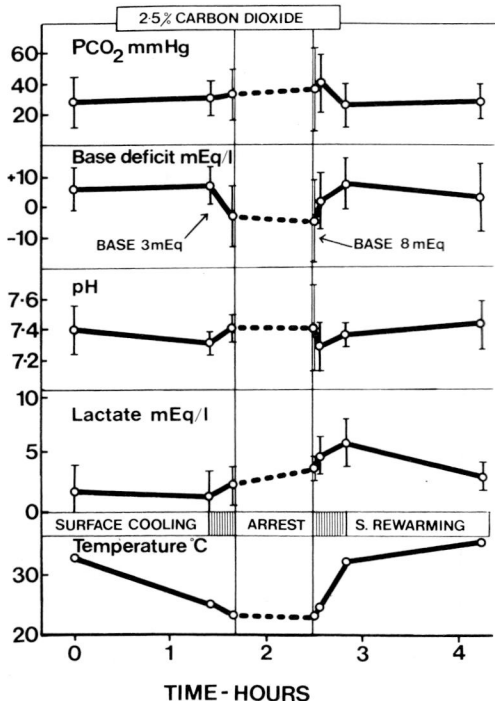

Figure 2-25 Metabolic accompaniments of profound hypothermia in infancy (mean ± 2 SD). Note the appearance of lactic acid during the period of arrest and then its accentuation during washout at the time of reperfusion and rewarming. Corresponding changes in base deficit and pH are noted.
Reproduced with permission from Barratt-Boyes.[B20]

keep the $PaCO_2$ at about 30 mmHg (see "Arterial Carbon Dioxide Pressure" in section on Externally Controlled Variables). It could be argued that higher levels are desirable to raise the $PaCO_2$ toward 70 mmHg, a level that has been shown to improve cerebral blood flow,[L5] but the lower pH

that would then result is probably disadvantageous at low temperatures.[H5]

Cooling and Rewarming Techniques and Duration of Bypass

A water bed, when compared with the less efficient water blanket used previously,[B9] has almost doubled the rate of surface cooling. It is possible with this technique to surface cool rapidly to low temperatures, particularly as efficient cooling continues after the ice bags have been removed, and the heart is being exposed. In contrast to earlier reports[B5,B9] ice bags are not now removed, and the thoracotomy not begun until at least 24°C is reached. By the time the heart has been cannulated the temperature will have fallen to about 21°C. Similarly, the rewarming period is more efficient as the water bed (at 40°C) contributes during core rewarming and after perfusion has been stopped, until the skin incision is closed. For these reasons rewarming perfusion is now continued only until the temperature has reached 35°C.

These factors have reduced the total operating time to approximately 4 hours in 4-kg infants. They have also reduced CPB time to a minimum, namely about 5 minutes for cooling perfusion and 30 minutes for rewarming perfusion.

Positioning of Arterial Cannula

The danger of entrapment of air in the left heart after the repair has been completed and as CPB is being discontinued is well recognized. Also, as previously noted, air may enter the ascending aorta through the arterial cannulation site during circulatory arrest because the vascular bed is largely exsanguinated and the purse-string stitch may not be airtight. Positioning of the aortic cross-clamp distal (downstream) to the arterial cannulation site throughout the arrest period prevents air from reaching the cerebral vessels and also allows easy aspiration, through the arterial line connector, of the blood used to flush air from the left ventricle.

APPENDIX

APPENDIX **2A**

EQUATIONS

The equation derived from the data in Figure 2-1 is

$$\log_{10}\dot{V}_{O_2} = -.69 \pm .061 + .043 \pm .0021 \cdot temperature$$ **(2A-1)**

where P for intercept and slope $< .0001$, SD of regression $= .12$, and $r^2 = .80$.

Correlation (r^2) of the data in Figure 2-2a to a linear model[S17] was .39; to a log-log model,[H4] .54; to Arrhenius'[P8] equation (log $\dot{V}_{O_2}$ proportional to 1/flow), .52; and to a hyperbolic model, .69. The equation for Figure 2-2 is

$$1/\dot{V}_{O_2} = .0062 \pm .00024 + .0044 \pm .00020/flow$$ **(2A-2)**

where $\dot{V}_{O_2}$ is oxygen consumption ($ml \cdot min^{-1} \cdot m^{-2}$) at 37°C; flow is perfusion flow rate ($l \cdot min^{-1} \cdot m^{-2}$) during CPB; P for intercept and slope $< .0001$; SD of regression $= .0024$; and $r^2 = .69$.

The equation represented by the nomogram in Figure 2-3 is

$$1/\dot{V}_{O_2} = .168 \cdot 10^{-.0387 \cdot T} + .0378 \cdot \dot{Q}^{-1} \cdot 10^{-.0253 \cdot T}$$ **(2A-3)**

This was derived as follows. The relationship between $\dot{V}_{O_2}$ and $\dot{Q}$ at 37°C was established from published animal experimental data (Fig. 2-2 and equation 2A-2). Fox and colleagues at UAB[F5] established these relationships at 20°C in humans during CPB. The equation is

$$1/\dot{V}_{O_2} = .0284 + .0118 \cdot \dot{Q}^{-1}$$ **(2A-4)**

In mating these for the curves at intermediate temperatures, the first coefficient in equation 2A-3 (relating to maximum oxygen consumption at limit less flow) followed Q_{10}, which happened to be 2.4. The second coefficient (relating flow slope change to temperature) followed a Q_{10} of 1.8. Both the experimental data at 37°C and the data of Fox and colleagues at 20°C are described by equation 2A-3.

The logistic equation for Figure 2-5 is

$$Z = -7.3 \pm 1.56 + .08 \pm .026 \cdot TCA \qquad (2A\text{-}5)$$

where TCA is total circulatory arrest time (minutes), P for intercept $< .0001$, and P for TCA $= .002$. Also, among the 211 patients without such events, total circulatory arrest time was 42 ± 14.0 (SD) minutes, compared to 59 ± 10.2 for the eight patients with such events ($P = .0008$).

REFERENCES

A

1. Andersen MN, Senning A: Studies in oxygen consumption during extracorporeal circulation with a pump-oxygenator. *Ann Surg* 148:59, 1958.
2. Ames A III, Wright RL, Kowada M, Thurston JM, Majno G: Cerebral ischemia. II. The no-reflow phenomenon. *Am J Pathol* 52:437, 1968.
3. Almond CH, Jones JC, Snyder HM, Grant SM, Meyer BW: Cooling gradients and brain damage with deep hypothermia. *J Thorac Cardiovasc Surg* 48:890, 1964.
4. Alivisatos CN, Filippakis M: Quelques données expérimentales sur l'arrêt provisoire de la circulation afférente du foie. *J Chir* (Paris) 101:191, 1971.
5. Andreasen AT, Watson F: Experimental cardiovascular surgery: 'The azygos factor.' *Br J Surg* 39:548, 1952.
6. Addonizio VP Jr, Strauss JF III, Colman RW, Edmunds LH Jr: Effects of prostaglandin E_1 on platelet loss during in vivo and in vitro extracorporeal circulation with a bubble oxygenator. *J Thorac Cardiovasc Surg* 77:119, 1979.
7. Addonizio VP Jr, Macarak EJ, Nicolaou KC, Edmunds LH, Colman RW: Effects of prostacyclin and albumin on platelet loss during in vitro simulation of extracorporeal circulation. *J Am Soc Hema* 53:1033, 1979.
8. Addonizio VP Jr, Smith JB, Strauss JF III, Colman RW, Edmunds LH Jr: Thromboxane synthesis and platelet secretion during cardiopulmonary bypass with bubble oxygenator. *J Thorac Cardiovasc Surg* 79:91, 1980.
9. Addonizio VP Jr, Macarak EJ, Niewiarowski S, Colman RW, Edmunds LH Jr: Preservation of human platelets with prostaglandin E_1 during in vitro simulation of cardiopulmonary bypass. *Circ Res* 44:350, 1979.
10. Addonizio VP Jr, Strauss JF III, Macarak EJ, Colman RW, Edmunds LH Jr: Preservation of platelet number and function with prostaglandin E_1 during total cardiopulmonary bypass in rhesus monkeys. *Surgery* 83:619, 1978.
11. Aljama P, Bird PAE, Ward MK, Feest TG, Walker W, Tanboga H, Sussman M, Kerr DNS: Haemodialysis-induced leucopenia and activation of complement: Effects of different membranes. *Proc Eur Dial Trans Nephrol* 15:144, 1978.
12. Alon L, Turina M, Gattiker R: Membrane and bubble oxygenator: A clinical comparison in patients undergoing aorto-coronary bypass procedures. *Herz* 4:56, 1979.
13. Aberg T, Ahlund P, Kihlgren M: Intellectual function late after open-heart operation. *Ann Thorac Surg* 36:680, 1983.

B

1. Bigelow WG, Lindsay WK, Greenwood WF: Hypothermia—its possible role in cardiac surgery: An investigation of factors governing survival in dogs at low body temperatures. *Ann Surg* 132:849, 1950.
2. Bigelow WG, Lindsay WK, Harrison RC, Gordon RA, Greenwood WF: Oxygen transport and utilization in dogs at low body temperatures. *Am J Physiol* 160:125, 1950.
3. Boerema I, Wildschut A, Schmidt WJH, Broekhuysen L: Experimental researches into hypothermia as an aid in the surgery of the heart. *Archivum Chirurgicum Neerlandicum* 3:25, 1951.
4. Bigelow WG, Callaghan JC, Hopps JA: General hypothermia for experimental intracardiac surgery. *Ann Surg* 132:531, 1950.
5. Barratt-Boyes BG, Simpson MM, Neutze JM: Intracardiac surgery in neonates and infants using deep hypothermia. *Circulation* 61,62(suppl III):III-73, 1970.
6. Burton AC: Human calorimetry. II. The average temperature of the tissues of the body. *J Nutr* 9:261, 1935.
7. Brunberg JA, Reilly EL, Doty DB: Central nervous system consequences in infants of cardiac surgery using deep hypothermia and circulatory arrest. *Circulation* 49,50(suppl II):II-11, 1973.
8. Bergouignan M, Fontan F, Trarieux M, Julien J: Syndromes choreiformes de l'enfant au décours d'interventions cardio-chirurgicales sous hypothermie profonde. *Rev Neurol* (Paris) 105:48, 1961.
9. Barratt-Boyes BG, Neutze JM, Clarkson P, Shardey GC, Brandt PWT: Repair of ventricular septal defect in the first two years of life using profound hypothermic-circulatory arrest techniques. *Ann Surg* 184:376, 1976.
10. Belsey RHR, Keen G, Skinner DB: Profound hypothermia in cardiac surgery. *J Thorac Cardiovasc Surg* 56:497, 1968.
11. Bernhard WF, McMurrey JD, Curtis GW: Feasibility of partial hepatic resection under hypothermia. *N Engl J Med* 253:159, 1955.
12. Bjork VO: Brain perfusions in dogs with artificially oxygenated blood. *Acta Chir Scand* 96(suppl):137, 1948.
13. Brown IW, Smith WW, Emmons WO: An efficient blood heat exchanger for use with extracorporeal circulation. *Surgery* 44:372, 1958.
14. Bharadwaj BB, Chong G: Effects of extracorporeal circulation on structure, function, and population distribution of canine blood platelets. Presented at the Combined Meeting of the Royal Australasian College of Surgeons and Royal Australasian College of Physicians, Sydney, Australia, February 24–29, 1980.
15. Backmann F, McKenna R, Cole ER, Najafi H: The hemostatic mechanism after open-heart surgery. I. Studies on plasma coagulation factors and fibrinolysis in 512 patients after extracorporeal circulation. *J Thorac Cardiovasc Surg* 70:76, 1975.
16. Birek A, Duffin J, Glynn MFX, Cooper JD: The effect of sulfinpyrazone on platelet and pulmonary responses to onset of membrane oxygenator perfusion. *Trans Am Soc Artif Intern Organs* 22:94, 1976.
17. Boucher JK, Rudy LM, Edmunds LH: Organ blood flow during cardiopulmonary bypass. *J Appl Physiol* 36:86, 1974.
18. Bixler TJ, Magee PG, Flaherty JT, Gardner TJ, Gott VL:

Beneficial effects of pulsatile perfusion in the hypertrophied ventricle during ventricular fibrillation. *Circulation* 60:1, 1979.

19. Ballinger WF II, Wollenweider H, Templeton JU III, Pierucci L Jr: Acidosis of hypothermia. *Ann Surg* 154:517, 1961.

20. Barratt-Boyes BG: The technique of intracardiac repair in infancy using deep hypothermia with circulatory arrest and limited cardiopulmonary bypass, in MI Ionescu, GH Wooler (eds): *Current Techniques in Extracorporeal Circulation.* London: Butterworth, 1976, pp 197–228.

21. Baue AE, Nusbaum M, Anstadt G, Blakemore WS: The pattern of lymphatic flow during extracorporeal circulation. *J Thorac Cardiovasc Surg* 50:648, 1965.

22. Breckenridge IM, Digerness SB, Kirklin JW: Validity of concept of increased extracellular fluid after open heart surgery. *Surgical Forum* 20:169, 1969.

23. Bennett EV Jr, Fewel JF, Ybarra J, Grover FL, Trinkle JK: Comparison of flow differences among venous cannulas. *Ann Thorac Surg* 36:59, 1983.

C

1. Civalero LA, Moreno JR, Senning A: Temperature conditions and oxygen consumption during deep hypothermia. *Acta Chir Scand* 123:179, 1962.

2. Cheng H-C, Kusunoki T, Bosher LH Jr, McElvein RB, Blake DA: A study of oxygen consumption during extracorporeal circulation. *Trans Am Soc Artif Intern Organs* 5:273, 1959.

3. Cohen ME, Olszowka JS, Subramanian S: Electroencephalographic and neurological correlates of deep hypothermia and circulatory arrest in infants. *Ann Thorac Surg* 23:238, 1977.

4. Clarkson PM, MacArthur BA, Barratt-Boyes BG, Whitlock RM, Neutze JM: Developmental progress following cardiac surgery in infancy using profound hypothermia and circulatory arrest. *Circulation* 62:855, 1980.

5. Chiang J, Kowada MD, Ames A III, Wright RL, Majno G: Cerebral ischemia. III. Vascular changes. *Am J Pathol* 52:455, 1968.

6. Crafoord C, Norberg B, Senning Å: Clinical studies in extracorporeal circulation with a heart-lung machine. *Acta Chir Scand* 112:200, 1957.

7. Cohen M, Lillehei CW: A quantitative study of the 'azygos factor' during vena caval occlusion in the dog. *Surg Gynecol Obstet* 98:255, 1954.

8. Chien S: Present state of blood rheology, in K Messmer and H Schmid-Schonbein (eds): *Hemodilution: Theoretical Basis and Clinical Application.* New York: Karger, Basel, 1972, pp 1–45.

9. Cohn LH, Angell WW, Shumway NE: Body fluid shifts after cardiopulmonary bypass. I. Effects of congestive heart failure and hemodilution. *J Thorac Cardiovasc Surg* 62:423, 1971.

10. Chenoweth DE, Cooper SW, Hugli TE, Stewart RW, Blackstone EH, Kirklin JW: Complement activation during cardiopulmonary bypass: Evidence for generation of C3a and C5a anaphylatoxins. *N Engl J Med* 304:497, 1981.

11. Craddock PR, Fehr J, Dalmasso AP, Brigham KL, Jacob HS: Pulmonary vascular leukostasis resulting from complement activation by dialyzer cellophane membranes. *J Clin Invest* 59:879, 1977.

12. Craddock PR, Fehr J, Brigham KL, Kronenberg RS, Jacob HS: Complement and leukocyte-mediated pulmonary dysfunction in hemodialysis. *N Engl J Med* 296:769, 1977.

13. Clark RE, Beauchamp RA, Magrath RA, Brooks JD, Ferguson TB, Weldon CS: Comparison of bubble and membrane oxygenators in short and long perfusions. *J Thorac Cardiovasc Surg* 78:655, 1979.

14. Chen RYZ, Wicks AE, Chien S: Hemoconcentration induced by surface hypothermia in infants. *J Thorac Cardiovasc Surg* 80:236, 1980.

15. Clark RE, Dietz DR, Miller JG: Continuous detection of microemboli during cardiopulmonary bypass in animals and man. *Circulation* 54(suppl III):III-74, 1976.

16. Clowes GHA Jr, Neville WE, Sabga G, Shibota Y: The relationship of oxygen consumption, perfusion rate, and temperature to the acidosis associated with cardiopulmonary circulatory bypass. *Surgery* 44:220, 1958.

17. Cordell AR, Spencer MP, Meredith JH: Studies of peripheral vascular resistance associated with total cardiopulmonary bypass. I. Peripheral resistance under conditions of normothermia and normotension. *J Thorac Cardiovasc Surg* 40:421, 1960.

18. Cleland J, Pluth JR, Tauxe WN, Kirklin JW: Blood volume and body fluid compartment changes soon after closed and open intracardiac surgery. *J Thorac Cardiovasc Surg* 52:698, 1966.

19. Chiu RC, Samson R: Complement (C3,C4) consumption in cardiopulmonary byass, cardioplegia, and protamine administration. *Ann Thorac Surg* 37:229, 1984.

D

1. Drew CE, Keen G, Benazon DB: Profound hypothermia. *Lancet* I:745, 1959.

2. Dillard DH, Mohri H, Hessel EA II, Anderson HN, Nelson RJ, Crawford EW, Morgan BC, Winterscheid LC, Merendino KA: Correction of total anomalous pulmonary venous drainage in infancy utilizing deep hypothermia with total circulatory arrest. *Circulation* 35,36(suppl I):I-105, 1967.

3. Donald DE, Kerr FWL: The response of dogs to perfusion and arrest of circulation at near zero cerebral temperatures. *J Surg Res* 4:243, 1964.

4. Dickinson DF, Sambrooks JE: Intellectual performance in children after circulatory arrest with profound hypothermia in infancy. *Arch Dis Child* 54:1, 1979.

5. Dennis C, Spreng DS Jr, Nelson GE, Karlson KE, Nelson RM, Thomas JV, Eder WP, Varco RL: Development of a pump-oxygenator to replace the heart and lungs: An apparatus applicable to human patients and application to one case. *Ann Surg* 134:709, 1951.

6. Donald DE, Harshbarger HG, Hetzel PS, Patrick RT, Wood EH, Kirklin JW: Experiences with a heart-lung bypass (Gibbon type) in the experimental laboratory: Preliminary report. *Proc Staff Meet Mayo Clin* 30:113, 1955.

7. Diesh G, Flynn PJ, Marable SA, Mulder DG, Schmutzer KJ, Longmire WP Jr, Maloney JV Jr: Comparison of low (azygos) flow and high flow principles of extracorporeal circulation employing a bubble oxygenator. *Surgery* 42:67, 1957.

8. DeBakey MD: Simple continuous flow blood transfusion instrument. *New Orleans Med Surg J* 87:386, 1934.

9. Davis FM, Parinelazhagan KN, Harris EA: Thermal balance during cardiopulmonary bypass with hypothermia in man. *Br J Anaesth* 49:1127, 1977.

10. Davies GC, Sobel M, Salzman EW: Elevated plasma fibrinopeptide A and thromboxane B_2 levels during cardiopulmonary bypass. *Circulation* 61:808, 1980.

11. DeVenuto F, Friedman HI, Neville JR, Peck CC: Appraisal of hemoglobin solution as a blood substitute. *Surg Gynecol Obstet* 149:417, 1979.

12. Dunn J, Kirsh MM, Harness J, Carroll H, Straker J, Sloan H:

Hemodynamic, metabolic, and hematologic effects of cardiopulmonary bypass. *J Thorac Cardiovasc Surg* 68:138, 1974.

13. Davis FM: Radial artery cannulation: Influence of catheter size and material on arterial occlusion. *Anaesth Intens Care* 6:49, 1978.

14. Donald DE, Fellows JL: Relation of temperature, gas tension and hydrostatic pressure to the formation of gas bubbles in extracorporeally oxygenated blood. *Surgical Forum* 10:589, 1959.

15. D'Amato HE, Hegnauer H: Blood volume in hypothermic dogs. *Am J Physiol* 173:703, 1963.

E

1. Egerton N, Egerton WS, Kay JH: Neurologic changes following profound hypothermia. *Ann Surg* 157:366, 1963.

2. Edmunds LH Jr, Saxena NC, Hillyer P, Wilson TJ: Relationship between platelet count and cardiotomy suction return. *Ann Thorac Surg* 25:306, 1978.

3. Ellison N, Behar M, MacVaugh H III, Marshall BE: Bradykinin, plasma protein fraction and hypotension. *Ann Thorac Surg* 29:15, 1980.

4. Ennema JJ, Mook PH, Elstrodt JM, Wildevuur RH: A new hollow fiber membrane oxygenator with an integral heat exchanger: A hematological evaluation in dogs. *Thorac Cardiovasc Surg* 31:359, 1983.

F

1. Fuhrman GJ, Fuhrman FA: Oxygen consumption of animals and tissues as a function of temperature. *J Gen Physiol* 42:715, 1959.

2. Fuhrman FA: Oxygen consumption of mammalian tissues at reduced temperatures, in RD Dripps (ed): *The Physiology of Induced Hypothermia*. Washington, DC: National Academy of Sciences, National Research Council, 1956, pp 50–51.

3. Field J II, Belding HS, Martin AW: An analysis of the relation between basal metabolism and summated tissue respiration in the rat. I. The post-pubertal albino rat. *J Cellular Comparative Physiol* 14:143, 1939.

4. Fuhrman FA, Fuhrman GJ, Farr DA, Fail JH: Relationship between tissue respiration and total metabolic rate in hypo and normothermic rats. *Am J Physiol* 201:231, 1961.

5. Fox LS, Blackstone EH, Kirklin JW, Stewart RW, Samuelson P: Relationship of whole body oxygen consumption to perfusion flow rate during hypothermic cardiopulmonary bypass. *J Thorac Cardiovasc Surg* 83:239, 1982.

6. Folkerth TL, Angell WW, Fosburg RG, Oury JH: Effect of deep hypothermia, limited cardiopulmonary bypass, and total arrest on growing puppies, in *Recent Advances in Studies on Cardiac Structure and Metabolism,* vol 10. Baltimore: University Park, 1975, pp 411–421.

7. Fisk GC, Wright JS, Turner BB, Baker DeC, Hicks RG, Lethlean AK, Stacey RB, Lawrence JC, Lawrie GM, Kalnins I, Rose M: Cerebral effects of circulatory arrest at 20°C in the infant pig. *Anaesth Intens Care* 2:33, 1974.

8. Fisk GC, Wright JS, Hicks RG, Anderson RM, Turner BB, Baker W, Lawrence JC, Stacey RB, Lawrie GM, Kalnins I, Rose M: The influence of duration of circulatory arrest at 20°C on cerebral changes. *Anaesth Intens Care* 4:126, 1976.

9. Frey MV, Gruber M: Untersuchungen über den Stoffwechsel isolierter Organe: Ein Respirations-Apparat für isolierte Organe. *Arch F Physiol* 9:519, 1885.

10. Friedenberg WR, Myers WO, Plotka ED, Beathard JN, Kummer DJ, Gatlin PF, Stoiber DL, Ray JF III, Sautter RD: Platelet

dysfunction associated with cardiopulmonary bypass. *Ann Thorac Surg* 25:298, 1978.

11. Feijen J: Thrombogenesis caused by blood: Foreign surface interaction, in RM Kenedi, JM Courtney, JDS Gaylor, T Gilchrist (eds): *Artificial Organs*. Baltimore: University Park, 1977, pp 235–247.

12. Fountain SW, Martin BA, Musclow CE, Cooper JD: Pulmonary leukostasis and its relationship to pulmonary dysfunction in sheep and rabbits. *Circ Res* 46:175, 1980.

13. Friedli B, Kent G, Olley PM: Inactivation of bradykinin in the pulmonary vascular bed of newborn and fetal lambs. *Circ Res* 33:421, 1973.

14. Fox LS, Blackstone EH, Kirklin JW, Bishop SP, Bradley EL: Relationship of brain blood flow and oxygen consumption to perfusion flow rate during hypothermic cardiopulmonary bypass. *J Thorac Cardiovasc Surg* 87:658, 1984.

G

1. Guiot G, Rougerie J, Dubost C, Blondeau P: Le 'grand froid' en neurochirurgie: Possibilités et perspectives d'avenir. *Neurochirurgie* 6:332, 1960.

2. Ginsberg MD, Myers RE: The topography of impaired microvascular perfusion in the primate brain following total circulatory arrest. *Neurology* 22:998, 1972.

3. Gowing NFC, Dexter D: The effects of temporary renal ischemia in normal and hypothermic rats. *J Pathol Bact* 72:519, 1956.

4. Gibbon JH Jr: The maintenance of life during experimental occlusion of the pulmonary artery followed by survival. *Surg Gynecol Obstet* 69:602, 1939.

5. Gibbon JH Jr: Application of a mechanical heart and lung apparatus to cardiac surgery, in *Recent Advances in Cardiovascular Physiology and Surgery*. Minneapolis: University of Minnesota, 1953, pp 107–113.

6. Gibbon JH Jr: (1954) Personal communication.

7. Grant JA, Dupree E, Goldman AS, Schultz DR, Jackson AL: Complement-mediated release of histamine from human leukocytes. *J Immunol* 114:1101, 1975.

8. Goldstein IM, Brai M, Osler AG, Weissmann G: Lysosomal enzyme release from human leukocytes: Mediation by the alternate pathway of complement activation. *J Immunol* 111:33, 1973.

9. Giron F, Birtwell WC, Soroff HS, Deterling RA: Hemodynamic effects of pulsatile and nonpulsatile flow. *Arch Surg* 93:802, 1966.

10. German JC, Chalmers GS, Hirai J, Mukherjee ND, Wakabayashi A, Connolly JE: Comparison of nonpulsatile and pulsatile extracorporeal circulation on renal tissue perfusion. *Chest* 61:65, 1972.

11. Gall WE, Clarke WR, Doty DB: Vasomotor dynamics associated with cardiac operations. I. Venous tone and the effects of vasodilators. *J Thorac Cardiovasc Surg* 83:724, 1982.

12. Govier AV, Reves JG, McKay RD, Karp RB, Zorn GL, Morawetz RB, Smith LR, Adams M, Freeman AM: Factors and their influence on regional cerebral blood flow during nonpulsatile cardiopulmonary bypass. *Ann Thorac Surg* 38:592, 1984.

H

1. Horiuchi T, Koyamada K, Matano I, Mohri H, Komatsu T, Honda T, Abe T, Ishitoya T, Sagawa Y, Matsuzawa K, Matsumura M, Tsuda T, Ishizawa E, Ishikawa S, Suzuki H, Saito Y:

Radical operation for ventricular septal defect in infancy. *J Thorac Cardiovasc Surg* 46:180, 1963.

2. Hikasa Y, Shirotani H, Satomura K, Muraoka R, Abe K, Tsushimi K, Yokota Y, Miki S, Kawai J, Mori A, Okamoto Y, Koie H. Ban T, Kanzaki Y, Yokata M: Open heart surgery in infants with the aid of hypothermic anesthesia. *Archiv Japan Chirurgie* 36:495, 1967.

3. Hamilton DI, Shackleton J, Rees GJ, Abbott T: Experience with deep hypothermia in infancy using core cooling, in BG Barratt-Boyes, JM Neutze, and EA Harris (eds): *Heart Disease in Infancy*. Baltimore: Williams & Wilkins, 1973, pp 52–64.

4. Harris EA, Seelye ER, Squire AW: Oxygen consumption during cardiopulmonary bypass with moderate hypothermia in man. *Br J Anaesth* 43:1113, 1971.

5. Harris EA: Metabolic aspects of profound hypothermia, in BG Barratt-Boyes, JM Neutze, and EA Harris (eds): *Heart Disease in Infancy*. Baltimore: Williams & Wilkins, 1973, p 65.

6. Harris EA, Seelye ER, Barratt-Boyes BG: Respiratory and metabolic acid-base changes during cardiopulmonary bypass in man. *Br J Anesth* 42:912, 1970.

7. Harden A, Pampiglione G, Waterston DJ: Circulatory arrest during hypothermia in cardiac surgery: An EEG study in children. *Br Med J* 2:1105, 1966.

8. Hallenbeck JM, Bradley ME: Experimental model for systematic study of impaired microvascular reperfusion. *Stroke* 8:23, 1977.

9. Hallenbeck JM: Prevention of postischemic impairment of microvascular perfusion. *Neurology* (Minneapolis) 27:3, 1977.

10. Haka-Ikse K, Blackwood MJA, Steward DJ: Psychomotor development of infants and children after profound hypothermia during surgery for congenital heart disease. *Dev Med Child Neurol* 20:62, 1978.

11. Huguet C, Nordlinger B, Bloch P, Conard J: Tolerance of the human liver to prolonged normothermic ischemia. *Arch Surg* 113:1448, 1978.

12. Harris EA, Seelye ER, Barratt-Boyes BG: On the availability of oxygen to the body during cardiopulmonary bypass in man. *Br J Anesth* 46:425, 1974.

13. Hallowell P, Austen WG, Laver MB: Influence of oxygen flow rate on arterial oxygenation and acid-base balance during cardiopulmonary bypass with use of a disc oxygenator. *Circulation* 35:119, 1967.

14. Hine IP, Wood WG, Mainwaring-Buton RW, Butler MJ, Irving MH, Booker B: The adrenergic response to surgery involving cardiopulmonary bypass, as measured by plasma and urinary catecholamine concentrations. *Br J Anaesth* 48:355, 1976.

15. Han P, Turpie AGG, Butt R, LeBlanc P, Genton E, Gunstensen S: The use of β-thromboglobulin release to assess platelet damage during cardiopulmonary bypass. Presented at the Combined Meeting of the Royal Australasian College of Surgeons and Royal Australasian College of Physicians, Sydney, Australia, February 24–29, 1980.

16. Hugli T: Chemical aspects of the serum anaphylatoxins. *Contemporary Topics in Molecular Immunology* 7:181, 1978.

17. Hairston P, Manos JP, Graber CD, Lee WH Jr: Depression of immunologic surveillance by pump-oxygenator perfusion. *J Surg Res* 9:587, 1969.

18. Habal SM, Weiss MB, Spotnitz HM, Parodi EN, Wolff M, Cannon PJ, Hoffman BF, Malm JR: Effects of pulsatile and nonpulsatile coronary perfusion on performance of the canine left ventricle. *J Thorac Cardiovasc Surg* 72:742, 1976.

19. Holobut W, Modrzejewski E, Stazka W: Irrigation sanguine et consommation d'oxygène de divers organes en température normale et en hypothermie. *J Physiol* (Paris) 61:507, 1969.

20. Hammerschmidt DE, White JG, Craddock PR, Jacob HS: Corticosteroids inhibit complement-induced granulocyte aggregation: A possible mechanism for their efficacy in shock states. *J Clin Invest* 63:798, 1979.

21. Hammerschmidt DE, Stroncek DF, Bowers TK, Lammi-Keefe CJ, Kurth DM, Ozalins A, Nicoloff DM, Lillehei RC, Craddock PR, Jacob HS: Complement activation and neutropenia occurring during cardiopulmonary bypass. *J Thorac Cardiovasc Surg* 81:370, 1981.

22. Harker LA, Malpass TW, Branson HE, Hessel EA II, Slichter SJ: Mechanisms of abnormal bleeding in patients undergoing cardiopulmonary bypass: Acquired transient platelet dysfunction associated with selective alpha-granule release. *Blood* 56:824, 1980.

23. Harlan BJ, Kyger ER III, Reul GJ Jr, Cooley DA: Needle suction of the aorta for left heart decompression during aortic cross-clamping. *Ann Thorac Surg* 23:259, 1977.

24. Hope AF, Heyns AduP, Lotter MG, van Reenen OR, de Kock F, Badenhorst PN, Pieters H, Kotze H, Meyer JM, Minnaar PC: Kinetics and sites of sequestration of indium 111-labeled human platelets during cardiopulmonary bypass. *J Thorac Cardiovasc Surg* 81:880, 1981.

J

1. Jones RE, Donald DE, Swan HJC, Harshbarger HG, Kirklin JW, Wood EH: Apparatus of the Gibbon type for mechanical bypass of the heart and lungs: Preliminary report. *Proc Staff Meet Mayo Clin* 30:105, 1955.

2. Jorgensen L, Hovig T, Towsell HC, Mustard JF: Adenosine diphosphate-induced platelet aggregation and vascular injury in swine and rabbit. *Am J Pathol* 61:161, 1970.

3. Jacobs LA, Klopp EH, Seamone W, Topaz SR, Gott VL: Improved organ function during cardiac bypass with a roller pump modified to deliver pulsatile flow. *J Thorac Cardiovasc Surg* 58:703, 1969.

4. Jynge P, Hearse DJ, Braimbridge MV: Myocardial protection during ischemic cardiac arrest. *J Thorac Cardiovasc Surg* 73:848, 1977.

5. Jacob HS, Craddock PR, Hammerschmidt DE, Moldow CF: Complement-induced granulocyte aggregation: An unsuspected mechanism of disease. *N Engl J Med* 302:789, 1980.

K

1. Kirklin JW, Dawson B, Devloo RA, Theye RA: Open intracardiac operations: Use of circulatory arrest during hypothermia induced by blood cooling. *Ann Surg* 154:769, 1961.

2. Kent B, Peirce EC II: Oxygen consumption during cardiopulmonary bypass in the uniformly cooled dog. *J Appl Physiol* 37:917, 1974.

3. Kramer RS, Sanders AP, Lesage AM, Woodhall B, Sealy WC: The effect of profound hypothermia on preservation of cerebral ATP content during circulatory arrest. *J Thorac Cardiovasc Surg* 56:699, 1968.

4. Kirklin JW, DuShane JW, Patrick RT, Donald DE, Hetzel PS, Harshbarger HG, Wood EH: Intracardiac surgery with the aid of a mechanical pump-oxygenator system (Gibbon type): Report of eight cases. *Proc Staff Meet Mayo Clin* 30:201, 1955.

5. Kirklin JW, Theye RA: Whole-body perfusion from a pump oxygenator for open intracardiac surgery, in JH Gibbon Jr (ed):

Surgery of the Chest. Philadelphia: WB Saunders, 1962, pp 694–707.

6. Kalter RD, Saul CM, Wetstein L, Soriano C, Reiss RF: Cardiopulmonary bypass: Associated hemostatic abnormalities. *J Thorac Cardiovasc Surg* 77:428, 1979.

7. Kusserow B, Larrow R, Nichols J: Perfusion- and surface-induced injury in leukocytes. *Fed Proc* 30:1516, 1971.

8. Kusserow BK, Machanic B, Collins FM Jr, Clapp JF III: Changes observed in blood corpuscles after prolonged perfusions with two types of blood pumps. *Trans Am Soc Artif Intern Organs* 11:122, 1965.

9. Kirklin JW: A letter to Helen. *J Thorac Cardiovasc Surg* 78:643, 1979.

10. Kirklin JK, Westaby S, Blackstone EH, Kirklin JW, Chenowith DE, Pacifico AD: Complement and the damaging effects of cardiopulmonary bypass. *J Thorac Cardiovasc Surg* 86:845, 1983.

11. Kirklin JK, Chenoweth DE, Naftel DC, Blackstone EH, Kirklin JW, Bitran DD, Curd JG, Reves JG, Samuelson PN: Effects of protamine administration after cardiopulmonary bypass on complement, blood elements, and the hemodynamic state. Annals of Thoracic Surgery (in press).

L

1. Lewis FS, Taufic M: Closure of atrial septal defects wih the air of hypothermia: Experimental accomplishments and the report of one successful case. *Surgery* 33:52, 1953.

2. Levin MB, Theye RA, Fowler WS, Kirklin JW: Performance of the stationary vertical-screen oxygenator (Mayo-Gibbon). *J Thorac Cardiovasc Surg* 39:417, 1960.

3. Lee WH Jr, Krumbhoar D, Fonkalsrud EW, Schjeide OA, Maloney JV Jr: Denaturation of plasma proteins as a cause of morbidity and death after intracardiac operations. *Surgery* 50:29, 1961.

4. Lambert CJ, Marengo-Rowe AJ, Leveson JE, Green RH, Theile JP, Geisler GF, Adam M, Mitchel BG: The treatment of postperfusion bleeding using epsilon-aminocaproic acid, cryoprecipitate, fresh-frozen plasma, and protamine sulfate. *Ann Thorac Surg* 28:440, 1979.

5. Larson CP Jr: Anesthesia and control of the cerebral circulation, in EJ Wylie, EK Ehrenfeld (eds): *Extracranial Occlusive Cerebrovascular Disease: Diagnosis and Management.* Philadelphia: WB Saunders, 1970, Chapter 8.

6. Lowenstein E, Johnston WE, Lappas DG, D'Ambra MN, Schneider RC, Daggett WM, Akins CW, Philbin DM: Catastrophic pulmonary vasoconstriction associated with protamine reversal of heparin. *Anesthesiology* 59:470, 1983.

M

1. Martin AW, Fuhrman FA: The relationship between summated tissue respiration and metabolic rate in the mouse and dog. *Physiol Zool* 28:18, 1955.

2. Moffitt EA, Kirklin JW, Theye RA: Physiologic studies during whole-body perfusion in tetralogy of Fallot. *J Thorac Cardiovasc Surg* 44:180, 1962.

3. Messmer BJ, Schallberger U, Gattiker R, Senning Å: Psychomotor and intellectual development after deep hypothermia and circulatory arrest in early infancy. *J Thorac Cardiovasc Surg* 72:495, 1976.

4. Martin RR: Alterations in leukocyte structure and function due to mechanical trauma, in NHC Hwang, DR Gross, DJ Patel (eds): *Quantitative Cardiovascular Studies: Clinical and Re-*

search Applications of Engineering Principles. Baltimore: University Park, 1979, pp 419–454.

5. Mortensen JD: *Evaluation of ASAIO Blood Damage Test,* vol 1. Salt Lake City, Utah: Utah Biomedical Test Laboratory, University of Utah Research Institute: 1977.

6. Monti R: Extracorporeal Oxygenators, in NHC Hwang, DR Gross, DJ Patel (eds): *Quantitative Cardiovascular Studies: Clinical and Research Applications of Engineering Principles.* Baltimore: University Park, 1979, pp 593–617.

7. Many M, Soroff HS, Birtwell WC, Giron F, Wise H, Deterling RA: The physiologic role of pulsatile and nonpulsatile flow. II. Effects on renal function. *Arch Surg* 95:762, 1967.

8. Maddoux G, Pappas G, Jenkins M, Battock D, Trow R, Smith SC Jr, Steele P: Effect of pulsatile and nonpulsatile flow during cardiopulmonary bypass on left ventricular ejection fraction early after aortocoronary bypass surgery. *Am J Cardiol* 37: 1000, 1976.

9. Mavroudis C: To pulse or not to pulse. *Ann Thorac Surg* 25:259, 1978.

10. McGoon DC, Moffitt EA, Theye RA, Kirklin JW: Physiologic studies during high flow, normothermic, whole body perfusion. *J Thorac Cardiovasc Surg* 39:275, 1960.

11. Molina JE, Einzig S, Mastri AR, Bianco RW, Marks JA, Rasmussen TM, Clack RM: Brain damage in profound hypothermia: Perfusion versus circulatory arrest. *J Thorac Cardiovasc Surg* 87:596, 1984.

12. Mills NL, Ochsner JL: Massive air embolism during cardiopulmonary bypass. *J Thorac Cardiovasc Surg* 80:708, 1980.

N

1. Norwood WI, Norwood CR, Castaneda AR: Cerebral anoxia: Effect of deep hypothermia and pH. *Surgery* 86:203, 1979.

2. Nagaoka H, Katori M: Inhibition of kinin formation by a kallikrein inhibitor during extracorporeal circulation in open-heart surgery. *Circulation* 52:325, 1975.

3. Nakayama K, Tamiya T, Yamamoto K, Izumi T, Akimoto S, Hashizume S, Iimori T: High-amplitude pulsatile pump in extracoropreal circulation with particular reference to hemodynamics. *Surgery* 54:798, 1963.

4. Nieminen MT, Philbin DM, Rosow CE, Lowenstein E, Triantafillou A, Levine FH, Buckley MJ: Temperature gradients and rewarming time during hypothermic cardiopulmonary bypass with and without pulsatile flow. *Ann Thorac Surg* 35:488, 1983.

5. Nordstrom L, Fletcher R, Pavek K: Shock of anaphylactoid type induced by protamine: A continuous cardiorespiratory record. *Acta Anaesth Scand* 22:195, 1978.

O

1. Olsson Y, Hossmann K-A: The effect of intravascular saline perfusion on the sequelae of transient cerebral ischemia. *Acta Neuropathol* 17:68, 1971.

2. Oh TE, Davis NJ: Radial artery cannulation. *Anaesth Intens Care* 3:12, 1975.

3. Ogata T, Ida Y, Nonoyama A, Takeda J, Sasaki H: A comparative study on the effectiveness of pulsatile and non-pulsatile blood flow in extracorporeal circulation. *Nippon Geka Hokan* 29:59, 1960.

P

1. Penrod KE: Oxygen consumption and cooling rates in immersion hypothermia in the dog. *Am J Physiol* 157:436, 1949.

2. Pappas G, Winter SD, Kopriva CJ, Steele P: Improvement of myocardial and other vital organ functions and metabolism with a simple method of pulsatile flow (IABP) during clinical CPB. *Surgery* 77:34, 1975.

3. Philbin DM, Levine FH, Emerson CW, Buckley MJ, Coggins CH, Moss J, Slater E: The renin-catecholamine vasopressor response to cardiopulmonary bypass with pulsatile flow. *Circulation* (abstr) 59,60:(suppl II):II-34, 1979.

4. Pruitt KM, Stroud RM, Scott JW: Blood damage in the heart-lung machine (35651). *Proc Soc Exp Biol Med* 137:714, 1971.

5. Parker DJ, Cantrell JW, Karp RB, Stroud RM, Digerness SB: Changes in serum complement and immunoglobins following cardiopulmonary bypass. *Surgery* 71:824, 1972.

6. Panossian A, Hagstrom JWC, Nealsen SL, Veith FJ: Secondary nature of surfactant changes in postperfusion pulmonary damage. *J Thorac Cardiovasc Surg* 57:628, 1969.

7. Pang LM, Stalcup SA, Lipset JS, Hayes CJ, Bowman FO Jr, Mellins RB: Increased circulation bradykinin during hypothermia and cardiopulmonary bypass in children. *Circulation* 60:1503, 1979.

8. Paneth M, Sellers R, Gott VL, Weirich WL, Allen P, Read RC, Lillehei CW: Physiologic studies upon prolonged cardiopulmonary bypass with the pump-oxygenator with particular reference to (1) acid-base balance, (2) siphon canal drainage. *J Thorac Surg* 34:570, 1947.

9. Pacifico AD, Digerness S, Kirklin JW: Acute alterations of body composition after open intracardiac operations. *Circulation* 41:331, 1970.

10. Perkowski SZ, Havill AM, Flynn JT, Gee MH: Role of intrapulmonary release of eicosanoids and superoxide anion as mediators of pulmonary dysfunction and endothelial injury in sheep with intermittent complement activation. *Circ Res* 53:574, 1983.

R

1. Ross DN: Hypothermia. II. Physiological observations during hypothermia. *Guy's Hospital Report* 103:116, 1954.

2. Reilly EL, Brunberg JA, Doty DB: The effect of deep hypothermia and total circulatory arrest on electroencephalogram in children. *Clin Neurophysiol* 36:661, 1974.

3. Rittenhouse EA, Mohri H, Reichenbach DD, Merendino KA: Morphological alterations in vital organs after prolonged cardiac arrest at low body temperature. *Ann Thorac Surg* 13:564, 1972.

4. Rudy LW Jr, Heymann MA, and Edmunds H Jr: Distribution of systemic blood flow during cardiopulmonary bypass. *J Appl Physiol* 34:194, 1973.

5. Reeves RB: Temperature induced changes in blood acid-base status: pH and P_{CO_2} in a binary buffer. *J Appl Physiol* 40:752, 1976.

6. Reeves RB: Temperature induced changes in blood acid-base status: Donnan r_{cl} and red cell volume. *J Appl Physiol* 40:762, 1976.

7. Rahn H, Reeves RB, Howell BJ: Hydrogen ion regulation, temperature and evolution. *Am Rev Respir Dis* 112:165, 1975.

8. Rosenthal TB: The effect of temperature on the pH of blood and plasma in vitro. *J Biol Chem* 173:25, 1948.

9. Ryhanen P, Herva E, Hollmen A, Nuutinen L, Pihlajaniemi R, Saarela E: Changes in peripheral blood leukocyte counts, lymphocyte subpopulations, and in vitro transformation after heart valve replacement. *J Thorac Cardiovasc Surg* 77:259, 1979.

10. Rosomoff HL, Holaday DA: Cerebral blood flow and cerebral oxygen consumption during hypothermia. *Am J Physiol* 179:85, 1954.

11. Reed CC, Romagnoli A, Taylor DE, Clark DK: Particulate matter in bubble oxygenators. *J Thorac Cardiovasc Surg* 68:971, 1974.

12. Reid DJ, Digerness S, Kirklin JW: Changes in whole body venous tone and distribution of blood after open intracardiac surgery. *Am J Cardiol* 22:621, 1968.

13. Rosenkranz ER, Utley JR, Menninger FJ III, Dembitsky WP, Hargens AR, Peters RM: Interstitial fluid pressure changes during cardiopulmonary bypass. *Ann Thorac Surg* 30:536, 1980.

14. Reves JG, Karp RB, Buttner EE, Tosone S, Smith LR, Samuelson PN, Kreusch GR, Oparil S: Neuronal and adrenomedullary catecholamine release in response to cardiopulmonary bypass in man. *Circulation* 66:49, 1982.

15. Rogers K, Milne B, Salerno TA: The hemodynamic effects of intra-aortic versus intravenous administration of protamine for reversal of heparin in pigs. *J Thorac Cardiovasc Surg* 85:851, 1983.

S

1. Swan H, Zeavin I, Blount SG Jr, Virtue RW: Surgery by direct vision in the open heart during hypothermia. *JAMA* 153:1081, 1953.

2. Sealy WC, Brown IW, Young WG: A report on the use of both extracorporeal circulation and hypothermia for open heart surgery. *Ann Surg* 147:603, 1958.

3. Shapiro H, Stoner EK: Body temperature and oxygen uptake in man. *Ann Phys Med* 8:250, 1966.

4. Setiey A, Challamel MJ, Champsaur G, Samuel D, Courjon J: Effects of profound hypothermia with circulatory and intraoperative electroencephalogram of the infant. *Société de EEG et de Neurophysiologie de Langue Française* 5:103, 1975.

5. Stewart RW, Blackstone EH, Kirklin JW: Neurological dysfunction after cardiac surgery, in L Parenzan, G. Crupi, G Graham (eds): *Congenital Heart Disease in the First Three Months of Life. Medical and Surgical Aspects.* Bologna, Italy: Patron Editore 1981, p 431.

6. Subramanian S, Vlad P, Fischer L, Cohen ME: Sequelae of profound hypothermia and circulatory arrest in the corrective treatment of congenital heart disease in infants and small children, in BSL Kidd, RD Rowe (eds): *The Child with Congenital Heart Disease at Surgery.* Mt, Kisco, New York: Futura 1976, p 421.

7. Stevenson JG, Stone EF, Dillard DH, Morgan BC: Intellectual development of children subjected to prolonged circulatory arrest druing hypothermic open heart surgery in infancy. *Circulation* 49,50:(suppl II):II-54, 1974.

8. Seelye ER, Harris EA, Squire AW, Barratt-Boyes BG: Metabolic effects of deep hypothermia and circulatory arrest in infants during cardiac surgery. *Br J Anaesth* 43:449, 1971.

9. Senning Å: Ventricular fibrillation during extracorporeal circulation: Used as a method to prevent air-embolisms and to facilitate intracardiac operations. *Acta Chir Scand* 171(suppl):1, 1952.

10. Shepard RB: Whole body oxygen consumption during hypoxic hypoxemia and cardiopulmonary bypass circulation. *Proceedings of the Tenth International Symposium on Space Technology and Science,* Tokyo, 1973, pp 1307–1318.

11. Swan H: *Thermoregulation and Bioenergetics: Paterns for Vertebrate Survival.* New York: Elsevier, 1974, pp 183–187.

12. Solen KA, Whiffen JD, Lightfoot EN: The effect of shear,

specific surface, and air interface on the development of blood emboli and hemolysis. *J Biomed Mater Res* 12:381, 1978.

13. Scott J: Mechanism of gamma globulin denaturation. Doctoral dissertation, UAB, 1970.

14. Singh RKK, Barratt-Boyes BG, Harris EA: Does pulsatile flow improve perfusion during hypothermic cardiopulmonary bypass? *J Thorac Cardiovasc Surg* 79:827, 1980.

15. Sink JD, Chitwood R Jr, Hill RC, Wechsler AS: Comparison of nonpulsatile and pulsatile extracorporeal circulation on renal cortical blood flow. *Ann Thorac Surg* 29:57, 1980.

16. Sade RH, Bartles DM, Dearing JP, Campbell LJ, Loadholt CB: A prospective randomized study of membrane vs. bubble oxygenators in children. *Ann Thorac Surg* 29:502, 1980.

T

1. Theye RA, Kirklin JW: Vertical film oxygenator performance at 30°C and oxygen levels during rewarming. *Surgery* 54:569, 1963.

2. Theye RA, Kirklin JW, Fowler WS: Performance and film volume of sheet and screen vertical-film oxygenators. *J Thorac Cardiovasc Surg* 43:481, 1962.

3. Theye RA, Donald DE, Jones RE: The effect of geometry and filming surface on the priming volume of the vertical-film oxygenator. *J Thorac Surg* 43:473, 1962.

4. Turley K, Graham B, Roizen M, Ebert PA: Catecholamine response to deep hypothermia and total circulatory arrest. *Circulation* (abstr) 59,60:(suppl II):II-169, 1979.

5. Tan C-K, Glisson SN, El-str AA, Ramakrishnaiah KB: Levels of circulating norepinephrine and epinephrine before, during, and after cardiopulmonary bypass in man. *J Thorac Cardiovasc Surg* 71:928, 1976.

6. Tamari Y, Aledort L, Puszkin E, Degnan TJ, Wagner N, Kaplitt MJ, Peirce EC II: Functional changes in platelets during extracorporeal circulation. *Ann Thorac Surg* 19:639, 1975.

7. Tsiao C, Lin CY, Glgov S, Replogle RL: Disseminated leukocyte injury during open-heart surgery. *Arch Pathol* 95:357, 1973.

8. Taylor KM, Bain WH, Maxted KJ, Hutton MM, McNab WY, Caves PK: Comparative studies of pulsatile and nonpulsatile flow during cardiopulmonary bypass. I. Pulsatile system employed and its hematologic effects. *J Thorac Cardiovasc Surg* 75:569, 1978.

9. Trinkle JK, Helton NE, Wood RE, Bryant LR: Metabolic comparison of a new pulsatile pump and a roller pump for cardiopulmonary bypass. *J Thorac Cardiovasc Surg* 58:562, 1969.

10. Trinkle JK, Helton NE, Bryant LR, Griffen WO: Pulsatile cardiopulmonary bypass: Clinical evaluation. *Surgery* 68:1074, 1970.

11. Taylor KM, Bain WH, Maxted KJ, Hutton MM, McNab WY, Caves PK: Comparative studies of pulsatile and nonpulsatile flow during cardiopulmonary bypass. II. The effects on adrenal secretion of cortisol. *J Thorac Cardiovasc Surg* 75:574, 1978.

12. Taylor KM, Wright GS, Bain WH, Caves PK, Beastall GS: Comparative studies of pulsatile and nonpulsatile flow during cardiopulmonary bypass. III. Response of anterior pituitary gland to thyrotropin-releasing hormone. *J Thorac Cardiovasc Surg* 75:579, 1978.

13. Turina M, Housman LB, Intaglietta M, Schauble J, Braunwald NS: An automatic cardiopulmonary bypass unit for use in infants. *J Thorac Cardiovasc Surg* 63:263, 1972.

14. Tanaka T, Bennett LR, Maloney JV, Jr: Ascorbic acid as an antisludging agent in extracorporeal circulation. *Surgical Forum* 14:275, 1963.

15. Treasure T, Naftel DC, Conger KA, Garcia JH, Kirklin JW, Blackstone EH: The effect of hypothermic circulatory arrest time on cerebral function, morphology, and biochemistry. *J Thorac Cardiovasc Surg* 86:761, 1983.

V

1. Venugopal P, Olszowka J, Wagner H, Vlad P, Lambert E, Subramanian S: Early correction of congenital heart disease with surface-induced deep hypothermia and circulatory arrest. *J Thorac Cardiovasc Surg* 66:375, 1973.

2. Vogt MT, Farber E: Reversible and irreversible cellular and mitochondrial metabolic alterations. *Am J Pathol* 53:1, 1968.

3. Verska JJ: Control of heparinization by activated clotting time during bypass with improved postoperative hemostasis. *Ann Thorac Surg* 24:170, 1977.

W

1. Weiss M, Piwnica A, Lenfant C, Sprovieri L, Laurent D, Blondeau P, Dubost C: Deep hypothermia with total circulatory arrest. *Trans Am Soc Artif Intern Organs* 6:227, 1960.

2. Wakusawa R, Shibata S, Saito H, Chiba T, Hosoi N, Sasaki T, Okada K, Hosoi Y: Clinical experience in 525 cases of open-heart surgery under simple profound hypothermia. *Jpn J Anesth* 18:240, 1968.

3. Wolin LR, Massopust LC Jr, White RJ: Behavioral effects of autocerebral perfusion, hypothermia and arrest of cerebral blood flow in the rhesus monkey. *Exp Neurol* 39:336, 1973.

4. Weiss M, Weiss J, Cotton J, Nicolas T, Binet JP: A study of the electroencephalogram during surgery with deep hypothermia and circulatory arrest in infants. *J Thorac Cardiovasc Surg* 70:316, 1975.

5. Wright JS, Hicks RG, Newman DC: Deep hypothermic arrest: Observations on later development in children. *J Thorac Cardiovasc Surg* 77:467, 1979.

6. Ward JP: Determination of the optimum temperature for regional renal hypothermia during temporary renal ischaemia. *Br J Urol* 47:17, 1975.

7. Warden HE, Cohen M, Read RC, Lillehei CW: Controlled cross circulation for open intracardiac surgery. *J Thorac Surg* 28:331, 1954.

8. Wallach R, Karp RB, Reves JG, Oparil S, Smith LR, James TN: Pathogenesis of paroxysmal hypertension developing during and after coronary artery bypass surgery: A study of hemodynamic and humoral factors. *Am J Cardiol* 46:559, 1980.

9. Ward CA, Ruegsegger B, Stanga D, Zingg W: Reduction in platelet adhesion to biomaterials by removal of gas nuclei. *Trans Am Soc Artif Intern Organs* 20:77, 1974.

10. Wilson JW: Pulmonary morphologic changes due to extracorporeal circulation: A model for 'the shock lung' at cellular level in humans, in BK Forscher, RC Lillehei, SS Stubbs (eds): *Shock in Low- and High-Flow States: Proceedings of a Symposium at Brook Lodge, Augusta, Michigan.* Amsterdam: Excerpta Medica, 1972, pp 160–171.

11. Wilkens H, Regelson W, Hoffmeister FS: The physiologic importance of pulsatile blood flow. *N Engl J Med* 267:443, 1962.

12. Wesolowski SA, Sauvage LR, Pinc RD: Extracorporeal circulation: The role of the pulse in maintenance of the systemic circulation during heart-lung bypass. *Surgery* 37:663, 1955.

13. Wright G, Sanderson JM: Brain damage and mortality in dogs following pulsatile and non-pulsatile blood flows in extracorporeal circulation. *Thorax* 27:738, 1972.

14. Williams GD, Seifen AB, Lawson NW, Norton JB, Readinger

RI, Dungan TW, Callaway JK: Pulsatile perfusion versus conventional high-flow nonpulsatile perfusion for rapid core cooling and rewarming of infants for circulatory arrest in cardiac operation. *J Thorac Cardiovasc Surg* 78:667, 1979.

15. Waldo AL, MacLean WA: *Diagnosis and Treatment of Cardiac Arrhythmias Following Open Heart Surgery: Emphasis on the Use of Atrial and Ventricular Epicardial Wire Electrodes.* Mt. Kisco, New York: Futura, 1980.

16. Walker DR, Blackstone EH, Kirklin JW, Karp RB, Kouchoukos NT, Pacifico AD, Shealy A, Roe CR, Bradley EL: The effect of micropore filtration of the arterial return during cardiopulmonary bypass: A randomized clinical study. (1976) Unpublished data.

17. Wells FC, Coghill S, Caplan HL, Lincoln C, Kirklin JW: Duration of circulatory arrest does influence the psychological development of children after cardiac operation in early life. *J Thorac Cardiovasc Surg* 86:823, 1983.

Z

1. Zingg W, Kantor S: Observations on the temperature in the brain during extracorporeal differential hypothermia. *Surgical Forum* 11:192, 1960.

3

MYOCARDIAL PROTECTION DURING CARDIAC SURGERY WITH CARDIOPULMONARY BYPASS

HISTORICAL NOTE

In the early years of cardiac surgery, little mention was made of the possibility that the existence of low cardiac output early postoperatively was related to perioperative myocardial necrosis, or infarction. Indeed, in two reviews of the complications of open heart operations published in 1965[W1] and 1966,[R1] early postoperative low cardiac output was discussed extensively, but no mention was made of myocardial necrosis as a complication of the surgery or as a cause of low cardiac output. Then, in 1967, Taber and colleagues described scattered small areas of myocardial necrosis, estimated to involve about 30% of the left ventricular myocardium, in a group of patients dying early after cardiac operations, and implicated this as the etiology of the patients' low cardiac output.[T1] Najafi and colleagues showed in 1967 that acute diffuse subendocardial myocardial infarction was found frequently in patients dying early after valve re-

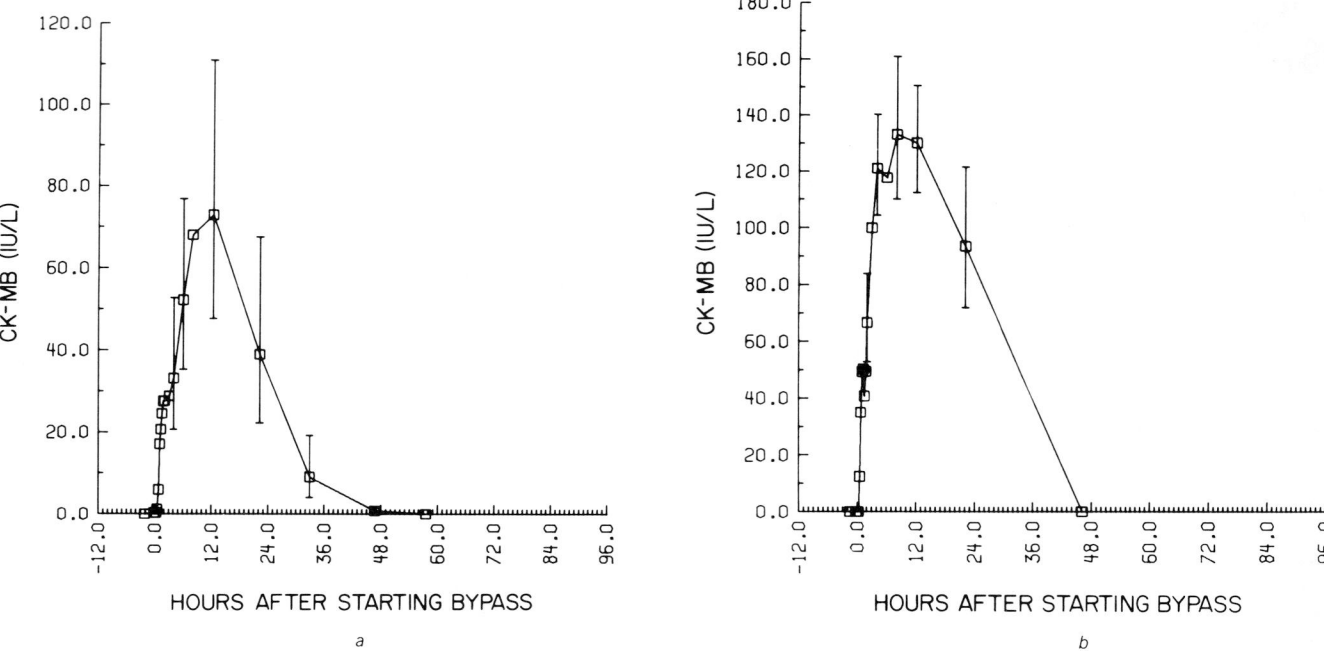

Figure 3-1 Perioperative MB isoenzyme of creatine kinase (CK-MB) plasma concentration in atrial septal defect repair using cold ischemic arrest.[P11] Data points are for the geometric mean, with asymmetric standard errors shown at selected time intervals after the start of cardiopulmonary bypass.
(a) Thirteen adult patients.
(b) Six children.

placement and suggested that this was related to methods of intraoperative management of the myocardium.[H1,N1] They discussed the possibility that disturbances of the myocardial oxygen supply-demand ratios might be implicated and that proper perfusion of the subendocardial layer of the myocardium was a particular problem during cardiopulmonary bypass (CPB).

When coronary artery bypass grafting began in the early 1970s, cardiologists and cardiac surgeons soon noted that a disturbingly high proportion of their surgical patients had developed a transmural myocardial infarction perioperatively (immediately before, during, or within 24 hours of operation).[A1,B1] Although first widely publicized in connection with coronary artery bypass grafting, the development of transmural myocardial infarction was soon shown to be a complication of cardiac surgery in general. In 1973, in a consecutive series of patients with normal coronary arteries who underwent various open cardiac operations, Hultgren and colleagues documented a 7% incidence of acute transmural myocardial infarction.[H2] At that time, these authors recognized that "there is clearly an urgent need to further improve the protection of the heart during [cardiac] surgery." Various autopsy studies have confirmed that acute transmural myocardial infarction as well as scattered myocardial necrosis and confluent subendocardial necrosis can occur after cardiac surgery despite the presence of normal coronary arteries.[R2] The rarely occurring extreme form of ischemic damage, "stone heart,"[C1] was recognized at about that time and has been confirmed to be essentially a massive myocardial infarction.[K1,L1]

In recent years, the development of knowledge in this area has been facilitated by improved methods of identifying myocardial necrosis during life and, to some degree at least, quantitating its extent. The electrocardiographic criteria for diagnosing transmural myocardial infarction and ischemic changes have been clarified[R3] and applied to postoperative patients. The appearance of cardiac-specific enzymes in plasma has been shown to correlate well with other evidence of myocardial necrosis,[D1,O1,R4] and their concentrations have been shown to correlate directly with the amount of muscle that has become necrotic, as judged by other criteria.[G1] However, some controversy continues in this area.[K2,K8] Radionucleotide imaging has also been useful in identifying the presence and extent of perioperative myocardial infarctions.[R5,R6]

With these methods, a number of clinical studies have supported the finding of autopsy studies that myocardial necrosis is an important and frequent complication of conventional cardiac surgery. In 1973, the frequency of myocardial necrosis in patients convalescing well was demonstrated in a study of isolated aortic valve replacement.[S1] Although the hospital mortality was low (2%), 15% of the patients developed electrocardiographic evidence of transmural myocardial infarction, and 70% developed isoenzymatic evidence of myocardial necrosis. In 1974, it was shown that, even after the short and simple operation for repair of an uncomplicated atrial septal defect, 12 (92%) of 13 adult patients and all 6 children developed isoenzymatic evidence of myocardial necrosis (Fig. 3-1).[P1] Myocardial necrosis was demonstrated by enzymatic methods in children undergoing surgery for a number of different congenital cardiac defects.[N2]

In 1974, data were collected that indicated that early postoperative cardiac output was inversely proportional to the extent of myocardial necrosis and, thus, that the amount of myocardial necrosis was a determinant of the early postoperative condition of the patient and of the probability of survival.[P2]

THE NEED FOR SPECIAL MEASURES

The normal human heart is perfused by blood that is ejected from the left ventricle and leaves the aorta via its first branches, the right and left coronary arteries. The blood is continuously modified by the organism so as to be correct in its composition and free of damaging materials, such as gaseous or particulate microemboli. The amount and distribution of the myocardial blood flow (and thus the myocardial oxygen supply) is continuously regulated, in part in response to myocardial oxygen demand. This flow is determined by the coronary perfusing pressure (aortic pressure), tension in the various layers of the myocardium (related in part to ventricular wall thickness and size), and coronary vascular resistance. The ratio between the flow to the inner one-fourth of the myocardium (the *subendocardial layer*) and that to the outer one-fourth (the *subepicardial layer*) in normal hearts with intact circulation is about 1 or a little larger. While blood flow to the subepicardial layer occurs in both systole and diastole, that to the subendocardial layer of the left ventricle occurs essentially only during diastole, since intramyocardial tension during systole closes the branches of the coronary arteries that pass perpendicularly through the myocardium to arborize in the subendocardium. The well-known vulnerability to ischemia of the left ventricular subendocardial layer in shock, ventricular hypertrophy, and coronary artery disease, as well as during cardiac surgery, is dependent in part on this relationship.

The heart is deprived of most of these protective regulatory factors during CPB. For the most part, blood passes in a retrograde fashion into the most proximal part of the aorta from an arterial cannula that is usually in the distal part of the ascending aorta. The determinants of the rate and distribution of coronary blood flow are quite abnormal during conventional CPB. The arterial pressure-pulse is narrow (essentially nonpulsatile), and the mean arterial blood pressure is highly variable. The heart is usually more or less empty and thus smaller than usual, which increases intramyocardial tension and tends to decrease flow to the subendocardial layer.[A2] Steed, Buckberg, and colleagues have shown that this state of the empty, beating heart in dogs on CPB increases transmural and subendocardial vascular resistance by 25% at normothermia and by 50% at 28°C.[S2] The effect is particularly powerful in the small heart, resistance to subendocardial flow rising 210% in puppy hearts. Ventricular fibrillation increases intramyocardial tension still more. Vascular resistances throughout the body are altered during CPB, presumably by the abnormal hemodynamic state and by circulating vasoactive agents (see Chapter 2, Section 2), and the coronary vascular resistance is surely no exception

to this. Furthermore, the perfusate is diluted blood of variable composition with highly abnormal physiochemical properties (see Chapter 2, Section 2). For example, it is heparinized and consequently has a rapid sedimentation rate and an increased tendency toward sludging. The blood may contain microemboli of several kinds. Thus, there is no reason to assume that the empty, beating, perfused human heart on CPB is well protected.

Many cardiac operations can be performed with the heart perfused and beating, but all are facilitated by having the aorta cross-clamped and the heart bloodless and quiet because of the cessation of coronary blood flow. Such a procedure imposes global myocardial ischemia. Since nearly all surgeons accept the need in most cardiac operations for the improved exposure that comes with at least intermittent aortic cross-clamping, the aim of proper myocardial protection during this period is to prevent the damage that would otherwise occur as a result of the myocardial ischemia and to some extent from CPB itself.

DAMAGE FROM GLOBAL MYOCARDIAL ISCHEMIA

Much of the damage from myocardial ischemia is evident only during or after reperfusion. However, one form of damage evident during the ischemic period itself is *ischemic contracture*,[H3] or *myocardial rigor*,[G7] which is an ischemic time-dependent sequence of mechanical and biochemical events that occur when the concentration of intracellular adenosine triphosphate (ATP) falls below a critical level.[H3,J4,V1] Ischemic contracture is rarely seen clinically. In spite of the confusion in the literature,[K1,L1] it is *not* the laboratory analogue of the clinical phenomenon called *stone heart*,[C1] which occurs *with reperfusion*.

The more clinically relevant phenomena that follow the global myocardial ischemia of aortic cross-clamping during CPB are (1) myocardial edema, (2) functional depression without permanent structural damage, or (3) myocardial cell death. Although ameliorated by the use of cold cardioplegia and modern methods of reperfusion, these same events may occur with whatever methods of myocardial protection are used.

Myocardial Edema

Some myocardial edema develops after CPB without aortic cross-clamping, from the same factors that produce increased interstitial fluid throughout the body. However, myocardial edema is more prominent after episodes of myocardial ischemia, and thus is present to some degree in most hearts after aortic cross-clamping. Ischemia induces not only the tendency toward interstitial edema upon reperfusion but also cellular edema and swelling. Cellular swelling results in part from depletion of energy stores and failure of active membrane transport of small molecules, particularly sodium, potassium, and chloride.[L7] It results also from intracellular production of new osmotically active molecules by ischemic metabolic conversion of osmotically less active larger molecules.[T10]

When sufficiently severe, myocardial edema reduces ventricular diastolic function by reducing compliance (distensibility). This tends to reduce stroke volume and cardiac output.

Temporary Functional Depression without Permanent Structural or Biochemical Damage

Even short periods of aortic cross-clamping with any method of myocardial protection are probably followed by temporary functional depression without permanent structural or biochemical damage.[L6] However, such depression has been difficult to define and quantitate.

Myocardial Necrosis

Because it is irreversible, myocardial cell death, or myocardial necrosis, is the most important sequel of global myocardial ischemia. However, under some circumstances, myocardial cell death is difficult to identify after ischemia without reperfusion. Thus, with routine light microscopy, no change can be detected in the structure of irreversibly damaged cells from regions of myocardium rendered temporarily ischemic for 60 minutes but nonreperfused,[J2] although special techniques do demonstrate discrete loss of glycogen.[J2] The loss of glycogen has been also shown by Moulder, Blackstone, and colleagues to occur after global ischemia.[M1] Electron microscopy shows uniform and readily recognizable changes, including relaxation of myofibrils, prominent I bands, virtual absence of glycogen, and margination of nuclear chromatin.

Other phenomena related to cell death occur during the ischemic period. Lactate accumulates in the tissue and intracellular pH falls[N3] as tissue Po_2 falls with ischemia and energy depletion. Adenosine triphosphate (ATP) levels fall as the ischemic time lengthens,[H3] and irreversible myocardial damage is associated with very low levels of ATP.[S15] The calcium content of isolated mitochondria also falls during the ischemic period.[C2]

After temporary ischemia for as short a time as 20 minutes *and reperfusion*, irreversibly damaged myocardial cells show prominent changes even when studied by light microscopy, including disruption of the regular myofibrillar pattern and the presence of prominent contraction bands[M2] (a certain indicator of cell death). During cardiac surgery, reperfusion of a heart that has been severely damaged by ischemia may produce a sudden massive palpable contracture[C1,H3,K1,L1] (localized or global "stone heart") that may seem to be ventricular fibrillation but that is not. This is not the true contracture of ischemia (see above) but is a phenomenon of reperfusion of a ventricle that has been ischemic. This contracture may be the gross analogue of the contraction bands observed microscopically. With reperfusion, calcium accumulations become abnormally high in the mitochondria.[I1,S3] This process is secondary to an accelerated entry of calcium ions into the cells, resulting from loss of membrane selective permeability in the presence of a reduced capacity for the control of cytolitic calcium by the sodium-calcium pump, and is believed to be the result of low levels of ATP.[N8]

The incidence and extent of ischemic myocardial necrosis are related in an important way to the duration of the global myocardial ischemia. Using a nonglobal ischemic model (temporary ligation of the left circumflex artery) in the dog at 37°C, Jennings and colleagues found that 20 minutes of temporary ischemia produces cell death in some areas of the ischemic myocardium, that more and more cells are irreversibly injured by ischemic periods up to 60 minutes, and that at 60 minutes essentially all cells in the area are necrosed (Fig. 3-2).[J1] Earlier studies by Blumgart and associates[B2] are compatible with these data. Similar data are not available for global myocardial ischemia, but presumably a similar relationship exists between ischemic time and the proportion of myocardial cells dying. When myocardium is hypothermic during the ischemic period, the proportion of cells dying from any given ischemic time is certainly less, but, again, these interrelationships have not been clearly defined.

It is also clear from Buckberg's work[F1] that, after a period of global ischemia, some myocardial cells are damaged, but not fatally, and that under proper circumstances of reperfusion they will recover from the damage and survive, while under improper ones they will die. It is also evident that myocardial damage from global ischemia may not be maximal immediately after reperfusion, using heterotopic intra-abdominal rat heart transplantation. Casale and colleagues found mitochondrial enzymatic markers of myocardial ischemic injury and light microscopic signs of damage to be maximal, not early after cold cardioplegic arrests and reperfusion, but 1 to 2 days later.[C16] They found gradual improvement over the subsequent 10 to 12 days. These findings are compatible with the clinical observation that cardiac performance is often less good 24 to 48 hours after operation than immediately after operation, and that after appropriate support cardiac performance may improve after that time.

THE IMPORTANCE OF PERIOPERATIVELY PRODUCED MYOCARDIAL NECROSIS

There is considerable evidence that perioperatively produced myocardial cell death results in lower cardiac output than would otherwise be present and that this, in turn, results in a higher proportion of hospital deaths, greater morbidity, and increased need for support mechanisms such as intra-aortic balloon pulsation and catecholamine infusions. In a group of patients undergoing mitral valve replacement with simple cold ischemic arrest (UAB), the greater the myocardial necrosis developing postoperatively, the lower the cardiac output (Fig. 3-3). The lower the cardiac output, the greater the need for support mechanisms such as an intra-aortic balloon pump and catecholamine infusions, and the greater the probability of hospital death (Fig. 3-4). Richardson and colleagues showed in patients undergoing combined aortic valve replacement and coronary artery bypass grafting that hospital mortality was significantly higher in those who developed a perioperative myocardial infarction than in those who did not (Table 3-1).[R7]

Although unproven, it seems likely that the development

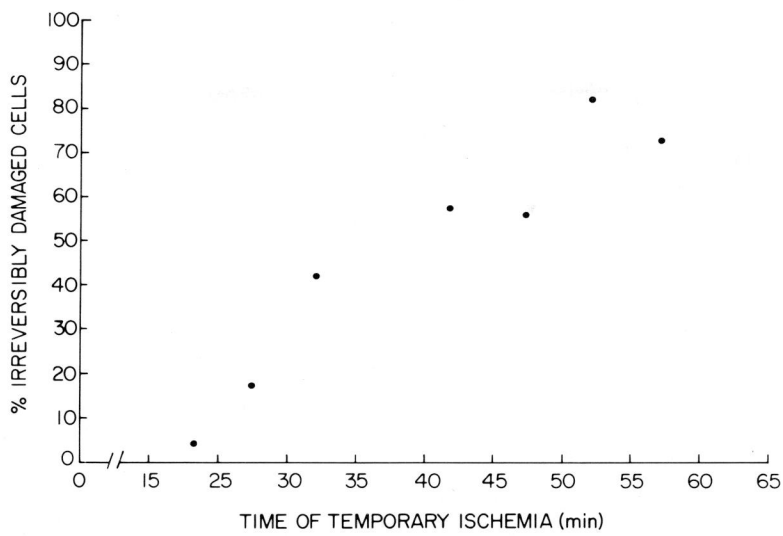

Figure 3-2 Relationship of extent of irreversible myocardial cell damage to time of temporary regional (left circumflex artery) ischemia in dogs at 37°C.

Modified from Jennings et al.[J2]

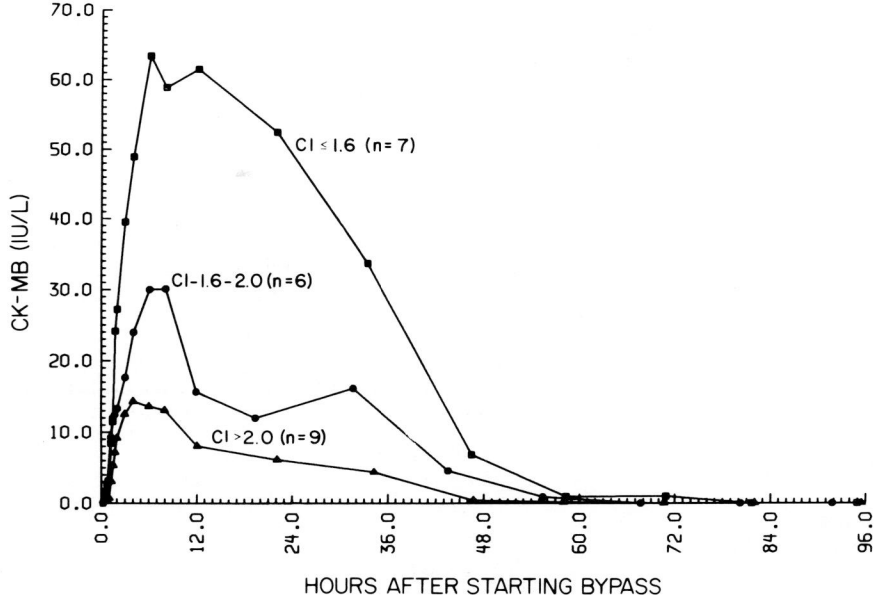

Figure 3-3 Blood CK-MB isoenzyme levels in the hours after the start of CPB and cardiac index 4–6 hours postoperatively in 22 consecutive patients undergoing isolated mitral valve replacement in 1975 with simple cold ischemic arrest.[P11] Geometric mean values are portrayed. Note the very high levels of CK-MB in patients with low cardiac output ($\geq$1.6) and the low levels in patients with higher cardiac output (>2.0). The overall correlation of CK-MB (duration, peak, and integrated area) and cardiac index is $r = -.4$, $P = .04$.

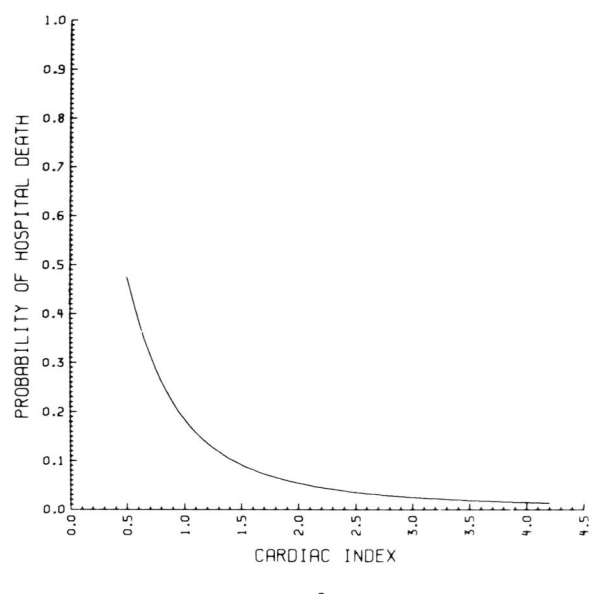

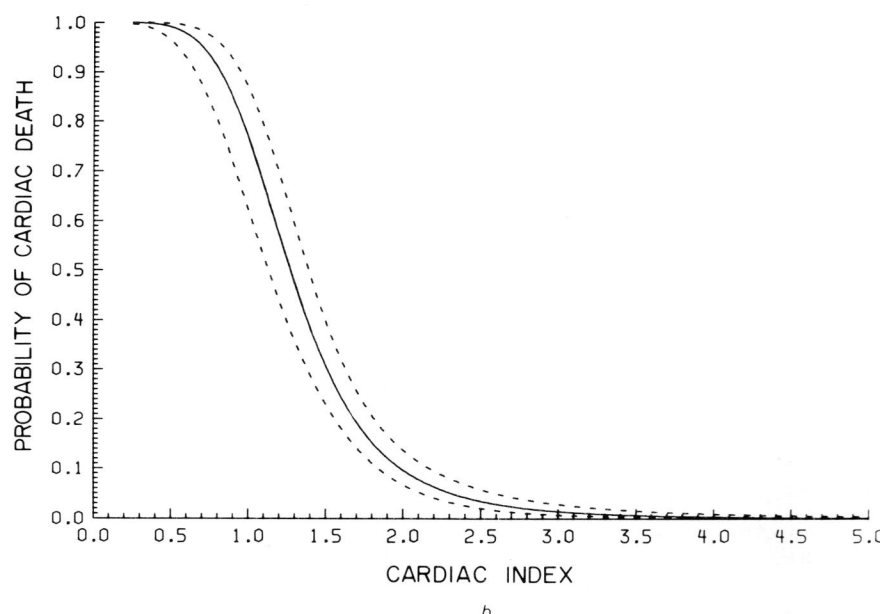

Figure 3-4

(*a*) The relationship between the early postoperative cardiac index and the probability of hospital death in patients undergoing mitral valve surgery (*P* < .05) (UAB, 1972–1973, cold ischemic arrest or intermittent ischemic arrest).

(*b*) Probability of acute cardiac death from early postoperative low cardiac output related to the cardiac index in 139 infants and children undergoing open intracardiac repair (UAB, 1972–1973). The dashed lines encompass the 70% confidence limits.

Part *a* reproduced with permission from Appelbaum et al.;[A3] see publication for data, equation, and statistics. Part *b* reproduced with permission from Parr et al.,[P3] and the American Heart Association, Inc.; see publication for data, equation, and statistics.

Table 3-1 Combined aortic valve replacement and coronary artery bypass grafting from May 1970 to June 1977 at UAB.[R7]

Perioperative Myocardial Infarction (by ECG)	No. of Patients	Hospital Deaths[a]		
		No.	%	CL
Definite	23	4	17%	9%–29%
Probable	66	3	5%	2%–9%
None	116	3	3%	1%–3%
Total	205	10	4.9%	3.3%–7.0%
$P_{(x^2)}$			.01	

KEY: CL, 70% confidence limits.

[a] Two additional patients died during operation and could not be evaluated.

of perioperative myocardial necrosis (infarction) predisposes the patient to ventricular electrical instability as well as to low cardiac output and hospital death.

The development of poor left ventricular function late postoperatively certainly follows extensive perioperative myocardial necrosis. Some patients with persisting symptoms of heart failure 1–2 years after valve replacement have been found at autopsy to have extensive left ventricular subendocardial scarring believed to be the result of extensive perioperative myocardial infarctions.

METHODS OF PREVENTING ISCHEMIC MYOCARDIAL DAMAGE

A number of methods of myocardial protection during cardiac surgery have been used through the years, and most of them are still used, although some infrequently.

Normothermic, Perfused, Empty, Beating Heart

In spite of the surgical disadvantages, the earliest intracardiac operations were performed on normothermic, perfused, empty, beating hearts, and, even as late as 1975, this technique was acclaimed as the optimal method for cardiac surgery.[B3] Earlier studies in experimental animals had been interpreted as showing "normal left ventricular function" after 30 minutes to 3 hours of CPB with the heart perfused, empty, and beating.[E1,N4]

Present information indicates that the method is not ideal. First, water tends to accumulate in the myocardium during CPB. Buckberg and colleagues found that, as a result, ventricular distensibility in dogs is decreased by nearly 50% after 3 hours of CPB with the heart perfused, empty, and beating.[F2] In addition, the distribution of coronary blood in the normothermic, beating, empty (and thus small) heart is abnormal (see section on the need for special measures). Also, the change in myocardial compressive forces and left ventricular wall geometry with the empty beating heart have been shown recently to markedly impede intracoronary collateral flow supplying potentially ischemic areas of myocardium.[M3]

In addition, the perfusate entering the arterial system (and, thus, the heart) from the pump-oxygenator is heparinized, diluted blood with abnormal physicochemical properties. Unless the oxygenator is a true biological membrane, oxygenation changes protein structure and gives the perfusate certain toxic properties, and, for a variety of reasons, vasoactive substances tend to accumulate in the perfusate (see Chapter 2, Section 2). Also, as mentioned above, the distribution of the coronary blood is abnormal.

Individual Normothermic or Moderately Hypothermic Coronary Artery Perfusion

Surgery on the aortic valve is possible with a perfused, empty, beating heart by the technique of individual coronary artery perfusion.[L2,M4] After CPB is established, the aorta is cross-clamped (stopping the retrograde flow of blood into the aortic root and then into the ostia of the right and left coronary arteries) and an incision made into the first part of the ascending aorta just as it emerges from the heart. Small individual cannulae are placed into the ostia of the right and left coronary arteries, and, usually by way of separate pumps and lines for each, blood is infused into both.

The cannulae inserted into the coronary ostia are at least 3–4 mm long, and some types are longer. Therefore, in some patients, the tip may extend beyond the bifurcation of the left main coronary artery, so that only the left anterior descending or circumflex artery is perfused. In about 1% of people, these two arteries arise separately from the aortic sinus, making proper individual cannulation more difficult. There is a higher than normal incidence of left dominant systems in patients with aortic stenosis secondary to congenital bicuspid valves, and, in such left dominant systems, the left main coronary artery is shorter than normal,[H4,K4,M5] again making individual coronary perfusion more difficult. In about 50% of people, the conus artery supplying the infundibulum of the right ventricle arises separately from the aortic sinus and is not perfused by a cannula inserted into the right coronary ostium. Also, mechanical injury to the coronary ostia can result in intraoperative myocardial infarction and late coronary ostial stenosis.[C4,H5,L3,M6,R8,S4,Y1]

The method is not without periods of global myocardial ischemia. An ischemic interval occurs between aortic cross-clamping and the initiation of right and left coronary artery perfusion. This interval varies, depending on the sequences elected by the surgeon, but can seldom be reduced below 2–3 minutes. If exposure for the operation is hampered by leakage of blood around the cannulae, coronary perfusion may have to be discontinued for short periods during the procedure. Further, patients with aortic valve disease generally have important left ventricular hypertrophy, which makes subendocardial ischemia more likely.

Perhaps the most detrimental aspect of individual coronary perfusion is the fixed flow delivered by individual pumps. Thus, there is no compensation for either the change in coronary resistance with time or the phase of the cardiac cycle. In addition, the optimum flow has been uncertain.

In spite of these problems, the clinical results of aortic valve replacement using this technique have been reasonably satisfactory. McGoon and colleagues[M7] reported a series of 100 consecutive cases of isolated aortic valve replacement with no hospital deaths, proof that the method, properly used, can provide good results. Only one of those patients required perioperative catecholamine support.[M8]

Later, Spanos, Brown, and McGoon[S5] showed that when ventricular fibrillation persisted throughout the period of coronary perfusion, the risk of perioperative infarction and death was higher than if the heart was beating. This would be expected from knowledge of subendocardial blood flow during ventricular fibrillation.[B4,H6] The incidence of transmural myocardial infarction when individual coronary artery perfusion is used for aortic valve replacement was shown by Sapsford and colleagues in a randomized study to be 15%, with isoenzymatic evidence of myocardial necrosis in 70% of patients, proportions as high as in the patients randomized to cold ischemic arrest.[S1] Although some surgeons continue to use individual coronary artery perfusion routinely for aortic valve surgery, no randomized studies have established its superiority over other methods, nor have they presented evidence that the incidence and extent of myocardial necrosis with it is minimal.

Individual coronary perfusion may still have a place under special circumstances (GLH). The flow rate during this kind of perfusion is particularly important. At GLH, when this technique was in general use, individual coronary artery perfusion was begun at a perfusion pressure of 110 mmHg, measured just downstream from the individual coronary pump. This arbitrary "standard" flow (one that gives a perfusion pressure, measured at this point, of 110 mmHg) was then increased by 25%. The reasons for this procedure are as follows.

Figure 3-5 shows the relationship between total coronary vascular resistance and total (right plus left) coronary arterial flow at 30°C.[B5,H7] There is a clear negative correlation between resistance and flow. The polynomial fit (curved line) indicates that resistance tends toward a minimal value as flow increases. This tendency is a well-known property of isolated vascular beds[B6] and results from dilatation of resistance vessels, and possibly recruitment of previously unperfused regions, as flow is increased. The scatter of points is partly due to variation in the capacity of the coronary bed from one patient to another. It might be surmised that oxygen delivery to outlying myocardial cells improves as resistance falls and, from Figure 3-5, that optimal conditions are approached, in a patient at 30°C, at a total coronary flow of around 250 ml · min^{-1}. Other lines of evidence suggest that this is so. Figure 3-6 shows (1) that oxygen consumption ($\dot{V}O_2$) increased significantly with flow up to 125% of standard flow (as described above) but that at 150% there was no further increase; (2) that lactate flux was negative (with the myocardium putting lactate *into* the blood) at 75% of standard flow, indicating myocardial anoxia, but essentially zero at flows higher than this; and (3) that nonesterified fatty acid flux was significantly negative at 75%, indicating myocardial anoxia, but positive at 100% of standard flow. The conclusion is that 125% of standard flow provides optimal conditions.

In the patients studied, coronary flow at 125% of standard averaged 203 ml · min^{-1}, with a range of 154–266 ml · min^{-1}. It seems that optimal metabolism and optimal resistance (Figs. 3-5, 3-6) are reached at about the same flow, and that this is comfortably below the flow of 300 ml · min^{-1}, above which Isom and colleagues[11] demonstrated histological evidence of myocardial damage resulting from coronary perfusion.

Why not define the standard in flow units rather than that at a pressure of 110 mmHg? The appropriate absolute flow depends on the capacity of the coronary vascular bed, and ths varies not only with the size of the patient but also with pathologic changes in the heart. No correlation has been demonstrable, in hearts with such pathologic conditions, between coronary resistance and body size.[H7] The flow cannot, therefore, be set according to the size of the patient. The alternative is to define flow in terms of perfusion pressure.

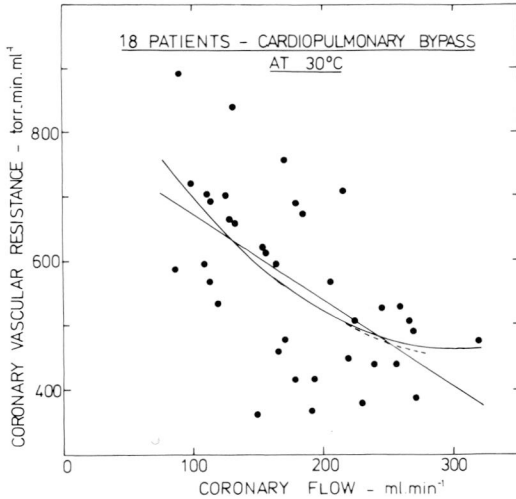

Figure 3-5 Combined (right and left) coronary vascular resistance in relation to total coronary flow delivered by roller pumps in 18 patients during cardiopulmonary bypass at 30°C. The straight line is the linear regression through the data. The curve is the regression calculated from a binomial equation to the second power of flow. The dashed tail shows the effect of omitting the extreme right-hand data point.
Reproduced with permission from Harris et al.[H7]

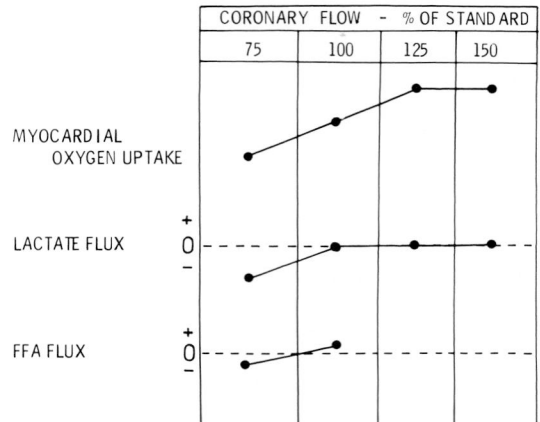

Figure 3-6 Qualitative diagram illustrating significant changes in myocardial O_2 uptake and in lactate and fatty acid flux as coronary flow is increased at 30°C.
Reproduced with permission from Harris et al.[H7]

Pressure measured near the *cannular* tips fluctuates very much more than line pressure, even at a steady flow. Doubtless this is due to the damping induced by the long coronary line and the air-buffered aneroid manometer used to measure line pressure. Thus, in practice, it is difficult and unreliable to set flow according to the actual coronary perfusion pressure. Therefore, the flow is defined by the pressure just downstream from the pump. This information is all relevant to optimal flow rates for infusion of cold cardioplegic solutions.

Continuous Coronary Perfusion with Ventricular Fibrillation

In continuous coronary perfusion with ventricular fibrillation, the fibrillation can be maintained by an electrical current, which is necessary when the perfusion is at 37°C; or it may be spontaneously or electrically induced and maintained by moderately hypothermic (28–32°C) coronary perfusion. The coronary perfusion can be through the intact aortic root (as in coronary artery bypass grafting) or by individual coronary perfusion cannulae during aortic valve replacement.

A number of theoretical objections can be raised to the method, one of which is that perfusion of the subendocardium is impaired during CPB and ventricular fibrillation. However, good clinical results have been obtained using normothermic CPB and electrically maintained ventricular fibrillation, moderate hypothermia and ventricular fibrillation sustained only by the hypothermia, or profound cardiac hypothermia and ventricular fibrillation. Aikins has reported excellent results from coronary artery bypass grafting using the latter method.[A8] Time constraints apply to this method, as to most others, but they have not been defined. No clinical studies have defined a particularly low incidence of myocardial cell death with this method, and the surgical conditions with it are not optimal.

Intermittent Cardiac Ischemia with Moderate Cardiac Hypothermia

The use of intermittent cardiac ischemia with moderate cardiac hypothermia generally consists of conducting CPB with the perfusate temperature at 28–32°C. Thereby the patient's heart soon reaches this temperature. The surgeon works on or in the heart intermittently for periods of 15–30 minutes, during which time the ascending aorta is cross-clamped (to stop coronary perfusion) or individual perfusion into the coronary ostia is interrupted. Between these periods, the aortic clamp is released (or individual coronary perfusion resumed) for 3–5 minutes, and, when the technique is used optimally, the heart is made to beat (not fibrillate) during this interval. This was the method most commonly used in the 1960s and early 1970s and is used by some today. While it has never been shown to be associated with a low incidence of myocardial necrosis, the clinical results can be good. McGoon's data confirm this.[M8] His analysis of one group of patients, those receiving valved extracardiac conduits, indicated no relationship between the proportion of nonsurvivors in the experience and the cumulative aortic cross-

clamp time. However, since 35% of the 468 patients had low cardiac output postoperatively[M8] (in which subset the mortality was 52%), the method must have been producing myocardial necrosis.

The method does not provide optimal surgical exposure. Unless the heart is electrically fibrillated just before the cross-clamping, it continues to beat during much of the ischemic period, making precise repair difficult. Each time coronary perfusion is recommenced, coronary (and perhaps systemic) air embolization is likely to occur, even when precautions against it are taken. A considerable amount of blood comes into the heart during the periods of coronary perfusion, stressing the intracardiac sucker systems and thereby increasing blood damage and interfering with the smooth and efficient flow of the operation. Moreover, each time the coronary arteries are perfused, a reperfusion injury may occur.

This method, with or without moderate hypothermia, continues to be used with success by some surgeons for coronary artery bypass grafting. Reduto and colleagues showed no difference in left ventricular performance early after coronary artery bypass grafting regardless of whether this or cold cardioplegic myocardial protection was used.[R17]

Profoundly Hypothermic Cardiac Ischemia

In profoundly hypothermic cardiac ischemia, the heart is profoundly cooled by the perfusate and/or by filling the pericardium with very cold saline solution.[B7,C5,G2,H8,K5,P4,S6] In clinical practice, myocardial temperature is generally about 22°C with these methods.[C6] Generally, the heart does not become electromechanically quiescent until 20–30 minutes after aortic cross-clamping. Most surgeons have believed that these methods allow 45–60 minutes of safe global ischemia.

This technique provides better operating conditions than do those discussed earlier, an important consideration, and many good results have been obtained by surgeons using it. However, in a randomized study of patients undergoing aortic valve replacement, it has been shown to result in as much myocardial necrosis as does individual coronary perfusion.[S1] The necrosis occurs in part because it is technically impossible to cool the whole myocardium by this technique, particularly when it is hypertrophied.

Profoundly hypothermic cardiac ischemia may be preferred for infant cardiac surgery in which profound hypothermia and total circulatory arrest are used (GLH). Part of the rationale for this preference is that no perfusate passes through the heart to rewarm or inadequately reperfuse it during total circulatory arrest, as may happen when cardiopulmonary bypass is continued. An experimental study indicates that the hearts of neonates perform better early after aortic cross-clamping when simple cold ischemic arrest is used than when cold cardioplegic arrest is employed.[L8]

Cold Cardioplegic Myocardial Protection

For a detailed discussion of cold cardioplegic myocardial protection, see "Technique of Myocardial Protection with Cold Cardioplegia."

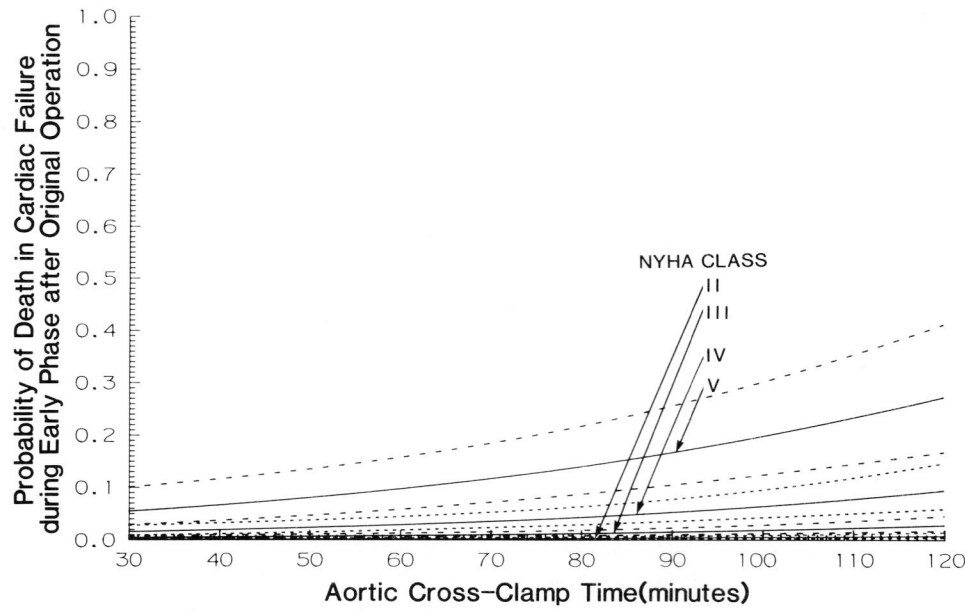

Figure 3-7 Probability of death with cardiac failure during the early phase (in hospital and for approximately 6 months thereafter) after primary aortic valve replacement. The probabilities are stratified according to the preoperative NYHA functional class (class V indicates emergency operation for shock or severe acidosis). The depiction is as in Figure 3-7. The findings are based on a study of 1,533 patients undergoing primary valve replacement (UAB, 1975–July 1979).

Reproduced with permission from Blackstone et al.;[B19] see original publication for equations and statistics.

TECHNIQUE OF MYOCARDIAL PROTECTION WITH COLD CARDIOPLEGIA

Present Concepts

Extensive laboratory and clinical research indicates that proper use of cardioplegia (the induction of electromechanical arrest) and profound cardiac cooling greatly extends the safe time of global cardiac ischemia, although the time limits have not been exactly defined. The clinical data indicate that there is little myocardial necrosis or permanent functional damage after total myocardial ischemia for up to 120 minutes (Fig. 3-7) (1) if the myocardial reserves preoperatively are good, that is, New York Heart Association (NYHA) functional class I, II, or III; (2) if oxygen consumption has been reduced by nearly immediate (or with a delay of no more than 2 minutes[F6]) and continuing cessation of electromechanical activity and rapid cooling of the heart; (3) if the myocardium throughout the ischemic period is 15–20°C;[B20] and (4) if the coronary arteries are reperfused with the cold cardioplegic solution about every 30 minutes for its washout effect as well as for its effect in maintaining cold cardioplegia.[C13,C14] However, information from myocardial ultrastructure and high-energy phosphate studies in humans indicates that such protection is less complete when the aortic cross-clamp time exceeds 120 minutes.[B16,C14] Furthermore, decreasing preoperative myocardial reserves such as are presumed to exist in patients preoperatively in NYHA functional classes III, IV, and especially V appear to decrease the safe time limits of cold cardioplegia, and the data suggest that only about 80 minutes are allowed in patients with advanced heart failure, that is, in NYHA class V.

Regardless of the protective effect of cold cardioplegia, the global ischemic time should be limited as much as possible by the performance of operations in an efficient manner.

History and Hypotheses

Cardioplegia as an aid to intracardiac exposure during cardiac surgery was introduced by Melrose and colleagues in 1955, during the early days of intracardiac surgery,[M9] using a hyperosmolar solution that was subsequently shown to be damaging and a cause of late cardiomyopathy. It was therefore soon discontinued and other noncardioplegic techniques substituted. However, particularly important studies by Bretschneider and colleagues concerning cardioplegia, hypothermia, and myocardial metabolism were reported in the late 1960s and the 1970s and summarized in 1975,[B8] and clinical reports concerning cardioplegia again began to appear in the late 1960s.[R9,R10,S7] The method was not then widely adopted, perhaps because the clinical results were not obviously superior to results being obtained by other methods. In 1972, Kirsch, Rodewald, and Kalmar published their results using normothermic cardioplegia.[K6] Again, they were no better than those obtained by many surgeons with traditional methods.

In the early 1970s, evidence was appearing, as noted above, that myocardial damage was common after cardiac surgery. New studies showed that the colder the heart during the ischemic period, the better the myocardial protection.[H9]

Then several groups showed experimentally that abruptly stopping the electromechanical activity of the heart at the onset of ischemia, combined with myocardial cooling, provided better myocardial protection than either method did alone.[E2,G3,H9,H10,J3,K7,S8] A number of nonconcurrent, nonrandomized clinical studies were soon reported that indicated that cardioplegia plus profound myocardial cooling (cold cardioplegia) provided better and longer myocardial protection and better clinical results than did any of the methods used previously.[A4,A5,A7,C7,E3,F3,F4,R7,R11,T4] Conti and colleagues showed in a randomized clinical study of patients undergoing coronary artery bypass grafting that cold cardioplegia provided better functional protection of the heart and provoked less myocardial necrosis than did cold ischemic arrest.[C6] Braimbridge and colleagues, studying myocardial biopsy specimens with quantitative birefringance (a measurement of ATP activity), found a higher incidence of endomyocardial damage with continuous coronary perfusion than with cold cardioplegia in patients undergoing valve surgery.[B9]

The hypothesis underlying the use of cold cardioplegic myocardial preservation is that it reduces myocardial oxygen demand during the ischemic period of cross-clamping to such low levels that the myocardial energy stores are sufficient to maintain cell structure and the energy-dependent cell membrane pumps that preserve transcellular gradients of sodium, potassium, calcium, and magnesium.[B10,B18,K8] Thus, myocardial cell viability and function are preserved.

During aortic cross-clamping, myocardial energy is derived primarily from anerobic metabolism of myocardial glycogen and glucose. This small energy output of anaerobiasis is sufficient to maintain myocardial viability during relatively prolonged ischemia if the energy demands are sufficiently low.[B8] When the heart is electromechanically quiescent, the energy demands are determined primarily by myocardial temperature and to some extent by resting wall tension. Thus, at 22°C, myocardial oxygen consumption in the electromechanically quiescent heart is $0.3 \ ml \cdot 100 \ g^{-1} \cdot min^{-1}$, while at 37°C it is $1 \ ml \cdot 100 \ g^{-1} \cdot min^{-1}$. In contrast, while the heart at 22°C is beating or fibrillating, oxygen consumption is approximately $2 \ ml \cdot 100 \ g^{-1} \cdot min^{-1}$.[B4]

The most commonly used cardioplegic agent at present is potassium, in concentrations of $15-35 \ mmol \ (mEq) \cdot l^{-1}$. Potassium in this concentration blocks the initial fast (inward sodium current) phase of myocardial cellular depolarization. Even in the presence of this concentration of potassium, electromechanical activity can persist or return in the presence of agents, such as catecholamines, that open the later slow (inward calcium and sodium current) phase of myocardial cellular depolarization, on which potassium has no effect.

Myocardial Temperature

Hearse and colleagues have shown that the protective effect of cold during global myocardial ischemia varies inversely with myocardial temperature. The relationship was maintained at the lowest temperature tested (12°C), but the improvement in protection with each degree of additional cool-

ing was most marked down to 22°C.[H9] Tyers and colleagues reported evidence of low-temperature injury in rat hearts cooled to 4°C,[T7] and Balderman and colleagues have found in humans that extreme myocardial hypothermia (6–10°C) during global ischemia was associated with significant reduction in ventricular function after reperfusion.[B17] The matters remain controversial, however. Schragge, Digerness, and Blackstone (UAB), using an isolated rat heart preparation, found no evidence of cold damage with temperatures as low as 2°C;[S14] and Rosenfeldt and colleagues, in Melbourne, in both experimental and clinical studies, found no evidence of myocardial damage in hearts cooled to 4–10°C but did find damage at −3°C.[R15]

These findings, combined with extensive clinical experience, indicate that the cardioplegic solution should be at 4°C, that the myocardial temperature should be lowered to 12–15°C with this perfusate, and that the heart should be kept at 15–20°C throughout the ischemic period.

Cardioplegic Solution

The solution must be cold when infused (about 4–8°C); must be cardioplegic; should produce no direct cell membrane damage; should minimize intracellular ionic changes (particularly increased free calcium concentration,[F5,K9,S9] which increases energy use in the myocardial cell); and should minimize changes in myocardial water content.

The ingredients of cardioplegic solutions vary. A concentration of potassium of about $30 \ mEq \cdot l^{-1}$ is safe and effective in producing cardioplegia.[C3,C6,G3,G4,M10,T6] Sodium, in a concentration at the lower end of the physiologic range, is usually included because marked extracellular hyponatremia increases calcium conductance, which is disadvantageous during and immediately after the ischemic period.[L4] However, some surgeons[B8,K6,R11] use a low concentration of sodium in the cardioplegic solution. This practice is based on the experimental work of Reidemeister and colleagues,[R9] which showed that reduction in sodium concentration arrests the heart through an inhibition of membrane excitation and may render less sodium available for cellular entry and, therefore, for cellular damage during ischemia. On some grounds, a solution without calcium ions might seem desirable. However, experimental evidence indicates that perfusates without calcium are dramatically harmful to cell membranes,[H11,Y2,Z1] probably because at least some calcium is necessary for maintenance of the structural integrity of the cell membrane.[C8] Reintroduction of calcium following an interval of calcium-free perfusion results in immediate biochemical and functional myocardial damage. This phenomenon, described first by Zimmerman and Hulsman,[Z2] is known as the *calcium paradox*. Langer has shown that as little as $0.05 \ mmol \cdot l^{-1}$ ($0.1 \ mEq \cdot l^{-1}$) in the cardioplegic solution can prevent such damage.[L9] Therefore, a free ionic concentration of calcium of about $0.25 \ mm \cdot l^{-1}$ ($0.5 \ mEq \cdot l^{-1}$) is desirable. The solution may be made slightly hyperosmotic (330–350 mosmol $\cdot \ l^{-1}$) by adding mannitol. Osmolarity in this range has been shown to retard the development of interstitial and intracellular edema during and after the period of ischemia.[P5,P6] Magnesium, in concentrations of 15 $mEq \cdot l^{-1}$, is recommended by Hearse and colleagues, since it produces cardioplegia by blocking calcium entry into the cell.[H15]

Some buffering capacity probably should be present, because the continuing (albeit small) metabolic activity during ischemia tends gradually to increase intracellular and extracellular acidosis, which is detrimental to function and to recovery from ischemia. Buffering capacity can be achieved by incorporating a bicarbonate-carbonate buffer. Tris(hydroxymethyl)aminomethane (TRIS) may be used, but it may have a positive ionotropic effect independent of any pH change, due probably to an increased release of tissue catecholamines and/or increased sensitivity of myocardial cells to catecholamines,[B11] although the experimental results from Follette, Buckberg, and colleagues[F1] deny this. Since TRIS is eliminated rather slowly, in part because of its intracellular as well as extracellular distribution,[H12,N5,R12] its possible ionotropic action could increase myocardial energy use during the ischemic arrest period and during reperfusion. Histidine is theoretically a superior buffer in this situation, since it remains active at low temperatures,[S13] while TRIS does not. Experiments by Tait and colleagues indicate that in fact myocardial protection is improved by using histidine as the buffer in the cardioplegic solution,[T8] as recommended by Bretschneider.[B18]

The solution may contain $500 \text{ mg} \cdot dl^{-1}$ of glucose, a concentration similar to that in the whole body perfusate (see Chapter 4). Its advantages are controversial.

Procaine produces cardioplegia when introduced into the heart in high concentrations and is said to have a membrane-stabilizing effect. The effect of procaine on the myocardial cell persists despite its washout by collateral flow.[B10] Its advantages are controversial, and it is not at present approved for intravenous use by the Federal Drug Administration in the United States.

Albumin may be beneficial in a physiologic concentration because of its role in preventing interstitial edema and because it has some buffering capacity. An albumin-containing solution may be used for infants and children, and a non–colloid-containing one for adults (UAB) (Table 3-2).

The St. Thomas's Hospital solution[J3] may be used because

Table 3-3 St. Thomas's cardioplegic solution (GLH). (St. Thomas Hospital, London, England)

Substance	Content ($mmol \cdot l^{-1}$)
Sodium chloride	144.3
Potassium chloride	19.6
Magnesium chloride	15.7
Calcium chloride	2.2
Procaine hydrochloride	0.05

it is simple to prepare and sterilize and is clinically satisfactory (GLH) (Table 3-3).

Modifications of the Cardioplegic Solution

Modified Blood as the Cardioplegic Solution
There has been considerable enthusiasm for using pump-oxygenator blood modified by adding an appropriate amount of K^+ as the cardioplegic solution.[C17,C18,E5,F4,F7,F10,I2,R18,S16,T9] However, the matter remains controversial, with some clinical studies showing no difference between blood and crystalloid cardioplegic solutions[N10] or an actual advantage of crystalloid cardioplegic solutions.[B15] Certainly, cardioplegic solutions containing red blood cells allow greater oxygen consumption by the arrested heart than do those without the cells, and this appears to be the only advantage of blood cardioplegia.[B25]

Currently, crystalloid cardioplegic solutions continue to be used (UAB, GLH). A clear solution may avoid some capillary blockage that could occur from sludging of red blood cells. The oxygenator blood probably contains considerable endogenously created catecholamines,[T2,T3] which might increase transmembrane calcium influx and thereby increase energy use during ischemia[F5,K9,S9] and might provoke additional damage during reperfusion.[K10,S3,S10,S11,T5,W2] Asanguineous cardioplegia interferes less with visibility during cardiac surgery.

Oxygenated Crystalloid Solutions
It is possible by simple techniques to oxygenate the crystalloid cardioplegic solution. Balderman and colleagues have shown better myocardial protection with oxygenated solutions than with simple aerated solutions.[B21] Oxygenated solutions may be incorporated safely into the clinical situation, provided a bubble trap is placed in the cardioplegic line to the patient (UAB).

Verapamil
A number of studies suggest the value of verapamil as an enhancement to cold cardioplegia, presumably because of its effect in blocking the slow-channel transport of calcium into the cell during reperfusion,[L14,N9,R14] and in preserving high energy stores.[B24] The verapamil is given as pretreatment; in some patients, it is added to the cardioplegic solution;[H16,L10] and in others, it is given just before reperfusion.[B22] Such an adjuvant is said to be particularly useful in neonatal hearts,[L10] in women undergoing coronary artery bypass grafting,[H16] and in other high-risk situations. The data are sufficiently suggestive of benefit that verapamil can be con-

Table 3-2 Solutions for cardioplegia (UAB).

Substance	Content ($mEq \cdot l^{-1}$)	Substance	Content ($g \cdot l^{-1}$)
With Albumin			
Sodium	100	Glucose	5
Potassium	30	Albumin	50
Chloride	84	Mannitol	5
Bicarbonate-carbonate (5:1)	28		
Calcium (total)	1.4		
Without Albumin			
Sodium	110	Glucose	5
Potassium	30	Mannitol	9.9
Chloride	85		
Bicarbonate-carbonate	27		
Calcium	1		

NOTE: Osmolarity = 330–350; pH = 7.5–7.55 at 37°C; Pco_2 = 40.

sidered for routine use in some manner in conjunction with cold cardioplegia (UAB).

Other Calcium Channel Blockers

Nifedipine probably has a beneficial effect similar to that of verapamil as an additive to the cardioplegic solution.[C10,M12] Clark and colleagues have demonstrated experimentally the beneficial effects of nifedipine used in this manner.[C11] Their randomized clinical trial suggested an advantage in using nifedipine in the cardioplegic solution but was not conclusive in this regard.[C12] Lidoflazine, another calcium channel blocking agent, has also been shown experimentally to be beneficial as a pretreatment.[K13]

Propranolol

Many studies have suggested that propranolol in the cardioplegic solution has additional beneficial effect.[K12]

Cortisone

Because of its presumed membrane-stabilizing effects, cortisone is included in many cardioplegic solutions.[A6]

Glutamate

The amino acid L-glutamate has been shown experimentally to improve aerobic and anaerobic metabolism when used to enrich a blood cardioplegic solution.[H18,L11,L12,R20,R22,R23] A clinical study also supports the advantage of using glutamate in this setting.[R19]

Warm Blood Induction of Cardioplegia

Rosenkranz, Buckberg, and colleagues have demonstrated experimentally that the warm blood induction of cardioplegia for the first 5 minutes after placing the aortic cross-clamp optimizes the conditions for recovery of function in the postischemic period. The use of this method, combined with the experimentally demonstrated advantages of a brief initial reperfusion with warm blood cardioplegic solution,[F8,L13] has been shown clinically to be advantageous when coronary artery bypass grafting is done for patients in cardiogenic shock.[R19] This method may therefore be useful in this setting, although as yet it is not widely used.

Oxygen-Free Radical Scavengers

Ischemic and reperfusion injuries involve the interaction of hydrogen ions and oxygen-free radicals.[H17] Within 5 seconds of the onset of myocardial ischemia, there is a rapid decrease in myocardial pH.[C15,G8] With the decrease in molecular oxygen that occurs simultaneously, there is an increased production of highly cytotoxic oxygen-free radicals.[D3,F9,P10] Superoxide anion scavengers, such as superoxide dismutase, in combination with the hydroxyl radical scavenger mannitol, have been shown experimentally to be beneficial.[S18,G9] These may become clinically useful.

Technique of Inducing and Maintaining Cold Cardioplegia

The perfusionist may be held responsible for the infusion of the cardioplegic solution (UAB). The pump-oxygenator is

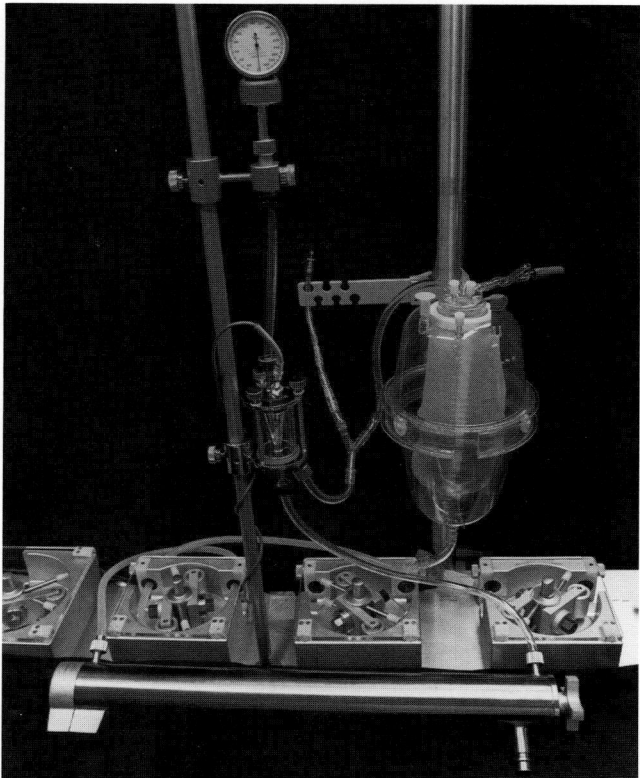

Figure 3-8 Pump-oxygenator assembly for infusion of the cardioplegic solution by the perfusionist (UAB). The cardioplegic solution is placed in (1) the commercially available reservoir. (2) A line from it passes through (3) the roller pump and (4) the heat exchanger. Cold water (4°C) circulates through the heat exchanger, and, since the cardioplegic solution is continuously recirculated, its temperature is 4–7°C. The solution is pumped through (5) a bubble trap containing (6) a thermistor for monitoring temperature and a manometer (7 is the line to it) for measuring pressure in the infusion line. (8) The line to the patient, shown with (9) the aortic cardioplegic needle on it, is kept clamped during recirculation back to the reservoir. When a cardioplegic infusion is desired, the perfusionist shifts this clamp to the recirculation line and increases (3) pump speed appropriately.

assembled with a separate small heat exchanger in a recirculating line with its own pump and reservoir and a thermistor probe incorporated within a bubble trap (Fig. 3-8). Before its infusion, the cardioplegic solution is recirculated and brought to about 5°C.

Alternatively, the cardioplegic solution may be infused by the anesthesiologist from a 1-liter plastic bag pressurized by an inflatable cuff (GLH). The bags are immersed in an iced water bucket before use. Standard intravenous tubing containing a bubble trap constitutes the infusion line (Fig. 3-9).

Cardiopulmonary bypass is begun at a temperature of about 34°C (see Chapter 2), and the perfusate temperature is made as cold as possible after the flow rate has been stabilized. A fine myocardial thermistor may routinely be introduced, just to the right or left of the lower one-third of the left anterior descending coronary artery into the anterior

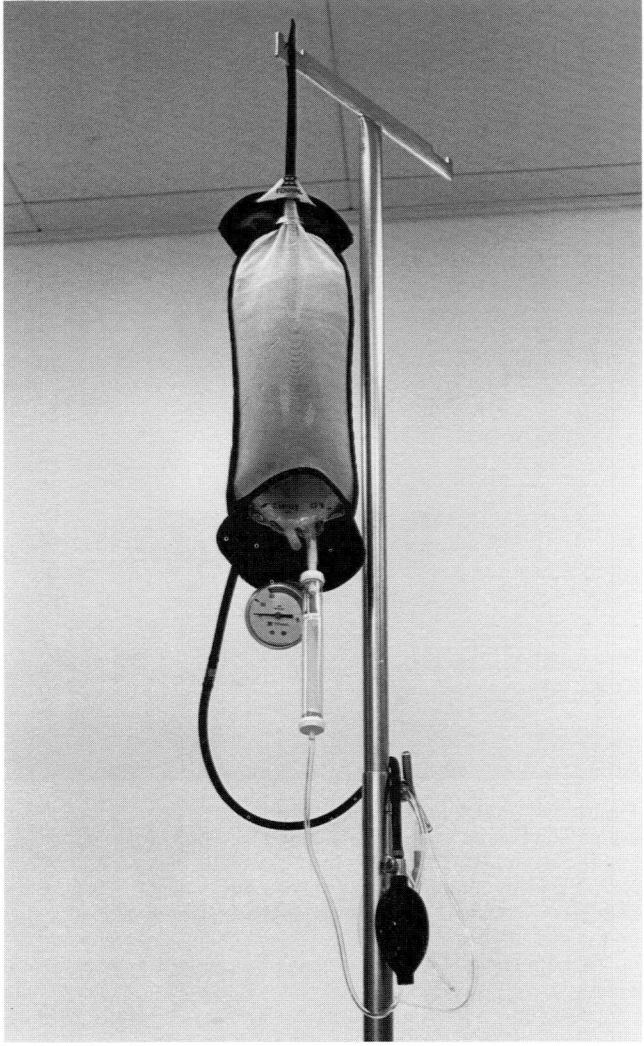

Figure 3-9 The cardioplegic infusion system in use at GLH. The 1-liter cardioplegic solution bag is removed from iced water immediately before use and is pressurized with an appropriately shaped cuffed bag that incorporates a pressure gauge. A standard intravenous set delivers the solution to the patient.

portion of the ventricular septum for continuous recording of myocardial temperature (GLH). However, it must be remembered that this temperature does not represent that of the entire myocardium and that under some circumstances significant temperature gradients exist during clinical use of cold cardioplegia. Nevertheless, after experience has been gained with a particular method, myocardial temperature during cardioplegia can be reasonably predicted, and its measurement may be omitted under usual circumstances (UAB). A catheter for the introduction of cold (4°C) saline solution for external cooling is positioned behind the heart. The saline solution may be sucked out intermittently (UAB), or it may be removed through a suction catheter and controlled by the perfusionist via a separate suction pump (GLH).

During this phase, the heart is beating, and the left atrial pressure is maintained as low as is possible.

The cardioplegic line is filled, and a short needle is positioned in the proximal ascending aorta through a previously placed purse-string suture of 4-0 polypropylene (Fig. 2-19) and secured. Alternatively, the needle may be positioned in the ascending aorta before CPB is begun (UAB). The aortic cross-clamp is applied, momentarily reducing the whole body perfusion flow to $0.5\ l \cdot min^{-1} \cdot m^{-2}$, in part to assist accurate placement of the clamp. The left ventricle, if distended, is quickly emptied by suction on the cardioplegic line or the left ventricular vent.

Infusion of the cold cardioplegic solution is begun *immediately* thereafter. The perfusionist may set the initial flow rate at $500\ ml \cdot min^{-1} \cdot m^{-2}$ (in order to distend the aortic root and close the aortic valve) and then, in about 5 seconds, at $450\ ml \cdot min^{-1} \cdot m^{-2}$ ($300\ ml \cdot min^{-1} \cdot m^{-2}$ for children less than 15 years old) (UAB). The surgeon continually monitors pressure in the ascending aorta, either digitally or by inserting a recording needle, attempting to keep it at about 70 mmHg by increasing or decreasing the cardioplegic flow as needed. The concepts of cardioplegic flow presented under "Individual Coronary Artery Perfusion with Normothermia or Moderate Hypothermia" apply here. Thus, greater reliance is placed on the aortic root perfusion pressure during the infusion than on the flow rate. The cardioplegic infusion may be continued for 3 minutes or until $450\ ml \cdot m^{-2} \times 3$ of solution ($300\ ml \cdot m^{-2} \times 3$ in children less than 15 years old) has been infused, whichever occurs first (UAB). Alternatively, the initial infusion is 1 liter in adults, approximately 500 ml in children, and approximately $15\ ml \cdot kg^{-1}$ in infants (GLH). Ideally, myocardial temperature should be lowered to about 12°C by the end of the infusion. The cardioplegic efflux from the coronary sinus may be allowed to return to the pump-oxygenator via the venous cannulae, except in infants and young children, in whom, through the opened right atrium, it is aspirated from the coronary sinus with a high-powered sucker and discarded (UAB). The cardioplegic efflux may be allowed to escape from the right atrium by loosening one of the caval cannula purse-string sutures (caval tapes are in place) and discarded (GLH). A method of scavenging the cardioplegic solution from the right heart has been shown to be effective in preventing patient hyperkalemia during the cardiac reperfusion period.[K14]

External cardiac cooling is begun promptly to keep the heart cold during cross-clamping. Some portions of the heart may not cool as rapidly as the septum, especially in the presence of coronary artery occlusions, and the cold irrigation facilitates cooling of these areas.

Rewarming of the myocardium must be minimized during cardioplegia. Rewarming occurs in part from direct heat transference from the surrounding lungs and mediastinal tissues. It also results from the collateral coronary flow[B12] from mediastinal branches that join the coronary arteries. This bleeds back from both the coronary ostia and the coronary sinus and may be large in patients with extensive coronary artery disease, cyanotic heart disease or extensive pericardial adhesions. In addition, excessive flow may pass through bronchial and large aortopulmonary collateral arteries, particularly in patients with cyanotic congenital heart disease, which produces a large return to the left atrium via the pulmonary veins. This blood passes into the aortic root and may produce sufficient pressure to perfuse the coronary arteries. If systemic venous blood in any amount is allowed to enter the right atrium, the coronary arteries may be perfused in a retrograde fashion via the coronary sinus.

The interplay of these factors necessitates constant observation of the heart, including its temperature and intracavitary pressures, and the manipulation of a number of variables. Thus,

1. The nasopharyngeal temperature (and that of the whole body perfusate) ideally should be kept between 20°C and 25°C. The lower the temperature, the more effective the myocardial cooling but the longer the period of rewarming CPB necessary to avoid a significant postbypass fall in temperature.

2. The CPB flow may be reduced (to less than $1.5 \, l \cdot min^{-1} \cdot m^{-2}$) to reduce collateral flow. Occasionally, the latter may be so large as to provoke the early reappearance of electromechanical activity and to interfere with surgical exposure. It may also then overdistend the right atrium if caval tapes have been used. For this reason, if, in an operation such as coronary artery bypass grafting procedures, caval taping is used (GLH), the inferior vena cava tape must be released after the cardioplegic infusion is completed so that coronary sinus return is picked up by the inferior vena caval line.

3. Systemic venous return should be totally diverted from the right atrium, either by attaining a zero or negative venous pressure with a properly positioned single two-stage venous cannula (UAB; see Chapter 2, Section 3), or by using two venous cannulae with caval taping (GHL).[B23]

4. The flow rate of the cold pericardial irrigation should be increased (to about 500 ml every 15 minutes) if the heart begins to warm too promptly. If a corrugated rubber or plastic foam sheet is used to insulate the heart from the lungs (GLH), the cold pericardial irrigation is surprisingly effective.[R16]

5. The left atrial vent (when present) must be run at an appropriate level to keep the left atrium and aorta empty; or intermittent suction must be placed on the cardioplegic needle in the ascending aorta to decompress the left heart.

6. Further infusions of cardioplegic solution at 4°C are given. The solution should be *reinfused* about every 30 minutes,[F2,N6] but if electrical activity returns or the temperature rises above 20°C before 30 minutes have elapsed, reinfusion is begun promptly. This procedure not only reduces the cardiac temperature again toward 8°C and produces total cardioplegia by reestablishing the buffered ionic milieu of the solution, but it also washes out blood that has entered the coronary arteries. Before reinfusion, the heart is returned to its normal position to allow the aortic valve to be competent and to prevent kinking of the left coronary artery.

7. The deliberate rewarming of the patient by the perfusate toward the end of the intracardiac procedure should be delayed until about 5 minutes before the aortic cross-clamp is removed, to prevent premature myocardial rewarming.[B17]

Coronary air embolization will occur each time the cardioplegic solution is reinfused if the heart has been opened, unless positive steps can be taken to avoid it. When the aortic root is accessible from below (e.g., when a ventricular septal defect is being repaired), air embolization can be minimized by filling the aortic root with fluid and rendering the aortic valve incompetent as the cardioplegic infusion begins. In some operations, for example, mitral valve surgery, there is no way of avoiding some coronary air embolization. Aortic valve surgery is discussed in "Technique in Patients with Aortic Valve Incompetence." Coronary air embolization may occur, even when the heart is not opened, should air enter the aorta around the cardioplegic needle when suction is applied to it inappropriately.

Technique in Patients with Aortic Valve Incompetence

In patients with aortic incompetence of any more than a very mild degree, and usually when aortic valve replacement is to be done for any cause, the cardioplegic solution is injected into the left and right coronary arteries individually through cannulae in their ostia. In one method, a Y connector is placed on the cardioplegic line (UAB). One arm of the Y connector is connected to the cardioplegic needle and the other to an O-ring coronary perfusion cannula. After establishing CPB, the perfusate temperature is reduced. The cardioplegic needle is placed in the ascending aorta, and the line to the O-ring cannula is clamped. The aorta is cross-clamped, the left ventricle emptied by suction on the left ventricular vent, external cardiac cooling begun, the aortic needle vent line clamped, and the aortic root opened transversely just downstream of the commissural attachments of the aortic cusps. The line to the O-ring cannula is filled, the cannula is inserted into the left coronary ostium, and three-fourths of the usual dose is given (see the discussion of dose under "Technique of Inducing and Maintaining Cold Cardioplegia"). The cannula is then inserted into the right coronary ostium, and about one-third of the usual dose is given. Subsequent reperfusions are performed in a similar manner.

Alternatively, individually placed coronary cannulae may be used (GLH). For this, King cannulae,[K11] held in place with a stay stitch passed around each line and secured with a rubber snugged from outside the aortic wall,[B13] are used. To prevent air embolization into the anteriorly placed right coronary artery, only the left coronary cannula is attached to a Y connector and infused at full pressure (70 mmHg, monitored by a needle in the tubing just proximal to the Y connector). The other opening of the Y connector is occluded with a finger, and with the right hand the heart is gently massaged. Usually, blood mixed with cardioplegic solution rapidly backfills the right coronary cannula, which is then connected to the Y connector without entrapping air. The infusion is now continued through both coronary arteries. When completed, the cannulae are left in position but disconnected from the Y connector and thus allowed to bleed back freely.

When a subsequent infusion is required, the left and sometimes both lines are already filled with blood, and air entrapment is easily avoided by using the same sequence described above. Precautions to avoid infusing only one branch of the left coronary artery are as necessary here as when using continuous coronary perfusion, and three cannulae may sometimes be necessary (GLH).

When aortic incompetence is mild in patients requiring aortic valve replacement or other operations, the initial cardioplegic infusion may be administered in the usual way, with a single needle into the aortic root proximal to the clamp (GLH). The left atrial line (with its tip in the left ventricle) is disconnected from the pump tubing and allowed to discharge into the pericardial space; in this way, significant reflux into the left ventricle is immediately apparent. If the infusion maintains an adequate pressure in the aortic root, and thus confirms that runoff is minimal, the left atrial vent line is clamped, the infusion continued, and the left ventricle gently massaged manually during the infusion period. This prevents left ventricular distention and assists in perfusing the coronary arteries. If runoff is excessive, the aortotomy is made and the cold-cardioplegic infusion given directly into the coronary ostia.

Technique in Patients Undergoing Coronary Artery Bypass Grafting

The cold cardioplegic reinfusions may be given directly into the aortic root. Alternatively, after the first aortic root infusion, the cardioplegic solution may be administered through the vein graft after each distal anastomosis (UAB); this procedure is advantageous in delivering the cardioplegic solution beyond areas of high-grade obstructive lesions in the coronary arterial tree.[R19] Experimental studies by Singh and colleagues identified no detrimental effect on vein patency or histologic appearance due to this alternative practice.

Myocardial Reperfusion after the Ischemic Period

The importance of the reperfusion phase is emphasized by the numerous studies quoted earlier, and by Follette, Buckberg, and colleagues' experimental demonstration of the favorable effect of modifying the reperfusate after an ischemic injury.[F1]

In preparation for myocardial reperfusion after the ischemic period, hemoglobin (Hb) level and base deficit are measured about 30 minutes before the estimated time of removal of the aortic cross-clamp. If the Hb level is less than 10 g · dl^{-1}, an appropriate amount (usually 250–500 ml) of packed red cells is added to the CPB circuit. Any base deficit is corrected with an appropriate amount of sodium bicarbonate. These maneuvers facilitate oxygen transport to the myocardium and prevent the deleterious effect of acidosis during myocardial reperfusion.[P7,S9,W3]

As the aortic cross-clamp is released after the repair (with a de-airing aortic stab wound or suction on the needle used for cardioplegic injections), the CPB flow rate is manipulated so that the arterial blood pressure is about 55 mmHg. After about 1 minute, the perfusate temperature is raised to 39°C, and thereafter arterial blood pressure is kept at about 80 mmHg, even if pharmacologic intervention (nitroprusside or Neo-Synephrine) is required. The maintenance of arterial blood pressure at 80 mmHg is necessary because some studies have shown that severe postischemic edema results when the reperfusion pressure is 100 mmHg after global ischemia.[E4] The intravenous infusion of nitroglycerine during this period has been found to be advantageous, probably because it produces some coronary vasodilation.

The left heart should be full of blood before the aorta is unclamped to prevent a significant amount of air from appearing in the aorta and to prevent coronary air embolization. As the aortic cross-clamp is released, the surgeon should palpate the heart frequently until it is beating well. Any evidence of right or left ventricular overdistention must immediately be relieved through the vent line or by the insertion of a large needle directly into the ventricle. Ventricular fibrillation, should it occur, is not allowed to persist, for a beating heart is preferable, and electrical defibrillation is usually possible even in a cold heart. The details of de-airing are described in Chapter 2.

If the cardioplegic infusions have been allowed to enter the CPB circuit, serum potassium levels of 6–7 mEq · l^{-1} may infrequently (in adults) exist at this stage. This is managed by a bolus injection of 400 mg of glucose per kilogram of body weight (as 50% glucose) and 0.2 units of soluble insulin per kilogram of body weight given 5 minutes after releasing the aortic clamp. As earlier studies suggest that both whole body intracellular potassium[P8] and circulating insulin levels[C3] are abnormally low at this point, these maneuvers are not unreasonable.

For 5 minutes or more after removal of the aortic cross-clamp, abnormalities of AV conduction, bizarre electrocardiographic patterns, and marked bradycardia are often present. These conditions result primarily from the potassium used for cardioplegia, but bizarre rhythms that persist for longer than a few minutes may signify errors in technique, particularly those resulting in coronary air embolism. These abnormalities disappear spontaneously, but this phase must end before the de-airing process can be effective or CPB discontinued. These effects may be due to inadequate protection of the sinus node and other conducting tissues, although they may be more frequent when procaine-containing solutions have been used. In patients with coronary artery disease, persistent bradycardia may also be related to preoperative beta-blockade treatment. These bradyarrhythmias are treated by promptly pacing the heart (atrially, or sequentially if necessary) at an adequate rate before discontinuing CPB.

OTHER MEASURES FOR THE PREVENTION OF MYOCARDIAL DAMAGE

Anesthetic and Supportive Management

Roe has shown that important myocardial necrosis can develop between induction of anesthesia and the start of CPB in as many as 30%–40% of patients undergoing coronary artery bypass grafting when anesthetic and supportive management is suboptimal,[R13] while Lell and colleagues have shown that this proportion can fall to 3% under optimum circumstances.[L5] No doubt patients other than those undergoing coronary artery bypass grafting are also at risk of developing myocardial damage during this period, particularly those with marked ventricular hypertrophy. Proper intraoperative management before and after CPB involves avoiding situations that increase myocardial oxygen demand (such as arterial hypertension, tachycardia, and increased endogenous catecholamine secretion due to anxiety and excitement); avoiding high ventricular end-diastolic pressures, with their detrimental effect on perfusion of the subendocardium;[H13] and provision of an optimal myocardial oxygen supply by maintaining adequate arterial oxygen levels and a ventricular preload that will result in a good cardiac output (see Chapter 4).

Early Postoperative Management

Important perioperative myocardial necrosis can develop after CPB, either before or after the patient leaves the operating room. Such necrosis may be precipitated by imbalances between myocardial oxygen demand and supply, as described under "Anesthetic and Supportive Management," and the same general measures described there are applicable early postoperatively. The use of catecholamines for the treatment of low cardiac output early after CPB can result in myocardial necrosis.[H14,M11,P9] The demonstration of the effectiveness and physiologic advantages[C10,D2,G6,N7] of intra-aortic balloon pulsation in treating many kinds of low cardiac output[B14,G5,K3,S12] makes this technique theoretically more desirable than the use of catecholamines (see Chapter 5).

SPECIAL SITUATIONS AND CONTROVERSIES

Myocardial Protection for Cardiac Operations in Neonates and Infants

Controversy continues about optimal methods for myocardial protection for cardiac operations in very young patients. In part, this is because (1) the myocardium of premature infants, neonates and young infants is different from that of mature patients; (2) the large number of different types of operations for the many types of congenital heart disease makes comparisons of different types of myocardial protection difficult; (3) the frequent use of ventriculotomies, atriotomies, and aortotomies introduces the possibility that cut coronary arteries and air embolization may play as important a role in producing myocardial damage as does the period of global myocardial ischemia.

Simple cold ischemic arrest may be preferred for all operations done with profoundly hypothermic total circulatory arrest (GLH). Experience at GLH has suggested that the use of cold cardioplegia with circulatory arrest techniques is associated with low postoperative cardiac output. It is to be noted that with circulatory arrest techniques (Chapter 2, Section 4), the cardioplegic solution is not washed out from the coronary bed by retrograde flow and remains in contact with the endothelium in undiluted form for the duration of the arrest period. Ebert and colleagues believe that profound myocardial cooling by the perfusate with or without a brief

period of ischemic arrest is safer for all infants than the use of cold cardioplegia.[E6]

Alternatively, cold cardioplegia may be used as a routine in essentially all operations in neonates and infants as well as in older patients (UAB). The study of Kirklin et al. showed that the use of cold cardioplegia was associated with a lesser hospital mortality than was intermittent aortic cross-clamping (Fig. 3-10) when cardiac ischemic times longer than about 40 minutes were required in infants less than 3 months of age.[K15] However, Bull et al. concluded from their study of mortality after pediatric cardiac surgery in general that there is no difference in mortality between the two methods.[B26]

Certainly, the immature myocardium presents special problems for myocardial protection, and, as suggested in earlier chapters, modifications of current techniques will probably be required.

Cardioplegia by Retrograde Coronary Sinus Infusion

Recent information and experiences suggest reconsideration of infusion of the cold cardioplegic solution retrograde into the coronary sinus. Albertal and colleagues have reported informally on the excellent results of this technique in all types of adult cardiac surgery. After the initial cardioplegic dose through the Foley catheter in the first portion of the coronary sinus, the solution is continuously infused at a low flow rate.[A9]

Retrograde perfusion of the coronary sinus by blood was used by Gott and colleagues in 1957.[G12] Subsequently several groups have shown that retroperfusion of the heart with blood or other nutrient media provides effective metabolic support.[B27,G11,H19,L15,L16,R24] Menasche and colleagues reported favorably on retroperfusing the cold cardioplegic solution through the coronary sinus in patients.[M13] More recently Gundry and colleagues concluded, from an animal study, that administration of the cardioplegic solution through the coronary sinus provides superior cooling and myocardial protection distal to coronary artery obstructions, when compared with the administration through the aortic root.[G10]

Situations in Which Cold Cardioplegia May Not Be an Ideal Technique

The cold cardioplegic technique may be used for essentially all cardiac operations, including those in infants (UAB). In a few very special situations, such as reoperation for replacement of a valved extracardiac conduit, dissection of the ascending aorta may be difficult. Since no intracardiac exposure is necessary, the operating is done without any aortic cross-clamping or cold cardioplegia (and for the same reasons, a single venous cannula is used).

In some additional situations, cold cardioplegia may not be considered the ideal technique (GLH). These situations are described below.

Moderate Aortic Incompetence Associated with Important Mitral Valve Disease

Patients with moderate aortic incompetence associated with important mitral valve disease require mitral valve repair or

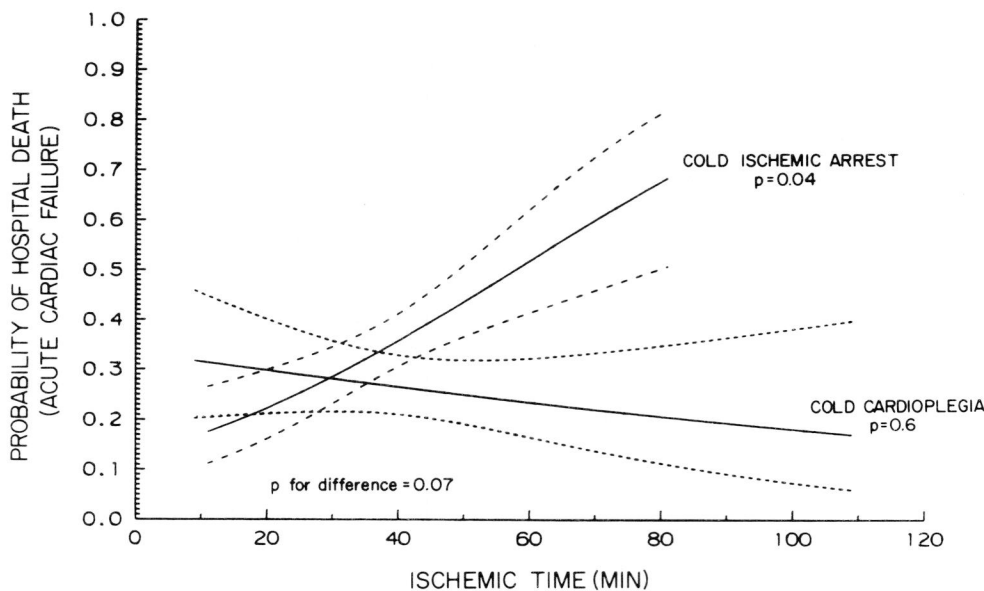

Figure 3-10 The effect of ischemic (aortic cross-clamp) time on the probability of hospital death with acute cardiac failure in infants less than 3 months of age undergoing open intracardiac repair. The solid lines indicate the point estimate, the dashed lines the 70% confidence limits. Note that, with a single period of cold ischemic arrest, a higher probability was evident when the cross-clamp time was about 35 minutes. With cold cardioplegia, there was no relationship between cross-clamp time and the probability of hospital death with cardiac failure. Note also that, when the cross-clamp time was less than 40 minutes, there was no difference between the two methods that could not be explained by chance.

Reproduced with permission from Kirklin JK et al[K15]; see original publication for equations and statistics.

replacement but not aortic valve replacement. When cold cardioplegia is used during the mitral valve surgery, the atonic left ventricle is liable to overdistend when the aortic cross-clamp is released, due to the runoff through the aortic valve. While a rise in left ventricular diastolic pressure can be controlled by increased suction on the left ventricular vent (when a left atrial vent is used, it is vital under such circumstances that its tip lie in the left ventricle), systemic blood flow and aortic pressure can be insufficient to maintain satisfactory coronary perfusion pressure despite an increase in total perfusion flow or the use of agents to increase peripheral vascular resistance. A vicious circle rapidly develops: the greater the perfusion flow, the greater the runoff through the vent line. If this situation develops, it can be controlled only by cross-clamping the aorta above the incompetent valve. The aortic valve must then be rendered competent, either by a "Frater stitch" (UAB; see below) or by valve replacement (GLH), or the myocardium can be revascularized by individual cannulation and perfusion of the coronary arteries (GLH).

At GLH, for these reasons, such patients are managed by elective artificial coronary artery perfusion (at 28°C with a beating heart). This procedure, of course, requires a deliberate aortic incision for cannulation and perfusion of the coronary arteries, following which the mitral valve is repaired or replaced and the left atrium closed. The beating, perfused heart is allowed to fill with blood by raising the right atrial pressure, and, when all air is excluded from the left heart, the left ventricle is contracting vigorously, the aortotomy has been closed, and the coronary cannulae has been removed, the cross-clamp is released. Despite the aortic incompetence, the ventricle will not overdistend, and CPB can be discontinued without problems. This form of management is considered in any patient with aortic incompetence that is likely to embarrass the left ventricle at the end of CPB but that is not per se severe enough to require aortic valve replacement (GLH).

An alternative method of managing this situation involves cross-clamping the aorta, opening the aortic route, and infusing the cold cardioplegic solution directly into the coronary ostia, as described under "Technique in Patients with Aortic Valve Incompetence" (UAB). After mitral replacement has been completed, the incompetent aortic valve is made temporarily competent by placing a "Frater stitch" through the central point of the leading edge of each leaflet and closing the aortotomy around the two ends of the untied suture, on which gentle traction is placed. The valve is then competent when the aortic cross-clamp is removed. After the heart is beating, the stitch is pulled out.

Mitral Valve Repair
Reconstructive techniques for correction of mitral incompetence[C9] are aided by careful preliminary examination of the mitral valve with the left ventricle in a normal tonic state. If the ventricle is atonic—and this is the case when a cold cardioplegic technique is used—the mitral valve can be

made to prolapse easily into the left atrium, and it is difficult to assess accurately the degree of leaflet prolapse, the length of chordae, or the type of repair required. A compromise may be adopted under such circumstances (GLH). The aorta is cross-clamped at 30°C, the heart is allowed to beat or fibrillate (the heart is evacuated via the left atrial vent), and the mitral valve is examined through the opened left atrium. Once the morphology has been accurately assessed and the repair decided on, the cold cardioplegic solution is injected into the aortic root in the usual way, and the pericardium is irrigated with cold electrolyte solution. The repair is then performed. It may be necessary to test the competence of the repaired valve with the ventricle again in tone; if so, the aortic clamp must be released and the heart kept fibrillating for a short period while this is done.

Active Rheumatic Pericarditis Necessitating Multiple Valve Surgery

Patients with active rheumatic pericarditis necessitating multiple valve surgery present special problems because of their extensive and very vascular pericardial adhesions, which, if divided, cause excessive bleeding and which contribute an excessive collateral coronary flow. Such patients are critically ill, usually with aortic and mitral incompetence. If cold cardioplegia is to be used, a low flow, profoundly hypothermic perfusion, and repeated cardioplegic infusions are necessary. Overall management is considered to be more satisfactory when conventional individual continuous coronary perfusion is used (GLH).

Short Procedures

There are a number of operations that can be accomplished within about 10 minutes, in which, it can be argued, elaborate maneuvers to protect the myocardium are of doubtful benefit because these measures in themselves necessitate a longer period of CPB, with its own potential problems (GLH). Such procedures include single coronary vein grafting, open mitral valvotomy, pulmonary valvotomy, valvotomy for congenital noncalcific aortic stenosis, and, possibly, surgery to correct uncomplicated atrial septal defect. In doubtful cases, the valve lesion or septal defect is exposed first using aortic cross-clamping with moderate or profound cardiac cooling (GLH). Should it then be apparent that repair will take longer than anticipated, the cold cardioplegic solution is infused before proceeding. Otherwise, the repair is completed expeditiously without infusing cardioplegic solution.

Combinations of Methods

In special situations, such as when a long or complex operation is being performed or the patient is at increased risk of hospital death, the use of combinations of methods for myocardial protection may be tempting. However, such combinations have usually proved to be disadvantageous. For example, the use of intermittent myocardial perfusion with blood combined with cold cardioplegia has not been an improvement over the standard method of cold cardioplegia. It may in fact produce more damage.

REFERENCES

A

1. Assad-Morell JL, Wallace RB, Elveback LR, Gau GT, Connolly DC, Barnhorst DA, Pluth JR, Danielson GK: Serum enzyme data in diagnosis of myocardial infarction during or early after aorta-coronary saphenous vein bypass graft operations. *J Thorac Cardiovasc Surg* 69:851, 1975.

2. Archie JP, Jr: Determinants of regional intramyocardial pressure. *J Surg Res* 14:338, 1973.

3. Appelbaum A, Kouchoukos NT, Blackstone EH, Kirklin JW: Early risks of open heart surgery for mitral valve disease. *Am J Cardiol* 37:201, 1976.

4. Adams PX, Cunningham JN Jr, Trehan NK, Brazier JR, Reed GE, Spencer FC: Clinical experience using potassium-induced cardioplegia with hypothermia in aortic valve replacement. *J Thorac Cardiovasc Surg* 75:564, 1978.

5. Adappa MG, Jacobson LB, Hetzer R, Hill JD, Kamm B, Kerth WJ: Cold hyperkalemic cardiac arrest versus intermittent aortic crossclamping and topical hypothermia for coronary bypass surgery. *J Thorac Cardiovasc Surg* 75:171, 1978.

6. Appelbaum A, Gotsman MS, Raz S, Ovil Y, Bosman JB: Protective effect of hydrocortisone on the myocardium during anoxic arrest. *Isr J Med Sci* 17:8, 1981.

7. Alfieri O, Vermeulen FEE, Kanepen PJ, De Geest R, Husymans HA, van Riempst ALEMSS: Extensive myocardial revascularization: Influence of cardioplegia on operative results. *Thorac Cardiovasc Surg* 28:343, 1980.

8. Akins CW: Noncardioplegic myocardial preservation for coronary revascularization. *J Thorac Cardiovasc Surg* 88:174, 1984.

9. Albertal, J: (1984) Personal communication.

B

1. Brewer DL, Bilbro RH, Bartel AG: Myocardial infarction as a complication of coronary bypass surgery. *Circulation* 47:58, 1973.

2. Blumgart HL, Gilligram DR, Schlesinger MJ: Experimental studies on the effect of temporary occlusion of coronary arteries. *Am Heart J* 22:374, 1941.

3. Buckberg GD, Olinger GN, Mulder DG, Maloney JV Jr: Depressed postoperative cardiac performance: Prevention by adequate myocardial protection during cardiopulmonary bypass. *J Thorac Cardiovasc Surg* 70:974, 1975.

4. Buckberg GD, Brazier JR, Nelson RL, Goldstein SM, McConnell DH, Cooper N: Studies of the effects of hypothermia on regional myocardial blood flow and metabolism during cardiopulmonary bypass. I. The adequately perfused beating, fibrillating, and arrested heart. *J Thorac Cardiovasc Surg* 73:87, 1977.

5. Barratt-Boyes BG, Harris EA, Kenyon AM, Lindop CR, Seelye ER: Coronary perfusion and myocardial metabolism during open-heart surgery in man. *J Thorac Cardiovasc Surg* 72:133, 1976.

6. Burton AC: Physiology and biophysics of the circulation. Chicago: Year Book, 1965, p 81.

7. Brody WR, Reitz BA: Topical hypothermic protection of the myocardium. *Ann Thorac Surg* 20:66, 1975.

8. Bretschneider J, Hubner G, Knoll D, Lohr B, Nordbeck H, Spiekerman PG: Myocardial resistance and tolerance to ischemia: Physiological and biochemical basis. *J Cardiovasc Surg* 16:241, 1975.

9. Braimbridge MV, Chayen J, Bitensky L, Hearse DJ, Jynge P, Cankovic-Darracott S: Cold cardioplegia or continuous coronary perfusion? Report on preliminary clinical experience as assessed cytochemically. *J Thorac Cardiovasc Surg* 74:900, 1977.

10. Buckberg GD: A proposed "solution" to the cardioplegic controversy. *J Thorac Cardiovasc Surg* 77:803, 1979.

11. Beierholm EA, Grantham RN, O'Keefe DD, Laver MB, Daggett WM: Effects of acid-base changes, hypoxia, and catecholamines on ventricular performance. *Am J Physiol* 228:1555, 1975.

12. Brazier J, Hottenrott C, Buckberg G: Noncoronary collateral myocardial blood flow. *Ann Thorac Surg* 19:426, 1975.

13. Barratt-Boyes BG: A method for preparing and inserting a homograft aortic valve. *Br J Surg* 52:847, 1965.

14. Buckley MJ, Leinbach RC, Kastor JA, Laird JD, Kantrowitz AR, Madras PN, Sanders CA, Austen WG: Hemodynamic evaluation of intra-aortic balloon pumping in man. *Circulation* 41(suppl II):II-130, 1970.

15. Buttner EE, Karp RB, Reves JG, Oparil S, Brummett C, McDaniel HG, Smith LR, Kreusch G: A randomized comparison of crystalloid and blood-containing cardioplegic solutions in 60 patients. *Circulation* 69:973, 1984.

16. Balderman SC, Bhayan JN, Binette P, Chan A, Gage AA: Perioperative preservation of myocardial ultrastructure and high-energy phosphates in man. *J Thorac Cardiovasc Surg* 82:860, 1981.

17. Borst HG, Iversen ST: Myocardial temperatures in clinical cardioplegia. *Thorac Cardiovasc Surg* 28:1, 1980.

18. Bretschneider HJ: Myocardial protection. *Thorac Cardiovasc Surg* 28:295, 1980.

19. Blackstone EH, Kirklin JW: Death and other time-related events after valve replacement. (1985) Unpublished study.

20. Balderman SC, Binette JP, Chan AWK, Gage AA: The optimal temperature for preservation of the myocardium during global ischemia. *Ann Thorac Surg* 35:605, 1983.

21. Bodenhamer RM, DeBoer LWV, Geffin GA, O'Keefe DD, Fallon JT, Aretz TH, Haas GS, Daggett WM: Enhanced myocardial protection during ischemic arrest: Oxygenation of a crystalloid cardioplegic solution. *J Thorac Cardiovasc Surg* 85:769, 1983.

22. Bolling SF, Schirmer WJ, Gott VL, Flaherty JT, Bulkley BH, Gardner TJ: Enhanced myocardial protection with verapamil prior to postischemic reflow. *Surgery* 94:283, 1983.

23. Bennett EV Jr, Fewel JG, Grover FL, Trinkle JK: Myocardial preservation: Effect of venous drainage. *Ann Thorac Surg* 36:132, 1983.

24. Balderman SC, Chan AK, Gage AA: Verapamil cardioplegia: Improved myocardial preservation during global ischemia. *J Thorac Cardiovasc Surg* 88:57, 1984.

25. Bing OHL, LaRai PJ, Stroughton FJ, Weintraub RM: Mechanism of myocardial protection during blood-potassium cardioplegia: A comparison of crystalloid red cell and methemoglobin solutions. *Circulation* 70(suppl 1):1–84, 1984.

26. Bull C, Cooper J, Stark J: Cardioplegia protection of the child's heart. *J Thorac Cardiovasc Surg* 88:287, 1984.

27. Bates RJ, Toscano M, Balderman SC, Anagnostopoulos CE: The cardiac veins and retrograde coronary venous perfusion (collective review). *Ann Thorac Surg* 23:83, 1977.

C

1. Cooley DA, Reul GJ, Wukasch DC: Ischemic contracture of the heart: "Stone heart." *Am J Cardiol* 29:575, 1972.

2. Chance B: The energy-linked reactions of calcium with mitochondria. *J Biol Chem* 240:2729, 1965.

3. Chiu RC, McArdle HA: Levels of plasma cyclic AMP and insulin in cardiac surgery. *J Thorac Cardiovasc Surg* 75:286, 1978.

4. Chawla SK, Najafi H, Javid H, Serry C: Coronary obstruction secondary to direct cannulation. *Ann Thorac Surg* 23:135, 1977.

5. Cohn LH, Collins JJ Jr: Local cardiac hypothermia for myocardial protection. *Ann Thorac Surg* 17:135, 1974.

6. Conti VR, Bertranou E, Blackstone EH, Kirklin JW, Digerness SB: Cold cardioplegia vs. hypothermia as myocardial protection: Randomized clinical study. *J Thorac Cardiovasc Surg* 76:577, 1978.

7. Craver JM, Sams AB, Hatcher CR Jr: Potassium-induced cardioplegia: Additive protection against ischemic myocardial injury during coronary revascularization. *J Thorac Cardiovasc Surg* 76:24, 1978.

8. Carafoli E: The interaction of Ca^{2+} with mitochondria, with special reference to the structural role of Ca^{2+} in mitochondrial and other membranes. *Mol Cell Biochem* 8:133, 1975.

9. Chatterjee S, Rosenswig J: Evaluation of intra-aortic balloon counterpulsation. *J Thorac Cardiovasc Surg* 61:405, 1971.

10. Clark RE, Ferguson BA, West PN, Shuchleik RC, Henry PD: Pharmacologic preservation of the ischemic heart. *Ann Thorac Surg* 24:307, 1977.

11. Clark RE, Christlieb IY, Spratt JA, Henry PD, Fischer AE, Williamson JR, Sobel BE: Myocardial preservation with nifedipine: A comparative study at normothermia. *Ann Thorac Surg* 31:3, 1981.

12. Clark RE, Christlieb IY, Fergusion TB, Weldon CS, Marbarger JP, Biello DR, Roberts R, Ludbrook PA, Sobel BE: The first American clinical trial of nifedipine in cardioplegia. *J Thorac Cardiovasc Surg* 82:848, 1981.

13. Conti VR, Kao RL: Metabolic and functional effects of carbohydrate substrate with single-dose and multiple-dose potassium cardioplegia. *Ann Thorac Surg* 36:320, 1983.

14. Chambers DJ, Darracott-Cankovic S, Braimbridge MV: Clinical and quantitative birefringence assessment of 100 patients with aortic clamping periods in excess of 120 minutes and hypothermic cardioplegic arrest. *Thorac Cardiovasc Surgeon* 31:266, 1983.

15. Cobbe SM, Poole-Wilson PA: The time of onset and severity of acidosis in myocardial ischemia. *J Mol Cell Cardiol* 12:745, 1980.

16. Casale AS, Bolling SF, Ru J, Flaherty JT, Bulkley BH, Jacobus WE, Gardner TJ: Progression and resolution of myocardial reflow injury. *J Surg Res* 37:94, 1984.

17. Catinella FP, Knoff EA, Cunningham JN Jr: Preservation of myocardial ATP during cardioplegia: Comparison of techniques. *J Cardiovasc Surg* 25:296, 1984.

18. Catinella FP, Cunningham JN Jr, Spencer FC: Myocardial protection during prolonged aortic cross-clamping. *J Thorac Cardiovasc Surg* 88:411, 1984.

D

1. Dixon SH Jr, Limbird LE, Roe CR, Wagner GS, Oldham HN Jr, Sabiston DC Jr: Recognition of postoperative acute myocardial infarction: Application of isoenzyme techniques. *Circulation* 47, 48(suppl III):III-137, 1973.

2. Dilley RB, Ross J Jr, Bernstein EF: Serial hemodynamics during intra-aortic balloon counterpulsation for cardiogenic shock. *Circulation* 47, 48(suppl III):III-99, 1973.

3. Demopoulos HB, Flamm ES, Pietronigro DD, Seligman ML: The free radical pathology and the microcirculation in the major central nervous system disorders. *Acta Physiol Scand [Suppl]* 492:91, 1980.

E

1. Ebert PA, Greenfield LJ, Austen WG, Morrow AG: Experimental comparison of methods for protecting the heart during aortic occlusion. *Ann Surg* 155:25, 1962.

2. Engelman RM, Levitsky S, O'Donoghue MJ, Auvil J: Cardioplegia and myocardial preservation during cardiopulmonary bypass. *Circulation* 58(suppl I):I-107, 1978.

3. Ellis RJ, Born M, Feit T, Ebert PA: Potassium cardioplegia: Early assessment by radionuclide ventriculography. *Circulation* 58(suppl I):I-57, 1978.

4. Engelman RM, Chandra R, Baumann FG, Goldman RA: Myocardial reperfusion: A cause of ischemic injury during cardiopulmonary bypass. *Surgery* 80:266, 1976.

5. Engelman RM, Rousou JH, Lemeshow S, Dobbs WA: The metabolic consequences of blood and crystalloid cardioplegia. *Circulation* 64(suppl II):II-67, 1981.

6. Ebert, PA: (1983) Personal communication.

F

1. Follette DM, Fey K, Livesay J, Nelson R, Maloney JV Jr, Buckberg GD: Reducing reperfusion injury with hypocalcemic, hyperkalemic, alkalotic blood during reoxygenation. *Surgical Forum* 29:284, 1978.

2. Follette DM, Fey K, Mulder DG, Maloney JV Jr, Buckberg GD: Prolonged safe aortic clamping by combining membrane stabilization, multidose cardioplegia and appropriate pH reperfusion. *J Thorac Cardiovasc Surg* 74:682, 1977.

3. Fisk RL, Gelfand ET, Callaghan JC: Hypothermic coronary perfusion for intraoperative cardioplegia. *Ann Thorac Surg* 23:58, 1977.

4. Follette DM, Mulder DG, Maloney JV Jr, Buckberg GD: Advantages of blood cardioplegia over continuous coronary perfusion or intermittent ischemia: Experimental and clinical study. *J Thorac Cardiovasc Surg* 76:604, 1978.

5. Fleckenstein A: Drug-induced changes in cardiac energy. *Adv Cardiol* 12:183, 1974.

6. Freedman BM, Pasque MK, Pellom GL, Deaton DW, Frame JR, Wechsler AS: Effects of delay in administration of potassium cardioplegia to the isolated rat heart. *Ann Thorac Surg* 37:309, 1984.

7. Feindel CM, Tait GA, Wilson GJ, Klement P, MacGregor DC: Multidose blood versus crystalloid cardioplegia: Comparison by quantitative assessment of irreversible myocardial injury. *J Thorac Cardiovasc Surg* 87:585, 1984.

8. Follette DM, Fey K, Buckberg GD, Helly JJ Jr, Steed DL, Foglia RP, Maloney JV Jr: Reducing postischemic damage by temporary modification of reperfusate calcium, potassium, pH, and osmolarity. *J Thorac Cardiovasc Surg* 81:493, 1981.

9. Fridovich I: Hypoxia and oxygen toxicity. *Adv Neurol* 26:255, 1979.

10. Fremes SE, Christakis GT, Weisel RD, Mickle DAG, Madonik MM, Ivanov J, Harding R, Seawright SJ, Houle S, McLaughlin PR, Baird RJ: A clinical trial of blood and crystalloid cardioplegia. *J Thorac Cardiovasc Surg* 88:726, 1984.

G

1. Gray RJ, Shell WE, Conklin C, Ganz W, Shah PK, Miyamoto AT, Matloff JM, Swan HJC: Quantification of myocardial injury during coronary artery bypass graft. *Circulation* 58(suppl II):II-38, 1978.

2. Griepp RB, Stinson EB, Shumway NE: Profound local hypothermia for myocardial protection during open-heart surgery. *J Thorac Cardiovasc Surg* 66:731, 1973.

3. Gay WA, Ebert PA: Functional, metabolic, and morphologic effects of potassium-induced cardioplegia. *Surgery* 74:184, 1973.

4. Gay WA: Potassium-induced cardioplegia. *Ann Thorac Surg* 20:95, 1975.

5. Gold HK, Leinbach RC, Buckley MJ, Mundth ED, Daggett WM, Austen WG: Refractory angina pectoris: Follow-up after intra-aortic balloon pumping and surgery. *Circulation* 54(suppl III):III-41, 1976.

6. Gill CC, Wechsler AS, Newman GE, Oldham HN Jr: Augmentation and redistribution of myocardial blood flow during acute ischemia by intraaortic balloon pumping. *Ann Thorac Surg* 16:445, 1973.

7. Gott VL, Dutton RC, Young WP: Myocardial rigor mortis as an indicator of cardiac metabolic function. *Surgical Forum* 13:172, 1962.

8. Garlick PB, Radda GK, Seeley PJ: Studies of acidosis in the ischemic heart by phosphorus nuclear magnetic resonance. *Biochem J* 184:547, 1979.

9. Gardner TJ, Stewart JR, Casale AS, Downey JM, Chambers DE: Reduction of myocardial ischemic injury with oxygen-derived free radical scavengers. *Surgery* 94:423, 1983.

10. Gundry SR, Kirsh MM: A comparison of retrograde cardioplegia versus antegrade cardioplegia in the presence of coronary artery obstruction. *Ann Thorac Surg* 38:124, 1984.

11. Gundry SR: Modification of myocardial ischemia in normal and hypertrophied hearts utilizing diastolic retroperfusion of the coronary veins. *J Thorac Cardiovasc Surg* 83:659, 1982.

12. Gott VL, Gonzalez JL, Zuhdi MN: Retrograde perfusion of the coronary sinus for direct-vision aortic surgery. *Surg Gynecol Obstet* 104:319, 1957.

H

1. Henson DE, Najafi H, Callaghan R, Coogan P, Julian OC, Eisenstein R: Myocardial lesions following open heart surgery. *Arch Pathol Lab Med* 88:423, 1969.

2. Hultgren HN, Miyagawa M, Buch W, Angell WW: Ischemic myocardial injury during cardiopulmonary bypass surgery. *Am Heart J* 85:167, 1973.

3. Hearse DJ, Garlick PB, Humphrey SM: Ischemic contracture of the myocardium: Mechanisms and prevention. *Am J Cardiol* 39:986, 1977.

4. Hutchins GM, Nazarian IH, Bulkley BH: Association of left dominant coronary arterial system with congenital bicuspid aortic valve. *Am J Cardiol* 42:57, 1978.

5. Hazan E, Rioux C, Dequirot A, Mathey J: Postperfusion steno-

sis of the common left coronary artery. *J Thorac Cardiovasc Surg* 69:703, 1975.

6. Hottentrot C, Maloney JV Jr, Buckberg GD: Studies of the effects of ventricular fibrillation on the adequacy of regional myocardial flow. I. Electrical vs. spontaneous fibrillation. *J Thorac Cardiovasc Surg* 68:615, 1974.

7. Harris EA, Parimelazhagan KN, Seelye ER, Barratt-Boyes BG: Optimization of coronary perfusion rate during cardiac surgery in man. *J Thorac Cardiovasc Surg* 77:662, 1979.

8. Hufnagel CA, Conrad PW, Schanno J, Pifarre R: Profound cardiac hypothermia. *Ann Surg* 153:790, 1961.

9. Hearse DJ, Stewart DA, Braimbridge MV: Cellular protection during myocardial ischemia: The development and characterization of a procedure for the induction of reversible ischemic arrest. *Circulation* 54:193, 1976.

10. Harlan BJ, Ross D, Macmanus Q, Knight R, Luber J, Starr A: Cardioplegic solutions for myocardial preservation: Analysis of hypothermic arrest, potassium arrest, and procaine arrest. *Circulation* 58(suppl I):I-114, 1978.

11. Holland CE, Olson RE: Prevention by hypothermia of paradoxical calcium necrosis in cardiac muscle. *J Mol Cell Cardiol* 7:917, 1975.

12. Holmdahl MH, Nahas GG: Volume of distribution of C^{14}-labeled tris (hydroxymethyl) aminomethane. *Am J Physiol* 202:1011, 1962.

13. Hoffman JIE: Determinants and prediction of transmural myocardial perfusion. *Circulation* 58:381, 1978.

14. Haft JI, Kranz PD, Albert FJ, Fani K: Intravascular platelet aggregation in the heart induced by norepinephrine: Microscopic studies. *Circulation* 46:698, 1972.

15. Hearse DJ, Stewart DA, Brainbridge MV: Myocardial protection during ischemic cardiac arrest: Importance of magnesium in cardioplegic infusates. *J Thorac Cardiovasc Surg* 75:877, 1978.

16. Hicks GL Jr, Salley RK, DeWeese JA: Calcium channel blockers: An intraoperative and postoperative trial in women. *Ann Thorac Surg* 37:319, 1984.

17. Hess ML, Manson NH, Okabe E: The role of free radicals in the pathophysiology of ischemic heart disease. *Can J Physiol Pharmacol* 60:1382, 1982.

18. Haas GS, DeBoer LWV, O'Keefe DD, Bodenhamer RM, Geffin GA, Drop LJ, Teplick RS, Daggett WM: Reduction of postischemic myocardial dysfunction by substrate repletion during reperfusion. *Circulation* 70(suppl I), I-65, 1984.

19. Hochberg MS, Austen WG: Selective retrograde coronary venous perfusion (collective review). *Ann Thorac Surg* 29:578, 1980.

I

1. Isom OW, Kutin WD, Falk EA, Spencer FC: Patterns of myocardial metabolism during cardiopulmonary bypass and coronary perfusion. *J Thorac Cardiovasc Surg* 66:705, 1973.

2. Iverson LIG, Young JN, Ennix CL Jr, Ecker RR, Moretti RL, Lee J, Hayes RL, Farrar MP, May RD, Masterson R, May IA: Myocardial protection: A comparison of cold blood and cold crystalloid cardioplegia. *J Thorac Cardiovasc Surg* 87:509, 1984.

J

1. Jennings RB, Sommers HM, Smyth GA, Flack HA, Linn H: Myocardial necrosis induced by temporary occlusion of a coronary artery in the dog. *Arch Pathol Lab Med* 70:82, 1960.

2. Jennings RB, Sommers HM, Herdson PB, Kaltenback JP: Ischemic injury of myocardium. *Ann NY Acad Sci* 156:61, 1969.

3. Jynge P, Hearse DJ, Braimbridge MV: Myocardial protection during ischemic cardiac arrest. *J Thorac Cardiovasc Surg* 73:848, 1977.

4. Jones RN, Attarian DE, Currie WD, Olsen CO, Hill RC, Sink JD, Wechsler AS: Metabolic deterioration during global ischemia as a function of time in the intact normal dog heart. *J Thorac Cardiovasc Surg* 81:264, 1981.

K

1. Katz AM, Tada M: The "stone heart" and other challenges to the biochemist. *Am J Cardiol* 39:1073, 1977.

2. Kirklin JW: *Nature of the Problem.* New York: *In:* Cardioplegia Workshop. An International Exchange of Ideas, June 23, 1979, Travenol Laboratories Inc., Publishers, Deerfield, Illinois, 1979, p 1.

3. Kantrowitz A, Tjonneland S, Freed PS, Phillips SJ, Butner AN, Sherman JL Jr: Initial clinical experience with intra-aortic balloon pumping in cardiogenic shock. *JAMA* 203:113, 1968.

4. Kronzon I, Deutsch P, Glassman E: Length of the left main coronary artery: Its relation to the pattern of coronary arterial distribution. *Am J Cardiol* 34:787, 1974.

5. Koster JK Jr, Cohn LH, Collins JJ Jr, Sanders JH, Muller JE, Young E: Continuous hypothermic arrest versus intermittent ischemia for myocardial protection during coronary revascularization. *Ann Thorac Surg* 24:330, 1977.

6. Kirsch U, Rodewald G, Kalmar P: Induced ischemic arrest: Clinical experience with cardioplegia in open-heart surgery. *J Thorac Cardiovasc Surg* 63:121, 1972.

7. Kay HR, Levine FH, Fallon JT, Grotte GJ, Butchart EG, Rao S, McEnany MT, Austen WG, Buckley MJ: Effect of cross-clamp time, temperature, and cardioplegic agents on myocardial function after induced arrest. *J Thorac Cardiovasc Surg* 76:590, 1978.

8. Kirklin JW, Conti VR, Blackstone EH: Prevention of myocardial damage during cardiac operations. *N Engl J Med* 301:135, 1979.

9. Katz AM, Repke DI: Calcium-membrane interactions in the myocardium: Effects of ouabain, epinephrine and 3',5'-cyclic adenosine monophosphate. *Am J Cardiol* 31:193, 1973.

10. Kloner RA, Ganote CE, Wahlen DA, Jennings RB: Effect of a transient period of ischemia on myocardial cells. II. Fine structure during the first few minutes of reflow. *Am J Pathol* 74:399, 1974.

11. King BJ: An improved coronary artery perfusion cannula. *J Thorac Cardiovasc Surg* 45:667, 1963.

12. Kanter KR, Flaherty JT, Bulkley BH, Gott VL, Gardner TJ: Beneficial effects of adding propranolol to multidose potassium cardioplegia. *Circulation* 64(suppl II):II-84, 1981.

13. Kates RA, Dorsey LM, Kaplan JA, Hatcher CR Jr, Guyton RA: Pretreatment with lidoflazine, a calcium-channel blocker: Useful adjunct to heterogenous cold potassium cardioplegia. *J Thorac Cardiovasc Surg* 85:278, 1983.

14. Kopman EA, Ferguson TB: Scavenging of cardioplegic solution from right heart to prevent hyperkalemia. *J Thorac Cardiovasc Surg* 86:153, 1983.

15. Kirklin JK, Blackstone EH, Kirklin JW, McKay R, Pacifico AD, Bargeron LM Jr: Intracardiac surgery in infants under age 3 months: Incremental risk factors for hospital mortality. *Am J Cardiol* 48:500, 1981.

L

1. Lie JT, Sun SC: Ultrastructure of ischemic contracture of the left ventricle ('stone heart'). *Mayo Clin Proc* 51:785, 1976.

2. Littlefield JB, Lowicki EM, Muller WH Jr: Experimental left coronary artery perfusion through an aortotomy during cardiopulmonary bypass. *J Thorac Cardiovasc Surg* 40:685, 1960.

3. Lesage CH Jr, Vogel JHK, Blount SG Jr: Iatrogenic coronary occlusive disease in patients with prosthetic heart valves. *Am J Cardiol* 26:123, 1970.

4. Langer GA: Kinetic studies of calcium distribution in ventricular muscle of the dog. *Circ Res* 15:393, 1964.

5. Lell WA, Walker DR, Blackstone EH, Kouchoukos NT, Allarde R, Roe CR: Evaluation of myocardial damage in patients undergoing coronary artery bypass procedures with halothane-N_2O anesthesia and adjuvants. *Anesth Analg* 56:556, 1977.

6. Lucas SK, Elmer EB, Flaherty JT, Prodromos CC, Bulkley BH, Gott VL, Gardner TJ: Effects of multiple-dose potassium cardioplegia on myocardial ischemia, return of ventricular function, and ultrastructural preservation. *J Thorac Cardiovasc Surg* 80:102, 1980.

7. Leaf A: Maintenance of concentration gradients and regulation of cell volume. *Ann NY Acad Sci* 72:396, 1959.

8. Laks H: (1984) Personal communication.

9. Langer GA: (1977) Personal communication.

10. Lupinetti FM, Hammon JW Jr, Huddleston CB, Boucek RJ Jr, Bender HW Jr: Global ischemia in the immature canine ventricle: Enhanced protective effect of verapamil and potassium. *J Thorac Cardiovasc Surg* 87:213, 1984.

11. Lazar HL, Buckberg GD, Manganaro AM, Becker H, Maloney JV Jr: Reversal of ischemic damage with amino acid substrate enhancement during reperfusion. *Surgery* 80:702, 1980.

12. Lazar HL, Buckberg GD, Manganaro AM, Becker H: Myocardial energy replenishment of secondary blood cardioplegic with amino acids during reperfusion. *J Thorac Cardiovasc Surg* 80:350, 1980.

13. Lazar HL, Buckberg GD, Manganaro A, Becker H, Mulder DG, Maloney JV Jr: Limitation imposed by hypothermia during recovery from ischemia. *Surgical Forum* 31:312, 1980.

14. Lange R, Ingwall J, Hale SL, Alker KJ, Braunwald E, Kloner RA: Preservation of high-energy phosphates by verapamil in reperfused myocardium. *Circulation* 70:734, 1984.

15. Lolley DM, Hewitt RL, Drapanas T: Retroperfusion of the heart with a solution of glucose, insulin and potassium during anoxic arrest. *J Thorac Cardiovasc Surg* 67:364, 1974.

16. Lolley DM, Hewitt RL: Myocardial distribution of asanguinous solutions retroperfused under low pressure through the coronary sinus. *J Cardiovasc Surg* (Torino) 21:287, 1980.

M

1. Moulder PV, Blackstone EH, Eckner FAO, Lev M: Pressure derivative loop for left ventriculur resuscitation. *Arch Surg* 96:323, 1968.

2. Martin AM Jr, Hackel DB: An electron microscopic study of the progression of myocardial lesions in the dog after hemorrhage shock. *Lab Invest* 15:243, 1966.

3. Miyamoto ATM, Robinson L, Matloff JM, Norman JR: Perioperative infarction: Effects of cardiopulmonary bypass on collateral circulation in an acute canine model. *Circulation* 58(suppl I):I-147, 1978.

4. Muller WH Jr, Warren WD, Dammann JF Jr, Beckwith JR,

Wood JE Jr: Surgical relief of aortic insufficiency by direct operation on the aortic valve. *Circulation* 21:587, 1960.

5. Murphy ES, Rosch J, Rahimtoola SH: Frequency and significance of coronary arterial dominance in isolated aortic stenosis. *Am J Cardiol* 39:505, 1977.

6. Midell AI, DeBoer A, Bermudez G: Postperfusion coronary ostial stenosis: Incidence and significance. *J Thorac Cardiovasc Surg* 72:80, 1976.

7. McGoon DC, Pestana C, Moffitt EA: Decreased risk of aortic valve surgery. *Arch Surg* 91:779, 1965.

8. McGoon DC: *Alternatives to Cardioplegia.* New York: *In:* Cardioplegia Workshop. An International Exchange of Ideas, June 23, 1979, Travenol Laboratories Inc., Publishers, Deerfield, Illinois, 1979, p 23.

9. Melrose DG, Dreyer B, Bentall HH, Baker JBE: Elective cardiac arrest. Preliminary communication. *Lancet* 2:21, 1955.

10. Mundth ED, Goel IP, Morgan RJ, McEnany MT, Austen WG: Effect of potassium cardioplegia and hypothermia on left ventricular function in hypertrophied and non-hypertrophied hearts. *Surgical Forum* 26:257, 1975.

11. Mueller HS, Evans R, Ayres SM: Effect of dopamine on hemodynamics and myocardial metabolism in shock following acute myocardial infarction in man. *Circulation* 57:361, 1978.

12. Macgovern GJ, Dixon CM, Burkholder JA: Improved myocardial protection with nifedipine and potassium-based cardioplegia. *J Thorac Cardiovasc Surg* 82:239, 1981.

13. Menasche P, Kural S, Fauchet M: Retrograde coronary sinus perfusion: A safe alternative for ensuring cardioplegic delivery in aortic valve surgery. *Ann Thorac Surg* 34:647, 1982.

N

1. Najafi H, Henson D, Dye WS, Javid H, Hunter JA, Callaghan R, Eisenstein R, Julian OC: Left ventricular hemorrhagic necrosis. *Ann Thorac Surg* 7:550, 1969.

2. Neutze JM, Drakely MJ, Barratt-Boyes BG, Hubbert K: Serum enzymes after cardiac surgery using cardiopulmonary bypass. *Am Heart J* 88:425, 1974.

3. Neely JR, Liedtke AJ, Whitman JT, Rovelto MJ: Relationship between coronary flow and adenosine triphosphate production from glycolysis and oxidative metabolism, in DE Roy, P Harris (eds): *The Cardiac Sarcoplasm*, vol 8. Baltimore: University Park, 1975, p 301.

4. Nelson RL, Goldstein SM, McConnell DH, Maloney JV Jr, Buckberg GD: Studies of the effects of hypothermia on regional myocardial blood flow and metabolism during cardiopulmonary bypass. V. Profound topical hypothermia during ischemia in arrested hearts. *J Thorac Cardiovasc Surg* 73:201, 1977.

5. Nahas GG: The pharmacology of tris (hydroxymethyl) aminomethane (tham). *Pharmacol Rev* 14:447, 1962.

6. Nelson R, Fey K, Follette D, Livesay JJJ, DeLand EC, Maloney JV Jr, Buckberg GD: The critical importance of intermittent infusion of cardioplegic solution during aortic cross-clamping. *Surgical Forum* 27:241, 1977.

7. Nicholas AB, Pohost GM, Gold HK, Leinbach RC, Beller GA, McKusick KA, Strauss HW, Buckley MJ: Left ventricular function during intra-aortic balloon pumping assessed by multigated cardiac blood pool imaging. *Circulation* 58(suppl I):I-176, 1978.

8. Nayler WB, Poole-Wilson PA, Williams A: Hypoxia and calcium. *J Mol Cell Cardiol* 11:683, 1979.

9. Nayler WG, Ferrari R, Williams A: Protective effect of pretreatment with verapamil, nifedipine and propranolol on mitochon-

drial function in the ischemic and reperfused myocardium. *Am J Cardiol* 46:242, 1980.

10. Nwaneri NJ, Levitsky S, Silverman NA, Feinberg H: Induction of cardioplegia with blood and crystalloid potassium solutions during prolonged aortic cross-clamping. *Surgery* 94:836, 1983.

O

1. Oldham HN Jr, Roe CR, Young WG Jr, Dixon SH Jr: Intraoperative detection of myocardial damage during coronary artery surgery by plasma creatine phosphokinase isoenzyme analysis. *Surgery* 74:917, 1973.

P

1. Pagliero M, Blackstone EH, Kirklin JW: Myocardial damage after cardiac surgery. (1976) Unpublished data.

2. Pagliero M, Blackstone EH, Conti VR, Kirklin JW: Myocardial damage after mitral valve replacement. (1976) Unpublished data.

3. Parr GVS, Blackstone EH, Kirklin JW: Cardiac performance and mortality early after intracardiac surgery in infants and young children. *Circulation* 51:867, 1975.

4. Pupello DF, Blank RH, Bessone LN, Connar RG, Carlton LM Jr: Local deep hypothermia for combined valvular and coronary heart disease. *Ann Thorac Surg* 21:508, 1976.

5. Powell WH, DiBona DR, Flores J, Frega N, Leaf A: Effects of hyperosmotic mannitol in reducing ischemic cell swelling and minimizing myocardial necrosis. *Circulation* 53(suppl I):I-45, 1976.

6. Powell WJ, DiBona DR, Flores J, Leaf A: The protective effect of hyperosmotic mannitol in myocardial ischemia and necrosis. *Circulation* 54:603, 1976.

7. Poole-Wilson PA, Langer GA: Effect of pH on ionic exchange and function in rat and rabbit myocardium. *Am J Physiol* 229:570, 1975.

8. Pacifico AD, Digerness S, Kirklin JW: Acute alterations of body composition after open intracardiac operations. *Circulation* 41:331, 1970.

9. Piscatelli RL, Fox LM: Myocardial injury from epinephrine overdosage. *Am J Cardiol* 21:735, 1968.

10. Pryor WA: The role of free radical reactions in biological system, in WA Pryor (ed): *Free Radicals in Biology*. New York: Academic, 1976, pp 1–49.

11. Pagliero KM, Blackstone EH, Kirklin JW: (1975) Unpublished observations.

R

1. Rosky LP, Rodman T: Medical aspects of open-heart surgery. *N Engl J Med* 274:833, 1966.

2. Roberts WC, Bulkley BH, Morrow AG: Pathologic anatomy of cardiac valve replacement: A study of 224 necropsy patients. *Prog Cardiovasc Dis* 15:539, 1973.

3. Rose GA, Blackburn H: *Cardiovascular Survey Methods: Belgium*. Geneva: World Health Organization, 1968, p 137.

4. Roe CR, Wagner GS, Young WG Jr, Curtis SE, Cobb FR, Irvin RG: The relationship of creatine kinase isoenzyme MB to the postoperative electrocardiographic diagnosis in patients undergoing coronary artery bypass surgery. *Circulation*, in press.

5. Righetti A, Crawford MH, O'Rourke RA, Hardarson T, Schelbert H, Daily PO, DeLuca A, Ashburn W, Ross J Jr: Detection of perioperative myocardial damage after coronary artery bypass graft surgery. *Circulation* 55:173, 1977.

6. Righetti A, O'Rourke RA, Schelbert H, Henning H, Hardarson T, Daily PO, Ashburn W, Ross J Jr: Usefulness of preoperative and postoperative Tc-99m (Sn)-pyrophosphate scans in patients with ischemic and valvular heart disease. *Am J Cardiol* 39:43, 1977.

7. Richardson JV, Kouchoukos NT, Wright JO III, Karp RB: Combined aortic valve replacement and myocardial revascularization: Results in 220 patients. *Circulation* 59:75, 1979.

8. Reed GE, Spencer FC, Boyd AD, Engelman RM, Glassman E: Late complications of intraoperative coronary artery perfusion. *Circulation* 47,48(suppl III):III-80, 1973.

9. Reidemeister JC, Heberer G, Bretschneider HJ: Induced cardiac arrest by sodium and calcium depletion and application of procaine. *Int Surg* 6:535, 1967.

10. Reidemeister JC, Heberer G, Gehl H, Thiele P: Klinische Ergebnisse mit der Kardioplegic durch extrazellularen Natriumund Calciumentzug und Procaingabe. *Langenbecks Arch Chir* 319:701, 1967.

11. Roe BB, Hutchinson JC, Fishman NH, Ullyot DJ, Smith DL: Myocardial protection with cold ischemic potassium-induced cardioplegia. *J Thorac Cardiovasc Surg* 73:366, 1977.

12. Robin ED, Wilson RJ, Bromberg PA: Intracellular acid-base relations and intracellular buffers. *Ann NY Acad Sci* 92:539, 1961.

13. Roe CR: Myocardial damage during induction of anesthesia. (1976) Unpublished data.

14. Robb-Nicholson C, Currie WD, Wechsler AS: The effects of verapamil in the myocardial tolerance to ischemic arrest. *Circulation* 58(suppl II):II-119, 1978.

15. Rosenfeldt FL, Arnold M, Fambiatos A, Stirling GR: Myocardial damage due to profound local hypothermia: Fact or fiction. Presented at a combined meeting of Royal Australasian College of Surgeons and Physicians, Sydney, February 24–29, 1980.

16. Rosenfeldt FL, Watson DA: Local cardiac hypothermia: Experimental comparison of Shumway's technique and perfusion cooling. *Ann Thorac Surg* 27:17, 1979.

17. Reduto LA, Lawrie GM, Reid JW, Whissenand HH, Noon GP, Kanon D, DeBakey ME, Miller RR: Sequential postoperative assessment of left ventricular performance with gated cardiac blood pool imaging following aortocoronary bypass surgery. *Am Heart J* 101:59, 1981.

18. Roberts AJ, Moran JM, Sanders JH, Spies SM, Lichtenthal PR, Kaplan KJ, Michaelis LL: Clinical evaluation of the relative effectiveness of multidose crystalloid and cold blood potassium cardioplegia in coronary artery bypass graft surgery: A non-randomized matched-pair analysis. *Ann Thorac Surg* 33:421, 1982.

19. Rosenkranz ER, Buckberg GD, Laks H, Mulder DG: Warm induction of cardioplegia with glutamate-enriched blood in coronary patients with cardiogenic shock who are dependent on inotropic drugs and intraaortic balloon support. *J Thorac Cardiovasc Surg* 86:507, 1983.

20. Rosenkranz ER, Okamoto F, Buckberg GD, Vinten-Johansen J, Edwards H, Bugyi H: Advantages of glutamate-enriched cold blood cardioplegia in energy-depleted hearts. *Circulation* 66 (suppl II):II-151, 1982.

21. Rosenkranz ER, Vinten-Johansen J, Buckberg GD, Okamoto F, Edwards H, Bugyi H: Benefits of normothermic induction of blood cardioplegia in energy-depleted hearts with maintenance of arrest by multidose cold blood cardioplegic infusions. *J Thorac Cardiovasc Surg* 84:667, 1982.

22. Robertson JM, Vinten-Johansen J, Buckberg GD, Rosenkratz

ER, Maloney JV Jr: Safety of prolonged aortic clamping with blood cardioplegia. *J Thorac Cardiovasc Surg* 88:395, 1984.

23. Rosenkratz ER, Okamoto F, Buckberg GD, Vinten-Johansen J, Robertson JM, Bugyi H: Safety of prolonged aortic clamping with blood cardioplegia. *J Thorac Cardiovasc Surg* 88:402, 1984.

24. Rhodes GR, Syracuse DC, McIntosh CL: Evaluation of regional myocardial nutrient perfusion following selective retrograde arterialization of the coronary vein. *Ann Thorac Surg* 25:329, 1978.

S

1. Sapsford RN, Blackstone EH, Kirklin JW, Karp RB, Kouchoukos NT, Pacifico AD, Roe CR, Bradley EL: Coronary perfusion versus cold ischemic arrest during aortic valve surgery: A randomized study. *Circulation* 49:1190, 1974.

2. Steed D, Follette D, Foglia R, Buckberg G: Unavoidable subendocardial underperfusion during bypass, especially in infants. *Circulation* 55,56(suppl III):III-248, 1977 (abstr).

3. Shen AC, Jennings RB: Myocardial calcium and magnesium in acute ischemic injury. *Am J Pathol* 67:417, 1972.

4. Sharratt GP, Rees P, Conway N: Myocardial infarction complicating aortic valve replacement. *J Thorac Cardiovasc Surg* 71:869, 1976.

5. Spanos PK, Brown AL Jr, McGoon DC: The significance of intraoperative ventricular fibrillation during aortic valve replacement. *J Thorac Cardiovasc Surg* 73:605, 1977.

6. Schraut W, Lamberti JJ, Kampman K, Anagnostopoulos C, Replogle R, Glagov S: Does local cardiac hypothermia during cardiopulmonary bypass protect the myocardium from long-term morphological and functional injury? *Ann Thorac Surg* 24:315, 1977.

7. Sondergaard T, Senn A: Klinische Erfahrungen in der Kardioplegie nach Bretschneider. *Langenbecks Arch Chir* 319:661, 1967.

8. Schaff HV, Dombroff R, Flaherty JT, Bulkley BH, Hutchins GM, Goldman RA, Gott VL: Effect of potassium cardioplegia on myocardial ischemia and post arrest ventricular function. *Circulation* 58:240, 1978.

9. Sperelakis N, Schneider J: A metabolic control mechanism for calcium ion influx that may protect the ventricular myocardial cell. *Amer J Cardiol* 37:1079, 1976.

10. Shen AC, Jennings RB: Kinetics of calcium accumulation in acute myocardial ischemic injury. *Amer J Pathol* 67:441, 1972.

11. Sharma GP, Varley KG, Kim SE, Barwinski J, Cohen M, Dhalla NS: Alterations in energy metabolism and ultrastructure upon reperfusion of the ischemic myocardium after coronary occlusion. *Amer J Cardiol* 36:234, 1975.

12. Scanlon PJ, O'Connell J, Johnson SA, Moran JM, Gunnar R, Pifarre R: Balloon counterpulsation following surgery for ischemic heart disease. *Circulation* 54(suppl III):III-90, 1976.

13. Swan H: Thermoregulation and bioenergetics: Patterns for vertebrate survival. New York: Elsevier, 1974, pp 183–187.

14. Shragge BW, Digerness SB, Blackstone EH: Complete recovery of myocardial function following cold exposure. *Circulation* 58(suppl II):II-97, 1978 (abstr).

15. Schaper J, Mulch J, Winkler B, Schaper W: Ultrastructural, functional, and biochemical criteria for estimation of reversibility of ischemic injury: A study on the effects of global ischemia on the isolated dog heart. *J Mol Cell Cardiol* 11:521, 1979.

16. Shapira N, Kirsh M, Jochim K, Behrendt DM: Comparison of the effect of blood cardioplegia to crystalloid cardioplegia on human myocardial contractility. *J Thorac Cardiovasc Surg* 80:647, 1980.

17. Singh AK, Capone RJ, O'Shea P, Karlson KE: Long-term changes in canine vein graft after infusion of cardioplegic solution. *Circulation* 68(suppl II):II-112, 1983.

18. Stewart JR, Blackwell WH, Crute SL, Loughlin V, Greenfield LJ, Hess ML: Inhibition of surgically induced ischemia/reperfusion injury by oxygen free radical scavengers. *J Thorac Cardiovasc Surg* 86:262, 1983.

T

1. Taber RE, Morales AR, Fine G: Myocardial necrosis and the postoperative low-cardiac-output syndrome. *Ann Thorac Surg* 4:12, 1967.

2. Tan CK, Glisson SN, El-Etr AA, Ramakrishnaiah KB: Levels of circulating norepinephrine and epinephrine before, during, and after cardiopulmonary bypass in man. *J Thorac Cardiovasc Surg* 71:928, 1976.

3. Taylor KM, Morton IJ, Brown JJ, Bain WH, Caves PK: Hypertension and the renin-angiotensin system following open-heart surgery. *J Thorac Cardiovasc Surg* 74:840, 1977.

4. Tyers GFO, Manley NJ, Williams EH, Shaffer CW, Williams DR, Kurusz M: Preliminary clinical experience with isotonic hypothermic potassium-induced arrest. *J Thorac Cardiovasc Surg* 74:674, 1977.

5. Trump BF, Mergner WJ, Kahng MW, Saladino AJ: Studies on the subcellular pathophysiology of ischemia. *Circulation* 53(suppl I):I-17, 1976.

6. Todd GJ, Tyers GFO: Potassium-induced arrest of the heart: Effect of low potassium concentration. *Surgical Forum* 26:255, 1975.

7. Tyers GFO, Williams EH, Hughs HC, Todd GJ: Effect of perfusate temperature on myocardial protection from ischemia. *J Thorac Cardiovasc Surg* 73:766, 1977.

8. Tait GA, Booker PD, Wilson GJ, Coles JG, Steward DJ, MacGregor DC: Effect of multidose cardioplegia and cardioplegic solution buffering on myocardial tissue acidosis. *J Thorac Cardiovasc Surg* 83:824, 1982.

9. Takamoto S, Levine FH, LaRaia PJ, Adzick NS, Fallon JT, Austen WG, Buckley MJ: Comparison of single-dose and multiple-dose crystalloid and blood potassium cardioplegia during prolonged hypothermic aortic occlusion. *J Thorac Cardiovasc Surg* 79:19, 1980.

10. Tranum-Jensen J, Janse MJ, Fiolet JWT, Krieger WJG, D'Alnoncourt CH, Durrer D: Tissue osmolality, cell swelling, and reperfusion in acute regional myocardial ischemia in the isolated porcine heart. *Circ Res* 49:364, 1981.

V

1. Van Trigt P, Jones RN, Olsen CO, Peyton RB, Currie WD, Pellon GL, Wechsler AS: Sonomicrometric determination of ischemic contracture of the left ventricle. *J Thorac Cardiovasc Surg* 83:298, 1982.

W

1. Williams JF Jr, Morrow AG, Braunwald E: The incidence and management of "medical" complications following cardiac operations. *Circulation* 32:608, 1965.

2. Whalen DA, Hamilton DG, Ganote CE, Jennings RB: Effect of a transient period of ischemia on myocardial cells. *Amer J Pathol* 74:381, 1974.

3. Williamson JR, Schaffer SW, Ford C, Safer B: The cellular basis of ischemia and infarction. I. Contribution of tissue acidosis to ischemic injury in the perfused rat heart. *Circulation* 53(suppl I):I-3, 1976.

Y

1. Yates JD, Kirsch MM, Sodeman TM, Walton JA Jr, Brymer JF: Coronary ostial stenosis: A complication of aortic valve replacement. *Circulation* 49:530, 1974.

2. Yates JC, Shalla NS: Structural and functional changes associated with failure and recovery of hearts after perfusion with Ca^{2+}-free medium. *J Mol Cell Cardiol* 7:91, 1975.

Z

1. Zimmerman AN, Daems W, Hulsmann WC, Snijder J, Wisse E, Durrer D: Morphological changes of heart muscle caused by successive perfusion with calcium-free and calcium-containing solutions (calcium paradox). *Cardiovasc Res* 1:201, 1967.

2. Zimmerman AN, Hulsmann WC: Paradoxical influence of calcium ions on the permeability of the cell membranes of the isolated rat heart. *Nature* 211:646, 1966.

4

ANESTHESIA FOR CARDIOVASCULAR SURGERY

Anesthetic management of patients undergoing cardiac surgery follows the same principles that govern general surgery. At the preoperative visit to the patient, the anesthesiologist collates the information provided by the history, physical examination, and laboratory results, and decides on the best form of anesthetic management. A successful outcome depends on carrying out these plans in an orderly sequence. Coordination and communication between the anesthesiologist and the surgical team are essential, for in this way even the most difficult problems in the operating room and postoperatively can be handled in a calm, efficient manner by an experienced team working together on a daily basis. After the operation, the anesthesiologist becomes an essential member of the team responsible for intensive care management.

This chapter was contributed by William A. Lell, M.D., J. G. Reves, M.D., and Paul N. Samuelson, M.D., Division of Cardiovascular Anesthesiology, Department of Anesthesiology, School of Medicine and the Medical Center of the University of Alabama at Birmingham.

In order to formulate a simple yet effective management protocol, the anesthesiologist must understand the patient's pathologic and pathophysiologic condition and the cardiovascular and other effects and potentially harmful interactions of anesthetic and adjuvant agents used in the perioperative period. Ideally, the patient's records should contain an outline of the planned operative procedure, for this assists in the formulation of management that will complement and expedite the operation.

SECTION 1

TYPICAL PROTOCOLS FOR ANESTHESIA AND SUPPORTIVE CARE FOR CARDIOVASCULAR OPERATIONS

Although each patient presents individual problems that directly affect anesthetic management and supportive care, a typical protocol can be presented. Management must, however, be individualized and based on careful evaluation of each patient's disease.

PATIENTS UNDERGOING CORONARY ARTERY BYPASS GRAFTING AND OTHER PROCEDURES FOR ISCHEMIC HEART DISEASE

Procedures

At the preoperative visit, current medications are checked. Resting, pain-free heart rate and blood pressure are recorded, and, when available, heart rate–systolic pressure product exercise-induced angina is noted. Evidence of pulmonary venous hypertension and congestive heart failure is sought. Patients with coronary artery disease are often anxious, and calm discussion by the anesthesiologist of the premedication, anesthetic management, and other aspects of the operation is important in preventing excessive catecholamine release. The patient should be sedated the night before the operation.

Premedication, given 1 hour before induction, usually consists of diazepam ($0.15 \text{ mg} \cdot \text{kg}^{-1}$) administered orally and morphine ($0.1 \text{ mg} \cdot \text{kg}^{-1}$) and scopolamine ($0.2–0.5 \text{ mg}$) given intramuscularly. The patient is transferred to the anesthetic room (GLH) or directly to the operating room (UAB). Interventions before induction are limited to placement of a blood pressure cuff, ECG leads, and a single peripheral intravenous infusion line, since complex, painful maneuvers may precipitate ischemia. Following induction with diazepam ($0.5 \text{ mg} \cdot \text{kg}^{-1}$),[S1] muscle relaxation is achieved with pancuronium ($0.1 \text{ mg} \cdot \text{kg}^{-1}$) and ventilation controlled for at least 4 minutes with 50% N_2O in oxygen and 0.5%–1% halothane or 1.0%–2.0% enflurane. A thiopentone, suxamethonium, d-tubocurarine, N_2O-oxygen sequence, with or without halothane or omnopon, may be preferred (GLH). Pancuronium may transiently increase blood pressure and heart rate but frequently does not in β-adrenergic–blocked patients. Once the patient is asleep, arterial and venous cannulae, including an internal or external jugular venous cannula, are inserted (UAB).

Before and after orotracheal intubation, all or some of the following interventions may be necessary to control the determinants of myocardial oxygen supply and demand:

1. Administration of crystalloid fluid to ensure adequate circulatory blood volume, cardiac output, and coronary perfusion.
2. Adjustment of the inspired concentration of halothane or enflurane in part to control myocardial contractility.
3. Administration of additional agents (diazepam, fentanyl, droperidol, propranolol, atropine) in part to control blood pressure and heart rate.
4. Administration of vasodilators (sodium nitroprusside, nitroglycerin) to control ventricular wall tension (afterload).
5. Administration of vasoconstrictors (methoxamine or phenylephrine) to increase aortic pressure and thus coronary blood flow.

The reduced plasma volume,[C1] present in many patients with ischemic heart disease, may cause hypotension during anesthetic induction. During the operation, the inspired concentration of halothane or enflurane is adjusted to provide a depth of anesthesia compatible with the changing levels of operative stimulation.[R1] The inspired concentration is kept lower in patients with documented abnormal left ventricular function or when systolic blood pressure falls, particularly if these events are associated with a mean left atrial pressure greater than 15 mmHg during operation. The inspired concentration of nitrous oxide and oxygen is maintained at 50% except in those patients who have developed severe ventricular dysfunction, in whom the oxygen concentration is increased.

If hypertension or tachycardia persist despite the use of additional anesthetic drugs, additional vasodilators, propranolol, or both are administered. Vasoconstrictors and inotropic drugs are sometimes used to correct hypotension unresponsive to volume administration or cessation of cardiac manipulation.

As the operation is ending, preload, as estimated by mean left atrial pressure (P_{LA}), is adjusted to an optimum level by infusion of whole blood, packed red blood cells, fresh frozen plasma, or 5% albumin (depending on the patient's hemoglobin level at that time). For patients with normal or near normal left ventricular function, this means a mean P_{LA} of 10–12 mmHg, and for those with poor left ventricular function, a mean P_{LA} of 15–20 mmHg. Heart rate is adjusted to about 90 beats per minute, using atrial pacing if necessary (see Chapter 5). Afterload reduction with sodium nitroprusside is generally continued if mean arterial blood pressure is greater than 100 mmHg.

In the closing stages of the operation, the anesthetic and relaxant drugs may be managed so that their effect continues into the first hour or two of convalescence in the intensive care unit, with a view to extubation a few hours later (UAB).[L1] Relaxants may be reversed at the end of operation in all patients, and some may be extubated before leaving the operating room (GLH).

The effectiveness of these simple methods of management in minimizing the incidence of perioperative myocardial necrosis has been documented.[L2,M20,R1]

Rationale

The management of patients during myocardial revascularization is directed toward preventing myocardial damage from the ischemic heart disease or from inadequacies of anesthetic or surgical management. Thus, anesthetic management is designed to provide an optimum myocardial oxygen demand-supply ratio.[P6,R2,R3] While this is important in every cardiac surgical patient, it is often critically important in the prevention of myocardial necrosis or acute functional impairment in patients with coronary artery disease.

Myocardial oxygen demand is directly related to heart rate, myocardial contractility, wall tension (afterload),[B1,S28] *and myocardial temperature* (see Chapter 3). Tachycardia increases myocardial oxygen demand. Catecholamine release (or administration) increases contractility and, thus, myocardial oxygen demand. Systemic arterial hypertension increases intraventricular pressure, thus increasing left ventricular systolic wall tension and myocardial oxygen demand. High left atrial pressure is associated with increased left ventricular volume, and, thus, wall tension and oxygen demand by the La Place relationship.

Myocardial oxygen supply is directly related to arterial oxygen content (in turn dependent on blood hemoglobin level and arterial oxygen tension) *and coronary blood flow* (in turn dependent on aortic diastolic pressure for the left ventricular subendocardial layer and aortic systolic and diastolic pressure for the outer layer). Coronary blood flow is also related inversely to coronary vascular resistance, but this is largely beyond control in the patient with extensive coronary artery disease. However, a fall in vascular resistance of the normal myocardium secondary to increased metabolic demands or selective vasodilation, in the face of a relatively fixed cardiac output, may result in decreased perfusion of areas supplied by stenotic coronary arteries. This is pertinent to the use of inotropic and vasodilator agents in patients with ischemic heart disease. By increasing the metabolic demands of normal tissue, inotropic agents may shunt blood away from jeopardized myocardium, causing ischemia. By lowering perfusion pressure or by selectively dilating vessels supplying normal myocardium, vasodilators may predispose the patient to intercoronary steal syndrome.[C2] Coronary collateral flow supplies some oxygen but is not at present controllable during operation. A blood hemoglobin level of about $10-12$ g $\cdot$ dl^{-1} and the maintenance of normal systemic blood pressure with a low left atrial pressure (14 mmHg) are optimal for myocardial oxygen delivery. A high left atrial pressure in these patients indicates increased left ventricular cavity pressure during diastole, which can result in a reduction of the left ventricular myocardium perfusion gradient (approximated by arterial pressure minus left atrial pressure).

The effects of various anesthetic and adjuvant agents on the determinants of myocardial oxygen supply and demand are discussed in detail in Sections 4 and 5. It is important to remember that all interventions entail risks. The use of potent and potentially harmful pharmacologic agents must, therefore, be selective. Transient alterations in hemodynamic variables may be better tolerated than the complications resulting from aggressive polypharmacy. Unfortunately, the lack of a single reliable index of myocardium ischemia necessitates the use of multiple variables in assessing the need for interventions. For example, detection of ST segment deflection in the absence of hemodynamic changes in heart rate, systolic pressure, or left atrial pressure may represent a nonspecific finding that does not require treatment. On the other hand, ischemia associated with hemodynamic changes may be present without detectable ST segment deflection. Rarely, the only manifestation of ischemia may be a rise in left atrial pressure. In contrast, some patients develop segmental ischemia that is not reflected by such global measurements as increased left atrial pressure. Obviously, in assessing the need for interventions, decisions must be based on the composite picture rather than on any single variable.

PATIENTS UNDERGOING SURGERY FOR VALVULAR HEART DISEASE

Procedures

Preoperative data are gathered as described above. Generally, such data indicate premedication similar to that given to patients with ischemic heart disease (see "Patients Undergo-

ing Coronary Artery Bypass Grafting for Ischemic Heart Disease"). Patients with pulmonary venous hypertension are transported to the operating room with the head of the bed elevated and breathing supplemental oxygen. In the operating room, a peripheral intravenous line is started, and the electrocardiogram and blood pressure are monitored (by cuff). Anesthesia is induced with $0.3-0.5$ mg $\cdot$ kg^{-1} of diazepam administered intravenously as a bolus and 50% nitrous oxide in oxygen administered by mask. Neuromuscular blockade is effected with 0.1 mg/kg of pancuronium bromide, and the patient is ventilated for 4 minutes. Simultaneously, monitoring devices are placed as described for patients with ischemic heart disease. Orotracheal intubation is performed following the administration of 4% topical lidocaine spray to the larynx, and anesthesia is maintained with 50% nitrous oxide in oxygen and incremental doses of fentanyl as needed.

As the patient is positioned and prepared, and during incision and sternotomy, fentanyl is titrated to a total dose of $10-15$ μg $\cdot$ kg^{-1}, as tolerated hemodynamically. Fluid administration is governed by the patient's history, response to the anesthetic agents, and central venous pressure until the heart can be visualized and a more accurate assessment of the filling pressures obtained with knowledge of left atrial pressure. Interventions, including vasodilator therapy, are used to reduce overload while maintaining coronary perfusion pressure. Pulse rate is maintained fast enough to ensure adequate cardiac index and ventricular function but not so fast that blood flow across stenotic valves is hindered or myocardial oxygen consumption is dangerously increased.

Additional neuromuscular blockade is used as needed and is added before CPB. Sodium nitroprusside (and, rarely, a vasoconstrictor) may be necessary to regulate perfusion pressure on bypass (see Section 3).

Anesthesia following CPB usually involves ventilation with oxygen alone and perhaps additional doses of fentanyl or morphine. Arterial blood samples are taken to monitor ventilation, acid-base status, hemoglobin level, and serum potassium concentration. Measurements of systemic, right atrial, and left atrial (and at times pulmonary artery) pressures and, when necessary, thermodilution cardiac output guide the management of preload, afterload, heart rate, contractility, and cardiac output. After the operation and appropriate cardiovascular stabilization, the patient is transferred to the intensive care unit to be ventilated and awakened from anesthesia without reversal of neuromuscular blocker or narcotic.

Rationale

Patients with aortic stenosis frequently have a long asymptomatic period and thus present for surgery with marked left ventricular hypertrophy with or without congestive heart failure. They may also have concomitant coronary artery disease (see Chapter 12). Anesthetic management is influenced by the presence of the thick, noncompliant left ventricle with outflow obstruction. Thus, the ventricle requires a high filling pressure. Heart rate must be kept within a relatively narrow range near normal, fast enough to maintain cardiac output but not so fast that myocardial oxygen consumption becomes excessive. Mild vasodilation may be helpful in patients with aortic stenosis (especially those with left ventricular dysfunction) to increase cardiac output, but care must be taken to maintain arterial pressures consistent with adequate coronary artery perfusion, especially in the presence of coronary artery disease.[C14,G8]

Patients with aortic regurgitation may be acutely or chronically ill. Those with acute disease due to bacterial endocarditis, aortic dissection, or dehiscence of a previously inserted aortic prosthetic valve frequently have more marked congestive heart failure, related in part to the normal size of the left ventricle. The chronic form of aortic regurgitation due to rheumatic heart disease is usually better tolerated because of the larger ventricular volume; however, when congestive heart failure is present in patients with aortic regurgitation, compensation has reached its limit. The specific considerations for anesthetic management include minimizing regurgitant (backward) flow and maximizing forward flow. Regurgitant flow into the ventricle is decreased by shortening the diastole by increasing the heart rate, or at least avoiding bradycardia. A high systolic pressure suggests the need for vasodilatation,[S30] but excessive vasodilatation may lower coronary artery perfusion pressure below safe levels.

Mitral stenosis is usually associated with slow deterioration in cardiac function, frequently accelerated by atrial fibrillation. There may be a rise in pulmonary vascular resistance resulting finally in right heart failure with or without tricuspid regurgitation. The major hemodynamic problems are decreased left ventricular filling and reduced cardiac output. To achieve adequate left ventricular filling, high left atrial pressure and volume are required. The anesthetic considerations include maintenance of this volume and filling pressure, and of a heart rate slow enough to permit adequate left ventricular diastolic filling time. It may be necessary to slow a rapid ventricular rate (see Section 5). Rarely, nitrous oxide may cause deterioration in cardiac performance presumably related to an increase in the pulmonary vascular resistance.

Mitral regurgitation, like aortic regurgitation, may be acute or chronic. The acute form may be secondary to bacterial endocarditis, chordal rupture, or dehiscence of a previously placed prosthetic device. The chronic form is usually secondary to rheumatic heart disease and occasionally to the floppy valve syndrome. The important pathophysiologic manifestation of this lesion is a volume overload of the left ventricle that is generally well tolerated because of increased compliance of the left atrium until the onset of congestive heart failure with severe pulmonary venous hypertension. Improved hemodynamic performance may be achieved with judicious vasodilation to decrease the backward regurgitant flow and increase the forward ejection from the left ventricle.[S30] Again, decreasing the systemic arterial pressure lower than that consistent with coronary perfusion must be avoided. Maintenance of a normal or slightly increased heart rate also aids in minimizing the regurgitant flow.

Patients may present with a mixed lesion (stenosis and incompetence) of a single valve, with multiple valve lesions, or with concomitant coronary artery disease. Although these factors may complicate the anesthetic plan, they can be controlled through the judicious use of anesthetic and adjuvant agents.

INFANTS AND CHILDREN UNDERGOING OPEN OPERATIONS FOR CONGENITAL HEART DISEASE

Hypothermic Cardiopulmonary Bypass

Most operations for repair of congenital heart disease, including those in small infants, may be performed during moderately or profoundly hypothermic CPB without total circulatory arrest (UAB) (see Chapter 2, Section 3). Following appropriate preoperative evaluation, the infant or small child is premedicated with 6–8 mg · kg^{-1} of pentobarbital, 0.1 mg · kg^{-1} of morphine, and 0.01 mg · kg^{-1} of scopolamine given intramuscularly approximately 1–1.5 hours before surgery. The infant is then brought into the operating room, and, if the infant is asleep, anesthesia is induced with low-dose halothane and oxygen with or without nitrous oxide (depending on the patient's oxygen saturation) by mask in a "steal" fashion. When anesthetized, the infant is placed on the operating room table. If the patient is not asleep from the premedication and is uncooperative during mask induction, or the pulmonary blood flow is excessively low, anesthetic induction is accomplished with 5 mg · kg^{-1} of intramuscular ketamine; then the patient is placed on the operating room table. A warming blanket is used under all patients 15 kg in weight. An intravenous route is established, and neuromuscular blockade is effected with 0.1 mg · kg^{-1} of pancuronium bromide. Mask ventilation for 4 minutes is followed by placement of an orotracheal tube. During this period, the electrocardiogram is monitored, and blood pressure is measured, first by cuff and then by indwelling arterial catheter. Heart sounds and ventilation are monitored. Following endotracheal intubation, a nasopharyngeal temperature probe is positioned. In those rare patients in whom the operation is to be done during total circulatory arrest, ice bags are placed around the patient following intubation and during placement of devices so that the nasopharyngeal temperature is usually 30°C by the time the incision is made.

Anesthesia is maintained with halothane, oxygen, and 10–20 μg · kg^{-1} of fentanyl in a titrated fashion, beginning just before the skin incision. Halothane or nitrous oxide is discontinued if hemodynamic instability occurs. Intravenous fluids are administered to maintain adequate preload, as judged by atrial pressures. Peripheral vasoconstrictors may be needed to minimize right-to-left shunting in some instances. Additional neuromuscular blockade is used as needed and given routinely immediately before CPB. Sodium nitroprusside (or, rarely, an α-constrictor) may be necessary to regulate perfusion pressure on CPB, particularly during the periods of cooling and rewarming.

Anesthesia following CPB usually involves ventilation with heated, humidified oxygen alone and perhaps additional doses of fentanyl. Arterial blood samples are taken to monitor ventilation, acid-base status, hemoglobin level, and potassium concentration. Measurements of systemic, right atrial, and left atrial (and at times pulmonary artery and/or ventricular) pressures and, when needed, thermodilution cardiac output, guide the management of preload, afterload, heart rate, and contractility.

At the conclusion of the operation, the orotracheal tube is replaced by a properly sized nasotracheal tube fixed with a Tunstall connector (Figure 4-1*a*) or some other similar device (Fig. 4-1*b*). A nasogastric tube is also positioned. The

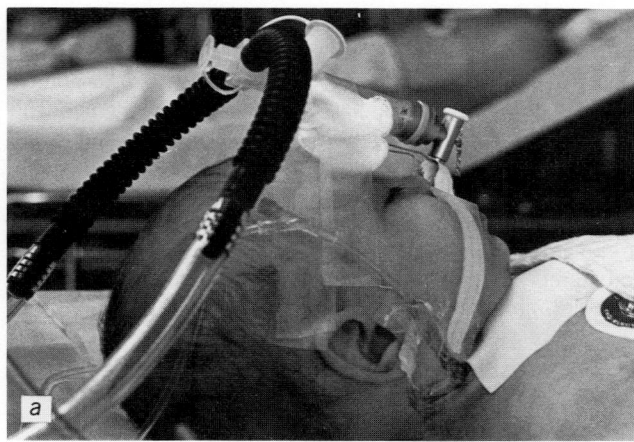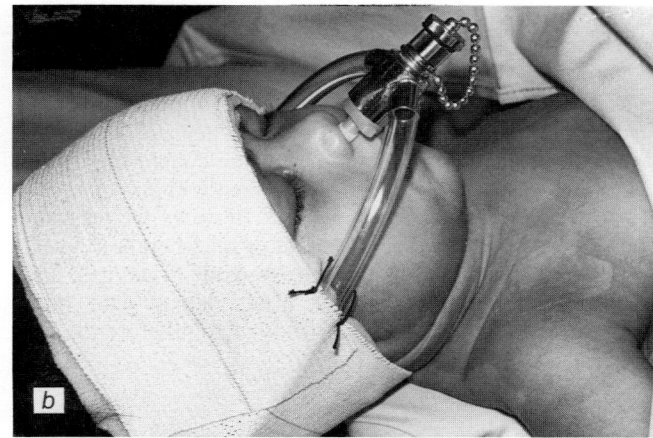

Figure 4-1
(*a*) Infant with nasotracheal tube in place and secured with a Tunstall adapter to hold the assembly securely on the forehead (UAB). This arrangement has proved satisfactory in minimizing inadvertent extubations and facilitates nursing care, including tracheal toilet.
(*b*) Infant with nasotracheal tube connector (GLH). This system has a low dead space and incorporates a suction catheter guide,[K15] which allows tracheal toilet to be carried out without interrupting positive pressure ventilation.

patient is then transferred to the intensive care unit, where he or she is ventilated and allowed to awaken from anesthesia without reversal of the activity of the neuromuscular blocker or narcotic.

Surface-Induced Deep Hypothermia with Circulatory Arrest and Limited Cardiopulmonary Bypass

Procedures
In infants weighing 8 kg and under, the correction of cardiac defects may be accomplished during circulatory arrest after cooling the patient to an appropriate temperature (GLH);[B17] or this method may be used only in infants weighing less than 2–3 kg and in a few special situations (UAB) (see Chapter 2).

A mixture containing 25 mg of pethidine hydrochloride, 6.25 mg of promethazine hydrochloride, and 6.25 mg of chlorpromazine is given intramuscularly as premedication. A face mask and oxygen supply should be available, as this premedication occasionally causes transient apnea. The patient is then disturbed as little as possible and usually arrives in the operating room already asleep. Anesthesia is induced by face mask, using equal parts of nitrous oxide and oxygen with 0.5%–1% halothane. The infant is then placed on a circulating water blanket, ECG monitoring is started, and an intravenous route is established. Either *d*-tubocurarine (0.5⁻¹ mg · kg⁻¹) or pancuronium (0.1 mg · kg⁻¹) is administered to facilitate endotracheal intubation and to prevent shivering during cooling. A nasotracheal tube of proper diameter and length[N3] (Fig. 4-2) is introduced initially (rather than using an orotracheal tube, which is changed at the conclusion of the procedure) and fixed in position as shown in Figure 4-1*b*. By decreasing the systemic vascular resistance, *d*-tubocurarine is thought to decrease temperature gradients in the tissues during cooling. Pancuronium is used in patients with low pulmonary blood flow, as it maintains systemic vascular resistance and minimizes right-to-left shunting.

Anesthesia is maintained with 50% nitrous oxide in oxygen and 0.5% halothane. Nasopharyngeal and rectal temperature probes are inserted, and surface cooling is initiated by circulating water at 0–4°C through the water blanket and placing plastic bags of crushed ice around the body.

Pressure monitoring lines are now introduced. Halothane is discontinued at about 30°C unless the arterial pressure remains above 80 mmHg. Serious arrhythmias during the cooling phase are uncommon and occur only at low temperatures. Should they occur and not respond to immediate electrical cardioversion, cooling is stopped, and the chest is opened. Otherwise, the ice bags are removed when the

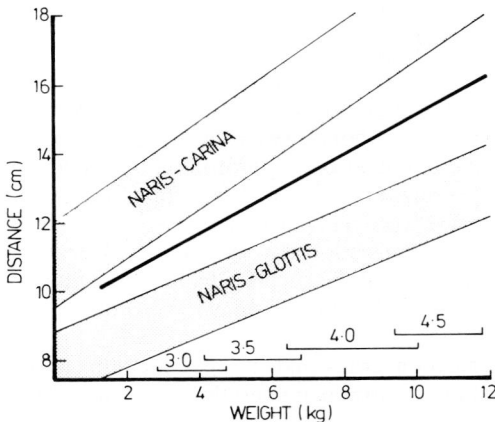

Figure 4-2 The relationship of naris-trachea distances and tracheal tube size (in millimeters of internal diameter) to body weight in infants with congenital cardiac lesions.

Heavy line, naris to mid-trachea; shaded areas, 75% confidence intervals for naris to carina and naris to glottis.

Reproduced with permission from Neutze et al.[N3]

nasopharyngeal temperature reaches 25°C, and the operation is begun.

The prime of the infant extracorporeal circuit is described in Chapter 2, Section 4, as are the details of perfusion cooling, rewarming, and decannulation. The heparin is neutralized with protamine sulphate, and at the conclusion of the operation the muscle relaxant is reversed with an appropriate dose of atropine and neostigmine. Between the termination of core rewarming and the end of the operation, anesthesia is maintained with 50% nitrous oxide in oxygen, and rewarming is completed with the water blanket. The endotracheal tube connector (Fig. 4-1b) is affixed before the patient leaves the operating room.

Rationale

Usually, patients with congenital heart disease come to operation in a relatively stable condition. A preexisting knowledge of the variable effects of drugs on systemic and pulmonary vascular resistance and cardiac contractility helps in designing an anesthetic plan. It is important with small infants and children to realize that the margin of error is small. Extreme vigilance and preparedness are the keynotes of management. The diagnosis of variations from normal that can result in a rapid deterioration of the patient's status and their prompt treatment are essential, but transient variations need not be treated, and unnecessary drugs provide their own complications.

Ventilation is important, as decreases in PaO_2 and high airway pressures both increase the pulmonary vascular resistance. At times, increased airway pressure is unavoidable because of low lung compliance. In such situations, the intravascular volume must be maintained or elevated so that the pulmonary vasculature remains distended and the systemic vascular resistance is preserved or increased to minimize right-to-left shunting before repair.

INFANTS AND CHILDREN UNDERGOING CLOSED CARDIOVASCULAR OPERATIONS

Procedures

The closed cardiovascular operations performed on infants and children can be divided into three categories: systemic-pulmonary artery shunts, repair of coarctation of the aorta, and closure of patent ductus arteriosus. Particular attention is paid to preoperative pulmonary status, for this may affect postoperative recovery. The anesthetic should facilitate early ambulation and recovery, and the anesthesiologist should bear in mind that, with palliative procedures, persistent cardiovascular pathology may have important effects on convalescence.

Premedication drugs and dosages are similar or slightly lower than those for open operations, and anesthetic induction and maintenance are also similar. Blood pressure is usually monitored with the aid of a Doppler pulse detector, and an arterial line is inserted only if there has been preexisting severe respiratory dysfunction or severe congestive heart failure or if a complex procedure is planned.

Body temperature is manipulated as a clinical tool. To protect the spinal cord, it may be intentionally lowered in infants with coarctation of the aorta and poorly developed collateral circulation. Similarly, in patients with poor pulmonary collateral circulation and unstable hemodynamics who might benefit from a reduction in oxygen requirement, mild hypothermia may be used during the construction of a systemic-pulmonary artery shunt or the creation of an atrial septal defect in transposition of the great vessels. In other circumstances, in neonates, and attempt is made to maintain body temperature near normal because of the adverse effects hypothermia might have on an already elevated pulmonary vascular resistance.

Following the surgical procedure, the neuromuscular blocker and, at times, the narcotic are reversed with atropine and neostigmine, and the patient is extubated in the operating room.

Rationale

Although early extubation facilitates the care and recovery of most infants undergoing closed cardiovascular procedures, occasionally infants need to remain intubated and ventilated during the early postoperative period. Such patients include those who have undergone complicated procedures with extensive blood and fluid replacement, those with severe preoperative respiratory dysfunction, those who remain hypothermic at the end of the procedure, and those who, because of their anatomy, require continued evaluation of the adequacy of a surgical shunt.

The premature infant undergoing ligation of a patent ductus arteriosus presents a different situation. The infant has minimal anesthetic requirements. Maintenance of body temperature is particularly important, and excessively high inspired oxygen concentration must be avoided. Fentanyl and pancuronium may be used, and the patient is ventilated with an FIo_2 (obtained with air mixture or nitrous oxide) similar to or slightly greater than that which resulted in appropriate arterial blood gas levels preoperatively. The neuromuscular blocker is not reversed after surgery, and the infant is transported to the high-risk nursery with the endotracheal tube in place. The adequacy of pulmonary function is then assessed, and weaning from the ventilator is performed over some days.

PATIENTS UNDERGOING OPERATIONS ON THE DESCENDING THORACIC AORTA

Anesthetic management of patients undergoing reconstruction of the descending thoracic aorta is directed toward minimizing respiratory and cardiovascular dysfunction resulting from patient positioning and cross-clamping of the proximal aorta. The left lateral decubitus position can result in impaired ventilation of the dependent lung secondary to restriction of chest wall movement, downward pressure of the mediastinum, and limitation of diaphragmatic motion. The resulting ventilation-perfusion abnormalities predispose the patient to hypoxemia, particularly obese patients and those with preexisting lung dysfunction. Collapse of the exposed lung by surgical retraction, and the use of a double lumen endobronchial tube to facilitate surgical exposure and prevent contamination of the dependent lung may also result in severe hypoxia.[D1] Hypoxemia may also occur secondary to prolonged pulmonary venous hypertension associated with aortic cross-clamping. Therefore, every effort should be made to minimize mechanical compression of the dependent lung and excessive retraction of the exposed lung. Selection of tidal volume, rate, pattern of ventilation, and FI_{O_2} is based on arterial blood gas levels. Severe hypoxia in association with collapse of the exposed lung may be corrected by transient clamping of the left pulmonary artery, but this is rarely necessary when anesthesia is maintained with a potent inhalation agent in a high inspired concentration of oxygen. Pulmonary venous hypertension should be avoided by monitoring left atrial pressure or pulmonary capillary wedge pressure and the use of methods described below.

Clamping of the proximal descending aorta results in impairment of distal flow and deterioration of left ventricular function secondary to a marked increase in left ventricular afterload.[K1,M19] Methods designed to provide proximal decompression while maintaining distal flow include (1) cross-clamping with vasodilator therapy, (2) partial CPB with or without an oxygenator, and (3) insertion of a temporary silastic shunt.

Cross-clamping with vasodilator therapy is simple and effective in controlling proximal hypertension. However, overuse of vasodilators may result in reduction of pressure-dependent distal collateral flow.[G9]

Partial CPB using femoral artery and vein cannulation provides an effective means of regulating proximal and distal pressure and perfusion. Such a system requires an oxygenator in the circuit. Alternatively, left atrial-femoral artery cannulation can be used and an oxygenator avoided. Cross-clamping the descending aorta in effect divides the circulation into proximal and distal segments. Perfusion of the proximal segment is a function of cardiac output, whereas distal perfusion depends on pump flow. The goal of this technique is to maintain both proximal and distal flow by balancing the preload of the heart with that of the pump. This is achieved by adjusting venous return to the pump. Excessive pump venous return is reflected by a rise in pump reservoir level, a decrease in right atrial or pulmonary artery occluded pressure, and a decrease in radial artery pressure and cardiac output. Inadequate pump venous return is reflected by proximal venous and arterial hypertension and a fall in reservoir level, necessitating a reduction in pump-dependent distal perfusion. The effectiveness of this technique in maintaining distal and proximal flow is limited by the adequacy of venous drainage and cardiac performance. Inadequate venous return may in part be compensated for by adding perfusate to the pump reservoir or by the use of a left atrial vent. Inadequate cardiac performance may necessitate the use of vasodilator or, rarely, inotropic agents. Advantages of the partial bypass method are (1) flexibility in providing proximal and distal perfusion, (2) the capability of retrieving blood when hemorrhage is excessive, and (3) the ability to control body temperature for additional organ protection. Disadvantages are (1) the complexity of the system, (2) the need for an experienced perfusionist, and (3) the necessity of systemic heparinization, which may potentiate external or intrapulmonary hemorrhage.

The use of a temporary silastic shunt is an effective means of providing blood flow to the descending thoracic aorta during aortic cross-clamping while at the same time providing proximal aortic decompression without the use of vasodilators. Distal flow is limited by the internal diameter of the shunt, but various diameters are available. The main advantage of this method is its simplicity, for perfusion equipment and personnel are not required, and systemic heparinization is avoided. Such simplicity is particularly advantageous in traumatized patients with multiple injuries. Disadvantages are occasional technical difficulties in placement of the shunt and the inability to retrieve excessive blood loss.

Ultimately, the method selected depends on the individual patient's needs. A young patient with normal pulmonary and cardiovascular function may tolerate aortic cross-clamping for repair of an aortic tear without complication, while an elderly patient with preexisting pulmonary and cardiac disease undergoing resection of a dissecting aneurysm may require more complex management.

Potential problems common to all patients undergoing reconstruction of the thoracic aorta include (1) large-volume blood loss, (2) neurologic deficit secondary to inadequate spinal cord perfusion, and (3) renal failure secondary to suboptimal fluid management and/or impaired renal perfusion. Anesthesia personnel must be prepared to deal with the complications of massive transfusion. Monitoring right atrial or left atrial or pulmonary artery wedge pressure is useful in guiding volume replacement. Total body hypothermia may be effective in minimizing neurologic and renal dysfunction. A decrease in nasopharyngeal temperature to 34–35°C is commonly observed with the chest cavity open. In selected cases, active cooling to 32°C with a heat exchanger may be desirable. Overcooling may result in impairment of cardiac performance. The use of mannitol and steroids to prevent organ damage during aortic cross-clamping remains controversial.

PATIENTS UNDERGOING PERICARDIECTOMY FOR CONSTRICTIVE PERICARDITIS AND PERICARDIAL TAMPONADE

Decreased cardiac output resulting from acute tamponade or a chronic constrictive process often requires surgical intervention. Cardiac output is reduced because there is inadequate diastolic filling of the ventricles. When the volume in the pericardium, the compliance of the pericardium, or both cause the intrapericardial pressure to exceed the intraventricular pressure, inadequate ventricular filling, decreased ventricular end-diastolic transmural pressure, and reduced cardiac output result.[M18,R4,S2] Normal compensatory mechanisms include an increase in heart rate and an increase in venous pressure. It is possible to have right without left ventricular tamponade, and vice versa, if pericardial compliance is such that the ventricular filling pressure of either ventricle is less than the pericardial pressure.[R4]

Regardless of the cause of cardiac tamponade, the principles of anesthetic approach are the same. The venous pressure, stroke volume, heart rate, and myocardial contractility must all be preserved. A suitable anesthetic regimen is ketamine induction (1 mg · kg^{-1}) and pancuronium (0.1 mg · kg^{-1}) with nitrous oxide in oxygen for maintenance. Positive pressure ventilation in the presence of cardiac tamponade depresses cardiac output, and maintenance of spontaneous breathing until the chest is opened should be considered.[M18,S37] Except in constrictive pericarditis,[V1] the cardiac performance immediately improves with pericardiotomy and should be continuously monitored with systemic arterial pressure, central venous pressure, and, on occasion, pulmonary artery catheters. In cases of uremic pericardial effusion, there are the additional anesthetic considerations for hemodialysis-dependent patients, which include drug metabolism, anemia, and fluid and electrolyte administration.[K2,P1] Drugs that are primarily excreted in the urine should be avoided, fluid must be administered cautiously, and serum potassium must be followed closely.

ANESTHESIA FOR PACEMAKER INSERTION

Preoperative evaluation of patients for pacemaker insertion or pulse generator change often documents degenerative diseases of the cardiovascular and other organ systems. It may be necessary, therefore, to treat not only cardiac dysfunction but also failure of other systems.

General anesthesia may be necessary in pediatric patients, occasionally in uncooperative adult patients, and in operations for placement of epicardial electrodes. Otherwise, local anesthesia with appropriate analgesic supplements is preferred for this relatively atraumatic procedure, performed often in elderly patients. With the patient aware, assessment of the level of consciousness provides information, not only of cerebral perfusion, but also of the adequacy of cardiac output in general. The avoidance of general anesthesia eliminates many potentially harmful drug interactions (see ''Drug Interactions'' in Section 5), and the incidence of postoperative nausea and vomiting is less, so patients can more quickly resume oral intake and medications, a distinct advantage for the diabetic patient.

The term *anesthesia standby* is a misnomer. Anesthesia personnel take an active role in patient management, including positioning, monitoring, and, if necessary, resuscitation or administration of a general anesthetic. Great care should be taken to prevent displacement of a temporary pacing electrode during patient positioning. The pulse generator should be readily accessible. It is important to remember that the pacing electrode is a direct conduit to the heart; therefore, the pacing system must be isolated electrically to prevent transfer of a fibrillating current. The patient is monitored with a blood pressure cuff and ECG electrodes. Palpation of a carotid or temporal pulse permits detection of arrhythmias and loss of capture. The pulse and the level of consciousness should be evaluated frequently. Most patients complain of some discomfort during pacemaker insertion. This is usually related to prolonged immobilization on a hard surface. Occasionally, analgesics are required for such discomfort, but, since most pacemaker patients are elderly with minimal re-

serves and altered pharmacokinetics, analgesic agents must be given in small, titrated doses. Fentanyl, in incremental doses of 10–20 μg, is recommended. Following its use, respiration should be closely monitored. Supplemental oxygen may be given with or without nitrous oxide for additional analgesia. Drugs that alter the level of consciousness should generally be avoided. Some sedative hypnotics are myocardial depressants (e.g., barbiturates) or alter systemic vascular resistance (e.g., droperidol, phenothiazines), resulting in hypotension that is poorly tolerated by elderly patients. Many patients experiencing pain demonstrate paradoxical excitement when given sedative hypnotics. Furthermore, these drugs are not readily reversible should excessive depression develop. Kindness and reassurance may be more effective and safer than pharmacologic interventions.

SECTION 2
OPERATIVE MONITORING

The technique of inserting arterial and venous monitoring lines is detailed in Chapter 2, as is the use of left and right atrial pressure lines. Also, both atrial pressures can be assessed by the surgeon during operation by palpation of these chambers, and left atrial pressure can be indirectly assessed by palpation of the tension in the pulmonary artery. Pulmonary artery pressure can be monitored by a Swan-Ganz catheter, but in operations done through a median sternotomy, direct insertion of the monitoring lines is preferred because it is simpler and safer.

Cardiac output is measured using a thermodilution technique in which a catheter of known length is inserted into the right atrium via the appendage, and a fine thermistor probe is inserted into the pulmonary artery via the right ventricle.

During operation, pressure signals are electronically transduced, and wave forms are displayed continuously on an oscilloscope. A strip chart recorder provides permanent records. The pressure wave form confirms the position of the catheter tip and reveals line damping. In addition to the oscilloscope display, the systolic, diastolic, or mean arterial pressure and the left- and right-sided venous pressures are displayed digitally (Fig. 4-3).

The electrocardiogram is monitored throughout and aids in assessing not only rhythm but also myocardial injury. The presence of Q waves does not necessarily signify necrosis. Specific criteria in terms of duration must be met, and even then, their presence or absence may not correlate with autopsy findings.[H11] Factors limiting the specificity of ST segment change as a clinical marker of myocardial ischemia include (1) the presence of ventricular arrhythmias or intraventricular conduction disturbances; (2) ST segment deflection secondary to therapy with such drugs as digitalis or electrolyte abnormalities such as hypokalemia, hyperventilation, and hypothermia; and (3) preexisting ST segment changes associated with aneurysm, pericarditis, or myocardiopathies.[F9,H10] ST segment monitoring should not, therefore, be used as the only marker of ischemia.

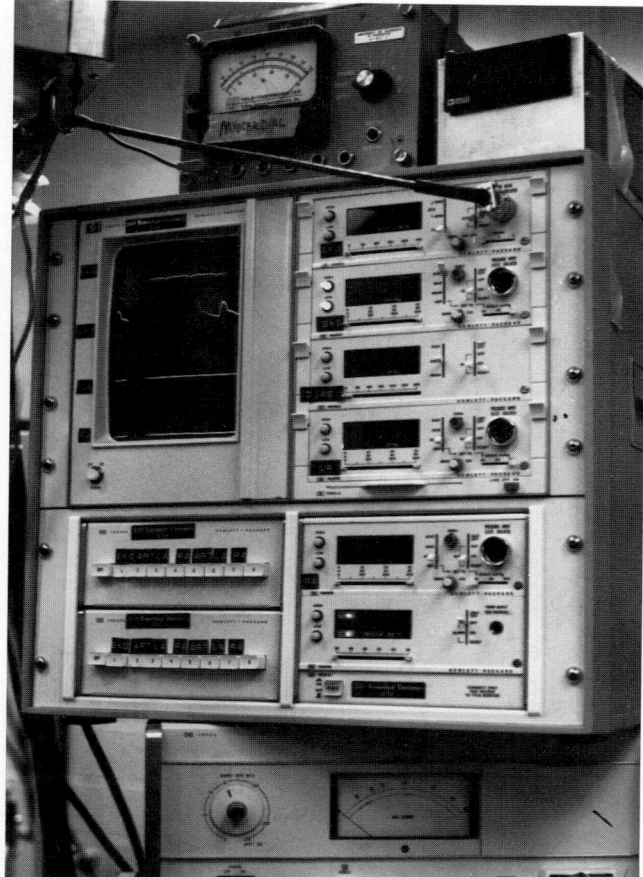

Figure 4-3 Monitoring equipment in the operating room includes an oscilloscope to visualize ECG and pulse tracings and a digital display of hemodynamic variables. Also continuously monitored is nasopharyngeal temperature; and, during cardiopulmonary bypass, septal myocardial temperature is measured.

Table 4-1 ACT protocol for heparin and protamine administration.

1. Measure ACT.
   a. Clear arterial line by withdrawing 10 ml.
   b. Withdraw into new syringe 2 ml of whole blood and place in BD tube no. XF534.
   c. Start timer.
   d. Mix thoroughly by inverting for 10 seconds.
   e. Place in heat block.
   f. Invert every 20 seconds.
   g. Stop timer when first clearly defined clot appears.
2. Determine heparin dosage before bypass.
   a. Measure control ACT after sternotomy; plot value on graph.
   b. Give 3 mg · kg^{-1} of heparin 10–15 minutes before cannulation after checking with surgeon.
   c. Measure ACT 2 minutes after heparin administration; plot value.
   d. Draw straight line between two plots that intersects 8-minute line on graph.
   e. Determine total dosage of heparin from extrapolated value at 8 minutes.
   f. If required, just before arterial cannulation, give heparin in addition to the 3 mg · kg^{-1} of heparin already given to produce ACT of 480 seconds.
   g. Before bypass, measure ACT 1 minute after additional heparin administration; plot corrected curve.
   h. Instruct surgeon when "safe" to cannulate.
3. Determine supplemental heparin dosage on bypass.
   a. Measure ACT at 30-minute intervals during bypass; plot value.
   b. If ACT < 8 minutes, give appropriate supplemental heparin (extrapolated dose).
4. Determine protamine dosage.
   a. Measure ACT at end of bypass; plot value.
   b. Multiply calculated amount of heparin (mg · kg^{-1}) present by 1.5 mg to get protamine dose to reverse effects of remaining heparin.
   c. Give calculated protamine dose.
   d. Measure ACT 15 minutes after protamine administration.
   e. If necessary, give more protamine to restore ACT to control value.
5. Keep all ACT samples until after the procedure, and note if fibrinolysis has occurred.

Urinary output is measured via an indwelling catheter. A gradual decline is not uncommon during CPB, but this decline should reverse when CPB is terminated. Abrupt cessation of urinary output during CPB is unusual and suggests poor renal perfusion.

Blood samples are taken intermittently for measurement of potassium, blood gases, and pH. Body temperature is measured by a nasopharyngeal thermistor probe.

Brain function is not monitored as a rule, although a "cerebral function monitor" is used in some institutions.[B13,M14]

The measurement of activated clotting times and the calculation of a heparin dose response curve enable the heparin and protamine doses to be individualized for each patient[B15] (Table 4-1). First, a base line, or control, activated clotting time (ACT) is established after sternotomy. Then heparin (3 mg · kg^{-1}) is given, and after 2 minutes the ACT is again determined and plotted on the record (Fig. 4-4). The two points thus obtained allow a dose response line to be plotted. If the line does not intersect the 8-minute mark, additional

heparin is given until an 8-minute ACT is achieved. Cannulation is then effected. The ACT is monitored during CPB at 30–60-minute intervals, and additional heparin is administered if the ACT drops below 8 minutes.

To calculate the appropriate protamine dose, the ACT is measured at the termination of CPB. The ACT value is plotted on the dose response line, and the amount of heparin remaining is determined. This amount is multiplied by 1.5 to calculate the dose of protamine. When using this ACT protocol, no heparin is added in the pump prime or the pump perfusate during CPB, except when blood is in the initial prime or during a blood addition (see Chapter 2).

Myocardial temperature is monitored, in association with the use of cold cardioplegia, with a calibrated thermistor probe. A thermistor electrogram probe is often used (see Chapter 3). The probe is inserted to a depth of 1 cm into the septal myocardium. Site selection may be modified by coronary anatomy and the presence of septal scarring secondary to previous infarction. Monitoring the electrogram facilitates

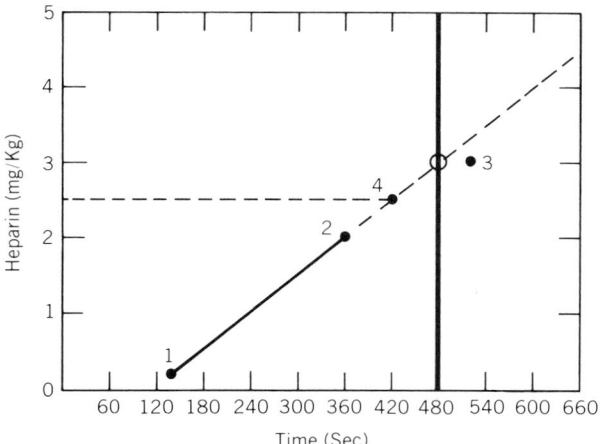

Figure 4-4 This graph is used to determine heparin and protamine dosages (see Table 4-1). Along the vertical axis is the dosage of heparin (in mg · kg^{-1}); activated clotting time (in seconds) is plotted along the horizontal axis. The closed circle 1 represents "control" ACT in a hypothetical case. Closed circle 2 is the ACT after administration of 2 mg · kg^{-1} of heparin. The open circle is drawn where a line (dose response line) between points 1 and 2 intersects 480 seconds. The open circle represents the total dose of heparin required to attain an ACT of 480 seconds. Therefore, an additional 1 mg · kg^{-1} (total of 3 mg · kg^{-1}) is required before cannulation is effected. The closed circle 3 is the ACT after all heparin is given; it falls safely beyond 480. Closed circle 4 is the ACT measured at termination of CPB and is equivalent to 2.5 mg · kg^{-1} of heparin. Since the action of heparin is reversed with a 1.5:1-ratio protamine-heparin dosage, the protamine reversal dosage for this patient is 3.75 mg · kg^{-1}. A final ACT should be obtained 15 minutes after reversal, and the measured value should coincide with that represented by closed circle 1.

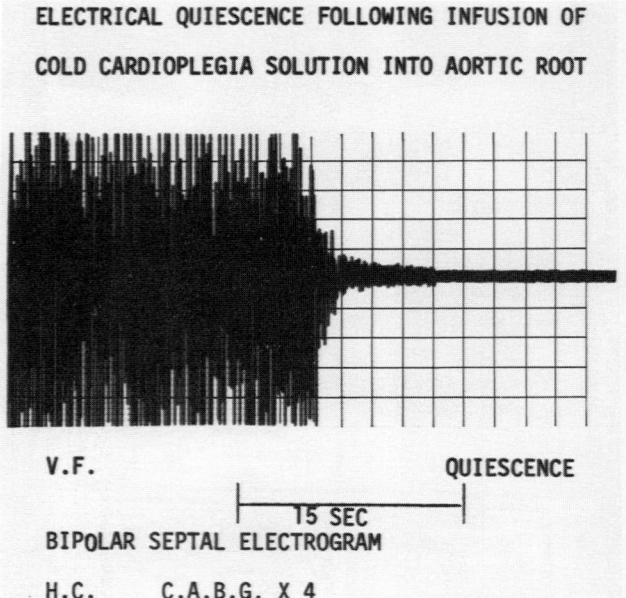

Figure 4-5 Continuous tracing of myocardial septal electrogram during infusion of hypothermic (7°C) cardioplegic solution into the aortic root. Note the rapid conversion from ventricular fibrillation to electrical quiescence.

CABG, coronary artery bypass grafting; VF, ventricular fibrillation.

probe placement in viable myocardium rather than scar tissue. Both the septal myocardial temperature and electrogram are displayed continuously on an oscilloscope with digital readout. Figure 4-5 shows a typical septal electrogram recorded simultaneously with the root infusion of cold potassium cardioplegic solution. There is rapid cessation of electrical activity associated with the fall in septal temperature. Figure 4-6 illustrates changes in myocardial, nasopharyngeal, and perfusate temperature during a myocardial revascularization procedure. The initial gradual decline in myocardial temperature with perfusate cooling is followed by a rapid fall with the aortic root infusion of cold cardioplegic solution. Failure to observe this increased rate of cooling suggests (1) improper thermistor placement, (2) inadequate cardioplegic infusion rate, (3) aortic insufficiency, or (4) severe proximal coronary stenosis. A rapid rise in myocardial temperature after initial cooling suggests (1) thermistor displacement, (2) nonocclusive cross-clamp, (3) extensive noncoronary collateral flow, or (4) inadequate cardiac decompression. When possible, corrective steps are taken. Following release of the aortic cross-clamp, there is a rapid rise in septal temperature associated with a return of electrical and mechanical activity.

SECTION 3
ANESTHETIC MANAGEMENT DURING CARDIOPULMONARY BYPASS

INITIATION OF CARDIOPULMONARY BYPASS

Following documentation of adequate heparinization with the accelerated clotting time (ACT) (Fig. 4-4), the anesthesiologist informs the surgeon that he or she may proceed with cardiac cannulation. Placement of the arterial cannula first provides the means of transfusing from the pump reservoir should hypovolemia occur during subsequent venous cannulation. Transient supraventricular arrhythmias are not uncommon during venous cannulation, particularly in hypovolemic patients. These arrhythmias are best treated by initiating CPB rather than by pharmacologic or electrical cardioversion.

As CPB is begun, the anesthesiologist checks jugular and systemic arterial pressure measurements and, on occasion, arterial blood gas analysis to make sure venous return to the pump and oxygenated arterial return to the patient are adequate. An additional dose of muscle relaxant is administered to prevent shivering during core cooling. Supplemental diazepam or thiopental may be given to ensure anesthesia and perhaps for a cerebral protective effect during subsequent low-flow perfusion. During the cooling phase, pulsatile flow is maintained by manipulation of venous return in order to allow the beating heart to eject with a left atrial pressure of

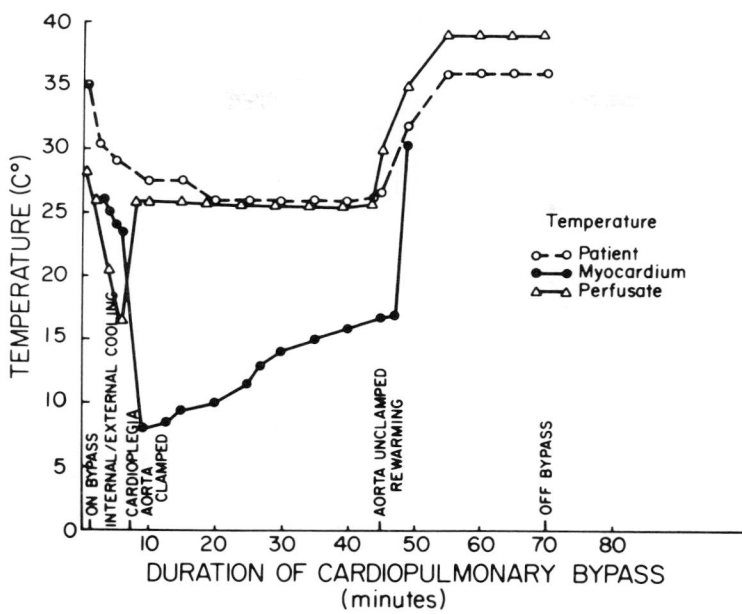

Figure 4-6 Simultaneous plots of nasopharyngeal (patient), septal myocardial (myocardium), and CPB perfusate temperatures during CPB (UAB). Note the gradual myocardial rewarming despite relatively low perfusion temperature and external (pericardial) cooling with iced saline solution.

4–6 mmHg. Once total CPB is established at full flow, mechanical ventilation is terminated, and the lungs are maintained at zero airway pressure. As hypothermic perfusion progresses and cardiac contraction becomes ineffective, surgeon and anesthesiologist must remain alert for signs of left heart distention, particularly in patients with aortic insufficiency or increased pulmonary collaterals.

Following initial myocardial cooling with the perfusate, the aorta is cross-clamped, and cold cardioplegia is instituted. During infusion of the cold cardioplegic solution, the anesthesiologist monitors (1) myocardial temperature to assess adequacy of cooling, (2) the ECG to document electrical quiescence, (3) left atrial pressure to detect ventricular distention secondary to infusion of solution through an incompetent aortic valve, and often (4) pressure in the isolated aortic root into which the cardioplegic solution is infused. Failure to note the rapid fall in myocardial temperature and cessation of electrical activity with infusion of cold cardioplegic solution suggests the need for corrective measures (see Chapter 3).

DISCONTINUATION OF CARDIOPULMONARY BYPASS

Successful weaning from CPB requires coordination and communication among anesthesiologist, surgeon, and perfusionist. A number of preliminary conditions must be met. First, the period of reperfusion following cardioplegia should have rewarmed the heart so that it is in a stable rhythm and capable of ejecting. Initial washout of cardioplegic solution and metabolic waste products is facilitated by maintaining a perfusion gradient of 75–80 mmHg across the myocardium. Perfusion pressure may be enhanced by increasing pump flow or the selective use of a vasoconstrictor such as phenylephrine or methoxamine. Optimal transmural flow occurs when ventricular distention is prevented by the use of left atrial pressure monitoring and judicious use of a ventricular vent. Overuse of the vent may result in an empty heart with impairment of subendocardial perfusion. Therefore, the perfusionist adjusts pump inflow and return to maintain left atrial pressure in the range of 2–6 mmHg.

Rhythm disturbances during myocardial perfusion are common. Atrial, ventricular, or sequential pacing is often required. The serum potassium level must be known.[B21] Rarely, antiarrhythmic agents such as lidocaine, procainamide hydrochloride, propranolol, or verapamil may be required. Many of the arrhythmias are self-limited and disappear spontaneously as reperfusion progresses. Persistent ventricular arrhythmias suggest myocardial damage, coronary air embolism, or inadequate surgical repair.

The next requirement before discontinuing CPB is complete evacuation of intracardiac air (see Chapter 2). Air evacuation is facilitated by intermittent positive pressure ventilation to drive air out of the pulmonary veins. Following reperfusion, the transient use of an inotropic agent may also assist by enhancing myocardial ejection.

Suture lines should be checked for hemostasis and significant bleeding points controlled before discontinuing bypass. The nasopharyngeal temperature should be stabilized at

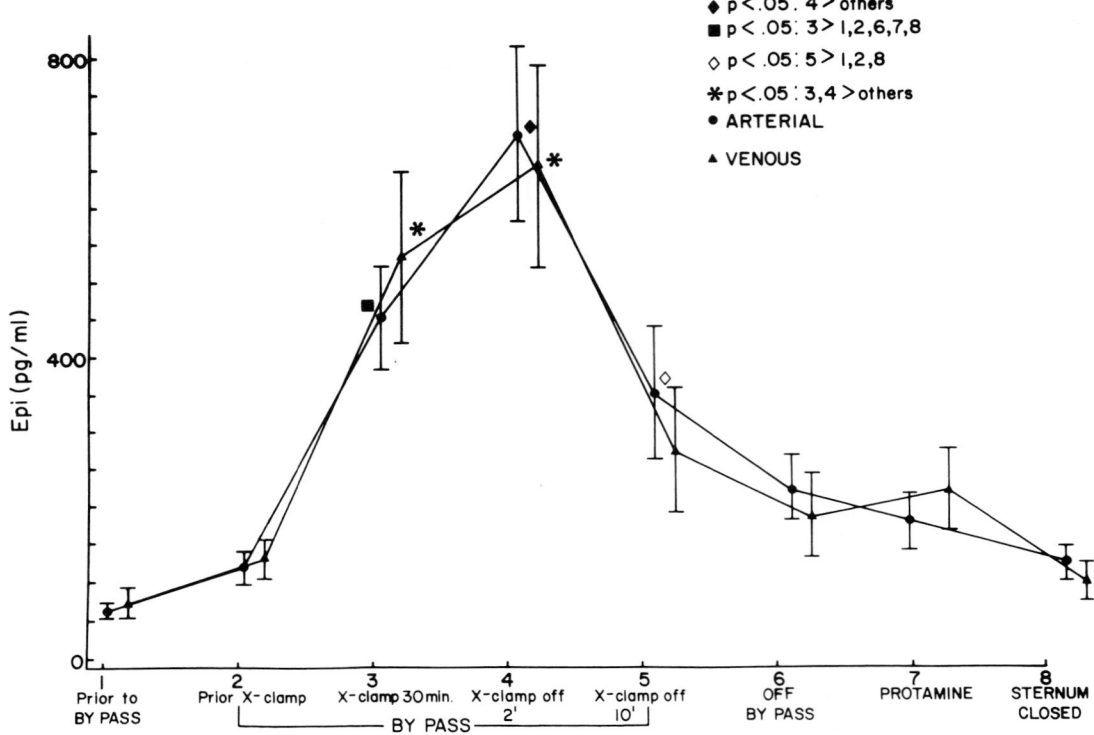

Figure 4-7 Plasma epinephrine concentration is plotted at various times during surgery ($n = 28$, mean ± SE). Note the significantly elevated epinephrine level at the end of aortic cross-clamping. Reproduced with permission from Reves et al.,[R15] and the American Heart Association, Inc.

37°C. Augmentation of pump flow and/or the use of vasodilators[N2] may facilitate the final stages of rewarming.

Once these preliminary steps of reperfusion, de-airing, and rewarming are completed, weaning from CPB begins. Electrical pacing is frequently used via epicardial wires to maintain an optimal heart rate. Preload is adjusted to maintain ventricular filling pressure in the range of 10–14 mmHg. The exact pressure selected depends on the compliance and function of the ventricles. The judicious use of peripheral vasodilators permits transfer of volume from the pump oxygenator to the patient without cardiac distention. Once optimal heart rate and preload are achieved, CPB is stopped and the lines are clamped. While the surgeon is assessing the surgical field and the repair and venous decannulation is being done, filling pressures are maintained by the intermittent infusion of perfusate from the pump oxygenator reservoir via the aorta. In most patients, nothing further need be done. However, in those with inadequate cardiac performance, as manifested by persistence of left or right atrial pressure > 14 mmHg, systolic arterial blood pressure < 80 mmHg, and cardiac index < 2.0 l · m^{-2}, CPB is reinstituted and the adequacy of the repair assessed. If the repair is satisfactory, drugs that reduce afterload or increase contractility may be required to maintain cardiac output during and after weaning from CPB. The endogenous epinephrine plasma level rises during CPB and reaches its peak at the end of aortic cross-clamping[R15,W8] (Fig. 4-7). Vasodilators such as nitroprusside (0.5–1.0 μg · kg^{-1} · min^{-1}) may be required to reduce sys-

temic impedance at this time. Nitroglycerin given intravenously is very useful during this period both as a coronary vasodilator and to control left atrial pressure. Vasodilator therapy may be used to lower the blood pressure during rewarming and as an adjunct to protecting suture lines and controlling hemorrhage.

Following decannulation, protamine is administered. The ACT is measured shortly before discontinuing CPB, and from that measurement the equivalent in circulating heparin (mg · kg^{-1}) is estimated (Fig. 4-4). The protamine reversal dose is 1.5 times that value. Traditionally, protamine has been given intravenously.

Reactions to protamine after the administration of heparin and CPB have always been recognized as possible. In recent years, the occurrence of sudden hypotension, elevated right atrial and pulmonary artery pressure, and usually abrupt reduction of left atrial pressure 2–5 minutes after the administration of protamine has become clearly recognized as a syndrome that is sometimes fatal.[L17,S38] It is controversial whether the administration of protamine slowly or rapidly, or by the left atrial or intra-aortic route[F12,R17] rather than into peripheral veins or the right atrium reduces the incidence and severity of this syndrome. In any event, it seems clear that complement is activated through the classical pathway when protamine is administered under these circumstances.[B19,B20,K17] This process is likely to be related to the syndrome that sometimes occurs.

Any residual blood in the pump reservoir is washed and

transfused, and administered to the patient as needed. Whole blood, plasma, packed cells, or a 5% albumin solution is infused to maintain filling pressures and a hemoglobin concentration of 10–12 g%. During the post-CPB period, "limits" at which the heart performs best are established, and this information is transmitted to the intensive care unit personnel for their use.

SECTION 4
ANESTHETIC DRUGS

Today, a single drug is seldom used as the sole anesthetic agent, but, rather, a group of drugs, each with particular pharmacologic characteristics best suited for the individual patient's requirements, is selected. The agents are blended to provide *balanced anesthesia,* a term coined by Lundy in 1926.[L3] A combination of various anesthetic drugs is used "in a small enough amount so that they produce no unsatisfactory effect."[L3] Balanced anesthesia provides sleep, amnesia, analgesia, muscle relaxation, and obtundation of sympathetic and other autonomic nervous system reflexes. The rationale for using a variety of drugs is simply that, with a combination of specific drugs, lower doses of each may be used to achieve the therapeutic goals. For example, the effective dose to achieve sleep with thiopental is relatively low, but much more is required to obtain muscle relaxation, and this amount results in severe myocardial depression and other unwanted effects. The combination of thiopental with a muscle relaxant such as succinylcholine allows small appropriate doses of both to be used without undesirable side effects. Thus, balanced anesthesia usually consists of an induction agent, a muscle relaxant, maintenance anesthetics,

and possibly vasoactive drugs. The purpose of this section is to review the pharmacology of drugs used during anesthesia for cardiac surgery and to discuss the potential for perioperative drug interactions.

INDUCTION AGENTS

The anesthetic induction agents, thiopental, droperidol, ketamine, diazepam, and midazolam, have distinctly different cardiovascular and anesthetic effects (Table 4-2). Thiopental is the oldest and still the most commonly administered intravenous induction agent. Transient direct myocardial depression with resultant diminished cardiac output and systemic blood pressure are its primary hemodynamic effects.[F1,S3,W1] The short action resulting from rapid redistribution makes supplementation with repeated thiopental or other anesthetic agents essential. Thiopental must be used carefully, if at all, in patients with reduced cardiac output.

Droperidol alone, or in a combination with fentanyl, as Innovar, decreases blood pressure through α-adrenergic blockade, with resultant systemic arterial vasodilatation.[F2,G1,M1,S4,S5,T1,W2] It may also decrease left ventricular end-diastolic pressure (by decreasing venous tone), which lowers blood pressure because of a decrease in cardiac output.[M21] There may be an associated increase in heart rate, which increases myocardial oxygen consumption (MvO_2) and coronary blood flow.[S5] The α-adrenergic blocking effect of droperidol may be useful in blocking the sympathetic response to intubation and surgical stimulation. However, serious hypotension may occur during induction in hypovolemic patients or patients with impaired venous return.

Ketamine is unique among anesthetic intravenous induction agents, since it produces sympathetic-nervous-system–

Table 4-2 Hemodynamic effects of anesthetic drugs.

Drug	Hemodynamic Effect					
	CI	BP	Rs	P_{LVED}	HR	Contractility
d-Tubocurarine	↓	↓	↓	↓	↑	←→
Diazepam	↓	↓	↓	↓	←→	←→
Dimethyl tubocurarine	↑	←↑→	←↓→	←↓→	↑	←→
Droperidol	←↑→	↓	↓	↓	↑	←→
Enflurane	↓	↓	↓	←↓→	←↓→	↓
Fentanyl	←→	↓	↓	←→	←→	←→
Halothane	↓	↓	←↓→	←↑→	←↕→	↓
Innovar	←↑→	↓	↓	↓	←→	←→
Ketamine	↑	↑	↑	↑	↑	↑
Methoxyflurane	↓	↓	↓	←→	←→	↓
Midazolam	←→	←→	←↓→	↓	↑	←↓→
Morphine	←↑→	←↓→	↓	←↑→	↓	←→
Nitrous oxide	↓	←↓→	←↑→	↑	←↓→	↓
Pancuronium	↑	↑	←→	↓	↑	?
Succinylcholine	↓	←↓→	↓	↓	↕	?
Thiopental	←↓→	←→	↑	←→	↑	↓

KEY: ↑, increase; ↓, decrease; ←→, no change; ?, insufficient data; CI, cardiac index; BP, blood pressure; Rs, systemic vascular resistance; P_{LVED}, left ventricular end-diastolic pressure; HR, heart rate.

mediated cardiovascular stimulation rather than depression, and has been recommended for induction of cardiac patients for this reason.[C3,C4,P1,R5] It increases heart rate, venous pressure, myocardial contractility, cardiac output, blood pressure, and systemic and pulmonary vascular resistance.[N1,T1,T3,V2] Hypertension, tachycardia, and delirium may occur.[C5,N1] The use of diazepam before and concurrently with ketamine administration ameliorates the tachycardia and hypertension produced by ketamine alone.[D2]

In contrast to the cardiovascular depression from thiopental and droperidol and the stimulation from ketamine are the hemodynamic effects of the two benzodiazepine derivatives, diazepam and midazolam. Diazepam, in a variety of dosages from sedative ($0.05-0.10$ mg $\cdot$ kg^{-1}) to fully hypnotic ($0.5-0.6$ mg $\cdot$ kg^{-1}), produces very little change in measured and derived cardiovascular data.[C6,J1,R6,S1,S31] Despite the stability of diazepam's hemodynamic effects, there is some evidence that diazepam increases coronary blood flow.[C6,I1] Midazolam (0.2 mg $\cdot$ kg^{-1}) also has relatively minor cardiovascular effects.[R7,S31] In patients with impaired left ventricular performance (elevated left ventricular end-diastolic pressure), cardiac function is improved after diazepam[C7] and midazolam.[R7] Disadvantages of diazepam induction are its relatively slow onset (1 minute) compared to that of thiopental (30 seconds), transient pain at the site of injection, and some incidence of thrombophlebitis. Because midazolam is water soluble, induction is faster and less painful[R8,S31] with a lower incidence of thrombophlebitis than with diazepam. The serum half-life of diazepam is $21-37$ hours, and it has at least one neuropharmacologically active metabolite (desmethyldiazepam). These characteristics account for the prolonged sedative and amnesic effects[K3] that are beneficial postoperatively.

AGENTS FOR MAINTENANCE OF ANESTHESIA

The most frequently used inhalation agent for anesthetic maintenance is nitrous oxide (N_2O). Because of its low anesthetic potency, N_2O is seldom used alone without a narcotic or some other inhalation drug. Nitrous oxide has little cardiovascular effect but may cause a sympathetic response in normal patients.[S6] In patients with cardiac disease, N_2O in conjunction with other agents may depress cardiac output.[B2,K4,L4,M2,S4,S7,W3] Nitrous oxide is rapidly eliminated by the lungs with minimal biotransformation.

The halogenated inhalation anesthetic drugs are all direct myocardial depressants. They include methoxyflurane, halothane, enflurane, and isoflurane. Methoxyflurane was the first available for clinical use and has been used routinely in at least one major cardiac surgical center.[E1] Methoxyflurane decreases blood pressure and cardiac index without changing heart rate.[B3,H1,L5,W4] Its disadvantages include slow uptake and distribution and high fat solubility, resulting in prolonged emergence compared to that of enflurane and halothane.[E2] A significant amount of methoxyflurane is metabolized, and the fluoride released can lead to renal failure. Halothane, in dose-related fashion, decreases myocardial contractility and, to a lesser extent, peripheral resistance and heart rate.[B3,B4,L6,M3,S8,S9,S12] Animal data indicate

that there is also a dose-dependent and equally distributed decrease in myocardial blood flow.[A1,M4,M5,W5] During experimentally induced canine myocardial ischemia, halothane decreases ST elevations,[B5] but myocardial oxygen tension and blood flow to the ischemic zone are reduced and ischemic regional contractility decreased.[L7,R9] Halothane does not protect the ischemic heart if the decrease in perfusion pressure is greater than the decrease in heart rate.[K16] Although oxygen supply to normal myocardium is diminished, metabolism is not altered.[M4,M5] Enflurane is a potent myocardial depressant with myocardial metabolic effects similar to those of halothane.[M6] It decreases cardiac index, blood pressure, systemic vascular resistance, and heart rate.[D3,G2,K5] The autonomic response to CO_2 is better with enflurane than with equipotent dosages of halothane.[M7] Myocardial depression with enflurane is dose related, and at higher doses it causes unacceptable depression not seen with halothane.[C8,C9,E3] Therefore, theoretically it has a small safety margin. An apparent advantage of enflurane over halothane is its relatively greater compatibility with epinephrine[J2,H2] and less potential for arrhythmias due in part to different effects on AV conduction.[A2,A3] Both drugs have relatively similar uptake and distribution,[E2] but at the same inspired concentration, halothane is roughly twice as potent an anesthetic as enflurane. Isoflurane lies between halothane and enflurane in potency.[S33] Its hemodynamic effects include a modest increase in heart rate and decreased systemic resistance and blood pressure.[S34] Isoflurane does not appear to have as great a negative inotropic effect as either halothane or enflurane and has a greater safety margin.[W10] It might, therefore, be more useful in patients with impaired ventricular performance. Since isoflurane is newly released, much may yet be learned about its role in cardiac anesthesia.

Narcotic drugs are used to supplement general anesthesia and sometimes for the induction of anesthesia. Morphine in relatively large dosages ($1-4$ mg $\cdot$ kg^{-1}) is useful for induction and maintenance of anesthesia, particularly in patients with pulmonary venous hypertension and low cardiac output.[L8] Hemodynamic effects of morphine induction include a variable (increase or decrease) change in heart rate, decreased systemic vascular resistance, and little change in cardiac output.[A4,L4,L9,S10,W3] Because of greater systemic arterial and venous dilatation, fluid and blood requirements are greater with morphine at these doses than with halothane ($1.0\%-1.5\%$).[S11] The autonomic nervous system response is preserved with morphine, which may be an advantage in valvular-heart–diseased patients with depressed ventricular function.[L8] However, because of the increases in oxygen consumption associated with reflex tachycardia and hypertension, the preservation of autonomic nervous response is not desirable in ischemic heart disease.[R10] Morphine in much smaller doses (0.1 mg $\cdot$ kg^{-1}) is used as a supplement to N_2O-O_2 relaxant anesthesia at GLH in those patients in whom halothane produces undesirable hypotension, bradycardia, or both. In this dose, the hemodynamic side effects of morphine are minimal. Fentanyl is a synthetic narcotic with a shorter duration of action than that of morphine, permitting more rapid emergence and earlier extubation.[R11] The cardiovascular effects of fentanyl are similar of those of morphine,[S12,S13] but volume requirements are less with fentanyl because venodilatation is minimal.[R12,S12] Fentanyl is administered in the operating room to minimize the hypertension that may occur with the transition from the operating room to the intensive care unit.[R13] There is increasing evidence that fentanyl in dosages of about 100 μg · kg^{-1} (roughly equivalent to 1 mg · kg^{-1} of morphine) as the sole anesthetic is a satisfactory induction and maintenance agent superior to morphine with regard to hemodynamic and fluid requirements.[L15,S12,S13] Sufentanil, another new synthetic narcotic, appears to be superior to high-dose fentanyl in patients with ischemic heart disease because it maintains greater hemodynamic stability and has greater potency.[D9]

MUSCLE RELAXANTS

Neuromuscular blocking agents, or muscle relaxant drugs, are of two types: depolarizing and nondepolarizing. There are many muscle relaxants available, but only four need be considered here: succinylcholine, which is depolarizing, and d-tubocurarine, dimethyltubocurarine, and pancuronium, which are nondepolarizing. Succinylcholine has only modest cardiovascular effects, any of which are biphasic, dose-related, and age-related.[G3] The predominant effects are slight decreases in heart rate, systemic resistance, and blood pressure that are all very transient.[G3,L16] Pancuronium and d-tubocurarine have more pronounced hemodynamic effects. Pancuronium increases heart rate, systemic blood pressure, and sometimes cardiac output.[H3,K6,L10,L11,M8,S1,S14] Although pancuronium increases AV conduction, it may be used without causing rapid ventricular response in patients with atrial fibrillation.[S25] There are conflicting data on systemic vascular resistance, but it is probably not markedly altered. On the other hand, d-tubocurarine significantly decreases the systemic vascular resistance, blood pressure, cardiac output, and ventricular filling pressures.[H3,L10,M9,S14] The circulatory effects of d-tubocurarine are dose-related and dependent on the volume status of the patient as well as concurrent anesthetic administration. The mechanism of decreased systemic resistance and hypotension is ganglionic blockade and histamine release.[M9] Dimethyltubocurarine does not share the ganglionic blockade and histamine-releasing properties of d-tubocurarine[M10,M15] and is devoid of many of the hemodynamic effects of d-tubocurarine.[F3,S14–16,Z1] Because of the relatively small hemodynamic changes with dimethyltubocurarine, it may gain more widespread use for cardiac anesthesia.

SECTION 5
ADJUVANT DRUGS

Adjuvant drugs are used during cardiac surgery to (1) support the failing heart and circulation, (2) control autonomic nervous system reflexes, and (3) reverse the effects of anesthetic drugs. The last two uses are exemplified in morphine anesthesia (1 mg · kg^{-1}): vasoconstrictor, as well as a relatively large fluid volume, may be required during induction to maintain the blood pressure; then, when surgery is begun, a vasodilator may be required to control the hypertensive (sympathetic)[H4] response to incision and sternotomy. The optimal anesthetic management plan minimizes adjuvant drug usage and dosage.

VASODILATORS

The vasodilators most commonly used are sodium nitroprusside, nitroglycerin, trimethaphan, and phentolamine (Table 4-3). One indication for the use of these drugs is impaired cardiac performance with heart failure, in which the vasodilators act to reduce left ventricular afterload, or impedance to ventricular ejection (Fig. 4-8). A vasodilator may be used alone or in combination with a positive inotropic drug. A second indication is increased systemic vascular resistance resulting from sympathetic reflexes during anesthesia and surgery. Commonly, systemic vascular resistance and blood pressure rise following intubation, sternotomy, and other stimulation. Vasodilators can be used to reduce persistent elevations of vascular resistance. A third indication, for the use of nitroglycerin, is the need to improve myocardial blood flow, particularly during myocardial reperfusion after a period of aortic cross-clamping. In such cases, nitroglycerin is often combined with phenylephrine to increase the perfusion pressure.

Sodium nitroprusside is often used intravenously when the primary indication is increased systemic vascular resistance.

Table 4-3 Vascular actions of intravenous vasodilators.

| Vasodilator | | Site of Prominent | | |
Generic Name	Trade Name	Vasodilatation	Onset	Duration
Sodium nitroprusside	Nipride	Arterial and venous	30 s	2–4 min
Nitroglycerin	Nitroglycerin	Venous	1–2 min	10 min
Diazoxide	Hyperstat	Arterial	1–2 min	4–12 h
Trimethaphan	Arfonad	Arterial and venous	1–2 min	4–8 h
Hydralazine	Apresoline	Arterial	10–20 min	3–4 h
Reserpine	Serpasil	Arterial	1.5 h	8–24 h
Phentolamine	Regitine	Arterial and venous	1–2 min	20 min

KEY: min, minutes; s, seconds.
SOURCE: Modified from Braunwald[B6] and Reves.[R13]

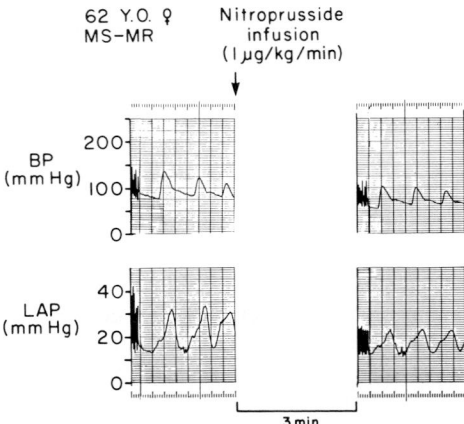

Figure 4-8 Nitroprusside infusion to reduce afterload and increase cardiac output in a 62-year-old woman with combined mitral stenosis and regurgitation (MS-MR) before cardiopulmonary bypass (UAB). The rhythm is atrial fibrillation. Note the significant drop in LAP 3 minutes after the start of nitroprusside infusion. Cardiac index improved from 1.8 to 2.1 $1 \cdot min^{-1} \cdot m^{-2}$ with the reduction in afterload.

BP, blood pressure; LAP, left atrial pressure.

Its rapid action, short duration, and preferential effect on the arterial resistance vessels are advantageous in this situation (Table 4-3). Because of its potency and cyanide production, intravenous nitroprusside must be administered with a constant and accurate infusion system, such as the commercially available IMED 922[1] or IVAC 530.[2] The total fatal nitroprusside dosage in three reported cases was approximately $10-15 mg \cdot kg^{-1}$,[D4,D5,M11] but it is prudent to stay below $1.5 mg \cdot kg^{-1}$.[V3] Infusion rates probably should be limited to less than $8-10 \mu g \cdot kg^{-1} \cdot min^{-1}$,[12] so as not to overwhelm the hepatic rhodanese-thiosulfate detoxification system. Early signs of cyanide toxicity are a systemic metabolic acidosis and an increase in mixed venous oxygen content. Should this unusual combination of laboratory values occur during large doses of nitroprusside therapy, the therapy should be discontinued.

Sublingual or intravenously[3] administered nitroglycerine dilates primarily the venous compliance vessels, causing a reduction in venous return and left ventricular end-diastolic volume. Some systemic arterial dilatation also occurs.[B6] Nitroglycerin, then, is the drug of choice in patients with pulmonary venous hypertension and a relatively low arterial pressure, and in cases of myocardial ischemia with elevated preload, in which preferential dilatation of the capacitance vessels, as well as favorable myocardial blood flow redistribution, is desired.[C2,K7,L12,M17]

Whereas nitroprusside and nitroglycerin both act directly

on the vascular smooth muscles to decrease resistance, phentolamine and trimethaphan reduce the systemic vascular resistance by alpha-adrenergic blockade and ganglionic blockade, respectively. Although used successfully in the past for postoperative afterload reduction,[K8] trimethaphan, by virtue of its ganglionic blockade, has many general effects. One particularly undesirable effect is cycloplegia, making neurological evaluation difficult.

A problem with vasodilators is that, in hypovolemic patients or those with normal ventricular function, they may cause reflex increases in heart rate and contractility and an undesirable increase in myocardial oxygen consumption.[B7,P2] Care should be used in administering vasodilators to patients who may be hypovolemic. These reflex changes are seldom observed in patients with abnormal ventricular function and pulmonary venous hypertension.[P7]

VASOCONSTRICTORS

The indications for drugs with predominant vasoconstrictive properties are few.[R1] Hypovolemia from any cause is best treated by volume replacement, but this treatment may be aided, particularly in emergency situations, by judicious administration of peripheral arterial and venous vasoconstrictors. Vasoconstrictors are very occasionally used before bypass in cyanotic patients with congenital heart disease to decrease right-to-left shunting when systemic resistance falls below a fixed high pulmonary arterial outflow tract resistance. Rarely, peripheral resistance drops because of drug or blood hypersensitivity reactions, and vasoconstrictors are useful in emergencies to restore perfusion pressure. As indicated earlier, the combination of a pure vasoconstrictor, such as phenylephrine, and intravenously administered nitroglycerin is often useful during the period of myocardial reperfusion after aortic cross-clamping.

The vasoconstrictors are sympathomimetic drugs that possess primarily α-1 adrenergic agonist properties[4] (Table 4-4). The vascular response to α-1 adrenergic stimulation is vasoconstriction, usually in both the arterial and venous circulations. If pure vasoconstriction without direct cardiac (β-1) response is desired, then either methoxamine or phenylephrine is administered. If, in addition to a predominantly α-adrenergic effect, some β-adrenergic cardiac response is desired to increase heart rate and myocardial contractility, then ephedrine, dopamine, epinephrine, or, rarely, norepinephrine might be used.

INOTROPIC DRUGS

Inotropic drugs have been less commonly used during cardiac anesthesia since the advent of cold cardioplegia.[R1] The

---

[1]IMED model no. 922, IMED Corporation, San Diego, Calif., 92121.

[2]IVAC model no. 530, IVAC Corporation, La Jolla, Calif., 92131.

[3]Available from G. Pohl-Boskamp, D-2214 Hohenlockstedt, West Germany, as Nitrolingual in 1-ml ampules containing 5 mg of nitroglycerin.

---

[4]Cardiovascular adrenergic stimulation consists of α-1 responses, consisting of arterial and venous vasoconstriction; β-1 responses, including increased myocardial contractility, sinoatrial rate (automaticity), conduction velocity of myocardial nervous tissue, and cardiac metabolism; and β-2 responses, consisting of weak systemic and pulmonary artery vasodilation and bronchodilation.[H12,V4]

Table 4-4 Adrenergic receptor stimulation and dosages of vasoconstrictors.

| Vasoconstrictor | | Activity | | | | | |
| | | Vascular | | Cardiac | | | |
Generic Name	Trade Name	α_1	β_2	β_1	Onset	Duration	Initial Adult Dosage
Methoxamine	Vasoxyl	+ + + +	0	0	+ +	+ +	0.5–2-mg bolus
Phenylephrine	Neo-Synephrine	+ + + +	0	0	+ +	+ + +	0.1–0.5-mg bolus
Norepinephrine	Levophed	+ + + +	+	+ +	+ + + +	+	Titrate with infusion
Ephedrine	Ephedrine	+ + +	0	+ +	+ +	+ + + +	2.5–5-mg bolus

KEY: The number of + 's denotes increasing activity or time; α, α-adrenergic; β, β-adrenergic.

most common indication for inotropic support is transiently depressed cardiac output immediately after CPB. Occasionally, inotropic drugs are indicated before CPB, such as in patients with mitral incompetence and reduced cardiac output unresponsive to vasodilator therapy.

Catecholamines adversely affect the myocardial oxygen supply-demand ratio and, when given for more than a brief period, may aggravate myocardial necrosis.[B8] Thus, when prolonged administration seems necessary, counterpulsation with an intra-aortic balloon should be considered, followed by gradual discontinuation of the inotropic drugs. Measurement of cardiac index after CPB can be helpful in making such a decision. Cardiac output is usually at least 25% higher in the operating room with the chest open than it is a few hours later. Thus, in adults, when heart rate, preload, and afterload are optimal and cardiac index is less than about 2.0 $l \cdot min^{-1} \cdot m^{-2}$ after CPB, inotropic support and then intra-aortic balloon pumping should be considered.

When inotropic support is indicated, one or two bolus administrations of relatively short-acting drugs, such as calcium chloride or ephedrine, commonly suffice; the anesthesiologist must remember that calcium is dangerous if the serum potassium is low. If myocardial dysfunction persists, continuous infusions of epinephrine, dopamine, dobutamine, or isoproterenol may be required (Table 4-5). Most of these drugs act predominantly on the β-1 adrenergic receptors and cause increased myocardial contractility, heart rate, AV conduction, and cardiac metabolism (glycogenolysis, adenyl cyclase activity, and cyclic 3'-5' AMP). The β-2 effect on systemic and pulmonary vasculature is one of weak vasodilatation. Catecholamines predispose patients anesthetized with halothane and other inhalation agents to arrhythmias. The following is a list of the catecholamines in order of increasing potential to cause supraventricular arrhythmia: dobutamine, dopamine, epinephrine, isproterenol.[H5,J3,M12,Z2] The relative potential for ventricular arrhythmias during in-

Table 4-5 Adrenergic receptor stimulation of inotropic drugs.

| Inotropic Drug | | Receptor Activity | | | |
| | | Vascular | | Cardiac | |
Generic Name	Trade Name	α	β_2	β_1	Comments
Epinephrine	Adrenalin	+ + +	+	+ +	Relative α and β effects are dose related (β in low doses and α in higher doses). Given by infusion (may be given by bolus injection).
Dopamine	Inotropin	+ +	+	+ +	Relative α and β effects are dose related, as are those of epinephrine, but splanchnic and renal vasoconstriction is avoided. Used in patients with compromised renal function. Given by infusion.
Dobutamine	Dobutrex	+	+	+ + +	Theoretically, has primarily β effects on myocardial contractility, with little other β cardiac effect. Given by infusion.
Ephedrine	Ephedrine	+ + +	0	+ +	β effects are primarily secondary to release of norepinephrine. Lasts 5–10 min after bolus injection. Tachyphylaxis may occur.
Isoproterenol	Isuprel	0	+ + + +	+ + + +	Has pure β effects. High dosages lead to ventricular irritability. Given by infusion.
Calcium chloride	Calcium	0	0	0	Is a rapid-acting positive inotropic drug and not adrenergic. Useful in patients on propranolol to increase contractility. Given by bolus injection.
Digoxin	Lanoxin, Digitoxin	0	0	0	Has delayed onset of inotropic action and low therapeutic safety ratio, which makes acute use inappropriate in most cases. Mechanism of action does not involve β system. Given by bolus injection.

KEY: The number of + 's denotes increasing activity or time; α, α-adrenergic; β, β-adrenergic.

halation anesthesia and low cardiac output is less clear, but enflurane appears to sensitize the heart less than other potent inhalation anesthetics.

Dopamine is a preferred inotropic agent. It is the natural precursor of norepinephrine and epinephrine, and has dose-related α- and β-adrenergic agonist properties. Its actions are direct as well as indirect, by the release of norepinephrine at adrenergic terminals. Through its β-1 effect, dopamine increases contractility and heart rate; and through α-adrenergic stimulation, it causes systemic peripheral vasoconstriction. The unique effect of dopamine is the dilatation of renal and mesenteric vascular beds by stimulation of postulated dopaminergic receptors.[G4] However, there is a tendency toward greater α-stimulation with higher doses of dopamine, and heart rate also increases in a dose-related fashion.[B9,S19] Dopamine is particularly suitable for inotropic support in patients with renal dysfunction. It may also be given in low dose ($2.5 \ \mu g \cdot kg^{-1} \cdot min^{-1}$) to stimulate renal blood flow and thus urine flow. There is some evidence to support its use in patients with pulmonary artery hypertension, since dopamine does not significantly increase pulmonary vascular resistance.

Dobutamine is a new synthetic inotropic drug[T4] that appears to be relatively specific for contractility, with minimal effects on heart rate and conduction.[S17,T4] However, there is a dose-related increase in heart rate when dobutamine is used after cardiac surgery.[S18] Comparative human studies have shown that tachycardias and arrhythmias are less prevalent with dobutamine than with isoproterenol, and that the α-adrenergic effects are minimal.[K10,S18]

Isoproterenol is the only drug available that has pure β-adrenergic effects. It is used when an increase in contractility, heart rate, and peripheral vasodilatation are desirable. Isoproterenol increases myocardial oxygen consumption,[K9] and the associated vasodilation and tachycardia may decrease oxygen supply. Its most serious side effect is its arrhythmic property, which is dose-related.

Epinephrine, like dopamine, has dose-related effects on α- and β-adrenergic receptors. In low dosage, the β effects predominate, but in higher dosages α-adrenergic effects are prominent, resulting in vasoconstriction and increased systemic vascular resistance (Fig. 4-9).

The combination of catecholamines with vasodilators may further increase cardiac output by reducing left and right ventricular afterload while augmenting myocardial contractility.[S19,S20] This combination is particularly appropriate if higher doses of the inotropic drugs are necessary with the attendant increases in vascular resistance. In such situations, the intra-aortic balloon pump should be considered.

Calcium increases myocardial contractility directly, whereas all other inotropic drugs probably indirectly augment contractility by increasing the intramyocardial cellular calcium level.[E4] Intravenous calcium chloride increases the extracellular-intracellular concentration gradient, resulting in almost immediate inotropic effects. The positive inotropic effects of Ca^{2+} peak in 1 minute and last 10–15 minutes.[D6] The predominant effect of Ca^{2+} is increased contractility, which is dose-related,[B10] resulting in increased cardiac index despite a decrease in heart rate.[D6] The blood pressure increases, but systemic vascular resistance is decreased.[D6,S21]

Calcium in doses of $10 \ mg \cdot kg^{-1}$ may be safely given after bypass to increase contractility in high-calcemic or normocalcemic patients.[W6] Doses as high as $1.5 \ mg \cdot kg^{-1} \cdot min^{-1}$ are recommended only in patients with hypocalcemia and when Ca^{2+} ion concentration can be monitored.[D7] The initial Ca^{2+} concentration is an important determinant of the circulatory response to calcium infusion.[D11] Although calcium can be used to replenish lowered Ca^{2+} or for brief inotropic therapy, prolonged infusion predisposes patients to elevated Ca^{2+} levels and arrhythmias for as long as 20 hours after surgery.[W6] Calcium chloride should not be administered within 10 minutes of releasing the aortic cross-clamp to reperfuse the myocardium. Administration via a peripheral vein carries a very high risk of skin necrosis around the infusion site; a central large vein must therefore be used.

Digitalis is a weakly positive inotropic drug with a nonadrenergic mechanism of action. Digitalis glycosides increase the amount of calcium released intracellularly for excitation-contraction coupling through membrane changes.[L13] The peak inotropic effects vary with the glycoside preparation, ouabain being the most rapid (5–10 minutes) and digitalis leaf the slowest (60 minutes).[F4] Inotropic effects from intravenous digoxin occur within 10 minutes and continue to increase over succeeding hours.[F4] The pharmacokinetic data reveal that all glycosides have prolonged serum half-life—which, for digoxin, is 34 hours—and excretion is primarily via the kidneys.[D8] Thus, in choosing digoxin for inotropic support, its relatively slow onset, long duration, and relatively weak effect must be considered. Intraoperatively, other inotropic drugs, such as calcium or infusions of catecholamines, are more commonly used than digoxin. Digitalization is best accomplished in the recovery period because intraoperative hypokalemia and alkalosis sensitize patients to the toxic arrhythmic effects of digitalis,[H6] and these conditions can be better controlled postoperatively. Digitalis remains useful for intraoperative control of rhythm disturbances.

ANTIARRHYTHMIC DRUGS

During anesthesia and operation, rhythm disturbances are frequent. Those due to handling of the heart are generally benign and self-limited. Arrhythmias that result from electrolyte imbalance, pH fluctuations, or the interaction of various drugs[K11,P3] should respond to correction of the underlying cause, although some require specific therapy. Digitalis decreases the ventricular response in patients with supraventricular tachyarrhythmias (Table 4-6). It decreases the rate of sinoatrial node firing, the refractory period, and the conduction velocity of the atrioventricular node and enhances the automaticity of the His-Purkinje system.[L14] The potassium concentration should be known for giving digoxin, to prevent possible toxicity, and in those patients on preoperative digitalis therapy, the serum digoxin level should be determined on the day before operation so that an overdose is not given. (Digoxin toxicity can produce a supraventricular arrhythmia.)

Propranolol is an antiarrhythmic drug with two modes of action. It is a β-adrenergic blocker and has membrane effects

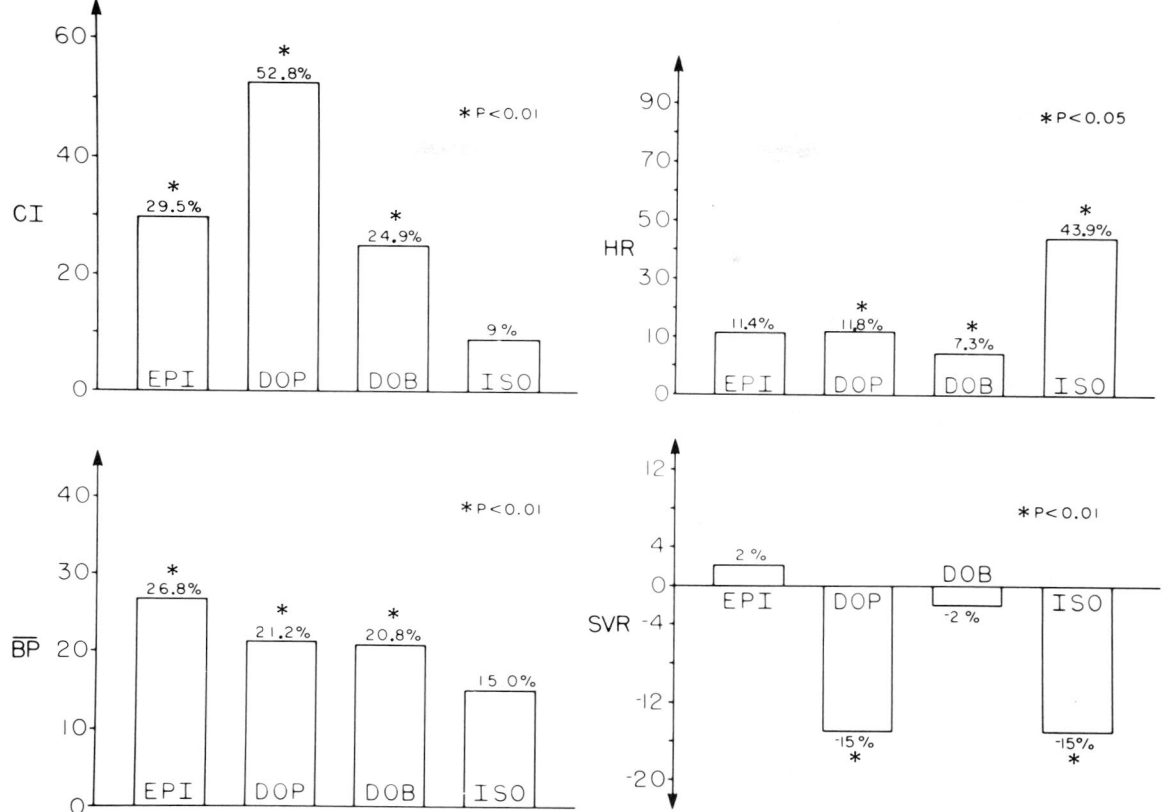

Figure 4-9 Hemodynamic changes (percent change from control) with four catecholamine infusions during surgery in patients after CPB. Although the data, with the exception of the isoproterenol group, were obtained in patients with an acceptable cardiac index, the hemodynamic changes are representative pharmacologic responses of these drugs at roughly equipotent dosages 10 minutes after infusion. The drugs and infusion dosages (in $\mu g \cdot kg^{-1} \cdot min^{-1}$) are epinephrine (EPI), 0.04; dopamine (DOP), 10; dobutamine (DOB), 1; isoproterenol (ISO), 0.02.

CI, cardiac index; HR, heart rate; BP, mean systemic blood pressure; SVR, systemic vascular resistance.

Redrawn from data by Tinker[T5] and Steen.[S29]

similar to those of quinidine. Propranolol slows the spontaneous SA node firing, decreases the atrial and AV node conduction velocity, and depresses the spontaneous automaticity of most of the conduction tissue.[B11,L4] The most prominent hemodynamic effects of intravenous propranolol administration are slowing of the heart rate with lower doses, and decreased contractility and cardiac output with higher doses. In patients with rapid heart rates, cardiac output often improves as heart rate slows and ventricular filling time increases. The usual intravenous dose is 0.25–1 mg, administered slowly (up to a maximum of 0.1 mg $\cdot$ kg^{-1}) while watching for bradycardia, decreased cardiac output, and brochospasm. The onset of action is rapid, and the effect persists for 2–8 hours.[L14] Primary indications for the use of propranolol are sinus and junctional tachycardias and, occasionally, digitalis toxicity. Doses of 0.1 mg $\cdot$ kg^{-1} significantly lower the temperature at which the heart fibrillates during induced hypothermia;[W9] propranolol can therefore be used intraoperatively to delay the onset of ventricular fibrillation associated with hypothermia.[S22]

Lidocaine (lignocaine) is a local anesthetic drug with prominent antiarrhythmic properties. It raises the threshold potential to electrical stimulation (decreases ventricular excitability) and is the drug of choice for the treatment of ventricular arrhythmias.[H3] In contrast to digoxin, propranolol, and procainamide, lidocaine does not change atrioventricular conduction. In therapeutic doses, it has no signficant cardiovascular effects,[G5] though higher doses may decrease myocardial contractility, heart rate, and systemic pressure.[A5] An intravenous bolus of 1 mg $\cdot$ kg^{-1}, followed by a second or third dose, may be required to obtain therapeutic levels. To maintain a therapeutic serum level (2–4 μg $\cdot$ ml^{-1}), an infusion of 20–25 μg $\cdot$ kg^{-1} $\cdot$ min^{-1} may be required,[H3] since a single bolus administration lasts for only about 20 minutes.[L14] Toxicity is manifested by muscular twitching, which can be masked by general anesthesia and muscle relaxants. Lidocaine must also be given cautiously in patients with third-degree heart block, as it can abolish the idioventricular pacemaker and produce asystole.

Procainamide (Pronestyl) is similar in its antiarrhythmic

Table 4-6 Activity and uses of antiarrhythmic drugs.

Generic Name (Trade Name)	Mechanism of Action	Cardiovascular Effects	Principal Indication	Intravenous Dosage	Comments
Digoxin (Lanoxin)	Decreases AV conduction. Decreases SA node rate. Increases ventricular automaticity.	Increases myocardial contractility. May decrease systemic resistance. Blood pressure response is variable.	Slow ventricular response to supraventricular tachyarrhythmias	0.125–0.25-mg bolus	Relatively slow action. K^+ and Ca^{2+} must be normal. Toxicity causes serious arrhythmias because of increased automaticity in His-Purkinje tissue.
Propranolol (Inderal)	β-adrenergic blockade effects decrease atrial automaticity. Decreases AV conduction. Membrane effects decrease excitability.	Decreases heart rate, myocardial contractility, cardiac output, and blood pressure.	Sinus tachycardia, slow ventricular response to supraventricular tachyarrhythmias	0.25–1-mg bolus	May depress cardiac output. Causes bronchospasm and AV block.
Lidocaine (Xylocaine)	Decreases ventricular excitability.	Has little effect in therapeutic concentrations.	Premature ventricular contractions, ventricular tachyarrhythmias	1-mg · kg^1 bolus; 20–50 μg · kg^{-1} · min^{-1} infusion.	Toxic dosage produces seizure activity. May abolish idioventricular pacemaker in third-degree block.
Procainamide (Pronestyl)	Decreases cardiac excitability. Has variable effect on refractory period. Decreases SA node rate. May slow AV and His-Purkinje conduction.	Causes minimal changes with moderate dosages. Decreases contractility and vasodilatation.	Broad spectrum use: premature atrial contractions, paroxysmal atrial tachycardia, atrial fibrillation, premature ventricular contractions, and ventricular tachycardia.	100-mg bolus slowly, repeated up to 1 g	May decrease blood pressure. Toxic dosage widens QRS complex. May cause ventricular fibrillation or asystole.
Atropine	Blocks parasympathetic inhibition of SA node.	Increases heart rate and cardiac output.	Sinus bradycardia	0.6–1-mg bolus	Small dose may cause bradycardia. Larger doses may cause junctional rhythms, sinus tachycardia, and premature ventricular contractions.
Verapamil	Blocks Ca^{2+} channel. Slows AV conduction.	Causes hypotension. Decreases myocardial contractility.	Supraventricular tachyarrhythmias	0.15 mg · kg^{-1}–10 mg · kg^{-1} IV bolus over 1–2 min	Causes transient hemodynamic changes, and, with conversion to sinus rhythm, may produce increased blood pressure and cardiac output.

and cardiovascular effects to quinidine. Both drugs directly depress excitability, conduction velocity, and contractility of the heart.[F5] Procainamide is used for the treatment of ventricular irritability that does not respond to lidocaine and for control of supraventricular arrhythmias (e.g., paroxysmal atrial tachycardia, atrial flutter, and atrial fibrillation) if pacing or electrical countershock fails or is not available. Rarely, vagolytic effects of procainamide may paradoxically potentiate supraventricular arrhythmias such as paroxysmal atrial tachycardia.[W7] The effective intravenous dose for treatment of ventricular arrhythmias is approximately 4–10 mg · kg^{-1}.[G6] Despite the fact that procainamide is a negative inotropic drug and possesses the ability to cause mild systemic vasodilation,[H7] 100-mg increments at 5-minute intervals may be given without seriously disturbing hemodynamic conditions.[G6] Fifty percent of procainamide is excreted unchanged by the kidneys; thus, the dosage must be reduced in patients with renal impairment.[D10] Oral procainamide (available in slow-release capsules as Procan SR) is used as maintenance therapy once intravenous lidocaine is discontinued. Oral quinidine (also available in slow-release capsules) can be used instead.

Atropine is an anticholinergic drug that competitively blocks postganglionic parasympathetic cholinergic receptors. Atropine blocks vagal (parasympathetic) effects on heart rate and conduction. The most common use of atropine is the treatment of sinus bradycardia resulting from excessive vagal stimulation or from high doses of propranolol (or other β-blocker therapy). Atropine sulfate given intravenously has dose-related cardiovascular effects. When a low dose (< 0.2 mg in an adult) is administered to patients with normal sinus rhythm, the heart rate slows, with little change in blood pressure, cardiac index, systemic vascular resistance, and PR interval.[F6,G7] The effects of atropine may vary with the underlying anesthetic agent,[J4] but generally it produces an increase in heart rate and blood pressure in higher doses.[C10] When treating bradyarrhythmias, doses of > 0.6 mg are used in normal-sized adults, and appropriately smaller doses in children and infants.

Verapamil is a calcium channel blocker with a narrow but important antiarrhythmic potential.[E6] Intravenous verapamil is highly effective in the treatment of paroxysmal supraventricular tachyarrhythmias in nonsurgical[B17,S35,S36] as well as postoperative patients.[W11] The hemodynamic effects of intravenous verapamil are a transient decrease in systemic vascular resistance, blood pressure, and left ventricular systolic function and an increase in left ventricular end-diastolic pressure, with no significant change in heart rate, cardiac output, and pulmonary artery pressure.[S37] The interaction of verapamil and anesthetic drugs has not been completely studied, but it is clear that combinations of verapamil with halothane, enflurane, and isoflurane result in additive cardiovascular depression and AV block.[R16]

DRUG INTERACTIONS

Propranolol and related drugs are often part of the medical management of patients with ischemic heart disease because of their β-adrenergic–blocking properties. The negative inotropic effects of propranolol could interact with the effects of halogenated anesthetics to produce synergistic myocardial depression.[S23] There is ample evidence from clinical practice, however, that it is safe and in fact advisable to continue propranolol therapy up to the time of operation.[C11,C12,K12,K13] Data that reveal the brief half-life of oral propranolol (3–6 hours)[E5,S24] and the abolition of negative chronotropic and inotropic effects within 24–48 hours of drug discontinuation[F7] also indicate that the drug may be discontinued safely the day of surgery with the expectation of little pharmacologic interaction during and immediately after operation. The propranolol dose is tapered to 80–160 mg daily if the patient's condition allows, and propranolol is discontinued on the morning of operation. The other β-adrenergic drugs[F10,F11]—nadolol, metoprolol, sotalol hydrochloride, timolol maleate, practolol, pindolol, oxprenolol hydrochloride, and atenolol—appear to also be safe in the perioperative period. Of particular note is the half-life of elimination, which ranges from the relatively short (oral oxprenolol, 2 hours) to long (sotalol, 5–13 hours).[F10] Naturally, drugs with greater half-life have a greater potential for perioperative drug interactions.

The group of drugs called calcium antagonists or slow channel blockers is also used in patients with ischemic heart disease and hypertension. These drugs include verapamil, nifedipine, diltiazem hydrochloride, and lidoflazine. The efficacy of nifedipine and verapamil for coronary artery spasm angina[A6,J5,P8] and verapamil for supraventricular arrhythmias clearly demonstrates that these drugs are useful during the perioperative period. Potential for additive myocardial depression and hypotension exists when Ca^{2+} entry blockers and anesthetic drugs are combined.[R16] Verapamil and inhalation drugs produce cardiovascular depression, as does the combination of nifedipine and halothane.[T6] Thus, care must be given to the dose of inhalation anesthetic agents administered to patients maintained on Ca^{2+} entry blocking drugs.

Digitalis and other antiarrhythmic drugs, such as procainamide and quinidine, may present some drug interaction problems. Digitalis in combination with potassium-wasting diuretics may result in digitalis toxicity, usually manifested as (1) premature ventricular contractions, (2) paroxysmal atrial tachydardia with block, or (3) Mobitz type 1 atrioventricular block. Because of electrolyte changes, particularly potassium changes during bypass, digitalis is often withheld for 36 hours before cardiac surgery, although this occasion-

ally can lead to rapid ventricular response rates in patients with atrial fibrillation,[S25] necessitating the intraoperative administration of digoxin. Presumably, discontinuing digitalis before cardiac surgery reduces the incidence of cardiac arrhythmias during and after surgery. A reasonable compromise is to continue digitalis in patients requiring rate control of supraventricular tachyarrhythmias; but its discontinuation 36 hours before surgery in prophylactic digitalization is not practiced.

Both procainamide and quinidine are continued up to operation in their usual doses despite the fact that they potentiate the neuromuscular blockade of nondepolarizing muscle relaxants and depolarizing agents.[M13,S26] The anesthesiologist must be aware of this relationship and administer muscle relaxants accordingly. The degree of neuromuscular blockade can be monitored with commercially available devices. Postoperative administration of quinidine or procainamide in patients emerging from neuromuscular blockade can result in respiratory paresis.

There are many antihypertensive medications, with varied actions. Drugs such as reserpine, hydralazine, methyldopa, quanethidine, and clonidine hydrochloride should all be continued up to the day of surgery, since well-controlled hypertensive patients do better during anesthesia than do partially controlled or uncontrolled patients.[F8,P4] Moreover, the danger of rebound hypertension exists in patients in whom clonidine is abruptly withdrawn.[H8] The one group of antihypertensive drugs that should be discontinued 2 weeks before surgery (and replaced with others) are the monoamine oxidase inhibitors. These drugs are used mainly as antidepressants; a partial list appears in Table 4-7. Monoamine oxidase inhibitors alter the function of the normal adrenergic terminal. The result is an alteration in synthesis of catecholamines and their metabolites that may lead to unusual interactions with drugs (particularly with narcotics and catecholamines) and tyramine-containing foods. Severe hypertension, hypotension, and unpredictable adrenergic drug effects have all been encountered in patients on these drugs undergoing anesthesia.[K14]

Diuretics are used to assist the treatment of hypertension by counteracting the compensatory sodium retention that accompanies antihypertensive therapy. Because they reduce blood volume, they are also important in treating congestive heart failure. There are three classes of diuretics: (1) thiazides (e.g., hydrochlorothiazide), which block sodium reabsorption in the distal tubules; (2) potent, or loop, diuretics (e.g., furosemide and ethacrynic acid), which inhibit sodium reabsorption in both the ascending Henle's loop and in the proximal tubule; and (3) potassium sparing diuretics (e.g., spironolactone and triamterene), which reduce both sodium reabsorption and potassium secretion. All these drugs in high doses may cause extracellular fluid depletion, which, combined with the vasodilatation of most anesthetic drugs, can result in hypotension. This is a more common problem with the potent diuretics, in patients with coronary artery disease who may already have reduced plasma volume,[C1] and in infants. Another potential drug interaction problem is the potassium-wasting effects of hydrochlorothiazide and loop diuretics when combined with digitalis, for a low potassium level predisposes patients to digitalis toxicity,

Table 4-7 Operative and postoperative drug interaction problems.

Drug Group	Drug	Interacting Drug	Complications	Recommendations
Adrenergic blockers	Propranolol	Halogenated inhalation anesthetics (methoxyflurane, halothane, enflurane)	Potentiation of myocardial depression, resistance to agonist drugs	Taper to 80 mg · d^{-1} if possible, but do not discontinue.
Digitalis	Digoxin (many others)	Insulin; diuretics and diuresis on bypass	Nitroglycerin digitalis toxicity manifested by arrhythmias	Measure serum glucose level. Discontinue 24 h before day of surgery. Monitor serum K$^+$ during operation.
Antiarrhythmics	Quinidine, procainamide	Nondepolarizing muscle relaxants (curare, pancuronium) and depolarizing muscle relaxants (succinylcholine)	Neuromuscular paralysis due to potentiation of muscle relaxants	Continue drug, but administer relaxants cautiously and monitor neuromuscular blockade with appropriate device.
Antihypertensives	Methyldopa	Any anesthetic that causes increased capacitance or vasodilatation	Hypotension	Continue drug. Monitor volume status carefully, and give volume when necessary or adrenergic agonist if hypotension occurs.
	Monoamine oxidase inhibitors (phenelzine, nialamide, isocarboxazid pazyline)	Opiods, sympathomimetic amines	Hypertension, possibly hypotension, unpredictable hemodynamic responses to adjuvant vasoactive drugs	Discontinue 2 wk before surgery.
Diuretics	Chlorothiazide, hydrochlorothiazide, furosemide, ethacrynic acid	Anesthetic drugs that cause increased capacitance or vasodilatation	Hypotension	Continue drugs. Monitor K$^+$ volume status carefully.
Tricyclic antidepressants	Amitriptyline, imipramine, doxepin, desipramine, nortriptyline, protriptyline	Sympathomimetic amines	Tachycardia, hypertension	Taper if possible. Administer adrenergic drugs cautiously.
		Anesthetic drugs	Hypotension	Monitor volume status. Treat hypotension with volume if possible.
Antibiotics	Tetracyclines	Methoxyflurane	Nephrotoxicity	Continue drug. Avoid methoxyflurane if possible; otherwise, retract dose to minimum required.
	Neomycin, kanamycin, gentamycin, polymycin, streptomycin, colistin, tetracycline (others)	Depolarizing muscle relaxants (succinylcholine) and nondepolarizing (curare, pancuronium) muscle relaxants	Neuromuscular paralysis due to potentiation of muscle relaxants	Continue drug. Use muscle relaxants with caution, and monitor neuromuscular blockade with appropriate devices.
Hepatic enzyme inducers	Diphenylhydantoin, phenobarbital, trimethodione ethanol (others)	Methoxyflurane		Continue and restrict halothane to smallest possible dose for shortest time required.

as previously mentioned. Diuretic therapy should be continued up to the day of surgery in patients with signs and symptoms of pulmonary venous hypertension, but in other patients, it should be discontinued 1–2 days before operation so that plasma volume may increase.

Because of the prevalence of mental depression in patients with severe cardiac disease, some are treated with tricyclic antidepressants (Table 4-7). These drugs have three principal actions: (1) sedation, (2) peripheral and central anticholinergic effects, and (3) inhibition of the amine pump responsible for norepinephrine reuptake at the adrenergic nerve terminal.[H9] It is the last action that probably accounts for their antidepressant activity. However, their anticholinergic and adrenergic effects are responsible for the undesirable cardiovascular and perioperative drug interaction problems. The anticholinergic effects of tricyclic therapy result in a sustained increase in heart rate and a transient decrease in AV conduction.[B12] Myocardial depression is a transient feature of initiating tricyclic therapy. Potential drug interaction problems include tachycardia and hypotension

with anesthetic induction, and hypertension and tachycardia with adjuvant administration of sympathomimetic amines.[B16] Therefore, the use of tricyclic antidepressants should be tapered off or discontinued before cardiac surgery in all patients except those in whom they are absolutely essential. They may be reinstituted during the postoperative hospital course for appropriate psychiatric indications.

Antibiotics may present some serious drug interaction problems. Tetracyclines, when combined with methoxyflurane, predispose patients to high-output renal failure. The "mycins"[5] and tetracyclines potentiate the neuromuscular blocking effects of both the depolarizing and nondepolarizing muscle relaxants.[P5] This drug interaction is potentially lethal, since respiratory paralysis and apnea may occur. Par-

---

[5] "Mycins" include neomycin, streptomycin, gentamicin, kanamycin, vancomycin, paraomymycin, viomycin, polymyxin, coliatin, lincomycin, and clindamycin.

enteral administration of these antibiotics potentiates the neuromuscular blockade of muscle relaxants (depolarizers and nondepolarizers) given during anesthesia.

Most drugs are biotransformed to some degree by the liver microsomal enzymes. These enzymes are induced by many drugs; the prototypes are anticonvulsants (e.g., phenobarbital and diphenylhydantoin), but many other chronically administered drugs produce hepatic microsomal enzyme induction. This is clinically significant because it means that higher doses of anesthetic drugs are generally required and because anesthetic-induced organotoxicity is based on metabolism of at least two drugs: methoxyflurane and halothane. Methoxyflurane following high dose and/or duration may result in a syndrome of high-output vasopressin-resistant renal failure. This has been correlated with high serum inorganic fluoride levels (> 50–60 $\mu mol \cdot l^{-1}$) produced by methoxyflurane metabolism. The renal failure is a result of direct fluoride toxicity of the renal tubules.[C13] There is evidence that drug therapy with the potential for enzyme induction and biotransformation increases the serum fluoride level. The inhalation agents enflurane and isoflurane are also metabolized, resulting, however, in serum inorganic fluoride levels much lower than that resulting from methoxyflurane. To eliminate fluoride tubular toxicity, the dose of methoxyflurane is limited,[S27] and probably this drug should not be administered to patients suspected to have enzyme induction. Although some aspects of halothane liver toxicity remain an enigma,[R14] it appears that biotransformation of halothane in the liver[M16] to a free radical–containing compound (trifluoroacetoaldehyde) in certain predisposed individuals causes hepatic damage. The potential for development of this extremely rare occurrence may be expected to increase in patients with hepatic enzyme induction. Hepatic enzyme–inducing drugs may be continued up to the time of surgery, but an awareness of the risk of potential complications must enter into the choice of anesthetic agents. Usually, the indications for the use of certain anesthetic drugs, such as halothane, far outweigh the risks.

REFERENCES

A

1. Amory DW, Steffenson JL, Forsyth RP: Systemic and regional blood flow changes during halothane anesthesia in the rhesus monkey. *Anesthesiology* 35:81, 1971.

2. Atlee JL, Rusy BF: Atrioventricular conduction times and atrioventricular nodal conductivity during enflurane anesthesia in dogs. *Anesthesiology* 47:498, 1977.

3. Atlee JL, Rusy BF, Kreul JF, Eby T: Supraventricular excitability in dogs during anesthesia with halothane and enflurane. *Anesthesiology* 49:407, 1978.

4. Arens JF, Benbow BP, Ochsner JL, Theard R: Morphine anesthesia for aortocoronary bypass procedure. *Anesth Analg* 51:901, 1972.

5. Austen WG, Moran JM: Cardiac and peripheral vascular effects of lidocaine and procainamide. *Am J Cardiol* 16:701, 1965.

6. Antman E, Muller J, Goldberg S, MacAlpin R, Rubenfire M, Tabatznik B, Liang C-S, Heupler F, Achuff S, Reichek N, Geltman E, Kerin NZ, Neff RK, Braunwald E: Nifedipine therapy for coronary-artery spasm: Experience in 127 patients. *N Engl J Med* 302:1269, 1980.

B

1. Braunwald E: The determinants of myocardial oxygen consumption. *Physiologist* 12:65, 1969.

2. Bahlman SH, Eger EI II, Smith NT, Stevens WC, Shakespeare TF, Sawyer DC, Halsey MJ, Cromwell TH: The cardiovascular effects of nitrous oxide-halothane in man. *Anesthesiology* 35:274, 1971.

3. Black GW, McArdle L: The effects of methoxyflurane (penthrane) on the peripheral circulation in man. *Br J Anaesth* 37:947, 1965.

4. Bahlman SH, Eger EI II, Halsey MJ, Stevens WC, Shakespeare TF, Smith NT, Cromwell TH, and Fourcade H: The cardiovascular effects of halothane in man during spontaneous ventilation. *Anesthesiology* 36:494, 1972.

5. Bland JHL, Lowenstein E: Halothane-induced decrease in experimental myocardial ischemia in the non-failing canine heart. *Anesthesiology* 45:287, 1976.

6. Braunwald E: Vasodilator therapy: A physiologic approach to the treatment of heart failure. *N Engl J Med* 297:331, 1977.

7. Bhatia SK, Frohlich ED: Hemodynamic comparison of agents useful in hypertensive emergencies. *Am Heart J* 85:367, 1973.

8. Braunwald E, Maroko PR: The reduction of infarct size: An idea whose time (for testing) has come. *Circulation* 50:206, 1974.

9. Beregovich J, Bianchi C, Rubler S, Lomnitz E, Cagin N, Levitt B: Dose-related hemodynamic and renal effects of dopamine in congestive heart failure. *Am Heart J* 87:550, 1974.

10. Bristow MR, Daniels JR, Kernoff RS, Harrison DC: Effect of D600, practolol and alterations in magnesium on ionized calcium concentration-response relationships in the intact dog heart. *Circ Res* 41:574, 1977.

11. Berkowitz WD, Wit AL, Lau SH, Steiner C, Damato AN: The effects of propranolol on cardiac conduction. *Circulation* 40:855, 1969.

12. Burckhardt D, Raeder E, Muller V, Imhof P, Neubauer H: Cardiovascular effects of tricyclic and tetracyclic antidepressants. *JAMA* 239:213, 1978.

13. Branthwaite MA: Prevention of neurological damage during open-heart surgery. *Thorax* 30:258, 1975.

14. Branthwaite MA: Factors affecting cerebral activity during open-heart surgery. *Anesthesiology* 28:619, 1973.

15. Bull BB, Huse WM, Brauer FS, Korpman RA: Heparin therapy during extracorporeal circulation. II. The use of a dose-response curve to individualize heparin and protamine dosage. *J Thorac Cardiovasc Surg* 69:685, 1975.

16. Boakes AJ, Laurence DR, Teoh PC, Barar FSK, Benedikter LT, Prichard BNC: Interactions between sympathomimetic amines and antidepressant agents in man. *Br Med J* [Clin Res] 1:311, 1973.

17. Brichard G, Zimmerman PE: Verapamil in cardiac dysrhythmias during anaesthesia. *Brit J Anaesth* 42:1005, 1970.

18. Barratt-Boyes BG, Neutze JM, Seelye ER, Simpson M: Com-

plete correction of cardiovascular malformations in the first year of life. *Prog Cardiovasc Dis* 15:229, 1972.

19. Best N, Sinosich MJ, Teisner B, Grudzinskas JG, Fisher M: Complement activation during cardiopulmonary bypass by heparin-protamine interaction. *Br J Anaesth* 56:339, 1984.

20. Best N, Teisner B, Grudzinskas JG, Fisher MM: Classical pathway activation during an adverse response to protamine sulphate. *Br J Anaesth* 55:1149, 1983.

21. Buttner EE, Reves JG, Karp RB, Zorn G: Reperfusion K⁺ and cardiac activity after cold cardioplegia. *Anesthesiology* 55:A21, 1981.

C

1. Cohn LH, Klovekorn P, Moore FD, Collins JJ: Intrinsic plasma volume deficits in patients with coronary artery disease. *Arch Surg* 108:57, 1974.

2. Chiariello M, Gold HK, Leinbach RC, Davis MA, Maroko PR: Comparison between the effects of nitroprusside and nitroglycerin on ischemic injury during acute myocardial infarction. *Circulation* 54:766, 1976.

3. Corssen G, Domino EF: Dissociative anesthesia: Further pharmacologic studies and first clinical experience with the phencyclidine derivative CI-581. *Anesth Analg* 45:29, 1966.

4. Corssen G, Allarde R, Brosch F, Arbenz G: Ketamine as the sole anesthetic in open-heart surgery: A preliminary report. *Anesth Analg* 49:1025, 1970.

5. Corssen G, Moustapha IF, Varner E: *The Role of Dissociative Anesthesia with Ketamine in Cardiac Surgery: A Preliminary Report Based on 253 Patients* (abstr). Singapore: Fourth Asian and Australian Congress of Anesthesiologists. 1974, p 136.

6. Cote P, Gueret P, Bourassa MG: Systemic and coronary hemodynamic effects of diazepam in patients with normal and diseased coronary arteries. *Circulation* 50:1210, 1974.

7. Cote P, Campeau L, Bourassa MG: Therapeutic implications of diazepam in patients with elevated left ventricular filling pressure. *Am Heart J* 91:747, 1976.

8. Claverly RK, Smith NT, Jones CW, Prys-Roberts C, Eger EI: Ventilatory and cardiovascular effects of enflurane anesthesia during spontaneous ventilation in man. *Anesth Analg* 57:610, 1978.

9. Claverly RK, Smith NT, Prys-Roberts C, Eger EI, Jones CW: Cardiovascular effects of enflurane anesthesia during controlled ventilation in man. *Anesth Analg* 57:619, 1978.

10. Carrow DJ, Aldrete JA, Masden RR, Jackson D: Effects of large doses of intravenous atropine on heart rate and arterial pressure of anesthetized patients. *Anesth Analg* 54:262, 1975.

11. Caralps JM, Mulet J, Wienke R, Moran JM, Pifarre R: Results of coronary artery surgery in patients receiving propranolol. *J Thorac Cardiovasc Surg* 67:526, 1974.

12. Coltart DJ, Cayen MN, Stinson EB, Goldman RH, Davies RO, Harrison DC: Investigation of the safe withdrawal period for propranolol in patients scheduled for open heart surgery. *Br Heart J* 37:1228, 1975.

13. Cousins MJ, Mazze RI, Kosek JC, Hitt BA, Love FV: The etiology of methoxyflurane nephrotoxicity. *J Pharmacol Exp Ther* 190:530, 1974.

14. Cohn JN, Franciosa JA: Vasodilator therapy of cardiac failure. *N Engl J Med* 297:27, 1977.

D

1. Das BB, Fenstermacher JM, Keats AS: Endobronchial anesthesia for resection of aneurysms of the descending aorta. *Anesthesiology* 32:152, 1970.

2. Dhadphale PR, Jackson APF, Alseri S: Comparison of anesthesia with diazepam and ketamine vs. morphine in patients undergoing heart-valve replacement. *Anesthesiology* 51:200, 1979.

3. Dobkin AB, Heinrich RG, Israel JS, Levy AA, Neville JF, Ounkasem K: Clinical and laboratory evaluation of a new inhalation agent: Compound 347 (CHF₂-O-CF₂CHF Cl). *Anesthesiology* 29:275, 1968.

4. Davies DW, Greiss L, Kadar D. Steward DJ: Sodium nitroprusside in children: Observations on metabolism during normal and abnormal responses. *Can Anaesth Soc J* 22:553, 1975.

5. Davies DW, Kadar D, Stewart DJ, Munro IR: A sudden death associated with the use of sodium nitroprusside for induction of hypotension during anesthesia. *Can Anaesth Soc J* 22:547, 1975.

6. Denlinger JK, Kaplan JA, Lecky JH, Wollman H: Cardiovascular responses to calcium administered intravenously to man during halothane anesthesia. *Anesthesiology* 42:390, 1975.

7. Drop LJ, Laver MB: Low plasma ionized calcium and responses to calcium therapy in critically ill man. *Anesthesiology* 43:300, 1975.

8. Doherty JE, Kane JJ: Digitalis glycosides: Recent advances in clinical pharmacology and treatment. *S Med J* 70:470, 1977.

9. deLange S, Boscoe MJ, Stanley TH: Comparison of sulfentanyl-O₂ and fentanyl-O₂ for coronary artery surgey. *Anesthesiology* 56:112, 1982.

10. Drayer DE, Lowenthal DT, Woosley RL, Nies AS, Schwartz A, Reidenberg MM: Cumulation of N-acetylprocainamide, an active metabolite of procainamide, in patients with impaired renal function. *Clin Pharmacol Ther* 22:63, 1977.

11. Drop LJ, Scheidegger D: Plasma ionized calcium concentration. *J Thorac Cardiovasc Surg* 79:425, 1980.

E

1. Estafanous FG, Viljoen JF: Effect of induction of anesthesia and ventilation on ECG signs of ischemia in patients with acute coronary artery insufficiency. *Anesth Analg* 53:610, 1974.

2. Eger EI: *Anesthetic Uptake and Action.* Baltimore: Williams & Wilkins, 1974, chapter 4.

3. Eger EI, Smith NT, Stoelting RK, Cullen DJ, Kadis LB, Whitcher CE: Cardiovascular effects of halothane in man. *Anesthesiology* 32:396, 1970.

4. Entman ML: Calcium and cardiac contractility. *Am J Med Sci* 259:164, 1970.

5. Evans GH, Shand DG: Disposition of propranolol VI: Independent variation in steady-state circulating drug concentrations and half-life as a result of plasma drug binding in man. *Clin Pharmacol Ther* 14:494, 1973.

6. Ellrodt G, Chew CYC, Singh BN: Therapeutic implications of slow-channel blockade in cardiocirculatory disorders. *Circulation* 62:669, 1980.

F

1. Filner BE, Karliner JS: Alterations of normal left ventricular performance by general anesthesia. *Anesthesiology* 45:610, 1976.

2. Ferrari HA, Gorten RJ, Talton IH, Cannent R, Goodrich JK: The action of droperidol and fentanyl on cardiac output and related hemodynamic parameters. *South Med J* 67:49, 1974.

3. Fogdall RP, DeMaster RJ: Comparative effects of metocurine, *d*-tubocurarine, and pancuronium on the peripheral circulation during cardiopulmonary bypass. *ASA Proceedings,* 1977.

4. Forester W, Lewis RP, Weissler AM, Wilke TA: The onset and magnitude of the contractile response to commonly used digitalis glycosides in normal subjects. *Circulation* 49:517, 1974.

5. Federman J, Vlietstra RE: Clinical pharmacology: Series on pharmacology in practice. II. Antiarrhythmic drug therapy. *Mayo Clin Proc* 54:531, 1979.

6. Fielder DL, Nelson DC, Andersen TW, Gravenstein JS: Cardiovascular effects of atropine and neostigmine in man. *Anesthesiology* 30:637, 1969.

7. Faulkner SL, Hopkins JT, Boerth RC, Young JL, Jellett LB, Nies AS, Bender HW, Shand DG: Time required for complete recovery from chronic propranolol therapy. *N Engl J Med* 289:607, 1973.

8. Foex P, Prys-Roberts C: Anaesthesia and the hypertensive patient. *Br J Anaesth* 46:575, 1974.

9. Fozzard HA, Das Gupta DS: ST-segment potentials and mapping: Theory and experiments. *Circulation* 54:533, 1976.

10. Frishman W: Clinical pharmacology of the new beta-adrenergic blocking drugs. I. Pharmacodynamic and pharmacokinetic properties. *Am Heart J* 97:663, 1979.

11. Frishman W, Silverman R: Clinical pharmacology of the new beta-adrenergic blocking drugs. 2. Physiologic and metabolic effects. *Am Heart J* 97:797, 1979.

12. Frater RWM, Oka Y, Hong Y, Tsubo T, Loubser PG, Masone R: Protamine-induced circulatory changes. *J Thorac Cardiovasc Surg* 87:687, 1984.

G

1. Graves CL, Downs NH, Browne AB: Cardiovascular effects of minimal analgesic quantities of innovar, fentanyl, and droperidol in man. *Anesth Analg* 54:15, 1975.

2. Graves CL, Downs NH: Cardiovascular and renal effects of enflurane in surgical patients. *Anesth Analg* 53:898, 1974.

3. Graf K, Strom G, Wahlin A: Circulatory effects of succinylcholine in man. *Acta Anaesthesiol Scand,* 1963, p 6.

4. Goldberg LI: Cardiovascular and renal actions of dopamine: Potential clinical applications. *Pharmacol Rev* 24:1, 1972.

5. Grossman JI, Cooper JA, Frieden J: Cardiovascular effects of infusion of lidocaine on patients with heart disease. *Am J Cardiol* 24:191, 1969.

6. Giardina EV, Heissenbuttel RH, Bigger JT: Intermittent intravenous procaine amide to treat ventricular arrhythmias: Correlation of plasma concentration with effect on arrhythmia, electrocardiogram, and blood pressure. *Ann Intern Med* 78:183, 1973.

7. Gravenstein JS, Andersen TW, DePadua CB: Effects of atropine and scopolamine on the cardiovascular system in man. *Anesthesiology* 25:123, 1964.

8. Grose R, Nivatpumin T, Katz S, Yipintsoi T, Scheuer J: Mechanism of nitroglycerin effect in valvular aortic stenosis. *Am J Cardiol* 44:1371, 1979.

9. Gelman S, Reves JG, Fowler K, Samuelson PN, Lell WA, Smith LR: Regional blood flow during cross-clamping of the thoracic aorta and infusion of sodium nitroprusside. *J Thorac Cardiovasc Surg* 85:287, 1983.

H

1. Hudon F, Jacques A, Dery R, Roux J, Mehard J: Respiratory and haemodynamic effects of methoxyflurane anaesthesia. *Can Anaesth Soc J* 10:442, 1963.

2. Horrigan RW, Eger EI, Wilson C: Epinephrine-induced arrhythmias during enflurane anesthesia in man: A nonlinear dose-response relationship and dose-dependent protection from lidocaine. *Anesth Analg* 57:547, 1978.

3. Harrison GA: The cardiovascular effects in some relaxant properties of four relaxants in patients about to undergo cardiac surgery. *Br J Anaesth* 44:485, 1972.

4. Hasbrouch JD: Morphine anesthesia for open-heart surgery. *Ann Thorac Surg* 10:364, 1970.

5. Holloway GA, Frederickson EL: Dobutamine: A new beta agonist. *Anesth Analg* 53:616, 1974.

6. Harrison DC, Kerber RE, Alderman EL: Pharmacodynamics and clinical use of cardiovascular drugs after cardiac surgery. *Am J Cardiol* 26:385, 1970.

7. Hoffman BF, Rosen MR, Wit AL: Electrophysiology and pharmacology of cardiac arrhythmias. VII. Cardiac effects of quinidine and procaine amide B. *Am Heart J* 90:117, 1975.

8. Hansson L, Hunyor SN, Julius S, Hoobler SW: Blood pressure crisis following withdrawal of clonidine (Catapres, Catapresan), with special reference to arterial and urinary catecholamine levels, and suggestions for acute management. *Am Heart J* 85:605, 1973.

9. Hollister LE: Tricyclic antidepressants: Part I. *N Engl J Med* 299:1106, 1978.

10. Holland RP, Brooks H: TQ-ST segment mapping: Critical review and analysis of current concepts. *Am J Cardiol* 40:110, 1977.

11. Horan LG, Flowers HC, Johnson JC: Significance of the diagnostic Q wave in myocardial infarction. *Circulation* 43:428, 1971.

12. Hoffman BB, Lefkowitz RJ: Alpha-adrenergic receptor subtypes. *N Engl J Med* 302:1390, 1980.

I

1. Ikram H, Rubin AP, Jewkes RF: Effect of diazepam on myocardial blood flow of patients with and without coronary artery disease. *Br Heart J* 35:626, 1973.

2. Ivankovich AD: Sodium nitroprusside: Metabolism and general considerations. *Int Anesthesiol Clin* 16:1, 1978.

J

1. Jackson APF, Dhadphale PR, Callaghan ML, Alseri S: Haemodynamic studies during induction of anaesthesia for open-heart surgery using diazepam and ketamine. *Br J Anaesth* 50:375, 1978.

2. Johnston RR, Eger EI, Wilson C: A comparative interaction of ephinephrine with enflurane, isoflurane and halothane in man. *Anesth Analg* 55:709, 1976.

3. Joas TA, Stevens WC: Comparison of the arrhythmic doses of epinephrine during forane, halothane and fluroxene anesthesia in dogs. *Anesthesiology* 35:48, 1971.

4. Jones RE, Duetsch S, Turndorf H: Effects of atropine on cardiac rhythm in conscious and anaesthetized man. *Anesthesiology* 22:67, 1961.

5. Johnson SM, Mauritson DR, Willerson JT: Comparison of verapamil and nifedipine in the treatment of variant angina pectoris: Preliminary observation in 10 patients. *Am J Cardiol* 47:1295, 1981.

K

1. Kouchoukos NT, Lell WA, Karp RB, Samuelson PN: Hemodynamic effects of aortic clamping and decompression with a temporary shunt for resection of the descending thoracic aorta. *Surgery* 85:25, 1979.

2. Konchigeri HN, Levitsky S: Anesthetic considerations for pericardectomy in uremic pericardial effusion. *Anesth Analg* 55:378, 1976.

3. Kaplan SA, Jack ML, Alexander K, Weinfeld H: Pharmacokinetic profile of diazepam in man following single intravenous and oral and chronic oral administration. *J Pharm Sci* 62:1789, 1973.

4. Kerr F, Irving JB, Ewing DJ, Kirby BJ: Nitrous-oxide analgesia in myocardial infarction. *Lancet* 56:63, 1972.

5. Karliczek G, Hempelmann G, Piepenbrock S: Hemodynamic changes of enflurane (ethrane) in open cardiac surgery. *Acta Anaesthesiol Belg* 2:276, 1974.

6. Kelman GR, Kennedy BR: Cardiovascular effects of pancuronium in man. *Br J Anaesth* 43:335, 1971.

7. Kaplan JA and Jones EL: Vasodilator therapy during coronary artery surgery. *J Thoac Cardiovasc Surg* 77:301, 1979.

8. Kouchoukos NT, Sheppard LC, Kirklin JW: Effect of alterations in arterial pressure on cardiac performance early after open intracardiac operations. *J Thorac Cardiovasc Surg* 64:563, 1972.

9. Kones RJ: The catecholamines: Reappraisal of their use for acute myocardial infarction and the low cardiac output syndromes. *Crit Care Med* 1:203, 1973.

10. Kersting F, Follath F, Moulds R, Mucklow J, McCloy R, Seares J, Dollery C: A comparison of cardiovascular effects of dobutamine and isoprenaline after open heart surgery. *Br Heart J* 38:622, 1976.

11. Katz RL, Bigger JT: Cardiac arrhythmias during anesthesia and operation. *Anesthesiology* 33:193, 1970.

12. Kaplan JA, Dunbar RW, Bland JW, Sumpter R, Jones EL: Propranolol and cardiac surgery: A problem for the anesthesiologist? *Anesth Analg* 54:571, 1975.

13. Kaplan JA, Dunbar RW: Propranolol and surgical anesthesia. *Anesth Analg* 55:1, 1976.

14. Katz RL: Hazardous effects of drugs in hypertensive patients scheduled for elective surgery. *Cardiovascular Medicine*, 3:1185, 1978.

15. Kerr DR, Vonwiller JB, Abrahams N: The stocks suction bullet. *Anaesth Intensive Care* 6:185, 1978.

16. Kissin I, Stanbridge R, Bishop SP, Reves JG: Effect of halothane on myocardial infarct size in rats. *Can Anaesth Soc J* 28:239, 1981.

17. Kirklin JK, Chenoweth DE, Naftel DC, Blackstone EH, Kirklin JW, Bitran DD, Curd JG, Reves JG, Samuelson PN: Effects of Protamine administration after cardiopulmonary bypass on complement, blood levels, and the hemodynamic state. (1985) Personal communication.

L

1. Lell WA, Samuelson PN, Reves JG, Strong SD: Duration of intubation and ICU stay after open heart surgery. *South Med J* 72:773, 1979.

2. Lell WA, Walker DR, Blackstone EH, Kouchoukos NT, Allarde R, Roe CR: Evaluation of myocardial damage in patients undergoing coronary-artery bypass procedures with halothane-N₂O anesthesia and adjuvants. *Anesth Analg* 56:556, 1977.

3. Lundy JS: Balanced anesthesia. *Minn Med* 9:399, 1926.

4. Lappas DG, Buckley MJ, Laver MB, Daggett WM, Lowenstein E: Left ventricular performance and pulmonary circulation following addition of nitrous oxide to morphine during coronary artery surgery. *Anesthesiology* 43:61, 1975.

5. Libonati M, Cooperman LH, Price HL: Time-dependent circulatory effects of methoxyflurane in man. *Anesthesiology* 34:439, 1971.

6. Lundborg RO, Rahimtoola SH, Swan HJC: Halothane administration and left ventricular function in man. *Anesth Analg* 46:377, 1967.

7. Lowenstein E, Poex P, Francis CM, Davies WL, Yusuf S, Ryder WA: Narrowed coronary arteries, halothane, and paradox. *Anesthesiology* 51(suppl 3):62, 1979 (abstr).

8. Lowenstein E, Hallowell P, Levine FH, Daggett WM, Austen WG, Laver MB: Cardiovascular response to large doses of intravenous morphine in man. *N Engl J Med* 281:1389, 1969.

9. Lappas DG, Geha D, Fischer JE, Laver MB, Lowenstein E: Filling pressures of the heart and pulmonary circulation of the patient with coronary-artery disease after large intravenous doses of morphine. *Anesthesiology* 42:153, 1975.

10. Loh L: The cardiovascular effects of pancuronium bromide. *Anaesthesia* 25:356, 1970.

11. Lyons SM, Clarke RS: A comparison of different drugs for anesthesia in cardiac surgical patients. *Br J Anaesth* 44:575, 1972.

12. Ludbrook PA, Byrne JD, Kurnik PB, McKnight RC: Influence of reduction of preload and afterload by nitroglycerin on left ventricular diastolic pressure-volume relations and relaxation in man. *Circulation* 56:938, 1977.

13. Lee KS, Klaus W: The subcellular basis for the mechanism of inotropic action of cardiac glycosides. *Pharmacol Rev* 23:293, 1971.

14. Lucchesi BR: Antiarrhythmic drugs, in MJ Antonaccio (ed): *Cardiovascular Pharmacology*, New York: Raven, 1977, p 269.

15. Lunn JD, Stanley TH, Eisele J, Webster L, Woodward A: High dose fentanyl anesthesia for coronary artery surgery: Plasma fentanyl concentration and influence of nitrous oxide on cardiovascular responses. *Anesth Analg* 58:390, 1979.

16. Lupprian KG, Churchill-Davidson HC: Effect of suxamethonium on cardiac rhythm. *Br Med J* 2:1774, 1960.

17. Lowenstein E, Johnston WE, Lappas DG, D'Ambra MN, Schneider RC, Daggett WM, Akins CW, Philbin DM: Catastrophic pulmonary vasoconstriction associated with protamine reversal of heparin. *Anesthesiology* 59:470, 1983.

M

1. MacDonald HR, Braid DP, Stead BR, Crawford IC, Taylor SH: Clinical and circulatory effects of neuroleptanalgesia with dehydrobenzperidol and phenoperidine. *Br Heart J* 28:654, 1966.

2. McDermott RW, Stanley TH: The cardiovascular effects of low concentrations of nitrous oxide during morphine anesthesia. *Anesthesiology* 44:89, 1974.

3. Mahaffey JE, Aldinger EE, Sprouse JH, Darby TD, Thrower WB: The cardiovascular effects of halothane. *Anesthesiology* 22:982, 1961.

4. Merin RG: Myocardial metabolism in the halothane-depressed canine heart. *Anesthesiology* 31:20, 1969.

5. Merin RG, Kumazawa T, Luka NL: Myocardial function and metabolism in the conscious dog and during halothane anesthesia. *Anesthesiology* 44:402, 1976.

6. Merin RG, Kumazawa T, Luka NL: Enflurane depresses myocardial function, perfusion, and metabolism in the dog. *Anesthesiology* 45:501, 1976.

7. Marshall BE, Cohen PJ, Klingenmaier CH, Neigh JL, Pender JW: Some pulmonary and cardiovascular effects of enflurane

(ethrane) anesthesia with varying $PaCO_2$ in man. *Br J Anaesth* 43:996, 1971.

8. Miller RD, Eger EI II, Stevens WC, Gibbons R: Pancuronium-induced tachycardia in relation to alveolar halothane, dose of pancuronium, and prior atropine. *Anesthesiology* 42:352, 1975.

9. Munger WL, Miller RD, Stevens WC: The dependence of *d*-tubocurarine-induced hypotension on alveolar concentration of halothane, dose of *d*-tubocurarine, and nitrous oxide. *Anesthesiology* 40:442, 1974.

10. McCullough LS, Stone WA, Delaunois AL, Reier CE, Hamelberg: The effect of dimethyl tubocurarine iodine on cardiovascular parameters, postganglionic sympathetic activity and histamine release. *Anesth Analg* 51:554, 1972.

11. Michenfelder JD, Tinker JH: Cyanide toxicity and thiosulfate protection during chronic administration of sodium nitroprusside in the dog: Correlation with a human case. *Anesthesiology* 47:441, 1977.

12. Munson ES, Tucker WK: Doses of epinephrine causing arrhythmia during enflurane, methoxyflurane, and halothane anesthesia in dogs. *Can Anaesth Soc J* 22:495, 1975.

13. Miller RD, Way WL, Katzung BG: The potentiation of neuromuscular blocking agents by quinidine. *Anesthesiology* 26:1036, 1967.

14. Maynard D, Prior PF, Scott DF: Device for continuous monitoring of cerebral activity in resuscitated patients. *Br Med J* 29:545, 1969.

15. McCullough LS, Reier CE, Delaunois AL, Gardier RW, Homelberg W: The effects of *d*-tubocurarine on spontaneous postganglionic sympathetic activity and histamine release. *Anesthesiology* 33:328, 1970.

16. McLain GE, Sipes IG, Brown BR: An animal model of halothane hepatotoxicity: Roles of enzyme induction and hypoxia. *Anesthesiology* 51:321, 1979.

17. Mikolich JR, Nicoloff NB, Robinson PH, Logue RB: Relief of refractory angina with continuous intravenous infusion of nitroglycerin. *Chest* 77:375, 1980.

18. Moller CT, Schoonbee CG, Rosendorff C: Haemodynamics of cardiac tamponade during various modes of ventilation. *Br J Anaesth* 51:409, 1979.

19. Moreno NN, DeCampo T, Kaiser GA, Pallares VS: Technical and pharmacologic management of distal hypotension during repair or coarctation of the aorta. *J Thorac Cardiovasc Surg* 80:182, 1980.

20. McDaniel HG, Reves JG, Kouchoukos NT, Smith LR, Rodgers WJ, Samuelson PN, Lell WA: Detection of myocardial injury after coronary artery bypass grafting using a hypothermic, cardioplegic technique. *Ann Thorac Surg* 33:139, 1982.

N

1. Nishimura K, Kitamura Y, Hamai R, Kitamura E, Fujimori M: Pharmacological studies of ketamine hydrochloride in the cardiovascular system. *Osaka City Med J* 19:17, 1973.

2. Noback CR, Tinker JH: Hypothermia after cardiopulmonary bypass in man: Amelioration by nitroprusside-induced vasodilation during rewarming. *Anesthesiology* 53:277, 1980.

3. Neutze JM, Moller CT, Harris EA, Horsburgh MP, Wilson MD: in *Intensive Care of the Heart and Lungs*. 3rd edition. Blackwell Scientific Publications, Oxford, 1982, p 281.

P

1. Posner MA, Reves JG, Lell WA: Aortic valve replacement in a hemodialysis-dependent patient: Anesthetic considerations—a case report. *Anesth Analg* 54:24, 1975.

2. Palmer RF, Lasseter KC: Nitroprusside and aortic dissecting aneurysm. *N Engl J Med* 294:1403, 1976.

3. Pratila MG, Pratilas V: Anesthetic agents and cardiac electromechanical activity. *Anesthesiology* 49:338, 1978.

4. Prys-Roberts C, Meloche R, Foex P: Studies of anaesthesia in relation to hypertension. I. Cardiovascular responses of treated and untreated patients. *Br J Anaesth* 43:122, 1971.

5. Pittinger C, Adamson R: Antibiotic blockade of neuromuscular function. *Ann Rev Pharmacol* 12:169, 1972.

6. Philips PA, Marty AT, Miyamoto AM: A clinical method for detecting subendocardial ischemia after cardiopulmonary bypass. *J Thorac Cardiovasc Surg* 67:30, 1975.

7. Parmley WW, Chatterjee K: Vasodilator therapy for chronic heart failure. *Cardiovasc Med* 1:17, 1976.

8. Pepine CJ, Feldman RJ, Whittle J: Effect of diltiazem in patients with variant angina: A randomized double-blind trial. *Am Heart J* 101:719, 1981.

R

1. Reves JG, Samuelson PN, Lell WA, McDaniel HG, Kouchoukos NT, Rogers WJ, Smith LR, Carter MR: Myocardial damage in coronary artery bypass surgical patients anaesthetized with two anaesthetic techniques: A random comparison of halothane versus enflurane. *Can Anaesth Soc J* 27:238, 1980.

2. Reves JG, Samuelson PN, Lell WA, Allarde RR, Younes HJ, Oget S: Anesthesia for coronary artery surgery: An evolution in anesthetic management. *Ala J Med Sci* 14:392, 1977.

3. Reves JG, Samuelson PN, Younes HJ, Lell WA: Anesthetic considerations for coronary artery surgery. *Anesthesiology Review* 4:19, 1977.

4. Reddy PS, Curtiss EI, O'Toole JD, Shaver JA: Cardiac tamponade: Hemodynamic observations in man. *Circulation* 48:265, 1978.

5. Radnay PA, Arai T, Nagashima H: Ketamine-gallamine anesthesia for great-vessel operations in infants. *Anesth Analg* 53:365, 1974.

6. Rao S, Sherbaniuk RW, Prasad K, Lee SJK, Sproule BJ: Cardiopulmonary effects of diazepam. *Clin Pharmacol Ther* 14:182, 1973.

7. Reves JG, Samuelson PN, Lewis S: Midazolam maleate induction in patients with ischaemic heart disease: Haemodynamic observations. *Can Anaesth Soc J* 26:402, 1979.

8. Reves JG, Corssen G, Holcomb C: Comparison of two benzodiazepines for anaesthesia induction: Midazolam and diazepam. *Can Anaesth Soc J* 25:211, 1978.

9. Reves JG, Mardis M, Erdmann W, Karp RB: Effects of halothane on normal and ischemic canine myocardial Po_2. American Society of Anesthesiologists Annual Meeting, 1977. *Abstracts of Scientific Papers*, p 253.

10. Reves JG, Lell WA, McCracken LE, Kravetz RA, Prough DS: Comparison of morphine and ketamine anesthetic technics for coronary surgery: a randomized study. *South Med J* 71:33, 1978.

11. Romagnoli A: Duration of action of fentanyl. *Anesthesiology* 39:568, 1973 (letter).

12. Romagnoli A, Keats AS, Ott E: Contrasting systemic vascular effects of morphine and fentanyl in man. American Society of Anesthesiologists Annual Meeting, 1977. *Abstracts of Scientific Papers*, p 527.

13. Reves JG, Sheppard LC, Wallach R, Lell WA: Therapeutic uses of sodium nitroprusside and an automated method of administration. *Int Anesthesiol Clin* 16:51, 1978.

14. Reves JG. Halothane hepatitis. *Postgrad Med* 56:65, 1974.

15. Reves JG, Karp RB, Buttner EE, Tosone S, Smith LR, Samuelson PN, Kreusch GR, Oparil S: Neuronal and adrenomedullary catecholamine release in response to cardiopulmonary bypass in man. *Circulation* 66:49, 1982.

16. Reves JG, Kissin I, Lell WA, Tosone S: Calcium entry blockers: Uses and implication for anesthesiologists. *Anesthesiology* 57:504, 1982.

17. Rogers K, Milne B, Salerno TA: The hemodynamic effects of intra-aortic versus intravenous administration of protamine for reversal in pigs. *J Thorac Cardiovasc Surg* 85:851, 1983.

S

1. Samuelson PN, Lell WA, Kouchoukos NT: Hemodynamics during diazepam induction of anesthesia for coronary artery bypass grafting. *South Med J* 73:332, 1980.

2. Shabetai R, Fowler NO, Guntheroth WG: The hemodynamics of cardiac tamponade and constrictive pericarditis. *Am J Cardiol* 26:480, 1970.

3. Sonntag H, Hellberg K, Schenk HD, Donath U, Regensburger D, Kettler D, Duchanova H, Larsen R: Effects of thiopental on coronary blood flow and myocardial metabolism in man. *Acta Anaesthesiol Scand* 19:69, 1975.

4. Stoelting RK, Gibbs PS, Creasser CW, Peterson C: Hemodynamic and ventilatory responses to fentanyl, fentanyl-droperidol, and nitrous oxide in patients with acquired valvular heart disease. *Anesthesiology* 42:319, 1975.

5. Sonntag H, Heiss HW, Knoll D, Regensburger D, Schenk HD, Bretschneider HJ: Myocardial blood flow and myocardial oxygen consumption in patients during induction of anesthesia with droperidol-fentanyl or ketamine. *Z Kreislaufforsch* 61:1092, 1972.

6. Smith NT, Eger EI II, Stoelting RK, Whayne TF, Cullen D, Kadis LB: The cardiovascular responses to the addition of nitrous oxide to halothane in man. *Anesthesiology* 32:410, 1970.

7. Stoelting RK, Reis RR, Longnecker DE: Hemodynamic responses to nitrous oxide-halothane and halothane in patients with valvular heart disease. *Anesthesiology* 37:430, 1972.

8. Severinghaus JW, Cullen SC: Depression of myocardium and body oxygen consumption with fluothane. *Anesthesiology* 19:165, 1958.

9. Sonntag H, Merin RG, Donath U, Radke J, Schenk HD: Myocardial metabolism and oxygenation in man awake and during halothane anesthesia. *Anesthesiology* 51:204, 1979.

10. Stoelting RK, Gibbs PS: Hemodynamic effects of morphine and morphine-nitrous oxide in valvular heart disease and coronary artery disease. *Anesthesiology* 38:45, 1973.

11. Stanley TH, Gray NH, Isern-Amaral JH, Patton C: Comparison of blood requirements during morphine and halothane anesthesia for open-heart surgery. *Anesthesiology* 41:34, 1974.

12. Stanley TH, Webster LR: Anesthetic requirements and cardiovascular effects of fentanyl-oxygen and fentanyl-diazepam-oxygen anesthesia in man. *Anesth Analg* 57:411, 1978.

13. Sonntag H, Donath U, Hillebrand W, Merin RG, Radke J: Left ventricular function in conscious man and during halothane anesthesia. *Anesthesiology* 48:320, 1978.

14. Stoelting RK: The hemodynamic effects of pancuronium and *d*-tubocurarine in anesthetized patients. *Anesthesiology* 36:612, 1972.

15. Stoelting RK: Hemodynamic effects of dimethyltubocurarine during nitrous oxide-halothane anesthesia. *Anesth Analg* 53:513, 1974.

16. Savarese JJ, Ali HH, Antonio RP: The clinical pharmacology of metocurine: Dimethyltubocurarine revisited. *Anesthesiology* 47:277, 1977.

17. Sonnenblick EH, Frishman WH, LeJemtel TH: Dobutamine: A new synthetic cardioactive sympathetic amine. *N Engl J Med* 300:17, 1979.

18. Sakamoto T, Yamada T: Hemodynamic effects of dobutamine in patients following open heart surgery. *Circulation* 55:525, 1977.

19. Stemple DR, Kleiman JH, Harrison DC: Combined nitroprusside-dopamine therapy in severe chronic congestive heart failure. *Am J Cardiol* 42:267, 1978.

20. Stephenson LW, Edmunds H, Raphealy R, Morrison DF, Hoffman WS, Rubis LJ: Effects of nitroprusside and dopamine on pulmonary arterial vasculature in children after cardiac surgery. *Circulation* 60 Suppl I:I–104, 1979.

21. Stanley TH, Isern-Amaral J, Liu W, Lunn JK and Gentry S: Peripheral vascular versus direct cardiac effects of calcium. *Anesthesiology* 45(1):46, 1976.

22. Slocum HC, Lell WA: The effect of propranolol on ventricular fibrillation and myocardial cooling in patients undergoing myocardial revascularization. American Society of Anesthesiologists Annual Meeting, 1978. *Abstracts of Scientific Papers*, p 513.

23. Slogoff S, Keats AS, Hibbs CW, Edmonds CH, Bragg DA: Failure of general anesthesia to potentiate propranolol activity. *Anesthesiology* 47:504, 1977.

24. Shand DG, Rangno RE: The disposition of propranolol. I. Elimination during oral absorption in man. *Pharmacology* 7:159, 1972.

25. Samuelson PN, Reves JG, Less WA: The effect of pancuronium bromide on ventricular response in patients with atrial fibrillation. *Ala J Med Sci* 16:2, 1979.

26. Schmidt JL, Nicholas AV, Sadove MS: The effect of quinidine on the action of muscle relaxants. *JAMA* 183:669, 1963.

27. Samuelson PN, Merin RG, Taves DR, Freeman RB, Calimlim JF, Kumazawa T: Toxicity following methoxyflurane anaesthesia. IV. The role of obesity and the effect of low dose anaesthesia on fluoride metabolism and renal function. *Can Anaesth Soc J* 23:465, 1976.

28. Sonnenblick EH, Ross J Jr, Braunwald E: Oxygen consumption of the heart: New concepts of its multifactoral determination. *Am J Cardiol* 22:328, 1968.

29. Steen PA, Tinker JH, Pluth JR, Barnhorst DA, Tarhan S: Efficacy of dopamine, dobutamine, and epinephrine during emergence from cardiopulmonary bypass in man. *Circulation* 57:378, 1978.

30. Stone JG, Hoar PF, Calabro JR, dePetrillo MA, Bendixen HH: Afterload reduction and preload augmentation improve the anesthetic management of patients with cardiac failure and valvular regurgitation. *Anesth Analg* 59:737, 1980.

31. Samuelson PN, Reves JG, Kouchoukos NT, Smith LR, Dole K: Hemodynamic response to anesthetic induction with midazolam or diazepam in patients with ischemic heart disease. *Anesth Analg* 60:802, 1981.

32. Singh BN, Collett JT, Chew CYC: New perspectives in the pharmacologic therapy of cardiac arrhythmias. *Prog Cardiovasc Dis* 22:243, 1980.

33. Stevens WC, Dolan WM, Gibbons RT, White A, Eger EI II, Miller RD, deJong RH, Elashoff RM: Minimum alveolar concentration (MAC) of isoflusane with and without nitrous oxide in patients of various ages. *Anesthesiology* 42:197, 1975.

34. Stevens WC, Cromwell TH, Halsey MJ, Eger EI II, Shakespeare TF, and Bahlman SH: The cardiovascular effects of a new inhalation anesthetic, forane, in human volunteers at constant arterial carbon dioxide tension. *Anesthesiology* 35:8, 1971.

35. Soler-Soler J, Sagrista-Sauleda J, Cabrera A, Sauleda-Pares J, Iglesias-Berenque J, Permanyer-Miralda G, Roca-Llop J: Effect of verapamil in infants with paroxysmal supraventricular tachycardia. *Circulation* 59:876, 1979.

36. Singh BN, Roche AHG: Effects of intravenous verapamil on hemodynamics in patients with heart disease. *Am Heart J* 94:593, 1977.

37. Stanley TH, Weidauer HE: Anesthesia for the patient with cardiac tamponade. *Anesth Analg* 52:110, 1973.

38. Stefaniszyn HJ, Novick RJ, Salerno TA: Toward a better understanding of the hemodynamic effects of protamine and heparin interaction. *J Thorac Cardiovasc Surg* 87:678, 1984.

T

1. Tarhan S, Moffitt EA, Lundborg RO, Frye RL: Hemodynamic and blood gas effects of Innovar in patients with acquired heart disease. *Anesthesiology* 34:250, 1971.

2. Tweed WA, Minuck M, Mymin D: Circulatory responses to ketamine anesthesia. *Anesthesiology* 37:613, 1972.

3. Tweed WA, Mymin D: Myocardial force-velocity relations during ketamine anesthesia at constant heart rate. *Anesthesiology* 41:49, 1974.

4. Tuttle RR, Mills J: Dobutamine development of a new catecholamine to selectively increase cardiac contractility. *Circ Res* 36:185, 1975.

5. Tinker JH, Tarhan S, White RD, Pluth JR, Barnhorst DA: Dobutamine for inotropic support during emergence from cardiopulmonary bypass. *Anesthesiology* 44:281, 1976.

6. Tosone S, Reves JG, Kissin I, Smith LR, Lell WA: Nifedipine and halothane interaction: Hemodynamic depression in dogs. *Anesth Analg* 61:218, 1982.

V

1. Viola AR: The influence of pericardiectomy on the hemodynamics of chronic constrictive pericarditis. *Circulation* 48:1038, 1973.

2. Virtue RW, Alanis JM, Mori M, Lafargue RT, Metcalf DR: An anesthetic agent: 2-orthochlorophenyl, 2-methylamino cyclohexanone HCl (CI-581). *Anesthesiology* 28:823, 1967.

3. Vesey CJ, Cole PV, Simpson PJ: Cyanide and thiocyanate concentrations following nitroprusside infusion in man. *Br J Anaesth* 48:651, 1976.

4. Vanhoutte PM: Introductory Remarks: Alpha- and beta-adrenergic receptors and the cardiovascular system. *J Cardiovasc Pharmacol* 3:(suppl 1):1, 1981.

W

1. Walker PF, Fahmy NR, Lappas DG: Pulmonary and systemic circulatory effects of thiopental in patients with coronary artery disease. American Society of Anesthesiologists Annual Meeting, 1976. *Abstracts of Scientific Papers*, p 375.

2. Whitwam JG, Russell WJ: The acute cardiovascular changes and adrenergic blockade by droperidol in man. *Br J Anaesth* 43:581, 1971.

3. Wong KC, Martin WE, Hornbein TF, Freund FG, Everett J: The cardiovascular effects of morphine sulfate with oxygen and with nitrous oxide in man. *Anesthesiology* 38:542, 1973.

4. Walker JA, Eggers GWN Jr, Allen CR: Cardiovascular effects of methoxyflurane anesthesia in man. *Anesthesiology* 23:639, 1962.

5. Webb GE, Jones D, Grover FL, Zauder HL: Regional myocardial flow during halothane anesthesia. American Society of Anesthesiology Annual Meeting, 1976. *Abstracts of Scientific Papers*, p 585.

6. Westhorpe RN, Varghese Z, Petrie A, Wills MR, Lumley J: Changes in ionized calcium and other plasma constituents associated with cardiopulmonary bypass. *Br J Anaesth* 50:951, 1978.

7. Wu D, Denes P, Bauernefeind R, Kehoe R, Amat-Y-Leon F, Rosen KM: Effects of procainamide on atrioventricular nodal re-entrant paroxysmal tachycardia. *Circulation* 57:1171, 1978.

8. Wallach R, Karp RB, Reves JR, Oparil S, Smith LR, James TN: Pathogenesis of paroxysmal hypertension developing during and after coronary artery bypass surgery: A study of hemodynamic and humoral factors. *Am J Cardiol* 46:559, 1980.

9. Warner WA, Anton AH, Andersen TW, Swofford JL: Ventricular fibrillation and catecholamine responses during profound hypothermia in dogs. *Anesthesiology* 33:43, 1970.

10. Wolfson B, Hetrick WD, Lake CL, Siker ES: Anesthetic indices: Further data. *Anesthesiology* 48:187, 1978.

11. Waldo AL, Plumb VJ, Zorn GL, Kouchoukos NT, Karp RB: The use of verapamil in the treatment of supraventricular tachyarrhythmias following open heart surgery: An overview. *Excerpta Medica* p 101, 1980.

Z

1. Zaidan J, Philbin DM, Antonio R, Savarese J: Hemodynamic effects of metocurine in patients with coronary artery disease receiving propranolol. *Anesth Analg* 56:255, 1977.

2. Zahed B, Miletich DJ, Ivankovich AD, Albrecht RF, Toyooka ET: Arrhythmic doses of epinephrine and dopamine during halothane, enflurane, methoxyflurane, and fluroxene anesthesia in goats. *Anesth Analg* 56:207, 1977.

5

POSTOPERATIVE CARE

The primary determinants of the success of a cardiac operation are events in the operating room. However, every surgical patient requires postoperative care. Unfortunately, all interventions, all invasive monitoring, and some noninvasive monitoring (e.g., the making of an electrocardiogram without proper grounding) impose some risks to the patient. They must, therefore, be used only when the need is greater than their inherent risks.

After open intracardiac operations, the combination of the basic cardiac disease, the cardiac trauma of the operation, the repair itself, and the whole body response to cardiopulmonary bypass (CPB), profound hypothermia, and total circulatory arrest create special problems. Those problems related to the cardiac trauma (see Chapter 3) and to the repair are complex and must be understood if postoperative care is to be appropriate. The problems related to CPB per se are extremely complex (see Chapter 2) and are incompletely understood. The added complexities produced by hypothermia and by total circulatory arrest (see Chapter 2) must also be appreciated, although they too are not yet fully understood. Many conceptual, scientific, and management errors are made by failing to realize that a human being during and for a time after CPB is in a special biological situation to which the knowledge and rules applied to other humans may or may not apply.

Fortunately, in spite of these problems, many cardiac operations are now almost without risk (risk approaches zero). Postoperative care can and should be quite simple for patients undergoing these operations. Yet certain situations still entail an appreciable probability of hospital death or morbidity, and in these situations extensive monitoring and interventions may be needed.

The patient may be considered a complex integrated system composed of a number of separate but interrelated subsystems (i.e., cardiovascular, pulmonary, renal, nervous, and alimentary). The care of such a patient can be accomplished effectively utilizing a "subsystems analysis" (alternatively, at GLH, a "systems analysis") approach.[K3] This analysis begins in the operating room as CPB is discontinued (see Chapters 2 and 4) and continues into the early and late postoperative period.

SECTION 1
NORMAL CONVALESCENCE AFTER CARDIAC SURGERY

An *uncomplicated, or normal, convalescence* is devoid of any findings or events that increase the probability of hospital death, important complications, or a suboptimal late result. As long as this pattern of normal convalescence continues, monitoring, testing, and interventions can safely be minimized. Alertness to deviations from the pattern of an uncomplicated convalescence is required, since deviations are an indication for closer observation and possibly more intensive treatment.

EVALUATION OF THE PATIENT

The patient convalescing normally—that is, without complications—after cardiac surgery usually appears at a glance to be doing well. Although there is always pain, which varies in intensity from patient to patient, there is no restlessness, agitation, or anxiety. The eyes and skin look normal, and the pulse is full but may be rapid. Breathing is neither labored nor excessively rapid. The patient is oriented and lucid and, whether an infant or an adult, exhibits generally appropriate behavior.

CARDIOVASCULAR SUBSYSTEM

Adequacy of Cardiac Output

Convalescence can be considered normal when the cardiac output is adequate for the metabolic needs of the body. This point can be determined either by measuring the cardiac output or by assessing its adequacy or both. Most commonly, such evaluations are made clinically without actually measuring cardiac output. This is a time-honored and usually reliable method. Cardiac output is measured in most infants and in seriously ill patients, since this provides additional information of importance in treatment and in evaluation of the completeness of the repair (see below).

Complete assessment of the adequacy of cardiac output early postoperatively would require information about the quantity and distribution of blood flow to each organ and subsystem and their venous blood and tissue oxygen levels. Such information, of course, is not available, but various indirect methods of assessment are commonly and effectively used. Probably the most reliable and simplest of these is evaluation of the pedal pulses as absent (0) or present (in strengths 1–4, with 4 being normal), and of the temperature of the skin of the foot as being cool, tepid, or warm by simple examination or (GLH) with a thermistor probe strapped to the pulp of the big toe. A study of cardiac surgery in infants less than 3 months old indicated that these simple observations reliably predicted the probability of hospital death from cardiac causes and thus were good evaluators of the adequacy of the cardiac output.[K4] Early postoperative oliguria suggests inadequate cardiac output and thus is an indication for treatment of the cardiovascular subsystem (see "Renal Subsystem"). In infants, oliguria is a fairly sensitive indicator, but, in adults, it is less sensitive, and treatment of the cardiovascular subsystem is often indicated in the absence of oliguria. Hyperkalemia rising over a 4-hour period (with sampling every 2 hours) to a level above 5 mEq·l^{-1} is a most sensitive indicator of a falling cardiac output in infants, and thus an indication for intensifying treatment. Hyperkalemia is usually accompanied by a fall in pedal skin temperature, but it precedes the appearance of a base deficit or arterial hypotension.

Mixed venous oxygen levels (generally expressed as oxygen tension, $P\bar{v}O_2$, or as saturation, $S\bar{v}O_2$) are another useful index of the adequacy of cardiac output because they reflect to some extent mean tissue oxygen levels.[K1] When they are below 28 mmHg, the cardiac output is likely to be inadequate

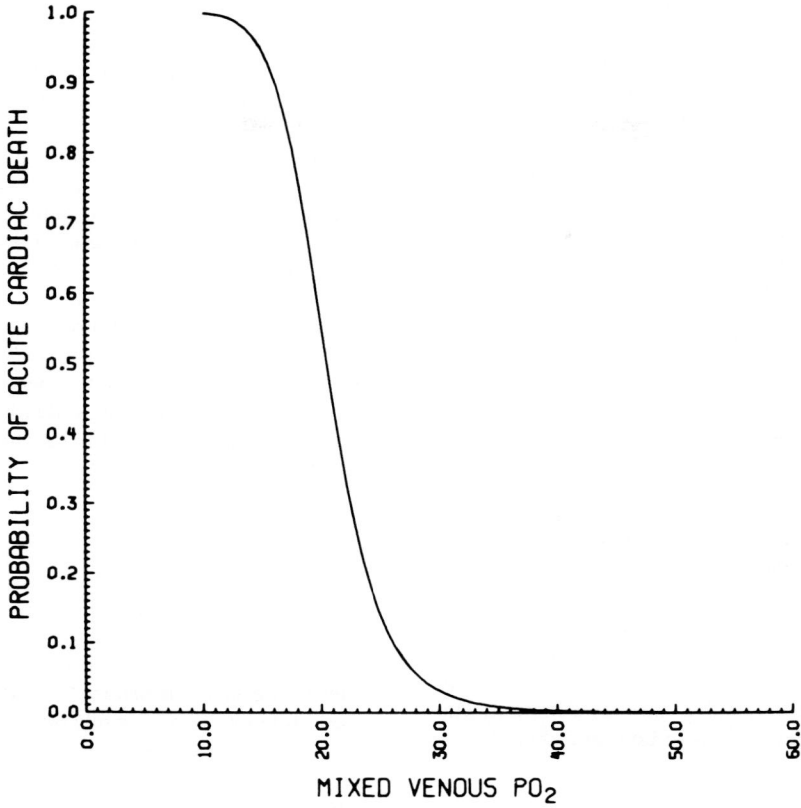

Figure 5-1 The relationship of mixed venous Po_2 ($P\bar{v}O_2$) to the probability of acute cardiac death in infants and children. Convalescence cannot be considered normal if the value is less than about 28 mmHg.

Reproduced with permission from Parr et al.,[P4] and the American Heart Association, Inc.

for the metabolic needs of the patient, and when they are below about 23 mmHg, the inadequacy is severe and the probability of cardiac death high (Fig. 5-1).

When the cardiac output and $P\bar{v}O_2$ are considered together, a more reliable idea of the adequacy of the performance of the cardiac subsystem is possible than when either is considered alone. When cardiac output is above the minimal levels described for normal convalescence (see "Cardiac Output"), and $P\bar{v}O_2$ is moderately or severely depressed, the cardiac performance is inadequate in spite of the cardiac output. If the hemoglobin level is above an arbitrary minimal acceptable level of about 9.5 g · dl^{-1}, this inadequacy is due either to excessively high oxygen consumption ($\dot{V}O_2$) caused by a large metabolic demand, or to a cardiac output that is in fact low even though above an arbitrary minimal acceptable level (about 2.0 l · min^{-1} · m^{-2}; see "Cardiac Output"). When $P\bar{v}O_2$ is above a minimal acceptable level ($\geq$ 28 mmHg) but the cardiac output is below the minimum level, cardiac performance is liable to be inadequate. When cardiac output is inadequate, peripheral areas of the microcirculation are not perfused, and the result is low oxygen consumption ($\dot{V}O_2$) and a $P\bar{v}O_2$ that is higher than anticipated.[K1] This failure to perfuse most of the microcirculation results in an abnormally low $\dot{V}O_2$ when normalized for

the existing body temperature, and if it continues for more than a few hours, it is a fatal condition. These data imply that a $P\bar{v}O_2$ above the minimal acceptable level is not reassuring unless $\dot{V}O_2$ is known to be more or less normal for temperature (130–155 ml · min^{-1} · m^{-2} at 37°C).

Cardiac Output

Cardiac output itself can be measured in both infants and adults after cardiac surgery, although debates continue as to the accuracy of the methodology. The indicator dilution method is used, with indocyanine green[P4] or thermodilution.[M4] A certain level of cardiac output, somewhat variable from patient to patient, is known to be in general adequate to meet metabolic needs, and thus to be associated with a low (< 5%) probability of cardiac death in acute cardiac failure or in subacute multisubsystem failure.[1] Dietzman and col-

---

[1] Death with acute cardiac failure usually occurs within the first few postoperative days, after a period of, and presumably related to, low and inadequate cardiac output. Cardiac death with subacute multisubsystem failure usually occurs a week or more after operation and is associated with low cardiac output and important renal, hepatic, and often cerebral and pulmonary dysfunction secondary to it. Car-

leagues presented data in 1969 that demonstrated the relationship between cardiac output and survival.[D1] Thus, in adults a cardiac index of 1.6 $1 \cdot min^{-1} \cdot m^{-2}$ or greater during the first few hours in the intensive care unit and an index of 2.0 on the morning after operation can be considered criteria of normal convalescence[2] (Fig. 5-2a and b). This index, of course, is considerably below the accepted range of normal, which is 2.5–4.4.[B4] Infants and small children appear to require a somewhat higher cardiac index (2.0–2.2) for normal convalescence (Fig. 5-3). This requirement may be related to the inadequacy of body surface area as a normalizing factor. When cardiac index is below these values, or when pharmacologic or invasive supports are required to maintain them, convalescence is no longer uncomplicated.

Basic Importance of Cardiac Output after Cardiac Surgery

The paradox that many very small infants as well as adults convalesce normally after CPB, which is known to have important damaging effects (see Chapter 2), is probably explained by the body's ability rapidly to correct the results of these damaging effects. This ability is enhanced by vigorous cardiac performance and is reduced by low cardiac output. Thus, postoperative seizures, oliguria, hyperkalemia, hemoconcentration, fluid retention, pulmonary dysfunction, and other phenomena have been shown to be more likely to occur when cardiac performance is reduced.

Arterial Blood Pressure

Early postoperatively, arterial blood pressure is an insensitive guide to cardiac performance, chiefly because the systemic vascular resistance is usually high. This resistance results in a normal or high arterial blood pressure even when cardiac output is low. Patients with cyanotic congenital heart disease tend to have a lower arterial blood pressure early postoperatively than do others, even when cardiac performance is good. This lower pressure is probably related to the preoperative development of abnormally large systemic arteries and a low systemic vascular resistance as a response to chronic hypoxia and polycythemia. Arterial hypotension is, however, always an indication for intense evaluation, and the patient cannot be considered to be convalescing normally when mean arterial blood pressure is less than 10% below normal for the patient's age (Table 5-1).

Arterial hypertension is present early after open heart surgery in many normally convalescing patients. It results from a high systemic vascular resistance, the precise cause of which no doubt varies from patient to patient.[E5] It may be related in many patients to increased levels of circulating catecholamines,[W9] plasma renin,[R1] or angiotensin II.

---

diac deaths may also be with arrhythmias, for example, deaths from important supraventricular or ventricular arrhythmias, usually tachyarrhythmias, not preceded by low cardiac output.

[2] The units will not be repeated but will be understood to apply to all numerical statements of the level of cardiac output expressed as cardiac index.

Cardiac Rhythm

Sinus rhythm is optimal postoperatively, and with this rhythm a wide range of heart rates at various ages is compatible with survival (Table 5-2). Junctional (nodal) rhythm[3] reduces cardiac output by 10%–15%, compared with sinus rhythm, but since it is usually transient and its effects are easily overcome by atrial pacing (unless the rate is fast),[H8] its presence does not connote added risk. Atrial fibrillation is common postoperatively and, if it was not present preoperatively, is usually transient and the ventricular rate is usually easily controlled with digitalis. Atrial fibrillation, therefore, does not make convalescence abnormal. Unifocal, isolated premature ventricular contractions occurring outside the T waves fewer than six times per minute are not known to increase the risk of cardiac death and are compatible with normal convalescence. Other arrhythmias indicate an abnormal convalescence.

RENAL SUBSYSTEM

Convalescence after cardiac surgery can be considered uncomplicated when urine volume is greater than 500 ml $\cdot$ 24 $h^{-1} \cdot m^{-2}$ or 167 ml $\cdot$ 8 $h^{-1} \cdot m^{-2}$, or 20 ml $\cdot h^{-1} \cdot m^{-2}$. These criteria are arbitrary.[4] The Boston Children's Hospital uses 1 ml $\cdot kg^{-1} \cdot h^{-1}$, while Srinivasan and colleagues[S4] and the Great Ormond Street Children's Hospital use 0.5 ml $\cdot kg^{-1} \cdot h^{-1}$ as their lower limit of acceptable urine flow. Convalescence cannot be considered normal when the urine is pink but without red blood cells early postoperatively, for this indicates an inordinate and potentially dangerous amount of hemolysis (free plasma hemoglobin levels > 40 mg $\cdot dl^{-1}$). Also, the convalescence is abnormal when solute excretion is insufficient to keep the serum potassium level below 5 mEq $\cdot l^{-1}$, the blood urea nitrogen (BUN) level below 40 mg $\cdot dl^{-1}$, and the creatinine level below 1.0 mg $\cdot dl^{-1}$ as the upper limits of normal.[S4]

PULMONARY SUBSYSTEM

In the first few days after operation, the normally convalescing patient often has mild pulmonary dysfunction by clinical criteria: mild tachypnea, some increase in the amount of clear or mucoid tracheobronchial fluid cleared by coughing, and moderate widening of the difference between alveolar and arterial oxygen tension, $(A-a)Po_2$.[H10] By the third postoperative day, pulmonary function should be improving, and

---

[3] Junctional (or AV nodal) rhythm is less efficient than sinus rhythm because atrial contribution to ventricular filling is absent in the former. When sinus rhythm is present, the atrial contraction gives an "atrial kick" to the last moments of ventricular filling, quickly increasing the ventricular distention (and thus the preload) and, in turn, the stroke volume.

[4] Many physiologic variables need, of course, to be normalized to body size. Usually, body surface area, expressed in square meters (m^2), is used. A few variables are normalized to body weight in kilograms (kg).

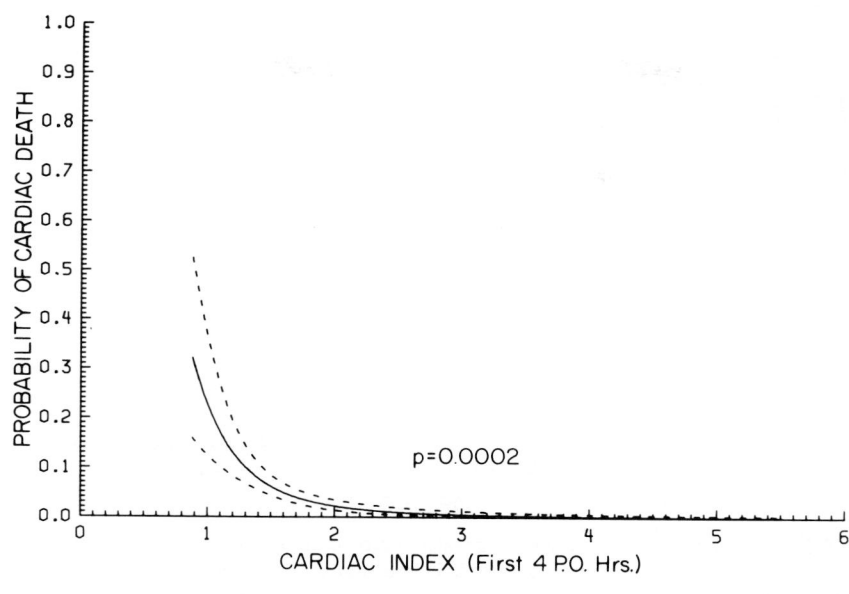

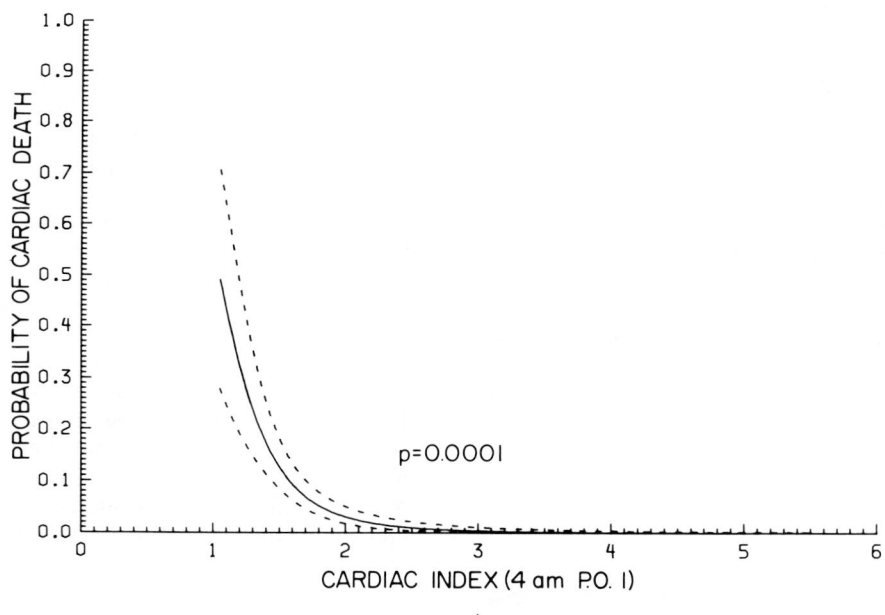

Figure 5-2

(*a*) The relationship of cardiac output in the early hours after mitral valve replacement to the probability of cardiac death (UAB, 1975–1979). The solid line is the point estimate, and the dotted lines are the 70% confidence limits. This graph illustrates the fact that convalescence cannot be considered to be normal when cardiac index is less than about 1.6 $l \cdot min^{-1} \cdot m^{-2}$.[C4]

(*b*) The presentation is the same as in *a*. This graph illustrates that convalescence cannot be considered to be normal 24 hours after operation when the cardiac index is less than about 2.0 $l \cdot min^{-1} \cdot m^{-2}$.[C4]

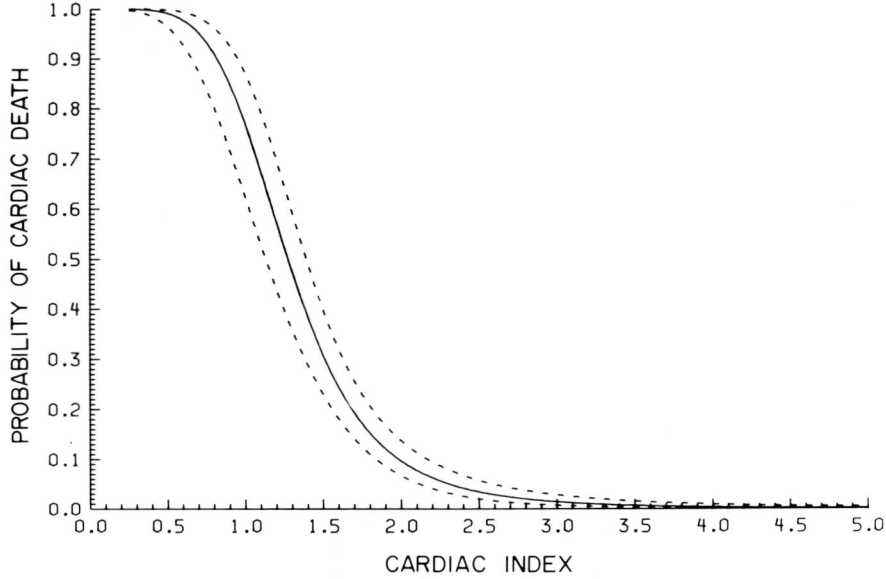

Figure 5-3 The relationship of early postoperative cardiac output (average of all early postoperative values) to the probability of cardiac death in infants and small children. This graph suggests that convalescence cannot be considered normal in infants and small children unless cardiac output is about 2.0–2.2 $l \cdot min^{-1} \cdot m^{-2}$, somewhat higher than the value for adults.
Reproduced with permission from Parr et al.,[P4] and the American Heart Association, Inc.

these clinical findings should be absent by the fifth postoperative day.

These mild manifestations of pulmonary dysfunction are in part the effects of a mild decrease in lung compliance, which in turn is in part related to a mild increase in extravascular lung water. Humans on CPB by current techniques increase their extracellular fluid volume in an amount that is directly proportional to the length of time on CPB.[C1,C5,P1] Part of this fluid comes to reside in the lungs. These pulmonary effects may be caused by leukocyte aggregation and sequestration in the lung (see Chapter 2, Section 2).

Alveolar ventilation in a normally convalescing patient is adequate to prevent respiratory acidosis. In the absence of metabolic alkalosis (pH > 7.4), this means that arterial carbon dioxide pressure ($PaCO_2$) in adults is < 45 mmHg, in young children < 50 mmHg, and in small infants < 55 mmHg. Values higher than these indicate inadequate alveolar ventilation.

This pattern of normal convalescence was studied carefully in 1976 by Rea and colleagues[R2] in 10 patients with preoperatively normal lung function undergoing coronary artery bypass grafting (GLH). No patient required assisted ventilation postoperatively. A bloodless pump-oxygenator prime was used, and no donor blood was added to the perfusate at any stage. The relatively minor changes in arterial PO_2, venous admixture, and arteriovenous oxygen content difference that occurred postoperatively (Fig. 5-4a) largely disappeared by the tenth postoperative day. The increase of minute ventilation and changes of breathing pattern (increased frequency and decreased tidal volume) tended to

Table 5-1 Normal values for blood pressure according to age.

Age (years) ≤ <	Systolic Pressure/ Diastolic Pressure (mmHg)	Mean[a] (mmHg)	10% > Mean Normal Value (mmHg)	10% < Mean Normal Value (mmHg)
0.5	80/46	57	63	51[b]
0.5---1.0	89/60	70	77	63
1.0---2.0	99/64	76	84	68
2.0---4.0	100/65	77	85	69
4.0---12.0	105/65	78	86	70
12.0---15.0	118/68	85	94	74
15.0	120/70	87	96	78

SOURCE: Modified from Nadas et al.[N2]

[a]The mean arterial blood pressure has been calculated as the diastolic pressure plus one-third of the pulse pressure.

[b]40 mmHg in infants < 1 month of age.

Table 5-2 Ranges of heart rate during sinus rhythm in normally convalescing patients

Age (yr) ≤ <	Heart Rate (beats $\cdot$ min^{-1})
1/12	120–190
1/12---6/12	110–180
6/12---12/12	100–170
1---3	90–160
3---6	80–150
6---15	80–140
15	70–130

SOURCE: Adapted from Kirklin et al.[K2]

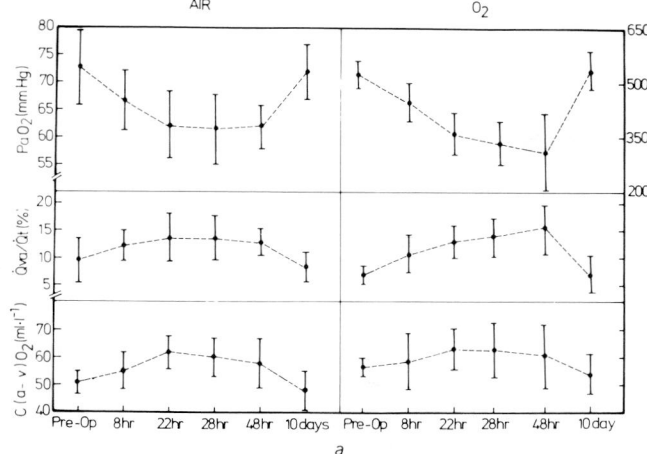

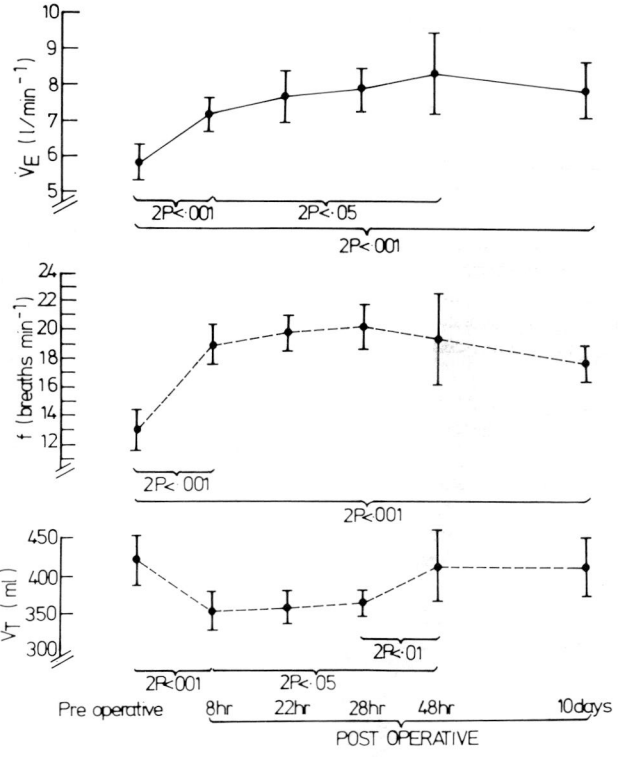

Figure 5-4

(*a*) Arterial oxygen tension (PaO₂), venous admixture (Q̇va/Q̇t), and arteriovenous oxygen content difference (C(a-v)O₂) measured pre-operatively and at each of the postoperative studies in 10 adults undergoing operation with CPB.

(*b*) Pre- and postoperative values for minute ventilation (V̇E), frequency (f), and tidal volume (VT) in the same patients. Air- and O₂-breathing results have been combined, and mean values for the group at each time are shown.

Reproduced with permission from Rea et al.[R2]

persist at 10 days postoperatively (Fig. 5-4*b*) and presumably reflected a decrease in lung and/or thoracic compliance. The venous admixture was considered likely due to an increase in the amount of lung with no ventilation or a critically low ventilation-perfusion ratio. The fall in functional residual capacity demonstrated in this study and the subsequent occurrence of airway closure may be one way in which this increase is produced.

The variability of the usual response of the pulmonary subsystem to CPB and cardiac surgery in different disease states is illustrated by a study by Lell and colleagues (UAB).[L2] They found that, using consistent criteria for extubation, 96% of patients undergoing coronary artery bypass grafting were extubated by the twentieth postoperative hour, but 82% of patients undergoing valve surgery and only 42% of those undergoing correction of congenital heart disease were extubated by this time.

Differences in CPB technique and in the type of patient may account for differences in post-CPB lung function reported in other studies.[E3,F3,H9,M3] The type of oxygenator and filters used; the type of prime, including the volume of homologous blood; the length of time on bypass; the degree of hypothermia; and the degree of preoperative lung damage are all important in determining the magnitude of the pulmonary dysfunction usually present in the postoperative period. Thus, Ratliff and colleagues[R3] examined, by electron and light microscopy, lung biopsy specimens taken 5 minutes before and 5 minutes after the end of CPB. They concluded that the state of the lungs before operation was a critical factor in the degree of post-CPB respiratory pathology and that a healthy lung was more resistant to the trauma of CPB than a previously injured one. Connell and colleagues[C8] described the pulmonary pathological changes in 37 patients who had undergone CPB using a bubble oxygenator and a diluted blood prime. Lung biopsy specimens (for electron microscopy) were taken 5 minutes before the start and approximately 1 hour after the end of CPB. The specimens taken postoperatively revealed extensive occlusion of the capillary bed by aggregates of leukocytes in various stages of disintegration. There was perivascular edema and swelling of the endothelium and overlying alveolar epithelium. The removal of leukocyte aggregates from the circuit by Dacron wool filters reduced these pulmonary changes.[C8] Rabelo and associates[R4] concluded that the use of a bloodless prime or autologous blood led to less lung damage than when homologous blood was used, and Hill and colleagues[H9] showed that a membrane oxygenator may produce less lung damage than a bubble oxygenator.

METABOLIC SUBSYSTEM

Metabolic acidosis, reflected in a reduction of buffer base (*base deficit*) of more than 2 mEq · l⁻¹, may be present in the first few hours after CPB but does not necessarily imply inadequate cardiac performance. During and immediately following CPB, some areas of the microcirculation are either poorly perfused or nonperfused. As recovery proceeds, washout of these areas brings lactic acid and other fixed acids into the circulation, the so-called washout acidosis.

Metabolic acidosis persisting for more than about 2 hours after the end of the operation indicates that convalescence is complicated by inadequate tissue perfusion, usually secondary to low cardiac output. Unfortunately, absence of metabolic acidosis is not strong evidence of an adequate cardiac output.

CPB causes retention of water and sodium and depletion of whole body potassium. Thus, total body water and extracellular (primarily interstitial) fluid are increased. In good-risk patients, the increase in body weight evident in the intensive care unit (usually about 5% above preoperative weight), which results from the increased extracellular fluid, is independent of the amount of crystalloid solution administered in the operating room.[S13] This is because under these circumstances the excess fluid is rapidly excreted by the kidneys. The renal excretion of excess fluid in normally convalescing patients brings body weight back to normal or subnormal levels within about 5 days. Intracellular potassium decreases during CPB.[P1] This process releases considerable amounts of potassium from cells (living or dead) during and in the early hours after operation, and is probably the reason that acute renal failure early after cardiac surgery is so often characterized by a rapid increase of serum potassium. A satisfactory explanation of this phenomenon of sodium and water accumulation and potassium depletion during CPB is not available (see Chapter 2), but it is associated with high levels of circulating antidiuretic hormone and aldosterone. These changes are of course characteristic of the metabolic response to trauma. Because of overriding water retention, the serum sodium level is commonly low despite sodium retention.

Body temperature is a result of many metabolic and physiologic processes. In the first few postoperative hours, it may be as low as 32°C because of incomplete rewarming after an intraoperative period of profound hypothermia. Normally, the temperature returns to about 37°C within 4–6 hours. Failure to do so suggests inadequate cardiac performance.[P6]

Varying degrees of hyperthermia (with a central body temperature up to 39.5°C, or 103.1°F) are nearly always present during the first 48 postoperative hours, even in normally convalescing patients.[L1] A rise of central body temperature above this point (≥ 39.5°C) early postoperatively may indicate an exacerbation of the poorly understood syndrome of hyperthermia and increased capillary permeability with marked increase in extravascular lung water, pulmonary dysfunction (and sometimes elevation of pulmonary artery pressure), and a tendency toward hemoconcentration. This combination of findings, part of what has been termed the *postperfusion syndrome*, is related to damage to the blood received in its passage through the pump-oxygenator (see Chapter 2). The hyperthermia is often accompanied by leukocytosis and the appearance of immature white blood cells, even without infection.[D2] The maximum body temperature most commonly occurs about 10 hours after operation. Wedley and colleagues have shown a high mortality (53%) in patients with a central body temperature > 41°C (105.8°F) early postoperatively.[W1] Their studies suggest that increased heat production is the primary cause of the hyperthermia, although inability to lose heat because of surface vasoconstriction in association with low cardiac output is present in some patients.

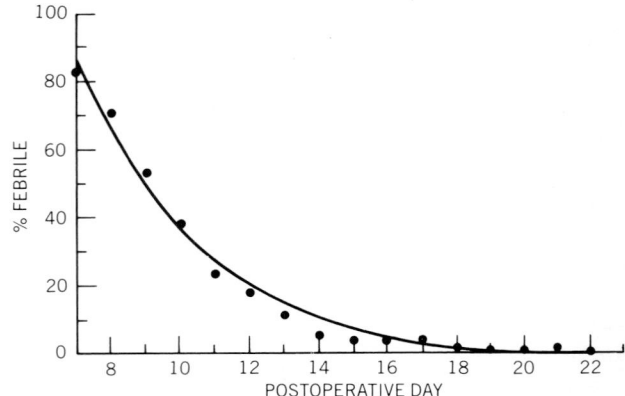

Figure 5-5 The proportion of patients febrile (temperature ≥ 37.8°C) after the sixth postoperative day, starting with the group febrile on the sixth day. Note the continuation of fever in some patients to nearly 3 weeks after surgery.

Reproduced with permission from Livelli et al.,[L1] and the American Heart Association, Inc.

Normally convalescing patients may continue to have pyrexia to 39.5°C (103.1°F) for the first 6 postoperative days and even reach 40.0°C (104°F) without infection.[B1] After the sixth postoperative day, the temperature trend is downward in normally convalescing patients, generally reaching 37.8°C (100°F) by the eighth postoperative day and being consistently less than 37.2°C (99°F) by the tenth postoperative day. The proportion of patients with fever steadily declines after the sixth postoperative day (Fig. 5-5). Unexplained postoperative fever in normally convalescing patients is probably the result of changes in blood components produced by their passage through a pump-oxygenator (see Chapter 2, Section 2) and perhaps in part from the effects of administering homologous blood. Livelli and colleagues have shown that it is unlikely that subclinical pulmonary atelectasis accounts for such fever.[L1] Patients convalescing normally are generally afebrile by 14 days postoperatively.

NEUROLOGIC SUBSYSTEM

Changes in intellectual performance do not occur after uncomplicated and well-managed CPB.[W2] Neither do seizures, athetoid movements, or visual field defects. However, some subtle and transient abnormalities occur with sufficient frequency in the first few days after CPB that they, unfortunately, must at present be considered part of "normal" convalescence. These abnormalities include mild mental confusion and mild hallucinations, which may in part be due to fibrin, platelet, or other microemboli, and inability to focus the eyes appropriately, which may result from changes in lens tension. These symptoms rapidly subside during normal convalescence.

Delerium, major halucinatory and delusional experiences, and frankly psychotic behavior are uncommon and are a departure from normal convalescence. When such symptoms become major, they are probably multifactorial in origin, with the patient's behavioral characteristics, environment during the first few postoperative days, preexisting physical state, and psychological conditioning or lack thereof playing a role in association with the effects of CPB noted above.

Localized neurologic defects, such as hemiplegia and visual field defects, are not part of normal convalescence and are assumed to result from specific discrete embolic (air or paticulate) events rather than to part of the postperfusion state. Seizures can hardly be considered a part of normal convalescence, but they seldom have ominous long-term implications.[S3] They seem to be more likely to occur when total circulatory arrest is used as a part of the support technique (see Chapter 2). Choreiform movements and grossly inappropriate behavior are more major neurological complications, which also occur more often when total circulatory arrest is used (see Chapter 2).[S3] These complications usually, but not always, clear without demonstrable sequelae.

GASTROINTESTINAL SUBSYSTEM

Abnormalities of function of the gastrointestinal tract, including the liver and pancreas, are not clinically detectable when convalescence is normal.

Mild retrosternal pain on swallowing without the characteristics of esophageal reflux may result from sterile pericarditis affecting the contiguous portion of the esophagus. This pain gradually subsides and is not considered a complication.

Minor or major abnormalities of function and structure of the gastrointestinal subsystem may occur during the postoperative period when convalescence is not normal. Such abnormalities are usually the result of low cardiac output, embolic events, a severe tendency to bleed, or the effects of antibiotics on the intestinal flora.

POSTOPERATIVE BLEEDING

A tendency to bleed always results from CPB as it is currently performed, with essentially all clotting factors being abnormal (see Chapter 2). Thus, some bleeding always occurs in the early postoperative hours, with resultant drainage from the pericardial and/or pleural tubes. Convalescence is considered normal when drainage from the chest is less than the criteria for reoperation (see section ''Early Postoperative Bleeding'' in Section 3).

SECTION 2
PATIENT MANAGEMENT PROTOCOLS FOR THE SUBSYSTEMS

CARDIOVASCULAR SUBSYSTEM

Normally Convalescing Patients

Ventricular Preload
When the patient is convalescing normally, precise adjustment of ventricular preload is not necessary. However, it is prudent to keep the higher of the two ventricular end-

Table 5-3 Patient management protocol for augmentation of blood volume early postoperatively after open intracardiac operations. All doses for augmentation of blood volume are prescribed with a stop order, to take effect when the higher of the two atrial pressures exceeds a stated limit (usually 15 mmHg but adjusted according to the patient's circumstances).

Blood Hemoglobin Concentration (g · dl⁻¹ blood)		Fluid (generally given in doses of 10% of estimated blood volume[a])
≤	<	
	9.5	Packed red blood cells
9.5	11.5	Whole blood
11.5		5% albumin solution, fresh-frozen plasma, or SPPS[b]

[a] Blood volume (ml) is estimated to be 0.08 × body weight (kg) in children < 12 years old, and 0.065 × body weight (kg) in older persons.

[b] Stable plasma protein solution (SPPS) is possibly the best available long-acting plasma expander (GLH). It contains 85% albumin and 15% globulin in a 5% balanced electrolyte solution and produces minimal side effects. It entails no risk of hepatitis but contains no coagulation factors. It should be used in conjunction with fresh-frozen plasma or freeze-dried plasma to supplement coagulation factors.

diastolic pressures at 8–10 mmHg[5] in the early hours after operation. To do this, fluid is administered intravenously until the desired atrial pressure is reached. The type of fluid is determined by the blood hemoglobin concentration at that time (Table 5-3), although the need for blood must be balanced against the disadvantages of whole blood administration. Although albumin is specified (UAB), the much less expensive substance hydroxyethyl starch has been shown to be a satisfactory substitute.[K6,M5] In the normally convalescing patient, administration of more than 500 ml · m⁻² of blood is usually unwise.

Ventricular Afterload
In the normally convalescing patient, precise adjustment of ventricular afterload[6] is usually unnecessary. However, the

---

[5] When the atrioventricular valves are normal, and when the atria are functioning normally as reservoirs (they are not, for example, after an atrial switch operation by Mustard's or Senning's technique[P5]), ventricular end-diastolic pressure is assumed to be the same as the mean pressure in the corresponding atrium. Therefore, mean atrial pressure is measured in order to know ventricular end-diastolic pressure. In the absence of pulmonary vascular disease and important pulmonary congestion or edema, pulmonary artery diastolic pressure is a reasonable approximation of left atrial pressure. Right atrial pressure is always monitored, either directly or via an internal jugular catheter. Left atrial pressure is measured routinely in the operating room, but sometimes the line is removed before closing the chest. These atrial pressures are measured at the end of expiration. When positive end-expiratory pressure (PEEP) is being used, its amount is subtracted from the observed atrial pressures to obtain the approximate *transmural pressure*, which is the ventricular filling pressure.

[6] Left ventricular afterload is related to the systemic arterial blood pressure (see footnote 10). Because of the many determinants of the presence and degree of systolic amplification, the systolic blood pressure at the radial artery has a variable relationship to the systolic pressure in the ascending aorta. The mean arterial blood pressure at the radial artery has a predictable relationship with the cen-

tendency toward arterial hypertension is present in most patients convalescing normally after cardiac surgical procedures, in part because of increased systemic arteriolar resistance.[G6] High aortic wall tension (related to intraluminal blood pressure) may tear an aortic suture line or produce bleeding through stitch holes or between sutures. Thus, when an aortic suture line is present, undue elevation of arterial blood pressure is avoided by pharmacologic means. Furthermore, the increased metabolic demands from a large left ventricular afterload may exacerbate any latent myocardial ischemia.[F5]

An appropriate criterion for treatment in this setting is a mean arterial blood pressure 10% above the normal value (Table 5-1). However, the subject's preoperative blood pressure must be taken into account, and, in order to avoid cerebral complications, markedly hypertensive patients must not be rendered hypotensive. Sodium nitroprusside or nitroglycerin is generally used for this purpose (see Appendix 5A), the latter particularly when myocardial ischemia is present, since nitroglycerin decreases coronary resistance. Other alternatives are diazoxide or phentolamine (see Appendix 5A), or the long-acting drug phenoxybenzamine hydrochloride (GLH), when prolonged vasodilator therapy is needed.

Increased Venous Tone
Early after operations using CPB, increased venous tone is often present in normally convalescing patients.[G6,R5] The saphenous vein at the ankle may feel cordlike upon palpation. By about 6–12 hours after operation, venous tone has begun to decrease, causing atrial pressures to fall. As indicated earlier, increasing the blood volume to combat the pressure decrease is generally not necessary in normally convalescing patients.

Myocardial Contractility
In normally convalescing patients, myocardial contractility requires no treatment.

Heart Rate and Rhythm
The development of atrial fibrillation or junctional rhythm requires treatment in normally convalescing patients. When the ventricular rate is less than 85 beats · min^{-1} with atrial fibrillation (usually in elderly patients, those with long-standing valvar heart disease, or those who have been on digoxin), ventricular pacing at 100 beats per minute is begun. If the ventricular rate with atrial fibrillation is between 85 and 100 beats per minute, no treatment is indicated. If it is between 100 and 110 beats per minute, a maintenance program of digoxin is begun (see Appendix 5B). If the ventricular rate is greater than 110 beats per minute, it is controlled by administration of digoxin intravenously (see Appendix 5B). It is prudent to increase heart rate in normally convalescing patients with slow sinus or junctional rhythm (< 70

beats per minute in adults, < 100 beats per minute in infants) in order to minimize the number of atrial and ventricular premature contractions. For this, atrial pacing[F1] via the two atrial wires placed at surgery is used (see Chapter 2).

Hematocrit
The normally convalescing patient tolerates well some reduction of hematocrit (or blood hemoglobin concentration) because of good cardiac reserve. However, when, as a result of the hemodilution techniques used during CPB, the hemoglobin is less than 9.0 g · dl^{-1}, one or two doses of packed red blood cells are given (Table 5-3).

Low Cardiac Output

Causes
Low cardiac output can be caused by low preload or high afterload, which are easily corrected. More important causes include (1) structural abnormalities (incomplete or inadequate repair), (2) cardiac tamponade, and (3) postrepair depression of myocardial function with or without myocardial necrosis.

Incomplete or inadequate repair must always be considered as a possible cause of low cardiac output because prompt reoperation may be indicated. In the operating room, pressures are measured to assess possible residual valvar or ventricular outflow stenosis, and artificial valve function is assessed by palpation. Pressures are also measured early postoperatively via polyvinyl catheters left at the time of surgery. When the operation involves repair of a septal defect, any possible residual left-to-right shunt is searched for in the Intensive Care Unit. The simplified shunt equation[7] may be (UAB) used to obtain the pulmonary-systemic blood flow ratio (Q̇p/Q̇s), measuring oxygen saturation in blood sampled through the indwelling polyvinyl catheters (see Chapter 2) from the right atrium, pulmonary artery, and systemic artery while FIO_2 is 0.5 or less.

A residual left-to-right shunt can also be identified by the contour of the indicator-dilution curve used to measure cardiac output. If a shunt is suspected and a pulmonary artery catheter is in place, it can be verified by double indicator-dilution curves obtained by injecting indocyanine green into the left atrium and sampling from the radial and pulmonary arteries.[W8] Very early appearing dye is seen in the curve from the pulmonary artery. The proportion of shunted blood is determined by dividing the area of the early appearing pulmonary curve by that of the curve from the radial artery. Q̇p/Q̇s is calculated as follows:

$$\dot{Q}p/\dot{Q}s = \frac{\text{Pulmonary blood flow}}{\text{Systemic blood flow}} = \frac{1}{\text{one} - \text{shunt proportion}}$$

---

tral aortic mean and systolic pressure. Therefore, mean arterial blood pressure is used (via a monitoring needle in the radial or femoral artery) in regulating left ventricular afterload. Right ventricular afterload is, of course, related to these pressures in the pulmonary artery.

[7]

$$\dot{Q}p/\dot{Q}s = \frac{S\bar{a}O_2 - S\bar{v}O_2 \text{ (RA)}}{S\bar{a}O_2 - S\bar{v}O_2 \text{ (PA)}} \qquad (5\text{-}1)$$

where $S\bar{a}O_2$ is the percent oxygen saturation of arterial blood, $S\bar{v}O_2$ (RA) that of blood withdrawn from right atrium, and $S\bar{v}O_2$ (PA) that of blood withdrawn from pulmonary artery.

Alternatively (GLH), echocardiograms are taken of atria, ventricles, and great arteries after the injection of a bolus of saline solution or blood into a peripheral vein (for right-to-left shunting) or the left atrium (for left-to-right shunting). A residual right-to-left shunt (through an overlooked patent foramen ovale, for example) can easily be detected by injecting dye into the right atrium and sampling from the radial artery.[W8] When cardiac performance is suboptimal and important residual ventricular outflow tract obstruction, AV valve or prosthetic valve dysfunction, or residual shunting with $\dot{Q}p/\dot{Q}s > 2.0$ are present, consideration is given to prompt reoperation although the need for this is uncommon.

Early postoperatively, a very significant right-to-left shunt may occur through an incompletely closed atrial communication if the surgery has temporarily compromised the right ventricle (e.g., after VSD repair). This may disappear as right ventricular compliance returns to normal and not be replaced by a significant left-to-right shunt.

Acute pericardial tamponade can occur early postoperatively. However, if hemostasis in the operating room is sufficiently precise, and if reoperation is performed promptly when indicated, early postoperative pericardial tamponade will be rare. Thus, emphasis is on precise hemostasis in the operating room and *early* reentry when chest drainage violates certain criteria (see Section 3). Nonetheless, cardiac tamponade must always be considered as a possible cause of postoperative low cardiac output, and unless it can be excluded with confidence (such as by echocardiography) in a patient with importantly reduced cardiac output, reoperation is indicated.

Following an early period of adequate and stable cardiac output, cardiac tamponade is a likely cause of rapid deterioration that cannot be easily explained otherwise, that is, when the repair is good and there is no reason to suspect myocardial damage. It is usually associated with rapidly rising right and left atrial pressures that often, but not always, become equal. Often, drainage from the chest tubes is initially brisk and then ceases, and serial chest roentgenograms show progressive widening of the heart and superior mediastinal shadows. Arterial pressure falls, and a paradoxical pulse may be replaced by a narrow pulse pressure. Characteristically, the arterial pressure shows a minimal response to a bolus injection of an inotrope. The diagnosis can often be confirmed, and alarming deterioration at least temporarily reversed, by gently irrigating the chest tubes with small amounts of saline solution using a meticulous sterile technique. This may unblock the chest tubes and produce a sudden gush of blood and a prompt rise in blood pressure. In patients who collapse from acute tamponade, which can occur very rapidly, all the drainage tubes should be totally removed (provided both pleura are intact) so that the stab wounds can drain blood freely into a dressing (GLH). In this way, some decompression is provided while the patient is being transferred to the operating room.

Acute myocardial necrosis should now be an uncommon occurrence, although it was frequent in earlier times (see Chapter 3). It can result from inadequate intraoperative myocardial protection, from inadequate myocardial revascularization in patients with coronary artery disease, and from early postoperative acute depression of the myocardial oxygen supply-demand ratio, most commonly the result of acute hypotension.

Occasionally, temporary functional myocardial depression, without myocardial necrosis, occurs even after operations performed in an entirely acceptable fashion, and may last 6–18 hours. Such depression is usually self-limited and may not always warrant intensive treatment.

Whatever the cause of the low cardiac output, one ventricle is often primarily affected and becomes the limiting factor. This ventricle's end-diastolic pressure (and thus the mean pressure in the corresponding atrium) becomes higher than that in the other ventricle.[8] This phenomenon is an important guide to the possible specific cause of low cardiac output.

Treatment

Experience indicates that it is worthwhile to treat intensively patients with low or inadequate cardiac output early after cardiac surgery, because cardiac performance often improves after one or two days, and this allows a good recovery from the operation. The treatment is directed at increasing the cardiac output by manipulation of preload,[9]

---

[8]Abnormal differences between left and right atrial pressures (normally, the mean left atrial pressure is 2–5 mmHg higher than the right) are the steady state result of a change in the relative performance of the two ventricles, resulting in a transient period in which the net forward flow from the two ventricles is different. After a variable number of heart beats in this imbalanced state, equal forward flow from the two ventricles again exists, in large part because of the Frank-Starling phenomenon. Observation of the atrial pressures can allow inferences concerning the events leading to the new steady state and may be helpful therapeutically. These events may be acute or chronic ones occurring preoperatively or acute ones occurring intraoperatively or postoperatively. Each ventricle, of course, has its own unique stroke volume and its own unique determinants of stroke volume, except for heart rate, which is shared by both. This means that each has its unique set of characteristics determining preload (see footnote 9), afterload (see footnote 10), and contractility (see footnote 11). These variables of relative stroke volumes and relative determinants of stroke volume are the determinants of the relationship between the two atrial pressures at any moment. (The absolute level of atrial pressure in any given patient is determined by the blood volume. Differences between the two atrial pressures are greater when their levels are high). If left or right atrial pressure is abnormally high relative to the other, acutely or chronically, it can be assumed that the stroke volume of its corresponding ventricle is greater than that of the other (from shunting or valvar incompetence), that the distensibility of its ventricle is less than that of the other (preload effect), that one of its determinants of systolic ventricular wall stress has increased relative to that of the other (afterload effect), or that its contractility relative to that of the other is reduced (see footnote 11).[B9]

[9]*Preload* is the length of the sarcomeres at the end of diastole. In the intact ventricle, this length is dependent on the change in ventricular volume between the end of systole and the end of diastole. The volume change is determined by the end-diastolic transmural pressure; ventricular compliance; the curvature of the ventricular wall, as determined by ventricular volume at the end of diastole (the La Place effect); the thickness of ventricular wall; and the transmural geometric arrangement of ventricular fibers. Transmural pressure is simply the difference between intraventricular pressure and in-

afterload,[10] contractile state,[11] and heart rate and at improving tissue oxygen levels.

When cardiac output is low, preload is made appropriate by increasing blood volume (Table 5-3) until the higher of the two atrial pressures is about 15 mmHg. If the wall thickness of the left ventricle is unusually great or its contractility and/ or compliance is decreased, it may be helpful to raise mean left atrial pressure to 20 mmHg. When the right ventricle is the limiting one, right atrial pressure usually can advantageously be raised only to about 18 mmHg. Above this level, a descending limb on the Starling curve seems to become apparent, and cardiac output falls.

When left ventricular performance is the limiting one and systemic arterial blood pressure is more than 10% above normal (Table 5-1), left ventricular afterload should be reduced to between normal and 10% above normal with vasodilating agents (see Appendix 5A). Rarely, in patients

---

trapericardial pressure. Only transmural pressure and compliance are likely to change acutely (intraoperatively or early postoperatively).

Acute differences from the usual sarcomere length or stretch at the end of diastole are usually related to changes in transmural pressure or compliance. Alternatively, the stretch of the sarcomeres at the end of diastole of one ventricle may be different from that of another ventricle subjected to the same transmural pressure, this difference being related to a chronic change in the weight of ventricular muscle (either because of differences in thickness or length) or in the shape of the ventricle.

In practice, in most patients with normal atrioventricular valves, acute changes in preload are equated with acute changes in mean left (in the case of the left ventricle) or right (in the case of the right ventricle) atrial pressure.

[10] In the intact ventricle, *afterload* is defined as the systolic wall stress. This is the analogue of the load which resists shortening in the isolated papillary muscle. Other things being equal, increased afterload results in decreased stroke volume. In the intact ventricle, afterload is related to (1) the intraventricular pressure during systole and (2) ventricular volume (by the La Place effect), thickness, length, and shape. Not only does the pressure within the ventricle vary during systole, but the thickness of the ventricle also varies. Hood, Rackley, and colleagues have demonstrated that in most hearts the ventricular wall is considerably thicker at mid-systole than at other phases of the cycle.[H1] If thickening fails to occur, systolic wall stress (per unit of cross-sectional area) is increased. If the ventricle becomes small and thick very early in systole, such as in severe mitral incompetence, the systolic wall stress is less.

In practice, acute changes in systolic blood pressure in the left or right ventricle, and thus (with nonobstructed ventricular outflow tracts) acute changes in systolic pressure in the aorta and the pulmonary artery, are related to acute changes in afterload in that ventricle.

[11] When a change in stroke volume cannot be explained in terms of change in end-diastolic fiber length or in the load which resists shortening, it is believed to result from a change in the *contractile state*. Contractility in a given ventricle can be acutely depressed or increased. When we attempt to compare the contractility of one ventricle with that of another, problems arise. A papillary muscle that is twice as thick as others might appear to have twice the contractility when studied in the usual way. In the ventricle, and at least theoretically in papillary muscle, data interpreted in terms of contractility must be normalized according to the muscle thickness and length.

---

with severe long-standing mitral valve disease or congenital heart disease with pulmonary vascular obstructive changes, right ventricular dysfunction associated with elevated pulmonary artery pressure may limit cardiac performance. Reduction of right ventricular afterload with vasodilating agents is occasionally dramatic in its increase of right ventricular, and thus cardiac, stroke volume. Nitroprusside ($0.5–3$ $\mu g \cdot kg^1 \cdot min^{-1}$), nitroglycerin ($0.5–3$ $\mu g \cdot kg^{-1} \cdot min^{-1}$), or phentolamine ($1.5–2$ $\mu g \cdot kg^{-1} \cdot min^{-1}$) may be effective in this setting.[K2] In infants, maintaining near-anesthesia for 24 to 48 hours with morphine or another intravenously administered agent may minimize paroxysms of pulmonary artery hypertension and increased right ventricular afterload.[L4]

Heart rate is adjusted to optimal levels when necessary by atrial pacing, by ventricular pacing when atrial fibrillation is present, or by AV sequential pacing when AV dissociation is present. When tachyarrhythmias are present, pharmacologic means of control may be employed (see below).

If these relatively simple measures do not bring cardiac output to an adequate level, the decision is made to use catecholamines or intra-aortic balloon pumping (IABP) (see Appendix 5D). The former is chosen in infants and children, in adults without major myocardial necrosis and with only mild or moderate impairments, and in adults with a contraindication to IABP. If catecholamines are indicated, initially dopamine may be infused at 2.5 $\mu g \cdot kg^{-1} \cdot min^{-1}$ (UAB) (see Appendix 5C; Chapter 4, "Inotropic Drugs"; and Table 4-5). This dose can be increased up to 15 $\mu g \cdot kg^{-1} \cdot min^{-1}$ if needed, although if a favorable response is not obtained at 10 $\mu g \cdot kg^{-1} \cdot min^{-1}$, it is not likely to be obtained at higher doses. Dopamine has the advantage of augmenting renal blood flow in addition to increasing cardiac contractility.[H4] Dopamine does increase ventricular automaticity (and thus the probability of ventricular arrhythmias), but to a lesser extent than does isoproterenol. At low doses ($2–4$ $\mu g \cdot kg^{-1} \cdot min^{-1}$), systemic peripheral vascular resistance is decreased or unchanged, while higher doses (> 6 $\mu g \cdot kg^{-1} \cdot min^{-1}$) increase peripheral resistance.[G3] When dopamine is not effective, dobutamine is gradually added in similar doses. Dobutamine, although more expensive than dopamine, does appear to augment myocardial blood flow more than does dopamine.[F6] Epinephrine and norepinephrine are rarely used because of their powerful peripheral vasoconstricting effect in this situation. Isoproterenol may be the preferred initial agent (GLH) (see Appendix 5C) and probably is superior in the presence of predominantly right ventricular dysfunction and decreased or normal heart rate because of its favorable effect on pulmonary vascular resistance. When a satisfactory response has been obtained from catecholamine infusion, 4–8 hours later, an aggressive and persistent effort is begun *gradually* to reduce and finally discontinue them.

In adults, if adjustment of preload, afterload, and heart rate and modest doses of catecholamines do not result in adequate cardiac performance, and the left ventricle is the limiting factor in cardiac performance, intra-aortic balloon pumping is initiated promptly (see Appendix 5D). If a strong suspicion of myocardial necrosis exists or if ventricular electrical instability is present, IABP is preferable to catecholamine infusion as *initial* treatment.

When the right ventricle is the limiting factor in cardiac performance in the operating room and the pulmonary artery pressure is elevated, consideration may be given to pulmonary artery counterpulsation.[F7,M6,M7,O3] For this, a 20-mm Dacron tube is attached end-to-side to the proximal pulmonary artery and the intra-aortic balloon catheter is passed through it and as far distally as it goes easily. Part of the balloon remains in the Dacron tube. Experience with this technique for support of the right ventricle has been unsatisfactory (UAB).

While efforts are being made to increase cardiac output, efforts are also directed at increasing tissue and mixed venous oxygen levels by attention to the other variables represented in the Fick equation.[12] The blood hemoglobin is kept between 12 and 14 $g \cdot dl^{-1}$ by administration of packed red blood cells or whole blood, and PaO_2 is kept at 100–200 mmHg by increasing the fractional concentration of oxygen in the inspired air. Unduly high oxygen consumption ($\dot{V}o_2$) is prevented while the patient is on the ventilator by the use of sedative or paralyzing drugs to prevent restlessness and agitation. Hyperthermia (rectal or central temperature greater than 40°C) is treated vigorously (see "Hyperthermia," under "Metabolic Subsystem").

When cardiac performance is unsatisfactory or when the risk of inadequate cardiac performance is increased because of the preoperative condition of the patient, the severity of the cardiac malformation or disease, or the nature of the operative procedure, certain general measures are important. The patient remains intubated, with the respirations controlled by the ventilator. Adults are continuously sedated with intermittent doses of morphine or diazepam (Valium), because restlessness increases oxygen consumption and

other metabolic demands. In neonates and infants, and particularly those in whom paroxysms of pulmonary artery hypertension or bronchospasm are anticipated, continuous, pharmacologically induced muscle paralysis or, alternatively, continuous anesthesia can be useful. For anesthesia, a continuous infusion of morphine,[L4] or of sublimaze (Fentanyl) in a dose of 0.33 $\mu g \cdot kg^{-1} \cdot min^{-1}$ (UAB), may be used. Hyperthermia is treated intensively (see "Hyperthermia" under the section on the metabolic subsystem).

Cardiac Arrhythmias

Postoperative morbidity and mortality can result from cardiac arrhythmias. These arrhythmias may occur either when the cardiac subsystem has been otherwise functioning normally or as a complication of low cardiac output. Atrial and ventricular pacing wires, routinely placed at operation (see Chapter 2) and left for 5–10 days postoperatively, are of utmost importance in the diagnosis[W3] and treatment[F1,W4] of postoperative arrhythmias.[W5]

Ventricular Electrical Instability

An important arrhythmia, ventricular electrical instability, includes premature ventricular contraction (PVC) and ventricular tachycardia. However, controversy exists concerning the proportion of patients with PVCs and some types of ventricular tachycardia who are at risk of developing ventricular fibrillation. In spite of this, it currently is prudent to assume that such arrhythmias place the patient at an increased risk of sudden death from ventricular fibrillation. Therefore, to detect such arrhythmias, the electrocardiogram is monitored continuously for at least the first 48 hours after operation.

When intermittent ventricular electrical instability appears (PVCs more than six times per minute and other arrhythmias as described in Appendix 5E), lidocaine (see "Antiarrhythmic Drugs" in Chapter 4 and Table 4-6) is administered as an intravenous bolus. The usual adult dose is 50 mg. If this is not effective, it is repeated twice, at 3–5-minute intervals. At the same time, the adequacy of the ventricular rate and the serum potassium (K^+) level are also considered. If hypokalemia ($K^+ < 4.0$ mEq $\cdot l^{-1}$) is present, 5 mEq of K^+ as KCl are given as an intravenous bolus, and a maintenance program is begun (see Appendix 5E). When the ventricular rate is less than 100 beats per minute, pacing should be used to increase it to 100–120 beats per minute. This alone may be effective prophylaxis against further PVCs.

If continuous ventricular electrical instability (ventricular tachycardia) develops, initial treatment is more vigorous. If the hemodynamic state is good, lidocaine is used initially, but if a favorable response is not quickly obtained, electroversion of some type is promptly performed. Usually, DC cardioversion is the method of choice. The first shock is given at 100 watt-seconds, and if this is ineffective, 200 watt-seconds are used. Alternatively, if the ventricular tachycardia is at a rate of less than about 150 beats per minute and the hemodynamic state is good, simple under- or overdrive ventricular pacing via the wires left at operation may restore the pretachycardic rhythm (sinus or atrial fibrillation). When

---

[12] The Fick equation states

$$\dot{Q} = \frac{\dot{V}o_2}{CaO_2 - C\bar{v}O_2} (1 \cdot min^{-1}) \qquad (5-2)$$

where $\dot{Q}$ is cardiac output in $1 \cdot min^{-1}$, $\dot{V}o_2$ is oxygen consumption in $ml \cdot min^{-1}$, CaO_2 is arterial O_2 content in $ml \cdot l^{-1}$, and $C\bar{v}O_2$ is mixed venous O_2 content in $ml \cdot l^{-1}$.

The oxygen content of blood consists of combined plus dissolved oxygen:

$$Co_2 = \frac{1.38 \cdot (Hb) \cdot So_2}{100} + 0.03 \, Po_2 \, (ml \cdot l^{-1}) \qquad (5-3)$$

where (Hb) is hemoglobin concentration in $g \cdot l^{-1}$, So_2 is O_2 saturation as a percentage of capacity, Po_2 is O_2 tension in mmHg, 1.38 is effective O_2 capacity of 1 g of hemoglobin in $ml \cdot g^{-1}$, and 0.03 is solubility of O_2 in blood at 37°C in $ml \cdot l^{-1}$ $mmHg^{-1}$.

Rearranging equation 5-2 and substituting for CaO_2 from equation 5-3,

$$C\bar{v}O_2 = \frac{1.38 \cdot (Hb) \cdot SaO_2}{100} + 0.03 \, PaO_2 - \frac{\dot{V}o_2}{\dot{Q}} \qquad (5-4)$$

For a given $\dot{V}o_2$, equation 5-4 indicates that to increase $C\bar{v}O_2$ there must be an increase in SaO_2, PaO_2, Hb, or $\dot{Q}$. $C\bar{v}O_2$ varies directly with $P\bar{v}O_2$, and $P\bar{v}O_2$ varies directly with cellular Po_2 unless there is shunting in the peripheral circulation. Thus, to maximize tissue oxygen supply, there must be an increase of one or more of the following: PaO_2 (and thus SaO_2), Hb, or $\dot{Q}$.

ventricular tachycardia appears and the hemodynamic state is poor, DC cardioversion should be performed immediately.

When the initial treatment with lidocaine is ineffective, the possibility that the diagnosis may not be ventricular electrical instability should be considered. A number of supraventricular arrhythmias associated with aberrant conduction may mimic wide QRS complex ventricular arrhythmias. Thus, expert cardiac electrophysiologic consultation should be sought.

When control is obtained by these initial measures, procainamide therapy is begun (see Appendix 5E). If the tendency toward ventricular electrical instability is strong, a continuous lidocaine infusion is begun at a dose of 20–50 μg · kg^{-1} · min^{-1} and continued until several doses of procainamide have been given. After 2–3 days, the procainamide is changed to procaine SR (given every 6–8 hours in a dose twice that of the procainamide), quinidine, or disopyramide (norpace). The serum level of the antiarrhythmic agent is measured before hospital dismissal. The usual practice is to continue the antiarrhythmic agent for 6 weeks after the patient leaves the hospital, but this may not always be appropriate. If the arrhythmia was only PVCs in the early hours after operation and ventricular function is good, or if after a few days of therapy, provocative electrophysiologic testing (via the temporary wires left at operation) by rapid pacing or the introduction of premature beats at selected intervals does not initiate sustained ventricular tachycardia, consideration is given to discontinuing the antiarrhythmic treatment before hospital dismissal.

Atrial Arrhythmias
Various atrial arrhythmias may complicate the postoperative period. Atrial fibrillation is treated initially with digitalis (see Appendix 5B). If it persists until the seventh postoperative day in patients who have not been in atrial fibrillation preoperatively, DC electroversion should usually be carried out. Atrial flutter, formerly a difficult arrhythmia postoperatively, is now routinely treated by rapid atrial pacing (via the two implanted atrial wires) at the so-called critical pacing rate (see Appendix 5F) and, after about 20 seconds, sudden cessation of pacing. Usually this stops the flutter. Digoxin is begun and continued for 6 weeks. Procainamide is begun (see Appendix 5E) and continued for 8 weeks; one of the longer-acting antiarrhythmic agents is substituted if long-term drug therapy is indicated. Paroxysmal atrial contractions (PACs) may trigger or lead to atrial fibrillation, and, therefore, an attempt is made to suppress them with atrial pacing, procainamine, or quinidine. Paroxysmal atrial tachycardia (PAT) is usually first treated by rapid atrial pacing and then sudden cessation (see Appendix 5F). If this is unsuccessful, carotid massage may break the rhythm, but this maneuver should be accompanied by administration of a vasoconstrictor. Propranolol may be given intravenously in doses of 0.5 mg every 2 minutes to a total intravenous dose of 4 mg, or verapamil may be infused slowly in a dose of 0.075 mg · kg^{-1} to a maximum dose of 5 mg. (These drugs may also be used to slow the ventricular rate in atrial fibrillation when it has not responded to full digitalization.)[P7] If PAT is recurrent or refractory to treatment, continuous rapid atrial pacing at about 100 beats faster than the intrinsic

atrial rate is employed to produce and sustain 2:1 block. Patients who have had PAT should generally receive digoxin for about 6 weeks.

When the onset of a supraventricular tachyarrhythmia is accompanied by important hemodynamic deterioration, prompt cardioversion (synchronous) is indicated if atrial wires are not in place.

RENAL SUBSYSTEM

Normally Convalescing Patients

Only preventive measures are used in normally convalescing patients. Most of these measures are incorporated in the perfusion techniques (see Chapter 2, Section 3) and also include maintenance of adequate cardiac output and a few special measures in patients with preoperatively impaired renal function (Appendix 5G).

As a guide to the continuing evaluation of the renal subsystem (see Section 1) a urinary catheter is inserted in the operating room preoperatively and left for about 48 hours to monitor urine flow. Serum potassium is measured every 4 hours during the first 24 postoperative hours and, if the patient is still in the Intensive Care Unit, every 8 hours for at least the next 48 hours. Serum creatinine and BUN levels are measured each morning for at least the first 48 hours.

Acute Renal Failure after Cardiac Surgery

Incidence
Acute renal failure is rare in adults, occurring in less than 0.1% of patients undergoing such operations as coronary artery bypass grafting, but it occurs in 2%–10% of infants undergoing open intracardiac operations.[C6,S4] It is nearly always associated with low cardiac output but rarely may occur when the other criteria of cardiac subsystem performance are satisfactory.[B5,H2,S4] The criteria for normal convalescence, and thus the absence of acute renal failure, are described in Section 1.

Characteristics
Acute renal failure may develop within 12–18 hours after operation. Its first manifestation is oliguria of increasing severity that is resistant to measures to increase cardiac output, to dopamine, and to furosemide and that results in a very rapidly rising serum potassium level (probably because of the acute loss of potassium from hemolyzing red blood cells and from the whole body loss of intracellular potassium that characterizes the perioperative period in patients who have been on CPB) and in more slowly rising BUN and creatinine levels. Although this form of acute renal failure is rarely the primary mode of death, it complicates recovery in a major way unless prompt and effective interventions are made.

A less lethal form of renal failure becomes apparent on the third or fourth postoperative day. This manifests itself by a progressive rise in BUN and creatinine levels, which peak at 80–120 and 5–8 mg · dl^{-1}, respectively, about 7–10 days postoperatively. There is often little or no oliguria, and hyperkalemia greater than 5 mEq · l^{-1} does not develop. Spontaneous resolution usually follows; and as long as the patient's clinical condition is satisfactory, urine flow is adequate, and BUN and creatinine levels do not continue to rise, dialysis is not indicated.

Incremental Risk Factors

Acute reduction in cardiac output early after the repair is the commonest and most important risk factor for the development of acute renal failure. However, there are additional risk factors.

Young age is a risk factor for acute renal failure. Following cardiac surgery in infants, when cardiac output is reduced, an incidence of acute renal failure as high as 8%–10% has been reported.[C6,S4] This complication is particularly high in neonates.[R6] The incidence seems to vary considerably among institutions and can be rare (GLH). One reason for the apparently increased incidence in infants with low early postoperative cardiac output is the immaturity of the kidney in infants and young children, with less ability than the adult kidney to concentrate urine. Compared to older patients, infants may develop more tissue hypoxia during and early after CPB, with a resultant increased production of potassium, urea nitrogen, and other substances, some of which may be nephrotoxic. Uric acid levels, for example, were shown by Hencz and colleagues to rise to nephrotoxic levels ($10 \text{ mg} \cdot \text{dl}^{-1}$) in some patients within 24 hours of operation, and the levels were significantly ($P = .001$) higher in patients less than 3 years of age than in older children.[H3]

Renal failure is more likely to occur after operations for cyanotic heart disease.[T1] A renal lesion is known to exist in many such patients preoperatively.

Preoperative impairment of renal function considerably increases the risk of acute renal failure early postoperatively.[A3,H2] Therefore, a part of the preoperative evaluation should be the determination of renal function.

A long period of CPB increases the risk of renal failure.[R6] This has been clearly demonstrated by a prospective study[K8] and is probably at least in part related to the damaging effects of cardiopulmonary bypass. The additional risk from profound hypothermia and total circulatory arrest is not known, nor is that of long periods of reduced flow during hypothermic CPB. However, flows $\geq 1.6 \text{ l} \cdot \text{min}^{-2}$ at $28°C$ and mean arterial blood pressure $\geq 30 \text{ mmHg}$ during CPB at moderate hypothermia seem adequate to minimize acute renal failure.[H2]

A high plasma hemoglobin level ($> 40 \text{ mg} \cdot \text{dl}^{-1}$) during and early after CPB probably increases the risk of acute renal failure. The suggestion that a whole blood prime increases risk is supported by several studies.[G2,W6]

Aminoglycosides (e.g., gentamicin) and some other antibiotics may increase the risk of this complication.

When oliguria occurs early postoperatively, cardiac preload and afterload are made optimal, and the administration of dopamine at $2.5 \text{ μg} \cdot \text{kg}^{-1} \cdot \text{min}^{-1}$ is begun. If these measures do not suffice, Lasix ($1 \text{ mg} \cdot \text{kg}^{-1}$) is administered intravenously. If a good response is obtained with Lasix, this dosage is repeated every 6–12 hours for 3 days. There is, however, no firm evidence that Lasix prevents progression of acute renal failure in such situations. If a response to Lasix is not obtained, the dose is doubled, then quadrupled,

and then $8 \text{ mg} \cdot \text{kg}^{-1}$ is given. When serum K^+ rises above $5.5 \text{ mEq} \cdot \text{l}^{-1}$, glucose-insulin solution is given intravenously, and K-exalate enemas are used (see Appendix 5H).

Unless oliguria and hyperkalemia respond to treatment within a few hours, and especially in infants, the nephrologist should proceed immediately with dialysis (see Appendix 5I). Peritoneal dialysis is nearly always the method used early postoperatively.[N3] Frequently, after 6–24 hours of peritoneal dialysis, the patient (usually an infant) begins to make urine as the general condition improves. Shortly thereafter, the dialysis can be discontinued.

In older patients, often with some preexisting renal disease, recovery from renal failure is less rapid, but many of these patients too can be maintained in good condition by dialysis until cardiac and renal function improve and ultimately recover fully.[G7,S4]

PULMONARY SUBSYSTEM

Normally Convalescing Patients

Patients are extubated early after cardiac surgery, as soon as the effects of the anesthetic agents have disappeared, when normal convalescence is likely. In patients undergoing closed operations, including infants, this usually means extubation in the operating room (see Chapter 4). Following open operations of an uncomplicated nature, such as repair of simple congenital lesions and coronary artery bypass grafting or isolated valve replacement or valvotomy, in infants as well as adults, the patient is usually extubated in the operating room after the effects of the anesthetic agents have been reversed (GLH) or within 4–8 hours postoperatively (UAB). Following complex open operations, ventilation is generally continued overnight. In any event, patients are not extubated until the appropriate criteria are met (see Appendix 5J).

While intubated, the patient is ventilated with a volume- or pressure-controlled respirator, which provides intermittent positive pressure breathing (IPPB). The circuit is modified to allow the patient to breathe spontaneously between periods of intermittent mandatory ventilation (IMV) from the ventilator. The IMV is reduced gradually to 6 machine-produced breaths per minute when spontaneous breathing is sufficient to allow it, not only to accustom the patient to breathing normally but also to gain the hemodynamic advantages of the negative intrapleural pressures that develop during spontaneous inspiration. Positive end-expiratory pressure (PEEP) may be used as a routine (UAB), or on indication (GLH), with a setting of 8 cm H_2O for adults and children over 12 years of age, and 4 cm H_2O for younger patients. Unless the hemodynamic state is suboptimal, PEEP does not alter it, even in infants.[L3] PEEP is used because of studies that suggest the existence of larger lung volumes and few perfused but nonventilated alveoli during ventilation; and smaller alveolar-arterial oxygen differences, P(A-a)O_2, after extubation when it is used.[A4] PEEP is contraindicated in patients with chronic obstructive lung disease (to avoid air-trapping and rupturing a bulla, with consequent pneumothorax) and in infants and children who have undergone an atrial switch operation, Fontan's operation, or a superior vena cava–to–right pulmonary artery anastomosis (Glenn's operation) (to avoid still further elevation of jugular venous pressure).

Continuous positive airway pressure (CPAP)[G4,S8] may be used in infants once their cardiovascular state is stable, obviating the need for IPPB and IMV (GLH). Should IPPB be required initially, the infant is transferred to IMV and someties to CPAP for several hours before extubation (see Appendix 5J).

While the patient is intubated and ventilated, the inspired gases are warmed and humidified. Appropriate aspiration of the trachea, turning of the patient, and chest physiotherapy are carried out (see Appendix 5J). Varying degrees of pulmonary atelectasis occur with sufficient frequency postoperatively to be considered part of normal convalescence. Particularly common is left lower lobe collapse. This is self-limiting and manageable by appropriate physiotherapy, which continues throughout the hospital stay.

When Convalescence Is Complicated

Reintubation
When the patient truly meets the criteria for extubation, reintubation is usually not necessary. However, reintubation is indicated when (1) the Pco$_2$ rises to a level > 50 mmHg over a 4-hour period, (2) there are signs of falling cardiac output, (3) the patient shows signs of exhaustion from breathing spontaneously, and (4) there are excessive pulmonary secretions, with ineffective coughing (the latter two are frequently combined). When the situation is borderline, proper management requires careful observation by senior members of the team.

Prolonged Intubation
A prolongation of the period of endotracheal intubation and IPPB or IMV is necessary when (1) criteria for extubation are not met, (2) neurologic complications are present, (3) severe dysfunction of the cardiac subsystem is present, or (4) persistent chest drainage or a residual cardiac defect make early return to the operating room a likely possibility. Prolonged intubation (beyond about 48 hours), although sometimes necessary, entails problems necessitating very fastidious care of the patient. All the details of care described in Appendix 5J must be practiced. In infants particularly, a pneumothorax occasionally develops from the positive pressure breathing and usually requires urgent aspiration and underwater drainage. Bronchospasm may become a particular problem, probably as a reflex response to the proteinaceous tracheobronchial fluid often present under these circumstances. The administration of nebulized Bronchosol (isoetharine) every hour can be helpful. In extreme cases, aminophylline is given as a continuous intravenous infusion in 10% dextrose in a dose of 0.15 mg · kg^{-1} · min^{-1}. An initial loading dose of about 4 mg · kg^{-1} is given over a 20-minute period.

In those unusual circumstances in which intubation is necessary for more than about 10 days, consideration is given to tracheostomy. This procedure has disadvantages but is sometimes very helpful in weaning the patient from the ventilator. In neonates and infants, tracheostomy is now very

rarely performed, because it is most difficult to manage in this age group. Moreover, nasotracheal intubation has few complications in infants even over periods of months provided the noncuffed tube is of the proper diameter and length (see Chapter 4, Fig. 4-2). In older infants, attempts to wean are continued for at least 3 weeks before resorting to tracheostomy. In children and adults, the disadvantages are fewer, and tracheostomy is seriously considered after 10 days.

Pulmonary Edema without Left Atrial Hypertension
In the early hours after CPB, pulmonary edema without left atrial hypertension may develop. During CPB, changes occur in the alveoli and small pulmonary vessels, and vasoactive polypeptides accumulate in the circulating blood (see Chapter 2). Probably as a result, pulmonary vessels become permeable, resulting in interstitial pulmonary edema and accumulation in the alveoli of protein-containing fluid. It is likely that these phenomena occur to some extent in all patients after CPB. Usually the pulmonary edema is not detectable by ordinary means, although a mild decrease in lung compliance and a widened alveolar-arterial oxygen difference are often present (Fig. 5-4). Occasionally, frank pulmonary edema or hemorrhage without left atrial hypertension is seen immediately after discontinuing CPB. This complication may clear completely within 1–2 hours or may continue into the postoperative period, when a chest roentgenogram will show patchy opacities representing widespread interstitial and alveolar edema and hemorrhage, and frothy or bloody fluid may be aspirated from the tracheobronchial tree in association with often severe cyanosis and a low PaO$_2$. Infants and cyanotic patients seem to be affected more often than others, but, rarely, this complication may follow seemingly straightforward operations.

The syndrome may not be manifest immediately after operation in mild cases, and the results of an early postoperative chest roentgenogram may be quite normal, although the PaO$_2$ progressively falls. Then, 48–72 hours after operation, the patient may begin to cough up thick tracheobronchial secretions. Often, seemingly paradoxically, dyspnea and tachypnea begin to lessen when this fluid appears in the tracheobronchial tree. Presumably, at this time, protein-rich fluid, which since CPB or soon thereafter has been in the alveoli and interstitium of the lung, begins to be moved by ciliary action out of the alveoli and terminal bronchioles and into the larger airways.

The treatment of this syndrome is not specific. When it is apparent in the operating room or early after operation, the FIo$_2$ is appropriately adjusted upward if the P(A-a)O$_2$ is large. Particular attention is given to tracheal suctioning. When hemoconcentration develops along with the syndrome, from the leakage of plasma from the intravascular space into the interstitial space of the lungs and all other organs and at times into the pleural and peritoneal spaces, administration of concentrated serum albumin seems helpful in counteracting this trend (see Appendix 5K). Diuretics may be useful to the extent that they reduce extracellular fluid volume and, in turn, extravascular lung water.

Associated with this syndrome, ascites often develops, particularly in infants, and a small-diameter plastic drainage catheter is then inserted. Relieving peritoneal pressure usually dramatically improves inferior vena caval return. This catheter can be used for peritoneal dialysis should there be associated renal failure with high BUN and/or potassium levels. Small pleural catheters are also inserted to remove pleural fluid, since this may dramatically improve PaO_2 even when the effusion is relatively small.

Delayed Interstitial Pulmonary Edema

Three to 6 days after operation, interstitial pulmonary edema may develop insidiously. This delayed edema is manifested by insidiously developing orthopnea and paroxysmal nocturnal dyspnea, and it occurs primarily in patients predisposed to the development of left atrial and pulmonary venous hypertension by marked left ventricular hypertrophy or poor left ventricular function. Often, the left atrial pressure has been moderately elevated (14–17 mmHg) earlier in the postoperative period. Twenty-four to 48 hours after CPB, fluid that accumulated in the interstitial space during and soon after CPB[C1,P1] returns to the vascular space. Presumably, whatever osmotic and other forces originally caused it to accumulate in the interstitium have dissipated, thus releasing it. Blood volume is thereby increased, the hematocrit and hemoglobin concentrations fall, and, under such circumstances, the renal response is subnormal, and the usual diuresis and control of blood volume do not follow. In this setting, left ventricular end-diastolic, left atrial, and pulmonary venous pressures rise and symptoms may develop. Weight gain and other evidences of fluid retention may be absent. The patient must be watched carefully for this syndrome postoperatively, and its presence should be suspected when a previously normally convalescing patient begins to complain of cough when lying down or of shortness of breath at night. Treatment with furosemide (Lasix) intravenously provides dramatic relief and confirms the diagnosis.

Pulmonary Embolism

The incidence of pulmonary embolism as a cause of morbidity and mortality after CPB is generally not appreciated. It is rare in patients who have been on continuous oral anticoagulants since about 48 hours postoperatively. In patients not on anticoagulants, the surgeon must be alert for the signs of deep venous thrombosis and should begin administering oral anticoagulants whenever there is a suspicion of such a pathologic condition. When the thrombosis is acute in onset, continuous intravenous heparin therapy (administered by a low-flow pump at a dose in adults of 10,000 units twice daily, after an initial bolus dose of 10,000 units) is begun immediately and continued for 2–3 days, until the oral anticoagulant has become effective.

Should massive pulmonary embolism occur, the treatment is urgent pulmonary embolectomy. Multiple recurrent small pulmonary emboli produce a clinical picture of excessive dyspnea when the patient begins to exercise, followed by continuous dyspnea at rest. Signs of deep venous thrombosis may or may not be evident, but oral anticoagulation should be commenced and continued for about 3 months.

Pleural Effusion

Unless the pleura has been opened (in which case effusion may represent postoperative bleeding that has drained in-

completely from the pleural cavity), pleural effusion is not a part of normal convalescence. An effusion appearing after 1 week suggests an underlying pathologic condition in the lung and, after 3 weeks, a postcardiotomy syndrome.

METABOLIC SUBSYSTEM

Normally Convalescing Patients

Because of the increase in extracellular fluid and total exchangeable sodium and the decrease in exchangeable potassium that develop during CPB, early postoperative fluid administration must be precise. On the basis of early work by Sturtz and colleagues,[S2] a standardized approach to fluid administration has been developed that seems to meet the requirements. For approximately 48 hours after operation, no sodium is administered, and minimal amounts of water (as 5% glucose in water) are given intravenously (see Appendix 5L). Larger amounts of water are disadvantageous because they result in higher urine volumes and an increased potassium loss if renal function is good, and fluid overload if renal function is impaired. A modest amount of potassium (10 $mEq \cdot m^{-2} \cdot d^{-1}$) is given on the day of surgery because large amounts generally are not needed in normally convalescing patients, in spite of the decrease in total exchangeable potassium, and because larger amounts simply escape in the urine.[B3] In the first 3 postoperative days, hypokalemia is not treated unless it becomes very severe (serum potassium level < 2.5 $mEq \cdot l^{-1}$) (UAB). Alternatively, the intravenous potassium dose may be adjusted on the basis of blood samples taken every 4–8 hours to keep the serum potassium level above 4 $mEq \cdot l^{-1}$ (GLH). If there are ventricular ectopic beats, the level is increased to between 4.5 and 5.0 $mmol \cdot l^{-1}$. Liquids are taken orally a few hours after extubation, and intravenous administration can then cease by the second postoperative day. Renal ability to excrete sodium may be impaired for some days after operation even in normally convalescing patients,[P2] and a diet low in sodium is therefore needed until daily weighing indicates that the patient's weight is less than it was preoperatively.

When extubation is delayed beyond the second postoperative day, an adequate caloric intake must be assured. Once bowel sounds are present, caloric needs can be met through nasogastric tube feedings using an appropriate high-caloric formula. Rarely, intravenous hyperalimentation is required.

In infants, more exacting management is required for several reasons. First, care must be taken to avoid fluid overload from the solution used to keep the pressure-recording lines patent. Second, because the infant's energy requirements are relatively large, 10% glucose is more appropriate than 5%. In addition, there is some evidence that infants may require small amounts of sodium from the beginning of the postoperative phase. Finally, infants tend to develop hyperkalemia very rapidly when oliguria develops. Thus, a special protocol may be used for infants (see Appendix 5L) in which 250 ml $\cdot$ m^{-2} of balanced salt solution is included each day (UAB).

In infants, oral feeding is not begun until 8 hours after extubation. Small feedings of glucose water every 4 hours are then given, and if they are well tolerated after two or three feedings, an appropriate formula low in sodium is started. If the mother is breast-feeding the infant, this is resumed as soon as the baby is strong enough. The child must be picked up and held for the feedings, and burped thereafter. If the infant is too weak to suck, gavage feedings are given through a nasogastric tube.

Gavage feedings are required in any infant who has been intubated for longer than 2 days. The fluid is placed in an open syringe or burette attached to the tube and allowed to run in slowly by gravity (see Appendix 5M). If gavage feeding is necessary for more than a few days, the baby's caloric and other metabolic needs must be calculated and a determined effort made to meet them.

As indicated earlier, some metabolic acidosis (base deficit of 2 mEq $\cdot$ l^{-1})[A5] may be present during the early hours after intracardiac surgery even when the patient is convalescing normally. It is left untreated if the arterial pH is ≥ 7.4 and PaCO$_2$ is ≥ 30 mmHg. If the PaCO$_2$ is < 30 mmHg, the base deficit is treated *before* adjusting the PaCO$_2$ appropriately upward. When pH is < 7.4, the base deficit is treated (Appendix 5N). However, if convalescence is otherwise normal, treatment is delayed for 4–8 hours in adults and 2–4 hours in infants, by which time it may have cleared spontaneously. In infants particularly, it is best to avoid this additional sodium load whenever possible. A mild metabolic alkalosis may be present 24 hours after operation in normally convalescing patients, probably related in part at least to the sodium load contained in the anticoagulant solution of the banked blood. Such metabolic alkalosis is self-correcting under these circumstances and is not treated.

When Convalescence Is Complicated

Metabolic Acidosis

When cardiac output in inadequate or acute cardiac failure has occurred, metabolic acidosis often develops. It is treated with sodium bicarbonate (see Appendix 5N).

Metabolic Alkalosis

When large amounts of homologous blood containing sodium citrate have been transfused, metabolic alkalosis can occur. Metabolism of the citrate leaves bicarbonate as the only anion available to balance the sodium ions. The situation may be exacerbated after 2–4 days by the migration of hydrogen ions from the cells, for the hydrogen ions are replaced by potassium ions, and serum potassium falls, sometimes precipitously (in association with potassium loss in the urine). Relatively large amounts of potassium chloride must be given under such circumstances (up to 200 mEq in 24 hours), but the dose should be titrated against 4-hourly serum potassium measurements. The alkalosis is associated with a fall in serum chloride and a compensatory rise in PaCO$_2$. Provided renal function is adequate, the situation corrects itself. If it continues to worsen, hydrochloric acid should be given intravenously (see Appendix 5O).

Hyperthermia

Body temperature may become severely elevated in the first 48 postoperative hours, particularly in infants, as discussed earlier. Such hyperthermia is usually a manifestation of a profound reaction to CPB, although infection, reaction to homologous blood, and brain stem damage are other possible etiologic factors. The identification and vigorous treatment of hyperthermia are important because the prognosis for patients is poor without them.[W1]

Whenever the usually monitored rectal temperature becomes abnormally high during the first 48 postoperative hours ($\geq 39.5°C$, or $103.1°F$), an esophageal thermistor should be introduced because central (core) temperature may be considerably higher than rectal temperature under these circumstances. When the central temperature exceeds $39.5°C$, vigorous antipyretic measures are initiated (Appendix 5P).

Hypoglycemia

During the first 48 postoperative hours, hypoglycemia may develop, particularly in infants less than 3 months old. Therefore, blood glucose is routinely measured twice daily in neonates. As a precaution against hypoglycemia, 10% dextrose in water may be used in maintenance fluids for infants (UAB) (see Appendix 5L). When hypoglycemia (blood glucose level < 80 mg $\cdot$ dl^{-1}) does occur, 50 mg $\cdot$ kg^{-1} of glucose is given (1 ml $\cdot$ kg^{-1} of 50% dextrose mixed with an equal amount of 5% glucose in water and administered intravenously over a 15-minute period). Blood glucose levels are measured 30 minutes later and at 4-hour intervals for 24 hours. Hypoglycemia is not seen in the first 12–24 hours postoperatively and rarely thereafter when heparinized blood is used in the machine prime (GLH), for each unit contains an additional 2,500 mg $\cdot$ dl^{-1} of glucose (see Chapter 2, Section 4).

Acute Adrenal Insufficiency

A rare complication of open heart operations, acute adrenal insufficiency, has been found by Alford and colleagues in 5, or 0.1%, of 4,364 patients.[A1] Symptoms generally appear between the fourth and tenth postoperative days and consist of abdominal and flank pain, abdominal distention, altered mental status, fever, and occasionally shock. When this diagnosis is suspected, a single low serum cortisol determination makes probable the diagnosis. The diagnosis is highly likely if the serum cortisol level remains low 60 minutes after administration of 25 units of intravenous or intramuscular ACTH. Later, confirmatory evidence of acute adrenal insufficiency should be obtained.[A1] Prompt treatment with intravenous cortisol and saline solutions results in rapid clearing of the symptoms. Lifetime oral treatment is indicated subsequently. The cause is probably hemorrhagic infarction of the adrenal gland.[A1] This could have been precipitated by CPB, and the tendency toward it may be aggravated by postoperative anticoagulant therapy.

NEUROLOGIC SUBSYSTEM

Normally Convalescing Patients

No treatment is necessary for the neurologic subsystem in normally convalescing patients.

When Convalescence Is Complicated

Neurological damage or dysfunction is now uncommon. When present, either generalized or focal signs of central nervous system damage are present immediately after operation. These are accompanied by cerebral edema, which progresses over a matter of a few hours. The administration of dexamethasone is begun as soon as significant damage is identified, in an intravenous dose of 4 mg in adults and continued every 6 hours for 48 hours. If there is improvement, the dose can be reduced over the next 5 days and then stopped. If there is no improvement, a higher dose should be continued for a further 3 days before abandoning this treatment. A flaccid decorticate state in adults indicates a poor prognosis, whereas children may make a dramatic recovery.

Seizures require treatment. They occur primarily in infants and children (see Chapter 2) and must be controlled pharmacologically (see Appendix 5Q). Seizures are usually related to the use of CPB with total circulatory arrest, but metabolic derangements may be associated with seizures and, if present, should be treated (see Appendix 5Q). Seizures usually do *not* indicate permanent brain damage, and usually, after the seizure activity subsides, the child is normal as far as can be determined.

More serious and more infrequent are choreoathetoid movements, which seem only to occur in infants and children (see Chapter 2). Their pharmacologic control and management are difficult. Thus, a pediatric neurologist should participate in the care of such a child. However, the symptoms usually regress and eventually disappear.

GASTROINTESTINAL SUBSYSTEM

Normally Convalescing Patients

No special treatment is required while the patient is intubated, except that a nasogastric tube is in place to avoid gastric distention from swallowed air. Sips of fluid are allowed by mouth 4–8 hours after extubation, provided cardiac and pulmonary function are normal.

Patients with a history of peptic ulcer disease are given 300 mg of cimetidine every 6 hours (by mouth or intravenously) during the postoperative hospitalization.

When Convalescence Is Complicated

Abdominal Distention
Occasionally, gas in the gastrointestinal tract produces abdominal distention within 24–48 hours of operation. Bowel sounds can be heard initially. Although not part of normal convalescence, this complication is usually benign and subsides after another day or so in response to fasting, the use of glycerine suppositories, and the application of heat to the abdomen. A rectal examination should be performed to exclude fecal impaction as a possible cause of the distention. If the distention does not promptly subside, other causes must be considered. The distention could be due to the oral administration of procainamide or cephalosporins, and these drugs may need to be administered by another route. *Mediastinitis* and an infected median sternotomy incision may be causative and should be sought. Abdominal disten-

tion may be the first sign of postoperative acute pancreatitis. When combined with marked weakness and fever, particularly in a patient on Coumadin (sodium warfarin), postoperative adrenal insufficiency must be excluded as a possible cause by appropriate tests (see section on Metabolic Subsystem).

Candida Esophagitis
Occasionally, substernal pain and dysphagia become prominent 3–7 days after operation, and when oral candidiasis is present, candida esophagitis is nearly certainly the cause[G5] and can be diagnosed by means of radiologic study of the barium-filled esophagus.[O1] When candida esophagitis appears, antibiotic therapy is stopped unless it is essential. Every 2–6 hours, 500,000–1,000,000 units of Nystatin are given orally, preferably in methylcellulose to increase viscosity.[G5] Treatment is continued for 1–3 weeks.

Watery Diarrhea
As a complication of cardiac surgery, watery diarrhea may accompany or follow abdominal distention or appear de novo toward the end of the first week. Should it become frequent and explosive, with passage of mucus and blood, it has ominous implications. The oral administration of lincomycin can be causative (GLH), and this drug must be avoided.[S9] Any other oral antibiotics should also be discontinued when diarrhea develops. The diarrhea may be caused by ischemia of the bowel secondary to a long period of low cardiac output, and this ischemia may lead to small or large bowel infarction,[A2] or it may be a form of ulcerative colitis and proctitis. The diagnosis can be made by sigmoidoscopy and colonoscopy. If the bowel ischemia and ulceration progress, laparotomy and bowel resection are required, but even with such treatment, the prognosis is poor.

Massive Gastrointestinal Bleeding
After open intracardiac operations, massive gastrointestinal bleeding is rare. When it does occur, it is usually the result of a postoperative bleeding diathesis, prolonged low cardiac output, or acute or chronic peptic ulceration, the latter particularly in patients on cortisone. Later in the postoperative period, anticoagulants may cause bleeding from peptic ulceration. A gastroenterologist is consulted to locate the site of bleeding. If it is coming primarily from the stomach, antacids, and cimetidine are used. Operation is rarely necessary.

Jaundice
Convalescence may be complicated by jaundice, with 23% of patients having a serum bilirubin concentration ≥ 3 mg · dl.[C11] The jaundice is moderate or severe (bilirubin concentration 6 mg · dl) in only 6% of patients. Chu and colleagues have shown that the severity of preoperative right atrial hypertension, hypoxia during operation, early postoperative hypotension, and the amount of blood transfused perioperatively all increased the probability of postoperative jaundice.[C11] In their analysis, whether or not halothane was used and the duration of cardiopulmonary bypass were not risk factors.

Provided that postoperative cardiac output is good, the hepatic dysfunction can be expected to improve gradually and disappear, but when cardiac output is low, the prognosis is poor. Frank hepatic necrosis may develop when cardiac output is acutely and severely reduced. The only useful treatment is that directed at improving cardiac performance and supplying adequate parenteral nutritional support.

Abdominal Emergencies

Such abdominal emergencies as perforated peptic ulcer, acute cholecystitis, and acute appendicitis can, of course, occur. The existence of these and other abdominal emergencies must be considered in any patient who complains of abdominal pain and tenderness.

SECTION 3
SPECIAL SITUATIONS AND CONTROVERSIES

EARLY POSTOPERATIVE BLEEDING

A bleeding tendency of some degree develops in all patients who have been on CPB, as most of the clotting factors are abnormal for a time. In spite of this, good hemostasis can be obtained in the operating room in almost all patients, although great patience and care are often required. Special hematologic investigation and treatment are seldom needed, and minimal blood administration is required in the operating room and intensive care unit in most uncomplicated cases. Any blood left in the pump-oxygenator after decannulation is either pumped into standard plastic blood collection bags and subsequently infused into the patient or placed in a device that packs and washes the red blood cells for intravenous infusion.

One important aspect of preventing continuous bleeding after CPB is avoiding having to infuse large volumes of homologous (banked) blood. This is achieved by making suture lines secure before discontinuing CPB, filling the patient with as much of the perfusate as possible before removing the arterial cannula, and stopping important bleeding after CPB as promptly as possible.

When the operation is a secondary one, or the patient is polycythemic, the likelihood of early bleeding is increased. In these situations, fresh frozen plasma (2 units, or about 500 ml, in adults) is given prophylactically immediately after CPB. Platelet concentrates are frequently administered under these circumstances, but there is little evidence that they are effective,[S12] except in preoperatively cyanotic patients.[W11] When the threat of serious bleeding is particularly great, the administration of fresh whole blood is optimal. The giving of banked blood is delayed if possible until the wound is dry, and a blood hemoglobin level as low as 6–7 g · dl^{-1} is acceptable if the hemodynamic state is reasonably good. Then, when hemostasis is secure, packed red blood cells or whole blood can be given.

Drainage from the chest tubes is monitored postoperatively. Uncommonly, the drainage is excessive, and then prompt reoperation is indicated. Under proper circumstances, reoperation should be necessary in only 1% or 2% of patients. In most circumstances when rigorous criteria for reoperation are applied, reentry is carried out within 3–4

hours of the patient's leaving the operating room, while the patient is in good condition, and without the disadvantages of infusing large volumes of homologous blood. A less strict protocol should be used when bleeding is anticipated from adhesions from previous surgery, particularly when there is no sign of a pericardial collection or impending tamponade.

The indications for prompt reentry are

1. Excessive bleeding from the chest tubes, as defined in Table 5-4. Drainage in excess of these criteria means that bleeding will probably continue and reach clearly excessive total amounts (in adults ≥ 1,500 ml total) within 12 hours. Exceptions to prompt reentry when this criterion is met are rare and are generally limited to patients in whom prolonged efforts at hemostasis have been made already and a bleeding diathesis is present, suture lines are known to be secure, and tamponade is not present.

2. Marked widening of the cardiac silhouette in the portable chest film 8–24 hours after operation. Such widening nearly always indicates the retention of some clots and blood in the pericardium. Even if the patient's condition is good, elective reoperation and evacuation of blood and clots are usually advisable.

3. Sudden increase (300 ml · h^{-1} or more in adults) in chest drainage that has been small in the first few postoperative hours. Such an increase usually results from bleeding from an incision in the heart or great arteries.

4. Evidence of acute cardiac tamponade (see "Low Cardiac Output," in Section 2).

POSTOPERATIVE PERICARDIAL EFFUSION

Most patients have some pericardial fluid early after open heart operation. Weitzman and colleagues found by echocardiographic study that 103 (84%; CL, 80%–88%) of 122 consecutive patients had pericardial effusions.[W10] Important pericardial effusions, detected by echocardiography 4 to 10 days postoperatively, are more common in patients in whom early postoperative bleeding was excessive.[S15] Effusions reach their maximum size in most patients on the tenth postoperative day and generally spontaneously regress after that time.

Most pericardial effusions are asymptomatic and require no particular treatment. Cardiac tamponade develops in only 1% of patients with pericardial fluid[W10] (see "Delayed Cardiac Tamponade").

DELAYED CARDIAC TAMPONADE

Several days to several weeks after the operation, cardiac tamponade may develop. Although this is uncommon, the incidence is greater among patients who are being treated with anticoagulants. If unrecognized, delayed tamponade can cause serious morbidity and mortality.[E2,H5,H6,M1] Clinical signs and symptoms may be subtle, but one or more of the following are usually present: progressive and unexplained weakness and lethargy; progressive dyspnea on exertion and orthopnea; unexplained hepatomegaly, ascites, or peripheral edema; elevated jugular venous pressure; pulsus

Table 5-4 Chest drainage criteria for reentry.

Preoperative Weight (kg)	Chest Drainage Indicating Reoperation				
	Hourly Amount (ml · h⁻¹)			Total Amount (ml)	
	No. of Successive Hours[a]			Hour No.[b]	
	1	2	3	4	5
5.0	70	60	50	120	130
6.0	70	60	50	130	155
7.0	70	60	50	150	180
8.0	90	70	50	175	200
9.0	90	80	60	195	230
10.0	100	90	65	220	260
12.0	130	100	80	260	300
14.0	150	120	90	300	360
16.0	170	140	100	350	400
18.0	195	150	120	390	460
20.0	200	175	130	450	520
25.0	270	220	160	540	650
30.0	325	260	195	650	770
35.0	380	300	230	760	900
40.0	430	350	260	800	1,035
45.0	500	400	300	975	1,150
50.0	500	400	300	1,000	1,200

[a]Reoperation is advisable if the patient has bled the amount indicated in any 1 hour (column 1), the lesser amount in column 2 during each of any 2 successive hours, or the still smaller amount (column 3) in each of any 3 successive hours.

[b]Reoperation is advisable if the patient has bled in total the amount indicated by the end of the fourth or fifth postoperative hour.

paradoxus; widening of the cardiac silhouette by chest x-ray; and unexplained prerenal azotemia.[K2] Important delayed cardiac tamponade rarely occurs before the seventh postoperative day, and a chest roentgenogram (which should be taken routinely the day before hospital dismissal or the seventh postoperative day, whichever comes first) usually shows enlargement of the cardiac silhouette before symptoms appear. Cardiac tamponade may, however, not become apparent until as late as 4 months after operation.[O2]

Pericardial fluid collections, suggested by the chest roentgenogram, may be confirmed by echocardiography. Right heart catheterization can be done, seeking equalization of right atrial, right ventricular end-diastolic, and pulmonary capillary wedge pressures. Contrast injection may identify fluid or a clot adjacent to the right atrium. However, since the probability of the accumulation of pericardial fluid is so great with positive roentgenographic and echocardiographic findings, invasive studies are rarely used.

Treatment consists of pericardial decompression, by either pericardiocentesis or surgical drainage. Drainage is generally effected under local anesthesia through a small (2-cm) reopening of the incision just below the xiphoid process and aspiration of the fluid with an ordinary surgical sucker.[H7] A chest tube is generally not required.

CHYLOTHORAX

Effused chyle may be present in the thoracic cavity after the repair of coarctation of the aorta; after Blalock-Taussig or, less frequently, gortex interposition shunts (see Chapter 23);

or, rarely, after the repair of patent ductus arteriosus.[C10,H11] In such instances, chylothorax probably results from cutting large tributaries of the thoracic duct or, less frequently, from injury to the thoracic duct itself. More complex and difficult to manage are the chylothoraces (and, on occasion, the pericardial accumulations of chyle with tamponade) that follow operations through a median sternotomy incision, such as the venous switch procedures for transposition of the great arteries (see Chapter 39), superior vena cava–right pulmonary artery anastomoses, and the Fontan procedure for tricuspid atresia (see Chapter 26). The chylothorax probably results from the combination of the inevitable transection of very small lymph channels (probably in the thymus gland) and the elevation of superior vena caval pressures which follow these procedures.

The chylothorax may develop immediately after operation, in which case it may not be recognized initially, since the fluid may appear to be serous. In the majority of such cases, the chylous drainage subsides spontaneously, and continuation of effective tube drainage is all that is necessary. Chylothorax may not develop for a week or more. In that case, needle aspirations repeated every 3–4 days usually constitute adequate treatment. Late-appearing chylothoraces are particularly likely to subside without operation, and the aspirations can be continued on an outpatient basis.

In early-appearing and persistingly massive chylothorax, the outlook with conservative treatment is less favorable. Malnutrition resistant to therapy rapidly develops, and surgical intervention is indicated if such drainage persists for more than about 7 days. The hemithorax in which the chyle is accumulating is entered through a posterolateral thoracotomy incision. The chylous leakage is sometimes easily seen and is oversewn. Unfortunately, the source is often not found, and watertight oversewing is not always possible. Under such circumstances, the thoracic duct can be sought behind the esophagus; if identified, it is doubly ligated, and this usually solves the problem. Even if these procedures are apparently successful, and certainly if they cannot be accomplished, the pleural space is scarified, and three properly placed intrapleural tubes are left for at least 96 hours, to ensure that the lung remains expanded and becomes adherent to the chest wall. Fibrin glue placed on the parietal pleura may enhance adherence.[S10] A good result is usually obtained from a combination of these maneuvers.

Rarely, after cardiac operations, chyle accumulates in the pericardial space, with or without chylothorax. This problem was first reported after operations with cardiopulmonary bypass by Thomas and McGoon[T3] and has subsequently been reported by others. It has been reported after the Waterston anastomosis,[H12,J1] in which, of course, the pericardium is opened. It has also been reported after a Blalock-Taussig shunt in which the pericardium was not opened.[F4] This is a difficult problem, and initial management consists of wide and prompt operative drainage of the pericardium into the pleural spaces by making large pericardial windows and then draining both pleural spaces with chest tubes. Following this, the measures described above are used.

Careful attention to the nutrition of the patient is important during the period of chylous drainage, but special diets designed to minimize the drainage are usually not helpful. Fortunately, chylothoraces have never been reported to become infected.

PROPHYLAXIS AGAINST INFECTION

A precise aseptic technique by the surgical, anesthetic, and perfusionist team is an essential part of the prophylaxis against infection in open cardiac operations. The large number of people involved and the length and complexity of the operations make bacterial contamination more likely than in shorter and simpler procedures. Infection inside or around the heart, particularly when prostheses have been used, is a major threat to the patient's life. Therefore, prophylactic antibiotic therapy is recommended after cardiac operations. Reported studies support the effectiveness of antibiotics as prophylaxis against infection in this setting.[F2,M2]

Adequate blood levels of antibiotics should be present during operation and while any intravascular or endotracheal device is in place.[B6] Administration is therefore commenced at induction of anesthesia, an additional dose is given before CPB, and a dose is given immediately after CPB. An appropriate intermittent dosage schedule is continued through the fourth postoperative day or for 24 hours after removal of the last intravascular or endotracheal device. The drug and dosage vary according to the most prevalent organisms and their susceptibility. At present, cephalosporins are recommended every 6 hours in a dose of 1 gm for adults and 12.5 $\mu g \cdot kg^{-1}$ in infants less than two years old.

All intravascular and endotracheal devices should be removed as early postoperatively as possible for many reasons, including minimizing the risk of infection. Infection is

also minimized by simplifying postoperative care, early transfer out of the intensive care unit, early ambulation and oral alimentation, and early hospital dismissal.

Corticosteroids greatly increase the risk of sternal wound infection. These drugs must therefore be discontinued completely or reduced to the lowest possible dose for several weeks (ideally, 6 or more) before operation. For similar reasons, in patients for whom renal transplant surgery is a planned part of management, the cardiac surgery should be performed first so that corticosteroids are not used postoperatively. Whenever corticosteroids must be used postoperatively, cephalosporins should be continued for about 3 weeks (until wound healing is adequate).

INFECTED MEDIAN STERNOTOMY WOUND

Fortunately, important complications of the median sternotomy wound are uncommon. Usually, these complications are in the form of mediastinitis and sternal dehiscence. In a prospective study by Breyer, the incidence was 0.8%,[B8] but the incidence has been reported to be 1.5% by Culliford and colleagues,[C13] and as high as 8% when bilateral internal mammary artery to coronary artery bypass grafting is performed.[C13]

Occasionally, a small localized subcutaneous collection of serum or necrotic fat may suggest a wound infection when in fact none is present. These minor complications occur in about 2% of patients.[B8] Such collections should be left alone until it becomes clear that a wound infection is present. Even when a small amount of frank pus drains from the wound, mediastinitis should not be assumed to be present unless the sternum has become unstable or drainage can be shown to be coming through the sternum from the retrosternal area. Further, very occasionally, the dehiscence is a sterile one.

Imperfect aseptic technique in the operating room is the basic cause of infected median sternotomy wounds. An undrained retrosternal hematoma is an incremental risk factor.[C13] This is a reason for leaving the pericardium open after cardiac operations so that retrosternal bleeding falls into the pericardial space and is aspirated by the pericardial drainage tubes. Prolonged operative time is also a risk factor for the development of mediastinal infections.[E9] Inaccurate and insecure sternal closure increases the incidence of important sternal infections.[S14]

The diagnosis of an infected wound should be made before there is extensive breakdown of the wound skin edges. Computed tomography (CT) scans may be helpful and should be obtained when the diagnosis is uncertain, but it must be remembered that at least edema and some hemorrhage in the anterior mediastinum is usually present in normally convalescing patients and is seen by CT scan. However, the diagnosis through CT scanning of retrosternal abscess or sternal disruption is usually indicative of mediastinitis.[K5]

Unusual fever and malaise, sternal tenderness, and, most important, persistent severe central chest pain not relieved by the usual analgesics suggest the possibility of an important sternotomy infection despite the absence of obvious inflammatory changes in the skin. Under these circumstances, the wound is examined twice daily for evidence of sternal instability or drainage coming through the sternum, and repeated blood and wound cultures are taken. Antibiotics are generally not begun until infection is confirmed, and they should be specific for the organisms involved.

As soon as the diagnosis of an infected median sternotomy incision is made, the patient is returned to the operating room and anesthetized, and a formal operation is undertaken.[S16] The entire median sternotomy incision is reopened, and all the sternal wires, other suture material, and necrotic tissue are removed. Usually, the infection is most marked immediately in front of and behind the sternum, and minimal around the heart itself. Although a few small fragments of sternum may be removed, extensive debridement of the sternum is not performed. Loculations of fluid around the heart are broken up and aspirated. The wound is thoroughly irrigated first with warm saline solution and then with dilute Betadine (providone-iodine) solution. Two small (16 F) chest tubes are left anteriorly for the postoperative continuous infusion of dilute Betadine or antibiotic solution, and two larger tubes (20 or 24 F) are left posteriorly for aspiration of fluid. Generally, the sternum is closed by rewiring, and the tissues anterior to it, including the skin, are closed en bloc by vertical mattress sutures.

If the sternum and adjacent tissue are very necrotic and badly infected, it may be appropriate to close only the skin and to apply a bulky dressing. In 72–96 hours, the patient is returned to the operating room, the chest tubes removed, the wound is cleansed and irrigated, and the described closure made secondarily. If the wound has not become clear within this period, the secondary closure may be carried out 10 days to 2 weeks later, although use of musculocutaneous flaps to aid in closure may then be necessary.[P8]

When the wound has been closed at the initial debridement, it is irrigated continuously with $1–2 \text{ ml} \cdot \text{kg}^{-1} \cdot \text{h}^{-1}$ of dilute (0.5%) Betadine or antibiotic solution through the anterior tubes and suction is continuously applied to the dependent tubes.[T2] Full-strength Betadine must be avoided because it injures tissue.[K7] When an antibiotic solution is used for irrigation, the level of the agent in the solution should be the same as the level in blood during maximal parenteral treatment. *An input-output chart must be maintained.* If the balance becomes positive, infusion is stopped until the fluid is recovered. Irrigations are not effective after 3–4 days, since by then the tubes have become sequestered from the retrosternal space. They are therefore removed at that time.

Fortunately, such a program is highly effective, and unless other problems are present, recovery is nearly always complete.[B7]

Sternal nonunion occurs occasionally in the absence of wound infection in patients with repetitive coughing spells produced by chronic bronchitis, emphysema, asthma, or bronchopneumonia. When there is obvious sternal mobility, the sternum should be rewired as soon as the patient's general condition permits. About 10 heavy-gauge wires should be used that encircle, rather than pierce, the sternal fragments.

POSTPERFUSION SYNDROMES

The postperfusion syndromes are complex and not yet fully understood. Whether they are totally part of the body's re-

sponse to the damaging effects of CPB (see Chapter 2, Section 2) or whether there are multiple etiologies is not certain.

A cytomegalic postperfusion syndrome has been described that consists of an infection with cytomegalic virus transmitted in homologous blood.[W7] The larger the volume of blood used, the greater the incidence of infection.[C9] This infection produces a moderate pyrexia, beginning at about the end of the first week, associated with a "flulike illness," the patient complaining of weakness, malaise, muscle pains, and sweating. The differential white blood count shows a lymphocytosis and atypical mononuclear cells. The disease can be confirmed by demonstrating a rise in complement-fixing special antibody, and the virus can be isolated from the urine, although this is technically difficult. The Paul-Bunnell test is negative, excluding infectious mononucleosis (which can present an identical clinical picture) as a possible diagnosis. While the fever and symptoms usually persist for about 2 weeks, the disease is self-limiting, and no treatment is required. Depression is a common sequel.

The postcommissurotomy syndrome was described by Soloff and associates in 1953, when it was noted to follow closed mitral valve surgery.[S6] Subsequently, it became clear that this syndrome was not related to rheumatic fever and could occur after any operation that involved opening the pericardium, hence the name *postpericardiotomy syndrome*,[11] also called the *postcardiotomy syndrome*. When Ito and colleagues coined the term *postpericardiotomy syndrome*, they suggested that the syndrome was due to an immunologic reaction to damaged autologous tissue in the pericardial cavity. Subsequent work at the same institution[E6,E7,E8] has confirmed an "autoimmune theory" of etiology. Apparently, heart-reactive antibodies appear in significant titers in a majority of patients undergoing cardiac surgery, but the titer is particularly higher in patients who develop this syndrome.[E6,E7]

Whether there are single or multiple etiologies, it is a fact that, in many patients, symptoms appear a few weeks to a few months after cardiac operation. Nishimura and colleagues found the median postoperative time of onset to be 4 weeks.[N4] The most striking symptom is chest pain, both a central ache from pericarditis and severe pleuritic pain from pleuritis. There may be no associated fever, but pericardial and pleural friction rubs are usually present and, often, pericardial and pleural effusions. These are usually minor but may be major, and delayed pericardial tamponade can occur. There are no specific changes in the formed blood elements. While the disease is self-limiting, its duration is highly variable, the median duration being 22 days and the range 2–100 days in the study by Nishimura and colleagues.[N4] Recurrences are not uncommon, appearing in 21% of patients in the Mayo Clinic series.[N4] In some of the patients, the recurrences were as long as 30 months after a previous episode. The syndrome usually recurs should reoperation be required.

The pain and effusions are often relieved by bed rest and aspirin. Although these symptoms are dramatically resolved by prednisone, steroids should be avoided whenever possible because of their side effects. However, when symptoms persist, and once the diagnosis is secure and infection has been excluded, prednisone may be given initially in high dosage (40 mg daily), gradually reduced, and completely discontinued within 4–8 weeks. Subsequent courses may be necessary.

SECTION 4

AUTOMATED CARE IN THE CARDIOVASCULAR SURGERY INTENSIVE CARE UNIT

Since most treatment decisions in the Intensive Care Unit are based on the use of numerical data and an orderly set of rules and logic,[K3] automation can be used for making, displaying, and storing observations and for intervening in some situations via a closed-loop computer system. These concepts were described in 1968,[S1] but the bedside hardware and computers have been continuously modified. Today, computers remain cost effective and useful to the surgical faculty, house staff, and nurses (UAB). There are studies and opinions to the contrary,[E4] but these reflect a difference in orientation and goals and, thus, a different method of using automated care.

The Intensive Care Unit computer (UAB) does the following:

1. Using the patient's age, height, weight, and hemoglobin level, the computer calculates and prints out preoperative orders, directions for assembly and priming of the pump-oxygenator, and postoperative orders.

2. Every 2 minutes, the computer automatically measures, numerically displays, and records systemic and pulmonary artery systolic, diastolic, and mean blood pressures; right and left atrial pressures; heart rate; chest tube drainage; urine flow; and temperature.

3. Using the chest tube drainage data and the rules and logic described under ''Early Postoperative Bleeding,'' the computer displays the message *consider reoperation* when such consideration is indicated.

4. The computer receives and uses densitometer data to inscribe indicator dilution curves for indocyanine green

and to calculate and display cardiac output, cardiac index, and stroke volume. The computer also uses densitometer data to calculate residual left-to-right shunts.

5. The computer stores and displays data on arterial blood gas and hemoglobin levels and calculates the base excess or deficit. When metabolic acidosis is present, the computer calculates the dose of bicarbonate required, using the rules and logic in Appendix 5N, and displays it.

6. The computer calculates the appropriate concentration and drip rate of infusion of any catecholamine desired for the patient, usng the rules and logic in Appendix 5C, and displays it.

7. The computer regulates the infusion of nitroprusside by a closed-loop system, having been programmed with the desired mean arterial blood pressure and other relevant information, using the rules and logic in Appendix 5A.[S5,S7] Studies indicate that this method of continuously maintaining a desired blood pressure is more effective than a manual method.

8. The computer calculates the type and amount of fluid to be given intravenously after surgery, according to the rules and logic in Appendix 5L, and prints it out.

9. The computer prints out the antibiotic orders, including dosages, according to the presence of drug allergies.

10. The computer determines the patient's estimated blood volume and prints it out as described for use with Table 5-3.

11. On request, the computer displays all recent data in a tabular form for review, with the time interval between measurements (5 minutes, 15 minutes, 30 minutes, or 1 hour) being selected by the reviewer.

While all these tasks can be done by medical and nursing staff, the computer is faster and more accurate and does not suffer from fatigue. It is likely that more efficient management of intensive care by computer results in earlier discharge from the Intensive Care Unit, now usually on the morning after operation. Also, requirements for resident house staff are reduced, and nurses spend a higher proportion of their time actually caring for patients.

APPENDIXES

APPENDIX 5A

PATIENT MANAGEMENT PROTOCOL FOR REDUCING ARTERIAL BLOOD PRESSURE

Sodium nitroprusside is administered intravenously (IV) continuously or intermittently as required. It acts directly on arterial, and to a lesser extent venous, smooth muscle, and thus decreases systemic and pulmonary vascular resistance and systemic venous tone. Its onset and end of action are immediate. The dose is $1–10 \ \mu g \cdot kg^{-1} \cdot min^{-1}$ (doses larger than this are *not* used), regulated to maintain a mean arterial blood pressure 10% above the normal value for the patient's age. In patients with thick left ventricular walls or coronary artery disease, concern about the coronary perfusion pressure makes a mean arterial blood pressure 20% above normal desirable

(or 150 mmHg in adults). Fifty or 100 μg of sodium nitroprusside are dissolved in 250 ml of 5% glucose in water. The drug may be administered with a servo-pump using a closed-loop system[S1] under computer control (UAB)[S5,S7] or using a slow-infusion Harvard pump (GLH). When nitroprusside is being administered, means should be available for measuring blood nitroprusside levels, since values > 10 $\mu g \cdot dl^{-1}$ are potentially toxic.[C7,P3] Toxicity is manifested by signs of intracellular suppression of oxygen consumption (elevation of mixed venous oxygen levels, narrowing of arterial-venous oxygen difference, and metabolic acidosis) and by anorexia, muscular spasms, disorientation, and convulsions. The toxicity is due largely to the formation of cyanide, the major metabolic product of sodium nitroprusside.[P3,C2] Toxicity is treated by IV infusion over a 15-minute period of 150 $\mu g \cdot kg^{-1}$ of a 25% solution of sodium thiosulfate (10 $\mu g \cdot kg^{-1} \cdot min^{-1}$), which is always available in the Intensive Care

Unit. This complication has not occurred (UAB, GLH), probably because sodium nitroprusside is seldom used for more than 24 hours and seldom at a dose > 6 $\mu g \cdot kg^{-1} \cdot min^{-1}$.

Nitroglycerin decreases venous tone but also decreases coronary resistance.[B2,C3,G1] It is therefore particularly useful when myocardial ischemia is present.[E1] Infusion rates of 0.5–3.0 $\mu g \cdot kg^{-1} \cdot min^{-1}$ are recommended.[K2] Nitroglycerin is absorbed into the polyvinyl tubing used for IV infusion, and the concentration reaching the patient is less than planned until the tubing becomes saturated. Nitroglycerin is not as effective as nitroprusside in lowering arterial pressure.

A single-dose, longer-acting drug, diazoxide, is available although seldom used. The dose is 3–5 $\mu g \cdot kg^{-1}$. Phentolamine (Regitine) is another vasodilator used on occasion. It has an α-adrenergic receptor blocking effect, produces direct smooth muscle relaxation, and reduces pulmonary vascular resistance.[N1] Its recommended infusion rates are 1.5–2 $\mu g \cdot kg^{-1} \cdot min^{-1}$.[K2]

Phenoxybenzamine (Dibenzyline) is a noncompetitive blocker of α-receptors with a prolonged (12–24-hour) effect and a delayed (30–60-minute) onset. It acts on both arterial and venous vessels and has no significant side effects. It is administered IV in a dose of 1 $mg \cdot kg^{-1}$, with the solution diluted in 20–50 ml of normal saline solution and infused slowly over about 15 minutes. The disadvantage of phenoxybenzamine is that its α-blocking effect is complete and permanent for at least 12 hours; thus, the drug is not used until the need for prolonged afterload reduction has been established by the patient's response to a sodium nitroprusside infusion over about a 12-hour period. Rather than continue infusing sodium nitroprusside at a relatively high rate, phenoxybenzamine may be substituted (GLH), and the dose repeated in 12–15 hours, when it is clear that its effect is wearing off. Alternatively, conventional afterload reducing agents are used in this setting (UAB).

APPENDIX **5B**

PATIENT MANAGEMENT PROTOCOL FOR ACUTE DIGITALIZATION

ATRIAL FIBRILLATION

When the ventricular rate is ≥ 110 beats per minute and no contraindication to digitalis exists, *small doses of digoxin* are given by the following schedule until the ventricular rate is 110 beats per minute.

1. When the rate is between 110 and 120 beats per minute, give a dose of 0.15 mg intravenously (IV) for adults and 10% of the estimated digitalizing dose to children.

2. When the rate is between 120 and 140 beats per minute, give an initial dose of 0.2 mg IV for adults and 15% of the estimated digitalizing dose to children.

3. When the rate exceeds 140 beats per minute, give an initial dose of 0.25 mg IV for adults and 20% of the estimated digitalizing dose to children.

4. Usually, several subsequent doses 2–3 hours apart are required, and the dose must be reassessed at each interval on the basis of ventricular rate.

5. When the ventricular rate is controlled, begin oral maintenance doses of digoxin 6–12 hours after the last IV dose (the usual oral maintenance dose is 0.25 mg daily for adults; for children, see section on sinus rhythm below).

When ventricular rate is not controlled by the time the estimated digitalizing dose has been administered (which can occur in patients in atrial flutter-fibrillation or in those receiving catecholamines), further digoxin should be given with caution to guard against the occurrence of digitalis toxicity before rate control is achieved. In this situation, verapamil is useful, and can be started in a dose of 80 mg by mouth every 8 hours.

SINUS RHYTHM

The digoxin dose cannot be titrated by heart rate, as in atrial fibrillation. Therefore, when digitalization is indicated, one-third of the *estimated digitalizing dose of digoxin* is given, usually IV, and this dose is generally repeated 3 hours later. Six hours later, a maintenance schedule is begun, usually with one-twelfth of the estimated digitalizing dose given twice daily. The estimated digitalizing dose of digoxin, when no digitalis has been given in the past 10 days, may be considered 0.9 $mg \cdot m^{-2}$ IV and 1.6 $mg \cdot m^{-2}$ orally (UAB).

Alternatively, the digitalizing dose in infants may be considered 50 $\mu g \cdot kg^{-1}$ IV, and the maintenance dose 10–15 $\mu g \cdot kg^{-1} \cdot d^{-1}$ (GLH).

Unless required for control of ventricular rate, digoxin should be discontinued 36–48 hours before operation. In all infants on digoxin preoperatively, serum digoxin levels should be measured the day before operation (GLH).

APPENDIX **5C**

PATIENT MANAGEMENT PROTOCOL FOR INFUSION OF CATECHOLAMINES

The rate of infusion is calculated and recorded in micrograms per kilogram body weight per minute ($\mu g \cdot kg^{-1} \cdot min^{-1}$). Using a microdrip apparatus, the number of drops per minute equals the number of milliliters per hour. The formula for milliliters per hour (drops per minute) as a function of infusion rate ($\mu g \cdot kg^{-1} \cdot min^{-1}$), body weight (kg), and concentration of catecholamine is

$$ml \cdot h^{-1} \text{ (or drops per minute)} = \frac{\text{infusion rate } (\mu g \cdot kg^{-1} \cdot min^{-1}) \times \text{weight (kg)} \times 60}{\text{concentration } (\mu g \cdot ml^{-1})}$$

The drug is diluted in 5% glucose and water, except in infants weighing less than 13 kg, for whom it is diluted in 10% glucose in water. A dilution is chosen that results in a drip rate of 3 $ml \cdot h^{-1}$ or greater (drip rates lower than this cannot be managed with precision, and the line may clot) but lower than 20–30 $ml \cdot h^{-1}$ in adults and lower than 10 $ml \cdot h^{-1}$ in infants (to avoid excess fluid administration).

First, the rate of drug infusion ($\mu g \cdot kg^{-1} \cdot min^{-1}$) is selected, and then the drip rate selected. The concentration of drug needed in the solution may be found by solving the equation above or with a graph (Fig. 5C-1) and tables (Tables 5C-1 and 5C-2). At UAB, the concentration is determined by computer.

For each drug, a "standard" rate of infusion ($\mu g \cdot kg^{-1} \cdot min^{-1}$) based on past experience has been determined. Infusion rates are altered according to the hemodynamic state and the response of the individual patient to the infusion. "Standard" rates of infusion should, however, be exceeded only under special circumstances.

The "standard" rates of infusion are

Dopamine	10.0 $\mu g \cdot kg^{-1} \cdot min^{-1}$
Isoproterenol	0.1 $\mu g \cdot kg^{-1} \cdot min^{-1}$
Epinephrine	0.1 $\mu g \cdot kg^{-1} \cdot min^{-1}$
Norepinephrine	0.1 $\mu g \cdot kg^{-1} \cdot min^{-1}$

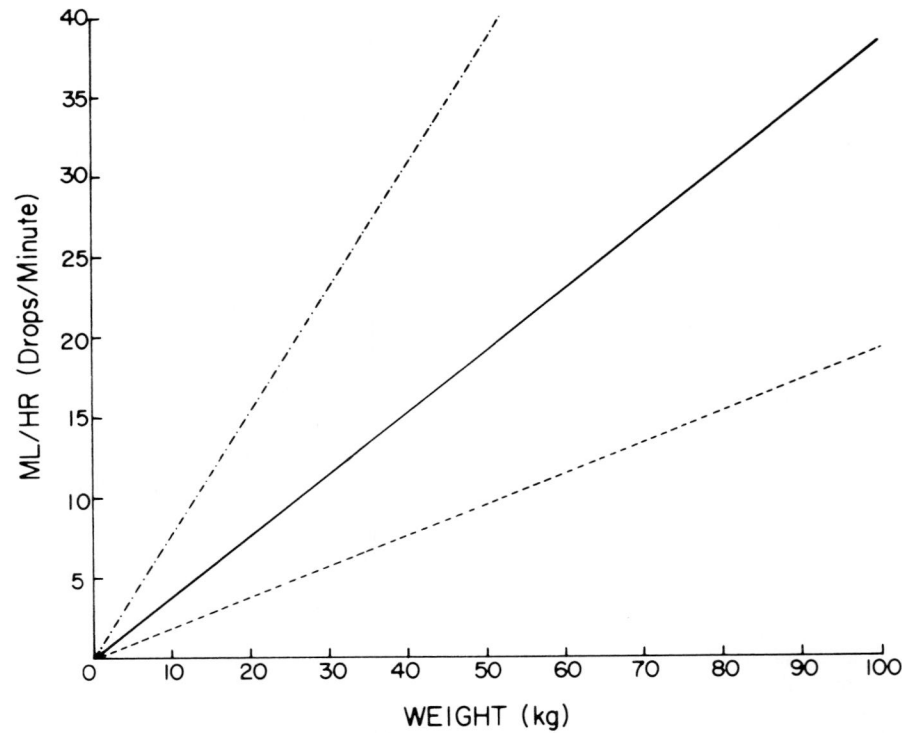

Figure 5C-1 Nomogram of drip rate (drops per minute) related to patient body weight for three different dose schedules ($\mu g \cdot kg \cdot min^{-1}$) of catecholamines. The desired drip rate is selected, and the concentration of the drug and its dose schedule determined from Table 5C-1 or 5C-2.

Table 5C-1 Representative data for dopamine and dobutamine.

Adults and children weighing > 13 kg:

1. Concentration 400 mg (10 ml) in 250 ml of 5% dextrose in water (5% glucose)
   a. _ _ _ _ _, 5 $\mu g \cdot kg^{-1} \cdot min^{-1}$
   b. _____, 10 $\mu g \cdot kg^{-1} \cdot min^{-1}$ ("standard")
   c. _._._._, 20 $\mu g \cdot kg^{-1} \cdot min^{-1}$

2. Concentration 800 mg (20 ml) in 250 ml of 5% dextrose in water (5% glucose)
   a. _ _ _ _ _, 10 $\mu g \cdot kg^{-1} \cdot min^{-1}$ ("standard")
   b. _____, 20 $\mu g \cdot kg^{-1} \cdot min^{-1}$
   c. _._._._, 40 $\mu g \cdot kg^{-1} \cdot min^{-1}$

3. Concentration 1,600 mg (40 ml) in 250 ml of 5% dextrose in water (5% glucose)
   a. _ _ _ _ _, 20 $\mu g \cdot kg^{-1} \cdot min^{-1}$
   b. _____, 40 $\mu g \cdot kg^{-1} \cdot min^{-1}$
   c. _._._._, not usually used

Infants and small children weighing < 13 kg:

1. Concentration 200 mg (5 ml) in 250 ml of 5% dextrose in water (10% glucose)
   a. _ _ _ _ _, not usually used
   b. _____, 5 $\mu g \cdot kg^{-1} \cdot min^{-1}$
   c. _._._._, 10 $\mu g \cdot kg^{-1} \cdot min^{-1}$ ("standard")

2. Concentration 400 mg (10 ml) in 250 ml of 5% dextrose in water (10% glucose)
   See 1 under "adults and children weighing > 13 kg."

NOTE: The dashed, solid, and dash-dot lines refer to the drip rate–body weight lines in Figure 5C-1.

An alternative to a microdrip apparatus is a constant-infusion pump (Harvard) (GLH). The infusion rate is a function of the pump setting and the dilution (Table 5C-3).

Dopamine has the advantage of augmenting renal blood flow in addition to increasing cardiac contractility.[H4] Dopamine does increase ventricular automaticity (and thus the probability of ventricular arrhythmias) but to a lesser extent than does isoproterenol. At

Table 5C-2 Representative data for epinephrine and norepinephrine.

Adults and children weighing > 13 kg:

1. Concentration 4 mg in 250 ml (5% glucose)
   a. _ _ _ _ _, 0.05 $\mu g \cdot kg^{-1} \cdot min^{-1}$
   b. _____, 0.1 $\mu g \cdot kg^{-1} \cdot min^{-1}$ ("standard")
   c. _._._._, 0.2 $\mu g \cdot kg^{-1} \cdot min^{-1}$

2. Concentration 8 mg in 250 ml (5% glucose)
   a. _ _ _ _ _, 0.1 $\mu g \cdot kg^{-1} \cdot min^{-1}$ ("standard")
   b. _____, 0.2 $\mu g \cdot kg^{-1} \cdot min^{-1}$
   c. _._._._, 0.4 $\mu g \cdot kg^{-1} \cdot min^{-1}$

Infants and small children weighing < 13 kg:

1. Concentration 2 mg in 250 ml (10% glucose)
   a. _ _ _ _ _, 0.025 $\mu g \cdot kg^{-1} \cdot min^{-1}$ (not usually used)
   b. _____, 0.05 $\mu g \cdot kg^{-1} \cdot min^{-1}$
   c. _._._._, 0.1 $\mu g \cdot kg^{-1} \cdot min^{-1}$ ("standard")

2. Concentration 4 mg in 250 ml (10% glucose)
   See 1 under "adults and children weighing > 13 kg."

NOTE: The dashed, solid, and dash-dot lines refer to the drip rate–body weight lines in Figure 5C-1.

Table 5C-3 Isoproterenol concentrations delivered by a constant infusion pump (Harvard model 2620) (GLH). The inotrope is diluted in a 50-ml syringe containing 5% or 10% glucose solution. For dopamine (and dobutamine) the concentrations are increased × 100. Thus, at a 97-ml · h^{-1} infusion rate, 200 mg of dopamine in a 50-ml syringe delivers 6,400 μg · min^{-1}.

Fluid Infused (ml · h^{-1})	Concentrations of Isoproterenol (μg/min)		
	2,000 μg per 50-ml Syringe	1,000 μg per 50-ml Syringe	500 μg per 50-ml Syringe
97	64.0	32.0	16.0
69	44.0	22.0	11.0
49	32.8	16.4	8.20
35	23.6	11.8	5.90
25	16.8	8.40	4.20
18	12.0	6.00	3.00
13	8.40	4.20	2.10
9.2	6.00	3.00	1.50
6.5	4.40	2.20	1.10
4.7	3.12	1.56	0.78
3.3	2.24	1.12	0.56
2.4	1.60	0.80	0.40
1.7	1.12	0.56	0.28
1.2	0.80	0.40	0.20
0.8	0.56	0.28	0.14
0.6	0.40	0.20	0.10
0.45	0.296	0.148	0.074
0.32	0.212	0.106	0.053
0.25	0.152	0.076	0.038
0.16	0.108	0.054	0.027

low doses (2–4 μg · kg^{-1} · min^{-1}), systemic peripheral vascular resistance is decreased or unchanged, while higher doses (> 6 μg · kg^{-1} · min^{-1}) increase peripheral resistance.[G3]

APPENDIX **5D**

PATIENT MANAGEMENT PROTOCOL FOR INTRA-AORTIC BALLOON PUMPING

Intra-aortic balloon pumping (IABP) utilizes the principle of diastolic counterpulsation, which augments diastolic coronary perfusion pressure, reduces systolic afterload, favorably affects the myocardial oxygen supply-demand ratio, and augments cardiac output. IABP is used in adult patients with inadequate cardiac performance not responsive to optimized preload, afterload, and heart rate and to moderate doses (≤ 10 μg · kg^{-1} · min^{-1}) of dopamine. It is used in preference to catecholamines postoperatively for patients with severe left ventricular dysfunction, with or without evidence of myocardial necrosis, and for patients with evidence of myocardial necrosis and inadequate cardiac output or severe ventricular arrhythmias.

The balloon made for percutaneous insertion is now usually used (UAB, GLH). Because of the risk of vascular complications in women and other patients with small femoral arteries,[S11,G8] the percutaneous technique is modified slightly for use in the operating room (see section on "Open Technique using the Balloon for Per-

cutaneous Insertion"). The older open technique is now uncommonly used, but since it is the basic technique it is described first.

Since important aortoiliac occlusion greatly increases the risk of vascular complications when the femoral route is used for insertion[G8] or makes the use of this route impossible, the balloon is inserted into the ascending aorta through a purse-string suture when needed.

OPEN TECHNIQUE

Both groins are prepared and draped before any operation in which IABP may be required. Either before the sternotomy incision, or when it has been determined that IABP is needed, the common femoral artery is dissected out just below the inguinal ligament and encircled proximally with a length of umbilical tape, which is then threaded through a rubber "snugger." Small arterial branches are occluded with loops of 0 silk. Fifty milligrams of heparin are now given intravenously, if the patient is not already heparinized. After the size of the artery is judged, the intra-aortic balloon is selected (20, 30, or 40 ml).

The tip of the balloon catheter is held at the level of the suprasternal notch, and a tie is placed on the shaft at the level of the inferior edge of the skin incision in the groin to mark the length of the catheter to be inserted. Air is extracted from the balloon using a three-way stopcock. The femoral artery is opened between arterial clamps by a small transverse incision and the balloon catheter is threaded carefully through this incision until it is in proper position. The umbilical tape is snugged down around the artery for hemostasis. The balloon is purged of air, and counterpulsation is begun. One or two fine interrupted sutures are used to close the incision around the balloon shaft and the umbilical tape is removed. The wound is closed in layers and the shaft of the balloon is sutured tightly to the skin. Anticoagulants are not used with the balloon in place (UAB), but alternatively, low-molecular-weight dextran may be infused hourly (GLH).

IABP is begun at 1:1 ratio with ventricular systole, a process requiring electrocardiographic and arterial pressure pulse signals. Often the patient's hemodynamic state improves promptly, and if this occurs, consideration is given to weaning the patient from IABP as early as 6–12 hours after insertion. If catecholamines have also been required, they are reduced to 5 μg · kg^{-1} · min^{-1} of dopamine or less as rapidly as possible. If the hemodynamic conditions remain good, the IABP ratio is progressively reduced to 1:8 (or 1:3 with some systems). In most postoperative patients, the final reduction can be reached within 12–48 hours. The balloon can then be removed.

The circulation in the leg distal to the site of balloon insertion is observed systematically. If signs of ischemia appear, generally the balloon is removed. If this is not possible but the patient appears salvageable, a femoro-femoral crossover graft or reinsertion of the balloon into the ascending aorta is considered.

REMOVAL BY AN OPEN TECHNIQUE

Removal of the intra-aortic balloon pump is carried out under the same sterile conditions. The previous incision is reopened, and the femoral artery is again exposed proximal and distal to the arteriotomy. The distal femoral artery is clamped in order to prevent thrombotic material from passing distally, and the balloon is expeditiously removed as the proximal clamp is placed. The proximal clamp is intermittently released to allow free bleeding and to expel any thrombotic material. A Fogarty catheter is used if a strong pulsatile flow is not obtained. The distal clamp is now intermittently opened to allow vigorous back-bleeding. If this does not occur, a Fogarty catheter is used to retrieve distal thrombi. The arteriotomy is closed with a few interrupted sutures and the clamps are removed. The adequacy of perfusion to the leg is determined by palpation of the pulse in the distal femoral artery in the wound and the distal pulses in the feet. The wound is closed without drainage.

OPEN TECHNIQUE USING THE BALLOON FOR PERCUTANEOUS INSERTION

When the open technique is employed using the balloon for percutaneous insertion in the operating room, the common femoral artery is exposed through a small vertical incision. The needle through which the guide wire is to be inserted is introduced percutaneously just inferior to the incision and passed into the *common* femoral artery under direct vision. Thereafter, the technique of inserting the dilators over the guide wire and the intra-aortic balloon through the dilator is the same as the standard percutaneous technique. The positioning of the balloon and its management are the same as described above. In patients at great risk of the need of a balloon after cardiopulmonary bypass, it is advantageous to insert the guide wire before cardiopulmonary bypass. Once the balloon is in place, the small incision over the femoral artery may be closed. No stitches are placed in the artery.

CLOSED TECHNIQUE FOR REMOVAL

When the intra-aortic balloon for percutaneous insertion has been inserted as just described, it is removed by a closed method. Although objections have been raised to the use of this method,[C12] most of the problems with it have occurred when the balloon inadvertently was inserted through the superficial, rather than the common, femoral artery. After removing the balloon percutaneously, firm pressure is applied to the groin and held for 1 hour. If the circulation to the leg does not remain entirely satisfactory or if a hematoma becomes apparent, prompt exploration in the operating room is indicated.

INSERTION AND REMOVAL THROUGH THE ASCENDING AORTA

The insertion of the balloon pump through the ascending aorta is usually performed before discontinuing cardiopulmonary bypass. A pledgetted mattress suture of 2-0 or 3-0 polypropylene is placed in the mid portion of the ascending aorta. A tie is placed on the shaft of the intra-aortic balloon to indicate the point that should be level with the aortic wall when the balloon is in proper position. A stab wound is made and controlled digitally, and the balloon introduced through it passed into the descending aorta. Proper position is verified by seeing an appropriate effect on the arterial pressure pulse when pumping is begun.

The balloon shaft is usually brought out through the lower end of the incision. When pumping is no longer needed, the patient is returned to the operating room, and median sternotomy reopened, and another pledgetted mattress suture placed outside the original one. As the balloon is removed, the stab wound is controlled digitally, and the pledgetted mattress suture is tied down.

APPENDIX **5E**

CERTAIN ASPECTS OF THE PATIENT MANAGEMENT PROTOCOL FOR VENTRICULAR ELECTRICAL INSTABILITY[13]

DEFINITIONS

1. Intermittent electrical instability:
   a. Nonconsecutive ventricular premature (ectopic) beats (6 or more per minute) of one morphology (uniform)
   b. Consecutive ventricular ectopic beats (2 or more) or paroxysmal ventricular tachycardia existing < 1 minute with maintenance of cardiac output
   c. Multiform premature ventricular beats (2 or more per minute)
   d. Premature ventricular beat interrupting the T wave of a preceding beat (i.e., coupling interval/QT interval is < 1)
2. Continuous electrical instability:
   a. Ventricular tachycardia persisting > 1 minute
   b. Ventricular tachycardia of any duration associated with reduction of cardiac output

IMMEDIATE INTERVENTION FOR VENTRICULAR ELECTRICAL INSTABILITY

1. Give lidocaine as an intravenous (IV) bolus injection (the dose is $1 \mu g \cdot kg^{-1}$ for adults and children, although in adults the usual dose is 50 mg) if the arrhythmia is PVC or ventricular tachycardia (VT) with a good hemodynamic state. If there is VT and reduction of cardiac output, use *immediate DC cardioversion* (100 and then 200 watt-seconds).
2. Draw a blood sample for determination of serum K^+; when the result is available, treat hypokalemia (K^+ concentration < 4.0 $mEq \cdot l^{-1}$) if present:
   a. Administer 5 mEq K^+ as an IV bolus.
   b. Administer 20 mEq K^+ in 50 ml 5% glucose over 1 hour; then obtain repeat serum K^+ level measurement and treat until the serum level is satisfactory (at least 3.5 $mEq \cdot l^{-1}$ and preferably 4.0 $mEq \cdot l^{-1}$).
   c. Double the IV maintenance K^+ dose.
   d. Recheck the serum K^+ level the next morning. If it is < 4.0 $mEq \cdot l^{-1}$ on either of these measurements, order oral K^+ supplement as 20% KCl, 10 ml twice a day in orange juice (60-mEq approximate daily dose).
3. When the ventricular rate is less than 80–90 beats per minute, initiate pacing. If basic rhythm is sinus or AV junctional, use atrial pacing. When cardiac rhythm is other than sinus or AV junctional, or atrial pacing fails to result in 1:1 AV conduction, use ventricular pacing (with the ventricular wire electrode attached to negative pole of pacer). In the presence of second- or third-degree AV block, consider AV sequential pacing.

INTERVENTIONS AFTER CONTROL OF THE URGENT SITUATION

1. If the arrhythmia recurs promptly or has been difficult to control, begin continuous IV lidocaine infusion in a dose of 20–50 μg ·

---

[13] This protocol was initially constructed (UAB) by Drs. A.D. Pacifico and A.L. Waldo.

Table 5E-1   Outline of the dosage, levels, and pharmacology of the major antiarrhythmic agents.[W5]

Characteristic	Quinidine	Procainamide	Propranolol	Lidocaine	Disopyramide
Route of administration	Oral, IM	Oral, IM, IV	Oral, IV	IV	Oral
Dosage					
Total daily oral	1.2–2.4 g	1.0–4.0 g	10–280 mg		400–800 mg
Frequency (usual)	Every 6 h	Every 3–4 h	Every 4–6 h		Every 6 h
Initial IV		$1.0\ \mu g \cdot kg^{-1} \cdot 5\ min^{-1}$ $\times$ 5–10; total,	$0.25\ mg \cdot 2$–$5\ min^{-1}$; total, 2.5 mg	$1\ mg \cdot kg^{-1} \cdot 3$–5 $min^{-1} \times 3$–4	
Maintenance IV		20–$80\ \mu g \cdot kg^{-1} \cdot min^{-1}$		20–$50\ \mu g \cdot kg^{-1} \cdot min^{-1}$	
Plasma level					
Peak, single oral dose	1.5–2 h	1–1.5 h	1–4 h		2 h
Plateau, chronic oral dose	36–48 h	18–24 h	2–3 d		36–48 h
Effective concentration	2.5–$8.0\ mg \cdot l^{-1}$	4–$10\ mg \cdot l^{-1}$	$100\ ng \cdot l^{-1}$; usual range, 40–$80\ ng \cdot l^{-1}$	2–$5\ \mu g \cdot ml^{-1}$	2–$4\ mg \cdot l^{-1}$
Half-life	6–7 h	3–5 h	3.5–6 h	15–30 min[a] 1–5 h[b]	6–7 h
Binding to protein	60%	15%	90%	10%	50%
Metabolism	Hydroxylation; liver	Hydrolysis; liver; plasma	Hydroxylation; liver	Oxidative deethylation; hydrolysis; liver	Dealkylation
Renal excretion of unmetabolized drug	20%–50%	50%–60%	1%	10%	50%

[a]Single dose.

[b]Chronic dose.

$kg^{-1} \cdot min^{-1}$, or 0.02–$0.05\ mg \cdot kg^{-1} \cdot min^{-1}$. To calculate the number of drops per minute of a solution of 2 g of lidocaine in 250 ml of solution,

$$\text{drops per minute} = \frac{\text{dose} \times \text{weight (kg)} \times 60}{4}$$

2. Begin procainamide 500 mg IM followed by 500 mg orally every 4 hours (the dose is generally $50\ mg \cdot kg^{-1} \cdot 24\ h^{-1}$ in divided doses). The interval may need shortening to 3 hours, and/or the dose may need to be increased to 750 mg to obtain control. After 2 days, the serum level is measured.

GUIDELINES FOR ADMINISTRATION OF PROCAINAMIDE, PROCAINE SR, QUINIDINE, AND DISOPYRAMIDE

See Table 5E-1.

1. If the procainamide dose is 750 mg every 3 hours, the quinidine dose is greater than 400 mg every 6 hours, or the disopyramide (Norpace) dose is greater than 200 mg every 6 hours, a daily representative segment of ECG lead II should be placed in the progress notes to document the QT interval.

2. Indicators of drug toxicity (when present, reduce antiarrhythmic drug dosage):

   a. QT prolongation > 25%

   b. QRS prolongation beyond 0.115 seconds

Note that these indicators are not applicable if bundle branch block is present before initiation of drug therapy.

3. If renal dysfunction was present preoperatively or if oliguria is present, BUN and/or creatinine levels are measured daily and antiarrhythmic drug dosages are reduced in concert with serum drug levels obtained at appropriate intervals.

4. When treatment with procainamide is initiated in the early postoperative period and will probably need to be continued for more than 4–6 weeks thereafter, procaine SR, quinidine, or disopyramide usually should be substituted for the procainamide. Administration of these drugs is begun in the usual way, and procainamide is continued for only 2 doses beyond initiation of the new drug therapy.

5. Quinidine administration may produce an important idiosyncratic reaction, usually within the first 24 hours after onset of therapy, resulting in severe ventricular electrical instability. Continuous ECG monitoring is therefore mandatory when administration of this drug is begun in the postoperative period.

6. Due to a digoxin-quinidine interaction, a higher than usual digoxin level will result when quinidine is administered concurrently with digoxin. Thus, in order to avoid digitalis toxicity, the initial digoxin maintenance dose should be halved when these drugs are used together. Adjustment of the digoxin dose may be made, but only in concert with serum digoxin levels. Even if no signs of digitalis toxicity are present when these two drugs are administered together, the digoxin level should be measured 5 days after beginning concurrent therapy with these drugs or at the slightest suspicion of digitalis toxicity.

APPENDIX 5F

PATIENT MANAGEMENT PROTOCOL FOR RAPID ATRIAL PACING VIA ATRIAL WIRES

RAPID ATRIAL PACING

The technique of rapid atrial pacing is applied to *atrial flutter*, defined as a general atrial rate of 250–350 beats per minute, with a constant beat-to-beat cycle length that *can be interrupted* by rapid atrial pacing. This is rarely possible in *atrial flutter-fibrillation*, a more rapid type of atrial flutter, with a rate > 350 beats per minute, and is not possible in atrial fibrillation.

The ECG limb leads are placed on the patient for monitoring, and the two atrial wires are connected to the rapid atrial pacer. As the atrial pacing threshold is usually high during atrial flutter, the output is set between 10 and 20 mA. Bipolar atrial pacing is used because the stimulus artifact then rarely distorts the ECG tracing, and the atrial complex in the ECG is clearly seen so that atrial capture can be verified.

A relatively slow pacing rate is used first, since occasionally the ventricle may be paced inadvertently with the occurrence of rapid ventricular tachycardia, which is to be avoided. After this, there are several possible maneuvers for control of atrial flutter and its rapid ventricular response, as described by Waldo and MacLean.[W5]

Ramp Technique

Atrial pacing is begun at a rate 10 beats per minute faster than the atrial flutter rate. The rate of atrial pacing is then gradually increased. When the typical negative atrial complex in lead II changes to a positive atrial complex, atrial pacing is either abruptly stopped or gradually slowed down until the ventricular rate is considered satisfactory.

Constant Rate Technique

Pacing is initiated at a rate 10 beats per minute faster than the spontaneous atrial flutter rate. After pacing at this rate for about 30 seconds, pacing is either abruptly stopped or the pacing rate quickly slowed until the ventricular rate is considered satisfactory. If these maneuvers are unsuccessful in interrupting the atrial flutter, they are repeated with the initial atrial pacing rate increased in increments of 10 beats per minute.

CONTINUOUS RAPID ATRIAL PACING

When atrial flutter is interrupted by the procedures described above but recurs with clinically unacceptable frequency, continuous atrial pacing at 400–600 beats per minute is used. This results in continuing atrial fibrillation with variable AV block. The ventricular rate can then be controlled by digoxin.

When premature atrial beats are continuous or recurrent in spite of pharmacologic treatment, continuous atrial pacing at about 200–230 per minute usually results in their suppression and a 2:1 AV conduction ratio with an acceptable ventricular rate.

APPENDIX **5G**

PATIENT MANAGEMENT PROTOCOL FOR PROPHYLAXIS AGAINST RENAL FAILURE AFTER OPEN HEART SURGERY IN ADULTS WITH PREOPERATIVELY IMPAIRED RENAL FUNCTION

1. Shortly after CPB, mannitol (25% solution) is administered in a dose of $1 \text{ g} \cdot \text{kg}^{-1}$ body weight unless urine flow is large ($2 \times$ the minimal acceptable urine flow given in number 3, below) and the urine appears normal.
2. Shortly after CPB, a dopamine infusion is begun at $2.5 \mu\text{g} \cdot \text{kg}^{-1} \cdot \text{min}^{-1}$ and continued for about 36 hours to improve renal blood flow.
3. When urine flow is less than an *arbitrary minimal acceptable urine flow* ($500 \text{ ml} \cdot \text{m}^{-2} \cdot 24 \text{ h}^{-1}$, $167 \text{ ml} \cdot \text{m}^{-2} \cdot 8 \text{ h}^{-1}$, or $20 \text{ ml} \cdot \text{m}^{-2} \cdot \text{h}^{-1}$), cardiac output is augmented to its maximum by ad-

justing preload, afterload, and heart rate and by increasing the dose of dopamine up to $5 \mu\text{g} \cdot \text{kg}^{-1} \cdot \text{min}^{-1}$.
4. If these measures do not produce the minimal acceptable urine flow, furosemide (Lasix) is given as often as every 6 hours. A dose of $1 \text{ mg} \cdot \text{kg}^{-1}$ is given, which if ineffective may be doubled and then redoubled and finally given in a dose of $8 \text{ mg} \cdot \text{kg}^{-1}$.

APPENDIX **5H**

PATIENT MANAGEMENT PROTOCOL FOR A SERUM K$^+$ LEVEL $> 5.5 \text{ mEq} \cdot \text{l}^{-1}$ FROM ACUTE RENAL FAILURE

1. Stop all potassium administration and send another blood sample for immediate potassium-level determination.
2. Assess and augment cardiac performance if necessary; begin prophylaxis against acute renal failure (see Appendix 5G).
3. If the above measures do not promptly increase urine output and improve the hemodynamic state, or if, despite such improvements, the potassium level remains $> 5.5 \text{ mEq} \cdot \text{l}^{-1}$, *prompt peritoneal dialysis is indicated* (see Appendix 5I), especially in infants. Interim measures include the following:
   a. Give glucose and insulin solution intravenously (IV). For adults, mix 20 units of regular insulin in 50 ml of 50% dextrose and give IV over 10 minutes. For children and infants, mix 0.5 ml of regular insulin per kilogram of body weight in 2 ml of 25% dextrose per kilogram and give IV over 10 minutes.
   b. Administer a K-exalate enema. For adults, mix 50 g in 200 ml of sorbitol or 20% dextrose and give as a retention enema; hold for 30 minutes, then remove; repeat hourly as necessary. For children and infants, give $1 \text{ g} \cdot \text{kg}^{-1}$ and 10–50 ml of sorbitol as a retention enema (total volume of sorbitol may be increased up to about 150 ml for children up to about 10 years of age).
   c. Give $1 \text{ mEq} \cdot \text{kg}^{-1}$ sodium bicarbonate IV for infants and children. For adults, give 1 ampule (44 mEq) IV.
   d. If potassium levels exceed $6.5 \text{ mEq} \cdot \text{l}^{-1}$ (this stage should never be reached before peritoneal dialysis is begun) and the patient is not receiving digoxin, give $10 \text{ mg} \cdot \text{kg}^{-1}$ of calcium chloride for infants and small children and about $200 \text{ mg} \cdot \text{kg}^{-1}$ for adults IV in order to decrease the cardiovascular effects of hyperkalemia.
4. If severe oliguria or anuria is present and/or potassium levels are rapidly rising, emergency peritoneal dialysis is indicated.

APPENDIX **5I**

PATIENT MANAGEMENT PROTOCOL FOR THE TREATMENT OF ACUTE RENAL FAILURE IN INFANTS

1. Call a pediatric nephrologist for immediate consultation after the first 2 hours of oliguria (see criteria in ''Acute Renal Failure after Cardiac Surgery'').
2. If a pediatric nephrologist is not immediately available and indications for peritoneal dialysis are considered by the surgeon to be present:
   a. Prepare the skin of the abdomen with Betadine, using sterile gloves and a simple drape.

b. Nick the skin with a Bard-Parker no. 11 blade 1 cm below the umbilicus in the midline. If possible, nick the linea alba as well.

c. Insert a 16-gauge "angiocath" or "Jelco" plastic needle with an inner metal needle until it pierces the peritoneum. Pull out the inner metal needle. Some fluid is usually obtained. If the plastic needle advances easily, it is surely in the peritoneal cavity.

d. Insert a guide wire (Cobe femoral guide wire no. 15-210) through the plastic needle, and withdraw the plastic needle.

e. Remove the outer sheath from a Cobe femoral catheter, no. 200 (or a Trocath peritoneal dialysis catheter, pediatric no. V-4901 or adult size), and insert the catheter over the guide wire, directing it as much as possible toward the pelvis. About 2 inches of catheter should be in the peritoneal cavity.

f. Remove the guide wire. Place a skin stitch to secure the catheter.

3. Connect the dialysis catheter to a Y tube system, with one arm going to an elevated 2-liter bottle containing the dialysis fluid (kept between infusions in a 37°C water bath) and the other going to a drainage bag near floor level.

4. If a pediatric nephrologist is still not available, begin peritoneal dialysis. One of three solutions (1.5% glucose, 2.5% glucose, 4.25% glucose) is used, usually with $2\ mEq \cdot l^{-1}$ of K^+ and 1,000 units of heparin per 2-liter bottle; the 4.25% solution is usually used first, since the infant's extracellular fluid is usually greatly increased at this time, and this solution is most efficacious in removing fluid. The infusion dose is $20-30\ ml \cdot kg^{-1}$, administered over a few minutes. The *dwell time* is usually initially 1 hour (shorter dwell times, and thus more frequent infusions, remove fluid and electrolytes more rapidly). The drainage time varies between 10 and 30 minutes and is not predetermined; rather, drainage continues until the rate falls to a slow drip into the bag.

5. The pediatric nephrologist subsequently manipulates all the variables to achieve the desired goals of the peritoneal dialysis.

6. If the dialysis is necessary for more than 48 hours but is expected to become unnecessary after about another 48 hours, the catheter is removed and another inserted. If longer peritoneal dialysis is anticipated, an infant-sized Tenckhoff peritoneal dialysis catheter is inserted surgically.

7. The infant Tenckhoff catheter is inserted through a short (2-cm) midline incision made just below the umbilicus. Ideally, the tip lies in the pelvic cul de sac, but attention must be paid to keeping the omentum away from it. The peritoneum is closed snuggly, and then the peritoneal edges are stitched to the Dacron cuff on the catheter. The linea alba fascia likewise is carefully sutured. A small skin stab wound is made about 2 cm to the left, and the end of the catheter is pulled out through this. This leaves the second Dacron cuff in the subcutaneous tissue, more or less plugging the underside of the stab wound. The skin of the midline incision is closed.

APPENDIX **5J**

PATIENT MANAGEMENT PROTOCOL FOR AN INTUBATED PATIENT AFTER CARDIAC SURGERY

1. The ventilator is used with its air heating and humidifying devices and the valves for intermittent mandatory ventilation and positive end-expiratory pressure functioning.

2. The patient has a well-positioned and well-secured orotracheal tube in place or, in infants and young children (for greater security and comfort) and adults in whom postoperative ventilation for more than 24 hours is likely, a well-positioned and well-secured nasotracheal tube in place (see Chapter 4).

3. Initially, the fractional concentration of oxygen (FI_{O_2}) is set at 0.6, tidal volume (TV) at $10-15\ ml \cdot kg^{-1}$, and IMV at 10 breaths per minute (15 breaths per minute in children, 20 breaths per minute in young children, 25 breaths per minute in infants). End-inspiratory pressure should normally be $< 40\ cm\ H_2O$. In all situations, *visual, palpatory,* and *auscultatory observation* of the patient's chest must be used to confirm that TV is adequate for good air movement in and out of the lungs. These observations must be made whenever the patient becomes restless or agitated or there is any other reason to suspect inadequate gas exchange. Except in patients with chronic obstructive lung disease and those in whom an atrial switch or Glenn's or Fontan's operation has been done, PEEP of 8 cm H_2O (4 cm H_2O in patients ≤ 4 years old) may be used (UAB).

4. A supine portable chest roentgenogram is obtained upon arrival in the Intensive Care Unit and reviewed by a physician for placement of the tip of the endotracheal tube; the presence of pneumothorax, atelectasis, vascular congestion, or gastric distention; and the size of the mediastinal silhouette. The chest film is routinely repeated the first postoperative morning and again after all chest tubes have been removed. Otherwise, blood gases are routinely obtained every 4–6 hours during the first 24 hours after operation if the patient is intubated.

5. Turning of the patient and sterile suctioning of the airway are performed each hour to clear retained secretions and minimize atelectasis. Suctioning is performed after "hand-bagging" with 100% oxygen, hyperventilation for several breaths, and instillation of 1–5 ml of sterile saline solution down the endotracheal tube. Suctioning is followed again by "hand-bagging" with 100% oxygen. *The length of the endotracheal tube must be known*, so that the suctioning catheter can be passed with certainty beyond the tube into the trachea.

6. In patients without severe preoperative pulmonary dysfunction, criteria for extubation include the following:

a. Patient awake and alert, indicating recovery from anesthesia and ability to protect his or her airway

b. Satisfactory hemodynamic state

c. Absence of important bleeding from chest tubes

d. Arterial $Po_2 \geq 70$ mmHg (in the absence of intracardiac right-to-left shunting) on IMV of 6 breaths per minute and FI_{O_2} of 0.40

e. Spontaneous respiratory rate < 25 breaths per minute in adults, < 40 breaths per minute in young children, and < 50 breaths per minute in infants

f. Absence of increased work of breathing (use of accessory respiratory muscles)

g. Normal $PaCO_2$ and pH ($PaCO_2$ may be somewhat elevated, with a normal pH, if metabolic alkalosis is present)

7. When using continuous positive airway pressure in infants (GLH), the FI_{O_2} is set at 0.75 and the end-expiratory pressure at 6 mmHg. FI_{O_2} is reduced in steps to 0.40, provided PaO_2 remains between 50 and 70 mmHg. If PaO_2 falls below 50 mmHg, FI_{O_2} is increased. After the FI_{O_2} has been stabilized at 0.40, the pressure is gradually reduced to zero. The infant is then extubated, provided the PaO_2 is > 60 mmHg. After extubation, the infant is placed in a head box in which the gases are kept humidified and the FI_{O_2} as close to 0.70 as possible. FI_{O_2} is gradually reduced over the next 24 hours.

APPENDIX **5K**

PATIENT MANAGEMENT PROTOCOL FOR CONTROL OF HEMOCONCENTRATION

If the Hb level is ≥ 16 g% and there is evidence of plasma leakage from the intravascular space,

1. Give 20 ml · m^{-2} of 25% serum albumin in a syringe *slowly* (over 5 minutes) *if* P_{LA} is < about 15 mmHg. If P_{LA} > 15 mmHg, consider administering Lasix and then albumin.
2. Repeat Hb measurement in 1 hour.
3. When Hb measurement in step 2 is ≥ 16 g%, repeat steps 1 and 2.

APPENDIX **5L**

PATIENT MANAGEMENT PROTOCOL FOR INTRAVENOUS FLUIDS AFTER CARDIAC SURGERY

In adults and children (> 2 years of age or > 13 kg in weight),

1. Day of operation:
   a. 500 ml of 5% glucose in water · m^{-2} · 20 h^{-1}
   b. 10 mEq of K^{+} · m^{-2} · 20 h^{-1}
2. First and second postoperative days:
   a. 750 ml of 5% glucose in water · m^{-2} · 24 h^{-1}
   b. 20 mEq of K^{+} · m^{-2} · 24 h^{-1}
3. Third postoperative day:
   a. 750 ml of 5% glucose in water · m^{-2} · 24 h^{-1} ⎫
   b. 350 ml of 5% glucose in saline solution · m^{-2} · 24 h^{-1} ⎬ or 1,100 ml of 5% glucose in one-quarter–strength saline solution · m^{-2} · 24 h^{-1}
   c. 10 mEq of K^{+} · m^{-2} · 24 h^{-1} ⎭
4. If oral intake has not been established on the third postoperative day, consider gavage feeding or intravenous (IV) hyperalimentation.

In infants (< 2 years old or < 13 kg in weight),

1. Day of operation:
   a. Calculate patient's saline requirement.
      (1) 250 ml · m^{-2} · 24 h^{-1} are required.
      (2) If this is 75 ml or less for the individual patient, use only balanced salt solution for flushing[14] the arterial catheter; if it is 75–150 ml, use balanced salt solution for flushing the arterial and left atrial catheters; if it is > 150 ml, flush the arterial, left atrial, and right atrial (and, if present, pulmonary artery) catheters with balanced salt solution.
      (3) Give no additional sodium-containing fluids if step (2) supplies the patient's needs. Otherwise, subtract the amount in step (2) from the requirement and give the difference.
   b. Calculate patient's water requirement.
      (1) 500 ml · m^{-2} · 24 h^{-1} of 10% glucose in water are required.

---

[14] An automatic very slow (3 ml · h^{-1} or 72 ml · 24 h^{-1}) continuous infusion system for all devices attached to pressure transducers is used (UAB). The solution flushing the arterial needle must be a balanced salt solution, to prevent arterial spasm and pain. When salt restriction is important, as in infants, a glucose solution can be used for flushing the other pressure lines.

(2) Subtract 72 ml × the number of intracardiac recording catheters being flushed with 10% glucose in water from the amount in step (1), and order that amount.
   c. Give no potassium in the fluids.
2. Days thereafter:
   a. Calculate patient's saline requirement.
      (1) 250 ml · m^{-2} · 24 h^{-1} are required.
      (2) Proceed as in 1a.
   b. Calculate patient's water requirement.
      (1) 750 ml · m^{-2} · 24 h^{-1} 10% glucose are required.
      (2) Subtract 72 ml × the number of intracardiac catheters being flushed with 10% glucose in water from the amount in step (1), and order that amount.
   c. Give no potassium in the IV fluids.
3. If oral intake has not been established on the third postoperative day, consider gavage feeding or IV hyperalimentation.

Note that when medications such as lidocaine, catecholamines, and sodium nitroprusside are administered, the amount of fluid thereby infused must be determined and subtracted from the daily fluid requirement.

APPENDIX **5M**

PATIENT MANAGEMENT PROTOCOL FOR FEEDING AFTER INFANT CARDIAC SURGERY

Infants can rapidly develop a profoundly catabolic state after major surgery. Caloric intake should be raised to adequate levels as soon as possible after operation.

When respiratory assistance via an endotracheal tube continues into the third postoperative day, gavage feeding is begun unless specific contraindications exist. In extubated infants, weakness and underdevelopment may prevent proper feeding and result in aspiration, making intermittent gavage feeding necessary. The steps are as follows:

1. As a precaution, prepare the endotracheal suction catheter for immediate use.
2. Check to be certain that the nasogastric tube is in the stomach; if intermittent gavage is to be used, a feeding catheter is inserted for each feeding and then removed.
   a. Aspirate the tube. If stomach contents are not obtained or if large quantities of air with a little mucus are obtained, the tube is probably in the trachea.
   b. While listening over the stomach with a stethoscope, inject a little air and listen for the typical noise.
   c. Persistent coughing suggests that the tube is in the trachea.
   d. Absence of a normal cry suggests the tube is in the trachea (steps a, b, and d apply to patients without an endotracheal tube).
3. If these checks indicate that the tube is in the stomach and if aspiration does not reveal > 10–15 ml of fluid in the stomach, then initial feedings can be begun. These feedings are injected slowly over 2–3 minutes or allowed to enter by gravity, preferably with the infant sitting upright. Otherwise, the infant is placed on his or her right side with the head inclined at at least a 15° angle.
4. The gavage feeding is given *every 3 hours* on the following schedule:
   a. Give sterile water, 10–15 ml × 1.

b. If well tolerated, give 10% dextrose in water, 30 ml × 1.

c. If well tolerated and if the residual is less than 5 ml, give Lanolac or SMA-20, 30 ml × 8, and, if well tolerated, full-strength Lanolac or SMA-20 in increasing amounts.

5. If needed,

a. Consider giving SMA-27 (27 calories per ounce) if diarrhea is not present.

b. Consider continuous drip infusion to avoid a bolus effect. (Residual fluid in the stomach is aspirated and measured every 2 hours.)

APPENDIX **5N**

PATIENT MANAGEMENT PROTOCOL FOR METABOLIC ACIDOSIS

INDICATION

Metabolic acidosis exists if the base deficit (by the Astrup's equation) is > 2 mEq $\cdot$ l^{-1} and pH is < 7.35 or $PaCO_2$ is < 30 mmHg.

RATIONALE

Treatment is directed only at the extracellular fluid, and a conservative dose of $NaHCO_3$ is given, since more can easily be administered if needed.

Extracellular fluid volume = 30% body weight (kg)

Base deficit (mEq $\cdot$ l^{-1}) $\cdot$ 0.3 $\cdot$ body weight (kg)
= total extracellular base deficit

TREATMENT

1. Administer $NaHCO_3$ so as to give an amount of Na$^+$ (mEq) equal to one-half the total extracellular base deficit.

2. Remeasure the base deficit in ½ hour and repeat treatment if indicated.

Note that in acute reduction of cardiac output or cardiac arrest, much larger doses of $NaHCO_3$ are indicated (44 mEq of sodium for adults, 1 mEq $\cdot$ kg^{-1} for infants and children).

APPENDIX **5O**

PATIENT MANAGEMENT PROTOCOL FOR SEVERE METABOLIC ALKALOSIS

INDICATION

Blood pH > 7.60 and/or base excess > 5.0 mEq $\cdot$ l^{-1}. Some surgeons use total base excess > 50 mEq.

Total base excess (mEq) = base excess (mEq $\cdot$ l^{-1})
$\times$ 0.3(l $\cdot$ kg^{-1}) $\times$ body weight (kg)

RATIONALE

Cardiac surgical patients who develop severe metabolic alkalosis are usually slow to convalesce and resume normal alimentation and are frequently on moderate or large diuretic programs. This complication may be more common in infants. The condition is associated with a volume-contracted state (dehydration), with potassium and chloride depletion, and, in the more severe form, with hypercapnia. The major complications of severe alkalemia include a leftward shift of the oxyhemoglobin dissociation curve, with attendant tissue hypoxia, peripheral and central chemoreceptor depression, hypoventilation, and hypoxemia; refractory cardiac arrhythmias; excessive myocardial contractility, with attendant increase in oxygen consumption; tetany; and altered calcium metabolism. Mild forms of metabolic alkalosis may be corrected with volume expansion and replacement of potassium and chloride. Severe alkalemia (pH $\geq$ 7.60) mandates aggressive therapy. The administration of hydrochloric acid corrects metabolic alkalosis directly without dependence on renal or hepatic metabolic function. Complications of hemolysis and tissue necrosis are not a problem if central venous administration of dilute hydrochloric acid is used. However, because of the respiratory depression (CO_2 retention and hypoxia) caused by metabolic alkalosis, the too rapid administration of hydrochloric acid may produce inappropriate hyperventilation and hypocapnia with an intracellular-extracellular H$^+$ dysequilibrium. With the concomitant correction of saline and potassium chloride deficits, IV infusion of hydrochloric acid is a safe and desirable therapy for severe metabolic alkalosis.

TREATMENT

1. Use an internal jugular or right atrial line for infusion.

2. Prepare 0.15N hydrochloric acid in sterile water (12.5 ml concentrated hydrochloric acid [36%–38%] diluted to a volume of 1,000 ml with sterile water). One liter of 0.15N HCl contains 150 mEq of H$^+$ and 150 mEq of Cl$^-$.

3. Determine the amount of hydrochloric acid required for correction of the metabolic alkalosis. Calculate the chloride deficit and the total base excess by the formulae:

Cl$^-$ deficit = 0.3 × body weight (kg)
× Cl$^-$ concentration (mEq $\cdot$ l^{-1})

Total base excess (mEq) = 0.3 × body weight (kg)
× base excess (mEq $\cdot$ l^{-1})

4. Administer the chloride deficit as 0.15N HCl over a 16–24-hour period. The maximum infusion rate should be about 0.2 mEq H$^+$ $\cdot$ kg^{-1} $\cdot$ h^{-1}. The infusion continues until the base excess is within an acceptable range, that is, < 5 mEq $\cdot$ l^{-1}. As a check, the total base excess should be reduced to between 0 and about 1 mEq $\cdot$ kg^{-1}. (Infusion tubing should be changed every 12 hours and the acid infused from a glass container, since the effect of hydrochloric acid on plastic is uncertain.)

5. Correct the patient's volume deficit based on current and previous body weight by volume expansion with saline solution. Administer the maintenance daily IV fluids and sodium and potassium requirements and replace any prior deficits. Correct potassium deficit and maintain potassium level greater than 3.5 mEq $\cdot$ l^{-1}.

6. Monitor arterial blood gases and electrolytes every 4–6 hours and BUN and creatinine levels once or twice daily.

APPENDIX **5P**

PATIENT MANAGEMENT PROTOCOL FOR HYPERTHERMIA

INDICATION

Rectal temperature is $\geq$ 101°F (38.3°C).

RATIONALE

Moderate hyperthermia increases metabolic demands and, thus, myocardial oxygen consumption. Severe hyperthermia (central temperatures $\geq$ 106°F [41.1°C]) may permanently and severely damage the brain.

TREATMENT

1. Rectal temperature $\geq$ 101°F: give acetaminophen as a rectal suppository every 4 hours. The dose in infants and children is 10 mg · kg^{-1} (rounded to the nearest 30 mg), and, in adults, 650–1,300 mg.

2. Rectal temperature $\geq$ 103°F:

   a. Insert esophageal temperature probe for continuous monitoring of central temperature and intensify efforts to improve cardiac output. Check for possible transfusion reaction.

   b. Esophageal temperature $\geq$ 103:

      (1) Give Tylenol (acetaminophen) as in step 1.

      (2) Give dexamethasone, 0.25 mg · kg^{-1} IV, then 0.1 mg · kg^{-1} IV every 6 hours × 4.

      (3) Use a cooling blanket or cold syringing and a fan or ice bags applied to the body until central temperature < 102°F.

      (4) Give sodium nitroprusside, 1 μg · kg^{-1} · min^{-1}, to increase peripheral heat loss if arterial pressure remains acceptable with this drug.

      (5) Abolish muscular heat production, particularly when the infant is restless, by paralyzing the child with pancuronium (0.1 mg · kg^{-1}).

      (6) Continue efforts to improve cardiac output.

APPENDIX 5Q

PATIENT MANAGEMENT PROTOCOL FOR SEIZURES IN INFANTS AND CHILDREN AFTER CARDIAC SURGERY

GENERAL COMMENTS

Generalized or focal seizures are an infrequent but potentially serious occurrence following cardiac surgery in infants and children. In such cases, a number of etiologies are possible (e.g., metabolic; infectious; cerebral edema, embolism or hemorrhage; decreased cerebral perfusion), but in any given case, a single specific causative factor may not be identified. The protocol below outlines the basic evaluation to identify possible correctable causes and describes a treatment regimen. The following generalizations are useful:

1. In infants and small children, whether the seizure is generalized or focal is not helpful diagnostically.

2. Respiratory arrest, discoordinate respiratory activity, or sudden inability to adequately mechanically ventilate can be an indication of seizural activity in infants. Additional evidence of seizures is usually present on detailed evaluation.

3. After initial control of seizures, anticonvulsant therapy should be continued through the recovery period. Decisions regarding long-term therapy are made before hospital discharge.

4. The majority of children having a seizure in the early postoperative period will not have a chronic seizure disorder.

5. In some circumstances, the possibility of the seizure's being due to meningitis, septicemia, or urinary tract infection should be considered.

6. Choreiform movements may indicate cerebral damage.

7. Because of its potential to cause cardiorespiratory depression and its short duration of action, diazepam (Valium) is best avoided as an anticonvulsant unless the patient is being artificially ventilated.

INITIAL EVALUATION AND TREATMENT

1. At the onset of a seizure, arterial blood gases and pH; serum glucose, calcium, and electrolytes; cardiac index; and body temperature are determined.

2. Interventions are made in an attempt to correct:

   a. pH < 7.25 or > 7.50; PaCO$_2$ < 25 mmHg; PaO$_2$ < 80 mmHg; and base deficit > 10–15 mEq · l^{-1}. (In some patients, prompt control of seizures will correct low values.)

   b. Serum glucose level < 40 mg · dl^{-1} in infants and < 60 mg · dl^{-1} in older children (see "Hypoglycemia," in Section 2).

   c. Serum calcium level < 7 mg · dl^{-1} in infants and < 8 mg · dl^{-1} in older children.

   d. Serum Na level < 125 mEq · l^{-1}. The usual management in this situation is restriction of salt and water intake.

   e. Cardiac index < 2.0 l · min^{-1} · m^{-2}.

   f. Body temperature > 101.5°F.

INITIAL ANTICONVULSANT THERAPY

When the seizure activity is first noted, steps are taken to terminate seizures or, if seizures are no longer present, to prevent their recurrence while the chemical and other variables are being determined.

1. Give

   a. 1 ml of paraldehyde IM in infants < 1 year of age and an additional 0.5–1.0 ml for each year of age > 1 (maximum, 5.0 ml); or 0.1–0.2 mg · kg^{-1} of diazepam IV and

   b. 15 mg · kg^{-1} of phenobarbital IV given over 5–10 minutes as a loading dose.

2. If seizures are not controlled by these measures, a further dose of paraldehyde may be given in ½–1 hour, or further diazepam (if the patient is being ventilated) may be used. (The full effect of the loading dose of phenobarbital may not be apparent for several hours, but if at this stage problems continue, consider giving a further 5 mg · kg^{-1}.)

3. If there has been spontaneous termination of seizural activity but prevention of recurrences is desired, omit step 1a and proceed to step 1b.

4. Continuing major seizures will rarely be a problem. If they are, a loading dose of phenytoin (Dilantin) (20 mg · kg^{-1} orally) is given, followed by maintenance with 3–4 mg · kg^{-1} · d given orally.

5. An alternative, especially when seizures interfere with effective ventilatory support, is paralysis with pancuronium.

MAINTENANCE ANTICONVULSIVE THERAPY

The administration of phenobarbital (2.5 mg · kg^{-1} · 12 h^{-1}) can be instituted 12–24 hours after giving the initial loading dose.

REFERENCES

A

1. Alford WC Jr, Meador CK, Mihalevich J, Burrus GR, Glassford DM Jr, Stoney WS, Thomas CS Jr: Acute adrenal insufficiency following cardiac surgical procedures. *J Thorac Cardiovasc Surg* 78:489, 1979.

2. Aldrete JS, Han SY, Laws HL, Kirklin JW: Intestinal infarction complicating low cardiac output states. *Surg Gynecol Obstet* 144:371, 1977.

3. Abel RM, Buckley MJ, Austen WG, Barratt GO, Beck CH Jr, Fisher JE: Etiology, incidence, and prognosis of renal failure following cardiac operations. *J Thorac Cardiovasc Surg* 71:323, 1976.

4. Ashbaugh DG, Petty TL: Positive end-expiratory pressure. *J Thorac Cardiovasc Surg* 65:165, 1979.

5. Astrup P, Andersen OS, Jorgenson K, Engel K: The acid-base metabolism: A new approach. *Lancet*:1035, 1960.

B

1. Bell DM, Goldmann DA, Hopkins CC, Karchmer AW, Moellering RC Jr: Unreliability of fever and leukocytosis in the diagnosis of infection after cardiac valve surgery. *J Thorac Cardiovasc Surg* 75:87, 1978.

2. Becker LC, Fortuin NJ, Pitt B: Effect of ischemia and antianginal drugs on the distribution of radioactive microspheres in the canine left ventricle. *Circ Res* 28:263, 1971.

3. Breckenridge IM, Deverall PB, Kirklin JW, Digerness SB: Potassium intake and balance after open intracardiac operations. *J Thorac Cardiovasc Surg* 63:305, 1972.

4. Barratt-Boyes BG, Wood EH: Cardiac output and related measurements and pressure values in the right heart and associated vessels. *J Lab Clin Med* 51:72, 1958.

5. Bourgeois BFD, Donath A, Paunier L, Rouge J-C: Effects of cardiac surgery on renal functions in children. *J Thorac Cardiovasc Surg* 77:283, 1979.

6. Burke JF: The effective period of preventive antibiotic action in experimental incisions and dermal lesions. *Surgery* 50:161, 1961.

7. Bryant LR, Spencer FC, Trinkle JK: Treatment of median sternotomy infection by mediastinal irrigation with an antibiotic solution. *Ann Surg* 169:915, 1969.

8. Breyer RH, Mills SA, Hudspeth AS, Johnston FR, Cordell AR: A prospective study of sternal wound complications. *Ann Thorac Surg* 37:412, 1984.

9. Berglund E: Ventricular function: VI. Balance of left and right ventricular output: relation between left and right atrial pressures. *Am J Physiol* 178:381, 1954.

C

1. Cohn LH, Angell WW, Shumway NE: Body fluid shifts after cardiopulmonary bypass. I. Effects of congestive heart failure and hemodilution. *J Thorac Cardiovasc Surg* 62:423, 1971.

2. Cottrell JE, Casthely P, Brodie JD, Patel K, Klein A, Trundorf H: Prevention of nitroprusside-induced cyanide toxicity with hydroxocobalamin. *N Engl J Med* 298:809, 1978.

3. Chiariello M, Gold HK, Leinbach RC, Davis MA, Maroko PR: Comparison between the effects of nitroprusside and nitroglycerin on ischemic injury during acute myocardial infarction. *Circulation* 54:766, 1976.

4. Conti VR, Wideman F, Blackstone EH, Kirklin JW: Incremental risk factors in mitral valve replacement. (1979) Unpublished study.

5. Cleland J, Pluth JR, Tauxe WN, Kirklin JW: Blood volume and body fluid compartment changes soon after closed and open intracardiac surgery. *J Thorac Cardiovasc Surg* 52:698, 1966.

6. Chesney RW, Kaplan BS, Freedom RM, Haller JA, Drummond KN: Acute renal failure: An important complication of cardiac surgery in infants. *J Pediatr* 87:381, 1975.

7. Cole P: The safe use of sodium nitroprusside. *Anaesthesia* 33:473, 1978.

8. Connell RS, Page US, Bartley TD, Bigelow JC, Webb MC: The effect on pulmonary ultrastructure of Dacron-wool filtration during cardiopulmonary bypass. *Ann Thorac Surg* 15:217, 1973.

9. Caul EO, Clarke SKR, Mott MG, Perham TGM, Wilson RSE: Cytomegalovirus infections after open heart surgery. *Lancet* 1:777, 1971.

10. Cevese PG, Vecchioni R, D'Amico DF, Cordiano C, Biasiato R, Favia G, Farello GA: Postoperative chylothorax. *J Thorac Cardiovasc Surg* 69:966, 1975.

11. Chu C, Chang C, Liaw Y, Hsieh M: Jaundice after open heart surgery: A prospective study. *Thorax* 39:52, 1984.

12. Cutler BS, Okike O, Salm TJV: Surgical versus percutaneous removal of the intra-aortic balloon. *J Thorac Cardiovasc Surg* 86:907, 1983.

13. Culliford AT, Cunningham JN Jr, Zeff RH, et al.: Sternal and costochondral infections following open-heart surgery: A review of 2,594 cases. *J Thorac Cardiovasc Surg* 54:586, 1967.

D

1. Dietzman RH, Ersek RA, Lillehei CW, Castaneda AR, Lillehei RC: Low output syndrome: Recognition and treatment. *J Thorac Cardiovasc Surg* 57:138, 1969.

2. deVillota ED, Barat G, Astorqui F, Dimaso D, Aveloo F: Pyrexia following open heart surgery. *Anesthesia* 29:529, 1974.

E

1. Epstein SE, Kent DM, Goldstein RE, Borer JS, Redwood ER: Reduction of ischemic injury by nitroglycerin during acute myocardial infarction. *N Engl J Med* 292:29, 1974.

2. Engelman RM, Spencer FC, Reed GE, Tice DA: Cardiac tamponade following open-heart surgery. *Circulation* 41,42(suppl II):II-165, 1970.

3. Eltringham WK, Schroder R, Jenny M, Matoff JM, Zollinger RM Jr: Pulmonary arteriovenous admixture in cardiac surgical patients. *Circulation* 37,38(suppl II):II-207, 1968.

4. Edmunds LH, MacVaugh H III, Stevens J, Wechsler AB, Worthington GM: Evaluation of computer-aided monitoring of patients after heart surgery. *J Thorac Cardiovasc Surg* 74:890, 1977.

5. Estafanous FG, Tarazi RC: Systemic arterial hypertension associated with cardiac surgery. *Am J Cardiol* 46:685, 1980.

6. Engle MA, McCabe JC, Ebert PA, Zabriskie J: The postpericardiotomy syndrome and antiheart antibodies. *Circulation* 49:401, 1974.

7. Engle MA, Zabriskie JB, Senterfit LB, Gay WA, Jr, O'Loughlin JE, Ehlers KH: Viral illness and the postpericardiotomy syndrome: A prospective study in children. *Circulation* 62:1151, 1980.

8. Engle MA, Gay WA Jr, McCabe J, Longo E, Johnson D, Senterfit LB, Zabriskie JB: Postpericardiotomy syndrome in

adults: Incidence, autoimmunity and virology. *Circulation* 64(suppl II):II-58, 1981.

9. Engelman RM, Williams CD, Gouge TH, et al.: Mediastinitis following open-heart surgery: Review of two years' experience. *Arch Surg* 107:772, 1973.

F

1. Friesen WG, Woodson RD, Ames AW, Herr RH, Starr A, Kassebaum DG: A hemodynamic comparison of atrial and ventricular pacing in postoperative cardiac surgical patients. *J Thorac Cardiovasc Surg* 55:271, 1968.

2. Firor WB: Infection following open-heart surgery, with special reference to the role of prophylactic antibiotics. *J Thorac Cardiovasc Surg* 53:371, 1967.

3. Fordham RMM: Hypothermia after aortic valve surgery under cardiopulmonary bypass. *Thorax* 20:505, 1965.

4. Feteih W, Syamasundar R, Whisennand HH, Mardini MK, Lawrie GM: Chylopericardium: New complication of Blalock-Taussig anastomosis. *J Thorac Cardiovasc Surg* 85:791, 1983.

5. Fremes SE, Weisel RD, Baird RJ, Mickleborough LL, Burns RJ, Teasdale SJ, Ivanov J, Seawright SJ, Madonik M, Mickle DAG, Scully HE, Goldman BS, McLaughlin PR: Effects of postoperative hypertension and its treatment. *J Thorac Cardiovasc Surg* 86:47, 1983.

6. Fowler MB, Alderman EL, Oesterle SN, Derby G, Daughters GT, Stinson EB, Ingels NB, Mitchell RS, Miller DC: Dobutamine and dopamine after cardiac surgery: Greater augmentation of myocardial blood flow with dobutamine. *Circulation* 70(suppl I),1–103, 1984.

7. Flege JB Jr, Wright CB, Reisinger TJ: Successful balloon counterpulsation for right ventricular failure. *Ann Thorac Surg* 37:167, 1984.

G

1. Goldstein RE, Stinson EB, Scherer JL, Seningen RP, Grehl TM, Epstein SE: Intraoperative coronary collateral function in patients with coronary occlusive disease: Nitroglycerin responsiveness and angiographic correlations. *Circulation* 49:298, 1974.

2. German JC, Chalmers GS, Hirai J, Nrisingha MD, Wakabayashi A, Connolly JE: Comparison of nonpulsatile and pulsatile extracorporeal circulation on renal tissue perfusion. *Chest* 61:65, 1972.

3. Goldberg LI: Dopamine—clinical use of an endogenous catecholamine. *N Engl J Med* 291:707, 1974.

4. Gregory GA, Kitterman JA, Phibbs RH, Tooley WH, Hamilton WK: Treatment of the idiopathic respiratory-distress syndrome with continuous positive airway pressure. *N Engl J Med* 284:1333, 1971.

5. Gundry SR, Borkon AM, McIntosh CL, Morrow AG: Candida esophagitis following cardiac operation and short-term antibiotic prophylaxis. *J Thorac Cardiovasc Surg* 80:661, 1980.

6. Gall WE, Clarke WR, Doty DB: Vasomotor dynamics associated with cardiac operations. I. Venous tone and the effects of vasodilators. *J Thorac Cardiovasc Surg* 83:724, 1982.

7. Gailiunas P Jr, Chawla R, Lazarus JM, Cohn L, Sanders J, Merrill JP: Acute renal failure following cardiac operations. *J Thorac Cardiovasc Surg* 79:241, 1980.

8. Gottlieb SO, Brinker JA, Borkon AM, Kallman CH, Potter A, Gott VL, Baughman KL: Identification of patients at high risk for complications of intraaortic balloon counterpulsation: A multivariate risk factor analysis. *Am J Cardiol* 53:1135, 1984.

H

1. Hood WP Jr, Rackley CE, Rolett E: Wall stress in the normal and hypertrophied human left ventricle. *Am J Cardiol* 22:550, 1968.

2. Hilberman M, Myers BD, Carrie BJ, Derby G, Jamison RL, Stinson EB: Acute renal failure following cardiac surgery. *J Thorac Cardiovasc Surg* 77:880, 1979.

3. Hencz P, Deverall PB, Crew AD, Steel AE, Mearns AJ: Hyperuricemia of infants and children: A complication of open heart surgery. *J Pediatr* 94:774, 1979.

4. Hollenberg NK, Adams DF, Mendell P, Abrams HL, Merrell JP: Renal vascular responses to dopamine: Hemodynamic and angiographic observations in normal man. *Clin Sci* 45:733, 1973.

5. Hockberg MS, Merrill WH, Gruber H, McIntosh CL, Henry WL, Morrow AG: Delayed cardiac tamponade associated with prophylactic anticoagulants. *J Thorac Cardiovasc Surg* 75:777, 1978.

6. Hill JD, Johnson DC, Miller GE Jr, Kerth WJ, Gerbode F: Latent mediastinal tamponade after open heart surgery. *Arch Surg* 99:808, 1969.

7. Hardesty RL, Thompson M, Lerberg DB, Siewers RD, O'Toole JD, Salerni R, Bahnson HT: Delayed postoperative cardiac tamponade: Diagnosis and management. *Ann Thorac Surg* 26:155, 1978.

8. Harris PD, Malm JR, Bowman FO Jr, Hoffman BF, Kaiser GA, Singer DH: Epicardial pacing to control arrhythmias following cardiac surgery. *Circulation* 37,38 (suppl II):II-178, 1968.

9. Hill DG, de Lanerolle P, Kosek JC, Agiular MJ, Hill JD: The pulmonary pathophysiology of membrane and bubble oxygenators. *Trans Am Soc Artif Intern Organs* 11:165, 1975.

10. Hedley-Whyte J, Corning H, Laver MB, Austen WG, Bendixen HH: Pulmonary ventilation-perfusion relations after heart valve replacement or repair in man. *J Clin Invest* 44:406, 1965.

11. Higgins GB, Mulder DG: Chylothorax after surgery for congenital heart disease. *J Thorac Cardiovasc Surg* 61:411, 1971.

12. Hawker RE, Cartmill TB, Celermajer JM, Bowdler JD: Chylous pericardial effusion complicating aorta-right pulmonary artery anastomosis. *J Thorac Cardiovasc Surg* 63:491, 1972.

I

1. Ito T, Engle MA, Goldberg HP: Postpericardiotomy syndrome following surgery for non-rheumatic heart disease. *Circulation* 17:549, 1958.

J

1. Jacob T, de Leval M, Stark J, Waterston DJ: Chylopericardium as a complication of aorto-pulmonary shunt. *Arch Surg* 108:870, 1974.

K

1. Kirklin JW, Archie JP Jr: The cardiovascular subsystem in surgical patients. *Surg Gynecol Obstet* 139:17, 1974.

2. Kirklin JK, Daggett WM Jr, Lappas DG: Potoperative care following cardiac surgery, in RA Johnson, E Haber, WG Austen (eds): *The Practice of Cardiology.* Boston: Little, Brown, 1980, pp 1110–1132.

3. Kirklin JW, *Systems Analysis in Surgical Patients with Particular Attention to the Cardiac and Pulmonary Subsystems,* Macewen Memorial Lecture. Glasgow: University of Glasgow Press, 1970.

4. Kirklin JK, Blackstone EH, Kirklin JW, McKay R, Pacifico AD, Bargeron LM Jr: Intracardiac surgery in infants under age 3 months: Predictors of postoperative in-hospital cardiac death. *Am J Cardiol* 48:507, 1981.

5. Kay HR, Goodman LR, Teplick SK, Mundth ED: Use of computed tomography to assess mediastinal complications after median sternotomy. *Ann Thorac Surg* 36:706, 1983.

6. Kirklin JK, Lell WA, Kouchoukos NT: Hydroxyethyl starch versus albumin for colloid infusion following cardiopulmonary bypass in patients undergoing myocardial revascularization. *Ann Thorac Surg* 37:40, 1984.

7. Kratz JM, Metcalf JS, Sade RM: Pericardial injury by antibacterial irrigants. *J Thorac Cardiovasc Surg* 85:785, 1983.

8. Kirklin JK, Westaby S, Blackstone EH, Kirklin JW, Chenoweth DE, Pacifico AD: Complement and the damaging effects of cardiopulmonary bypass. *J Thorac Cardiovasc Surg* 86:845, 1983.

L

1. Livelli FD Jr, Johnson RA, McEnany MT, Sherman E, Newell J, Block PC, DeSanctis RW: Unexplained in-hospital fever following cardiac surgery. *Circulation* 57:968, 1978.

2. Lell WL, Samuelson P, Reves JG, Strong SD: Duration of intubation and ICU stay after open heart surgery. *South Med J* 72:773, 1979.

3. Levett JM, Culpepper WS, Lin CY, Arcilla RA, Replogle RL: Cardiovascular responses to PEEP and CPAP following repair of complicated congenital heart defects. *Ann Thorac Surg* 36:411, 1983.

4. Lynn AM, Opheim KE, Tyler DC: Morphine infusion after pediatric cardiac surgery. *Crit Care Med* 12:863, 1984.

M

1. Merrill W, Donahoo JS, Brawley RK, Taylor D: Late cardiac tamponade: A potentially lethal complication of open-heart surgery. *J Thorac Cardiovasc Surg* 72:919, 1976.

2. Myerowitz PD, Caswell K, Lindsay WG, Nicoloff DM: Antibiotic prophylaxis for open-heart surgery. *J Thorac Cardiovasc Surg* 73:625, 1977.

3. McLennan JR, Young WE, Sykes MK: Respiratory changes after open-heart surgery. *Thorax* 20:545, 1965.

4. Mathur M, Harris EA, Yarrow S, Barratt-Boyes BG: Measurement of cardiac output by thermodilution in infants and children after open heart operations. *J Thorac Cardiovasc Surg* 72:221, 1976.

5. Moggio RA, Rha CC, Somberg ED, Praeger PI, Pooley RW, Reed GE: Hemodynamic comparison of albumin and hydroxyethyl starch in postoperative cardiac surgery patients. *Crit Care Med* 11:943, 1983.

6. Moran JM, Opravil M, Gorman AJ, Rastegar H, Meyers SN, Michaelis LL: Pulmonary artery balloon counterpulsation for right ventricular failure: II. Clinical experience. *Ann Thorac Surg* 38:254, 1984.

7. Miller DC, Moreno-Cabral RJ, Stinson EB, et al: Pulmonary artery balloon counterpulsation for acute right ventricular failure. *J Thorac Cardiovasc Surg* 80:760, 1980.

N

1. Nickerson M: Drugs inhibiting adrenergic nerves and structures innervated by them, in LS Goodman, A Gilman (eds): *The Pharmacological Basis of Therapeutics* (ed 4). New York: Macmillan, 1970, p 559.

2. Nadas AS, Fyler DC: *Pediatric Cardiology*. Philadelphia: Saunders, 1972.

3. Norman JC, McDonald HP, Sloan H: The early and aggressive treatment of acute renal failure following cardiopulmonary bypass with continuous peritoneal dialysis. *Surgery* 56:240, 1964.

4. Nishimura RA, Fuster V, Burgert SL, Puga FJ: Clinical features and long-term natural history of the postpericardiotomy syndrome. *Int J Cardiol* 4:443, 1983.

O

1. Orringer MB, Sloan H: Monilial esophagitis: An increasingly frequent cause of esophageal stenosis. *Ann Thorac Surg* 26:364, 1978.

2. Ofori-Kraykye SK, Tyberg TI, Geha AS, Hammond GL, Cohen LS, Langou RA: Late cardiac tamponade after open heart surgery: Incidence, role of anticoagulants in its pathogenesis and its relationship to the postpericardiotomy syndrome. *Circulation* 63:1323, 1981.

3. Opravil M, German AJ, Krejcie TC, Michaelis LL, Moran JM: Pulmonary artery balloon counterpulsation for right ventricular failure: I. Experimental results. *Ann Thorac Surg* 38:242, 1984.

P

1. Pacifico AD, Digerness S, Kirklin JW: Acute alterations of body composition after open intracardiac operations. *Circulation* 41:331, 1970.

2. Pacifico AD, Digerness S, Kirklin JW: Sodium-excreting ability before and after intracardiac surgery. *Circulation* 41,42(suppl II):II-142, 1970.

3. Palmer RF, Lasseter KC: Drug therapy: Sodium nitroprusside. *N Engl J Med* 292:294, 1975.

4. Parr GVS, Blackstone EH, Kirklin JW: Cardiac performance and mortality early after intracardiac surgery in infants and young children. *Circulation* 51:867, 1975.

5. Parr GVS, Blackstone EH, Kirklin JW, Pacifico AD, Lauridsen P: Cardiac performance early after interatrial transposition of venous return in infants and small children. *Circulation* 49, 50(suppl II):II-163, 1974.

6. Philbin DM, Sullivan SF, Bowman FO Jr, Malm JR, Papper EM: Postoperative hypoxemia: Contribution of the cardiac output. *Anesthesiology* 32:136, 1970.

7. Plumb VJ, Karp RB, Kouchoukos NT, Zorn GL Jr, James TN, Waldo AL: Verapamil therapy of atrial fibrillation and atrial flutter following cardiac operation. *J Thorac Cardiovasc Surg* 83:590, 1982.

8. Pairolero PC, Arnold PG: Management of recalcitrant median sternotomy wounds. *J Thorac Cardiovasc Surg* 88:357, 1984.

R

1. Roberts AJ, Niarchos AP, Subramanian VA, Abel RM, Herman SD, Sealey JE, Case DB, White RP, Johnson GA, Laragh JH, Gay WA Jr: Systemic hypertension associated with coronary artery bypass surgery. *J Thorac Cardiovasc Surg* 74:846, 1977.

2. Rea HH, Harris EA, Seelye ER, Whitlock RML, Withy SJ: The effects of cardiopulmonary bypass upon pulmonary gas exchange. *J Thorac Cardiovasc Surg* 75:104, 1978.

3. Ratliff NB, Young WG Jr, Hackel DB, Mikat E, Wilson JW: Pulmonary injury secondary to extracorporeal circulation: An ultrastructure study. *J Thorac Cardiovasc Surg* 65:425, 1973.

4. Rabelo RC, Oliveira SA, Tanaka H, Weigl DR, Verginelli G, Zerbini EJ: The influence of the nature of the prime on postperfusion pulmonary changes. *J Thorac Cardiovasc Surg* 66:782, 1973.

5. Reid DJ, Digerness SB, Kirklin JW: Changes in whole body venous tone and distribution of blood after open intracardiac surgery. *Am J Cardiol* 22:621, 1968.

6. Rigden SPA, Barratt TM, Dillon MJ, deLaval M, Stark J: Acute renal failure complicating cardiopulmonary bypass surgery. *Arch Dis Child* 57:425, 1982.

S

1. Sheppard LC, Kouchoukos NT, Kurtts MA, Kirklin JW: Automated treatment of critically ill patients following operation. *Ann Surg* 168:596, 1968.

2. Sturtz GS, Kirklin JW, Burke EC, Power MH: Water metabolism after cardiac operations involving a Gibbon-type pump-oxygenator. II. Benign forms of water loss. *Circulation* 16:1000, 1957.

3. Stewart RW, Blackstone EH, Kirklin JW: Neurological dysfunction after cardiac surgery, in L Parenzan, G Crupi, G Graham (eds): *Congenital Heart Disease in the First 3 Months of Life: Medical and Surgical Aspects.* Bologna, Italy: Patron Editore, 1981, pp 99–109.

4. Srinivasan V, Levinsky L, Choh JH, Baliah T, Subramanian S: Renal failure following intracardiac surgery in infants—improved survival with early dialysis: Indications and results. (1981) Personal communication.

5. Sheppard LC, Shotts JF, Roberson NF, Wallace FD, Kouchoukos NT: Computer controlled infusion of vasoactive drugs in post cardiac surgical patients. *Proc IEEE 1979: Frontiers of Engineering in Health Care* (IEEE catalog no. 79CH1440-7).

6. Soloff LA, Zatuchui J, Janton OH, O'Neill TJE, Glover RP: Reactivation of rheumatic fever following mitral commissurotomy. *Circulation* 8:481, 1953.

7. Sheppard LC, Kouchoukos NT, Shotts JF, Wallace FD: Regulation of mean arterial pressure by computer control of vasoactive agents in postoperative patients. *Computers in Cardiology* (IEEE catalog no. 75CH1018-C), Rotterdam, The Netherlands, October 2–4, 1975, pp 91–94.

8. Stewart S III, Edmunds LH Jr, Kirklin JW, Allarde RR: Spontaneous breathing with continuous positive airway pressure after open intracardiac operations in infants. *J Thorac Cardiovasc Surg* 65:37, 1973.

9. Scott AJ, Nicholson GI, Kerr AR: Lincomycin as a cause of pseudomembranous colitis. *Lancet* 2:1232, 1973.

10. Stenzl W, Rigler B, Tscheliessnigg KH, Beitzke A, Metzler H: Treatment of Postsurgical Chylothorax with Fibrin Glue. *Thorac Cardiovasc Surg* 31:35, 1983.

11. Shahian DM, Neptune WB, Ellis FH, Maggs PR: Intraaortic balloon pump morbidity: A comparative analysis of risk factors between percutaneous and surgical techniques. *Ann Thorac Surg* 36:644, 1983.

12. Simon TL, Akl BF, Murphy W: Controlled trial of routine administration of platelet concentrates in cardiopulmonary bypass surgery. *Ann Thorac Surg* 37:359, 1984.

13. Stone JG, Hoar PF, Khambatta JH: Influence of volume loading on intraoperative hemodynamics and perioperative fluid retention in patients with valvular regurgitation undergoing prosthetic replacement. *Am J Cardiol* 52:530, 1983.

14. Sarr MG, Gott VL, Townsend TR: Mediastinal infection after cardiac surgery. *Ann Thorac Surg* 38:415, 1984.

15. Stevenson LW, Child JS, Laks H, Kern L: Incidence and significance of early pericardial effusions after cardiac surgery. *Am J Cardiol* 54:848, 1984.

16. Shumaker HB Jr, Mandelbaum I: Continuous antibiotic irrigation in the treatment of infection. *Arch Surg* 86:384, 1963.

T

1. Tanaka J, Yasui H, Nakano E, Sese A, Matsui K, Takeda Y, Tokunaga K: Predisposing factors of renal dysfunction following total correction of tetralogy of Fallot in the adult. *J Thorac Cardiovasc Surg* 80:135, 1980.

2. Thurer RJ, Bognolo D, Vargas A, Isch JH, Kaiser GA: The management of mediastinal infection following cardiac surgery: An experience utilizing continuous irrigation with povidone-iodine. *J Thorac Cardiovasc Surg* 68:962, 1974.

3. Thomas CS Jr, McGoon DC: Isolated massive chyloperi-cardium following cardiopulmonary bypass. *J Thorac Cardiovasc Surg* 61:945, 1971.

W

1. Wedley JR, Lunn HF, Vale RJ: Studies of temperature balance after open-heart surgery. *Crit Care Med* 3:134, 1975.

2. Walker DB, Blackstone EH, Kirklin JW, Karp RB, Kouchoukos NT, Pacifico AD, Shealy A, Roe CR, Bradley EL: The effect of micropore filtration of the arterial return during cardiopulmonary bypass: A randomized clinical study. (1977) Unpublished.

3. Waldo AL, Ross SM, Kaiser GA: The epicardial electrogram in the diagnosis of cardiac arrhythmias following cardiac surgery. *Geriatrics* 26:108, 1971.

4. Waldo AL, MacLean WAH, Karp RB, Kouchoukos NT, James TN: Sustained rapid atrial pacing to control supraventricular tachycardias following open heart surgery. *Circulation* 51,52 (suppl. II):II-13, 1975.

5. Waldo AL, MacLean WAH: *Diagnosis and Treatment of Cardiac Arrhythmias Following Open Heart Surgery: Emphasis on the Use of Atrial and Ventricular Epicardial Wire Electrodes.* New York: Futura, 1980.

6. Williams GD, Seifen AB, Lawson NW, Norton JB, Readinger RI, Dungan TW, Callaway JK: Pulsatile perfusion versus conventional high-flow nonpulsatile perfusion for rapid core cooling and rewarming of infants for circulatory arrest in cardiac operation. *J Thorac Cardiovasc Surg* 78:667, 1979.

7. Weller TH: The cytomegaloviruses: Ubiquitous agents with protean clinical manifestations. *N Engl J Med* 285:267, 1971.

8. Wood EH: Use of indicator-dilution technics, in *Congenital Heart Disease.* Washington, D.C.: American Association of Advanced Science, 1960, pp 209–240.

9. Wallach R, Karp RB, Reves JG, Oparil S, Smith LR, James TN: Pathogenesis of paroxysmal hypertension developing during and after coronary bypass surgery: A study of hemodynamic and humoral factors. *Am J Cardiol* 46:559, 1980.

10. Weitzman LB, Tinker WP, Kronzon I, Cohen ML, Glassman E, Spencer FC: The incidence and natural history of pericardial effusion after cardiac surgery: An echocardiographic study. *Circulation* 69:506, 1984.

11. Woods JE, Taswell HF, Kirklin JW, Owen CA Jr: The transfusion of platelet concentrates in patients undergoing heart surgery. *Mayo Clin Proc* 42:318, 1967.

6

SURGICAL CONCEPTS, RESEARCH METHODS, AND DATA ANALYSIS AND USE

Early in the development of cardiac surgery, surgeons, clinicians, and investigators made important contributions of new knowledge and their patient-care decisions using simply innovation and intuition. Now, more analysis and effort are required to identify the fundamental truths involved in patient-care decisions in this complex area, and still more to improve the results by the development of new knowledge, new inferences, and new techniques. The purpose of this chapter is to describe the concepts and methods underlying such analyses, the methods by which new knowledge and new inferences in cardiac surgery can be generated, and some of the methods of decision making in the practice of cardiac surgery itself.

SECTION **1**

SURGICAL SUCCESS AND FAILURE

Cardiac surgery is successful for a patient when the goal of cure or palliation has been achieved. *Cure* is the restoration of a functional capacity within normal limits for the patient's age and sex, and of a life expectancy equal to that of the general population of the patient's age, race, and sex.[1] *Palli-*

---

[1] Specifically, the 70% confidence limits of the survival rate or hazard function (see "Parametric Methods" under Section 4) overlap those of the matched population.

ation is the improvement of the patient's functional capacity, the lengthening of the patient's life expectancy, or both. To reach these goals, the patient must survive throughout the operation and the postoperative hospital stay, and complications must be avoided. The goal is a hospital mortality approaching zero.[2] It could also be said that the goal is to make the result of the operation as nearly deterministic and as little subject to the laws of chance as is possible. The phrase is *approaching zero,* rather than zero itself, because the results of very few, if any, cardiac operations are deterministic. Thus, in individual cases, more than one outcome is assumed to be possible, since not all factors relating to outcome are known and not all the human performances involved are perfect.

Surgical failure is failure to achieve cure or palliation for the patient. Surgical failures include such early postoperative events as hospital mortality, heart block, and infection. Surgical failures also include premature late death and other such time-related events as thromboembolism, periprosthetic leakage, and graft closure. In this text, some of the results of cardiac surgery are conceptualized in terms of surgical failure in order to emphasize the causes of the failure, the progress that has been made in reducing its incidence, and the steps that must be taken to further minimize it.

CAUSES OF SURGICAL FAILURE

Human error and lack of scientific progress are the causes of surgical failure. Human error is considered the cause when an error has been made in the use or application of available techniques and knowledge. Lack of scientific progress is the cause when the techniques and/or knowledge necessary to prevent the failure are not available.

Human Error

When a surgical failure is stated to be due to human error, it is psychologically traumatic for a surgical team and subjects them to the possibility of severe criticism from others. Nevertheless, many surgical failures are in fact due to human error. This does not mean that they are from carelessness, inattention, or poor preparation, although such factors increase the probability of error. Errors, or, perhaps better, imperfect performances, are a part of the cyclic nature of human activities and events, although their frequency varies from person to person and can be reduced by a variety of methods. There are many more errors than surgical failures because many errors in performance are tolerated by the patient without ill effect or are neutralized by a corrective action taken by a member of the surgical team.

Regarding the problem of human error, cardiac surgery is akin to the flying of aircraft, mining, athletics, and many other activities. A considerable literature has evolved in

these and other fields about the difficulties and dangers of identifying human error as a cause of accidents or failures and the need to do so. Some knowledge of the situations in which errors have been likely to occur in other kinds of work and of the general methods found useful in preventing them are of value to the cardiac surgeon. Common situations include poor preparation of personnel for the specific job at hand, incomplete or complex information received, inaccurate communication, inattention, boredom or fatigue during the performance of the task, and other results of inadequate emotional or physical conditioning.[E1,H5,L2,W2] The relevance of information on human error to cardiac surgery is obvious. Recognition of human fallibility should aid in efforts to improve the results of cardiac surgery.

Lack of Scientific Progress

As a cause of surgical failure, a lack of scientific progress may be evident in inadequacy of preoperative evaluation techniques, unavailability of an operation appropriate to the disease, or failure to disseminate available information so that it can become part of general scientific progress. For example, lack of scientific progress in minimizing the damaging effects of cardiopulmonary bypass may result in surgical failure. It is the accurate identification of the specific deficits in scientific progress that guides research.

Surgical failure could result because cure or palliation is unattainable. This simple explanation is often invoked, but its proof is difficult. Usually, the most that can be shown is that cure or palliation is unattainable by the methods used. It is a very serious matter to conclude that cure or palliation is truly unattainable; therefore this step should be taken with due caution.

MODES OF SURGICAL FAILURE

A surgical failure, such as hospital death or premature late death, may occur in a number of modes. Generally, the mode is a category, syndrome, or pattern describing the subsystem failure or event that appears to be associated with the death or other form of failure. Thus, hospital death early after a cardiac operation may be associated with the syndrome of acute cardiac failure (low cardiac output syndrome) or with pulmonary insufficiency or acute renal failure and so forth. The identification of mode of death, or the mode of other kinds of surgical failure, is important in all clinical studies because the incremental risk factors and true causes of failure are often different for different modes of failure.

Section 2
INCREMENTAL RISK FACTORS

Certain factors, or variables, can be shown to increase the probability of surgical failure. These can be considered cor-

---

[2] For the purposes of this text, this is defined as a hospital mortality rate with a lower 70% confidence limit less than 1% and upper 70% confidence limit less than 5%.

relations, or associations, with surgical failures, and they affect the degree of difficulty of preventing a surgical failure. Because surgical failure or success in a group of patients is dependent on multiple variables that interact with one another to increase the risk, these variables have been called *incremental risk factors*.[K3] Risk factors were probably first formally studied in the way presented here in the Framingham Arteriosclerosis Project.[G10,W1]

Incremental risk factors are not causes of surgical failure, but are associations and their identification through clinical experience, research, and development does aid in identifying these causes. This process leads to research and development of new knowledge and to altered patient management programs that ultimately reduce the risk of surgical failure by neutralizing risk factors. Also, identifying incremental risk factors aids in comparing experiences with different results in order to determine whether the differences are related to different methods or merely to the presence of fewer incremental risk factors in certain groups of patients.

SECTION 3
RESEARCH METHODS IN CARDIAC SURGERY

A number of research methods are used in generating new knowledge, inferences, and techniques in cardiac surgery.

EXPERIMENTAL STUDIES

Research may be conducted under highly controlled conditions without the constraints inherent in attempting to achieve surgical success in patients. Such experimental studies may be purely chemical or may involve in vitro studies of biological material. They may be conducted with excised and isolated organs, with isolated organs in situ, or with the entire organism of an experimental animal. Properly designed, they can provide the most reliable information and results least likely to be due to chance, and these can be used for testing hypotheses, forming inferences, and testing new methods, but their disadvantages are several. Generally, they can address well only one or a small number of points at a time and therefore are time-consuming and relatively expensive ways of generating new knowledge. Also, unless the hypotheses, inferences, or new methods being tested are carefully selected on the basis of considerable experience and knowledge of the subject in humans, unless the experimental animal has a considerable similarity to a human in the area under study, and unless experimental design is appropriate, the results, although reliable and unlikely to be due to chance, may not be relevant to the surgical problem.

Excellent texts concerning experimental design and other facets of laboratory research are available.[C1,C2,F1,L1] The proposal of the hypotheses and new methods to be tested, and the forming of inferences, are dependent on the skill and experience of the investigator and on the data and interpreta-

tions generated by clinical research and prospective clinical studies (see "Clinical Research"). Because of the time and expense involved in experimental studies, priorities must be established, a process also dependent on skill, experience, data, and interpretations.

CLINICAL RESEARCH

In clinical research, quantitative observations are made in a prospective way, usually by laboratory methods, of specific variables under relatively standardized conditions in humans. In contrast to the situation in experimental studies, variables usually cannot be manipulated solely for experimental purposes. The advantages of clinical research are that the data are numerical and are the result of methods specifically designed for and applied to the research at hand and that the observations are made in humans. When the patient care setting in which the research is done is appropriate, some hypotheses can be tested, inferences formed, and new methods evaluated. The limitations of the method are that only procedures believed to be therapeutic can be studied, that manipulation of variables only for testing a hypothesis is generally not possible, that uncontrollable variables may influence the results, and that information is frequently missing (e.g., surviving patients do not have autopsy).

A number of texts[C1,C2,F1,L1] are useful in planning clinical research studies, in which precise study design and protocols are as important as in laboratory research. An important requisite for clinical research in cardiac surgery is that the surgeon accept the responsibility for the patient's welfare *and* for the enthusiastic and proper conduct of the research. At times, a study may need, properly, to be aborted because it unexpectedly threatens the patient's welfare. On the other hand, lack of enthusiasm and lack of commitment by the surgeon to the need for the new knowledge can result in uncalled-for abortions of studies. Skill, experience, and prior knowledge from prospective clinical studies and from experimental studies are required for the planning of really useful clinical research studies. The establishment of priorities for this type of research is also essential, for the same reasons as in experimental studies and for the additional reason that the protection of the patient requires that only a very limited number of clinical research projects can be carried out in any one unit at any one time.

PROSPECTIVE CLINICAL STUDIES

Research may also be conducted on a well-defined group of patients treated by a protocol and be based on data collected in the course of the patients' study and care, rather than by laboratory methods specifically directed toward the research. The advantages of such prospective clinical studies are that they are generally highly relevant and yield information that, properly analyzed and interpreted, is immediately applicable both to patient care and to the formulation of new hypotheses and inferences and new methods for further testing and study. The disadvantages are that generally only correlations, rather than causative factors, are established; the number of patients (n) in the study is sometimes of necessity small; and unless the unit is organized specifically for high-quality clinical studies, there is a good deal of nonnumerical, missing, or inaccurate data.

Prospective clinical studies are of two types. One is a study of a group of patients treated by a predetermined protocol;[T4] the other is a study of a group of patients concurrently treated by assignment to one of several treatment protocols in a randomized fashion. In the first method, the setting of the protocol is essentially the rigorous definition of what is considered to be optimal treatment at that time. When true uncertainty exists concerning optimal treatment, the moral justification for a randomized study is present.

When surgeons practice with *standardized treatment protocols*, they themselves can use relatively simple methods to analyze in a rigorous way the results of their experience with the prospective studies. (Proper standardized treatment protocols, revised when new knowledge is available, also provide the basis for optimal patient care.) Unless special methods of analysis are used the disadvantages of single-protocol studies is that a large number of uncontrolled variables that may affect the results can escape notice. These include changes with time, variations in the patient population and the disease process, and changes in intraoperative and postoperative management even within the protocol. Furthermore, unless multivariate analysis is used, correlations between a variable and the result may be hidden by interactions between variables.

Randomized trials[G6,L6,W7] offer the best opportunity for making formal comparisons between various treatment protocols and deriving inferences. A major disadvantage is that true uncertainty as to the relative efficacy of treatment protocols is not common, and thus the moral justification for a randomized trial is often absent. Another disadvantage is that randomization does not assure absence of the same uncontrolled variables that can complicate single-protocol studies. Also, in the surgical setting, where the study should be done over a particularly short period of time, the n available for randomization may be undesirably small; and especially with a small n, the events by which treatment superiority are judged may be so infrequent or so frequent that they cannot be sensitive discriminators of the treatment modality. Still another disadvantage is that, as in other types of research, unless the hypotheses being tested are carefully selected and answerable by such a study, a randomized study will fail to provide clinically relevant new inferences and knowledge.

Methods for randomized studies are described in several texts and papers.[B1,B2,B3,F2,M1] Little is written about the most commonly used and often informative type of prospective study: that by single protocol. This is particularly unfortunate because failure to use proper methodology in these studies is common and highly detrimental to the development of new knowledge. This methodology is discussed in Appendix 6A.

COMPARISON BETWEEN NONRANDOMIZED PROSPECTIVE CLINICAL STUDIES

The informal comparison of early and/or late results obtained by different methods and institutions has been, and will probably continue to be, the most commonly used method of generating new information and testing new techniques in cardiac surgery. Its advantages are the ready availability of such data and its obvious relevance to the problems of clinical cardiac surgery. Unfortunately, the method has many disadvantages. Uncontrolled variables are usually numerous and unstated. When the comparisons are interinstitutional, the forms in which much of the information exists may be so dissimilar as to preclude comparisons. The data available may be summarized in such a way as to preclude valid comparisons. (A conflict does of course exist between the authors of scientific papers and the editors of journals, for the editors are interested in keeping all articles short and are apt to complain when there is "too much detail.") In the past, many comparisons of studies have been made in a superficial and nonrigorous manner without using appropriate statistical methods.

With good data and rigorous methodology, useful information can be obtained by this method.[G11] The data base is the same as described for prospective single-protocol clinical studies (see Appendix 6A). Appropriate methodology is described in Section 4.

RETROSPECTIVE CLINICAL STUDIES

A conglomerate of case reports forms the data base for retrospective clinical studies. Such studies begin with patients, or specimens or data from them, that are of interest because they have something in common (e.g., prosthetic endocarditis, complications of vein grafts, arrhythmias after cardiac surgery). The study in some manner analyzes these common phenomena. The advantage of this type of study is that the common phenomenon may be of great clinical interest. A major disadvantage of such studies is that the "denominator is unknown,"[S1] that is, the frequency and factors contributing to the phenomenon being studied are not known. While such studies are thus of limited value, retrospective, matched case-control studies can be valuable.[B28]

The methods are generally descriptive (see Section 4).

MATHEMATICAL MODELING

Cardiac surgical units infrequently have the expertise for mathematical modeling. However, when available, this method can provide new insights into cardiac surgical problems, and for that reason, it forms the basis of some commonly used methods (e.g., indicator dilution curves). Mathematical modeling is a process of rigorously and logically stating in symbolic terms interrelationships in either a static or a dynamic system.[M5] Its advantages are that all variables are specifically stated and that the system is a totally controlled one. Its disadvantages are that relevance is always questionable and that the phenomena being studied are often very complex and therefore the models tend to be complex and difficult for many to understand.

SECTION 4
METHODS OF DATA PRESENTATION, ANALYSIS, AND COMPARISON

THE NEED FOR STATISTICAL METHODS

Human populations are heterogeneous. There are immense differences between individuals, and these are reflected in differences in their susceptibility to disease, their ability to recover, and their response to treatment. No single surgeon, not even an entire team, sees more than a very small proportion of the population of individuals with a given condition. Yet, the practical aim of research is to use the available information, which has been gathered using small samples of subjects, to design and test treatment and to determine and predict results that will be applicable to an entire present or future population.

For example, a standard surgical method for replacing heart valves has a new competitor that its advocates claim is more successful. In order to investigate this, two groups of patients are operated on, using one of the methods for each group. The standard method has a failure rate of 40%, while the new method has a failure rate of 20%. As a record of actual events, these figures are unassailable. The problem lies in extrapolating from the sample to the entire population of valve replacement patients. Perhaps the new method is indeed better and will result in fewer failures if it is applied generally, perhaps the difference occurred merely because the patients in the second group were by chance more robust (fewer incremental risk factors), or perhaps some combination of these causes was operating.

For the results of surgical research to be meaningful, methods are required for inferring, from the results of treatments performed on a sample of patients, what might occur if similar treatments were broadly applied to a larger population of such individuals. The usual assumption is that the sample has been chosen at random from the population, and misleading inferences are made if such an assumption is untrue. This assumption has an important implication. If there has been formal or informal screening (or selection) of subjects entering a sample or study, the conclusions reached apply only to those patients who would pass the screening. Any extension of the results to a larger, less selected population requires additional information.

Where there are simple, well-defined questions to answer, such as whether one failure rate is really smaller than another, the statistical techniques are simple and fairly intuitive. Indeed, as evidence mounts, formal application of statistical techniques often becomes unnecessary. However, in cardiac surgery, information is of necessity often sought about complex relationships from information gathered from a relatively small number of patients. The statistical techniques necessary to do this are sophisticated and difficult to understand, and they make many assumptions about the processes involved. If not at least approximately true, these assumptions could result in erroneous conclusions. Statistical methods enable the making of a number of different types of inferential statements about the nature of a population from sample information. None of these statements describes the nature of the population with certainty and precision, because a degree of uncertainty is inherent when sampling from diversity.

The language of probability (''what might occur'') requires a few comments. When it is said that the probability of success for a valve replacement operation is 80%, it simply means that if the same operation was performed on a large group of patients similar to the sample studied, 80% of the operations would be successful and 20% would not. What is random is the particular individuals in whom the treatment will fail, for our state of knowledge from these data alone is insufficiently advanced for us to identify from these data alone *which* patients will experience treatment failure. One goal of surgical research is the reduction of this degree of uncertainty as to which patient will experience surgical failure by relating failure or success to other measured characteristics of the patient (incremental risk factors) in order to divide the population into more homogeneous subgroups in which the failure rate is either very close to zero or very close to one. Identifying where failures occur can be useful for decision making and may be an important step toward identifying the causes of failure.

While the surgeon generally cannot truly understand or evaluate statistical methods, the programmable hand-held calculator provides a ready means of analyzing data. Some useful programs for such analyses appear in Appendix 6B. Properly used, these calculators allow the surgeon to make quick and rather precise comparisons and evaluations of either published data or data from the surgeon's own experience and research. The use of such an instrument requires some understanding of methods of analysis and presentation of data, if only for the selection of the program appropriate for the job at hand. In part, this chapter is designed to fill that need and to make the surgeon aware of the fundamental assumptions underlying each statistical method. The surgeon's use of the programmable hand-held calculator and the information derived from it should be checked and evaluated at appropriate intervals by a colleague in statistics. Furthermore, the surgeon should be prepared to understand the implications and results of more sophisticated analyses made by statisticians and to interact with the statistician in forming inferences, in order that the results of surgical research receive the wisest possible interpretations and the most appropriate applications.

THE MEASURABLE CHARACTERISTICS FOR STATISTICAL ANALYSIS

A measurable characteristic of a subject—for example, age, weight, sex, number of children—is called a *variable* (or random variable or variate). The term is used to indicate the fact that the measurements vary (differ) from individual to individual. Characteristics of a *population,* or group of individuals, are called *parameters.* Parameters generally appear as constants when used in an equation.

SORTING AND TALLYING

A fundamental and often initial feature of exploration and presentation of data is the sorting of data and tallying of results in various forms.[T1] This basic step should, however, be deferred until all the data have been retrieved and verified (see Appendix 6A).

Sorting produces tables with "cells" or "bins." Adding down the columns produces column totals, and adding across, row totals. Together these are called *marginal totals.* Column and row totals should add up to the same number. If not, errors or inconsistencies are present, which must be identified and corrected. Unfortunately, a number of publications emerge with inconsistencies, which indicate lack of scientific rigor and may even raise questions about the author's conclusions.

A different method of sorting, particularly of continuous variables such as age or year of operation, that is sometimes helpful is decile sorting. In this method, the group is arranged in order by the variable and divided into 10 cells, each containing approximately the same number of cases. Within each cell, the proportion dying, or with thromboembolism, or with any other event, is determined. By this technique, trends can sometimes be identified that escaped notice in previous sortings.

PROPORTIONS AND CONFIDENCE LIMITS

In cardiac surgery, proportions, usually expressed as percentages, are used nearly every day to denote the hospital mortality rate for a given procedure, the incidence of complete heart block, the frequency with which saphenous vein grafts close off, or the 5- or 10-year survival rate after valve replacement. However, in the cardiac surgical literature, only recently has the degree of certainty of the proportion itself been expressed.

The inclusion of the degree of certainty implies that the information in scientific publications is not simply a record of achievement but an evaluation of a method in a manner that facilitates comparison of the experience with other experiences and estimation of what can be expected in future samples of the population of patients studied. Such inferences from the data necessitate the use of confidence limits.[N1,N2]

For example, if there is one hospital death in three operations for postinfarction ventricular septal defect (VSD), the proportion of hospital deaths (hospital mortality) was .33 (33%). This *was* the mortality in that experience, looking at it solely as a record of achievement. Likewise, if 10 deaths occurred among 30 such operations, or 100 occurred among 300, the mortality *was* also 33%. More sophistication is required when *inferences* are drawn from these data. Intuitively, there would be more confidence that the *true* or future

risk (experienced in an entire population, not just in the small sample studied) was near 33% on the basis of the experience with 300 operations than on the basis of three operations. Yet intuitively also one knows that *something* has been learned about the true or future risk from only three operations. For example, the true risk is not zero.

The questions "What is the true (or future) risk of the repair of postinfarction VSD?" and "Is the risk with this method higher or lower than that with another method?" are like the question seventeenth-century gamblers asked of the great Galileo, from which emerged the laws of chance,[G1] now known as the *theory of probability.* These laws are believed to apply to all things that can have more than one possible result; things with exactly one result are the limiting case of this theory, having a probability equal to 1, or certainty. More and more scientists believe that nearly all phenomena, including things in the physical world, behave in accordance with the theory of probability.[B21,H4] As has already been indicated, until the incidence of surgical failures is zero, the events and phenomena of cardiac surgery must also be considered to behave in accordance with this theory.

If this theory is applied hypothetically, it can be shown[G1] that if the "true risk" of death in the repair of postinfarction VSD by a method is 33% and samples of three patients are taken repeatedly, then zero deaths among the three would be experienced in 30% of samples taken, are death in 44% of samples, two deaths in 22% of samples and three deaths in 4% of samples. If larger samples are repeatedly taken, the results are less variable. For example, with samples of size 300, although the number of deaths experienced will still be quite variable, the proportion dying will be between 30% and 36% for 70% of samples taken.

Because of this random variability in the sample estimates of risk (the population parameter), it is impossible to estimate the parameter with certainty (that is, to know the true risk) from such sample information. However, the pattern of variability in repeated sampling is well understood, and in most situations it is possible to derive a formula for calculating an interval of values that would contain the parameter for a specified percentage, for example 70% of samples taken. A 70% confidence interval for the parameter (or risk) is obtained by applying this formula to the particular sample data available. The 70% confidence in the resulting interval is derived from the fact that a formula that works 70% of the time has been used; that is, 70% of the time it will contain the true risk. Anyone using 70% confidence intervals should be made aware of the fact that, on average, every third time an interval is calculated from a new sample, it will not contain the true incidence (or risk). Using 50% confidence intervals (limits), this will occur every second time. Users of confidence limits should also be aware of the fact that the confidence limits (intervals) for most proportions are asymmetric, in contrast to standard deviations, which are symmetric.

As the sample increases so that more information is available, the width of the interval decreases. In other words, a more precise estimate is obtained. With a more precise estimate, the observer may be less uncertain where the true parameter lies (what the true risk is). With a less precise estimate, the observer is more uncertain.[D1,J1,N1,N2]

As an extension of the facts relating to confidence intervals, it can be considered useful to express the degree of uncertainty (or certainty) in terms of specific confidence limits, wherein they could be termed *credibility limits*.

In using confidence limits, if great certainty of being correct in estimating a risk is desired, the broader 90% or 95% CLs are chosen, and the observer must compare nonoverlapping 90% or 95% CLs of various methods to be nearly certain that one of the methods is superior. For example, in comparing an extremely simple, satisfactory, and currently used surgical method with a new one that is expensive and complex, 95% CLs should be used to obtain as high a degree of certainty as possible that there is a true difference in results before changing. (A *P* value for the difference of .05 or less should also be sought in such situations as an indicator of a small likelihood that the difference is due to chance.) If, on the other hand, the method being used is complex and not very satisfactory and results are poor, and it is being compared with a very simple and inexpensive new method, a change should be made if there is even a small possibility that improvement will result. In making such a comparison, 50% CLs would be chosen, even though every second time the change is made, it would be to a method with no better true risk. (In such a situation, the change should be made if the *P* value for the difference is less than .2).

Most situations in cardiac surgery at the present seem to lie somewhere between these two extremes, and thus the use of 70% CLs for most comparisons seems reasonable. The interval is relatively narrow (specific), and it is reasonably sure that the truth is within the confidence limits; there is a 30% chance that it will not be. Also, the 70% CLs (actually 68.3% CLs) are equivalent to 1 standard deviation, which is generally used to describe the variability in the mean value of a continuous variable. When the 70% CLs of two proportions do not overlap, the *P* value for the difference between them is generally near .05 and is certainly less than .15. Thus, 70% CLs provide a simple, quick scanning method for use in looking at data or interpreting and comparing results.

Because the phrase *nonoverlapping confidence limits suggest with a stated degree of uncertainty that a difference exists* is cumbersome, the phrase *evident difference* may be used to express the same idea (UAB). Nonoverlapping confidence limits are easily visualized in a nomogram in which the confidence limits are displayed around the value expressing the association between variables. In this context, it can be said, with a stated degree of uncertainty, that the effect of the independent variable compared to a baseline value becomes *evident* at the point where the confidence limits just separate. However, in contrast to evident differences in a contingency table, this point displayed in a nomogram is not easily seen, nor does it appear in an equation. The point at which evident differences appear in equations can, however, be calculated mathematically (see Appendix 6C).

Methods have been developed for calculating the confidence limits for proportions.[B12,B18,B20,W3] These methods require a very large number of computations, and their precise everyday use requires a large computer. Confidence limits that closely approximate these can be easily and rapidly obtained with a programmable hand-held calculator (see Appendix 6B). Approximate confidence limits can also be obtained, less precisely, from one of several nomograms published in statistical texts.[D1]

POPULATION PARAMETERS, SAMPLE ESTIMATES, AND DESCRIPTORS

The word *population* refers to a group of subjects, for example, patients with coronary artery disease. Characteristics of a population are called *parameters*. Generally, the parameters are unknown, and research on samples of patients is undertaken so that important population parameters may be estimated. This section discusses methods of estimating parameters of continuously distributed variables. A more accurate description might be *more or less continuously distributed*, since many scientists argue that nothing in the universe is truly continuous.

The raw data used in estimating parameters are generally not published, because each patient or subject in a study is likely to be unique in regard to continuous variables, making any tabular presentation of the raw data for study or publication generally unwieldy unless the number of patients in the group is quite small. Summarizing statements may be made of the raw data by one of several techniques before the abstract process of estimating parameters begins.

The commonly used summarizing statement of the raw data is contained in a simple table, really a contingency table, described under "Sorting and Tallying." A *histogram* is a plot of such a table (Fig. 6-1*a*). Another method of constructing such a table is decile sorting, also described earlier. An alternative to grouping in "reasonable" groups (e.g., equally spaced) is to divide the patients into various percentiles, stating the value of the variable at these percentiles. The *median* is the fiftieth percentile. For consistency, one might also state the fifteenth and eighty-fifth percentile, for they correspond to 70% confidence limits. More commonly, twenty-fifth and seventy-fifth percentiles or tenth and ninetieth percentiles are used. A *cumulative distribution plot*, produced easily by computer but laboriously by hand, presents all the raw data in percentile form and is a very useful way of looking at it (Fig. 6-1*b*).

The simplest of the *abstract methods* is the *arithmetic average*, or *mean*, which is the summation of all elements in the continuous variable, such as age, pulmonary artery pressure, and so on, divided by the number of people or observations (*n*). The rationale for using the arithmetic average is that it provides an estimate of the *central tendency* of the data set and a characteristic or parameter of the population studied. If the data are distributed perfectly symmetrically, then the arithmetic average is exactly at the midpoint of the data range. It is also the most frequently occurring number (or *mode*), and half the patients are above the value and half below it (the *median*). The mean is the easiest statistic to calculate, since the others require that the data first be sorted. Unfortunately, the mean is not a robust measure of central tendency. If many infants and only one or two adults are in a study, the average age is greatly affected by the few adults. A more robust measure of central tendency is the

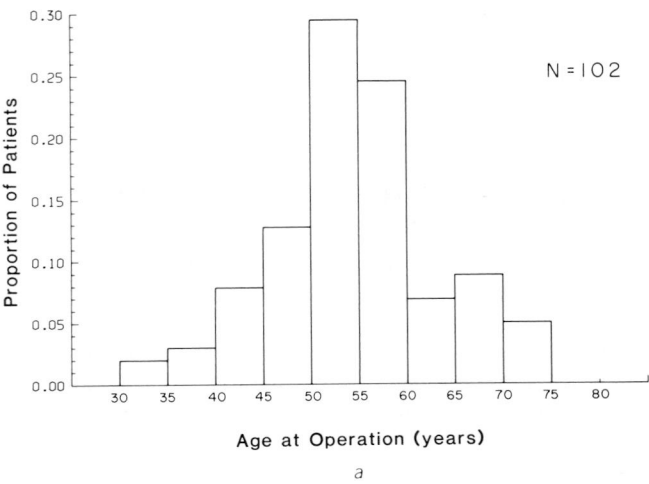

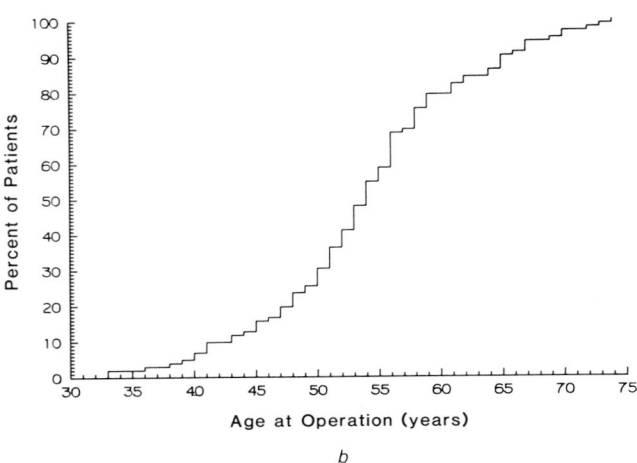

Figure 6-1

(a) Histogram of the age at operation of 102 patients undergoing coronary artery bypass grafting. Approximately 30% of the patients were 50–55 years of age at operation, 25% were 55–60, and lesser percentages of patients were older or younger.

(b) Cumulative distribution plot of the raw data used for Figure 6-1a. Age is shown on the horizontal axis. The vertical axis shows the percent of patients coming to operation at or younger than any given age on the horizontal axis. The vertical axis gives directly the percentile of patients coming to operation by a given age. The median is the fiftieth percentile. The S shape of this particular plot suggests a normal distribution; any other shape would suggest a different distribution.

median. The median is that value below which 50% of the patients lie and above which the other 50% lie.

The necessity for the sample data to be normally distributed for the mean to yield a reliable estimate of central tendency has been stated. This follows from an assumption that the data from the population being studied are symmetrically distributed in a bell-shaped curve. Whether the sample data are normally distributed (Fig. 6-2) may be tested by such statistics as the Shapiro-Wilk W statistic[S2] for a small n (say, 50 or less) and the Kolmogorov-Smirnov D statistic[S3] for

larger samples. The skewness of the data (rightward or leftward asymmetric tail) and their kurtosis (abnormal peakedness) are also tested.

The derivation of averages, or means, was begun by astronomers centuries ago. They thought that the scatter in their data was from observational errors or imprecision, and they used means, or averages, in an attempt to see true trends. Later, Gauss discussed and described the symmetric *normal distribution curve*[G2] (which actually was described by DeMoivre[D2] 300 years ago). An equation describes this curve and can be used to calculate the standard deviation.[G3] It has already been noted that the 70% confidence limits and one standard deviation are essentially the same. But this similarity of confidence limits and standard deviation occurs only when distribution is normal, and since in most proportions the distribution or curve is asymmetric, confidence limits, not standard deviation, must be used for them.

In addition to an estimation of the population mean, some measure of the *dispersion* (variance or spread) of the population is needed. This is used to determine whether an individual is "within the limits of normal" and is necessary for comparison statistics. One such measure is the standard deviation. The *standard deviation* refers to the variability from subject to subject, or the variability of individuals within the sample, or population. The standard deviation from the mean of an individual regarding a particular measured variable (commonly called Z) is often useful in cardiac surgery. This is calculated from the difference between the measurement for the individual and the mean value divided by the standard deviation. It may be a negative or positive value and has no units.

The *standard error* is a measure of the reliability with which the population mean is estimated from the sample mean, and it is needed for comparing one group to another. It is more appropriately, but infrequently, called the *standard deviation of the mean* and is obtained simply by dividing the standard deviation by the square root of n.

Other methods are available for expressing data that are skewed (not normally distributed). One is to resort to a purely *nonparametric* (without equations, coefficients, etc.)[F3,H1] description of the data (for example, using the median and its various percentiles). Another is to *transform* the data into a more normally distributed variable.[T1] For example, a logarithmic transformation is often useful, the resultant mean being called a *geometric mean*.

P VALUES

Use of the P value in making conclusions, inferences, and decisions under conditions of uncertainty is a relatively recent development in science. Its emergence was in large part the result of the need of biological scientists to examine the uncertainties generated by Darwin's *Origin of the Species*.[P1] P values, then, are almost a phenomenon of the twentieth century and have come into general use in the medical sciences only since about 1945.

In making inferences (or drawing conclusions) from data, a hypothesis is usually being tested. Generally, this involves testing the null hypothesis, which is that two data sets, for

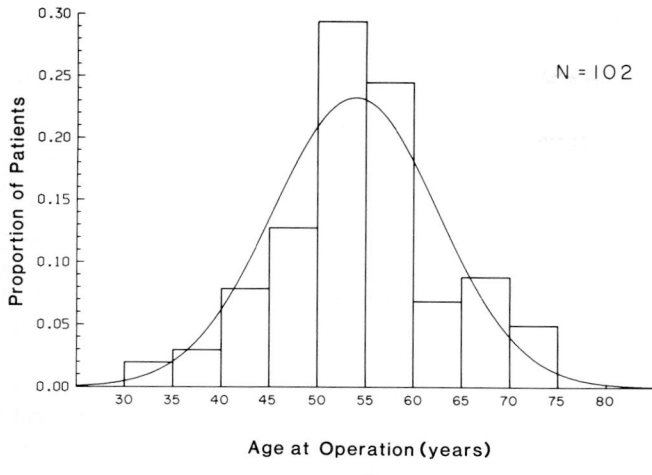

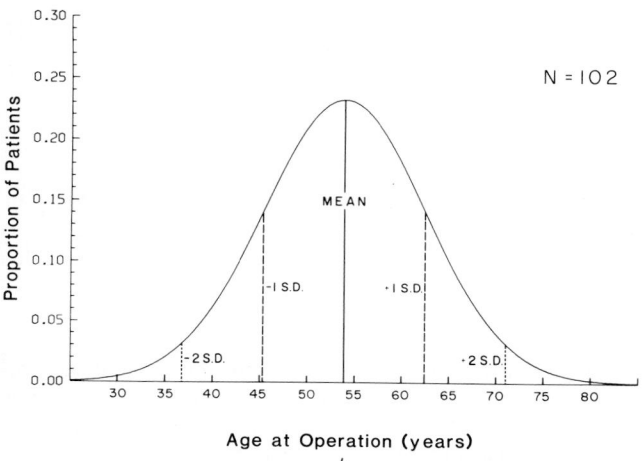

Figure 6-2

(a) The normal distribution curve fitted to the data in Figure 6-1. (b) Shown are the mean ± 1 and 2 standard deviations (SD). The point of inflection of the curve from concave to convex is 1 SD.

Table 6-1 Interpretation of P values, illustrating the proper use of symbols of inequality. Each P value can be unambiguously located in one of the four lines of the table. The top line contains all P values < .05. The fourth, or bottom, line contains all P values ≥ .2. The second line embraces all P values ≥ .05 but < .1.

P value		Interpretation of Null Hypothesis	Inferences about the Difference
≤	<		
	.05	Nearly certainly not true	Unlikely to be due to chance
.05---	.1	Probably not true	Probably not due to chance
.1---	.2	Possibly not true	Possibly not due to chance
.2		True	Likely to be due to chance

example, are not different. The P value is a measure of the evidence against the null hypothesis, and the smaller the P value, the greater the evidence against it.

In testing hypotheses, an incorrect conclusion (inference) can be made by rejecting the null hypothesis when it is true (type I error). An incorrect inference can also be made by not rejecting the null hypothesis when it is false (type II error). The null hypothesis is frequently rejected in laboratory and clinical investigations when P values are less than .05, and such P values indicate that the differences are unlikely to be due to chance. Alternatively, in clinical studies the null hypothesis may be rejected with P values up to .20 (UAB). The argument for this is primarily a desire to minimize type II errors, particularly since in clinical studies the use of too stringent criteria for rejecting the null hypothesis can lead to premature discounting of possibly important associations. In any event, rather than using < .05 or *"significant versus not significant,"* the explicit P value may

be stated and used evidentially in order to indicate the degree of certainty with which the null hypothesis is rejected (UAB) (Table 6-1). This is a practice of many statisticians[K4] and has become easy with the availability of hand-held calculators.

In clinical and laboratory medical research, the use of P values involves the following steps:[B4,D1]

1. The data samples are examined, including inspection of the confidence limits in the case of proportions and standard deviations or standard errors in the case of continuous variables (see "Population Parameters, Sample Estimates, and Descriptors").

2. The estimates of the parameters of the relevant data distributions are examined.

3. A null hypothesis or hypotheses and alternative hypotheses are proposed (e.g., the null hypothesis could be that the hospital mortality is no different with or without cardioplegia; and the alternative hypothesis could be that it is lower with cardioplegia).

4. A test statistic (an intermediate step in obtaining the P value) is calculated, which measures the distance (or interval or difference) between the parameters implied by the null hypothesis and the estimates of the parameters from the data.

5. Since a test statistic has a distribution, just as do population parameters, a determination can be made of the probability (P value) that a given test statistic is at least as extreme in relationship to (that is, as far from) the central tendency of the test statistic were the null hypothesis true as is the corresponding confidence interval. For this, the distance of the specific test statistic from that of the null hypothesis is determined in terms of the confidence interval. The area remaining in the more extreme portion of the curve is the P value.

6. On the basis of the P value, a decision is made whether to reject the null hypothesis, and, in the case of rejection, the degree of certainty of the decision is noted ($< 1 - P$).

7. Then a conclusion, or inference, is made on the basis of the decision.

In the case of a simple hypothesis, when the alternative hypothesis involves a change in only one direction (i.e., A is less than B), a one-tailed P value is used. When the alternative hypothesis involves a change in either direction (i.e., *A* is different than *B*), a two-tailed *P* value is used. The latter is used in this book unless otherwise stated.

The specific *P* value to be used in a decision-making process involving several alternatives (e.g., in patient care) should vary according to the circumstances, just as the confidence limits used for this process should vary (see ''Proportions and Confidence Limits''). For example, when one form of treatment (such as primary repair in infancy) is judged to be relatively inexpensive and expeditious treatment and is compared with an alternative treatment that is only a little less ideal in these regards (such as two-stage repair), the ideal treatment (one-stage repair) is desired unless the alternative treatment has a lower hospital mortality. A comparison is made of hospital mortality after the two forms of treatment. The null hypothesis is that the mortalities are the same. If the alternative treatment has a lower overall hospital mortality, it would be chosen if there is any reasonable possibility that this difference is not due to chance, since human life is at stake and the cost etc. of the two methods are similar. Thus, it could be chosen if the *P* value for the difference is, for example, < .2. However, when the alternative treatment is extremely expensive and requires a very prolonged course of treatment, it would be chosen only when it is unlikely that the difference is due to chance and nearly certain that the alternative treatment is safer, and thus it would be chosen only if the *P* value for the difference were < .05 (Table 6-1).

One of the most common situations in cardiac surgery in which *P* values are desired is the *simple contingency table*, in which two or more proportions are compared. The standard test is the *chi-square test*, which is appropriate when the sample size is large[B22] (see Appendix 6B). For practical purposes, when the number of events is two or less and the sample size or *n* (denominator) is small (< 100), Fisher's exact test is used[F7] (see Appendix 6B). In this situation, some investigators use corrected forms of the chi-square test[C7,C8,L3,L4,Y1] or other types of tests.[S5] When the contingency table contains more than two proportions for an ordered variable (such as NYHA functional class, pedal pulses, number of distal coronary anastomoses), additional insight is obtained by a logistic regression test for trend.[C9,R2]

When the comparison is between two continuous variables, their mean and standard errors are computed, and Student's *t* test is used for the comparison[S4] (see Appendix 6B). Since one of the assumptions in the *t* test is that the variability of the two distributions is equal, in practice this assumption is always tested by an *F* test[W4,W5] (see Appendix 6B). If the variability is found to be unequal, the Welch modification of the *t* test is used[W4,W5] (see Appendix 6B).

In some situations, a comparison is made between continuous variables in the same individual before and after some event or intervention. For this, the paired *t* test is used. In practice, the difference between each pair of observations is determined, and a mean difference ($\bar{x}$) and its standard error (SE) are calculated. The ratio of the mean divided by its standard error is used in a *t* test (see Appendix 6B).

When more than two means are being compared, an overall procedure can be used to test the hypothesis that all the means are similar. An analysis of variance is used to test the overall hypothesis (rather than using multiple two-sampled *t* tests, which introduces a large risk of falsely rejecting the null hypothesis[G7]). Additional special tests for contrasts among the means are made by such tests as Duncan's new multiple-range test.[D3]

P values are also obtained for the coefficients of multivariate linear and nonlinear regression equations.[E4,H7] In essence, these *P* values are obtained by a test that the parameter of interest is zero. In nonlinear regression equations, such as the logistic and Cox equations, the *P* values are obtained with the assumption that the *n* is infinitely large. They must therefore be used with caution.

P values as well as confidence limits (see ''Proportions and Confidence Limits'') can be used to identify ''evident differences,'' a different use of the *P* value than in the identification of the significance of a parameter. For example, once age has been identified as a risk factor, the surgeon may wish to know, with some stated degree of uncertainty, at what age, or point, old age evidently increases the risk of hospital death after valve replacement. The identification of this point with nonoverlapping confidence limits has already been described. Using confidence limits is probably the simplest and most direct method, requiring fewer assumptions than does the use of *P* values, but some prefer the use of *P* values. This method is similar to doing an analysis of contrasts following an analysis of variance. The details of the calculation for this use of *P* values are described in Appendix 6C.

One of the assumptions behind the calculation of the *P* value under many circumstances is that the test statistic is normally distributed. When this is not the case, it may be possible to transform the variable into one that results in a normally distributed test statistic or to use an appropriate alternative distribution for the test statistics. If such solutions are not possible, so-called nonparametric tests may be used to generate *P* values.[K5,W6]

NUMBERS

Since both hand-held calculators and large computers generate numerical information in the form of many digits, it is necessary to know how properly to compact and express (display) numerical data. Numerical data should be expressed in such a way as to connote its accuracy and its reproducibility. *Accuracy* is lack of systematic bias from the truth. *Reproducibility*, or precision, implies a narrow range of variability.

The way in which numerical results are expressed has certain implications. Thus, 493 implies that the precision, or reproducibility, and accuracy are such that the result is somewhere between 492.5 and 493.5. Similarly, 492.8 implies that the result is somewhere between 492.75 and 492.85, and 492.76 implies that the result is somewhere between 492.755 and 492.765. Thus, a numerical result is ordinarily interpreted as being accurate and reproducible within one-half unit of the last (rightmost) significant figure given.

In the number 493, the 4 is the first significant figure. The first *significant figure* is the first nonzero figure on the left side of the number. In this example, it is in the hundreds place. The *place* is the relationship of the number to the decimal point. The units place is the first to the left of the decimal point, the tens the second, the hundreds the third, and so on. The tenth place is the first to the right, the hundredth the second, and so on. In 0.04928, the 4 is still in the first significant figure but is in the hundredth place. The significant figure is independent of the decimal place.

In computation and computer storage, all digits should be retained. For displaying numbers, they should be rounded off so as to imply correctly their precision, or reproducibility.[E2] There are certain generally agreed upon rules for rounding off, although they are not easily found in print. The first step is the calculation of the standard error of the mean value or proportion. The place of the first significant figure of the standard error is determined. Then the mean or proportion is rounded off to that place. The same place is saved in confidence limits. One additional place is saved in the standard error (because the usual ± expression of the standard error is a form of shorthand, and saving the extra place helps in using the standard error to calculate the confidence limits). Exceptions to this are as follows: (1) if the first significant figure of the standard error is 1, then one additional place is saved; and (2) within a single contingency table, consistency in saving figures is desirable, so all numbers are rounded off to the place indicated by the majority of the numbers.

Rounding off, or removing nonsignificant places, is done as follows.[C3] If the numeral in the first place beyond (to the right of) the figure to be rounded off is greater than 5, round the figure up one and drop all other figures to the right. If this numeral is less than 5, simply drop it and all other figures to the right. If it is exactly 500 . . . 0, round up if the last significant figure is odd, and round down if it is even.

Numbers are often presented in tabular form indicating the distribution of data (e.g., patients or events) between the extremes of a continuous variable. Such tables should be prepared so that the positioning of any point along the continuous variable can be unambiguously determined. In this text, intervals between the extremes of the continuous variable are indicated by symbols of inequality. For example, in Table 6-1, any *P* value can be unambiguously located in one of the intervals indicated. This method of presentation is mathematically conventional.

AGES OF PATIENTS

In very young patients particularly, imprecise presentation of age can lead to erroneous conclusions. The problem lies in the fact that *1 month of age* means 28 days if the month is February, 30 if it is September, and 31 if it is July. Precise definition is possible by using the Julian date to calculate age in days given the data of birth and the date of event. The interval between any two events can be similarly calculated[F6] (see Appendix 6B). The day is the basic measure of

Table 6-2 The use of days to calculate months and years.

Time Period (days)	Time Period (months)	Time Period (years)
≤ <	≤ <	≤ <
30	1	1/12
30--- 91	1--- 3	1/12---3/12
91---182	3--- 6	3/12---6/12
182---365	6---12	6/12---1
365---730	12---24	1---2
730	24	2

time, and age in months or years is derived from age in days (Table 6-2). A *year* is defined as 365.2425 days. A *month* is defined as 365.2425/12, or 30.44, days.

MULTIVARIATE ANALYSIS

Multivariate analysis is a process in which all possible variables (theoretically, at least) related to an event or another variable are simultaneously examined to determine the combination that best explains (or is best related to) that event or other variable.[D4,L7] The importance of examining variables jointly rather than singly is well discussed by Breslow and Day.[B28] In this process, variables found to be not related to the event or other variable are dropped (the law of parsimony).[C6] The strength of the effect of each variable among the least number of common denominators and its significance (the degree of certainty that the variable is related to the event or other variable) are determined in relation to all other variables in the model. Because fitting such models is a trial-and-error process that is much more an art than a science, it should be pursued with a statistician.[H2] The search is for a good model that adequately explains most of the events or other variables. It is to be emphasized that these processes identify associations, not causal relationships.

Multivariate analysis models are generally empirical and additive in order to be mathematically tractable. Thus,

$$z = \beta_0 x_0 + \beta_1 x_1 + \cdots \beta_n x_n \qquad (6\text{-}1)$$

where z is the event or other variable or some special transformation of it, β is a regression coefficient (relating to the strength of the association), and x is a variable. The additive nature of the model assumes a certain type of symmetry in the effects of the explanatory variables. Often a better fit can be obtained if several of the variables are transformed, or measured on a different scale, for example, a logarithmic scale. New variables may have to be introduced that represent an interaction (multiplication) of one variable with another. For example, the effect of aortic cross-clamp time may be greater for older patients than for younger patients. Since these are empirical models, some test for lack of fit of the model to the data should be used (see Appendix 6D).

Although multivariate analysis is a very sophisticated analytical tool, the advantages to experienced groups of using it in the very early stages of the analysis of complex clinical problems in cardiac surgery are becoming apparent. The

Table 6-3 An example of tabular presentation of the logistic equation: incremental risk factors for hospital death after repair of AV septal defects (51 deaths among 310 patients).

Incremental Risk Factors	Logistic Coefficient ± SD	P Value
Date of operation (mo from 1/1/67)	−0.033 ± 0.0069	< .0001
Age at operation (mo)	−0.047 ± 0.0165	.004
Interaction of age with date of operation	0.00029 ± 0.000108	.008
Increasing severity of preoperative AV valve incompetence (0–5)	0.5 ± 0.22	.03
Increasing level of disability (NYHA class I–V)	0.9 ± 0.27	.001
Interventricular communication present	1.4 ± 0.50	.005
Presence of accessory valve orifice	1.8 ± 0.73	.01
Intercept	−2.0 ± 0.52	

SOURCE: Reproduced with permission from Studer et al.[S6]
KEY: SD, standard deviation; AV, atrioventricular.

variables to be analyzed must be selected according to a well-conceived plan by experienced senior investigators with clear concepts about the purposes of the analyses. The subsequent construction of simple contingency tables of variables found to be significant is one way of displaying the association of variables with an event by using raw data.

The methods for multivariate analysis of cardiac surgical data should result in equations that can be plotted as relatively simple nomograms. The immediate usability of Table 6-3, for example, is limited in considering the effects of age and date of operation on hospital mortality. In contrast, a nomogram (Fig. 6-3) makes it clear that the results have improved with time and that there is an interaction between age and date of operation such that in earlier years young age increased the risk but in recent years it did not.

Multivariate regression equations may be linear or nonlinear. In the former type, the coefficients are calculated directly from the data. In the latter, the coefficients are determined by an iterative procedure (a repetitive procedure in which an initial "guess" is made, then another, and then another, each being tested for goodness of fit to the data until the best fit or explanation of the data is obtained). The advent of the high-speed computer has made nonlinear regression analysis practicable.

A special and useful kind of multivariate regression analytic tool that requires a nonlinear fitting procedure is logistic analysis[B13,B14,B15,W1] (see Appendix 6D). Generally, as used in cardiac surgery, the probability of an event in a population (e.g., in-hospital death) is related to one or more variables. These variables can be continuous or discrete (e.g., total circulatory arrest: yes or no) or mixtures of the two. As indicated earlier, the implication is that results of cardiac surgery for an individual are to date *probabilistic* and follow the theory of probability (laws of chance). The more the determinants of the event under study are known, however, the less remains to be explained by chance. Also, the more infrequent are surgical failures (hospital death, saphenous vein bypass closure, and so forth) the more deterministic the situation becomes.

The nomogram of the logistic equation (Fig. 6-4) portrays relationships that are familiar to the cardiac surgeon and intuitively easily grasped.[K3] That is to say, as logit units are added (e.g., as minutes of aortic cross-clamp time accumulate or NYHA functional class increases), their effect on probability varies according to the starting position on the logit curve. Thus, if the relative absence of incremental risk factors places a person far to the left on the logit curve of Figure 6-4, the addition of 10 more minutes of cross-clamp time (1 logit unit) increases the risk only slightly. In contrast, if other risk factors place the patient at − 1 on the logit scale, the addition of 1 logit unit (e.g., 10 more minutes of cross-clamp time) increases the risk by 23%. In other words, the addition of 1 logit unit here has a much more powerful effect on the probability than it does farther to the left on the logit curve. This is the straw that breaks the camel's back.

Multivariate analysis is currently applied most commonly to the individual phases of time-related events (UAB) (see section on "Parametric Methods," under "Analysis of Time-Related Events").

ANALYSIS OF TIME-RELATED EVENTS

Analysis of time-related events (death, thromboembolic episodes, reoperation, freedom from symptoms, etc.) requires additional methods.[E3,G4] For complete understanding, multivariate methods are also required for determining incremental risk factors for the various time-phases of these time-related events. For the analysis of time-related events, abstractions by actuarial methods, logistic analysis, and parametric methods are generally used.

However, the raw data can be presented by a simple method (e.g., a crude life table or reduced sample method). For example, such a method begins with counting all the patients who have survived for a specific interval after an operation, say, 5 years. This number is then added to the total number of patients who died before that interval. Thus is obtained the denominator of the desired proportion, the numerator being the number of patients who have survived that interval. In this method, patients lost to follow-up in earlier years are not usable and thus are wasted, as are those operated upon less than 5 years ago. Since in any analysis each survival time period is composed in part of a different set of patients, nonsensical results can be obtained (e.g., 10-year survival may be higher than 5-year survival). The limitations of this method make it generally unsuitable, and it should rarely be used.

Actuarial Methods

Although cardiac surgeons now commonly use actuarial methods in studying their long-term results, they were introduced to the surgical literature by Berkson only in 1950.[B5] The method itself, however, is very old and dates back to Halley, in England, in 1693.[H2] Actuarial methods do not present raw data and are based on certain assumptions.[E3] Such methods have been most commonly used to estimate freedom from death (survival).

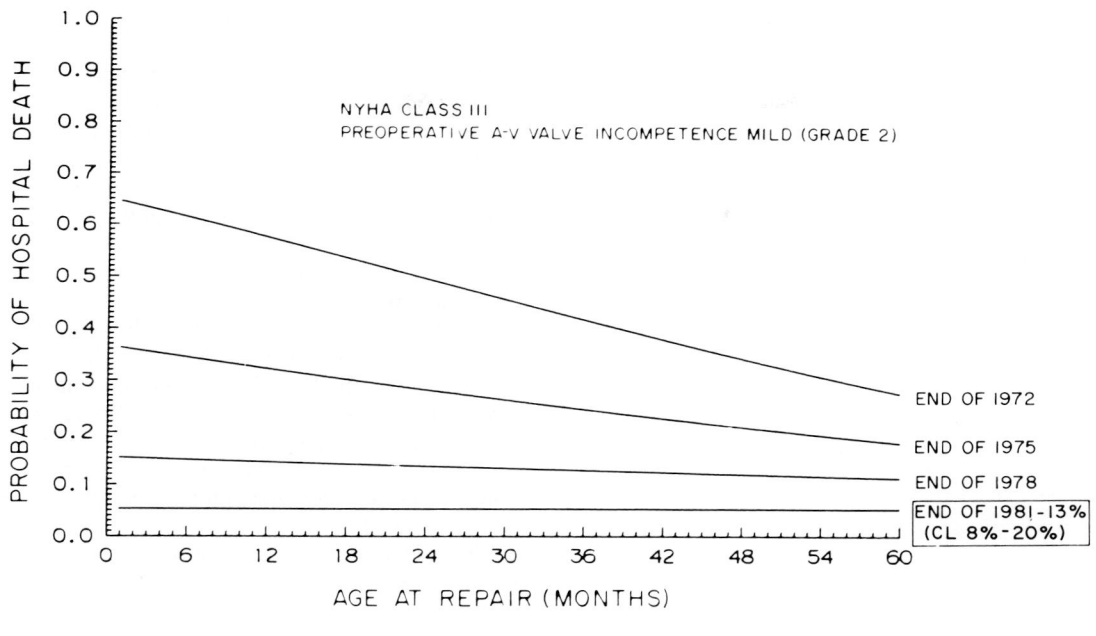

a

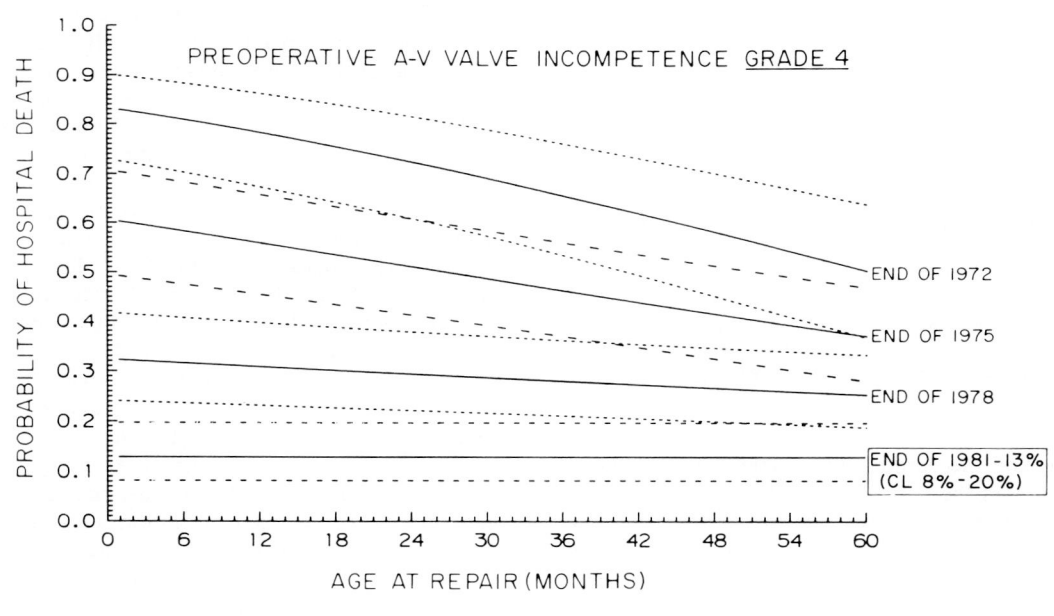

b

Figure 6-3 Examples of the useful plots that can be generated by some methods of multivariate analysis.

(*a*) Nomogram from the logistic equation in Table 6-3, for patients with interventricular communication with mild to moderate (grade 2) AV valve incompetence, no major associated cardiac anomaly, no accessory AV valve orifice, and NYHA class III preoperative status. Note: CL = 70% confidence limits.

(*b*) Nomogram for similar patients with severe (grade 4) AV valve incompetence. Dashed and dotted lines enclose the 70% confidence limits.

Reproduced with permission from Studer et al.[S6]

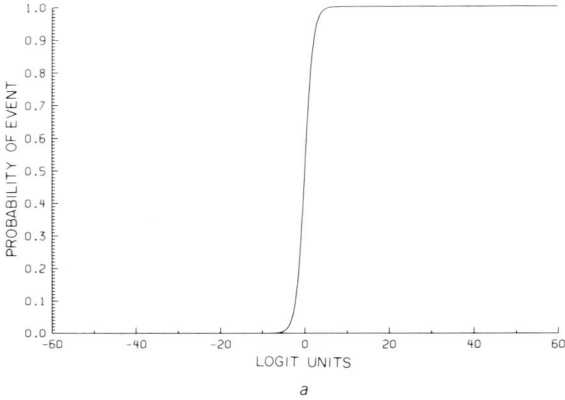

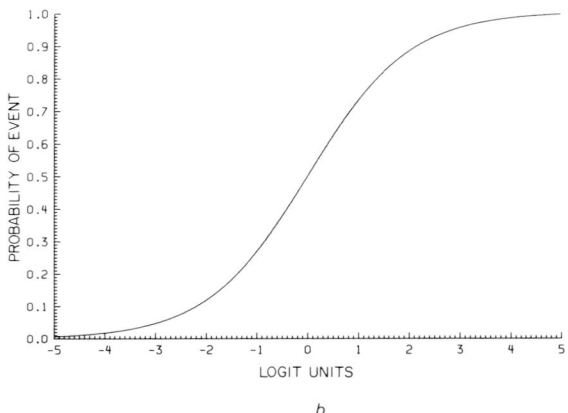

Figure 6-4 Nomograms of the logistic equation $P = 1/(1 + e^{-z})$. (a) The nomogram is presented with ± 60 logit units along the horizontal axis. The equation and the nomogram indicate a specific probability for each specific total logit unit.
(b) Nomogram of the same equation portrayed with ± 5 logit units along the horizontal axis. The same specific probability is denoted by each specific total logit unit, and the relationship between the two as portrayed in the nomogram only seems to be different.

In contrast to the crude life table, the actuarial method[B5,M2] uses all the patients, and thus all the information, in its calculations of survival. In this method, the time interval is subdivided, often into years. The probability of the occurrence of an event during each subdivision is calculated. The numerator is the number of patients experiencing the event during the period; the denominator is the number of patients entering the period (and thus exposed to risk during the period). Patients entering the subdivision who are untraced ("censored") after entering the interval are *assumed* to be at risk for one-half the interval. Thus, the denominator is the number of patients actually entering the interval minus half the number of patients censored. In the case of late death, the probability of surviving within the interval is 1.0 minus the probability of experiencing the event. Actuarial survival to the end of the total interval is calculated as the product of the probability of surviving all the preceding intervals. Thus, if there is 90% probability of surviving the first 5 years and 80% probability of surviving the 5- to 10-year interval, the probability of being alive after 10 years is 90% times 80%, or 72%.

More recently, Kaplan and Meier have reintroduced the product limit method of actuarial analysis,[B6,K2] which is applicable to small samples[K1] (see Appendix 6E). With this method, a new estimate of the probability of the event is made at that point in time when the event occurred, rather than at arbitrary subdivisions of time. The calculations are the same as for the actuarial method, except that the numerator is now generally only one patient, and the denominator is that number of patients who have not experienced the event and yet have been followed to that point in time. No estimate is possible after the last event, even though a large number of individuals may have been traced a long time thereafter. It is usual in graphic presentations to indicate this by extending a properly identified dashed line beyond the last event. It is also useful to indicate at various points along the actuarial plot the number of patients still being followed.

The degree of uncertainty of the actuarial estimate should be indicated. The traditional way of expressing the uncertainty is presenting the standard deviation of the estimate[G8] (standard error). However, since the actuarial estimate is a proportion, confidence limits are a more appropriate measure of the degree of uncertainty (see Appendix 6E).[A2,C4]

An operation can be said to result in a cure when the survival after the operation is the same as that of the general population matched with the patient group as to age, sex, and race. The data for the general population are readily obtained from population life tables and are considered so reliable that they have no confidence limits. By using some measure of uncertainty of the survival of patients, it can be determined whether survival is the same or different from that of the general population.[O1,P4] This method can of course be criticized but is useful[C10] (see Appendix 6F).

Actuarial methods have been used to express time-related events other than survival, such as prosthetic valve endocarditis, re-replacement of prosthetic devices, thromboembolism, and so forth. These results are generally presented as "free from" the event, although they can be presented as incidence by simply subtracting the actuarial estimate from 1. In these analyses, great care must be exercised in the clear definition of the event in question and the time at which patients not experiencing the event are considered untraced for it. For example, a patient dying without having experienced a thromboembolic event must be considered untraced after the date of death.

Actuarial analyses can be made of *compound* events, such as death *or* thromboembolism, rather than single ones.[D5] A patient is said to experience a compound event on the earliest date of occurrence of one of the events being considered. Such an analysis is generally presented as a complication-free rate. This concept has been used by Grunkemeier and colleagues[G12] in their presentation of cumulative complication-free curves. In such a representation, a series of compound-event actuarial curves (only the first event is single) is constituted in hierarchical order (generally starting with the most serious complication) and presented in a single graph in which all events add up (cumulate) to 100%. The choice of which cumulative complication-free series of curves to present depends on the purpose of the analysis.

Actuarial methods are inadequate for exploring the risk factors affecting survival. The best that can be done is to divide patients into subgroups, separately analyze the survival curves, and then compare them. This works reasonably well for dichotomous (yes-no) variables and ordered variables (e.g., NYHA classes I–V). An analysis of overlapping 70% confidence limits can then be used to examine differences between these curves. Alternatively, differences in the slopes of the survival curves can be described by a P value;[G5,M3,M4,P2,P3] a plot comparing P value and time is also possible,[F4] the P value between two actuarial curves being obtained at a number of points in time in the follow-up period (see Appendix 6B).

Logistic Analysis

Logistic analysis is most naturally applied to determine incremental risk factors for a yes-no time-related event at a particular point in time.[W1] Examples of such factors are periprosthetic leakage at any time in the follow-up period, survival for 5 years, heterograft degeneration within 10 years, and so forth. The methods are similar to those described previously.

Parametric Methods

Frustrations with the limitations of the actuarial and logistic methods have led to efforts to develop other parametric and semiparametric methods for the analysis and presentation of data concerned with time-related events.[B7,B8,C5,E3] Parametric methods have been used for such purposes in industry for some time to describe the life history of light bulbs, transistors, and so forth.[B9] However, the determination of risk factors has generally not been incorporated into the industrial models.

The proportional hazards linear model developed by Cox[C5] approaches the need for risk factor analysis of late results by generalizing the actuarial method to incorporate a parametric model of risk factors.[B12,C5,K1] It is based on the hazard function (discussed below). In the Cox model, an attempt is made to relate the hazard for a particular individual to incremental risk factors (see Appendix 6G). The time-related events are still presented actuarially (nonparametrically), and no inferences can be made about the shapes of their functions.

More recently, parametric methods to describe both the time-related event and incremental risk factors have been described for each time phase.[B29,H3,K1,T2,T3] These methods have become more important as it has become apparent that not all early deaths after cardiac surgery occur in the hospital but, rather, some occur in the early weeks after hospital dismissal. Emphasis must shift to analyses of the late results of cardiac surgery. By parametric analysis, a *survivorship function*, $S(t)$, which is similar to the traditional actuarial representation of the time-related event, can be calculated.[G4]

A *hazard function*, $\lambda(t)$, which is the instantaneous risk of an event's occurring in individuals not yet experiencing the event, can also be calculated (for example, see Chapter 7, Fig. 7-13). The hazard function is expressed as incidence per unit of time (usually the unit of time selected is the unit plotted on the horizontal axis), although the calculation is of instantaneous risk. (Analogously, instantaneous speed can be expressed as miles per hour.) The common practice in the surgical literature of presenting time-related events in terms of risk per patient-year assumes a constant hazard function, but the calculation supporting this is rarely made.

A first step in the parametric analysis is the plotting of cumulative hazard function from the negative logarithm of the actuarial curve.[B29,N3] Visual inspection of the cumulative hazard function plot may indicate one, two, or more phases. Mathematical models are derived to describe the resultant curve[B10,B11,H3,T2,T3] or its separate phases.[B8,B29,K11] Then, using the original data, coefficients and their degree of uncertainty in the mathematical models derived are estimated. Survivorship function and hazard function for the data set can now be calculated or plotted (an example is in the paper by Ivert and colleagues[I1]). Application of the proportional hazards concept of the Cox method to the parametric analysis allows identification of risk factors for each phase.[B29,H3]

The multivariate analysis for risk factors in time-related events is made simultaneously for each phase of the hazard function.[B29] The general methods are those described under "Multivariate Analysis." They are similar to the methods used in multivariate logistic analysis of the probability of an event and in the Cox proportional hazards model.

SECTION 5
DECISION MAKING FOR INDIVIDUAL PATIENTS

When cardiac surgery is advised, it is in anticipation of cure or palliation. In either case, operation should be advised only when life expectancy and functional capacity are better with operation than without. Thus, each patient care decisions involves a comparison, and ideally the comparison should be made with full knowledge of the degree of uncertainty imposed by the available data and their analysis. In fact, one goal of research is the provision of this information for decision making in as many areas of cardiac surgery as possible and with as high a degree of certainty as is possible.

When patients fall within well-defined categories for which reliable information is available, individual patient care decisions can be made largely on the basis of prior appropriate comparisons of the options. That is, the option can be chosen that has been shown to result in the lowest hospital mortality, the highest long-term survival, the least incidence of reoperation, and so on in patients like the one under consideration. One of the major goals of this text is the presentation of data in such a form that it can be used in such a way for individual patient care decisions. For this method to be applicable, the patient being considered must be like those for whom the options have been studied, and the options being considered must be those that have been studied and not ones merely similar to them.

When reliable information is not available or the patient or options being considered are different from those that have been studied, the same principles can be used, but only anecdotal information, judgments, and general knowledge of the area are available as a basis for the decision. Obviously, the degree of uncertainty is considerably greater. In such situations, a prospective clinical study of some type is needed to generate the information desired.

Some surgical failures are related to inadequacies of the decision-making process about the individual patient, either as a result of human error or of lack of scientific progress. For example, the decision not to operate on a patient in whom the risks and unknown factors without operation are known to be significantly greater than those with operation is a human error. To operate on a patient in whom an early fatal outcome after surgery is known with considerable certainty to be inevitable is also an error.

In most places in the world today, the resources available for cardiac surgery are insufficient for the surgical treatment of every patient potentially amenable to this kind of intervention. Thus, a process of *triage* (the sorting process used by military surgeons during combat) is consciously or unconsciously used, in which the resources are allocated for patients most likely to benefit from treatment. Recently, this process has come to be termed *cost containment.*[B16] Again, such decisions are best made when the potential benefits can be described factually and with knowledge of the degree of uncertainty attached to the conclusions. The special circumstances of each patient and the need for continued probing into the possibility and methods of extending and improving the results of cardiac surgery must also form part of each patient care decision.

SECTION 6
IMPROVING THE RESULTS OF CARDIAC SURGERY

When an individual surgeon or an institution is dissatisfied with the early or late results of surgical therapy, either in general or under specific conditions, then programmatic decisions should be made with the goal of improving the results. Generally, six steps are involved in a long-range program to improve surgical results:

1. Determine the degree of certainty that current results in the program under study are less than optimal (compared to those achieved by others or those theoretically possible). Confidence limits and *P* values are among the statistics useful in expressing the degree of certainty.

2. Determine incremental risk factors for the undesired event (factors associated with surgical failure or with increased difficulty of obtaining a good result).

3. Determine the true causes of the surgical failures. In gen-

eral, surgical failures are caused by a lack of scientific progress or by human error, but the specific lacks and errors must be pinpointed so that programs can be planned to overcome them.

4. Plan new research and development. Knowledge of incremental risk factors and of the true causes of surgical failures, along with general scientific knowledge related to cardiac surgery, should enable the planning of new research and development to improve results in the future.

5. Meantime, use knowledge of results and incremental risk factors to develop new interim patient management protocols based on available information.

6. When new knowledge has resulted from step 4, develop new patient management protocols and prospectively test them.

Much of this chapter has been devoted to the methods for accomplishing steps 1 and 2. Determining the true causes of surgical failure and identifying the mode of failure (e.g., hospital death with chronic pulmonary insufficiency, or late death with periprosthetic valve leakage) are difficult and somewhat subjective. Yet these are important steps in improving the results of cardiac surgery. The causes and mode of failure should be identified by a thoughtful review of the record of each case considered a failure conducted by a senior person, usually with another person experienced in such analyses. Care must be taken that no conscious or unconscious effort to "explain" the failure colors these determinations. Such determinations are surprisingly reproducible from observer to observer and by the same observer when the same clinical data are reviewed as unknowns at a later time. Such evaluations direct future research and development aimed at improving the results of cardiac surgery.

The planning of research and development, and their accomplishment, is simple to describe, but, of course, this process is a lifelong continuum for those seriously concerned with increasing the efficacy of the management of patients with heart disease. The studies required range from basic research at a cellular level to simple laboratory and clinical studies of a wide variety of matters. Since one institution can undertake only a small proportion of the necessary research, continued study of the results of such research by others, and of the general field of science, is required by each group if substantial progress is to be made.

In the interim, after clinical study of an entity such as unstable angina pectoris, mitral valve prolapse, or tetralogy of Fallot, revised patient management protocols should be designed and followed. The revised protocols should be designed to maximize the benefits to the patients of current information on techniques and results. For these reasons, this text presents the indications for operation after the results.

Finally, when as a result of research, new knowledge and techniques are available, a new management program is designed. Unless its benefits are instantly obvious, which is rare, prospective testing by some method is usually required to determine whether improvement has actually resulted. A useful hypothetical example of this process of improving surgical results has been published.[B25]

APPENDIXES

Appendix **6A**
TECHNIQUES OF PROSPECTIVE SINGLE-PROTOCOL CLINICAL STUDIES

A single–treatment protocol study requires that a protocol has been in effect during the period covered by the study (e.g., routine primary repair of the tetralogy of Fallot, routine immediate operation for all or defined subsets of acute aortic dissection, valve repair for defined subsets of mitral incompetence, and coronary artery bypass grafting for unstable angina pectoris). Since total adherence to the protocol during the time period of the study may not have occurred, it is of critical importance to identify the exceptions and to consider their possible effect on the conclusions drawn from the study.

Single-protocol studies are best reported as including all cases treated between more or less standard time frames, such as January 1, 1970, to January 1, 1977 (1970–1977). The beginning or termination of a study at nonstandard times is usually biased by knowledge of events just before or after those dates. The same is true when the study group is defined with 73 or 100 consecutive cases, for the question as to what events occurred in the cases just before or after this arbitrary number arises.

CONCURRENT DATA RECORDING

Data recording must be precise and detailed, and generally should be incorporated into the clinical record. Thus, clinical studies can only be as accurate and complete as are the data available in the patient's record. Therefore, the cardiothoracic surgeon and the team members seriously interested in scientific progress must make their preoperative, operative, and postoperative records in a sufficiently clear, precise, and extensive manner that data gathering from them can be complete and meaningful. The notes should emphasize description, and, although they may well contain the conclusions of the moment, it is the description of basic data that becomes useful in later analysis for clinical studies.

All information should be recorded in clearly defined objective terms. A preference may be held for using descriptive terms that are clearly defined (e.g., *absent, trivial, mild, moderate, severe*) (GLH). Alternatively, numerical coding may be used,[B27,F8] with clear definition of each numerical grade (UAB). Thus, pedal pulses, for example, may be recorded as 0, 1, 2, 3, or 4, with 4 indicating normal.

A part of many single-protocol studies is follow-up information.[B17] Ideally, follow-up data are recorded in the patient's ongoing clinical record. At times, they can only be obtained remotely. In such cases, a *short* conversational form letter to elicit *positive* responses is useful, and the letter is generally followed up by direct telephone contact with the patient. Information obtained directly from patients may be inferior to that obtained as a result of examination of the patient by an informed medical practitioner. The most important, and all too often forgotten, information to elicit in long-term follow-up is actual dates of events. This means, for example, that a letter to a patient's doctor should ask the last date the patient was seen, not the date of the doctor's response.

Data may be retrieved concurrently or at the end of the study ("retrolectively").[F5] In either case, particularly when the *n* is large, a precise methodology should be used to prevent repetitious handling of the patient's record and of data sheets and to assure complete and accurate data retrieval.

Insofar as possible, the documents from which data are to be extracted are reproduced (e.g., photocopied), organized in looseleaf ring binders (notebooks), and permanently stored. These documents may include the patient's admission slip for demographic data, any catheterization reports, the operative note, the discharge summary of the hospital course, any autopsy reports, and follow-up questionnaires. Particular studies will require other documents, such as electrocardiograms, the anesthesia record, and so forth. No attempt is made to organize the patients in these notebooks except by an arbitrary study number (which often corresponds roughly to some convenient order, such as alphabetical order or chronological order of operative date). Whatever shuffling and reordering may be necessary is done later by use of computer sorting routines. These notebooks are used in the initial stages by the senior investigators to purify the study group. If a patient does not fit into the study, the patient's records are merely removed from the notebook without altering the numbering sequence. At the end of the study, the notebooks are permanently stored for future reference. Index tabs are conveniently used to separate each patient's documents from others'. The tab bears the study number and the patient's name on front and back to provide viewing from both sides of the notebook.

DATA EXTRACTION

Once the cases are verified and as many of the documents entered in the notebooks as possible, a decision is made about the data desired for the analysis. In many instances, this will lead the investigator back to the original clinical chart for the extraction of additional information.

The data are now formally entered into the records to be used for the study. The accuracy of data entry is improved by recording insofar as possible only primary data (e.g., date of birth, date of operation) and not indexes derived or calculated from them (e.g., patient age at operation). Such indexes can later be calculated quickly and accurately. Insofar as possible, the data should also be coded in a way that is simple and self-documenting (using natural language). Such coding necessitates computer programs that can handle nonnumerical information. The records may be a separate data sheet or data card ("punch card") for each patient. In fact, this method is mandatory if noncomputer methods of sorting are to be flexible and easy. The often used longhand tabulation of the data from a group of patients on a single sheet of paper, with or without color-coded entries, precludes flexible sorting when a computer is not used. When computers are used, the records exist within the computer system and may be displayed or printed out in many different forms.

No matter what method is used, experience dictates that a final step of data verification be inserted before any analyses. This process is long and tedious and can be boring. It reveals *many* errors, however, and also allows one more review of each patient to detect missed information. The data are then checked for reasonableness, a process aided by computer. This is done quite simply by looking at the maximum, minimum, and average of each variable (though sometimes more sophisticated univariate analyses must be done) and by making simple scatter plots (e.g., age, height, and weight form a smooth scatter plot against one another) and cumulative distribution plots. Discrepancies and outliers are found and the data resolved. Although a controversial statistical point, the data should probably not be "doctored" by rejecting outliers, unless there is a reason to suspect that they are less reliable than the values obtained for other patients. It is often useful to list all patients with missing data so that any gaps can be filled in. Finally, an alphabetical list is made to make sure that patients do not have duplicate records, particularly if the same patients were subjects of a preceding study.

The process of data gathering and assembly is the most time-consuming step in a study. It is not unusual for this step to consume months or years of work.

An alternative to a retrolective[F5] method of data collection is to employ an ongoing data collection scheme whereby data are extracted and entered into a computer as each patient is operated on. Currently, such a scheme for a hospital or outpatient population is too expensive to be generally applicable. Further, the method of individual study projects described has other advantages:

1. Reasonable parsimony can be practiced regarding the number of data items collected in the study. In ongoing data collection, many more items than necessary are usually collected for fear of "missing something."

2. Current and consistent descriptions of morphology, results of special tests, surgical procedures, etc. can be used in recording data.

3. The time of a few individuals can be committed to an individual study project to ensure uniformity of data collection; too often in ongoing data collection studies, the least knowledgeable person is assigned to enter the data. In the individual study project method, the principal investigators are able to participate in data collection for each patient, as it is more manageable to put aside a block of time to review a large number of cases than to review individual cases day by day. As they participate in this process of looking at the original data, the investigators often perceive previously unappreciated patterns of morphology, morbidity, and other variables and events, and these become useful guides to the subsequent analyses.

4. From the point of view of the morale of support people, the study project method encourages the completion of explicitly identifiable studies. All too often, ongoing data collection encourages interminable data collection with few visible results to reward hard and often very tedious work.

ANALYSIS OF DATA

The first step in data analysis is generally the production of simple descriptive tables by the process of sorting and tallying. These tables, plus the experiences of the senior investigators, usually then lead directly to a multivariate analysis of the variables relating to the events of interest in the study (e.g., death and other time-related events such as heart block, recurrence of angina pectoris, and so forth). These variables are often usefully expressed as incremental risk factors (see Section 2).

Then, further analyses of various types are made as a basis for additional interpretations of the risk factors and events. At times, a single or two-variable, rather than multivariate, analysis is made for ease of interpretation and presentation. Generally, however, the effect of a single variable is best portrayed by solving the multivariate equation for it and plotting the result in a nomogram. The methods used are discussed in Section 4.

INTERPRETATION AND THE FRAMING OF HYPOTHESES

All steps in the research process have as their objective the generation of new knowledge. This goal is not reached by analysis of data

alone, but requires considerable time and intense concentration on the data by the senior investigators, a sequence often omitted. Additional analysis is often required as a part of this final step.

Appendix **6B**
PROGRAMS FOR PROGRAMMABLE HAND-HELD CALCULATORS

The easy availability of programmable hand-held calculators offers every surgeon a versatile and helpful tool for clinical and laboratory research. By providing the means for quick comparative analysis, it also encourages in surgeons the commendable habit of reading the cardiac surgical literature critically. This appendix describes some programs that are helpful in this regard. It also describes more sophisticated programs for use in special situations.

CONFIDENCE LIMITS FOR PROPORTIONS

A quadratic normal approximation to the binomial distribution containing a correction for continuity has been found to yield confidence limits about as accurate as those obtained using more complex F ratios,[B19] even when n is small.[B20]

The continuity correction (p') for the upper confidence limit of a proportion (p) is

$$p' = p + \frac{1}{2n} \qquad \textbf{(6B-1)}$$

and the sign of $\pm$ in equation 6B-3 is positive ($+$).

The continuity correction for the lower confidence limit of the proportion is

$$p' = p - \frac{1}{2n} \qquad \textbf{(6B-2)}$$

and the sign in equation 6B-3 is negative ($-$).

The upper (p_U) and lower (p_L) confidence limits are successively solved by substituting P' and K into the following quadratic equation:

$$CL = \frac{2np' + K[K \pm \sqrt{K^2 + 4np'(1 - p')}]}{2(n + K^2)} \qquad \textbf{(6B-3)}$$

The choice of K depends on the confidence coefficient desired. For 70% confidence limits, $K = 1.03643$; for 50% limits, $K = 0.67449$; for 90% limits, $K = 1.64485$; for 95% limits, $K = 1.95996$; and for 68.3% limits exactly corresponding to ± 1 standard deviation of p, $K = 1.0$. When $K = 1$, equation 6B-3 reduces to

$$CL = \frac{2np' + 1 \pm \sqrt{1 + 4np'(1 - p')}}{2(n + 1)} \qquad \textbf{(6B-4)}$$

In Figure 6B-1, the departure of the 70% confidence limits calculated by this simple normal approximation from those calculated using the more complex computer methodology is displayed. For a small n, the error results in an error of 1 percentage point in the confidence limits. As n becomes large, the difference approaches zero.

In presenting proportions and their confidence limits, each should be rounded to the first significant figure in the standard deviation of the proportion (equivalent to standard error):

$$SD = \sqrt{\frac{p(1 - p)}{n}} \qquad \textbf{(6B-5)}$$

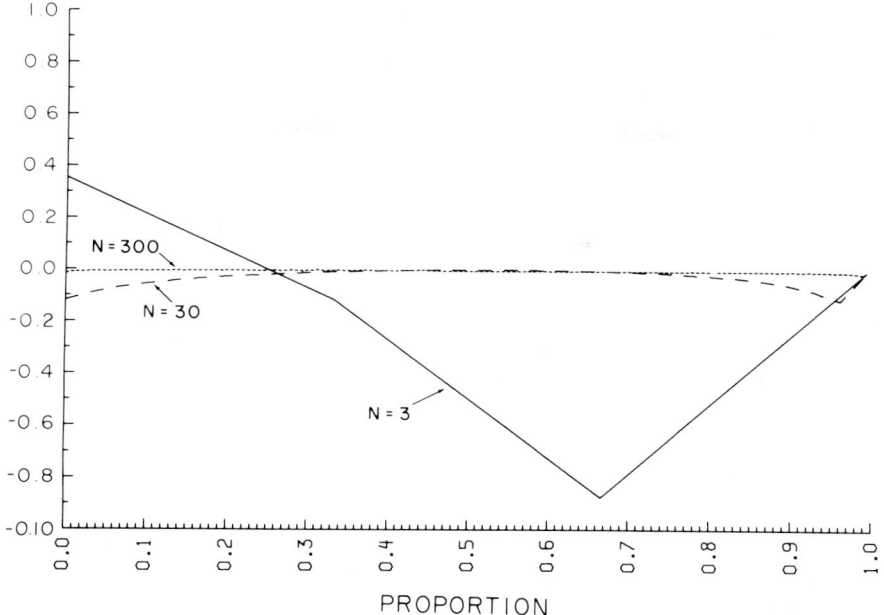

Figure 6B-1 Evaluation of quadratic approximation by hand-held calculator (equation 6B-3)[B20] to 70% confidence limits with results obtained by large computer calculation using the f distribution.[B19]

CONFIDENCE LIMITS FOR LOGISTIC PROBABILITY ESTIMATES

Probability estimates (P) are obtained from the logistic regression equation according to the following formulas:

$$P = \frac{1}{1 + e^{-z}} \tag{6B-6}$$

$$z = \beta_0 + \beta_1 x_1 + \cdots + \beta_k x_k \tag{6B-7}$$

where e is the base of the natural logarithms, β_0 is the intercept of the logistic equation, and $\beta_1 - \beta_k$ are logistic regression coefficients associated with the values for the incremental risk factors $x_1 - x_k$. Confidence limits for P are obtained by calculating the symmetric confidence limits for z in equation 6B-7, then transforming these limits to asymmetric probability limits using logistic equation 6B-6. To do this requires an estimate of the variance (Var) of z. This is found from the variance-covariance matrix (v) available from the computer analysis generating the regression coefficients:

$$\text{Var}(z) = \sum_{i=0}^{k} \sum_{j=0}^{k} v_i x_i v_j x_j \tag{6B-8}$$

where $x_0 = 1$ (i.e., it is the x associated with the intercept term). As an example of the use of equation 6B-8, Var_i may be designated as the diagonal elements of the variance-covariance matrix (i.e., the square of each coefficient's standard deviation) and Cov_{ij} as the off-diagonal elements representing the covariance between the ith and the jth coefficient:

$$\mathbf{Var}(z) = \text{Var}_0 + \text{Var}_1 x_1^2 + \cdots + \text{Var}_k x_k^2 \tag{6B-9}$$
$$+ 2(\text{Cov}_{0,1} x_1 + \cdots + \text{Cov}_{0,k} x_k)$$
$$+ 2(\text{Cov}_{1,2} x_1 x_2 + \cdots \text{Cov}_{1,k} x_1 x_k)$$
$$+ 2(\text{Cov}_{k-1,k} x_{k-1} x_k)$$

Then,

$$\underline{z} = z - K\sqrt{\text{Var}(z)} \tag{6B-10}$$

and

$$\bar{z} = z + K\sqrt{\text{Var}(z)} \tag{6B-11}$$

where $\underline{z}$ is the lower confidence limit and $\bar{z}$ the upper confidence limit of z, and K is derived from the confidence coefficient using the normal distribution. For example, if the equivalent of ± 1 SD is desired, $K = 1$; if 70% confidence limits are desired, $K = 1.03643$, and so forth, as for K in equation 6B-3 for the confidence limits for proportions. $\underline{z}$ and $\bar{z}$ are then transformed to probabilities using equation 6B-6.[K7]

TEST STATISTICS FOR 2 × 2 CONTINGENCY TABLES

Either the chi-square (χ^2) or Fisher's exact test is used to test contingency tables of the following form:

		Mortality		
		Survival	Dead	
Factor[a]	Present	a	b	$n_p = a + b$
	Absent	c	d	$n_a = c + d$
		$n_s = a + c$	$n_d = b + d$	n

[a]This can be any two attributes being tested.

In this table, n_p is the number of cases in which the factor is present and for which a survivors and b deaths have been observed; n_a is the number of cases in which the factor is absent and for which c survivors and d deaths have been observed; n_s is the total number of survivors, and n_d is the total number of deaths; n is the total number of cases observed and is equal to $a + b + c + d$, $n_p + n_a$, and $n_s + n_d$. Since this table has two rows and two columns for displaying the basic data, it is called a *two-by-two* (2×2) *contingency table*. The additional column to the right of the table and the lowest row contain what are known as *marginal totals*. The proportion of patients who died in the presence of the factor is $p_p = b/n_p$, and the proportion who died in the absence of the factor is $p_a = d/n_a$. The overall proportion of patients dying is $p = n_d/n$.

To test the null hypothesis (H_0) that the two mortality proportions are equal, the chi-square statistic is calculated as

$$\chi^2 = \frac{(p_p - p_a)^2}{p(1 - p)(1/n_p + 1/n_a)} \qquad \textbf{(6B-12)}$$

The P value for the difference between the two proportions p_p and p_a can be obtained from this statistic in one of two ways: (1) a χ^2 distribution table (or calculator program) can be used with 1 degree of freedom or (2) the square root of the χ^2 statistic can be taken and a normal distribution table (or program) used. Computationally, the latter method is considerably faster because of the availability of formulas that can closely approximate the normal distribution.

The test may not be accurate for small sample sizes, particularly when the number of events (e.g., deaths) is either very small (say, < 2) or large (say, within two of the marginal total). To determine whether or not the χ^2 test is likely to be accurate, Brownlee suggests multiplying the *smaller* of n_p and n_a by the *smaller* of n_s and n_d (i.e., the smaller row and column marginal totals) and dividing this product by n.[B22] If the result is greater than 3.5, then consider the test reliable; if it is not, then use Fisher's exact test.

Fisher's exact test[F7] utilizes the following formula:

$$P = \frac{[(a + b)! (c + d)! (a + c)! (b + d)!]}{a!b!c!d!n!} \qquad \textbf{(6B-13)}$$

where ! means factorial. This equation gives the probability of obtaining the particular contingency table observed; to obtain a P value, however, the probability of obtaining all the more extreme ("worse") tables must also be calculated and summed together. Each successive table is obtained in one of two ways: (1) if the quantity $ad - bc$ is negative, then a and d are decreased by 1 while b and c are increased by 1; (2) if the quantity is positive, then a and d are increased by 1 while b and c are decreased by 1. Another P is calculated with these new definitions of a, b, c, and d, and added to the one obtained above. This procedure is stopped after the calculation of a P with a, b, c, or d reduced to zero.

TEST STATISTICS FOR $2 \times k$ CONTINGENCY TABLE

If the factor in the above mortality table consists of more than two levels (as, for example, in comparing results from three or more institutions), then a $2 \times k$ chi-square test is performed to test the hypothesis that results are equal (homogeneous) across all the levels of the factor. (This is an *overall* test; it is not a test for trend or for interesting contrasts that might be hidden by an overall test). Such a table takes the following form:

| | Mortality | | |
	Survived	Dead	
Level 1	a_1	b_1	n_1
Level 2	a_2	b_2	n_2
Level 3	a_3	b_3	n_3
.	.	.	.
.	.	.	.
.	.	.	.
Level k	a_k	b_k	n_k
	n_s	n_d	n

Here, each level of the factor of interest is numbered from 1 to k, as are the marginal row totals. The *general* procedure is to calculate for each entry (usually called a *cell*) an expected a_i or b_i (where i ranges from $1-k$) on the assumption that the mortality is the same across all levels of the factor. For example, the overall mortality is n_d/n, and thus the number of deaths, f_1, expected for level 1 is $n_1 n_d/n$. A cell chi-square is then calculated for each cell in the table using the observed frequency (f) and the appropriate expected frequency (f_e):

$$\text{cell } \chi^2 = \frac{(f - f_e)^2}{f_e} \qquad \textbf{(6B-14)}$$

All cell χ^2 values are summed for the overall χ^2 test for the table. The cell χ^2 values are themselves of interest in spotting possible interesting deviations from expected frequencies; however, an overall χ^2 can also be calculated directly by the formula

$$\chi^2 = (n/n_s) \sum_{i=1}^{k} (a_i^2/n_i) + (n/n_d) \sum_{i=1}^{k} (b_i^2/n_i) - n \qquad \textbf{(6B-15)}$$

where Σ means *find the sum of* the indicated quantity for each entry $1-k$. The P value can be found using the χ^2 distribution table (or calculator program) with $k-1$ degrees of freedom.

CALCULATION OF MEAN, STANDARD DEVIATION, AND STANDARD ERROR

Most programmable hand-held calculators have the calculation of mean, standard deviation, and standard error as built-in functions. A separate program can be developed to simplify their use.

P VALUES FOR COMPARISONS OF MEAN VALUES

Sample means ($\bar{x}$) may be tested against a hypothesized value, against a population mean value, or against another sample mean using the t test.[S4]

Test against Hypothesized Value

A sample mean is tested against a specific hypothesized value (H_0) by the formula

$$t = \frac{(\bar{x} - H_0)}{\text{SD}/\sqrt{n}} \qquad \textbf{(6B-16)}$$

where t is the test statistic, SD is the sample standard deviation, and n is the sample size. A P value is obtained using a table (or calculator program) of the t distribution for $n-1$ degrees of freedom.

Paired t Test

In those situations in which pairs of observations are made before and after an intervention, the t test is used to test the null hypothesis that the mean of the differences before and after is zero. Equation 6B-16 is used, with $\bar{x}$ representing the mean difference and SD the standard deviation of the differences; n is the number of pairs of valves, and $H_0 = 0$.

Test for Two Sample Means

When two sample means ($\bar{x}_1$ and $\bar{x}_2$) are to be tested against a hypothesis (generally that the difference is zero), the standard t test assumes that the variability for each sample as reflected by the respective standard deviations (SD_1 and SD_2) is similar. This is tested using the F statistic:

$$F = \frac{SD_1^2}{SD_2^2} \qquad \text{(6B-17)}$$

where, arbitrarily, we select $SD_1 \geqslant SD_2$, and the P value is found in a table of the F distribution (or calculator program) with degrees of freedom being $n_1 - 1$ for the numerator and $n_2 - 1$ for the denominator.

The t test for two sample means when SD_1 and SD_2 can be considered equal is

$$t = \frac{\bar{x}_1 - \bar{x}_2 - H_0}{\sqrt{\left[\dfrac{SD_1^2(n_1 - 1) + SD_2^2(n_2 - 1)}{n_1 + n_2 - 2}\right]\left[\dfrac{1}{n_1} + \dfrac{1}{n_2}\right]}} \qquad \text{(6B-18)}$$

The P value is found using a table (or program) of the t distribution for $n_1 + n_2 - 2$ degrees of freedom.

When the two samples cannot be considered to have equal variation, Welch[W4,W5] has suggested using the formula

$$t = \frac{\bar{x}_1 - \bar{x}_2 - H_0}{\sqrt{\dfrac{SD_1^2}{n_1} + \dfrac{SD_2^2}{n_2}}} \qquad \text{(6B-19)}$$

The P value is found using a table (or program) of the t distribution for the nearest integer of degrees of freedom approximated by the formula

$$df \approx \frac{(SD_1^2/n_1 + SD_2^2/n_2)^2}{[(SD_1^2/n_1)^2/(n_1 - 1)] + [(SD_2^2/n_2)^2/(n_2 - 1)]} \qquad \text{(6B-20)}$$

OBTAINING *P* VALUES FOR COMPARISONS OF TWO TREATMENTS USING THE LOGISTIC EQUATION

Two treatments can be compared by a combined logistic analysis as a function of other variables within the logistic equation (e.g., as a function of age at operation, date of operation, aortic cross-clamp time, and so forth) using the formula

$$t = \frac{(z_1 - z_2 - H_0)}{\sqrt{Var(z_1) + Var(z_2)}} \qquad \text{(6B-21)}$$

where z_1 and z_2 are obtained by solving the logistic regression equation 6B-7 for the two differing treatments. The respective variances (Var) of z_1 and z_2 are obtained using equation 6B-8. Because of present uncertainty concerning the appropriate degrees of freedom to assign to t, a P value is estimated using a table (or program) of the normal distribution rather than the t distribution.

If alternative treatment probabilities are obtained by separate analyses, then the actual variance of each estimated probability (P) is required:

$$Var(P) = P^2(1 - P)^2 Var(z) \qquad \text{(6B-22)}$$

where $Var(z)$ is obtained using equation 6B-8. The arcsine–square root transform method can then be employed to obtain a test statistic:

$$t = (P_1' - P_2' - H_0)\sqrt{Var(P_1') - Var(P_2')} \qquad \text{(6B-23)}$$

where

$$P' = \sin^{-1}(\sqrt{P}) \qquad \text{(6B-24)}$$

$$Var(P') = \frac{1}{(4n_e)} \qquad \text{(6B-25)}$$

$$n_e = \frac{P(1 - P)}{Var(P)} \qquad \text{(6B-26)}$$

In equation 6B-24, $\sin^{-1}$ is the arcsine function (radians); in equations 6B-25 and 6B-26, n_e is an "effective" sample size. The P value is estimated, as above, using the normal distribution.

CONVERTING GREGORIAN CALENDAR DATES TO JULIAN DATES

A number of algorithms are available for converting Gregorian calendar dates (the conventional ones) to Julian dates. One such algorithm* is

$$JD = 1{,}721{,}060 + 365Y + 31(M - 1) + D \qquad \text{(6B-27)}$$
$$+ \ INT(Y'/4) - INT(Y'/100) + INT(Y'/400) - X$$

where Y is the year (e.g., 1980), M is the month (1–12), and D is the day of the month. For $M > 2$, $X = INT(0.4M - 2.3)$ and $Y' = Y$; for $M \leqslant 2$, $X = 0$ and $Y' = Y - 1$. INT( ) is the integer part of a number (any decimal fraction truncated). The interval in days between any two calendar dates is calculated by converting each date to its Julian date by equation 6B-27 and subtracting.

OTHER PROGRAMS

A number of specific task-oriented programs are helpful. For example, the Z value (see "Population Parameters, Sample Estimates, and Descriptors") for the normal cardiac valve diameter for a given patient's size can be calculated on a hand-held programmable calculator for any of the four valves using the patient's body surface area. Such programs are useful in valve repair and replacement and in the repair of tetralogy of Fallot.[B26] For a specific entity such as tetralogy of Fallot, a useful program is one that calculates the P value for the difference between predicted hospital mortalities for alternative treatment protocols.[K10] Which of these types of programs is useful varies from one cardiac surgical unit to another.

APPENDIX **6C**

EQUATIONS FOR CALCULATING EVIDENT DIFFERENCES

FINDING THE POINT AT WHICH THE EFFECT OF A VARIABLE IS EVIDENT USING NONOVERLAPPING CONFIDENCE LIMITS

Consider a simple linear relationship between effect x and outcome z:

$$z = \beta_0 + \beta_1 x \qquad \text{(6C-1)}$$

where the coefficients β_0, the intercept, and β_1, the slope, are determined from a regression analysis. The first requisite is to select a reference value of x, call it x_1; the object is to find a different x, call it x_2, at and beyond which the effect is evident, that is, different from that at x_1.

---

*Available from Hewlett-Packard Company as program 01366A, written by Moshe M. Brewer. User Library, Hewlett-Packard Co., Dept. 39UL, 1000 NE Circle Blvd., Corvallis, OR 97330.

The confidence limits for z at x_1, calculated from the variance of z (Var) and a confidence coefficient transformed to an appropriate t (e.g., $t \sim 1$ for 70% confidence limits) are calculated as follows:

$$\text{Var}[z(x_1)] = V_0 + V_1 x_1^2 + 2\,\text{Cov}_{0,1} x_1 \qquad \text{(6C-2)}$$

$$\text{CL}[z(x_1)] = z(x_1) \pm t\,\sqrt{\text{Var}[z(x_1)]} \qquad \text{(6C-3)}$$

where V_0 and V_1 are the variances of β_0 and β_1 (variance being the square of the standard deviation, SD) and $\text{Cov}_{0,1}$ is the covariance term between β_0 and β_1 ($\text{Cov}_{0,1}$ is related to the correlation, r, between β_0 and β_1 by the expression $\text{SD}_0 \text{SD}_1 r$). The confidence limits of the unknown x_2 are given by equations 6C-2 and 6C-3 with x_2 substituted for x_1.

Since the confidence limits of $z(x_2)$ must exactly equal one of those of $z(x_1)$, we can write, using equations 6C-2 and 6C-3

$$\text{CL}[z(x_1)] = \text{CL}[z(x_2)] = z(x_2) \pm t\,\sqrt{\text{Var}[z(x_2)]} \qquad \text{(6C-4)}$$

or

$$\text{CL}[z(x_1)] = \beta_0 + \beta_1 x_2 \pm t\,\sqrt{V_0 + V_1 x_2^2 + 2\,\text{Cov}_{0,2} x_2} \qquad \text{(6C-5)}$$

The only unknown in equation 6C-5 is x_2, which, in this case, can be found using the general solution for the roots of a quadratic equation. For uncomplicated situations that reduce to equation 6C-5, the four roots (two each for the $\pm$ expression) can be calculated using a hand-held calculator program. Two of the roots will simply yield x_1. Which of the other two roots is the desired x_2 is easily selected by inspection.

In more complex, multivariate cases, the equation must be solved for explicit values of all variables except x_2; thus, even a complex set of coefficients often can be reduced to the form of equation 6C-5. However, if higher-order terms in x (higher powers) are involved, it is probably easier to solve the resulting equation using an iterative method of solving nonlinear equations.

FINDING THE POINT AT WHICH THE EFFECT OF A VARIABLE IS EVIDENT USING P VALUES

If, instead of (or in addition to) determining an evident difference using nonoverlapping confidence limits, one wishes to detect an evident difference at some level of significance (P value), then equations 6C-1 and 6C-2 are used to define $z(x_1)$, $z(x_2)$, $\text{Var}[z(x_1)]$, and $\text{Var}[z(x_2)]$. Then the general equation for a test of significance is used:

$$\frac{z(x_1) - z(x_2)}{\sqrt{\text{Var}[z(x_1)] + \text{Var}[z(x_2)]}} = t \qquad \text{(6C-6)}$$

where t is the number of standard deviations represented by the selected P value. Expanding equation 6C-6

$$\frac{z(x_1) - (\beta_0 + \beta_1 x_2)}{\sqrt{\text{Var}[z(x_1)] + (V_0 + V_1 x_2^2 + 2\,\text{Cov}_{0,2} x_2)}} = t \qquad \text{(6C-7)}$$

yields an equation with only one unknown, x_2. In the simplest cases, equation 6C-7 can be solved using a solution for roots of a quadratic equation. Higher-order terms of x require the use of iterative methods.

Note that if equation 6C-2 represents a logistic equation, we recommend solving for evident differences in the logistic domain for consistency, since we recommend that confidence limits and P values for such equations be calculated in the logistic domain and transformed, if necessary, to probabilities as a final step.

LOGISTIC ANALYSIS

HISTORY

The logistic equation was introduced by Verhulst between 1835 and 1845 to describe the growth of the populations of France and Belgium.[V2,V3] Thus, it belongs to a large class of "growth equations." The logistic equation is the simplest of these equations that, when plotted, results in a curve of S shape.[T2] The equation arises naturally in the description of autocatalytic chemical reactions,[R1] characterized by an initial phase of increasingly rapid chemical conversion catalyzed by the products produced, followed by a decelerating phase as reactants are consumed (e.g., the hydrolysis of ethyl acetate to acetic acid and ethyl alcohol). Berkson introduced the logistic equation into bioassay.[B14] In 1955, Berkson dubbed the units of the logistic nomogram *logit units,* parallel to the probit units of another method of bioassay.[B13]

PRINCIPLES

Multivariate logistic regression *generalizes* the discriminant analysis of Fisher[F9] by embedding it within the logistic equation.[W1] Z, in logit units, is assumed to be related to a linear combination of incremental risk factors:

$$z = \beta_0 + \beta_1 x_1 + \beta_2 x_2 + \cdots \beta_k x_k \qquad \text{(6D-1)}$$

where β_0 is the intercept term (logit units when all the xs = 0), x_1–x_k are the numerical values of the independent variables, and β_1–β_k are coefficients, estimated from the data, that translate the values of the independent variables to logit units. Logit units are related to probabilities (P) by the logistic relationship

$$z = \ln\left[\frac{P}{(1 - P)}\right] \qquad \text{(6D-2)}$$

where ln stands for the natural logarithm. This form of the logistic equation makes clear why *log* is part of its name. Notice, also, that z is a function of the ratio of P, the probability of an event, and $1 - P$, the complementary probability that the event does not occur. Such a ratio has been called the *odds ratio,* and equation 6D-2 has been referred to as *log odds.*[C9] Equation 6D-2 is not computationally applicable to raw clinical data for which P is *exactly* 0 or 1 for each patient (e.g., when one is analyzing a dichotomous variable such as mortality). Thus, the computational form is a nonlinear equation obtained by exponentiating this equation:

$$P = \frac{1}{(1 + e^{-z})} \qquad \text{(6D-3)}$$

where P is the estimated probability using the maximum likelihood principle, and e is the base of the natural logarithms.[W1] In practice, the dependent variable is a dichotomous variable with the values 0 (no event) or 1 (event), and the independent variables are potential incremental risk factors. In this form, no restrictions are made on the distribution of the risk factors (x's); they may be any mix of continuous, discrete, or ordered variables.

COMPUTATIONAL CONSIDERATIONS

Except for situations in which the only variables considered are categorical, practically every patient has a different combination of values for the incremental risk factors. Thus, the fitting of the data to the logistic equation requires a large amount of computer data storage. Therefore, the use of large-scale statistical computation facilities is advised for logistic data analyses.

At least two widely distributed biological data analysis systems incorporate special facilities for logistic regression: SAS[H7] and BMDP.[E4] In addition, many available nonlinear least-squares regression packages can be adapted to logistic regression, since Bradley has shown that the maximum likelihood estimates can be obtained by iteratively reweighted least-squares techniques.[B24]

As with all nonlinear regression, the β's are estimated *iteratively*, starting with initial guesses and refining them. The best practice is always to start with initial guesses of zero for all β's, since guesses with an incorrect sign makes the computation unstable. This advice is *critical* in stepwise procedures (especially backwards elimination procedures), where there is a temptation to use preceding estimates for initial guesses.

It is essential to have available a program that permits some kind of automatic variable selection; otherwise, the labor of testing variable leads rapidly to discouragement. A number of schemes have been implemented to bring in variables in a stepwise fashion either on the basis of the P value for the slope or the improvement in the overall maximum likelihood. Similarly, backwards elimination schemes have been devised. An "all possible regression" scheme can also be used to resolve differences between forward stepwise and backwards elimination schemes.

A further refinement of logistic analysis, to make it usable, is the elimination of negative logistic coefficient signs whenever possible. This presents the final analysis in the form of incremental risk factors. Thus, dichotomous variables are recoded to change a negative sign on a coefficient to a positive one. Some continuous variables may need to be left with a negative coefficient. The interactions of continuous and discrete variables are also examined for sign. The model can sometimes be simplified by observing that an interaction term with an equal magnitude but opposite sign to a main effect can be recorded so as to eliminate a variable from the model.

Having made all these changes, the final model is fitted. This fitting produces the final estimated coefficients and a variance-covariance matrix. The latter is useful for establishing P values and for determining confidence limits for predicted probabilities (see Appendix 6-B). The goodness of fit of the model to the data can be determined by calculating the probability of the event for each person, stratifying the data set into deciles, and comparing the number of observed events with those calculated from the model. More formal methods of testing for goodness of fit have been described.[P5,P6]

Sometimes the "event" whose probability is being calculated does not take the convenient from of 0 and 1. Consider hospital mortality; it may occur in a multiplicity of modes (acute cardiac death, death from hemorrhage, death in renal failure, etc.), each of which is a dichotomous event. The data may need to be analyzed for more than one mode of death. Such analysis leads to the coding of multiple so-called competing events:[D6] alive, acute cardiac death, death in renal failure, and so forth. If the number of events is small compared to the overall sample size, one can analyze separately total mortality, cardiac mortality, and so forth. However, in general, the total calculated risk for a patient from the various modes is not guaranteed to add up to the overall probability. Hosmer has described the equations and has programmed the algorithm for performing a logistic regression simultaneously on multiple events.[H8] At present, his programs have limited distribution. They are, in fact, unnecessary, for an ordinary logistic regression program can be arranged to do the job.

Also, the event may not be dichotomous. Instead, there may be three or four possibilities (e.g., no, mild, moderate, or severe postoperative left AV valve incompetence). The logistic model can be modified to permit these possibilities to be analyzed.

APPENDIX **6E**

THE KAPLAN-MEIER ACTUARIAL METHOD AND ITS CONFIDENCE LIMITS

The product-limit[K2] actuarial estimate, $P(t_i)$, involves the following variables:

N is the original number of individuals at risk.

N_{ui} is the total accumulated number of individuals censored by t_i (i.e., not known to be dead or alive).

N_{pi} is the total number of individuals known to have been dead by t_{i-1} (the time of the most recent event prior to time t_i).

N_{di} is the number of individuals known to have died at time t_i.

(Note that by convention, if a patient is censored at exactly the same time as an observed event, then it is assumed that the event slightly preceded the censoring.)

Let

$$r_i = N - N_{ui} - N_{pi} - N_{di} \qquad (6E\text{-}1)$$

and

$$n_i = N - N_{ui} - N_{pi} \qquad (6E\text{-}2)$$

Thus, n_i is the number of patients at risk at time t_i, and r_i is the number at risk following events N_{di} occurring at time t_i. Then the probability of surviving at t_i is r_i/n_i. The product-limit estimate of survival is the continued product (designated mathematically by Π) of all the previous survival probabilities:

$$\hat{P}(t_i) = \prod_{k=1}^{i} r_k/n_k \qquad (6E\text{-}3)$$

An obvious difficulty arises when the last events occur in the last patients followed. Instead of letting $r = 0$, we let

$$r_{\text{final}} = \frac{n_{\text{final}}}{(N+1)\,\hat{P}(t_{i-1})} \qquad (6E\text{-}4)$$

where n_{final} is the number of patients at the final calculation and $\hat{P}(t_{i-1})$ is the survival probability up to the time of calculating the final estimate.

The formulae for determining the confidence limits were compiled at UAB by Malcolm Turner, professor of biostatistics and biomathematics. These confidence limits are *asymptotic*; that is, they are known to hold for large sample sizes and to be approximate for small ones. The confidence limits are based on both determining the standard deviation of actuarial estimates and selecting an appropriate statistical distribution for the estimates.

STANDARD DEVIATION

It has been customary to use the approximation to the standard deviation published in 1926 by Greenwood.[G8] In this age of high-speed computers and powerful hand-held calculators, the calculation of exact standard deviations by the maximum likelihood method is recommended.[C4] Kuzma has found that, while Greenwood's approximation is very close to the exact result much of the time, it *underestimates* the standard deviation when the censoring rate is high,[K6] as it is in general for cardiac surgery data.

Then the *maximum likelihood estimate* for the variance of $\hat{P}(t_i)$, σ^2, is:

$$\sigma^2 = \hat{P}^2(t_i) \cdot \left[\left(\prod_{k=1}^{i} \left\{ \frac{1}{r_k} - \frac{1}{n_k} + 1 \right\} \right) - 1 \right] \qquad (6E\text{-}5)$$

The standard deviation is the square root of σ^2. Since r_k and n_k are used in calculating $\hat{P}(t_i)$, the extra calculations involved in using this formula instead of that suggested by Greenwood are quite trivial.

STATISTICAL DISTRIBUTION

Probably the β approximation of the sampling distribution is superior; it involves ratios of F distributions. In practice, however, confidence limits based on the asymptotic normality of a logistic transformation of $\hat{P}(t_i)^{K7}$ and the exact variance of a product are used.[G9] These limits are quickly calculated, even using a hand-held programmable calculator. The derivation yields the following equations:

$$CL = \frac{\hat{P}(t_i)}{\hat{P}(t_i) + [1 - \hat{P}(t_i)]\exp[Ks(t_i)\text{sign}]} \quad \textbf{(6E-6)}$$

where K is the test statistic from the normal distribution corresponding to the confidence coefficient (see Appendix 6B); sign is -1 for the upper confidence limit and $+1$ for the lower confidence limits; and $s(t_i)$ is

$$s(t_i) = \frac{1}{1 - \hat{P}(t_i)} \sqrt{\left(\prod_{k=1}^{i} \left\{ \frac{1}{r_k} - \frac{1}{n_k} + 1 \right\} \right) - 1} \quad \textbf{(6E-7)}$$

COMMENT

Using the logistic transformation, exact standard deviations and confidence limits can be found for the actuarial method (using equally spaced time *intervals*),[B5] although the formulae are more complex than for the product-limit method.[C4] The complexity is particularly increased when one wishes, for example, to analyze only cardiac-related deaths, treating *known nonrelated* deaths as censored during the interval in which they occurred. This is one reason for preferring the product-limit method.

It is recommended that actuarial estimates and plots be presented with 70% (or, more exactly, 68.3%) confidence limits of the actuarial estimates to correspond to the equivalent of ± 1 standard deviation of the estimate. Those who consistently present *all* data to ± 2 SDs are advised to use 95% limits. The confidence limits are asymmetric about the actuarial estimate, as they should be, and are constrained within the range 0–1.

Appendix **6F**
COMPARISONS OF SURVIVAL WITH POPULATION LIFE TABLES

A life table for the general population can be constructed that matches at least the age characteristic (and generally also the sex and race characteristics, if desired) of the surgical group under study.[A1,E3] The government bureaus of many countries publish population life tables similar to *Vital Statistics of the United States*.[V1]

CONSTRUCTION OF A MATCHED POPULATION LIFE TABLE

To construct an age-normalized life table for a group of patients, the median age (T) at operation is determined, as is the survival to that median age in the general population, $S(T)$. The formula for the survival of the age-matched general population, $S_T(t)$, is

$$S_T(t) = \frac{S(t + T)}{S(T)} \quad \textbf{(6F-1)}$$

The construction of a curve matched for age, sex, and race begins by sorting the patients by sex and race. Then, weighting coefficients are formed based on the number of cases in each sex-race category:

$$\alpha_{\text{wm}} = \frac{n_{\text{wm}}}{N} \quad \textbf{(6F-2)}$$

$$\alpha_{\text{wf}} = \frac{n_{\text{wf}}}{N} \quad \textbf{(6F-3)}$$

$$\alpha_{\text{om}} = \frac{n_{\text{om}}}{N} \quad \textbf{(6F-4)}$$

$$\alpha_{\text{of}} = \frac{n_{\text{of}}}{N} \quad \textbf{(6F-5)}$$

where wm is white male; wf is white female; om is other (race) male; of is other (race) female; $n_{\text{wm}}-n_{\text{of}}$ are the number of patients in each category; and N is the total number of cases. Note that

$$n_{\text{wm}} + n_{\text{om}} + n_{\text{wf}} + n_{\text{of}} = N \quad \textbf{(6F-6)}$$

and

$$\alpha_{\text{wm}} + \alpha_{\text{wf}} + \alpha_{\text{om}} + \alpha_{\text{of}} = 1 \quad \textbf{(6F-7)}$$

Within each of these four subgroups of patients, the median age at operation is determined; call these T_{wm}, T_{wf}, T_{om}, and T_{of}. From the individual life tables for each sex-race group, the survival at that median age is determined; call these $S_{\text{wm}}(T_{\text{wm}})$, $S_{\text{wf}}(T_{\text{wf}})$, $S_{\text{om}}(T_{\text{om}})$, and $S_{\text{of}}(T_{\text{of}})$. Then the composite survival curve $S_c(t)$ is calculated, starting from the date of operation ($t = 0$) through as many years as desired:

$$S_c(t) = \alpha_{\text{wm}} \frac{S_{\text{wm}}(t + T_{\text{wm}})}{S_{\text{wm}}(T_{\text{wm}})} \quad \textbf{(6F-8)}$$
$$+ \alpha_{\text{wf}} \frac{S_{\text{wf}}(t + T_{\text{wf}})}{S_{\text{wf}}(T_{\text{wf}})}$$
$$+ \alpha_{\text{om}} \frac{S_{\text{om}}(t + T_{\text{om}})}{S_{\text{om}}(T_{\text{om}})}$$
$$+ \alpha_{\text{of}} \frac{S_{\text{of}}(t + T_{\text{of}})}{S_{\text{of}}(T_{\text{of}})}$$

Except for the first year of life, the United States life tables do not list survival by fractional years. This problem can be handled by linearly interpolating between the yearly survival figures. Let A represent an actual age between table entries A_L and A_H, with A_L the nearest entry in the life table such that $A_L \leqslant A$, and A_H the nearest entry in the life table such that $A \leqslant A_H$ (i.e., $A_L \leqslant A \leqslant A_H$). Then let F_A be the fraction of the time interval, I, between A_L and A:

$$F_A = \frac{(A - A_L)}{I} \quad \textbf{(6F-9)}$$

The survival is determined at both A_L and A_H from the life table, calling these $S(A_L)$ and $S(A_H)$, respectively (note that these would be taken from the sex-race tables if an age-sex-race matched table were being constructed). Then

$$S(A) = S(A_L) - [S(A_L) - S(A_H)]F_A \quad \textbf{(6F-10)}$$

Note that if $A = A_H$, then $F_A = 1$ and $S(A) = S(A_H)$; also, if $A = A_L$, then $F_A = 0$ and $S(A) = S(A_L)$.

COMPARISON OF THE SURGICAL LIFE TABLE TO THE MATCHED POPULATION LIFE TABLE

One method used to compare the surgical life table, $L(t)$, to a matched population life table, $S_c(t)$, is by use of the normal distribution statistic Z:

$$Z = \frac{L(t) - S_c(t)}{\text{SD of } L(t)} \qquad \textbf{(6F-11)}$$

where SD of $L(t)$ is the standard deviation of the parametric or nonparametric surgical survival probability at time t following operation. A P value can be found from tables of Z or appropriate computer or hand-held calculator programs for the normal distribution.[K8] A time-related P value results.

Another method is to compare observed late deaths and expected mortality using the chi-square statistic. In this method, the expected mortality is calculated for *each* patient using the appropriate sex and race life table as above to calculate the probability of dying over the actual interval of follow-up. Let A_O be a patient's age at operation and A_F be the patient's age at follow-up. Then

$$P_D = 1 - \frac{S(A_F)}{S(A_O)} \qquad \textbf{(6F-12)}$$

where P_D is the probability of dying between A_O and A_F, and $S(A_F)$ and $S(A_O)$ are the appropriate population survival figures for the ages A_F and A_O (interpolated, if need be). All these individual P_D's are summed to yield the expected deaths. From these, the chi-square statistic (χ^2 with one degree of freedom) can be calculated:

$$\chi^2 = \frac{(\text{observed deaths} - \text{expected deaths})^2}{\text{expected deaths}} \qquad \textbf{(6F-13)}$$

A P value is then obtained by consultation of χ^2 tables or by the appropriate computer or hand-held calculator program.[K9]

Alternatives to the schemes described above must be sought when incremental risk factors are identified that affect the long-term surgical results.[B23,H6,L5] Breslow has devised a scheme for using the results of Cox and completely parametric regression analyses and population life table comparisons to quantitate cure.[B23] He estimates a relative death rate: the ratio of the hazard of dying observed in the clinical data to that of the matched general population, taking into account the incremental risk factors. He then determines whether this ratio is significantly greater than unity; that is, whether the hazard function of dying is greater than that of the general population.

PROPORTIONAL HAZARDS LINEAR MODELS

The simplest and most commonly used version of the proportional hazards model is a linear relationship between $\log_e \lambda(t)$ (to avoid range restrictions) and the explanatory variables:

$$\log_e \lambda(t) = \log_e \lambda_0(t) + \beta_1 x_1 + \beta_2 x_2 + \cdots + \beta_k x_k \quad \textbf{(6G-1)}$$

where $\lambda_0(t)$ is an overall population hazard that is modified by the additional information provided by the explanatory variables. A positive β indicates that large values of x are linked to an increase in hazard; if β is negative, large values of x are associated with decreased hazard. The relationship (equation 6G-1) includes the important assumptions that the relative risk of death for two individuals depends only on the differences in values of their explanatory variables and that this relative risk does not change with time. In practical terms, relative risks should be fairly constant over the time period of interest. An advantage of the proportional hazards model is that confidence intervals for the β's and tests of no effect for a variable ($\beta = 0$) can be carried out without making assumptions about the average hazard, $\lambda_0(t)$. This means that statistical inferences about the β_i's can be made with no assumptions about the shapes of curves depicting the survivorship functions or the underlying hazard function. The only assumptions necessary concern the effect of the explanatory variables on the unknown hazard function. The resulting estimates are almost as accurate as those derived when the functional form of $\lambda_0(t)$ is known. However, if distinguishable phases of changing hazard are evident, the assumption that the explanatory variables are applicable and have the same strength of affect throughout time may not be valid.

Clearly, in practice, as with logistic regression, such simple relationships cannot be expected to fit the data exactly. Often a better fit can be obtained by measuring a variable on a different scale, for example, by taking logarithms or square roots of the original measurements for some variable. Often variables must be coded to allow for interactions between the effects of variables on survival. Sometimes the proportional hazards assumption of constant relative risks describes the situation well for some variables and not for others.[K1] Usually, in practice, fitting such models is an exploratory, trial-and-error process involving all these elements.

REFERENCES

A

1. Axtell LM: Computing survival rates for chronic disease patients: A simple procedure. *JAMA* 186:1125, 1963.

2. Anderson JR, Berstein L, Pike MC: Approximate confidence intervals for probabilities of survival and quantiles in life-table analysis. *Biometrics* 38:407, 1982.

B

1. Burdette WJ, Geham EA: *Planning and Analysis of Clinical Studies.* Springfield, Ill: Charles C Thomas, 1970.

2. Birnbaum Memorial Symposium: Medical research: Statistics and ethics. *Science* 198:677, 1977.

3. Byar DP, Simon RM, Friedewald WT, Schlesselman JJ, De-

Mets DL, Ellenberg JH, Gail MH, Ware JH: Randomized clinical trials: Perspectives on some recent ideas. *N Engl J Med* 295:74, 1976.

4. Barnett V: *Comparative Statistical Inference.* New York: Wiley, 1975.

5. Berkson J, Gage RP: Calculation of survival rates for cancer. *Mayo Clin Proc* 25:270, 1950.

6. Bohmer PE: Theorie de unabhangigen Wahrscheinlichkeiten. Rapports, Memoires et Proces-verbaux de Septieme Congres International d'Actuaires, Amsterdam 2:327, 1912.

7. Breslow NE: Analysis of survival data under the proportional hazards model. *Int Stat Rev* 43:45, 1975.

8. Bailey RC, Homer LD, Summe JP: A proposal for the analysis of kidney graft survival. *Transplantation* 24:309, 1977.

9. Buckland WR: *The Life Characteristic*. London: Charles Griffin, 1964.

10. Bertranou EG, Blackstone EH, Hazelrig JB, Turner ME, Kirklin JW: Life expectancy without surgery in tetralogy of Fallot. *Am J Cardiol* 42:458, 1978.

11. Berger TJ, Blackstone EH, Kirklin JW, Bargeron LM, Hazelrig JB, Turner ME: Survival and probability of cure without and with operation in complete atrioventricular canal. *Ann Thorac Surg* 27:104, 1979.

12. Breslow N: Covariance analysis of censored survival data. *Biometrics* 30:89, 1974.

13. Berkson J: Application of the logistic function to bioassay. *Journal of the American Statistical Association* 39:357, 1944.

14. Berkson J: Why I prefer logits to probits. *Biometrics* 7:327, 1951.

15. Berkson J: A statistically precise and relatively simple method of estimating the bioassay with quantal response, based on the logistic function. *Journal of the American Statistical Association* 48:565, 1953.

16. Bunker JP, Barnes DA, Mosteller F (eds): *Costs, Risks, and Benefits of Surgery*. New York: Oxford University, 1977.

17. Boice JD Jr: Follow-up methods to trace women treated for pulmonary tuberculosis, 1930–1954. *Am J Epidemiol* 107:127, 1978.

18. Brownlee KA: *Statistical Theory and Methodology in Science and Engineering* (ed 2). New York: Wiley, 1965, pp 91–95.

19. Ibid, pp 148–149.

20. Ibid, pp 149–150.

21. Bartlett MS: *Essays on Probability and Statistics*. New York: Wiley, 1962.

22. Brownlee KA: *Statistical Theory and Methodology in Science and Engineering* (ed 2). New York: Wiley, 1965, p 217.

23. Breslow NE: Analysis of survival data under the proportional hazards model. *Int Stat Rev* 43:45, 1975.

24. Bradley EL: The equivalence of maximum likelihood and weighted least squares estimates in the exponential family. *Journal of the American Statistical Association* 68:199, 1973.

25. Blackstone EH, Kirklin JW: Rational decision-making in pediatric cardiac surgery, in M Godman (ed): *Pediatric Cardiology*, vol 4. Edinburgh: Churchill Livingstone, 1981, pp 334–343.

26. Blackstone EH, Kirklin JW, Bertranou EG, Labrosse CJ, Soto B, Bargeron LM Jr: Preoperative prediction from cineangiograms of postrepair right ventricular pressure in tetralogy of Fallot. *J Thorac Cariovasc Surg* 78:542, 1979.

27. Bryant GD, Norman GR: Expressions of probability: Words and numbers. *N Engl J Med* 302:422, 1980 (letter to the editor).

28. Breslow NE, Day NE: *Statistical Methods in Cancer Research*. Vol 1: *The Analysis of Case Control Studies*. London: International Agency for Research on Cancer, 1980.

29. Blackstone EH, Naftel DC, Turner ME Jr: The decomposition of time-varying hazard into phases each incorporating a separate stream of concomitant information. *J Am Statist Assn* (in press).

C

1. Cochran WG, Cox GM: *Experimental Designs* (ed 2). New York: Wiley, 1957.

2. Cox DR: *Planning of Experiments*. New York: Wiley, 1958.

3. Croxton FE: *Elementary Statistics with Applications in Medicine and the Biological Sciences*. New York: Dover, 1953.

4. Chiang CL: *Introduction to Stochastic Processes in Biostatistics*. New York: Wiley, 1968.

5. Cox DR: Regression models and life tables. *J. Roy. Stat. Soc. B.* 34:187, 1972.

6. Crombie AC: *Medieval and Early Modern Science*. Vol 2: *Science in the Later Middle Ages and Early Modern Times: XIII–XVII Centuries*. Garden City, NY: Doubleday, 1959, pp 1–35.

7. Cochran WG: Some methods for strengthening the common χ^2 tests. *Biometrics* 10:417, 1954.

8. Cox MAA, Plackett RL: Small samples in contingency tables. *Biometrika* 67:1, 1980.

9. Cox DA: *The Analysis of Binary Data*. London: Methuen, 1970.

10. Califf R, Ornstein S, Kimm SY, Grufferman S, Lee K, Rosati R: Use of the age and sex specific population for analysis of survival in coronary disease. *Am J Cardiol* 50:1279, 1982.

D

1. Dixson WJ, Massey FJ Jr: *Introduction to Statistical Analysis* (ed 2). New York: McGraw-Hill, 1957.

2. DeMoivre A: *The Doctrine of Chances*. 1756. Reprint (ed 3). New York: Chelsea, 1967.

3. Duncan DB: T-tests and intervals for comparisons suggested by the data. *Biometrics* 31:339, 1975.

4. Draper NR, Smith H: *Applied Regression Analysis* (ed 2). New York: Wiley, 1981.

5. Duvoisim GE, Wallace RB, Ellis FH Jr, Anderson MW, McGoon DC: Late results of cardiac-valve replacement. *Circulation* 37, 38(suppl II):II-75, 1968.

6. David HA, Moeschberger ML: *The Theory of Competing Risks*. New York: Macmillan, 1978.

E

1. Eidelman D: Fatigue: Towards an analysis and a unified definition. *Med Hypotheses* 6:517, 1980.

2. Eisenhart C: Expression of the uncertainties of final results. *Science* 160:1201, 1968.

3. Elandt-Johnson RC, Johnson JL: *Survival Models and Data Analysis*. New York: Wiley, 1980.

4. Engelman L: Stepwise logistic regression, in WJ Dixon, MB Brown (eds): *BMDP Biomedical Computer Programs P-series, 1979*. Los Angeles: University of California 1979, pp 517.1–517.13.

F

1. Fisher RA: *Design of Experiments*. Edinburgh: Oliver and Boyd, 1935.

2. Feinstein AR: *Clinical Biostatistics*. St. Louis: Mosby, 1977.

3. Fraser DAS: *Nonparametric Methods in Statistics*. New York: Wiley, 1957.

4. Forsythe AB, Frey HS: Tests of significance from survival data. *Comput Biomed Res* 3:124, 1970.

5. Feinstein AR: Clinical biostatistics XX: The epidemiologic trohoc, the ablative risk ratio, and 'retrospective' research. *Clin Pharmacol Ther* 14:291, 1973.

6. Fliegel HF, Van Flandern TC: A machine algorithm for processing calendar dates. *Communications of the ACM* 11:657, 1968.

7. Fisher RA: *Statistical Methods for Research Workers*. 1925. Reprint (ed 14). New York: Hafner, 1970.

8. Feinstein AR: The Jones criteria and the challenges of clinimetrics. *Circulation* 66:1, 1982.

9. Fisher RA: The use of multiple measurements in taxonomic problems. *Ann Eugenics* 7:179, 1936.

G

1. Galilei, G: Sopra le scoperte dei dadi, as summarized in R Langley: *Practical Statistics Simply Explained*. New York: Dover, 1970.
2. Gauss CF: Theory of motion of the heavenly bodies moving about the sun in conic sections. 1809. Reprint. New York: Dover, 1963.
3. *Gauss's Work (1803–1826) on the Theory of Least Squares*, F Trotter (trans). Statistical Techniques Research Group, Technical Report No. 5. Princeton, NJ: Princeton University, 1957.
4. Gross AJ, Clark VA: *Survival Distributions: Reliability Applications in the Biomedical Sciences*. New York: Wiley, 1975.
5. Gehan EA: A generalized Wilcoxon test for comparing arbitrarily singly-censored samples. *Biometrika* 52:203, 1965.
6. Gehan EA, Freireich EJ: Non-randomized controls in cancer clinical trials. *N Engl J Med* 290:198–203, 1974.
7. Glantz SA: Biostatistics: How to detect, correct and prevent errors in the medical literature. *Circulation* 61:1, 1980.
8. Greenwood M: The natural duration of cancer. *Reports on Public Health and Medical Subjects* 33:1, 1926.
9. Goodman LA: The variance of the product of k random variables. *Journal of the American Statistical Association* 57:54, 1962.
10. Gordon T, Kannel WB: Multiple risk functions for predicting coronary heart disease: The concept, accuracy, and application. *Am Heart J* 103:1031, 1982.
11. Glass GV: Integrating findings: The meta-analysis of research, in L Shulman (ed): *Review of Research in Education*, vol 5. Itasca, Ill: FE Peacock, 1977.
12. Grunkemeier GL, Lambert LE, Bonchek LI, Starr A: An improved statistical method for assessing the results of operation. *Ann Thorac Surg* 20:289, 1975.

H

1. Hollander M, Wolfe DA: *Non-parametric Statistical Methods*. New York: Wiley, 1973.
2. Halley E: An estimate of the degrees of the mortality of mankind, drawn from curious tables of the births and funerals of the city of Breslau. *Philosophical Transactions of the Royal Society of London*. 17:596, 1693.
3. Hazelrig JB, Turner ME, Blackstone EH: Parametric survival analysis combining longitudinal and cross-sectional censored and interval censored data with concomitant information. *Biometrics* 38:1, 1982.
4. Heisenberg W: *Physics and Philosophy: The Revolution in Modern Science*. New York: Harper and Brothers, 1958.
5. Haddon W: The prevention of accidents, in DW Clark, B McMahon (eds): *Textbook of Preventive Medicine*. Boston: Little, Brown, 1967, pp 591–621.
6. Hakulinen T: On long-term relative survival rates. *J Chronic Dis* 30:431, 1977.
7. Harrell F: The LOGIST procedure, in *SAS Supplemental Library User's Guide*. Cary, NC: SAS Institute, 1980, pp 83–102.
8. Hosmer DW, Wang CY, Lin IC, Lemeshow S: A computer program for stepwise logistic regression using maximum likelihood estimation. *Comput Programs Biomed* 8:121, 1978.

I

1. Ivert TSA, Dismukes WE, Cobbs GC, Blackstone EH, Kirklin JW, Bergdahl LAL: Prosthetic valve endocarditis. *Circulation* 69:223, 1984.

J

1. Jaynes ET: Prior probabilities. *Transactions of Systems Science and Cybernetics* SSC-4:227, 1968.

K

1. Kalbfleisch JD, Prentice RL: *The Statistical Analysis of Failure-Time Data*. New York: Wiley, 1980.
2. Kaplan EL, Meier P: Nonparametric estimation from incomplete observations. *Journal of the American Statistical Association* 53:457, 1958.
3. Kirklin JW: A letter to Helen. *J Thorac Cardiovasc Surg* 78:543, 1979.
4. Kempthorne O: Of what use are tests of significance and tests of hypotheses? *Commun Statist Theor Meth A* 5:763, 1976.
5. Kruskal WH, Wallis WA: Use of ranks in one-criterion analysis of variance. *Journal of the American Statistical Association* 47:583, 1952.
6. Kuzma J: A comparison of two life table methods. *Biometrics* 23:51, 1967.
7. Ku HH: Notes on the use of propagation of error formulas. *Journal of Research of the National Bureau of Standards* 70C:263, 1966.
8. Kirklin JW, Kouchoukos NT, Blackstone EH, Oberman A: Research related to surgical treatment of coronary artery disease. *Circulation* 60:1613, 1979.
9. Katz NM, Blackstone EH, Kirklin JW, Pacifico AD, Bargeron LM Jr: Late survival and symptoms after repair of tetralogy of Fallot. *Circulation* 65:403, 1982.
10. Kirklin JW, Blackstone EH, Pacifico AD, Brown RN, Bargeron LM Jr: Routine primary repair vs. two-stage repair of tetralogy of Fallot. *Circulation* 60:373, 1979.
11. Kodlin D: A new response time distribution. *Biometrics* 23:227, 1967.

L

1. Lloyd LE: Techniques for efficient research. New York: Chemical, 1966.
2. Lawrence AC: Human error as a cause of accidents in gold mining. *Journal of Safety Research* 6:78, 1974.
3. Lewantin RC, Felsenstein J: The robustness of homogeneity tests in 2 × N tables. *Biometrics* 21:19, 1965.
4. Larntz K: Small-sample comparisons of exact levels for chi-square goodness-of-fit statistics. *Journal of the American Statistical Association* 73:253, 1978.
5. Lilienfeld DE, Pyne DA: On indices of mortality: Deficiencies, validity, and alternatives. *J Chronic Dis* 32:463, 1979.
6. Loop FD: A surgeon's view of randomized prospective studies. *J Thorac Cardiovasc Surg* 78:161, 1979.
7. Lew RA, Day CL Jr, Harrist TJ, Wood WC, Mihm MC Jr: Multivariate analysis: Some guidelines for physicians. *JAMA* 249:641, 1983.

M

1. Meier P: Statistics and medical experimentation. *Biometrics* 31:511, 1975.

2. Murphy RD, Papps PCH: *Construction of Mortality Tables from the Records of Insured Lives*. New York: The Actuarial Society of America, 1922.

3. Mantel N, Haenszel W: Statistical aspects of the analysis of data from retrospective studies of disease. *J Nat Cancer Inst* 22:719, 1959.

4. Mantel N: Evaluation of survival data and two new rank order statistics arising in its consideration. *Cancer Chemotherapy Reports* 50:163, 1966.

5. McIntosh JEA, McIntosh RP: *Mathematical Modelling and Computers in Endocrinology*. New York: Springer-Verlag, 1980, pp 1–73.

N

1. Neyman J: On the problem of confidence intervals. *Ann Math Stat* 6:111, 1935.

2. Neyman J: Outline of a theory of statistical estimation based on the classical theory of probability. *Philosophical Transactions Series A* 236:333, 1937.

3. Nelson W: Theory and applications of hazard plotting for censored failure data. *Technometrics* 14:945, 1972.

O

1. O'Neill TJ: Distribution-free estimation of cure time. *Biometrika* 66:184, 1979.

P

1. Pearson K: *Early Statistical Papers*. Cambridge, Mass: Cambridge University, 1956.

2. Prentice RL, Marek P: A qualitative discrepancy between censored data rank tests. *Biometrics* 35:861, 1979.

3. Peto R, Peto J: Asymptotically efficient rank invariant test procedures. *Journal of the Royal Statistical Society A* 135:185, 1972.

4. Prentice RL, Kalbfleisch JD, Peterson AV Jr, Flournoy N, Farewell VT, Breslow NE: The analysis of failure times in the presence of competing risks. *Biometrics* 34:541, 1978.

5. Pregibon D: Logistic regression diagnostics. *Ann Statist* 9:705, 1981.

6. Pregibon D: Goodness of link tests for generalized linear models. *Applied Statistics* 29:15, 1980.

R

1. Reed LJ, Berkson J: The application of the logistic function to experimental data. *Journal of Physical Chemistry* 33:760, 1929.

2. Rothman KJ, Boice JK Jr: *Epidemiologic Analysis with a Programmable Calculator*. Washington, DC: US Government Printing Office, 1979, pp 38–39, 137–140.

S

1. Spodick DH: Numerators without denominators: There is no FDA for the surgeon. *JAMA* 232:35, 1975.

2. Shapiro SS, Wilk MB: An analysis of variance test for normality (complete samples). *Biometrika* 52:591, 1965.

3. Stephens MA: Use of the Kolmogorov-Smirnov, Cramer–Von Mises and related statistics without extensive tables. *Journal of the American Statistical Association* 69:730, 1974.

4. "Student": The probable error of a mean. *Biometrika* 6:1, 1908.

5. Sokal RR, Rohlf FJ: *Biometry: The Principle and Practice of Statistics in Biological Research*. San Francisco: Freeman, 1969.

6. Studer M, Blackstone EH, Kirklin JW, Pacifico AD, Soto B, Chung GKT, Kirklin JK, Bargeron LM Jr: Determinants of early and late results of repair of atrioventricular septal (canal) defects. *J Thorac Cardiovasc Surg* 84:523, 1982.

T

1. Tukey JW: *Exploratory Data Analysis*. Reading, Mass: Addison-Wesley, 1977.

2. Turner ME, Pruitt KM: A common basis for survival, growth, and autocatalysis. *Mathematical Biosciences* 39:113, 1978.

3. Turner ME, Hazelrig JB, Blackstone EH: Bounded survival. *Mathematical Biosciences* 59:33, 1982.

4. Tukey J: Some thoughts on clinical trials, especially problems of multiplicity. *Science* 198:679, 1977.

V

1. *Vital Statistics of the United States*. Vol II: *Mortality*. Hyattsville, Md: US Department of Health, Education, and Welfare, Public Health Service, National Center for Health Statistics, 1976.

2. Verhulst PF: Notice sur la loi que la population suit dans son accroissement. *Mathématique et Physique* 10:113, 1838.

3. Verhulst PF: Recherches mathématiques sur la loi d'accroissement de la population. *Nouv Mém Acad Roy Sci Belleslett, Bruxelles* 18:1, 1845.

W

1. Walker SH, Duncan DB: Estimation of the probability of an event as a function of several independent variables. *Biometrika* 54:167, 1967.

2. Wigglesworth EC: A teaching model of injury causation and a guide for selecting countermeasures. *Occupational Psychology* 46:69, 1972.

3. Weast RC, Selby SM (eds): *Handbook of Tables for Mathematics*. Cleveland: CRC, 1975.

4. Welch BL: The significance of the difference between two means when the population variances are unequal. *Biometrika* 29:350, 1937.

5. Welch BL: The generalization of 'Student's' problem when several different population variances are involved. *Biometrika* 34:28, 1947.

6. Wilcoxon F: Individual comparisons by ranking methods. *Biometrics Bulletin* 1:80, 1947.

7. Weinstein MC: Allocation of subjects in medical experiments. *N Engl J Med* 291:1278, 1974.

Y

1. Yates F: Contingency tables involving small numbers and the χ^2 test. *Journal of the Royal Statistical Society* 1(suppl):217, 1934.

ISCHEMIC
HEART DISEASE

PART II

7

STENOTIC ARTERIOSCLEROTIC CORONARY ARTERY DISEASE

DEFINITION

Stenotic arteriosclerotic coronary artery disease is a narrowing of the coronary arteries due to atherosclerosis, which limits the flow of blood to the myocardium. Initially, the disease limits the normal response to stimuli that tend to increase coronary blood flow, but when sufficiently advanced, it reduces the blood flow through the affected artery even at rest. In its most severe form, it occludes the coronary artery.

HISTORICAL NOTE

The development of coronary cinearteriography by Sones,[S1] at the Cleveland Clinic, in the early 1960s made possible the direct identification of stenotic and obstructive arteriosclerotic lesions in the coronary arteries and laid the basis for coronary artery surgery. Previously, sporadic surgical efforts had been made to improve coronary blood flow, but they were almost blind ones because of the lack of precise anatomic diagnosis. In 1951, Vineberg, in Montreal, reported the direct implantation of an internal mammary artery into the myocardium,[V1] a procedure that the Cleveland Clinic group showed years later brought new blood to the left ventricular myocardium.[E4] However, the new blood flow was too small in amount and limited in distribution to be effective. In 1954, Murray and associates obviously were thinking about a direct surgical approach to coronary artery disease when they reported experimental studies of the anastomosis of the internal mammary artery to a coronary artery.[M7] Shortly thereafter, Longmire and colleagues, at the University of California in Los Angeles, reported a series of patients in whom direct-vision coronary endarterectomy was carried out without cardiopulmonary bypass (CPB).[L9] Then CPB began to be used to facilitate the operation, and Senning reported patch grafting of a stenotic coronary artery in 1961.[S17] At about this time, Effler and colleagues, at the Cleveland Clinic, began their consistent efforts to achieve myocardial revascularization by a direct surgical attack on stenotic coronary lesions demonstrated by Sones through coronary arteriography.[E2,S16]

In May 1967, Favaloro and Effler, at the Cleveland Clinic, began performing reversed saphenous vein bypass grafting, and by January 1971, this group had performed 741 such operations.[L3] Favaloro, now in Buenos Aires, described the technique of the operation from the Cleveland Clinic in 1969.[F4] Even earlier, Garrett, at that time working with DeBakey in Houston, successfully performed a reversed saphenous vein coronary artery bypass graft to the left anterior descending artery in an unplanned way;[G6] at restudy seven years later the vein graft was still open.

Progress was rapid after this early era. In 1968, Green, in New York, reported the anastomosis of the distal end of the left internal mammary artery to the anterior descending artery,[G7] using the dissecting microscope, and Edwards and colleagues (along with Kerr, now at GLH) also began using this procedure at UAB in 1969.[E3] In 1971, Flemma, Johnson, and Lepley, in Milwaukee, described the technique and advantages of sequential grafting, in which one vein was used for several distal anastomoses.[F6] The advantages of this technique were further amplified by the reports of Bartley, Bigelow, and Page[B2] in 1972 and Sewell in 1974.[S2] Thus, within a very short time, the foundations were laid for the rapid spread throughout the world of the operation of coronary artery bypass grafting (CABG).

MORPHOLOGY

Development of Coronary Artery Stenosis

The arteriosclerotic process in the coronary arteries, as in other blood vessels, consists of focal intimal accumulations of lipids, complex carbohydrates, blood and blood products, fibrous tissue, and calcium deposits, associated with changes in the media. The lipoid foci are associated with or converted into plaques of fibrous or hyaline connective tissue, although current thinking suggests that at least some atherosclerotic plaques result from the organization of thrombi.[R7]

The fibrolipoid plaques may become very thick and encroach upon the lumen of the artery to produce a stenotic lesion. Probably episodically, and at times over a period of years, new layers develop on the luminal side of the plaque, resulting in further narrowing and sometimes complete coronary occlusion. Newly formed very small blood vessels form around and within the atheroma. Hemorrhage may occur suddenly within a plaque (the mechanism of its development is debated), and occasionally this may suddenly increase the degree of coronary stenosis and precipitate acute myocardial infarction or unstable angina pectoris. Gradual regression of plaque swelling, seen clinically as regression of stenoses in a few patients,[S36] and the development of collateral coronary blood flow can result in at least partial spontaneous restoration of regional myocardial blood flow.

Thrombosis occasionally complicates the coronary arteriosclerotic process, generally when there is luminal narrowing. Sudden complete obstruction may result, and it is generally now agreed that acute thrombotic occlusion is the genesis of acute myocardial infarction in most patients. Rapid recanalization frequently follows this process.

Platelet aggregation within the lumen of an already narrowed coronary artery may induce the thrombosis or may per se suddenly narrow the lumen and provoke an acute myocardial infarction or unstable angina. Platelet aggregation may play a role in the development of the atherosclerotic plaque itself. Moreover, platelet aggregation releases thromboxane A_2, an extremely potent vasoconstrictor. Thus, the interrelationships among atherosclerotic narrowing, platelet aggregation, and coronary spasm may be important.

The arteriosclerotic process usually affects multiple coronary arteries. Gensini has reported that 40% of patients with coronary artery disease sufficient to lead to cineangiographic study have significant stenoses in all three major coronary arteries, while 30% have two vessels involved.[G9] Ninety-five percent of patients with complete occlusions of one artery have important stenoses in at least one of the other two arteries. In a recent study at GLH in which 324 men under 60 years of age had coronary angiography performed routinely 4 weeks after surviving a first myocardial infarction, 37% had a score of 10.1–15 (equivalent to triple-vessel disease), 52% had a score of 5.1–10 (equivalent to double-vessel disease), and only 11% had a score of less than 5 (equivalent to single-vessel disease).

The disease usually involves the proximal portion of the larger coronary arteries, particularly at or just beyond the sites of branching. Thus, coronary artery stenoses in the main trunks of the left anterior descending (LAD) artery, circumflex (Cx) artery, and right coronary arteries (RCA) often involve the first of the secondary branches (that is, the first diagonal branch of the LAD artery, the obtuse marginal branch of the Cx artery, and the posterior descending branch [PDA] of the RCA). When the disease is more extensive in the main trunks, the origins and first portions of more distal secondary branches may be involved. Diffuse distal disease, at least severe enough to render the patient unsuitable for CABG, is extremely uncommon.

The right coronary and the left anterior descending systems are more frequently involved in the atherosclerotic obstructive process than is the circumflex artery. In 10%–20% of patients with important coronary artery stenoses, the left main coronary artery is involved with an important stenosis.

Occasionally, a major coronary artery may lie beneath a muscle bridge. This is most common in the mid third of the LAD artery, but sometimes one or all of the obtuse marginal branches of the circumflex artery are buried in muscle throughout their course. Almost always these portions of artery are free of atheroma.

Myocardial Infarction and Its Morphologic Sequelae

When myocardial blood flow is sufficiently impaired in relationship to myocardial oxygen demands, myocardial necrosis occurs. The resultant infarction may be subendocardial and not involve the entire thickness of the ventricular wall. In its most extreme form, subendocardial infarction may be diffuse and result from triple-vessel disease, but more often subendocardial infarcts are regional and result primarily from the stenotic lesion in one or two vessels. They are generally less extensive than so-called transmural infarcts. A *transmural* myocardial infarction involves the entire thickness of the ventricular wall. It is usually the result of a sudden increase in luminal narrowing or the complete obstruction of the artery supplying that area, or a sudden generalized increase in myocardial oxygen demand in the presence of a severely stenotic coronary artery. Although the categorization of acute infarctions as subendocardial or transmural is convenient, most so-called transmural myocardial infarcts are not homogenous but contain islands of viable muscle of varying number and size.

The process of infarction is complex. Animal studies indicate that some myocardial cells die after 20 minutes of complete coronary occlusion and that after 60 minutes of complete occlusion, there is extensive myocardial cell death.[S14] However, probably within minutes of the onset of the episode of acute ischemia, some reperfusion occurs within the ischemic area of myocardium, particularly in the border zone. If this spontaneous reperfusion occurs within 3–4 hours, the amount of necrosis is restricted, at times considerably so;[T4] infarct size is reduced; and mortality is decreased.[B27] The complexity of the process is evidenced by the fact that, in addition to these beneficial effects, spontaneous reperfusion can lead to hemorrhage, edema, and ventricular electrical instability.[C14,K15]

Healing of the acute myocardial infarction leaves a scarred

area of myocardium. Usually this scarred area is a mixture of fibrous tissue and viable myocardial cells in varying proportions. Such scarring is evident from intraoperative inspections of areas of previous infarction and from the change from akinesia to hypokinesia or normal wall motion in some left ventricular wall segments when patients go from a symptomatic to an asymptomatic state after percutaneous transluminal coronary angioplasty or coronary artery bypass grafting. When the scar is virtually all fibrous tissue, it is usually large and termed a left ventricular *aneurysm* (see Chapter 8).

These morphologic changes may be self-aggravating because of their effect on the circulation to the subendocardial layer, and repeated infarctions may occur and add still more scarring. In aggregate, myocardial scarring leads to left ventricular systolic and diastolic dysfunction and, ultimately, if the patient survives long enough, to the syndrome of chronic congestive heart failure with elevated right atrial and jugular venous pressure, hepatomegaly, and fluid retention. More commonly, however, patients with severe ischemic left ventricular dysfunction die of another infarction or of sudden ventricular fibrillation.

Sudden Death

Severe triple-vessel coronary artery disease results more frequently in sudden death *without* evidence of myocardial necrosis than in fatal acute myocardial infarction.[B17] Presumably, sudden death without infarction is from sudden ventricular fibrillation, precipitated by acute thrombosis, sudden increase in severity of the stenotic lesion, embolism of transient platelet aggregates, massive catecholamine release, or as yet unknown mechanisms.[J4]

CLINICAL FEATURES AND DIAGNOSTIC CRITERIA

Routine Methods

Coronary artery disease is usually first suspected with the development of the symptom complex of angina pectoris or of an acute myocardial infarction; occasionally because of electrocardiographic evidence of the relics of a silent acute myocardial infarction or because of a positive electrocardiographic response to a graded exercise test; or because of sudden death with resuscitation. Rarely, coronary artery disease is first suspected because of cardiomegaly and symptoms of chronic congestive heart failure without any other obvious cause.

The exact nature, location, duration, and severity of any chest pain is determined by careful questioning of the patient. Its precipitating causes and maneuvers that relieve it are noted, as are any recent changes in the pain pattern. The findings on physical examination are usually not specific.

Many noninvasive tests, beginning with a chest roentgenogram and an electrocardiogram at rest and during exercise and extending to include more complex methods, are currently used to identify and quantitate the coronary artery disease and its sequelae. Such tests cannot as yet accurately define the extent or distribution of the anatomic coronary

disease. From a surgical standpoint, therefore, properly performed coronary arteriography remains the definitive diagnostic procedure. This could change as new noninvasive methods and methods that enable the surgeon to define stenotic lesions in the operating room with reasonable accuracy are perfected.[S22]

Methods of evaluating left ventricular (LV) function are also necessary. These may be based in part on historical data, physical findings, and the chest x-ray film. Noninvasive and/or invasive special study methods may be used. Even when complex study methods are employed, the results must be interpreted with knowledge of the simple but reliable clinical data. An ejection fraction (EF) of 0.35 has a different implication when accompanied by minimal LV enlargement as seen on the chest roentgenogram than when enlargement is marked; and an EF of 0.30 is much more ominous when accompanied by important elevation of jugular and right atrial pressure with hepatomegaly and fluid retention than when these variables are normal. Exercise capacity may be variable in patients with similar EFs, and the variations are prognostically important. It should be noted, however, that heart size can be deceptive, for it can remain normal in the presence of severe LV dysfunction.

Such important associated conditions as arterial hypertension, diabetes, and a history of myocardial infarction, smoking, or a particularly stressful occupation or life-style should be noted. Since arteriosclerosis is the cause of the coronary artery disease, a history suggesting transient cerebral ischemic attacks and the finding of carotid bruits must be carefully pursued. Intermittent claudication and diminished femoral, popliteal, or pedal pulses are looked for. The thoracic and abdominal aorta are examined for possible aneurysm. Renal function is evaluated.

Coronary Arteriography

The coronary angiograms must provide definitive information. Their quality must be sufficient to permit detailed assessment from several angles of both coronary ostia and all the major and minor branches of both left and right coronary arteries. However, angiography is currrently not a perfect method. The severity of a visualized stenotic lesion may be underestimated by coronary arteriography. The diameter of vessels distal to a stenosis is often underestimated, and small distal size on cineangiography should not be a contraindication to operation. Levin and colleagues found that bypass grafts could be successfully placed in 73% of vessels considered to be inadequate because of severe distal narrowing or absence of filling on the arteriogram.[L23]

Assessment of the coronary arteries at operation by external palpation or probing of the open vessel cannot substitute for good coronary arteriograms. However, when the arteries cannot be adequately filled by contrast media, or for some reason the study that is available is incomplete and cannot be repeated (this should be uncommon), the intraoperative observations can be used to supplement the findings from the angiographic studies. In fact, the surgeon should assess all branches carefully at the time of the operation, rather than assuming that the coronary arteriogram is a totally precise diagnostic tool (see "Strategy of the Operation," "The Management of Less Than 50% Narrowings in Patients Already Committed to Operation," and "The Importance of Complete Revascularization").

The techniques of coronary arteriography at GLH and UAB, while differing in some details, are representative of most generally accepted practices (see Appendix 7A).

Recording and Reporting Data from Coronary Arteriography

Whatever the techniques used for coronary arteriography, the methods of recording and analyzing the data are critically important.

A 75% cross-sectional area loss (50% diameter loss) is considered a significant but moderate stenosis, while a 90% cross-sectional area (67% diameter) loss is considered severe (Fig. 7-1). Some groups have considered significant only those lesions with a 70% or more diameter loss (90% or more cross-sectional area loss).[H8,K17,W7]

It is conventional to classify the extent of significant coronary artery stenoses as single-vessel, double-vessel, or triple-vessel disease, usually with left main coronary artery disease as a separate category. In this chapter, the terms *single-*, *double-*, and *triple-vessel disease* are used, for the most part, to comply with this convention and allow comparison with other data reported in the literature. However, these terms have been quite properly criticized[G20,G21,S31] because they give no indication of the amount of left ventricular myocardium made ischemic by the lesions. For example, a stenosis in the LAD has a different significance when it lies at the origin of a large first diagonal artery than when it involves the mid third of the artery beyond its major septal and diagonal branches. A single stenosis in the proximal portion of the Cx artery varies in significance depending on whether this artery is dominant. Single-vessel disease involving the right coronary artery has a different implication from that involving the anterior descending artery. Many other examples can be given of the inadequacies of this type of terminology. Obviously, the relating of the results of medical or surgical treatment to the functionally important amount of coronary artery disease will be imprecise until the simpler terms are abandoned in favor of a correct manner of recording and quantitating the obstructions to myocardial perfusion by some sort of myocardial perfusion score. This has recently been documented by two studies showing more precise prediction of survival by a myocardial perfusion scoring system than by the simpler system.[G22,P11]

Only a few systems have been described to obviate these shortcomings. They include Gensini's rather complex scheme, which takes into account the severity of the stenoses, the various segments of the coronary artery tree involved, and the area of myocardium usually perfused by them;[G20,G21,G23] a simple scheme from the Massachusetts General Hospital;[J8] and the recent but incomplete method of the Coronary Artery Surgery Study (CASS) of the United States National Heart, Lung, and Blood Institute (NHLBI), dividing the coronary arteries into a total of 27 specified segments. Some so-called myocardial jeopardy scores have attempted to do the same thing but suffer from the assumption that akinetic areas cannot be revascularized.[R10]

A realistic and practicable myocardial perfusion scoring system has been in continuous use at GLH since 1972[B33] and is recommended for general use (see Appendix 7B). A diagram made by the reporting radiologist is displayed at the time of operation, when it functions as an accurate guide to the surgeon. It can also be used for computer storage of arteriographic information.

Whatever the recording and reporting methods, they are not a substitute for the personal review of the cineangiograms by the surgeon before making the decision for or against operation and again immediately before the operation. Ideally, the cineangiograms should be reviewed again after the operation to correlate the surgical and angiographic findings.

Tests for Global and Segmental Left Ventricular Function

Resting Global Left Ventricular Systolic Function

The global left ventricular systolic function can be estimated by global ejection fraction, usually obtained from quantitative angiographic measurements of end-diastolic and end-systolic volumes. This may be done by integration from the right anterior oblique (RAO) projection (GLH), but possible errors are introduced by reliance on single-plane (rather than biplane) angiocardiography for assessment of LV function.

An ejection fraction > 0.50 is considered normal (more strictly, ≥ 0.60 is normal; < 0.60 and ≥ 0.50, borderline normal or mildly depressed, depending on age); < 0.50 and ≥ 0.40, mildly depressed; < 0.4 and ≥ 0.30, moderately depressed; and < 0.30, severely depressed. When the EF is abnormal at rest, additional information can be obtained by noting the EF after a ventricular ectopic beat, for then the ventricle is responding to the stress of increased ventricular filling. If quantitative angiocardiography is not done, a subjective estimate of the EF can be made from the left ventriculogram. Echocardiographic and radioisotopic imaging

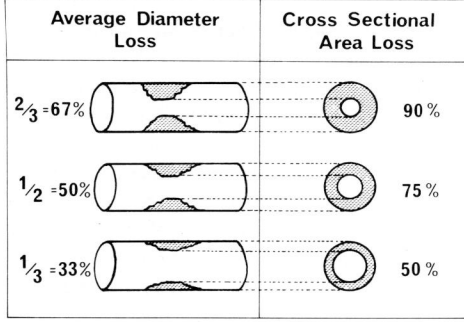

Average Diameter Loss	Cross Sectional Area Loss
²⁄₃ = 67%	90%
¹⁄₂ = 50%	75%
¹⁄₃ = 33%	50%

Figure 7-1 Diagrammatic presentation of the relationship between the two methods of estimating the severity of coronary artery stenosis. Reports from UAB use diameter loss, while those from GLH use cross-sectional area loss.

Reproduced with permission from Brandt et al.[B33]

methods can also be used for these assessments (see "Methodology").

Resting Global Left Ventricular Diastolic Function
The left ventricular end-diastolic pressure measured before and after performing the ventriculogram to some extent reflects resting left ventricular diastolic function. More sophisticated methods of studying diastolic function are available but are generally not used in making individual patient care decisions.

Resting Segmental Left Ventricular Systolic Wall Function
Compared to resting global systolic function, the resting segmental left ventricular systolic wall function is a more refined and in some ways informative determination.[A3,G8,Z2] It can be studied informally by viewing the cineangiogram, but more precise methods are usually used. For example, the left ventricular outline may be divided into five segments[A5] (anterobasal, anterolateral, apical, diaphragmatic, and posterobasal) and the motion of each segment recorded visually as normal, hypokinetic, akinetic, or dyskinetic (GLH). Biplane cineangiography and 10 segments may be used (UAB),[R10] and in some institutions still different numbers of segments are used. Ideally, the coronary artery distribution to each of the segments in the individual patient should also be noted. This information can be correlated with the areas of myocardial scarring as assessed electrocardiographically. However, the addition of a jeopardy score,[J8,K17,R10] based on an assumption that severely hypokinetic or akinetic areas are already irreversibly damaged and therefore *not* in jeopardy, is *not* a valid guide to the selection of the arteries that should be bypassed. Akinetic and dyskinetic areas *do* improve in function after the grafting of the coronary arteries to such areas in some patients.

Global and Segmental Left Ventricular Function during Stress
Electrocardiographic stress testing is an indirect study of global and segmental left ventricular functions. Sophisticated studies during exercise have added a new dimension to the understanding of ischemic heart disease and the effect of CABG but are not a necessary part of preoperative evaluation in most patients.

Other Variables
Cardiac output, measured at cardiac catheterization by the Fick or other indicator dilution methods; left ventricular end-diastolic pressure; pulmonary artery pressure; and right ventricular and right atrial pressures are also helpful in evaluating left ventricular performance, particularly in patients on the border of operability.

Methodology
The evaluation of left ventricular performance is a rapidly changing area. Currently, indexes of both systolic and diastolic left ventricular function at rest can be obtained by echocardiographic techniques. Combined studies using angiocardiography and echocardiography can be particularly useful in providing complete information.[H1,H3,J3,R2] Quantitative radionuclide angiography using either first-pass or equilibration (gated) techniques provides information concerning both global and regional LV function and can be used when the patient is at rest or during exercise.[H1,P9,S11,S12,S13] Myocardial perfusion imaging with thallium 201 can be used to define areas of myocardial ischemia that appear as cold spots in the scan. Future developments in instrumentation and in computer analysis of scintillation data can be expected to refine these techniques, which are particularly attractive because they are essentially noninvasive and suitable for exercise studies.

NATURAL HISTORY

Great gaps exist in the knowledge of the natural history of persons with arteriosclerotic coronary artery disease. Many of these gaps will be permanent, since the withholding of at least medical treatment is no longer justifiable. The closest approach to natural history comes from the data gathered in patients seen and treated medically before about 1970. Unfortunately, many studies from that earlier era suffer from the disadvantage that patients were not categorized according to the anatomic extent of their disease and left ventricular function. Since about 1970, patients generally have been categorized, but medical treatment has become more effective and no doubt has changed the life history.

From the standpoint of finding a reference point for the results of surgery for ischemic heart disease, a further complexity is that in nearly all studies since 1970, patients have quite properly been allowed to *cross over* to surgical treatment during the study period. Thus, virtually all currently available information compares the results of surgery, not with natural history or the results of medical treatment, but with medical treatment in a situation in which surgery was available and allowed if the situation warranted it. This matter becomes particularly important in interpreting the results of randomized trials.

Survival According to Anatomic Extent of Disease

The proportion of patients with stable or unstable angina pectoris, acute myocardial infarction and death, sudden or otherwise, tends to vary with the anatomical extent of the disease. Unfortunately, information concerning events other than survival is particularly incomplete, and even the survival data are compromised by variable criteria as to what constitutes a significant stenosis and no doubt also by poor-quality angiography in a number of the earlier studies. The far from satisfactory classification of patients into single-, double-, or triple-vessel disease categories is also to be noted, as well as the fact that nearly all the large natural history studies have been carried out in *symptomatic* patients, generally with angina.

When important ($\geq 50\%$ reduction of diameter) narrowing is limited to one major coronary artery and left ventricular function is not severely depressed, survival is similar to that of an age- and sex-matched general population, with about

95% of patients alive 5 years later (Fig. 7-2). However, recalculation on the data presented by Mock and colleagues from the CASS Registry (in which approximately 20% of the patients crossed over to surgery during the study period and were then censored from the actuarial analysis) indicates a difference ($P < .0001$) between the 97% 4-year survival of patients without significant ($\geq 70\%$ diameter reduction) coronary artery stenosis and that of 92% in patients with single-vessel disease.[M19] It is a reasonable assumption that in this and all other similar situations, survival would have been worse had crossover not been allowed. Friesinger and colleagues also found a similarly high survival rate in patients with single-vessel disease.[F9] Patients with very proximal (proximal to the first septal artery) isolated left anterior descending coronary artery stenosis have a 90% 5-year survival rate, compared with 98% for those with more distal lesions.[C25] The strategic importance of severe proximal LAD stenosis is also evident from the fact that the response of ejection fraction to exercise in patients without previous infarction is generally normal in patients with single- or double-vessel disease not involving the proximal LAD artery and usually abnormal when an important proximal LAD artery stenosis exists alone or in combination with other lesions.[K21] Conversely, the prognosis is better ($P = .03$) for patients with single-vessel disease in the right coronary artery than for those with disease in other vessels.[C25] The 5-year survival rate is 96% in patients with right coronary disease, compared with 92% in patients with left coronary disease.

When there are also mild ($< 50\%$) stenoses in other arteries associated with an important stenosis in a single major artery, life expectancy is further reduced (Fig. 7-3), possibly because of the known tendency of such lesions to progress.

When important stenoses are present in two of the three major coronary arteries (LAD, Cx, and/or RCA) and left ventricular function is not known to be severely depressed, the 5-year survival with medical treatment alone has been estimated to be as low as 70%.[P13] Mock and colleagues reported from the CASS Registry, in which approximately 40% of the patients crossed over to surgery during the study period and were censored, that about 85% of patients treated nonsurgically were alive 4 years later.[M19] This survival rate is lower than that of the general population (Fig. 7-2). When very proximal LAD artery stenosis is part of the double-vessel disease, survival may be reduced further. Thus, the European Coronary Surgery Study Group, in which surgical crossover occurred but censoring was not done, found in patients under 65 years of age with normal or only mildly depressed left ventricular function that 5-year survival with double-vessel disease that included an important proximal LAD artery lesion was 82% (similar to that for triple-vessel disease) when initial assignment was to medical treatment, whereas in its absence, survival was 96%.[E5,V2] Similarly, Chaitman and colleagues reported that in the CASS Registry sponsored by the United States National Institutes of Health (NIH), patients with severe proximal stenoses in the LAD and Cx arteries had a 5-year survival rate of 55%, compared to that of 70% for similar patients in whom the LAD artery lesion was in the mid portion of the artery (P for difference

$= .001$).[C27] It was also found that the patients with proximal LAD and Cx artery disease varied in their 5-year survival from 76% to 30% depending on their myocardial perfusion score, emphasizing again the imprecision of categorizing patients simply as having single-, double-, or triple-vessel disease. Data from Duke University suggest that survival is poorer when a total occlusion of the RCA is associated with a severe lesion of the LAD artery.[M10] Stenoses of less than 50% diameter reduction in the third artery probably unfavorably affect the outlook of patients with double-vessel disease, but secure information in this regard is not available.

When important disease is present in the three major arteries, 5-year survival of patients is clearly less than that of an age- and sex-matched general population. According to Proudfit and colleagues, only 50% of patients survived 5 years with nonsurgical treatment. According to the United States Veterans Administration Cooperative Study (in which surgical crossover was allowed and occurred), when resting left ventricular function was not severely depressed, about 75% of patients initially assigned to medical treatment survived about 5 years (Fig. 7-2). This percentage includes patients with a left main stenosis. According to the European Coronary Surgery Study Group, which also allowed crossover to surgery, about 85% of surgically untreated patients under 65 years of age with triple-vessel disease (excluding those with left main stenosis) and with normal or only mildly depressed resting left ventricular function lived 5 years.[V2] The 4-year survival of patients with 70% diameter narrowing in all three major coronary arteries was 68% in the CASS Registry, in which approximately 50% of the patients crossed over to surgery during the study period.[M19] The variation in these surgical figures emphasizes the wide range of stenotic coronary artery disease included under the heading of triple-vessel disease, and the effect of other variables. Also, in triple-vessel disease, severe proximal LAD stenoses appear to be critically important. Schuster and colleagues found that 92% of their 77 autopsied cases of death from recent acute myocardial infarction had triple-vessel disease, with proximal LAD artery stenosis accounting for 30% of the critical narrowings.[S27] Yet acute thrombotic occlusions were present in the proximal LAD artery in 61% of the cases. In other words, once it occludes, the fatal potential of a critical proximal LAD stenosis seems greater than that of other stenoses in patients with triple-vessel disease.

When the left main coronary artery has a significant ($\geq 50\%$ diameter) narrowing, survival for 5 years without surgical treatment occurs in less than two-thirds,[C12] and perhaps as few as 50%,[P13] of those affected (Fig. 7-2). According to the European Study, about 60% live 5 years when initially assigned to medical treatment and resting left ventricular function is initially normal or only mildly depressed.[V2] Presumably, the prognosis is worse when extensive triple-vessel coronary artery disease is associated with the left main lesion, or when left main ostial stenosis is combined with RCA ostial stenosis, as happens occasionally, particularly in women.[L6]

In all anatomic subsets, left ventricular function also affects survival and should be included in all estimates of prognosis.[C29]

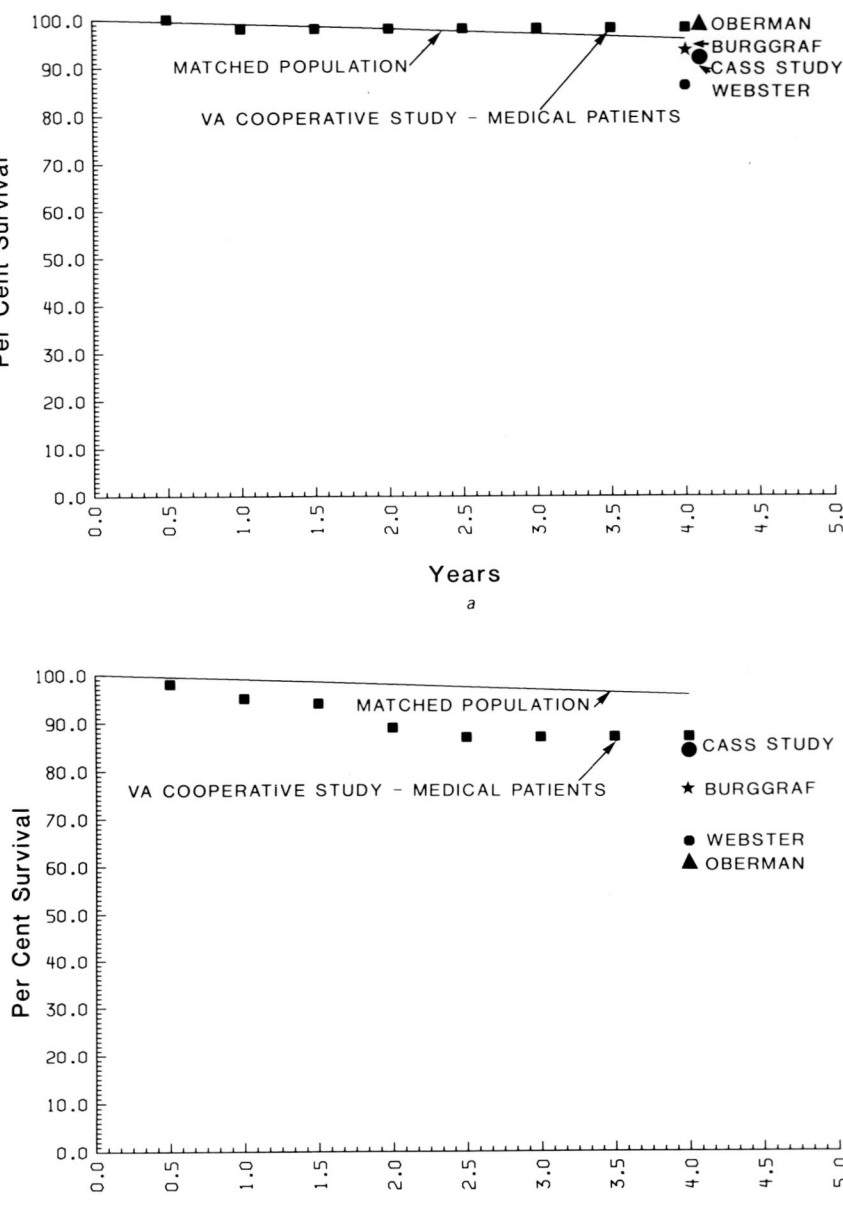

Figure 7-2 Actuarial analysis of the 4-year survival of medically treated men with coronary artery disease, stable angina pectoris of at least 6 months' duration, and somewhat less than severe LV dysfunction in the United States Veterans Administration Cooperative Study (solid squares).[R5] For comparison, the solid line depicts the survival of a population matched for age and sex taken from the 1976 United States Life Tables. Shown also are the data for other groups of medically treated patients published earlier by Oberman and colleagues,[O2] Burggraf and colleagues,[B15] and Webster and colleagues.[W3] The lower survival rates of the last three groups may be due to less restrictive selection of patients than for the Veterans Administration group and to better medical treatment in the more recent Veterans Administration group. Data from the CASS study, in which important stenosis meant a 70% diameter reduction, are also shown.[M19] These data include patients with all types of ventricular function, treated medically in the current era. The left main coronary artery data from the CASS study refer to left main coronary artery plus triple-vessel disease.

(a) Single-vessel disease.

(b) Double-vessel disease.

Reproduced with permission from Kirklin et al.,[K7] and the American Heart Association, Inc.

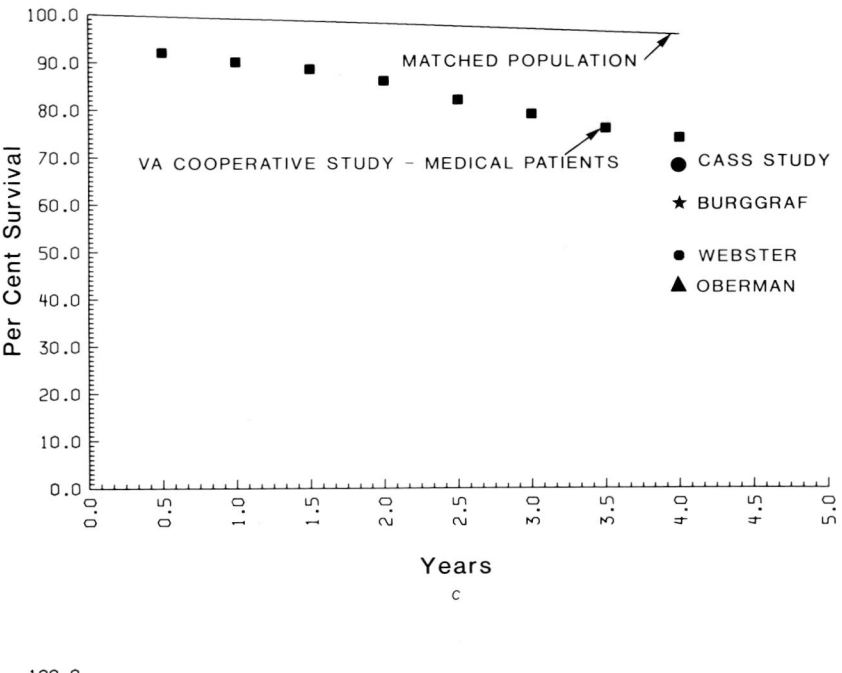

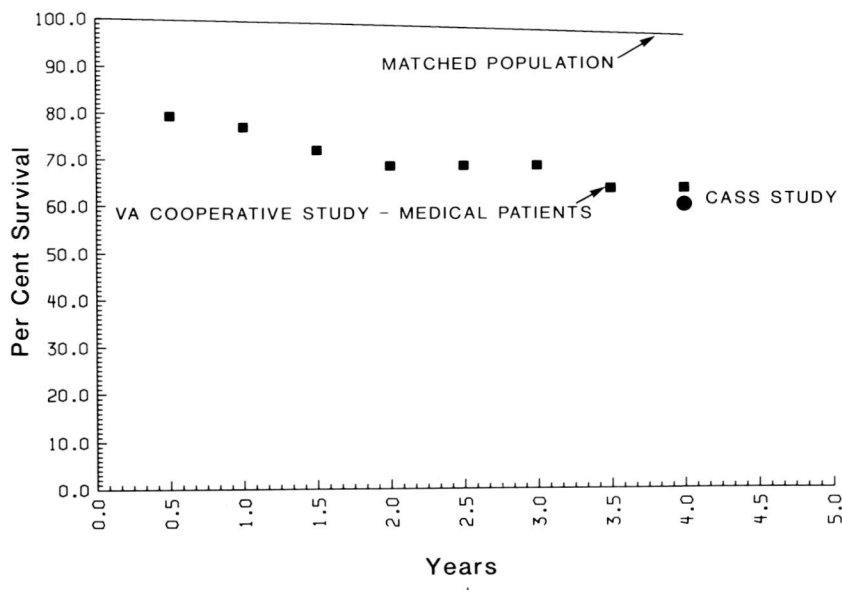

Figure 7-2 (*continued*)
(*c*) Triple-vessel disease.
(*d*) Left main coronary artery disease.

Survival According to Left Ventricular Structure and Function

Left ventricular function and left ventricular morphologic relics of previous overt or silent myocardial infarctions have a dominantly important effect on the survival as well as the functional capacity of patients with ischemic heart disease. Thus, the 5-year survival in the CASS randomized trial was 95% in patients initially assigned to medical treatment (al-lowed to cross over to surgery when indicated) and with ejection fractions greater than 0.50; in this group there was no additional effect of the number of vessels diseased.[C31] However, in the CASS Registry, the number of diseased vessels did affect the prognosis of patients with essentially normal left ventricular function[M19] (Table 7-1). The attractive implication that surgery can be delayed in patients with normal left ventricular function, since their prognosis with initial medical treatment is so good, should, however, be

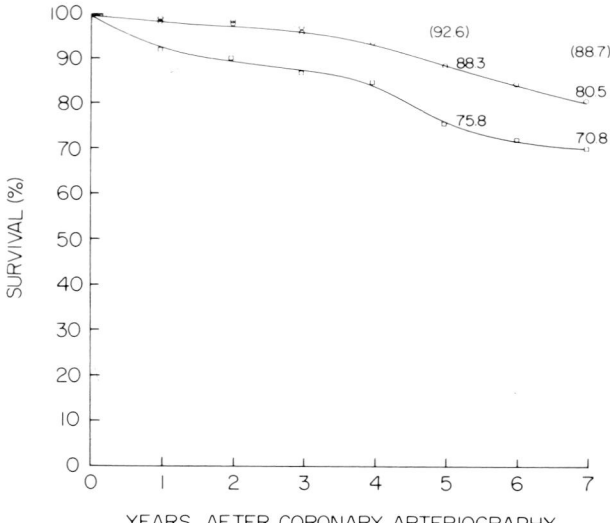

Figure 7-3 Survival of nonsurgical patients with single-vessel disease (⩾ 50% diameter narrowing). The dotted line with open circles portrays cardiac deaths in patients with isolated single-vessel disease. The solid line with open circles represents all deaths in patients with isolated single-vessel disease. The solid line with open squares represents all deaths in patients with single-vessel disease plus moderate (30%–50%) narrowings in other vessels.

Reproduced with modifications and permission from Bruschke et al.,[B10] and the American Heart Association, Inc.

accepted with caution. Surgery, ideally at least, should not be delayed until the prognosis without surgery is poor because of a severely damaged left ventricle.

In randomized trials of treatment in patients asymptomatic after recurrent myocardial infarction at GLH, and more recently in patients after one myocardial infarction and with significant (⩾ 75% cross-sectional area loss) coronary artery disease (excluding left main coronary artery disease), late survival of those initially assigned to medical treatment (but allowed to cross over to surgery if indicated) was again not related to the extent of coronary artery disease expressed as myocardial score, but was related to left ventricular function.[N4] Similarly, Hammermeister and colleagues found that when left ventricular systolic function was moderately im-

paired (EF 0.3–0.5) 5-year survival with nonsurgical treatment was only 72%, but that when function was normal or very mildly depressed, it was 92%.[H6,H8] Other studies have substantiated the importance of left ventricular function to survival.

Progression of Stenotic Coronary Artery Disease

The natural history of patients with a given anatomic extent of coronary artery disease and a given state of left ventricular function depends not only on these variables at some instant but also on their dynamic progression. There is a tendency for both the number and severity of stenotic coronary arterial lesions to progress with time,[B32,M9] but the details of such progression and the factors affecting it are incompletely understood.[S36] Further, to some extent progression is unpredictable, and many of the usually accepted risk factors for the *presence* of coronary artery disease have not been helpful in predicting rate of *progression*.[B31,K16,S36]

In symptomatic patients, new coronary artery disease seems to appear within 2 years in about 50% of cases.[S36] During that period, about 20% of stenoses progress, with the tendency to progression being considerably greater in lesions that had ⩾ 95% diameter reduction at the first observation.[B31,S36]

Patients with persistent or increasing angina tend to have high rates of progression of their stenoses over a 2-year period.[S36] Young patients with coronary arteriosclerosis tend to show more rapid progression than do older ones.[B32,K16,M9] Some evidence exists that more severe lesions progress more rapidly than do mild narrowings, as indicated earlier.[B31] Obese patients seem to experience more rapid progression of lesions than do others.[S36]

As the coronary artery disease progresses with time, left ventricular function tends to deteriorate.[B31]

Evolution of Left Ventricular Dysfunction

Ischemic Dysfunction
Left ventricular performance is adversely affected by important coronary arterial stenoses, even in the absence of fixed morphologic damage from myocardial infarction. The first indications of dysfunction are localized abnormalities of regional wall motion (left ventricular systolic function) during

Table 7-1 The association of left ventricular systolic function (as estimated by global ejection fraction) and extent of severe (⩾ 70% diameter reduction) coronary artery disease with 4-year survival in patients treated medically in the current era. These data must be interpreted in light of the fact that during the study period approximately 20%, 30%, and 45% of patients with single-, double-, and triple-vessel disease, respectively, crossed over to surgical treatment.

Ejection Fraction ⩽ <	Single-Vessel Disease 4-Yr Survival				Double-Vessel Disease 4-Yr Survival				Triple-Vessel Disease 4-Yr Survival				P (χ²) for Difference
	n	No.	%	CL	n	No.	%	CL	n	No.	%	CL	
0.50	761	723	95%	94%–96%	415	386	93%	91%–94%	227	186	82%	79%–85%	< .0001
0.35---0.50	184	167	91%	88%–93%	144	120	83%	79%–87%	88	62	71%	65%–76%	.0001
0.35	57	42	74%	66%–80%	57	32	56%	48%–64%	69	35	51%	44%–58%	.03
P (χ²)	< .0001				< .0001				< .0001				

SOURCE: Recalculated from data presented from the CASS study by Mock et al.[M19]

KEY: CL, 70% confidence limits.

exercise or other forms of stress.[S3] These abnormalities are the result of transient myocardial ischemia, which can be demonstrated as myocardial perfusion defects during exercise.[S4,S5] Exercise-induced electrocardiographic changes also reflect these transient myocardial perfusion abnormalities, which may be so severe as to cause hypotension during exercise testing.[B34] When these regional abnormalities are sufficiently extensive, global left ventricular systolic function during exercise becomes abnormal and falls during exercise.[B39,H1,J1,R2,S4] In contrast, global left ventricular systolic function rises during exercise in normal individuals, except in old age. Related to this decrease in function in some patients, left ventricular end-diastolic volume responds abnormally to exercise by increasing more than 50% above resting value.[B3,H1,J1,R2] These transient abnormalities of regional myocardial perfusion and wall motion occasionally occur at rest, most commonly in patients with unstable angina.[K3]

Abnormalities of left ventricular diastolic function, even at rest and in the absence of resting systolic dysfunction, can be demonstrated in most patients.[M23,R16] These abnormalities take the form of reduced peak left ventricular filling rate and increased time to peak filling rate.[B41,R16] These phenomena are the clinical reflection of the laboratory demonstration that hypoxia impairs the rate of diastolic relaxation of papillary muscle,[F13] related to the fact that myocardial relaxation during early diastole is an active, energy-dependent process. The diastolic abnormalities in patients may also reflect the lack of a rise in early diastolic coronary blood flow and lack of its impact on early left ventricular relaxation in patients with coronary artery stenoses.

In aggregate, these purely ischemic abnormalities of left ventricular systolic and diastolic function may be severe enough, particularly during stress, to result in considerably increased left ventricular end-diastolic pressure. This may produce dyspnea and even transient paroxysmal nocturnal dyspnea, as well as angina, during severe ischemic episodes. Further evidence that these abnormalities of left ventricular systolic and diastolic function can be the result of myocardial ischemia alone is provided by their reversal after successful percutaneous transluminal coronary angioplasty[B40,B54] or after the CABG operation (see "Left Ventricular Dysfunction").

Dysfunction from Myocardial Scarring
Myocardial scarring from overt or silent myocardial infarction usually impairs left ventricular function. In the scarred areas, which contain variable amounts of muscle (except in the case of aneurysms, discussed in Chapter 8), myocardial perfusion is often impaired and wall motion abnormal during rest as well as exercise. (As noted, the presence of these abnormalities *at rest* is not per se evidence of myocardial scarring and irreversible damage.) Global left ventricular systolic function at rest may be normal when the scar is small and the rest of the left ventricle is well perfused. More commonly, resting global left ventricular ejection fraction is depressed, and moderate (EF ≤ 0.40) or severe (EF ≤ 0.30) depression implies considerable myocardial scarring.

Myocardial scars from previous myocardial infarctions result also in abnormalities of left ventricular diastolic func-

tion.[S22,S33] Both clinical and experimental studies indicate that the increase in left ventricular and end-diastolic volume, which results from both the diastolic and systolic abnormalities of function, is directly related to scar size.[F12]

Patients whose left ventricular function is severely depressed from myocardial scarring exhibit morphologic, physiologic, and functional variability. Some have moderately increased left ventricular end-diastolic pressure at rest and a considerably reduced exercise capacity but only a mildly increased cardiac size by chest x-ray. These patients have moderate scarring and considerable ischemic dysfunction in scarred or nonscarred parts of the ventricles and can often be helped by operation. Some have chronic symptoms of pulmonary venous hypertension and can possibly still be helped by operation. A few have moderate or severe cardiomegaly, reduced cardiac output, importantly elevated right atrial and jugular venous pressure, hepatomegaly, and fluid retention. Patients in the latter group have advanced left ventricular dysfunction from very extensive myocardial scarring, and they generally cannot be improved by operation unless the scar is discrete, is full thickness (aneurysm), and can be resected (see Chapter 8).

Effect of Chronic Stable Angina Pectoris on Natural History

The natural history of patients with chronic stable angina pectoris is determined primarily by the extent of the atherosclerotic occlusive coronary artery disease and by the left ventricular function. Whether the presence of angina pectoris (in contrast to an asymptomatic state) affects the prognosis imposed by a given extent of coronary artery disease and left ventricular dysfunction is not known with certainty. One point of view is that it would be surprising if the presence of angina did affect prognosis, since even myocardial ischemia severe enough to cause frank and sometimes massive infarction may be unaccompanied by pain of any kind. Supporting this point of view is a study from the CASS registry; it indicates that among patients with LMCA disease, symptomatic and asymptomatic patients had similar survival rates and in both instances surgically treated patients had a significantly better survival than did medically treated ones.[D12] Another point of view is that it would be surprising if angina did not adversely affect prognosis, for angina implies insufficient myocardial blood flow, which is not measured by angiography. A carefully performed retrospective study by Cohn and colleagues suggests that, other things being equal, the prognosis with nonsurgical treatment *is* less favorable in patients *with* angina pectoris than in asymptomatic patients.[C15] However, in that study, asymptomatic patients with triple-vessel disease had a mortality rate of about 5% per year, not very different from that reported by others for triple-vessel disease in patients with angina.

Effect of Unstable Angina Pectoris on Natural History

Patients with severely *unstable angina pectoris* (also called intermediate coronary syndrome,[B35] preinfarction angina, acute coronary insufficiency, or coronary failure) either of new onset or representing a changing pattern in previously stable angina, seem to have a less favorable life history without operation than do patients with similar coronary and left ventricular abnormality but either without symptoms or with chronic stable angina pectoris. This conclusion is supported by the NIH Cooperative Study on unstable angina.[R3] Among patients in that study treated medically, 20% of those with single-vessel disease, 33% with double-vessel disease, and 50% with triple-vessel disease had symptoms of such severity in the subsequent 3 years that operation became necessary. Nonetheless, 3-year survival of patients initially treated medically was 90%.

In a GLH study of 158 patients with unstable angina admitted to the coronary care unit between 1967 and 1971, 20 (13%) experienced myocardial infarctions from 48 hours to 3 weeks after hospital admission, and of these, 3 died. Three other patients died without developing infarction, for a total mortality of 4%. The subsequent mortality was about 5% per annum. Survival at 3 years was 82% and at 5 years 75%.[H9] These results parallel those of the NIH study.[R3]

Although unstable angina pectoris is often an indication that the underlying coronary artery disease has progressed,[T8] periods of unstable angina may represent, not changes in the basic coronary arteriosclerotic disease, but, rather, transient changes in neurohumeral mechanisms and responses. These changes may result in acute but reversible occlusion of a major artery by platelet aggregates or other types of thrombi, in either unstable angina[V5] or frank infarction.[D5] The products of platelet aggregation may provoke coronary spasm or transient increases in myocardial oxygen consumption. Therefore, the clinical event of unstable angina itself is not necessarily an indication for surgical treatment.

Effect of Acute Myocardial Infarction on Natural History

Death from ischemic heart disease is commonly related in one way or another to myocardial infarction. The other mode of death is "sudden death" without evidence of myocardial necrosis even in those who are resuscitated and survive. The latter occurs primarily in patients with extensive triple-vessel coronary artery disease and seems to result from acute ventricular fibrillation precipitated by factors other than acute myocardial necrosis[B37,R14] (see "Sudden Death").

There is increasing evidence that most acute myocardial infarctions are associated with acute thrombotic occlusion of the artery supplying the infarcted area.[D5,R18,R19,R20] Reduto and colleagues found this in 26 (81%, CL 71%–89%) of 32 patients with acute infarction, and the other 6 had severe proximal stenosis with poor distal flow.[R18] The cause of the acute occlusion remains controversial. Transient neurohumeral changes may lead to platelet aggregation and thrombosis. Internal disruption of an atherosclerotic plaque can occur and lead to platelet aggregation and thrombosis.

Overall, 15% to 30% of patients die during an acute myocardial infarction.[S4] Some patients die of uncontrolled ventricular electrical instability, but in the current era, many

deaths are due to inadequate cardiac output often associated with pulmonary venous hypertension.

Hospital (or < 30-day) survival after acute myocardial infarction is probably determined primarily by the extensiveness of the myocardial necrosis (size of the infarct).[C17,M2] The early (hospital) mortality is generally less than 5% when the infarct is small, as suggested by low peak serum glutamic-oxaloacetic transaminase (SGOT) levels (less than 120 units)[T5] or normal cardiac output and left atrial pressure. When the infarct is large, as suggested by peak SGOT levels greater than 240 units, clinical evidence of low cardiac output, or severely reduced (< 1.6) cardiac index, the mortality is 15%–50%. Thus, the deaths are usually in patients whose ejection fractions after the acute infarction are less than 0.30[S24] and in whom, at autopsy, infarction involves 40% or more of the left ventricle.[P4] If the acute infarction is not the patient's first one, the involved area of left ventricle may contain a combination of old (scar) and new infarct. However, the clinical response to a given degree of acute myocardial necrosis is variable and depends at least on the amount of already developed collateral circulation, the morphologic and functional status of the remainder of the left ventricle, and the rapidity and extent of spontaneous reperfusion of the infarcted area.[H11] Animal studies suggest that when the clinical course is favorable after an acute infarction, some areas of abnormal myocardial contraction normalize as coronary blood flow increases during the recovery phase.[G20]

Many types of analyses have been made of predictors of early death after acute myocardial infarction, that of Forrester and colleagues also being correlative.[F10] Marmor and colleagues find that early recurrence of chest pain after infarction, a nontransmural infarct, female sex, and obesity predispose patients to early death after acute infarction.[M21] Swan has observed that patients with acute myocardial infarctions associated with RCA occlusions have a generally better probability of survival than do others.[S35]

Acute myocardial infarction also alters the natural history in patients who survive the acute episode, in that only 70%–80% of early survivors are alive 2 years after the infarction.[B20,K12] Furthermore, a large proportion of these deaths occur within the first few months after hospital discharge.[D3,E7] The postinfarction scar results in reduced global systolic function, and the magnitude of the reduction in function is directly related to the size of the infarct.[H17] The scar may also affect remote regions of the left ventricle, resulting in left ventricular wall thinning and dilation out of proportion to the increase in mass.[P10] The postinfarction ventricle also has a tendency toward severe ventricular electrical instability.

These considerations make it evident that size of the infarct is related to late survival, as well as to survival of the acute episode.[B38,M13,S25] Thus, most deaths occur in patients whose ejection fraction after recovery from the acute episode is less than 0.40. Many of the deaths are sudden or associated with demonstrated severe electrical instability.[H12] Factors responsible for sudden ventricular electrical instability in this setting are numerous, but platelet aggregation on a stenotic lesion has been demonstrated to be one reversible factor.[K14]

Recently, it has been shown that study by electrophysiologic programmed stimulation (EPS) early after the acute infarction can identify the patients with moderately or severely impaired left ventricular function who are at particular risk of dying in the first year after recovery from the infarct. Ventricular electrical instability, demonstrated by EPS, was present in 38 patients studied early after myocardial infarction by Richards and colleagues, and 10 (26%, CL 18%–36%) of these died within 1 year; death occurred suddenly in 8.[R15] Instability was not present among 127 patients tested, and only 7 (6%, CL 3%–8%) died within 1 year (*P* for difference = .0002). Cohen and colleagues found that ventricular electrical instability leading to ventricular tachyarrhythmia was more common late after infarction when the ventricular septum had been involved.[C30]

Previous infarctions and older age also increase the risk of death in the first few years after a myocardial infarction,[N3] although the risks seem less currently than in earlier eras.[B21,N4] The extent of the coronary artery disease is also related to prognosis after an acute myocardial infarction. At UAB, Rogers and colleagues found 100% survival for 3 years after acute infarction in patients with single-vessel disease and only 75% in patients with triple-vessel disease.[R10] Other factors no doubt relate the prognosis of patients who have survived an acute myocardial infarction. For example, patients who have had acute pulmonary edema in the course of their acute infarction have a significantly increased risk of recurrent infarction and death, even though after the infarction they have good left ventricular function.[W10]

TECHNIQUE OF OPERATION

Most patients coming to the CABG operation have extensive triple-vessel coronary artery disease, and most of the discussion concerns the operation in these circumstances. In patients with single- or double-vessel disease when only a few coronary artery anastomoses are required, the planning and execution of the operation is much simpler than when there are many stenosed coronary arteries requiring grafts.

Preoperative Preparation

Many patients come to coronary artery bypass grafting taking propranolol or calcium channel blocking agents, and there are many reasons for continuing these up to the time of operation. Several studies have shown a tendency for patients to develop an acute myocardial infarction when propranolol is stopped. Boudoulas and associates have shown a significant increase in adrenergic tone in most patients the day before operation, the effects of which are well controlled by propranolol.[B29] Propranolol lessens the incidence of intraoperative ventricular arrhythmias[S19] and does not compromise left ventricular function.[R6] The dose of propranolol is not changed unless it exceeds 160 mg per day. Since Wechsler has shown an increased need for perioperative catecholamine support when a dose of 300–400 mg of propranolol is maintained up to operation,[W5] the patient is hospitalized for 2–3 days before operation when the daily dose

exceeds 160 mg. The dose is then reduced in one or two steps to 160 mg per day. If angina worsens, then the attempt to reduce the dose is abandoned. Similar plans are followed for other β-blocking agents as well as for calcium channel blockers.

Digoxin is discontinued 36 hours before operation unless there is atrial fibrillation with a rapid ventricular rate (see Chapter 4). If digoxin is recommenced within the first 2 days after operation, the patient is considered to have already received one-half of the estimated digitalizing dose (see Chapter 5).

The immediately preoperative medication and the management of the patient in the operating room are of vital importance to successful CABG and are detailed in Chapter 5.

Preparations in the Operating Room

The anesthetic methods described in Chapter 4, used precisely and intelligently, suffice. Insertion of a Swan-Ganz catheter or other devices before anesthetizing the patient or preoperative intra-aortic balloon pumping is rarely necessary. After the patient's anesthetic and supportive management have begun and the devices have been inserted into the arm (see Chapter 2), the skin is prepared over the chest, abdomen, groin, and the complete circumference of both legs, including the feet. Draping includes covering the toes with a sterile glove and placing sterile and waterproof drapes beneath the legs. The drapes are arranged so that the genitalia and pubis are out of the sterile field. The lines to the pump oxygenator for cardiopulmonary bypass (CPB) are secured in place (see Chapter 2, Section 3).

Strategy of the Operation

The strategy of the CABG operation currently recommended is directed toward obtaining *complete revascularization* by bypassing all significant stenosis (≥ 50% diameter reduction) in all coronary arterial trunks and branches, except those of trivial (≤ 1.1 mm in diameter) size. Since five or more individual conduits cannot conveniently be used, at least some of the grafts must have *sequential anastomoses* (side-to-side or skip anastomoses). Thus, any argument concerning sequential versus single anastomoses on a vein segment is largely academic. However, studies have indicated that anastomotic patency rates are at least as high with the sequential technique as with the method of using a single distal anastomosis per conduit. To increase the likelihood that the entire graft will remain patent, the *distal end-to-side anastomosis* of a sequential graft is made whenever possible to a relatively large artery with a severe proximal stenosis and a good runoff.

Although a number of different strategies have been used during the development of the CABG operation at UAB and at GLH and at present some surgeon-to-surgeon variability exists, the currently recommended strategy involves the use of the internal mammary artery (IMA) to the LAD artery and one to three segments of saphenous vein to the remaining coronary arteries requiring revascularization. Generally one vein segment revascularizes the first and second diagonal arteries, and either one or two vein graft segments are used to revascularize the circumflex and right coronary systems. If anastomoses to several small branches of these two systems are required, the tendency is to use a single vein graft with multiple sequential anastomoses. At the other extreme, if only a large marginal branch of the circumflex artery and the distal right coronary artery are to be revascularized, separate vein graft segments are used for each. The details of the graft placements are individualized for the patient's pathologic condition, but in dealing with extensive disease many of the operations are similar.

Generally, the distal anastomoses to the circumflex and right coronary system are made first, then those to the diagonal system, and finally the IMA anastomosis to the LAD artery. An alternative method involves making the proximal anastomoses first (see "Proximal Anastomosis First versus Distal Anastomosis First" in section on Special Situations and Controversies), but this technique is recommended for special situations only.

In patients with extensive triple-vessel coronary artery disease, the cineangiogram provides the most important information for planning the operation, but the surgeon may elect to open vessels suspected of having important stenosis from either the cineangiogram or observations at operation. A few errors will inevitably be made as to which vessels should be grafted. The surgeon must decide which error is more acceptable: opening and grafting a vessel that does not need it or failing to open and graft a vessel with an important stenosis.

After taking down the IMA (if it is to be used), removing the saphenous vein, and establishing CPB and cold cardioplegia, all arteries on the back of the heart which are to be bypassed are opened, and sequential anastomoses are done, beginning with the distal end-to-side anastomosis. In patients with extensive triple-vessel disease, this generally means the first and second marginal branches of the circumflex artery and the distal RCA or, if it is stenosed, the posterior descending artery and one or two marginal branches of the posterolateral segment are grafted. An infusion of cold cardioplegic solution is again administered into the aortic root, and then the arteries on the front of the heart are exposed and inspected and all to be bypassed are opened. A vein graft is anastomosed end-to-side to the most distal diagonal artery to be revascularized and side-to-side to the more proximal ones. As the last step, the end of the internal mammary artery is anastomosed to the LAD artery.

After completion of the distal anastomoses, the removal of the aortic cross-clamp, and the beginning of rewarming of the patient, the vein grafts are routed to the aorta. The vein graft to the diagonal arteries is brought through the transverse sinus, and that to RCA and Cx artery systems to the right and posteriorly around the right atrium to the right lateral aspect of the ascending aorta (UAB) (Fig. 7-4a). If a separate (third) vein has been used for the Cx artery system, it is brought through the transverse sinus. The proximal anastomoses are then all made to the right lateral aspect of the ascending aorta. Alternatively, the vein segment to the diagonal artery system is brought over the pulmonary trunk to the anterior aspect of the aorta for proximal anastomosis

(Fig. 7-4b); the vein segment to the RCA and Cx artery systems is brought to the right and anterior to the right atrium to the anterior aspect of the aorta (GLH). All the proximal anastomoses are then made to the anterior aspect of the aorta. If a separate (third) vein segment is used for the Cx artery system, it is brought over the pulmonary trunk (GLH).

The IMA graft must course smoothly and without tension to the LAD artery. The vein segment must not only be anastomosed proximally and distally with precision, but throughout its course it must lie smoothly without kinks, tension, or redundancy. The achievement of such precision and smoothness is facilitated by the method described of selecting and opening *all* the arteries to be grafted by a vein segment before performing any of the sequential anastomoses. The placement of incisions in the arteries is dictated primarily by the pathologic condition but to some extent by the optimal course of the sequential graft. Because the elasticity and natural curves of prepared veins vary widely, the vein segment is distended with cold cardioplegic solution each time it is fitted between two sequential anastomoses or between the first distal anastomosis, and again is distended with blood when fitting it for the aortic anastomosis. This allows not only precise selection of the proper point of incision on the vein for the sequential anastomosis but also selection of a routing for the vein that is harmonious with its natural curves. The vein graft is distended by infusing the cold cardioplegic solution (UAB) under about 100 mmHg pressure through the small cannulae tied into the proximal end of the vein, during which process 25–50 ml of the solution is infused through already made anastomoses into the regional myocardium. The cardioplegic solution is not damaging to the vein graft.[S38] Alternatively, a fine bulldog clamp is placed immediately proximal to the anastomosis and the vein distended with a cold, balanced salt solution (GLH).

Removal and Preparation of the Vein Graft

Whenever possible, a single, long segment (usually 65–75 cm) of the greater saphenous vein is removed from the leg. If two vein segments are to be used, about 25–30 cm of vein are needed for the arteries on the front of the heart (the LAD artery system) and about 35 cm for those on the back of the heart (the Cx artery and RCA systems). If two separate vein segments are to be used for the back of the heart, about 22 cm of length are generally needed for the marginal Cx branches and about 18 cm for the right coronary artery and its branches. As long as the external diameter of the vein is greater than about 3.5 mm, vein width is probably not an important consideration. Large veins reduce in size as time passes after insertion, and thus adaptation to function seems to occur.[S29] Veins of poor wall quality are to be avoided when possible, as experience in peripheral vascular surgery indicates that they have a particular propensity to failure.

It is generally agreed that the details of removal and storage of the vein until its insertion are important in minimizing damage to the vein, including intimal disruption, deposition of platelets and leukocytes on the intima, contraction damage to smooth muscle mechanisms, and disruption of extracellular matrix.[C20,G10,G15,L15,L17,S34] Overdistention of the

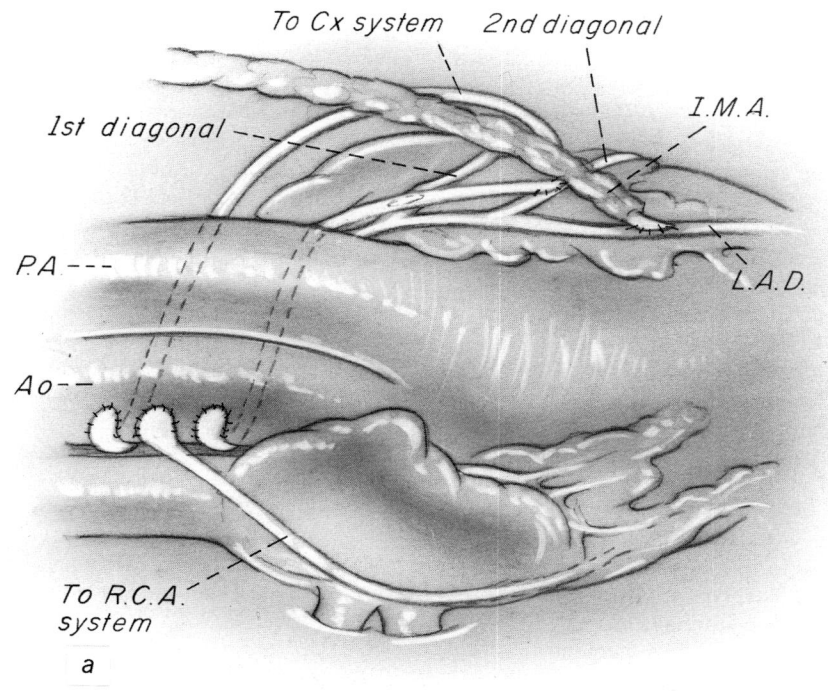

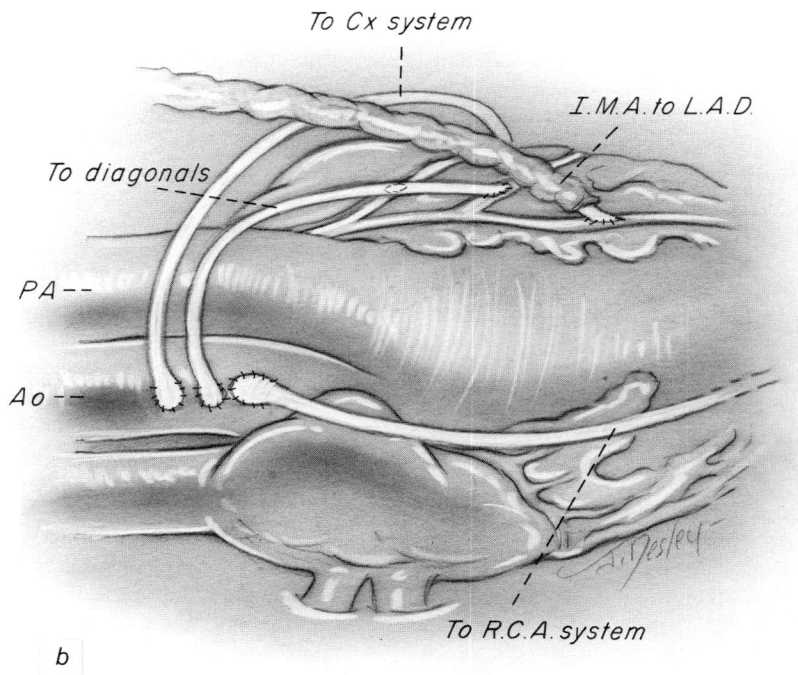

Figure 7-4

(*a*) One configuration of the IMA and vein grafts for coronary artery bypass grafting of extensive triple-vessel coronary artery disease (UAB). The IMA is anastomosed to the LAD artery. The vein graft to the diagonal branches of the LAD (the "front of the heart") is anastomosed to the inferior aortic opening, and passes through the transverse sinus.[G12] The vein anastomosed to the middle opening passes to the right of the right atrium and goes to the RCA (or its branches). The superiorly positioned vein goes to the Cx marginal branches. Occasionally (see text) only a single vein is used for the RCA and Cx systems.

(*b*) Configuration at GLH when the IMA and three vein grafts are used.

Ao, aorta; PA, pulmonary artery.

vein,[H14] storage at room temperature,[L15] and venous spasm[L15] are probably disadvantageous. There is no consensus as to the optimal methods of protection, and relatively simple methods can be used. As soon as the skin incision has been made, a gauze sponge saturated with warm papaverine in normal saline solution (60 mg in 500 ml solution) is placed over the saphenous vein. As soon as the vein is removed, it is flushed and then distended with the warm (37°) solution to which has been added 2 ml (2000 units) of heparin per 100 ml of solution. After the preparation of the vein is completed, it is again distended with a cold solution of the same composition and stored in the cold solution at about 4°C (UAB).

The right or left greater saphenous vein is chosen for removal, following preoperative examination of both legs with the patient standing erect. The presence of superficial varicosities need not indicate an unusable greater saphenous vein. However, wound healing may be poor in such extremities, and, if possible, a leg without varicosities is chosen. Multiple large varices in the saphenous vein do, however, render it unsuitable. The vein from one leg may be found to be too short or to have segments too narrow or too thick-walled for use. Then an additional segment of appropriate length is removed from the other leg. Rarely, adequate segments of greater saphenous vein cannot be found, and then the lesser saphenous vein is exposed and used if it proves of adequate diameter. On rare occasions, suitable segments of vein cannot be found in the legs by any method. The cephalic vein can then be taken from wrist to shoulder, but its walls are usually thinner than those of the leg veins. One or both internal mammary arteries may be employed in some such situations.

The leg is abducted anterolaterally, and the knee is flexed about 45° and supported, avoiding occlusion of the popliteal vessels. The greater saphenous vein may be initially exposed by a skin incision just anterior to the medial malleolus, or the dissection may be begun in the groin, depending on the clinical estimation of the size of the vein in the lower leg. After the skin incision is made, the desired plane is achieved by bluntly dissecting down to the vein with the tips of the curved Mayo scissors. The skin is undermined with scissors by staying just superficial to the saphenous vein and spreading the tips of the scissors over the vein. The undermined skin is incised with the scissors (UAB) or a knife (GLH) directly over the vein and the creation of flaps is avoided. This dissection is continued over the course of the vein until the desired length is exposed. The vein may divide just below the knee and become confluent again just above the knee. Either of the two branches may be the larger vessel, but it is generally better to pursue the anterior branch, which is the true saphenous vein, unless the posterior one is obviously better. The greater saphenous vein often gives off a superficial branch 8–10 cm above the knee, which continues to run parallel although superficial to the saphenous vein and eventually joints it just below the femoral vein. Occasionally, the superficial branch is the larger vessel and should be used. The saphenous vein usually becomes too large and undesirable for bypass purposes just before its penetration of the fascia lata and termination in the femoral vein. Therefore, dissection is usually not carried into this area.

When the usable vein has been exposed and measured for length, the proximal (femoral vein) end is isolated and di-

vided between ligatures. A vascular clamp is placed on the vein graft, to mark what will become the *distal* end of the graft. The vein is removed from above downward, being retracted anteriorly so that there is just enough tension to expose the branches. The branches are ligated and divided, and adequate length (1–2 mm) is left between tie and vein to ensure that the vein is not narrowed and beyond the ligature to ensure its permanence. Care is taken to preserve the saphenous nerve. Following ligation and division of all branches and removal from its bed, the saphenous vein is divided between ligatures at its lower end, just superior to the medial malleolus.

The vein is removed to a preparation table, and a tapered "Christmas tree" connector[1] or an Aldrete round-ended cystic duct needle is inserted into the open proximal end and secured with a ligature. The vein is flushed with the cold heparinized solution. The vein is distended moderately (< 150 mmHg pressure) with the solution, any unsecured branches are ligated, and any constricting advential bands are removed. Alternatively, the vein is threaded and concertinaed over a long (6-cm) smooth, blunt-ended needle (GLH). Vein distention to test for leaks can then be begun near the new distal end. The needle is gradually withdrawn as the vein distends, and any untied small branches are ligated serially. This method avoids excessive intravenous pressure. Once prepared, the untwisted vein is laid on the table and distended moderately while a straight marking line is drawn along its length with an indelible blue surgical pencil. The vein is moderately distended with the solution via the proximal cannula and clamped at each end and placed in a similar cold (10°C) solution until used.

When the small saphenous vein must be taken, the knee and hip of the leg are partly flexed. With the plantar surface of the foot flat against the surface of the operating table, the foot is brought up close to the lateral aspect of the gluteal muscle mass and the leg rotated medially. The operating table can be rolled away from the operator. Alternatively, the patient can be initially positioned on the face for removal of the short saphenous vein and subsequently repositioned and redraped in a supine position. The incision is begun just lateral to the Achilles tendon, and the vein is exposed from below upward, as previously described. The sural nerve lies parallel to the vein and is preserved.

All the leg incisions are closed with continuous absorbable Dexon suture material. This is done as soon as the vein is prepared, even if the patient is now on CPB (UAB). Alternatively, closure may be deferred until after CPB (GLH). The subcutaneous tissue is closed in one or two layers, depending on the depth of the incision, in order to eliminate all dead space, and the skin is closed with a subcuticular (actually, deep intradermal) continuous suture of 3-0 Dexon.

Preparation and Use of the Internal Mammary Artery

Usually, the IMA pedicle is mobilized immediately after splitting the sternum, before opening the pericardium, and before giving heparin. A standard sternal spreader may be

---

[1] Leur-Lock catheter tip no. 3092 by Becton-Dickenson, Rutherford, N.J. 07070.

used to separate widely the divided sternal edges, tilting the spreader to elevate and rotate the left-sided sternal fragment. Alternatively, the Favaloro retractor is used (UAB). The operating table is rotated to the left to expose better the undersurface of the left sternal fragment and the left IMA. The pedicle to be dissected consists of the IMA, the internal mammary vein, fat, and some muscle and pleura. A diathermy cut is made down the sternal side of the artery and vein, about 5 mm from the IMA along the full length from the sixth intercostal space to the first rib. The dissection is begun at the sixth space, where there are no branches. The pedicle is freed from the underlying sixth costal cartilage. Through blunt dissection with a dissector and scissors, the intercostal arteries are identified in turn as they arise from the lateral aspect of the pedicle. They are occluded with clips or ties on the artery end and by diathermy on the chest wall end, and divided. The IMA must not be grasped with instruments, but only gently retracted.

The pedicle is freed in this fashion up to the first rib and then wrapped in a papaverine-soaked gauze swab (20 mg of papaverine diluted in 20 ml of saline solution). The distal end of the pedicle is not divided until the patient is heparinized and everything is in readiness for CPB. At this time, the pedicle is tied distally at the sixth intercostal space, transected, and free bleeding is allowed from the proximal end. If the IMA is of good quality and the bleeding is brisk, the graft is considered to be satisfactory and a very light bulldog clamp is placed on the distal end of the pedicle. The pedicle is sprayed with dilute papaverine and left lying loosely anterior to the lung.

After completing the distal vein anastomoses and opening the LAD artery, the IMA pedicle is brought into the surgical field. The other elements of the pedicle are dissected away from a 1-cm segment of the internal mammary artery just proximal to the place where it will be transected for a proper fit to the LAD artery. The IMA is generally dilated with a 1.0-mm and then a 1.5-mm dilator and is then sharply divided obliquely. The anastomosis to the LAD artery is made with interrupted 7-0 silk or polypropylene double-armed sutures, passing the stitches from inside-out in both the IMA and the LAD artery. After the anastomosis is completed, the important step of tacking the pedicle to the cardiac surface with a few interrupted sutures is performed, to prevent any tension on the suture line. Finally the pericardium is cut down transversely on the left side to allow the pedicle to pass smoothly to the LAD artery.

The Distal Anastomoses

The epicardium is incised over the area of the coronary artery that has been selected for the anastomoses, using a no. 15 Bard-Parker blade on the scalpel. Some use special scalpels with a completely rounded end. The anterior surface of the artery is cleared by gentle transverse brushing with the scalpel. Careful inspection of the artery will then reveal, even with cardioplegia, a thin central line, which is red or translucent and indicates the lumen. The anterior wall of the artery is opened longitudinally over this line, caressed gently with the scalpel so as not to damage the posterior wall. Occasionally, when the anterior wall of the artery cannot be placed under proper tension, it may be opened by stabbing

with a special small sharp-pointed scalpel. The blade must enter the artery obliquely, so that it does not penetrate the back wall. The incision is enlarged with fine, angled scissors to a length of 4–6 mm. The epicardial incision must extend beyond each angle of the arteriotomy, to facilitate the anastomosis. Generally the artery is sized by passing measured probes into it, and proximal and distal patency is assessed.

The vein is opened longitudinally for all sequential anastomoses by a similar technique, at precisely the place that has been determined by vein distention to be the correct location of the anastomosis. The incision is made about 10%–20% longer than that in the artery, and the suture bites in the vein are placed slightly farther apart than those in the artery, to make the desirable ''cobra head'' of the vein over the artery. When the end of the vein is being prepared for the most distal anastomosis, it is cut in a beveled fashion (Fig. 7-5) so that the circumference of the opening is somewhat larger than that of the opening in the artery.

The technique of anastomosis utilizes one double-armed 6-0 polypropylene suture placed as a continuous stitch. Stitches in the artery classically go from intima to adventitia (inside to outside), and the stitch pierces the intima near the vessel edge but often emerges through periarterial fat or muscle 2–3 mm away from the edge. Stitches in the vein go from outside to inside. The stitches through vein-artery are made separately unless it is very convenient to place them with one ''bite.'' Even then, the vein and artery wall are held apart as each ''bite'' is made, so that the needle point is visualized after it has pierced one vessel and before it pierces the other, to be certain that the stitch is accurate and no extraneous tissue has been caught.

Although the actual sequence of the stitching varies from one location on the heart to another, and occasionally varies in the same location because of special conditions of exposure or arterial pathology, certain general principles are followed. When the vein and artery are to approach and depart from the end-to-side (Fig. 7-6) or side-to-side (Fig. 7-7) anastomosis *parallel one to the other*, the suturing is generally begun 2–3 mm *away* from the arterial (and venous) angles so that the knot is kept away from the angle. When the vein is to *cross* the artery transversely, rather than running parallel to it, or approaches it at an angle for an end-to-side anastomosis, the stitch is begun by passing the suture first *through* an angle of the *vein*, so that the only stitch requiring a judgment of distances is that next passed through the arterial wall (Fig. 7-8). This arterial stitch is placed precisely at the point where the vein angle should rest to provide the proper predeter-

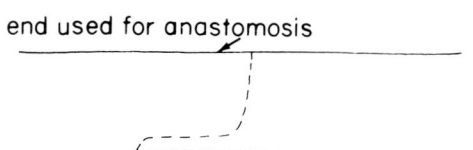

end used for anastomosis

Figure 7-5 Transection of the vein for end-to-side anastomosis to the coronary artery. Normally the circumference of the vein opening is 10%–20% larger than that of the opening in the artery, providing a large hood of vein over the distal anastomosis. If the vein is a little smaller than usual, it may be cut as for a proximal anastomosis (Fig. 7-10*b*) to provide a large enough hood.

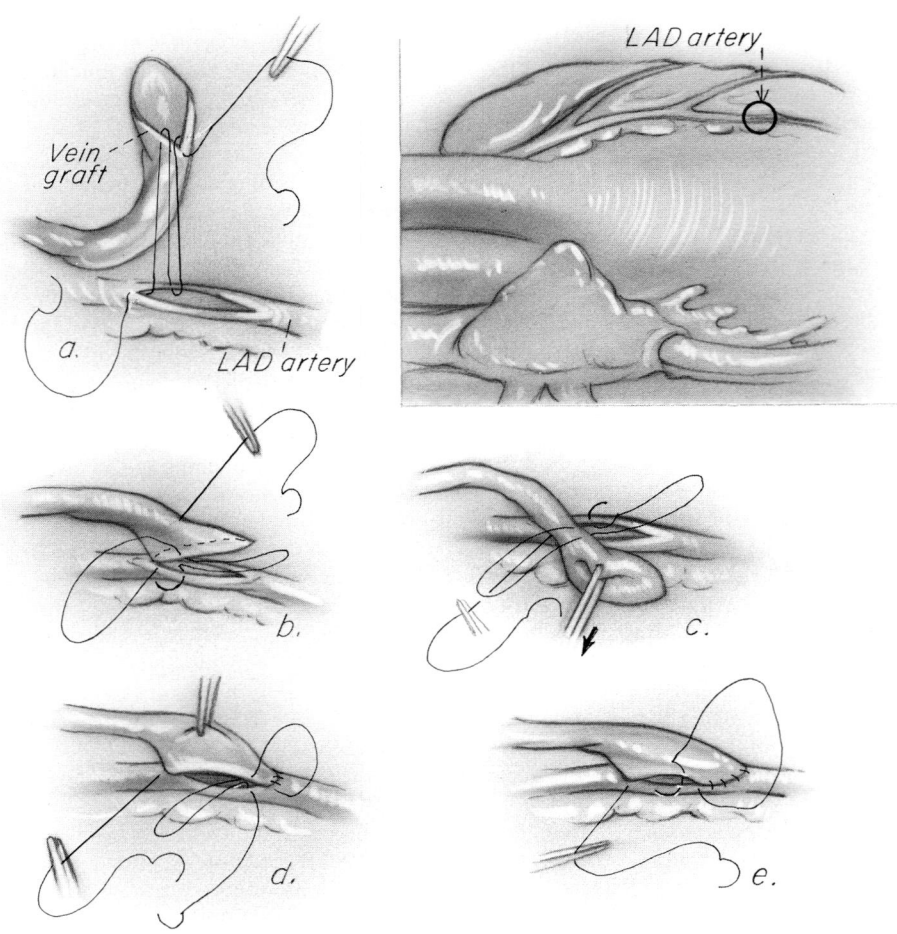

Figure 7-6   The distal anastomoses between the vein graft and the left anterior descending artery. In this and subsequent figures, the orientation is indicated by the upper right-hand drawing. (a) The vein graft is anastomosed slightly obliquely to the artery. The drawing shows the first stitch starting through the angle of the vein graft. (b) The suture line continues beyond the proximal angle of the arteriotomy. (c) The other arm of the suture has been placed from outside in through the vein and then inside out through the artery. (d, e) The suture is continued and tied to the other suture arm. This general method applies to all end-to-side anastomoses. Note that the knot is away from the angles of the arteriotomy.

mined angle of approach. In a side-to-side anatomosis, the other vein angle must rest at the corresponding point on the opposite wall of the artery so that the vein goes straight across the artery. In other words, the angles of approach and departure must be the same. The same principles apply when the vein crosses the artery diagonally. In both the parallel and crossing vein artery configurations, the sequence of subsequent suturing varies depending on location and exposure problems but is designed to provide good exposure of each stitch that is placed.

Generally the suturing is done from the outside in a more or less conventional manner. That is, the stitch passes first from outside in on the vein and them from inside out on the artery. Occasionally, exposure and suturing are easier if the stitching is done from the inside of the vessels. For this, the

vein lies alongside or transverse to the artery with the incision turned up. The suturing goes from inside out on the artery and outside in on the vein (Fig. 7-9). After doing one side, or going around one angle, in this way, the surgeon continues suturing in the more classic manner from the outside.

After suturing is completed, the vein may be distended by injecting cardioplegic solution through the proximal vein cannula as the 6-0 polypropylene suture is snugged up until there is no leakage and tied (UAB).

The Proximal Anastomoses

After completion of the distal anastomoses, release of the aortic cross-clamp, and beginning of the rewarming of the

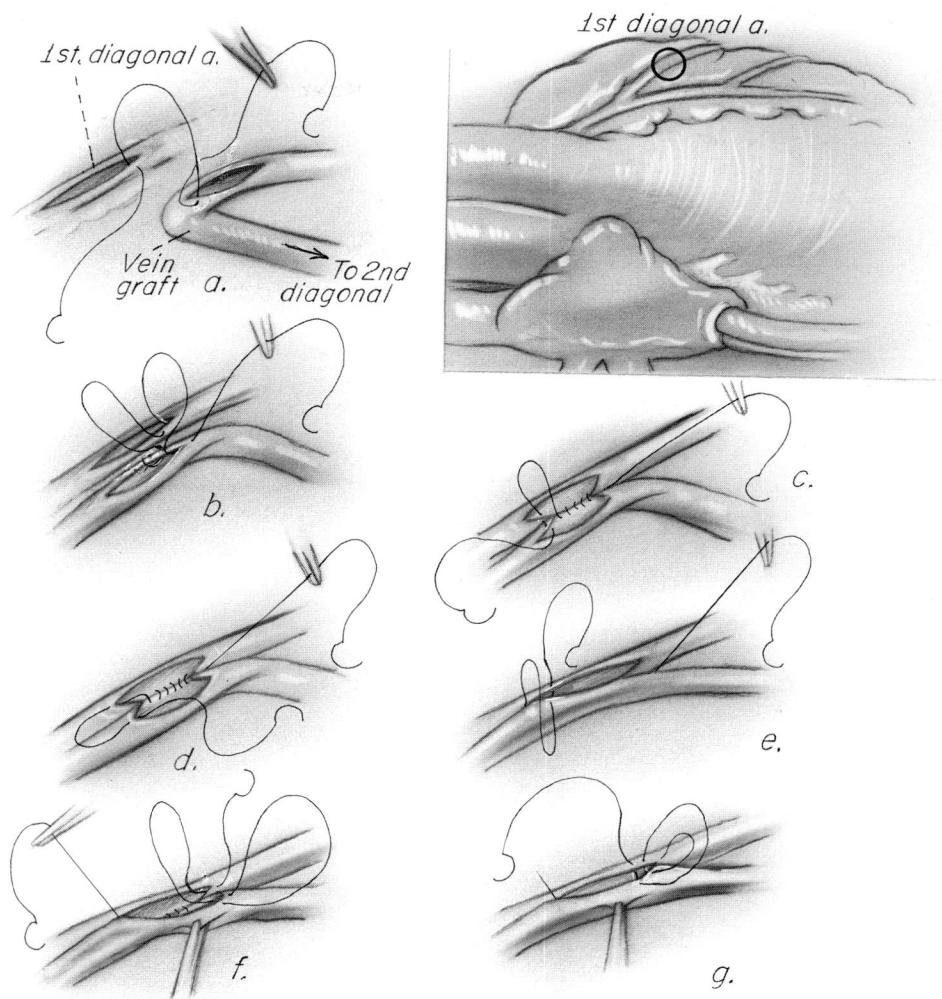

Figure 7-7 Parallel sequential side-to-side anastomosis of the vein graft to the first diagonal artery. (a) The anastomosis is begun just off the angle of the vein graft. (b, c) The anastomosis is continued from within the lumina and (d, e) carried around the proximal angle of the arteriotomy, with separate bites taken into the vein and artery. (f) The other arm of the suture is passed from outside in through the vein and (g) then used to go around the distal angle of the arteriotomy and continued to complete the suture line.

patient with the perfusate, the proximal anastomoses are made. The vein segments are appropriately routed to the area of anastomosis on the ascending aorta (see Fig. 7-4). Each vein segment is distended as described earlier, to determine precisely its proper course and length and the proper point for the proximal anastomosis marked with a light bulldog clamp.

For exteriorizing the right lateral aspect of the ascending aorta, a side-biting clamp[2] with a long flat blade is positioned (Fig. 7-10a). A longitudinal slit about 3 mm in length is made

at the site of each proximal anastomosis. A special punch[3] with the 4.9-mm diameter blade is slipped completely and freely into the aorta through each slit and closed so as to punch out a circular piece of aorta at each site (Fig. 7-10a). The proximal end of the vein graft is cut slightly obliquely, and an incision is made on the down side so as to form a hood (Fig. 7-10b). As in all anastomoses in which the "cobra head" effect is desired, the circumference of this hooded end of the vein graft is made about 10%–20% longer than that of the circular opening in the aorta, and the stitches are placed

---

[2]Ochsner aortic clamp no. 37-1026 by Codman, Randolph, Mass. 02368.

[3]Goosen aortic punch no. DP-05 by Deknatal, Queens Village, N.Y. 11429.

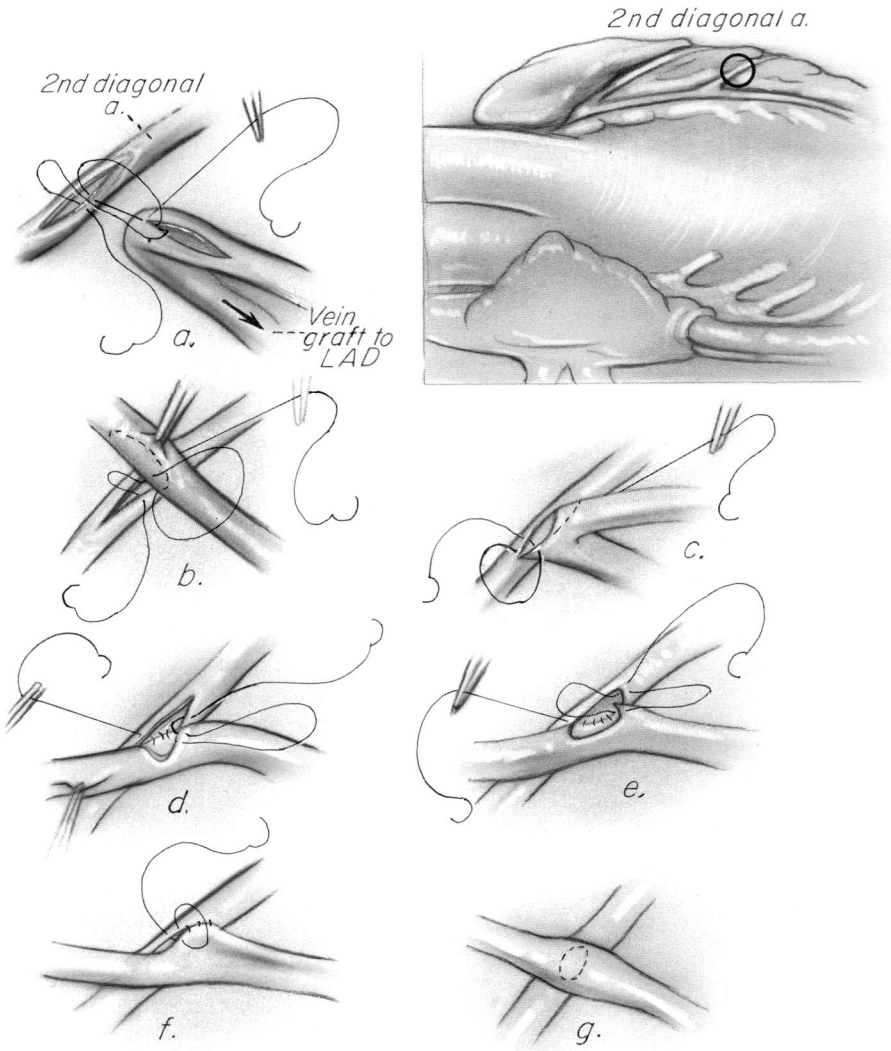

Figure 7-8   Transverse sequential side-to-side anastomosis as, for example, to the second diagonal artery. (a) The first stitch is placed through the angle of the vein graft and (b, c) continued. (d) With the other arm of the suture, a stitch is taken from outside in through the vein, and (e, f) with this arm, the anastomosis is completed. (g) The vein lies smoothly across the artery without distortion or narrowing.

a little farther apart on the vein graft than on the aortic opening. The anastomosis is then made with continuous 5-0 polypropylene sutures.

Alternatively, the two grafts that pass from left to right in front of the main pulmonary artery are anastomosed to the most anterior part of the aorta after exteriorizing this portion of the aorta with a side-biting clamp and excising an appropriately sized segment of aortic wall with a punch or knife to match the vein diameter (GLH). This clamp is then removed, and the graft that approaches from the right is joined to the right anterolateral aspect of the aorta, exteriorized with a separate clamp. A longer, almost vertical aortotomy is made without excising any aortic wall.

Summary of the CABG Operation with the Distal Anastomoses Done First

While the median sternotomy incision is being made, the saphenous vein is removed, most conveniently from the left leg. The IMA is mobilized after splitting the sternum. As the vein is being prepared, the usual purse-string sutures are placed and preparations made for CPB (see Chapter 2). A left atrial pressure monitoring line is placed (UAB) (see Chapter 2). *The heart is not examined digitally or manipulated in any way.* The phase of the operation should be accomplished within 15–20 minutes.

CPB is established, with two venous cannulae (GLH) or

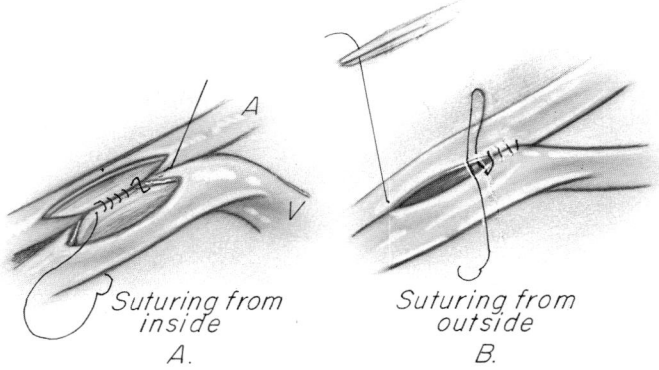

Figure 7-9 A part of an anastomosis can often more conveniently be made by suturing from inside the lumina of the vein and artery.
(*a*) An entirely accurate anastomosis can be constructed in this manner. When such a suture line is carried around an angle of the arteriotomy, separate bites must be made into the vein and artery.
(*b*) The more conventional method of suturing is from the outside.

with one (UAB) (see Chapter 2). The perfusate temperature is taken as low as possible, external cardiac cooling is begun, the aorta is cross-clamped, and the cold cardioplegic solution is injected (see Chapter 3). The cardioplegic solution is reinfused after about 30 minutes or when myocardial electrical activity resumes. When myocardial temperature is measured, additional cardioplegic solution is given whenever it reaches 20°C (GLH). As indicated earlier, the cold cardioplegic solution used to distend the vein graft after each distal anastomosis (UAB) distributes to the myocardium in that region and contributes to the myocardial protection. The perfusate temperature is brought to 25°C. Gentle suction may be placed on the aortic needle vent to decompress the left side of the heart (UAB).

The distal anastomoses are now made. Those of the vein segment to the LAD artery system are generally made first, and then the arteries to the back of the heart are bypassed. The reverse order is used when the IMA is used to revascularize the LAD or diagonal coronary arteries. The aortic clamp is released, and rewarming is begun. The proximal anastomoses are then made.

CPB is discontinued, and the operation is completed in the usual manner (see Chapter 2).

Summary of the CABG Operation with the Proximal Anastomoses Done First

The CABG operation is the same regardless of which anastomoses are done first until the heparin is given. Then a side-biting clamp is placed on the right lateral aspect of the ascending aorta, as described earlier (Fig. 7-11). Properly positioned, the clamp exteriorizes a sufficient cuff of aorta without interfering with the hemodynamic state. Punched out openings are made, and an end-to-side anastomosis is made between the end of a vein graft and each of these openings. After removing the side-biting clamp, the inferior vein segment (or the two most inferior vein segments if three

are to be used) is passed through the transverse sinus with the aid of the clamp and without rotating the graft. A small 5-0 silk stitch has previously been placed and tied at a convenient place to the left of the proximal portion of the LAD artery. The vein graft, with a bulldog clamp on its distal end, is now distended by arterial blood pressure and is occluded with a small, light bulldog clamp at the point that lies opposite the stitch. The superior vein graft is passed to the right of the right atrium and similarly measured to a stitch previously placed near the origin of the posterior descending coronary artery (PDA).

CPB is established, and aortic cross-clamping, external cardiac cooling, and cold cardioplegia provide exposure and myocardial protection, as described in "Summary of the CABG Operation with the Distal Anastomoses Done First." The diagonal branches and LAD are examined, and appropriate arteriotomies are made, as described earlier. The vein graft is distended by infusing the cardioplegic solution into the aortic root, the point on the vein previously identified is placed at the marking stitch, and the point on the vein related to the arteriotomy on the first diagonal artery is noted. The vein is incised at that point, and the side-to-side anastomosis is made. The cardioplegic solution is reinfused as the suture is tied, and as the infusion of the cardioplegic solution distends the vein graft, the point on the vein for the next incision is selected. The incision is made, and the anastomosis performed. This sequence continues until grafting to the LAD artery system is complete.

Then the heart is tilted up, and, with the other vein graft, anastomoses are similarly made to the distal right coronary artery or its branches and to the marginal branches of the circumflex artery. As is the case when the distal anastomoses are made first, the anastomoses on the back of the heart are made initially when the IMA is used for the LAD system.

The aortic clamp is then released, rewarming having begun as the last distal anastomosis was made. The operation is completed as usual.

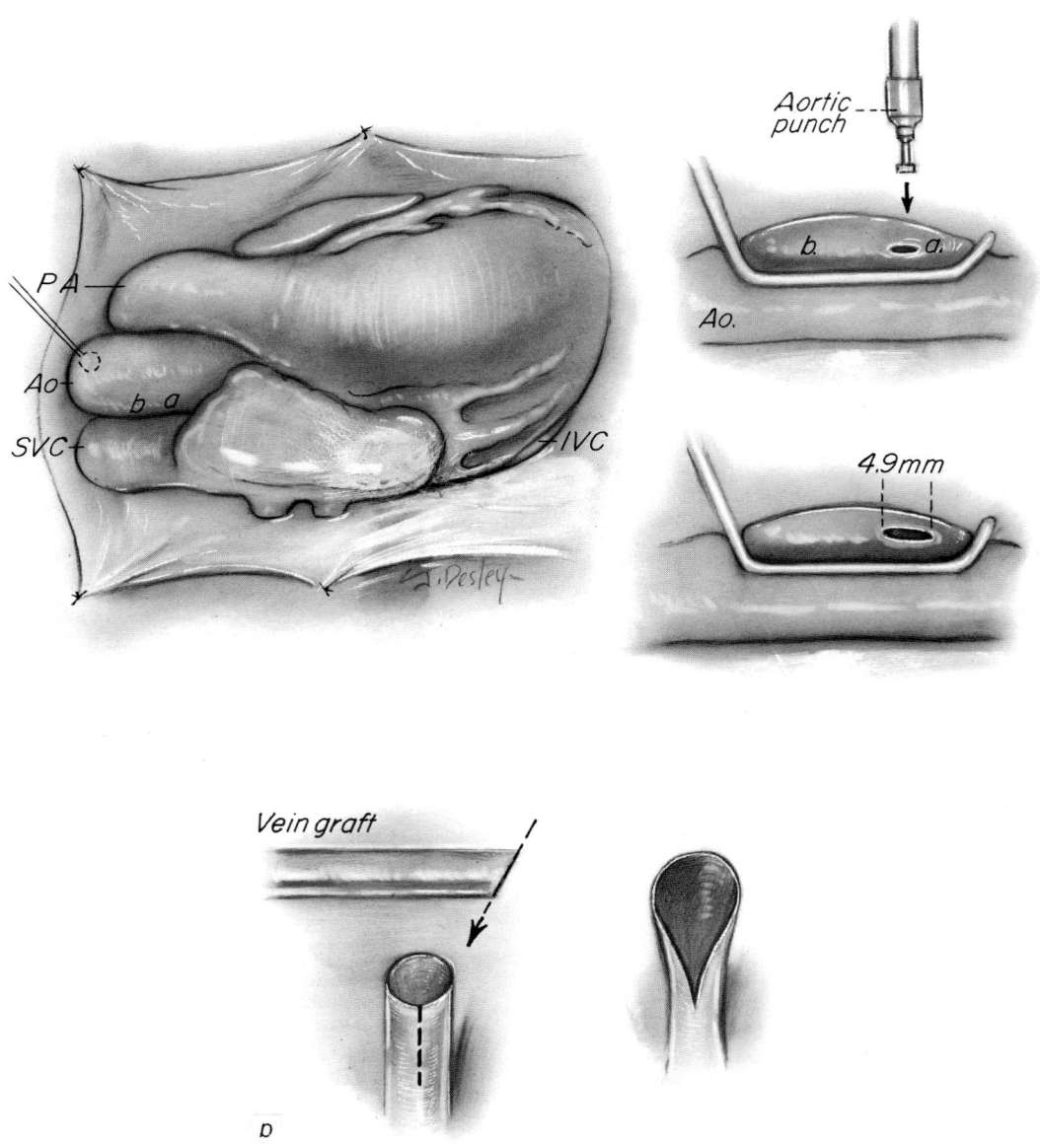

Figure 7-10 The proximal anastomoses when the distal anastomoses are made first.

(a) Preparation for the proximal vein graft anastomosis to the right lateral aspect of the ascending aorta (UAB). The sites for the proximal anastomoses are selected (a) for the vein segment to the LAD artery system and (b) for the segment to the RCA and Cx artery systems. The side-biting clamp is placed on the right lateral aspect of the ascending aorta (to exteriorize the area where the anastomoses will be made). A longitudinal incision is made at a and b. The punch is used to remove a more or less circular piece of wall.

(b) The proximal end of the vein graft is prepared by amputating the distal few millimeters with a slightly oblique cut. An incision is then made down the back of the graft of sufficient length that the circumference of the vein graft opening is 10%–20% larger than that of the opening in the aorta. This allows the end of the vein graft to open out in a "cobra head" configuration.

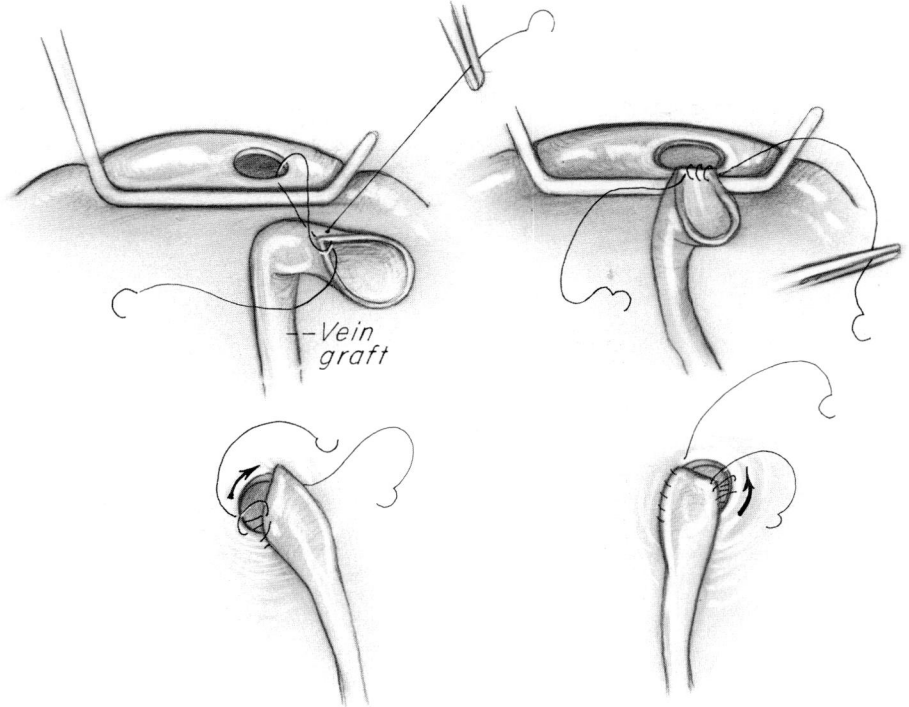

Figure 7-10 (*continued*)
(c) The proximal end of the vein is anastomosed to the punched-out opening with continuous 5-0 polypropylene as illustrated.

Ao, aorta; IVC, inferior vena cava; PA, pulmonary artery; SVC, superior vena cava.

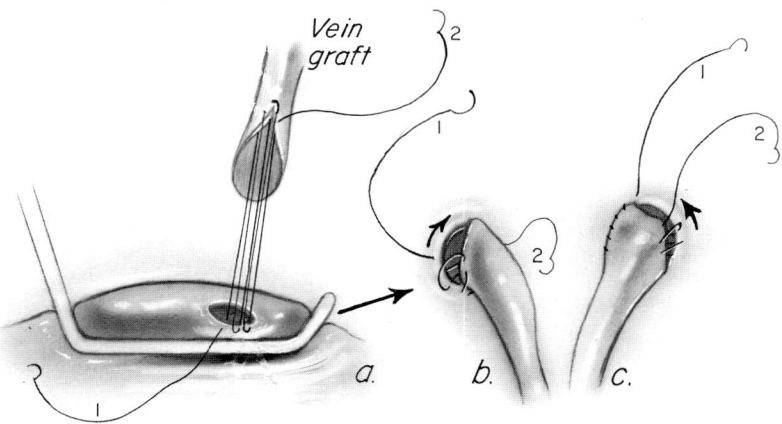

Figure 7-11   When the proximal anastomosis is made before CPB, the first three or four stitches are placed with the vein at a distance. The sutures are pulled up, and the suturing is continued about halfway around with the same end of the suture (1). This end is then dropped, the other end (2) is picked up, and the remainder of the anastomosis is made, sewing from outside in on the aorta, if the aorta is of good quality. Occasionally, the aorta is of poor quality; then (2) a mattress stitch is placed in the vein to reverse the direction of suturing, and the sewing is continued outside in through the vein and inside out through the aorta.

CABG Reoperation

The technique of CABG reoperation is similar to that of the original operation, with a few important differences. The sternotomy is made with the oscillating saw (see Chapter 2 for the technique). Usually, vein grafts from the leg and the internal mammary artery are needed, and these are prepared in the same manner as when the operation is a primary one. The dissection proceeds in general as described in Chapter 2. However, for this operation, the heart must be completely liberated from the pericardium, and the functioning vein or IMA grafts dissected out without damaging them. Grafts originally routed over the pulmonary trunk tend to adhere to the pericardium and are looked for as the mobilization proceeds in that area. Well-functioning vein grafts appear soft and very similar to when first inserted, even after 5–10 years. Nonfunctioning grafts are usually fibrotic throughout. The IMA graft usually remains soft and pliable. As much as is easily possible of the dissection is done before establishing CPB, but a considerable portion of the dissection, including the ligation of the posterobasal, apical, and lateral aspects of the left ventricle, is usually performed after CPB has been established.

Cannulation is accomplished as usual for the operation of CPB, and with the perfusate at 34°C, the remainder of the liberation of the heart is accomplished by sharp dissection. No matter what the usual preference of the surgeon, it is distinctly advantageous to make the distal anastomoses first in reoperations, because there is greater uncertainty as to which vessels will be available for grafting. Because of the epicardial reaction usually present, the arteries to be grafted must be located by identifying the most subtle evidence of their presence. The distal anastomoses are made during cold cardioplegia by the usual techniques. After releasing the aortic cross-clamp, the proximal anastomoses are made during rewarming, as described earlier. The routing and location of the proximal anastomoses depends on the areas of ascending aorta available after the previous CABG operation, and the same general principles apply as for the primary operation.

SPECIAL FEATURES OF POSTOPERATIVE CARE

Most patients are extubated either in the operating room (GLH) or a few hours postoperatively (UAB) and are discharged from the Intensive Care Unit the following morning. Discharge from the hospital to outpatient supervision may occur on the sixth or seventh postoperative day (UAB), and dismissal home from the surgeon's care on the tenth or twelfth day. Thus, postoperative care is simple in most patients (see Chapter 5).

Occasionally, 8–12 hours after operation, arterial blood pressure may fall to levels 10%–20% below normal, while pedal pulses remain full and cardiac index is greater than 2.0. No treatment or a low-dose (2.5 $\mu g \cdot kg^{-1} \cdot min^{-1}$) infusion of dopamine is indicated.

Oral propranolol may be given in a dose of 5 mg every 6 hours beginning 6 hours postoperatively, and this regimen continued until discharge as a prophylaxis against supraventricular tachyarrhythmias.[W9] Alternatively, no prophylactic medication may be given (UAB). Digitalis is not routinely used prophylactically, because it may produce atrial and ventricular arrhythmias. Other drugs or combinations of drugs may prove to be superior to propranolol alone. For example, improved suppression has been reported to result from combining digoxin (begun on postoperative day 1) and propranolol (begun on postoperative day 2 in doses of 30 mg every 8 hours).[R17]

Coumadin has in the past been given on the evening of postoperative day 2 and continued during the period of hospitalization, controlled by daily measurement of prothrombin time, because removal of the saphenous vein from the leg predisposes the patient to deep vein thrombosis and embolization.

Currently, Coumadin is not administered and the aspirin-dipyridamole protocol evolved by Chesebro and colleagues is used for its antiplatelet effect.[C16,C18,C33] In this protocol, 100 mg of dipyridamole is given orally 4 times a day, beginning 2 days before the operation. On the day of operation, 100 mg is given orally at 5 a.m., and through a nasogastric tube 1 hour after operation. Administration of dipyridamole (75 mg) and aspirin (325 mg) is given by nasogastric tube 7 hours after operation and is continued by mouth 3 times a day thereafter. Although perioperative bleeding seems somewhat increased with the use of this protocol, major complications are not encountered. The patient is advised to continue this protocol for 1 year. However, in patients with a history of bleeding peptic ulcer disease the protocol is discontinued after 90 days, and in patients with a strong ulcer diathesis it is discontinued at hospital dismissal, these drugs probably being most important perioperatively and early after operation.[D11]

Occasionally in a patient undergoing CABG, intra-aortic balloon pumping (see Chapter 5) is required for a few hours to a few days after operation. The indication is usually low cardiac output with high left atrial pressure or, occasionally, the occurrence of intractable ventricular arrhythmias intraoperatively or early postoperatively. This intervention is required in about 1% of patients (in the 1977 UAB experience, in 9 of 750 patients that could be analyzed for this event).

EARLY RESULTS

Hospital Mortality

The hospital mortality for the primary CABG operation has always been low but in the current era approaches zero.[M26] (See Chapter 6, "Causes of Surgical Failure," for the definition of a hospital mortality approaching zero.) Thus, in the earlier combined GLH-UAB experience (UAB, 1974–1978;[K10] GLH, 1974–1979), 55 patients (1.5%, CL 1.3%–1.7%) died among 3,467 undergoing the primary CABG operation as an isolated procedure. Acute cardiac failure was the commonest mode of death. In the current era (UAB, 1977–1981; GLH, 1980–1982; see Tables 7-2, 7-3), 36 patients (0.8%, CL 0.7%–1.0%) died in the combined experience with 4,271 primary, isolated CABG operations.

Table 7-2 Hospital mortality after primary CABG operations (UAB; 1977–1981; $n = 3872$).

Category of CABG	n	Hospital Deaths		
		No.	%	CL
Isolated	3610	26	0.72%	0.58%–0.90%
With LV resection	177	8	4.5%	2.9%–6.8%
With valve surgery for ischemic mitral incompetence	51	8	16%	10%–23%
With closure of post-infarction VSD	16	3	19%	8%–34%
With operation for ventricular tachycardia	18	1	6%	1%–18%
Total	3872	46	1.19%	1.01%–1.40%
P (χ^2)			< .0001	

KEY: CABG, coronary artery bypass grafting; CL, 70% confidence limits; LV, left ventricular; VSD, ventricular septal defect.

Incremental Risk Factors for Hospital and Early-Phase Death

The determination of incremental risk factors for hospital and early-phase death for the CABG operation in the current era is handicapped by the very small number of deaths. For example, in the GLH multivariate logistic analysis of the 1980–1981 experience, many variables could not be analyzed, since no deaths occurred, whether the variable was yes or no. Some institution-to-institution variability must exist, and the composition of the patient populations of various institutions must also vary. Thus, the very large collaborative studies provide interesting general information from pooled data[K17] but may not reflect results under optimal conditions or in a specific institution.

Rather than considering hospital deaths and late deaths, it is advantageous to examine the entire time-related incidence of death, beginning with the completion of cardiopulmonary bypass and extending to the furthest point of follow-up. Therefore, the incremental risk factors across this entire spectrum of time are presented under "Late Results."

Perioperative Myocardial Infarction

Electrocardiographically identifiable perioperative myocardial infarctions occur in about 5% of patients undergoing the CABG operation.[C26] The percentage was higher in the early experiences with the operation and can be considerably lower under optimal circumstances.

Electrocardiographically identifiable perioperative myocardial infarctions occurred in 2.4% of patients in the UAB

Table 7-3 Univariate analysis of association of hospital (30-day) mortality with a number of the variables present in patients undergoing isolated, primary CABG operations (GLH, 1980–1982).

Variable	Category	n	Hospital Deaths			P Value (χ^2)
			No.	%	CL	
Age (yr)	20–59	443	2	0.5%	0.1%–1%	.002
	60–79	218	8	3.7%	2.4%–5.5%	
Sex	Male	541	8	1.5%	1.0%–2.2%	.9
	Female	120	2	1.7%	0.6%–3.9%	
Angina severity[a]	0–1	21	0	0%	0%–9%	
	2–3	214	2	0.9%	0.3%–2%	.8
	4	426	8	1.9%	1.2%–2.8%	
Angina pattern	Stable	584	9	1.5%	1%–2.3%	.9
	Unstable	72	1	1%	0.2%–5%	
Diabetes (frank)	Present	29	3	10%	5%–20%	
	Absent	611	7	1.1%	0.7%–1.8%	.02
Hypertension	Present	225	6	2.7%	1.6%–4.3%	.09
	Absent	436	4	0.9%	0.5%–1.7%	
Myocardial score	5–11.9	370	4	1.1%	0.5%–2.0%	.3
	12–14.5	287	6	2.1%	1.2%–3.4%	
Left main stenosis	Present	127	4	3%	2%–6%	.09
	Absent	534	6	1.1%	0.7%–1.8%	
LVEDP (mmHg)	< 15	356	5	1.4%	0.8%–2.5%	
	15 < 25	147	1	0.7%	0.1%–2.3%	.6
	≥ 25	52	2	4%	1%–9%	
Ejection fraction	≥ 50	491	7	1.4%	0.9%–2.2%	
	30–49	98	2	2%	0.7%–4.8%	.9
	< 30	28	1	4%	0.5%–12%	
End-diastolic volume (ml)	< 200	491	7	1.4%	0.9%–2.2%	
	200 < 300	68	0	0%	0%–3%	.6
	≥ 300	12	1	8%	1%–26%	
No. of distal anastomoses	1–3	464	7	1.5%	0.9%–2.3%	
	4–6	197	3	1.5%	0.7%–3.0%	.9
Total cases		661	10	1.5%	1.0%–2.2%	

KEY: CL, 70% confidence limits. LVEDP—left ventricular end diastolic pressure

[a] Canadian Heart Association criteria.

experience, 1973–1978,[K10] and in 2.0% (CL 0.3%–6.7%) of 50 consecutive and representative patients studied in 1978.[M16] A somewhat larger number of patients, up to 15%, have isoenzymatic evidence of some myocardial necrosis without electrocardiographic evidence of a transmural infarction. Thus, in the 1980–1981 GLH experience, the aspartate aminotransferase was $\geqslant$ 100 units^{-1} (normal range 10–50 units^{-1}) on the first postoperative day in 10% of patients. Current anesthesia and supportive techniques (see Chapter 4) and current techniques of myocardial protection (see Chapter 3) have effected a reduction in the incidence and extent of myocardial necrosis.[C10]

Perioperative myocardial infarction occurs occasionally during and after all kinds of operations using CPB and is not unique to the CABG operation. The magnitude of the additional contribution of the coronary artery disease and the CABG operation is problematic. While graft occlusion to the infarcted area is sometimes found at autopsy in patients dying in hospital after CABG, at other times the grafts are patent.[B22,B23] Complete revascularization per se has not reduced the incidence of perioperative myocardial infarction.[B23] Perhaps long CPB time may contribute to the development of early postoperative myocardial necrosis.[B23,C26] This would not be surprising, in view of the known generalized damaging effects of CPB (see Chapter 2). Perioperative infarction is more likely to occur when the CABG operation is done in patients with cardiomegaly than when it is done in those with a normal-sized left ventricle.[C26] This relationship, however, is true in cardiac surgery in general (see Chapter 3).

Depending on its extensiveness, perioperative infarction may or may not be clinically significant. In most cases, it is not associated with a postoperative decrease in ejection fraction.[D10] When extensive, it clearly increases the risk of hospital death.[C9,C26] It may permanently depress left ventricular function.[B24] It has not been demonstrated clearly that perioperative infarction adversely affects late results in patients surviving the early postoperative period.[C26]

LATE RESULTS

CABG favorably affects the incidence and severity of angina pectoris and the need for medication up to a minimum of 10 years after operation. At least in patients with left main or extensive triple-vessel coronary artery disease and with less than severe resting left ventricular dysfunction, CABG also favorably affects longevity and may do so in some subsets of patients with double-vessel disease and impaired left ventricular function. CABG also improves left ventricular function. Late results in patients operated on in the current era are better than those from an earlier era.[M26]

Survival

Even in an earlier era, about 90% of patients who survived the immediate postoperative period (30 days) survived 5 or more years after the CABG operation (Table 7-4). This survival rate is a little lower than that of an age-, sex-, and race-matched general population.[K7] The operation was therefore

Table 7-4   Late survival in hospital survivors of CABG operations according to various categories of disease and compared with matched population.

| Category | Survival (%) at 5 Years | | P value |
	Surgical Treatment ($\pm$ SE)	Matched Population	
Single-vessel	94.8 ± 2.63	94.9	.7
Double-vessel	88.5 ± 2.47	95.0	.003
Triple-vessel	89.8 ± 1.89[a]	95.0	.001
Left main	87.6 ± 3.90[a]	94.4	.05

SOURCE: Reproduced with slight modification from Kirklin et al.[K7]
KEY: SE, standard error.
[a] P for differences between these categories > .6.

considered palliative, but not curative, in spite of the finding of Greene and colleagues that late survival was the same as that of matched cohorts of the general population.[G18] The fact that about 65%–70% of patients survived 10 or more years after the CABG operation[M24,S39] is remarkable, considering that the operation was performed in an early era. However, Lawrie and colleagues reported a 10-year survival of only 48% in triple-vessel disease, 69% in double-vessel disease, 78% for single-vessel disease, but 67% for left main coronary artery disease.[L13] All these results are probably *not* representative of those obtainable currently, since hospital mortality was often high in these earlier patients, revascularization was often incomplete, and reoperation was seldom advised.

In the current era, since about 1977, considering all patients undergoing coronary artery bypass grafting with or without associated surgical procedures for ischemic heart disease (see Table 7-2), the actuarial 5-year survival from the moment in the operating room when cardiopulmonary bypass is discontinued is about 85% (Fig. 7-12). Hazard function analysis (see Chapter 6 "Parametric Methods" in Section 4, for methodology) for the instantaneous incidence (risk) of death across time (Fig. 7-13) shows an early phase of rapidly declining hazard (instantaneous risk) ending at about 6 months, an intermediate phase of low constant hazard, and a late phase of slowly increasing hazard beginning about 3.5 years after operation.

Incremental Risk Factors for Premature Late Death

Extent of the Coronary Artery Disease
A most important fact is that, in the current era, the extensiveness of the coronary artery disease, including multivessel and left main coronary artery disease, is not identified by multivariate analysis as a risk factor for premature death in any time-related postoperative phase to date (Table 7-5). Also, neither the extent of the coronary artery disease (Table 7-6) nor the number of distal anastomoses (Table 7-7) are related to in-hospital mortality in simple contingency table analysis (UAB). Likewise, these variables were not related to the hospital mortality in the GLH multivariate analysis (Table 7-8).

In view of the similar experiences at GLH and UAB and in

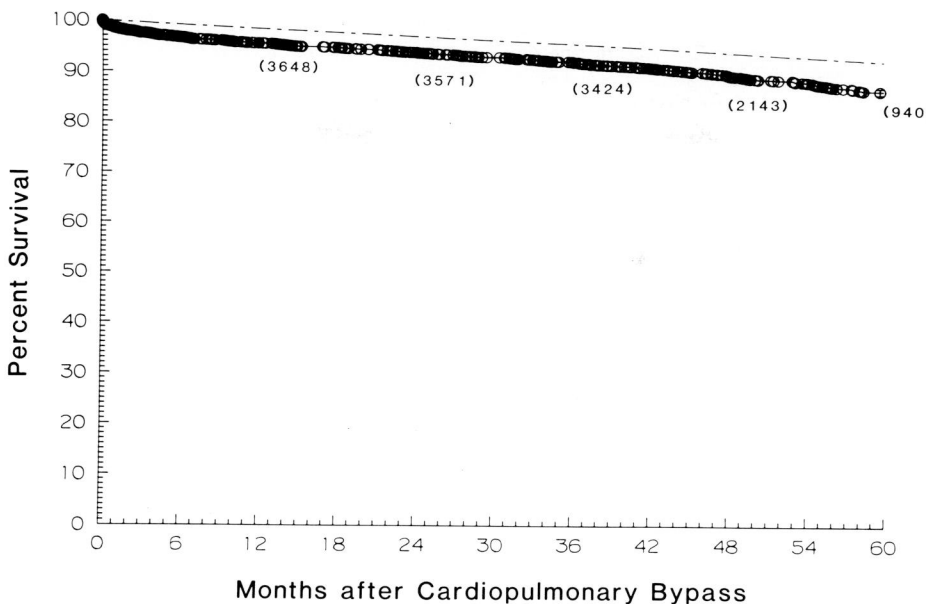

Figure 7-12 Actuarial survival rate (in this and Figures 7-13, 7-14, and 7-15 from the time CPB was discontinued in the operating room) after primary, isolated, or combined CABG (UAB; 1977–1981; $n = 3872$; 460 deaths; see Table 7-2 for patient categories). The numbers in parentheses are the numbers of traced patients at each follow-up period. The 70% confidence limits are enclosed by the vertical bars (barely visible). Each patient death is represented by a circle. The dashed line represents an age-, sex-, and race-matched general population from the 1976 United States Life Tables.

Reproduced with permission from Kirklin et al.,[K23] and the American College of Cardiology.

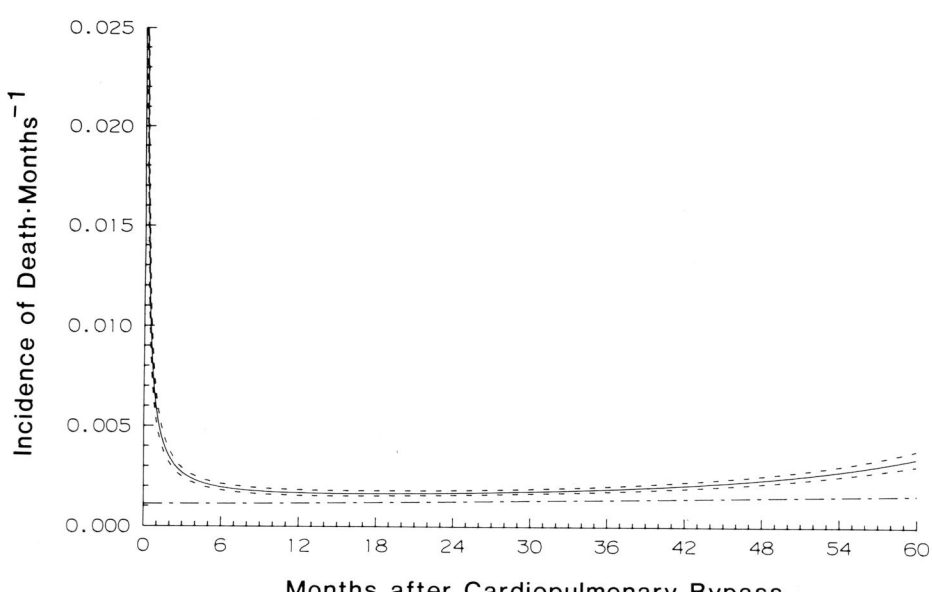

Figure 7-13 Hazard function (instantaneous risk of death per month, shown along the vertical axis) after primary isolated and combined CABG (UAB, 1977–1981; $n = 3827$; 460 deaths; see Table 7-2 for patient categories). Presentation is as in Figure 7-12.

Reproduced with permission from Kirklin et al.,[K23] and the American College of Cardiology.

Table 7-5 Risk factors for premature death after primary, isolated, or combined CABG operations (UAB; 1977–1981; n = 3,872, 460 deaths; see Table 7-2 for patient categories).[K23] Twenty-nine preoperative and intraoperative variables, including those describing the extensiveness of the coronary artery disease and the presence or absence of left main coronary artery disease, were entered. Only those shown in the table had a P value < .20 and were retained.

| | Hazard Phase | | | | | |
| | Early | | Intermediate | | Late | |
Incremental Risk Factor	Coefficient ± SD	P value	Coefficient ± SD	P value	Coefficient ± SD	P value
CASS LV score (5–30)	0.11 ± 0.032	.001	0.11 ± 0.026	< .0001		
Left ventricular end-diastolic pressure (mm Hg)			0.066 ± 0.0113	< .0001		
Age at operation (years)	0.08 ± 0.023	.0003			0.072 ± 0.0164	< .0001
Aortic cross-clamp time (minutes)	0.018 ± 0.0053	.0008				
Left ventricular resection	1.5 ± 0.38	.0001			1.1 ± 0.39	.006
Valve surgery for ischemic mitral incompetence	1.6 ± 0.51	.0009				
Operation for intractable ventricular tachycardia			1.5 ± 0.59	.01	1.8 ± 0.86	.04
Earlier date of operation (months)	−0.020 ± 0.0113	.08				
Intercept	−9.9		−8.6		−7.9	

KEY: SD, standard deviation.

an earlier era,[K10] this matter is not considered controversial, although some have reported a different finding.[K18] However, diffuse coronary arterial disease probably prevents any important increase in myocardial perfusion after the CABG operation in some patients and may be a risk factor, although this is seldom analyzed in reported data and, fortunately, is uncommon. Diffuse disease is the likely reason for the appearance of diabetes as an incremental risk factor in the GLH multivariate analysis (Table 7-8) and in the analyses of Salomon and colleagues[S40] and Johnson and colleagues.[J15]

Hacker and colleagues,[H13] Nomay and colleagues,[N6] and Phillips and associates[P7] also found no relationship between the number of diseased coronary arteries and 5-year survival. Essentially the same findings have been reported from a continuing analysis of the Veterans Administration Cooperative Study.[D6] Phillips' study also found no relationship between the Massachusetts General Hospital myocardial perfusion score and survival.[P7] Loop and colleagues found that the presence of left main coronary artery disease, either with or without other important coronary artery disease, does not increase the risk of premature death in the late postoperative period after a proper operation.[L5] These facts all support the idea that the CABG operation is effective in

Table 7-6 Hospital mortality after primary CABG operations (UAB; 1977–1981).

| Vessel Disease | n | Hospital Deaths | | |
		No.	%	CL
Without left main	3031	21	0.69%	0.54%–0.89%
With single-vessel disease	334	2	0.6%	0.2%–1.4%
With double-vessel disease	1099	8	0.7%	0.5%–1.1%
With triple-vessel disease	1559	11	0.7%	0.5%–1.10%
Vessel disease unknown	39	0	0%	0%–5%
With left main	548	5	0.9%	0.5%–1.6%
With no other disease	11	0	0%	0%–16%
With single-vessel disease	43	0	0%	0%–4%
With double-vessel disease	167	2	1.2%	0.4%–2.8%
With triple-vessel disease	317	3	0.9%	0.4%–1.9%
Vessel disease unknown	10	0	0%	0%–17%
Left main unknown	31	0	0%	0%–6%
Total	3610	26	0.72%	0.58%–0.90%
P (χ^2)				.99

KEY: CL, 70% confidence limits.

Table 7-7 Relationship of hospital death to number of distal anastomoses performed in primary CABG operations without associated procedures (UAB; 1977–1981, n = 3,610, 26 events).

| Number of Distal Anastomoses | % of 3610 | No. | Hospital Deaths | | |
			n	%	CL
1	3%	115	0	0%	0%–1.7%
2	13%	460	3	0.7%	0.3%–1.3%
3	25%	907	3	0.33%	0.14%–0.67%
4	30%	1.088	9	0.8%	0.5%–1.2%
5		672	6	0.9%	0.5%–1.4%
6		265	4	1.5%	0.8%–2.7%
7	29%	77	1	1.3%	0.2%–4.4%
8		22	0	0%	0%–8%
9		3	0	0%	0%–47%
10		1	0	0%	0–85%
P (χ^2)					0.8

KEY: CL, 70% confidence limits.

Table 7-8 Incremental risk factors for hospital death in the GLH CABG experience (1980–1982; 10 deaths in 661 patients), determined by multivariate logistic analysis. The variables analyzed are in Appendix 7C. CPB time and age were significant also as continuous variables but fitted the model best when expressed as in the table.

Incremental Risk Factor	Logistic Coefficient ± SD	P-value
CPB time ≥ 135 min	2.5 ± 0.69	.0003
Age ≥ 60 yr	1.9 ± 0.82	.021
Frank diabetes	2.0 ± 0.80	.013
Intercept	12.62	

KEY: CPB, cardiopulmonary bypass; SD, standard deviation.

increasing myocardial blood flow and improving life expectancy, since without operation the subgroups with more extensive coronary artery disease have had significantly worse 5-year survival rates (see ''Natural History'').

The experience of some other groups is different and suggests that more extensive coronary artery disease decreases 5-year survival after operation.[L11,S8] Using logistic multivariate analysis techniques, Hoffman and colleagues have, for example, found that more extensive coronary artery disease is a significant incremental risk factor for premature death.[H3] However, at least in a univariate analysis, the differences were small, and only double-vessel, triple-vessel, and left main coronary artery disease were considered. These findings do not argue persuasively against the ideas presented above.

Femaleness
Being female is not a risk factor in either the GLH (Table 7-8) or the UAB experience (Table 7-5), in contrast to the findings of some studies.[K17,K18] Perhaps femaleness does not constitute a risk because of the near routine use of complete revascularization even when anastomoses must be made to vessels between 1.0 and 1.5 mm in diameter.

Angina
The type and severity of angina is no longer a risk factor (Table 7-8), as has also been found by others.[B14,C13,K10,K18,R3]

Left Ventricular Dysfunction
Current techniques have neutralized the incremental risk in the early phase of anything less than severely depressed left ventricular dysfunction. In some experiences (GLH), even severe dysfunction is not a risk factor (Table 7-8). This is all the more significant when it is appreciated that operation is advised (GLH, UAB) even when left ventricular dysfunction is severe, but not in the face of right heart failure (characterized by a right atrial pressure > 15 mmHg, hepatomegaly, ascites, and peripheral edema).

However, left ventricular dysfunction is an incremental risk factor for death across time after CABG (Table 7-5), whether this is expressed as ejection fraction or left ventricular CASS score.[C31] Thus, with normal left ventricular function, 5-year survival is approximately 95% no mater how extensive the coronary artery disease (Fig. 7-14); and even

with very poor left ventricular function, it is approximately 60%. Faulkner and colleagues and Kennedy and colleagues have reported similar findings.[F7,K17]

A few studies have found no relationship between the degree of left ventricular dysfunction and the probability of premature late death.[C36,P7] However, studies do demonstrate increasing probability of premature late death with increasingly severe preoperative left ventricular dysfunction.[H3,K8,L3,L12,L13,S7,V4] Using logistic multivariate analysis, Hoffman and colleagues found that preoperatively poor left ventricular function (assessed both globally and segmentally from cineangiograms) is a significant determinant of 5-year survival after CABG.[H3] In a univariate analysis in this study, when left ventricular function was normal, moderately, and severely impaired, 5-year survival was 92.3%, 89.2%, and 69.6%, respectively.

However, as noted earlier, in spite of the unfavorable effect of poor left ventricular function on survival, as long as right heart failure is not present, survival with surgical treatment is surprisingly good and probably better than that with medical treatment. Also, Faulkner and colleagues found the 2-year actuarial survival to be 83% in patients with ejection fractions less than 0.30 who were treated surgically, and 47% in those treated medically.[F7] Coles and colleagues found an 80% 5-year survival rate among a group of patients with poor left ventricular function whose preoperative ejection fractions averaged 0.28.[C22]

Older Age
Older age continues to be a risk factor in all studies. In the GLH analysis (Tables 7-3, 7-8) and the UAB experience (Table 7-5), as well as in the CASS Registry study,[K17,K18] this risk was evident beyond 60 years of age. It affects both the early and the late phase (Fig. 7-15). However, the early mortality remains quite low, even in patients in the eighth decade of life, but 5-year survival is more significantly affected by this variable. Hoffman and colleagues also found older age to be an incremental risk factor for premature death within 5 years of the CABG operation, patients aged 40–50 years at operation having a 5-year survival of 90.8% and those over 50 years of age one of about 82%.[H3]

Aortic Cross-Clamp Time
Longer aortic cross-clamp times increase the risk of death in the early phase. However, this increase is very small in the range of cross-clamp times used in patients undergoing isolated coronary artery bypass grafting (Table 7-9). Correspondingly, the cardiopulmonary bypass time is an incremental risk factor when it is longer than 135 minutes (Table 7-8), but cardiopulmonary bypass times are rarely longer than 100 minutes for isolated CABG operations.

Earlier Date of Operation
The safety of the CABG operation continues to improve. Thus, an earlier date of operation is an incremental risk factor (Table 7-5).

Preoperatively Important Ventricular Arrhythmias
The existence of important ventricular arrhythmias preoperatively is an incremental risk factor for premature late death.

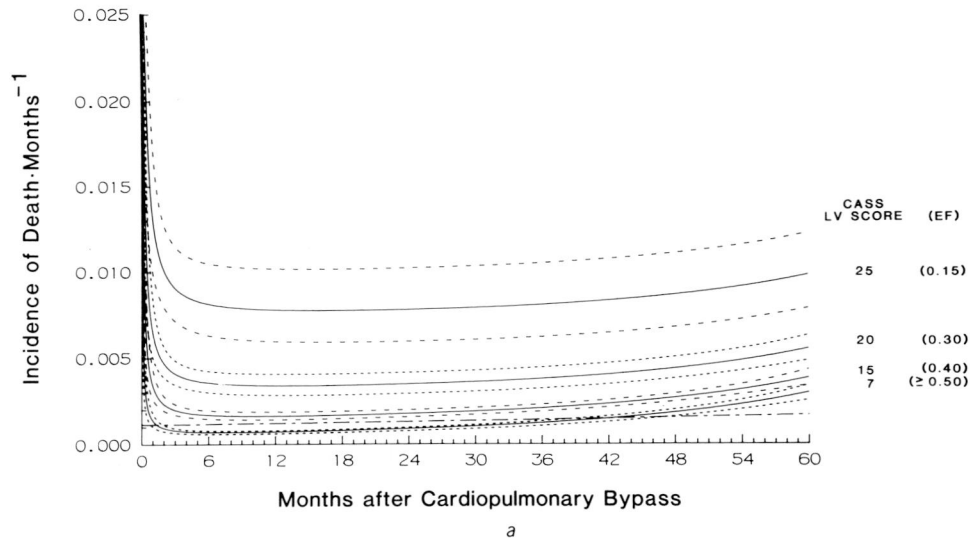

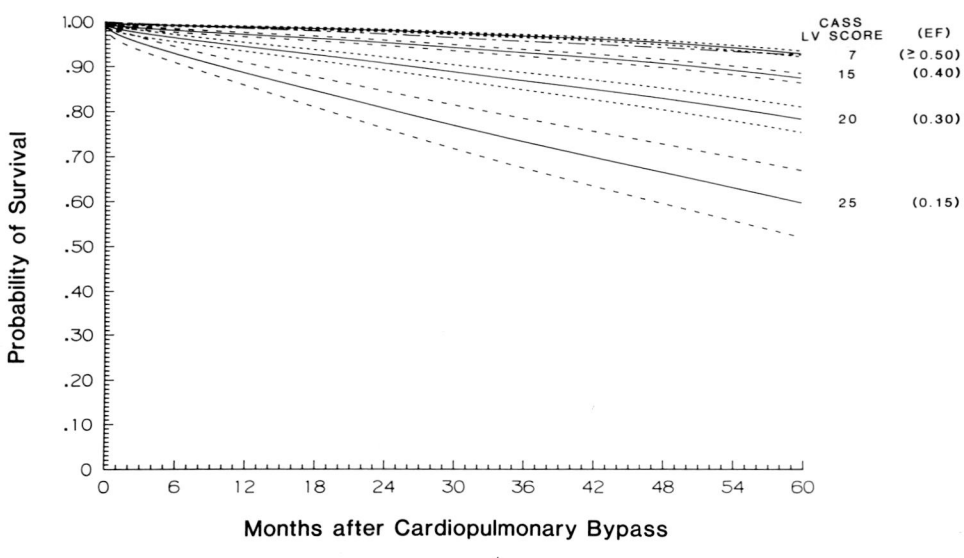

Figure 7-14 Effect of left ventricular function (expressed as CASS LV score and, in parentheses, LV ejection fraction) on survival after CABG (UAB; 1977–1981; data base and presentation as in Fig. 7-13). These nomograms are solutions of the multivariate equation in Table 7-5. The values for ejection fraction are obtained from a regression analysis of the relationship of ejection fraction to CASS LV score in the 3872 patients ($r = .73$). LV resection, surgery for ischemic mitral incompetence, and surgery for intractable ventricular tachycardia were set at no, age was set at 56 years (median value for $n = 3610$), and aortic cross-clamp time at 50 minutes (median value). Left-ventricular end diastolic pressure was set at the median value for each of the four specific CASS LV scores (10 mmHg, 13 mmHg, 17 mmHg, and 22 mmHg for LV scores of 7, 15, 20, and 25, respectively).

(a) Hazard function (instantaneous risk, or incidence, of death per month).

(b) Parametric estimates of survival.

Reproduced with permission from Kirklin et al.,[K23] and the American College of Cardiology.

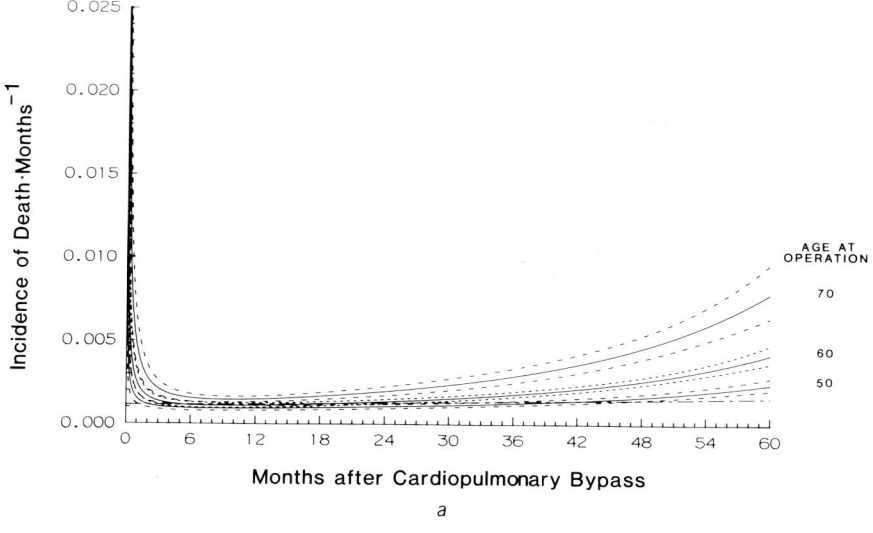

a

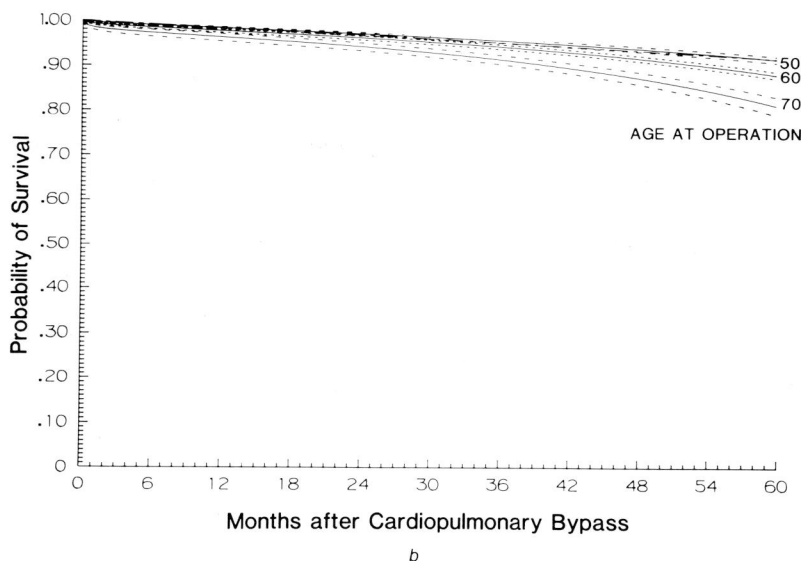

b

Figure 7-15   Effect of age on survival after CABG (UAB; 1977–1981; data base and depiction as in Fig. 7-13). These nomograms are solutions of the multivariate equation in Table 7-5. LV resection, surgery for ischemic mitral incompetence, and surgery for intractable ventricular tachycardia were set at no, and aortic cross-clamp time was set at 50 minutes (median value for n = 3610). LV end-diastolic pressure was set at 13 (median value), and LV score at 10 (median value).
(*a*) Hazard function (instantaneous risk, or incidence, of death per month).
(*b*) Parametric estimates of survival.

This risk is separate from (or perhaps additive to) the increased risk posed by the important left ventricular dysfunction usually present in such patients.[N6] Such relationships are not surprising, in view of the effect of this variable on the natural history after acute myocardial infarction (see "Effect of Acute Myocardial Infarction on Natural History").

Preoperative Myocardial Infarction
When considered as a single variable, preoperative myocardial infarction is an incremental risk factor, particularly when there were multiple infarctions. However, this factor drops out in multivariate analysis,[H3] probably because the effect of previous myocardial infarctions is through their influence on left ventricular function.

Perioperative Myocardial Infarction
Several studies have documented an adverse effect of perioperative myocardial infarction on late survival,[O3,N6,S45] although Jones and colleagues could not demonstrate one.[J2] Small amounts of perioperative myocardial necrosis would

Table 7-9 Digital nomogram (a solution of the multivariate equation in Table 7-5) demonstrating the relationship between aortic cross-clamp time and the mortality within 48 hours and within 2 weeks (the equation was solved for a median age of 56 years, a median CASS score of 10, and a median left ventricular end-diastolic pressure of 13; operation for intractable ventricular tachycardia and valve surgery for ischemic mitral incompetence were entered as no; left ventricular resection was entered as yes in 5% of cases; the operation date was 1981). In virtually all operations for isolated CABG, the cross-clamp time is between 30 and 90 minutes.

| Aortic Cross-Clamp Time (min) | Estimated Mortality | | | |
| | 48 Hours | | 2 Weeks | |
	%	CL	%	CL
30	0.13%	0.08%–0.20%	0.29%	0.20%–0.44%
60	0.22%	0.14%–0.32%	0.48%	0.33%–0.68%
90	0.36%	0.24%–0.54%	0.79%	0.54%–1.13%
120	0.61%	0.39%–0.97%	1.31%	0.85%–2.00%

KEY: CL, 70% confidence limits.

not be expected to influence late results. However, a sizable perioperative infarction worsens left ventricular function and must affect late results.

Completeness of Revascularization
Zorn, at UAB, has shown that patients with triple-vessel disease and normal or mildly impaired left ventricular function have a 5-year survival of 96% after relatively complete revascularization, whereas those with incomplete revascularization have one of 88% (P = .005) (Fig. 7-16).[Z3] Similar results have been presented by Loop and associates,[L3] Stiles and colleagues,[S8] Lawrie and colleagues,[L12] and Cukingnan and associates.[C11]

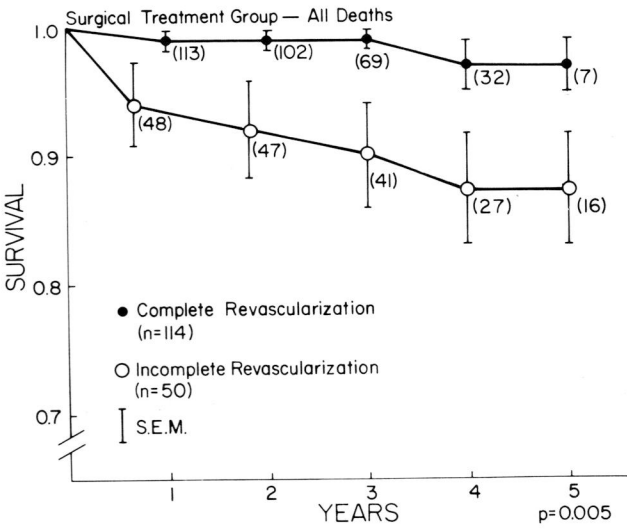

Figure 7-16 Five-year survival rate after CABG in patients with triple-vessel disease and no or mild left ventricular dysfunction, according to whether all important stenoses were bypassed (UAB). Used with permission from Zorn.[Z3]

Complete evaluation of this variable is handicapped by the wide variety of definitions of complete revascularization. This problem is evidenced by the detailed multivariate analysis of their experience by Lawrie and colleagues.[L19] They found no effect on 5-year survival of the *preoperative* extent of the coronary artery disease. There was a strong effect of residual (unbypassed) stenoses of a *major* coronary artery (i.e., left main, LAD, Cx, or right coronary) with the effect being the strongest in patients with poor left ventricular function and/or triple-vessel disease. These researchers emphasize that it remains to be proven whether residual stenoses in smaller arteries (such as the second or third diagonal branches or marginal branches of the posterolateral segment) adversely affect survival and symptomatic results.

Non-Use of the Internal Mammary Artery
A high patency rate has long been known to be characteristic of the IMA when it is used for anastomosis to the LAD artery.[G26,G27,T9] Reservations concerning its efficacy have remained. However, a study from the Cleveland Clinic clearly establishes the fact that, other things being equal, survival after the CABG operation is enhanced when the internal mammary artery is used as the conduit to the LAD artery.[L27] Conversely, failure to use the internal mammary artery when grafting of the LAD is required is a risk factor for premature late death.

Preoperatively Elevated Serum Cholesterol Levels
A higher proportion of premature deaths is associated with preoperatively elevated serum cholesterol levels. However, the levels of triglycerides, the presence of diabetes, and a history of smoking are not significant determinants of late survival.[H3]

History of Stroke
Not surprisingly, a history of stroke appears to severely reduce 5-year survival.[H3] This effect is probably related to the widespread atherosclerosis that is likely to be present in such patients, rather than to their cardiac status.

Method of Myocardial Protection
The method used to protect the myocardium during surgery has not been demonstrated to affect long-term survival.

Comparisons of Survival after Surgical versus Medical Treatment

The most reliable comparisons are those in which a randomized trial has been directed specifically to the hypothesis being tested. Unfortunately, a limited amount of information is available from such trials comparing survival after surgical versus medical treatment. Therefore, informal comparisons must, in some instances, be made between well-studied surgical groups of patients and those treated by other methods. The following inferences can be drawn from the information currently available.

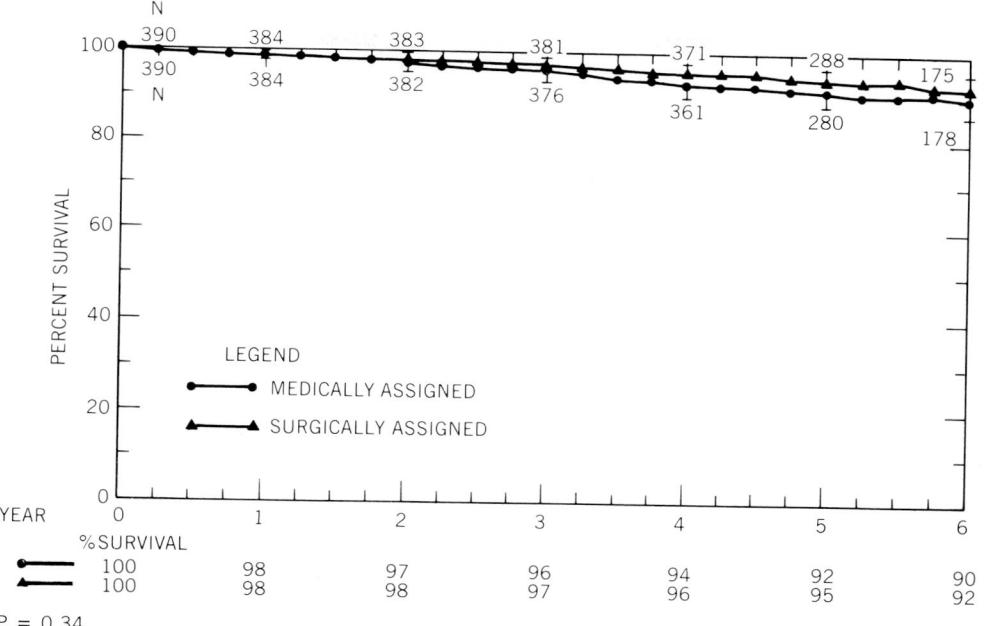

Figure 7-17 Actuarial survival of all patients randomly assigned to initial medical treatment or to initial surgical treatment in the CASS randomized trial. The patients, less than 66 years of age, were either asymptomatic after a previous myocardial infarction or had mild stable angina (class I or II). Seventy-two percent of the patients had normal or near normal left ventricular function at rest; 30% had a severe proximal lesion in the anterior descending coronary artery.
Reproduced with permission from CASS Principal Investigators and Their Associates,[C31] and the American Heart Association, Inc.

Patients with Good Left Ventricular Function
In general, patients with good left ventricular function who have stable and mild or moderate angina or who are asymptomatic after an acute myocardial infarction have a good (about 90%) 5-year survival rate, whether treated initially by the CABG operation or initially assigned to medical treatment. As a general statement, this is the most important inference to be drawn from the CASS randomized trial[C31] (Fig. 7-17). This finding is amplified in another report from that trial, which indicates that the 5-year survival *free* of nonfatal myocardial infarction is also similar.[C32]

The design of the CASS randomized trial allowed crossover to surgery of patients assigned to medical treatment when, in the judgment of the cardiologist, this best served the patient's well-being. Most of the crossovers were for worsening angina. Even in the case of single-vessel disease, 10% of patients crossed over to surgery within 5 years, and in the case of three-vessel disease, 38% (Fig. 7-18). These facts emphasize that the comparison is not between 1) surgical and 2) medical treatment but between 1) initial surgical treatment and 2) initial medical treatment and CABG at a later time when indicated.

This inference about patients with good left ventricular function is tenable also in the context of the European randomized trial of surgical treatment,[E12] which included only patients with good (EF > 0.50) left ventricular function and mild or moderate angina and which also allowed crossover. In that study, when double- or triple-vessel disease did not include a severe proximal left anterior descending artery lesion, initial assignment to surgical treatment did not improve survival.

Patients with Impaired Left Ventricular Function
No randomized trial has been directed specifically at patients with impaired left ventricular function, and no cases of this type were included in the European trial.[E12] Only 27% of the patients in the CASS randomized trial had something less than good left ventricular function, but the original randomization process was stratified by LV function, and thus some information is available. Patients with chronic, stable, mild, or moderate angina and an LV ejection fraction less than 0.50 had a better 5-year survival rate (96%) when assigned to surgical treatment than that (85%) of patients assigned initially to medical treatment with the opportunity for crossover to surgery[C31] (Fig. 7-19). The *P* value, .057, indicates that probably this difference is *not* due to chance and that probably it would appear in another similar group managed in an identical fashion. Further support for these inferences comes from a recent analysis of the CASS randomized trial, in which it is shown that the *7-year* survival of patients with an LV injection fraction of < .50 assigned to initial surgical treatment was 84% compared with 70% for those initially assigned to medical treatment (*P* = .01).[P14] Again, it is to be noted that many of the patients initially assigned to medical treatment and retained in this category crossed over to surgery during the study period.

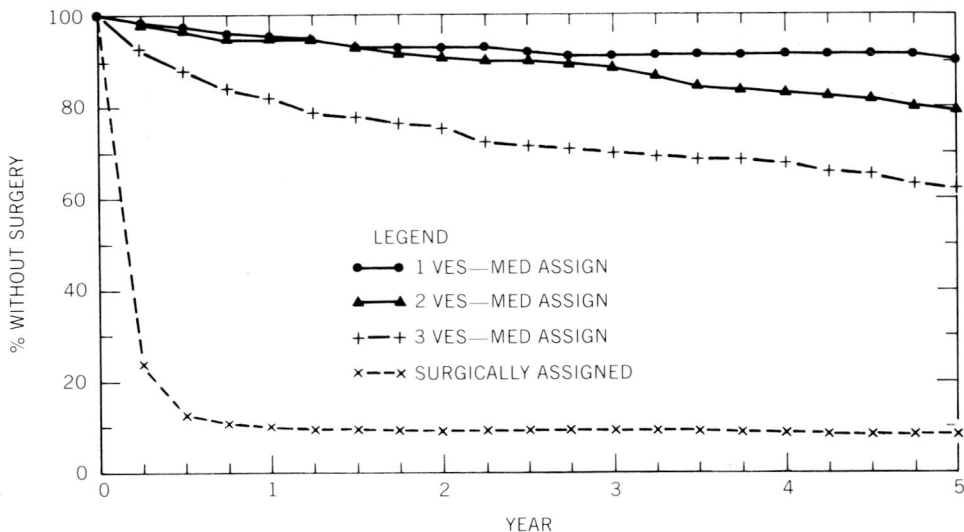

Figure 7-18 Actuarial depiction of crossovers (shown as the inverse percent without surgery) from assigned treatment in the CASS randomized trial.[C31] Crossovers to surgery of patients initially assigned to medical treatment are indicated by the solid lines, stratified by number of vessels with 70% or greater stenoses.

Reproduced with permission from CASS Principal Investigators and Their Associates,[C31] and the American Heart Association, Inc.

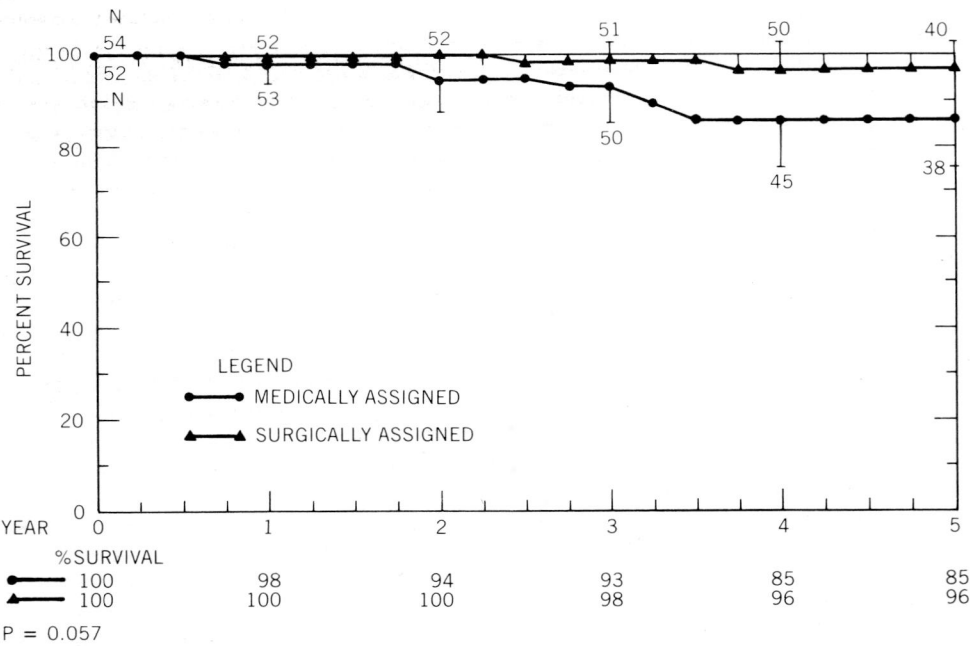

Figure 7-19 Actuarial depiction of survival in patients (group B) with impaired LV function (EF < 0.50) in the CASS randomized trial.[C31]

Reproduced with permission from CASS Principal Investigators and Their Associates,[C31] and the American Heart Association, Inc.

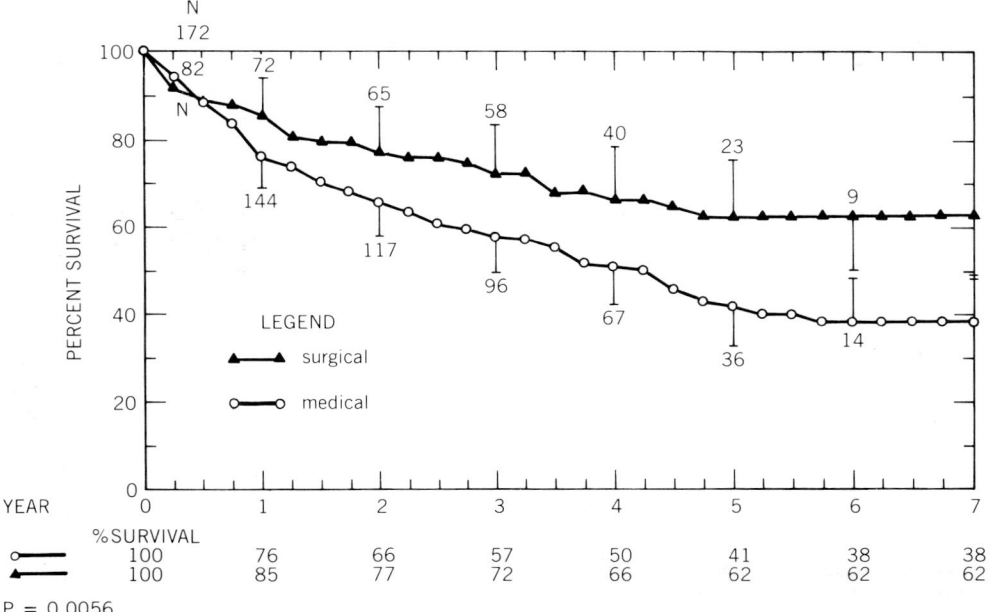

Figure 7-20   Survival rates in patients with coronary artery disease and ejection fractions less than 0.25, with initial treatment by coronary artery bypass grafting and with initial medical treatment. Reproduced with permission from Alderman et al.,[A9] and the American Heart Association, Inc.

Patients with more severe left ventricular dysfunction have a better 5-year survival rate with CABG than with medical treatment. Informal comparison of UAB results (Fig. 7-14) with those of initial assignment to medical treatment in the CASS registry[A9,M19] supports this conclusion, as do comparisons of patients in the CASS registry (Fig. 7-20). Whether this is true of patients whose LV function is severely depressed (EF < 0.30) is not known, but an informal comparison with data from the CASS registry[A9,M19] suggests that it is, at least in patients with triple-vessel disease.

Patients with Left Main Coronary Artery Disease
Even when left ventricular function is good, patients with left main coronary artery disease have a better 5-year survival rate when treated surgically than when treated medically.[D12] This inference is supported by the United States Veterans Administration randomized trial of coronary surgery[R5] and, with a lesser degree of certainty (P = .12), perhaps related to the small number of cases in the European trial.[E12] Patients with left main coronary artery disease were not included in the CASS randomized trial. The inference is true also when left ventricular function is impaired.

The improved results with surgical treatment are particularly marked when the left main coronary artery disease is associated with extensive triple-vessel disease.[T3,V2] The increased 5-year survival rate obtained by surgical, compared with medical, treatment is particularly great and evident when the left main diameter stenosis is 75% or greater, left ventricular function is depressed, and the functional status of the patient is impaired.[C29,T7]

Patients with Proximal High-Grade Stenoses of the Left Anterior Descending Artery
Patients with important ($\geqslant$ 50%) stenosis in the proximal anterior descending coronary artery, as a part of triple- or double-vessel disease, have a better prognosis when treated surgically than when initially assigned to medical treatment[E12] (Fig. 7-21). This finding was not supported by the CASS randomized study.

Informal comparisons in patients with single-vessel disease fail to define clearly better survival with surgical than with initially medical treatment.

Patients with Triple-Vessel Disease
When triple-vessel coronary artery disease without severe proximal LAD artery disease is associated with good left ventricular function, the 5-year survival rates with surgical and with initially medical treatment are similar in randomized trials (see "Patients with Good Left Ventricular Function" in earlier part of section on Comparisons of Survival after Surgical versus Medical Treatment).

Informal comparisons from nonrandomized trials[H6,R5,V2] give variable results, but the largest study with a 5-year follow-up found that, in the overall setting described above, the surgical and medical groups had 5-year survival rates of 94.9% and 84.8%, respectively (P < .001). This is supported by the recent data from the Seattle Heart Watch.[D2] When triple-vessel coronary artery disease is associated with moderately impaired left ventricular function (EF 0.3–0.5), the 5-year survival rate after the CABG operation was a little lower in one informal comparison than in the European

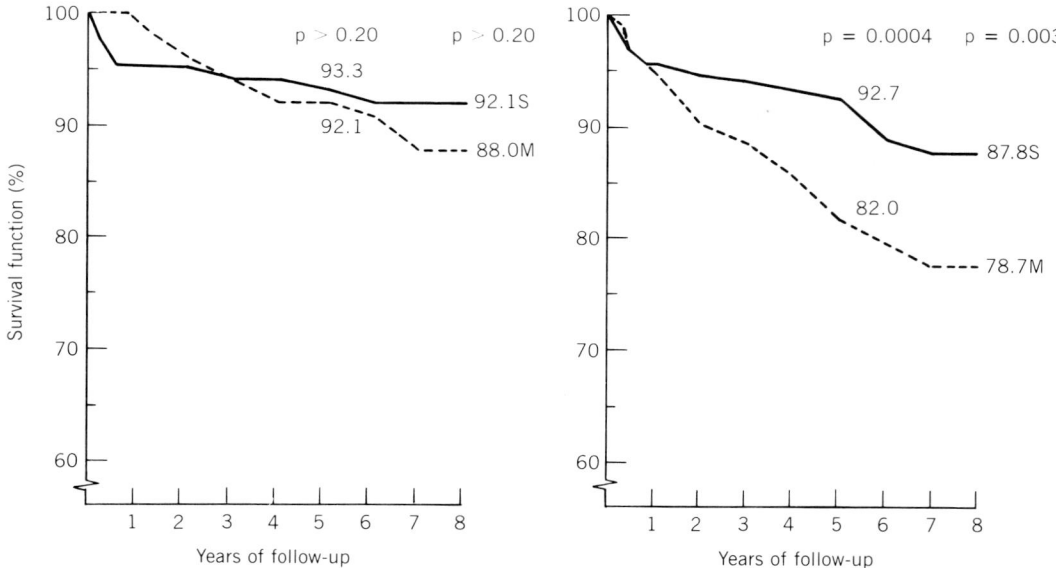

Figure 7-21 Survival curves for patients with double- or triple-vessel disease and good left ventricular function, stratified as to initial medical (dashed line) versus initial surgical (solid line) treatment. Patients without important proximal stenosis in the left anterior descending artery are depicted on the left. On the right are those with important proximal LAD stenosis.

Reproduced with permission from the European Coronary Surgery Study Group Report.[E12]

study (about 90%), but the survival rate with medical treatment was considerably less.[H6]

Patients with Double-Vessel Disease

In general, in patients less than 65 years of age and with normal or mildly reduced left ventricular function at rest and without severe proximal LAD artery disease, the surgical treatment of double-vessel coronary artery disease has not been shown to result in higher survival rates at 5-year follow-up (91.6% for surgery, 87.5% for medicine, $P = .67$, in the European study[V2]). The data are controversial for patients with double-vessel disease and *moderately impaired left ventricular function* (EF 0.3–0.5), but Hammermeister and colleagues found the 5-year survival rate to be about 85% with either surgical or medical treatment.[H6] The effect of severe proximal LAD artery disease in this subset was discussed above.

Patients with Single-Vessel Disease

No studies present convincing evidence that patients less than 65 years of age and with normal or mildly impaired left ventricular function and single-vessel coronary artery disease have a better 5-year survival rate with surgical than with medical treatment.[B26,C25] The 5-year survival rate in the European study was about 95% with either form of treatment,[V2] as it was in the UAB study.[K7] Concern remains that this conclusion may not be valid when the single-vessel disease involves the proximal LAD artery with a 50% or greater diameter narrowing, particularly since about half the patients presenting with postinfarction left ventricular aneurysm have this disease.

Patients with Severe or Unstable Angina

Inasmuch as no incremental risk of the severity or type of angina has been found to be related to the early results of CABG (Table 7-8), the presence of these symptoms thus does not adversely affect the surgical results in any of the preceding comparisons of surgical and medical treatment. Since severe angina (Canadian angina class III or IV) or persistently unstable angina are themselves indications for surgical treatment, probably no randomized trial and no specific comparison of patients treated surgically with those treated medically are possible. However, the informal comparison from the CASS registry indicates that in patients with preoperatively severe angina, survival after the CABG operation is higher than with medical treatment.[R24]

Asymptomatic Patients

The foregoing comparisons of survival following medical versus surgical treatment cannot be assumed to be the same in *asymptomatic patients*. This conclusion is supported by the GLH randomized trial of initial assignment to surgical versus medical treatment in asymptomatic patients following recurrent myocardial infarctions, for this shows no difference in 5-year survival rates in the two groups, despite the fact that most of these patients had triple-vessel disease and a reduced ejection fraction.[N4] However, in the nonrandomized study from the Seattle Heart Watch, surgery did improve the survival rate in essentially asymptomatic patients when triple-vessel disease was associated with a reduced ejection fraction.[H6,H8] Also, data from the CASS registry indicate that in the case of patients with LMCA disease, asymptomatic patients have a significantly better 5-year survival when treated surgically than when treated medically.[D12]

Modes of Premature Late Death

Most late deaths are from cardiac causes, specifically myocardial infarction or ventricular electrical instability. Thus, in Zorn's combined group of patients with complete or incomplete revascularization, five (71%, CL 45%–90%) of seven late deaths were from myocardial infarction. The incremental risk factors affecting the probability of late myocardial infarction are thus probably the same ones that affect overall late survival.

Myocardial Infarction

None of the large randomized studies, including the CASS randomized trial, has shown a reduction in nonfatal myocardial infarctions with surgical, compared with medical, treatment.[C32] Also, in the GLH trial, the incidence of infarction on follow-up was similar in the two groups.[N4] However, in a small subset of the European multicenter trial for the treatment of patients with double- or triple-vessel disease and stable angina, Yacoub and colleagues found 92% of patients surgically treated free of late infarction at 6 years, compared with 54% of the medical group. Also, at UAB, in an earlier era and by nonrandomized study, in patients with preoperative ejection fraction ≤ 0.35, the CABG operation increased ($P = .001$) the proportion (51%) alive and free of myocardial infarction at 7 years, compared with medical treatment.[P12]

Relief of Angina Pectoris

The efficacy of CABG in relieving angina pectoris, and its superiority over medical treatment in this regard, has been demonstrated by several randomized studies.[K9,M2,V2] Sixty percent to 95% of patients are reported to be free of angina pectoris 1–5 years after operation. As the follow-up period lengthens, the proportion of angina-free patients gradually declines,[A1,A2,C8,T2] no doubt partly from reduction in graft flow and graft closure, but also from progression of disease in ungrafted vessels. However, 46% of patients undergoing the CABG operation were asymptomatic 10 years later, in the experience of Mather and colleagues, compared with 3% of patients randomized to medical treatment.[M24] Schaff and colleagues found 66% of their patients either without symptoms or with mild symptoms 10 years after operation.[S39] The more complete the revascularization and the higher the proportion of open anastomoses, the higher the proportion of patients free of angina.[C11,F2] In fact, the data indicate that a patient *will* be free of angina after operation unless the revascularization has been incomplete or graft closure has occurred. The dominant importance of graft patency is evident in the data of Gould and colleagues, who showed that patients with all of their multivessel grafts patent experienced at least 7 more years of symptomatic relief of angina than did their counterparts with all grafts occluded.[G24]

Hamby and colleagues found that 83% of their patients with recurrent angina had graft closure, progression of native coronary disease or incomplete revascularization.[H2] In the study by Campeau and colleagues, the return of angina in patients angina free at the end of 1 year was about 5% per postoperative year.[C8] In years 6 and 7, it became about 12% per year. The most significant correlate of the recurrence of angina in their study was progression of disease in the native coronary circulation. This was presumably primarily in ungrafted vessels, since other studies have shown progression of disease distal to a graft to be uncommon unless important stenoses were there at the time of operation.

It is possible that the rate of return of angina will be lower in patients currently being operated on, as a result of the many other events that already have been shown to be different in patients operated on in the current era.

Functional Status

Maximal exercise capacity of patients is improved in at least the first few years after CABG,[B12,B13,F3,K11,L7,O1,S9,S10] and electrocardiographic abnormalities during exercise are usually significantly reduced.[S9] The degree of recovery and the ultimate exercise capacity reached after operation depends on preoperative left ventricular function, the completeness of revascularization, and graft patency. It has been clearly demonstrated that, from 3–10 years postoperatively, the maximal exercise capacity of patients is significantly more improved by CABG than by medical treatment.[M24,V2]

The mechanisms of improvement in functional capacity after CABG are probably complex. Improved left ventricular function occurs and must contribute to the improved functional capacity (see "Gainful Employment"). However, Serruys and colleagues found an increase in maximal heart rate, presumably secondary to increased myocardial blood flow, to be a determinant of increased functional capacity, as well as an increase in cardiac output.[S9] These results are consistent with the variable exercise performance observed in patients with similar and severe left ventricular dysfunction, accounted for by variability in heart rate and arterial-venous oxygen differences.[H15] As would be expected, the increase in functional capacity, as evidenced by an increase in cardiac output with exercise postoperatively, is considerably greater in patients with complete, as opposed to incomplete, revascularization (26% versus 6%; $P = .0001$).[H18]

Gainful Employment

Currently, in North America, fewer than two-thirds of patients return to gainful employment after a successful CABG operation,[B11,R4,S6] although the proportion of patients with few or no symptoms is considerably larger. Fowler and colleagues have stressed[F2] that most patients are unemployed for reasons other than current functional status. Among their patients, only 14% were unemployed because of disability associated with coronary artery disease, although, overall, 48% were unemployed. In spite of this seemingly unimpressive record, the randomized study of Frick and colleagues indicates the superiority of surgical over medical treatment in this regard, as only 26% of medically treated patients were working at 2-year follow-up, compared with 60% of surgically treated patients.[F3]

In order for the maximal socioeconomic benefits to be

achieved from the operation of CABG, better rehabilitation programs and some attitudinal changes on the part of patients, doctors, employers, and government are required.

Use of Medication

Nearly all studies report a decrease in the use of vasodilators and β-blocking agents after operation. The cooperative randomized study by the European Coronary Surgery Study Group, for example, found about 70% of patients randomized to medical treatment taking β-blockers during the first 3 years of follow-up, in contrast to 25% of the surgical patients.[V2]

Left Ventricular Function and Regional Myocardial Perfusion

Improvements in global and regional myocardial perfusion and wall function brought about by the CABG operation result in improved exercise tolerance.[K3,K4] Direct information about myocardial perfusion and wall function, therefore, provide important objective information related to the effectiveness of the operation.

Preoperatively Normal Resting Left Ventricular Systolic Function
In patients with normal preoperative resting LV systolic function, including patients with mild dysfunction (EF ≥ 0.40), function usually remains essentially normal 5 years postoperatively. However, an interesting sequence of changes begins at operation. Roberts and colleagues have shown that, with current methods of myocardial protection and perioperative management, 2 hours after operation, left ventricular ejection fraction is reduced by about 10%. Within 24 hours of operation, it rises to the preoperative level, and 7 days after operation is usually higher than preoperatively.[R11] Rubenson and colleagues also have shown that segmental wall function may be better 6 weeks after the CABG operation than it is 1 week postoperatively.[R13]

More insight into the effect of CABG on left ventricular function in patients with preoperatively normal resting left ventricular function is obtained from studies during exercise or other forms of stress, such as rapid atrial pacing. The fall in ejection fraction with exercise that is characteristic of ischemic heart disease is gone 2 weeks after operation in most such patients, with the ejection fraction rising normally with exercise (Fig. 7-22).[H1,K2,N2] This favorable response to stress can be brought about only by the CABG operation[S32] (or percutaneous transluminal coronary dilation) and does not result from collateral circulation even when it is extensive.[S18] Furthermore, patients who continue to have angina after operation (presumably from an incomplete operation) do not have this response and continue to have a fall in ejection fraction with exercise;[N2] and when global and segmental function during exercise is not improved early (3 months) after operation, one or more vein grafts are usually found to be blocked or stenosed.[L18] Most patients with preoperatively abnormal increases in LV end-diastolic volume greater than 50% have normal increase with exercise 2 weeks after operation.[H1] Presumably, these favorable early

postoperative responses continue long-term after operation until there is progression of the native coronary arterial disease or graft closure.

Exercise-induced regional wall motion dysfunction, nearly always present preoperatively, even in the presence of normal left ventricular function at rest, disappears within 2 weeks of operation in most patients.[H1,M1]

Preoperatively Depressed Resting Left Ventricular Systolic Function
Several studies confirm that preoperatively depressed resting global left ventricular systolic function (estimated by ejection fraction or by d_p/d_t) is less depressed as early as 2 weeks after successful CABG.[B4,C3,C4,C5,H4] Improvement has also been demonstrated 6 months to several years after operation. Five years or more after operation, resting global left ventricular function maintains its improvement in some patients, but in some, it is again depressed and may be even worse than preoperatively.[T1] Those patients with worsened left ventricular function have a lower graft patency rate.[T1]

In patients with preoperatively depressed resting function, the response of the ejection fraction to exercise often becomes normal within 2 weeks of operation, and when it fails to do so, the revascularization usually is incomplete.[H1,H4] Thus, Hellman and colleagues have demonstrated that 16 of 19 post-CABG patients with preoperative resting ejection fractions < 0.40 showed similar or increased ejection fractions with exercise early postoperatively (± 2 weeks) and no deterioration of regional wall motion[H4] (Fig. 7-22b). Three of four patients with an abnormal response to exercise were shown by coronary arteriography to have incomplete revascularization.

When preoperative left ventricular function is moderately depressed (EF between 0.30 and 0.40), myocardial scarring can be expected to be present. The variable amount of viable muscle scattered through the scarred areas (except in the case of a true left ventricular aneurysm) can respond to increased blood flow, and if the muscle in the area of scarring is sufficient, regional myocardial perfusion and segmental wall can improve. This, plus the improvement in ischemic but nonscarred areas, accounts for the improved global function observed in many patients.

When preoperative left ventricular dysfunction is severe (EF < 0.30), the greater amount of myocardial scarring no doubt still further limits recovery of left ventricular function. Surprisingly, however, even in some of these patients, improvement in regional and global left ventricular function occurs with the CABG operation, and symptoms of pulmonary venous hypertension may regress. Hellman and colleagues found improvement in resting ejection fraction (0.29, 0.21, and 0.28) in all three patients with ejection fractions < 0.25 preoperatively, and all three showed an increased ejection fraction with exercise postoperatively.

Regional Wall Segment Abnormalities
Left ventricular wall segments that *preoperatively exhibit normal contraction at rest* usually (95% of the time, according to Zir and colleagues[Z2]) have normal contraction 1–2 years after operation.[W6] Left ventricular wall segments that are hypokinetic, akinetic, or even *dyskinetic at rest preoper-*

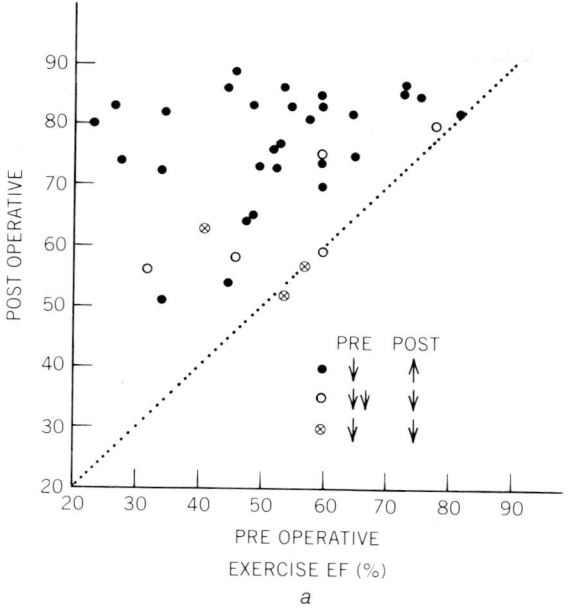

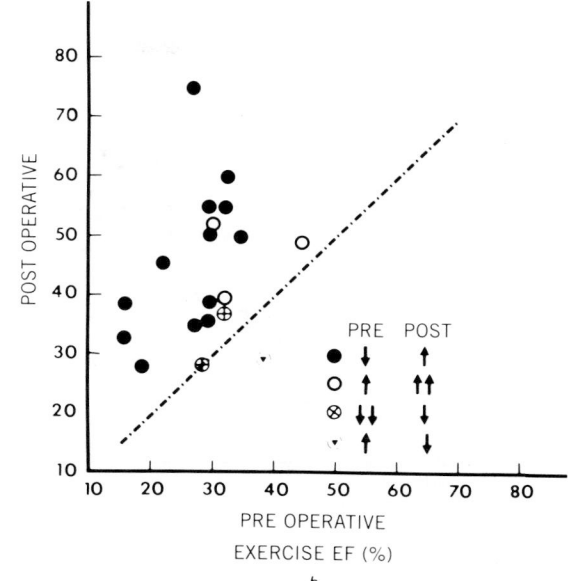

Figure 7-22

(a) A comparison of postoperative exercise ejection fraction (vertical axis) to preoperative exercise EF in patients with coronary artery disease and preoperatively normal or mildly depressed global LV function. Closed circles represent patients with a decrease in EF preoperatively and an increase postoperatively. Open circles represent those with a marked decrease in EF preoperatively and a continued but minor decrease postoperatively. Crossed circles represent those with a minor decrease both preoperatively and postoperatively.

(b) A comparison of postoperative exercise ejection fraction to preoperative exercise EF in patients with coronary artery disease, and preoperatively poor LV function. Closed circles represent patients with a decrease in EF preoperatively and an increase postoperatively. Open circles represent patients with a slight increase preoperatively and a more marked increase postoperatively. Crossed circles represent those with a marked decrease preoperatively and a minor decrease postoperatively. The circle with a triangle represents one patient with an increase in EF preoperatively and a decrease postoperatively.

Reproduced with permission from Hellman et al.[H1]

atively often function better after CABG.[C4,C21,W6] Zir and colleagues found improvement 1–2 years postoperatively in 25% of their patients, operated on in an earlier era.[Z2] It is interesting that some of the segments that improved were in an area of perioperative infarction. Improvement in segmental wall motion 12 months after CABG operation has also been observed even in areas of scarring from previous myocardial infarction.[M18] Brundage and colleagues showed that 19 of 29 left ventricular wall segments with reversible asynergy preoperatively at rest had improved and often normal function late postoperatively.[B51] All of these segments had improved perfusion during exercise after surgery and were supplied by a patent bypass graft. Nine of the 10 segments in which abnormal wall motion persisted postoperatively continued to have exercise-induced perfusion deficits. This finding supports the idea that viable muscle cells are scattered through hypokinetic and at times even akinetic and dyskinetic segments and that wall motion in such segments can be improved by the CABG operation. When wall segment contraction does not occur after the CABG operation, incomplete revascularization is the cause in some patients.[C21]

Improvement in regional myocardial perfusion after the CABG operation is associated with improved segmental wall motion.[K3] Even resting regional perfusion defects (at least in patients with unstable angina) have improved after the CABG operation in 65% of patients.[K3] The preoperative resting perfusion defects must have been due only to ischemia; or the scarred areas contained considerable amounts of muscle that were revascularized. Most of the patients without improvement had occluded grafts to the area. Also, Wainwright and colleagues have shown that when the CABG operation is incomplete (specifically, when a stenotic first diagonal branch of the LAD artery is not grafted), regional myocardial perfusion defects usually persist in the area supplied by the ungrafted vessel.[W4]

Significantly, improvement in regional perfusion and segmental wall motion, as well as a significant increase in global ejection fraction at rest, has been demonstrated after CABG in regions of apparent old infarction.[K3] This finding, in combination with those of other studies,[C2,Z1] again supports the idea that such areas contain some viable muscle and that improved perfusion by CABG can result in improved function.

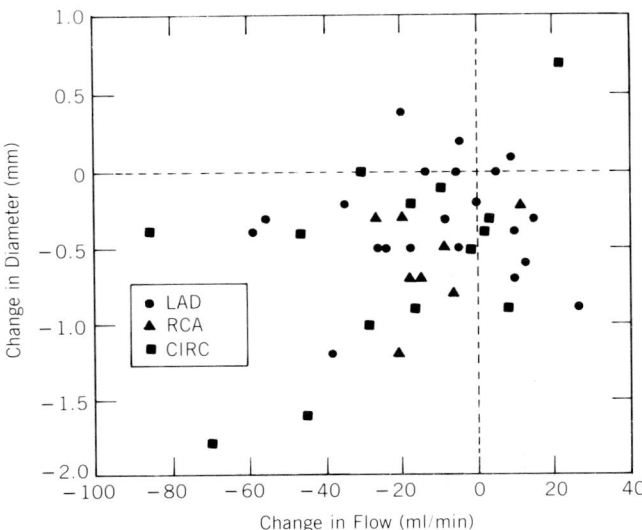

Figure 7-23 Relationship between change in saphenous vein bypass graft flow and change in diameter between early (2 weeks) and late (average 1.5 years) postoperative study by roentgenographic methods. In general, a decrease in diameter correlates with a decrease in flow.

CIRC, circumflex coronary artery; LAD, left anterior descending coronary artery; RCA, right coronary artery.

Reproduced with permission from Weisz et al.[W1]

Vein Graft Function

That a patent vein graft serves as a conduit for coronary blood flow to the myocardium cannot be doubted. Many intraoperative measurements have been made of flow through coronary artery bypass grafts, but the relationship of these flows to those existing postoperatively is uncertain. Not unexpectedly, in the few studies done late postoperatively, flow is largest in vein grafts to the LAD artery system. Thus, Hamby and colleagues, using a roentgen densiometric method, found at 2 weeks after operation a mean flow of 79 ml · min^{-1} in grafts to the LAD artery (range 39–179), and of 65 and 68 ml · min^{-1} in those to the RCA and Cx artery, respectively.[H2] The flow through the graft in the early postoperative period is not related to graft size, measured by cineangiographic techniques, and is presumably determined primarily by the size of the arterial bed distal to the anastomosis.[W1] An average of 2.5 years later, some vein grafts (35% of the total) showed an important (average, 45%) reduction in flow, compared with the early postoperative study. Thirty-five percent showed only a mild decrease during this period, and 30% showed no change. Such reductions of flow probably result in part from the morphologic changes in the graft; thus, Weisz and colleagues found the change in graft flow to be associated with a similar directional change in graft caliber (Fig. 7-23).[W1] However, at this time, the diameter of the vein graft usually still remains larger than that of the artery to which it is anastomosed.[W1]

The coronary flow reserve (ability to increase flow in response to increased myocardial oxygen demand or pharmacologic vasodilation) is improved by CABG over that of

stenotic coronary arteries, but is not normal. This has previously been determined from measurements made in the operating room after the CABG procedure.[B53,G25,S43] It has recently been confirmed in postoperative patients by Bates and colleagues, who found, however, some overlap between the values in postoperative patients and those in normal individuals.[B52] The ability to increase coronary flow is absent when there is a stenotic coronary lesion beyond the graft.

In general, a patent anastomosis between a vein graft and a coronary artery perfuses that segment of myocardium to which the native artery has supplied blood.[K4] However, about 25% of anastomoses distribute blood well beyond the segment of myocardium that would have been expected to be supplied by the native vessel.[M4] In about two-thirds of such situations, the area unexpectedly perfused by the anastomosis is in the distribution of an occluded native vessel to which there was a nonobstructed graft. Significantly, segmental contractility was often improved postoperatively in the unexpectedly perfused area, even when its own native vessel and graft were occluded. These kinds of phenomena probably explain the rather frequent finding of a functionally excellent result in spite of the presence of one or two occluded anastomoses.

Vein Graft Structure and Patency

Intimal Hyperplasia
Diffuse intimal thickening, so-called intimal hyperplasia, is a universal finding in vein grafts that have been in place for more than 1 month.[B7,B19,M5,S30,V3] The data indicate that this process is not a progressive one.[S30] The thickness of the intimal hyperplasia seems to be inversely related to the flow in the graft, and the process appears to result in a matching of vein lumen size to that of the coronary arteries supplied by the graft. Intimal hyperplasia is thus best considered as a remodeling process.[S30,V3] The adventitia thickens rather quickly, but this usually does not produce luminal narrowing. Hyperplasia of smooth muscle cells and some fibrosis occur in the media.[B8,K6,U1,V3]

As a result of these changes, most grafts show an angiographically detectable diffuse reduction in caliber so that by 1 year after implantation they tend to approximate the diameter of the size of the recipient coronary artery. This diffuse and even narrowing is not related to occlusion rates.[S30] By increasing the velocity of flow, it may be beneficial, particularly when the vein is large initially.[B36,S29]

Although these phenomena described as occurring within the graft are universal, only about 30% of grafts patent 1 year after operation have intimal hyperplasia sufficiently gross to be demonstrable by cineangiography.[G4,P3] The incidence rises to 45% by 5 years.[G4] Absence of cineangiographically evident intimal hyperplasia at 1 year is a good prognostic sign, for only about 10% of such grafts have evident intimal hyperplasia 5 years postoperatively.

Early Events
The highest rate of anastomotic closure occurs during the first few postoperative weeks, with 80%–95% of vein graft anastomoses patent at that time. Those that have closed have usually done so because of anastomotic thrombosis or

Table 7-10 Association of late (1-year) graft patency after CABG operation with a regimen of preoperative and postoperative dipyridamole and aspirin (compared with administration of a placebo) and with coronary artery size.

Coronary Artery Internal Diameter (mm)		DIP and ASA				Placebo				P for difference
			Anastomosis Patent				Anastomosis Patent			
≤	<	n	No.	%	CL	n	No.	%	CL	
	1	9	6	67%	44%–85%	15	6	40%	25%–57%	.21
1	---1.5	128	120	94%	91%–96%	113	80	71%	66%–75%	< .0001
1.5	---2.0	98	90	92%	88%–95%	38	20	53%	43%–62%	< .0001
2.0		15	14	93%	79%–99%	19	18	95%	83%–99%	0.9
$P (\chi^2)$				.04				.001		

SOURCE: Modified from Chesebro JH and colleagues.[C18]

KEY: ASA, aspirin; CL, 70% confidence limits; DIP, dipyridamole.

technical problems at the *distal* anastomosis.[B5,L10] Technical problems include luminal constrictions at the anastomosis and are more common in anastomoses to small arteries. Such technical problems should now be rare. Anastomotic thrombosis is more common[B18] and can result from a thrombotic tendency within the graft or from limited distal runoff. Uncommonly, a dissecting hematoma may develop at the anastomotic site,[B5] narrowing the coronary artery and predisposing the patient to early anastomotic closure or thrombosis. It is in part because of this possibility that great care must be taken at operation when opening the coronary artery, lest the back wall inadvertently be incised and the stage set for arterial dissection. A thrombotic tendency in the graft may result from morphologic changes in the vein graft, particularly if the graft is removed and prepared in a suboptimal manner.[G10] Endothelial cell loss and exposure of the basement membrane and collagen appear promptly after some methods of graft preparation and predispose the graft to the early accumulation of platelets, fibrin, and thrombus.[B7,B19,F5,J5,R9] In view of these phenomena, it is not surprising that platelet regeneration (and thus survival) times are significantly shorter in patients with occluded grafts than in normal persons or patients with patent grafts.[L4]

Recent studies indicate the possibility of minimizing early graft closure by better vein graft preservation during removal and storage of the graft (as brief as this period is) before insertion and by pharmacologic interventions designed to minimize platelet aggregation and deposition on the vein intima intra- and postoperatively. As indicated earlier, LoGerfo's studies demonstrate the possibility that vein damage can be minimized, and presumably late patency rates increased, by preventing spasm during removal and storage by the use of papaverine and by preserving intima and media by keeping the vein graft cold and somewhat distended with a tissue-culture medium or blood until insertion.[L15] Following a successful experimental study,[J11] Chesebro and colleagues, in a randomized study in patients, found a beneficial effect from a regimen of antiplatelet drugs begun preoperatively.[C16] Dipyridamole was instituted 2 days before operation and aspirin 7 hours after operation, and both were continued late postoperatively. Within one month of operation, only 8% of treated patients showed graft occlusion, compared to 21% of patients in the placebo group ($P = .003$), while at 6 months the occlusion rates reached 10% and 38%,

respectively ($P = .000001$). As the postoperative interval increased further, the graft occlusion rate in the placebo group increased, but it remained the same in the treatment group, and the results continued to be significantly different at 1 year[C18,C33] (Table 7-10). The failure of other studies to show a beneficial result may be in part because, in them, the treatment was not begun until after operation.[P2]

Late Events

With time, the intima in some areas of the graft develop plaques that are morphologically indistinguishable from the fibrous plaques of arteriosclerosis.[B7,B8,B9,G3] Graft flow is thereby reduced, and graft failure probably ultimately results in many patients. Smith and Gear found frank atherosclerotic lesions only in grafts that had been in place for more than 3.5 years.[S30] However, after 10 years most vein grafts have undergone at least some arteriosclerotic changes, Campeau and colleagues finding this to be the case in 82 (62%, CL 57%–67%) of 132 grafts patent one year postoperatively.[C35]

Late anastomotic and graft closures occur at a rate of about 0.4%–3% of grafts per year.[H2,K5] Guthaner and colleagues found that 34 (87%, CL 79%–93%) of 39 grafts patent at one year were still patent 5 or more years later.[G4] Loop and associates report that 87% of grafts patent at an initial catheterization about 1 year after surgery were still open 4½ years after CABG.[L3] The commonest cause of late closure seems to be accelerated atherosclerosis within the vein graft itself.[B7,C7] Campeau and colleagues found the cumulative graft patency rate at 10 years to be 45%.[C28]

Anastomotic strictures appear to be the morphologic explanation for some late graft closures, but whether as an isolated process or as a localized manifestation of arteriosclerosis is not certain. Proximal graft stenosis existed in about 20% of grafts studied at 1 year by Guthaner and colleagues;[G4] more than half of these grafts did not change by 5 years after operation, but 25% of the veins with proximal stenoses were occluded 5 years postoperatively. Distal stenoses of some degree were present in about 50% of patients studied 1 year after operation. These remained unchanged over the next 5 years in most instances.[G4] However, new stenosis developed in about 10% of patients without stenoses in the distal suture line 1 year after operation.[G4] The type of anastomosis must determine whether adverse local rheological factors are present to accelerate the development of atheroma. Unfortunately, there is no information as to the influence of the type of anastomosis (oblique end to side, T shaped end to side, parallel or transverse side to side) on the incidence of local atherosclerosis and late stricture.

Incremental Risk Factors for Graft Closure

Whatever the basic process leading to early or late graft closure, the incremental risk factors associated with these events have been only partially clarified.[P5,R8] It is not even certain whether local factors or general systemic factors are primarily involved.[P5,R8]

One local factor documented as a risk for anastomotic or graft closure, even in the current era, is *small size of the coronary artery*[C18,S26] (Table 7-10). The incremental nature of risk factors is evident in the data of Chesebro and colleagues.[C18] With the dipyridamole-aspirin program, only a diameter of 1 mm or less was a risk factor; without these agents, increments of risk for graft closure occurred also with those less than 2.0 mm in diameter. However, anastomoses to vessels as small as 1 mm have patency rates generally at or above 50% at 1 year.

In any event, the use of sequential grafting, rather than only 1 distal anastomosis on each vein segment, has *not* increased the incidence of anastomotic or graft closure.[B43] In fact, there is some evidence that patency rates are increased, especially in anastomoses to small arteries.[B16] Meurala and colleagues found 85% of anastomoses open 2 years after operation in vein segments with a single distal anastomosis, and 97% (CL 92%–99%) in those with multiple distal anastomoses (P for difference = .04).[M17] This may be related to the greater flow through the proximal portion of vein segments that have multiple rather than one, distal anastomoses to the lesser tendency toward intimal hyperplasia of vein segments with large flow velocity.[F11]

Progression of Native Coronary Artery Disease after the CABG Operation

Arteriosclerosis has a tendency to progress with time. The effect of the CABG operation, both on grafted and ungrafted arteries, has not been fully described, but some trends are evident. The known tendency of the cineangiogram to underestimate the extent and severity of the coronary artery disease invokes caution in interpreting these data.

Important Stenoses

Fifty percent to 95% of important coronary artery stenoses proximal to a vein graft become more severe or totally obstructive within 5 years of the CABG operation.[B6,G4,L2] Important stenoses distal to the anastomosis have a strong tendency to obstruct within 5 years[G4,N1] (but grafts should have been placed *beyond* such lesions). Important stenoses in ungrafted vessels also progress after operation, presumably at about the same rate as in the natural history of coronary artery disease (see "Progression of Stenotic Coronary Artery Disease").

Controversy continues as to whether in fact important stenoses progress more rapidly in grafted than in ungrafted vessels. Some data suggest that the former is in fact the case.[E11,N1] Other information suggests that progress is at the same rate in both,[B6,G4] and Palac and colleagues provide data that support this idea. They found a 36% incidence of significant progression over a 5-year period of stenoses in grafted arteries and the same incidence in the ungrafted arteries of patients who had been randomized to medical treatment.[P5]

Lesser Stenoses

The incidence and rate of progression of lesser stenoses proximal to a vein graft remains uncertain. Lesser stenoses distal to a functioning vein graft tend to remain unchanged.[G4,I1] However, one study reported considerable progression of distal arterial stenoses when the vein graft to the artery was nonfunctioning.[N1]

Lesser stenoses in ungrafted arteries progress in severity with less frequency than do important stenoses, but 25%–50% of such lesions progress within 5 years.[G4,L2] Thus, in a group of patients undergoing the CABG operation, Laks and colleagues found progression of the proximal stenosis in 16 (27%, CL 20%–34%) of 60 nonbypassed RCAs with less than 50% narrowings in a mean follow-up period of 20 months.[L2] Two (3%, CL 1%–8%) of the 60 had progressed to complete obstruction.

New Stenoses

New stenoses do appear in apparently nonstenotic arteries that were not grafted.[B6,H2] Palac and colleagues, in following patients randomized to surgical versus medical treatment, found new lesions within 5 years in about 15% of both groups.[P5]

Ventricular Arrhythmias

Successful coronary artery bypass grafting, with relief of myocardial ischemia and its symptoms, generally does not decrease the frequency or severity of exercise-induced or resting ventricular arrhythmias,[D1,G1,L1] including ventricular tachycardia and fibrillation, although reports to the contrary are in the literature.[B1,C1,E1,R1] This lack of a favorable effect is related to the fact that in most patients with serious ventricular arrhythmias, ventricular scars, rather than exercise-induced myocardial ischemia, are the origin of the arrhythmias (see detailed discussion in Chapter 48).

The failure of simple CABG operations to abolish serious ventricular electrical instability is particularly unfortunate, since exercise-induced ventricular tachycardia or ventricular fibrillation carries a poor prognosis in patients with coronary artery disease,[L1] and sudden death is a common mode of death late after the CABG operation. Therefore, when operation is contemplated in patients with these arrhythmias, consideration should be given to surgical procedures directed specifically at the ventricular arrhythmia, even in the absence of LV aneurysm (see Chapter 48).

Exceptions to these general statements are the few patients without ventricular scars or aneurysm in whom life-threatening ventricular arrhythmias occur purely on the

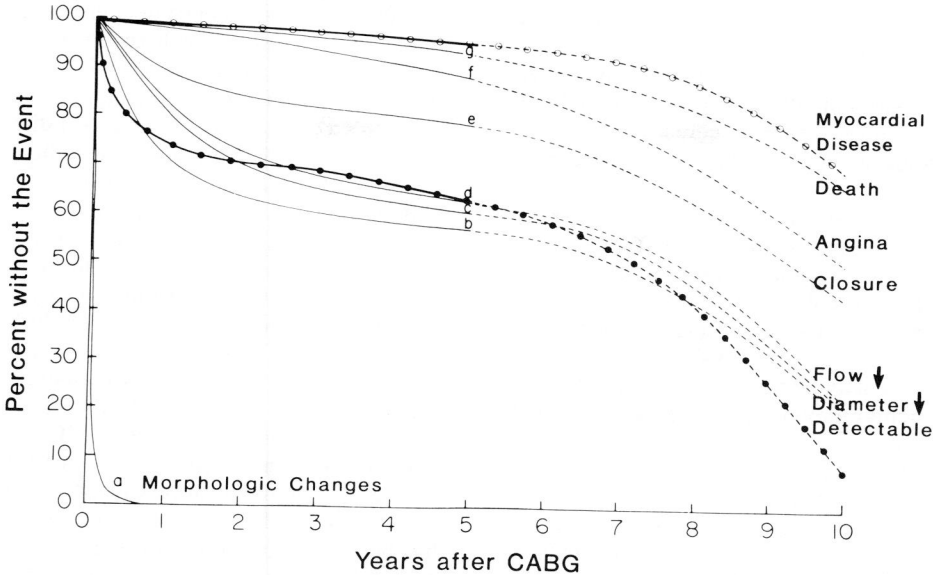

Figure 7-24 A composite, nonrigorous presentation of time-related events in patients undergoing the CABG operation with complete revascularization of extensive triple-vessel coronary artery disease, assuming no reoperations were done. The graph is based on currently available information. The dashed sections of the curves represent extrapolations for the most part. *Percent without the event* refers to patients in the case of return of angina pectoris and death and to individual anastomoses or vein grafts in the case of cineangiographically visible morphologic vein graft changes, reduction in vein graft diameter, reduction in vein graft flow, and individual vein graft (anastomosis) closure. The progression of myocardial disease is presumed to occur primarily in patients with preoperatively moderate or severe LV dysfunction and would be expected to increase the death rate only in such patients. Likewise, important new proximal disease can occur only in ungrafted vessels and thus only in patients with less than extensive triple-vessel disease preoperatively. (*a*) Morphologic vein graft changes (intimal hyperplasia). (*b*) Cineradiographically visible morphologic vein graft changes. (*c*) Reduction in vein graft diameter. (*d*) Important reduction in vein graft flow. (*e*) Individual vein graft (anastomosis) closure (the early decline in patency is primarily from thrombotic occlusion; that after 5 years is primarily from accelerated atherosclerosis). (*f*) Return of angina pectoris. (*g*) Death.

o–o–o, progressive myocardial disease, applicable only to patients with preoperatively moderate or severe left ventricular dysfunction; ●–●–●, important new proximal disease, applicable only to patients with less than extensive triple-vessel disease at the time of operation and not to patients described by the other lines.

basis of reversible left ventricular myocardial ischemia. In them, CABG can relieve the arrhythmic tendency.

Time-Related Postoperative Events

The postoperative, time-related phenomena are interrelated, but only a tentative general representation of them can be made at this time (Fig. 7-24).

When complete revascularization is performed for extensive triple-vessel coronary artery disease with or without left main coronary artery disease and most of the left ventricular wall is still composed by viable muscle, in the early weeks after operation the myocardium is presumably completely perfused, myocardial blood flow reserve is probably present, and global and regional myocardial response to stress is normal. However, about 5%–15% of graft anastomoses close in these first few weeks after operation as the result of a thrombotic process. Angina pectoris can be expected to be absent at rest or with exercise, and maximal exercise capacity

should be near normal. Medication should be unnecessary. The saphenous vein graft has begun to undergo a remodeling process in its new environment. After about 1 year, this progress is evident cineradiographically in about 30% of grafts. Five years after the operation, about 15% more of the graft anastomoses are closed as a result of various processes. By 5 years after the operation, angina pectoris will have returned in about 10%–20% of the patients, and 5%–10% of them will have died. At 10 years, none of the grafts and graft anastomoses will have closed, largely as the result of an accelerated arteriosclerotic process. A return of angina pectoris can probably be expected in about 50% of patients initially surviving CABG, and death in about 30%. There is a vague suggestion, under present circumstances, that death follows the return of angina pectoris by about 3–5 years, unless a new intervention is undertaken.

When the operation has been done for double-vessel or single-vessel disease, the consequences of graft narrowing or closure are less global, and new stenoses or progression in the severity of minor stenoses becomes an additional variable affecting the postoperative course. About 25% of patients can be expected to develop these new complications within 3 years of the operation, 30% at 5 years, and perhaps 75% at 10 years. If left untreated, these new lesions interact with developing graft lesions to affect the late postoperative course.

When left ventricular dysfunction is moderately or severely impaired preoperatively because of ventricular scarring, the experience with valvar heart disease suggests the possibility that the left ventricular dysfunction may progress postoperatively, even in the absence of further ischemic injury. The time course of this is slow in valvar heart disease, and probably also in ischemic heart disease, and thus the progression in dysfunction may have little effect until 5–10 years postoperatively.

Much of this natural history after the initial CABG operation can be modified by a CABG reoperation. In patients in whom distal vessels are still available for grafting—and this is usually the case—and left ventricular function is reasonably well preserved, the time-related course illustrated in Figure 7-24 may be set back to zero time.

INDICATIONS FOR OPERATION

Chronic Stable Angina

CABG is indicated for relief of chronic stable angina that is not relieved by the use of β-blocking drugs, calcium antagonists, and long-acting nitrates, and when it is interfering with the patient's life-style. Such a patient is advised to undergo coronary angiography with a view to operation. When chronic stable angina is relieved by drugs, no invasive study or treatment is advised (GLH). Alternatively, before committing patients with chronic stable angina to a continuing program of noninvasive treatment, exercise testing, and if the results are positive, arteriography may be advised (UAB). A positive exercise test with ST segment depression > 2 mm, combined in some patients with hypotension almost always indicates severe left main or triple-vessel coronary artery disease and is considered an indication for particularly prompt cineangiography.

A tight (> 75%) left main arterial stenosis or tight proximal stenosis of all three major branches is an indication for very urgent operation. Should extensive triple-vessel disease with important proximal LAD stenoses or left main coronary artery disease with 50% or greater narrowing be present, CABG is advised. If triple-vessel disease without important proximal LAD stenosis is present and left ventricular function is good (EF ≥ 0.50), initial assignment to medical therapy with periodic reevaluation is generally advisable (see "Comparisons of Survival after Surgical versus Medical Treatment"). When, with this pathologic condition, left ventricular function is impaired, initial treatment with CABG is indicated. Severe impairment of left ventricular function does not contraindicate the operation. Should significant single- or double-vessel disease be demonstrated, intensification of medical treatment or percutaneous transluminal coronary angioplasty (PTCA) is generally advised initially. The effectiveness of the latter procedure in obtaining early and intermediate-term (1–2 years) improvement in many

(± 50%) patients has been demonstrated.[K19] An exception is double-vessel disease with severe proximal LAD stenosis, which is an indication for operation. Should left ventricular function be impaired, an indication for CABG is generally considered present in double-vessel disease.

In all current discussions of the indications for CABG, the potential of PTCA must be considered. Currently, PTCA, in expert hands and in properly selected cases, is initially successful in about 85% of the patients.[J14] Intermediate-term failures (within 1–2 years) do occur, probably in at least 10% of the patients and perhaps in as many as 40%.[J16] The more limited the disease, the greater should be the consideration given to PTCA in preference to CABG. However, PTCA may prove to be satisfactory treatment in at least some subsets of patients with multiple-vessel disease. Hartzler and colleagues report that 69 (86%, CL 81%–90%) of 80 such patients were improved after PTCA,[H16] and Dorros and colleagues report initial success in 74%.[D9] However, in patients with multivessel disease, the mortality from the procedure has been 3.2% in the CASS Registry experience, compared with 1.5% with single-vessel disease.[M25] Currently, reliable comparisons between the results of the CABG operation and PTCA cannot be made and, as Mock and colleagues have stated, such a comparison may not be possible for a considerable period of time unless an appropriate randomized trial is conducted.[M27]

Unstable Angina

Unstable angina (crescendo angina, or the intermediate coronary syndrome) can be considered an indication for the CABG operation on a semiurgent basis when full medical treatment (bed rest, effective β-blockade, one or two vasodilators, and calcium channel blocker therapy) fails to prevent recurrent rest pain over a period of about 7 days. Cineangiography is performed, and operation is undertaken promptly, provided the sequence persists. A modest rise in serum enzymes (CPK) during this period is not a contraindication to operation, although ECG changes of full-thickness infarction may be considered a contraindication (GLH). Alternatively, the development of infarction may be considered an indication for emergency operation (UAB).

This is a controversial area, as the hospital mortality and early infarction rates among patients hospitalized for unstable angina in the past have been similar (about 2% and 10%, respectively) with medical and surgical treatment.[R3,B44] With the excellent results now being obtained by CABG operations in unstable angina,[J13] and even in patients with frank acute myocardial infarction, there is an increasing tendency to proceed with operation in the conditions described above.

PTCA is an alternative to CABG for unstable angina, but it may be less effective than in patients with chronic stable angina.[D7]

Acute Myocardial Infarction

The presence of acute myocardial infarction has not generally been an indication for urgent CABG. However, invasive treatments (e.g., administration of thrombolytic agents) and CABG operation are advised in patients at high risk of dying

Table 7-11 CABG operations within 1 month of acute myocardial infarction in patients without acute ventricular rupture or mitral incompetence (UAB; 1981–1983).

Interval Since Acute Infarction (days)			Hospital Deaths		
≤ <	n	No.	%	CL	
1	21[a]	1	5%	0.6%–15%	
1--- 2	1	1	0%	0%–85%	
2--- 7	11	0	0%	0%–16%	
7---30	28	3	11%	5%–20%	
Uncertain	16	1	6%	0.8%–20%	
Total	77	5	6%	4%–11%	
$P(x^2)$			0.7		

KEY: CL, confidence limits.

[a] Three were within 6 hours of infarction.

with their acute infarction and in those in whom recovery from the acute event is complicated. This is because of reports in which operation done within 4–8 hours of the onset of pain has been associated with a lowering of mortality and lessened impairment of left ventricular structure and function.[B28,B30,J7] The early results of operative intervention have been encouraging (Table 7-11), but a final evaluation of these programs awaits further information about early and late results, particularly as to preservation of left ventricular structure and function (see "CABG for Acute Myocardial Infarction").

Severe Ventricular Electrical Instability

Important ventricular arrhythmias late after myocardial infarction, even without LV aneurysm, are an indication for operation. The operation must include a procedure directed against the electrical instability (see Chapter 48, section 4 on "Ventricular Tachycardia in Ischemic Heart Disease"). Because of the prognostic importance of a positive electrophysiologic programmed stimulation test, particularly after acute myocardial infarction (see "Dysfunction from Myocardial Scarring"), this predictor of death from ventricular electrical instability may per se become an indication for operation.

Summary

All decisions for or against operation must be made concerning an individual patient after considering his or her special situation and the manner in which it may affect the decision. The evaluation of any incremental risk factors for a poor early or late result is an important part of these considerations.

The coronary artery disease is *rarely if ever too extensive* or diffuse to allow the CABG operation when the technique used allows multiple anastomoses to very distal vessels if use of the central arteries is denied. The angiographic prediction of diffuse nongraftable coronary artery disease or severe distal arterial disease rendering the arteries nonbypassable has been shown to be completely unreliable.[L25] Left ventricular dysfunction adds to the case for surgery, unless it is so severe that elevated right atrial pressures ≥ 15 mmHg,

hepatomegaly, and fluid retention are present (a rare occurrence). Old age is a relatively mild contraindication to the CABG operation. Operation is advised for individuals in their seventies and eighties if their general health is good and if the indications are persuasive. The presence of other important arteriosclerotic lesions is not a contraindication, but special problems may exist in patients with such lesions.

Operation is not indicated in patients with coronary artery spasm as the only abnormality. It may be indicated rarely when there is severe muscle bridging of the LAD artery associated with classic effort angina and positive results of an exercise test, including evidence of ischemia in the area of LAD artery distribution in an exercise thallium study (GLH).

SPECIAL SITUATIONS AND CONTROVERSIES

The Internal Mammary Artery for the CABG Operation

Although the internal mammary artery was used for coronary artery bypass grafting very early in the development of coronary artery surgery,[E3,G7] most surgeons have not seriously considered its use until recent years. In part this has been because of the rather tedious dissection required for mobilizing the IMA pedicle. In part it has been because of uncertainty as to the flow capabilities of the IMA as a graft. In part it has been because the early results of saphenous vein bypass grafts have been favorable. Recently, however, there has been clear demonstration, not only of the better patency rates of the IMA compared with the saphenous vein conduits, but also better survival when the IMA is used as the conduit to the LAD artery.[G28,L27,O4]

The internal mammary artery, used as a pedicle graft, is the only satisfactory alternative to autogenous saphenous vein for the CABG operation. Arm veins have proved to be relatively unsatisfactory.[S44] Other conduits, such as excised segments of radial or splenic arteries, homologous saphenous and umbilical veins, and Gore-Tex (polytetrafluoroethylene) tubes are unsuitable because of low patency rates.

A pedicled IMA graft has higher early and late patency rates than does a saphenous vein graft.[B48,S41] Thus, the Cleveland Clinic reported 54 (93%, CL 85%–96%) of 58 IMA grafts to the LAD artery patent about 3 years after operation,[L3] a higher rate than for isolated saphenous vein grafts to the LAD artery.[L8] The CASS report also shows a higher patency rate for IMA grafts (96%) than for vein anastomoses (87%–91%).[N5] This is partly because the artery does not change histologically or progressively narrow from intimal hyperplasia. Also, atherosclerosis is uncommon in the IMA, both in situ and up to 10 years after being placed as a conduit to the LAD artery. Grondin and colleagues found atheromatous changes in only one (5%, CL .7%–17%) of patent IMA grafts in place for 10 years.[G28]

As has already been discussed (see "Non-Use of the Internal Mammary Artery" in section on Late Results), survival is better when the IMA is used to the LAD artery than when vein grafts are used. Also, Lytle and colleagues have found remarkable 7-year and 9-year survival rates of 97% and 90% respectively in a small group of patients in whom only bilateral internal mammary artery grafting was performed.[L26]

These results were obtained even though revascularization was probably incomplete in many of the patients.

There are disadvantages to the use of the IMA. The incidence of reentry for postoperative bleeding (about 12%) is probably higher than that after the use of saphenous vein grafts.[L26] There is also a suggestion that sternal healing may be impaired when both are mobilized, and that when just one IMA is used and mediastinitis occurs treatment must include the use of muscle pedicle flaps.[N7]

Currently, as discussed in "Technique of Operation," the IMA graft is used whenever a stenotic lesion in the LAD artery requires bypass grafting (GLH and UAB). Thus, it is used currently in nearly all CABG operations. It is not used when the IMA is small or atherosclerotic, when there is extensive arteriosclerosis in the brachiocephalic vessels, or when the operation is done in a patient in cardiogenic shock.

Currently in some cardiac surgical centers, the IMA is used for sequential as well as individual grafting.[K22,T10,T11] Bilateral internal mammary grafting is also employed by several groups.[T10,L26] The role of these more extensive uses of the IMA has not yet been clearly defined.

Important Coronary Artery Disease

Generally, a reduction of diameter of about 50% (equivalent to a 75% reduction in cross-sectional area) is considered an important (critical) coronary artery stenosis, that is, one associated with a functionally significant reduction in blood flow and diminished myocardial perfusion.[G13,M8,S21] The matter remains controversial, however, as evidenced by the selection of a *70%* diameter narrowing as critical by CASS study of the NHLBI. Such matters are important in comparing the results of treatment by different methods or institutions.[H8,W7]

Assessment of importance is further complicated by the possibility that the numerical value may be different for different arteries. Recent studies at UAB by Rafflenbeul, Urthaler, Lichtlen, and James indicate that, while a 50% reduction in diameter does seem critical for the LAD artery, in the right coronary artery a 40% reduction in diameter (about 60% reduction in cross-sectional area) is associated with sufficient reductions of blood flow to cause angina, segmental wall motion abnormalities, and the development of collateral arteries.[R12]

Determining importance is further complicated when a coronary artery stenosis has considerable length, as well as when there are multiple lesions in series.[F8,K15] This matter is addressed in the GLH myocardial scoring system (Appendix 7B).

Management of Less Than 50% Narrowings in Patients Already Committed to Operation

Occasionally, when on the basis of the number and distributions of severe stenoses a patient is advised to undergo CABG, a major vessel or branch with a narrowing that is less than critical may also be bypassed (UAB). This policy is adopted because the degree of narrowing may be underestimated by cineangiography[W8] and because such lesions tend to progress in severity (see "Progression of Native Coronary Artery Disease after the CABG Operation" in section on Late Results). Alternatively, such vessels may not be bypassed, because about 75% of such stenoses do not show progression within a few years (GLH). Moreover, it may be felt that the progression in vessels with less than 50% stenosis is greater in *grafted* vessels than in those not grafted[C23] and that development and progression of stenosis in a vein graft may be more frequent and rapid than in a stenosis in the host artery (GLH).

If subcritical stenoses are bypassed, there is concern that, when the first side-to-side anastomosis of a sequential vein graft is to a large artery with a stenosis less than 50%, the flow may go from proximal artery to distal graft (rather than from proximal aortic anastomosis to artery), which may predispose that segment of graft to closure between the aorta and the first of the sequential anastomoses. The UAB experience has given some anecdotal support to this idea, and the demonstration of continued myocardial perfusion by the native coronary artery in spite of a patent graft distal to the stenosis[K3] also is compatible with this concern. The experimental studies of Furuse and colleagues[F1] and Kakos and colleagues[K1] did, however, show that flow from vein graft *to* an unobstructed coronary artery was 75%–90% of the total flow in the distal coronary artery. One option in such circumstances may be to commit a separate vein graft to the less than critically narrowed bypassed artery, so that only this one anastomosis could be lost from competitive flow (UAB).

The First Septal Branch of the Left Anterior Descending Artery

Occasionally a large first septal artery has an important orifice stenosis or originates from a stenosed segment of the LAD artery. Direct bypass grafting to such a septal artery has been successfully accomplished by some surgeons.[B25,M3,S20] This is theoretically desirable, since a large septal artery may be responsible for 15% of the myocardial blood flow.[J6] In a small series of 13 patients, Bedard reported 86% patency of the graft to the septal artery at about 6 months.[B25] An indirect technique has also been used, combining endarterectomy of the septal artery and adjacent LAD artery and bypass grafting to this area of the LAD artery,[B25,P1] but Bedard reported that only 40% of 15 patients had good flow into the septal artery after this procedure.

The procedure is difficult to perform, partly because of the proximal position of the artery and the fat surrounding it and also because massive bleeding that is difficult to control can occur from the right ventricular cavity during its dissection.[M3] This procedure continues to be controversial, but it may be practiced when indicated (UAB).

Proximal Anastomosis First versus Distal Anastomosis First

There is no necessarily correct order of performance of the proximal and distal anastomoses. When the proximal anastomosis is performed first, CPB time can be shortened by doing these anastomoses before cannulation and CPB but with the patient heparinized. After the side-biting clamp is removed, the vein grafts are distended by arterial blood pressure, making the estimation of the proper length of the vein graft to the first distal anastomosis quite reliable. Performing the proximal anastomoses first allows easy distention of the vein graft, by briefly infusing cold cardioplegic solution into the aortic root and through the proximal anastomosis into the graft, between the making of each sequential anastomosis. This maneuver also has the advantage of delivering the cold cardioplegic solution to previously ischemic areas. Also, when the aortic cross-clamp is finally removed after the ischemic period required for the distal anastomosis, the myocardium is immediately fully reperfused.

A disadvantage to performing the proximal anastomoses first is that the lie of the proximal portion of the vein is established *before* the surgeon examines the entire surface of the heart and determines the exact positions, sizes, and accessibility of those coronary arteries with significant stenoses. However, in practice, the proximal anastomoses, once made, allow considerable flexibility in the routing of the vein. For example, when the vein segment originally destined to go to the right of the right atrium and back of the heart is chosen to go instead to the circumflex artery only, it can be rerouted through the transverse sinus to the circumflex artery. Another disadvantage of the technique used when the proximal anastomoses are made first is that the periodic distention of the vein by the infusion of the cardioplegic solution into the aortic root may be incomplete because of mild aortic incompetence. This interferes with precise sizing of vein segments between sequential anastomoses. A final disadvantage is that CPB is discontinued after a shorter interval of myocardial reperfusion than when the distal anastomoses are done first.

The advantages of making the distal anastomoses first include complete flexibility in the sequencing of the distal anastomoses and routing of the vein graft. The sizing of graft length between the proximal and distal anastomoses can be made precise by distending the vein graft with blood or saline injected into the proximal end. The period of myocardial perfusion while the proximal anastomoses are being made allows very smooth and easy discontinuation of CPB in nearly all cases. Both methods give excellent results, which is why surgeon-to-surgeon variability in this matter persists.

The Incision in the Vein for a Side-to-Side Anastomosis

A longitudinal incision in the vein, and a so-called diamond anastomosis,[G2] is preferred in all circumstances, whether the vein and artery are parallel to one another at the anastomosis or cross at right angles or obliquely. When the circumference of the longitudinal incision in the vein is 10%–20% longer than that of the artery, when the vein approaches the artery at the angle "it wishes" and leaves at a corresponding angle, and when the anastomosis is neatly made, the vein seems simply to lie over the artery after the anastomosis is completed, and is not distorted. A transverse venotomy is less flexible and more difficult to use.

Endarterectomy

While some surgeons use endarterectomy frequently, particularly in the distal RCA, the preference is to use the more distal branches for anastomosis, rather than to endarterectomize the parent trunk and graft to it.

Some surgeons report lower graft patency rates through endarterectomized arteries. Yeh and colleagues reported a graft patency rate of 64% when endarterectomy was done to the artery grafted, compared with 92% when endarterectomy was not used.[Y1] However, many studies[C6,H5,K13,Y2] suggest that patency rates and flow of grafts to endarterectomized arteries compare favorably with those to nonendarterectomized arteries. Whether perioperative myocardial infarction is more likely to occur when endarterectomy is employed is controversial,[M6] as is the relative completeness of revascularization achieved with the two techniques.

The Importance of Complete Revascularization

The definition and importance of complete revascularization remain controversial, even though Sheldon and colleagues, as long ago as 1972, and Assad-Morell and associates, in 1975, demonstrated the advantages of complete revascularizations.[A4,S15]

The phrase *complete revascularization* is defined differently by different groups. A practical definition is that it is the making of an anastomosis beyond every stenosis $\geqslant 50\%$ (or beyond the most distal of a series of stenoses) in each involved coronary arterial trunk or branch $\geqslant 1$ mm–1.25 mm in diameter. A more meaningful definition would relate the coronary pathologic condition to the left ventricular wall segments and could be stated as the revascularization of all areas of myocardium by the making of anastomoses beyond all stenoses with a myocardial value $\geqslant 1.0$.

Complete revascularization is feasible in nearly all patients, but in patients with extensive triple-vessel disease it may require four to eight distal anastomoses. It is uncommon for disease to extend so far distally that anastomoses cannot be made beyond it. Complete revascularization is made difficult but not impossible when large branches, most commonly the first diagonal and first Cx marginal branches, are intramyocardial. Such branches can usually be located by observing the very light color over them, in contrast to the darker brown of the myocardium. It is difficult and time-consuming, and at times impossible, to obtain complete revascularization when an area is supplied by multiple small branches rather than one or two large ones.

Other arguments against attempts at complete revascularization include the contention that sequential anastomoses to smaller arteries jeopardize the end-to-side anastomosis to the larger vessel, that the small artery is likely to occlude at the anastomotic site or that the anastomosis itself is more likely to become stenotic, that its use is unnecessary for obtaining good results, and that it takes longer.

The advantages of complete revascularization probably outweigh the disadvantages. Certainly, with proper techniques, hospital mortality is not adversely affected by the making of many distal anastomoses.[G11] There is no evidence that the incidence of perioperative myocardial infarction is increased by increasing the number of distal anastomoses, and it may in fact be decreased by complete revascularization. There is an impressive amount of evidence that patients with complete revascularization have a significantly lower incidence of persistent angina pectoris postoperatively, better improvement in left ventricular function, better exercise capacity,[H19] and better 5-year survival rates than do patients with incomplete revascularization.[B45,C19,J10,L12,T6] Hellman and colleagues, for example, have shown that among eight patients with preoperative ejection fractions ≥ 0.40, postoperative persistence of segmental wall motion abnormalities, and abnormal response of ejection fraction to exercise, seven had incomplete revascularization.[H1] Long-term survival rates are higher with complete revascularization (Fig. 7-16).

An interesting challenge to the concept of complete revascularization is posed by the possible role of percutaneous transluminal coronary dilation in patients with more than simple single-vessel disease. If this procedure can in fact relieve symptoms and prolong productive life for a considerable period of time in a high proportion of such patients, the concept of complete revascularization may not be valid. Also in support of this challenge, Lytle and colleagues reported a 5-year actuarial survival rate of 97% of patients with multivessel disease treated only by bilateral internal mammary artery grafting.[L24] Symptomatic relief was said to be as good as in complete revascularization.

CABG for Acute Myocardial Infarction

Until recently, most institutions have avoided CABG operations in patients with acute myocardial infarction. This was partly because of poor results from this practice in an earlier era and partly because of concern as to the safety of cardiac catheterization during or early after an acute myocardial infarction. Also, the risk of dying from an acute myocardial infarction seemed to be lessening.

Interest in the possible role of the CABG operation in acute myocardial infarction has increased in recent years. This is related to the demonstrated safety of cardiac catheterization during or soon after an acute myocardial infarction;[D5,R10] renewed interest in invasive treatments of all kinds for acute myocardial infarction, not only to save life but also to decrease left ventricular damage;[S35] and the demonstration by several groups,[D4,J7,R10] particularly Berg and colleagues,[B28,B42] that the risk of CABG can be low even in the presence of an acute infarction. Selinger, Berg, and colleagues have recently reported only two hospital deaths (2%, CL .7%–5%) among 101 patients undergoing the CABG operation within 12 hours after the onset of acute myocardial infarction.[S28]

This aggressive approach to acute myocardial infarction has arisen in part also because of recent support for the old concept that most acute infarctions are associated with complete occlusion of the major vessel to that area (see "Effect of Acute Myocardial Infarction on Natural History"). The occlusions are probably acute and in many cases reversible with intracoronary administration of thrombolytic agents.[G19,M14,R18,R19,R20] However, because a significant atherosclerotic stenotic lesion is present at the point of thrombosis in nearly all patients,[M22] the recurrence rate of occlusion is considerable. Under such circumstances, concomitant percutaneous transluminal coronary angioplasty is undertaken;[G14] should this not relieve the stenosis, and particularly when there are other significant lesions, CABG may be indicated.[L16,M15,S35] The risk of these interventions after the use of intracoronary thrombolytic agents[K20] is low, although bleeding is troublesome in some of the operations. Sterling and colleagues reported 1 death (2%) among 41 patients treated by intracoronary thrombolysis with streptokinase followed within 3 to 10 days by CABG and noted no problems different from those of elective CABG and overall good results.[S42]

Currently, patients may be considered for urgent operation when the hemodynamic state is unstable, chest pain persists or recurs after the infarction,[M21] or there is other evidence of poor prognosis (UAB). The hospital mortality is low when CABG is done early after acute infarction (Table 7-11). Jones and colleagues reported no deaths (0%, CL 0%–2%) among 110 patients undergoing urgent CABG operations within 1 month of an acute myocardial infarction.[J12] These experiences, plus the reports of DeWood and associates[D4] and Phillips and colleagues[P6] indicate that the risk of CABG is low no matter what the interval since the acute infarction, unless acute or chronic cardiogenic shock is present.

However, other details of the early results of aggressive treatment (thrombolysis therapy, percutaneous transluminal coronary angioplasty, and CABG) are not yet clearly defined. Substantial improvements in regional wall motion and an apparent reduction in size of the infarct have been demonstrated with intracoronary streptokinase infusion.[M15] However, intracoronary thrombolysis with streptokinase has been successful in only about 85% of patients,[M12] and it has been suggested that this intervention can produce worsening of the patient's condition from large hemorrhage into the infarction.[M11] Emergency percutaneous transluminal coronary angioplasty has at least the same failure rate (15%–20%) when performed in patients with acute myocardial infarction, as it does in patients with chronic stable angina. Furthermore, Jones and colleagues reported a significantly higher incidence of new infarctions, use of inotropic agents, and ventricular arrhythmias when CABG is done as an emergency after a failed percutaneous transluminal angioplasty than when done primarily.[J14]

The real place of the aggressive approach to acute myocardial infarction depends in part on demonstrated reduction in the extent of the infarction and the resultant scarring, and thus a reduction in the incidence and severity of late sequelae, such as ventricular electrical instability, sudden death, recurrent infarction, heart failure, and left ventricular aneurysm. To achieve this, the interventions must occur within a certain time after an acute infarction. Several considerations suggest that this time frame extends to about 8 hours after the infarction occurs. The extent of infarction in humans appears to reach a maximum within 7–18 hours.[S37]

Experimental studies indicate that a favorable effect results if myocardial reperfusion is accomplished within 4–8 hours after onset of infarction[B30] and if cold cardioplegic myocardial protection is used during the operation.[W11] Phillips and colleagues did emergency CABG operations within an average of 6 hours after the onset of the infarction and found a significant ($P < .05$) increase in ejection fraction from an immediate preoperative average of 0.35 to 0.47 some weeks after the CABG operation, and decreased end-systolic and end-diastolic left ventricular volumes.[P6]

The mechanism of improvement in left ventricular function is not yet clear, particularly in view of some of the findings after successful acute coronary recanalization with streptokinase. Reduto and colleagues found *no* immediate change in left ventricular function immediately after acute recanalization in the 18 (69%, CL 57%–79%) of 26 patients who responded to intracoronary streptokinase infusion; however, 7 (39%, CL 25%–54%) of the 18 showed important improvement in systolic function 10 days later.[R18] Thus, the improvements from reperfusion, in this setting, need not necessarily occur immediately but may appear gradually thereafter. This phenomenon has been observed experimentally.[R21] However, Rentrop and colleagues found most of the improvement to occur immediately after reperfusion.[R22] In any event, when persistent total occlusion of the coronary artery persists, the acute dysfunction persists. When the vessel is or becomes patent, function can be expected to improve.[F14]

There is probably also benefit from emergency CABG operations done for continuing angina or shock, more than 8 hours after an acute infarction. The myocardium lost as a result of the infarction cannot be reclaimed, but further loss of myocardium may be prevented and the probability of long-term survival improved.

Reoperation after the CABG Operation

Since symptoms tend to recur with time (Fig. 7-24), reoperation may have to be considered at some time in many patients who have undergone the CABG operation. The incidence of reoperation after the initial CABG operation is variable and depends at least upon the indications for the original CABG procedure, the technique and completeness of revascularization, and the pharmacologic interventions perioperatively. The incidence can be as high as 5%–10% within 5 postoperative years.[L24] It can be as low as 2.2% within 5 years (Fig. 7-25). It is important to note that the instantaneous risk of reoperation begins to rise about 3.5 years after the original CABG operation when vein grafts have been used exclusively (Fig. 7-26).

The reasons for the return of symptoms and thus the need for reoperation may be graft closures, progression of the native coronary artery disease, or incomplete revascularization at the original operation. Deferral of the original CABG operation as long as is safe helps to defer reoperation.

Once symptoms return, the control of myocardial ischemia by medical measures for as long as is safe and judicous use of percutaneous transluminal coronary angioplasty for localized graft or native vessel stenosis may allow reoperation also to be deferred for a time. Thus, Douglas and colleagues found PTCA useful in about 80% of patients with stenosis at the distal anastomosis over a follow-up period of about 11 months.[D8] Success was achieved in only about half the patients in whom the stenosis was at the proximal anastomosis.

The technique of CABG reoperation is described under "Technique of Operation." The postoperative care and course are similar to those after primary CABG operations. The amount of postoperative bleeding and the incidence of important myocardial necrosis are the same as after the primary CABG operation.[R23]

The early results are good, but the hospital mortality is

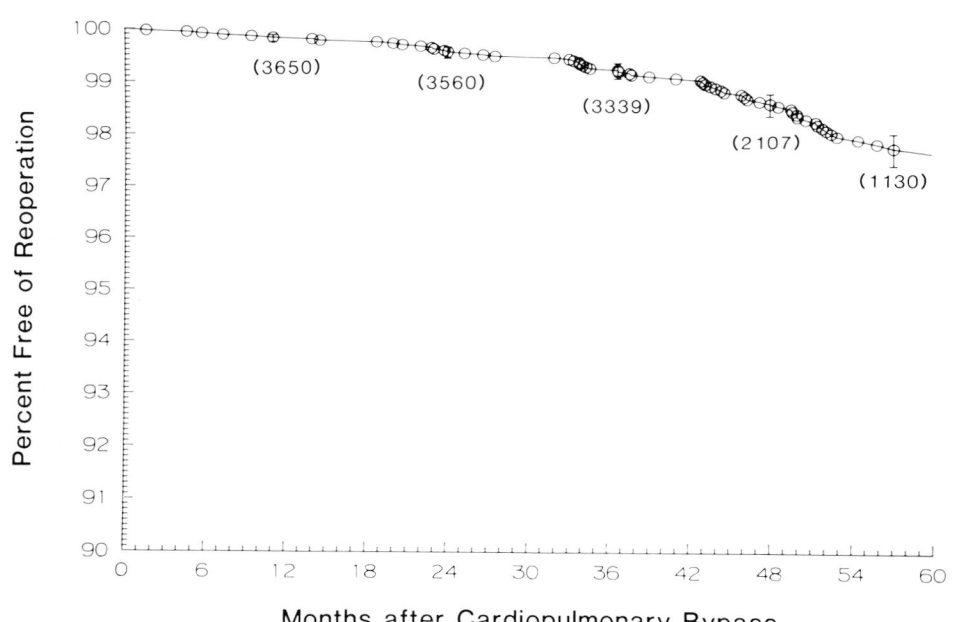

Figure 7-25 Actuarial incidence of coronary artery bypass graft reoperations (UAB; primary operation 1977–1981; $n = 3872$, 72 reoperations). Note the expanded vertical scale. The actuarial freedom from reoperation at 5 years is 97.8% (CL 97.4%–98.0%).

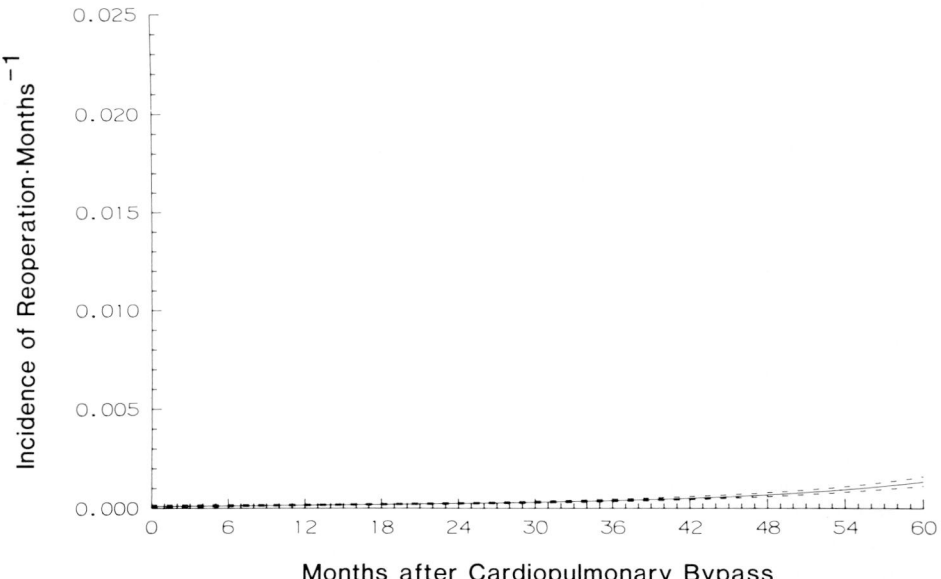

Figure 7-26 Hazard function (instantaneous risk per month) of reoperation after coronary artery bypass grafting. (Data base is the same as in Figure 7-25.)

higher than that of the primary operation, being 4% (CL 2%–7%) for the first reoperation (Table 7-12). The experience of Loop and colleagues,[L20] Quazi and colleagues,[Q1] and Foster and colleagues[F15] support these conclusions.

The symptomatic results are good if satisfactory revascularization can be accomplished. In a small group of 5 patients, Winkler and colleagues found 4 (80%, CL 47%–97%) to have good symptomatic relief;[W2] Quazi and colleagues found 33 (85%, CL 76%–91%) of 39 to be asymptomatic or improved by operation.[Q1] Loop and colleagues also reported excellent long-term results, with an 89% 5-year survival rate.[L20] No appreciable difference has been noted whether the reoperation was for graft failure, incomplete revascularization, or progressive arteriosclerosis, but eventually progressive and diffuse coronary arteriosclerosis will probably be shown to be a risk factor for premature death after reoperations.

Combined Carotid and Coronary Artery Disease

Significant stenosis of the aortic arch branches (usually at the origin of the internal carotid artery but sometimes more proximally in the innominate or common carotid arteries or the vertebral artery) is known to occur in only a small percentage of patients who undergo CABG (1.3% of the Cleveland Clinic patients[H10]).

Carotid artery disease is associated more commonly with left main coronary artery stenosis than with other subsets of coronary artery disease. In the UAB experience, the incidence of left main coronary artery disease has been 37% (27/73), in patients with combined carotid and coronary artery disease compared to a 14.2% incidence in all CABG patients;[S23] and at GLH, the incidence of associated carotid artery disease has been 50% among patients with left main coronary artery disease (Table 7-13), compared to 19% among other patients undergoing the CABG operation. There may also be a higher incidence of triple-vessel disease, of significantly depressed left ventricular function, and of women among patients with the combined diseases. Finally, patients undergoing combined coronary and carotid artery surgery tend to be older than those undergoing the isolated CABG operation.[J9,L14]

The preoperative examination may suggest the presence of carotid artery stenoses by a history of transient ischemic attacks or frank stroke or by a bruit over the carotid arteries. When the latter is found without symptoms, carotid arterio-

Table 7-12 Hospital death after primary and secondary CABG operations, (UAB; 1977–1981; see Table 7-2 for details of the primary group).

		Hospital Deaths		
Category[a]	n	No.	%	CL
Primary CABG	3851	38	0.99%	0.82%–1.18%
First CABG reoperation	80	3	4%	2%–7%
CABG after Vineberg or patch-graft arteriography	4	0	0%	0%–38%
CABG after aneurysmectomy	1	1	100%	15%–100%
Third CABG reoperation	1	0	0%	0%–85%
Total	3937	42	1.07%	0.90%–1.26%
P (χ²)			< .0001	

[a] All cases, including those with concomitant ventricular and vascular procedures. In the reoperation group, many of the original operations had been done elsewhere.

Table 7-13 Findings in the 38 patients receiving carotid artery surgery within 6 months of CABG operation (GLH; 1973–1982). The hospital mortality refers to deaths within 30 days of either procedure. There was no mortality in the interval between operations. In four instances, valve replacement surgery was combined with the coronary artery surgery.

		n	% of 38	Hospital Deaths
Myocardial score	12–13.9	18	47%	1
	10–11.9	10	26%	1
	8– 9.9	6	16%	0
	< 8	2	5%	0
	Not known	2	5%	0
Left main stenosis	≥ 75%	19	50%	1

		Hospital Death			Postoperative Stroke (n)	
	n	n	%	CL	Carotid Operation	CABG Operation
Staged procedure	31	0	0%	0%–6%	3 (1)[a]	4 (1)
Simultaneous procedure	7	2	29%	10%–55%	0	2 (1)
Total	38	2				

	n	Vertebral Disease	No. Symptoms	Hospital Death	Major Stroke
Bilateral carotid	17[b]	6	3	1	2
Unilateral carotid	21	2	8	1	1
Total	38	8	11	2	3

[a] Figures in parentheses are major strokes. The others were transient ischemic events.

[b] Includes one innominate artery stenosis.

grams are done only after noninvasive testing gives positive results, although this policy is controversial.[K18] Obviously, significant carotid occlusive disease may be present without signs or symptoms and be undiagnosed.

The surgical strategy for the combination of coronary and carotid artery disease when both carry an indication for operation is controversial. Two separate, staged procedures may be done, with either the carotid endarterectomy or the CABG operation being done first; or both procedures can be performed in a combined operation. The staged operation is advantageous because it carries a low mortality and morbidity. Thus, in the GLH experience, there have been no hospital deaths, and in the Cleveland Clinic experience, a 1.7% mortality[H10] from the two-stage procedure. In the absence of routine carotid and coronary arteriography in patients undergoing either operation, however, such figures must be interpreted with care. There is a risk of myocardial infarction at the time of carotid endarterectomy, but with current management this is small (6% in the GLH series).

Repair of both lesions can be done simultaneously, either routinely[E6] or selectively in those with angiographically severe coronary artery disease[C24] (including severe left main coronary artery stenosis) or in patients with bilateral carotid stenosis, in whom the more critical carotid stenosis has been relieved at an earlier operation.[H10,U2] The mortality of the combined operation has varied from 2%–10%. Combining three large series from Cleveland, Dallas, and Milwaukee provides a total of 500 such operations with a 5% hospital mortality and a stroke incidence of about 5%.[J9,L14,U3] At UAB, where the simultaneous repair is used in only selected

cases and less frequently now than earlier, this procedure has carried 19% mortality when a left main stenosis > 50% was present but only 4% when it was absent (*P* = .06).[S23] This is comparable to other results in the current era, illustrated by the hospital mortality of 4 deaths (3%) among 132 patients selected to receive the combined procedure by Jones and colleagues.[J17]

When a simultaneous procedure is required, the carotid endarterectomy may be done before CPB is begun (GLH) or during CPB (UAB). In either situation, the carotid artery is exposed while the saphenous vein is removed and the sternotomy made. The heart is prepared for cannulation, and heparin is given. When the carotid endarterectomy is done before CPB, it is accomplished at this point. The neck wound is not closed until after CPB and the administration of protamine. Alternatively, CPB is established at 30°C, a pulsatile and normal or near normal arterial blood pressure maintained by keeping the left atrial pressure at 6–8 mmHg, and endarterectomy performed. Thereafter the CABG operation is carried out as usual (UAB). The latter method would appear to offer maximal protection against cerebral or myocardial infarction. Neither type of infarction has been experienced in a small group of patients at UAB managed by this method.

In any case, a combination of severe coronary and carotid artery disease unfavorably affects the long-term prognosis. Loop and colleagues reported a 5-year survival rate of 80% in patients undergoing stimultaneous combined carotid and coronary operations, compared to 93% for patients undergoing the isolated CABG operation.[L22]

APPENDIXES

CORONARY ARTERIOGRAPHY

Reliable and accurate arteriography depends on experienced skillful personnel using appropriate equipment and techniques. Cineangiographic techniques are preferred over serial large-film studies since modern image intensifiers are capable of detailed resolution of vessels less than 0.5 mm in diameter.

EQUIPMENT AND METHODOLOGY

The production of good cineangiographic detail requires a high-powered generator and x-ray tube capable of delivering at least 1,000 mA on cine mode at 50 frames per second and killivolts in the range of 60–85 with short exposure times (1–3 msec). Cine processing must be carefully controlled to ensure consistent results. Equipment must permit a wide range of easily achieved projections not only around the transverse body plane but also with cranial and caudal angulation of up to 40° of any of the transverse body plane views (Fig. 7A1). Studies indicate that without craniocaudal (in which the x-ray beam enters the back of the patient and courses toward the feet) and caudocranial (in which the x-ray beam enters the back of the patient and courses toward the head) views, incomplete and inaccurate diagnosis result in at least half the patients studied.[A6] It has become clear that diagnostic accuracy was compromised by the limitations of the conventional cineangiographic system, usually consisting of a fixed ceiling-suspended image intensifier with no ability to angle the x-ray beam. Without the ability to angle the x-ray beam, standard or nonangled views are characterized by overlapping of arteries and foreshortening of segments, resulting in an obscuration of the origin of branches, complete masking of some specific lesions, or significant underestimation of a lesion. The implications of these problems for the results of surgical management are obvious.

The first angled coronary arteriographic view was a caudocranial left anterior oblique (half-axial) view, designed to profile the left main, proximal, and mid-left anterior descending artery and its branches. With the advent of x-ray tube–image intensifier configurations with triaxial motion capability (U or C arms with all the movements in the arms or some movements in both the arms and the table; see Fig. 7A-1), angled views were additionally designed to profile the left main coronary artery; the circumflex-marginal system; the mid LAD artery, including its septal and diagonal branches; and the distal right coronary artery. A number of publications describe the methodology and advantages of these views.[A7,A8,B46,B47,E8,E9,E10,G16,G17,M20,P8]

ARTERIOGRAPHIC TECHNIQUE

In many patients, the proximal left coronary artery is oriented approximately in the transverse body plane as it bifurcates into the anterior descending and circumflex arteries or divides into three or even four branches. A shallow left anterior oblique (LAO) view (about 40° left of sagittal) profiles the origin of the left main coronary artery but views the distal left main coronary artery and proximal anterior descending artery end on or superimposes these vessels on intermediate and proximal circumflex arteries. A deep diaphragm inspiratory effort by the patient helps to reveal these branch origins by lowering the cardiac apex. In addition, if the x-ray beam is angled 30–40° toward the head (40° LAO with 30–40° cranial tilt), these

difficulties are minimized or overcome. Steeper degrees of LAO and even lateral projection with cranial tilting may be required to profile the origin of each branch in some cases. If the proximal left coronary artery and its branches pass upward in their initial course, a caudally tilted version of the LAO to lateral series may be required to display the left main coronary artery and its proximal branch origins.

In right anterior oblique projection, the left coronary orifice is viewed *en face* and is not readily assessed. However, the mid and distal portions of the left main coronary artery are usually well seen in this view, which is approximately at right angles to that obtained in the cranially tilted LAO projection, the two views allowing a more accurate assessment of the severity of moderate lesions than is possible from one view. The addition of cranial tilt to a shallow RAO (or frontal) projection helps to profile the origin and demonstrate the proximal parts of those intermediate and proximal diagonal branches that tend to arc upward in relationship to the anterior descending artery, while caudal tilt with steeper degrees of RAO better separates those branches that tend to lie below the level of the anterior descending artery in the transverse body plane.

The more distally arising branches of anterior descending and circumflex arteries are more readily demonstrated. Each cine run should be panned if necessary to show all parts of the distal coronary tree. The cine runs should be long enough to show vessels that are occluded proximally and fill only slowly by collaterals, sometimes requiring 15 or more seconds to fill.

The proximal right coronary artery is usually well assessed with 50° LAO and 30° RAO views. Occasionally additional views are required for tortuosities. A lateral view usually gives the most accurate profile of the origin and can be added if a moderate orificial lesion is suspected. The distal RCA and its branching pattern at the crux inferiorly may require special projections. If the heart lies horizontally, the conventional LAO view shows the posterior descending branch end on, and its origin and quality can be shown in LAO only by cranially tilted views. A shallower LAO (about 30°) will help to show the crux clear of the right diaphragm if the patient cannot depress it sufficiently. Cranial tilting of the RAO projection is also helpful if the posterior descending and inferior surface (posterolateral segment) left ventricular branches are superimposed in the transverse plane RAO view.

Extensive knowledge of the congenital variations of origin and distribution that can occur in the coronary tree is essential if the radiologist is to avoid errors of interpretation and incomplete demonstration of the coronary tree.

The views and positions that have proved particularly useful are summarized and illustrated in Figures 7A-1–7A-6.

JUDGMENT OF SEVERITY OF DISEASE

The patient is given oral nitroglycerin to obtain maximal dilatation of the coronary arteries and to minimize arterial spasm. This permits a better appreciation of the severity of a moderate (50% diameter loss) stenosis. Severe ($\geq$ 70% diameter loss) or mild (< 50% diameter loss) stenoses are readily assessed when the lesion is localized and the adjacent vessel is obviously healthy and of normal calibre. A moderate localized lesion in a *diffusely diseased* vessel is difficult to evaluate, and an inexperienced or uncritical assessment may result in underestimation of severity. Diffuse narrowing without marked local stenoses is particularly difficult to grade, and attention to vessel wall quality and absolute size of the vessels is necessary.

Areas of localized muscle bridging can be identified as relatively short segments in which the lumen constricts during systole but returns to a normal diameter during diastole.

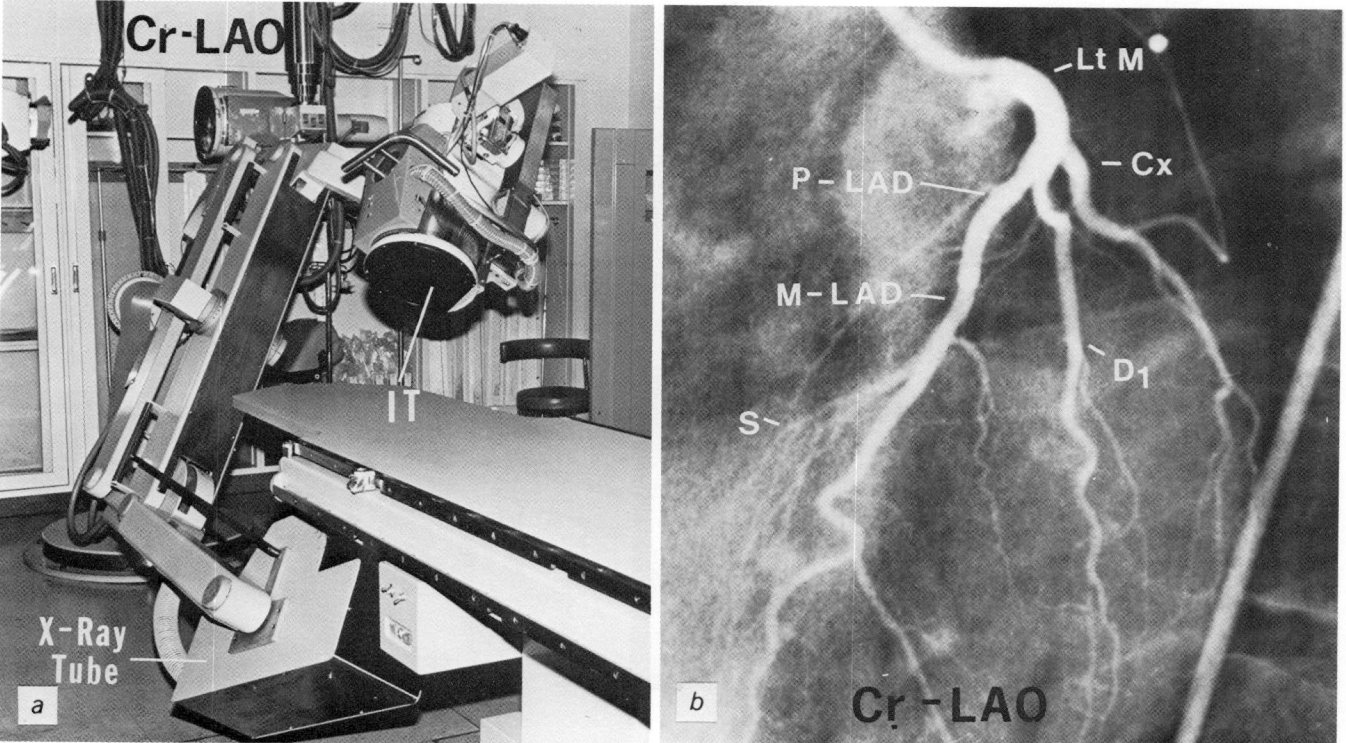

Figure 7A-1 Caudocranial (CR) left anterior oblique (LAO), or half-axial, view (UAB).
(a) The image intensifier (IT) is moved left and angled so the x-ray beam passes in a caudocranial direction (cranial angulation) toward the head.
(b) Selective left coronary arteriogram. The Cr-LAO view profiles the left main (Lt M), proximal left anterior descending (P-LAD), mid-left anterior descending (M-LAD), and first diagonal (D1) arteries. Septal arteries (S) course to the patient's right. The proximal circumflex artery (Cx) is also seen.

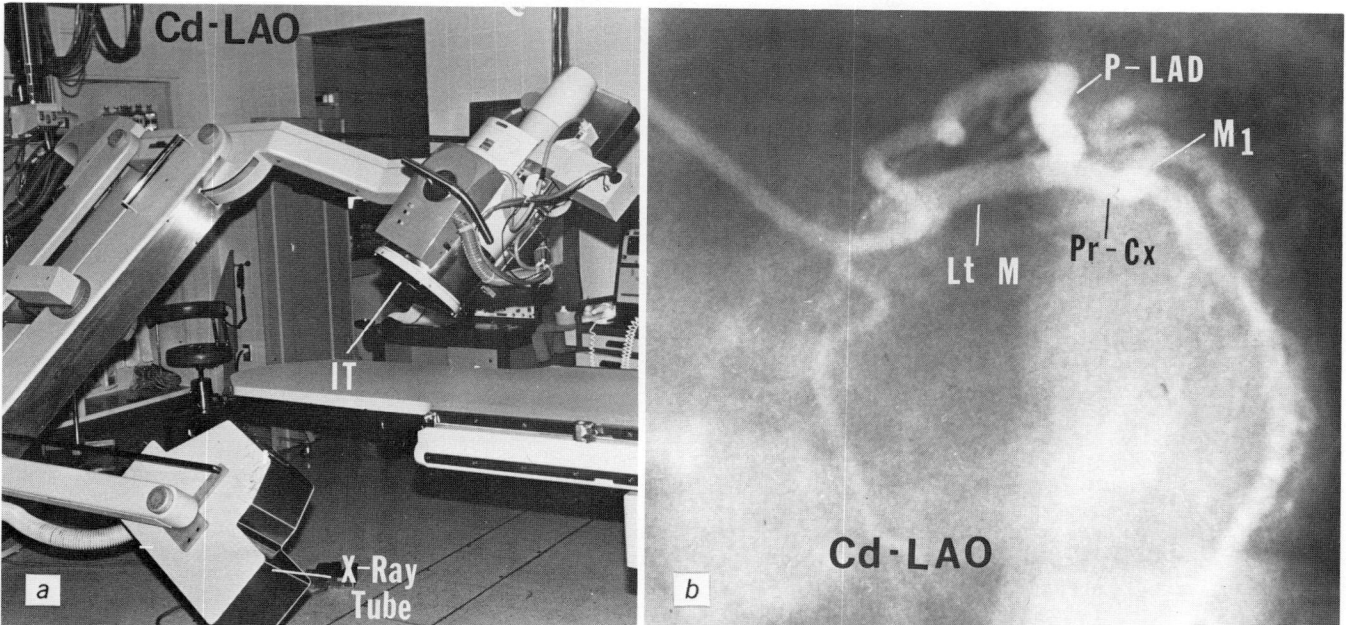

Figure 7A-2 Craniocaudal (Cd) LAO, or "weeping willow," view (UAB).
(a) The image intensifier (IT) is moved left and angled so the x-ray beam passes in a craniocaudal direction (caudal angulation) toward the feet.
(b) Selective left coronary arteriogram. The Cd-LAO view profiles the left main (Lt M), origin and trunk of the proximal (P) LAD artery, and origin and trunk of the proximal circumflex (Pr-Cx) artery. The origin of the first marginal (M1) artery is usually well seen.

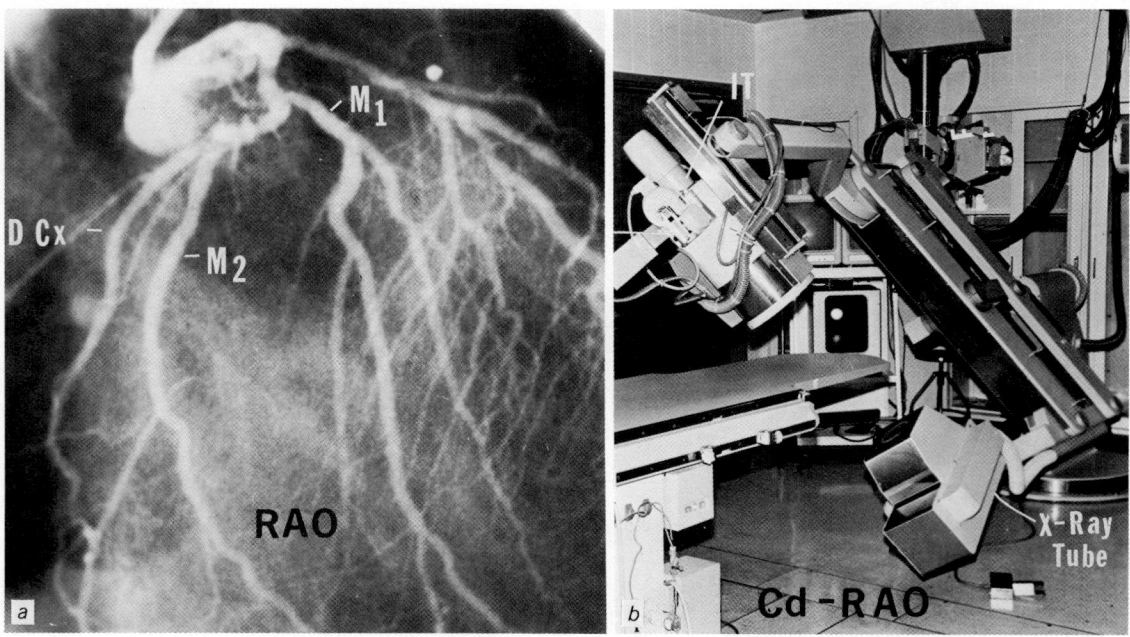

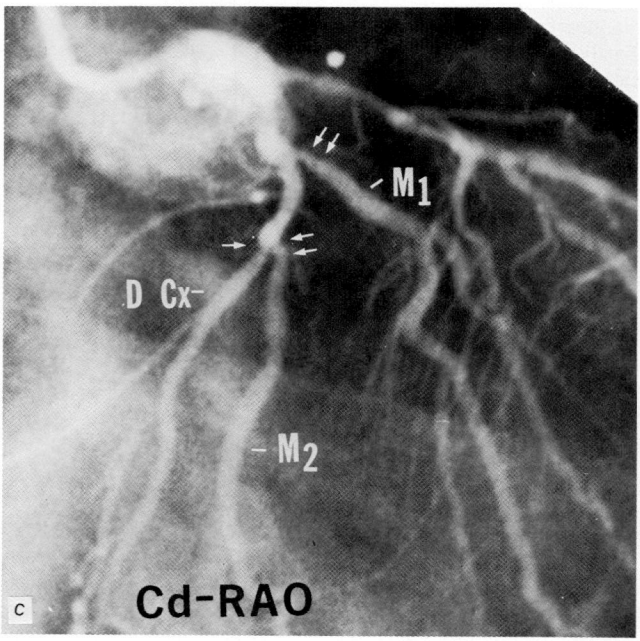

Figure 7A-3 Advantages of the caudal (Cd) right anterior oblique (RAO) view in profiling the circumflex-marginal artery system.

(a) Standard RAO view with selective left coronary arteriogram. A questionable lesion exists at the origin of the first marginal (M1) artery. The origins of the second marginal (M2) and distal circumflex (D-Cx) arteries appear normal.

(b) The image intensifier (IT) is moved right and angled caudally.

(c) Selective coronary arteriogram in caudal RAO view. The origin of the first marginal (M1) artery shows a 50%–60% stenosis (double vertical arrows), the origin of the second marginal (M2) artery a 50%–60% stenosis (double horizontal arrows), and the origin of the distal circumflex (D-Cx) artery a 40% stenosis (arrow).

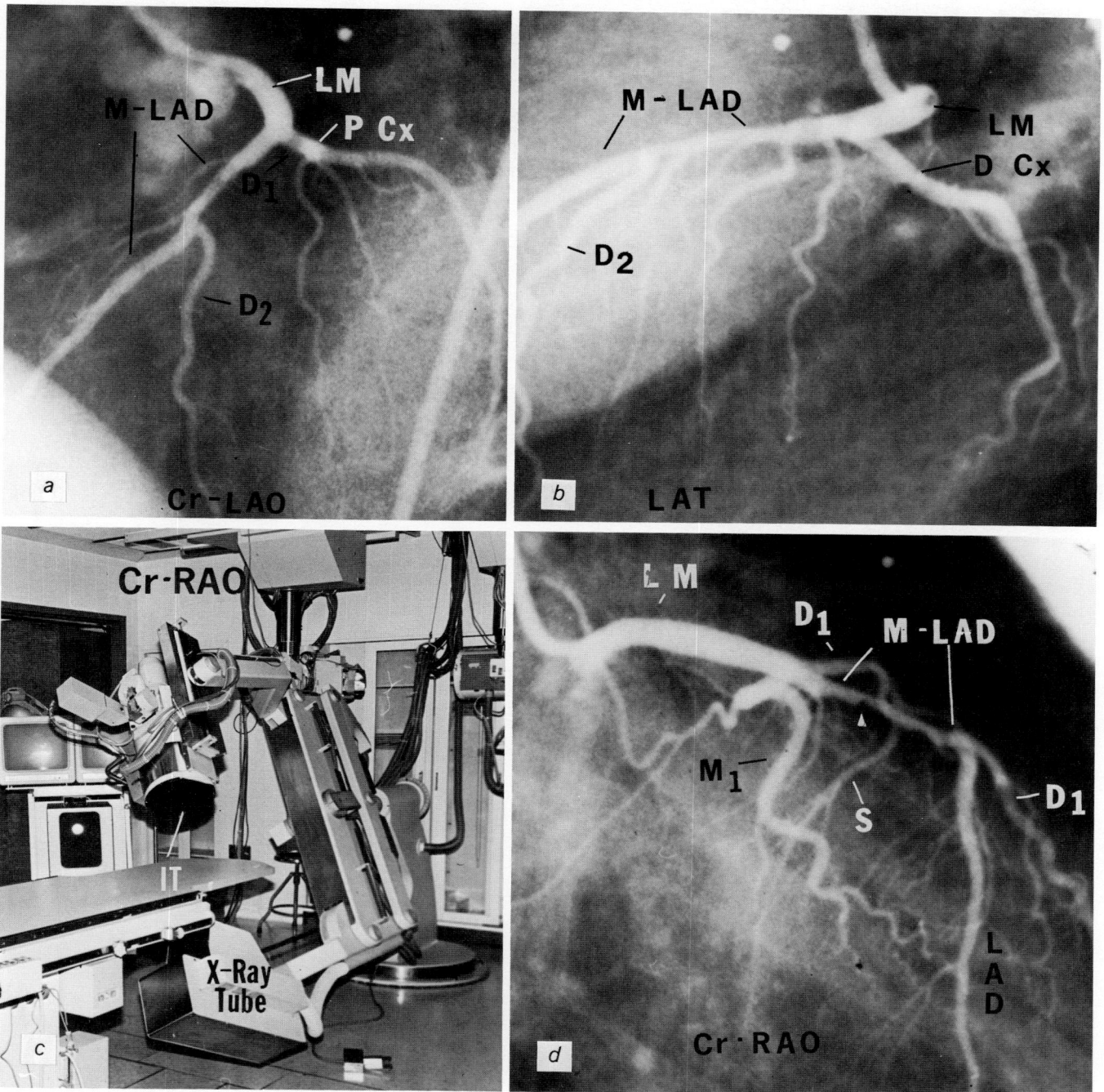

Figure 7A-4 Advantages of the cranial (Cr) RAO view (UAB).

(a) Cr-LAO (half-axial) view of a selective left coronary arteriogram.

(b) Lateral view. Is there significant disease in the mid-left anterior descending (M-LAD) artery in either view? The obvious answer is no.

(c) Cranial RAO view. The image intensifier (IT) is moved right and angled cranially.

(d) The Cr-RAO view unmasked diffuse disease in the mid-left anterior descending artery as well as a discrete high-grade lesion (arrowhead). This degree of disease was not seen in the standard RAO view.

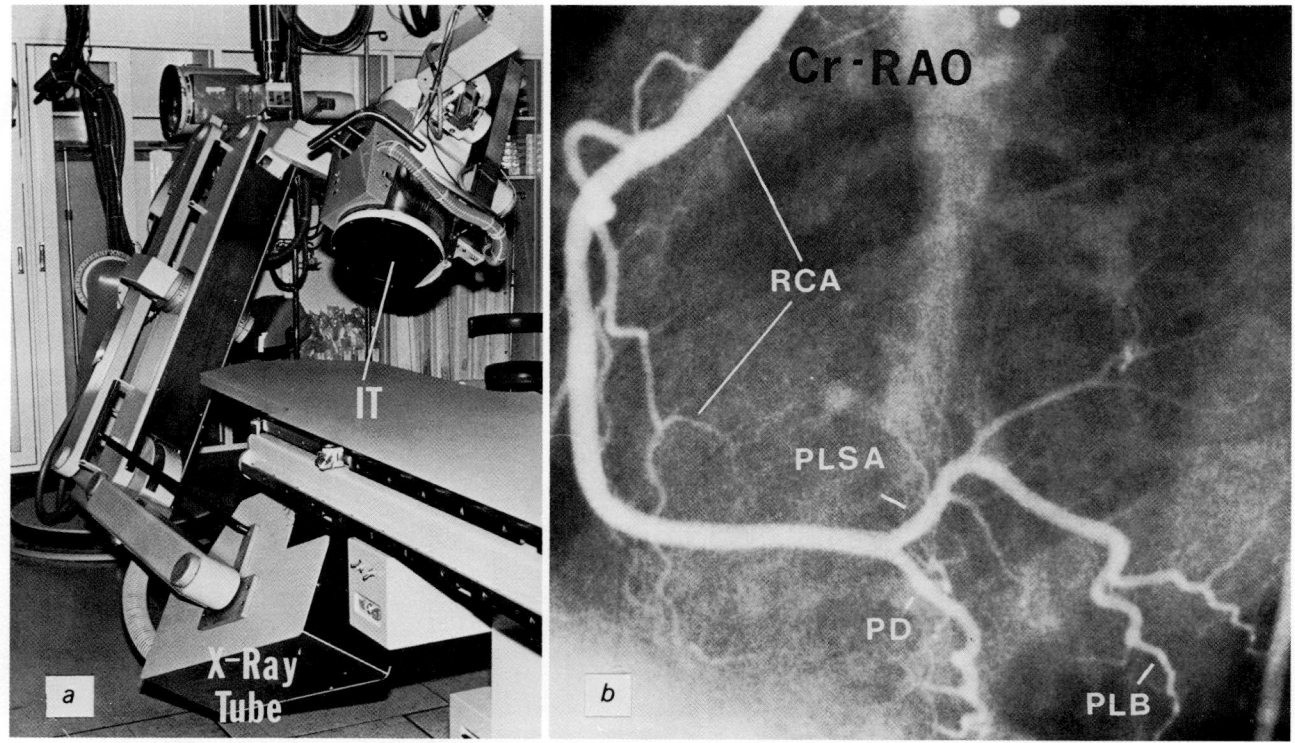

Figure 7A-5 Cranial (Cr) LAO view in a right coronary arteriogram (UAB).
(a) The image intensifier (IT) is moved left and angled cranially.
(b) The right coronary artery (RCA) is well visualized. There is improved visualization of the distal right coronary artery (RCA), posterior descending (PD) artery, posterolateral segment artery (PLSA), posterolateral branch (PLB) artery, and their origins compared with the standard LAO and lateral views.

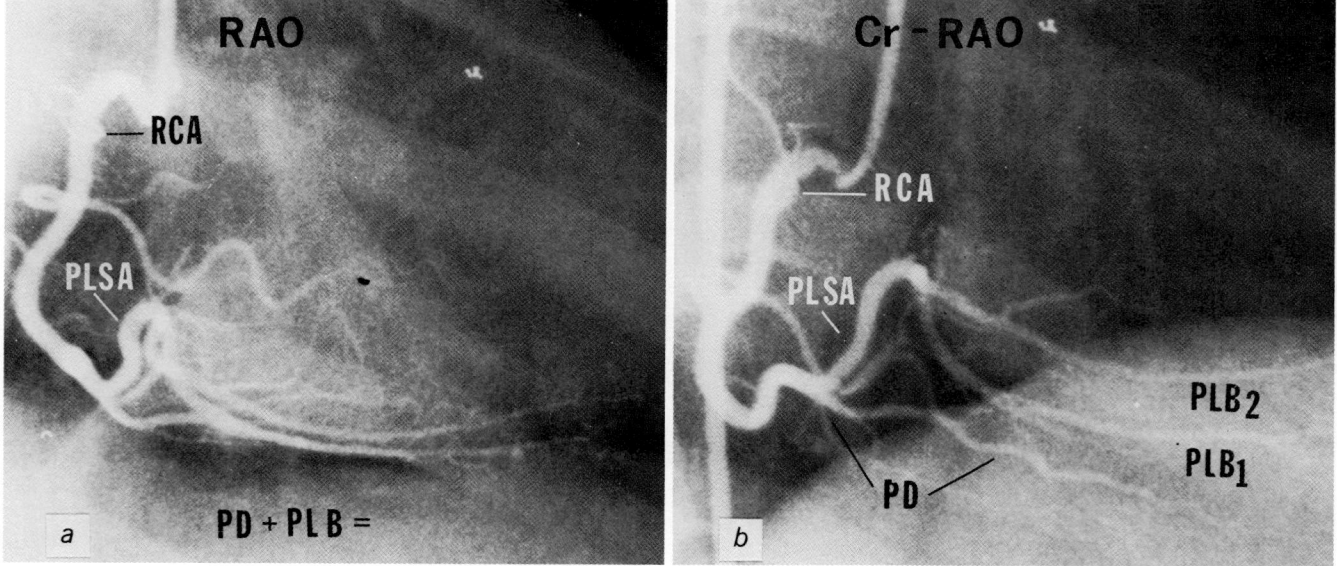

Figure 7A-6 Advantage of the cranial (Cr) RAO view in visualizing the distal branches of the RCA (UAB).
(a) Selective right coronary arteriogram in the standard RAO view. The posterior descending (PD) and posterolateral branch (PLB) arteries are superimposed, and the posterolateral segment artery (PLSA) is foreshortened.
(b) Cranial RAO view (see Figure 7A-4c). This view produces a stair-step effect, resulting in an uncovering of the posterior descending artery and two posterolateral branch arteries (PLB ± 1 and ± 2). The posterolateral segment artery is shown in better profile as well.

Finally, a reproducible judgment regarding the relative importance of each branch can be included in the assessment (see Appendix 7B).

APPENDIX **7B**

MYOCARDIAL PERFUSION SCORING SYSTEM FOR CORONARY ARTERIOGRAPHY

At GLH, a preprinted background for the myocardial perfusion scoring system views the heart from the apex, the free wall of the left ventricle being flattened into a semicircle so that the curved perimeter represents the atrioventricular groove, while the septum is drawn as a central oblong. The LV free wall is divided into diagonal, obtuse marginal, and inferior (diaphragmatic or posterolateral) segments of fixed size and the septum into anterior and posterior portions of variable size (Fig. 7B-1). Each left ventricular myocardial segment is given a numerical value, for a total of 15.[F9] When, for example, two equal-sized arteries go to a segment, one-half of the numerical value of that segment is assigned to each artery as its *myocardial value*. The right ventricle is shown as a triangular area divided into conal, anterior, and inferior segments.

A 75% cross-sectional area (50% diameter) loss is considered a significant but moderate stenosis, while a 90% cross-sectional area (67% diameter) loss is considered severe (Fig. 7B-3). Some clinicians have considered only those lesions with a 70% or more diameter loss (greater than 90% cross-sectional area loss) significant.[H8,K17,W7]

For scoring purposes, the grade of severity of arterial obstruction is related to the myocardial value of the particular branch as shown in Table 7B-1. The total score for each patient is recorded. A score of < 5 corresponds approximately to single-vessel disease, of 5 < 10 to double-vessel disease, and of 10–15 to triple-vessel disease. Representative diagrams are shown in Figures 7B-2 and 7B-3.

A diagram of each patient's coronary tree is drawn freehand on a preprinted background (Fig. 7B-2) by the reporting radiologist; the stenoses are then indicated by crosses, and the degree of stenosis by an adjacent number (Fig. 7B-2).

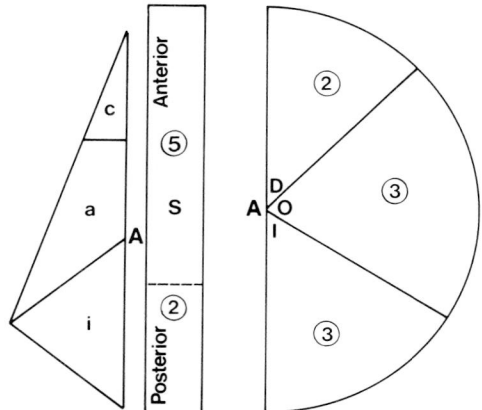

Figure 7B-1 Diagrammatic presentation of the segments of left and right ventricles, including the ventricular septum (GLH). The myocardial value of each left ventricular segment is indicated by the encircled numbers.

A, apex; D, LV diagonal area; O, LV obtuse marginal area; I, LV inferior (diaphragmatic area); a, RV anterior area; c, RV conus area; i, RV inferior area; S, septum; anterior, portion of septum supplied by LAD artery; posterior, portion of septum supplied by posterior descending artery.

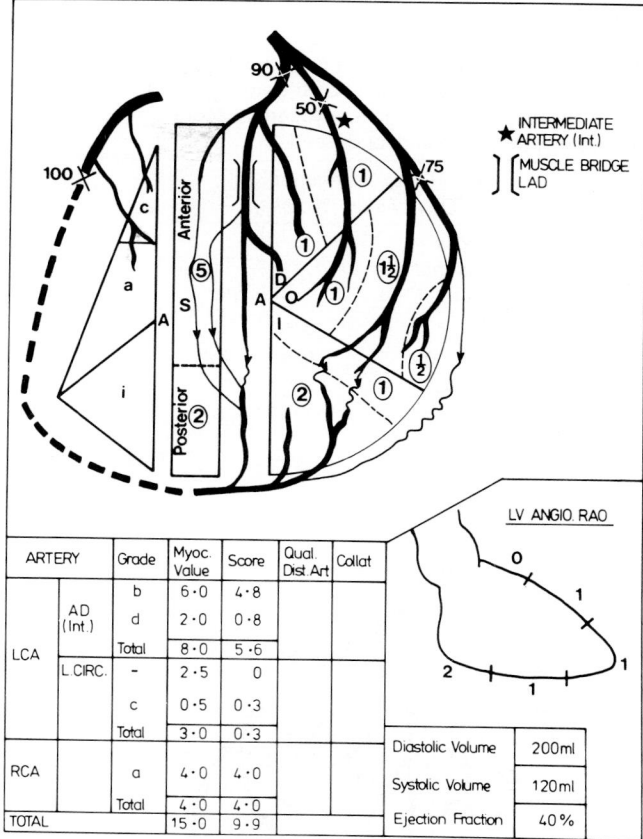

ARTERY		Grade	Myoc. Value	Score	Qual. Dist Art	Collat
LCA	A.D. (Int.)	b	6·0	4·8		
		d	2·0	0·8		
		Total	8·0	5·6		
	L.CIRC.	–	2·5	0		
		c	0·5	0·3		
		Total	3·0	0·3		
RCA		a	4·0	4·0		
		Total	4·0	4·0		
TOTAL			15·0	9·9		

Diastolic Volume	200ml
Systolic Volume	120ml
Ejection Fraction	40%

Figure 7B-2 Diagrammatic presentation of a coronary arteriogram in a right dominant coronary tree. The myocardial areas are subdivided as shown in Appendix 7B, Figure 7B-1. The distribution of arteries supplying these segments is sketched in to facilitate the assessment of the myocardial value of each artery or group of arteries. In this example, the proximal RCA is occluded. Its distal branches, distributed to an average amount of the posterior septum (myocardial value = 2) and two-thirds of the inferior LV area ("posteriolateral segment" area with myocardial value = 2, total value = 4) fill by collateral arteries from left coronary branches (shown by finer interconnecting lines with arrows indicating direction of flow). An intermediate (or first diagonal) artery supplies the basal half of the diagonal area and the apical one-third of the obtuse marginal area (total myocardial value = 2). The first marginal branch supplies most of the obtuse marginal segment (1 μ) but also the left one-third of the inferior area (1).

Sites of stenosis are indicated by a cross, and the degree of stenosis (cross-sectional area loss) by an adjacent number. Beneath the diagram, the score is calculated according to the grade of stenosis and the myocardial value of each branch (see Appendix 7B, Table 7B-1). In addition to the myocardial score, the RAO LV angiogram is also recorded, dividing the profile into five segments. The segmental wall motion is indicated by the number alongside each segment.

AD, anterior descending artery; Int, intermediate (first diagonal) artery; LCA, left coronary artery; L Circ, left circumflex artery; RAO, right anterior oblique; RCA, right coronary artery; 0, normal contraction; 1, hypokinesia; 2, akinesia; 3, dyskinesia.

Table 7B-1 Table for computing the myocardial score of a stenosed coronary artery according to the grade of arterial obstruction and its myocardial value (see text). The myocardial value is directly proportional to the amount of left ventricle myocardium perfused by (assigned to) each artery were it unobstructed. If two similar stenoses are present in series or if a stenosis is more than 1 cm long, the grade is increased by one but not to grade a. The score for each artery is entered separately in the boxes provided beneath the diagram and summated to give the total myocardial score. The larger the score, the greater the amount of potentially ischemic myocardium. By this system, the score cannot exceed 15.

Grade	Cross-sectional Area	Diameter	Myocardial Value									
a	100%	100%	1	2	3	4	5	6	7	8	9	10
b	90% < 100%	67% < 100%	0.8	1.6	2.4	3.2	4	4.8	5.6	6.4	7.2	8
c	75% < 90%	50% < 67%	0.6	1.2	1.8	2.4	3	3.6	4.2	4.8	5.4	6
d	50% < 75%	33% < 50%	0.4	0.8	1.2	1.6	2	2.4	2.8	3.2	3.6	4
e	< 50%	< 33%	0.2	0.4	0.6	0.8	1	1.2	1.4	1.6	1.8	2

Grade of Arterial Obstruction (% Loss)

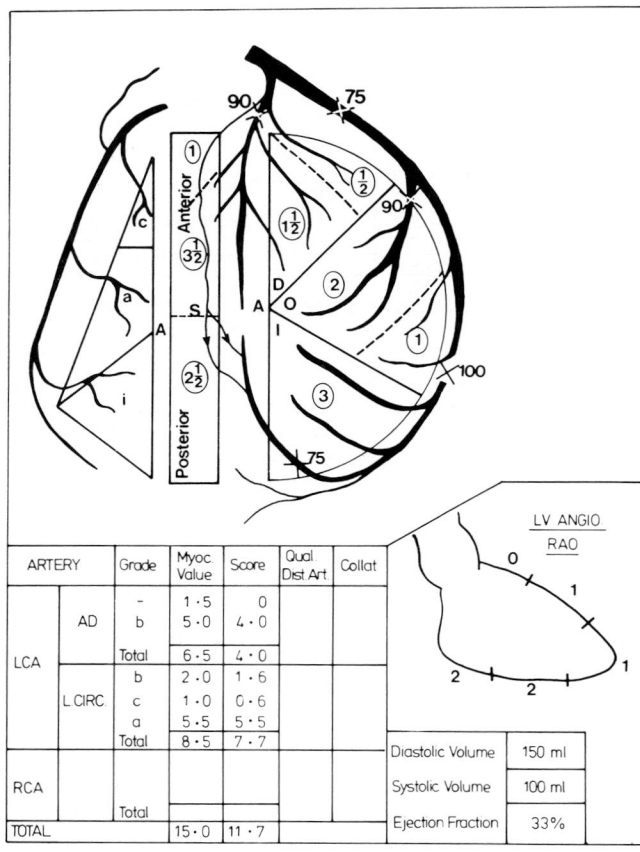

Figure 7B-3 Diagrammatic presentation in a diseased left dominant coronary tree. The LAD artery is shorter than average, while the posterior descending artery is correspondingly longer and arises from the circumflex artery (value = 2.5). The right coronary artery is small and does not supply the left ventricle. Even severe narrowing or occlusion of the RCA would not affect the myocardial score.

APPENDIX **7C**

MULTIVARIATE LOGISTIC ANALYSIS OF INCREMENTAL RISK FACTORS FOR HOSPITAL DEATH AFTER CABG (GLH)

Table 7C-1 Variables fitted to the model for hospital deaths (10) using logistic regression analysis of 661 patients undergoing CABG (GLH; 1980–1982).

Variable	Decrease in χ^2
Bypass time ≥ 135 min	16.20
Bypass time (continuous)	13.15
Endarterectomy	9.65
Age ≥ 60 yr	9.50
Aortic clamp time ≥ 85 min	8.37
Frank diabetes	7.42
Age (continuous)	5.10
Aortic clamp time (continuous)	5.05
Internal mammary artery graft	3.59
Hypertension	2.85
Ejection fraction (continuous)	2.43
Left main stenosis	2.34
Cardioplegia	2.30
Left ventricular end-diastolic pressure (continuous)	1.46
Left ventricular end-systolic volume (continuous)	1.43
Number of occluded arteries (0–7)	1.16
Number of proximal anastomoses (1–5)	1.05
Angina severity (0–4)	0.88
Number of distal anastomoses (1–7)	0.86
Myocardial score (continuous)	0.76
Preoperative ventricular tachycardia	0.66
Enzyme level day 1 (AST ≥ 100)	0.60
Emergency operation	0.57
Number of preoperative infarcts (1–4)	0.41
Left ventricular end-diastolic volume (continuous)	0.24
Grade of dyspnea (0–4)	0.04
Sex	0.02
Angina pattern (stable, unstable)	0.01

NOTE: A number of other variables with no hospital deaths could not be fitted.

REFERENCES

A

1. Adam M, Mitchell BF, Gambert CJ, Geisler GF: Long-term results with aorto-to-coronary artery bypass grafts. *Ann Thorac Surg* 14:1, 1972.

2. Anderson RP, Rahimtoola SH, Bouchek LI, Starr A: The prognosis of patients with coronary artery disease after coronary bypass operations. *Circulation* 50:274, 1974.

3. Ashburn WL, Braunwald E, Simon AL, Peterson KL, Gault JH: Myocardial perfusion imaging with radioactive-labeled particles injected directly into the coronary circulation of patients with coronary artery disease. *Circulation* 44:851, 1971.

4. Assad-Morell JL, Frye RL, Connolly DC, Davis GD, Pluth JR, Wallace RB, Barnhorst DA, Elveback LR, Danielson GK: Aorto-coronary artery saphenous vein bypass surgery: Clinical and angiographic results. *Mayo Clin Proc* 50:379, 1975.

5. Austen WG, Edwards JE, Frye RL, Gensini GG, Goh VL, Griffith LSC, McGoon DC, Murphy ML, Roe BB: AHA committee report: A reporting system on patients evaluated for coronary artery disease. *Circulation* 51(suppl):5, 1975.

6. Aldridge HE: Special projections: A generation of coronary arteriography. *Cleve Clin Q* 49:145, 1979.

7. Aldridge HE, McLoughlin JM, Taylor KW: Improved diagonals in coronary arteriography with routine use of 110° oblique views and cranial and caudal angulations: Comparison with standard transverse oblique views in 100 patients. *Am J Cardiol* 36:468, 1975.

8. Arani DT, Bunnell IL, Greene DG: Lordotic right posterior oblique projections of the left coronary artery: A special view for special anatomy. *Circulation* 52:504, 1975.

9. Alderman EL, Fisher LD, Litwin P, Kaiser GC, Myers WO, Maynard C, Levine F, Schloss M: Results of coronary artery surgery in patients with poor left ventricular function (CASS). *Circulation* 68:785, 1983.

B

1. Bryson AL, Parisi AF, Schnechter E, Wolfson S: Life-threatening ventricular arrhythmias induced by exercise: Cessation after coronary artery bypass surgery. *Am J Cardiol* 32:995, 1973.

2. Bartley TD, Bigelow JC, Page US: Aortocoronary bypass grafting with multiple sequential anastomoses to a single vein. *Arch Surg* 105:915, 1972.

3. Berger HJ, Reduto LA, Johnstone DE, Borkowski H, Sands JM, Cohen LS, Langou RA, Gottschalk A, Zaret BL, Pytlik L: Global and regional left ventricular response to bicycle exercise in coronary artery disease. *Am J Med* 66:13, 1979.

4. Bourassa MG, Lesperance J, Campeau L, Saltiel J: Fate of left ventricular contraction following aortocoronary venous grafts: Early and late postoperative modifications. *Circulation* 46:724, 1972.

5. Bulkley BH: Why coronary bypass grafts fail: Early and late pathologic changes. *J Cardiovasc Med* Nov: 1027, 1980.

6. Bourassa MG, Lesperance J, Corbara F, Saltiel J, Campeau L: Progression of obstructive coronary artery disease 5 to 7 years after aortocoronary bypass surgery. *Circulation* 58(suppl I):I-100, 1978.

7. Bulkley BH, Hutchins GM: Accelerated "atherosclerosis": A morphologic study of 97 saphenous vein coronary artery bypass grafts. *Circulation* 55:163, 1977.

8. Barboriak JJ, Pintar K, Korns ME: Atherosclerosis in aortocoronary vein grafts. *Lancet* 2:621, 1974.

9. Barboriak JJ, Pintar K, Van Horn DL, Batayias GE, Korns ME: Pathologic findings in the aortocoronary vein grafts: A scanning electron microscopic study. *Atherosclerosis* 29:69, 1978.

10. Bruschke AVG, Proudfit WL, Sones FM Jr: Progress study of 590 consecutive nonsurgical cases of coronary artery disease followed 5–9 years. I. Arteriographic correlations. *Circulation* 47:1147, 1973.

11. Barnes GK, Ray MJ, Oberman A, Kouchoukos NT: Changes in working status of patients following coronary bypass surgery. *JAMA* 238:1259, 1977.

12. Bartel AG, Behar VS, Peter RH, Orgain ES, Kong Y: Exercise stress testing in evaluation of aortocoronary bypass surgery. *Circulation* 48:141, 1973.

13. Balcon R, Honey M, Richards AF, Sturridge MF, Walsh W, Wilkinson RK, Wright JEC: Evaluation by exercise testing and atrial pacing of aorto-coronary bypass surgery. *Br Heart J* 36:841, 1974.

14. Brawley RK, Merrill W, Gott VL, Donahoo JS, Watkins L Jr, Gardner TJ: Unstable angina pectoris: Factors influencing operative risks. *Ann Surg* 191:745, 1980.

15. Burggraf GW, Parker JO: Prognosis in coronary artery disease: Angiographic, hemodynamic, and clinical factors. *Circulation* 51:146, 1975.

16. Bigelow JC, Bartley TD, Page US, Krause AH Jr: Long-term follow-up of sequential aortocoronary venous grafts. *Ann Thorac Surg* 22:507, 1976.

17. Braum RS, Alvarez H III, Cobb LA: Survival after resuscitation from out-of-hospital ventricular fibrillation. *Circulation* 50:1231, 1974.

18. Brody WR, Angell WW, Kosek JC: Histologic fate of the venous coronary artery bypass in dogs. *Am J Pathol* 66:111, 1972.

19. Barboriak JJ, Van Horn DL, Pintar K, Batayias GE, Korns ME: Late lesions in aorta-coronary artery vein grafts. *J Thorac Cardiovasc Surg* 71:673, 1976.

20. Bigger JT Jr, Heller CA, Wenger TL, Weld FM: Risk stratification after acute myocardial infarction. *Am J Cardiol* 42:202, 1978.

21. Barratt-Boyes BG: Cardiothoracic surgery in the Antipodes. *J Thorac Cardiovasc Surg* 78:804, 1979.

22. Bulkley BH, Hutchins GM: Myocardial consequences of coronary artery bypass surgery: The paradox of necrosis in areas of revascularization. *Circulation* 56:906, 1977.

23. Baur HR, Peterson TA, Arnar O, Gannon PG, Gobel FL: Predictors of perioperative myocardial infarction in coronary artery operation. *Ann Thorac Surg* 31:36, 1981.

24. Brewer DL, Bilbro RH, Bartel AG: Myocardial infarction as a complication of coronary bypass surgery. *Circulation* 48:58, 1973.

25. Bedard P, Keon WJ, Brais M, Goldstein W: First septal artery: Direct or indirect grafting. *Circulation* 61,62(suppl I):I-116, 1980.

26. Bourassa MG: The role of bypass surgery in isolated left anterior descending artery stenosis or occlusion. *Circulation* 61:875, 1980 (editorial).

27. Baughman BL, Maroko PR, Vatner SF: Effects of coronary artery reperfusion on myocardial infarct size and survival in conscious dogs. *Circulation* 63:317, 1981.

28. Berg R Jr, Kendall RW, Duvoisin GE, Ganji JH, Rudy LW, Everhart FJ: Acute myocardial infarction: A surgical emergency. *J Thorac Cardiovasc Surg* 70:432, 1975.

29. Boudoulas H, Snyder GL, Lewis RP, Kates RE, Karayannacos PE, Vasko JS: Safety and rationale for continuation of propranolol therapy during coronary bypass operation. *Ann Thorac Surg* 26:222, 1978.

30. Bolooki H: Myocardial revascularization after acute infarction. *Am J Cardiol* 36:395, 1975.

31. Bruschke AVG, Wijers TS, Kolsters W, Landmann J: The anatomic evolution of coronary artery disease demonstrated by coronary arteriography in 256 nonoperated patients. *Circulation* 63:527, 1981.

32. Bemis CE, Gorlin R, Kemp HG, Herman MV: Progression of coronary artery disease: A clinical angiographic study. *Circulation* 47:455, 1973.

33. Brandt PWT, Partridge JB, Wattie WJ: Coronary arteriography: A method of presentation of the arteriogram report and a scoring system. *Clin Radiol* 28:361, 1977.

34. Bruce RA, De Rouen TA, Hammermeister KE: Noninvasive screening criteria for enhanced 4-year survival after aortocoronary bypass surgery. *Circulation* 60:638, 1979.

35. Bertolasi CA, Tronge JE, Riccitelli MA, Villamayor RM, Zuffardi E: Natural history of unstable angina with medical or surgical therapy. *Chest* 70:596, 1976.

36. Bourassa MG, Campeau L, Lesperance J, Grondin CM: Changes in graft and coronary arteries after saphenous vein aortocoronary bypass surgery: Results at repeat angiography. *Circulation* 65(suppl II):II-90, 1982.

37. Baum RS, Alvarez H III, Cobb LA: Survival after resuscitation from out-of-hospital ventricular fibrillation. *Circulation* 50:1231, 1974.

38. Borer JS, Rosing DR, Miller RH, Stark RM, Kent KM, Bacharach SL, Green MV, Lake CR, Cohen H, Holmes D, Donohue D, Epstein SE: Natural history of left ventricular function during 1 year after acute myocardial infarction: Comparison with clinical, electrocardiographic and biochemical determinations. *Am J Cardiol* 46:1, 1980.

39. Borer JS, Bacharach SL, Green MV, Kent KM, Epstein SE, Johnston GS: Real-time radionuclide cineangiography in the noninvasive evaluation of global and regional left ventricular function at rest and during exercise in patients with coronary artery disease. *N Engl J Med* 296:839, 1977.

40. Bonow RO, Kent KM, Rosing DR, Lipson LC, Bacharach SL, Green MV, Epstein SE: Improved left ventricular diastolic filling in patients with coronary artery diseases after percutaneous transluminal coronary angioplasty. *Circulation* 66:1159, 1982.

41. Bonow RO, Bacharach SL, Green MV, Kent KM, Rosing DR, Lipson LC, Leon MB, Epstein SE: Impaired left ventricular diastolic filling in patients with coronary artery disease: Assessment with radionuclide angiography. *Circulation* 64:315, 1981.

42. Berg R Jr, Selinger SL, Leonard JJ, Grunwald RP, O'Grady WP: Immediate coronary artery bypass for acute evolving myocardial infarction. *J Thorac Cardiovasc Surg* 81:493, 1981.

43. Brower RW, van Eijk KF, Spek J, Bos E: Sequential versus conventional coronary artery bypass graft surgery in matched patient groups. *Thorac Cardiovasc Surg* 29:158, 1981.

44. Brown CA, Hutter AM, De Sanctis RW, Gold HK, Leinbach RC, Roberts-Niles A, Austen WG, Buckley MJ: Prospective study of medical and urgent surgical therapy in randomizable patients with unstable angina pectoris: Results of in-hospital and chronic mortality and morbidity. *Am Heart J* 102:959, 1981.

45. Buda AJ, Macdonald IL, Anderson MJ, Strauss HD, David TE, Berman ND: Long-term results following coronary bypass operation: Importance of preoperative factors and complete revascularization. *J Thorac Cardiovasc Surg* 82:383, 1981.

46. Bunnell IL, Greene DG, Tandon RN, Arani DT: The half axial projection: A new look at the proximal left coronary artery. *Circulation* 48:1151, 1973.

47. Begmans RF: Oblique, caudal and cranial x-ray beam angulation with coronary angiography: A schematic approach to the optimum visualization of the coronary arteries. *Medicamundi* 21:114, 1976.

48. Barner HB, Swartz MT, Mudd JG, Tyras DH: Late patency of the internal mammary artery as a coronary bypass conduit. *Ann Thorac Surg* 34:408, 1982.

49. Batist G, Blaker M, Kosinski E, Brown E, Christlieb R, Leland S Jr, Neptune W: Coronary bypass surgery in juvenile onset diabetes. *Am Heart J* 106:51, 1983.

50. Brindis RG, Brundage BH, Ullyot DJ, McKay CW, Lipton MJ, Turley K: Graft patency in patients with coronary artery bypass operation complicated by perioperative myocardial infarction. *JACC* 3:55, 1984.

51. Brundage BH, Massie BM, Botvinick EH: Improved regional ventricular function after successful surgical revascularization. *JACC* 3:902, 1984.

52. Bates ER, Vogel RA, LeFree MT, Kirlin PC, O'Neill WW, Pitt B: The chronic coronary flow reserve provided by saphenous vein bypass grafts as determined by digital coronary radiography. *Am Heart J* 108:462, 1984.

53. Bittar N, Kroncke GM, Dacumos GC, Rowe GG, Young WP, Chopra PS, Folts JD, Kahn DR: Vein graft flow and reactive hyperemia in the human heart. *J Thorac Cardiovasc Surg* 64:855, 1972.

54. Bonow RO, Vitale DF, Bacharach SL, Frederick TM, Kent KM, Green MV: Asynchronous left ventricular regional function and impaired global diastolic filling in patients with coronary artery disease: reversal after coronary angioplasty. *Circulation* 71:297, 1985.

C

1. Cline RE, Armstrong RG, Stanford W: Successful myocardial revascularization after ventricular fibrillation induced by treadmill exercise. *J Thorac Cardiovasc Surg* 65:802, 1973.

2. Conde CA, Meller J, Espinoza J, Donoso E, Dack S: Disappearance of abnormal Q waves after aortocoronary bypass surgery. *Am J Cardiol* 36:889, 1975.

3. Chatterjee K, Swan HJC, Parmley WW, Sustaita H, Marcus H, Matloff J: Depression of left ventricular function due to acute myocardial ischemia and its reversal following aortocoronary saphenous vein bypass. *N Engl J Med* 286:117, 1972.

4. Chatterjee K, Swan HJC, Parmley WW, Sustaita H, Marcus H, Matloff J: Influence of direct myocardial revascularization on left ventricular asynergy and function in patients with coronary artery disease, with and without previous myocardial infarction. *Circulation* 47:276, 1973.

5. Chatterjee K, Matloff JM, Swan HJC, Ganz W, Kaushik VS, Magnusson P, Henis MM, Forrester JS: Abnormal regional metabolism and mechanical function in patients with ischemic heart disease: Improvement after successful regional revascularization by aortocoronary bypass. *Circulation* 52:390, 1975.

6. Cheanvechai C, Groves LK, Reyes EA, Shirey EK, Sones FM Jr: Manual coronary endarterectomy. *J Thorac Cardiovasc Surg* 70:524, 1975.

7. Campeau L, Lesperance J, Corbara F, Hermann J, Grondin CM, Bourassa MG: Aortocoronary saphenous vein bypass graft changes 5 to 7 years after surgery. *Circulation* 58(suppl I):I-170, 1978.

8. Campeau L, Lesperance J, Hermann J, Corbara F, Grondin CM, Bourassa MG: Loss of the improvement of angina between 1 and 7 years after aortocoronary bypass surgery. *Circulation* 60(suppl I):I-1, 1979.

9. Chaitman BR, Bourassa MG, Heitz A, Campeau L: Influence of left ventricular function and other parameters on early and late mortality following coronary artery bypass surgery. *Can J Surg* 20:119, 1977.

10. Conti VR, Bertranou EG, Blackstone EH, Kirklin JW, Digerness SB: Cold cardioplegia versus hypothermia for myocardial protection: Randomized clinical study. *J Thorac Cardiovasc Surg* 76:577, 1978.

11. Cukingnan RA, Carey JS, Wittig JH, Brown BG: Influence of complete coronary revascularization on relief of angina. *J Thorac Cardiovasc Surg* 79:188, 1980.

12. Cohen MV, Cohn PF, Herman MV, Gorlin R: Diagnosis and prognosis of main left coronary artery obstruction. *Circulation* 45,46(suppl I):I-57, 1972.

13. Cohn LH, Alpert J, Koster JK Jr, Mee RBB, Collins JJ Jr: Changing indications for the surgical treatment of unstable angina. *Arch Surg* 113:1312, 1978.

14. Corbalan R, Verrier RL, Lown B: Differing mechanisms for ventricular vulnerability during coronary occlusion and release. *Am Heart J* 92:223, 1976.

15. Cohn PF, Harris P, Barry WH, Rosati RA, Rosenbaum P, Waternaux C: Prognostic importance of anginal symptoms in angiographically defined coronary artery disease. *Am J Cardiol* 47:233, 1981.

16. Chesebro JH, Clements IP, Fuster V, Elveback LR, Smith HC, Bardsley WT, Frye RL, Holmes DR Jr, Vlietstra RE, Pluth JR, Wallace RB, Puga FJ, Orszulak TA, Piehler JM, Schaff HV, Danielson GK: A platelet-inhibitor-drug trial in coronary-artery bypass operations: Benefit of perioperative dipyridamole and aspirin therapy on early postoperative vein-graft patency. *N Engl J Med* 307:73, 1982.

17. Chapman BL: Relation of cardiac complications to SGOT level in acute myocardial infarction. *Br Heart J* 34:890, 1972.

18. Chesebro JH, Clements IP, Fuster V, Elveback LR, Holmes DR, Pluth JR: Benefit of perioperative dipyridamole plus aspirin therapy for late postoperative aortocoronary vein graft patency. *Circulation* 66(suppl II):II-94, 1982.

19. Campeau L: Survival following aortocoronary bypass graft surgery. *Cleve Clin Q* 45:160, 1978.

20. Catinella FP, Cunningham JN, Srungaram RK, Baumann FG, Nathan IM, Glassman EA, Knopp EA, Spencer FC: The factors influencing early patency of coronary artery bypass vein grafts. *J Thorac Cardiovasc Surg* 83:686, 1982.

21. Chesebro JH, Ritman EL, Frye RL, Smith HC, Connolly DC, Rutherford BD, Davis GD, Danielson GK, Pluth JR, Barnhorst DA, Wallace RB: Videometric analysis of regional left ventricular function before and after aortocoronary artery bypass surgery. *J Clin Invest* 58:1339, 1976.

22. Coles JG, Del Campo C, Ahmed SN, Corpus R, MacDonald AC, Goldbach MM, Coles JC: Improved long-term survival following myocardial revascularization in patients with severe left ventricular dysfunction. *J Thorac Cardiovasc Surg* 81:846, 1981.

23. Cosgrove DM, Loop FD, Saunders CL, Lytle BW, Kramer JR: Should coronary arteries with less than fifty percent stenosis be bypassed? *J Thorac Cardiovasc Surg* 82:520, 1981.

24. Craver JM, Murphy DA, Jones EL, Curling PE, Bone DK, Smith RB III, Perdue GD, Hatcher CR Jr, Kandrach M: Concomitant carotid and coronary artery reconstruction. *Ann Surg* 195:712, 1982.

25. Califf RM, Tomabechi Y, Lee KL, Phillips H, Pryor DB, Harrell FE Jr, Harris PJ, Phil D, Peter RH, Behar VS, Kong Y, Rosati RA: Outcome in one-vessel coronary artery disease. *Circulation* 64:283, 1983.

26. Chaitman BR, Alderman EL, Sheffield LT, Tong T, Fisher L, Mock MB, Weins RD, Kaiser GC, Roitman D, Berger R, Gersh B, Schaff H, Bourassa MG, Killip T: Use of survival analysis to determine the clinical significance of new Q waves after coronary bypass surgery. *Circulation* 67:302, 1983.

27. Chaitman BR, Davis K, Bourassa MG, Fisher LD, Fray D, Rogers WJ, Tyras KH, Mock M, Killip T: Prognostic importance of left main non-equivalent coronary disease (CASS). *Circulation* 66(suppl II):II-10, 1982 (abstr).

28. Campeau L, Enjalbert M, Lesperance J, Vaislic C, Grondin CM, Bourassa MG: Atherosclerosis and late closure of aortocoronary saphenous vein grafts: Sequential angiographic studies at 2 weeks, 1 year, 5 to 7 years, and 10 to 12 years after surgery. *Circulation* 68(suppl II):II-1, 1983.

29. Chaitman BR, Fisher LD, Bourassa MG, Davis K, Rogers WJ, Maynard C, Tyras DH, Berger RL, Judkins MP, Ringqvist I, Mock MB, Killip T: Effect of coronary bypass surgery on survival patterns in subsets of patients with left main coronary artery disease. *Am J Cardiol* 48:765, 1981.

30. Cohen M, Wienar I, Pichard A, Holt J, Smith H, Gorlin R: Determinants of ventricular tachycardia in patients with coronary artery disease and ventricular aneurysm: Clinical, hemodynamic and angiographic factors. *Am J Cardiol* 51:61, 1983.

31. CASS Principal Investigators and Their Associates: Coronary Artery Surgery Study (CASS): A randomized trial of coronary artery bypass surgery: Survival data. *Circulation* 68:939, 1983.

32. CASS Principal Investigators and Their Associates: Myocardial infarction and mortality in the coronary artery surgery (CASS) randomized trial. *New Engl J Med* 310:750, 1984.

33. Chesebro JH, Fuster V, Elveback LR, Clements IP, Smith HC, Holmes DR Jr, Bardsley WT, Pluth JR, Wallace RB, Puga FJ, Orszulak TA, Piehler JM, Danielson GK, Schaff HV, Frye RL: Effect of dipyridamole and aspirin on late vein-graft patency after coronary bypass operations. *New Engl J Med* 310:209, 1984.

34. Cobanoglu A, Freimanis I, Grunkemeier G, Lambert L, Anderson V, Nunley D, Garcia C, Starr A: Enhanced late survival following coronary artery bypass graft operation for unstable versus chronic angina. *Ann Thorac Surg* 37:52, 1984.

35. Campeau L, Enjalbert M, Lespérance J, Bourassa MG, Kwiterovich P Jr, Wacholder S, Sniderman A: The relation of risk factors to the development of atherosclerosis in saphenous-vein bypass grafts and the progression of disease in the native circulation. *NEJM* 311:1329, 1984.

36. Cosgrove DM, Loop FD, Lytle BW, Baillot R, Gill CC, Golding LAR, Taylor PC, Goormastic M: Primary myocardial revascularization. *J Thorac Cardiovasc Surg* 88:673, 1984.

D

1. deSoyza N, Murphy ML, Bissett JK, Kane JJ, Doherty JE III: Ventricular arrhythmias in chronic stable angina pectoris with surgical or medical treatment. *Ann Intern Med* 89:10, 1978.

2. DeRouen TA, Hammermeister KE, Dodge HT: Comparisons of the effects on survival after coronary artery surgery in subgroups of patients from the Seattle Heart Watch. *Circulation* 63:537, 1981.

3. De Feyter PJ, van Eenige MJ, Dighton DH, Visser FC: Prognostic value of exercise testing, coronary angiography and left ventriculography 6–8 weeks after myocardial infarction. *Circulation* 66:527, 1982.

4. DeWood MA, Spores J, Notske RN, Lang HT, Shields JP, Simpson CS, Rudy LW, Grunwald R: Medical and surgical management of myocardial infarction. *Am J Cardiol* 44:1356, 1979.

5. DeWood MA, Spores J, Notske R, Mouser LT, Burroughs R, Golden MS, Lang HT: Prevalence of total coronary occlusion during the early hours of transmural myocardial infarction. *N Engl J Med* 303:897, 1980.

6. Detre K, Peduzzi P, Murphy M, Hultgreen H, Thomsen J, Oberman A, Takaro T: Effect of bypass surgery on survival in patients in low- and high-risk subgroups delineated by the use of simple clinical variables. *Circulation* 63:1329, 1981.

7. David PR, Waters DD, Scholl JM, Crepeau J, Szlachcic J, Lesperance J, Hudon G, Bourassa MG: Percutaneous transluminal coronary angioplasty in patients with variant angina. *Circulation* 66:695, 1982.

8. Douglas JS Jr, Gruentzig AR, King SB III, Hollman J: Long-term results of percutaneous transluminal angioplasty for aortocoronary saphenous vein graft stenosis. *Circulation* 66(suppl II):II-124, 1982 (abstr).

9. Dorros G, Stertzer SH, Cowley M, Kent K, Williams D: Complex transluminal coronary angioplasty: Multivessel disease and multiple dilations. *Circulation* 66(suppl II):II-329, 1982 (abstr).

10. Detre KM, Peduzzi P, Hammermeister KE, Murphy ML, Hultgren HN, Takaro T: Five-year effect of medical and surgical therapy on resting left ventricular function in stable angina: Veterans Administration Cooperative Study. *Am J Cardiol* 53:444, 1984.

11. Dewanjee MK, Tago M, Josa M, Fuster V, Kaye MP: Quantification of platelet retention in aortocoronary femoral vein bypass graft in dogs treated with dipyridamole and aspirin. *Circulation* 69:350, 1984.

12. Deumite NJ, Chaitman BR, Davis KB, Killip T, Frommer PL, Rogers WJ: Asymptomatic left main coronary artery disease (CASS). *JACC* 5:518, 1985 (abstr).

E

1. Ecker RR, Mullins CB, Grammer JC, Rea WJ, Atkins JM: Control of intractable ventricular tachycardia by coronary revascularization. *Circulation* 44:666, 1971.

2. Effler DR, Sones FM Jr, Favaloro R, Groves LK: Coronary endarterectomy with patch-graft reconstruction: Clinical experience with 34 cases. *Ann Surg* 162:590, 1965.

3. Edwards WS, Jones WB, Dear HD, Kerr AR: Direct surgery for coronary artery disease: Techniques for left anterior descending coronary artery bypass. *JAMA* 211:1182, 1970.

4. Effler DB, Sones FM Jr, Groves LK, Suarez E: Myocardial revascularization by Vineberg's internal mammary artery implant: Evaluation of postoperative results. *J Thorac Cardiovasc Surg* 50:527, 1965.

5. European Coronary Surgery Study Group: Prospective randomized study of coronary artery bypass surgery in stable angina pectoris: A progress report on survival. *Circulation* 65(suppl II):II-78, 1982.

6. Ennix CL Jr, Lawrie GM, Morris GC Jr, Crawford ES, Howell JF, Reardon MJ, Weatherford SL: Improved results of carotid endarterectomy in patients with symptomatic coronary disease: An analysis of 1,546 consecutive carotid operations. *Stroke* 10:122, 1979.

7. Epstein SE, Palmeri ST, Patterson RE: Evaluation of patients after acute myocardial infarction: Indications for cardiac catheterization and surgical intervention. *New Engl J Med* 307:1487, 1982.

8. Eldh P, Silverman JF: Methods of studying the proximal left anterior descending coronary artery. *Radiology* 113:738, 1974.

9. Elliott LP, Bream PR, Soto B, Russell RO Jr, Rogers WJ, Mantle MA, Hood WP Jr: The significance of the caudal-left anterior oblique view in analyzing the left main coronary artery and its major branches. *Radiology* 139:39, 1981.

10. Elliott LP, Green CE: The importance of angled right anterior oblique views in improving visualization of the coronary arteries. I. Caudocranial view. *Radiology* 142:631, 1982.

11. Enjalbert M, Campeau L, Lesperance J, Bourassa MG: Progression of coronary artery disease 10 years after aortocoronary bypass surgery. *Circulation* 66(suppl II):II-246, 1982 (abstr).

12. European Coronary Surgery Study Group: Long-term results of prospective randomized study of coronary artery bypass surgery in stable angina pectoris. *Lancet:* 1173, November 27, 1982.

13. Elayda MA, Hall RJ, Gray AG, Mathur VS, Cooley DA: Coronary revascularization in the elderly patient. *JACC* 3:1398, 1984.

F

1. Furuse A, Klopp EH, Brawley RK, Gott VL: Hemodynamics of aorto-to-coronary artery bypass: Experimental and analytical studies. *Ann Thorac Surg* 14:282, 1972.

2. Fowler BN, Jacobs ML, Zir L, Dinsmore RE, Vezerides MP, Daggett WM: Late graft patency and symptom relief after aorta-coronary bypass graft. *J Thorac Cardiovasc Surg* 79:288, 1980.

3. Frick MH, Harjola PT, Valle M: Work status after coronary bypass surgery: A prospective randomized study with ergometric and angiographic correlations. *Acta Med Scand* 206:61, 1979.

4. Favaloro RG: Saphenous vein graft in the surgical treatment of coronary artery disease: Operative technique. *J Thorac Cardiovasc Surg* 58:178, 1969.

5. Ferrans VJ, Jones M, Roberts WC: The pathology of saphenous vein aortocoronary bypass grafts, in V Gallucci, RM Bini, G Thiene (eds): *Proceedings of the International Symposium on Selected Topics in Cardiac Surgery.* Bologna, Italy: Patron Editore, 1980, p 423.

6. Flemma RJ, Johnson WD, Lepley D Jr: Triple aorto-coronary vein bypass as treatment for coronary insufficiency. *Arch Surg* 103:82, 1971.

7. Faulkner SL, Stoney WS, Alford WC, Thomas CS, Burrus GS, Frist RS, Page HL: Ischemic cardiomyopathy: Medical versus surgical treatment. *J Thorac Cardiovasc Surg* 74:77, 1977.

8. Feldman RL, Nichols WW, Pepine CJ, Conetta DA, Conti CR: The coronary hemodynamics of left main and branch coronary stenoses: The effects of reduction in stenosis diameter, stenosis length, and number of stenoses. *J Thorac Cardiovasc Surg* 77:377, 1979.

9. Friesinger GC, Page EE, Ross RS: Prognostic significance of coronary arteriography. *Trans Assoc Am Physicians* 83:78, 1970.

10. Forrester JS, Diamond GA, Swan HFC: Correlative classification of clinical and hemodynamic function after acute myocardial infarction. *Am J Cardiol* 39:137, 1977.

11. Faulkner SL, Fisher RD, Conkle DM, Page DL, Bender HW: Effect of blood flow rate on subendothelial proliferation in venous autografts used as arterial substitutes. *Circulation* 51,52(suppl I):I-163, 1975.

12. Fletcher PJ, Pfeffer JM, Pfeffer MC, Braunwald E: Left ventricular diastolic pressure-volume relations in rats with healed myocardial infarction: Effects on systolic function. *Circ Res* 49:618, 1981.

13. Frist WH, Palacious I, Powell WJ Jr: Effect of hypoxia on myocardial relaxations in isometric cat papillary muscle. *J Clin Invest* 61:1218, 1978.

14. Ferguson DW, Kirchner P, Kioschos JM, Marcus ML, White CW: Heterogeneity of left ventricular improvement in acute myocardial infarction: Role of persistent total coronary occlusion. *Circulation* 66(suppl II):II-87, 1982 (abstr).

15. Foster ED, Fisher LD, Kaiser GC, Myers WO, Principal investigators of CASS and their associates: Comparison of operative mortality and morbidity for initial and repeat coronary artery bypass grafting: The Coronary Artery Surgery Study (CASS) registry experience. *Ann Thorac Surg* 38:563, 1984.

G

1. Guinn GA, Mathur VS: Surgical versus medical treatment for stable angina pectoris: Prospective randomized study with 1- to 4-year follow-up. *Ann Thorac Surg* 22:524, 1976.

2. Grow JB Sr, Brantigan CO: The diamond anastomosis: A technique for creating a right angle side-to-side vascular anastomosis. *J Thorac Cardiovasc Surg* 69:188, 1975.

3. Griffith LSC, Bulkley BH, Hutchins GM, Brawley RK: Occlusive changes at the coronary artery-bypass graft anastomosis: Morphologic study of 95 grafts. *J Thorac Cardiovasc Surg* 73:668, 1977.

4. Guthaner DF, Robert EW, Alderman EL, Wexler L: Long-term serial angiographic studies after coronary artery bypass surgery. *Circulation* 60:250, 1979.

5. Grondin CM, Campeau L, Lesperance J, Solymoss C, Vouhe P, Castonguay YR, Meere C, Bourassa MG: Atherosclerotic changes in coronary vein grafts six years after operation: Angiographic aspect in 110 patients. *J Thorac Cardiovasc Surg* 77:24, 1979.

6. Garrett HE, Dennis EW, DeBakey ME: Aortocoronary bypass with saphenous vein graft: Seven-year follow-up. *JAMA* 223:792, 1973.

7. Green GE, Stertzer SH, Reppert EH: Coronary arterial bypass grafts. *Ann Thorac Surg* 5:443, 1968.

8. Griffith LSC, Achuff SC, Conti CR, Humphries JO, Brawley RK, Gott VL, Ross RS: Changes in intrinsic coronary circulation and segmental ventricular motion after saphenous vein coronary bypass graft surgery. *N Engl J Med* 288:589, 1973.

9. Gensini GG: *Coronary Arteriography*. Mt. Kisco, NY: Futura, 1975.

10. Gundry SR, Jones M, Ishihara T, Ferrans VJ: Intraoperative trauma to human saphenous veins: Scanning electron microscopic comparison of preparation techniques. *Ann Thorac Surg* 30:40, 1980.

11. Geisler GF, Adam M, Mitchel BF, Lambert CJ, Thiele JP: Treatment of severe coronary artery disease with 5, 6 and 7 saphenous vein bypasses: Review of 131 consecutive patients. *Ann Thorac Surg* 24:246, 1977.

12. Grondin CM, Limet R: Vein grafts to left-sided arteries: Passage through the transverse sinus. *Ann Thorac Surg* 21:348, 1976.

13. Gould KL, Schelbert HR, Phelps ME, Hoffman EJ: Noninvasive assessment of coronary stenoses with myocardial perfusion imaging during pharmacologic coronary vasodilation. V. Detection of 47 percent diameter stenosis with intravenous nitrogen-13 ammonia and emission-computer tomography in intact dogs. *Am J Cardiol* 43:200, 1979.

14. Gruentzig AR, Senning A, Siegenthaler, WE: Nonoperative dilation of coronary artery stenosis: Percutaneous transluminal coronary angioplasty. *N Engl J Med* 301:62, 1979.

15. Gundry SR, Jones M, Ishihara T, Ferrans VJ: Optimal preparation techniques for human saphenous vein grafts. *Surgery* 88:785, 1980.

16. Guthaner D, Wexler L: New aspects of coronary angiography. *Radiol Clin North Am* 18:501, 1980.

17. Green CE, Elliott LP: The importance of angled right anterior oblique views in improving visualization of the coronary arteries. II. Craniocaudal view. *Radiology* 142:637, 1982.

18. Greene DG, Bunnell IL, Arani DT, Schimert G, Lajos TZ, Lee AB, Tandon RN, Zimdahl WT, Bozer JM, Kohn RM, Visco JP, Dean DC, Smith GL: Long-term survival after coronary bypass surgery: Comparison of various subsets of patients with general population. *Br Heart J* 45:417, 1981.

19. Ganz W, Buchbinder N, Marcus H, Mondkar A, Maddahi J, Charuzi Y, O'Connor L, Shell W, Fishbein M, Kass RA, Miyamoto A, Swan HJC: Intracoronary thrombolysis in evolving myocardial infarction. *Am Heart J* 101:4, 1981.

20. Gibbons EF, Hogan RD, Franklin TD, Nolting M, Weyman AE: The natural history of regional dysfunction in a canine preparation of chronic infarction. *Circulation* 71:394, 1985.

21. Gensini GG: A more meaningful scoring system for determining the severity of coronary heart disease. *Am J Cardiol* 51:606, 1983.

22. Gensini G, Giambartolomei A, Esente P, Archambault T, Shaw C: Natural history of coronary artery disease, angiographic findings in 830 patients: Importance and significance of the angiographic coronary score. *Circulation* 66(suppl II):II-369, 1982 (abstr).

23. Gensini GG: Coronary arteriography, in E Braunwald (ed): *Heart Disease: A Textbook of Cardiac Medicine*. Philadelphia: Saunders, 1980.

24. Gould BL, Clayton PD, Jensen RL, Liddle HV: Association between early graft patency and late outcome for patients undergoing artery bypass graft surgery. *Circulation* 69:569, 1984.

25. Greenfield JC, Rembert JC, Young WG, Oldham HN, Alexander JA, Sabiston DC: Studies of blood flow in aorta-to-coronary venous bypass grafts in man. *J Clin Invest* 51:2724, 1972.

26. Geha AS, Krone RJ, McCormick JR, Baue AE: Selection of coronary bypass: anatomic, physiological, and angiographic considerations of vein and mammary artery grafts. *J Thorac Cardiovasc Surg* 70:414, 1975.

27. Greene GE: Internal mammary artery-to-coronary artery anastomosis: Three-year experience with 165 patients. *Ann Thorac Surg* 14:260, 1972.

28. Grondin CM, Campeau L, Lespérance J, Enjalbert M, Bourassa MG: Comparison of late changes in internal mammary artery and saphenous vein grafts in two consecutive series of 10 years after operation. *Circulation* 70(Suppl I) I-208, 1984.

H

1. Hellman CK, Kamath ML, Schmidt DH, Anholm J, Balu F, Johnson WD: Improvement in left ventricular function after myocardial revascularization: Assessment by first-pass rest and exercise nuclear angiography. *J Thorac Cardiovasc Surg* 79:645, 1980.

2. Hamby RI, Aintablian A, Handler M, Voleti C, Weisz D, Garvey JW, Wisoff G: Aortocoronary saphenous vein bypass grafts: Long-term patency, morphology and blood flow in patients with patent grafts early after surgery. *Circulation* 60:901, 1979.

3. Hoffmann RG, Blumlein SL, Anderson AJ, Barboriak JJ, Walker JA, Rimm AA: The probability of surviving coronary bypass surgery: 5-year results from 1,718 patients. *JAMA* 243:1341, 1980.

4. Hellman C, Schmidt DH, Kamath ML, Anholm J, Blau F, Johnson WD: Bypass graft surgery in severe left ventricular dysfunction. *Circulation* 62(suppl I):I-103, 1980.

5. Hochberg MS, Merrill WH, Michaelis LL, McIntosh CL: Results of combined coronary endarterectomy and coronary bypass for diffuse coronary artery disease. *J Thorac Cardiovasc Surg* 75:38, 1978.

6. Hammermeister KE, DeRouen TA, Dodge HT: Effect of coronary surgery on survival in asymptomatic and minimally symptomatic patients. *Circulation* 61,62(suppl I):I-98, 1980.

7. Hung J, Kelly DT, Baird DK, Hendel PN, Leckie BD, Grant AF, Uren RF: Aorta-coronary bypass grafting in patients with severe left ventricular dysfunction. *J Thorac Cardiovasc Surg* 79:718, 1980.

8. Hammermeister KE, DeRouen TA, Dodge HT: Comparison of survival of medically and surgically treated coronary disease patients in Seattle Heart Watch: A nonrandomized study. *Circulation* 65(suppl II):II-53, 1982.

9. Heng MK, Norris RM, Singh BN, Partridge JB: Prognosis in unstable angina. *Br Heart J* 38:921, 1976.

10. Hertzer NR, Loop FD, Taylor PC, Beven EG: Staged and combined surgical approach to simultaneous carotid and coronary vascular disease. *Surgery* 84:803, 1978.

11. Harper RW, Gold HK, Leinbach RC: Acute myocardial infarction, in E Haber, PH Johnston, WG Austen (eds): *The Practice of Cardiology*. Boston: Little, Brown, 1980, p 310.

12. Hamer A, Vohra J, Hunt D, Sloman G: Prediction of sudden death by electrophysiologic studies in high-risk patients surviving acute myocardial infarction. *Am J Cardiol* 50:223, 1982.

13. Hacker RW, Torka M, von der Emde J: Life expectancy after coronary artery bypass surgery. *Thorac Cardiovasc Surg* 29:212, 1981.

14. Hasse J, Graedel E, Hofer H, Guggenheim R, Amsler B, Mihatsch MJ: Morphologic studies in saphenous vein grafts for aorto-coronary bypass surgery. II. Influence of a pressure-limited graft dilation. *Thorac Cardiovasc Surg* 29:38, 1981.

15. Higginbotham MB, Morris KG, Conn EH, Coleman RE, Cobb FR: Determinants of variable exercise performance among patients with severe left ventricular dysfunction. *Am J Cardiol* 51:52, 1983.

16. Hartzler GO, Rutherford BD, McConahay DR, McCallister SH: Simultaneous multiple lesion coronary angioplasty: A preferred therapy for patients with multiple vessel disease. *Circulation* 66(suppl II):II-5, 1982 (abstr).

17. Horton PD, Jennings HS, Kronenberg MW, Privette DC, Friesinger GC: The effect of myocardial infarct size on left ventricular exercise performance. *Circulation* 66(suppl II):II-264, 1982 (abstr).

18. Hossack KF, Bruce RA, Ivey TD, Kusumi F: Changes in cardiac functional capacity after coronary bypass surgery in relation to adequacy of revascularization. *JACC* 3:47, 1984.

19. Hossack KF, Bruce RA, Ivey TD, Kusumi F, Kannagi T: Improvement in aerobic and hemodynamic responses to exercise following aorta-coronary bypass grafting. *J Thorac Cardiovasc Surg* 87:901, 1984.

I

1. Itscoitz SB, Redwood DR, Stinson EB, Reis RL, Epstein SE: Saphenous vein bypass grafts: Long-term patency and effect on the native coronary circulation. *Am J Cardiol* 36:739, 1975.

J

1. Jengo JA, Oren V, Conant R, Brizendine M, Nelson T, Uszler JM, Mena I: Effects of maximal exercise stress on left ventricular function in patients with coronary artery disease using first-pass radionuclide angiocardiography. *Circulation* 59:60, 1979.

2. Jones EL, Craver JM, King SB III, Douglas JS, Bradford JM, Brown CM, Bone DK, Hatcher CR Jr: Clinical, anatomical, and functional descriptors influencing morbidity, survival, and adequacy of revascularization following coronary bypass. *Ann Surg* 192:390, 1980.

3. Jengo JA, Mena I, Blaufuss A, Criley JM: Evaluation of left ventricular function (ejection fraction and segmental wall motion) by single-pass radioisotope angiography. *Circulation* 57:326, 1978.

4. Johnson RA, Haber E, Austen WG: *The Practice of Cardiology*. Boston: Little, Brown, 1980.

5. Jones M, Conkle DM, Ferrans VJ, Robert WC, Levine FH, Melvin DB, Stinson EB: Lesions observed in arterial autogenous vein grafts: Light and electron microscopic evaluation. *Circulation* 47,48(suppl III):III-198, 1973.

6. James TN, Burch GE: Blood supply of the human interventricular septum. *Circulation* 17:391, 1958.

7. Jones EL, Douglas JS Jr, Craver JM, King SB III, Kaplan JA, Morgan EA, Hatcher CR Jr: Results of coronary revascularization in patients with recent myocardial infarction. *J Thorac Cardiovasc Surg* 76:545, 1978.

8. Johnson RA, Zir LM, Harper RW, Leinbach RC, Hutter AM Jr, Pohost GM, Block PC, Gold HK: Patterns of haemodynamic alteration during left ventricular ischaemia in man: Relation to angiographic extent of coronary artery disease. *Br Heart J* 41:441, 1979.

9. Johnson WD in MJ Koplitt, JB Borman (eds): *Cardiac Surgery Update in Jerusalem, 1982* (in press).

10. Jones EL, Craver JM, Guyton RA, Bone DK, Hatcher CR, Reichwald N: Importance of complete revascularization in performance of the coronary bypass operation. *Am J Cardiol* 51:7, 1983.

11. Josa M, Lie JT, Bianco RL, Kaye MP: Reduction of thrombosis in canine coronary bypass vein grafts with dipyridamole and aspirin. *Am J Cardiol* 47:1248, 1981.

12. Jones EL, Waites TF, Craver JM, Bradford JM, Douglas JS, King SB, Bone DK, Dorney ER, Clements SD, Thompkins T, Hatcher CR: Coronary bypass for relief of persistent pain following acute myocardial infarction. *Ann Thorac Surg* 32:33, 1981.

13. Jones EL, Waites TF, Craver JM, Bone DK, Hatcher CR, Thompkins T: Unstable angina pectoris: Comparison with the national cooperative study. *Ann Thorac Surg* 34:427, 1982.

14. Jones EL, Craver JM, Gruntzig AR, King SB III, Douglas JS, Bone DK, Guyton RG, Hatcher CR Jr: Percutaneous translu-

minal coronary angioplasty: Role of the surgeon. *Ann Thorac Surg* 34:493, 1982.

15. Johnson WD, Pedraza PM, Kayser KL: Coronary artery surgery in diabetics: 261 consecutive patients followed four to seven years. *Am Heart J* 104:823, 1982.

16. Jutzy KR, Berte LE, Alderman EL, Ratts J, Simpson JB: Coronary restenosis rates in a consecutive patient series one year post successful angioplasty. *Circulation* 66(suppl II):II-331, 1982 (abstr).

17. Jones EL, Craver JM, Michalik RA, Murphy DA, Guyton RA, Bone DK, Hatcher CR, Reichwald NA: Combined carotid and coronary operations: Where are they necessary? *J Thorac Cardiovasc Surg* 87:7, 1984.

K

1. Kakos GS, Oldham HN Jr, Dixon SH Jr, Davis RW, Hagen P, Sabiston DC Jr: Coronary artery hemodynamics after aorto-coronary artery vein bypass: An experimental evaluation. *J Thorac Cardiovasc Surg* 63:849, 1972.

2. Kent KM, Borer JS, Green MV, Bacharach SL, McIntosh CL, Conkle DM, Epstein SE: Effects of coronary artery bypass on global and regional left ventricular function during exercise. *N Engl J Med* 298:1434, 1977.

3. Kolibash AJ, Goodenow JS, Bush CA, Tetalman MR, Lewis RP: Improvement of myocardial perfusion and left ventricular function after coronary artery bypass grafting in patients with unstable angina. *Circulation* 59:66, 1979.

4. Kolibash AJ, Lewis RP, Goodenow JS, Bush CA, Tetalman MR: Extensive myocardial blood flow distribution through individual coronary artery bypass grafts. *Chest* 77:17, 1980.

5. Kouchoukos NT, Karp RB, Oberman A, Russell RO Jr, Allison HW, Holt JH Jr: Long-term patency of sahenous veins for coronary bypass grafting. *Circulation* 56,57(suppl III):III-189, 1977.

6. Kern WH, Dermer GB, Lindesmith GG: The intimal proliferation in aortic-coronary saphenous vein grafts: Light and electron microscopic studies. *Am Heart J* 84:771, 1972.

7. Kirklin JW, Kouchoukos NT, Blackstone EH, Oberman A: Research related to surgical treatment of coronary artery disease. *Circulation* 60:1613, 1979.

8. Keon WJ, Bedard P, Akyurekli Y, Brais M, Berkman F, Tan KW, Morton BC: Five years' experience with aortocoronary bypass grafting. *Can Med Assoc J* 114:312, 1976.

9. Kloster FE, Kremkau EL, Ritzmann LW, Rahimtoola SH, Rosch J, Kanorek PH: Coronary bypass for stable angina: A prospective randomized study. *New Engl J Med* 300:149, 1979.

10. Kouchoukos NT, Oberman A, Kirklin JW, Russell RO Jr, Karp RB, Pacifico AD, Zorn GL: Coronary bypass surgery: Analysis of factors affecting hospital mortality. *Circulation* 62(suppl I): I-84, 1980.

11. Knoebel SB, McHenry PL, Phillips JF, Lowe DK: The effect of aortocoronary bypass grafts on myocardial blood flow reserve and treadmill exercise tolerance. *Circulation* 50:685, 1974.

12. Kannel WB, Sorlie P, McNamara PM: Prognosis after initial myocardial infarction: The Framingham Study. *Am J Cardiol* 44:53, 1979.

13. Kamath ML, Schmidt DH, Pedraza PM, Blau FM, Sampathkumar A, Grzelak LL, Johnson WD: Patency and flow response in endarterectomized coronary arteries. *Ann Thorac Surg* 31:28, 1981.

14. Kowey PR, Verrier RL, Lown B, Handin RI: Influence of intracoronary platelet aggregation on ventricular electrical properties during partial coronary artery stenosis. *Am J Cardiol* 51:596, 1983.

15. Karayannacos PE, Talukder N, Nerem RM, Roshon S, Vasko JS: The role of multiple, noncritical arterial stenoses in the pathogenesis of ischemia. *J Thorac Cardiovasc Surg* 73:458, 1977.

16. Kramer JR, Matsuda Y, Mulligan JC, Aronow M, Proudfit WL: Progression of coronary atherosclerosis. *Circulation* 63:519, 1981.

17. Kennedy JW, Kaiser GL, Fisher LD, Maynard C, Fritz TC, Myers W, Mudd JG, Ryan TJ, Coggin J: Multivariate discriminant analysis of the clinical and angiographic predictors of operative mortality from the collaborative study in coronary artery surgery (CASS). *J Thorac Cardiovasc Surg* 80:876, 1980.

18. Kennedy JW, Kaiser GC, Fisher LD, Fritz JK, Myers W, Mudd JG, Ryan TJ. Clinical and angiographic predictors of operative mortality from the collaborative study in coronary artery surgery (CASS). *Circulation* 63:793, 1981.

19. Kent KM, Bentivoglio LG, Block PC, Cowley MJ, Dorros G, Gosselin AJ, Gruntzig A, Myler RK, Simpson J, Stertzer SH, Williams DO, Fisher L, Gillespie MJ, Detre K, Kelsey S, Mullin S, Mock MB: Percutaneous transluminal coronary angioplasty: Report from the Registry of the National Heart, Lung, and Blood Institute. *Am J Cardiol* 49:2011, 1982.

20. Krebber HJ, Mathey D, Kuck KJ, Kalmar P, Rodewald G: Management of evolving myocardial infarction by intracoronary thrombolysis and subsequent aorto-coronary bypass. *J Thorac Cardiovasc Surg* 83:186, 1982.

21. Katz RJ, Wasserman AG, Leiboff RH, Bren GB, Varghese PJ, Ross AM: The importance of left anterior descending stenosis in the ejection fraction response to exercise radionuclide ventriculography. *Circulation* 66(suppl II):II-63.

22. Kabbani SS, Hanna ES, Bashour TT, Crew JR, Ellertson DG: Sequential internal mammary–coronary artery bypass. *J Thorac Cardiovasc Surg* 86:697, 1983.

23. Kirklin JW, Blackstone EH, Rogers WJ: The plights of the invasive treatment of ischemic heart disease. *JACC* 5:158, 1985.

24. Kaiser GC, Davis KB, Fisher LD, Myers WO, Foster ED, Passamani ER, Gillespie MJ: Survival following CABG in patients with severe angina pectoris (CASS): An observational study. Presented at the Tenth Annual Meeting of the Western Thoracic Surgical Association, Maui, Hawaii, June 20–23, 1984.

L

1. Lehrman KL, Tilkian AG, Hultgren HN, Fowles RE: Effect of coronary arterial bypass surgery on exercise-induced ventricular arrhythmias: Long-term follow-up of a prospective randomized study. *Am J Cardiol* 44:1056, 1979.

2. Laks H, Kaiser GC, Mudd JG, Halstead J, Pennington G, Tyras D, Codd J, Barner HB: Revascularization of the right coronary artery. *Am J Cardiol* 43:1109, 1979.

3. Loop FD, Cosgrove DM, Lytle BW, Thurer RL, Simpfendorfer C, Taylor PC, Proudfit WL: An 11-year evolution of coronary artery surgery (1967–1978). *Ann Surg* 190:444, 1979.

4. Latour J-G, Trudel J-R, Campeau L, Cote P, Bourassa MG, Corbara F, Solymoss CB: Platelet regeneration time and late occlusion of aortocoronary saphenous vein bypass grafts. *Can Med Assoc J* 122:1390, 1980.

5. Loop FD, Lytle BW, Cosgrove DM, Sheldon WC, Irarrazaval M, Taylor PC, Groves LK, Pichard AD: Atherosclerosis of the left main coronary artery: 5-year results of surgical treatment. *Am J Cardiol* 44:195, 1979.

6. Lavine P, Kimbiris D, Segal BL, Linhart JW: Left main coronary artery disease: Clinical arteriographic and hemodynamic appraisal. *Am J Cardiol* 30:791, 1972.

7. Lapin ES, Murray JA, Bruce RA, Winterscheid L: Changes in maximal exercise performance in the evaluation of saphenous vein bypass surgery. *Circulation* 47:1164, 1973.

8. Lytle BW, Loop FD, Thurer RL, Groves LK, Taylor PC, Cosgrove DM: Isolated left anterior descending coronary atherosclerosis: Long-term comparison of internal mammary artery and venous autografts. *Circulation* 61:869, 1980.

9. Longmire WP Jr, Cannon JA, Kattus AA: Direct-vision coronary endarterectomy for angina pectoris. *N Engl J Med* 259:993, 1958.

10. Lawrie GM, Lie JT, Morris GC Jr, Beazley HL: Vein graft patency and intimal proliferation after aortocoronary bypass: Early and long-term angiopathologic correlations. *Am J Cardiol* 38:856, 1976.

11. Lawrie GM, Morris GC Jr: Factors influencing late survival after coronary bypass surgery. *Ann Surg* 187:665, 1978.

12. Lawrie GM, Morris GC Jr, Howell JF, Tredici TD, Chapman SW: Improved survival after 5 years in 1,144 patients after coronary bypass surgery. *Am J Cardiol* 42:709, 1978.

13. Lawrie GM, Morris GC Jr, Calhoon JH, Safi H, Zamora JL, Beltengady M, Baron A, Silvers A, Chapman DW: Clinical results of coronary bypass in 500 patients at least 10 years after operation. *Circulation* 66(suppl I):I-1, 1982.

14. Loop FD in MJ Kaplitt, JB Borman (eds): *Cardiac Surgery Update in Jerusalem, 1982* (in press).

15. LoGerfo FW, Quist WC, Cantelmo NL, Haudenschild CC: Integrity of vein grafts as a function of initial intimal and medial preservation. *Circulation* 68(suppl II):II-117, 1983.

16. Lee G, Low RI, Takeda P, Joe P, DeMaria AN, Amsterdam EA, Lui H, Dietrich P, Lee K, Mason DT: Importance of follow-up medical and surgical approaches to prevent reinfarction, reocclusion, and recurrent angina following intracoronary thrombolysis with streptokinase in acute myocardial infarction. *Am Heart J* 104:921, 1982.

17. LoGerfo FW, Quist WC, Crawshaw HM, Haudenschild CC: An improved technique for preservation of endothelial morphology in vein grafts. *Surgery* 90:1015, 1981.

18. Lim YL, Kalff V, Kelly MJ, Mason PJ, Currie PJ, Harper RW, Anderson ST, Federman J, Stirling GR, Pitt A: Radionuclide angiographic assessment of global and segmental left ventricular function at rest and during exercise after coronary artery bypass graft surgery. *Circulation* 66:972, 1982.

19. Lawrie GM, Morris GC, Silvers A, Wagner WF, Baron AE, Beltangady SS, Glaeser DH, Chapman DW: The influence of residual disease after coronary bypass on the 5-year survival rate of 1274 men with coronary artery disease. *Circulation* 66:717, 1982.

20. Loop FD, Cosgrove DM, Kramer JR, Lytle BW, Taylor PC, Golding LAR, Groves LK: Late clinical and arteriographic results in 500 coronary artery reoperations. *J Thorac Cardiovasc Surg* 81:675, 1981.

21. Lytle BW, Cosgrove DM, Saltus GL, Soto JM, Taylor PC, Loop FD: Multivessel coronary revascularization without saphenous vein: Long-term results of bilateral mammary artery grafting. *Circulation* 66(suppl II):II-93, 1982 (abstr).

22. Loop FD, Hertzer NR, Beven EG, Taylor PC, Lytle BW, Cosgrove DM: Intermediate-term results of combined (simultaneous) carotid endarterectomy and coronary artery surgery. *Circulation* 66(suppl II):II-92, 1982 (abstr).

23. Levin DC, Cohon LH, Doster JK Jr, Collins JJ Jr: Accuracy of angiography in predicting quality and caliber of the distal coronary artery lumen in preparation for bypass surgery. *Circulation* 66(suppl II):II-93, 1982 (abstr).

24. Laird-Meeter K, Van Den Brand MJBM, Serruys PW, Penn OCKM, Haalebos MMP, Bos E, Hugenholtz PG: Reoperation after aortocoronary bypass procedure: Results in 53 patients in a group of 1041 with consecutive first operations. *Br Heart J* 50:157, 1983.

25. Levin DC, Cohn LH, Koster JK Jr, Collins JJ Jr: The reliability of angiography in predicting quality and caliber of the distal coronary artery lumen in preparation for bypass surgery. *Circulation* 68(suppl II):II-185, 1983.

26. Lytle BW, Cosgrove DM, Saltus GL, Taylor PC, Loop FD: Multivessel coronary revascularization without saphenous vein: Long-term results of bilateral internal mammary artery grafting. *Ann Thorac Surg* 36:540, 1983.

27. Loop FD, Lytle BW, Cosgrove DM, Stewart RW, Goormastic M, Williams GW, Golding LAR, Gill CC, Taylor PC, Sheldon WC, Proudfit WL: Influence of the internal mammary graft on postoperative cardiac events and 10-year survival. *N Engl J Med* (in press).

M

1. Marshall RC, Berger HJ, Costin JC, Freedman GS, Wolberg J, Cohen LS, Gottschalk A, Zaret BL: Assessment of cardiac performance with quantitative radionuclide angiography: Sequential left ventricular ejection fraction, normalized left ventricular ejection rate, and regional wall motion. *Circulation* 56:820, 1977.

2. Mathur VS, Guinn GA: Prospective randomized study of coronary bypass surgery in stable angina pectoris: The first 100 patients. *Circulation* 51,52(suppl I):I-133, 1975.

3. Moran JM, Michaelis LL, Sanders JH, Roberts AJ: Revascularization of "neglected" coronary arteries. *Surgery* 86:852, 1979.

4. McNamara JJ, Bjerke HJ, Chung GKT, Dang CR: Blood flow in sequential vein grafts. *Circulation* 60(suppl I):I-33, 1979.

5. Minick CR, Stemerman MB, Insull W Jr: Role of endothelium and hypercholesterolemia in intimal thickening and lipid accumulation. *Am J Pathol* 95:131, 1979.

6. Miller DC, Stinson EB, Oyer PE, Reitz BA, Jamieson SW, MorenoCabral RJ, Shumway NE: Long-term clinical assessment of the efficacy of adjunctive coronary endarterectomy. *J Thorac Cardiovasc Surg* 81:21, 1981.

7. Murray G, Porcheron R, Hilario J, Roschlau W: Anastomosis of a systemic artery to the coronary. *Can Med Assoc J* 71:594, 1954.

8. McMahon MM, Brown BG, Cukingnan R, Rolett EL, Bolson E, Frimer M, Dodge HT: Quantitative coronary angiography: Measurement of the "critical" stenosis in patients with unstable angina and single-vessel disease without collaterals. *Circulation* 60:106, 1979.

9. Marchandise B, Bourassa MG, Chaitman BR, Lesperance J: Angiographic evaluation of the natural history of normal coronary arteries and mild coronary atherosclerosis. *Am J Cardiol* 41:216, 1978.

10. Mittler BS, Lee KL, Rosati RA: Surgical vs medical treatment in patients with totally occluded right and sub-totally-occluded left anterior descending coronary arteries. *Circulation* 51,52(suppl II):II-91, 1975 (abstr).

11. Mathey DG, Schofer J, Kuck KH, Beil U, Kloppel G: Transmural, haemorrhagic myocardial infarction after intracoronary streptokinase. *Br Heart J* 48:546, 1982.

12. Messmer BJ, Merx W, Meyer J, Bardos P, Minale C, Effert S: New developments in medical-surgical treatment of acute myocardial infarction. *Ann Thorac Surg* 35:70, 1983.

13. Moss AJ, Davis HT, De Camilla J, Bayer LW: Ventricular ectopic beats and their relation to sudden and nonsudden cardiac death after myocardial infarction. *Circulation* 60:998, 1979.

14. Markis JE, Malagold M, Parker JA, Silverman KJ, Barry WH, Als AV, Paulin S, Grossman W, Braunwald E: Myocardial salvage after intracoronary thrombolysis with streptokinase in acute myocardial infarction. *N Engl J Med* 305:977, 1981.

15. Mathey DG, Rodewald G, Rentrop P, Leitz K, Merx W, Messmer BJ, Rutsch W, Bucherl ES: Intracoronary streptokinase thrombolytic recanalization and subsequent surgical bypass of remaining atherosclerotic stenosis in acute myocardial infarction: Complementary combined approach affecting reduced infarct size, preventing reinfarction, and improving left ventricular function. *Am Heart J* 102:1194, 1981.

16. McDaniel HG, Reves JG, Kouchoukos NT, Smith LR, Rogers WJ, Samuelson PN, Lell WA: Detection of myocardial injury after coronary artery bypass grafting using a hypothermic, cardioplegic technique. *Ann Thorac Surg* 33:139, 1982.

17. Meurala H, Hekali M, Valle MH, Frick MH, Harjola PT: The effect of sequential versus single vein aortocoronary bypass surgery on resting left ventricular function. *Thorac Cardiovasc Surg* 30:99, 1982.

18. Mintz LJ, Ingels NB, Daughters GT, Stinson EB, Alderman EL: Sequential studies of left ventricular function and wall motion after coronary arterial bypass surgery. *Am J Cardiol* 45:210, 1980.

19. Mock MB, Ringqvist I, Fisher LD, Davis KB, Chaitman BR, Kouchoukos NT, Kaiser GC, Alerman E, Ryan TJ, Russell RO, Mullin S, Fray D, Kilip T III: Survival of medically treated patients in the Coronary Artery Surgery Study (CASS) Registry. *Circulation* 66:562, 1982.

20. Miller RA, Felix WG, Leighton RF: Angulated views in coronary arteriography. *Am J Roent* 134:407, 1980.

21. Marmor A, Geltman EM, Schechtman K, Sobel BE, Roberts R: Recurrent myocardial infarction: Clinical predictors and prognostic implications. *Circulation* 66:415, 1982.

22. Mathey DG, Kuch KH, Tilsner V, Krebber HJ, Bleifield W: Nonsurgical coronary artery recanalization in acute transmural myocardial infarction. *Circulation* 63:489, 1981.

23. Mann T, Goldberg S, Mudge GH, Grossman W: Factors contributing to altered left ventricular diastolic properties during angina pectoris. *Circulation* 59:14, 1979.

24. Mathur VS, Guinn GA: Prospective randomized study to evaluate coronary bypass surgery: 10 year (yr) followup: *Circulation* 66(suppl II):II-219, 1982 (abstr).

25. Mock M, Holmes D Jr, Vlietstra R, Detre K, Gersh B, Orszulak T, Schaff H, Piehler J, VanRaden M, Passamani E, Kent K, Kelsye S, Gruentzig A: Percutaneous transluminal coronary angioplasty (PTCA) in patients 60 years of age registered in the NHLBI Registry. *Circulation* 66(suppl II):II-329, 1982 (abstr).

26. Miller DC, Stinson EB, Oyer PE, Jamieson SW, Mitchell RS, Reitz BA, Baumgartner WA, Shumway NE: Discriminant analysis of the changing risks of coronary artery operations: 1971–1979. *J Thorac Cardiovasc Surg* 85:197, 1983.

27. Mock MB, Reeder GS, Schaff HV, Holmes DR Jr, Vlietstra RE, Smith HC, Gersh BJ: Percutaneous transluminal coronary angioplasty versus coronary artery bypass: Isn't it time for a randomized trial? *N Engl J Med* 312:916, 1985.

N

1. Nitter-Hauge S, Levorstad K: Does aortocoronary saphenous vein bypass surgery change the native coronary arteries? *Acta Med Scand* 207:189, 1980.

2. Newman GE, Rerych SK, Jones RH, Sabiston DC Jr: Noninvasive assessment of the effects of aorto-coronary bypass grafting on ventricular function during rest and exercise. *J Thorac Cardiovasc Surg* 79:617, 1980.

3. Norris RM, Caughey DE, Deeming LW, Mercer CJ, Scott PJ: Coronary prognostic index for predicting survival after recovery from acute myocardial infarction. *Lancet* 2:485, 1970.

4. Norris RM, Agnew TM, Brandt PWT, Graham KJ, Hill DG, Kerr AR, Lowe JB, Roche AGH, Whitlock RML, Barratt-Boyes BG: Coronary surgery after recurrent myocardial infarction: Progress of a trial comparing surgical with nonsurgical management for asymptomatic patients with advanced coronary disease. *Circulation* 63:785, 1981.

5. National Heart Lung and Blood Institute Coronary Artery Surgery Study. *Circulation* 63(suppl I):I-1 1981.

6. Namay DL, Hammermeister KE, May SZ, DeRouen TA, Dodge HT, Namay K: Effect of perioperative myocardial infarction on late survival in patients undergoing coronary artery bypass surgery. *Circulation* 65:1066, 1982.

7. Nkongho A, Luber JM, Bell-Thomson J, Green GE: Sternotomy infection after harvesting of the internal mammary artery. *J Thorac Cardiovasc Surg* 88:788, 1984.

O

1. Olinger GN, Bonchek LI, Keelan MH Jr, Tresch DD, Siegel R, Bamrah V, Tristani FE: Unstable angina: The case for operation. *Am J Cardiol* 42:634, 1978.

2. Oberman A, Jones WB, Riley CP, Reeves TJ, Sheffield LT, Turner ME: Natural history of coronary artery disease. *Bull NY Acad Med* 48:1109, 1972.

3. Oberman A, Kouchoukos NT, Makar YN, Russell RO Jr, Sheffield LT, Ray M, Allen RE, Kitts JR: Perioperative myocardial infarction after coronary bypass surgery. *Cleve Clin Q* 45:172, 1978.

4. Okies JE, Page US, Bigelow JC, Krause AH, Salomon NW: The left internal mammary artery: The graft of choice. *Circulation* 70(suppl I):I-213, 1984.

P

1. Parsonnet V, Gilbert L, Gielchinsky I, Bhaktan K: Endarterectomy of the left anterior descending and mainstem coronary arteries: A technique for reconstruction of inoperable arteries. *Surgery* 80:662, 1976.

2. Pantely GA, Goodnight SH Jr, Rahimtoola SH, Harlan BJ, DeMots H, Calvin L, Rosch J: Failure of antiplatelet and anticoagulant therapy to improve patency of grafts after coronary artery bypass: A controlled randomized study. *N Engl J Med* 301:962, 1979.

3. Palac RT, Meadows WR, Hwang MH, Loeb HS, Pifarre R, Gunnar RM: Risk factors related to progressive narrowing in aorto coronary vein grafts studied 1 and 5 years after surgery. *Circulation* 66(suppl I):I-40, 1982.

4. Page DL, Caulfield JB, Kastor JA, De Sanctis RW, Sanders CA: Myocardial changes associated with cardiogenic shock. *N Engl J Med* 285:133, 1971.

5. Palac RT, Hwang MH, Meadows WR, Croke RP, Pifarre R, Loeb HS, Gunnar RM: Progression of coronary artery disease in medially and surgically treated patients 5 years after randomization. *Circulation* 64(suppl II):II-17, 1981.

6. Phillips SJ, Kongtahworn C, Zeff RH, Benson M, Iannone L, Brown T, Gordon DF: Emergency coronary artery revascularization: A possible therapy for acute myocardial infarction. *Circulation* 60:241, 1979.

7. Phillips HR, Johnson RA, Hindman MA, Wagner GS, Harris PJ, Dinsmore RE, Gold HK, Leinbach RC, Hutter AM Jr, Erdman AJ III, Daggett WM Jr, Buckley MJ: Aortocoronary bypass grafting in patients without left main stenosis: Relation of risk factors to early and late survival. *Br Heart J* 45:549, 1981.

8. Paulin S: Tilted views in cardiac angiography. *Medicamundi* 24:2, 1979.

9. Papapietro SE, Yester MV, Logic JR, Tauxe WN, Mantle JA, Rogers WJ, Russell RO Jr, Rackley CE: Method for quantitative analysis of regional left ventricular function with first-pass and gated blood pool scintigraphy. *Am J Cardiol* 47:618, 1981.

10. Pfeffer JM, Pfeffer MA, Mirsky I, Steinberg CR, Braunwald E: Progressive ventricular dilatation and diastolic wall stress in rats with myocardial infarction and failure. *Circulation* 66(suppl II):II-66, 1982 (abstr).

11. Phillips HR, Hindman MC, Califf RM, Lee KL, Harrell FE Jr, Behar VS, Wagner GS, Johnson RA, Rosati RA: Prognostic value of a coronary artery jeopardy score. *Circulation* 66(suppl II):II-369, 1982 (abstr).

12. Pigott JD, Kouchoukos NT, Oberman A, Cutter G: Late results of medical and surgical therapy for patients with coronary artery disease and depressed ejection fraction. *Circulation* 66(suppl II):II-220, 1982 (abstr).

13. Proudfit WJ, Bruschke AVG, MacMillan JP, Williams GW, Sones FM Jr: Fifteen-year survival study of patients with obstructive coronary artery disease. *Circulation* 68:986, 1983.

14. Passamani E and CASS Principal Investigators: Coronary artery surgery study (CASS): A randomized trial of coronary artery bypass surgery. Survival in low ejection fraction patients. (1985) Personal Communication.

Q

1. Quazi A, Garcia JM, Mispireta LA, Corso PJ: Reoperation for coronary artery disease. *Ann Thorac Surg* 32:16, 1981.

R

1. Ricks WB, Winkle RA, Shumway NE, Harrison DC: Survival management of life-threatening ventricular arrhythmias in patients with coronary artery disease. *Circulation* 56:38, 1977.

2. Rerych SK, Scholz PM, Newman GE, Sabiston DC Jr, Jones RH: Cardiac function at rest and during exercise in normals and in patients with coronary artery disease: Evaluation by radionuclide angiography. *Ann Surg* 187:449, 1978.

3. Russell RO Jr, and Unstable Angina Study Associates: Unstable angina pectoris: National Cooperative Study Group to Compare Surgical and Medical Therapy. II. In-hospital experience and initial follow-up results in patients with one, two and three vessel disease. *Am J Cardiol* 42:839, 1978.

4. Rimm AA, Barboriak JJ, Anderson AJ, Simon JS: Changes in occupation after aortocoronary vein-bypass operation. *JAMA* 236:361, 1976.

5. Read RC, Murphy ML, Hultgren HN, Takaro T: Survival of mean treated for chronic stable angina pectoris. A Cooperative Randomized Study. *J Thorac Cardiovasc Surg* 75:1, 1978.

6. Reduto LA, Berger HJ, Geha A, Hammond G, Cohen LS, Gottschalk A, Zaret BL: Radionuclide assessment of ventricular performance during propranolol withdrawal prior to aortocoronary bypass surgery. *Am Heart J* 96:714, 1978.

7. Roberts WC: Does thrombosis play a major role in the development of symptom-producing atherosclerotic plaques? *Circulation* 48:1161, 1973.

8. Rimm AA, Blumlein S, Barboriak JJ, Anderson AJ, Walker JA,

Johnson WD: The probability of closure in aortocoronary vein bypass grafts. *JAMA* 236:2637, 1976.

9. Reichle FA, Stewart GJ, Essa N: A transmission and scanning electron microscopic study of luminal surfaces in Dacron and autogenous vein bypasses in man and dog. *Surgery* 74:945, 1973.

10. Rogers WJ, Smith LR, Oberman A, Kouchoukos NT, Mantle JA, Russell RO Jr, Rackley CE: Surgical vs. nonsurgical management of patients after myocardial infarction. *Circulation* 61,62(suppl I):I-67, 1980.

11. Roberts AJ, Spies SM, Meyers SN, Moran JM, Sanders JH Jr, Lichtenthal PR, Michaelis LL: Early and long-term improvement in left ventricular performance following coronary bypass surgery. *Surgery* 88:467, 1980.

12. Rafflenbeul W, Urthaler F, Lichtlen P, James TN: Quantitative difference in "critical" stenosis between right and left coronary artery in man. *Circulation* 62:118, 1980.

13. Rubenson DS, Tucker CR, London E, Miller DC, Stinson EB, Popp RL: Two-dimensional echocardiographic analysis of segmental left ventricular wall motion before and after coronary artery bypass surgery. *Circulation* 66:1025, 1982.

14. Roberts WC and Buja LM: The frequency and significance of coronary arterial thrombi and other observations in fatal acute myocardial infarction: A study of 107 necropsy patients. *Am J Med* 52:425, 1972.

15. Richards DA, Cody DV, Denniss AR, Russell PA, Young AA, Uther JB: Ventricular electrical instability: A predictor of death after myocardial infarction. *Am J Cardiol* 51:75, 1983.

16. Reduto LA, Wickemeyer WJ, Young JB, Del Ventura LA, Reid JW, Glaeser DH, Quinones MA, Miller RR: Left ventricular diastolic performance at rest and during exercise in patients with coronary artery disease. *Circulation* 63:1228, 1981.

17. Roffman JA, Fieldman A: Digoxin and propranolol: The prophylaxis of supraventricular tachydysrhythmias after coronary artery bypass surgery. *Ann Thorac Surg* 31:496, 1981.

18. Reduto LA, Smalling RW, Freund GC, Gould KL: Intracoronary infusion of streptokinase in patients with acute myocardial infarction: Effects of reperfusion on left ventricular performance. *Am J Cardiol* 48:403, 1981.

19. Rentrop P, Blanke H, Dostering K, Karsch KR: Acute myocardial infarction: Intracoronary application of nitroglycerin and streptokinase in combination with transluminal recanalization. *Clin Cardiol* 2:354, 1979.

20. Rentrop P, Blanke H, Karsch KR, Kiaser H, Kostering H, Leitz K: Selective intracoronary thrombolysis in acute myocardial infarction and unstable angina pectoris. *Circulation* 63:307, 1981.

21. Ross J, Theroux P, Sasayma S, McKown D, Franklin D: Late recovery of cardiac function after coronary artery reperfusion. *Circulation* 51(suppl II):II-21, 1975 (abstr).

22. Rentrop KP, Blanke H, Karsch KR: Effects of nonsurgical coronary reperfusion on the left ventricle in human subjects compared with conventional treatment. *Am J Cardiol* 49:1, 1982.

23. Reves JG, Karp RB, Buttner EE, Tosone S, Smith R, Samuelson PN, Kreusch GR, Oparil S: Neuronal and adrenomedullary catecholamine release in response to cardiopulmonary bypass in man. *Circulation* 66:49, 1982.

S

1. Sones FM Jr, Shirey EK: Cine coronary arteriography. *Mod Concepts Cardiovasc Dis* 31:735, 1962.

2. Sewell WH: Improved coronary vein graft patency rates with side-to-side anastomosis. *Ann Thorac Surg* 17:538, 1974.

3. See JR, Cohn PF, Holman BL, Roberts BH, Adams DF: Angiographic abnormalities associated with alterations in regional myocardial blood flow in coronary artery disease. *Br Heart J* 38:1278, 1976.

4. Sharma B, Goodwin JF, Raphael MJ, Steiner RE, Rainbow RG, Taylor SH: Left ventricular angiography on exercise: A new method of assessing left ventricular function in ischemic heart disease. *Br Heart J* 38:59, 1976.

5. Sharma B, Taylor SH: Localization of left ventricular ischemia in angina pectoris by cineangiography during exercise. *Br Heart J* 37:963, 1975.

6. Seymmes JC, Lenkei SCM, Berman ND: Influence of aortocoronary bypass surgery on employment. *Can Med Assoc J* 118:268, 1978.

7. Seybold-Epting W, Oglietti J, Wukasch DC, Reul GJ Jr, Hall RJ, Hallman GL, Cooley DA: Early and late results after surgical treatment of preinfarction angina. *Ann Thorac Surg* 21:97, 1976.

8. Stiles QR, Lindesmith GG, Tucker BL, Hughes RK, Meyer BW: Long-term follow-up of patients with coronary artery bypass grafts. *Circulation* 54(suppl III):III-32, 1976.

9. Serruys PW, Rousseau MF, Cosyns J, Ponlot R, Brasseu LA, Detry J-MR: Hemodynamics during maximal exercise after coronary bypass surgery. *Br Heart J* 40:1205, 1978.

10. Siegel W, Loop FD: Comparison of internal mammary artery and saphenous vein bypass grafts for myocardial revascularization: Exercise test and angiographic correlations. *Circulation* 53,54(suppl III):III-1, 1976.

11. Schelbert HR, Verba JW, Johnson HD, Brock GW, Alazraki NP, Rose FJ, Ashburn WL: Nontraumatic determination of left ventricular ejection fraction by radionuclide angiocardiography. *Circulation* 51:902, 1975.

12. Steele P, Kirch D, Matthews M, Davies H: Measurement of left heart ejection fraction and end-diastolic volume by a computerized, scintigraphic technique using a wedged pulmonary arterial catheter. *Am J Cardiol* 34:179, 1974.

13. Steele P, Kirch D, LeFree M, and Battock D: Measurement of right and left ventricular ejection fractions by radionuclide angiocardiography in coronary artery disease. *Chest* 70:51, 1976.

14. Sommers HM, Jennings RB: Experimental acute myocardial infarction. *Lab Invest* 13:1491, 1964.

15. Sheldon WC, Rincon G, Effler DB, Proudfit WL, Sones FM Jr: Vein graft surgery for coronary artery disease: Survival and angiographic results among the first one thousand patients. *Circulation* 45,46(suppl II):II-110, 1972 (abstr).

16. Sheldon WL, Sones FM Jr, Shirey EK, Fergusson DJG, Favaloro RG, Effler DB: Reconstructive coronary artery surgery: Postoperative assessment. *Circulation* 39,40(suppl I):I-61, 1969.

17. Senning A: Strip grafting in coronary arteries: Report of a case. *J Thorac Cardiovasc Surg* 41:542, 1961.

18. Sasto M, Schwartz F: Regional myocardial function at rest and after rapid ventricular pacing in patients after myocardial revascularization by coronary bypass graft or by collateral vessels. *Am J Cardiol* 43:920, 1979.

19. Slogoff S, Keats AS, Ott E: Preoperative propranolol therapy and aortocoronary bypass operation. *JAMA* 240:1487, 1978.

20. Stoney WS, Vernon RP, Alford WC Jr, Burrus GC, Thomas CS Jr: Revascularization of the septal artery. *Ann Thorac Surg* 21:2, 1976.

21. Selwyn AP, Steiner R, Kivisaari A, Fox K, Forse G: Krypton-81m in the physiologic assessment of coronary arterial stenosis in man. *Am J Cardiol* 43:547, 1979.

22. Sahn DJ, Barratt-Boyes BG, Graham K, Kerr AR, Roche AHG, Hill DG, Brandt PWT, Copeland JG, Mammana R, Temkia LP, Glenn W: Ultrasonic imaging of coronary arteries in open chest humans: Evaluation of coronary atherosclerotic lesions during cardiac surgery. *Circulation* 66:1034, 1982.

23. Schwartz RL, Garrett JR, Karp RB, Kouchoukos NT: Simultaneous myocardial revascularization and carotid endarterectomy. *Circulation* 66(suppl I):I-97, 1982.

24. Shah PK, Pichler M, Bergman DS, Singh BN, Swan HFC: Left ventricular ejection fraction determined by radionuclide ventriculography in early stages of first transmural myocardial infarction. *Am J Cardiol* 45:542, 1980.

25. Silverman KJ, Becker LC, Bulkley BH, Burow RD, Mellits ED, Kallman CH, Weisfeldt ML: Value of early thallium-201 scintigraphy for predicting mortality in patients with acute myocardial infarction. *Circulation* 61:996, 1980.

26. Sharma GVRK, Khuri SF, Folland ED, Josa M, Parisi AF: Lack of benefit from aspirin-dipyridamole therapy in aortocoronary vein graft patency. *Circulation* 66(suppl II):II-94, 1982.

27. Schuster EH, Griffith LS, Bulkley BH: Preponderance of acute proximal left anterior descending coronary arterial lesions in fatal myocardial infarction: A clinicopathologic study. *Am J Cardiol* 47:1189, 1981.

28. Selinger SL, Berg R Jr, Leonard JJ, Grunwald RP, O'Grady WP: Surgical treatment of acute evolving anterior myocardial infarction. *Circulation* 64(suppl II):II-28, 1981.

29. Simon R, Amende I, Oelert H, Hetzer R, Borst HG, Lichtlen PR: Blood velocity, flow and dimensions of aortocoronary venous bypass grafts in the postoperative state. *Circulation* 66(suppl 1):34, 1982.

30. Smith SH, Geer JC: Morphology of saphenous vein-coronary artery bypass grafts: 7–116 months postoperative. *Arch Pathol Lab Med* 107:13, 1983.

31. Selzer A: On the limitation of therapeutic intervention trials in ischemic heart disease: A clinician's viewpoint. *Am J Cardiol* 49:252, 1982.

32. Sigwart U, Grbic M, Essinger A, Bischof-Delaloye A, Sadeghi H, Rivier J: Improvement of left ventricular function after percutaneous transluminal coronary angioplasty. *Am J Cardiol* 49:651, 1982.

33. Swan HFC, Forrester JS, Diamond G, Chatterjee K, Parmley WWL: Hemodynamic spectrum of myocardial infarction and cardiogenic shock: A conceptual model. *Circulation* 45:1097, 1972.

34. Stanley JC, Sottiurai V, Fry RE, Fry WJ: Comparative evaluation of vein graft preparation media: Electron and light microscopic studies. *J Surg Res* 18:235, 1975.

35. Swan HFC: Thrombolysis in acute myocardial infarction: Treatment of the underlying coronary artery disease. *Circulation* 66:914, 1982.

36. Shub C, Vlietstra RE, Smith HC, Fulton RE, Elveback LR: The unpredictable progression of symptomatic coronary artery disease: A serial clinical-angiographic analysis. *Mayo Clin Proc* 56:155, 1981.

37. Smith JL, Jaffe AS, Baird T, Galie E, Sobel BE, Geltman EM: The interval of evolution of infarction in patients assessed by positron emission tomography. *Circulation* 66(suppl II):II-87, 1982 (abstr).

38. Singh AK, Capone RJ, O'Shea P, Karlson KE: Long-term

changes in canine vein graft following infusion of cardioplegic solution. *Circulation* 66(suppl II):II-135, 1982 (abstr).

39. Schaff HV, Gersh BJ, Pluth JR, Danielson GK, Orszulak TA, Puga FJ, Piehler JM, Frye RL: Survival and functional results after coronary artery bypass grafting: Results 10 to 12 years postoperatively in 500 patients. *Circulation* 66(suppl II):II-246, 1982 (abstr).

40. Salomon NW, Page US, Okies JE, Stephens J, Krause AH, Bigelow JC: Diabetes mellitus and coronary artery bypass. *J Thorac Cardiovasc Surg* 85:264, 1983.

41. Singh RN, Sosa JA, Green GE: Long-term fate of the internal mammary artery and saphenous vein grafts. *J Thorac Cardiovasc Surg* 86:359, 1983.

42. Sterling RP, Walker WE, Weiland AP, Freund GC, Fuentes F, Smalling RW, Gould KL: Early bypass grafting following intracoronary thrombolysis with streptokinase. *J Thorac Cardiovasc Surg* 87:487, 1984.

43. Stinson EB, Olinger GN, Glancy DL: Anatomical and physiological determinants of blood flow through aortocoronary vein bypass grafts. *Surgery* 74:390, 1973.

44. Stoney WS, Alford WC, Burrus GR, Glassford DM Jr, Petracek MR, Thomas CS: The fate of arm veins used for aorta-coronary bypass grafts. *J Thorac Cardiovasc Surg* 88:522, 1984.

45. Schaff HV and CASS Registry Associates: Detrimental effect of perioperative myocardial infarction on late survival after coronary artery bypass. *J Thorac Cardiovasc Surg* 88:972, 1984.

T

1. Tyras DH, Ahmad N, Kaiser GC, Barner HB, Codd JE, Willman VL: Ventricular function and the native coronary circulation five years after myocardial revascularization. *Ann Thorac Surg* 27:547, 1979.

2. Tecklenberg PL, Aldermann EL, Miller DC, Shumway NE, Harrison DG: Changes in survival and symptom relief in a longitudinal study of patients after bypass surgery. *Circulation* 51,52(suppl I):I-98, 1975.

3. Takaro T, Hultgren HN, Lipton MJ, Detre KM and Participants in VA Study Group: The VA Cooperative randomized study of surgery for coronary arterial occlusive disease. II. Subgroup with significant left main lesions. *Circulation* 54(suppl III):III-107, 1976.

4. Theroux P, Ross J Jr, Franklin D, Kemper WS, Sasayama S: Coronary arterial reperfusion. III. Early and late effects on regional myocardial function and dimensions in conscious dogs. *Am J Cardiol* 38:599, 1976.

5. Thanavaro S, Krone RJ, Kleiger RE, Province MA, Miller JP, De Mello VR, Oliver GC: In-hospital prognosis of patients with first nontransmural and transmural infarction. *Circulation* 61:29, 1980.

6. Tyras DH, Barner HB, Kaiser GC, Codd JE, Laks H, Pennington DG, Willman VL: Long-term results of myocardial revascularization. *Am J Cardiol* 44:1290, 1979.

7. Takaro T, Peduzzi P, Detre KM, Hultgren HN, Murphy ML, Bel-Kahn J, Thomsen J, Meadows WR: Survival in subgroups of patients with left main coronary artery disease. *Circulation* 66:14, 1982.

8. Taeymans Y, Moise A, Theroux P, Descoings B, Lesperance J, Waters DD, Bourassa MG: Unstable angina pectoris as an indicator of progression of coronary artery disease. *Circulation* 66(suppl II):II-17, 1982 (abstr).

9. Tector AJ, Schmahl TM, Janson B, Kallies JR, Johnson G: The internal mammary artery graft: Its longevity after coronary bypass. *JAMA* 246:2181, 1981.

10. Tector AJ, Schmahl TM: Techniques for multiple internal mammary artery bypass grafts. *Ann Thorac Surg* 38:281, 1984.

11. Tector AJ, Schmahl TM, Canino VR, Kallies JR, Sanfilipo D: The role of the sequential internal mammary artery graft in coronary surgery. *Circulation* 70(Suppl I):I-222, 1984.

U

1. Unni KK, Kottke BA, Titus JL, Frye RL, Wallace RB, Brown AL: Pathologic changes in aortocoronary saphenous vein grafts. *Am J Cardiol* 34:526, 1974.

2. Urschel HC, Razzuk MA, Gardner MA: Management of concomitant occlusive disease of the carotid and coronary arteries. *J Thorac Cardiovasc Surg* 72:829, 1976.

3. Urschel HC in MJ Kaplitt, JB Borman (ed): *Cardiac Surgery Update in Jerusalem, 1982* (in press).

V

1. Vineberg AM, Miller G: Internal mammary coronary anastomosis in the surgical treatment of coronary artery insufficiency. *Can Med Assoc J* 64:204, 1951.

2. Varnauskas E, Olsson SB, Carlström E, Peterson LE: Prospective randomized study of coronary artery bypass surgery in stable angina pectoris: Second interim report by the European Coronary Surgery Study Group. *Lancet*:491, September 6, 1980.

3. Vladover Z, Edwards JE: Pathologic changes in aortic-coronary arterial saphenous vein grafts. *Circulation* 44:719, 1971.

4. Vlietstra RE, Assad-Morell JL, Frye RL, Elveback LR, Connolly DC, Ritman EL, Pluth JR, Barnhorst DA, Danielson GK, Wallace RB: Survival predictors in coronary artery disease: Medical and surgical comparisons. *Mayo Clin Proc* 52:85, 1977.

5. Vetrovec GW, Cowley MJ, Overton H, Richardson DW: Intracoronary thrombus in syndromes of unstable myocardial ischemia. *Am Heart J* 102:1202, 1981.

W

1. Weisz D, Hamby RI, Aintablian A, Voletic C, Fogel R, Wisoff BG: Late coronary bypass graft flow: Quantitative assessment by roentgendensitometry. *Ann Thorac Surg* 28:429, 1979.

2. Winkle RA, Alderman EL, Shumway NE, Harrison DC: Results of reoperation for unsuccessful coronary artery bypass surgery. *Circulation* 51,52(suppl I):I-61, 1975.

3. Webster JS, Moberg C, Rincon G: Natural history of severe proximal coronary artery disease as documented by coronary cineangiography. *Am J Cardiol* 33:195, 1974.

4. Wainwright RJ, Brennand-Roper DA, Maisey MN, Sowton E: Exercise thallium-201 myocardial scintigraphy in the follow-up of aortocoronary bypass graft surgery. *Br Heart J* 43:56, 1980.

5. Wechsler A: Assessment of prospectively randomized patients receiving propranolol therapy before coronary bypass operation. *Ann Thorac Surg* 30:128, 1980.

6. Wolf NM, Kreulen TH, Bove AA, McDonough MT, Kessler KM, Strong M, Lemole G, Spann JF: Left ventricular function following coronary bypass surgery. *Circulation* 58:63, 1978.

7. Whalen RE, Harrell FE Jr, Lee KL, Rosati RA: Survival of coronary artery disease of patients with stable pain and normal left ventricular function treated medically or surgically at Duke University. *Circulation* 65(suppl II):II-49, 1982.

8. Waller BF, Roberts WC: Amount of narrowing by atherosclerotic plaque in 44 nonbypassed and 52 bypassed major

epicardial coronary arteries in 32 necropsy patients who died within 1 month of aortocoronary bypass grafting. *Am J Cardiol* 46:956, 1980.

9. Williams JB, Stephenson LW, Holford FD, Langer T, Dunkman WB, Josephson ME: Arrhythmia prophylaxis using propranolol after coronary artery surgery. *Ann Thorac Surg* 34:435, 1982.

10. Warnowicz MA, Parker H, Cheitlin MD: Prognosis of patients with acute pulmonary edema and normal ejection fraction after acute myocardial infarction. *Circulation* 67:330, 1983.

11. Wood D, Roberts C, Van Devanter SH, Kloner R, Cohn LH: Limitation of myocardial infarct size after surgical reperfusion for acute coronary occlusion. *J Thorac Cardiovasc Surg* 84:353, 1982.

Y

1. Yeh TJ, Heidary D, Shelton L: Y-grafts and sequential grafts in coronary bypass surgery: A critical evaluation of patency rates. *Ann Thorac Surg* 27:409, 1979.

2. Yacoub MH, Fawzy E, Anyanwu H, Towers M: Combined gas endarterectomy and coronary artery bypass graft. *Circulation* 52(suppl I):I-182, 1975.

3. Yacoub MH, Ashraf MH, Pillai R, Qureshi S, Towers M: Effect of myocardial revascularization on the incidence and severity of myocardial infarction in patients with stable angina: A prospective randomized study. *Circulation* 66(suppl II):II-245, 1982 (abstr).

Z

1. Zeft HJ, Friedberg HD, King JF, Manley JC, Juston JH, Johnson WD: Reappearance of anterior QRS forces after coronary bypass surgery: An electrovectorcardiographic study. *Am J Cardiol* 36:163, 1975.

2. Zir LM, Dinsmore R, Vexeridis M, Singh JB, Harthorne JW, Daggett WM: Effects of coronary bypass grafting on resting left ventricular contraction in patients studied 1 to 2 years after operation. *Am J Cardiol* 44:601, 1979.

3. Zorn, GL: The value of complete revascularization in the coronary operation. (1980) Unpublished data.

8

LEFT VENTRICULAR ANEURYSM

DEFINITION

A postinfarction aneurysm of the left ventricle (LV) is a well-delineated transmural fibrous scar, virtually devoid of muscle, in which the characteristic fine trabecular pattern of the inner surface of the wall has been replaced by smooth fibrous tissue. In such areas, the wall is usually thin, and both inner and outer surfaces bulge outward. During systole, the involved wall segments are akinetic (without movement) or dyskinetic (characterized by paradoxical movement).

Scars and infarcts that are excised are not considered aneurysms. Unlike aneurysms, they are not discrete, and with scars and infarcts, the LV wall is not thin but is usually predominately muscle.

The definition of *aneurysm* and the criteria for the separation of aneurysm from other types of LV scars are controversial, and some clinicians have adopted a broader, nonmorphologic definition than the one set forth above. Thus, Johnson and colleagues define aneurysm as "a large single

area of infarction (scar) that causes the left ventricular ejection fraction to be profoundly depressed (to approximately 0.35 or lower)."[J1] While realistically the definition of LV aneurysm is less important to the surgeon than are the criteria for and results of surgical excision of left ventricular scars, the lack of uniformity of definition complicates almost all discussions of this entity.

HISTORICAL NOTE

Although John Hunter and others had recognized very early that aneurysms of the left ventricle occurred, it was not until the 1880s that the relationship among stenotic coronary artery disease, myocardial infarction, myocardial fibrosis, and left ventricular aneurysm was recognized.[C1,L1,M1,T1,Z1] Until about 1950, very few cases were diagnosed during life, but after that time, the ability to diagnose LV aneurysms improved. In 1966, Gorlin showed that a strong suspicion of aneurysm could be obtained in 75% of the patients with this complication of myocardial infarction based on the history, physical examination, and apex cardiographic, electrocardiographic, and radiologic studies.[G1]

The surgical treatment of postinfarction left ventricular aneurysm probably began in 1944, when Beck reinforced such a lesion with fascia lata in an effort to reduce expansile pulsation and prevent rupture. A closed ventriculoplasty, done with a special side-biting left ventricular clamp, was reported in 1955 by Likoff and Bailey.[L2] A few years later, Bailey reported five survivors among six patients treated by this method. Cooley, in Houston, Texas, reported the first successful open excision of a left ventricular aneurysm, using cardiopulmonary bypass (CPB), in 1958.[C2]

MORPHOLOGY

Gross Pathology

The wall of a mature aneurysm is a white fibrous scar, visible externally, on the cut surface, and endocardially. Characteristically, the aneurysmal portion of the LV wall is thin, the endocardial surface is smooth and nontrabeculated, and the area is rather clearly demarcated. In over half the patients with classic LV aneurysms, varying amounts of mural thrombi are intimately attached to the endocardial surface. The mural thrombus may calcify. The overlying pericardium is usually densely adherent to the epicardial surface of the aneurysm,[D1,P1] and this, too, may calcify.

Such classic LV aneurysms are at one end of the spectrum of postinfarction left ventricular scars. At the other end are the diffuse, scattered, at times sparse, punctate scars, frequently visible at operation in areas of previous myocardial infarction. These scars are not transmural, and the left ventricular wall is not thin. The endocardium beneath retains its trabeculations, and the area of scarring is not clearly demarcated from the rest of the wall. Mural thrombi are not commonly present, and the pericardium is not commonly adherent to the area.

Between these two extremes is a continuous spectrum of postinfarction LV scarring, which is to be anticipated from the fact that, in an area of myocardial infarction, the myocardial necrosis rarely involves an entire area homogeneously (see "Myocardial Infarction and Its Morphologic Sequelae" in Chapter 7).

Microscopic Pathology

A mature aneurysm consists almost entirely of hyalinized fibrous tissue. However, a small number of viable muscle cells are regularly seen.[G1] Fibrous tissue of the type present in aneurysms takes at least 1 month to form, although collagen is present within 10 days of infarction. Thus, when an aneurysm is said to be present (on the basis of wall thinning and dilatation) within 1 week or so of a first infarction, the wall is composed largely of necrotic muscle and is not therefore by definition a true (mature) aneurysm.

Location

About 85% of left ventricular aneurysms are located anterolaterally near the apex. Very few are confined to the lateral (obtuse marginal) area, and only 5%–10% are posterior, near the base of the heart. Posterior, or inferior, aneurysms (i.e., those occurring in the diaphragmatic surface of the left ventricle) are in some ways different from apical and anterolateral aneurysms. Nearly half of the posterior aneurysms are false aneurysms (see "False Left Ventricular Aneurysm" in section on Special Situations and Controversies), whereas nearly all anterolateral and apical aneurysms are true aneurysms.[B7] True posterior wall postinfarction aneurysms are associated with a high incidence of postinfarction mitral incompetence secondary to ischemic papillary muscle involvement (see Chapter 10).[B7,V1]

Coronary Arteries

About half the patients undergoing resection of classic LV aneurysms or scars have stenotic coronary artery disease only in the left anterior descending (LAD) coronary artery (UAB).[L3,R1,S1] More often, however, multivessel disease is present.[B1,D1,D2,F1,K1,R2] Cooperman and colleagues found that about 75% of their patients had multivessel disease,[C7] and in the GLH experience of surgically treated true aneurysms, 78% of the patients had multivessel disease.[B10] Almost two-thirds of the GLH patients had a myocardial score ≥ 10 (see Chapter 7, Appendix 7B for a description of the myocardial scoring method). The left anterior descending artery was involved in 98% of those cases, and in 83% of these, the lesion was a total occlusion. The left main coronary artery was involved in 6.4% of the cases (half were totally occluded), and the right coronary artery and the circumflex artery or its branches were each involved in about two-thirds of the cases. The discrepancy between single- and multiple-vessel disease incidence may be related to the definition of LV aneurysm used; whether the source of the material was clinical, surgical, or postmortem; and, in the case of surgical material, case selection. A patient with single-vessel disease is more apt to survive an acute infarction and appear in a surgical series than is a patient with multiple-vessel disease.

It has been suggested that patients who develop left ventricular aneurysms have poor intercoronary collateral arteries.[B2,C3] The speculation is that a rich collateral blood supply to an area of myocardial infarction tends to increase the number and size of the islands of viable myocardial cells in the area and to decrease the probability that the necrosis is extensive enough to result in a thin-walled transmural scar (aneurysm).

Left Ventricle

Postmortem studies indicate that most patients with classic LV aneurysms have increased cardiac volume and weight.[D1,G2,P1] The increase in volume is in part the result of simple thinning and bulging of the aneurysmal portion of the LV wall. However, the nonaneurysmal portions of the LV also increase in volume and thickness secondary to the hemodynamic stress placed on them by the akinesia of the aneurysm and by LaPlace's law.

Klein and colleagues have shown that inactivation (by akinesis or dyskinesis) of at least 20% of the left ventricular wall area is required for left ventricular enlargement to be stimulated.[C4,K1] The larger the akinetic or dyskinetic area, the greater the enlargement of the rest of the ventricle.

The time course of these events has not been clearly defined. This is unfortunate, since it is probably the enlargement of the rest of the ventricle that allows safe excision of the aneurysm.

CLINICAL FEATURES AND DIAGNOSTIC CRITERIA

The morphologic diagnosis of postinfarction LV aneurysm can be made with assurance only at operation or autopsy. This is because the akinetic or dyskinetic segmental wall motion of a left ventricular aneurysm can be mimicked by scars or early infarcts, which are not morphologically aneurysms. Thus, Froehlich and colleagues found no aneurysm at operation in 3 (17%, CL 7%–31%) of 18 patients with a preoperative diagnosis of aneurysm and only a questionable aneurysm, which was plicated, in an additional 4 patients (22%, CL 12%–37%).[F6]

A patient with an aneurysm of significant size may present because of dyspnea that has persisted from the time of infarction and that frequently progresses to congestive heart failure requiring medication for its control[R1] (Table 8-1). Angina pectoris alone or with the symptoms of heart failure is often present. From 15%–30% of patients have symptoms related to ventricular arrhythmias.[G6] Despite the fact that about half the aneurysms contain clot, thromboembolism occurs in only a small proportion of patients.[B10]

On physical examination, palpation over the heart usually demonstrates a diffuse sustained apical systolic thrust and a double impulse, and on auscultation there is usually a third heart sound and often also a fourth (atrial) sound. There may be an apical pansystolic murmur if mitral incompetence coexists. A chest roentgenogram and fluoroscopy may show an external bulge or convexity when the aneurysm is large enough and profiled.

Table 8-1 Symptoms in patients operated on for left ventricular aneurysm (GLH; 1969–1981).

Symptoms	n	% of 145
Severe angina[a] alone	45	31
Mild angina[a] alone	8	5.5
CHF alone	30	21
CHF + severe angina	27	19
CHF + mild angina	12	8
VT ± other symptoms	22	15
Mild effort dyspnea	1	0.7
Total	145	100

Modified from Barratt-Boyes et al.[B10]

KEY: CHF, congestive heart failure (severe dyspnea, orthopnea, paroxysmal nocturnal dyspnea, fluid retention, hepatomegaly); VT, ventricular tachycardia (two or more episodes of documented VT or ventricular fibrillation despite treatment with antiarrhythmic drugs).

[a]Mild = Canadian Heart Association class 1 or 2; severe = class 3 or 4.

Methods of left ventricular imaging, namely, left ventriculography, two-dimensional echocardiography, and radionuclide cardiac blood pool imaging, are all useful diagnostic techniques, but the preoperative or premortem diagnosis of aneurysm is still sometimes made incorrectly. Ventriculography is probably the most sensitive of the methods. When there is akinesia or, less often, dyskinesia, of the wall segment during systole, a permanent outward bulging or convexity,[G1,H3] thinning of the wall and lack of inner wall trabeculation, and clear demarcation of the area from the remaining ventricle, the diagnosis is probably correct. Wall thinning and even bulging of the contrast-medium–lined cavity can be undetected when there is extensive smooth clot; and it is frequently difficult to define the margins of an area with akinesia. The confident identification of significant mural thrombi adds to the probability of aneurysm, as does the presence of calcification in the wall. Right heart catheterization is useful, for it enables calculation of cardiac output. From the left heart study, the left ventricular end-diastolic pressure, ejection fraction, and end-diastolic volume are measured or calculated.

A coronary angiogram is always made.

NATURAL HISTORY

Time Course

About 10%–30% of patients with an acute myocardial infarction develop an LV aneurysm over a period of 2–8 weeks.[A3,N1] Such development cannot occur, of course, when the area of myocardial necrosis is massive and prevents survival. When the necrosis is transmural and involves most of the myocardial cells in a large area, but the area is sufficiently small to allow survival (this probably means < 40% of the LV wall area), the stage is set for aneurysm formation. While the occurrence of a large myocardial infarction is a prerequisite for aneurysm development, other conditions such as augmented segmental LV performance in adjacent areas are also required.[A3] Probable aggravating factors are hypertension[M5] and steroid therapy.[B9]

Survival

The 3-year survival rate of surgically untreated patients with aneurysm, dated from the time of acute infarction, may be as low as 25%[C4,N1] (Fig. 8-1) or as high as 79%[F10] (in contrast to 80% for patients in whom acute infarction does not result in an aneurysm) and the 5-year survival rate as low as 10%[S2] or as high as 70%.[F10]

The adverse effects of LV aneurysms on life-style and survival depend in great part on their extent and size,[F3,G1] and thus the magnitude of their geometric effects on the other parts of the LV wall. Patients with few symptoms, such as mild dyspnea only, generally have smaller aneurysms and a considerably better prognosis without surgical treatment than do those with symptoms of congestive heart failure (Fig. 8-2).[G6]

Poor LV systolic function, expressed as poor global ejection fraction or as segmental wall motion abnormalities in the

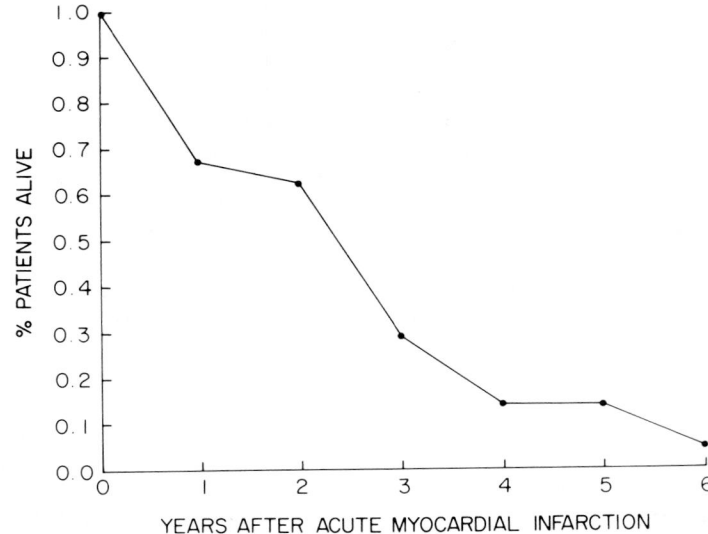

Figure 8-1   Length of survival, dated from the acute myocardial infarction, in 21 necropsy patients with classic left ventricular aneurysm.
Reproduced with modification from Cabin and Roberts.[C4]

nonaneurysmal portion of the ventricle, decreases survival time in patients treated nonsurgically.[G6] In fact, when functional status and left ventricular function are taken into account, there is probably no difference in survival of patients with ischemic heart disease with or without aneurysms.[F10]

Symptoms

The course during life of patients with LV aneurysm is frequently characterized by increasing impairment of LV function leading to chronic congestive heart failure and ultimately death.[C4,C7,H3] About half the patients, however, have only angina, and in such patients recurrent infarction is common. A smaller number of patients, about 10%, have a life-threatening ventricular arrhythmia (see "Special Situations and Controversies").

Effect on Left Ventricular Function

Aneurysms adversely affect LV function (and thus produce the chronic congestive heart failure characteristic of the natural history) by several mechanisms:[K5] (1) loss of contractile tissue in the area of aneurysm reduces segmental and global LV ejection fraction, (2) the resultant increase in ventricular size increases systolic wall stress (and myocardial oxygen consumption) by LaPlace's law, and (3) paradoxic expansion

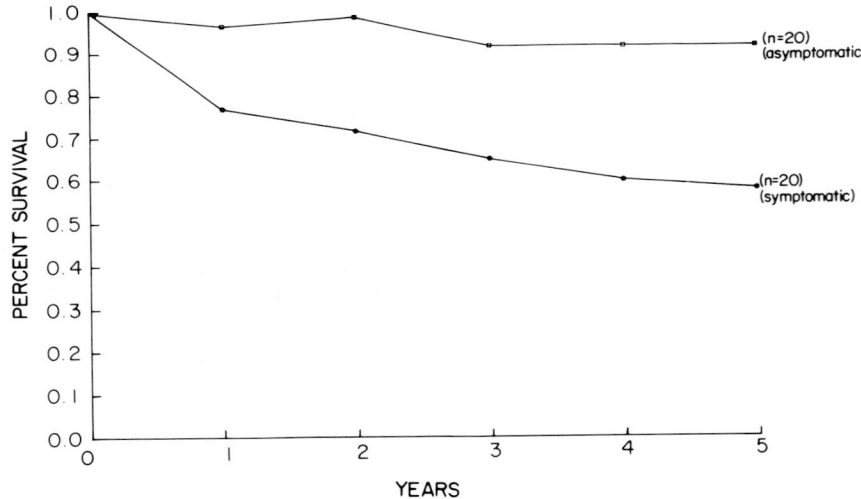

Figure 8-2   Five-year survival rate without surgery of 20 patients with few or no symptoms with left ventricular aneurysm and 20 symptomatic patients.
Adapted from Grondin et al.[G6]

of the aneurysm reduces forward stroke volume and ejection fraction, as proven experimentally by Austen and colleagues.[A1]

Complexities in Analysis of Natural History

The fact that important but dissimilar segmental wall abnormalities can result from scars or recent infarcts that are not morphologically LV aneurysms complicates the analysis of the natural history of patients with LV aneurysm. For example, Parmley and colleagues showed that the degree of paradoxic movement was least when a true, fibrous LV aneurysm was present and greatest when the "aneurysm" was acute and largely muscular.[P2] The latter condition is better termed an area of acute myocardial infarction. In such cases, according to Parmley and colleagues, the reduction in ejection fraction is greater than with a fibrous-walled aneurysm, other things being equal.

Since reports of natural history may include different kinds of ventricular scars within the category of ventricular aneurysm, it would be more useful to describe the natural history of the entire spectrum of postinfarction ventricular scars, varying from punctate, small scars scattered through an area of healed myocardial infarction that retains some contractile power, through larger scars composed partly of viable myocardial cells and partly of akinetic or dyskinetic fibrous tissue, to left ventricular aneurysms. In a way, Bruschke and colleagues acknowledge these difficulties by avoiding the term *aneurysm* in reporting a 5-year survival rate without operation of 69% in patients with left ventricular akinetic areas, 54% in patients with dyskinetic areas but good contractility in the rest of the ventricle, and 36% in patients with a dyskinetic area and a dilated and poorly contracting ventricle.[B3]

TECHNIQUE OF OPERATION

Most patients undergoing resection of postinfarction LV aneurysms or other scars also require the coronary artery bypass graft (CABG) operation. The following discussion is additive to the description of coronary artery bypass grafting in Chapter 7.

The preoperative and operating room preparations, removal and preparation of the vein graft, and median sternotomy are accomplished as described previously. The pericardial adhesions over the left ventricle are not disturbed at this point. Generally the distal anastomoses are made first, but if for some reason the proximal anastomoses are to be placed first, this is done now. Any adhesions that block the transverse sinus may be freed in order to pass one or more of the saphenous vein grafts through the sinus in the usual way.

Cardiopulmonary bypass at 34°C is established, using double venous cannulation and caval taping (GLH) or a single venous cannula (UAB). A left atrial or left ventricular vent is not inserted. If the adhesions are flimsy and can be separated with minimal manipulation of the left ventricle, the dissection is done at this point. Otherwise, it is deferred until the aorta is cross-clamped, lest mural thrombi in the left ventricle be dislodged by the operative manipulations and embolized. The cardioplegic needle is inserted, external cardiac

cooling is begun, the perfusate temperature is taken to as low a temperature as possible, the aorta is cross-clamped, and the cold cardioplegic solution is infused (see Chapter 3 for a discussion of the remainder of the myocardial protection techniques utilized). As the patient's body temperature approaches 25°C, the perfusate temperature is stabilized at that temperature.

When the adhesions are flimsy, they are mobilized over the entire aneurysm, but if the aneurysm is densely adherent to the pericardium, the left ventricle is separated from the aneurysm without disturbing these adhesions (Fig. 8-3). The junction of aneurysm and ventricle is incised at some convenient point. Loose thrombi are sought and removed. When the aneurysm contains considerable clot and debris, a sponge is tucked inside the ventricle over the aortic and mitral valves, which are at the bottom of the field, to prevent loss of debris into aorta and left atrium. This is removed after the dissection is completed, and a small vent sucker is placed through the incision into the ventricle and across the mitral valve into the left atrium. The suction is managed so as to maintain a pool of blood within the open ventricle, in order that air cannot enter the aorta or the coronary ostia. The incision is carried around the entire aneurysm, leaving a thin rim of tough scar to facilitate closure. The surgeon should bear in mind in performing this resection that a classic aneurysm has a smooth endocardial surface, and thus all the left ventricular free wall with a smooth endocardium should be removed. Additional endocardial tissue may be removed, and other procedures done, when the patient has a history of life-threatening ventricular arrhythmias (see "Intractable Ventricular Tachyarrhythmias" in section on Special Situations and Controversies). When large amounts of clot have required removal and fragments may have broken off, the ventricular cavity is inspected and irrigated to remove any debris. Otherwise, this is not done, in order to avoid the entrance of air into the aortic root and coronary ostia. If the aneurysm has been left adherent to the pericardium, thrombotic material is removed from its wall (this can be done later, during rewarming, after the ventricle is closed), and the avascular fibrous tissue is left attached to the pericardium.

The left ventricle is now reconstructed. A line of closure is selected that distorts the ventricle the least. Usually, a stay suture is placed at each end of the proposed closure. If the edges are tough and the aneurysm moderate in size, closure may be by two rows of a simple over-and-over stitch with 0 or 1 polypropylene on a large heavy needle. Otherwise, Teflon felt strips and a continuous horizontal mattress stitch are used, reinforced by a second over-and-over row (Fig. 8-3).

Just before this closure is completed, the ventricle is filled with cold saline solution. After the closure is completed, suction is placed on the needle vent in the ascending aorta (see Chapter 2). The venous line is intermittently occluded a few times to drive some blood through the lungs and into the left atrium and ventricle. A no. 14 needle is inserted momentarily into the apex of the left ventricle as the anesthesiologist inflates the lung to evacuate any bolus of air that may be present. Then another cold cardioplegic infusion is given into the ascending aorta.

The distal vein grafts to coronary artery anastomoses are now made (see "Technique of Operation" in Chapter 7). The LAD artery and second and third diagonal arteries are often obliterated and not graftable, and even if open, they are not grafted if they supply only an area of full-thickness scar. The first diagonal artery is frequently included among the vessels grafted. With strong suction on the aortic needle vent, the aortic cross-clamp is released, and rewarming is begun. The heart must be de-aired at this point (see Chapter 2), before removing the aortic cross-clamp and performing the proximal anastomoses. The proximal anastomoses are then made, and the operation is completed as described earlier.

SPECIAL FEATURES OF POSTOPERATIVE CARE

The postoperative care is the same as that for other patients after open heart surgery (see Chapter 5) and particularly after coronary artery bypass grafting.

EARLY RESULTS

Hospital Mortality

Before about 1977, most cardiac surgical units reported a hospital mortality of 10%–20% for left ventricular aneurysmectomy.[B1,C5,C7,L3,M2,R1,S2] The UAB mortality was 11%,[R1] and the GLH experience was similar (Table 8-2). However, even in that era, better results were obtained in some units.[M3,R2] As demonstrated by the more recent GLH experience (Table 8-3) and the still more recent UAB experience (Table 8-4), current results are better. Hospital mortality in the combined GLH-UAB recent series (27 deaths among 334 patients) is 8.1% (CL 6.5%–9.9%). It does not approach zero primarily because of the poor left ventricular function present preoperatively in some patients and the inability to identify precisely left ventricular dysfunction so severe as to be incompatible with survival. The reduction in mortality in the current era is related to improved myocardial protection, more complete myocardial revasculariza-

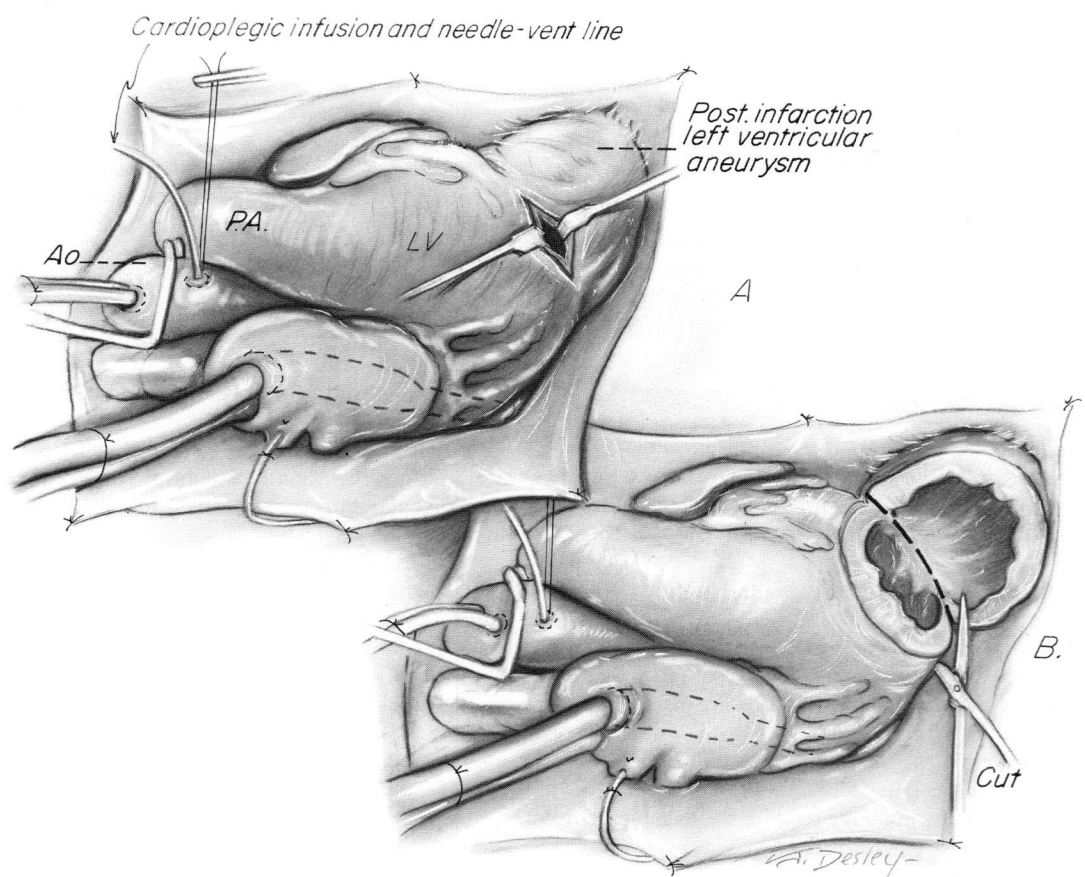

Figure 8-3 The technique of left ventricular aneurysmectomy.
(a) Without mobilizing the aneurysm from the pericardium and after cross-clamping the aorta and injecting the cardioplegic solution, an incision is made into the junction between the left ventricle and the aneurysm.
(b) The left ventricle is cut away from the aneurysm, which is left in place, adherent to the pericardium.

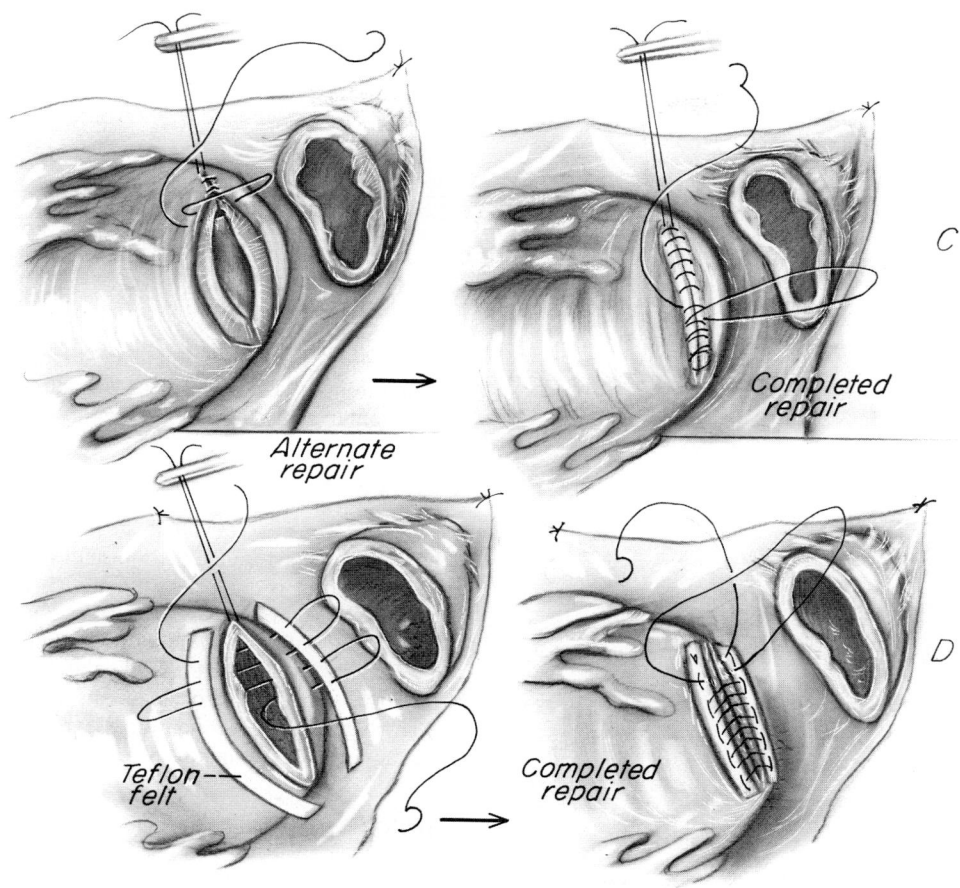

Figure 8-3 (*continued*)

(*c*) When the edges of the left ventriculotomy are fibrous and tough, a simple through-and-through two-row closure is made with 0 or 1 polypropylene.

(*d*) When the edges are more muscular or the resection is particularly large, felt strips are used, with two rows of sutures.

Ao, aorta; PA, pulmonary artery.

Table 8-2 Early and late results (follow-up 1–121 months, mean 39 months) from resection or plication of left ventricular aneurysms, scars, and infarcts (GLH; 1969–1982).[B10]

		Hospital Deaths			Late Deaths			Late Survivors		
	n	No.	%	CL	No.	%[a]	CL	No.	%[b]	CL
True LVA	145	22	15%	12%–19%	44	36%	31%–41%	79	54%	50%–59%
Scar or infarct	24	3	12%	6%–24%	9	43%	30%–56%	12	50%	38%–62%
LVA + valve surgery	7	1	14%	2%–41%	5	83%	54%–98%	1	14%	2%–41%
LVA or infarct + VSD surgery	3	0	0%	0%–47%	1	33%	4%–76%	2	67%	24%–96%
False LVA	2	0	0%	0%–61%	1	50%	7%–93%	1	50%	7%–93%
Total	181	26	14%	12%–18%	60	39%	34%–43%	95	52%	48%–57%

KEY: LVA, left ventricular aneurysm; VSD, ventricular septal defect.

[a] Percent of hospital survivors.

[b] Percent of those who underwent operation originally (*n*).

Table 8-3 The influence of year of operation on hospital death following surgery for left ventricular aneurysm and scar or infarcts (GLH; 1969–1982).

Era (year)		LVA				Scar or Infarct				Total			
			Hospital Deaths				Hospital Deaths				Hospital Deaths		
≤ <	n	No.	%	CL	n	No.	%	CL	n	No.	%	CL
1969 --- 1975	21	7	33%	22%–47%	4	1	25%	3%–63%	25	8	32%	21%–44%
1975 --- 1982	124	15	12%	9%–16%	20	2	10%	3%–22%	144	17	12%	9%–15%
Total	145	22	15%	12%–19%	24	3	12%	6%–24%	179	25	14%	11%–17%
P			.01								.02	

KEY: CL, 70% confidence limits; LVA, left ventricular aneurysm.

Table 8-4 Hospital mortality after left ventricular aneurysmectomy in the current era (UAB; 1977–1981). Results of primary isolated CABG operations in the same years are shown for comparison.

Category		Hospital Deaths		
	n	No.	%	CL
Primary isolated CABG	3608	26	0.72%	0.58%–0.90%
LV Aneurysmectomy	210	12	5.7%	4.1%–7.9%
Isolated with or without CABG	175	8	4.6%	3.0%–6.8%
With MVR or MVA	8	1	12%	2%–36%
With surgical treatment of ventricular tachycardia	13	1	8%	1%–24%
With surgical treatment of VSD	6	1	17%	2%–46%
Other	8	1	12%	2%–36%

KEY: CABG, coronary artery bypass grafting; CL, 70% confidence limits; LV, left ventricular; MVA, mitral valve annuloplasty; MVR, mitral valve replacement; VSD, ventricular septal defect.

Table 8-5 Incremental risk factors for hospital death after resection or plication of left ventricular aneurysm (n = 145; GLH; 1969–1981).[B10] (The variables tested and the details of the logistic regression method are in the original paper[B10]). The same variables were significant when the patients with left ventricular scars as well as aneurysms were included.

Variable	Coefficient ± SD	P value
NYHA class (0, 1, or 4)[a]	1.4 ± 0.35	< .00001
Myocardial score (0–15)	0.6 ± 0.20	.0001
Date of operation (before January 1974)	3.4 ± 0.97	.0001
Furosemide (frusemide) > 80 mg (0 or 1)[b]	1.2 ± 0.63	.06
Intercept	10.66	

NOTE: In this table and in Table 8-12, a positive coefficient signifies an increased probability of death and a negative coefficient the opposite.
KEY: SD, standard deviation.
[a] 0 = class I, II, III; 1 = class IV; 4 = class V.
[b] 0 = no, 1 = yes.

tion,[B10,J2] better protection against embolization, and the introduction of direct surgical measures against intractable ventricular arrhythmias (see Chapter 48).

Mode of Death

The mode of hospital death in the past decade has usually been acute heart failure. About half of these deaths occur in the operating room or within hours of leaving it and the others from persistent low cardiac output with or without myocardial infarction and with or without graft occlusion at autopsy.[B10] Intractable ventricular arrhythmias have been the other chief cause of death, usually in patients operated on for ventricular tachycardia. Severe cerebral damage from entrapped clot or air has also occurred.

Table 8-6 Hospital mortality related to the extent of occlusive coronary artery disease in patients undergoing left ventricular aneurysmectomy (GLH; 1969–1982; missing values existed in cases not included).

Extent of Coronary Artery Disease	Total		Hospital Deaths		
	n	% of n Total	No.	%	70% CL
Single vessel	31	22%	2	6%[a]	2%–15%
Double vessel	38	27%	6	16%	10%–24%
Triple vessel	62	44%	12	19%[a]	14%–26%
Left main	9	6%	2	22%	8%–45%
Total	140		22	16%	12%–20%
P(χ²)				.4	

Extent of Coronary Artery Disease	Total		Hospital Deaths		
	n	% of n Total	No.	%	70% CL
Myocardial score < 10	55	39%	6	11%	7%–17%
Myocardial score 10–12	61	43%	8	13%	9%–19%
Myocardial score > 12	25	18%	8	32%	21%–44%
Total	141		22	16%	12%–19%
P(χ²)				.04[b]	

[a] Single- versus triple-vessel disease: P(χ²) = .1 or .09 (Fisher).
[b] Myocardial score < 10 vs > 12: P(χ²) = .02.

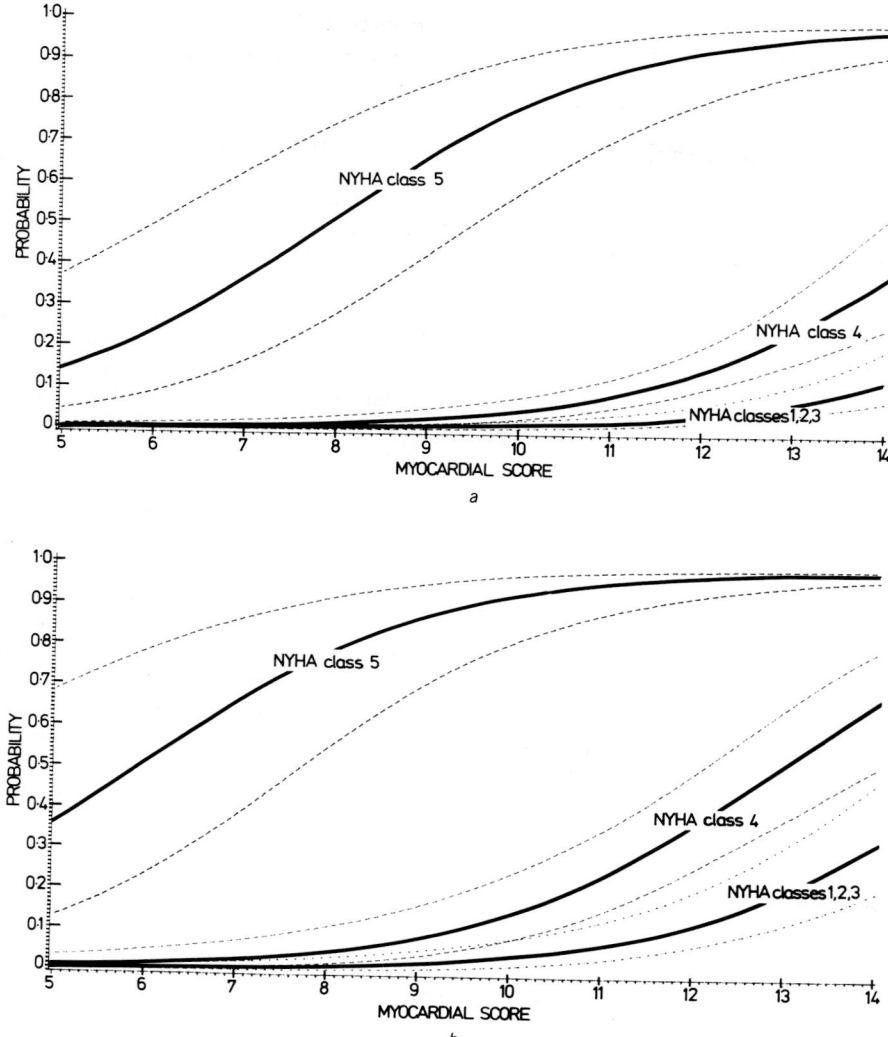

Figure 8-4 Nomogram of the GLH multivariate logistic equation for hospital deaths after left ventricular aneurysmectomy (Table 8-5). The dashed lines enclose the 70% confidence limits. The interacting incremental risks of a high myocardial score and poor functional status, related at least in part to poor left ventricular function, are well demonstrated.
(a) With ≤ 80 mg furosemide (frusemide) daily.
(b) With > 80 mg furosemide daily.
Reproduced with permission from Barratt-Boyes et al.[B10]

Incremental Risk Factors for Early Death

Extent of Occlusive Coronary Artery Disease
The more extensive the occlusive coronary artery disease, the greater the hospital mortality after left ventricular aneurysmectomy, even when complete revascularization is attempted (Tables 8-5, 8-6).[B10] However, the effect is not evident unless the coronary artery disease is very extensive, as for example disease with a myocardial score of about 10 or more in the GLH system[B8] (Fig. 8-4). Such a relationship has not always been found by others.[R1,R4,W4] This may relate to the fact that most other reports have used the simple

classification of single-, double-, or triple-vessel disease or used only univariate analysis. Thus, single-vessel, double-vessel, triple-vessel, and left main coronary artery disease did not appear as risk factors in the GLH multivariate[B10] or simple contingency table analysis (Table 8-6). Similarly, in the current UAB experience, this less precise way of expressing the extent of the coronary artery stenoses showed that a relationship was only possibly present (Table 8-7). Analysis of the UAB experience did indicate that it is the overall extent of the coronary disease, not the presence or absence of left main coronary artery disease, that is important (Table 8-7). Brawley and colleagues found the presence

Table 8-7 Hospital mortality after left ventricular aneurysmectomy (plication in six patients), related to the number of stenosed coronary arteries (UAB; 1977–1981). For this analysis, a vessel was considered severely stenosed if the luminal diameter was reduced by 70% or more, except for the left main coronary artery, in which severe stenosis was defined as a narrowing of 50% or more.

Number of Severely Stenosed Coronary Arteries	n	Hospital Deaths		
		No.	%	CL
Without Left Main Disease				
0	1	0		
1	58	2	3%	1%–8%
2	69	2	3%	1%–7%
3	69	6	9%	5%–14%
Total	210	12	5.7%	4.1%–7.9%
With Left Main Disease	13	2	15%	5%–33%
+ 1	1	0		
+ 2	6	0		
+ 3	6	2		
Total	210	12	5.7%	4.1%–7.9%
$P(\chi^2)$			.18	
P(logistic)			.07	

KEY: CL, 70% confidence limits.

NOTE: A two-variable logistic analysis was made of hospital death related to (1) the number of severely diseased arteries (0,1,2, or 3) and (2) the presence of left main coronary artery disease (yes or no). P for variable 1 = .08; P for variable 2 = .21.

of circumflex artery stenosis to increase the early risks of left ventricular aneurysmectomy,[B5] and this was true also in the GLH analysis[B10] ($P = .07$).

Left Ventricular Dysfunction

As in other kinds of surgery for ischemic heart disease, preoperative global left ventricular dysfunction adversely affects the hospital mortality after left ventricular aneurysmectomy.[N4] The evidence for this is both direct and indirect.

Part of the indirect evidence is the fact that poor preoperative functional status, which probably reflects at least in part poor global left ventricular function, is clearly an important independent risk factor (Table 8-5), a fact also suggested by contingency table analysis of the GLH experience (Table 8-8) and by the experience of others.[R4,W5] In the GLH analysis, NYHA class included symptoms of either heart failure or angina; therefore, the analysis is not specific for heart failure. However, the presence of severe fluid retention certainly reflects poor left ventricular function, and the GLH analysis clearly established poor LV function as an incremental risk factor (Tables 8-5, 8-9). The finding of preoperatively elevated left ventricular end-diastolic pressure as a risk factor by univariate analysis[K6] supports these ideas, although it dropped out in favor of other variables in the GLH multivariate analysis. A low cardiac index preoperatively has been found to be a risk factor for hospital death by several groups,[C7,M2,S10] again indirect evidence of the unfavorable effect of poor left ventricular function.

Table 8-8 Hospital mortality related to NYHA functional class of patients undergoing operation for left ventricular aneurysm and scar or infarcts (GLH; 1969–1982).

NYHA Class	LVA				Scar or Infarct			
		Hospital Deaths				Hospital Deaths		
	n	No.	%	CL	n	No.	%	CL
I	0				0			
II	39	2	5%	2%–12%	7	0	0%	0%–24%
III	52	5	10%	5%–15%	7	0	0%	0%–24%
IV	48	10	21%	15%–29%	9	2	22%	7%–45%
V	6	5	83%	54%–98%	1	1	100%	15%–100%
Total	145	22	15%	12%–19%	24	3	12%	6%–24%
$P(\chi^2)$			.0001				.02	

KEY: CL, 70% confidence limits; LVA, left ventricular aneurysm.

Table 8-9 Hospital mortality related to preoperative diuretic dose in patients undergoing left ventricular aneurysmectomy (GLH; 1969–1982).

Preoperative Dose of Diuretic (Furosemide) (mg daily)	LVA				Scar or Infarct			
		Hospital Deaths				Hospital Deaths		
	n	No.	%	CL	n	No.	%	CL
≤ 80	112	11	10%	7%–14%	17	1	6	0.8%–19%
> 80	33	11	33%	24%–44%	7	2	29%	10%–55%
Total	145	22	15%	12%–19%	24	3	12%	6%–24%
$P(\chi^2)$			.0009					

KEY: CL, 70% confidence limits; LVA, left ventricular aneurysm.

The segmental wall function of the nonaneurysmal portion of the left ventricle was not related to the probability of hospital death in the GLH multivariate analysis.[B10] This may be because the method of assessing the segmental wall function was not sufficiently sensitive, but Fontan and colleagues also found the ejection fraction of the nonaneurysmal portion of the left ventricle unrelated to the probability of hospital death after resection.[F5] However, Keifer and colleagues reported a hospital mortality of 6.5% after left ventricular aneurysmectomy in patients with ejection fractions of the nonaneurysmal portion of the ventricle of 35% or greater and a left ventricular end-diastolic pressure less than 25 mmHg; otherwise, the hospital mortality was 27%.[K8] Muller and colleagues found absence of septal motion a risk factor.[M3] This all suggests that the severity and extent of wall motion abnormalities of the nonaneurysmal part of the ventricle may in fact be incremental risk factors.

The interrelated effects of left ventricular dysfunction (as estimated by the patient's functional status) and the extent of the occlusive coronary artery disease are well demonstrated in the GLH analysis[B10] (Fig. 8-4). The adverse effect of a larger myocardial score is evident only when the score is 12 or greater in patients in NYHA class I, II, or III; in patients in class IV or V, a myocardial score of 9 is already an evident incremental risk. When there is less extensive obstructive coronary artery disease (myocardial score of less than 9), even NYHA class IV does not increase the probability of hospital death.

Date of Operation
The effect of the era in which the operation was done, as mentioned earlier, is supported by the multivariate analysis of the GLH experience (Table 8-5). Thus, in the more recent experiences, the risk of hospital death is less.

Variables Apparently Not Related to Early Risks
As in the isolated CABG operation, increasing the number of distal anastomoses does not increase the probability of hospital death, other things being equal (Tables 8-5, 8-10). Older age is not demonstrated to be a risk factor, but age over 70 years may increase risk. The interval between the acute infarction and aneurysm resection does not affect hospital mortality.[C7]

Ventricular Arrhythmias

In the early experience with left ventricular aneurysmectomy, the early postoperative course was complicated by important ventricular arrhythmias in about half of the patients.[F7] Current surgical approaches in patients with preoperative life-threatening arrhythmias have decreased the morbidity and mortality from this problem (see Chapter 48).

LATE RESULTS
Survival

Among patients leaving the hospital alive after left ventricular aneurysmectomy, 70%–85% survived at least 3 years,[B10,C2] 70%–75% survived at least 5–6 years,[B1,F5,F7,L4,O1] (Fig. 8-5) but only about 45% remained alive 8 years after operation in the GLH experience[B10] (Fig. 8-6, Table 8-11). These survival rates are generally considered better than those with nonsurgical treatment.[C6,F5,G6]

Comparing resection for left ventricular aneurysm to isolated CABG, other variables being equal, the resection of a left ventricular aneurysm appears to increase the risk of death in both the early and late phase (Fig. 8-7a) and result in a 5-year survival rate of about 73%, compared to 83% for isolated CABG (Fig. 8-7b). Presumably this is related to the effect of the resection or reconstruction on left ventricular structure and function.

The survival figures given above are an oversimplification because of the differing results in some subsets of patients with left ventricular aneurysm.[B10] Thus, at GLH, the late survival rate was higher among hospital survivors of aneurysmectomy whose only preoperative symptom was angina than it was among those whose symptom was congestive heart failure (Fig. 8-8). In fact, patients with angina with or without a history of congestive heart failure had better late survival rates than those with congestive heart failure alone (Table 8-11). Burton and colleagues reported similar findings.[B1] Presumably the adverse effect of a history of congestive heart failure without angina is that this syndrome is usually found in patients with advanced left ventricular dysfunction.[C7]

Mode of Premature Late Death

The late deaths are due to recurrent myocardial infarction in about 33% of cases and to recurrent and progressive congestive heart failure without reinfarction in another 33%. The remaining deaths are due either to ventricular arrhythmia (about 20%) or other cardiac or noncardiac illnesses.[B10]

Table 8-10 Hospital mortality after left ventricular aneurysmectomy, related to the number of concomitantly made distal anastomoses beyond stenosed coronary arteries (UAB; 1977–1981).

Number of Distal Anastomoses	n	Hospital Deaths		
		No.	%	CL
0	33	1	3%	0.4%–10%
1	47	4	9%	4%–15%
2	46	2	4%	1%–10%
3	44	2	5%	2%–10%
4	28	1	4%	0.5%–12%
5	10	2	20%	7%–41%
6	2	0	0%	0%–61%
Total	210	12	5.7%	4.1%–7.9%
$P(\chi^2)$			.5	
P(logistic)			.6	

KEY: CL, 70% confidence limits.

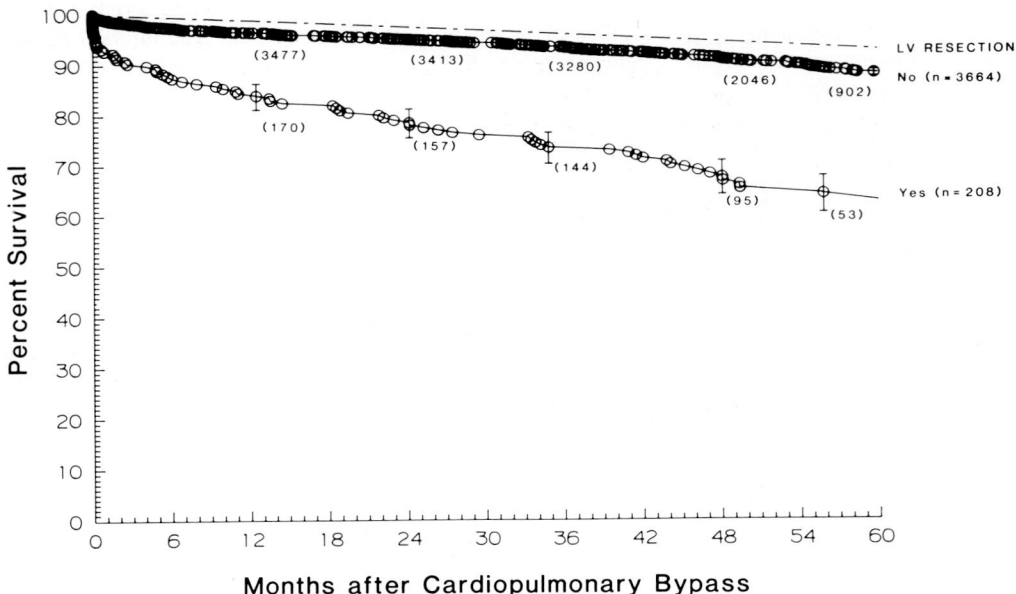

Figure 8-5   Actuarial survival curve of patients undergoing left ventricular resection for aneurysm and coronary artery bypass grafting compared to that of patients in whom no left ventricular resection was done (UAB; 1977–1981; presentation and data base are as described in Chapter 7, Fig. 7-12).

Incremental Risk Factors for Premature Late Death

Extent and Location of Coronary Artery Disease

Extensive coronary artery disease was a risk factor for premature late death in some earlier reports,[F1,G5,L4] and this may have been related to less complete concomitant revascularizations. In the earlier[R1] and current UAB experience (see Chapter 7, Table 7-5) and in the multivariate analysis of the GLH experience[B10] (Table 8-12), the extent of the coronary artery disease was not a risk factor for premature late death after surgical treatment.

The specific presence of important right coronary artery stenosis was an incremental risk factor ($P = .001$) in the GLH multivariate analysis[B10] (Fig. 8-9).

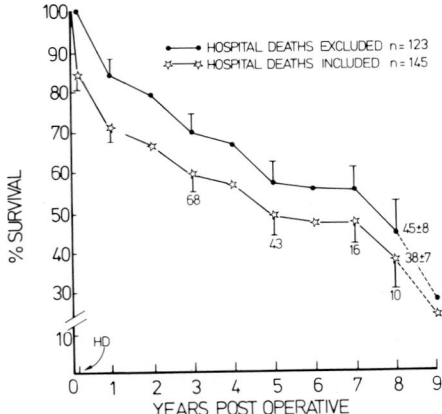

Figure 8-6   Actuarial survival curves for patients with left ventricular aneurysms (GLH; 1969–1982). The numbers of patients at risk are noted.

Reproduced with permission from Barratt-Boyes et al.[B10]

Preoperative Nonaneurysmal Left Ventricular Function

Impaired systolic function (contractility) of the posterior basal segment of the left ventricle was an incremental risk factor for premature late death in the GLH multivariate analysis[B10] (Table 8-12, Fig. 8-10) and was equally significant when inferior aneurysms were excluded from the analysis. The results of other studies[B1,M6] are in accord with these findings. It is to be expected that the late result is strongly related to the function of the basal segments, in view of the fact that the anterior-apical area (the usual site of aneurysm resection) uniformly is akinetic after resection. As is also to be expected, impaired septal systolic function is also a risk factor.[M3] This was not assessed in the GLH analysis.

Extent and Quality of Myocardial Revascularization

In the GLH multivariate analysis, the greater the number of distal anastomoses, the greater the probability of late survival (Table 8-12), although the completeness of the revascularization per se was not a risk factor. Cosgrove and colleagues from the Cleveland Clinic reported a 7-year survival rate after LV aneurysmectomy of 65% in patients with multiple-vessel disease undergoing concomitant complete revascularization, compared to 50% for those with incomplete revascularization ($P = .005$).[C9]

Preoperative Congestive Heart Failure versus Angina

Burton and colleagues found that congestive heart failure, rather than angina, as the indication for operation, was a risk factor for premature late death.[B1] Similar findings have been reported by Rittenhouse and colleagues.[R4] As noted earlier, the GLH experience is similar (Table 8-11), although in the

Table 8-11 Hospital, late, and total mortality after left ventricular aneurysmectomy, according to preoperative symptoms (GLH; 1969–1982). Note the marked and evident difference ($P < .001$) in total deaths between patients with angina alone and those with CHF alone.

Symptoms	Total Patients	Hospital Deaths			Late Deaths			Total Deaths			Late Survival		
		n	%	CL	n	%[a]	CL	n	%[b]	CL	n	%[a]	CL
Angina alone	53	4	8%	4%–13%	11	22%	16%–30%	15	28%	22%–36%	38	78%	70%–84%
CHF alone	30	8	27%	18%–37%	17	77%	64%–87%	25	83%	73%–91%	5	23%	13%–36%
CHF + mild angina	12	2	17%	6%–35%	0	0%	0%–17%	2	17%	6%–35%	10	100%	83%–100%
CHF + severe angina	27	3	11%	5%–21%	8	33%	22%–46%	11	41%	30%–53%	16	67%	54%–78%
Mild effort dyspnea	1	0	0%	0%–86%	0	0%	0%–86%	0	0%	0%–86%	1	100%	15%–100%
VT ± other symptoms	22	5	23%	13%–36%	8	47%	32%–62%	13	59%	46%–71%	9	53%	38%–68%
Total	145	22	15%	12%–19%	44	36%	31%–41%	66	46%	41%–51%	79	64%	59%–69%
$P(\chi^2)$			.22			< .001						< .001	

KEY: CHF, congestive heart failure; CL, 70% confidence limits; VT, intractable ventricular tachycardia.

[a] Percent of hospital survivors.

[b] Percent of total patients.

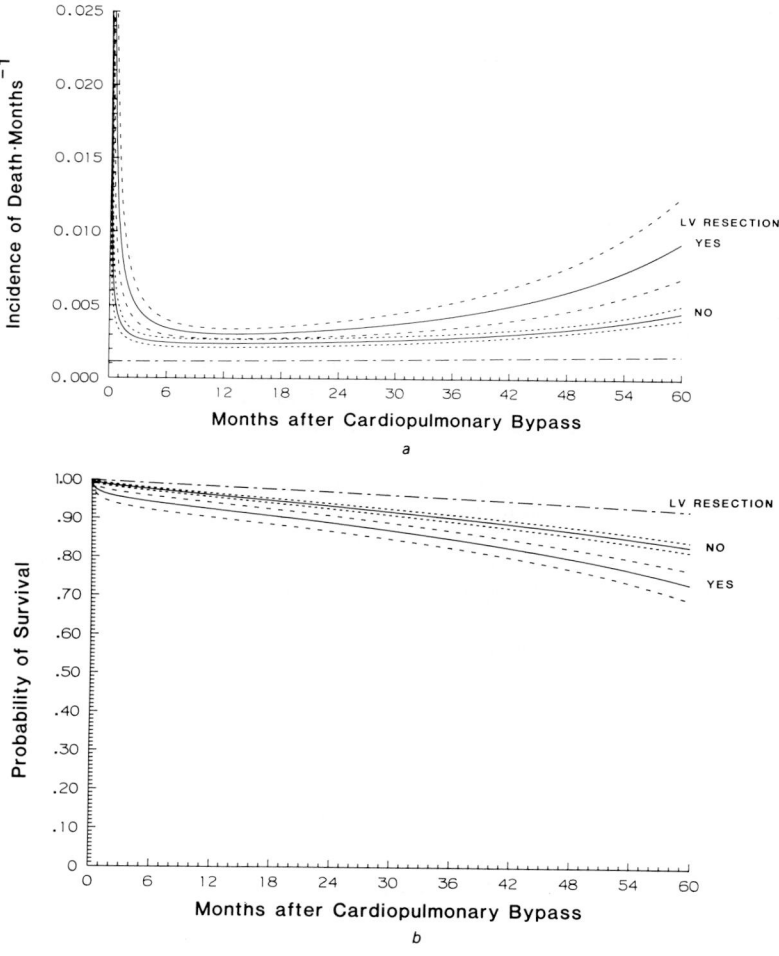

Figure 8-7 Effect of left ventricular resection for aneurysm, along with coronary artery bypass grafting, on survival (UAB; 1977–1981; data base and depiction are as in Chapter 7, Fig. 7-13). These nomograms are solutions of the multivariate equation in Chapter 7, Table 7-5. Operation for intractable ventricular tachycardia and operation for ischemic mitral incompetence were entered no. The following mean values of the other parameters in patients undergoing LV resection were entered in the equations for both LV resection yes and no: CASS LV score 15, LV end-diastolic pressure, 20, aortic cross-clamp time 50 minutes.
(a) Hazard function (instantaneous risk, or incidence, of death per month).
(b) Parametric estimates of survival.
Reproduced with permission from Kirklin et al.,[K9] and the American College of Cardiology.

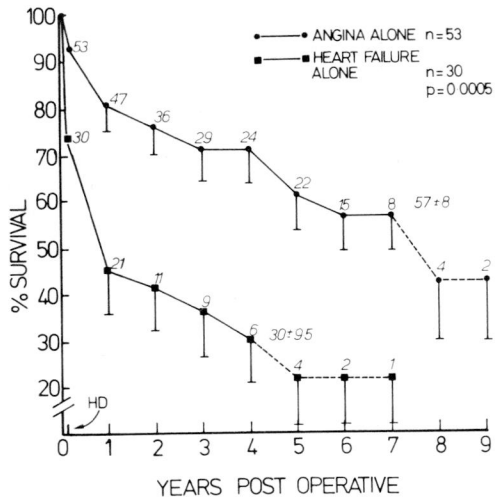

Figure 8-8 Actuarial survival curves for surgically treated patients with isolated left ventricular aneurysm, comparing those with congestive heart failure as the only symptom with those complaining only of angina (GLH; 1969–1981). The numbers of patients at risk are noted.

Reproduced with permission from Barratt-Boyes et al.[B10]

multivariate analysis, only a history of angina was retained (as a variable *increasing* the probability of late survival) (Fig. 8-11).

Preoperative Life-Threatening Ventricular Electrical Instability

Although not identified as a risk factor in the GLH multivariate analysis, the univariate analysis (Table 8-11) suggests that intractable preoperative ventricular tachycardia may be an incremental risk factor for premature late death. Also, Frank and colleagues treated by aneurysmectomy 13 patients with aneurysms and life-threatening ventricular arrhythmias;[F7] 4 died in hospital of ventricular tachyarrhythmias, and 2 died suddenly a few years later. One survivor still had life-threatening ventricular tachycardia, 4 had other

Table 8-12 Incremental risk factors by proportional hazards regression analysis for premature late death after 30 days following surgery for true left ventricular aneurysm (GLH; 1969–1982).[B10]

Variable	Coefficient ± SD	P Value
RCA stenosis	1.72 ± 0.50	.001
Contr 5	1.17 ± 0.44	.008
Angina	−0.54 ± 0.21	.01
Number of grafts	−0.51 ± 0.21	.02

KEY: Contr 5, contractility of posterior basal segment of left ventricle (RAO ventriculogram); RCA, right coronary artery; SD, standard deviation (so-called standard error).

NOTE: RCA stenosis of ⩾ 75% cross-sectional area loss was no-yes; Contr 5 was 0 for normal or hypokinetic, 1 for akinetic or dyskinetic; for angina, 0 indicated none, 1 mild, and 2 severe; the number of grafts was 0–4. The details of the analysis are in the published paper.[B10]

complex arrhythmias, and only 2 were free of arrhythmias.[F7] Direct operations for arrhythmias will no doubt improve this situation in the future.

Symptomatic Results

Most long-term survivors have a reasonable period of marked symptomatic improvement after LV aneurysmectomy. In the GLH series, 79 surviving patients were followed up to 122 months (mean 45 months). Although preoperatively 72% were in NYHA classes III, IV, or V, at last follow-up only 12% were in these classes. Donaldson and colleagues reported 18 (62%, CL 51%–72%) of 29 hospital survivors of resection of symptomatic aneurysms to be asymptomatic an average of 18 months after operation,[D3] and Fontan reported 64% to be well an average of 36 months after operation.[F5] Crosby and colleagues found 95% of hospital survivors to be in NYHA functional class I or II an average of 40 months after operation, with the proportion in full and gainful employment in the 61 hospital survivors increasing from 33% preoperatively to 63% postoperatively.[C10] Exercise testing has confirmed the functional improvement that many patients experience after LV aneurysmectomy.[B14]

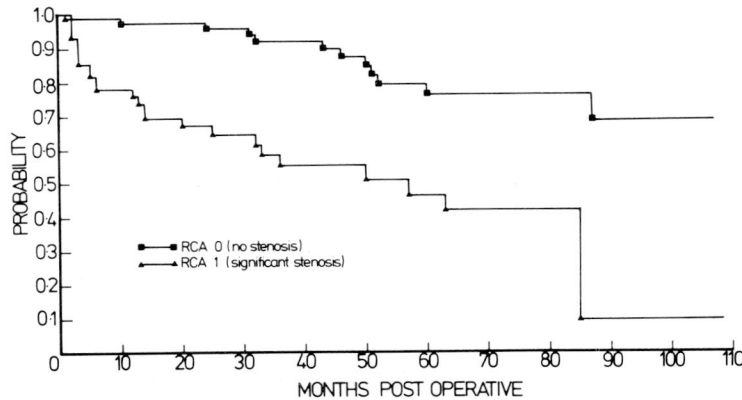

Figure 8-9 Actuarial survival curves for patients with and without significant (⩾ 75% area reduction) stenosis of the right coronary artery.

Reproduced with permission from Barratt-Boyes et al.[B10]

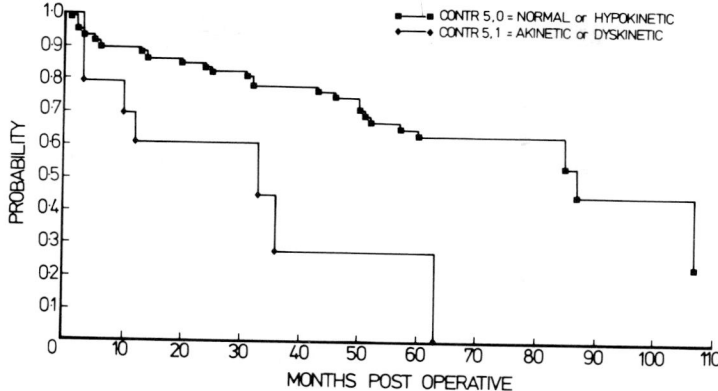

Figure 8-10 Actuarial survival curves for hospital survivors of left ventricular aneurysmectomy for isolated LV aneurysm according to the contractility of the posterior basal segment of the left ventricle. The analyses for this and Figures 8-8 and 8-9 are based on Table 8-12, with standardization for number of grafts = 0, angina = 0, contractility 5 = 0, and RCA stenosis = 0. The standardization was omitted for the variable displayed in the figure.
Reproduced with permission from Barratt-Boyes et al.[B10]

Even the difficult preoperative symptom of life-threatening ventricular tachyarrhythmias has been relieved in 52% of hospital survivors by simple aneurysmectomy and coronary artery bypass grafting.[C9]

Reoperation may be necessary either because of recurrent angina or, rarely, because of the occurrence of LV aneurysm or the appearance of mitral regurgitation. Reoperation was required in 5% of the GLH patients.[B10]

Late Postoperative Global Left Ventricular Performance

The resection of classic large LV aneurysms itself may improve resting global left ventricular performance.[C1,D6, M7,S5] A reduction in end-diastolic pressure is well correlated with the clinical improvement in some patients.[S5] Harman and colleagues (UAB) demonstrated in 1969 in three patients with single-vessel LAD artery disease and classic aneurysm that simple resection, without coronary artery bypass grafting, increased left ventricular ejection fraction, stroke volume, and stroke work, as well as cardiac index, and reduced left ventricular end-diastolic pressure and volume.[H1] Two of three patients were also relieved of angina pectoris. The data indicate that the resection and resultant decrease in LV volume decreases wall forces according to LaPlace's law. The decreased tension (afterload) during systole probably increases the rate of fiber shortening, thus increasing stroke volume, and decreases myocardial oxygen consumption, thus decreasing angina pectoris (see Chapter 5, footnote 10). Autoregulatory mechanisms then decrease LV end-diastolic pressures. The overall result is improved cardiac performance and relief of the symptoms of heart failure and often of angina pectoris.

Left ventricular performance is not demonstrably improved in all patients by aneurysmectomy with or without bypass grafting, and some patients with clear symptomatic improvement are without objective evidence of improvement in LV global function.[F6] Possible mechanisms for the failure of LV function to improve demonstrably in some patients include incomplete aneurysm resection (Froehlich

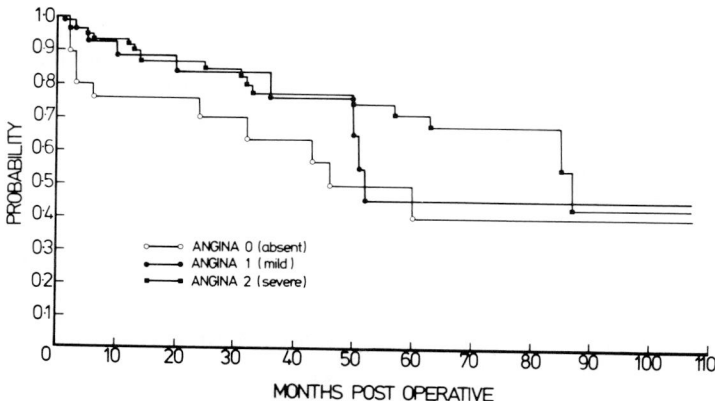

Figure 8-11 Actuarial survival curves for patients with varying grades of angina preoperatively.
Reproduced with permission from Barratt-Boyes et al.[B10]

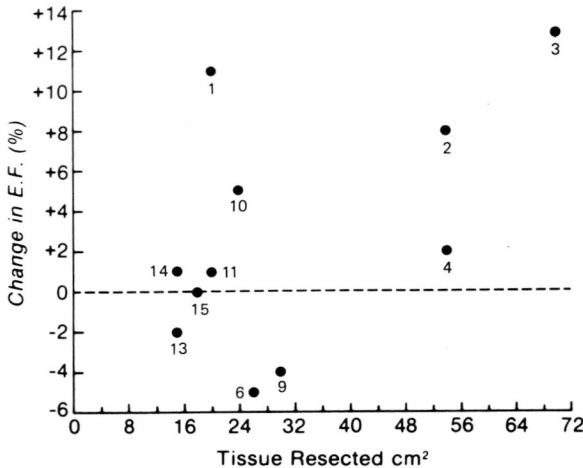

Figure 8-12   Relationship between size of resected left ventricular wall (aneurysm), on the horizontal axis, and change in resting ejection fraction, on the verticle axis, after left ventricular aneurysmectomy with or without bypass grafting. Although the number of patients is small, the data suggest that ejection fraction is increased postoperatively only when the aneurysm resection is large.
Reproduced with permission from Froehlich et al.[F6]

and colleagues found in most of their patients that only 50% of the noncontractile area visualized by left ventriculography was resected[F6]); small size of the aneurysm and thus small changes by LaPlace's law after resection (see Fig. 8-12); size of the akinetic scar resulting from resection (see "Late Postoperative Segmental Left Ventricular Wall Motion"); and intraoperative damage to nonaneurysmal portions of the ventricle.

It is also possible that current techniques of studying LV function do not identify the small increases in LV function that allow symptomatic improvement. However, in a careful study, Dymond and colleagues found no improvement in exercise left ventricular ejection fraction or exercise stroke volume index, even though the resting values for these variables were improved.[D6] They noted particularly that postoperative exercise function remained abnormal even in patients with single-vessel coronary artery disease.

Late Postoperative Segmental Left Ventricular Wall Motion

The area of scar produced by the suture line after aneurysmectomy is always akinetic,[S5] which detracts significantly from global LV performance. The extent of this area of akinesia is variable and may in part be related to incomplete aneurysm resection, but it seems always present and is always a significant detractor from global LV function.[S9]

The postoperative segmental left ventricular wall motion of the parts uninvolved by the postresection scar is probably determined by the same factors operative after simple coronary artery bypass grafting in addition to those resulting from reduction in the left ventricular volume by LaPlace's law, incident to the aneurysmectomy, as described under "Late Postoperative Global Left Ventricular Performance." Also, Shaw and colleagues found the postoperative segmental wall motion of these areas well correlated ($r = .76$) with

the patient's preoperative functional class,[S5] and thus presumably with preoperative segmental wall motion.

INDICATIONS FOR OPERATION

A large left ventricular aneurysm in a symptomatic patient, particularly one with angina pectoris, is an indication for operation. Appropriate coronary artery bypass grafting is indicated at the time of aneurysmectomy, as described in Chapter 6.

In view of the high risk of operation in patients with advanced chronic congestive heart failure, operation is not recommended in such a setting when the known risk factors are highly unfavorable to survival. From Figure 8-4 it is apparent that a patient with an LV aneurysm, in NYHA class V, with a myocardial score of 8 (double-vessel disease) or more, and requiring more than 80 mg furosemide (frusemide) daily for severe congestive heart failure has a probability of hospital death of 80% (CL 55%–90%), while if the myocardial score is 11 or greater, the risk approaches 100%. In both these circumstances, operation is probably contraindicated. The risk is lower when the congestive heart failure is less severe (as evidenced by a daily furosemide dosage less than 80 mg and a NYHA class IV or less), and in such circumstances operation is advised. In borderline cases, akinesia or dyskinesia of the posterior-basal segment of the left ventricle is recognized as an additional risk factor, and its presence may weigh against a decision for operation. The same is true for significant right coronary artery stenosis.

When the left ventricular aneurysm is small or moderate sized, it is not per se an indication for operation. This conclusion is in part based on the fact that many preoperatively diagnosed aneurysms are not found to be aneurysms at operation or autopsy. Patients in such situations are advised about operation on the basis of their coronary artery disease and left ventricular function, as described in Chapter 6, rather than on the basis of the small or moderate-sized aneurysm. In this regard, it is noteworthy that an aneurysm that remains small 1 year after the infarction is unlikely to enlarge progressively thereafter, and embolization from it is unlikely.

When the indications for resection of an LV aneurysm are present, there is no reason to defer the operation for maturation of the aneurysm. Thus, Walker and colleagues report 1 hospital death (5%, CL 0.6%–16%) among 20 patients undergoing the operation within 8 weeks of the acute infarction. Six of the patients underwent early operation because of recurrent ventricular tachycardia. The long-term results were excellent, with an actuarial survival rate of 92%.[W4]

LV scars encountered in the operating room during surgery for coronary artery disease may require excision if they clearly contain little muscle and are of significant size. Usually, they are best left undisturbed.

SPECIAL SITUATIONS AND CONTROVERSIES

Alternative Methods of Left Ventricular Reconstruction

Stoney and colleagues have suggested a method of reconstruction involving inversion of the cut end of the left ventricular free wall against the septum.[S11] This could be an important modification with regard to postoperative left ventricular function, since Hutchings and Brawley have presented data that suggest that the ideal ventricular closure produces more curvature of the ventricular wall than does the classic one.[H7]

Intractable Ventricular Tachyarrhythmias

Although intractable ventricular tachyarrhythmias do occur in patients with ischemic heart disease in the absence of areas of left ventricular scarring, they occur more often in patients with LV aneurysms or extensive fibrosis. However, only a minority of patients with left ventricular aneurysm develop intractable ventricular tachycardia.[C11] Most who do develop such an arrhythmia have poor global LV function,[A2] and it has recently been suggested that ventricular tachyarrhythmias are particularly likely to occur when the ventricular septum has been involved in the infarction. As a corollary, poor left ventricular function and nonresponsiveness to drug therapy for ventricular tachycardia have been identified as risk factors of sudden cardiac death,[S13] and these are then indications for surgical treatment.

The effect of left ventricular aneurysmectomy, with or without coronary artery bypass grafting, on important preoperative ventricular tachyarrhythmias is variable. Buda and associates[B4] state that "left ventricular aneurysmectomy without mapping techniques for refractory life-threatening ventricular arrhythmias produced a satisfactory clinical result in the majority of cases." Yet, 7 (13%, CL 8%–19%) of 56 patients so treated surgically by them died in the early postoperative period of recurrent ventricular arrhythmias, and 20 surviving patients (36%, CL 29%–43%) of the original 56 had sufficiently severe ventricular tachyarrhythmias to require continuing drug therapy. Disappointing results have also been experienced by others,[S8] including ourselves (see Chapter 48, "Indirect Operations for Ventricular Tachycardia" in Section 4). This has stimulated the adoption of epicardial and/or endocardial mapping and programmed electrophysiologic stimulation,[F2,G3,K2,S1,S3,S4,W1] and, when indicated, the addition to aneurysmectomy of left ventricular endomyocardial incision or excision.

The extended operations for ventricular tachycardia in patients with LV aneurysm are based on the fact that these disturbances are probably *reentrant arrhythmias*.[B12,H5,K3,K7] *Automatic ventricular tachycardia*, the type generally occurring perioperatively or with an acute infarction, is currently not amenable to surgical therapy. Knowledge of the mechanisms of reentrant arrhythmias has been developed only since about 1970.[M4,S7,W2] An important tool for surgical treatment, programmed electrical stimulation was developed by Durrer and Roos in 1967[D4] and is today used to identify patients with refractory, sustained, reentrant ventricular tachycardia.[H5,J3] The induction of sustained ventricular tachycardia verifies the tachycardia as being life-threatening, as has become evident in patients recovering from acute myocardial infarction (see Chapter 7). Epicardial and particularly endocardial mapping during sinus rhythm and during ventricular tachycardia can identify ventricular tissue likely to be responsible for reentrant ventricular tachycardia by finding pacing-induced fragmentation of impulse wave fronts and variously depressed and rapid conduction.[E1,E2,W3] The endocardial mapping is of particular importance in directing the surgery, and currently it is believed (UAB) that the area of earliest endocardial activation during ventricular tachycardia is over the reentrant circuit (see Chapter 48, Section 4).

These extended operations more often eliminate important ventricular tachyarrhythmias than do simple aneurysmectomy or scar excision,[F8,F9,G7,M8,O2] but the precise indications for them, the preferred techniques, and the details of the results are only now becoming clear. Originally, interruption of the reentrant pathway by a nontransmural endocardial encircling ventriculotomy was used.[G4] After opening the ventricle, through the myocardial scar or aneurysm, the endocardial scar is usually observed to be more extensive than the transmural scar and often to involve the septum, which of course is not resectable. When endocardial mapping identifies the areas that are appropriate substrate for the reentrant, sustained ventricular tachycardia (usually, in fact, such areas are primarily in the borders between the scar and good muscle), the encircling ventriculotomy is made about 5 mm deep from within the ventricle, just outside the junction between scar and muscle. The incision is closed with a running suture. The method has some effectiveness[A2] (see Chapter 48, "Special Situations and Controversies" in Section 4), but there is evidence that it has a damaging effect on LV function. Because of this, Ostermeyer and colleagues now recommend a *partially* encircling procedure in which primarily the septal portion of the scar is encircled.[O2,O3]

Endocardial excision is practiced instead by Harken and colleagues[H4,H5] and is becoming more generally accepted. After opening the ventricle through the scar, these authors identify the endocardial focus of the reentrant arrhythmia as the earliest site of electrophysiologic breakthrough, and excise it as part of an endocardial peel from an area 2–3 cm back from and all around the ventriculotomy or aneurysmectomy edge. Harken and associates reported 2 hospital deaths (7%, CL 2%–15%) among 30 patients treated by aneurysmectomy and such "directed" endocardial resection, compared to 7 deaths from intractable ventricular tachyarrhythmias and 1 from other causes for a total of 8 (42%, CL 29%–57%) among 19 patients treated by simple aneurysmectomy.[H4] Twenty-seven (90%) of the 30 patients treated by directed endocardial resection were free of inducible ventricular tachycardia postoperatively; in the simple aneurysmectomy group, only 4 (21%) of 19 were free of important recurrent ventricular tachycardia postoperatively ($P < .0001$). Less favorable results have been reported in patients whose ventricular tachyarrhythmia seems to originate in the scarred ventricular septum.[G7] This again emphasizes the strategic role of this area of the left ventricle in prognosis for ischemic heart disease.

With only an intermediate-term follow-up, the results have been encouraging.[A2] Among 53 patients (UAB; August 1978–October 1982) and with most (35%) of the operations being a limited myotomy with endocardial excision, 50% of patients were alive at 48 months; 15% had died in hospital. However, virtually all patients followed this long had either recurrence of ventricular tachycardia or were in NYHA class III or IV

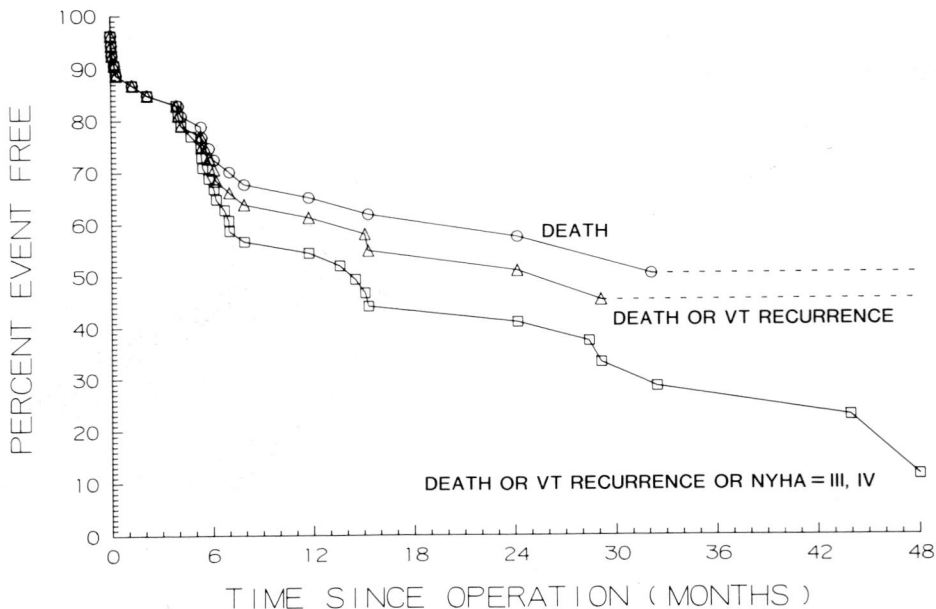

Figure 8-13 Cumulative actuarial events after surgery directed toward intractable ventricular tachycardia, including events in hospital after the operation (UAB; August 1978–October 1982; *n* = 52).

(Fig. 8-13). Current methods—particularly with improved intraoperative mapping and use of the cryoprobe—are producing more efficacious and less traumatic operations and improved late results (see Chapter 48, Section 4, for a detailed discussion of these matters).

False Left Ventricular Aneurysms

The aneurysms discussed in this chapter, so-called true aneurysms, are formed by scarring, thinning, and stretching of an infarcted area of left ventricular wall. This process produces a wide-mouthed aneurysm. In contrast, a *false aneurysm* develops after acute rupture of an infarcted area of left ventricle. While such ruptures are usually fatal, when the pericardium is sufficiently adherent to the epicardium, the rupture may result only in a localized hemopericardium. The persistent communication of the hemopericardium with the left ventricular cavity results in gradual expansion of the hemopericardium into a large false aneurysm whose wall is composed of pericardium and adhesions[C8,R3] and whose mouth is usually narrow.[V1] Such aneurysms have a strong tendency to rupture,[V2] in contrast to so-called true aneurysms. False aneurysms are much more likely to occur posteriorly (on the diaphragmatic surface of the left ventricle) or laterally than are true aneurysms.

Resection of a false left ventricular aneurysm is clearly advisable[H2] with or without coronary artery bypass grafting. The resection may pose formidable problems when the false sac extends anteriorly beneath the sternum. It is then necessary to begin partial CPB via cannulae introduced into the femoral artery and vein. The heart is fibrillated electrically or by profoundly hypothermic CPB as the sternum is opened and the false sac entered. Blood from this sac is returned to the circuit by open heart suckers while a second venous cannula is inserted into right atrium to pick up the superior

vena caval return. The operation can then proceed in a formal way. The edematous, thick adhesions forming the sac can be a source of copious bleeding.

Postinfarction Left Ventricular Free Wall Rupture

Acute rupture of the ventricle occasionally complicates full-thickness acute myocardial infarction.[N2] Hatcher and colleagues in 1970 reported the results of one of the first successful operations for this condition.[H8] Occasionally, in this condition, the rupture is massive and death quickly results from exsanguination.[B13] Usually the cardiac rupture is not a "blowout" phenomenon but a more gradual process that begins with small endocardial tears. These allow the formation of a hematoma, which gradually dissects the area of necrosis into the pericardium, resulting in sudden fatal pericardial tamponade.[K4] The result can be seen by echocardiography. The diagnosis can be confirmed by pericardiocentesis, and the patient should then be taken to the operating room for prompt surgical treatment. Usually the rest of the left ventricle is in good condition, and surgical salvage is possible.[F4]

Ideally, a coronary arteriogram should be made, and if this is to be done, an intra-aortic balloon should be inserted first. Immediately after this, the patient is taken to the operating room.

On CPB, the infarct is excised, and the ventricle is closed using Teflon reinforcement, as for other types of ventricular resection for ischemic heart disease. Coronary artery bypass grafting is added when appropriate.

When surgical treatment is properly and appropriately applied, long-term survival is possible.[B11] Piffare and colleagues report four patients preoperatively in shock who survived with long-term good results.[P4] Nunez and colleagues report a good result in four of seven patients; they covered the ventricular tear and the surrounding myocardium with a wide Teflon patch.[N3]

Congenital Left Ventricular Aneurysm

An isolated congenital ventricular aneurysm is usually a long, finger-shaped projection from the LV, although it may communicate with both ventricles[S12] and is therefore generally called a *congenital diverticulum*. It is a rare lesion,[D5] only 12 cases having been reported before the GLH case report in 1959.[L5] Its wall consists of endocardium, myocardium (which may be scanty or thick, particularly at the distal blind end), and epicardium, and it may contain thrombus. Rupture is not uncommon, probably because of a sphincter-like obstruction of the proximal intramural portion that produces high distal pressures.[L5] The diverticulum usually projects downward into the epigastrium and is palpable beneath the skin. Surgical excision is required and can be undertaken without CPB.[H6,L5]

Traumatic Left Ventricular Aneurysm

Rarely, violent nonpenetrating trauma to the chest produces such a severe contusion of the heart that a localized (and probably false) aneurysm forms.[S6] The aneurysm, which is usually well localized and may be very thin walled,[B6] may be detected within 6 weeks of the trauma[P3] or not until several years later. Because of its thin wall and liability to rupture, a posttraumatic LV aneurysm should be resected.

REFERENCES

A

1. Austen WG, Tsunekawa T, Bender HW, Ebert PA, Morrow AG: The acute hemodynamic effects of left ventricular aneurysm. *J Surg Res* 2:161, 1962.

2. Arciniegas JG, Klein H, Karp RB, Kouchoukos NT, James TN, Kirklin JW, Waldo AL: Surgical treatment of life-threatening ventricular tachyarrhythmias. *Circulation* 62(suppl III):III-42, 1980 (abstr).

3. Arvan S, Badillo P: Contractile properties of the left ventricle with aneurysm. *Am J Cardiol* 55:338, 1985.

B

1. Burton NA, Stinson EB, Oyer PE, Shumway NE: Left ventricular aneurysm: Preoperative risk factors and long-term postoperative results. *J Thorac Cardiovasc Surg* 77:65, 1979.

2. Banka VS, Bodenheimer MM, Helfant RH: Determinants of reversible asynergy: Effect of pathologic Q waves, coronary collaterals, and anatomic location. *Circulation* 50:714, 1974.

3. Bruschke AVG, Proudfit WL, Sones FM Jr: Progress study of 590 consecutive nonsurgical cases of coronary disease followed by 5–9 years. II. Ventriculographic and other correlations. *Circulation* 47:1154, 1973.

4. Buda AJ, Stinson EB, Harrison DC: Surgery for life-threatening ventricular tachyarrhythmias. *Am J Cardiol* 44:1171, 1979.

5. Brawley RK, Schaff H, Stevens R, Ducci H, Gott VL, Donahoo JS: Influence of coronary artery anatomy on survival following resection of left ventricular aneurysms and chronic infarcts. *J Thorac Cardiovasc Surg* 763:120, 1977.

6. Berkoff HA, Rowe GG, Crummy AB, Kahn DR: Asymptomatic left ventricular aneurysm: A sequela of blunt chest trauma. *Circulation* 55:545, 1977.

7. Buehler DL, Stinson EB, Oyer PE, Shumway NE: Surgical treatment of aneurysms of the inferior left ventricular wall. *J Thorac Cardiovasc Surg* 78:74, 1979.

8. Brandt PWT, Partridge JB, Wattie WJ: Coronary arteriography: A method of presentation of the arteriogram report and a scoring system. *Clin Radiol* 28:361, 1977.

9. Bulkley BH, Roberts WC: Steroid therapy during acute myocardial infarction: A cause of delayed healing and of ventricular aneurysm. *Am J Med* 56:244, 1974.

10. Barratt-Boyes BG, White HD, Agnew TM, Pewberton JR, Wild C: The results of surgical treatment of left ventricular aneurysms: An assessment of the risk factors affecting early and late mortality. *J Thorac Cardiovasc Surg* 87:87, 1984.

11. Baudouy PY, Menashe P, Kural S, Wolff M, Piwnica A: Acute left ventricular rupture secondary to myocardial infarction: Report of long-term survival after early surgical repair. *Thorac Cardiovasc Surg* 30:409, 1982.

12. Boineau JP, Cox JL: Rationale for a direct surgical approach to control ventricular arrhythmias. *Am J Cardiol* 49:381, 1982.

13. Balakumaran K, Verbaan CJ, Essed CE, Nauta J, Bos E, Haalebos MMP, Penn O, Simoons ML, Hugenholtz PG: Ventricular free wall rupture: sudden, subacute, slow, sealed and stabilized varieties. *Eur Heart J* 5:282, 1984.

14. Balu V, Hook N, Dean DC, Naughton J: Effect of left ventricular aneurysmectomy on exercise performance. *Int J Cardiol* 5:210, 1984.

C

1. Cohnheim J, Schulthess-Rechberg AV: Über die folgen der kranzarterienverschliessung für das Hertz. *Virchows Arch [A]* 85:503, 1881.

2. Cooley DA, Henly WS, Amad KH, Chapman DW: Ventricular aneurysm following myocardial infarction: Results of surgical treatment. *Ann Surg* 150:595, 1959.

3. Cheng TO: Incidence of ventricular aneurysm in coronary artery disease: An angiographic appraisal. *Am J Med* 50:340, 1971.

4. Cabin HS, Roberts WC: True left ventricular aneurysm and healed myocardial infarction: Clinical and necropsy observations including quantification of degrees of coronary arterial narrowing. *Am J Cardiol* 46:754, 1980.

5. Cooley DA, Hallman GL: Surgical treatment of left ventricular aneurysm: Experience with excision of postinfarction lesions in 80 patients. *Prog Cardiovasc Dis* 11:222, 1968.

6. Cullhed I, Delius W, Bjork L, Hallen A, Nordgren L: Resection of left ventricular aneurysm: Late results. *Acta Med Scand* 197:241, 1975.

7. Cooperman M, Stinson EB, Griepp RB, Shumway NE: Survival and function after left ventricular aneurysmectomy. *J Thorac Cardiovasc Surg* 69:321, 1975.

8. Chesler E, Korns ME, Semba T, Edwards JE: False aneurysm

of the left ventricle following myocardial infarction. *Am J Cardiol* 23:76, 1969.

9. Cosgrove DM, Loop FD, Irarrazaval MG, Groves LK, Taylor PC, Golding LA: Determinants of long-term survival after ventricular aneurysmectomy. *Ann Thorac Surg* 26:257, 1978.

10. Crosby IK, Wellons HA Jr, Martin RP, Schuch D, Muller WH Jr: Employability: A new indication for aneurysmectomy and coronary revascularization. *Circulation* 62(suppl I):I-79, 1980.

11. Cohen M, Wienar I, Pichard A, Holt J, Smith H, Gorlin R: Determinants of ventricular tachycardia in patients with coronary artery disease and ventricular aneurysm: Clinical, hemodynamic and angiographic factors. *Am J Cardiol* 51:61, 1983.

D

1. Dubnow MH, Burchell HB, Titus JL: Postinfarction ventricular aneurysm: A clinicomorphologic and electrocardiographic study of 80 cases. *Am Heart J* 70:753, 1965.

2. Davis RW, Ebert PA: Ventricular aneurysm: A clinical-pathologic correlation. *Am J Cardiol* 29:1, 1972.

3. Donaldson RM, Honey M, Balcon R, Banim SO, Sturridge MF, Wright JEC: Surgical treatment of postinfarction left ventricular aneurysm in 32 patients. *Brit Heart J* 38:1223, 1976.

4. Durrer D, Roos JP: Epicardial excitation of the ventricles in a patient with W.P.W. syndrome. *Circulation* 35:15, 1967.

5. Davila JC, Enriquez F, Bergoglio S, Voci G, Wells CRE: Congenital aneurysm of the left ventricle. *Ann Thorac Surg* 1:697, 1965.

6. Dymond DS, Stephens JD, Stone DL, Elliott AT, Rees GM, Spurrell RAJ: Combined exercise radionuclide and hemodynamic evaluation of left ventricular aneurysmectomy. *Am Heart J* 104:977, 1982.

E

1. El-Sherif N, Hope RR, Scherlag NJ, Lazzara R: Re-entrant ventricular arrhythmias in the late myocardial infarction period. II. Patterns of initiation and termination of re-entry. *Circulation* 55:702, 1977.

2. El-Sherif N, Scherlag NJ, Lazzara R, Hope RR: Re-entrant arrhythmias in the later myocardial period. I. Conduction characteristics in the infarct zone. *Circulation* 55:686, 1977.

F

1. Fisher VJ, Alvarez AJ, Shah A, Dolgin M, Tice DA: Left ventricular scars: Clinical and haemodynamic results of excision. *Br Heart J* 36:132, 1974.

2. Fontaine G, Frank R, Guiraudon G, Vedel J, Grosgogeaf Y, Cabrol C: Surgical treatment of resistant re-entrant ventricular tachycardia by ventriculotomy: A new application of epicardial mapping. *Circulation* 49,50(suppl III):III-82, 1974 (abstr).

3. Feild BJ, Russell RO Jr, Dowling JT, Rackley CE: Regional left ventricular performance in the year following myocardial infarction. *Circulation* 46:679, 1972.

4. Friedman HS, Juhn LA, Katz AM: Clinical and electrocardiographic features of cardiac rupture following acute myocardial infarction. *Am J Med* 50:709, 1971.

5. Fontan F: The prognostic value of pre-operative left ventricular performance in left ventricular resection. *Thorac Cardiovasc Surg* 27:281, 1979.

6. Froehlich RT, Falsetti HL, Doty DB, Marcus ML: Prospective study of surgery for left ventricular aneurysm. *Am J Cardiol* 45:923, 1980.

7. Frank G, Klein H, Bednarska E, Gahl K, Flohr E, Trieb G, Borst HG: Results after resection of postinfarction left ventricular aneurysms. *Thorac Cardiovasc Surg* 28:423, 1980.

8. Fontaine G, Guiraudon G, Frank R, Fillette F, Cabrol C, Grosgogeat Y: Surgical management of ventricular tachycardia unrelated to myocardial ischemia or infarction. *Am J Cardiol* 49:397, 1982.

9. Frank G, Klein H, Lichtlen P, Borst HG: Direct surgical therapy of ventricular arrhythmias in coronary heart disease. *Thorac Cardiovasc Surg* 29:315, 1981.

10. Faxon DP, Ryan TJ, Davis KB, McCabe CH, Myers W, Lesperance J, Shaw R, Tong TG: Prognostic significance of angiographically documented left ventricular aneurysm from the Coronary Artery Surgery Study (CASS). *Amer J Cardiol* 50:157, 1982.

G

1. Gorlin R, Klein MD, Sullivan JM: Prospective correlative study of ventricular aneurysm: Mechanistic concept and clinical recognition. *Am J Med* 42:512, 1967.

2. Gross H, Schwedel JB: The clinical course in ventricular aneurysm. *NY State J Med* 41:488, 1941.

3. Gallagher JJ, Oldham HN, Wallace AG, Peter RH, Kasell J: Ventricular aneurysm with ventricular tachycardia: Report of a case with epicardial mapping and successful resection. *Am J Cardiol* 35:696, 1975.

4. Guiraudon G, Fontaine G, Frank R, Escande G, Etievent P, Cabrol C: Encircling endocardial ventriculotomy: A new surgical treatment for life-threatening ventricular tachycardias resistant to medical treatment following myocardial infarction. *Ann Thorac Surg* 26:438, 1978.

5. Graber JD, Oakley CM, Pickering BN, Goodwin JF, Raphael MJ, Steiner RE: Ventricular aneurysm: An appraisal of diagnosis and surgical treatment. *Brit Heart J* 34:830, 1972.

6. Grondin P, Kretz JG, Bical O, Donzeau-Gouge P, Petitclerc R, Campeau L: Natural history of saccular aneurysms of the left ventricle. *J Thorac Cardiovasc Surg* 77:57, 1979.

7. Guiraudon G, Fontaine G, Frank R, Leandri R, Barra J, Cabrol C: Surgical treatment of ventricular tachycardia guided by ventricular mapping in 23 patients without coronary artery disease. *Ann Thorac Surg* 32:439, 1981.

H

1. Harman MA, Baxley WA, Jones WB, Dodge HT, Edwards S: Surgical intervention in chronic postinfarction cardiac failure. *Circulation* 39,40(suppl I):I-91, 1969.

2. Harper RW, Sloman G, Westlake G: Successful surgical resection of a chronic false aneurysm of the left ventricle. *Chest* 67:359, 1975.

3. Herman MV, Heinle RA, Klein MD, Gorlin R: Localized disorders in myocardial contraction: Asynergy and its role in congestive heart disease. *N Engl J Med* 277:222, 1967.

4. Harken AH, Horowitz LN, Josephson ME: Comparison of standard aneurysmectomy and aneurysmectomy with directed endocardial resection for the treatment of recurrent sustained ventricular tachycardia. *J Thorac Cardiovasc Surg* 80:527, 1980.

5. Harken AH, Horowitz LN, Josephson ME: The surgical treatment of ventricular tachycardia. *Ann Thorac Surg* 30:499, 1980.

6. Hertzeanu H, Deutsch V, Yahini JH, Lieberman Y, Neufeld HN: Left ventricular aneurysm of unusual aetiology: Report of two cases. *Thorax* 31:220, 1976.

7. Hutchins GM, Brawley RK: The influence of cardiac geometry on the results of ventricular aneurysm repair. *Am J Pathol* 99:221, 1980.

8. Hatcher CR, Mansour K, Logan WD: Surgical complications of myocardial infarction. *Circulation* 45:1231, 1972.

J

1. Johnson RA, Daggett WM Jr: Heart failure resulting from coronary artery disease, in RA Johnson, E Haber, WG Austen (eds): *The Practice of Cardiology*. Boston: Little, Brown, 1980, p 345.

2. Jones EL, Craver JM, Hurst JW, Bradford JA, Bone DK, Robinson PH, Cobbs BW, Thompkins TR, Hatcher CR: Influence of left ventricular aneurysm on survival following the coronary bypass operation. *Ann Surg* 193:733, 1981.

3. Josephson ME, Harken AH, Horowitz LN: Long-term results of endocardial resection for sustained ventricular tachycardia in coronary disease patients. *Am Heart J* 104:51, 1982.

K

1. Kitamura S, Kay JH, Krohn BG, Magidson O, Dunne EF: Geometric and functional abnormalities of the left ventricle with a chronic localized noncontractile area. *Am J Cardiol* 31:701, 1973.

2. Kastor JA, Spear JF, Moore EN: Localization of ventricular irritability by epicardial mapping. *Circulation* 45:952, 1972.

3. Kastor JA: How should refractory ventricular tachycardia be treated? *Am J Cardiol* 44:1213, 1979.

4. Kendall RW, DeWood MA: Postinfarction cardiac rupture: Surgical success and review of the literature. *Ann Thorac Surg* 25:311, 1978.

5. Klein MD, Herman MV, Gorlin R: A hemodynamic study of left ventricular aneurysm. *Circulation* 35:614, 1967.

6. Kapelnaski DP, Al-Sadir J, Lambert JJ, Anagnostopoulos CE: Ventriculographic features predictive of surgical outcome for left ventricular aneurysm. *Circulation* 58:1167, 1978.

7. Kastor JA, Horowitz LN, Harken AH, Josephson ME: Clinical electrophysiology of ventricular tachycardia. *N Engl J Med* 304:1004, 1981.

8. Kiefer SK, Flaker GC, Martin RH, Curtis JJ: Clinical improvement after ventricular aneurysm repair: Prediction by angiographic and hemodynamic variables. *JACC* 2:30, 1983.

9. Kirklin JW, Blackstone EH, Rogers WJ: The plights of the invasive treatment of ischemic heart disease. *JACC* 5:158, 1985.

L

1. Loeb J: Über partielle erweichende myocarditis (malacia cordis). Dissertation. University of Würzburg, Würzburg, West Germany: 1880.

2. Likoff W, Bailey CP: Ventriculoplasty: Excision of myocardial aneurysm, report of a successful case. *JAMA* 158:915, 1955.

3. Loop FD, Effler DB, Navia JA, Sheldon WC, Groves LK: Aneurysms of the left ventricle: Survival and results of a ten-year surgical experience. *Ann Surg* 178:399, 1973.

4. Lee DC-S, Johnson RA, Bocher CA, Wexler LF, McEnany MT: Angiographic predictors of survival following left ventricular aneurysmectomy. *Circulation* 56(suppl II):II-12, 1977.

5. Lowe JB, Williams JCP, Robb D, Cole D: Congenital diverticulum of the left ventricle. *Br Heart J* 21:101, 1949.

M

1. Marie R: Anévrisme de la pointe du coeur. *Bulletin de la Société Anatomique de Paris* pp 11–13, 1896.

2. Moran JM, Scanlon PJ, Nemickas R, Pifarre R: Surgical treatment of postinfarction ventricular aneurysm. *Ann Thorac Surg* 21:107, 1976.

3. Mullen DC, Posey L, Gabriel R, Singh HM, Flemma RJ, Lepley D Jr: Prognostic considerations in the management of left ventricular aneurysms. *Ann Thorac Surg* 23:455, 1977.

4. Moe GK, Mendez C: The physiologic basis of reciprocal rhythms. *Prog Cardiovasc Dis* 8:461, 1966.

5. Mourdjinis A, Olsen E, Raphael MJ: Clinical diagnosis and prognosis of ventricular aneurysm. *Br Heart J* 30:497, 1968.

6. Marco JD, Kaiser GC, Barnes HE, Codd JE, Willman VL: Left ventricular aneurysmectomy. *Arch Surg* 111:419, 1975.

7. Martin JL, Untereker WJ, Harken AH, Horowitz LN, Josephson ME: Aneurysmectomy and endocardial resection for ventricular tachycardia: Favorable hemodynamic and antiarrhythmic results in patients with global left ventricular dysfunction. *Am Heart J* 103:960, 1982.

8. Mason JW, Stinson EB, Winkle RA, Griffin JC, Oyer PE, Ross DL, Derby G: Surgery for ventricular tachycardia: Efficacy of left ventricular aneurysm resection compared with operation guided by electrical activation mapping. *Circulation* 65:1148, 1982.

N

1. Nagle RE, Williams DO: Natural history of ventricular aneurysm without surgical treatment. *Br Heart J* 36:1037, 1974 (abstr).

2. Norris RM, Sammel NL: Predictors of late hospital death in acute myocardial infarction. *Prog Cardiovasc Dis* 23:129, 1980.

3. Nunez L, de la Llana R, Sendon JL, Coma J, Aguado MG, Larrea JL: Diagnosis and treatment of subacute free wall ventricular rupture after infarction. *Ann Thorac Surg* 35:525, 1983.

4. Novick RJ, Stefaniszyn HJ, Morin JE, Symes JF, Sniderman AD, Dobell ARC: Surgery for postinfarction left ventricular aneurysm: prognosis and long-term follow-up. *Can J Surg* 27:161, 1984.

O

1. Okies JE, Dietl C, Garrison HB, Starr A: Early and late results of resection of ventricular aneurysm. *J Thorac Cardiovasc Surg* 75:255, 1978.

2. Ostermeyer J, Breithardt G, Kolvenbach R, Borggrefe M, Seipel L, Schulte HD, Bircks W: The surgical treatment of ventricular tachycardias. *J Thorac Cardiovasc Surg* 84:704, 1982.

3. Ostermeyer J: (1984) Personal communication.

P

1. Phares WS, Edwards JE, Burchell HB: Cardiac aneurysms: Clinicopathologic studies. *Proceedings of the Staff Meetings of the Mayo Clinic* 28:264, 1953.

2. Parmley WW, Chuck L, Kivowitz C, Matloff JM, Swan HJC: In vitro length-tension relations of human ventricular aneurysms: Relation of stiffness to mechanical disadvantage. *Am J Cardiol* 32:889, 1973.

3. Pupello DF, Daily PO, Stinson EB, Shumway NE: Successful repair of left ventricular aneurysm due to trauma. *JAMA* 211:826, 1970.

4. Pifarre R, Sullivan JH, Grieco J, Montoya A, Bakhos M, Scanlon PF, Gunar RM: Management of left ventricular rupture complicating myocardial infarction. *J Thorac Cardiovasc Surg* 86:441, 1983.

R

1. Rogers WJ, Oberman A, Kouchoukos NT: Left ventricular aneurysmectomy in patients with single vs. multivessel coronary artery disease. *Circulation* 58(suppl I):I-50, 1978.

2. Rao G, Zikria EA, Miller WH, Samandani SR, Ford WB: Experience with sixty consecutive ventricular aneurysm resections. *Circulation* 49,50(suppl II):II-149, 1974.

3. Roberts WC, Morrow AG: Pseudoaneurysm of the left ventricle: An unusual sequence of myocardial infarction and rupture of the heart. *Am J Med* 43:639, 1967.

4. Rittenhouse EA, Sauvage LR, Mansfield PB, Smith JC, Davis CC, Hall DG, O'Brien MA: Results of combined left ventricular aneurysmectomy and coronary artery bypass: 1974 to 1980. *Am J Surg* 143:575, 1982.

S

1. Sbokos CG, Monro JL, Ross JK: Elective operations for postinfarction left ventricular aneurysms. *Thorax* 31:55, 1976.

2. Schlichter J, Hellerstein HK, Katz LN: Aneurysm of the heart: A correlative study of one hundred and two proved cases. *Medicine* 33:43, 1954.

3. Spurrell RAJ, Yates AK, Thorburn CW, Sowton GE, Duechar DC: Surgical treatment of ventricular tachycardia after epicardial mapping studies. *Br Heart J* 37:115, 1975.

4. Spielman SR, Michelson EL, Horowitz LN, Spear JF, Moore EN: The limitations of epicardial mapping as a guide to the surgical therapy of ventricular tachycardia. *Circulation* 57:666, 1978.

5. Shaw RC, Connors JP, Hieb BR, Ludbrook PA, Krone R, Kleiger RE, Ferguson TB, Weldon CS: Postoperative investigation of left ventricular aneurysm resection. *Circulation* 56(suppl II):II-7, 1977.

6. Singh R, Molan SP, Schrank JP: Traumatic left ventricular aneurysm: Two cases with normal coronary arteriograms. *JAMA* 234:412, 1975.

7. Sasyniuk BJ, Mendez C: A mechanism for re-entry in canine ventricular tissue. *Circ Res* 28:3, 1971.

8. Sami M, Chaitman BR, Bourassa MG, Charpin D, Chabot M: Long-term follow-up of aneurysmectomy for recurrent ventricular tachycardia or fibrillation. *Am Heart J* 96:303, 1978.

9. Sesto M, Schwartz F, Thiedemann KL, Flameng W, Schlepper M: Failure of aneurysmectomy to improve left ventricular function. *Br Heart J* 41:79, 1979.

10. Swan HJC, Magnusson PT, Buchbinder NA, Mattoff JM, Gray RJ: Aneurysm of the cardiac ventricle: Its management by medical and surgical intervention. *West J Med* 129:26, 1978.

11. Stoney WS, Alford WC Jr, Burrus GR, Thomas CS Jr: Repair of anteroseptal ventricular aneurysm. *Ann Thorac Surg* 15:394, 1973.

12. Skapinker S: Diverticulum of the left ventricle of the heart. *Arch Surg* 63:629, 1951.

13. Swerdlow CD, Winkle RA, Mason JW: Determinants of survival in patients with ventricular tachyarrhythmias. *New Engl J Med* 308:1436, 1983.

T

1. Tantin LF: De quelques lésions des arteres coronaires comme causes d'altération du myocarde. *Thèse Paris,* 1878.

V

1. Van Tassel RA, Edwards JE: Rupture of heart complicating myocardial infarction: Analysis of 40 cases including nine examples of left ventricular false aneurysm. *Chest* 61:104, 1972.

2. Vlodaver Z, Coe JI, Edwards JE: True and false left ventricular aneurysms: Propensity for the latter to rupture. *Circulation* 51:567, 1975.

W

1. Wittig JH, Boineau JP: Surgical treatment of ventricular arrhythmias using epicardial, transmural, and endocardial mapping. *Ann Thorac Surg* 20:117, 1975.

2. Wellens HJJ: Observations on the pathophysiology of ventricular tachycardia in man. *Arch Intern Med* 135:473, 1975.

3. Waldo AL, Arciniegas JG, Klein H: Surgical treatment of life-threatening ventricular arrhythmias: The role of intraoperative mapping and consideration of the presently available surgical techniques. *Prog Cardiovasc Dis* 23:247, 1981.

4. Walker WE, Stoney WS, Alford WC, Burrus GR, Glassford DM, Thomas CS: Results of surgical management of acute left ventricular aneurysm. *Circulation* 62(suppl I):II-75, 1980.

5. Walker WE, Stoney WS, Alford WC, Burrus GR, Frist RA, Glassford DM, Thomas CS: Techniques and results of ventricular aneurysmectomy with emphasis on anteroseptal repair. *J Thorac Cardiovasc Surg* 76:824, 1978.

Z

1. Ziegler E: *Über die Urasachen der Nierenschrumpfung nebst bemerkungen fiber die Unterschiedung Verschiedener Formen de Nephritis.* Freiburg, West Germany: 1879, pp 586–623.

9

POSTINFARCTION VENTRICULAR SEPTAL DEFECT

DEFINITION

Postinfarction ventricular septal defect (VSD) is a defect developing in the ventricular septum as a result of rupture of an acute myocardial infarct.

HISTORICAL NOTE

In 1847, Latham first described a postinfarction VSD at autopsy, but it was not until 1923 that Brum made the diagnosis clinically.[B2] In 1957, Cooley and colleagues first reported the surgical repair of a postinfarction VSD, 11 weeks after the myocardial infarction.[C1] The patient died 6 weeks later. The first long-term survivor of repair of such a lesion was the first patient we reported from the Mayo Clinic in 1963.[P1]

MORPHOLOGY

The postinfarction VSD is most commonly (in about 60% of cases) located in the anterior or apical portion of the ventricular septum,[S4] in association with atheromatous narrowing or occlusion of the anterior descending coronary artery and a full-thickness anterior myocardial infarction. About 20% of patients have a VSD in the posterior or inlet portion of the ventricular septum in association with lesions in the posterior descending coronary artery and an inferior myocardial infarction.

In fact, when ventricular septal rupture occurs, it is usual to find occlusive disease in both the anterior descending and posterior descending coronary arteries. The VSDs may be multiple, and they may develop, not simultaneously, but within several days of each other.

Particularly, the posterior VSD may be accompanied by important mitral valve incompetence secondary to papillary muscle infarction or dysfunction (see Chapter 10). In those patients who survive the early period of ventricular septal rupture, the remainder of the infarcted septum and ventricular wall may become aneurysmal.[S2] This is said to be the case in about 40% of patients with postinfarction VSD.[J1]

CLINICAL FEATURES AND DIAGNOSTIC CRITERIA

The first sign of septal rupture, in a patient who has recently sustained a myocardial infarct, is the development of a pansystolic murmur, usually at the left lower sternal border with or without radiation to the axilla and of varying intensity. If the murmur is overlooked or its significance ignored, most patients with ventricular septal rupture die undiagnosed. The chest roentgenogram gives evidence of pulmonary venous hypertension and a large pulmonary blood flow.

A systolic murmur can result from acute mitral incompetence secondary to myocardial infarction as well as from postinfarction VSD, and the two may coexist. Therefore, after recognizing the new murmur, a Swan-Ganz catheter is introduced promptly at the bedside, and samples are obtained from the right atrium, pulmonary artery, and radial artery to document the presence of a left-to-right shunt, which is usually large (pulmonary-systemic blood flow ratio, or $\dot{Q}_p/\dot{Q}_s$, of 2 or more). Pulmonary artery wedge (reflecting left atrial) pressure and pulmonary artery pressure are both usually elevated.

Once a left-to-right shunt is confirmed and proper preparations are made (see "Preoperative Preparation"), coronary arteriography, cardiac catheterization, and, if the patient's condition allows it, left ventriculography are carried out urgently. The coronary arteriogram locates significant obstructive coronary artery lesions, so that appropriate coronary artery bypass grafting (CABG) procedures can be carried out at the time of operation. Cardiac catheterization confirms and quantitates the presence of a left-to-right shunt and measures pulmonary artery pressures and resistances. The left ventriculogram determines the location and number of VSDs, defines left ventricular function, and assesses any mitral incompetence; however, if the patient is critically ill, the left ventriculogram (which in this setting may acutely depress ventricular function) is omitted.

NATURAL HISTORY

Studies by Oyamata and Queen,[O1] Jonas and colleagues,[J2] and others indicate that postinfarction ventricular septal defect complicates approximately 1%–2% of cases of acute myocardial infarction.

Septal perforation occurs, on the average, 2–3 days after the acute myocardial infarction[S3] but may occur at any time within the first 2 weeks of the infarction. It is followed by severely reduced cardiac output and all its sequelae.

Early death is frequent. Only about 75% of patients survive the first 24 hours after the event, and only 50% survive the first week.[O1,S1] Less than 30% survive 2 weeks, and only 20% survive more than 30 days (Fig. 9-1). Thus, the risk of death is highest immediately after a postinfarction ventricular septal rupture and gradually declines thereafter (Fig. 9-1c).

TECHNIQUE OF OPERATION

Preoperative Preparation

Since most patients with this complication are seriously ill and require operation early after septal rupture, their management before operation is of critical importance.

Once the diagnosis of acute postinfarction VSD is confirmed by the findings with the Swan-Ganz catheter, which is inserted upon the first suspicion that a VSD may have developed, the decision is made to proceed promptly with further study and surgery. (The only exception to this is the rare patient with minimal hemodynamic disturbance.) An intra-aortic balloon is inserted immediately because of the tendency of these patients to deteriorate very rapidly.[G1] The patient is then taken to the cardiac catheterization laboratory for the special studies described earlier (see "Clinical Features and Diagnostic Criteria"), with the intra-aortic balloon

in place and functioning. Once the studies have been completed, operation is undertaken, for any improvement afforded by intra-aortic balloon pumping is only temporary.[B3,D1]

Initial Steps of the Operation

After the usual initial preparations in the operating room (see Chapter 2), a median sternotomy incision is made. The heart is disturbed as little as possible before establishing CPB because of the unstable hemodynamic state of the patient. While making the median sternotomy incision, a long segment of saphenous vein is removed and prepared in the usual manner (see Chapter 7). Because of the length and complexity of the operation, the surgical plan must be an efficient one so that the aortic cross-clamp and cardiopulmonary bypass (CPB) times are within reasonable limits.

CBP is promptly established using two venous cannulae and caval tapes. The perfusate temperature is lowered to as cold as is possible, external cardiac cooling is begun, the aorta is cross-clamped, the cold cardioplegic solution is injected, and the perfusate temperature is stabilized at 25°C. The usual cardioplegic reinfusions are made (see Chapter 3). The caval tapes are snugged. A left atrial vent may be inserted but is not necessary or recommended.

Repair of Ventricular Septal Defect

Attention is now turned to the VSD, which is nearly always approached through the left ventricle, as described in 1969 by Kay[K2] and Dubost[D3] and subsequently by Kitamura and associates,[K3] Javid and colleagues,[J1] and others.[D2,K1] The repair itself is a modification of the double-patch method of Iben and colleagues.[D1,G5,I1]

When the VSD is located anteriorly, it is approached through the anterolateral infarct (or aneurysm) that is nearly always present (Fig. 9-2). The defect in the septum is usually found immediately beneath this. It is repaired using a knitted Dacron velour patch, lined if possible with pericardium to make it immediately leakproof. The patch is sewn into place on the left ventricular side with pledgetted mattress sutures placed well back from the edge and close together and with the pledgets on the right ventricular side of the defect (Fig. 9-2). The infarction (or aneurysm) is excised, and care is taken

---

Figure 9-1 Survival without surgical treatment of patients with ventricular septal rupture after acute myocardial infarction, based on an actuarial analysis of all proven cases (n = 139) reported in the literature until 1977. The solid line represents the actuarial incidence, and the dashed lines enclose the 70% confidence limits.
(a) Interval in months between perforation and death.
(b) Interval in days between perforation and death. Note that half of the patients are dead within 7 days of perforation.
(c) Hazard function, or instantaneous risk of death, each day after septal rupture. Note that the hazard function is greatest early after rupture and declines steadily thereafter.

Reproduced with permission from Berger et al;[B4] data and references available upon request.

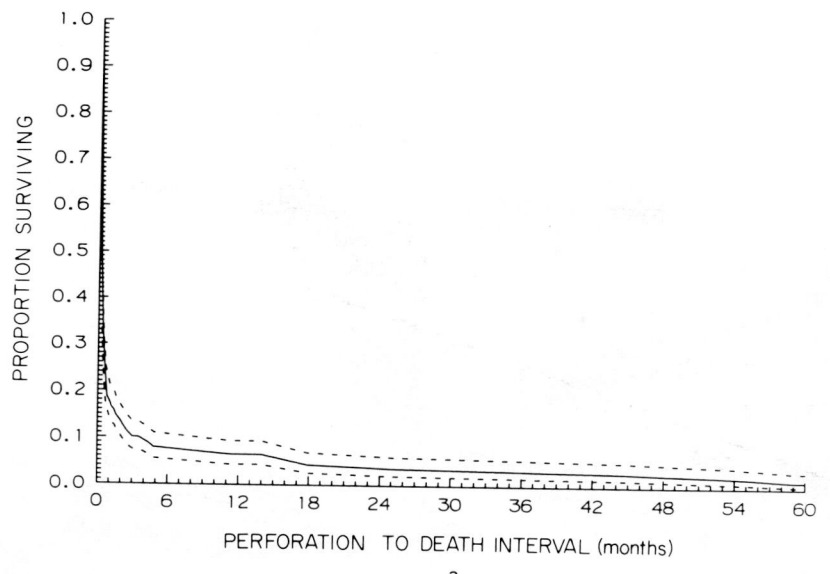

a

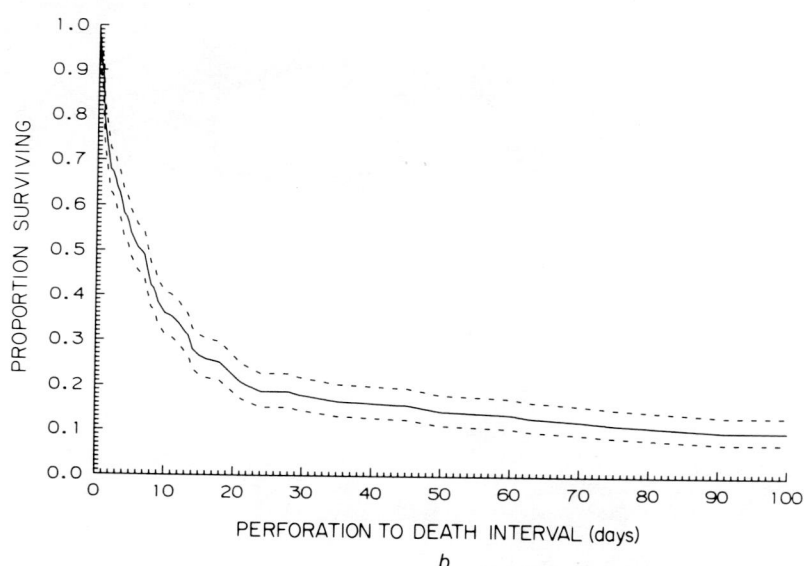

b

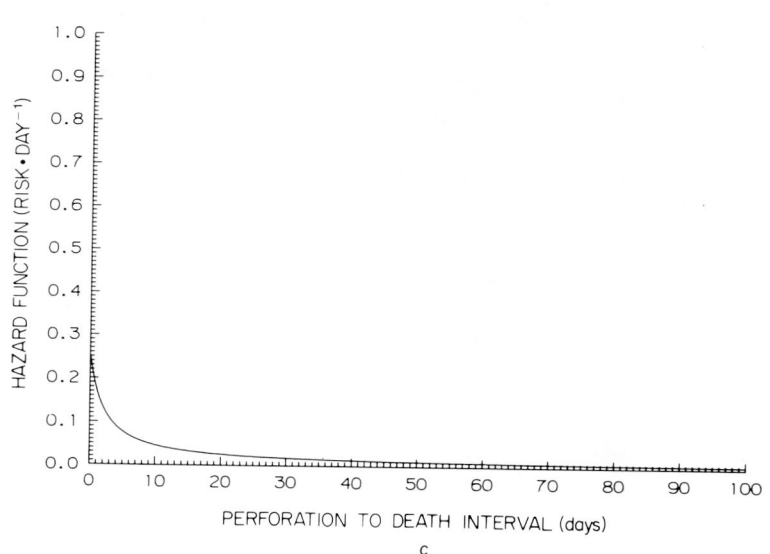

c

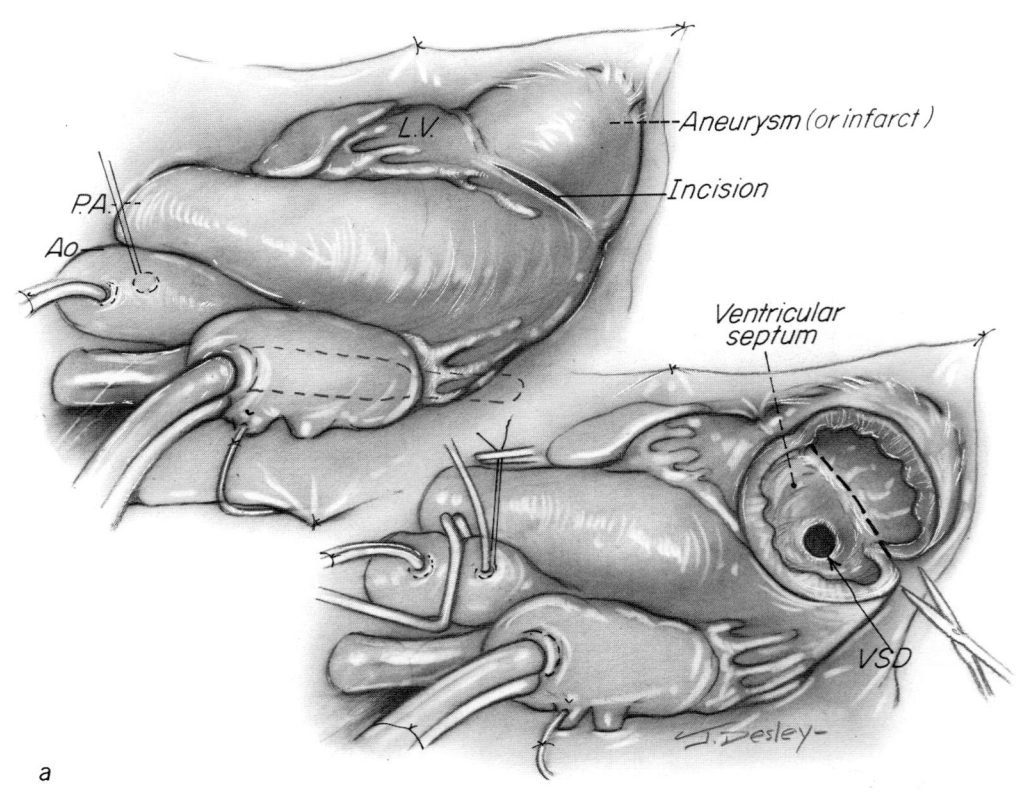

L.V.

Aneurysm (or infarct)

P.A.

Incision

Ao.

Ventricular septum

J. Desley-

VSD

a

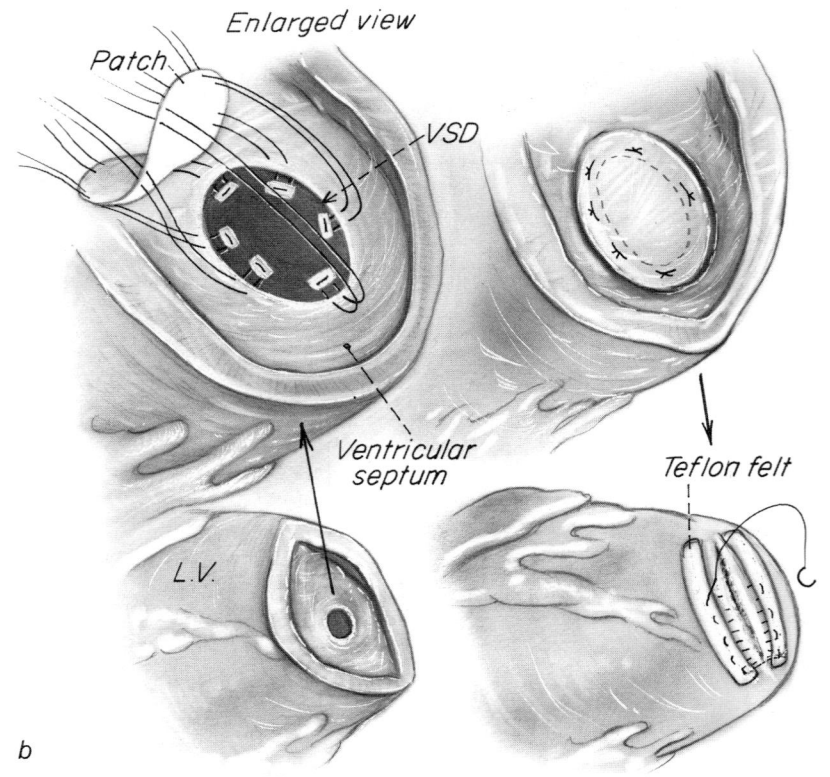

Enlarged view

Patch

VSD

L.V.

Ventricular septum

Teflon felt

b

Figure 9-2 Repair of anteriorly located postinfarction VSD.
(a) The incision is made through the anterolateral infarct that is usually present or, if some weeks have elapsed, through the scar or edge of the aneurysm that has formed. The illustration shows a single venous cannula being used, which works satisfactorily. Alternatively, two venous cannulae with direct caval insertion and tourniquets may be used (GLH).
(b) Since the edges of the VSD are friable if the operation is done early after septal perforation, as it should be, large felt pledgets (on the right ventricular side) are used with the mattress sutures for securing the septal patch (see the text for details; the sutures are placed closer together and further from the edge than shown). The ventriculotomy is closed as is any other left ventricular incision or postresectional defect (see Chapter 8).

Ao, aorta; LV, left ventricle; PA, pulmonary artery; VSD, ventricular septal defect.

---

not to damage the anterolateral papillary muscle of the mitral valve. Unless the infarct is a small one, it may be necessary to close the left ventricle after infarctectomy with a patch, also sewn into place with pledgetted mattress sutures. This patch is lined on the ventricular side with pericardium in order to make it absolutely leakproof.

When the VSD is in the apical portion of the septum and is associated with an apical myocardial infarction, the operation most expeditiously consists of amputation of the apex of the ventricle, including the involved portion of the ventricular septum (Fig. 9-3). As a beginning, the left ventricle is

opened through the infarct, and when examination of the septum indicates that the VSD is immediately adjacent to the apical infarct, the apex of the heart is excised, including the involved portion of the septum. This, of course, opens into the right ventricular cavity as well. Utilizing strips of felt on each side of the septum and on the right and left ventricular sides of the incision, heavy mattress sutures are placed that simultaneously close the interventricular communication and the opening into both ventricles.

Posterior VSDs are more difficult to expose and repair. Again, they are approached through an incision in the necrotic posterior left ventricular infarct, and for this the heart is dislocated forward from the pericardium. If the VSD is relatively small, the necrotic tissue, including the infarcted wall and adjacent septum, can be excised, and this usually includes the overlying occluded posterior descending artery. The septal patch is then sewn to the free wall of the right ventricle with interrupted mattress sutures to obliterate the VSD, supported on the septal and free wall side by felt strips. A patch of pericardially lined Dacron may then be needed to close the left ventricle after excision of the infarct. When a posterior VSD is large, two patches must be employed, one to close the VSD and the other to close the left ventricle after excision of the infarct[D1] (Fig. 9-4). The patch for the VSD is placed as usual on the left ventricular side of the septum, held in place by pledgetted mattress sutures with the pledgets on the right ventricular side of the septum. The

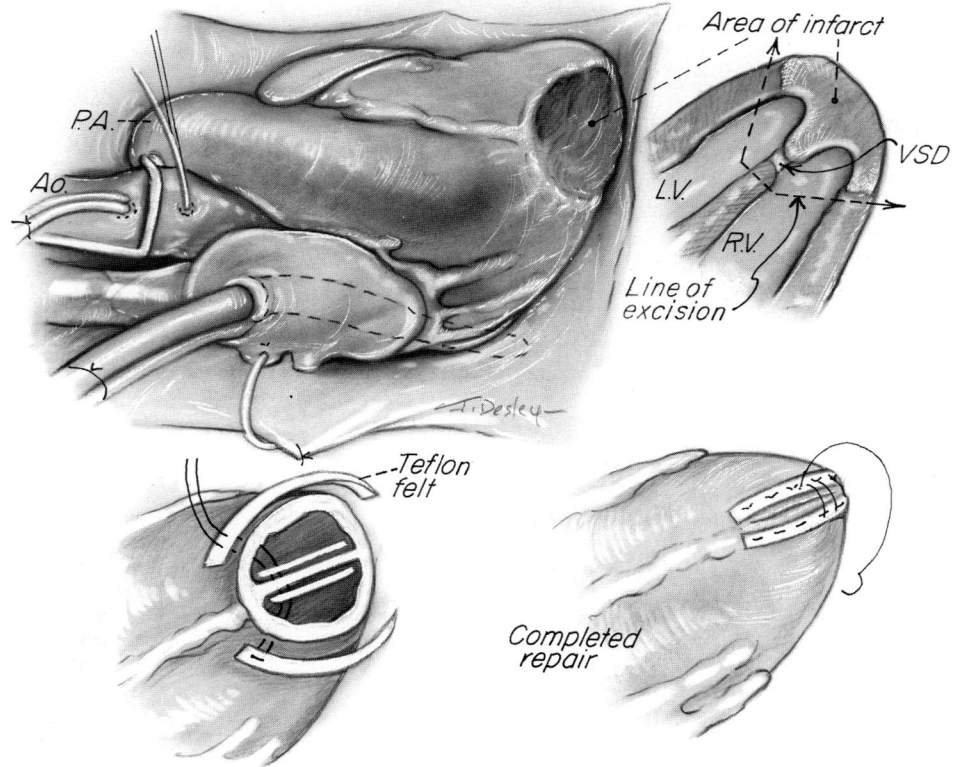

Figure 9-3 Repair of postinfarction VSD located in the apical portion of the septum. The resected area, beyond the line of excision, includes the apical transmural infarct and the apical portion of septum containing the VSD.

Ao, aorta; LV, left ventricle; PA, pulmonary artery; RV, right ventricle; VSD, ventricular septal defect.

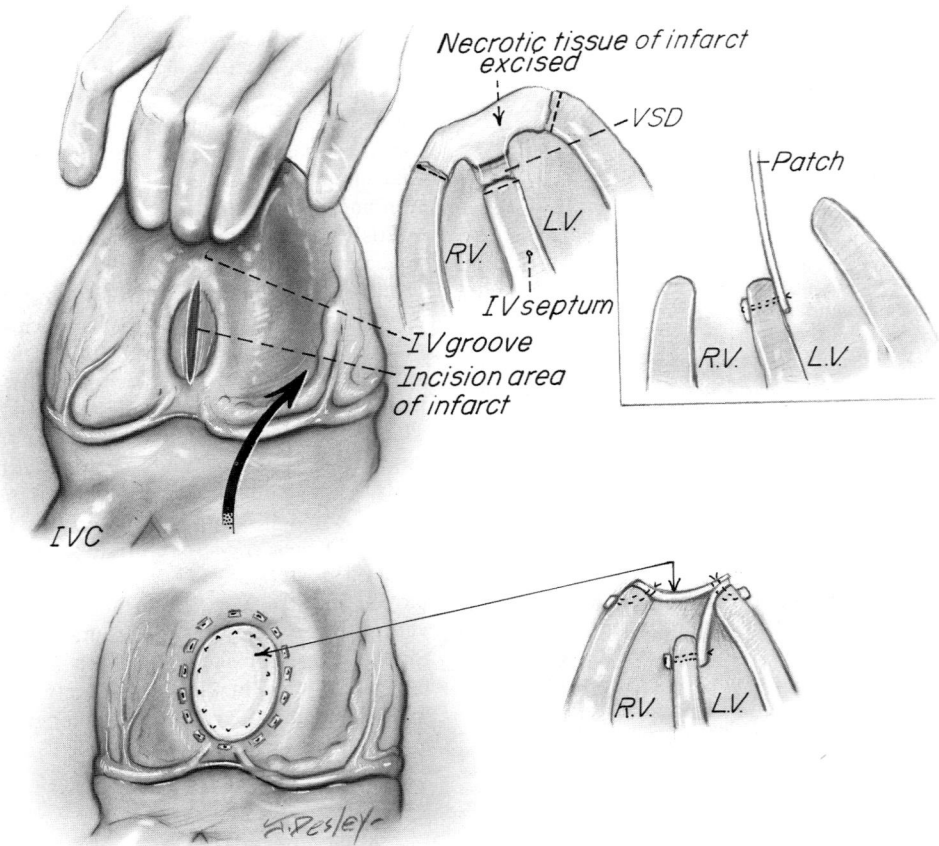

Figure 9-4 Repair of postinfarction VSD located posteriorly in the septum, usually associated with infarction on the posterior (diaphragmatic) surface of the left ventricle.

IVC, inferior vena cava; LV, left ventricle; RV, right ventricle; VSD, ventricular septal defect.

patch is then sewn to the posterior right ventricular free wall (Fig. 9-4), again with a felt strip externally to complete the closure of the interventricular communication. The patch for closure of the left ventricle is attached to the patch already in position and to the free wall of the left ventricle, mattress sutures over felt strips again being used.

Associated Procedure

Occasionally, important mitral incompetence may be associated with acute septal rupture, particularly when the infarction is posterior. The mitral valve must be replaced under such circumstances. This is usually best done through the left ventriculotomy incision using interrupted pledgetted mattress sutures, with the pledgets on the ventricular side of the anulus (see Chapter 10).

When a left ventricular aneurysm is associated with postinfarction septal perforation, it is excised as the initial step in the operation.[F1] Then, after repair of the VSD, the aneurysm is generally repaired as usual (see Chapter 8). However, improvisation in the repair is sometimes necessary.

Rarely, patients with postinfarction VSD are found also to have free wall perforation of the infarct. In surgical patients, the perforation is usually small and is taken care of by the excision of the infarct. The possibility of such an associated lesion lends obvious urgency to such situations.

Coronary Artery Bypass Grafting Procedure

In complex situations requiring coronary artery bypass grafting, only the classically indicated bypass grafts are placed. The distal anastomoses are now carried out (see Chapter 7). When they are completed, the aortic clamp is released as strong suction is placed on the aortic needle vent after the apex of the left ventricle is aspirated for air and the caval tapes are released. Suction is continued on the needle vent while the proximal anastomoses are made in the usual fashion (see Chapter 7).

Completion of the Operation

The remainder of the operation is completed in the usual manner, with particular care to hemostasis. Left atrial, right atrial, and pulmonary arterial catheters are left, as well as two right atrial and two right ventricular myocardial wires, so that atrioventricular sequential pacing is possible if needed. Intra-aortic balloon pumping is resumed during the rewarming phase of CPB and is continued into the postoperative period.

SPECIAL FEATURES OF POSTOPERATIVE CARE

The postoperative care of the patient is conducted as described in Chapter 5. Intra-aortic balloon pumping is continued in a one-to-one mode until cardiac output is adequate; it is then gradually discontinued and the balloon removed (see Chapter 5). Because the patients are often critically ill in the early postoperative period, with low cardiac output and often complicating arrhythmias, a full therapeutic regimen is required.

Using the technique described in Chapter 5 (see ''Low Cardiac Output'' in Section 2), measurements are made to detect residual shunt, which can be present because of the friability of the septum and relative insecurity of the repair. If the $\dot{Q}_p/\dot{Q}_s$ is 2.0 and the hemodynamic state is poor, prompt reoperation is considered.

EARLY RESULTS

Hospital Mortality

Hospital mortality after repair has generally been about 35%. Twelve (39%) of 31 patients in the combined GLH-UAB experience have died (Table 9-1). A similar overall hospital mortality (34%) has been recorded from the Massachusetts General Hospital by Daggett and colleagues.[D1] This high mortality is related to the usually poor preoperative state of the patients and the marked depression of ventricular function.

The results of operation have been improved in recent years by various technical and supportive measures now in use. Thus, in a collective review, Brandt and colleagues[B1] found that the hospital mortality was significantly lower after 1970 compared to before. Likewise, Daggett and colleagues reported a hospital mortality of 47% before 1973, which was reduced to 18% after that date.[D1] Also, Miyamoto and colleagues reported 2 deaths (25%, CL 9%–50%) among 8 patients operated on since January 1980.[M2] Also in the current era (UAB; 1977–1981), 3 deaths (19%, CL 8%–

34%) occurred among 16 patients operated on for closure of a postinfarction VSD and CABG. The improved recent results are related to the increased use of intra-aortic balloon pumping for support before, during, and early after operation; the approach to the VSD by an incision through the infarct; the greater use of prosthetic materials to replace necrotic muscle and to close the defect securely; and improvements in the techniques of myocardial protection.

Incremental Risk Factors for Early Death

An important risk factor is the *interval* between the perforation of the septum and the operative intervention. Intervention very early after perforation is associated with a higher risk than that carried out 3 weeks or more after the event.[C2] Thus, Brandt and colleagues in their collective review noted that since 1970, 22 (41%, CL 33%–49%) of 54 patients operated on within 3 weeks of septal rupture died in hospital. In contrast, only 3 (6%, CL 3%–11%) of 51 patients died in hospital when the operation could be carried out after an interval of 3 or more weeks ($P < .0001$). The same trend is evident in the experiences at UAB and GLH (Table 9-1) and at Massachusetts General Hospital (MGH).[D1] This trend persists in the experience of MGH in the current era (1975–1982), with a 30% (CL 20%–43%) hospital mortality when repair was done within 3 weeks of rupture and 0% (CL 0%–32%) when operation was done after a longer interval.[D5] No doubt it is not early operation per se that accounts for the high mortality, but rather the acutely ill condition of the patients who come to surgery soon after septal rupture.[G3] However, as emphasized long ago by Graham and colleagues, the important thing is that some patients who would otherwise die do survive an early repair.[G2]

The *functional status* of the patient is an important determinant of hospital survival.[L1] Thus, patients in shock before operation have had a very high hospital mortality rate,[M1] 73% (CL 53%–76%) in the experience of MGH.[R1] Gaudiani and colleagues have shown by multivariate analysis that poor cardiac performance and multiple subsystems failure (as evidenced by obtunded sensorium) are highly significant incremental risk factors for early death.[G3] In large measure, this is the result of very poor left ventricular performance.[F2,G2]

Table 9-1 Relationship of interval between septal perforation and operation to hospital mortality (UAB; 1967–July 1979 and GLH; 1970–1981).

Interval between Perforation and Repair (days)		No. of Patients			Hospital Deaths				
≤ <		UAB	GLH	Total	UAB	GLH	Total	%	CL
	7	7	2	9	5	1	6	67%	44%–85%
7 --- 14		4	0	4	3	0	3	75%	37%–97%
14		12	6	18	1	2	3	17%	7%–31%
Total		23	8	31	9	3	12	39%	29%–50%
P (Fisher)							.004		

KEY: CL, 70% confidence limits.

Table 9-2 Relationship of age to hospital mortality after repair of septal perforation (same patients as in Table 9-1).

Age (years)		No. of Patients			Hospital Deaths				
≤	<	UAB	GLH	Total	UAB	GLH	Total	%	CL
	60	9	1	10	1	0	1	10%	1%–30%
60 --- 70		11	5	16	5	2	7	44%	29%–60%
70		3	2	5	3	1	4	80%	47%–97%
Total		23	8	31	9	3	12	39%	29%–50%
P (Fisher)								.03	

KEY: CL, 70% confidence limits.

Old age has been an incremental risk factor in the experience at UAB and GLH (Table 9-2), the risk being particularly high in patients over the age of 70 years. This is no doubt related to the tendency of the elderly to have widespread arteriosclerosis and depressed ventricular, pulmonary, and renal function.

The experience of several groups suggests a higher hospital mortality when the *location* of the postinfarction ventricular septal defect is in the posterior (inferior) portion of the septum.[D1,D4,G3,K4] The extent of the coronary artery disease has not been related to the probability of postoperative early death.[R1]

LATE RESULTS

About 75% of hospital survivors are alive 5 years later. In the Massachusetts General Hospital series, 21 (81%, CL 69%–89%) of 26 hospital survivors survived the follow-up period of somewhat less than 5 years,[D1] and Gaudiani and colleagues reported an 89% 5-year survival rate.[G3] Most of the deaths were from conditions unrelated to the heart. The 8-year actuarial survival rate is 63% of those coming to operation.[K4]

The functional status of most patients surviving the hospital period is good.[G4] Thus, again in the Massachusetts General Hospital series, 8 (42%, CL 29%–57%) of the 19 long-term survivors were in NYHA class I, and 10 (53%, CL 38%–66%), were in NYHA class II.

A residual VSD has been noted early or late postoperatively in 10%–25% of patients.[B1] This may be due to the reopening of a closed defect, to the presence of an overlooked VSD, or to the development of a new septal rupture in the early postoperative period. Reoperation is required for closure of such residual defects when $\dot{Q}_p/\dot{Q}_s$ is greater than about 2.0.

INDICATIONS FOR OPERATION

The presence of a postinfarction VSD is almost always an indication for operation, since all of them produce large left-to-right shunts. The only question is the timing of operation. The relative safety of repair of postinfarction VSD 2–3 weeks or more after perforation is apparent from the information already presented. By then, the edges of the defect have become tougher, and repair is more securely and safely accomplished. Therefore, when the hemodynamic state of the patient is good, repair should be initially delayed. The criteria for deferment include an adequate cardiac output and no suggestion of cardiogenic shock, absence of symptoms of pulmonary venous hypertension or easy control of initial symptoms of this type with digitalis and diuretics, absence of fluid retention or its easy control by digitalis and diuretics, and good renal function with normal BUN and creatinine levels. The natural history of the disease suggests that such circumstances are uncommon.

In the vast majority of cases, septal perforation leads rapidly to a deteriorating hemodynamic state, with cardiogenic shock, marked and intractable symptoms of pulmonary venous hypertension, and fluid retention. Immediate preoperative preparation, study, and urgent operation are then indicated. Even if these signs are absent and renal function deteriorates, as evidenced by rising BUN and creatinine levels, surgical intervention should be undertaken promptly. The increased surgical risk of early repair is accepted because of the very great risk without surgery under such circumstances.

Delayed detection and referral for surgical treatment of desperately ill patients may make recovery so unlikely that it is wise to allow the natural history of the disease to unfold without surgical intervention. Such a situation would occur, for example, when the surgeon sees the patient only after profound shock has led to neurologic unresponsiveness, to ischemic loss of limb or bowel, or to severe impairment of renal function with markedly elevated BUN and creatinine levels.

REFERENCES

B

1. Brandt B III, Wright CB, Ehrenhaft JL: Ventricular septal defect following myocardial infarction. *Ann Thorac Surg* 27:580, 1979.

2. Brunn F: Zur Diagnostic der erworbenen Ruptur der Kammerscheidowand des Horzons. *Wien Arch Med* 6:533, 1923.

3. Buckley MJ, Mundth ED, Daggett WM, Gold HK, Leinbach RC, Austen WG: Surgical management of ventricular septal defects and mitral regurgitation complicating acute myocardial infarction. *Ann Thorac Surg* 16:598, 1973.

4. Berger TJ, Blackstone EH, Kirklin JW: Unpublished study (1978).

C

1. Cooley DA, Belmonte BA, Zeis LB, Schnur S: Surgical repair of ruptured interventricular septum following acute myocardial infarction. *Surgery* 41:930, 1957.

2. Campion BC, Harrison CE Jr, Giuliani ER, Schattenberg TT, Ellis FH Jr: Ventricular septal defect after myocardial infarction. *Ann Intern Med* 70:251, 1969.

D

1. Daggett WM, Guyton RA, Mundth ED, Buckley MJ, McEnany MT, Gold HK, Leinbach RC, Austen WG: Surgery for post-myocardial infarct ventricular septal defect. *Ann Surg* 186:260, 1977.

2. Daggett WM, Burwell LR, Lawson DW, Austen WG: Resection of acute ventricular aneurysm and ruptured interventricular septum after myocardial infarction. *N Engl J Med* 283:1507, 1970.

3. Dubost C: Discussion of paper by Iben AB.[11] *Ann Thorac Surg* 8:252, 1969.

4. Donahoo JS, Brawley RK, Taylor D, Gott VL: Factors influencing survival following post-infarction ventricular septal defects. *Ann Thorac Surg* 19:648, 1975.

5. Daggett WM, Buckley MJ, Akins CW, Leinbach RC, Gold HK, Block PC, Austen WG: Improved results of surgical management of postinfarction ventricular septal rupture. *Ann Surg* 196:269, 1982.

F

1. Freeny PC, Schattenberg TT, Danielson GK, McGoon DC, Greenberg BH: Ventricular septal defect and ventricular aneurysm secondary to acute myocardial infarction. *Circulation* 43:360, 1971.

2. Firt P, Hejnal J, Kramar R, Fabian J: Surgical treatment of postinfarction ventricular septal rupture. *J Cardiovasc Surg* 25:25, 1984.

G

1. Gold HK, Leinbach RC, Sanders CA, Buckley MJ, Mundth ED, Austen WG: Intraaortic balloon pumping for ventricular septal defect or mitral regurgitation complicating acute myocardial infarction. *Circulation* 47:1191, 1973.

2. Graham AF, Stinson EB, Daily PO, Harrison DC: Ventricular septal defects after myocardial infarction: Early operative treatment. *JAMA* 225:708, 1973.

3. Gaudiani VA, Miller DC, Stinson EB, Oyer PE, Reitz BA, Moreno-Cabral RJ, Shumway NE: Post-infarction ventricular septal defect: An argument for early operation. *Surgery* 89:48, 1981.

4. Giuliani ER, Danielson GK, Pluth JR, Odyniec NA, Wallace RB: Postinfarction ventricular septal rupture: Surgical considerations and results. *Circulation* 49:455, 1974.

5. Gonzalez-Lavin L, Zajtchuk R: Surgical considerations in the treatment of acute acquired ventricular septal defect. *Thorax* 26:610, 1971.

H

1. Hill JD, Lary D, Kerth WJ, Gerbode F: Acquired ventricular septal defects: Evolution of an operation, surgical technique, and results. *J Thorac Cardiovasc Surg* 70:440, 1975.

I

1. Iben AB, Pupello DF, Stinson EB, Shumway NE: Surgical treatment of postinfarction ventricular septal defects. *Ann Thorac Surg* 8:252, 1969.

J

1. Javid H, Hunter JA, Najafi H, Dye WS, Julian OC: Left ventricular approach for the repair of ventricular septal perforation and infarctectomy. *J Thorac Cardiovasc Surg* 63:14, 1972.

2. Jonas V, Hyncik V, Shlumsky J, Chlumska A: Eight-year survival after perforation of ventricular septum in myocardial infarction. *Acta Univer Carol [Med]* 16:133, 1970.

K

1. Kouchoukos NT: Infarction ventricular septal defect, in LH Cohn (ed): *Modern Techniques in Surgery*. Mt. Kisco, NY: Futura, 1979, p 9-1.

2. Kay JH: Discussion of paper by Iben AB.[11] *Ann Thorac Surg* 8:252, 1969.

3. Kitamura S, Mendez A, Kay JH: Ventricular septal defect following myocardial infarction. *J Thorac Cardiovasc Surg* 61:186, 1971.

4. Keenan DJM, Monro JL, Ross JK, Manners JM, Conway N, Johnson AM: Acquired ventricular septal defect. *J Thorac Cardiovasc Surg* 85:116, 1983.

L

1. Loisance DY, Cachera JP, Poulain H, Aubry PH, Juvin AM, Galey JJ: Ventricular septal defect after acute myocardial infarction: Early repair. *J Thorac Cardiovasc Surg* 80:61, 1980.

M

1. Matsui K, Kay JH, Mendez M, Pubiate P, Vanstrom N, Yokoyama T: Ventricular septal rupture secondary to myocardial infarction. *JAMA* 245:1537, 1981.

2. Miyamoto AT, Lee ME, Kass RM, Chaux A, Sethna D, Gray R, Matloff JM: Post-myocardial infarction ventricular septal defect. *J Thorac Cardiovasc Surg* 86:41, 1983.

O

1. Oyamada A, Queen FB: Spontaneous rupture of an interventricular septum following acute myocardial infarction with some clinicopathological observations of survival in five cases. Pre-

sented at the Pan-Pacific Pathology Congress, Tripler U.S. Army Hospital, Honolulu, Hawaii, October 12, 1961.

P

1. Payne WS, Hunt JC, Kirklin JW: Surgical repair of ventricular septal defect due to myocardial infarction: Report of a case. *JAMA* 183:603, 1963.

R

1. Radford MJ, Johnson RA, Daggett WM, Fallon JT, Buckley MJ, Gold HK, Leinbach RC: Ventricular septal rupture: A review of clinical and physiologic features and an analysis of survival. *Circulation* 64:545, 1981.

S

1. Sanders RJ, Kern WH, Blount SG, Jr: Perforation of the interventricular septum complicating myocardial infarction: A report of eight cases, one with cardiac catheterization. *Am Heart J* 51:736, 1956.
2. Schlichter J, Hellerstein HK, Katz LN: Aneurysm of the heart: A correlative study of one hundred and two proved cases. *Medicine* 33:43, 1954.
3. Selzer A, Gerbode F, Kerth WJ: Clinical, hemodynamic, and surgical considerations of rupture of the ventricular septum after myocardial infarction. *Am Heart J* 78:598, 1969.
4. Swithinbank JM: Perforation of the interventricular septum in myocardial infarction. *Br Heart J* 21:562, 1959.

10

MITRAL INCOMPETENCE FROM ISCHEMIC HEART DISEASE

DEFINITION

Mitral incompetence secondary to coronary artery disease may be due to papillary muscle infarction and rupture, in which case the lesion and cause are obvious. In some patients with mitral incompetence, muscle ischemia or fibrosis may not be recognized by the surgeon at operation or by the pathologist in excised surgical specimens or even at autopsy, and the ischemic origin of the incompetence may not be evident on morphologic grounds. Ischemic mitral incompetence is nonetheless probable when there is a clear history of the onset of mitral incompetence or a systolic murmur soon after a documented myocardial infarction.

Mitral incompetence may develop and be severe early after myocardial infarction (*acute* ischemic mitral incompetence) or it may not become symptomatic until later (*chronic* ischemic mitral incompetence). Occasionally, mitral incompetence is *periodic* in nature and varies as left ventricular function changes.

HISTORICAL NOTE

Mitral incompetence from ruptured papillary muscle has been recognized for a long time as a rare and frequently catastrophic complication of acute myocardial infarction.[B3,S1] A case was identified at autopsy at the Johns Hopkins Hospital in 1935,[S2] but apparently the diagnosis was correctly made antemortem only in 1948.[D1] Mitral incompetence, without papillary muscle rupture, occurring as an acute or chronic complication of ischemic heart disease with or without myocardial infarction was described in 1963 by Burch and colleagues, from New Orleans.[B2]

The first successful surgical correction of papillary muscle rupture was reported by Austen and colleagues, from Massachusetts General Hospital in 1965.[A1]

MORPHOLOGY

Acute Mitral Incompetence Complicating Myocardial Infarction

Of patients with acute myocardial infarction, 0.4%–5% die from sudden and severe mitral incompetence from total rupture of a papillary muscle.[W1] Death occurs within hours of the event, as half of both leaflets are then flail, and incompetence is massive and often silent.

The rupture of the body of the papillary muscle may remain incomplete for some days. Under such circumstances, the elongation of the papillary muscle results in some leaflet prolapse during valve closure, but the regurgitation is less massive. Alternatively, and less commonly, one or more of multiple heads of a papillary muscle (usually the posteromedial papillary muscle, which is more prone to such an arrangement) becomes detached. In this event, the prolapse may be confined to a portion of one leaflet, and the mitral regurgitation is again less severe.

Most commonly, the posteromedial papillary muscle is the one that ruptures. Related to this is the fact that when a transmural myocardial infarction exists with acute papillary muscle rupture, it is usually sited inferiorly.[E1] In about 20% of cases of acute papillary muscle rupture, the anterolateral papillary muscle is involved. This lesser incidence in the anterolateral papillary muscle may be related to its receiving blood supply both from the diagonal branches of the left anterior descending artery and the marginal branches of the circumflex artery. The posteromedial papillary muscle is supplied only by the posterior descending branch of the right coronary artery. The myocardial infarction is primarily subendocardial in about half the cases of papillary muscle rupture and is transmural in the others.[N2] Furthermore, the myocardial infarction is often small.[N2]

When infarction is present, it may be either full thickness or subendocardial, and in the majority of cases it is not massive and not therefore associated with a markedly reduced ejection fraction. However, in some instances, papillary muscle rupture is associated with the development either of a postinfarction ventricular septal defect[R1] or a free wall rupture.[V1] Severe (≥ 75% diameter reduction) coronary artery stenosis was limited to one vessel in half of the patients reported from the Mayo Clinic,[N2] and only 3 of 14 patients had triple-vessel disease.

Chronic Mitral Incompetence from Ischemic Heart Disease

In mitral incompetence of ischemic origin, the pathologic condition of the primary mitral valve is confined to the papillary muscles. The valve leaflets remain normal unless one portion has been flail for some time. Then it will become stretched, redundant, and diffusely thickened.

Partial papillary muscle rupture or infarction without rupture during acute myocardial infarction generally produces less severe immediate incompetence, and patients may survive to have important chronic mitral incompetence. However, the necrotic muscle is entirely replaced by scar tissue within 4–6 months,[M2] and in chronic cases the shriveled nubbin of tissue may provide insufficient evidence to distinguish the pathologic state from that of idiopathic chordal rupture. Alternatively, it can be postulated that as a result of ischemia only the chords may rupture at their origin from the papillary muscle, which is otherwise intact, although presumably scarred. As idiopathic chordal rupture can of course occur in the presence of coronary artery disease, it is difficult to differentiate this from ischemic chordal rupture. The ischemic etiology is probable if the regurgitation is known to have begun soon after the myocardial infarct or if there is hypokinesia or akinesia in that portion of left ventricular free

wall from which the affected papillary muscle arises (and preferably appropriate ECG changes of infarction). However, the situation is compounded by the knowledge that in occasional proven cases of papillary muscle rupture, there is no free wall infarct.

Mitral incompetence may be present intermittently or constantly in patients with ischemic heart disease.[B2,R1] In many of them, the papillary muscle ischemia was insufficient at the time of myocardial infarction to produce rupture. Instead, the papillary muscle becomes fibrosed, noncontractile, thinned, and usually elongated (papillary muscle dysfunction). There may then be leaflet prolapse with intact chordae. This seems to be the pathologic state in about 50% of patients who come to operation within 2 months of the myocardial infarction and in about 80% of those who come to operation after a longer interval.[R1] It is thus the usual cause of chronic ischemic mitral incompetence. In such instances, free wall infarction is almost invariably present, and it may be massive enough to result in a left ventricular aneurysm. The site of origin of the papillary muscles predicts that the aneurysm will involve either the inferior or the lateral free wall. When there is papillary muscle dysfunction, the degree of regurgitation is a function of lack of papillary muscle contraction and papillary muscle elongation; of the papillary muscle's lying within an aneurysm relative chordal shortening, or simply of alteration in alignment of papillary muscle and leaflet.[B2]

It is postulated that chronic mitral incompetence can occur in patients with ischemic heart disease from relative ischemia of a papillary muscle. This can occur episodically with or without episodes of angina, and the resultant loss of papillary muscle contraction presumably can produce sudden and reversible mitral incompetence that may be severe enough to precipitate left ventricular failure.[B2,B4] This is the likely explanation of the fluctuating apical systolic murmurs that occur in some patients with ischemic heart disease.

Secondary Effects of Mitral Incompetence

The morphologic and functional effects of acute and chronic mitral incompetence on the cardiac chambers, the lungs, and other organs are those of mitral incompetence in general (see Chapter 11). In acute mitral incompetence, the left atrium is small, and the mitral ring is not dilated, while in the more chronic forms, these structures usually dilate.

CLINICAL FEATURES AND DIAGNOSTIC CRITERIA

Acute Mitral Incompetence Complicating Myocardial Infarction

Papillary muscle rupture presents as an acute event within a few hours to 14 days of an episode of myocardial infarction. The onset is usually characterized by pulmonary edema or hypotension or both, most commonly 2–7 days after the acute infarction.[N2,V1,W1] It is signaled by worsening of the patient's clinical condition. Profound shock indicates gross mitral regurgitation from total rupture, and less severe signs indicate lesser degrees of mitral regurgitation from partial rupture. As pointed out by Buckley and colleagues,[B1] papillary muscle dysfunction (rather than rupture) is also a cause of acute severe regurgitation. A new apical systolic murmur can be heard, provided there is an adequate cardiac output and the regurgitation is not too gross. The murmur is frequently absent in total rupture and usually present in partial rupture.[V1] An apical third heart sound is usual, and pulmonary edema is common on the chest x-ray film. The heart is usually normal in size or only slightly enlarged, and the left atrium is small.

The introduction of a Swan-Ganz catheter can give important information, as it can exclude the presence of left-to-right shunting and, when in the wedged pulmonary artery position, the tracing may show a prominent V wave. Left ventriculography via retrograde aortic catheterization may be performed to confirm the diagnosis of mitral regurgitation (or ventricular septal defect or occasionally both) and to define the areas of impaired left ventricular contraction or aneurysm formation. However, in critically ill patients, the left ventriculogram is omitted when the precatheterization studies make the diagnosis of acute mitral incompetence and only coronary arteriography is done. When the patient is seriously ill, an intra-aortic balloon catheter is introduced before cardiac catheterization and is left in position until operation.

Two-dimensional echocardiography now is a particularly valuable diagnostic tool in this clinical setting.[N2] It is often helpful in making the important distinction between papillary muscle rupture and papillary muscle dysfunction. In the latter, the findings are those of large transmural acute myocardial wall motion abnormalities. The papillary muscle itself may appear hypokinetic and echo dense, resulting in echocardiographically visible improper coaptation of the mitral leaflet.[G2] When there has been papillary muscle rupture, the mitral leaflet becomes flail and extends into the left atrial during systole.[N2] The ruptured portion of papillary muscle may be directly visualized as a separate mass attached to the chordae.[E1,M4,N2]

Chronic Mitral Incompetence from Ischemic Heart Disease

Usually the patient presents with gradually increasing mitral regurgitation; and when the murmur dates from a myocardial infarction, the ischemic etiology is obvious. There may be cardiac enlargement, including left atrial enlargement; hypokinesia; or akinesia at the site of papillary muscle involvement or sometimes a left ventricular aneurysm. Other diagnostic criteria are the same as in other types of chronic mitral incompetence (see Chapter 11).

NATURAL HISTORY

Acute Mitral Incompetence Complicating Myocardial Infarction

Only about 25% of patients treated nonsurgically survive more than 24 hours after total rupture of a papillary muscle.[S1,V1] Survival after partial papillary muscle rupture is bet-

ter, as over 70% of patients survive the first 24 hours, and about 50% survive more than 1 month to become examples of chronic ischemic mitral incompetence.

Chronic Mitral Incompetence from Ischemic Heart Disease

The impact of chronic mitral incompetence on the natural history of patients with coronary artery disease has not been fully determined. Mild or moderate mitral incompetence without partial papillary muscle rupture is episodic in some patients, presumably as a result of changing myocardial ischemia and ventricular function. Persistent and severe mitral incompetence, often but not always associated with moderate or severe left ventricular dysfunction,[R1,V2] must worsen the already limited prognosis of patients with poor left ventricular function (see Chapter 7, "Incremental Risk Factors for Death as a Time-Related Event after CABG" in Late Results). The available information suggests that severe left ventricular dysfunction alone, in patients with coronary artery disease, imposes a 5-year survival rate of only about 50% and that, when important mitral incompetence is added, the devolutionary cycle is even more rapid.

TECHNIQUE OF OPERATION

Acute Mitral Incompetence Complicating Myocardial Infarction

In critically ill subjects with this complication of acute myocardial infarction, intra-aortic balloon pumping is begun as soon as the acute catastrophe has been recognized and is continued until the patient is on cardiopulmonary bypass (CPB).[B1]

The patient is prepared and draped for a coronary artery bypass graft (CABG) operation, and the sternotomy, removal of the sphaenous vein, and preparation for CPB are accomplished expeditiously. With CPB established, the aorta is cross-clamped, the cold cardioplegic solution is infused, and the distal coronary anastomoses are performed (see Chapter 7). (The proximal anastomoses may be performed first, on CPB, and then the distal anastomoses.) Certainly the distal anastomoses must be completed before the valve procedure. In the presence of an acute myocardial infarction, there is a real danger of left ventricular rupture during dislocation of the heart and retraction for distal anastomoses to obtuse marginal vessels, and this risk is significantly increased when the ventricle contains a rigid prosthesis.

The approach to the mitral valve is via the left atrium in the usual fashion. When there is acute papillary muscle rupture, the mitral valve is replaced with either a prosthetic or bioprosthetic valve (see Chapter 11). As the mitral ring tissue is not thickened and may be more friable than normal, great care must be taken to obtain adequate bites of tissue when placing the ring sutures and not to exert excessive traction on the stitches as the valve is lowered into position, lest they begin to pull through the tissues. Pledgetted or nonpledgetted simple interrupted sutures are preferred.

When the chordal mechanism is intact and there is annular dilation, annuloplasty using a Carpentier ring can be considered as an alternative to valve replacement (see Chapter 11). Leaflet prolapse secondary to chordal lengthening from acute ischemia of the papillary muscle with severe left ventricular dysfunction from infarction[B1] is not suitable for correction by chordal shortening techniques.

Chronic Mitral Incompetence from Ischemic Heart Disease

The variability with time in the magnitude of chronic mitral incompetence in some patients with ischemic heart disease can make surgical decisions difficult during the CABG operation. Patients with moderate (grade 3 on the basis of 1–6) mitral incompetence by cineangiography preoperatively may have only a small regurgitant jet palpable at operation, and a patient with mild (grade 1 or 2) incompetence at preoperative study may have a moderate regurgitant jet palpable at operation. In general, when at operation the incompetence is estimated to be grade 3 or more on the basis of the palpation of the regurgitant jet from outside or from within the left atrium (see Chapter 11), the mitral valve is exposed by the usual left atrial approach (see Chapter 11). This should be done after completing the distal anastomoses (see Chapter 11 for details of the combined mitral and CABG operation). Usually in this situation of periodic mitral incompetence, the valve is delicate and normal in appearance when exposed. An annuloplasty, using the Carpentier-Edwards annuloplasty ring, is usually performed (see "Special Situations and Controversies").

When mitral incompetence is severe and a dominant part of the patient's presentation, the details concerning valve replacement or repair depend on the mechanism of incompetence. When incompetence is associated with an inferior or lateral left ventricular aneurysm, the affected papillary muscle is excised along with the aneurysmal sac. Mitral valve replacement is then the appropriate treatment and is performed through the left ventricular exposure provided by the aneurysmectomy.[N1] (See Chapter 8 for details of the aneurysmectomy and CABG procedure.)

Generally the mitral valve is exposed through the usual left atrial approach. When there is a localized area of flail posterior cusp secondary to rupture of one head of the papillary muscle or to chordal rupture, a U-shaped (or rectangular) resection of the portion of leaflet combined with annuloplasty is appropriate (see Chapter 11), but when the anterior leaflet is involved, such a repair is not satisfactory, and valve replacement must be done.

When in doubt as to whether mitral valve surgery is required, a situation that should be uncommon, CPB may be discontinued to assess myocardial behavior and the degree of mitral incompetence. If cardiac output is clearly satisfactory, left atrial pressure is normally related to right atrial pressure, and there is neither a palpable nor a recordable systolic left atrial wave or thrill, then mitral valve surgery is clearly not required. An inadequate cardiac output accompanied by the signs of residual mitral incompetence, is an indication for recommencing CPB to allow mitral valve replacement or repair.

SPECIAL FEATURES OF POSTOPERATIVE CARE

The usual management protocols are followed (see Chapter 5). Since patients in this category are apt to have low cardiac output postoperatively, catecholamine support and intra-aortic balloon pumping are required more often than after other kinds of operation.

EARLY RESULTS

Acute Mitral Incompetence Complicating Myocardial Infarction

When operation is required in the early postinfarction period, the risks are considerable. Buckley and colleagues report two deaths (40%, CL 14%–71%) among 5 patients operated on within 7 days of the acute infarction, 1 (50%) among 2 operated on 7–14 days later, and none among 2 operated on 14–19 days later, for a total mortality of 3 (33%, CL 15%–56%) among 9.[B1] No hospital deaths (0%, CL 0%–38%) occurred among 4 patients operated on by Buckley and colleagues for acute papillary muscle rupture. Three (60%, CL 29%–86%) deaths occurred among 5 patients in whom acute papillary muscle dysfunction was found at operation (P [Fisher] for difference = .12). This possible difference in hospital mortality could be related to the fact that the latter group had a higher proportion of patients with extensive transmural myocardial infarctions and thus poor left ventricular function (ejection fraction less than 0.35).[R1] The deaths were all related to acute cardiac failure (low cardiac output).

In the GLH experience, there was one hospital death (17%, CL 2%–46%) among six patients with severe mitral incompetence operated on less than 6 weeks (2 days to 5 weeks) from the onset of infarction. The death occurred in a patient with a large false left ventricular aneurysm secondary to left ventricular rupture, which was excised (Table 10-1). All four patients with papillary muscle rupture survived, while one of two with papillary muscle dysfunction did not.

Chronic Mitral Incompetence from Ischemic Heart Disease

At UAB between 1975 and July 1979, 29 patients with chronic mitral incompetence from ischemic papillary muscle dysfunction or rupture[1] underwent mitral valve replacement with or without coronary artery bypass grafting, and five (17%, CL 10%–28%) have died in hospital. Twenty-eight of the 29 patients underwent simultaneous coronary artery bypass grafting, with the same five deaths (18%, CL 19%–28%). The results are similar in the slightly more current era (UAB, 1977–1981), 8 hospital deaths (16%, CL 10%–23%) having occurred among 51 patients undergoing valve surgery for ischemic mitral incompetence and CABG. This is a considerably higher hospital mortality (P for difference = .001) than that for the combined procedure when the mitral replacement is for rheumatic disease or mitral prolapse (Table 10-2). This idea is supported by an analysis of this same experience for the incremental risk factors for postoperative

---

[1] In this chapter the phrase "papillary muscle dysfunction" is used synonomously with "ischemic mitral incompetence."

Table 10-1 Mitral valve replacement for ischemic mitral incompetence (GLH; 1968–1982). Eighteen of the 24 patients had concomitant CABG operation. Three of the 6 without the CABG operation had single-vessel disease to an area of aneurysm resection.

Variable	n	Hospital Deaths		
		No.	%	CL
NYHA Class				
II	2		0%	0%–61%
III	7		0%	0%–24%
IV	15[a]	2	13%	4%–29%
Total	24	2	8%	3%–19%
Time Postinfarction				
< 6 weeks	6	1	17%	2%–46%
≥ 6 weeks	18	1	6%	0.7%–18%
Total	24	2		
LV Aneurysm				
Yes	5	1	20%	3%–53%
No	19	1	5%	0.7%–17%
Total	24	2		
Age (year)				
< 60	11		0%	0%–16%
≥ 60 (60–73)	13	2	15%	5%–33%
Total	24	2		

KEY: CL, 70% confidence limits; LV, left ventricular.

[a] Includes five emergency operations with one death.

Table 10-3 Incremental risk factors for hospital death with acute or chronic heart failure after isolated or combined primary mitral valve replacement (UAB; January 1975–July 1979; $n = 445$; 15 events; see Chapter 11, Appendix 11A, for details).

Incremental Risk Factors	Logistic Regression Coefficient ± SD	P Value
NYHA functional class (I–V)	2.8 ± 0.78	.0001
Papillary muscle dysfunction	3.6 ± 1.34	.004
Age (yr)	0.08 ± 0.048	.03
Atrial fibrillation	2.9 ± 1.21	.02
If noncardioplegia: date of operation (mo since January 1, 1975)	−0.27 ± 0.008	.008
If cardioplegia: body surface area (m²)	−12 ± 6.6	.10
Intercept	−2.8, if noncardioplegia, −17	

KEY: SD, standard deviation.

probability of hospital survival after mitral replacement and CABG for ischemic mitral incompetence.[R1] Hospital mortality was 28% when ejection fraction was greater than 0.35, and 40% when it was ≤ 0.35; whether the operation was done early or late after myocardial infarction and the extent of the coronary artery disease did not affect the hospital mortality.

Concomitant left ventricular aneurysmectomy, along with coronary artery bypass grafting and mitral valve replacement, decreases the probability of hospital survival, although this was not evident in the GLH experience (Table 10-1). Miller and colleagues found the hospital mortality to be 56% (CL 34%–76%) in this subset, compared to 13% (CL 6%–25%) when LV aneurysmectomy was not necessary (*P* = .02).[M1]

in-hospital cardiac death, which shows the presence of ischemic papillary muscle dysfunction to be a highly significant risk factor (Table 10-3), even when the preoperative clinical status (NYHA functional class) is taken into account. Presumably, this is related to the particularly poor left ventricular function present preoperatively in many of the patients with ischemic mitral incompetence, produced by both muscle ischemia and volume overload.

As corroboration of this, Radford and colleagues, at Massachusetts General Hospital, found that preoperative left ventricular ejection fraction was the main determinant of the

LATE RESULTS

When the operation is done acutely for rupture of a papillary muscle, the late results are often good. Thus, all five GLH

Table 10-2 Hospital mortality of patients with papillary muscle rupture or dysfunction undergoing primary replacement of the mitral valve plus CABG, compared to that of patients with other types of mitral valve incompetence undergoing similar combined surgery (UAB; 1975–July 1979).

Pathology of Mitral Incompetence	n	Hospital Deaths			
		No.	%	CL	
Rheumatic	34	1	3%	0.4%–10% ⎤	1/52, 1.9%[a]
Mitral prolapse	18	0	0%	0%–10% ⎦	(0.2%–6.4%)
Endocarditis	3	1	33%	4%–76%	
Papillary muscle dysfunction	28	5	18%[a]	10%–28%	
Ruptured chordae	9	1	11%	1%–33%	
Unable to classify	4	0	0%	0%–38%	
Total	96	8	8.3%	5.4%–12.3%	

KEY: CL, 70% confidence limits.

NOTE: When patients with ruptured chordae and unclassifiable pathologic condition are assumed to have an ischemic basis for mitral valve disease and are added to those with papillary muscle dysfunction, *P* = .03 for the difference from the first two groups.

[a] *P* (Fisher) for difference = .02.

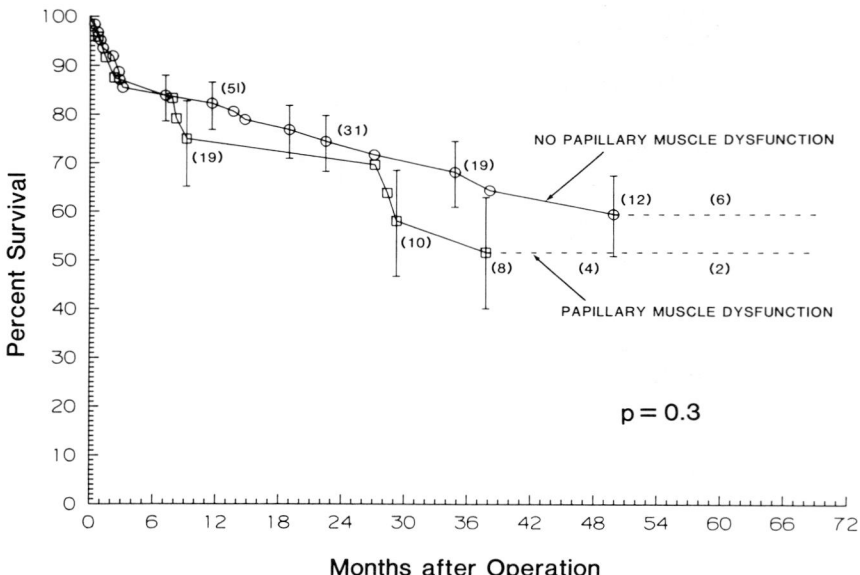

Figure 10-1 Actuarial survival rates for hospital survivors (23 of 28 patients operated on; see Table 10-1) of primary mitral valve replacement and coronary artery bypass grafting in patients with ischemic mitral incompetence (papillary muscle dysfunction), compared with that in patients with nonischemic incompetence (UAB; 1975–July 1979).

hospital survivors were alive and well (median follow-up 4 years) as were the 4 patients reported by Buckley and colleagues[B1] (follow-up of 4–14 months). Their ultimate prognosis may, however, be limited by their underlying coronary and myocardial disease. Thus, Morrow and colleagues found in four patients undergoing only mitral valve replacement 3–15 months after papillary muscle rupture[C1] that left ventricular end-diastolic pressure remained elevated 11 months postoperatively because of left ventricular dysfunction.[M2]

The late results of combined mitral valve replacement and CABG for ischemic heart disease and chronic ischemic mitral incompetence are somewhat less good than when the combined operation is done for patients with mitral incompetence of other etiology. Thus, among those in the former category operated upon at UAB 1975–July 1979, the 3-year survival rate was 50% (Fig. 10-1); most of the late deaths occurred in the first postoperative year. The 3-year survival rate was 65% for the latter group. The 3-year survival results are similar to those reported by Miller and colleagues.[M1] These differences are probably due to a higher proportion of patients with ischemic mitral incompetence having important and irreversible left ventricular dysfunction.

These late results are distinctly inferior to those for isolated nonischemic mitral valve disease treated by valve replacement or for uncomplicated ischemic heart disease treated by CABG. Thus, the 3-year survival rate is 80% for all patients ($n = 445$) undergoing primary mitral replacement at UAB during that time (see Chapter 11) and is 92% for patients undergoing only triple-vessel bypass grafting (see Chapter 7).

As is the case with hospital mortality, late survival within the group is also highly dependent on preoperative left ventricular function. Radford and colleagues found the 3-year survival rate of hospital survivors to be 100% when

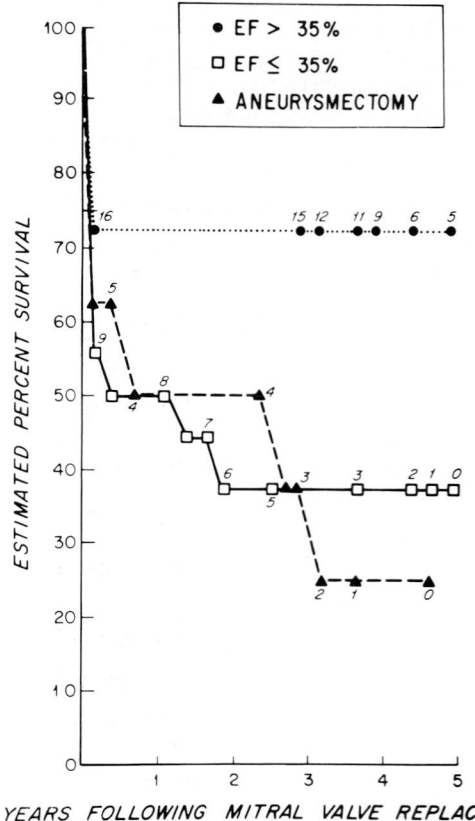

YEARS FOLLOWING MITRAL VALVE REPLACEMENT

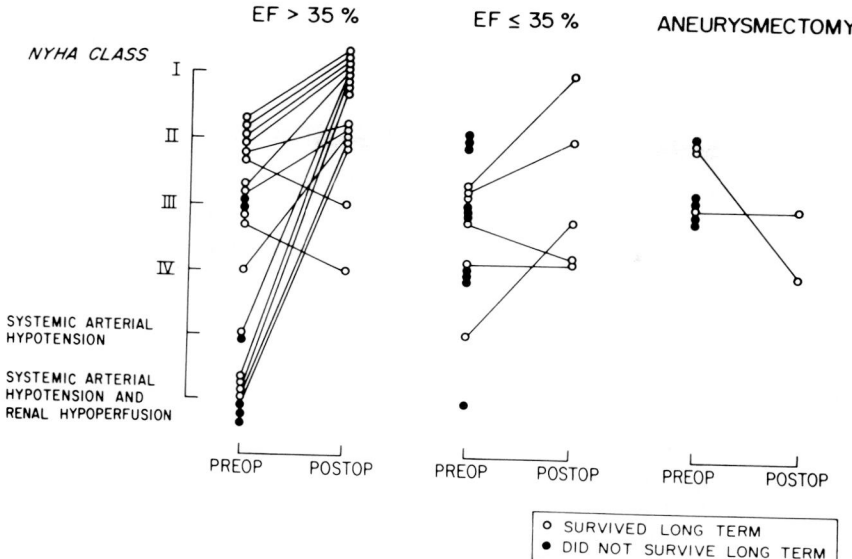

Figure 10-3 Functional status after valve replacement for ischemic mitral incompetence. The degree of heart failure (NYHA functional class) before operation and during the follow-up period is shown. The follow-up heart failure status is unknown for three patients who are known to be long-term survivors; these patients are designated by preoperative symbols that are unconnected to postoperative symbols. Systemic arterial hypotension and renal hypoperfusion represent more advanced heart failure than implied by NYHA class IV and are similar to the symptoms for class V in the modification of NYHA class used at UAB and GLH.

EF, left ventricular ejection fraction; NYHA, New York Heart Association.

Reproduced with permission from Radford et al.,[R1] and the American Heart Association, Inc.

preoperative left ventricular ejection fraction was > 35% and about 60% when it was ≤ 35% (Fig. 10-2).[R1]

No difference in late survival (or symptomatic results) has been demonstrated between mitral valve replacement and repair.[M3] Possibly the strikingly better late results with repair reported by Kay and associates are related to case selection.[K1]

In the combined UAB and GLH experience, eight patients left the hospital after combined mitral valve replacement, left ventricular aneurysmectomy, and CABG, and only two (25%, CL 9%–50%) remained alive on follow-up. Most deaths occurred in the first postoperative year. Miller and colleagues also found unfavorable late results in this group, only 35% (CL 4%–25%) of hospital survivors being alive 3 years later.[M1] Karp and colleagues, in a study at UAB of a longer experience with valve replacement as an isolated or combined procedure, found preoperative left ventricular an-

eurysm a very significant incremental risk factor for premature late death.[K2]

Symptomatic relief is generally good in survivors after mitral valve replacement and CABG for ischemic mitral incompetence, with most patients experiencing considerable relief of their symptoms of heart failure.[R1] Most are in NYHA class I or II 3–5 years after operation (Fig. 10-3). The less favorable results in such patients reported earlier by Glancy and colleagues[G1] may be related to the fact that the operation consisted only of mitral valve replacement. Again, the less favorable result in patients undergoing left ventricular aneurysmectomy plus mitral replacement and coronary revascularization is evident in the data of Radford and associates, for none of the three long-term survivors in this category had symptomatic improvement from that operation (Fig. 10-3).

INDICATIONS FOR OPERATION

When a patient with an acute myocardial infarction suddenly develops acute mitral incompetence, operation is advisable, recognizing that hospital mortality under such circumstances may be 30% or greater. As in acute perforation of the ventricular septum (see Chapter 9), if possible, operation should be done before severe hemodynamic deterioration occurs. When the hemodynamic state is reasonably good, one option is to delay operation about 2 weeks to 2 months. However, Nishimura and colleagues, from the Mayo Clinic, report sudden deterioration followed by death in five patients whose condition had initially stabilized with medical therapy. This indicates that all patients with papillary muscle rupture com-

Figure 10-2 Survival following mitral valve replacement, usually with coronary artery bypass grafting, for patients with ischemic mitral incompetence. Hospital mortality is included. The numbers in small type are the numbers of patients alive at the time indicated. Points are plotted at times that correspond to a death or a change in the number of patients at risk of death. The minimum follow-up period was 32 months. Standard error of percent was 9.5% at all follow-up intervals for the group with EF > 35%, varied from 12.1%–12.5% for the group with EF ≤ 35%, and varied from 15.3%–17.7% for the aneurysmectomy group.

EF, left ventricular ejection fraction.

Reproduced with permission from Radford et al.,[R1] and the American Heart Association, Inc.

plicating acute myocardial infarction should have prompt investigation and operation. Operation should be avoided when the patient is moribund (see Chapter 9, ''Indications for Operation'').

The indications for operation in chronic mitral incompetence resulting from ischemic heart disease are less well defined. Uncommonly and particularly when the mitral incompetence developed acutely from partial rupture of a papillary muscle after myocardial infarction, the mitral incompetence per se dominates the clinical picture and causes the symptoms and disability.[R1] Then the decision for operation on the mitral valve is straightforward and is made based on the usual indications (see Chapter 11).

More often, the patient with the usual symptoms of ischemic heart disease has some signs of left ventricular failure and clinical and angiographic evidence of mitral incompetence. As already mentioned, the incompetence often fluctuates in degree, but it may be constant and moderate or severe. In the latter circumstances, operation is advisable and includes replacement or repair of the mitral incompetence (see ''Special Situations and Controversies''). When the incompetence is variable with time, it is more difficult to know when mitral valve surgery should be done at the time of coronary artery bypass grafting. This is particularly so since the effect of coronary artery bypass grafting alone on this kind of mitral incompetence is not known. However, if at operation mitral incompetence greater than grade 3 (on a basis of 1–6, 6 being the most severe) is identified on palpa-

tion inside (see Chapter 11) or outside the left atrium, mitral repair or replacement is believed to be indicated.

SPECIAL SITUATIONS AND CONTROVERSIES
Repair or Replacement of the Mitral Valve

Until recently, the policy has been to replace the valve routinely when operation on it has been felt to be indicated in ischemic heart disease. This has also been the policy at Massachusetts General Hospital.[A1,B1,R1] The experience of Kay and colleagues[K1] has caused a revision of concepts, and a reparative operation is now preferred unless (1) the operation is done for acute severe mitral incompetence complicating acute myocardial infarction, when valve replacement is done to ensure a completely competent valve, and (2) partial rupture has resulted in chronic mitral incompetence with ruptured chordal attachment to the anterior leaflet or to more than half of the posterior leaflet.

When a reparative operation is selected and no specific pathologic condition, such as ruptured chordae or ruptured papillary muscle, is found, an annuloplasty by the Carpentier ring is performed (see Chapter 11). If ruptured chordae to less than one-half the posterior leaflet are found, annuloplasty plus rectangular valve excision and repair are done. The long-term results of this protocol have not been established, but good long-term results have been reported by Kay and colleagues.[K1]

REFERENCES

A

1. Austen WG, Sanders CA, Averill JH, Friedlich AL: Ruptured papillary muscle: Report of a case with successful mitral valve replacement. *Circulation* 32:597, 1965.

B

1. Buckley MJ, Mundth ED, Daggett WM, Gold HK, Leinbach RC, Austen WG: Surgical management of ventricular septal defects and mitral regurgitation complicating acute myocardial infarction. *Ann Thorac Surg* 16:598, 1973.
2. Burch GE, De Pasquale NP, Phillips JH: Clinical manifestations of papillary muscle dysfunction. *Arch Intern Med* 112:158, 1963.
3. Breneman GM, Drake FH: Ruptured papillary muscle following myocardial infarction with long survival: Report of two cases. *Circulation* 25:862, 1962.
4. Brody W, Criley JM: Intermittent severe mitral regurgitation: Hemodynamic studies in a patient with recurrent acute left-sided heart failure. *N Engl J Med* 283:673, 1970.

C

1. Cohen LS, Morrow AG, Braunwald NS, Roberts WC, Braunwald E: Severe mitral regurgitation following acute myocardial infarction and ruptured papillary muscle: Hemodynamic findings and results of mitral valve replacement in four patients. *Circulation* 35,36(suppl II):II-87, 1967 (abstr).

D

1. Davidson S: Spontaneous rupture of a papillary muscle of the heart: A report of three cases and a review of the literature. *Mt Sinai J Med* 14:941, 1948.

E

1. Erbel R, Schweizer P, Bardos P, Meyer J: Two-dimensional echocardiographic diagnosis of papillary muscle rupture. *Chest* 79:595, 1981.

G

1. Glancy DL, Stinson EB, Shepherd RL, Itscoitz SB, Roberts WC, Epstein SE, Morrow AG: Results of valve replacement for severe mitral regurgitation due to papillary muscle rupture or fibrosis. *Am J Cardiol* 32:313, 1973.
2. Godley RW, Weyman AE, Feigenbaum H, Rogers EW, Green D: Patterns of mitral leaflet motion in patients with probable papillary muscle dysfunction. *Am J Cardiol* 43:411, 1979 (abstr).

K

1. Kay JH, Zubiate P, Mendez MA, Vanstrom N, Yokoyama T, Gharavi MA: Surgical treatment of mitral insufficiency secondary to coronary artery disease. *J Thorac Cardiovasc Surg* 79:12, 1980.

2. Karp RB, Cyrus RJ, Blackstone EH, Kirklin JW, Kouchoukos NT, Pacifico AD: The Bjork-Shiley valve. *J Thorac Cardiovasc Surg* 81:602, 1981.

M

1. Miller DC, Stinson EB, Rossiter SJ, Oyer PE, Reitz BA, Shumway NE: Impact of simultaneous myocardial revascularization on operative risk, functional result, and survival following mitral valve replacement. *Surgery* 84:848, 1978.
2. Morrow AG, Cohen LS, Roberts WC, Braunwald NS, Braunwald E: Severe mitral regurgitation following acute myocardial infarction and ruptured papillary muscle. *Circulation* 37,38 (suppl II):II-124, 1968.
3. Merin G, Giuliani ER, Pluth JR, Wallace RB, Danielson GK: Surgery for mitral valve incompetence after myocardial infarction. *Am J Cardiol* 32:322, 1973.
4. Mintz GS, Victor MF, Kotler MN, Parry WR, Segal BL: Two-dimensional echocardiographic identification of surgically correctable complications of acute myocardial infarction. *Circulation* 64:91, 1981.

N

1. Najafi H, Javid H, Hunter JA, Goldin MD, Serry C, Dye WS: Mitral insufficiency secondary to coronary heart disease. *Ann Thorac Surg* 20:529, 1975.
2. Nishimura RA, Schaff HV, Shub C, Gersh BJ, Edwards WE, Tajik AJ: Papillary muscle rupture complicating acute myocardial infarction: Analysis of 17 patients. *Am J Cardiol* 51:373, 1983.

R

1. Radford MJ, Johnson RA, Buckley MJ, Daggett WM, Leinbach RC, Godl HK: Survival following mitral valve replacement for mitral regurgitation due to coronary artery disease. *Circulation* 60: (suppl I):I-39, 1979.

S

1. Sanders RJ, Neubuerger KT, Ravin A: Rupture of papillary muscles: Occurrence of rupture of the posterior muscle in posterior myocardial infarction. *Dis Chest* 36:316, 1957.
2. Stevenson RR, Turner WJ: Rupture of a papillary muscle in the heart as a cause of sudden death. *Bulletin of the Johns Hopkins Hospital* 57:235, 1935.

V

1. Vlodaver Z, Edwards JE: Rupture of ventricular septum or papillary muscle complicating myocardial infarction. *Circulation* 55:815, 1977.
2. Vismara LA, Miller RR, DeMaria A, Mason DT, Amsterdam EA: Mitral regurgitation in patients with coronary artery disease: Relation to extent of myocardial dysfunction. *Am J Cardiol* 33:175, 1974 (abstr).

W

1. Wei JY, Hutchins GM, Bulkley BH: Papillary muscle rupture in fatal acute myocardial infarction: A potentially treatable form of cardiogenic shock. *Ann Intern Med* 90:149, 1979.

ACQUIRED VALVULAR HEART DISEASE

PART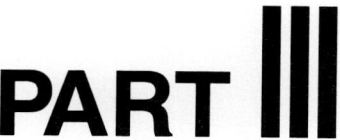

11

MITRAL VALVE DISEASE WITH OR WITHOUT TRICUSPID VALVE DISEASE

DEFINITION

This chapter describes the surgical aspects of acquired mitral valve disease, excluding congenital mitral stenosis and incompetence (see Chapter 36) and some aspects of ischemic mitral incompetence (see Chapter 10). Associated or secondary tricuspid valve disease is also considered.

HISTORICAL NOTE

One of the first to write about the possibility of treating mitral valve disease surgically was Sir Lauder Brunton,[B1] in his "preliminary note" published in *The Lancet* in 1902. Cutler, then at Western Reserve University Medical School and later the Mosley Professor of Surgery at the Harvard Medical School and the Peter Bent Brigham Hospital in Boston, subsequently did further experimental work related to treating mitral stenosis surgically, as did others. He and Levine in 1923 reported a case operated on through a median sternotomy incision in which a special curved knife was inserted through the left ventricular apex to cut a stenotic mitral valve.[C1] In 1925, Souttar digitally opened a stenotic mitral valve through the left atrial appendage.[S1] An effective surgical approach to mitral stenosis began with Harken[H1] and Bailey[B2] in the United States and Brock in London.[B28] Harken had been doing animal experiments regarding mitral valve surgery at the Boston City Hospital in 1939 before serving with the United States Army in World War II, during which time he became well-known for the successful removal of missiles and shell fragments from the heart. After the war, he continued his work on mitral valve surgery at the Boston City and Peter Bent Brigham Hospitals in Boston. Bailey was working primarily at Hahnemann Hospital in Philadelphia. Although their techniques and terminology were somewhat different, their approaches to opening the stenotic mitral valve through the left atrial appendage were similar. Many useful technical modifications were subsequently added to the operation of closed mitral commissurotomy, one of the most important of which was Tubb's transventricular dilator used with digital control by a finger inserted through the left atrial appendage.[A6] Because the results were satisfactory and frequently very good with these simple closed methods, it was not until about 1970 that most surgeons had abandoned them for an open operation with cardiopulmonary bypass (CPB).

Although a few ingenious closed methods of surgically improving mitral incompetence were reported in the early 1950s, particularly by Bailey, Nichols, Davila, and Glover,[B29,D9,N3] an effective open approach to this problem was first made with CPB by Lillehei in 1957[L5] and independently by Merendino in the same year.[M4] McGoon described an effective repair for mitral incompetence from ruptured chordae in 1960.[M3] In subsequent years, a number of surgeons have contributed technical advances in the repair of mitral valve incompetence, particularly Carpentier, working with Dubost and colleagues in Paris.

A number of surgeons realized very early the need for replacement of at least some diseased mitral valves. However, Starr and Edwards, from the University of Oregon Medical Center in Portland, first reported successful mitral valve replacement in 1961.[S2]

MORPHOLOGY

Mitral stenosis is a result of rheumatic heart disease, as is mixed stenosis and incompetence. Pure mitral incompetence may be rheumatic in origin but is often the result of some other pathologic process. Tricuspid valve disease usually takes the form of secondary functional tricuspid incompetence, but rheumatic disease may make the tricuspid valve stenotic and incompetent.

Mitral Stenosis

In clinically important mitral stenosis, some degree of *commissural fusion* and *leaflet thickening* are the dominant features. The characteristic fusion of the edges of the mitral leaflets in the commissural areas is a complex process, involving the coapting edges of commissural, posterior (mural), and anterior (septal) leaflets at both the anterolateral and posteromedial commissures. The valve leaflets are thickened to varying degrees, particularly at their free edges and at the sites of fusion. Calcification often occurs in older patients, beginning at the commissures but extending sometimes into the anulus posteriorly.

The *chordae tendinae* are variably involved by the rheumatic process. Occasionally, in the presence of severe mitral stenosis, the chordae are nearly normal in appearance, and opening the valve commissure results in a wide orifice. More commonly, some degree of chordal thickening, fusion, and shortening is present in each commissural area. This process is extreme in some patients, particularly those in whom restenosis develops after an earlier commissurotomy, and results in an obstructing, tough, subcommissural mass on either side of the narrow orifice. This advanced pathologic condition may be purely rheumatic in origin or in part a result of the hemodynamic and (in the case of restenosis) surgical trauma. It may remain as an obstructive lesion even after commissurotomy.

The *left atrium* is enlarged, but usually not severely, in pure mitral stenosis, and its wall is thickened.

The *left ventricular* volume and mass are normal or slightly abnormally small.[K1] When fibrosis and particularly calcification involve the mitral anulus, regional wall motion at the base of the left ventricle is impaired, but overall left ventricular systolic and diastolic function are often normal in surgical patients. However, left ventricular function may be significantly impaired in those coming to operation late in the life history of the disease (see also "Left Ventricular Function: Mitral Stenosis" in section on Late Results).

Due to spasm in the pulmonary arterioles, the *pulmonary vascular resistance* may increase in patients with severe mitral stenosis. This is presumed to be a reflex from left atrial enlargement. This phenomenon is confined to severe stenosis but is otherwise unpredictable. Organic pulmonary vascular disease is most commonly found in young Polynesian and Asian patients as well as in a small proportion of patients with long-standing mitral stenosis. Rarely, the vascular disease may progress to obliteration of pulmonary arterioles. The rise in pulmonary vascular resistance produces a rise in pulmonary artery pressure and right ventricular pressure out of proportion to the valve stenosis and the left atrial pressure increase, which leads to right ventricular hypertrophy and finally secondary tricuspid incompetence.

Mitral Stenosis and Incompetence

Mixed stenosis and incompetence is always primarily rheumatic in origin. The stenosis is produced by varying degrees of commissural fusion and chordal thickening. The incompetence results from fibrous retraction of the central unfused portion of the leaflets and either chordal shortening or elongation. Shortening restricts leaflet motion and increases the gaping central orifice, while elongation allows cusp prolapse. Occasionally, chordae can rupture as a result of the rheumatic process per se. Endocarditis on a rheumatic stenotic valve adds incompetence by eroding either leaflet or chordal tissue.

Mitral Incompetence

Incompetence can be due to rheumatic valve disease, but it has numerous other causes and corresponding morphologic patterns.

Rheumatic Mitral Incompetence
Mitral incompetence can occur as a severe lesion (sometimes combined with aortic incompetence) during the acute rheumatic process in association with an extensive myocarditis and sometimes pericarditis and pancarditis. Annular dilatation is the primary cause of the incompetence, with the valve leaflets frequently showing edema only and virtually normal chordae. Following remission of the acute process, the incompetence may spontaneously regress, presumably because the myocarditis heals, the heart becomes smaller, and the annular dilation regresses. In most cases, however, there is progressive leaflet thickening, particularly of the posterior cusp, which becomes retracted and rolled with shortening of chordae. The anterior leaflet is less thickened, and the major chordae are frequently elongated, allowing leaflet prolapse. The posterior chordae may also elongate, and occasionally one or more may rupture. The commissural leaflets are obliterated and fused, but the commissures remain more or less open. Calcification is uncommon. Annular dilatation is almost invariable and progressive, and produces increasing incompetence.

Mitral Valve Prolapse
Prolapse of a mitral valve leaflet, occurring as an isolated abnormality (Barlow's syndrome,[B5] floppy valve, or myxomatous valve degeneration) is a relatively common and complex entity, well described elsewhere,[B6,D8,J1] which relatively uncommonly in its severe form results in important mitral incompetence (10% of cases[M6]). Nonetheless, in the United States at least, mitral valve prolapse has been reported to be the commonest cause of surgically treated isolated mitral valve incompetence.[R15] The basic pathologic condition is mitral leaflet redundancy and myxomatous leaflet thickening, resulting at least in part from acid mucopolysaccharide replacement of the collagen of the leaflets. The redundant and elongated leaflets no longer meet properly so as to support each other during systole, and they begin to overshoot into the left atrium during systole. Not only is the valve thereby rendered incompetent, but abnormal strain is placed on the chordae. They elongate, and ultimately many of them rupture, producing more incompetence. Calcifications may occur in the mitral anulus in this setting but do not appear to contribute to the mitral valve dysfunction.[B34]

Idiopathic and more or less localized chordal rupture is usually a variant of the mitral valve prolapse syndrome, in which a considerable portion of the leaflet tissue is uninvolved by the myxomatous process. Usually, the posteromedial portion of the posterior leaflet is involved, and after chordal rupture this becomes redundant and flail. More extensive posterior chordal ruptures sometimes occur. Localized chordal rupture can also occur in patients with Marfan's syndrome.

Ischemic Papillary Muscle Dysfunction, or Rupture
Papillary muscle dysfunction or rupture, from myocardial infarction or ischemic fibrosis, can produce severe mitral incompetence. This is the subject of Chapter 10.

Infective Endocarditis
Endocarditis is a relatively uncommon cause of pure mitral incompetence compared to its etiologic frequency in aortic incompetence. When the aortic valve is infected and incompetent, vegetations may drop down onto and infect the central portion of the anterior mitral leaflet, producing perforation and mitral incompetence. In the absence of aortic valve disease, a normal or abnormal mitral valve may become infected,[B4] with destruction of cusps or chordae or both.

Mitral Annular Calcification

Mitral annular calcification frequently occurs in older patients without evident disease of the leaflets or chordae. In such situations, it is usually associated with calcific deposits in the aortic valve cusps and in the coronary arteries.[R15] It is probably a manifestation of atherosclerosis.

Secondary, or Functional, Tricuspid Incompetence

When tricuspid incompetence develops purely as a consequence of important disease on the left side of the heart or of pulmonary arterial hypertension, the anulus dilates, but the leaflets and chordae remain delicate and normal in appearance. The septal leaflet portion of the anulus lengthens very little, as it is fixed between the right and left trigones and the atrial and ventricular septa. The remaining two-thirds of the anulus lengthens greatly, particularly that part giving origin to the posterior leaflet.[C10]

Rheumatic Tricuspid Stenosis and Incompetence

Surgically significant rheumatic tricuspid valve disease does not occur alone but in association with mitral valve disease and sometimes aortic valve disease. Usually rheumatic tricuspid disease results in an incompetent valve with variable amounts of stenosis. Rarely there may be virtually pure stenosis. The orifice size is larger than that in mitral stenosis, even when hemodynamically there is severe obstruction to flow, for the vis a tergo of blood reaching the right atrium is less than that of blood reaching the left atrium, and therefore the hemodynamic effects of moderate tricuspid stenosis are the equivalent of tight mitral stenosis.

Usually all commissures are equally fused, with diffuse but moderate leaflet thickening, particularly around the stenotic orifice. Chordal thickening and agglutination is mild, and calcification absent. In dominant rheumatic tricuspid incompetence, the leaflet changes are less marked, often with minimal peripheral commissural fusion, particularly of the anteroseptal commissure. There may be elongation of the chordae to the anterior leaflet, and annular dilatation is commonly present.

CLINICAL FEATURES AND DIAGNOSTIC CRITERIA

Mitral Stenosis

In most patients, mitral stenosis can be diagnosed clinically on the basis of the history, physical examination, chest x-ray, and electrocardiogram. The *auscultatory findings* are particularly secure evidence of mitral stenosis when they include a loud first sound, an opening snap, and the characteristic diastolic rumble with a presystolic crescendo when sinus rhythm is present. In severe stenosis, the mid-diastolic murmur occupies more than half of diastole, and the opening snap is early.

In patients being considered for operation because of important mitral stenosis, the *chest x-ray* nearly always shows some left atrial enlargement, although it is often only about grade 2 (on the basis of 1–6, 6 being the most severe). The left atrial appendage may or may not appear prominent along the left upper border of the cardiac silhouette. The left ventricle is normal in size, but the right ventricle and pulmonary artery are usually somewhat enlarged. When pulmonary vascular resistance is elevated, the main pulmonary artery segments and hilar arteries are more enlarged, and once tricuspid incompetence occurs, there is considerable right atrial and right ventricular enlargement. The lung fields also show varying degrees of pulmonary venous hypertension on the plain chest roentgenogram (large pulmonary veins in upper lung fields, interstitial pulmonary edema, Kerley B lines, or alveolar pulmonary edema).

The *electrocardiogram* is of course not diagnostic but often shows P-wave abnormalities characteristic of left atrial enlargement (P mitrale) or atrial fibrillation, and evidence of right ventricular hypertrophy when pulmonary hypertension is present.

M-mode echocardiography can usually identify mitral stenosis and leaflet thickening but does not allow a reliable estimate of its severity. Two-dimensional echocardiography, on the other hand, demonstrates the degree of stenosis and leaflet mobility and thickening. The echocardiographic observations, along with the findings described above, are usu-ally sufficient to make a secure diagnosis in doubtful cases, and cardiac catheterization is unnecessary.

Cardiac catheterization is usually necessary when a diastolic murmur is not audible or is unduly short, which can occur when there is a low cardiac output or in obese patients. The pulmonary capillary wedge pressure is measured to determine the severity of the pulmonary venous hypertension, and the gradient between the capillary wedge pressure (which is similar to left atrial pressure) is compared to the directly measured left ventricular diastolic pressure. A resting end-diastolic gradient of 10 mmHg or more indicates important mitral stenosis. Exercise studies are helpful in borderline cases, and if the pulmonary artery wedge pressure measurement is in doubt, a direct left atrial pressure is obtained by transseptal puncture. The mitral valve area is calculated from Gorlin's modified orifice equation.[C2] Most symptomatic patients have a mitral valve area of 0.5–0.8 $cm^2 \cdot m^{-2}$, but occasionally the calculated area in patients whose symptoms are from mitral stenosis is as large as 1 $cm^2 \cdot m^{-2}$. Coronary arteriography, and thus catheterization, is indicated in patients over about 40 years of age.

In summary, these findings, combined with a reliable history of increasing dyspnea, orthopnea, and paroxysmal nocturnal dyspnea, make tight mitral stenosis highly likely. Hemoptysis may occur.

The patient with far-advanced mitral stenosis, with low cardiac output and chronic congestive heart failure secondary to a high pulmonary vascular resistance, is seldom seen today. Usually such a patient is a woman, with marked mitral facies, peripheral coldness, cyanosis, hepatic enlargement and pulsation, a high jugular venous pressure with waves of tricuspid incompetence, and sometimes ascites and peripheral edema.

In a patient coming to surgery for mitral stenosis, the possibility of left atrial myxoma must always be considered. Since mitral commissurotomy is now routinely done by open techniques, special studies directed at this possibility are not necessary as a routine. Echocardiography (M mode and two dimensional) can detect a left atrial myxoma[N1] and is the type of screening performed when further information as to this possibility is needed. (See Chapter 50, Section 1, "Cardiac Myxomas.")

Mitral Incompetence

As is the case with mitral stenosis, important mitral incompetence can usually be diagnosed on the basis of the history, physical examination, chest x-ray, and electrocardiogram. The classical *apical systolic murmur* of mitral incompetence is pansystolic and loudest at the apex and radiates to the left axilla and left lung base. However, when the incompetence is the result primarily of prolapse of the posterior leaflet, the regurgitant jet is directed toward the roof (superior aspect) of the left atrium and is transmitted to the aortic root. Therefore, the murmur is maximal in the aortic area parasternally and may radiate into the carotid arteries. As a result of the large and rapid mitral valve flow during diastole, a left ventricular filling sound (S_3) and a diastolic rumble often exist. Two important signs of the severity of the stenosis are the presence of an overactive left ventricular impulse at the apex (from left ventricular enlargement) and of a precordial lift, the latter the result of systolic pulsation in the enlarged left atrium.

In severe chronic mitral incompetence, the *chest x-ray* is usually highly characteristic. The left atrium is in general more markedly enlarged than in patients with mitral stenosis, and the left atrial appendage is usually prominent. The left ventricle may be enlarged, and there may be varying degrees of right atrial enlargement, depending on the amount of associated tricuspid incompetence.

The *electrocardiogram* may remain normal even in the presence of severe mitral incompetence. However, a pattern of left ventricular hypertrophy is common.

Echocardiography can show leaflet prolapse, and color and doppler echocardiography are becoming useful in assessing the presence and magnitude of incompetence.

Left *ventriculography* demonstrates the regurgitant process at the mitral valve and can show leaflet prolapse, although not always its exact site. The degree of incompetence can usually be estimated with reasonable accuracy, although if left atrial or left ventricular enlargement is severe, the estimate is less valid. Fairly accurate calculations of regurgitant flow can be made from measurements of left ventricular stroke volume by quantitative left ventriculography and of forward flow by some measurement of cardiac output.[R12]

In *acute mitral incompetence*, the presentation is different. The left atrium and left ventricle are normal in size or only slightly enlarged. The chest x-ray is dominated by signs of pulmonary venous hypertension, and the left atrial pressure is high, as is the V wave.

NATURAL HISTORY

Mitral Stenosis

Rheumatic mitral stenosis develops relatively slowly after the initial rheumatic involvement of the valve. In New England, the average age of the initial attack of rheumatic fever has been 12 years, the average age of onset of clinical signs of mitral stenosis 20 years, and the onset of symptoms 31 years.[B3] Progression of the valvular fibrosis and calcification is related in part to repeated episodes of rheumatic fever, but mechanical trauma and deposition of platelets and other blood substances resulting from the stenosis-induced alterations of flow patterns also play a role.[S3] It is this progression that ultimately leads to increasing symptoms, although in the final stages, left ventricular function may also deteriorate.

Once symptoms develop after the so-called latent period, their progression to a state of total disability (NYHA class IV) has been estimated to take another 7–10 years[R2,W2] (Fig. 11-1). The average age of death of patients with surgically untreated mitral stenosis has been estimated variously to be between 40 and 50 years.[R1,R2]

This general pattern of evolution is considerably shorter in some parts of the world and in some races. Thus, a markedly accelerated evolution of signs, symptoms, and disability has been experienced by Polynesians in New Zealand, blacks in south central Alabama, Eskimos in Alaska, and Asians. Many reports suggest that, in addition to possible genetic

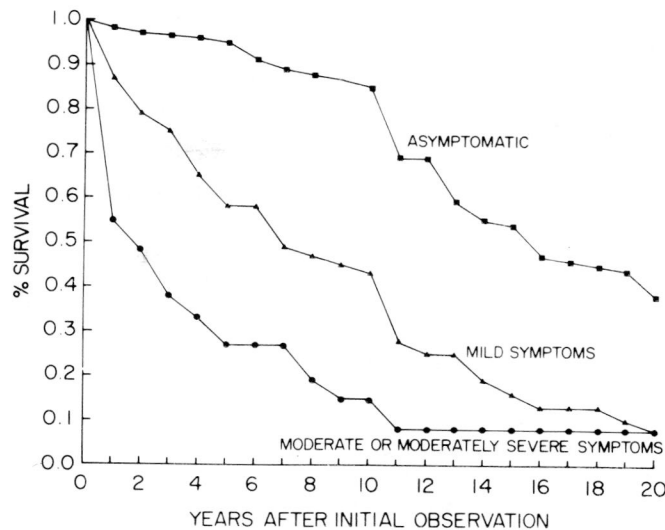

Figure 11-1 The survival of patients with nonsurgically treated mitral stenosis, according to their symptomatic status at the time of initial observation.
Modified from data of Rowe et al.[R1]

factors affecting these time variables, economic underdevelopment may also play a role.[A4,A5,B25,C8,M7,R10]

Certain other events, or complications, tend to occur during the lifetime of surgically untreated mitral stenosis that in turn may alter the natural history of the disease. Atrial fibrillation usually develops eventually. It often occurs first in paroxysmal form. The first paroxysm may initiate symptoms because the patient with mitral stenosis is particularly sensitive to the loss of the atrial contribution to ventricular filling and to shortening of the ventricular filling time such as occurs in the tachycardia of atrial fibrillation. Although originally incited by left atrial hypertension and hypertrophy, atrial fibrillation eventually becomes fixed and intractable because of disintegration of the architecture of atrial muscle.[B26] Because atrial fibrillation reduces cardiac output and elevates left atrial pressure, it accelerates the devolutionary course of patients with mitral stenosis. Both because of this and because the appearance of atrial fibrillation indicates in general a relatively advanced stage of the disease, atrial fibrillation is an incremental risk factor for premature death of these patients. Olesen found that as a group, their 10-year and 20-year survival rates were 25% and 10%, respectively, whereas in patients in sinus rhythm at initial observation, the rates were 46% and 29%.[O1]

As the disease state progresses, there develops in many patients a reduced systolic function generally due to an increased afterload. Left ventricular muscle function, however, has generally been found to be normal.[G6]

Systemic arterial emboli, the majority of which go to the brain, can suddenly complicate or terminate the life of patients with mitral stenosis. Most of these originate in the left atrial appendage or left atrium, and yet no residual thrombus may be left in the heart after embolization. Also, some patients with large left atrial thrombi never have had demonstrable embolization. Left atrial thrombosis and embolization are much more common when atrial fibrillation is present but are not unknown in patients in sinus rhythm. It has been estimated that at least 10% of surgically untreated patients suffer arterial embolization during their lifetime, and the occurrence of a massive cerebral embolus may suddenly terminate the life of a previously mildly symptomatic patient.[S3]

Infectious endocarditis is unusual in patients with mitral stenosis.[R1]

Massive pulmonary hemorrhage may very occasionally develop in patients otherwise mildly symptomatic from mitral stenosis. That it is indeed related to the presence of mitral stenosis is strongly suggested by its prompt and long-standing remission after surgical relief of the stenosis.[R11]

In fact, all the foregoing is really *not* the natural (i.e., untreated) history of mitral stenosis. It is rather the spectrum of mitral stenosis in *surgically untreated* patients receiving the medical treatment that was available in the mid portion of the twentieth century. The end stage of the disease in many of these patients was characterized by cardiac cachexia, a state uncommonly seen before diuretic therapy became available. The true natural history of mitral stenosis in the first 25 years of the twentieth century must have been very different from that portrayed here, with the interval between onset of symptoms and death very much shorter and the patterns of death different.

Likewise, evolution of the rheumatic disease complex is different in patients whose mitral stenosis has been treated surgically than in those treated medically. The course of the disease varies because the increased length of life imparted by the operation (see "Late Results") allows a considerably greater proportion of patients with mitral stenosis to develop hemodynamically significant rheumatic aortic valve disease and important tricuspid incompetence (Fig. 11-2).

Mitral Incompetence

The natural history of mitral incompetence is difficult to define because (1) the etiology is variable, (2) the age at onset is variable, (3) mitral incompetence may be mild and non-progressive for many years, and (4) left ventricular function, an important determinant of symptoms and survival, deteriorates at a variable rate.

Rheumatic Mitral Incompetence

Surgically untreated but hemodynamically important rheumatic mitral incompetence seems to have a survival curve surprisingly similar to that of mitral stenosis,[M2,R2] and this curve is different in different environmental and genetic situations, as it is in mitral stenosis. In San Francisco, the survival of such patients 5 years after initial evaluation was 80%, and 10-year survival 60%; in Venezuela, 5-year survival of such patients was only 46%.[M1] As in mitral stenosis, most patients develop symptoms in adult life, but in the same geographical areas where severe mitral stenosis appears in the young, accelerated forms of rheumatic mitral regurgitation also occur, with severe symptoms by the age of 10 years.[S4]

Mitral Valve Prolapse

Mitral incompetence from mitral valve prolapse (variously termed *myxomatous mitral valve degeneration, floppy valves, the symptom-complex of mid-systolic click and late systolic murmur,* and *Barlow's syndrome*) has a complex natural history which entails more than simply leakage at the mitral valve. Serious and rarely fatal arrhythmias may occur in patients with only mild leakage,[P3] and psychiatric disturbances may occur. In such patients, other symptoms may be

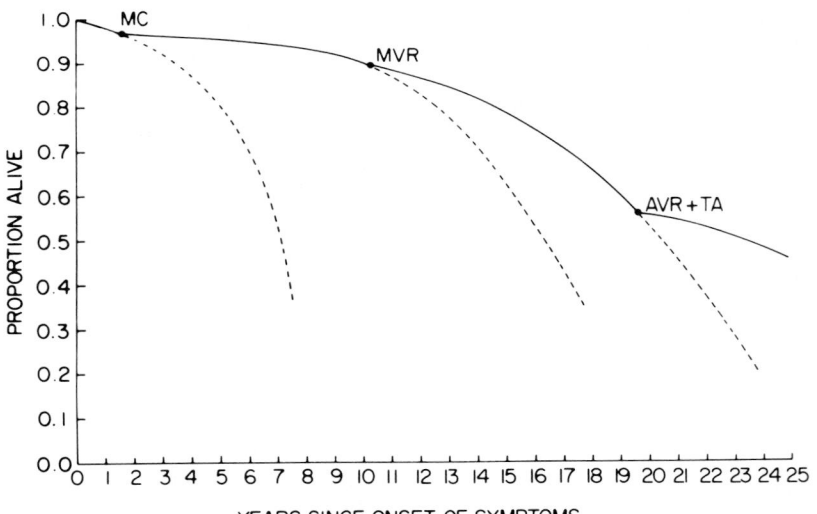

Figure 11-2 Schematic representation of the subsequent life history after the initial development of symptoms of a large group of patients with mitral stenosis. The solid circles indicate a surgical procedure. The dashed lines represent estimated survival of patients not receiving the surgical procedure.

AVR, aortic valve replacement; MC, mitral commissurotomy; MRV, mitral valve replacement; TA, tricuspid annuloplasty.

present that mimic thyrotoxicosis, hyperadrenergic states, or hypoglycemia,[B14,B15,C3,F2] and the patients often have higher than normal catecholamine levels and other evidences of high adrenergic tone.[B14] All this is further complicated by the fact that patients with hyperthyroidism have a higher than usual incidence of mitral prolapse.[C12] However, once important mitral incompetence appears, it tends to progress just as it does in patients with rheumatic mitral incompetence. Presumably, as prolapse worsens, the support in systole provided by the closing of the two leaflets against each other (the stacked rifle effect) is lost. This puts an abnormally large load on the chordae, which elongate, thin, and eventually rupture. This process worsens the incompetence and accelerates the natural history of the disease.

Ruptured Chordae Tendinae

Patients with mitral incompetence and ruptured chordae tendinae may have an insidious, slow development of symptoms. In such patients, ruptured chordae of the anterior or posterior leaflet or both are often found at operation, and the mitral valve leaflets have the appearance of myxomatous degeneration referred to previously. This particular group of patients probably represents a subgroup of individuals with mitral valve prolapse. In fact, ruptured chordae may be present in patients with mitral valve prolapse without any important symptoms. Thus, Grenadier and colleagues found 8% of 134 patients with mitral valve prolapse to have ruptured chordae and few or no symptoms.[G5]

In contrast, mitral incompetence produced acutely by chordal rupture, in patients previously without symptoms or incompetence, presents differently. It appears predominately in middle-aged males.[S4] Often it is a complication in the life history of patients with mid-systolic clicks but without previous evidence of mitral incompetence. The anterior mitral leaflet and its chordae are frequently entirely normal, and the disease process may be limited to the medial aspect of the posterior mitral leaflet. In this group of patients with acutely appearing and severe symptoms, presumably initiated by the sudden chordal rupture, the left atrium and left ventricle are small, the left atrial pressure is high and the V wave markedly accentuated, and clinical and radiologic evidence of pulmonary venous hypertension is marked. As time passes, these findings change. Moderate left ventricular and left atrial enlargement develop,[T2] and symptoms may lessen with appropriate medical management. The patient gradually regains a feeling of well-being. One year later, left atrial and left ventricular enlargement may not have progressed, and left ventricular and left atrial adaptation to the sudden volume overload seems to have occurred. Years may now pass before the self-aggravating tendency of mitral incompetence results in an increased mitral regurgitant volume. After this, the classic natural history of important mitral incompetence evolves.

In other patients with acutely appearing severe symptoms, the symptoms improve only mildly with intense medical treatment. In this group, although most patients survive, left ventricular and left atrial enlargement progress steadily in the months after onset. Such patients have a very large mitral regurgitant flow. When untreated surgically, these patients progress through the life history of severe mitral in-

competence more rapidly than do most individuals and are dead within 2–5 years. In a few of them, the symptoms and signs very rapidly worsen and require urgent surgical intervention.

Bacterial Endocarditis

Bacterial endocarditis on a mildly abnormal mitral valve may produce acute mitral incompetence. The natural history of that condition is similar to that described for acute chordal rupture, except that the early mortality is higher. Uncommonly, death is related to uncontrolled infection.

TECHNIQUE OF OPERATION

Mitral Commissurotomy

After the usual preparations and a median sternotomy incision, pericardial stay sutures are placed, and the left atrial catheter is inserted (UAB) (see Chapter 2). Chamber size is evaluated. By palpation posteriorly, against the back wall of the left arium, and then over the roof of the left atrium under the ascending aorta, a regurgitant mitral jet of incompetence is sought. Either during this exploratory phase or just before inserting the right atrial cannula, a palpating finger is inserted into the right atrium through the right atrial appendage to identify any tricuspid stenosis or incompetence that may be present.

The aortic cannula is inserted, venous cannulation is accomplished, with a single venous cannula (UAB) or bicaval cannulation (GLH), cardiopulmonary bypass (CPB) is established, and the perfusate temperature is made very cold (see Chapter 2 for details of these procedures). Left atrial venting may be omitted (UAB), or during the cooling phase, a vent (incorporating a pressure-monitoring line) may be inserted through the base of the right superior pulmonary vein and advanced only a centimeter or so in case clot is present in the atrium (GLH). A cardioplegic needle is placed in the ascending aorta (see Chapter 3). The aorta is cross-clamped, the cold cardioplegic solution is injected, and the perfusate temperature is stabilized at 25°C. The left atrium is opened vertically from the right side. This may be done after developing the interatrial groove in instances of minimal left atrial enlargement (GLH), or the incision may be started very medially on the right superior pulmonary vein without dissecting the groove (UAB). The incision is medial to the left atrial vent if one is used. Superiorly, the incision can be extended beneath the superior vena cava, after the right pulmonary artery is dissected away from the superior aspect of the left atrium; inferiorly, it may be extended by cutting behind the freed inferior vena caval junction with the right atrium. A Cooley left atrial retractor or a Deaver retractor is inserted. The tip of the previously inserted left atrial vent (GLH), or, alternatively, an intracardiac sump sucker placed through the incision (UAB), is positioned in the orifice of the left pulmonary vein to keep the operative field dry (Fig. 11-3). The mitral valve is examined to determine its suitability for commissurotomy, and a judgment is made as to whether, after the commissurotomy, the leaflets will be sufficiently pliable to open adequately at a low left atrial pressure.

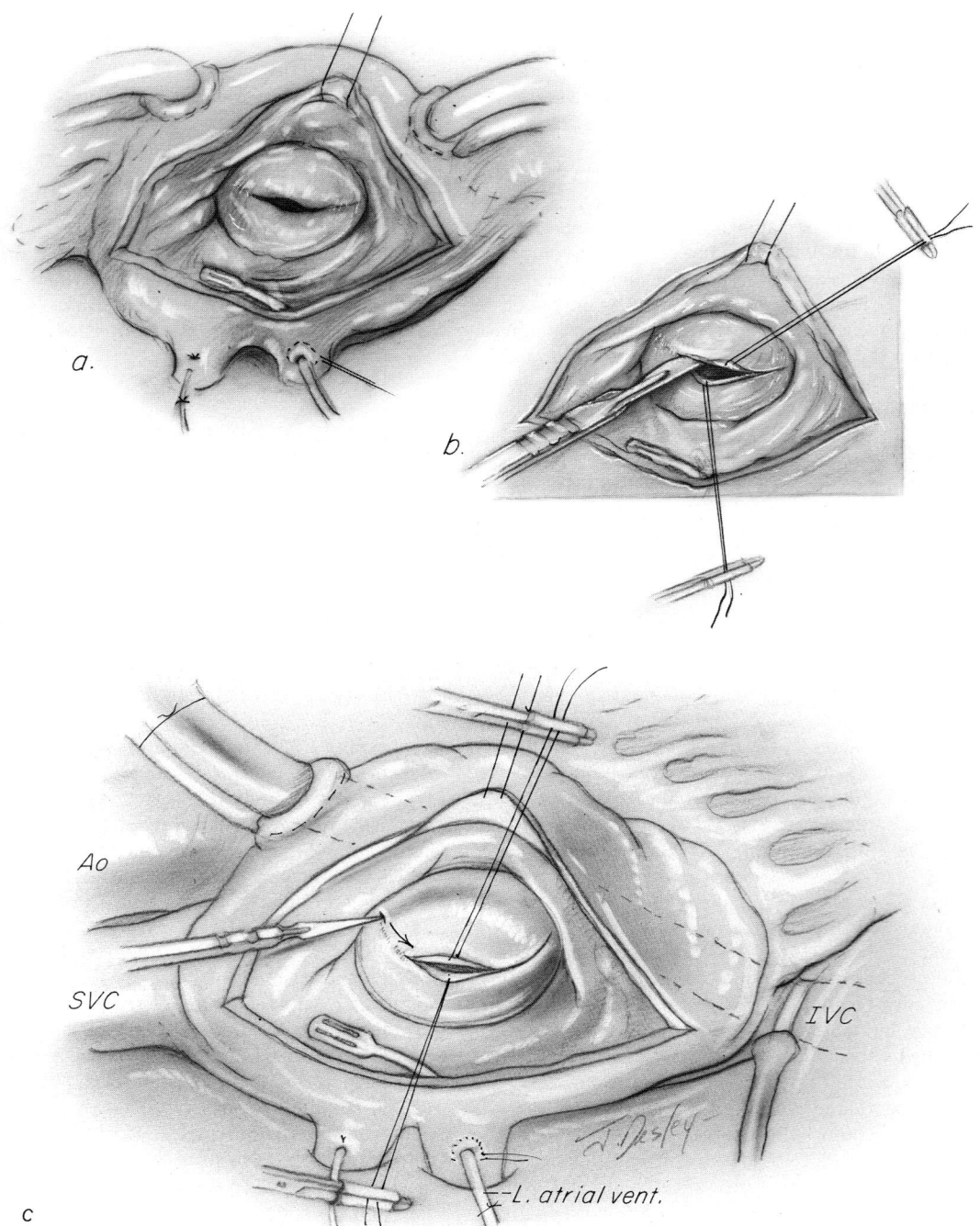

Figure 11-3

(a) The exposure for open mitral commissurotomy is with a median sternotomy incision and opening the left atrium from the right side, in front of the right pulmonary veins. The Cooley left atrial retractor is positioned (not shown).

(b) With traction on the stay sutures shown, the valve is well exposed for commissurotomy. With care, the anterolateral commissure is incised with the knife (GLH); the line to be incised is located by staying in the leaflet tissue overlying the *center* of the underlying nest of chordae to the anterolateral papillary muscle (see the text for details). Note that the correctly placed incision curves anteriorly. As the incision is made, the chordae beneath the commissure are visualized and used as a guide for keeping the incision in the leaflet tissue over the middle of the chordal network.[R14]

(c) Alternatively, the incision may be begun on the anulus, at the point indicated by the arrow, and carried centrally (see text) (UAB). After the commissurotomy is made, fused chordae are split downward toward the papillary muscle, and, when necessary, this splitting is carried into the papillary muscle itself. A similar procedure is carried out at the posteromedial commissure.

Ao, aorta; IVC, inferior vena cava; SVC, superior vena cava.

If commissurotomy is decided on, a fine stay suture may be placed in the mid portion of the free edge of the anterior leaflet and one placed similarly in the posterior leaflet (UAB). With retraction on these, the leaflets and their commissures are placed on some tension. With a sharp-pointed scalpel (no. 11 Bard-Parker blade), a stab incision is made in the fused anterolateral commissure, right at the anulus, as recommended by Carpentier (UAB). The incision is extended with the knife toward the valve orifice, in the groove of the commissural fusion. After the incision is 3–4 mm long, the fan of underlying chordae is well seen through the incision, making it easy to stay in the middle of the commissural tissue over the center of the fan.[R14] The incision is carried into the valve orifice. Alternatively, a blunt-ended, long-handled hook is placed beneath each leaflet, and by trial and error, these hooks are positioned exactly in the spot that provides the best exposure for division of each commissure (GLH). With the scalpel, an incision is made at the anterolateral commissure which begins at the orifice and is extended toward the anulus. The surgeon takes care to follow the true line of commissure, which extends more anteriorly than might be thought (Fig. 11-3). With either method, when fused chordae are present beneath the commissure, they can usually be separated with the knife or scissors (Fig. 11-3); and when appropriate, the incision is carried down into the center of the papillary muscle, dividing it into anterior and posterior halves.

The posteromedial commissure is usually less well defined and fused for a shorter distance than is the anterolateral commissure. By one of the techniques just described, this commissural leaflet tissue is incised. Chordae are often more importantly fused beneath this commissure and their separation by sharp dissection may be needed, together with longitudinal division of the papillary muscle.

A firm plastic catheter with multiple side holes (a 24 Fr chest drainage tube is ideal) is now placed through the valve into the left ventricle and tied to the left atrial vent snare to hold it in position (GLH). This acts to frustrate the valve, and the side holes lying in left atrium are an additional safeguard to prevent ejection by the left ventricle into the aorta until de-airing is complete. The left atrium is closed with a continuous 000 polypropylene suture but with the loops left loose where the frustrator exits through the left atrial incision. The left atrial vent is turned off during this procedure to allow the left heart to fill with blood. If return to the left atrium is inadequate, right atrial pressure is raised by returning blood to the patient. The left ventricular apex is needled for air without dislocating the heart (using a large needle and 20-ml syringe). With the patient head down, the aortic cross-clamp is released while suction is applied to the aortic vent needle. The heart is defibrillated and the ventricle allowed to eject into the left atrium and pericardium until all air is clearly excluded. The frustrator is then removed and the left atrial suture pulled tight and tied. The frustrator is particularly valuable when there is any aortic incompetence, as it allows the ventricle to return to a strong beat without any risk of overdistention.

Alternatively, after the commissurotomy is completed, the left atrium is completely closed before the aortic cross-clamp is released; the sump sucker is removed and the left atrium

filled with saline solution just before the suture line is completed (UAB). The closure with 3-0 polypropylene suture is started at the superior angle, carried partway down, and held. With another suture, the closure is begun at the inferior angle and carried superiorly until the other suture is reached. The closure must be done precisely, as it is difficult to see the angles later. The venous line is momentarily clamped, and, while the lungs are compressed, a 13-gauge needle is inserted into the gently elevated apex of the left ventricle to remove any air. Suction is placed on the needle vent in the ascending aorta, the aortic clamp is released, and rewarming is begun. The left ventricle is carefully observed for any distention, and if distention occurs, a 13-gauge needle is inserted into the right ventricle and across the septum into left ventricle. After a good cardiac action has returned, the usual further de-airing procedures are followed (see Chapter 2).

As rewarming progresses, two right atrial and one right ventricular myocardial wires are placed. Before decannulation, palpation over the left atrium should have given no evidence of more than trivial mitral incompetence. After CPB is discontinued, the right (and at GLH also the left) atrial polyvinyl catheter is inserted, or, if preferred, a catheter can be brought out from the pulmonary artery by way of the right ventricle.

Mitral Incompetence Repair

The most difficult part of the repair of mitral incompetence is the determination of whether repair will provide an acceptable result. The circumstance under which repair can be most confidently performed is that of ruptured chordae to a limited portion of the posterior leaflet with an essentially normal anterior leaflet. The next is rheumatic mitral incompetence in childhood, when frequently distortion of the valve is insufficient to require valve replacement. The third is rheumatic, noncalcific, nearly pure mitral incompetence in the adult. Rarely, incompetence due to bacterial endocarditis, with resultant chordal rupture or a perforated cusp, lends itself to repair.[B32] An approach to the repair of mitral incompetence which is more enthusiastic than that (UAB and GLH) just described has been presented by Carpentier.[C9]

When the cause of the incompetence is *ruptured chordae to the posteromedial portion of the posterior leaflet*, the mitral valve is exposed as described for mitral commissurotomy. A rectangular excision is made of this area of posterior leaflet and its ruptured chordae (Fig. 11-4).[C4] After suture reconstruction of this area, the Carpentier mitral anuloplasty ring of proper size is selected and sewn into place (Fig. 11-4), either routinely (UAB) or only if the anulus is dilated (GLH).

When repair, rather than replacement, is done for *rheumatic mitral incompetence in adults*, annuloplasty has been the technique employed in most cases. Generally, the Carpentier technique including the ring has been used for annuloplasty (Fig. 11-4*d*). When annuloplasty is necessary in young children with years of growth ahead, the annuloplasty ring is not employed. Instead, a so-called asymmetric measured annuloplasty is done by the technique described by Reed and colleagues[R4] (Fig. 11-5). This operation, like most repairs of mitral incompetence, is based on the fact that the central portion of the anterior leaflet of the mitral valve is usually pliable and of good quality. This area, indicated by the *x* in Figure 11-5*c*, forms the line of closure of the repaired valve, both in the Reed repair and after insertion of the Carpentier ring. When more extensive revisions of the valve have been needed, valve replacement has been done. Carpentier describes and uses techniques for the shortening of chordae and the reimplantation of partially ruptured papillary muscles.[C4] These techniques have been used to only a limited extent at GLH and UAB.

The determination of the competence of the repaired valve while the left atrium is still open is an imprecise matter. After use of many different methods, including saline injection under pressure into the left ventricle, and Yacoub's maneuver[Y1] of perfusion of warm blood into the aortic root proximal to the cross-clamp through the cardioplegic needle so that the function of the repaired valve can be inspected with the heart beating, the conclusion has been reached that careful examination of the valve leaflets after the repair and an evaluation of their opposing surfaces is the most reliable method (GLH, UAB). If all this is satisfactory, the heart is closed and de-aired, and CPB is discontinued. If careful palpation over the posterior and superior aspects of the left

atrium reveals no mitral regurgitation and the hemodynamic state is good, probably important residual mitral incompetence is not present. If this is the case, CPB can be resumed to complete rewarming. Otherwise, after CPB is resumed, the mitral valve is replaced.

Mitral Valve Replacement

Procedure
Mitral valve replacement begins with exposure of the mitral valve as described for mitral commissurotomy using one or two valve hooks to display the leaflets. The incision is begun with the knife in the center of the anterior mitral leaflet approximately at the 12-o'clock position, about 2 mm from the anulus because at that point the leaflet tissue is nearly always pliable and easily accessible (Fig. 11-6). The incision is carried from this point leftward and rightward, either with the knife or scissors. When necessary, exposure can be improved by traction on a pledgetted mattress suture placed in the anulus with the pledget on the atrial side. The continuation of the incision through the anterolateral commissural tissue can be facilitated by first cutting the chordae underlying this commissure. The incision is then carried toward and through the posteromedial commissural tissue. The resec-

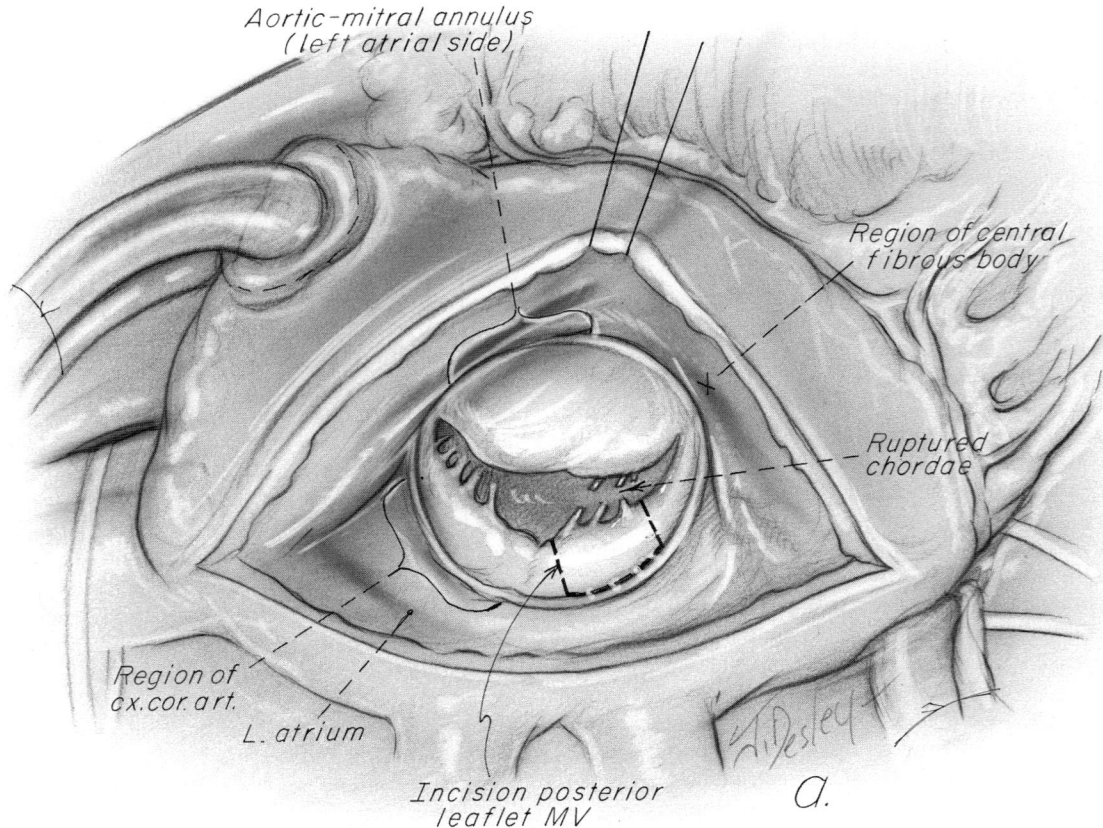

Figure 11-4 Repair of mitral incompetence from ruptured chordae to the posteromedial aspect of the posterior leaflet.
(a) After the pathologic condition of the valve is determined by careful study, the prolapsing portion is circumscribed by the placement of a 5-0 silk stitch at the free edge on each side of the flail portion and a similar pair at the anulus.

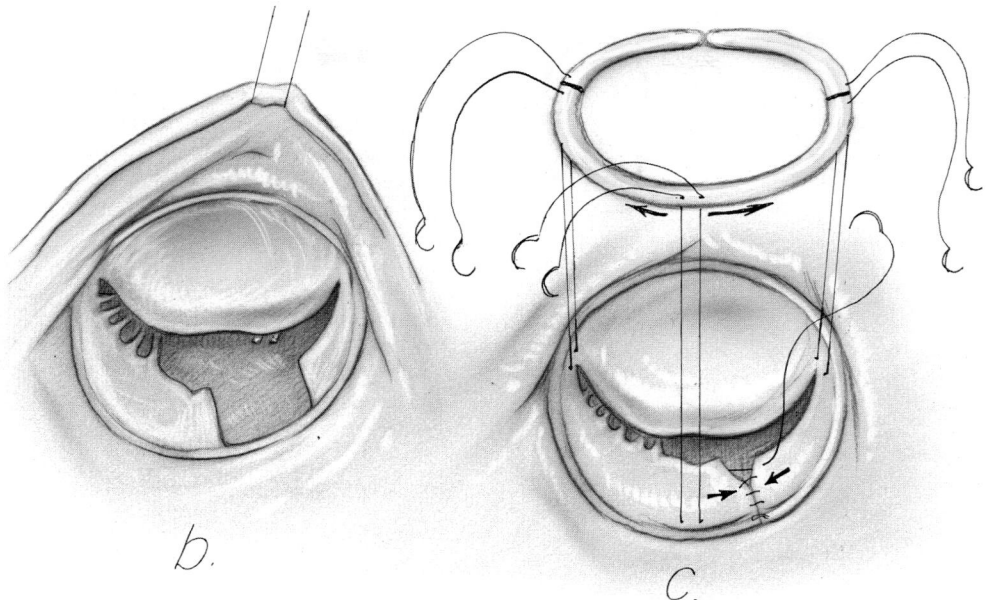

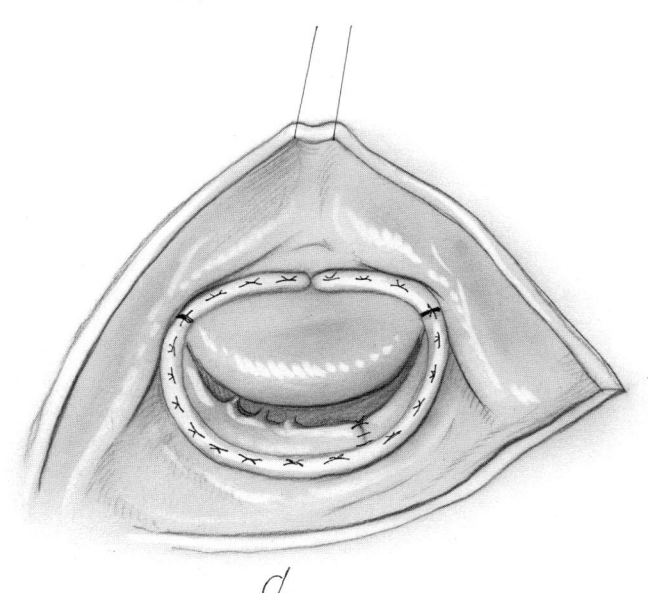

Figure 11-4 (*continued*)
(*b*) The rectangular segment of the prolapsing leaflet tissue is excised back to the anulus, with the lines of excision straight, *not* convex outward.
(*c*) A localized annuloplasty is made by the placement of a figure-of-eight stitch of a 2-0 Dacron polyester suture in the anulus so as to bring back together the base of the posterior leaflet tissue. The posterior leaflet is reconstructed with a continuous fine polypropylene suture or with fine, simple interrupted sutures. The Carpentier-Edwards flexible mitral annuloplasty ring is then inserted.
(1) The first step is the placement of two temporary stay sutures in the anulus, positioned precisely just anterior to each commissure. The ring sizer is then used to select the proper-sized ring (usually 32 mm). The sizer has two notches, corresponding to the two commissures, which are helpful in selecting the proper size. Also, the area of the sizer should be about that of the anterior leaflet.
(2) A double-arm mattress suture is placed at the base of each commissural leaflet and passed through the sewing ring in the marked point. A third mattress suture is placed at the very center of the base of the posterior leaflet and passed through the very center of the posterior half of the sewing ring. Similarly placed interrupted mattress sutures are placed, proceeding anteriorly from each commissural suture. Similarly, sutures are placed in the base of the posterior leaflet, proceeding in either direction from the centrally placed suture to plicate the posterior leaflet. The sewing ring is lowered into position, and the sutures are tied.
(*d*) The ring has been lowered into position and the sutures have been tied.

tion is facilitated by keeping the incisions through the commissural areas close to the anulus so that the anterior and posterior leaflets stay together. Again, the underlying chordae are cut just ahead of the incision to allow better exposure. The incision is carried now onto the posterior leaflet from either side. The secondary chordae tethering the posterior leaflet to the underlying ventricular myocardium are cut, and when subannular calcification is present and can be excised without disturbing the anulus or the myocardium, it is removed. Otherwise, it is left because too bold efforts to remove calcification may damage the circumflex coronary artery or precipitate postrepair ventricular rupture.

The prosthetic valve or bioprosthesis may be sewn into place with interrupted simple sutures of 00 silk (GLH) or, with a continuous suture of 0 of braided polyester fibers (Dacron) (UAB) (Fig. 11-6). A recent study indicates that both methods are associated with an extremely low incidence of periprosthetic leakage.[D2] The continuous technique is simple, economical in terms of time, and effective (see "Periprosthetic Leakage" in section on "Late Results"). The technique employing interrupted pledgetted mattress Dacron sutures with the pledgets on the atrial side is used occasionally (UAB). It may be chosen when heavy calcification remains in some areas of the anulus or when exposure is particularly difficult. With this technique, all the sutures are placed in the heart first and then passed through the valve sewing ring. The valve can then be lowered into position and the sutures tied.

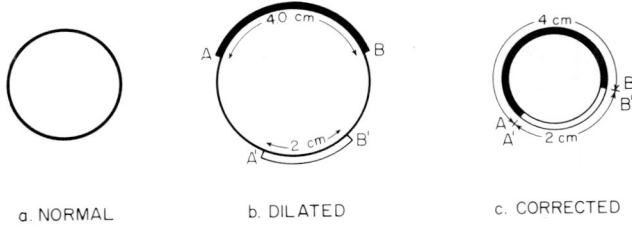

a. NORMAL   b. DILATED   c. CORRECTED

a

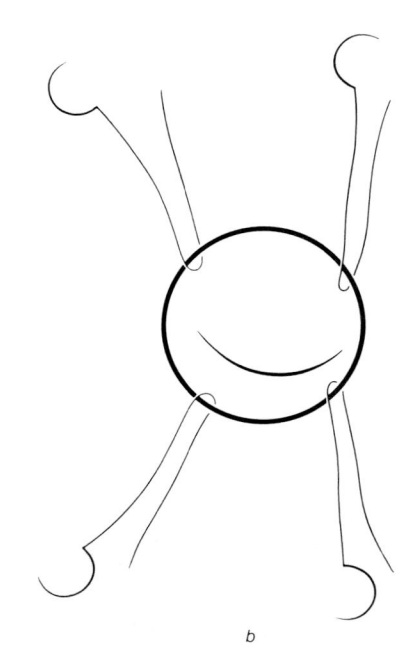

b

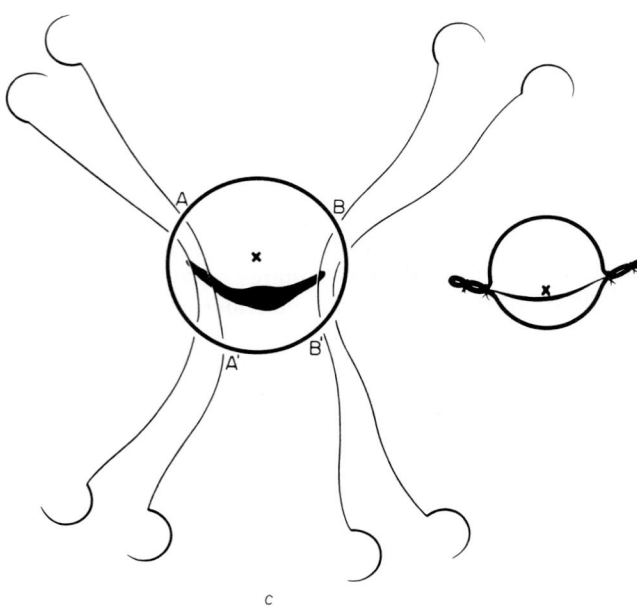

c

After completing valve insertion, a Foley catheter is passed through the valve into the left ventricle to act as a frustrator, and the balloon may be partially inflated (GLH). The steps for exiting from the left heart and de-airing are exactly as described for mitral stenosis. The Foley catheter is not deflated and withdrawn until the heart contraction is stable. Alternatively, after the valve is inserted, the left atrium is simply closed, and the remainder of the operation is conducted as under "Mitral Commissurotomy" (UAB).

The Device

A vital and difficult part of mitral valve replacement is selection of the appropriate replacement device. The considerations in doing this are summarized in "Choice of the Replacement Device" in the section on Special Situations and Controversies.

Tricuspid Annuloplasty

When evaluation before CPB indicates important tricuspid incompetence, two venous cannulae are used. The tricuspid procedure may be done during continuing cold cardioplegia with the addition of external cardiac cooling (UAB); or rewarming of the patient with the perfusate may be started, the aortic clamp released with suction on the aortic vent needle after the left heart has been carefully de-aired, and the tricuspid annuloplasty or replacement done in the beating, perfused heart (GLH).

After the mitral operation is completed, the right atrium is opened with the usual oblique incision (Fig. 11-7). The Carpentier tricuspid annuloplasty ring is nearly always employed.[C10] The annular length of the entire base of the tricuspid septal leaflet (or the area of the anterior leaflet) is measured with a sizer or calipers, and on the basis of this, the proper-sized ring is selected. The ring is a modified oval, corresponding with the configuration of the tricuspid anulus, with a gap in the portion designed to overlie the atrioventricular node and bundle so that the conducting tissue is not compromised. The ring corrects incompetence by returning

---

Figure 11-5 Reed's measured annuloplasty.

(*a*) According to Reed and colleagues,[R4] mitral annuloplasty in adults should leave an anular circumference of 6–7 cm in order that the resultant mitral orifice area be greater than 2.5 cm^2. The shortening of the circumference is accomplished along the posterior leaflet.

(*b*) The first step in the repair is placement of four marking sutures in the anulus about 1 cm anterior and posterior to each commissure. These provide reference points for measurements and facilitate placement of the annuloplasty sutures.

(*c*) After measuring, the annuloplasty sutures of heavy Dacron polyester are placed. The first stitch (A-A') is taken through the anulus at a point 8 mm anterior to the line of interception of the anterolateral commissure with the anulus. The suture is continued through the anulus posteriorly at a point (A') 1 cm anterior to the center of the posterior leaflet anulus. A second annuloplasty suture is placed between the suture A-A' and the anterolateral commissure. From A, a distance of 4 cm is measured along the anulus of the anterior leaflet to point B, where a third suture is placed. This suture then passes through the anulus of the posterior leaflet at B', 2 cm to the right of A'. A fourth suture is placed between B-B' and the posteromedial commissure. The stay sutures are removed, and the annuloplasty sutures are tied.

the anulus to slightly less than its original size by plicating that portion of the anulus at the base of the posterior (posteroinferior) leaflet and at the commissure between that and the anterior leaflet. Thus the ring effectively "bicuspidizes" the tricuspid valve. The sutures do not plicate the anulus at the attachment of the septal leaflet or over the major part of the attachment of the large anterior leaflet. It is unwise to select too small a ring in the belief that it will be more effective, since it distorts and narrows the orifice and may pull away subsequently. Because the tissues around the tricuspid valve are usually tenuous, the sutures must take adequate bites, beginning in the atrial wall and passing into the deeper part of the anulus itself, carefully avoiding leaflet tissue.

Interrupted mattress sutures of 00 silk or Dacron are used (GLH), placed first through host tissue and then through the cloth of the undersurface of the ring. The ring is not lowered into position until all sutures are in place. The first stitch is positioned exactly at the midpoint of the septal leaflet anulus, and only two further mattress stitches are needed for this septal portion of the ring. Five or six mattress stitches are needed in that portion of anulus to be plicated, and these are passed through the cloth of the Carpentier ring close together (marking stitches are present on the ring cloth to guide the surgeon). The remainder of the ring, corresponding to about half its circumference, is attached to the anulus at the base of the anterior cusp with at the most four fairly widely spaced mattress sutures. The ring is now lowered into

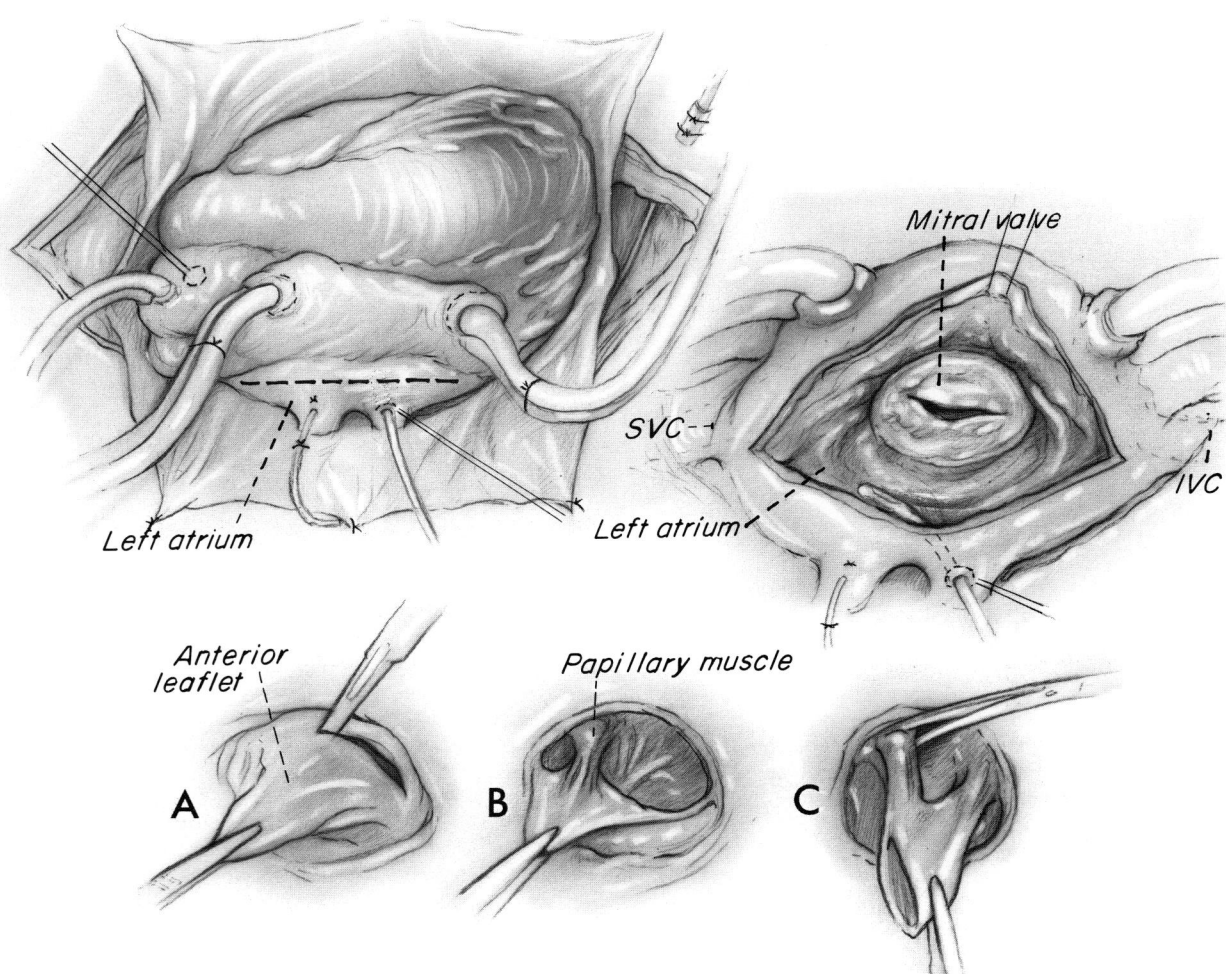

Figure 11-6 Mitral valve replacement, through a median sternotomy incision and opening into left atrium from the right side anterior to the right pulmonary veins (see legend of Fig. 11-3 for details). A Cooley left atriotomy retractor is used (not shown).
(a) As described in the text, the incision is begun with the knife anteriorly and about 2 mm from the anulus, where nearly always the leaflet is pliable and relatively free of disease.
(b) As the incision is carried leftward with the knife or scissors toward the anterolateral commissure, the underlying papillary muscle and fused chordae come into view and are cut.
(c) As the incision is carried across the anterolateral (illustrated here) and posteromedial commissural areas, the chordae are cut near the papillary muscle and care is taken to stay close to the anulus so that the valve is kept in one piece. This greatly facilitates the rest of the valve excision.

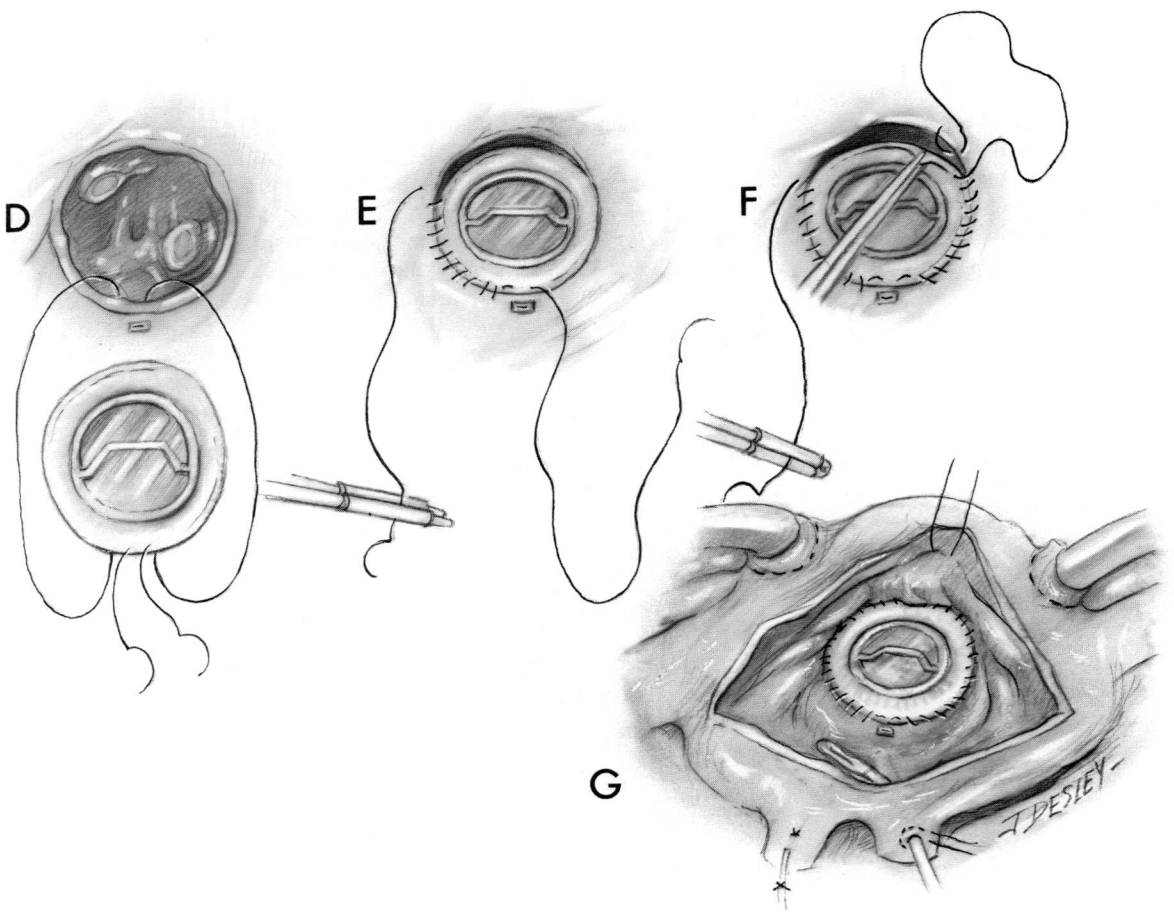

Figure 11-6 *(continued)*

(*d*) When a *continuous suture technique* with 0 Dacron polyester is chosen, it is begun as a pledgetted mattress suture at the 6-o'clock position.

(*e*) After the suture line is passed through the valve the valve is lowered into place and the suture line is carried up and to the left, passing the stitches through the prosthesis and then to anulus. The surgeon can roll the valve into the atrium for ease of placement of some of these stitches. The stitches should be securely but not too deeply placed, lest the underlying noncoronary and left coronary cusps of the aortic valve be damaged. When well past the region of the anterolateral commissure, the suture end is held.

(*f*) With the other end of the suture, the suture line is carried to the right and up, extending from anulus to valve. The sutures should be secure but, in the region formerly occupied by the posteromedial commissure, not be too deep lest the underlying AV node be damaged.

(*g*) The suture line is completed by the tying together of the two suture ends.

(*h*) When an *interrupted suture line technique is chosen* the first suture is placed at the anterolateral commissure at the 10-o'clock position. Each stitch (0 silk, GLH) is passed first through the sewing ring of the valve (the valve remains outside the chest, being held by the assistant with the aid of a valve holder) and then through the valve ring of the patient, with the needle held in reverse (backhand) fashion and passed from the left ventricular to the left atrial side. Each stitch passes just inside the host valve ring, and emerges through the adjacent portion of the atrial wall; care is taken that it not pass deep enough to damage the underlying circumflex coronary artery. Suturing continues in a counterclockwise direction around exactly half the circumference of the host valve ring (to the 4-o'clock position), as well as around half the circumference of the sewing ring of the prosthesis. When the sutures are placed between the 6-o'clock and 4-o'clock positions, the needle is best passed forehand. The two ends of each of these sutures are clipped together with a hemostat just after the suture is placed, the handle of the hemostat is threaded onto a large "safety pin" outside the chest, to prevent the sutures from becoming crossed when they are tied later. With all the posterior sutures in position, the safety pin is closed.

(*i*) The valve is now held by the assistant to the surgeon's left. Suturing recommences at the 10-o'clock position, with the stitches again passed first through the prosthetic valve ring and then through the host tissue from left ventricle to left atrium in a clockwise direction and with the needle reversed for the latter. Along the base of the left and noncoronary aortic leaflets (the region of the aortic mitral anulus) the stitches must not pass too deeply; in fact, only ring tissue is picked up at these points. Suturing continues to about the 1-o'clock position (and thus involves a further quarter of the circumference of host and prosthetic valve rings). The ends of the sutures are now gathered together with separate hemostats, as before.

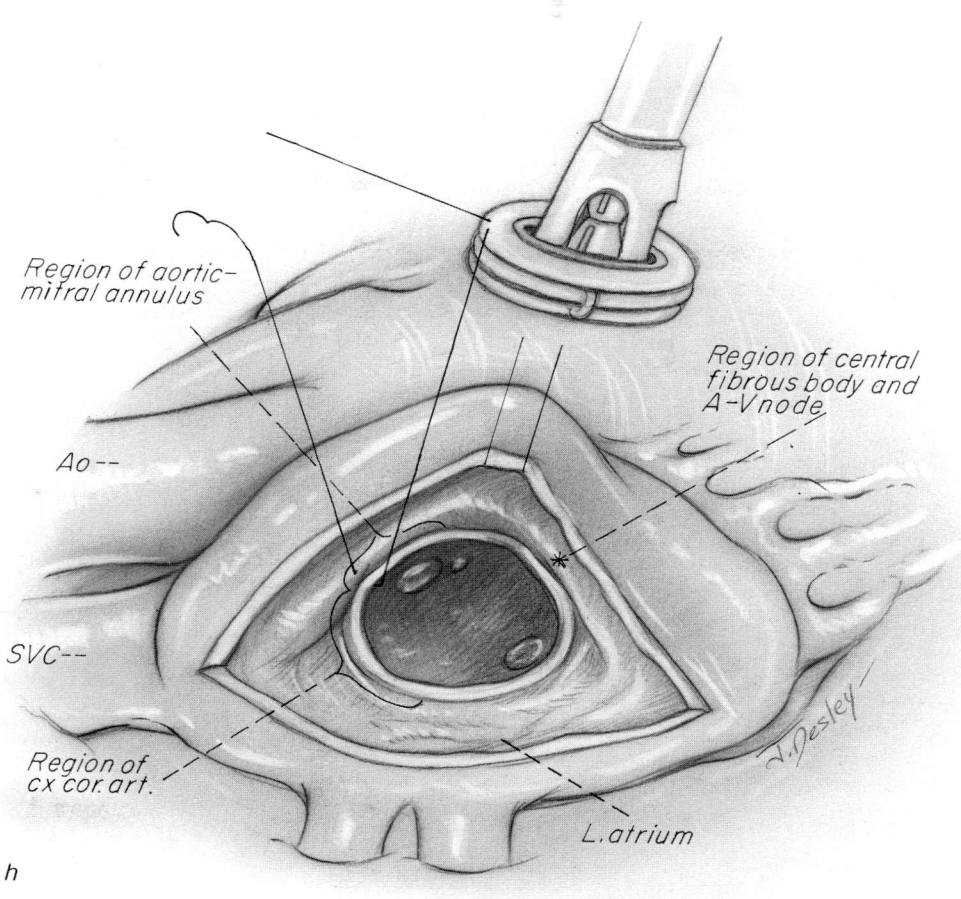

h

Region of aortic-
mitral annulus

Ao--

SVC--

Region of
cx cor. art.

Region of central
fibrous body and
A-V node

L. atrium

J. Desley

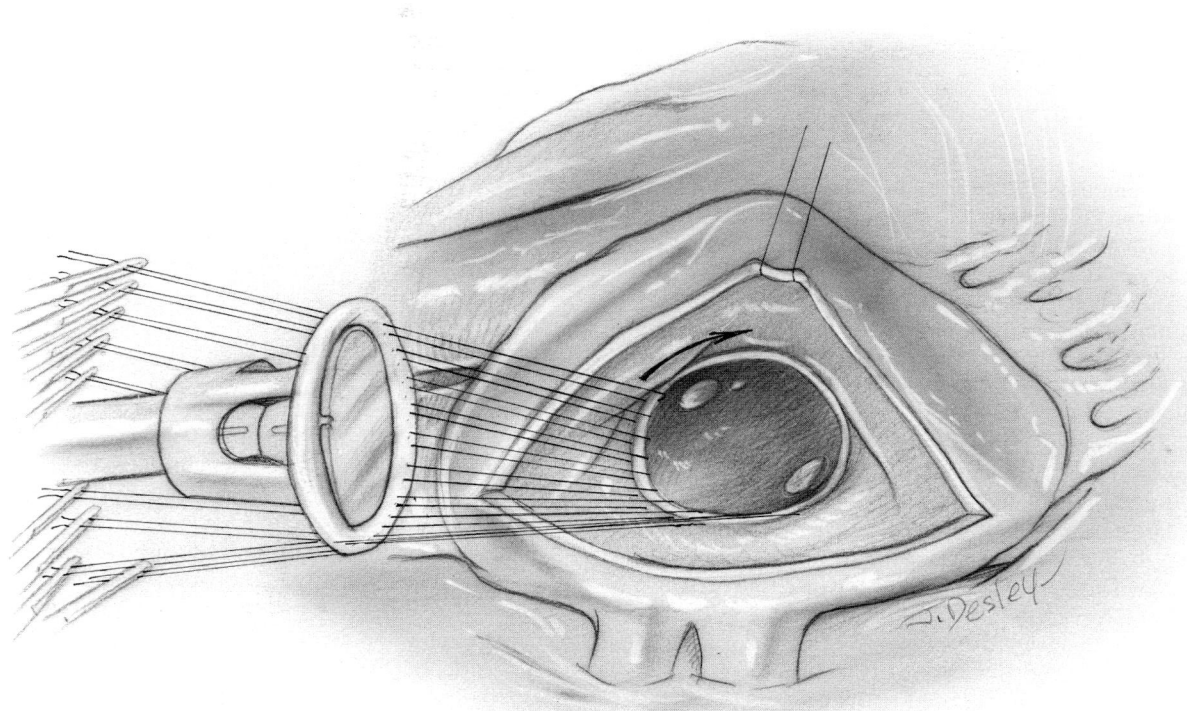

i

J. Desley

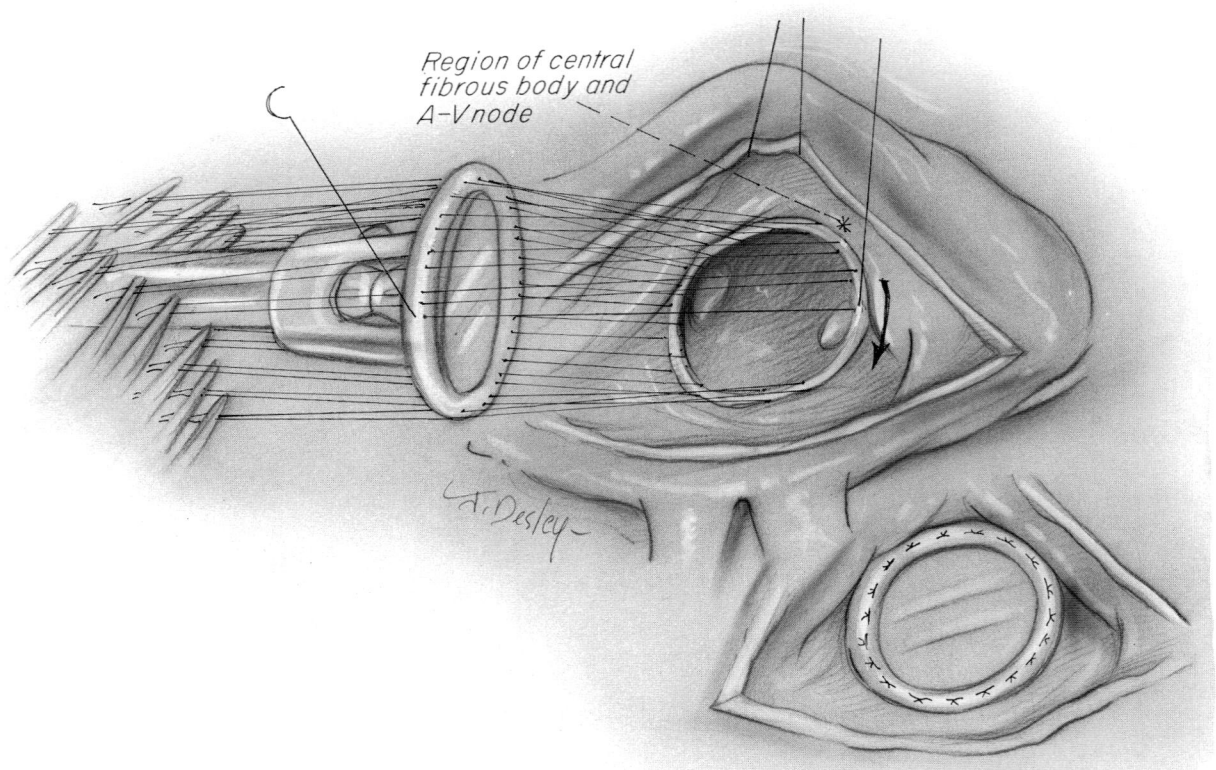

Region of central fibrous body and A-V node

Figure 11-6 *(continued)*

(*j*) Sutures in the final quarter of the circumference are placed first into the host ring tissue and from the left atrial to the left ventricular side with the needle reversed (backhand) and then into the valve sewing ring. They must not be placed too deeply at the site of the bundle of His (between the 2- and 3-o'clock positions). The suture ends are also clamped together with hemostats, to form a third group. Alternatively (UAB), the stitches are held by the assistant's hand as they are being inserted, and when half are in place, the ends emerging from the valve ring are gathered together in a clamp, and the other ends in a second clamp. This process is repeated after the second half of the sutures are placed. After the valve is lowered into position, the stitches are tied. This technique is illustrated in Chapter 12 for aortic valve replacement.

Ao, aorta; IVC, inferior vena cava; SVC, superior vena cava.

position along the sutures, with great care taken not to pull upward strongly on them lest they tear out.

Alternatively, three or four interrupted pledgetted mattress Dacron sutures may be placed along the inferior one-half of the septal leaflet anulus, inferior and anterior to the conduction tissue, and then through the annuloplasty ring (UAB). A 3-0 polypropylene suture is placed through the anulus just on the anterior leaflet side of the anteroseptal commissure and then through the other open end of the ring, and another similar suture is placed through the anulus just anterior to the posteroseptal commissure. A stay suture is placed through the anulus at the commissure between anterior and posterior leaflets and through the ring at the marker. The ring is lowered into place, the interrupted sutures are tied, the two polypropylene sutures are tied, and the valve is sewn in the rest of the way with continuous polypropylene sutures, beginning with the superior stitch (Fig. 11-7). As described above, most of the ring is attached to that part of the anulus occupied by the anterior leaflet, and the plication in the region of the posterior leaflet is accomplished by placing the stitches rather wide apart in the anulus and close together in the sewing ring.

With the sewing ring inserted, the right atrium is closed with continuous polypropylene sutures. Air is aspirated from the right ventricle and the pulmonary artery. The left heart is de-aired, and the operation is completed as described under "Mitral Commissurotomy."

Tricuspid Replacement

When tricuspid replacement is elected, the leaflets are excised, and a 2–3-mm fringe of leaflet tissue is left on the anulus. Interrupted pledgetted mattress sutures are placed in the anulus along the area occupied by the septal leaflet. Either a continuous polypropylene suture or interrupted pledgetted mattress sutures may be used for the remainder of the insertion (UAB). Alternatively, simple interrupted sutures of 0 silk may be used throughout (GLH) (for further details, see Chapter 27, "Tricuspid Valve Replacement and Atrial Septal Defect Repair" in section on Technique of Operation).

The device for tricuspid replacement is controversial, as is that for mitral replacement, and the data base for the selection less satisfactory (see Chapter 14, "Choice of Tricuspid

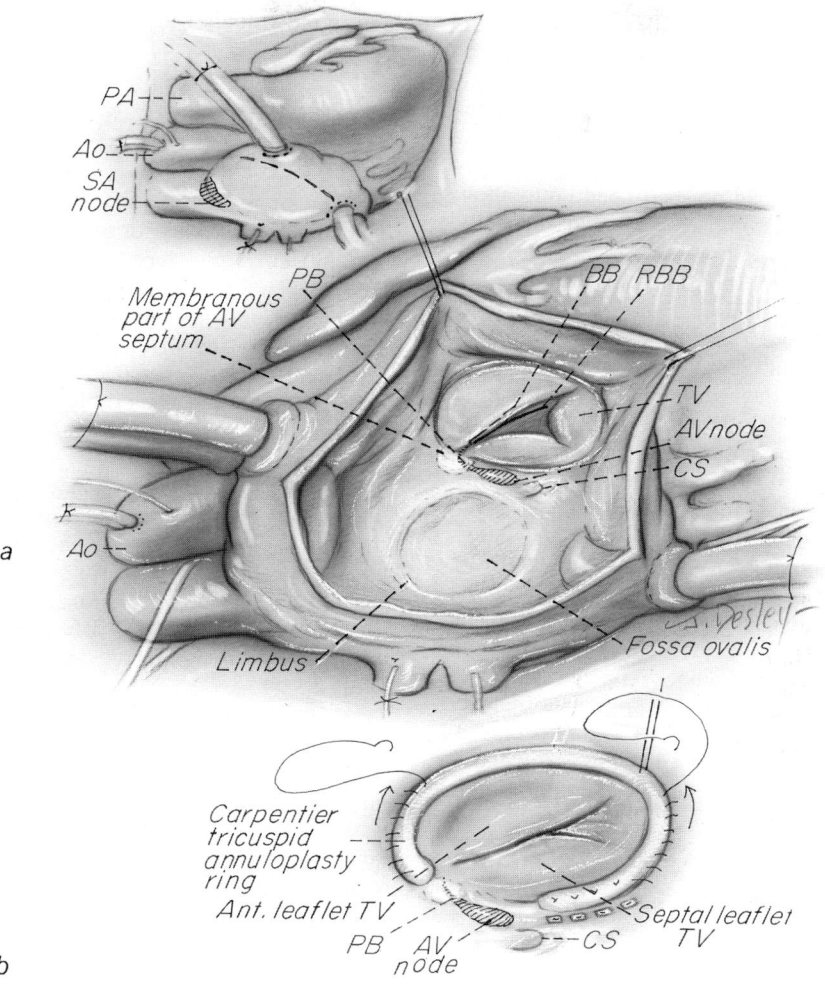

Figure 11-7 Tricuspid annuloplasty.

(a) The exposure is through the usual oblique right atriotomy.

(b) Stay sutures provide excellent exposure, and retractors are not needed. The surgeon identifies the anteroseptal tricuspid valve commissure, the membranous part of this atrioventricular septum, and the coronary sinus orifice. The surgeon can then mentally visualize the location of the atrioventricular node and the penetrating portion of the bundle of His. Using the appropriate sizers, notched at points corresponding to the anteroseptal and posteroseptal commissures at either end of the septal tricuspid leaflet, a proper-sized open, flexible Carpentier-Edwards tricuspid annuloplasty ring is selected. The ring is sewn into place with interrupted sutures (see text) or with interrupted pledgetted mattress sutures along the inferior aspect of the septal leaflet and continuous sutures elsewhere (see the figure), as described in the text. In either case, a stay suture is first placed through the anulus at the junction of the anterior and posterior leaflets and then through the marker on the annuloplasty ring, as shown.

Ao, aorta; AV node, atrioventricular node; BB, bundle branch; CS, coronary sinus; PB, penetrating bundle; RBB, right bundle branch; SA node, sinoatrial node; TV, tricuspid valve.

Reproduced with permission from Bharati et al.[B27]

Valve Prosthesis'' in section on Special Situations and Controversies).

Combined Mitral Replacement and Coronary Artery Bypass Grafting

The primary considerations in the combined operation are the planning of the operation so that bypass time and myocardial ischemic (aortic cross-clamp) time are minimized and the need to tilt the heart up *after* the valve is inserted is minimal (see "Mitral Valve Replacement" in section on Technique of Operation). Two good methods are available and can be recommended.

In one method (UAB and GLH), the operation is begun by first performing the distal anastomoses as described in Chapter 7. Then, after the administration of an additional dose of cardioplegia, the left atrium is opened from the right side, and the mitral valve operation performed. The left atrium is closed. After aspirating air from the tip of the left ventricle and with strong suction on the aortic needle vent, the aortic clamp is removed, and rewarming is begun. The vein grafts are routed as usual and anastomosed to the openings in the exteriorized portion of the aorta. After the side-biting clamp is removed, the usual de-airing procedures are carried out. The operation is completed in the usual manner. Unless urgently indicated, the heart should not be tipped up to allow inspection of the posterior anastomoses, lest ventricular rupture be produced.

In an alternative method, the proximal anastomoses are made before CPB as described in Chapter 7. Then CPB is begun, cold cardioplegia is established, and the distal anastomoses are performed as usual. Care is taken that the vein graft coursing to the right of the right atrium is a little more redundant than usual, in order that it is not damaged by retraction during the mitral insertion. Particular care is taken that the anastomoses are hemostatic, again to avoid the potentially dangerous maneuver of tilting up the heart *after* the mitral replacement device is inserted. Small bulldog clamps are placed very proximally on each vein graft (they must be removed later, a minute or so after release of the cross-clamp) to prevent the air that enters the aortic root during mitral replacement from entering the vein graft. After the infusion of another dose of the cold cardioplegic solution, the left atrium is opened, and mitral valve repair or replacement is carried out as usual. After the left atrium is closed, and with suction on the aortic needle vent, the aortic clamp is released. After rewarming and de-airing, the operation is completed as usual.

SPECIAL FEATURES OF POSTOPERATIVE CARE

In both the operating room and the Intensive Care Unit, patients may display a large V wave in the left atrial pressure pulse. In such situations, this is *not* a reliable indicator of mitral valve incompetence. The height of the V wave is related primarily to the level of mean left atrial pressure,[B11] and in patients who have just undergone mitral valve replacement, the mean left atrial pressure is usually somewhat elevated and the V wave high.

Patients undergoing mitral valve replacement (including those receiving heterografts) are begun on anticoagulant therapy with Coumadin (sodium warfarin) the evening of postoperative day 2 (the day of surgery being considered postoperative day 0). For adults with a normal prothrombin time, the initial dose is generally 7.5–15 mg (UAB) and is followed by daily doses guided while in hospital by daily measurements of prothrombin time. A second dose of 10 mg may be given 12 hours after the first dose, with a subsequent 24-hour gap before beginning daily doses (GLH). The goal is a prothrombin activity about 20%–30% of normal or a prothrombin time about twice the control value. When a prosthetic valve has been inserted, this program is continued indefinitely, and the patient is told of its extreme importance. When a heterograft is inserted or annuloplasty or valvotomy performed, anticoagulation is continued only through the eighth postoperative week. However, when a prosthetic valve has not been used, anticoagulation is discontinued at hospital dismissal in very young children, in very old people, and in individuals with serious bleeding problems.

EARLY RESULTS

Hospital Mortality

Mitral Commissurotomy (Valvotomy)
The hospital mortality for open mitral commissurotomy (valvotomy) currently approaches zero.[G1,H5] For example, at GLH one hospital death occurred (0.6%, CL 0.1%–2.2%) among 154 patients undergoing this operation in the years 1968–1976;[S10] and in the present era at UAB, there have been no deaths (0%, CL 0%–1.8%) in 105 patients treated by open commissurotomy (Table 11-1). This is lower than the mortality for closed commissurotomy.[G1,H11,S10]

Repair of Mitral Incompetence
The hospital mortality after repair of mitral incompetence may be slightly higher. Between 1967 and 1980, in 108 patients, it was 3.7% (CL 1.0%–6.7%) and is similar in the current era (Tables 11-1, 11-2) (UAB). Between 1972 and 1983, it was 0% (CL 0%–4%) in 43 patients (GLH). These results are comparable to those reported by other groups.[C4,D5]

Primary Isolated Mitral Valve Replacement
The hospital mortality for mitral valve replacement is probably higher than that for reparative operations and varies between 2.7% (CL 1.7%–4.1%) and 6.9% (CL 4.9%–9.5%) (Tables 11-2, 11-3, 11-4). The difference may relate to variability in the preoperative functional state of the patient. The hospital mortality tends to be higher in patients undergoing associated procedures along with primary mitral valve replacement and in those who have had previous mitral operations (Tables 11-3, 11-4, 11-5). These results in a current era are better than reported from an earlier era, between 1972 and 1973, by Appelbaum and colleagues[A1] and from other institutions at that time.[B5,C5,H4,L3] However, unusually good results were achieved from 1970 to 1974 (GLH; Table 11-6), achieved using a stented aortic homograft valve.[H15]

Mode of Death

Usually the mode of postoperative hospital death is acute or chronic heart failure (Table 11-7). The deaths associated with acute cardiac failure (low cardiac output) occurred within about 96 hours of operation, and the postoperative course was characterized by all the features of this syndrome. Death with subacute heart failure usually occurred 10–21 days after operation, after a postoperative course characterized by stable but low cardiac output and consequent widespread subsystem failure, often including cool and rarely frankly ischemic extremities, abdominal distention and occasionally frankly ischemic bowel, gastrointestinal bleeding, jaundice, poor renal function, and mental confusion. Infection may occur as a terminal event. Primary infection is the mode of death in about 10% of patients who fail to survive, but, overall, hospital death from infection is uncommon, occurring in 0.4% of patients undergoing

Table 11-1 Hospital mortality after isolated and combined mitral valve surgery (UAB; 1975–July 1979; n = 669).

Surgery[a]	n	No.	%	CL	
				Hospital Deaths	
Primary MVR	479	27	5.6%[b]	4.5%–6.9%	
Secondary MVR	30	3	10%	4%–19%	
Tertiary MVR	8	2	25%	9%–50%	
Quaternary MVR	1	0	0%	0%–86%	
Mitral annuloplasty	46	2	4%	1%–10% }	2/151, 1.3%[b]
Mitral commissurotomy (open)	105	0	0%	0%–1.8% }	CL 0.4%–3%
Total	669	34	5.1%	4.2%–6.1%	

KEY: CL, 70% confidence limits; MVR, mitral valve replacement.

NOTE: *P* for a table of primary, secondary, tertiary, and quaternary MVR (χ^2) = .05.

[a] Includes those with associated procedure, except those with associated aortic and tricuspid valve replacement (2 patients, 0 deaths) and MVR as part of repair of important congenital heart disease.

[b] *P* for difference (χ^2) = .03; P (Fisher) = .02.

Table 11-2 Hospital mortality after isolated procedures on the mitral valve (UAB; 1975–July 1979; n = 339).

Surgery	n	No.	%	CL	
				Hospital Deaths	
Primary MVR	263	7	2.7%[a]	1.7%–4.1%	
Secondary MVR	18	2	11%	4%–24%	
Tertiary MVR	4	2	50%	18%–82%	
Quaternary MVR	1	0	0%	0%–10%	
Mitral annuloplasty	19	0	0%	0%–10% }	0/113, 0%[a]
Mitral commissurotomy (open)	94	0	0%	0%–2% }	CL 0%–2%
Total	399	11	2.8%	1.9%–3.9%	

KEY: CL, 70% confidence limits; MVR, mitral valve replacement.

NOTE: *P* for a table of primary, secondary, tertiary, and quaternary MVR (χ^2) < .0001.

[a] *P* for difference (Fisher) = .08.

Table 11-3 Hospital mortality after mitral valve replacement, isolated and combined with other procedures, including primary and repeated operations (GLH; 1976–1980).

Surgery	n	No.	%	CL
			Hospital Deaths	
MVR, isolated	174	12	6.9%	4.9%–9.5%
MVR + tricuspid surgery	43	2	5%	2%–11%
MVR + CABG ± tricuspid surgery	37	4	11%	6%–19%
MVR + other cardiac surgery	8	1	12%	2%–36%
Total	262	19	7.3%	5.6%–9.3%

KEY: CABG, coronary artery bypass graft; CL, 70% confidence limits; MVR, mitral valve replacement.

isolated or combined mitral valve replacement. Massive hemorrhage, usually from left atrioventricular or ventricular rupture, is currently a rare cause of death, as are valve thrombosis (disc valves with improper anticoagulation) and neurologic damage (from escaped left atrial thrombus or cerebral air embolism).

Incremental Risk Factors for Hospital Death after Mitral Valve Replacement

Important preoperative functional impairment, as reflected by the preoperative NYHA functional class, is an important incremental risk factor for hospital death (Table 11-8, Fig. 11-8). This is reflected in the contingency tables of the recent experiences (UAB, Table 11-9; GLH, Table 11-10). The fallacy of comparing results without knowledge of risk factors is evident from Tables 11-9 and 11-10: there is a significant difference in overall mortality between the two tables but no significant difference (70% confidence limits overlapping) when a comparison is made according to preoperative NYHA class. The effect of the preoperative functional state is also reflected in other earlier experiences.[B7,B17,C5,S8]

This effect is probably a reflection of the basic incremental risk of *decreased left ventricular systolic and diastolic func-*

Table 11-4 Hospital mortality after primary and repeated operations on the mitral valve (mitral valve replacement with or without tricuspid surgery, with or without coronary artery bypass grafting, with or without other cardiac surgery except aortic valve replacement; GLH; 1976–1980.)

Surgery	n	Hospital Deaths No.	%	CL
No previous MV surgery	174	12	6.9%	4.9%–9.5%
Previous MV repair	38	5	13%	7%–21%
Previous MV replacement	50	2	4.0%	1%–9%
Total	262	19	7.3%	5.6%–9.3%
$P(\chi^2)$			.25	

KEY: CL, 70% confidence limits; MV, mitral valve.

Table 11-5 Hospital mortality in various categories of patients after primary isolated or combined replacement of the mitral valve (UAB; 1975–July 1979; $n = 445$).

Surgery	n	Hospital Deaths No.	%	CL	
MVR, isolated	314	7	2.2%	1.4%–3.5%	
No previous surgery	263	7	2.7%	1.7%–4.1%	
Previous closed mitral surgery	28	0	0%	0%–7%	12/349[b]
Previous open mitral surgery	23	0	0%	0%–8%	3.4%
MVR + TVA	35	5	14%	8%–23%	2.4%–4.7%
No previous surgery	26	3	12%	5%–22%	
Previous closed mitral surgery	8	2	25%	9%–50%	
Previous open mitral surgery	1	0	0%	0%–85%	
MVR + CABG	89	8	9%	6%–13%	
No previous surgery	85	8	9%	6%–14%	
Previous closed mitral surgery	4	0	0%	0%–38%	8/96[b]
Previous open mitral surgery					8%
MVR + TVA + CABG	7	0	0%	0%–24%	5%–12%
No previous surgery	5	0	0%	0%–32%	
Previous closed mitral surgery	2	0	0%	0%–61%	
Previous open mitral surgery					
Total[a]	445	20	4.5%	3.5%–5.8%	

KEY: CABG, coronary artery bypass grafting; CL, 70% confidence limits; MVR, mitral valve replacement; TVA, tricuspid valve annuloplasty.

[a] Thirty-four patients (from the $n = 479$) with a heterogeneous variety of associated conditions, previous kinds of cardiac surgery, or concomitant procedures different from those listed have been excluded (seven deaths).

[b] P for difference = .04.

Table 11-6 Hospital deaths after mitral valve replacement without tricuspid valve surgery or coronary artery bypass grafting, including primary and repeated operations (GLH).

NYHA Class	Stented Homograft Valves[a] n	Hospital Deaths No.	%	CL	Starr or Porcine Valves[b] n	Hospital Deaths No.	%	CL
I					7	0	0%	0%–24%
II	1	0	0%	0%–85%	29	0	0%	0%–6%
III	37	0	0%	0%–5%	62	3	5%	2%–10%
IV, V	91	5	5.5%	3.1%–9.2%	71	9	12.7%	8.5%–18.1%
Total	129	5	3.9%	2.2%–6.5%	169[c]	12	7.1%[c]	5.1%–9.8%

KEY: CL, 70% confidence limits.

[a] Operation 1970–1974.

[b] Operation 1976–1980.

[c] Total excludes 5 patients without NYHA class.

Table 11-7 Mode of death following primary mitral valve replacement (UAB; 1975–July 1979; n = 445).

Mode of Death	Total[a] (n = 445) n		No Cardioplegia (n = 215) n		Cardioplegia (n = 230) n	
Acute cardiac failure	10 ⎫		7 ⎫		3 ⎫	
Subacute cardiac failure	5 ⎬	15	3 ⎬	10	2 ⎬	5
Infection	2 ⎭	(75% of 20)	1 ⎭	(83% of 12)	1 ⎭	(62% of 8)
Hemorrhage	1		1		1	
Valve thrombosis	1				1	
Neurologic damage	1				1	
Total	20		12		8	

[a] n = 445 is a subset of the 479 in Table 11-2; however, it includes only primary replacement either isolated or with primary CABG and/or primary tricuspid annuloplasty in patients without associated cardiac anomalies with no previous surgery or with previous closed or open mitral surgery as their only previous surgery.

tion. This thesis is supported by the tendency of patients dying after mitral valve replacement to have lower preoperative cardiac indexes and higher left ventricular end-diastolic pressures than those surviving (Table 11-11).

Papillary muscle rupture and/or dysfunction was a risk factor for hospital death after mitral valve replacement in the UAB 1975–July 1979 experience. This may in fact represent again the effect of left ventricular dysfunction, in this instance dysfunction from ischemic left ventricular scarring (see Chapter 10).

Atrial fibrillation is probably a risk factor for hospital death, even though few hospital deaths are related to thromboembolism (Table 11-7).[C5] Possibly the presence or absence of atrial fibrillation refines the estimate of the degree and duration of left ventricular dysfunction obtained from the NYHA functional class, and this may be the reason for its being related to the probability of hospital death. The same reasoning applies to the presence of *left atrial thrombosis* as a possible risk factor.

Older age at operation has been an incremental risk factor, both in our experience (Table 11-8) and in that of others.[C5,S8]

Table 11-8 Incremental risk factors for all hospital deaths after isolated or combined primary mitral valve replacement (UAB; 1975–July 1979; n = 445, 20 events; see Appendix 11A for details of the analysis).

Incremental Risk Factors for Hospital Death	Coefficient	P Value
NYHA functional class	1.8 ± 0.52	.0004
Papillary muscle rupture and/or dysfunction	2.2 ± 0.95	.02
Age at operation (yr)	0.07 ± 0.033	.05
Preoperative atrial fibrillation	1.7 ± 0.94	.07
Left atrial thrombus	1.1 ± 0.81	.16
If noncardioplegia:		
Date of operation (mo since January 1, 1975)	-0.12 ± 0.054	.03
If cardioplegia:		
Body surface area (m²)	-6 ± 2.9	.03
Ischemic time (min)	0.033 ± 0.0161	.04
Preoperative atrial fibrillation	2.5 ± 1.78	.17
Intercept	-9	

This is probably because of the adverse general effect of old age on organ and subsystem function. The increased risk becomes evident at about 65 years of age when cold cardioplegia is used (Fig. 11-9) and 55 years without it.

When cold cardioplegia is used, the *aortic cross-clamp (ischemic) time* is also a risk factor (Fig. 11-8).

Other Incremental Risk Factors for Early Death after Mitral Valve Surgery

Mitral valve replacement probably has a higher risk than does mitral valve repair in the current era (Tables 11-1, 11-2), just as in our earlier Mayo Clinic experience. It is possible that the resection of the mitral valve itself produces some disturbance of left ventricular function and thus adversely affects hospital mortality, other things being equal. It was at one time presumed that the fixation of the anulus by the rigid ring of the prosthesis was disadvantageous to left ventricular function, but in an experimental study in *normal* dogs we were unable to demonstrate this.[T3] Also, the favorable experiences with the Carpentier annuloplasty ring casts doubt on this hypothesis.

The *type of prosthesis* has been suggested as being an important contributor to the increased risk of replacement over repair, the "high profile" of the caged-ball valve being alleged to be an incremental risk factor because of its supposed detrimental effect on left ventricular function. On the contrary, the achievement of superior results at GLH in the 1970–1973 era using a stented aortic homograft valve (Table 11-6) strongly suggests that a nonobstructive device with a central orifice flow pattern is optimal. Otherwise, this hypothesis has never been supported by appropriate data.

Under some circumstances, *mitral re-replacement* can be carried out at a risk no greater than that of primary valve replacement (Table 11-4). However, a second or third re-replacement probably does impose a higher probability of hospital death (Tables 11-1, 11-2). This may be because patients undergoing these have more advanced disability and because technical surgical errors are most difficult to avoid in these situations. A *previous closed or open mitral reparative operation* may not be an incremental risk factor for primary mitral valve replacement.

Tricuspid annuloplasty need not increase the risk of mitral

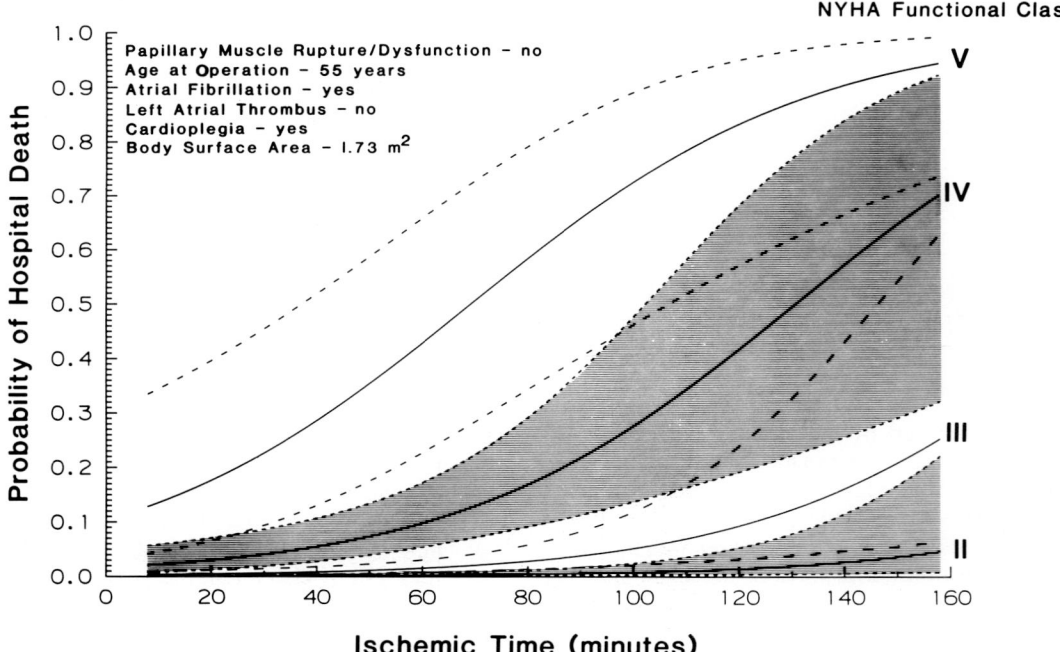

Papillary Muscle Rupture/Dysfunction – no
Age at Operation – 55 years
Atrial Fibrillation – yes
Left Atrial Thrombus – no
Cardioplegia – yes
Body Surface Area – 1.73 m^2

Figure 11-8 The interrelationship of the effect of aortic cross-clamp (ischemic) time and preoperative NYHA functional class on hospital mortality after isolated or combined primary mitral valve replacement using cold cardioplegic myocardial protection. The nomogram is based on the multivariate analysis shown in Table 11-8 (UAB; 1975–July 1979; n = 445; 20 events). The other values used in the equation are in the upper left corner of the figure. The mean value for age at operation among the 445 patients was 55 years, and that for body surface area was 1.73 m^2. The 70% confidence limits are indicated by the dashed lines, and those around NYHA classes II and IV are crosshatched for ease of viewing. Note that with 60 minutes of ischemic time, the increased risk is evident only for NYHA classes IV and V and that the increased risk of long cross-clamp (ischemic) time is only evident for functional classes IV and V.

Table 11-9 Hospital death according to NYHA functional class following primary replacement of the mitral valve, with or without associated procedures (UAB; 1975–July 1979; n = 441, the NYHA class being undetermined in four patients, with no deaths). NYHA class V includes patients undergoing emergency operation because of shock.

NYHA Class	n	No.		%	CL
			Hospital Deaths		
I	8	0		0%	0%–21%
II	30	0	2.4%	0%	0%–6%
III	333	9	CL 1.6%–3.6%	2.7%	1.8%–4.0%
IV	65	8	16%	12%	8%–18%
V	5	3	CL 11%–22%	60%	29%–86%
Total	441	20		4.5%	3.5%–5.8%
P (logistic)			< .0001		

KEY: CL, 70% confidence limits.

Table 11-10 Hospital mortality for patients with primary and repeated mitral valve replacement, with or without associated cardiac surgery, related to NYHA class and type of valve disease. The table excludes nine patients, zero deaths, not coded for NYHA class (GLH; 1976–1980).

NYHA Class	Mitral Stenosis		Hospital Deaths		Mitral Incompetence		Hospital Deaths		Mixed Lesions		Hospital Deaths		Total		Hospital Deaths	
	n	No.	%	CL	n	No.	%	CL	n	No.	%	CL	n	No.	%	CL
I	1	0	0%	0%–85%	6	0	0%	0%–27%	2	0	0%	0%–61%	9	0	0%	0%–19%
II	9	0	0%	0%–19%	28	0	0%	0%–7%	5	1	20%	3%–53%	42	1	2%	0.3%–7%
III	13	1	8%	1%–24%	64	3	5%	2%–9%	22	2	9%	3%–20%	99	6	6%	4%–10%
IV	15	0	0%	0%–12%	55	6	11%	7%–17%	10	1	10%	1%–30%	80	7	9%	5%–13%
V	7	3	43%	20%–68%	16	2	12%	4%–27%					23	5	22%	12%–34%
Total	45	4	9%	5%–16%	169	11	6.5%	4.6%–9.1%	39	4	10%	5%–18%	253	19	7.5%	5.8%–9.6%
$P(\chi^2)$		.01				.25				.85				.05		

Table 11-11 Variables associated with hospital death after primary replacement of the mitral valve (UAB; 1975–July 1979; n = 445).

Single Continuous Variable	No. of Patients for Whom Data Are Available	Survivors		Hospital Deaths		P Value
		No.	Mean ± SE	No.	Mean ± SE	
Age	445	425	52.9 ± 0.64	20	64 ± 2.1	.0001
Date of operation (mo since January 1, 1975)	445	425	27.1 ± 0.78	20	22 ± 4.2	.21
Preoperative CI	275	266	2.54 ± 0.046	9	1.65 ± 0.150	.0005
Preoperative LVEDP	303	290	10.9 ± 0.43	13	14.9 ± 1.86	.05

KEY: CI, cardiac index; LVEDP, left ventricular end diastolic pressure; SE, standard error.

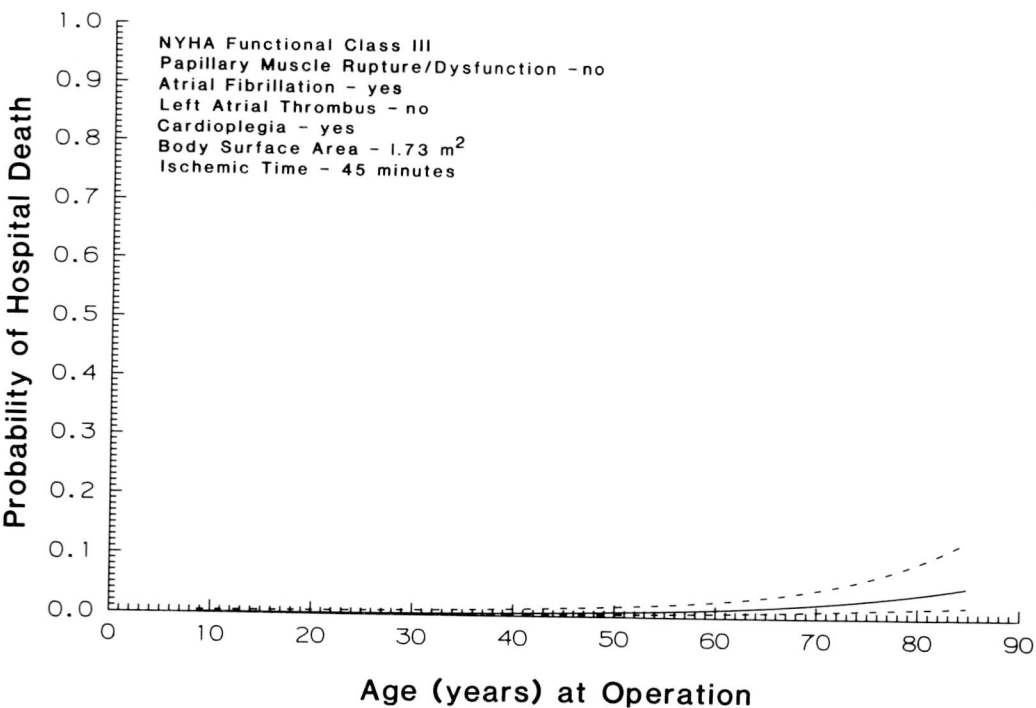

NYHA Functional Class III
Papillary Muscle Rupture/Dysfunction – no
Atrial Fibrillation – yes
Left Atrial Thrombus – no
Cardioplegia – yes
Body Surface Area – 1.73 m^2
Ischemic Time – 45 minutes

Figure 11-9 The effect of age at operation on the probability of hospital death after mitral valve replacement. The presentation is as in Figure 11-8. Mean ischemic time in the series is 45 minutes. Note that although there is an evident increase in risk with older age over about 60 years, even at 80 years under these conditions the risk is between 2% and 12%.

valve replacement, as is evident in the GLH experience (Table 11-3) and from the absence of this as a risk factor in the UAB multivariate analysis (Table 11-8). In an earlier era, when *tricuspid valve replacement* was more frequently performed, this procedure did increase the risk of hospital death.[B20,J2,S12] For example, Boyd and colleagues experienced six hospital deaths (14%, CL 8%–21%) in 44 patients undergoing mitral replacement and tricuspid annuloplasty and 20 deaths (33%, CL 27%–41%) in 60 patients undergoing mitral and tricuspid replacement (*P* = .02).[B21]

The *addition of coronary artery bypass grafting* (CABG) is not itself an incremental risk factor, as is evident from the multivariate analysis (Table 11-8) and from the contingency table analysis of the GLH experience (Table 11-3). This fact is not apparent from a *superficial* examination of the experiences (Table 11-5), in which CABG seems to about double the risk of primary mitral valve replacement. However, a closer look at the recent experience with the 96 patients undergoing primary mitral valve replacement plus CABG shows that the patients with ischemic papillary muscle dysfunction or rupture (from ischemic heart disease, discussed in Chapter 10) are responsible for the higher mortality of the patients receiving concomitant CABG (Table 11-12).

Other than ischemic papillary muscle dysfunction, none of the other *types of mitral pathology* affects the hospital mortality of mitral valve replacement currently (Table 11-13). Also, in contrast to the earlier experience of others, the functional mitral lesion (incompetence, stenosis, or mixed) does not influence mortality (Tables 11-10, 11-14, 11-15, 11-16). However, preoperative mitral incompetence (as opposed to mitral stenosis) remains a potential incremental risk factor for hospital death, but one that is currently indemonstrable because of the generally improved results of mitral valve surgery. The potential risk of preoperative mitral incompetence is indicated by the data from an earlier era.[C5] It is further supported by the fact that currently the presence preoperatively of important mitral incompetence does tend to depress the cardiac output early postoperatively (Table 11-17), probably in the current era a more sensitive indicator of its effect than is hospital death.

LATE RESULTS

Late survival and functional status are the results of the interactions of a number of variables: (1) the mechanical, or

Table 11-12 Hospital mortality according to pathologic basis of the mitral valve incompetence after primary replacement of the mitral valve and coronary artery bypass grafting (UAB; 1975–July 1979; *n* = 65).

Pathologic Basis	n	No.	%	CL	
				Hospital Deaths[a]	
Rheumatic disease	4	0	0%	0%–38% ⎱	0/22, 0%[c]
Mitral prolapse	18	0	0%	0%–10% ⎰	CL 0%–8%
Ischemic papillary muscle dysfunction or rupture	29	5	17%	10%–28%[c]	
Ruptured chordae, nonischemic	8	1[b]	12%	2%–36%	
Bacterial endocarditis	3	1[b]	33%	4%–76%	
Unknown	3	0	0%	0%–47%	
Total	65	7	11%	7%–16%	

KEY: CL, 70% confidence limits.

NOTE: When patients with a rupture of the chordae that was presumably nonischemic in origin are assumed to have an ischemic basis for their mitral valve disease and are added to those with papillary muscle dysfunction, *P* = .06 for the difference from the first two groups.

[a] Mode of death was acute (four patients) or chronic (one patient) cardiac failure *except* as indicated.

[b] Mode of death was infection.

[c] *P* for difference = .05.

Table 11-13 Hospital mortality according to the pathologic basis of the mitral disease (stenosis or incompetence or both) after primary replacement of the mitral valve (UAB; 1975–July 1979; *n* = 445).

Pathologic Basis	n	Hospital Deaths			Hospital Deaths (Cardiac)		
		No.	%	CL	No.	%	CL
Rheumatic disease	258	9	3.5%	2.3%–5.1%	5	1.9%	1.1%–3.3%
Mitral prolapse	93	4	4%	2%–8%	4	4%	2%–8%
Ischemic papillary muscle dysfunction or rupture	30	5	17%	9%–27%	5	17%	9%–27%
Ruptured chordae, nonischemic	26	1	4%	0.5%–12%	0	0%	0%–7%
Bacterial endocarditis	17	1	6%	1%–19%	0	0%	0%–11%
Unknown	21	0			0		
Total	445	20	4.5%	3.5%–5.8%	14	3.1%	2.3%–4.2%
P			.03[a]			.0005	

[a] *P* = .95 when the 30 patients with papillary muscle dysfunction or rupture are excluded.

Table 11-14 Hospital mortality according to the functional lesion after primary mitral valve replacement (UAB; 1975–July 1979; n = 445).

Lesion	n	Hospital Deaths					Hospital Deaths (Cardiac)			
		No.	%	CL			No.	%	CL	
Incompetence	209	12	5.7%	4.1%–7.9%			9	4.3%	2.9%–6.3%	
Stenosis	121	5	4.1%	2.3%–6.9%	3.3%		4	3.3%	1.7%–5.9%	2.1%
Mixed	115	3	2.6%	1.1%–5.2%	CL 2.2%–5.0%		1	0.9%	0.1%–2.9%	CL 1.2%–3.6%
Total	445	20	4.5%	3.5%–5.8%			14	3.1%	2.3%–4.2%	
P			.4					.24		

KEY: CL, 70% confidence limits.

Table 11-15 Hospital mortality for patients undergoing mitral valve replacement and tricuspid valve surgery with or without coronary artery bypass grafting, including primary and repeated operations (GLH; 1976–1980). The table excludes one patient without NYHA class.

NYHA Class	Mitral Stenosis				Mitral Incompetence + Mixed Lesions				Total			
		Hospital Deaths				Hospital Deaths				Hospital Deaths		
	n	No.	%	CL	n	No.	%	CL	n	No.	%	CL
I					2	0	0%	0%–61%	2	0	0%	0%–61%
II	1	0	0%	0%–85%	5	0	0%	0%–32%	6	0	0%	0%–27%
III	3	0	0%	0%–47%	13	1	8%	1%–24%	16	1	6%	0.8%–20%
IV	3	0	0%	0%–47%	11	1	9%	1%–28%	14	1	7%	0.9%–22%
V	1	0	0%	0%–85%	3	0	0%	0%–47%	4	0	0%	0%–38%
Total	8	0	0%	0%–21%	34	2	6%	2%–13%	42	2	5%	2%–11%

Table 11-16 Hospital mortality for patients undergoing mitral valve replacement and coronary artery bypass grafting with or without tricuspid surgery, including primary and repeated operations (GLH; 1976–1980). The table excludes three patients without NYHA class.

NYHA Class	Mitral Stenosis				Mitral Incompetence + Mixed Lesions				Total			
		Hospital Deaths				Hospital Deaths				Hospital Deaths		
	n	No.	%	CL	n	No.	%	CL	n	No.	%	CL
I												
II	2	0	0%	0%–61%	3	1[a]	33%	4%–76%	5	1	20%	3%–53%
III	1	0	0%	0%–85%	13	1[b]	8%	1%–24%	14	1	7%	0.9%–22%
IV	2	0	0%	0%–61%	9	1[c]	11%	1%–33%	11	1	9%	1%–28%
V					4	1[c]	25%	3%–63%	4	1	25%	3%–63%
Total	5	0	0%	0%–32%	29	4	14%	7%–24%	34	4	12%	6%–20%

KEY: CL, 70% compliance limits.
[a] Cause of death: cerebral air embolism.
[b] Cause of death: left ventricular tear.
[c] Cause of death: low cardiac output.

hemodynamic, function of the repaired or replaced mitral valve, which may change with time; (2) the extent of secondary left ventricular cardiomyopathy, the amount of its regression after relief of the mitral valve abnormality, and its possible progression evolving late postoperatively; (3) possible secondary pulmonary vascular disease and/or secondary *right* ventricular cardiomyopathy and their regression or persistence; (4) the presence, progression, or development of other valvar or coronary artery disease; and (5) accidents, such as valve thrombosis or deterioration, thromboem-

bolism, bleeding as a result of Coumadin, therapy, and prosthetic infection.

Mitral Commissurotomy

The late results depend primarily on the magnitude of increase in effective mitral valve orifice area (and thus the decrease in flow resistance) produced by the operation, the secondary effects of the increase, and the durability of the effect. Although open commissurotomy more often re-

Table 11-17 Factors influencing early postoperative (4 hours) cardiac index, obtained by multivariate analysis using catheterization and operative information ($n = 226$ patients with measurement of cardiac index) (UAB; 1975–July 1, 1979; $n = 445$; see Appendix 11-B for details). A negative coefficient indicates that cardiac index is lower when the variable is present or as the value of the variable increases.

Variable	Coefficient ± SD	P Value	Single-Variable r Value (P value)
Preoperative cardiac index	0.28 ± 0.065	<.0001	.33(<.0001)
Prosthesis valve diameter	0.06 ± 0.02	.004	.07(.16)
Preoperative atrial fibrillation	−0.26 ± 0.097	.008	−.21(<.0001)
Mitral incompetence present	−0.22 ± 0.104	.03	−.05(.3)
Date of operation	0.008 ± 0.0030	.01	.01(.8)
Age at operation	−0.011 ± 0.0044	.02	−.31(<.0001)
Systolic arterial pressure at catheterization	−0.005 ± 0.0021	.02	−.14(.02)
NYHA class	−0.19 ± 0.092	.04	−.21(<.0001)
Intercept	1.7		

sults in a very wide opening of the valve than does closed commissurotomy, the results of both methods are in many ways similar and depending in part on the pathologic condition of the valve.

The increase in calculated mitral valve area (or orifice size) produced by commissurotomy varies markedly and depends not only on the surgical opening but in part on leaflet pliability and the extent of subvalvar obstruction from fused chordae.[A3] Feigenbaum and colleagues found that closed mitral commissurotomy, usually with a transventricular dilator, on the average increased mitral valve area by 1.3–2.6 cm[2], with postoperative mitral valve areas ranging from 0.7–5.8 cm[2]. Younger patients tend to have a better functional result[C8] and to experience greater increases in calculated valve area than do older patients,[F3] perhaps because younger patients tend to have more pliable valves.

A secondary effect of the increased orifice size is a lowering of left atrial pressure, although this pressure frequently remains above the normal value. It is usually about 20 mmHg at rest preoperatively and on the average falls to 12 mmHg after operation. However, on exercise it generally increases to an average value of 17 mmHg.[F3] Left ventricular end-diastolic pressure often is modestly higher after commissurotomy.[F3]

Cardiac output is usually increased by operation, and the amount of increase at rest and exercise correlates well with the increase in calculated valve area.[F3] Pulmonary vascular resistance usually falls, especially in young patients. Pulmonary artery pressure falls, and the fall is well correlated with the fall in left atrial pressure and pulmonary vascular resistance.

Important symptomatic improvement is brought about by these striking primary and secondary effects of mitral commissurotomy. Most patients are in NYHA class I or II 1 year after operation, with the symptomatic improvement paralleling the hemodynamic changes.[H10]

Reoperation and survival rates depend on the initial improvement resulting from the operation and its durability (or freedom from restenosis). In the early era of digital mitral commissurotomy, the nonactuarial 10-year survival rate without reoperation was 57%, with severe preoperative dis-

ability, older age, mitral valve calcification, and associated mitral incompetence adversely affecting the results.[E3] Twenty percent of the patients required reoperation within the 10-year period, and another 23% died. Most of the 10-year survivors without reoperation were still symptomatically improved. Even better results from closed mitral commissurotomy have recently been reported by Commerford and colleagues.[C14] The overall actuarial survival at 12 years in their experience was 78%. Survival was adversely affected by immobility of the mitral valve, advanced symptomatology, and pulmonary hypertension. Likewise, a recent report by Rutledge and colleagues also confirms the very good late results from closed mitral commissurotomy.[R16]

In the current era of open mitral commissurotomy, the long-term results are better, although at least part of the improvement is the result of the use of valve *replacement* within the follow-up period of 1 month to 9.5 years. For example, 5 (3%, CL 2%–6%) of 153 patients required valve replacement within 6 months of valvotomy.[S10] The 10-year survival rate without reoperation was 86% in a report from Gross and colleagues.[G1] 91% of patients who have not had reoperation are in NYHA class I or II an average of 48 months postoperatively (Fig. 11-10),[S10] and similar results are reported by others.[G1,H5,V1] Residual mitral gradients and mitral incompetence account for most poor late results. Poor preoperative condition, atrial fibrillation, and mild preoperative mitral incompetence are strong risk factors for a poor late result; and previous mitral valve surgery, elevated pulmonary vascular resistance, and mitral calcification are lesser risk factors.[S10]

In spite of the excellent early and interim results in the current era, the durability of the results is limited. The scarring from the rheumatic process in the valve seems gradually to progress with time, and eventually most patients return with restenosis or newly developed incompetence. This return of symptoms may begin as long as 20 years after the commissurotomy. However, *persistent* mitral stenosis and mitral incompetence are more common causes of unsatisfactory late results.[H8,S10]

Effective mitral commissurotomy reduces the incidence of

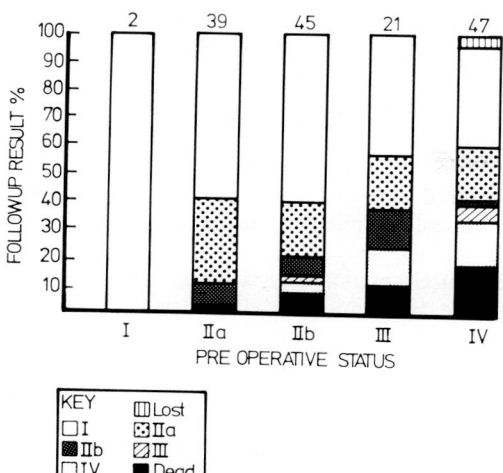

Figure 11-10 Comparison of preoperative and postoperative status in 123 surviving patients an average of 48 months following open mitral valvotomy (GLH; 1968–1976).

Class IIa, breathlessness with unusually strenuous activity; class IIb, breathlessness with ordinary activity.

Reproduced with permission from Smith et al.[S10]

thromboembolic complications.[H10] Gross and colleagues report an annualized incidence of 0.3% per year in the first 10 years after operation.[G1] However, the protection is not complete and is variable.[S10] Further, atrial fibrillation and older age increase the likelihood of a late postoperative thromboembolic event.[S10]

The late results are summarized in Figure 11-11, which shows that 88% of patients were alive 8 years postoperatively, but 16.1% of them required mitral valve replacement and an additional 8.3% experienced an embolic event.

Repair of Mitral Incompetence

The late results of repair of mitral incompetence are variable and depend at least on the repair techniques and the basic pathologic condition for which the repair was done.[C9] However, with modern techniques, the functional results are generally excellent. Thus, Lessana and colleagues report that 89% of 116 patients undergoing Carpentier-type repairs were in NYHA class I an average of 38 months after repair, and 9% were in NYHA class II.[L10]

There is an incidence of immediately unsatisfactory results in the operation room, necessitating immediate valve replacement because of continuing mitral incompetence. Duran reports such results in 7.8% (CL 6.0%–10.1%) of cases in his large experience.[D5]

In patients in whom the repair seemed satisfactory in the operating room, there is an incidence of later unsatisfactory results. Lessana and colleagues report that 5 (19%, CL 11%–31%) of 26 patients studied by left ventriculography about 1 year after a Carpentier-type repair had important mitral incompetence.[L6] In an intermediate-term follow-up, Duran reports that 9 (12%, CL 8%–18%) of 72 patients recatheterized an average of 2.5 years after repair with his flexible ring (which probably gives results similar to those obtained with the Carpentier ring) had severe persisting or recurrent incompetence. Kronzon and colleagues report that 10 of 11 patients had no Doppler echocardiographic evidence of regurgitation after the Carpentier repair.[K9] Yacoub, however, using slightly different methods for mitral repair in a group of 82 patients with mitral incompetence from floppy valves, found that only 2 (2%, CL 0.8%–6%) required reoperation within a follow-up period of 8 years.[Y1] Also, Adebo and Ross found a failure rate within 6 years of only 6.7% among 84 patients surviving repair by the Carpentier methods.[A7] In summary, it appears that valve repair fails within about 5

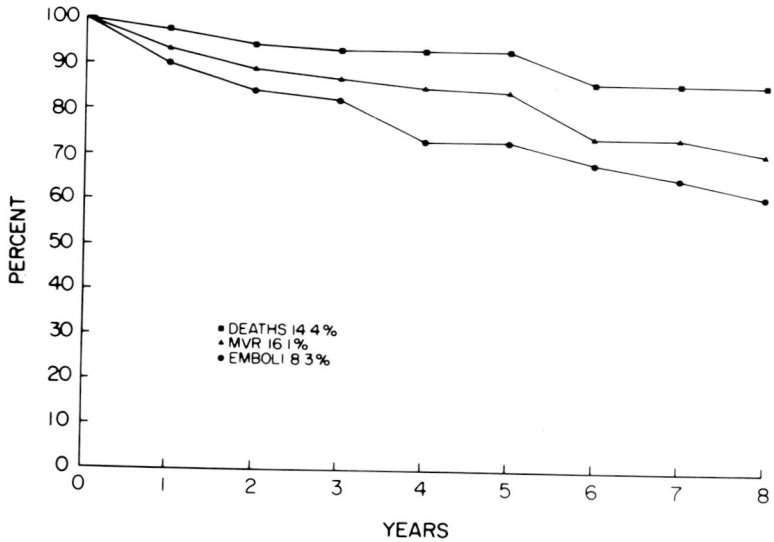

Figure 11-11 Cumulative complication-free rates of three late events (death, mitral valve replacement, and emboli) after open mitral valvotomy at GLH.

MVR, mitral valve replacement.

Reproduced with permission from Smith et al.[S10]

years in 10%–20% of patients with various types of preoperative incompetence.

Good results have also been obtained with other techniques; thus, after the Wooler repair there has been an 18% (CL 14%–23%) incidence of reoperation for valve replacement within 10 years.[P1]

Reed has reported late follow-up data as long as 17 years after mitral repair by his technique of asymmetric measured annuloplasty.[R6,R8] Among the 111 hospital survivors of repair for pure rheumatic mitral incompetence, there were 9 late deaths; the actuarial survival rate at 17 years was 86%. This corresponds to Yacoub's actuarial survival rate of 81% at 9 years after repair.[Y1] Reoperation was necessary in the follow-up period in 11 patients (10%, CL 7%–14%). Thus, again, 80%–90% of the patients experienced intermediate-term good results. Among a subset of 20 children followed from 5–12 years after repair by Reed and colleagues,[R7] 16 (80%, CL 67%–90%) showed marked and sustained improvement, and 3 (15%, CL 7%–28%) required reoperation.

In most series, the best results have been in patients with rupture of chordae to the medial portion of the posterior leaflet.[S9] Ellis and colleagues reported that 23 (88%, CL 78%–95%) of 26 hospital survivors in this category had sustained functional improvement up to 7 years after repair.[E2] In Carpentier's entire group of patients whose mitral incompetence was from systolic leaflet eversion or prolapse, which included also ruptured chordae and very elongated chordae to the anterior leaflet, 95% were without reoperation over an 8 year follow-up.[C4] Of 93 patients with follow-up over 2 years, 58% (CL 52%–64%) were without a murmur, 37%

(CL 31%–42%) had a grade 1–3/6 murmur (grade 1 being the softest and 6 being the loudest), and 5% (CL 3%–9%) had loud murmurs suggesting the later requirement of reoperation. Thus, in about 90% of this group, a good 10-year result could be anticipated. It is noteworthy that Orszulak and colleagues recently reported equally good results in patients with ruptured chordae to the anterior leaflet, using techniques basically similar to those used for the posterior leaflet.[O3]

When mitral annuloplasty successfully relieves mitral incompetence, the changes in left ventricular performance are the same as after mitral valve replacement.[L6]

Patients undergoing mitral valve repair generally do not receive long-term anticoagulation therapy, and most are free of late thromboembolic complications. Duran found 93% of patients free of thromboembolism within the first 4.5 years after repair, an incidence similar to that for heterograft replacement, in his experience.[D5]

Mitral Valve Replacement

Survival
About 90% of hospital survivors of isolated mitral valve replacement survive at least 3 years (80% when mitral replacement with associated procedures is included), 80% of patients at least 5 years (Figs. 11-12, 11-13), about 60% at least 10 years, and about 45% at least 15 years.[B7,K2,L1,T4,W1] Although no precise comparisons have been made, these survival rates are better than those for the various diseases leading to mitral replacement but worse than that of the gen-

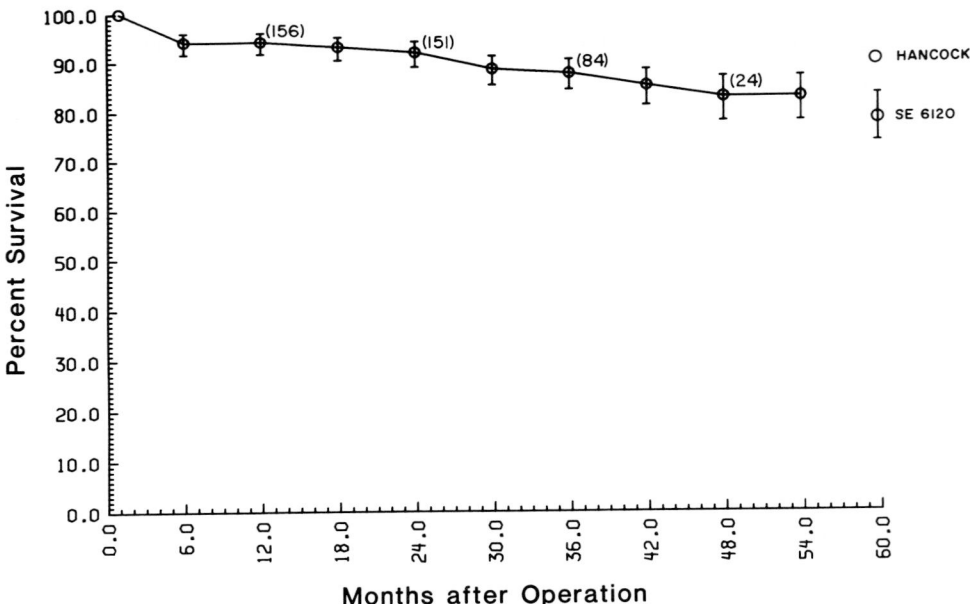

Figure 11-12   Late survival rate among patients leaving the hospital alive after mitral valve replacement with the Bjork-Shiley prosthesis.[K2] The 5-year survival rate with the Hancock bioprosthesis[D1] and the Starr-Edwards model 6120 ball valve prosthesis[M2] are seen to be similar. The vertical bars represent the 70% confidence limits. The figures within parentheses are the number of patients followed beyond the specified interval.

Reproduced with permission from Karp et al.[K2]

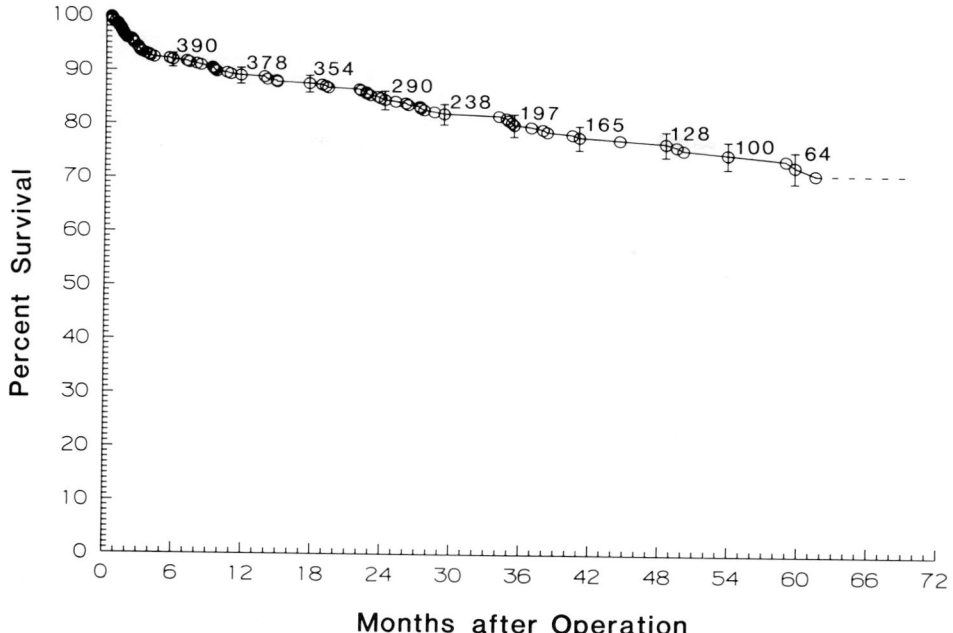

Figure 11-13 Actuarial late survival rate of hospital survivors of primary mitral valve replacement with or without associated procedures (UAB; 1975–July 1979; $n = 445$).

eral population, so the operations are palliative rather than curative. About 50% of the late deaths are with heart failure and about 20% with late complications (thromboembolism, valve thrombosis or degeneration, infection, etc.) of the operation or the device inserted.[T4]

Incremental Risk Factors for Premature Late Death
The presence of severe preoperative symptoms, as evidenced by NYHA classes III and IV, increases the risk of premature death.[C4,L4,S8] Thus, the 4-year survival rate is about 90%–95% for patients preoperatively in NYHA class I and II, 85% for those in class III, and 60% for those in class IV[K2,W1] (Fig. 11-14). As with early in-hospital death, the basic incremental risk factor is probably *preoperative left ventricular dysfunction*, which, when advanced, seems largely irreversible. This same conclusion is suggested by the deleterious effect on late survival of a preoperatively low cardiac index[G2] or, in the case of mitral incompetence, a preoperatively low ejection fraction.[P5]

Older age at operation is probably an incremental risk for premature late death,[G2,P5,S8,W1] although the effect of old age is at least partly from noncardiac causes.

Neither the *functional mitral lesion* nor *mitral pathologic conditions* other than *ischemic mitral incompetence* (discussed in Chapter 10) have been conclusively demonstrated to be risk factors for premature late death after mitral valve replacement.[M5,S8] Ischemic mitral incompetence is a risk factor for premature late death after mitral valve replacement, as reported by Kay and colleagues[K10] and Blackstone and Kirklin.[B35] For the reasons described under "Left Ventricular Dysfunction: Mitral Incompetence," preoperative mitral incompetence would be expected to have an adverse effect on long-term survival (Fig. 11-15).[C5,L4]

A *previous valve replacement* does appear to be an incremental risk affecting late survival.[K2] Indeed, Grunkemeier and colleagues find that any previous cardiac operation increases the risk of premature death.[G2]

The *device inserted* does not seem to affect survival (considering only the Bjork-Shiley valve, Starr-Edwards silastic ball valve model 6120, and the stent-mounted porcine heterograft),[K2] although Cohn and colleagues concluded that a difference does exist.[C6] The mode of late death, however, does differ with the different devices. Acute hemodynamic deterioration leading to death as a result of valve thrombosis (so-called valve encapsulation) seems to be limited to the Bjork-Shiley valve. This important complication occurred within 4.5 years of operation in 12% of patients receiving a mitral Bjork-Shiley prosthesis.[K2] It may occur at any time postoperatively and seems *more* likely to occur very late postoperatively. Sudden cessation of anticoagulation or suboptimal long-term anticoagulant programs no doubt contribute to the occurrence of the problem. The Starr-Edwards silastic ball valve prosthesis may have a slightly higher proportion of late deaths from thromboembolism than do the other devices.

The stent-mounted xenograft bioprosthesis has as its special cause of death valve degeneration, usually with the development of stenosis from calcification, incompetence from cusp rupture, or both. The data of Lipson and colleagues indicate that early postoperatively in patients averaging 53 years of age, the average heterograft bioprosthetic orifice size was 2.2 cm² (with a mean valve gradient at rest of 6 mmHg) but that by 9 years after operation, orifice size has been reduced to 1.7 cm² ($P < .01$).[L7] Usually, these changes are recognized and lead to valve re-replacement rather than death, but degeneration is a disadvantage of the porcine het-

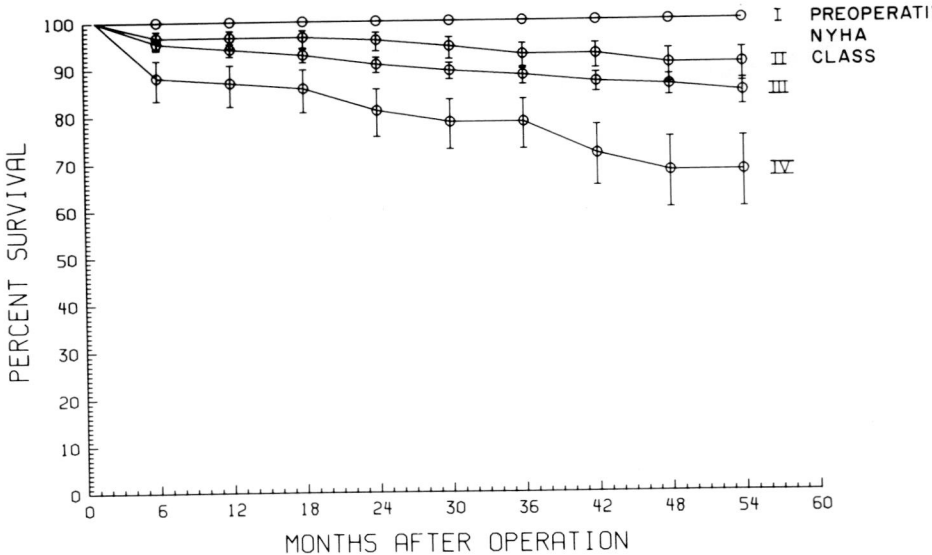

Figure 11-14 The representation is as in Figure 11-12 except that the actuarial survival rate has been separately calculated for each preoperative NYHA functional class.

Reproduced with permission from Karp et al.[K2]

erograft valve (and the Ionescu-Shiley stent-mounted bovine pericardial valve as well). Some of the factors in this degeneration process are becoming known, and perhaps related to this is a suggestion in the analyses of the Henry Ford Hospital experience that this complication is less frequent in the valves processed in recent years than in those processed earlier.[M11] Certainly this complication develops more rapidly in younger patients (Fig. 11-16), probably because of their higher calcium turnover.[S5] About 40% of patients less than

21 years of age at the time of insertion require reoperation within 4 years, compared to 13% of those over that age (Fig. 11-17). In the group less than 21 years of age, only 40% are event free 4 years after valve replacement (Fig. 11-18). About 35% of patients less than 30 years of age required reoperation within 5 years (Fig. 11-19).[W1] Magilligan finds in the current analysis of the Henry Ford experience that 50% of porcine valves have failed within 9 years in patients less than 35 years of age at the time of insertion, compared to

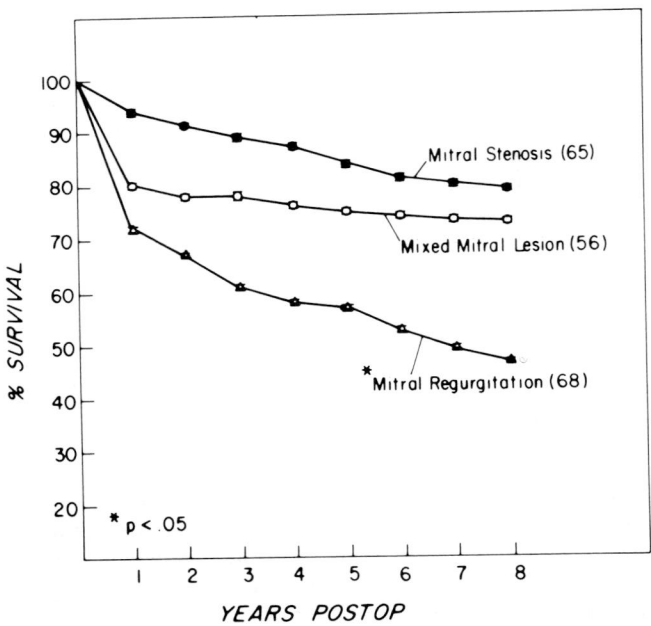

Figure 11-15 Late survival rate after mitral valve replacement, based on preoperative functional valve lesion.

Reproduced with permission from Chaffin et al.[C5]

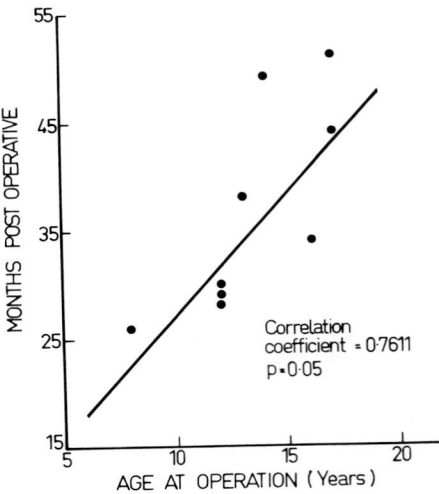

Figure 11-16 A correlation between age at bioprosthetic valve insertion and the time interval before its removal by reoperation in nine patients less than 21 years of age at the time of insertion of a mitral porcine bioprosthesis with or without associated cardiac procedures (GLH). The probability that the line of best fit is significantly different from a line of zero slope is .05.

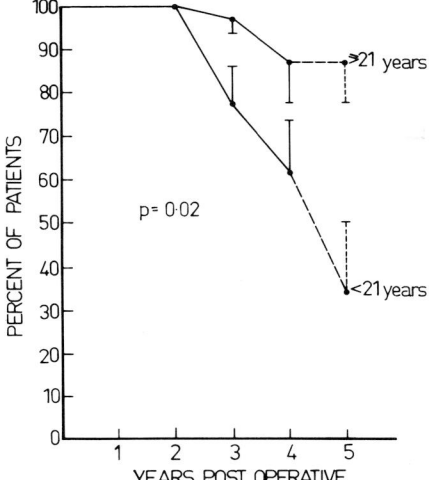

Figure 11-17 Actuarial reoperation rates (expressed as percent of patients free of reoperation) after valve replacement in relationship to age at operation. The series includes other simultaneous cardiac surgery, including aortic valve replacement. The bars represent the standard error in one direction (equivalent to the 70% confidence limits) (GLH; 1976–1980).

10% in patients over this age.[M11] Premature valve degeneration leads not only to unsatisfactory valve function and reoperation but also to premature late death (Fig. 11-18).

Symptomatic Results

Symptoms are lessened and functional capacity is significantly increased in most patients after mitral valve replacement. Thus, in those receiving Bjork-Shiley or heterograft valves, about 75% of patients preoperatively in NYHA class III or IV improved to class I or II after recovery from operation.[K2,W1]

The symptomatic and functional status over time has not been described actuarially to our knowledge. Clearly, however, some patients have striking symptomatic improvement for some years and then gradually again develop important symptoms and disability in spite of good function of the device inserted. This sequence is usually the result of the progression of a secondary cardiomyopathy that was present before operation or the progression of other valve lesions. This deterioration can also result from prosthesis complications.

Hemodynamic State

A transvalvar end-diastolic gradient is present in most patients after valve replacement,[G3,H6,J1] and the magnitude of the gradient depends on the patient's size and physical activity (that is, on the cardiac output at rest and during exercise), the size of the device inserted, and the type of device. When a device *larger* than the 29-mm size can be used, gradients are small. However, when a 29-mm, 27-mm or 25-mm device is used, gradients are nearly always present (Table 11-18). Zero pressure fixation techniques[B30] may improve the performance of the porcine valve in the future by making the leaflets more pliable.

In spite of these gradients, the function of the left atrioven-

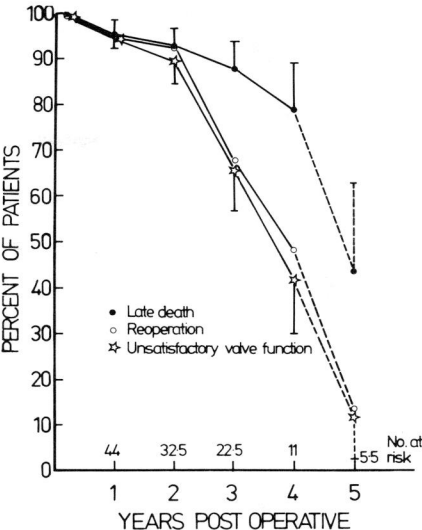

Figure 11-18 Cumulative complication-free rates depicting freedom from events (late death, reoperation, and unsatisfactory valve function) of patients under 21 years of age following mitral valve replacement with a porcine bioprosthetic valve. The series includes other simultaneous cardiac surgery, including aortic valve replacement. The number of patients at risk at each interval is noted. The bars represent the standard error in one direction (GLH; 1976–1979).

tricular valve is usually greatly improved after mitral valve replacement. Thus, to the extent allowed by left ventricular performance (see below), many favorable secondary effects occur. Left atrial pressure is reduced, cardiac output, both at rest and during exercise, is generally increased,[H6] and *pulmonary artery pressure* and pulmonary vascular resistance are decreased both early and late postoperatively.[H6]

Left Ventricular Function: Mitral Stenosis

Preoperatively, most patients with mitral stenosis have normal left ventricular function and ejection fractions[H13] but do not increase their cardiac output under stress, such as when left ventricular afterload is acutely reduced by the infusion of sodium nitroprusside.[B24] These findings support the idea that the major cause of chronically reduced cardiac output in these patients is obstructive mitral stenosis.[B24,H3,H12] However, some patients with mitral stenosis preoperatively have minor posterobasal regional wall contraction abnormalities, perhaps from a rigid mitral valve complex.[H3] As a group, the patients tend to have relatively normal left ventricular ejection fraction, volumes (end-diastolic and end-systolic diameters), and wall thickness. This state continues into the late postoperative period.[S6]

A small proportion of patients with apparently isolated mitral stenosis, usually older ones, have significantly reduced ejection fractions.[B24,C11] Such patients have severe posterobasal segmented wall contraction abnormalities,[H3] sometimes anterolateral segmental contraction abnormalities, and occasionally diffuse hypokinesis.[B24,C11,H14] The anterolateral segmental contraction abnormalities may be due to papillary muscle scarring and immobilization. Diffuse hypokinesis may result from scarring and decreased left ven-

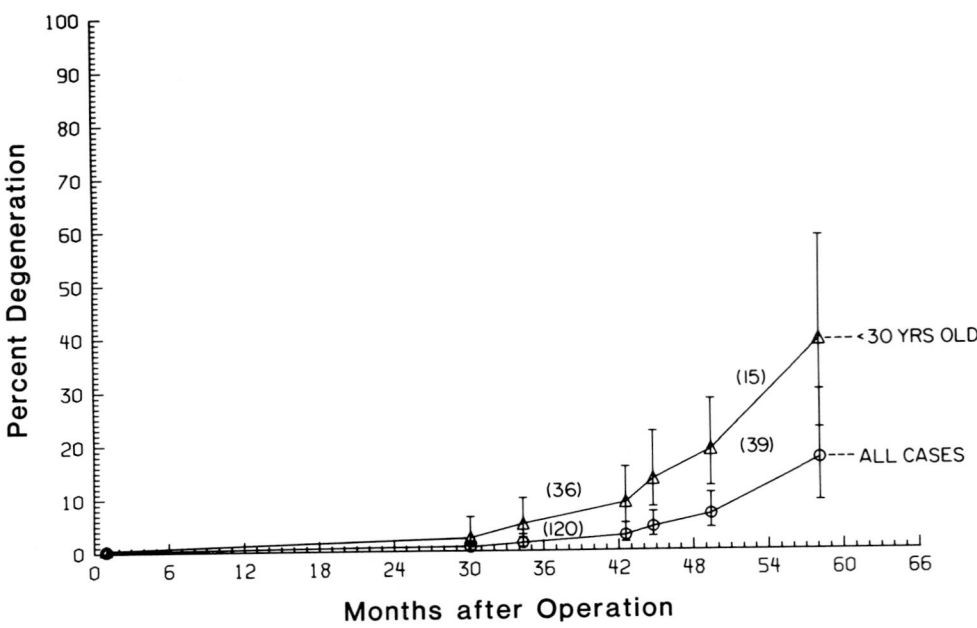

Figure 11-19 Actuarial incidence of hemodynamically important degeneration, in bioprostheses use or for aortic and/or mitral replacements, in all patients and in those less than 30 years old at the time of implantation. Vertical bars represent 70% confidence limits.
Reproduced with permission from Williams et al.[W1]

tricular compliance, secondary to chronic low cardiac output and low coronary blood flow. The response of the left ventricle of such patients to corrective mitral valve surgery has not been defined clearly, although cardiac index increases and left atrial and pulmonary artery pressure decrease in response to the acute surgical reduction of the mitral valve gradient.

Left Ventricular Function: Mitral Incompetence
The sudden ablation of mitral incompetence by mitral valve replacement triggers a particularly complex response.[K4,R5] To a considerable degree, the complexity is related to the fact that left ventricular afterload (see Chapter 5, footnote 10) is reduced in patients with mitral incompetence by the ejection of part of the left ventricular stroke volume into the low pressure left atrium.[B13,E1,U1] As a result, the left ventricle becomes small and thick walled very early during systole in this situation, and this sequence contributes to the reduced afterload through the reduction in wall stress, in part from the more favorable relationships in the Laplace's law that result.[B36,H2] Because of this, the symptoms remain mild in many patients with long-standing mitral incompetence and markedly enlarged hearts, and left ventricular ejection fraction is maintained by and is dependent on the abrupt reduction in afterload early in systole. Indeed, the ejection fraction can even increase during exercise.[P2] Left ventricular contractility is nonetheless often reduced preoperatively,[E1] but this is masked by the afterload-reducing effect of the mitral incompetence. Thus, unless ejection fraction is greater than 0.65–0.7 preoperatively in patients with mitral incompetence, it cannot be concluded that left ventricular contractility is normal.[E1]

After valve replacement for mitral incompetence, left ventricular afterload is suddenly increased, and ejection fraction is reduced in most patients (Fig. 11-20).[B12,P5,R5,S6] However, the response is dependent to some extent on the preoperative state of the left ventricle. If the ventricle is normal, such as in acute experimental regurgitation, the sudden correction of mitral incompetence immediately increases forward cardiac output, in spite of an increased afterload.[S16] In patients in whom the left ventricle is more than moderately enlarged by the time of operation (with an echocardiographically determined end-diastolic diameter greater than 7 cm or an end-systolic diameter greater than 5 cm[S6]), a condition no doubt accompanied by decreased left ventricular contractility and increased myocardial degenerative changes,[A6,F1] ejection fraction is markedly reduced 2 weeks after valve replacement and usually continues to deteriorate still further in the last postoperative period. In such patients, left ventricular size is usually reduced early postoperatively (end-diastolic volume is less,[B12,S6] end-systolic volume is about the same[B12,S6]). However, late postoperatively (6–12 months after operation) left ventricular size again *increases* in most patients.[B12,S6] Left ventricular wall hypertrophy does not regress.[S6] In such patients, not only do the preoperative left ventricular structural and contractile abnormalities not regress after valve replacement, but in fact they *progress* and account for many of the recurrences of symptoms 2–5 years postoperatively and many of the deaths 2–10 years after operation.

When preoperative left ventricular enlargement is only mild or moderate (with an end-diastolic diameter of 7.0 cm or less and an end-systolic diameter of 5.0 cm or less, as determined by echocardiography[S6]), ejection fraction again is re-

Table 11-18 Hemodynamic conditions after the insertion of various mitral valve replacement devices in adults.

Devices and Standard Values	Diastolic LA → LV Gradient (mmHg)		Effective Orifice Area (cm²)		Effective Orifice Area Index (cm²·m⁻²)	
	Rest	Exercise	Rest	Exercise	Rest	Exercise
25 mm Devices[B33,C15,H16,L7,L8,M9,S5,S14]						
Bjork-Shiley[a]	4					
St. Jude[a]	1 (2)	6.2 (2)	2.1 (2)	2.3 (2)	1.2 (2)	1.3 (2)
Standard orifice Hancock heterograft valve[b]	12 (8)		1.76 (12)		1.95 (2)	
Ionescu-Shiley heterograft pericardium[a]	9 (4)		1.35 (4)			
27 mm Devices[B33,C15,C16,G3,H16,H17,J1,L7,L8,N4,P6,S5,S15]						
Bjork-Shiley[a]	6					
St. Jude[a]	3 (12)	3 (10)	2.1 (5)	3.6 (10)	1.4 (5)	2.3 (10)
Starr-Edwards 6120 (2M)[b]	8 (40)	12.0 (9)	1.68 (25)	2.15 (4)		
Standard orifice Hancock heterograft valve[b]	9 (10)	24 (2)	1.46 (7)		1.40 (2)	
Carpentier-Edwards heterograft valve[b]	7 (3)	20.0 (2)	1.68 (3)	2.42 (2)	1.13 (3)	1.64 (2)
Ionescu-Shiley heterograft pericardium[a]	6 (8)		1.33 (13)			
29 mm Devices[B33,C15,G3,H9,H16,H17,J1,L7,L9,N4,P6,S5,S14,S15]						
Bjork-Shiley Standard[a]	4 (26)	10 (26)	1.85 (20)	4 (20)		
St. Jude[a]	2 (48)	7 (8)	2.92 (41)	3.32 (25)	1.8 (16)	
Starr-Edwards 6120 (3M = 28 mm)[b]	7 (28)		1.65 (14)			
Standard orifice Hancock heterograft valve[a]	5 (43)	14 (2)	2.20 (60)		1.37 (3)	
Carpentier-Edwards heterograft valve[b]	3 (13)		3.0 (13)			
Ionescu-Shiley heterograft pericardium[a]	5 (7)		1.35 (11)			
Standard Values						
Normal			4–6		3	
Severe stenosis	> 12		< 1		< 0.6	
Desired postoperative value	< 10	< 15	> 1.5		> 0.9	

KEY: LA → LV, left atrium to left ventricle.

NOTE: The numbers in parentheses are the total numbers of patients observed.

[a] Acceptable devices.

[b] Devices of borderline acceptability.

duced early and late after operation but is usually still within the normal range (Fig. 11-21). In only 2 (with values of 0.43 and 0.49) of 12 such patients studied by Schuler and colleagues was it less than 0.5.[S6] The left ventricular enlargement also regresses after operation, both end-diastolic and end-systolic diameters returning to normal (Fig. 11-22).[B12,S6] Left ventricular wall hypertrophy regresses toward normal. Thus, structural left ventricular wall abnormalities regress at least to some extent and more or less permanently after mitral valve replacement for mitral incompetence, provided they had not become severe by the time of operation, and in this group, left ventricular contractility is probably normal or near normal preoperatively and remains so after operation.[K3,S6]

Thromboembolism

About 90% of patients are free of major or minor thromboembolic complications 5 years after mitral valve replacement, and this proportion is about the same in patients receiving the Bjork-Shiley prosthesis[K2] and on anticoagulation as in those receiving the stent-mounted heterograft, only a few of which were on long-term anticoagulation.[W1] Thus Dalby and colleagues have noted a similar thromboembolic rate in anticoagulated patients receiving a prosthetic device (in their case Starr-Edwards ball valve prosthesis) and in those receiving a stent-mounted heterograft without long-term anticoagulation.[D3] In Starr's recent experience, 95% of patients receiving this device were free of thromboembolic complications 5 years postoperatively.[T4] However, Miller

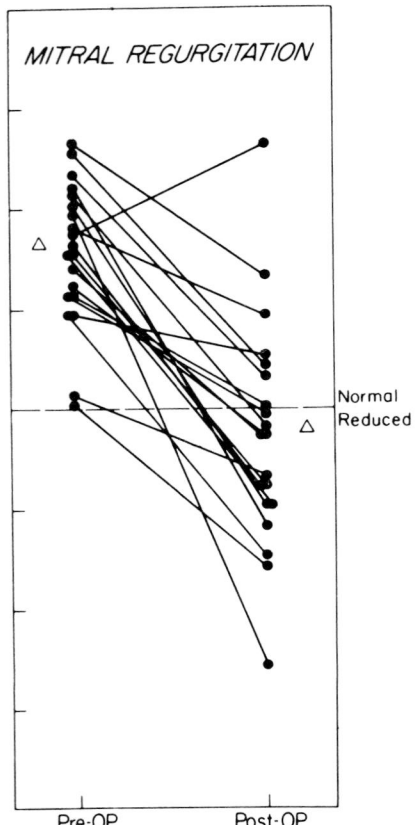

Figure 11-20 Ventricular systolic function (expressed as ejection fraction) before and early after mitral valve replacement for mitral incompetence. Individual values are shown, and mean values are expressed by Δ. After operation, nine patients with mitral regurgitation had an ejection fraction below normal. The lower limit of normal (0.50) is represented by a broken line.
Reproduced with permission from Boucher et al.[B12]

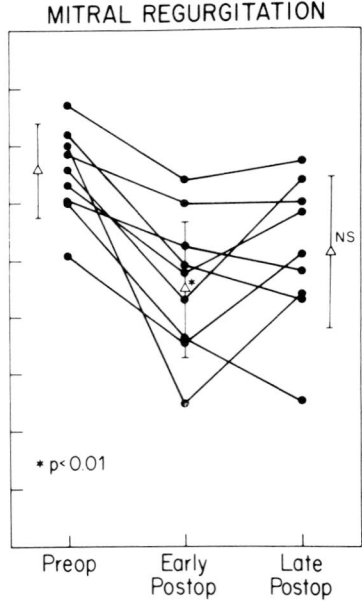

Figure 11-21 The representation is as in Figure 11-20 but shows only the nine patients with mitral regurgitation who also had late postoperative scans. Mean values (Δ) ±1 standard deviation are shown. In these patients, the mean ejection fraction decreased early postoperatively ($P < .01$) and did not change significantly between the early and late postoperative scans.
NS, not significant.
Reproduced with permission from Boucher et al.[B12]

and colleagues report a higher incidence of thromboembolic complications, only 55% of patients with the Starr Edwards model 6120 prosthesis being free of thromboembolism at 10 years.[M8] Borkon and colleagues found 87% of patients receiving the Hancock stent-mounted heterograft free of thromboembolic complications 5 years after operation.[B19] In other reports, the proportion free of thromboembolism has been a little lower (about 80%–85%).[B7,L1,M2] In general, about one-fourth of the thromboembolic events are *fatal* ones.[K2] The risk of thromboembolism does not seem to decrease with time.[K2]

The probability of having a late thromboembolic complication may be increased by older age ($P = .15$, UAB) and by the presence of atrial fibrillation.[H7,W1]

Acute Thrombotic Occlusion
The actuarial incidence of acute thrombotic occlusion in patients receiving Bjork-Shiley valves in the mitral position[K2] has been 13% at 4.5 years (CL 5%–27%) Fig. 11-23). The episode was a fatal one in 80% of these patients. The Starr-Edwards model 6120 ball valve prosthesis is not without this

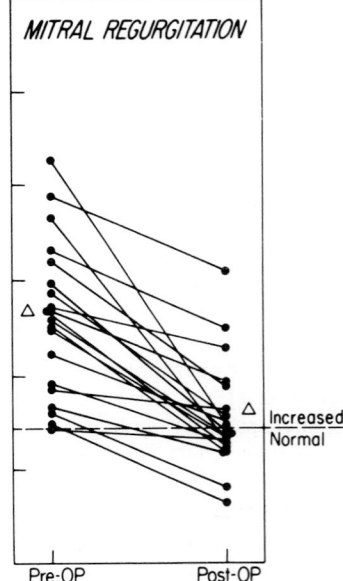

Figure 11-22 The representation is as in Figure 11-20 but shows end-diastolic volume. Preoperatively, end-diastolic volume was above the range of normal in all but one patient. Postoperatively, it decreased in all patients, becoming normal in 11 patients. The upper limit of normal (72 ml/m²) is represented by a broken line.
Reproduced with permission from Boucher et al.[B12]

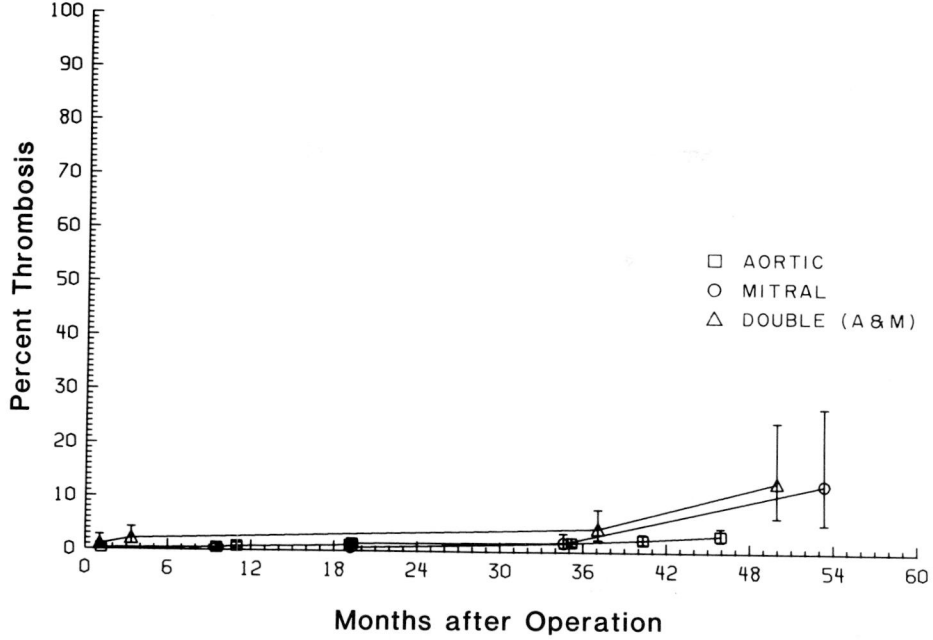

Figure 11-23 Actuarial incidence of acute valve thrombosis for aortic, mitral, and double valve replacement with the Bjork-Shiley prosthesis. The number of valves inserted was 643. Reproduced with permission from Karp et al.[K2]

complication, but it is much less frequent than with the Bjork-Shiley valve.[M8]

Acute thrombotic occlusion occurs primarily but not exclusively in patients in whom anticoagulant therapy is suboptimal. It produces such a characteristic clinical syndrome that upon its appearance emergency operation should be advised *without* the delay inherent in performing special studies.[C7] With such a program, many such patients may survive.[C7]

Patients with this catastrophic complication usually become symptomatic only 1–3 days before admission and present principally with extreme dyspnea and orthopnea. The patient may have noticed a decrease in the intensity of the prosthetic valve sounds at about the time symptoms began. Important chest pain is experienced by many. Signs of shock are usually present. Although incompetence is often present, an apical systolic murmur is rarely heard. Although the fluoroscopic finding of limited disc movement supports the diagnosis, an echocardiogram is said to be diagnostic.[B18] Cardiac catheterization usually gives conclusive evidence of mitral obstruction, but the patient may be too ill to allow this to be done.

Complications of Long-Term Anticoagulation
By 5 years after operation, actuarially about 95% of patients on long-term anticoagulant therapy after valve replacement are free of a major anticoagulant complication, but only about 50% are free of a major or *minor* one (Fig. 11-24).[K2] In Starr's recent experience, bleeding as a complication of long-term coagulation occurred at a rate of 4.4% per patient year.[T4] No late deaths have been attributed to this by Karp and colleagues.[K2]

Prosthetic Valve Endocarditis
An uncommon complication of mitral valve replacement, prosthetic valve endocarditis, is nevertheless very serious, as over half the patients developing it ultimately die as a result.[D2,I2] This condition strongly predisposes the patient to periprosthetic leakage.[D2] When prosthetic valve endocarditis appears within 3–6 months of operation, it is probably related to events in the operating room.[I2] When it develops later than that, it is probably from a new transient bacteremia.

Infection in mitral prostheses behaves in general as does infection in aortic replacement devices (prosthetic valve endocarditis is discussed in detail in Chapter 12).

Periprosthetic Leakage
The incidence of periprosthetic leakage in uninfected patients approaches zero when the suture techniques described in this chapter are used.[D2] When the continuous suture line is made with 00 (rather than 0) polypropylene, the risk of dehiscence is increased to about 10% within 4 years of operation.[D2] Preoperative infectious endocarditis increases the risk of mitral prosthesis dehiscence.[R17] Annular calcification also increases somewhat the risk of periprosthetic leakage.[D2] In an era in which various suture techniques were used (1975–July 1979) 13 (2.9%, CL 2.1%–3.9%) of 452 patients required reoperation for periprosthetic leakage (UAB).

Chronic Hemolysis
Well-functioning stent-mounted heterografts and homografts produce little or no chronic hemolysis.[A2] The Bjork-Shiley prosthesis in the mitral position produces, on the average, very mild or no chronic hemolysis. Ahmad and colleagues

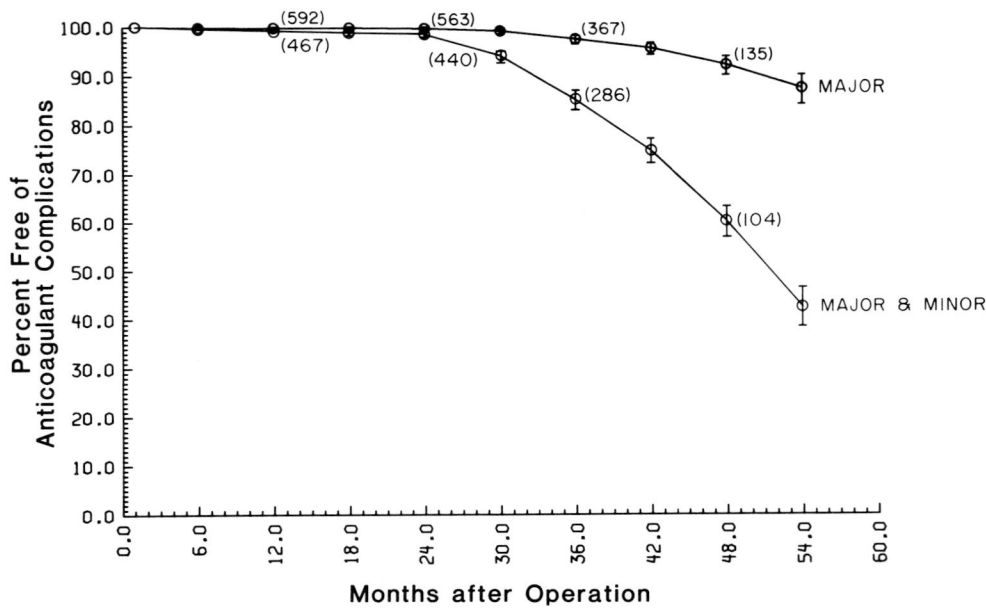

Figure 11-24 Complications of anticoagulants in patients receiving aortic and/or mitral Bjork-Shiley prostheses. A major complication is one requiring hospitalization and/or transfusions. Reproduced with permission from Karp et al.[K2]

found that 35% of patients with this device had mild chronic hemolysis, with red cell half-life of 21–25 days (normal 27 ± 3 days, severe reduction less than 15 days), serum lactate dehydrogenase (LDH) less than 400 IU per liter at 25°C (normal 50–200), hemosiderinuria low or absent, serum haptoglobin normal (50–250 mg · dl^{-1}), schistocytes less than 10 per 1,000 red cells (normal), and reticulocytes less than 3% (normal 0.2–2%).[A2] One patient had severe chronic hemolysis without obvious cause. Very similar results are reported by Slater and colleagues.[S11]

The Starr-Edwards silastic ball, non–cloth-covered valve model 6120 is said to produce only mild chronic hemolysis.[L1] In contrast, with the *composite seat* Starr-Edwards mitral prosthesis (model 6310), 65% of patients have mild or moderate hemolysis, and only 15% are without some hemolysis.

When periprosthetic leakage is present, hemolysis may be severe with any device, the red cell trauma and fragmentation being extreme under these circumstances. An unusually small mechanical prosthesis also may result in severe hemolysis.[N2]

Pulmonary Vascular Resistance
Pulmonary artery pressure is elevated preoperatively in many patients with mitral stenosis or mitral incompetence. This is the combined result of simple back pressure from an elevated left atrial pressure, and of elevated pulmonary vascular resistance. The latter may have both a dynamic element, immediately reduced by reducing left atrial pressure,[D4] and an organic element from pulmonary vascular disease, which may or may not slowly regress after operation.

When even severe pulmonary hypertension is present pre-operatively, it will very likely regress toward normal after mitral valve replacement (Fig. 11-25). Kaul and colleagues reported on 30 patients with average preoperative pulmonary artery pressures of 110 mmHg systolic and 74 mmHg mean.[K5] Their symptomatic improvement was striking. Restudy an average of 5.5 years after mitral valve replacement showed average systolic pulmonary artery pressure to be 48 mmHg and mean to be 31 mmHg. This fall often occurs soon after valve replacement, and thus it seems related largely to sudden reduction of left atrial pressure and to reversal of the severe spastic pulmonary vasoconstriction that accompanies left atrial hypertension in some patients (Fig. 11-26).[B16] Although this initial reduction appears rapidly in most patients,[D4] pulmonary vascular resistance sometimes continues to fall further in the months after operation. The changes are similar, whether the operation was done for stenosis or incompetence.[B16]

Summary
The complex spectrum of late results is summarized actuarially in a 5-year follow-up (Fig. 11-27). The overall survival rate was 71.5% (late death occurred in 28.5% of the patients), with 88% of the surviving patients free of reoperation, 97.5% free of embolization, 99% free of endocarditis and hemorrhage, and 99% free of important hemorrhagic problems. The cumulative incidence of event-free survival was 56% (± 7.7). When patients under 21 years of age are excluded (Fig. 11-28), there is a marked reduction in the proportions needing reoperation, related to the less rapid deterioration of porcine heterografts in older patients. The late death rate is also reduced, and the incidence of event-free survival rises to 67% (± 7%).

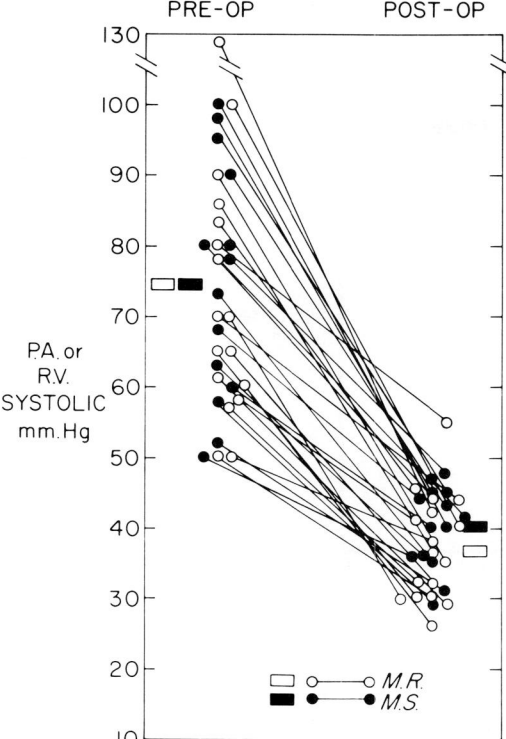

Figure 11-25 Comparison of preoperative and postoperative pulmonary arterial (PA) or right ventricular (RV) systolic pressures in patients with predominant mitral regurgitation (MR) and mitral stenosis (MS). The horizontal bars represent the mean values in each group.

Reprinted from Braunwald et al. by permission of *The New England Journal of Medicine*, 273:509, 1965.[B16]

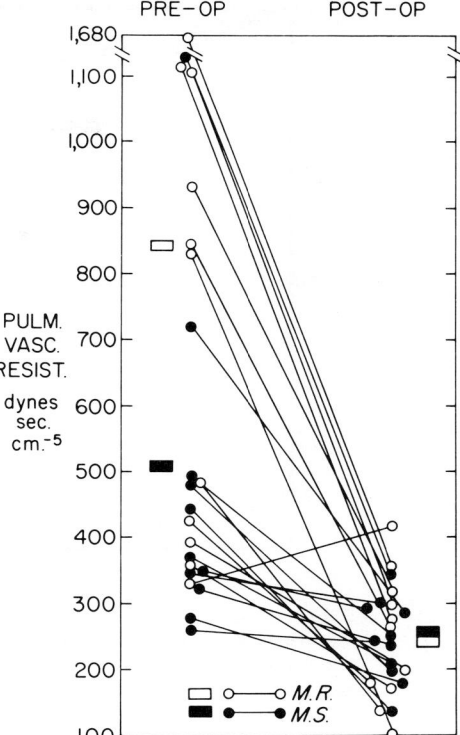

Figure 11-26 The representation is as in Figure 11-25 but shows pulmonary vascular resistance (pulm. vasc. resist.).

Reprinted from Braunwald et al. by permission of *The New England Journal of Medicine*, 273:509, 1965.[B16]

Mitral Valve Surgery in Patients with Tricuspid Disease

Incidence of Tricuspid Surgery

In the recent era (Table 11-5), 35 (9.9%, CL 8.3%–11.8%) of 353 patients undergoing primary mitral replacement also underwent tricuspid annuloplasty, and 2 (0.6%, CL 0.2%–13.4%) underwent tricuspid replacement for rheumatic stenosis and incompetence (UAB). Further, 38 (14%, CL 12%–17%) of 262 patients undergoing isolated mitral valve replacement (primary and repeated operation, including other cardiac surgery) underwent simultaneous tricuspid valve annuloplasty, and 9 (3.4%, CL 2.3%–5%) underwent tricuspid valve replacement (GLH). Of 154 patients undergoing open mitral commissurotomy, 13 (8%, CL 6%–11%) required tricuspid valve surgery, only 1 (0.6%, CL 0.1%–2% of 154) of whom required it for tricuspid stenosis (GLH).[S10] A somewhat higher incidence (22.3%, CL 20.7%–23.9%) of tricuspid valve surgery is reported by Boyd and colleagues,[B21] whose paper suggests that their indications were more liberal. A proportion similar to that at GLH and UAB was reported in the combined Madrid-Montreal experience.[G4]

Prognosis of Surgically Untreated Tricuspid Incompetence

Patients with functional tricuspid incompetence secondary to mitral valve disease who do *not* undergo repair of the incompetence at the time of mitral valve surgery have a variable course late postoperatively.[B23] Probably depending in part on the surgeon's indication for not repairing the tricuspid valve at the original mitral valve operation, 6% (CL 4%–9%)[S10] to 35%[S13] (CL 23%–49%) have moderate or severe incompetence late postoperatively. In most of these patients, the tricuspid incompetence is a persistence of that present preoperatively, but in a few it is a worsening of that present preoperatively in spite of surgically improved mitral valve function. This may be due in part to the presence of organic rheumatic tricuspid leaflet damage combined with a marked increase in cardiac output in those patients whose cardiac output preoperatively was limited by the mitral rather than the tricuspid lesion.

Experimental work by Tsakiris and colleagues, at the Mayo Clinic, has shown that perfect tricuspid leaflet closure in systole depends on proper systolic shortening in the circumference of the tricuspid anulus.[T1,T5] Simon and colleagues have shown a considerable increase postoperatively in systolic shortening in those patients whose tricuspid incompetence lessens after mitral valve surgery and no change in those in whom it persists or worsens.[S13]

The incremental risk factors for persisting or worsening

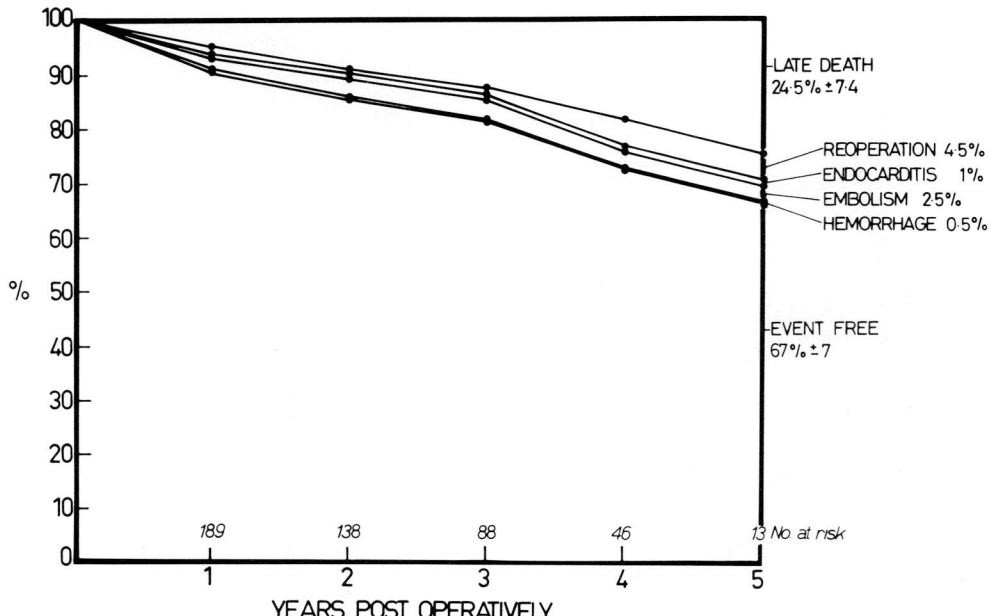

Figure 11-27 Cumulative complication-free rates in 245 hospital survivors of mitral valve replacement with prosthetic valves (45% of patients) and porcine bioprostheses (55% of patients) with or without tricuspid valve surgery. Only the patients with prosthetic valves received long-term anticoagulation therapy. The patients include those with first operations or reoperations, and those with other simultaneous cardiac procedures except surgery on the aortic valve, a left ventricular aneurysm, or an ascending aortic aneurysm. The ± indicates the standard error (GLH; 1976–1979).

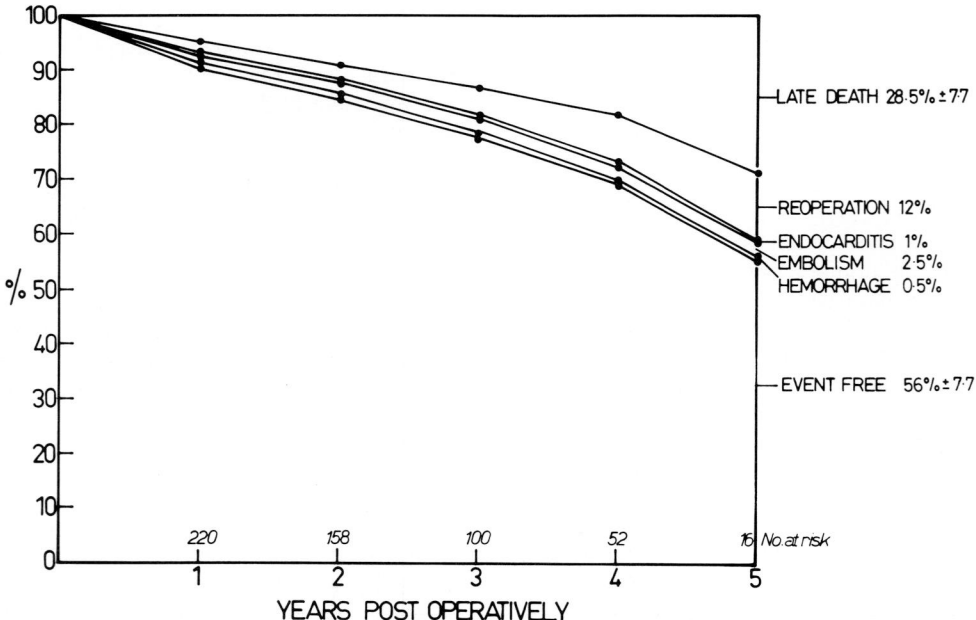

Figure 11-28 Cumulative complication-free rates, as in Figure 11-27 but excluding patients under 21 years of age. The numbers of patients at risk are noted. The proportions are given ± standard error (essentially the 70% confidence limits) (GLH; 1976–1979).

tricuspid incompetence after mitral valve repair or replacement *without surgery* to the tricuspid valve are several:

1. Persistent or recurrent mitral disease predisposes the patient to tricuspid incompetence. Thus, four of the five patients requiring subsequent tricuspid valve surgery late after open commissurotomy also required mitral valve replacement (GLH).

2. The more severe the unrepaired tricuspid incompetence, the more likely it is to persist or increase late after mitral valve surgery. Thus, tricuspid incompetence judged mild at operation rarely persists or progresses after adequate mitral valve surgery, whereas moderate or severe incompetence may do so.[B22]

3. Long-standing and perhaps irreversible right ventricular enlargement, secondary to mitral or pulmonary vascular disease, probably predisposes the patient to persistent tricuspid incompetence. Such situations probably interfere with systolic shortening of the tricuspid anulus. Thus, tricuspid incompetence that does not disappear promptly with intensive decongestive treatment preoperatively and is therefore fixed, rather than variable, is more likely to persist late postoperatively if not repaired.[C10]

4. Organic tricuspid incompetence (usually associated with some stenosis) is more likely to persist than is functional incompetence.

Thus, when Duran and colleagues ignored functional tricuspid incompetence present at the time of mitral valve surgery, tricuspid incompetence was absent late postoperatively in 8 (100%, CL 79%–100%) of 8 patients with low pulmonary vascular resistance postoperatively but in none (0%, CL 9%–19%) of 9 with high pulmonary vascular resistance late postoperatively ($P < .0001$).[D7] In all, Duran and colleagues found untreated functional tricuspid incompetence to disappear in 8 (47%, CL 32%–62%) of 17 patients undergoing mitral valve surgery. In contrast, they found ignored *organic* tricuspid incompetence to disappear in 0 (0%, CL 0%–13%) of 14 patients undergoing mitral valve surgery ($P = .003$).[D7]

Results of Tricuspid Repair or Replacement
Chapter 14 contains a full discussion of the results of tricuspid valve repair and replacement.

INDICATIONS FOR OPERATION
Mitral Stenosis

When the opening snap is prominent and when calcification cannot be demonstrated fluoroscopically, good results from mitral commissurotomy can usually be obtained. Under these circumstances, moderate symptoms (NYHA functional class II) and evidence of severe mitral stenosis are indications for operation. Particularly in young women, one acute episode of important paroxysmal nocturnal dyspnea or pulmonary edema in the presence of at least moderate mitral stenosis is an indication for operation when commis-

surotomy is very likely the operation that will be done. Surgical intervention is indicated particularly before the onset of atrial fibrillation.[S10] Operation is also advisable whenever there is a significant increase in pulmonary vascular resistance, even in the absence of symptoms. Even asymptomatic patients with multiple episodes of arterial emboli are advised to undergo operation if commissurotomy seems very likely.

When a mitral valve replacement seems likely (because of absence of an opening snap, heavy mitral valve calcification, severe subvalvar disease,[A3] previous commissurotomy, or associated mitral incompetence), a more symptomatic state is demanded as the indication for operation, because of the added long-term imponderables introduced by the device inserted. Therefore, more severe chronic symptoms (NYHA functional class III) or several acute episodes of symptoms of pulmonary venous hypertension are required as indications for operation.

Advanced disability, associated tricuspid valve disease, and associated coronary artery disease are not contraindications to operation, nor is severe pulmonary hypertension.

Mitral Incompetence

The decision about operation is often more difficult in patients with mitral incompetence than in those with mitral stenosis because (1) prediction of repair rather than replacement is made with less certainty, and (2) only mild symptoms may coexist with long-standing disease and gradually deteriorating left ventricular function. Thus, whereas in mitral stenosis the diagnosis and symptoms are generally all that is needed for decision making, in mitral incompetence, special attention must also be paid to the status of the left ventricle.

In patients with chronic mitral incompetence and in NYHA functional class I or II, left ventricular enlargement *less* than grade 3 (on the basis of 1–6, 6 being extreme enlargement)—as judged primarily by physical examination, chest roentgenogram, and echocardiogram—supports advice to continue nonsurgical treatment. When in this clinical setting the left ventricular enlargement is grade 3 or more, the secondary left ventricular cardiomyopathy of mitral incompetence has usually become prominent, portending its progression to an irreversible state. Operation is then advisable even in the absence of disabling symptoms. The role of left atrial enlargement per se in decision making is uncertain. It is likely that more than moderate left atrial dilatation has a deleterious effect after valve replacement, and its presence therefore argues in favor of operation.

When the patient is in NYHA functional class III or IV because of mitral incompetence, operation is clearly indicated. Currently, even advanced disability is not a contraindication to operation, although it is recognized that the secondary left ventricular cardiomyopathy associated with and in part responsible for this state has a deleterious effect on the early and late results of operation. The natural history without operation is even worse.

The decision about operation is somewhat more difficult in patients with acute mitral incompetence from nonischemic chordal rupture. If the symptoms of pulmonary venous hypertension come promptly under control by medical management (as is often the case), operation should be deferred and the patient reevaluated at frequent intervals (see "Natural History"). Thereafter, the criteria used in chronic mitral incompetence apply. However, if the holosystolic murmur radiates into the aortic area and the neck and there is other evidence that the ruptured chordae are to the posterior leaflet, the indications for operation should be somewhat liberalized by the knowledge that a reparative operation (rather than valve replacement) can probably be done.

When mitral incompetence develops acutely as a result of native valve bacterial endocarditis, the situation is similar. If symptoms are initially mild or moderate and come under good control, together with the infection, continuing in-hospital medical treatment is indicated. However, surveillance must be close, because rapid progression in the severity of the incompetence is possible. If this is suspected, operation is urgently indicated before hemodynamic deterioration occurs. Acute pulmonary edema, paroxysmal nocturnal dyspnea, or rising BUN or creatinine levels are an indication for urgent operation. Systemic embolization during treatment or continuing activity of infection in spite of intense antibiotic treatment also indicate the probable need for operation.

Mitral Valve Disease with Tricuspid Incompetence

Operation is rarely advised primarily for tricuspid incompetence, but often repair of the tricuspid incompetence must be considered at operation. The decision for or against repair can be a difficult one to make. One reason is that estimation of the presence and magnitude of the tricuspid incompetence preoperatively and intraoperatively is difficult. Fournier and colleagues,[F4] Carpentier,[C10] and Duran[D7] have emphasized their view that digital estimation at operation, with a finger through the right atrial appendage, is unreliable in determining this. However, information of some value can be obtained in this manner if (1) care is taken to assure a good hemodynamic state when the observation is made, (2) the observer is experienced in detecting the relatively low-velocity and thus difficult-to-feel regurgitant stream of tricuspid incompetence, and (3) it is recognized that the presence and degree of tricuspid incompetence is quite variable with time in a given patient. Another reason this decision is difficult is variability in the late results of ignoring the tricuspid incompetence at the time of mitral valve surgery (see "Prognosis of Surgically Untreated Tricuspid Incompetence" in section on Late Results).

The patient should come to the operating room after a careful preoperative evaluation over a period of time. Tricuspid annuloplasty is generally not indicated when tricuspid incompetence is variable preoperatively and is absent during periods of good medical control of heart failure, organic tricuspid disease is excluded by digital examination of the valve at operation, a good repair or replacement can be done for the mitral disease, and pulmonary vascular resistance is low. Usually the surgeon finds no or grade 1, 2, or 3 tricuspid incompetence (grade 6 being severe) by digital examination at surgery under these circumstances. If the incompetence is more severe under these circumstances, annuloplasty is indicated. When the tricuspid incompetence

has been important and constant preoperatively, repair at surgery is indicated, as has been stressed by Carpentier.[C10] Usually under these circumstances, the surgeon finds tricuspid incompetence greater than grade 3 by digital examination, and the left-sided disease is long-standing, with the possibility of irreversible left ventricular dysfunction. When organic (rheumatic) tricuspid disease is present, it virtually always requires repair (or, uncommonly, replacement).

In any case, if tricuspid incompetence has been left unrepaired, right atrial pressure is the same or higher than left immediately after cardiopulmonary bypass (CPB), and the tricuspid incompetence is assessed digitally as grade 3 or more, tricuspid annuloplasty is indicated *if* temporary acute right ventricular dysfunction (usually from right coronary air embolization) can be excluded. This exclusion is made by resuming CPB; a vasoconstrictor (see Chapter 4) is then given to assure a normal arterial blood pressure, the heart is "unloaded," and CPB is continued for 5–10 minutes. CPB is then discontinued, and if unrepaired important tricuspid incompetence persists and right atrial pressure is the same as or greater than left (indicating that the right ventricular performance, not the left, is the limiting factor), tricuspid valve repair should be done.

CHOICE OF THE REPLACEMENT DEVICE

Some surgeons routinely use one device or another for mitral valve replacement, and the valve of choice varies widely. It cannot be said that there is a consensus in the surgical world about this matter. Lefrak and Starr summarize this field in their monograph.[L1] The trade-off in the choice is primarily between the durability of most of the prosthetic devices versus the lack of need of long-term anticoagulation in most patients with a bioprosthesis; and between the proven, long-term performance of the Starr-Edwards model 6120 ball valve prosthesis and the Bjork-Shiley valve[B8] versus the possibly improved hemodynamic and thromboembolic performance of the relatively new St. Jude valve. In the case of prostheses, the advantage of durability is tempered by the need for long-term anticoagulation and its attendant risks; and in the case of the bioprostheses, the advantage of the freedom from need for anticoagulation is tempered by the tendency of the bioprostheses to degenerate. This is compounded by the more rapid degeneration of bioprostheses in the young[A8,A9] (Figs. 11-19, 11-29), in whom their use would otherwise be particularly attractive, and by the fact that advanced age and atrial fibrillation increase the probability of thromboembolism in the unanticoagulated patient with a bioprosthesis. Also, Warnes and colleagues have reported that bioprostheses degenerate more rapidly in the mitral position than in the aortic position.[W3] Bioprostheses are in a state of evolution, and continuing improvements will probably lead to better durability of these devices.[C13]

Starr-Edwards Silastic Ball Valve Prosthesis (Model 6120)

When a prosthesis rather than a bioprosthesis is indicated for mitral valve replacement, the Starr-Edwards silastic ball valve prosthesis has been commonly recommended and con-

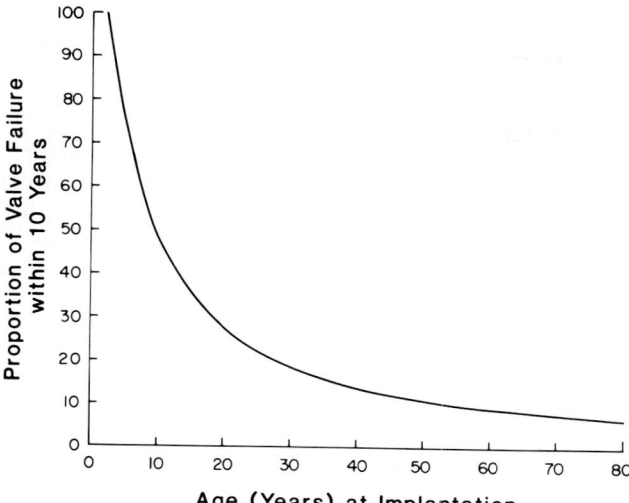

Figure 11-29 Free-hand representation, based on studies from UAB, GLH,[W1] Sanders and associates,[S5] Lakier and colleagues,[L2] Borkon and colleagues,[B19] and Magilligan[M11] of the relationship of age at implantation of heterograft valves to the proportion of patients with hemodynamically important valve degeneration within 10 years of implantation.

tinues to be used (GLH) on the basis of a long experience with it. The 5M (34-mm) size is inserted whenever possible, but the 4M (32-mm) size is acceptable. Although the 3M (28-mm) and even the 2M (27-mm) sizes are said to perform in a hemodynamically satisfactory fashion, they are not recommended for use in adults (Table 11-18). There is no firm evidence that the projection of the valve cage into the left ventricle is functionally disadvantageous, and this device is virtually free of the complications of intraoperative sticking and late acute thrombotic occlusion or encasement. Its thromboembolic tendency is probably greater than that of other prosthetic valves.[M8] Horstkotte and colleagues found in a randomized trial that thromboembolic complications were greater when the Starr-Edwards prosthesis was used in the mitral position than when the Bjork-Shiley device was used.[H19]

Bjork-Shiley Valve

The Bjork-Shiley disc valve functions well in the mitral position; even the 25-mm size has satisfactory hemodynamic function, and the 27-mm and 29-mm sizes have excellent function (Table 11-18). Sizes of Bjork-Shiley valves smaller than these should not be used in the mitral position in adults. The Bjork-Shiley valve has two disadvantages. One is its tendency to stick in the closed position as the heart is being closed and CPB is being discontinued, unless special measures are taken to prevent this. The other disadvantage is its tendency toward acute thrombotic encasement late postoperatively (see "Acute Thrombotic Occlusion" in section on Late Results). The acute intraoperative sticking of the valve in the closed position may be due to a mechanical factor, such as the wedging of chordae or suture ends between the disc and the seat of the disc. However, it seems sometimes

due simply to surface tension forces generated particularly when there is some left ventricular distention before the heart begins to beat. Because of this problem, especially when the Bjork-Shiley valve is used, the frustrator used at GLH or a small catheter through the valve should be removed only after an excellent cardiac action has been re-established and CPB is nearly complete. The Bjork-Shiley valve is oriented in most cases so that the larger opening is posterior and inferior.[B8] The Bjork-Shiley valve may be used routinely in adults or only when the orifice is too small for a 4M Starr-Edwards silastic ball valve. It is particularly useful when valve replacement is mandatory in infants and children.

St. Jude Valve

The St. Jude valve has very good hemodynamic performance[H9] (Table 11-18) and can also be used for adults routinely (UAB) or when a device smaller than the 4M Starr-Edwards valve is required for mitral replacement (GLH). The durability and the frequency of sticking and late thrombotic encasement of this valve are not yet known, but thromboembolic complications appear to be minimal.[C17,H9] Hemolysis may be greater than with the Bjork-Shiley valve.[H9]

Biological Valves

When biological valves are used for mitral valve replacement, permanent anticoagulant therapy has usually not been prescribed. Marshall and colleagues found no greater rate of thromboembolism in unanticoagulated patients with a porcine bioprosthesis in the mitral position than in anticoagulated patients with a Bjork-Shiley device.[M10]

However, the matter of anticoagulation for patients with bioprostheses in the mitral position remains controversial. Chesebro and colleagues found a higher rate of thromboembolism after bioprosthetic mitral replacement than after aortic valve replacement; and they found the rate after mitral replacement reduced by long-term antithrombotic therapy.[C18] Bioprostheses have the disadvantages that they deteriorate in time, becoming stenotic because of valvar calcification or incompetent because of cusp rupture. The deterioration is particularly rapid in young patients[A8] (Fig. 11-29) and in patients with chronic renal failure. When the patient is in sinus rhythm and over the age of 60–65 years, the considerations in favor of the bioprosthesis are persuasive. In women who wish to have children and in persons involved in physically hazardous occupations or hobbies, a bioprosthesis is often used, with the realization that its replacement with a prosthetic device will probably be needed within 10–15 years. A bioprosthesis would not be used in the mitral position in infants and children because of the high probability of deterioration within a few years (Fig. 11-29).

The Carpentier-Edwards stent-mounted, glutaraldehyde-treated porcine valve is used when a bioprosthesis is indicated, or the Hancock heterograft valve may be used. When the mitral annular orifice is smaller than 29 mm, necessitating a 27-mm or 25-mm stent-mounted porcine valve, the device can be expected to be somewhat stenotic (Table 11-18).

Therefore, under these conditions, the less-obstructive Ionescu-Shiley heterograft pericardial valve (Table 11-18) is indicated (GLH) or the recently developed Carpentier-Edwards model of this type.

The stent-mounted antibiotic-treated homograft aortic valve was used almost exclusively for mitral valve replacement (GLH) between 1968 and 1974. The very low hospital mortality and the good early results, enhanced by the low gradient across this device, were encouraging. However, incompetence occurred, on longer follow-up, due to detachment of the aortic wall remnant from the rigid stent pillars,[H15] and this valve was not used after 1976. Subsequent experimental studies led to the development of an acetal copolymer stent with flexible pillars,[P4] but the more recent use of this stent in a limited number of patients has indicated that the problem persists. Thus, the relatively friable antibiotic-treated homograft tissue is apparently unsuited to mounting on a frame for use in the mitral (and aortic) positions.

SPECIAL SITUATIONS AND CONTROVERSIES

Mitral Repair or Replacement

Some surgeons routinely replace, rather than repair, the mitral valve for incompetence. By preference the valve is repaired whenever possible, primarily because of the good results of repair and the long-term risks and imponderables associated with any of the available replacement devices (UAB, GLH). Occasionally the incompetence may persist or recur, but the risk of reoperation for valve replacement, should this be indicated later, is not increased when a repair has been done previously.

Essentially the same reasoning and policy applies to mitral commissurotomy for mitral stenosis. Commissurotomy and preservation of the valve is done whenever an effective opening, leaflet pliability, and trivial or no incompetence afterward indicate a high probability of at least 5 years of palliation from the operation (GLH, UAB). The open, rather than the closed, method of commissurotomy is chosen because of the ease of converting to replacement if indicated and the belief that with it, the opening can be better and more accurately placed.[S10] The GLH experience since 1958 provides useful information as to the proportion of patients with mitral stenosis in whom commissurotomy rather than replacement is feasible, since it contains a largely unselected patient population. Among 220 patients operated on between 1968 and 1976, 154 (70%, CL 66%–73%) had commissurotomy, while the remaining 66 (30%, CL 27%–34%) had valve replacement.[S10] Most (46 of 66) of the replacements were done because of moderate or severe calcification, and a few (3) because of stiffened but noncalcified leaflets. Some (10) replacements were done because of marked subvalvar obstruction by fused chordae. Three were done because of associated incompetence.

Preservation of the Chordae of the Posterior Leaflet during Valve Replacement

Resection of the posterior leaflet is controversial, as leaving it in situ allegedly reduces the tendency to postrepair ventricular rupture. Leaving the leaflet has also been said to minimize the depression of left ventricular function that seems to accompany mitral valve replacement.[L11] At the Mayo Clinic before 1967, we from time to time followed the practice of leaving the posterior leaflet, but there was no indication that cardiac performance was better in such patients.[R9] Furthermore, experimental studies at that time did not support the idea.[R18] The idea of leaving the leaflet has recently again been supported by Hetzer and colleagues[H18] and David and colleagues.[D10] This practice has not been readopted currently (UAB, GLH).

Giant Left Atrium

Massive enlargement of the left atrium has long been known to develop in patients with long-standing severe mitral incompetence.[D11,O2,P7] Surgical reduction in its size has been recommended[J3] since the early days of cardiac surgery but has not been generally adopted (GLH, UAB). Kawazoe and colleagues have used a special plication procedure designed to reduce bronchial compression and improve left ventricular performance.[K8] Their experience suggests that it is effective in doing this. It remains controversial as to whether it need be adopted.

Alternative Surgical Approaches to the Mitral Valve

Occasionally in large patients with small left atria, the exposure is not optimal with the approach described under "Technique of Operation." The superior approach through the most superior aspect of the left atrium, where it appears in the transverse sinus, is an attractive alternative[R13,S7] and is used on occasions (UAB). The superior vena cava is mobilized and retracted to the right, and the aorta retracted to the left (after cross-clamping the aorta and injecting the cardioplegic solution, since the retraction may make the aortic valve incompetent). The transverse incision is made *superiorly*, not anteriorly, as far from the aortic root origin as possible. The mitral valve is found to be very accessible. Often only stay sutures are required for retraction. Since the valve is easily accessible and strong retraction is not required, the study of the competence of the valve after commissurotomy or repair is easier. The closure of this incision must be accurate, catching all layers, including endocardium, with each stitch. Hemostasis should be secure before discontinuing cardiopulmonary bypass.

An approach through the right atrium and across the atrial septum can be used, but it is often unsatisfactory. The exposure is small, and retraction is impeded by concern about injury to the AV node.

A right thoracotomy was employed by Lillehei and colleagues in their first open operations for mitral valve disease,[L5] and it continues to be used by some surgeons. With this approach, the incision is through the left atrium just behind the interatrial groove, as in the median sternotomy. Its chief disadvantages are the limited field provided by the anterolateral interspace approach (with the patient positioned obliquely) and the relative inaccessibility of the ascending aorta both for cannulation and for infusion of the cardioplegic solution. The arterial cannula may have to be positioned in the left external iliac (or femoral) artery.

A left thoracotomy has been used in the past. Venous cannulation is difficult, and this approach cannot currently be recommended.

Method of Tricuspid Annuloplasty

As in the case of mitral incompetence, several techniques have been used for the repair of tricuspid incompetence. Sutures have been used to narrow the anulus by plication of that portion of the anulus occupied by the posterior leaflet.[B21,K7] The deVega technique,[D6] basically two nearly encircling sutures to narrow the anulus, has been popular, but it is no longer used because of late recurrences of the incompetence due to the cutting through or breaking of the sutures (UAB, GLH). The Carpentier technique is reproducible and generally gives good results both early and late postoperatively.

Combined Mitral Replacement and Coronary Artery Bypass Grafting

The experience at the Massachusetts General Hospital supports the idea that the coronary artery bypass graft operation should be done, in addition to mitral valve replacement, in those patients with combined disease; the hospital mortality was 8% for patients in whom both mitral valve replacement and CABG were done and 28% for those with associated coronary artery disease in which *only* valve replacement was done (*P* for difference = .002).[C5] These findings are similar to those of Salomon and colleagues, who also found surgically untreated coronary artery disease to be an incremental risk factor for hospital death after mitral valve replacement.[S8]

Left Ventricular Rupture as a Complication of Mitral Valve Replacement

Massive intrapericardial hemorrhage may occur shortly after discontinuing CPB or in the Intensive Care Unit a few hours later. This complication is usually from left ventricular rupture in or near the atrioventricular groove posteriorly. Virtually all patients die when the rupture occurs postoperatively but some may be saved when the rupture occurs while the chest is open.[B10]

The causes of this dreaded complication are several, but the commonest are undue traction on the anulus during excision of the mitral valve or insertion of the prosthesis, tearing of the anulus by already placed sutures when the heart is manually tilted up after the mitral prosthetic device is in place, and penetration of stitches into the left atrioventricular groove posteriorly.[B29] These are particularly dangerous problems, since the surgeon is usually unaware of producing them during the operation, which may have been a technically very easy one. Roberts and Morrow, in the initial report on this matter, indicated that the complication can also result from perforation of the ventricular wall as a papillary muscle is excised and from perforation of the atrioventricular groove as a calcific deposit is being removed.[R3] Because of this potential problem, the surgeon must be very gentle in all the maneuvers during mitral valve replacement. The heart should *not* be tipped up for air evacuation or ligation of the left atrial appendage or for routine inspection on the back of the heart after the prosthesis is inserted. Excising only the chordae tendinae, rather than including the whole of the papillary muscle, and simply leaving in place deeply embedded calcific deposits in the anulus and placing sutures on the atrial side of them should remove these as causes of rupture.

Left ventricular rupture can occur in the mid portion of the posterior wall, rather than in the region of the AV valve anulus.[K6] Whether the mechanism of this type of rupture is different is not certain, but it can be caused by penetration of a pillar of a stented valve. It seems to occur primarily in women with small left ventricles.

Once massive hemorrhage has occurred, CPB must be reinitiated as quickly as possible, while the hemorrhage is controlled digitally to the extent possible. A premature attempt to suture it will surely end in the death of the patient. After establishing CPB, cross-clamping the aorta, and giving the cold cardioplegic solution, the left atrium is reopened and the valve removed. Then, with multiple large felt-pledgetted sutures, the rupture is closed as carefully as possible from within the left ventricle and from without if necessary. Even though every attempt is made to avoid the proximal circumflex artery, it may be compromised by these sutures, so the area of the circumflex artery must be carefully inspected *before reinserting the valve*. If it is compromised, a saphenous vein bypass graft to a large marginal branch must be placed. Then the valve is reinserted and the remainder of the procedure completed as usual. Great care must be taken with myocardial protection throughout this procedure.

Management of Mitral Prosthetic Infection

It is assumed that mitral prosthetic infection that becomes evident within 3–6 months of implantation of the device originated at the operation. Because of its highly lethal implications and the strong tendency for periprosthetic leakage to occur, intense antibiotic treatment followed in most patients by early prosthetic replacement are indicated. The organism and its antibiotic sensitivity should, of course, be identified, and highly specific therapy used. In the usual circumstances in which the response to antibiotics is excellent, no evidence of peripheral embolization exists, and there is no suspicion of periprosthetic leakage, reoperation may be deferred and the patient followed closely under hospital conditions that allow immediate reoperation should any of these complications occur.

When mitral prosthetic infection becomes apparent for the first time more than 6–12 months postoperatively, it is more likely to have resulted from intercurrent bacteremia related to a dental procedure, urinary tract infection, and the like. The same protocols for management apply, but probably more patients will respond well to intense medical treatment alone than with infections occurring within the first year after operation.

Management of Periprosthetic Leakage

Proper intraoperative and perioperative techniques against infection and a proper suture technique must be used in order to prevent periprosthetic leakage.[D2]

Periprosthetic leakage should be suspected in any patient who redevelops symptoms after mitral valve replacement, has more than the usual amount of hemolysis, or develops prosthetic valve infection. The auscultatory findings are notoriously unreliable, and in an ill patient, no apical systolic murmur may be heard when the periprosthetic leakage is severe, and an apical systolic murmur may be present without periprosthetic leakage. Cinefluorographic study of prosthetic motion is helpful, particularly when it can be compared with a similar study made early after operation. The definitive study is left ventriculography.

Mild periprosthetic leakage without infection is usually stable and does not progress. Important periprosthetic leakage is an indication for reoperation. If infection is almost certainly not present and the leakage is very localized, one or two pledgetted mattress sutures usually suffice to close the leakage permanently. Otherwise, re-replacement is indicated.

APPENDIXES

APPENDIX 11A
MULTIVARIATE ANALYSIS OF HOSPITAL DEATH (UAB)

The factors examined in the multivariate logistic analysis for all postoperative hospital deaths and hospital deaths in acute or chronic heart failure after mitral valve replacement were:

Demographic
    Age (years) at operation
    Body surface area (m²) at operation
    Date (months since January 1, 1975) of operation
Preoperative
    NYHA functional class (I–V)
    Old myocardial infarct
    Admission cardiac rhythm (sinus, atrial fibrillation, other)
Operative
    CABG performed (yes, no)
    Tricuspid annuloplasty performed (yes, no)
    Lesion (stenosis, regurgitation, mixed)
    Mitral pathologic condition (rheumatic, mitral prolapse, papillary muscle dysfunction, ruptured chordae, active endocarditis, other)
    LA thrombus found at operation (yes, no)
    Cold cardioplegia used (yes, no)
    Cumulative cardiac ischemic (aortic cross-clamp) time (minutes)
    Surgeon

Postoperative
    First cardiac index within 4 hours of operation
    Cardiac index at 0400 hours on postoperative day 1

APPENDIX 11B
MULTIVARIATE ANALYSIS OF POSTOPERATIVE CARDIAC INDEX (UAB)

For the multivariate analysis of factors relating to early postoperative cardiac index, all the variables listed in Appendix 11A were included in the analysis in addition to the following:

Demographic
    Sex
Preoperative
    Preoperative cardiac index
    Systolic arterial pressure
    Left ventricular end-diastolic pressure
Operative
    Size of device inserted
    Operative assessment of left atrial size
    Coronary arterial system into which bypass grafts were placed

---

REFERENCES

A

1. Appelbaum A, Kouchoukos NT, Blackstone EH, Kirklin JW: Early risks of open heart surgery for mitral valve disease. *Am J Cardiol* 37:201, 1976.

2. Ahmad R, Manohitharajah SM, Deverall PB, Watson DA: Chronic hemolysis following mitral valve replacement. *J Thorac Cardiovasc Surg* 71:212, 1976.

3. Akins CW, Kirklin JK, Block PC, Buckley MJ, Austen WG: Preoperative evaluation of subvalvular fibrosis in mitral stenosis: A predictive factor in conservative versus replacement surgical therapy. *Circulation* 60(suppl I)I-71, 1979.

4. Angelino PF, Levi V, Brusca A, Actis-Dato A: Mitral commissurotomy in younger age group. *Am Heart J* 51:916, 1956.

5. Al-Bahrani IR, Thamer MA, Al-Omeri MM, Al-Naaman YD: Rheumatic heart disease in the young in Iraq. *Br Heart J* 28:824, 1966.

6. Austen WG, Wooler GH: Surgical treatment of mitral stenosis by the transventricular approach with a mechanical dilator. *N Engl J Med* 263:661, 1960.

7. Adebo OA, Ross JK: Conservative surgery for mitral valve disease: Clinical and echocardiographic analysis of results. *Thorax* 38:565, 1983.

8. Antunes MJ, Med M, Santos LP: Performance of glutaraldehyde-preserved porcine bioprosthesis as a mitral valve substitute in a young population group. *Ann Thorac Surg* 37:387, 1984.

9. Antunes MJ: Bioprosthetic valve replacement in children—Long-term follow-up of 135 isolated mitral valve implantations. *Eur Heart J* 5:913, 1984.

B

1. Brunton L, Edin MD: Preliminary note on the possibility of treating mitral stenosis by surgical methods. *Lancet* Feb 8, 1902, p 352.

2. Bailey CP: The surgical treatment of mitral stenosis (mitral commissurotomy). *Diseases of the Chest* 15:377, 1949.

3. Bland EF, Jones TD: Rheumatic fever and rheumatic heart disease: A twenty-year report on 1000 patients followed since childhood. *Circulation* 4:836, 1951.

4. Buchbinder NA, Roberts WC: Left-sided valvular active infective endocarditis. *Am J Med* 53:20, 1972.

5. Barlow JB, Pocock WA, Marchand P, Denny M: The significance of late systolic murmurs. *Am Heart J* 66:443, 1963.

6. Braunwald E: *Heart Disease: A Textbook of Cardiovascular Medicine.* Philadelphia: Saunders, 1980.

7. Barnhorst DA, Oxman HA, Connolly DC, Pluth JR, Danielson GK, Wallace RB, McGoon DC: Long-term follow-up of isolated replacement of the aortic or mitral valve with the Starr-Edwards prosthesis. *Am J Cardiol* 35:228, 1975.

8. Bjork VO, Book K, Holmgren A: The Bjork-Shiley mitral valve prosthesis. *Ann Thorac Surg* 18:379, 1974.

9. Bjork VO: Left ventricular rupture after mitral valve replacement. *Ann Thorac Surg* 31:101, 1981 (editorial).

10. Bjork VO, Henze A, Rodriguez L: Left ventricular rupture as a complication of mitral valve replacement. *J Thorac Cardiovasc Surg* 73:14, 1977.

11. Book K, Holmgren A, Szamosi A: The left atrial V-wave after mitral valve replacement. *Scand J Thorac Cardiovasc Surg* 9:9, 1975.

12. Boucher CA, Bingham JB, Osbakken MD, Okada RD, Strauss HW, Block PC, Levine FH, Phillips HR, Pohost GM: Early changes in left ventricular size and function after correction of left ventricular volume overload. *Am J Cardiol* 47:991, 1981.

13. Braunwald E: Mitral regurgitation: Physiologic, clinical and surgical considerations. *N Engl J Med* 281:425, 1969.

14. Boudoulas H, Reynolds JC, Mazzaferri E, Wooley CF: Metabolic studies in mitral valve prolapse syndrome: A neuroendocrine-cardiovascular process. *Circulation* 61:1200, 1980.

15. Barlow JB, Pocock WA: The problem of nonejection clicks and associated mitral systolic murmurs: Emphasis on the billowing mitral leaflet syndrome. *Am Heart J* 90:639, 1975.

16. Braunwald E, Braunwald NS, Ross J Jr, Morrow AG: Effects of mitral valve replacement on the pulmonary vascular dynamics of patients with pulmonary hypertension. *N Engl J Med* 273:509, 1965.

17. Barnhorst DA, Oxman HA, Connolly DC, Pluth JR, Danielson GK, Wallace RB, McGoon DC: Isolated replacement of the mitral valve with the Starr-Edwards prosthesis: An eleven-year review. *J Thorac Cardiovasc Surg* 71:230, 1976.

18. Bernal-Ramirez JB, Phillips JH: Echocardiographic study of malfunction of the Bjork-Shiley prosthetic heart valve in the mitral position. *Am J Cardiol* 40:449, 1977.

19. Borkon AM, McIntosh CL, Von Rueden TJ, Morrow AG: Mitral valve replacement with the Hancock bioprosthesis: Five-to-ten–year follow-up. *Ann Thorac Surg* 32:127, 1981.

20. Baxter RH, Bain WH, Rankin RJ, Turner MA, Escarous AE, Thomson RM, Lorimer AR, Lawrie TDV: Tricuspid valve replacement: A five-year appraisal. *Thorax* 30:158, 1975.

21. Boyd AD, Engelman RM, Isom OW, Reed GE, Spencer FC: Tricuspid annuloplasty. *J Thorac Cardiovasc Surg* 68:344, 1974.

22. Breyer RH, McClenathan JH, Michaelis LL, McIntosh CL, Morrow AG: Tricuspid regurgitation. *J Thorac Cardiovasc Surg* 72:867, 1976.

23. Braunwald NS, Ross J, Morrow AG: Conservative management of tricuspid regurgitation in patients undergoing mitral valve replacement. *Circulation* 35(suppl I):I-31, 1967.

24. Bolen JL, Lopes MG, Harrison DC, Alderman EL: Analysis of left ventricular function in response to afterload changes in patients with mitral stenosis. *Circulation* 52:894, 1975.

25. Borman JB, Stern S, Shapira T, Milvidsky H, Braun K: Mitral valvotomy in children. *Am Heart J* 61:763, 1961.

26. Bailey GWH, Braniff BA, Hancock EW, Cohn KE: Relation of left atrial pathology to atrial fibrillation in mitral valvular disease. *Ann Intern Med* 69:13, 1968.

27. Bharati S, Lev M, Kirklin JW: *Cardiac Surgery and the Conduction System.* New York: Wiley, 1983.

28. Baker C, Brock RC, Campbell M: Valvulotomy for mitral stenosis: Report of six successful cases. *Br Med J* 1:1283, 1950.

29. Bailey CP, Bolton HE, Redondo-Ramirez HP: Surgery of the mitral valve. *Surg Clin North Am* 32:1807, 1952.

30. Broom ND, Thomson FJ: The influence of fixation conditions on the performance of glutaraldehyde-treated porcine aortic valves: towards a more scientific basis. *Thorax* 166, 1979.

31. Barratt-Boyes BG, Roche A, Agnew TM, Cole D, Kerr A, Monro JL, Lowe JB, Brandt PWT: Homograft valves. *Med J Aust* 2(suppl):38, 1972.

32. Barratt-Boyes BG: Surgical correction of mitral incompetence resulting from bacterial endocarditis. *Br Heart J* 25:415, 1963.

33. Becker RM, Strom J, Fishman W, Oka Y, Lin YT, Yellin EL, Trater RWM: Hemodynamic performance of the Ionescu-Shiley valve prosthesis. *J Thorac Cardiovasc Surg* 80:613, 1980.

34. Byram MT, Roberts WC: Frequency and extent of calcific deposits in purely regurgitant mitral valves: Analysis of 108 operatively excised valves. *Am J Cardiol* 52:1059, 1983.

35. Blackstone EH, Kirklin JW: Death and other time related events after valve replaced (1985) *Circulation* (in press).

36. Bove AA, Lazarow N, Kontos GJ, Owen RM, Mock MB: Temporal nonuniformity of left ventricular contraction in chronic mitral regurgitation. *JACC* 5:486, 1985 (abstract).

C

1. Cutler EC, Levine SA: Cardiotomy and valvulotomy for mitral stenosis: Experimental observations and clinical notes concerning an operated case with recovery. *The Boston Medical and Surgical Journal* 188:1023, 1923.

2. Cohen MV, Gorlin R: Modified orifice equation for the calculation of mitral valve area. *Am Heart J* 84:839, 1972.

3. Criley JM, Lewis KB, Humphries JO, Ross PS: Prolapse of the mitral valve: Clinical and cineangiographic findings. *Br Heart J* 28:488, 1966.

4. Carpentier A, Relland J, Deloche A, Fabiani J-N, D'Allaines C, Blondeau P, Piwnica A, Chauvaud S, Dubost C: Conservative management of the prolapsed mitral valve. *Ann Thorac Surg* 26:294, 1978.

5. Chaffin JS, Daggett WM: Mitral valve replacement: A nine-year follow-up of risks and survivals. *Ann Thorac Surg* 27:312, 1979.

6. Cohn LH, Sanders JH, Collins JJ Jr: Actuarial comparison of Hancock porcine and prosthetic disc valves for isolated mitral valve replacement. *Circulation* 54(supp: III):III-60, 1976.

7. Copans H, Lakier JB, Kinsley RH, Colsen PR, Fritz VU, Barlow JB: Thrombosed Bjork-Shiley mitral prostheses. *Circulation* 61:169, 1980.

8. Cherian G, Vytilingam KL, Sukumar JP, Gopinath N: Mitral valvotomy in young patients. *Br Heart J* 26:157, 1964.

9. Carpentier A, Chauvaud S, Fabiani JN, Deloche A, Relland J, Lessana A, de'Allaines C, Blondeau P, Piwnica A, Dubost C: Reconstructive surgery of mitral valve incompetence: Ten-year appraisal. *J Thorac Cardiovasc Surg* 79:338, 1980.

10. Carpentier A, Deloche A, Hanania G, Forman J, Sellier PH, Piwnica A, Dubost CH: Surgical management of acquired tricuspid valve disease. *J Thorac Cardiovasc Surg* 67:53, 1974.

11. Curry GC, Elliott LP, Ramsey HW: Quantitative left ventricular angiocardiographic findings in mitral stenosis. *Am J Cardiol* 29:621, 1972.

12. Channick BJ, Adlin EV, Marks AD, Denenberg BS, McDonough MT, Chakko CS, Spann JF: Hyperthyroidism and mitral-valve prolapse. *N Engl J Med* 305:497, 1981.

13. Carpentier A, Dubost C, Lane E, Nashef A, Carpentier S, Relland J, Deloche A, Fabiana J, Chauvaud S, Perier P, Maxwell S: Continuing improvements in valvular bioprostheses. *J Thorac Cardiovasc Surg* 83:27, 1982.

14. Commerford PJ, Hastie T, Beck W: Closed mitral valvotomy: Actuarial analysis of results in 654 patients over 12 years and analysis of preoperative predictors of long-term survival. *Ann Thorac Surg* 33:473, 1982.

15. Chaux AC, Gray RJ, Matloff JM, Feldman H, Sustaita H: An appreciation of the new St. Jude valvular prosthesis. *J Thorac Cardiovasc Surg* 81:202, 1981.

16. Chaitman BR, Bonan R, Lepage G, Tubau JF, David PR, Dyrda I, Grondin CM: Hemodynamic evaluation of the Carpentier-Edwards porcine xenograft. *Circulation* 60:1170, 1979.

17. Chaux A, Czer LSC, Matloff JM, DeRobertis MA, Stewart ME, Bateman TM, Kass RM, Lee ME, Gray RJ: The St. Jude medical bileaflet valve prosthesis. *J Thorac Cardiovasc Surg* 88:706, 1984.

18. Chesebro JH, Fuster V, Fisher LD, Danielson GK, Pluth JR, Orszulak TA, Schaff HV, Piehler JM, Puga FJ: Thromboembolism after biologic prosthetic heart valve replacement. *JACC* 5:459, 1985 (abstract).

D

1. Davila JC, Magilligan DJ Jr, Lewis JW Jr: Is the Hancock porcine valve the best cardiac valve substitute today? *Ann Thorac Surg* 26:303, 1978.

2. Dhasmana JP, Blackstone EH, Kirklin JW, Kouchoukos NT: Factors associated with periprosthetic leakage following primary mitral valve replacement: With special consideration of the suture technique. *Ann Thorac Surg* 35:170, 1983.

3. Dalby AJ, Firth BG, Forman R: Preoperative factors affecting the outcome of isolated mitral valve replacement: A 10 year review. *Am J Cardiol* 47:826, 1981.

4. Dalen JE, Matloff JM, Evans GI, Hoppin FG Jr, Bhardwaj P, Harken DE, Dexter L: Early reduction of pulmonary vascular resistance after mitral-valve replacement. *N Engl J Med* 277:387, 1967.

5. Duran CG, Pomar JL, Revuelta JM, Gallo I, Poveda J, Ochoteco A, Ubago JL: Conservative operation for mitral insufficiency. *J Thorac Cardiovasc Surg* 79:326, 1980.

6. De Vega NG: La anuloplastia selectiva, regulable y permanente. *Rev Esp Cardiol* 25:555, 1972.

7. Duran CMG, Pomar JL, Colman T, Figueroa A, Revuelta JM, Ubago JL: Is tricuspid valve repair necessary? *J Thorac Cardiovasc Surg* 80:849, 1980.

8. Devereux RB, Perloff JK, Reichek N, Josephson ME: Mitral valve prolapse. *Circulation* 54:3, 1976.

9. Davila JC, Glover RP: Circumferential suture of the mitral valve for the correction of regurgitation. *Am J Cardiol* 2:267, 1958.

10. David TE, Druck MM, Burns RJ: Mitral valve replacement for mitral regurgitation with and without preservation of chordae tendinae. *J Thorac Cardiovasc Surg* 88:718, 1984.

11. DeSanctis RW, Dean DC, Bland FE: Extreme left atrial enlargement. *Circulation* 29:14, 1964.

E

1. Eckbert DL, Gault JH, Bouchard RL, Karliner JS, Ross J Jr: Mechanics of left ventricular contractions in chronic mitral regurgitation. *Circulation* 47:1252, 1973.

2. Ellis FH Jr, Frye RL, McGoon DC: Results of reconstructive operations for mitral insufficiency due to ruptured chordae tendineae. *Surgery* 59:165, 1966.

3. Ellis LB, Benson H, Harken DE: The effect of age and other factors on the early and late results following closed mitral valvuloplasty. *Am Heart J* 75:743, 1968.

F

1. Fuster V, Danielson GA, Robb RA, Broadbent JC, Brown AL Jr, Elveback LR: Quantitation of left ventricular myocardial fiber hypertrophy and interstitial tissue in human hearts with chronically increased volume and pressure overload. *Circulation* 55:504, 1977.

2. Fontana ME, Pence HL, Leighton RF, Wooley CF: The varying clinical spectrum of the systolic click-late systolic murmur syndrome: A postural auscultatory phenomenon. *Circulation* 41:807, 1970.

3. Feigenbaum H, Linback RE, Nasser WK: Hemodynamic studies before and after instrumental mitral commissurotomy. *Circulation* 38:261, 1968.

4. Fournier C, Gay J, Gerbaux A: Évolution à long terme des insuffisances tricuspides non opérées après correction chirurgicale des valvulopathies mitrales et mitro-aortiques. *Arch Mal Coeur* 68:907, 1975.

G

1. Gross RI, Cunningham JN Jr, Snively SL, Catinella FP, Nathan IM, Adams PX, Spencer FC: Long-term results of open radical mitral commissurotomy: Ten-year follow-up study of 202 patients. *Am J Cardiol* 47:821, 1981.

2. Grunkemeier GL, Macmanus Q, Thomas DR, Starr A: Regression analysis of late survival following mitral valve replacement. *J Thorac Cardiovasc Surg* 75:131, 1978.

3. Glancy DL, O'Brien KP, Reis RL: Hemodynamic studies in patients with 2M and 3M Starr-Edwards prostheses: Evidence of obstruction to left atrial emptying. *Circulation* 39–40(suppl I): I-113, 1969.

4. Grondin P, Meere C, Limet R, Lopez-Bescos L, Delcan JL, Rivera R: Carpentier's annulus and De Vega's annuloplasty. *J Thorac Cardiovasc Surg* 70:852, 1975.

5. Grenadier E, Alpan G, Keidar S, Palant A: The prevalence of ruptured chordae tendineae in the mitral valve prolapse syndrome. *Am Heart J* 105:603, 1983.

6. Gash AK, Carabello BA, Cepin D, Spann JF: Left ventricular ejection performance and systolic muscle function in patients with mitral stenosis. *Circulation* 67:148, 1983.

H

1. Harken DW, Ellis LB, Ware PF, Norman LR: The surgical treatment of mitral stenosis. I. Valvuloplasty. *N Engl J Med* 239:801, 1948.

2. Hood WP Jr, Rackley CE, Rolatt EL: Wall stress in the normal and hypertrophied human left ventricle. *Am J Cardiol* 22:550, 1968.

3. Heller SJ, Carleton RA: Abnormal left ventricular contraction in patients with mitral stenosis. *Circulation* 42:1099, 1970.

4. Hammermeister KE, Fisher L, Kennedy JW, Samuels S, Dodge HT: Prediction of late survival in patients with mitral valve disease from clinical, hemodynamic, and quantitative angiographic variables. *Circulation* 54:341, 1978.

5. Halseth WL, Elliott DP, Walker EL, Smith EA: Open mitral commissurotomy. *J Thorac Cardiovasc Surg* 80:842, 1980.

6. Hawe A, Frye RL, Ellis FH Jr: Late hemodynamic studies after mitral valve surgery. *J Thorac Cardiovasc Surg* 65:351, 1973.

7. Hetzer R, Hill JD, Kerth WJ, Ansbro J, Adappa MG, Rodvien R, Kamm B, Gerbode F: Thromboembolic complications after mitral valve replacement with Hancock xenograft. *J Thorac Cardiovasc Surg* 75:651, 1978.

8. Higgs LM, Glancy DL, O'Brien KP, Epstein SE, Morrow AG: Mitral restenosis: An uncommon cause of recurrent symptoms following mitral commissurotomy. *Am J Cardiol* 26:34, 1970.

9. Hortskottle D, Haesten K, Herzen JA, Seipel L, Birchs W, Loogen F: Preliminary clinical and hemodynamic results after mitral valve replacement using St. Jude Medical prostheses in comparison with the Bjork-Shiley valve. *Thorac Cardiovasc Surg* 29:93, 1981.

10. Housman LB, Bonchek L, Lambert L, Grunkemeier G, Starr A: Prognosis of patients after open mitral commissurotomy. *J Thorac Cardiovasc Surg* 73:742, 1977.

11. Hoeksema TD, Wallace RB, Kirklin JW: Closed mitral commissurotomy: Recent results in 291 cases. *Am J Cardiol* 17:825, 1966.

12. Horwitz LD, Mullins CG, Payne RM, Curry GC: Left ventricular function in mitral stenosis. *Chest* 64:609, 1973.

13. Halperin Z, Karasik A, Lewis BS, Geft IL, Gotsman MS: Echocardiographic left ventricular function in mitral stenosis. *Isr J Med Sci* 14:841, 1978.

14. Holzer JA, Karliner JS, O'Rourke RA, Peterson KL: Quantitative angiographic analysis of the left ventricle in patients with isolated rheumatic mitral stenosis. *Br Heart J* 35:497, 1973.

15. Heng MK, Barratt-Boyes BG, Agnew TM, Brandt PWT, Kerr AR, Graham KJ: Isolated mitral replacement with stent-mounted antibiotic-treated aortic allograft valves. *J Thorac Cardiovasc Surg* 74:230, 1977.

16. Horstkotte D, Haersten K, Herzer JA, Siepel L, Birchs W, Loogen F: Preliminary results in mitral valve replacement with the St. Jude medical prosthesis: Companion with the Bjork-Shiley valve. *Circulation* 64(suppl II):II-209, 1981.

17. Horowitz MS, Goodman DJ, Fogarty TJ, Harrison DC: Mitral valve replacement with the glutaraldehyde-preserved porcine heterograft. *J Thorac Cardiovasc Surg* 67:885, 1974.

18. Hetzer R, Bougioukas G, Franz M, Borst HG: Mitral valve replacement with preservation of papillary muscles and chordae tendineae: Revival of a seemingly forgotten concept. I. Preliminary clinical report. *Thorac Cardiovasc Surg* 31:291, 1983.

19. Horstkotte D, Haerten K, Herzer JA, Loogen F, Scheibling R, Schulte HD: Five-year results after randomized mitral valve replacement with Bjork-Shiley, Lillehei-Kaster, and Starr-Edwards prostheses. *Thorac Cardiovasc Surg* 31:106, 1983.

I

1. Ionescu M, Smith DR, Hasan SS, Chidambaram M, Tandon AP: Clinical durability of the pericardial xenograft valve: Ten years' experience with mitral replacement. *Ann Thorac Surg* 34:265, 1982.

2. Ivert TSA, Dismukes WE, Cobbs CG, Blackstone EH, Kirklin JW, Bergdahl LAL: Prosthetic valve endocarditis. *Circulation* 69:223, 1984.

J

1. Johnson AD, Daily PO, Peterson KL, LeWinter M, DiDonna GJ, Blair G, Niwayama G: Functional evaluation of the porcine heterograft in the mitral position. *Circulation* 50,51(suppl I):I-40, 1975.

2. Jugdutt BI, Fraser RS, Lee SJK, Rossall RE, Callaghan JC: Long-term survival after tricuspid valve replacement. *J Thorac Cardiovasc Surg* 74:20, 1977.

3. Johnson J, Danielson GK, MacVaugh H III, Joyner CR: Plication of the giant left atrium at operation for severe mitral regurgitation. *Surgery* 61:118, 1967.

K

1. Kennedy JW, Yarnall SR, Murray JA, Figley MM: Quantitative angiocardiography. IV. Relationships of left atrial and ventricular pressure and volume in mitral valve disease. *Circulation* 41:817, 1970.

2. Karp RB, Cyrus RJ, Blackstone EH, Kirklin JW, Kouchoukos NT, Pacifico AD: The Bjork-Shiley valve: Intermediate-term follow-up. *J Thorac Cardiovasc Surg* 81:602, 1981.

3. Kennedy JW, Doces JG, Stewart DK: Left ventricular function before and following surgical treatment of mitral valve disease. *Am Heart J* 97:592, 1979.

4. Kirklin JW: Replacement of the mitral valve for mitral incompetence. *Surgery* 72:827, 1972.

5. Kaul TK, Bain WH, Jones JV, Lorimer AR, Thomson RM, Turner MA, Escarous A: Mitral valve replacement in the presence of severe pulmonary hypertension. *Thorax* 31:332, 1976.

6. Katske G, Golding LR, Tubbs RR, Loop FD: Posterior midventricular rupture after mitral valve replacement. *Ann Thorac Surg* 27:130, 1979.

7. Kay JH, Maselli-Campagna G, Tsuji HK: Surgical treatment of tricuspid insufficiency. *Ann Surg* 162:53, 1965.

8. Kawazoe K, Beppu S, Takahara Y, Nakajima N, Tanaka K, Ichihashi K, Fujita T, Manabe H: Surgical treatment of giant left atrium combined with mitral valvular disease. *J Thorac Cardiovasc Surg* 85:885, 1983.

9. Kronzon I, Mercurio P, Winer HE, Colvin S: Echocardiographic evaluation of Carpentier mitral valvuloplasty. *Am Heart J* 106:362, 1983.

10. Kay PH, Nunley DL, Grunkemeier GL, Pinson CW, Starr A: Late results of combined mitral valve replacement and coronary bypass surgery. *JACC* 5:29, 1985.

L

1. Lefrak EA, Starr A: *Cardiac Valve Prostheses.* New York: Appleton-Century-Crofts, 1979, p 110.

2. Lakier JB, Khaja F, Magilligan DJ Jr, Goldstein S: Porcine xenograft valves: Long-term (60–89 month) follow-up. *Circulation* 62:313, 1980.

3. Litwak RS, Silvay J, Gadboys HL, Lukban SB, Sakurai H, Castro-Blanco J: Factors associated with operative risk in mitral valve replacement. *Am J Cardiol* 23:335, 1969.

4. Lepley D Jr, Flemma RJ, Mullen DC, Motl M, Anderson AJ, Weirauch E: Long-term follow-up of the Bjork-Shiley prosthetic valve used in the mitral position. *Ann Thorac Surg* 30:164, 1980.

5. Lillehei CW, Gott VL, Dewall RA, Varco RL: Surgical correction of pure mitral insufficiency by annuloplasty under direct vision. *The Journal-Lancet* 77:446, 1957.

6. Lessana A, Herreman F, Boffety C, Cosma H, Guerin F, Kara M, Degeorges M: Hemodynamic and cineangiographic study before and after mitral valvuloplasty (Carpentier's techniques). *Circulation* 64(suppl II):II-195, 1981.

7. Lipson LC, Kent KM, Rosing DR, Bonow RO, McIntosh CL, Condit J, Epstein SE, Morrow AG: Long-term hemodynamic assessment of the porcine heterograft in the mitral position. *Circulation* 64:397, 1981.

8. Lurie AJ, Miller RR, Maxwell KS, Grehl TM, Vismara LA, Hurley AJ, Mason DT: Hemodynamic assessment of the glutaraldehyde-preserved porcine heterograft in the aortic and mitral position. *Circulation* 56:104, 1977.

9. Levine FM, Carter JE, Buckley MJ, Daggett WM, Akins CW, Austen WG: Hemodynamic evaluation of Hancock and Carpentier-Edwards bioprosthesis. *Circulation* 64(suppl II)II-192, 1981.

10. Lessana A, Viet TT, Ades F, Kara SM, Ameur A, Ruffenach A, Guerin F, Herreman F, Degeorges M: Mitral reconstructive operations: A series of 130 consecutive cases. *J Thorac Cardiovasc Surg* 86:553, 1983.

11. Lillehei CW, Levy MJ, Bonnabeau RC: Mitral valve replacement with preservation of papillary muscles and chordae tendinae. *J Thorac Cardiovasc Surg* 47:532, 1964.

M

1. Munoz S, Gallardo J, Diaz-Gorrin JR, Medina O: Influence of surgery on the natural history of rheumatic mitral and aortic valve disease. *Am J Cardiol* 35:234, 1975.

2. Macmanus Q, Grunkemeier GL, Lambert LE, Starr A: Non–cloth-covered caged-ball prostheses: The second decade. *J Thorac Cardiovasc Surg* 76:788, 1978.

3. McGoon DC: Repair of mitral insufficiency due to ruptured chordae tendineae. *J Thorac Cardiovasc Surg* 39:357, 1960.

4. Merendino KA, Bruce RA: One hundred seventeen surgically treated cases of valvular rheumatic heart disease: With a preliminary report of two cases of mitral regurgitation treated under direct vision with the aid of a pump-oxygenator. *JAMA* 164:749, 1957.

5. Miller DC, Stinson EB, Rossiter SJ, Oyer PE, Reitz BA, Shumway NE: Impact of simultaneous myocardial revascularization on operative risk, functional result, and survival following mitral valve replacement. *Surgery* 84:848, 1978.

6. Mills P, Rose J, Hollingsworth J, Amara I, Craige E: Long-term prognosis of mitral-valve prolapse. *N Engl J Med* 297:13, 1977.

7. Manteuffel-Szoege L, Nowicki J, Wasniewska M, Sitkowski W, Turski C: Mitral commissurotomy: Results of 1700 cases. *J Cardiovasc Surg* 11:350, 1970.

8. Miller DC, Oyer PE, Stinson EB, Reitz BA, Jamieson SW, Baumgartner WA, Mitchell RS, Shumway NE: Ten-to-fifteen–year reassessment of the performance characteristics of the Starr-Edwards Model 6120 mitral valve prosthesis. *J Thorac Cardiovasc Surg* 85:1, 1983.

9. McIntosh CL, Michaelis LL, Morrow AG, Itscoity SB, Redwood DR, Epstein SE: Atrioventricular valve replacement with the Hancock porcine xenograft: A 5-year clinical experience. *Surgery* 78:768, 1975.

10. Marshall WG, Kouchoukos NT, Karp RB, Williams JB: Late results after mitral valve replacement with the Bjork-Shiley and porcine prostheses. *J Thorac Cardiovasc Surg* 85:902, 1983.

11. Magilligan DJ Jr: (1983) Personal communication.

N

1. Nasser WK, Davis RH, Dillon JC, Tavel ME, Helmen CH, Feigenbaum H, Fisch C: Atrial myxoma. I. Clinical and pathologic features in 9 cases. II. Phonocardiographic, echocardiographic, hemodynamic, and angiographic features in 9 cases. *Am Heart J* 83:694, 1972.

2. Nevaril CG, Lynch EC, Alfrey CP Jr, Hellums JD: Erythrocyte damage and destruction induced by shearing stress. *J Lab Clin Med* 71:784, 1968.

3. Nichols HT: Mitral insufficiency: Treatment by polar cross fusion of the mitral annulus fibrosus. *J Thorac Cardiovasc Surg* 33:102, 1957.

4. Nicoloff DM, Emery RW, Arom KV, Northup WF, Jorgenson CR, Wang Y, Lindsay WG: Clinical and hemodynamic results with the St. Jude medical cardiac valve prosthesis. *J Thorac Cardiovasc Surg* 82:674, 1981.

O

1. Olesen KH: The natural history of 271 patients with mitral stenosis under medical treatment. *Br Heart J* 24:349, 1962.

2. Owen I, Fenton WJ: A case of extreme dilatation of the left auricle of the heart. *Transactions of the Clinical Society of London* 34:183, 1901.

3. Orszulak TA, Schaff HV, Danielson GK, Piehler JM, Pluth JR, Puga FJ, McGoon DC, Frye RL: Late results of repair of ruptured chordae. *J Thorac Cardiovasc Surg* (in press).

P

1. Pakrashi BC, Mary DA, Elmufti ME, Wooler GH, Ionescu MI: Clinical and haemodynamic results of mitral annuloplasty. *Br Heart J* 36:768, 1974.

2. Peter CA, Austin EH, Jones RH: Effect of valve replacement from chronic mitral insufficiency on left ventricular function during rest and exercise. *J Thorac Cardiovasc Surg* 82:127, 1981.

3. Pocock WA, Barlow JB: Postexercise arrhythmias in the billowing posterior mitral leaflet syndrome. *Am Heart J* 80:740, 1970.

4. Pohlner PG, Thomson FJ, Hjelems E, Barratt-Boyes BG: Experimental evaluation of aortic homograft valves mounted on flexible support frames and comparison with glutaraldehyde-treated porcine valves. *J Thorac Cardiovasc Surg* 77:287, 1979.

5. Phillips HR, Levine FH, Carter JE, Boucher CA, Osbakken MD, Okada RD, Akins CW, Daggett WM, Buckley MJ, Pohost GM: Mitral valve replacement for isolated mitral regurgitation: Analysis of clinical course and late postoperative left ventricular ejection fraction. *Am J Cardiol* 48:647, 1981.

6. Pyle RB, Mayer JE Jr, Lindsay WG, Jorgensen CR, Wang Y, Nicoloff DM: Hemodynamic evaluation of Lillehei Kaster and Starr-Edwards prostheses: *Ann Thorac Surg* 26:336, 1978.

7. Parsonnet AE, Bernstein A, Martland HS: Massive left auricle

with special reference to its etiology and mechanism: Report of case. *Am Heart J* 31:438, 1946.

R

1. Rowe JC, Bland EF, Sprague HB, White PD: The course of mitral stenosis without surgery: Ten- and twenty-year perspectives. *Ann Intern Med* 52:741, 1960.

2. Rapaport E: Natural history of aortic and mitral valve disease. *Am J Cardiol* 35:221, 1975.

3. Roberts WC, Morrow AG: Causes of early postoperative death following cardiac valve replacement: Clinicopathologic correlations in 64 patients studied at necropsy. *J Thorac Cardiovasc Surg* 54:422, 1967.

4. Reed GE, Tice DA, Clauss RH: Asymmetric exaggerated mitral annuloplasty: Repair of mitral insufficiency with hemodynamic predictability. *J Thorac Cardiovasc Surg* 49:752, 1965.

5. Rankin JS, Nicholas LM, Kouchoukos NT: Experimental mitral regurgitation: Effects on left ventricular function before and after elimination of chronic regurgitation in the dog. *J Thorac Cardiovasc Surg* 70:478, 1975.

6. Reed GE: Repair of mitral regurgitation: An 11-year experience. *Am J Cardiol* 31:494, 1973.

7. Reed GE, Kloth HH, Kiely B, Danilowicz DA, Rader B, Doyle EF: Long-term results of mitral annuloplasty in children with rheumatic mitral regurgitation. *Circulation* 49,50(suppl II):II-189, 1974.

8. Reed GE, Pooley RW, Moggio RA: Durability of measured mitral annuloplasty. *J Thorac Cardiovasc Surg* 79:321, 1980.

9. Rouleau CA, Frye RL, Ellis FH Jr: Hemodynamic state after open mitral valve replacement and reconstruction. *J Thorac Cardiovasc Surg* 58:870, 1969.

10. Roy SB, Gopinath N: Mitral stenosis. *Circulation* 38(suppl V):V-68, 1968.

11. Ramsey HW, De La Torre A, Bartley TD, Linhart JW: Intractable hemoptysis in mitral stenosis treated by emergency mitral commissurotomy. *Ann Intern Med* 67:588, 1967.

12. Rackley CE, Hood WP Jr: Quantitative angiographic evaluation and patho-physiologic mechanisms in valvular heart disease. *Prog Cardiovasc Dis* 15:427, 1973.

13. Richi AA, Sade RM, May MG, Hohn AR: Repair of left atrial abnormalities in children by the superior approach. *Ann Thorac Surg* 31:433, 1981.

14. Rusted IE, Sheifley CH, Edwards JE, Kirklin JW: Guides to the commissures in operations upon the mitral valve. *Proc Staff Meet Mayo Clin* 26:297, 1951.

15. Roberts WC: Morphologic features of the normal and abnormal mitral valve. *Am J Cardiol* 51:1005, 1983.

16. Rutledge R, McIntosh CL, Morrow AG, Picken CA, Siwek L, Zwischenberger JB, Schier JJ: Mitral valve replacement after closed mitral commissurotomy. *Circulation* 66(suppl I):I-162, 1982.

17. Rizzoli G, Russo R, Resta M, Valfre C, Mazzucco A, Brumana T, Aru G, Livi U, Gallucci V: Mitral valve prosthesis dehiscence necessitating reoperation: An analysis of the risk factors involved. *Thorac Cardiovasc Surg* 31:91, 1983.

18. Rastelli G, Kirklin JW: Hemodynamic state early after prosthetic replacement of mitral valve. *Circulation* 34:448, 1966.

S

1. Souttar HS: The surgical treatment of mitral stenosis. *Br Med J* 2:603, 1925.

2. Starr A, Edwards ML: Mitral replacement: Clinical experience with a ball valve prosthesis. *Ann Surg* 154:726, 1961.

3. Selzer A, Cohn KE: Natural history of mitral stenosis: A review. *Circulation* 45:878, 1972.

4. Selzer A, Katayama F: Mitral regurgitation: Clinical patterns, pathophysiology and natural history. *Medicine* 51:337, 1972.

5. Sanders SP, Levy RV, Freed MD, Norwood WI, Castaneda AR: Use of Hancock porcine xenografts in children and adolescents. *Am J Cardiol* 46:429, 1980.

6. Schuler G, Peterson KL, Johnson A, Francis G, Dennish G, Utley J, Daily PO, Ashburn W, Ross J Jr: Temporal response of left ventricular performance to mitral valve surgery. *Circulation* 59:1218, 1979.

7. Saksena DS, Tucker BL, Lindesmith GG, Nelson RM, Stiles QR, Meyer BW: The superior approach to the mitral valve. *Ann Thorac Surg* 12:146, 1971.

8. Salomon NW, Stinson EB, Griepp RB, Shumway NE: Patient-related risk factors as predictors of results following isolated mitral valve replacement. *Ann Thorac Surg* 24:519, 1977.

9. Selzer A, Kelly JJ Jr, Kerth WJ, Gerbode F: Immediate and long-range results of valvuloplasty for mitral regurgitation due to ruptured chordae tendineae. *Circulation* 45,46(suppl I):I-52, 1972.

10. Smith WM, Neutze JM, Barratt-Boyes BG, Lower JB: Open mitral valvotomy: Effect of preoperative factors on result. *J Thorac Cardiovasc Surg* 82:738, 1981.

11. Slater SD, Sallam IA, Bain WH, Turner MA, Lawrie TDV: Haemolysis with Bjork-Shiley and Starr-Edwards prosthetic heart valves: A comparative study. *Thorax* 29:624, 1974.

12. Sanfelippo PM, Giuliani ER, Danielson GK, Wallace RB, Pluth JR, McGoon DC: Tricuspid valve prosthetic replacement. *J Thorac Cardiovasc Surg* 71:441, 1976.

13. Simon R, Oelert H, Borst H-G, Lichtlen PR: Influence of mitral valve surgery on tricuspid incompetence concomitant with mitral valve disease. *Circulation* 62(suppl I):I-152, 1980.

14. Strom J, Becker RM, Frishman W, Salazar C, Oku Y, Bassell G, Lin YT, Frater RW: Hemodynamic evaluation of the Ionescu-Shiley bovine heterograft valve. *Am J Cardiol* 41:421, 1978.

15. Sala A, Schoevaerdts JC, Jaumin P, Ponlot R, Chalant CM: Review of 387 isolated mitral valve replacements by the model 6120 Starr-Edwards prosthesis. *J Thorac Cardiovasc Surg* 84:744, 1982.

16. Spratt JA, Olsen CO, Tyson GS Jr, Glower DD Jr, Davis JW, Rankin JS: Experimental mitral regurgitation: Physiological effects of correction on left ventricular dynamics. *J Thorac Cardiovasc Surg* 86:479, 1983.

T

1. Tsakiri AG, Mair DD, Seki S, Titus JL, Wood EH: Motion of the tricuspid valve annulus in anesthetized intact dogs. *Circ Res* 36:43, 1975.

2. Taylor RR, Hopkins BE: Left ventricular response to experimentally induced chronic regurgitation. *Cardiovasc Res* 6:404, 1972.

3. Tsakiris AG, Rastelli GC, Banchero N, Wood EH, Kirklin JW: Fixation of the annulus of the mitral valve with a rigid ring: Hemodynamic studies. *Am J Cardiol* 20:812, 1967.

4. Teply JF, Grunkemeier GL, Sutherland HD, Lambert LE, Johnson VA, Starr A: The ultimate prognosis after valve replacement: An assessment at twenty years. *Ann Thorac Surg* 32:111, 1981.

5. Tsakiri AG, Sturm RE, Wood EH: Experimental studies on the mechanisms of closure of cardiac valves with use of roentgen videodensitometry. *Am J Cardiol* 32:136, 1973.

U

1. Urschel CW, Covell JW, Sonnenblick EH, Ross J Jr, Braunwald E: Myocardial mechanics in aortic and mitral valvular regurgitation: The concept of instantaneous impedance as a determinant of the performance of the intact heart. *J Clin Invest* 47:867, 1968.

V

1. Vega JL, Fleitas M, Martinez R, Gallo JI, Gutierrez JA, Colman T, Duran CMG: Open mitral commissurotomy. *Ann Thorac Surg* 31:266, 1981.

W

1. Williams JB, Karp RB, Kirklin JW, Kouchoukos NT, Pacifico AD, Zorn GL Jr, Blackstone EH, Brown RN, Piantadosi S, Bradley EL: Considerations in selection and management of patients undergoing valve replacement with glutaraldehyde-fixed porcine bioprostheses. *Ann Thorac Surg* 30:247, 1980.

2. Wood P: An appreciation of mitral stenosis. *Br Med J* 1:1051, 1954.

3. Warnes CA, Scott ML, Silver GM, Smith CW, Ferrans VJ, Roberts WC: Comparison of late degenerative changes in porcine bioprostheses in the mitral and aortic valve position in the same patient. *Am J Cardiol* 51:965, 1983.

Y

1. Yacoub M, Halim M, Radley-Smith R, McKay R, Nijveld A, Towers M: Surgical treatment of mitral regurgitation caused by floppy valves: Repair versus replacement. *Circulation* 64(suppl II):II-210, 1981.

12

AORTIC VALVE DISEASE

DEFINITION

This chapter describes the surgical aspects of aortic valve disease, excluding congenital aortic stenosis in infants and children (see Chapter 32) and aortic incompetence with ventricular septal defect (see Chapter 20) or sinus of Valsalva aneurysm (see Chapter 21).

HISTORICAL NOTE

In 1947, Smithy (who died of mitral stenosis at age 45) and Parker, at the University of South Carolina in Charleston,

first reported an experimental study of aortic valvotomy.[S2] Apparently, before that time, surgeons did not seriously contemplate the surgical treatment of aortic valve disease. In the early 1950s, Bailey and colleagues, in Philadelphia, used closed methods—either a dilator introduced transventricularly or a digital approach through a "poncho" sewn onto the ascending aorta—in clinical attempts to relieve severe aortic stenosis.[B2,B3] Modest success in some patients was obtained by them and by us.[E3]

In 1951, Hufnagel, in Washington, D.C., developed a ball valve prosthesis for rapid insertion into the descending thoracic aorta.[H1,H2] (From his work with Gross in the development of the coarctation operation, he was well aware of the risk of paraplegia with aortic cross-clamping; see Chapter 34.) The prosthesis could be rapidly inserted because of its multiple point fixation rings, placed outside the aorta and around each end of the prosthesis within the aorta. He, we,[E4] and others obtained fairly good palliation of severe aortic incompetence in some patients with this device. However, the upper body signs of aortic incompetence became very severe. In the early 1950s, Bailey developed and actually used in patients a number of ingenious but quite unsuccessful closed methods of overcoming aortic incompetence.[B1]

A more effective approach to the surgical treatment of aortic valve disease in adults began with the advent of clinical cardiopulmonary bypass (CPB) through a pump-oxygenator in 1954 and 1955 (see Chapter 2). At first, aortic valvotomy and the removal of calcific deposits were all that could be done.[H11,K11] Then Bahnson and, independently, Hufnagel[H9] developed a single-leaflet prosthesis, which became commercially available and was used considerably by us and others.[H11,M17] Generally, the leaflets were used for partial replacement of the aortic valve, but they could be used together for total aortic valve replacement. Probably the first single-unit prosthesis for total aortic valve replacement was the Teflon sleeve prosthesis developed and first used by McGoon at the Mayo Clinic in 1961.[M6] Although this device was used successfully (at least in terms of early results) by us at the Mayo Clinic for a short time, initial competence was sometimes not achieved, and this made the hospital mortality appreciable. The introduction of the ball valve prosthesis for aortic valve replacement by Harken and Starr in 1960 established aortic valve surgery on a firm basis.[H10,S16] A number of different kinds of prosthetic valves have subsequently appeared.

The 1956 report of Murray[M15] showed that the semilunar aortic valve could be used as a valve transplant in the descending thoracic aorta in patients with aortic incompetence, and a subsequent report[K13] included a 6-year follow-up. The first orthotopic insertion of a homograft valve using the modern double suture line technique was performed at GLH in August 1962.[B28] Ross, in London, working independently, carried out a similar procedure in July of that year[R3,R10] using a single suture line technique described by Duran and Gunning.[D7] At first, the valves were collected aseptically and implanted within a few days or weeks, but, for logistic reasons, this technique was soon replaced by unsterile collection and sterilization by either betapropiolactone or ethylene oxide. The homografts were then stored either in Hanks' balanced salt solution at 4°C or by freeze-drying.[B27] In 1968, because of a relatively high incidence of cusp rupture with these techniques, antibiotic sterilization was introduced at GLH;[B6] unfortunately, our experience at the Mayo Clinic and early at UAB continued with sterilization chemically or by irradiation.[H12,K12,P7]

Other biological valves soon began to be used. Senning and colleagues, in Zurich, replaced the aortic valve clinically with individual leaflets made of the patients' own fascia lata.[S17] A high late postoperative incidence of bacterial endocarditis caused this method to be abandoned. Use of autologous fascia lata mounted on a frame was described by Ionescu and Ross[I4] but was also abandoned because of late dehiscence. Allograft dura mater valves preserved in glycerol were used for aortic valve replacement by Zerbini and colleagues, in Brazil.[P5]

The first stent-mounted porcine aortic valves were sterilized and preserved in a special formaldehyde solution and implanted by Binet in Paris in 1965.[B19] They were used at UAB for a short period but were not satisfactory, as they degenerated rapidly, with dehiscence of the commissures from the frame. The glutaraldehyde-preserved stent-mounted porcine valves were introduced by Carpentier, in Paris, in 1968.[C3] Bovine pericardium, glutaraldehyde-treated and frame-mounted, was introduced by Ionescu at Leeds, England, in 1971.[I5]

MORPHOLOGY

Aortic Stenosis

Adult aortic stenosis in developed countries most commonly results from the calcareous degeneration of congenitally malformed and bicuspid valves. As seen at operation, *calcific aortic stenosis in a congenitally bicuspid valve* presents a mountainous mass of calcium within the leaflets that often extends into the anulus. The subannular extension in the region of the rightward portion of the right coronary cusp and commissure between it and the noncoronary cusp (beneath which is the membranous septum) leads to complete heart block in some patients. The orifice is small, often eccentrically located, and usually fixed. Because of this, there is usually some valvar incompetence. The commissure between the left coronary and noncoronary cusps is often well formed, but usually that between the left and right coronary cusps is represented only by a heavily calcified central buttress between these cusps.

Rheumatic aortic stenosis has an entirely different appearance. The basic tricuspid architecture of the valve is preserved. The cusps are fused along the commissures by the rheumatic process, resulting in a somewhat cone-shaped valvar mass with a narrow orifice in the middle. The cusps are usually somewhat thickened and cartilaginous. A little calcification may be present. Truly isolated rheumatic aortic stenosis is uncommon (Table 12-1), as the mitral valve usually is also affected, albeit subclinically.

Occasionally in patients over about 60 years of age, a severe systolic pressure gradient is present across a three-

Table 12-1 Etiology of isolated aortic stenosis in adults presenting for their first operation (GLH; 1962–1981). Ten of the total gave a history of bacterial endocarditis.

Etiology	No.		%
Congenital	460		61.3%
Calcified		456	
Noncalcified		4	
Rheumatic	95		12.6%
Atheromatous	182		24.2%
Calcific (uncertain etiology)	14		1.9%
Total	751		100%

cusped valve without commissural fusion. The leaflets are a little thickened generally, and fine coarse calcific particles and atheromatous deposits fill the aortic side of the belly of the cusps. This severely restricts valve motion, and a functionally important stenosis results. This is assumed to be *arteriosclerotic aortic stenosis*.

Aortic Incompetence

The morphologic characteristics of aortic incompetence depend on a widely varied etiology (Table 12-2). *Rheumatic aortic incompetence* results from a different response of the valve to the rheumatic process than occurs when stenosis develops. Commissural fusion is not present, and the leaflets are only a little thickened. The major pathologic process appears to be a cicatricial shortening of the distance between the free edge of the cusps and their annular attachment. As time passes, the aortic root widens in response to the aortic regurgitation, increasing the valvar incompetence still further.

Annular ectasia can produce severe valvular incompetence even though the cusps are normal, and this morphologic basis for the incompetence is becoming more common in surgical series.[O6] This is most commonly due to medionecrosis of the ascending aorta and can be associated with Marfan's syndrome. The process begins in the sinuses of Valsalva, and at this stage incompetence is usually not present. With time, the process extends to involve the proximal ascending aorta, producing a symmetric, pear-shaped aneurysmal enlargement. Incompetence now appears and progresses because the dilatation of the aortic wall at commissural level tightens the free leaflet edges, which can no longer coapt during diastole. The aortic anulus is not primarily involved, although it, too, dilates in response to the increasing regurgitation. The aneurysmal process eventually involves the entire ascending aorta but nearly always stops abruptly before the innominate artery origin, although the remainder of the arch usually shows medionecrosis. The aneurysms are thin walled with a smooth lining. Acute or chronic localized or extending dissections may begin within them and extend proximally and distally, although most acute aortic dissections occur in the absence of a medionecrotic root aneurysm. With proximal extension of such a dissection, the commissural attachment of the valve becomes separated from the outer aortic wall so that the valve prolapses centrally and acute incompetence occurs (see Chapter 54).

The less common *atherosclerotic ascending aortic aneurysm* produces valvar incompetence in a similar fashion, but these aneurysms display severe intimal atheroma and are not usually associated with dissection. *Syphilitic ascending aortic aneurysm* is also accompanied by aortic incompetence, exacerbated by a valvulitis that produces cusp edge thickening and retraction.

Bacterial endocarditis is a fairly frequent cause of aortic incompetence. It may occur on a structurally normal valve or on congenitally or rheumatically deformed valves. Incompetence may result from a destroyed commissural area, with leaflet prolapse, or from a perforation in the cusp belly. An infected pannus may appear below the cusps, or there may be extensive destruction of the aortic root, with a periaortic root abscess sometimes extending onto the anterior mitral leaflet.

A congenitally *bicuspid or unicuspid valve* can produce incompetence due to prolapse of the free edge of a redundant leaflet.[R8] In such cases, the incompetence may be aggravated by bacterial endocarditis or by an attempt at valvotomy (see Chapter 32).

An *aortitis* occurs in some patients with rheumatoid arthritis, ankylosing spondylitis,[S4] and Reiter's disease. This may lead to aneurysmal dilation of the ascending aorta and aortic valvar incompetence.[K10] The aortitis is characterized by a dense adventitial inflammatory fibrosis involving the sinuses of Valsalva and proximal aorta, particularly adjacent to the commissures.[B18] The process may extend below the base of the aortic valve to form a characteristic subvalvar ridge and may involve the base of the anterior mitral leaflet or even the adjacent ventricular septum, causing conduction disturbances. In rheumatoid arthritis in particular, the leaflets may be thickened and shortened and show rheumatoid nodules histologically.[R11]

Other rare causes of aortic valve incompetence are spontaneous cusp rupture,[O2] rupture due to severe closed chest trauma,[M7,R13] and severe long-standing systemic hypertension with aortic root dilatation (annular ectasia). Recent studies have indicated that, in patients with long-standing hypertension and in some others, the valvar incompetence

Table 12-2 The etiology of isolated aortic incompetence, including cases of ascending arch aneurysm, in patients presenting for their first operation (GLH; 1962–1981).

Etiology	No.		%
Rheumatic fever	217		46.5%
Alone		173	
+ BE		44	
Medionecrosis	84		18.0%
Alone		19	
+ Dissection		25	
+ Aneurysm		40	
Congenital (bicuspid)	63		13.5%
Alone		33	
+ BE		30	
Bacterial endocarditis	60		12.8%
(on "normal" valve)			
Syphilis	10		2.1%
Alone		6	
+ Aneurysm		4	
Atheromatous aneurysm	4		0.9%
Aortitis	10		2.1%
Reiter's disease		2	
Ankylosing spondylitis		2	
Rheumatoid arthritis		6	
Spontaneous cusp rupture	6		1.3%
Hypertension	4		0.9%
Uncertain	9		1.9%
Total	467		100%

KEY: BE, bacterial endocarditis.

[a] Twenty-one showed calcification.

may be the result of typical myxoid degeneration of the valve.[A5,L11,T8]

Occasionally, the etiology of the incompetence may not be apparent. Some instances of incompetence are probably related to the arthropathies with minimal joint involvement, or to hypertension, psoriasis, giant cell aortitis,[G9] or Takyashu's disease.

Combined Aortic Stenosis and Incompetence

The etiology and morphology of aortic stenosis and incompetence are similar to those for the stenotic group (Table 12-3). In some cases, an episode of endocarditis produces incompetence in a previously stenotic valve.

CLINICAL FEATURES AND DIAGNOSTIC CRITERIA

Aortic Stenosis

Patients with aortic stenosis are usually symptomatic when first seen (Table 12-4), but they may present in an asymptomatic state, being referred because of a cardiac murmur. The classic triad of effort dyspnea, angina, and syncope is present in about one-third of the patients. Angina pectoris is present as the only symptom or combined with others in 50%–70% of patients.[B7,B8,B9,E1,L1] The angina pectoris in aortic stenosis *without* coronary artery disease has been thought to be the result of increased myocardial oxygen consumption related to the increased left ventricular (LV) systolic pressure and increased left ventricular mass. However, Basta and colleagues did not find a difference at rest in the hemodynamic variables or in left ventricular wall thickness or volume of patient with angina pectoris, as opposed to those without it.[B7,B10,M3] From 30%–50% have frank or incipient syncope. Symptoms of pulmonary venous hypertension (dyspnea, orthopnea, paroxysmal nocturnal dyspnea, or frank pulmonary edema) are present in 30%–40% of cases, either alone or with other symptoms. A very few patients (10%) survive these symptoms long enough to develop secondary right ventricular failure. They present with a clinical picture dominated by elevated right atrial and jugular venous pressure, hepatomegaly, cardiac cachexia, and, rarely, tricuspid incompetence.

Table 12-3 The etiology of combined (balanced) aortic stenosis and incompetence in patients presenting for their first aortic valve replacement (GLH; 1962–1981).

Etiology	No.		%
Congenital (bicuspid)	43[a]		51%
Calcified		41	
Noncalcified		2	
Rheumatic fever	39[a]		46%
Syphilis (without aneurysm)	1		1%
Aortitis (rheumatoid arthritis)	1		1%
Uncertain	1		1%
Total	85		100%

[a]Eight of these 82 patients also had endocarditis.

Table 12-4 Symptoms present in 1273 patients with isolated aortic valve disease before their first aortic valve replacement (GLH; 1962–1981).

Symptoms	Aortic Stenosis		Aortic Incompetence		Mixed Stenosis and Incompetence	
	No.	%	No.	%	No.	%
None	7	0.9%	18	4.5%	2	2.2%
Angina	512	65.2%	80	20.1%	47	52.2%
Syncope	379	48.3%	4	1.0%	21	23.2%
Dyspnea (effort)	381	48.5%	125	31.4%	38	42.2%
Orthopnea	20	2.5%	11	2.8%	2	2.2%
PND or pulmonary edema	218	27.8%	129	32.4%	33	36.7%
Systemic venous congestion	83	10.6%	102	25.6%	12	13.3%
Other	1	0.1%	5	1.3%	0	0%
Angina + syncope + dyspnea	264	33.6%	3	0.8%	14	15.6%
Total	785		398		90	

KEY: PND, paroxysmal nocturnal dyspnea.

On physical examination, a diagnosis of important aortic stenosis can often be made with reasonable certainty when in addition to the presence of an aortic ejection murmur (usually best heard in the second right intercostal space beside the sternum and conducted to the carotids but often well heard also at the apex and in the second left intercostal space) the arterial pulse is of small volume with a slow upstroke. Support for the diagnosis may be obtained from expiratory splitting of the second heart sound and from evidence of left ventricular hypertrophy provided by the character of the apex beat and the electrocardiogram. When in addition the chest x-ray or cinefluoroscopy shows calcification of the aortic valve and the convexity along the upper part of the left ventricular silhouette produced by left ventricular hypertrophy, the diagnosis of calcareous aortic stenosis becomes a near certainty.[E1] Usually, but not always, the electrocardiogram gives evidence of left ventricular hypertrophy, with or without inverted T waves in V_6 (so-called strain pattern).

At times, the physical findings are less diagnostic. Systemic hypertension or, in the older patient, inelasticity of aortic and arterial walls may alter the character of the arterial pulse wave and prevent the development of a clinically recognizable slow upstroke. Absence of the aortic component may prevent assessment of the respiratory behavior of the second heart sound while, in those with right or left bundle-branch block, splitting of this sound is of no value as a guide to the severity of aortic stenosis. Moreover, in the older patient especially, the character of the cardiac apex may be unreliable as a clinical guide to the presence and degree of left ventricular hypertrophy. The electrocardiogram also at times fails to show the degree of left ventricular hypertrophy to be expected in severe aortic stenosis and, indeed, in an occasional patient with this condition, the electrocardiogram remains strictly normal and without any evidence of left ventricular involvement. Finally, in the terminal stages of low output heart failure, the aortic murmur may be so faint as not to direct attention to the presence of aortic stenosis, particularly in adult patients in whom the heart sounds are distant, either because of thickness of the chest wall or inelastic and voluminous lungs.

When the clinical findings are classic, the diagnosis of severe aortic stenosis can be made with a high degree of confidence, and special studies are not needed.[E1] However, in patients over about 40 years of age, coronary arteriography is performed when operation is being considered, since coronary artery disease coexists in a considerable proportion of these patients whether or not they have angina.[B10,M3] At the time of coronary arteriography, the systolic pressure gradient across the aortic valve is measured. (Basta and colleagues recommend coronary arteriography only when the patient has angina pectoris, since they conclude from their experience that patients without this symptom rarely have coronary artery disease.) Cardiac output can be measured, and the valve area calculated by the Gorlin equation. A valve area less than $0.8 \text{ cm}^2 \cdot \text{m}^{-2}$ represents significant stenosis.

When the clinical findings are atypical but the diagnosis of important aortic stenosis is being considered, retrograde arterial catheterization and measurements of the aortic valve gradient are indicated.

Aortic Incompetence

Patients with aortic incompetence more frequently present without symptoms than do those with aortic stenosis, perhaps because of the more dramatic physical and radiologic findings of this condition and because of its relatively long asymptomatic phase. In most patients, the dominant symptoms are those of pulmonary venous hypertension (dyspnea, orthopnea, paroxysmal nocturnal dyspnea, or pulmonary edema). Angina pectoris is often part of the presenting complaint but is the chief complaint in less than one-quarter of the cases[B7,G2,S3] (Table 12-4) and tends to be more common in older patients. Coronary artery disease is present in about 20% of the patients with angina pectoris.[B7] Syncope (dizziness) is quite rare.

In severe aortic incompetence, the left ventricular apex is usually displaced and overactive in character. The carotid and other pulses are jerky to palpation in moderate incompetence and collapsing or "water hammer" in severe incompetence due to the wide pulse pressure and the rapid rise and fall of the pulse wave. Blood pressure measured by the Korotkof sounds may reach 200–250 mmHg systolic and 50–0 mmHg diastolic. Usually, the brachial or radial pulse pressure measured by an arterial needle is less than by Korotkof sounds, and the central aortic pulse pressure is less still. These phenomena (including the systolic amplification observed between central aortic and radial artery blood pressure) are related to the standing waves created by the pulsatile ejection of an unusually large left ventricular stroke volume into the aorta and the remainder of the arterial tree. If the cardiac output is low with severe cardiac failure, these phenomena are minimized.

Auscultation in the aortic area reveals an early diastolic murmur that radiates toward the apex of the heart. Often a systolic click or ejection murmur is also present. At the apex, there is frequently a mid-diastolic murmur due to fluttering of the anterior mitral leaflet produced by a prominent regurgitant jet (Austin Flint murmur). This may be difficult

to distinguish from mitral stenosis, although in the latter an opening snap is often present. When mitral stenosis coexists, the electrocardiogram usually shows p-mitrale, and the left atrium is enlarged. Two-dimensional echocardiography is most useful in making the distinction between mitral stenosis and merely an Austin-Flint murmur. The chest x-ray confirms left ventricular enlargement; the left atrium is usually normal or slightly enlarged. Radiological evidence of pulmonary venous hypertension may or may not be present. Enlargement of the shadow of the ascending aorta to the right suggests an accompanying aneurysm of the ascending aorta, but an aneurysm can be present without this sign. The electrocardiogram gives evidence of left ventricular enlargement, often with the high-peaked T waves and prominent Q waves of left ventricular volume overload. T-wave inversion and ST-segment depression is seldom present until the left ventricle is very large. In severe and long-standing pure aortic incompetence, the electrocardiogram may show p-mitrale.

The diagnosis of aortic valve incompetence can usually be made on the clinical findings, but other abnormalities in the aortic root allowing a rapid aortic runoff (such as ruptured aneurysm of the sinus of Valsalva and large patent ductus arteriosus with pulmonary valve incompetence) cannot be entirely eliminated without special studies. The diagnosis can be firmly established and the degree of aortic incompetence quantitated by cineangiography using an aortic root contrast injection in the right anterior oblique projection.[B27] In patients over the age of about 40 years, coronary arteriography also is indicated.

Combined Aortic Stenosis and Incompetence

While many patients with severe aortic stenosis have mild incompetence and a few with severe incompetence have some stenosis, there remains a small group of patients in whom the lesions appear virtually balanced. The symptoms in such patients are generally similar to those of aortic stenosis (Table 12-4). This may in fact be a particularly unfavorable group because there is both a volume and pressure overload on the left ventricle.

NATURAL HISTORY

Aortic Stenosis

Unfortunately, the natural history of surgically untreated adults with aortic valve disease is incompletely known, and a general concept about this requires a number of assumptions.

Grant has reported that 35% of symptomatic, surgically untreated patients with aortic stenosis are alive at the end of 10 years.[G1] Wood stated that 46% of such patients were alive 1–7 years later.[W3] Frank and Ross report that, of 12 surgically untreated patients with severe aortic stenosis, only 18% were alive 5 years later.[F1] On the basis of their data, Ross and Braunwald conclude that average survival after onset of angina or syncope is 3 years, and after the onset of congestive failure about 1.5 years.[R1]

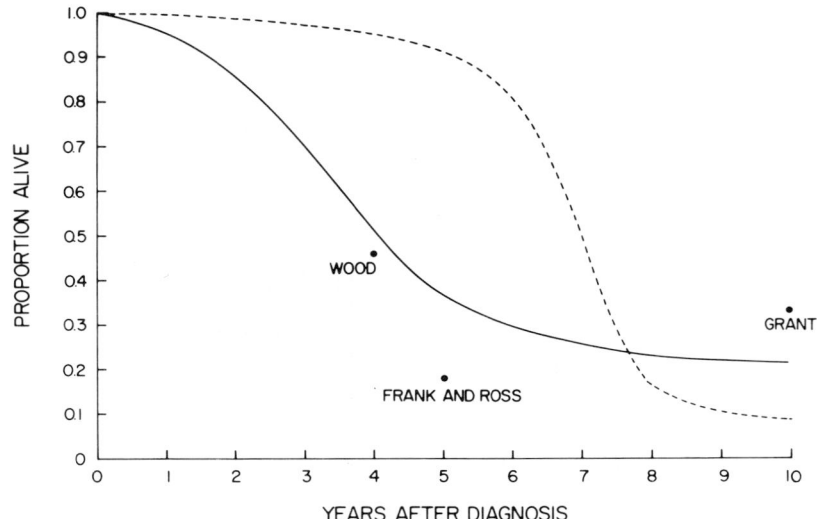

Figure 12-1 Freehand and nonrigorously derived survival curves for patients with surgically un-treated severe aortic stenosis and severe aortic incompetence. The survival of such patients with aortic stenosis reported by Wood,[W3] Frank and Ross,[F1] and Grant[G1] are shown as discrete solid circles.

KEY: ---------, aortic incompetence; ————, aortic stenosis.

While it is impossible to assemble rigorously such dispar-ate data, a likely survival curve for adult patients with se-vere, surgically untreated aortic stenosis is shown in Figure 12-1. The deaths within the first year or two are likely to be sudden, presumably associated with ventricular fibrillation (15%–20% of all deaths in aortic stenosis are sudden[F1]), or after a few hours or days of acute pulmonary edema, from sudden left ventricular failure. Most surgically untreated pa-tients die in the latter mode within about 5 years of diag-nosis. Beyond 5 years of follow-up, some die of gradually worsening cardiac failure, with low cardiac output and gradually worsening symptoms of pulmonary venous hyper-tension. Moderate pulmonary artery hypertension develops in some patients exhibiting these findings, and in a few, typi-cal symptoms and signs of *right* ventricular failure become prominent.

The left ventricle progressively hypertrophies in the pres-ence of important aortic stenosis, and the myocardial cells hypertrophy. The resultant thickening of the left ventricular wall keeps left ventricular afterload (systolic wall stress; see Chapter 5, footnote 10) more or less normal, and left ventric-ular systolic function is preserved. Left ventricular com-pliance, however, decreases, and thus diastolic function is decreased. At a more advanced stage, hypertrophy and wall thickness increase less than does left ventricular systolic pressure (afterload mismatch[R2]), and the resulting increase in afterload impairs systolic function of the left ventricle. Indexes of systolic function (ejection fraction, end-systolic volume, left ventricular fractional shortening, velocity of cir-cumferential shortening) decline, cardiac output decreases gradually or acutely, and left ventricular end-diastolic pres-sure increases. Contractility is preserved initially, but in the later stages of the life history of the patient becomes re-duced. By this time, the condition is very advanced, and chronic heart failure is present.

Occasionally, complete heart block develops in patients with extensive calcification of the stenotic aortic valve. This may be the result of gradually increasing pressure on the bundle of His by calcific deposits beneath the commissural area between the noncoronary and right coronary cusps.[W6] However, complete heart block sometimes occurs in pa-tients with calcific aortic stenosis without calcific pressure on the bundle of His,[L5] and it is hypothesized that pressure in the left ventricle may play a role in this. Very rarely, surgical relief of the aortic stenosis relieves the heart block.[P4]

Aortic Incompetence

The fate of patients with aortic incompetence depends primarily on the severity of the incompetence.[H6] Mild or moderate aortic incompetence appears to affect activity and life expectancy very little.

Severe aortic incompetence may have a long latent period of 3–10 years in which left ventricular enlargement is only mild and symptoms are absent or mild.[S1] Bonow and col-leagues have shown that 81% of asymptomatic patients with normal left ventricular systolic function are alive and with-out the need of aortic valve replacement 5 years later and that when operation is indicated because of the development of symptoms or increasing left ventricular enlargement, the response to surgery is in all ways satisfactory.[B42] The pa-tient's life-style may partly determine when left ventricular enlargement begins to progress, but the timing of this is probably determined primarily by the rapidity of the worsen-ing of the aortic incompetence.[B15] This idea is consistent with an early finding with quantitative angiocardiography that in patients with aortic incompetence, the LV end-diastolic volume was directly related to the magnitude of the aortic regurgitant flow.[M5]

Not only does heart size increase as time passes, but the systolic function of the left ventricle decreases as well. Henry and colleagues found that in the asymptomatic stage of the disease, this decrease continues rather regularly. For example, the rate of increase in echocardiographically determined left ventricular end-systolic dimension (indicating decreased systolic function) was about 7 mm per year.[H7]

As the severity of the aortic incompetence increases to 50% or more of forward flow and cardiomegaly and loss of systolic function worsen,[C20] symptoms of effort intolerance and angina develop. Resting ejection fraction is well maintained during this time,[K4] and left ventricular end-diastolic pressure may remain low.[L2] In most patients, eventually a loss of left ventricular reserve develops, and left ventricular end-diastolic pressure may then rise rapidly. Croft and colleagues present data which indicate that when left ventricular function begins to deteriorate, the deterioration then often progresses rapidly.[C20] With this, symptoms of pulmonary venous hypertension appear, sometimes suddenly. These may rapidly progress to a fatal outcome. Even if they regress temporarily under treatment, they indicate an advanced stage of aortic incompetence and a poor prognosis without surgical treatment.

Should the patient escape catastrophic symptomatology, left ventricular functional and structural deterioration proceed. Ejection fraction at rest becomes reduced, and there is a lack of increase in left ventricular stroke work in response to a stress such as afterload increase by an infusion of angiotensin. Symptoms worsen, and in most patients, once this stage is reached, death comes within 6–18 months (Fig. 12-1).

Most patients with aortic incompetence live long enough to develop considerable left ventricular enlargement and severe left ventricular hypertrophy.[S8] Rarely, these patients may develop secondary right ventricular failure and chronic congestive heart failure. Rarely, complete heart block may occur. Once advanced symptoms develop, death within 2–3 years is the rule.

The left ventricle responds to the incompetence by a change in its ultrastructure and by increasing its left ventricular volume, mass, and wall thickness.[P2] Left ventricular compliance decreases, and thus diastolic function is compromised.[C11] For a time, left ventricular systolic function is preserved by compensatory processes. Although left ventricular systolic function declines as the incompetence worsens, symptoms are minimal and exercise tolerance is maintained for some time. In time, however, the systolic function declines to such a state that it worsens during stress (such as exercise or isoproterenol infusion). Symptoms then worsen, and the decline continues.

In a group of 180 patients with isolated severe aortic incompetence of rheumatic origin referred to GLH between 1958 and 1967, the factors that increased the risk of death without operation were heart failure, ventricular premature beats, marked cardiomegaly (cardiothoracic ratio > 0.6) and extreme left ventricular hypertrophy in the electrocardiogram.[S8]

When severe aortic incompetence develops acutely, as from bacterial endocarditis, the natural history is much less favorable.[R16] Only 10%–30% survive more than 1 year after onset.[D5,H6,T2]

In a few patients in whom the incompetence is due to a congenitally bicuspid valve or rheumatic valvulitis, the gradual onset of leaflet calcification converts the mild-to-moderate incompetence to a dominant stenosis or a balanced lesion.

TECHNIQUE OF OPERATION

Aortic Valve Replacement

Initial Steps of the Operation

After the usual preparations and the making of the median sternotomy incision (see Chapter 2), cardiopulmonary bypass (CPB) is established at 34°C, using a large, two-stage single venous cannula (UAB) or, alternatively, two venous cannulae (GLH). Although the operation is sometimes performed without a vent, generally one is introduced into the left atrium from the right side (see Chapter 2) and advanced into left ventricle, using, if necessary, the right hand behind the heart to palpate the vent through the back wall of left atrium and help guide it through the mitral valve (rather than into the left pulmonary veins). A multiholed curved cannula[1] may be used (UAB), or, alternatively, one incorporating a pressure-monitoring line (GLH). The cardioplegic needle, on one arm of a Y assembly on the cardioplegic infusion line, is positioned in the ascending aorta. The assembly has been previously filled with cardioplegic solution. The other arm of the Y assembly, now clamped, is connected to an O ring cannula to be used later for direct cardioplegic infusion into the coronary ostia (see Chapter 3). External cardiac cooling is begun.

The temperature of the whole body perfusate is now lowered maximally. The aorta is cross-clamped, the perfusate temperature is adjusted to 25°C, and suction on the left ventricular vent is increased until the aortic root becomes empty, and the transverse aortotomy is made.

The initial aortotomy is best considered as the anterior portion of an incision for transecting the aorta and is made about 14 mm downstream to the origin of the right coronary artery (Fig. 12-2a). Its precise location is very important, not only in terms of surgical exposure, but also in terms of ease and security of closure, avoidance of damage to the right coronary artery or its ostium, and facilitation of aortic root enlargement (see "Small Aortic Root" in section on Special Situations and Controversies) should that be necessary. Exposure for this incision is facilitated by the first assistant's retracting the fat pad along the right atrioventricular groove, over the aortic root. The pulmonary artery may also need to be elevated from the aorta to avoid incising it. The initial incision is made directly anteriorly with the scissors, the collapsed state of the aorta facilitating this. Once this incision is made, the inside of the aortic root is visualized, and the decision is finalized as to whether a homograft valve will be used or prosthesis inserted.

If a homograft is to be used, the extension of the transverse portion of the aortotomy is kept 12 mm above the top of the commissures (Fig. 12-2b) to allow room to sew on the

---

[1] Made by the Sarns Company, Ann Arbor, Michigan 48106.

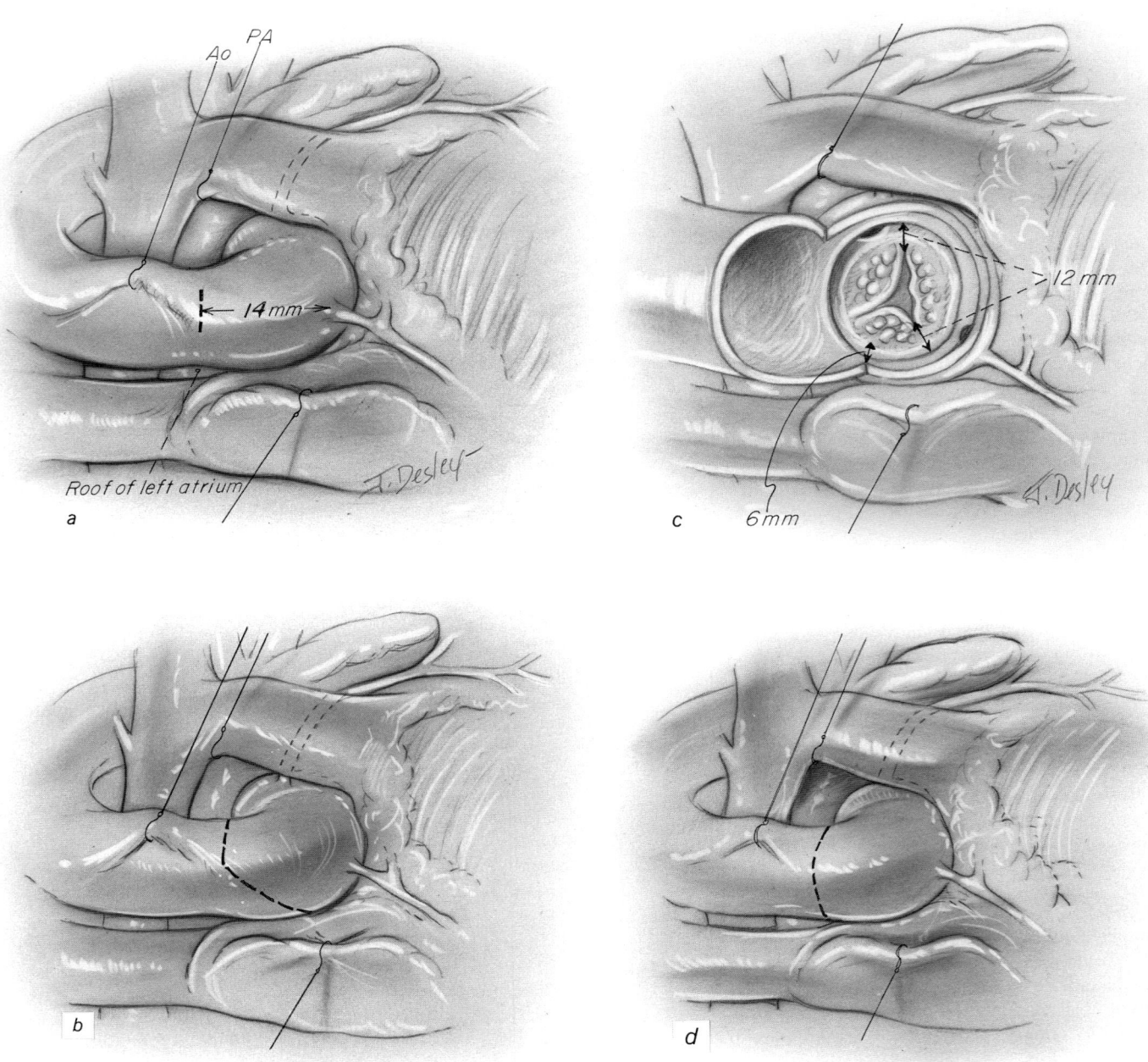

Figure 12-2 General techniques for aortic valve replacement.

(a) The initial incision into the ascending aorta is the same whether a homograft or prosthesis is used. Lengthened just a little, it suffices for infusing the cold cardioplegic solution directly into the coronary ostia, evaluating the aortic valve, and deciding on the procedure to be used.

(b) The incision is extended into the middle of the noncoronary sinus of Valsalva if the decision is for homograft replacement of the aortic valve.

(c) The aortic root is now open, and the aortic valve is exposed. Note that 12 mm of aortic wall remain above the commissure between left and right coronary cusps and that the incision into the noncoronary sinus stops 6 mm short of the nadir of the noncoronary cusp. The heavily calcified aortic valve is visible.

(d) The incision is extended as a transverse one if the decision has been made to use prosthetic replacement of the valve.

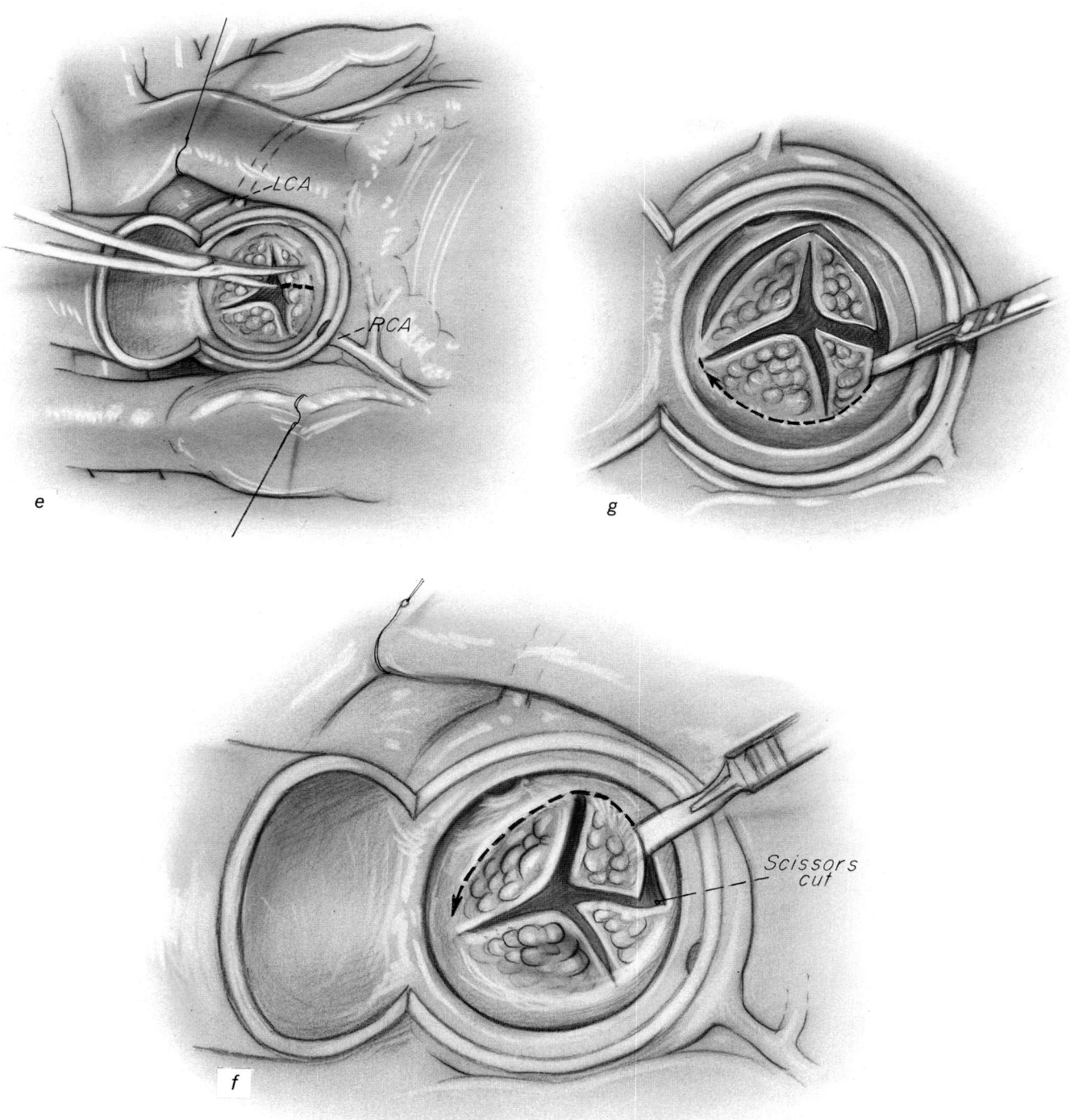

Figure 12-2 *(continued)*

(e) A scissors cut is made in the right coronary cusp, extending to but *not* into the aortic wall.

(f) The valve excision is then begun with the knife, incising the hinge line of the right coronary cusp. This incision is carried around nearly to the commissure between left and noncoronary cusps.

(g) Going back to the original scissors cut, the dissection is now carried in the opposite direction.

Ao, aorta; LCA, left coronary artery, PA, pulmonary artery; RCA, right coronary artery.

aortic buttresses of the graft above each commissure, and the incision is curved downward *exactly into the center* of the noncoronary sinus of Valsalva, stopping 6 mm above the nadir of the noncoronary cusp (Fig. 12-2*c*).

If a prosthesis is to be used, the incision is extended to the left about 5 mm downstream to the left coronary–right coronary cusp commissure and to the right, heading for a point about 5 mm downstream to the left coronary–noncoronary cusp commissure (Fig. 12-2*d*). The incision should be carried *nearly to but not beyond that point,* because if aortic root enlargement is needed, the aortic root incision is extended down into that commissural area (see "Small Aortic Root" in section on Special Situations and Controversies). Two traction sutures, *engaging only aortic adventitia,* are placed on the upstream side of the incision, one tied to the pericardial edge on the right and one to the edge on the left. Often a single traction suture is placed on the downstream side as well.

Just after the opening of the aorta and before the completion of the aortotomy and the placement of traction sutures, the cold cardioplegic solution is infused directly into the left and right coronary ostia, simultaneously (GLH) or sequentially (UAB) by clamping the arm of the Y to the cardioplegic needle and using the O ring cannula to infuse the solution first into the left coronary ostium and then into the right (see Chapter 3). This method of infusing the cold cardioplegic solution directly into the coronary ostia may be used routinely because enough incompetence is nearly always present that aortic root infusion is unsatisfactory (UAB). Alternatively, but only in patients with calcareous aortic stenosis without evident incompetence, a trial infusion of the solution can be made through the cardioplegic needle, which is positioned in the ascending aorta, before making the aortotomy (GLH). The left ventricle is gently massaged to prevent overdistention as the infusion proceeds, but if a satisfactory aortic root pressure is not achieved, this is promptly abandoned. In any case, the cold cardioplegic solution is reinfused every 30 minutes.

The aortic valve is now removed. Unless the aortic valve disease is noncalcific, a short strip of narrow packing gauze is inserted through the valve orifice into the left ventricle (and some foolproof system is used for ensuring its removal) to entrap any small calcific fragment that may escape during valvectomy. Neat, complete removal of the valve, particularly when heavily calcified, without damage to the anulus, ventricular septum, or aortic wall is one of the critically important parts of the operation. Usually, in more or less the mid portion of the right coronary cusp, there is an area where an initial scissors cut can be made from the free edge to the anulus (Fig. 12-2*e*). This allows entry of a knife blade to incise precisely along the annular attachment of the right coronary cusp toward the left coronary cusp–right coronary cusp commissure. This commissure may also be calcified, but the incision can usually be carried between it and the aortic wall, often with the scissors. The incision is then carried along the left coronary cusp's attachment to the anulus (Fig. 12-2*f*), stopping at a point about two-thirds of the way to the left coronary cusp–noncoronary cusp commissure (because its continuance beyond that point has a tendency to carry the incision *into* the aortic wall or anulus). Returning

now to the right coronary cusp, the incision is extended toward the right coronary cusp–noncoronary cusp commissure (Fig. 12-2*g*). In this area and in this commissure, the calcification is often especially abundant, and it may extend into the underlying ventricular septum or, especially at the commissure, into the aortic wall or underlying membranous septum. Thus, in dissecting this area, great care must be taken in deciding whether to cut through the cusp attachment to the anulus and aortic wall or to go around some of the calcific material and leave it for later piece-by-piece removal. To the extent possible, one-piece removal is preferable, but perforation of septum, anulus, or aortic wall should not be risked. The incision is carried down between the noncoronary cusp and anulus, stopping about two-thirds of the way to the commissure between the noncoronary and left coronary cusps. The latter commissural area, which is one of particular risk of annular and/or aortic wall perforation during the valvectomy, can then be approached with excellent visibility from both sides, and the incision is carried through this area with good upward traction on the valve.

After the valve is excised, the bed is examined, and any loose calcific particles are removed. Small remaining fragments are grasped with the thumb forceps or a small rongeur and gently removed with a twisting motion *if* it appears that this will not damage the anulus.

The downstream area of aorta near the cross-clamp is now irrigated and examined for any loose calcific fragments. The valve bed is wiped with gauze and irrigated with cold saline solution to remove any tiny fragments there. The left ventricular vent is turned off (so it will not suck fragments into the inaccessible depths of the ventricle), and the gauze strip carefully removed from the left ventricular cavity. Usually it has trapped a few small calcific fragments. The left ventricular cavity is then vigorously irrigated and aspirated with the high-pressure sucker and inspected for fragments. Usually none are found. The precautionary processes against calcific embolization now complete, the left ventricular vent is again activated. This may be a convenient time for cold cardioplegic reinfusion.

Insertion of an Aortic Valve Homograft
The aortic ring is now carefully sized with an obturator, and the aortic diameter at commissural level is also estimated. The proper-sized banked homograft valve (sized during processing at both anulus and commissural level) is selected; the diameter at both levels should be 2 mm less than in the host. When there is excessive dilatation of the host ring in association with a normal diameter at valve commissural level, as is the case often in chronic severe aortic incompetence, the aortic root is tailored down to an appropriate size (GLH; see "Large Aortic Root" in section on Special Situations and Controversies). Alternatively, this finding may be considered to indicate use of a prosthesis (UAB).

The processing of the homograft and its preparation for final trimming are described in Appendix 12C. At the operating table, the homograft valve is trimmed of excess tissue after the creation of an exactly straight lower margin 2 mm below the nadir of each aortic cusp (Fig. 12-3*a*). The cardiac muscle here is cut to leave a sewing edge 2–3 mm thick (strong enough to hold sutures well but not so bulky as to

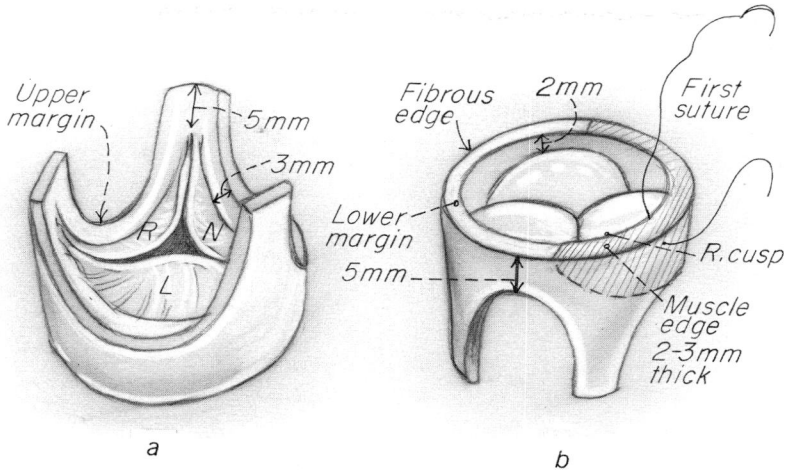

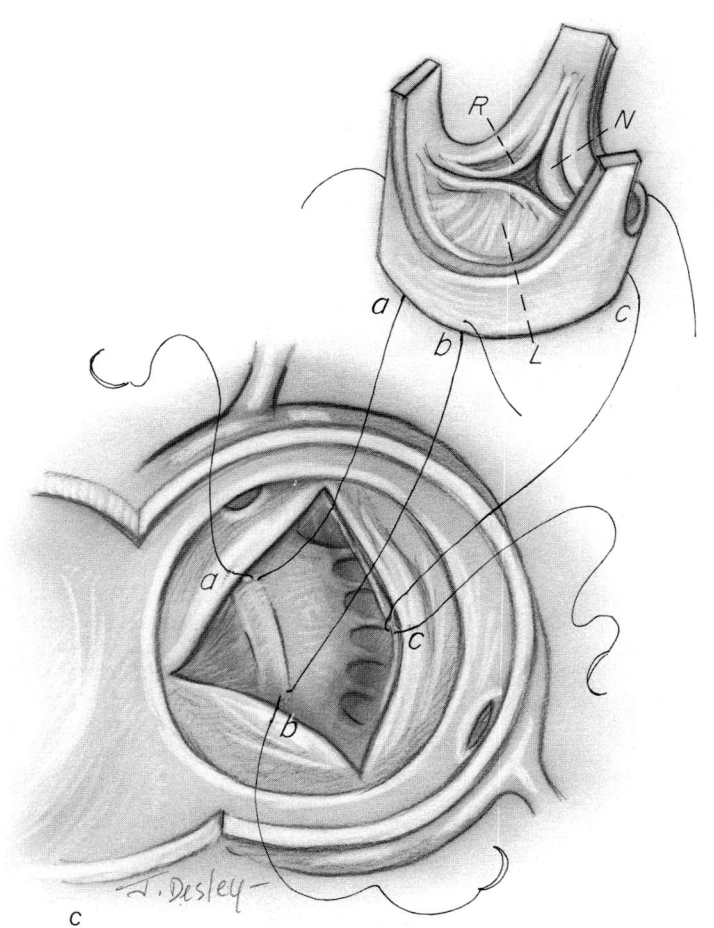

Figure 12-3 Homograft replacement of the aortic valve.

(a) The homograft has been precisely trimmed (see the text).

(b) The homograft valve has been turned upside down, and the first stitch has been placed (see the text).

(c) Three sutures have been placed, passing beneath the cusp remnant (see the text), and the valve is about to be lowered along them into the aortic root.

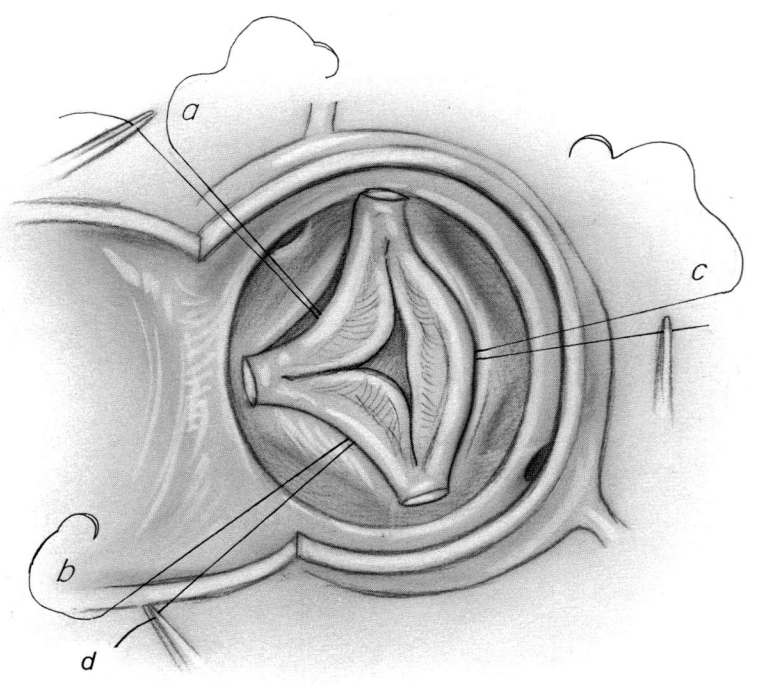

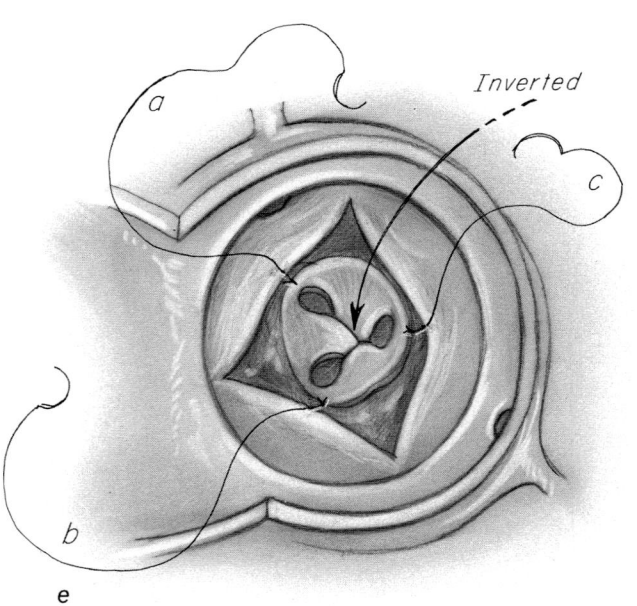

Inverted

(f) An over-and-over continuous first row of silk sutures is placed. The suture line beneath the noncoronary and left cusp base is completed first, with full thickness of the graft muscle picked up with each stitch and the needle entering 2 mm from the edge and emerging 0.5 mm from the edge (on the leaflet side) to allow the graft to seat well when turned upward. The muscle is never squeezed with forceps, as this crushes it; and the stitches are held at just enough tension to make them hemostatic without allowing them to cut through the tissue. This completed suture is tied to the stay stitch beneath the left coronary cusp, and this second stitch continues the suture line between left and right cusp bases, the sutures placed this time in backhand fashion (from graft to host). The third segment (beneath right and noncoronary cusps) is completed by passing the sutures forehand from host to graft for its first half, where the suture line must cross above the center of the membranous ventricular septum, thus making it easier to avoid the bundle of His. For the second half of this suture line, the stitches are more easily passed from graft to host through the base of the noncoronary cusp remnant. The completed suture line is now examined to ensure that it is secure. If gaps are found, they are closed with additional interrupted sutures.

(g) One pillar of the valve is pulled up to return the homograft to its correct position.

(h) Each of the three mattress sutures is in place. The correctness of the homograft position is now verified (see the text).

Figure 12-3 *(continued)*
(d) The homograft is in place in the aortic root.
(e) The homograft is inverted, and the previously placed sutures are tied.

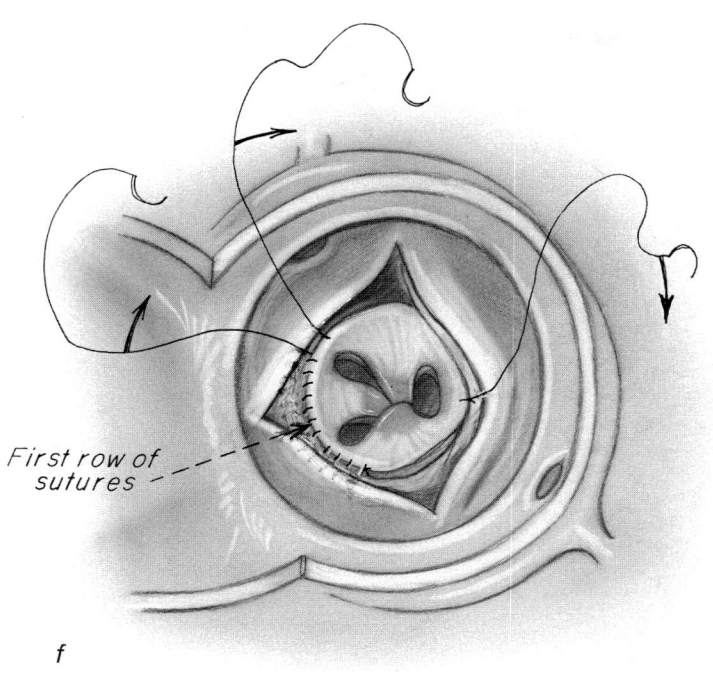

First row of
sutures

f

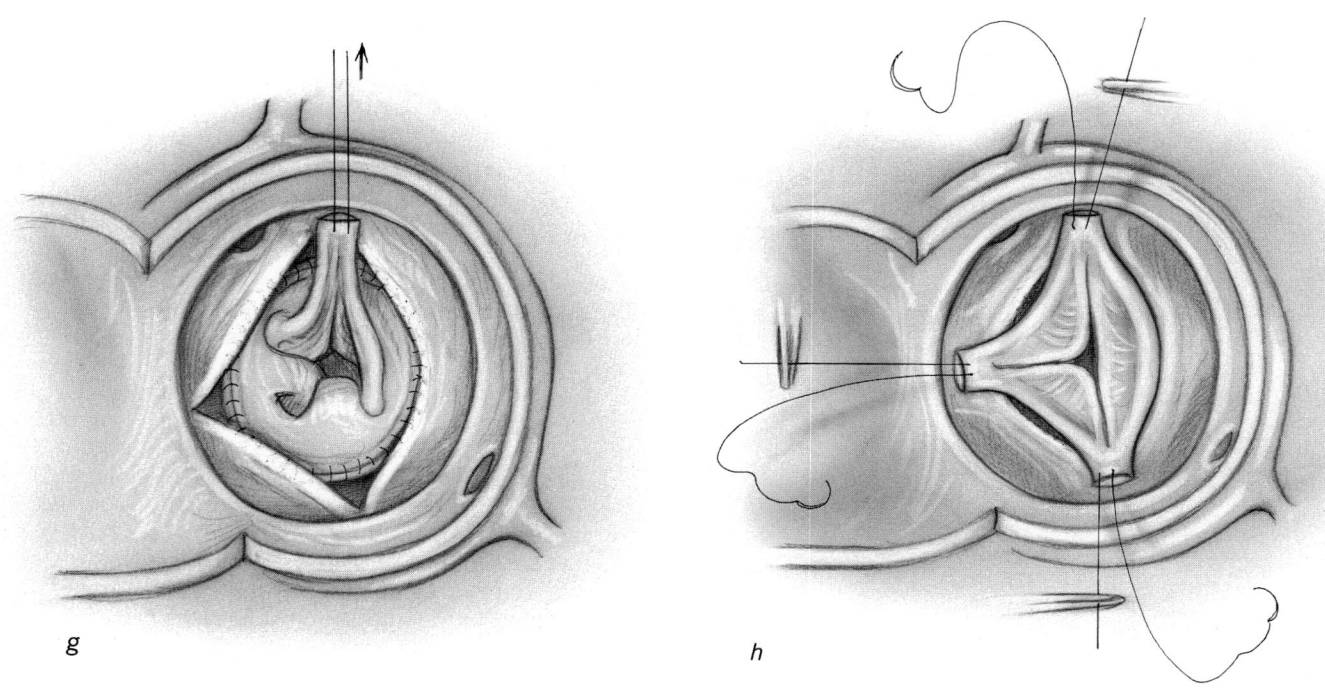

g

h

Figure 12-3 *(continued)*

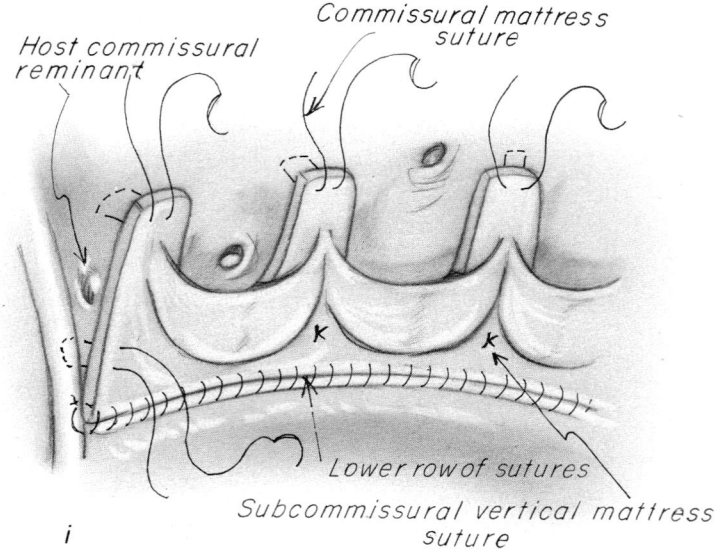

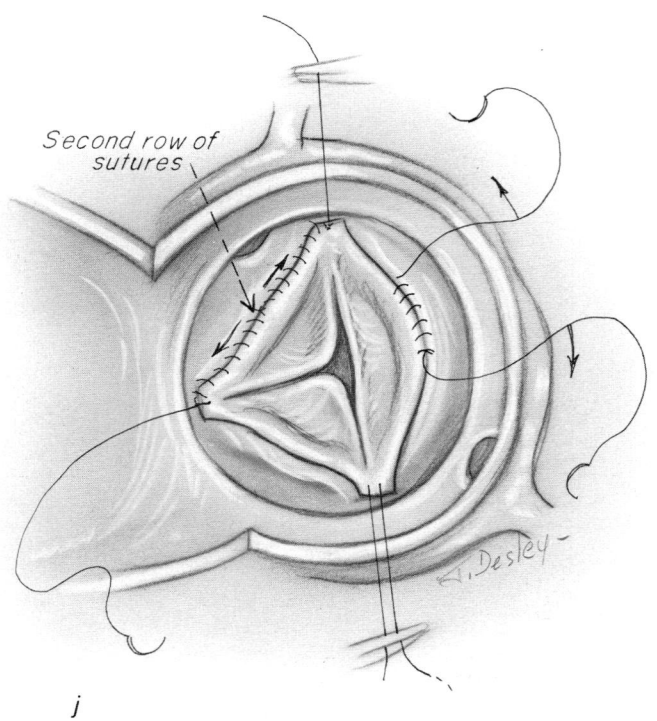

Figure 12-3 (continued)

(i) The subcommissural vertical mattress sutures are placed and tied (GLH).

(j) The second row of sutures is begun in the left coronary sinus (see the text). Next, the suture line is placed in the right coronary sinus. This and the suture line for the noncoronary sinus may be placed by beginning with one of the commissural sutures rather than with a new suture at the bottom of the sinus, as illustrated.

prove obstructive, since the valve will be subsequently turned upward on this suture line). The upper margin, consisting of aortic wall, is cut away 3 mm from the cusp attachment but 5 mm at the top of each commissure (Fig. 12-3a).

The first of three guiding stay sutures is now placed immediately beneath the original right cusp (easily recognized as the leaflet that originates entirely from muscle). The suture is passed from the outside wall of the graft 2 mm from the edge to emerge from the inside wall of the graft 0.5 mm from the edge (Fig. 12-3b). It is then passed through the host's tissue beneath the nadir of the left cusp remnant, stitching from below upward (Fig. 12-3c). (If the nadir of the left cusp remnant lies less than 6 mm from the left coronary ostium, the suture is placed correspondingly further beneath the ostium; otherwise, the upper valve suture line will cover the ostium.) The short end of this suture is tagged, and both ends are placed on the drapes in proper position to avoid subsequent twisting. The other two stay sutures are positioned similarly beneath the nadir of the two remaining homograft and host cusps.

With the ends of the three stay sutures positioned across the drapes 120° apart to avoid twisting, the valve graft is lowered into position along them (Fig. 12-3d), with gentle traction applied to their *long* ends and the valve turned inside out as it is lowered so that the circular lower graft ring now presents to the surgeon within the host valve ring (Fig. 12-3e). The fit should be exact. The three stay sutures are tied down in turn and their short ends retagged. The homograft now lies with the muscular portion of its ring positioned posteriorly and leftward overlying the fibrous anterior mitral leaflet base, while its fibrous portion lies anteriorly and rightward, extending across the membranous ventricular septum. The homograft has thus been rotated 120° counterclockwise (viewed from above) so that the original right cusp becomes the new left cusp. This rotation avoids the sewing of muscle to muscle anteriorly and probably results in a more secure suture line. The long ends of the three stay sutures are now used to create a continuous over-and-over suture line (whip stitch) that follows a *straight* line between the starting points beneath the nadir of each cusp remnant (Fig. 12-3*f*).

The homograft valve is now pulled upward into its correct position, with care taken not to grasp the delicate cusp tissue. A mattress suture is placed through the graft aortic wall remnant at the top of each commissure and into virtually full thickness of host aortic wall (Fig. 12-3*g*). The correct points for the mattress suture lie about 5 mm above the top of each host commissure, and care must be taken that the homograft commissure lies straight and that the graft aortic wall does not bow centrally (Fig. 12-3*h*). The ends of each commissural mattress suture are tagged, but they are not tied, for it is convenient to be able to manipulate the graft away from the host aortic wall later when placing both the subcommissural mattress sutures and parts of the upper suture line.

At this stage, the position of the leaflets is carefully assessed. They must coapt easily centrally, and the three cusp edges must all be at the same level. If this is not the case, the valve needs to be repositioned (or, if too small, replaced with a larger valve). The usual error is to have placed the suture line along the host's left sinus too low, or, less often, along the right sinus too high, or both, so that the left cusp ends up too low and prolapses centrally.

Three vertical subcommissural mattress sutures are now positioned and tied in order to obliterate most of the dead space between graft and host (GLH; Fig. 12-3*i*). These sutures seat the graft firmly against the aortic wall. Those beneath the left–noncoronary commissure and the right-left commissure are placed by working from within the lumen (and tied inside), while the third is more easily placed (by a right-handed surgeon) by working between graft and host.

The second (upper) row of continuous sutures is now begun at the bottom of the left sinus. The aortic wall of the graft is picked up first, using a double-ended 3-0 silk suture, then the host aortic wall directly beneath the left coronary ostium. The whip stitch proceeds first along the rightward edge of the sinus, taking good bites of the graft and host aortic wall and being pulled tight enough so that it will be hemostatic, and then along the leftward edge (Fig. 12-3*j*). Each of these sutures is tied to the commissural mattress stitch after it, too, has been tied down. It is often convenient to pull the graft away from the host wall during the positioning of some of the sutures and to use the silk stitch itself for retraction to improve exposure for the exact positioning of the next stitch; for this reason, silk, rather than a polypropylene, suture is used (GLH). These sutures must be placed with absolute accuracy to avoid narrowing the coronary ostium. There is frequently annoying backflow of blood from the left coronary ostium, which obscures the field. This is overcome by placing an obturator (such as the cuffed King coronary cannula[B28]) into the ostium or by temporarily reducing the perfusion flow rate to 0.5 1 · min^{-1} · m^{-2} during this part of the procedure. In addition, blood may appear through the valve from the left ventricle when the left ventricular vent suction becomes ineffective because the closely approximated homograft leaflets prevent air entering the left ventricle. This does not occur if the pressure-monitoring side-arm on the left ventricular vent line is left open to air (see Chapter 5). Otherwise, a fine catheter is positioned through the leaflets with its tip in the left ventricle.

With the left sinus suture line completed, the right (anterior) sinus is completed next and finally, the noncoronary sinus. For both of these, it is convenient to use the long end of the commissural suture, starting the right sinus suture line at its leftward end; but a double-ended suture can be used, beginning at the bottom of each sinus (as described for the left). Traction on the suture itself is particularly important for exposure inferior and to the right of the right coronary ostium, and here it is again helpful to pull the graft away from the aortic wall by loosening the mattress suture (not yet tied) at the top of the right coronary–noncoronary commissure. When the upper suture line is completed, it is examined carefully to confirm that it will be hemostatic; and if there are gaps, they are closed with additional interrupted sutures.

Insertion of a Prosthesis

If a prosthesis is to be used instead of a nonstented homograft, the appropriate and correctly sized replacement device is selected after the aortic valve is excised. It should be as large as possible, but prostheses should not fit too tightly into the aortic root (see "Small Aortic Root" in section on Special Situations and Controversies).

In selecting a replacement prosthesis, many of the same considerations apply as in mitral replacement (see Chapter 11), except that (1) the Bjork-Shiley valve in the aortic position is less subject to acute thrombotic prosthetic occlusion than it is in the mitral position (see Chapter 11); (2) the Starr-Edwards ball valve prosthesis is less desirable in the aortic position, because the ball in the open position in a relatively small aortic root can be obstructive; and (3) a small aortic anulus can pose special problems (see "Small Aortic Root" in section on Special Situations and Controversies). In general, when in an adult the aortic root can accept a 23-mm or larger prosthesis, any of the standard replacement devices may be selected. The Bjork-Shiley, St. Jude, or Starr-Edwards (GLH) devices or a stent-mounted heterograft is generally used when a prosthesis is selected.

The standard method of insertion of the mechanical prosthesis or bioprosthesis is with simple interrupted sutures of 2-0 Dacron polyester sutures (Fig. 12-4*a*). If the aortic root is quite large, the insertion is sometimes done with interrupted pledgetted mattress sutures (UAB), leaving the pledgets on the aortic side. With both methods, each suture is placed through both anulus and valve as the replacement proceeds. After all sutures are placed, the valve is lowered into position, and the sutures are tied (Fig. 12-4*b*).

Completing the Operation

Rewarming of the patient with the perfusate is begun as the last sutures are being placed or tied, and the rate of administration of the external cardiac cooling fluid is increased to insulate the heart from the rewarming as much as possible. The aortotomy is closed with a simple over-and-over stitch of 3-0 or 4-0 polypropylene suture (UAB) or of 3-0 silk (GLH). One stitch is begun as a pledgetted mattress suture at the posterior rightward angle and then held at the mid portion. The other is begun similarly at the anterior leftward end and carried to the midpoint, where it is tied to the first stitch. In persons over about 60 years of age and in others in whom the aorta is thin, soft, or friable, continuous everting mattress sutures of 3-0 polypropylene placed over felt strips on each side of the aortotomy are substituted for the whip stitch (UAB).

The heart is gently elevated, and a large venting needle is inserted into the apex as the anesthesiologist gives positive pressure to the lungs. Alternatively, the left atrium is first aspirated for air with a syringe and large needle through the base of the right superior pulmonary vein, and the front of the left ventricular apex is aspirated without dislocating the heart (GLH). Strong suction is now placed on the needle vent in the ascending aorta, the suction on the ventricular vent is decreased, the operating table is tilted head down (GLH), and the aortic clamp is released. The surgeon keeps a hand continuously on the heart, so if there is any left ventricular distention the surgeon can direct the perfusionist to increase the left ventricular vent suction until distention is no longer present. If ventricular fibrillation is felt or seen on the electrocardiogram, the heart is defibrillated.

Once the heart is beating, the very important de-airing protocol (see Chapter 2) is followed. Two right atrial and ventricular temporary pacemaking wires are inserted. When rewarming is complete and the hemodynamic state is good, CPB is discontinued as usual (see Chapter 2).

Aortic Valve Replacement and Coronary Artery Bypass Grafting

The preparation and draping of the patient, and the simultaneous making of the incision and removal and preparation of the saphenous vein are the same as in the operation of simple CABG (see Chapter 7). A left atrial pressure-monitoring line is placed. The purse-string sutures for aortic cannulation are placed, with care taken that they are far enough distally (downstream) from the aortic valve that there is room both for the aortotomy and the proximal vein graft anastomoses.

Cardiopulmonary bypass (CPB) is established, and the operative procedure begins exactly as does that for isolated aortic valve replacement, through the excision of the aortic valve and selection of the replacement device. A left ventricular vent is not always placed (UAB). The distal vein graft anastomoses are now performed. Additional infusions of cardioplegic solution may be given through the vein graft after each distal anastomosis (UAB) or intermittently through the coronary perfusion cannulae left in place in the aortic root (GLH). The aortic valve replacement is now completed, the aortotomy closed, the aortic cross-clamp released, and rewarming begun. The veins are routed and sized for proximal anastomoses. By now, the heart is usually beating well, and the usual de-airing procedures are accomplished. The proximal anastomoses are performed next exactly as described in Chapter 7. CPB is discontinued and the operation completed as usual.

Some surgeons prefer a technique in which the proximal anastomoses are made first, before CPB. This technique can result in a shorter CPB time but is more cumbersome. After

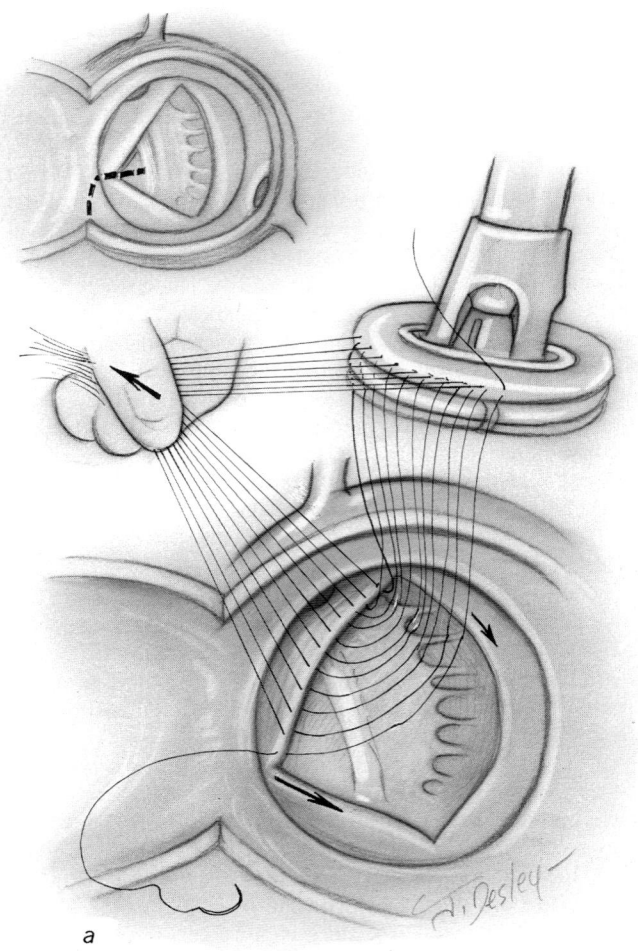

a

Figure 12-4   Replacement of the aortic valve with a mechanical prosthesis or bioprosthesis.
(*a*) Interrupted Dacron sutures are being placed for insertion of the prosthesis. They are first placed in the area of the left coronary sinus, then in that of the contiguous one-half of the noncoronary sinus, and then tagged. The placement of sutures is begun again at the leftward end of the right coronary sinus and carried around clockwise. After all the sutures are placed, the prosthesis is slid down the sutures and into place. (The insert shows the extension of the aortotomy incision down through the commissure between left and noncoronary cusps, as is done if aortic root enlargement is needed; see "Special Situations and Controversies").

heparinizing the patient, the proximal aorta–vein graft anastomoses are performed (see Chapter 7). These are placed more downstream on the aorta than usual to allow room for a second aortic cross-clamp. The heart is cannulated using a single venous cannula, and CPB is established and perfusion cooling begun. The aorta is cross-clamped in the usual place, just upstream from the aortic cannula, and the usual aortotomy incision is made. The cold cardioplegic solution is infused directly into each coronary ostium as described earlier. Now a second aortic cross-clamp is placed just distal (downstream) to the transverse aortotomy. This isolates the

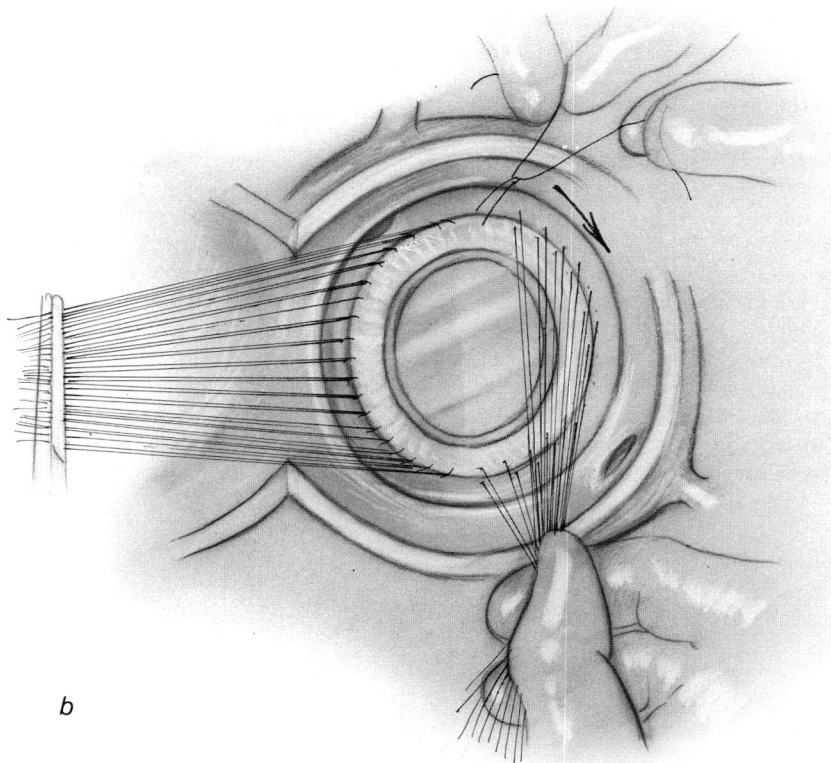

b

Figure 12-4 *(continued)*
(*b*) The prosthesis is in place, and the sutures are being tied. After the sutures have been tied, and if a Bjork-Shiley prosthesis has been used, the prosthesis is examined to determine that disc motion is unimpeded both below and above the device. If it is not, with the anulus supported by traction on the uncut sutures, the prosthesis is rotated into a position in which the disc motion is entirely free. The sutures are then cut.

segment of ascending aorta from which the two vein grafts arise and into which the needle vent, which serves as the pathway of infusion of the cold cardioplegic solution and later for air venting, has been positioned. The whole body perfusate temperature has now been stabilized at about 24°C, since external cardiac cooling is not in use. The anastomoses of the vein graft to the front of the heart are made and then those to the back of the heart, as described in Chapter 7. As usual, the cold cardioplegic solution is infused as the anastomotic sutures are being tied and for measuring the position on the vein of each subsequent anastomosis. When the anastomoses are complete, a small bulldog clamp is placed on each vein graft right next to the aorta to keep it from filling with air. The aortic clamp farthest upstream is then removed. Now the exposure and stay sutures are arranged for the aortic valve replacement, and the operation continues and is completed as described earlier for isolated aortic valve replacement.

Composite Graft Replacement of Aortic Valve and Ascending Aorta

The composite graft operation is most frequently performed for aortic annular ectasia with aortic valve incompetence,

and the technique for that setting, using the inclusion method, is described here. Occasionally composite graft replacement is performed in the setting of acute or chronic aortic dissection with aortic valve incompetence and the technique of the distal anastomosis may then be somewhat different (see Chapters 54 and 55, in sections on Technique of Operation).

The early steps of the composite graft operation are in some ways different from those of simple aortic valve replacement. The arterial cannulation is often through the femoral (UAB) or right external iliac artery (GLH), but when the aneurysm stops short of the innominate artery origin, the distal ascending or proximal transverse arch can be cannulated in the usual fashion. The conduit is selected and preclotted before CPB is established, as a 27-mm valve within a 30-mm, low-porosity, woven Dacron tube fits virtually all patients with this condition. A commercially available composite woven Dacron graft with a preattached Bjork-Shiley or St. Jude aortic valve prosthesis is used (UAB), or the conduit-valve device can be constructed by the surgeon using a Bjork-Shiley, Starr-Edwards, or stented heterograft valve (GLH).

A limited dissection is done to allow safe placement of the aortic cross-clamp just proximal to the innominate artery and the laying of a Teflon felt strip around the aorta. This procedure involves cleanly separating the right and contiguous portion of the main pulmonary artery from the back of the aorta and aneurysm if possible. The felt strip is placed around the aorta as soon as the dissection is completed, or, if this is not easy, just after starting CPB.

CPB is established at 34°C using single (UAB) or double (GLH) venous cannulation and a left atrial vent. External cardiac cooling is begun, and the perfusate temperature is lowered as rapidly as possible. When the heart begins to be ineffective or develops ventricular fibrillation, the aorta is cross-clamped just proximal to the innominate artery and the perfusate temperature taken to 25°C. The aneurysm is opened longitudinally in its mid portion, stay sutures are applied (Fig. 12-5), and the cardioplegic solution is infused directly into the coronary ostia. The aortic valve is excised, and the valved portion of the composite conduit is sewn into place using closely placed interrupted sutures. When the

valved conduit is constructed by the surgeon, the sewing ring of the prosthesis may be tacked inside the Dacron graft with three stay sutures, and the interrupted sutures may be used to position the valve passed through both the sewing ring and the Dacron (GLH). The stay sutures are then cut and removed.

The anastomosis of the coronary ostia to holes in the side of the graft is the part of the operation most vulnerable to problems, both early (massive hemorrhage) and late (false aneurysm formation). Therefore, the most secure method possible is used. A hole about 1.5 cm in diameter is cut in the graft opposite the ostium of the left coronary artery and a comfortable distance downstream from the prosthetic valve. The anastomosis to the aortic wall around the left ostium is made with interrupted horizontal pledgetted mattress sutures of 5-0 polypropylene or Dacron polyester sutures, placed with pledgetts on the aortic side. Alternatively, a felt strip may be used (Fig. 12-5). The first mattress suture is

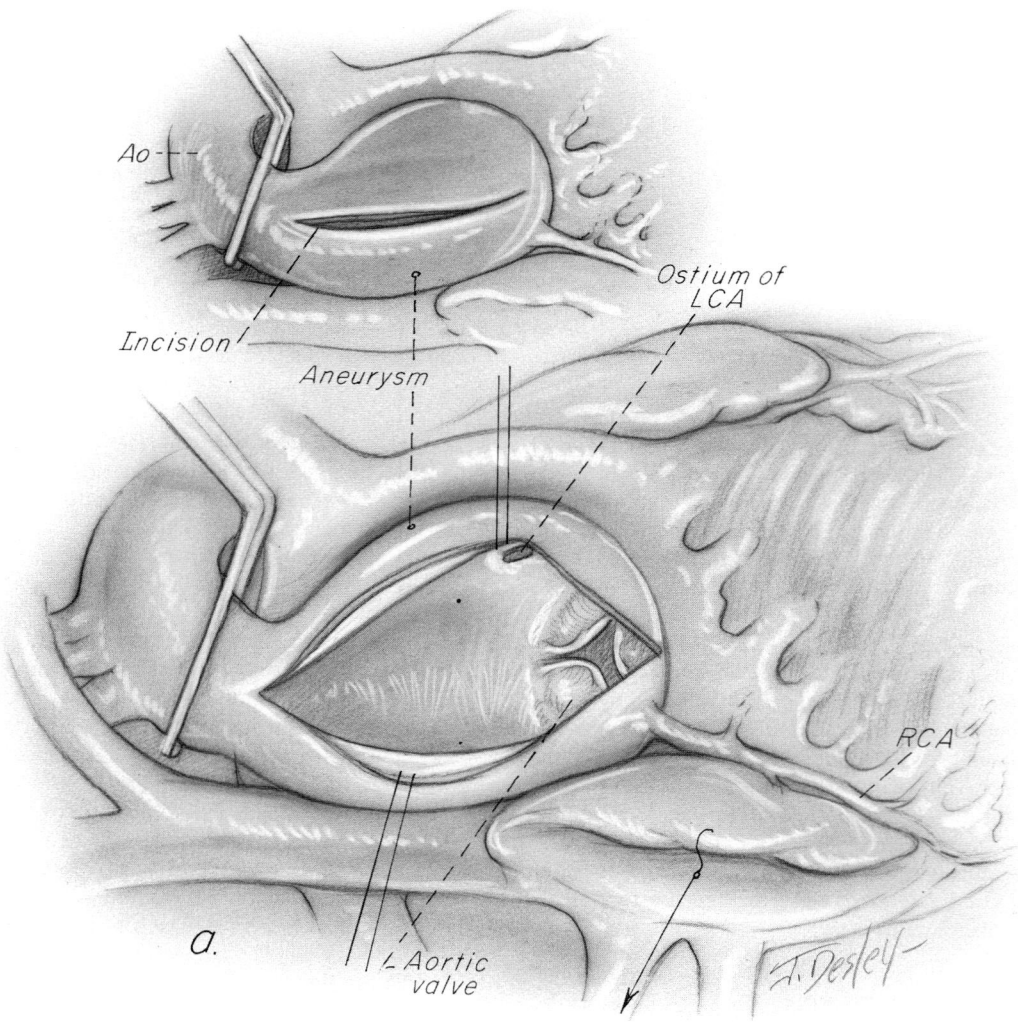

Figure 12-5 Replacement of aortic valve and ascending aorta using the inclusion technique. (a) After CPB is established, the aortic clamp is placed, and the aneurysm is opened longitudinally (see the inset). The ostia of the left and right coronary arteries are identified, usually displaced somewhat downstream to their normal position. The cold cardioplegic solution is given.

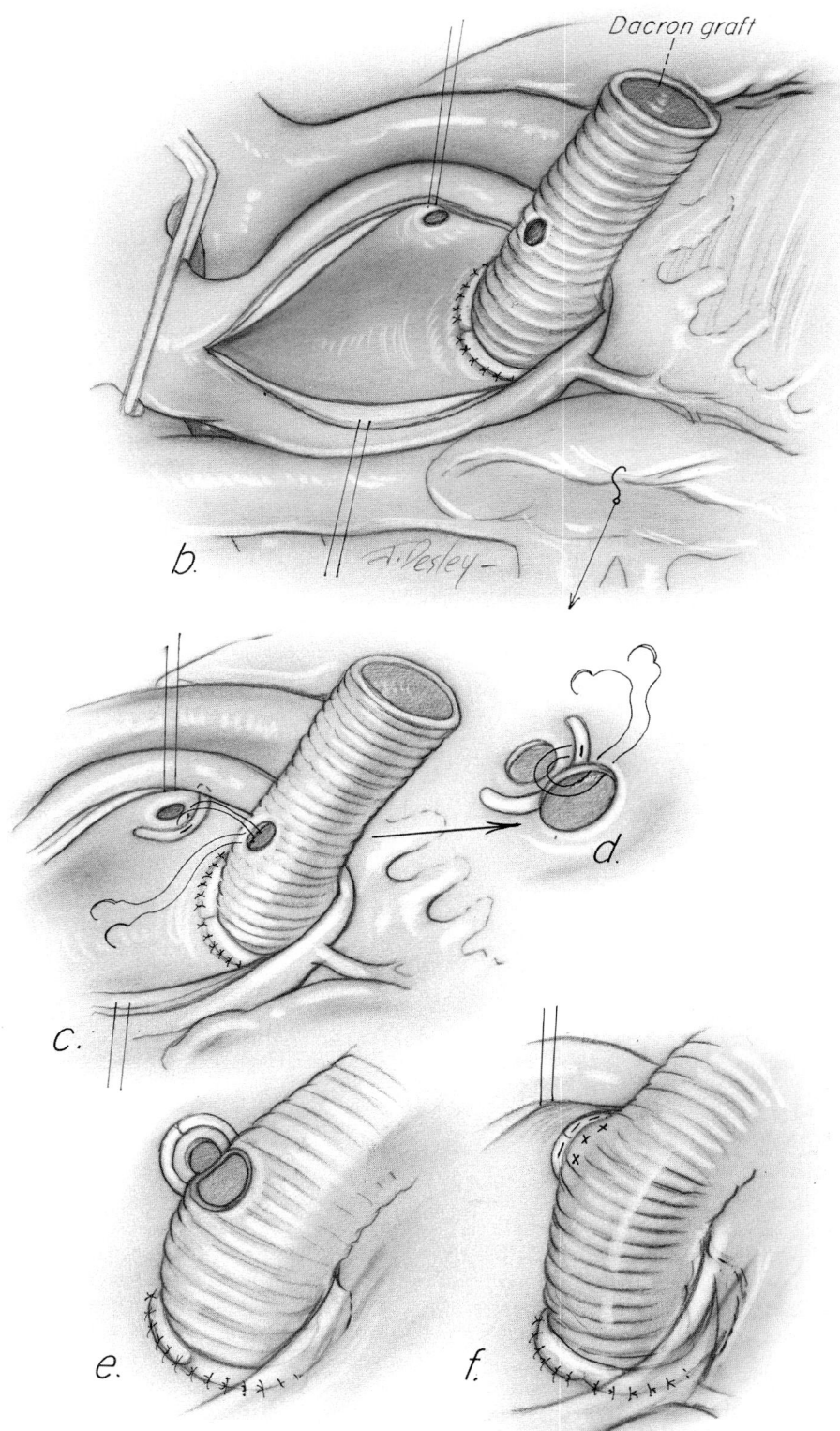

Figure 12-5 *(continued)*

(*b*) After excising the aortic valve, the Dacron graft with the attached Bjork-Shiley valve is sutured into place. A hole has been cut in the graft preparatory to suturing this around the ostium of the left coronary artery.

(*c*) The anastomosis is begun between the graft and the aortic wall around coronary ostium (see the text for details). (*d*) Interrupted everting mattress sutures are used, supported by felt strips on the aortic side. (*e*) The anastomosis is partially complete. (*f*) The anterior row of sutures has been placed.

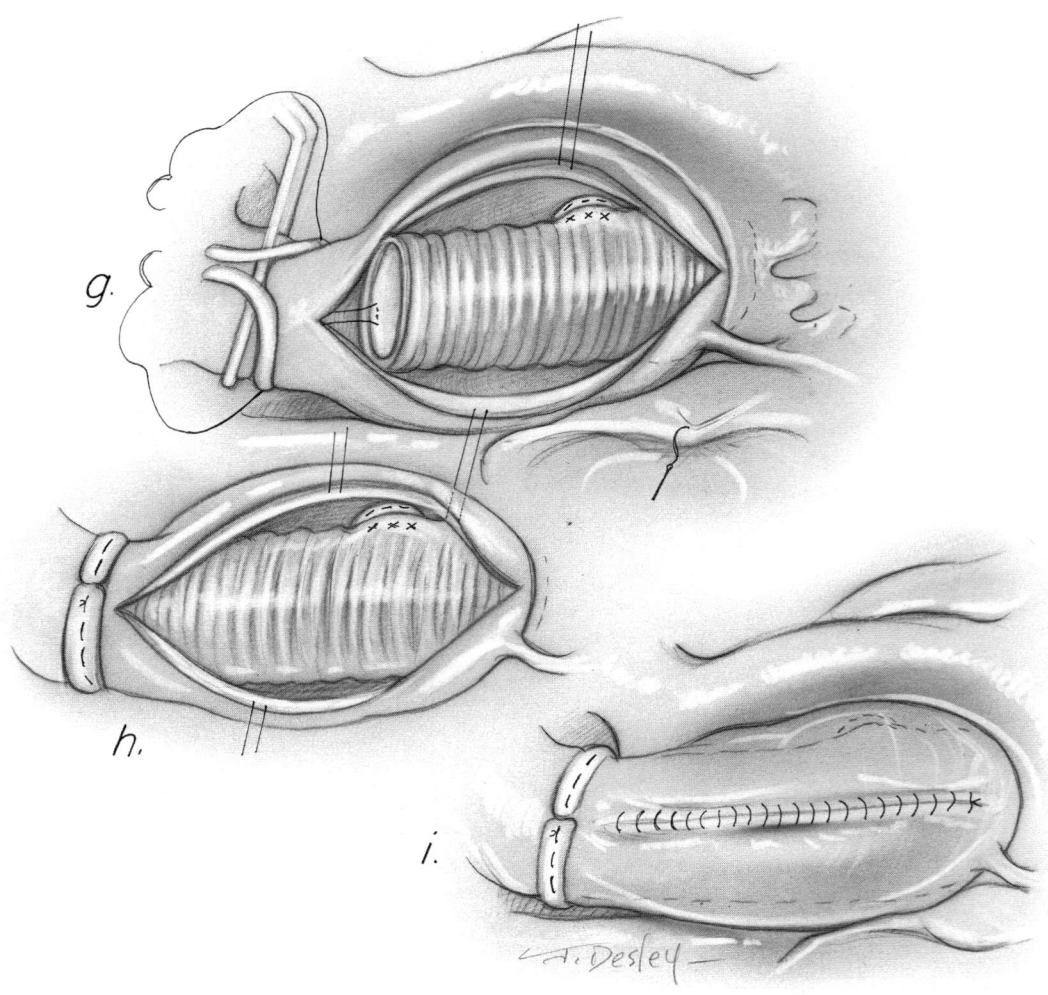

Figure 12-5 *(continued)*
(g) After felt strips are placed around the aorta, the distal anastomosis is begun with a continuous everting mattress suture. *(h)* The distal anastomosis has been completed. The clamp is removed, and the suture lines are inspected for leakage.
(i) After any important leaks are controlled, the aneurysm wall is wrapped around the graft for additional hemostasis.

placed in the middle of the posterior portion. Two or three are then placed on either side, and then all of these sutures are tied down. The remainder of the interrupted mattress sutures are placed and tied. A similar anastomosis is made to the aortic wall around the right coronary ostium. Alternatively, simple mattress sutures may be placed over felt strips.

The graft is cut to an appropriate length, and preparations are made for the distal anastomosis. With a 2-0 or 3-0 polypropylene suture, an everting horizontal mattress stitch is begun through the bottom (6-o'clock) angle of the graft. The surgeon brings the stitch through the aorta and felt strip already in position, retrieving one arm to the left of the aorta and one to the right and taking care that they pass through the aorta close together. Using one arm of the suture and then the other, the surgeon continues the suture line anteriorly as a horizontal mattress stitch through felt and aorta

and through graft (everting it). The suture ends are tied to each other anteriorly. Alternatively, interrupted pledgetted mattress sutures or polypropylene or Dacron polyester may be used, placed with the pledgets outside the aorta.

With a needle vent through the distal suture line, or through the aorta just beyond it, the aortic cross-clamp is released. Important bleeding from any of the four suture lines should be controlled with additional sutures. Control of bleeding is extremely difficult in the case of the suture lines around the coronary ostia, which underscores the importance of their accurate placement initially. Once bleeding is controlled, the aneurysm wall is trimmed back and sutured snugly around the graft using a vertical anterior suture line of 3-0 polypropylene. This final wrapping must not be done before the aortic clamp is released and the anastomoses tested for leaks, for not only must the wrapping not be relied on to control major bleeding, but also, if sewn around a slack tube graft, it may compress and kink it. This can jam the Bjork-Shiley disc or compromise the space around the cage and ball of a Starr-Edwards prosthesis. The remainder of the operation is completed as usual.

SPECIAL FEATURES OF POSTOPERATIVE CARE

In general, postoperative care after adult aortic valve surgery is the same as after other types of cardiac surgery (see Chapter 5). Patients receiving a prosthetic aortic valve are begun on Coumadin (sodium warfarin) anticoagulant therapy on the evening of the second postoperative day, and this is continued for the rest of their lives, while those receiving stent-mounted heterografts are anticoagulated for only 6–8 weeks after operation. The details of the anticoagulant program are the same as for mitral valve replacement (see Chapter 11). Homograft valve patients do not receive any anticoagulants.

The thick-walled hypertrophied left ventricle secondary to aortic valve disease requires a higher than usual filling pressure to distend it. Thus, a mean left atrial pressure of 8–10 mmHg, considered quite adequate under many circumstances, may be inadequate to develop optimal left *ventricular preload* (see Chapter 5, "Ventricular Preload" in section 2, Patient Management Protocols for the Subsystems, and footnote 9) early after operation in patients with significant left ventricular hypertrophy. Also, the reduction in myocardial compliance that occurs during cardiac surgery further increases the disparity between the usual mean left atrial pressure (left ventricular filling pressure) and optimal preload.

For these reasons, in the early hours after adult aortic valve surgery, particularly for severe aortic stenosis, unless cardiac performance is already optimal, left atrial pressure should be maintained at 15–18 mmHg by appropriate fluid infusion (see Chapter 5, Table 5-3, for description of appropriate fluid).

This need is often less when operation has been done for aortic incompetence. Here, the sudden reduction in left ventricular stroke volume by the ablation of the aortic regurgitant flow improves left ventricular performance in relationship to right (see Chapter 5). Thus, mean left atrial pressure may not be as elevated early postoperatively as when the operation has been done for aortic stenosis.

EARLY RESULTS

Hospital Mortality

The hospital mortality of primary isolated aortic valve replacement, the commonest subset of aortic valve replacements, seems to have been low from its inception. Thus, at GLH, it was 4.4% in the first 90 patients operated on[B30] and averaged 6% between 1962 and 1966 (Table 12-5); and in our early Mayo Clinic experience with the first 132 patients undergoing aortic valve replacement with the Starr-Edwards prosthesis, hospital mortality was 3% (CL 1.5%–5%).[M18] Also, there are several older reports in the literature of modest-sized series of aortic valve replacement without mortality.[K8,M14] No doubt, however, the early experiences contained fewer high-risk patients than did the later ones, for example, the GLH 1977–1981 experience.

Even in the current era, the overall hospital mortality of isolated, primary aortic valve replacement does not approach zero (see Chapter 6 for definition), although it is 2.0% (CL 1.4%–2.9%; see Table 12-6). The failure of the mortality to approach zero is probably related to the fact that some patients still come to operation very ill and with advanced left ventricular dysfunction and that some are quite elderly. Without such patients, the risk of primary isolated aortic valve replacement does approach zero (see "Incremental Risk Factors for Hospital Death").

Mode of Hospital Death

Among patients in the current era undergoing primary aortic valve replacement with or without associated procedures, the commonest mode of hospital death is postoperative acute cardiac failure (Table 12-7). The next commonest is hemorrhage.[C4] A multivariate analysis (UAB) shows that the incremental risk factors for hospital death associated with massive hemorrhage were severe preoperative functional disability (NYHA functional class), old age, and the presence of aortic incompetence (Table 12-8). Presumably, the first two factors render the tissue friable, which predisposes it to slight tearing and thus bleeding along suture lines. If the correlation between aortic incompetence and death with hemorrhage is not a spurious correlation, it may be that the thin aortic anulus in such patients predisposes the tissue to tearing and subsequent hemorrhage with suture placement. The precise operative techniques described in this chapter,

Table 12-5 Total experience of primary isolated aortic valve replacement. (GLH; August 1962–January 1981).

	Elective				Emergency[a]				Total			
		Hospital Deaths				Hospital Deaths				Hospital Deaths		
Year of Operation	n	No.	%	CL	n	No.	%	CL	n	No.	%	CL
1962–1966	310	18	5.8%	4.4%–7.5%	7	1	14%	2%–44%	317	19	6.0%	4.6%–7.7%
1967–1971	347	24	6.9%	5.5%–8.6%	19	7	37%	24%–51%	366	31	8.5%	7.0%–10.3%
1972–1976	309	12	3.9%	2.8%–5.4%	20	4	20%	10%–33%	329	16	4.9%	3.6%–6.4%
1977–1981	241	12	4.9%	3.5%–6.9%	20	6	30%	19%–44%	261	18	6.9%	5.3%–8.9%
Total	1207	66	5.5%	4.8%–6.2%	66	18	27%	21%–34%	1273	84	6.6%	5.9%–7.4%

KEY: CL, 70% confidence limits.

[a] In this and subsequent tables (GLH), *emergency* includes patients requiring operation within 24 hours of being referred to the surgeon. It does not include all class V patients.

Table 12-6 Early results of primary aortic valve replacement with or without associated procedures (UAB; 1975–July 1, 1979; n = 842).

| Category | n | Hospital Deaths | | |
		No.	%	CL
Isolated AVR	489	10	2.0%	1.4%–2.9%
AVR + CABG	251	9	3.6%	2.4%–5.2%
AVR + resection AAA	63	3	5%	2%–9%
AVR + CABG + resection AAA	12	2	17%	6%–35%
AVR + resection LVA	1	0	0%	0%–85%
AVR + CABG + resection LVA	2	0	0%	0%–61%
AVR + CABG + resection AAA & LVA	1	0	0%	0%–85%
AVR + previous AV repair	9	0	0%	0%–19%
AVR + resection AAA + previous AV repair	4	0	0%	0%–38%
AVR + resection AAA + CABG + previous AV repair	1	0	0%	0%–85%
AVR + previous LV myomectomy	1	0	0%	0%–85%
AVR + other concomitant or previous operation	8	0	0%	0%–21%

P = .21
P = .7
P = .001

KEY: AAA, ascending aortic aneurysm; AV, aortic valve; AVR, aortic valve replacement; CABG, coronary artery bypass grafting; CL, 70% confidence limits; LV, left ventricle; LVA, left ventricular aneurysm.

Table 12-7 Mode of hospital death after primary aortic valve replacement (UAB; 1975–July 1, 1979; n = 842).

Mode of Hospital Death	Non-cardioplegia (n = 422)	Cold Cardioplegia (n = 420)	Total (n = 842)
Acute cardiac failure	7	5	12
Hemorrhage	0	6	6
Infection	1	2	3
Pulmonary thrombo-embolism	0	1	1
Other	2	0	2
Total	10	14	24

Table 12-8 Multivariate analysis of death from hemorrhage after primary isolated or combined aortic valve replacement in the cold cardioplegic group (UAB; 1975–July 1, 1979; n = 420; 6 events; see Appendix 12A for other variables entered).

Incremental Risk Factors for Hospital Death from Hemorrhage	Logistic Coefficient ± SD	P Value
NYHA functional class (I–V)	1.5 ± 0.51	.003
Age at operation (yr)	0.13 ± 0.065	.04
Presence of aortic incompetence	2.2 ± 1.17	.06
Intercept	−19	

developed in part in response to this information, should minimize the occurrence of important bleeding.

Incremental Risk Factors for Hospital Death

The *preoperative functional status* of the patient expressed as the NYHA functional class is a risk factor (Table 12-9), as is evidenced by the very similar UAB (Table 12-10, Fig. 12-6) and GLH (Table 12-11) experiences in this regard. Barnhorst and colleagues also identified the higher NYHA classes as risk factors for hospital death in their review of our initial Mayo Clinic experience with valve replacement.[B4,B5]

The preoperative functional status must reflect *left ventricular function*, which, along with other determinants of cardiac performance, such as maximal heart rate, are the real risk factors reflected in the associations shown. The preoperative functional status would be a more refined esti-

Table 12-9 Multivariate analysis of hospital death from all causes after primary isolated or combined aortic valve replacement (UAB; 1975–July 1, 1979; n = 842; see Appendix 12B for details).

Incremental Risk Factor for Hospital Death from All Causes	Logistic Coefficient ± SD	P value
NYHA functional class (I–V)	1.2 ± 0.28	<.0001
Age at operation (year)	0.04 ± 0.021	.06
Presence of aortic incompetence	1.0 ± 0.48	.03
If noncardioplegia:		
Add to intercept	−3.7 ± 1.15	.001
Ischemic time (minutes)	0.052 ± 0.0157	.001
Intercept	−10.0	

KEY: SD, standard deviation.

Table 12-10 The relationship of preoperative NYHA functional class to hospital mortality after primary isolated or combined aortic valve replacement (UAB; 1975–July 1, 1979; n = 842).

NYHA Class	n^a	Hospital Deaths		
		No.	%	CL
I	35	0	0%	0%–5%
II	256	2	0.8%	0.3%–1.8%
III	435	11	2.5%	1.8%–3.6%
IV	97	7	7%	5%–11%
V^b	14	4	29%	15%–46%
P			< .0001	

11/111, 10% (CL 7%–14%)

KEY: CL, 70% confidence limits.

^{a}Five patients could not be categorized.

^{b}Indicates patients coming to the operating room in acute severe hemodynamic deterioration.

mate of these if previous episodes of overt left ventricular failure and the amount of drug therapy required to control symptoms were also taken into account. Direct measurements reflecting left ventricular function should also refine this variable, and adding the response to objective exercise testing allows even closer correlation. This has been demonstrated by studies from the United States National Institutes of Health[B16,H4] that emphasize that evaluation of left ventricular systolic function is incomplete without assessment of reserves by testing of exercise capacity. Thus, although in their experience depressed left ventricular systolic function was found to be an incremental risk factor for postoperative in-hospital acute cardiac death after valve replacement for aortic incompetence, its predictive capability was refined by the addition of a graded exercise test.

Older age at operation is an incremental risk factor for in-

hospital death after aortic valve replacement[L10] (Table 12-9), as it is in the case of most operations. However, it is not a strong risk factor,[C19] the risk at age 40 being about 1% and at age 75 about 5% (Fig. 12-7). Its effect in part is because of the increased risk of massive hemorrhage in older patients (Table 12-8). The precise surgical techniques described in this chapter should neutralize this effect.

Aortic incompetence (as opposed to pure aortic stenosis or mitral stenosis and incompetence) has been an incremental risk factor for in-hospital death after aortic valve replacement. This is apparent in both the UAB experience (Table 12-9) and at GLH (Table 12-12). This incremental effect of aortic incompetence on risk is particularly evident in patients with advanced heart failure (Table 12-12). This all relates to the probability that patients coming to operation with aortic valve incompetence have more severe left ventricular dysfunction than those being operated on for aortic stenosis.

The *method of myocardial protection* is a risk factor, although it is difficult to demonstrate its effect when the aortic cross-clamp times are relatively short (< 80 minutes). Thus, continuous coronary artery perfusion was used until about July 1978 (GLH), and the results as a whole are only possibly better with cold cardioplegia (Table 12-13). A randomized study at UAB in 1973 showed no difference in hospital mortality or the extent of myocardial necrosis between continuous coronary perfusion and cold ischemic cardiac arrest[S18] for simple aortic valve replacement in which cross-clamp times were relatively short (see Chapter 3). However, the lack of use of cold cardioplegia *was* a risk factor demonstrated in the multivariate analysis of the 1975–July 1979 UAB experience, the incremental risk of simple cold ischemic arrest being particularly evident when long periods of arrest were used (Table 12-9). Lytle and colleagues have shown by multivariate analysis that the use of cold cardio-

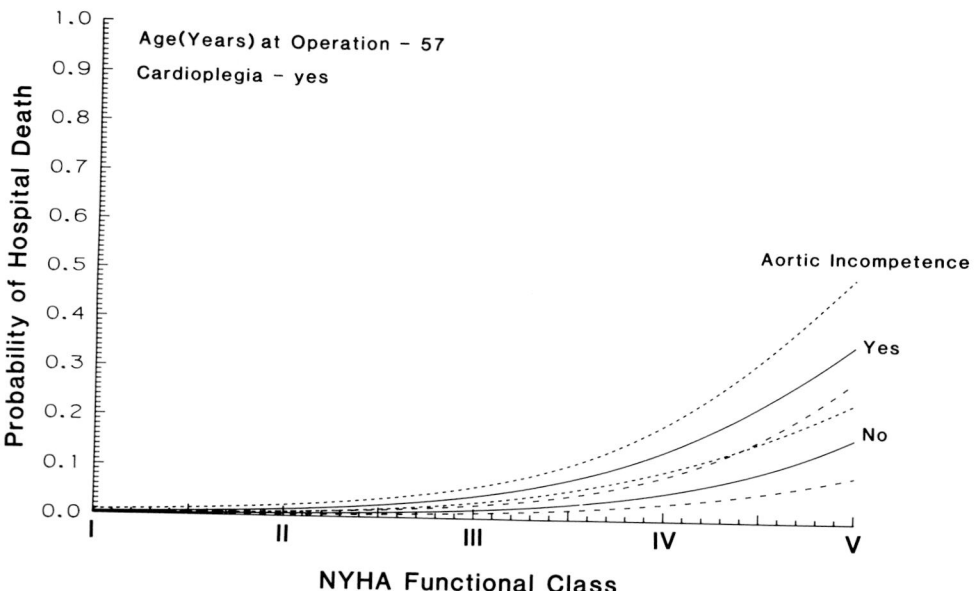

Figure 12-6 Nomogram of univariate logistic analysis of the relationship of preoperative functional class to probability of hospital death from all causes after primary isolated or combined aortic valve replacement (UAB; 1975–July, 1979; n = 842).

Table 12-11 Hospital mortality after aortic valve replacement with and without associated procedures (GLH; 1976–1981).

NYHA Class	Primary Operation				Repeat Operation				Total			
		Hospital Deaths				Hospital Deaths				Hospital Deaths		
	n	No.	%	CL	n	No.	%	CL	n	No.	%	CL
I	28	1	4%	0.5%–12%	34	1	3%	0.4%–10%	62	2	3%	1%–7%
II	140	3	2.1%	0.9%–4.3%	24	1	4%	0.5%–13%	164	4	2.4%	1.2%–4.4%
III	125	8	6%	4%–10%	31	0	0%	0%–6%	156	8	5.1%	3.3%–7.7%
IV	42	3	7%	3%–14%	16	3	19%	8%–34%	58	6	10%	6%–16%
V	21	8	38%	26%–52%	8	4	50%	27%–73%	29	12	41%	31%–53%
Total	356	23	6.5%	5.1%–8.1%	113	9	8%	5%–12%	469	32	6.8%	5.6%–8.2%

KEY: CL, 70% confidence limits.

NOTE: Six patients in whom the NYHA class is not known are excluded.

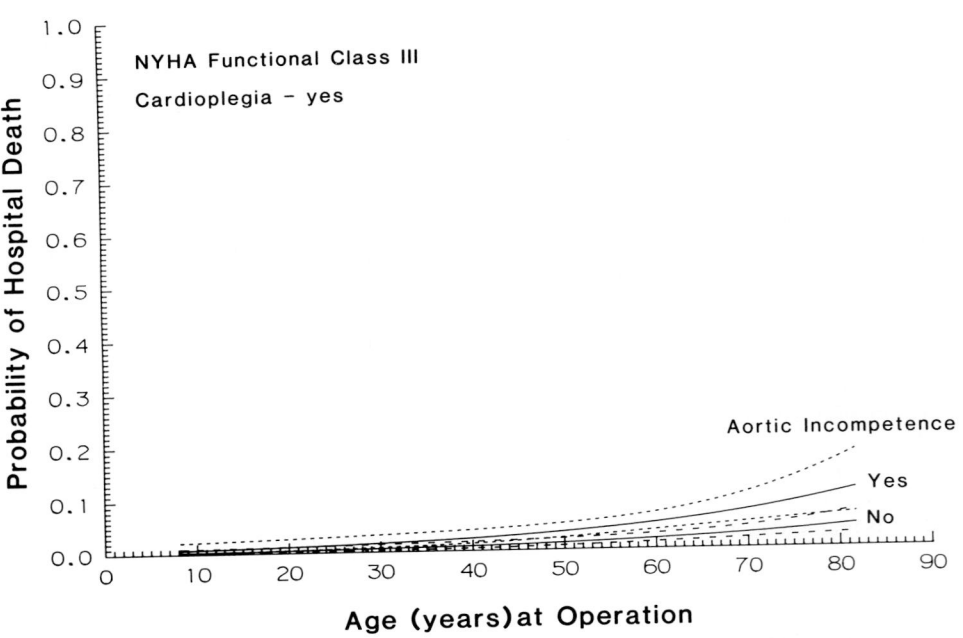

Figure 12-7 Nomogram of univariate logistic analysis of the relation of age at operation to probability of hospital death from all causes after primary isolated or combined aortic valve replacement (UAB; 1975–July 1979; $n = 842$).

Table 12-12 Hospital mortality after primary and repeat isolated aortic valve replacement (GLH; 1976–1981).

NYHA Class	Aortic Stenosis With or Without Incompetence				Aortic Incompetence				Total			
		Hospital Deaths				Hospital Deaths				Hospital Deaths		
	n	No.	%	CL	n	No.	%	CL	n	No.	%	CL
I	5	0	0%	0%–32%	16	0	0%	0%–11%	21	0	0%	0%–9%
II	89	1	1.1%	0.1%–3.8%	36	3	8%	4%–16%	125	4	3.2%	1.6%–5.8%
III	66	5	8%	4%–13%	41	1	2%	0.3%–8%	107	6	6%	3%–9%
IV	17	2	12%	4%–26%	20	2	10%	3%–22%	37	4	11%	6%–19%
V	3	0	0%	0%–47%	18	8	44%	30%–59%	21	8	38%	26%–52%
Total	180	8	4.4%[a]	2.9%–6.6%	131	14	11%[a]	8%–14%	311	22	7.1%	5.6%–8.9%
$P(\chi^2)$		.17				<.0001				<.0001		
Excluding class V	177	8	4.5%	2.9%–6.8%	113	6	5%	3%–8%	290	14	4.8%	3.5%–6.5%

KEY: CL, 70% confidence limits.

[a] $P(\chi^2)$ for difference .03.

Table 12-13 The effect of two forms of myocardial protection on hospital mortality after primary isolated aortic valve replacement (GLH; 1962–1981).

| Myocardial Protection | Elective | | | | Emergency | | | | Total | | | |
| | | Hospital Deaths | | | | Hospital Deaths | | | | Hospital Deaths | | |
	n	No.	%	CL	n	No.	%	CL	n	No.	%	CL
Coronary perfusion	1071	61	5.7%	5.0%–6.5%	53	15	28%	22%–36%	1124	76	6.8%	6.0%–7.6%
Cold cardioplegia	134	5	3.7%	2.1%–6.3%	11	2	18%	6%–38%	145	7	4.8%	3.0%–7.4%
P			.3				.5				.3	

KEY: CL, 70% confidence limits.

plegia did decrease hospital mortality in patients undergoing combined aortic valve replacement and coronary artery bypass grafting.[L10] A separate analysis (UAB) shows, however, that even with cold cardioplegia, the risk of aortic cross-clamp times over about an hour may ($P = .17$) interact with the risk of the increased risk of preoperative functional status (Fig. 12-8).

Successive aortic valve *re-replacements* with or without associated procedures carry an increased risk of hospital death, particularly after the first re-replacement[W1] (Table 12-14). This is in part because of the conditions leading to re-replacement and in part because of the technical problems involved. The risk is particularly increased in severely affected patients (NYHA classes IV and V) (Table 12-11), a point that has been emphasized by Jacobs and colleagues and Parr and colleagues.[J1,P3] With each prosthetic re-replacement the incidence of valve dehiscence is higher (UAB and GLH), emphasizing the need for making the first valve replacement as permanent as possible.

The *replacement device* used for aortic valve replacement may be a risk factor. The GLH experience suggests that bioprostheses and mechanical prostheses may be incremental risk factors, compared with the homograft valve inserted freehand (Tables 12-15, 12-16). This may be related to the improved systolic and diastolic performance of the homograft. Neither the mechanical prosthesis nor the bioprosthesis is superior as a risk factor in hospital mortality.

Associated coronary artery disease, for which concomitant coronary artery bypass grafting (CABG) is done, has not increased the in-hospital risk of aortic valve replacement (Tables 12-6, 12-17) and was not identified as a risk factor in the multivariate analysis (Table 12-9). On the contrary, when the concomitant procedure of CABG is not done in patients with combined aortic valve and coronary artery disease, the hospital mortality for aortic valve replacement is increased, as evidenced by the Stanford experience, in which without the CABG operation it was 8.3% in those with coronary artery disease and 2.2% in those without it ($P < .05$).[M9]

Associated ascending aortic aneurysm, treated by concomitant resection of ascending aorta, has not in recent years been an incremental risk factor (Tables 12-6, 12-9).

Native aortic valve endocarditis might seem to be an in-

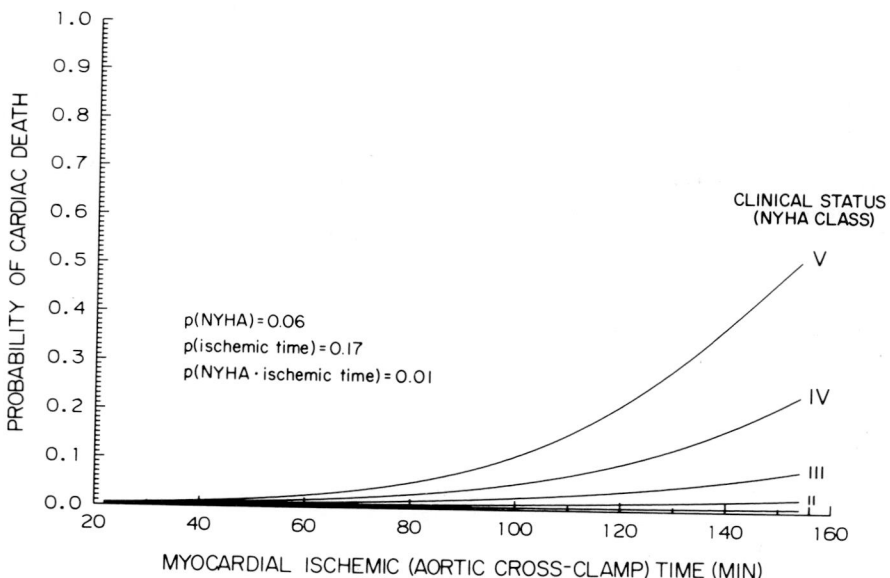

Figure 12-8 Two-variable analysis of the relationship of preoperative clinical status and myocardial ischemic time to probability of cardiac death after primary or repeated isolated or combined aortic valve replacement using cold cardioplegic myocardial protection (UAB; 1975–July 1979; $n = 1,042$ patients; 543 of these were operated on using cold cardioplegia, 534 with complete data and thus analyzed; 6 events).

Table 12-14 Early results of isolated and combined aortic valve replacement (UAB; 1975–July 1, 1979; $n = 1042$).[W1]

Category	n	Hospital Deaths			Probability of Hospital Death (from Logistic Equation[a])	
		No.	%	CL	%	CL
Initial AVR	842	24	2.9%	2.3%–3.6%	2.7%	2.2%–3.3%
First RRP	181	7	3.9%	2.4%–6.0%	5.1%	4.0%–6.5%
Second RRP	18	3	17%	7%–31%	9%	6%–15%
Third RRP	1	0	0%	0%–85%	16%	8%–30%
Total	1042	34	3.3%	2.7%–3.9%		
P (logistic)			0.03			

KEY: AVR, aortic valve replacement; CL, 70% confidence limits; RRP, re-replacement.

[a] $Z = -4.2 \pm 0.44 + 0.64 \pm 0.03 \cdot$ replacement number.

Table 12-15 The relationship of the type of valve replacement to hospital mortality after primary isolated aortic valve replacement (GLH; 1962–1981).

Replacement Valve	n	Hospital Deaths		
		No.	%	CL
Homograft	1106	68	6.1%	5.4%–7.0%
Porcine or prosthetic	157	16	10%	8%–13%
P			.08	

KEY: CL, 70% confidence limits

cremental risk factor in patients undergoing aortic valve replacement. Of 14 patients in the population described by Table 12-6 who had native valve endocarditis, 2 (14%, CL 5%–31%) died in hospital postoperatively, compared with 22 (2.7%, CL 2.1%–3.4%) of 828 without it ($P = .06$). However, one death was of a patient in preoperative NYHA class V; and one was among the 10 patients in NYHA class IV. Two others who lived were preoperatively in NYHA class II or III. Also, by multivariate analysis of the UAB experience, native valve endocarditis was *not* identified as an incremental risk factor. Thus, the apparent risk is from advanced disability and heart failure, not endocarditis per se. These

ideas are supported by the low hospital mortality (4%) obtained by Bortolotti and colleagues in a group of 23 patients undergoing aortic valve replacement because of active infective endocarditis.[B37]

Morbidity

Uncommonly, complete heart block is produced by the operation of aortic valve replacement for severely calcareous aortic stenosis. Such stenosis is usually the result of trauma to the bundle of His incident to removal of calcium close to the membranous septum and right trigone beneath the noncoronary cusp–right coronary cusp commissure. Although this complication may very occasionally be unavoidable, care in removing calcium from these areas and rigorous avoidance of suture penetration of the anulus in the contiguous half of the noncoronary and right coronary cusps should reduce its incidence to a very low level.

Neurologic deficits, some massive and fatal, were common in the early days of aortic valve replacement. In the current era, they are rare, occurring in less than 1% of patients. This low incidence is due to the development of techniques for avoiding the loss of any tiny calcific fragments during valve resection and replacement and to improved techniques for de-airing of the heart after closing the aorta.

LATE RESULTS

Survival

The 5-year survival rate of hospital survivors of aortic valve replacement is about 85% (Figs. 12-9, 12-10). At UAB, the 4.5-year actuarial survival rate after aortic valve replacement with the Bjork-Shiley prosthesis has been 86% (CL 83%–88%),[K1] and 87% (CL 84%–90%) at 3 years with the porcine bioprosthesis.[W1] This experience is similar to that reported by others with the Bjork-Shiley prosthesis,[C4] with the Starr-Edwards model 1200 ball valve prosthesis,[M1] with the porcine prosthesis,[D1] and with the bovine pericardial xenograft valve.[I6]

In spite of the improvement in life expectancy afforded by aortic valve replacement, the operation is in general palliative rather than curative. This is apparent in the GLH homo-

Table 12-16 Hospital mortality after primary and repeated aortic valve replacement, with or without concomitant procedures, except excision of ascending arch aneurysm, 30 cases with 6 deaths. (GLH; 1976–1981).

NYHA Class	Homograft				Bioprosthesis				Mechanical Prosthesis				Total			
		Hospital Deaths				Hospital Deaths				Hospital Deaths				Hospital Deaths		
	n	No.	%	CL	n	No.	%	CL	n	No.	%	CL	n	No.	%	CL
I	28	1	4%	0.5%–12%	12	0	0%	0%–15%	19	0	0%	0%–10%	59	1	1.7%	0.2%–5.7%
II	115	2	1.7%	0.6%–4.1%	13	2	15%	5%–33%	32	0	0%	0%–6%	160	4	2.5%	1.3%–4.5%
III	93	3	3.2%	1.4%–6.4%	14	1	7%	0.9%–22%	43	4	9%	5%–16%	148	8	5.4%	3.5%–8.1%
IV	25	2	8%	3%–18%	8	0	0%	0%–21%	15	3	20%	9%–36%	48	5	10%	6%–17%
V	14	4	29%	15%–46%	3	2	7%	24%–96%	5	2	40%	14%–71%	22	8	36%	25%–50%
Total	275	12	4.4%	3.1%–6.0%	50	5	10%	6%–16%	114	9	8%	5%–11%	439	26	5.9%	4.8%–7.3%

KEY: CL, 70% confidence limits.

NOTE: Six patients without NYHA classification are not included. The P value of .04 for the difference between homograft mortality of 4.4% and combined mechanical and biprosthesis mortality of 9% is similar to that obtained by multivariate logistic analysis.

Table 12-17 Primary and repeated aortic valve replacement (GLH; 1976–1981).

| | Aortic Stenosis | | | Aortic Incompetence | | | Aortic Stenosis and Incompetence | | | Total | | | |
| | | Hospital Deaths | | | Hospital Deaths | | | Hospital Deaths | | | Hospital Deaths | | |
Procedure	n	No.	%	n	No.	%	n	No.	%	n	No.	%	CL
AVR alone	162	7	4.3%	131	14	10.7%	18	1	5.5%	311	22	7.1%	5.6%–8.9%
AVR + CABG + other	58	2	3.4%	18	1	6%	2	0	0%	78	3	4%	2%–8%
AVR + AAA + CABG	1	0	0%	27[a]	6	22%	0	0	0%	28[a]	6	21%	13%–32%
AVR + other	6	0	0%	10	0	0%	0	0	0%	16	0	0%	0%–11%
Total	227	9	4.0%	186[b]	21	11.3%	20	1	4.5%	433	31	7.2%[c]	5.9%–8.7%

KEY: AAA, ascending aortic aneurysm; AVR, aortic valve replacement; CABG, coronary artery bypass graft. CL, 70% confidence limits.
NOTE: Six patients without NYHA class and 36 patients undergoing prosthetic valve re-replacement are excluded.
[a] Includes 6 emergency operations with 4 deaths.
[b] Includes 25 emergency operations with 12 deaths; with these excluded, the hospital mortality is 5.6% (70% CL 3.7%–8.1%).
[c] Without emergency operations, hospital mortality is 4.7% (70% CL 3.6%–6.0%).

graft experience in patients 40 years of age and over (Fig. 12-11a) but less apparent in patients over the age of 65 years of operation (Fig. 12-11b). Barnhorst and colleagues, at the Mayo Clinic, also demonstrated this by showing that the 8-year survival rate of about 70% for patients undergoing aortic valve replacement was less than that for an age-, sex-, and race-matched general population.[B5]

Modes of Premature Late Death

About 50% of late deaths are related to the cardiac condition but presumably unrelated to the specific device used.[B5,K1,W1] Sudden death without obvious cause occurs in 10%–20% of cases. Conceivably, in patients with mechanical prostheses, sudden death could be caused by emboli, but the frequency of sudden death in patients with homografts and almost certain absence of embolism confirms the impression that this is not the case. Five to 20% of late deaths are related to coronary artery disease, and most of the remainder of the cardiac deaths are caused by unresolved left ventricular secondary cardiomyopathy.

About 25% of late deaths are related to the replacement device, but with at least some devices, the frequency of such deaths may have lessened in recent years.[T4] These modes of late death include thromboembolism and anticoagulation-induced hemorrhage (5%–15%), prosthetic thrombosis, failure of other forms of device (prosthesis or bioprosthesis) (1%–5% but highly variable and time related), prosthetic valve endocarditis (5%–10% but time related), and paravalvular leakage.

Interestingly, with the use of homografts, only two modes of death are related to the replacement device: incompetence from leaflet rupture (8% of the total deaths) and homograft valve endocarditis (4%). The commonest modes have been sudden death (25%) and death from coronary artery disease (myocardial infarction, 19%).

Incremental Risk Factors for Premature Late Death

Important preoperative left ventricular dysfunction is a risk factor for premature late death after aortic valve replacement. Cunha and colleagues demonstrated directly that this is the case when they showed that patients with aortic incompetence and decreased left ventricular systolic function have a significantly increased probability of premature late death (Fig. 12-12a).[C10] They also showed that the functional status (NYHA functional class) refined still further the predictive value of poor left ventricular systolic function (Fig. 12-12b). Louagie and colleagues have also shown that poor preoperative functional status is a risk factor for premature late death after valve replacement for aortic incompetence.[L12] Lytle and colleagues by multivariate analysis also identified preoperatively poor left ventricular function as a risk factor for premature late death.[L10] Bonow and col-

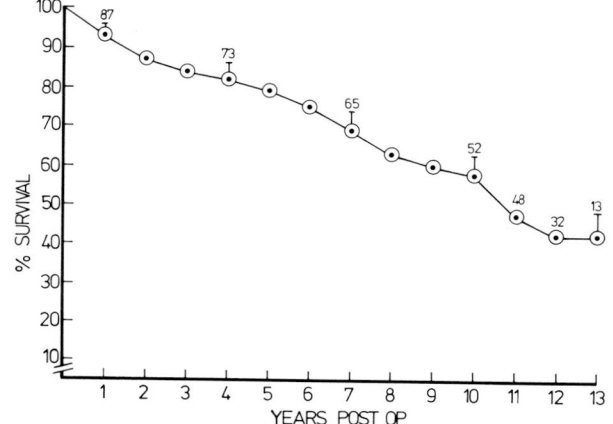

Figure 12-9 The 13-year actuarial survival of 91 hospital survivors of isolated aortic valve replacement with an antibiotic-treated homograft (GLH; 1968–1971). The patients have been detailed in earlier publications.[B25,B31] The bars represent one standard error (equivalent to 70% confidence limits).

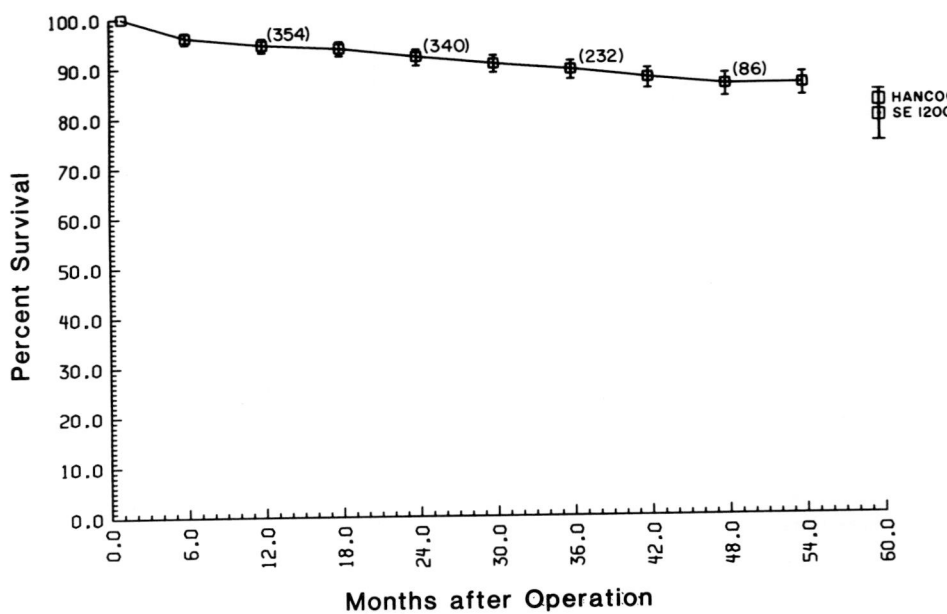

Figure 12-10   Late survival after aortic valve replacement with Bjork-Shiley valve at UAB compared to the report of Macmanus and associates[M1] for the Starr-Edwards (SE) non–cloth-covered prosthesis and the report of Davila and colleagues[D1] for the Hancock xenograft. Vertical bars represent 70% confidence limits. The figures within parentheses are the number of patients followed byeond the specified interval. Thirty-day mortality is not included.

Reproduced with permission from Karp et al.[K1]

leagues showed significantly decreased late survival in patients with preoperatively impaired systolic function[B16,B35] (Fig. 12-13).

A multivariate proportional hazards analysis of the UAB experience with both the Bjork-Shiley valve[K1] and the porcine heterograft valve[W2] indicates that poor preoperative functional status, as reflected in the higher NYHA functional classes, and no doubt reflecting severe left ventricular dys-

function, is a risk factor for premature late death, and actuarial survival data stratified according to preoperative NYHA functional status support this inference (Fig. 12-14). The classic study of 1975 by Barnhorst and colleagues, of the Mayo Clinic, also showed patients in NYHA class IV to have a worse prognosis, particularly in the first 2 years after operation,[B5] and similar conclusions have been reached in other studies.[C9,G4,K1,W2] The fact that marked preoperative

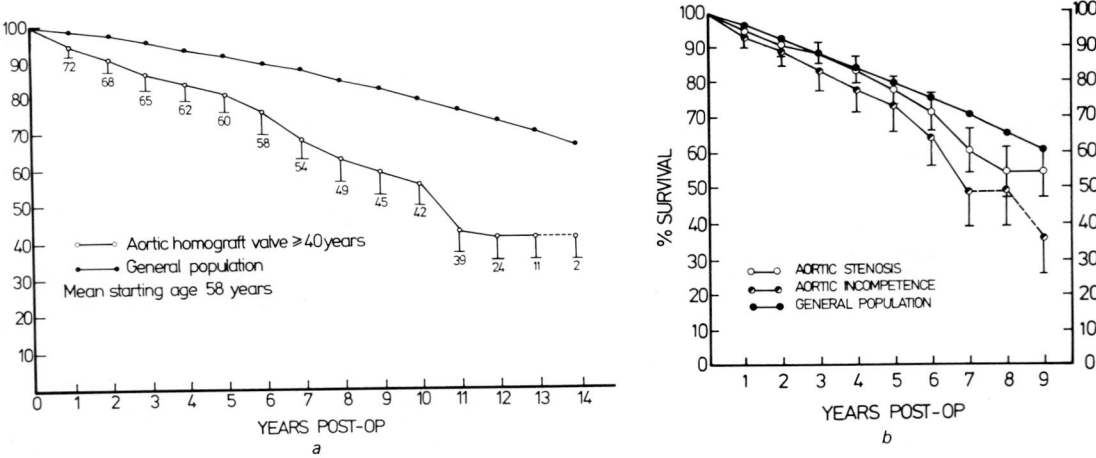

Figure 12-11   Survival after freehand aortic homograft valve replacement compared with general New Zealand population matched for age, sex, and race (GLH).
(a) Patients ≤ 40 years from the same data set as in Figure 12-8.
(b) Patients ≤ 65 years of age with isolated aortic valve replacement operated on between 1968 and 1978 using tissue or prosthetic valves. The mean age of the aortic valve patients was 68 years and of the general population, 70 years.

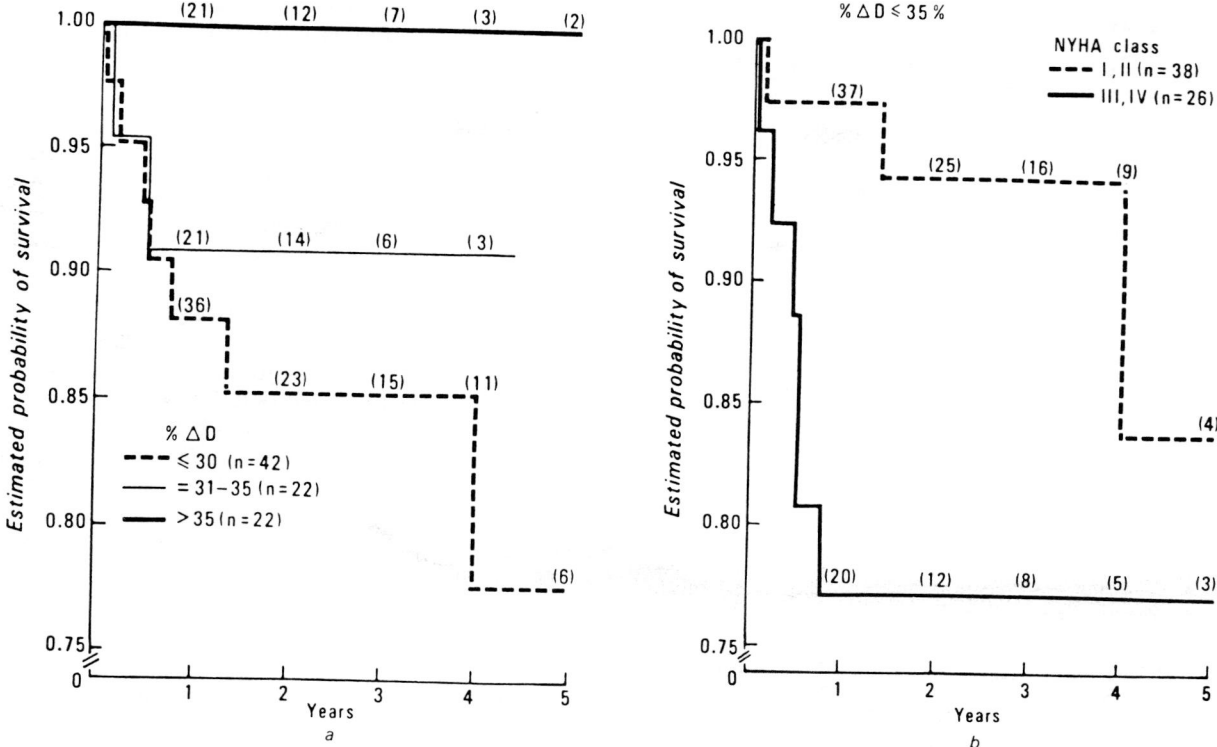

Figure 12-12 Late survival after replacement of the aortic valve for incompetence.
(a) Relationship between probability of survival after valve replacement for aortic insufficiency and preoperative percent change of left ventricular dimension (%ΔD), an index of systolic function. Patients with low values have significantly decreased probability of survival (P < .05). Numbers in parentheses are numbers of patients.
(b) Relationship between preoperative NYHA functional classification and probability of survival after valve replacement for aortic insufficiency in patients with percent change of left ventricular dimension (%ΔD) of 35% or less. Functional class improved predictive ability of percent change of dimension. Patients in functional class I or II have longer survival than those in class III or IV (P = .05). Numbers in parentheses are numbers of patients.
Reproduced with permission from Cunha et al.[C10]

cardiomegaly adversely affects late survival[B5,S8] supports these findings.

Important *preoperative ventricular arrhythmias* are an incremental risk factor for premature late death after aortic valve replacement.[A1,K1,S8] Presumably, these arrhythmias result from advanced secondary left ventricular cardiomyopathy, not reversed by the valve replacement. This is supported by the finding of Gradman and colleagues that significant left ventricular arrhythmias occur more frequently in patients with depressed left ventricular ejection fractions.[G13]

The development of left bundle-branch block following aortic valve replacement may be an incremental risk for premature late death, as reported by Thomas and colleagues.[T5] Further, sudden death occurred more frequently (P < .025) in those patients with left bundle conduction defects.

Preoperative aortic incompetence has a detrimental effect on long-term survival.[A1,B5,C9] This again may be related to the larger proportion of patients in this subset (compared to patients with aortic stenosis) who have developed advanced left ventricular dysfunction by the time of operation.

Not unexpectedly, both *older age*[C9,W2] and *concomitant*

untreated coronary artery disease[C9,K1,W2] adversely affect long-term survival.

The *type of replacement device used* has infrequently been demonstrated to be a determinant of the probability of premature late death. In the Cleveland Clinic experience, patients in whom bioprostheses were used for atrioventricular valve replacement and who were not anticoagulated had higher survival and event-free survival rates than did those receiving mechanical prostheses; their survival rates were also higher than those who were anticoagulated and received bioprostheses.[L10] The better 5-year survival with a Hancock porcine bioprosthesis reported by Copeland and colleagues, of Stanford,[C9] and by Ionescu for the pericardial xenograft valve[I6] may prove to be true differences.

The *type of myocardial protection* used almost certainly has an effect on late survival, for it is probable that direct coronary artery perfusion techniques were associated with a relatively high incidence of myocardial damage, particularly of the subendocardium, in these hypertrophied hearts and that this contributed to late cardiomyopathy. In the UAB experience, simple cold ischemic cardiac arrest increased late survival over that obtained with direct coronary artery

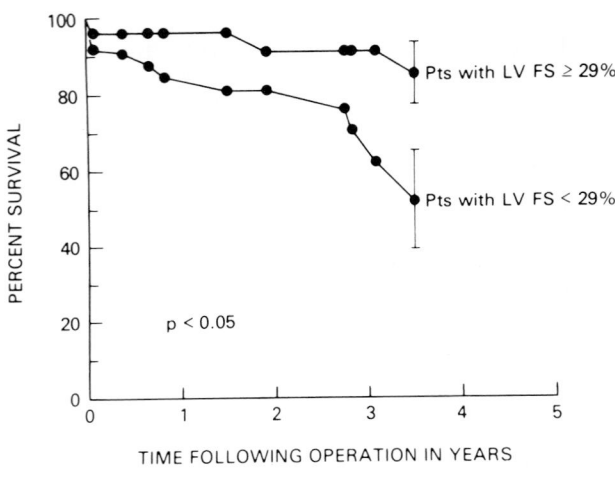

a

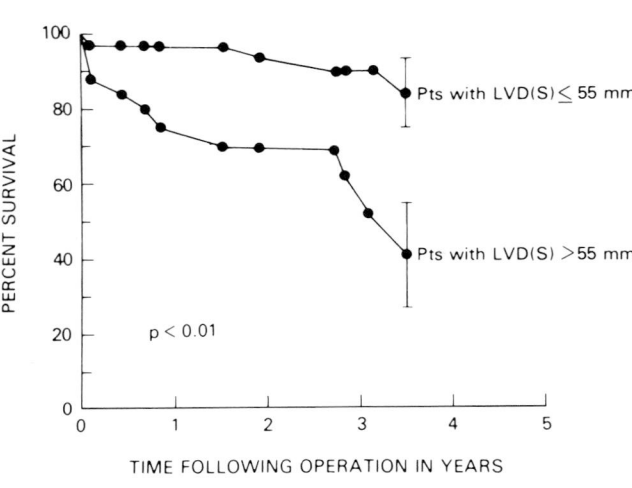

b

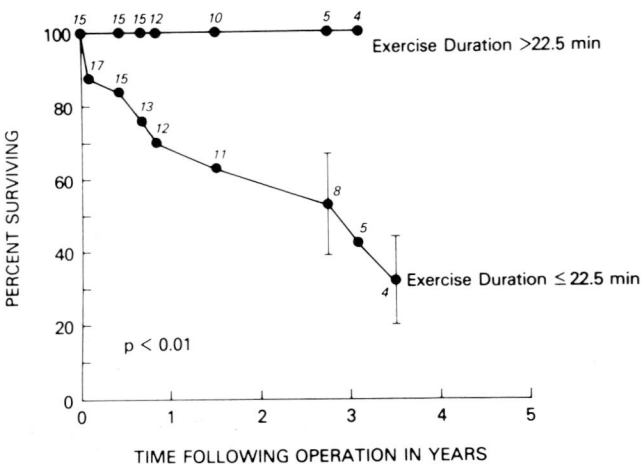

c

perfusion.[K1,W2] It is likely that cold cardioplegic myocardial preservation will further improve late results.

Symptomatic Results

Although premature late death does occur in some patients after aortic valve replacement, the functional status of most surviving patients is good. In fact, about 90% of patients traced 5–10 years (specifically, 8 years in the cases of Copeland and associates[C9]) are in NYHA functional class I or II. About 70% of patients preoperatively in NYHA class IV become class I or II postoperatively, as do about 80% of those preoperatively in class III and 90% of those preoperatively in class II, according to the UAB experience.[K1,W1]

Exercise capacity tested objectively can be near normal after valve replacement. This has been shown to occur, for example, in patients with aortic stenosis, depressed preoperative exercise capacity by objective testing but near-normal resting left ventricular end-diastolic pressure.[K5] In other situations, for example, in patients with aortic incompetence and preoperatively increased left ventricular end-diastolic pressure, exercise capacity is improved after operation but remains subnormal.[K5]

Left Ventricular Structure and Function

After successful aortic valve replacement, improvement in left ventricular structure and function may or may not occur. The outcome is determined in part at least by the aortic valve lesion and its particular effect on the myocardium, and on the extent of the secondary cardiomyopathy at the time of operation.

Aortic Stenosis

As aortic stenosis progresses and symptoms develop, the left ventricle is gradually (chronically) changed, both morphologically and in terms of systolic and diastolic function, as noted earlier.[R2]

The amount of *increase* in left ventricular mass that has developed by the time of operation has complex interrelationships with the systolic wall function and the reversibility of the hypertrophy postoperatively. Thus, Schwartz and colleagues found good systolic function and only hypertrophic myocardial cells when LV mass was < 200 g · m^{-2}. When LV mass was between 200 and 300 g · m^{-2}, degenerative changes were present but were mild. When it was > 300 g · m^{-2}, they found that systolic function was markedly depressed and multiple degenerative changes in ultrastructure

---

Figure 12-13 Late survival after replacement of the aortic valve for incompetence.

(*a*) Survival in patients stratified according to left ventricular fractional shortening (LVFS).

(*b*) Survival in patients subgrouped on the basis of preoperative left ventricular and systolic dimensions (LVD(S)).

(*c*) Survival in patients with subnormal (<29%) preoperative left ventricular fractional shortening, subgrouped on the basis of tested duration of exercise.

Parts *a*, *b* reproduced with permission from Bonow et al.,[B35] part *c* reproduced with permission from Bonow et al.,[B16] and the American Heart Association, Inc.

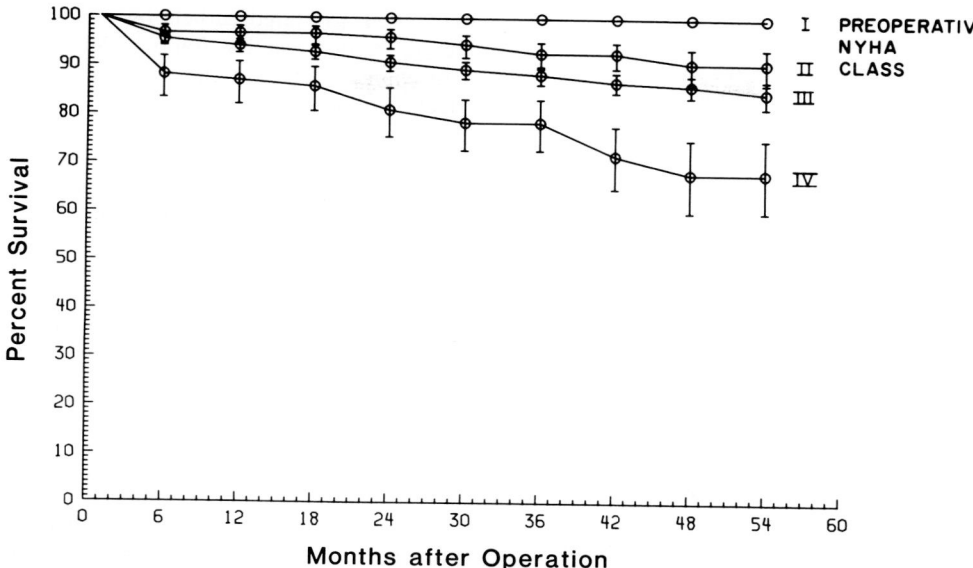

Figure 12-14 Late survival after aortic valve replacement with Bjork-Shiley prosthesis (UAB) by preoperative NYHA functional class (*n* = 642). The presentation is as in Figure 12-7. Reproduced with permission from Karp et al.[K1]

had occurred (mitochondrial changes, disruption of sarcomeric units, nonoriented growth of fiber components, disappearance of organelles).[S7] These degenerative changes have also been studied and described in detail by Maron and colleagues.[M2] Probably they are the morphologic basis for the loss of inotropic (contractile) strength and for irreversibility. The hypertrophy of myocardial cells (increased myocardial cell diameter) is a determinant of the decreased diastolic function of the left ventricle found in aortic stenosis.[S12] Myocardial fibrosis exerts little effect.

The morphologic response of the ventricle to the sudden reduction of afterload (specifically, that component of afterload that is the left ventricular pressure during systole) produced by valve replacement varies according to the nature and extent of the chronic changes present at the time of operation.[S6] When (as is usual) the left ventricular mass, as well as wall thickness, has increased by the time of operation but left ventricular end-diastolic pressure is still low (LV hypertrophy has been appropriate to maintain a relatively normal LV wall stress in the face of increased LV systolic pressure), left ventricular mass and wall thickness regress substantially after operation from an average of 206 g · m^{-2} to 133 g · m^{-2} (*P* < .05).[K5] However, normal LV mass is rarely attained.[K5,M10,P1] Significant reduction in LV mass after operation has been shown to occur at least in some patients with preoperatively elevated LV end-diastolic pressure.[S5] Presumably, these are patients in whom LV decompensation has occurred by the time of operation because of hypertrophy insufficient to maintain normal LV wall stress (afterload mismatch) rather than by reduced inotropic state (reduced contractile function). In the latter, irreversible left ventricular damage may be present, regression of left ventricular mass may fail to occur, and, indeed, ventricular function may worsen in the months after operation, with a poor late result.

The functional response of the left ventricle to aortic valve replacement also varies. Ejection fraction remains normal or supranormal postoperatively[K5,M10,S5] in patients in whom preoperative left ventricular systolic function (estimated, for example, by ejection fraction, mean circumferential fiber shortening rate, or end-systolic volume[B24]) has remained normal by virtue of appropriate left ventricular hypertrophy.[S5] The hypertrophy has maintained a relatively normal left ventricular wall stress (which, other things being equal, is inversely related to wall thickness) and a relatively normal left ventricular end-diastolic pressure in the face of high left ventricular systolic pressure. However, in some patients, the disease state has progressed to the point that the severely elevated left ventricular systolic pressure is not compensated by adequate left ventricular hypertrophy and increased wall thickness (afterload mismatch;[C1,R2] Fig. 12-15), ejection fraction is reduced, and end-diastolic pressure may be severely elevated. This condition does not imply a reduction of the inotropic state (or unit functional capacity) of the ventricle, and when the left ventricular systolic pressure is suddenly reduced by replacement of the stenotic aortic valve, afterload mismatch is gone, ejection fraction rises to normal, and left ventricular end-diastolic pressure falls to normal.[C1,K5,K6] A certain degree of regression of left ventricular hypertrophy also follows.[C1,K5] In contrast, when the secondary left ventricular cardiomyopathy has progressed to the stage that the inotropic state of the myocardium has become depressed, ejection fraction does not rise appreciably after operation,[C1] and the long-term prognosis after valve replacement is poor.

Loss of *left ventricular diastolic function* also results from left ventricular hypertrophy and myocardial cell hypertrophy in patients with severe aortic stenosis.[G7,S12] The increased diastolic stiffness of the ventricle regresses after successful valve replacement, but not to normal.

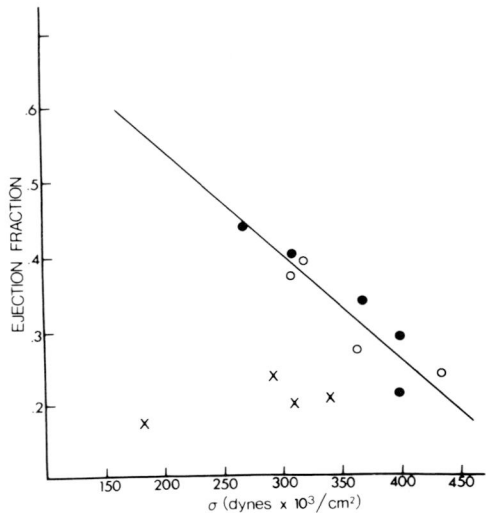

Figure 12-15   Ejection fraction in patients undergoing aortic valve replacement for severe aortic stenosis and congestive heart failure plotted against mean circumferential left ventricular wall stress (σ). Group 1 (closed circles) consists of patients doing well after operation, and group 2 (X's) of those doing poorly. Group 2 patients fell below and to the left of group 1 patients, indicating lower ejection fraction despite less σ. This is consistent with the concept that left ventricular performance (ejection fraction) was depressed in group 1 patients due to afterload mismatch and in group 2 patients due to myocardial failure (depressed inotropic state).

Modified with permission from Carabello et al.,[C1] and the American Heart Association, Inc.

Aortic Incompetence

Clearly, some patients die within a few months to a few years because of intractable heart failure after apparently successful aortic valve replacement for chronic aortic incompetence,[B4,H5,I1] and at least in them, preoperatively impaired left ventricular systolic and diastolic function is not improved by operation. Under other circumstances, left ventricular structure and function can be nearly normal late postoperatively.[G3] That this at least is possible under proper circumstances is suggested by the experimental study of left ventricular volume overload by Papdimitriou and colleagues.[P2] They found that within 6 months of closure of a previously created large systemic arteriovenous fistula, and thus removal of the volume overload, LV volume and systolic function were normal, myocardial ultrastructure was virtually normal, and LV mass was reduced toward normal but not quite to normal.

The increased left ventricular mass associated with aortic incompetence is reduced late postoperatively, but not to normal,[O6] when the hemodynamic response to aortic valve replacement for aortic regurgitation is good (with a decrease in LV end-diastolic volume and an increase in resting ejection fraction to normal).[K5,M5] Left ventricular mass *fails* to regress when aortic valve replacement is done so late in the course of the disease that left ventricular systolic function remains depressed[C14] and diastolic function (expressed in the left ventricular pressure-volume characteristics and in left ventricular end-diastolic volume) remains highly abnormal.

Preoperatively normal left ventricular systolic function

(estimated, as stated earlier, by a number of methods, including resting ejection fraction, left ventricular fractional shortening, velocity of circumferential shortening, left ventricular end-systolic volume, and, more informatively, exercise ejection fraction and end-systolic volume) remains normal late postoperatively after successful aortic valve replacement for aortic incompetence, unless myocardial damage has been produced intraoperatively. Yet truly normal preoperative left ventricular systolic function is present in less than 10% of patients with symptomatic aortic incompetence.[B17]

Preoperatively impaired resting or stressed left ventricular systolic function generally returns toward normal late after aortic valve replacement, but often not to normal.[B17,C5,K5] Thus, the response of left ventricular systolic function (ejection fraction or end-systolic volume) to exercise usually remains abnormal postoperatively. The regression toward normal is affected by the duration of the preoperative left ventricular dysfunction, and when it has been present for more than one year regression is less likely to occur.[B43] When in addition to impaired left ventricular systolic function there is marked limitation in exercise capacity, the return toward normal is particularly incomplete.[B16] Severe preoperative reduction in left ventricular systolic function during stress, even in patients with only mild symptoms, is often irreversible.[B16,G3,O1] In fact, some such patients have worse LV systolic function late postoperatively than before operation and may show a progressive deterioration in left ventricular systolic function and an increase in left ventricular diastolic volumes, leading to death with heart failure a few months to a few years after operation.

Knowledge about preoperative and postoperative left ventricular diastolic function in patients with aortic incompetence is less complete. In part, this is because diastolic function is difficult to study. LV end-diastolic wall thickness is abnormally great preoperatively and usually does not regress postoperatively.[S12] This important determinant of diastolic behavior[G8] thus is unchanged by operation. Schwarz and colleagues found elastic stiffness of the left ventricle increased preoperatively and unchanged by operation in patients with aortic incompetence.[S12]

Preoperatively large left ventricular end-diastolic volume (affected by diastolic function but by other things as well) decreases after aortic valve replacement in most but not all patients. Kennedy and colleagues found regression of the large LV end-diastolic volume in all five of their patients operated on for aortic incompetence.[K5] Gaasch and colleagues and Schuler and colleagues found a decrease in volume within 10 days of valve replacement, with some further regression in size late postoperatively.[G4,S9] The occurrence and magnitude of regression of left ventricular end-diastolic volume depends on the stage of the morphologic and functional left ventricular systolic and diastolic damage sustained before operation, reflected in part by the preoperative functional state of the patient. Thus, Bonow and colleagues found that left ventricular end-diastolic dimensions fell strikingly and occasionally to near-normal values in patients with good exercise tolerance, all of whom had important cardiomegaly preoperatively; whereas in patients with impaired exercise ability, some hearts were larger postop-

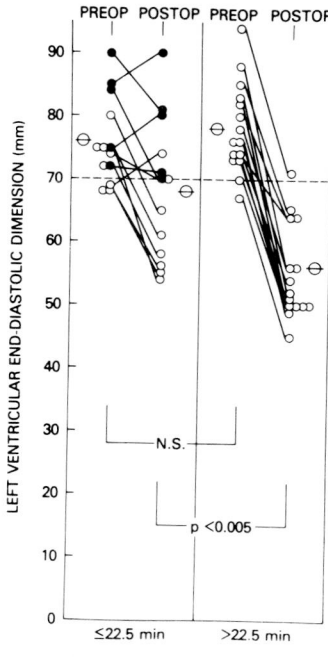

Figure 12-16 Changes in echocardiographic left ventricular end-diastolic dimension as a result of operation in symptomatic patients undergoing valve replacement for aortic incompetence, according to preoperative exercise duration. Patients who completed stage 1 before operation (< 22.5 minutes) had a greater decrease in diastolic size than did patients who could not complete stage 1 (≤ 22.5 minutes). The dashed line at 70 mm indicates the value of postoperative diastolic dimension above which patients have been shown to be at high risk of subsequent death from congestive heart failure.

KEY: open circle, alive; closed circle, late death from congestive heart failure.

Reproduced with permission from Bonow et al.,[B16] and the American Heart Association, Inc.

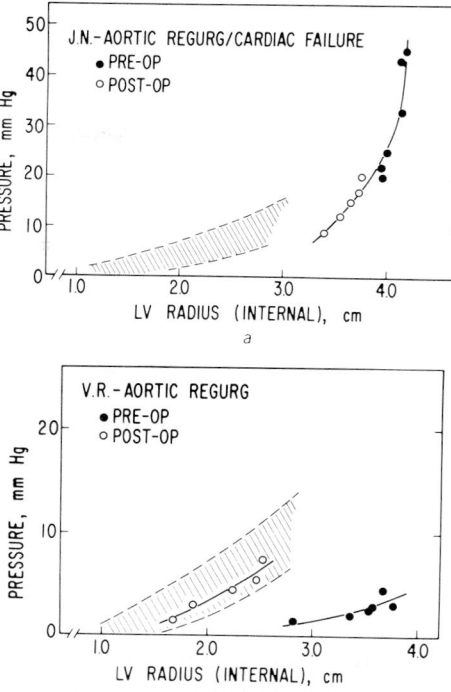

Figure 12-17 Left ventricular internal radius is plotted on the horizontal axis with corresponding measurements of LV pressure on the vertical axis throughout the diastolic filling period in preoperative study (closed circles) and postoperative study approximately 1 year after aortic valve replacement for aortic incompetence (open circles). The cross-hatched area defines the range of pressure-radius values observed in a previously studied group of patients with normal LV function without valvular regurgitation.
(a) A patient with preoperatively depressed inotropic state.
(b) A patient with normal preoperative inotropic state.

Reproduced with permission from Gault et al.,[G3] and the American Heart Association, Inc.

eratively, and few regressed in size late postoperatively[B16] (Fig. 12-16). Failure of LV end-diastolic volume to regress toward normal indicates irreversible morphologic and functional left ventricular damage and suggests that the long-term result of operation will be poor.[H4]

In summary, in the volume overloaded left ventricle of aortic incompetence, irreversible structural and functional changes develop when the increase in left ventricular mass reaches a certain stage.[K6] In contrast to the course of the disease in aortic stenosis, the patient may remain relatively well even when the stage of irreversibility is approaching. In fact, more advanced impairment of left ventricular systolic function is present in patients in a given NYHA functional class with aortic incompetence than in those with aortic stenosis.[H3] Thus, LV systolic function during stress such as exercise becomes to some extent at least irreversibly impaired quite early in the life history of patients with aortic incompetence. By the time exercise ability has become impaired, the diastolic properties of the left ventricle may have become irreversibly impaired, and fixed cardiomegaly may be present. This was clearly defined by Gault and colleagues[G3] (Fig. 12-17).

The foregoing applies to patients without periprosthetic leakage late postoperatively. The hemodynamic and functional variables after operation are very sensitive to the left ventricular volume overload of periprosthetic leakage. Thus, Schwarz and colleagues found such patients to have significantly reduced LV systolic function late postoperatively, compared to patients without periprosthetic leakage.[S10]

Left Ventricular–Aortic Pressure Gradients

Gradients are rare after freehand aortic homograft valve replacement[B25,B31] but are present after mechanical prosthetic or bioprosthetic aortic valve replacement in virtually all patients (Fig. 12-18). Their magnitude varies greatly and is determined primarily by the characteristics of the prosthesis itself, the size of the device relative to the size of the patient, the cardiac output (and thus whether the study was done during rest, exercise, or pharmacologic stimulation of output), and abnormal developments in or around the replacement device.

Nonetheless, virtually all mechanical prostheses[B13] and

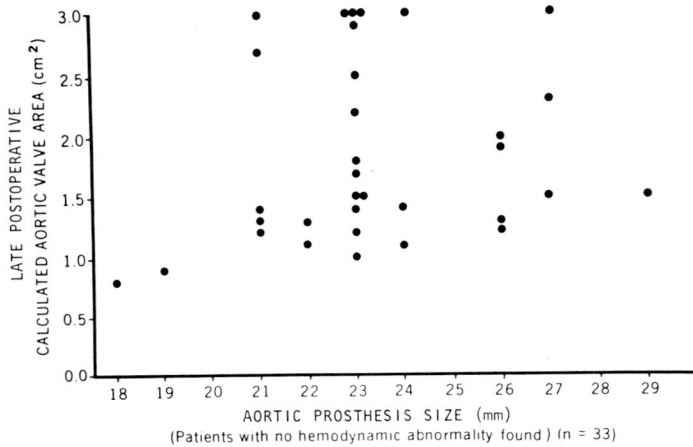

Figure 12-18 Late postoperative effective valve orifice area (calculated aortic valve area) after aortic valve replacement with prostheses of different types and sizes. Only patients thought to have no prosthetic complications are included. Note the wide variability of the values for any given prosthetic size.[B13]

bioprostheses larger than the 21-mm size can provide satisfactory performance in most adults (Fig. 12-19). However, the small (10-mmHg) resting gradients associated with even the 25- or 27-mm Bjork-Shiley valve regularly become 30–50 mmHg during periods of increased cardiac output.[T3] Most 21-mm size mechanical prostheses[B12] and bioprostheses[C7] (Fig. 12-20) are quite obstructive, particularly during periods of increased cardiac output (Table 12-18). Among the 21-mm mechanical prostheses, the St. Jude valve performs the best in this regard,[W7] and among the bioprostheses of this size,

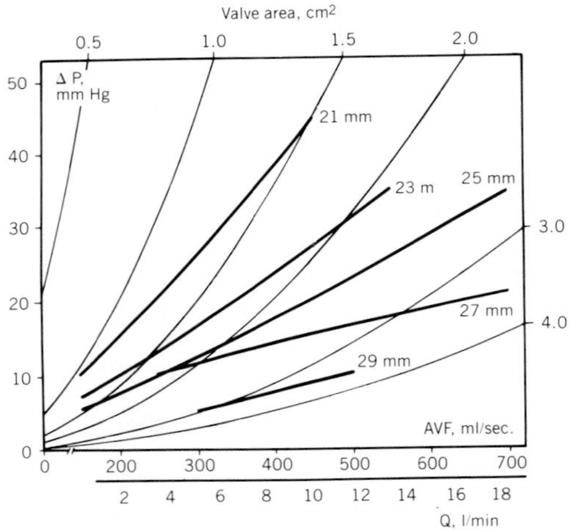

the Ionescu-Shiley heterograft pericardial bioprosthesis and the Hancock modified orifice prosthesis have the lowest gradients. In the 19-mm sizes, in general, only the Ionescu-Shiley bioprosthesis performs satisfactorily (Table 12-18, Fig. 12-20). However, in small patients (with their smaller cardiac output), some 19-mm devices may perform satisfactorily in this regard (Fig. 12-21).

Because of the variability in the gradients usually present across the prostheses used for aortic valve replacement, abnormal gradients may be difficult to identify. However, such abnormalities do develop from fibrous ingrowth below or above the device, dense clot around the valve (thrombotic encasement), or leaflet calcification of a bioprosthesis.[B13,B32] Gradients of 85–100 mmHg may be produced, but they can be much lower and more difficult to define as abnormal when cardiac output is reduced by these developments.

Chronic Hemolysis

Patients with homograft valves sewn freehand into the aortic root do not have abnormal red blood cell hemolysis, even when there is a paravalvar or central leak; neither do those with well-functioning stent-mounted heterografts. At least a small increase in hemolysis is produced by all well-functioning prosthetic valves, with the disc-type valve producing less than the ball valves.[D2] Thus, 50% of patients with the Bjork-Shiley aortic valve prosthesis in place have normal serum LDH activity and haptoglobin levels.[B12] Patients with well-functioning prosthetic aortic valves in general have normal hemoglobin concentrations. Only with the Lillehei-Kastor valve do the acceptable-sized but small valves have more hemolysis than the larger ones.[D2]

Periprosthetic and/or intraprosthetic leakage produces increased amounts of hemolysis, and the magnitude of the increase of hemolysis is related to the amount of regurgitation (Fig. 12-22).[B12] Thrombotic narrowing of a prosthetic orifice also increases hemolysis significantly.

Figure 12-19 Relationship (thick lines) between mean pressure differences (ΔP) across five sizes of the Bjork-Shiley aortic prosthesis (n = 90) and mean aortic valve flow (AVF) or cardiac output (Q). Thin lines indicate the calculated valve area in square centimeters according to Gorlin's formula. The valves were distributed as follows: 21-mm size, 12 patients; 23-mm size, 26 patients; 25-mm size, 33 patients; 27-mm size, 12 patients; and 29-mm size, 7 patients.

Reproduced with permission from Bjork et al.[B12]

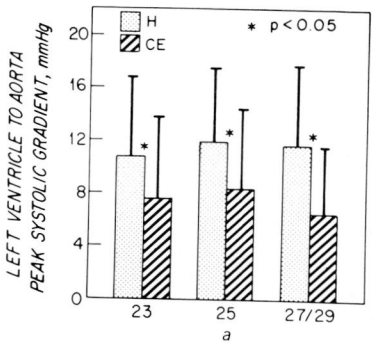

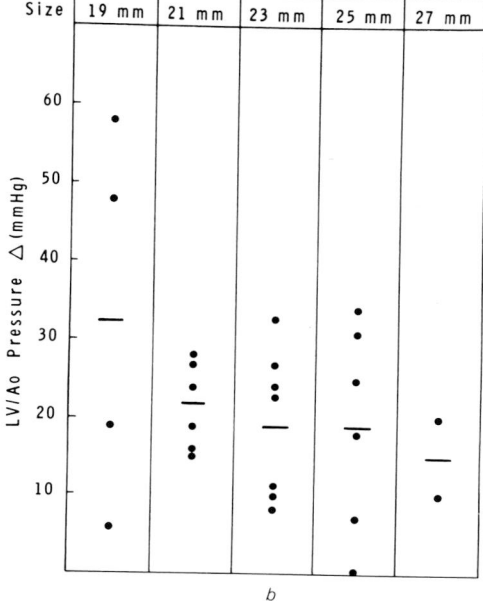

Figure 12-20 Postoperative left ventricular-aortic peak pressure gradients across stent-mounted porcine heterografts in the aortic position, according to valve size (external stent diameter).
(*a*) Comparison of Hancock (H) and Carpentier-Edwards bioprostheses. The Hancock bioprostheses were standard ones, except for the 23-mm size, which was the modified-orifice type. Zusman and colleagues[Z1] reported similar mean gradients for the 23-mm modified-orifice Hancock bioprosthesis, and the same gradient for the 21-mm device.
(*b*) Postoperative left ventricular-aortic peak pressure gradients across the standard Hancock bioprosthesis. The horizontal lines represent mean values. The mean value for calculated valve area (cm^2) for the 19-mm size was 0.98, for the 21-mm size 1.03, for the 23-mm size 1.2, for the 25-mm size 1.44, and for the 27-mm size 1.61.

Part *a* reproduced with permission from Levine et al.,[L3] and the American Heart Association Inc.; part *b* reproduced with permission from Jones et al.[J2]

Periprosthetic Leakage

After homograft aortic valve replacement, periprosthetic leakage has not been experienced since 1968 (GLH, UAB). However, earlier in the GLH experience with homografts sewn freehand into the aortic root, this was relatively common. It was abolished by compartmentalizing and obliterating the dead space between graft and host by the use of subcommissural vertical mattress sutures.[B33,G10]

With the use of mechanical prostheses or bioprostheses, important periprosthetic leakage is uncommon in the absence of infection,[J1] although minor leakage may occur. Periprosthetic leakage usually becomes evident in the early months after operation.[R17] At GLH amongst 147 aortic valve replacements with prosthetic or bioprosthetic valves over a 4-year period (1976–1979), only 1 patient (0.7%, CL 0.1%–2.3%) and at UAB 10 (1.2%, CL 0.8%–1.7%) among 842 (1975–July 1979) have required reoperation for perivalvar leakage. Shean and colleagues reported an incidence of minor periprosthetic leakage of 17% in the Massachusetts General Hospital series.[S14] In addition, 6% (CL 5%–7%) had clinically recognizable hemolysis. When periprosthetic leakage develops and infection is not present, the area of dehiscence is usually small and can be repaired with one or two pledgetted mattress sutures.

Central Leakage

In the early experience with homograft aortic valves, central leakage occurred in some patients with very large aortic roots, which resulted in overstretching of the leaflets and central leakage.[B25] It is also probable that this phenomenon increased the risk of leaflet rupture because the leaflets do not support each other centrally in the closed position and stresses are therefore greater. The proportion of patients free of moderate or severe important homograft valve incompetence during the era of antibiotic sterilization and storage in nutrient medium is shown in Fig. 12-23. The decrease in this proportion in cases with very large aortic root (internal diameter at the valve anulus > 30 mm) is evident, and this has also been observed by Khanna and associates.[K9] The freehand-sewn homograft is therefore not suitable in such cases. However, moderate enlargement of the aortic root can be well managed by aortic root tailoring.[B27]

In the current era, then, important late incompetence in a homograft aortic valve is nearly always a result of cusp rupture. Ninety-five percent of patients with small or normal-sized aortic roots (there is no difference between the two) are free of this important aortic incompetence 5 years after insertion, 75% are free of it 10 years after insertion, and 42% are free of it 13 years postoperatively. There was no difference in the incidence of important incompetence in those less than 20 years of age compared to those over 20 years of age. An additional group of patients have mild (10%) or trivial (33%) incompetence 6 years postoperatively (Fig. 12-24).

The importance of the method of handling and preserving homograft valves is evident from the fact that leaflet rupture (sometimes associated with patchy calcification) has not been a catastrophic event in the era described above, and incompetence may remain mild for as long as 5 years before progressing. In contrast, progression is more rapid, and rupture more common and earlier in appearance, with chemical treatment of the valve[B6,B25] (GLH) or irradiation (UAB). The differences relate to the more active host tissue reaction onto and into the leaflet with antibiotic sterilization,[G11] a process that protects the leaflet from rupture. The current method for handling homografts, at GLH and more recently at UAB, involves use of an altered antibiotic combination and freezing and storage in liquid nitrogen after 48 hours (see Appen-

Table 12-18 Hemodynamic conditions after the insertion of various aortic valve replacement devices in adults.

Devices and Standard Values	Systolic LV Aortic Gradient (mm Hg)		Effective Orifice Area (cm²)[a]		Effective Orifice Area Index (cm² · m⁻²)[b]	
	Rest	Exercise	Rest	Exercise	Rest	Exercise
21-mm Devices[A4,B23,B36,B38−41,C7,C15−18,H5,J2,L7−9,M12,N4,N5,P8,R14,R15,S21,T5,W7,W8,Z1]						
Bjork-Shiley standard type[b]	25 (33)	41 (20)	1.28 (10)			
Bjork-Shiley concave-convex[a]	6 (5)		1.4 (10)	1.5 (10)		
St. Jude[a]	6 (5)		2.47 (15)		1.61 (15)	
Starr-Edwards 1260[b] (8A = 21 mm)	11 (28)	63 (1)	1.11 (17)			
Standard orifice Hancock heterograft valve[b]	20 (18)	51 (12)	1.15 (32)		0.8 (15)	
Modified orifice Hancock heterograft[a]	9 (46)	18 (7)	1.51 (33)	1.23 (7)	1.6 (7)	
Carpentier-Edwards heterograft valve[b]	13 (5)	16 (1)	1.31 (5)	0.98 (1)	0.83 (5)	0.68 (1)
Ionescu-Shiley heterograft pericordium[b]	8 (6)	13 (6)	1.23 (15)	1.8 (6)		
19-mm Devices[C15,J2,M4,R14,S11,T5,T6,W7,Z1]						
Bjork-Shiley standard type[b]	16 (24)		1.06 (24)		0.62 (24)	
St. Jude[a]	15 (9)	32 (6)	1.27 (9)	1.16 (5)	0.85 (9)	0.71 (5)
Standard orifice Hancock heterograft valve[b]	34 (8)	38 (7)	0.98 (7)			
Modified orifice Hancock heterograft[b]	19 (6)	70 (1)	0.90 (1)		0.89 (1)	
Ionescu-Shiley heterograft pericardium[b]	8 (3)	12 (3)	1.1 (3)	1.3 (3)		
Standard Values						
Normal			2–4		2	
Severe stenosis			< 1		0.67	
Desired postoperative value	≤ 10	≤ 30	≥ 1.35		≥ 0.90	

KEY: LA, left atrium; LV, left ventricle.

NOTE: The numbers in parentheses are the total numbers of patients observed.

[a] Acceptable devices.

[b] Devices of borderline acceptability.

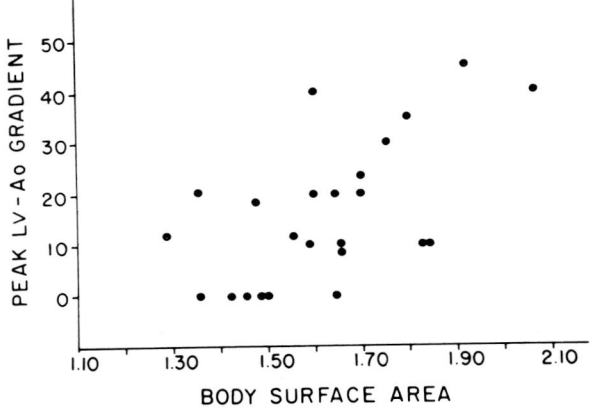

Figure 12-21 The relationship of peak left ventricular (LV) aortic (Ao) gradient to body surface area (m²) in patients in whom a 19-mm Bjork-Shiley valve has been inserted. The data indicate to us that use of the 19-mm size Bjork-Shiley valve is generally appropriate only when the patient's body surface area is less than 1.5 m². Reproduced with permission from Schaff et al.[S11]

dix 12C). Animal experiments at GLH[A3] have demonstrated that with the new method there is better preservation of the acid mucopolysaccharide and ground substance of the leaflets and an improved host tissue ingrowth comparable to that achieved with fresh, untreated leaflets, in which complete host tissue replacement can occur.[G12] This method has been used with success by O'Brien, in Brisbane,[O5] and it is anticipated that the incidence of cusp rupture will be lower with it.

The matter of central leakage through stent-mounted glutaraldehyde-preserved porcine heterografts has been less well studied. An estimate of the late failure rate of porcine heterografts is presented in Chapter 11, Figure 11-29, but the degree of uncertainty in that estimate is considerably greater than in the case of homografts. Also, the heterograft failures are from the development of calcific stenosis as well as incompetence.

Mechanical prostheses develop important central leakage only when there is mechanical failure of the device (such as poppet escape) or suture, or tissue or thrombotic encroach-

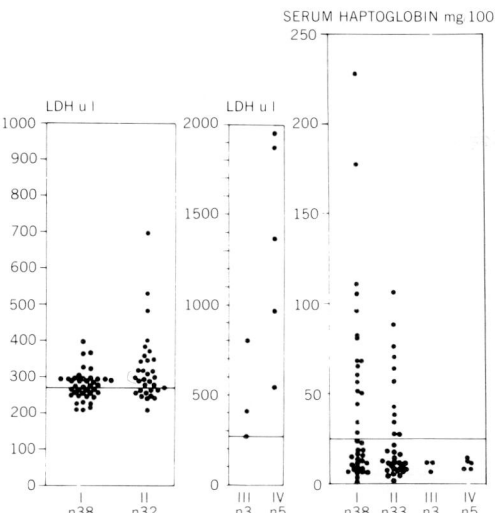

Figure 12-22 Relationship of serum lactic dehydrogenase activity and haptoglobin to the grade of aortic regurgitation after operation. Horizontal lines equal upper (LDH) and lower (haptoglobin) normal ranges.

Reproduced with permission from Bjork et al.[B12]

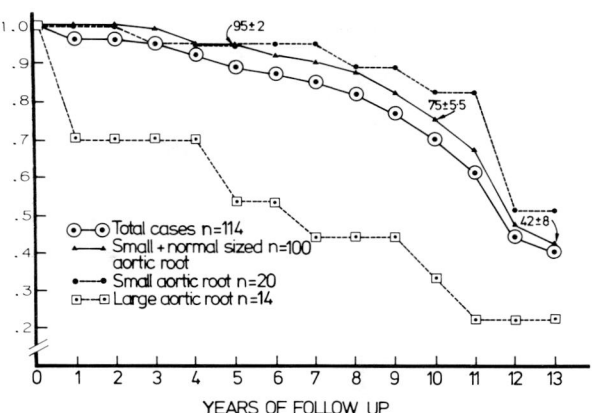

Figure 12-23 The proportion of patients free of important (moderate or severe) homograft valve incompetence (GLH; antibiotic sterilization with PSKA and nutrient medium storage at 4°C; see Appendix C). Ninety patients had isolated aortic valve disease, and 31 had multivalve disease, as detailed in an earlier publication.[B25] One hundred fourteen patients left hospital alive. Two patients were lost to follow-up at 54 and 74 months. The other 48 survivors were followed for 132–162 months (average 12 years). Of the 29 instances of incompetence occurring in the 100 patients with small or normal-sized roots, 24 were presumed or proven cusp rupture, 4 others were related to homograft valve endocarditis, and 1 was due to leaflet malposition related to technical error at insertion. For small and normal-sized aortic roots compared with large aortic roots, $P = .0006$.

ment into the seating area of the device. The incidence of this, though not rigorously studied, is low.

Prosthetic, or Homograft, Valve Endocarditis

Prosthetic endocarditis is an uncommon but very serious complication of aortic valve replacement, since only about 60% of patients are long-term survivors of this complication.

The incidence of prosthetic (and homograft) valve endocarditis (PVE) is difficult to estimate for several reasons. Most series are relatively small, and the differences are frequently statistically not significant. This is the case in the differences between the overall incidence at GLH and UAB. Differences in incidence result also from the fact that frequently follow-up data are incomplete, nonactuarial methods are used, studies are often only retrospective, and too restrictive criteria are used in diagnosing PVE.

Incremental risk factors have now been identified that increase the probability of prosthetic valve endocarditis.[13] The strongest is the presence of native valve endocarditis (Table 12-19), which increases fivefold the probability of prosthetic valve endocarditis. At least at UAB, being black and being male also increased the probability of PVE. Longer elapsed time of cardiopulmonary bypass was a weak incremental risk factor.

Of great importance is the replacement device itself. The homograft valve has a low incidence of PVE[C12] (Fig. 12-25), whereas the mechanical prosthesis has the highest incidence. To discuss further this difference, the time course of PVE must be considered. Examination of the actuarial incidence of PVE indicates that a large proportion of patients develop it within the first 3 months of valve replacement[13] (Fig. 12-26). A hazard function analysis (UAB) indicates that the mechanical prosthesis gives the highest early risk of PVE (Fig. 12-27). A similar analysis (GLH) experience indicates

that there is no early phase of PVE when the homograft is used (Fig. 12-28). An early phase is clearly evident at GLH when mechanical or bioprostheses are used. Thus, the homograft is highly resistant to the surface contamination that must be etiologic to this phase. The bioprosthesis falls between the mechanical prosthesis and the homograft valve in this regard (UAB and GLH). However, Cohn and colleagues report the incidence of PVE to be higher with bioprostheses than with mechanical valves,[C21] and the explanation for this difference is not apparent.

The time course of PVE is also different in patients with and without native valve endocarditis, which predisposes patients to a high incidence of PVE early after operation. The organisms involved in the early phase of postoperative PVE are strikingly different from those in native valve endocarditis in general. Rather than being primarily streptococcal in origin, they are due most commonly to staphylococci, gram negative cocci, or mixed organisms.[13] Rarely, a fungal infection occurs, and this is almost always lethal. The late phase of PVE is frequently caused by the streptococcus. The implication of all of this information is that the early phase of PVE very likely results from operating room contamination, and the late phase from transient bacteremias.

When prosthetic valve endocarditis occurs, either in the early or late postoperative period, intense and appropriate antibiotic treatment is indicated. As long as there is no evidence of incompetence at the replacement device, medical treatment should be continued, as good results can be obtained in many patients. Unfortunately, most patients de-

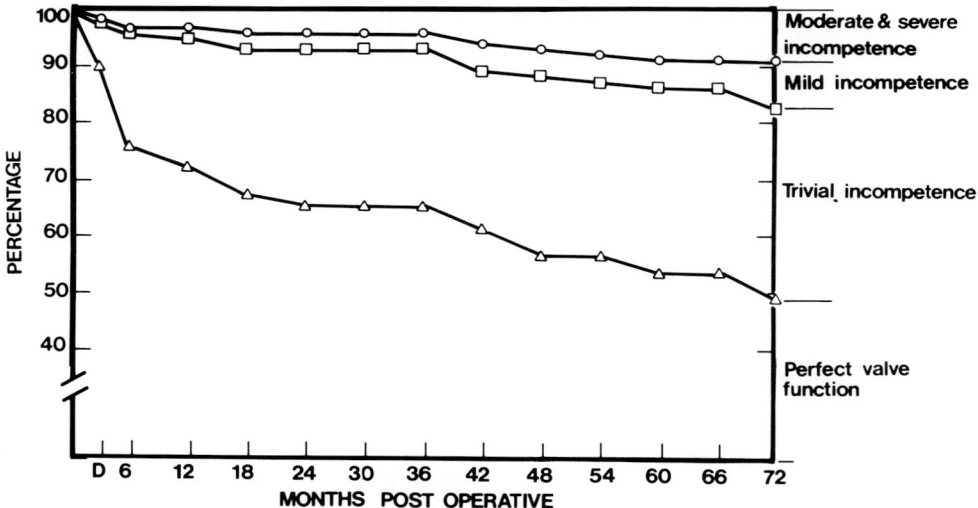

Figure 12-24   Actuarial incidence of homograft aortic valve incompetence in patients leaving hospital (GLH). Both the rate of appearance of incompetence and its severity are portrayed. Those beneath the lowest line had no diastolic aortic murmur.

Reproduced with permission from Barratt-Boyes et al.,[B25] and the American Heart Association, Inc.

velop incompetence at the replacement device. Under such circumstances, although intense antibiotic treatment is the basic method of management, replacement of the device is nearly always required because of a rapidly progressive periprosthetic leak and the threat of or actual acute hemodynamic deterioration. Tissue destruction is usually marked, and the surgical challenge formidable. Special surgical procedures are sometimes necessary because of extensive annular destruction by infection (see "Surgical Problems of Native Aortic Valve Endocarditis"). A hospital mortality for these operations is about 25%, and recurrence and reoperation are not uncommon.[12] Clearly, the emphasis must be on prevention by scrupulous operating room technique, such as described in Chapter 2, and appropriate antimicrobial prophylaxis. In this regard, it is prudent to don a second pair of gloves when tying down a group of interrupted valve sutures.

Thromboembolism

Thromboembolic complications are quite rare in nonanticoagulated patients following freehand insertion of antibiotic sterilized homografts in the aortic root. Tiny platelet emboli probably occur during the early healing phase, as they have been recognized in the retinal vessels, where they rarely cause transient episodes of blindness or aphasia.[B32] It is probable that thromboembolism does not occur following this period even when there is later leaflet rupture or calcification. The one exception is endocarditis.

After replacement of the aortic valve with a Bjork-Shiley prosthesis, the freedom from a thromboembolic event among patients on chronic anticoagulant therapy is 88% at 4 years (Fig. 12-29), not significantly different from that in patients undergoing mitral replacement.[K1] This is similar to the incidence after use of the Starr-Edwards valve in the

Table 12-19   Multivariate analysis (Cox proportional hazard method) of incremental risk factors for postoperative prosthetic valve endocarditis (UAB; 1975–July 1, 1979; n = 1465, 53 events).[13]

Incremental Risk Factor	Cox Coefficient ± SD	P value	Increase in Incidence
Presence of native valve endocarditis (all degrees of activity)	1.7 ± 0.40	<.0001	5 times
Blacks	1.3 ± 0.33	.0003	4 times
Mechanical prostheses	1.0 ± 0.38	.005	3 times
Males	0.7 ± 0.33	.04	2 times
Longer elapsed time of cardiopulmonary bypass (min)[a]	0.006 ± 0.0033	.09	120 min vs. 60 min = 1.4 times

[a]Or cardiac ischemic time (P = .03).

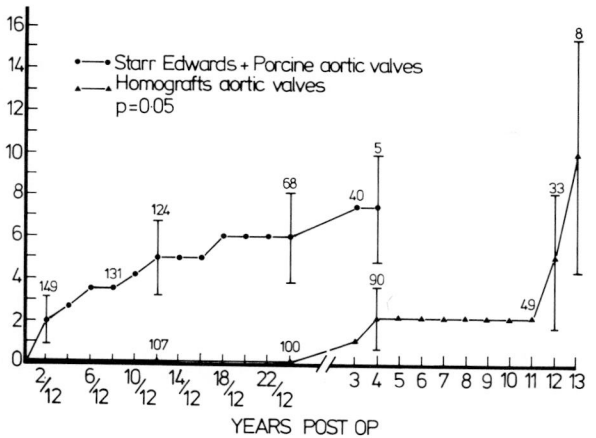

Figure 12-25 Actuarial incidence of postoperative endocarditis on the various types of aortic valve replacement devices used at GLH. The Starr-Edwards and porcine valves were inserted between 1976–1981, and the antibiotic-treated homograft valves between 1968–1971 (same series as Fig. 12-9). The vertical bars represent one standard error.

current era, an incidence significantly less than that in earlier years.[T4] The incidence of thromboembolism does not decrease with time and appears to be about 2% per year expressed actuarially; McGoon and colleagues report 60% of patients with aortic valve replacement with a Starr-Edwards ball valve prosthesis to be free of thromboembolism at 10 years and 54% at 15 years.[M19]

Likewise, the actuarial freedom from thromboembolism after aortic valve replacement with a stent-mounted heterograft (90% at 3 years[W2]) in patients without chronic anticoag-

ulant treatment is similar to that for heterograft mitral replacement and to that for Bjork-Shiley aortic valve replacement. As in the mitral experience with heterografts, older age and atrial fibrillation increase the risk of postoperative thromboembolism in patients with heterograft replacement of the aortic valve.[W2]

The incidence of prosthetic thrombosis or encapsulation with the Bjork-Shiley valve, an acute catastrophic complication, is 3% at 4 years, appreciably less than in the mitral position (see Chapter 11, Fig. 11-23). The incidence of thromboembolism does not decrease with time and appears to be about 2% per year expressed actuarially.[T4]

Late Postoperative Bleeding

A significant complication of the chronic anticoagulation required with a mechanical prosthesis is late postoperative bleeding. The actuarial incidence (GLH) has been 9% at 4 years, including 4 fatal bleeding episodes among 173 patients followed up to 4 years. Starr's group has noted a threefold increase, from 1.3% to 4.3% per patient year ($P < .001$), in the incidence of hemorrhage in the recent era,[T4] probably related to more strenuous efforts to maintain effective anticoagulation.

Postoperative Aortic Root Aneurysms

Three unsuspected small aneurysms were found among 100 patients studied by aortography 6–9 months after aortic valve replacement by Bjork and colleagues.[B11] One was in the aortotomy suture line, and two seemed to originate from the left coronary sinus. One false aneurysm and one dissecting aneurysm, both large and symptomatic and presenting 6

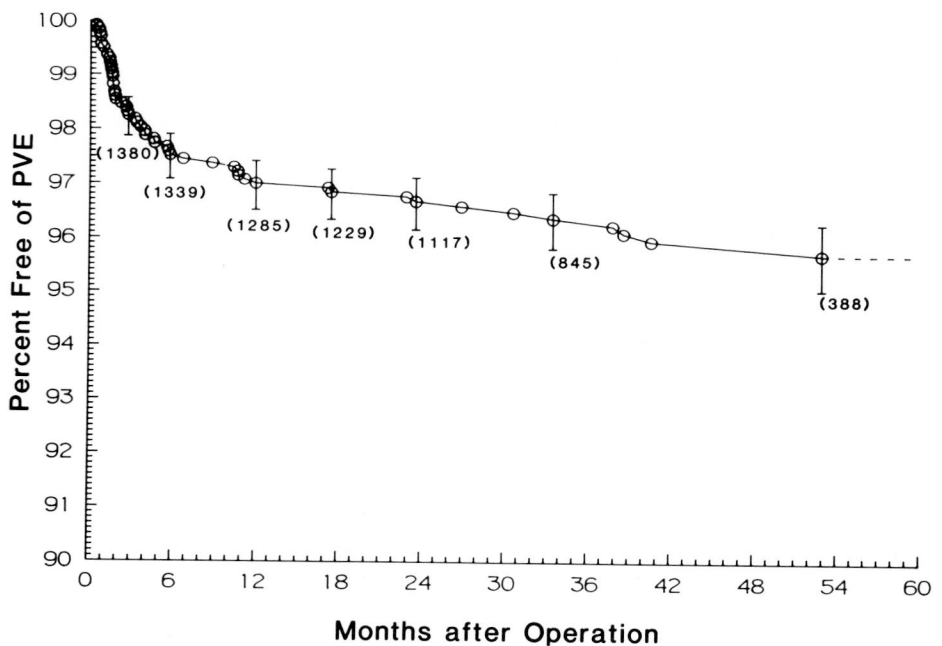

Figure 12-26 Actuarial time related incidence of patients free of prosthetic valve endocarditis (PVE) (UAB; 1975–July 1979; all single- and multiple-valve replacements; $n = 1465$; 53 events). The site of valve replacement did not affect the incidence.

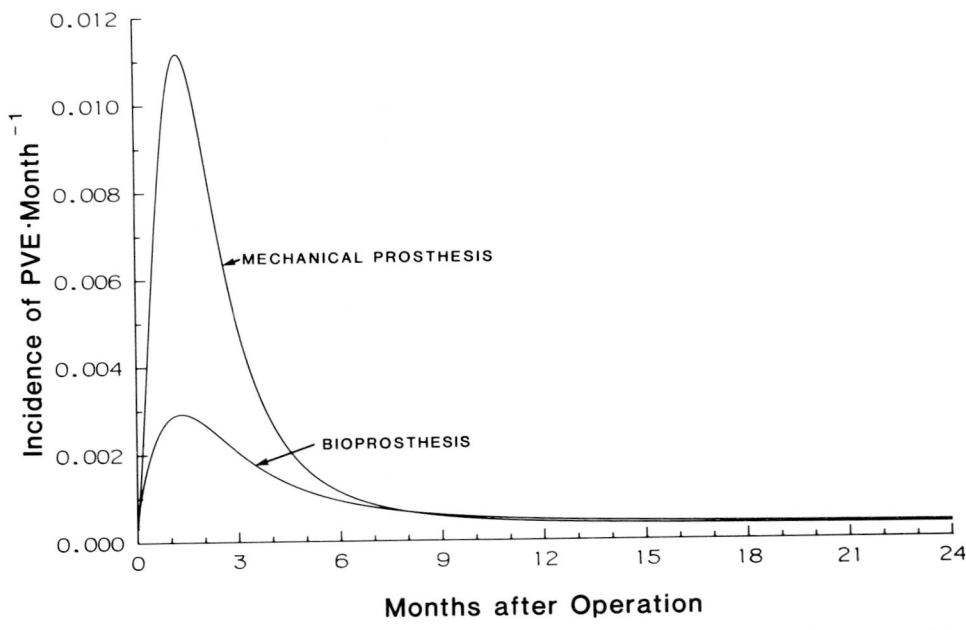

Figure 12-27 Hazard function analysis (see Chapter 6) of the time-related instantaneous risks (vertical axis) of developing prosthetic valve endocarditis (PVE) after valve replacement. The data have been stratified into patients with mechanical prostheses versus those with bioprostheses.[13]

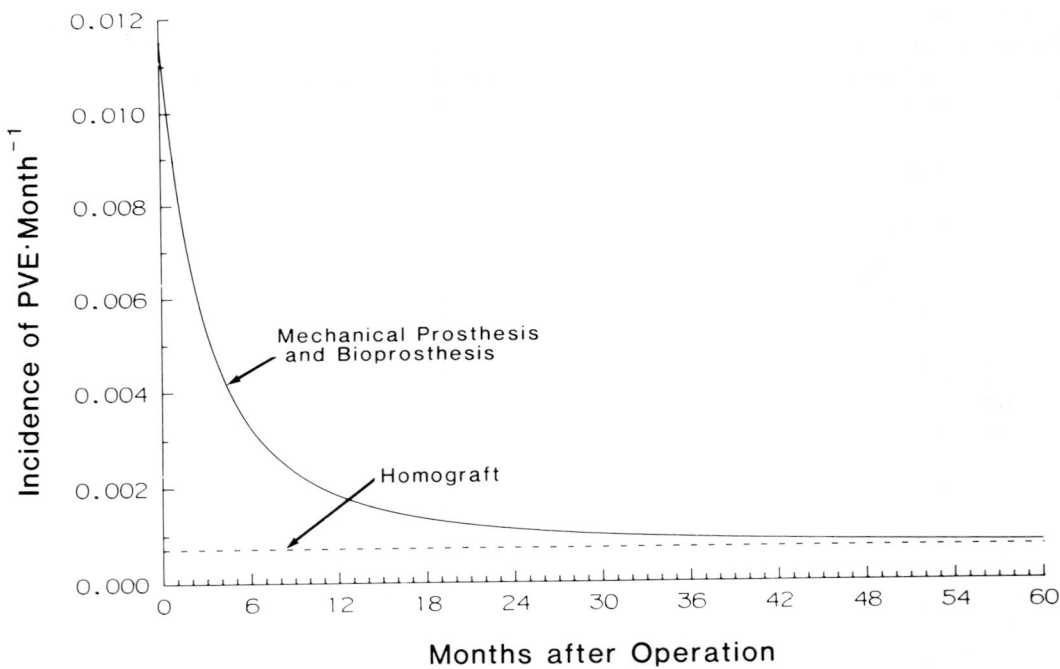

Figure 12-28 Hazard function analysis of prosthetic valve endocarditis. The presentation is the same as in Figure 12-26. The patients are stratified into those receiving homografts versus those receiving mechanical prostheses and bioprostheses (GLH; prostheses 1976–1980, n = 147, 11 events; homografts 1968–1981, n = 71, 4 events).

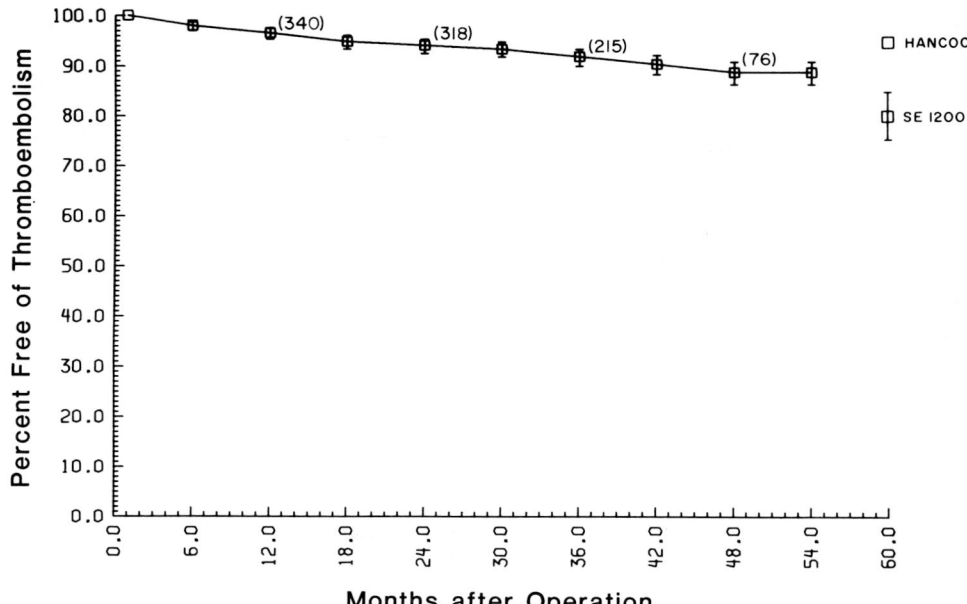

Figure 12-29 *Freedom from thromboembolism among patients having aortic valve replacement with a Bjork-Shiley prosthesis. For comparison, values from the literature at the 5-year (60-month) point are presented for the Starr-Edwards prosthesis (SE 1200) and for the Hancock bioprosthesis in patients without anticoagulation.*
Reproduced with permission from Karp et al.[K1]

and 8 years after operation, have been seen at UAB. Both arose from the aortotomy suture line. Thus, at operation, a very secure full thickness closure must always be obtained, not only to prevent bleeding, but also to prevent late aneurysm formation.

INDICATIONS FOR OPERATION

Aortic Stenosis

Patients with calcific aortic stenosis usually present because of symptoms. When in such patients the presence of important stenosis is confirmed by clinical findings or the measurement of a peak pressure gradient across the aortic valve of 50 mmHg or more, operation is clearly indicated. This becomes apparent from a comparison of the survival of surgically untreated patients (see Fig. 12-1) with that of those treated surgically (Figs. 12-9, 12-10).

The presence of severe left ventricular hypertrophy and symptoms indicative of increasing pulmonary venous hypertension make operation urgent, particularly when there are signs and symptoms of left ventricular failure, including pulsus alternans or the presence of right heart failure. Virtually no patient with severe aortic stenosis is considered inoperable, with the possible exception of elderly patients (> 75 years of age) in severe heart failure and with associated coronary artery disease.

Occasionally there is the dilemma of the patient with absent or trivial symptoms. When the stenosis is clearly important on clinical findings and there is a peak systolic gradient of 75 mmHg or more, operation is advised, in part because of

the risk of sudden death. When the stenosis on hemodynamic measurement is less than severe (gradient < 50 mmHg or valve area ≤ 0.8 cm$^2 \cdot$ m^{-2}), the presence of significant and particularly progressive left ventricular hypertrophy on the electrocardiogram and of heavy aortic valve calcification make important stenosis more likely and thereby indicate operation. A positive graded exercise test lends weight to the decision for operation.

Some patients with moderate aortic stenosis, on cardiac catheterization, are found to have severe coronary artery disease. In them, particularly if there is effort angina, coronary artery bypass grafting is the major indication for operation, but the aortic valve is replaced at the same time. The rationale for this is supported by data from the Mayo Clinic showing important progression of untreated aortic stenosis within a few years in this situation.[F4]

The urgency of operation in patients with important aortic stenosis and syncope or near syncope as the only complaint has been debated. While this symptom does not generally make operation urgent, it does make it advisable.

Aortic Incompetence

Decisions concerning the need for operation have in the past been more difficult in patients with aortic incompetence than in those with stenosis because the asymptomatic phase of gradually developing but important aortic incompetence is usually longer than that of aortic stenosis (see Fig. 12-1). However, once symptoms develop in aortic incompetence, the left ventricle has usually already become very large, and the devolutionary course rather far advanced. Thus, patients with important aortic incompetence first seen in a symptomatic state are advised to undergo operation promptly. Even when left ventricular hypertrophy is massive and symptoms of right heart failure are present, operation is advisable because relief of symptoms for some years is possible even though in such situations late postoperative death often occurs because of irreversible secondary cardiomyopathy.

Asymptomatic patients with aortic incompetence present a more difficult problem. It is important to recall that, even in them, when left ventricular enlargement reaches a certain point, the secondary cardiomyopathy may not be completely reversible, and thereby the long-term results of operation will be less satisfactory. Therefore, even in apparently asymptomatic patients, operation becomes advisable when the cardiothoracic ratio exceeds 55% (alternatively stated (UAB), when the left ventricle is enlarged grade 3 or more on a scale of 1–6). As in aortic stenosis, graded exercise testing is helpful in assessing the patient's true symptomatic state.

A more objective way of following asymptomatic patients with chronic severe aortic incompetence has been provided by Henry and colleagues[H7] using serial echocardiographic indexes of left ventricular systolic function. Their data indicate that operation should be urgently advised for patients whose left ventricular end-systolic dimension reaches 55 mm and electively advised when it reaches 50 mm. A generally similar conclusion about operation in asymptomatic patients was reached by Herreman and colleagues. They used an ejection fraction less than 40% and a mean velocity of circumferential fiber shortening less than 0.6 circumferences per second as their left ventricular systolic function indexes of the need for surgery.[H8]

CHOICE OF THE REPLACEMENT DEVICE

In patients over about 15 years of age, the operation for aortic valve disease is nearly always aortic valve replacement. Not only must this fact be taken into account in the indications for operation, but the valve replacement device itself must also be considered.

The late results with *antibiotic sterilized, nutrient-medium–stored homograft* sewn freehand into the aortic root serve as a reference point for those of prostheses and those with newer methods of homograft preparation, which presumably should considerably delay the appearance of cusp rupture. Earlier at GLH and at UAB, various methods of sterilizing the homograft were used, all to various degrees more damaging to the homograft than is the antibiotic method. Other than late prosthetic endocarditis, the only late complication of the homograft is cusp rupture, with resultant homograft incompetence, occurring in about 4% of patients within 5 years of insertion and 20% of patients within 10 years (Fig. 12-23). Elective reoperation is required for cusp rupture, but this can be accomplished at about the same risk as the original operation (Tables 12-11, 12-14). There are no late thromboembolic complications (other than rare transient episodes of platelet emboli) and, since anticoagulation is not required, no bleeding complications. The homograft has been immune to early endocarditis even when used in patients with native valve endocarditis, and accelerated degeneration has not been experienced by young patients.

Currently, therefore, the aortic valve homograft, processed and stored as described in Appendix 12C and inserted as described in this chapter, is considered the optimal replacement device for patients less than 45 years of age and for all patients with native valve endocarditis (GLH, UAB). It is used nearly routinely (GLH) at all ages when contraindications are not present. Heavy calcification of the leaflets of the patient's valve extending into the anulus is not a contraindication, since it is possible to enucleate this material.

An aortic homograft, inserted freehand in the manner described, is contraindicated in circumstances that predispose the patient to progressive dilatation of the aortic sinus or root, since this produces overstretching of the homograft leaflets and central incompetence. Thus, any form of ascending arch aneurysm, aneurysms of the sinus of Valsalva, or medionecrotic root ectasia are contraindications. The same is true for aortic incompetence due to ankylosing spondylitis, Reiter's disease, and similar conditions. Medionecrotic root ectasia must be clearly distinguished from annular ectasia secondary to aortic incompetence, for in the latter, the aortic tissues are normal or fibrotic and will not continue to dilate once the incompetence is corrected and the aortic root has, when necessary, been tailored to a more normal size. The aortic homograft inserted freehand is probably a poor choice in a dilated, thin-walled ascending aorta in an elderly patient with a large aortic ring (> 30mm), as it is likely that medionecrosis is present and the aorta will continue to dilate, and in the large and grossly distorted root occasionally associated with a bicuspid valve. The homograft valve may also be disadvantageous in the presence of severe and poorly controlled hypertension, which places unusual stress on the valve leaflets and may therefore predispose the patient to leaflet rupture.[L6]

The *stent-mounted glutaraldehyde-preserved porcine heterograft valve* also does not require that the patient be anticoagulated. Its use is undesirable in patients less than 45 years of age because of the risk of accelerated degeneration (see Chapter 11, Fig. 11-29). It is susceptible to early prosthetic endocarditis, although less so than mechanical prostheses. The reoperation rate at 10 years (see Chapter 11, Fig. 11-29) is probably not significantly different than that with homografts, and for this reason, stent-mounted porcine heterograft valves can be recommended routinely for patients over 60 years of age and for patients over 45 years of age when anticoagulants are particularly contraindicated (UAB). Chronic renal failure, with high calcium turnover, is probably a contraindication, as is inability to use at least a 21-mm, and preferably a 23-mm, device. Other bioprostheses, such as those made with heterograft bovine pericardial tissue, may be recommended by some surgeons in such situations. Newer heterograft valves, such as those processed under low pressures,[B31] will probably broaden the indications for use of bioprostheses.

The *Bjork-Shiley prosthesis* and the *St. Jude prosthesis* are used for many patients less than about 60 years of age in whom chronic and lifelong anticoagulation is not unusually disadvantageous (UAB). Generally, these are patients without a history of peptic ulcer disease who are not exposed to situations with more than the usual risk of trauma, and who prefer the risks of anticoagulation to the anxiety, discomfort, and risk of possible second operation. Other prostheses may be recommended by other surgeons in such situations.

Unusually small or large aortic roots may modify these general indications (see "Special Situations and Controversies").

SPECIAL SITUATIONS AND CONTROVERSIES

Combined Aortic Valve and Coronary Artery Disease

Incidence

The importance of coexisting coronary artery disease in patients treated surgically for aortic valve disease was first stressed by Linhart and Wheat in 1967.[L4] Now it is realized that coronary artery disease coexists in 25%–50% of patients with aortic valve disease.[B7,B8] Miller and colleagues found that absence of angina pectoris in such patients is not a reliable indicator of absence of significant coronary artery disease.[M9] Thus, it is not surprising that in the era when CABG is performed along with aortic valve replacement when coronary artery disease is also present, 20%–30% of patients undergoing aortic valve replacement have concomitant CABG (Tables 12-6, 12-17).

The idea that coronary artery disease coexisting with aortic valve disease can be important to the patient is indicated by the fact that 5%–20% of the late deaths after aortic valve replacement in an early era were attributed to coronary artery disease and that failure of left ventricular function to improve after valve replacement for aortic stenosis has been correlated with residual coronary artery disease in some patients.[T1]

Management

Secure proof of the beneficial effect of performing CABG as well as aortic valve replacement in patients with both diseases is lacking. Proof is particularly lacking for patients with single- or double-vessel disease in the absence of angina. However, now that it is possible to perform the combined operation without an increased hospital mortality (Tables 12-6, 12-17), and in the absence of proof that CABG in the absence of angina may be detrimental in the long run, it is considered prudent, routinely, to do CABG to all coronary arteries meeting the criteria generally used in isolated coronary artery disease (see Chapter 7).

Combined Aortic Incompetence and Ascending Aortic Aneurysm

About 5%–10% (Tables 12-6, 12-17) of patients undergoing aortic valve replacement in the current era have an ascending aortic aneurysm requiring a concomitant surgical procedure. Most of these are aneurysms, which begin in the aortic sinuses of Valsalva but gradually or rapidly extend until the entire ascending aorta is involved. The aneurysmal enlargement usually stops abruptly just before the innominate artery. Within such an aneurysm, there may be an entirely unexpected chronic dissection, sometimes extending far beyond the confines of the aneurysm.

Acute or chronic aortic dissection and syphilitic aortitis may cause aortic incompetence and ascending aortic aneurysm. They are considered in Chapters 54 and 55.

There has been controversy concerning the surgical aspects of this challenging entity since the first successful surgical cases of Groves and colleagues, Wheat and colleagues, and Bloodwell and associates.[B21,G6,W5] The early operation of simultaneous but separate replacement of the aortic valve and ascending aorta was associated with a significant risk of bleeding from the exposed graft and its suture lines, and the procedure did not exclude the aneurysmal sinuses of Valsalva. This led to the introduction by Bentall and colleagues and by Edwards and Kerr (UAB) of an intra-aneurysmal operation consisting of aortic valve replacement, composite valve graft reconstruction with implantation of coronary ostia into the side of the graft, and wrapping of the graft with the remnants of aneurysm.[B22,E2]

The risk of the composite graft operation has been about 5% in recent years (Table 12-6). However, a recent experience from Stanford with the original classic operation has had a similar low hospital mortality (1 death in 23 patients; 4%; CL 0.6%–14%).[M8]

The late results of the two methods have not been adequately compared. An excellent follow-up report from Stanford shows the 5-year and 10-year survival rates of patients leaving the hospital alive after the classic operation to be 77% and 57%, respectively;[M8] only 1 of 20 late deaths seemed related to complications in the aortic root. No reoperations have been required for recurrent aneurysms of the sinuses of Valsalva or ascending aorta. However, the Mayo Clinic has reported several expanding sinus of Valsalva aneurysms late after this procedure that did require reoperation.[M13] Following the composite graft reconstruction, some late reoperations have also been required for false aneurysms arising from the anastomosis of the coronary ostia to the graft,[K6] and in two GLH patients, the graft was found to be detached from the distal suture line at late follow-up.

Currently, for cases with annulo-aortic ectasia, the composite graft technique is used, with particular care given to the coronary ostial anastomosis. When the sinuses of Valsalva are not aneurysmally enlarged, the classic method is used. It should be noted that severe aortic incompetence due to medionecrotic dilatation may occasionally require aortic valve replacement only (when the aorta has not reached aneurysmal proportions).

Other Techniques of Using Aortic Valve Homografts

Khanna and colleagues have found that insertion of a homograft without the 120° rotation described here also gives satisfactory results.[K9]

Yacoub and Ross have recommended using a graft of intact proximal aorta and valve as a tubular conduit replacement for both valve and ascending aorta when an aneurysm is present.[G9,R12] The host coronary ostia are sewn to appropriate openings in the graft as for the Bentall operation. This technique raises concern about the long-term fate of an unsupported tubular aortic homograft, with its recognized propensity for calcification, in such situations.

A complete homograft tube has been used by some as routine in the operation of aortic valve replacement, in contrast to the recommended technique of excising the upper aortic wall from each sinus of the graft. This is considered inappropriate, for the aortic wall of the graft usually calcifies and may then encroach upon the coronary ostia.

A stented, antibiotic-treated aortic homograft is a theoretical alternative to freehand insertion.[P6] Unfortunately, the antibiotic-treated homograft tissue becomes detached from the pillars of the stent even when the pillars are flexible. In contrast to glutaraldehyde-treated aortic wall tissue, antibiotic-treated tissue is too friable to withstand the stresses involved.

Aortic Valve Replacement with Pulmonary Valve Autograft

Ross and colleagues in London have a long experience with aortic valve replacement by pulmonary valve autograft combined with right ventricular outflow tract reconstruction by a variety of methods.[G5,R3] In a long-term follow-up study of 188 patients, Gula and associates report autograft failure with at least moderate regurgitation in 10% of patients by 10 years after operation.[G5] Somerville and colleagues report trivial aortic incompetence in an additional 30% of patients by this time.[S15] Antibiotic-treated homografts have given the best results in the right ventricular outflow reconstruction necessitated by this technique.

Continuous Suture Technique for Prosthesis or Bioprosthesis

A continuous suture technique is practiced with satisfaction by some surgeons.[C6] In contrast to the situation in mitral replacement, all the stitches must be placed with the prosthesis at a distance and then pulled up, creating the risk that some of the stitches may cut through a friable anulus. The continuous suture technique described by Fernandez has the prosthesis held in situ in the subcoronary position as the stitches are placed,[F2] but this technique is possible only when the aortic root is large.

Nonuse of the Left Ventricular Vent

It is possible to perform aortic valve replacement without a vent in the left atrium or left ventricle when a well-positioned venous cannula and cold cardioplegia are used, and this technique may be chosen on occasion (UAB). It is particularly useful in patients with extensive adhesions, in whom access to the right side of the left atrium is difficult. Occasional aspiration of blood from the left ventricle through the aortic root is required, and for this reason, this technique should not be used for homograft aortic valve replacement.

Large Aortic Root

When the aortic root is large but not over 30 mm in internal diameter, the root may be tailored to a size that will accom-

modate a homograft (GLH), or another valve replacement device may be used (UAB). Tailoring is accomplished by extending the incision in the noncoronary sinus across the base of the noncoronary cusp into the mitral-aortic anulus (Fig. 12-30). The incision lies immediately posterior to the right trigone (avoiding the bundle of His, which penetrates this structure) and extends for about 8 mm into the mitral-aortic anulus, which overlies and is loosely attached to the left atrial wall. The left atrium is loosely dissected away as deeply as possible first, but whether this chamber is entered at the lowest point of the incision is not important. A parallel incision is next made posteriorly and tapered so as to remove an ellipse of aortic root with its widest point at ring level and with the ends at the mitral-aortic anulus and the sinus wall superiorly. The exact amount of aortic wall to be removed to reduce the diameter appropriately can be calculated, but it can also be judged visually as long as it is remembered that further reduction in circumference occurs when the sutures are placed several millimeters from the edge and tied down. The posterior edge of the area of excision must not be too close to the left coronary ostium because room must be left for the commissure of the homograft valve to be sewn into position. The lowest part of the defect so created is closed using interrupted figure-eight 3-0 silk sutures that pick up good bites of tissue (avoiding deep placement into the right trigone), including the adjacent left atrial wall if it has been opened. Where the left atrium has been dissected off the bottom of the sinus, it is picked up by each suture so that the left atrium is drawn against the suture line when the stitches are tied. The suture line is completed at this stage only to the nadir of the excised noncoronary cusp in order to maintain good exposure for positioning of the homograft. It is convenient to leave the last figure-eight suture long so that it can be used later for the continuous whip stitch that closes the rest of the aortotomy; actually, the next 8 mm or so of the sinus wall require approximation in this fashion before the upper (second) row of homograft sutures can be positioned in the base of the new noncoronary sinus.

Small Aortic Root

Some adult patients have a smaller than usual aortic anulus and/or a narrow waist to the aorta just at the level of the commissural attachment of the cusps. (True congenital subvalvar or supravalvar aortic narrowing is considered in Chapter 32.)

The freehand aortic homograft is the best device in the small aortic root, as appropriate-sized homografts to a minimum internal diameter of 16 mm are available in graft banks (GLH and UAB) and can be inserted with no resulting gradient.

This simple solution, of using whatever size of replacement device is needed, is not acceptable when prostheses are used, for with many prostheses, the use of a size smaller than 23 mm results in considerable obstruction (Table 12-18). Replacement device mismatch is a serious iatrogenic disease that produces persisting or increasing left ventricular dysfunction, hemolysis, and a very difficult reoperation.[J2,S11] Only in small and rather inactive patients should a 19-mm device be used, and it should be a pericardial bioprosthesis

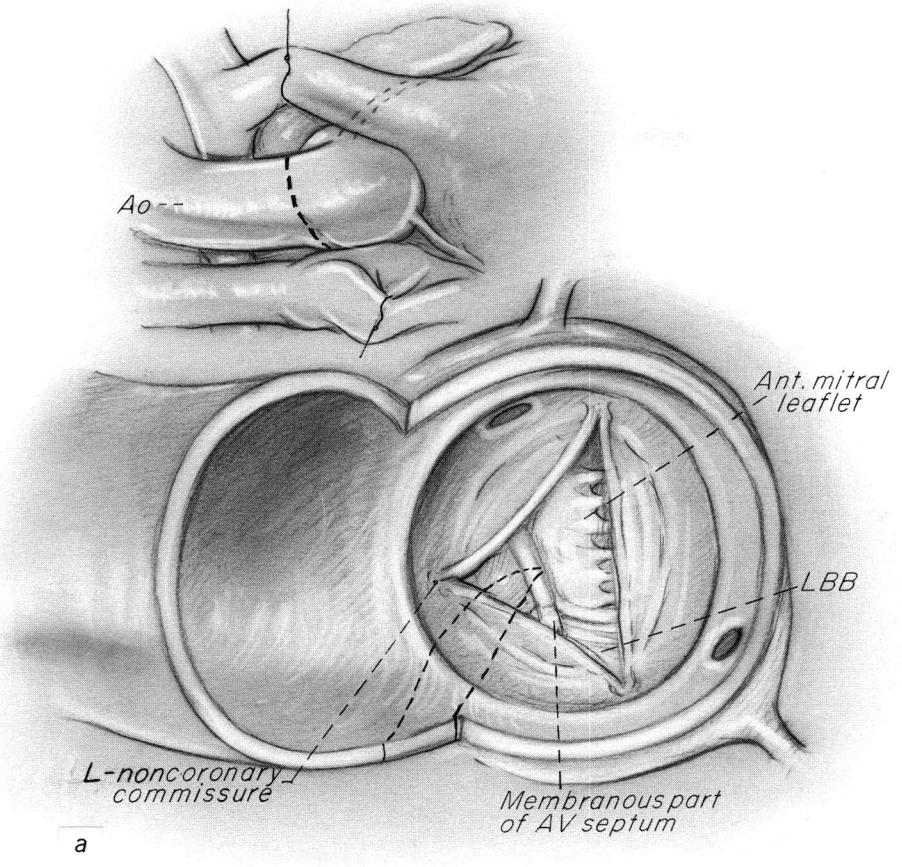

Ao

Ant. mitral
leaflet

LBB

L-noncoronary
commissure

Membranous part
of AV septum

a

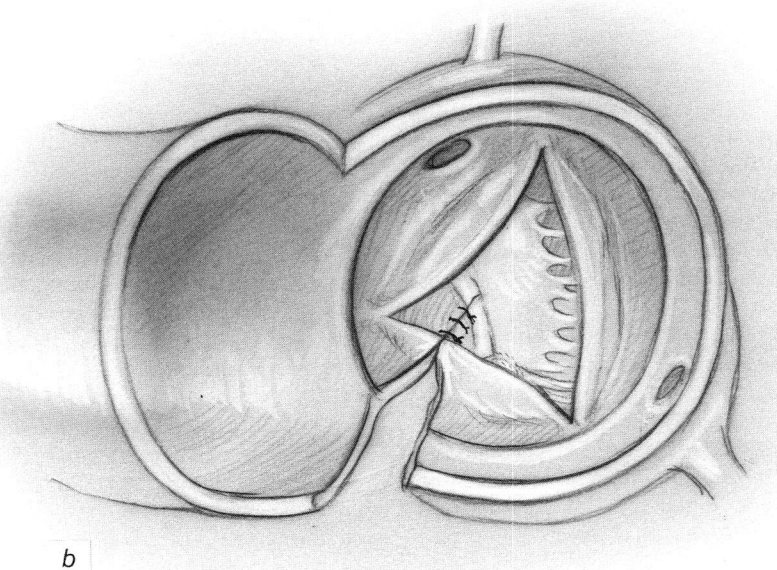

b

Figure 12-30 Tailoring the large aortic root.
(a) The dashed line shows the area to be excised between the mid portion of the noncoronary sinus
and the commissure between the noncoronary and left coronary cusp.
(b) Interrupted 4-0 silk or prolene sutures are placed from within to narrow the aortic anulus. An
additional stitch is now placed from the outside, tied, and one end left long. This end can be seen
in c.

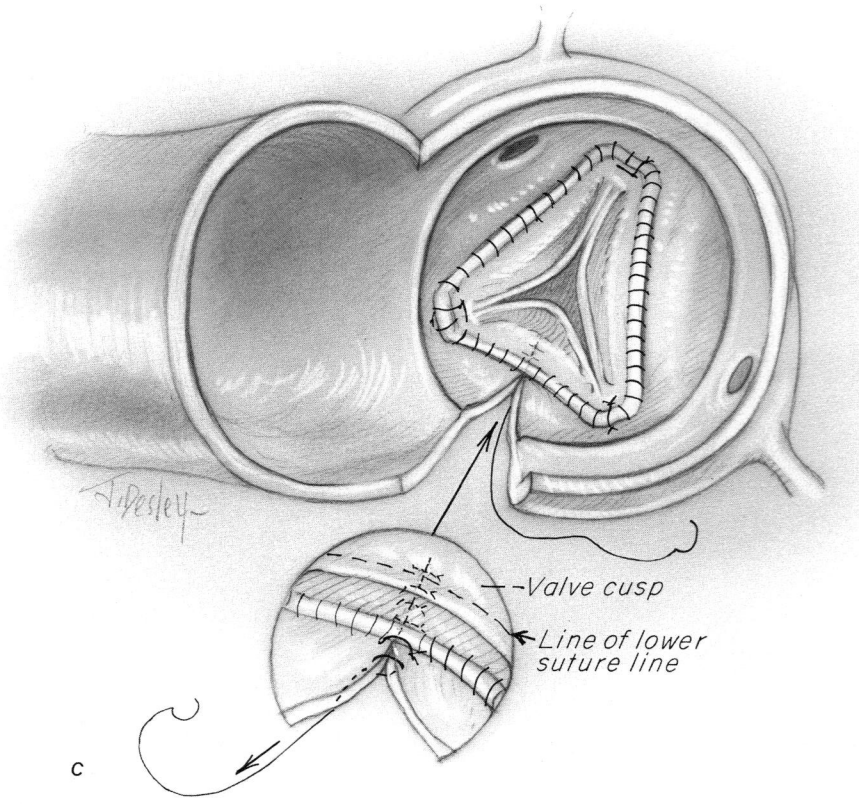

Figure 12-30 *(continued)*
(c) The homograft valve has been placed, and the insert shows its relationship to the previously placed sutures. The end that has been left long is used to begin the closure of the aortotomy with a whipstitch.
LBB, left bundle branch.

or a St. Jude mechanical prosthesis (Table 12-18). A 21-mm standard[B36] or modified orifice Hancock porcine bioprosthesis, a 21-mm Bjork-Shiley convexo-concave type,[A11] or a St. Jude valve[W7] is acceptable only if the patient is not large and active. Otherwise, with aortic roots of this size and if a prosthesis is to be used, the aortic root must be enlarged by one of several methods.

The simplest technique for use in patients with a small aortic anulus is the *positioning* of the replacement device in part *in a supraannular position.* Such positioning takes advantage of the bulging of particularly the noncoronary sinus of Valsalva. A replacement device one size larger than the aortic anulus can be used by suturing it to the anulus along the left and right sinuses and in the supraannular position along the noncoronary sinus. In that area, pledgetted mattress sutures are placed from outside in.[D8,G14,O4]

Another method of aortic root enlargement is *supraannular enlargement* with a patch graft into the noncoronary sinus of Valsalva. A patch of pericardium has the advantage of ease of handling and insertion, and with it, the suture line is easily made hemostatic. The study by Piehler and colleagues of patients followed nearly 20 years has shown that the pericardial patch in this position does not become aneurysmal.[P9] Alternatively, a knitted Dacron velour patch with pericardium on the inner surface may be used. Woven Dacron patches, preclotted or not, can also be used, but the suture line tends to be less hemostatic initially with these. The method of supraannular enlargement became an obvious one, once the surgical treatment of congenital supravalvar aortic stenosis had been developed (see Chapter 32); it was used earlier at the Mayo Clinic and has been used at GLH and UAB for many years. It was also described by Najafi in 1969.[N1]

Another method is *supraannular and annular enlargement* by similar patch graft enlargement but carried across the anulus and into the aortic-mitral anulus below it. This again became obvious after the development of the technique of tailoring the aortic root before homograft insertion,[B27] for aortic root patch graft enlargement is just the opposite, and this method has been used (UAB and GLH) for selected cases for many years. This method also was described by Nicks and associates;[N2] a slight modification has recently been described by Blank and colleagues;[B14] and good results with it have been published by Maron and colleagues.[M2]

Enlargement of the supraannular and annular area can also be achieved by extending the aortotomy through the left coronary–noncoronary commissural area and into the underlying aortic-mitral anulus,[M4,M11,M12,R7,S13] and this is currently the preferred method for aortic root and annular enlargement for prosthetic aortic valve replacement. When the valve has been excised and the need for aortic root enlargement has been determined, the aortotomy incision (which has been made as shown in Fig. 12-2d) is extended posteroinferiorly directly through the left coronary–noncoronary commissural area (Fig. 12-4a), across the anulus, and into the base of the aortic-mitral anulus where it adheres to the left atrial wall. The incision does not reach the hinge point of the mitral leaflet. The left atrium is first dissected away and may or may not be opened as the incision is made. A broad, teardrop-shaped patch, generally about 4 cm wide, is fashioned. A narrow felt strip is laid along the incision outside the aortic wall. Beginning at the midpoint of the bottom of the incision, about seven or eight interrupted horizontal mattress sutures of a 3-0 Dacron suture are placed through felt strip, aorta, and patch with particular care, as it is difficult to see this area again after the stitches are tied and the aortic clamp is removed. The valve is sewn into place using interrupted horizontal mattress sutures in the region of the patch, bringing these in from the outside to secure valve against patch. The remainder of the aortotomy is closed by sewing the rest of the patch in place with continuous horizontal mattress sutures over felt strips in order to be sure that the suture line is hemostatic.

The anulus and subvalvar left ventricular outflow tract can also be enlarged by the operation of *aortoventriculoplasty*. In this a longitudinal, anteriorly placed aortotomy incision is carried to the patient's left of the origin of the right coronary artery into both the right ventricular free wall and the ventricular septum and inserting a double patch graft for enlargement of both. This was described by Konno and colleagues[K2] and by Rastan and associates[R4,R5] (see Chapter 32, Fig. 32-21). While this method has a place in the treatment of the tunnel type of congenital subaortic stenosis (see Chapter 32), it is a more complex procedure than is usually needed for aortic valve replacement. Also, the mortality has been 24% (CL 14%–37%) in the early experience of Rastan and colleagues[R4] but only 4% (CL 1%–10%) in their more recent experience.[V1] Misbach and colleagues have reported 14 such procedures with no (0%, CL 0%–13%) mortality.[M16]

The use of a *left ventricular apico-abdominal aortic valved conduit*[C8,N3] should not be considered the primary approach to the problem of small anulus or aortic root in patients requiring valve replacement. When the patient is facing a second or third replacement, however, and has no periprosthetic leakage, the use of such a conduit may be preferable to aortic root enlargement.

Functional Mitral Incompetence Associated with Aortic Valve Disease

Important organic mitral incompetence may coexist with severe aortic valve disease, and repair or replacement of both valves is then the proper surgical procedure (see Chapter 13). However, mitral incompetence which is grade 2 or 3 (on the basis of 1–6) may occur in the presence of aortic valve disease, even when the mitral leaflets are normal, presumably because of annular dilation. Under such circumstances, the mitral incompetence is usually abolished or considerably reduced by aortic valve replacement.[A2] Therefore, when this situation is encountered, the surgeon should either palpate or visualize the mitral valve at operation (the superior approach is often optimal for this; see Chapter 11) and, if it seems structurally normal and the incompetence no more than grade 3, should not repair or replace it. In borderline cases, it is best to discontinue CPB and reassess mitral valve function with the heart beating and ejecting. If mitral incompetence is then significant, CPB is recommended, and the mitral valve is repaired with a Carpentier ring. It rarely requires replacement.

Surgical Problems of Native Aortic Valve Endocarditis

The primary treatment of aortic native valve endocarditis is appropriate, intense, and prolonged antibiotic treatment. However, beginning with the report of successful surgical treatment of acute aortic valve endocarditis by Wallace and colleagues[W4] it has become apparent that surgical intervention is required in a number of patients.

Knowledge of a number of factors is helpful in making this decision for surgical intervention:

1. Well-treated native valve endocarditis per se does not increase the risk of hospital death after valve replacement (Table 12-20), although it does increase the risk of postoperative prosthetic valve endocarditis unless a homograft is used.[I2] Therefore, when severe aortic incompetence appears in the course of well-treated endocarditis, there should be no reluctance to proceed with operation, and whenever possible, a homograft should be used for valve replacement.[O3]

2. Acute hemodynamic deterioration (NYHA class V) increases the risk of hospital death after aortic valve replacement (Tables 12-10, 12-11). Therefore, when dyspnea, rising BUN and creatinine levels, or other evidence of decreasing cardiac function appears in the course of antibiotic treatment of native aortic valve endocarditis with aortic incompetence, operation should be carried out promptly before acute hemodynamic deterioration occurs.

3. Patients with infective endocarditis who have developed acute hemodynamic deterioration with extreme heart failure (NYHA class V) are nonetheless more likely ($P <$ .01) to survive with surgical than with continued medical treatment, regardless of whether or not the programmed course of antibiotic treatment has been completed.[O3]

4. Continued infection (as evidenced by persistent marked fever beyond 1 week from the beginning of antibiotic administration) is associated with an increased incidence of extension of infection beyond the valve (infected pannus or root abscess) and increased hospital mortality. Thus, evidence of persistent infection is an indication for early operation and excision of the infected valve focus.

5. Hospital mortality is probably higher in native valve endocarditis when the infecting organism is a staphylococcus,[R9] and thus earlier operation may be considered.

Table 12-20 The relationship of prosthetic valve endocarditis and preoperative functional class to hospital mortality after aortic valve re-replacement (UAB; 1975–July 1, 1979; n = 200).[W1]

| | With PVE (n = 27) | | | | Without PVE (n = 173) | | | | |
| | | Hospital Deaths | | | | Hospital Deaths | | | P for |
NYHA Class	n	No.	%	CL	n	No.	%	CL	Difference
I	2	0	0%	0%–61%	58	0	0%	0%–3%	1.0
II	2	0	0%	0%–61%	57	1	2%	0.2%–6%	1.0
III	10	1	10%	1%–30%	44	3	7%	3%–13%	.7
IV	12	4	33%	18%–52%	10	1	10%	1%–30%	.22
Unknown	1	0			4	0			
Total	27	5	19%	11%–29%	173	5	2.9%	1.6%–4.9%	.0005

KEY: CL, 70% confidence limits; PVE, prosthetic valve endocarditis.

NOTE: Within any given NYHA functional class, risk is not affected by the presence of PVE.

When operation is indicated in the course of antibiotic treatment of acute native aortic valve endocarditis, the surgical procedure is often uncomplicated, since the infection remains limited to the valve leaflets, and standard techniques can be used. Infrequently, annular or subannular myocardial abscesses complicate the situation. Most often they can be evacuated after the aortic valve is excised. Every attempt is made to use a freehand homograft, which can usually be fashioned and sutured to cover the infected area; sometimes abscess spaces are plicated or a patch is placed over them[B34] before the valve is inserted. In those unusual circumstances in which the distortion of the aortic root is so severe as to preclude use of a homograft, a bioprosthesis is sewn into place with interrupted pledgetted mattress sutures that at the same time obliterate cavity spaces. At times, the mattress sutures achieve a better purchase in the areas if they are introduced from the outside of the aortic root and the pledgets are left in place outside the aorta. A bioprosthesis is selected because it is more resistant than are mechanical prostheses to the early phase of prosthetic valve endocarditis.

Rarely, abscess formation and tissue destruction are so extensive around the aortic root that there is true left ven-tricular–aortic discontinuity and a very hazardous situation. Two radical options can then be considered. One is translocation of the aortic valve, with closure of the coronary ostia, insertion of a prosthesis in the ascending aorta, and coronary artery bypass grafting from the downstream aorta (or innominate artery) to the right, anterior descending, and large circumflex marginal coronary arteries.[B20,D3,D4,R6] A second option, after valve excision and debridement of the annular abscesses, is use of a composite valve conduit (as for aortic incompetence and aneurysm of the ascending aorta) or a homograft valve and ascending aorta,[D9] with the valve sunk into the left ventricular outflow tract by suturing it to the mitral-aortic anulus posteriorly and to the right, the ventricular septum anteriorly, and the left ventricular myocardium to the left.[F3] The coronary artery ostia are anastomosed to the side of the graft, and the distal anastomoses are completed as described earlier (see "Composite Graft Replacement of Aortic Valve and Ascending Aorta" in section on Technique of Operation). Both of these procedures are extensive, and although success can be achieved in very seriously ill patients, the risks are high. Thus, the mortality was 25% (CL 3%–63%) in the recent Stanford experience with translocation.[R6]

APPENDIXES

APPENDIX **12A**

MULTIVARIATE ANALYSIS OF INCREMENTAL RISK FACTORS FOR HOSPITAL DEATH FROM HEMORRHAGE

The logistic multivariate analysis of incremental risk factors for hospital death from hemorrhage (UAB; n = 420; see Table 12-8), included the following variables:

Age

Race

Sex

NYHA functional class (I–IV, classic; or I–V, UAB)

Veterans Administration patient (yes or no)

Type of aortic valve lesion (stenosis, mixed, incompetence; and presence [yes or no] of any but mild incompetence)

Date of operation

Myocardial ischemic (cross-clamp) time

Size of replacement device inserted

Use of a biological valve (yes or no)

Concomitant coronary artery bypass grafting (yes or no and number of distal anastomoses)

Concomitant replacement of the ascending aorta

Variables with a P value < .20 were rejected in the final model.

APPENDIX **12B**
MULTIVARIATE ANALYSIS OF INCREMENTAL RISK FACTORS FOR HOSPITAL DEATH FROM ALL CAUSES

The logistic multivariate analysis of incremental risk factors for hospital death from all causes (UAB; $n = 842$; 24 events; see Table 12-9), included the following variables:

Age

Race

Sex

NYHA functional class (I–IV and again with I–V)

Emergency operation (yes or no)

Veterans Administration patient (yes or no)

Previous aortic valve repair (yes or no)

APPENDIX **12C**
METHOD OF HOMOGRAFT VALVE PREPARATION

COLLECTION TECHNIQUE

The aortic root and valve and the ascending and transverse aorta are most conveniently obtained at autopsy (usually a coroner's autopsy) in a clean condition (GLH). Alternatively (UAB), they may be removed along with the heart through a median sternotomy incision aseptically and in an operating room from a subject who is serving as a cadaver kidney donor (and usually also as a corneal donor and occasionally as a pancreas donor). The considerable length of aorta is harvested because the homograft bank is also the source of valved extracardiac conduits for ventriculo-pulmonary artery reconstruction.

When the aortic homograft is removed as part of kidney harvesting, this is done immediately after removal of the kidneys. The donor has been completely screened prior to the procedure and has met the stringent health and age requirements for donating organs. The heart and ascending and transverse arches are removed in exactly the same manner as for cardiac transplantation. Gentle rinsing with saline solution removes blood from the cardiac chambers and aorta. The heart and 200 ml of saline solution are placed sequentially in a plastic bag, a second bag, a lid-sealed plastic container, another bag, and an ice-filled chest. The temperature is thus maintained at 4°C during rapid transfer to the organ bank.

When the homograft is removed at autopsy, the thorax is opened in the usual manner. With clean, sterile scissors, the pericardium is opened, and the heart is removed by cutting across the major vessels. Both atria may be opened, the incision extending into the atrial appendage, providing a good view of the mitral and tricuspid valves from above. The aortic valve may be seen by looking down the aorta. The myocardium can be examined by a series of slices across the apex. The slices should extend no further than 2 cm below the mitral leaflet. The coronary arteries may be cut in the usual manner, with multiple transverse cuts. Care must be exercised as the ostia are approached, and at this stage, the cuts should expose only the lumen of the coronary artery. A clean, long knife may be passed into the right ventricle from the amputated apex up through the pulmonary artery. The ventricle and pulmonary artery may be laid open for examination. The heart is then placed in a sterile container in modified Hanks' solution at 4°C for transport.

Alternatively, the heart is removed at the start of the postmortem and placed in a sterile bag for transfer. A person skilled in valve removal under sterile conditions then dissects the aortic valve out completely with a portion of septum and the entire mitral septal leaflet. The remainder of the heart is returned to the postmortem.

Blood is collected from the donor heart at postmortem and tested for hepatitis B antigen by radioimmunoassay. Valves from antigen-positive donors are discarded.

Valves removed at autopsy are acceptable from donors up to 60 years of age, provided the body has been refrigerated and autopsy performed within 24 hours of death. Exceptions are death from endocarditis, septicemia, and hepatitis. Carcinoma is not a contraindication, but most coroner's autopsy subjects will have died from trauma. The valve leaflets must be free of significant atheroma and any calcification, normally formed and tricuspid, and free of major fenestrations that might weaken the commissural attachment of the leaflets.

DISSECTION TECHNIQUE

Prompt dissection of the homograft from the fresh heart in an aseptic environment with normal surgical discipline is important. The dissection is done under a laminar flow cabinet. First, the epicardium is raised and dissected from the aorta down to the aortic root. A heavy artery forcep provides useful countertraction. The coronary arteries are identified and cut about 3 mm from the ostia, and the aorta is dissected from the pulmonary artery. Once the septal myocardium is identified, cutting in a downward direction may be much bolder. Continuing with dissection toward the left atria will expose the mitral leaflet; this should be dissected from the atrial wall as closely as possible. The same procedure is followed for the right atrium and the tricuspid leaflets. Great care is required not to cut through the membranous septum. Another hazard is accidentally cutting the sinus of Valsalva in a specimen in which this structure is very large. The valve may now be cut clear of the cardiac mass. The aorta is left long distally so that the homograft may be used as a valved extracardiac conduit, and the aortic root is trimmed proximally at a level 1 cm below the lower point of the aortic cusp attachment. The aortic root is reduced by trimming away excess myocardium. This is done by gently placing the moistened gloved finger through the valve from below. The myocardium rests against the finger and can be trimmed with scissors. The thickness of the myocardium should be reduced to about 5 mm. The valve is now vigorously rinsed in modified Hanks' solution.

VALVE INSPECTION AND SIZING

A pair of dissecting forceps is passed carefully through the valve, the cut aortic wall is grasped, and the valve is turned inside out. The leaflets are now carefully examined. Fenestrations are usually acceptable unless severe, but any congenital variation, unless mild, is not. Unfortunately, many variations are not seen until this stage is reached. In cases of death by trauma, damage to the leaflets and myocardium should be looked for. Any leaflet atheroma is also unacceptable. After examination of the leaflets, the homograft is uninverted.

The valve ring is rinsed again in Hanks' solution, and a moist obturator is passed into the anulus. Sizing is most easily done before trimming the aortic root, since the mitral leaflet remnant can be grasped with forceps and the anulus lifted as the obturator is passed inside. The anulus must not be stretched. The aorta is sized in a similar manner. These details are recorded, together with the valve number, date and time after death of dissection, cause of donor death, and brief comment concerning any defects in the graft. A strip of tissue is cut from the aorta and divided into nine pieces. The valve is again rinsed in Hanks' solution. When the valve is moved up and down in the solution, the movement of the leaflets can be observed. The valve is placed in a jar of sterile antibiotic Hanks' solution, and six pieces of aortic tissue are added. The remaining three pieces are put into another sterile jar, and about 10 ml of the final rinse is added. The two jars are immediately transferred to the bacteriology department for gram stain and culture.

PREPARATION OF ANTIBIOTIC SOLUTION

Suitable dilutions* of the appropriate antibiotics[S20] are prepared freshly in sterile distilled water and added aseptically to 1 litre of modified Hanks' solution.† The prepared solution is dispensed into suitable jars for allograft storage, for example, wide-mouthed 200-ml jars fitted with lids that provide an airtight seal. This solution is stable for 1 week when stored at 4°C; and pH should lie between 6.8 and 7.0.

PROCESSING OF ALLOGRAFTS

The valve is stored at 4°C and after 24 hours is transferred to fresh antibiotic solution. After a further 24 hours, it is transferred to 150 ml of tissue culture medium 199,‡ sealed, and may be (GLH) stored at 4°C for another 24 hours or, alternatively (GLH, UAB), frozen at this point after insertion into an appropriate container along with a balanced salt solution containing supplemental amino acids, vitamins, and glucose to which has been added dimethyl sulfoxide (DMSO) to a 10% concentration and fetal calf serum to a 10% concentration.

MICROBIOLOGICAL CULTURE OF ALLOGRAFTS

The pieces of tissue not exposed to antibiotics, and the samples of fluid in which each homograft was rinsed are placed in thioglycollate broth§ and Sabouraud dextrose broth with antibiotics.‖ Broth cultures are incubated at 37°C, except for one Sabouraud dextrose broth, which is kept at 27°C for 6 weeks. Broths showing visible growth of microorganisms are subcultured at 3 days onto appropriate solid media and incubated aerobically, anaerobically, and in 7% carbon dioxide. Those not showing growth are subcultured at 7 days and kept for a further 5 weeks. When each homograft is transferred to fresh antibiotic solution at 24 hours, two of the pieces treated with it are placed in two thioglycollate broths. At 48 hours, when each homograft is frozen, two pieces are again placed in thioglycollate broths and one piece in Sabouraud dextrose broth without antibiotics. Thioglycollate broths are incubated at 37°C for 1 week and, if the results are negative, a further 5 weeks. The Sabouraud dextrose broth is incubated at 27°C for 6 weeks.

All microorganisms isolated are identified according to the method of Cowan and Steel[C12] and tested for sensitivity to the antibiotics used in the disinfecting solution by Stokes' disc diffusion method.[S19]

STORAGE OF ALLOGRAFTS IN LIQUID NITROGEN

Allografts are frozen in a freezing chamber (CRFC-1-Linde)². Freezing is controlled at −1°C per minute to −40°C, at which temperature the homograft is transferred to its permanent storage in liquid nitrogen. It may be stored indefinitely. This is the method developed and used at the Department of Cardiac Surgery, Prince Charles Hospital, Brisbane, by O'Brien.[O5] Should any of the cultured aortic wall fragments prove to be contaminated, the valve is discarded.

PREPARATION FOR INSERTION

When needed, the frozen homograft in its container is removed from its storage position in the liquid nitrogen, and the container is placed in a 6-quart transport container containing 2 liters of saline solution at 42°C. After arrival in the operating room, the transport person scrubs and dons gown and gloves in the usual way. The homograft is gently removed from its container and placed in 42°C tissue culture fluid with 10% DMSO. The homograft is then passed through three successive gentle rinses and warming, each for 1 minute, and each with decreasing concentrations of DSMO. Then a final warm rinse in pure tissue culture medium is allowed.

The valve is now ready for final trimming for its use as a replacement for the aortic valve (see Chapter 12) or as a valved extracardiac conduit (see Chapter 23).

---

*Antibiotic solution (CLPVA) (μg/l modified Hanks' solution): Cefoxitin, 240; lincomycin, 120; polymyxin B, 100; vancomycin hydrochloride, 50; amphotericin B, 25.

†Modified Hanks' solution: sodium chloride (NaCl), 8.0 g; potassium chloride (KCl), 0.4 g; magnesium sulphate ($MgSO_4 \cdot 7H_2O$), 0.1 g; magnesium chloride ($MgCl_2 \cdot 6H_2O$), 0.1 g; $Na_2HPO_4 \cdot 12H_2O$, 0.12 g; KH_2PO_4, 0.06 g; dextrose, 1.0 g; sodium bicarbonate ($NaHCO_3$), 0.35 g; water for injection, 1.0 liter.

‡Tissue culture medium 199 (TC 199) is supplied by Grand Island Biological Company (GIBCO), Grand Island, New York, as 100-ml bottles of 10 × concentrate with Hanks' salts and L-glutamine. This concentrate is diluted to 1 liter, and 0.35 g of sodium bicarbonate is added.

§Thioglycollate broth (as for cerebrospinal and blood culture): Baltimore Biological Laboratories (BBL) thioglycollate without indicator, 30 g; distilled water, 1 liter; normal saline solution, 5 ml; liquid Roche, 0.5 g. This is dispensed in 20-ml volumes into 25-ml McCarney bottles.

‖Sabouraud dextrose broth: GIBCO animal tissue polypeptone, 10 g; dextrose, 40 g; distilled water, 1 liter. Sabouraud dextrose broth with antibiotics is prepared in the same way but with the following antibiotics added: chloramphenicol, 100 mg/l; gentamicin, 40 mg/l.

²Made by a Division of Union Carbide, Danbury, Connecticut 06817.

REFERENCES

A

1. Acar J, Luxereau PH, Ducimetiere P, Cadilhac M, Jallut H, Vahanian A: Prognosis of surgically treated chronic aortic valve disease. *J Thorac Cardiovasc Surg* 82:114, 1981.

2. Austen WG, Kastor JA, Sanders CA: Resolution of functional mitral regurgitation following surgical correction of aortic valvular disease. *J Thorac Cardiovasc Surg* 53:255, 1967.

3. Armiger LC, Gavin JB, Barratt-Boyes BG: Histological assessment of orthotopic aortic valve leaflet allografts: Its role in selecting graft pre-treatment. *Pathology* 15:67, 1983.

4. Aberg B, Holmgren A: Haemodynamic evaluation of the Convexo-Concave Bjork-Shiley prosthesis in patients with narrow aortic annulus. *Scand J Thor Cardiovasc Surg* 15:111, 1981.

5. Allen WM, Matloff JM, Fishbein MC: Myxoid degeneration of the aortic valve and isolated severe aortic regurgitation. *Am J Cardiol* 55:439, 1985.

B

1. Bailey CP, Likoff W: The surgical treatment of aortic insufficiency. *Ann Intern Med* 42:388, 1955.

2. Bailey CP, Glover RP, O'Neill TJE, Redondo-Ramirez HP: Experience with the experimental surgical relief of aortic stenosis: A preliminary report. *J Thorac Surg* 20:516, 1950.

3. Bailey CP, Redondo-Ramirez HP, Larzelere HB: Surgical treatment of aortic stenosis. *JAMA* 150:1647, 1952.

4. Barnhorst DA, Oxman HA, Connolly DC, Pluth JR, Danielson GK, Wallace RB, McGoon DC: Long-term follow-up of isolated replacement of the aortic or mitral valve with the Starr-Edwards prosthesis. *Am J Cardiol* 35:228, 1975.

5. Barnhorst DA, Oxman HA, Connolly DC, Pluth JR, Danielson GK, Wallace RB, McGoon DC: Isolated replacement of the aortic valve with the Starr-Edwards prosthesis: A 9 year review. *J Thorac Cardiovasc Surg* 70:113, 1975.

6. Barratt-Boyes BG: Long-term follow-up of aortic valvar grafts. *Br Heart J* 33(suppl):60, 1971.

7. Basta LL, Raines D, Najjar S, Kioschos JM: Clinical, haemodynamic, and coronary angiographic correlates of angina pectoris in patients with severe aortic valve disease. *Br Heart J* 37:150, 1975.

8. Bonchek LI, Anderson RP, Rosch J: Should coronary arteriography be performed routinely before valve replacement? *Am J Cardiol* 31:462, 1973.

9. Baker C, Somerville J: Clinical features and surgical treatment of fifty patients with severe aortic stenosis. *Guy's Hosp Reports* 108:101, 1959.

10. Baxter RH, Reid JM, McGuiness JB, Stevenson JG: Relation of angina to coronary artery disease in mitral and in aortic valve disease. *Br Heart J* 40:918, 1978.

11. Bjork VO, Henze A, Jereb M: Aortographic follow-up in patients with the Bjork-Shiley aortic disc valve prosthesis. *Scand J Thor Cardiovasc Surg* 7:1, 1973.

12. Bjork VO, Henze A, Holmgren A: Five years' experience with the Bjork-Shiley tilting-disc valve in isolated aortic valvular disease. *J Thorac Cardiovasc Surg* 68:393, 1974.

13. Baxley WA, Karp RB, Dye LE: Evaluation of patients for malfunction of mechanical aortic valve prostheses (1983) unpublished study.

14. Blank RH, Pupello DF, Bessone LN, Harrison EE, Sbar S: Method of managing the small aortic annulus during valve replacement. *Ann Thorac Surg* 22:356, 1976.

15. Bolen JL, Holloway EL, Zener JC, Harrison DC, Alderman EL: Evaluation of left ventricular function in patients with aortic regurgitation using afterload stress. *Circulation* 53:132, 1976.

16. Bonow RO, Borer JS, Rosing DR, Henry WL, Pearlman AS, McIntosh CL, Morrow AG, Epstein SE: Preoperative exercise capacity in symptomatic patients with aortic regurgitation as a predictor of postoperative left ventricular function and long-term prognosis. *Circulation* 62:1280, 1980.

17. Borer JS, Rosing DR, Kent KM, Bacharach SL, Green MV, McIntosh CJ, Morrow AG, Epstein SE: Left ventricular function at rest and during exercise after aortic valve replacement in patients with aortic regurgitation. *Am J Cardiol* 44:1297, 1979.

18. Bulkley BH, Roberts WC: Ankylosing spondylitis and aortic regurgitation: Description of the characteristic cardiovascular lesion from study of eight necropsy patients. *Circulation* 48:1014, 1973.

19. Binet JP, Duran CG, Carpentier A, Langlois J: Heterologous aortic valve transplantation. *Lancet* 2:1275, 1965.

20. Buckley MJ, Mundth ED, Daggett WM, Austen WG: Surgical management of the complications of sepsis involving the aortic valve, aortic root, and ascending aorta. *Ann Thorac Surg* 12:391, 1971.

21. Bloodwell RD, Hallman GL, Cooley DA: Aneurysm of the ascending aorta with aortic valvular insufficiency. *Arch Surg* 92:588, 1965.

22. Bentall HH, DeBono A: A technique for complete replacement of the ascending aorta. *Thorax* 23:338, 1968.

23. Bjork VO, Henze A, Holmgren A, Szamosi A: Evaluation of the 21 mm Bjork-Shiley tilting disc valve in patients with narrow aortic roots. *Scand J Thorac Cardiovasc Surg* 7:203, 1973.

24. Borow K, Green LH, Mann T, Sloss LJ, Collins JJ, Jr, Cohn L, Grossman W: End systolic volume as a predictor of postoperative left ventricular function in volume overload from valvular regurgitation. *Circulation* 55,56(suppl III):III-40, 1977 (abstr).

25. Barratt-Boyes BG, Roche AHG, Whitlock RML: Six year review of the results of free-hand aortic valve replacement using an antibiotic sterilized homograft valve. *Circulation* 55:353, 1977.

26. Bahnson HT, Spencer FC, Busse EFG, Davis FW Jr: Cusp replacement and coronary artery perfusion in open operations on the aortic valve. *Ann Surg* 152:494, 1960.

27. Barratt-Boyes BG: A method for preparing and inserting a homograft aortic valve. *Br J Surg* 52:847, 1965.

28. Barratt-Boyes BG: Homograft aortic valve replacement in aortic incompetence and stenosis. *Thorax* 19:131, 1964.

29. Brandt PWT, Roche AHG, Barratt-Boyes BG, Lowe JB: Radiology of homograft aortic valves. *Thorax* 24:129, 1969.

30. Barratt-Boyes BG, Lowe JB, Cole DS, Kelly DT: Homograft valve replacement for aortic valve disease. *Thorax* 20:495, 1965.

31. Barratt-Boyes BG: Cardiothoracic surgery in the Antipodes. *J Thorac Cardiovasc Surg* 78:804, 1979.

32. Barratt-Boyes BG, Roche AHG, Brandt PWT, Smith JC, Lowe JB: Aortic homograft valve replacement: A long-term follow-up of an initial series of 101 patients. *Circulation* 40:763, 1969.

33. Barratt-Boyes BG, Roche AHG: A review of aortic valve homografts over a six and one-half year period. *Ann Surg* 170:483, 1969.

34. Bailey WW, Ivey TD, Miller DW Jr: Dacron patch closure of aortic annulus mycotic aneurysms. *Circulation* 66(suppl I):I-127, 1982.

35. Bonow RO, Rosing DR, Kent KM, Epstein SE: Timing of operation for chronic aortic regurgitation. *Am J Cardiol* 50:325, 1982.

36. Borkon AM, McIntosh CL, Jones M, Lipson LC, Kent KM, Morrow AG: Hemodynamic function of the Hancock standard orifice aortic valve bioprosthesis. *J Thorac Cardiovasc Surg* 82:601, 1981.

37. Bortolotti U, Milano A, Livi U, Russo R, Valfre C, Mazzucco A, Gallucci V: Aortic valve replacement in active infective endocarditis. *Thorac Cardiovasc Surg* 29:303, 1981.

38. Behrendt DM, Austin WG: Current status of prostheses for heart valve replacement. *Progress in Cardiovascular Disease* 15:369, 1973.

39. Becker RM, Strom J, Frishman W, Oha Y, Lin YT, Yellin EL, Frater RW: Hemodynamic performance of the Ionescu-Shiley valve prosthesis. *J Thorac Cardiovasc Surg* 80:613, 1980.

40. Bjork VO, Holmgren A, Olin C, Ovenfors CO: Clinical and haemodynamic results of aortic valve replacement with the Bjork-Shiley tilting disc valve prosthesis. *Scand J Thorac Cardiovasc Surg* 5:177, 1971.

41. Bjork VO: A new central flow tilting disc valve prosthesis: One year's clinical experience with 103 patients. *J Thorac Cardiovasc Surg* 60:355, 1970.

42. Bonow RO, Rosing DR, McIntosh CL, Jones M, Maron BJ, Lan KKG, Lakatos E, Bacharach SL, Green MV, Epstein SE: The natural history of asymptomatic patients with aortic regurgitation and normal left ventricular function. *Circulation* 68:509, 1983.

43. Bonow RO, Rosing DR, Maron BJ, McIntosh CL, Jones M, Bacharach SL, Green MV, Clark RE, Epstein SE: Reversal of left ventricular dysfunction after aortic valve replacement for chronic aortic regurgitation: influence of duration of preoperative left ventricular dysfunction. *Circulation* 70:570, 1984.

C

1. Carabello BA, Green LH, Grossman W, Cohn LH, Koster JK, Collins JJ Jr: Hemodynamic determinants of prognosis of aortic valve replacement in critical aortic stenosis and advanced congestive heart failure. *Circulation* 62:42, 1980.

2. Carpentier A, Deloche A, Relland J, Fabiani JN, Forman J, Camilleri JP, Soyer R, Dubost C: Six-year follow-up of glutaraldehyde-preserved heterografts. *J Thorac Cardiovasc Surg* 68:771, 1974.

3. Carpentier A, Lemaigre G, Robert L, Carpentier S, Dubost C: Biological factors affecting long-term results of valvular heterografts. *J Thorac Cardiovasc Surg* 58:467, 1969.

4. Cheung D, Flemma RJ, Mullen DC, Lepley D Jr, Anderson AJ, Weirauch E: Ten-year follow-up in aortic valve replacement using the Bjork-Shiley prosthesis. *Ann Thorac Surg* 32:138, 1981.

5. Clark DG, McAnulty JH, Rahimtoola SH: Valve replacement in aortic insufficiency with left ventricular dysfunction. *Circulation* 61:411, 1980.

6. Cleland J: A universally applicable continuous suture technique for insertion of aortic valve prostheses. *Ann Thorac Surg* 19:719, 1975.

7. Cohn LH, Sanders JH Jr, Collins JJ Jr: Aortic valve replacement with the Hancock porcine xenograft. *Ann Thorac Surg* 22:221, 1976.

8. Cooley DA, Norman JC: Severe intravascular hemolysis after aortic valve replacement. *J Thorac Cardiovasc Surg* 74:322, 1977.

9. Copeland JG, Griepp RB, Stinson EB, Shumway NE: Long-term follow-up after isolated aortic valve replacement. *J Thorac Cardiovasc Surg* 74:875, 1977.

10. Cunha CLP, Giuliani ER, Fuster V, Seward JB, Brandenburg RO, McGoon DC: Preoperative M-mode echocardiography as a predictor of surgical results in chronic aortic insufficiency. *J Thorac Cardiovasc Surg* 79:256, 1980.

11. Covell JW, Ross J Jr: Nature and significance of alterations in myocardial compliance. *Am J Cardiol* 32:449, 1973.

12. Clarkson PM, Barratt-Boyes BG: Bacterial endocarditis following homograft replacement of the aortic valve. *Circulation* 42:987, 1970.

13. Cowan ST, Steel KJ: Manual for the identification of medical bacteria. 2nd ed. Cambridge University Press, 1974.

14. Carroll JD, Gaasch WH, Zile MR, Levine HJ: Serial changes in left ventricular function after correction of chronic aortic regurgitation: Dependency on early changes in preload and subsequent regression of hypertrophy. *Am J Cardiol* 51:476, 1983.

15. Craver JM, King SB, Douglas JS, Franch RH, Jones EH, Morris DC, Kopchak J, Hatcher CR: Late hemodynamic evaluation of Hancock modified orifice aortic bioprosthesis. *Circulation* 60(Suppl. I):I-93, 1979.

16. Chaitman BR, Bonan R, Lepage G, Tubau JF, David PR, Dyrda I, Grondin CM: Hemodynamic evaluation of the Carpentier-Edwards porcine xenograft. *Circulation* 60:1170, 1979.

17. Cohn LH, Koster JK, Mee RBB, Collins Jr JJ: Long-term follow-up of the Hancock bioprosthetic heart valve: A 6-year review. *Circulation* 60(Suppl. I):I-87, 1979.

18. Chaux AC, Gray RJ, Matlogg JM, Feldman H, Sustaita H: An appreciation of the new St. Jude valvular prosthesis. *J Thorac Cardiovasc Surg* 81:202, 1981.

19. Craver JM, Goldstein J, Jones EL, Knaff WA, Hatcher CR Jr: Clinical, hemodynamic, and operative descriptors affecting outcome of aortic valve replacement in elderly versus young patients. *Ann Surg* 199:733, 1984.

20. Croft CH, Heck Heidi, de Castro C, Floresca M, Lipscomb K, Hillis LD, Firth BG: Chronic aortic regurgitation: Relationship of temporal changes in severity of regurgitation to left ventricular dysfunction. *JACC* 5:486, 1985 (abstr).

21. Cohn LH, Allred EN, DiSesa VJ, Sawtelle K, Shemin RJ, Collins JJ Jr: Early and late risk of aortic valve replacement. *J Thorac Cardiovasc Surg* 88:695, 1984.

D

1. Davila JC, Magilligan DJ Jr, Lewis JW Jr: Is the Hancock porcine valve the best cardiac valve substitute today? *Ann Thorac Surg* 26:303, 1978.

2. Dale J, Myhre E: Intravascular hemolysis in the late course of aortic valve replacement: Relation to valve type, size and function. *Am Heart J* 96:24, 1978.

3. Dismukes WE, Karchmer AW, Buckley MJ: Prosthetic valve endocarditis: Analysis of 38 cases. *Circulation* 48:365, 1973.

4. Danielson GK, Titus JL, DuShane JW: Successful treatment of aortic valve endocarditis and aortic root abscesses by insertion of prosthetic valve in ascending aorta and placement of bypass grafts to coronary arteries. *J Thorac Cardiovasc Surg* 67:443, 1974.

5. Degeorges M, Delzant JF: Elements de pronostic de l'in-

suffisance aortique isolee recueillis chez 206 malades ages de moins de 50 ans. *Sem Hop Paris* 42:1171, 1966.

6. Donaldson RM, Florio R, Rickards AF, Bennett JG, Yacoub M, Ross DN, Olsen E: Irreversible morphological changes contributing to depressed cardiac function after surgery for chronic aortic regurgitation. *Br Heart J* 48:589, 1982.

7. Duran CG, Gunning AJ: A method for placing a total homologous aortic valve in the subcoronary position. *Lancet* 2:488, 1962.

8. David TE, Uden DE: Aortic valve replacement in adult patients with small aortic annuli. *Ann Thorac Surg* 36:577, 1983.

9. Donaldson RM, Ross DM: Homograft aortic root replacement for complicated prosthetic valve endocarditis. *Circulation* 70 (suppl I):I-178, 1984.

E

1. Eddleman EE, Frommeyer WB, Lyle DP, Bancroft WH, Turner ME: Critical analysis of clinical factors in estimating severity of aortic valve disease. *Am J Cardiol* 31:687, 1973.

2. Edwards WS, Kerr AR: A safer technique for replacement of the entire ascending aorta and aortic valve. *J Thorac Cardiovasc Surg* 59:837, 1970.

3. Ellis FH Jr, Kirklin JW: Aortic stenosis. *Surg Clin N Amer* 35:1029, 1955.

4. Ellis FH Jr, Kirklin JW: Aortic insufficiency. *Surg Clin N Amer* 35:1035, 1955.

F

1. Frank S, Ross J Jr: The natural history of severe, acquired valvular aortic stenosis. *Am J Cardiol* 19:128, 1967.

2. Fernandez J: Insertion of Bjork-Shiley aortic prosthesis by continuous suture technique. *Ann Thorac Surg* 17:587, 1974.

3. Frantz PT, Murray GF, Wilcox BR: Surgical management of left ventricular-aortic discontinuity complicating bacterial endocarditis. *Ann Thorac Surg* 29:1, 1980.

4. Frye, RL: (1984) Personal communication.

G

1. Grant RT: After histories for ten years of a thousand men suffering from heart disease: A study in prognosis. *Heart* 16:275, 1933.

2. Goldschlager N, Pfeifer J, Cohn K, Popper R, Selzer A: The natural history of aortic regurgitation. *Am J Med* 54:577, 1973.

3. Gault JH, Covell JW, Braunwald E, Ross J Jr: Left ventricular performance following correction of free aortic regurgitation. *Circulation* 47:773, 1970.

4. Gaasch WH, Andrias CW, Levine HJ: Chronic aortic regurgitation: The effect of aortic valve replacement on left ventricular volume, mass and function. *Circulation* 58:825, 1978.

5. Gula G, Wain WH, Ross DN: Ten years' experience with pulmonary autograft replacements for aortic valve disease. *Ann Thorac Surg* 28:392, 1979.

6. Groves LK, Effler DB, Hawk WA, Gulati K: Aortic insufficiency secondary to aneurysmal changes in the ascending aorta: Surgical management. *J Thorac Cardiovasc Surg* 48:362, 1964.

7. Gaasch WH, Levine JH, Quinones MA, Alexander JK: Left ventricular compliance: Mechanism and clinical implications. *Am J Cardiol* 38:645, 1976.

8. Grossman W, McLaurin LP, Moos SP, Stefadouros M, Young DT: Wall thickness and diastolic properties of the left ventricle. *Circulation* 49:129, 1974.

9. Gula G, Pomerance A, Bennet M, Yacoub MH: Homograft replacement of aortic valve and ascending aorta in a patient with non-specific giant cell aortitis. *Br Heart J* 39:581, 1977.

10. Gonzalez-Lavin L, Barratt-Boyes BG: Surgical considerations in the treatment of ventricular septal defects associated with aortic valvular incompetence. *J Thorac Cardiovasc Surg* 57:422, 1969.

11. Gavin JB, Herdson PB, Monro R, Barratt-Boyes BG: Pathology of antibiotic treated human heart valve allografts. *Thorax* 28:473, 1973.

12. Gavin JB, Barratt-Boyes BG, Hitchcock GC, Herdson PB: The histopathology of 'fresh' human aortic valve allografts. *Thorax* 28:482, 1973.

13. Gradman AH, Harbison MA, Berger HJ, Geha AS, Shaw RK, Crocco CJ, Stoterau S, Pytlik L, Zaret BL: Ventricular arrhythmias late after aortic valve replacement and their relation to left ventricular performance. *Am J Cardiol* 48:824, 1981.

14. Girardet RW, Wheat MW Jr: Technique of aortic valve replacement. *J Thorac Cardiovasc Surg* 71:446, 1976.

H

1. Hufnagel CA: Aortic plastic valvular prosthesis. *Bull Georgetown Univ M Center* 4:128, 1951.

2. Hufnagel CA, Harvey WP: The surgical correction of aortic regurgitation. *Bull Georgetown Univ M Center* 6:60, 1953.

3. Hirshfeld JW Jr, Epstein SE, Roberts AJ, Glancy DL, Morrow AG: Indices predicting long-term survival after valve replacement in patients with aortic regurgitation and patients with aortic stenosis. *Circulation* 50:1190, 1974.

4. Henry WL, Bonow RO, Borer JS, Ware JH, Kent KM, Redwood DR, McIntosh CL, Morrow AG, Epstein SE: Observations on the optimum time for operative intervention for aortic regurgitation. I. Evaluation of the results of aortic valve replacement in symptomatic patients. *Circulation* 61:471, 1980.

5. Hannah H, Reis RL: Current status of porcine heterograft prostheses: A 5-year appraisal. *Circulation* 54(suppl III):III-27, 1976.

6. Hegglin R, Scheu H, Rothlin M: Aortic insufficiency. *Circulation* 37,38(supp V):V-77, 1968.

7. Henry WL, Bonow RO, Rosing DR, Epstein SE: Observations on the optimum time for operative intervention for aortic regurgitation. II. Serial echocardiographic evaluation of asymptomatic patients. *Circulation* 61:484, 1980.

8. Herreman F, Ameur A, de Vernejoul F, Bourgin JH, Gueret P, Guerin F, Degeorges M: Pre- and postoperative hemodynamic and cineangiocardiographic assessment of left ventricular function in patients with aortic regurgitation. *Am Heart J* 98:63, 1979.

9. Hufnagel CA, Conrad PW: The direct approach for the correction of aortic insufficiency. *JAMA* 178:275, 1961.

10. Harken DE, Soroff HS, Taylor WJ, Lefemine AA, Gupta SK, Lunzer S: Partial and complete prostheses in aortic insufficiency. *J Thorac Cardiovasc Surg* 40:744, 1960.

11. Hurley PJ, Lowe JB, Barratt-Boyes BG: Debridement valvotomy for aortic stenosis in adults: A follow-up of 76 patients. *Thorax* 22:314, 1967.

12. Hoeksima TD, Titus JL, Giuliani ER, Kirklin JW: Early results of use of homografts for replacement of the aortic valve in man. *Circulation* 35,36(suppl I):I-9, 1967.

I

1. Isom OW, Dembrow JM, Glassman E, Pasternack BS, Sackler JP, Spencer FC: Factors influencing long-term survival after isolated aortic valve replacement. *Circulation* 49,50(suppl II):II-154, 1974.

2. Ionescu MI, Tandon AP: Long-term clinical and hemodynamic evaluation of the Ionescu-Shiley pericardial xenograft valve. *Thorax Chirurgie* 26:250, 1978.

3. Ivert TSA, Dismukes WE, Cobbs GC, Blackstone EH, Kirklin JW, Bergdahl LAL: Prosthetic valve endocarditis. *Circulation* 69:223, 1984.

4. Ionescu MI, Ross DN: Heart-valve replacement with autologous fascia lata. *Lancet* 2:1, 1969.

5. Ionescu MI, Pakrashi BC, Holden MP, Mary DH, Wooler GH: Results of aortic valve replacement with frame-supported fascia lata and pericardial grafts. *J Thorac Cardiovasc Surg* 64:340, 1972.

6. Ionescu MI, Tandon AP: The Ionescu-Shiley pericardial xenograft heart valve, in MI Ionescu (ed): *Tissue Heart Valves*. London: Butterworth, 1979.

J

1. Jacobs ML, Fowler BN, Vezeridis MP, Jones N, Daggett WM: Aortic valve replacement: A 9-year experience. *Ann Thorac Surg* 30:439, 1980.

2. Jones EL, Craver JM, Morris DC, King SB, Douglas JS Jr, Franch RH, Hatcher CR Jr, Morgan EA: Hemodynamic and clinical evaluation of the Hancock xenograft bioprosthesis for aortic valve replacement (with emphasis on management of the small aortic root). *J Thorac Cardiovasc Surg* 75:300, 1978.

K

1. Karp RB, Cyrus RJ, Blackstone EH, Kirklin JW, Kouchoukos NT, Pacifico AD: The Bjork-Shiley Valve. *J Thorac Cardiovasc Surg* 81:602, 1981.

2. Konno S, Imai Y, Iida Y, Nakajima M, Tatsuno K: New method for prosthetic valve replacement in congenital aortic stenosis associated with hypoplasia of the aortic valve ring. *J Thorac Cardiovasc Surg* 70:909, 1975.

3. Krayenbuehl HP, Turina M, Hess OM, Rothlin M, Senning A: Pre- and postoperative left ventricular contractile function in patients with aortic valve disease. *Br Heart J* 41:204, 1979.

4. Kennedy JW, Twiss RD, Blackmon JR, Dodge HT: Quantitative angiocardiography. III. Relationships of left ventricular pressure, volume, and mass in aortic valve disease. *Circulation* 38:838, 1968.

5. Kennedy JW, Doces J, Stewart DK: Left ventricular function before and following aortic valve replacement. *Circulation* 56:944, 1977.

6. Kouchoukos NT, Karp RB, Blackstone EH, Kirklin JW, Pacifico AD, Zorn GL: Replacement of the ascending aorta and aortic valve with a composite graft. *Ann Surg* 192:403, 1980.

7. Kouchoukos NT, Kerr AR, Sheppard LC, Ceballos RC, Kirklin JW: Heterograft replacement of the mitral valve: Clinical, hemodynamic, and pathological features. *Circulation* 41,42(suppl II):II-20, 1970.

8. Karp RB, Lell W: Evaluating techniques of myocardial preservation for aortic valve replacement: Operative risk. *J Thorac Cardiovasc Surg* 72:206, 1976.

9. Khanna SK, Ross JK, Monro JL: Homograft aortic valve replacement: Seven years' experience with antibiotic-treated valves. *Thorax* 36:330, 1981.

10. Kawasuji M, Hetzer R, Oelert H, Stauch G, Borst HG: Aortic valve replacement and ascending aorta replacement in ankylosing spondylitis: Report of three surgical cases and review of the literature. *Thorac Cardiovasc Surg* 30:310, 1982.

11. Kirklin JW, Mankin HT: Open operation in the treatment of calcific aortic stenosis. *Circulation* 21:578, 1960.

12. Karp RB, Kirklin JW: Replacement of diseased aortic valves with homografts. *Ann Surg* 169:921, 1969.

13. Kerwin AJ, Lenkei SC, Wilson DR: Aortic valve homograft in the treatment of aortic insufficiency: Report of nine cases with one followed for six years. *N Engl J Med* 266:852, 1962.

L

1. Lewes D: Diagnosis of aortic stenosis. *Br Med J* 8:211, 1951.

2. Lewis RP, Bristow JD, Griswold HE: Exercise hemodynamics in aortic regurgitation. *Am Heart J* 80:171, 1970.

3. Levine FH, Carter JE, Buckley MJ, Daggett WM, Akins CW, Austen WG: Hemodynamic evaluation of Hancock and Carpentier-Edwards bioprostheses. *Circulation* 64(suppl II):II-192, 1981.

4. Linhart JW, Wheat MW Jr: Myocardial dysfunction following aortic valve replacement. *J Thorac Cardiovasc Surg* 54:259, 1967.

5. Lev M: The normal anatomy of conduction system in man and its pathology in A-V block. *Ann NY Acad Sci* III:817, 1964.

6. Layton C, Monro J, Brigden W, McDonald A, McDonald L, Weaver J: Systemic hypertension after homograft aortic valvar replacement. A cause of late homograft failure. *Lancet* 2:1343, 1973.

7. Lillehei CW: Worldwide experience with the St. Jude medical prosthesis. *Contemporary Surg* 20:17, 1973.

8. Lee G, Grehl TM, Jaye JA, Kaku RF, Harter W, DeMaria AN, Mason DT: Hemodynamic assessment of the new aortic Carpentier-Edwards bioprosthesis. *Cathet Cardiov Diagn* 4:373, 1978.

9. Levine FH, Buckley MJ, Austen WG: Hemodynamic evaluation of the Hancock-Modified orifice bioprosthesis in the aortic position. *Circulation* 58(suppl I):I-33, 1978.

10. Lytle BW, Cosgrove DM, Loop FD, Taylor PC, Gill CC, Golding LAR, Goormastic M, Groves LK: Replacement of aortic valve combined with myocardial revascularization: Determinants of early and late risk for 500 patients, 1967–1981. *Circulation* 68:1149, 1983.

11. Lakier JB, Copans H, Rosman HS, Lam R, Fine G, Khaja F, Goldstein S: Idiopathic degeneration of the aortic valve: A common cause of isolated aortic regurgitation. *JACC* 5:347, 1985.

12. Louagie Y, Brohet C, Robert A, Lopez E, Jaumin P, Schoevaerdts J-C, Chalant C-H: Factors influencing postoperative survival in aortic regurgitation. *J Thorac Cardiovasc Surg* 88:225, 1984.

M

1. Macmanus Q, Grunkemeier GL, Lambert LE, Starr A: Non–cloth-covered caged-ball prostheses: The second decade. *J Thorac Cardiovasc Surg* 76:788, 1978.

2. Maron BJ, Ferrans VJ, Roberts WC: Myocardial ultrastructure in patients with chronic aortic valve disease. *Am J Cardiol* 35:725, 1975.

3. Moraski RE, Russell RO Jr, Mantle JA, Rackley CE: Aortic

stenosis, angina pectoris, coronary artery disease. *Cath and Cardiovasc Diag* 2:157, 1976.

4. Morris DC, King SB III, Douglas JS Jr, Wickliffe CW, Jones EL: Hemodynamic results of aortic valvular replacement with the porcine xenograft valve. *Circulation* 56:841, 1977.

5. Miller GAH, Kirklin JW, Swan HJC: Myocardial function and left ventricular volumes in acquired valvular insufficiency. *Circulation* 31:374, 1965.

6. McGoon DC: Prosthetic reconstruction of the aortic valve. *Proc Staff Mtgs Mayo Clin* 36:88, 1961.

7. McIlduff JB, Foster ED: Disruption of a normal aortic valve as a result of blunt chest trauma. *J Trauma* 18:373, 1978.

8. Miller DC, Stinson EB, Oyer PE, Moreno-Cabral RJ, Reitz BA, Rossiter SJ, Shumway NE: Concomitant resection of ascending aortic aneurysm and replacement of the aortic valve. *J Thorac Cardiovasc Surg* 79:388, 1980.

9. Miller DC, Stinson EB, Oyer PE, Rossiter SJ, Reitz BA, Shumway NE: Surgical implications and results of combined aortic valve replacement and myocardial revascularization. *Am J Cardiol* 43:494, 1979.

10. Mirsky I, Henschke C, Hess OM, Krayenbuehl: Prediction of postoperative performance in aortic valve disease. *Am J Cardiol* 48:195, 1981.

11. Manouguian S, Seybold-Epting W: Patch enlargement of the aortic valve ring by extending the aortic incision into the anterior mitral leaflet: new operative technique. *J Thorac Cardiovasc Surg* 78:402, 1979.

12. Mori T, Kawashima Y, Kitamura S, Nakano S, Kawachi K, Nakata T: Results of aortic valve replacement in patients with a narrow aortic annulus: Effects of enlargement of the aortic annulus. *Ann Thorac Surg* 31:111, 1981.

13. McCready RA, Pluth JR: Surgical treatment of ascending aortic aneurysms associated with aortic valve insufficiency. *Ann Thorac Surg* 28:307, 1979.

14. McGoon DC, Moffett EA: Total prosthetic reconstruction of the aortic valve. *J Thorac Cardiovasc Surg* 45:162, 1963.

15. Murray G: Homologous aortic valve segment transplant as surgical treatment for aortic and mitral insufficiency. *Angiology* 7:466, 1956.

16. Misbach GA, Turley K, Ullyot DJ, Ebert PA: Left ventricular outflow enlargement using the Konno procedure. *J Thorac Cardiovasc Surg* 84:696, 1982.

17. McGoon DC, Mankin HT, Kirklin JW: Results of open heart operation for acquired aortic valve disease. *J Thorac Cardiovasc Surg* 45:47, 1963.

18. McGoon DC, Ellis FH Jr, Kirklin JW: Late results of operation for acquired aortic valvular disease. *Circulation* 31,32(suppl I):I-108, 1965.

19. McGoon MD, Fuster V, McGood DC, Pumphrey CW, Pluth JR, Elveback LR: Aortic and mitral valve incompetence: Long-term follow-up (10 to 19 years) of patients treated with the Starr-Edwards Prosthesis. *JACC* 3:930, 1984.

N

1. Najafi H, Ostermiller WE, Hushang J: Narrow aortic root complicating aortic valve replacement. *Arch Surg* 99:690, 1969.

2. Nicks R, Cartmill T, Bernstein L: Hypoplasia of the aortic root. *Thorax* 25:339, 1970.

3. Norman JC, Nihill MR, Cooley DA: Valved apico-aortic composite conduits for left ventricular outflow tract obstructions. *Am J Cardiol* 45:1265, 1980.

4. Nitter-Hauge S, Enge I, Sembe BKH, Hall KV: Primary clinical experience with the Hall-Kaster valve in the aortic position. *Circulation* 60(suppl II):II-55, 1979.

5. Nicoloff DM, Emery RW, Arom KV, Northup WF, Jorgenson CR, Wang Y, Lindsay WG: Clinical and hemodynamic results with the St. Jude medical cardiac valve prosthesis. *J Thorac Cardiovasc Surg* 82:674, 1981.

O

1. O'Toole JD, Geiser EA, Reddy PS, Curtiss EI, Landfair RM: Effect of preoperative ejection fraction on survival and hemodynamic improvement following aortic valve replacement. *Circulation* 58:1175, 1978.

2. O'Brien KP, Hitchcock GC, Barratt-Boyes BG, Lowe JB: Spontaneous aortic cusp rupture associated with valvular myxomatous transformation. *Circulation* 37:273, 1968.

3. Ormiston JA, Neutze JM, Agnew TM, Lowe JB, Kerr AR: Infective endocarditis: A lethal disease. *Aust NZ J Med* 11:620, 1981.

4. Olin CL, Bomfim V, Halvazulis V, Holmgren AG, Lamke BJ: Optimal insertion technique for the Bjork-Shiley valve in the narrow aortic ostium. *Ann Thorac Surg* 36:567, 1983.

5. O'Brien, KP: (1983) Personal communication.

6. Olson LJ, Subramanian R, Edwards WD: Surgical pathology of pure aortic insufficiency: A study of 225 cases. *Mayo Clin Proc* 59:835, 1984.

P

1. Pantely G, Morton M, Rahimtoola SH: Effects of successful, uncomplicated valve replacement on ventricular hypertrophy, volume, and performance in aortic stenosis and in aortic incompetence. *J Thorac Cardiovasc Surg* 75:383, 1978.

2. Papadimitriou JM, Hopkins BE, Taylor RR: Regression of left ventricular dilation and hypertrophy after removal of volume overload. *Circ Res* 35:127, 1974.

3. Parr GVS, Kirklin JW, Blackstone EH: The early risks of re-replacement of aortic valves. *Ann Thorac Surg* 23:319, 1977.

4. Pakrashi BC, Mary DAS, Garcia JB, Ionescu MI: Recovery from complete heart block following aortic valve replacement. *Arch Surg* 108:373, 1974.

5. Puig LB, Verginelli G, Belotti G, Kawabe L, Frack CRR, Pileggi F, Decourt LV, Zerbini EJ: Homologous dura mater cardiac valve. Preliminary study of 30 cases. *J Thorac Cardiovasc Surg* 64:154, 1972.

6. Pohluer PG, Thomson FJ, Hjelius E, Barratt-Boyes BG: Experimental evaluation of aortic homograft valves mounted on flexible support frames and comparison with glutaraldehyde treated porcine valves. *J Thorac Cardiovasc Surg* 77:287, 1979.

7. Pacifico AD, Karp RB, Kirklin JW: Homografts for replacement of the aortic valve. *Circulation* 45,46(suppl I):I-36, 1972.

8. Pyle RB, Mayer Jr JE, Lindsay WG, Jorgensen CR, Wang Y, Nicoloff DM: Hemodynamic evaluation of Lillehei-Kaster and Starr-Edwards prostheses. *Ann Thorac Surg* 26:336, 1978.

9. Piehler JM, Danielson GK, Pluth JR, Orszulak TA, Puga FJ, Schaff HV, Edwards WD, Shub C: Enlargement of the aortic root or annulus with autogenous pericardial patch during aortic valve replacement. *J Thorac Cardiovasc Surg* 86:350, 1983.

R

1. Ross J Jr, Braunwald E: Aortic stenosis. *Circulation* 38(suppl V):V-61, 1968.

2. Ross J Jr: Afterload mismatch and preload reserve: A conceptual framework for the analysis of ventricular function. *Prog Cardiovasc Dis* 18:255, 1976.

3. Ross DN: Replacement of aortic and mitral valve with a pulmonary autograft. *Lancet* 2:956, 1967.

4. Rastan H, Koncz J: Plastische Erweiterung der linken Ausflussbahn: Eine neue Operationsmethode. *Thorax-chirurgie* 23:169, 1975.

5. Rastan H, Abu-Aishah N, Rastan D, Heisig B, Koncz J, Bjornstad PG, Beuren AJ: Results of aortoventriculoplasty in 21 consecutive patients with left ventricular outflow tract obstruction. *J Thorac Cardiovasc Surg* 75:659, 1978.

6. Reitz BA, Stinson EB, Watson DC, Baumgartner WA, Jamieson SW: Translocation of the aortic valve for prosthetic valve endocarditis. *J Thorac Cardiovasc Surg* 81:212, 1981.

7. Rittenhouse EA, Sauvage LR, Stamm SJ, Mansfield PB, Hall DG, Herndon PS: Radical enlargement of the aortic root and outflow tract to allow valve replacement. *Ann Thorac Surg* 27:367, 1979.

8. Roberts WC, Morrow AG, McIntosh CL, Jones M, Epstein SE: Congenitally bicuspid aortic valve causing severe, pure aortic regurgitation without superimposed infective endocarditis. *Am J Cardiol* 47:206, 1981.

9. Richardson JV, Karp RB, Kirklin JW, Dismukes WE: Treatment of infective endocarditis: A 10 year comparative analysis. *Circulation* 58:589, 1978.

10. Ross DN: Homograft replacement of the aortic valve. *Lancet* 2:487, 1962.

11. Roberts WC, Kehoe JA, Carpenter DF, Golden A: Cardiac valvular lesions in rheumatoid arthritis. *Arch Intern Med* 122:141, 1980.

12. Ross DN, Martelli V, Wain WH: Allograft and autograft valves used for aortic valve replacement, in MI Ionescu (ed): *Tissue Heart Valves.* London: Butterworth 1979.

13. Rehr RB, Mack M, Firth BG: Aortic regurgitation and sinus of Valsalva–right atrial fistula after blunt thoracic trauma. *Br Heart J* 48:420, 1982.

14. Rossiter SJ, Miller DC, Stinson EB, Oyer PE, Reity BA, Moreno-Cabral RJ, Mace JA, Robert EW, Tsagari TJ, Sutton RB, Alderman EL, Shumway NE: Hemodynamic and clinical comparisons of the Hancock modified orifice and standard orifice bioprostheses in the aortic position. *J Thorac Cardiovasc Surg* 80:54, 1980.

15. Rothkopf M, Davidson T, Lipscomb K, Narahara K, Hillis LD, Willerson JT, Estrera A, Platt M, Mills L: Hemodynamic evaluation of the Carpentier-Edwards bioprosthesis in the aortic position. *Am J Cardiol* 44:209, 1979.

16. Rapaport E: Natural history of aortic and mitral valve disease. *Am J Cardiol* 35:221, 1975.

17. Rizzoli: G, Russo R, Valente S, Mazzucco A, Valfre C, Brumana T, Aru G, Rubino M, Rocco F, Gallucci V: Dehiscence of aortic valve prostheses: analysis of a ten-year experience. *Int J Cardiol* 6:207, 1984.

S

1. Spagnuolo M, Kloth H, Taranta A, Doyle E, Pasternack B: Natural history of rheumatic aortic regurgitation: Criteria predictive of death, congestive heart failure and angina in young patients. *Circulation* 44:368, 1971.

2. Smithy HG, Parker EF: Experimental aortic valvulotomy, preliminary report. *Surg Gynec Obstet* 34:625, 1947.

3. Segal J, Harvery WP, Hufnagel C: A clinical study of one hundred cases of severe aortic insufficiency. *Am J Med* 21:200, 1956.

4. Spangler RD, McCallister BD, McGoon DC: Aortic valve replacement in patients with severe aortic valve incompetence associated with rheumatoid spondylitis. *Am J Cardiol* 26:130, 1970.

5. Schwarz F, Flameng W, Thormann J, Sesto M, Langebartels F, Hehrlein F, Schlepper M: Recovery from myocardial failure after aortic valve replacement. *J Thorac Cardiovasc Surg* 75:854, 1978.

6. Smith N, McAnulty JH, Rahimtoola SH: Severe aortic stenosis with impaired left ventricular function and clinical heart failure: Results of valve replacement. *Circulation* 58:255, 1978.

7. Schwarz F, Schaper J, Flameng W, Hehrlein FW: Correlation between left ventricular function and myocardial ultrastructure in patients with aortic valve disease. *Circulation* 53,54(suppl II):II-67, 1976 (abstr).

8. Smith HJ, Neutze JM, Roche AHG, Agnew TM, Barratt-Boyes BG: The natural history of rheumatic aortic regurgitation and the indications for surgery. *Br Heart J* 38:147, 1976.

9. Schuler G, Person KL, Johnson AD, Grancis G, Ashburn W, Dennish G, Daily PO, Ross J Jr: Serial noninvasive assessment of left ventricular hypertrophy and function after surgical correction of aortic regurgitation. *Am J Cardiol* 44:585, 1979.

10. Schwarz F, Flameng W, Langebartels F, Sesto M, Walter P, Schlepper M: Impaired left ventricular function in chronic aortic valve disease: Survival and function after replacement by Bjork-Shiley prosthesis. *Circulation* 60:48, 1979.

11. Schaff HV, Borkon AM, Hughes C, Achuff S, Donahoo JS, Gardner TJ, Watkins L Jr, Gott VL, Morrow AG, Brawley RK: Clinical and hemodynamic evaluation of the 19 mm Bjork-Shiley aortic valve prosthesis. *Ann Thorac Surg* 32:50, 1981.

12. Schwarz F, Flameng W, Schaper J, Hehrlein F: Correlation between myocardial structure and diastolic properties of the heart in chronic aortic valve disease: effects of corrective surgery. *Am J Cardiol* 42:895, 1978.

13. Seybold-Epting W, Hoffmeister HE: Clinical experience with enlargement of the aortic annulus by extension of the aortic incision into the anterior mitral leaflet. *Thorac Cardiovasc Surg* 28:420, 1980.

14. Shean FC, Austen WG, Buckley MJ, Mundth ED, Scannell JG, Daggett WM: Survival after Starr-Edwards aortic valve replacement. *Circulation* 44:1, 1971.

15. Somerville J, Saravalli O, Ross D, Stone S: Long-term results of pulmonary autograft for aortic valve replacement. *Br Heart J* 42:533, 1979.

16. Starr A, Edwards ML, McCord CW, Griswold HE: Aortic replacement: Clinical experience with a semirigid ball-valve prosthesis. *Circulation* 27:779, 1963.

17. Senning A: Fascia lata replacement of aortic valves. *J Thorac Cardiovasc Surg* 54:465, 1967.

18. Sapsford RN, Blackstone EH, Kirklin JW, Karp RB, Kouchoukos NT, Pacifico AD, Roe CR, Bradley EL: Coronary perfusion versus cold ischemic arrest during aortic valve surgery: A randomized study. *Circulation* 49:1190, 1974.

19. Stokes HJ: *Clinical Bacteriology* (ed 3). London: Edward Arnold, 1968.

20. Strickett MG, Barratt-Boyes BG, MacCulloch D: Disinfection of human heart valve allografts with antibiotics in low concentration. *Pathology* 15:457, 1983.

21. Strom J, Becker RM, Frishman W, Salazar C, Oku Y, Bassell G, Lin YT, Frater RW: Hemodynamic evaluation of the Ionescu-Shiley bovine heterograft valve. *Am J Cardiol* 41:421, 1978.

T

1. Thompson R, Yacoub M, Ahmed M, Seabra-Gomes R, Rickards A, Towers M: Influence of preoperative left ventricular function on results of homograft replacement of the aortic valve for aortic stenosis. *Am J Cardiol* 43:929, 1979.
2. Tompsett R, Lubash GD: Aortic valve perforation in bacterial endocarditis. *Circulation* 23:662, 1961.
3. Thormann J, Gottwik M, Schlepper M, Hehrlein F: Hemodynamic alterations induced by Isoproterenol and pacing after aortic valve replacement with the Bjork-Shiley or St. Jude Medical prosthesis. *Circulation* 63:895, 1981.
4. Tepley JF, Grunkemeier GJ, Sutherland HD, Lambert LE, Johnson VA, Starr A: The ultimate prognosis after valve replacement: An assessment at twenty years. *Ann Thorac Surg* 32:111, 1981.
5. Thomas JL, Dickstein RA, Parker FB Jr, Potts JL, Poirier RA, Fruehan CT, Rich RH: Prognostic significance of the development of left bundle conduction defects following aortic valve replacement. *J Thorac Cardiovasc Surg* 84:382, 1982.
6. Tandon AP, Smith DR, Whitaker W, Ionescu MI: Long-term hemodynamic evaluation of aortic pericardial xenograft. *Br Heart J* 40:602, 1978.
7. Turie AJ, Miller RR, Maxwell KS, Grehl TM, Vismara LA, Hurley EJ, Mason DT: Hemodynamic assessment of the glutaraldehyde-preserved porcine heterograft in the aortic and mitral positions. *Circulation* 56(suppl II):II-104, 1977.
8. Tonnemacher D: Myxomatous degeneration of the aortic valve is a common cause of severe pure aortic regurgitation. *JACC* 5:505, 1985 (abstr).

V

1. Vogt J, Rupprath G, de Vivie ER, Beuren AJ: Hemodynamic findings before and after aortoventriculoplasty (AVP). *Thorac Cardiovasc Surg* 29:381, 1981.

W

1. Wideman FE, Blackstone EH, Kirklin JW, Karp RB, Kouchoukos NT, Pacifico AD: The hospital mortality of re-replacement of the aortic valve: Incremental risk factors. *J Thorac Cardiovasc Surg* 82:870, 1981.
2. Williams JB, Karp RB, Kirklin JW, Kouchoukos NT, Pacifico AD, Zorn GL Jr, Blackstone EH, Brown RN, Piantadosi S, Bradley EL: Considerations in selection and management of patients undergoing valve replacement with glutaraldehyde-fixed porcine bioprostheses. *Ann Thorac Surg* 30:247, 1980.
3. Wood P: Aortic stenosis. *Am J Cardiol* 1:553, 1958.
4. Wallace AG, Young WG, Osterhout S: Treatment of acute bacterial endocarditis by valve excision and replacement. *Circulation* 31:450, 1965.
5. Wheat MW Jr, Wilson JR, Bartley TD: Successful replacement of the entire ascending aorta and aortic valve. *JAMA* 188:717, 1964.
6. Warshawsky H, Abramson W: Complete heart block in calcareous aortic stenosis. *Ann Intern Med* 27:1040, 1947.
7. Worthaum DC, Major MD, Tri TB, Bowen TE: Hemodynamic evaluation of the St. Jude medical valve prosthesis in the small aortic annulus. *J Thorac Cardiovasc Surg* 81:615, 1981.
8. Winter TQ, Reis RL, Glancy L, Roberts WC, Epstein SE, Morrow AG: Current status of the Starr-Edwards cloth-covered prosthetic cardiac valves. *Circulation* 45,46(suppl I):I-14, 1972.

Z

1. Zusman DR, Levine FH, Carter JE, Buckley MJ: Hemodynamic and clinical evaluation of the Hancock modified-orifice aortic bioprosthesis. *Circulation* 64(suppl II):II-189, 1981.

13

COMBINED AORTIC AND MITRAL VALVE DISEASE WITH OR WITHOUT TRICUSPID VALVE DISEASE

DEFINITION

Acquired diseases of both the aortic and mitral valves severe enough to require simultaneous surgery (replacement, repair, or valvotomy) are considered in this chapter. Since tricuspid valve disease may form a part of this spectrum and require simultaneous surgery, it is also considered in this context.

HISTORICAL NOTE

As in isolated aortic and mitral valve disease, the surgical treatment of patients with a combination of these lesions began in the early 1950s by closed methods. In 1955, Likoff and colleagues reported 74 patients who had undergone simultaneous closed repair of aortic and mitral stenosis by Bailey and Glover, in Philadelphia.[L1] Lillehei and colleagues

were the first to report simultaneous repairs of both valves by open techniques using cardiopulmonary bypass (CPB), in 1958.[L2] In 1963, soon after introduction of durable prosthetic valves, Cartwright and colleagues first reported simultaneous aortic and mitral valve replacement.[C1] Starr and colleagues in 1964 reported 13 patients who had undergone multiple valve replacements, including one who received prosthetic aortic, mitral, and tricuspid valves.[S1]

MORPHOLOGY

The morphology of the diseases involving mitral, aortic, and tricuspid valves is described in Chapters 11 and 12. While in the vast majority of patients multivalvular disease is purely rheumatic, each valve may manifest a separate pathologic condition, for example, rheumatic aortic valve disease and mitral incompetence from bacterial endocarditis, idiopathic chordal rupture, or ischemic papillary muscle dysfunction.

The effect of combined disease on the morphology of the left ventricle is of great importance. Thus, at the extremes, combined aortic and mitral incompetence imposes a very large volume overload on the left ventricle, and left ventricular volume and wall thickness increase severely; and combined aortic and mitral stenosis result in a small, thick-walled, and noncompliant left ventricle.

CLINICAL FEATURES AND DIAGNOSTIC CRITERIA

In general, the clinical criteria and noninvasive diagnostic tests are the same for mitral and aortic valve disease when they are combined rather than isolated, but the need for the additional data provided by cardiac catheterization and angiocardiography is more frequent.

One lesion is usually dominant, and it may modify the clinical signs of the less dominant one. A frequent problem is the assessment of the severity of the second lesion, for if it is in fact mild, or even mild to moderate, it may not require simultaneous correction. In some instances, it is possible to obtain reliable information on the second lesion during the operation by palpating an atrial chamber to detect systolic pulsation, feeling the valve directly with the finger before beginning CPB, or actually exposing the valve. Thus, in selected instances, it is not necessary to obtain all the information preoperatively.

In patients over 40 years old, coronary angiography is indicated routinely, and the valve lesions are assessed simultaneously.

Dominant Aortic Stenosis

The auscultatory signs of moderate mitral stenosis may be masked by dominant aortic stenosis, and transmission of the systolic murmur to the apex may confuse the assessment of mitral incompetence. Two-dimensional echocardiography of the mitral valve displays leaflet thickness, motion and orifice size, and thus the severity of mitral stenosis. The severity of pure mitral stenosis associated with aortic stenosis can be verified by pressure measurements (left atrium to left ventricle) on the operating table, although varying cardiac output sometimes makes interpretation difficult. In questionable cases, the valve may be palpated on CPB, often most easily by the superior approach to the left atrium (see Chapter 11).

The most convincing sign of significant mitral incompetence associated with aortic stenosis is a right parasternal systolic lift, especially if associated with an apical third heart sound when the venous and hepatic pulses do not indicate important tricuspid incompetence. More than modest (at UAB, $\geq$ grade 3 on the basis of 1–6) left atrial enlargement on the posteroanterior chest x-ray and also p-mitrale in the electrocardiogram strongly suggest significant associated mitral valve disease. Two-dimensional echocardiography does not help in identifying mitral incompetence. The assessment of severity of associated mitral incompetence may be difficult and may require both left ventriculography and palpation at operation.

Dominant Aortic Incompetence

As noted in Chapter 12, a diastolic murmur that is actually an Austin-Flint murmur can simulate mitral stenosis, the absence of which can be confirmed by echocardiography. When in addition to a mid-diastolic murmur there is an opening snap, left atrial enlargement more than grade 2, and p-mitrale, important mitral stenosis is usually present.

As with dominant aortic stenosis, the severity of associated mitral incompetence requires careful assessment, particularly since it is not infrequently secondary to left ventricular enlargement or dysfunction. If it is less than grade 3 in severity, it usually regresses after the aortic incompetence is corrected. When the left ventricle is severely enlarged, it is likely that both aortic and mitral incompetence are severe.

Dominant Mitral Stenosis

Aortic incompetence may be associated with mitral stenosis, and when the regurgitant flow is moderate or large, its presence and severity are readily assessed clinically by the character of the arterial pulse and by the blood pressure. At times, however, what seems to be something less than grade 3 (on the basis of 1–6) incompetence becomes clearly moderate or severe after surgical relief of the mitral stenosis. In any case, the magnitude of aortic incompetence cannot be assessed reliably at operation. Visual inspection of the aortic valve at operation may provide information about the extent of the rheumatic condition but not about magnitude of leakage. Thus, when severity is in doubt preoperatively, aortography is indicated.

Moderate (grade 3 or less) associated aortic stenosis can usually be identified clinically by the characteristic physical findings (see Chapter 12), and the left ventricular-aortic gradient can be measured at operation but with the disadvantage that flow may not be known. Therefore, a pressure gradient obtained at cardiac catheterization and, using it and the aortic valve flow, an estimation of orifice size are frequently needed in this situation.

Dominant Mitral Incompetence

The same considerations discussed for dominant mitral stenosis apply to aortic valve disease associated with dominant mitral incompetence.

Dominant Tricuspid Valve Disease

In uncommon cases of dominant tricuspid stenosis or incompetence, accurate clinical assessment of the downstream lesions in mitral and aortic valves is seldom possible. Under such circumstances, preoperative cardiac catheterization is nearly always needed.

NATURAL HISTORY

Consideration of the natural history of combined aortic and mitral valve disease is complicated by the same variability in the dominance of one lesion over the other that makes diagnosis and decision making difficult. For example, in rheumatic aortic valve disease, the mitral valve is virtually always involved, although the lesions—either stenosis or incompetence—may be so mild as not to require surgery until many years after replacement of the aortic valve. The double valve surgery in such patients is, of course, sequential and not simultaneous. Patients with rheumatic mitral valve disease often have only mild rheumatic aortic valve disease at the time of their original mitral operation. The longer such a patient survives, the more likely a mild rheumatic aortic lesion is to become important, aided perhaps by the development of calcification, and require operation (see Chapter 11).

Simultaneously developing important aortic and mitral valve disease usually results from a particularly severe and prolonged attack of rheumatic fever or from recurrent attacks, and there may be a florid myocarditis and pericarditis as well. Regurgitant combined valve lesions may mature particularly rapidly such that surgery may be required by the second decade of life.

When dominant aortic stenosis coexists with mitral stenosis, the prognosis may be worse than that of isolated aortic stenosis. When severe aortic and mitral incompetence coexist, the protective effect of the reduction of left ventricular afterload by mitral incompetence (see Chapter 11), combined with the tendency of patients with aortic incompetence to remain asymptomatic even though there is advanced left ventricular dysfunction (see Chapter 12), makes it particularly likely that patients with this combination will remain virtually asymptomatic well beyond the stage when left ventricular dysfunction remains reversible. When dominant mitral stenosis coexists with important aortic stenosis, survival is shorter than that for isolated mitral stenosis, with sudden death a particular risk.

TECHNIQUE OF OPERATION

Combined Aortic and Mitral Valve Replacement without Associated Procedures

The preparations for operation are described in Chapter 2. Both groins are draped into the sterile field, to provide easy access to the femoral artery should intra-aortic balloon pumping be required.

After the chest and pericardium are opened and the left atrial pressure monitoring line is inserted, the aortic cannulation purse-string suture is placed, followed by those for the cardioplegic needle and then those for the venous cannulae (see Chapter 2).

A systematic evaluation is then made, by inspection, palpation, and pressure measurements, of the morphologic effects and thrills created by the aortic and mitral valves and of the various chamber sizes. The tricuspid valve is palpated with a finger inserted through the right atrial appendage, either at this time or just before inserting the venous cannula. Then the patient is heparinized, and the aortic cannula is inserted. The procedure varies from this point on, depending on whether two prostheses are to be used (UAB, occasionally GLH) or the aortic valve replacement will be with a homograft (the usual procedure at GLH).

In any case, the large two-stage single venous cannula is inserted, and cardiopulmonary bypass is begun at 34°C (UAB). Alternatively, two venous cannulae are used, and the cavae are taped (GLH). If repair or replacement of the tricuspid valve is to be included in the operative procedure, two venous cannulae are of course mandatory, and they may be (UAB) inserted directly into the cavae (see Chapter 2, "Preparation for Cardiopulmonary Bypass" in Section 3).

With the usual precautions, a left atrial vent may be inserted through a stab wound just behind the proposed incision and allowed to lie in the atrium rather than being advanced into the ventricle (GLH). Alternatively, a suction line may be inserted later into the left atrium through the atriotomy incision and removed when the left atrium is closed, and the aortic valve replacement performed without a vent (UAB) (see Chapter 12). The perfusate temperature is now lowered rapidly. The aorta is cross-clamped, and the aortic and left atrial vents are used to empty the heart, after which the aortic root is opened as for aortic valve replacement. The cold cardioplegic solution is infused into coronary ostia as in isolated aortic valve replacement (see Chapter 12). The whole body perfusate temperature is adjusted to 25°C.

The aortic valve is excised at this time (see Chapter 12), and if a prosthesis is to be used to replace both valves, the aortic prosthesis is chosen and set aside. The left atrium is now opened from the right side, and the same exposure obtained as for isolated mitral valve surgery. Unless the left atrium is large, the usually marked left ventricular hypertrophy often present in combined aortic and mitral valve disease can make exposure difficult, and in such situations, the left atriotomy is extended beneath the superior and inferior vena cavae. The mitral valve is excised and the replacement device inserted (see Chapter 11, section on Technique of Operation). If a left atrial vent has been inserted through a stab wound, its tip is advanced into the replacement valve, and the left atrium is closed.

Returning now to the aortic root, the surgeon inserts the usual stay sutures (see Chapter 12, section on Technique of Operation), and external cardiac cooling is begun. The cardioplegic solution is reinfused into the coronary ostia, the aortic valve is excised, and the replacement device is sewn into place. The cardioplegic solution may again be infused partway through this procedure. The aortic root is closed, and the remainder of the operation is carried out as described in Chapter 12, with an important proviso. The surgeon must be very aware of the risk of atrioventricular rupture from the tilting up of the tense or beating heart that contains aortic and mitral prostheses (see "Mode of Hospital Death"). Therefore, while the cross-clamp is still in place, the left ventricle is aspirated through its tip by gently tilting up the heart and then suturing the needle hole immediately. If for any reason further aspirations are needed after the aortic cross-clamp has been released, they are done via the right ventricle and across the septum *without* tilting up the heart (see Chapters 2 and 12).

When homograft replacement of the aortic valve is combined with mitral valve replacement, the aortic homograft valve is inserted *first* because previous excision of the anterior mitral leaflet and the presence of the sewing ring of the mitral prosthesis immediately below the mitral-aortic anulus make placement of the lower continuous aortic homograft valve suture line much more difficult. Also, when a Starr-Edwards mitral prosthesis is used, the cage within the left ventricle would prevent inversion of the homograft valve into the ventricle. A left atrial vent line, preferably with its tip in the left ventricle, is essential to keep the aortic root entirely free of blood, and the left atriotomy is not made until homograft valve replacement is completed and the aortotomy is closed. During the aortic valve replacement, the pericardium is irrigated with cold saline solution.

After closure of the aortotomy, the left atrium is opened, and the mitral valve is replaced. The atriotomy is closed and the de-airing routine carried out as after isolated aortic valve replacement (see Chapter 2, "De-airing the Heart" in Section 3).

Combined Aortic Valve Replacement and Mitral Valve Repair

The same sequence described for prosthetic replacement of the aortic and mitral valve may be used for combined aortic valve replacement and mitral valve repair (UAB). The mitral procedure may be commissurotomy or repair of mitral incompetence (see Chapter 11). Alternatively, the mitral procedure may be done first, and after the left atrium is closed and external cardiac cooling is begun, the aortic root is opened and the valve replacement is done (GLH).

Combined Aortic, Mitral, and Tricuspid Valve Surgery

After the aortic and mitral procedures are completed, including closure of the aortotomy and the atriotomy, and with two caval cannulae in place and the tapes snugged down, the tricuspid valve procedure is undertaken. There are two alternative protocols: (1) tricuspid valve surgery under cold cardioplegia and (2) tricuspid valve replacement with a rewarmed beating heart.

Tricuspid valve surgery under cold cardioplegia (UAB) is usually possible when *prosthetic* aortic and mitral replacements are used. Such replacements can be completed in less than 80 minutes, and the tricuspid procedure (repair or replacement) takes 15–30 minutes, resulting at most in 110 minutes of aortic cross-clamping. Core rewarming is not begun during the later stages of the surgery on the last of the two (aortic or mitral) valves. Instead, an additional dose of cold cardioplegic solution is given through the aortic needle vent, as the aortic valve is now competent. The right atrium is opened through the usual oblique incision (see Chapter 11). The rate of infusion of the cold saline solution into the pericardium for external cardiac cooling is now increased, and the perfusate temperature is now raised to begin rewarming the patient. Tricuspid valve annuloplasty or replacement is carried out according to the indications and techniques described in Chapter 11. The right atrium is closed, and the caval tapes are loosened. The remainder of the operation proceeds exactly as already described for double valve replacement.

Tricuspid valve replacement with a rewarmed beating heart is used routinely at GLH after double valve replacement surgery (in part because the aortic homograft valve

freehand insertion takes longer than the insertion of a prosthesis) and at UAB when aortic cross-clamp time is likely to exceed 140 minutes because of other associated problems or procedures. Core rewarming is begun during the later stages of the aortic and mitral surgery, and with the aortic cross-clamp released, the heart is de-aired and defibrillated and allowed to eject by the return of blood to the patient and the temporary reduction of CPB flow. Suction is applied to the aortic needle vent during this procedure and can be continued (at about 150 ml/min) during the tricuspid surgery, although this is not necessary if the left heart has been properly de-aired. The caval tapes are snugged down, and the right atrium is opened. Coronary sinus return is aspirated with a pump sucker, the tip of which is in the sinus orifice. The tricuspid valve is repaired or replaced, the atriotomy closed, and CPB gradually discontinued, with suction reapplied to the aortic needle vent to evacuate any residual air.

Aortic and Mitral Valve Replacement and Coronary Artery Bypass Grafting

The combination of aortic and mitral valve replacement and coronary artery bypass grafting (CABG) is performed in a manner similar to that described for combined aortic valve replacement and CABG (see Chapter 12). The same dilemma exists as to the advantages of performing the distal anastomoses first versus the shorter CPB time of performing the proximal anastomoses first, off CPB. Generally, the technique most familiar to the surgeon is the one that should be employed.

After establishing CPB with a single venous cannula, the aorta is cross-clamped, the aortic root opened transversely, and the cold cardioplegic solution infused directly into the coronary ostia. The distal coronary anastomoses are made (see Chapter 7). The left atrium is opened from the right side, the mitral valve replaced, and the left atrium closed. The aortic valve replacement is then carried out, and the operation essentially completed as described under "Combined Aortic and Mitral Valve Replacement without Associated Procedures." However, after the heart has been de-aired CBP is not discontinued but rather the proximal vein graft anastomoses are made (see Chapter 7, "The Proximal Anastamoses" in Technique of Operation) CPB is then discontinued, and the operation completed as usual. If 5 or 6 distal CABG anastomoses are needed in addition to combined aortic and mitral valve replacement, and if the operation is well organized and performed efficiently, the aortic cross-clamp time should be less than 150 minutes, which is acceptable, but it should not be longer. If it appears that the cross-clamp time may be longer than this, and particularly when tricuspid valve surgery must be added, it is prudent not to attempt complete revascularization but to accept graft placement only to key arteries, and to perform the tricuspid procedure in the rewarming beating heart.

SPECIAL FEATURES OF POSTOPERATIVE CARE

The postoperative care of patients who have undergone combined aortic and mitral valve surgery is the same as that for other patients undergoing cardiac surgery with the aid of cardiopulmonary bypass, and this is described in Chapter 5. The comments concerning appropriate left atrial pressure in patients undergoing isolated aortic valve replacement (see Chapter 12, section on Special Features of Postoperative Care) also apply to those undergoing combined aortic and mitral valve replacement.

EARLY RESULTS

Hospital Mortality

The hospital mortality for combined aortic and mitral valve surgery was appreciable in earlier eras, with mortality rates as high as 20% having been reported. It has become considerably lower in the recent era (since about 1975), being about 8% even when all cases with or without associated procedures are included (Tables 13-1, 13-2). When only primary isolated aortic and mitral valve replacement is considered, an improvement in the recent era has also been evident (Table 13-3), the hospital mortality in 1975–1981 being 4.5% (CL 2.9%–6.7%), no greater than that for aortic valve replacement and mitral repair (Table 13-4).

Mode of Hospital Death

The commonest mode of death is cardiac failure,[H1,R1] just as in the case of isolated aortic and mitral valve replacement, and this mode accounted for 78% of the deaths in the combined GLH-UAB experience (Table 13-5). Somewhat more than half of the instances of cardiac failure were acute and occurred within 48 hours of operation; the remainder were subacute, with death occurring more than 48 hours after surgery and usually with multiple subsystem failure.

Hemorrhage was the next most common mode of death in the UAB-GLH experience (Table 13-5), and in contrast to the isolated aortic valve replacement and isolated mitral valve experiences, left ventricular (or atrioventricular groove) rupture was the mode of death in 9% of the fatalities. Fourteen percent of hospital deaths were by rupture in the experience of Melvin and associates,[M1] and Aberg found this complication to account for 29% of the hospital deaths in Bjork's unit after combined mitral and aortic valve replacement. Tearing of the left ventricle or the atrioventricular grooves may occur when the heart is tilted up for any reason

or simply from pulling on the mitral or aortic anulus during placement of the sutures, presumably because of the fixation of the atrioventricular groove by two rigid devices close together. The complication has not occurred in double valve replacement when a homograft has been used in the aortic position (GLH). The death from hemorrhage from pericardial adhesions in a patient with acute rheumatic pancarditis emphasizes the importance of mobilizing the heart as little as possible under such circumstances.

Incremental Risk Factors for Hospital Death

The presence of *advanced symptoms*, which probably reflects advanced left ventricular dysfunction, increase the risk of hospital death after combined aortic and mitral valve replacement (Fig. 13-1). This increase is less evident in the multivariate analysis of hospital deaths from cardiac causes (Table 13-6) and in a simple contingency table (Table 13-7) than it is in the case of mitral (see Chapter 11) and aortic (see Chapter 12) valve replacement, but has recently been reaffirmed by a study of all patients undergoing valve replacement of any type in that era.[B2] The effect is also evident in the GLH experience (Table 13-8). The high proportion of class V patients at GLH is mainly the result of the often fulminating nature of the rheumatic process in Polynesian and Asian patients and the frequency of acute bacterial endocarditis. The finding by Melvin and colleagues that preoperative left atrial pressure over 30 mmHg was an incremental risk factor for hospital death[M1] probably reflects the same impairment of left ventricular function as do these clinical correlates.

Polynesians and Asians appear to be at greater risk of hospital death after aortic valve replacement. In fact, 61% of the deaths at GLH occurred in these racial groups; their mean age at death was 25.7 years.

Important preoperative mitral incompetence is an incremental risk factor for hospital death after combined aortic and mitral valve replacement (Table 13-6). It appears as a more significant risk factor here than in isolated mitral valve replacement, probably again because the overall risks are greater in double valve replacement, and the effect of mitral incompetence is therefore more visible. The most lethal combined lesion is probably mitral incompetence plus aortic incompetence. In the current era at GLH, 10 (77%) of the 13 hospital deaths occurred in such patients.

Table 13-1 Hospital mortality for all patients undergoing primary or secondary simultaneous combined aortic and mitral valve surgery (replacement or repair) with or without tricuspid valve surgery or other associated procedures (GLH; 1970–1982).

	1970–1976				1976–1982				Total			
		Hospital Deaths				Hospital Deaths				Hospital Deaths		
Type of Surgery	n	No.	%	CL	n	No.	%	CL	n	No.	%	CL
AVS + MVS	88	15	17%	13%–22%	130	12	9%	7%–13%	218	27	12%	10%–15%
AVS + MVS + TVA	7	1	14%	2%–41%	28	1	4%	0.5%–12%	35	2	6%	2%–13%
AVS + MVS + TVR	18	3	17%	7%–31%	6	0	0%	0%–27%	24	3	12%	6%–24%
Total	113[a]	19	17%	13%–21%	164[b]	13	8%	6%–11%	277	32	11.6%	9.5%–13.9%

Coronary artery perfusion techniques were used up to November 1978 and cold cardioplegia thereafter.

KEY: AVS, aortic valve surgery; CL, 70% confidence limits; MVS, mitral valve surgery; TVA, tricuspid valve annuloplasty; TVR, tricuspid valve replacement.

[a]Includes one patient undergoing resection of ascending aortic aneurysm, who died.

[b]Includes seven patients undergoing CABG, with two deaths.

Table 13-2 Hospital mortality of combined aortic and mitral valve replacement with or without associated procedures, such as coronary artery bypass grafting and resection of ascending aorta (UAB; 1967–1981).

| Type of Surgery | n | Hospital Deaths | | |
		No.	%	CL
1967–1975				
Primary	292	44	15.1%	12.9%–17.6%
AVR + MVR	250	35	14.0%	11.7%–16.6%
AVR + MVR + TVA	4	0	0.0%	0.0%–37.6%
AVR + MVR + TVR	38	9	23.7%	16.2%–32.9%
After a previous valve replacement	8	2	25.0%	8.5%–49.6%
Total	300	46	15.3%	13.1%–17.8%
1975–1981				
Primary	266	20	7.5%	5.8%–9.6%
AVR + MVR	219	13	5.9%	4.3%–8.1%
AVR + MVR + TVA	38	4	10.5%	5.4%–18.4%
AVR + MVR + TVR	9	3	33.3%	15.3%–56.0%
After a previous valve replacement	50	6	12.0%	7.2%–18.7%
Total	316	26	8.2%	6.6%–10.1%

KEY: AVR, aortic valve replacement; CL, 70% confidence limits; MVR, mitral valve replacement; TVA, tricuspid valve annuloplasty; TVR, tricuspid valve replacement.

NOTE: In this and other tables of the UAB 1975–1981 experience, for homogeneity of the subset, 11 patients (2 deaths) undergoing primary repair with coronary perfusion as the method of myocardial protection are excluded, as are 2 (0 deaths) patients undergoing double valve replacement after a previous valve replacement.

Table 13-3 Hospital mortality of combined aortic and mitral valve replacement without associated procedures (UAB; 1967–1981).

| Type of Surgery | n | Hospital Deaths | | |
		No.	%	CL
1967–1975				
Primary	284	42	14.8%	12.6%–17.3%
AVR + MVR	242	33	13.6%	11.3%–16.3%
AVR + MVR + TVA	4	0	0.0%	0.0%–37.6%
AVR + MVR + TVR	38	9	23.7%	16.2%–32.9%
After a previous valve replacement	8	2	25.0%	8.5%–49.6%
Total	292	44	15.1%	12.9%–17.5%
1975–1981				
Primary	220	15	6.8%	5.1%–9.1%
AVR + MVR	178	8	4.5%	2.9%–6.7%
AVR + MVR + TVA	34	4	11.8%	6.1%–20.4%
AVR + MVR + TVR	8	3	37.5%	17.4%–61.6%
After a previous valve replacement	44	6	13.6%	8.2%–21.2%
Total	264	21	8.0%	6.2%–10.1%

KEY: AVR, aortic valve replacement; CL, 70% confidence limits; MVR, mitral valve replacement; TVA, tricuspid valve annuloplasty; TVR, tricuspid valve replacement.

NOTE: The same 13 patients are excluded as on Table 13-2.

Associated coronary artery disease is still an incremental risk factor in this subset of patients (Table 13-6). In the current era (1975–1981) at UAB, essentially all such patients received concomitant coronary artery bypass grafting, and their increased risk (Table 13-9) suggests that it is the additional procedure, rather than the presence of coronary disease, that is the risk factor. This risk may be related to the increased duration of CPB in such circumstances and is an argument for limiting the grafts to major arteries rather than attempting complete revascularization in patients with combined double valve and coronary artery disease.

Date of operation is related to hospital mortality, as already indicated. The improvements over time are related to improved methods of myocardial protection and improved surgical techniques.

Older types of myocardial protection increased the risk of

Table 13-4 Simultaneous aortic valve replacement and mitral valve repair with and without associated procedures (UAB; 1975–July 1979). During this period, there were no cases of aortic valve repair and mitral replacement or of repair of both valves.

| Type of Surgery | n | Hospital Deaths | |
		No.	%
Primary AVR + OMC	13[a]	0	0%
Primary AVR + OMC + OTC	1	0	0%
Primary AVR + OMA	3[b]	0	0%
Primary AVR + MVRP + CABPG	7[c]	1	14%
Primary AVR + repair of mitral perforation from bacterial endocarditis	1	0	0%
Secondary AVR + primary MVRP	2[d]	0	0%
Total	27	1	4% (CL 0.5%–12%)
P (χ^2)			0.7

KEY: AVR, aortic valve replacement; CL, 70% confidence limits; MVR, mitral valve replacement; MVRP, mitral valve repair (annuloplasty and/or commissurotomy); OMA, open mitral annuloplasty; OMC, open mitral commissurotomy; OTC, open tricuspid commissurotomy.

[a] In three, an annuloplasty was also done; in another, a closed mitral commissurotomy had been done previously; in another, WPW pathways were mapped and interrupted.

[b] One also had tricuspid annuloplasty.

[c] Three had mitral annuloplasty; three (one death) had mitral commissurotomy; one had commissurotomy and annuloplasty.

[d] One had mitral commissurotomy; one had annuloplasty.

Table 13-5 Mode of hospital death in the current era after mitral and aortic valve surgery with or without tricuspid valve operations and associated cardiac procedures. The UAB data correspond to Table 13-2; the GLH data correspond to Table 13-1.

| Mode of Death | UAB, 1975–1981 (n = 266) | GLH, 1976–1982 (n = 164) | Total (n = 430) | |
			No.	% of 33
Cardiac				
Acute cardiac failure	10	6	16	48%
Subacute cardiac failure	7	3	10	30%
Hemorrhage				
Atrioventricular rupture	2	1	3	9%
Aortic root tear	1		1	3%
Pericardial adhesions		1	1	3%
Unknown origin		1	1	3%
Coma		1	1	
Total	20[a]	13[b]	33[c]	

[a] 7.5%, CL 5.8%–9.8% of n.

[b] 7.9%, CL 5.7%–10.7% of n.

[c] 7.7%, CL 6.3%–9.2% of n.

hospital death. Thus, hospital mortality associated with the use of coronary perfusion at UAB for combined aortic and mitral valve replacement was significantly higher than that associated with cold cardioplegia (14.6% compared to 8.5%; $P = .04$). This is nearly identical to the experience at GLH (Table 13-10). Parr and colleagues reported similar findings.[P1] The use of simple cold ischemic arrest can be associated with a low mortality (Table 13-11). In part, this has been the result of keeping cross-clamp times below about 70 minutes by employing modifications of the technique described here. This corresponds to the experience of Lemole and colleagues, who achieved a mortality of 3% by

carefully planning the operation under simple cold ischemic arrest so that the cross-clamp time was relatively short.[L3]

It is interesting that longer aortic cross-clamp time was only possibly ($P = .15$) an incremental risk factor in this experience. This is probably because short cross-clamp times (< 60 minutes), with their very low risks, were missing from this experience, and thus the presumed incremental risk of longer cross-clamp times was not highlighted.

Concomitant tricuspid valve repair is probably not a risk factor currently, although *replacing the tricuspid valve* may add to the risk of operation (Tables 13-1, 13-2, 13-3, 13-12). A similar significant increase in risk from the addition of tricus-

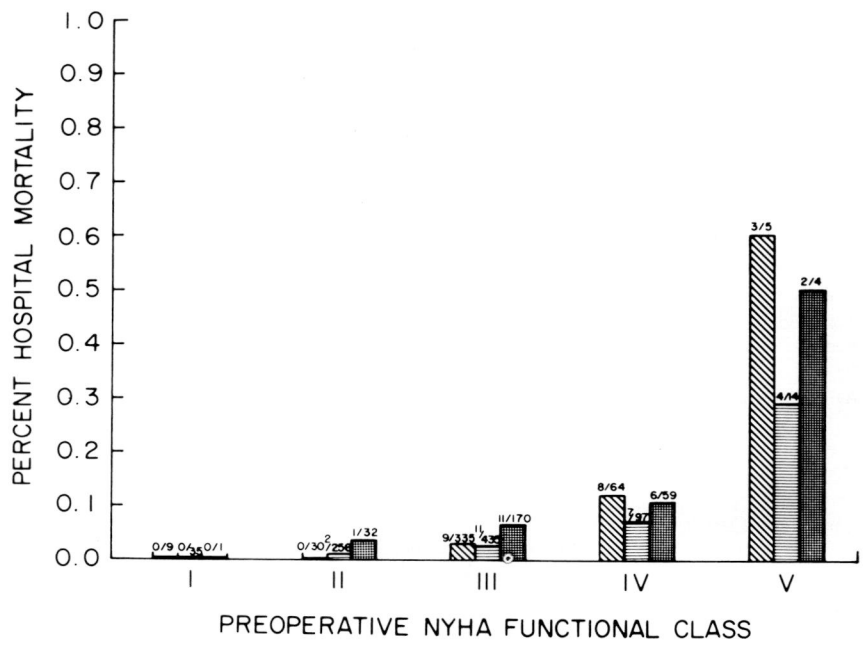

Figure 13-1   A comparison of hospital mortality by preoperative NYHA functional class, according to whether isolated mitral valve replacement (UAB; 1975–July 1, 1979; diagnonal hatching), aortic valve replacement (UAB; 1975–July 1, 1979; horizontal hatching), or combined aortic and mitral valve replacement (UAB; 1975–1981; stippling) was done.

Table 13-6   Incremental risk factors for cardiac mode of hospital death after simultaneous primary aortic and mitral valve replacement with or without associated procedures or tricuspid valve surgery (UAB; 1975–1981; n = 266).

Incremental Risk Factors	Logistic Coefficient ± SD	P Value
Higher NYHA functional class	0.8 ± 0.53	.15
Mitral incompetence	2.4 ± 0.86	.004
Associated coronary artery disease	1.8 ± 0.82	.03
Female sex	2.9 ± 0.91	.002
Duration of symptoms (months)	−0.028 ± 0.0126	.03
Longer ischemic (cross-clamp) time	0.020 ± 0.0140	.15
Tricuspid annuloplasty	1.3 ± 0.81	.11
Tricuspid replacement	3.2 ± 1.13	.005
Intercept	−10	

NOTE: 17 events; see Appendix 13A for details of the analysis.

pid valve replacement to combined aortic and mitral valve replacement was reported by Middell and colleagues[M2] in an earlier period. The possibly lower mortality at GLH (Table 13-1) could be related to the preference for a stented aortic or pulmonary homograft valve, which has no gradient, rather than a prosthetic or bioprosthetic device used (Tables 13-2, 13-3).

A previous valve operation was not per se an incremental risk factor (Tables 13-2, 13-3, 13-13). Certainly this is true of a previous valve repair (Table 13-6), and it is probably true when there has been a previous single valve replacement. Probably more than one previous valve replacement is a risk factor, particularly in patients with advanced disability.

Mitral valve replacement, rather than repair, in association with aortic valve replacement, is not an incremental risk factor (Tables 13-4, 13-14).

Table 13-7 Hospital mortality after primary combined aortic and mitral valve replacement, with or without tricuspid valve surgery or other procedures, according to preoperative functional class (UAB; 1975–1981; n = 266).

NYHA Class	n	Hospital Deaths No.	%	CL
I	1	0	0%	0%–85%
II	32	1	3.1%	0.4%–10.2%
III	170	11	6.5%	4.5%–9.0%
IV	59	6	10.2%	6.1%–16%
V[a]	4	2	50.0%	17.7%–82.3%
Total	266	20	7.5%	5.8%–9.6%
P(logistic)			.02	

KEY: CL, 70% confidence limits.

[a] Includes only patients in shock and in acute hemodynamic deterioration at the time of emergency operation, not all patients undergoing emergency operations.

Table 13-8 Hospital mortality after a consecutive series of 95 primary or secondary double or triple valve operations with or without other procedures (GLH; 1976–1980).

NYHA Class	n	Hospital Deaths No.	%	CL
I	2	0	0%	0%–61%
II	15	0	0%	0%–12%
III	41	1	2%	0.3%–8%
IV	21	4	19%	10%–32%
V[a]	16	5	31%	18%–47%
Total	95	10	11%	7%–15%

KEY: CL, 70% confidence limits.

[a] Includes patients undergoing emergency operation and those with end-stage cardiac disease (uncontrollable heart failure, low cardiac output, severe renal failure, cardiac cachexia).

Table 13-10 Hospital mortality related to method of myocardial support (GLH; 1970–1982). The presentation is as in Table 13-1.

Method of Myocardial Support during CPB	n	Hospital Deaths No.	%	CL
Coronary artery perfusion (1970–November 1978)	177	25	14%	11%–17%
Cold cardioplegia (December 1978–December 1981; St. Thomas's solution)	100	7	7%	4%–11%

KEY: CL, 70% confidence limits.

Table 13-11 Hospital death after combined aortic and mitral valve replacement with or without tricuspid valve surgery or other procedures (UAB; 1975–1981). The presentation is as in Table 13-2.

Method of Myocardial Protection during CPB	n	Hospital Deaths No.	%	CL
Cardioplegia	171	13	7.6%	5.5%–10.3%
Cold ischemic arrest (one or two periods)	95	7	7.4%	4.6%–11.3%
Total	266	20	7.5%	5.8%–9.6%

KEY: CL, 70% confidence limits.

Table 13-12 Hospital mortality after simultaneous combined aortic and mitral valve replacement, according to concomitant tricuspid procedures (UAB; 1975–1981; n = 266). The presentation is as in Table 13-2.

Tricuspid Procedure	n	Hospital Deaths No.	%	CL
None	219	13	5.9%	4.3%–8.1%
Annuloplasty	38	4	10.5%	5.4%–18.4%
Replacement	9	3	33.0%	15.3%–56%
Total	266	20	7.5%	5.8%–9.6%

KEY: CL, 70% confidence limits.

Table 13-9 Hospital mortality for primary aortic and mitral valve replacement without tricuspid valve surgery, according to associated procedures (UAB; 1967–1981). The presentation is as in Table 13-2.

Type of Surgery	1970–1975 Hospital Deaths n	No.	%	CL	1976–1981 Hospital Deaths n	No.	%	CL	Total Hospital Deaths n	No.	%	CL
AVR + MVR	243	33	14%	11%–16%	180	8	4%[a]	3%–7%	423	4	9.7%	8.2%–11.40%
AVR + MVR + CABG	6	2	33%	12%–62%	36	5	14%[a]	8%–22%	42	7	17%	11%–25%
AVR + MVR + Res AAA					2	0	0%	0%–61%	2	0	0%	0%–61%
AVR + MVR + other	1	0	0%	0%–85%	1	0	0%	0%–85%	2	0	0%	0%–61%
Total	250	35	14%	12%–17%	219	13	6%	4%–8%	469	48	10.2%	8.8%–11.9%

KEY: AVR, aortic valve replacement; CL, 70% confidence limits; CABG, coronary artery bypass grafting; MVR, mitral valve replacement; Res AAA, resection of abdominal aortic aneurysm.

[a] P for difference (χ^2) = .03.

Table 13-13 Hospital mortality after combined aortic and mitral valve surgery, in the case of primary operations and reoperations following previous cardiac surgery on one or more heart valves. The presentation is as in Table 13-1 (GLH; 1970–1982).

		1970–1975 Hospital Deaths				1976–1981 Hospital Deaths				Total Hospital Deaths		
	n	No.	%	CL	n	No.	%	CL	n	No.	%	CL
Primary operation	87	15	17%	13%–22%	114	9	8%	5%–11%	201	24	12%	10%–15%
Reoperation	26	4	15%	8%–26%	50	4	8%	4%–14%	76	8	11%	7%–15%
Total	113	19	17%	13%–21%	164	13	8%	6%–11%	277	32	11.6%	9.5%–13.9%

KEY: CL, 70% confidence limits.

Table 13-14 Hospital mortality according to type of combined mitral and aortic valve surgery. The presentation is as in Table 13-1 (GLH; 1970–1982).

Type of Surgery		1970–1975 Hospital Deaths				1976–1981 Hospital Deaths				Total Hospital Deaths		
	n	No.	%	CL	n	No.	%	CL	n	No.	%	CL
Mitral + aortic replacement	88[a]	15	17%	13%–22%	118[b]	11	9%	7%–13%	206	26	13%	10%–15%
Mitral repair[c] + aortic replacement	25	4	16%	8%–27%	42	2	5%	2%–11%	67	6	9%	5%–14%
Aortic valvotomy + mitral replacement	0	0	0		4	0	0%	0%–38%	4	0	0%	0%–38%
Total	113	19	17%	13%–21%	164	13	8%	6%–11%	277	32	11.6%	9.5%–13.9%

KEY: CL, 70% confidence limits.
[a] Includes one patient undergoing associated ascending aortic aneurysm resection, with one death.
[b] Includes seven patients undergoing CABG, with two deaths.
[c] Includes mitral valvotomy.

Table 13-15 Hospital mortality after double or triple valve surgery according to whether the procedure was an elective one or an emergency (GLH). The presentation is as in Table 13-1.

Type of Surgery		1970–1975 Hospital Deaths				1976–1981 Hospital Deaths				Total Hospital Deaths		
	n	No.	%	CL	n	No.	%	CL	n	No.	%	CL
Elective operation	100	12	12%	9%–16%	141	9	6%	4%–9%	241	21	8.7%	6.8%–11.0%
Emergency operation	13	7	54%	36%–71%	23	4	17%	9%–29%	36	11	31%	22%–40%
Total	113	19	17%	13%–21%	164	13	8%	6%–11%	277	32	11.6%	9.5%–13.9%
P												.0014

KEY: CL, 70% confidence limits.

Emergency operations have carried a higher risk than elective ones. Thus 21 (8.7%, CL 6.8%–11%) of 241 patients (GLH) died after elective aortic and mitral valve surgery, with or without tricuspid surgery, but after emergency operation 11 (31%, CL 22%–40%) of 36 died (Table 13-15). The increased risk may be the result of the very poor clinical status of the patients in whom it is required.

LATE RESULTS

Survival

The 5-year survival rate of patients leaving the hospital alive after primary aortic and mitral valve replacement has been 70% (in contrast to 80% for isolated aortic or mitral valve replacement) and the 10-year survival rate 50% (Fig. 13-2). The lower late survival rate is reflected also in the mul-

tivariate analysis of all patients receiving Bjork-Shiley valves, in which double-valve replacement, in contrast to single aortic or mitral valve replacement, was an incremental risk factor.[K1]

Incremental Risk Factors for Premature Late Death

Poor preoperative condition of the patient (NYHA class IV or IV) adversely affects long-term survival after combined mitral and aortic valve replacement (Table 13-16, Fig. 13-3). Thus, the 5-year survival is 80% for those preoperatively in NYHA class II and 50% for those in class IV. Presumably, as in other types of heart disease, the patients with more advanced symptoms and disability preoperatively have more advanced left ventricular dysfunction, and this probably accounts for the poorer long-term survival of these patients.

Preoperatively *important mitral or aortic valve incompetence* is an incremental risk factor for premature late death

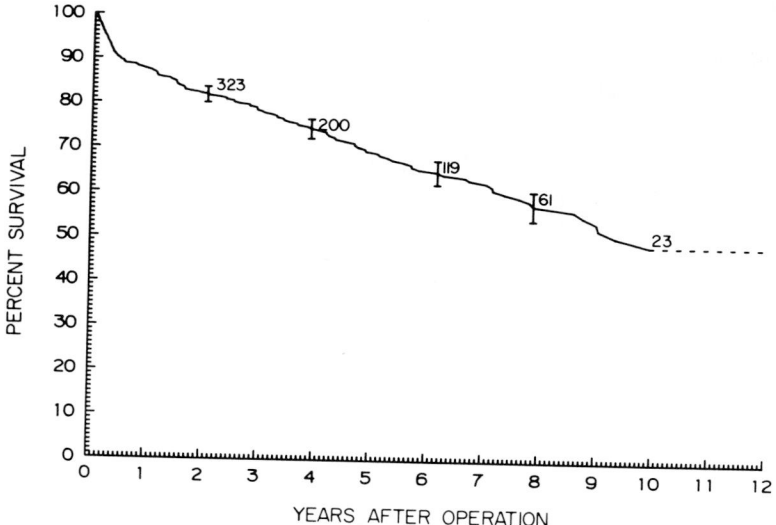

Figure 13-2 Actuarial survival after simultaneous aortic and mitral valve replacement with or without tricuspid valve surgery or other associated procedures. The bars enclose the 70% confidence limits (±1 standard deviation). The dashed lines indicate traced patients without further events (UAB; 1967–1981; n = 503 hospital survivors only).

Table 13-16 Simultaneous primary aortic and mitral valve replacement, with or without associated procedures or tricuspid valve surgery (UAB; 1967–1981).

Incremental Risk Factor	Coefficient	P Value
NYHA class (I–V)	0.46814	.0008
Black	0.73041	.0008
Body surface area	1.20530	.0011
Age	0.01677	.0164
Aortic valve incompetence	0.32381	.0805
Mitral valve incompetence	0.33425	.0911

NOTE: The analysis of late deaths includes 147 events in 503 hospital survivors (see Appendix 13B for details of the analysis).

(Table 13-16). This risk is no doubt related to the impaired left ventricular function so frequently present in both these conditions. When mitral and aortic valve incompetence coexist, the effect is particularly unfavorable, and the 5-year survival is 50%, compared to 75% for those without such a condition (Fig. 13-4).

Symptomatic Results

Among 503 hospital survivors, 171 (34%) are alive and well and in NYHA class I at follow-up (Fig. 13-5), including 28% of those preoperatively in NYHA class IV. Altogether, 323 (64% of the 503 hospital survivors) are alive and in NYHA

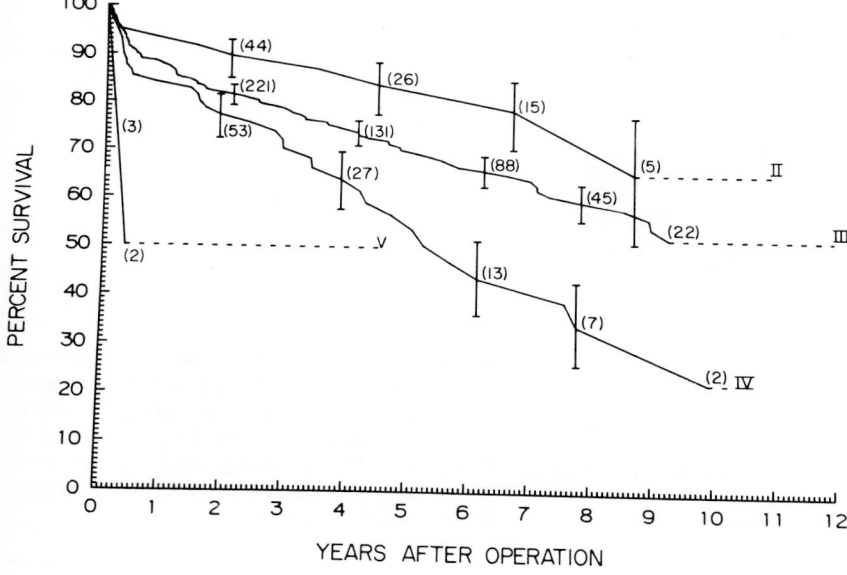

Figure 13-3 Actuarial survival after simultaneous aortic and mitral valve replacement, according to preoperative NYHA functional class (UAB; 1967–1981). The presentation and data base are as in Figure 13-2.

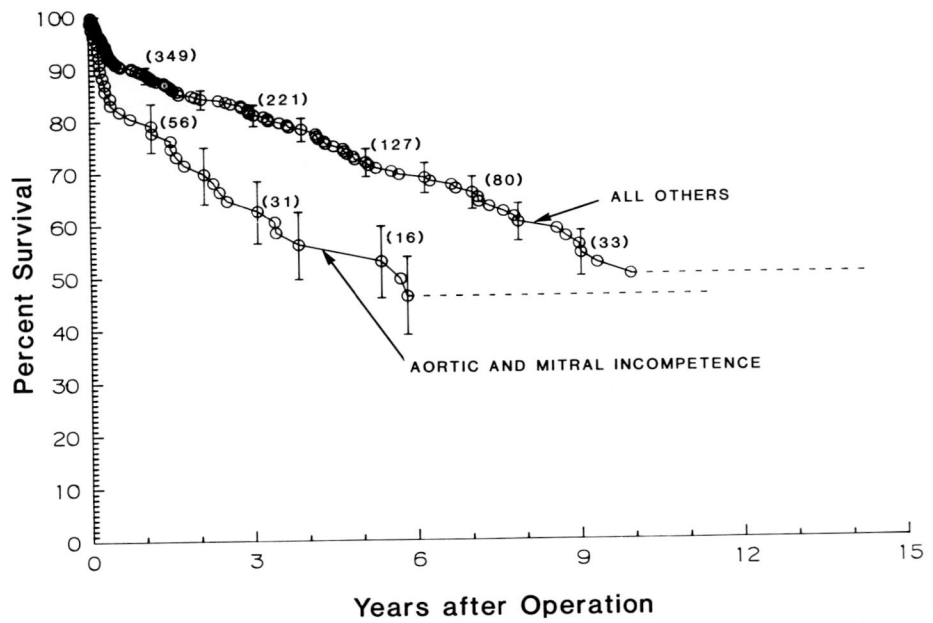

Figure 13-4 Actuarial survival after simultaneous aortic and mitral valve replacement, according to whether or not both the mitral and aortic lesions were incompetent. The presentation and data base are as in Figure 13-2 (UAB; 1967–1981).

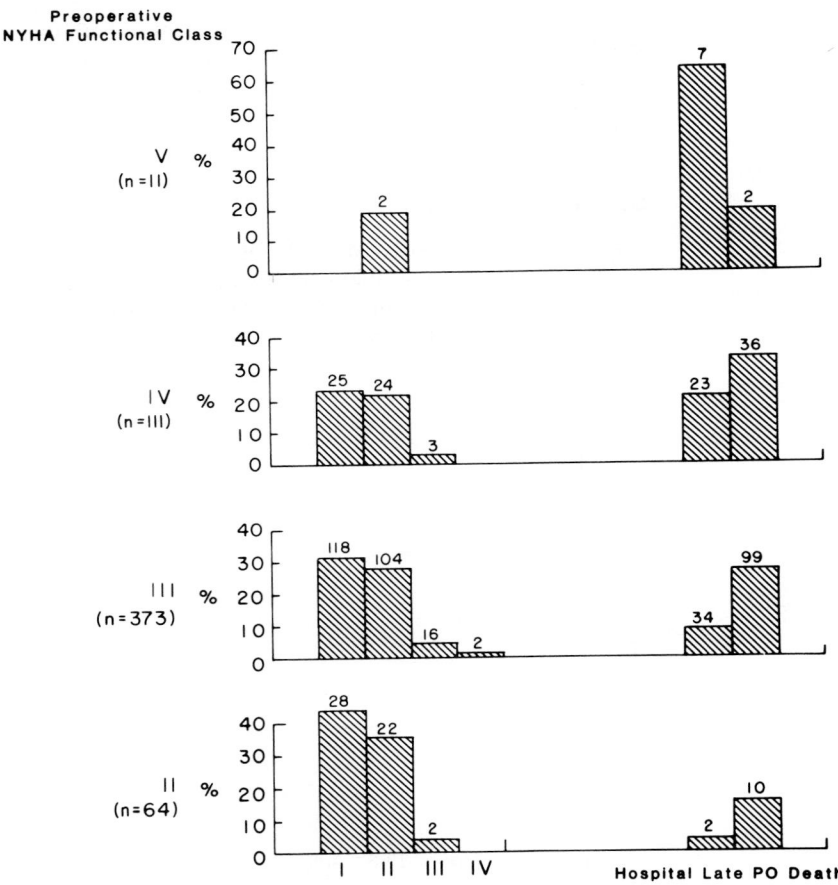

Figure 13-5 Clinical status late after combined aortic and mitral valve replacement, according to preoperative NYHA functional class (UAB; 1967–1981). The presentation and data base are as in Figure 13-2. The two categories of postoperative (PO) death are hospital (lefthand columns) and late (righthand columns).

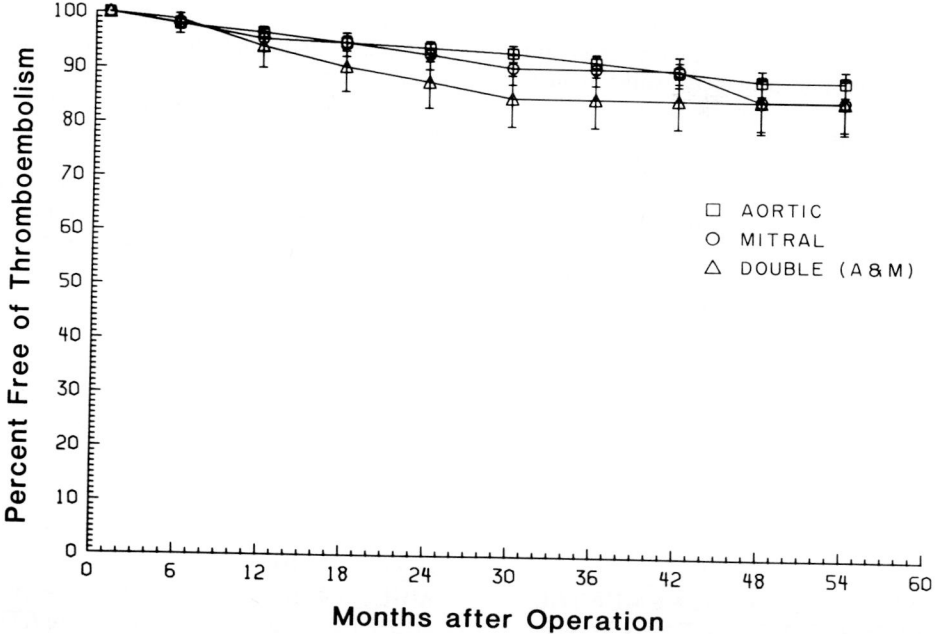

Figure 13-6 Percent of patients free of thromboembolism among patients having double valve replacement, compared to those among patients having isolated aortic and isolated mitral valve replacement.

Reproduced with permission from Karp et al.[K1]

class I or II at follow-up. This corresponds roughly to Aberg's report from Stockholm, in which 81% of patients undergoing combined aortic and mitral replacement were improved by one functional class after operation.[A1]

Thromboembolism

With the Bjork-Shiley valve, the rate of freedom from thromboembolism for double valve replacement is similar to that for isolated aortic or mitral replacement (Fig. 13-6).[K1] Thus, at 36 months, 88% of patients with combined aortic and mitral valve replacement are free from thromboemboli. Presumably, these same figures apply when the double replacement is with the Starr-Edwards silastic ball valve. In patients with both valves replaced by a stent-mounted porcine heterograft, most of whom were not anticoagulated, the proportion with thromboembolism has been similar.[W1]

Complications of Anticoagulant Treatment

Complications related to anticoagulant therapy are the same as described for other patients on anticoagulants after valve replacement (see Chapters 11 and 12).

Hemolysis

With two mechanical prostheses, hemolysis is greater than with one. It is generally not of sufficient magnitude to be a clinical problem.

INDICATIONS FOR OPERATION

Aortic and mitral valve replacement may be required when the patient's symptoms are significant (NYHA class III or greater) despite an appropriate and intense medical regimen. Such an approach, more conservative than that with isolated mitral or aortic valve replacement, is indicated by the higher early and late risks of double valve replacement and the probable increased late morbidity when there are two, rather than one, artificial devices in situ. However, it is unwise to insist on severe limitations (NYHA class IV) before recommending double or triple valve surgery, and it is particularly important to avoid being forced to operate on emergency and class V patients, for then the early and late risk becomes very high. An exception is formed by patients with combined aortic and mitral incompetence, and they are advised to have operation when left ventricular enlargement is ≥ grade 3 (on the basis of 1–6), even though symptoms are mild.

Patients with active rheumatic carditis, severe aortic and mitral incompetence, and critical heart failure must be operated on when it is clear that the acute rheumatic episode is not subsiding. Patients with severe aortic and mitral incompetence and active bacterial endocarditis, in whom neither the infection nor the heart failure can be controlled medically, must also undergo operation without delay.

CHOICE OF THE REPLACEMENT DEVICE

Two mechanical prostheses or bioprostheses devices may be used in those patients in whom both aortic and mitral valve replacement is deemed necessary (UAB). The argument in favor of mechanical prostheses has been that no more anti-coagulants are required for one prosthetic valve than for two, and a second device of that type is appropriate and, indeed, as good as or better than a tissue valve in the second site. In favor of this approach is the decreased likelihood of a second operation for valve failure and the apparent absence of a clinically important increase in risk of either thrombo-embolism or hemolysis with two devices rather than one. When anticoagulants are contraindicated, bioprostheses may be used in both aortic and mitral positions (UAB).

A freehand aortic homograft, along with a mechanical prosthesis or bioprosthesis in the mitral position, may be used routinely in the aortic position unless contraindicated for the reasons outlined in Chapter 12 (GLH). An aortic homograft may be considered significantly superior to other devices in terms of the risk of thromboembolism, the ab-sence of a gradient, and the removal of increased risk of atrioventricular rupture (GLH). For these reasons, the prob-able need for reoperation is accepted.

APPENDIXES

APPENDIX 13A
MULTIVARIATE ANALYSIS OF INCREMENTAL RISK FACTORS FOR HOSPITAL DEATH WITH SIMULTANEOUS PRIMARY AORTIC AND MITRAL VALVE REPLACEMENT

In the logistic multivariate analysis of incremental risk factors for in-hospital cardiac death in patients with simultaneous primary aortic and mitral valve replacement with or without procedures on the tricuspid valve and other associated procedures (UAB; 1975–1981; $n = 266$; 17 cardiac deaths), the following variables were analyzed. Factors not appearing in the final model were associated with P values $> .2$.

Demographic
    Age
    Body surface area
    Sex
    Race
    Veterans Administration patient

Era
    Date of operation
    Method of myocardial preservation

Preoperative medical status
    Atrial fibrillation
    History of coronary artery disease
    NYHA functional class (I–V)
    Duration of complaint
    Previous valve repair

Valve related
    Mitral valve lesion (stenosis, incompetence, both)
    Aortic valve lesion (stenosis, incompetence, both)
    Active infection of valve at time of surgery
    Aortic valve morphology
    Mitral valve morphology

Operative
    Xenograft prosthesis
    Concurrent tricuspid valve annuloplasty
    Concurrent tricuspid valve replacement
    Ischemic time
    Surgeon
    Concurrent CABG

APPENDIX 13B
MULTIVARIATE ANALYSIS OF INCREMENTAL RISK FACTORS FOR LATE DEATH AFTER SIMULTANEOUS PRIMARY AORTIC AND MITRAL VALVE REPLACEMENT

In the Cox multivariate analysis of incremental risk factors for late death after hospital dismissal from all causes after simultaneous primary aortic and mitral valve replacement (UAB; 1967–1981; $n = 569$; 503 hospital survivors; 147 late deaths), the following variables were analyzed. Factors not appearing in the final model were associ-ated with P values $> .2$.

$$
\begin{aligned}
\text{Observations used in analysis} &= 497 \\
\text{Missing values} &= 6 \\
\text{Hospital deaths} &= \underline{66} \\
&\ 569
\end{aligned}
$$

Demographic
    Age
    Body surface area
    Sex
    Race

Preoperative medical status
    Atrial fibrillation
    History of coronary artery disease
    NYHA functional class (I–V)
    Duration of complaint
    Previous valve repair

Valve related
    Mitral valve lesion (stenosis, incompetence, both)
    Aortic valve lesion (stenosis, incompetence, both)
    Active infection of valve at time of surgery
    Aortic valve morphology
    Mitral valve morphology

Operative
    Xenograft prosthesis
    Concurrent tricuspid valve annuloplasty
    Concurrent tricuspid valve replacement
    Ischemic time

REFERENCES

A

1. Aberg B: Surgical treatment of combined aortic and mitral valve disease. *Scand J Thorac Cardiovasc Surg* (suppl 25)1980:1.

B

1. Bigelow JC, Herr RH, Wood JA, Starr A: Multiple valve replacement: Review of five years' experience. *Circulation* 38:656, 1968.
2. Blackstone EH, Kirklin JW: Death and other time-related events after valve replacement. (1985) Unpublished study.

C

1. Cartwright RS, Giacobine JW, Ratan RS, Ford WB, Palich WE: Combined aortic and mitral valve replacement. *J Thorac Cardiovasc Surg* 45:35, 1963.

H

1. Hurley EJ, Angell WW, Dor V, Reeves MM, Shumway NE: Multiple valve replacement. *Arch Surg* 94:163, 1967.

K

1. Karp RB, Cyrus RJ, Blackstone EH, Kirklin JW, Kouchoukos NT, Pacifico AD: The Bjork-Shiley valve. *J Thorac Cardiovasc Surg* 81:602, 1981.

L

1. Likoff W, Berkowitz D, Denton C, Goldberg H: A clinical evaluation of the surgical management of combined mitral and aortic stenosis. *Am Heart J* 49:394, 1955.
2. Lillehei CW, Gott VL, DeWall RA, Varco RL: The surgical treatment of stenotic and regurgitant lesions of the mitral and aortic valves by direct vision utilizing a pump-oxygenator. *J Thorac Surg* 35:154, 1958.
3. Lemole GM, Cuasay R: Improved technique of double valve replacement. *J Thorac Cardiovasc Surg* 71:759, 1976.

M

1. Melvin DB, Tecklenberg PL, Hollingsworth JF, Levine FH, Glancy DL, Epstein SE, Morrow AG: Computer-based analysis of preoperative and postoperative prognostic factors in 100 patients with combined aortic and mitral valve replacement. *Circulation* 47, 48(suppl III):III-56, 1973.
2. Midell AL, DeBoer A: Multiple valve replacement: An analysis of early and late results. *Arch Surg* 104:471, 1972.

O

1. Okies JE, Phillips SJ, Chaitman BR, Starr A: Technical consideration in multiple valve and coronary artery surgery. *J Thorac Cardiovasc Surg* 67:762, 1974.

P

1. Parr GVS, Fox S, Waldhausen JA, Pierce WS, O'Neill MJ Jr: Improving results in combined aortic and mitral valve replacement using cold potassium cardioplegia. J Cardiovasc Surg 20:457, 1979.

R

1. Rostad H, Simonsen S, Nitter-Hauge S: Combined aortic and mitral valve replacement: A randomized study comparing the Bjork-Shiley and Lillehei-Kaster disc valve. *Thorac Cardiovasc Surg* 27:308, 1979.

S

1. Starr A, Edwards M, McCord CW, Wood J, Herr R, Griswold HE: Multiple-valve replacement. *Circulation* 29:30, 1964.

T

1. Terzaki AK, Cokkinos DV, Leachman RD, Meade JB, Hallman GL, Cooley DA: Combined mitral and aortic valve disease. *Am J Cardiol* 25:588, 1970.

W

1. Williams JB, Karp RB, Kirklin JW, Kouchoukos NT, Pacifico AD, Zorn GL Jr, Blackstone EH, Brown RN, Piantadosi S, Bradley EL: Considerations in selection and management of patients undergoing valve replacement with glutaraldehyde-fixed porcine bioprostheses. *Ann Thorac Surg* 30:247, 1980.

14

TRICUSPID VALVE DISEASE

DEFINITION

This chapter discusses incompetence and stenosis of the tricuspid valve in those uncommon situations in which it occurs as an isolated lesion and some aspects of tricuspid valve disease associated with mitral or combined mitral and aortic valve disease not detailed in Chapters 11 and 13.

Tricuspid valve disease may be associated with various conditions discussed in other chapters, including atrioventricular canal defect, in Chapter 19; ventricular septal defect (straddling tricuspid valve), in Chapter 20; congenital pulmonary atresia and intact ventricular septum, in Chapter 25; Ebstein's disease, in Chapter 27; and right atrial myxomas, in Chapter 50. Various rare examples of isolated tricuspid valve disease of surgical significance are not discussed, including tricuspid valve dysfunction secondary to chronic cor pulmonale,[K2,K3] inferior myocardial infarction,[C2,M3,Z1] the administration of methysergide,[B2] scleroderma,[S3] lupus erythematosus,[G1] and hypereosinophilic syndrome.[C3,S4,V1]

MORPHOLOGY

Because of the infrequency of tricuspid valve disease, and the paucity of specific information about it, some comments about diagnosis, indications, and treatment are included in this section.

Tricuspid Valve Endocarditis

Acute tricuspid valve endocarditis is rare and appears to be nearly confined to persons habitually engaged in the intravenous self-administration of drugs.[A1] The organism most commonly involved is *Pseudomonas aeruginosa,* and the second commonest is *Staphylococcus aureus.* A variety of gram-negative bacilli may be involved. Rarely, *Candida albicans* is the infective agent.

When endocarditis develops, tricuspid valve function is usually rapidly destroyed, and the classic signs and symptoms of tricuspid valve incompetence develop. Frequently, pulmonary symptoms and signs secondary to septic pulmonary emboli are marked.[R1] The illness is usually only 1–3 weeks in duration before the presentation of the patient for medical care.

The *diagnosis* can be strongly suspected from a history of drug abuse, evidence of systemic infection, elevated jugular venous pressure, pulsatile neck veins, and pulsatile liver. These features, combined with positive results of blood cultures (often in those taken from the right ventricle or pulmonary artery) and echocardiography,[K1] are usually sufficient to establish the diagnosis.

Because of the high incidence of recurrence of the situation leading to the original infection, most replacement devices inserted in the tricuspid position become reinfected and fail. Therefore, the infected valve is excised to control the infection, and no replacement device is inserted.[A2,A3,M1,S1,W1]

In view of the total absence of tricuspid valve function, the right atrial pressure must be kept high (20–25 mmHg) in the early postoperative period.

The *hospital mortality* of this simple operation carries a significant risk because of the important residual hemodynamic defect. Thus, 6 (10%, CL 6%–15%) of 61 cases collected in a recent report died in hospital after operation,[A1] a higher risk than that of single or double left-sided valve replacement.

The *late results* are of course those of persistent free tricuspid incompetence. Willerson and colleagues, in Dallas, found both early and late postoperatively that such patients are unable to increase cardiac output with exercise and that, even with mild exercise, signs of elevated right atrial pressure, fatigue, and, interestingly, tachypnea develop.[W2] It is surprising that many such patients can survive and manage reasonably well, at least for 5–10 years.[A1] However, within this period, at least 20% require tricuspid valve replacement to control these symptoms.[A1]

The *indications* for tricuspid valve excision without replacement are tricuspid valve endocarditis in habitually drug-abusing patients or in any other uncommon situation in which reinfection seems inevitable. Once this risk is removed, tricuspid replacement is indicated.

Traumatic Rupture of the Tricuspid Valve

Tricuspid incompetence is an uncommon result of severe, nonpenetrating chest injury, and in this setting is due to rupture of one or more of the papillary muscles or chordae of the tricuspid valve. Usually it is the anterior tricuspid leaflet that becomes flail. In patients who survive the initial trauma, the tricuspid incompetence, despite the fact that it is severe, may be tolerated for many months or years.[B1,M2] This is an example of the much slower development of the deleterious effects of ventricular volume overload on the right side of the heart compared with the left. (Other examples include atrial septal defect and natural or iatrogenically produced severe pulmonary valvular incompetence.)

The *diagnosis* of tricuspid incompetence after injury is usually easily established by the presence of signs of severe tricuspid incompetence (see "Clinical Features and Diagnostic Criteria"). Occasionally, the relationship of these findings to a history of injury is not obvious, and since in patients with tricuspid incompetence, right-to-left shunting may occur across a patent foramen ovale, the diagnosis of Ebstein's malformation may be mistakenly made.

The *natural history* of surgically untreated severe tricuspid incompetence of traumatic or other origin is as inevitably unfavorable as that of severe left-sided atrioventricular valve incompetence. However, rather than a 2–5-year progression to severe disability or death, in patients with severe isolated tricuspid incompetence, the interval is frequently 5–10 years.[B1,M2,S2]

Treatment consists of tricuspid valve replacement. The results are those of tricuspid valve replacement in general.

Carcinoid Tricuspid Valve Disease

The rare carcinoid tumors originate from Kulchitsky's cells in the gastrointestinal tract, which produce serotoxin (*t*-hydroxytryptamine), a substance inactivated in the liver. However, carcinoid tumors that metastasize to the liver produce serotoxin there; and in carcinoid tricuspid valve disease, the powerful substance passes into the pulmonary and to a lesser extent (since a good deal of it is inactivated in the lungs) the systemic circulation. Thereby, the carcinoid syndrome may be produced, with bronchospasm, diarrhea, nausea, malabsorption, flushing, and telangiectasia.

Although the mechanism is not entirely clear, these patients also develop cicatricial deformity of the tricuspid and pulmonary valves. Carpena and colleagues describe the tricuspid commissures as fused, the chordae tendinae as thickened and fused, and the leaflets as thickened and shortened.[C1] Both tricuspid stenosis and incompetence result. Microscopically, a deposition of loose or compact fibrous tissue can be seen on both surfaces of the tricuspid leaflets.

When symptoms of the tricuspid disease become severe, tricuspid valve replacement is indicated. Probably a prosthesis (rather than a heterograft or homograft) is the proper replacement device in this setting.

Palliation has been good in the few patients in whom replacement (sometimes accompanied by pulmonary valvotomy) has been accomplished.[H1,H2]

Tricuspid Valve Disease in Multivalvular Disease

Tricuspid valve disease, including incompetence, stenosis and incompetence, and, uncommonly, stenosis alone, are most commonly associated with rheumatic involvement of the mitral valve, the mitral and aortic valves combined, or, rarely, the aortic valve alone. The tricuspid valve disease in this circumstance may be rheumatic in origin, but at other times it appears to be functional and the result of right ventricular dilation. Tsakiris and colleagues and Tei and colleagues have shown that the tricuspid anulus shortens during systole when the tricuspid valve is competent.[T1,T2] When right ventricular dilation develops, the anulus dilates and the tricuspid fails to shorten during systole.[U1] In patients with severe tricuspid incompetence preoperatively that persists after isolated mitral valve replacement, the failure of the tricuspid annular shortening has no doubt persisted. However, in many patients requiring tricuspid valve surgery for incompetence late after mitral valve operations, the tricuspid incompetence initially was mild. Thus, King and colleagues have reported that 66% of patients returning for tricuspid valve surgery late after mitral valve replacement had only mild tricuspid valve insufficiency at the time of the initial valve operation.[K4] This course of events is related in some patients to failure of the mitral valve operation, as evidenced by the fact that concomitant mitral valve surgery was necessary in 53% of the patients reported by King and colleagues[K4] (see also "Reoperation" in section on Late Results). Some other aspects of these matters are discussed in conjunction with a presentation of the results of mitral valve surgery (see Chapter 11, "Prognosis of Surgically Untreated Tricuspid Incompetence" in section on Late Results).

CLINICAL FEATURES AND DIAGNOSTIC CRITERIA

Moderate degrees of *tricuspid stenosis* can be overlooked, particularly if the patient is in atrial fibrillation. If sinus rhythm is present, there will be a dominant *a* wave in the jugular venous pulse (immediately preceding the carotid pulse). Other signs include a mid-diastolic, often high-pitched murmur maximal over the lower left sternal edge that increases on inspiration; and there may be a tricuspid opening snap. The murmur may be confused with an aortic early diastolic murmur (as its timing may be relatively early) or with a conducted mitral diastolic murmur. The liver is enlarged but not pulsatile (unless, as rarely occurs, from a very forceful atrial contraction when a presystolic pulse is felt).

The history and physical signs are sufficient to establish the diagnosis of important *tricuspid incompetence*. The jugular venous pulse shows a dominant fused c and v wave followed by a sharp, deep *y* descent. The murmur is pansystolic and often high-pitched and increases on inspiration, and the enlarged liver shows systolic pulsation. In advanced cases, there are other signs of right heart failure, with peripheral edema and ascites. The mitral or aortic valve disease signs may confuse the findings, and severe right heart failure may of course occur under such conditions without tricuspid valve disease.

The chest x-ray shows right atrial enlargement, and the electrocardiogram shows a prominent P wave unless atrial fibrillation is present. Two-dimensional echocardiography is helpful in establishing the presence of leaflet thickening. Cardiac catheterization with simultaneous measurement of right atrial and right ventricular pressure identifies a diastolic gradient (> 4 mm) across the valve in cases of stenosis. Tricuspid incompetence can be demonstrated cineangiographically but is difficult to grade, and interpretation may be confounded by the intermittent slippage of the injection catheter through the valve. Doppler and color echocardiography may be helpful in estimating the amount of incompetence.

Final surgical evaluation of the tricuspid valve is made at the time of operation (see Chapter 11, "Mitral Valve Disease with Tricuspid Incompetence" in section on Special Situations and Controversies). In multivalve disease, this is particularly important, as occasionally even experienced observers may fail to recognize important disease preoperatively. The accuracy of the intraoperative evaluation may be improved by the use of contrast echocardiography.[G2]

TECHNIQUE OF OPERATION

Tricuspid valve *repair* is described previously in the discussion of mitral valve surgery (see Chapter 11, "Tricuspid Annuloplasty" in section on Technique of Operation and "Method of Tricuspid Annuloplasty" in section on Special Situations and Controversies). It usually entails the use of a Carpentier ring with or without valvotomy. Tricuspid valve *replacement* is also described in Chapter 11 but details are in the discussion of Ebstein's malformation (see Chapter 27, "Tricuspid Valve Replacement and Atrial Septal Defect Closure" in section on Technique of Operation).

SPECIAL FEATURES OF POSTOPERATIVE CARE

Chronic anticoagulation is used when a prosthetic valve has been used. Coumadin administration is begun on the evening of postoperative day 2 (see Chapter 11, "Special Features of Postoperative Care"). In most such patients, of course, there is an additional prosthetic valve in position in either mitral or aortic position or both, which also requires anticoagulation.

Because of the risk of the appearance of complete heart block in the latter part of the hospital stay, electrocardiographic monitoring should be continued until a stable rhythm is established at an adequate heart rate.

EARLY RESULTS

Hospital Mortality

The hospital mortality of tricuspid valve surgery varies widely, and may be between 0%–33%.

Incremental Risk Factors for Hospital Death

Type of Operation
The simplest operation, tricuspid valve excision, has an appreciable mortality of 10% (6 of 61 cases,[H1] CL 6%–15%). Isolated tricuspid valve replacement or repair has a low hospital mortality (0% CL 0%–19%, Table 14-1).

Associated Cardiac Procedures
Tricuspid repair (annuloplasty) combined with mitral valve surgery has a hospital mortality of 5% (CL 3%–8%) in the current era, not evidently different from that of isolated tricuspid surgery (Table 14-1; see also Chapter 11, Table 11-5); also, tricuspid repair is not an incremental risk factor when added to the operation of mitral valve replacement (see Chapter 11, Table 11-8). Tricuspid repair combined with aortic and mitral valve surgery carries a variable and low risk of hospital death (Tables 14-1, 14-2; see also Chapter 13, Table 13-2). However, tricuspid repair is an incremental risk factor for a cardiac mode of hospital death (see Chapter 13, Table 13-6), an association more related to the type of patient requiring the procedure than to the procedure itself.

Tricuspid valve replacement, in combination with mitral and/or aortic valve surgery, carries a variable risk. When a mechanical valve or a heterograft prosthesis is used in combination with mitral and/or aortic valve replacement, the mortality may be as high as 33% (see Chapter 13, Table 13-2). When a stent-mounted large homograft aortic or pulmonary valve is used for the tricuspid replacement in combination with mitral and/or aortic valve surgery, the mortality has been 6%, no different from that of annuloplasty (Table 14-1).

Tricuspid valve surgery in association with aortic valve surgery (without mitral valve surgery) has carried a high mortality (Table 14-1). This may partly be related to the older age of the patients with this combination (Table 14-3) and also to the fact that this unusual combination always signifies advanced aortic valve disease. Mortality may also be increased by other associated nonvalve procedures (Table 14-1).

Table 14-1 Hospital death after tricuspid valve surgery for acquired tricuspid valve disease (GLH; 1965–1982; n = 246 operations in 230 patients).

	1965–1973				1973–1982												Total			
	TV Replacement				TV Replacement				TV Annuloplasty				Total							
Category of Patient		Hospital Deaths				Hospital Deaths				Hospital Deaths				Hospital Deaths				Hospital Deaths		
	n	No.	%	CL	n	No.	%	CL	n	No.	%	CL	n	No.	%	CL	n	No.	%	CL
TVS alone	3	0	0%	0%–47%	5	0	0%	0%–32%	1	0	0%	0%–85%	6	0	0%	0%–27%	9	0	0%	0%–19%
TVS + MVS	30	10	33%	24%–44%	39	2	5%	2%–12%	80	4	5%	3%–9%	119	6	5%	3%–8%	149	16	11%	8%–14%
TVS + MVS + AVS	12	5	42%	25%–60%	17	1	6%	0.8%–19%	32	2	6%	2%–14%	49	3	6%	3%–12%	61	8	13%	9%–19%
TVS + AVS	1	0	0%	0%–85%	1	1	100%	85%–100%	2	1	50%	7%–93%	3	2	67%	24%–96%	4	2	50%	18%–82%
TVS + excision AAA[a]									2	1	50%	7%–93%	2	1	50%	7%–93%	2	1	50%	7%–93%
TVS + MVS + CABG									5	1	20%	3%–53%	5	1	20%	3%–53%	5	1	20%	3%–53%
Total	46	15	33%	25%–41%	62	4	6%	3%–11%	122	9	7%	5%–11%	184	13	7.1%	5.1%–9.6%	230	28	12%	10%–15%
$P(\chi^2)$		.5				.002				.03				.0002				.08		

KEY: AAA, ascending aortic aneurysm; AVS, aortic valve surgery; CABG, coronary artery bypass graft; CL, 70% confidence limits; MVS, mitral valve surgery; TVS, tricuspid valve surgery; TV, tricuspid valve.

NOTE: The replacement device was a stented homograft semilunar valve in 91 operations, a porcine bioprosthesis in 20, and a prosthesis in 9. Tricuspid annuloplasty (not done before 1973) was by the De Vega method in 18 operations and by a Carpentier ring in 108.

[a] One also had aortic valve replacement; one aortic valve replacement with mitral valve replacement.

Table 14-2 Tricuspid valve surgery as part of simultaneous multivalve operations (GLH; 1973–1982).

		Hospital Deaths		
Type of Surgery	n	No.	%	CL
Triple valve replacement	13	1	8%	1%–24%
Double valve replacement + repair of third valve	31	1	3%	0.4%–11%
Single valve replacement + repair of two other valves	6	1	17%	2%–46%
Double valve replacement	44	3	7%	3%–13%
Single valve replacement + repair of one other valve	78	7	9%	6%–14%
Double valve repair	18	0	0%	0%–10%
Total	190	13	6.8%	4.9%–9.3%
$P(\chi^2)$		0.6		

KEY: CL, 70% confidence limits.

Clinical Condition of the Patient

Older age is probably an incremental risk factor for tricuspid valve surgery (Table 14-3). Likewise, the hospital mortality is higher in patients with advanced disability (Table 14-4), as it is in other operations for valvular disease, an association also found by Baughman and colleagues.[B3] These investigators also found pulmonary artery hypertension to be a risk factor.[B3]

Complete Heart Block

Rarely at operation, but in about 5% of patients within the first 5 postoperative weeks, complete heart block develops after tricuspid valve surgery, or a very slow ventricular response continues in patients who remain in atrial fibrillation or junctional rhythm (see "Late Complete Heart Block" in section on Late Results).

Table 14-3 The relationship between age at operation and hospital death after tricuspid valve surgery (GLH; 1973–1982; n = 198 operations in 184 patients).

Age (yr)		TV Alone				TV + MV				TV + MV + AV				TV + AV				Total			
			Hospital Deaths				Hospital Deaths				Hospital Deaths				Hospital Deaths				Hospital Deaths		
≤	<	n	No.	%	CL	n	No.	%	CL	n	No.	%	CL	n	No.	%	CL	n	No.	%	CL
	10					1	0	0%	0%–85%	1	0	0%	0%–85%					2	0	0%	0%–61%
10	20					21	1	5%	0.6%–15%	11	1	9%	1%–28%					32	2	6%	2%–14%
20	30	2	0	0%	0%–61%	32	1	3%	0.4%–10%	12	1	8%	1%–26%	1	0	0%	0%–85%	47	2	4%	1%–10%
30	40	1	0	0%	0%–85%	30	0	0%	0%–6%	11	1	9%	1%–28%	2	0	0%	0%–61%	44	1	2%	0.3%–8%
40	50	3	0	0%	0%–47%	19	1	5%	0.7%–17%	5	1	20%	2.6%–53%					27	2	7%	2%–17%
50	60					14	1	7%	0.9%–22%	6	0	0%	0%–27%					20	1	5%	0.6%–16%
60	70	1	0	0%	0%–85%	16	3	19%	8%–34%	5	0	0%	0%–32%	1	1	100%	85%–100%	23	4	17%	9%–29%
70	80					2	0	0%	0%–61%					1	1	100%	85%–100%	3	1	33%	4%–76%
Total		7	0	0%	0%–24%	135	7	5.2%	3.2%–8.0%	51	4	8%	4%–14%	5	2	40%	14%–71%	198	13	6.6%	4.7%–8.9%
$P(\chi^2)$							.32				9				.17				.09 (logistic)		

KEY: AV, aortic valve surgery; CL, 70% confidence limits; MV, mitral valve surgery; TV, tricuspid valve surgery.

Table 14-4 The relationship between hospital mortality and NYHA class after isolated or multivalve tricuspid valve surgery in two eras (GLH; 1965–1982; *n* = 246 operations).

| | 1965–1973 | | | | 1973–1982 | | | | Total | | | |
| | Hospital Deaths | | | | Hospital Deaths | | | | Hospital Deaths | | | |
NYHA Class	n	No.	%	CL	n	No.	%	CL	n	No.	%	CL
I												
II					1	0	0%	0%–85%	1	0	0%	0%–85%
III	1	0	0%	0%–85%	18	1	6%	0.7%–18%	19	1	5%	0.7%–17%
IV	30	5	17%	9%–27%	109	2	1.8%	0.6%–4.3%	139	7	5%	3.1%–7.7%
V[a]	17	10	59%	43%–73%	70	10	14%	10%–20%	87	20	23%	18%–29%
Total	48	15	31%	24%–40%	198	13	6.6%	4.7%–8.9%	246	28	11%	9%–14%
P(logistic)		.004				.01				.003		

KEY: CL, 70% confidence limits.

NOTE: Multivariate logistic test for era and NYHA class: P(era) = .0001
P(NYHA) = .0002

[a]Includes patients requiring hospitalization and intense decongestive therapy for up to 4 weeks preoperatively because of gross heart failure. Among the 87 class V patients, 22 required emergency operation.

LATE RESULTS

Survival

Premature late death in patients who have undergone operations on the tricuspid valve, most of whom have undergone multivalve procedures, occurs with about the same frequency as after other operations for multivalvular disease. Thus, the 9-year actuarial survival rate for patients after tricuspid valve replacement has been 52% (Fig. 14-1) and after either tricuspid valve replacement or repair 55% (Fig. 14-2). Survival rates are similar after tricuspid procedures as a part of a single, double, and triple valve operation.

Mode of Premature Late Death

Following tricuspid valve surgery, most late deaths are related to advanced ventricular dysfunction or arrhythmias.

Endocarditis and cerebrovascular accidents are uncommon causes. Recurrent moderate or severe tricuspid stenosis or incompetence due to malfunction of the replacement devices or failed annuloplasty are uncommon causes of late death. Thus, in the combined GLH-UAB late follow-up, the incidence of these complications related to the tricuspid valve repair or replacement was similar and accounted for 9 (11%, CL 8%–16%) of the late deaths, or a 3.2% (CL 2%–5%) mortality from them among the 284 patients followed over a period of nearly 10 years.

Functional Status

The late functional status of most patients undergoing tricuspid valve surgery is influenced more by the multivalvular nature of most of the procedures than by the tricuspid repair or replacement itself. Nonetheless, most patients are considerably improved by the surgical procedure. Thus, in both the GLH and UAB follow-up groups, 42% were in New York

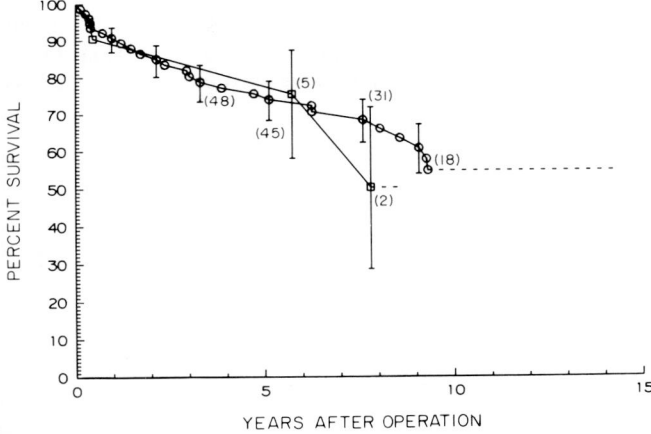

Figure 14-1 Actuarial survival of patients leaving the hospital alive after tricuspid valve replacement (UAB). The squares represent patients having only tricuspid valve replacement (*n* = 21). The circles represent patients having tricuspid and mitral valve replacement with or without aortic valve replacement (*n* = 77) (UAB; 1967–1981).

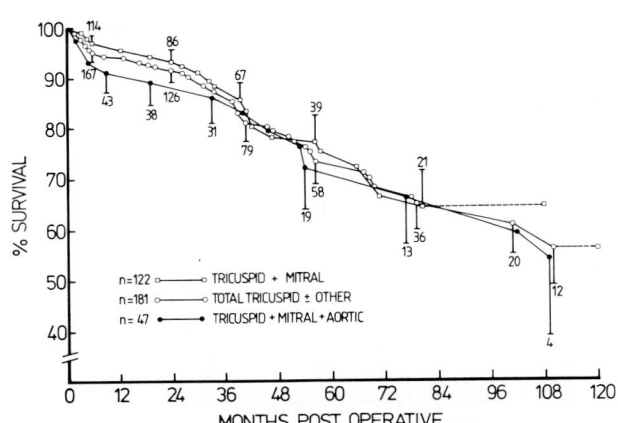

Figure 14-2 Actuarial survival of patients leaving the hospital alive after tricuspid valve surgery (replacement or repair) with or without other valve surgery (GLH; 1965–1982; *n* = 193 operations in 181 traced patients).

Table 14-5 NYHA class at last follow-up compared to preoperative NYHA class in patients undergoing tricuspid valve surgery with or without other valve or nonvalve cardiac surgery (GLH; 1965–1982; maximum follow-up 10 years; mean 46 months, SD ± 35.7).

NYHA Class at Follow-Up	Preoperative NYHA Class					
	Total	I	II	III	IV	V
I	103	0	1	6	62	34
II	32	0	0	6	16	10
III	12	0	0	1	7	4
IV	33	0	0	2	22	9
V	5	0	0	0	2	3
NA	61	0	0	4	30	27
Total	246	0	1	19	139	87

KEY: NA, hospital death or untraced.

Heart Association (NYHA) class I late postoperatively. This is more impressive when it is realized that, of the 103 patients in class I late postoperatively, 34 were preoperatively in class V, 62 in class IV, and 6 in class III (GLH; Table 14-5). In both series, less than 15% were in class IV late postoperatively.

Late Complete Heart Block

Complete heart block occasionally develops late after tricuspid valve replacement operations and occurred in 6 (6%, CL 3%–9%) of 108 patients (GLH). Five of the 6 patients had associated mitral valve replacement, and the association of delayed development of complete heart block with combined mitral and tricuspid valve replacement has also been observed at UAB. This association is undoubtedly related to the interposition of the atrioventricular node between the two replacement devices. In all, about 10% of patients (UAB, GLH) receiving both tricuspid and mitral replacement required insertion of a pacemaker late postoperatively because of heart block (Table 14-6), and up to 10 years postoperatively the actuarial incidence is 25% (Fig. 14-3). None of the patients (UAB, GLH) receiving tricuspid replacement as an isolated procedure had this complication (P for difference = .16). The late development of complete heart block

is uncommon after tricuspid annuloplasty, this occurring in 2 (1.6%, CL 0.5%–4%) of 122 patients undergoing tricuspid annuloplasty procedures (GLH).

Pulmonary Embolization

As a complication of tricuspid valve surgery, pulmonary embolization is rare. Only 1 of 106 patients had probable large pulmonary emboli on follow-up (UAB); since that patient had also deep vein thrombophlebitis in one leg, it is not certain that the emboli originated from the tricuspid replacement device.

Symptoms of Systemic Venous Hypertension

The majority of patients remain free of systemic venous hypertension late postoperatively. However, peripheral edema and hepatomegaly, with or without ascites, were present at follow-up in 28 (29%) of 97 patients after tricuspid replacement with mechanical or bioprostheses in whom these features were assessed (UAB). These symptoms could be the results of either a functional or an organic obstruction of the tricuspid replacement device, of residual left-sided cardiac failure with or without left-sided valvular disease, or of important residual pulmonary hypertension (high pulmonary vascular resistance). In this regard Silver and colleagues report higher right atrial pressures after tricuspid valve replacement than before in patients with Ebstein's anomaly, but also marked symptomatic improvement in cardiac function.[S6]

Reoperation

Most patients who have undergone tricuspid valve replacement are free of the need for reoperation up to 10 years later. Thus, 96% of patients receiving mechanical prostheses or heterograft valves are free of tricuspid reoperation at 5 years, and 89% at 9 years (Fig. 14-4). The proportions are not significantly different when stent-mounted homograft semilunar valves are used (Table 14-7); actuarially, about 80% are reoperation free 8 years postoperatively (Fig. 14-5).

Reoperation for tricuspid valve dysfunction may be less

Table 14-6 Late results of tricuspid valve replacement (UAB; 1967–1981; n = 106 in 103 patients).

Category of Patient	Hospital Survivors (n)	Late Death			Reoperation for TV Problem			Late Pacemaker Insertion[a]		
		No.	%	CL	No.	%	CL	No.	% of n	CL
TVR alone	21	4	19%	10%–32%	2	10%	3%–21%	0/20	0%	0%–9%
TVR + MVR	34	11	32%	23%–44%	1	3%	0.4%–10%	3/32	9%	4%–18%
TVR + MVR + AVR	43	15	35%	27%–44%	1	2%	0.3%–8%	3/40	8%	3%–15%
TVR + other[b]	5	2	40%	14%–71%	1	20%	3%–53%	0/5	0%	0%–32%
Total	103	32	31%	26%–36%	5	5%	3%–8%	6/97	6%	4%–10%

KEY: AVR, aortic valve replacement; CL, 70% confidence limits; MVR, mitral valve replacement; PVR, pulmonary valve replacement; TV, tricuspid valve; TVR, tricuspid valve replacement.

NOTE: The median follow-up time was 7.0 years (6.6 months to 14.4 years); the median age at operation was 43 years (5.7–76 years).

[a] n = 97 for hospital survivors without pacemakers. In addition, two patients had pacemakers preoperatively, and four had pacemakers implanted during initial hospitalization (three were TVR + MVR + AVR, one was TVR + MVR).

[b] Two patients had TVR + AVR, two had TVR + orthotopic or heterotopic PVR, and one had TVR + AVR + PVR.

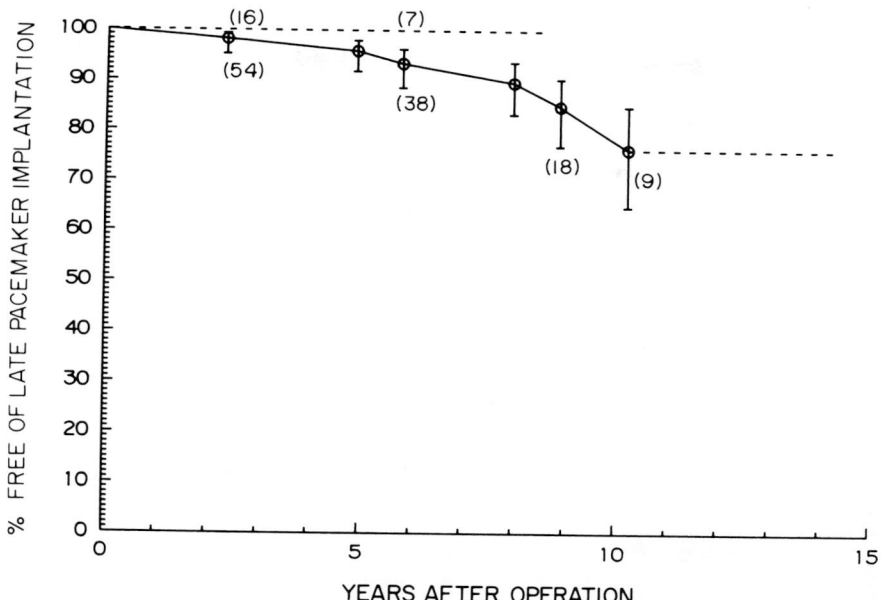

Figure 14-3 Actuarial analysis of the percent of patients free of pacemaker implantation late postoperatively. The circles represent patients undergoing tricuspid and mitral valve replacement with or without aortic replacement, who left the hospital alive without a pacemaker (*n* = 73 traced patients). The dashed lines represent those undergoing only tricuspid valve replacement (*n* = 20 traced patients) (UAB; 1967–1981).

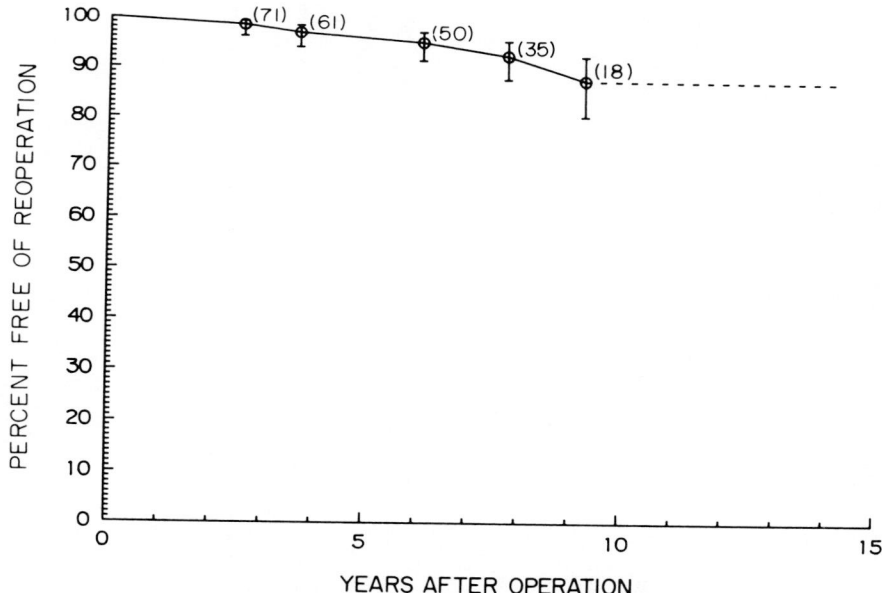

Figure 14-4 Actuarial analysis of the percent of patients free of tricuspid reoperation after tricuspid valve replacement (UAB; 1967–1981; *n* = 98).

Table 14-7 Incidence of tricuspid valve dysfunction at late follow-up after tricuspid valve surgery (GLH; 1965–1982).

Device Used and Type of Dysfunction	n	Recurrent Tricuspid Dysfunction									Reoperation[a]			Associated Lesions								
		Severe			Moderate			Total						MVD			AVD			PH		
		No.	%	CL	No.	%	CL	No.	%	CL	No.	%	CL	No.	%	CL	No.	%	CL	No.	%	CL
Homograft valve,[b]	75	15	20%	15%–26%	3	4%	2%–8%	18	24%	19%–30%	12	16%	12%–22%	10	13%	9%–19%	2	2.7%	0.9%–6.2%	5	7%	4%–11%
incompetence and		14	19%	14%–24%	3	4%	2%–8%	17	23%	17%–29%	11	15%	10%–20%	10	13%	9%–19%	2	2.9%	0.9%–6.2%	5	7%	4%–11%
stenosis		1*	1.3%	0.2%–4.5%	0	0%	0%–2.6%	1	1.3%	0.2%–4.5%	1	1.3%	0.2%–4.5%	0	0%	0%–2.6%	0	0%	0%–2.6%	0	0%	0%–2.6%
Carpentier Ring, incompetence[d]	84	5	6%	3%–10%	5	6%	3%–10%	10	12%	8%–17%	3	6%	3%–10%	3	6%	3%–10%	0	0%	0%–2.3%	1	1.2%	0.2%–4.0%
De Vega repair, incompetence[e]	14	0	0%	0%–13%	0	0%	0%–13%	0	0%	0%–13%	0	0%	0%–13%	0	0%	0%–13%	0	0%	0%–13%	0	0%	0%–13%
Porcine valve, stenosis[f]	15	1	7%	0.9%–21%	0	0%	0%–12%	1	7%	0.9%–21%	1	7%	0.9%–21%	1	7%	0.9%–21%	0	0%	0%–12%	0	0%	0%–12%
Bjork-Shiley valve, stenosis[g]	3	1	33%	4%–76%	0	0%	0%–47%	1	33%	4%–76%	0	0%	0%–47%	0	0%	0%–47%	0	0%	0%–47%	1	0%	0%–47%
Braunwald-Cutter valve, stenosis	1	0	0%	0%–85%	1	100%	15%–100%	1	100%	15%–100%	0	0%	0%–85%	0	0%	0%–85%	0	0%	0%–85%	0	0%	0%–85%
Star-Edwards valve, stenosis	1	0	0%	0%–85%	0	0%	0%–85%	0	0%	0%–85%	0	0%	0%–85%	0	0%	0%–85%	0	0%	0%–85%	0	0%	0%–85%
Total	193	22	11%	9%–14%	9	4.7%	3.1%–6.8%	31	16%	13%–19%	16	8.3%	6.2%–10.9%	14	7.3%	5.3%–9.7%	2	1.0%	0.3%–2.4%	7	3.6%	2.3%–5.6%
$P(\chi^2)$															.3			.8			.06	

KEY: AVD, aortic valve disease; CL, 70% confidence limits; MVD, mitral valve disease; PH, pulmonary hypertension.

NOTE: An associated lesion is one present when the tricuspid valve dysfunction was identified late postoperatively. This was either native aortic or mitral valve disease not evident or mild at the time of tricuspid valve surgery or malfunction or failure of the repair or replacement of one of those valves performed at the time of tricuspid valve surgery. Late postoperatively, the mitral valve disease was severe in two patients, moderate in six, and mild in six. Aortic valve disease was severe incompetence in both. In three of the seven patients with residual severe pulmonary hypertension, it was not associated with residual left-sided valve disease.

[a] On the tricuspid valve.
[b] Duration of follow-up 67 ± 41.5 mo.
[c] Valve diameter 23 mm.
[d] Duration of follow-up 35 ± 24.2 mo.
[e] Duration of follow-up 20 ± 11.8 mo.
[f] Duration of follow-up 31 ± 18.1 mo.
[g] Duration of follow-up 34 ± 27.7 mo.

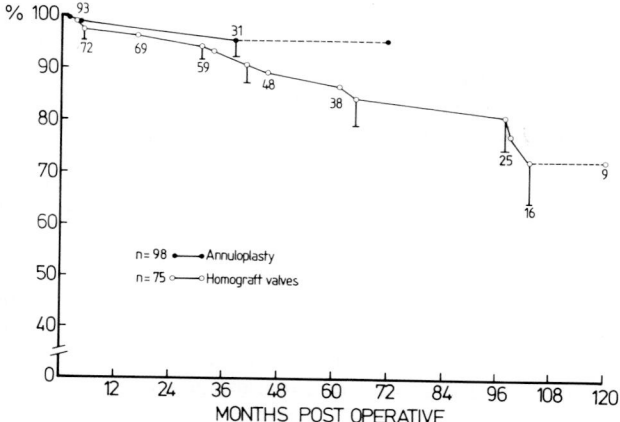

Figure 14-5 Actuarial analysis of the percent of patients free of tricuspid reoperation after tricuspid valve repair or replacement with stent-mounted homograft semilunar valves (GLH; 1965–1982; n = 173).

frequent following annuloplasty, 97% of this group being free of reoperation 3 years postoperatively (Fig. 14-5).

Tricuspid Valve Function after Repair or Replacement

Annuloplasty

At least with the Carpentier ring technique, annuloplasty of the tricuspid valve has good results on intermediate term follow-up in most patients (GLH; Table 14-7), with an actuarial absence of recurrent incompetence in 87% of patients at 3 years postoperatively (Fig. 14-6). At the time of reoperation in 3 of these patients, the Carpentier ring, sewn in with a continuous suture, had partly dehisced. Carpentier and colleagues found late postoperatively that no tricuspid incompetence was present in 17 (68%, CL 56%–79%) of 25 patients with preoperatively moderate or severe tricuspid incompetence, and mild incompetence in 7 (28%, CL 18%–40%).

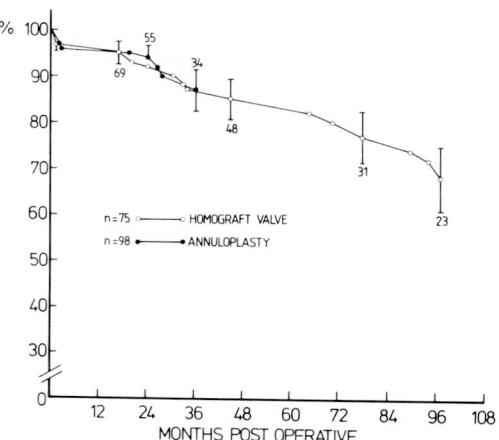

Figure 14-6 Actuarial analysis of the percent of patients free of significant (moderate and severe) tricuspid valve dysfunction after stented semilunar homograft valve replacement and tricuspid Carpentier or De Vega annuloplasty (GLH; 1965–1982; n = 173).

Only 1 patient had moderate incompetence late postoperatively, and that patient had severe incompetence preoperatively.[C4] A small experience with the De Vega annuloplasty (GLH; 18 patients) has also had good results (Table 14-7).

However, there are risk factors for persisting tricuspid incompetence after repair. Thus, recurrence is more likely when recurrent mitral disease or severe residual pulmonary hypertension coexist (Table 14-7). Duran and colleagues found that when functional tricuspid incompetence was repaired, 31 (89%, CL 80%–94%) of 35 patients with low late postoperative pulmonary vascular resistance (< 6 units · m^2) had no tricuspid regurgitation, while this was true of only 6 (43%, CL 27%–60%) of 14 patients with high pulmonary vascular resistance (P [Fisher] $= .001$).[D1]

Stent-mounted Aortic and Pulmonary Homograft Valves

No gradient is present across stent-mounted aortic and pulmonary homograft valves (Fig. 14-7), in contrast to the other types of tricuspid replacement devices. At GLH, 80% of the stent-mounted homograft valves have been pulmonary and 20% aortic, and the two behave similarly. Eighty-eight per-

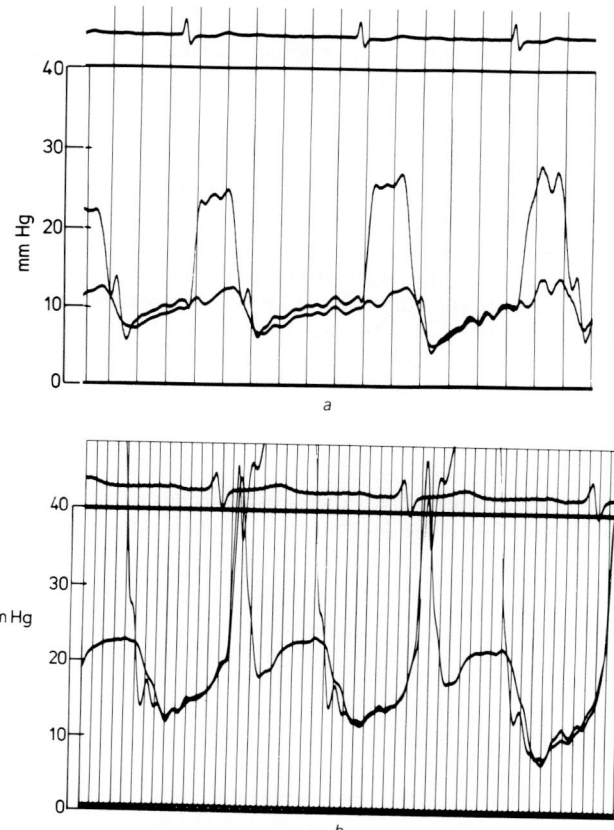

Figure 14-7 Simultaneous right ventricular–right atrial pressure curves in two patients at follow-up cardiac catheterization following tricuspid valve replacement with stented homograft semilunar valves (GLH). Both tracings show equalization of right ventricular diastolic and right atrial pressures.
(a) Pulmonary homograft valve on 30-mm stent.
(b) Aortic homograft valve on 30-mm stent.

Table 14-8 Causes of incompetence in 12 patients among 75 receiving stent-mounted aortic and pulmonary homograft valves in the tricuspid position and followed for a mean of 48 months (maximum 168 months) (GLH; 1970–1982).

Cause of Incompetence	n	% of 12	Comment
Bacterial endocarditis	3	25	Left-sided valves infected in all three
Perivalvar leak	1	8	Present from time of insertion; reoperation at 2/12 years
Leaflet rupture	4	33	Leaflet calcification in two (aged 38 and 60 years)
Retracted leaflets	3	25	Probably due to poor stent-mounting technique
Aortic wall detachment from stent post	1	8	Identical to that occurring with stented homograft in mitral position[H3]

cent of patients are free of homograft valve failure at 36 months after operation, and at 8 years postoperatively 69% are still free of valve dysfunction (Fig. 14-6). The causes of incompetence include leaflet rupture, retracted leaflets, and bacterial endocarditis (Table 14-8). Thirteen of the 17 instances of tricuspid valve failure occurred when important left-sided valve disease or residual pulmonary hypertension was also present (Table 14-7).

Stent-mounted Heterograft Valves
Presumably, gradients of 4–10 mmHg exist across the stent-mounted heterograft valve in the tricuspid position. These bioprostheses seem to degenerate at about the same rate and with the same age-related incidence in the tricuspid position as they do in the mitral and aortic positions (see Chapter 11, Fig. 11-29). In the combined UAB-GLH experience with 33 bioprostheses in the tricuspid position, 3 patients have undergone reoperation, 2 of whom were less than 20 years of age and required reoperation at 2.6 and 3.7 years after insertion (Tables 14-7, 14-9).

Mechanical Prostheses
The Starr-Edwards ball valve prosthesis has performed well in the tricuspid position. Thus, only 1 of 46 patients required reoperation over a median follow-up period of 7 years (UAB;

Table 14-9). No instances of acute or recurrent occlusion or encapsulation were seen, although one Braunwald-Cutter valve required reoperation 8 years postoperatively for encapsulation (Table 14-9). The Bjork-Shiley valve has also performed well in the tricuspid position, although, as do all mechanical prostheses, it no doubt has a gradient in virtually all cases. One Bjork-Shiley valve required reoperation for thrombotic encapsulation (UAB) (Table 14-9). P'eterffy and Bjork reported this complication in two of five patients undergoing tricuspid valve replacement with this device.[P1] The St. Jude medical valve appears to exhibit optimal hemodynamic performance in the tricuspid position; Singh and colleagues reported no diastolic gradient in six patients with this device and a gradient of 2 mm in one patient.[S5]

INDICATIONS FOR OPERATION

Patients with isolated tricuspid valve disease should in general be operated on when their functional status is unsatisfactory (NYHA class III or IV). Information concerning the indications for operation in the various morphological subsets of isolated tricuspid valve disease is presented under the section on Morphology.

Tricuspid incompetence secondary to left heart disease can be severe, and the indications for its surgical treatment are given in Chapters 11 and 13 (see sections on Indications for Operation). Rheumatic tricuspid incompetence and/or stenosis is never isolated, but, rarely, only the tricuspid disease may require surgical treatment. The indications for this is functional disability equivalent to NYHA class III or IV.

It bears repeating that annuloplasty, rather than replacement, is indicated unless the leaflets are so distorted that competence cannot be achieved.

CHOICE OF TRICUSPID VALVE PROSTHESIS

When tricuspid replacement is necessary, a stent-mounted human semilunar valve seems to be ideal. Gradients are not present when a valve of at least 28 mm internal diameter is used. Premature degeneration in the young has not been

Table 14-9 Reoperations on tricuspid replacement device (UAB; 1967–1981).

Replacement Device	n[a]	Reoperation		Indication
		Age of Patient[b]	Interval[c] (yr)	
Starr-Edwards ball valve	46	43	9.3	Prosthetic valve endocarditis
Bjork-Shiley valve	23	39	6.1	Thrombotic encapsulation
Braunwald-Cutter ball valve	8	15	7.8	Thrombotic encapsulation
Heterograft valves	29	9	3.7	Heterograft degeneration
Heterograft valves	29	18	2.6	Heterograft degeneration

NOTE: Three reoperations were at UAB; three patients survived. Two reoperations elsewhere; both patients died at reoperation.

[a]Number of devices inserted into tricuspid position.

[b]Age (years) at initial valve replacement operation.

[c]Interval between initial replacement and re-replacement.

observed. Late malfunction has occurred no more frequently than with other devices and may be less. When this device is not available, a large heterograft valve may be used in pa-tients over about 50 years of age. In patients younger than this, a large St. Jude, Starr-Edwards, or Bjork-Shiley valve is indicated.

APPENDIX

APPENDIX **14A**
STENT-MOUNTING THE HUMAN SEMILUNAR VALVE

The method of valve collection trimming, and antibiotic sterilization and storage is detailed in Chapter 12, Appendix 12C. Large-diameter (> 28 mm) aortic and pulmonary valves are suitable.

The uncovered stents (Fig. 14A-1) are different in shape for the aortic and pulmonary valves. The covered stent is shown in Figure 14A-2. Metal stents are preferable, for a valve mounted on a metal stent can be deep-frozen with liquid nitrogen for permanent storage without altering the physical properties of the stent. The behavior of plastics after deep-freezing and thawing is uncertain, and a pliable plastic stent has no advantage in the low-pressure tricuspid position.

The valve chosen must be free of significant fenestrations at the commissures and other structural abnormalities. Dilated sinuses and large discrepancies between annular and commissural diameters make the valve unsuitable. Under meticulous aseptic technique, the selected valve is trimmed, with a scalloped upper margin 3 mm above the leaflets and a strictly transverse lower margin 2 mm below the nadir of each cusp. The myocardial remnants are trimmed to reduce their thickness to about 2 mm; using a shaving motion with a scalpel while inserting a finger through the valve to steady it is the easiest way to do this.

The valve is now fitted to a stent that has an internal diameter 2 mm larger than the internal diameter of the anulus of the valve. The leaflets are gently closed to confirm that there is adequate central leaflet coaptation. If the gap between the aortic wall and the stent is too wide, a smaller stent is substituted. It is important not to use too small a stent, since a valve that is cramped into a stent will be stenotic. The top of the valve commissures should be 2–3 mm below the top of each stent post, with each commissure in the middle of each stent post. The stent posts are asymmetric, in line with the usual valve geometry, and the valve is tried in various positions before deciding on the optimum siting of each commissure. When a good valve-to-stent fit is found, the valve is tacked in position with fine temporary sutures at the top of each post and beneath the nadir of each cusp.

The valve anulus is now sutured to the stent with a 5/0 polypropylene monofilament whip stitch. The stent is turned upright, and the

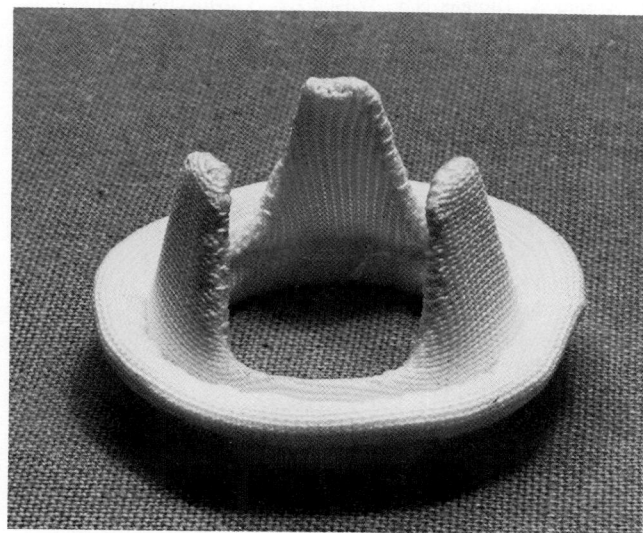

Figure 14A-2 Cloth-covered stent ready for the mounting of the aortic or pulmonary valve homograft.

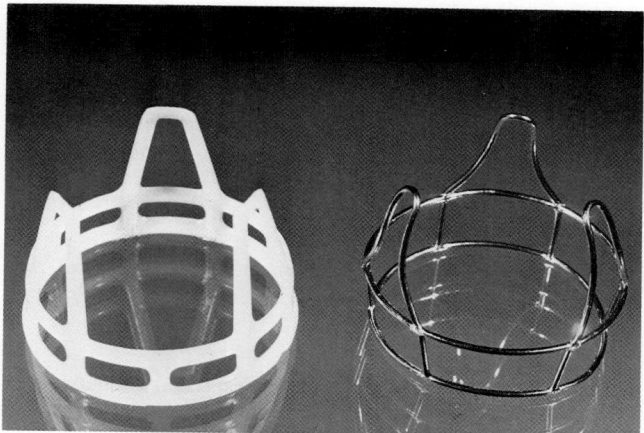

Figure 14A-1 Acetal copolymer pulmonary valve stent (left) and uncovered stainless steel aortic valve stent (right). The diameter of the anulus of the aortic valve stent is less than the remainder of the stent, while for the pulmonary valve it is slightly greater.

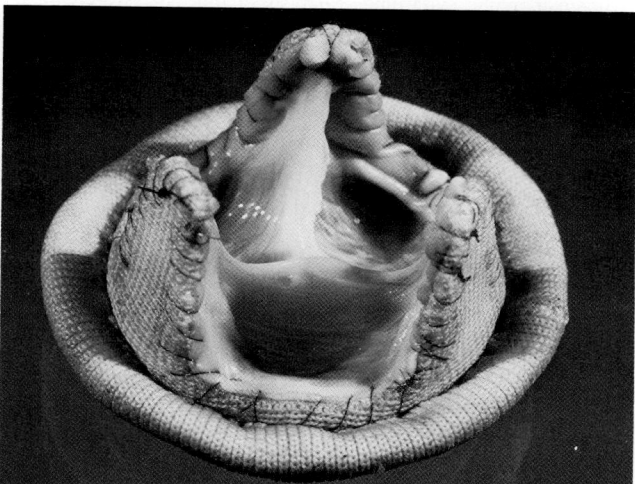

Figure 14A-3 The upper scalloped suture line is completed as a simple whip stitch.

leaflets are temporarily held closed by lightly packing with moist cotton wool. The aortic wall remnant usually requires further trimming with scissors, and the position of the commissures may need readjusting. One or two mattress sutures are placed to tack adventitia of the valve to the center of each stent post. The upper suture line is now completed as a simple whip stitch (Fig. 14A-3). More elaborate suturing is not recommended, since it weakens the relatively delicate aortic (or pulmonary) wall remnant of the valve.

The mounted valve is tested for competency by pouring Hanks'

solution through the valve into a Latex tube secured around the ring of the stent with a pipe cleaner. The tubing is squeezed to pressurize the leaflets. Incompetent valves must be remounted or discarded. Satisfactory valves are either stored in Hanks' solution at 4°C or deep-frozen.

All the aortic wall trimmings and some of the rinsing Hanks' solution are cultured. The valve should not be used until negative culture results are confirmed.

REFERENCES

A

1. Arbulu A, Asfaw I: Tricuspid valvulectomy without prosthetic replacement. *J Thorac Cardiovasc Surg* 82:684, 1981.

2. Arbulu A, Thomas NW, Wilson RF: Valvulectomy without replacement: A lifesaving operation for tricuspid Pseudomonas endocarditis. *J Thorac Cardiovasc Surg* 64:103, 1972.

3. Arneborn P, Bjork VO, Rodriguez L, Svanbom M: Two-stage replacement of tricuspid valve in active endocarditis. *Br Heart J* 39:1276, 1977.

B

1. Beasley K: Traumatic tricuspid insufficiency. *Tex Med* 69:71, 1973.

2. Barrillon A. Baragan J: Methysergide and tricuspid valve lesions. *Circulation* 58:578, 1978 (letter to the editor).

3. Baughman KL, Kallman CH, Yurchak PM, Daggett WM, Buckley MJ: Predictors of survival after tricuspid valve surgery. *Am J Cardiol* 54:137, 1984.

C

1. Carpena C, Kay JH, Mendez AM, Redington JV, Zubiate P, Zucker R: Carcinoid heart disease: Surgery for tricuspid and pulmonary valve lesions. *Am J Cardiol* 32:229, 1973.

2. Collins P, Daly JJ: Tricuspid incompetence complicating acute myocardial infarction. *Postgrad Med J* 53:51, 1977.

3. Chusid MJ, Dale DC, West BC, Wolffe SM: The hypereosinophilic syndrome: Analysis of fourteen cases with review of the literature. *Medicine* 54:1, 1975.

4. Carpentier A, Deloche A, Hanania G, Forman J, Sellier PH, Piwnica A, Dubost CH: Surgical management of acquired tricuspid valve disease. *J Thorac Cardiovasc Surg* 67:53, 1974.

D

1. Duran CMG, Pomar JL, Colman T, Figueroa A, Revuelta JM, Ubago JL: Is tricuspid valve repair necessary? *J Thorac Cardiovasc Surg* 80:849, 1980.

G

1. Gibson R, Wood P: The diagnosis of tricuspid stenosis. *Br Heart J* 17:552, 1955.

2. Goldman M, Mindich B, Guarino T, Fuster V: Intraoperative contrast echo: A new method to evaluate tricuspid regurgitation. *JACC* 5:459, 1985 (abstr).

H

1. Honey M, Paneth M: Carcinoid heart disease: Successful tricuspid valve replacement. *Thorax* 30:464, 1975.

2. Hendel N, Leckie B, Richards J: Carcinoid heart disease: Eight-year survival following tricuspid valve replacement and pulmonary valvotomy. *Ann Thorac Surg* 30:391, 1980.

3. Heng MK, Barratt-Boyes BG, Agnew TM, Brandt PWT, Kerr AR, Graham KG: Isolated mitral valve replacement with stent-mounted antibiotic-treated aortic allograft valves. *J Thorac Cardiovasc Surg* 74:230, 1977.

K

1. Kisslo J, Von Ramm OT, Haney R, Jones R, Juk SS, Behar VS: Echocardiographic evaluation of tricuspid valve endocarditis: An M-mode and two-dimensional study. *Am J Cardiol* 38:502, 1976.

2. Keller BD, Boal BH, Lewin A, Kaltman AJ: Development of tricuspid valvular regurgitation during the course of chronic cor pulmonale. *Chest* 57:196, 1970.

3. Khosla SN, Arora BS: Tricuspid incompetence in chronic cor pulmonale. *J Assoc Physicians India* 20:571, 1972.

4. King RM, Schaff HV, Danielson GK, Gersh BJ, Phil D, Orszulak TA, Piehler JM, Puga FJ, Pluth JR: Surgery for tricuspid regurgitation late after mitral valve replacement. *Circulation* 70(suppl I):I-193, 1984.

M

1. Michl L, Shumacker HB, Hobbs D: Tricuspid valvulectomy. *Surg Gynecol Obstet* 137:590, 1973.

2. Marvin RF, Schrank JP, Nolan SP: Traumatic tricuspid insufficiency. *Am J Cardiol* 32:723, 1973.

3. McAllister RG, Friesinger GC, Sinclair-Smith BC: Tricuspid regurgitation following inferior myocardial infarction. *Arch Intern Med* 136:95, 1976.

P

1. P'eterffy A, Bjork VO: Surgical treatment of Ebstein's anomaly. *Scand J Thorac Cardiovasc Surg* 13:1, 1979.

R

1. Reisberg BE: Infective endocarditis in the narcotic addict. *Prog Cardiovasc Dis* 22:193, 1979.

S

1. Sethia B, Williams BT: Tricuspid valve excision without replacement in a case of endocarditis secondary to drug abuse. *Br Heart J* 40:579, 1978.

2. Stephenson LW, MacVaugh H III, Kastor JA: Tricuspid valvular incompetence and rupture of the ventricular septum caused by nonpenetrating trauma. *J Thorac Cardiovasc Surg* 77:768, 1979.

3. Sackner MA, Heinz ER, Steinberg AJ: The heart in scleroderma. *Am J Cardiol* 17:542, 1966.

4. Solley GO, Maldonado JE, Gleich GJ, Giuliani ER, Hoagland HC, Pierre RV, Brown AL Jr: Endomyocardiopathy with eosinophilia. *Mayo Clin Proc* 51:697, 1976.

5. Singh AK, Christian FD, Williams DO, Georas CS, Riley RR, Nanian KB, Karlson KE: Follow-up assessment of St. Jude medical prosthetic valve in the tricuspid position: Clinical and hemodynamic results. *Ann Thorac Surg* 37:324, 1984.

6. Silver MA, Cohen SR, McIntosh CL, Cannon RO III, Roberts WC: Late (5 to 132 months) clinical and hemodynamic results after either tricuspid valve replacement or annuloplasty for Epstein's anomaly of the tricuspid valve. *Am J Cardiol* 54:627, 1984.

T

1. Tsakiris AG, Mair DD, Seki S, Titus JL, Wood EH: Motion of the tricuspid valve annulus in anesthetized intact dogs. *Circ Res* 36:43, 1975.

2. Tei C, Pilgrim JP, Shah PM, Ormiston JA, Wong M: The tricuspid valve annulus: study of size and motion in normal subjects and in patients with tricuspid regurgitation. *Circulation* 66:665, 1982.

U

1. Ubago JL, Figuero A, Ochoteco A, Colman T, Duran RM, Duran CG: Analysis of the amount of tricuspid valve anular dilatation required to produce functional tricuspid regurgitation. *Am J Cardiol* 52:155, 1983.

V

1. Van Slyck EJ, Adamson TC: Acute hypereosinophilic syndrome: Successful treatment with vincristine, cytarabine, and prednisone. *JAMA* 242:175, 1979.

W

1. Wright JS, Glennie JS: Excision of tricuspid valve with later replacement in endocarditis of drug addiction. *Thorax* 33:518, 1978.

2. Willerson JT: (1981) Personal communication.

Z

1. Zone DD, Botti RE: Right ventricular infarction with tricuspid insufficiency and chronic right heart failure. *Am J Cardiol* 37:445, 1976.

CONGENITAL HEART DISEASE

PART IV

15

ATRIAL SEPTAL DEFECT AND PARTIAL ANOMALOUS PULMONARY VENOUS CONNECTION

DEFINITION

An atrial septal defect (ASD) is a hole of variable size in the atrial septum. A patent foramen ovale that is functionally closed by the overlapping limbic tissue superiorly and the valve of the fossa ovalis inferiorly (in response to the normal left-to-right atrial pressure gradient) is excluded. Partial anomalous pulmonary venous connection (PAPVC) is a condition in which some but not all of the pulmonary veins of one or both lungs connect to the right atrium or its tributaries, rather than to the left atrium. ASDs generally allow left-to-right shunting at atrial level. PAPVCs may occur as isolated lesions or combined with ASDs. These two groups of anomalies are considered together in this chapter. Total anomalous pulmonary venous connection is considered in Chapter 16.

ASDs commonly occur in association with other cardiac anomalies, and these are considered in chapters dealing with those anomalies.

HISTORICAL NOTE

The clinical recognition of an ASD has been possible only in about the last 50 years. Thus, among the 62 recorded autopsy cases of ASD analyzed by Roesler in 1934, only one had been correctly diagnosed during life.[R1] By 1941, Bedford and colleagues were able to make the diagnosis clinically in a number of patients.[B4] When cardiac catheterization came into general use in the late 1940s and early 1950s, a secure diagnosis became possible. The first description of PAPVC is said to be that by Winslow[B7] in 1739 or Wilson in 1798.[M6] The first diagnosis of PAPVC during life appears to have been made by Dotter in 1949.[D6]

A number of ingenious closed methods for repair of ASDs and related conditions were proposed and studied experimentally in the very productive and expansive surgical era following the end of the World War II in 1945. Probably the first clinical trial was Murray's closure of an ASD in a child by external suturing in Toronto in 1948.[M3] Several other closed methods had clinical trials, including Bailey's atrio-septo-pexy[B3] and Søndergard's purse-string suture closure.[S2] However, the very limited applicability of these methods was always apparent, and they were soon discarded.

The technique of hypothermia induced by surface cooling and inflow stasis (see Chapter 2, "Historical Note") for the repair of ASDs was introduced in the early 1950s. Lewis and Taufic reported the first successful open repair of an ASD with this method in 1953.[L1] At about the same time, Gross invented the ingenious atrial well technique, a semiopen technique in which a rubber, open-bottomed well or cone was sutured to an incision in a clamp-exteriorized portion of the right atrial wall.[G3,K2] When the clamp was released, the blood rose into the well, and through this pool of blood, the surgeon could place sutures under direct or patch closure of the defect. Gibbon, in 1953, started the era of open heart surgery when he successfully repaired an ASD in a young woman using a pump-oxygenator.[G1] Although these three methods of hypothermia and inflow stasis, the atrial well, and cardiopulmonary bypass were all used in the late 1950s and gave similar early results, by the

late 1960s, almost all surgeons used cardiopulmonary bypass exclusively for these repairs.

The first reported treatment of any kind of PAPVC was by lobectomy in 1950.[D5] In that same year, Neptune and associates reported repair by a closed technique in 17 patients with PAPVC of the right lung to the right atrium associated with ASD.[N3] It is not certain who first repaired the sinus venosus syndrome, but the malformation was clearly illustrated by Bedford and Sellors in 1957.[B1] The repair of PAPVC to the inferior vena cava (IVC) performed by us at the Mayo Clinic in 1960 was described by Zubiate and Kay in 1962[Z1] and by us at UAB in 1971.[M9] The correction of anomalous connection of the left pulmonary veins to the left innominate vein and other forms of PAPVC was described by us in 1953[G5,K3] and later.[K6]

MORPHOLOGY

Types of Atrial Septal Defects

The normal atrial septum is illustrated from the right atrial (RA) side in Figure 1-1 (Chapter 1). Defects can occur nearly anywhere in this septum (Table 15-1). Although the morphology of these defects has been known since the early descriptions by Rokitansky,[R2] the advent of open heart surgery brought emphasis to their surgically important aspects. The paper by Lewis and colleagues[L4] and that by Bedford and colleagues[B1] are excellent examples of this (Fig. 15-1).

Fossa Ovalis Type of Atrial Septal Defect

The commonest atrial septal defect is the fossa ovalis type (also called a foramen ovale type or ostium secundum defect). This lies within the perimeter inscribed by the limbus anteriorly, superiorly, and posteriorly (Fig. 15-2). The smallest are essentially valvular incompetent foramina ovale, which occur beneath the superior limbus, between it and the valve (floor) of the fossa ovalis. The floor of the fossa ovalis (the remnant of the septum primum) may in this situation have multiple fenestrations of various sizes (Fig. 15-3). When more of the floor of the fossa ovalis is absent, a larger fossa ovalis defect is present. When all fossa ovalis tissue is absent, the ASD is confluent with the orifice of the inferior vena cava. The eustachian valve of the inferior vena cava then overhangs the ASD and must not be mistaken for its inferior edge at operation. The size of this type of ASD is

---

Table 15-1 Types of atrial septal defects (UAB classification).

Fossa ovalis ASD[a]

Posterior ASD

Absence of the atrioventricular septum (ostium primum ASD)

Coronary sinus ASD

Subcaval ASD (sinus venosus ASD)

Confluent ASDs

KEY: ASD, atrial septal defect.

NOTE: An alternative (GLH) classification includes fossa ovalis, posterior, and most confluent defects under "ostium secundum ASDs."

[a]Varies in size from small, valvular, incompetent, foramen ovale type of ASD to complete absence of fossa ovalis tissue with resultant ASD extending to the inferior vena cava.

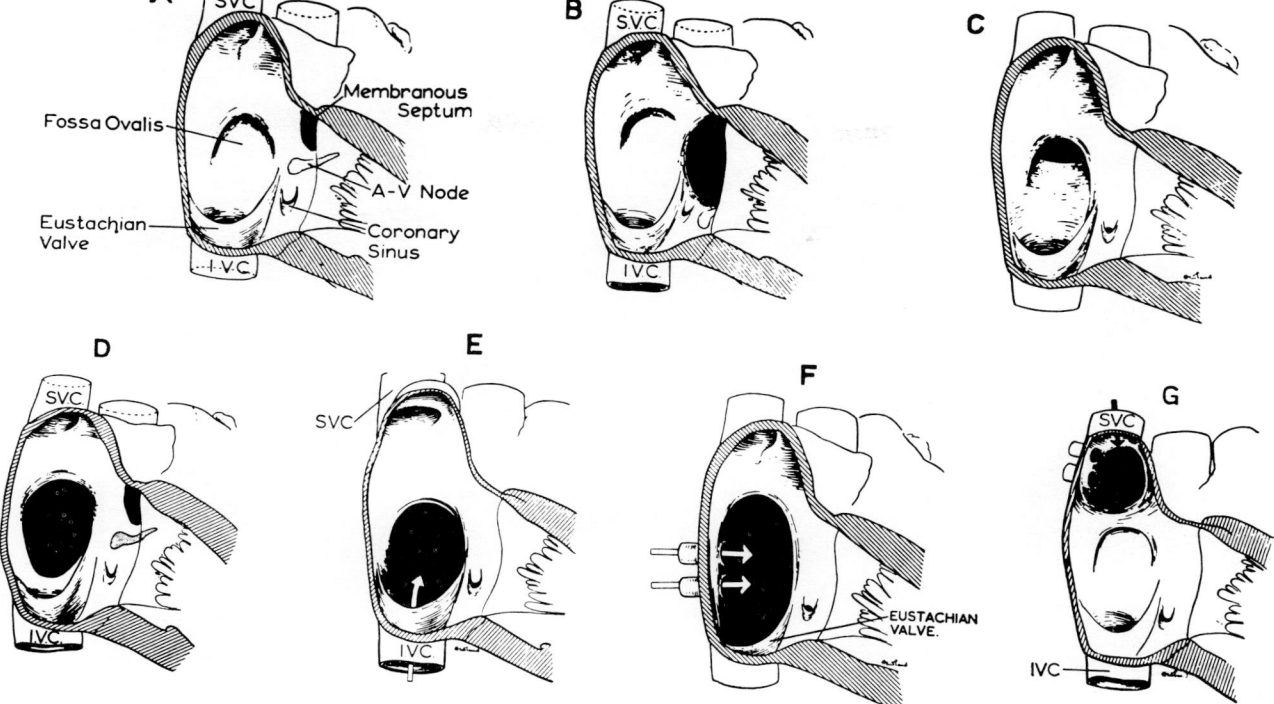

Figure 15-1 Anatomy of atrial septal defects, viewed from the right atrium, as accurately depicted and described in 1957 by Bedford and colleagues. The terminology is theirs.
(*a*) Normal atrial septum.
(*b*) AV type of defect.
(*c*) Widely patent foramen ovale.
(*d*) Fossa ovalis defect with complete septal rim.
(*e*) Low fossa ovalis defect astride inferior caval orifice with large eustachian valve.
(*f*) Large fossa ovalis defect without any posterior septal rim; pseudoanomalous right pulmonary veins.
(*g*) Superior caval type of defect, showing entrance of right upper pulmonary veins.
Reproduced with permission from Bedford et al.[B1]

also affected by any hypoplasia of the limbus that may be present. When the limbus is quite hypoplastic anteriorly, there is only a thin rim of tissue above the atrioventricular (AV) valves (formerly this was called an *intermediate defect* and was sometimes confused with an ostium primum defect). The limbus may also be hypoplastic superiorly or posteriorly.

The inferior vena caval–right atrial junction is normally partly to the left of the plane of the limbus, so that when the valve of the fossa ovalis is absent and the ASD extends to the IVC, the caval ostium overrides (or straddles) the defect onto the left atrium. This results in some right-to-left shunting of IVC blood to left atrium in virtually all patients with a large fossa ovalis type of ASD.[K8,M5,S11] Also, the position of the normally connected right pulmonary veins next to the atrial septal remnant results in preferential left-to-right shunting of their venous drainage.[B10,S11]

Posterior Atrial Septal Defect

A defect may exist in the most posterior and inferior part of the atrial septum, with absence, hypoplasia, or anterior displacement of the posterior limbus, and is termed a posterior ASD. The orifices of the right pulmonary veins usually open directly into the area of the defect, but true anomalous pulmonary venous connection of the right lung frequently coexists. In the pure form of this type of ASD, the tissue of the fossa ovalis (including the posterior limbus) is present, and the ASD is an oval one posterior to this (Fig. 15-4).

Ostium Primum Atrial Septal Defect

An ASD occurs anterior to the fossa ovalis (and the anterior limbus) when the atrioventricular septum is *absent*. Such defects are called *AV canal defects*, or *ostium primum atrial septal defects*, and are considered in Chapter 19. When essentially the entire atrial septum is absent (common atrium), the defect includes absence of the atrioventricular septum (see Chapter 19, "Atrial Septal Deficiency and Interatrial Communication" in section on Morphology).

Coronary Sinus Atrial Septal Defect

Coronary sinus ASDs are part of the unroofed coronary sinus syndrome. When the sinus is completely unroofed and no partition is present to separate it from the left atrium, the ostium of the coronary sinus is a hole in the atrial septum that allows free communication between left and right atria (see Chapter 18). Occasionally, there may be a fenestration

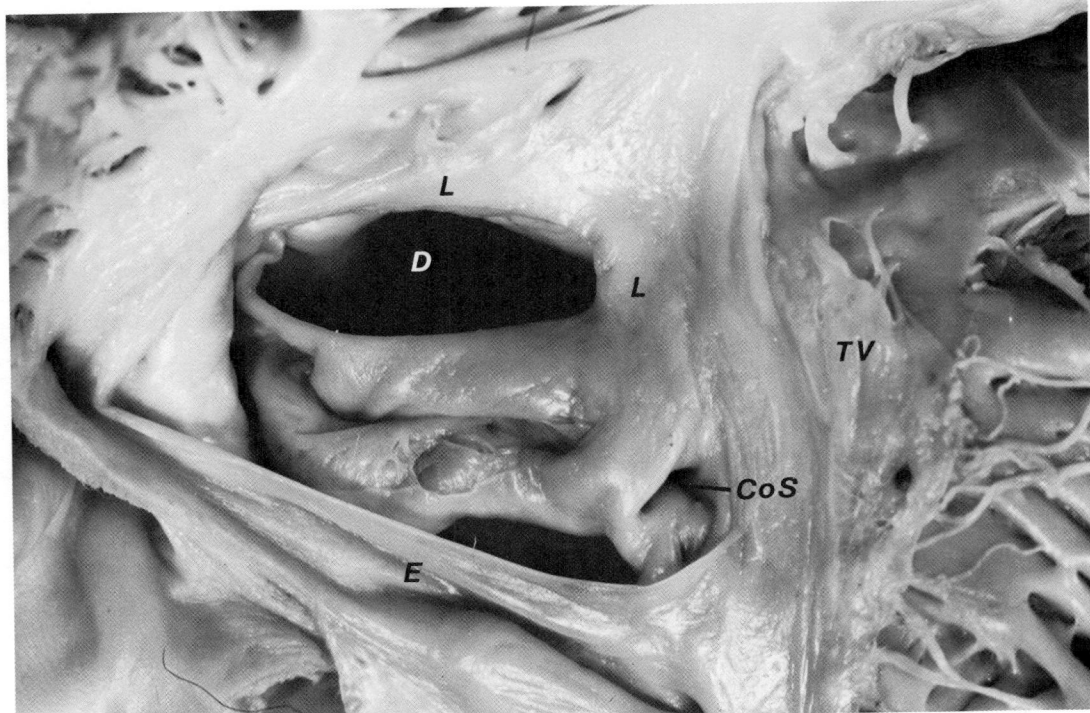

Figure 15-2 Specimen with fossa ovalis type of ASD, viewed in anatomic orientation with the superior vena cava above and the inferior vena cava and its eustachian valve below (GLH). The limbus forms the anterior, superior, and posterior rim of the defect, and the remnants of the floor (valve) of the fossa ovalis the inferior rim.

CoS, coronary sinus; D, atrial septal defect; E, eustachian valve; L, limbus; TV, septal leaflet of tricuspid valve.

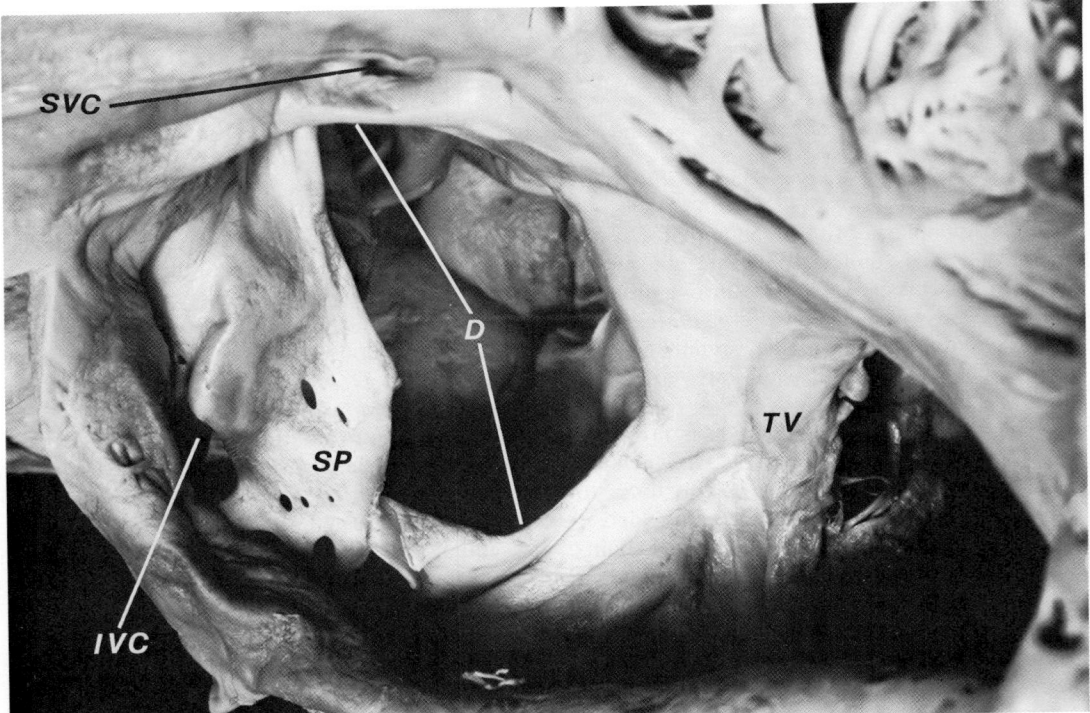

Figure 15-3 Specimen with large fossa ovalis type of ASD viewed from the opened right atrium in the same orientation as Figure 15-2 (GLH). The thin remnant of the septum primum shows numerous perforations.

D, defect; IVC, inferior vena cava; SP, septum primum; SVC, superior vena cava; TV, tricuspid valve.

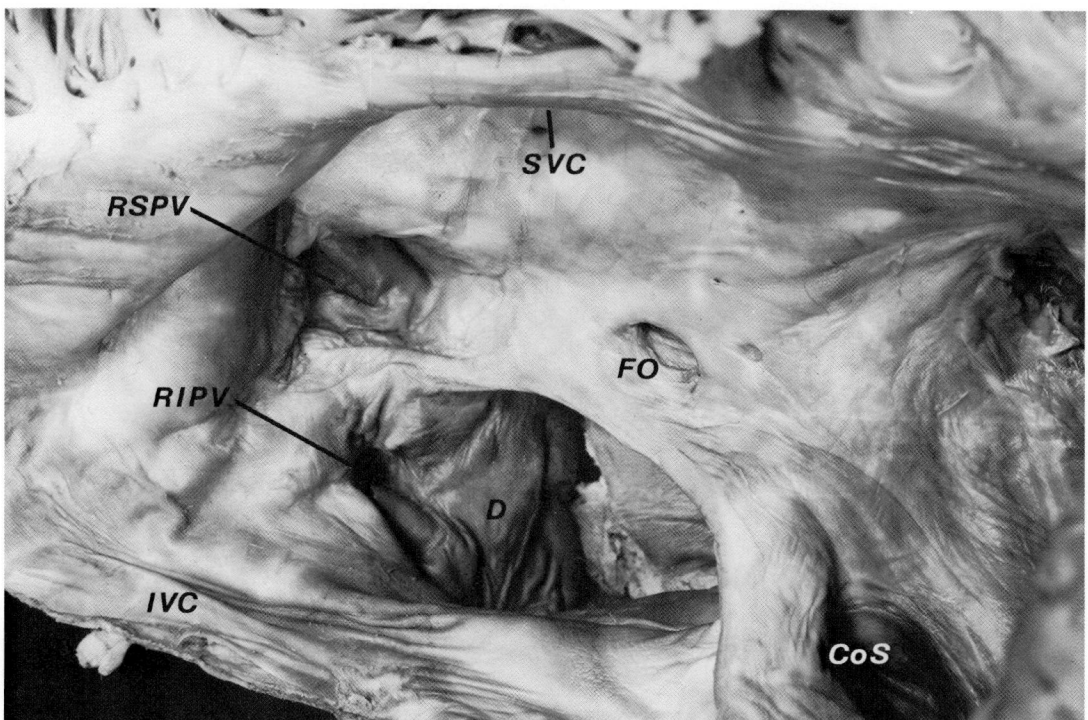

Figure 15-4 Specimen with large posterior ASD viewed from opened right atrium (GLH). The orientation is as in the other anatomic figures. The fossa ovalis is intact, but there is a patent foramen ovale. The right inferior pulmonary vein certainly drains anomalously but is probably normally connected. The right superior pulmonary vein is anomalously connected to the right atrium.

CoS, coronary sinus; D, atrial septal defect; FO, fossa ovalis; IVC, inferior vena cava; RIPV, right inferior pulmonary vein; RSPV, right superior pulmonary vein.

in this partition in the mid portion of the coronary sinus (this has been seen particularly in hearts with tricuspid atresia), or, rarely, the fenestration may be nearly at the ostium of the coronary sinus (Fig. 15-5).

Subcaval Atrial Septal Defect
The subcaval ASD (sinus venosus defect, superior vena caval defect), which occurs in the sinus venosus syndrome is located immediately beneath the orifice of the superior vena cava (SVC), superior to the limbic tissue, and is almost always associated with anomalous pulmonary venous connection of the right superior pulmonary vein to the SVC near or at the SVC–right atrial junction. The lower margin of the defect is a sharply defined crescentic edge of atrial septum, while its upper margin is devoid of septum, being continuous with the posterior SVC wall, which in turn is continuous with the upper edge of left atrium.

Confluent Atrial Septal Defects
Large ASDs may represent a confluence of two of the above defects. Thus, a fossa ovalis defect coexisting with absence of the posterior limbus can present as a very large ASD with no septal remnant posteriorly. Another confluent defect occasionally seen is a combination of a coronary sinus and fossa ovalis defect.

Types of Partial Anomalous Pulmonary Venous Connections

Sinus Venosus Syndrome
Probably the commonest type of anomalous pulmonary venous connection is that present in the sinus venosus syndrome, in which it coexists with a subcaval ASD. In this syndrome, the right upper and middle lobe pulmonary veins (right superior pulmonary vein) attach to the low SVC or the SVC-RA junction, an arrangement that is present in about 95% of patients with a subcaval ASD.[C3,L7,S10] Most commonly the anomalous connection is by way of two anomalous veins (from upper and middle lobes) one superior to the other, but there may be three or, rarely, four, and in such instances the uppermost vein may enter the SVC near the azygous vein entry. Very uncommonly, only part of the right superior vein connects anomalously, the inferior (right middle lobe) portion of that vein connecting to left atrium; and rarely, also both the right superior and right inferior pulmonary veins connect anomalously to the low SVC and/or the SVC–right atrial junction (Fig. 15-6).

The lowermost part of the SVC that receives the anomalous veins is usually wider than normal. It may, however, be relatively small, particularly when there is also a well-formed left SVC, which is not uncommon.[T5] The SVC typically overrides the ASD to some extent and enters partly

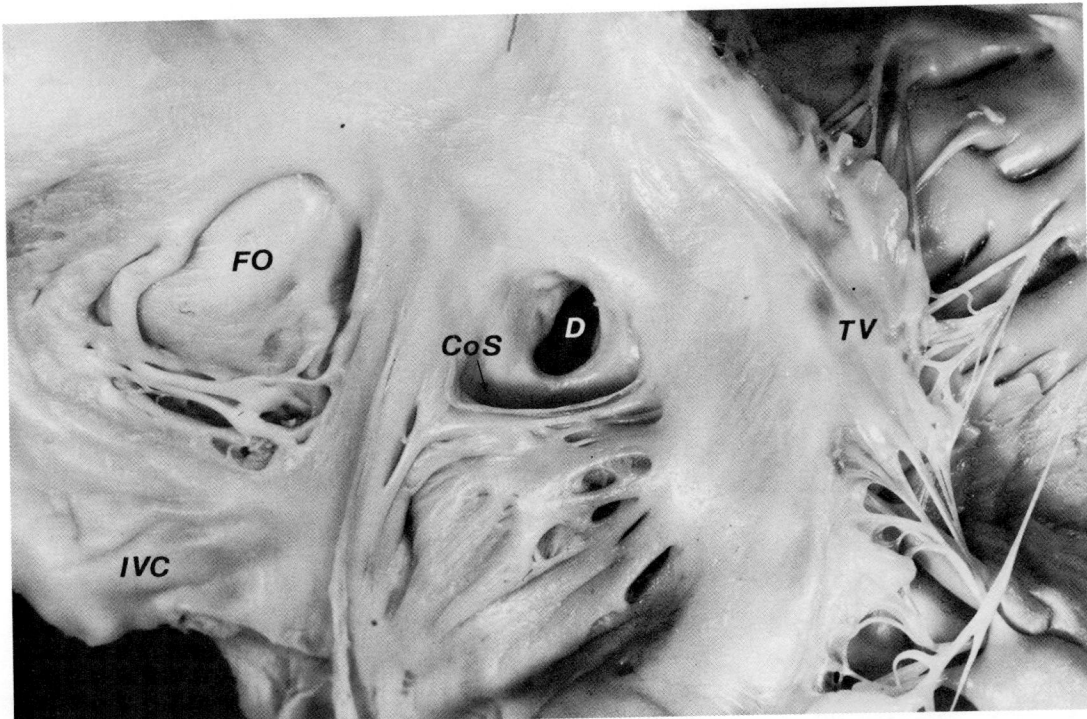

Figure 15-5 An unusual example of a small coronary sinus ASD that is near the ostium (GLH). Other anomalies present were a patent foramen ovale, a ventricular septal defect, mild aortic incompetence and possible mitral incompetence.

CoS, coronary sinus; D, defect; FO, fossa ovalis; IVC, inferior vena cava; TV, tricuspid valve.

into the left atrium, resulting in a right-to-left shunt of some superior caval blood to left atrium. In a few patients, the overriding of the SVC is severe enough to produce a large right-to-left shunt and marked cyanosis,[S7] and it may be complete, so that the superior vena cava drains directly and completely into the left atrium.[P6]

Rarely, the typical high, subcaval ASD is present without the anomalous pulmonary venous connection; the right pulmonary veins connect to the left atrium, but more superiorly than normal.

Right Superior Vein to Superior Vena Cava
Occasionally, the entire right superior pulmonary vein connects to the SVC without an associated subcaval ASD. The connection is then almost always well above (superior to) the SVC–right atrial junction. In such instances, the lower part of the SVC is not dilated. Very rarely, even when no subcaval ASD is present, the connection may be in the typical low position of the sinus venosus syndrome. Occasionally, only a *portion* of the right superior pulmonary vein draining one or two segments of the right upper lobe connects directly to the SVC. The PAPVC may be isolated or associated with a fossa ovalis ASD.

Right Pulmonary Veins to Right Atrium
The right pulmonary veins may connect directly to the right atrium, either in toto (in which case they may connect as two or three separate veins) or only via the superior (or, rarely,

the inferior) right pulmonary vein. This anomaly may exist as an isolated one, without an ASD or with only a patent foramen ovale, in which case the plane of the atrial septum is altered from coronal to near sagittal due to leftward displacement of its lateral attachment. The plane of the right pulmonary vein is in fact little altered from normal. Since in such situations the posterior limbus is present, the veins are clearly anomalously connected to the right atrium. In ASDs with absence of the posterior limbus (posterior ASD) and at times in large fossa ovalis ASDs, the point of division between right and left atrium posteriorly can be questionable, and thus the atrial connection of the right pulmonary veins in this area is debatable. However, in such defects true anomalous connection of the right pulmonary veins can be present (Fig. 15-4).[M8,S6]

Right Pulmonary Veins to Inferior Vena Cava
An anomalous right pulmonary vein, generally draining the entire right lung but occasionally only the middle and lower lobe, may descend toward the diaphragm more or less parallel to the pericardial border, but with a crescentic (scimitar) shape, and then curve sharply to the left just above or below the right atrial-IVC junction.[K4] The anomalous pulmonary venous trunk usually passes anterior to the hilum of the right lung but may occasionally be posterior to it. The entrance into the IVC is just superior to the hepatic vein orifices. The atrial septum may be intact, or a fossa ovalis ASD may be present. Occasionally, the anomalous vein connects also to

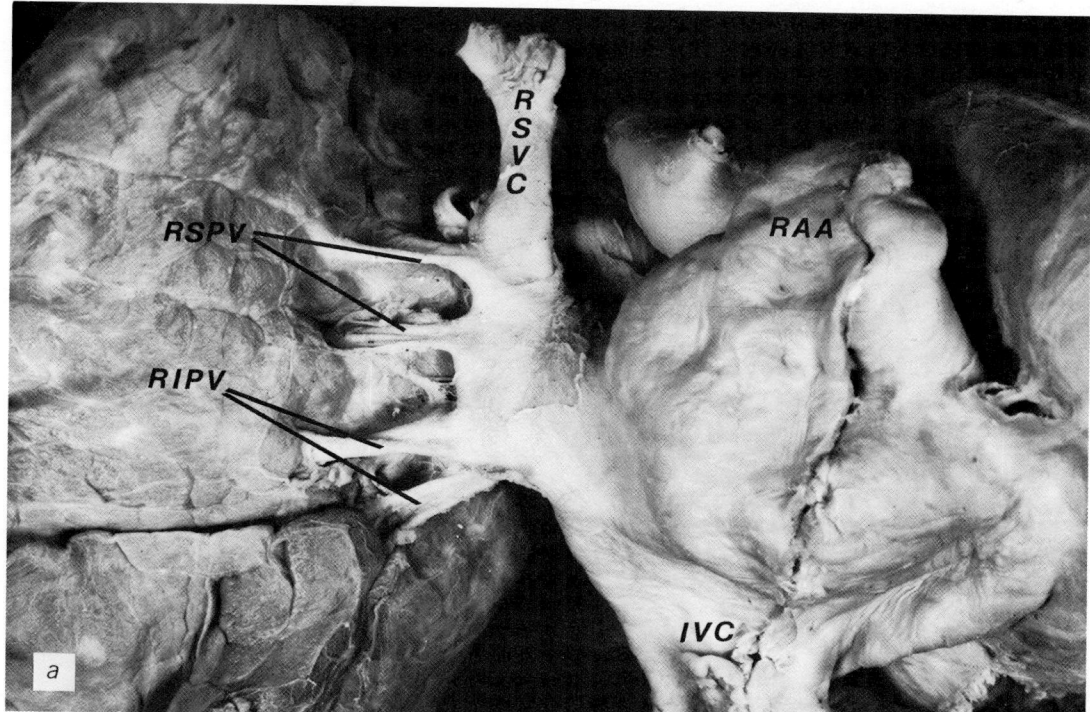

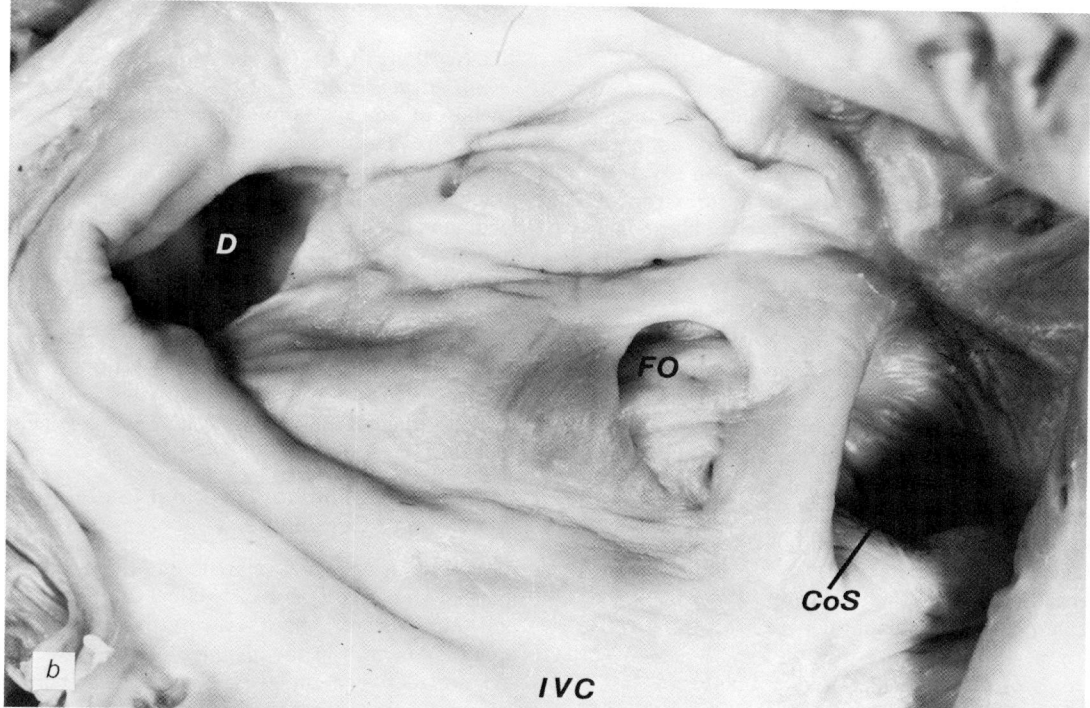

Figure 15-6

(a) Specimen with sinus venosus syndrome, with the typical subcaval ASD, but with both the right superior and right inferior pulmonary veins entering the superior vena cava–right atrial junction (GLH). In addition, the left pulmonary veins form a common channel connected to the left atrium and the right SVC. There was also a left superior vena cava and mitral atresia.

(b) Interior of right atrium showing the subcaval ASD high in the septum and the enlarged coronary sinus ostium to which is connected the left superior vena cava.

CoS, coronary sinus; D, atrial septal defect; FO, fossa ovalis; IVC, inferior vena cava; RAA, right atrial appendage; RIPV, right inferior pulmonary vein; RSPV, right superior pulmonary vein; SVC, superior vena cava.

Table 15-2   Patients with anomalous pulmonary venous connection of the entire right lung to the inferior vena cava (scimitar syndrome) (GLH; 1970–1983).

Age at Presentation	Status of Right Lung Cardiac Position	RPA	Anomalous Arterial Supply to Right Lung	Other Anomalies	Operation
3 wk	Severe hypoplasia Dextroposition	Absent	Yes	Anomalous LPA,[a] LSVC to coronary sinus, ASD, small PDA	None
4 mo	Severe hypoplasia Dextroposition	Absent	Yes	ASD, small PDA	None
8 mo	Normal Dextrocardia	Normal	No	None	Closure ASD, correction APVC to IVC
16 mo	Severe hypoplasia Dextroposition	Tiny	Yes	Large VSD, LSVC to coronary sinus, IVC to azygous vein	Closure VSD, ligation RPA
4 yr	Severe hypoplasia Dextroposition	Absent	Yes	Large VSD, moderate PDA	Closure VSD and PDA
40 yr	Normal Levocardia	Normal	No	None	Closure ASD, correction APVC to IVC

KEY: APVC, anomalous pulmonary venous connection; ASD, atrial septal defect; CS, coronary sinus; LPA, left pulmonary artery; LSVC, left superior vena cava; PDA, patent ductus arteriosus; RPA, right pulmonary artery; VSD, ventricular septal defect.

NOTE: Only the 8-mo- and 40-yr-old patients in the table are included in the data analysis in this chapter.

[a] Posterior to trachea and left main bronchus.

the *left* atrium,[G6,M10] and, rarely, the scimitar syndrome can exist with connection of the anomalous vein *only* to the left atrium.[M11] Pulmonary venous *drainage* is then normal. (Rarely, the left lung may connect via a scimitar-shaped vein to the IVC.)[D7,M12]

The right-sided scimitar syndrome occurs as an isolated lesion in a minority of cases (Table 15-2). In most instances, anomalies of the right lung are also present. Most common among these is right lung hypoplasia, which when severe is associated with a marked mediastinal shift and dextroposition of the heart, the entire heart lying in the right chest. The blood supply to the hypoplastic right lung comes mainly from a branch of the abdominal aorta in the region of the coeliac axis, which ascends through the inferior pulmonary ligament to supply the lower lobe or, more often, the entire right lung. A small pulmonary artery may be present, but often the central and hilar portions of the right pulmonary artery are absent (Table 15-2). Occasionally there may be a true right lower lobe bronchopulmonary sequestration, with secondary intrapulmonary cyst formation.

Frequently, there are associated cardiac anomalies, and diaphragmatic anomalies occurred in about 20% of the cases reviewed by Kiely and associates.[K4] These included herniation of the right lung through the foramen of Bockdalek and abnormal attachments of the diaphragm.

Rare Connections of the Right Pulmonary Veins
Rarely, the right pulmonary veins may connect anomalously to the azygous vein or coronary sinus with or without a fossa ovalis ASD.

Anomalous Left Pulmonary Venous Connections
The left pulmonary veins may connect to the left innominate vein by way of an anomalous vertical vein.[S8] The anomalous drainage is usually from the entire left lung but may be from only the left upper lobe.[B7] A fossa ovalis ASD coexists in some patients, and in others the atrial septum is intact.[H8]

On rare occasions, the left pulmonary veins connect anomalously to the coronary sinus, a right-sided superior vena cava, or the right atrium.

Bilateral Partial Anomalous Pulmonary Venous Connection
Partial but bilateral anomalous pulmonary venous connection is rare. The commonest variant is probably that in which the atrial septum is intact, the left superior pulmonary vein attaches to the left innominate vein by way of an anomalous vertical vein, and the right superior pulmonary vein attaches to the SVC–right atrial junction. Another form is that in which a common pulmonary venous chamber (see Chapter 16 for definition) is present and some veins from both lungs connect to it (two cases at GLH, one at UAB). All but one lobe or only one lobe from each side may connect to the sinus. The common venous sinus may connect to the right atrium or the left innominate vein (one case of each at GLH).

The Cardiac Chambers in Atrial Septal Defect and Related Conditions

Typically, in ASD and related conditions, the right atrium is markedly enlarged (at least grade 3 or 4, on the basis of 1–6) and thick-walled. The left atrium is not enlarged. This discrepancy occurs in the absence of any flow or pressure restriction between the two, because the right atrial wall is inherently more distensible than the left atrial wall.

The right ventricular diastolic size is increased, often markedly, because of the volume overload imposed by the left-to-right shunt. Whereas normal right ventricular diastolic dimensions are between 0.6 and 1.4 cm $\cdot$ m^{-2}, those in patients with large left-to-right shunts at atrial level are on the average 2.66 cm $\cdot$ m^{-2} and may be as large as 4 cm $\cdot$ m^{-2}.[P2] Consequently, the cardiac apex is often formed by the right ventricle.

Morphologically, the left ventricle is normal or slightly

decreased in size. However, important left ventricular dynamic abnormalities are present in most patients with ASD (see "Mitral Valve Prolapse").

The Mitral Valve and Atrial Septal Defects

Mitral Prolapse

Mitral valve prolapse occurs in association with the fossa ovalis type of ASD, the sinus venosus syndrome,[T5] and probably other types of ASDs and related conditions that result in left-to-right shunts at atrial level. The likely incidence of true prolapse is about 20%;[L3] it increases with age and with the pulmonary-to-systemic blood flow ratio ($\dot{Q}p/\dot{Q}s$).[L3,S4] Schreiber and colleagues have considerably clarified a previously confused subject by relating mitral valve prolapse to the abnormalities of left ventricular shape[S4] demonstrated to be present in patients with ASD.[L2,L8,W2] The alteration in left ventricular configuration results from a leftward shift of the ventricular septum, a process that begins as a slight decrease in the normal rightward convexity and progresses with time to flattening and then reversal, with a resultant central bulge into the left ventricle. This process is a response to the right ventricular enlargement, which is secondary to the volume overload of this chamber in ASD. This etiologic basis of the mitral valve prolapse is supported by the fact that it is decreased in degree or abolished in most cases by closure of the ASD and return of the left ventricular geometry to normal.[A3,S4]

Mitral Incompetence

Mitral prolapse in ASD can lead to mitral incompetence, as does idiopathic mitral prolapse. The true incidence of incompetence in unselected patients varies, since older patients and those with larger pulmonary blood flows have a higher incidence of this abnormality as well as of prolapse per se. The incidence of mitral incompetence severe enough to require correction at the time of ASD repair may be as low as 2% (GLH, 8 in 395 cases) and as high as 10%. It occurred in 6% of operated cases at the Mayo Cinic. The data of Leachman and colleagues strongly suggest that this type of mitral prolapse can also precipitate chordal rupture, as it can in Barlow's syndrome.[L3]

Cleft Mitral Leaflets

Cleft anterior or posterior mitral leaflets that cause mitral incompetence are said to occur occasionally in patients with ASDs.[D1,G4,H4] However, judging from some of the illustrations of such "clefts," they may in fact simply be spaces between commissural and main leaflets in prolapsed valves.

The Lungs

The pulmonary arteries are considerably dilated and elongated when pulmonary blood flow is large. This involves even the smallest branches, which tend to compress the smaller airways, with resultant retention of secretions and bronchiolitis.

Hypertensive pulmonary vascular disease (see Chapter 20, "Pulmonary Vascular Disease" in section on Morphology) develops uncommonly in patients with ASD, and then usually in the third or fourth decade of life. This contrasts sharply with ventricular septal defects, AV canal, and patent ductus arteriosus, in which pulmonary vascular disease is present early in life. In ASD, the pulmonary vascular disease is due mainly to secondary thrombosis in the dilated pulmonary artery branches, with changes in the intima and media of the vessels usually playing a minor role, although Haworth has suggested that an increase in pulmonary arterial smooth muscle can be the only finding.[H10]

Associated Cardiac Conditions

ASDs and related conditions may coexist with nearly all varieties of congenital heart disease, but such cases are not considered here unless the left-to-right shunt at atrial level is the dominant hemodynamic lesion. The spectrum of cardiac anomalies coexisting with ASD as the dominant lesion is wide (Table 15-3).

Valvular heart disease may coexist with hemodynamically significant ASDs. Six cases with moderate or severe rheumatic mitral stenosis and a hemodynamically significant ASD (Lutembacher's syndrome) were included among 443 patients with an ASD at GLH (1957–1983). Eleven cases of moderate or severe mitral incompetence were included, in three of which the incompetence was rheumatic in origin. Both mitral stenosis and incompetence increase the left-to-right shunting.

Tricuspid incompetence of variable severity frequently complicates ASDs in older patients with heart failure, the mechanism generally being right ventricular and tricuspid annular dilation. In ten of 443 patients undergoing repair of ASD (GLH), the tricuspid incompetence required surgical treatment.

Other Associated Conditions

Rarely, ASD may occur in patients with Marfan's syndrome, Turner's syndrome, Noonan's syndrome, and the Holt-Oram syndrome (one each in the GLH experience).

Table 15-3 Associated cardiac anomalies in 443 patients with ASD or PAPVC as their major cardiac anomaly (GLH; 1957–1983).

Anomaly	n	% of 443	Hospital Deaths
Left superior vena cava	24	5%	1
Mild or moderate PS	16	4%	0
Peripheral PA stenoses	4	1%	0
Azygous extension IVC	4	1%	0
Small VSD	2	0.01%	0
Small PDA	2	0.01%	0
Mild coarctation	2	0.01%	1
Small coronary–MPA fistula	2	0.01%	0
Anomalous right subclavian artery	2	0.01%	0
Dextrocardia (isolated)	1	0.005%	0

KEY: IVC, inferior vena cava; MPA, main pulmonary artery; PA, pulmonary artery; PDA, patent ductus arteriosus; PS, pulmonary stenosis; VSD, ventricular septal defect.

NOTE: Since some patients had more than one anomaly, the figures are not cumulative.

CLINICAL FEATURES AND DIAGNOSTIC CRITERIA

The symptoms, clinical features, and signs in ASD and related conditions producing left-to-right shunting at atrial level are related largely to the size of the left-to-right shunt.[1] Thus, in general, when $\dot{Q}p/\dot{Q}s$ is less than 1.5, there are neither signs nor symptoms of the shunt, and this is often true with a $\dot{Q}p/\dot{Q}s$ up to 1.8. When $\dot{Q}p/\dot{Q}s$ is larger than this, signs of the shunt are present, and symptoms usually appear eventually (see "Natural History"). Infants present an exception to these generalizations, for in them the clinical features are often atypical; for example, the splitting of the second heart sound is unrelated to $\dot{Q}p/\dot{Q}s$.[H1]

Symptoms

Symptoms may be absent for several decades, but when they occur, they consist of effort breathlessness and a tendency toward recurrent respiratory tract infections. Palpitation from paroxysmal atrial tachycardia or atrial fibrillation may occur, the latter later in life. Older adults with long-neglected heart disease may present with chronic congestive heart failure with fluid retention, hepatomegaly, and severe cardiac cachexia. Occasionally in an infant with ASD and a large left to right shunt, often in association with partial anomalous pulmonary venous connection, there may be congestive heart failure with tachypnea, but this is uncommon. In such infants, other associated lesions may contribute to the heart failure.

Atypical presentations occur occasionally. An unequivocal history of cyanosis rarely may bring a patient with an uncomplicated atrial septal defect to medical attention,[I1] as it did in one of the 340 patients in the UAB surgical series. He was a 12-year-old child with normal pulmonary artery pressure, a large fossa ovalis ASD extending to the inferior vena cava, and considerable right-to-left shunting from the inferior vena cava to the left atrium. This coincides with the occasional finding of bilateral shunting in patients with otherwise uncomplicated ASDs.[G8] Patients with coexisting right-to-left shunts tend to be in the older age group.[G8] For the same anatomic reasons (see "Morphology"), the patient

may present with paradoxical emboli or cerebral infarctions; two patients (1%) in the UAB series presented in this way, one being 33 years old and the other 38. Both had normal pulmonary artery pressures. This presentation occurred in 9 (2%) of the Mayo Clinic series of 546 patients.[R5] Uncommonly, the presentation may be modified by the presence of severe pulmonary hypertension, in which case cyanosis, effort intolerance, and hemoptysis may be present.

Signs

The clinical signs that are diagnostic of a large ($\dot{Q}p/\dot{Q}s > 1.8$–2) shunt at atrial level are an overactive left parasternal systolic lift, fixed splitting of the second heart sound throughout the respiratory cycle (this is absent when the large $\dot{Q}p/\dot{Q}s$ is from partial anomalous pulmonary venous connection with an intact atrial septum), a soft pulmonary mid-systolic flow murmur (in the second and third left intercostal spaces), and a mid-diastolic tricuspid flow murmur (in the fourth and fifth left intercostal spaces) present in borderline situations only on inspiration. This last sign may, however, be absent occasionally, particularly in older patients, even with a larger shunt. In addition, a very large shunt produces a more marked left-sided precordial right ventricular lift, occasionally some prominence of the left anterior chest wall, and leftward displacement of the cardiac apex. Many of the patients are shorter and thinner than their peers.

When congestive heart failure is present, the jugular venous pressure is elevated, the liver is enlarged, and there is gross cardiomegaly. Tricuspid incompetence produces systolic liver pulsation and a greater tendency to ascites and peripheral edema.

Significant pulmonary hypertension is evident clinically by accentuation of the second heart sound and a more marked right ventricular and pulmonary artery lift. Sometimes there is a pulmonary incompetent murmur, and there may also be evidence of tricuspid incompetence.

Chest X-ray

The chest x-ray reflects the large $\dot{Q}p/\dot{Q}s$. The right atrium and right ventricle are large. The main pulmonary artery shadow in the upper left portion of the cardiac silhouette is enlarged, and the right and left pulmonary arteries are enlarged to the periphery of the lung field. The shadow of the transverse aortic arch is abnormally small. In patients with congestive heart failure, there may be interstitial pulmonary edema and areas of pulmonary consolidation and/or atelectasis. These signs are probably secondary to compression of the smaller airways by the enormously enlarged small pulmonary vessels.

Some suggestions as to the specific anatomic diagnosis may be contained in the chest x-ray. Occasionally the right superior pulmonary vein can be identified lying more superiorly than is normal (Fig. 15-7), leading to suspicion of the sinus venosus syndrome. A crescentic shadow more or less parallel to the right heart border (Fig. 15-8) suggests the diagnosis of anomalous pulmonary venous connection of the right pulmonary veins to the inferior vena cava (scimitar syndrome).

---

[1] Left-to-right shunting across a nonrestrictive (< 2 cm in an adult) ASD under ordinary circumstances is a function of the relative compliance (reflected in the diastolic pressures) of right and left ventricles. The right ventricular compliance in particular is unpredictable, one factor making for variability of $\dot{Q}p/\dot{Q}s$ from one patient to another. A very compliant distensible right ventricle (in association with a normal pulmonary vascular bed) will allow a very large shunt; a less compliant one (such as may result from pulmonary hypertension or from morphologic right ventricular changes that occur later in life[J1,P5]) allows a more modest shunt. Left ventricular compliance tends to decrease with age, and this tends to increase $\dot{Q}p/\dot{Q}s$ as patients get older. Shunting will be increased by systemic hypertension when this results in a decreased left ventricular compliance. Mitral incompetence or stenosis increases $\dot{Q}p/\dot{Q}s$. When the ASD is small and flow is restrictive, it limits the left-to-right shunting. Even then, mitral stenosis may elevate the left atrial pressure sufficiently that a large left-to-right shunt results (along with a soft continuous murmur because of flow through all phases of the cardiac cycle).

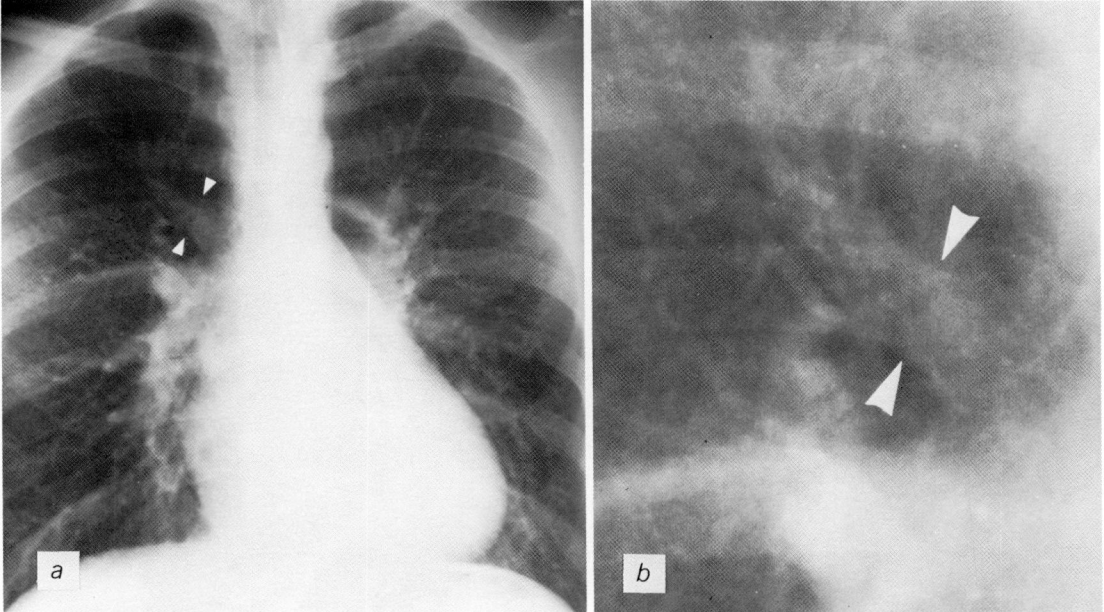

Figure 15-7 Chest x-ray of a patient with the sinus venosus syndrome (UAB). The arrow indicates the right superior pulmonary vein.
(a) Ordinary view.
(b) Magnification copy.

Electrocardiogram

The electrocardiogram almost always shows the pattern of incomplete right bundle-branch block and a clockwise frontal loop. Left axis deviation and a counterclockwise loop strongly suggest an AV canal defect, but this pattern does occur in about 10% of patients with fossa ovalis ASDs.

Two-dimensional Echocardiography

The clinical diagnosis of ASD can be confirmed by visualizing the defect directly using two-dimensional echocardiography.[L2,S12] The echocardiogram also gives indirect evidence of ASD by its demonstration of right ventricular volume overload, which includes increased right ventricular diastolic size and abnormal (flat or paradoxic) septal motion.[M4,T4]

Cardiac Catheterization and Cineangiography

When the diagnosis of a typical and apparently uncomplicated ASD has been made by noninvasive methods in children, adolescents, and young adults, cardiac catheterization is not required. It then becomes the surgeon's responsibility to determine at operation the type of ASD and the presence or absence of any anomalous pulmonary venous connections. Cardiac catheterization and appropriate cineangiography are indicated in infants (because of possible associated anomalies), in many adults (for assessment of possible pulmonary hypertension and the status of the mitral valve), and in any patient in whom the noninvasive tests suggest PAPVC. Coronary arteriography is performed in patients over 40 years of age.

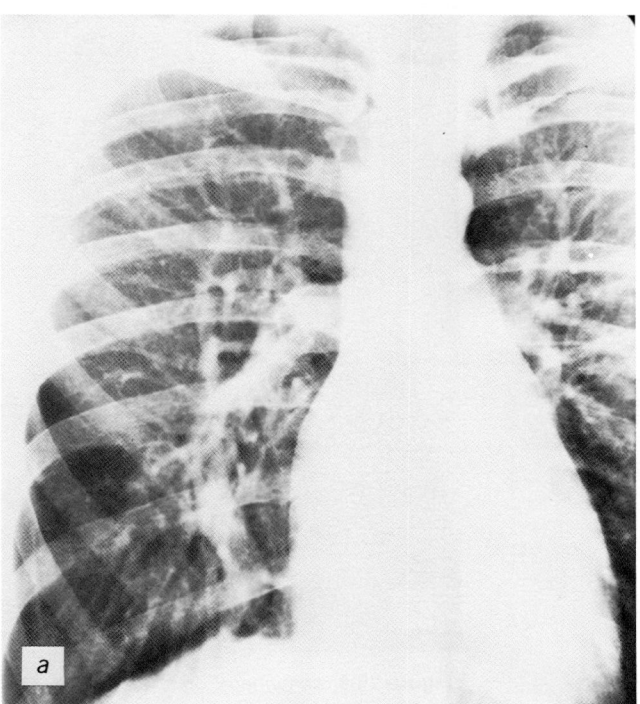

Figure 15-8 Partial anomalous pulmonary venous connection of the right pulmonary veins to the inferior vena cava in a patient with scimitar syndrome (UAB).
(a) Plain chest roentgenogram, frontal view. The crescentic shadow of the anomalous pulmonary vein is evident.

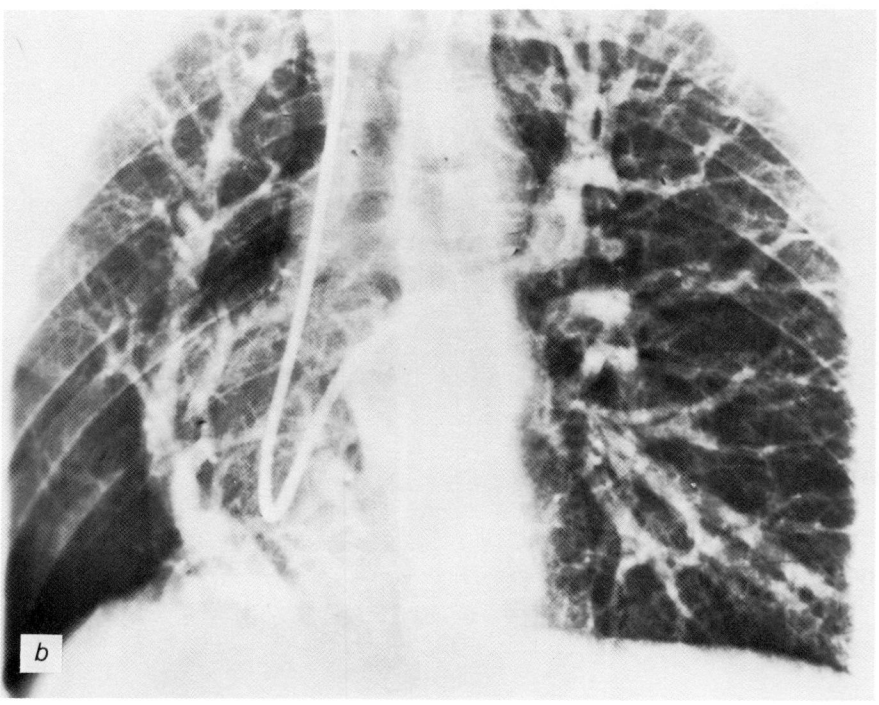

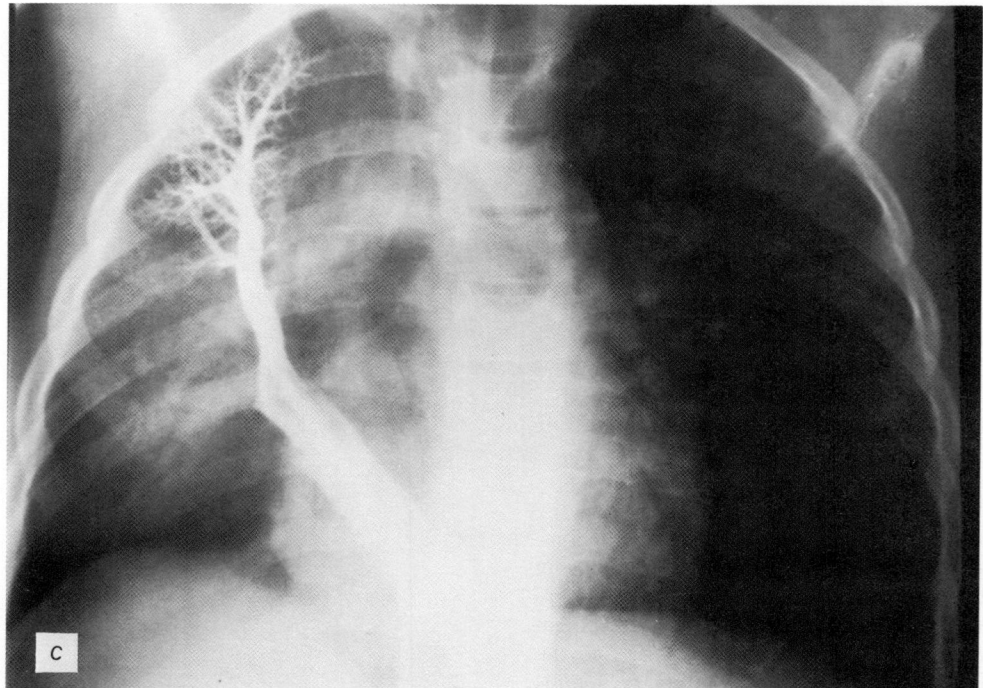

Figure 15-8 (*continued*)
(*b*) Levophase of a pulmonary angiogram, showing the anomalous pulmonary vein draining into the inferior vena cava.
(*c*) Selective angiogram into the anomalous pulmonary vein.

The assessment of operability in patients with pulmonary hypertension is a particular problem, since even in Eisenmenger syndrome, with shunt reversal at atrial level, the pulmonary artery pressure is rarely more than two-thirds that of systemic pressure. (There is no transmission of systemic pressure across the defect, as is the case with large defects at ventricular or ductus level; see Chapter 20.) A patient with pulmonary vascular resistance greater than 12 units · m² is inoperable.

When the resting pulmonary vascular resistance is elevated to 6–12 units · m², the assessment of operability requires calculation of pulmonary and systemic vascular resistance on exercise as well. Characteristic findings of inoperability would be a Q̇p/Q̇s of 1.5 at rest and 0.85 on exercise in association with a fall in systemic arterial oxygen saturation (measurements of the arterial oxygen saturation alone at rest and on exercise will indicate the need for more elaborate studies). These findings indicate that the pulmonary vascular resistance is unchanged or higher during exercise, and systemic vascular resistance lower. Such patients are not improved by operation, and indeed their life may be shortened by it.

Cardiac catheterization and angiography are also useful in defining the anatomic details of the related conditions that can cause shunting at atrial level. Increased oxygen saturation of blood in the low SVC gives presumptive evidence of the diagnosis of the sinus venous syndrome, and this becomes virtually certain if the catheter can be passed through a subcaval ASD into the left atrium. An indicator dilution curve obtained after injection of dye into the SVC may show some right-to-left shunting, which is generally completely absent in patients with a fossa ovalis ASD (in whom there may be right-to-left shunting from the inferior vena cava). In addition, curves obtained after injection into the right pulmonary artery generally show a much larger left-to-right shunt (as a result of the anomalously draining right pulmonary veins) than those obtained after injection into the left pulmonary artery. The identification of the specific anatomic details of the sinus venosus syndrome is best accomplished by cineangiography after right pulmonary artery injection, for the typical location and drainage of the right superior pulmonary vein can then be seen. Pulmonary artery injection may confirm anomalous connection of the right pulmonary veins to right atrium or inferior vena cava (Fig. 15-8), of the left veins to the left innominate or other veins, or of bilateral anomalous connections.

When anomalous connection of the right pulmonary veins to the inferior vena cava is demonstrated, an aortogram should also be done to define any anomalous systemic arteries from the abdominal or thoracic aorta to the right lower lobe. If the right lung is small, if the right lower lobe is contracted or seems otherwise abnormal on the chest x-ray, or if the patient gives a history of hemoptysis or recurrent pulmonary infections, bronchoscopy or bronchography are also indicated.

Calculations of Q̇p/Q̇s are of particular importance in patients with isolated PAPVC of only a part of one lung. An operation is not indicated when the ratio is < 1.8. However, even when only the right superior pulmonary vein is involved and the atrial septum is intact, the shunt may be greater than this, presumably because right atrial and caval pressures are distinctly lower than left atrial pressures, producing a larger than usual pulmonary venous gradient.[H2]

NATURAL HISTORY

The natural history of persons born with ASDs and related conditions producing left-to-right shunts at atrial level is not known with precision, but its general characteristics have been described.[C4,C5]

Survival

Although a large isolated ASD is an important congenital cardiac malformation, it is not immediately lethal. Important symptoms may develop in the first year of life[D2,H5,N1,S5] but probably in only about 1% of infants born with this malformation.[A1] However, the experience of Hunt and colleagues suggests that up to 10% of the infants who are symptomatic from ASDs die when treated nonsurgically.[H7]

This suggests that only 0.1% of those born with ASD die of it in infancy. However, an ASD causes death even less frequently in the first and second decades of life. A few (probably 5%–15% of those born with large ASDs[C4]) die in the third and fourth decade of life with severe pulmonary hypertension and Eisenmenger's syndrome. In the UAB surgical series, 14% of patients catheterized had pulmonary hypertension with a mean pulmonary artery pressure > 25 mmHg. In the GLH surgical series, the pulmonary artery systemic pressure was > 50 mmHg in 13% of catheterized patients and in 11% of the total series (Fig. 15-9). The incidence of a significant increase in pulmonary vascular resistance (4 units · m²) was 4.5% and was very rare (1%) below 20 years of age. However, in a few areas in which individuals reside in high altitudes, the incidence of pulmonary hypertension is higher. Cherian and his colleagues report pulmonary hyper-

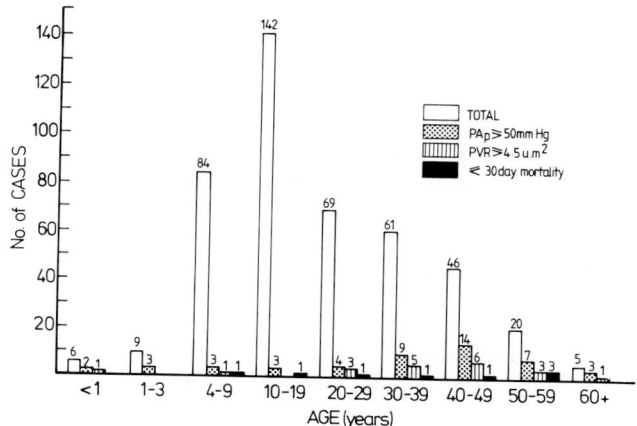

Figure 15-9 Histogram showing the frequency of pulmonary hypertension and increased pulmonary vascular resistance (PVR) in a series of surgically treated ASDs (GLH; n = 442). Of these patients, 371 were catheterized, and in the remaining 71, the pulmonary artery systolic pressure (PAₚ) was assumed to be less than 50 mmHg and the PVR less than 4.5 units · m².

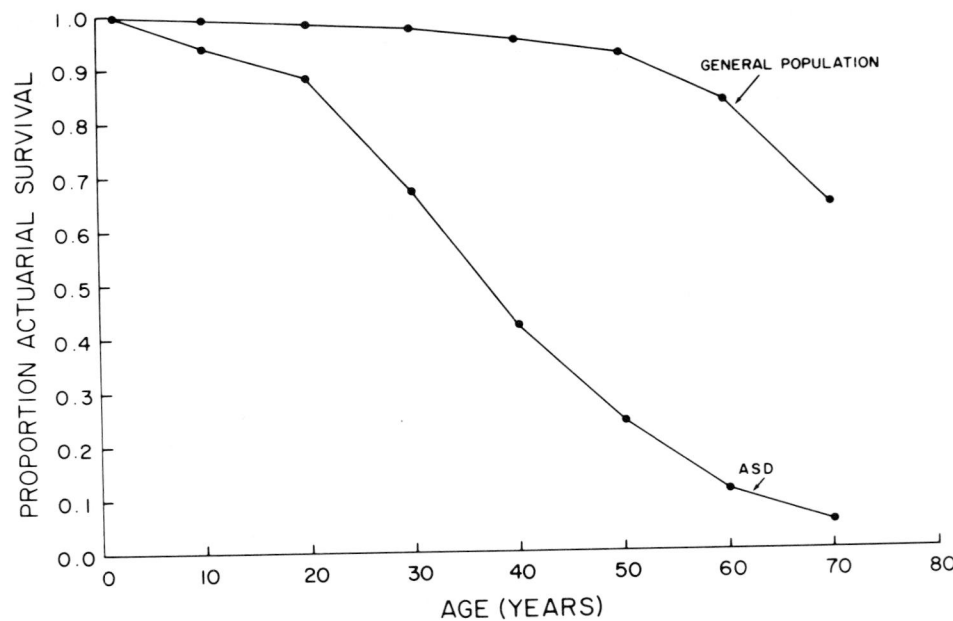

Figure 15-10 Plot of Campbell's actuarial survival computations of the life expectancy of surgically untreated patients with atrial septal defects who reach the age of 1 year.[C5] It is based on three sets of collected data. There is some spread between the three sets of data, indicating confidence limits of modest width around the point estimates (they cannot be calculated from the data). The life expectancy of the general population 1 year old is also from Campbell and is very close to that computed from United States life tables (UAB). The data (see "Natural History") suggest that 99.9% of patients born with ASD reach the first year of life unless unrelated conditions cause their death.

tension in 13% of patients in their region of India who are less than 10 years of age.[C6]

Premature late death with congestive heart failure occurs in an increasing proportion with age after the fifth decade of life, so most individuals with large ASDs die in chronic congestive heart failure if they do not succumb to other illnesses. Even so, probably no more than 25% of persons born with a large ASD die of it, since the lethal manifestations of the disease tend to occur so late in life that other unrelated conditions may cause death first.

Campbell, in 1970, published the most detailed study available of the survival of patients with ASD treated nonsurgically.[C5] The transformation of this into the conventional actuarial plot and its comparison with the life expectancy of the general population provide good insight into the life expectancy of patients with ASD (Fig. 15-10).

The natural history of patients with the sinus venosus syndrome[H8] and most other types of partial anomalous pulmonary venous connections and ASD[B8,S9] is similar to that of patients with large fossa ovalis ASD. Thus, patients with the sinus venosus syndrome in the fourth to sixth decades of life have presented in chronic congestive heart failure or with severe pulmonary hypertension from pulmonary vascular disease.

The natural history of the scimitar syndrome is not clear. Presumably those patients without important anomalies of the right lung and with a large left-to-right shunt have a life history similar to that of patients with a large fossa ovalis ASD, while those with right lung hypoplasia often have a life history dominated more by their pulmonary pathology, including hemoptysis and recurrent pulmonary infections.

When there is isolated PAPVC of part of one lung and the $\dot{Q}p/\dot{Q}s$ is less than 1.8, life expectancy may well be normal. Rarely, paradoxical emboli are seen in patients with the sinus venosus syndrome (from the SVC) as well as in those with fossa ovalis ASDs (from the IVC).

Functional Status

Most patients are asymptomatic through the first and second decades of life, although many are shorter and slighter than their peers. Effort intolerance and easy fatigability may develop in the second or third decades of life or as late as the fifth or sixth decade. This progresses gradually to fluid retention, hepatomegaly, and elevated jugular venous pressure, and leads to gradually increasing disability. These phenomena are well exemplified in the surgical experience, in which preoperative New York Heart Association (NYHA) functional class and age at operation are moderately well correlated ($r = .61$, $P < .05$) (Table 15-4). When heart failure becomes advanced, both mitral and tricuspid incompetence are likely to have developed.

Spontaneous Closure

Spontaneous closure of a hemodynamically significant and isolated ASD does occur in the first year of life,[M3] and Cockerham and colleagues found this in 22% of 87 patients. They

Table 15-4 Relationship between NYHA functional class and age at operation (UAB; 1967–1969; *n* = 340).

Preoperative NYHA Class	Age (yr) at Operation		
	Mean	Median	Range
I	16	12	3.3–63
II	32	30	4.2–72
III	50	54	0.9–68
IV	51	57	2.2–66

found smaller left-to-right shunts in patients whose defects subsequently closed.[C7] Spontaneous closure is uncommon after the first year of life.[C1,G2,H1,M1,M2] Spontaneous closure of an ASD producing marked right ventricular enlargement and symptoms seems particularly uncommon.

Changes in Q̇p/Q̇s with Time

It has already been noted that decreasing left ventricular compliance increases Q̇p/Q̇s in patients with ASD, and this may occur as the fifth and sixth decades are reached. Systemic arterial hypertension accelerates this process and may unmask an ASD that was not the source of a significant shunt before the onset of a decrease in left ventricular compliance. It is also likely that most ASDs actually increase in size as time passes; this has been clearly demonstrated in the case of the patent foramen ovale.[H11] The direct relationship between Q̇p/Q̇s and the tendency toward mitral valve prolapse also supports the concept that the shunt increases with age.[S4] These increases in Q̇p/Q̇s with time do not occur when the shunt is from anomalous pulmonary venous connection without ASD.

Q̇p/Q̇s decreases when pulmonary hypertension develops. The mechanism for this is the decrease in right ventricular compliance that accompanies right ventricular hypertrophy (see footnote 1).

Right Ventricular Function

Right ventricular volume overload and consequent increased right ventricular diastolic dimensions are characteristic of patients with a hemodynamically significant ASD or PAPVC. The ventricular septum is displaced posteriorly under such circumstances.[W2] However, systolic anterior motion of the septum occurs.[H3,P1,W2] These features are well tolerated by the right ventricle for many years (much longer than is the case for the volume overloaded *left* ventricle and probably longer than that of the volume overload produced by acute tricuspid or pulmonary valve incompetence), but eventually right ventricular failure occurs, with decreased right ventricular ejection fraction and hypokinesia. Doty and colleagues have demonstrated loss of coronary reserve in patients with ASD and volume-induced right ventricular hypertrophy,[D8] and this contributes further to the development of right ventricular failure. Associated with this, the signs and symptoms of elevated systemic venous pressure (peripheral edema, elevated jugular venous pressure and hepatome-

galy, and finally ascites) develop, often with tricuspid incompetence.

These phenomena have been documented by several studies. Liberthson and colleagues found increased right ventricular volume but normal (64%) ejection fraction, in 9 asymptomatic patients with a mean age of 25 years; whereas 11 symptomatic patients with a mean age of 52 years had diffuse right ventricular hypokinesia and ejection fraction averaging 36% in addition to increased right ventricular volume.[L5] Perhaps related to this is the fact that adult patients with ASD but without pulmonary artery hypertension occasionally have marked pulmonary valve incompetence,[L6] which disappears after repair of the ASD.

Left Ventricular Function

Most adult patients with hemodynamically significant ASD or PAPVC have normal left ventricular systolic dimensions but have subnormal diastolic dimensions.[B6,P11,T3] Some loss of left ventricular functional reserve is present in most adult patients and in some children with ASD. Thus, in contrast to normal persons, such individuals do not increase left ventricular ejection fraction during maximal exercise[B6] (Fig. 15-11),

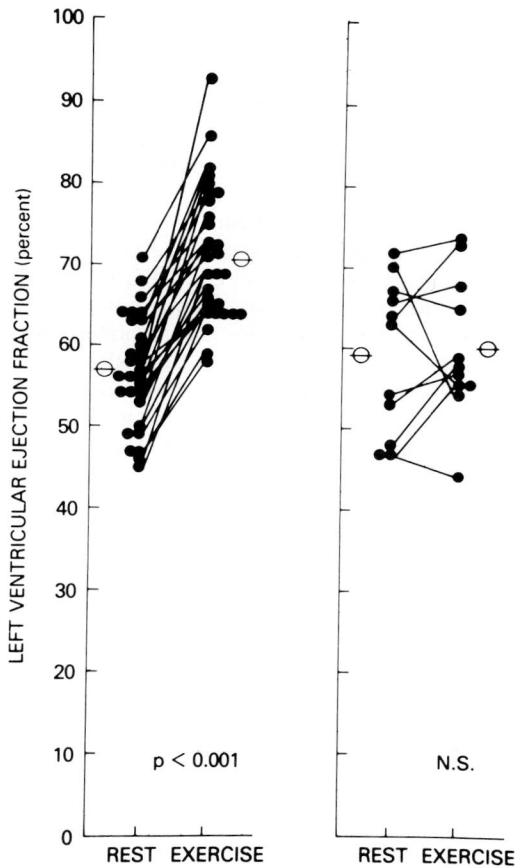

Figure 15-11 The normal response of increased left ventricular ejection fraction with maximal exercise (left). In contrast (right), adult patients with ASDs generally do not increase ejection fraction with maximal exercise.

Reproduced with permission from Bonow et al.,[B6] and the American Heart Association, Inc.

although resting left ventricular ejection fractions are usually within normal limits.[B6,P1] Also, Popio and colleagues reported abnormal sequences of left ventricular contraction.[P1]

These preoperative left ventricular abnormalities are convincingly ascribed by Bonow and colleagues to the effects of the volume-overloaded *right* ventricle. Other studies have established that, even in the absence of symptoms of systemic venous hypertension from right ventricular failure, left ventricular structure and function in patients with ASDs are influenced by the increased right ventricular volume rather than changes in *left* ventricular compliance per se.[K1,L8,W2]

Atrioventricular Valvular Dysfunction

As discussed earlier, important mitral incompetence is present in 2.5%–10% of adults with large ASDs, and both mitral and tricuspid incompetence sometimes become prominent in older patients in whom the syndrome of chronic congestive heart failure develops. When the tricuspid valve is viewed at operation, it does not appear to be intrinsically abnormal. Presumably, the incompetence develops because of annular dilation and a lack of proper shortening of the tricuspid anulus during systole[T1,T2] secondary to the right ventricular enlargement that has developed from the long-standing volume overload.

Supraventricular Arrhythmias

After the third decade of life, supraventricular arrhythmias complicate the natural history of patients with large ASDs and related conditions in increasing numbers as the years pass. Most commonly, this begins with paroxysmal atrial fibrillation, which gradually becomes permanent. Thus, atrial fibrillation was present in 15 (20%, CL 15%–26%) of 75 patients over the age of 40 years operated on by Magilligan and colleagues.[M6] Of 19 patients preoperatively in NYHA class III or IV, 47% (CL 34%–64%) had this arrhythmia, compared with 11% (CL 6%–17%) of 56 in class I or II. St. John Sutton and colleagues found 56% of their patients over the age of 60 years at the time of operation to have atrial fibrillation.[S1]

Systemic Arterial Hypertension

Adult patients with hemodynamically important ASDs are likely to have systemic arterial hypertension. This fact has been established by St. John Sutton and colleagues, at the Mayo Clinic.[S1] They found that 25 (38%) of their 66 patients had systemic arterial blood pressures above 150/90, a significantly higher proportion ($P < .01$) than in an age-matched general population. As noted, this relationship may in part be due to the effect of the hypertension on the size of the shunt.

TECHNIQUE OF OPERATION

Repair of Fossa Ovalis Type of Atrial Septal Defect

Anesthetic management, positioning and preparation of the patient, the median sternotomy incision, preparations for cardiopulmonary bypass (CPB), and the details of CPB are discussed in detail in Chapters 2 and 4. However, an alternative to the midline skin incision may be used in girls, in which a bilateral fourth interspace submammary skin incision is made and a skin flap raised superiorly and inferiorly before the sternum is incised vertically in the usual way (GLH). In young women with breast development, a right anterolateral fifth intercostal space incision may be used if there is concern by the patient about the cosmetic effects of a midline scar (GLH).

In children and young adults with uncomplicated ASDs, a left atrial line as a routine is considered unnecessary (UAB), or, alternatively, may be considered necessary because of the known tendency of the left atrial pressure to be considerably higher than the right after repair (GLH).

After making the incision and placing pericardial stay sutures, the intrapericardial anatomy is assessed. The characteristically large right atrium and right ventricle of ASD are noted, as well as the normal-sized left atrium and left ventricle. A left superior vena cava in the fold of Marshall or a left vertical vein without a connection to the coronary sinus, which may be above the left pulmonary veins, is sought. The external position and connections of the right and left superior and inferior pulmonary veins are noted. Often the ASD can be palpated through the atrial wall. In older children and adults, the interior of the right atrium may be examined digitally with the left index finger passed through the right atrial appendage, under tourniquet control, just before inserting the caval cannula. The ASD, the position of the orifices of the pulmonary veins, and any mitral or tricuspid incompetence can be evaluated in this way.

The patient is heparinized and the arterial cannula inserted. Two venous cannulae are used, and both are inserted through the right atrial appendage using an unsutured purse-string controlled with a Rumell tourniquet (GLH), or, alternatively, direct caval cannulation with the special metal cannulae is employed (UAB) (see Chapter 2, Fig. 2-20).

CPB is established at 34°C. As soon as the perfusion is well-established, the perfusate temperature is made as cold as possible. The cardioplegic needle may be placed in the ascending aorta now (GLH), or it may have been placed before CPB (UAB) (see Chapter 3). After a few minutes, the heart is cool, and the aorta is cross-clamped, the cold cardioplegic solution injected, and external cardiac cooling begun. Rewarming of the patient with the perfusate is begun (see Chapter 2), now that the heart is cold and isolated. The caval tapes are snugged, and the right atrium is opened obliquely (Fig. 15-12). The oblique atriotomy incision is subsequently extended into the appendage if cannulation has been through it, cutting the purse-string and freeing the caval lines to retract out of the surgical field (GLH). A left atrial suction line is never inserted through the left atrial wall in this condition, as it is not necessary and imposes a remote risk of cerebral air embolism.

A few fine silk stay sutures are placed on the edges of the atriotomy incision. Blood in the left atrium is sucked out only enough to expose clearly the edges of the ASD, as the evacuation of more blood than this from the left side of the heart needlessly exposes the patient to the risk of air entrapment and subsequent air embolization. Doubt about mitral valve function imposes an exception to this policy, for under

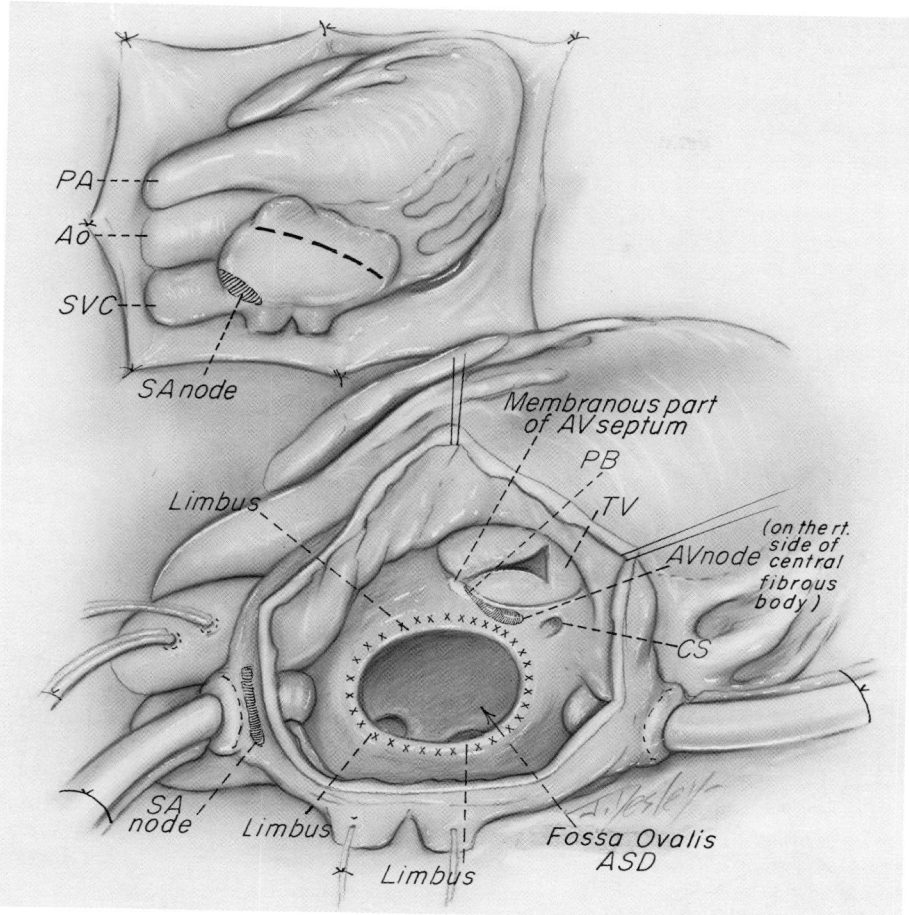

Figure 15-12   The usual oblique right atriotomy incision is made. The vulnerability of the sinus node in the superior aspect of the crista terminalis is evident. It is important to note the proximity of the suture bites (x's) in the anterior limbic tissue to the AV node, lying in the muscular portion of the atrioventricular septum, just inferior to the membranous portion.

Ao, aorta; ASD, atrial septal defect; AV, atrioventricular; CS, coronary sinus; PA, pulmonary artery; PB, penetration of bundle; SA, sinoatrial; SVC, superior vena cava; TV, tricuspid valve.

Reproduced with permission from Bharati et al.[B9]

such circumstances the mitral valve must be carefully examined. The entire right atrial internal anatomy is examined, particularly to identify the limbus anteriorly, superiorly, and inferiorly and the location and rim of the ASD. The relationships of the defect to the ostium of the coronary sinus, the membranous portion of the atrioventricular septum, and the commissural area between the septal and anterior tricuspid leaflets are studied, as these serve as guides to the location of the AV node and penetrating portion of the bundle of His (Fig. 15-12). Possible fenestrations in the valve (floor) of the fossa ovalis are sought, particularly between it and the limbus anteriorly, and inferiorly adjacent to the inferior vena cava. When fenestrations are present among thin tissue, they may be joined to the main defect by the excision of sufficient tissue to create an edge strong enough to hold sutures well (GLH), or the fenestrated tissue may be simply imbricated into the suture line (UAB).

Usually, the ASD is closed directly (see "Special Situations and Controversies"). The suturing is begun at the inferior angle (Fig. 15-13), by the placement of a half purse-string stitch of 4-0 or 3-0 polypropylene, and care is taken to catch good, substantial anterior and posterior limbic tissue with the first and last bites of the half purse-string stitch (Fig. 15-13). This stitch must be inferior to any remaining fenestrations. Great care is taken to avoid confusing the eustachian valve of the inferior vena cava with the remnant of the floor of the fossa ovalis. Such an error would result in the connection of the inferior vena cava to the *left* atrium and can occur when the operation is being done under circulatory arrest and there is no IVC cannula. After this half purse-string stitch is tied, the ASD assumes a slitlike appearance. The suture line is now carried superiorly, catching tough limbic tissue anteriorly and posteriorly. The sutures must not be placed too far from the edge anteriorly, lest the AV node be damaged. Before the last few stitches are pulled up, a clamp or tissue forceps is placed in the aperture, and the anesthesiologist inflates the lung to expel any air from the left atrium. The suture line is snugged while lung inflation is maintained, and an additional bite is taken with the stitch, which is then tied. After the right atrium is sucked dry, once

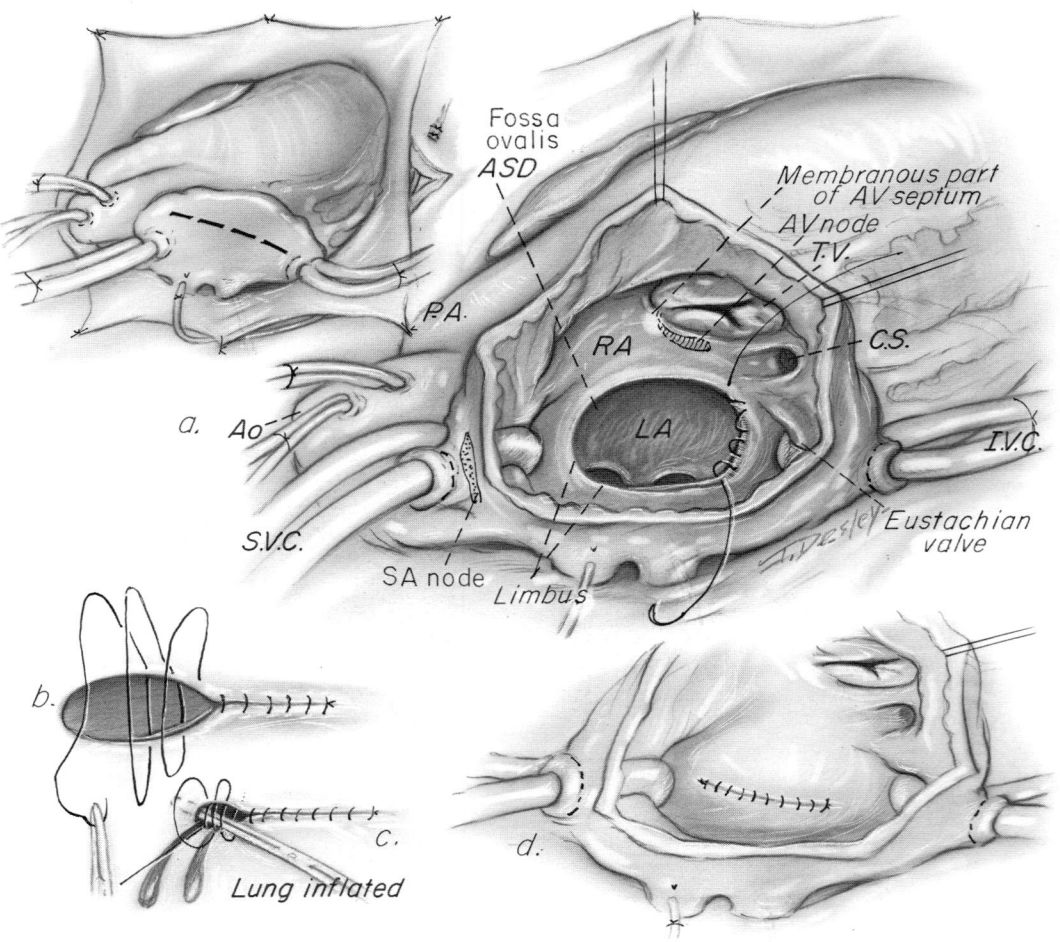

Figure 15-13

(*a*) After the exposure is arranged and all the structures are examined, the first stitches are taken in the form of a half purse-string, as shown. If the ASD extends to the inferior vena cava (IVC), the initial stitches are in the floor of the IVC. The eustachian valve is first identified so that it is not erroneously included.

(*b*) After the first stitch is tied, the large ASD becomes almost slitlike.

(*c*) Before tying the last stitch, the anesthesiologist places positive pressure on the lung to express any air from the left atrium.

(*d*) Completed repair.

Ao, aorta; ASD, atrial septal defect; CS, coronary sinus; IVC, inferior vena cava; PA, pulmonary artery; RA, right atrium; SVC, superior vena cava; TV, tricuspid valve.

again the lungs are inflated to drive left atrial blood through, and thus identify, any defects in the suture line. If any are seen, they are closed with a few interrupted sutures. The right atrium is then closed. The caval tapes are released, the apex of the upturned left ventricle is aspirated for air, strong suction is placed on the aortic needle vent, and the aortic clamp is released. Generally, it has been in place about 10 minutes for this procedure.

After a good cardiac action has developed, the usual de-airing procedures are carried out. Atrial wires are placed routinely (GLH), or, alternatively, they may be omitted in young patients (UAB). CPB is now discontinued, with care taken not to overdistend the left side of the heart in the

process. Even when a left atrial catheter is not left for the postoperative period, left atrial pressure is measured at this time (or estimated by palpation of the pulmonary artery), and it will be noted that it is 5–15 mmHg higher than right atrial pressure. This increase is related to the small size and decreased compliance of the left ventricle compared to that of the right (see footnote 1 and Chapter 5, footnote 8). The remainder of the operation is completed as usual.

Repair of Posterior Atrial Septal Defect

If the defect is a pure posterior ASD, closure by direct suture is possible in a manner similar to that described under "Re-

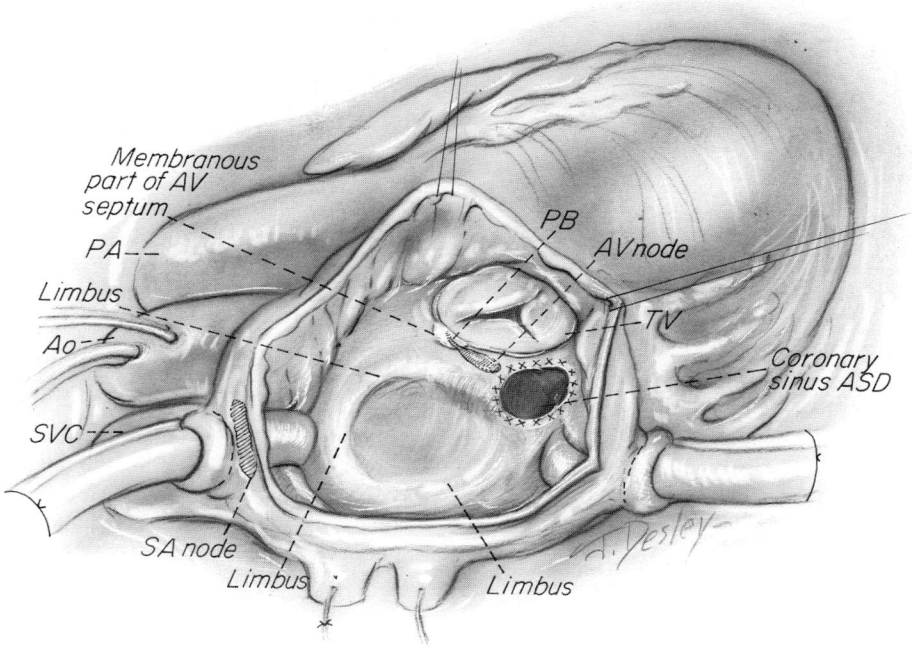

Figure 15-14   Repair of coronary sinus type of ASD. The proximity of this type of ASD to the AV node is shown. The *x*'s indicate the suture siting for the patch repair, which must be close to the edge of the defect to avoid the AV node.

Ao, aorta; ASD, atrial septal defect; AV, atrioventricular; PA, pulmonary artery; PB, penetrating bundle; SA, sinus node; SVC, superior vena cava.

Reproduced with permission from Bharati et al.[89]

pair of Fossa Ovalis Type of ASD." If the posterior ASD is confluent with a fossa ovalis ASD, the defect is too large for direct closure. Thus, a patch of pericardium or knitted Dacron velour is used.

Repair of Coronary Sinus Type of Atrial Septal Defect

Since the coronary sinus type of ASD is close to the AV node (Fig. 15-14), stitches must be placed close to the edge of the defect superiorly, in tissue that may not be very strong. For these reasons, closure with a patch is generally advisable.

Repair of Sinus Venosus Syndrome

The preparation and positioning of the patient are performed as usual for repair of sinus venosus syndrome. After the sternotomy incision is made, the pericardium is cleared of the pleural reflections bilaterally, and a large piece of it is taken out and set aside between moist towels.[2] After the remaining pericardium is widely opened, stay sutures are

placed, and the anatomy is examined. The right superior pulmonary vein is easily seen, attached to the low SVC or SVC–right atrial junction. The size of the SVC is noted, as is the possible presence of a left SVC, in which case the right-sided SVC is likely to be small. The right atrium and right ventricle are usually considerably enlarged.

The purse-string sutures are placed as usual, including those for direct caval cannulation. That for SVC cannulation is placed on the anterior aspect of the SVC cephalad to the area of abnormal connection of the right superior pulmonary vein.

Cardiopulmonary bypass (CPB) is then established. The perfusate from the pump-oxygenator is promptly cooled, and the heartbeat soon becomes ineffective. The caval tapes are secured. (In infants, the repair may be done with a single venous cannula and total circulatory arrest).

If the heartbeat has become ineffective, the atriotomy is made, and aortic cross-clamping and infusion of the cold cardioplegic solution is deferred until the exposure is obtained. Otherwise, the heart is arrested before the atriotomy is made. When the aorta is cross-clamped, the perfusate temperature is stabilized at 25°C.

When the configuration of the superior pulmonary vein is usual and the SVC–right atrial junction is widened, the right atrium is opened through the usual oblique incision beginning at the base of the right atrial appendage and extending down toward the IVC cannula (Fig. 15-16). Stay sutures are

---

[2] A special technique for using a pericardial patch was developed many years ago (GLH) and has had long use at both GLH and UAB (Fig. 15-15). It greatly facilitates trimming the patch and beginning its insertion.

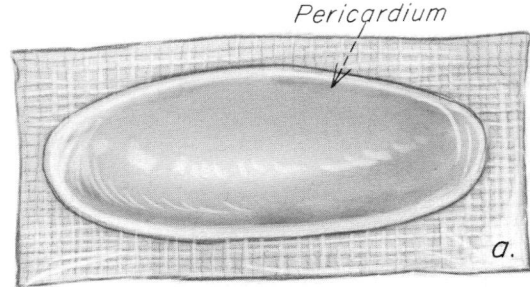

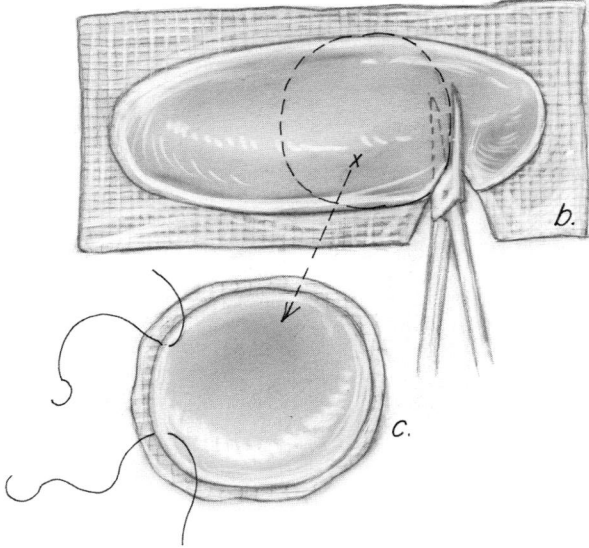

Figure 15-15 A useful technique that facilitates handling of a pericardial patch and avoids the need for stay sutures.
(a) The piece of excised pericardium is flattened onto a piece of wet toweling with its shiny serosa uppermost.
(b) The pericardium and toweling are both cut to the appropriate shape.
(c) A suture can now be positioned without distorting the pericardium. Pericardium and toweling are both lowered into the heart, and the cloth is not withdrawn until the pericardial patch is appropriately positioned.

placed. A pump sump sucker is placed across the foramen ovale into the left atrium (or through a stab wound made there for it) (UAB), or, alternatively, no left atrial vent may be used (GLH). When the lower SVC is small (as it may be, particularly when there is a large left SVC) or the anomalous pulmonary veins are three or four in number and some enter the SVC more superiorly than usual, a vertical atriotomy is made posteriorly and extended into the SVC posterior to the sinus node and just in front of the anomalous veins (Fig. 15-17), in preparation for a V-Y–plasty enlargement of the SVC (GLH).

The repair directs the pulmonary venous drainage through the ASD into the left atrium while closing the interatrial communication (Fig. 15-16). This is done with a pericardial baffle, which forms approximately the anterior half of this internal conduit. The width of the pericardial patch should be about one and one-half times the diameter of the ASD,

and its length about one and one-quarter times the estimated length of the distances from the superior edge of the anomalous vein to the inferior edge of the ASD. This assures an adequate pulmonary venous pathway and does not obstruct the SVC.

When a V-Y–plasty has been elected (GLH), the plastic enlargement of the SVC is usually carried out before the release of the aortic cross-clamp (Fig. 15-17). Otherwise, after the repair is made, the sump (if used) is removed and the defect made for it is closed. Rewarming is begun, and with suction on the needle vent in the ascending aorta, the aortic clamp is released. The right atriotomy incision is closed. The operation is completed as usual (see Chapter 2).

Repair of Anomalous Connection of Right Pulmonary Veins to Right Atrium

The operation begins exactly as described for the sinus venosus syndrome, including the opening of the right atrium through the usual oblique incision. The interior of the right atrium is examined, the anomalous connections of the right pulmonary veins and the normal connection to the left atrium of the left pulmonary veins are confirmed, and any defects in the atrial septum are identified.

When the atrial septum is intact, the repair can often be accomplished by making a longitudinal incision in the atrial septum next to the atrial wall posteriorly and resuturing the septum to the lateral right atrial wall in front of the right pulmonary vein orifices. Alternatively, and particularly when the geometry in the right atrium does not lend itself to this simple repair, the fossa ovalis and posterior limbic tissue may be excised and a pericardial or knitted Dacron patch used for the reconstruction (Fig. 15-18).

Figure 15-16 Repair of sinus venous syndrome, consisting typically of a subcaval atrial septal defect associated with partial anomalous pulmonary venous connection of the right superior pulmonary vein to the low superior vena cava.
(a) The usual oblique atriotomy incision (dashed line) is far removed from the sinus node.
(b) Representation of the interior of the right atrium and superior vena cava, shown diagrammatically as if the anterior right atrial wall were cut away. The subcaval atrial septal defect is superior to the limbus. At times, the superior vena cava overrides the defect to drain in part directly into the left atrium. The atrial septal defect is far removed from the tricuspid valve and atrioventricular node. The anterior (leftward) point of the suture line for the pericardial patch will be at a. The first stitch for the insertion of the pericardial patch is shown.
(c) The pericardial patch is being sewn into place with continuous 4-0 polypropylene suture. The x's indicate the siting of sutures yet to be placed.
(d) The convex pericardial roof of the tunnel has been completed, beneath which blood from the anomalously connected right superior pulmonary vein drains into the left atrium. The pathway from the superior vena cava to the right atrium is unobstructed (in this depiction, the atriotomy incision is depicted as it actually is). When the superior vena cava is cannulated directly, as shown, exposure is good through this oblique incision.

Ao, aorta; ASD, atrial septal defect; CS, coronary sinus; PA, pulmonary artery; RSPV, right superior pulmonary vein; SYC, superior vena cava; TV, tricuspid valve.

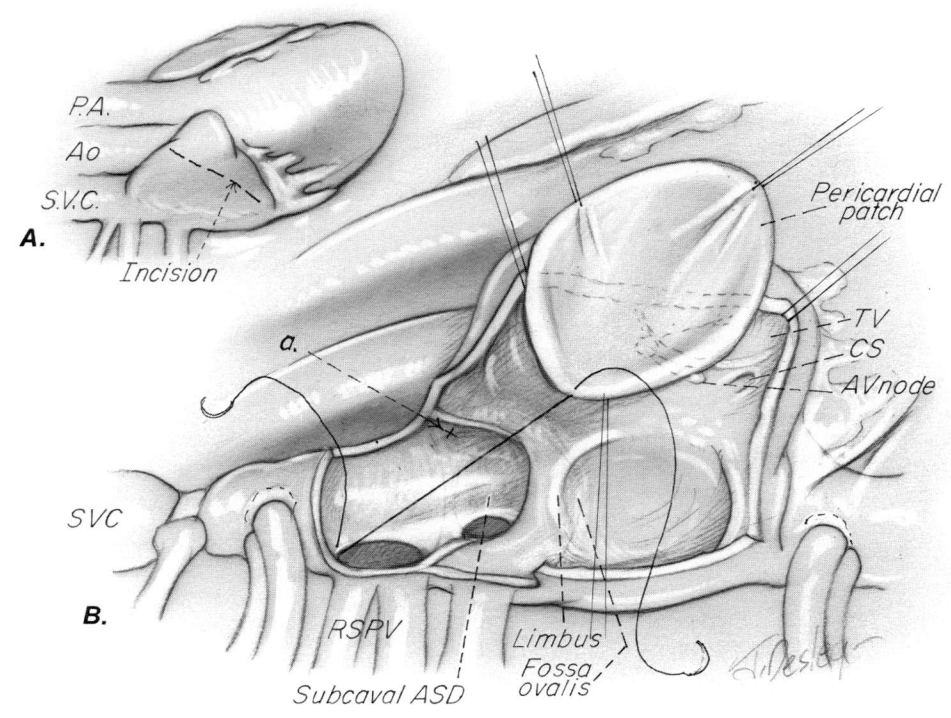

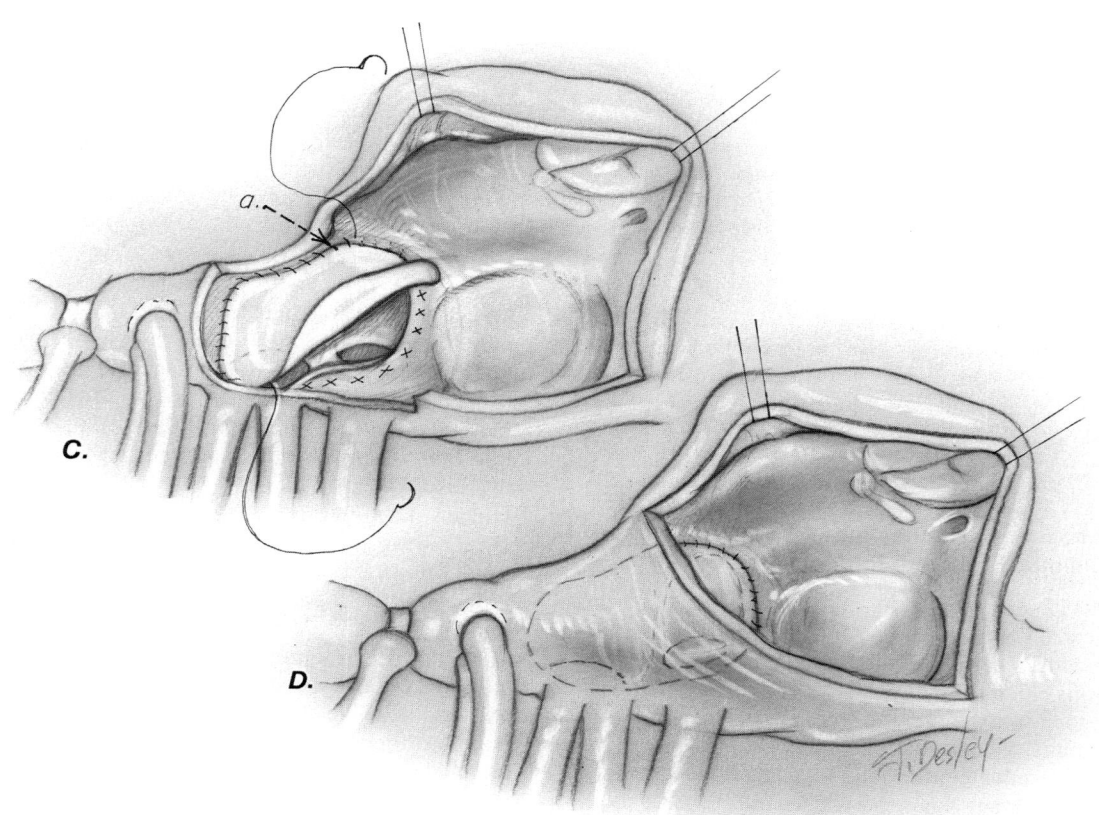

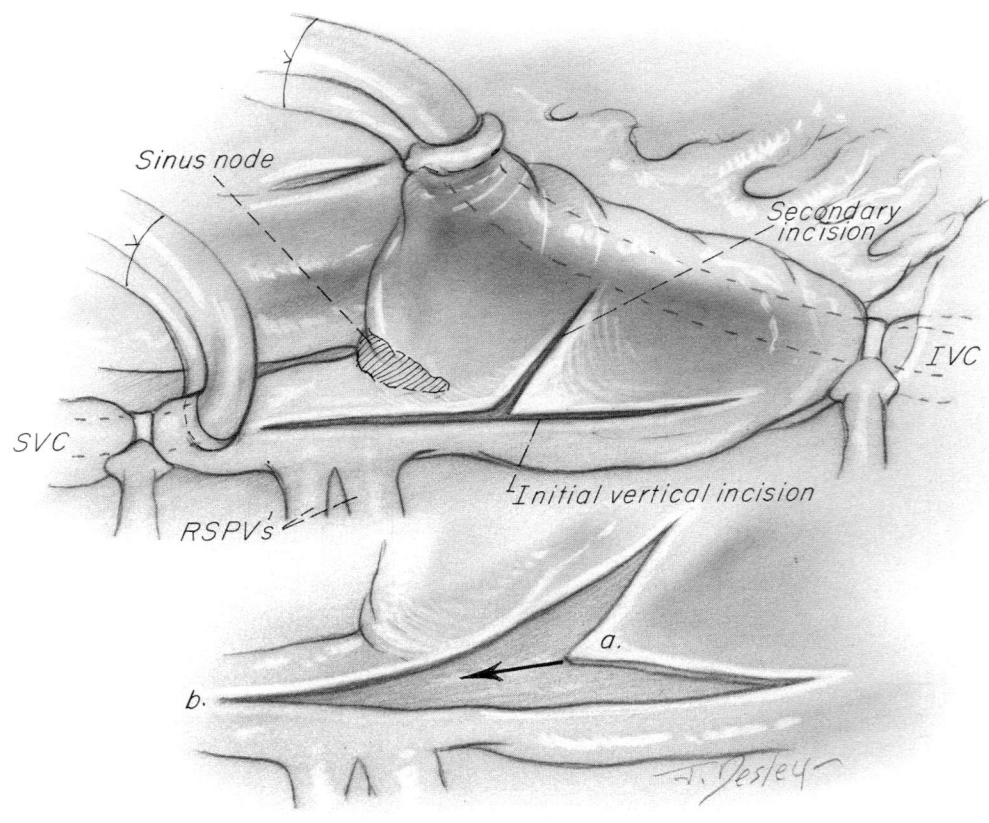

Figure 15-17   V-Y atrioplasty technique for enlargement of SVC (GLH). The initial incision is vertical (longitudinal) and does not cross the SVC-RA junction unless it is thought that SVC enlargement will be required. In such cases, the secondary incision is then added to create a V flap of right atrial wall. The SVC is enlarged by advancing the tip of the V flap (a) to the apex of the SVC incision.

IVC, inferior vena cava; RSPV, right superior pulmonary vein; SVC, superior vena cava.

When an ASD is present, the repair is similar. When the defect is large and of the fossa ovalis or confluent type, a patch is used, in a fashion similar to that shown in Figure 15-18c and d. Occasionally, and particularly when the associated ASD is a posterior one, repair by direct suture is possible.

Repair of Anomalous Connection of Right Pulmonary Veins to Inferior Vena Cava

The initial stages of the operation proceed as described for the sinus venosus syndrome. An internal conduit is then constructed within the right atrium to conduct the right pulmonary venous blood from its entrance into the inferior vena cava across the atrial septum into the left atrium.

In small infants, the entire repair may be done during profoundly hypothermic total circulatory arrest. In older patients, part of the repair can be performed during profoundly hypothermic total circulatory arrest (UAB), or, alternatively, the entire repair can be performed during conventional CPB at 25°C. In the latter case, the IVC tape may be passed inferior (caudad) to the entrance of the anomalous pulmonary vein into the IVC and the right-angled metal cannula used to cannulate the IVC inferior to this point. This possibility depends on the entrance of the anomalous vein at the right atrial–IVC junction. If this is not possible, the common femoral or external iliac vein may be cannulated for IVC return (GLH).

In any case, CPB is established with two venous cannulae, and if part of the repair is to be made with total circulatory arrest, the IVC tape is placed on the cardiac side of the IVC entrance of the anomalous vein. The aorta is cross-clamped, and the cold cardioplegic solution is infused. After the caval tapes have been tightened, the right atrium is opened with the usual oblique incision, carried right down to the IVC. If present, the valve of the fossa ovalis is completely excised to create a large ASD (Fig. 15-19). The pericardial patch is trimmed according to the measurements made, and stay sutures are applied at the four corners.

Total circulatory arrest is established with the patient at 20°C when this modality is used, and the IVC cannula is removed. Otherwise, the repair proceeds during CPB. The

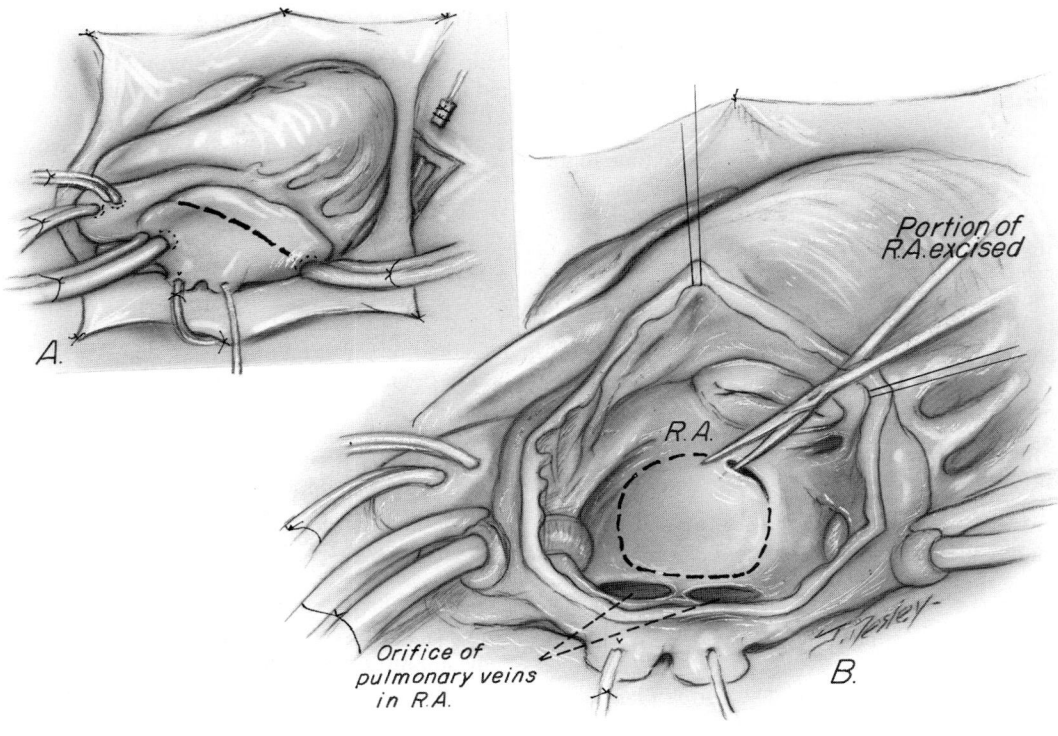

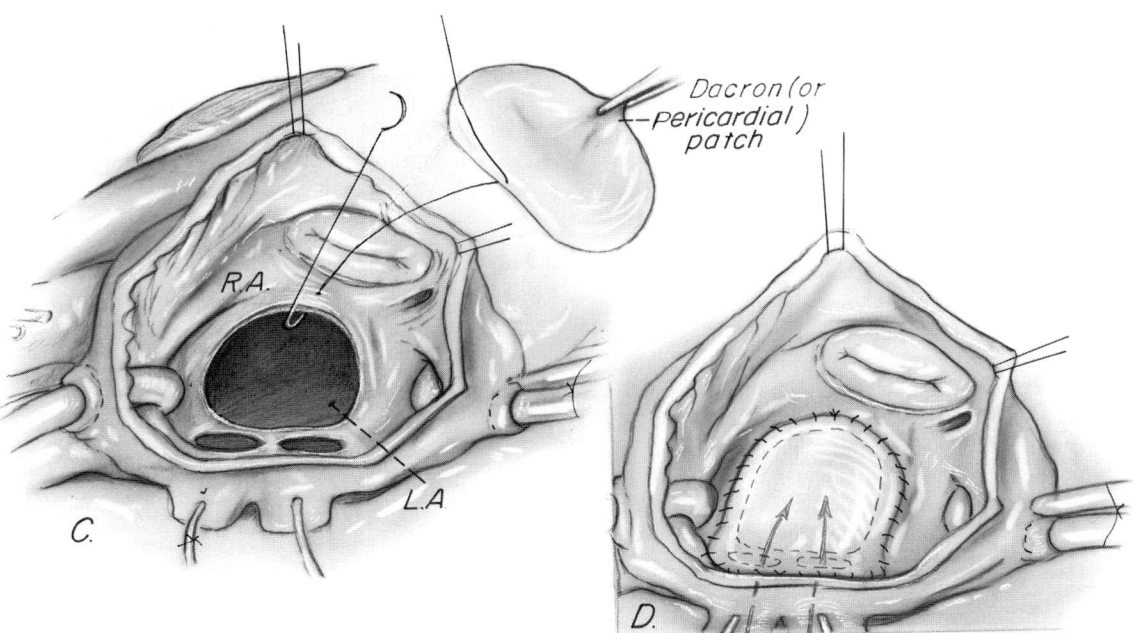

Figure 15-18 The repair of anomalous connection of the right superior and inferior pulmonary veins to right atrium without an ASD.

(a) The right atrial incision is the usual oblique one, as is indicated by the dashed line.

(b) The fossa ovalis and posterior limbus are excised.

(c, d) The repair is made by replacing the excised portion of the atrial septum with a patch, brought to the right of the right pulmonary vein orifices.

LA, left atrium; RA, right atrium.

pericardial patch is sewn into place so as to form the anterior wall of a conduit between the entrance of the anomalous vein and the defect created in the atrial septum (Fig. 15-19). If the repair has been done during total circulatory arrest, the IVC cannula is reinserted, the caval tape re-tightened, CPB re-established, and rewarming of the patient with the perfusate begun. The anomalous vein is observed from time to time to be certain that pressure in it is not elevated, for its drainage is now temporarily obstructed by the IVC tape. The right atrium is closed, and the caval tapes are promptly released. The apex of the left ventricle is aspirated for air, and with suction on the aortic needle vent, the aortic clamp is released. Drainage of the anomalous pulmonary vein is now unobstructed. The remainder of the procedure is completed as usual.

Repair of Anomalous Connection of Left Pulmonary Veins to Left Innominate Vein

When the atrial septum is intact or there is only a valvular competent foramen ovale, the operation is by a closed technique. The left chest is entered through a posterolateral incision. The anomalous left vertical vein is dissected up to the left innominate vein. The left superior and inferior veins are dissected and mobilized as much as possible. A tape is placed around the left pulmonary artery. The pericardium is opened, usually behind the phrenic nerve, and a large window is made. A clamp is placed across the very base of the left atrial appendage, and most of the appendage is amputated. The left pulmonary artery is temporarily occluded, the left vertical vein is ligated flush with the left innominate vein, a clamp is placed across its proximal portion, and it is divided as far distally (downstream) as possible. With great care taken to avoid any rotation, the vein is positioned and anastomosed to the base of the left atrial appendage. At least part of the anastomosis is made with interrupted sutures to avoid any possible purse-string effect. Before releasing the clamps, care is taken that no air is in the vein.

When there is an associated fossa ovalis ASD, both the anomalous left pulmonary venous connection and the ASD should be repaired. (The first patient undergoing repair of this anomaly, reported from the Mayo Clinic in 1953,[K3] required later closure of the ASD, at which time the previously made anastomosis was functioning well.) This can all be accomplished through a median sternotomy incision with CPB.

The anastomosis between the vertical vein and the left atrial appendage can be modified when CPB is used. Ports and colleagues[P4] make a long incision in the lateral aspect of the left atrial appendage, carrying it down onto the left atrium. The anomalous vein is cut transversely, and then a T extension is made posteriorly. The end-to-side anastomosis is then a very wide one. Alternatively, a side-to-side vertical vein to left atrial anastomosis is made, ligating the vertical vein at its junction with the innominate vein (GLH).

Repair of Other Anomalous Pulmonary Venous Connections

Bilateral PAPVCs and rare right or left anomalous connections require individual techniques, using the principles described for the standard repairs.

Treatment of Associated Mitral or Tricuspid Valve Disease

Mitral stenosis is treated by valvotomy and mitral and tricuspid incompetence, whenever possible, by annuloplasty (see Chapter 11, "Mitral Incompetence Repair" in section on Technique of Operation). Should mitral valve replacement be required, great care is required, since the anulus tends to be very friable.

SPECIAL FEATURES OF POSTOPERATIVE CARE

The convalescence of most children and adolescents who have had repair of an uncomplicated ASD, and also of most adults operated on before they have reached NYHA functional class IV, is uneventful. Thus, they are extubated in the operating room or within a few hours of leaving it. The arterial blood pressure is monitored until the next morning via an arterial needle and right atrial (or, alternatively, (GLH) both right and left atrial) pressure via the usual polyvinyl catheter (see Chapter 2).

Occasionally older patients have unusually high left atrial pressures (20–25 mmHg) in the early hours after repair, presumably because systolic and diastolic left ventricular functions are more than usually impaired by the aging process or by coexisting coronary artery disease, systolic arterial hypertension, or by residual significant mitral incompetence that has been underestimated preoperatively. In contrast to a few examples reported in the literature,[B2,B5] in which urgent reoperation was performed and the ASD reopened because of severe left heart failure with pulmonary edema, in 30 years of experience with this malformation at GLH, the Mayo Clinic, and UAB, no ASD has had to be reopened. A part of the explanation for this may be that closure of the ASD has not been recommended when the *primary* problem was left ventricular cardiomyopathy. However, because of

---

Figure 15-19 Repair of the scimitar syndrome.

(a) The usual oblique right atriotomy incision is made, extending it to the inferior vena cava (IVC).

(b) The valve (floor) of the fossa ovalis is excised, as shown by the dashed circle, creating an atrial septal defect that extends nearly to the IVC.

(c) Stay sutures are placed as shown to mark out the proposed suture line. The distance from the inferior aspect of the orifice of the anomalous vein entrance into the IVC to the superior limbus is measured. The width of the fossa ovalis is measured. The pericardial patch is trimmed in a rectangular shape, the length of which is about 1.25 times the measured length and whose width is about 1.5 times the width of the fossa ovalis. A pledgetted mattress suture of 4-0 or 3-0 prolene is placed at the inferior aspect of the orifice of the anomalous pulmonary vein in the IVC, after this orifice and that of the hepatic vein are positively identified. The suture line between the patch and the floor of the IVC is carried to the patient's left and then up toward and onto anterior limbus, where it is held. With the other arm of the original suture, the patch is attached above the orifice of the anomalous vein as the suture line is carried superiorly. The patch is then attached successively to the posterior limbus, the superior limbus, and the anterior limbus and tied there to the other end of the suture.

(d, e) The patch now forms approximately one-half of an intra-atrial internal conduit conducting right pulmonary vein blood across the defect created in the fossa ovalis into the left atrium.

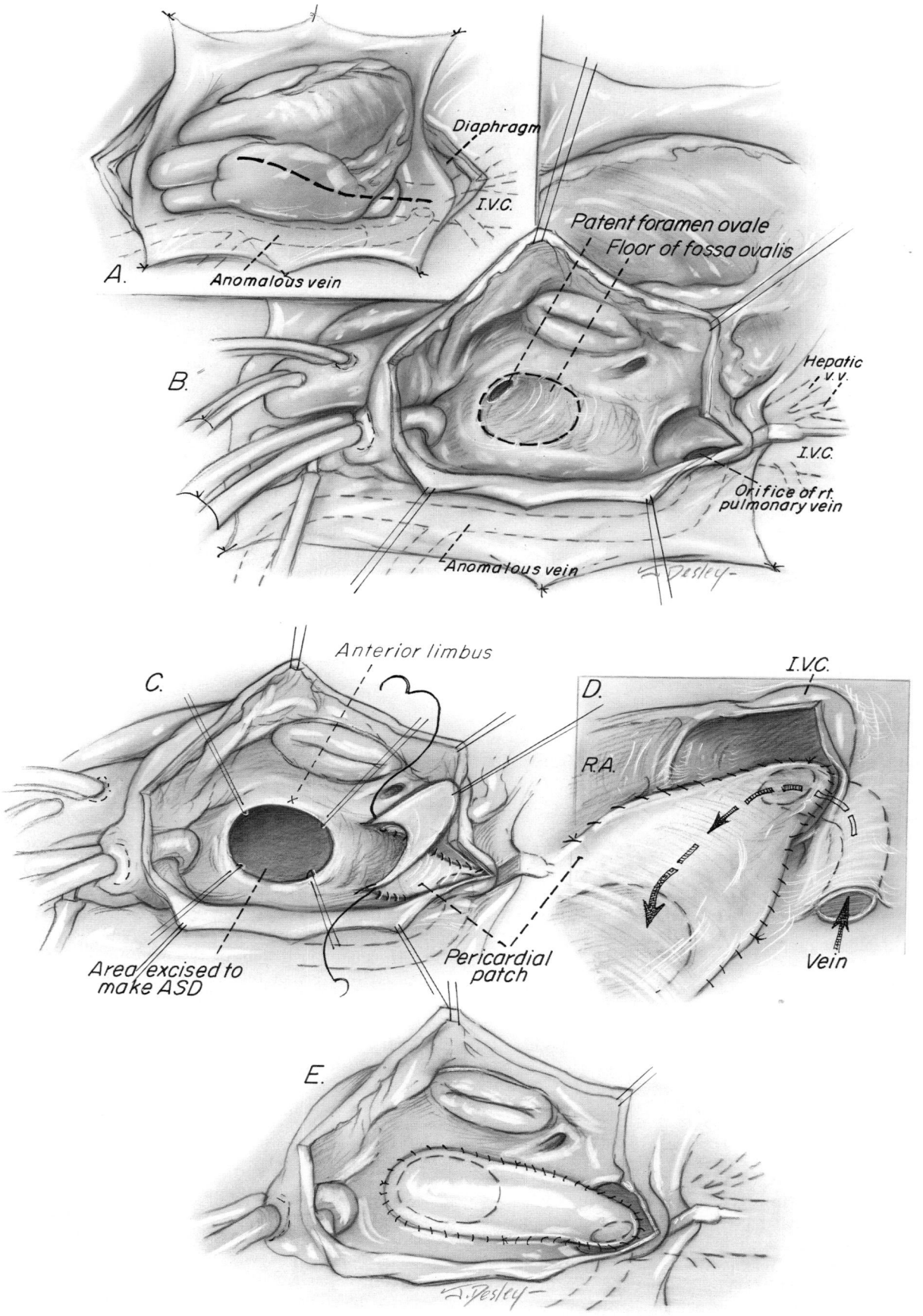

A.

Diaphragm

I.V.C.

Anomalous vein

B.

Patent foramen ovale

Floor of fossa ovalis

Hepatic v. v.

I.V.C.

Orifice of rt. pulmonary vein

Anomalous vein

C.

Anterior limbus

Area excised to make ASD

Pericardial patch

D.

I.V.C.

R.A.

Vein

E.

these considerations, left atrial pressure is routinely monitored intraoperatively and for about 24 hours postoperatively in older patients. Occasionally, when mitral incompetence has been underestimated preoperatively and there are signs of severe pulmonary venous hypertension postoperatively, an urgent left ventricular angiogram may be required. If the angiogram shows important residual mitral regurgitation, reoperation may be necessary to repair or replace the mitral valve.

All patients over 35 years of age at operation receive Coumadin (sodium warfarin) prophylactically, beginning on the evening of the second postoperative day and continuing for 8–12 weeks after the repair (UAB). The rationale is that there is an important incidence of both pulmonary and systemic arterial embolization after repair in patients over about 35 years of age.[H2] The incidence is particularly high in elderly patients in atrial fibrillation (see "Late Results"), and in them permanent anticoagulation is usually warranted.

EARLY RESULTS

Hemodynamic Results

Striking changes occur immediately after closure of an uncomplicated atrial septal defect. Mean pressure in the ascending aorta increases, as does mean aortic blood flow.[S13] Of course, there is an immediate reduction in pulmonary blood flow.[L9] Right atrial pressure decreases, and left atrial pressure increases, Søndergard and colleagues finding an average immediate rise of 8 mmHg.[S13]

Hospital Mortality

The hospital mortality for repair of ASDs and related conditions has approached zero for many years in most cardiac surgical centers throughout the world. Even in the early years of cardiac surgery, between 1954 and 1965, 696 patients underwent repair of the ASD by us at the Mayo Clinic, with 22 hospital deaths (3.2%),[R5] and in that era at GLH there were three hospital deaths (2.5%) among the first 122 patients undergoing repair, including those with PAPVC.[B11] In the current era, in the combined UAB-GLH experience, five deaths (1.0%, CL 0.5%–1.6%) have occurred among 518 patients undergoing repair of ASD alone (Tables 15-5, 15-6); and one death (0.7%, CL 0.1%–2.5%) has occurred among patients undergoing repair of PAPVC with or without ASD (Tables 15-6, 15-7).

Mode of Hospital Death

The modes of death are variable, and most not relevant to current experience. However, they do serve to emphasize some of the risks that have been overcome in time with improved knowledge, technique, and experience. Among the six deaths in the combined GLH-UAB experience with repair of ASD and PAPVC in the current era, one (operation in 1969) was from a profound neurologic deficit, probably from cerebral air embolism; three were from multiple sub-

Table 15-5 Hospital mortality after repair of isolated atrial septal defect (UAB; 1967–1979).

| Location (Type) of ASD[a] | n[b] | Hospital Deaths | |
		No.	%
Fossa ovalis	317	3	0.9%
Posterior (absence of posterior limbus)	12		0%
Confluent (fossa ovalis plus absence of posterior limbus)	7		0%
Not classified	4		0%
Total	340[c]	3	0.9%(CL 0.4%–1.8%)

KEY: ASD, atrial septal defect; CL, 70% confidence limits.

[a] The isolated sinus venosus ASDs are in Table 15-9. All patients with coronary sinus ASDs had major associated cardiac anomalies and appear in Chapter 18.

[b] Excludes patients with ASD and partial or total anomalous pulmonary venous connection, AV canal defects, major associated cardiac malformations, or associated coronary artery bypass grafting (13 patients, no deaths) or valve replacement for unrelated mitral valve disease (10 patients, no deaths).

[c] Females 236, males 104. Age range 11/12–72 years.

system failure secondary to low cardiac output in older patients with advanced heart failure preoperatively; one in another patient in advanced heart failure preoperatively was from uncontrolled supraventricular tachycardia on the second postoperative day. One 19-year-old girl with a history of severe drug abuse died on the fifth postoperative day, of renewed acute drug abuse, after four days of normal convalescence.

Incremental Risk Factors for Hospital Death

Advanced chronic congestive heart failure, as reflected in the preoperative NYHA functional class, is an incremental risk factor for hospital death (Table 15-8). However, the difference in risk is not evident until the disability is severe and the NYHA functional class is IV or V. Even then, current risks can be expected to be less than 10%. Advanced and probably irreversible right ventricular dysfunction is the basis of the increased risk in such situations.

The anatomic details of the malformation have not increased the risk of repair (Tables 15-5, 15-6, 15-7, 15-9). Neither very young age (Table 15-10) nor old age (Table 15-11) has increased the risk; this was also the situation in our earlier experience at the Mayo Clinic[D3] as well as later experiences at that institution.[H2,S1]

Morbidity

This is rare in the current era, but that occurring earlier provides a warning as to potential problems. Three patients operated on before 1973 (UAB) had neurologic complications, including the child who died. In the other two patients, such complications were transient. Presumably, they resulted from air embolization. Early reoperation for postoperative bleeding has been rare (1.5% in the UAB experience).

Table 15-6 Technique and hospital mortality after repair of ASD and PAPVC (GLH; 1957–1983). (Ostium secundum includes foramen ovale, confluent, and posterior ASDs).

Type of Defect	Year of Operation									
	1957–1968						1968–1983			
				Hospital Deaths				Hospital Deaths		
	Atrial Well	CPB	Total	No.	%	CL	CPB	No.	%	CL
OS	162	18	180	3	1.7%	.7%–3.3%	178	2[a]	1.1%	0.4%–2.7%
OS + PAPVC	17	3	20	1	5%	.6%–16%	17	0	0%	0%–11%
Isolated PAPVC							3	0	0%	0%–47%
Sinus venosus syndrome	23	0	23	2	9%	3%–19%	22	0	0%	0%–8%
Total	202[b]	21	223	6	2.7%	1.6%–4.3%	220	2	0.9%	0.3%–2.1%
$P(\chi^2)$				.12				.9		

KEY: CL, 70% confidence limits; CPB, cardiopulmonary bypass; OS, ostium secundum; PAPVC, partial anomalous pulmonary venous connection.

NOTE: The table includes all patients in whom the ASD was the dominant lesion or of equal significance to any associated lesions, 17 patients undergoing simultaneous surgery for unrelated mitral valve disease (3 deaths), and 2 undergoing simultaneous coronary artery bypass grafting (no deaths).

[a] Both patients required mitral valve surgery for severe regurgitation.

[b] Includes two atrioseptopexies.

Table 15-7 Hospital death after repair of partial anomalous pulmonary venous connection according to morphologic category (UAB; 1967–1981 and GLH; 1957–1983).

Category of Partial Anomalous Pulmonary Venous Connection	UAB			GLH			Total		
		Hospital Deaths			Hospital Deaths			Hospital Deaths	
	n	No.	%	n	No.	%	n	No.	%
Sinus venosus syndrome	56	1	2%	45	2	4%	101	3	3%
Part or all of right superior pulmonary veins to SVC without subcaval ASD	9		0%	3		0%	12		0%
Right superior and inferior pulmonary veins to RA	5		0%	23	1	4%	28	1	4%
Posterior ASD (absent posterior limbus) and anomalous connection right pulmonary veins to RA	7		0%	7		0%	14		0%
Right pulmonary veins to IVC (scimitar syndrome)	10		0%	2		0%	12		0%
Right pulmonary veins to coronary sinus				1		0%	1		0%
Left pulmonary veins to left innominate vein	3		0%	2		0%	5		0%
Bilateral but subtotal anomalous pulmonary venous connections	4		0%	2		0%	6		0%
Total	94	1	1%(CL .1%–4%)	85	3	3.5%(CL 1.6%–7.0%)	179	4	2.2%(CL 1.1%–4%)
$P(\chi^2)$		.99			.99			.98	

KEY: ASD, atrial septal defect; CL, 70% confidence limits; IVC, inferior vena cava; RA, right atrium; SVC, superior vena cava.

NOTE: Only three patients in the GLH series had no ASD. The three deaths in the GLH group were all before 1966.

Table 15-8 Preoperative status and hospital death after repair of atrial septal defect (UAB; 1967–1979; n = 340).

Preoperative NYHA Class (mean age in yr)	n	Hospital Deaths		
		No.	%	
I (16)	171	1	0.6%	⎱
II (32)	112	1	0.9%	⎰ 2/324, .6%, CL .2%–1.5%[a]
III (50)	41		0%	
IV (51)	13	1	8%	CL 1%–24%[a]
Unknown	3			
Total	340	3	0.9%	(CL 0.4%–1.8%)
$P(\chi^2)$		0.06		

KEY: CL, 70% confidence limits.

[a] P for difference (Fisher) = .11.

Table 15-9 Details of sinus venosus syndrome and hospital mortality after repair (UAB; 1967–1981).

Details of Sinus Venosus Syndrome	n	Hospital Deaths	
		No.	%
Typical	52	1[a]	2%
Without anomalous pulmonary venous connection	2		0%
With upper portion of right superior PV anomalously connected and inferior part to LA	1		0%
With right superior and inferior PV to low SVC	1		0%
Total	56	1	1.8%(CL .2%–6%)

KEY: ASD, atrial septal defect; CL, 70% confidence limits; LA, left atrium; PV, pulmonary vein; SVC, superior vena cava.

[a] 69-year-old man, in NYHA Class IV, with associated tricuspid incompetence; death with sepsis and multiple subsystem failure.

Table 15-10 ASD repair in patients under 2 years of age (GLH; 1957–1983). All have survived.

Age at Operation months	Type of Defect	Associated Anomalies
2	OS, APVC all R lung to RA	Moderate or severe PS
2	OS, APVC all R lung to RA	Mild coarctation of the aorta, mild aortic stenosis, anomalous R subclavian artery, LSVC
3	OS	Small PDA
5	OS	Large Morgagni hernia, small VSD, LSVC, isolated dextrocardia
6	OS, APVC all R lung to RA	
8	OS, APVC all R lung to IVC	Severe bronchiolitis
15	OS	
22	OS, APVC all R lung to RA	

KEY: APVC, anomalous pulmonary venous connection; IVC, inferior vena cava; LSVC, left superior vena cava; OS, ostium secundum ASD (see Table 15-1); PDA, patent ductus arteriosus; PS, pulmonary stenosis; R, right; RA, right atrium; VSD, ventricular septal defect.

NOTE: Congestive heart failure, recurrent respiratory infections, and growth retardation were present in all instances. Profound hypothermia and total circulatory arrest were used in those under 12 months of age.

LATE RESULTS

Survival

The long-term survival of patients whose ASD or PAPVC is repaired in the first few years of life is probably that of a matched general population, although this has not been proven. When operation is performed later in childhood or in early adult life, survival is probably very near to that of the matched general population, although this also has not been demonstrated.

Even in older patients, repair of ASD improves life expectancy, but survival is not that of a general population matched with the patient group as to age and sex. Thus, St.

John Sutton and associates found the 10-year survival rate to be 64% after repair of ASD in patients over 60 years of age, significantly better than that of similar patients treated nonsurgically (Fig. 15-20) but not as good as that of a matched general population.[S1]

Mode of Premature Late Death

In patients operated on at an older age (60 years or more), a neurologic mode of late death (cerebrovascular accident) is the commonest, occurring in 60% of the patients, and most have systemic arterial hypertension.[S1] The pathologic condition was intracerebral hemorrhage in those in whom autopsy

Table 15-11 Age and hospital mortality after repair of atrial septal defect (UAB; 1967–1979).

Age years ≤ <	n	Hospital Deaths No.	Hospital Deaths %
2	1[a]		0%
2--- 5	19		0%
5---10	71	1	1.4%
10---20	82	1	1.2%
20---30	40		0%
30---40	27		0%
40---50	39		0%
50---60	34	1	2.9%
60---70	26		0%
70---80	1		0%
Total	340	3	.9%(CL .4%–1.8%)
$P(\chi^2)$			.9

KEY: CL, 70% confidence limits.

[a] Eleven months old.

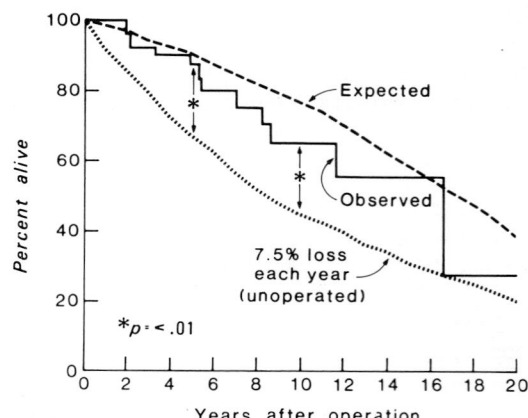

Figure 15-20 Late survival of patients over the age of 60 years after undergoing repair of ASD (hospital survivors only) compared to the survival of an age- and sex-matched general population (expected) and to that of patients of the same age treated nonsurgically (unoperated).

was done, in the experience of St. John Sutton and colleagues.[S1] The next commonest cause of premature late death in those operated on at age 60 and over is chronic congestive heart failure, which is particularly likely to occur among those with important heart failure preoperatively.[S1]

Symptomatic Results

In asymptomatic children, there is of course no change in symptoms from operation. Symptomatic infants undergoing repair of ASD have experienced complete relief of symptoms,[P3] and older symptomatic patients show improvement nearly routinely.[D4,R3,S3] Thus, Forfang and colleagues found that closure of the ASD in patients over 40 years of age improved the symptomatic state by one NYHA functional class in every patient.[F1] They, as well as other groups, found that arrhythmic symptoms regress less frequently than do others.

Even among patients operated on when over 60 years of age, the functional and symptomatic improvement is striking.[N2] St. John Sutton and colleagues found that 87% of their patients in this category were improved at least one NYHA functional class. Among the 31 patients preoperatively in NYHA class III or IV, only 2 (6%) remained severely disabled.[S1]

This striking symptomatic improvement, even in older patients whose cardiomegaly does not always regress, is documented in the studies by Pearlman and colleagues.[P2] They found excellent exercise treadmill performance and normal maximal oxygen consumption in all 14 consecutive patients studied late after repair of ASD, despite the fact that nine had persistently large right ventricular diastolic dimensions.

Incremental Risk Factors for Disability or Premature Late Death

No preoperative findings predispose patients to a poor long-term result except advanced preoperative symptoms, and even when this is present, considerable improvement usually results from the operation.[S1] St. John Sutton and colleagues found that, provided the pulmonary-systemic blood flow is greater than 1.5, neither preoperative pulmonary artery hypertension nor elevated pulmonary vascular resistance increases the risk of a poor late result (presupposing that the operation has not been performed in patients with a resistance above 12 units · m²).[S1] This is so despite the fact that in older patients the pulmonary vascular resistance is known not to decrease postoperatively.[G7]

The anatomic defect producing the left-to-right shunt at atrial level has not affected the late results significantly. Thus, the same survival rates and, with few exceptions, the same functional results apply throughout the group.[K7] Thus, Trusler and colleagues have reported good functional results in 29 patients followed 2–14 years after repair of the sinus venosus syndrome by techniques similar to those described here, with 25 being asymptomatic and 4 having mild symptoms.[T5] Among 18 of their patients undergoing late cardiac catheterization after this type of repair, only 1 had a gradient (6 mm) between SVC and right atrium.

Late Changes in Right Ventricular Function

Right ventricular diastolic dimensions are decreased strikingly after operation[B6] (Fig. 15-21) but still are above normal in many patients.[L5,M13,S4] This is consistent with Young's early observation that some children had important residual cardiomegaly years after complete repair of their ASD,[Y1] which he correctly ascribed to the secondary cardiomyopathy resulting from the chronic right ventricular volume overload. Pearlman and associates have shown an effect of age at operation in this regard;[P2] seven (64%, CL 44%–81%) of 11 patients 10 years of age or less at operation had normal or near normal right ventricular diastolic volumes late postoperatively, while only 3 (21%, CL 10%–38%) of 14 patients over the age of 25 years at operation had this finding (P [Fisher] for difference = .04).

In adult patients with preoperatively decreased right ventricular wall motion and ejection fraction, most of whom have elevated right atrial pressure and are importantly asymptomatic, the reduction in right ventricular size after surgical repair is less, and ejection fraction, although larger than preoperatively, remains abnormally low (47% in the experience of Liberthson and colleagues[L5]). Such patients are improved by operation but do not become asymptomatic. The analogies between this and the response to surgery of the volume overloaded *left* ventricle are apparent (see Chapter 12, "Left Ventricular Structure and Function" in section on Late Results).

Late Changes in Left Ventricular Function

Postoperatively, in contrast to the preoperative condition, the left ventricular ejection fraction increases normally with maximal exercise (Fig. 15-22). Thus, even in patients who have undergone repair of their ASD in adult life, exercise ejection fraction is normal after repair. This favorable change is the result of ablation of the right ventricular volume overload by closure of the ASD.

Also, left ventricular diastolic dimensions, when abnormally small preoperatively, increase to normal within 6 months of operation.[B6,W1] The abnormalities of left ventricular geometry present preoperatively are also corrected by the repair of the ASD.

Cardiac Conduction and Arrhythmias

The closure of atrial septal defects in children has been shown to improve atrioventricular (AV) conduction, decrease AV nodal refractory periods, and improve sinus node function in most patients early postoperatively.[B13] Presumably this is the result of reduction in right ventricular and right atrial volume after ablation of the left-to-right shunt at atrial level. However, Bolens and colleagues also found loss of sinus node function after operation and an atrial ectopic rhythm.[B13] This may have been the result of direct surgical damage to the sinus node.

Little specific information is available on arrhythmias late after repair of ASDs in infants and children. Presumably these are uncommon. Most adult patients with atrial fibrillation preoperatively continue to have it late postoperatively.

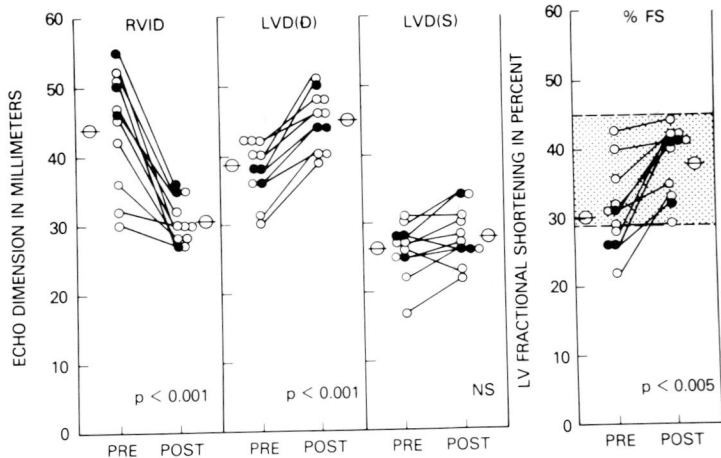

Figure 15-21 Effect of atrial septal defect repair on echocardiographic right ventricular internal dimension (RVID) at end diastole, left ventricular dimension (LVD) at end diastole (D) and end systole (S), and left ventricular fractional shortening (%FS). The normal range of fractional shortening (29%–45%) is indicated by the stippled area. Open circles with bars indicate mean values. Three symptomatic patients with the marked fall in ejection fraction during exercise are represented by the solid symbols.

Reproduced with permission from Bonow et al.,[B6] and the American Heart Association, Inc.

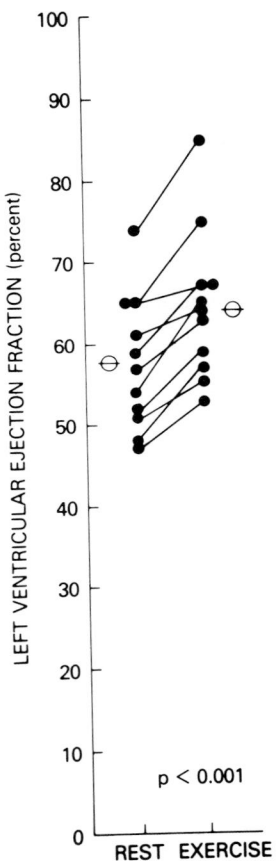

Figure 15-22 Left ventricular ejection fractions at rest and during exercise after repair of atrial septal defect. Open circles with bars indicate mean values.

Reproduced with permission from Bonow et al.,[B6] and the American Heart Association, Inc.

Furthermore, at least in patients over about 40 years of age, nearly half of those *not* in atrial fibrillation preoperatively develop it late postoperatively.[H2,M16]

Essentially these same findings apply after the repair of PAPVC, particularly of the sinus venosus syndrome, so that the pessimistic view expressed by Clark and colleagues[C2] is not justified. Twenty-three (79%, CL 69%–87%) of the 29 patients followed by Trusler and colleagues after repair of the sinus venosus syndrome were in sinus rhythm late postoperatively, and six were in junctional rhythm (one of whom had it preoperatively). Also, the incidence of changed rhythms after the repair has been found to be very little different in patients with fossa ovalis ASDs compared to those with sinus venosus syndrome. Twenty-six (84%, CL 74%–91%) of 31 patients undergoing repair of the sinus venosus syndrome had no change in their preoperative rhythm during the first 7 days after operation, compared to 190 (92%, CL 89%–94%) of 207 such patients undergoing repair of fossa ovalis defects ($P[\chi^2] = .16$).[R4] Similar findings were reorted by Trusler and colleagues,[T5] but they found that 4 of 29 children had sick sinus syndrome or junctional rhythm late postoperatively, all 4 of whom had an atriotomy incision across the caval-atrial junction.[T5]

Postoperative Embolization

Both systemic and pulmonary emboli tend to occur. Hawe and colleagues, studying 587 patients who were hospital survivors of the repair of ASD at the Mayo Clinic between 1953 and 1963, found postoperative embolization as late as 11 years after repair.[H2] They also found a higher incidence in those over the age of 40 years, especially in the older patients with atrial fibrillation (Fig. 15-23).

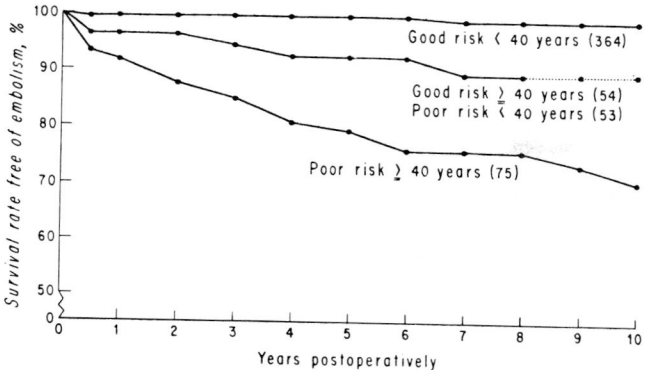

Figure 15-23 Actuarial estimate of survival rate free of embolization in hospital survivors of repair of ASD. Good risk patients had neither preoperative embolization, preoperative pulmonary hypertension, nor postoperative atrial fibrillation. Poor risk patients had one or more of these. Good risk patients 40 or more years of age and poor risk patients less than 40 years of age are combined in a single line because their curves were not significantly different. The numbers in parentheses represent the number of patients in the group initially.

Reproduced with permission from Hawe et al.,[H2] and the American Heart Association, Inc.

Reoperation for Recurrent ASD

Recurrent ASD has required reoperation in about 2% of patients (Table 15-12). Recurrence of the ASD is particularly likely to occur in older patients in congestive heart failure preoperatively. In one infant operated on using circulatory arrest, reoperation was required because the IVC was misdirected to the left atrium (GLH).

Reoperation is likewise rarely necessary after repair of PAPVC. One of 56 hospital survivors required reoperation for partial patch dehiscence resulting in partial SVC obstruction and diversion of SVC largely to the left atrium (UAB). At reoperation, an entirely new patch was placed with a good result. Two of 12 patients required reoperation following repair of the scimitar syndrome because of stenosis of the surgically created channel (UAB). Both had right lung hypoplasia with a $\dot{Q}p/\dot{Q}s$ of 1.6.

Reoperation has a very low risk, no deaths having occurred (GLH and UAB) but when a stenosis occurs beneath a pericardial or Dacron tunnel, it may be difficult to relieve.

INDICATIONS FOR OPERATION

The presence of an uncomplicated ASD or of PAPVC with evidence of right ventricular volume overload is an indication for operation. This generally means ASDs and related anomalies with a pulmonary-systemic blood flow ratio ($\dot{Q}p/\dot{Q}s$) of 2 or more and at times, if the anomaly is uncomplicated, of > 1.5. An exception is those cases of scimitar syndrome with severe hypoplasia of the right lung and a $\dot{Q}p/\dot{Q}s$ < 2. Surgery (usually lobectomy or pneumonectomy with ligation of the anomalous arterial supply) may be required in some patients with such hypoplasia, because of complications of bronchopulmonary sequestration. Isolated PAPVC of a part of one lung without an ASD is not an indication for operation when the $\dot{Q}p/\dot{Q}s$ is < 1.8, particularly since the shunt under such circumstances does not increase with age. Isolated PAPVC of a whole lung is an indication for repair, however, since whenever an entire lung drains anomalously and the atrial septum is intact, only the opposite correctly draining lung can return oxygenated blood to the systemic circuit. Thus, should this normal lung be importantly compromised (e.g., by pneumonia, pneumothorax, or atelectasis from inhaled foreign body or tumor) potentially fatal anoxia occurs.

The optimal age for operation is < 5 years of age (GLH) and can be considered 1–2 years of age because of the deleterious effects of longer periods of right ventricular volume overload (UAB). However, the opportunity to intervene surgically as early as this is not always present, since the diagnosis is often made later in life. Very young or very old age is not a contraindication to operation.

Pulmonary vascular disease of sufficient severity to raise the pulmonary vascular resistance to 7–12 units · m^2 at rest and to prevent its decrease with exercise is a contraindication to operation. Such conditions are usually present with a resting $\dot{Q}p/\dot{Q}s$ of < 1.5 in patients with an elevated pulmo-

Table 15-12 Reoperations following repair of ASD and/or PAPVC using cardiopulmonary bypass (GLH; 1957–1983).

Age/Sex	CHF	Size of Defect	Initial Repair	Operation Dates First	Second
46 yr/female	Yes	Very large confluent	Ivalon patch	1962	1964
49 yr/female	Yes (+ TI)	Large FO	Direct suture	1966	1967
2 mo/male	Yes	Large FO + PAPVC	Pericardial patch[a]	1972	1972 (3 days postoperatively)
57 yr/female	Yes	Moderate FO	Pericardial patch[b]	1974	1982
75 yr/male	Yes (+ TI)	Moderate FO	Direct suture	1982	1982 (12 days postoperatively)

KEY: CHF, preoperative congestive heart failure; FO, fossa ovalis defect; PAPVC, partial anomalous pulmonary venous connection; TI, tricuspid incompetence.

[a] Misdirection of inferior vena cava to left atrium using profoundly hypothermic circulatory arrest technique.

[b] Localized dehiscence affecting one-third of the suture line; repaired at reoperation.

nary artery pressure but may be present with a $\dot{Q}p/\dot{Q}s$ of 2 (see "Cardiac Catheterization and Cineangiography" in section on Clinical Features and Diagnostic Criteria).

Associated tricuspid and/or mitral incompetence (present particularly in older patients) is not a contraindication to operation. If significant, such conditions are repaired at the time of closure of the ASD. Grading of mitral regurgitation angiographically is difficult when there is major runoff from left to right atrium through the ASD, and of course the regurgitation becomes more important when the ASD is closed. For these reasons, moderate mitral regurgitation is usually an indication for mitral valve repair.

SPECIAL SITUATIONS AND CONTROVERSIES

The Need for Cold Cardioplegic Myocardial Protection

The repair of uncomplicated ASDs was done safely before the advent of cold cardioplegic myocardial protection and requires only a very short time inside the heart. These facts can be used to support doing the operation with simple ischemic arrest. However, as discussed in Chapter 3, when done in that way, even this simple operation can result in some myocardial necrosis. Further, the risk of air embolism can be reduced to an absolute minimum with cold cardioplegia, and the operation can be performed more perfectly and more elegantly (and thus more safely) with it. Moreover, this modality adds no more than a few minutes to the operative procedure, and it may minimize the risk of right ventricular functional damage. For these reasons, its use is advocated.

Direct Suture versus Patch Repair

Cardiac surgeons vary as to the frequency with which a patch (usually pericardium or knitted Dacron velour) is used to close ASDs. For example, this was done in 17% of cases in the Mayo Clinic experience,[S2] in approximately 30% in the GLH experience, and in 3% at UAB. Provided a patch is used when the defect is particularly large or the tissues are unduly friable, there appears to be no difference in end re-

sults, including early or late thromboembolic complications.[H2] Under such circumstances, the ease and simplicity of direct suture recommend its use in most patients.

Patch Material in the Atrial Septum

Pericardium is the material of choice for interatrial patches when a regurgitant jet may strike it, as after repair of AV canal defects (prosthetic patches may produce severe hemolysis under these circumstances), when it forms part of the wall of an intracardiac conduit whose exact contour (position) is primarily determined by the pressure on the two sides, or when it is sewn to a very delicate area. In situations other than these, Dacron patches are a suitable alternative.

Superior Vena Caval Obstruction After Repair of the Sinus Venosus Syndrome

Left postoperative narrowing of the superior vena cava is rare after the repair of the sinus venosus syndrome by the techniques described. For this reason there seems little to recommend the more complex repairs that have been reported,[W3,W4] particularly when their long-term results are not yet known in a sizable group of patients.

In those rare cases in which at operation the SVC compartment is found to be too small following placement of the ASD patch in front of the ostia of the anomalous pulmonary veins, the SVC needs to be enlarged. The insertion of a pericardial patch for this purpose is undesirable, for it may lead to postoperative SVC stenosis. Such stenosis occurred in 1 of 4 such patients in Trusler's series who were re-catheterized late postoperatively[T5] and in 6 of 14 patients reported by Friedlo and colleagues[F2] in whom the type of repair used had produced a much smaller SVC before patching than was the case with Trusler's patients. Moreover, the late retraction and thickening of a pericardial patch could compromise the sinus node, as the suture line inevitably lies close to this structure. Fortunately, it is possible to use as an alternative, the lateral right atrial wall employing a V-Y atrioplasty technique (see "Repair of Sinus Venosus Syndrome" in section on Technique of Operation).

REFERENCES

A

1. Adams CW: A reappraisal of life expectancy with atrial shunts of the secundum type. *Diseases of the Chest* 48:357, 1965.

2. Alpert JS, Dexter L, Vieweg WVR, Haynes FW, Dalen JE: Anomalous pulmonary venous return with intact atrial septum. *Circulation* 56:870, 1977.

3. Angel J, Soler J, Del Castillo HG, Anivarro I, Batlle-Diaz J: The role of reduced left ventricular end diastolic volume in the apparently high prevalence of mitral valve prolapse in atrial septal defect. *Eur J Cardiol* 11:341, 1980.

B

1. Bedford DE, Sellors TH, Somerville W, Belcher JR, Besterman EMM: Atrial septal defect and its surgical treatment. *Lancet* 1957:1255.

2. Beyer J: Atrial septal defect: Acute left heart failure after surgical closure. *Ann Thorac Surg* 25:36, 1978.

3. Bailey CP, Nichols HT, Bolton HE, Jamison WL, Gomez-Almedia M: Surgical treatment of forty-six interatrial septal defects by atrio-septo-pexy. *Ann Surg* 140:805, 1954.

4. Bedford DE, Papp C, Parkinson J: Atrial septal defect. *Br Heart J* 3:37, 1941.

5. Beyer J, Brunner L, Hugel W, Kreuzer E, Reichart B, Sunder-Plassmann L, Klinner W: Acute left heart failure following repair of atrial septal defects. *Thoraxchirurgie* 23:346, 1975.

6. Bonow RO, Borer JS, Rosing DR, Bacharach SL, Green MV, Kent KM: Left ventricular functional reserve in adult patients with atrial septal defect: Pre- and postoperative studies. *Circulation* 63:1315, 1981.

7. Brody H: Drainage of the pulmonary veins into the right side of the heart. *Arch Path* 33:221, 1942.

8. Babb JD, McGlynn TJ, Pierce WS, Kirkman PM: Isolated partial anomalous venous connection: A congenital defect with late and serious complications. *Ann Thorac Surg* 31:540, 1980.

9. Bharati S, Lev M, Kirklin JW: *Cardiac Surgery and the Conduction System.* New York: Wiley, 1983.

10. Bowes DE, Kirklin JW, Swan HJC: Effect of large atrial septal defects in dogs. *Am J Physiol* 179:620, 1954.

11. Barratt-Boyes BG. The results of repair of atrial septal defect using the atrial well method. *Ann R Coll Surg Engl* 33:209, 1963.

12. Brandenburg RO Jr, Holmes DR Jr, Brandenburg RO, McGoon DC: Clinical follow-up study of paroxysmal supraventricular tachyarrhythmias after operative repair of secundum type atrial septal defect in adults. *Am J Cardiol* 51:273, 1983.

13. Bolens M, Friedli B: Sinus node function and conduction system before and after surgery for secundum atrial septal defect: An electrophysiologic study. *Am J Cardiol* 53:1415, 1984.

C

1. Cayler GG: Spontaneous functional closure of symptomatic atrial septal defects. *N Engl J Med* 276:65, 1967.

2. Clark EB, Rolad JMA, Varghese PJ, Neill CA, Haller JA: Should the sinus venosus type ASD be closed? A review of the atrial conduction defects and surgical results in twenty-eight children. *Am J Cardiol* 35:127, 1975 (abstr).

3. Cooley DA, Ellis PR, Bellizi ME: Atrial septal defects of the sinus venosus type: Surgical considerations. *Diseases of the Chest* 39:158, 1961.

4. Craig AJ, Selzer A: Natural history and prognosis of atrial septal defect. *Circulation* 37:805, 1968.

5. Campbell M: Natural history of atrial septal defect. *Br Heart J* 32:820, 1970.

6. Cherian G, Uthaman CB, Durairaj M, Sukumar IP, Krishnaswami S, Jairaj PS, John S, Krishnaswami H, Bhaktaviziam A: Pulmonary hypertension in isolated secundum atrial septal defect: High frequency in young patients. *Am Heart J* 105:950, 1983.

7. Cockerham JT, Martin TC, Gutierrez FR, Harmann AF Jr, Goldring D, Strauss AW: Spontaneous closure of secundum atrial septal defect in infants and young children. *Am J Cardiol* 52:1267, 1983.

D

1. Davies RS, Green DC, Brott WH: Secundum atrial septal defect and cleft mitral valve. *Ann Thorac Surg* 24:28, 1977.

2. Dimich I, Steinfeld L, Park SC: Symptomatic atrial septal defect in infants. *Am Heart J* 85:601, 1973.

3. Daicoff GR, Brandenburg RO, Kirklin JW: Results of operation for atrial septal defect in patients forty-five years of age and older. *Circulation* 35(suppl I):I-143, 1967.

4. Dave KS, Pakrashi BC, Wooler GH, Ionescu MI: Atrial septal defect in adults. *Am J Cardiol* 31:7, 1973.

5. Drake EH, Lynch JP: Bronchiectasis associated with anomaly of the right pulmonary vein and right diaphragm. *J Thorac Surg* 19:433, 1950.

6. Dotter CT, Hardisty NM, and Steinberg I: Anomalous right pulmonary vein entering the inferior vena cava: Two cases diagnosed during life by angiocardiography and cardiac catheterization. *Am J Med Sci* 218:31, 1949.

7. D'Cruz IA, Arcilla RA: Anomalous venous drainage of the left lung into the inferior vena cava: A case report. *Am Heart J* 67:539, 1964.

8. Doty DB, Wright CB, Hiratzka LF, Eastham CL, Marcus ML: Coronary reserve in volume-induced right ventricular hypertrophy from atrial septal defect. *Am J Cardiol* 54:1059, 1984.

F

1. Forfang K, Simonsen S, Andersen A, Efskind L: Atrial septal defect of secundum type in the middle-aged. *Am Heart J* 94:44, 1977.

2. Friedlo B, Guierra R, Davignon A, Foavon JC, Stanley P: Surgical treatment of partial anomalous pulmonary venous drainage: A long-term follow-up study. *Circulation* 45:159, 1972.

G

1. Gibbon JH: Application of a mechanical heart-lung apparatus to cardiac surgery. *Minn Med*, p 171, 1954.

2. Giardina ACV, Raptoulis AS, Engle MA, Levin AR: Spontaneous closure of atrial septal defect with cardiac failure in infancy. *Chest* 75:395, 1975.

3. Gross RE, Pomeranz AA, Watkins E Jr, Goldsmith EI: Surgical closure of defects of the interauricular septum by use of an atrial well. *N Engl J Med* 247:455, 1952.

4. Goodman DJ, Hancock EW: Secundum atrial septal defect associated with a cleft mitral valve. *Br Heart J* 35:1315, 1973.

5. Geraci JE, Kirklin JW: Transplantation of left anomalous pulmonary vein to left atrium: Report of case. *Proc Staff Meet Mayo Clin* 28:472, 1953.

6. Gazzaniga AB, Matloff JM, Harken DE: Anomalous right pulmonary venous drainage into the inferior vena cava and left atrium. *J Thorac Cardiovasc Surg* 57:251, 1969.

7. Gault JH, Morrow AG, Gay WA Jr, Ross J Jr: Atrial septal defect in patients over the age of 40 years: Clinical and hemodynamic studies and the effects of operation. *Circulation* 37:261, 1968.

8. Galve E, Angel J, Evangelista A, Anivarro I, Permanyer-Miralda G, Soler-Soler J: Bidirectional shunt in uncomplicated atrial septal defect. *Br Heart J* 51:480, 1984.

H

1. Hoffman JIE, Rudolph AM, Danilowicz D: Left-to-right atrial shunts in infants. *Am J Cardiol* 30:868, 1972.

2. Hawe A, Tastelli GC, Brandenburg RO, McGoon DC: Embolic complications following repair of atrial septal defects. *Circulation* 39,40(suppl I):I-185, 1969.

3. Hagan AD, Francis GS, Sahn DJ, Karliner JS, Friedman WF, O'Rourke RA: Ultrasound evaluation of systolic anterior septal motion in patients with and without right ventricular volume overload. *Circulation* 50:248, 1974.

4. Hara M, Char F: Partial cleft of septal mitral leaflet associated with atrial septal defect of the secundum type. *Am J Cardiol* 17:282, 1966.

5. Hastreiter AR, Wennemark JT, Miller RA, Paul MH: Secundum atrial septal defects with congestive heart failure during infancy and early childhood. *Am Heart J* 64:467, 1962.

6. Hairston P, Parker EF, Arrants JE, Bradham RR, Lee WH Jr: The adult atrial septal defect: Results of surgical repair. *Ann Surg* 179:799, 1974.

7. Hunt CE, Lucas RV Jr: Symptomatic atrial septal defect in infancy. *Circulation* 47:1042, 1973.

8. Hickie JB, Gimlette TMD, Bacon APC: Anomalous pulmonary venous drainage. *Br Heart J* 18:365, 1956.

9. Hynes KM, Frye RL, Brandenburg RO, McGoon DC, Titus JL, Giuliani ER: Atrial septal defect (secundum) associated with mitral regurgitation. *Am J Cardiol* 34:333, 1974.

10. Haworth SG: Pulmonary vascular disease in atrial septal defect in childhood. *Am J Cardiol* 51:265, 1983.

11. Hagen PT, Scholz DG, Edwards WD: Incidence and size of patent foramen ovale during the first 10 decades of life: An autopsy study of 965 normal hearts. *Mayo Clin Proc* 59:17, 1984.

I

1. Ikaheimo MJ, Pokela RE, Karkola PJ, Takkunen JT: Cyanotic ostium secundum atrial septal defect without pulmonary hypertension and clinical signs of heart disease: Report of two cases. *Chest* 84:598, 1983.

J

1. Joffe HS: Effect of age on pressure flow dynamics in secundum atrial septal defect. *Br Heart J* 51:469, 1984.

K

1. Kelly DT, Spotnitz HM, Beiser GD, Pierce JE, Epstein SE: Effects of chronic right ventricular volume and pressure loading on left ventricular performance. *Circulation* 44:403, 1971.

2. Kirklin JW, Ellis FH Jr, Barratt-Boyes BG: Technique for repair of atrial septal defect using the atrial well. *Surg Gynecol Obstet* 103:646, 1956.

3. Kirklin JW: Surgical treatment of anomalous pulmonary venous connection (partial anomalous pulmonary venous drainage). *Proc Staff Meet Mayo Clin* 28:476, 1953.

4. Kiely B, Filler J, Stone S, Doyle EF: Syndrome of anomalous venous drainage of the right lung to the inferior vena cava. *Am J Cardiol* 20:102, 1967.

5. Kalke BR, Carlson RG, Ferlic RM, Sellers RD, Lillehei CW: Partial anomalous pulmonary venous connections. *Am J Cardiol* 20:91, 1967.

6. Kirklin JW, Ellis FH Jr, Wood ED: Treatment of anomalous pulmonary venous connections in association with interatrial communications. *Surgery* 39:389, 1956.

7. Kyger ER, Frazier OH, Cooley DA, Gillette PC, Reul GJ, Saniford FM, Wukasch DC: Sinus venosus atrial septal defect: Early and late results following closure in 109 patients. *Ann Thorac Surg* 25:44, 1978.

8. Kirklin JW, Swan HJC, Wood EH, Burchell HB, Edwards JE: Anatomic, physiologic, and surgical considerations in repair of interatrial communications in man. *J Thorac Surg* 29:37, 1955.

L

1. Lewis FJ, Taufic M: Closure of atrial septal defects with the aid of hypothermia: Experimental accomplishments and the report of the one successful case. *Surgery* 33:52, 1953.

2. Lieppe W, Scallion R, Behar VS, Kisslo JA: Two-dimensional echocardiographic findings in atrial septal defect. *Circulation* 56:447, 1977.

3. Leachman RD, Cokkinos DV, Cooley DA: Association of ostium secundum atrial septal defects with mitral valve prolapse. *Am J Cardiol* 38:167, 1976.

4. Lewis FJ, Taufic M, Varco RL, Niazi S: The surgical anatomy of atrial septal defects: Experiences with repair under direct vision. *Ann Surg* 142:401, 1955.

5. Liberthson RR, Boucher CA, Strauss HW, Dinsmore RE, McKusick KA, Pohost GM: Right ventricular function in adult atrial septal defect. *Am J Cardiol* 47:56, 1981.

6. Liberthson RR, Buckley MJ, Boucher CA: Pulmonary regurgitation in large atrial shunts without pulmonary hypertension. *Circulation* 54:966, 1976.

7. Lewis FJ: High defects of the atrial septum. *J Thorac Cardiovasc Surg* 36:1, 1958.

8. Levin AR, Liebson PR, Ehlers KH, Diamant B: Assessment of left ventricular function in secundum atrial septal defect: Evaluation by determination of volume, pressure and external systolic time indices. *Pediatr Res* 9:894, 1975.

9. Lucas CL, Wilcox BR, Coulter NA: Pulmonary vascular response to atrial septal closure in children. *J Surg Res* 18:571, 1975.

M

1. Menon VA, Wagner HR: Spontaneous closure of secundum atrial septal defect. *New York State J Med* 1975:1068.

2. Mody MR: Serial hemodynamic observations in secundum atrial septal defect with special reference to spontaneous closure. *Am J Cardiol* 32:978, 1973.

3. Murray G: Closure of defects in cardiac septa. *Ann Surg* 128:843, 1948.

4. Meyer RA, Schwartz DC, Benzing G III, Kaplan S: Ventricular septum in right ventricular volume overload: An echocardiographic study. *Am J Cardiol* 30:349, 1972.

5. Marshall HW, Helmholz HF, Wood EH: Physiologic consequences of congenital heart disease, in *Handbook of Physiology: Circulation*, vol. 1. Washington, DC: American Physiologic Society, 1962, p 417.

6. Magilligan DJ Jr, Lam CR, Lewis JW Jr, Davila JC: Late results of atrial septal defect repair in adults. *Arch Surg* 113:1245, 1978.

7. McCotter RE: Three cases of the persistence of the left superior vena cava. *Anat Rec* 10:377, 1916.

8. McCormack RJM, Pickering D: A rare type of atrial septal defect. *Thorax* 23:350, 1968.

9. Murphy JW, Kerr AR, Kirklin JW: Intracardiac repair for anomalous pulmonary venous connection of right lung to inferior vena cava. *Ann Thorac Surg* 11:38, 1971.

10. Mohiuddin SM, Levin HS, Runco V, Booth RW: Anomalous pulmonary venous drainage: A common trunk emptying into left atrium and inferior vena cava. *Circulation* 34:46, 1966.

11. Morgan JR, Forker AD: Syndrome of hypoplasia of the right lung and dextroposition of the heart: Scimitar sign with normal pulmonary venous drainage. *Circulation* 43:27, 1971.

12. Mardini MK, Sakati NA, Nyhan WI: Anomalous left pulmonary venous drainage to the inferior vena cava and through the pericardium phrenic vein to the innominate vein: Left-sided scimitar syndrome. *Am Heart J* 101:860, 1981.

13. Meyer RA, Korfhagen JC, Covitz W, Kaplan S: Long-term follow-up study after closure of secundum atrial septal defect in children: An echocardiographic study. *Am J Cardiol* 50:143, 1982.

N

1. Nakamura F, Houck A, Nadas A: Atrial septal defect in infants. *Pediatrics* 34:101, 1964.

2. Nasrallah AT, Hall RJ, Garcia E, Leachman RD, Cooley DA: Surgical repair of atrial septal defect in patients over 60 years of age, long-term results. *Circulation* 53:329, 1976.

3. Neptune WB, Bailey CP, Goldberg H: The surgical correction of atrial septal defects associated with transposition of the pulmonary veins. *J Thorac Cardiovasc Surg* 25:623, 1953.

P

1. Popio KA, Gorlin R, Teichholz LE, Cohn PF, Bechtel D, Herman MV: Abnormalities of left ventricular function and geometry in adults with an atrial septal defect. *Am J Cardiol* 36:302, 1975.

2. Pearlman AS, Borer JS, Clark CE, Henry WL, Redwood DR, Morrow AG, Epstein SE, Burn C, Cohen E, McKay FJ: Abnormal right ventricular size and ventricular septal motion after atrial septal defect closure. *Am J Cardiol* 41:295, 1978.

3. Phillips SJ, Okies JE, Henken D, Sunderland CO, Starr A: Complex of secundum atrial septal defect and congestive heart failure in infants. *J Thorac Cardiovasc Surg* 70:696, 1975.

4. Ports TA, Turley K, Brundage BH, Ebert PA: Operative correction of total left anomalous pulmonary venous return. *Ann Thorac Surg* 27:246, 1979.

5. Perloff JK: Ostium secundum atrial septal defect: Survival for 87 and 94 years. *Am J Cardiol* 53:388, 1984.

6. Park H-M, Summerer MH, Preuss K, Armstrong WF, Mahomed Y, Hamilton DJ: Anomalous drainage of the right superior vena cava into the left atrium. *JACC* 2:358, 1983.

R

1. Roesler H: Interatrial septal defect. *Arch Intern Med* 54:339, 1954.

2. Robitansky CF: *Die Defect der Scheidewande des Herzens.* Vienna: Wilhelm Braumuller, 1875, p 153.

3. Richmond DE, Lowe JB, Barratt-Boyes BG: Results of surgical repair of atrial septal defects in the middle-aged and elderly. *Thorax* 24:536, 1969.

4. Rouse RG, MacLean WH, Kirklin JW: (1979) Unpublished study.

5. Rahimtoola SH, Kirklin JW, Burchell HB: Atrial septal defect. *Circulation* 37,38(suppl V):V-2, 1968.

6. Ruschhaupt DG, Khoury L, Thilenius OG, Replogle RL, Arcilla RA: Electrophysiologic abnormalities of children with ostium secundum atrial septal defect. *Am J Cardiol* 53:1643, 1984.

S

1. St. John Sutton MG, Tajik AJ, McGoon DC: Atrial septal defect in patients ages 60 years or older: Operative results and long-term postoperative follow-up. *Circulation* 64:402, 1981.

2. Søndergard T: Closure of atrial septal defects: Report of three cases. *Acta Chir Scand* 107:492, 1954.

3. Saksena FB, Aldridge HE: Atrial septal defect in the older patient. *Circulation* 42:1009, 1970.

4. Schreiber TL, Feigenbaum H, Weyman AE: Effect of atrial septal defect repair on left ventricular geometry and degree of mitral valve prolapse. *Circulation* 61:888, 1980.

5. Spangler JG, Feldt RH, Danielson GK: Secundum atrial septal defect encountered in infancy. *J Thorac Cardiovasc Surg* 71:398, 1971.

6. Sturm JT, Ankeney JL: Surgical repair of inferior sinus venosus atrial septal defect. *J Thorac Cardiovasc Surg* 78:570, 1979.

7. Shapiro EP, Al-Sadir J, Campbell NPS, Thilenius OG, Anagnostopoulos CE, Harp P: Drainage of right superior vena cava into both atria. *Circulation* 63:712, 1981.

8. Snellen HA, Van Ingen HC, Hoefsmit ECM: Patterns of anomalous pulmonary venous drainage. *Circulation* 38:45, 1968.

9. Saalouke MG, Shapiro ST, Perry LW, Scott LP: Isolated partial anomalous pulmonary venous drainage associated with pulmonary vascular obstructive disease. *Am J Cardiol* 39:439, 1977.

10. Swan HJC, Kirklin JW, Becu LM, Wood EH: Anomalous connection of right pulmonary veins to superior vena cava with interatrial communications: Hemodynamic data in eight cases. *Circulation* 16:54, 1957.

11. Silver AW, Kirklin JW, Wood EH: Demonstration of preferential flow of blood from inferior vena cava and from right pulmonary veins through experimental atrial septal defects in dogs. *Circ Res* 14:413, 1956.

12. Shub C, Dimopoulos IN, Seward JB, Callahan JA, Tancredi RG, Schattenberg TT, Reeder GS, Hagler DJ, Tajik AJ: Sensitivity of two-dimensional echocardiography in the direct visualization of atrial septal defect utilizing the subcostal approach: Experience with 154 patients. *JACC* 2:127, 1983.

13. Søndergard T, Paulsen PK: Some immediate hemodynamic consequences of closure of atrial septal defects of the secundum type. *Circulation* 69:905, 1984.

T

1. Tsakiri AG, Mair DD, Seki S, Titus JL, Wood EH: Motion of the tricuspid valve annulus in anesthetized intact dog. *Circ Res* 36:43, 1975.

2. Tsakiri AG, Sturm RE, Wood EH: Experimental studies on the mechanisms of closure of cardiac valves with use of roentgen videodensitometry. *Am J Cardiol* 32:136, 1973.

3. Tikoff G, Schmidt AM, Kuida H, Hecht HH: Heart failure in atrial septal defect. *Am J Med* 39:533, 1965.

4. Tajik AJ, Gau GT, Ritter DG, Schattenberg TT: Echocardiographic pattern of right ventricular diastolic volume overload in children. *Circulation* 46:36, 1972.

5. Trusler GA, Kazenelson G, Freedom RM, Williams WG, Rowe RD: Late results following repair of partial anomalous pulmonary venous connection with sinus venosus atrial septal defect. *J Thorac Cardiovasc Surg* 79:776, 1980.

W

1. Wanderman KL, Ovsyshcher I, Gueron M: Left ventricular performance in patients with atrial septal defect: Evaluation with noninvasive methods. *Am J Cardiol* 41:487, 1978.

2. Weyman AE, Wann S, Feigenbaum H, Dillon JC: Mechanism of abnormal septal motion in patients with right ventricular volume overload: A cross-sectional echocardiographic study. *Circulation* 54:179, 1976.

3. Williams WH, Zorn-Chilton S, Raviele AA, Michalik RE, Guyton RA, Dooley KJ, Hatcher CR Jr: Extracardiac atrial pedicle conduit repair of partial anomalous pulmonary venous connection to the superior vena cava in children. *Ann Thorac Surg* 38:345, 1984.

4. Warden HE, Gustafson RA, Zarnay TJ, Neal WA: An alternative method for repair of partial anomalous pulmonary venous connection to the superior vena cava. *Ann Thorac Surg* 38:601, 1984.

Y

1. Young D: Later results of closure of secundum atrial septal defect in children. *Am J Cardiol* 31:14, 1973.

Z

1. Zubiate P, Kay JH: Surgical correction of anomalous pulmonary venous connection. *Ann Surg* 156:234, 1962.

16

TOTAL ANOMALOUS PULMONARY VENOUS CONNECTION

DEFINITION

Total anomalous pulmonary venous connection (TAPVC) is a cardiac malformation in which there is no direct connection between any pulmonary vein and the left atrium but, rather, all the pulmonary veins connect to the right atrium or one of its tributaries. A patent foramen ovale or an atrial septal defect is present in essentially all persons with TAPVC who survive after birth.

This chapter concerns TAPVC as it occurs in hearts with concordant atrioventricular and ventriculoarterial connections without other major cardiac anomalies except patent ductus arteriosus. TAPVC as it occurs in persons with atrial isomerism is considered in Chapter 46.

HISTORICAL NOTE

Total anomalous pulmonary venous connection was apparently first described by Wilson in 1798.[W1] Muller, then at the University of California Medical Center in Los Angeles, reported the first successful surgical approach in patients with total anomalous pulmonary venous connection in 1951.[M1] His correction was partial, achieved by anastomosing the common pulmonary venous sinus to the left atrial appendage using a closed technique. In 1956, Lewis and Varco,[L1] at the University of Minnesota, reported successful open repair of this malformation using moderate hypothermia induced by surface cooling and temporary occlusion of venous inflow to the heart. In the same year, we reported the successful repair of TAPVC using cardiopulmonary bypass (CPB).[B1] This report also described a successful operation several years earlier by the atrial well technique of Gross.[G1]

Subsequently, it became apparent that the mortality for repair of TAPVC in infants using conventional cardiopulmonary bypass was strikingly higher than that for older patients,[B2,C1,M2,S1] and attempts to improve the results by staged operation or by palliative measures were not successful.[M3] However, successes were reported from time to time, even for critically ill infants with infradiaphragmatic drainage.[W2]

Improvement in intraoperative techniques did eventually bring substantial improvements in the results in infants. Thus, Dillard achieved good results by the use of profound hypothermia and total circulatory arrest without cardiopulmonary bypass,[D1] and in 1971 Malm and associates reported good results in a small group of young infants using standard, normothermic cardiopulmonary bypass.[G2] Profound hypothermia, limited cardiopulmonary bypass, and total circulatory arrest were used at GLH in 1969 and achieved striking improvements in results.[B3,B4]

MORPHOLOGY

Pulmonary Venous Anatomy

TAPVC is supracardiac in about 45% of cases, cardiac in about 25% of cases, infracardiac in about 25% of cases, and mixed in about 5% of cases.[B5,B6,D2,D3] The connection in supracardiac TAPVC is usually to a left vertical vein draining into the left innominate vein, less often to the superior vena cava, usually at its junction with the right atrium, and rarely to the azygos vein. In cardiac TAPVC, the connection is usually to coronary sinus and less often to right atrium directly. The commonest sites of connection in patients with infracardiac (infradiaphragmatic) drainage are the portal vein (65% of cases, according to Duff and colleagues[D4]) and the ductus venosus; less common are the gastric vein, the right or left hepatic vein, and the inferior vena cava. In the commonest connections in mixed TAPVC, the left lung (usually the upper lobe) drains to a left vertical vein and the remainder of both lungs to the coronary sinus.

No matter what the final connection or termination may be, the individual right and left pulmonary veins nearly always converge to form a *common pulmonary venous sinus,* which in turn connects to the systemic venous system in one of the ways noted above. A common pulmonary venous channel may be absent in some cases with cardiac or mixed connections. Because this sinus is usually posterior to the pericardium, the pericardium is cut first and then the wall of the venous sinus when at operation the surgeon opens the common pulmonary venous sinus. The long axis of the sinus is usually oriented transversely, with the pulmonary veins of the left lung converging to form its left extremity and those from the right lung to form its right extremity. When the drainage is infracardiac, the right and left pulmonary veins slope downward to converge into a vertical sinus, the entire arrangement having a Y,[C2] T, or tree shape.[K2,T1] The intrapericardial portion of this type of common sinus, before it

pierces the diaphragm, may be very short. The apparent absence of a common sinus in some patients with a cardiac connection may be an illusion caused by a defect in the anterior wall of the sinus that is the orifice connecting it to the coronary sinus or right atrium.

Pulmonary venous obstruction is a severe associated condition usually resulting from a stenosis involving the vein connecting the common pulmonary venous sinus to the systemic venous system. For example, a localized stenosis may occur at the junction of the left vertical vein with either the left innominate vein or the common pulmonary venous sinus, or at the junction of a connecting vein that joins the superior vena cava. Such a localized stenosis may occur where the common pulmonary venous sinus joins the coronary sinus or, rarely, at the coronary sinus ostium.[A3] Alternatively, in the common "snowman" type of supracardiac drainage, a severe obstruction may be due to the so-called vascular vice, in which the left vertical vein passes posterior to the left pulmonary artery rather than anterior to it and is compressed between it and the left main bronchus. In infracardiac drainage, the connecting vein may be similarly narrowed at its junction with the portal vein or ductus venosus, or it may be compressed where it penetrates the diaphragm. In those varieties of infracardiac drainage in which the ductus venosus is not available to bypass the liver, the portal sinusoids offer additional important obstruction to venous return. Finally, pulmonary venous obstruction may be the result simply of the length of a comparatively narrow connecting vein. Significant pulmonary venous obstruction of these various types exists in all patients with infracardiac connection and in almost all with connections to the azygos vein, in 65% of those to the superior vena cava, in 40% of those to the left innominate vein, and in 40% of the mixed type.[D3] It is less common in patients with a cardiac connection. These types of pulmonary venous obstruction are corrected by the surgical repair.

Rarely, pulmonary venous obstruction is the result of stenoses of the individual pulmonary veins at or close to their connections to the common pulmonary venous sinus.[G3] (See further discussion of this in Chapter 37.)

Cardiac Chamber and Septal Anatomy

An atrial septal defect or patent foramen ovale is virtually always present, but in the review of Delisle and associates, one of the 93 autopsy cases was an 11-year-old with an intact atrial septum and multiple ventricular septal defects,[D3] and Hastreiter and colleagues presented a 6-week-old patient with TAPVC to the ductus venosus, a patent ductus, and a closed foramen ovale.[H1] It has been stated in the past that the atrial communication in TAPVC is usually of adequate size and not obstructive.[B2,G3] In fact, in the recent GLH experience, the defect was small in about half the infants operated on. It is important to note that there is frequently no pressure gradient between the two atria even when the defect is small.[E1,W3]

The right atrium is enlarged and thick-walled in patients with TAPVC, and anatomic studies have shown that the left atrium is abnormally small.[B5,B7] Cineangiographic studies by Mathews and colleagues have also shown left atrial volume

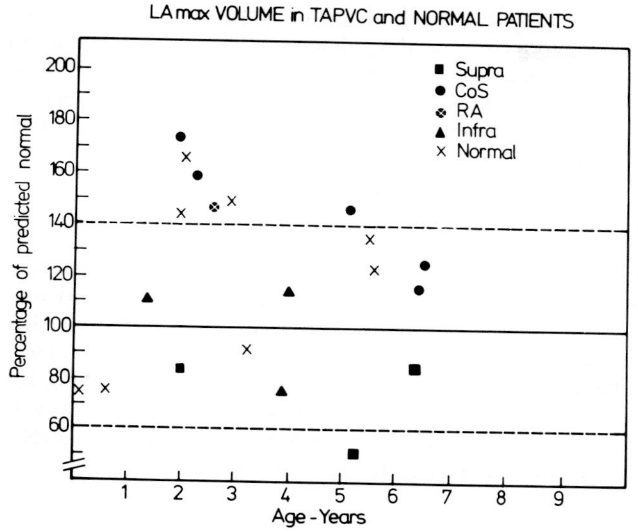

LA max VOLUME in TAPVC and NORMAL PATIENTS

Figure 16-1 Left atrial size late after repair of TAPVC. Left atrial maximal volumes are presented as a percentage of predicted normal volume in 12 patients with TAPVC and eight patients with normal left heart chambers. The horizontal broken lines indicate ± 2 SD of normal.

CoS, coronary sinus; Infra, infracardiac; RA, right atrial; Supra, supracardiac type of TAPVC.

Reproduced with permission from Whight et al.[W3]

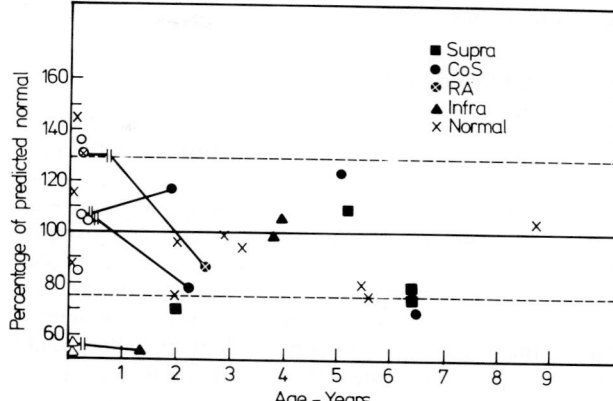

Figure 16-2 Preoperative left ventricular end-diastolic volume (LVEDV) as a percentage of predicted normal LVEDV in 7 patients with TAPVC (open symbols), late postoperative LVEDV in 12 patients after operation (solid symbols), and LVEDV in 10 patients with normal left heart chambers. The horizontal broken lines indicate ± 2 SD of normal.

— ‖   ‖ — time of surgery; CoS, coronary sinus; Infra, infracardiac; RA, right atrial; Supra, supracardiac type of TAPVC.

Reproduced with permission from Whight et al.[W3]

to be abnormally small (53% of the predicted normal).[M4] These investigators noted that the left atrial appendage was normal in size and believed that the left atrial smallness could be explained by the absence of the pulmonary vein component. In addition, in patients with TAPVC to the right atrium, the posterior attachment of the atrial septum is shifted to the left, so the septum lies nearer the sagittal than, as usual, to the coronal plane. Postoperative cineangiographic studies of infants at GLH have shown left atrial volumes to be highly variable, 4 of 12 being larger than normal (all with the original anomalous drainage to the coronary sinus or right atrium) and one (originally with TAPVC to the superior vena cava) being smaller than normal. Seven were within normal range (Fig. 16-1).[W3] Probably, the incorporation of the pulmonary venous sinus, and the coronary sinus in some types, does generally bring left atrial size, which was small before repair, to normal for age postoperatively. However, some functional abnormality is present early and late postoperatively, perhaps based on abnormally low compliance of part of the atrium, since left atrial pressure tracings are often abnormal both early[P1] and late postoperatively.[W3]

Anatomic studies have shown that the left ventricle may be small but is usually normal in size.[B5] Thus, Haworth and Reid's quantitative study showed the inflow measurements of the left ventricle to be normal in eight of nine infants dying with TAPVC but abnormally small in one.[H2] In this infant, the weight of the free left ventricular wall plus that of the septum was less than these weights in a normal fetus at full term. In all nine infants, the thickness of the left ventricular free wall was normal. In a quantitative pathologic study,

Bove and colleagues also found the mass of the left ventricle to be normal in the infants with TAPVC studied by them at autopsy.[B8] However, they found the left ventricular cavity small because of leftward displacement of the septum secondary to the right ventricular pressure-volume overload (see Chapter 15, "Mitral Prolapse," in section on Morphology). This small size may explain the finding by Nakazawa and colleagues that angiocardiographically determined left ventricular end-diastolic volume (LVEDV) was 79% less than normal ($P = .009$) in a group of infants with TAPVC and severe pulmonary hypertension.[N1] Hammon and colleagues also reported small LVEDV in infants with TAPVC.[H3] Both small and normal left ventricular volumes have been observed by cineangiographic study in patients with TAPVC preoperatively (GLH; Fig. 16-2).[W3]

The right ventricle varies in size, depending on the presence or absence of pulmonary venous stenosis and the point at which the anomalous pulmonary veins connect. When the drainage was infradiaphragmatic, Haworth and Reid found that the right ventricle was neither dilated nor hypertrophied. In cases in which the venous return was to a supradiaphragmatic site, the septum and the right ventricle were hypertrophied, and the ventricle was dilated.[H2]

Pulmonary Vasculature

As might be anticipated from the fact that most infants with TAPVC have marked pulmonary hypertension, structural changes can usually be found in the lungs of even the youngest infants dying with the malformation.[N2] Haworth and Reid demonstrated increased pulmonary arterial muscularity in all infants dying with this malformation, including an 8-day-old infant, as shown by increase in arterial wall thickness and by extension of muscle into smaller and more peripheral arteries than normal.[H2] Vein wall thickness was increased in all but the youngest child.

Associated Conditions

Most infants presenting with severe symptoms from TAPVC have either no associated defect or a small or large patent ductus arteriosus. Patent ductus arteriosus is present in nearly all infants coming to operation in the first few weeks of life with pulmonary venous obstruction and overall in about 15% of cases. Ventricular septal defects occasionally occur. However, over one-third of patients coming to autopsy have other major associated cardiac anomalies.[D3] TAPVC may be associated with tetralogy of Fallot, double-outlet right ventricle, interrupted aortic arch (one such instance has been successfully corrected at GLH[B9]), and other lesions. The combination of TAPVC with other major cardiac anomalies is especially likely to occur when there is atrial situs ambiguus (see Chapter 46).[B5,D3,S2]

CLINICAL FEATURES AND DIAGNOSTIC CRITERIA

Presentation

Usually patients with TAPVC present as seriously and often critically ill infants in the first few weeks or first month of life.[C3] The diagnosis has been frequently missed in the past because of the lack of florid signs and symptoms. It is now appreciated that TAPVC must be suspected in any neonate who has unexplained tachypnea, for tachypnea is the cardinal symptom of this anomaly. In the first two weeks of life, there are other causes of tachypnea, which may be impossible to distinguish clinically from TAPVC, particularly a diffuse pneumonic process and retention of fetal lung fluid.[S3] Meconium aspiration and myocarditis may also lead to confusion. Respiratory distress syndrome should not be difficult to differentiate because of its classic radiologic features: prematurity and intercostal and sternal indrawing. Cyanosis is usually unimpressive in TAPVC unless there is a combination of marked pulmonary venous obstruction and a widely open ductus arteriosus that allows a right-to-left shunt.

Examination

On examination, the heart is not particularly overactive. There may be an unimpressive precordial systolic murmur and gallop sound (the latter often proves to be a tricuspid flow murmur). The second heart sound is usually single or narrowly split. These symptoms and signs accompany presentation in infancy. In older children, the signs are those of a large atrial septal defect unless there is a rise in pulmonary vascular resistance.

Chest X-ray

On chest x-ray the heart size is usually near normal if there is pulmonary venous obstruction, but it may be large when there is a high pulmonary blood flow. The latter is associated with plethora, but the more common pulmonary venous obstruction is evident as a diffuse haziness or gives the appearance of ground glass in its severe forms (Fig. 16-3a). This sign is reduced when the pulmonary circuit can decompress via a patent ductus arteriosus. Older infants with TAPVC to the left innominate vein have a characteristic "figure of eight" or "snowman" configuration on the chest x-ray (Fig. 16-3b).[S3]

Echocardiography

Echocardiographic features of TAPVC have been described.[P2] The combination of criteria for right ventricular diastolic overload and an echo-free space posterior to the left atrium appear to be specific for the anomaly. Two-dimensional echocardiography is becoming remarkably accurate in assessing the morphology of TAPVC.[S9] However, cardiac catheterization and high-quality angiocardiography are currently indicated for definitive diagnosis.

Cardiac Catheterization and Cineangiography

The definitive diagnosis of TAPVC in infants is made by cardiac catheterization and angiocardiography. Angiocardiograms obtained by pulmonary artery or pulmonary vein injections define the malformation, identify the site of drainage, and often localize the site of pulmonary venous obstruction. This study is diagnostic in nearly all patients.[G3]

When the connection is to a left vertical vein, the common pulmonary venous sinus and vertical vein can usually be demonstrated (Fig. 16-4a). When the anomalous connection is to the coronary sinus, it appears as an ovoid opacification over the left side of the spine within the right atrial contour.[R1] When it is infradiaphragmatic, the descending vein can usually be demonstrated, although its precise infradiaphragmatic connection may not be seen (Fig. 16-4b). Tynan and associates have pointed out that in the neonate umbilical vein catheterization allows direct injection of a contrast medium into the anomalous connecting infradiaphragmatic vein and a very precise diagnosis of its connections.[T1] Where injections of contrast medium are made into the main pulmonary artery and there is a patent ductus arteriosus, virtually all the contrast medium will pass down the descending aorta; hence, the injection must be repeated more distally in the left pulmonary artery.

The site of pulmonary venous obstruction may be identified as a discrete narrowing on the angiocardiogram, or by slow clearing of dye from the lungs or slow filling of the area to which the connection is made. The presence of pulmonary venous obstruction is established by demonstrating a gradient between the left atrial and pulmonary artery wedge pressures. In the common left vertical vein drainage, it is usually possible to pass a catheter retrogradely from the innominate vein into the common pulmonary venous chamber and to localize the site of obstruction on catheter withdrawal.

In TAPVC, the right atrium is theoretically a common mixing chamber.[B10] This situation is reflected in the frequent finding of close similarity of the oxygen content and saturations from the right atrium, left atrium, pulmonary artery, and systemic artery.[F1] There is considerable deviation from this pattern, however, because of the streaming of the sys-

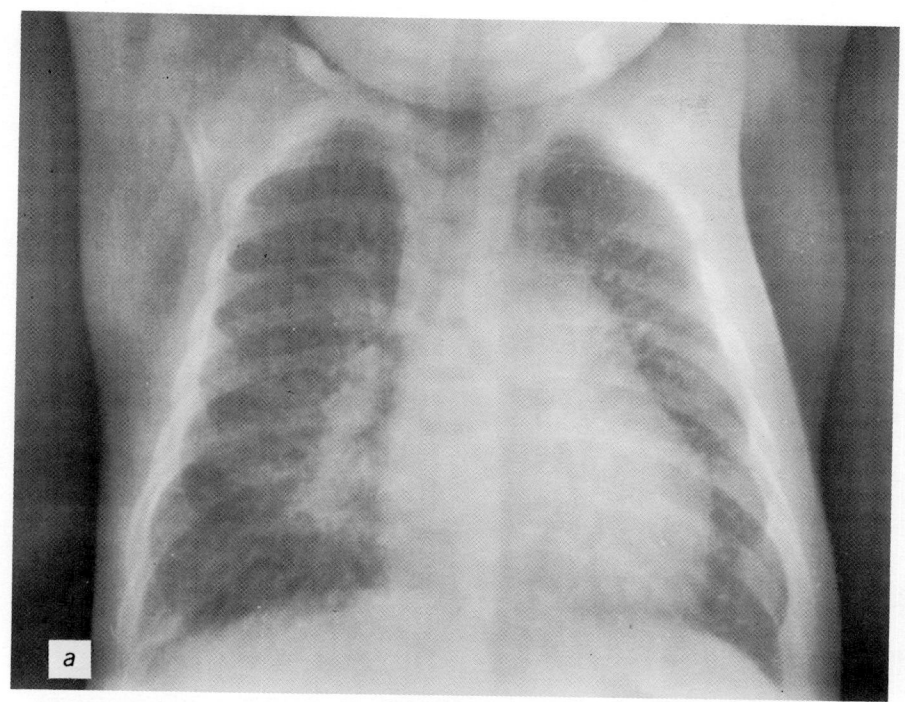

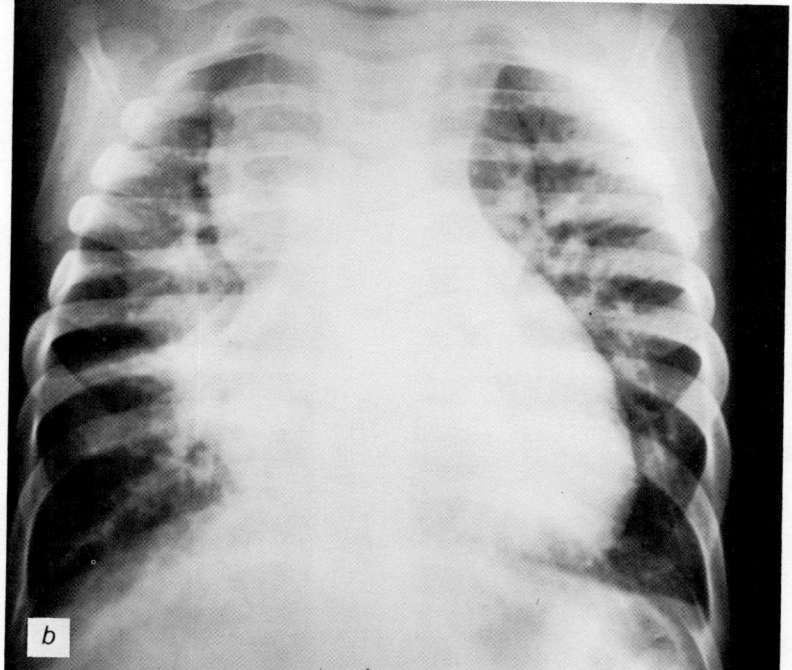

Figure 16-3

(a) Chest x-ray of a 2.5-month-old infant with infradiaphragmatic TAPVC (UAB). Note the mild cardiac enlargement and the evidence of pulmonary venous hypertension.

(b) "Snowman," or "figure of 8," in the chest x-ray of a 1-year-old patient with TAPVC to the left innominate vein (UAB). The shadow above the heart on the left is the large left vertical vein. That on the right is cast by the large superior vena cava.

503

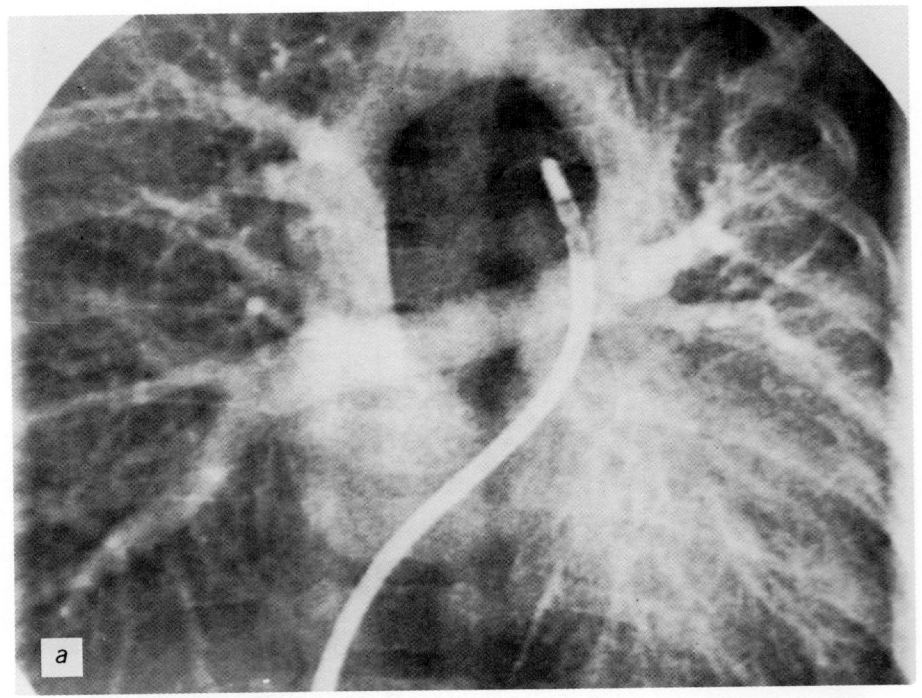

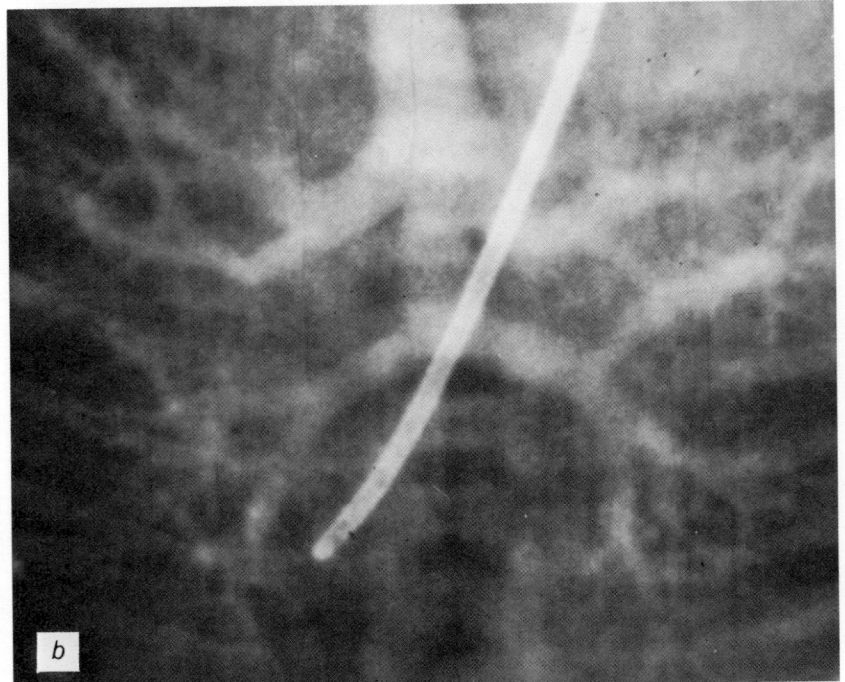

Figure 16-4 Angiocardiogram of infants with TAPVC (UAB).
(*a*) TAPVC to left innominate vein.
(*b*) TAPVC draining infradiaphragmatically.

temic venous return in the right atrium, inferior vena caval blood tending to pass through the foramen ovale and mitral valve and superior vena caval blood through the tricuspid valve. Thus, in infracardiac TAPVC, systemic arterial saturation is typically higher than pulmonary artery saturation.

Since TAPVC has this common mixing chamber, in most patients who have lived beyond infancy a direct relationship exists between the magnitude of pulmonary blood flow and the arterial oxygen saturation, assuming a constant oxygen consumption and blood hemoglobin level. This relationship was formulated into a nomogram by Burchell (Fig. 16-5).[B10] Since the pulmonary-systemic blood flow ratio ($\dot{Q}p/\dot{Q}s$) in such patients is determined primarily by the magnitude of the pulmonary blood flow, and since pulmonary vascular resistance is inversely related to pulmonary blood flow in such patients, the arterial oxygen saturation is a rough guide to the patient's operability vis-à-vis the pulmonary vascular disease. When in children and adults the arterial oxygen saturation is less than about 80%, the $\dot{Q}p/\dot{Q}s$ is likely to be less than 1.4 and the pulmonary vascular resistance greater than 10 units · m².

NATURAL HISTORY

TAPVC is a relatively uncommon anomaly, accounting for only about 1.5%–3% of cases of congenital heart disease.[B5,K1]

Infants born with TAPVC have a generally unfavorable prognosis, only about 20% surviving the first year of life.[B7,B11,K3] In fact, only about 50% survive beyond the age of 3 months, death occurring in the first few weeks or months of life in most neonates with this condition who develop tachypnea, cyanosis, and clinical evidence of low cardiac output. Such infants usually have pulmonary venous obstruction, long pulmonary venous pathways, and a small patent foramen ovale.[B7] Survival past the critical first few weeks and months of life does not portend a favorable prognosis, since only about half the patients surviving to age 3 months survive to the age of 1 year (see below).

Infants who survive the first few weeks of life usually have cardiomegaly and a large pulmonary blood flow, with mild cyanosis. Most of them have some degree of pulmonary artery hypertension.[G3] Their clinical syndrome includes tachypnea, recurrent episodes of severe pulmonary congestion, failure to thrive, fluid retention, and hepatomegaly.

Those with TAPVC who survive the first year of life without surgical treatment usually have a large atrial septal defect. Characteristically, they exhibit significant physical underdevelopment similar to that of patients with other kinds of large left-to-right shunts, mild cyanosis, and mild exercise intolerance (see Chapter 15, ''Survival,'' in section on Natural History). Similar to patients with large atrial septal defects, they tend to have a stable hemodynamic state for 10–20 years, with little change in pulmonary vascular resistance and thus little change in pulmonary artery pressure, blood flow, and arterial oxygen levels.[G3] In the second decade of life, pulmonary vascular disease develops in some patients, and there is increasing cyanosis as pulmonary blood flow diminishes (Eisenmenger's complex).

In order to quantitate the natural history as well as possible, data from 183 collected autopsied cases of surgically untreated TAPVC have been analyzed.[L2] Median survival age among these 183 cases was 2 months, the shortest survival being 1 day and the longest 49 years. Ninety percent of the deaths occurred in the first year of life. Obstruction of the pulmonary venous pathway significantly reduced survival ($P < .0001$) (Fig. 16-6), the median survival being 3

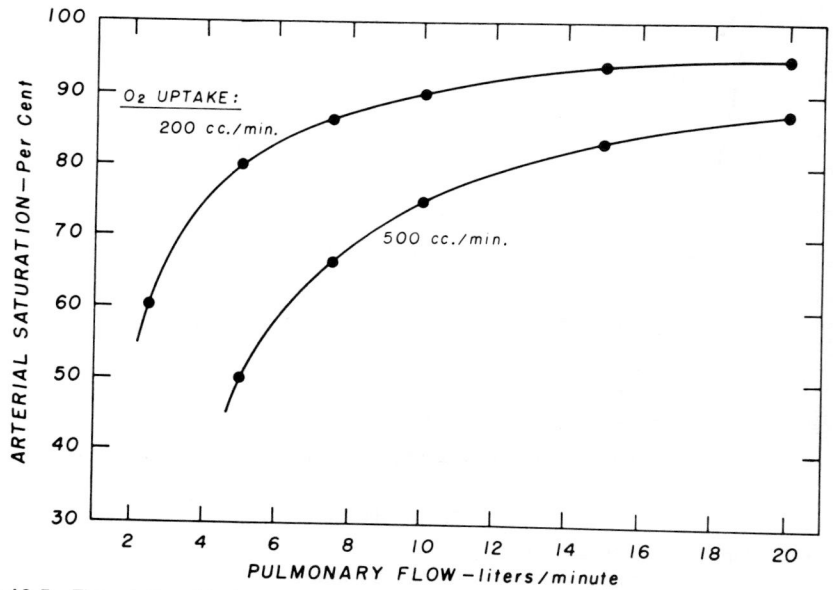

Figure 16-5 The relationship between arterial oxygen percent saturation and pulmonary blood flow in persons with common mixing chambers, formulated on theoretical grounds by Burchell.[B10] The upper curve is at rest, the lower at moderate exercise. The systemic blood flow may be assumed to be 2.5 l · min⁻¹.

Reproduced with permission from Burchell.[B10]

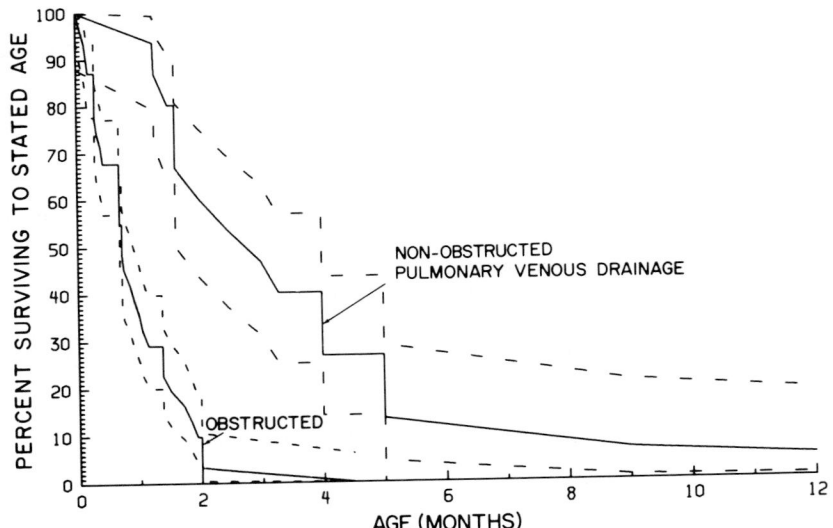

Figure 16-6   Actuarial survival of surgically untreated patients with TAPVC, according to clearly present or clearly absent obstruction to pulmonary venous drainage, based on 31 cases among 183 in which the autopsy protocol was clear in this regard.[L2] The dashed lines represent the 70% confidence limits (*P* for difference < .0001).

weeks in the obstructed group and 2.5 months in the nonobstructed group. Patients with supracardiac and cardiac connections have a similar history, with median survival times of 2.5 and 3 months, respectively, whereas those with infracardiac connections died earlier, with a median survival time of 3 weeks. Only 3 patients had mixed connections, and they died at 3.3, 5, and 5 months, respectively. The unfavorable effect of infracardiac TAPVC is confirmed by parametric analysis (Fig. 16-7). Such analysis also indicates that the presence of an atrial septal defect (rather than a patent foramen ovale) increases survival, particularly when the connection is not infracardiac. Thus, in the group with supracardiac or cardiac connections, less than 20% of those with only a patent foramen ovale lived 12 months, whereas nearly 40% of those with an atrial septal defect survived to this age.

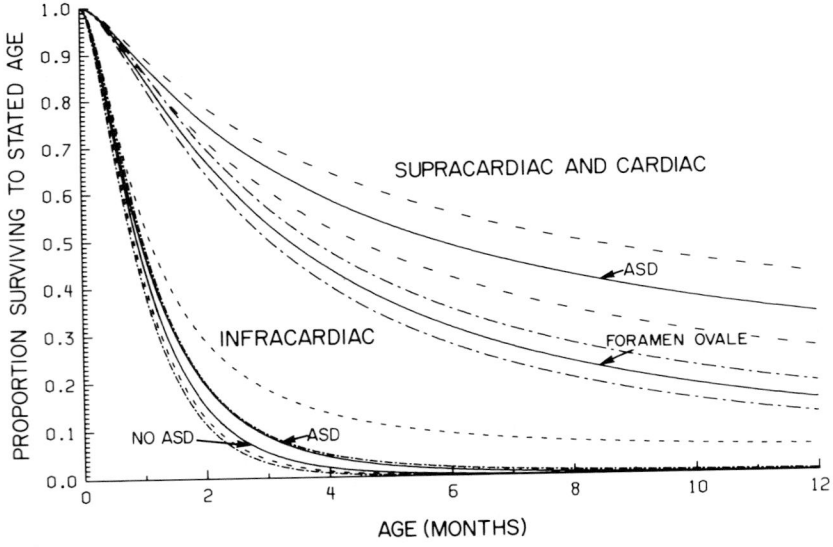

Figure 16-7   Nomogram of the equation relating survival of surgically untreated patients (*n* = 183) with TAPVC to the type of connection and the presence or absence of an atrial septal defect.[L2] The survival was not different for the supracardiac and cardiac types. The solid lines represent the probabilities, the dashed lines the 70% confidence limits. The separation into atrial septal defect and foramen ovale groups was based simply on the words used in the autopsy protocol, under the presumption that atrial septal defect denoted larger holes.

TECHNIQUE OF OPERATION

The technique of profound hypothermia, limited cardiopulmonary bypass (CPB), and total circulatory arrest may be used routinely in infants (GLH); alternatively, profoundly hypothermic total circulatory arrest may be used selectively (in infants < 2.5 kg in weight, in patients with infradiaphragmatic connections, and, some with supradiaphragmatic connections) and CPB at 25°C used otherwise (UAB; see Chapter 2, Sections 3 and 4). The ascending aorta is usually very small, and the aortic cannulation must be done precisely. The ductus arteriosus must be dissected and closed routinely in infants (see Chapter 20, Fig. 20-40), even though it was not visualized in the preoperative studies.[B16,F3] This is usually accomplished during the period of immersion cooling (GLH) or just after CPB is established and before profound cooling is begun (UAB).

Total Anomalous Pulmonary Venous Connection to Left Innominate Vein

After establishing CPB and while cooling with CPB is under way, the posterior pericardial attachments of the heart are cut (Fig. 16-8). The common pulmonary venous sinus, lying behind the pericardium, is identified after tilting the heart up, out of the pericardial space, so as to visualize the retrocardiac portion of the pericardium. The right pulmonary artery, running parallel and just cephalad to the sinus, is also identified to avoid confusing these two structures. The vertical vein draining the common pulmonary venous sinus to the left innominate vein can sometimes be seen inside the pericardium, but usually the pericardium on the left must be retracted toward the patient's right and the persistent left vertical vein identified beneath the mediastinal pleura. The vein is isolated (Fig. 16-8). A ligature is tied on the tip of the left atrial appendage for leftward retraction.

When profoundly hypothermic total circulatory arrest is to be used and the baby's body temperature reaches 18–20°C, which is usually about the time these preparations have been completed, the aorta may simply be cross-clamped and total circulatory arrest established (GLH). Alternatively, the cold cardioplegic solution may be injected just before arrest is established (UAB) (see Chapter 3). When the repair is to be done during CPB, the perfusate temperature is stabilized at 25°C and the flow reduced to $1.6 \ 1 \cdot min^{-1} \cdot m^{-2}$ after the aorta is cross-clamped. The persistent vertical vein is doubly ligated. The common pulmonary venous sinus is opened. The posterior left atrial wall is opened (Fig. 16-8). An anastomosis is then made between the common pulmonary venous sinus and the left atrium (Fig. 16-8). The sutures must be placed precisely and rather close together, to avoid postoperative bleeding. The continuous portion of the suture line must not be pulled up so tightly as to purse-string the anastomosis and narrow it.

The right atrium is opened (if this has not already been done), and the foramen ovale closed. The atrium is closed. If a single venous cannulae has been used, it is reinserted and CPB is reestablished. Rewarming is begun, the aortic cross-clamp removed with strong suction on the needle vent, and the remainder of the operation is completed as usual, including the de-airing procedure (see Chapter 2, Section 3).

Total Anomalous Pulmonary Venous Connection to Superior Vena Cava

A common pulmonary venous sinus is usually present in TAPVC to the superior vena cava, providing free communication between right and left pulmonary veins. When during cooling the presence of this sinus is confirmed, as described under "Total Anomalous Pulmonary Venous Connection to Left Innominate Vein," the perfusate temperature is stabilized at 25°C (or, after the patient's nasopharyngeal temperature has reached 18–20° C, total circulatory arrest is established), the aorta is cross-clamped, the cold cardioplegic infusion is given (UAB), and the usual right atrial incision is made. The connection into the lower part of the superior vena cavae is identified, and palpation is performed with a right-angled clamp to confirm the anatomic details. An anastomosis is made between the common pulmonary venous sinus and the left atrium as described in Figure 16-8. This may be facilitated by actually disconnecting the sinus from the superior vena cavae by cutting across the connection. The resultant opening in the sinus is extended in both directions before making the sinus-to-left-atrial anastomosis. The site of connection into the superior vena cava is then easily closed from within the right atrium using a pericardial or Dacron patch. The right atrium is then closed, rewarming is begun, the aortic clamp is released with strong suction on the aortic needle vent, and the remainder of the operation is completed as usual.

Total Anomalous Pulmonary Venous Connection to Coronary Sinus

To repair TAPVC to the coronary sinus, the operation proceeds as already described for other types of TAPVC. After the aorta is clamped, the right atrium is opened by the usual oblique incision and stay sutures are applied to the edges of the incision. The repair most used in the past has included excision of both the roof of the coronary sinus, so that it communicates freely with left atrium, and the fossa ovalis. The resulting large defect was then closed with a patch of pericardium or Dacron. Because of the occurrence of late postoperative stenosis with this technique, the repair described by Van Praagh and colleagues is now used.[V1] The foramen ovale may have to be enlarged so as to obtain an adequate exposure within the left atrium (Fig. 16-9). The wall between the coronary sinus and left atrium is incised. The incision is enlarged as much as possible in both directions. The foramen ovale and coronary sinus ostium are now closed separately (Fig. 16-9). The pulmonary venous drainage is now into the left atrium through the surgically unroofed coronary sinus. The remainder of the operation is completed as described for the other types of TAPVC.

Total Anomalous Pulmonary Venous Connection to Right Atrium

The repair most used in the past to correct TAPVC to the right atrium has been an intra-atrial one, in which the fossa

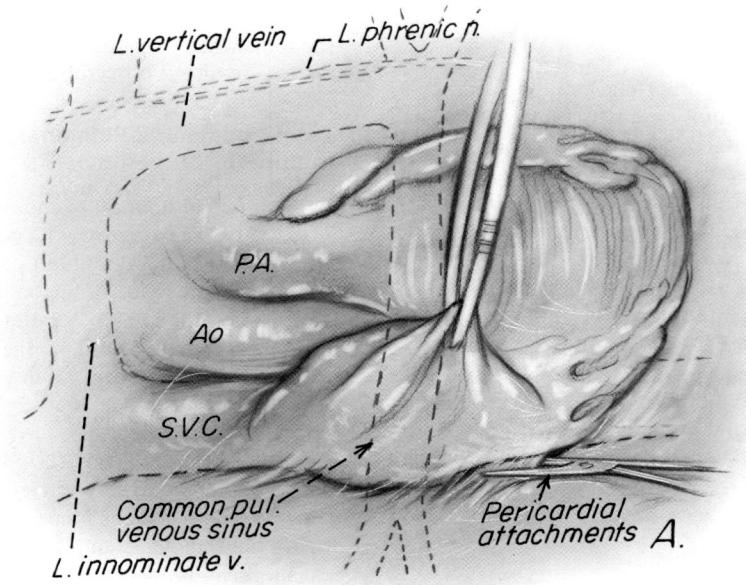

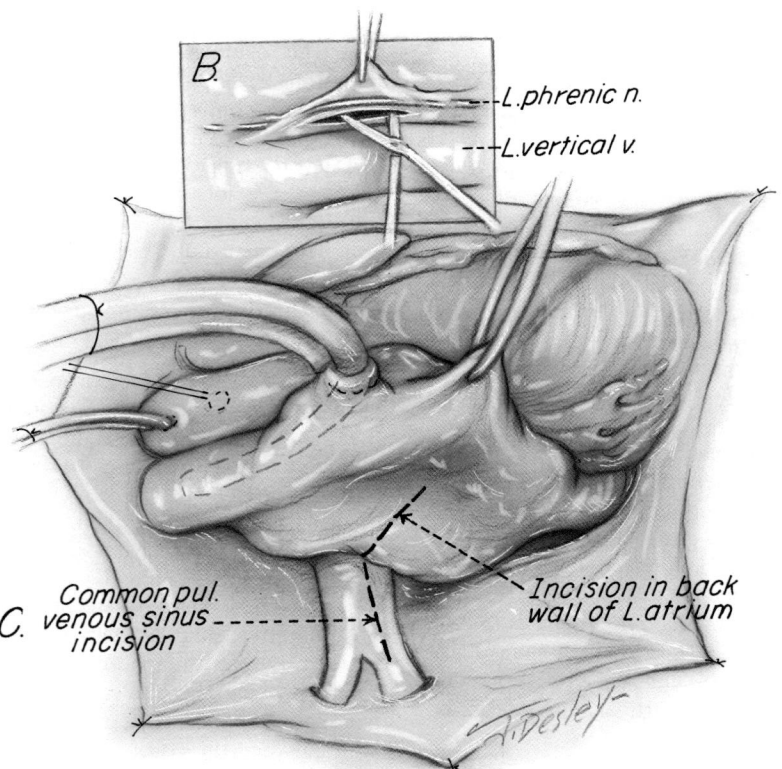

Figure 16-8 Repair of TAPVC to the left innominate vein.

(*a*) The posterior pericardial attachments of the heart are cut, allowing the cavae and atria to be lifted completely free of the common pulmonary venous sinus, which is behind the pericardium.

(*b*) The left vertical vein is exposed, preferably from within the pericardium. If extrapericardial exposure is required, the phrenic nerve is elevated off the pericardium and vein. This dissection must be done sharply and with perfect exposure and visibility, since damage to this vein might necessitate its premature ligation. In this case, the common pulmonary venous sinus would have to be opened immediately to prevent severe pulmonary venous hypertension. Also, the dissection must identify the site of connection of the uppermost left pulmonary vein, so that the vertical vein may be ligated *superior* to that point.

(*c*) The pericardium over the common pulmonary venous sinus and the anterior wall of the sinus are

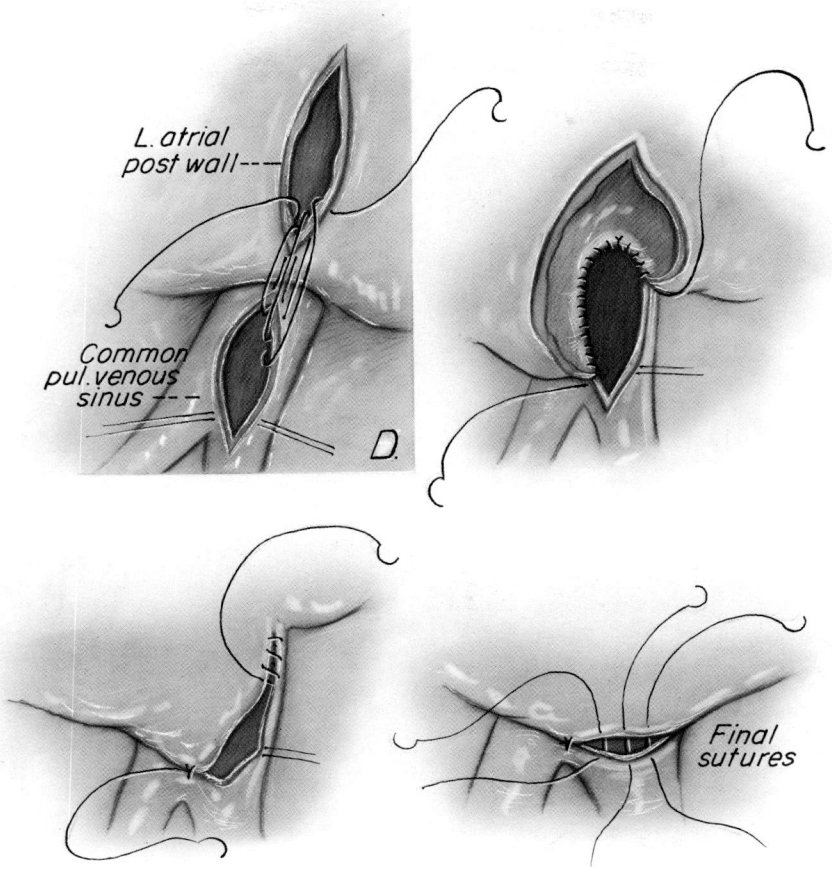

Figure 16-8 (*continued*)

opened parallel to the long axis of the sinus. The incision should be made over the full length of the sinus. The orifices of the left and right pulmonary veins are located and inspected, and care is taken to avoid damage to them. A corresponding incision is made more or less transversely in the back wall of the left atrium. The back of the left atrium is made taut by the surgeon's tugging to the patient's left on the previously placed ligature on the left atrial appendage. The incision may need to be carried onto the base of the left atrial appendage to gain sufficient length. It is carried to the atrial septum on the right, but care is taken not to enter the septum itself. When in doubt about initial placement of the left atrial incision, it is helpful to pass a small curved clamp through an incision in the right atrial wall and through the foramen ovale, so that its tip tents the back wall of the left atrium outward.

(*d*) Traction sutures of 5-0 silk are placed on inferior and superior lips of the incision into the common pulmonary venous sinus; both the sinus wall and the posterior pericardium are caught with these sutures and with the suture line. The anastomosis is begun at the point shown, with the first stitch placed from outside to inside in the atrial wall, allowing the suture line to be made from inside the vessels, as illustrated. The suture line is carried toward and around the left-sided angle of the incisions and along most of the superior side. The previously held other end of the double-armed 4-0 or 5-0 polypropylene stitch then is used to approximate, in similar fashion, the inferior edge. Here the stitches are placed from outside to inside on the sinus and from inside to outside on the atrial wall. The suture line is carried nearly to the right-sided angle. The suture line is then completed, either with a few interrupted stitches or as a continuous suture.

Ao, aorta; PA, pulmonary artery; SVC, superior vena cava.

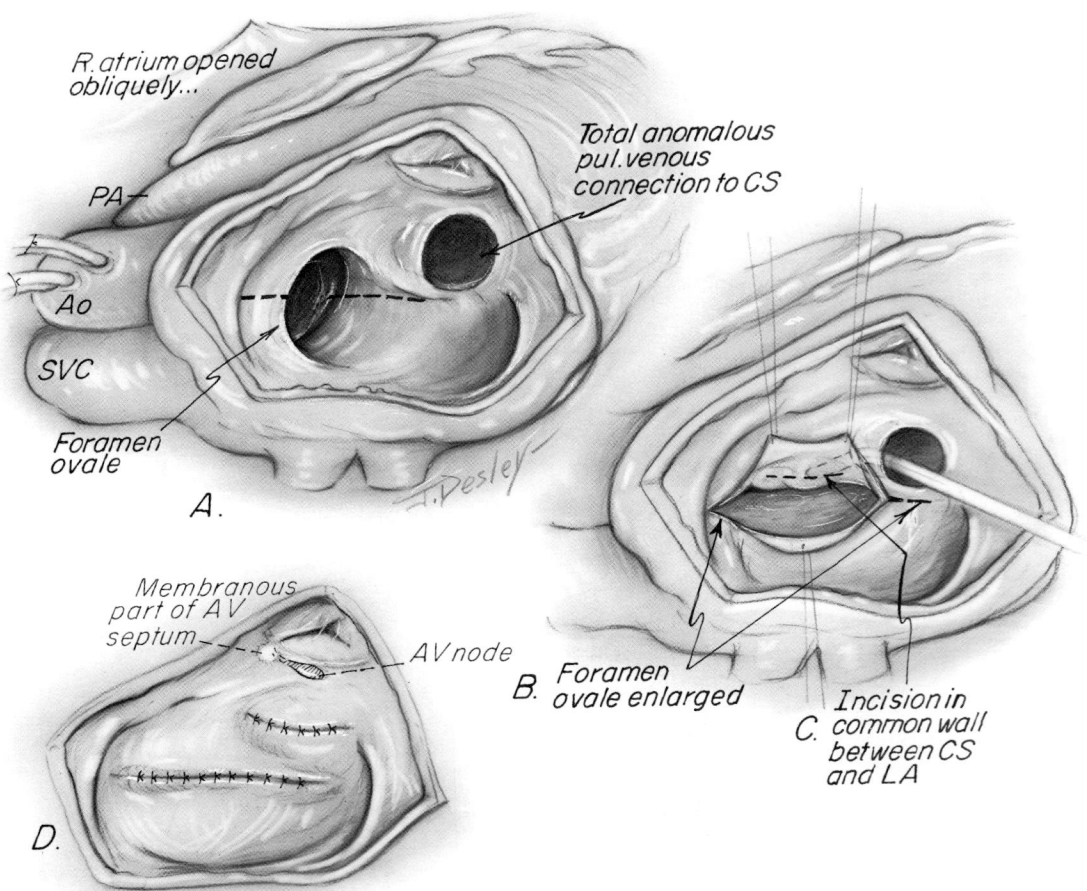

Figure 16-9 Repair of TAPVC to the coronary sinus.
(*a*) After the usual preparations, the right atrium is opened obliquely, and the exposure is arranged.
(*b*) The foramen ovale is enlarged cephalad and at times caudad to attain adequate visibility within the left atrium.
(*c*) An opening is made with a scalpel in the common wall between the coronary sinus and left atrium, after the wall has been tented up with a right-angled forcep as shown. This opening is enlarged downward and to the left; care must be taken *not* to go outside the heart in the process. If such occurs, the opening must be closed at this point from within the heart by a few sutures, because the area is difficult to expose from outside the heart. The incision is carried anteriorly and to the right to within a few millimeters of the ostium of the coronary sinus.
(*d*) After the surgical unroofing of the coronary sinus is completed, the foramen ovale and ostium of the coronary sinus are closed, usually individually, with interrupted or continuous suture. As in other operations in this area, the suture line should start inferiorly just below the last tiny coronary vein entering the sinus and, as it proceeds superiorly, should be made with only shallow bites and preferably kept within the coronary sinus ostium to avoid that portion of the AV node that may project into the ostium.
Ao, aorta; AV, atrioventricular; CS, coronary sinus; LA, left atrium; PA, pulmonary artery; SVC, superior vena cava.

ovalis is excised and a baffle of pericardium (or Dacron) is placed so as to divert the pulmonary venous blood across the large defect in the atrial septum and into the left atrium. Because of the occasional occurrence of late stenosis when this technique has been used, whenever possible the common pulmonary venous sinus is anastomosed to the back of the left atrium directly, in a manner similar to the repair employed for TAPVC to the left innominate vein. Since the heart cannot be rotated up off the common sinus, the repair

is made from within the left atrium or the anomalous connection is severed so that the anastomosis can be made from behind the heart.[B1]

The initial stages of the operation are the same as described for other types of TAPVC. The right atrium is opened obliquely, and stay sutures are applied. The anomalous connection is explored with an instrument to verify the presence of a confluent pulmonary venous sinus. The foramen ovale is then enlarged, and working through it an incision is made in the posterior left atrial wall. The heart is rotated up and to the right, and the point at which the opening is to be made in the common pulmonary venous sinus marked with a suture. Working again from within the heart and through the left atrial posterior wall incision, the anterior wall of the common sinus is incised. This opening is enlarged and anastomosed to the left atrial incision, still working from within the atria. The enlarged foramen ovale is closed by direct suture. The original connection of the common pulmonary venous sinus to the right atrium is closed with a relatively small pericardial patch; it must be remembered that the pulmonary venous pathway from the right lung is beneath the patch. Alternatively, as described for the repair of TAPVC to the superior vena cavae, the common pulmonary venous sinus can be detached from the right atrium, the opening in the common pulmonary venous sinus enlarged and used for anastomosis to the left atrium, and the resulting defect in the posterior atrial wall closed. The remainder of the operation is completed in the usual manner.

Total Anomalous Pulmonary Venous Connection to Infradiaphragmatic Vein

In TAPVC to an infradiaphragmatic vein, the distal (inferior) portion of the common pulmonary venous sinus is vertical, and proximally (superiorly) it forms a Y or T connection with the left and right pulmonary veins. Therefore, after the initial stages of the operation have been performed as described for the other types of TAPVC, the aorta clamped and the cold cardioplegic solution infused if it is to be used, the heart is tilted up and to the right. The common pulmonary venous sinus is opened by a vertical or oblique incision that may extend into the left or right upper pulmonary vein or both[T2] (Fig. 16-10). The posterior wall of the left atrium is opened more vertically than usual. The anastomosis is constructed. The common pulmonary venous sinus may be ligated routinely (GLH), and as this is done, the point of entry of the lowermost veins from the right and left lungs must be identified to ensure that the ligature lies inferior to them. If the surgical opening into the sinus has been placed partly inferior to the lower limit of the posterior left atrial wall, the vein is divided between sutures just above the diaphragm to allow it to ascend further into the chest. Alternatively, it may at times be elected not to ligate or divide the sinus,[J1] since the sinus connects to a high-resistance system infradiaphragmatically (UAB). Finally, the right atrium is opened, the foramen ovale closed, and the remainder of the operation completed as described for the other types of TAPVC.

Miscellaneous Types of Total Anomalous Pulmonary Venous Connection

Some rare types of TAPVC do occur, such as to the azygos vein. When at operation the connection cannot readily be found or dissected out, the common pulmonary venous sinus is opened first and the connection identified from within it.

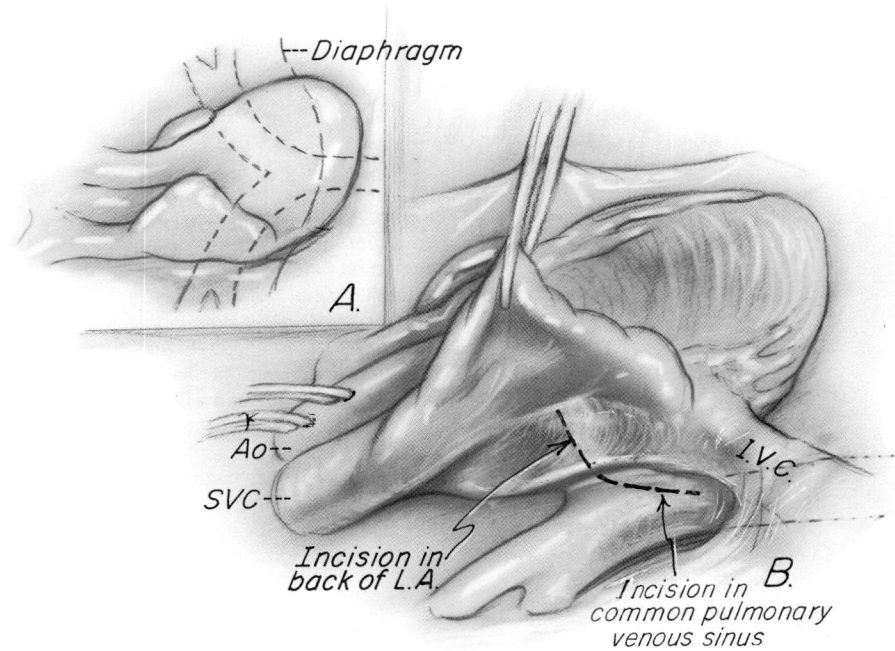

Figure 16-10 Repair of TAPVC draining infradiaphragmatically.
(a) The schematic representation of the configuration of the confluence of the pulmonary veins indicates the vertical (rather than transverse) course of the common pulmonary venous sinus.
(b) The incision in the common pulmonary venous sinus often must be extended onto the left or right pulmonary vein for its length to be adequate. The incision in the back of the left atrium should be as vertical as possible.

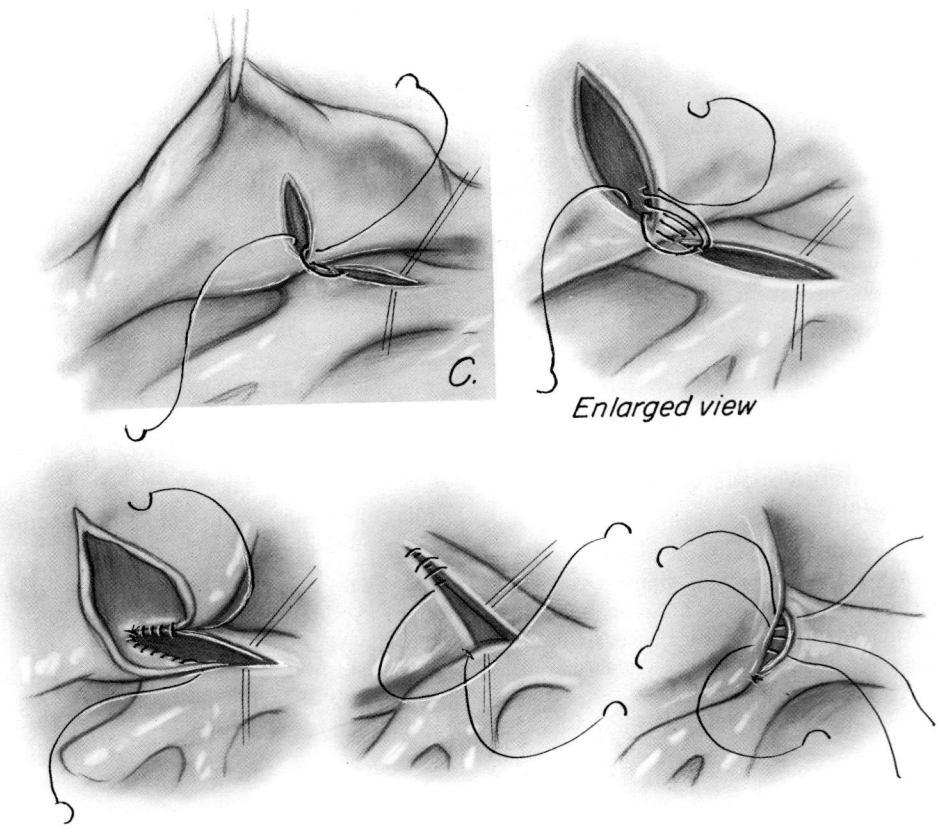

C.

Enlarged view

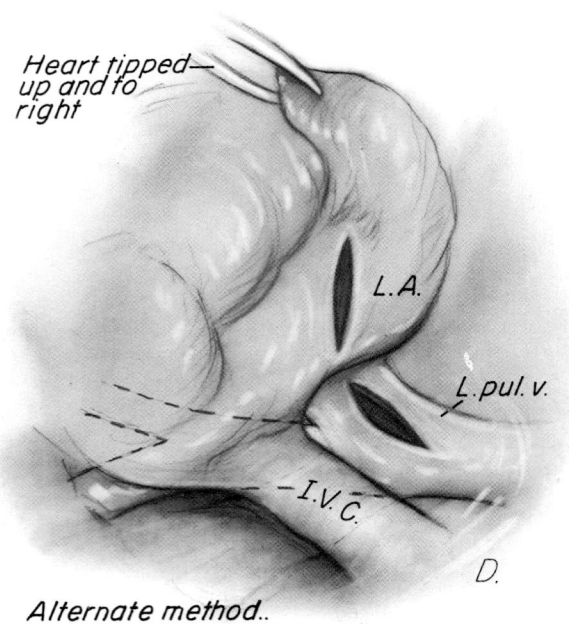

Heart tipped up and to right

L.A.

L.pul.v.

I.V.C.

D.

Alternate method..

Figure 16-10 (continued)

(c) From the same exposure as in Figure 16-8, the suture line is begun by placing a stitch from outside to inside at the midpoint of the left side of the atriotomy incision, then inside to outside at a similar point in the opening into the common pulmonary venous sinus, then from outside to inside in the atrium, as shown. Working from inside the vessels, the suture line is carried cephalad, around the superior angle, and a few stitches down the right side. The other arm of the suture is now passed from outside to inside the atrium, forming a mattress stitch; then inside to outside on the sinus wall; and then outside to inside on the atrial wall, working caudad. This suture line is carried caudad and around the inferior angle, working from inside the vessels. When the right side is reached, the suture line is continued similarly from outside the vessels. The last few stitches can be made with interrupted sutures.

(d) Alternatively, but less satisfactorily, the heart is tipped up and to the right. After the common pulmonary venous sinus and left atrium are opened, the anastomosis is made. With this approach, particular care must be taken not to tear the common pulmonary venous sinus or left atrium by too strong traction on the sutures.

Ao, aorta; IVC, inferior vena cava; LA, left atrium; L pul v, left pulmonary vein; SVC, superior vena cava.

512

After the connection is closed, the usual anastomosis is made between the common pulmonary venous sinus and the left atrium.

Mixed Total Anomalous Pulmonary Venous Connection

Patients with mixed TAPVCs present a particular diagnostic challenge as well as a surgical one. The management of each patient must be individualized and based on analysis of the particular mixture presented. The techniques used for correction of some forms of partial anomalous pulmonary venous connection apply to repair of the mixed type (see Chapter 15). In some small babies in whom an extensive operation would be required for complete one-stage repair, the use of subtotal repair can be successful, leaving unrepaired, for example, anomalous connection of the left upper lobe to the left innominate vein.

SPECIAL FEATURES OF POSTOPERATIVE CARE

The overall management of patients after correction of TAPVC is accomplished in the usual way (see Chapter 5). The relationship between left and right atrial pressures is of

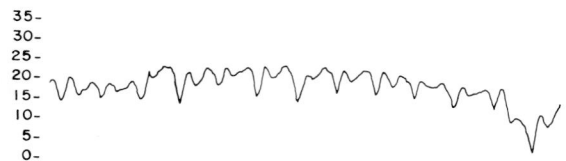

Right Atrial Pressure (mm Hg)

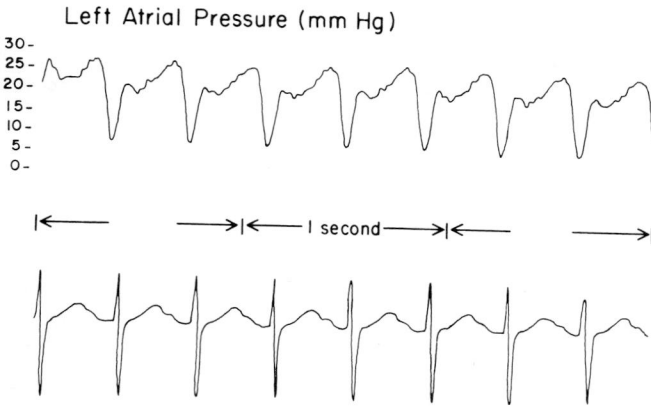

Left Atrial Pressure (mm Hg)

Electrocardiogram

Figure 16-11   Left and right atrial pressure pulses and electrocardiogram in an infant a few hours after repair of TAPVC. The left atrial pressure pulse is characterized by a rapid Y descent, probably because of low left atrial compliance. The right atrial pressure pulse has an essentially normal contour, because of its large size and normal compliance. The electrocardiogram shows that the Y descent coincides with the opening of the mitral valve.

Reproduced with permission from Parr et al.[P1]

particular importance in the postoperative management of this condition. Left atrial pressure may be significantly higher than right atrial pressure when the pulmonary artery pressure falls immediately after repair and particularly when a relatively small and noncompliant left atrium is acting more like a conduit than a reservoir.[P1] The left atrial pressure pulse after operation is then characterized by a steep Y descent (Fig. 16-11). A small or borderline-sized left ventricle contributes to this situation.

Unfortunately, in infants and particularly neonates who present for operation in a critical condition with pulmonary venous obstruction, the pulmonary artery pressure and resistance may remain very high in the early postoperative period, which in part may reflect the damaging effects of CPB (see Chapter 2) and postoperative acidemia. The right atrial and right ventricular end-diastolic pressures are then higher than left atrial pressure, and right ventricular stroke volume is reduced. When this condition is present, acidemia must be vigorously treated, and, in particular, the $PaCO_2$ should be kept low by hyperventilation.[D7] Drugs that dilate the pulmonary vascular bed specifically, such as tolazoline hydrochloride, prostacyclin ($PG1_2$), and possibly dopamine, may be beneficial (GLH), since vasospasm probably plays an important role in the pulmonary artery hypertension. Tolazoline hydrochloride is given initially as a bolus dose of 2 $mg \cdot kg^{-1}$, followed by a continuous infusion ($1-2$ $mg \cdot kg^{-1} \cdot h^{-1}$),[S10] but the exact dose of prostacyclin remains uncertain. The dose of both drugs may need to be lowered if the blood pressure falls unduly. Alternatively, in this setting the use of muscle paralysis or continuous light anesthesia with sublimaze (see Chapter 5, Section 2, "Treatment," under section on Low Cardiac Output) is used (UAB).

EARLY RESULTS

Hospital Mortality

The hospital mortality for the repair of TAPVC in the first year of life remains appreciable and does not approach zero. It is 17% (CL 11%–25%) in the combined UAB-GLH experience (Tables 16-1, 16-2), similar to the hospital mortality of 14% (CL 6%–26%) reported by Turley and associates.[T2] Thus, the hospital mortality of 10 deaths (16%, CL 11%–22%) among the 64 patients in the three series combined probably fairly represents current risks.[B12]

Theoretically, the hospital mortality should approach zero in this completely corrective operation in which the ventricles are not opened. However, the severity of the condition in most infants presenting for treatment, combined with the small size of most of the patients and the relative rarity of the condition (and thus the infrequency of the operation in any one center) makes this situation very sensitive to even small errors. As an index of the severity of the condition, both left and right ventricular functions, judged by ejection fraction, have been shown to be depressed compared to normal ($P <$ .001 in both instances) in infants seriously ill with TAPVC and marked pulmonary hypertension,[H3,N1] and myocardial necrosis may be present preoperatively. Some of these neonates are so critically ill that they require intubation immediately upon hospital admission.

Table 16-1 Hospital mortality after repair of TAPVC according to type of drainage.

Type	GLH (1969–1977)				UAB (1974–1977)				Total						
		Hospital Deaths				Hospital Deaths				Hospital Deaths					
	n	No.	%	CL	n	No.	%	CL	n	No.	%	CL			
Supracardiac															
LVV	3	1	33%	4%–76%	8	2	25%	9%–50%	11	3	27%	12%–47% }			
RSVC	2	1	50%	7%–93%	1	0	0%	0%–86%	3	1	33%	4%–76% } 4/15			
Azygos vein					1	0	0%	0%–86%	1	0	0%	0%–86% }			$P(x^2) = .07$
Cardiac															P(maximum
CoS	9	0	0%	0%–19%	2	0	0%	0%–61%	11	0	0%	0%–16% }			likelihood
RA	1	0	0%	0%–86%	1	0	0%	0%–86%	2	0	0%	0%–61% } 0/13			$x^2) = .04$
Infracardiac	6	1	17%	2%–46%	4	0	0%	0%–38%	10	1	10%	1%–30% }			
Mixed	2	0	0%	0%–86%	2	2	100%	39%–100%	4	2	50%	18%–82% }			
Total	23	3	13%	6%–25%	19	4	21%	11%–35%	42	7	17%	11%–25%			
$P(x^2)$											.25				
P(maximum likelihood x^2)											.17				

KEY: CL, 70% confidence limits; CoS, coronary sinus; LVV, left vertical vein; RA, right atrium; RSVC, right superior vena cava.

Although the hospital mortality for the repair of TAPVC in infants was very high before the 1970s,[D4] that for those few patients who survived beyond the first year of life without severe pulmonary vascular disease has been relatively low since the early days of cardiac surgery (Table 16-3).[B1,C1,G4] This is not of much practical importance, however, since virtually all operations for this condition are now done in the first year of life. Thus, the remainder of the discussion concerns primarily this group.

Mode of Death

In the combined UAB-GLH group operated on in the first year of life, six of the seven deaths were from acute cardiac failure, and one was from severe pulmonary dysfunction.

Incremental Risk Factors for Hospital Death

Although a formal approach to determining incremental risk factors by multivariate analysis has not been taken for TAPVC, due to the small number of cases and their

Table 16-3 Hospital mortality after repair of TAPVC in patients ≥ 2 years of age (UAB, GLH).

Age (years)			Hospital Deaths		
≤	<	n	No.	%	
2 ---	6	6	1[a]	17%	
6 ---	11	3	1[b]	25%	
11 ---	21	2		0%	
21[c]		3		0%	
Total		14[d]	2	14%	(CL 5%–31%)
$P(x^2)$				.6	

KEY: CL, 70% confidence limits.

[a] Mixed type; death with postperfusion syndrome.

[b] Patient died an arrhythmic death, with small posterior myocardial infarction, possibly from damage to a circumflex marginal branch by the repair.

[c] Ages 24, 37, 49 years.

[d] One additional patient, not included, with severe and inoperable pulmonary vascular disease was also operated on at GLH inadvisably; he died.

Table 16-2 Hospital mortality after repair of TAPVC according to age.

Age (months)	GLH (1969–1977)				UAB (July 1974–July 1977)				Total			
		Hospital Deaths				Hospital Deaths				Hospital Deaths		
≤ <	n	No.	%	CL	n	No.	%	CL	n	No.	%	CL
1	8	2	25%	9%–50%	9	3	33%	15%–56%	17	5	29%	17%–45%
1 --- 3	2	0	0%	0%–61%	6	0	0%	0%–27%	8	0	0%	0%–21%
3 --- 6	8	1	12%	2%–36%	3	1	33%	4%–76%	11	2	18%	6%–38%
6 --- 12	5	0	0%	0%–32%	1	0	0%	0%–85%	6	0	0%	0%–27%
12												
Total	23	3	13%	6%–25%	19	4	21%	11%–35%	42	7	17%	11%–25%
$P(x^2)$											.19	
P(maximum likelihood x^2)											.08	
P(logistic)											.15	

KEY: CL, 70% confidence limits.

Table 16-4 Hospital mortality after repair of TAPVC, excluding mixed types (UAB; July 1974–July 1977).[K4]

Preoperative Condition		Hospital Deaths		
	n	No.	%	CL
Critical				
Intubated	4	2	50%	18%–82% ⎫
Not intubated	6	0	0%	0%–27% ⎬ P (Fisher) = .04
Noncritical	7	0	0%	0%–24% ⎭
Total	17	2	12%	4%–26%

KEY: CL, 70% confidence limits.

heterogeneity, a poor preoperative state of the patient is clearly an important incremental risk factor (Table 16-4). This judgment is supported by the experience of Hammon and colleagues[H3] and by the overall experience at GLH and UAB with cardiac surgery in infants less than 3 months old.[B17,K8] The experience of Turley and colleagues[T2] and that of Bove and colleagues indicate that, particularly when preoperative acidosis is present, a poor preoperative state predisposed infants with infracardiac TAPVC to hospital death after repair.[B16] There is thus a strong argument for operation before acute deterioration occurs, regardless of age.

Pulmonary venous obstruction is clearly the most important anatomic incremental risk factor for early death in surgically untreated patients (Fig. 16-6) and as such is responsible for the critical preoperative state found in many infants.[M7,T2]

The *type of TAPVC* influenced hospital mortality in the GLH-UAB experience (Table 16-1). The striking feature is the absence of hospital deaths among those with cardiac connections. The occurrence of two deaths among four patients with mixed TAPVC suggests that this type carries a higher mortality, perhaps because it presents difficult technical problems. Turley and colleagues also had the highest mortality in the mixed group,[T2] although, in contrast to their experience and that of many others, the risk in the UAB-GLH series was not increased in the patients with infradiaphragmatic connection.

In the combined GLH-UAB experience, *young age* is only possibly a risk factor (Table 16-2). Turley and colleagues also emphasized that very young age does not appreciably increase the risk of repair of TAPVC,[T2] although Mazzucco and colleagues found neonatal age to be a possible risk factor.

In the UAB and GLH infant experience, high *preoperative pulmonary artery pressure and resistance* were not incremental risk factors, no doubt because young infants usually have reversible, although often severe, pulmonary vascular disease.[K4,W3] However, it is difficult to deny that the high pulmonary vascular resistance of the neonate, persisting into the early postoperative period, may contribute to low cardiac output and hospital death.[N2] This situation in infants is different from experiences in older patients,[G4,L3] in whom moderate or severe pulmonary vascular disease does increase the risk of operation.

In two of the three hospital deaths at GLH and in one of the four at UAB, a *small left ventricle* may have contributed to the poor hemodynamic state leading to death. However, small left ventricular size should not be considered a contraindication to operation.

Major associated cardiac anomalies increase the surgical risk, particularly if left uncorrected.[M7] One death is thought to be related to the presence of an uncorrected ventricular septal defect (GLH).

Attempts to enlarge the left atrium by shifting the atrial septum to the right have not improved hospital mortality (10 patients at UAB).[K4] This added surgical complexity is therefore not advisable.

LATE RESULTS

Unless failure of the repair complicates the late postoperative period, the late results of the operation are excellent, and the operation can be considered curative.

Survival

At UAB since January 1967, 35 infants have survived the hospital period, and only 2 of those (6%, CL 2%–13%) died late postoperatively, both after reoperation for anastomotic stricture. Autopsy in one patient, who had a pulmonary artery systolic pressure of 120 mmHg (and a systemic pressure of 75 mmHg) after re-repair, showed marked pulmonary arteriolar hypertrophy and pulmonary vein fibrosis. At GLH since January 1969, 20 infants have survived the hospital period, and 4 (20%, CL 10%–33%) died from 6 weeks to 6 months postoperatively. Two of the 4 deaths were from complications related to the operation: a posttracheotomy tracheal stenosis in one, and a postrepair pulmonary venous stenosis in the other. Thus, in the combined series, 6 (11%, CL 7%–17%) of 55 patients died late postoperatively.

When the operation is done in childhood, the results are also good if pulmonary vascular disease has not developed. Gomes and associates,[G4] reporting in 1970 the long-term results of patients operated on at the Mayo Clinic before that time, found that 1 (2%, CL 0.3%–7%) of 49 patients died suddenly 2 years after operation, presumably of an arrhythmia; the other 48 were alive and well 1–14 years (average 8 years) after operation.

Functional Status

The functional result in most surviving patients who had their repair in infancy is excellent. At GLH, all 16 surviving patients are known to be asymptomatic and growing normally, although revision of the repair of the atrial septal defect was required in one child, in whom the initial repair had partially diverted the inferior vena cava into left atrium. Sinus rhythm is present in all but one patient, who had a slow junctional rhythm preoperatively and postoperatively.

Hemodynamic Result

Pulmonary artery pressure was normal in all 15 surviving patients who were recatheterized 2–78 months (average 40 months) after repair (GLH), except in the patient with junctional rhythm, in whom it was mildly elevated.[W3] Cardiac index was normal, varying between 2.9 and 5.2 $1 \cdot min \cdot m^{-2}$ (average 3.7 $1 \cdot min \cdot m^{-2}$) in the 14 patients in whom it was measured.

Right ventricular volume, variable but often increased preoperatively, is normal or only mildly enlarged late postoperatively.[H3] Left ventricular end-diastolic volume, normal or abnormally small preoperatively, increases to normal late postoperatively.[H3] Left ventricular systolic function, often markedly depressed before operation, returns to normal late postoperatively (Fig. 16-12).[H3] Part of the explanation for this return to normal may be the improved left ventricular geometry resulting from the reduction in right ventricular size (see Chapter 15, "Late Changes in Left Ventricular Function," in section on Late Results).

Postoperative Pulmonary Venous Obstruction

Although uncommon, postoperative pulmonary venous obstruction is the most frequent mode of surgical failure. Postoperative pulmonary venous obstruction may be found at a number of different sites either singly or in combination (Table 16-5). Postoperative pulmonary venous obstruction usually manifests itself within 6 months of operation by the development of recurrent dyspnea and signs of pulmonary venous congestion on the chest x-ray. Prompt restudy is indicated. The restudy should include an attempt to enter the pulmonary veins retrogradely from the left atrium to make a direct left atrial (or pulmonary vein) angiogram as well as to determine the pressures across the site of the anastomosis. Pulmonary vein stenosis may not be amenable to surgical relief (see Chapter 37). When a surgically correctable obstruction is demonstrated, reoperation is required promptly, since death may occur soon after the stricture develops. However, the results are frequently disappointing, with a high early mortality and a significant chance of a second restenosis, as reported by Breckenridge and colleagues.[B13]

Most anastomoses between the pulmonary venous sinus and the left atrium grow normally. All such anastomoses have been recatheterized (GLH), and none had a significant gradient across the anastomosis (Table 16-6).[W3] Further, in one patient in whom the anastomosis was reexamined at a re-repair of the atrial septal defect, the anastomosis site was not apparent, both the left atrium and common pulmonary venous sinus forming a single new, large left atrial compartment. This suggests that if the initial anastomosis is large

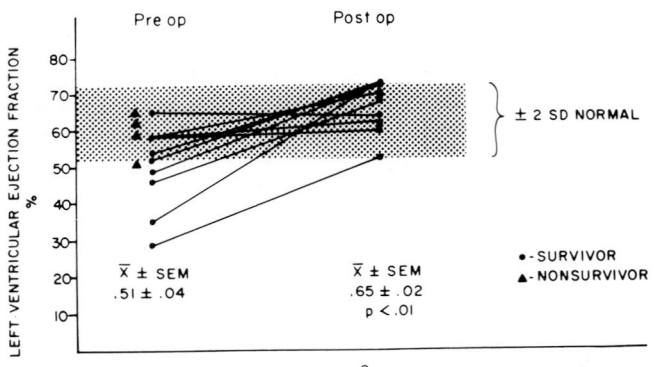

a

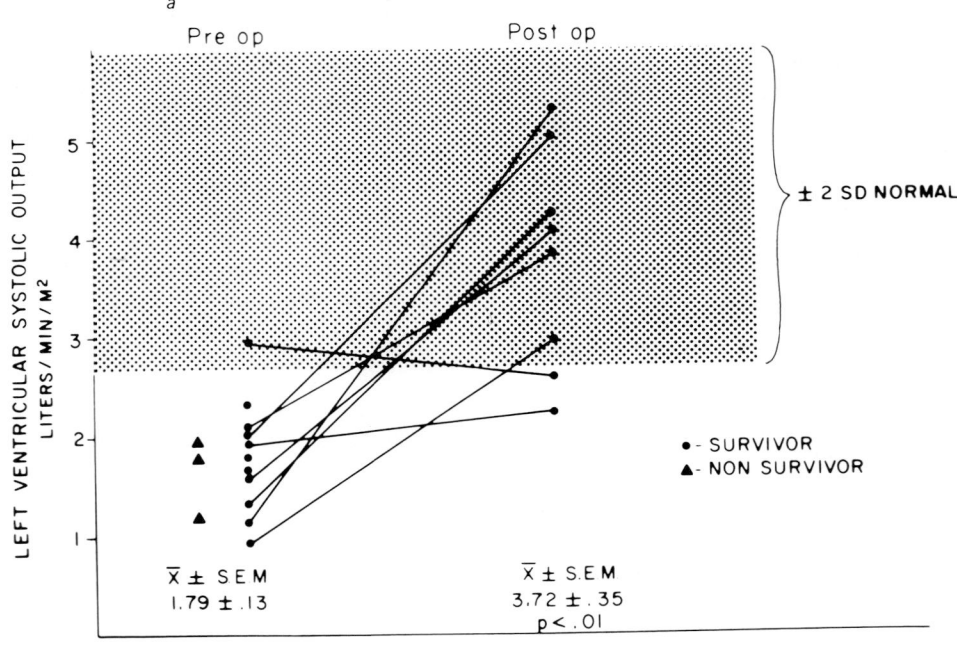

b

Figure 16-12 Depressed preoperative left ventricular systolic function returning to normal late after repair of TAPVC in infancy.
(*a*) Changes in left ventricular ejection fraction.
(*b*) Changes in left ventricular systolic output.
Reproduced with permission from Hammon et al.[H3]

Table 16-5 Sites of postoperative pulmonary venous obstruction after repair of TAPVC.

Stricture at pulmonary venous sinus–left atrial anastomosis

Stricture or stenosis at intra-atrial repair site

Stenosis at junction of pulmonary venous sinus to coronary sinus

Stenosis of pulmonary veins

NOTE: Strictures are related to the operation. Stenoses are naturally occurring.

enough, there is in most patients subsequent further enlargement with growth. However, anastomotic strictures have occurred in growing infants after repair of supracardiac or infracardiac drainage (Table 16-6). The exact incidence of anastomotic stricture is uncertain, since most reports fail to distinguish a true anastomotic stricture from one occurring after repair of cardiac TAPVC by the older technique, in which there is no such anastomosis. Moreover, because few patients have been catheterized routinely postoperatively, most incidence figures relate to patients who have become severely symptomatic postoperatively and either die or are reoperated on.[R2] Overall, there appears to be a 6%–14% chance of severe stricture formation when operation is performed in the first year of life (Table 16-6). These strictures all appeared within 1–6 months of operation, and in almost all cases, the initial repair was performed in the first month of life (Table 16-7). Despite theoretical considerations that favor the use of interrupted sutures,[S4] there is no correlation between stricture formation and the method of suturing (the GLH infants all had a continuous suture line, and in the UAB infants, half the suture line was interrupted). It is likely that the open technique of anastomosis is preferable to the use of clamps;[B13] for example, Davignon[D5] in 1972 reported anastomotic stenosis in three of five infants in whom clamps

Table 16-6 Incidence of stricture formation at the anastomosis between the common pulmonary venous sinus and left atrium after repair of the supracardiac and infracardiac varieties of TAPVC in infants in the first year of life.

| Source | n | Late Anastomotic Stricture | |
		No.	%
GLH, 1969–1977[W3]	8	0	0%
UAB, 1967–July 1977[A1,K4]	32	3	9%
GOS, 1963–January 1970[B2]	11	1	9%
GOS, May 1971–February 1973[B13]	11	2	18%
Cooley et al, 1955–1964[C1]	16[a]	1	6%
Total	78	7	9% (CL 6%–14%)
$P(\chi^2)$			.7

KEY: CL, 70% confidence limits; GOS, Great Ormond Street Hospital, London.

NOTE: n refers to the number of hospital survivors. Except in the GLH patients, in whom routine postoperative cardiac catheterization was performed, the data concern patients dying or requiring reoperation for stricture formation. The 70% confidence limits of the individual proportions all overlap; this overlap and the P value make institutional differences in incidence unlikely.

[a] This may include some infants with a cardiac connection.

were used. An adequate size for the new junction is the primary consideration, and clamps undoubtedly limit its size.

As already suggested, pulmonary venous obstruction may follow repair of cardiac TAPVC with the older technique of an intra-atrial patch of pericardium or Dacron. As with anastomotic stricture, the incidence of this complication is difficult to ascertain from the literature, partly because survival after repair of cardiac drainage was inexplicably rare in reports as late as 1974.[A1,B2] In the UAB experience, the only two infants surviving an intracardiac repair of this type of TAPVC before 1974 developed obstruction; in one, pericardium was used to construct an intra-atrial tunnel, and in the other, the atrial septum was repositioned to the right of the junction of a common pulmonary venous sinus with the right atrium.[A1] In the GLH experience, of 11 infants surviving repair of cardiac drainage, one developed a stricture between the pericardial patch and the opened coronary sinus (Fig. 16-13).[W3] This stricture was due partly to inadequate opening of the coronary sinus into the left atrium and partly to thickening of the pericardial patch. Neirotti, in Buenos Aires, noted a similar complication after repair of coronary sinus TAPVC using pericardium.[N3] To prevent such problems, the techniques of repair described earlier in this chapter are now used.

Late stenosis of the anomalous connection of the pulmonary venous sinus to the coronary sinus, well away from the surgical area, occurred in one infant (GLH) with coronary sinus drainage.[W3] Such stenosis may develop according to a mechanism similar to that of the prenatal development of pulmonary venous obstruction or to that of late pulmonary vein orifice stenosis.

Late stenosis in the pulmonary veins themselves may occur, either at the ostium where they join the common sinus or over a greater length, and thus may be combined with other sites of stenosis. In all, this complication was present in three of the five patients with postoperative pulmonary venous obstruction in the GLH-UAB experience (Table 16-7). Freidli and colleagues[F2] and Fleming and colleagues[F3] reported similar cases in infants with infradiaphragmatic drainage. In one infant (UAB), late pulmonary vein stenosis was due mainly to thickened endocardium at the ostium that was successfully excised. In most instances, however, the pulmonary vein stenosis is due at least in part to diffuse fibrosis. Thus, while pulmonary vein stenosis has long been recognized as a rare cause of pulmonary venous obstruction preoperatively in TAPVC, it is now apparent that it is an important cause of postoperative pulmonary venous obstruction in this condition, regardless of the type of connection.[T2] It is tempting to postulate that pulmonary vein stenosis is a part of the TAPVC disease complex that may very rarely be present at birth or soon afterward but that appears more commonly at 3–6 months of age. Presumably, such stenosis is becoming more apparent now that more infants are surviving primary repair, for the early literature provides very few examples.[G3,L4] In this connection it is of interest that 10 of 16 infants who were recatheterized (GLH) showed small mean gradients between the wedge pulmonary artery pressure and the left ventricular diastolic (or direct left atrial) pressure; these appeared to result from a slower Y descent

Table 16-7 Causes of postoperative pulmonary venous obstruction (GLH; 1969–1977, cases 1–3 and UAB; July 1974–July 1977, cases 4–5).

Case No.	Causes of PVO	Age at Repair (months)	Type of TAPVC	Age at Death or Re-repair (months)	Attempted or Actual Re-repair
1	Pulmonary vein stenosis	0.3	CS	4.5	Yes
2	Stenosis of ostium between pulmonary venous sinus and coronary sinus; and pulmonary vein stenosis	4.5	CS	10.5	No
3	Postrepair stenosis (coronary sinus)	3.5	CS	5.0	No
4	Pulmonary vein stenosis	0.5	IC	2.1	Yes
5	Anastomotic stricture (common pulmonary venous sinus to left atrium)	0.2	LVV	1.8	Yes

KEY: CS, TAPVC to coronary sinus; IC, infracardiac pulmonary venous connection; LVV, TAPVC via left vertical vein; PVO, pulmonary venous obstruction; TAPVC, total anomalous pulmonary venous connection.

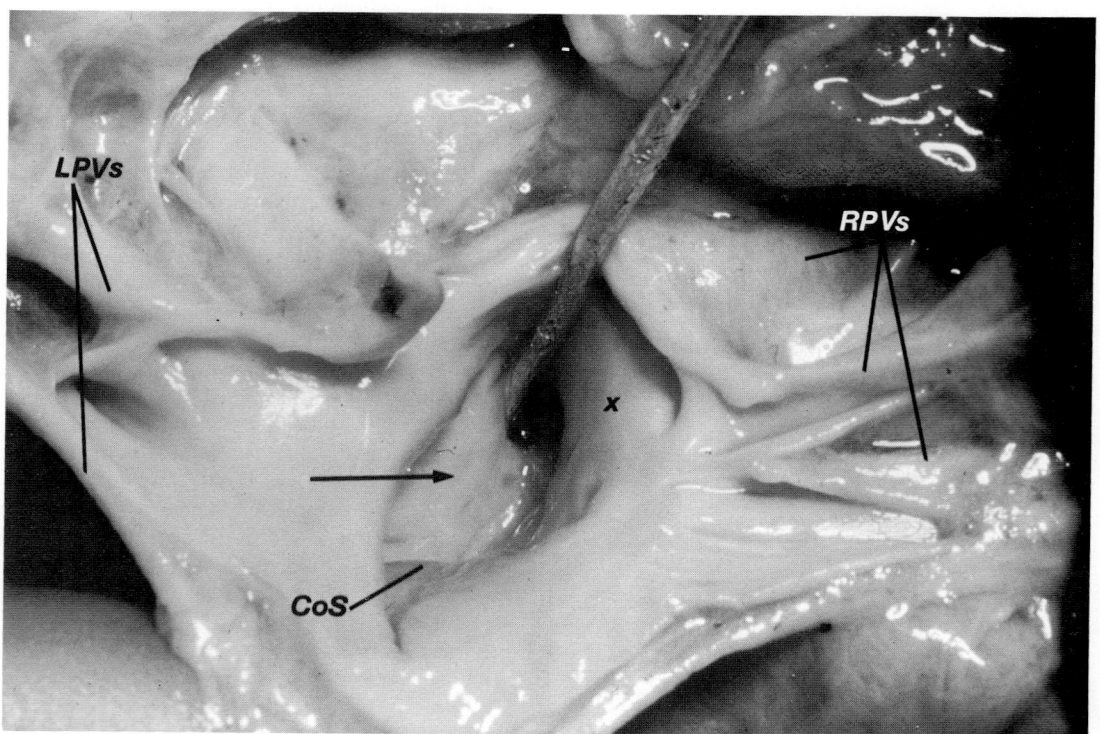

Figure 16-13 Photograph of autopsy specimen following repair of TAPVC to coronary sinus TAPVC using the conventional operation with a pericardial patch (GLH). The operation was performed at 3 months of age, and death occurred 6 weeks later from stenosis at the repair site. The specimen has been opened from behind. The probe lies in the stenotic surgically created ostium (3.5-mm diameter) between the coronary sinus and the pericardial patch (x). The arrow indicates a still intact portion of the roof of the coronary sinus that forms one boundary to the stenosis.

CoS, coronary sinus; LPV, left pulmonary veins; RPV, right pulmonary vein.

Reproduced with permission from Whight et al.[W3]

and a higher Y point in the wedged pulmonary artery pressure than in the pressures from the other sites. Such findings are believed to be due to mild narrowing or reduced compliance of the pulmonary veins and reduced compliance of the left atrium.[W3] (See Chapter 37 for further discussion of pulmonary venous stenosis.)

INDICATIONS FOR OPERATION

Investigation must be undertaken promptly in any infant, no matter how tiny, who develops symptoms and signs suggestive of the diagnosis of TAPVC, since procrastination leads to death in babies with obstructive TAPVC, and indeed in some without it, or to admission to hospital in a semi-moribund state, which seriously increases the risk of operation (see Table 16-4).

Operation should be undertaken immediately, once the diagnosis has been made, in any infant with obstructive TAPVC. This policy sometimes leads to surgical intervention in the first few days or week of life, frequently in the first month of life, and nearly always before 6 months of age. In neonates with nonobstructive TAPVC, an initial balloon septostomy and decongestive therapy may produce a prompt and obvious favorable response, but even then operation should be done in the first 3 months of life.

In infants in whom the diagnosis is made between 6 and 12 months of age, operation should be undertaken promptly, since the risk of operation is very low and even infants who appear to be doing well are at risk of dying before the age of 1 year.[B11,K3,L2]

Rarely, individuals survive into childhood or early adult life with TAPVC and are first seen for surgical consideration at that time. Operation is advisable if severe pulmonary vascular disease has not developed. The criteria of operability with regard to the pulmonary vascular disease are similar to those for patients with atrial septal defect (see Chapter 15, section on Indications for Operation). However, they are more difficult to apply in patients with TAPVC because of the systemic arterial desaturation present, as a result of the common mixing chamber. When pulmonary vascular resistance is less than 6 units · m^2 and $\dot{Q}p/\dot{Q}s$ is 2 or greater in such patients, operation is advisable. When the resistance is higher than this or the $\dot{Q}p/\dot{Q}s$ lower, the patient must be studied during moderate exercise. If the pulmonary vascular resistance stays the same or rises so that pulmonary flow cannot increase significantly, the $\dot{Q}p/\dot{Q}s$ falls because of the rise in systemic blood flow induced by exercise and made possible by an increased right-to-left shunt at atrial level. If, as a result of these changes during exercise, $\dot{Q}p/\dot{Q}s$ becomes less than about 1.2–1.4, the long-term results of operation are usually unsatisfactory, and repair is not advisable. Otherwise, it should be done.

SPECIAL SITUATIONS AND CONTROVERSIES

Mixed Total Anomalous Pulmonary Venous Connection

Repair of mixed TAPVC has been associated with high mortality in the literature, but the two patients with it in the GLH series survived, and there are several other reports of successful corrections.[B13,D6,G4,K5,W4] Better results will no doubt be obtained generally in the future, based on more precise preoperative cineangiocardiographic study and more precise surgical correction. Occasionally in infants with mixed TAPVC, as noted earlier, subtotal correction may be appropriate at the first operation.

Delayed Operation

Some centers have advised balloon atrial septostomy and hospital treatment for several months before the undertaking of surgical correction of TAPVC in very young infants.[M5] Mullins and colleagues reported clinical improvement and survival for several months in 9 of 12 infants treated in this way.[M6] One, however, died 1 week after balloon septostomy. Serratto and colleagues reported initially satisfactory results in infants without pulmonary venous obstruction.[S5]

The usefulness of balloon atrial septostomy in delaying operation in the sick young infant is severely limited because such babies usually have pulmonary venous obstruction that is unaffected by balloon septostomy. An exception may be those with drainage to the coronary sinus, but in this group, balloon septostomy will destroy the valve of the fossa ovalis and make direct suture repair using the Van Praagh technique[V1] difficult or impossible. Further, the present relatively low hospital mortality rates, even in very young infants, and the great risks inherent in allowing possible clinical deterioration of the patient during any kind of procrastination indicate that prompt surgical intervention is preferable to balloon septostomy combined with decongestive therapy.

Partial or Staged Corrections

In the early experience with surgical correction of TAPVC, staging of the repair was adopted by some centers in an effort to reduce what was then a high mortality rate.[B2,M3] Having found some degree of pulmonary venous congestion and pulmonary edema in 41 of 45 postoperative deaths among patients operated on before 1968, Mustard and associates recommended not interrupting at the initial operation the left vertical vein or the infradiaphragmatic connection if present.[M2] However, the mortality rate was high even with this staged procedure. At the Hospital for Sick Children, Great Ormond Street, London, an approach adopted at one time was ligation of the anomalous connection at the time of repair if tolerated but deferral of closure of the interatrial communication until a second operation if its patency persisted.[S6] Examples of spontaneous closure of the interatrial communication several years after the initial operation were documented.[S6] Again, however, the staged approach did not result in a marked reduction in hospital mortality.[B2]

With the present results with one-stage complete repair, total correction at one operation is advisable.

Operative Exposure

Correction of TAPVC by anastomosis of the common pulmonary venous sinus to the left atrium has been carried out from a variety of exposures. In our early cases, in 1955–1956 at the Mayo Clinic, the right atrium and then the atrial septum were opened, followed by an incision for the anastomosis in the back of the left atrium. The common pulmonary venous sinus was visualized through this incision and incised, and the anastomosis was performed between it and the left atrium. This anastomosis was carried across the septum and onto the back of the right atrium when necessary, and a new septum was inserted to the right of the anastomosis. Cooley and Ochsner later described this same approach.[C5] This approach continues to be used in some centers[H4] but is considered less desirable than that described in this text (UAB, GLH).

A left posterolateral thoracotomy was employed in Muller's first partial correction.[M1] Roe more recently recommended this exposure in the repair of supracardiac TAPVC using CPB.[R3] The majority of surgeons have, however, adopted exposure through a median sternotomy for all types of TAPVC.

Shumacker and King described carrying a transverse right atriotomy onto the lateral left atrial wall.[S7] This procedure permitted the left atrial–pulmonary venous trunk anastomosis to be accomplished essentially from outside the heart. Williams and associates described elevation of the apex of the heart to gain exposure for construction of the left atrial–pulmonary venous sinus anastomosis from outside the heart.[W5] Tucker and associates described exposing the structures for the anastomosis of the common pulmonary venous sinus to the left atrium through the transverse sinus between the aorta and the superior vena cava.[T3]

After some experience with these various procedures, the method described in this chapter, which achieves exposure without elevation of the apex or use of a large right atrial–left atrial incision, evolved.[K6] By the incision of the posterior pericardial attachments, the heart and cavae are easily elevated and retracted to the left to bring the posterior left atrium and pulmonary venous sinus into good view. Moreover, with this method there is virtually no risk of kinking or twisting of the anastomosis.

Surgical Enlargement of the Left Atrium

Trusler and colleagues found in dogs that a decrease in atrial volume of more than 50% resulted in a significant reduction in cardiac output.[T4] Brighton and coworkers, using a mechanical model, obtained a substantial improvement in cardiac output by adding a flexible atrium to the inlet of their artificial heart.[B14] Suga, in studying the effect of atrial compliance on cardiac performance with an electrical model, found cardiac performance to be markedly improved by increasing atrial compliance while maintaining constant ventricular contractility.[S8] Analysis suggested that increased atrial compliance facilitated the reservoir function of the atrium and the maintenance of a relatively high mean atrial

pressure during ventricular filling. When these facts are combined with the preoperatively observed small size of the left atrium in patients with TAPVC, its enlargement by the shifting of the atrial septum to the right has long been attractive.[G5,K7]

However, in the UAB experience, there was no significant difference in survival with and without left atrial enlargement.[K4] These findings may be due to the fact that surgical efforts to improve the left atrial size are not very effective or the possibility that adequate left atrial enlargement may result in any case from incorporation of the common pulmonary venous sinus into the left atrium by the repair.[M4,W3] Also, the lack of left atrial reservoir function may in fact rarely be critical early or late postoperatively if other aspects of the situation favor survival.

Support System during Repair

The dissection and suturing behind the heart required for repair of TAPVC in small babies is greatly facilitated by the use of profound hypothermia and total circulatory arrest. A not unimportant advantage of preliminary surface cooling to low temperatures (as in the GLH technique) is the ease of exposure of the aorta for cannulation that the low intravascular pressures allow. In TAPVC in the tiny infant, the aorta is very small and hidden by the very large and hypertrophied right ventricular outflow tract. Retraction of this tract for exposure and cannulation of the aorta at normothermia can precipitate severe persistent hypotension.

However, Turley and colleagues, in San Francisco, reported comparable results using more or less conventional CPB, but with a single right atrial venous cannula. After closure of the foramen ovale, the repair behind the heart can be made during CPB.

It has been noted that in some very sick infants, during the process of core cooling, the heart becomes very hard in ventricular fibrillation soon after the start of CPB. It may then quickly become extensively hemorrhagic in the subepicardial (and probably also subendocardial) layers (UAB). In this setting, the heart may have received ischemic injury preoperatively, and such injury, combined with the heart's small size (see Chapter 3), would make it prone to further ischemic injury during this phase of the operation. The thickness of the ventricular wall and the small left ventricular volume (due in part also to the smallness of the infant and in part to the small left ventricular volume usually present in this malformation) may increase wall tension markedly and severely limit the perfusion of the inner layers of both right and left ventricles.[A2,B15] This phenomenon is an argument in favor of a technique in which the heart continues to beat and is filled throughout the surface cooling process (GLH) or, if cooling is done with CPB, of inducing cold cardioplegia *before* ventricular fibrillation or myocardial hardness develops.

REFERENCES

A

1. Appelbaum A, Kirklin JW, Pacifico AD, Bargeron LM Jr: The surgical treatment of total anomalous pulmonary venous connection. *Israel J Med* 11:89, 1975.
2. Archie JP Jr: Determinants of regional intramyocardial pressure. *J Surg Res* 14:338, 1973.
3. Arciniegas E, Henry JG, Green EW: Stenosis of the coronary sinus ostium. *J Thorac Cardiovasc Surg* 79:303, 1980.

B

1. Burroughs JT, Kirklin JW: Complete surgical correction of total anomalous pulmonary venous connection: Report of three cases. *Proc Staff Meet Mayo Clin* 31:182, 1956.
2. Behrendt DM, Aberdeen E, Waterston DJ, Bonham-Carter RE: Total anomalous pulmonary venous drainage in infants. I. Clinical and hemodynamic findings, methods, and result of operation in 37 cases. *Circulation* 46:347, 1972.
3. Barratt-Boyes BG, Simpson M, Neutze JM: Intracardiac surgery in neonates and infants using deep hypothermia with surface cooling and limited cardiopulmonary bypass. *Circulation* 43,44(suppl I):I-25, 1971.
4. Barratt-Boyes BG: Primary definitive intracardiac operations in infants: Total anomalous pulmonary venous connection, in JW Kirklin (ed): *Advances in Cardiovascular Surgery.* New York: Grune & Stratton, 1973, p 127.
5. Bharati S, Lev M: Congenital anomalies of the pulmonary veins. *Cardiovasc Clin* 5:23, 1973.
6. Brody H: Drainage of the pulmonary veins into the right side of the heart. *Arch Path Lab Med* 33:221, 1942.
7. Burroughs JT, Edwards JE: Total anomalous venous connection. *Am Heart J* 59:913, 1960.
8. Bove KE, Geiser EA, Meyer RA: The left ventricle in anomalous pulmonary venous return. *Arch Path Lab Med* 99:522, 1975.
9. Barratt-Boyes BG, Nicholls TT, Brandt PWT, Neutze JM: Aortic arch interruption associated with patent ductus arteriosus, ventricular septal defect and total anomalous pulmonary venous connection: Total correction in an eight day old infant using profound hypothermia and limited cardiopulmonary bypass. *J Thorac Cardiovasc Surg* 63:367, 1972.
10. Burchell HB: Total anomalous pulmonary venous drainage: Clinical and physiologic patterns. Staff Meetings of the Mayo Clinic 31:161, 1956.
11. Bonham-Carter RE, Capriles M, Noe Y: Total anomalous pulmonary venous drainage. *Br Heart J* 31:45, 1969.
12. Buckley MJ, Behrendt DM, Goldblatt A, Laver MB, Austin WS: Correction of total anomalous pulmonary venous drainage in the first month of life. *J Thorac Cardiovasc Surg* 63:269, 1972.
13. Breckenridge IM, de Leval M, Stark J, Waterston DJ: Correction of total anomalous pulmonary venous drainage in infancy. *J Thorac Cardiovasc Surg* 66:447, 1973.
14. Brighton JA, Wade ZA, Pierce WS, Phillips WM, O'Bannon W: Effect of atrial volume on the performance of a sac-type artificial heart. *Trans Am Soc Artif Intern Organs* 19:567, 1973.
15. Barnard RJ, Buckberg GD, Manganaro AJ: Ventricular volume a major determinant of minimum subendocardial vascular resistance. *Circulation* 58(part 2):87, 1978 (abstr).

16. Bove EL, de Leval MR, Taylor JFN, Macartney FJ, Szarnicki RJ, Stark J: Infradiaphragmatic total anomalous pulmonary venous drainage: Surgical treatment and long-term results. *Ann Thorac Surg* 31:544, 1981.
17. Barratt-Boyes BG: Corrective surgery for congenital heart disease in infants with the use of profound hypothermia and circulatory arrest techniques. *Aust NZ J Surg* 47:737, 1979.

C

1. Cooley DA, Hallman GL, Leachman RD: Total anomalous pulmonary venous drainage: Correction with the use of cardiopulmonary bypass in 62 cases. *J Thorac Cardiovasc Surg* 51:88, 1966.
2. Cooley DA, Balas PE: Total anomalous pulmonary venous drainage into the inferior vena cava: Report of successful surgical correction. *Surgery* 51:798, 1962.
3. Carter REB, Capriles M, Noe Y: Total anomalous pulmonary venous drainage: A clinical and anatomical study of 75 children. *Br Heart J* 31:45, 1969.
4. Castaneda AR: (1980) Personal communication.
5. Cooley DA, Ochsner A Jr: Correction of total anomalous pulmonary venous drainage: Technical considerations. *Surgery* 42:1014, 1957.

D

1. Dillard DH, Mohri H, Hessel EA II, Anderson HN, Nelson RJ, Crawford EW, Morgan BC, Winterscheid LC, Merendino KA: Correction of total anomalous pulmonary venous drainage in infancy utilizing deep hypothermia with total circulatory arrest. *Circulation* 35,36(suppl I):I-105, 1967.
2. Darling RC, Rothney WB, Craig JM: Total pulmonary venous drainage into the right side of the heart. *Lab Invest* 6:44, 1957.
3. Delisle G, Ando M, Calder AL, Zuberbuhler JR, Rochenmacker S, Alday LE, Mangini O, Van Praagh S, Van Praagh R: Total anomalous pulmonary venous connection: Report of 93 autopsied cases with emphasis on diagnostic and surgical considerations. *Am Heart J* 91:99, 1976.
4. Duff DF, Nihill MR, McNamara DG: Infradiaphragmatic total anomalous pulmonary venous return: Review of clinical and pathological findings and results of operation in 28 cases. *Br Heart J* 39:619, 1977.
5. Davignon A: Cure du retour veineux anormal total du nourisson: Pont de vue de médicin. Journées de Cardiologie Pediatrique, Château de Feillac, October 7, 1972.
6. de Leval M, Stark J, Waterston DJ: Mixed type of total anomalous pulmonary venous drainage: Surgical correction in 3 infants. *Ann Thorac Surg* 16:464, 1973.
7. Drummond WH, Gregory GA, Heymann MA, Phibbs RA: The independent effects of hyperventilation, tolazoline and dopamine on infants with persistent pulmonary hypertension. *J Pediatr* 98:603, 1981.

E

1. El-Said GM, Mullins CE, McNamara DG: Management of total anomalous pulmonary venous return. *Circulation* 45:1240, 1972.

F

1. Friedlich A, Bing RJ, Blount SG Jr: Physiological studies in congenital heart disease. IX. Circulatory dynamics in the anomalies of venous return to the heart including pulmonary arteriovenous fistula. *Bull Johns Hopkins Hosp* 86:20, 1950.

2. Friedli B, Davignon A, Stanley P: Infradiaphragmatic anomalous pulmonary venous return: Surgical correction in a newborn infant. *J Thorac Cardiovasc Surg* 62:301, 1971.

3. Fleming WH, Clark EB, Dooley KJ, Hofschire PJ, Ruckman RN, Hopeman AR, Sarafian L, Mooring PK: Late complications following surgical repair of total anomalous pulmonary venous return below the diaphragm. *Ann Thorac Surg* 27:435, 1979.

G

1. Gross RE, Watkins E Jr, Pomeranz AA, Goldsmith EI: A method for surgical closure of interauricular septal defects. *Surg Gynecol Obstet* 96:1, 1953.

2. Gersony WM, Bowman FO Jr, Steeg CN, Hayes CJ, Jesse MJ, Malm JR: Management of total anomalous pulmonary venous drainage in early infancy. *Circulation* 43,44(suppl I):I-19, 1971.

3. Gathman GE, Nadas AS: Total anomalous pulmonary venous connection: Clinical and physiologic observations of 75 pediatric patients. *Circulation* 42:143, 1970.

4. Gomes MMR, Feldt RH, McGoon DC, Danielson GK: Total anomalous pulmonary venous connection: Surgical considerations and results of operation. *J Thorac Cardiovasc Surg* 60:116, 1970.

5. Goor DA, Yellin A, Frand M, Smolinsky A, Neufeldt H: The operative problem of small left atrium in total anomalous pulmonary venous connection: Report of 5 patients. *Ann Thorac Surg* 72:245, 1976.

H

1. Hastreiter AR, Paul MH, Molthan ME, Miller RA: Total anomalous pulmonary venous connection with severe pulmonary venous obstruction. *Circulation* 25:916, 1962.

2. Haworth SG, Reid L: Structural study of pulmonary circulation and of heart in total anomalous pulmonary venous return in early infancy. *Br Heart J* 39:80, 1977.

3. Hammon JW Jr, Bender HW Jr, Graham TP Jr, Boucek RJ Jr, Smith CW, Erath HG Jr: Total anomalous pulmonary venous connection in infancy: Ten years' experience including studies of postoperative ventricular function. *J Thorac Cardiovasc Surg* 80:544, 1980.

4. Hawkins JA, Clark EB, Coty DB: Total anomalous pulmonary venous connection. *Ann Thorac Surg* 36:548, 1983.

J

1. Jegier W, Charrette E, Dobell ARC: Infradiaphragmatic anomalous pulmonary venous drainage. *Circulation* 35:396, 1967.

K

1. Keith JD, Rowe RD, Vlad P: Heart disease in infancy and childhood, (ed 2). New York: Macmillan, 1967, p 493.

2. Kawashima Y, Matsuda H, Nakano S, Miyamoto IC, Fujino M, Kozaka T, Manabe H: Tree-shaped pulmonary veins in intracardiac total anomalous pulmonary venous drainage. *Ann Thorac Surg* 23:436, 1977.

3. Keith JD, Rowe RD, Vlad P, O'Hanley JH: Complete anomalous pulmonary venous drainage. *Am J Med* 16:23, 1954.

4. Katz NM, Kirklin JW, Pacifico AD: Concepts and practices in surgery for total anomalous pulmonary venous connection. *Ann Thorac Surg* 25:479, 1978.

5. Klint R, Weldon C, Hartmann A Jr, Schad N, Hernandez A, Goldring D: Mixed-type total anomalous pulmonary venous drainage. *J Thorac Cardiovasc Surg* 63:164, 1972.

6. Kirklin JW: Surgical treatment of total anomalous pulmonary venous connection in infancy, in BG Barratt-Boyes, JM Neutze, EA Harris (eds): *Heart Disease in Infancy: Diagnosis and Surgical Treatment.* Edinburgh: Churchill Livingstone, 1973, p 89.

7. Kirklin JW: Corrective surgical treatment of cyanotic congenital heart disease, in AD Bass, GK Moe (eds): *Congenital Heart Disease.* Washington, DC: American Association for the Advancement of Science, 1960, p 329.

8. Kirklin JK, Blackstone EH, Kirklin JW, McKay R, Pacifico AD, Bargeron LM Jr: Intracardiac surgery in infants under age 3 months: Incremental risk factors for hospital mortality. *Am J Cardiol* 48:500, 1981.

L

1. Lewis FJ, Varco RL, Taufic M, Niazi SA: Direct vision repair of triatrial heart and total anomalous pulmonary venous drainage. *Surg Gynecol Obstet* 102:713, 1956.

2. LaBrosse CJ, Blackstone EH, Turner ME Jr, Kirklin JW: The natural history of total anomalous pulmonary venous connections. (1978) Unpublished study.

3. Leachman RA, Cooley DA, Hallman G, Simpson JW, Dear WE: Total anomalous pulmonary venous return: Correlation and hemodynamic observations and surgical mortality in 58 cases. *Ann Thorac Surg* 7:5, 1969.

4. Lucas RV, Anderson RC, Amplatz K, Adamas P Jr, Edwards JE: Congenital causes of pulmonary venous obstruction. *Pediatr Clin North Am* 10:781, 1963.

M

1. Muller WH: The surgical treatment of transposition of the pulmonary veins. *Ann Surg* 134:683, 1951.

2. Mustard WT, Keon WJ, Trusler GA: Transposition of the lesser veins (total anomalous pulmonary venous drainage). *Prog Cardiovasc Dis* 11:145, 1968.

3. Mustard WT, Keith JD, Trusler GA: Two-stage correction for total anomalous pulmonary venous drainage in childhood. *J Thorac Cardiovasc Surg* 44:477, 1962.

4. Mathew R, Thilenius OG, Replogle RL, Arcilla RA: Cardiac function in total anomalous pulmonary venous return before and after surgery. *Circulation* 55:361, 1977.

5. Miller WW, Rashkind WJ, Miller RA, Hastreiter AR, Green EW, Golinko RJ, Young D: Total anomalous pulmonary venous return: Effective palliation of critically ill infants by balloon atrial septostomy. *Circulation* 35,36(suppl II):II-189, 1967 (abstr).

6. Mullins CE, El-Said GM, Neches WH, Williams RL, Vargo TA, Nihill MR, McNamara DG: Balloon atrial septostomy for total anomalous pulmonary venous return. *Br Heart J* 35:752, 1973.

7. Mazzucco A, Rizzoli G, Fracasso A, Stellin G, Valfre C, Pellegrino P, Bartolotti U, Gallucci V: Experience with operation for total anomalous pulmonary venous connection in infancy. *J Thorac Cardiovasc Surg* 85:686, 1983.

N

1. Nakazawa M, Jarmakini JM, Gyepes MT, Prochazka JV, Yabek SM, Marks RA: Pre- and postoperative ventricular function in

infants and children with right ventricular volume overload. *Circulation* 55:479, 1977.

2. Newfeld EA, Wilson A, Paul MH, Reisch JS: Pulmonary vascular disease in total anomalous pulmonary venous drainage. *Circulation* 61:103, 1980.

3. Neirotti, R: (1981) Personal communication.

P

1. Parr GVS, Kirklin JW, Pacifico AD, Blackstone EH, Lauridsen P: Cardiac performance in infants after repair of total anomalous pulmonary venous connection. *Ann Thorac Surg* 17:561, 1974.

2. Paquet M, Gutgesell H: Electrocardiographic features of total anomalous pulmonary venous connection. *Circulation* 51:599, 1975.

R

1. Rowe RD, Glass IH, Keith JD: Total anomalous pulmonary venous drainage at cardiac level: Angiocardiographic differentiation. *Circulation* 23:77, 1961.

2. Riker WL, Idriss FS, Aubert J, Midell A: The surgical treatment of total anomalous pulmonary venous drainage. *J Pediatr Surg* 5:444, 1970.

3. Roe BB: Posterior approach to correction of total anomalous pulmonary venous return. *J Thorac Cardiovasc Surg* 59:748, 1970.

S

1. Sloan H, Mackenzie J, Morris JD, Stern A, Sigmann J: Open heart surgery in infancy. *J Thorac Cardiovasc Surg* 44:459, 1962.

2. Stanger P, Rudolph AM, Edwards JE: Cardiac malpositions. *Circulation* 56:159, 1977.

3. Swischuk LE: Radiology of the newborn and young infant. Baltimore: Williams & Wilkins, 1973, p 40.

4. Sauvage LR, Harkins HN: Growth of vascular anastomoses: An experimental study of the influence of suture type and suture method with a note on certain mechanical factors involved. *Bull Johns Hopkins Hosp* 91:276, 1952.

5. Serratto M, Bucheleres HG, Bicoff P, Miller RA, Hastreiter AR: Palliative balloon atrial septostomy for total anomalous pulmonary venous connection in infancy. *J Pediatr* 73:734, 1968.

6. Silove ED, Behrendt DM, Aberdeen E, Bonham-Carter RE: Total anomalous pulmonary venous drainage. II. Spontaneous functional closure of interatrial communication after surgical correction in infancy. *Circulation* 46:357, 1972.

7. Shumacker HB Jr, King H: A modified procedure for complete repair of total anomalous pulmonary venous drainage. *Surg Gynecol Obstet* 112:763, 1961.

8. Suga H: Importance of atrial compliance in cardiac performance. *Circ Res* 35:39, 1974.

9. Smallhorn JF, Sutherland GR, Tommasini G, Hunter S, Anderson RH, Macartney FJ: Assessment of total anomalous pulmonary venous connection by two-dimensional echocardiography. *Br Heart J* 46:613, 1981.

10. Shinebourne EA, DelTorso S, Miller GAH, Jones ODH, Capuani A, Lincoln C: Total anomalous pulmonary venous drainage (TAPVD): Medical aspects and surgical indications, in L Parenzan, G Crupi, G Graham (eds): *Congenital Heart Disease in the First Three Months of Life*. Bologna: Patron Editore, p 447.

T

1. Tynan M, Behrendt D, Urquhart W: Portal vein catheterisation and selective angiography in diagnosis of total anomalous pulmonary venous connection. *Br Heart J* 36:115, 1974.

2. Turley K, Tucker WY, Ullyot DJ, Ebert PA: Total anomalous pulmonary venous connection in infancy: Influence of age and type of lesion. *Am J Cardiol* 45:92, 1980.

3. Tucker BL, Lindesmith GG, Stiles QR, Meyer BW: The superior approach for correction of the supracardiac type of total anomalous pulmonary venous return. *Ann Thorac Surg* 22:374, 1976.

4. Trusler GA, Bull RC, Hoeskema T, Mustard WT: The effect on cardiac output of a reduction in atrial volume. *J Thorac Cardiovasc Surg* 46:109, 1963.

V

1. Van Praagh R, Harken AH, Delisle G, Ando M, Gross RE: Total anomalous pulmonary venous drainage to the coronary sinus: A revised procedure for its correction. *J Thorac Cardiovasc Surg* 64:132, 1972.

W

1. Wilson J: A description of a very unusual formation of the human heart. *Philos Trans R Soc Lond* 88:346, 1798.

2. Woodwark GM, Vince DJ, Ashmore PG: Total anomalous pulmonary venous return to the portal vein: Report of a case of successful surgical treatment. *J Thorac Cardiovasc Surg* 45:662, 1963.

3. Whight CH, Barratt-Boyes BG, Calder L, Neutze JM, Brandt PWT: Total anomalous pulmonary venous connection: Long-term results following repair in infancy. *J Thorac Cardiovasc Surg* 75:52, 1978.

4. Wukasch DC, Deutsch M, Reul GJ, Hallman GL, Cooley DA: Total anomalous pulmonary venous return: A review of 125 patients treated surgically. *Ann Thorac Surg* 19:622, 1975.

5. Williams GR, Richardson WR, Campbell GS: Repair of total anomalous pulmonary venous drainage in infancy. *J Thorac Cardiovasc Surg* 47:199, 1964.

17

COR TRIATRIATUM

DEFINITION

Classic cor triatriatum, or cor triatriatum sinister, is a rare congenital cardiac anomaly in which all the pulmonary veins enter the common pulmonary venous chamber, located behind the heart and separated from the true left atrium, a distal chamber containing the atrial appendage and mitral valve, by a diaphragm in which there are one or more restrictive ostia.

Some types of complex congenital heart disease may bear similarities to cor triatriatum, and conceptualizing the repair of such lesions may be aided by considering them atypical forms of cor triatriatum. For example, the pulmonary veins may connect to the left atrium more superiorly than usual and into a portion of the left atrium separated from the rest by a nonrestrictive waist. Such incomplete absorption of the pulmonary veins could be considered a forme fruste cor triatriatum. Another example is the anomaly in which the pulmonary veins enter a chamber behind the heart that opens into the right atrium, with or without openings into the left atrium as well.[T1] This anomaly could also be considered a forme fruste cor triatriatum or a variety of total anomalous pulmonary venous connection to the right atrium.

Cor triatriatum dexter is a term used to describe the partially divided right atrium present in some cardiac malformations. This condition is considered later (see Chapter 26, "Morphology") and is unrelated to cor triatriatum sinister.

HISTORICAL NOTE

Cor triatriatum was apparently first described in 1868 by Church.[C1] The name *cor triatriatum* was applied to the malformation by Borst in 1905.[B1] The angiographic diagnosis seems first to have been made in our cases at the Mayo Clinic and described by Miller and colleagues in 1964.[M1] The first surgical correction is believed to have been performed by Vineberg in 1956[V3] and shortly thereafter by Lewis.[L2]

MORPHOLOGY

It is unfortunate that cor triatriatum was first defined as "an abnormal septum in the left atrium,"[C1] because the description obscures the surgically important concepts about cor triatriatum.

Relationship of Cor Triatriatum to Total and Partial Anomalous Pulmonary Venous Connection and Unroofed Coronary Sinus Syndrome

In hearts with atrioventricular (AV) concordant connection and normally positioned ventricles (D-loop in situs solitus), the left atrium contains the left atrial appendage and empties into the left ventricle through the mitral valve. An atrial septum, with or without a foramen ovale, separates the left atrium from the right atrium. In cor triatriatum, the right and left pulmonary veins do not join the left atrium but enter a chamber generally posterior and a little superior or medial to the left atrium that is analogous to the common pulmonary venous sinus of total anomalous pulmonary venous connection (TAPVC), described in Chapter 16. Indeed, Van Praagh and Orsini termed this chamber the *common pulmonary vein chamber of cor triatriatum*,[V1] and Marin-Garcia and colleagues used similar terminology.[M2] In classic cor triatriatum, this proximal common pulmonary venous chamber connects directly with the left atrium by way of one or more

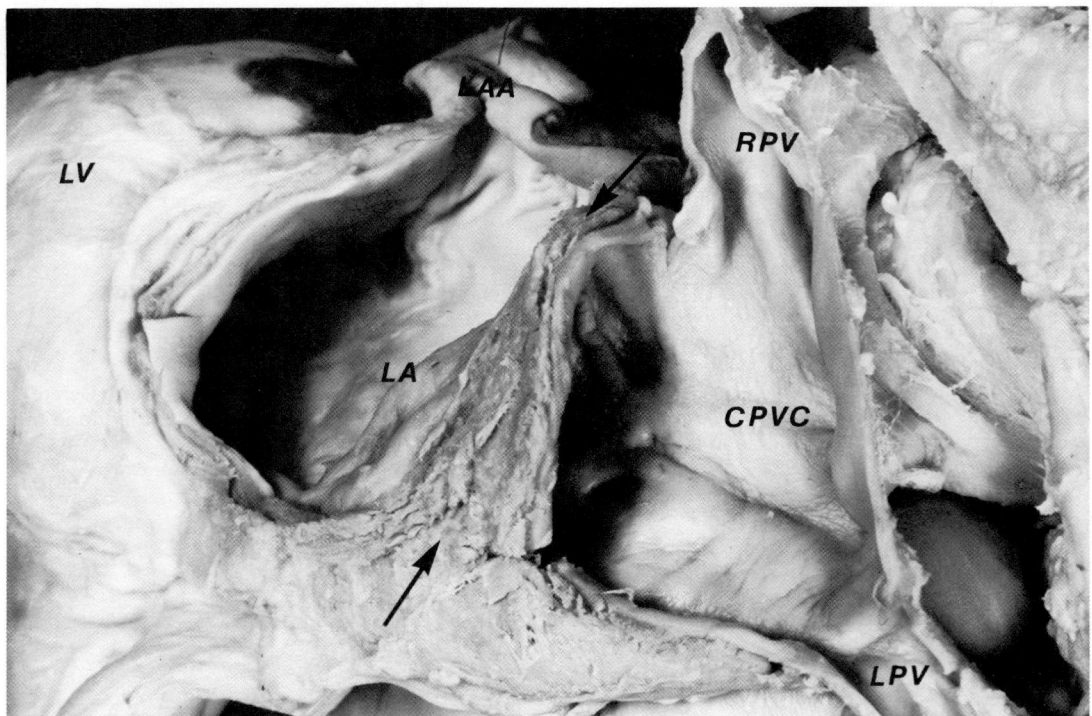

Figure 17-1 An autopsy specimen of cor triatriatum showing the opened common pulmonary venous chamber (proximal chamber) separated by a thick diaphragm (between the arrows) from the opened left atrium (distal chamber) (GLH). The diaphragm has a restrictive orifice (not seen here) in its center. The relation of this anomaly to total anomalous pulmonary venous connection is evident from this specimen.

CPVC, common pulmonary venous chamber; LA, left atrium; LAA, left atrial appendage; LPV, left pulmonary veins; LV, left ventricle; RPV, right pulmonary veins.

holes of restrictive size in the common wall (or membrane or diaphragm).

Many authors in the past considered this entire complex a left atrium divided into an upper chamber and a lower chamber by an anomalous membrane with an aperture. Thus emerged the unfortunate phrase "subdivided left atrium."[R1,T1] A more useful concept is that the proximal chamber is analogous to the common pulmonary venous sinus of TAPVC and the distal chamber is the true left atrium. Thus, cor triatriatum is an example of total anomalous pulmonary venous *connection* with normal *drainage* to the left atrium.

The usefulness of these concepts is supported also by cases of cor triatriatum associated with partial anomalous pulmonary venous connection. In 1976, Thilenius and associates described a subset of cor triatriatum in which only the right pulmonary veins opened into the common pulmonary venous chamber (or proximal chamber), the left pulmonary veins connecting to the left atrium. Van Praagh and Corsini reported anomalous pulmonary venous connection of the left upper lobe to the left innominate vein (rather than the proximal chamber) as an accompaniment of cor triatriatum;[V1] and Somerville[S1] and Richardson and colleagues[R1] reported cases of cor triatriatum in which the entire left lung connected anomalously to the left innominate vein. Lam and

colleagues in 1962[L1] also noted the relation of cor triatriatum to anomalous pulmonary venous connection in their cases.

Lam and colleagues reported cases in which all the pulmonary veins drained into the common pulmonary venous chamber (proximal chamber) and from there only into the right atrium, and the orifice of the coronary sinus was not visualized as such.[L1] Instead, an atrial septal defect (ASD) was present posteroinferiorly in the septum (coronary sinus type of ASD; see Chapter 15, section on Morphology). The surgical management of complex cases of this type that have in addition a persistent left superior vena cava attached to the upper left corner of the left atrium (or distal chamber) just superior and posterior to the left atrial appendage is facilitated by visualizing them as having both cor triatriatum emptying into the coronary sinus and unroofed coronary sinus (see Chapter 18). Understanding of these complex situations, many of which occur in patients with atrial isomerism (see Chapter 46), is enhanced by realizing that they can be termed total anomalous pulmonary venous connections.

Morphology of Classic Cor Triatriatum

Typically, in classic cor triatriatum, the common pulmonary venous chamber (proximal chamber) is somewhat larger

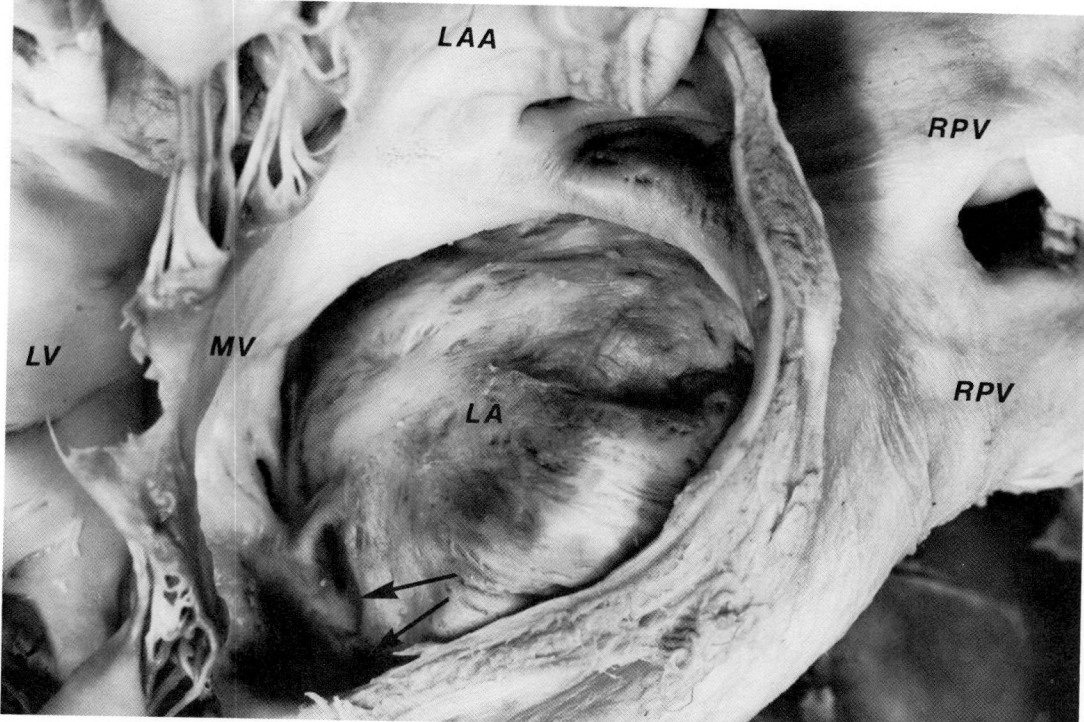

Figure 17-2 An autopsy specimen in which only the left atrium and left ventricle have been opened (GLH). The arrows indicate the two small openings in the diaphragm that communicate with the common pulmonary venous chamber, to which all the pulmonary veins are attached.

LA, left atrium; LAA, left atrial appendage; LV, left ventricle; MV, mitral valve; RPV, right pulmonary vein.

than the left atrium (distal chamber). The common wall between them, which may have one or more openings in it, is usually rather thick and fibromuscular (Fig. 17-1). Occasionally, rather than being an aperture in the common wall or diaphragm, the connection may be tubular.[M2,R1]

The common pulmonary venous chamber is usually thick-walled, whereas the left atrium containing the mitral valve and left atrial appendage is thin-walled (Fig. 17-2). Despite the high pressure in the proximal chamber, the pulmonary veins are not dilated. The entry of the right pulmonary veins to the common pulmonary venous chamber bears the same relationship to the right atrium and superior vena cava as in the normal heart (Fig. 17-3). The right ventricle is usually enlarged, but this enlargement depends on the presence and degree of left-to-right shunting at atrial level. The left ventricle is usually normal in size or small.

The fossa ovalis is usually located in the septum between the common pulmonary venous chamber and the right atrium[N1] but occasionally is in the septum between the left and right atria. In about 70% of cases, there is an interatrial communication, usually a stretched patent foramen ovale.

Associated Anomalies

In addition to partial anomalous pulmonary venous connection and unroofed coronary sinus with a left superior vena cava joining the left atrium, anomalies that may be associated with cor triatriatum are ventricular septal defect, coarctation of the aorta, AV canal defect, tetralogy of Fallot, and, rarely, asplenia and polysplenia.[M2]

CLINICAL FEATURES AND DIAGNOSTIC CRITERIA

Infants with classic cor triatriatum, with a small opening between the common pulmonary venous chamber and the left atrium, usually present with evidence of low cardiac output, including pallor, tachypnea, poor peripheral pulses, and growth failure.[W1] When there is associated left-to-right shunting because of an opening of the proximal chamber into the right atrium or because of associated partial anomalous pulmonary venous connection, evidence of pulmonary overcirculation and venous obstruction may be present in the chest x-ray, and right ventricular enlargement is prominent.

In children and young adults, the classic presentation is with the signs and symptoms of pulmonary venous hypertension. However, just as does mitral stenosis, cor triatriatum may present with less classic symptoms.[S1]

The diagnosis can be strongly suspected by study with M-mode echocardiography and confirmed by study with two-dimensional echocardiography.[N2,O2] Cardiac catheterization and cineangiographic studies are no longer considered necessary unless the presence of major associated cardiac anomalies is suspected (UAB). However, further evidence

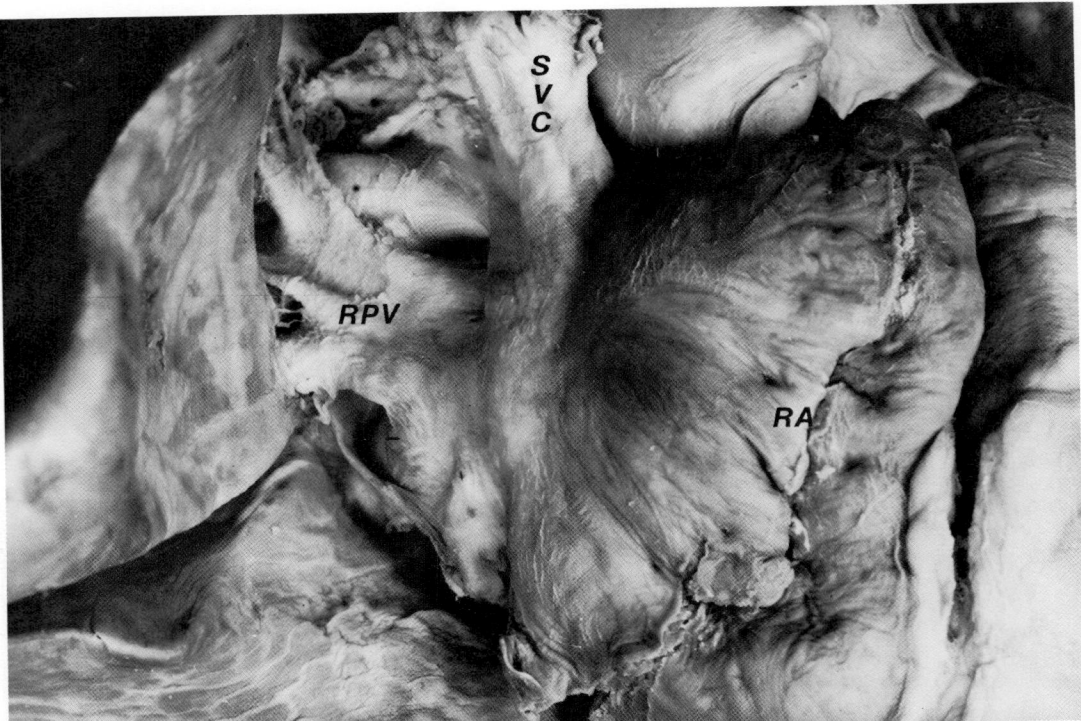

Figure 17-3 The same specimen as in Figure 17-2, oriented anatomically with the great vessels at the top (GLH). The specimen is viewed from in front, and an incision made in the right atrium has been closed. Note the normal relationship between the right pulmonary veins and the superior vena cava and right atrium.

RA, right atrium; RPV, right pulmonary veins; SVC, superior vena cava.

may be obtained from selective cineangiographic studies and pressure measurements in the common pulmonary venous chamber and the left atrium. If the catheter cannot be manipulated into the proximal and distal chambers from the right atrium, sometimes an arterial catheter can be advanced into the left ventricle and retrogradely across the mitral valve and into the distal and then the proximal chamber.[V2] Gradients of 20–25 mmHg have been demonstrated between the two chambers.[V2]

NATURAL HISTORY

The natural history of classic cor triatriatum depends on the effective size of the hole in the partition (diaphragm) between the common pulmonary venous chamber and the left atrium. When the hole is small, the infant becomes critically ill in the early months of life and, without surgical treatment, dies at that young age.[J1,O1,P1,W1] If the orifice is larger, the patient presents in childhood or young adulthood with the signs, symptoms, and prognosis without surgical treatment of mitral stenosis.[B2]

In most patients, the hole in the common wall is severely restrictive, and about 75% of persons born with classic cor triatriatum die in infancy. However, when the common pul-

monary venous chamber communicates with the right atrium through a fossa ovalis ASD, the prognosis is better because the proximal chamber decompresses into the right atrium.

TECHNIQUE OF OPERATION

Typical Cor Triatriatum

The enlargement of the common pulmonary venous chamber in typical cor triatriatum unassociated with other cardiac anomalies makes the surgical approach through an incision in its right side attractive, and under such circumstances this approach is recommended. The common pulmonary venous chamber may not be enlarged to the right, and the right atrium may be enlarged; in such a situation, an approach through the right atrium is preferable.

After the usual preparations, moderately hypothermic cardiopulmonary bypass (CPB) is established, using two venous cannulae as a precaution against surgical inconvenience should the foramen ovale be patent. The cold cardioplegic solution is injected into the aortic root. Alternatively, profound hypothermia, total circulatory arrest, in simple aortic clamping without cardioplegia, is used in infants (GLH). The common pulmonary venous chamber is opened through a vertical incision anterior to the right pulmonary veins, exactly as for mitral valve surgery (see Chapter 11, section on Technique of Operation). After the insertion of an appropriately sized Richardson retractor or a similar instrument, the diaphragm is exposed, and the hole or holes in it are identified. A preliminary incision out from the holes in the diaphragm improves exposure for the definitive excision. The orifices of the pulmonary veins on both sides are located. The position of the atrial septum is also identified, if necessary by opening the right atrium and inserting a curved clamp to displace the atrial septum into either the left atrium or the common pulmonary venous chamber. Most of the diaphragm (the common wall between the proximal and distal chambers) is now excised to make an opening as large as possible. This procedure is usually easily and quickly done.

When an approach through the right atrium is indicated, the foramen ovale is situated between the common pulmonary venous chamber and the right atrium. This opening is enlarged to provide good exposure within the common pulmonary venous chamber. The procedure described above is carried out and the opening in the atrial septum closed.

The cardiotomy is closed, having been filled with blood or saline solution before the last few sutures were placed. With suction on the aortic needle vent, the aortic clamp is released. Rewarming of the patient with the perfusate has usually been begun about 5 minutes before this. After good cardiac action has commenced, the usual de-airing procedures are carried out (see Chapter 2, Section 3). When rewarming is completed, CPB is discontinued, decannulation effected, and the remainder of the operation completed in the usual manner (see Chapter 2, Section 3).

Cor Triatriatum Associated with a Large Defect between the Common Pulmonary Venous Chamber and the Right Atrium

Compared to classic cases of cor triatriatum, cases associated with a large defect between the common pulmonary venous chamber and the right atrium are characterized by less marked enlargement of the proximal chamber but considerable right atrial enlargement. The surgical approach is therefore best made, at least initially, through the right atrium.

After CPB has been established using two venous cannulae, and the aorta cross-clamped and the heart cooled and arrested by the cold cardioplegic solution, the usual oblique right atriotomy incision is made (see Chapter 15, Fig. 15-12). The anatomy is now systematically and precisely defined, as it must be in all complex anomalies. Within the right atrium, the characteristic structures are identified, including the tricuspid valve, the atrioventricular septum, the location of the AV node and bundle of His (see Chapter 1, Figs. 1-1, 1-14), the ostium of the coronary sinus, the orifices of the cavae and the eustachian valve, and, most important, the limbus and the fossa ovalis. The proximal chamber, which may have a small or large opening into the left atrium, is identified by the location of the orifices of all pulmonary veins entering it. The left atrial appendage and mitral valve allow identification of the left atrium. A persistent left

superior vena cava may connect to the upper left corner of the left atrium.

The large defect between the common pulmonary venous chamber and the right atrium may be posterior, with absence of the posterior limbus. In such a situation, repair is rather simple, effected by excising most of the diaphragm between the proximal and distal chambers, closing any interatrial communication, and closing the large defect. The large defect may be located more anteriorly in the region usually occupied by the orifice of the coronary sinus. When in such a case a left superior vena cava coexists attached to the superior left corner of the left atrium, a baffle must be used to partition the two atria in such a way that the left superior vena cava drains into the right atrium and the pulmonary veins into left atrium via the common pulmonary venous chamber (see Chapter 18, Fig. 18-1). If no left superior vena cava is present, the large anteriorly placed defect in the atrial septum is closed after it is ascertained that there is a large communication between the common pulmonary venous chamber and the left atrium.

Without precise analysis of the anatomic details and a proper concept of cor triatriatum, an effective repair cannot be planned.

SPECIAL FEATURES OF POSTOPERATIVE CARE

For patients with cor triatriatum, postoperative care is as usual (see Chapter 5).

EARLY RESULTS

No (0%, CL 0%–24%) hospital deaths occurred among three patients with classic cor triatriatum repaired by us at the Mayo Clinic 1955–1967[M1] and four patients (aged 2, 6, and 11 months and 3 years) operated on at UAB 1967–July 1984. Carpena and colleagues reported no deaths among four patients operated on at the Buffalo Children's Hospital.[C2]

Infants coming to operation in NYHA class V can be expected to have a high mortality. Thus, one such patient, ventilated preoperatively and undergoing an emergency repair, died early after a technically complete and satisfactory correction (GLH).

Complex cor triatriatum can be successfully repaired. In one critically ill young infant, presenting with signs of low cardiac output, the common pulmonary venous chamber drained to the left atrium through a 3-mm perforation and opened into the right atrium through a large aperture in the region of the posterior limbus, and the right atrium opened into left atrium through a patent foramen ovale 3 mm in diameter (UAB). This patient's malformation was the same as that described in several patients by Niwayama.[N1] Another patient, 3 years old, had a large and nonrestrictive orifice between the superiorly placed common pulmonary venous chamber and the left atrium, a large left superior vena cava attached to the upper left corner of the left atrium and absence of the coronary sinus with a large coronary sinus atrial septal defect (unroofed coronary sinus syndrome) along with tetralogy of Fallot (UAB). Both patients survived repair and are well.

LATE RESULTS

The six patients with classic or complex cor triatriatum are without symptoms (UAB). The life expectancy after repair of classic cor triatriatum should approach that of the general population, especially when the operation is done in infancy. However, Richardson and colleagues reported one late death in their group of eight hospital survivors, from pulmonary vein stenosis (see Chapter 37).[R1] The association of pulmonary vein stenosis with cor triatriatum suggests again the interrelationship between cor triatriatum and total anomalous pulmonary venous connection (see Chapter 16, "Postoperative Pulmonary Venous Obstruction" in section on Late Results).

Another unfavorable late event may be restenosis of the orifice between the common pulmonary venous chamber and the left atrium.[J1] Such restenosis may be the result of an inadequate original operation in which something less than complete resection was made of the common wall between the two chambers.

INDICATIONS FOR OPERATION

Classic cor triatriatum, with a restrictive aperture in the partition between the proximal common pulmonary venous sinus (or chamber) and the distal left atrium, is an urgent indication for operation. Since 75% of patients with such malformations die in infancy, symptoms usually develop early, and operation is necessary in the first year of life. When older patients present with chronic symptoms, operation is also urgently indicated.

In complex cor triatriatum, when the common pulmonary venous chamber opens into the right atrium and a restrictive opening or no opening is present between the common pulmonary venous chamber and the left atrium and only a small patent foramen ovale between the right atrium and the left atrium, a large left-to-right shunt, combined with very restricted left atrial and left ventricular inflow, produces severe symptoms in the early months of life, and operation is indicated on an urgent basis.

REFERENCES

B

1. Borst H: Ein Cor triatriatum. *Zentralbl Allg Pathol* 16:812, 1905.
2. Belcher JR, Somerville W: Cor triatriatum (stenosis of the common pulmonary vein). *Br Med J* 1:1280, 1951.

C

1. Church WS: Congenital malformation of the heart: Abnormal septum in left auricle. *Trans Pathol Soc London* 19:188, 1867/1868.
2. Carpena C, Colokathis B, Subramanian S: Cor Triatriatum. *Ann Thorac Surg* 17:325, 1974.

G

1. Gibson DG, Honey M, Lennox SC: Cor triatriatum: Diagnosis by echocardiography. *Br Heart J* 36:835, 1974.

J

1. Jorgensen CR, Ferlic RM, Varco RL, Lillehei CW, Eliot RS: Cor triatriatum: Review of the surgical aspects with a follow-up report on the first patient successfully treated with surgery. *Circulation* 36:101, 1967.

L

1. Lam CR, Green E, Drake E: Diagnosis and surgical correction of 2 types of triatrial heart. *Surgery* 51:127, 1962.
2. Lewis FJ, Varco RL, Taufic M, Niazi SA: Direct vision repair of triatrial heart and total anomalous pulmonary venous drainage. *Surg Gynecol Obstet* 102:713, 1956.

M

1. Miller GAH, Ongley PA, Anderson MW, Kincaid OW, Swan HJC: Cor triatriatum: Hemodynamic and angiocardiographic diagnosis. *Am Heart J* 68:298, 1964.
2. Marin-Garcia J, Tandon R, Lucas RV Jr, Edwards JE: Cor triatriatum: Study of 20 cases. *Am J Cardiol* 35:59, 1975.

N

1. Niwayama G: Cor triatriatum. *Am Heart J* 59:291, 1960.
2. Nimura Y, Matsumoto M, Beppu S, Matsuo H, Sakakibara H, Abe H: Noninvasive preoperative diagnosis of cor triatriatum with ultrasonocardiotomogram and conventional echocardiogram. *Am Heart J* 88:240, 1974.

O

1. Oelert H, Breckenridge IM, Rosland G, Stark J: Surgical treatment of cor triatriatum in a 4½-month-old infant. *Thorax* 28:242, 1973.
2. Ostman-Smith I, Silverman NH, Oldershaw P, Lincoln C, Shinebourne EA: Cor triatriatum sinistrum: Diagnostic features on cross sectional echocardiography. *Br Heart J* 51:211, 1984.

P

1. Perry LW, Scott LD, McClenathan JE: Cor triatriatum: Preoperative diagnosis and successful repair in a small infant. *J Pediatr* 71:840, 1967.

R

1. Richardson JV, Doty DB, Siewers RD, Zuberbuhler JR: Cor triatriatum (subdivided left atrium). *J Thorac Cardiovasc Surg* 81:232, 1981.

S

1. Somerville J: Masked cor triatriatum. *Br Heart J* 28:55, 1966.

T

1. Thilenius OG, Bharati S, Lev M: Subdivided left atrium: An expanded concept of cor triatriatum sinistrum. *Am J Cardiol* 37:743, 1976.

V

1. Van Praagh R, Corsini I: Cor triatriatum: Pathologic anatomy and a consideration of morphogenesis based on 13 postmortem cases and a study of normal development of the pulmonary vein and atrial septum in 83 human embryos. *Am Heart J* 78:379, 1969.

2. van der Horst RL, Gotsman MS: Cor triatriatum: Angiographic diagnosis by retrograde catheterization of the dorsal accessory chamber. *Br J Radiol* 44:273, 1971.

3. Vineberg A, Gialloreto O: Report of a successful operation for stenosis of common pulmonary vein (cor triatriatum). *Can Med Assoc J* 74:719, 1956.

W

1. Wolfe RR, Ruttenberg HD, Desilets DT, Mulder DE: Cor triatriatum. *J Thorac Cardiovasc Surg* 56:114, 1968.

18

UNROOFED CORONARY SINUS SYNDROME

DEFINITION

The unroofed coronary sinus syndrome is a spectrum of cardiac anomalies in which part or all of the common wall between the coronary sinus and the left atrium is absent.

Hearts with atrial isomerism and a left-sided superior vena cava (SVC) entering a left-sided atrium are included in this chapter for completeness, recognizing the controversy concerning proper classification of such anomalies (see later section on "Atrial Isomerism" and Chapter 46).

HISTORICAL NOTE

The unroofed coronary sinus syndrome did not come to the attention of cardiac pathologists before the era of cardiac catheterization and cardiac surgery. Winter, a radiologist at Hahnemann Hospital, in Philadelphia, provided a pathologic paper in 1954 that mentions persistent left superior vena cava (LSVC) attached to the left atrium,[W1] and Friedlich and colleagues reported four instances of LSVC entering the left atrium, as identified at cardiac catheterization.[F1] An isolated case was also presented by Tuchman and colleagues in 1956.[T1] Campbell and Deuchar, in 1954, referred to instances of LSVC attached to the left atrium, although they did not have such an example in their own series of LSVC. They appreciated that in such cases there was no true coronary sinus. The understanding of the morphology of the syndrome came from the classic paper by Raghib, Edwards, and colleagues in 1965.[R2] The descriptive phrase "unroofed coronary sinus" was first used by Helseth and Peterson in 1974.[H2]

In cyanotic patients with a communication between the left and right SVC, the LSVC was first tied off (appropriately) by Hurwitt and colleagues in 1955[H1] and then by Davis and colleagues in 1959.[D1] Taybi and colleagues, in 1965, reported a ligation and mentioned "transferring the left SVC to the right atrium," but presumably this was unsuccessful, since no further details are given.[T2] The first report of successful repair was ours from the Mayo Clinic in 1963.[R1] In this case, a tunnel was constructed from the posterior wall of the left atrium. In the same journal,[M2] we described the insertion of a large pericardial atrial baffle that totally corrected anomalous connection of both the superior vena cava and the inferior vena cava (IVC) to a left-sided atrium. This procedure was used at GLH in two patients with the unroofed coronary sinus syndrome in 1970 and was also described by Helseth and Peterson, in 1974.[H2]

533

MORPHOLOGY

Completely Unroofed Coronary Sinus with Persistent Left Superior Vena Cava

In one form of the unroofed coronary sinus syndrome, the coronary sinus does not exist because the common wall between it and the left atrium is absent. A persistent LSVC, which normally becomes continuous with the coronary sinus, connects to the left upper corner of the left atrium. The place of connection of the LSVC to the left atrium appears to be constant and lies between the opening of the left atrial appendage anteriorly and slightly superiorly and the opening of the left pulmonary veins posteriorly and inferiorly. The pulmonary veins may enter the left atrium more superiorly than usual in this form of the syndrome. The aperture of a coronary sinus atrial septal defect is present in the posteroinferior region of the atrial septum, in the usual position of the ostium of the coronary sinus (see Chapter 15, Figs. 15-5, 15-14). The atrial septal defect (ASD) is separated from the atrioventricular (AV) valve ring by a remnant of atrial septum (in contrast to an ostium primum ASD), while its inferior margin is formed by the atrial wall where it joins the inferior vena cava. There may be a separate foramen ovale ASD or a single large confluent ASD, formed by the confluence of both defects. The coronary sinus ASD may be confluent with an ostium primum ASD, or there may be a common atrium.

As the coronary sinus does not exist, the individual coronary veins drain separately into the inferior aspect of the left atrium. Some also drain into the right atrium.

Of considerable surgical importance is the fact that the left innominate vein is absent in 80%–90% of cases with the unroofed coronary sinus syndrome and LSVC.[Q1,R1] The right SVC is frequently small and it may be absent. The inferior vena cava not infrequently crosses to the left side below the diaphragm to enter the left hemiazygous vein, which joins the LSVC. The hepatic veins usually enter the inferior aspect of the right atrium, but they too may enter the inferior left atrial wall. When all the systemic veins enter a morphologically left atrium, total anomalous systemic venous connection is present.

Completely Unroofed Coronary Sinus without Persistent Left Superior Vena Cava

In some cases, the syndrome is characterized by a completely unroofed coronary sinus without a persistent LSVC. Such cases consist of a classic coronary sinus type of ASD and the total absence of the coronary sinus due to the absence of the partition between it and the left atrium.

Partially Unroofed Mid-portion of the Coronary Sinus

Another form of the syndrome is characterized by a partially unroofed mid-portion of the coronary sinus (also called bi-atrial opening of coronary sinus or coronary sinus–to–left atrial window or fenestration). In this anomaly, only an aperture is present in the mid-portion of the wall between the coronary sinus and the left atrium. Through this aperture, a left-to-right or right-to-left shunt occurs, depending on whether obstructions are present to left atrial or right atrial outflow.[F2]

When this rare form of the unroofed coronary sinus syndrome occurs as an isolated lesion, there may be a large left-to-right shunt.[A1,M1] It has also been reported as a major cardiac anomaly associated with tricuspid atresia, recognized only after the Fontan repair has elevated the right atrial pressure and produced a right-to-left shunt.[F2,R3]

When such mid-portion unroofing occurs in the presence of an LSVC, there is a right-to-left shunt into left atrium.

Partially Unroofed Terminal Portion of the Coronary Sinus

Particularly in the presence of AV canal defects, the coronary sinus ostium may open into the left atrium rather than the right. Also, a localized unroofing of the sinus may occur just before it enters the ostium of the coronary sinus, resulting in a coronary sinus ASD with preservation of the coronary sinus. Such an anomaly can be called unroofing (or absence) of the terminal portion of the coronary sinus.

Relationship of Unroofed Coronary Sinus Syndrome to Cor Triatriatum and Atrioventricular Canal Defects

As indicated, when the completely unroofed coronary sinus with persistent LSVC is present, both left and right pulmonary veins may enter the left atrium more superiorly than usual. Sometimes this condition is accompanied by a mild or moderate narrowing between the portion of the left atrium to which the pulmonary veins are attached (the common pulmonary venous chamber) and that to which the LSVC and left atrial appendage and mitral valve are attached. Such a malformation can be interpreted as forme fruste cor triatriatum (see Chapter 17, "Relationship of Cor Triatriatum to Total and Partial Anomalous Pulmonary Venous Connection and Unroofed Coronary Sinus Syndrome" in section on Morphology). Furthermore, the common pulmonary venous chamber may be posterior as well as superior to the left atrium, and efforts surgically to partition the coronary sinus from the left atrium by creating a tunnel that crosses the posteroinferior atrial wall may obstruct pulmonary venous flow to the mitral valve (see "Special Situations and Controversies").

Unroofed coronary sinus syndrome has as its commonest major associated cardiac anomaly an AV canal defect, not infrequently with a common atrium (see Chapter 19). Interestingly, AV canal defects are more commonly associated with persistent LSVC than are other kinds of ASDs.

Atrial Isomerism

Many patients with an LSVC connecting to the left side of the atria have atrial isomerism (see Chapter 46), and the majority of such patients have an AV canal defect. Thus, in an autopsy series of 26 hearts with LSVC connecting to the left-sided atrium, only 3 are examples of the classic unroofed coronary sinus syndrome (GLH). Twenty-three hearts had atrial isomerism, 17 with bilateral morphologically right atria (most with asplenia) and 6 with bilateral morphologically left atria (most with polysplenia). Of the 23, 20 had an AV canal defect in addition to numerous other cardiac anomalies. When bilateral morphologically right atria are present, the left-sided SVC enters the left-sided right atrium behind a typical crista terminalis and is not therefore an example of unroofed coronary sinus, despite the fact that the coronary sinus is usually absent. When bilateral morphologically left atria are present, the left-sided SVC may or may not be part of an unroofed coronary sinus syndrome. In such cases, the coronary sinus is, however, frequently absent.

CLINICAL FEATURES AND DIAGNOSTIC CRITERIA

Usually, the diagnosis of unroofed coronary sinus syndrome is only suspected, not confirmed, before operation. However, the demonstration of an LSVC by catheter passage or cineangiogram provides suspicion of the diagnosis, which is confirmed, if the LSVC can also be shown to drain into the left atrium. The diagnosis of partially unroofed mid-portion of the coronary sinus can be made by cineangiography after injection into the right atrium when right atrial pressure is higher than left (such as after the Fontan operation). Konstam and colleagues have pointed out that radionuclide angiography can be used to make the diagnosis, since intravenous injections into the left arm will show much larger right-to-left shunting than those into the right arm.[K1]

Generally, however, the diagnosis must be made by the surgeon after viewing of the external and internal morphology of the heart at operation.

NATURAL HISTORY

Cyanosis from right-to-left shunting dominates the clinical picture of isolated completely unroofed coronary sinus with persistent LSVC and determines its natural history. The cyanosis has been mild in the UAB cases, all of whom were less than 17 years old, but was severe in some older patients reported in the literature.

Cerebral embolization and cerebral abscess complicate the life history in 10%–25% of such patients (Table 18-1). This situation is similar to that in other types of right-to-left shunting. Presumably, life expectancy is considerably reduced by these complications and the other problems associated with increasing cyanosis and polycythemia.

TECHNIQUE OF OPERATION

Isolated Completely Unroofed Coronary Sinus with Persistent Left Superior Vena Cava

The anesthesia and preparation of the patient for repair of isolated completely unroofed coronary sinus with persistent LSVC is as usual (see Chapter 2). When the diagnosis is known preoperatively, the anesthesiologist inserts a pressure-monitoring line into the *left* external or, preferably, internal jugular vein. After the sternotomy has been made, a large piece of pericardium is removed and set aside (see Chapter 15, footnote 15-2). The LSVC is temporarily oc-

Table 18-1 Some details of eight patients (UAB; 1967–1977) with isolated completely unroofed coronary sinus with left superior vena cava.[Q1] (The figures are not cumulative.)

Data	No. of Patients
Age	
1–11 yr	8
History	
Brain abscess or TIA	2
Mild arterial desaturation	8
Anatomy	
LSVC to upper corner of LA	8
LSVC to innominate vein	1
Coronary sinus type ASD	4
Isolated	2
With foramen ovale	2
Confluent ASD (coronary sinus plus fossa ovalis type)	4
Management	
Ligation of LSVC and closure of ASD	1
Roofing of coronary sinus	
With posterior wall of LA	4
With pericardium	2
With opened Dacron tube	1

KEY: ASD, atrial septal defect; LA, left atrium; LSVC, left superior vena cava; RA, right atrium; TIA, transient ischemic attacks.

cluded, and if there is no rise in jugular vein pressure, it may simply be ligated and the atrial septal defect repaired (see "Special Situations and Controversies"). Otherwise, a pericardial baffle repair is required.

The operation may be done routinely with cardiopulmonary bypass (CPB) at 25°C and the usual direct caval cannulation (see Chapter 2, section 3); the return from the LSVC is picked up with a pump-oxygenator sump sucker (UAB). Alternatively, in infancy a single venous cannula and repair during profoundly hypothermic total circulatory arrest may be used (GLH).

After aortic cross-clamping and the injection of the cold cardioplegic solution (see Chapter 3) or after simple aortic cross-clamping if the repair is to be done during profoundly hypothermic total circulatory arrest (GLH), the right atrium is opened through the usual oblique incision. The orifices of the three cavae are identified with certainty. The fossa ovalis is excised and the orifices of the four pulmonary veins identified. The positions of the mitral and tricuspid valves are noted. Any remaining atrial septum is now excised, except for the anterior limbus, which is preserved as a protection for the AV node and bundle of His (see Chapter 1, Figs. 1-1, 1-14). Stay sutures are placed to mark the corners of the proposed suture line, which lies anterior to the orifices of the pulmonary veins; behind the orifices of the SVC, IVC, and LSVC; and between the AV valves (Fig. 18-1). The pericardial baffle is cut to proper shape and size and then sewn into place with continuous polypropylene sutures. It is best to begin this suture line with a double-armed suture just posterior to the orifice of the LSVC (and thus posterior to the left atrial appendage but anterior to the left pulmonary veins) and to carry one arm along the left lateral atrial wall in front of the pulmonary veins and the mitral valve to the limbus and the other arm rightward along the superior wall of the atrium below the orifice of the right SVC and then along the right lateral wall of the right atrium in front of the right pulmonary veins. The suture line then curves beneath the IVC orifice and passes up to the anterior limbus.

When the unroofed coronary sinus syndrome is an isolated anomaly, rewarming of the patient with CPB is begun as the suture line is being completed. With suction applied to the aortic vent needle, the aortic clamp is released after the repair is completed. The right atrium is closed. After good cardiac action is obtained, the usual de-airing procedures are carried out (see Chapter 2, Section 3), and the operation is completed as usual.

Partially Unroofed Mid-portion of the Coronary Sinus

The repair of a partially unroofed mid-portion of the coronary sinus is made through a right atrial approach. The important step is defining the aperture, which is done by passing a small forceps into the coronary sinus, through the defect, and into the left atrium, verifying that the tip has in fact entered the left atrium. The closure usually can be made

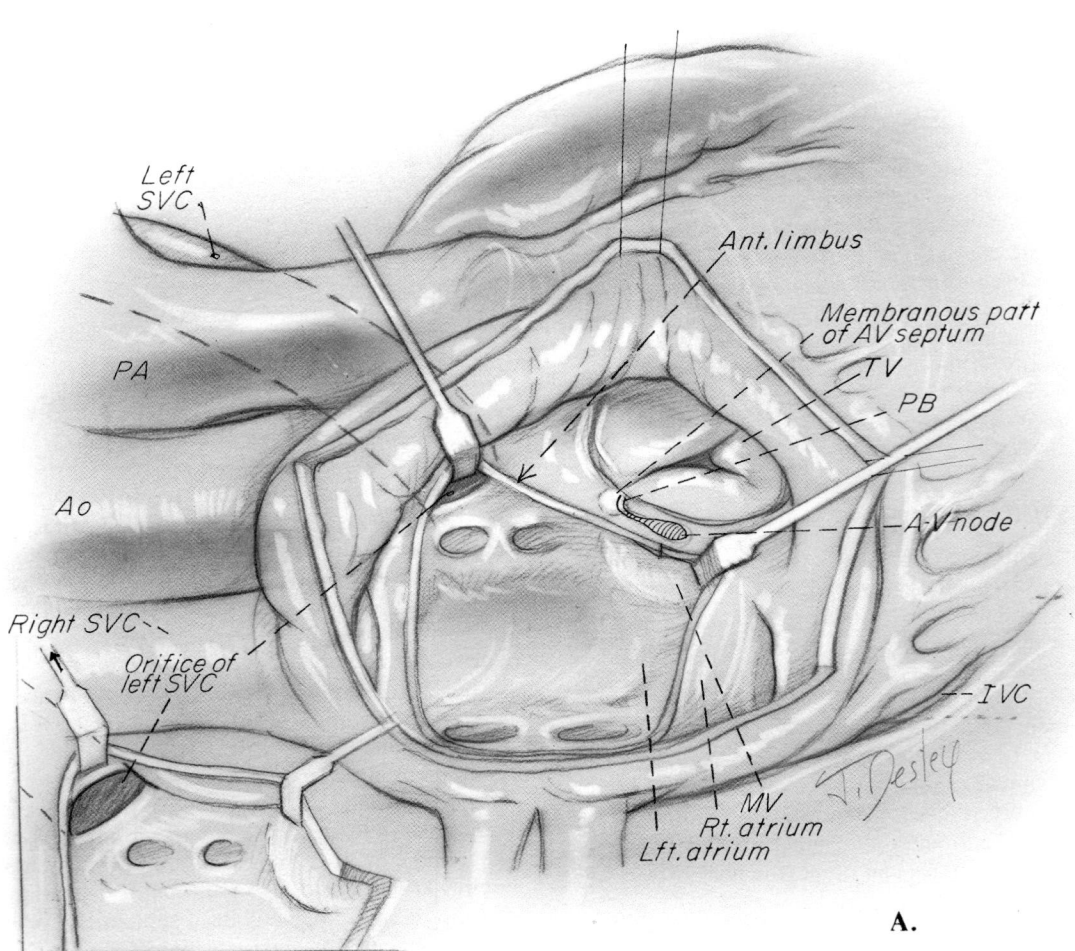

Figure 18-1 The technique of repair of unroofed coronary sinus with large persistent left superior vena cava entering the upper left corner of the left atrium. The exposure is through an oblique right atriotomy incision.

(a) The atrial septum has been excised, with care taken to preserve the anterior limbus as a protection for the atrioventricular node and the bundle of His. The orifice of the right and left pulmonary veins are visible. Anterosuperior to the orifices of the left pulmonary veins is the orifice of the left superior vena cava, and just inferior to that (not visible) is the left atrial appendage. A half purse-string stitch is placed just anterior and superior to the left superior pulmonary vein and to the right superior pulmonary vein. A similar gathering half purse-string suture is placed in the tissue just posterior to the usual location of the coronary sinus (not shown) and anterior and superior to the orifice of the inferior vena cava. These gathering sutures are initial preparations for the pathway to be made by the insertion of the patch.

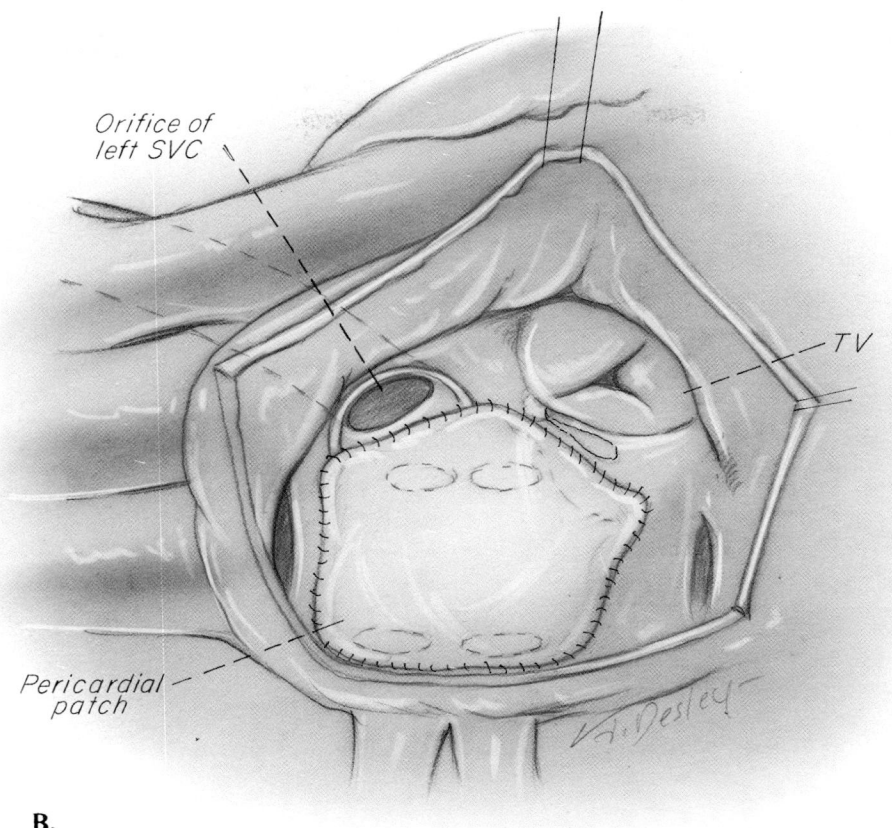

B.

Figure 18-1 (continued)
(b) The pericardial patch, trimmed so as to fit snugly, is sewn into place. The three caval orifices drain into the right atrium, and the pulmonary veins now drain into the left atrium and through the mitral valve.

Ao, aorta; AV node, atrioventricular node; IVC, inferior vena cava; MV, mitral valve; PA, pulmonary artery; PB, penetrating bundle; SVC, superior vena cava; TV, tricuspid valve.

from within the coronary sinus, whether or not there is a left SVC. Alternatively, the repair can be made from the left atrial side, approached through an opening in the atrial septum.

Partially Unroofed Terminal Portion of the Coronary Sinus

A partially unroofed terminal portion of the coronary sinus occurs primarily in association with AV canal defects. The coronary sinus ostium is simply left draining into the left atrium by the repair (see Chapter 19).

Unroofed Coronary Sinus Syndrome with Left Superior Vena Cava and Atrioventricular Canal Defect

For unroofed coronary sinus syndrome with LSVC and AV canal defect, the repair is made exactly as described for uncomplicated cases except that, rather than being attached to the limbus, the pericardial baffle is attached to the crest of the ventricular septum and AV valves (partial AV canal de-

fect) or to the top of the Dacron patch used to close the interventricular communication (complete AV canal defect) (Fig. 18-2, and see Chapter 46, Fig. 46-2).

Completely Unroofed Coronary Sinus Associated with Other Complex Cardiac Anomalies

No description can be given of the details of the repair of the complex anomalies in which the unroofed coronary sinus syndrome is but a part of the malformation. Such cases are often unique, and the surgeon must study the malformation in detail and plan the repair according to the findings. The general comments concerning complex cor triatriatum apply (see Chapter 17).

EARLY RESULTS

The risk of repairing unroofed coronary sinus syndrome, either isolated or combined with other specific malformations, is low, 1 death (4%, CL 0.6%–14%) having occurred in

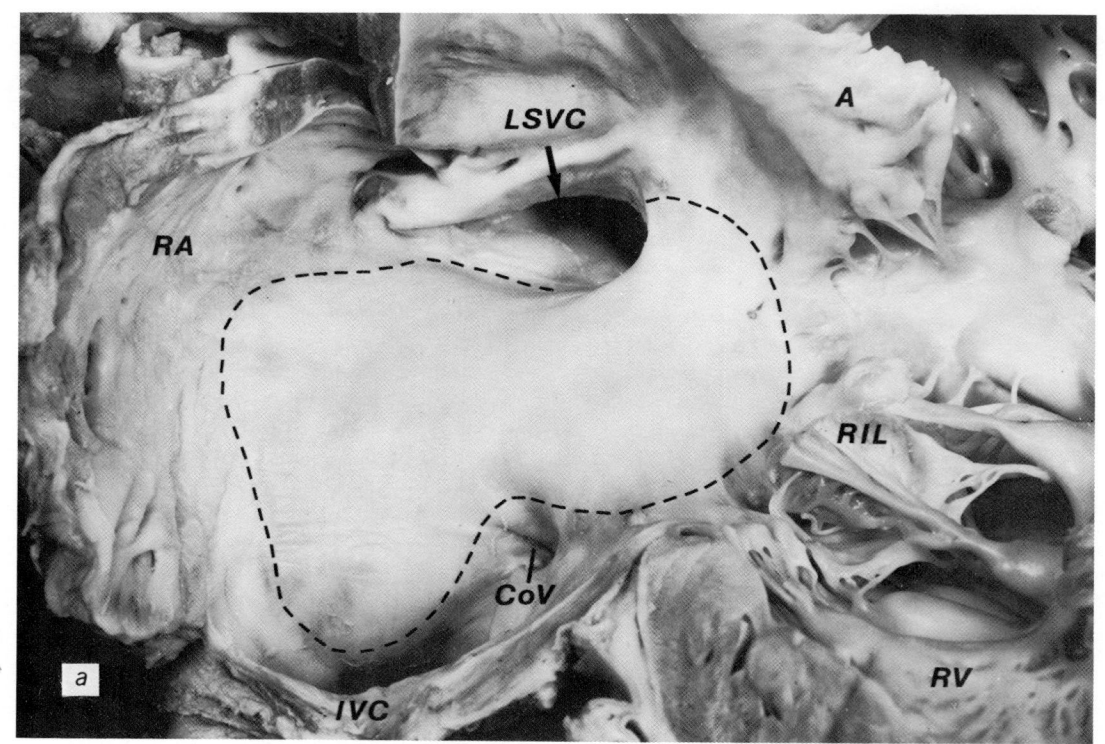

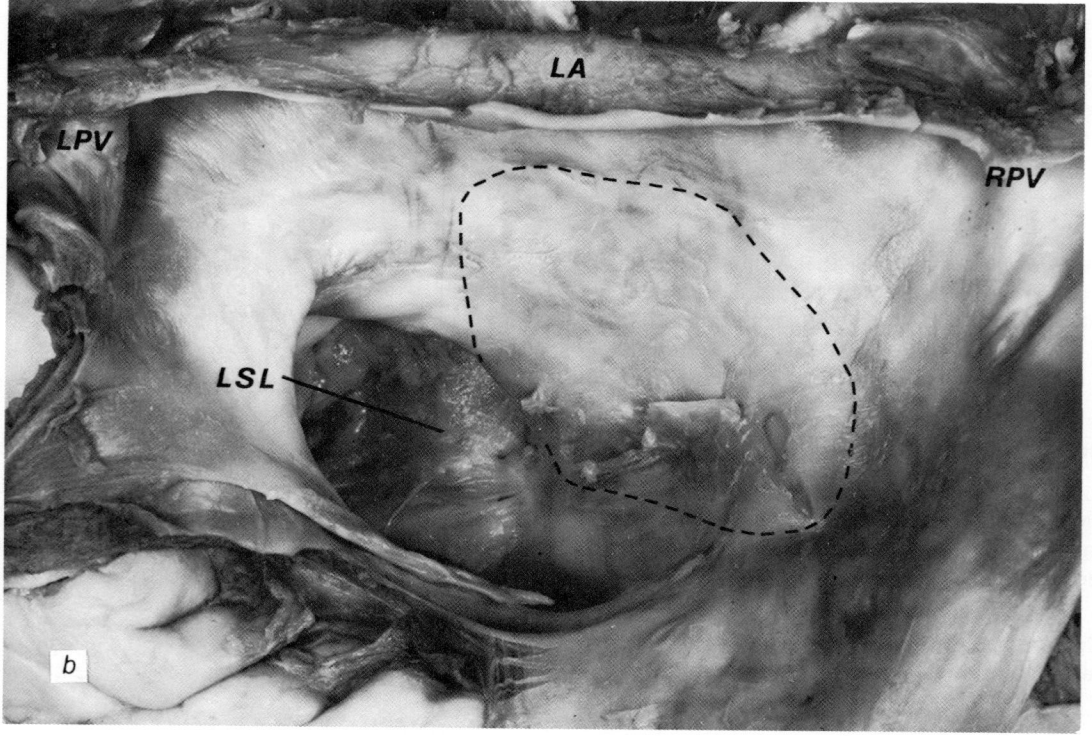

Table 18-2   Repair of unroofed coronary sinus syndrome (UAB; 1967–October 1977).

Category	n	No. of Hospital Deaths
Completely unroofed CS and persistent LSVC	13	0
Isolated	8	0
With TF	1	0
With common atrium (no interventricular communication)	4	0
Completely unroofed CS without persistent LSVC with TF	1	0
Unroofed Distal CS		
With partial AV canal defect	3	
With complete AV canal defect	1	0
Complex[a] unroofed CS		
With common atrium, complete AV canal, DORV, polysplenia	2	0
With common atrium, complete AV canal, DORV, PS, TASVC, hypoplastic LV, asplenia	1	1
With TAPVC, polysplenia	1	1
With dextroversion, isolated ventricular inversion, polysplenia	1	0
With situs inversus totalis, complete AV canal, DORV, PS	1	1

KEY: AV, atrioventricular; CL, 70% confidence limits; CS, coronary sinus; DORV, double-outlet right ventricle; LV, left ventricle; LSVC, left superior vena cava (right superior vena cava with situs inversus totalis); PS, pulmonary stenosis; TAPVC, total anomalous pulmonary venous connection; TASVC, total anomalous systemic venous connection; TF, tetralogy of Fallot.

[a]With atrial situs ambiguus or inversus.

the 23 patients in the UAB experience (Tables 18-1, 18-2) and the GLH experience combined.

When the syndrome is part of a complex anomaly associated with atrial isomerism, the risk has in the past been much higher. Three (50%, CL 24%–76%) of six patients in the UAB 1967–1977 experience died (Table 18-2). Better understanding of the morphology and improved intraoperative methods, including avoidance of the tunnel repair (see "Spe-

---

Figure 18-2   Autopsy specimen showing a pericardial baffle that completely corrects an unroofed coronary sinus syndrome (LSVC to LA) in association with a common atrium and partial AV canal defect (GLH). The operation was performed on a patient 20 months of age; the child died at 13 years of age, probably from arrhythmia. In both views, the pericardial baffle suture line is identified by a dashed line.
(a) Exposure from the opened right atrium and right ventricle. The baffle suture line passes behind the left superior vena caval ostium to reach the ventricular septal crest between the right and left AV valves and then behind the inferior vena caval ostium. There is no right SVC in this heart.
(b) Viewed from the opened left atrium.

A, anterior leaflet right AV valve; CoV, opening of large coronary vein into atrium; IVC, inferior vena cava; LA, left atrium; LPV, left pulmonary veins; LSL, left superior AV valve leaflet; RIL, right inferior AV valve leaflet; RPV, right pulmonary veins.

cial Situations and Controversies"), should improve these results considerably in the current era (for further details see Chapter 46).

LATE RESULTS

No late deaths occurred after repair of uncomplicated unroofed coronary sinus syndrome in the UAB experience, but one of the patients in the UAB 1967–1977 series required reoperation after 8 years because of tunnel obstruction. At GLH, there was one late death 10 years postoperatively unrelated to the repair; at autopsy, the repair was in excellent condition (Fig. 18-2). The living patients are without symptoms, including the one requiring reoperation.

INDICATIONS FOR OPERATION

When the diagnosis of isolated completely unroofed coronary sinus with persistent LSVC is made, operation is advisable because of arterial desaturation, the risk of cerebral emboli, and the good results of operation. The indications for repair of the rare isolated completely unroofed coronary sinus without persistent LSVC (coronary sinus ASD) are the same as for other types of ASD[L1] (see Chapter 15). When unroofed coronary sinus is associated with other major cardiac anomalies, the associated anomaly usually presents a clear indication for operation.

SPECIAL SITUATIONS AND CONTROVERSIES

Tunnel Repair

A tunnel repair was used in the first reported case of unroofed coronary sinus syndrome repair[R1] and has subsequently been used for most cases at UAB[Q1] and by others.[S2] The hospital mortality in the noncomplex cases has been low (Table 18-2), but the operation can be difficult and in complex cases the tunnel can obstruct pulmonary venous access to the mitral valve. Obstruction is particularly likely to occur when there is an associated forme fruste cor triatriatum. Because of these difficulties, as well as the favorable GLH and, in complex cases, UAB experience with the baffle repair described here, the tunnel repair is no longer used (GLH, UAB).

Ligation of the Left Superior Vena Cava

Some surgeons ligate the LSVC even when jugular vein pressure rises as high as 30 mmHg when the LSVC is occluded and report no ill effects late postoperatively, although venous engorgement, facial edema, and chylothorax may be early complications.[D2] Such ligation is not practiced at either UAB or GLH.

REFERENCES

A

1. Allmendinger P, Dear WE, Cooley DA: Atrial septal defect with communication through the coronary sinus. *Ann Thorac Surg* 17:193, 1974.
2. Asano K, Sakurai Y, Matsuzawa H: Surgical correction of common atrium with anomalously connected persistent left superior vena cava. *Jpn Heart J* 10:545, 1969.

C

1. Campbell M, Deuchar DC: The left-sided superior vena cava. *Br Heart J* 16:423, 1954.

D

1. Davis WH, Jordaan FR, Snyman HW: Persistent left superior vena cava draining into the left atrium, as an isolated anomaly. *Am Heart J* 57:616, 1959.
2. de Leval MR, Ritter DG, McGoon DC, Danielson GK: Anomalous systemic venous connection: Surgical considerations. *Mayo Clin Proc* 50:599, 1975.

F

1. Friedlich A, Bing RJ, Blount SG Jr: Circulatory dynamics in the anomalies of venous return to the heart including pulmonary arteriovenous fistula. *Bull Johns Hopkins Hosp* 86:20, 1956.
2. Freedom RM, Culham JAG, Rowe RD: Left atrial to coronary sinus fenestration (partially unroofed coronary sinus): Morphological and angiocardiographic observations. *Br Heart J* 46:63, 1981.

H

1. Hurwitt ES, Escher DJW, Citrin LI: Surgical correction of cyanosis due to entrance of left superior vena cava into left auricle. *Surgery* 38:903, 1955.
2. Helseth HK, Peterson CR: Atrial septal defect with termination of left superior vena cava in the left atrium and absence of the coronary sinus. *Ann Thorac Surg* 17:186, 1974.

K

1. Konstam MA, Levine BW, Strauss HW, McKusick KA: Left superior vena cava to left atrial communication diagnosed with radionuclide angiography and with differential right-to-left shunting. *Am J Cardiol* 43:149, 1979.

L

1. Lee ME, Sade RM: Coronary sinus septal defect: Surgical considerations. *J Thorac Cardiovasc Surg* 78:563, 1979.

M

1. Mantini E, Grondin CM, Lillehei CW, Edwards JE: Congenital anomalies involving the coronary sinus. *Circulation* 33:317, 1966.
2. Miller GAH, Ongley P, Rastelli GC, Kirklin JW: Surgical correction of total anomalous systemic venous connection: Report of a case. *Mayo Clin Proc* 40:532, 1965.

Q

1. Quaegebeur J, Kirklin JW, Pacifico AD, Bargeron LM Jr: Surgical experience with unroofed coronary sinus. *Ann Thorac Surg* 27:418, 1979.

R

1. Rastelli GC, Ongley PA, Kirklin JW: Surgical correction of common atrium with anomalously connected persistent left superior vena cava: Report of a case. *Mayo Clin Proc* 40:528, 1965.
2. Raghib G, Ruttenberg HD, Anderson RC, Amplatz K, Adams P Jr, Edward JE: Termination of left superior vena cava in left atrium, atrial septal defect, and absence of coronary sinus. *Circulation* 31:906, 1965.
3. Rose AG, Beckman CB, Edwards JE: Communication between coronary sinus and left atrium. *Br Heart J* 36:182, 1974.

S

1. Shumacker HB Jr, King H, Waldhausen JA: The persistent left superior vena cava: Surgical implications, with special reference to caval drainage into the left atrium. *Ann Surg* 165:797, 1967.
2. Sherafat M, Friedman S, Waldhausen JA: Persistent left superior vena cava draining into the left atrium with absent right superior vena cava. *Ann Thorac Surg* 11:160, 1971.

T

1. Tuchman H, Brown JF, Huston JH, Weinstein AB, Rowe GC, Crumpton CW: Superior vena cava draining into left atrium. *Am J Med* 21:481, 1956.
2. Taybi H, Kurlander GJ, Lurie PR, Campbell JA: Anomalous systemic venous connection to the left atrium or to a pulmonary vein. *Am J Roent* 94:62, 1965.

W

1. Winter FS: Persistent left superior vena cava. *Angiology* 5:90, 1954.

19

ATRIOVENTRICULAR CANAL DEFECTS

DEFINITION

Atrioventricular (AV) canal defects are characterized by a deficiency or absence of septal tissue immediately above and below the normal level of the atrioventricular valves, in the region normally occupied by the atrioventricular septum, in hearts with two ventricles. The atrioventricular valves are always abnormal to a varying degree.

These defects have also been called atrioventricular defects, atrioventricular septal defects, endocardial cushion defects, ostium primum atrial septal defects (when there is no interventricular communication), and common AV orifice (when there is only a single AV valve orifice).

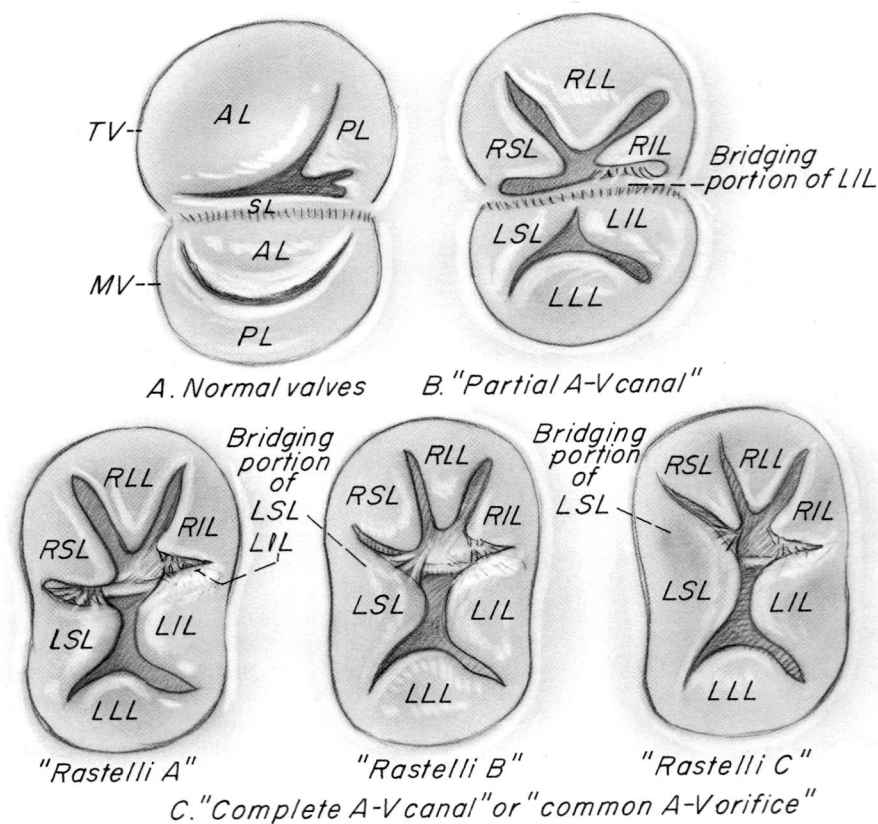

Figure 19-1 Diagrammatic representation of the AV valves viewed from the atrial side (surgical orientation).

(a) Normal, with anterior and posterior mitral valve leaflets and septal, anterior, and posterior tricuspid valve leaflets.

(b) The leaflets in partial AV canal defects. The left superior, left inferior, and left lateral leaflets form the left AV valve; the right superior, right inferior, and right lateral leaflets form the right AV valve.

(c) The leaflets in complete AV canal defects are similar to those in b. However, the left superior and left inferior leaflets are not connected. The left inferior leaflet usually bridges a little (grade 1 or 2, on the basis of 1–5) across the crest of the ventricular septum. The left superior leaflet may bridge little or not at all (grade 0 or 1, Rastelli type A) or moderately (grade 2 or 3, Rastelli type B), or markedly (grade 4 or 5, Rastelli type C).

AL, anterior leaflet; LIL, left inferior leaflet; LLL, left lateral leaflet; LSL, left superior leaflet; PL, posterior leaflet; RIL, right inferior leaflet; RLL, right lateral leaflet; RSL, right superior leaflet; SL, septal leaflet.

Reproduced with permission from Kirklin et al.[K13]

HISTORICAL NOTE

Morphology

Although apparently Abbott had recognized the "ostium primum atrial septal defect" and the "common atrioventricular canal defect,"[A2] it was Rogers and Edwards[R4] who in 1948 recognized that morphologically these defects were similar. This concept was further elaborated by Wakai and Edwards in 1956[W1] and 1958.[W2] The terms *partial* and *complete atrioventricular canal defects* were introduced by these investigators, who realized nonetheless that not all cases fit these definitions. During this period, Lev was formulating his concepts of the ostium primum ASD (or partial AV canal) and the common AV orifice (or complete AV canal), and he

described the position of the AV node and bundle of His in these malformations.[L4] Wakai and Edwards,[W1,W2] and later Bharati and Lev,[B5] became dissatisfied with trying to compress all cases into two categories and added the terms *intermediate* and *transitional*. During this period, Van Mierop's scholarly studies added a great deal of knowledge to the overall anatomic features of the AV canal (endocardial cushion) defects.[V3,V6]

By the early 1960s, surgical treatment of these defects provided a stimulus to further morphologic studies. In 1966, Rastelli, with us at the Mayo Clinic, described in more detail the morphology of the AV valve leaflets in cases with common AV orifice.[R3] The error made in this study was to compress into the designation *common anterior leaflet* a leaflet that was in fact divided in two by a commissure (i.e., the divided common anterior leaflet of type A). The description by Rastelli and associates of the AV valve leaflets was accepted for some years, but in 1976 a publication by Ugarte and colleagues emphasized the idea of leaflets *bridging* the ventricular septum,[U1] a concept also held by Lev. Meanwhile, at GLH we realized in the late 1960s, on the basis of anatomic and cineangiographic studies[B10] and in accordance with the description of Baron and colleagues[B4] and Van Mierop and colleagues,[V3] that the basic defect in these malformations was *absence of the atrioventricular septum*. This concept is particularly important, since the atrioventricular septum can be identified in the left ventriculogram in the right anterior oblique projection. These concepts were further expanded by Piccoli and colleagues,[P5,P6] who began to consider all the variations of the defect as part of a spectrum (Fig. 19-1).

Surgical Treatment

In 1952, at the University of Minnesota Hospitals in Minneapolis, after a long period of laboratory investigation, Dennis and Varco attempted for the first time a cardiac operation in a human being using a pump-oxygenator. The preoperative diagnosis was atrial septal defect, and at operation they thought they had closed the defect. The patient died, and autopsy showed the true diagnosis to be partial AV canal defect.[E6] In 1954, we successfully repaired a partial AV canal through the atrial well of Gross[K6,W3] and in 1955 began repairing AV canal defects by open cardiotomy and use of the pump-oxygenator.[K10,R2]

The first successful repair of a complete AV canal defect was performed by Lillehei and colleagues[L1] in 1954, using cross-circulation and direct suture of the atrial rim of the septal defect to the crest of the ventricular septum. The early experiences[C1,E1,L2] with complete AV canal defects were all associated with a high hospital mortality, often related to complete heart block, postrepair left AV valve regurgitation, or the creation of subaortic stenosis.[S4] Interestingly, in many of these early operations a two-patch technique was used. In 1958, Lev's description[L4] of the location of the bundle of His provided the basis for techniques of repair that avoid heart block. In 1959, Dubost and Blondeau reported their early experience in Paris[D2] and emphasized that the "cleft" in the "mitral leaflet" need not be sutured in repairing partial AV canal defects. In 1962, Maloney and associates[M1] described two cases in which a single patch was used to close both defects and the valve tissue was correctly suspended from the patch. This technique was again described by Gerbode in 1962[G2] and led to a decrease in hospital mortality.[R1] McGoon recognized the importance of "taking from the tricuspid valve" to leave sufficient tissue from which to create an adequate left AV valve. These technical advances allowed repair of even the more complex variants of the defect.[P1,R5,Z1] Subsequently, good results were obtained in patients over about 2 years of age,[G1,H1,K1,M2,M4,V1] but results in infants remained relatively poor.[B1,B2,R1] Between 1968 and 1971, we successfully repaired this anomaly in four severely ill infants at GLH,[B12] and subsequently, improved results in infants have been reported by many

Table 19-1 Morphologic characteristics of AV canal defects.

Size of interatrial communication: 0, 1, 2, 3, 4, or 5[a]
Size of interventricular communication: 0, 1, 2, 3, 4, or 5[b]
  Beneath LSL: 0, 1, 2, 3, 4, or 5
  Beneath LIL: 0, 1, 2, 3, 4, or 5
  Beneath LSL-LIL connection: yes or no
LSL-LIL connection: 0, 1, 2, 3, 4, or 5[c]
Degree of bridging of LSL: 0, 1, 2, 3, 4, or 5[d]
Degree of bridging of LIL: 0, 1, 2, 3, 4, or 5
Common AV valve orifice: yes or no
Accessory orifice: yes or no
Major associated cardiac anomalies

KEY: LIL, left inferior leaflet; LSL, left superior leaflet.

[a]0, condition in which the characteristic atrioventricular septal deficiency is present but the AV valves are adherent to the edges of the defect and there is no interatrial communication; 5, common atrium.

[b]5, very large communication but not common ventricle.

[c]0, separate LSL and LIL, such as in common AV orifice; 1 and 2, narrow connections (deep cleft in anterior mitral leaflet); 3 and 4, broad connection (shallow cleft or notch); 5, no cleft, anterior mitral leaflet.

[d]0 and 1, Rastelli type A; 2 and 3, type B; 4 and 5, type C.

others.[A1,B2,B3,C3,C5,M3,M5] More recently, Carpentier has correctly emphasized that generally the left AV valve functions best when repaired as a three-leaflet valve.[C6] As a result of these advances, the risks of operation for nearly all types of AV canal defect are now low.[B1,C2,S2]

MORPHOLOGY

General Morphologic Characteristics

The AV canal defects have as defining characteristics a deficiency or absence of the atrioventricular septum, resulting in an ostium primum defect immediately above the AV valves and a deficiency (or scooped-out area) in the inlet (basal) portion of the ventricular septum immediately below the AV valves. These deficiencies vary in size and may or may not result in interatrial and/or interventricular communications, depending on the configuration and attachments of the AV valves (Tables 19-1, 19-2, 19-3). While the basic defect in these malformations is absence of the AV

Table 19-2 Interatrial communication present in AV canal defects (UAB; 1967–1982; n = 310).[S2]

Interatrial Communication	Incidence No.	% of 310
0[a]	2	0.6%
1	2	0.6%
2	27	8.7%
3	35	11.3%
4	223	71.9%
5[b]	21	6.8%

[a]The atrial septum was deficient in the usual area (of the atrioventricular septum), but the interatrial communication was closed by adherence of the AV valve leaflets to the edges of the ostium primum defect.

[b]Common atrium.

Table 19-3 Interventricular communication present in AV canal defects.[S2]

Interventricular Communication	Beneath LSL		Beneath LIL	
	No.	% of 310	No.	% of 309[a]
0	158	51%	176	57%
1	3	1.0%	3	1.0%
2	9	2.9%	9	2.9%
3	4	1.3%	16	5.2%
4	9	2.9%	22	7.1%
5[b]	127	41%	82	27%

KEY: LIL, left inferior leaflet; LSL, left superior leaflet.

[a] Data not available for one patient.

[b] 5, very large communication but not common ventricle.

septum,[B3,B4,B10] there is no way of knowing whether the ventricular septal or atrial septal deficiency, or the AV valve abnormality is the result only of AV septal absence.

The atrioventricular valves are also abnormal. Five or more leaflets of variable size are usually present (Fig. 19-1), but there is often variability in the completeness of commissures and prominent crenations in the leaflets (Fig. 19-2a,b,c). For example, among the 43 hearts with all types of AV canal defects and two ventricles in the GLH autopsy series in which the number of leaflets could be accurately assessed, 10 (23%) had 4 leaflets, 18 (42%) 5, 14 (33%) 6, and 1 (2%) 7. When a large interventricular communication was present (complete AV canal defect), the commonest number of leaflets was 5 (16/28 or 57%).

The left superior leaflet (LSL) and the left inferior leaflet

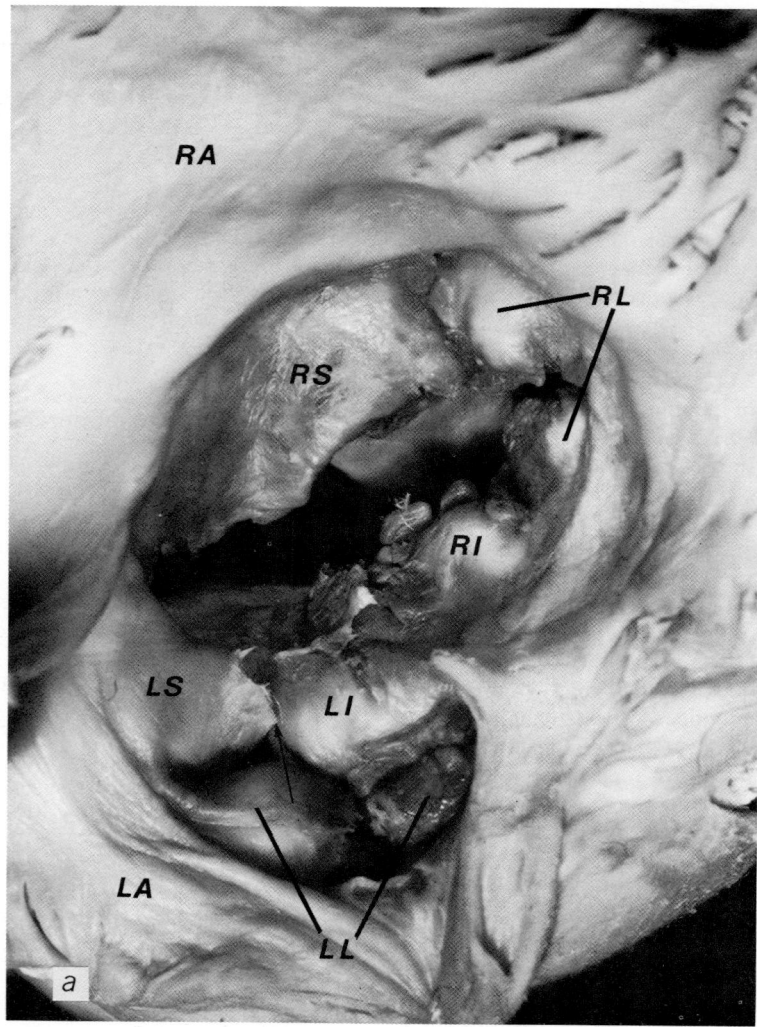

Figure 19-2 The AV valves in AV canal defects viewed from the atrial aspect in a series of fixed specimens (GLH).
(a) Specimen with partial AV canal defect in which the left superior and left inferior leaflets are adherent to the crest of the ventricular septum and there is no interventricular communication. The arrow marks the line of closure between the left superior and left inferior leaflets, formerly called *the cleft in the anterior mitral leaflet*. Note that, as usual, the left superior leaflet does not bridge the septum (there is no leaflet tissue in the position of the superior portion of the normal tricuspid septal leaflet). In this heart, as is not uncommon, there are two left lateral and two right lateral leaflets.

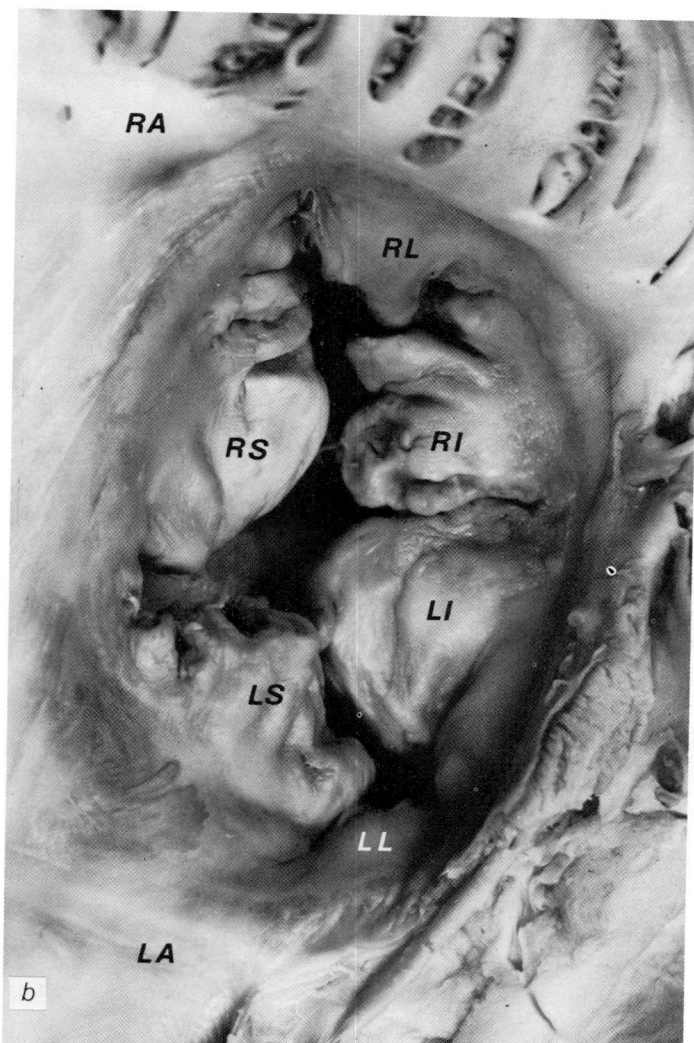

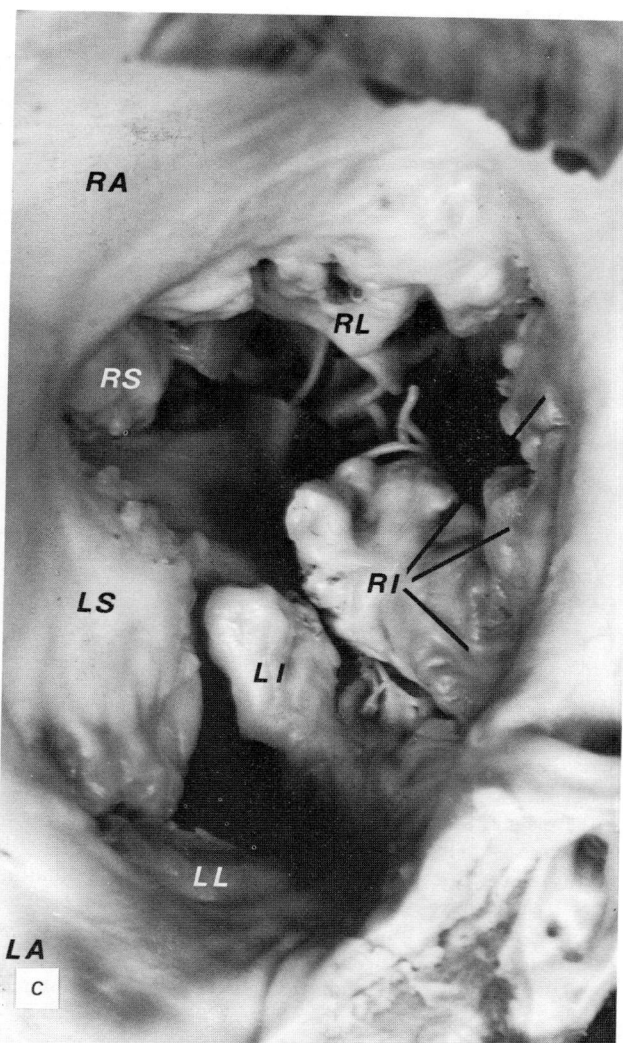

Figure 19-2 (continued)

(b) Specimen with complete AV canal defect in which there are interventricular communications beneath the left superior and left inferior leaflets. The left superior leaflet does not bridge the crest of the septum. The right superior leaflet is characteristically large. The left inferior leaflet is bridging (grade 2) and very distinct from the right inferior leaflet.

(c) Specimen of a complete AV canal defect in which the left superior leaflet markedly bridges the crest of the septum. Correspondingly, the right superior leaflet is small. The left superior leaflet is characteristically larger than the left inferior leaflet.

LA, left atrium; LI, left inferior leaflet; LL, left lateral leaflet; LS, left superior leaflet; RA, right atrium; RL, right lateral leaflet; RS, right superior leaflet.

(LIL) are particularly variable in size, their connections one to the other (Table 19-4), and their degree of bridging across the crest of the ventricular septum (Table 19-5, Figs. 19-1, 19-2). There may be one or two AV valve orifices (Table 19-6).

Hearts with AV canal defects are also characterized by absence of the usual wedged position of the aortic valve above the AV valves. Instead, the aortic valve is elevated and deviated anteriorly.[G6,P5,V3,V5,V6] The details of the aortic-mitral fibrous continuity often differ from those in the normal heart. Thus, the continuity was abnormal in over half of 21 specimens with normally related great arteries in the GLH

autopsy series; the continuity was to the base of the non-coronary cusp in only 5 (24%) and to both the noncoronary and right coronary cusps in 7 (33%). In addition, the left ventricular (LV) inflow tract is shortened in relationship to the length of the outflow portion,[G3,P5,V3,V5] and there is a related reduction in the length of the diaphragmatic wall of the left ventricle.[G7] The left ventricular outflow tract is also narrowed, although rarely is the narrowing sufficient to be of hemodynamic importance.[P7]

AV canal defects include a spectrum of malformations. At one end is the simplest type, in which there is an interatrial communication but no interventricular communication and a

Table 19-4 Left superior and left inferior leaflet connections present in AV canal defects.[S2]

Degree of LSL-LIL Connection	No Interventricular Communication (n = 154)		Interventricular Communication (n = 156)	
	No.	% of 154	No.	% of 156
0	2	1.3%	139	89%
1	55	36%	11[a]	7%
2	82	53%	5[a]	3%
3	9	6%		
4	5	3%		
5	1	0.6%		
Connected, unknown degree			1[a]	

KEY: LIL, left inferior leaflet; LSL, left superior leaflet.

[a] Among these 17, in 4 the LSL and LIL were connected but free floating, with large interventricular communications beneath them and their connections (Bharati type C[B9]). In 11, very small interventricular communications were present beneath the LSL and/or LIL. In 2, no interatrial communication was present.

connection of variable width between the left superior and left inferior leaflets. This anomaly is called a *partial AV canal defect* or *ostium primum defect*. At the other end of the spectrum is the most extreme form, with large deficiencies in the atrial and ventricular septa, a common AV valve orifice, and large interatrial and interventricular communications. This malformation is called a *complete AV canal defect*. Because a continuous spectrum of gradations lies between these two extremes, some anomalies have been grouped under the phrase *intermediate AV canal defects*. Added complexity is provided by the occurrence of a large variety of major and minor associated cardiac anomalies (Tables 19-7, 19-8, 19-9). In addition, Down's syndrome is common, particularly in patients with an interventricular communication.

Since it has proved virtually impossible to subdivide the

Table 19-5 Left superior leaflet bridging present in AV canal defects.[S2]

Bridging of LSL	Without Interventricular Communication (n = 154)		With Interventricular Communication (n = 156)		
	No.	% of 153[a]	No.	% of 154[b]	
0	150	98%	65	42%	} Rastelli type A
1	3	2.0%	23	15%	
2			5	3.2%	} Rastelli type B
3			10	6.5%	
4			8	5.2%	} Rastelli type C
5			43	28%	

KEY: LSL, left superior leaflet.

[a] Data not available for one patient.

[b] Data not available for two patients.

Table 19-6 Type of AV valve orifices in AV canal defects.[S2]

Type of AV Valve Orifice	Incidence	
	No.	% of 310
Two AV valves	171[a]	55%
Common AV valve	139	45%

[a] This includes the 154 patients without interventricular communications; 11 with small interventricular communications beneath the LSL and/or LIL; 4 with connected but free-floating and connected LSL and LIL (see Table 19-4); and 2 with no interatrial communication but large interventricular communication (*not* AV canal type VSDs).

spectrum of AV canal defects into satisfactory, noncontroversial subgroups, this chapter describes cases by their morphologic and functional variables. Problems in diagnosis, surgical treatment, and results can then be analyzed in a clearer and more meaningful way.[S2] The older, imprecise terms continue to be useful as shorthand; and, in this chapter, *partial AV canal* refers to a malformation with two AV orifices and no interventricular communication, while *complete AV canal* refers to a defect with a common AV orifice and large (grade 2 or more) interventricular communication.

Atrial Septal Deficiency and Interatrial Communications

Ostium Primum Atrial Septal Defect
Almost always, there is an interatrial communication from the *deficiency of the atrioventricular septum* and possibly because of a deficiency of adjacent atrial septal tissue also: the so-called ostium primum atrial septal defect (Fig. 19-3). The defect is bounded below by the inferiorly displaced AV valve leaflets and above by a crescentic ridge of atrial septum that fuses with the AV valve ring only at its extremities.

Table 19-7 Major associated cardiac anomalies in AV canal defects.[S2]

Major Associated Cardiac Anomalies	Incidence	
	No.	% of 310
Without major associated cardiac anomalies	237	76%
Patent ductus arteriosus	31	10.0%
Tetralogy of Fallot	20	6.5%
Completely unroofed coronary sinus with left SVC	9	2.9%
Situs ambiguus	7	2.3%
DORV without PS	6	1.9%
Additional VSDs	5	1.6%
DORV + PS	3	1.0%
Situs inversus totalis	3	1.0%
TAPVC	2	0.6%
LV outflow obstruction	2	0.6%
TGA	1	0.3%
PS, supravalvar mitral stenosis, Ebstein's malformation, coarctation, isolated dextrocardia	1 each	0.3%

KEY: DORV, double-outlet right ventricle; LV, left ventricular; PS, pulmonary stenosis; SVC, superior vena cava; TAPVC, total anomalous pulmonary venous connection; TGA, transposition of the great arteries.

Table 19-8 Minor associated cardiac anomalies in AV canal defects.[S2]

Minor Associated Cardiac Anomalies	Without Interventricular Communication (n = 154)			With Interventricular Communication (n = 156)		
	No.	% of 154	CL	No.	% of 156	CL
(Sizable) ASD[a]	17	11%	8%–14%	32	21%	17%–24%
Left SVC without unroofed coronary sinus	10	6%	4%–9%	7	4%	3%–7%
Partially unroofed CS	5	3%	1%–5%	2	1%	0.4%–3%
Azygos extension of IVC	4	3%	1%–5%	3	1%	0.6%–3%
IVC to lower left common atrium				1	1%	0.1%–2%
Bilateral IVCs	1	1%	0.1%–2%			
TASVC to common atrium				1	1%	0.1%–2%
Right PVs to RA	1	1%	0.1%–2%			
Anomalous origin LAD from RCA (TF)				1	1%	0.1%–2%
Origin stenosis LPA (not TF)	1	1%	0.1%–2%			
Wolff-Parkinson White syndrome	1	1%	0.1%–2%			
Spontaneous heart block	1	1%	0.1%–2%			
CAD requiring CABG	1	1%	0.1%–2%			

KEY: ASD, atrial septal defect; CABG, coronary artery bypass grafting; CAD, coronary artery disease; CL, 70% confidence limits; CS, coronary sinus; IVC, inferior vena cava; LAD, anterior descending coronary artery; LPA, left pulmonary artery; PV, pulmonary vein; RA, right atrium; RCA, right coronary artery; SVC, superior vena cava; TASVC, total anomalous systemic venous connection; TF, tetralogy of Fallot.

[a] Does not include patent foramen ovale.

Generally, there is little atrial septal tissue at the superior point of fusion of the atrial septum with the valve ring, adjacent to the aorta, but more tissue is usually present inferiorly, adjacent to the coronary sinus (Fig. 19-4). The distance between the crescentic atrial margin of the defect and the AV valves (and thus the size of the interatrial communication) is variable. In most cases, the fossa ovalis is normally formed, and there is a patent foramen ovale or an associated fossa ovalis type of ASD. Usually, the interatrial communication is moderate in size. When the interatrial communication is small, the atrial septal deficiency is restricted to the area normally occupied by the atrioventricular septum. The communication may be made still smaller by fusion of the base of the left superior or inferior leaflet or both to the edge of the atrial septum superiorly and inferiorly. Rarely, there may be an accessory "parachute" of fibrous tissue

Table 19-9 Conditions associated with AV canal defects in hearts with two ventricles (GLH autopsy series of nonsurgical and surgical cases; the number with Down's syndrome may not be representative, in view of case selection).

Associated Condition	No.	% of Total
Down's syndrome	9	13%
Trisomy E	3	4%
Asplenia	19	28%
Polysplenia	4	6%
Other complex congenital heart disease	18	26%

narrowing or obstructing the defect. Under such circumstances, a pressure difference exists between the two atria.

Common Atrium
There may, however, be associated deficiencies in the anterior limbus or fossa ovalis, resulting in a larger interatrial communication, and occasionally the entire limbus and the fossa ovalis are absent, along with the atrioventricular septum. The condition is then termed common atrium (Tables 19-1, 19-2).[E3,G5,R6,R7]

Absence of Interatrial Communication
Rarely, AV valve tissue is attached completely to the edge of the atrial septum, and no interatrial communication exists in spite of the deficiency in the septum (Table 19-2).[P5,S2] In this unusual variant, the characteristic deficiency of the inlet (basal) portion of the ventricular septum is also present and is associated with a large interventricular communication beneath the leaflets. The functionally left AV valve, consisting only of those portions of the left superior and left inferior leaflets on the *left* side of their attachment to the atrial septum, tends to be competent. When viewed from the ventricular side, the appearance is typical of a complete AV canal defect. It is quite distinct from the so-called *AV canal type of ventricular septal defect* (VSD), which is not related to a deficiency of the atrioventricular septum (see "Ventricular Septal Defect of the AV Canal Type" later in this section on Morphology and Chapter 20, "VSD Beneath Tricuspid Septal Leaflet" in section on Morphology).

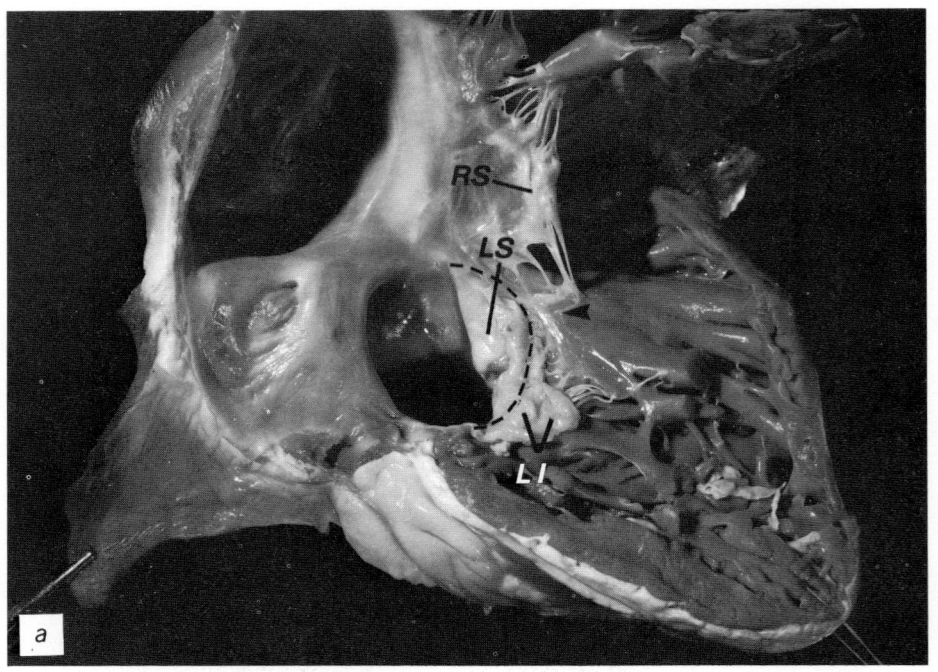

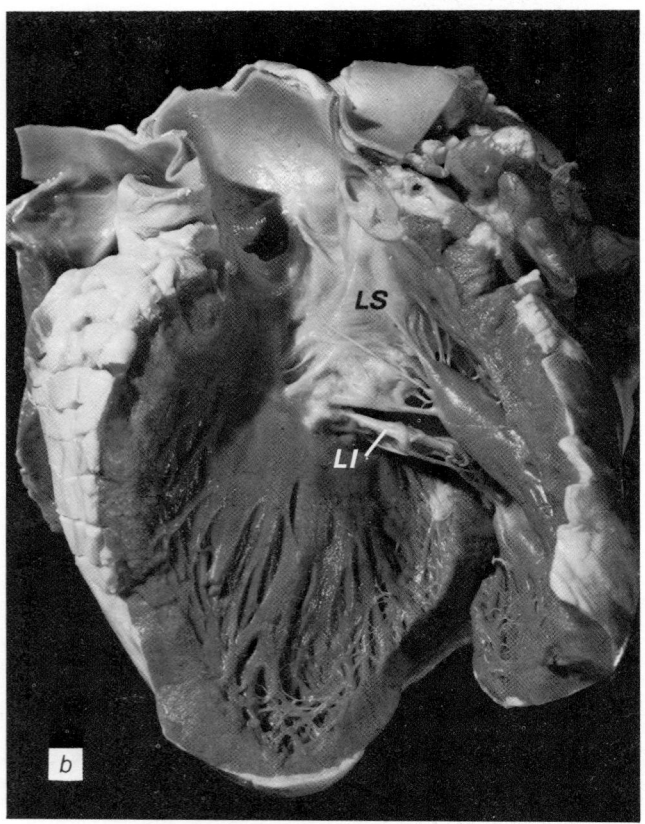

Figure 19-3 Partial AV canal defect.
(a) View from the right atrium and right ventricle. The large ostium primum type of atrial septal defect is seen above the AV valve leaflets. No interventricular communication is present beneath the leaflets. The deficiency of the basal (inlet) portion of the ventricular septum is, however, apparent. The left superior leaflet is attached firmly by fibrous tissue to the crest of the septum (denoted by the dashed line) and does not bridge onto the right ventricular side. There is thus a bare area on the right side of the superior aspect of the ventricular septum (arrow). The left inferior leaflet bridges onto the right ventricular side. The right superior leaflet is clearly visible, but the right lateral and inferior leaflets are not in the photograph. (b) Left ventricular outflow view. The left superior and left inferior leaflets are firmly attached to the crest of the ventricular septum. The narrowing and elongation of the left ventricular outflow tract is apparent. This figure makes clear why, in describing the position of the two leaflets attached to the ventricular crest, the terms *superior* and *inferior* are preferable to *anterior* and *posterior*, terms that lead to confusion with normally arising mitral leaflets.

LI, left inferior leaflet; LS, left superior leaflet; RS, right superior leaflet.

Reproduced with permission from Dr. Maurice Lev.

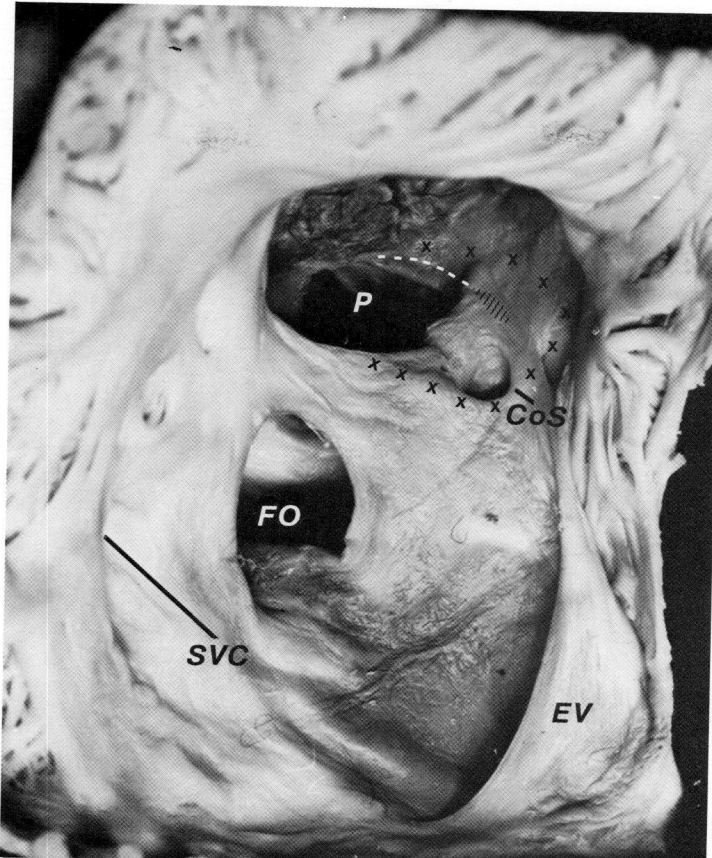

Figure 19-4 Right atrial view of a specimen of a partial AV canal defect (GLH). The coronary sinus ostium is seen inferior and posterior to the ostium primum defect in the atrial septum. The approximate position of the AV node and His bundle is shown as a dotted line. The placement of the inferior part of the patch suture line is shown as a dashed line.

CoS, coronary sinus ostium; EV, eustachian valve of inferior vena cava; FO, fossa ovalis; OP, ostium primum; SVC, superior vena cava.

Ventricular Septal Deficiency and Interventricular Communications

Partial AV Canal Defect

A deficiency of the inlet portion of the ventricular septum immediately beneath the AV valves of variable extent is also a constant finding. There is usually no interventricular communication when the left superior and inferior leaflets are connected and attached to the downwardly displaced crest of the septum throughout its length (Figs. 19-3, 19-5), the situation usually described as a partial AV canal defect. Occasionally one or several small interventricular communications are present beneath the attachment of the AV valve to the septum (Table 19-3, Fig. 19-5b).

Complete AV Canal Defect

With ventricular septal deficiency similar to that in a partial AV canal defect, a moderate or large interventricular communication may be present, and usually, in such cases, the left superior and inferior leaflets are separate. This anomaly is described as a *complete AV canal defect* (Fig. 19-5c).

Often the communication is particularly large beneath the left superior leaflet and smaller beneath the left inferior leaflet while in about 5% of cases there is a large interventricular communication beneath the LSL and none beneath the LIL. Rarely (0.5% of cases), there is no VSD beneath the LSL and a large one beneath the LIL.

A remnant of the membranous ventricular septum may be present (Fig. 19-5b). This was the case in 8 (30%) of 27 GLH autopsy specimens of AV canal with normally related great arteries. In 19, the membranous septum was not identified.

AV Valves

The attachments of the AV valves to the crest of the ventricular septum in partial AV canal defects, as well as their chordal attachments in complete AV canal defects, are displaced toward the apex of the heart because of the deficiency of the inlet (basal) portion of the septum. This alters the orientation of the AV orifices relative to the aortic orifice, (that is, the aortic valve is no longer wedged between the AV

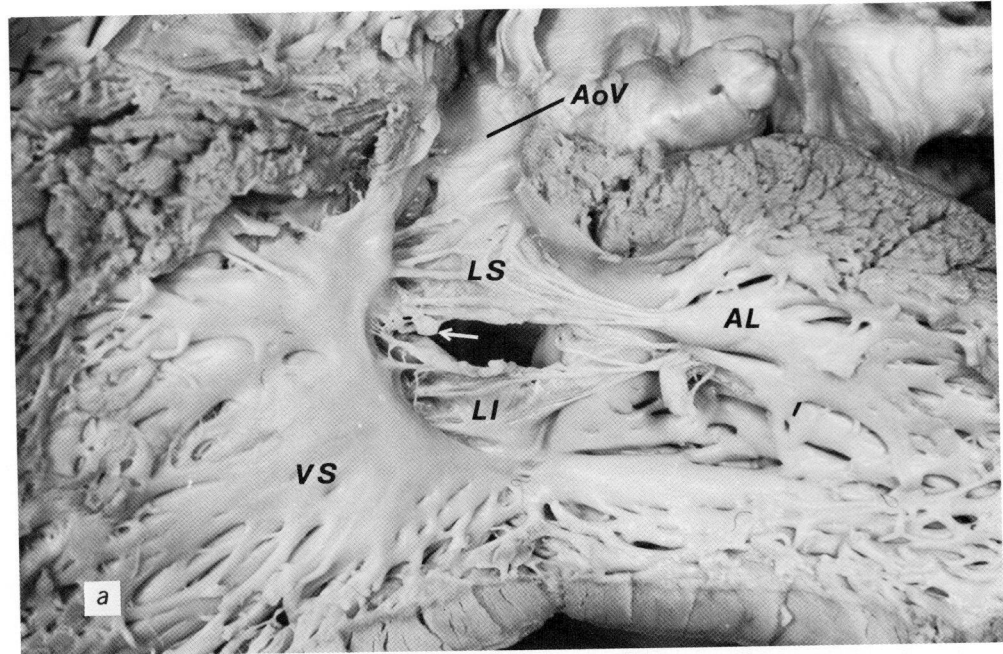

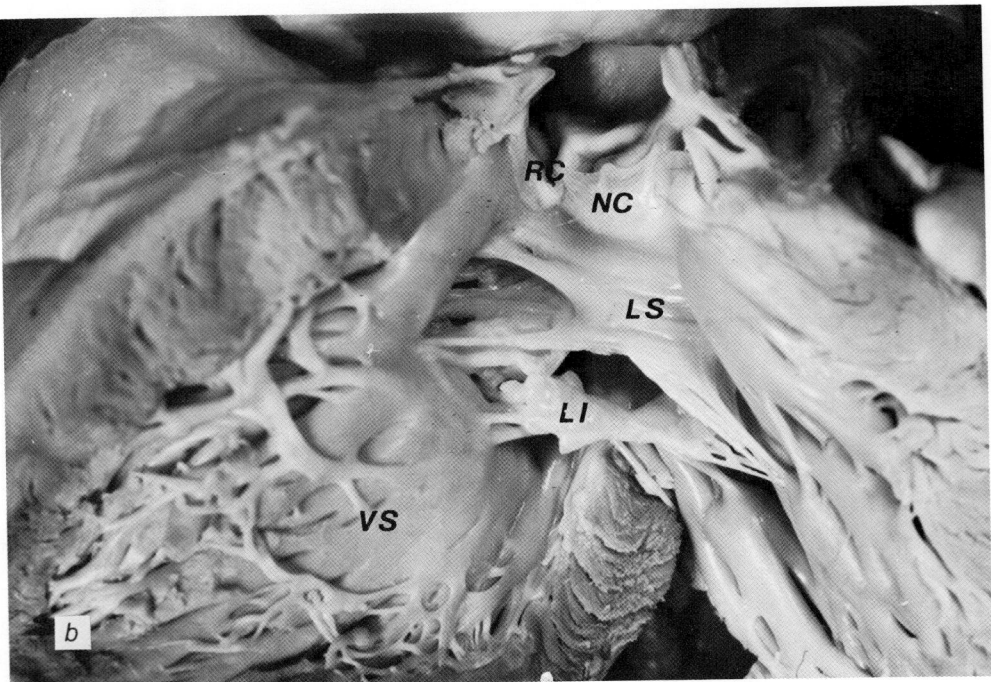

Figure 19-5 Left ventricular aspect of AV canal defects.
(a) Partial AV canal defect viewed from the opened left ventricle (GLH). The left superior and left inferior leaflets are completely attached to the crest of a deficient ventricular septum. The area of contact or closure between the left superior and left inferior leaflets (formerly called *the cleft in the anterior mitral leaflet*) is indicated by the arrow. In this specimen, only the anterior papillary muscle is present (parachute mitral valve).
(b) Intermediate type of AV canal defect from the left ventricular view (GLH). Numerous small interventricular communications between thick short chordae tether both the left superior and left inferior leaflets to the ventricular crest. Fibrous tissue extending from the superior leaflet to below the right coronary aortic cusp represents a remnant of membranous septum.

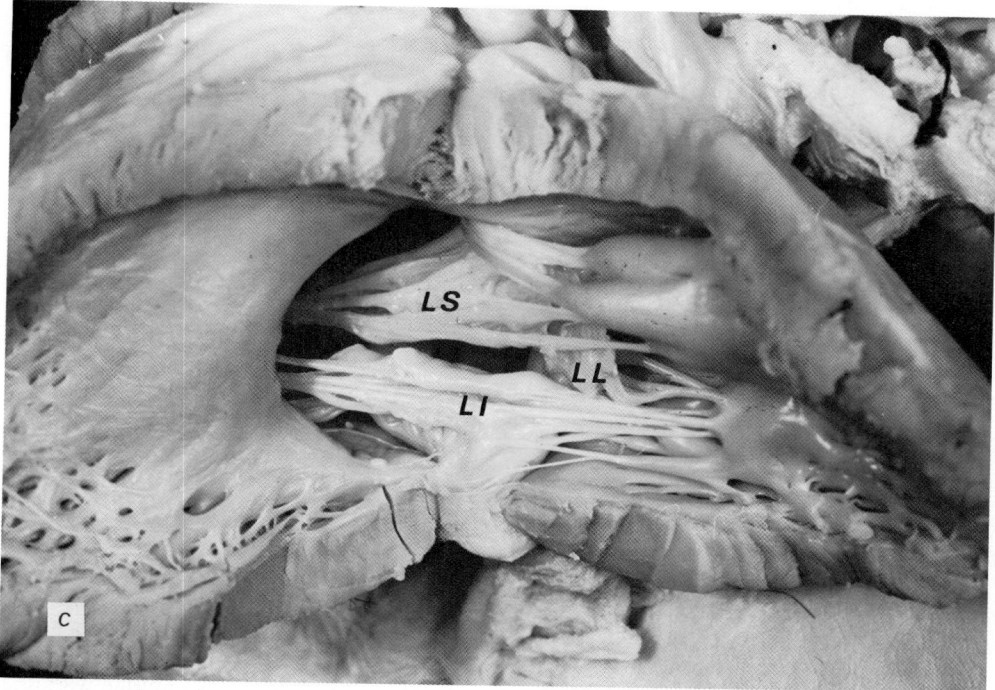

Figure 19-5 *(continued)*

(c) Complete AV canal defect viewed from the left ventricular aspect (GLH). The left superior and left inferior bridging leaflets are free floating, and there is a large interventricular communication between them and the underlying crest of the ventricular septum (GLH). This specimen also has double-outlet right ventricle.

AL, anterior papillary muscle; AoV, aortic valve; LI, left inferior leaflet; LL, left lateral leaflet; LS, left superior leaflet; NC, noncoronary aortic leaflet; R, right coronary aortic cusp; VS, septal surface of left ventricle.

valves) and provides an important diagnostic criterion of this lesion angiocardiographically.[B6,B7,B10]

Two AV Valve Orifices

Typically, when two AV valve orifices are present, the left superior and left inferior leaflets are joined together to a variable extent anteriorly, near the crest of the ventricular septum, by leaflet tissue (Figs. 19-1, 19-3). Thus, together they resemble an anterior (septal) mitral leaflet with a cleft, but in fact the left AV valve is tricuspid and differently oriented from the normal valve (Figs. 19-1, 19-2). The connection between superior and inferior leaflets may be only a thin strand of tissue (complete cleft), but more commonly it is 2–4 mm or more wide (Table 19-4). This connection, too, is usually fused to the crest of the ventricular septum in partial AV canal defects. Rarely, the separation into LSL and LIL is represented only by a notch in the center of the free edge of a nearly normal "anterior mitral leaflet."

When the LSL and LIL are nearly completely separated (connection grades 1 and 2; see Table 19-4), an appreciable gap may occur during systole, producing incompetence, and when the valve is incompetent, the leaflet tissue forming the margin is usually thickened and rolled. Occasionally, chordae pass from the opposing edges of the LSL and LIL to the muscular ventricular septum beneath.[E2]

The left lateral leaflet is usually smaller than the other two

leaflets and triangular. An accessory orifice (double left AV valve orifice) is present in the commissure on one side of the left lateral leaflet in about 5% of cases (Table 19-10).

In aggregate, these left AV valve leaflet anomalies may make the valve incompetent to a variable degree, sometimes severely (Table 19-11). The exact mechanism of severe left AV valve incompetence is frequently not evident but at least in some cases appears to be deficiency of leaflet tissue, particularly in the LIL. The jet of incompetence is usually directed into the right atrium. Rarely, the left AV valve is stenotic, but this usually occurs when the left ventricle is hypoplastic.[B17]

The right AV valve is also abnormal when there are two

Table 19-10 Double left AV valve orifice in AV canal defect.[S2]

Left AV Valve Orifice	Without Interventricular Communication (n = 154)		With Interventricular Communication (n = 156)	
	No	% of 154	No.	% of 156
Single	149	97%	147	94%
Double	5	3%[a]	9	6%[a]

[a] $P(\chi^2)$ for difference = .28.

Table 19-11   Preoperative AV valve incompetence in patients with AV canal defect without major associated cardiac anomalies.[S2]

AV Valve Incompetence	Total		Without Interventricular Communication		With Interventricular Communication	
	No.	% of 305[a]	No.	% of 154	No.	% of 151[a]
0	29	10%	15	10%	14	9%
1	39	13%	26	17%	13	9%
2	85	28%	48	31%	37	25%
3	98	32%	41 ⎱ 65/154	27%	57 ⎱ 87/151	38%
4	43	14%	16 ⎰ 42%[b]	10%	27 ⎰ 58%[b]	18%
5	11	4%	8	5%	3	2%
Total	305		154		151	

[a] No information on five patients.

[b] $P(\chi^2)$ for difference = .007.

AV orifices, although less attention has been paid to it. It may consist of three leaflets—the right superior leaflet (RSL), the right lateral leaflet (RLL), and the right inferior leaflet (RIL)—or of two or four leaflets (Figs. 19-1, 19-2). Leaflet tissue attached completely or by chordae to the crest or right side of the crest of the septum, and thus contributing to closure of the right AV valves, is considered to represent bridging of the *left* superior or inferior leaflet (Fig. 19-1). Usually, in cases without an interventricular communication, the LSL does not bridge at all (previously, this finding has been interpreted as absence or hypoplasia of the superior part of the tricuspid septal leaflet) and the LIL bridges moderately (Fig. 19-2a). In spite of the abnormalities of the right AV valve, incompetence is rare (unless right heart failure develops).

Common AV Valve Orifice
When there is a common AV valve orifice and a large interventricular communication (complete AV canal defect), the LSL and LIL are separate, and a bare area is exposed on the crest of the ventricular septum (Figs. 19-1, 19-5c, 19-6). The LSL may be entirely on the left ventricular side of the septum or may to a variable degree bridge the septum and extend onto the right ventricular side (Figs. 19-2b, c, Table 19-5). This variability formed the basis for the classification of Rastelli and colleagues into types A, B, and C.[R3] The chordal attachments of the right ventricular extremity of the LSL vary according to the degree of bridging (Fig. 19-7).[P6] When there is no bridging, the chordal attachments are to the ventricular crest (Fig. 19-7a). With mild bridging, they are to the medial papillary muscle in the right ventricle; with moderate bridging, to an accessory (often large) apical papillary muscle (Fig. 19-7b); and with marked bridging, to the normally positioned (although often bifid) anterolateral papillary muscle of the right ventricle (Fig. 19-7c). When the LSL bridges the septum moderately or markedly and extends into the right ventricle, it is usually unattached to the underlying ventricular crest (free floating), but it may occasionally be attached by chordae (tethered) to the ventricular crest. The length of the chordal or fibrous attachments to the right side or crest of the ventricular septum

varies according to the size of the interventricular communication or the position of the leaflet.

The LIL typically bridges moderately, but it too varies in this respect. It is not uncommon for a bridging inferior leaflet to be attached to the underlying ventricular crest either completely or by short, thick chordae with interchordal spaces.

The chordal attachments of the leftward components of the common AV valve in the left ventricle are usually relatively normal, although the posterior papillary muscle is displaced more laterally than normal and a third papillary muscle may be present.[C6] There may be only one papillary muscle producing a "parachute" type valve that is difficult to repair.[C6] This was the case in 7 (13%) of the 53 cases in the GLH autopsy series, in 14% of the specimens described by David and colleagues,[D5] and in 4% of 155 surgical cases reported by Ilbawi and colleagues.[I1]

The right ventricular portion of the common AV valve has superior, lateral, and inferior leaflets, but, as in the partial AV canal defects, they vary considerably in number and size (Fig. 19-2). When the bridging of the LSL is absent or mild, the right superior leaflet is large, while with more extensive bridging the right superior leaflet is smaller.[P6]

When the leaflets of the common AV valve close appropriately during ventricular systole, AV valve incompetence is absent or mild. However, important left AV valve incompetence may be present (Table 19-11). The precise mechanism of the incompetence is often not clearly understood. Accessory orifices seem to predispose the patient both to incompetence and stenosis.

Unusual AV Valve Combinations
Other unusual combinations of size, connections, attachments, and degree of bridging of the AV valve leaflets in the spectrum of AV canal defects prompted Wakai and Edwards[W1,W4] and Bharati and colleagues[B9] to use a transitional or intermediate category. Rarely, in patients with two AV valve orifices with no VSD beneath the LSL and LIL, these leaflets are connected only by a fibrous strand adherent to the ventricular septal crest (Tables 19-4, 19-6), forming what Bharati and colleagues have called a *"pseudomitral" leaflet*, rather than an *"anterior mitral leaflet with a cleft."*[B9] In

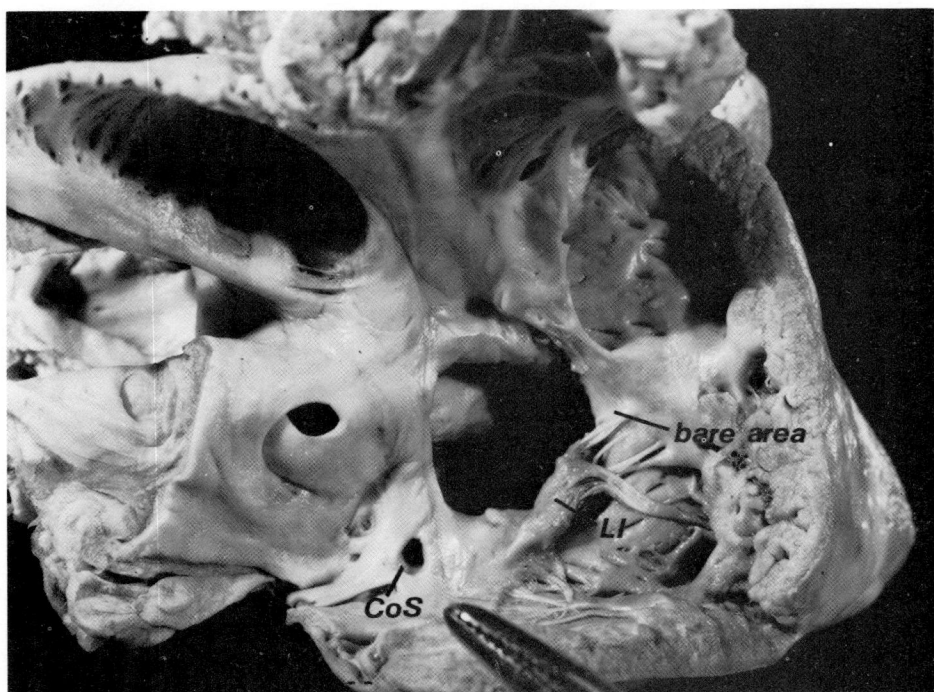

Figure 19-6 Complete AV canal defect viewed from the right ventricular side in a specimen in which the left inferior leaflet bridges over the crest of the septum onto the right ventricular side (GLH). The left superior leaflet (poorly seen) does not bridge, resulting in a bare area of the crest of the ventricular septum on the right side, where in a normal heart the superior aspect of the septal leaflet touches the septum. A small fossa ovalis atrial septal defect is also present.

CoS, coronary sinus; LI, left inferior leaflet.

such patients, deficiency of the LIL tissue and severe left AV valve incompetence are common. Occasionally, when the LSL and LIL are connected and thus two AV valve orifices are present, one or multiple small interchordal interventricular communications are present beneath the leaflets (Tables 19-3, 19-6), and occasionally one or two larger holes may be present (Figs. 19-5b, 19-8). In about 1% of cases, the connected LSL and LIL have large interventricular communications beneath them; then the connection is a thin strand of valve tissue, beneath which there is also a large interventricular communication (Fig. 19-9), but two AV valve orifices can be said to be present (Table 19-6). Bharati and Lev have referred to this also as *intermediate type C*.[B9]

At GLH in the past, the term *intermediate AV canal* has been used when the interventricular communication is, in toto, restrictive (small or moderate), the term *partial* being reserved for defects without any interventricular communication and *complete* for defects with large interventricular communications and equalized ventricular pressures.

Ventricles

The left ventricular outflow tract is characteristically elongated and narrowed (Fig. 19-10) in all types of AV canal defect, as discussed earlier (see "General Morphologic Characteristics"). In the AV canal defect with large inter-ventricular communications, the left ventricle may be abnormally large.[T6] However, its size is variable, both absolutely and in relationship to the right ventricle.[B5] In the severely right dominant type of AV canal defect, the left ventricle may be severely hypoplastic[S2] (Fig. 19-11). In such cases, the atrial septum may be displaced leftward in relationship to the plane of the ventricular septum, in which case it over-rides the left AV valve to a varying degree, and may be associated with hypoplasia of both left atrium and left ventricle.[T2,U1]

The right ventricle has no specific anomalies but is usually enlarged from the left-to-right shunt. Its size is also variable, and occasionally it is significantly hypoplastic.[T6]

The relative and absolute sizes of the two ventricles and their function must be evaluated in each patient being considered for operation. Severe left or right ventricular dominance can increase the risk of surgical repair and may render the situation uncorrectable.[F4,S2,T6]

Left Ventricular Outflow or Inflow Obstruction

Important left ventricular outflow tract obstruction occurs occasionally (about 1% of cases)[S2] in all types of AV canal defects.[P7,S4,T2] It is surprising that it is not more frequent, in view of the elongation and narrowing of this area in affected hearts.[E7] The LV obstruction may be a morphologically discrete subaortic stenosis[B15,S3,T5] or may be due to excres-

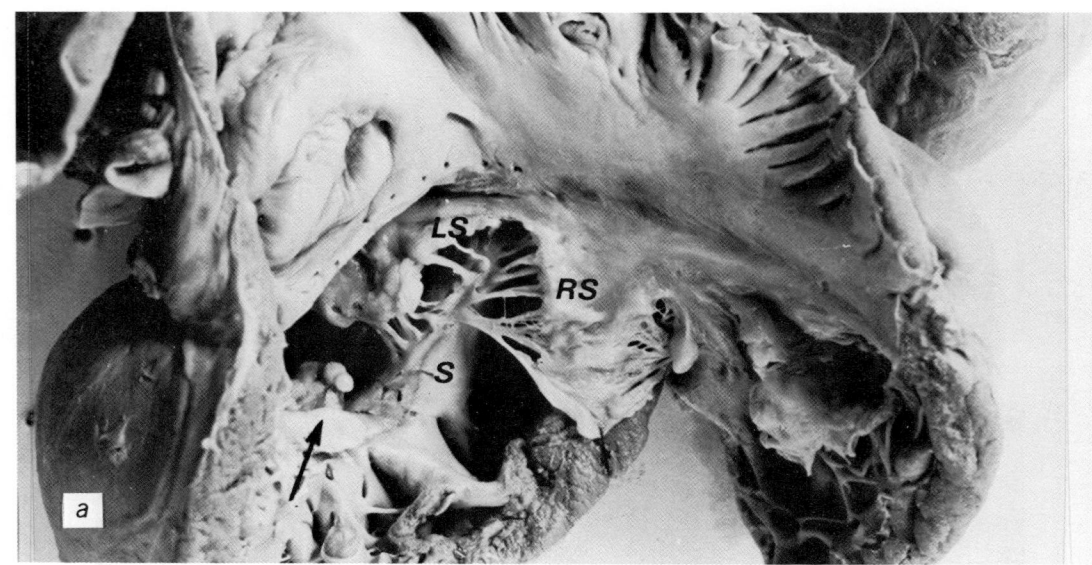

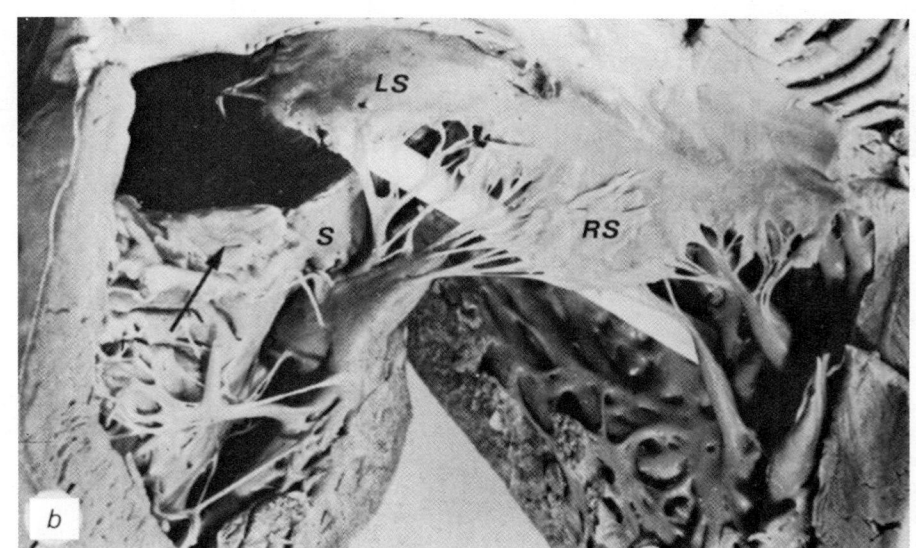

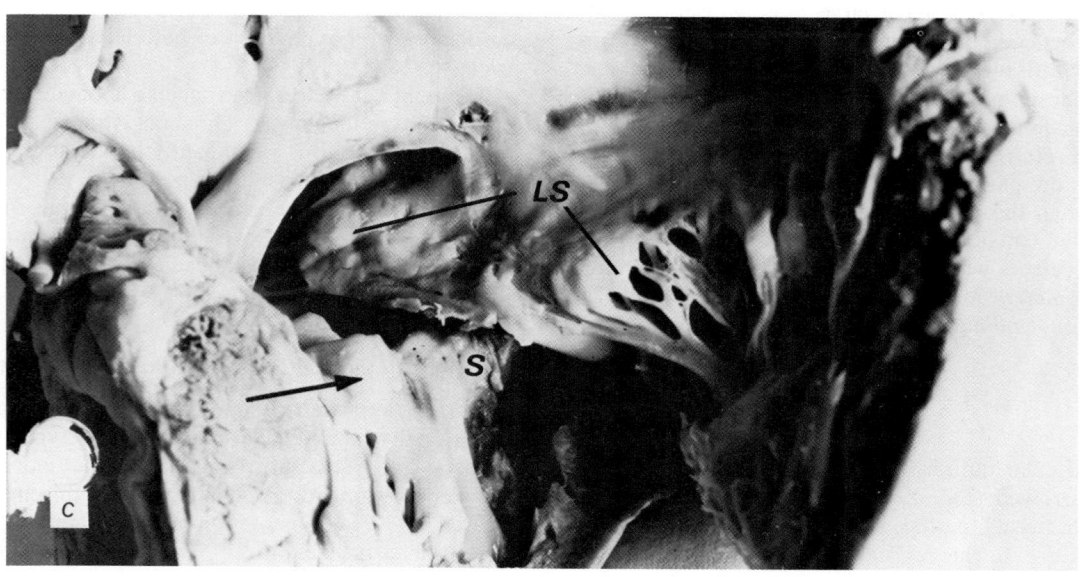

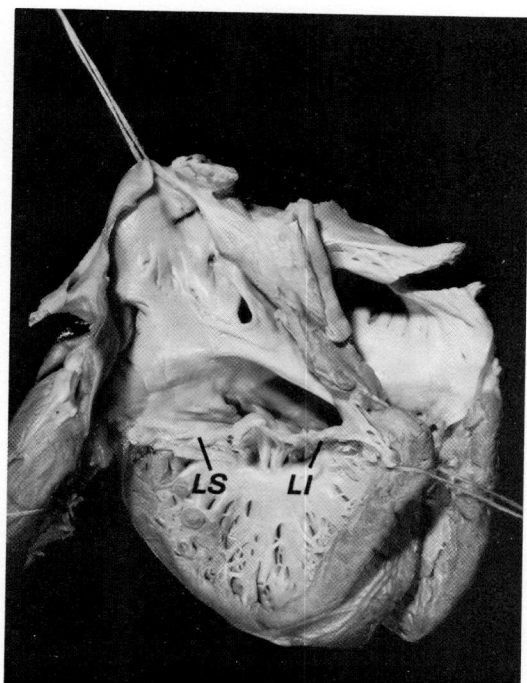

Figure 19-8   Intermediate type[B9] of AV canal defect, left ventricular aspect. The left superior leaflet is connected to the left inferior leaflet by leaflet tissue, resulting in two AV valve orifices; yet there are interventricular communications between short, thick chordae connecting the leaflets and their connection to the underlying ventricular septum. The left superior and inferior leaflets, particularly the latter, are deficient of valve tissue.

LI, left inferior leaflet; LS, left superior leaflet.

Reproduced with permission from Bharati et al.[B9]

cences of AV valve tissue heaped up in the left ventricular outflow tract.[P7,T5] It may also result from abnormally positioned papillary muscles.[P7] Occasionally, its presence is overlooked preoperatively, and it becomes apparent only after operation.

Important left ventricular inflow obstruction may occur rarely.[P7] This may be from simple narrowing of the AV valve entrance into the left ventricle, usually associated with marked right ventricular dominance. It may be related to the

Figure 19-7   Complete AV canal defects with varying degrees of bridging of the left superior leaflet.
(a) Nonbridging (bridging-0) left superior leaflet (Rastelli type A). This surgical specimen (the patch having been removed) is viewed from the right atrium. The arrow marks the mildly bridging left inferior leaflet.
(b) Moderate (grade 2 or 3) bridging of the left superior leaflet. Chordae from its right ventricular extremity go to a papillary muscle in right ventricle. The arrow indicates the bridging portion of the left inferior leaflet. (Rastelli and associates termed this *type B*, but it is just part of the spectrum from bridging-0 through bridging-5.)
(c) Marked (grade 5) bridging of the left superior leaflet (Rastelli type C). The arrow marks the bridging part of the left inferior leaflet.
LS, left superior leaflet; RS, right superior leaflet; S, ventricular septal crest.
Reproduced with permission from Rastelli et al.[R3]

presence of an accessory AV valve orifice on the left side, or it may result from cor triatriatum (Chapter 17) or a supravalvar fibrous ring.[T8]

Conduction System

The defect in the atrioventricular septum often displaces the coronary sinus ostium inferiorly (and it may appear to lie in the left atrium, especially when the ostium primum atrial defect is particularly large). The atrioventricular node is displaced inferiorly (caudally) and lies in the posterior right atrial wall, between the orifice of the coronary sinus and the ventricular crest (Figs. 19-12, 19-13),[L4] in what has been termed the nodal triangle.[T7] The bundle of His passes forward and superiorly from the node to the ventricular crest, reaching it where the crest fuses posteriorly with the AV valve ring (Fig. 19-4). It then courses along the *top* of the ventricular septum, beneath the bridging portion of the left inferior leaflet, giving off the left bundle branches. As it reaches the midpoint of the crest of the ventricular septum, it becomes the right bundle branch, which continues along the crest a little farther before it descends toward the muscle of Lancisi and moderator band. These anatomic findings have been supported by electrophysiologic studies at the time of operation.[K3,K4,K5] This morphology of the conduction system is a determinant of the electrocardiographic pattern usually seen in AV canal defects[F2] and is of obvious surgical importance.[T7]

Major Associated Cardiac Anomalies

Table 19-7 gives the incidence of the major cardiac anomalies associated with AV canal defects. A *patent ductus arteriosus* is present in about 10% of patients with AV canal defects, being particularly common in those with an interventricular communication.

Typical *tetralogy of Fallot* is present in about 10% of cases with complete AV canal defects.[B13] In the spectrum of tetralogy of Fallot, about 1% have associated complete AV canal defects.[K11] The LSL bridges markedly, and the interventricular communication beneath it is large and subaortic.[D4,F3,L8,T3] Rarely, the LSL and LIL are connected by a fibrous (or valvar) band, beneath which also is a large interventricular communication. The right ventricular outflow tract has the typical tetralogy morphology (see Chapter 23), which may be so severe that pulmonary atresia is present. A localized narrowing in that portion of the left ventricular outflow tract just upstream from the recess formed by the subaortic deficiency of the ventricular septum further complicates the situation in rare cases.

Double-outlet right ventricle without pulmonary stenosis complicates complete AV canal defects in about 2% of cases.[B11,B13,R3,S2,S7,T3] As in tetralogy of Fallot, usually the deficiency of the ventricular septum is large and subaortic beneath the extensively bridging LSL. However, occasionally the interventricular communication is far from the aortic and pulmonary valves and is "noncommitted."[B11] Rarely, the Taussig-Bing type of double-outlet right ventricle is present.[B13,S7] Double-outlet right ventricle combined with severe pulmonary stenosis coexists with complete AV canal defects in about 1% of cases.[S2] These combinations of double-outlet

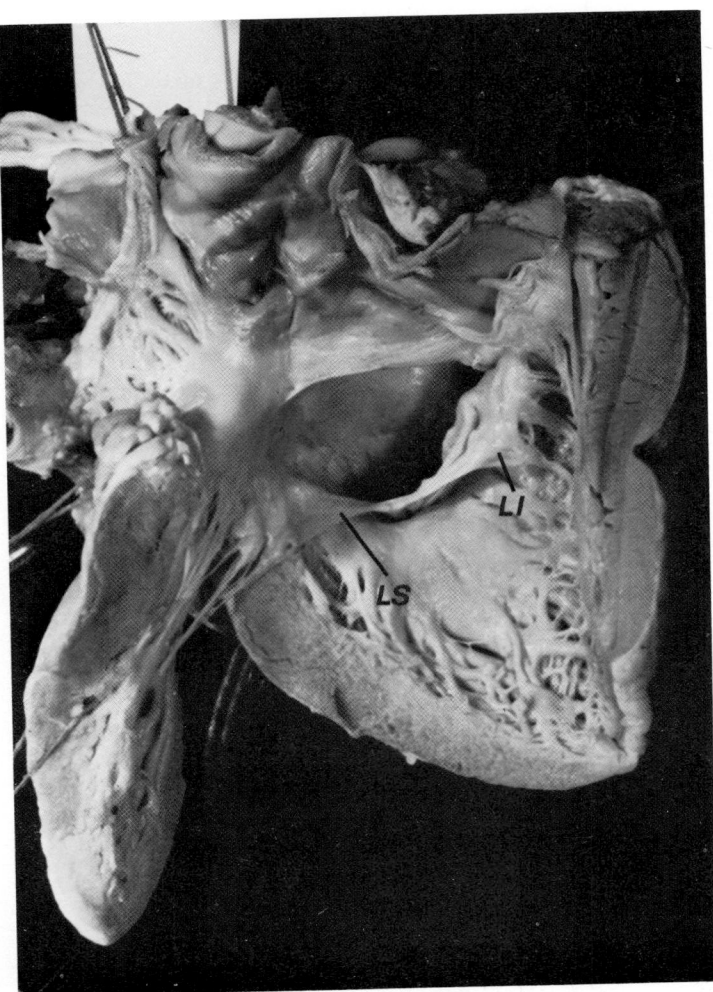

Figure 19-9 Intermediate type of AV canal defect viewed from the left ventricular aspect. The left superior and left inferior leaflets are connected by leaflet tissue, and thus two AV valve orifices are present. However, the interventricular communication is large, and neither the connection nor the leaflets are attached to the underlying ventricular septum.

LI, left inferior leaflet; LS, left superior leaflet.

Reproduced with permission from Bharati et al.[B9]

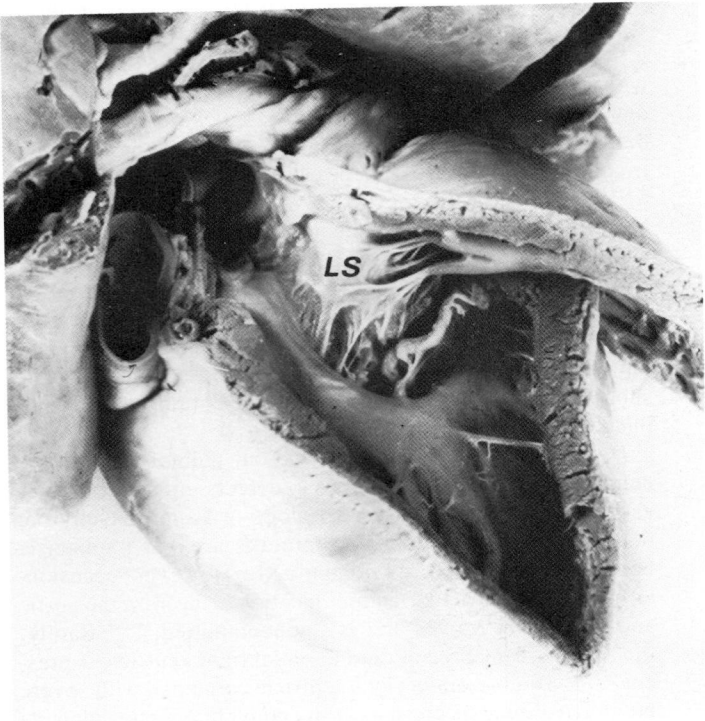

Figure 19-10 Complete AV canal defect with no bridging of the left superior leaflet and connection of the leaflet to the underlying ventricular septum by long chordae. The narrowness of the left ventricular outflow tract is apparent.

LS, left superior leaflet.

Reproduced with permission from Rastelli et al.[R3]

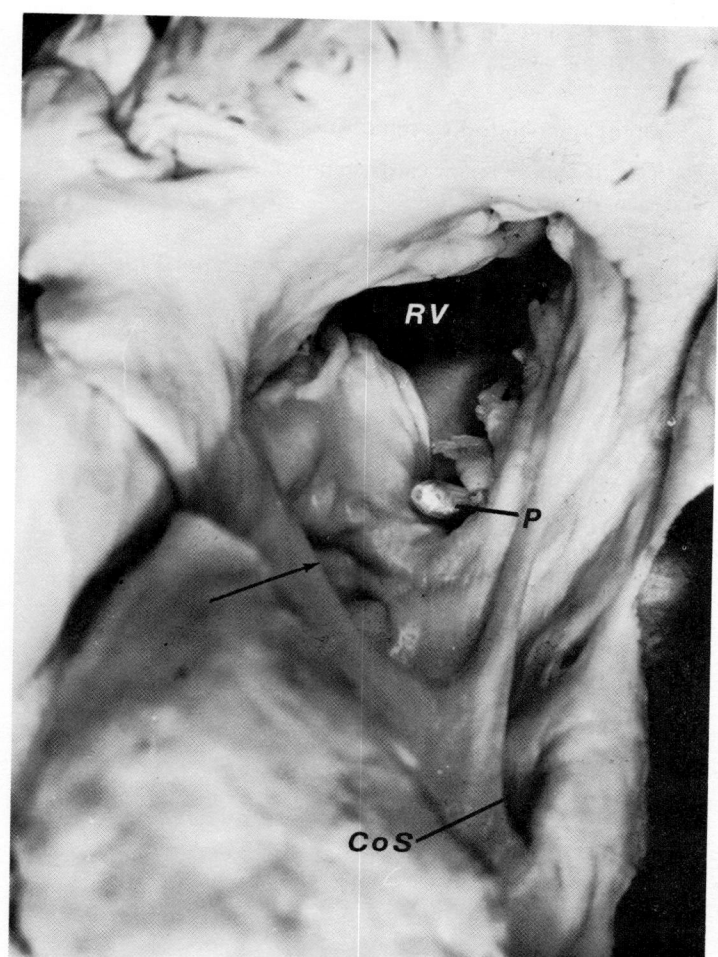

Figure 19-11 Complete AV canal defect with hypoplasia of the left ventricle and a dominant right ventricle (GLH). The specimen is viewed from its right atrial aspect, and a probe passes into the left ventricular cavity. The common AV valves open almost entirely into the right ventricle. The arrow indicates the superior margin of the ostium primum atrial septal defect.

CoS, coronary sinus; P, probe; RV, right ventricle.

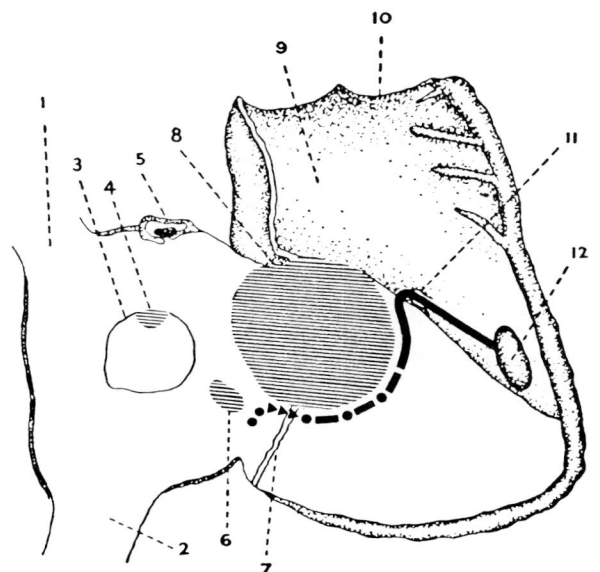

Figure 19-12 Diagrammatic sketch of the course of the AV node, His bundle, and right bundle branch in common AV canal defect, right atrial and ventricular view. (The sinoatrial node is normal.)

●, AV node; ▲, penetrating portion of the AV bundle; ● ■■■ ●, branching portion of the AV bundle; ■■■■, right bundle branch; 1, superior vena cava; 2, inferior vena cava; 3, limbus; 4, patent foramen ovale; 5, cut edge of atrial appendage; 6, entry of coronary sinus; 7, base of AV valve; 8, combined patency of atrial and ventricular septa; 9, infundibulum; 10, base of pulmonary valve; 11, muscle of Lancisi; 12, cut edge of moderator band.

Reproduced with permission from Lev.[L4]

right ventricle and AV canal defect with large interventricular communication frequently also have situs ambiguus or situs inversus, common atrium, completely unroofed coronary sinus with left superior vena cava, azygous extension of the inferior vena cava, or total anomalous pulmonary venous connection.[P3,S7]

Very rarely, *transposition of the great arteries* (discordant ventriculoarterial connection) is associated (Table 19-7).[B13]

Completely unroofed coronary sinus with persistent left superior vena cava (see Chapter 18) attached to left atrium occurs in about 3% of patients with an interventricular communication and in about 3% without, and is more frequent when common atrium is present.[Q1] A *partially unroofed* distal end of the coronary sinus, resulting in the drainage of the coronary sinus into the left atrium, occasionally occurs[Y1] but is a minor and unimportant associated anomaly.

Minor Associated Cardiac Anomalies

Table 19-8 lists minor cardiac anomalies associated with AV canal defects.

Ventricular Septal Defect of the AV Canal Type

It is important to note that a so-called *isolated* AV canal type of VSD (see Chapter 20) occurs without any of the features of an AV canal defect, as defined in this chapter, except that it involves the inflow portion of the ventricular septum be-

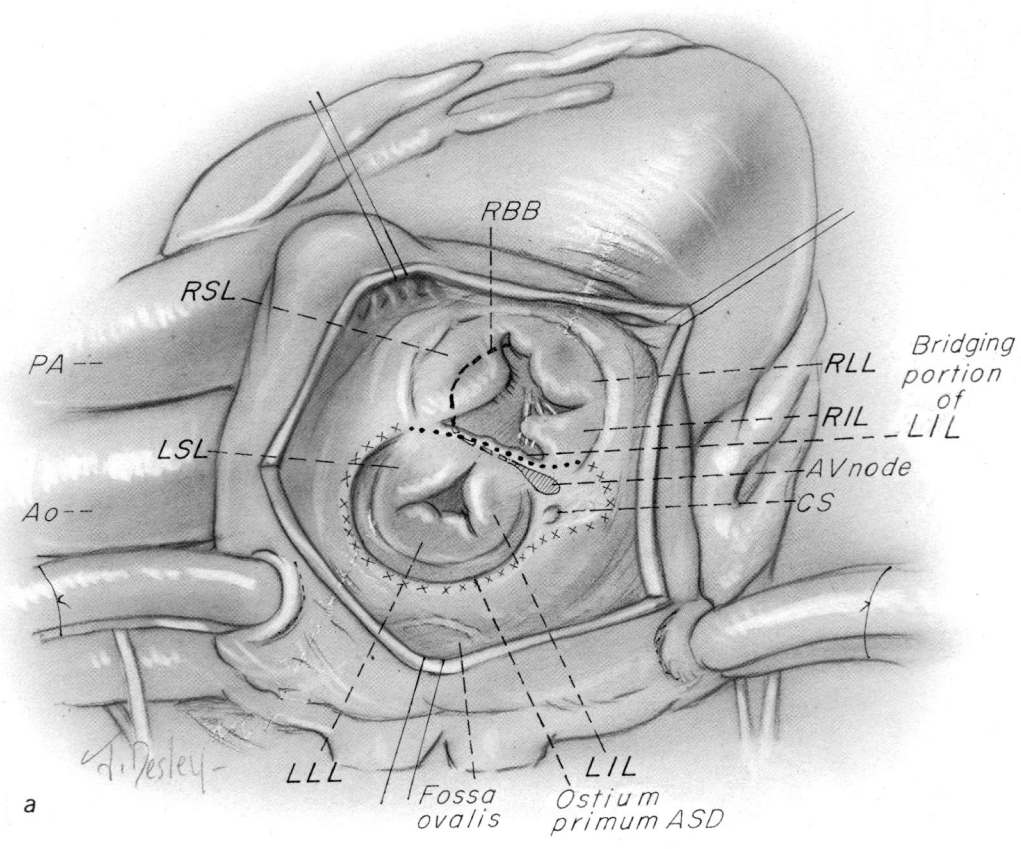

Figure 19-13   The conduction system and suture siting in AV canal defects. The conduction system itself is in the same position in all types of AV canal defects, but the surgical problem is somewhat different in defects without an interventricular communication than in those with one. (The stippled x's represent stitches for repair in the right ventricular aspect of the septum, beneath leaflet tissue. Stitches in the septal and atrial wall tissue are represented by the solid x's, and suture siting in leaflet tissue is represented by a dotted line.)
(a) Partial AV canal defect (AV canal defect without an interventricular communication). The AV node lies on the right side of the inferior (caudad) atrial septal remnant, at its junction with the floor of the right atrium over the crux cordis. The node pierces the abnormally formed central fibrous body to become the short penetrating portion of the His bundle. This structure immediately becomes the branching bundle, which gives off the left bundle branches earlier than normal as it travels along the crest of the ventricular septum. In its course, it is covered by the fibrous tissue that fuses the left inferior and left superior leaflets to the septal crest. At about the mid-portion of the crest of the septum, the branching bundle becomes the right bundle branch, which proceeds as illustrated.
Reproduced with permission from Bharati et al.[B19]

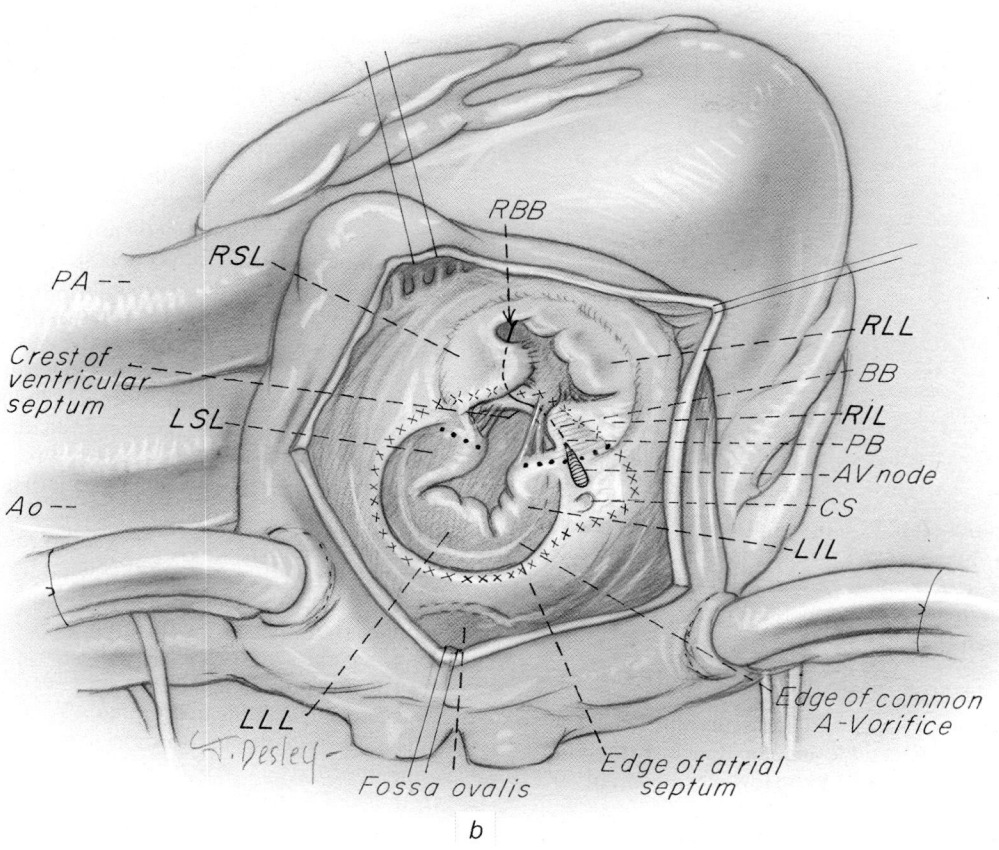

b

Figure 19-13   *(continued)*
(*b*) Complete AV canal defect (AV canal defect with common AV valve orifice and interventricular communication). The conduction system is in the same basic position as in the specimen in part *a*. However, the bundle of His is exposed as it passes along the crest of the septum.

Ao, aorta; ASD, atrial septal defect; AV, atrioventricular; BB, branching portion of bundle of His; CS, coronary sinus ostium; LIL, left inferior leaflet; LLL, left lateral leaflet; LSL, left superior leaflet; PA, pulmonary artery; PB, penetrating portion of bundle of His; RBB, right bundle branch; RIL, right inferior leaflet; RLL, right lateral leaflet; RSL, right superior leaflet.

neath the septal tricuspid valve leaflet and usually also the area of the membranous ventricular septum. The atrioventricular septum is, however, intact, and the mitral and tricuspid rings and aortic orifice lie in normal positions. This feature allows them to be readily differentiated angiographically from AV canal defects. Interestingly, in isolated AV canal–type VSD, the anterior mitral leaflet is occasionally cleft.

CLINICAL FEATURES AND DIAGNOSTIC CRITERIA

Pathophysiology

Shunts
Left-to-right shunting is present in AV canal defects unless severe pulmonary vascular disease has developed or important pulmonary stenosis coexists. When there is no interven-

tricular communication, the shunt is at atrial level and usually large. It may, however, be small or moderate, and in such cases a pressure gradient can be demonstrated between left and right atria. When the shunt is large and left AV valve incompetence is mild or absent, the hemodynamic state of the patient is identical to that in isolated ASD (see Chapter 15, "Clinical Features and Diagnostic Criteria"). Only right ventricular stroke volume is increased. When important left AV valve incompetence is present, the left-to-right shunt becomes much larger; in fact, the incompetent jet usually goes directly from left ventricle to right atrium. Left as well as right ventricular stroke volume is increased, and marked cardiomegaly and heart failure develop early in life.

When a large interventricular communication is also present (complete AV canal defect), the left-to-right shunt is large, and right ventricular and pulmonary artery pressures approach or equal systemic pressures (Table 19-12). Pulmonary vascular resistance rises rapidly and is usually

Table 19-12 Preoperative pulmonary artery–aortic pressure ratios in patients without major associated cardiac anomalies.[S2]

PA/AO Pressure Ratio	Without Interventricular Communication (n = 140)		With Interventricular Communication (n = 97)	
≤ <	No.	% of 97[a]	No.	% of 74[b]
0.3	65	67% ⎱ 85/97	5	7% ⎱ 12/74
0.3 --- 0.5	20	21% ⎰ 88%	7	9% ⎰ 16%
0.5 --- 0.7	5	5%	10	14%
0.7 --- 0.9	6	6% ⎱ 7/97	29	39% ⎱ 52/74
0.9	1	1% ⎰ 7%	23	31% ⎰ 70%

[a] Data not available for 43 patients.

[b] Data not available for 23 patients.

significantly elevated after 12 months of age and sometimes before.[N1] When present, AV valve incompetence adds greatly to the ventricular volume overload. For some reason, however, the overload usually seems to enlarge the right ventricle more than the left.

AV Valve Incompetence

About 10% of patients with or without interventricular communications have no detectable incompetence of the common or left AV valve (Table 19-11). However, in about 40% of patients with partial AV canal and in 60% of those with complete AV canal, AV incompetence is moderate or severe. A not uncommon site of incompetence is through the commissure between left superior and left inferior leaflets (the "mitral cleft"), particularly near the leaflet hinge or base, and, partly for this reason, the regurgitant flow frequently goes directly into the right atrium. Under such circumstances, the left atrium remains small and the right becomes large, but when the interatrial communication is smaller or the incompetence is sited elsewhere, the regurgitation may enter the left atrium, which enlarges.

While the precise mechanism of AV valve incompetence is often unclear, it apparently varies considerably, as would be expected from the variations in the number, size, and configuration of the leaflets and their chordal attachments.

Symptoms and Physical Findings

Patients without an interventricular communication (partial AV canal defect or ostium primum ASD) and with absent or mild left AV valve incompetence often present in the first decade of life, but they may remain asymptomatic well beyond that age. Their clinical presentation (symptoms and physical findings) are virtually identical to those of patients with the more common fossa ovalis type of ASD (see Chapter 15) except that they may have an apical systolic murmur if mild left AV valve incompetence is present, and the electrocardiographic finding is of left axis deviation and a counterclockwise frontal plane loop.[O1,T1]

When there is moderate or severe (grade 3, 4, or 5) left AV valve incompetence in patients with AV canal defects,

symptoms occur earlier, and progressive severe heart failure may require treatment in infancy.[B12] In addition to the usual signs of ASD, the heart is more active in association with a loud apical pansystolic murmur, and the apex of the left ventricle may be palpable. Tachypnea and hepatomegaly are often evident.

In patients with complete AV canal defect, presentation is usually in the first year of life, and frequently in the first months, due to progressive severe heart failure, which may not be controllable medically. There is associated tachypnea, poor peripheral perfusion, and failure to thrive. Occasionally, heart failure is minimal early in life, and presentation may be delayed until some years later, by which time there is almost always severe hypertensive pulmonary vascular disease and Eisenmenger's syndrome (see Chapter 20, "Clinical Features" in section on Clinical Features and Diagnostic Criteria). On physical examination, cardiomegaly with increased ventricular activity is apparent. The second heart sound at the base is split and is usually fixed, with accentuation of the second component due to the elevated pulmonary artery pressure. A systolic murmur is audible over the left precordium from the shunt at ventricular level and is increased in intensity and nearer the apex when there is significant AV valve incompetence. A mid-diastolic flow murmur is characteristically widely heard both over the lower left precordium and at the apex secondary to the large diastolic flow across the malformed AV valve leaflets (consequent upon both the left-to-right shunt and any AV valve incompetence).

In those patients with morphology intermediate between the partial and complete AV canal defects, the clinical features depend on the size of the interventricular communication and the severity of the left AV valve incompetence.

Chest X-ray

In patients without an interventricular communication or important left AV valve incompetence, the chest x-ray is the same as in other large ASDs. When moderate or severe left AV valve incompetence is present, the roentgenogram usually shows marked cardiomegaly, with evidence of left ventricular, right ventricular, and right atrial enlargement and marked pulmonary plethora. Left atrial enlargement is not apparent unless the ostium primum defect is restrictive.

In the complete AV canal defect, cardiomegaly and pulmonary plethora are evident in infants and young children presenting with heart failure. In those patients surviving beyond this age, severely increased pulmonary vascular resistance usually dominates the situation, and the heart is less enlarged, central pulmonary arteries are large, and the lung fields are clear.

Electrocardiogram

The electrocardiographic findings are rather specific.[D3] They usually indicate marked right ventricular hypertrophy and may show left ventricular hypertrophy as well. The PR interval is frequently prolonged. Of considerable diagnostic significance is the vectorcardiogram.[T1] Ongley and colleagues conclude that a counterclockwise frontal plane loop anterior and to the right strongly suggests, but does not prove, the diagnosis.[O1]

Two-Dimensional Echocardiogram

In AV canal defects without an interventricular communication or important left AV valve incompetence, a two-dimensional echocardiogram, together with the clinical presentation, chest x-ray, and electrocardiogram, is diagnostic, and cardiac catheterization and a cineangiogram are not necessary. In all other situations, although a two-dimensional echocardiogram can display well the morphology of the AV canal defect, cineangiographic study is still indicated before operation, particularly to define possible associated major cardiac anomalies (present in 25% of cases) and to assess the details of any AV valve incompetence and of the interventricular communications.

Cardiac Catheterization and Cineangiogram

The direction and magnitude of shunting; pulmonary and systemic pressures, resistances, and flows; and right and left ventricular pressures are measured and calculated from data obtained at the time of cardiac catheterization (see Chapter 20, "Cardiac Catheterization" in section on Clinical Features and Diagnostic Criteria).[F1,P2]

Cineangiographic studies are particularly useful in AV canal defects. The basic angiocardiographic features of AV canal defects were well described by Baron and colleagues in 1964[B4,B6] and further refined by the work of Brandt and colleagues,[B10] Bargeron and colleagues,[S8] and McCartney and colleagues in London.[M12]

Both oblique[B10] and axial[B7] views are used. Adequate cineangiographic studies demonstrate the absence of the atrioventricular septum and the deficiency of the inlet portion of the ventricular septum, the elongation of the left ventricular outflow tract in relationship to the inflow tract, the elevation and anterior displacement of the aortic valve vis-à-vis the AV valves, and the changed relationship of the anterior components of the left AV valve to the aorta. This is well portrayed by Baron and colleagues[B4] (Fig. 19-14) and described by line drawings (Fig. 19-15) and representative cineangiograms (Fig. 19-16). The changed left AV valve relationship to the aorta results in a change in the direction of left AV valve movement. The interatrial and interventricular shunting can also be demonstrated in cineangiographic studies. The presence of one or two AV valve orifices is also well established. With high-quality studies, the leaflets of the left AV valve often can be visualized in motion to determine the degree, location, and mechanism of valvar incompetence. The relative sizes of the two ventricles and of the AV orifices are determined.

Special Situations and Associated Defects

The presence of a common atrium can now generally be identified preoperatively by a two-dimensional echocardiogram and/or a cineangiocardiogram, which shows the nearly complete absence of both the atrial septum and the atrioventricular septum. The finding of mild arterial desaturation in a patient with the clinical findings of an AV canal defect without an interventricular communication or pulmonary artery hypertension suggests the presence of a common atrium.[D3,F1,M8,R6,R7] The presence of a left superior vena cava in such a setting suggests both unroofed coronary sinus syndrome and common atrium, since they frequently coexist.[Q1,R7] In patients with common atrium and situs ambiguus, even more complex associations occur,[S5] including double-outlet right ventricle,[P3] partial or total anomalous pulmonary venous connection,[D1] and azygous extension of the inferior vena cava (see Chapter 46).[K7,T4]

A patent ductus arteriosus can be identified on aortographic study. Likewise, associated anomalies, such as tetralogy of Fallot, double-outlet right ventricle, transposition of the great arteries, and other VSDs, are identified by a combination of two-dimensional echocardiography and cineangiocardiography.

Assessment of functionally important left ventricular outflow tract obstruction is more difficult. Narrowing of this tract is an inherent part of the AV canal defect, but it rarely results in a systolic pressure gradient. Variations in the size and attachment of the left superior leaflet are occasionally seen cineangiocardiographically, as are abnormal positions of papillary muscles[P4,S4] and muscular subaortic narrowings, but it is hazardous to predict gradients on the basis of these morphologic appearances, and a significant pressure gradient between left ventricle and aorta must be demonstrated before surgical relief is contemplated. Even though there is no gradient preoperatively, an otherwise proper repair can result in an important left ventricular–aortic gradient in a few patients.[L9]

NATURAL HISTORY

The life history of patients with surgically untreated AV canal defects depends on the morphologic and functional details of their malformation. When there is a *partial AV canal defect, only mild left AV valve incompetence,* and no major associated cardiac anomaly, the life history without surgical treatment is similar to that of patients with large fossa ovalis ASDs (see Chapter 15). A relatively small number of patients develop important pulmonary vascular disease in their twenties, thirties, and forties.[P2] At GLH, only 5 (8%, CL 5%–14%) among 61 such patients had pulmonary vascular resistance greater than 5 units · m² at presentation. As in other types of large ASD, the symptomatic deterioration of patients in adult life often coincides with the development of atrial fibrillation. This relationship is evident from Somerville's data,[S6] which show that the proportion with supraventricular arrhythmia increases with age (Fig. 19-17).

Patients with a *partial AV canal defect* but *with moderate or severe left AV valve incompetence* have a very different natural history. Because of the nonrestrictive interatrial communication present, severe left atrial and pulmonary venous hypertension are absent, but the left-to-right shunt is large and pulmonary artery pressure usually at least moderately elevated. Probably at least 20% of such patients are severely symptomatic in infancy, and without surgical treatment, many of these die in the first decade of life.

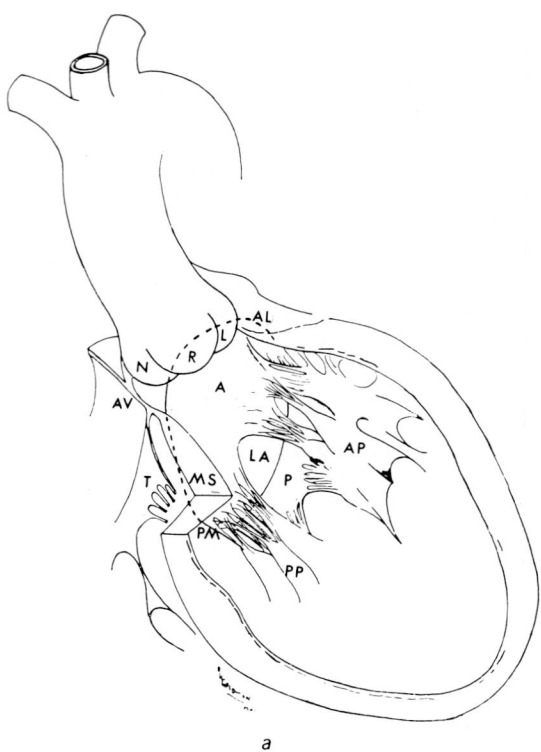

a

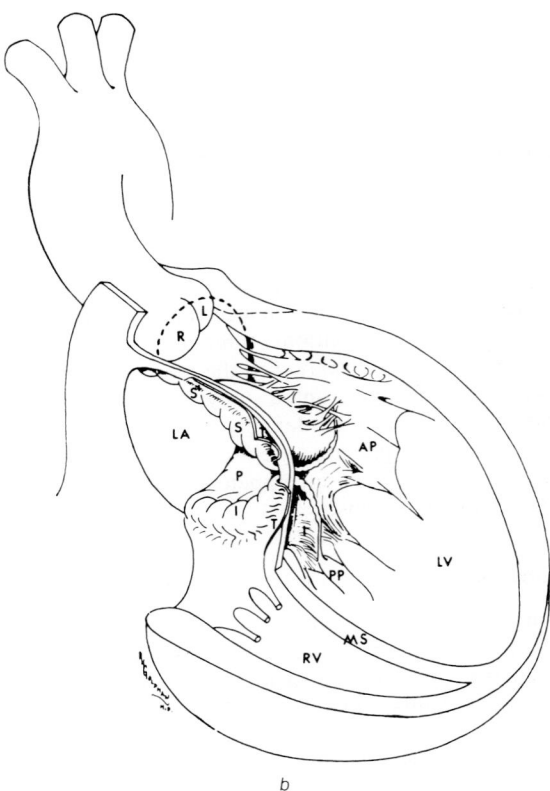

b

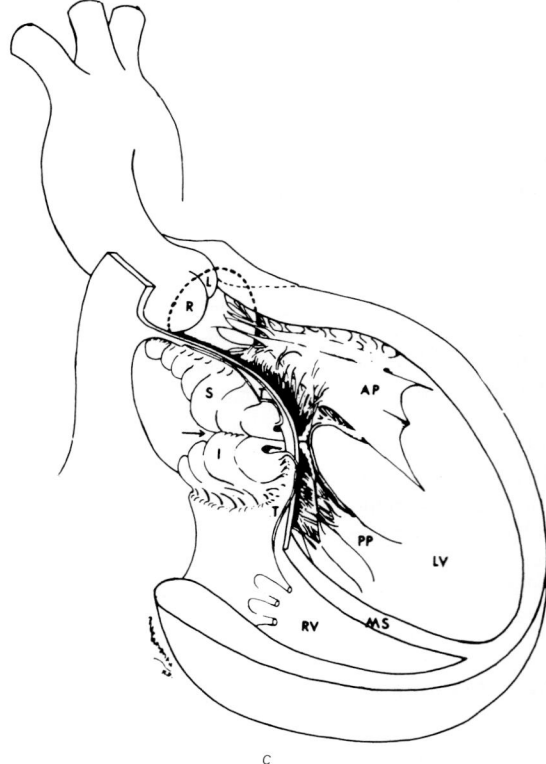

c

Figure 19-14 Diagrams of the altered attachment of the anterior mitral and septal leaflets in AV canal defect compared with the normal heart. The heart is shown in its in vivo position as seen in a frontal angiocardiogram. The right ventricle and most of the ventricular septum and right atrium have been removed. The dashed line indicates the portion of the line of attachment of the mitral valve that is hidden by other structures.

(*a*) Normal heart. The attachment of the anterior mitral leaflet begins at the anterolateral commissure and runs anteriorly for a short distance along the free wall of the left ventricle. It is then continuous with the root of the aorta in relationship to the adjacent portion of the left coronary and noncoronary aortic cusps. The line of attachment proceeds downward along the atrioventricular septum to the posteromedial commissure. The attachment of the mitral valve to the atrioventricular septum is profiled in the right anterior oblique view (see Fig. 19-15).

(*b* and *c*) Partial AV canal defect shown in diastole (*b*) and systole (*c*). The scooped-out crest of the basal portion of the ventricular septum is shown considerably thinner than it actually is. The right AV valve leaflets are shown only at their sites of attachment. The diastolic figure depicts the left superior and left inferior leaflets as open. The line of attachment of these leaflets to the root of the aorta is nearly normal, but it then passes along the superior rim of the scooped-out ventricular septal crest. The left superior leaflet is displaced upward into the left ventricular outflow tract, narrowing this portion of the chamber. The left inferior leaflet is folded back against the left ventricular aspect of the sinus septum. In the systolic figure, left superior and inferior leaflets are closed. The increased left ventricular pressure balloons them toward the atria. The arrow marks their point of coaptation.

A, anterior mitral leaflet; AL, anterolateral commissure of mitral valve; AP, anterior papillary muscle; I, left inferior leaflet of AV valve; L, left coronary aortic cusp; LA, left atrium; LV, left ventricle; MS, muscular ventricular septum; N, non-coronary aortic cusp; P, posterior mitral leaflet; PM, posteromedial commissure of mitral valve; PP, posterior papillary muscle; R, right aortic cusp; S, left superior leaflet of AV valve; T, tricuspid valve.

Reproduced with permission from Baron et al.[B4]

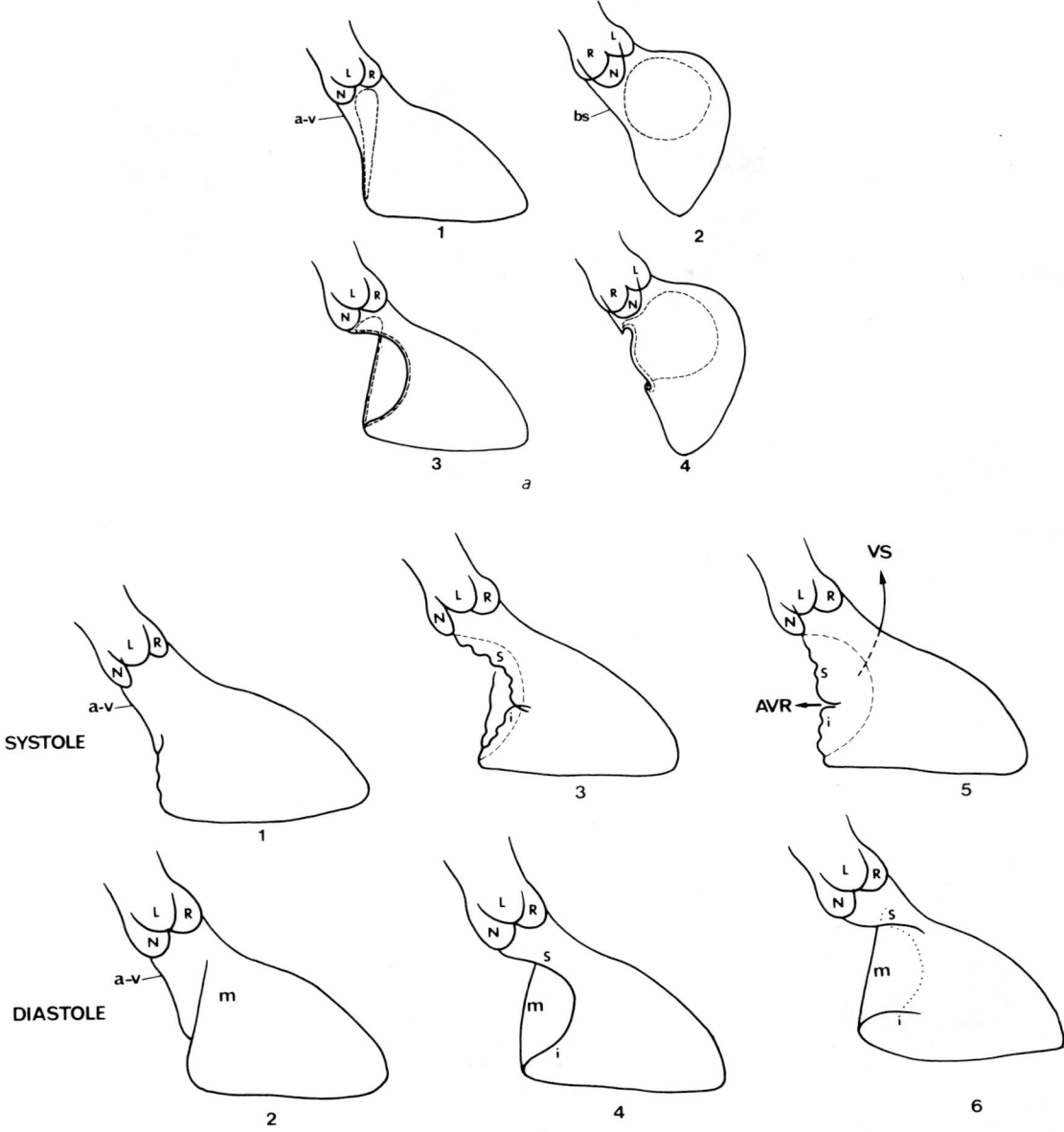

Figure 19-15 Diagrammatic representations of cineangiocardiograms of a normal heart and hearts with AV canal defects, in oblique and axial views (GLH).

(a) The mitral valve orifice and leaflet attachments (interrupted line) in RAO and LAO projections. (1) The normal mitral orifice is approximately profiled in 40° RAO projection but is overlapped by the left ventricular (LV) outflow tract. The rightward posterior border of the normal LV outflow tract is formed by atrioventricular septal tissue (a-v), not mitral valve. (2) In 50° LAO projections, the rightward anterior margin of the normal outflow tract consists of the basal ventricular sinus septum, membranous above, muscular below. Again, the mitral valve attachments do not reach the septal margin. (3,4) In AV canal defects, absence of the atrioventricular septum and adjacent deficiency of the basal (inlet) ventricular septum modify the left AV valve attachments and the position and shape of the left AV orifice and LV outflow tract. (b) LV cineangiocardiograms in 40° RAO projections. (1,2) The normal features can be compared with those of (3,4) the typical partial AV canal and (5,6) the complete AV canal in systole and diastole. In the normal heart, mitral leaflets contribute only to the lowest portion of the rightward posterior LV outflow margin in systole, the relatively immobile atrioventricular septum (a-v), forming the remainder of this margin throughout the cardiac cycle. In diastole, the line of attachment (m) of the mural (posterior) leaflet of the mitral valve can be identified, since contrast is trapped between the leaflet and the adjacent LV wall. In AV canal defects, the rightward posterior margin of the LV outflow tract consists of mobile leaflet tissue: left superior leaflet (s) above and left inferior leaflet (i) below. The atrioventricular septum is absent. The mural leaflet attachment lies in relatively normal position. When there is complete attachment of the left superior and inferior leaflets to the septal crest (dashed line), the LV outflow tract deformity is well marked in systole, and the position of the septal crest can be identified in diastole, contrast being trapped between the open leaflets and the septum. When there is a large interventricular communication with superior and inferior leaflets that are free-floating or attached to the septal crest by thin chordae only (5,6), the systolic deformity may be less marked and the septal crest may be invisible, since contrast is washed away by nonopaque inflow. The RAO view separates an AV regurgitant stream (AVR) from an interventricular shunt (VS).

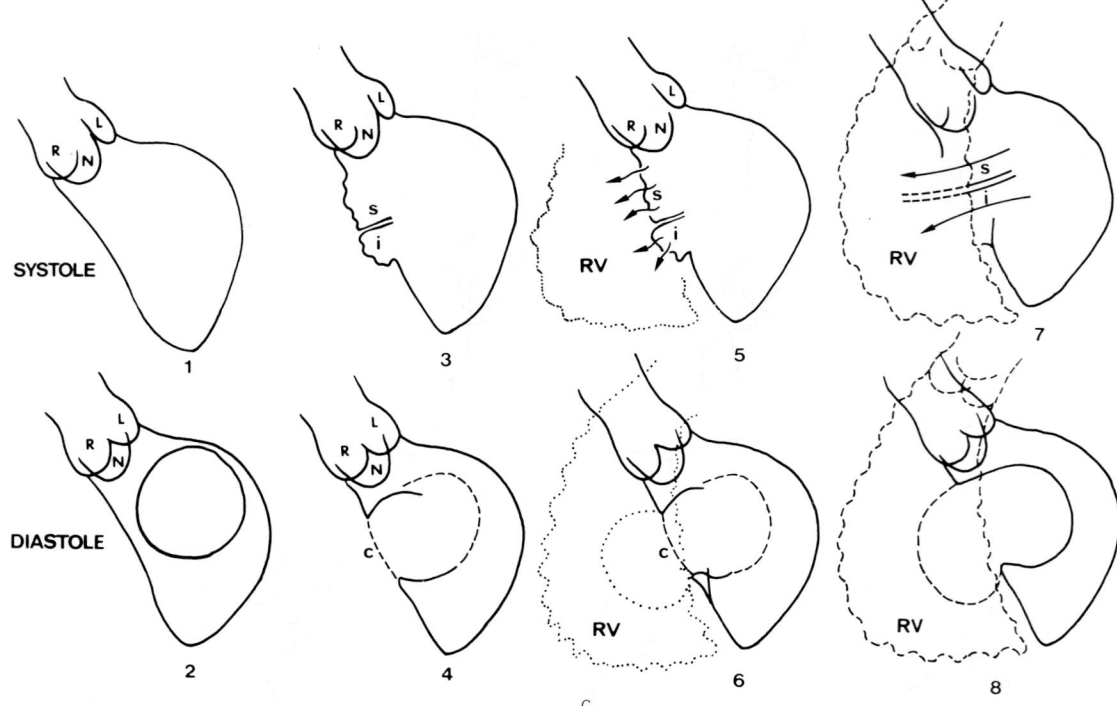

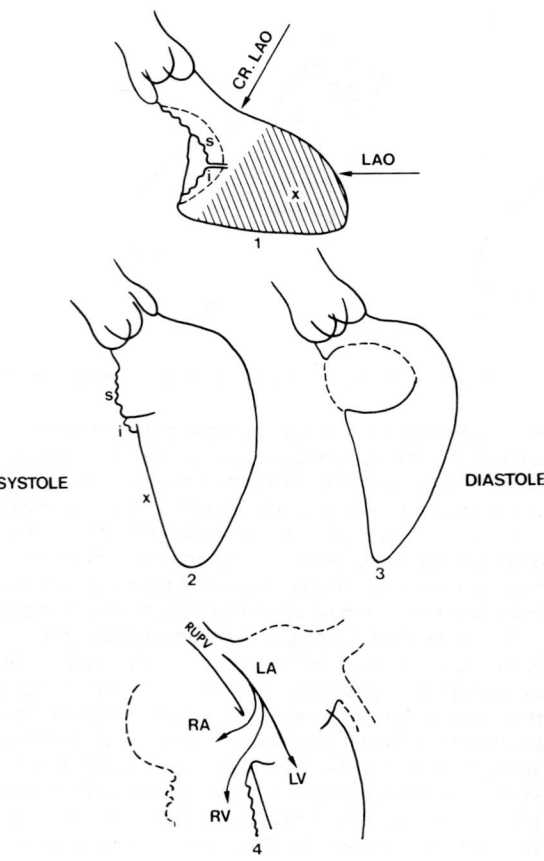

Figure 19-15 *(continued)*

(c) LV cineangiocardiograms in 50° LAO projection. (1,2) In the normal heart, the septal margin of the LV outflow tract is uninterrupted in systole and diastole. In AV canal defect (3–8), the septal margin is interrupted by the defect in the basal ventricular septum, the defect being continuous with the left AV orifice. (3,4) When the left superior and inferior leaflets are completely attached to the septal crest, as in partial AV canal, leaflet tissue bulges into the defect in systole, and the position of the septal crest (c) can be identified in diastole. (7,8) When there is a large interventricular communication, systolic flow to the right ventricle can be observed passing beneath the left superior (upper arrow) or left inferior (lower arrow) leaflets. In diastole, a common AV orifice is identified. (5,6) In some cases, attachments to the septal crest are present but leave smaller interventricular communications. AV valve regurgitation tends to obscure valve detail as the overlying atria opacify.

(d) LV or left atrial cineangiocardiograms of AV canal defect in 50° LAO with cranial angulation (axial, hepatoclavicular, or four-chamber view). (1) Arrows in the 40° RAO view illustrate why conventional LAO (part c) shows the full height of the AV orifice, providing the best separation of left superior from left inferior leaflets. The cranially tilted version of LAO (CR LAO) foreshortens the AV orifice, and tends to superimpose these leaflets. (2,3) However, the characteristic deformity of septal and AV orifice anatomy seen in the conventional LAO can be appreciated in the axial LAO views which are shown in both systole and diastole. In addition, the mid muscular and apical parts of the sinus septum are better separated from the basal defect so that additional muscular defects in the cross hatched area (e.g., at x) may be identified. AV valve regurgitation will again obscure detail, but partial separation of atria from ventricles improves differentiation of regurgitation from interventricular shunting. With a left atrial (LA), or right upper pulmonary venous (RUPV) injection in 50° LAO with cranial angulation (4) contrast flow (arrows) early in the sequence shows the position of the atrial septal defect adjacent to the AV valves. Contrast enters right atrium, right ventricle, and left ventricle. Cranial angulation rarely achieves a perfect profile of the AV ring and ventricular opacification obscures detail later in the sequence.

a-v, atrioventricular septum; AVR, AV regurgitant stream; bs, basal portion of ventricular septum; c, septal crest; i, left inferior leaflet; L, left coronary sinus of the aortic root; LA, left atrium; LV, left ventricle; m, line of attachment of posterior mitral leaflet; N, noncoronary sinus of the aortic root; R, right coronary sinus of the aortic root; RA, right atrium; RV, right ventricle; s, left superior leaflet; VS, ventricular shunt.

Patients with a *complete AV canal defect* have a still more unfavorable natural history. Since no group of infants known to have this lesion has been followed from birth without surgical intervention, the ideal data base for delineation of their natural history does not exist. The closest approach to such an analysis was in the prospective study of 56,109 live births by Mitchell and colleagues,[M11] which included 10 infants judged to have isolated complete AV canal defect (excluding 4 stillbirths with the malformation), 4 of whom died within the first 3 years of life. This information is inconclusive, however, because of the small number of patients involved; the failure to obtain a positive diagnosis by surgery, autopsy, or cardiac catheterization in all patients in the study; and the use of surgical intervention in some cases. Also, the specific ages of the six survivors were not given.

In the absence of a definitive prospective study, an approximation of the survival history of complete AV canal defect has been constructed from 39 patients in two reports of autopsies.[B8] This analysis indicates that about 80% of patients unoperated on die by age 2 years (Fig. 19-18). A child who has survived to 1 year of age has only about a 15% chance of living to age 5 years. Those patients who die in the first 1–2 years of life usually do so with congestive heart failure, with or without recurrent pulmonary infections, as a result of the large left-to-right shunt and the moderate-to-severe AV valve incompetence present in 60% of the pa-

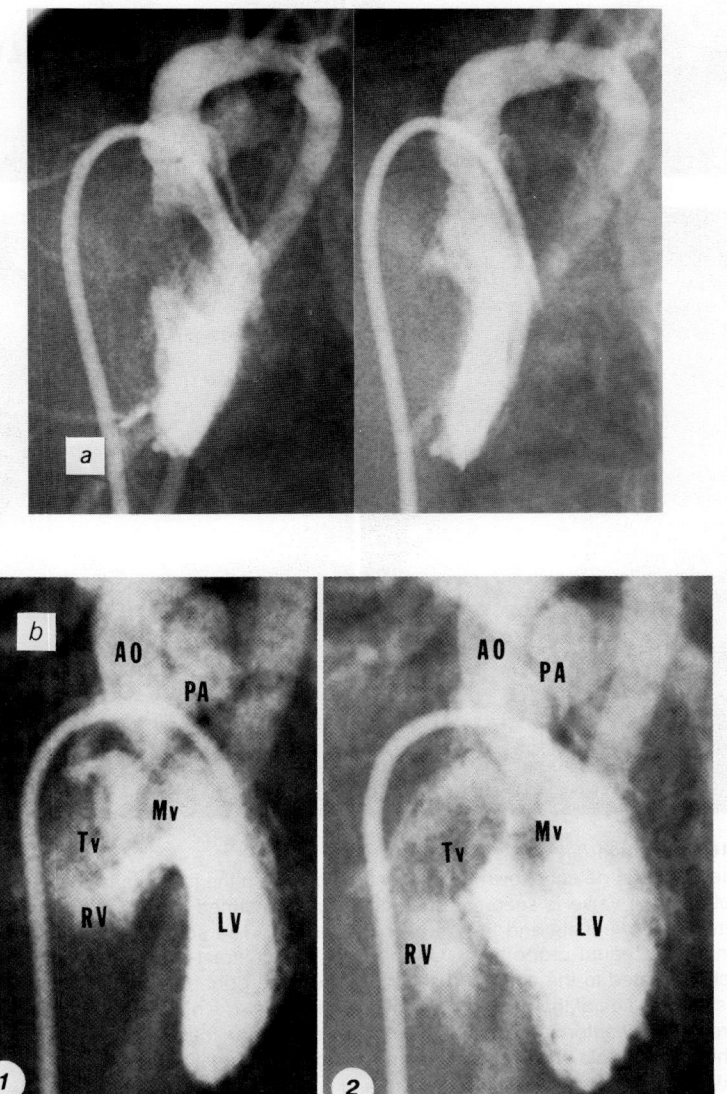

Figure 19-16 Cineangiograms in patients with AV canal defects.
(a) Partial AV canal defect shown by left ventriculogram in the four-chamber position (UAB). Diastolic frame (left) and systolic frame (right). Loss of the straight line contour from the aortic valve to the crux cordis indicates absence of the major part of the AV septum.
(b) AV canal defect with two AV valve orifices and an interventricular communication (UAB).

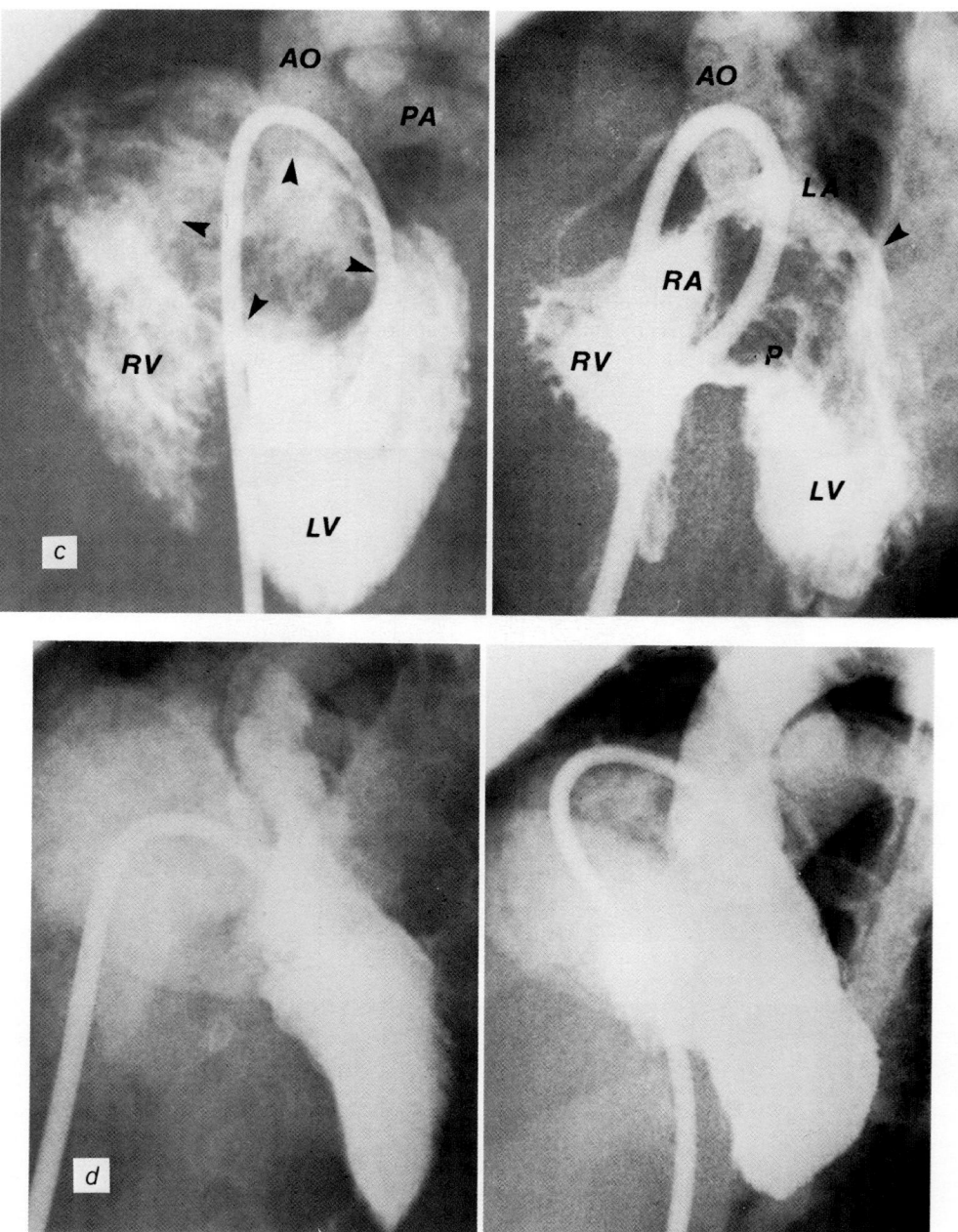

Figure 19-16 (*continued*)

(*c*) Complete AV canal defect shown by left ventriculogram in the four-chamber view (UAB). On the left, the anulus of the valve is seen as a negative shadow formed by the accumulation of contrast medium between the leaflets and the free ventricular wall. The anulus includes the right and left ventricles in almost equal proportions. On the right, the contrast medium outlines the left lateral leaflet, which is related to the aorta and separated from the right anterior leaflet by a commissure, which marks the position of the papillary muscle of the conus. The outline of the left anterior leaflet is separated from the left anterior leaflet by a commissure, marking the position of the anterior papillary muscle of the left ventricle. This represents an example of Rastelli type A defect.

(*d*) Partial AV canal defects with moderate (left) and severe (right) incompetence of the left AV valve (UAB). The contrast medium has passed from the left ventricle into the right atrium through the incompetent valve.

Ao, aorta; LA, left lateral leaflet; LV, left ventricle; Mv, left AV valve; PA, pulmonary artery; RA, right anterior leaflet; RV, right ventricle; Tv, right AV valve.

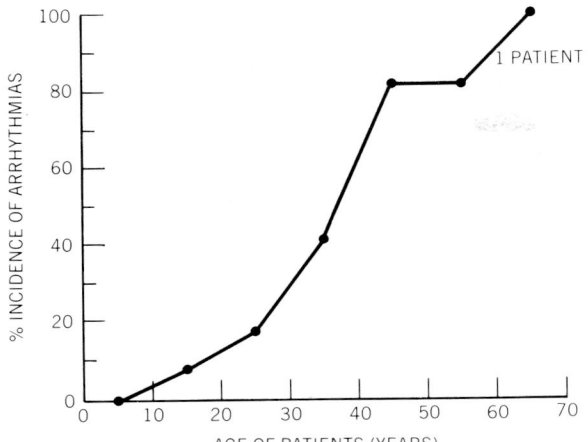

Figure 19-17 Incidence of cardiac arrhythmias in surgically untreated patients with a partial AV canal defect according to the age of the patient. The increased incidence in older patients is striking. Reproduced with permission from Somerville.[S6]

tients with this lesion.[S2] After the first 1–2 years of life, valve incompetence and increasing pulmonary vascular disease become the dominant factors in the natural history. Newfeld and colleagues[N1] have shown histologically that advanced pulmonary vascular disease (Heath-Edwards grade 3 and 4; see Chapter 24) is occasionally present in such infants even in the first year of life. However, over the age of 1 year, it is present in nearly 90% of cases (seven of their eight specimens).

A corroboration of these features of the natural history of AV canal defects is given in Figure 19-19. About 30% of the patients with complete AV canal defects come forward for operation by the age of 12 months and 70% by 2 years, whereas of those with partial AV canal defects only 5% do so at 12 months, 30% at 4 years, and 50% at 10 years.

Another aspect of the natural history of patients with AV canal defects is the tendency of their offspring to have similar defects or other congenital cardiac malformations. Emanuel and colleagues have shown that 14% of offspring of mothers with AV canal defects have congenital heart disease.[E5] Half have tetralogy of Fallot and the other half AV canal defects. This incidence is much higher than the 2%–4% incidence among children of parents with other types of congenital heart disease.

TECHNIQUE OF OPERATION

Surgical treatment of AV canal defects is directed toward (1) closure of the ASD, which is virtually always present; (2) closure of the interventricular communication if one is present; (3) avoidance of damage to the AV node and bundle of His; and (4) maintenance or creation of two competent, nonstenotic AV valves.

There continues to be considerable variability in the techniques used in the repair. Variations include the use of one patch[R1] or of two in repairing the malformation when there is a large interventricular communication, and dividing a markedly bridging left superior leaflet (LSL)[R5] or leaving it in-

tact.[B16,S2] In addition, the AV node and bundle of His may be avoided by staying on the left ventricular and left atrial side[M13] or by staying on the right side.[S2] The contiguous surfaces of the LSL and left inferior leaflet (LIL) may be sutured together,[R2] or the left AV valve may be left as a tricuspid structure under ordinary circumstances.[C6] An accessory orifice may be left alone, or the leaflet tissue may be split so that a double orifice becomes a single one.[G4] The patch may be attached to leaflet tissue by simple sutures or by pledgetted mattress sutures with some sort of sandwich method.[C8,S2] An assortment of techniques has been employed to establish AV valve competence.[C6] The methods described in this chapter are the products of experience (UAB and GLH) and have improved the surgical results.[S2] They avoid functionally important damage to the conduction system, provide complete and permanent closure of interatrial and interventricular communications, and are suitable for the many variations within the spectrum of AV canal defects. They are well adapted to cases with major associated cardiac anomalies. They retain AV valve competence when it is present, minimize the incidence of valve repair dehiscence, and generally abolish or lessen AV valve incompetence,[S2] although in this regard the results are imperfect, particularly in patients without interventricular communications.

Repair of Complete AV Canal Defect with Little or No Bridging of the Left Superior and Left Inferior Leaflets: Rastelli Type A

After the usual preparations, a median sternotomy incision is made, a large piece of pericardium is removed and set aside between wet towels, and pericardial stay sutures are applied. The external cardiac anatomy is evaluated, and a left superior vena cava is searched for. If one is present, there is a 50% chance of associated unroofed coronary sinus syndrome. Purse-string sutures are placed.

The repair may be performed with the technique of limited cardiopulmonary bypass (CPB) with a single venous cannula, profound hypothermia, and total circulatory arrest without the use of cardioplegia when the patient is less than 8 kg in weight, and standard cardiopulmonary bypass in larger patients (GLH). Alternatively, in infants and older children, hypothermic CPB at 25°C and cold cardioplegia may be used (UAB). In this method, the cavae are cannulated directly with special, thin-walled, metal, right-angled cannulae (see Chapter 2, Fig. 2-20). The CPB flow rate is reduced to 1.6–2.0 $1 \cdot min^{-1} \cdot m^{-2}$ when the patient's temperature reaches 25°C. Short periods of flow at 0.5 $1 \cdot min^{-1} \cdot m^{-2}$ or of total circulatory arrest are occasionally used if visibility is not otherwise excellent. As cooling proceeds, the right atrium is opened widely, and a pump sump sucker is passed through the foramen ovale into the left atrium. Stay sutures are applied, the aorta is cross-clamped, and the cold cardioplegic solution is injected. The injection is repeated every 20–30 minutes (see Chapter 3). The repair can be expected to require 30–70 minutes inside the heart.

The malformation is now examined carefully, and each morphologic detail is noted (Fig. 19-20a). Cold saline solution is injected once or twice through the valve, and the

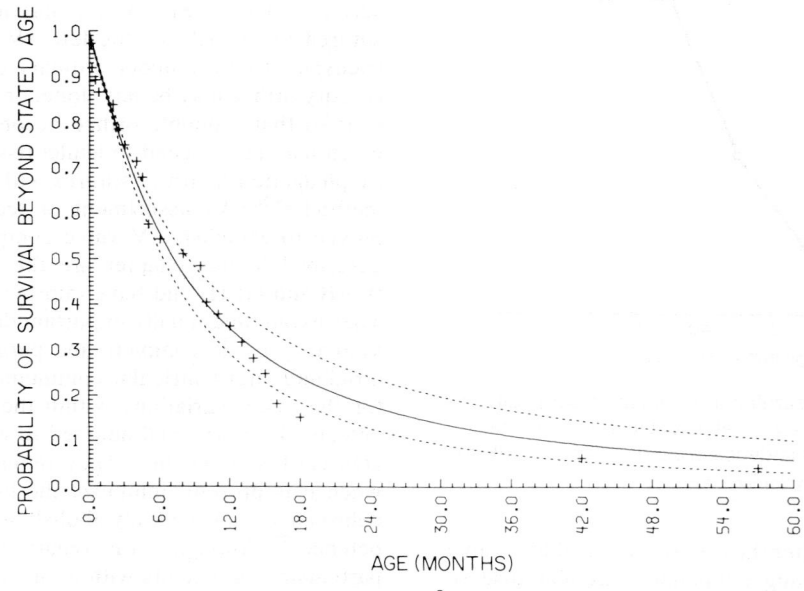

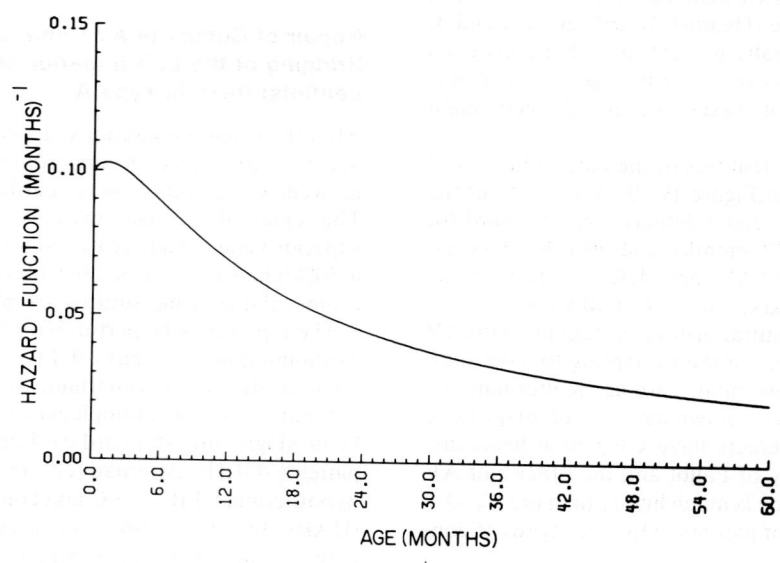

Figure 19-18 Life expectancy without surgery in complete AV canal defects.
(a) The plus signs represent the nonparametric estimates. The solid line, enclosed within its 70% confidence limits (dotted lines), is a nomogram of the equation describing survival. Note that the probability of surviving beyond 6 months is 50% and that for surviving beyond a year is only 30% (see the original source for equation and statistics.)
(b) Hazard function according to age. Note that the risk of dying from a complete AV canal defect is highest in the first few months of life.

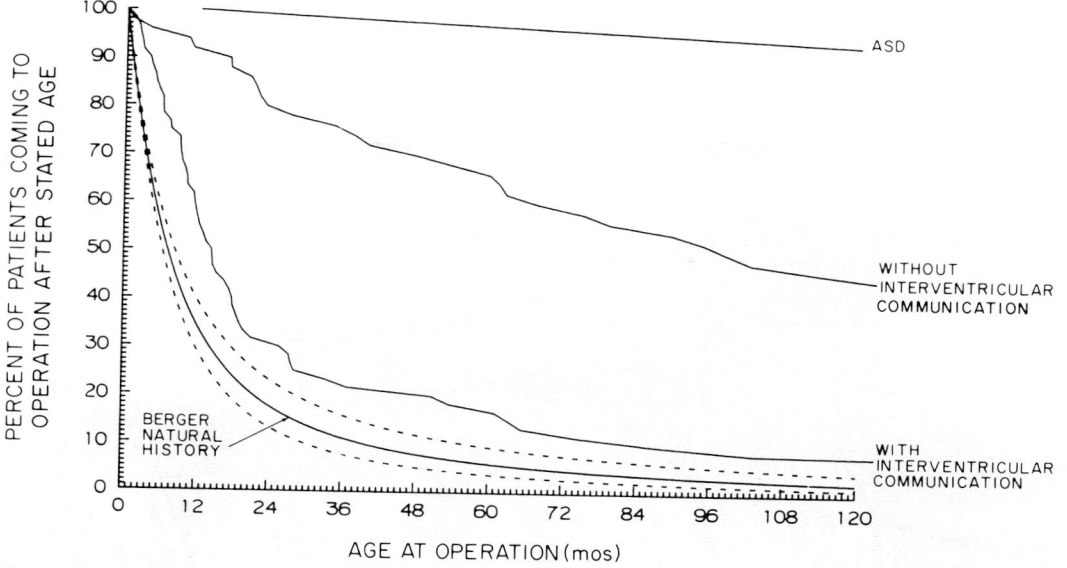

Figure 19-19   Percent of patients coming to operation for AV canal defects after the stated age (along the horizontal axis), according to whether there was an interventricular communication (UAB; 1977–1982). The patients were without major associated cardiac anomalies, and are depicted by the jagged solid lines. For comparison, using the vertical axis to represent percent survival at a stated age, along the horizontal axis, the natural history of patients with atrial septal defect (see Chapter 15, "Survival" in section on Natural History) is depicted by the straight solid line; and that of patients with complete AV canal defects by the Berger Natural History line.

Reproduced with permission from Kirklin et al.[K13]

closure pattern and any regurgitant leaks are studied. This information is used later if incompetence is known to be present. The morphology of the left superior and left inferior leaflets is carefully noted, particularly in regard to its effect on the closing pattern, and the surface of the opposing leaflets are carefully studied (Fig. 19-20b). The most anterior (rightward) point of the LSL-LIL opposing edges is found, and a double-armed 6-0 polypropylene suture placed through it (Fig. 19-20b). Leaflet stay and marking sutures are placed, measurements are made, and the Dacron interventricular patch is trimmed.

The preclotted Dacron interventricular patch is now sutured to the right side of the crest of the ventricular septum with continuous 5-0 polypropylene suture (Fig. 19-20c,d). The chordae of the right superior leaflet (RSL) and right inferior leaflet (RIL) stay on the right ventricular side of the patch. Those of the LSL and LIL are on the left ventricular side, and some may be cut if they interfere with the suturing, since the anterior edges of these leaflets will be sutured to the Dacron patch. When this phase is completed, the anterior edge of the LSL-LIL is sutured to the edge of the Dacron patch, with the chordal attachments of these leaflets to the ventricular crest kept taut so that the leaflets are suspended at the correct height (Fig. 19-20e). Great care is taken that the alignment of the leaflets is perfect and that there is no distortion. Then the pericardial interatrial patch is trimmed to the appropriate shape and size, and the first part of its insertion is accomplished (Fig. 19-20f). As an alternative to the continuous mattress suture which encloses the anterior edges of the LSL and LIL between the Dacron patch below and pericardial patch above, interrupted

mattress sutures of 5-0 or 6-0 Dacron may be more conveniently used.

Saline solution is again injected through the left-sided portion of the AV valves (two orifices are present, now that the interventricular patch is in place), in order to study its closure pattern and competence. A few additional "tailoring sutures" are placed without tension between the LSL and LIL near the patch if needed to prevent systolic eversion or prolapse. Usually they are not required. If a central leak (at the point of junction of LSL, LIL, and left lateral leaflet [LLL]) persists, an annuloplasty stitch is placed in the region of the commissure between the LSL and LLL. If necessary and if the orifice is large enough, a similar stitch can be placed at the LLL-LIL commissure, the surgeon being certain not to approach the AV node. This part of the operation is critically important and requires patience and ingenuity. The assessment of both left and right AV valves at this point includes a consideration of their size. The diameter of each is estimated with Hegar dilators and considered acceptable if within 1 standard deviation of normal for the size of the patient (Fig. 19-21).

The repair is completed by the suturing of the rest of the pericardial interatrial patch in place, the suture line passing *around* the AV node and bundle of His and not across them (Fig. 19-20g). The right-sided leaflets are not sutured to the patch. They close competently without this. If any commissural tissue between the LSL and the RSL or the LIL and the RIL is cut, the right side of this (as well as the left side) is sutured to the patch.

As this suture line is being completed, the CPB perfusate temperature may be increased to begin rewarming the pa-

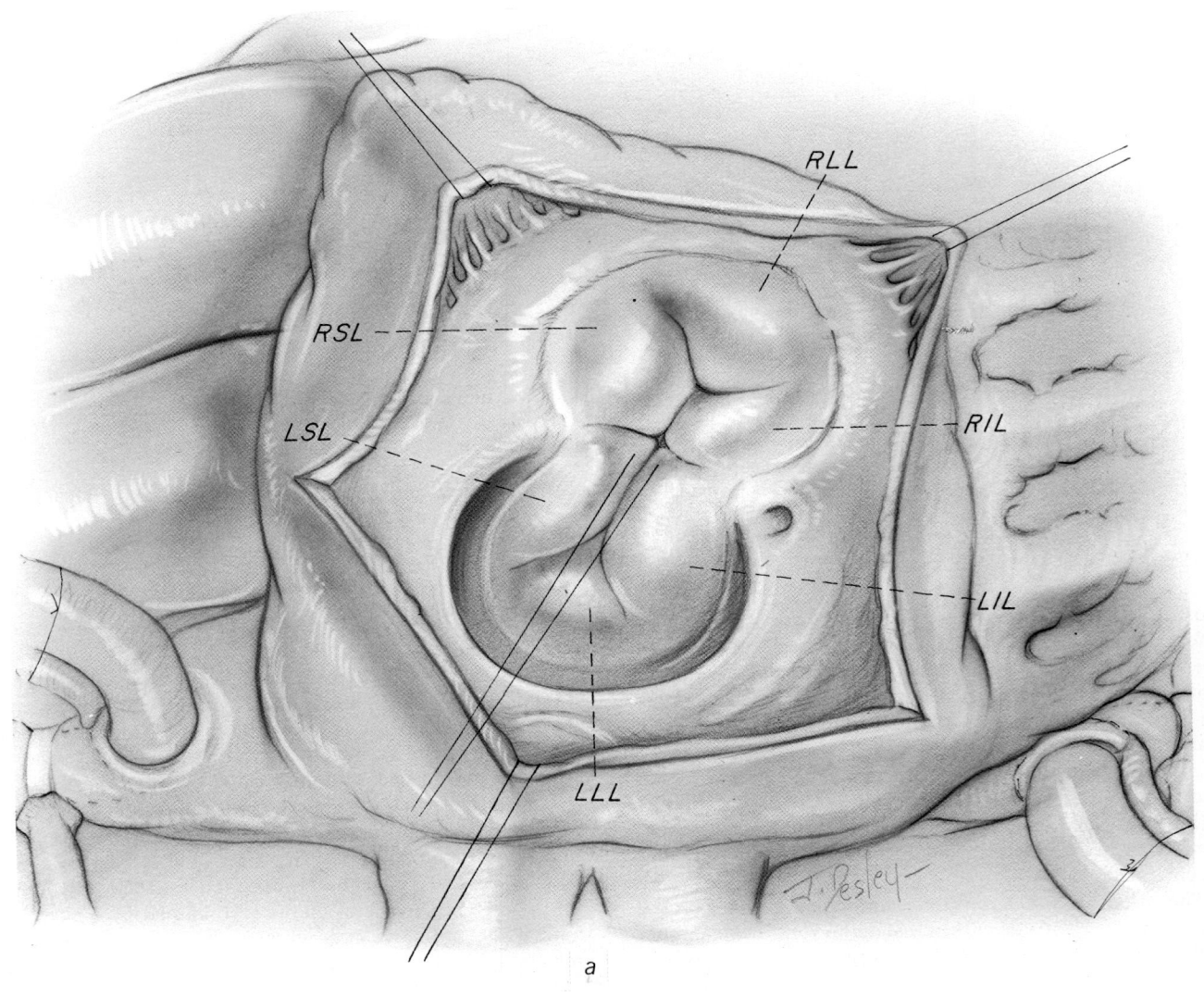

Figure 19-20 Repair of complete AV canal defect.
(a) After the atrium is opened, the leaflets are often closed exactly as they are in systole. If, instead, they are open, saline solution is injected into the ventricle to close them. At this point, the morphology of the leaflets, particularly their closure pattern, is carefully studied, and the information obtained is used to plan the repair of any incompetence that may be present. A fine (6-0 polypropylene) suture is placed between the left superior leaflet (LSL) and left inferior leaflet (LIL) in the position shown, and left loose.
LLL, left lateral leaflet; RIL, right inferior leaflet; RLL, right lateral leaflet; RSL, right superior leaflet.

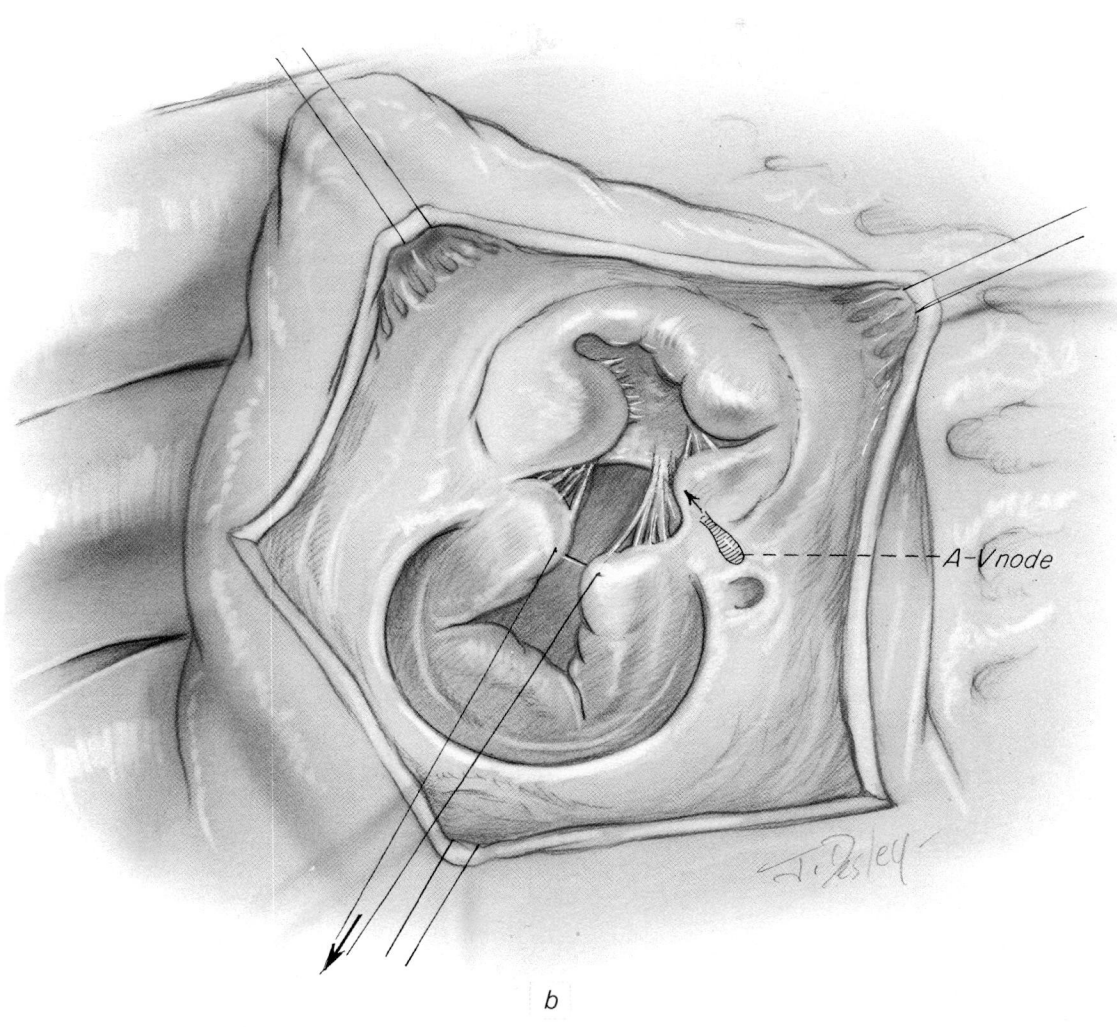

A-V node

Figure 19-20 (*continued*)
(*b*) The leaflets are allowed to collapse in the open position, and the details of the atrial and ventricular septal deficiencies and of the interatrial and interventricular communications are studied. The position of the coronary sinus is carefully noted, and the positions of the unseen AV node and bundle of His are visualized by the surgeon from a knowledge of the anatomy.

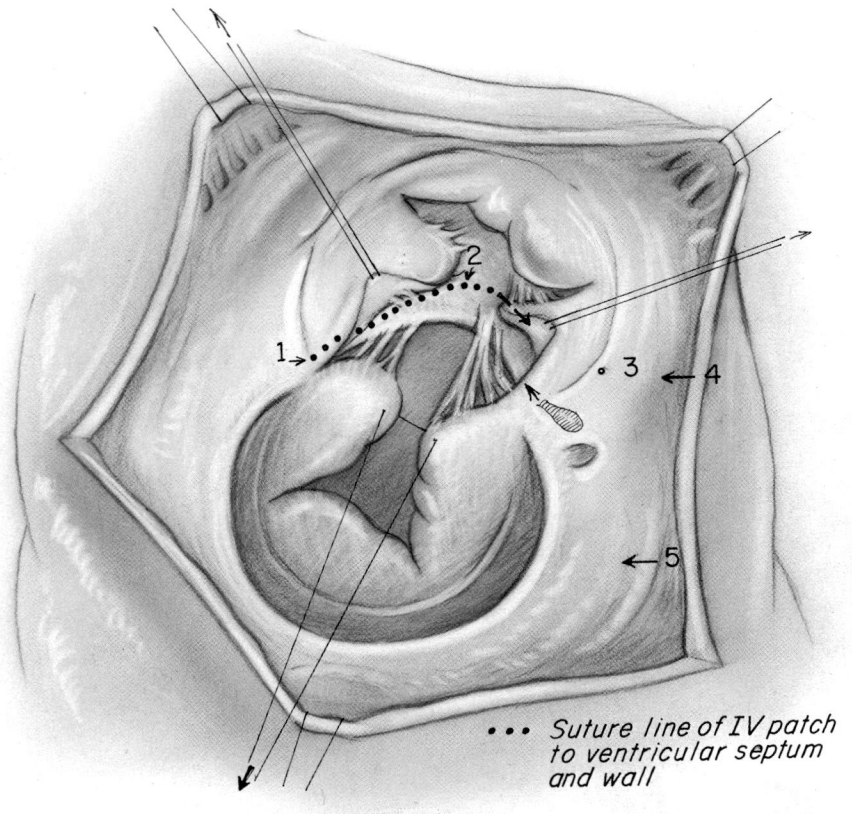

• • • *Suture line of IV patch
to ventricular septum
and wall*

c

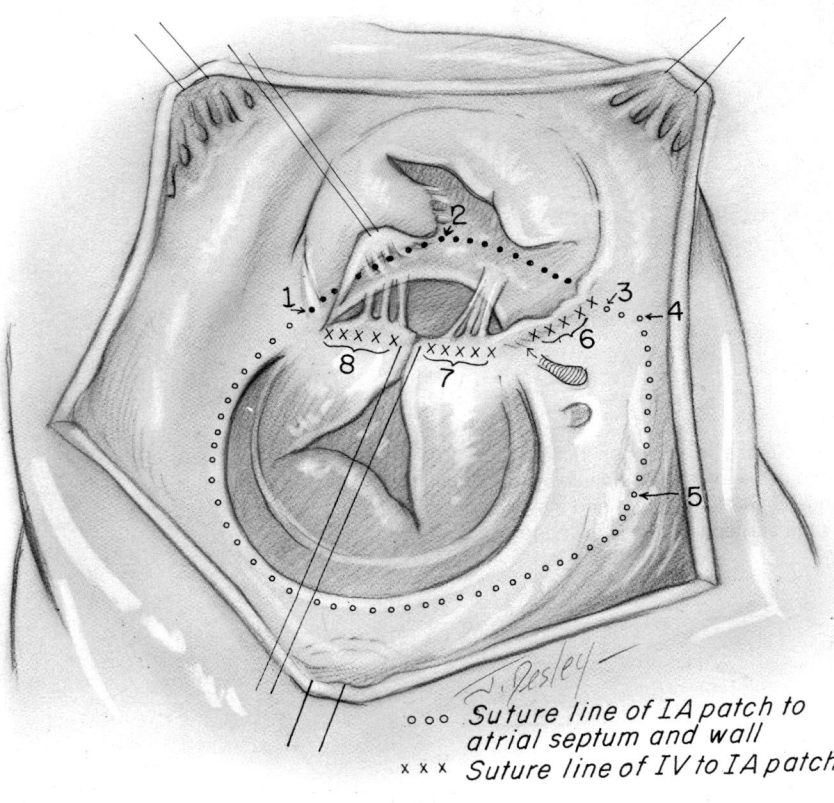

∘∘∘ *Suture line of IA patch to
atrial septum and wall*
✕ ✕ ✕ *Suture line of IV to IA patch*

d

Figure 19-20 (*continued*)

(*c*) A 5-0 silk stay suture is placed at point 2, the suture is then stretched toward the left leaflets, marked to the length between point 2 and the leaflets held with their chordae taut, removed, and used in cutting the interventricular Dacron patch to a proper width. The suture line of the interventricular patch to the ventricular septum and free wall is now visualized by the surgeon. As shown, this suture line lies on the right ventricular side of all of the chordae from the left-sided leaflets, including those from any bridging components of the LIL. The suture line goes beneath the right inferior leaflet (RIL), well away from the crest of the ventricular septum. The suture line begins at point 1. A stay suture is placed through the base of the RIL at point 3, where the suture line between interventricular patch and ventricle also ends by coming through the base of the RIL. Points 4 and 5 on the right atrium are on the suture line between the interatrial patch and the atrium.

(*d*) Point 6 is the area along which the base of the right inferior leaflet (RIL) is sandwiched between the interatrial and interventricular patches (the RIL has been removed here by the artist to facilitate visualization). Areas 7 and 8 are the portions of the LIL and LSL that are sandwiched between the interventricular and interatrial patches. Note that the suture lines completely avoid the AV node and bundle of His, the bundle lying in the muscle of the ventricular crest *beneath* valvar tissue. A 4-0 or 5-0 polypropylene suture is placed through the anulus at the base of any commissural tissue between the LSL and RSL at point 1. This suture will be used to begin suturing the Dacron patch to the ventricular septum. A marking suture of 5-0 polypropylene is placed through the base of the RIL leaflet at point 3. A fine silk stitch is placed and tied at point 4 and at point 5 to mark these locations. The position of the suture line between the Dacron patch and the ventricular septum, and the pericardial patch and the atrial wall and septum can now be visualized, as well as that between the interventricular and interatrial patches. The latter suture line will enclose the base of the LSL and LIL leaflets, as in a sandwich.

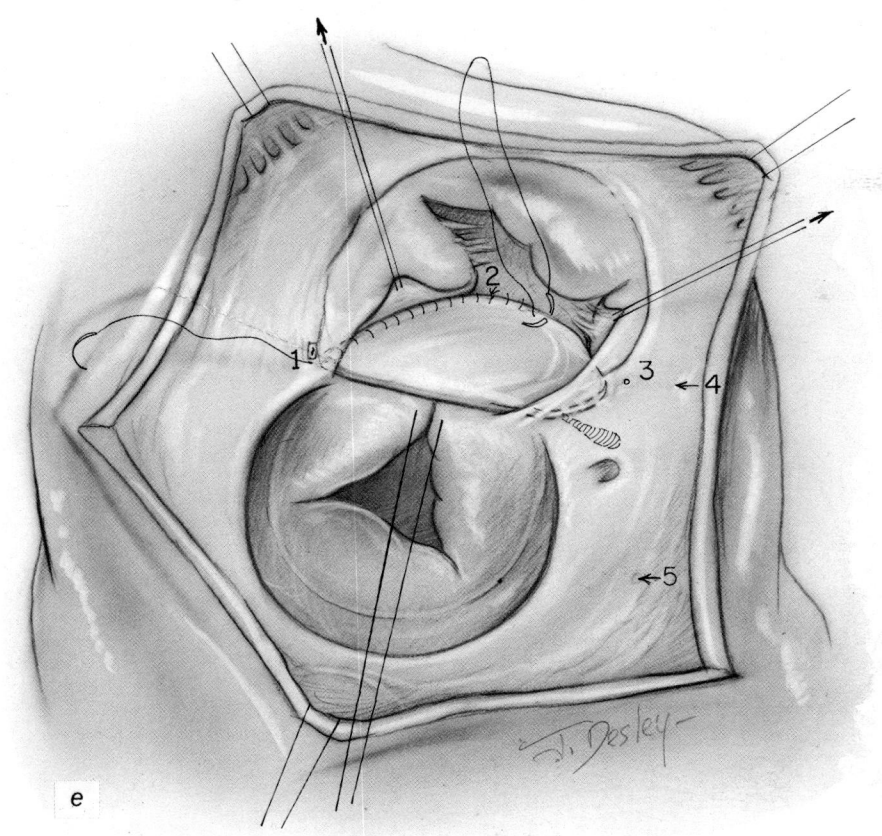

e

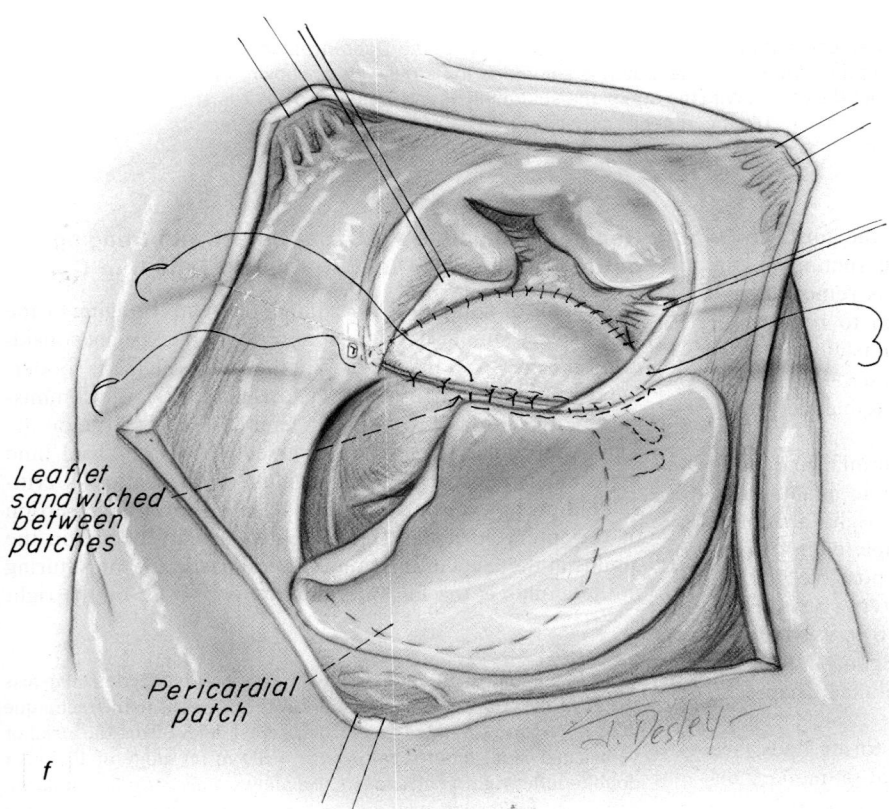

Leaflet
sandwiched
between
patches

Pericardial
patch

f

Figure 19-20 (*continued*)

(*e*) After the Dacron patch has been trimmed according to measurements to fit precisely into position, it is sutured in place with the pledgetted mattress stitch previously placed at point 1. Note that the suture line is well on the right ventricular side of the crest of the ventricular septum, as illustrated in part *d*. The suture line is approaching point 3, which previously was marked with a stay suture.

(*f*) The pericardial patch has now been cut according to measurements that have been made, and a new continuous mattress suture line is begun in the base of the RIL opposite point 3 (see part *e*). This suture passes through the pericardial patch and base of the RIL, catches the Dacron patch, returns through tne base of the leaflet to pass through the pericardial patch, and so on. After this suture line is completed, the pericardial patch is turned upward so that the left AV valve can be inspected. The stay suture previously placed between the anterior edge of the coapting surfaces of the LSL and LIL is passed through the edge of the Dacron patch at the appropriate point. A number of fine interrupted simple stitches are placed between the anterior aspect of these leaflets and the Dacron patch so as to perfectly align them. The previous suture used for the horizontal mattress stitches is now continued in the same manner through the pericardial patch, the base of the leaflets, and the Dacron patch, sandwiching the leaflet securely between the two patches in areas 7 and 8. (See text for currently preferred alternative suture technique.) After this suture line is completed, the pericardial patch is turned upward again, and the leaflets are closed by the injection of saline solution. If incompetence is present, the maneuvers described in the text are used to minimize or ablate the incompetence.

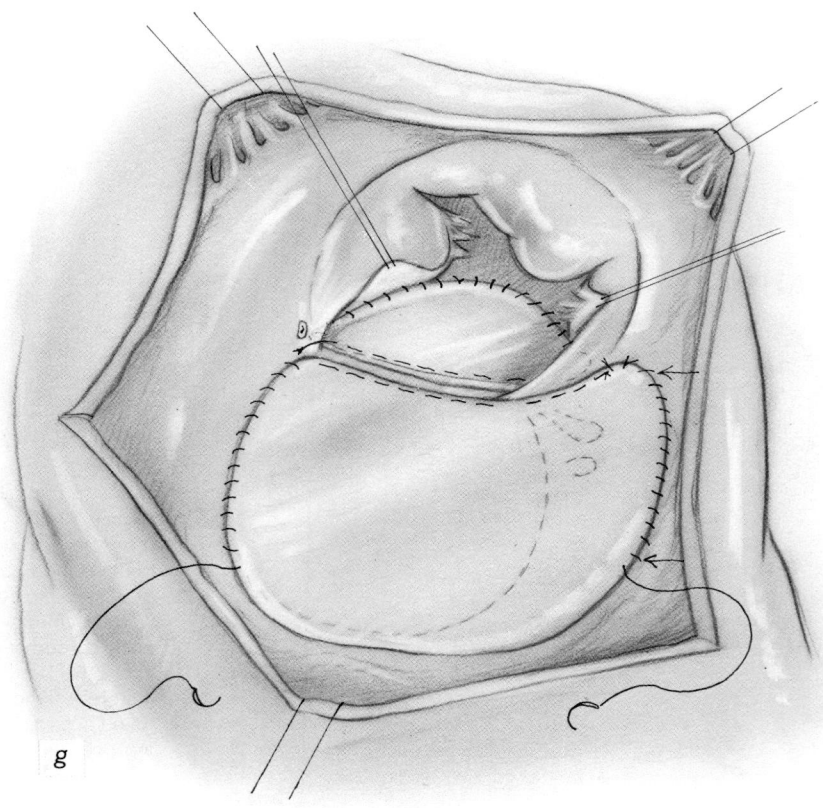

Figure 19-20   *(continued)*

(g) With the previously held suture that has completed the attachment of the Dacron patch to the ventricular septum, shown in part *f*, the pericardial patch is sutured to the atrial wall as shown, well away from the AV node and bundle of His. With the arm of the suture left after tying the two sutures at point 1, the pericardial patch is sutured to the superior aspect of the rim of the atrial septal defect. When this suture line is finished, the repair has been completed.

Reproduced with permission from Kirklin et al.[K13]

tient (UAB). When rewarming is complete, the aortic cross-clamp is released, with continuous strong suction on the aortic needle vent. The transseptal sump is removed, and the foramen ovale closed, with care taken to trap no air in the left side of the heart. The right atrium is closed. After good cardiac action has returned, the usual de-airing procedures are carried out (see Chapter 2). The remainder of the operation proceeds as usual.

Alternatively, when profound hypothermia and total circulatory arrest are used for the operation in infants, total circulatory arrest is continued until the right atrium is closed, provided the procedure can be completed in 45 minutes arrest time, which is almost always possible (GLH). Otherwise, the sequence described in Chapter 2, Section 4 is adopted. The single venous cannula is then reinserted, the heart is de-aired, CPB for rewarming is begun, and the remainder of the procedure proceeds as usual (see Chapter 2, Section 4).

Left atrial and right atrial pressure-monitoring lines (see Chapter 2) are left routinely, and if residual pulmonary artery hypertension is present, leaving a pulmonary artery line is also advantageous.

Repair of Complete AV Canal Defect with Bridging of the Left Superior Leaflet: Rastelli Type B or C

The repair of complete AV canal defect with bridging of the LSL is very similar to that just described, but special consideration is given to the LSL. Whether the bridging is moderate (Rastelli type B) or marked (Rastelli type C), the commissure between it and the RSL is generally only a little on the right ventricular side of the intersection of the atrial (and ventricular) septum with the anulus. This location is critically important, because, again, the suturing for the insertion of the interventricular Dacron patch usually begins in the anulus at the level of this commissural tissue.[1] If the suturing in the anulus is too far anterior, that is, too far on the right

---

[1]The beginning of the suture line with a half-pledgetted mattress suture at the commissural area is entirely analogous to the technique used in repairing isolated ventricular septal defect from the atrial or ventricular side, or in repairing the VSD in tetralogy of Fallot or double-outlet right ventricle. Its use allows a measure of standardization in the repair techniques and helps make the operation efficient and accurate.

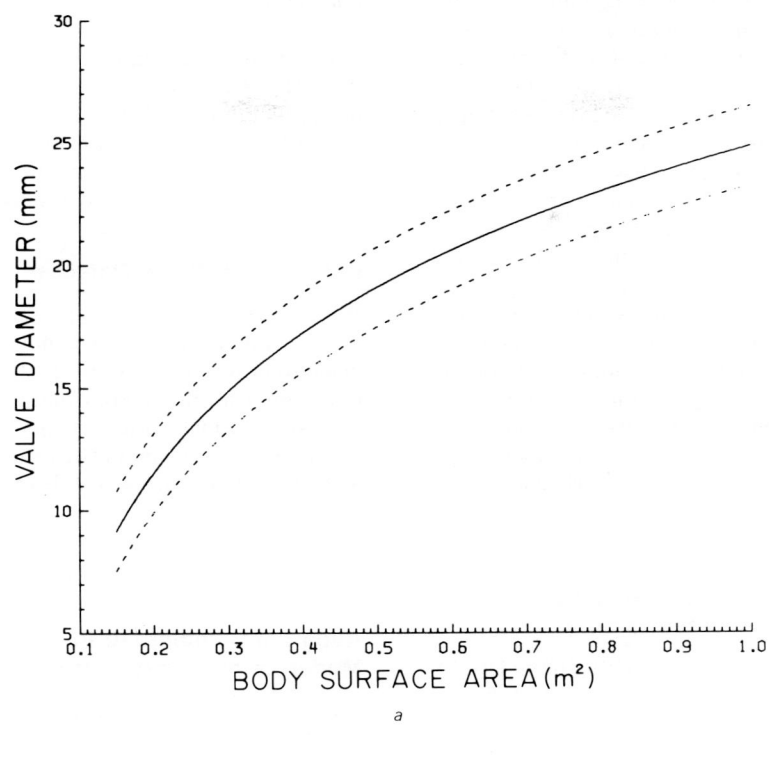

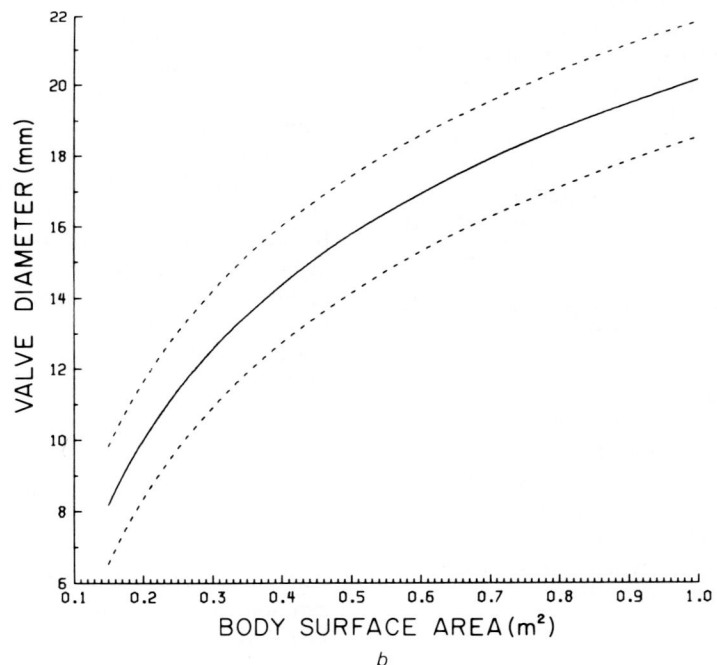

Figure 19-21 Nomograms of normal (*a*) tricuspid and (*b*) mitral valve diameter, according to the body size of the patient. The dashed lines enclose the 70% confidence limits.

Calculated from the data of Rowlatt et al.[R8]

ventricular side of the junction of anulus with atrial septum, either by error or because the LSL-RSL commissure is far anterior, the *right AV valve orifice will be too narrow*. Narrowing of the orifice can also be produced by attaching the interventricular Dacron patch *too far to the right of the crest of the septum* with the first superior (cephalad) few stitches.

Either the chordae going from the right extremity of the LSL to the right ventricular papillary muscle are covered by the interventricular patch (which is acceptable only if it does not narrow the right AV valve orifice), the patch is slid *beneath them*, or they are cut. Most often, the patch is placed beneath them (on their posterior or leftward side), but some of the chordae must usually be cut for surgical exposure. Since the whole anterior edge of the LSL is later attached to the patch, there is no functional harm in cutting the chordae. Incising the LSL from its free edge to the anulus is rarely necessary, although in extreme cases in which a small right AV valve would otherwise result, it may be done, with both divided edges later sutured onto the interventricular Dacron patch (GLH).

Repair of Partial AV Canal Defect with Little or No Left AV Valve Incompetence

The repair of partial AV canal defect with little or no left AV valve incompetence is similar to that just described, but no interventricular Dacron patch is required. After CPB has been established, the intra-atrial exposure arranged, and the cold cardioplegic solution given, the morphology is studied. The attachments of the LSL and LIL to the crest of the ventricular septum are probed to be certain there are no small interventricular communications. If the preoperative studies have shown no left AV valve incompetence, nothing is done to the valve, and generally the same policy is followed if mild incompetence has been demonstrated. Alternatively, if mitral incompetence is demonstrated to be occurring through the periphery (septal extremity) of the LSL-LIL commissure in association with thickening and rolling of the margins, the margins may be approximated in this area with interrupted 5-0 silk sutures (GLH). An annuloplasty stitch may also be placed opposite the LSL-LIL commissure.

The interatrial pericardial patch is sewn into place in a way that is analogous to that used in repairing a complete AV canal defect (Fig. 19-20). Small pledgetted mattress sutures of 5-0 or 6-0 Dacron are passed from the right ventricular side through the base of the RIL and the bridging part of the LIL, and through the pericardial patch. The patch is sewn to the fibrous, valvar tissue attached to the crest of the ventricular septum in this reinforced manner, analogous to its suturing to the top of the Dacron patch (Fig. 19-22).

Repair of AV Canal Defect with Small Interchordal Interventricular Communications

When two AV valve orifices are present but small interventricular communications exist between thick short chordae attaching the left superior leaflet to the crest of the ventricular septum, the repair is simple. The interventricular communication is simply closed by the taking of the anterior portion of the pericardial patch just to the right side of the septal crest.

When the interventricular communications are beneath the LIL, the same maneuver may be followed. However, because of the bundle of His, care must be taken to keep the suture line well away from the crest of the septum and to attach the patch in the same manner as the interventricular patch is attached in the repair of complete AV canal defects.

Repair of AV Canal Defect with Common Atrium

When a common atrium is present with an AV canal defect, either with or without a communication, special effort is made to ensure that there is no left superior vena cava or, if one is present, that there is not a completely unroofed coronary sinus, which would change the repair (see Chapter 18).

The repair is accomplished by the sewing of an appropriately larger pericardial patch to the atrial wall on the left atrial side of the orifice of the inferior vena cava, to the right of the right pulmonary veins, and beneath the superior vena cava (where there is usually a small septal remnant).

Repair of Complete or Partial AV Canal Defect with Moderate or Severe Left AV Valve Incompetence

The repair of an AV canal defect with moderate or severe left AV valve incompetence remains extremely controversial, since results seem to vary, even with the same techniques, from one institution to another.

One view is that the relief of important incompetence in patients with complete AV canal defects can often be accomplished by appropriate repair, but less predictively in patients with partial AV canal defects, and that some special methods described for producing competence[C6] are unreliable (UAB). In this view, each case with important left AV valve incompetence must be evaluated individually by careful study of the two-dimensional echocardiogram, the cineangiogram, and the valve at operation. Depending on the findings, the repair is planned. About the only tools thought to be available, in this view, are (1) remodeling of the leaflet closure by suturing of portions of the LSL and LIL together in areas where regurgitation is demonstrated ("closure of the cleft") or by plicating them, although this must be done thoughtfully to prevent narrowing the orifice or later dehiscence, and (2) narrowing of the anulus. The latter is accomplished by annuloplasty at the commissures on both sides of the left lateral leaflet and by making the edge of the pericardial patch along LSL-LIL complex *shorter* than the combined length of the base of the leaflets. The latter maneuver can sometimes be facilitated by suturing the patch to the LSL-LIL 5–15 mm *away from* (on the orifice side of) their attachment to the crest of the septum. Leaflet tissue between the crest and this suture line functionally then becomes interventricular septum.

Alternatively, other special maneuvers may correct severe incompetence, even in partial AV canal defects (GLH). Thus, in this view, the edges of the leaflets are felt to be thickened invariably and to hold sutures well. When simple

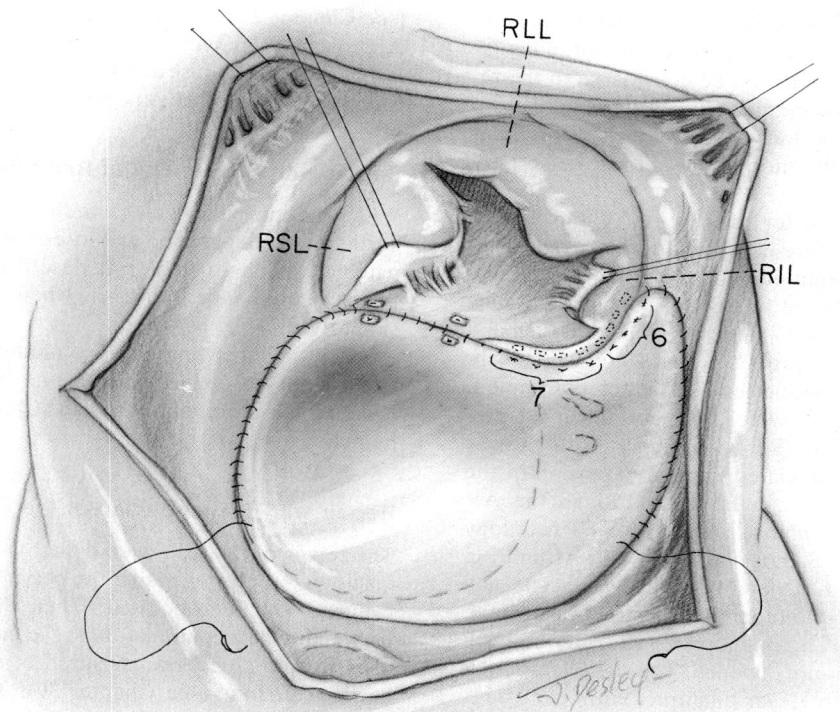

Figure 19-22   The repair of the partial AV canal defect. This repair is analogous to that described for complete AV canal defects in Figure 19-20f, except that the attachment of the left-sided AV valve leaflets to the crest of the ventricular septum obviates the need for a Dacron interventricular patch. The pericardial patch is attached along area 6 by the placement of pledgetted sutures in the ventricular free wall, through the right inferior leaflet (RIL), and through the pericardial patch. In area 7, the pledgetted mattress sutures are only in the base of the bridging portion of the left inferior leaflet (LIL) because the septal tissue beneath it contains the bundle of His. This situation is again analogous to that depicted in Figure 19-20f for complete AV canal defects, except that in the latter repair, the sutures are passed through the Dacron patch. Several additional pledgetted mattress sutures are placed to begin the attachment of the pericardial patch to the right side of the crest of the ventricular septum, superior to area 7, where damage to the bundle of His will not occur. Then an over and over continuous stitch is used to seal this part of the suture line.

RIL, right inferior leaflet; RLL, right lateral leaflet; RSL, right superior leaflet.

Reproduced with permission from Kirklin et al.[K13]

maneuvers fail, in this view, better results may be obtained by detaching the LSL-LIL complex from the ventricular crest in patients with the partial AV canal defect and reattaching it to a pericardial or Dacron patch at a higher level as for a complete AV canal repair,[C6] again shortening the ring at this point.

Right AV Valve

In hearts with or without interventricular communications, the right AV valve rarely requires attention. The repair leaves this valve without a complete "septal leaflet," but in this and other situations, this condition does not result in incompetence. The RSL and RIL (and the RLL) are well supported by chordae, and this, combined with their closure against the Dacron patch or bare ventricular septum, generally makes the valve competent.

LSL-RSL and LIL-RIL Commissures

Generally, repairs of LSL-RSL and LIL-RIL commissures can be made without disturbing the commissural leaflet tissue in these areas. Occasionally, however, these commissural leaflet areas are larger than usual and handicap exposure. Then they may be incised back to the anulus, *once it is certain that this is the commissural tissue*. The tissue on the left ventricular side is incorporated into the repair along with the LSL or LIL. That on the right side should be reattached to the patch with a few sutures at the end of the repair.

Repair with Tetralogy of Fallot

In tetralogy of Fallot, the large VSD extends subaortically. The LSL bridges moderately (grade 3) or markedly (grades 4 or 5) and is not attached to the crest of the ventricular septum. Any of the types of right ventricular outflow tract obstruction associated with tetralogy of Fallot may be present (see Chapter 23), but anterior deviation of the infundibular septum is always present and must be considered in the repair. Preoperative cineangiographic studies are necessary to indicate the surgically important details of right ventricular outflow obstruction and the morphology of the pulmonary arteries.

The operation is begun as for repair of the complete AV canal defect. However, before heparinization, if a right ventricular outflow patch is required, an appropriately sized woven Dacron tube is preclotted (UAB), or adequate pericardium is removed (GLH) (see Chapter 23, "General Plan and Details Common to All Approaches" in section on Technique of Operation). The preclotted VSD patch is trimmed, with a wide superior aspect, which is important in the prevention of *left* ventricular outflow obstruction.

Usually, the anteriorly deviated parietal extension of the infundibular septum (band) can be seen through the AV valve (see Chapter 23, "Repair of Uncomplicated Tetralogy of Fallot with Pulmonary Stenosis via the Right Atrium" in section on Technique of Operation), and it is cut and mobilized. Other muscular infundibular obstructions can be visualized and resected. The pulmonary valve can be visualized, and fused commissures opened. The right ventricular outflow tract is sized with Hegar dilators.

The interventricular communication is closed by the suturing into place of the Dacron patch from this right atrial approach, sequencing the repair exactly as described for other complete AV canal defects. This sequencing is basically the same as for the repair of a typical VSD in the tetralogy. Familiarity with the atrial approach for the repair of isolated VSD (see Chapter 20) and for the repair of the VSD in simple tetralogy of Fallot (see Chapter 23), as well as familiarity with the repair of uncomplicated complete AV canal defects are important preparations for this. Stay sutures are placed as usual for transatrial repair. One important stay suture is at the area where the infundibular septum meets the septal band (trabecula septomarginalis). The repair is begun at the AV valve anulus superiorly, where the atrial septal remnant meets the anulus. This point is generally about at the commissural area between the bridging LSL and the RSL. Care must be taken that the repair does not begin too far anteriorly, in which case the right side of the surgically partitioned AV valve orifice will be too small. Because of the dextroposed aorta, the attachment of the VSD patch to the tissue over the aortic root (and beneath the commissural tissue and RSL) is particularly important. The patch is generally beneath (on the *left* ventricular side of) the chordae attached to the right extremity of the bridging LSL and beneath this leaflet itself. Since this leaflet is to be attached to the VSD patch, some or all of these chordae may be cut to facilitate exposure. The suture line is then carried down toward the base of the RIL as described earlier for the usual complete AV canal defect. The remainder of the AV canal defect is repaired as described earlier.

The right ventricular outflow tract is again sized with Hegar dilators. If it is adequate nothing further is done. Otherwise, the right ventricular outflow tract is enlarged by the incision of the infundibulum and, if necessary, the pul-

monary ring and the positioning of an outflow tract patch (see Chapter 23, "General Plan and Details Common to All Approaches" in section on Technique of Operation; "Post Repair $P_{RV/LV}$: Its Use and Predictions" in section on Special Situations and Controversies).

Repair with Double-Outlet Right Ventricle

When the interventricular communication is large and subaortic, the configuration and insertion of the interventricular patch is similar to that just described for the tetralogy of Fallot. Pulmonary stenosis, when coexisting, is treated similarly.

When the interventricular communication is *not* subaortic and cannot be converted into one by septal excision (see Chapter 40), a Fontan repair (see Chapter 26) is necessary if pulmonary stenosis coexists.

Repair with Transposition of the Great Arteries

The repair of the AV canal defect is completed in the usual fashion up to the point that the pericardial interatrial patch is trimmed and incorporated. Then the pericardial patch is trimmed to be a combination of the one usually used and that used for interatrial transposition of venous return by Mustard's technique (see Chapter 39). The patch is sewn into place as a baffle for effecting an atrial "switch" but connected to the upper edge of the interventricular patch and base of RIL, as described, rather than to the anterior limbus.

As an alternative, the usual repair of the AV canal defect can be carried out, and an arterial switch operation performed (see Chapter 39). This may be particularly advisable if the right AV valve has been left somewhat small.

Repair with Left Ventricular Outflow Tract Obstruction

Left ventricular outflow tract obstruction, an uncommon concomitant or late postoperative complication of AV canal defects, has a variable morphology and thus a variable surgical treatment. When it results from valvar excrescences protruding into the left ventricular outflow tract, or when the morphology is that of discrete subvalvar stenosis, the obstruction can be excised through the aortic root (see Chapter 32). Occasionally, it results from diffuse subvalvar narrowing. For this situation, a right ventriculotomy incision is made, and then the LV outflow tract is entered through an incision in the infundibular septum *exactly parallel* to the LV outflow tract. This incision is best made after the opening of the aortic root and the insertion of an instrument or a finger to protect the aortic valve cusps. Through the LV outflow tract incision, part of the obstructing muscle can be excised. The entire area is then enlarged by closing the septal incision with a patch of woven Dacron (see Chapter 32, Fig. 32-22).

The encroachment of the left AV valve on the left ventricular outflow tract (Figs. 19-5a, 19-10) plays a role in all types of left ventricular outflow tract obstruction in AV canal defects. Consequently, left AV valve replacement may accentuate or produce subaortic stenosis. The left AV valve replacement prosthesis can be kept away from the subaortic area by a rectangular piece of Dacron attached to the anulus of the left AV valve in the subaortic area. The prosthesis is then sutured to this artificial mitral-aortic anulus and to the natural anulus for the rest of the circumference.

SPECIAL FEATURES OF POSTOPERATIVE CARE

The usual care, as described in Chapter 2, is accorded patients after repair of AV canal defects, but certain features require emphasis. Because of the complexity of the repair and in spite of the generally good results now obtained, constant vigilance must be exercised to detect any important imperfections in the repair. Thus, the use of an indicator-dilution curve is advantageous a few hours after the patients' return to the intensive care unit, to verify complete closure of the interatrial and interventricular communications. A left atrial pressure more than 6 mmHg higher than right atrial pressure raises the possibility of either severe left AV valve incompetence or stenosis, although it can result simply from the small size and low compliance of the left ventricle (see Chapter 5, footnote 8). The height of the V wave is *not* helpful, because, as in all circumstances, this correlates more with the height of the mean left atrial pressure than with the degree of incompetence.

If the condition of the patient is not optimal and important residual left AV valve incompetence is suspected, and particularly if deterioration continues over several hours, left ventriculographic studies (or some other reliable method of quantitating left AV valve incompetence) should be considered. Indirect indications, both in the operating room and early postoperatively (including absence of a murmur) are not reliable. If severe incompetence is demonstrated, reoperation is indicated. Likewise, if the patient's condition is unsatisfactory and a large residual left-to-right shunt is present, reoperation is indicated.

When the patient does not thrive and convalesce normally, left ventriculographic studies before hospital dismissal are indicated. Since left AV valve repair failure predisposes the patient to death within the first year after operation, consideration should be given to early reoperation if severe incompetence is found.

EARLY RESULTS

The early results have been excellent for 20 years for the repair of partial AV canal defects without important left AV valve incompetence[M7,R2] and for those few patients with complete AV canal defects who reach the age of 2–5 years without important AV valve incompetence and without severe pulmonary vascular disease.[M2] When operation was required in infancy or when significant AV valve incompetence was present, the results in earlier years were suboptimal, but in recent years, the hospital mortality in this group has also been low.[B12,M6,S2]

Hospital Mortality

Currently, the risk of hospital death approaches zero for most patients with *uncomplicated partial AV canal defect*

(without accessory AV valve orifice or major associated cardiac anomaly and with little or no left AV incompetence) even when they are importantly symptomatic. Thus, when New York Heart Association (NYHA) class is III, hospital mortality under such circumstances currently is estimated to be 0.6% (CL 0.2%–1.4%; Fig. 19-23). It is a little higher (4%, CL 2%–7%) when considerable preoperative left AV valve incompetence (grade 4) is present. This is consistent with the actual UAB and GLH experiences in the current era (see later discussion of *date of operation* in "Incremental Risk Factors for Hospital Death").

Currently, the risk of hospital death after *repair of complete AV canal defects* does not approach zero, probably because operation is so frequently required in the first year of life in babies seriously ill and with morphologically difficult complete AV canal defects (Table 19-13). However, results have improved over those obtained earlier, and the estimated risk of hospital death in the current era when AV valve incompetence is absent or mild is 5% (CL 3%–10%) and 13% (CL 8%–20%) when it is more severe (Fig. 19-24). These estimates are compatible with current experiences, in which there is no incremental risk of young age (Table 19-14).

Hospital mortality is increased under many circumstances, as is indicated in the discussion of incremental risk factors, and these result in an increased risk in patients with many types of major associated cardiac anomalies (Table 19-15).

Mode of Death

Approximately three-fourths of the hospital deaths are in acute cardiac failure (Table 19-16).

Incremental Risk Factors for Hospital Death

The *date of operation* is in most institutions an important determinant of risk, as the results have improved with time.[B1,S2] For example, at UAB, results in recent years have been demonstrated (Table 19-17) to be better than in earlier years (Figs. 19-23, 19-24; Tables 19-14, 19-18). Improved results in recent years have been due largely to improved intraoperative management.

Age at operation has been an incremental risk factor in the past[B3,M2] (Table 19-17), but currently, under appropriate circumstances, it is not (Figs. 19-23, 19-24).[B1,S2] It is not certain from the total combined UAB-GLH experience (Table 19-19) that this would be the case if a large number of infants operated on in the first 3 months of life was included. Very young age continues to pose special problems, and the neutralization of its incremental risk requires special knowledge of the malformation and infant cardiac surgery in general.

Severe preoperative AV valve incompetence increases the risk of operation (Table 19-17, Fig. 19-25, Table 19-20), no doubt because it increases the probability of valve repair failure. This in turn affects cardiac performance adversely and contributes to hospital mortality. Thus, one factor contributing to the lower hospital mortality in recent years has been the improvement of surgical methods for managing the incompetence.

Increasing levels of disability preoperatively, as reflected

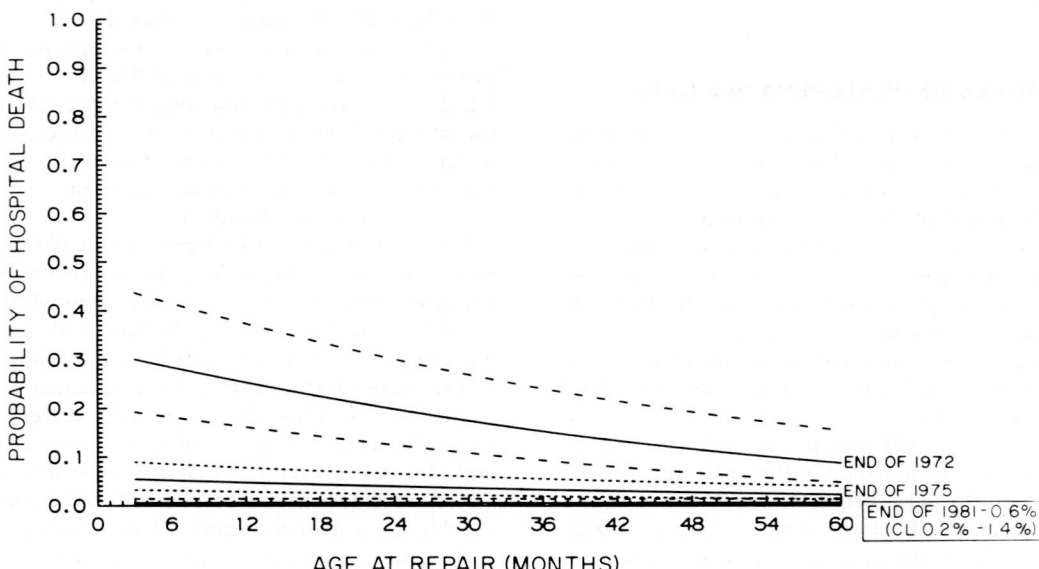

Figure 19-23 Probability of hospital death according to age at operation after repair of partial AV canal defects. (See Table 19-17 for the logistic equation for which this nomogram is a solution under the conditions specified: date of operation, end of 1972, 1975, and 1981; preoperative left AV valve incompetence grade 2; NYHA class III; no accessory valve orifice.) The dashed lines are the 70% confidence limits around the solid lines. Note the mortality of 0.6% in 1981 (representing the current era), unaffected by age.

Reproduced with permission from Studer et al.[S2]

Table 19-13 Hospital and late mortality and reoperation after repair of complete AV canal defects (GLH; 1971–1983).

Age at Operation (months)			Hospital Deaths			Late Deaths	Reoperation
≤	<	n	No.	%	CL		
1 --- 3		2	1	50%	7%–93%	0	0
3 --- 6		5	2	40%	14%–71%	0	0
6 --- 12		6	0	0%	0%–27%	1	1
12 --- 24		2	0	0%	0%–61%	0	0
24 --- 60		4	0	0%	0%–38%	0	1
60 --- 72		2	2	100%	39%–100%	0	0
Total		21	5	24%	14%–37%	1	2(12%;[a] CL 4%–27%)
$P(\chi^2)$				.04			

KEY: CL, 70% confidence limits.

NOTE: The hospital mortality has been similar throughout the period. The one late death was with left AV valve stenosis. Both reoperations were for left AV valve incompetence, one from extensive late chordal rupture of the left superior and inferior leaflets and the other from detachment of the leaflets from the pericardial patch.

[a] Percentage of 16 hospital survivors.

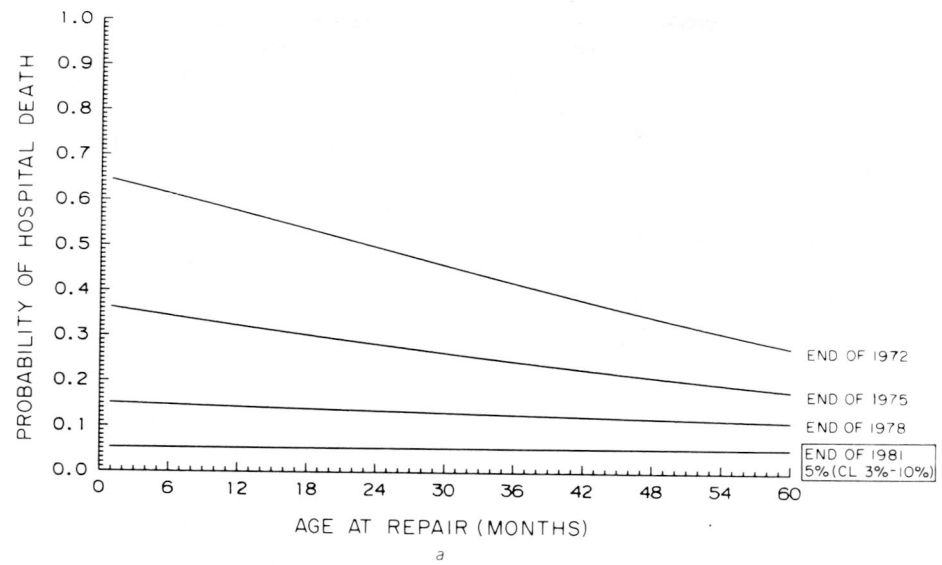

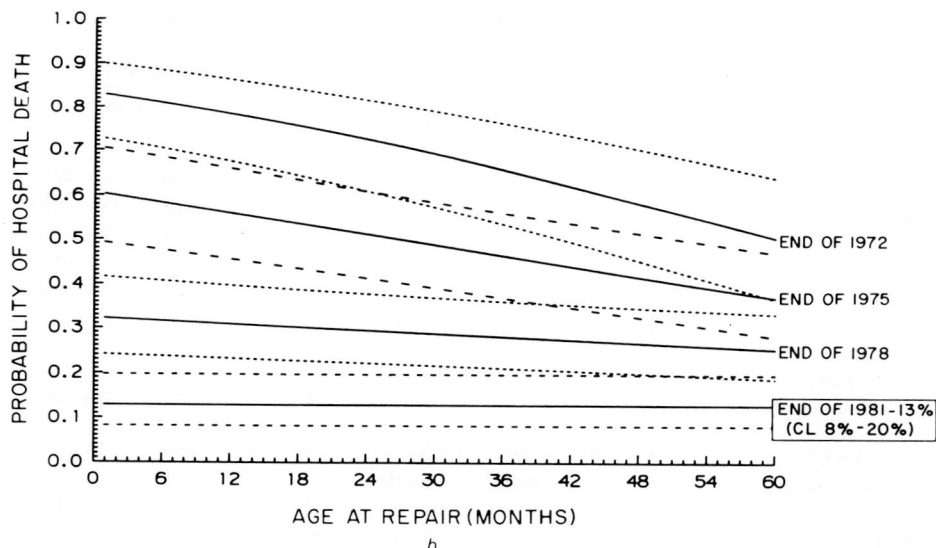

Figure 19-24 Probability of hospital death after repair of complete AV canal defects. The presentation is as in Figure 19-23.

(a) Patients with grade 2 AV valve incompetence and in NYHA class III. Note that by 1981 hospital mortality was 5% and unaffected by age at operation (70% confidence limits are available in the original source but not shown).

(b) Patients with important (grade 4) AV valve incompetence and in NYHA class III. Note that by the end of 1981 hospital mortality was 13%, and unaffected by age at operation.

Reproduced with permission from Studer et al.[S2]

Table 19-14 Hospital mortality in the current era after repair of AV canal defects without major associated cardiac anomalies (UAB; 1981).[S2]

Age (months)	Without Interventricular Communication				With Interventricular Communication			
		Hospital Deaths				Hospital Deaths		
≤ <	n	No.	%	CL	n	No.	%	CL
3	1	0	0%		1	0	0%	
3 --- 6	0				2	0	0%	
6 --- 12	1	0	0%		5	0	0%	
12 --- 24	1	0	0%		3	1	33%	
24 --- 48	1	0	0%		2	0	0%	
48	6	0	0%		3	1	33%	
Total	10	0	0%	0%–17%	16	2	12%	4%–27%
$P(\chi^2)$							.6	

KEY: CL, 70% confidence limits.

Table 19-15 Hospital mortality in patients with major associated cardiac anomalies (UAB; 1967–1982).

Major Associated Cardiac Anomaly[a]	Without Interventricular Communication				With Interventricular Communication			
		Hospital Deaths				Hospital Deaths		
	n	No.	%	CL	n	No.	%	CL
DQRV without PS					6	2	33%	12%–62%
DORV + PS					3	3	100%	53%–100%
TF					20	6	30%	19%–44%
TGA					1	0	0%	0%–85%
TAPVC					2	1	50%	7%–93%
PS	1	0	0%	0%–85%				
LV outflow obstruction	2	1	50%	7%–93%				
Supravalvular MS					1	0	0%	0%–85%
Completely unroofed CS	5	0	0%	0%–32%	4	1	25%	3%–63%
Ebstein's malformation	1	1	100%	15%–100%				
Additional VSDs	1	0	0%	0%–85%	4	3	75%	37%–97%
PDA	2	0	0%	0%–61%	29	12	41%	31%–53%
Coarctation					1	1	100%	15%–100%
Dextrocardia with situs solitus					1	1	100%	15%–100%
Situs ambiguus	1	0	0%	0%–85%	6	2	33%	12%–62%
Situs inversus	1	0	0%	0%–85%	2	1	50%	7%–93%
Total patients	14	2	14%	5%–31%	59	22	37%	30%–45%

KEY: CL, 70% confidence limits; CS, coronary sinus; DORV, double-outlet right ventricle; LV, left ventricular; MS, mitral stenosis; PDA, patent ductus arteriosus; PS, pulmonary stenosis; TAPVC, total anomalous pulmonary venous connection; TF, tetralogy of Fallot; TGA, transposition of the great arteries; VSD, ventricular septal defect.

[a] Categories are not mutually exclusive.

Table 19-16 Mode of death after repair of AV canal defects of all types, with or without associated cardiac anomalies (UAB; 1967–1982; n = 310).

Mode of Death	No.	% of 51
Cardiac	39	76%
Acute cardiac failure	35	69%
Chronic cardiac failure with multiple subsystem failure	3	6%
Arrhythmic death	1	2%
Pulmonary dysfunction	6	12%
Hemorrhagic pulmonary edema without elevated left atrial pressure	1	2%
Hemorrhage[a]	2	4%
Sepsis	1	2%
Metabolic[b]	1	2%
Sudden[c]	1	2%
Total	51	100%

[a] One patient died acutely with hemorrhagic diathesis; one died of prolonged hemorrhagic diathesis on postoperative day 8.

[b] Severe hyperpyrexia and hyperkalemia with good hemodynamic conditions.

[c] On the third postoperative day (patient was 10 years old, with severe pulmonary vascular disease).

in the NYHA functional class, increases hospital mortality (Table 19-17, Fig. 19-25, Table 19-21). This has been true in many other types of cardiac surgery and in infant cardiac surgery in general.[K12]

The *presence of an interventricular communication* (i.e., complete AV canal as opposed to a partial AV canal) has increased the hospital mortality through the years (Tables 19-17, 19-20, 19-22), although as preoperative and intraoperative methods have improved, these differences in hospital mortality have become smaller. The size of the interventricular communication has not been a risk factor,[S2] although it may be doubted that small interventricular com-

munications between thick chordae impose the same risks as large ones.

If it is chosen to classify cases of AV canal defect according to whether there is a *common AV valve orifice* or two AV valve orifices, it is again true that the complete AV canal defect (that with a common AV valve orifice, in this context) carries a higher risk of hospital death after repair than does the partial AV canal defect with two AV valve orifices (Table 19-22). The repair is certainly more complex in patients with a common AV valve orifice and large interventricular communication.

The presence of an *accessory left AV valve orifice* has increased the risk of hospital death in the past[C2,S2] (Table 19-17), probably because these valves tend to be narrow or incompetent or both, particularly after repair. Current surgical techniques may reduce these risks.

Hypoplasia of left or right ventricles, particularly of the former, which is more common and often more severe, is an important risk factor for hospital death after complete repair (Table 19-23, Fig. 19-26).[S2] Clearly, the risk of hospital death becomes excessive when the RV/LV ratio exceeds about 2.0 (significant LV hypoplasia). Under such circumstances, anatomic repair is contraindicated.

Heart Block

Since Lev described in 1958 the architecture of the conduction system in AV canal defects, surgically induced permanent complete heart block has been avoidable. In fact, its incidence has approached zero. At GLH, the second patient operated on in 1959 developed permanent complete heart block, but this has not occurred since then, regardless of the presence of associated defects or left AV valve replacement (0 in 103, 0%, CL 0%–1.9%). At UAB, the experience has been similar (Table 19-24). Currently, the presence of associated cardiac anomalies does not increase the risk of heart block.

When left AV valve replacement is required in AV canal defects, heart block has occurred more frequently (at UAB

Table 19-17 Incremental risk factors for hospital death after repair of AV canal defects of all types (UAB; 1967–1982; 51 deaths among 310 patients).[S2]

Incremental Risk Factors[a]	Logistic Coefficient ± SD	P Value
Date of operation (months from January 1, 1967)[b]	−0.033 ± 0.0069	< .0001
Age at operation (months)[b]	−0.047 ± 0.0165	.004
Interaction of age with date of operation[b]	0.00029 ± 0.000108	.008
Increasing severity of left AV valve incompetence (0–5)[b]	0.5 ± 0.22	.03
Increasing level of disability (NYHA class I–V)[b]	0.9 ± 0.27	.001
Interventricular communication present	1.4 ± 0.50	.005
Accessory valve orifice present	1.8 ± 0.73	.01
Intercept	−2.0 ± 0.52	

[a] Does not include variables from preoperative catheterization or cineangiographic studies.

[b] Use only if major associated cardiac anomaly is *not* present.

Table 19-18 Hospital death according to age, after primary repair of partial AV canal defects without major associated cardiac anomalies (GLH, UAB). Patients with common atrium are included.

| Age (years) | | UAB (1967–1982) | | | | GLH (1959–1982) | | | | Total | | | |
| | | | Hospital Deaths | | | | Hospital Deaths | | | | Hospital Deaths | | |
≤	<	n	No.	%	CL	n	No.	%	CL	n	No.	%	CL
	3/12	1	0	0%	0%–85%	1	0	0%	0%–85%	2	0	0%	0%–61%
3/12 ---	6/12	4	2	50%	18%–82%					4	2	50%	18%–82%
6/12 ---	1	3	0	0%	0%–47%	1	0	0%	0%–85%	4	0	0%	0%–38%
12 ---	2	8	1	12%	2%–36%	3	0	0%	0%–47%	11	1	9%	1%–28%
2 ---	4	12	1	8%	1%–26%	1	0	0%	0%–85%	13	1	8%	1%–24%
4 ---	5	6	0	0%	0%–27%	5	1	20%	3%–53%	11	1	9%	1%–28%
5 ---	10	33	1	3%	0.4%–10%	22	0	0%	0%–8%	55	1	2%	0.2%–6%
10 ---	20	34	0	0%	0%–6%	22	0	0%	0%–8%	56	0	0%	0%–3%
20 ---	30	15	0	0%	0%–12%	8	1	12%	2%–37%	23	1	4%	0.6%–14%
30		24	0	0%	0%–8%	10	1	10%	1%–30%	34	1	3%	0.4%–10%
Total		140	5	3.6%	2.0%–6.0%	73[a]	3	4%	2%–8%	213	8	3.8%	2.4%–5.6%
$P(\chi^2)$				.0003				.5				.0006	
P(logistic)				.08									

KEY: CL, 70% confidence limits.

[a] At GLH, 1967–1983, 1 hospital death (2%, CL 3%–8%) occurred, in 1969, among 42 patients.

in 4 of 20 patients, 20%, CL 10%–33%).[S2] This increased incidence is due to the fact that in this malformation sutures placed in the left AV valve ring at about the 2-o'clock position overlie the AV node. A fringe of AV valve tissue must be left in this area so the valve replacement sutures can be placed in the fringe and, more anteriorly, in the interatrial pericardial patch rather than the anulus. With these precautions, complete heart block should be avoidable in such situations.

LATE RESULTS

Unless there has been failure of the AV valve repair or significant pulmonary vascular disease, the late results of operation have been good and essentially curative in all varieties of AV canal defects.

Survival

Late survival has been closely related to the severity preoperatively of AV valve incompetence, and not to the presence of an interventricular communication or major associated cardiac anomalies (Table 19-25, Fig. 19-27). In fact, among 19 late deaths occurring in 258 traced hospital survivors, 14 were related to failure of the AV valve repair and 2 were in patients with persistent severe pulmonary vascular disease (UAB).[S2] The effect of failure of the AV valve repair is particularly evident from the actuarial plot of survival in patients with and without AV valve repair failure (Fig. 19-28).

Functional Status

Most long-term survivors are in excellent health. Eighty-eight percent of surviving patients in the UAB experience are in NYHA functional class I, and 11% are in class II.

Table 19-19 Hospital death according to age after repair of complete AV canal defects without major associated cardiac anomalies (UAB, GLH).

| Age (years) | | UAB (1967–1982) | | | | GLH (1959–1982) | | | | Total | | | |
| | | | Hospital Deaths | | | | Hospital Deaths | | | | Hospital Deaths | | |
≤	<	n	No.	%	CL	n	No.	%	CL	n	No.	%	CL
	3/12	7	3	43%	20%–68%	4	3	75%	37%–97%	11	6	55%	35%–73%
3/12 ---	6/12	10	2	20%	7%–41%	5	2	40%	14%–71%	15	4	27%	14%–43%
6/12 ---	1	19	5	26%	15%–41%	8	0	0%	0%–21%	27	5	19%	11%–29%
1 ---	2	29	8	28%	18%–30%	3	0	0%	0%–47%	32	8	25%	17%–35%
2 ---	4	9	1	11%	1%–33%	4	0	0%	0%–38%	13	1	8%	1%–24%
4 ---	10	6	2	33%	12%–62%	7	3	43%	20%–68%	13	5	38%	23%–57%
10		7	1	14%	2%–41%	1	0	0%	0%–85%	8	1	12%	2%–36%
Total		87	22	21%	14%–29%	32	8	25%	17%–35%	119	30	25%	21%–30%
$P(\chi^2)$				.8				.05				.14	

KEY: CL, 70% confidence limits.

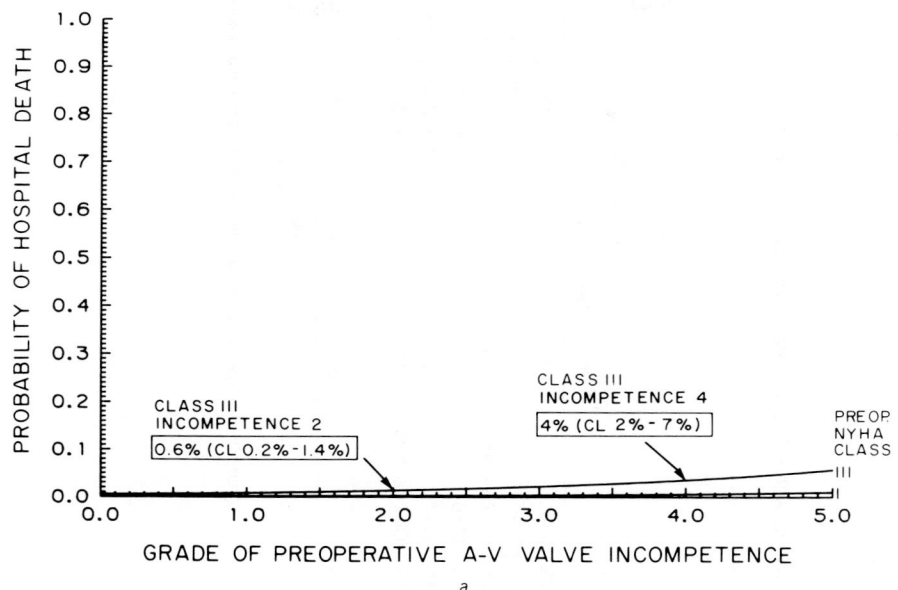

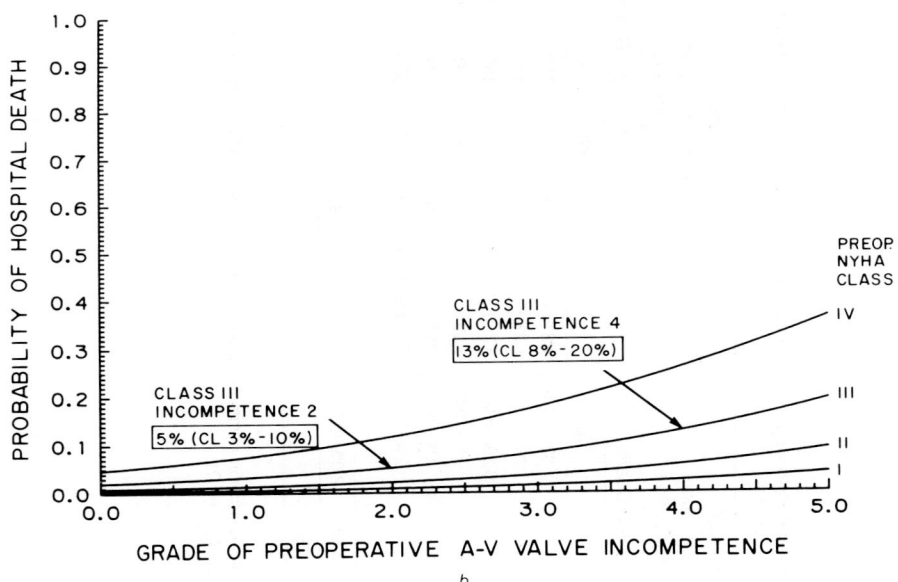

Figure 19-25 Hospital mortality in the current era (date of operation, end of 1981) according to the NYHA class and severity (grade) of preoperative AV valve incompetence (from Table 19-17). The 70% confidence limits are available in the original source but not shown.

(a) Patients with partial AV canal defects. Only NYHA classes I and III are shown.

(b) Patients with complete AV canal defects.

Reproduced with permission from Studer et al.[S2]

Table 19-20 Hospital mortality related to degree of preoperative left AV valve incompetence in patients with AV canal defects without major associated cardiac anomalies (UAB; 1967–1982; n = 237).[S2]

Grade of Preoperative AV Valve Incompetence	Without Interventricular Communication					With Interventricular Communication					Total				
	n	Hospital Deaths No.	%	CL	Grouped	n	Hospital Deaths No.	%	CL	Grouped	n	Hospital Deaths No.	%	CL	Grouped
0	13	0	0%	0%–14%	1/81	9	1	11%	1%–33%	5/40	22	1	5%	0.6%–15%	6/121
1 mild	25	0	0%	0%–7%	1.2%[a] (CL 0.2%–4.1%)	8	1	12%	2%–36%	12%[b] (CL 7%–20%)	33	1	3%	0.4%–10%	5.0%[c] (CL 3.0%–7.9%)
2 } Moderate	43	1	2%	0.3%–8%		23	3	13%	6%–25%		66	4	6%	3%–11%	
3	35	2	6%	2%–13%	4/59	35	10	29%	20%–39%	17/56	70	12	17%	12%–23%	21/115
4 } Severe	16	1	6%	1%–20%	7%[a] (CL 3%–12%)	18	6	33%	21%–48%	30%[b] (CL 24%–38%)	34	7	21%	13%–30%	18%[c] (CL 14%–23%)
5	8	1	12%	2%–36%		3	1	33%	4%–76%		11	2	18%	6%–38%	
Unknown						1	0				1	0			
Total	140	5	3.6%	2.0%–6.0%		97	22	23%	18%–28%		237	27	11%	9%–14%	
P(logistic)			.06					.07					.005		

KEY: CL, 70% confidence limits.

NOTE: Of 140 patients without an interventricular communication, 59 (42%, CL 38%–47%) had left AV incompetence ⩾ grade 3; of 97 patients with an interventricular communication, 56 (58%, CL 53%–64%) had this (1 unknown). $P(\chi^2) = .01$.

[a] $P(\text{Fisher}) = .1$.

[b] $P(\chi^2) = .04$.

[c] $P(\chi^2) = .001$.

Table 19-21 Hospital mortality according to preoperative functional class in patients with AV canal defects without major associated cardiac anomalies (UAB; 1967–1982; $n = 237$).

Preoperative NYHA Class	Without Interventricular Communication				With Interventricular Communication				Total			
		Hospital Deaths				Hospital Deaths				Hospital Deaths		
	n	No.	%	CL	n	No.	%	CL	n	No.	%	CL
I	46	0	0%	0%–4%	17	1	6%	1%–19%	63	1	1.6%	0.2%–5.3%
II	60	0	0%	0%–3%	36	6	17%	10%–26%	96	6	6%	4%–10%
III	27	5	19%	11%–29%	34	10	29%	21%–40%	61	15	25%	19%–32%
IV	7	0	0%	0%–24%	10	5	50%	30%–70%	17	5	29%	17%–45%
V												
Total	140	5	3.6%	2.0%–6.0%	97	22	23%	18%–28%	237	27	11%	9%–14%
P(logistic)		.01				.006				< .001		

KEY: CL, 70% confidence limits.

AV Valve Repair Failure

Only routine left ventriculographic studies immediately after operation and again 1–12 months postoperatively allow a precise estimate of the proportion of patients in whom the repair has failed to achieve a reasonably competent and non-stenotic left AV valve. However, some reasonably reliable estimates are possible. Criteria of AV valve repair failure used in an earlier study[S2] are shown in Table 19-26.

About 10% of patients with partial AV canal defects have AV valve repair failure early or late postoperatively; thus, in the combined UAB-GLH series of 210 traced patients, 22 (11%, CL 8%–13%) had this complication (GLH data in Table 19-27). McMullan and colleagues reported an incidence of 25% (CL 21%–30%) in an early experience at the Mayo Clinic,[M7] and other similar experiences are reported in the literature.[L6,L7] It is noteworthy that AV valve repair failure occasionally occurred in patients who preoperatively had no more than mild incompetence (Table 19-28).

At UAB, 15 (10%, CL 7%–13%) of 156 patients with the complete AV canal defect had this complication. However, the multivariate analysis and most surgeons' experiences show that the risk of AV valve repair failure is greater in patients with partial AV canal defects than in those with complete ones.

In all subsets, left AV valve repair failure is more likely to occur when preoperative AV valve incompetence is severe (Tables 19-28, 19-29, Fig. 19-29).

The current risks of AV valve repair failure, with techniques used up until 1982, are less than in earlier experiences,[S2] in part because of the use of reinforced leaflet attachment methods[B18,R9] (Table 19-29).

Pulmonary Hypertension

When important pulmonary hypertension is present preoperatively, it can be expected to regress postoperatively if the pulmonary blood flow was large and the patient was less than about 2 years of age at the time of operation.[B1,C2,C5,L3] No doubt these interrelationships are the same as those described in more detail for patients with ventricular septal defects (see Chapter 20, Figs. 20-35, 20-36, 20-37, 20-38, 20-39).

Table 19-22 Hospital mortality according to anatomic category in patients with AV canal defects without major associated cardiac anomalies (UAB; 1967–1982; $n = 237$).

Category	n	Hospital Deaths			P for Difference
		No.	%	CL	
Absence of interventricular communication	140	5	3.6%	2.0%–6.0%	
Presence of interventricular communication	97	22	23%	18%–28%	
Total	237	27	11%	9%–14%	< .0001
Two AV valve orifices	154[a]	8	5.2%	3.4%–7.8%	
Common AV valve orifice	83	19	23%	18%–29%	
Total	237	27	11%	9%–14%	< .0001

KEY: CL, 70% confidence limits.

NOTE: The phrase *partial AV canal defect* may mean the absence of an interventricular communication or the presence of two AV valve orifices. Note that the number of patients with partial AV canal defects varies depending on which definition is chosen.

[a] Fourteen patients with two AV valve orifices had interventricular communications (three died).

Table 19-23 Hospital mortality after repair of AV canal defects of all types in patients with reviewed cineangiograms (UAB; 1967–1982; n = 142).

RV/LV Ratio	LV/RV Ratio (Inverted RV/LV Ratio)	n	No.	%	CL
					Hospital Deaths
0.7	1.4	1		0%	⎫
0.8	1.25	6	2	33%	⎬ 4/21 = 19%(CL 10%–32%)
0.9	1.1	14	2	14%	⎭
1.0		24	3	12%	⎫
1.1		20	2	10%	⎪ $P(\chi^2)$ = .8
1.2		19	3	16%	⎪
1.3		16	1	6%	⎬ 17/102 = 17%(CL 13%–21%)
1.4		17	5	29%	⎪
1.5		6	3	50%	⎭
1.6					
1.7		1		0%	⎫
1.8		4	2	50%	⎪ $P(\chi^2)$ = .0001
1.9					
2.0		7	3	43%	
2.1					
2.2					
2.3					
2.4					11/19 = 58%(CL 43%–71%)
2.5		4	4	100%	⎬
.					
.					
3.0		2	1	50%	
.					
.					
4.0		1	1	100%	⎭
Total		142	32	23%	

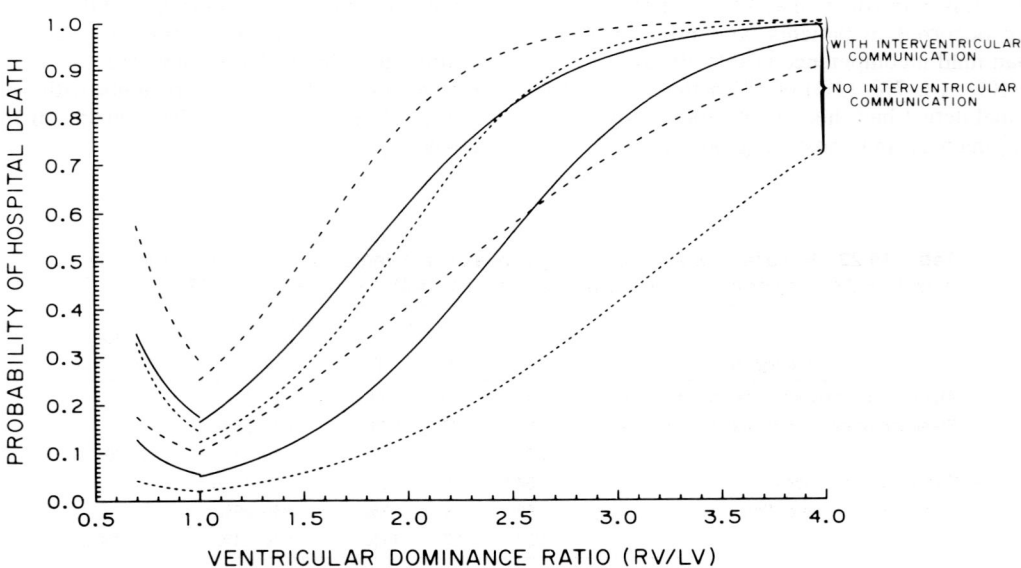

Figure 19-26 Nomogram of hospital mortality after repair of AV canal defects according to the ventricular dominance (see the original source for details of variables examined and of the logistic regression equation for the nomogram).

Reproduced with permission from Studer et al.[S2]

Table 19-24 Complete heart block after repair in patients with AV canal defects without major associated cardiac anomalies (UAB; 1967–1982).[S2]

Category	n	No.	%	CL	
		Complete Heart Block			
Without interventricular communication	135	0	0%	0%–1.4%	
With interventricular communication	96	1[a]	1.0%	0.1%–3.5%	P = .4
Total[b]	231	1	0.4%	0.06%–1.5%	

KEY: CL, 70% confidence limits.

[a] Date of operation October 27, 1976.

[b] Seventy-two additional patients had major associated cardiac anomalies; three developed heart block. Six additional patients had primary AV valve replacement; one developed heart block. One additional patient had heart block preoperatively.

INDICATIONS FOR OPERATION

The presence of an AV canal defect indicates for operation, since an important hemodynamic derangement is nearly always present, and spontaneous repair does not occur.

In partial AV canal defects, pulmonary hypertension is usually absent, and the optimal age for operation is 2–4 years (GLH) or, alternatively, 1–2 years (UAB). This indication is the same as for patients with fossa ovalis types of atrial septal defects (see Chapter 15). When congestive heart failure or severe growth failure is evident earlier in life, opera-

Table 19-25 Incremental risk factors for late death among hospital survivors of the repair of AV canal defects of all types (UAB; 1967–1982; 19 deaths, 258 traced hospital survivors).[S2]

Incremental Risk Factor	Cox Coefficient ± SD	P Value
Severe preoperative AV valve incompetence (grades 0–5)	0.5 ± 0.22	.03
Poor preoperative functional status (NYHA class I–IV)	0.7 ± 0.27	.008
Accessory AV valve orifice	1.4 ± 0.77	.06
Down's syndrome	1.5 ± 0.71	.04

tion is indicated at that time. Under such circumstances, moderate or severe left AV valve repair failure is usually present, and pulmonary artery pressure may be increased.

Operation is indicated in the first year of life for complete AV canal defects. When the infant's general condition is good, the repair can be done electively at about 6 months of age. When refractory congestive heart failure or severe growth failure is evident at an earlier age, repair must be done at that time.

Major associated cardiac anomalies change both the indications and timing for operation. Thus, the management of patients in such categories must be individualized (see "Major Associated Cardiac Anomalies" in Special Situations and Controversies).

The presence of Down's syndrome may alter the indications for operation (GLH).

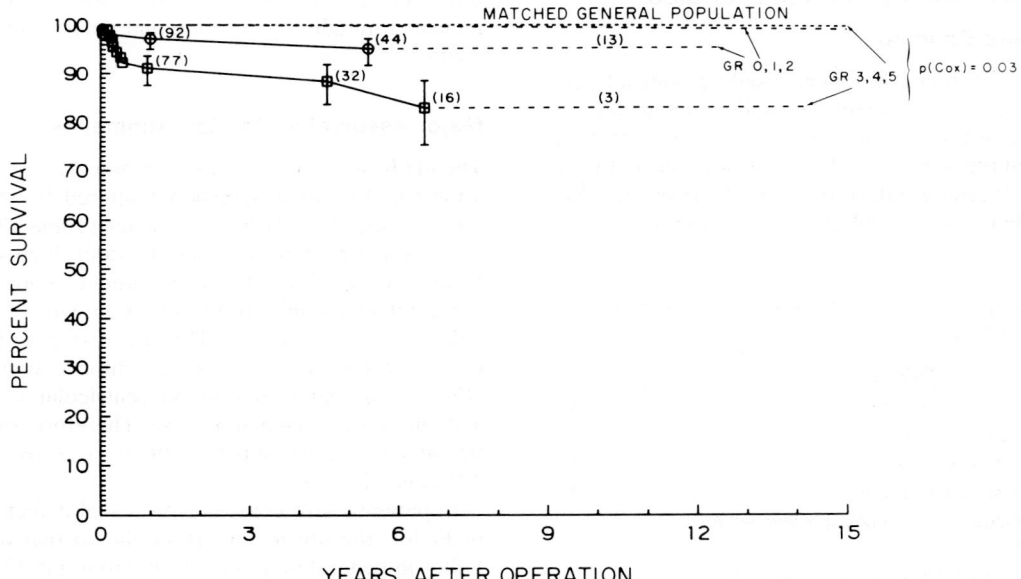

Figure 19-27 Actuarial survival of hospital survivors after repair of AV canal defects according to preoperative grade of AV valve incompetence (grades 0, 1, and 2, compared to grades 3, 4, and 5). The two interrupted lines at the top are the two age-, sex-, and race-matched general populations, matched separately for comparison with the two groups of patients. The vertical bars enclose 1 standard deviation (70% confidence limits). The numbers in parentheses are traced cases at the indicated time interval. The dashed extensions of the solid lines represent traced patients with no late deaths.

Reproduced with permission from Studer et al.[S2]

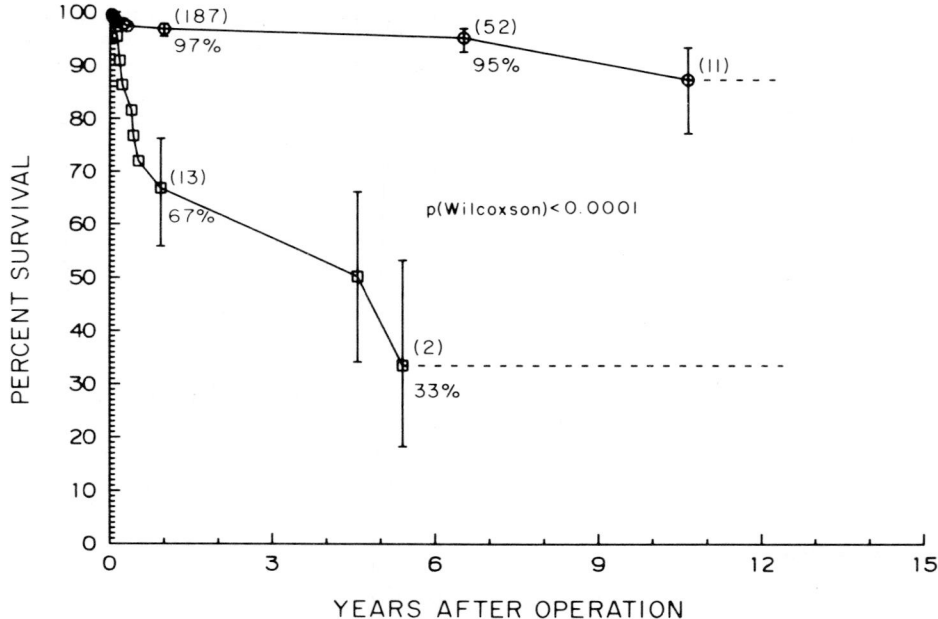

Figure 19-28 Actuarial survival of hospital survivors (*n* = 259) of repair of AV canal defects according to whether failure of the AV valve repair occurred. The open squares represent patients with AV valve repair failure (*n* = 23) and the open circles those without AV valve repair failure (*n* = 236, with one untraced patient). The two deaths after 5 postoperative years in the latter group were of patients with known severe preoperative and postoperative pulmonary vascular disease. Presentation is as in Fig. 19-27.

Reproduced with permission from Studer et al.[S2]

SPECIAL SITUATIONS AND CONTROVERSIES

Pulmonary Artery Banding

Pulmonary artery banding has been used episodically for many years as initial management for small infants with complete AV canal defects, and in recent years some excellent results have been reported.[E4,W5] This approach has not been used in the last decade at GLH and UAB.[K9] However, Silverman and colleagues, as well as Williams and associates, have demonstrated that very sick, small infants can be well managed initially by banding and deferral of repair for 1–2 years.[S10,W5]

Major Associated Cardiac Anomalies

The life history, indications, techniques, and results of operation for AV canal defects are altered by the presence of major associated cardiac anomalies (Table 19-15).

For some reason, associated patent ductus arteriosus increases hospital mortality in patients with complete AV canal defects, similar to the situation with ventricular septal defects (see Chapter 20). This increase does not seem to be due to technical problems but, rather, to the incremental effect of the patent ductus on ventricular volume overload and pulmonary vascular disease. Therefore, operation is particularly urgent when patent ductus arteriosus coexists with AV canal defects.

In patients with complete AV canal defects and tetralogy of Fallot, the life history is similar to that for tetralogy of Fallot in general unless there is important AV valve incompetence as well, when the combined malformation is much more serious. Very cyanotic infants with complete AV canal defect and tetralogy of Fallot should undergo a palliative shunting operation (see Chapter 23) unless AV valve incompetence is severe. In that case, primary repair is indicated. If a palliative operation is not required in early infancy and repair can be done electively, the age of about 2–3 years seems optimal for this. Hospital mortality to date has been

Table 19-26 Categories comprising the event AV valve repair failure (UAB; 1967–1982).[S2]

Category	n
Left AV valve replacement at first repair	6
Left AV valve repair later (21 days–14 years)	14
Re-repair for left AV valve incompetence	3
Death with valve dehiscence at autopsy	2
Death with other findings indicating postoperative left AV valve incompetence	2
Certain angiographic or clinical evidence of postoperative left AV valve incompetence	5
Total	32[a]

KEY: CL, 70% confidence limits.

NOTE: The incidence of AV valve repair failure (32 among 310 patients; 10%, CL 9%–12%) is probably less than the true incidence, because of imprecision in identifying this in patients dying in hospital.

[a] Seventeen patients had no interventricular communication; 15 had an interventricular communication.

Table 19-27 Preoperative and late postoperative degree of left AV valve (mitral) incompetence in the first 56 hospital survivors of repair of the partial AV canal defect (GLH). Those patients with moderate or severe incompetence late postoperatively were considered to have AV valve repair failure.

% of Total	Degree of Mitral Incompetence Preoperatively	No.	No.	Degree of Mitral Incompetence Postoperatively	% of Total
12% (CL 8%–19%)	Severe	7	1[a]	Severe	2% (CL 0.2%–6%)
12% (CL 8%–19%)	Moderate	7	1	Moderate	7% (CL 4%–13%)
			3		
75% (CL 68%–81%)	None or mild		6	None or mild	91% (CL 85%–95%)
		42	6		
			39		
		56	56		

KEY: CL, 70% confidence limits.

[a] Required later valve replacement.

high (30%; see Table 19-13), and although current risks may be closer to 10%,[B16] they continue to reflect the risks inherent in repair of tetralogy of Fallot (see Chapter 23) in addition to those imposed by the complexity of the combined repair. The long-term results of operation are similar to those for the repair of tetralogy of Fallot in general.

When complete AV canal with subaortic VSD is combined with double outlet right ventricle without pulmonary stenosis, the life history and indications for operation are the same for complete AV canal defect. In complete AV canal defect and double-outlet right ventricle with pulmonary stenosis the management problem is often further complicated by atrial isomerism with further associated cardiac anomalies (see chapter 46).[L5,P3] Although the mortality has been high (33%; see Table 19-15), with currently used techniques it may prove to be lower (see Chapter 40). The late results are similar to those for isolated complete AV canal defect. If pulmonary stenosis coexists, the indications and strategy of operation are the same as for complete AV canal defect with tetralogy of Fallot.

Septal Patches

There have been several reports of near fatal hemolysis from a left AV valve's regurgitant jet striking a synthetic interatrial patch after repair of AV canal defects.[H2,S1,V4] Therefore, for maximal safety, this patch should be made of pericardium.

Kawashima and colleagues reported aneurysm formation in pericardial patches used to close ventricular septal defects,[K2] although this has not been reported after repair of complete AV canal. For this reason, however, it is safest to use Dacron, Teflon, or Gore-Tex patches to close a sizable interventricular communication.

McGoon Method of Avoiding Heart Block

McGoon has for years used with success a method that basically involves keeping the suture line on the *left* and superior sides of the conduction tissue, rather than on the right side and inferiorly, as described. The patch is sutured to the LSL-LIL complex on the *left* side of its attachment to the crest of the ventricular septum. Inferiorly, the suture line goes then to the *edge* of the ostium primum defect, posterior and central (in relationship to the orifice) to the AV node and bundle of His, and posteriorly along the atrial septal edge. As Figure 19-13 shows, this method keeps the suture line to the *left* of and away from the AV node and bundle of His.

Table 19-28 AV valve repair failure after repair of all types of AV canal defects (UAB; 1967–1982).

Preoperative Left AV Valve Incompetence		n	Repair Failure		
			No.	%	CL
0		29	1	3%	0.4%–11%
1	Mild	39	0	0%	0%–5%
2	Moderate	85	4	5%	2%–8%
3		98	13	13%	10%–18%
4	Severe	43	8	19%	12%–27%
5		11	6	55%	35%–73%
	Total	305[a]	32	10.5%	8.7%–12.6%
$P(\chi^2)$				< .0001	
P(logistic)				< .0001	

KEY: CL, 70% confidence limits.

[a] In five patients, assessment of preoperative AV valve function was not available.

Table 19-29 Incremental risk factors for left AV valve repair failure (UAB; 1967–1982; 32 instances among 310 patients).

Incremental Risk Factor	Logistic Coefficient ± SD	P Value
Severity of preoperative left AV valve incompetence (grade 0–5)	0.6 ± 0.23	.006
Poor preoperative functional status (NYHA class I–V)	0.6 ± 0.24	.01
No interventricular communication	0.43 ± 0.162[a]	.008
In presence of interventricular communication, failure to use reinforced leaflet attachment[b]	1.6 ± 0.58	.004
Intercept	−6.4	

[a] Add to above coefficient before multiplying by grade of incompetence.

[b] Double-patch sandwich method or pledgetted mattress sutures for patch attachment of left superior and left inferior leaflets.

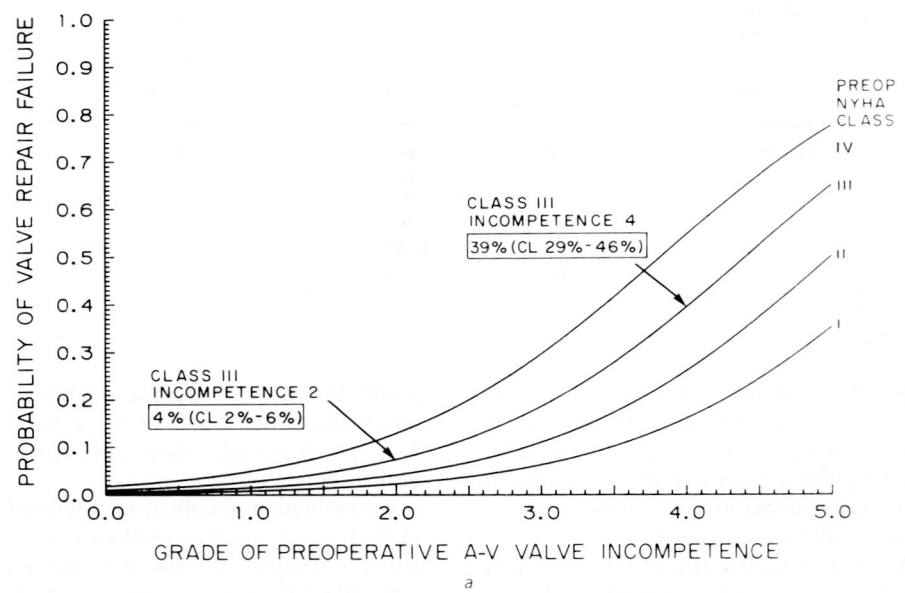

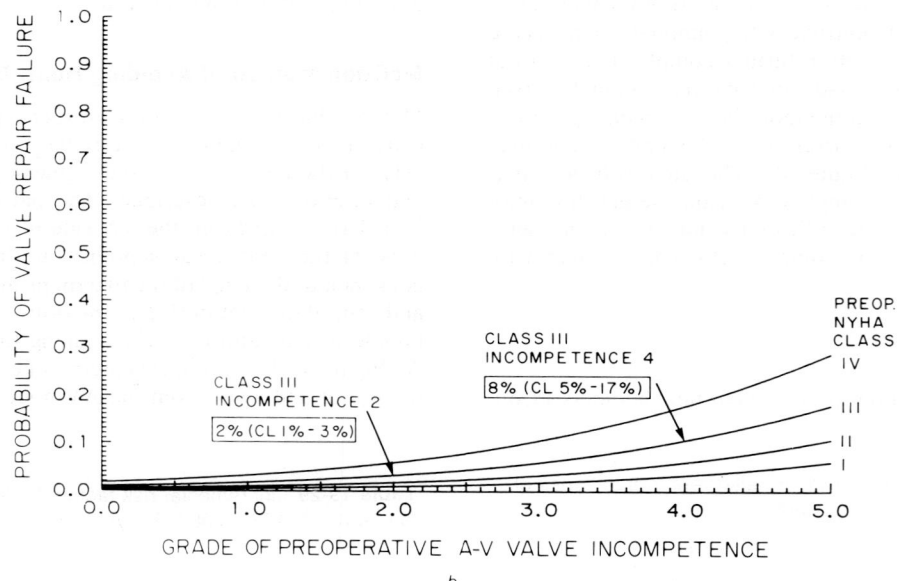

Figure 19-29 Probability of AV valve repair failure after repair of AV canal defects according to grade of preoperative AV valve incompetence and preoperative NYHA functional class. Seventy-percent confidence limits are not shown but are available in the original source (from the multivariate logistic analysis shown in Table 19-28).

(*a*) Patients with partial AV canal defects.

(*b*) Patients with complete AV canal defects.

Reproduced with permission from Studer et al.[S2]

REFERENCES

A

1. Alfieri O, Subramanian S: Successful repair of complete atrioventricular canal with undivided anterior common leaflet in a 6 month old infant. *Ann Thorac Surg* 19:92, 1975.

2. Abbott ME: *Atlas of Congenital Cardiac Disease.* New York: The American Heart Association, 1936, pp 34–35 and 50–51.

B

1. Bender HW, Hammon JW, Hubbard SG, Muirhead J, Graham TP: Repair of A-V canal malformation in the 1st year of life. *J Thorac Cardiovasc Surg* 84:515, 1982.

2. Bailey LL, Takeuchi Y, Williams WG, Trusler GA, Mustard WT: Surgical management of congenital cardiovascular anomalies with the use of profound hypothermia and circulatory arrest: Analysis of 180 consecutive cases. *J Thorac Cardiovasc Surg* 71:485, 1976.

3. Berger TJ, Kirklin JW, Blackstone EH, Pacifico AD, Kouchoukos NT: Primary repair of complete atrioventricular canal in patients less than 2 years old. *Am J Cardiol* 41:906, 1978.

4. Baron MG, Wolf BS, Steinfeld L, Van Mierop LHS: Endocardial cushion defects: Specific diagnosis by angiocardiography. *Am J Cardiol* 13:162, 1964.

5. Bharati S, Lev M: The spectrum of common atrioventricular orifice (canal). *Am Heart J* 86:533, 1973.

6. Baron MG: Abnormalities of the mitral valve in endocardial cushion defects. *Circulation* 45:672, 1972.

7. Bargeron LM, Jr, Elliott LP, Soto B, Beam PR, Curry GC: Axial cineangiography in congenital heart disease. Section I. *Circulation* 56:1075, 1977.

8. Berger TJ, Blackstone EH, Kirklin JW, Bargeron LM, Jr, Hazelrig JB, Turner ME Jr: Survival and probability of cure without and with surgery in complete atrioventricular canal. *Ann Thorac Surg* 27:104, 1979.

9. Bharati S, Lev M, McAllister HA, Jr, Kirklin JW: Surgical anatomy of the atrioventricular valve in the intermediate type of common atrioventricular orifice. *J Thorac Cardiovasc Surg* 79:884, 1980.

10. Brandt PWT, Clarkson PM, Neutze JM, Barratt-Boyes BG: Left ventricular cineangiocardiography in endocardial cushion defect (persistent common atrioventricular canal). *Australian Radiol* 16:367, 1972.

11. Barratt-Boyes BG, Calder AL: Double outlet ventricle: Classification and surgical management, in JC Davila (ed): *Second Henry Ford Hospital International Symposium on Cardiac Surgery.* New York: Appleton-Century-Crofts, 1977, p 285.

12. Barratt-Boyes BG: Correction of atrioventricular canal defects in infancy using profound hypothermia, in BG Barratt-Boyes, JM Neutze, EA Harris (eds): *Heart Disease in Infancy: Diagnosis and Surgical Treatment.* Edinburgh: Churchill Livingstone, 1973, p 110.

13. Bharati S, Kirklin JW, McAllister HA, Jr, Lev M: The surgical anatomy of common atrioventricular orifice associated with tetralogy of Fallot, double outlet right ventricle and complete regular transposition. *Circulation* 61:1142, 1980.

14. Becker AE, Anderson RH: Atrioventricular septal defects: What's in a name? *J Thorac Cardiovasc Surg* 83:461, 1982.

15. Ben-Shachar G, Moller JH, Cataneda-Zuniga W, Edwards JE: Signs of membranous subaortic stenosis appearing after correction of persistent common atrioventricular canal. *Am J Cardiol* 48:340, 1981.

16. Binet JP, Losay J, Hvass U: Tetralogy of Fallot with type C complete atrioventricular canal. *J Thorac Cardiovasc Surg* 79:761, 1980.

17. Bloom KR, Freedom RM, Williams CM, Trusler GA, Rowe RD: Echocardiographic recognition of atrioventricular valve stenosis associated with endocardial cushion defect: Pathologic and surgical correlates. *Am J Cardiol* 44:1326, 1979.

18. Bove EL, Sondheimer HM, Kavey R, Byrum CJ, Blackman MS: Results with the two-patch technique for repair of complete atrioventricular septal defect. *Ann Thorac Surg* 38:157, 1984.

19. Bharati S, Lev M, Kirklin JW: *Cardiac Surgery and the Conduction System.* New York: John Wiley & Sons, Publishers, 1983.

C

1. Cooley DA: Results of surgical treatment of atrial septal defects: Particular consideration of low defects including ostium primum and atrioventricular canal. *Am J Cardiol* 6:605, 1960.

2. Chin AJ, Keane JF, Norwood WI, Castaneda AR: Repair of complete common atrioventricular canal repair in infancy. *J Thorac Cardiovasc Surg* 84:437, 1982.

3. Cooper DKC, de Leval MR, Stark J: Results of surgical correction of persistent complete atrioventricular canal. *Thorac Cardiovasc Surg* 27:111, 1979.

4. Castaneda AR, Nicholoff DM, Moller JH, Lucas RV: Surgical correction of complete atrioventricular canal utilizing ball-valve replacement of the mitral valve: Technical considerations and results. *J Thorac Cardiovasc Surg* 62:926, 1971.

5. Culpepper W, Kolff J, Lim C-Y, Vitullo D, Lamberti J, Arcilla RA, Replogle R: Complete common atrioventricular canal in infancy: Surgical repair and postoperative hemodynamics. *Circulation* 58:550, 1978.

6. Carpentier A: Surgical anatomy and management of the mitral component of atrioventricular canal defects, in RH Anderson, EA Shinebourne (eds): *Pediatric Cardiology.* London: Churchill Livingstone, 1978, pp 477–490.

D

1. Danielson GK, McMullan MH, Kinsley RH, DuShane JW: Successful repair of complete atrioventricular canal associated with dextroversion, common atrium, and total anomalous systemic venous return. *J Thorac Cardiovasc Surg* 66:817, 1973.

2. Dubost C, Blondeau P: Canal atrio-ventriculaire et ostium primum. *J de Chirurgie* 78:241, 1959.

3. DuShane JW, Weidman WH, Brandenburg RO, Kirklin JW: Differentiation of interatrial communications by clinical methods: Ostium secundum, ostium primum, common atrium, and total anomalous pulmonary venous connection. *Circulation* 21:363, 1960.

4. d'Allaines C, Colvez P, Fevre C, Levasseur P, Facquet J, Dubost C: A rare congenital cardiopathy: Association of tetralogy of Fallot and complete A-V canal. *Arch Mal Coeur* 62:996, 1969.

5. David I, Castaneda AR, Van Praagh L: Potentially parachute mitral valve in common atrioventricular canal: Pathological anatomy and surgical importance. *J Thorac Cardiovasc Surg* 84:178, 1982.

E

1. Ellis FH, McGoon D, Kirklin JW: Surgical management of persistent common atrioventricular canal. *Am J Cardiol* 6:598, 1960.
2. Edwards JE: The problem of mitral insufficiency caused by accessory chordae tendineae in persistent common atrioventricular canal. *Proc Mayo Clin* 35:299, 1960.
3. Ellis FH Jr, Kirklin JW, Swan HJC, DuShane JW, Edwards JE: Diagnosis and surgical treatment of common atrium (cor triloculare-biventriculare). *Surgery* 45:160, 1959.
4. Epstein ML, Moller JH, Amplatz K, Nicoloff DM: Pulmonary artery banding in infants with complete atrioventricular canal. *J Thorac Cardiovasc Surg* 78:28, 1979.
5. Emanuel R, Somerville J, Inns A, Withers R: Evidence of congenital heart disease in the offspring of parents with atrioventricular defects. *Br Heart J* 49:144, 1983.
6. Edwards, JE: (1980) Personal communication.
7. Ebels T, Meijboom EJ, Anderson RH, Leeuwen MJM, Lenstra D, Eijgelaar A, Bossina KK, van der Heide JNH: Anatomic and functional "obstruction" of the outflow tract in atrioventricular septal defects with separate valve orifices ("Ostium Primum Atrial Septal Defect"): An echocardiographic study. *Am J Cardiol* 54:843, 1984.

F

1. Feldt, RH (ed): *Atrioventricular Canal Defects*. Philadelphia: Saunders, 1976.
2. Feldt RH, DuShane JW, Titus JL: The atrioventricular conduction system in persistent common atrioventricular canal defect. *Circulation* 42:437, 1970.
3. Fisher RD, Bone DK, Rowe RD, Gott VL: Complete atrioventricular canal associated with tetralogy of Fallot: Clinical experience and operative methods. *J Thorac Cardiovasc Surg* 70:265, 1975.
4. Freedom RM, Bini M, Rowe RD: Endocardial cushion defect and significant hypoplasia of the left ventricle: A distant clinical and pathological entity. *Eur J Cardiol* 7:263, 1978.

G

1. Gerbode F, Sanchez PA, Arguero R, Kerth WJ, Hill JD, deVries PA, Selzer A, Robinson SJ: Endocardial cushion defects. *Ann Surg* 166:486, 1967.
2. Gerbode F: Surgical repair of endocardial cushion defect. *Ann Chir Thorac Cardio-Vasculaire* 1:753, 1962.
3. Goor D, Lillehei CW, Edwards JE: Further observations on the pathology of the atrioventricular canal malformation. *Arch Surg* 97:954, 1968.
4. Gschnitzer F: Double mitral valve combined with an intermediate type of persistent atrioventricular canal: A contribution to surgical correction. *Thoraxchirurgie* 24:249, 1976.
5. Ghosh PK, Donnelly RJ, Hamilton DI, Wilkinson JL: Surgical correction of a case of common atrium with anomalous systemic and pulmonary venous drainage. *J Thorac Cardiovasc Surg* 74:604, 1977.
6. Goor DA, Lillehei CW: Atrioventricular canal malformations, in *Congenital Malformations of the Heart*. New York: Grune & Stratton, 1975, p 132.
7. Ibid, p 138.

H

1. Hardesty RL, Zuberbuhler JR, Bahnson HT: Surgical treatment of atrioventricular canal defect. *Arch Surg* 110:1391, 1975.

2. Hines GL, Finnerty TT, Doyle E, Isom OW: Near fatal hemolysis following repair of ostium primum atrial septal defect. *J Cardiovasc Surg* 19:7, 1978.

I

1. Ilbawi MN, Idriss FS, DeLeon SY, Riggs TW, Muster AJ, Berry TE, Paul MH: Unusual mitral valve abnormalities complicating surgical repair of endocardial cushion defects. *J Thorac Cardiovasc Surg* 85:697, 1983.

K

1. Kahn DR, Levy J, France NE, Chung KJ, Dacumos GC: Recent results after repair of atrioventricular canal. *J Thorac Cardiovasc Surg* 73:413, 1977.
2. Kawashima Y, Nakano S, Kato M, Danno M, Sato K, Manabe H: Fate of pericardium utilized for the closure of ventricular septal defect: Postoperative ventricular septal aneurysm. *J Thorac Cardiovasc Surg* 68:209, 1974.
3. Kaiser GA, Waldo AL, Bowman FO Jr, Hoffman BG, Malm JR: Specialized cardiac conduction system: Improved electrophysiologic identification at surgery. *Arch Surg* 101:673, 1970.
4. Krongrad E, Malm JR, Bowman FO Jr, Hoffman BF, Kaiser GA, Waldo AL: Electrophysiological delineation of the specialized A-V conduction system in patients with congenital heart disease. I. Delineation of the His bundle proximal to the membranous septum. *J Thorac Cardiovasc Surg* 67:875, 1974.
5. Krongrad E, Malm JR, Bowman FO, Jr, Hoffman BF, Waldo AL: Electrophysiological delineation of the specialized AV conduction system in patients with congenital heart disease. II. Delineation of the distal His bundle and the right bundle branch. *Circulation* 49:1232, 1974.
6. Kirklin JW, Daugherty GW, Burchell HB, Wood EH: Repair of the partial form of persistent common atrioventricular canal: So-called ostium primum type of atrial septal defect with interventricular communication. *Ann Surg* 142:858, 1955.
7. Krayenbugl CV, Lincoln JCR: Total anomalous systemic venous connection, common atrium, and partial atrioventricular canal. *J Thorac Cardiovasc Surg* 73:686, 1977.
8. Katz NM, Blackstone EH, Kirklin JW, Bradley EL, Lemons JE: Suture techniques for atrioventricular valves: An experimental study. *J Thorac Cardiovasc Surg* 81:528, 1981.
9. Kirklin JW, Blackstone EH: Management of the infant with complete atrioventricular canal. *J Thorac Cardiovasc Surg* 78:32, 1979.
10. Kirklin JW, DuShane JW, Patrick RT, Donald DE, Hetzel PS, Harshbarger HG, Wood EH: Intracardiac surgery with the aid of a mechanical pump-oxygenator system (Gibbon type): Report of eight cases. *Proc Staff Meet Mayo Clin* 30:201, 1955.
11. Kirklin JW, Blackstone EH, Pacifico AD, Brown RN, Bargeron LM Jr: Routine primary repair vs. two-stage repair of tetralogy of Fallot. *Circulation* 60:373, 1979.
12. Kirklin JK, Blackstone EH, Kirklin JW, McKay R, Pacifico AD, Bargeron LM Jr: Intracardiac surgery in infants under age 3 months: Incremental risk factors for hospital mortality. *Am J Cardiol* 48:500, 1981.
13. Kirklin JW, Pacifico AD, Kirklin JK: The surgical treatment of atrioventricular canal defects, in E Arciniegas (ed): *Pediatric Cardiac Surgery*. Chicago: Year Book Medical Publishers, Inc., 1985.

L

1. Lillehei CW, Cohen M, Warden HE, Varco RL: The direct-vision intracardiac correction of congenital anomalies by con-

trolled cross circulation: Results in thirty-two patients with ventricular septal defects, tetralogy of Fallot, and atrioventricularis communis defects. *Surgery* 38:11, 1955.

2. Levy MJ, Cuello L, Tuna N, Lillehei CW: Atrioventricularis communis. Clinical aspects and surgical treatment. *Am J Cardiol* 14:587, 1964.

3. Lillehei CW, Anderson RC, Ferlic RM, Bonnabeau RC, Jr: Persistent common atrioventricular canal: Recatheterization results in 37 patients following intracardiac repair. *J Thorac Cardiovasc Surg* 47:83, 1969.

4. Lev M: The architecture of the conduction system in congenital heart disease. I. Common atrioventricular orifice. *AMA Arch Pathol* 65:174, 1958.

5. Lev M, Liberthson RR, Eckner FAO, Arcilla RA: Pathologic anatomy of dextrocardia and its clinical implications. *Circulation* 37:979, 1968.

6. Levy S, Blondeau P, Dubost C: Long-term follow-up after surgical correction of the partial form of common atrioventricular canal (ostium primum). *J Thorac Cardiovasc Surg* 67:353, 1974.

7. Losay J, Rosenthal A, Castaneda AR, Bernhard WH, Nadas AS: Repair of atrial septal defect primum: Results, course, and prognosis. *J Thorac Cardiovasc Surg* 75:248, 1978.

8. Lev M, Agustsson MH, Arcilla R: The pathologic anatomy of common atrioventricular orifice associated with tetralogy of Fallot. *Am J Clin Pathol* 36:408, 1961.

9. Lappen RS, Muster AJ, Idriss FS, Riggs TW, Ilbawi M, Paul M, Bharati S, Lev M: Masked subaortic stenosis in ostium primum atrial septal defect: Recognition and treatment. *Am J Cardiol* 52:336, 1983.

M

1. Maloney JV Jr, Marable SA, Mulder DG: The surgical treatment of common atrioventricular canal. *J Thorac Cardiovasc Surg* 43:84, 1962.

2. McMullan MH, Wallace RB, Weidman WH, McGoon DC: Surgical treatment of complete atrioventricular canal. *Surgery* 72:905, 1972.

3. Mair DD, McGoon DC: Surgical correction of atrioventricular canal during the first year of life. *Am J Cardiol* 40:66, 1977.

4. Mills NL, Ochsner JL, King TD: Correction of type C complete atrioventricular canal: Surgical considerations. *J Thorac Cardiovasc Surg* 71:20, 1976.

5. Midgley FM, Galioto FM, Shapiro SR, Perry LW, Scott LP: Experience with repair of complete atrioventricular canal. *Ann Thorac Surg* 30:151, 1980.

6. McGoon DC, McMullan MH, Mair DD, Danielson GK: Correction of complete atrioventricular canal in infants. *Mayo Clin Proc* 48:769, 1973.

7. McMullan MH, McGoon DC, Wallace RB, Danielson GK, Weidman WH: Surgical treatment of partial atrioventricular canal. *Arch Surg* 107:705, 1973.

8. Munoz-Armas S, Gorrin JRD, Anselmi G, Hernandez PB, Anselmi A: Single atrium: Embryologic, anatomic, electrocardiographic and other diagnostic features. *Am J Cardiol* 21:639, 1968.

9. Mavroudis C, Weinstein G, Turley K, Ebert PA: Surgical management of complete atrioventricular canal. *J Thorac Cardiovasc Surg* 83:670, 1982.

10. Moreno-Cabral RJ, Shumway NE: Double-patch technique for correction of complete atrioventricular canal. *Ann Thorac Surg* 33:86, 1982.

11. Mitchell SC, Korones SB, Berendas HW: Congenital heart disease in 56,109 births: Incidence and natural history. *Circulation* 43:323, 1971.

12. McCartney FJ, Rees PG, Daly K, Piccoli GP, Taylor JFN, de Leval MR, Stark J, Anderson RH: Angiographic appearances of atrioventricular defects with particular reference to distinction of ostium primum atrial septal defects from common atrioventricular orifice. *Br Heart J* 42:640, 1979.

13. McGoon, DC: (1978) Personal communication.

N

1. Newfeld EA, Sher M, Paul MH, Nikaidoh H: Pulmonary vascular disease in complete atrioventricular canal defect. *Am J Cardiol* 39:721, 1977.

2. Nora JJ, Nora AH: The evolution of specific genetic and environmental counseling in congenital heart disease. *Circulation* 57:205, 1978.

O

1. Ongley PA, Pongpanich B, Spangler JG, Feldt RH: The electrocardiogram in atrioventricular canal, in RH Feldt (ed): *Atrioventricular Canal Defects*. Philadelphia: Saunders, 1976, p 51.

P

1. Pacifico AD, Kirklin JW: Surgical repair of complete atrioventricular canal and anterior common leaflet attached to an anomalous right ventricular papillary muscle. *J Thorac Cardiovasc Surg* 65:727, 1973.

2. Park JM, Ritter DG, Mair DD: Cardiac catheterization findings in persistent atrioventricular canal, in RH Feldt (ed): *Atrioventricular Canal Defects*. Philadelphia: Saunders, 1976, p 76.

3. Pacifico AD, Kirklin JW, Bargeron LM Jr: Repair of complete atrioventricular canal associated with tetralogy of Fallot or double-outlet right ventricle: Report of 10 patients. *Ann Thorac Surg* 29:351, 1980.

4. Pieroni DR, Homcy E, Freedom RM: Echocardiography in atrioventricular canal defects: A clinical spectrum. *Am J Cardiol* 35:54, 1975.

5. Piccoli GP, Gerlis LM, Wilkinson JL, Lozsadi K, McCartney FJ, Anderson RH: Morphology and classification of atrioventricular defects. *Br Heart J* 42:621, 1979.

6. Piccoli GP, Macartney FJ, Wilkinson JL, Gerlis LM, Anderson RH: Morphology and classification of complete atrioventricular defects. *Br Heart J* 42:633, 1979.

7. Piccoli GP, Wilkinson JL, Macartney FJ, Gerlis LM, Anderson RH: Left-sided obstructive lesions in atrioventricular septal defect. *J Thorac Cardiovasc Surg* 83:453, 1982.

Q

1. Quaegebeur J, Kirklin JW, Pacifico AD, Bargeron LM Jr: Surgical experience with unroofed coronary sinus. *Ann Thorac Surg* 27:418, 1979.

R

1. Rastelli GC, Ongley PA, Kirklin JW, McGoon DC: Surgical repair of complete form of persistent common atrioventricular canal. *J Thorac Cardiovasc Surg* 55:299, 1968.

2. Rastelli GC, Weidman WH, Kirklin JW: Surgical repair of the partial form of persistent common atrioventricular canal, with special reference to the problem of mitral valve incompetence. *Circulation* 31,32(suppl I):I-31, 1965.

3. Rastelli GC, Kirklin JW, Titus JL: Anatomic observations on complete form of persistent common atrioventricular canal with

special reference to atrioventricular valves. *Mayo Clin Proc* 41:296, 1966.

4. Rogers HM, Edwards JE: Incomplete division of the atrioventricular canal with patent interatrial foramen primum (persistent common atrioventricular ostium): Report of five cases and review of the literature. *Am Heart J* 36:28, 1948.

5. Rastelli GC, Ongley PA, McGoon DC: Surgical repair of complete atrioventricular canal with anterior common leaflet undivided and unattached to ventricular septum. *Mayo Clin Proc* 44:335, 1969.

6. Rastelli GC, Ongley PA, Kirklin JW: Common atrium with left superior vena cava. *Mayo Clin Proc* 40:528, 1965.

7. Rastelli GC, Rahimtoola SH, Ongley RA, McGoon DC: Common atrium: Anatomy, hemodynamics, repair and surgery. *J Thorac Cardiovasc Surg* 55:834, 1968.

8. Rowlatt JF, Rimoldi HJA, Lev M: The quantitative anatomy of the normal child's heart. *Pediatr Clin North Am* 10:499, 1963.

9. Rizzoli G, Mazzucco A, Brumana T, Valfre C, Rubino M, Rocco F, Daliento L, Frescura C, Gallucci V: Operative risk of correction of atrioventricular septal defects. *Br Heart J* 52:258, 1984.

S

1. Sayd HM, Dacie JV, Handley DA, Lewis SM, Cleland WP: Hemolytic anemia of mechanical origin after open heart surgery. *Thorax* 16:356, 1961.

2. Studer M, Blackstone EH, Kirklin JW, Pacifico AD, Soto B, Chung GKT, Kirklin JK, Bargeron LM Jr: Determinants of early and late results of repair of atrioventricular septal (canal) defects. *J Thorac Cardiovasc Surg* 84:523, 1982.

3. Spanos PK, Fiddler GI, Mair DD, McGoon DC: Repair of atrioventricular canal associated with membranous subaortic stenosis. *Mayo Clin Proc* 52:121, 1977.

4. Sellers RD, Lillehei CW, Edwards JE: Subaortic stenosis caused by anomalies of the atrioventricular valves. *J Thorac Cardiovasc Surg* 48:289, 1964.

5. Stanger P, Rudolph AM, Edwards JE: Cardiac malpositions. An overview based on study of sixty-five necropsy specimens. *Circulation* 56:159, 1977.

6. Somerville J: Ostium primum defects: Factors causing deterioration in the natural history. *Br Heart J* 27:413, 1965.

7. Sridaromont S, Feldt RH, Ritter DG, Davis GD, McGoon DC, Edwards JE: Double-outlet right ventricle associated with persistent common atrioventricular canal. *Circulation* 52:933, 1975.

8. Soto B, Bargeron LM Jr, Pacifico AD, Vanini V, Kirklin JW: Angiography of atrioventricular canal defects. *Am J Cardiol* 48:492, 1981.

9. Smallhorn JF, Tommasini G, Anderson RH, Macartney FJ: Assessment of atrioventricular septal defects by two dimensional echocardiography. *Br Heart J* 48:109, 1982.

10. Silverman N, Levitsky S, Fisher E, DuBrow I, Hastreiter A, Scagliotti D: Efficacy of pulmonary artery banding in infants with complete atrioventricular canal. *Circulation* 68(suppl II):II-148, 1983.

T

1. Toscano-Barbosa E, Brandenburg RO, Burchell HB: Electrocardiographic studies of cases with intracardiac malformations of the atrioventricular canal. *Proc Mayo Clin* 31:513, 1956.

2. Tenckhoff L, Stamm SJ: An analysis of 35 cases of the complete form of persistent common atrioventricular canal. *Circulation* 48:416, 1973.

3. Tandon R, Moller JH, Edwards JE: Tetralogy of Fallot associated with persistent common atrioventricular canal (endocardial cushion defect). *Br Heart J* 36:197, 1974.

4. Takanashi Y, Anzai N, Okada T, Sano A, Ando M, Konno S: Common atrium associated with anomalous high insertion of the inferior vena cava. *J Thorac Cardiovasc Surg* 69:912, 1975.

5. Taylor NC, Somerville J: Fixed subaortic stenosis after repair of ostium primum defects. *Br Heart J* 45:689, 1981.

6. Thanopoulos BD, Fisher EA, DuBrown IW, Hastreiter AR: Right and left ventricular volume characteristics in common atrioventricular canal. (1981) Personal communication.

7. Thiene G, Wenink ACG, Frescura C, Wilkinson JL, Gallucci V, Ho SY, Mazzucco A, Anderson RH: Surgical anatomy and pathology of the conduction tissues in atrioventricular defects. *J Thorac Cardiovasc Surg* 82:928, 1981.

8. Thilenius OG, Vitullo D, Bharati S, Luken J, Lamberti JJ, Tatooles C, Lev M, Carr I, Arcilla RA: Endocardial cushion defect associated with cor triatriatum sinistrum or supravalve mitral ring. *Am J Cardiol* 44:1339, 1979.

U

1. Ugarte M, de Salamanca FE, Quero M: Endocardial cushion defects: An anatomical study of 54 specimens. *Br Heart J* 38:674, 1976.

V

1. Vanetti A, Daumet P: Traitement chirurgical des formes sévères du canal atrioventriculaire. *Arch Mal Coeur* 68:719, 1975.

2. Van Praagh R, Cowin RD, Dahlquist E, Freedom RM, Mattioli L, Nebesar RA: Tetralogy of Fallot with severe left ventricular outflow tract obstruction due to anomalous attachment of the mitral valve to the ventricular septum. *Am J Cardiol* 26:93, 1970.

3. Van Mierop LHS, Alley RD, Kansel HW, Stranahan A: The anatomy and embryology of endocardial cushion defects. *J Thorac Cardiovasc Surg* 43:71, 1962.

4. Verdon TA Jr, Forrester RH, Crosby WH: Hemolytic anemia after open heart repair of ostium primum defects. *N Engl J Med* 269:444, 1963.

5. Van Mierop LHS, Alley RD: The management of the cleft mitral valve in endocardial cushion defects. *Ann Thorac Surg* 2:416, 1966.

6. Van Mierop LHS: Pathology and pathogenesis of endocardial cushion defect. Surgical implications, in JC Davila (ed): *Second Henry Ford Hospital International Symposium on Cardiac Surgery.* New York: Appleton-Century-Crofts, 1977, pp 201–207.

7. Villani M, Locatelli G, Tiraboschi R, Alfieri O, Parenzan L: Atrioventricular canal malformations: Recent surgical techniques. *Thorac Cardiovasc Surg* 27:116, 1979.

W

1. Wakai CS, Edwards JE: Development and pathologic considerations in persistent common atrioventricular canal. *Proc Mayo Clin* 31:487, 1956.

2. Wakai CS, Edwards JE: Pathology study of persistent common atrioventricular canal. *Am Heart J* 56:779, 1958.

3. Watkins E Jr, Gross RE: Experiences with surgical repair of atrial septal defects. *J Thorac Cardiovasc Surg* 30:469, 1955.

4. Williams RG, Rudd M: Echocardiographic features of endocardial cushion defects. *Circulation* 49:418, 1974.

5. Williams WH, Guyton RA, Michalik RE, Jones EL, Rhee KH, Plauth WH Jr, Hatcher CR Jr: Individualized surgical management of complete atrioventricular canal. *J Thorac Cardiovasc Surg* 86:838, 1983.

Y

1. Yokoyama M, Ando M, Takao A, Sakakibara S: The location of the coronary sinus orifice in endocardial cushion defects. *Am Heart J* 85:302, 1973.

Z

1. Zavanella C, Matsuda H, Subramanian S: Successful correction of a complete form of atrioventricular canal associated with tetralogy of Fallot. *J Thorac Cardiovasc Surg* 74:195, 1977.

20

VENTRICULAR SEPTAL DEFECT

SECTION 1
PRIMARY VENTRICULAR SEPTAL DEFECT

DEFINITION

A ventricular septal defect (VSD) is a hole or multiple holes in the ventricular septum. This chapter considers VSDs that occur as the primary lesion with or without major associated cardiac anomalies.

A VSD may not be the primary lesion, but, rather, part of another anomaly, such as tetralogy of Fallot, complete atrio-ventricular (AV) canal defect, anatomically corrected malposition of the great arteries, truncus arteriosus, tricuspid atresia, sinus of Valsalva aneurysm, interrupted aortic arch, and so forth. VSDs may be acquired. All of these types are discussed in other chapters.

HISTORICAL NOTE

In 1954, Lillehei, Varco, and their colleagues, at the University of Minnesota in Minneapolis, began to repair ventricular septal defects (VSDs) using normothermic, low-flow, *controlled cross-circulation* based on the so-called azygos-flow principle[A1,C1] with an adult human being as the oxygenator.[L1,W1] This was the beginning of the era of cardiac surgery using *cardiopulmonary bypass*, a term coined by Cooley a few years later. The paper by Lillehei and associates in 1955 contains some excesses of enthusiasm, such as "these observations would seem to deny the classical concept that the conduction system of the human or canine heart (atrioventricular node and bundle of His) is concentrated in a small localized discrète locus which is thereby very vulnerable to mechanical injury." However, their feat was remarkable, even in retrospect. Five of the first eight patients were in their first year of life, and only two (40%, CL 14%–71%) of the five died, a tribute to surgical skill, the lack of cardiac ischemia (the aorta was not cross-clamped), and the perfectness of their human oxygenator. The dramatic weight gain of the surgically cured infants with large VSDs was documented. Three other patients, aged 4, 5, and 5 years, also survived, one with multiple VSDs.

We reported in 1956 the cases of 20 patients with large VSDs who had undergone intracardiac repair with a *mechanical pump-oxygenator* at the Mayo Clinic beginning in March 1955.[D1] Normothermic flow rates of 70 ml · kg^{-1} · min^{-1} (about 2.1 l · min^{-1} · m^{-2}) were used, along with a pump sucker system to return intracardiac blood to the machine. The duration of cardiopulmonary bypass varied from 10–45 minutes. Four (20%, CL 10%–33%) of the 20 patients died in hospital.

Truex described the location of the specialized conduction tissue in hearts with VSDs.[T8] Lev, in a more detailed study, amplified on this topic,[L3] and his work was the basis on which we developed a surgical technique that avoided the production of heart block during the repair of VSDs.[K3]

Lillehei showed the feasibility of an atrial approach to VSDs in 1957.[S6] The technique of profound hypothermia and total circulatory arrest, with rewarming by a pump-oxygenator, was applied successfully to infants with VSD by Okamoto and colleagues.[O2] Sloan and colleagues reported the feasibility of primary repair of VSD in infants in 1967,[S2] as did we in 1961.[K12] Beginning in 1969 at GLH, we demonstrated that routine primary repair of VSD in sick, small infants was superior to pulmonary artery banding.[B7]

MORPHOLOGY

Size

VSDs are highly variable in size, and their division into groups is arbitrary but useful.

Large VSDs are approximately the size of the aortic orifice or larger. They offer little resistance to flow, and thus their VSD resistance index[1] is less than 20 units · m^2 in situations in which the calculation of the index is valid.[H6,S1] Right ventricular (RV) systolic pressure approximates left

---

[1]VSD resistance index $= \dfrac{P_{LV(peak)} - P_{RV(peak)}}{\dot{Q}p - \dot{Q}s} \times$ body surface area (BSA).

ventricular (LV) pressure, and the pulmonary-systemic flow ratio ($\dot{Q}p/\dot{Q}s$) is increased to a degree dependent on the level of the pulmonary vascular resistance.

Small VSDs are of insufficient size to raise right ventricular systolic pressure, and the $\dot{Q}p/\dot{Q}s$ is not increased above 1.75. They have a VSD resistance index greater than 20 units · m^2.[H6] Multiple small defects behave in aggregate as a large defect.

Moderate-sized VSDs, while still restrictive, are of sufficient size to raise RV systolic pressure to approximately half LV pressure and the $\dot{Q}p/\dot{Q}s$ to 3.5.

Location

VSDs can occur anywhere in the ventricular septum (Fig. 20-1). They may be perimembranous, subpulmonary, beneath the tricuspid septal leaflet, or in other locations. In addition, they may be confluent, and they may have straddling or overriding tricuspid valves.

Perimembranous Ventricular Septal Defect
Approximately 80% of the patients operated on for VSD have a defect that lies against the tricuspid anulus in the region of the anteroseptal commissure, immediately inferior to the infundibular septum and adjacent to or involving the membranous ventricular septum[B2] (Fig. 20-2). Such VSDs have been termed typical high, infracristal, or membranous

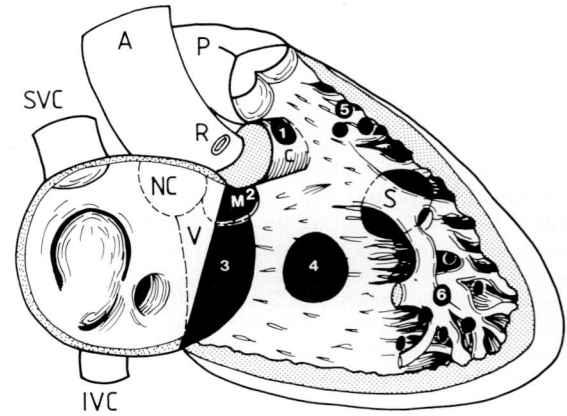

Figure 20-1 Schematic representation of the position of VSDs as seen from the right ventricular side of the septum. The front of the right ventricle and right atrium and the tricuspid valve have been removed (see the anatomic specimen, Chapter 1, Fig. 1-3, for morphologic detail). Shown are (1) a subpulmonary (conal) VSD; (2) a perimembranous VSD; (3) an AV canal VSD; (4, 5, 6) muscular VSDs in various parts of the septum (mid-muscular, high anterior, and apical, respectively). In positions 5 and 6, the VSDs tend to be small and multiple, and when most of this trabeculated area and the mid-muscular septum are peppered with holes, the term *Swiss-cheese* defect is used. A single large muscular defect shown between positions 5 and 6 is crossed by the septal band (S) and has, as a result, at least two openings on the right ventricular side.

A, aorta; c, conal septum; IVC, inferior vena cava; NC, noncoronary aortic cusp; M, membranous septum with ventricular and atrioventricular portions; P, pulmonary artery and valve; R, right coronary artery cut off at its origin; SVC, superior vena cava; V, muscular portion of atrioventricular septum.

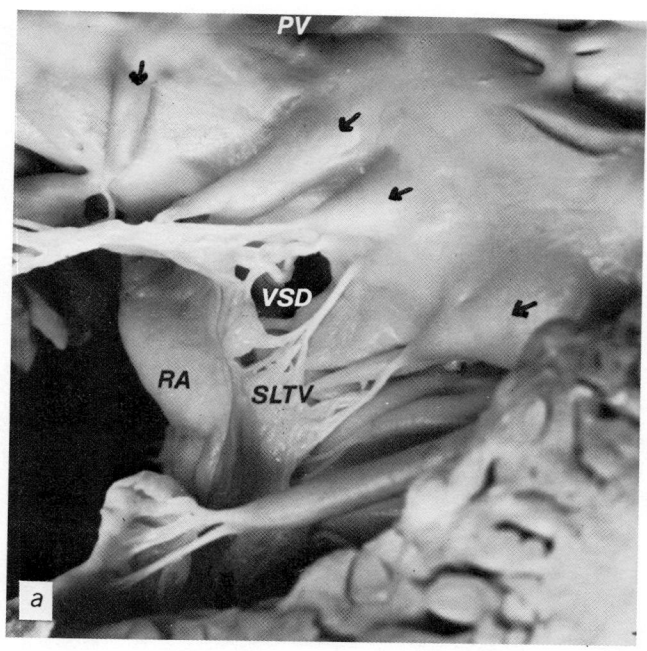

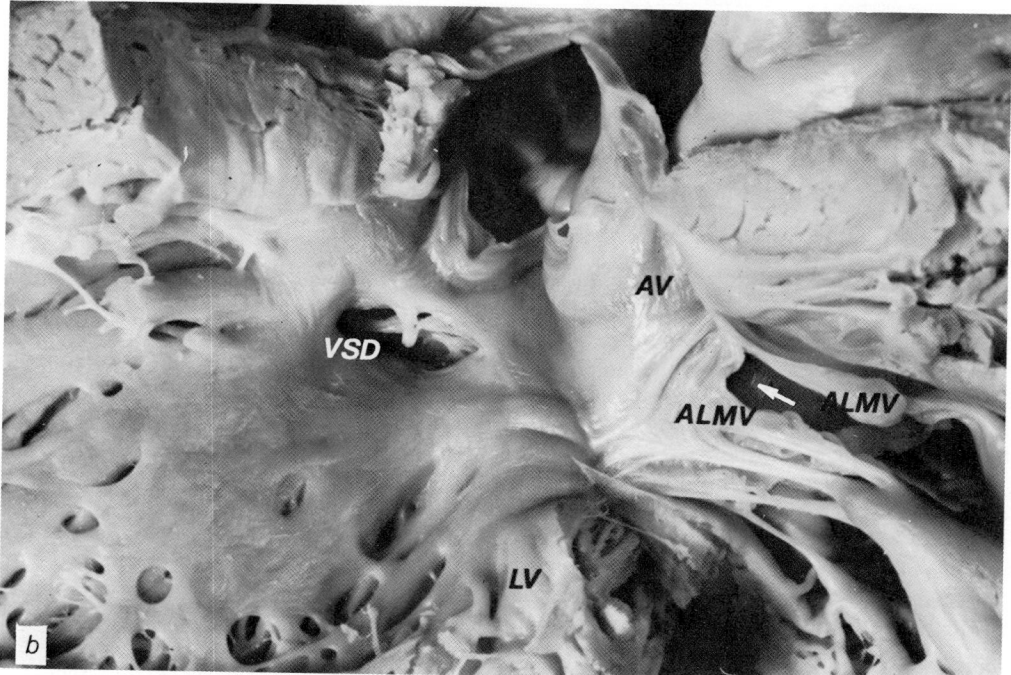

Figure 20-2 Perimembranous VSD.

(a) A perimembranous VSD of moderate size in the region of the anteroseptal commissure of the tricuspid valve, viewed from the right ventricle (GLH). The VSD extends inferiorly beneath the septal leaflet of the tricuspid valve and abuts the commissural area between the anterior and septal tricuspid leaflets and the remnant of the membranous septum. Numerous tricuspid chordae and papillary muscles (arrows) are present.

(b) The same defect viewed from the left ventricle. The VSD lies well below the noncoronary cusp of the aortic valve (AV). The arrow indicates a cleft in the anterior mitral leaflet.

ALMV, anterior mitral leaflet; AV, aortic valve; LV, left ventricle; PV, pulmonary valve; RA, right atrium; SLTV, septal leaflet of tricuspid valve.

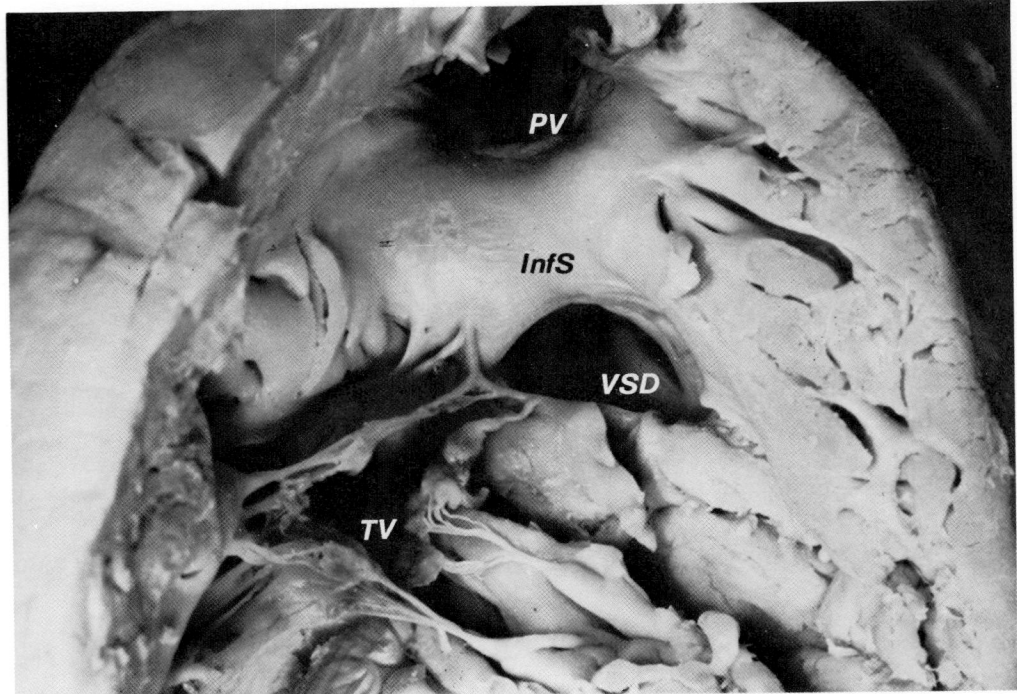

Figure 20-3 Perimembranous VSD viewed from the right ventricle (GLH). The VSD is at the anteroseptal commissure of the tricuspid valve and extends into the mid-portion of the muscular septum.

InfS, infundibular septum; PV, pulmonary valve; TV, tricuspid valve.

defects in the past but are now generally called *perimembranous VSDs*.[L7,S13]

These defects are variously related to the ventricular portion of the membranous septum. The latter may be absent, in which case the right trigone (beneath the nadir of the noncoronary aortic valve cusp) and base of the septal and anterior leaflets of the tricuspid valve are exposed and form the posteroinferior rim of the VSD. The bundle of His, as it penetrates the fibrous right trigone at the base of the noncoronary cusp, is intimately related to the posteroinferior angle of such a defect. This is associated with a deficiency in the posterior limb of the trabecula septomarginalis.[K14] Alternatively, remnants of the membranous septum may form the posteroinferior margin.

When viewed from the left ventricular side, these VSDs lie in the posterior part of the left ventricular outflow tract and characteristically beneath the commissure between right and noncoronary cusps of the aortic valve. They vary in size from a few millimeters to a diameter in excess of the aortic root and are almost always single.

A perimembranous VSD may extend inferiorly beneath the septal tricuspid leaflet (Fig. 20-2), forward into the muscular septum (Fig. 20-3), either above or below the papillary muscle of the conus, or superiorly toward the pulmonary valve in association with reduction in size of the infundibular septum.[S13] The aorta may override onto the right ventricle.

Characteristically, the medial papillary muscle joins the anteroinferior angle of the defect and receives chordae from the adjacent portions of the tricuspid anterior and septal leaflets. These chordae may be increased in number and abnormally positioned around the edges of a perimembranous defect, attached to the posterior edge, the superior edge (Fig. 20-4), or, most commonly, the anterior edge. A thick leash of chordae joining the center of the anterior edge of a large defect may produce an appearance on angiocardiography or even at surgery of a double defect. Sometimes chordae from the anterior leaflet attach to all three margins (Fig. 20-2), and the anterior leaflet then limits the shunt from left to right through the defect as well as hindering surgical repair.

Rarely, the ventricular portion of the membranous septum may be well-developed, thickened, and perforated by one or many holes, forming an "aneurysm of the membranous septum" that bulges toward the right in systole. This so-called *aneurysm* is simulated on angiography by the much more common tethered anterior leaflet. Accessory fibrous tissue, not part of the tricuspid valve mechanism, may lie along the posterior or superior margin of the defect. This phenomenon is most marked in the so-called *flap valve* VSD (see Chapter 23, Section 2).

The intimate association of the perimembranous VSD with the commissure between anterior and septal tricuspid leaflets sometimes results in adherence of the leaflet tissue to the edges of the defect and shunting directly from the left ventricle into the right atrium[B8] (Fig. 20-5). This so-called *left ventricular–right atrial defect*,[G4,P2,S8] which constitutes less than 5% of perimembranous VSDs, rarely involves the atrioventricular septum.

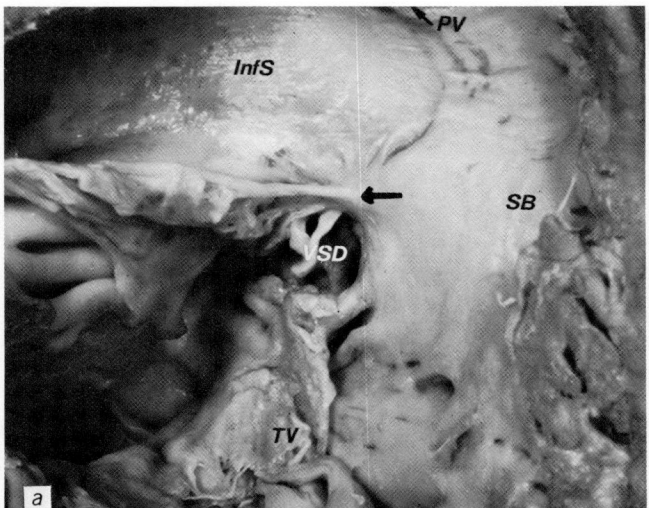

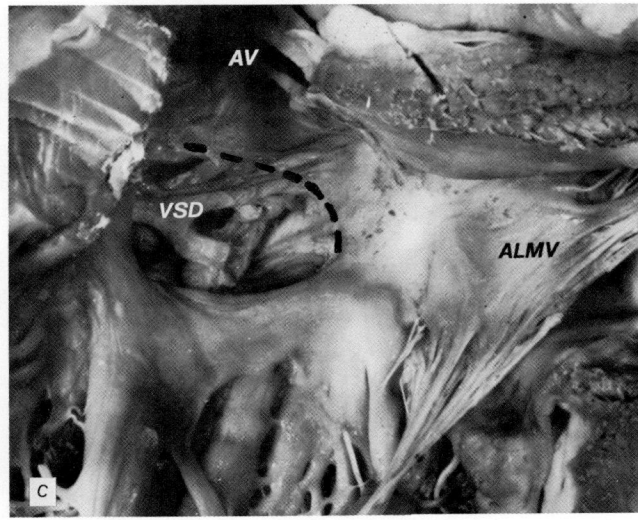

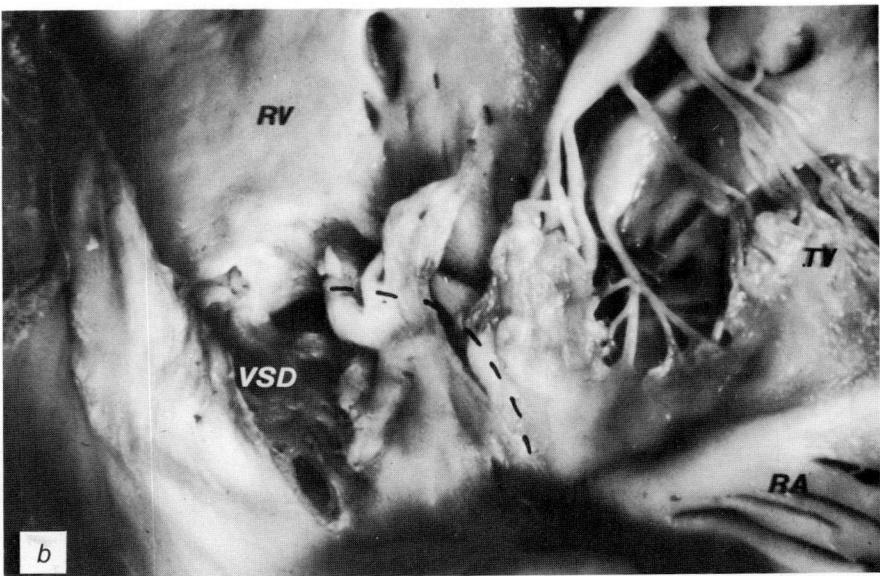

Figure 20-4 Perimembranous VSD associated with anomalous leaflet tissue (GLH).
(a) Viewed from the right ventricle. Note the chordal attachment (arrow) of the anterior tricuspid leaflet to the anterosuperior margin of the defect. The normal position of the infundibular septum between the two limbs of the trabecula septomarginalis, or septal band, is well seen.
(b) Viewed from the right atrium. The VSD is partly obscured by tricuspid leaflet tissue, but its extent is indicated by the dashed line.
(c) Viewed from left ventricle. The VSD is immediately beneath the aortic valve, and its extent is indicated by the dashed line. The abnormal tricuspid valve attachments are obvious, and on a angiocardiogram they are indistinguishable from an aneurysm of the membranous ventricular septum.

ALMV, anterior leaflet of the mitral valve; AV, aortic valve; InfS, infundibular septum; RA, right atrium; RV, right ventricle; SB, septal band, or trabecula septomarginalis; TV, tricuspid valve; VSD, ventricular septal defect.

Subpulmonary Ventricular Septal Defect
Five percent to 10% of patients treated surgically have a single subpulmonary VSD, usually of moderate or large size. These are also called conal, infundibular, supracristal, or intracristal defects. This defect is more common in Asian than in Caucasian or black people.[T7]

Most commonly, these defects are *subarterial,* lying immediately beneath the pulmonary and aortic valves (Fig. 20-

6).[S13] They may be circular, diamond-shaped, or oval, with the long axis lying transversely (Fig. 20-7). When viewed from the left ventricular aspect, they are in the outflow portion of the ventricular septum (Fig. 20-6), beneath the right coronary cusp or the commissure between it and the left cusp. The aortic and pulmonary valve cusps are separated by only a thin rim of fibrous tissue. The right aortic cusp and, less commonly, the noncoronary cusp may prolapse into the

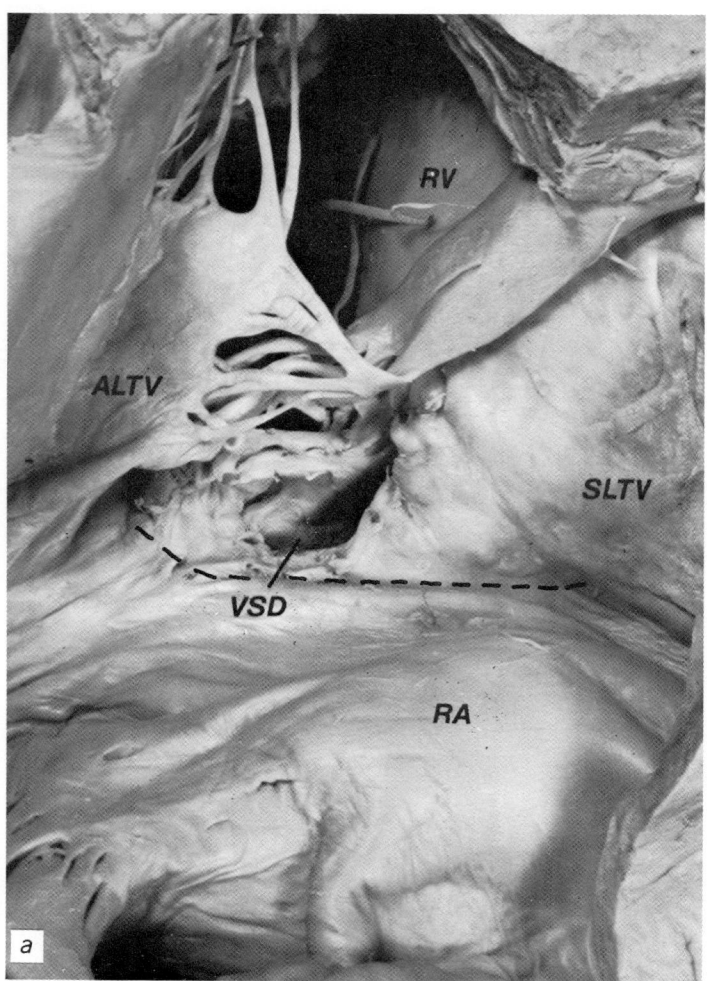

Figure 20-5 A variety of perimembranous VSD that ejects directly into the right atrium, a so-called left ventricular–right atrial defect (GLH).

(*a*) Viewed from the right atrium. The posterior part of the tricuspid anulus is marked by a dashed line. The tricuspid septal leaflet is anomalously adherent to the underlying ventricular septum and the edges of the VSD. The intact atrioventricular septum lies on the atrial side of the tricuspid ring (beneath the letters *VSD*). The bundle of His is along the posterior angle of the defect.

(*b*) Viewed from the left ventricle. The VSD is beneath the commissure between the right and noncoronary aortic cusps.

ALTV, anterior leaflet of the tricuspid valve; ALMV, anterior leaflet of the mitral valve; LV, left ventricle; NC, noncoronary aortic cusps; RA, right atrium; RV, right ventricle; SLTV, tricuspid septal leaflet; VSD, ventricular septal defect.

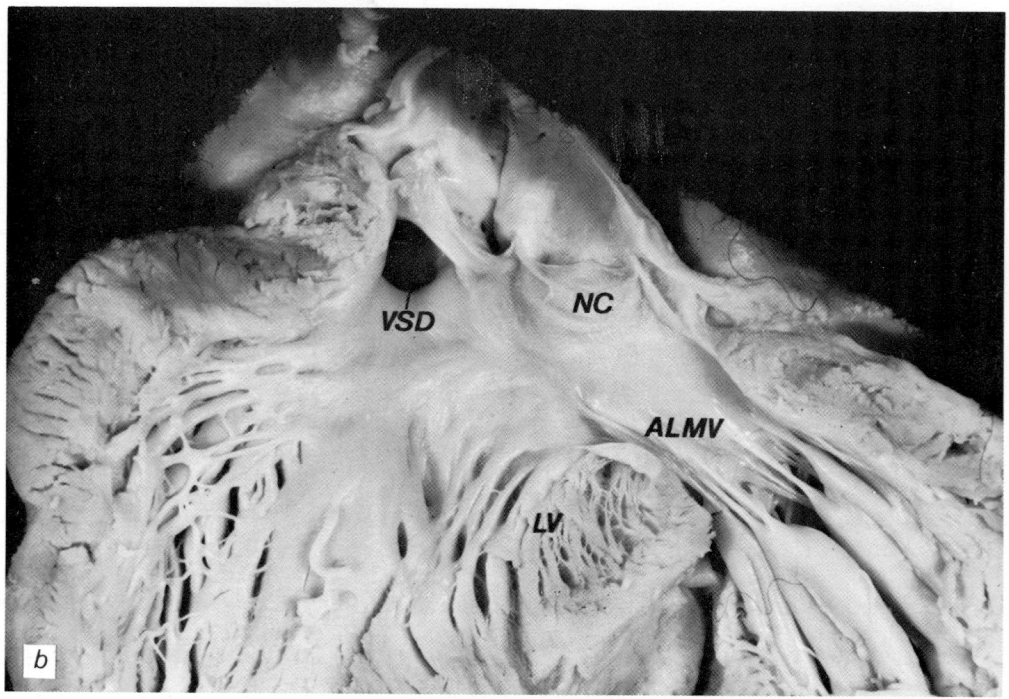

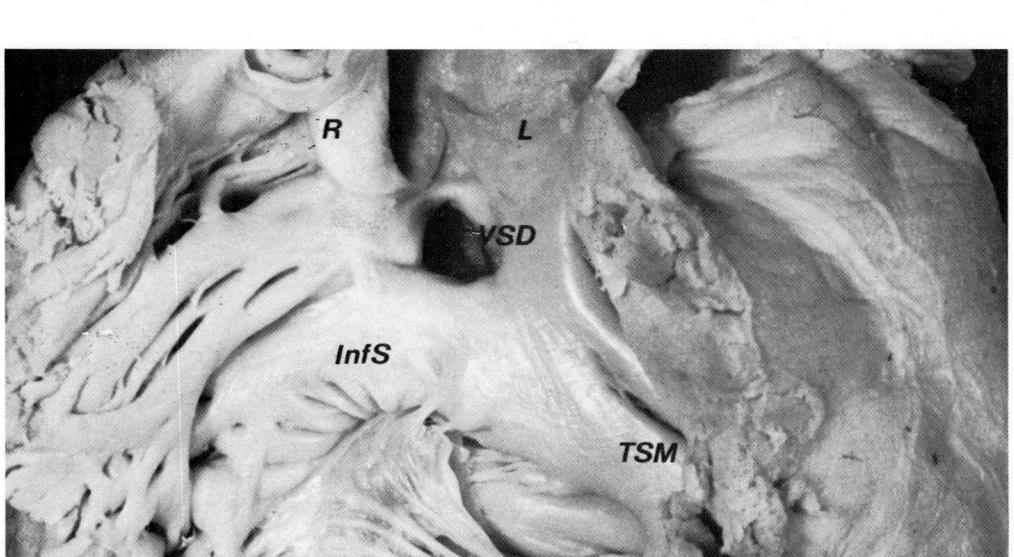

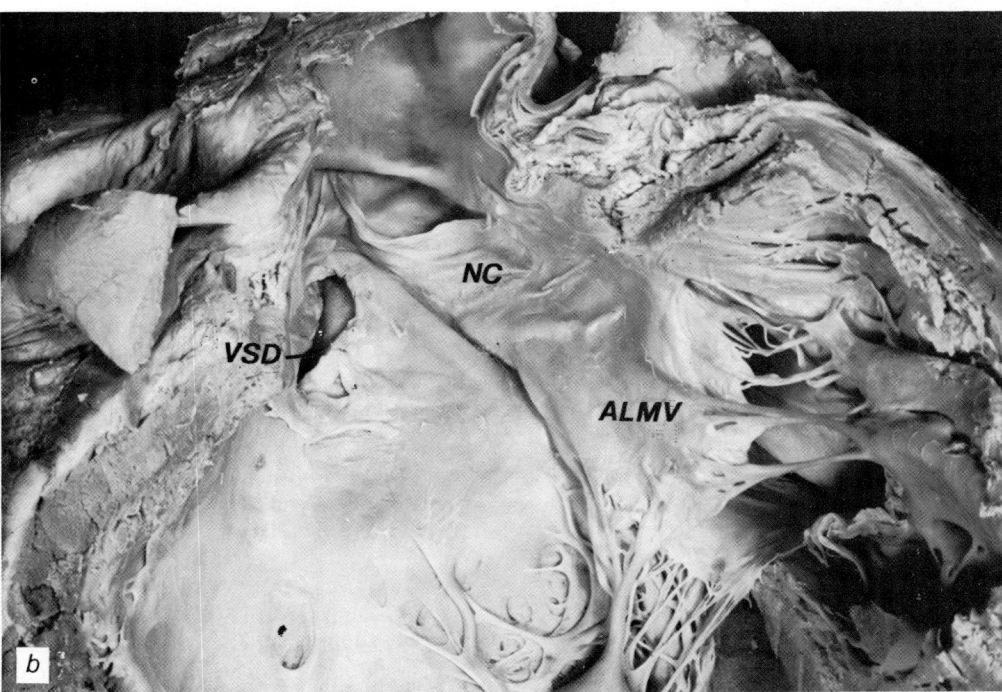

Figure 20-6 Subpulmonary, subarterial VSD (GLH).
(a) Viewed from the right ventricle. The inferior margin of the VSD is formed of thick infundibular septum. The superior margin of the VSD is formed by the confluent right pulmonary and right aortic cusps, which are separated by a thin ridge of fibrous tissue.
(b) Viewed from the left ventricle. The VSD is beneath the right coronary cusp of the aortic valve and is more anterior than a perimembranous VSD.

ALMV, anterior leaflet of the mitral valve; InfS, infundibular septum; L, left pulmonary cusp; LV, left ventricle; NC, noncoronary aortic cusp; R, right pulmonary cusp; TSM, trabecula septomarginalis; VSD, ventricular septal defect.

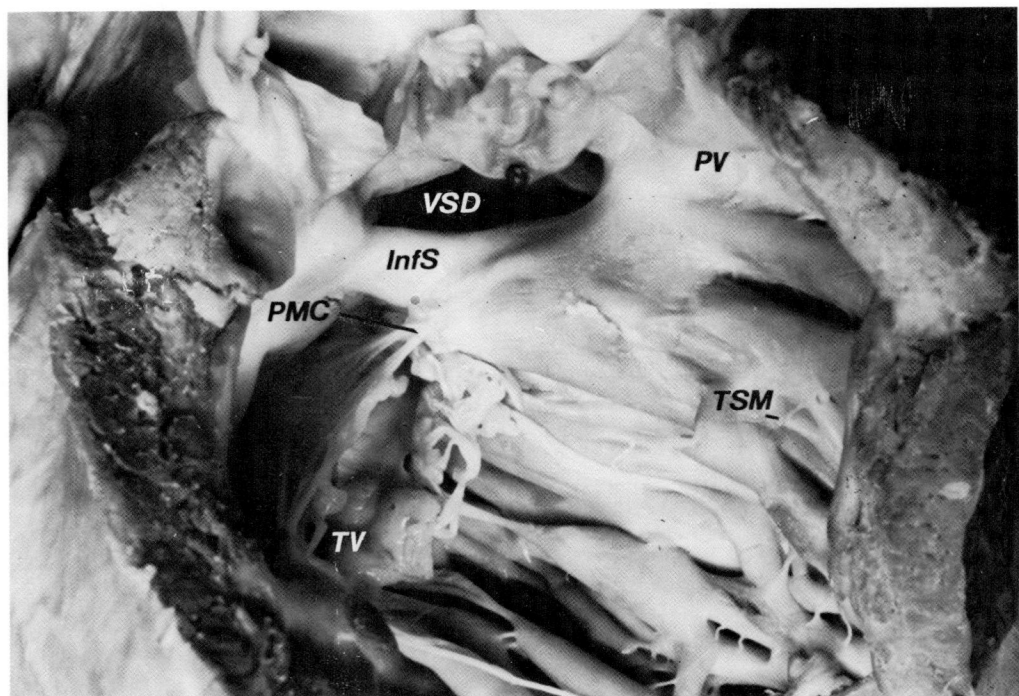

Figure 20-7 Subpulmonary, subarterial VSD viewed from the right ventricle (GLH). The VSD lies immediately beneath the pulmonary valve. Inferior to the defect are the infundibular septum and the trabecula septomarginalis. The tricuspid valve, papillary muscle of conus, and bundle of His are far from the defect.

InfS, infundibular septum; PMC, papillary muscle of conus; PV, pulmonary valve; TSM, trabecula septomarginalis; TV, tricuspid valve; VSD, ventricular septal defect.

upper margin of the defect, with or without aortic incompetence (see Section 2). Cusp prolapse occurred in 11 (39%) of 28 subarterial VSDs (GLH). The posteroinferior margin of these defects is usually well separated from the tricuspid valve anulus by a band of muscle and consequently is well above the bundle of His.

Occasionally, however, a particularly large subpulmonary VSD may reach the tricuspid anulus and be also perimembranous (Fig. 20-8). When the pulmonary artery overrides by more than 50% the superior margin of such a VSD and lies over the left ventricle, the condition is double-outlet left ventricle. When the aorta overrides into the right ventricle, the condition is double-outlet right ventricle with doubly committed VSD.

Some subpulmonary defects are *muscular* and lie in the substance of the infundibular septum, with a muscle bridge of infundibular septum superior to the defect (Fig. 20-9). Occasionally, the superiorly positioned muscular bridge may be displaced leftward into the aortic outflow tract, producing a muscular subaortic stenosis that lies above the VSD (Fig. 20-9). This anomaly is particularly common in association with interrupted aortic arch and occasionally with coarctation.[A7,D8,F4,V2]

Ventricular Septal Defect beneath Tricuspid Septal Leaflet
Five percent or less of surgical patients have a VSD beneath the tricuspid septal leaflet, the so-called *AV canal type of*

VSD.[N3] This defect involves the basal (inlet) sinus septum beneath the tricuspid septal leaflet. Its posterior margin is formed by the exposed AV valve ring, and its anterior margin is muscular and crescentic (Fig. 20-10). Superiorly, the defect extends to the membranous septum and thus is a variety of perimembranous VSD. The bundle of His lies along the posteroinferior rim of the defect, slightly on the left ventricular side, as in other perimembranous VSDs. The atrioventricular septum is intact, in contrast to the situation in hearts with AV canal defects (see Chapter 19). The anterior (septal) mitral leaflet may be cleft either partially or completely, and there may be associated mitral incompetence. (In Chapter 19, "Ventricular Septal Defect of the AV Canal Type" in section on Morphology are further comments on the AV canal type of VSD.)

A muscular VSD can occur beneath the tricuspid septal leaflet (Fig. 20-11). The posterior margin of such a defect is separated from the tricuspid ring by muscle. A muscular VSD must be distinguished from the AV canal type of VSD because the conducting tissue runs *superior* to a muscular defect.

Ventricular Septal Defects in Other Locations
VSDs in other locations are generally *muscular* VSDs, and the entire border consists of muscle. Such defects are frequently multiple and may be associated with perimembranous or subpulmonary VSDs. Single or multiple muscular de-

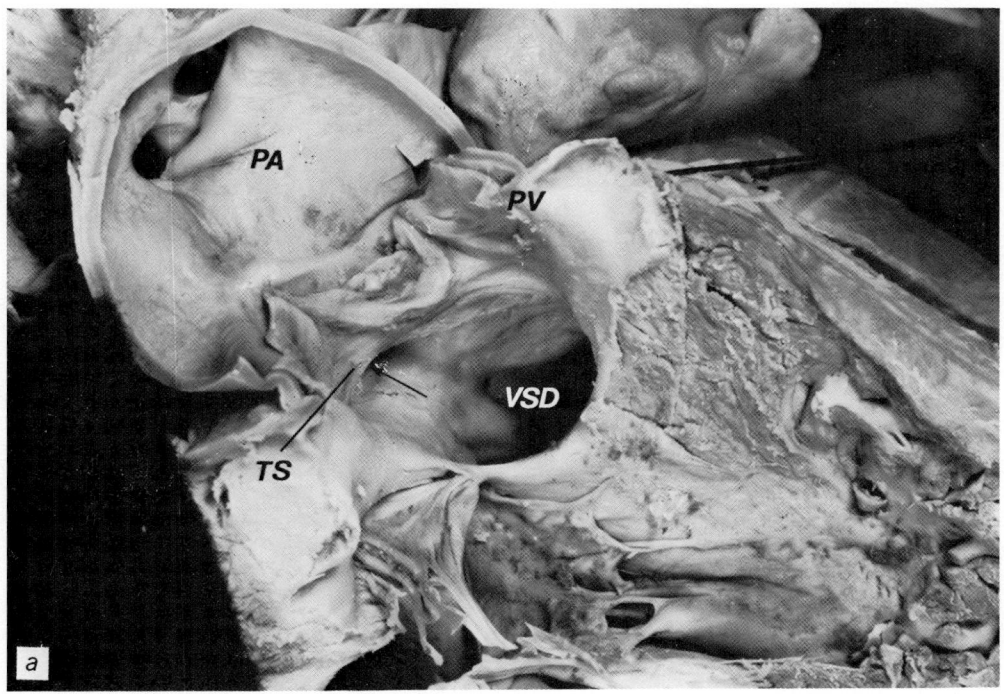

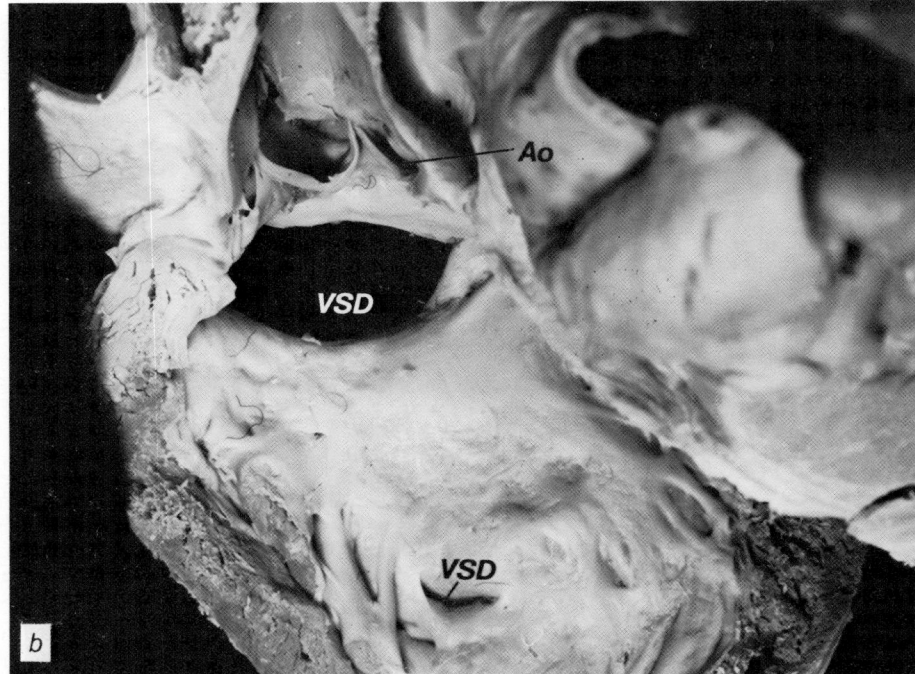

Figure 20-8 Large subpulmonary VSD extending downward to reach the tricuspid anulus (GLH). This type of VSD is also seen in double-outlet right ventricle with doubly committed VSD and in double-outlet left ventricle.

(*a*) Viewed from the right ventricle. At the superior margin of the VSD, the pulmonary and aortic leaflets are in fibrous continuity. The arrow points toward the aortic valve.

(*b*) Viewed from the left ventricle. Note the additional small muscular defect.

Ao, aorta; PA, pulmonary artery; PV, pulmonary and aortic leaflets; TS, infundibular septum; VSD, ventricular septal defect.

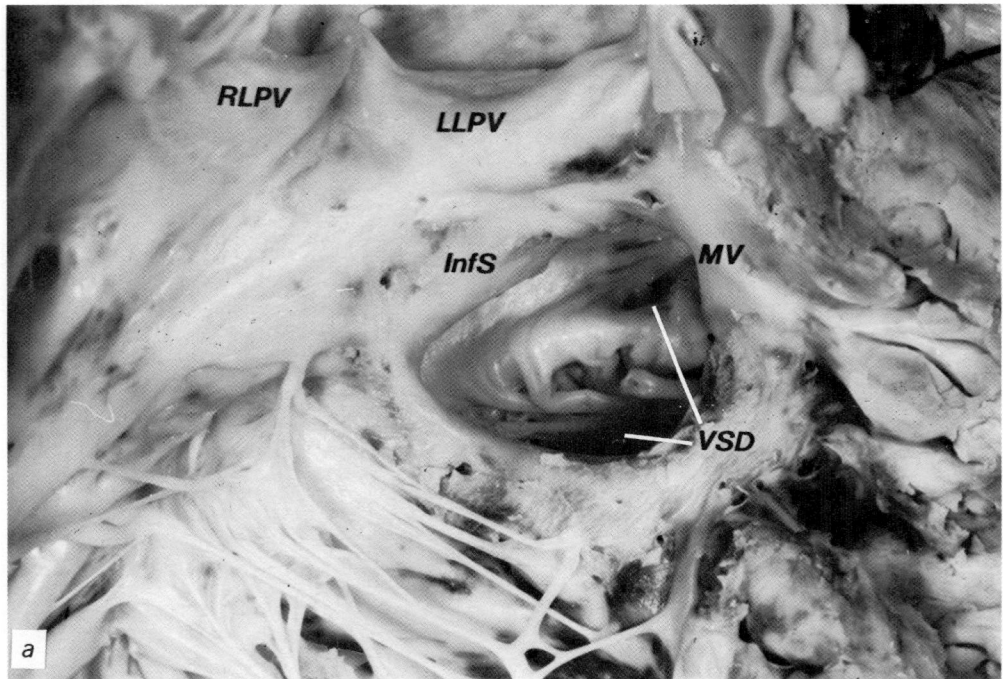

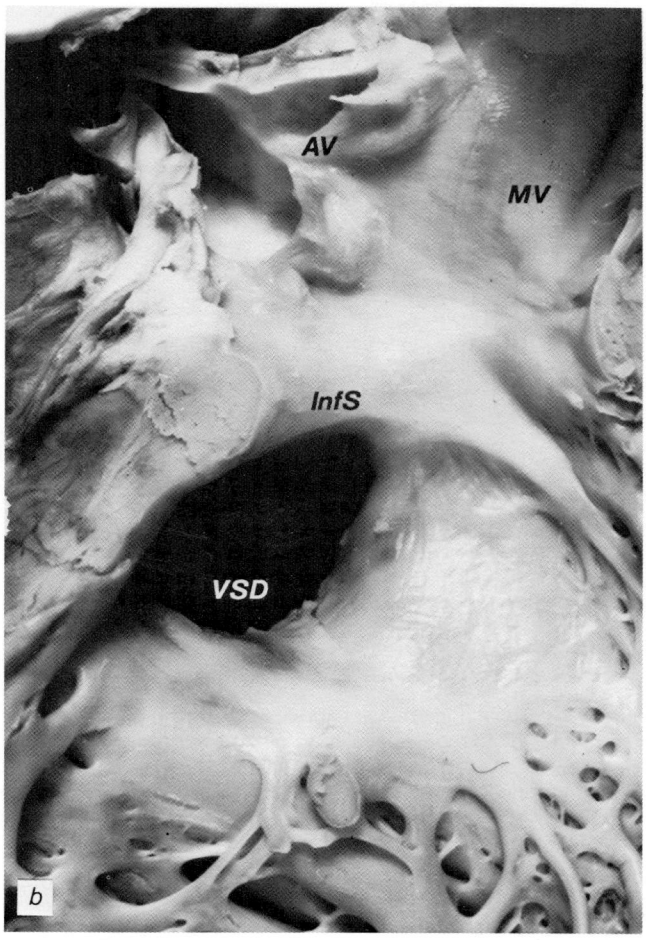

Figure 20-9 A subpulmonary, muscular VSD in association with a prominent muscle bridge of infundibular septum that separates the upper margin of the defect from the pulmonary and aortic valves (GLH).

(*a*) Viewed from the right ventricle. The VSD is completely surrounded by muscle, and a portion of the infundibular septum is between the defect and the pulmonary valve. The mitral valve is seen through the defect.

(*b*) Viewed from the left ventricle. The infundibular septum is displaced leftward beneath the aortic valve, producing subaortic stenosis that lies above (downstream to) the VSD.

AV, aortic valve; InfS, infundibular septum; LLPV, left leaflet of pulmonary valve; MV, mitral valve; RLPV, right leaflet of pulmonary valve; VSD, ventricular septal defect.

defects are relatively more common in infants requiring surgical treatment than in older children. For example, 16 (22%) of a group of 73 infants less than 2 years old in a surgical series had muscular defects (GLH).

Muscular defects can occur anywhere in the muscular septum (Fig. 20-1). Those in the mid-septum are the commonest (Fig. 20-12) and may be straddled by the septal band (trabecula septomarginalis); thus, even when single on the left ventricular side, they have at least two openings on the right side. Anterior muscular defects are nearly always multiple and most commonly are in the apical and infundibular portions of the septum. They may, however, extend all along the anterior part of the septum, from the apex to the infundibulum. Commonly, there are more openings on the left ventricular than on the right ventricular side.

A particularly important group of patients are those with many defects of variable size, not only along the anterior portion of the septum but throughout the mid-portion as

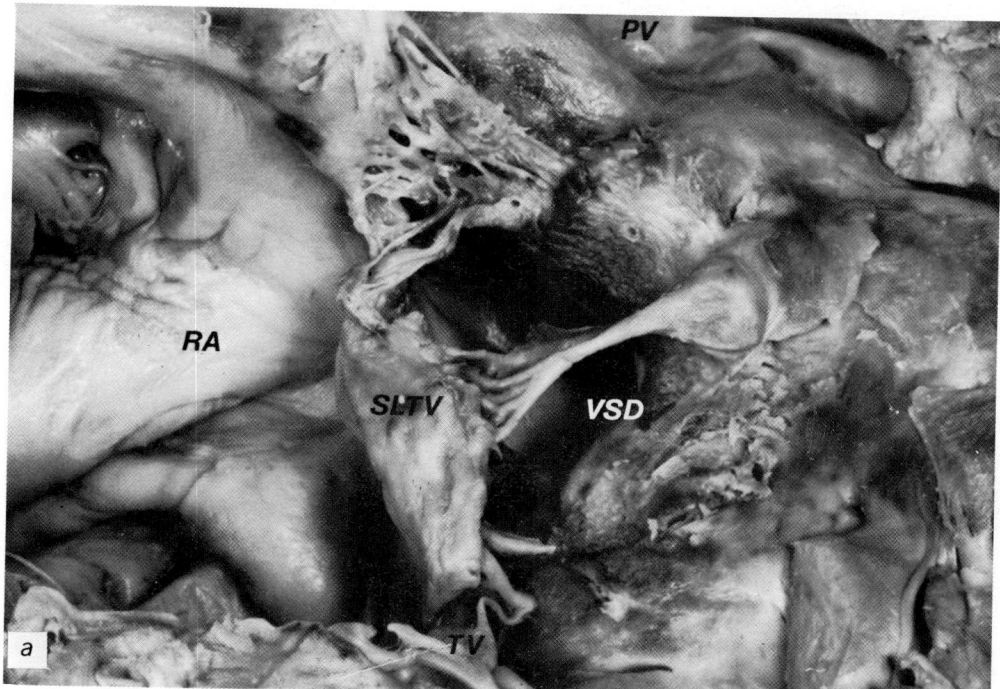

Figure 20-10 AV canal type of VSD beneath the septal leaflet of the tricuspid valve (GLH). The VSD is also perimembranous in position, and the posterior margin of the defect is formed by the tricuspid anulus.

(a) Viewed from right ventricle. Note the crescentic anterior margin of the defect. (A previously placed Dacron patch has been removed.)

(b) Viewed from left ventricle. Superiorly this defect reaches almost to the aortic valve, and posteriorly it extends to the mitral valve.

AV, aortic valve; MV, mitral valve; RA, right atrium; SLTV, septal leaflet of the tricuspid valve; TV, tricuspid valve; VSD, ventricular septal defect.

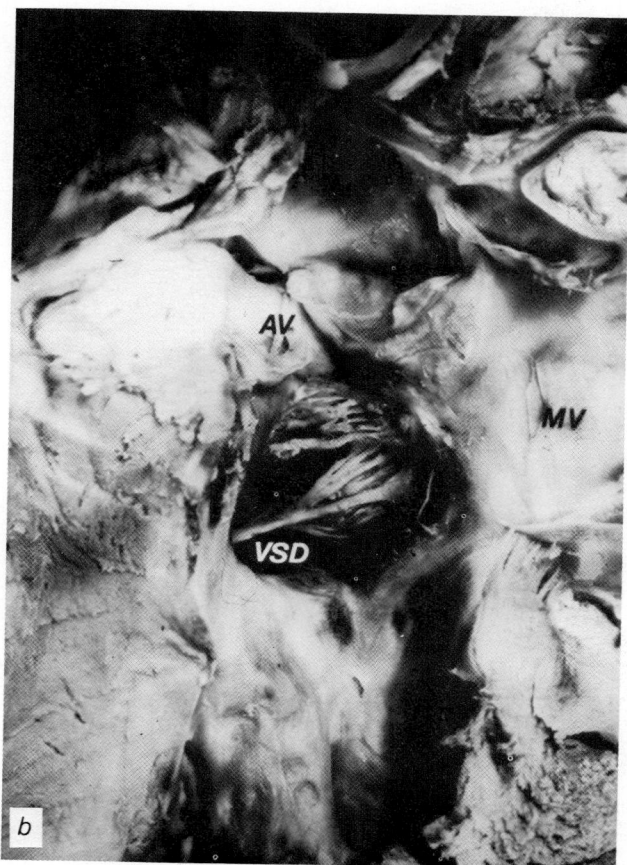

well, the so-called *Swiss-cheese defects* (Fig. 20-13). The defects often pass obliquely through the septum to appear on both sides of the septal band or in the anterior part of the septum. They may be associated with large or small perimembranous or subpulmonary defects. Major associated cardiac anomalies are rather common. For example, three of seven patients with Swiss-cheese defects also had severe coarctation of the aorta (GLH).

Confluent Ventricular Septal Defect

Some unusually large, single confluent VSDs involve more than one area of the septum. Rarely, a confluent VSD may involve most of the septum (Fig. 20-14), but hearts with such defects should not be classified as having a single ventricle.

Ventricular Septal Defect with Straddling or Overriding Tricuspid Valve

In rare instances, the tricuspid valve chordae may *straddle* the ventricular septum in association with a large defect resembling an AV canal type of VSD (Fig. 20-15).[L5,M7,R2] When the tricuspid valve is *overriding*, the anulus is over both ventricles. When overriding is severe, the tricuspid ring is

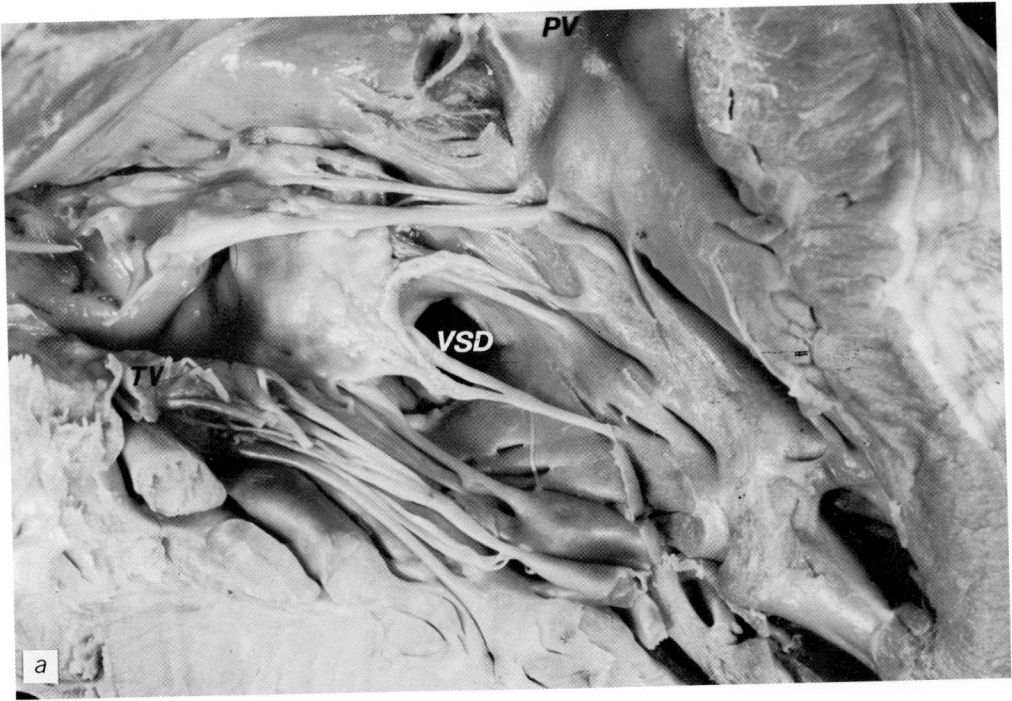

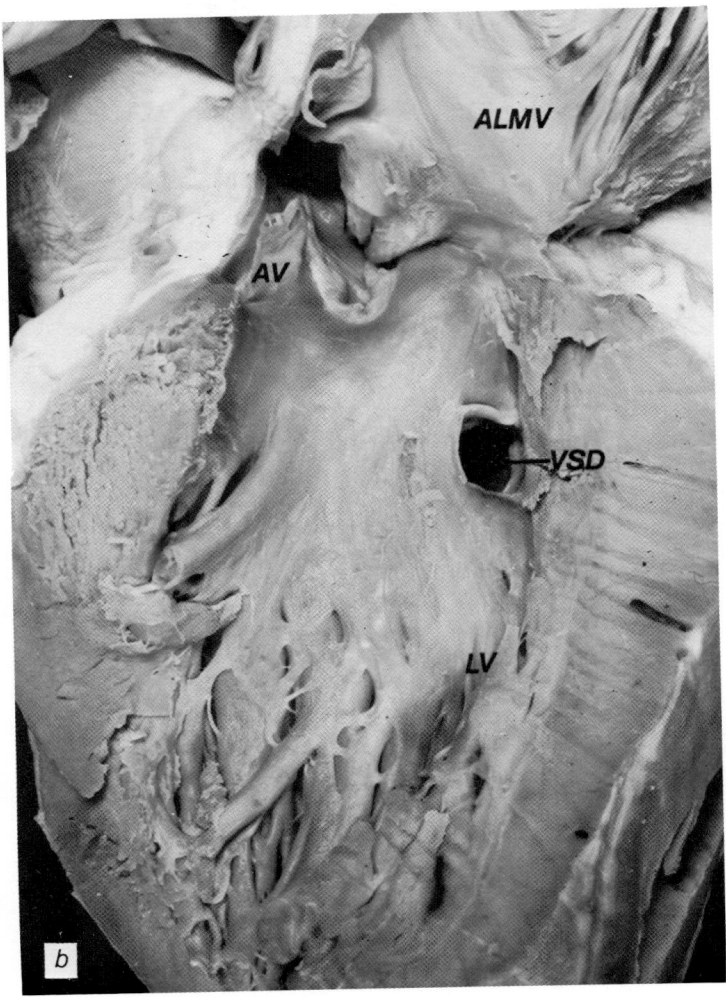

Figure 20-11 A single moderate-sized muscular (trabecular) VSD lying beneath the tricuspid septal leaflet (GLH).

(*a*) Viewed from the right ventricle. Note the septal muscle between the VSD and the tricuspid valve. The bundle of His lies superior to the VSD. This defect can easily be closed from a right atrial approach.

(*b*) Viewed from left ventricle. This defect (VSD) is in the posterior part of the nontrabeculated portion of the left side of the ventricular septum.

AV, aortic valve; ALMV, anterior leaflet of mitral valve; LV, left ventricle; PV, pulmonary valve; TV, tricuspid valve; VSD, ventricular septal defect.

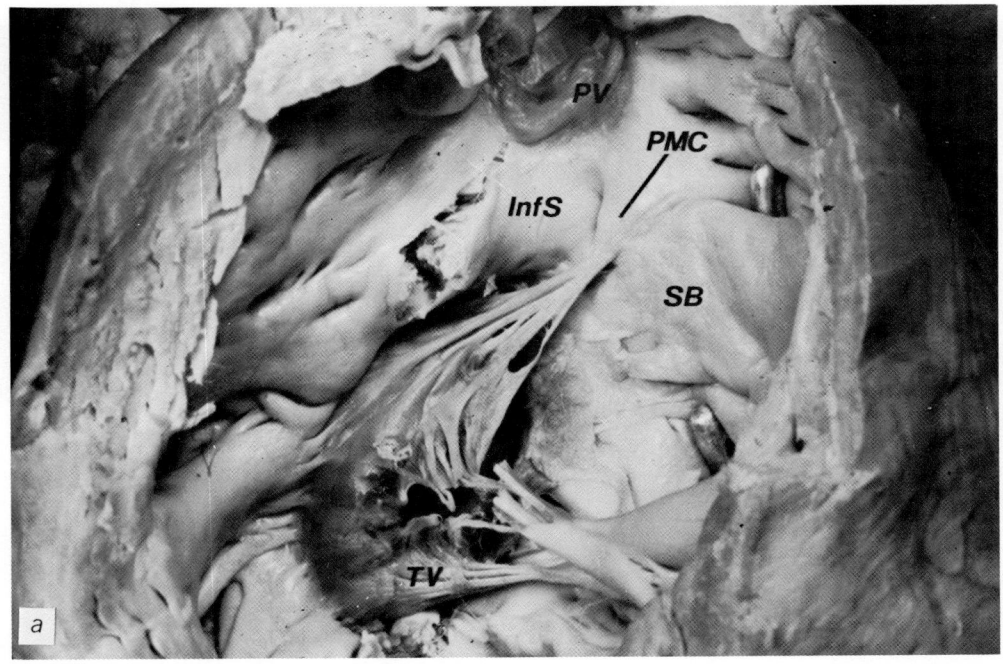

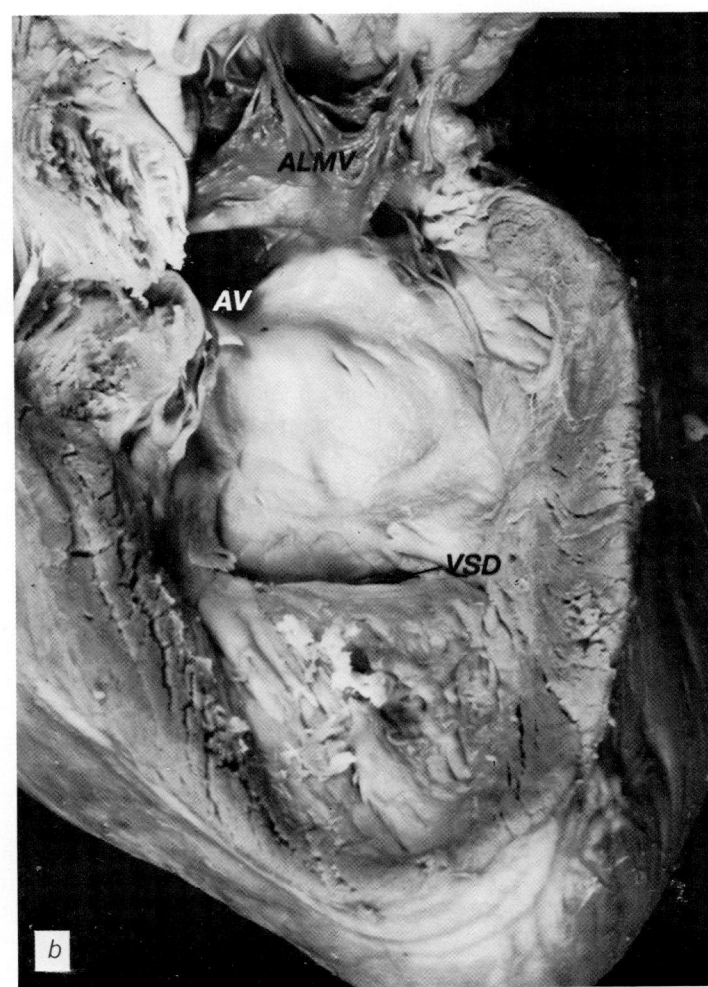

Figure 20-12 A mid-muscular VSD (GLH).

(a) Viewed from the right ventricle. The VSD is actually a single one but is covered by the septal band, or trabecula septomarginalis, and therefore has two openings into the right ventricle (see probes).

(b) Viewed from the left ventricle. The VSD, appearing more slitlike than it actually is, lies at the junction of the smooth and trabeculated portions of the septum. This defect can be closed from the right ventricle, provided the lower end of the septal band is detached (using a vertical incision parallel to the left anterior descending coronary artery) but may also be approached from left ventricle.

Ao, aorta; ALMV, anterior leaflet of mitral valve; InfS, infundibular septum, or crista supraventricularis; PMC, papillary muscle of conus; PV, pulmonary valve; SB, septal band or trabecula septomarginalis; TV, tricuspid valve; VSD, ventricular septal defect.

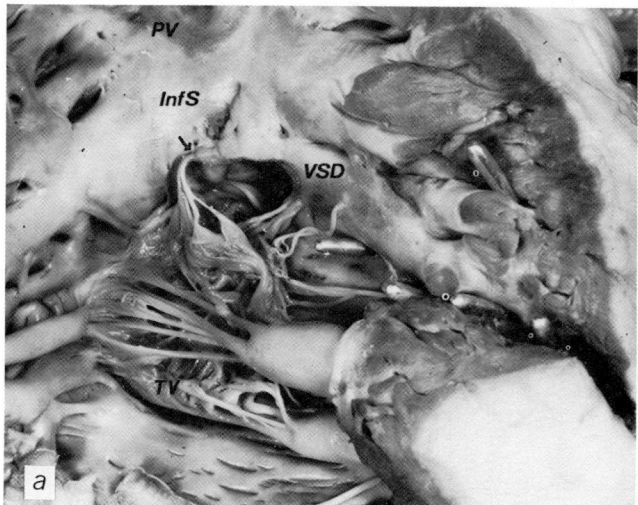

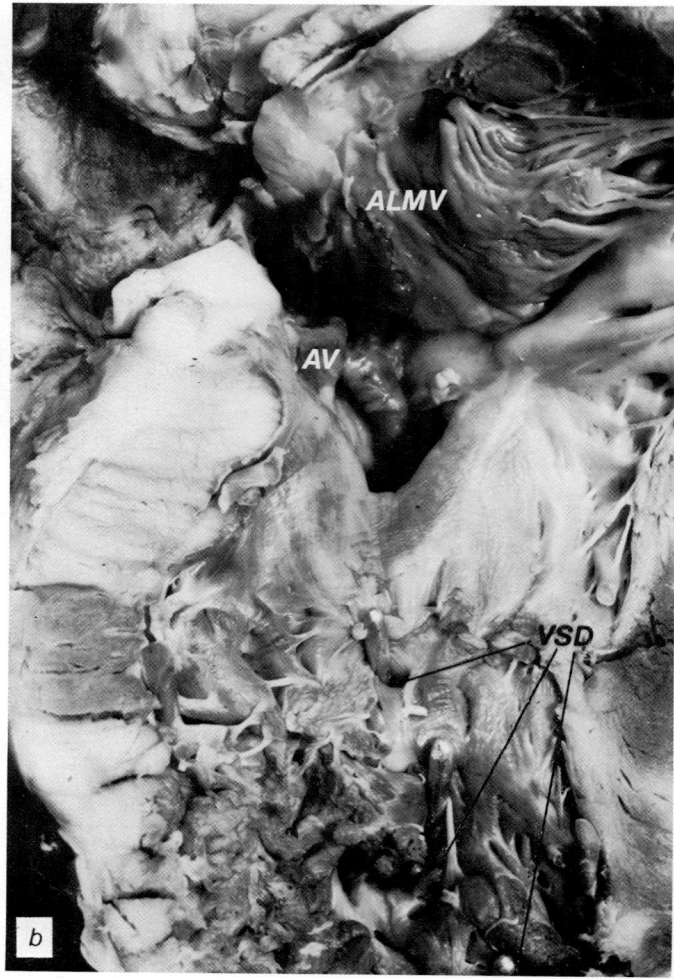

Figure 20-13 Swiss-cheese type of multiple VSDs associated with a large perimembranous defect (GLH).

(*a*) Viewed from the right ventricle. The perimembranous defect (VSD) shows anomalous chordal attachment from the tricuspid valve to the posterosuperior margin of the defect (arrow). The probes demonstrate five separate openings of small defects, one above and four below the trabecula septomarginalis.

(*b*) Viewed from the left ventricle. The perimembranous defect is seen. Probes demonstrate three separate openings of the Swiss-cheese defects, but many more lie in the grossly trabeculated lower portion of the septum.

AV, aortic valve; ALMV, anterior leaflet of mitral valve; InfS, infundibular septum; PV, pulmonary valve; TV, tricuspid valve; VSD, ventricular septal defect.

usually very large, and many of the chordae from it are attached to the left ventricular side of the septum (a combination of straddling and overriding).[B12] The plane of the septum is abnormal, and the VSD extends to the crux cordis. The right ventricle is often hypoplastic. The tricuspid valve may be incompetent. In this anomaly, the position of the AV node lies inferior to the VSD and more anterior than usual,[H14] and the risk of iatrogenic heart block is high. (A further discussion of ''Straddling and Overriding AV Valves'' is in Chapter 44 in the section on Special Situations and Controversies.)

Associated Lesions

Nearly half the patients undergoing surgical treatment for VSD have an associated lesion (Table 20-1).[B1,B3,R5]

A moderate- or large-sized *patent ductus arteriosus* is present in about 6% of the patients of all ages, but about 25% of infants in heart failure have an associated significant patent ductus (see Chapter 22).[B3] VSD occurs in combination with moderate or severe coarctation in about 5% of patients (see Chapter 34). This combination is also much more common among infants with large VSD coming to operation

when less than 3 months old, 5 (20%) of 20 such infants having such a combined lesion (GLH).

Congenital valvar or subvalvar *aortic stenosis* occurs in about 2% of patients requiring operation for VSD (Table 20-1). Subvalvar stenosis is more common[L8] and may also occur in association with VSD and infundibular pulmonary stenosis. The subvalvar stenosis is of two types. One is caused by a discrete fibromuscular bar that lies inferior (caudad or upstream) to the VSD. The other is located distal (downstream) to the VSD and, as noted earlier, often consists of a displacement of infundibular septal muscle into the left ventricular outflow tract. The latter type is often associated with aortic coarctation and interrupted arch (see Chapter 32 for more details).[A5,D7,M6,V2,V3] Subvalvar aortic stenosis may also occur after pulmonary artery banding.[F2]

Congenital mitral valve disease occurs in about 2% of patients (see Chapter 36).[B1] One of the *pulmonary arteries* may be *absent* or severely stenotic. Severe peripheral pulmonary artery stenoses occur rarely. Severe *positional cardiac anomalies*, such as isolated dextrocardia or situs inversus totalis, are uncommon in patients with VSD.

A number of minor anomalies may also be present in patients coming to operation for VSD (Table 20-2). While atrial

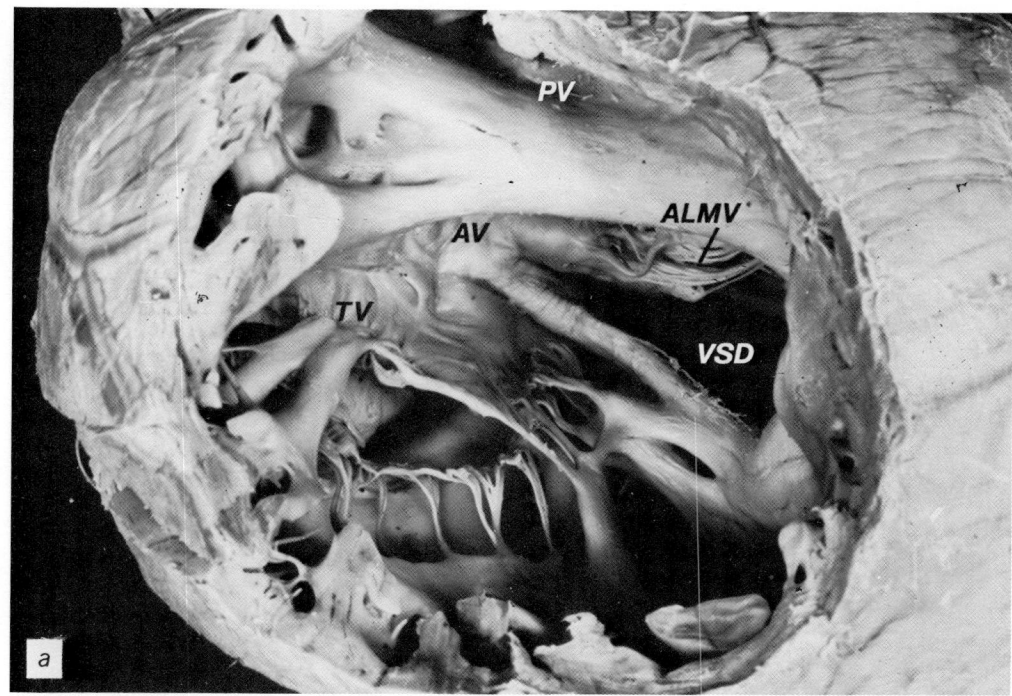

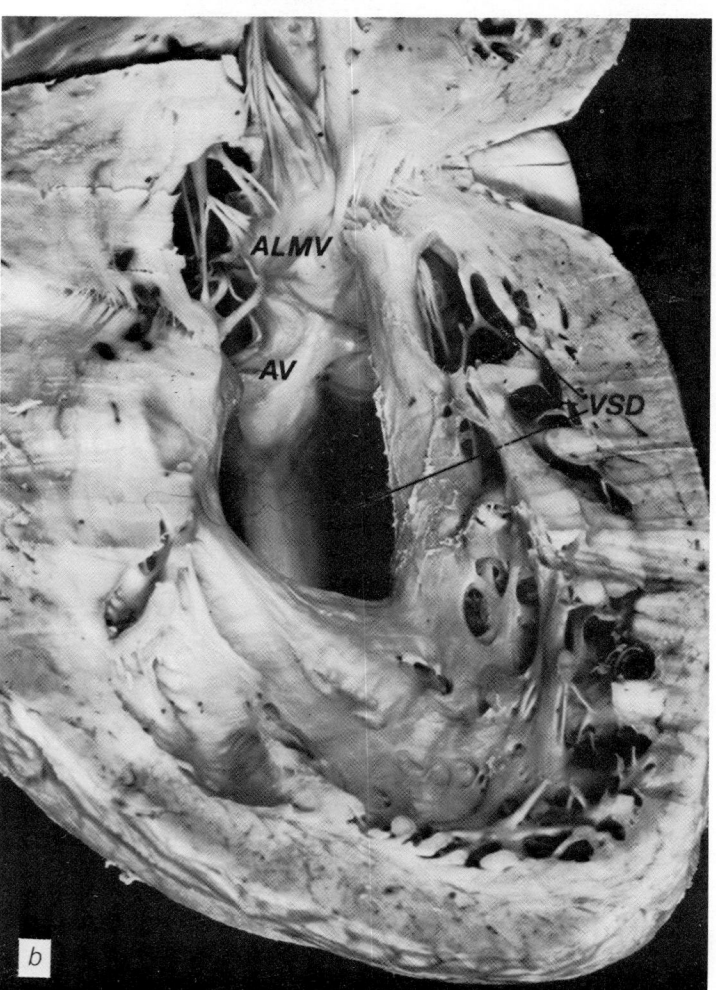

Figure 20-14 A large confluent VSD which is perimembranous and also occupies the upper half of the muscular septum beneath the infundibular septum. It is associated with Swiss-cheese VSDs (GLH).

(a) Viewed from right ventricle. The surgeon's initial impression would be that the patient had a single ventricle.

(b) Viewed from the left ventricle, the malformation is clearly not a single ventricle.

AV, aortic valve; ALMV, anterior leaflet of mitral valve; PV, pulmonary valve; TV, tricuspid valve; VSD, ventricular septal defect.

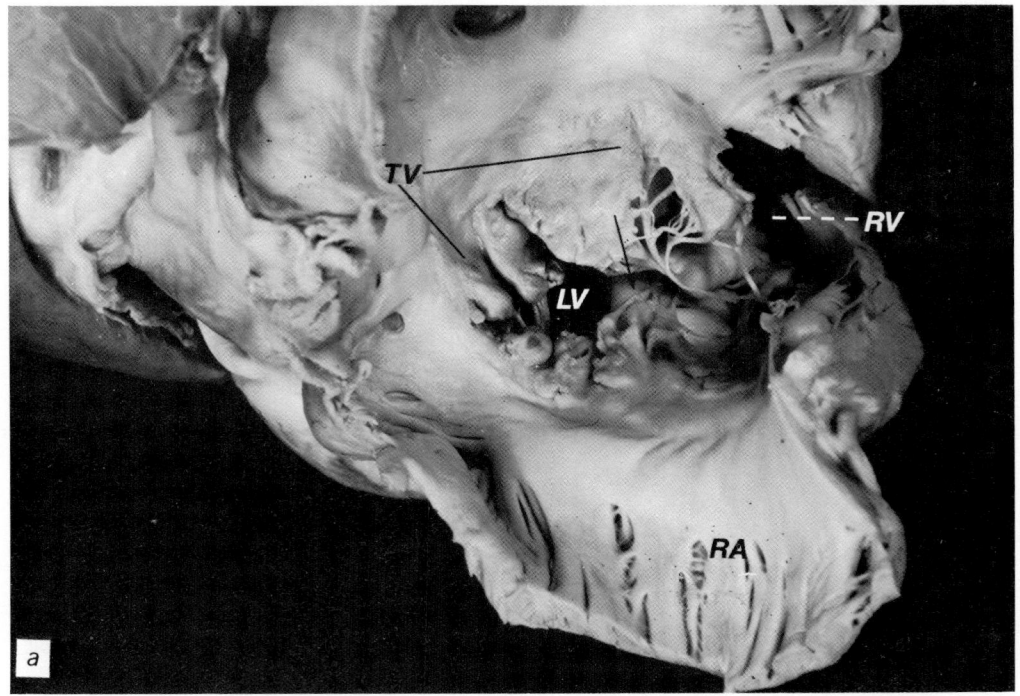

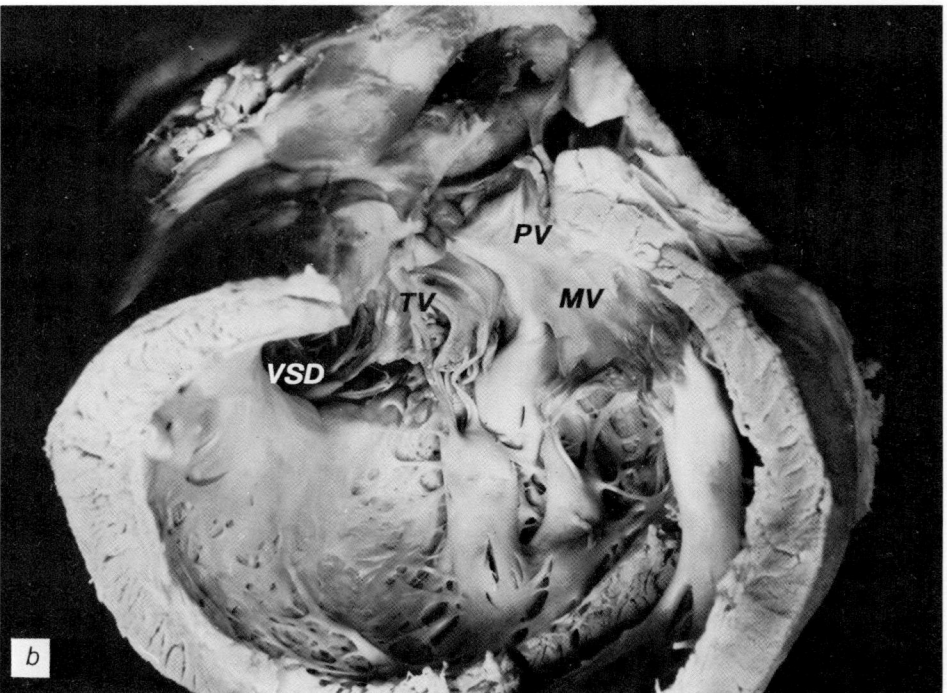

Figure 20-15 VSD and straddling tricuspid valve (GLH).
(*a*) Viewed from the right atrium. The crest of the ventricular septum forming the lower boundary of the defect (black arrow) crosses almost beneath the center of the large tricuspid orifice.
(*b*) Viewed from the left ventricle. The chordal attachments of the tricuspid valve cross the VSD to attach to the septal surface of the left ventricle. This heart also exhibits transposition of the great arteries, with the pulmonary artery above the left ventricle.

LV, left ventricle; MV, mitral valve; PA, pulmonary artery; RA, right atrium; RV, right ventricle; TV, tricuspid valve orifice.

Table 20-1 Major associated cardiac anomalies in surgical patients with primary VSD (GLH; 1956–1976; $n = 205$ and UAB; 1967–1979; $n = 312$).

Major Associated Anomaly	UAB n	UAB Hospital Deaths No.	UAB Hospital Deaths %	GLH n	GLH Hospital Deaths No.	GLH Hospital Deaths %
None	254	16	6.3%	172	9	5.2%
PDA	18	4	22%	9	0	0%
Coarctation of aorta or interrupted aortic arch						
Previously repaired[a]	5	2	40%	NT		
Plus unrepaired recoarctation	1	0	0%	NT		
Simultaneously repaired	3	2	67%	2	1	50%
Unrepaired	2	0	0%			
Mitral valve disease	4	1	25%	4	0	0%
Plus straddling and cleft mitral valve	1	0	0%			
Plus PDA	3	1	33%	NT		
Straddling tricuspid valve	4	0	0%	NT		
Tricuspid incompetence	2	0	0%	NT		
Positional cardiac anomalies				3	0	0%
Mesoposition of the heart	1	0	0%			
Dextrocardia, unrepaired coarctation of aorta	1	1	100%			
Situs inversus totalis	1	0	0%			
Plus PDA	1	1	100%			
Valvar aortic stenosis				3	2	67%
Subaortic stenosis	2	0	0%	5	1	20%
Plus PDA, coarctation of aorta repaired	1	1	100%	NT		
Severe stenosis of MPA				1	0	0%
Absence or severe stenosis of LPA or RPA	3	1	33%	2	0	0%
Absent LPA with PDA	1	0	0%			
Origin of RPA from ascending aorta	1	0	0%			
Anomalous pulmonary or systemic venous connection[b]	1	0	0%	2	0	0%
Hypoplastic RV, small tricuspid anulus	1	0	0%			
Unroofed coronary sinus	1	0	0%	NT		

KEY: LPA, left pulmonary artery; MPA, main pulmonary artery; NT, not tabulated; PDA, patent ductus arteriosus; RPA, right pulmonary artery; RV, right ventricle.

[a] Excludes those treated initially by coarctation repair plus pulmonary artery banding.

[b] Exclusive of persistent left superior vena cava.

septal defects in general are not considered major associated anomalies, they may coexist with a large VSD in small infants and be very important lesions.[B3]

Pulmonary Vascular Disease

The classic description of the pathology of hypertensive pulmonary vascular disease is that of Heath and Edwards.[H1] They defined grade 1 changes as being characterized by medial hypertrophy without intimal proliferation; grade 2 by medial hypertrophy with cellular intimal reaction; grade 3 by intimal fibrosis, as well as medial hypertrophy, possibly early generalized vascular dilation; grade 4 by generalized vascular dilation, areas of vascular occlusion by intimal fibrosis, and plexiform lesions; grade 5 by other dilation lesions such as cavernous and angiomatoid lesions; and grade 6 by necrotizing arteritis in addition to the characteristics of the grade 5 changes.

The pulmonary resistance in patients with large VSD (and those with large patent ductus arteriosus) has been positively correlated with the histologic severity of the hypertensive pulmonary vascular disease by Heath and colleagues.[H2] However, recent reanalysis of their data shows that the confidence limits are rather wide around the probability of severe pulmonary vascular disease as predicted from the pulmonary resistance (UAB; Fig. 20-16). Such results were not unexpected, since the Heath-Edwards classification is based on the most severe lesion seen, regardless of its frequency, and, as pointed out by Wagenvoort[W2,W3] and more recently by Yamaki and Tezuka,[Y1] the grading should include an assessment of the number of vessels affected. Moreover, the calculation of pulmonary vascular resistance is open to many errors.[H11]

A somewhat different view of hypertensive pulmonary vascular disease in infants with large VSD has been provided in recent years by Reid and colleagues.[H7] Others had pointed out earlier that intimal proliferation (and thus Heath-Edwards changes of grade 2 or greater) rarely develops in infants with large VSD until 1 or 2 years of age,[D6,W2] and yet infants occasionally do have severely elevated pulmonary

Table 20-2 Minor associated cardiac anomalies in surgical patients with large primary VSD (GLH; 1958–1976; and UAB; 1967–1976).

Minor Associated Anomaly	Number and % of 138 Patients[a] (UAB)	Number and % of 205 Patients[a] (GLH)	Number and % of 343 Patients (Combined Series)
None	73, 53%	111, 54%	184, 54%
Mild or moderate pulmonary stenosis	27, 20%	18, 9%	45, 13%
Atrial septal defect[b]	24, 17%	26, 13%	50, 15%
Persistent left superior vena cava	12, 9%	16, 8%	28, 8%
Dextroposition of the aorta	7, 5%	NT	NT
Aneurysm of membranous septum	2, 1%	3, 1%	5, 1%
Mild or moderate coarctation of aorta	2, 1%	6, 3%	8, 2%
Vascular ring	1, 0.7%	1, 0.5%	2, 1%
Right aortic arch	NT	4, 2%	NT
Tricuspid incompetence, mild	2, 1%	2, 1%	4, 1%
Mitral incompetence, mild		2, 1%	2, 1%
Pulmonary valve incompetence	1, 0.7%	3, 1%	4, 1%
Inferior vena cava draining via azygos vein		1, 0.5%	1, 0.3%
Hepatic veins entering right atrium directly	1, 0.7%		1, 0.3%
Congenital aneurysm of anterior RV wall		2, 1%	2, 1%
Anomalous RV muscle band without pulmonary stenosis	1, 0.7%		1, 0.3%
Anterior descending coronary artery arising from right coronary artery		1, 0.5%	1, 0.3%

KEY: NT, not tabulated; RV, right ventricle.

[a] Sum of percentages is > 100% because some patients had more than one minor associated condition.

[b] Exclusive of simple patent foramen ovale.

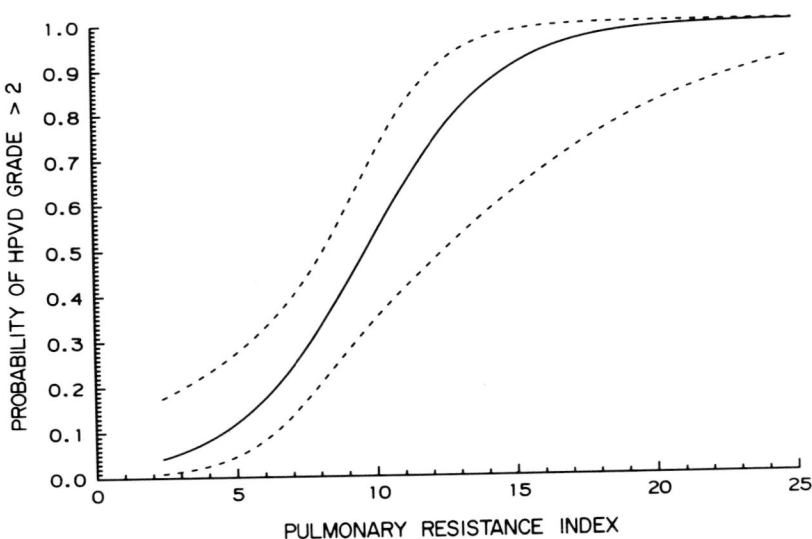

Figure 20-16 Probability of the occurrence of hypertensive pulmonary vascular disease greater than grade 2 in patients with VSD, given the total pulmonary resistance index (units·m²). Dotted lines enclose the 70% confidence limits ($P = .07$).

HPVD, hypertensive pulmonary vascular disease.

Data from Heath et al.[H2]

resistance. Reid and colleagues found that infants dying at 3–6 months of age with large VSD and high (> 8 units $\cdot$ m^2) pulmonary vascular resistance with intermittent right-to-left shunting have marked medial hypertrophy affecting both large and small pulmonary arteries, including those less than 200 micrometers (μm) in diameter.[H7] The usual number of intra-acinar vessels was present. In contrast, they found that infants (3–10 months old) with large VSD dying with a history of large pulmonary blood flow and congestive heart failure and normal or slightly elevated pulmonary vascular resistance have medial hypertrophy affecting mainly arteries larger than 200 μm. The intra-acinar vessels were fewer than usual. These histologic features have been shown by Rabinovitch and colleagues to correlate with the pulmonary hemodynamic findings after the repair of ventricular septal defects.[R6]

The histologic reversibility of pulmonary vascular disease after closure of the VSD has not been documented. The favorable results in infants may be from an increase in the number of arterioles and capillaries as growth proceeds. Presumably, pulmonary vascular disease of Heath and Edwards' grade 3 or greater severity is not reversible.

CLINICAL FEATURES AND DIAGNOSTIC CRITERIA

Clinical Features

In infants, signs and symptoms of heart failure, including tachypnea and liver enlargement often associated with growth failure, and the physical findings of a precordial pansystolic or more abbreviated systolic murmur and a hyperactive heart suggest the diagnosis of *large VSD*. An apical diastolic murmur suggests large flow across the mitral valve during diastole, the result of a large pulmonary blood flow. Cardiomegaly and evidence of large pulmonary blood flow are seen on the chest x-ray (Fig. 20-17). The electrocardio-

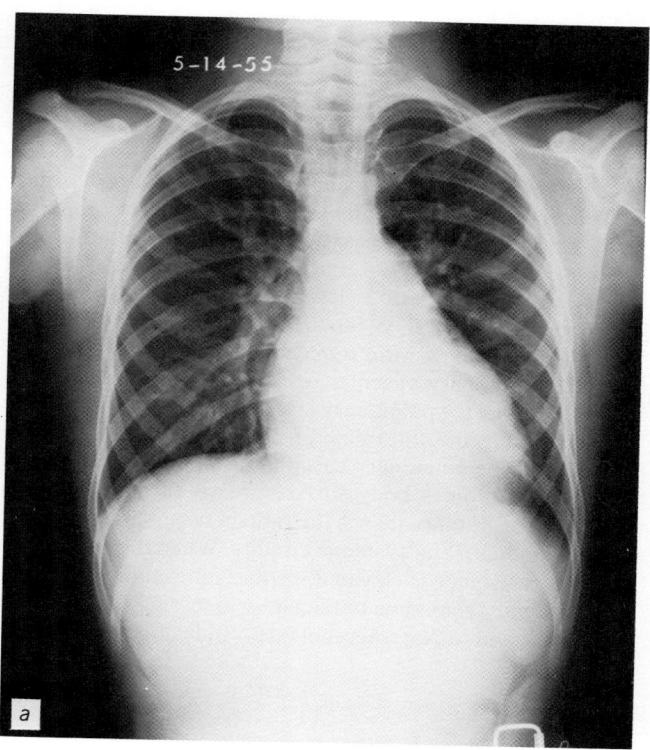
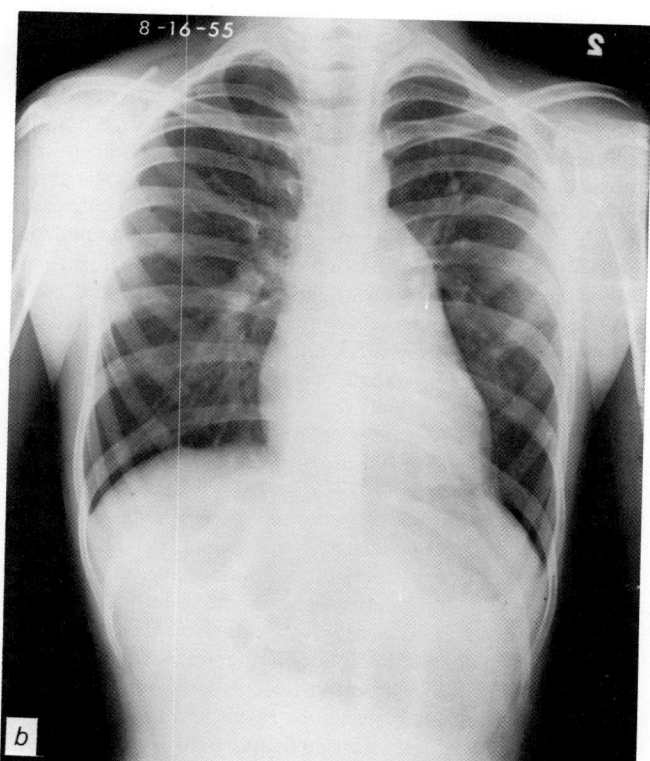

Figure 20-17   Chest x-rays in patients with VSD.
(*a*) Chest x-ray of an 11-year-old girl with a large VSD with a large left-to-right shunt, severe pulmonary hypertension, and low pulmonary vascular resistance. Cardiac enlargement and increased pulmonary vascularity are evident. The pulmonary artery is enlarged, and the aortic arch is small. Examination of this patient revealed an overactive heart with a systolic thrill and a loud (grade 4), long systolic murmur extending from the lower left sternal border to the apex and an apical diastolic murmur. The electrocardiogram showed evidence of left ventricular overwork.
(*b*) Chest x-ray of a 10-year-old girl with a large VSD, severe pulmonary hypertension, $\dot{Q}p/\dot{Q}s$ of 1.2, and pulmonary vascular resistance of 11 units·m^2. The cardiac size is normal, but the main pulmonary artery segment is enlarged. The pulmonary vascularity is not increased. Examination revealed a quiet heart, no thrill, a soft (grade 2) systolic murmur, and no apical diastolic murmur; closure of the pulmonic valve was loud and palpable. The electrocardiogram demonstrated right ventricular hypertrophy without evidence of left ventricular overwork.
Reproduced with permission from Kirklin et al.[K2]

gram (ECG) usually shows biventricular hypertrophy. In older patients with large VSD, the history is often nonspecific, but examination also shows evidence of left and right ventricular enlargement and a systolic murmur usually best heard in the third and fourth left interspaces. In patients with subpulmonary VSDs, the systolic murmur is maximal in the second and third interspaces, and in defects shunting mainly into the right atrium, in the fourth and fifth interspaces.

A *high pulmonary vascular resistance* from severe pulmonary vascular disease changes the hemodynamic state and the clinical findings in patients with large VSDs. A large left-to-right shunt is no longer present because the output resistances of the two pathways for left ventricular emptying are similar, and the shunt is bidirectional and of about equal magnitude in the two directions. The heart is not enlarged in volume and is not hyperactive. The systolic murmur (which is produced by the large flow across the VSD) is soft or absent, and no apical diastolic murmur is heard. The pulmonary component of the second sound at the base is loud and sometimes palpable. The chest x-ray reflects these features (Fig. 20-17b). The ECG shows severe right ventricular hypertrophy, rather than combined ventricular hypertrophy and evidence of left ventricular volume overload. When the pulmonary vascular disease is even more advanced, cyanosis develops (Eisenmenger's complex) because the shunt across the VSD becomes right-to-left as the right ventricular output resistance through the pulmonary vascular bed becomes higher than that through the VSD and the aorta.

Patients with *small VSDs* have small shunts and often have no abnormal signs or symptoms other than the pansystolic murmur. The chest x-ray and ECG both may be normal. When the defect is *moderate in size* and the shunt somewhat larger than that associated with small VSDs, the left ventricle is mildly or moderately enlarged, as shown by physical examination, chest x-ray, and ECG, and the volume of the right ventricle is increased.

When there is associated *pulmonary stenosis* or *aortic stenosis,* the diagnostic features are changed. Thus, with significant pulmonary stenosis, the pulmonary blood flow is reduced and the shunt may even be right-to-left. The degree of right ventricular hypertrophy is increased. With significant aortic stenosis, the load on the left ventricle is increased, and if the obstruction is cephalad to the VSD, the left-to-right shunt is also greater, resulting in more than the expected degree of left ventricular hypertrophy in the ECG. Coarctation of the aorta may also produce these features in older children.

Two-Dimensional Echocardiography

Two-dimensional echocardiography often identifies the defect in the ventricular septum and, in combination with the clinical criteria, may be sufficient for the diagnosis. Nonetheless, currently the definitive data from the surgical standpoint continue to be provided by cardiac catheterization and proper angiocardiography. These invasive studies are indicated to identify precisely the location, size, and number of the VSDs and any associated anomalies. Further, the preoperative sizing of VSDs is often important in arriving at

Table 20-3 Pulmonary vascular resistance.

≤	Units · m²	<
	Normal	4
4	Mildly elevated	6
6	Moderately elevated	10
10	Severely elevated	

management decisions, and the sizing can be a difficult matter. Sizing can be especially difficult when the VSD is associated with another lesion, such as coarctation or pulmonary stenosis. The most reliable way to size the defect is to measure its diameter at cineangiography. The VSD must be accurately profiled, and the measurement either corrected to allow for magnification or compared to aortic root diameter. In applying this method to perimembranous VSDs, the defect is smaller in a cranially tilted left anterior oblique projection (LAO) than in the conventional LAO position.

Cardiac Catheterization

Cardiac catheterization should include both right and left heart studies, the latter mainly to obtain left ventricular angiocardiograms. Basic data obtained at cardiac catheterization should include oxygen consumption; systolic, diastolic, and mean pulmonary, pulmonary artery wedge, and systemic arterial pressures; oxygen content and saturation in right atrial, pulmonary arterial, aortic or peripheral arterial blood, and, when possible, left atrial blood. The pulmonary ($\dot{Q}p$) and systemic ($\dot{Q}s$) blood flows and the pulmonary-systemic blood flow ratio ($\dot{Q}p/\dot{Q}s$) are calculated,[2] together with the pulmonary vascular resistance (Rpv) (Table 20-3). When left atrial (or pulmonary arterial wedge) pressure is not available, only the total pulmonary resistance (Rp) can be calculated. The pulmonary vascular (arteriolar) resistance in absolute units times body surface area is of more value in predicting operability than is the ratio between the resistance in the pulmonary and systemic circuits. When the pulmonary vascular resistance is elevated, further information concerning operability should be obtained by assessing the response to exercise and to isoproterenol (see "Indications for Operation").

---

[2] $$\dot{Q}p = \dot{V}o_2/(Cpvo_2 - Cpao_2) \text{ in } l \cdot m^{-1}$$

where pv is pulmonary vein and pa is pulmonary artery. $\dot{Q}p$ may be expressed as index ($l \cdot min^{-1} \cdot m^{-2}$) by dividing by body surface area (BSA) expressed in square meters.

$$\dot{Q}s = \dot{V}o_2/(Cao_2 - C\bar{v}o_2) \text{ in } l \cdot min^{-1}$$

where a is aorta or arterial and $\bar{v}$ is mixed venous.

$$\dot{Q}p/\dot{Q}s = (Cao_2 - C\bar{v}o_2)/(Cpvo_2 - Cpao_2).$$

Note that total oxygen consumption is not needed for this calculation.

$$Rpv = (Ppa - Pla)/\dot{Q}p \times BSA; \text{ Rpv is expressed in units} \cdot m^2$$

$$Rp = Ppa/\dot{Q}p \times BSA; \text{ Rp is expressed in units} \cdot m^2$$

Angiocardiography

The angiocardiographic assessment of VSDs is best performed using biplane cineangiographic techniques in appropriate *projections*.[B9,B13] Whereas the cardiologists and radiologists carry primary responsibility for these studies, appreciation of their findings and of their limitations is essential to the surgeon, who must also understand when the study is an incomplete one.

A summary of the surgically important features of cineangiograms of VSDs is presented in Figure 20-18, and representative cineangiograms of the various types of VSDs are shown in Figure 20-19.

NATURAL HISTORY

Spontaneous Closure

VSDs have a tendency to close spontaneously, and this fact is relevant to decisions about operation.[C10] Spontaneous clo-

sure can be complete by 1 year of age, or the defect may have only narrowed by then, with complete closure taking considerably longer. When the VSD is perimembranous in position, the mechanism of narrowing or closure of the defect is adherence of tricuspid leaflet or chordal tissue to the edges of the VSD.[S19] The phenomenon of spontaneous closure of narrowing of VSDs explains the infrequency with which large VSDs are encountered in adults. An inverse relation exists between the probability of eventual spontaneous closure and the age at which the patient is observed (Fig. 20-20).[B1,H6,K5] About 80% of persons with large VSDs seen at 1 month of age seem to experience eventual spontaneous closure, as do about 60% of those seen at 3 months of age, about 50% of those seen at 6 months of age, and about 25% of those seen at 12 months of age. This decreasing tendency to spontaneous closure of a VSD as the patient becomes older has also been confirmed by Beerman and colleagues, who found no instances of closure in patients whose VSDs were still open at 6 years of age.[B16]

The validity of these inferences about the tendency toward

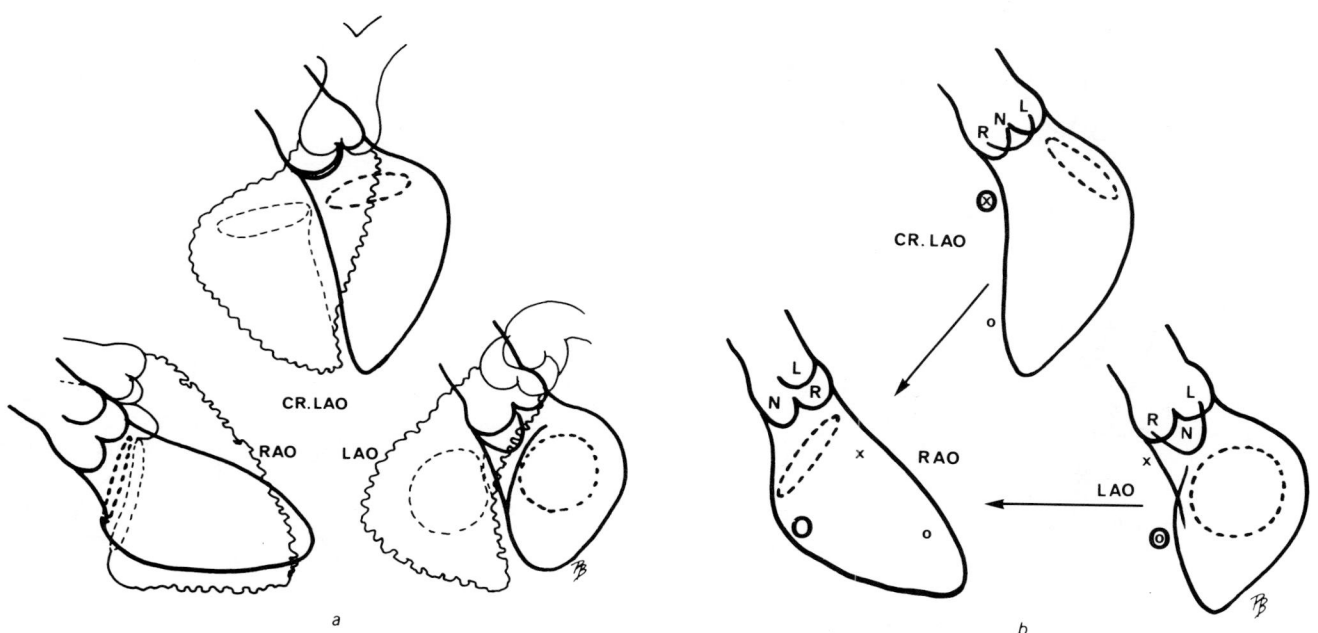

Figure 20-18 Line drawings of angiographic projections for VSD assessment.
(a) Interrelationships of the left ventricle and aortic root (thick line) with the right ventricle and pulmonary artery (thin line) in 40° right anterior oblique (RAO), 50° left anterior oblique (LAO), and 40° cranially tilted (CR.LAO) projections. The RAO view profiles the conal (infundibular) and high anterior parts of the right ventricular outflow septum below and in front of the right coronary sinus and profiles the atrioventricular septum beneath the noncoronary sinus of the aortic root. Both LAO views profile the sinus (apical trabecular) portion of the septum. The LAO view also partly profiles the RV outflow septum but superimposes it on the left ventricular outflow tract and aortic root. The CR.LAO projection views the RV outflow septum en face and superimposes it on the left ventricle. Because the orientation shows a horizontally lying heart, the LAO view depicts the full height (cranial to caudal) of the sinus (apical trabecular) portion of the venticular septum and atrioventricular valve rings (interrupted lines), while the CR.LAO view depicts the full length of the sinus septum from base to apex.
(b) Both cranially tilted (CR) and conventional LAO views are required for a complete assessment of the sinus septum. Basal (inlet) (O, x) VSDs are separated from more apical (o) VSDs by the CR.LAO projection, while high (x) VSDs are separated from low (O) VSDs by the LAO view.
L, left coronary; LV, left ventricle; N, noncoronary; R, right coronary; RV, right ventricle.
Reproduced with permission from Brandt et al.[B14]

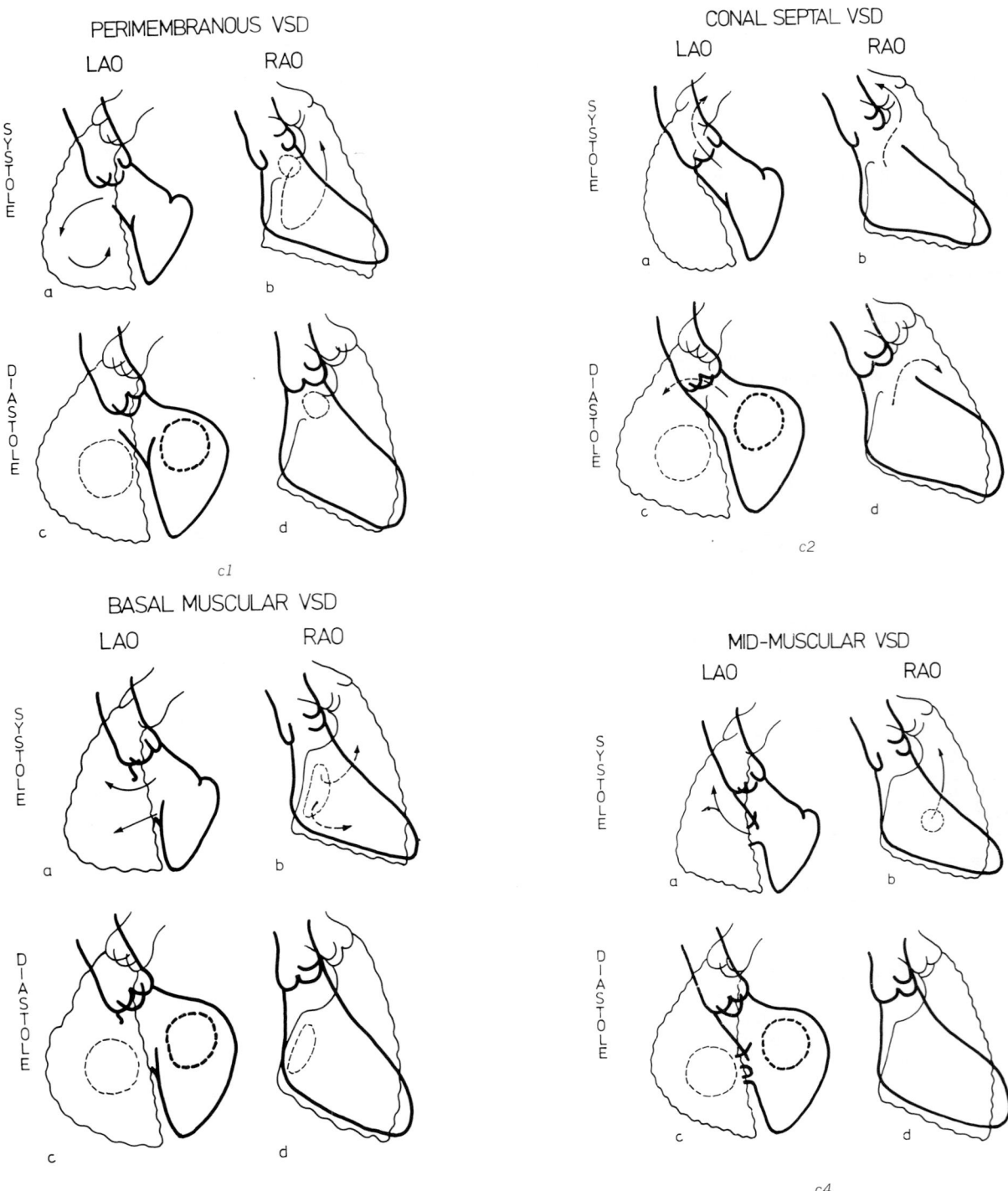

PERIMEMBRANOUS VSD

CONAL SEPTAL VSD

BASAL MUSCULAR VSD

MID-MUSCULAR VSD

620

HIGH ANTERIOR & APICAL MUSCULAR VSDs

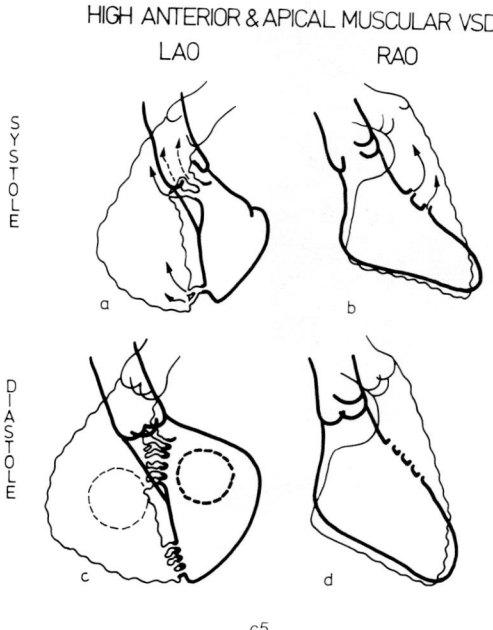

Figure 20-18 *(continued)*

(c) The anatomical and hemodynamic features of VSDs shown by left ventricular cineangiocardiograms. The LAO diagrams show a compromise between conventional and cranially tilted options. The left ventricle and aorta are shown by thick lines, the right ventricle and pulmonary artery by thin lines, and the atrioventricular valves and nonprofiled VSDs by interrupted lines.

(1) Perimembranous VSD. The LAO view profiles the VSD just beneath the parietal band at the upper margin of the basal (inlet) septum. The flow enters the base of the right ventricle above the tricuspid valve, filling the base before reaching the infundibulum. The tricuspid valve is well seen in diastole, and the lower margin of the defect can be accurately related to the tricuspid ring in LAO.

The RAO view does not profile the defect unless it extends into the conal septum. Note the intact atrioventricular septum beneath the noncoronary sinus of the aortic root. The shunt enters the right ventricular infundibulum, crossing but not interrupting the intact superior margin of the left ventricle, indicating intact conal and high anterior septal regions.

(2) Subpulmonary (subarterial or conal septal) VSD. The LAO view shows an intact septum from aortic valve to apex. The right

ventricular sinus usually fills only faintly by diastolic mixing from the infundibular region, and the tricuspid valve may not be shown. The defect is superimposed on the aortic root.

The RAO view profiles the defect beneath the contiguous parts of the aortic and pulmonary valves. Systolic streaming through the right ventricular infundibulum to the pulmonary artery is well shown, with some mixing to the more anterior part of the right ventricle in diastole, but the high anterior septal region is intact.

(3) Inlet (basal) septal VSD. The VSD is adjacent to the tricuspid valve (AV canal VSD) or separated from it by a rim of muscle (muscular VSD). These two types of VSDs are not readily distinguished radiologically.

In the LAO view, the defect is profiled between the AV valves, replacing the full height of the basal septum (conventional LAO view), perhaps extending into the adjacent middle portion of the ventricular septum but not into the apical region (cranially tilted LAO view). Contrast medium streams directly into the base of the right ventricular sinus in systole, providing a good depiction of the tricuspid orifice in diastole. Separate AV valves are present, in contrast to the finding in a complete AV canal defect (see Chapter 19).

In the RAO view, the VSD is not profiled. The intact atrioventricular septum distinguishes this defect from a true AV canal defect. Note the intact conal and high anterior septal regions.

(4) Mid-muscular VSD. The LAO views show an intact basal (inlet) septum and no extension into the apical region, though a small additional defect is seen in diastole, closing in systole. Some of the contrast medium streams directly into the right ventricular outflow during systole. The height of the defect from the floor of the ventricle (bottom of the AV valve) is appreciated in the LAO view, the separation from basal and apical regions in the cranially tilted LAO view. RAO features are as in parts 1 and 3.

(5) Multiple muscular anterior infundibular and apical VSDs. Muscular VSDs in these regions frequently coexist and, if numerous, form a continuous series throughout the trabeculated septum from high in the right ventricular infundibulum to the apical sinus septum. For clarity, only the highest and lowest are shown here.

In the LAO view, the intact basal and middle septal regions are profiled. The apical defects are profiled, but the high anterior defects are superimposed on the left ventricular outflow region. Contrast medium tends to stream to the right ventricular outflow tract without filling the basal parts.

In the RAO view, the high anterior defects are profiled, interrupting the superior margin of the left ventricle anterior to the intact conal septum. More defects are open in diastole than in systole.

621

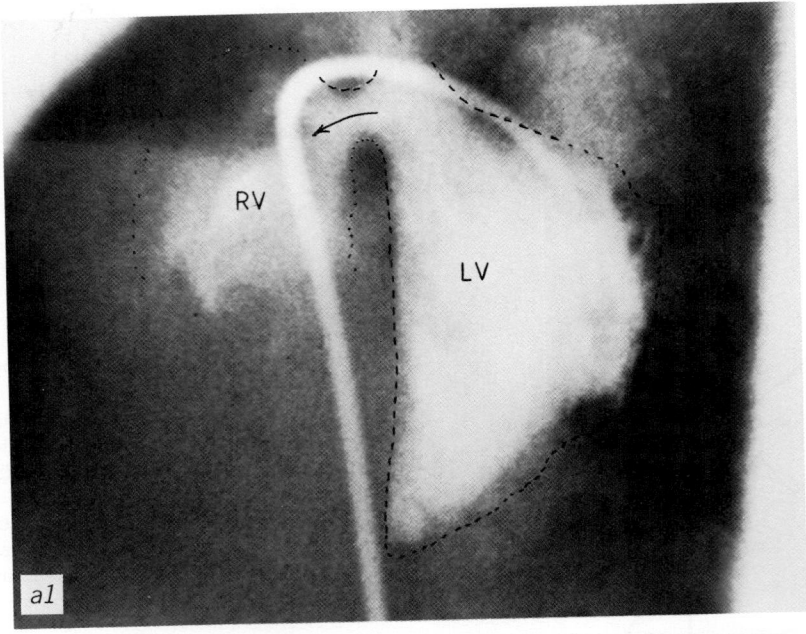

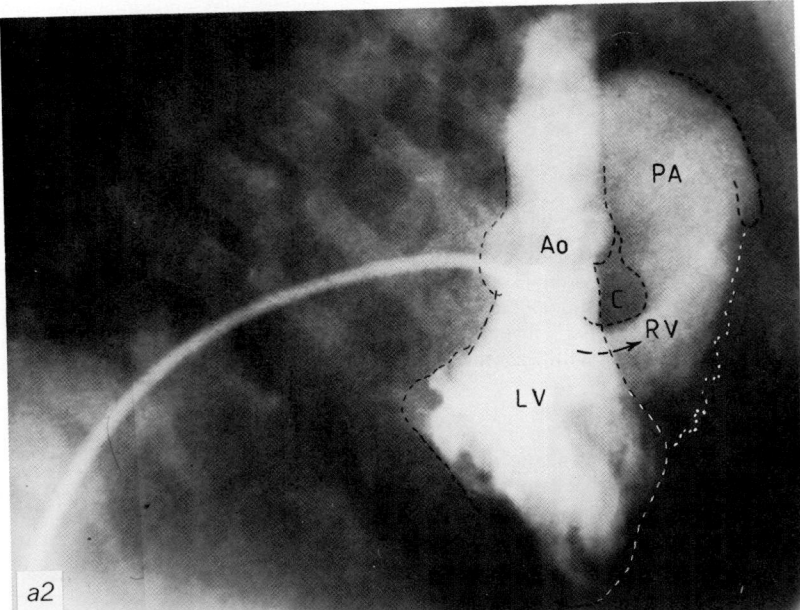

Figure 20-19 Cineangiocardiograms of patients with ventricular septal defect (GLH).
(a) Left ventricular cineangiocardiograms of a perimembranous VSD.

(1) Forty-degree cranially tilted 60° LAO projection, systolic frame, early in cineangiographic sequence. The VSD (arrow) lies in the basal part of the ventricular septum adjacent to the aortic root. No additional defects are seen in the middle and apical portions of the septum (catheter to left ventricle through atrial septum and mitral valve).

(2) Thirty-degree RAO projection, systolic frame, slightly later than 1 in cine sequence. The patient was positioned to achieve the cranial tilting of the simultaneously exposed LAO view shown in (1). Note the intact atrioventricular septum beneath the noncoronary aortic sinus and the intact conal septum (c). Contrast medium from the shunt through the nonprofiled VSD fills the right ventricular outflow tract, crossing (arrow) but not interrupting the high anterior margin of the left ventricle.

A, aortic valve; Ao, aorta; C, conal or infundibular septum; D, subpulmonary (conal) VSD; LV, left ventricle; P, pulmonary valve; PA or MPA, pulmonary artery; RV, right ventricle; V, atrioventricular septum.

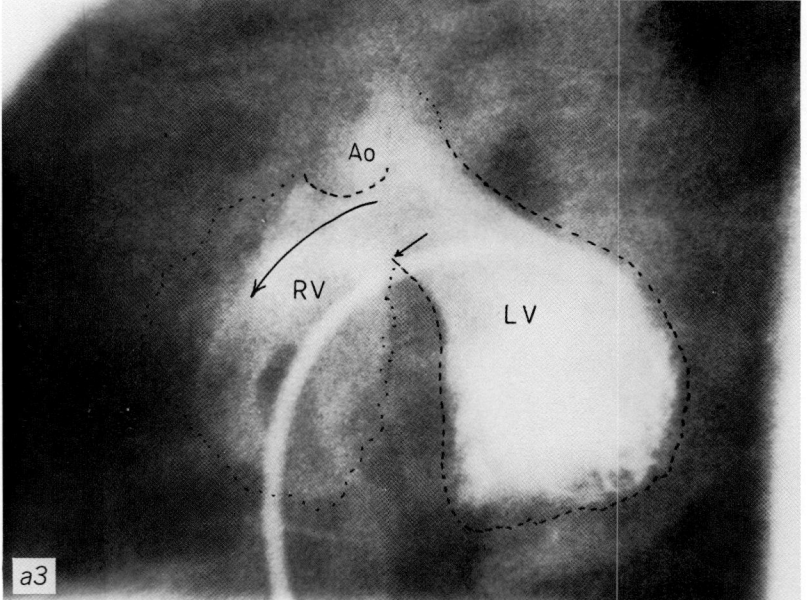

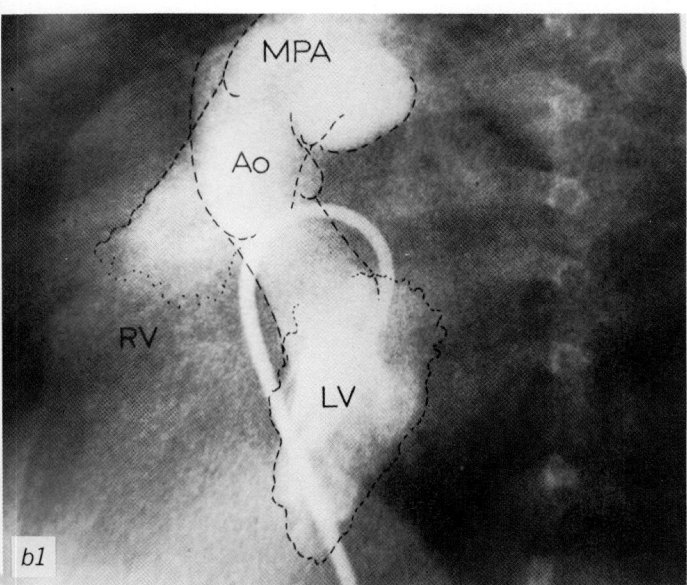

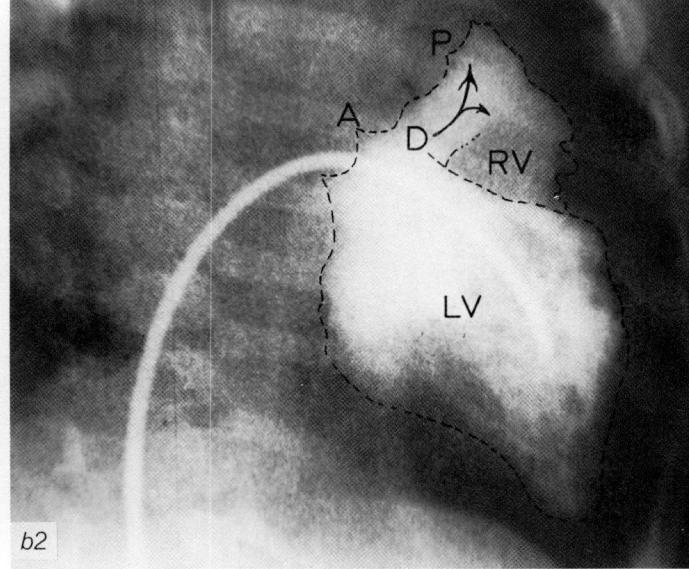

Figure 20-19 *(continued)*

(3) Fifty-degree LAO projection, systolic frame early in cine sequence (second injection). The perimembranous VSD is profiled as in (1) beneath the aortic root. The large arrow indicates flow into the base of the right ventricle above the tricuspid valve (identified in diastole but not illustrated). The downward extent of the VSD (small arrow) is accurately shown, and there are no additional defects lower in the basal sinus septum. Perimembranous defects are frequently small, of the dimensions profiled in cranially tilted LAO (1), compared with LAO.

(b) Left ventricular cineangiocardiograms of a subpulmonary (conal) VSD.

(1) Sixty-degree LAO projection, systolic frame early in cine sequence. Pulmonary arteries are filled by the shunt through the conal septal defect superimposed on the left ventricular outflow tract. Only a little contrast medium is seen in the right ventricular sinus, and the whole of the sinus septum is shown to be intact.

(2) Thirty-degree RAO projection, diastolic or very early systolic frame early in cine sequence. The subpulmonary (conal) VSD is profiled immediately beneath the contiguous parts of aortic and pulmonary valves still closed. Arrows show streaming from the VSD toward the pulmonary valve, with some filling of the remainder of the right ventricular infundibulum, but the high anterior left ventricular margin is intact.

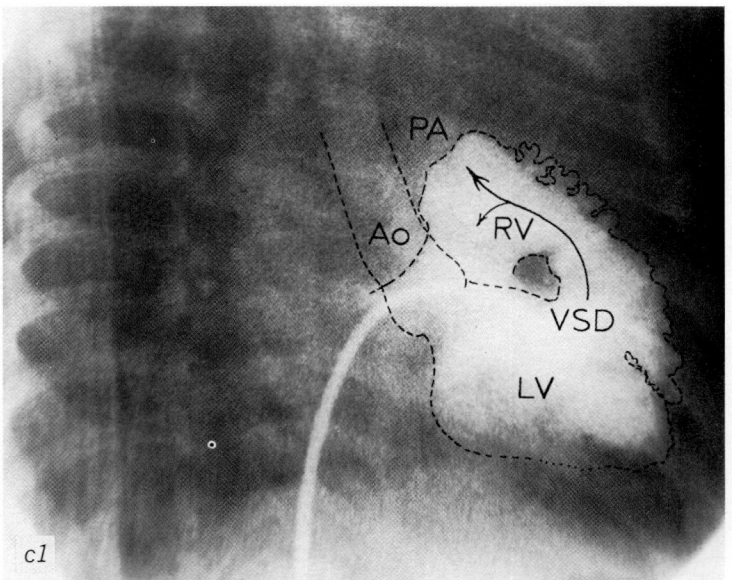

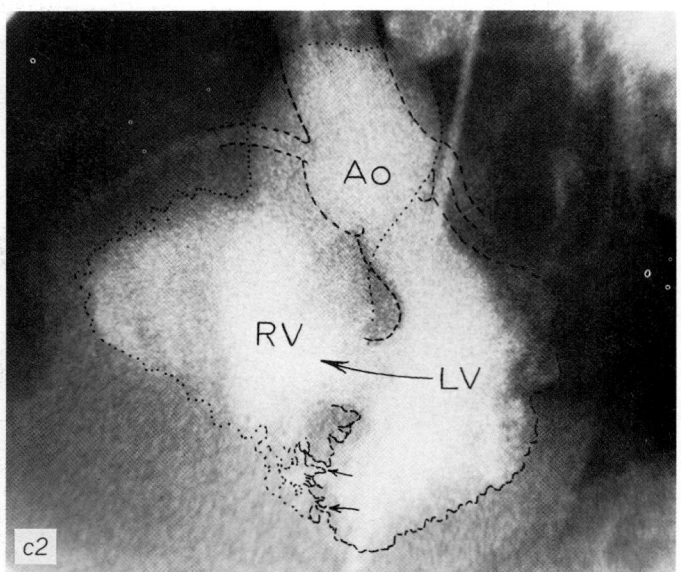

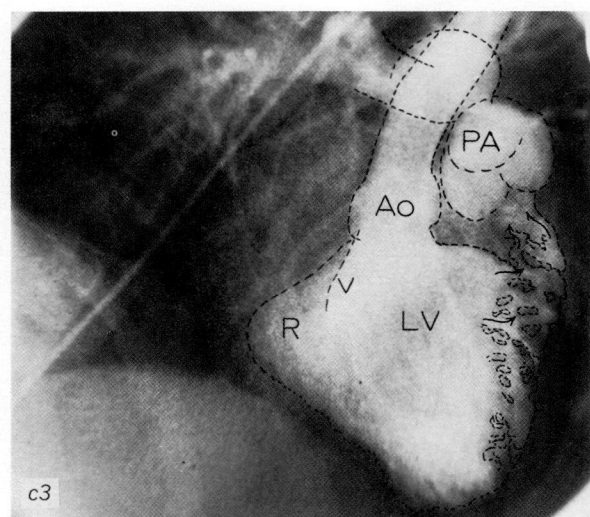

Figure 20-19 (*continued*)

(c) Left ventricular cineangiocardiograms of muscular VSDs.

(1) High anterior infundibular) muscular VSD. Thirty-degree RAO projection, diastolic or very early systolic cine frame early in sequence. The shunt through the large high anterior muscular VSD fills the anterior part of the right ventricular infundibulum. Arrows show that the main stream toward the pulmonary valve is still closed. There is a little mixing to the right ventricular sinus, but the conal (infundibular) septum is intact.

(2) Multiple muscular VSDs (Swiss-cheese septum). Forty-degree cranially tilted 60° LAO projection, systolic cine frame. A large mid-muscular VSD (large arrow), accompanied by numerous small apical defects (small arrows), is profiled, but the basal part of the ventricular septum beneath the aortic root is intact. In diastole (not illustrated), more numerous apical defects were apparent. Note the surgically banded pulmonary artery.

(3) Thirty-degree RAO projection, diastolic frame in the same patient as in (2). Numerous high anterior muscular VSDs (arrows) interrupt the LV margin. Note the intact conal septal margin of left ventricle near the aortic valve. Earlier in the sequence the intact atrioventricular septum was identified, but the base of the filled right ventricle overlaps the base of the left ventricle in this frame. Note that the position of the large mid-muscular VSD is incompletely evaluated. An LAO view would determine its height above the floor of the ventricles.

624

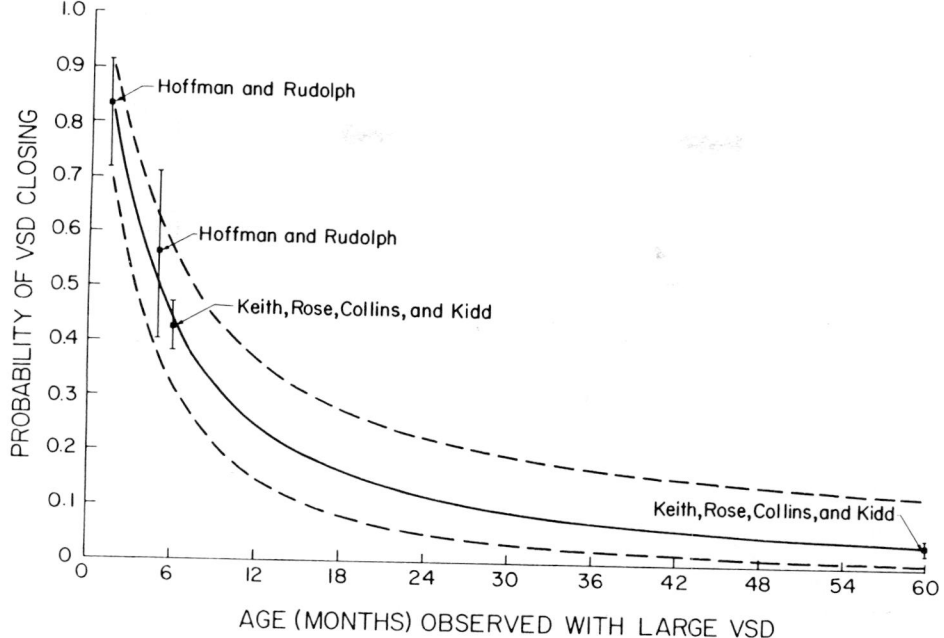

Figure 20-20 Probability of eventual spontaneous closure of a large VSD according to the age at which the patient is observed. The dotted lines enclose the 70% confidence limits. The specific ratios, with the 70% confidence limits, reported by Hoffman and Rudolph[H6] and Keith and associates[K5] are shown centered on the mean or assumed ages of patients in their reports. P for age < .0001. See original sources for equations and statistics.
Reproduced with permission from Blackstone et al.[B1]

spontaneous closure can be questioned. Hoffman and Rudolph's data, one of the sources for Figure 20-20, indicate that 80% of infants 6 weeks of age with large VSDs will experience spontaneous closure or reduction in size of the VSD.[H6] However, the size of the defects was not determined angiocardiographically, and in this age group the VSD resistance index may be misleading. Rowe found that none of 11 infants (mean age 46 days) with a VSD that was 80% or greater in diameter than that of the aorta showed subsequent reduction in size during the period of observation.[R4] Among 8 patients who had pulmonary artery banding at age 6 weeks or less for primary large VSD, only 1 (12%, CL 2%–36%) underwent spontaneous closure by the time of debanding (GLH). Admittedly, the milieu for spontaneous closure may be altered in patients who have undergone banding.

Pulmonary Vascular Disease

A large VSD predisposes the patient to the development of increased pulmonary vascular resistance from hypertensive pulmonary vascular disease, which tends to worsen as the person gets older.[A3,L2] Thus, the proportion of patients with large VSDs who have a severely elevated pulmonary vascular resistance (for definitions, see Table 20-3) is directly related to age (Fig. 20-21).

The statement that some infants less than 2 years of age with large VSDs have severely elevated pulmonary vascular resistance is doubted by some, but its occurrence is well documented.[B3] Seven (14%) of 50 patients between 1 and 13

months of age with large primary VSDs had pulmonary vascular resistance of 8 units · m² or more (GLH). Some infants and children with severely elevated pulmonary vascular resistance have not undergone the usual fall in pulmonary vascular resistance a few weeks to a few months after birth. Others have undergone this,[J5] but later in the first 2 years of life have developed a rapid increase in pulmonary vascular resistance.[H8]

Some infants with large VSDs, and most of those with moderate-sized ones, have normal or mildly elevated resistance, retain this through the first decade of life, and then if their VSD is still large, may or may not develop more severe pulmonary vascular changes as the years pass.[K2,K5]

Bacterial Endocarditis

In persons with VSD, bacterial endocarditis is rare, occurring at a rate of about 0.15%–0.3% per year.[C12,C13,G7,S7] Its incidence is greater in males, and in persons over the age of 20 years.[G7] Often a pulmonary process is the presenting feature, presumably developing from emboli secondary to right-sided bacterial vegetations. Prognosis with modern antibiotic treatment regimens is excellent.

Premature Death

Past experience and reports in the literature indicate that, without surgical treatment, some infants (about 9% of those with large VSDs) die with their large VSD in the first year of

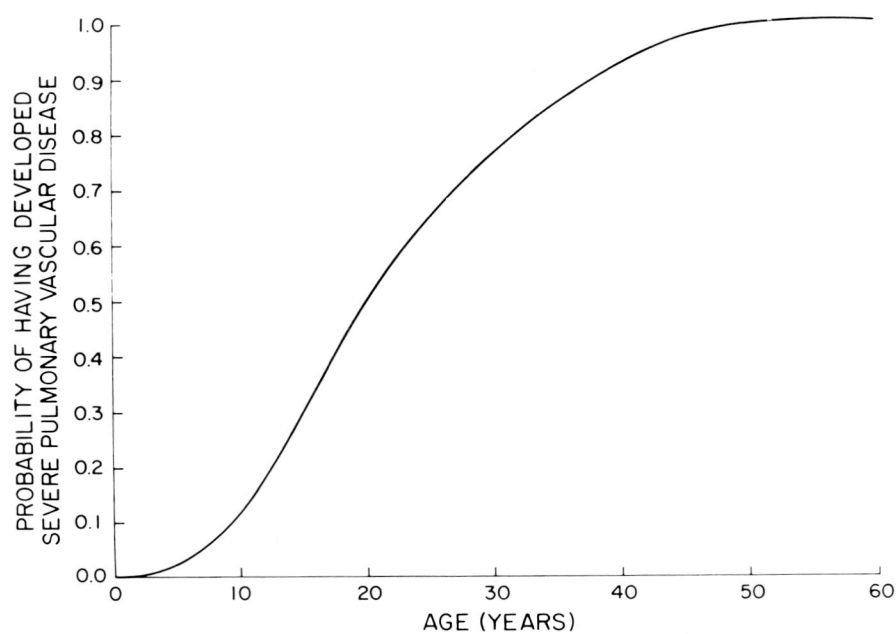

Figure 20-21 The probability of developing severe pulmonary vascular disease (pulmonary vascular resistance ≥ 8 units·m²) in patients with large ventricular septal defects according to age estimated, not formally calculated, from the data presented by Keith and colleagues.[K5]

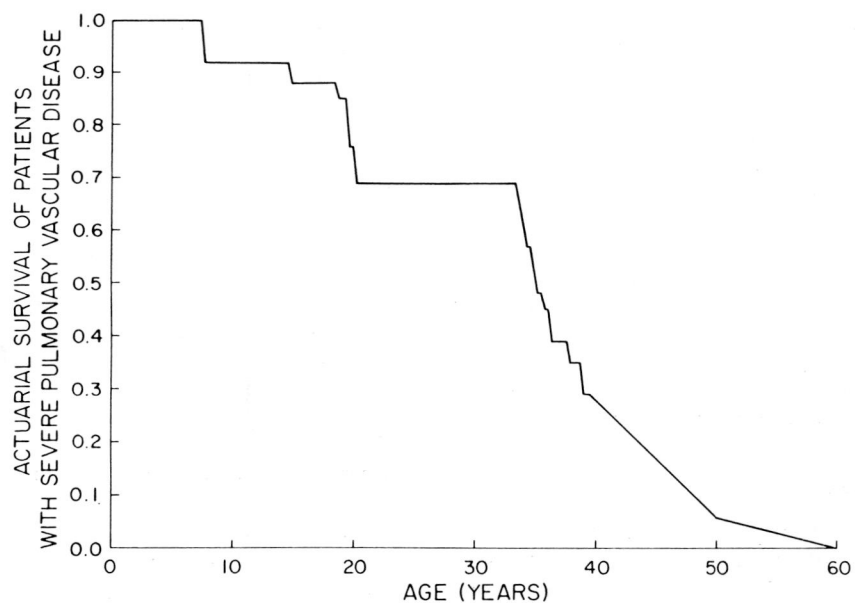

Figure 20-22 Actuarial survival after diagnosis of patients with large ventricular septal defects who had proven elevation of pulmonary vascular resistance to a level that made them inoperable (≥10 units·m²) demonstrated at cardiac catheterization at various ages. Note that fatalities begin to occur in the second decade of life, that about half of the patients were dead by age 35, and that a few survived until 50 years of age.

Modified from Clarkson et al.,[C2] and the American Heart Association, Inc.

life.[A2,K5] Death may result from congestive heart failure, which may develop very early but usually occurs at about 2–3 months of age, presumably because at that time the left-to-right shunt increases as the medial hypertrophy present in the small pulmonary arteries at birth regresses.[D6] Death also may result from recurrent pulmonary infections secondary to pulmonary edema from high pulmonary venous pressure. Death is most likely to occur in those infants with large VSDs who have associated conditions of major anatomic or functional significance, such as patent ductus arteriosus, coarctation of the aorta, or a large atrial septal defect.[B3]

After the age of 1 year, few if any patients die with their VSD until the second decade of life. By then, most patients whose VSDs have remained large develop pulmonary vascular disease and ultimately die with complications of their Eisenmenger's complex (Fig. 20-22).[C2] These include hemoptysis, polycythemia, cerebral abscess or infarction, and right heart failure.

Patients with *small* VSDs do not develop pulmonary vascular disease and are not likely to die prematurely. Their only real risk is bacterial endocarditis. The incidence of this complication is low,[S7] and it is generally well treated by antibiotics.

Clinical Course

Patients with small VSDs rarely have symptoms related to the defect. Those with large VSDs may have symptoms of intractable heart failure in the first few months of life, with poor peripheral pulses, inability to feed, sweating, and chronic pulmonary edema. About half the patients coming to operation in the first 2 years of life do so because of intractable heart failure (Table 20-4).[B3] During early life, rapid and labored respiration and recurrent pulmonary infections may occur secondary to high pulmonary venous pressure and chronic pulmonary edema. At any time in the first year of life, lobes of the lung may become chronically hyperinflated because of pressure of the large and tense pulmonary arteries on the bronchi, preventing complete escape of air during expiration.[O4] All this causes many babies with large VSDs to be small and physically underdeveloped. Such symptomatic patients who fail to respond well to medical management are at particular risk of dying in the first year of

life. Some babies who survive through the first year of life with large VSDs have controlled heart failure and failure to thrive in the second year of life as well.

Children and young adults with large VSDs are usually symptomatic and tend to be small both in height and weight. As pulmonary vascular disease develops, symptoms may regress.

Development of Aortic Incompetence

A small proportion of patients (probably about 5% in Caucasian and black races) develops aortic valve incompetence as a complication of their VSD (see Section 2). The incompetence is rarely present at birth but develops during the first decade of life. It gradually worsens, so that by the end of the second decade it is usually severe. As the incompetence increases, the shunt often decreases, due to occlusion of the VSD by the prolapsed aortic cusp.

Development of Infundibular Pulmonary Stenosis

A small proportion (5%–10%) of patients with large VSDs and large left-to-right shunt in infancy develop infundibular pulmonary stenosis.[G2,H9,K5] The mild and moderate infundibular pulmonary stenoses in those patients operated on for primary VSD (see Table 20-2), as well as some of the more important pulmonary stenoses (see Chapter 23), probably develop in this way. The stenosis may become severe enough to produce shunt reversal and cyanosis, and the condition then can properly be termed tetralogy of Fallot.[S17] Those who undergo the transformation probably are born with some anterior displacement of the infundibular septum and its extensions.

TECHNIQUE OF OPERATION

VSDs are repaired either through the right atrium, the right ventricle, or, in special circumstances, the left ventricle. In infants weighing less than about 8 kg, the repair is done under profound hypothermia to 18°C and total circulatory arrest (see Chapter 2, Section 4), using a single venous cannula and no cold cardioplegia, reserving conventional cardiopulmonary bypass (CPB) for patients larger than this (GLH). Alternatively, CPB at 25°C, with direct caval cannulation is used unless the infant weighs less than about 2.5 kg (see Chapter 2, Section 3), in which case profoundly hypothermic total circulatory arrest is used; cold cardioplegia is used in all cases (UAB).

After the usual anesthetic (see Chapter 4) and surgical preparations (see Chapter 2, Section 3), a median sternotomy incision is made. The presence of anomalies of pulmonary or systemic venous return is determined. The ductus arteriosus should be known from preoperative study to be open or closed; an open ductus during open cardiotomy, and particularly during total circulatory arrest, allows air to enter the aorta and later go to the brain, and during CPB increases intracardiac return and overdistends the pulmonary circulation. When a patent ductus is present, it is ligated from the

Table 20-4 Indications for repair of ventricular septal defect in patients operated on in the first 2 years of life.

Indication for VSD Repair	n	% of Total	Average Age and Range (mo)
Intractable congestive heart failure	30	53%	2.9, 1–7
Recurrent respiratory infections	3	5%	8, 6–9
Controlled congestive heart failure and failure to thrive	17	30%	11.4, 4–21
Increased pulmonary vascular resistance	7	12%	14.6, 10–19

SOURCE: Modified from Barratt-Boyes et al.[B3]

anterior approach, usually during cooling (see later discussion for details).

Repair of Perimembranous Ventricular Septal Defect

After CPB or circulatory arrest has been established, cooling begun, the aorta cross-clamped, and the cold cardioplegic solution injected (if it is to be used), the right atrium is opened obliquely, a pump sump sucker placed across the naturally present or surgically created foramen ovale, and the exposure arranged (UAB); this is done before aortic cross-clamping if the heart has become ineffective because of cooling (Fig. 20-23). Before the repair is started, the defect is carefully examined to establish that all margins can be seen and reached. In the rare circumstances in which this is not possible, a radial incision may be made in the tricuspid valve (see "Repair of AV Canal Type Ventricular Septal Defect") or a decision made to repair the VSD through the right ventricle. The relationship of the bundle of His to the posterior and inferior margin of the defect must be clearly understood in order to accomplish a safe repair (Fig. 20-27).

All perimembranous VSDs are repaired with a patch, sewn in place with continuous polypropylene sutures (UAB; Fig. 20-23). After the repair has been completed, the pump sump sucker is removed, the foramen ovale closed, and the aortic clamp released, with strong suction on the aortic needle vent. Rewarming of the perfusate is begun about 5 minutes before this. The right atrium is closed, and the remainder of the operation is completed as usual (see Chapter 2).

Alternatively, a right ventricular approach through a transverse incision is used as a routine (GLH). The repair is performed with interrupted sutures (GLH) (Fig. 20-24). Alternatively, when the ventricular approach is used, the technique of the repair and sequencing of the suturing may be identical to those used with the atrial approach (UAB; see the description in Chapter 23).

Repair of Subpulmonary Ventricular Septal Defect

An approach through a transverse incision in the infundibulum is used for subpulmonary VSDs (Fig. 20-25). Alternatively, when the main pulmonary artery and pulmonary ring are large (as a result of the left-to-right shunt), subarterial defects can be closed via a pulmonary arteriotomy just above the valve (GLH). Such defects are usually large enough to require a patch for closure.

Repair of AV Canal Type Ventricular Septal Defect

AV canal types of VSD are most easily repaired through the right atrium (Fig. 20-26), although of course repair is possible through the right ventricle. Such defects are nearly always repaired with a patch. The defects lie beneath the septal leaflet of the tricuspid valve, and care is taken to avoid damage to the leaflet or its chordae and to tailor the patch so that it is not too bulky beneath the septal leaflet. One method of avoiding damage to the septal leaflet and improving exposure is the temporary detachment of the base of the septal leaflet

and a portion of the anterior leaflet of the tricuspid valve and retraction of the leaflet anteriorly (Fig. 20-26).[H12]

Repair of Muscular Ventricular Septal Defect

A right-sided approach is used for repair of muscular VSDs whenever possible. Left ventriculotomy gives excellent exposure,[A4,B3] and, although Singh and colleagues have reported it not to be disadvantageous in infants,[S14] it can produce important left ventricular dysfunction early and late postoperatively.[G8]

Single or multiple defects in the inlet (basal) septum and mid-septum (see Fig. 20-12) are approached through the right atrium. When a single defect is slitlike or oval, direct suture (often in part at least with pledgetted mattress sutures) is satisfactory, but when it is large and circular, a patch is used. A cluster of defects in the mid-septum can be closed with a single patch or individually. However, when a mid-septal or basal muscular VSD coexists with a perimembranous VSD, a single patch is used to avoid damage to the bundle of His (Fig. 20-27).

VSDs with a single left ventricular opening but two or more openings into the right ventricle on both sides of the septal band are first examined through the right atrium. If by using curved forceps the position of the openings can be clearly defined, the repair may be done via a vertical right ventriculotomy close to the septum, centered over the defects. The defect is converted into a single right ventricular orifice by detaching the lower end of the septal band or trabecula septomarginalis and moderator band from the septum as the ventriculotomy is made and retracting them along with the free wall to the right. The VSD is closed with a patch. As the ventriculotomy is closed, the septal band falls back into place.

Multiple defects in the anterior portion of the septum may be closed through a high transverse ventriculotomy. Alternatively, at times the VSDs may be considered too numerous to close individually, and they are simply compressed and often totally closed by interrupted mattress sutures between a felt strip on the anterior ventricular wall (away from the left anterior descending coronary artery) and pledgets inside the right ventricle and inferior to the VSDs (UAB).[B5] This repair may be done from the right atrium or via a vertical right ventriculotomy.

Apical muscular VSDs can be exposed through the right atrium and tricuspid valve or via a low vertical right ventriculotomy. This can be extended around the apex for a short distance onto the posterior wall.

The rare Swiss-cheese septum may at times not be totally correctable. Its repair requires a left ventricular approach, and a patch over the entire muscular septum may be necessary. An associated perimembranous defect should be repaired through the right atrium, as its repair from the left ventricular side increases the risk of heart block. Incisions into both ventricles are avoided whenever possible. Great care is used in making and closing the left ventriculotomy incision so as not to damage coronary artery branches. A continuous mattress suture over fine Teflon felt strips plus an over-and-over stitch give a secure closure.

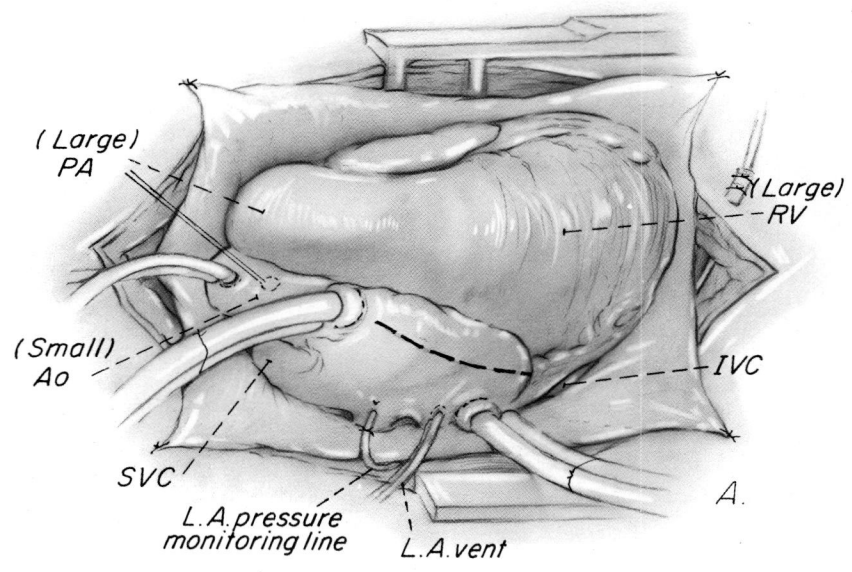

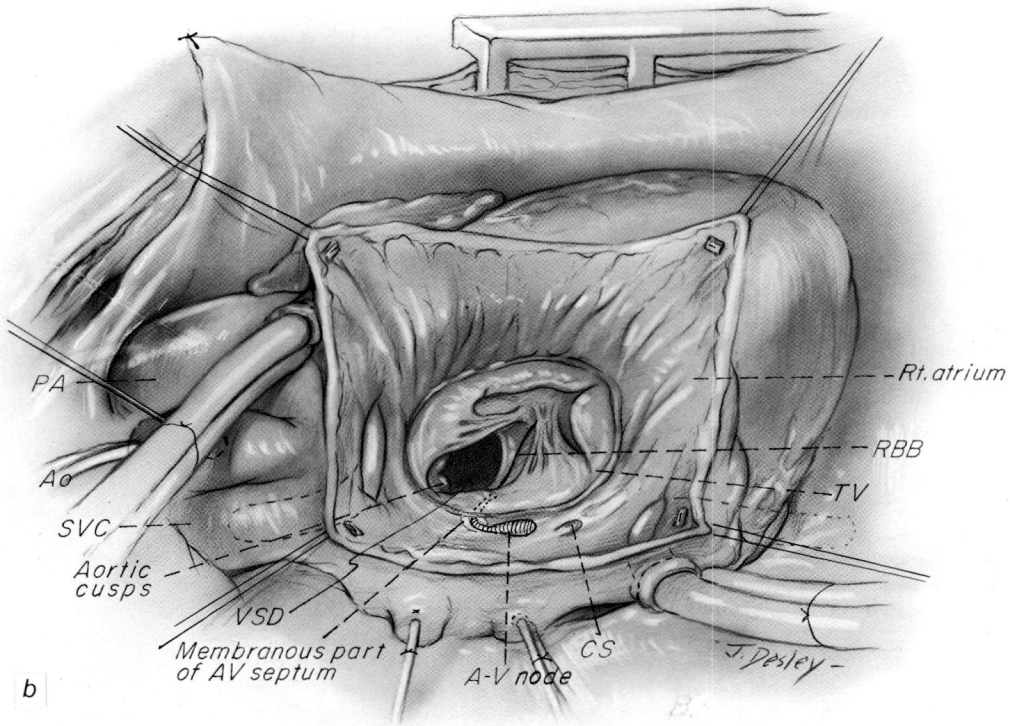

Figure 20-23 Repair of a perimembranous VSD from the right atrium.

(*a*) The dashed line indicates the right atriotomy incision, carried inferiorly toward the inferior vena cava cannula. Currently, caval cannulae are inserted directly into the superior and inferior vena cavae (UAB).

(*b*) Stay sutures have been placed. Note that initially the superior edge of this typical perimembranous defect is not visible. The AV node is in the muscular portion of the atrioventricular septum, just on the atrial side of the commissure between tricuspid septal and anterior leaflet. The bundle of His thus penetrates at the posterior angle of the VSD, where it is vulnerable to injury.

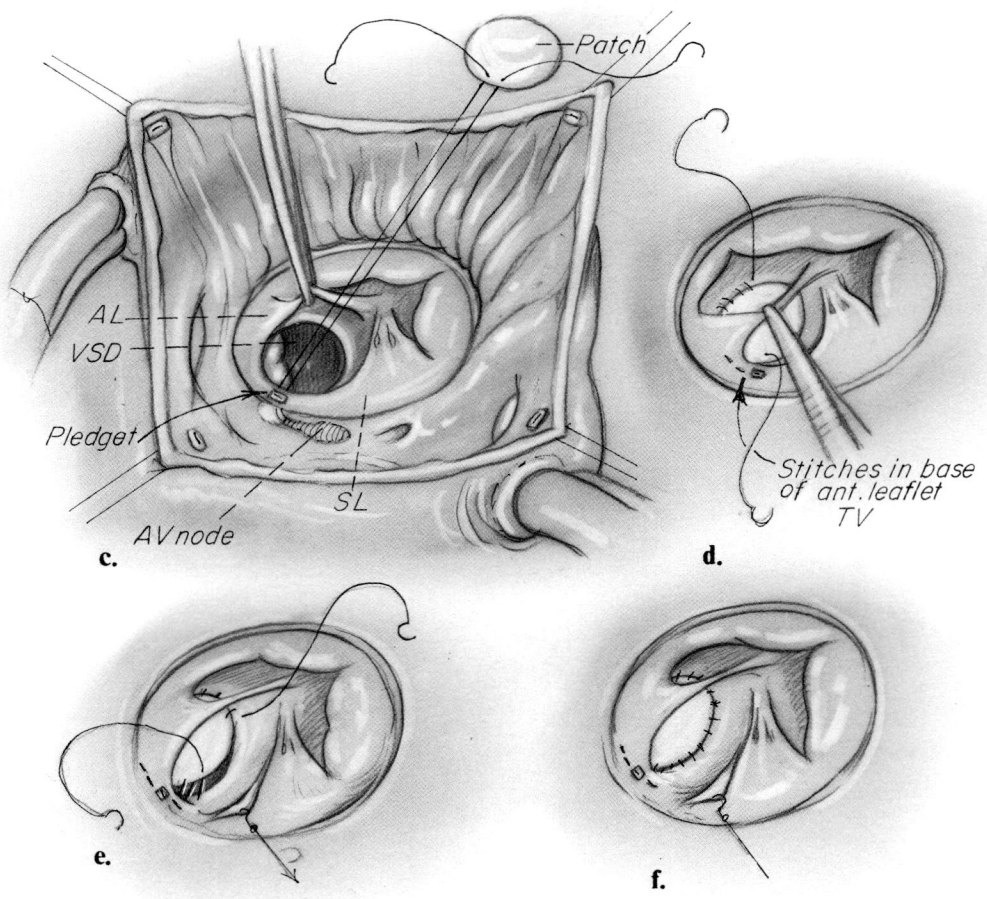

c.   AL

VSD

Pledget

AV node

SL

Patch

d. Stitches in base of ant. leaflet TV

e.

f.

Figure 20-23 (*continued*)

(*c*) The repair of the perimembranous VSD is begun by placing a mattress suture of 4-0 polypropylene with a small pledget through the base of the tricuspid valve commissural tissue between the septal and anterior leaflet, just above the posterior angle of the defect. A piece of knitted Dacron velour is trimmed to be slightly larger than the approximate size of the defect. One arm of the suture is passed through the Dacron patch, back through the base of the leaflet, and again through the leaflet and then the patch. At this point or after placing several more stitches, the sutures are snugged up as the patch is lowered into place.

(*d*) The suture line between the superior rim of the defect and patch is continued. Traction on the suture exposes the next area to be stitched and provides good visibility. The suture is passed behind any tricuspid chordae that overhang the defect. Care must be taken to visualize accurately the edge of the VSD that is formed by the ventriculo-infundibular fold and the parietal extension of the infundibular septum, which is just above the aortic valve.

(*e*) With the other arm of the suture, a stitch is made through the base of the tricuspid valve from ventricular to atrial side, then back from the atrial to the ventricular side of the leaflet, and through the patch. Stitches are now taken between ventricular septum and patch along the inferior edge of the defect. These stitches are placed 5–7 mm away from the edge of the defect in order to avoid the area most probably occupied by the bundle of His and more anteriorly 3–5 mm back from the edge.

(*f*) Again, care is taken to weave the stitches beneath any overhanging tricuspid chordae. The suturing between patch and septum is continued in this way until the previous suture is reached, and the two sutures are tied together.

Ao, aorta; AL, anterior leaflet; AV node, atrioventricular node; CS, coronary sinus; IVC, inferior vena cava; PA, pulmonary artery; RBB, right bundle branch; SVC, superior vena cava; TV, tricuspid valve.

While it is important to avoid residual shunts, multiple incisions and a prolonged search for a few small additional muscular VSDs are generally not advisable. Preoperative study should accurately delineate the size as well as the position of all the defects.

Closure of Associated Patent Ductus Arteriosus

When the operation is done during profoundly hypothermic total circulatory arrest, the dissection of the ductus is easy during cooling because the blood pressure is low (GLH). It is

therefore accomplished before cannulating the aorta and beginning CPB. When the repair is done during CPB, no attempt is made to dissect the ductus until CPB is established, for until then, the exposure can be difficult and the risk of serious hemorrhage from an error in dissection more than trivial (UAB). After establishing CPB, with the perfusate temperature at about 34°C and with the caval tapes still unsnugged (so that the heart will not distend) and the right atrial pressure at zero, the ductus is dissected. The heart must continue to beat; otherwise, a large shunt will rapidly overdistend the right heart and the lungs. If the heart does

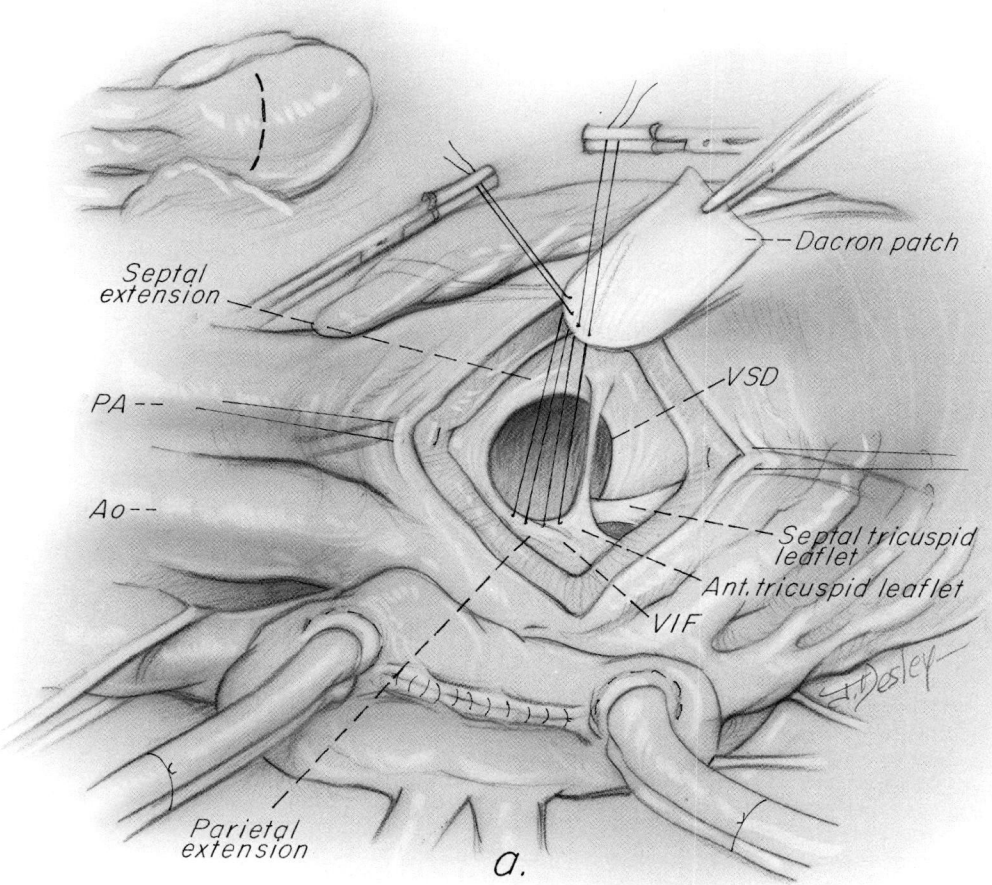

Figure 20-24   Repair of a perimembranous VSD from the right ventricle.
(a) When a ventricular approach is chosen, a limited transverse ventriculotomy is made low in the outflow tract (GLH). Note that the atrial septum has been examined via a right atriotomy, and an atrial septal defect or patent foramen ovale has been closed (usually done after the VSD closure is completed). The patch is cut as a rectangle, with only the two lower angles rounded off. The first stitch is placed as a mattress suture (using a single-armed suture), passed first through the patch as shown, then through the edge of the VSD along its posterior superior margin from below upward. A deep bite of muscular tissue is taken here, through the ventriculo-infundibular fold about 3 mm from the aortic ring between the nadir of the noncoronary and right aortic cusps. This stitch is then passed through from the patch. The two ends of this and subsequent sutures are clipped in a mosquito forceps and cut off. The second mattress stitch is placed more superiorly, in exactly similar fashion, from patch to VSD edge and then to patch. This second stitch must be at least 3 mm to the right ventricular side of the nadir of the noncoronary cusp (which identifies the position of the right trigone and the point of penetration of the bundle of His).

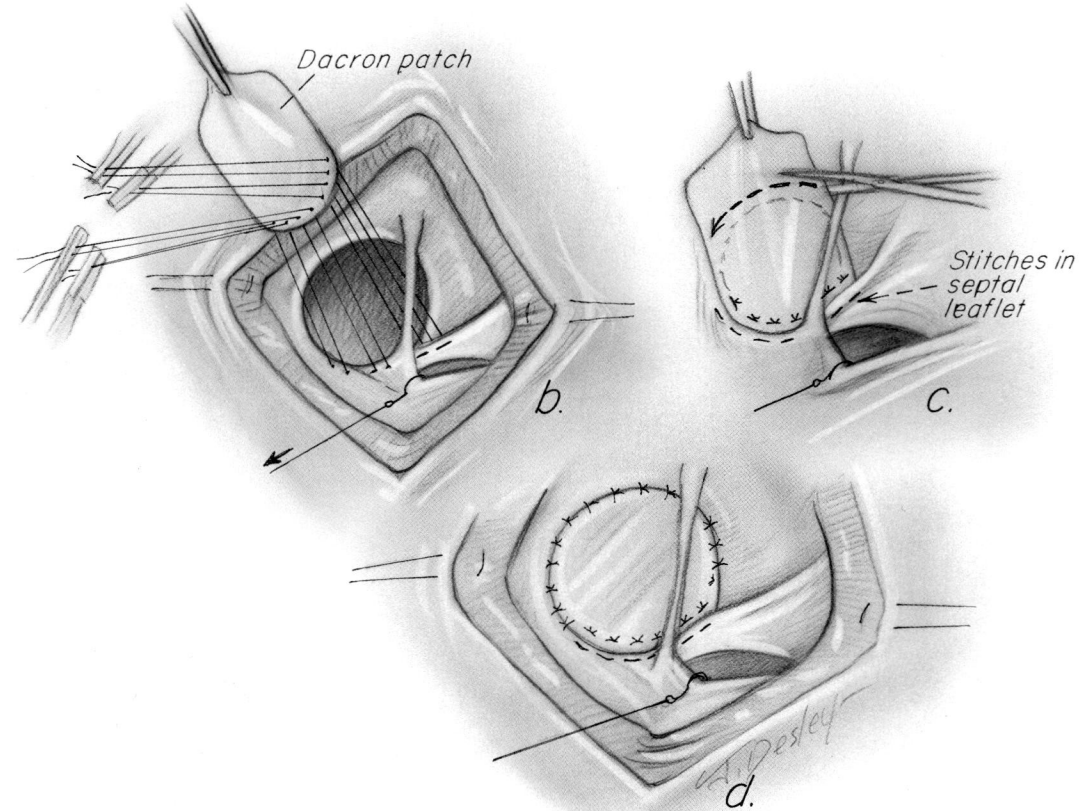

Dacron patch

Stitches in septal leaflet

b.

c.

d.

Figure 20-24 *(continued)*

(*b*) The third and fourth mattress stitches are placed on the other side of the original stitch, and usually are passed through the base of the anterior tricuspid leaflet (on the leaflet side of the tricuspid ring). The fifth stitch can either pick up the tissue at the anteroinferior margin of the defect, if the location of the right trigone indicates that the bundle of His is well below the inferior defect edge; or, when the bundle is at risk in this region, be placed through muscle on the right ventricular side about 2 mm from the defect edge, taking a deep bite of muscle, but not so deep that the needle penetrates to the left side of the septum (the stitch may always be placed in the latter position in a true perimembranous VSD [UAB]). There are tricuspid chordae along this margin (the papillary muscle of the conus and often a number of chordae), and the suture often needs to be threaded beneath them to avoid distorting them when the suture is tied down.

(*c*) With the first 5 or 6 sutures in position, the patch is carefully lowered into the defect and the sutures tied and cut. They must all be snug, and those in muscle must not be allowed to cut through. The superior margin of the patch is now fashioned to match exactly the superior margin of the defect. Occasionally, major chordae pass from the tricuspid valve to the anterior edge of anterosuperior angle of the defect and make exposure of the lower defect edge impossible from the ventricular approach. In such instances, the chord (including a button of muscle) is detached at its point of insertion into the defect edge before the patch sutures are placed (GLH). The detached chord is tagged with a fine polypropylene stitch placed through its base and is later resutured to the patch at a corresponding point.

(*d*) Suturing is completed now by returning to the posterosuperior angle. The stitches pass through the full thickness of the parietal extension of the infundibular septum after picking up the defect edge. Anteriorly, the sutures are continued as simple over-and-over interrupted stitches, first picking up deep bites of muscle on the right ventricular side of the defect edge. Superiorly, the final sutures pass through the full thickness of the infundibular septum, with care taken not to damage the base of the right coronary cusp. Once the patch has been lowered into position, each suture is tied and cut as it is positioned.

Ao, aorta; PA, pulmonary artery; VIF, ventriculo-infundibular fold; VSD, ventricular septal defect.

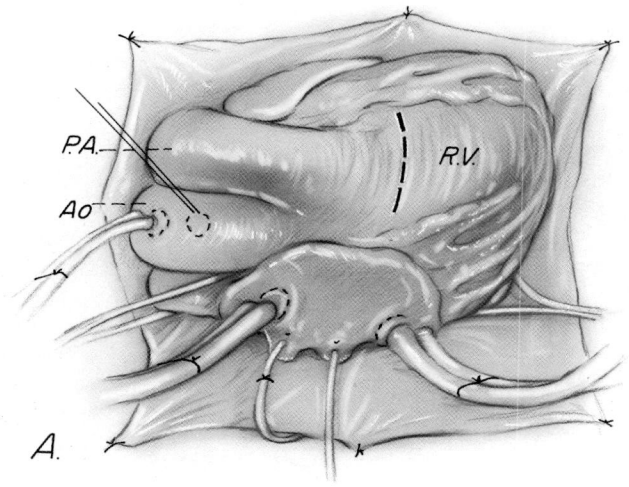

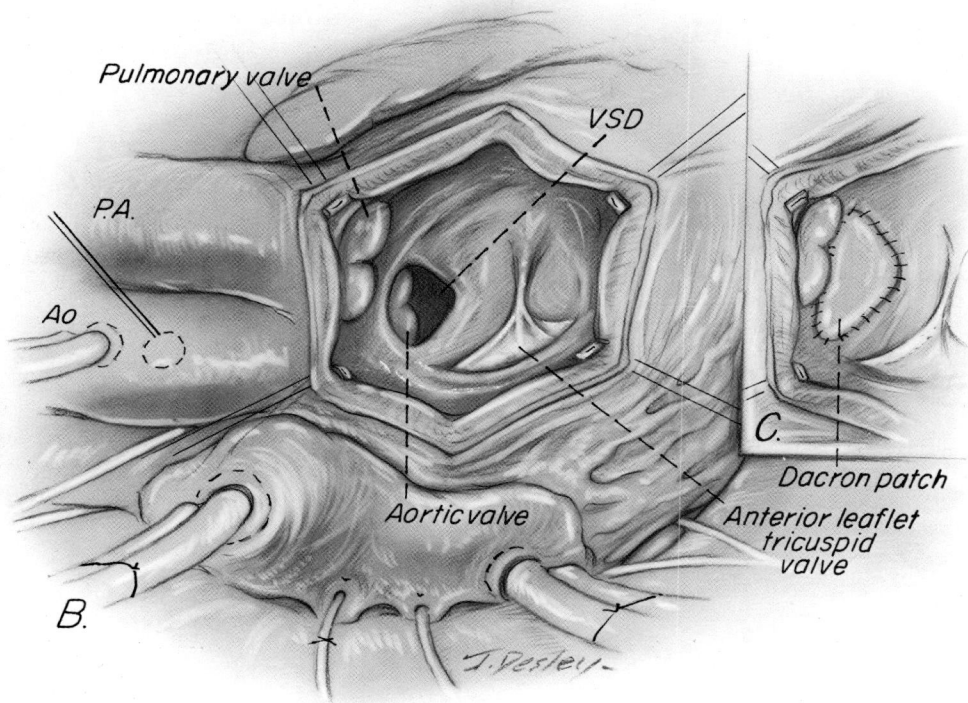

Figure 20-25 Repair of subarterial VSD.

(a) A subarterial (subpulmonary) VSD in the infundibular septum is usually approached through a transverse incision in the right ventricular infundibulum. The bundle of His is far posterior and is unrelated to the posterior inferior edge of the VSD.

(b) After exposure is obtained and the anatomy studied, an initial stitch is taken through the patch at the 6-o'clock position and then through the posterior angle of the defect from left ventricular to right ventricular side. This stitch is then continued through the patch and then the edge of defect, working to the surgeon's left and along the cephalad edge of the defect. Usually only a narrow fibrous rim separates the pulmonary valve anteriorly from the aortic valve posteriorly. Each stitch in this area must be placed with the aortic valve in view to avoid damaging its cusps. For better visualization, the valve can be closed occasionally by infusion of a little cardioplegic solution through the infusion needle present in the ascending aorta (not shown). When the fibrous ridge between aortic and pulmonary cusps is not sturdy enough to hold sutures, interrupted mattress sutures may be passed completely through the pulmonary artery wall at the base of the sinuses, with three or four sutures placed before any of them are pulled tight, tied, and cut (GLH). If the aortic sinus is prolapsing through a thinned area in the infundibular septum, the patch should be placed over this area. When the continuous suture line has been carried to about the 12-o'clock position, it is tagged. The other end of the original double-armed stitch is now used to go through the edge of defect and then the patch as the suture line is carried along the caudal edge of the defect, working anteriorly. The sutures are placed along the edge of the defect, since the bundle of His is posterior and inferior to the defect and well away from its edge.

(c) When the 12-o'clock position is reached, the two stitches are tied together to complete the repair.

Ao, aorta; PA, pulmonary artery; RV, right ventricle.

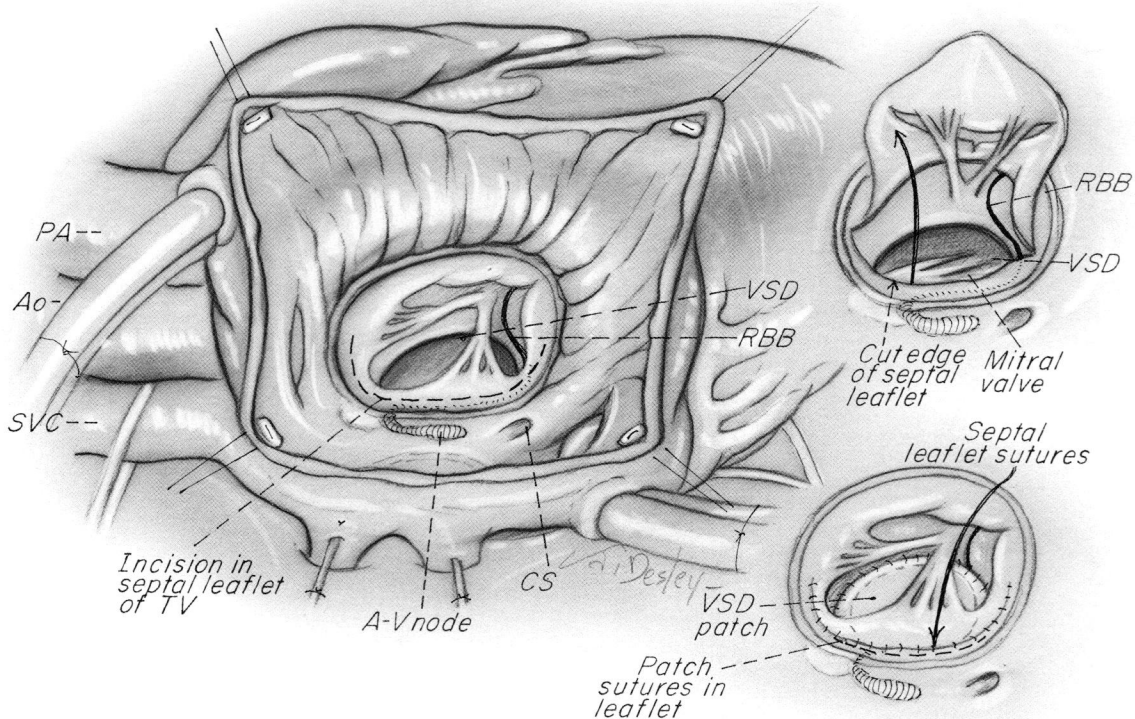

Figure 20-26 Repair of the AV canal type of VSD after incision and reflection of the septal and part of the anterior tricuspid leaflet. Most of these defects can be repaired simply through the uncut tricuspid valve. Occasionally, however, tricuspid chordae overhang the VSD in such a way as to make this difficult, and, in such cases, it is preferable to incise the leaflet along the base of the septal and anteroseptal commissural leaflets so as to detach these and reflect them anteriorly, as shown. This allows ready access to the VSD. As the incision is made, several pairs (on each side of the incision) of marking stitches of 5-0 silk are placed to aid accurate leaflet reconstruction after repair. In closing the VSD inferiorly, the stitches are kept well away from the edge of the VSD, as in the repair of other perimembranous VSDs (see Fig. 20-23), to avoid damaging the bundle of His. The patch is attached to the base of the septal leaflet behind the cut edge. The leaflet is reattached with continuous 6-0 polypropylene sutures.

Ao, aorta; AV, atrioventricular; CS, coronary sinus; PA, pulmonary artery; RBB, right bundle branch; SVC, superior vena cava; TV, tricuspid valve; VSD, ventricular septal defect.

fibrillate, CPB flows are immediately reduced while the dissection is rapidly completed.

With downward traction on the main pulmonary artery (Fig. 20-28),[K4] the ductus can usually be seen through its pericardial reflection and surrounding adventitial tissue. The left pulmonary artery and the undersurface of the aorta both proximal and distal to the ductus are clearly identified to prevent these structures from being damaged or ligated after being mistaken for the ductus. The delicate pericardial reflection and adventitial tissue on both sides of the ductus are sharply dissected from it. The adventitia of the ductus itself and of the adjacent pulmonary artery and aorta must not be entered. The recurrent laryngeal nerve is not seen. Only when the dissection is complete, the left pulmonary artery visualized, and the ductus identified with absolute certainty (a process that usually takes only a few minutes) is a fine right-angled clamp passed behind it to grasp the 2-0 silk ligature. One ligature is tied on the aortic end of the ductus while perfusion flows are reduced to lower intravascular pressures, and one is tied on the pulmonary end. If there is enough space, a transfixion ligature may be placed between these two ligatures. (A clip may be used instead to close the ductus; see Chapter 22, footnote 2.) The operation then proceeds as usual.

Pulmonary Artery Banding

Banding of the pulmonary artery is performed through a small left anterolateral thoracotomy. The pulmonary artery band is marked, according to Trusler's rule,[A6,T2] to a length of 20 mm plus the number of millimeters corresponding to the weight of the child in kilograms. (If the banding is done for transposition of the great arteries with a large VSD or some other complex cardiac anomaly with bidirectional

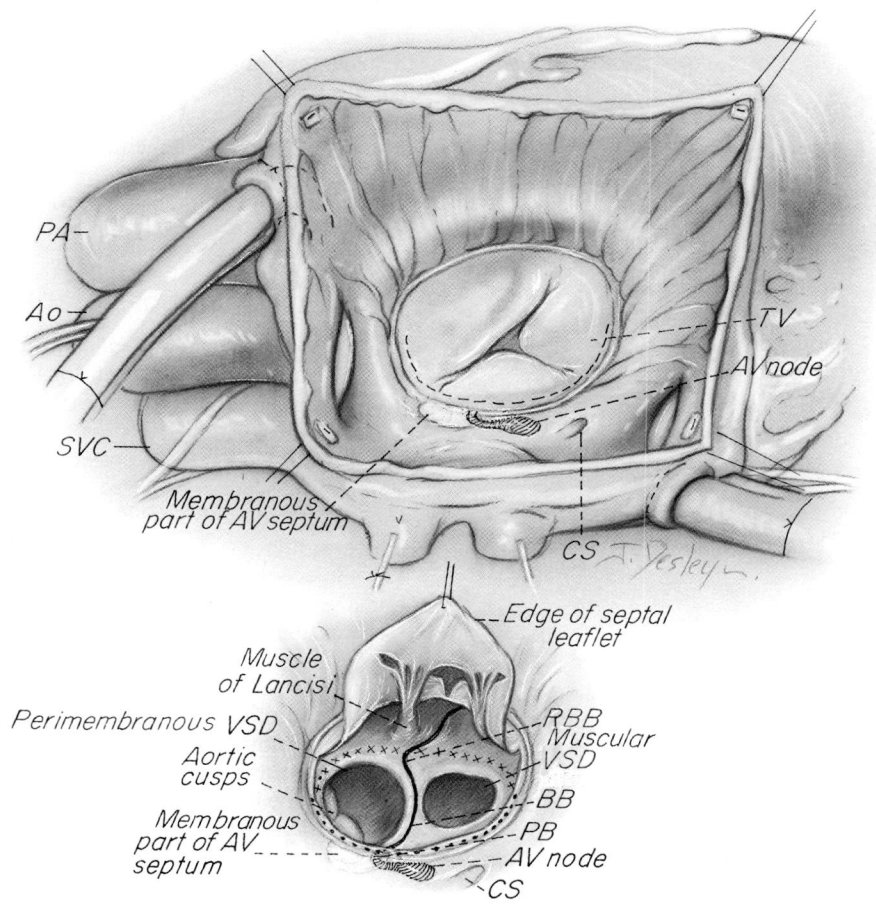

Figure 20-27 Repair of multiple (two) VSDs, one in the perimembranous position and one in the mid-muscular portion of the sinus septum. A radial incision has been made in the base of the septal leaflet and the commissural tissue on each side. As depicted, the bundle of His runs posteriorly and inferiorly to the perimembranous VSD and superiorly to the muscular one. Therefore, stitches cannot be placed in the muscle between the two defects without great risk of producing heart block, and both defects are closed as one by a patch.

Ao, aorta; AV node, atrioventricular node; BB, branching portion of His bundle; CS, coronary sinus orifice; PA, pulmonary artery; PB, penetrating portion of His bundle; RBB, right bundle branch; SVC, superior vena cava; TV, tricuspid valve; VSD, ventricular septal defect.

Reproduced with permission from Bharati et al.[B15]

shunting, the length is 24 mm plus the child's weight.) A 3–4 mm wide Teflon tape is used. A small incision is made in the pericardium, generally anterior to the phrenic nerve. The pulmonary artery is separated from the aorta by dissecting close to the *aorta*. A right-angled clamp is passed around and behind the aorta to grasp one end of the band and pull it through. The other end of the band is retrieved by a clamp passed through the transverse sinus. With the band now safely around the mid-portion of the main pulmonary artery, the marked points on the band are joined with a few interrupted sutures to produce the desired circumference of the pulmonary artery, and the excess band is trimmed away. If bradycardia or cyanosis develops, the band must be loosened a little. If the narrowing is insufficient, as judged by the pressure difference across the band (distal pulmonary

artery pressure should be less than 50% of systemic pressure), the band is tightened. A few stitches are placed between the band and the pulmonary artery adventitia in an effort to prevent the band's migration. The pericardium is closed.

Pulmonary Artery Debanding

When a Teflon band has been properly applied and is removed when the patient is 6 months or less of age, simple band removal is usually all that is necessary. When the patient is older, reconstruction of the pulmonary artery is usually required.

When profound hypothermia with surface cooling is employed, the band is dissected from the pulmonary artery be-

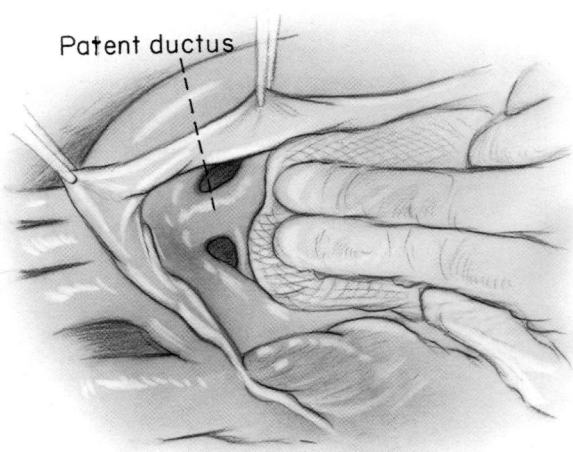

Patent ductus

Figure 20-28 Technique of exposure and closure of patent ductus arteriosus through a median sternotomy incision as a part of an open cardiac operation on cardiopulmonary bypass. See the text for details.

Reproduced with permission from Kirklin et al.[K4]

fore beginning cooling bypass or during the cooling bypass phase (GLH). The band can almost always be cut and removed without damaging the underlying artery; in fact, the tip of the left atrial appendage is more likely to suffer damage, since it is always adherent to the banded area. If CPB is employed, dissection is delayed until CPB has been established, when, if necessary, flows can be reduced to facilitate exposure and dissection (UAB).

In this situation, the VSD is usually repaired through the right ventricle (GLH). With the band removed, a transverse ventriculotomy is performed to expose the VSD if it is still open. It is closed using the techniques already described. The right ventricular infundibulum is carefully examined, for the excessive hypertrophy present may have produced an infundibular stenosis; if so, muscle is excised from this region. The interior of the main pulmonary artery is examined through the pulmonary valve, and a curved forcep is passed through the banded area and opened to further assess the diameter at this point. A similar assessment can be made when the VSD has been repaired through a right atrial approach (UAB). If the diameter appears adequate, nothing more need be done. If the residual stenosis is still significant, or if it is proved to be significant by pressure measurements after closing the right ventricle and discontinuing CPB (a sequence that should always be followed), the pulmonary artery is reconstructed. The most satisfactory technique is local excision of the short, narrowed, scarred segment of artery—except for the most posterior portion, which is left intact—and reanastomosis of the divided pulmonary artery using a continuous polypropylene suture.[D7] This technique can usually be employed even when the band lies very close to the pulmonary valve by extending the incision vertically into the most anterior sinus between the valve cusps to enlarge the diameter of the proximal end. A similar technique can be used to enlarge an orificial stenosis involving only one branch of the pulmonary artery. When the pulmonary

leaflets have become excessively thick, their edges may require excision. If an adequate diameter is not obtainable by the technique of excision and end-to-end anastomosis, a diamond-shaped patch must be inserted to enlarge adequately the stenotic area (using pericardium or preclotted woven Dacron). An extensive reconstruction (see Chapter 23, Figs. 23-32, 23-33, and 23-34) is required when the band constricts the origin of the pulmonary arteries.

SPECIAL FEATURES OF POSTOPERATIVE CARE

The general measures and management of complications described in Chapter 5 are used for the postoperative care of patients undergoing repair of primary VSD.

If the hemodynamic state is poor early postoperatively, an unusual occurrence, the possibility of residual left-to-right shunting must be considered, particularly if left atrial pressure is considerably higher than right.[3] The contour of an indicator-dilution curve, particularly one obtained with indicator injected into the left atrium and sampled from a systemic artery,[T1] is very helpful in establishing or eliminating this possibility. Also, the finding of a considerably higher oxygen content or saturation in blood from the pulmonary artery (withdrawn through a polyvinyl catheter left at operation) than in that from the right atrium establishes the existence of a shunt.[V4] The most precise method used in the Intensive Care Unit is the double-sampling dye curve method, in which indocyanine green is injected into the left atrium and samples taken from the radial artery and the pulmonary artery.[W5] Alternatively, contrast echocardiography or pulsed Doppler echocardiography can be used.[S18]

When a knitted Dacron or Teflon patch is used to close the VSD, considerable shunting may occur through the patch or between sutures for 12–24 hours after operation, and the demonstration of residual shunting does not necessarily indicate a need for reoperation. However, if the hemodynamic state remains poor, and if after 24 hours a $\dot{Q}p/\dot{Q}s$ of 2.0 or greater is calculated by the double-sampling dye curve

---

[3] When the two ventricles have equal stroke volumes (i.e., no shunts or valvular incompetence are present), the left and right atrial pressures are determined by the relative contractility, distensibility, and volume at zero pressure of the two ventricles.[B4] The greater each of these values is for a given ventricle, the better its performance and the lower its end-diastolic and (if the AV valves are not stenotic) its atrial pressure tend to be relative to that of the other ventricle. (For a more detailed discussion of these matters, see Chapter 5, footnote 8 in "Low Cardiac Output" in Section 2, Cardiovascular Subsystem.) After complete repair of a large VSD via the right atrium in a patient who preoperatively had a large left-to-right shunt and a large $\dot{Q}p/\dot{Q}s$, the atrial pressures are similar, or the right is slightly higher than the left. When the repair is via right ventriculotomy, the right atrial pressure may be 20%–30% higher than left. Unless the repair has been done through a left ventriculotomy incision, and in the absence of other left heart lesions (such as aortic stenosis or coarctation), a left atrial pressure considerably greater (> 6 mm) than right suggests a residual left-to-right shunt. The high left atrial pressure under such circumstances is related to the large left ventricular stroke volume.

Table 20-5 Effect of age on hospital mortality after primary repair of single large VSD without major associated cardiac anomalies (UAB; 1967–1979; n = 166).[R5]

Age at Operation (mo)		1967–1979				1974–1979			
			Hospital Deaths				Hospital Deaths		
≤	<	n	No.	%	CL	n	No.	%	CL
	3	14	2	14%	5%–31%	11	1[a]	9%	1%–28%
3	6	12	0	0%	0%–15%	10	0	0%	0%–17%
6	12	23	3	13%	6%–25%	14	0	0%	0%–13%
12	24	21	1	5%	1%–15%	11	0	0%	0%–16%
24	48	27	0	0%	0%–7%	15	0	0%	0%–12%
48		69	0	0%	0%–3%	33	0	0%	0%–6%
Total		166[b]	6	3.6%	2.1%–5.8%	94	1	1.1%	0.1%–3.6%
$P(\chi^2)$				.01				> .9	

KEY: CL, 70% confidence limits.

[a] A 1.2-month-old baby with preoperative seizures was admitted already intubated, and ventilated; the patient died on postoperative day 3 with acute cardiac failure.

[b] In the years 1967–1974, 5 hospital deaths (6.9%, CL 3.9%–11.5%) occurred among 72 patients.

method, urgent restudy by left ventriculography is indicated to confirm and localize the position of the recurrent or residual VSD. Prompt reoperation is indicated if a significant ($\dot{Q}p/\dot{Q}s > 2.0$) residual shunt is present, which should be rare.

If complete atrioventricular dissociation is present for a time after CPB but sinus rhythm reappears, a demand pacemaker attached to ventricular wires should be in place for a week postoperatively, since early postoperative AV dissociation may recur temporarily. When pacing is required, sequential AV pacing is used (see Chapter 47).

EARLY RESULTS

Hospital Mortality

The hospital mortality for the repair of uncomplicated VSDs, most of which are repaired in infancy, approaches zero in the current era in centers properly prepared for this type of surgery (Tables 20-5, 20-6; Fig. 20-29). The risk is higher when major associated cardiac anomalies coexist (see "Incremental Risk Factors for Hospital Death").

Mode of Death

Most patients who die early after repair of primary VSD have acute cardiac failure.[R5] Others generally die with severe pulmonary dysfunction.

Incremental Risk Factors for Hospital Death

It is difficult to identify risk factors for hospital death after the repair of VSD in current experiences because deaths are few. Studies of experiences extending back a number of years (GLH and UAB) do allow the identification of incremental risk factors (Table 20-7).

The risk of repair has decreased in recent years, and thus

early date of operation is an incremental risk factor (Tables 20-5, 20-7, 20-8, 20-9; Fig. 20-29). This improvement from an original risk of hospital death of 20% in the earliest era began in our experience at the Mayo Clinic in the early 1960s (Table 20-10). This type of improvement has, of course, been demonstrated in other centers.[R7]

In previous eras, *young age* increased the risk of operation (Tables 20-5, 20-6, 20-7, 20-9); the identification of young age as a risk factor has been confirmed by Rizzoli and colleagues[R7] and Yeager and colleagues.[Y3] This risk factor has been neutralized in recent years (Fig. 20-29).[R5] Young age is still an incremental risk factor when major associated anomalies coexist (Tables 20-7, 20-11; Fig. 20-30).

Multiple VSDs have increased the risk of operation in the past (Tables 20-7, 20-9), but the risk has declined considerably in the current era (Fig. 20-30) and is now not increased by young age. However, complicated multiple VSDs impose

Table 20-6 Hospital mortality after repair of single large primary VSD with or without major associated cardiac anomalies (GLH; 1969–1982).

Age at Operation (mo)			Hospital Deaths		
≤	<	n	No.	%	CL
	3[a]	20	3	15%	7%–28%
3	6	28	0	0%	0%–7%
6	12	37	1	3%	0.3%–9%
12	24	28	2	7%	2%–16%
24		71	2	2.8%	0.9%–6.6%
Total		184	8[b]	4.3%	2.8%–6.5%
$P(\chi^2)$				.10	

KEY: CL, 70% confidence limits.

[a] Details in Table 20-11.

[b] Six of the eight deaths were of patients with major associated cardiac anomalies.

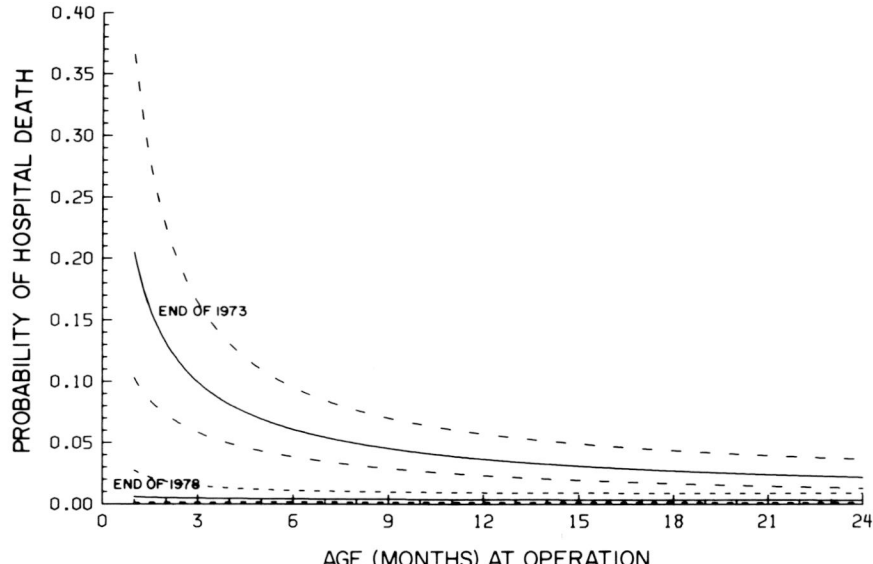

Figure 20-29 Hospital mortality after repair of single large VSDs without major associated cardiac anomalies, according to age and year at operation. The nomogram is from the logistic equation in Table 20-7. The dashed lines represent the 70% confidence limits.

Reproduced with permission from Rizzoli et al.[R5]

a higher risk of hospital death than do uncomplicated ones (Tables 20-12, 20-13), a finding that has been confirmed by others.[R7]

Major associated cardiac anomalies increase the risk of hospital death.[R7] The magnitude of the increased risk is, of course, determined by the specific associated anomaly. Coexisting patent ductus arteriosus and aortic coarctation increase the risk of repair of VSD less than do more serious

anomalies, such as congenital mitral valve disease (Tables 20-1, 20-7). Multiple VSDs impose a higher risk in the presence of major associated cardiac anomalies than do single VSDs (Fig. 20-31). The decrease in risk in the current era has not been apparent in the presence of most major associated anomalies (Table 20-7).

Neither the location of the VSD (Tables 20-14, 20-15) nor the surgical approach (Table 20-16) affects the risk of operation. Neither do previous pulmonary artery banding or such associated lesions as aortic incompetence and sinus of Valsalva aneurysm (Table 20-15).

Preoperative pulmonary artery pressure and pulmonary vascular resistance are not at present determinants of early mortality (although they do affect late results[B1]). This current situation is different from our earlier Mayo Clinic[C2,C3] experiences, no doubt because the upper limit of operable pulmonary vascular resistance is better understood and perioperative management has improved.

Table 20-7 Incremental risk factors for hospital death after repair of single and multiple VSDs with or without major associated cardiac anomalies (UAB; 1967–1979; n = 312, 30 hospital deaths).[R5]

Incremental Risk Factors	Logistic Coefficient ± SD	P Value
Young age (in months)	−2.2 ± 0.47	< .0001
Multiple VSDs (nontrabecular[a])	2.9 ± 1.20	.02
Multiple VSDs (all others)	2.2 ± 0.60	.0003
If no major associated cardiac anomaly		
Date of operation	−0.08 ± 0.020	.0001
Date of operation × age (in months)	0.015 ± 0.0058	.008
If major associated cardiac anomaly		
Mitral lesion	3.7 ± 1.61	.02
Major associated lesions other than PDA or simultaneously repaired coarctation of the aorta	1.8 ± 1.12	.10
Intercept	5.9[b]	

KEY: ln, natural logarithm; PDA, patent ductus arteriosus; SD, standard deviation; VSD, ventricular septal defect.

[a] Indicates that none of the VSDs were muscular.

[b] If a major associated cardiac anomaly, intercept is 1.8.

LATE RESULTS

Survival

Premature late death occurs rarely (in < 2.5% of patients) when pulmonary vascular resistance is low preoperatively. Presumably, the deaths are from arrhythmias, either ventricular fibrillation or the sudden development of heart block late postoperatively.

Patients with a high pulmonary vascular resistance preoperatively often die from progression of their pulmonary vascular disease (see later discussion in "Pulmonary Hypertension").

Table 20-8 Hospital mortality after repair of single and multiple VSDs with or without major or minor associated anomalies (GLH; 1958–1982, 20 deaths [5.5%] in 359 patients).

Category of VSD	1958–1965 Large VSD				1958–1965 Medium VSD				1958–1965 Small VSD				1958–1965 Total				1965–1982 Large VSD				1965–1982 Medium VSD				1965–1982 Small VSD				1965–1982 Total				$P(\chi^2)$
	n	No.	%	CL	n	No.	%	CL	n	No.	%	CL	n	No.	%	CL	n	No.	%	CL	n	No.	%	CL	n	No.	%	CL	n	No.	%	CL	
VSD (primary)	38	5	13%	7%–21%	18	2	11%	4%–24%	8	1ª	12%	2%–36%	64	8	12%	4%–8%	156	8	5.1%	3.3%–7.7%	45	0	0%	0%–4%	13	0	0%	0%–14%	214	8	3.7%	2.4%–5.6%	.21
VSD plus banded PA																	24	3	12%	6%–24%	2	0	0%	0%–61%					26	3	12%	5%–22%	.6
VSD plus AI	5	0	0%	0%–32%					2	1	50%	7%–93%	7	1	14%	2%–41%	17	0	0%	0%–11%	16	0	0%	0%–11%	8	0	0%	0%–21%	41	0	0%	0%–5%	
VSD plus S of V plus AI																	4	0	0%	0%–38%	2	0	0%	0%–61%	1	0	0%	0%–85%	7	0	0%	0%–24%	
Total	43	5	12%	7%–19%	18	2	11%	4%–24%	10	2	20%	7%–41%	71	9	13%	9%–18%	201	11	5.5%	3.8%–7.7%	65	0	0%	0%–3%	22	0	0%	0%–8%	288	11	3.8%	2.7%–5.4%	.08
$P(\chi^2)$	.4								.24				.9				.3												.11				

KEY: AI, aortic incompetence; CL, 70% confidence limits; PA, pulmonary artery; S of V, sinus of Valsalva aneurysm; VSD, ventricular septal defect.

NOTE: A two variable logistic test for the era (1958–1982) and VSD size shows early era ($P = .004$) and possibly large size of VSD ($P = .17$) to be incremental risk factors.

ª Severe associated valvar aortic stenosis.

Table 20-9 Hospital mortality according to age at primary repair of multiple VSDs without major associated cardiac anomalies (UAB; 1967–1979).[R5]

Age (mo)			1967–1979				1974–1979		
				Hospital Deaths				Hospital Deaths	
≤	<	n	No.	%	CL	n	No.	%	CL
	3	1	0	0%	0%–85%	1	0	0%	0%–85%
3 ---	6	4	2	50%	18%–82%	2	0	0%	0%–61%
6 ---	12	5	1	20%	3%–53%	3	0	0%	0%–47%
12 ---	24	7	3	43%	20%–68%	4	1	25%	3%–63%
24 ---	48	5	3	60%	29%–86%	1	0	0%	0%–85%
48		7	0	0%	0%–24%	3	0	0%	0%–47%
	Total	29	9	31%	21%–42%	14	1	7%	1%–22%
	$P(\chi^2)$				.22				.7

KEY: CL, 70% confidence limits.

[a] In the years 1967–1974, 8 hospital deaths (53%, CL 37%–69%) occurred among 15 patients.

Repair of VSD in the first year or two of life is curative for most patients, resulting in full functional activity and normal or near normal life expectancy.

Physical Development

A prominent feature of the late postoperative course following repair of large VSDs in infants is improved physical development,[R1] and an impressive increase in weight can also be demonstrated (GLH; Fig. 20-32a),[C11] as Lillehei and colleagues first showed in 1955. There is a less impressive increase in length (Fig. 20-32b) and in head circumference.[C11] This improved physical development is usually associated with complete relief of symptoms. Increase in weight postoperatively also occurs in children in whom a large VSD is repaired later in the first decade of life (Fig. 20-33).[C3]

Conduction Disturbances

Conduction disturbances are frequent after the repair of VSDs.

Right Bundle-Branch Block

Right bundle-branch block is present late postoperatively in most patients in whom VSDs are repaired via right ven-

triculotomy. In an infant series the incidence was 80% (CL 72%–86%) (GLH).[B3] On the basis of their studies, Gelband and colleagues concluded that the cause is the right ventriculotomy.[G3] However, Weidman and colleagues at the Mayo Clinic reported that 44% (CL 35%–54%) of 36 patients undergoing repair of perimembranous VSDs via right atriotomy developed new right bundle-branch block.[O3] Castaneda and colleagues reported right bundle-branch block in 34% (CL 26%–43%) of their infants undergoing repair via right atriotomy.[R1] Thus, in some patients, right bundle-branch block must result from damage to the right bundle by sutures along the inferior border of perimembranous VSDs.

Right Bundle-Branch Block and Left Anterior Hemiblock

A small proportion of patients develop the electrocardiographic pattern of right bundle-branch block and left anterior

Table 20-10 Hospital mortality after repair of large VSDs in our early era at the Mayo Clinic.[C3,K3]

Era	n	Hospital Deaths		
		No.	%	CL
1955–1960	241	50	20.7%	18.0%–23.8%
1960–1966	247	31	12.6%	10.3%–15.1%
Total	488	81	16.6%	14.8%–18.5%
$P(\chi^2)$				.02

KEY: CL, 70% confidence limits.

NOTE: Between 1962 and 1966, the hospital mortality in patients over the age of 6 months was 4.1% (CL 2.4%–6.5%).[C3]

Table 20-11 Hospital death after primary repair of single large VSD with or without major associated cardiac anomalies in patients less than 3 months old (GLH; 1969–1982).

Category of VSD	No.	Hospital Deaths	
VSD alone	4	0	
VSD plus large ASD	5	0	0/10 0%[a] CL 0%–17%
VSD plus partial anomalous pulmonary venous connection	1	0	
VSD and PDA (moderate or large)	4	0	
VSD plus severe coarctation of the aorta (simultaneous repair)	2	1	3/10 30%[a] CL 14%–51%
VSD plus moderate coarctation of the aorta (not repaired)	3	1	
VSD plus severe aortic stenosis (uncorrectable)	1	1	
Total	20	3(15%, CL 7%–28%)	

KEY: ASD, atrial septal defect; CL, 70% confidence limits; PDA, patent ductus arteriosus; VSD, ventricular septal defect.

[a] P(Fisher) = .11.

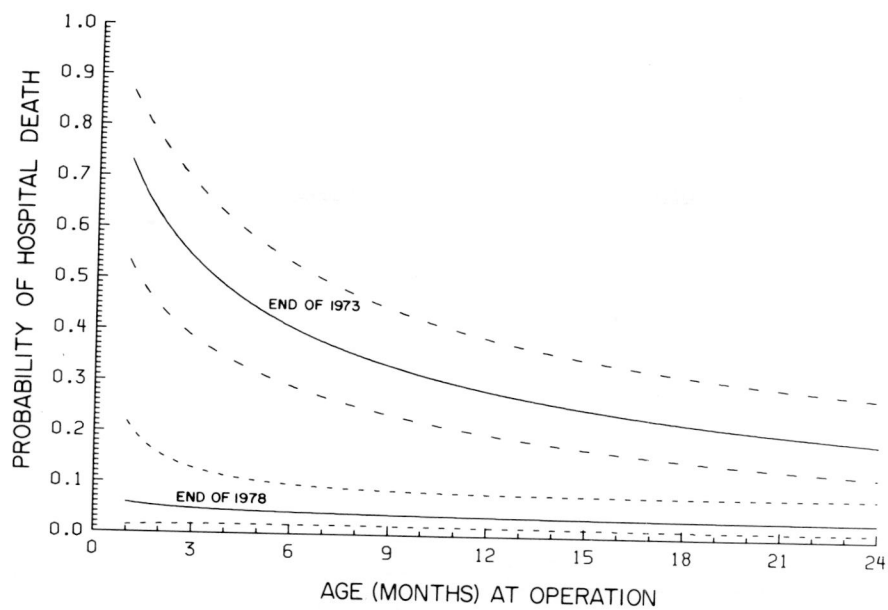

Figure 20-30 Hospital mortality after repair of multiple VSDs without major associated cardiac anomalies, according to age and year at operation. The presentation is as in Figure 20-29. Reproduced with permission from Rizzoli et al.[R5]

Table 20-12 Hospital mortality after primary repair of multiple VSDs without major associated lesions (UAB; 1967–1979).[R5]

Type of Multiple VSD	1967–1979				1974–1979			
		Hospital Deaths				Hospital Deaths		
	n	No.	%	CL	n	No.	%	CL
Nontrabecular[a]	6	0	0%	0%–27%	2	0	0%	0%–61%
Nontrabecular plus trabecular (1 or 2)	8	5	62%	38%–83% ⎱ 9/23	3	1	33%	4%–76%
Multiple (≥ 3) trabecular[b]	15	4	27%	14%–43% ⎰ 39% CL 27%–52%	9	0	0%	0%–19%
Total	29	9	31%	21%–42%	14	1	7%	1%–22%
P(χ²)				.04				.14

KEY: CL, 70% confidence limits; VSD, ventricular septal defect.
[a] Two (rarely 3) large single VSDs (e.g., one perimembranous and one subpulmonary), none of which are trabecular (muscular).
[b] With or without a large nontrabecular VSD.

Table 20-13 Hospital mortality after repair of muscular VSDs (GLH; 1958–1982).

Type of Muscular VSD	n	Hospital Deaths		
		No.	%	CL
Single	12	2	17%	6%–35%
Isolated	10	0	0%	0%–17%
Plus coarctation of the aorta (simultaneous repair)	1	1	100%	15%–100%
Plus scimitar syndrome plus mod PDA	1	1	100%	15%–100%
Two or more	7	2	29%	10%–55%
Isolated	4	0	0%	0%–38%
Plus debanding PA	1	0	0%	0%–85%
Plus debanding PA plus recurrent coarctation of the aorta[a]	2	2	100%	39%–100%
Swiss cheese	3	1	33%	4%–76%
Plus debanding PA	2	0	0%	0%–61%
Plus debanding PA plus previous coarctectomy	1	1	100%	15%–100%
Total	22	5	23%	13%–36%

KEY: CL, 70% confidence limits; PA, pulmonary artery; mod PDA, moderate-sized patent ductus arteriosus; VSD, ventricular septal defect.
[a] Recurrent coarctation of the aorta not repaired. One patient also had moderate aortic stenosis.

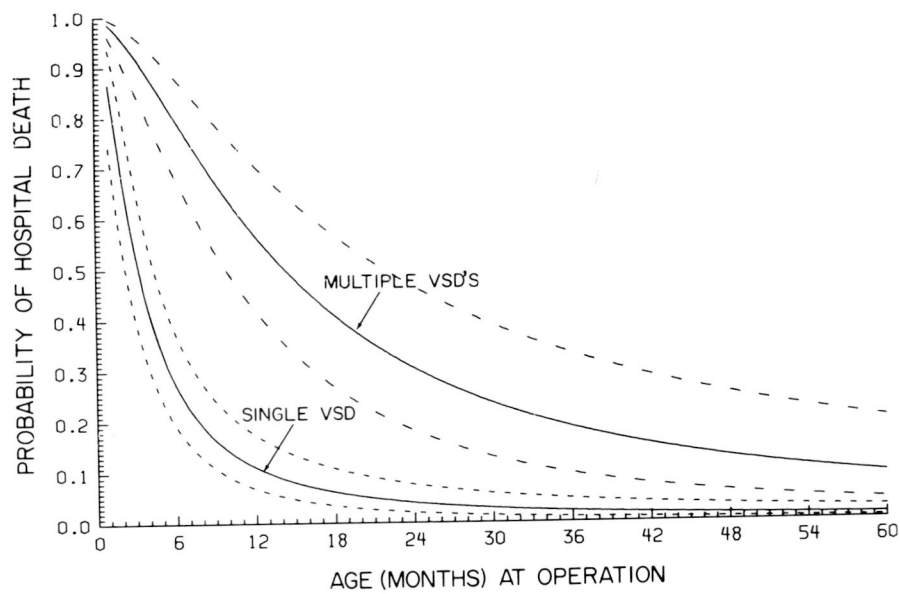

Figure 20-31 Hospital mortality after repair of VSDs with major associated cardiac anomalies, according to age and year at operation. The presentation is as in Figure 20-29. Reproduced with permission from Rizzoli et al.[R5]

hemiblock after repair of VSD. The incidence was 8% (CL 4%–14%) (GLH),[B3] 10% (CL 6%–16%) in another group of 68 patients repaired through a right ventriculotomy,[Z1] 17% (CL 11%–25%) in Castaneda's patients repaired via right atriotomy,[R1] and 12% (CL 7%–19%) in Lincoln's patients, 72% of whom were repaired through the right atrium.[L7] Such a combination of disturbances has not yet been proved to be a poor prognostic finding, but concern and some controversy has been expressed about it.[K10,Z1] Wolff and colleagues reported that this combination was associated with a significant incidence of late complete heart block and sudden death after repair of tetralogy of Fallot.[W4] However, Downing and colleagues, who found this combination in 6% (CL 4%–10%) of 109 patients undergoing repair of isolated VSD, observed no late complications of any kind in patients followed 1–10 years.[D5] The controversy may relate in part to the lack of homogeneity of this group of patients.[S10] That is, right bundle-branch block can result from damage to the main right bundle branch during repair, in which case its combination with left anterior hemiblock might be more hazardous than when right bundle-branch block results from disruption of a very peripheral branch of the right bundle's arborization secondary to a right ventriculotomy.[K11] Intracardiac recording techniques at cardiac catheterization can probably distinguish between these two groups and thus be of help prognostically.[S11]

Permanent Heart Block

The incidence of permanent heart block (complete atrioventricular dissociation, with independent atrial activity not conducted to the ventricles) after repair of single VSD approaches zero with present techniques (GLH, UAB). For

Table 20-14 Hospital mortality according to type of VSD after primary repair of single large VSD without major associated cardiac anomalies (UAB; 1967–1979).[R5]

Type of VSD	1967–1979				1974–1979			
		Hospital Deaths				Hospital Deaths		
	n	No.	%	CL	n	No.	%	CL
Perimembranous	140	6	4.3%	2.5%–6.9%	78	1	1.3%	0.2%–4.3%
Subpulmonary	10	0	0%	0%–17%	9	0	0%	0%–19%
AV canal	7	0	0%	0%–24%	4	0	0%	0%–38%
Muscular	7	0	0%	0%–24%	1	0	0%	0%–85%
Confluent	2	0	0%	0%–61%	2	0	0%	0%–61%
Total	166	6	3.6%	2.1%–5.8%	94	1	1.1%	0.1%–3.6%
$P(\chi^2)$			.89					

KEY: AV, atrioventricular; CL, 70% confidence limits.

Table 20-15 Hospital mortality after repair of VSDs of all types with or without major associated cardiac anomalies (GLH; 1958–1982).

Category of VSD	Type of VSD																											
	Perimembranous				Subpulmonary				AV Canal				Single or Multiple Muscular				Swiss Cheese				Total				
		Hospital Deaths				Hospital Deaths				Hospital Deaths				Hospital Deaths				Hospital Deaths				Hospital Deaths			
	n	No.	%	CL	n	No.	%	CL	n	No.	%	CL	n	No.	%	CL	n	No.	%	CL	n	No.	%	CL	$P(\chi^2)$
VSD, primary	233[a]	10	4.3%	2.9%–6.1%	23	2	9%	3%–19%	6	2	33%	12%–62%	16	2	12%	4%–27%					278	16	5.8%	4.3%–7.6%	.01
VSD plus banded PA	15	0	0%	0%–12%	4	0	0%	0%–38%	1	0	0%	0%–85%	3	2[b]	67%	24%–96%	3	1	33%	4%–76%	26	3	12%	5%–22%	.01
VSD plus AI	31	0	0%	0%–6%	17	1	6%	0.8%–19%													48	1	2%	0.3%–7%	.17
VSD plus S of V plus AI	6	0	0%	0%–27%	1	0	0%	0%–85%													7	0	0%	0%–24%	
Total	285	10	3.5%	2.4%–5.0%	45	3	7%	3%–13%	7	2	29%	10%–55%	19	4	21%	11%–35%	3	1	33%	4%–76%	359	20	5.6%	4.3%–7.1%	.0002
$P(\chi^2)$			.5				.9				.5				.03								.3		

KEY: AI, aortic incompetence; CL, 70% confidence limits; PA, pulmonary artery; S of V, sinus of Valsalva; VSD, ventricular septal defect.

[a] Includes 13 examples of confluent VSD.

[b] Both patients had severe recurrent coarctation of the aorta at the time of debanding, and one also congenital aortic stenosis.

Table 20-16 Hospital mortality related to the surgical approach after primary repair of single large VSDs without major associated cardiac anomalies (UAB; 1967–1979).[R5]

Surgical Approach	1967–1979				1974–1979			
		Hospital Deaths				Hospital Deaths		
	n	No.	%	CL	n	No.	%	CL
RA	105	2	1.9%	0.6%–4.5%	65	1	1.5%	0.2%–5.1%
RA → RV	4	0	0%	0%–38%	2	0	0%	0%–61%
RV	57	4	7%	4%–12%	27	0	0%	0%–7%
Total	166	6	3.6%	2.1%–5.8%	94	1	1.1%	0.1%–3.6%
$P(\chi^2)$		.23				> .9		

KEY: CL, 70% confidence limits; RA, right atrium; RV, right ventricle; RA → RV, RA approach aborted to RV approach.

example, heart block was present at death or hospital dismissal in 1 (0.4%, CL 0.05–1.3%) of 261 patients with single large VSDs with or without major associated cardiac anomalies, except straddling tricuspid valves (UAB). Four (67%, CL 8%–38%) of 6 patients with straddling tricuspid valve in the combined GLH-UAB series developed complete heart block. In our earlier experience at the Mayo Clinic, no instance occurred among the 146 patients with single large VSD operated on between 1962 and 1966. The incidence is a little higher after repair of multiple VSDs. Two (4%, CL 1%–

10%) of 47 patients undergoing repair of multiple VSDs developed complete heart block (UAB).[R5]

Cardiac Function

Late postoperative cardiac function is essentially normal when repair is done in the first 2 years of life by modern techniques through the right atrium or right ventricle. Cordell, Graham, and colleagues found left ventricular end diastolic volume, systolic output, and ejection fraction all to be

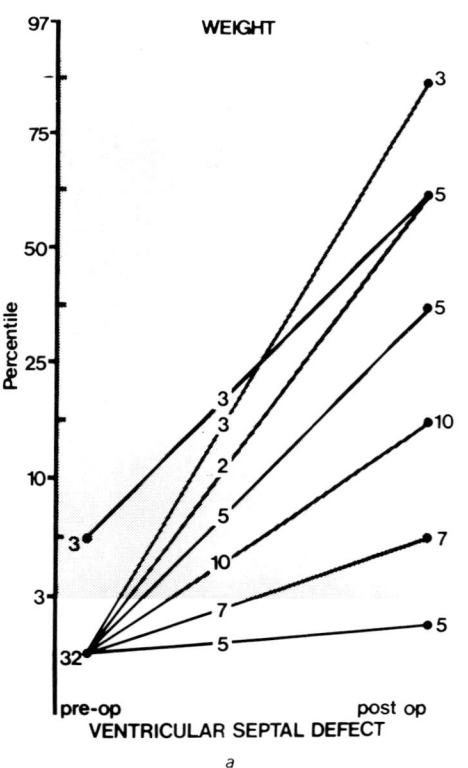

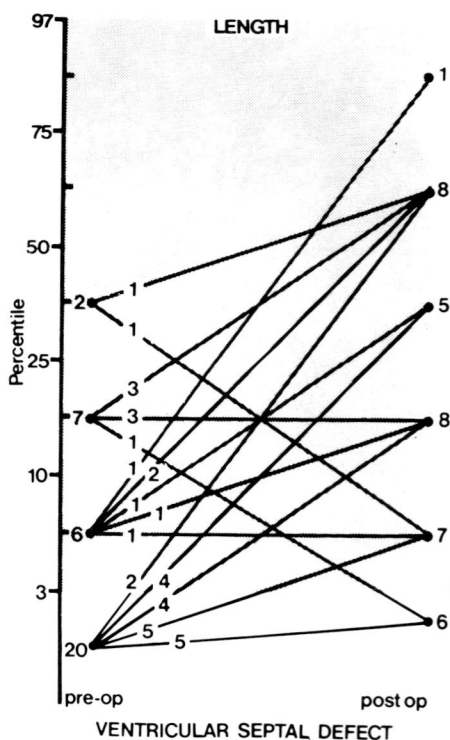

Figure 20-32 Changes in (a) weight and (b) length in infants after VSD closure.
Reproduced with permission from Clarkson et al.[C11]

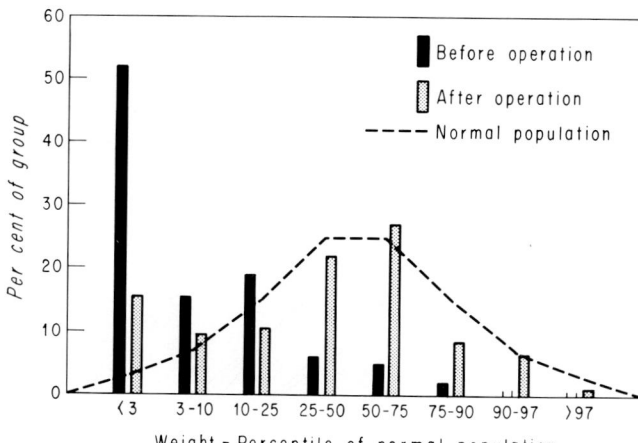

Figure 20-33 Changes in weight after repair of VSD in 96 patients 10 years old or less with Pp/Ps ≥ 0.45 and Rp/Rs < 0.75 preoperatively.

Reproduced with permission from Cartmill et al.[C3]

normal about a year after operation in a group of such patients (Fig. 20-34).[C4] Others have found persisting abnormalities of left ventricular size and function after repair of large VSDs at an older age, although all patients were asymptomatic.[J1,J2,M1] This information suggests that in general patients with large VSDs should be operated on before they are 2 years old, and preferably in the first year of life.

The experience with left ventricular function after left ventriculotomy for repairing VSDs in infants has been sobering, since in some patients cardiac output has been low and left atrial pressure high in spite of the absence of a shunt. One patient developed a large false aneurysm (UAB).

Residual Shunting

Postoperative left-to-right shunts large enough to require reoperation are uncommon when proper techniques are used. One of 138 patients (0.7%, CL 0.1%–2%) operated on for repair of a large VSD required reoperation (UAB) and this was for overlooked multiple muscular defect;[B1] and 3 (1.9%, CL 0.8%–4%) of 158 patients required reoperation (GLH). Castaneda reported that 1 patient out of 48 hospital survivors (2%, CL 0%–7%) required reoperation for residual VSD.[R1]

Small but hemodynamically insignificant residual VSDs cannot be entirely ignored, because of the theoretical possibility of bacterial endocarditis at such sites. An accurate estimation of their incidence would require routine postoperative left ventriculography, and this has not been done. However, among 35 patients recatheterized for reasons other than confirmation of the presence of a significant residual shunt, 3 (9%, CL 4%–17%) had small residual shunts detectable by oxygen saturation data (GLH). Four others (11%, CL 6%–20%) had shunts detected only by left ventricular cineangiography, in two of whom the shunting was through very small, unclosed muscular defects.

Pulmonary Hyperinflation Syndrome

When pulmonary hyperinflation syndrome is present in infants before repair of their VSD, it usually completely disappears within 1–2 months after repair.[O4]

Surgically Produced Aortic or Tricuspid Incompetence

As complications of repair of primary VSD, surgically produced aortic and tricuspid incompetence are rare. The first patient operated on in 1958 required reoperation in 1976 for surgically produced aortic incompetence (GLH). In patients operated on since then, none are known to have significant iatrogenic aortic incompetence (GLH and UAB).

The fact that surgically induced tricuspid incompetence is rare is surprising, considering how often abnormal chordae are attached around the defect. Such a complication has been recognized as important in only one patient (GLH and UAB), who had a large confluent defect extending from the perimembranous position to beneath the septal tricuspid leaflet, which was torn at its base and repaired during the operation.

Pulmonary Hypertension

When severe pulmonary hypertension persists after operation, it may worsen with the passage of time[F3] and cause premature late death, usually within 3–10 years of operation.[D2,F3,H3] About 25% of patients with preoperative pulmonary hypertension and high pulmonary vascular resistance (≥ 10 units · m²) die with pulmonary hypertension within 5 years of operation (Fig. 20-35).[B1] However, some patients with pulmonary hypertension and elevated pulmonary vascular resistance late postoperatively have neither progression nor regression of their disease for as long as 20 years, although they have some limitation in exercise tolerance.[D2,H10]

In general, the younger the child at the time of repair, the better are the child's chances of surviving and having an essentially normal pulmonary artery pressure 5 years and more later (Fig. 20-36).[B3,C8,D2,H8,L4,M2,S16,Y2] The lower the pulmonary vascular resistance at the time of repair, the better are the chances of having normal pulmonary artery pressure late postoperatively (Fig. 20-37). These two factors, age and preoperative pulmonary vascular resistance, interact in determining late postoperative pulmonary artery pressure (Fig. 20-38).

Surgical Cure

Combining the data on pulmonary artery pressure late postoperatively with the proportion of patients dying early and late postoperatively, chances of surgical cure (defined as surviving the early postoperative period and being alive late postoperatively with essentially normal pulmonary artery pressure) can be estimated for an individual patient (Fig. 20-39). If repair of a large VSD is performed in a patient at 6 months of age, there is at least a 95% chance of surgical cure, unless pulmonary vascular resistance is greater than 10 units · m² (which is rare at that age). This is supported by the studies by Rabinovitch and colleagues, which also find that

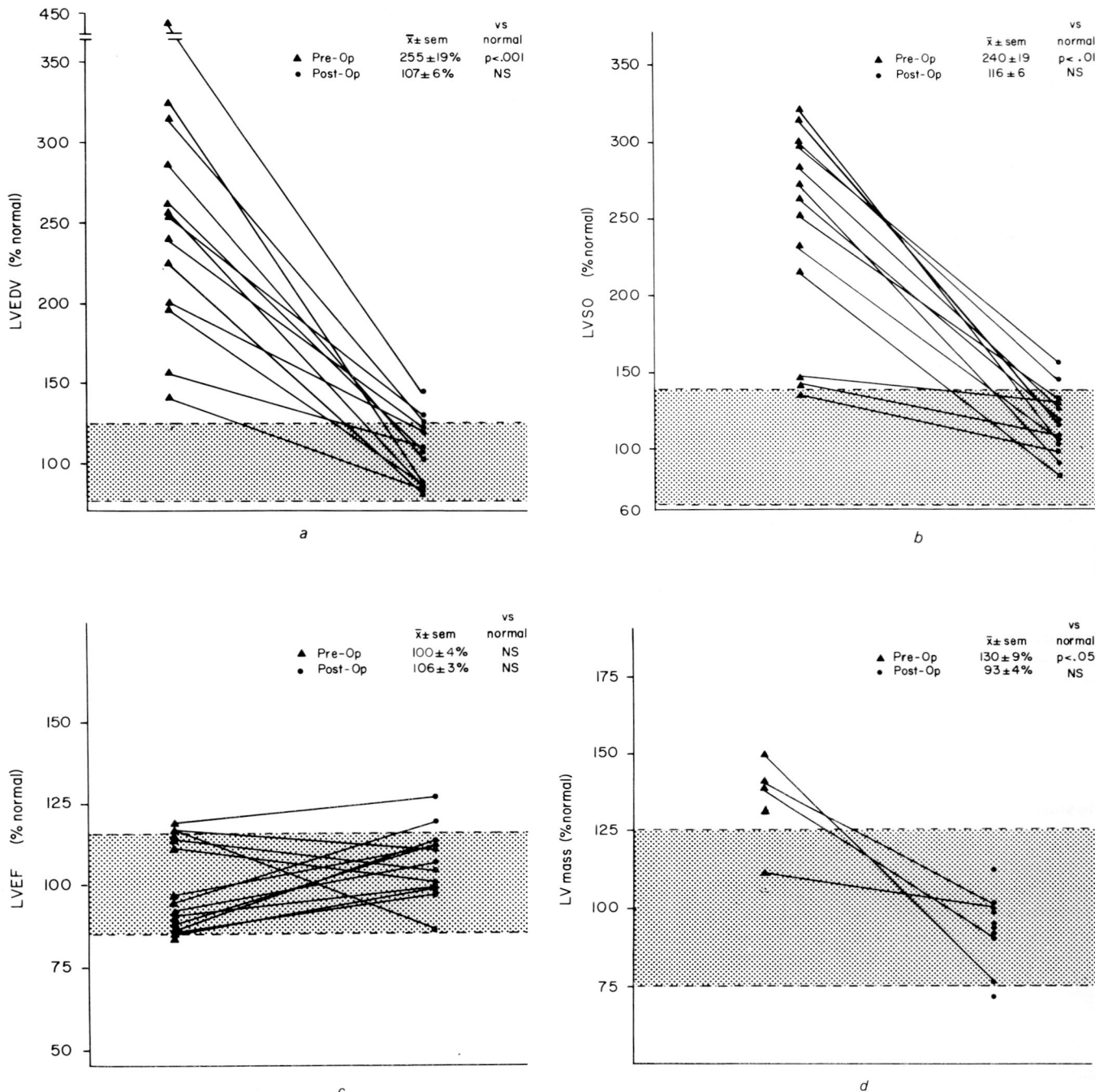

Figure 20-34 Preoperative and postoperative studies of cardiac function 1 year after repair of large VSDs in infants. Shaded areas represent the 95% confidence limits around the normal value.
(*a*) Left ventricular end-diastolic volume, large preoperatively, returns to normal.
(*b*) Left ventricular systolic output returns to normal with ablation of the shunt.
(*c*) Ejection fraction is normal preoperatively and postoperatively.
(*d*) Left ventricular mass returns to normal.

Reproduced with permission from Cordell et al.,[C4] and the American Heart Association, Inc.

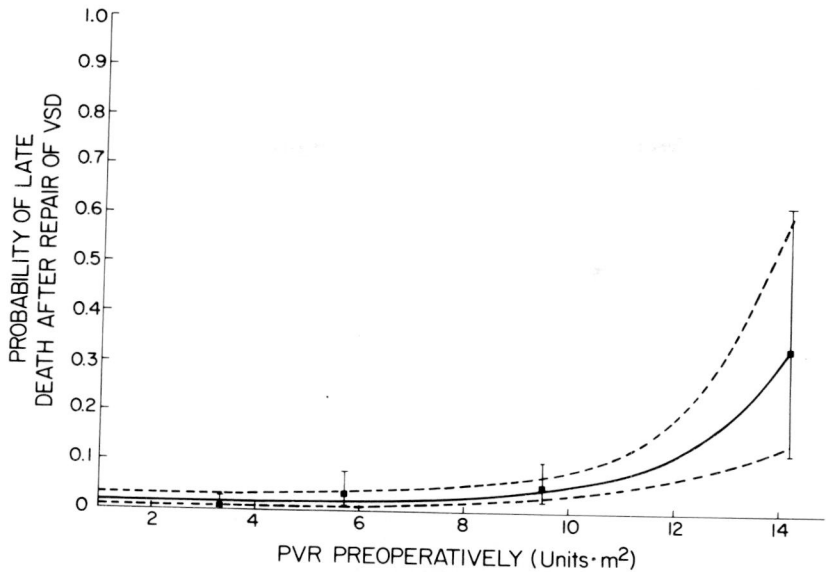

Figure 20-35 Probability of late death (within 5 years of operation) in patients who have survived the early postoperative period, according to pulmonary vascular resistance preoperatively. The dashed lines enclose the 70% confidence limits. The actual proportions of death obtained from Cartmill and associates[C3] are shown with their 70% confidence limits. *P* for PVR = .0002. The data, equations, and statistics are contained in the original source.

Reproduced with permission from Blackstone et al.[B1]

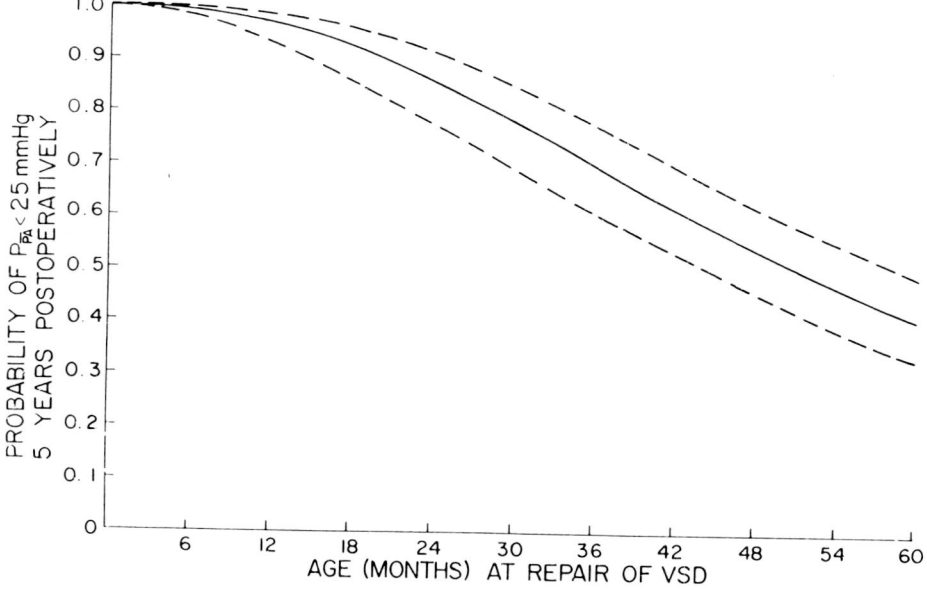

Figure 20-36 Probability of good late results (mean pulmonary artery pressure < 25 mmHg 5 years after repair) in patients leaving the hospital alive after operation and surviving 5 years, according to age (months) at the time of repair of a large VSD. The dashed lines enclose the 70% confidence limits. *P* for age < .0001. Equations and statistics are available on request; the analysis is based on the data of DuShane and Kirklin.[D2]

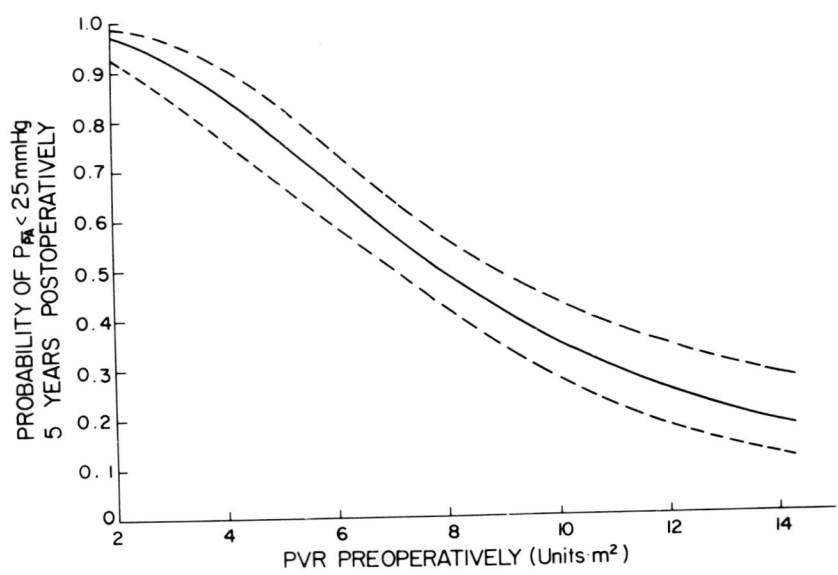

Figure 20-37 Probability of good late results (mean pulmonary artery pressure < 25 mmHg 5 years after repair) in patients leaving the hospital alive after operation and surviving 5 years, according to preoperative pulmonary vascular resistance. The dashed lines enclose the 70% confidence limits. *P* for PVR < .001. Equations and statistics are available on request; the analysis is based on the data of DuShane and Kirklin.[D2]

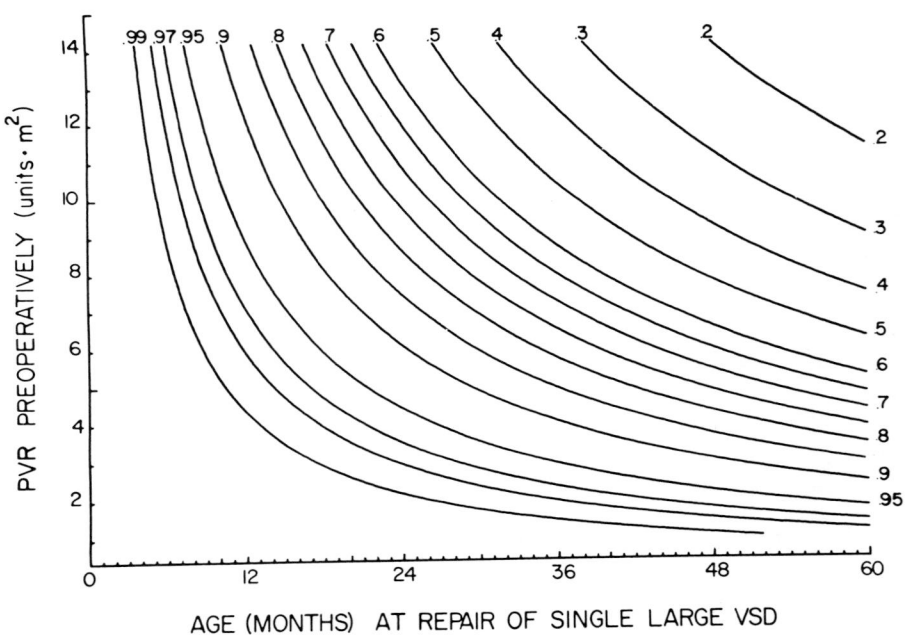

Figure 20-38 Probability of good late results (mean pulmonary artery pressure < 25 mmHg 5 years after repair) in patients leaving the hospital alive after operation and surviving 5 years (represented by the contoured lines) according to age at the time of repair of a large VSD and the preoperative level of pulmonary vascular resistance. Equations and statistics are available on request; the analysis is based on the data of DuShane and Kirklin.[D2]

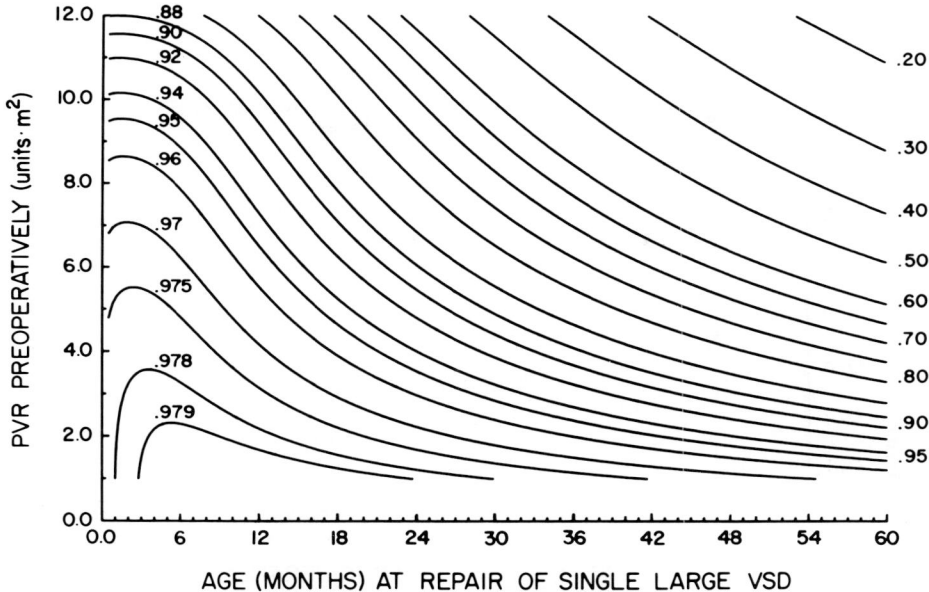

Figure 20-39 Probability of overall surgical cure (survival of the operation and at least 5 years postoperatively with a mean pulmonary artery pressure < 25 mmHg) of patients with a single large VSD (represented by the contoured lines) according to the combined effect of age at operation and preoperative pulmonary vascular resistance. This plot considers hospital mortality as of 1978. Note that when operation is performed in the first year of life and PVR is 6, over 95% of patients are cured. Equations and statistics are available on request; the analysis is based on the data of DuShane and Kirklin.[D2]

surgical cure is likely to result in any infant in whom the VSD is repaired before the age of 6–9 months, irrespective of the degree of pulmonary vascular disease.[R6] In a patient that is 2 years old, the chances of cure are this good only if preoperative pulmonary vascular resistance is less than about 5 units · m². In a patient operated on for repair of large VSD at 4 years of age, the chances are that good only if the resistance is normal preoperatively (which is unusual). This unfavorable effect of older age in such a setting has been confirmed by John and colleagues.[J4] This supports the practice of repair of large defects at least by age 12 months and can be used to predict the results of operation in individual patients.

INDICATIONS FOR OPERATION

When infants with large VSDs have severe and intractable heart failure or respiratory symptoms in the *first 3 months of life,* prompt primary repair of the VSD is indicated. Most such infants have major associated cardiac anomalies, which are repaired simultaneously when appropriate. Exceptions to this practice are made for the rare infants with Swiss-cheese septum, who present a special problem because of the higher risk of surgery and the need for a left ventriculotomy. In this setting in the first 3 months of life, pulmonary artery banding may be indicated; when there are no

complications from the band, repair of the Swiss-cheese septum and debanding are postponed until the age of 3–5 years. This general plan is also followed when Swiss-cheese septum coexists with aortic coarctation (see "VSD and Coarctation of the Aorta"). Other exceptions to primary repair in the first 3 months of life are infants with straddling tricuspid valve (see "Straddling Tricuspid Valve").

Operation is not advised electively in the first 3 months of life in infants without serious symptoms, in the hope that spontaneous closure or narrowing of the VSD may occur.

When severe symptoms, significant growth failure, or rising pulmonary vascular resistance are present in infants *older than 3 months of age,* prompt primary repair again is advised.

When an infant reaches *6 months* of age with a single, large VSD, the infant is rarely truly thriving. The probability of cure by spontaneous VSD closure has decreased significantly (Fig. 20-40). If the pulmonary vascular resistance is greater than 8 units · m², repair is advisable without undue delay, since delay lessens the chances of surgical cure (Fig. 20-38). If the pulmonary vascular resistance is low (< 4 units · m²) and the clinical condition reasonably good, operation can be deferred until about 12 months of age in the hope of spontaneous VSD narrowing or closure (Fig. 20-40), although the risks of repair are no less than at 6 months of age.

Patients with large VSDs who are first seen *after infancy*

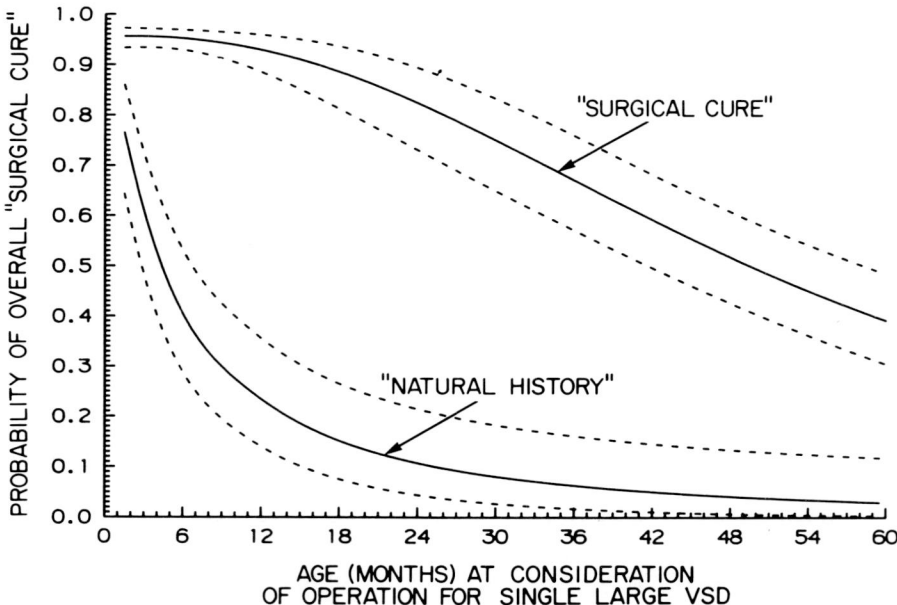

Figure 20-40 Probability of overall surgical cure (survival from the operation and at least 5 years postoperatively with a mean pulmonary artery pressure < 25 mmHg) according to age (months) at the time of repair for all patients with single large VSDs. The analysis is based on the data of DuShane and Kirklin.[D2] Also shown is the natural history, for which the vertical axis is the probability of long-term survival and ultimate spontaneous closure of the defect, and the horizontal axis the age at observation of a patient with a large VSD. Equations and statistics are available upon request.

are considered primarily on the basis of the extent of their pulmonary vascular disease.[K2] When the pulmonary vascular resistance is greater than 10 units · m², the resting pulmonary-systemic blood flow ratio ($\dot{Q}p/\dot{Q}s$) is less than 1.5, and the clinical data are also consistent with such a hemodynamic state (the systolic murmur is soft or absent, no apical diastolic flow murmur is present, the lung fields on the chest x-ray are not plethoric, the left ventricle is normal or near normal in size, and the ECG shows at least moderate right ventricular hypertrophy), operation is not advisable. Closure of the defect would deny right-to-left shunting during exercise, resulting in a lower exercise capacity and life expectancy with the defect closed than with it open. When pulmonary vascular resistance is elevated but within the operable range (5–10 units · m²), operation is usually advisable, even though the long-term results may be compromised by persisting and possibly increasing pulmonary vascular disease. However, some patients with resistance values at rest in this range have a fixed pulmonary vascular resistance that does not fall during stress. Therefore, in patients with borderline operability who are old enough to cooperate, measurement of pulmonary and systemic blood flow and resistances during moderate exercise is indicated. A $\dot{Q}p/\dot{Q}s$ of 1.5–1.8 at rest that becomes 1.0 or less during moderate exercise (from systemic peripheral vasodilation, increased systemic blood flow, and a fixed and high pulmonary vascular resistance preventing increased pulmonary blood flow) is an indication of inoperability. The simple finding of a significant fall in arterial oxygen saturation during exercise (from right-to-left

shunting across the VSD for the reasons described) also suggests inoperability, but a more complete investigation is required for a final decision. The response of pulmonary vascular resistance to inhalation of mixtures high in oxygen is not useful in determining operability in borderline situations.

In infants, study during exercise is not possible, and the resistance response to a continuous isoproterenol infusion is used instead. Even when the resistance is 12 units · m² at rest in small infants, if it falls to 8 units · m² with isoproterenol, the VSD may be considered operable.

A considerable number of children have a moderate-sized VSD, which is not sufficient to raise systolic pulmonary artery pressure above 40–50 mmHg, will not result in subsequent elevation of pulmonary vascular resistance, and yet produces a $\dot{Q}p/\dot{Q}s$ of up to 3, moderate cardiomegaly, and significant pulmonary plethora, with few if any symptoms. Such patients are kept under observation for about 5 years in the hope that there will be spontaneous reduction in size of the VSD. If there is no change on subsequent recatheterization, closure is indicated.

Young patients with small VSDs are not advised to undergo repair. When they reach about 10 years of age, the situation is controversial. In favor of avoiding operation is the possibility that the defect may still close spontaneously; that its only ill effect is possible bacterial endocarditis, which is easily treated; and that operation carries a small risk. In favor of repair is the possibility of bacterial endocarditis, with its morbidity and risk, however small; the very real psychological impact on the adolescent child and young adult of the defect; and the high probability of complete cure by operation. Each patient must therefore be considered according to the individual circumstances.

Subpulmonary defects constitute a special situation. Even though apparently small, they should not be left untreated in patients over 5 years of age if there is any aortic cusp deformity on cineangiography, lest aortic incompetence develop (see Section 2). They should be repaired promptly if an aortic diastolic murmur develops.

SPECIAL SITUATIONS AND CONTROVERSIES

Ventricular Septal Defect and Patent Ductus Arteriosus

The combination of large VSD and moderate or large patent ductus arteriosus is particularly likely to cause severe symptoms and require operation early in infancy.[B3] In the first 6–8 weeks of life in patients with a very large ductus and only a moderate-sized or small VSD, the ductus alone may be closed with a simple closed operation (see Chapter 22), since the VSD may narrow or close spontaneously. If this does not happen, the VSD is closed at an appropriate time. When the VSD is large, both it and the patent ductus are closed simultaneously if operation is required in early life. The risk of operation at present should not be higher than that for isolated VSD, but the technique is important.

Ventricular Septal Defect and Coarctation of the Aorta

The combination of VSD and aortic coarctation frequently causes severe symptoms in infancy. Both the coarctation and the VSD are variable in severity. Clearly, the worst combination is a large VSD and severe coarctation, but even a small VSD in association with significant coarctation may produce heart failure relatively early in life. Six of the nine patients with the latter combination required coarctation repair in the first 8 months of life (GLH).

Management options for this combination of defects include simultaneous repair of both lesions,[B3] initial repair of the coarctation alone,[N2] initial coarctation repair and pulmonary artery banding, or initial VSD closure alone.[R3] With a large VSD and severe coarctation, repair of the VSD first has certain theoretical advantages[R3] but has been practiced rarely under such circumstances. *Repair of the coarctation only* as the initial operation has the advantage of removing the afterload on the left ventricle and reducing the shunt through the defect. It also avoids a second operation if the VSD closes spontaneously.[N2] The mortality with repair of aortic coarctation has been high in the past (GLH; Table 20-17).[N2] More recent experience with this repair has been good (UAB; Table 20-18). Malm and associates also have had good results with this protocol, two (11%, CL 4%–28%) hospital deaths having occurred among 17 patients so treated. Four (27%, CL 14%–43%) of the 15 survivors required repair of the VSD in early infancy, and two (13%, CL 4%–29%) required it later. Nine (60%, CL 43%–75%) of the hospital survivors experienced spontaneous closure or narrowing of their VSD within the follow-up period (2–10 years).

The results have also been good in the current era with *initial coarctation repair and pulmonary artery banding* (GLH; Table 20-17).

Simultaneous repair of both the *coarctation* and *a large VSD* has in the past carried a high risk in the first 2 months of life.[B1,B3,N2] The only exception is the experience of Tiraboschi and colleagues, but only one of their four patients was less than 3 months old.[T10,T11] However, good results have been obtained in the current era. Thus, simultaneous repair of both defects has been performed in five infants (ages 3 weeks to 9 months) with one death (20%, CL 3%–53%), that of a 3-week-old infant (GLH).[B3]

Current protocols are as follows:

1. When the VSD is large, the coarctation severe, and the infant presents in the first 2 months of life with severe and intractable heart failure, which is the usual situation, the coarctation is repaired at urgent operation; the pulmonary artery may be banded (GLH), or alternatively, only

Table 20-17 Hospital mortality after the initial operation in infants with VSD and coarctation of the aorta (GLH; 1961–1978).

| Type of Operation | | 1961–1969 | | | | 1969–1978 | | |
| | | Hospital Deaths | | | | Hospital Deaths | | |
	n	No.	%	CL	n	No.	%	CL
Large VSD plus Severe Coarctation								
Coarctectomy plus VSD repair					2[c]	1	50%	7%–93%
Coarctectomy[a]	7	4	57%	32%–80%	5[c]	2	40%	14%–71%
Coarctectomy plus PA banding	4	2	50%	18%–82%	8[b,c]	0	0%	0%–21%
Large VSD plus Moderate Coarctation								
VSD repair	1	0	0%	0%–85%	6	1	17%	2%–46%
Small VSD plus Coarctation								
Coarctectomy	2	0	0%	0%–61%	7	0	0%	0%–24%
Total	14	6	43%	27%–60%	28	4	14%	7%–24%

KEY: CL, 70% confidence limits; PA, pulmonary artery; VSD, ventricular septal defect.
[a]In 1961–1971, 6 (50%, CL 32%–68%) of 12 infants so treated died.
[b]Seven had a subsequent second-stage VSD repair, with one death (Swiss-cheese septum).
[c]All < 3 months old at initial operation.

Table 20-18 Hospital mortality in VSD with coarctation of the aorta according to method of management (UAB; 1967–1981; age < 1 year).

Methods of Management of Cases with VSD (n = 20)	Overall Group		Resection and End-to-End Anastomosis		Subclavian Flap	
	No.	Hospital Deaths	No.	Hospital Deaths	No.	Hospital Deaths
Coarctation repair						
Without pulmonary artery banding	8	1	1	1	7	0
With pulmonary artery banding[a]	8	2	4	1	3	0
One-stage primary repair	3	1[b]	3	1		
Two-stage repair done during same hospitalization	1	0			1	0
Total	20	4 20% (CL 10%–33%)	8	3 38% (CL 17%–62%)	11	0 0% (CL 0%–16%)

KEY: CL, confidence limits; VSD, ventricular septal defect.

NOTE: Within each vertical column of hospital deaths, all CLs overlapped.

[a] One additional patient had patch graft repair and died of hemorrhage on postoperative day 3.

[b] Patient had multiple VSD.

coarctation repair is done, and the baby is closely followed (UAB). If severe heart failure persists, then the VSD is repaired a few days or a few weeks later, as may be required. In the absence of Swiss-cheese septum, if a band has been placed, it is removed and the VSD repaired at 6 months of age, thereby usually avoiding the need to reconstruct the pulmonary artery. When Swiss-cheese septum is present, debanding and repair are delayed if possible until the patient is about 5 years of age.

2. When the VSD is large, the coarctation is severe, and the infant presents beyond the first 2 months of life, simultaneous repair of both anomalies may be performed (GLH), or occasionally, the coarctation alone may be repaired and the plan outlined above followed (UAB).

3. When the coarctation is severe and the VSD is small, only the coarctation is repaired, and the results are those of coarctation repair in general (Table 20-17; see Chapter 34). Subsequent repair of the VSD is rarely required.

4. When the coarctation is moderate in severity and the VSD large, the VSD may be repaired initially, and the coarctation repair postponed until the patient is 6–12 months of age. The techniques of CPB are standard, perfusion of the lower body being quite satisfactory in this situation. Alternatively, if both lesions seem clearly in need of repair and the infant is older than 2 months of age, both lesions may be repaired simultaneously.

Straddling Tricuspid Valve

Surgical treatment is complicated when straddling tricuspid valve occurs as a major associated defect in patients with VSDs in the posterior (inlet) septum. In such patients, the tendency of the AV node to be anomalously positioned has resulted in a high incidence of heart block after repair. Occasionally, the straddling tricuspid valve is severely incompetent, and then it must be replaced as part of the repair. Also, when the straddling is great and 40%–50% or more of the valve is over the left ventricle, replacement may be necessary. In some cases, modifications of the technique of VSD repair may allow preservation of the tricuspid valve.[P4,T9] In one such modification, the VSD is repaired in the usual way, except that a slot is made in the patch for passage of the anomalous chordae tendinae crossing to a *left* ventricular papillary muscle (see Chapter 44, "Straddling and Overriding Atrioventricular Valves" in section on Special Situations and Controversies). Following such repair, the tricuspid valve function late postoperatively has seemed satisfactory. Alternatively, in repairing the VSD, the patch may be sutured on the left ventricular side of the septum beyond the anomalous papillary muscle to which the anomalous tricuspid septal leaflet chordae are attached. This minor septation of the left ventricle as part of the repair may not be possible if the papillary muscle also has chordae to the mitral valve.

Six such patients have undergone repair, and all have survived (GLH, UAB). Four of the six patients had complete heart block postoperatively.

Because of the possible need for valve replacement when straddling is present as a major associated lesion, VSD closure is delayed until 5–10 years of age whenever possible. When necessary, pulmonary artery banding is done in infancy.

Pulmonary Artery Banding

Civin and Edwards[C7] noted the good prognosis and freedom from pulmonary vascular disease of patients with single ventricle and moderate pulmonary stenosis, and, based on that observation, Muller and Dammann performed pulmonary artery banding in 1963.[M3] For many years thereafter, this procedure was used by many for infants who required operation for large VSD, thereby allowing deferral of the intracardiac repair until an older age.[M4,O1,P1]

The techniques of management have, however, so improved the results of primary repair that banding is now seldom indicated for isolated large VSDs. The reasons for the current policy are several. Hospital mortality of pulmonary artery banding has been significant, and a second opera-

Table 20-19 Hospital mortality after pulmonary artery banding for VSD (GLH; 1961–1978). Patients with coarctation of the aorta are included.

Type of VSD	n	Hospital Deaths			
		No.	%	CL	
Swiss Cheese	7	1	14%	2%–41%	} P = .7
Other	30	3	10%	4%–19%	
Total	37	4	11%	6%–19%	

KEY: CL, 70% confidence limits; VSD, ventricular septal defect.

tion, which carries an additional mortality, is always required.[G1,H4,H5] The hospital mortality reported in the literature for pulmonary artery banding in the first year of life is 16%.[K6,S3,S4,S5] The early mortality is independent of the type of VSD (GLH; Table 20-19). It is difficult to adjust the tightness of the band perfectly, and at times reentry a few days later is needed for modification of the tightness. Furthermore, good palliation is not always achieved by banding, and there may be a significant intermediate mortality before second-stage repair. Complications result from banding in some patients, including the development of infundibular and valvar pulmonary stenosis, subaortic stenosis,[F2] and migration of the band to the pulmonary artery bifurcation (Fig. 20-41). The hospital mortality from pulmonary artery debanding and VSD repair has been about 10% (Table 20-15), and the debanding operation is technically more demanding than is primary repair. Furthermore, restenosis of the pulmonary artery sometimes follows debanding and repair of the VSD, necessitating a third operation.[K6]

Pulmonary artery banding as an initial palliative procedure in the very young may still be appropriate in some centers.[S15] However, for a number of years there have been only two indications for pulmonary artery banding in infants with primary VSD (GLH, UAB): (1) severe heart failure from Swiss-cheese septum and (2) associated severe coarctation of the aorta and severe heart failure in the first 2 months of life (GLH).

Right Atrial versus Right Ventricular Approach for Perimembranous VSD

The right ventricular approach may be used almost exclusively for the repair of perimembranous VSDs and results in a low hospital mortality even in patients with a high pulmonary vascular resistance (GLH). It has the advantage that the nadir of the noncoronary cusp of the aortic valve, which is the area of the right trigone and bundle of His, can be accurately visualized, which may be helpful in choosing the suture technique that will minimize the incidence of heart block (GLH; Fig. 20-24). It has the disadvantage that it leaves a scar in the right ventricle and is associated with a higher incidence of complete right bundle-branch block than is an atrial approach.

The right atrial approach may be used almost exclusively, a practice that we began in about 1960 at the Mayo Clinic (UAB).[C3] An accurate repair can be obtained through a right atrial approach in nearly all cases. Associated infundibular

pulmonary stenosis can be excised. A right ventricular scar is avoided, and the incidence of right bundle-branch block is lower than with the transventricular approach.[H13] With the right atrial approach, however, all movements must be very precise to avoid damage to the tricuspid valve leaflets or chordae.

Continuous versus Interrupted Sutures for Repair

A simple continuous suture may be used for sewing in the VSD patch (UAB). The advent of monofilament sutures that can be pulled up snugly without tearing the friable muscle around the edge of the defect has made this practice simple and safe. Theoretically, tension on the sutures should be more even with a continuous technique with monofilament sutures than with interrupted sutures. Pulling through of one or two stitches could occur, and this is a disadvantage. Alternatively, interrupted silk sutures are used for patch closure of large perimembranous defects, but continuous sutures are used in large muscular and sometimes in large subpulmonary defects (GLH).

SECTION 2
VENTRICULAR SEPTAL DEFECT AND AORTIC INCOMPETENCE

DEFINITION

The ventricular septal defect (VSD) and aortic incompetence (AI) syndrome includes hearts in which aortic incompetence is of congenital origin, due usually to cusp prolapse or a bicuspid aortic valve. The VSD may be either subpulmonary or perimembranous but is always subaortic. This syndrome is related to congenital aneurysm of the sinus of Valsalva (Chapter 21) and tetralogy of Fallot with aortic incompetence (Chapter 23).

HISTORICAL NOTE

Initial description of the syndrome of VSD with AI due to a prolapsed aortic cusp is attributed to Laubry and Pezzi's publication in 1921.[L6] The first reports of operative correction were those of Garamella and colleagues[G6] and Starr and colleagues[S12] in 1960. Experience with this syndrome at GLH began in 1960. In a patient operated on in 1962, severe incompetence was virtually abolished by wedge resection of the prolapsed leaflet, and the incompetence remained mild on review 12 years later (GLH). Our experience at the Mayo Clinic began at about the same time.[K9] On review of this experience in 1963, of the 30 patients in whom the aortic valve cusps were reconstructed and repaired, 10 (33%, CL 24%–44%) still had important valve incompetence.[E2] This and other reports[T3] in which the results of cusp reconstruction were equally unsatisfactory led to the adoption (GLH and UAB) of aortic valve replacement using either a homograft[G5] or a prosthetic valve. During this period, operations for this syndrome were delayed beyond childhood whenever

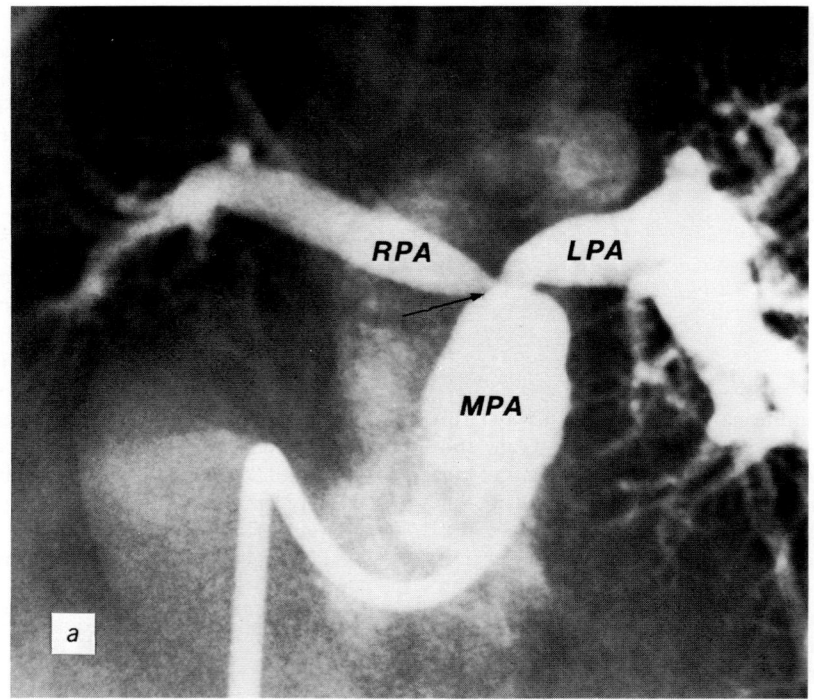

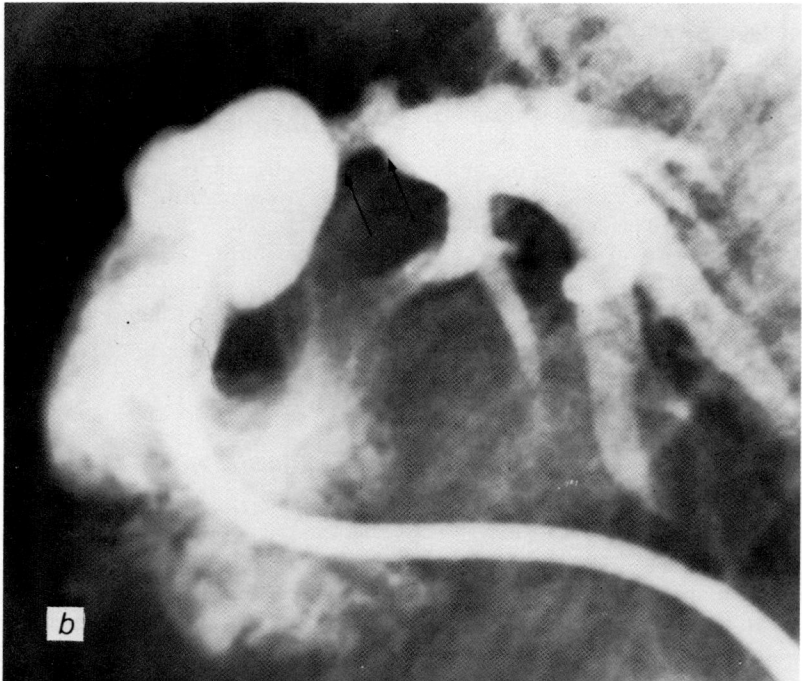

Figure 20-41 Cineangiogram of a 4-year-old patient who had previously undergone pulmonary artery banding (UAB).

(*a*) Pulmonary artery injection in the frontal view of the sitting-up position. The arrow indicates the position of the band at the bifurcation of the pulmonary trunk and the narrowing of the origin of the right and left pulmonary arteries.

(*b*) Lateral view. The width of the pulmonary band is indicated by the two arrows as well as by its migration to the pulmonary artery bifurcation.

LPA, left pulmonary artery; MPA, main pulmonary artery or pulmonary trunk; RPA, right pulmonary artery.

possible in order to avoid valve replacement in the young age group. Renewed interest in the use of leaflet reconstruction dates from the publications of Spencer and colleagues[S9] and Trusler and colleagues[T4] in 1973. Work by Sakakibara and associates, in Japan, has done much to elucidate the nature of the anomaly and document the good results obtained by closure of the VSD alone when the incompetence is mild.[T5,T6,T7]

MORPHOLOGY

The VSD in the VSD–aortic incompetence (AI) syndrome is always in the left ventricular outflow portion of the septum and is contiguous with the aortic valve. As already noted, AI is commonest in subpulmonary subarterial VSDs, which have no muscle present at the superior margin of the defect (Table 20-20). The adjacent right cusp of the aortic valve, and sometimes the adjacent portion of the noncoronary cusp, is exposed and unsupported. The VSD is characteristically semilunar or oval, with its long axis parallel to the aortic ring. It is usually large or at least moderate in size but is occasionally small. The infundibular septum may be underdeveloped and displaced anteriorly and leftward[V1] (as in tetralogy of Fallot), a feature responsible for the mild infundibular stenosis that may be present. Occasionally, the right ventricular trabecula near the junction of the infundibular septum and the free wall may contribute to the infundibular stenosis, as may hypertrophy of the moderator band at a lower level. Thus, Keane and colleagues found typical low-lying infundibular pulmonary stenosis (double-chambered right ventricle) in 14% of their patients.[K7]

Some patients with the syndrome of VSD and AI have perimembranous defects near the anteroseptal commissure of the tricuspid valve (in the so-called *infracristal position*). For some reason, the majority of patients with VSD and AI operated on at GLH have had their VSDs in this position, although in some, a narrow bar of muscle separated the VSD from the tricuspid valve.

The aortic root and valve exhibit a variety of anomalies. The aortic incompetence may be due to anomalies of a cusp or its commissural attachment, or to a deformed bicuspid valve. Usually, it is due to cusp prolapse, in which case the right aortic cusp, rarely the noncoronary cusp, and occasionally both are elongated and enlarged, both along the free margin and in the belly of the leaflet. The cusps may prolapse not only into but at times through the VSD (Table 20-21). Protrusion through the VSD increases during diastole and effectively plugs the defect, limiting the shunt even when the defect is large. Extensive cusp prolapse through a large VSD can also produce some obstruction to right ventricular outflow. In advanced cases, the center of the cusp's free margin is thickened and retracted, a feature that makes re-suspension of the leaflet relatively ineffective. In some cases, there is additional damage produced by endocarditis.

The sinus of Valsalva adjacent to the prolapsed leaflet is enlarged, often considerably. This is associated with asymmetric splaying and dilatation of the aortic ring, a feature aggravated by severe incompetence and volume changes in the left ventricle. It is virtually impossible to distinguish the junction between the prolapsed leaflet and the dilated sinus at cineangiography and at times at operation. The wall of the enlarged sinus may be thinned and aneurysmal adjacent to

Table 20-20 The type of ventricular septal defect and severity of aortic valve incompetence in a group of 86 Japanese patients with VSD and aortic incompetence.

Degree and Type of AI	Subpulmonary VSD		Perimembranous VSD		Total
	No.	% of Total	No.	% of Total	
Mild	35	88%	5	12%	40
With cusp prolapse					
Moderate	12	86%	2	14%	14
Severe	9	90%	1	10%	10
Without cusp prolapse	17	77%	5	23%	22
Total	73	85%	13	15%	86

KEY: AI, aortic incompetence; VSD, ventricular septal defect.

SOURCE: Modified from Tatsuno et al.[T7]

Table 20-21 Characteristics of surgical patients with VSD and aortic incompetence (GLH; 1960–1982; *n* = 48 and UAB; 1967–1976; *n* = 28).

Characteristics of Patients	GLH		UAB	
	No.	% of 48	No.	% of 78
VSD Position				
Subpulmonary	17	35%	23	82%
Perimembranous	31	65%	5	18%
VSD Size				
Small	10	21%	NT	
Moderate	16	33%		
Large	22	46%		
Aortic Cusp Anomaly				
Right cusp prolapse	37	77%	15	54%
Noncoronary cusp prolapse	5	10%	3	11%
Both cusps prolapsed	4	8%	8	29%
Bicuspid valve	2	4%	1	4%
Additional SBE	4	8%	NT	
Undefined			1	4%
Sinus of Valsalva				
Aneurysm (unruptured)	7	15%	NT	
Magnitude of AI				
Severe	25	52%	16	57%
Moderate	10	21%	6	21%
Mild	13	27%	6	21%
Magnitude of PS				
Mild to moderate	9	19	NT	
Aortic Valve Procedure[a]				
Reconstruction	26	54%	11	39%
Valve replacement	12	25%	12	43%
None	10	21%	5	18%

KEY: AI, aortic incompetence; NT, not tabulated; PS, pulmonary stenosis (infundibular) with gradient > 15 mmHg; SBE, bacterial endocarditis; VSD, ventricular septal defect.

NOTE: One (1.3%, CL 0.2%–4.4%) of the 76 patients died in hospital after repair. The mean age and range (years) was 15.4 (4/12 to 54, UAB) and 17.6 (2/12 to 44, GLH).

[a]All had repair of VSD.

the leaflet hinge and, rarely, may protrude into the right ventricle immediately above the prolapsed cusp. Such a finding indicates the close similarity between this condition and that of ruptured congenital aneurysm of the sinus of Valsalva with VSD (see ''Natural History'' and also Chapter 21).

The mechanism of the cusp prolapse and incompetence is uncertain. It may result from lack of support of the aortic sinus of Valsalva and anulus by the infundibular septum,[T6,V1] although since most large perimembranous defects are closely adjacent to the aortic ring and very few have associated incompetence, this cannot be the entire explanation. A structural defect in the base of the sinus itself may also play a role, particularly when the VSD is small.[E3] Hemodynamic influences during both systole and diastole aggravate the tendencies toward incompetence.[T6] Such influences are more marked once incompetence develops, resulting in progressive prolapse and distortion.

CLINICAL FEATURES AND DIAGNOSTIC CRITERIA

The potential for the development of aortic incompetence can be assessed by noting the possible presence of aortic leaflet prolapse at cineangiography. Thus, Tatsuno and colleagues[T7] found prolapse of the right aortic cusp in 10 (42%, CL 30%–54%) of 24 patients with a subpulmonary defect in whom aortic incompetence (AI) had not yet occurred. Leaflet prolapse was present in 11 (38%, CL 28%–49%) of 29 subpulmonary defects (GLH). The exact incidence of leaflet prolapse with or without AI in perimembranous defects is unknown, but it is clearly much less.

In patients with mild incompetence, such as younger patients, the signs of the VSD dominate the clinical picture, but as the AI increases, the shunt decreases. Such patients characteristically have a to-and-fro murmur, which may simulate the continuous murmur of patent ductus arteriosus but occasionally may be mistaken for that of isolated aortic incompetence or combined aortic incompetence and stenosis.

Studies in such patients should include right heart catheterization (for shunt calculation and measurement of pressures in the pulmonary artery and right ventricle), right ventriculography (for study of possible infundibular pulmonary stenosis), left ventriculography (for identification of the location and size of the VSD), and aortography (for estimation of the magnitude of the AI and the morphology of the aortic root). The finding of a normal aortic root diameter without cusp prolapse suggests that the incompetence is due to a bicuspid valve and may not be amenable to repair. The anatomical size of the VSD cannot be demonstrated angiographically when, as is frequent, it is occluded throughout the cardiac cycle by the prolapsed aortic cusp.

NATURAL HISTORY

The exact incidence of aortic valve incompetence among patients with VSD is uncertain. In the combined surgical series (UAB and GLH), it was 11%. In a review of 756 young patients with VSD studied at the Boston Children's Hospital between 1948 and 1962, Nadas and associates reported an incidence of 4.5%.[N1] The incidence is related in part to the age at which the population is studied, for this complication is rare before 2 years of age. It is also related to the frequency with which subpulmonary VSDs occur in the population studied, for AI is much more common with this type of defect.[D4,P3] The latter relationship explains the relatively high incidence of VSD and AI reported from Japan[K8,T7] and China.[L9]

The aortic valve incompetence in this syndrome does not usually appear until the individual is between 2 and 5 years of age. However, three patients operated on at 2, 3, and 7 months of age had associated mild AI and one operated on at 22 months of age had moderate aortic incompetence (GLH). Once aortic incompetence appears, it gradually increases and within 10 years is usually severe. This sequence is similar whether the VSD is subpulmonary or perimembranous.

The secondary effects of the aortic valve incompetence on the left ventricle are at least as marked as those of rheumatic aortic incompetence (see Chapter 12, ''Aortic Incompetence'' in section on Natural History) and may be more severe because of the additional volume load from the VSD. Pulmonary vascular resistance is seldom if ever elevated, presumably because functionally, at least, the VSD is usually not large.

Aneurysms of the sinuses of Valsalva also may develop as part of the natural history of patients with subpulmonary VSDs. This is a slower process than is the development of aortic valve incompetence, and Momma and colleagues did not observe sinus of Valsalva aneurysms in patients before the age of 10 years with subpulmonary VSDs.[M9] Most commonly the aneurysms are observed during the third decade, when they may be present in 10% of the patients whose subpulmonary VSDs are still open.[M9]

TECHNIQUE OF OPERATION

In patients in whom the aortic incompetence (AI) is trivial or mild, the VSD only is repaired. When the AI is significant (moderate or severe), the aortic valve is repaired or replaced.

When aortic incompetence is significant, after cannulating and establishing CPB the aorta is cross-clamped, the aortic root opened transversely, and myocardial protection arranged (see Chapter 3). In all instances, the aortic valve is examined to assess the feasibility of repair. If the leaflet edge is retracted and thickened or the valve bicuspid, repair is usually not possible. Otherwise, one or more leaflets are repaired by Trusler's method of plication (Fig. 20-42).[T4] When this procedure must be carried out at the commissure between right and left coronary cusps, the pulmonary artery must first be carefully dissected from the aortic root so that the sutures do not damage it. After completion of the repair, the Frater stitch is left in place temporarily, and the aortotomy is closed around it. A little traction on the Frater stitch keeps the valve securely competent during any subsequent aortic root injections of cardioplegic solution and later when the aortic cross-clamp is released. After the heart begins to beat, the Frater stitch is easily pulled out.

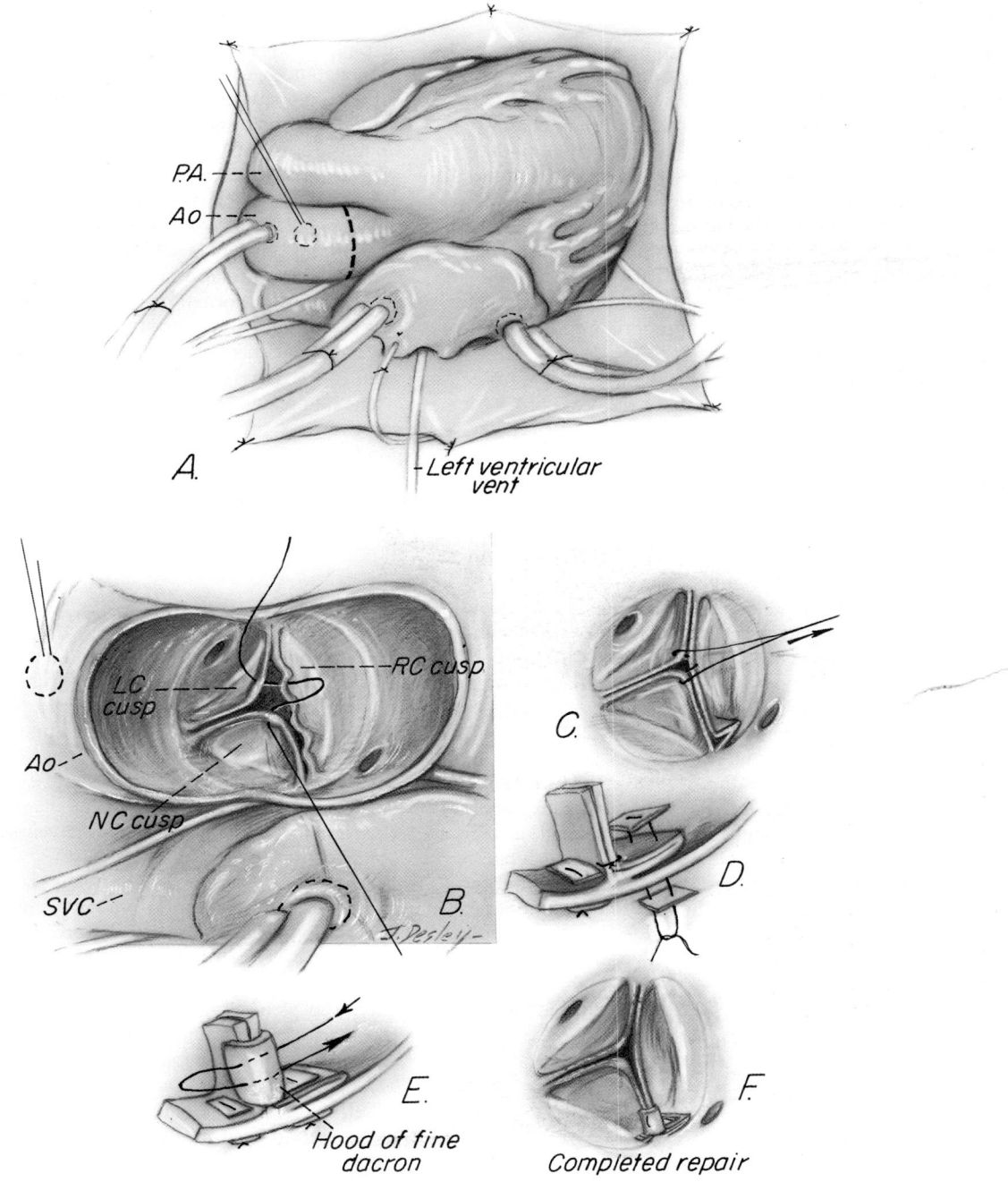

Figure 20-42 Repair of the prolapsed aortic valve cusp by Trusler's technique in patients with VSD and aortic incompetence.

(*a*) A transverse aortotomy incision is made at a level just downstream from the commissural attachments of the aortic valve.

(*b*) The Frater stitch of 5-0 polypropylene is placed through the midpoint of each cusp.

(*c*) Traction on this stitch allows identification of redundant or elongated free edges of a cusp, as shown here in the case of the right coronary cusp near its commissure with the noncoronary cusp.

(*d*) A 5-0 polypropylene stitch is placed between right and noncoronary cusps nearly at the aortic wall, thereby adjusting the length of each appropriately. The redundant portion of the right cusp is secured against the aortic wall with a pledgetted mattress stitch of 4-0 or 5-0 polypropylene, as has been done for the contiguous portion of the noncoronary cusp.

(*e*) A hood of fine Dacron cloth is sutured in place over the two cusps to further support the repair. Then the aortotomy is closed, and the Frater stitch is left and brought out between aortotomy closure stitches. This ensures aortic valve competence during further injections of cardioplegic solution and when the aortic clamp is released. The VSD is now repaired through a transverse right ventriculotomy incision. After this repair is completed, the aortic clamp is released, and the Frater stitch is removed after cardiac action resumes.

(*f*) The repair has been completed.

Ao, aorta; NC cusp, noncoronary cusp; PA, pulmonary artery; SVC, superior vena cava.

Modified from Trusler et al.[T4]

657

With the valve repair completed and the aorta closed, the right ventricle is opened through a transverse or vertical incision, depending on which cuts the fewest coronary arteries. Many surgeons recommend testing the competency of the repair at this stage by releasing the aortic clamp, but this maneuver is not usually necessary. Any infundibular stenosis is relieved by the excision of the trabecular muscle bands between the infundibular septum and the free wall of the right ventricle and, when necessary, the mobilization and excision of the parietal and septal extensions of the infundibular septum and portions of the moderator bands. The VSD is closed using the technique appropriate to the defect site, as described in Section I.

If the valve requires replacement, the right ventricle should be opened before valve insertion, the VSD repaired, the right ventricle closed, and then the aortic valve replacement inserted. This sequence is advised because occasionally it may be necessary to place the sutures from the prosthetic valve ring across the upper margin of the VSD patch where it extends between the base of the right and noncoronary leaflets (in the region normally occupied by the membranous septum). The sutures in this area should be securely buttressed with pledgets of Teflon felt. Although a freehand homograft has been used successfully for valve replacement under such circumstances,[G5] the degree of distortion of the aortic sinuses may make its placement difficult.[B10] At present, mechanical prostheses or bioprostheses are used (see Chapter 11, "Choice of the Replacement Device" in section on Special Situations and Controversies).

When there is also a true thin-walled aneurysm of the sinus of Valsalva at the base of the right aortic cusp and a VSD, the repair is more difficult, since the sinus must also be repaired. If the aortic valve requires excision and replacement, excision should include the base of the cusp and the thinned area of the sinus wall, which becomes continuous with the VSD and is incorporated in its closure. Again, under such circumstances, the prosthetic valve suture line will cross the Dacron patch. When the valve is suitable for plication, the base of the cusp is preserved and sutured back to the patch (see also Chapter 21).

RESULTS OF OPERATION

The *early* results of operation are good. Only one of the 76 patients operated on died in hospital (UAB and GLH; Table 20-21); there have been no instances of heart block and no recurrent VSDs.

The *late* results are influenced by the preoperative severity of the AI and the method of repair. When the AI is from cusp prolapse and is mild (or there is cusp prolapse without incompetence), closure of the VSD alone aborts progression of the incompetence or abolishes it.[C9,T6] Four of five patients treated in this manner have no murmur, and one has a grade 1/6 murmur (UAB). When the incompetence is moderate or severe, the operation is, not curative, but palliative. When the valve is suitable for reconstruction and a Trusler type repair is performed,[T4] the palliation is usually good,[M5] and Trusler and colleagues achieved such results in 12 of 13 children with cusp prolapse.[T4] Of 11 patients treated in this manner, 10 showed normal or decreased heart size after repair (UAB; 1967–1976). A diastolic murmur was present in all. Three patients have required reoperation and valve replacement (GLH-UAB).

The late results when the aortic incompetence was judged so severe as to require valve replacement have been less good. At UAB, one patient died of heart failure 6 years after the replacement. Dihiscence of the VSD repair required reoperation in two patients. Reoperation for replacement of a homograft was required in two patients.

INDICATIONS FOR OPERATION

When a child with a VSD first develops the murmur of aortic incompetence (AI), repair of the VSD should be promptly accomplished while the AI is still mild.[T6,T7] If cusp prolapse is demonstrated on the aortogram, without AI, in association with either a subpulmonary VSD or a perimembranous VSD, early repair is also indicated. Even if cusp prolapse has not occurred, a subpulmonary VSD of significant size should be closed before the patient is about 5 years old to prevent this complication.

When AI is moderate or severe and cusp prolapse is noted on the aortogram, operation should be undertaken promptly. Certainly, it should be done before the patient is 10 years old, since reconstruction of the valve is usually possible when operation is done in the first decade of life. Thereby, valve replacement is prevented or at least postponed. That this is true is suggested by the fact that at UAB the average age of the patients requiring replacement was 19.5 years, compared with 12.1 years for the remainder of the group. When the aortogram shows minimal enlargement of the sinuses and no cusp prolapse in the presence of severe AI, a bicuspid valve is probably present, and valve replacement may be required. Operation should therefore be postponed until significant symptoms develop or left ventricular enlargement itself indicates the need for operation (see Chapter 12, "Aortic Incompetence" in section on Indications for Operation).

REFERENCES

A

1. Andreasen AT, Watson F: Experimental cardiovascular surgery: 'The azygos factor.' *Br J Surg* 39:548, 1952.

2. Ash R: Natural history of ventricular septal defects in childhood lesions with predominant arteriovenous shunts. *J Pediatr* 64:45, 1964.

3. Auld PAM, Johnson AL, Gibbons JE, and McGregor M: Changes in pulmonary vascular resistance in infants and children with intracardiac left-to-right shunts. *Circulation* 27:257, 1963.

4. Aaron BL, Lower RR: Muscular ventricular septal defect repair made easy. *Ann Thorac Surg* 19:568, 1975.

5. Anderson RH, Lenox CC, Zuberbuhler JR: Morphology of ventricular septal defect associated with coarctation of aorta. *Br Heart J* 50:176, 1983.

6. Albus RA, Trusler GA, Izukawa T, Williams WG: Pulmonary artery banding. *J Thorac Cardiovasc Surg* 88:645, 1984.

7. Anderson RH, Lenox CC, Zuberbuhler JR: Morphology of ventricular septal defect associated with coarctation of aorta. *Br Heart J* 50:176, 1983.

B

1. Blackstone EH, Kirklin JW, Bradley EL, DuShane JW, Appelbaum A: Optimal age and results in repair of large ventricular septal defects. *J Thorac Cardiovasc Surg* 72:661, 1976.

2. Becu LM, Fontana RS, DuShane JW, Kirklin JW, Burchell HB, Edwards JE: Anatomic and pathologic studies in ventricular septal defect. *Circulation* 14:349, 1956.

3. Barratt-Boyes BG, Neutze JM, Clarkson PM, Shardey GC, Brandt PWT: Repair of ventricular septal defect in the first two years of life using profound hypothermia–circulatory arrest techniques. *Ann Surg* 184:376, 1976.

4. Berglund E: Ventricular Function. VI. Balance of left and right ventricular output: Relation between left and right atrial pressures. *Am J Physiol* 178:381, 1954.

5. Breckenridge IM, Stark J, Waterston DJ, Bonham-Carter RE: Multiple ventricular septal defects. *Ann Thorac Surg* 13:128, 1972.

6. Brandt PWT, Calder AL: Cardiac connections: The segmental approach to radiologic diagnosis in congenital heart disease. *Curr Probl Diag Radiol* 7:1, 1977.

7. Barratt-Boyes BG, Simpson M, Neutze JM: Intracardiac surgery in neonates and infants using deep hypothermia with surface cooling and limited cardiopulmonary bypass. *Circulation* 43(suppl I):I-25, 1971.

8. Braunwald E, Morrow AG: Left-ventriculo–right atrial communication: Diagnosis by clinical, hemodynamic, and angiographic methods. *Am J Med* 28:913, 1960.

9. Bargeron LM Jr, Elliott LP, Soto B, Beam PR, Curry GC: Axial cineangiography in congenital heart disease: Section 1. *Circulation* 56:1975, 1977.

10. Barratt-Boyes BG, Roche AHG, Whitlock RML: Six year review of the results of freehand aortic valve replacement using an antibiotic sterilized homograft valve. *Circulation* 55:353, 1977.

11. Binet JP, Conso JF, Langlois J, Pottemann M, Cloup M, Thibert M, Lucet P: Fermeture de certaines communications interventriculaires congénitales basses par le ventricule gauche. *Arch Mal Coeur* 63:1345, 1970.

12. Bharati S, McAllister HA Jr, Lev M: Straddling and displaced atrioventricular orifices and valves. *Circulation* 60:673, 1979.

13. Bergdahl LAL, Blackstone EH, Kirklin JW, Pacifico AD, Bargeron LM Jr: Determinants of early success in repair of aortic coarctation in infants. *J Thorac Cardiovasc Surg* 83:736, 1982.

14. Brandt PWT: Cineangiography of atrioventricular and ventriculoarterial connections, in MJ Godman (ed): *Pediatric Cardiology*, vol. 4. Edinburgh: Churchill Livingstone, 1980, p 191.

15. Bharati S, Lev M, Kirklin JW: *Cardiac Surgery and the Conduction System.* New York: John Wiley & Sons, 1983.

16. Beerman LB, Park SC, Fischer DR, Fricker FJ, Mathews RA, Neches WH, Lenox CC, Zuberbuhler JR: Ventricular septal defect associated with aneurysm of the membranous septum. *JACC* 5:118, 1985.

C

1. Cohen M, Lillehei CW: A quantitative study of the 'azygos factor' during vena caval occlusion in the dog. *Surg Gynecol Obstet* 98:225, 1954.

2. Clarkson PM, Frye RL, DuShane JW, Burchell HB, Wood EH, Weidman WH: Prognosis for patients with ventricular septal defect and severe pulmonary vascular obstructive disease. *Circulation* 38:129, 1968.

3. Cartmill TB, DuShane JW, McGoon DC, Kirklin JW: Results of repair of ventricular septal defect. *J Thorac Cardiovasc Surg* 52:486, 1966.

4. Cordell D, Graham TP Jr, Atwood GF, Boerth RC, Boucek RJ, Bender HW: Left heart volume characteristics following ventricular septal defect closure in infancy. *Circulation* 54:294, 1976.

5. Ching E, DuShane JW, McGoon DC, Danielson GK: Total correction of ventricular septal defect in infancy using extracorporeal circulation: Surgical considerations and results of operation. *Ann Thorac Surg* 12:1, 1971.

6. Cooley DA, Garrett HE, Howard HS: The surgical treatment of ventricular septal defect: An analysis of 300 consecutive surgical cases. *Prog Cardiovasc Dis* 4:312, 1962.

7. Civin WH, Edwards JE: Pathology of the pulmonary vascular tree. I. A comparison of the intrapulmonary arteries in Eisenmenger's complex and in stenosis of ostium infundibuli associated with biventricular origin of the aorta. *Circulation* 2:545, 1950.

8. Castaneda AR, Zamora R, Nicoloff DM, Moller JH, Hunt CE, Lucas RV: High-pressure, high-resistance ventricular septal defect: Surgical results of closure through right atrium. *Ann Thorac Surg* 12:29, 1971.

9. Chung KJ, Manning JA: Ventricular septal defect associated with aortic insufficiency: Medical and surgical management. *Am Heart J* 87:435, 1974.

10. Collins G, Calder L, Rose V, Kidd L, Keith J: Ventricular septal defect: Clinical and hemodynamic changes in the first five years of life. *Am Heart J* 84:695, 1972.

11. Clarkson PM: Growth following corrective cardiac operation in early infancy, in BG Barratt-Boyes, JM Neutze, EA Harris (eds): *Heart Disease in Infancy: Diagnosis and Surgical Treatment.* London: Churchill Livingstone, 1973, p 75.

12. Corone P, Doyan F, Gaudeau S, Guerin F, Vernant P, Ducam H, Rumeau-Rouquette C, Gaudeul P: Natural history of ventric-

ular septal defect: A study involving 790 cases. *Circulation* 55:908, 1977.

13. Campbell M: Natural history of ventricular septal defect. *Br Heart J* 33:246, 1971.

D

1. DuShane JW, Kirklin JW, Patrick RT, Donald DE, Terry HR Jr, Burchell HB, Wood EH: Ventricular septal defects with pulmonary hypertension: Surgical treatment by means of a mechanical pump-oxygenator. *JAMA* 160:950, 1956.

2. DuShane JW, Kirklin JW: Late results of the repair of ventricular septal defect in pulmonary vascular disease, in JW Kirklin (ed): *Advances in Cardiovascular Surgery.* New York: Grune & Stratton, 1973, p 9.

3. Dimich I, Steinfeld L, Litwak RS, Park S, Silvers N: Subpulmonic ventricular septal defect associated with aortic insufficiency. *Am J Cardiol* 32:325, 1973.

4. Downing JW, Kaplan S, Bove KE: Postsurgical left anterior hemiblock and right bundle branch block. *Br Heart J* 34:263, 1972.

5. Dammann JF Jr, Ferenze C: The significance of the pulmonary vascular bed in congenital heart disease. III. Defects between the ventricles or great vessels in which both increased pressure and blood flow may act upon the lungs, and in which there is a common ejectile force. *Am Heart J* 52:210, 1956.

6. Davis Z, McGoon DC, Danielson GK, Wallace RB: Removal of pulmonary artery band. *Is J Med Sci* 11:110, 1975.

7. Dirksen T, Moulaert AJ, Buis-Liem TN, Brom AG: Ventricular septal defect associated with left ventricular outflow tract obstruction below the defect. *J Thorac Cardiovasc Surg* 75:688, 1978.

E

1. Elliott LP, Bargeron LM Jr, Beam PR, Soto B, Curry GC: Axial cineangiography in congenital heart disease. II. Specific lesions. *Circulation* 56:1084, 1977.

2. Ellis H Jr, Ongley PA, Kirklin JW: Ventricular septal defect with aortic valvular incompetence. Surgical considerations. *Circulation* 27:789, 1963.

3. Edwards JE, Burchell HB: The pathologic anatomy of deficiencies between the aortic root and the heart including aortic sinus aneurysm. *Thorax* 12:125, 1957.

F

1. Friedman WF, Mehrizi A, Pusch AL: Multiple muscular ventricular septal defects. *Circulation* 32:35, 1965.

2. Freed MD, Rosenthal A, Plauth WH Jr, Nadas AS: Development of subaortic stenosis after pulmonary artery banding. *Circulation* 47,48(suppl 3):7, 1973.

3. Friedli B, Kidd BSL, Mustard WT, Keith JD: Ventricular septal defect with increased pulmonary vascular resistance: Late results of surgical closure. *Am J Cardiol* 33:403, 1974.

4. Freedom RM, Dische MR, Rowe RD: Pathologic anatomy of subaortic stenosis and atresia in the first year of life. *Am J Cardiol* 39:1035, 1977.

5. Fox KM, Patel RG, Graham RG, Taylor JFN, Stark J, de Leval MR, Macartney FJ: Multiple and single ventricular septal defect. A clinical and hemodynamic comparison. *Br Heart J* 40:141, 1978.

G

1. Girod DA, Hurwitz RA, King H, Jolly W: Recent results of two-stage surgical treatment of large ventricular septal defect. *Circulation* 49,50(suppl II):II-9, 1974.

2. Gasul BM, Dillon RF, Vrla V, Hait G: Ventricular septal defects: Their natural transformation into those with infundibular stenosis or into the cyanotic or non-cyanotic type of tetralogy of Fallot. *JAMA* 164:847, 1957.

3. Gelband H, Waldo AL, Kaiser GA, Bowman FO Jr, Malm JR, Hoffman BF: Etiology of right bundle-branch block in patients undergoing total correction of tetralogy of Fallot. *Circulation* 44:1022, 1971.

4. Gerbode F, Hultgren H, Melrose D, Osborn J: Syndrome of left ventricular–right atrial shunt: Successful surgical repair of defect in five cases, with observation of bradycardia on closure. *Ann Surg* 148:433, 1958.

5. Gonzalez-Lavin L, Barratt-Boyes BG: Surgical considerations of ventricular septal defect associated with aortic valve incompetence. *J Thorac Cardiovasc Surg* 57:422, 1969.

6. Garamella JJ, Cruz AB, Heupel WH, Dahl JC, Jensen NK, Berman R: Ventricular septal defect with aortic insufficiency: Successful surgical correction of both defects by the transaortic approach. *Am J Cardiol* 5:266, 1960.

7. Gersony WM, Hayes CJ: Bacterial endocarditis in patients with pulmonary stenosis, aortic stenosis, or ventricular septal defect. *Circulation* 56:84, 1977.

8. Griffiths SP, Turi GK, Ellis K, Krongrad E, Swift LH, Gersony WM, Bowman FO Jr, Malm JR: Muscular ventricular septal defects repaired with left ventriculotomy. *Am J Cardiol* 48:877, 1981.

H

1. Heath D, Edwards JE: The pathology of hypertensive pulmonary vascular disease: A description of six grades of structural changes in the pulmonary arteries with special reference to congenital cardiac septal defects. *Circulation* 18:533, 1958.

2. Heath D, Helmholz HF Jr, Burchell HB, DuShane JW, Edwards JE: Graded pulmonary vascular changes and hemodynamic findings in cases of atrial and ventricular septal defect and patent ductus arteriosus. *Circulation* 18:1155, 1958.

3. Hallidie-Smith KA, Hollman A, Cleland WP, Bentall HH, Goodwin JF: Effects of surgical closure of ventricular septal defects upon pulmonary vascular disease. *Br Heart J* 31:246, 1969.

4. Hunt CE, Formanek G, Levine MA, Castaneda A, Moller JH: Banding of the pulmonary artery: Results in 111 children. *Circulation* 43:395, 1971.

5. Henry J, Kaplan S, Helmsworth JA, Schreiber JT: Management of infants with large ventricular septal defects: Results with two-stage surgical treatment. *Ann Thorac Surg* 15:109, 1973.

6. Hoffman JIE, Rudolph AM: The natural history of ventricular septal defects in infancy. *Am J Cardiol* 16:634, 1965.

7. Hislop A, Haworth SG, Shinebourne EA, Reid L: Quantitative structural analysis of pulmonary vessels in isolated ventricular septal defects in infancy. *Br Heart J* 37:1014, 1975.

8. Hoffman JIE, Rudolph AM: Increasing pulmonary vascular resistance during infancy in association with ventricular septal defect. *Pediatrics* 38:220, 1966.

9. Hoffman JIE, Rudolph AM: The natural history of isolated ventricular septal defect, with special reference to selection of pa-

tients for surgery, in I Schulman (ed): *Advances in Pediatrics,* vol 17, 1970, p 57.

10. Hallidie-Smith KA, Edwards RE, Wilson R, Zeidifard E: Long-term cardiorespiratory assessment after surgical closure of ventricular septal defect in childhood. *Proc Br Cardiac Soc* 37:553, 1975 (abstr).

11. Hoffman JIE: Diagnosis and treatment of pulmonary vascular disease. *Birth Defects: Original Article Series* 8:9, 1972.

12. Hudspeth AS, Cordell AR, Meredith JH, Johnston FR: An improved transatrial approach to the closure of ventricular septal defects. *J Thorac Cardiovasc Surg* 43:157, 1962.

13. Hobbins SM, Izukawa T, Radford DJ, Williams WG, Trusler GA: Conduction disturbances after surgical correction of ventricular septal defect by the atrial approach. *Br Heart J* 41:289, 1979.

14. Ho SY, Milo S, Anderson RH, Macartney FJ, Goodwin A, Becker AE, Wenink ACG, Gerlis LM, Wilkinson JL: Straddling atrioventricular valve with absent atrioventricular connection. *Br Heart J* 47:344, 1982.

J

1. Jarmakani JMM, Graham TP Jr, Canent RV, Capp MP: The effect of corrective surgery on left heart volume and mass in children with ventricular septal defect. *Am J Cardiol* 27:254, 1971.

2. Jarmakani JM, Graham TP Jr, Canent RV Jr: Left ventricular contractile state in children with successfully corrected ventricular septal defect. *Circulation* 45,46(suppl I):I-102, 1971.

3. Johnson DC, Cartmill TB, Celermajer JM, Hawker RE, Stuckey DS, Bowdler JD, Overton J: Intracardiac repair of large ventricular septal defect in the first year of life. *Med J Aust* 2:193, 1974.

4. John S, Korula R, Jairaj PS, Muralidharan S, Ravikumar E, Babuthaman C, Sathyamoorthy I, Krishnaswamy S, Cherian G, Sukumar IP: Results of surgical treatment of ventricular septal defects with pulmonary hypertension. *Thorax* 38:279, 1983.

5. Juaneda E, Gittenberger de Groot A, Oppenheimer-Dekker A, Haworth SG: Pulmonary arterial development in infants with large perimembranous ventricular septal defects associated with overriding of the aortic valve. *Int J Cardiol* 7:223, 1985.

K

1. Kirklin JW, Harshbarger HG, Donald DE, Edwards JE: Surgical correction of ventricular septal defect: Anatomic and technical considerations. *J Thorac Surg* 33:45, 1957.

2. Kirklin JW, DuShane JW: Indications for repair of ventricular septal defects. *Am J Cardiol* 12:79, 1963.

3. Kirklin JW, McGoon DC, DuShane JW: Surgical treatment of ventricular septal defect. *Am J Cardiol* 12:79, 1963.

4. Kirklin JW, Silver AW: Technic of exposing the ductus arteriosus prior to establishing extracorporeal circulation. *Proc Mayo Clin* 33:423, 1958.

5. Keith JD, Rose V, Collins G, Kidd BSL: Ventricular septal defect: Incidence, morbidity, and mortality in various age groups. *Br Heart J* 33(suppl):81, 1971.

6. Kirklin JW, Appelbaum A, Bargeron LM Jr: Primary repair versus banding for ventricular septal defects in infants, in BSL Kidd, RD Rowe (eds): *The Child with Congenital Heart Disease after Surgery.* Mount Kisco, NY: Futura, 1976, p 3.

7. Keane JF, Fellows KE, Buckley L, Castaneda AR, Nadas AS: Ventricular septal defect with aortic regurgitation: A 33 year experience, in MJ Godman (ed): *World Congress of Paediatric Cardiology.* Edinburgh: Churchill Livingstone, 1981, p 292. (abstr).

8. Kawashima Y, Damno M, Shimizer Y, Matsuda H, Miyamoto T, Fujita T, Kozyka T, Manabe H: Ventricular septal defect associated wth aortic insufficiency. *Circulation* 47:1057, 1973.

9. Keck EWO, Ongley PA, Kincaid OW, Swan HJC: Ventricular septal defect with aortic insufficiency: A clinical and hemodynamic study of 18 proved cases. *Circulation* 27:203, 1963.

10. Kulbertus HE, Coyne JJ, Hallidie-Smith KA: Conduction disturbances before and after surgical closure of ventricular septal defect. *Am Heart J* 77:123, 1969.

11. Krongrad E, Hefler SE, Bowman FO Jr, Malm JR, Hoffman BF: Further observations on the etiology of the right bundle branch block pattern following right ventriculotomy. *Circulation* 50:1105, 1974.

12. Kirklin JW, DuShane JW: Repair of ventricular septal defect in infancy. *Pediatrics* 27:961, 1961.

13. Kirklin JK, Castaneda AR, Keane JF, Fellows KE, Norwood WI: Surgical management of multiple ventricular septal defects. *J Thorac Cardiovasc Surg* 80:458, 1980.

14. Kurosawa H, Becker AE: Modification of the precise relationship of the atrioventricular conduction bundle to the margins of the ventricular septal defects by the trabecula septomarginalis. *J Thorac Cardiovasc Surg* 87:605, 1984.

L

1. Lillehei CW, Cohen M, Warden HE, Ziegler NR, Varco RL: The results of direct vision closure of ventricular septal defects in eight patients by means of controlled cross circulation. *Surg Gynecol Obstet* 101:446, 1955.

2. Lucas RV Jr, Adams P Jr, Anderson RC, Meyne NG, Lillehei CW, Varco RL: The natural history of isolated ventricular septal defect: A serial physiologic study. *Circulation* 24:1372, 1961.

3. Lev M: The architecture of the conduction system in congenital heart disease. III. Ventricular septal defect. *Arch Pathol* 70:529, 1960.

4. Lillehei CW, Anderson RC, Eliot RS, Wang Y, Ferlic RM: Pre- and postoperative cardiac catheterization in 200 patients undergoing closure of ventricular septal defects. *Surgery* 63:69, 1968.

5. Liberthson RR, Paul MH, Muster AJ, Arcilla RA, Eckner FAO, Lev M: Straddling and displaced atrioventricular orifices and valves with primitive ventricles. *Circulation* 43:213, 1971.

6. Laubry C, Pezzi C: Traité des maladies Carpentales du Cocur, in Laubry C, Routier D, Soulie P: Les soufflés de (a maladie de Roger). *Rev Med Paris* 50:439, 1933.

7. Lincoln C, Jamieson S, Joseph M, Shinebourne E, Anderson RH: Transatrial repair of ventricular septal defects with reference to their anatomic classification. *J Thorac Cardiovasc Surg* 74:183, 1977.

8. Lauer RM, DuShane JW, Edwards JE: Obstruction of left ventricular outlet in association with ventricular septal defect. *Circulation* 22:110, 1960.

9. Lue HC, Shen CT, Wang NK, Wu JR, Chu SH, Hung CR: Ventricular septal defect and coronary cusp prolapse: An assessment of some special features in Chinese, in MJ Godman (ed): *World Congress of Paediatric Cardiology.* Edinburgh: Churchill Livingstone, 1981, p 291 (abstr).

M

1. Mason DT, Spann JF Jr, Zelis R, Amsterdam EA: Comparison of the contractile state of the normal, hypertrophied, and failing

heart in man, in N Alpert (ed): *Cardiac Hypertrophy.* New York: Academic, 1971, p 433.

2. Maron BJ, Redwood DR, Hirschfeld JW Jr, Goldstein RE, Morrow AG, Epstein SE: Postoperative assessment of patients with ventricular septal defect and pulmonary hypertension: Response to intense upright exercise. *Circulation* 48:864, 1973.

3. Muller WH Jr, Dammann JF Jr: The treatment of certain congenital malformations of the heart by the creation of pulmonic stenosis to reduce pulmonary hypertension and excessive pulmonary blood flow: A preliminary report. *Surg Gynecol Obstet* 95:213, 1952.

4. Menahem S, Venables AW: Pulmonary artery banding in isolated or complicated ventricular septal defects: Results and effects on growth. Br Heart J 34:87, 1972.

5. Moreno-Cabral RJ, Mamiya RT, Nakamura FF, Brainard SC, McNamara JJ: Ventricular septal defect and aortic insufficiency: Surgical treatment. *J Thorac Cardiovasc Surg* 73:358, 1977.

6. Moulaert AJ, Bruins CG, Oppenheimer-Dekker A: Anomalies of the aortic arch and ventricular septal defects. *Circulation* 53:1011, 1976.

7. Milo S, Ho SY, Macartney FJ, Wilkinson JL, Becker AE, Wenink ACG, deGroot ACG, Anderson RH: Straddling and overriding atrioventricular valves: Morphology and classification. *Am J Cardiol* 44:112, 1979.

8. McNicholas K, Stratford M, Hayes C, Gersony W, Ellis K, Bowman F, Malm J: Management of the infant with ventricular septal defect and coarctation of the aorta, in MJ Godman (ed): *World Congress of Paediatric Cardiology.* Edinburgh: Churchill Livingstone, 1981, p 127 (abstr).

9. Momma K, Toyama K, Takao A, Ando M, Nakazawa M, Hirosawa K, Imai Y: Natural history of subarterial infundibular ventricular septal defect. *Am Heart J* 108:1312, 1984.

N

1. Nadas AS, Thilenius OG, LaFarge CG, Hauck AJ: Ventricular septal defect with aortic regurgitation: Medical and pathologic aspects. *Circulation* 29:862, 1964.

2. Neches WH, Park SC, Lenox CC, Zuberbuhler JR, Siewers RD, Hardesty RL: Coarctation of the aorta with ventricular septal defect. *Circulation* 55:189, 1977.

3. Neufeld HN, Titus JL, DuShane JW, Burchell HB, Edwards JE: Isolated ventricular septal defect of the persistent common atrioventricular canal type. *Circulation* 23:685, 1961.

4. Nanton MA, Belcourt CL, Gillis DA, Krause VW, Roy DL: Left ventricular outflow tract obstruction owing to accessory endocardial cushion tissue. *J Thorac Cardiovasc Surg* 78:537, 1979.

O

1. Oldham HN Jr, Kakos GS, Jarmakani MM, Sabiston DC Jr: Pulmonary artery banding in infants with complex congenital heart defects. *Ann Thorac Surg* 13:342, 1971.

2. Okamoto Y: Clinical studies for open heart surgery in infants with profound hypothermia. *Arch Jpn Chir* 38:188, 1969.

3. Okoroma EO, Guller B, Maloney JD, Weidman WH: Etiology of right bundle-branch block pattern after surgical closure of ventricular septal defect. *Am Heart J* 90:14, 1975.

4. Oh KS, Park SC, Galvis AG, Young LW, Neches WH, Zuberbuhler JR: Pulmonary hyperinflation in ventricular septal defect. *J Thorac Cardiovasc Surg* 76:706, 1978.

P

1. Patel RG, Ihenacho HNC, Abrams LD, Astley R, Parsons CG, Roberts KD, Singh SP: Pulmonary artery banding and subsequent repair in ventricular septal defect. *Br Heart J* 35:651, 1973.

2. Perry EL, Burchell HB, Edwards JE: Congenital communication between the left ventricle and the right atrium: Co-existing ventricular septal defect and double tricuspid orifice. *Proc Staff Meet Mayo Clin* 24:198, 1949.

3. Plauth NH Jr, Braunwald E, Rockoff SD, Mason DT, Morrow AG: Ventricular septal defect and aortic regurgitation: Clinical, hemodynamic and surgical considerations. *Am J Med* 39:552, 1965.

4. Pacifico AD, Soto B, Bargeron LM Jr: Surgical treatment of straddling tricuspid valves. *Circulation* 60:655, 1979.

R

1. Rein JG, Freed MD, Norwood WI, Castaneda AR: Early and late results of closure of ventricular septal defect in infancy. *Ann Thorac Surg* 24:19, 1977.

2. Rastelli GC, Ongley PA, Titus JL: Ventricular septal defect of atrioventricular canal type with straddling right atrioventricular valve and mitral valve deformity. *Circulation* 37:816, 1968.

3. Rowe RD, Vlad P: Diagnostic problems in the newborn: Origins of mortality in congenital cardiac malformations, in BG Barratt-Boyes, JM Neutze, EA Harris (eds): *Heart Disease in Infancy: Diagnosis and Surgical Treatment.* London: Churchill Livingstone, 1973, p 3.

4. Rowe RD: Angiocardiography in the prognosis for young infants in congestive failure with ventricular septal defect: The value of defect/ascending aorta diameter ratio, in BG Barratt-Boyes, JM Neutze, EA Harris (eds): *Heart Disease in Infancy: Diagnosis and Surgical Treatment.* London: Churchill Livingstone, 1973, p 119.

5. Rizzoli G, Blackstone EH, Kirklin JW, Pacifico AD, Bargeron LM Jr: Incremental risk factors in hospital mortality after repair of ventricular septal defect. *J Thorac Cardiovasc Surg* 80:494, 1980.

6. Rabinovitch M, Keane JF, Norwood WI, Castaneda AR, Reid L: Vascular structure in lung tissue obtained at biopsy correlated with pulmonary hemodynamic findings after repair of congenital heart defects. *Circulation* 69:655, 1984.

7. Rizzoli G, Rubino M, Mazzucco A, Rocco F, Bellini P, Brumana T, Scutari M, Valfre C, Gallucci V: Progress in the surgical treatment of ventricular septal defect: An analysis of a twelve years' experience. *Thorac Cardiovasc Surg* 31:382, 1983.

S

1. Savard M, Swan JHC, Kirklin JW, Wood EH: Hemodynamic alterations associated with ventricular septal defects, in *Congenital Heart Disease.* Washington, DC: American Association for the Advancement of Science, 1960, p 141.

2. Sigmann JM, Stern AM, Sloan HE: Early surgical correction of large ventricular septal defects. *Pediatrics* 39:4, 1967.

3. Stark J, Tynan M, Aberdeen E, Waterston DJ, Bonham-Carter RE, Graham GR, Somerville J: Repair of intracardiac defects after previous constriction (banding) of the pulmonary artery. *Surgery* 67:536, 1970.

4. Subramanian S, Wagner HR: Pulmonary artery banding and debanding in patients with ventricular septal defect, in BG Barratt-Boyes, JM Neutze, EA Harris (eds): *Heart Disease in In-*

fancy: Diagnosis and Surgical Treatment. London: Churchill Livingstone, 1973, p 141.

5. Stark J, Hucin B, Aberdeen E, Waterston DJ: Cardiac surgery in the first year of life: Experience with 1,049 operations. *Surgery* 69:483, 1971.

6. Stirling GR, Stanley PH, Lillehei CW: Effect of cardiac bypass and ventriculotomy upon right ventricular function. *Surgical Forum* 8:433, 1957.

7. Shah P, Singh WSA, Rose V, Keith JD: Incidence of bacterial endocarditis in ventricular septal defects. *Circulation* 34:127, 1966.

8. Stahlman M, Kaplan S, Helmsworth JA, Clark LC, Scott HW Jr: Syndrome of left ventricular–right atrial shunt resulting from high inter-ventricular septal defect associated with defective leaflet of the tricuspid valve. *Circulation* 12:813, 1955.

9. Spencer FC, Doyle EF, Danilowicz DA, Bahnson HT, Weldon CS: Long-term evaluation of aortic valvuloplasty for aortic insufficiency and ventricular septal defect. *J Thorac Cardiovasc Surg* 65:15, 1973.

10. Steeg CN, Krongrad E, Davachi F, Bowman FO Jr, Malm JR, Gersony WM: Postoperative left anterior hemiblock and right bundle branch block following repair of tetralogy of Fallot: Clinical and etiological considerations. *Circulation* 51:1026, 1975.

11. Sung RJ, Tamer DM, Garcia OL, Castellanos A, Myerburg RJ, Gelband H: Analysis of surgically induced right bundle branch block pattern using intracardiac recording techniques. *Circulation* 54:442, 1976.

12. Starr A, Menasche V, Dotter D: Surgical correction of aortic insufficiency associated with ventricular septal defect. *Surg Gynecol Obstet* 111:71, 1960.

13. Soto B, Becker AE, Moulaert AH, Lie JT, Anderson RH: Classification of ventricular septal defects. *Br Heart J* 43:332, 1980.

14. Singh AK, de Leval MR, Stark J: Left ventriculotomy for closure of muscular ventricular septal defects. *Ann Surg* 186:577, 1977.

15. Sandrasagra FA, Hamilton DI, Wilkinson JL: Surgery of VSD in Infancy, in MJ Godman (ed): *World Congress of Paediatric Cardiology.* Edinburgh: Churchill Livingstone, 1981, p 289 (abstr).

16. Sigmann JM, Perry BL, Behrendt DM, Stern AM, Kirsh MM, Sloan HE: Ventricular septal defect: Results after repair in infancy. *Am J Cardiol* 39:66, 1977.

17. Somerville J: (1980) Personal communication.

18. Stevenson JG, Kawabori I, Stamm SJ, Bailey WW, Hall DG, Mansfield PB, Rittenhouse EA: Pulsed Doppler echocardiograph evaluation of ventricular septal defect patches. *Circulation* 70 (suppl I):I-38, 1984.

19. Sutherland GR, Godman MJ, Keeton BR, Shore DF, Bain HH, Hunter S: Natural history of perimembranous ventricular septal defects: a prospective echocardiographic haemodynamic correlative study. *Br Heart J* 51:682, 1984.

T

1. Theye RA, Kirklin JW: Physiologic studies early after repair of tetralogy of Fallot. *Circulation* 28:42, 1963.

2. Trusler GA, Mustard WT: A method of banding the pulmonary artery for large isolated ventricular septal defect with and without transposition of the great arteries. *Ann Thorac Surg* 13:351, 1972.

3. Tatooles CJ, Miller RA: Palliative surgery in infants with congenital heart disease. *Prog Cardiovasc Dis* 15:331, 1973.

4. Trusler GA, Moes CAF, Kidd BSL: Repair of ventricular septal defect with aortic insufficiency. *J Thorac Cardiovasc Surg* 66:394, 1973.

5. Tatsuno K, Konno S, Sakakibara S: Ventricular septal defect with aortic insufficiency: Angiocardiographic aspects and a new classification. *Am Heart J* 85:13, 1973.

6. Tatsuno K, Konno S, Ando M, Sakakibara S: Pathogenetic mechanisms of prolapsing aortic valve and aortic regurgitation associated with ventricular septal defect. *Circulation* 48:1028, 1973.

7. Tatsuno K, Ando M, Takao A, Hatsune K, Konno S: Diagnostic importance of aortography in conal ventricular septal defect. *Am Heart J* 89:171, 1975.

8. Truex RC: The sinoatrial node and its connections with the atrial tissues, in HJJ Wellens, KI Lie, MJ Janse (eds): *The Conduction System of the Heart.* Philadelphia: Lea & Febiger, 1976, p 209.

9. Tabry IF, McGoon DC, Danielson GK, Wallace RB, Tajik AJ, Seward JB: Surgical management of straddling valve. *J Thorac Cardiovasc Surg* 77:191, 1979.

10. Tiraboschi R, Villani M, Bianchi T, Locatelli G, Vanini V, Crupi G, Parenzan L: Trattamento chirurgico del difetto interventricolare associato a coartazione aortica. *G Ital Cardiol* 8:811, 1978.

11. Tiraboschi R, Alfieri O, Carpentier A, Parenzan L: One stage correction of coarctation of the aorta associated with intracardiac defects in infancy. *J Cardiovasc Surg* 19:11, 1978.

V

1. Van Praagh R, McNamara JJ: Anatomic types of ventricular septal defect with aortic insufficiency: Diagnostic and surgical considerations. *Am Heart J* 75:604, 1968.

2. Van Praagh R, Bernhard WF, Rosenthal A, Parisi LF, Fyler DC: Interrupted aortic arch: Surgical treatment. *Am J Cardiol* 27:200, 1971.

3. Vogel M, Freedom RM, Brand A, Trusler GA, Williams WG, Rowe RD: Ventricular septal defect and subaortic stenosis: An analysis of 41 patients. *Am J Cardiol* 52:1258, 1983.

4. Vincent RN, Lang P, Chipman CW, Castaneda AR: Assessment of hemodynamic status in the Intensive Care Unit immediately after closure of ventricular septal defect. *Am J Cardiol* 55:526, 1985.

W

1. Warden HE, Cohen M, Read RC, Lillehei CW: Controlled cross circulation for open intracardiac surgery. *J Thorac Surg* 28:331, 1954.

2. Wagenvoort CA, Neufeld HN, DuShane JW, Edwards JE: The pulmonary arterial tree in ventricular septal defect: A quantitative study of anatomic features in fetuses, infants, and children. *Circulation* 23:740, 1961.

3. Wagenvoort CA, Wagenvoort N: Primary pulmonary hypertension: A pathological study of the lung vessels in 156 clinically diagnosed cases. *Circulation* 42:1163, 1970.

4. Wolff GS, Rowland TW, Ellison RC: Surgically induced right bundle branch block with left anterior hemiblock: An ominous sign in postoperative tetralogy of Fallot. *Circulation* 46:587, 1972.

5. Wood EH: Use of indicator-dilution technics, in *Congenital Heart Disease.* Washington, DC: American Association for the Advancement of Science, 1960, pp 209–240.

Y

1. Yamaki S, Tezuka F: Quantitative analysis of pulmonary vascular disease in complete transposition of the great arteries. *Circulation* 54:805, 1976.
2. Yacoub MH, Radley-Smith R, deGasperis C: Primary repair of large ventricular septal defects in the first year of life. *G Ital Cardiol* 8:827, 1978.
3. Yeager SB, Freed MD, Keane JF, Norwood WI, Castaneda AR: Primary surgical closure of ventricular septal defect in the first year of life: Results in 128 infants. *JACC* 3:1269, 1984.

Z

1. Ziady GM, Hallidie-Smith KA, Goodwin JF: Conduction disturbances after surgical closure of ventricular septal defect. *Br Heart J* 34:1199, 1972.

21

CONGENITAL ANEURYSMS OF THE SINUS OF VALSALVA

DEFINITION

Congenital aneurysms of the sinuses of Valsalva are thin-walled, tubular, and narrow outpouchings, nearly always in the right sinus or adjacent half of the noncoronary sinus, with an entirely intracardiac course, that frequently rupture into the right heart chambers to form an aortocardiac fistula. Associated congenital cardiac defects are common, but apart from bacterial endocarditis, acquired heart disease is rare.

HISTORICAL NOTE

The syndrome of acute rupture of a congenital sinus of Valsalva aneurysm was apparently first described by Hope in 1839.[H3] A year later, Thurman[T2] published the first important paper on the subject. He discussed Hope's case and added five of his own, none of which had ruptured. Eighty years later, Abbott redescribed the clinical features of acute rupture and reported one such case, together with a description of the eight previously reported cases.[A2] In these earlier years,[S4] and even as late as 1937,[S5] the majority of ruptured and unruptured sinus of Valsalva aneurysms were considered syphilitic. Smith stated in 1914 that "the lesion which is usually syphilitic is not so rare as to be altogether devoid of clinical interest, but the diagnosis, perforating or otherwise, presents almost insurmountable difficulties."[S13] Jones and Langley reviewed the subject of congenital and acquired aneurysm in 1949.[J1] They accepted 25 cases as being of con-

genital origin and were able to enunciate most of the important features of the condition. Venning in 1951[V1] was possibly the first to diagnose acute rupture during life, although Oram and East claimed this distinction in 1955[O2] (as did Brown and associates[B4]). In the cases of Oram and East, cardiac catheterization confirmed the presence of a left-to-right shunt, although angiography was not performed. The earliest report of the use of aortography in diagnosis (of an unruptured aneurysm) is that of Falholt and Thomsen in 1953.[F1]

The first successful surgical repairs done with cardiopulmonary bypass (CPB) by us were in 1956 at the Mayo Clinic,[B1,M7] and Lillehei and Varco, at the University of Minnesota, carried out successful repairs that same year.[L1] Bahnson[S10] and Cooley[M2] also reported early successful cases. In 1957, both Morrow[M1] and Bigelow[B3] closed a ruptured congenital sinus aneurysm successfully using mild hypothermia with inflow stasis, but this technique was not used subsequently. There followed numerous reports of one or two successfully repaired patients using CPB, but in 1962 Dubost reported eight cases,[D2] and in 1963 Sellors reported six.[B2] A collective review in 1969 by Keiffer and Winchell[K2] reported 78 surgical and nonsurgical cases, in 59 of which the sinus aneurysm had ruptured into a cardiac chamber. Sakakibara and Konno noted the frequency of this lesion in Japan and its association with VSD and aortic incompetence, and were among the first to provide a comprehensive classification.[S1,S2,S3] Their first patient was repaired in 1960.[S14]

MORPHOLOGY

Morphology of the Aneurysm

The basic congenital lesion in congenital aneurysms of the sinuses of Valsalva is a thinning of the wall of the aortic sinus just above the anulus at the leaflet hinge.[E1] This thinning is believed to be a result of the absence of normal elastic and muscular tissue.[E3,V1] Such a finding is not uncommon in patients operated on for the combined lesions of ventricular septal defect (VSD) and aortic incompetence (AI) (see Chapter 20, Section 2) and no doubt does not always lead to aneurysm or fistula formation (see Chapter 20, "Natural History," in Section 2).

This weak area gradually gives way under aortic pressure to form an aneurysm resembling a wind sock, which ultimately ruptures into an adjacent low-pressure cardiac chamber (usually the right ventricle (Fig. 21-1) or right atrium). The thin-walled aneurysm characteristically has an intracardiac fistulous portion and a nipplelike projection into the cardiac chamber with one or more points of rupture at its apex (Fig. 21-2); rarely does it project outside the aortic root or heart. In about one-quarter of the patients, there is no wind-sock or any other suggestion of aneurysm formation but, rather, a direct fistulous communication between the aortic sinus and the heart.[N1] A typical wind-sock deformity may be more common in lesions originating from the right sinus and communicating with the right ventricle and a direct fistula more common in noncoronary sinus–to–right atrial lesions.[B1] In the rare instances of origin from the left sinus,[E4] there may be an obvious extracardiac aneurysm,[K1,K2,N1,S10] an exception to the usual situation in congenital sinus aneurysms. All of the surgical cases seen by us earlier at the Mayo Clinic, and throughout at UAB and GLH, have had an aneurysm, but a direct fistula has been present in those few examples in which the condition was recognized at birth or soon afterward.[D2,K2,P1]

The sinus origin of the aneurysm is the main determinant of the direction of protrusion and rupture of the aneurysm and thus of the chamber into which the aneurysm ruptures (Fig. 21-3; Tables 21-1, 21-2). Those aneurysms arising from the right sinus are the commonest,[G2,K2,J1,N1,O2,S8] and they

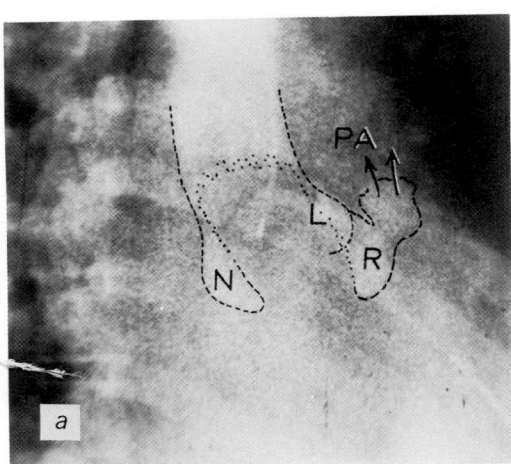

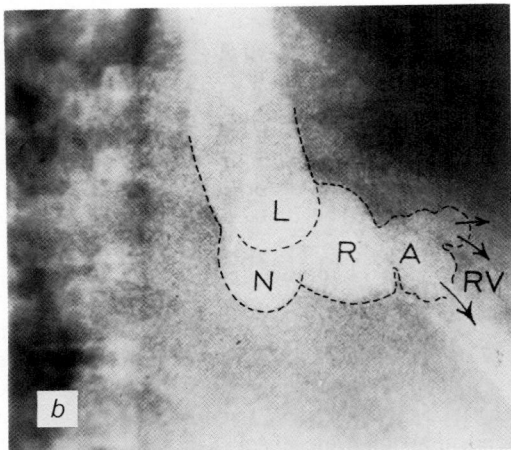

Figure 21-1 Cineangiograms in the right anterior oblique (RAO) projection of a patient with a right sinus of Valsalva aneurysm ruptured into the right ventricle (GLH); (a) is in systole and (b) in diastole. The noncoronary and left coronary sinuses and leaflets are normal. The right coronary sinus is enlarged, and there is a mobile wind-sock aneurysm protruding into the right ventricular infundibulum. The arrows indicate contrast medium shunting through holes in the aneurysm filling the right ventricular infundibulum in diastole and the main pulmonary artery in systole (when the aneurysm almost prolapses through the pulmonary valve). There is no aortic regurgitation, but the ruptured aneurysm is associated with a large perimembranous ventricular septal defect.

A, aneurysm; L, left coronary sinus; N, noncoronary sinus; PA, pulmonary artery; R, right coronary sinus; RV, right ventricular infundibulum.

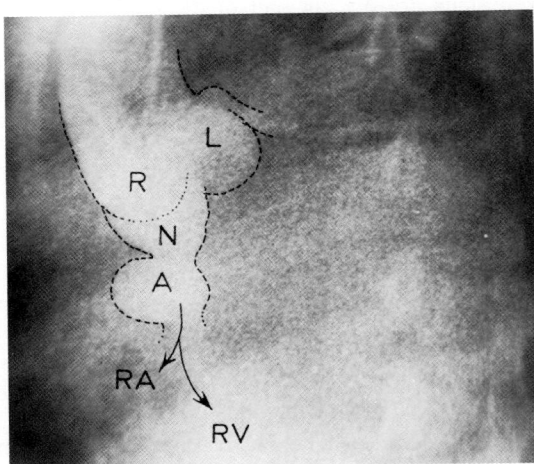

Figure 21-2 Cineangiogram in left anterior oblique (LAO) projection of a patient with an aneurysm and a fistula arising from the noncoronary sinus of Valsalva and rupturing into the right atrium (GLH). The aneurysm fills from the nadir of the noncoronary sinus. There is shunting of contrast medium to the right atrium, through the tricuspid valve, and to the right ventricle. The right and left coronary sinuses appear normal. There is no aortic regurgitation and no ventricular septal defect.

A, aneurysm; L, left coronary sinus; N, noncoronary sinus; R, right coronary sinus; RA, right atrium; RV, right ventricle.

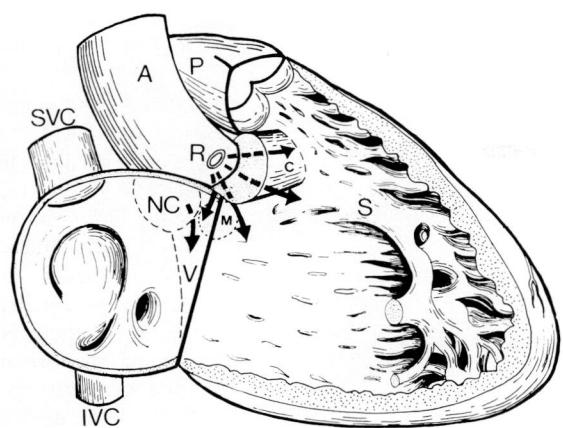

Figure 21-3 Diagrammatic representation of the structures depicted in a right anterior oblique (RAO) view of the heart. The arrows indicate the common sites of rupture of sinus of Valsalva aneurysms.

A, aorta; C, conal (infundibular) septum; IVC, inferior vena cava; M, membranous septum; NC, noncoronary sinus; P, pulmonary artery; R, right coronary sinus; S, septal band; SVC, superior vena cava; V, atrioventricular septum.

Table 21-2 Incidence of VSD and morphology of aneurysms of sinus of Valsalva in surgically treated patients (GLH; 1957–1980; $n = 10$ and UAB; 1967–1980; $n = 19$)

| | | Morphology of Sinus of Valsalva Aneurysm | | | |
| | | RCS → RV | | NCS → RA | |
VSD	n	No.	% of n	No.	% of n
Yes	17	15[a]	88%	2[b]	12%
No	12	5	42%	7	58%
Total	29	20	69%	9	31%

KEY: NCS → RA, noncoronary sinus aneurysm extending into right atrium; RCS → RV, right coronary sinus aneurysm extending into right ventricle; VSD, ventricular septal defect.

[a]One 26-year-old patient had rupture into the pulmonary artery rather than the right ventricle; he had also a mildly incompetent tricuspid aortic valve.

[b]Ruptured into the right ventricle rather than the right atrium.

usually arise from the left portion of the sinus, with the wind sock projecting into the adjacent outflow tract of the right ventricle just below the pulmonary valve.[S3] (This was termed *type I* by Sakakibera and Konno.[S3]) Uncommonly, the aneurysm originates more centrally from the right sinus and projects through the substance of the infundibular septum (Fig. 21-4), or it arises from the right portion of the right sinus and enters the right ventricle beneath the parietal band (parietal extension of the infundibular septum) in the region of the membranous ventricular septum. Aneurysms from the noncoronary sinus (Fig. 21-2) usually originate from its anterior portion and project into the right atrium (Fig. 21-5), but rarely they project and rupture into the right ventricle (Table 21-1). Rarely, rupture can occur simultaneously into both the right ventricle and the right atrium or into the muscular ventricular septum.[G1] Sinus of Valsalva aneurysms rupturing into areas adjacent to the tricuspid valve are also adjacent to the atrioventricular node and bundle and may be a cause of heart block[T1] or right bundle-branch block. Rarely, a right sinus aneurysm or noncoronary sinus aneurysm extends into

the left ventricle,[H4,S12,W2] and rarely an aneurysm has diffuse origin involving the whole of one sinus. Very rarely, aneurysms arise from the left coronary sinus or from the posterior portion of the noncoronary sinus, with rupture from these sites into the adjacent pericardium and left atrium.

Acquired aneurysms of the aortic sinuses of Valsalva (due to medionecrosis,[D3] syphilis,[S13] atherosclerosis,[D1] endocarditis,[S7] or penetrating injuries[M2]) are usually readily distinguishable from the congenital forms, which are the subject of this chapter, because they are more diffuse, involving more of the sinus or multiple sinuses and often the ascending aorta, and projecting therefore into the pericardium outside the heart. In fact, a congenital aneurysm is frequently diagnosed by exclusion of any other etiology as well as by the presence of its typically associated congenital cardiac lesions. Difficulties arise with mycotic aneurysms,[J1,V1] for endocarditis complicates about 5%–10% of congenital aneurysms,[N1] and with medionecrosis, for Marfan's syndrome and medionecrosis both occur in some patients with congenital sinus of Valsalva aneurysms.[A1,M3]

Associated Cardiac Anomalies

Associated congenital cardiac defects are present in the majority of patients. The most common—and seemingly part of the spectrum of sinus of Valsalva aneurysms—are ventricu-

Table 21-1 Ruptured congenital sinus of Valsalva aneurysms.[N1]

| | Termination | | | | | | | | | | | | | | |
| | RV | | RA | | RV + RA | | LV | | LA | | PA | | Pericardium | | Total | | |
Origin	n	% of n	n	% of n	n	% of n	n	% of n	n	% of n	n	% of n	n	% of n	n	% of 119	CL
RCS ($n = 80$)	57	71%	16	20%	2	3%	3	4%	0		1	1%	1	1%	80	67%	62%–72%
NCS ($n = 30$)	7	23%	21	70%	0		1	3%	1	3%	0		0		30	25%	21%–30%
LCS ($n = 9$)	3	33%	4	44%	0		1	11%	1	11%	0		0		9	8%	5%–11%
Total	67		41		2		5		2		1		1		119		

KEY: CL, 70% confidence limits; LA, left atrium; LCS, left coronary sinus; LV, left ventricle; NCS, noncoronary sinus; PA, pulmonary artery; RA, right atrium; RCS, right coronary sinus; RV, right ventricle.

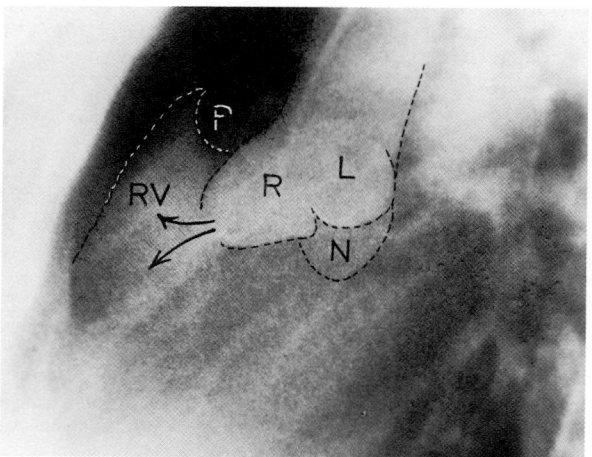

Figure 21-4 Cineangiogram in diastole (lateral projection) of a patient with an aneurysm of the right coronary sinus that protrudes into a right ventricular infundibulum filled by contrast medium shunting through the ruptured aneurysm (GLH). The pulmonary valve is still closed. The left coronary and noncoronary sinuses appear normal. There is no aortic regurgitation. At operation, this aneurysm arose from the center of the right sinus, with a prominent wind-sock aneurysm of the infundibular septum; immediately beneath it was a moderately sized ventricular septal defect.

L, left coronary sinus; N, noncoronary sinus; P, pulmonary valve; R, right coronary sinus; RV, right ventricular infundibulum.

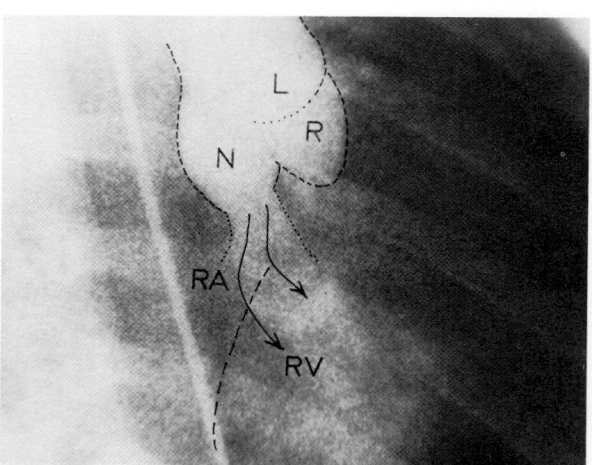

Figure 21-5 Cineangiogram in the right anterior oblique (RAO) projection (diastole) of a patient with a large aneurysmal connection of the noncoronary sinus to the right atrium (GLH). The contrast flow (arrows) was observed to enter the right atrium close to the tricuspid ring (dashed line) before passing through the tricuspid valve to right ventricle. The right and left coronary sinuses appear normal. There is no aortic regurgitation and no ventricular septal defect. At operation there was a 15-mm long wind-sock aneurysm projecting into the RA adjacent to the anteroseptal commissure of the tricuspid valve.

L, left coronary sinus; N, noncoronary sinus; R, right coronary sinus; RA, right atrium; RV, right ventricle.

lar septal defects (VSDs) aortic valve anomalies, and pulmonary stenoses. Less common associated malformations are coarctation of the aorta, patent ductus arteriosus, atrial septal defect, subaortic stenosis, and tetralogy of Fallot.

Ventricular Septal Defects

Ventricular septal defects occur in 30%–50% of reported patients with congenital sinus of Valsalva aneurysms,[N1,O1,S2,S3] but the incidence may be a little higher in patients treated surgically (Table 21-2). The proportion of patients with VSDs is higher when the aneurysm arises from the right sinus (Table 22-2). When the aneurysm arises from the left one-third of the right aortic sinus, the VSD is subaortic and is commonly immediately subpulmonary, with its upper margin formed by the confluent aortic and pulmonary valve rings. The VSD may lie within the substance of the muscle of the infundibular septum when it is associated with an aneurysm arising from the central third of the right sinus. When the aneurysm arises from the right third of the right sinus (or very rarely in the anterior portion of the noncoronary sinus),[E1,S2] the VSD is usually perimembranous in position.

As has been pointed out, the essential defect leading to the development of a congenital sinus of Valsalva aneurysm is deficiency of the aortic media immediately above the aortic anulus. When a VSD is also present, there is a similar absence of muscle below the aortic anulus. It is therefore to be expected that the two lesions will usually be sited in the manner described above. However, on rare occasions, a perimembranous VSD can occur in association with an aneu-

rysm arising from the central or left third of the right sinus, and Sakakibara considers this an example of the coincidental association of two independent malformations rather than a single developmental anomaly.[S2]

Aortic Valve Abnormalities and Incompetence

Aortic valve abnormalities and incompetence are common in patients with sinus or Valsalva aneurysms (Table 21-3). When a VSD is present, the aortic incompetence (AI) is nearly always from a prolapsed aortic cusp, similar to the finding in the syndrome of VSD and AI (see Chapter 20, Section 2). When a VSD is not present, the incompetence

Table 21-3 Aortic incompetence in patients undergoing repair of congenital aneurysms of the sinus of Valsalva (UAB; 1967–1980 and GLH; 1957–1980).

			Causes of Incompetence					
			Prolapsed Aortic Cusp		Others		Total	
Series	VSD	n	No.	% of n	No.	% of n	No.	% of n
UAB	Yes	10	6[a]	60%		0%	6	60%
	No	9		0%	5[b]	56%	5	56%
GLH		10					6[c]	60%
Total		29					17	59%

KEY: VSD, ventricular septal defect.

[a]Two had Trusler repair; four had valve replacement.

[b]Four had valve replacement; one had repair of avulsed commissure.

[c]Two had Trusler repair; two had valve replacement; two had no treatment.

usually is from other aortic valve abnormalities, including a bicuspid valve.

As in VSD and AI, cusp prolapse in patients with congenital aneurysms of the sinuses of Valsalva occurs most often when the VSD is subpulmonary but can occur also when it is perimembranous. There is a progressive prolapse of the aortic cusp into the defect and a progressive increase in the severity of the incompetence.[S2] If the aortic anulus remains intact at the base of a prolapsed cusp, a sinus of Valsalva aneurysm projects toward the ventricle superior to the anulus, and the cusp projects through the VSD inferior to the anulus. However, when the anulus does not remain intact, as is frequently the case, both structures form a single sac.[S1,S2,S3] Taguchi[T1] points out that prolonged incompetence produces a fixed fibrous deformity of the prolapsed leaflet.

The frequency of aortic leaflet prolapse in sinus of Valsalva aneurysms was undoubtedly underestimated in earlier reports, particularly when no aortograms were obtained and the aorta was not opened at operation. Aortic leaflet prolapse is also less common if only ruptured sinus aneurysm is considered. Thus, in Taguchi's series,[T1] which includes unruptured cases, aortic incompetence, albeit usually mild, was present in 75%, while in the Okada series[O1] from Japan, which includes only ruptured cases, the incidence was 17%. A complicating problem is the difficulty of determining what constitutes a true (unruptured) sinus aneurysm when there is a combination of VSD and AI. Aneurysmal enlargement of the aortic sinus is frequent in such a setting, and its distinction from unruptured sinus aneurysm is difficult on aortography and even at autopsy or operation. However, 7 (15%) of 48 surgical patients with VSD and AI had a distinct but unruptured sinus of Valsalva aneurysm (GLH; see Chapter 20, Table 20-21).

Pulmonary Stenosis

Important pulmonary stenosis is uncommon in patients with congenital aneurysms of the sinuses of Valsalva, but small gradients are common.[O1] Three (10%) of the 29 patients in the combined GLH-UAB surgical series had important stenosis. The stenosis may be valvar but is usually due either to projection of the wind sock itself in front of the infundibular septum[B1] or to a developmental anomaly of the right ventricular outflow similar to that present in tetralogy of Fallot and in the VSD-AI syndrome.

CLINICAL FEATURES AND DIAGNOSTIC CRITERIA

Unruptured congenital sinus of Valsalva aneurysms are silent lesions, and their diagnosis depends on aortograms usually obtained to demonstrate such associated symptomatic lesions as VSD or AI.

Rupture of a sinus aneurysm produces acute symptoms in about 35% of the patients experiencing it.[M6,N1,T1] In 45% of patients, quite amazingly, rupture is associated only with the gradual onset of effort dyspnea, and in 20% no symptoms develop. When acute symptoms are present, they consist of sudden breathlessness and pain, usually precordial and sometimes also epigastric, the latter probably due to acute hepatic congestion and the former simulating myocardial in-

farction, although radiation of the pain beyond the substernal area is said to be unusual.[O2] In a few patients, death occurs within days of rupture from right heart failure, but in most there is improvement during the so-called *latent period*,[O2] which may last for weeks, months, or years; this improvement may occur without decongestive therapy. The latent period is usually followed by recurrent dyspnea and the signs of right heart failure. The characteristic features at this final stage are those of aortic incompetence and tricuspid incompetence, an unusual combination.[O2,S8]

The infrequency of severe symptoms at the time of rupture may be related to the fact that the rupture is initially a small one in many patients. Studies by Sawyers in dogs indicated that symptoms were severe when the fistula was greater than 5 mm in diameter.[S8] There was, however, little correlation between the size of the fistulous opening found at operation and a history of acute symptoms in Taguichi's patients.[T1] Acute symptoms at the time of rupture may be less frequent when there is also a VSD[S2,T1] and more frequent when there is severe associated aortic valve incompetence.

Acute symptomatic ruptures may be precipitated by heavy exertion, but they have occurred also after serious automobile accidents and at the time of cardiac catheterization.[B1] Rarely, an episode of bacterial endocarditis may be the precipitating factor. Marfan's syndrome may also predispose the aneurysm to rupture.[S6]

Rupture is heralded not only by pain and dyspnea but also by the appearance of a characteristic murmur that is loud, harsh, superficial, and accompanied by a coarse thrill.[S9] The murmur is usually continuous with either systolic or diastolic accentuation, but it may be to and fro in nature, similar to that present in the VSD-AI syndrome. In the past, this murmur has been mistaken for that of a patent ductus arteriosus, but it is maximal at a lower site, usually the left second, third, or fourth intercostal space. With rupture into the sinus portion of the right ventricle or the right atrium, rather than into the right ventricular outflow tract, the murmur tends to be maximal at a lower level over the sternum or to the right of the lower sternum.[E2,M4,M5,S1] Rarely, the murmur of a ruptured sinus of Valsalva aneurysm may be systolic only,[B1] possibly because the communication is small.[H2] Alternatively, the murmur may be confined to diastole in those few instances in which rupture occurs into the high-pressure left ventricle[N1,W2] or in which right ventricular pressure is at systemic level, as in the neonate.[A1] When the murmur is continuous, its timing and accentuation are a function of several factors:[T1] the degree of associated aortic incompetence, the degree of any aortic systolic murmur, the functional size of the VSD, and the size of the rupture itself. Morch and associates assessed the various causes of murmurs which were believed to be continuous associated with signs of rapid aortic runoff in their adult patients[M6] and found that a ruptured sinus aneurysm (8 cases) was the second most common, after a patent ductus arteriosus (33 cases), followed by VSD and AI (3 cases), aortopulmonary window (3 cases), coronary arteriovenous fistula (1 case), and pulmonary arteriovenous fistula (1 case).

Other physical signs of ruptured aneurysms of the sinuses of Valsalva include widened aortic pulse pressure, suggesting mild to severe aortic incompetence. An elevated jugular venous pressure with a prominent V wave, suggesting tricuspid incompetence, may be due in some instances to the direct entrance of a fistula into the right atrium, but in most cases this sign is absent[B2] until the onset of right heart failure, when liver enlargement and pulsation also occur.

The chest x-ray does not show any enlargement of the aortic root. Plethora may be present, although the left-to-right shunt both through the fistula and any associated VSD is usually small. The electrocardiogram shows either left ventricular hypertrophy or combined ventricular hypertrophy. A right bundle-branch block has been described and is said to be commoner in those aneurysms with an intracardiac course close to the AV node and bundle. Complete heart block can also occur.

While the diagnosis is virtually certain on clinical grounds in patients with acute symptoms and the sudden appearance of a continuous murmur, two-dimensional and contrast echocardiography are used to verify the diagnosis.[T5,V2,W1] Cardiac catheterization and angiocardiography (Fig. 21-6) are generally performed to study the site of origin and termination of the fistula and the presence of associated lesions, particularly VSD, AI, and pulmonary stenosis. True VSD size cannot be estimated angiocardiographically when the right aortic cusp is prolapsed into the VSD. The degree of left-to-right shunting through the fistulous communication combined with any associated VSD is calculated, together with the pulmonary vascular resistance (see Chapter 20, "Cardiac Catheterization" in Section 1, Clinical Features and Diagnostic Criteria).

NATURAL HISTORY

No information is available on the frequency of rupture of a sinus aneurysm. It is likely that many sinus aneurysms fail to rupture during the patient's natural life span, and the unrup-

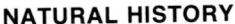

Figure 21-6 Cineangiograms of patients with aneurysms of the sinuses of Valsalva (UAB).

(a) Unruptured small aneurysm of the right sinus of Valsalva associated with aortic incompetence. The aortic root injection is seen in the left anterior oblique view in (1) systole and (2) diastole. The large right and noncoronary cusps of the aortic valve are displaced inferiorly.

(b) Ascending aortic aortogram in another patient, in (1) elongated right anterior oblique view and (2) long axial view. The right coronary cusp of the aortic valve is large and protrudes anteriorly and inferiorly. The rupture of the aneurysm of the right sinus of Valsalva into the right ventricle is indicated by the arrow. Some contrast medium refluxed from the aorta into the left ventricle, indicating mild aortic incompetence.

(c) Aneurysm of the noncoronary sinus of Valsalva in a different patient, rupturing (unusually) into right ventricle. The ascending aortogram is in (1) the elongated right anterior oblique view and (2) the long axial view. Contrast medium can be seen passing through the fistula into the right ventricle. The noncoronary cusp is large and displaced inferiorly. There is mild aortic incompetence.

Ao, ascending aorta; lc, left sinus of Valsalva; LV, left ventricle; nc, noncoronary sinus of Valsalva; rc, right sinus of Valsalva; RV, right ventricle.

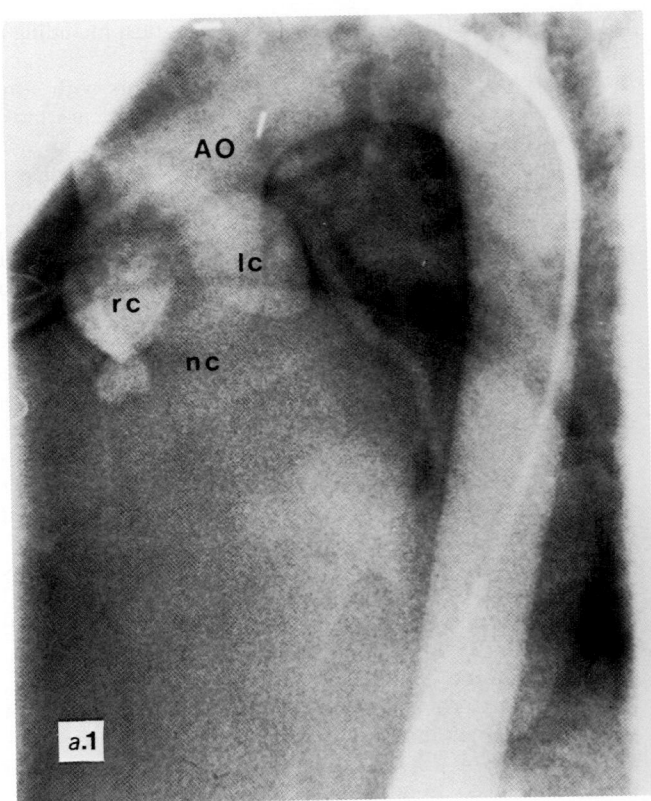

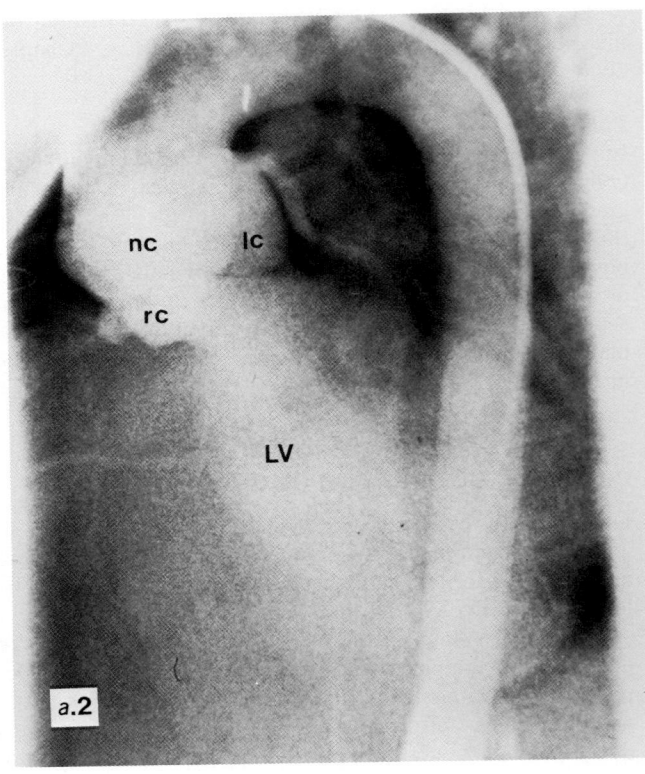

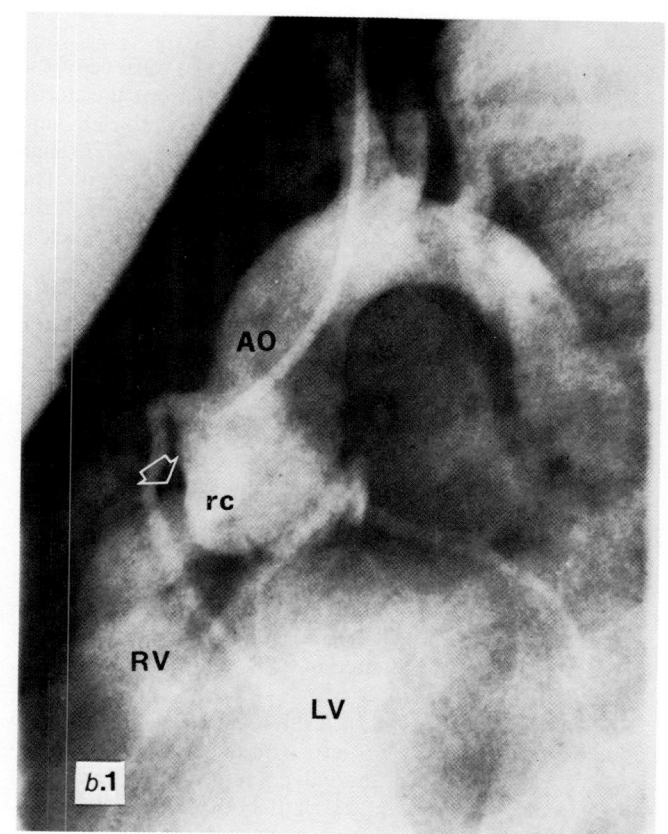

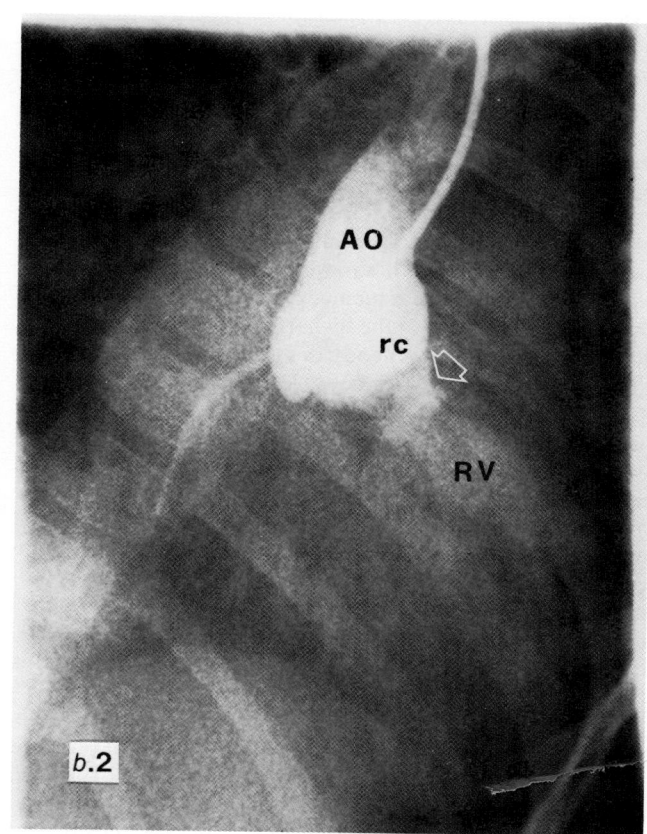

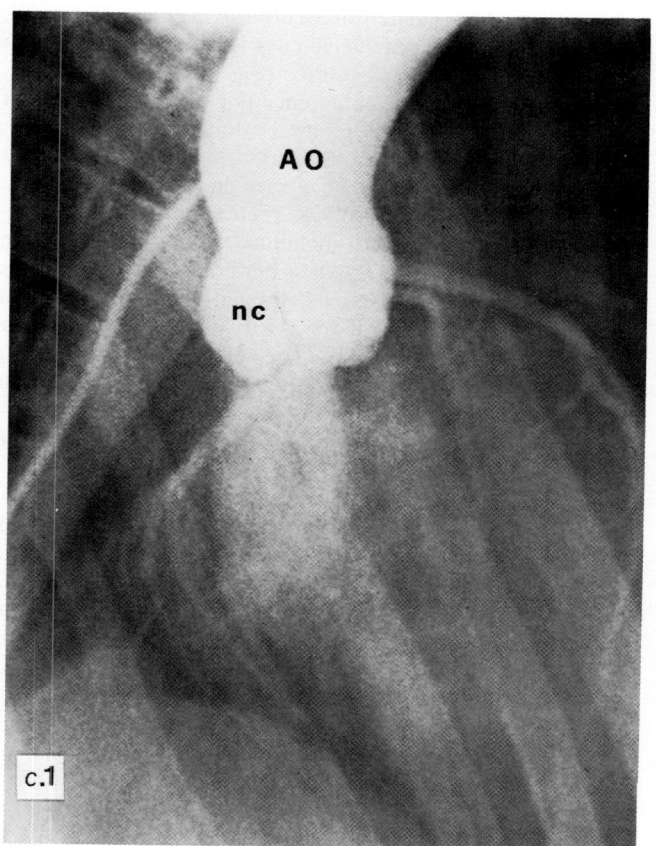

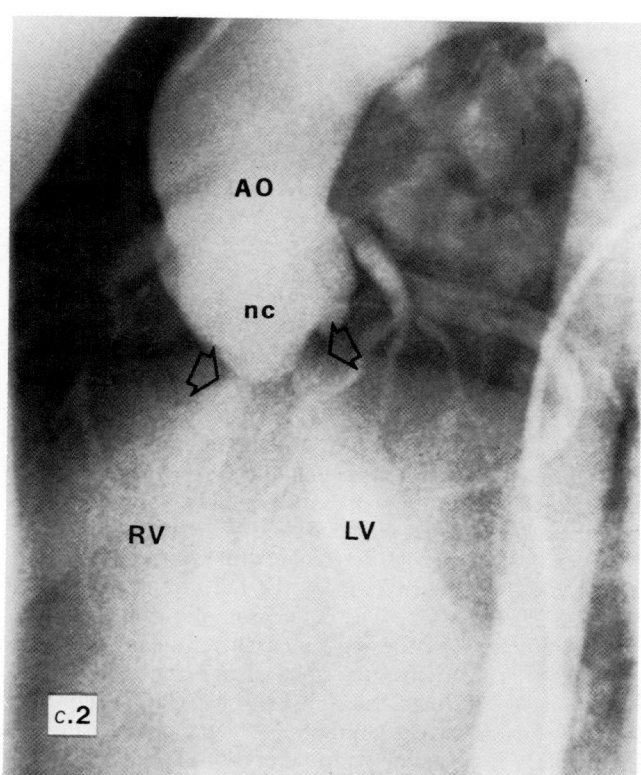

tured aneurysm is never identified. Eighty percent of patients with sinus of Valsalva aneurysms are males.[J1,S8]

When at birth there is a weakness in the aortic root immediately above the anulus, the pressure within the aorta gradually produces a thin-walled aneurysm that is asymptomatic until it finally ruptures into a low-pressure cardiac chamber. Uncommonly, a small fistulous connection may be present at birth[A1,D2,S1] that is well tolerated and not a cause of early death. The infrequency of rupture into the left ventricle is said to be due to the higher pressure in that chamber. Rupture occurs predominantly in the third and fourth decade of life, the average age of rupture being 31.2 years. The mean survival time after rupture in the review of Sawyers and associates was 3.9 years.[S8] If, however, two patients who lived 10 and 15 years were excluded, the average survival time fell to 1 year. In this regard, it is of interest that the mean age in the UAB surgical series was 27 ± 10.7 (standard deviation) years, almost identical to that of our earlier Mayo Clinic series.[B1] Death is usually due to congestive heart failure, but endocarditis complicates the syndrome in about 8% of patients[N1] and may also be a cause of death. Three (16%) of 19 surgical patients gave a history of bacterial endocarditis (UAB).

When present, AI becomes progressively more severe in association with an increase in the degree of leaflet prolapse into the subjacent VSD[S2] and the development of a fixed fibrous deformity of the leaflet.[T1] The VSD becomes occluded to an ever-increasing degree, and the left-to-right shunt decreases as the AI increases. In this way, even an anatomically large VSD becomes functionally small, and both pulmonary hypertension and an increase in pulmonary vascular resistance are rare.[N1]

TECHNIQUE OF OPERATION

The initial stages of the operation are the usual ones (see Chapter 2, Section 3). Before cardiopulmonary bypass (CPB) is begun, a finger inserted through the right atrium can usually palpate the wind sock of the ruptured aneurysm in the right atrium or, through the tricuspid valve, in the right ventricle. CPB is established at 34°C using two venous cannulae, and a vent is inserted into the left ventricle via the left atrium (see Chapter 2, Section 3). As in all situations characterized by a rapid aortic runoff, cooling must not be started nor must the heart be allowed to fibrillate until preparations for venting and aortic cross-clamping are complete. When they are, the perfusate temperature is taken as cold as possible, the aorta is cross-clamped, and the perfusate temperature is adjusted to 25°C. External cardiac cooling is begun.

The aorta is opened as for aortic valve replacement (see Chapter 12, Fig. 12-2). The cold cardioplegic solution is injected directly into the left and right coronary ostia (see Chapter 3). The origin of the sinus aneurysm, usually deep in the sinus, is identified, together with its relationship to the base of the cusp. The aortic valve is examined carefully, particularly if AI is known to be present. A VSD is always sought (since it can be overlooked at preoperative study if it is plugged completely or nearly so by a prolapsed aortic

valve cusp) by looking at the left ventricular surface of the ventricular septum immediately upstream from the aortic valve. When the sinus aneurysm has ruptured into right ventricle or right atrium, this chamber is then opened through the usual incision (the combined approach).[M5,S11,S14] The wind sock is opened widely so as to visualize through it the base of the aortic cusp, and then most of the wind sock is excised.

When no VSD is present, direct suture closure in a transverse direction relative to aortic flow with two rows of continuous polypropylene sutures is safe if the defect in the sinus is small and has strong fibrous margins. Otherwise, a Dacron patch (which may be lined with pericardium) is sewn into place with a continuous polypropylene suture to effect secure closure. In any case, care is taken not to catch the aortic cusp in the suture line. The right ventricle or atrium is closed. Returning to the aortic root, the cusps of the valve are inspected and then the aortotomy is closed. After the tip of the left ventricle is aspirated for air and suction is placed on the needle vent in the ascending aorta, the aortic clamp is released and rewarming is begun. The usual de-airing procedures and gradual termination of CPB follow (see Chapter 2, Section 3).

When a VSD is present, after the wind sock is excised, a double-barreled aperture is left, with the VSD below or upstream from the base of the valve and the sinus defect just downstream from it (Fig. 21-7). If both defects are small, they may be closed as one with horizontal pledgetted mattress sutures that sandwich the base of the valve cusp between the defect edges. When the defects are large or the edges soft, a single patch of Dacron is used to close both, and the base of the aortic valve cusp is attached to the patch with interrupted mattress sutures (Fig. 21-7).

When aortic valve incompetence is present as a result of cusp prolapse, a Trusler repair is done (see Chapter 20, "Technique of Operation" in Section 2). This repair is best deferred until the ruptured aneurysm and VSD (virtually always present when cusp prolapse is etiologic to the incompetence) have been repaired, including the attachment of the base of the cusp to the patch. Then, after the ventricle is closed, the cusp is reexamined through the aortotomy, and the Trusler repair done. If the AI is long-standing and the cusp very deformed, valve replacement is necessary. When important aortic incompetence occurs in sinus of Valsalva aneurysm without VSD, valve replacement is usually necessary. The considerations involved in selecting the device for replacement of the aortic valve and the technique of insertion are the same as for patients with ventricular septal defect and aortic incompetence (see Chapter 20, "Technique of Operation" in Section 2, Ventricular Septal Defect and Aortic Incompetence). The aortic valve should be excised and the bioprosthesis or prosthesis inserted after the repair of the sinus aneurysm through its chamber of entry. Because the tissues are usually normal and thus delicate, pledgetted mattress sutures should be used for the valve insertions.

Rarely, an unruptured congenital sinus of Valsalva aneurysm may be encountered during an operation for repair of aortic valve disease (with or without a VSD). Its orifice should be closed from the aortic side using an onlay Dacron

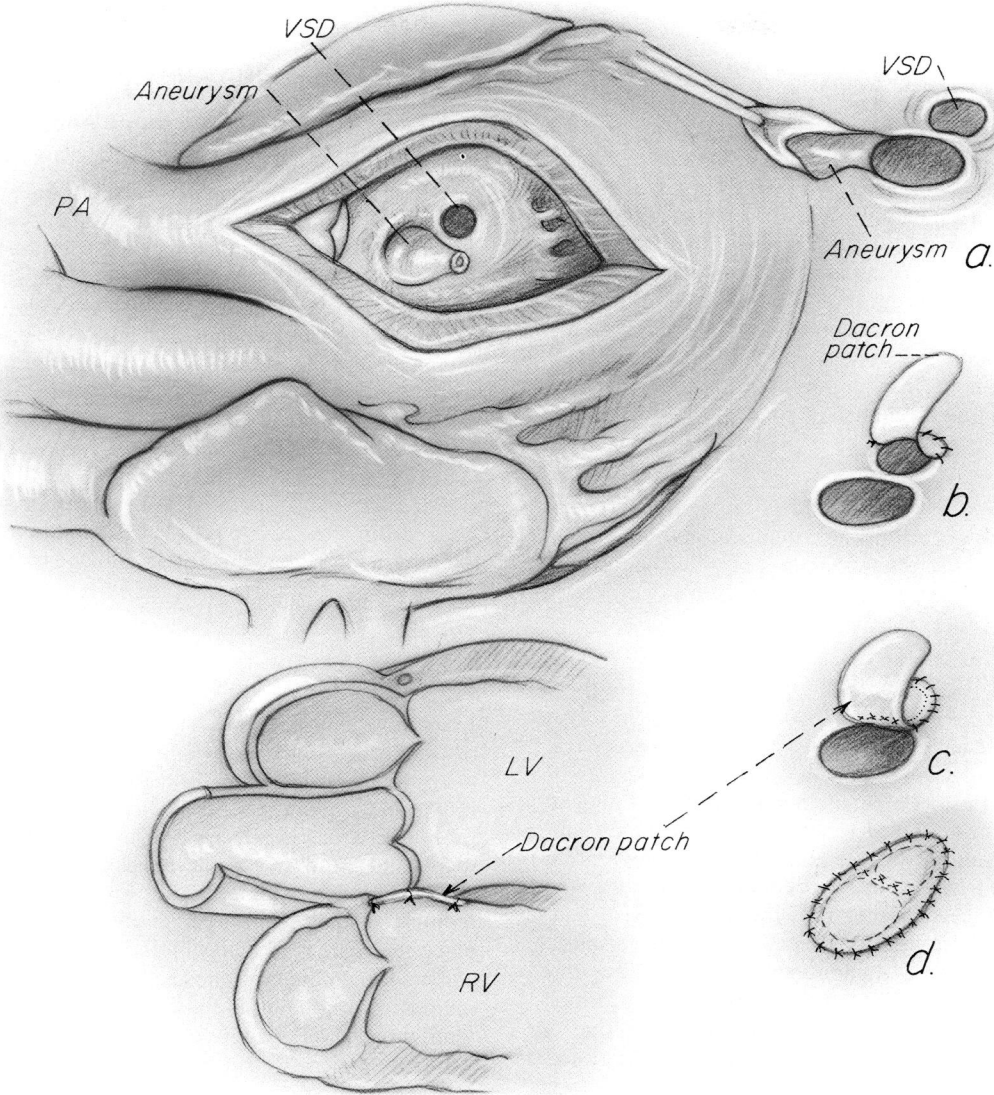

Figure 21-7 Repair of congenital aneurysm of the right sinus of Valsalva, ruptured into the right ventricle. A vertical ventriculotomy incision is shown, although the repair can be made through a transverse incision or, on occasion, through a right atriotomy incision. Not shown is the initial aortotomy.

(a) The wind sock aneurysm is excised, leaving the base of the aortic cusp as the divider between the VSD and the defect left after excision of the aneurysm.

(b) The two defects are closed as one with a knitted or double velour woven Dacron patch.

(c) When the repair reaches the base of the aortic valve cusp, the cusp is attached to the patch with interrupted sutures.

(d) The completed repair closes the defects of the VSD and the sinus of Valsalva aneurysm, and attaches the base of the aortic valve cusp to the patch.

LV, left ventricle; PA, pulmonary artery; RV, right ventricle; VSD, ventricular septal defect.

patch sewn to the margins of the aneurysm. No attempt is made to excise the aneurysm.

EARLY RESULTS

Hospital Mortality

The hospital mortality after repair of congenital aneurysms of the sinus of Valsalva with or without VSD or aortic valve incompetence approaches zero, with no (0%, CL 0%–6%) deaths in a series of 29 patients (GLH-UAB). Similarly, in our Mayo Clinic experience (1956–1967), there were no deaths; this experience was updated by Bonfils-Roberts and colleagues in 1971 in their report of 21 cases.[B1] A low mortality of 8 deaths (4.1%, CL 2.7%–6.1%) among 195 patients was reported by Okada and colleagues.[O1] The higher mortality reported by others[H1,N1] must not, therefore, be representative of what can be accomplished.

Complications

Heart block has not occurred as a complication of the repair of congenital aneurysms of the sinuses of Valsalva (GLH-UAB).

LATE RESULTS

When aortic valve incompetence is not present preoperatively, the late results are excellent.[T1] Thus, among 12 patients without aortic incompetence, no late deaths and no reoperations occurred (GLH-UAB). Life expectancy and late functional results are determined by the preoperative size of the left ventricle, as in other conditions with chronic rapid aortic runoff (see Chapter 12, "Incremental Risk Factors for Premature Late Death" in section on Late Results). Others[B1,H1] have reported uncommon instances of reoperation for recurrence of the VSD or fistulous communication.

When aortic incompetence was present initially, reoperation was required in four of 17 patients (GLH-UAB), and four late deaths occurred, one related to reoperation. Two late deaths were sudden and are believed related to the massive left ventricular enlargement that developed preoperatively in response to the great volume overload imposed by the combined aortic valve incompetence, ruptured aneurysm, and VSD (UAB).

Indications for Operation

When unaccompanied by VSD or aortic valve incompetence, unruptured congenital aneurysms of the sinus of Valsalva are rarely detected, although they may be encountered unexpectedly at operation for VSD and aortic valve incompetence. Management of such an isolated unruptured congenital aneurysm diagnosed preoperatively is controversial, but elective repair may be advised, as suggested by Mayer and colleagues (UAB).[M3]

When the congenital sinus of Valsalva aneurysm has ruptured or is associated with a VSD or with a VSD and aortic incompetence, prompt operation is advisable.

SPECIAL SITUATIONS AND CONTROVERSIES

Approach to the Ruptured Sinus Aneurysm

Originally, an approach solely through the chamber of entry was used, usually the right ventricle or right atrium.[B1,M7] The aortic runoff through the ruptured aneurysm can be controlled by opening the chamber early in the period of CPB and placing a clamp across the base of the aneurysm. Then, after the release of the aortic cross-clamp, cooling of the patient and heart can begin, and later the aorta can be cross-clamped and the cold cardioplegia solution injected into the aortic root as usual (see Chapter 3). The repair is accomplished as described. Some have used an approach through the aorta alone, but this approach is believed to be less satisfactory than the others (GLH, UAB). It is particularly to be avoided when an associated VSD is present; the repair of the VSD through the aortic root is in actuality a repair from the left ventricular side, which risks damage to the bundle of His during repair.

Aortic-Ventricular Tunnel

In its most characteristic form,[B6,C1,G3,L2,P2] the aortic orifice of the aortic-ventricular tunnel is anterior and downstream from the uppermost level of the aortic valve cusp attachment, and separated from the right sinus of Valsalva by a prominent transverse supravalvar ridge. It is visible externally, and the extracardiac bulge can often be seen on the chest x-ray. The tunnel passes directly downward to communicate usually with the left ventricle. The tunnel may displace the right ventricular infundibular septum and produce some subpulmonary stenosis. Rarely, the tunnel may communicate with the infundibulum of the right ventricle, rather than with the left ventricle.

In one patient,[B5] the orifice of the right coronary artery was shown to arise from the extracardiac portion of the tunnel. This finding, coupled with the demonstration of the existence of elastic fibers in the extracardiac portion of some of these tunnels, suggests that such tunnels may actually be examples of coronary artery fistulae.

Aortic-ventricular tunnels are usually present at birth and produce severe aortic regurgitation into the left ventricle. Severe congestive heart failure develops early, and death frequently occurs in the first few months of life.[L3,O3] In all these regards, aortic-ventricular tunnels are quite different from aneurysms of the sinuses of Valsalva.

Two-dimensional and pulsed Doppler echocardiography can make the diagnosis of aortic-ventricular tunnel, and at least in some patients can exclude aortic valve incompetence.[B7,F2] Cardiac catheterization and cineangiography are performed, to provide additional anatomic detail and exclude associated cardiac anomalies.

Urgent surgical treatment is indicated and consists of an aortic approach and closure of the aortic ostium by direct suturing or a patch.

In the report by Perez-Martinez, 5 (62%, CL 38%–83%) of 8 surgical patients survived. Turley and colleagues and Fripp and colleagues have reported successful repairs in neonates.[F2,T4] The late results may be marred by the development of aortic valve incompetence, which may necessitate repeated reoperations and ultimately aortic valve replacement.[R1,S15,S16]

REFERENCES

A

1. Ainger LE, Pate JW: Rupture of a sinus of Valsalva aneurysm in an infant: Surgical correction. *Am J Cardiol* 11:547, 1963.
2. Abbott ME: *Clinical and Developmental Study of a Case of Ruptured Aneurysm of the Right Anterior Aortic Sinus of Valsalva: Contributions to Medical and Biological Research*, vol. 2. New York: Paul B. Hoeber, 1919, p 899.

B

1. Bonfils-Roberts EA, DuShane JW, McGoon DC, Danielson GK: Aortic sinus fistula: Surgical considerations and results of operation. *Ann Thorac Surg* 12:492, 1971.
2. Besterman EMM, Goldberg MJ, Sellors TH: Surgical repair of ruptured sinus of Valsalva. *Br Med J* 2:410, 1963.
3. Bigelow WG, Barnes WT: Ruptured aneurysm of aortic sinus. *Ann Surg* 150:117, 1959.
4. Brown JW, Heath D, Whitaker W: Cardio aortic fistula: A case diagnosed in life and treated surgically. *Circulation* 12:819, 1955.
5. Bharati S, Lev M, Cassels DE: Aortico-right ventricular tunnel. *Chest* 63:198, 1973.
6. Bove KE, Schwartz DC: Aortico-left ventricular tunnel: A new concept. *Am J Cardiol* 19:696, 1967.
7. Bash SE, Huhta JC, Nihill MR, Vargo TA, Hallman GL: Aortico-left ventricular tunnel with ventricular septal defect: Two-dimensional/Doppler echocardiographic diagnosis. *JACC* 5:757, 1985.

C

1. Cooley RN, Harris LC, Rodin AE: Abnormal communication between the aorta and left ventricle: Aortico-left ventricular tunnel. *Circulation* 31:564, 1965.

D

1. DeBakey ME, Lowrie GM: Aneurysm of sinus of Valsalva with coronary atherosclerosis: Successful surgical correction. *Ann Surg* 189:303, 1979.
2. Dubost C, Blondeau P, Piwnica A: Right aorta-atrial fistulas resulting from a rupture of the sinus of Valsalva: A report on 6 cases. *J Thorac Cardiovasc Surg* 43:421, 1962.
3. DeBakey ME, Diethrich EB, Liddocoat JE, Kinard SA, Garrett HE: Abnormalities of the sinuses of Valsalva: Experience with 35 patients. *J Thorac Cardiovasc Surg* 54:312, 1967.

E

1. Edwards JE, Burchell HB: The pathological anatomy of deficiencies between the aortic root and the heart, including aortic sinus aneurysms. *Thorax* 12:125, 1957.
2. Evans JW, Harris TR, Brody DA: Ruptured aortic sinus aneurysm: Case report, with review of clinical features. *Am Heart J* 61:408, 1961.
3. Edwards JE, Burchell HB: Specimen exhibiting the essential lesion in aneurysm of the aortic sinus. *Proc Staff Meet Mayo Clin* 31:407, 1956.
4. Eliott RS, Wolbrink A, Edwards JE: Congenital aneurysm of the left aortic sinus: A rare lesion and a rare cause of coronary insufficiency. *Circulation* 28:951, 1963.

F

1. Falholt W, Thomsen G: Congenital aneurysm of the right sinus of Valsalva, diagnosed by aortography. *Circulation* 8:549, 1953.
2. Fripp RR, Werner JC, Whitman V, Nordenberg A, Waldhausen JA: Pulsed Doppler and two-dimensional echocardiographic findings in aortico-left ventricular tunnel. *JACC* 4:1012, 1984.

G

1. Gibbs NM, Harris EL: Aortic sinus aneurysms. *Br Heart J* 23:131, 1961.
2. Gerbode F, Osborne JJ, Johnston JB, Kerth WJ: Ruptured aneurysm of the aortic sinuses of Valsalva. *Am J Surg* 102:268, 1961.
3. Goor DA, Lillehei CW: *Congenital Malformations of the Heart*. New York: Grune & Stratton, 1975, p 301.

H

1. Howard RJ, Moller J, Castaneda AR, Varco RL, Nicoloff DM: Surgical correction of sinus of Valsalva aneurysm. *J Thorac Cardiovasc Surg* 66:420, 1973.
2. Hong PW, Lee SS, Kim SW, Cha HD: Unusual manifestations of aneurysm of the aortic sinus: A report of 2 cases. *J Thorac Cardiovasc Surg* 51:507, 1966.
3. Hope J: A treatise of diseases of the heart and great vessels (ed 3). London: John Churchill, 1839.
4. Heydorn WH, Nelson WP, Fitter JD, Floyd GD, Strevey TE: Congenital aneurysm of the sinus of Valsalva protruding into the left ventricle. *J Thorac Cardiovasc Surg* 71:839, 1976.

J

1. Jones AM, Langley FA: Aortic sinus aneurysms. *Br Heart J* 11:325, 1949.

K

1. Kay JH, Anderson RM, Lewis RR, Reinberg M: Successful repair of sinus of Valsalva–left atrial fistula. *Circulation* 20:427, 1959.
2. Kieffer SA, Winchell P: Congenital aneurysms of the aortic sinuses with cardio aortic fistula. *Chest* 38:79, 1960.

L

1. Lillehei CW, Stanley P, Varco RL: Surgical treatment of ruptured aneurysms of the sinus of Valsalva. *Ann Surg* 146:460, 1957.

2. Levy MJ, Lillehei CW, Anderson RC, Arnplatz K, Edwards JE: Aortico-left ventricular tunnel. *Circulation* 27:841, 1963.

3. Levy MJ, Schachner A, Blieden LC: Aortico–left ventricular tunnel. Collective review. *J Thorac Cardiovasc Surg* 84:102, 1982.

M

1. Morrow AG, Baker RR, Hanson HE, Mattingly TW: Successful surgical repair of a ruptured aneurysm of the sinus of Valsalva. *Circulation* 16:533, 1957.

2. Morris GC Jr, Foster RP, Dunn RJ, Cooley DA: Traumatic aortico-ventricular fistula: Report of two cases successfully repaired. *Am Surg* 24:883, 1958.

3. Mayer J, Wukasch DC, Hallman GL, Cooley DA: Aneurysm and fistula of the sinus of Valsalva. *Ann Thorac Surg* 19:170, 1975.

4. Magidson O, Kay JH: Ruptured aortic sinus aneurysms: Clinical and surgical aspects of seven cases. *Am Heart J* 65:597, 1963.

5. Morgan JR, Rogers AK, Fosburg RG: Ruptured aneurysms of the sinus of Valsalva. *Chest* 61:640, 1972.

6. Morch JE, Greenwood WF: Rupture of the sinus of Valsalva: A study of eight cases with discussion on the differential diagnosis of continuous murmurs. *Am J Cardiol* 18:827, 1966.

7. McGoon DC, Edwards JE, Kirklin JW: Surgical treatment of ruptured aneurysm of aortic sinus. *Ann Surg* 147:387, 1958.

N

1. Nowicki ER, Aberdeen E, Friedman S, Rashkind WJ: Congenital left aortic sinus–left ventricle fistula and review of aortocardiac fistulas. *Ann Thorac Surg* 23:378, 1977.

O

1. Okada M, Muranaka S, Mukubo M, Asada S: Surgical correction of the ruptured aneurysm of the sinus of Valsalva. *J Cardiovasc Surg* (Torino) 18:171, 1977.

2. Oram S, East T: Rupture of aneurysm of aortic sinus (of Valsalva) into the right side of the heart. *Br Heart J* 17:541, 1955.

3. Okoroma EO, Perry LW, Scott LP III, McClenathan JE: Aortico-left ventricular tunnel: Clinical profile, diagnostic features, and surgical considerations. *J Thorac Cardiovasc Surg* 71:238, 1976.

P

1. Perloff JK: Sinus of Valsalva–right heart communications due to congenital aortic sinus defects. *Am Heart J* 59:318, 1960.

2. Perez-Martinez V, Quero M, Castro C, Moreno F, Brito JM, Merino G: Aortico–left ventricular tunnel: A clinical and pathologic review of this uncommon entity. *Am Heart J* 85:237, 1973.

R

1. Ruschewski W, de Vivie ER, Kirchhoff PG: Aortico–left ventricular tunnel. *J Thorac Cardiovasc Surg* 29:282, 1981.

S

1. Sakakibara S, Konno W: Congenital aneurysms of sinus of Valsalva: A clinical study. *Am Heart J* 63:708, 1962.

2. Sakakibara S, Konno S: Congenital aneurysm of the sinus of Valsalva associated with ventricular septal defect: Anatomical aspects. *Am Heart J* 75:595, 1968.

3. Sakakibara S, Konno S: Congenital aneurysm of the sinus of Valsalva: Anatomy and classification. *Am Heart J* 63:405, 1962.

4. Scott RW: Aortic aneurysm rupturing into the pulmonary artery: Report of two cases. *JAMA* 82:1417, 1924.

5. Schuster NH: Aneurysm of the sinus of Valsalva involving the coronary orifice. *Lancet* 1:507, 1937.

6. Szweda JA, Drake EH: Ruptured congenital aneurysms of the sinuses of Valsalva: A report of 2 cases treated surgically. *Circulation* 25:559, 1962.

7. Shumacker HB Jr: Aneurysms of the aortic sinuses of Valsalva due to bacterial endocarditis, with special reference to their operative management. *J Thorac Cardiovasc Surg* 63:896, 1972.

8. Sawyers JL, Adams JE, Scott HW Jr: Surgical treatment for aneurysms of the aortic sinuses with aortico atrial fistula: Experimental and clinical study. *Surgery* 41:26, 1957.

9. Segal BL, Likoff W, Novack P: Rupture of a sinus of Valsalva aneurysm. *Am J Cardiol* 12:544, 1963.

10. Spencer FC, Blake HA, Bahnson HT: Surgical repair of ruptured aneurysm of sinus of Valsalva in two patients. *Ann Surg* 152:963, 1960.

11. Shumacker HB Jr, King H, Waldhausen JA: Transaortic approach for the repair of ruptured aneurysms of the sinuses of Valsalva. *Ann Surg* 161:946, 1965.

12. Shumacker HB Jr, Judson WE: Rupture of aneurysm of sinus of Valsalva into left ventricle and its operative repair. *J Thorac Cardiovasc Surg* 45:650, 1963.

13. Smith WA: Aneurysm of the sinus of Valsalva with report of two cases. *JAMA* 62:1878, 1914.

14. Sakakibara S, Konno S: Congenital aneurysm of the sinus of Valsalva: Criteria for recommending surgery. *Am J Cardiol* 12:100, 1963.

15. Somerville J, English T, Ross DN: Aorto–left ventricular tunnel: Clinical features and surgical management. *Br Heart J* 36:321, 1974.

16. Serino W, Andrade JL, Ross D, de Leval M, Somerville J: Aorto–left ventricular communication after closure: Late postoperative problems. *Br Heart J* 49:501, 1983.

T

1. Taguchi K, Sasaki N, Matasuura Y, Mura R: Surgical correction of aneurysm of the sinus of Valsalva: A report of 45 consecutive patients, including 8 with total replacement of the aortic valve. *Am J Cardiol* 23:180, 1969.

2. Thurman J: On aneurysms and especially spontaneous varicose aneurysms of the ascending aorta and sinuses of Valsalva, with cases. *Med Chir Tr London* 23:323, 1840.

3. Trusler GA, Moes, CAF, Kidd BSL: Repair of ventricular septal defect with aortic insufficiency. *J Thorac Cardiovasc Surg* 66:394, 1973.

4. Turley K, Silverman NH, Teitel D, Mavroudis C, Snider R, Rudolph A: Repair of aortico–left ventricular tunnel in the neonate: Surgical, anatomic and echocardiographic considerations. *Circulation* 65:1015, 1982.

5. Terdjman M, Bourdarias J-P, Farcot J-C, Gueret P, Dubourg O, Ferrier A, Hanania G: Aneurysms of sinus of Valsalva: Two-dimensional echocardiographic diagnosis and recognition of rupture into the right heart cavities. *JACC* 3:1227, 1984.

V

1. Venning GR: Aneurysms of the sinuses of Valsalva. *Am Heart J* 42:57, 1951.
2. Vered Z, Rath S, Benjamin P, Motro M, Neufeld HN: Ruptured sinus of Valsalva: Demonstration by contrast echocardiography during cardiac catheterization. *Am Heart J* 109:365, 1985.

W

1. Weyman AE, Dillon JC, Feigenbaum H, Chang S: Premature pulmonic valve opening following sinus of Valsalva aneurysm rupture into the right atrium. *Circulation* 52:556, 1975.
2. Warthen RO: Congenital aneurysm of the right anterior sinus of Valsalva (interventricular aneurysm) with spontaneous rupture into the left ventricle. *Am Heart J* 37:975, 1949.

22

PATENT DUCTUS ARTERIOSUS

DEFINITION

Patent ductus arteriosus (PDA) is an open communication that is usually between the upper descending thoracic aorta and the proximal portion of the left pulmonary artery and is the result of persistent patency of the fetal ductus arteriosus. When the aortic arch is right-sided, the ductus usually connects to the proximal right pulmonary artery. The ductus may at times connect with the adjacent subclavian or innominate arteries rather than the upper descending thoracic aorta.

This chapter is concerned chiefly with isolated PDA. Patent ductus is frequently associated with other anomalies, and in these settings it is discussed in other chapters (coarctation of the aorta, Chapter 34; ventricular septal defect, Chapter 20; and tetralogy of Fallot with pulmonary stenosis or pulmonary atresia, Chapter 23).

HISTORICAL NOTE

The ductus arteriosus apparently was first described by Galen (born in AD 131), and Harvey demonstrated its physiologic importance in the fetal circulation. Munro is generally considered the first person to have demonstrated, in 1888, in an infant cadaver, the feasibility of dissection and ligation of a persistently patent ductus arteriosus.[M1] In 1900, Gibson described the diagnostic continuous murmur of this anomaly.[G1] However, it was not until 1937 that John Strieder, in Boston, attempted to close a patent ductus arteriosus (PDA) surgically in a patient with fulminating bacterial endocarditis (or endarteritis); the patient died on the fourth postoperative day with gastric distention and aspiration of vomitus.[G2]

Cardiac surgery received a great impetus on August 26, 1938, when Robert E. Gross successfully ligated the PDA of a 7-year-old girl at the Boston Children's Hospital.[G3] Subsequently, he developed division rather than ligation of the PDA as the surgical method of choice.[G7,G8] The first successful repair of an infected PDA was reported by Touroff and Vesell in 1940,[T4] and these authors later reported the successful division of an infected PDA.[T3]

MORPHOLOGY

Morphology of Normal Ductal Closure

At birth, the fetal ductus arteriosus is patent. The ductus at birth "resembles a muscular artery with an intact, wavy internal elastic lamina, interrupted only underneath the intimal cushions. At those sites the elastic lamina is fragmented and is sometimes split up into several layers. The media is mainly composed of circularly arranged smooth muscle cells, with only minimal elastin fibers in between. The medial components may be widely separated, predominantly along the line of junction with intimal cushions, thereby creating large pools filled with a mucoid, slightly eosinophilic substance, the so-called mucoid lakes. In more advanced stages of anatomical closure, necrosis of cellular components of the media and a diffuse fibrous proliferation of the intima begin to appear."[G11]

Postnatal closure[C6] occurs in two stages. The first stage is complete within 10–15 hours after birth in full-term infants and is due to contraction of the smooth muscle in the media of the ductal wall, which produces shortening and an increase in wall thickness. This functional closure is assisted by approximation of the intimal cushions. The intimal cushions (or mounds or pillows)[J4] are swellings composed of longitudinally oriented smooth muscle cells that protrude into the lumen and lie between the endothelium and the internal elastic lamina and thus within the intima. They increase in thickness as the duct matures and are most prominent at the pulmonary end. Muscle contraction occurs both circumferentially from the circularly arranged smooth muscle cells that fill almost the entire media, as well as longitudinally from one or more longitudinally arranged bands of muscle in the inner media.[S4]

The second stage of closure is usually completed by 2–3 weeks. It is the result of diffuse fibrous proliferation of the intima, sometimes associated with necrosis of the inner layer of the media, and hemorrhage into the wall. The latter may be due to intimal tears producing a limited dissection of the ductus wall; there may also be small thrombi within the lumen, but gross luminal thrombus is rare.[C7] These changes result in permanent sealing of the lumen and produce the fibrous ligamentum arteriosus.

Closure usually begins at the pulmonary end and may remain incomplete at the aortic end, leaving an aortic ampulla from which the ligamentum arteriosum arises. Less commonly, there may be a ductus diverticulum arising from the proximal left pulmonary artery.

The ductus arteriosus is completely closed by 8 weeks of age in 88% of people with an otherwise normal cardiovascular system.[C3] When the process is delayed, the term *prolonged patency* of the ductus arteriosus is appropriate; when it ultimately fails, *persisting patency* of the ductus arteriosus exists. Ductus closure is mediated by the release of vasoac-

tive substances (acetylcholine, bradykinin, endogenous catecholamines, and probably others), by variations in pH, but chiefly by oxygen tension[M4] and prostaglandins (PGE$_1$, PGE$_2$ and prostacyclin PG$_{12}$).[C8] The oxygen tension and prostaglandins act in opposite directions, a rising PO$_2$ constricting the ductus and prostaglandins relaxing it, and the potency of both varies at different gestational ages.[H6] Thus, the ductus is considerably more sensitive to the PO$_2$ in the mature fetus and to PGE$_1$ in the immature fetus. The complex interplay of these factors is the reason that prolonged patency of the ductus is much more common in premature infants, particularly when there is associated respiratory distress syndrome (see "Special Situations and Controversies"). *Intermittent patency* of the ductus arteriosus has been documented, particularly when the ductus is long and narrow.[D3]

Position and Absence

It is noteworthy that at birth, usually in subjects with other cardiac anomalies, the ductus may be unilateral, bilateral, or, rarely, completely absent. It is absent in 35% of autopsy specimens (GLH) of tetralogy of Fallot with pulmonary stenosis and in 40% of those with tetralogy of Fallot and pulmonary atresia (see Chapter 23). It is rarely absent in patients with pulmonary atresia and an intact ventricular septum (4%) and in those with pulmonary atresia and other complex anomalies (15%).

Anatomic Details

Isolated Patent Ductus Arteriosus

The usual isolated PDA connects to and is in communication with the upper descending thoracic aorta 2–10 mm beyond the aortic origin of the left subclavian artery (Fig. 22-1). From the aorta, it passes centrally toward the origin of the left pulmonary artery from the pulmonary trunk, either directly or angling superiorly and hugging the undersurface of the distal aortic arch.

The PDA most commonly is from 5 to 10 mm in length, with a wide aortic orifice and a pulmonary orifice that is considerably narrower and is restrictive to flow. The PDA may be longer or shorter than this and may have a wide pulmonary as well as aortic orifice.

Patent Ductus Arteriosus as a Coexisting Anomaly

When other cardiac anomalies are present, the orientation of the ductus to the aortic arch varies, as does the flow pattern in fetal life.[C7] When, as in the normally developing heart, the ductus delivers approximately 55% of the combined ventricular output into the descending aorta,[H5] the ductus meets the aorta at a proximal acute angle (less than 40°),[C7,M5] and the distal angle is correspondingly obtuse (110°–160°, mean 134°)[C7] (Table 22-1). In striking contrast, when there is pulmonary atresia and the pulmonary circulation is ductus dependent, ductal flow in utero is from the aorta to the pulmonary artery; then the ductus becomes a downwardly directed branch of the distal aortic arch so that the proximal angle is much less acute and often obtuse[C7] and the distal angle is often acute[R5] (Fig. 22-2, Table 22-1) (see also Chapter 23, "Aortic Arch and Ductus Arteriosus" in Section 1, Mor-

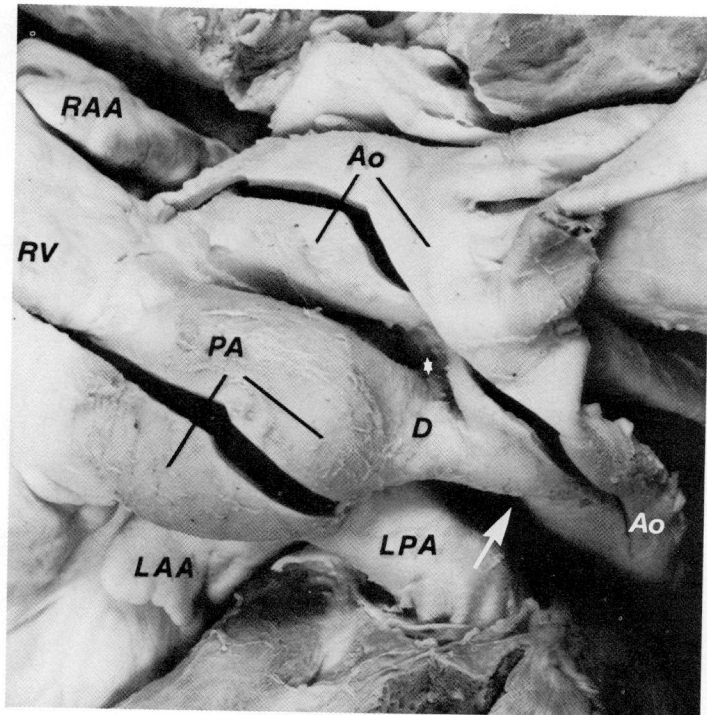

Figure 22-1 Specimen of isolated patent ductus arteriosus in an infant (GLH). The ductus passes from the junction of the pulmonary trunk and left pulmonary artery in an inferior and lateral direction to join the descending aorta. The angle between the superior border of the ductus (asterisk) and the aorta is acute and that between the lower border and aorta (arrow) is obtuse.

Ao, aorta; D, patent ductus arteriosus; LAA, left atrial appendage; LPA, left pulmonary artery; PA, pulmonary trunk; RAA, right atrial appendage; RV, right ventricle.

Reproduced with permission from Calder et al.[C7]

phology). When this is not the case, it is likely that the pulmonary atresia develops late in pregnancy.[S5] In aortic atresia and coarctation of the aorta, the distal angle is similar to normal, but the proximal angle in these shorter, broader examples of PDA is much less acute, probably because ductal flow enters both the ascending and descending aorta.[C7]

Both the diameter and length of a PDA vary widely. In fixed autopsy specimens, the range in otherwise normal hearts varied from 4 to 12 mm and the length from 2.5 to 8 mm. In pulmonary atresia, the ductus is usually longer and narrower[C7] (see Fig. 22-2). The lumen is usually narrower at the pulmonary end and wider at the aortic end.

Uncommonly, in the presence of a left aortic arch, the ductus may arise from an aortic diverticulum (thought to represent persistence of the most distal portion of the right fourth branchial arch), which projects from the medial aspect of the left arch just distal to the origin of the left subclavian artery.[G12] In the rare cases in which the ductus is bilateral, the right-sided PDA connects the right pulmonary artery to the innominate artery.

Table 22-1   Morphologic features of ductus arteriosus in fixed autopsy specimens (GLH).[C7]

Cardiac Diagnosis	n	Age		Ductal Status		Average Length (mm)	Average Width (mm)	Average prox angle[a] (deg)	Average distal angle[a] (deg)
		Range	Median	Open	Closed				
Normal[b]	13	SB–5 mo	2 d	10	3	8	5.9	29	134
Pulmonary atresia	32	SB–11 mo	8 d	13	19	9.7	3.7	83[c]	90[c]
Aortic atresia	13	2 d–11 wk	4 d	12	1	7.9	7.2	70[c]	127
Coarctation	14	3 d–6 mo	14 d	8	6	5.6	6.0	70[c]	139
Miscellaneous CHD	37	1 d–8 mo	23 d	18	19	7.1	4.6	52	124

KEY: CHD, congenital heart disease; SB, stillborn; deg, degrees.

[a]Angle between ductus and descending aorta.

[b]Normal hearts except for open ductus arteriosus.

[c]Difference from normal: $P < 0.001$.

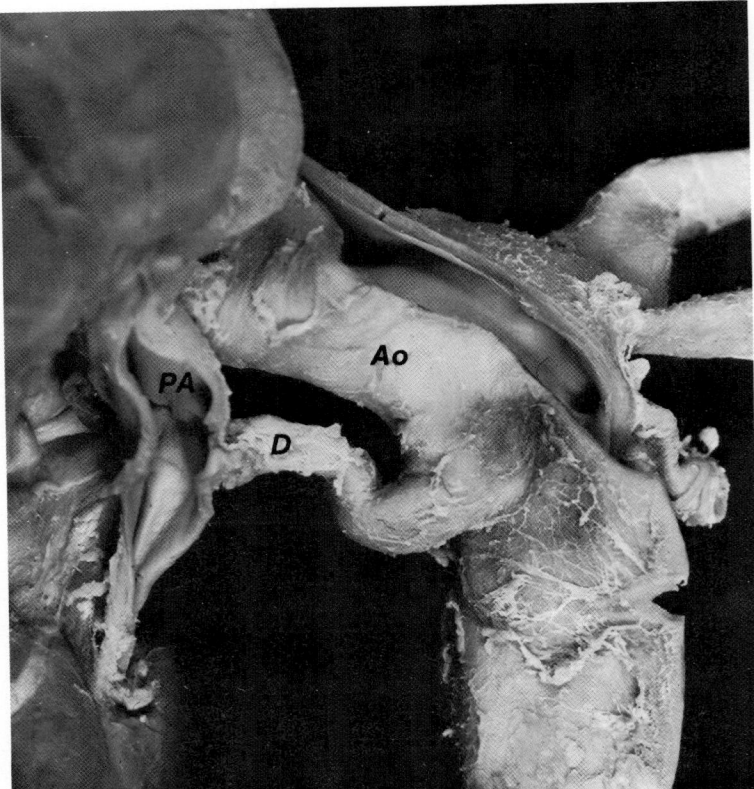

Figure 22-2   Specimen of patent ductus arteriosus in an infant with pulmonary atresia (GLH). Compared with the ductus in Figure 22-1, this ductus is long and relatively narrow and joins the aorta at a completely different angle. Thus the superior angle is obtuse and the inferior angle acute.

Ao, aorta; D, patent ductus arteriosus; PA, pulmonary artery.

Reproduced with permission from Calder et al.[C7]

With a right aortic arch a left-sided ductus is still more common. When there is a mirror-image branching of the right arch, the left PDA arises from the distal innominate (or proximal left subclavian artery) (see Chapter 23). Much less commonly, the right PDA persists in mirror image to the normal, passing from the right arch beyond the right subclavian artery to the right pulmonary artery origin. A PDA (or ligamentum arteriosus) arising from an aortic diverticulum or from an aberrant left subclavian artery is one form of vascular ring (see Chapter 38).

Histology

The histology of a persistent PDA is different from that of simple prolonged patency of the ductus.[G6] It is also different from that of its adjoining great arteries. A persisting PDA has a relatively thick intima with an unfragmented elastic lamina separating it from the media, an additional, pronounced wavy unfragmented subendothelial elastic lamina,[G6] and variable mucoid material in the media in which there is an intricate helicoid spiral muscular arrangement. The media contain variable amounts of elastic material that may form conspicuous lamellae so that the ductus wall then resembles the wall of the aorta (aortification).

Aneurysms of the Ductus Arteriosus

Aneurysms of the ductus arteriosus, which are rare lesions, appear to be of two types. One type is the so-called spontaneous infantile ductal aneurysm, which is present at birth or develops very shortly thereafter,[H4] and the other type develops in childhood or adult life.

The occurrence of the first type may not be suspected until autopsy after death from other causes.[D2] The aneurysm involves the entire length of the ductus arteriosus and is almost always associated with occlusion of the pulmonary artery end and a relatively narrow but patent aortic end. It usually contains thrombus and occasionally is a site of infection and embolism. Rarely it may be a true dissecting aneurysm of the ductal wall.[F2] This rare lesion presents most often in newborns with a history of respiratory difficulties.[H4] It produces a tumorlike shadow of variable size that projects beyond the mediastinum adjacent to the aortic knob in the posteroanterior chest film, but it may be discovered only incidentally at autopsy after death from other causes.[D2,F2] The aneurysm almost always regresses spontaneously within weeks or months, presumably as a result of complete thrombosis and organization, but progressive enlargement or the onset of hoarseness from recurrent laryngeal nerve involvement is an indication for surgical exploration and excision.[H4] Less marked dilatation of the ductus can be seen on the plain chest x-ray film as a fusiform shadow between 6 and 18 hours of birth, disappearing by 24–48 hours of age.[B7] It has been called the *ductus bump.*

The second type of ductal aneurysm occurs in childhood or adult life, is very rare, and is thought to be unrelated to the infantile form. The ductus may be patent at both ends, but usually the pulmonary artery end is closed.[G5,T6] There is a greater tendency for progressive enlargement, and death may occur from rupture.[C4]

CLINICAL FEATURES AND DIAGNOSTIC CRITERIA

The symptoms and signs in patent ductus arteriosus are the consequence of left-to-right shunting, and the magnitude of the shunt depends upon the size of the communication and the relationship between the systemic and pulmonary vascular resistances. In this regard, it is similar to the other types of high-pressure shunts, which include those across the ventricular septum and others from the aorta itself.

Large Patent Ductus Arteriosus

Aortic and pulmonary artery pressures are essentially equal when the PDA is large so that shunting is dependent upon changes in pulmonary vascular resistance, since systemic vascular resistance remains fairly constant after birth.[R6] As the neonatal pulmonary vascular resistance falls, left-to-right shunting rapidly increases and the infant develops severe congestive heart failure within a month or so of birth. There is tachypnea, tachycardia, sweating and irritability, poor feeding, and slow weight gain.[K1] Pulmonary edema and pneumonia or less severe and recurrent respiratory infection may occur.

On *examination*, there is an overactive precordium, sometimes with a systolic thrill,[A2] and evidence of cardiac enlargement with a thrusting left ventricular apical impulse. The pulse is jerky or frankly collapsing and the pulse pressure correspondingly wide; these features become more obvious when the heart failure is controlled medically. On *auscultation*, there is a systolic murmur maximal in the pulmonary area, with late systolic accentuation and minimal spillover into diastole.[R1] Occasionally, the murmur is continuous, but occasionally with severe heart failure no murmur is heard.[M2] The first and second heart sounds are accentuated, and there is a third sound at the apex or a prominent middiastolic mitral flow murmur.[R2] There is liver enlargement and elevated jugular venous pressure and frequently rales in the lung bases.

The *electrocardiogram* (ECG) shows left ventricular enlargement with deep Q waves and tall R waves in left ventricular leads. There may also be evidence of right ventricular hypertrophy with upright T waves in right precordial leads and evidence of left atrial enlargement with widened P waves. The *chest x-ray* shows marked cardiomegaly and plethora with or without interstitial or alveolar pulmonary edema. The main pulmonary artery segment is enlarged, as is the ascending aorta. The *echocardiogram* shows left atrial

enlargement, and the ductus itself may be visualized with 2D echocardiographic techniques.

In occasional infants with a large PDA the congestive heart failure may be less marked, presumably because the pulmonary vascular resistance does not fall to the same degree as usual. As with a large ventricular septal defect, there is in these infants a tendency to develop an increased pulmonary vascular resistance by the age of 2 years. The same may occur in those in whom the heart failure is controlled medically and the ductus is not closed surgically. These patients become asymptomatic and the left-to-right shunt diminishes. The murmur becomes purely systolic, the pulmonary component of the second heart sound is markedly accentuated, the apical middiastolic murmur disappears, and the pulse loses its jerky quality. Right ventricular hypertrophy becomes dominant in the electrocardiogram, the heart becomes smaller on the chest x-ray and pulmonary plethora disappears. Cyanosis develops as the pulmonary vascular resistance increases above the systemic vascular resistance (Eisenmenger's syndrome), usually by the age of 5 years or more. *Differential cyanosis* may be noted with blueness of the feet and sometimes the left hand, but not the face or right hand.

Moderate-Sized Patent Ductus Arteriosus

The left-to-right shunt in moderate-sized PDA is regulated by the size of the ductus arteriosus, and in this setting pulmonary artery pressure is only moderately elevated. As the neonatal pulmonary vascular resistance falls, the shunt increases and heart failure may occur; but by the second or third month of life, the compensatory left ventricular hypertrophy is usually associated with clinical improvement and stabilization of symptoms. Physical development may be somewhat retarded and breathlessness and fatigue may occur, but many persons with moderate-sized PDA remain essentially asymptomatic until the second decade of life or later.

On *examination*, the pulse is jerky, the precordium mildly overactive, and the left ventricle palpable at the apex in association with some cardiac enlargement. The classical continuous murmur is usually present to *auscultation* by the age of 2–3 months, although it varies in intensity.[L1] The murmur is usually loud and often masks the heart sounds. It is maximal in the pulmonary artery and radiates upward beneath the midthird of the clavicle. As described by Gibson in 1900,[G1] "it begins after the commencement of the first sound—it persists through the second sound and dies away gradually during the long pause. The murmur is rough and thrilling. It begins softly and increases in intensity so as to reach its acme at or immediately after the incidence of the second sound, and from that point gradually wanes until its termination." Substandard physical growth is common; Krovetz and Warden found body weight below the third percentile in 26% of 515 surgically proven cases.[K1] The *electrocardiogram* may be relatively normal during infancy, but some degree of left ventricular hypertrophy develops in older children. The *chest x-ray* shows moderate cardiac enlargement and plethora and a prominent ascending aorta (in contrast to the findings in patients with a large ventricular or atrial septal defect). In adults, the PDA may be calcified. It is rare for the pulmonary vascular resistance to rise, and Eisenmenger's syndrome does not develop.

Small Patent Ductus Arteriosus

The left-to-right shunt is small in early life, and the pulmonary vascular resistance falls rapidly to normal after birth. Left ventricular failure does not occur, and symptoms are absent in infancy and childhood. They may appear much later in life, but usually attention is drawn to the condition by the murmur that is detected on routine physical examination.

Physical development is normal unless there is maternal rubella. The pulse is normal and the precordium not overactive. By 2–3 months of age a short systolic murmur is usually replaced by a murmur that spills over into diastole, or it may be continuous in the second left intercostal space but less intense and with less radiation than when the ductus is moderate in size. The continuous murmur varies greatly in intensity between patients and in some is detectable only when the patient is sitting or standing upright. *Electrocardiogram* and *chest x-ray* are normal or nearly so.

Special Investigations

Most children and young adults with a PDA and a continuous murmur maximal in the second left intercostal space do not need invasive studies before an operation unless other defects are suspected. Cardiac catheterization and angiography are indicated, however, in most infants and in patients in whom the murmur is atypical, particularly if the findings suggest an elevated pulmonary vascular resistance.

NATURAL HISTORY

The incidence of isolated PDA in term infants is about 1 in 2,000 live births[M6] and accounts for 5%–10% of all types of congenital heart disease. It is twice as common in women as in men.[C2] A PDA may occur in siblings, suggesting a genetic factor in some cases. It is particularly common when the mother contracts rubella during the first trimester of pregnancy and may then be associated with multiple peripheral pulmonary artery stenoses and renal artery stenosis.

Because of the early introduction of surgical closure of a PDA and its antedating of other methods of proving the diagnosis, the natural history of patent ductus arteriosus is not completely documented.

Spontaneous Closure

Campbell's study led him to conclude that spontaneous closure of an isolated PDA occurs in 0.6% of patients per year and that this rate is fairly constant through the first four decades of life.[C2] If this is accepted, it means that in about 20% of patients with PDAs, it will have closed by the age of 60 years. His study concerned only patients diagnosed beyond 12 months of age and was based entirely on clinical findings, closure being assumed to have occurred when a typical murmur was no longer audible, regardless of the size

of the ductus or of the initial right-to-left shunt. The early GLH experience, which is incompletely documented, suggests that the closure rate is much lower than this, and it is generally agreed that spontaneous closure is uncommon beyond 3–5 months of age in full-term infants. Delayed closure of the ductus arteriosus in preterm infants is, however, common (see "Special Situations and Controversies").

Death

The death rate from untreated PDA is highest in infancy, and it has been estimated that 30% of patients born with an isolated PDA die in the first year of life.[C2,H2] In fact, the risk of death is highest in the first few months of life.

After infancy, the annual death rate of patients with untreated PDA falls dramatically to about 0.5% per year.[C2] By the third decade, the death rate has increased to about 1% per year, by the fourth decade to 1.8% per year, and in subsequent decades it may be as high as 4% per year.[C2] As a result of this, about 42% of patients with PDA will have died by 45 years of age. Most of the deaths in older patients are related to the development of intractable left ventricular failure, secondary to the long-standing volume overload.

Modes of Death

In infants with a large PDA, death is almost always due to congestive heart failure. Recurrent respiratory infection terminating in pneumonia is a less common cause. In those with a large PDA who survive infancy, subsequent death is usually due to right heart failure secondary to the development of severe pulmonary vascular disease by the second or third decade. The incidence of pulmonary vascular disease in patients with large PDA is similar to the incidence in patients with large ventricular septal defect (see Chapter 20).

In patients with a moderate-sized PDA, congestive heart failure can be a cause of death from the third and fourth decade onward. Excluding infants and death from pulmonary vascular disease, Campbell estimated that heart failure was the cause of death in 30% of patients.[C2]

Subacute bacterial endocarditis occurs mainly as a complication of small PDA and less often with a moderate-sized ductus. It rarely occurs when the ductus is large. In the preantibiotic years, endocarditis was responsible for about 45% of deaths in patients with surgically untreated PDA.[A1,C2,K2] After the advent of antibiotics, few patients died from this cause, but they remained subject to another episode.

TECHNIQUE OF OPERATION

Division of the Patent Ductus Arteriosus

Except in neonates and some infants, the patent ductus arteriosus (PDA) is divided rather than ligated.

Unless the patient is an infant in severe heart failure, an intra-arterial needle is unnecessary. After the usual induction of anesthesia and preparations for operation (see Chapter 4), the patient is positioned on the right side. A small pad or pillow may be placed under the midchest. The patient is far enough down from the head of the table for the second assistant to be to the surgeon's right and still be comfortably in the sterile field. The patient is positioned near the surgeon's side of the table but not so much so that the first assistant, across the table from the surgeon, cannot see in the field well and work comfortably. The surgical nurse is to the surgeon's left and, as usual, is an integral part of the surgical team.

A curving skin incision is made, centered about 1–2 cm below the tip of the scapula. In infants, the incision is really a lateral one, since only the latissimus dorsi and the posterior part of the serratus anterior muscles need be cut. In children, the incision is posterolateral, extending posterosuperiorly to overlie the lower 1 or 2 cm of the trapezius muscle, which is also incised (Fig. 22-3). In patients who are in the second or later decade of life, the incision extends from the anterior axillary line around the scapula and up midway between the spine and posterior scapular border over the lower 4 cm of the trapezius muscle. After incising the latissimus dorsi muscle (and trapezius if indicated), the scapula is elevated and the ribs are counted from the top down. Three criteria are used. The surgeon's left hand is passed under the serratus, and the most superior rib, the first, is identified by palpation. The serratus anterior attaches superiorly to the second rib, and with upward traction on the scapula elevator the prominent posterior border of this muscle is made taut, which allows identification of this attachment and thus of the second rib. The third criterion is that the second intercostal space is nearly always appreciably wider than the third. The second and third criteria for rib counting are more reliable than the first. The fifth rib is identified and scored. Only then are the posterior and midportion of the serratus anterior muscle divided so that the muscle incision may be directly over the fifth rib. The fourth interspace may be opened with the knife or diathermy while taking care not to damage the lung (GLH), or the chest may be entered through the superior part of the bed of the nonresected fifth rib (or the inferior part of the fourth rib) (UAB). In this latter method, the periostium over the rib is incised, and its superior part is elevated from the front and back with a periosteal elevator.

After extending the incision in the rib cage anteriorly and posteriorly, the rib spreader is placed with the ratcheted portion anteriorly (Fig. 22-3). At first the rib spreader is opened only partially, but as the intrathoracic operation proceeds it is gradually opened further to obtain wide exposure.

With a soft retractor on the lung, an incision is made in the mediastinal pleura over the upper descending thoracic aorta (Fig. 22-3b). (Gross made an anterolateral thoracotomy incision and placed the pleural incision midway between the phrenic and vagus nerve and retracted the vagus nerve posteriorly.[G3,G7,G8,G9] Exposure is less good with this method.) The pleural incision is made nearly as long as that for coarctation repair, and interrupted silk sutures are placed rather close together on the anterior and posterior pleural flaps. The soft retractor holding the lung is removed, a moist gauze is placed over the lung, and the anterior flap sutures are gathered into two groups and pulled taut by anchoring them to the ratcheted handle of the rib spreader or to the drapes.

This allows the anesthesiologist to inflate the left lung and to ventilate it as well as the right during the operation. The sutures on the posterior pleural flap may be similarly placed on tension.

These maneuvers also place tension on the tissues and the dissection is done sharply and under perfect control (Fig. 22-3c). The hemiazygous vein is divided between ligatures. The PDA is completely dissected by a standardized technique (Fig. 23-1d, e, f). In small infants, particular care is taken that the structure identified as the PDA connects the aorta and the pulmonary artery and is not the left pulmonary artery or the distal aortic arch. As the dissection proceeds, the recurrent laryngeal nerve is not dissected out, although it may be seen behind the areolar tissue just inferior and posterior to the PDA. If a tape or heavy ligature had been placed around the PDA to aid in the dissection, it is now removed.

In infants and young children, one straight and two angled fine-toothed Potts' patent ductus clamps are selected. In teenage children and adults, the longer-handled and less sharp-toothed DeBakey patent ductus clamps are used.[1] All three clamps are examined thoroughly by the surgeon to be sure they are in proper condition. If the Potts clamps are used, the ratchet on the clamp must be closed completely after placement for them to be safe. At about this time, and particularly in older children and adults, the anesthesiologist reduces the arterial blood pressure (see Chapter 4) and keeps the patient hypotensive until the clamps are removed. The role of the assistants during ductal division is explained to them, and they are asked to hold the clamps and get a comfortable feel for them. From this point on until the clamps are removed, the surgeon must not look anywhere but at the wound and must concentrate completely on the operation.

The straight clamp is placed completely across the aortic end of the PDA, making sure that its tip does not pick up the recurrent laryngeal nerve or other soft tissue deep to the ductus. This clamp, in the surgeon's left hand, is gently pulled anteriorly, and the angled ductus clamp is placed behind (lateral to) it, usually on the aorta contiguous with the PDA rather than on the ductus itself. The straight clamp is removed. With the clamp on the aortic origin of the PDA held in the surgeon's right hand, the other angled clamp is placed with the left hand on the pulmonary end of the ductus. The lappet of pericardium has earlier been dissected off from the PDA, and the clamp must catch only ductus and not any of the lappet or other fibrous tissue lest the ductus be held insecurely and retract within the pericardium. This clamp, like the clamp on the aortic end, is "squeezed" back onto the pulmonary artery as much as possible to give added length to the ductus. The ductus is divided midway between these clamps by Potts scissors; the clamp on the aortic end is positioned in the second assistant's hands and that on the pulmonary end in the first assistant's hands.

The aortic end of the PDA is oversewn with two rows of 5-0 polypropylene suture placed as a whip stitch (Fig. 22-3g). The pulmonary end is similarly closed. Although accurate

---

[1] The Potts' fine-toothed clamps are Muller no. (straight) CH6500 and (angled) CH5602. The DeBakey ones are Pilling no. (straight) 37-1160 and (angled) 37-1161.

suturing is of obvious importance, the widely separated placement of the clamps, so that a substantial cuff of ductus protrudes beyond them after ductus division, is the key to a safe repair.

The clamp is removed from the pulmonary end of the divided ductus, and a sponge is pressed firmly against the suture line by the first assistant. The clamp is removed from the aortic side, and a sponge is pressed against the aortic end of the divided ductus by the surgeon. The field is kept dry with a sucker held against the sponges until 5 minutes have passed. Unless the original placement of the clamps has been faulty and the cuff available for suturing too short or the suture closure grossly inaccurate, any bleeding that occurs as the clamps are removed stops within this period. If not, and if the suture line is basically as good as it should be, a stitch of 5-0 polypropylene suture catching simply the adventitia on both sides of the suture line nearly always suffices to control the bleeding.

A pledget of gel foam is left between the divided ends of the ductus to keep the suture lines from rubbing on each other. The mediastinal pleura is closed with interrupted 5-0 silk sutures, leaving a small opening at each end. In the unlikely event that there is bleeding from the suture lines after operation, this closure will tamponade the bleeding and save the patient's life during transport to the operating room for definitive control.

The rib spreader is removed, a small catheter is inserted into the posterior gutter through a stab wound in about the seventh interspace at the midaxillary line, and suction of about 15–25 cm of water is placed on it. The chest wall is closed, the anesthesiologist inflating the lung just before the ribs are pulled together. The muscles are closed individually with a running suture of a slowly absorbable synthetic material (polyglycolic acid), and the skin is sutured with the same type of suture in a subcuticular stitch. In infants, the chest tube is removed in the operating room.

Ligation of the Patent Ductus Arteriosus

In neonates and some infants, the PDA may be ligated rather than divided, since the vessels are pliable and yielding. The technique is basically that described by Blalock in 1946.[B6]

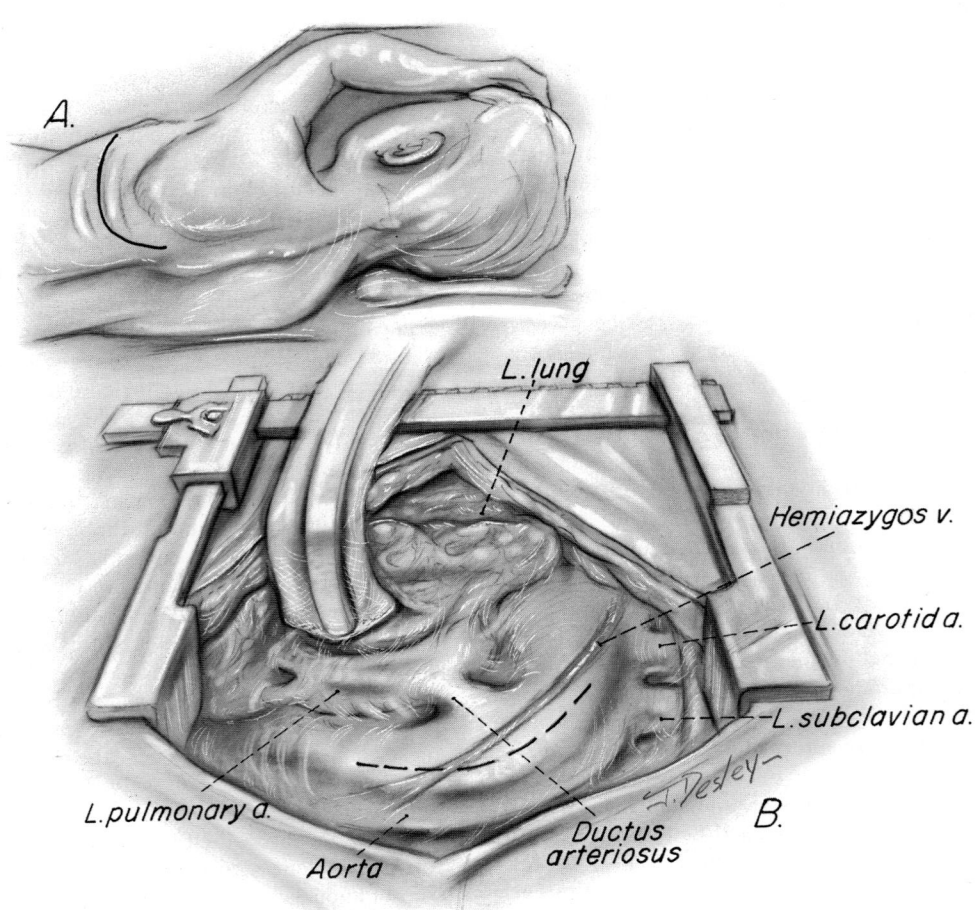

Figure 22-3 Closure of the PDA by division.
(a) The posterolateral incision is shown in a patient properly positioned for operation.
(b) The rib spreader has been placed and opened to its final width over a period of 5–10 minutes. The lung is gently retracted anteriorly, with a malleable retractor or the surgeon's hand. The dashed line shows the incision in the mediastinal pleura, which is made over the hemiazygos vein. Usually the vein is then ligated and divided.

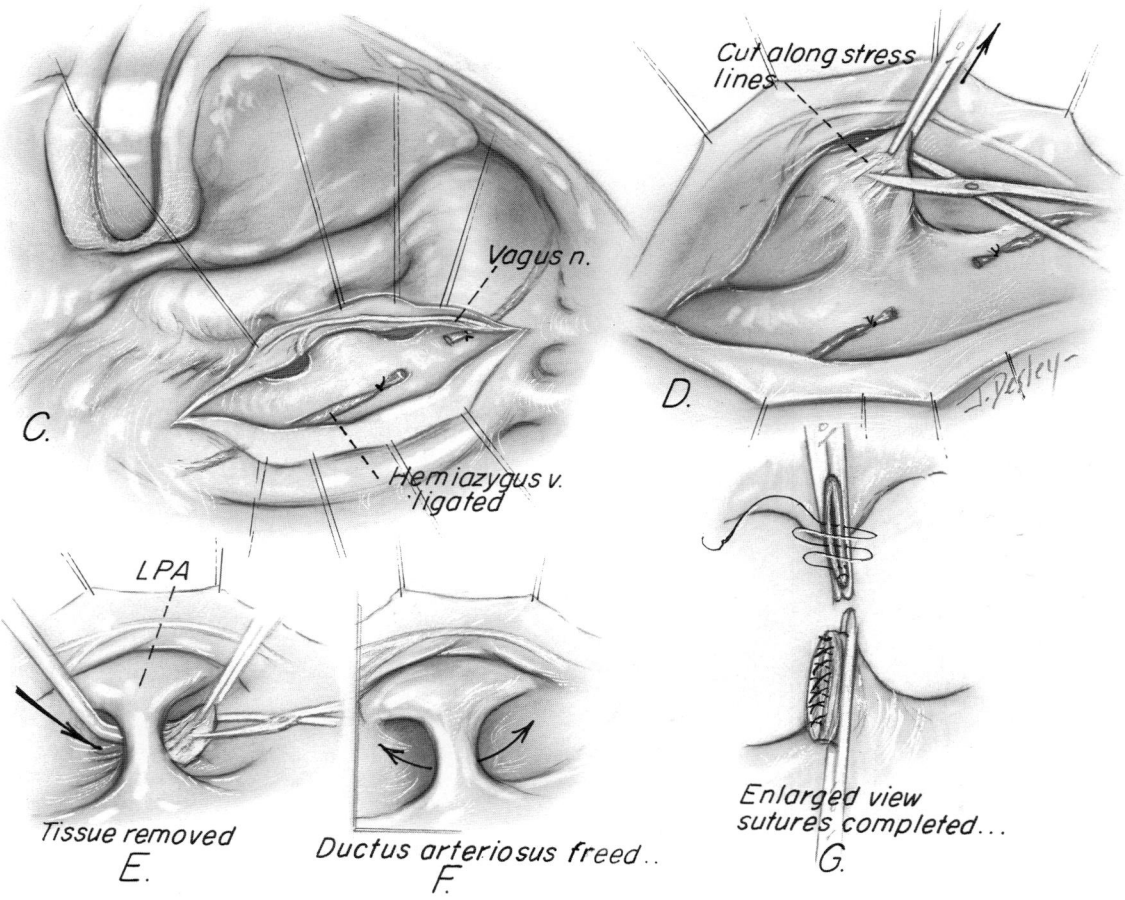

Vagus n.

Hemiazygus v. ligated

C.

Cut along stress lines

D.

LPA

Tissue removed
E.

Ductus arteriosus freed..
F.

Enlarged view sutures completed...
G.

Figure 22-3 *(continued)*

(c) The traction sutures on the mediastinal pleura are in place, and the malleable retractor will be removed.

(d) The areolar tissues and pericardial lappet anterior to the PDA are elevated by the assistant's tissue forceps, and the surgeon may retract the aortic adventitia toward him or herself to place tension on the tissue and develop the fine transverse *stress lines* that guide the dissection. These indicate that the tissue is under proper tension for safe dissection, with many little "snips" with the tips of scissors. Care is taken that the dissection leaves the adventitial layer of the PDA undisturbed.

(e) After the anterior surface of the ductus has been cleared far enough centrally that the junction of the PDA with the left pulmonary artery is visible, the superior and inferior ductal surfaces are similarly dissected. Then a right-angled clamp in the surgeon's right hand is passed behind the PDA, palpating above the ductus with the left index finger to guide the clamp. The clamp merely tents up the areolar tissue behind the ductus, which is then grasped with tissue forceps and cut away with little snips with the tips of the scissors.

(f) The maneuver illustrated in E, repeated several times, creates a space behind the PDA. The recurrent laryngeal nerve is usually not dissected but can be seen in the areolar tissue behind the space.

(g) The ductus has been divided between clamps (see text). The aortic end has been oversewn (see text), and the pulmonary end is being oversewn.

LPA, left pulmonary artery.

The operation proceeds exactly as described for ductal division until the PDA is completely dissected. Adventitial stitches are taken, with a double armed 5-0 polypropylene suture, into the accessible superior, inferior, and anterior aspects of the aortic wall contiguous with the PDA (Fig. 22-4). One end of the suture is passed beneath the ductus, and the ends are held. A similar purse-string type of stitch is placed at the pulmonary end. The aortic stitch is pulled up and tied snugly; then the suture at the pulmonary end is tied. A long length of ductus is now between these two tied stitches. Finally, a transfixion ligature at the middle of the PDA completes the repair (Fig. 22-4). The operation is completed as described for division of the PDA.

Closure of the Patent Ductus Arteriosus in Older Adults

When a PDA requires closure in the fifth or sixth decade of life, the aortic end is often calcified and the ductus is very short. An alternative technique using cardiopulmonary by-

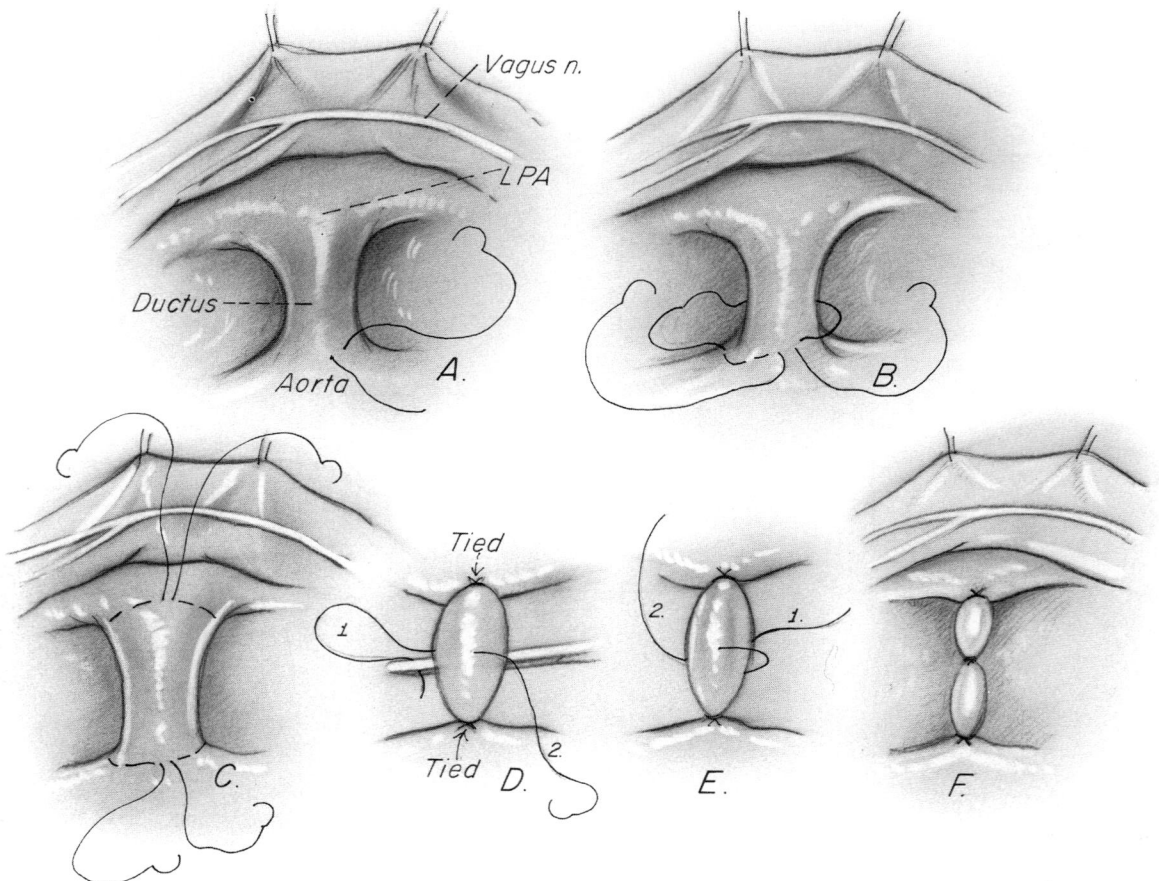

Figure 22-4   The technique for suture closure of the PDA.

(*a*) The dissection has been completed as shown in Figure 22-3. An adventitial purse-string stitch has been started around the aortic end of the ductus.

(*b*) The remainder of the adventitial stitches have been placed after one arm of the suture has been brought beneath the PDA.

(*c*) A similar purse-string stitch has been placed around the pulmonary end of the ductus.

(*d*) The two purse-string sutures have been snugly tied down. A transfixion ligature (1) has been placed through the ductus, the needle cut off, and the end brought beneath the ductus with a right angle clamp.

(*e*) In similar fashion, the other end (2) is brought beneath the ductus in the opposite direction.

(*f*) The transfixion ligature has been tied, leaving a space between it and the purse-string sutures at either end.

pass (CPB), described by Goncalves-Estella and colleagues[G4] and later by O'Donovan and Beck,[O1] is then useful.

With the usual preparations (see Chapter 2), a median sternotomy incision is made, and the usual stay sutures, recording catheters, and purse-string sutures are placed. The aorta and pulmonary trunk are dissected apart. CPB is established with a single venous cannula (see details in Chapter 2), and the water bath is made as cold as possible. The head of the table is lowered to place the patient in moderate Trendelenburg position. As the heart begins to slow from the cold perfusion, the ductus is obliterated by compressing the front wall of the left pulmonary artery (LPA) against it with the finger of the left hand. This is essential, for otherwise ductal flow into the pulmonary artery will overdistend the pulmo-

nary vascular bed and the right ventricle (this will not occur when the heart is ejecting adequately). When the temperature is 28°C, the aorta is cross-clamped and the cold cardioplegic solution is infused. The perfusion temperature is stabilized at 25°C, and the flow rate is reduced to 0.5 $l \cdot min^{-1} m^{-2}$. The finger is now removed, and the distal main pulmonary atery is opened anteriorly and the longitudinal incision continued into the LPA opposite the ductus. (In the event that external pressure on the LPA does not control ductal flow during CPB cooling, flows are temporarily reduced to a low level and the pulmonary artery incision is made so that the finger can be placed directly over the ostium of the ductus to control the flow from it into the LPA. CPB flows are then increased until cooling is completed.)

With the temperature stabilized at 25°C, the flow rate reduced to 0.5 l·min^{-1}m^{-2}, and the intracardiac sucker positioned within the LPA beyond the ductus to aspirate blood entering it, the ductal orifice is closed by placing and tying three pledgetted sutures of 3-0 polypropylene. This is readily accomplished because the pulmonary artery end of the ductus is very rarely calcified and the pulmonary artery tissues are strong enough to hold sutures well. The period of low flow perfusion is less than 10 minutes. Flows are then restored, the table leveled, and rewarming of the patient with the perfusate begun. Any leak from the ductus closure site is secured with additional sutures. The pulmonary arteriotomy is closed with a running stitch of fine polypropylene.

With strong suction on the aortic needle vent, the aortic clamp is released. The remainder of the operation is completed in the usual fashion.

Closure of the Patent Ductus Arteriosus in the Premature Infant

The technique of the perioperative management and the operation is quite different when surgical closure of the ductus is believed to be indicated in the premature infant, most of whom weigh about 1,000 g and some as little as 600 g (UAB). Precise management of ventilation, fluid administration, and body temperature, as well as a precise surgical technique, are essential for success.[S1]

The infant is intubated in the neonatal nursery, and proper position of the tube is verified by a chest x-ray. The patient, covered by a plastic wrap blanket and cloth cap, is transported to the operating room in a prewarmed (37°C) transport isolette, which is taken into the operating room.

The room is prewarmed to about 30°C, and the patient is placed on the right side on an infant operating table with overhead radiant warmers and a servocontrol set at 37°C. Alternatively, the operation may be undertaken in the Intensive Care nursery.[E7]

After preparation and draping, a short left lateral incision about 2.5 cm in length is made, cutting the latissimus dorsi and the posterior aspect of the serratus anterior muscles. The chest is entered through the fourth interspace, and a small rib spreader is put into place. With a narrow malleable retractor, the lung is held forward by the first assistant. The ductus is usually large but is variable in its position. It may course superiorly as well as anteriorly from the aorta and be immediately adjacent to the distal transverse aortic arch and easily mistaken for the arch. It may course directly anteriorly and be well inferior to the arch.

The friable, vascular tissue makes the usual complete dissection of the ductus inadvisable, and instead just two tissue planes are developed.[G10,K3,M3,T2] The mediastinal pleura is incised with fine scissors just superior to the aortic end of the ductus and then just inferior to it. The tissue plane superior to the ductus is developed by gently spreading fine scissors, as is that inferiorly. As the inferior tissue plane is developed, the back wall (or right side) of the ductus is seen. No attempt is made to pass an instrument around the back wall. Instead, a medium-sized hemoclip[2] on a holder is positioned well

---

[2] Ethicon Ligaclip LC 300.

across the ductus at its aortic end, and by closing the holder the ductus is closed. The adventia of the aorta may be grasped and gently retracted toward the surgeon as the clip is placed. A second one may be placed on the pulmonary end if desired.

A no. 12 catheter is brought out through a stab wound in the chest wall and placed on suction for closed drainage. The chest wall is closed with two pericostal sutures. The muscles are closed with a continuous suture of fine absorbable suture (polyglycolic acid) and the closure is completed with a subcuticular stitch of fine absorbable sutures.

The infant is transferred back to the high-risk nursery in the same prewarmed transfer isolette.

SPECIAL FEATURES OF POSTOPERATIVE CARE

The care is simple after division or ligation of patent ductus arteriosus and follows the principles described in Chapter 5. The patient is usually extubated in the operating room or a few hours after leaving it. The chest tube is removed in the operating room or a few hours after leaving it. The patient leaves the intensive care unit the following morning.

When the operation is done with cardiopulmonary bypass, the care is also simple and usual (see Chapter 5).

EARLY RESULTS

Hospital Mortality

Within 10 years of Gross and Hubbard's first successful case, the hospital mortality for surgical closure of uncomplicated PDA had become very low. Gross and Longino, in 1951, reported eight deaths (1.9%, CL 1%–3%) among their first 412 surgically treated cases.[G9] In 1955, Ash and Fischer reported no deaths (0%, CL 0%–1.6%) among 116 consecutive children (ages 4 months to 14 years) undergoing surgical closure of a PDA before 1955.[A2] Other similar experiences reinforce the idea that the operation has become very safe, and hospital mortality (UAB, GLH) in recent years has in fact approached zero (Tables 22-2, 22-3).

Incremental Risk Factors for Early Death

Because the inoperability of patients with essentially isolated PDA and severe pulmonary vascular disease became recognized in the early 1950s,[E4] because most patients are now operated in infancy or childhood (Fig. 22-5), and because as a result of early operation, the probability of early postoperative death approaches zero, no risk factors can be identified by study of the experiences of the last 15 or so years. Currently, neither associated congenital anomalies (Table 22-4), nor pulmonary hypertension (Table 22-5), nor mild or moderate increase of pulmonary vascular resistance (Table 22-6) increases the risk of hospital death. Also, early risks are very low no matter what technique is used (Table 22-7). However, by considering the entire span of time since Gross first successfully closed a PDA in 1938, certain incremental risk factors can be identified.

Table 22-2 The surgical experience and hospital mortality with closure of essentially isolated PDA (GLH; 1966–1984). The one hospital death (0.4%; CL 0.05%–1.4%) was after ductal repair, in 1968, in a 44-year-old man who also had mild aortic incompetence and a history of bacterial endocarditis 1 year before; death was from an arrhythmia on the third postoperative day. Only 11 of the 246 patients had ductal ligation (rather than division), and ductal patency recurred in one such patient.

Age ≤ <	n	% of Total	Heart Failure n	%	PAP > 20 mmHg n	%
Months						
1	1(0)	0.4%	1	100%	1	100%
1---3	3(0)	1.2%	3	100%	2	67%
3---6	18(0)	7.3%	15	83%	11	61%
6---12	3(0)	12.6%	25	81%	17	55%
Years						
1---5	89(0)	36.2%	18	20%	15	17%
5---10	70(0)	28.4%	3	4%	2	3%
10---20	20(0)	8.1%		0%		0%
20---30	6(0)	2.4%	1[a]	17%	1[a]	17%
30---40	2(0)	0.8%		0%		0%
40---50	2(1)*	0.8%		0%		0%
50---60	2(0)	0.8%	1[b]	50%		0%
60---70	2(0)	0.8%	1[b]	50%	1	50%
Total	246(1)	100%	68	28%	50	20%

KEY: ( ), hospital deaths; PAP, mean pulmonary artery pressure.
[a] Third reoperation (others done elsewhere).
[b] Chronic atrial fibrillation.

When *pulmonary vascular disease* is *severe* and the shunt is bidirectional or dominantly right to left, the risk is high; five of 14 such patients (36%, CL 21%–53%) died in the hospital in our early Mayo Clinic experience.[E4] Death was either from hemorrhage during the operation (from the pulmonary artery suture line, since the pulmonary artery pressure after closure is *higher* than systemic arterial pressure and the pulmonary artery is large and thin walled) or occurred suddenly some days later without any demonstrable cause.[E4] Probably the results would be the same today.

When pulmonary vascular disease is mild or moderate in severity, and thus when a large left-to-right shunt is present, there is no increased risk (Table 22-6). Even in the early era, 16 among 271 patients undergoing repair of PDA by us at the Mayo Clinic had severe pulmonary hypertension but with only mild or moderate pulmonary vascular disease and a large left-to-right shunt, and there were no (0%; CL 0%–11%) early or late deaths.[E4]

Even in the absence of severe pulmonary vascular disease, *older age* mildly increases the risk of surgical closure. This increase is from the technical problems posed by the friable and often calcified ductal wall in older patients and the tendency of the very long-standing volume overload of the left ventricle to predispose to fatal arrhythmias (see Table 22-2). The mildly increased risk in the older age group is illustrated by the report of Black and Goldman in 1972, describing one death (2%, CL 0.2%–6%) in 53 adults (age 14–55 years) undergoing surgical closure of a PDA. Death occurred at early reoperation for postoperative bleeding

Table 22-3 Hospital mortality after repair of isolated patent ductus arteriosus exclusive of preterm infants (UAB). The experience was studied in 1980; later the years 1982 and 1983 were added to identify any trends with time. The "Total" column is the combination of the two columns to the left. No deaths occurred in the overall experience, 1967–1984.

Age ≤ <	Year of Operation 1967–1979 n	Hospital Deaths (No.)	1982–1984 n	Hospital Deaths (No.)	Total n	Hospital Deaths (No.)
Months						
1	3		0			
1---3	9		4		13	
3---6	9		5		14	
6---12	17		7		24	
12---24	28		1		29	
24---48	38		9		47	
Years						
4---10	59		9		68	
10---20	24		3		27	
20---30	15		0		15	
30---40	2		1		3	
40---50	7		0		7	
50---60	6		1		7	
60---70	2		1		3	
70---80	1		0		1	
Total	220	0	41	0	261	0(0%; CL 0%–0.7%)

KEY: CL, 70% confidence limits.

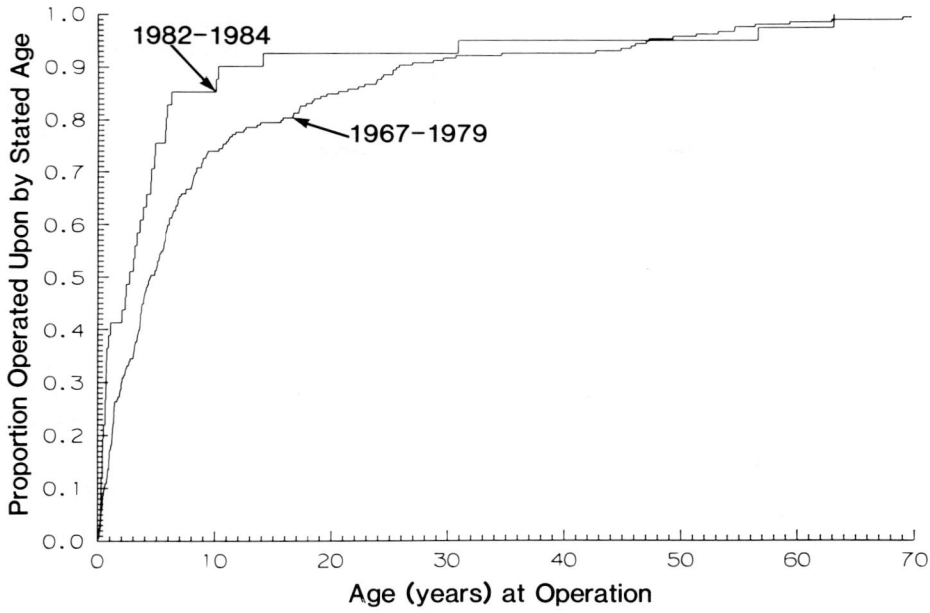

Figure 22-5 Proportion of patients receiving surgical closure of an essentially isolated PDA by a given age in the two time periods studied (UAB; 1967–1979 and 1982–1984). P for difference = .005. The proportions receiving operation by 1/2, 1, 2, 5, and 10 years of age are 0.10, 0.17, 0.30, 0.52, and 0.76, respectively, for the 1967–1979 group and 0.22, 0.39, 0.42, 0.76, and 0.85, respectively, for the 1982–1984 group.

from a tear in the aorta.[B3] In recent years, the technical problems in older patients have been eased by the use of an open technique under certain circumstances (see "Technique of Operation").

Left Vocal Cord Paralysis

Uncommonly, transient left vocal cord paralysis results from manipulation of the recurrent laryngeal nerve.

Phrenic Nerve Paralysis

Paralysis of the phrenic nerve with elevation of the hemidiaphragm is an uncommon complication of PDA closure. It usually occurs on the left side and nearly always in infants but is not necessarily thought to be due to surgical damage to the phrenic nerve since it may develop on the right side. It often regresses spontaneously but may complicate the early postoperative period.

Table 22-4 Associated anomalies in a surgical series of essentially isolated patent ductus arteriosus (GLH; 1966–1984). The categories are not mutually exclusive.

Associated Anomalies	No. of Cases
Mild congenital aortic stenosis and/or incompetence	5
Mild congenital mitral valve disease	5
Small VSD	8
Right or left pulmonary artery stenosis	3
Congenital complete heart block	1
Preterm infant	14[a]
Rubella syndrome	16[b]
Somatic congenital anomalies	9[b]
Congenital lobar emphysema	1
Laryngeal web	1

KEY: VSD, ventricular septal defect.

[a] Operation done in 4 patients at 2–5 months of age and in 10 between 1–13 years of age.

[b] Includes one example of Larsen's syndrome and one of Cornelia de Lang syndrome.

Table 22-5 Surgical closure of essentially isolated patent ductus arteriosus (GLH; 1966–1984): distribution of preoperative mean pulmonary artery pressure among patients in whom it was ≥ 20 mmHg. Cardiac catheterization was done in these 50 patients because there was a suggestion on clinical grounds that the pulmonary vascular resistance was elevated.

Mean Pulmonary Artery Pressure (mmHg) ≤ <	No. of Patients	% of Total
20---30	13	26%
30---40	7	14%
40---50	15	30%
50---60	12	24%
60---70	1	2%
Uncertain	2	4%
Total	50	100%

Table 22-6 Surgical closure of essentially isolated patent ductus arteriosus (GLH; 1966–1984): distribution of preoperative pulmonary vascular resistance among patients catheterized preoperatively (see Table 22-5).

Pulmonary Vascular Resistance (units · m²)		No. of Patients	% of Total
≤	<		
	2	8	16%
2	5	25	50%
5	7	10	20%
7			0%
NA		7	14%
Total		50	100%

KEY: NA, not available because oxygen consumption was not measured.

Chylothorax

Chylothorax is a rare complication of surgical ductal closure. Its management is discussed in Chapter 5, Section 3.

LATE RESULTS

Survival

Life expectancy is normal after surgical closure of an uncomplicated PDA in infancy or childhood. When moderate or severe pulmonary vascular disease has developed preoperatively, late deaths may result from its progression, as is the case in children with ventricular septal defect (see Chapter 20, "Pulmonary Hypertension" in Section 1, Late Results).

When the operation is performed in adults with advanced and long-standing chronic congestive heart failure, premature late death may not always be avoided. This is because the cardiomyopathy secondary to long-standing left ventricular volume overload is irreversible in some patients, in an entirely analogous way to the situation in patients with long-standing aortic valve incompetence (see Chapter 12, "Left Ventricular Structure and Function" in section on Late Results).

Symptomatic and Functional Status

The disappearance of the signs and symptoms of congestive heart failure are dramatic after surgical closure of a large PDA. Ash and Fischer recount that the marked hepato-megaly and splenectomy of a 3-year-old girl with cardiac cachexia and advanced heart failure from a large PDA were no longer detectable 3 hours after surgical closure of the ductus arteriosus and that the cardiac size on chest x-ray film had returned to near normal within 4 months.[A2]

Physical Development

It has been presumed that when a large isolated PDA is closed in infancy, the growth pattern becomes normal. However, retardation, particularly as regards height, tends to persist,[E6] particularly when the operation is delayed beyond infancy or the child has a rubella syndrome. The same may occur after repair of ventricular septal defect (see Chapter 20, "Physical Development" in Section 1, Late Results).

Recurrence of Ductal Patency

Currently, the incidence of recurrent or persisting ductal patency approaches zero when division or appropriate ligation techniques are used;[E2,L2] no cases of this have been recognized (UAB or GLH) since 1967, except in the one patient in whom simple ligation was used very early in this period (see Table 22-2). In an earlier era, it did occur. Jones reported 12 patients (20%, CL 14%–26%) with recurrent or persistent ductal patency out of 61 who had ductal ligation with heavy tape.[J1] Later, it became less common; Panagopoulos and colleagues reported only four cases (0.4%, CL 0.2%–0.8%) among 936 undergoing ductal closure, mostly by ligation.[P1] Trippestad and Efskind reported an incidence of 20 among 639 traced cases (3.1%, CL 2.4%–4.0%).[T5]

False Aneurysm

False aneurysm, a rare complication of surgical ductal closure, has not been encountered among patients in whom this procedure has been carried out at GLH or UAB; one successful repair has been performed (GLH) of a large false aneurysm (using femoro-femoral bypass and moderate hypothermia) that followed ductal closure elsewhere. This complication has usually occurred after ductal ligation rather than division,[P3,P4,R3] a fact that supports the use of division in most operations for closure of the patent ductus. Only two cases of false aneurysm have been reported after ductal division,[C1,H1] and these must have resulted from technical errors or infection.[R4]

The development of a false aneurysm is an indication for urgent reoperation.

INDICATIONS FOR OPERATION

The presence of *persisting patency* of the PDA (see "Morphology") is an indication for its surgical closure, and for at least 30 years it has been known that the optimal age for operating is during the first year of life.[A2] Patients, either term or preterm, with *prolonged patency of the ductus arteriosus* (see "Morphology") require surgical closure in very early life only when a large left-to-right shunt results in heart failure. In practice, this means that in term infants in the first

Table 22-7 Method of closure of isolated patent ductus arteriosus, exclusive of preterm infants (UAB). There were no hospital deaths.

Method of Closure of the Ductus	n	% of 261
Division	218	84%
Ligation	41	16%
Transpulmonary on cardiopulmonary bypass	2	0.8%
Total	261	100%

month of life surgical closure of a PDA is indicated only when symptoms of heart failure are present. The special situation in preterm infants is discussed in "Patent Ductus Arteriosus in Preterm Infants" in "Special Situations and Controversies."

Beyond the first month of life, prophylactic closure of the PDA is indicated. In the absence of symptoms, operation may be delayed until the age of about 6 months. However, surgical closure is indicated at any time before this when symptoms of heart failure or failure to thrive persist in spite of intense medical treatment.

Older age is not a contraindication to closure of an isolated PDA in the absence of severe pulmonary vascular disease.

Severe pulmonary vascular disease is a contraindication to surgical closure. The criteria of inoperability in this setting are the same as described for patients with ventricular septal defect (see Chapter 20, "Indications for Operation" in Section 1). In the case of patients with PDA, the ductus may be temporarily occluded at operation; if pulmonary artery pressure does not fall but remains severely elevated and no rise in aortic pressure occurs, it may be concluded that the shunt is *not* dominantly left to right. Closure of the ductus can therefore not reduce the pulmonary artery pressure nor the left atrial pressure and therefore cannot trigger a favorable change in pulmonary vascular resistance. Repair is contraindicated in this situation.

SPECIAL SITUATIONS AND CONTROVERSIES

Patent Ductus Arteriosus in Preterm Infants

Historical Note
In 1963, both Powell[P2] and, independently, De Cancq[D1] were apparently the first to close a PDA in a premature infant by operation. Subsequently, the improvement in the cardiovascular status of preterm infants after surgical closure of the PDA has been clearly demonstrated.[B2,J2]

Clinical Features and Diagnostic Criteria
The preterm infant with a PDA may have a continuous murmur, and under these circumstances the diagnosis of PDA is made with confidence.[C9,E5] The shunt is considered large enough to be important if there is pulmonary plethora and cardiomegaly on the chest x-ray film, if the peripheral pulses are bounding, or if by echocardiography the left atrium–aortic ratio is greater than or equal to 1.5.[J3]

A systolic murmur is less specific for PDA, but the diagnosis is made clinically if the murmur is associated with a hyperactive precordium, increased pulse pressure, or a positive chest x-ray or echocardiogram. A few preterm infants have these positive clinical and laboratory evidences of patent ductus arteriosus without a murmur being present.[M2,T1]

Natural History
A high proportion of preterm infants have prolonged patency of the ductus arteriosus after birth. Frequency increases with decreasing gestational age and with decreasing birth weight[H5] (Tables 22-8, 22-9). Thus, Siassi and colleagues report an incidence of PDA (based on the presence of a long

Table 22-8 A study of 69 consecutive preterm infants less than 2000 g birthweight who survived 30 or more hours, seen over a 6-month period (GLH, 1979); 9 who died less than 30 hours from birth were excluded (4 were less than 1000 g and died less than 8 hours of age; 4 of the 9 deaths were considered inevitable because of other complex anomalies). Indomethacin was not used in this group of infants, and no infant had surgical closure of the PDA. One of the 7 with a large shunt died at 14 days of age with a still patent ductus. There were 4 deaths in the other 25 infants at the ages of 4–40 days, with the ductus patent at autopsy in 1 only. In all late survivors the ductus was closed clinically.

Gestational Age (weeks)	n	Patent Ductus	
		n	%
26–30	13	10 (5)[a]	77% ⎤ 59%
31–32	24	12 (1)	50% ⎦ ⎤ P = .04
33–34	17	6	35% ⎤ 31% ⎦
35–36	15	4 (1)	27% ⎦
Total	69	32 (7)	46%

[a]Figures in parentheses are those with a large shunt.

systolic murmur) in 77% of premature infants with a gestational age of 28–30 weeks, 44% with a gestational age of 31–33 weeks, and 21% with a gestational age of 34–36 weeks.[S3] Birth weights of less than 1,000, 1,000–1,500, and 1,500–2,000 g were associated with a PDA incidence of 83%, 47%, and 27%, respectively.

The frequency of hemodynamically significant PDA is less, however, and is approximately 40% when the birth weight is less than 1,000 g and 10% when it is less than 1,750 g.[E5] A PDA has the same hemodynamic effects in preterm infants as in postnatal patients, as evidenced by collapsing pulses and radiographic evidence of increased pulmonary blood flow, left atrial enlargement, and cardiomegaly. Further, experimental studies in preterm lambs have shown that the left-to-right shunt through the open ductus is associated with reduced effective systemic blood flow and organ hypoperfusion.[B1] This has led to the speculation that necrotizing enterocolitis in preterm infants may be associated with a large patent ductus arteriosus.

There is a strong correlation between patency of the ductus arteriosus and idiopathic respiratory distress syndrome, although these are not thought to be causally related.[E1,E3,T1] There is also an association between fluid administration and ductal patency,[B5] and thus PDA is less frequent in neonatal units that restrict fluids in preterm infants.

Table 22-9 Further details of the data set in Table 22-8.

Birth Weight (g)	n	Patent Ductus	
		n	%
800–999	3	3(2)	100%
1000–1499	24	13(4)	54%
1500–1999	42	16(1)	38%
Total	69	32(7)	46%

Table 22-10 Hospital mortality after surgical closure of the ductus arteriosus in preterm infants (UAB; 1967–1979; 1982–1984). The experience was studied in 1979; later the years 1982 and 1983 were added to identify any trends with time. The weight of the infants varied between 600 and 1800 g.

Management of Ductus	n	Hospital Deaths		
		No.	%	CL
Ligation	71	14	20%	
Clip	32	7	22%	
Division[a]	1	1	100%	
Total	104	22	21%	17%–26%

KEY: CL, 70% confidence limits.

[a] Done by necessity, not election.

Technique of Operation
See earlier section, "Technique of Operation."

Special Features of Postoperative Care
Since surgical closure of the PDA is only one facet of the preterm infant's care, the patient is returned to care by the neonatologist in the neonatal intensive care unit. The chest tube may be left until mechanical ventilation of the infant is no longer necessary, because of the occasional development of a pneumothorax in preterm infants maintained on a ventilator.

Early Results
Overall hospital mortality is 10%–30%, that at UAB (Table 22-10) being representative. The tendency (UAB) in recent years has been to use the operation more frequently (Table 22-11), although this tendency may be related to the increasing number of even very small preterm infants being referred to specialized neonatal care services. The hospital mortality is not related to the interval between birth and operation (Table 22-12), but as in other circumstances in preterm infants is probably related to the birth weight and gestational age. Death may be from continuing respiratory distress, intracranial hemorrhage, or a diffuse coagulopathy,[B4] but it occurs rarely in the immediately perioperative period (Table

Table 22-11 Hospital mortality after surgical closure of the ductus arteriosus in preterm infants (UAB; 1967–1979; 1982–1984).

Year of Operation	n	Hospital Deaths		
		No.	%	CL
1974	4	0	0%	
1975	2	1	50%	7%–93%
1976	3	1	33%	4%–76%
1977	8	2	25%	9%–50%
1978	26	6	23%	14%–35%
1982	21	5	24%	14%–37%
1983	40	7	18%	11%–26%
Total	104	22	21%	17%–26%
$P(\chi^2)$			.8	

KEY: CL, 70% confidence limits.

Table 22-12 Hospital mortality after surgical closure of the ductus arteriosus in preterm infants (UAB; 1967–1979; 1982–1984).

Age at Operation (Days)	n	Hospital Deaths	
		No.	%
0	1	0	0%
1	9	3	33%
2	6	2	33%
3	5	2	40%
4	9	0	0%
5	9	3	33%
6	4	1	25%
7–13	25	3	12%
14–20	21	7	33%
21–45	15	1	7%
< 46	0		
Total	104	22	21%
$P(\chi^2)$			.28

22-13). There is no evidence that the incidence of intracranial hemorrhage is increased by surgical closure of the ductus.[S2]

There is usually an immediate improvement in the cardiac status, and the left atrial size is promptly reduced.[B4] At least one randomized study indicates overall benefit of early surgical closure of the PDA in preterm infants weighing less than 1,500 g and requiring mechanical ventilation.[C5] However, comparisons of medical versus surgical treatment are particularly difficult in this situation.

Late Results
Only one-half of the hospital survivors of the PDA operation are alive and well 1–5 years later.[B4] About one-third of the survivors have bronchopulmonary dysplasia on chest roentgenogram, with variable clinical findings. About one-sixth have more severe complications, such as retrolental fibroplasia, blindness, and cerebral palsy.[B4]

Indications for Operation
Indications for surgical PDA closure vary from respiratory distress (ventilator dependency and the need for high levels

Table 22-13 Day of death after surgical closure of the ductus arteriosus in preterm infants (UAB; 1967–1979; 1982–1984).

Postoperative Day	No. of Deaths
0 (day of surgery)	1[a]
1	2[b]
2	2
3	
4–10	2
10–20	2
> 20	13
Total	22

[a] Operation 1975.

[b] Operation 1978, 1983.

of oxygen in the inspired air in the absence of a significant shunt), to the demonstration of a large PDA (collapsing pulses, left atrial enlargement by echocardiography, and a large Q_P/Q_S by radionucleotide scanning), to none.

A selective protocol may be applied (UAB). Those patients weighing more than 1,600 g seldom require urgent PDA closure. In patients weighing 1,000–1,600 g with clinical evidence of PDA and/or respiratory distress, fluid restriction is initiated. If the signs begin to regress and the clinical and respiratory statuses improve within 24–72 hours, medical therapy is continued. Otherwise, the diagnosis of PDA is confirmed by Doppler echocardiography and/or radionucleotide scanning for Q_P/Q_S. If the shunt is large ($Q_P/Q_S > 3$), the ductus is closed surgically. The same protocol is followed in infants weighing less than 1,000 g, but only 18 hours are allowed for clinical improvement before proceeding with study and surgical repair.

A more conservative protocol may be followed (GLH). This is related to the following factors operating in the GLH environment that tend to lower the incidence of prolonged ductus patency with a shunt large enough to threaten survival:

1. Almost all infants are born within the hospital (rather than transferred after birth), this allowing consistent management.

2. Prenatal betamethasone is used. This drug significantly lowers the incidence of preterm infants of less than 34 weeks gestation with PDA requiring treatment.[C8]

3. Fluid intake is restricted whenever a significant shunt is suspected. As has been noted earlier, this simple therapy effectively reduces heart failure.[B5]

4. The numbers of infants seen with a birthweight of less than 1,000 g has been relatively small, and surgical intervention has not been considered appropriate in the first 24 hours of life in this group (GLH).

5. Indomethacin (0.2 mg·kg^{-1} body weight) is used.[F1,H3] This drug has been effective in closing the ductus in 75% of the preterm infants[E1] (see Tables 22-8, 22-9). Its possible toxic effects have not been considered a contraindication to its use.

6. A simple method of treatment is desirable since 80%–100% of PDAs in premature infants eventually close spontaneously.

REFERENCES

A

1. Abbott M: *Atlas of Congenital Heart Disease*. New York: American Heart Association, 1936.

2. Ash R, Fischer D: Manifestations and results of treatment of patent ductus arteriosus in infancy and childhood. An analysis of 138 cases. *Pediatrics* 16:695, 1955.

B

1. Baylen BG, Ogata H, Ikegami M, Jacobs HC, Jobe AH, Emmanouilides GC: Left ventricular performance and regional blood flows before and after ductus arteriosus occlusion in premature lambs treated with surfactant. *Circulation* 67:837, 1983.

2. Baylen BG, Emmanouilides GC: Patent ductus arteriosus in the newborn, in GA Gregory, DW Thibeault (eds): *Neonatal Pulmonary Care*, Menlo Park, CA: Addison-Wesley, 1979, p 318.

3. Black LL, Goldman BS: Surgical treatment of the patent ductus arteriosus in the adult. *Ann Surg* 175:290, 1972.

4. Brandt B, Marvin WJ, Ehrenhaft JL, Heintz S, Doty DB: Ligation of patent ductus arteriosus in premature infants. *Ann Thorac Surg* 32:167, 1981.

5. Bell EF, Warburton D, Stonestreet BS, Oh W: Effect of fluid administration on the development of symptomatic patent ductus arteriosus and congestive heart failure in premature infants. *N Engl J Med* 302:598, 1980.

6. Blalock A: Operative closure of the patent ductus arteriosus. *Surg Gynecol Obstet* 82:113, 1946.

7. Baden M, Kirks DR: Transient dilatation of the ductus arteriosus—the "ductus bump." *J Pediatr* 84:858, 1974.

C

1. Crafoord G: Discussion of paper by Gross RE: Complete division for the patent ductus arteriosus. *J Thorac Surg* 16:314, 1947.

2. Campbell M: Natural history of persistent ductus arteriosus. *Br Heart J* 30:4, 1968.

3. Christie A: Normal closing time of the foramen ovale and the ductus arteriosus. *Am J Dis Child* 40:323, 1930.

4. Cruickshank B, Marquis RM: Spontaneous aneurysms of the ductus arteriosus. *Am J Med* 25:140, 1958.

5. Cotton RB, Stahlman MT, Bender HW, Graham TP, Catterton WZ, Kovar I: Randomized trial of early closure of symptomatic patent ductus arteriosus in small preterm infants. *J Pediatr* 93:647, 1978.

6. Cassels DE: *The ductus arteriosus*. Springfield, Illinois: CC Thomas, 1973, p. 75.

7. Calder AL, Kirker JA, Netuze JM, Starling MB: Pathology of the ductus arteriosus treated with prostaglandins: Comparisons with untreated cases. *Pediatr Cardiol* 5:85, 1984.

8. Clyman RI, Heymann MA: Pharmacology of the ductus arteriosus. *Pediatr Clin North Am* 28:77, 1981.

9. Clarkson PM, Orgill AA: Continuous murmurs in infants of low birth weight. *J Pediatr* 84:208, 1974.

D

1. De Cancq HE Jr: Repair of patent ductus arteriosus in a 1417 g infant. *Am J Dis Child* 106:402, 1963.

2. Das JB, Chesterman JT: Aneurysms of the patent ductus arteriosus. *Thorax* 11:295, 1956.

3. DuBrow IW, Fisher E, Hastreiter A: Intermittent functional closure of patent ductus arteriosus in a ten-month old infant: Hemodynamic documentation. *Chest* 68:110, 1975.

E

1. Edmunds LH Jr: Operation or indomethacin for the premature ductus. *Ann Thorac Surg* 26:586, 1978.

2. Emmanouilides GC: Persistent patency of the ductus arteriosus

in premature infants, in *Seventy-fifth Ross Conference on Pediatric Research*, Palm Beach, FL: Dec 4–7, 1977.

3. Edmunds LH Jr, Gregory GA, Heymann MA, Kitterman JA, Rudolph AM, Tooley WH: Surgical closure of the ductus arteriosus in premature infants. *Circulation* 48:856, 1973.

4. Ellis FH Jr, Kirklin JW, Callahan JA, Wood EH: Patent ductus arteriosus with pulmonary hypertension. *J Thorac Surg* 31:268, 1956.

5. Ellison RC, Peckham GJ, Lang P, Talner NS, Lerer TJ, Lin L, Dooley KJ, Nadas AS: Evaluation of the preterm infant for patent ductus arteriosus. *Pediatrics* 71:364, 1983.

6. Engle MA, Holswade GR, Goldbert HP, Glenn F: Present problems pertaining to patency of the ductus arteriosus. I. Persistence of growth retardation after successful surgery. *Pediatrics* 21:70, 1958.

7. Eggert LD, Jung AL, McGough EC, Ruttenberg HD: Surgical treatment of patent ductus arteriosus in preterm infants. Four-year experience with ligation in the newborn intensive care unit. *Pediatr Cardiol* 2:15, 1982.

F

1. Friedman WF, Hirschlau MJ, Printz MP, Pitlick PT, Kirkpatrick SE: Pharmacologic closure of patent ductus arteriosus in the premature infant. *N Engl J Med* 295:526, 1976.

2. Falcone MW, Perloff JK, Roberts WC: Aneurysm of the non-patent ductus arteriosus. *Am J Cardiol* 29:422, 1972.

G

1. Gibson GA: Persistence of the arterial duct and its diagnosis. *Edinburgh Med J* 8:1, 1900.

2. Graybial A, Strieder JW, Boyer NH: An attempt to obliterate the patent ductus arteriosus in a patient with subacute bacterial endocarditis. *Am Heart J* 15:621, 1938.

3. Gross RE, Hubbard JP: Surgical ligation of a patent ductus arteriosus. Report of first successful case. *J Am Med Assoc* 112:729, 1939.

4. Goncalves-Estella A, Perez-Villoria J, Gonzalez-Reoyo F, Gimenez-Mendez JP, Castro-Cels A, Castro-Llorens M: Closure of a complicated ductus arteriosus through the transpulmonary route using hypothermia. *J Thorac Cardiovasc Surg* 69:698, 1975.

5. Graham EA: Aneurysm of the ductus arteriosus, with a consideration of its importance to the thoracic surgeon. *Arch Surg* 41:324, 1940.

6. Gittenberger-De Groot AC: Persistent ductus arteriosus: Most probably a primary congenital malformation. *Br Heart J* 39:610, 1977.

7. Gross RE: Complete surgical division of the patent ductus arteriosus. *Surg Gynecol Obstet* 78:36, 1944.

8. Gross RE: Complete division for the patent ductus arteriosus. *J Thorac Surg* 16:314, 1947.

9. Gross RE, Longino LA: The patent ductus arteriosus. Observations from 412 surgically treated cases. *Circulation* 3:125, 1951.

10. Gunning AJ: A simple, safe, surgical technique for closing the persistent ductus arteriosus in the preterm neonate. *Ann R Coll Surg Engl* 65:214, 1983.

11. Gittenberger-De Groot AC, Harinck ME, Becker AE: Histopathology of the ductus arteriosus after prostaglandin E₁ administration in ductus dependent cardiac anomalies. *Br Heart J* 40:215, 1978.

12. Grottman JH Jr, Harris CH, Hamilton LC: Congenital diverticula of the aortic arch. *N Engl J Med* 276:1178, 1967.

H

1. Hallman AL, Cooley DA: False aortic aneurysm following division and suture of a patent ductus arteriosus. Successful excision with hypothermia. *J Cardiovasc Surg* 5:23, 1964.

2. Hay JD: Population and clinic studies of congenital heart disease in Liverpool. *Br Med J* 2:661, 1966.

3. Heymann MA, Rudolph AM, Silverman NH: Closure of the ductus arteriosus in premature infants by inhibition of prostaglandin synthesis. *N Engl J Med* 295:530, 1976.

4. Heikkinen ES, Simila S, Laitinen J, Larmi T: Infantile aneurysm of the ductus arteriosus. *Acta Paediatr Scand* 63:241, 1974.

5. Heymann MA: In FH Adams, GC Emmanouilides (eds): *Heart Disease in Infants, Children and Adolescents* (ed 3). Baltimore: Williams and Wilkins, 1983, Chapter 11.

6. Heymann MA, Rudolph AM: Control of the ductus arteriosus. *Physiol Rev* 55:62, 1975.

J

1. Jones JC: Twenty-five years experience with the surgery of patent ductus arteriosus. *J Thorac Cardiovasc Surg* 50:2, 1965.

2. Jacob J, Gluck L, DiSessa T, Edwards D, Kulovich M, Kurlinski J, Merrit TA, Friedman WF: The contribution of PDA in the neonate with severe RDS. *J Pediatr* 96:79, 1980.

3. Johnson GL, Breart GL, Gewitz MH, Brenner JI, Lang P, Dooley KJ, Ellison RC: Echocardiographic characteristics of premature infants with patent ductus arteriosus. *Pediatrics* 72:846, 1983.

4. Jager BV, Wollenman OF Jr: An anatomical study of the closure of the ductus arteriosus. *Am J Pathol* 18:595, 1942.

K

1. Krovetz LJ, Warden HE: Patent ductus arteriosus. An analysis of 515 surgically proved cases. *Diseases of the Chest* 42:241, 1962.

2. Keys A, Shapiro MJ: Patency of the ductus arteriosus in adults. *Am Heart J* 25:158, 1943.

3. Kron IL, Mentzer RM Jr, Rheuban KS, Nolan SP: A simple, rapid technique for operative closure of patent ductus arteriosus in the premature infant. *Ann Thorac Surg* 37:422, 1984.

L

1. Levine SA, Geremia AE: Clinical features of patent ductus arteriosus with special reference to cardiac murmurs. *Am J Med Sci* 213:385, 1947.

2. Lucht U, Sondergaard T: Late results of operation for patent ductus arteriosus. *Scand J Thorac Cardiovasc Surg* 5:223, 1971.

M

1. Munro JC: Surgery of the vascular system. Ligation of patent ductus arteriosus. *Ann Surg* 46:335, 1907.

2. McGrath RL, McGuinness GA, Way GL, Wolfe RR, Nora JJ, Simmons MA: The silent ductus arteriosus. *J Pediatr* 93:110, 1978.

3. Mavroudis C, Cook LN, Fleischaker JW, Nagaraj HS, Shott RJ, Howe WR, Gray LA Jr: Management of patent ductus arteriosus in the premature infant: Indomethacin versus ligation. *Ann Thorac Surg* 36:561, 1983.

4. McMurphy DM, Heymann MA, Rudolph AM, Melmon KL: Developmental change in constriction of the ductus arteriosus:

Response to oxygen and vasoactive substances in the isolated ductus arteriosus of the fetal lamb. *Pediatr Res* 6:231, 1972.

5. Mancini AJ: A study of the angle formed by the ductus arteriosus with the descending thoracic aorta. *Anatomic Record* 109:535, 1951.

6. Mitchell SC, Korones SB, Berendes HW: Congenital heart disease in 56,109 births. Incidence and natural history. *Circulation* 43:323, 1971.

O

1. O'Donovan TG, Beck W: Closure of the complicated patent ductus arteriosus. *Ann Thorac Surg* 25:463, 1978.

P

1. Panagopoulos PH, Tatooles CJ, Aberdeen E, Waterston DJ, Bonham-Carter RE: Patent ductus arteriosus in infants and children: A review of 936 operations (1946–69). *Thorax* 26:1937, 1971.

2. Powell ML: Patent ductus arteriosus in premature infants. *Med J Aust* 2:56, 1963.

3. Payne RF, Jordan SC: Postoperative aneurysms following ligation of the patent ductus arteriosus. *Br J Radiol* 42:858, 1968.

4. Punsar S, Scheinin T, Tala P, Telivuo L: Postoperative aneurysm of the patent ductus arteriosus. *Ann Chir Gynaecol (Fenn)* 51:385, 1962.

R

1. Rowe RD, Lowe JB: Auscultation in the diagnosis of persistent ductus arteriosus in infancy: A study of 50 patients. *NZ Med J* 63:195, 1964.

2. Ravin A, Karley W: Apical diastolic murmur in patent ductus arteriosus. *Ann Intern Med* 33:903, 1950.

3. Ross RJ, Feder FP, Spencer FC: Aneurysms of the previously ligated patent ductus arteriosus. *Circulation* 23:350, 1961.

4. Rosenkrantz JG, Kelminson LL, Paton BC, Vogel JHK: False aneurysm after ligation of a patent ductus arteriosus. *Ann Thorac Surg* 3:353, 1967.

5. Rudolph AM, Heymann HA, Spitznas U: Hemodynamic considerations in the development of narrowing of the aorta. *Am J Cardiol* 30:514, 1972.

6. Rudolph AM: The changes in the circulation after birth: Their importance in congenital heart disease. *Circulation* 41:343, 1970.

S

1. Strange M, Philips J, Kirklin JK, Lell W, Cassady G: Perioperative management of the tiny infant undergoing ligation of the patent ductus arteriosus (PDA). Section on Anesthesiology, Program for Specific Sessions, American Academy of Pediatrics, Spring Meetings, 1984 (abstr).

2. Strange M, Myers G, Kirklin JK, Pacifico AD, Cassady G: Lack of effect of patent ductus arteriosus ligation on intraventricular hemorrhage in preterm infants. *Clin Res* 31:913 A, 1983.

3. Siassi B, Blanco C, Cabal LA, Coran AG: Incidence and clinical features of patent ductus arteriosus in low-birthweight infants: A prospective analysis of 150 consecutively born infants. *Pediatrics* 57:347, 1976.

4. Silver MM, Freedom RM, Silver MD, Olley PM: The morphology of the human newborn ductus arteriosus: A reappraisal of its structure and function with special reference to prostaglandin E_1 therapy. *Hum Pathol* 12:1123, 1981.

5. Santos MA, Moll JN, Drummond C, Aranjo WB, Romano N, Reiss NB: Development of the ductus arteriosus in right ventricular outflow tract obstruction. *Circulation* 62:818, 1980.

T

1. Thibeault DW, Emmanouilides GC, Nelson RJ, Lachman RS, Rosengart RM, Oh W: Patent ductus arteriosus complicating the respiratory distress syndrome in preterm infants. *J Pediatr* 86:120, 1975.

2. Traugott RC, Will RJ, Schuchmann GF, Treasure RL: A simplified method of ligation of patent ductus arteriosus in premature infants. *Ann Thorac Surg* 29:263, 1980.

3. Touroff ASW, Vesell H: Experiences in the surgical treatment of sub-acute streptococcus viridans endarteritis complicating patent ductus arteriosus. *J Thorac Surg* 10:59, 1940.

4. Touroff ASW, Vesell H: Subacute *Streptococcus viridans* endarteritis complicating patent ductus arteriosus: Recovery following surgical treatment. *JAMA* 115:1270, 1940.

5. Trippestad A, Efskind L: Patent ductus arteriosus. Surgical treatment of 686 patients. *Scand J Thorac Cardiovasc Surg* 6:38, 1972.

6. Tutassaura H, Goldman B, Moes CAF, Mustard WT: Spontaneous aneurysm of the ductus arteriosus in childhood. *J Thorac Cardiovasc Surg* 57:180, 1969.

23

VENTRICULAR SEPTAL DEFECT AND PULMONARY STENOSIS OR ATRESIA

TETRALOGY OF FALLOT

DEFINITION

The tetralogy of Fallot (TF) is a congenital cardiac malformation characterized by underdevelopment of the right ventricular infundibulum with anterior and leftward displacement of the infundibular (conal) septum and its parietal extension. The displacement of the infundibular septum is associated with right ventricular outflow (pulmonary) stenosis (or, in extreme forms, atresia) and a large malalignment-type ventricular septal defect (VSD). Typically, the VSD is subaortic in position, but it may be beneath both aorta and pulmonary artery (subpulmonary VSD). The right and left ventricles are the same thickness, and their systolic pressures are the same. The atrioventricular connection is concordant, and the aorta is biventricular in origin, overriding onto the right ventricle. (If the aorta arises mostly [more than 90%] from the right ventricle, the cardiac anomaly may be termed double outlet right ventricle with pulmonary stenosis [UAB], and then an intraventricular tunnel operation, rather than repair of the VSD, is usually required [see Chapter 40]. Alternatively [GLH], the malformation may be called double outlet right ventricle if the aorta arises more than 50% from right ventricle [see description of aorta in "Morphology"].)

HISTORICAL NOTE

The tetralogy of Fallot was first treated surgically by Blalock and Taussig in 1945 when they performed a palliative subclavian-pulmonary artery anastomosis.[B4] Other types of systemic-pulmonary artery anastomoses were introduced by Potts, Smith, and Gibson (1946),[P2] Waterston (1962),[W1] Klinner (1961),[K17,K23] Davidson (1955),[D9] Laks and Castaneda (1975),[L9] de Leval and colleagues,[D6] and no doubt others. Palliation by direct relief of the pulmonary stenosis with a closed technique was introduced by Sellors[S18] and Brock[B29] in 1948.

The tetralogy of Fallot was first successfully repaired by Lillehei and Varco, at the University of Minnesota in 1954, using "controlled cross-circulation" with another human being as the oxygenator.[L3] The first successful repair of the tetralogy of Fallot with a pump oxygenator was done by us at the Mayo Clinic in 1955.[K2] Warden, Lillehei, and colleagues introduced a patch enlargement of the right ventricular infundibulum,[W4] and we reported the use of transannular patching in 1959.[K3] The use of a right ventricular-pulmonary artery conduit for tetralogy of Fallot with pulmonary atresia was reported by us in 1965,[R1] and Ross and colleagues first reported the use of a valved extracardiac conduit for this purpose in 1966.[R23] It was recognized very early that repair of the tetralogy in infants carried a high mortality, and use of a two-stage repair soon evolved.[L14] In 1969 at GLH,[B9,B28] a policy of routine primary repair was first adopted and later shown to give good results. However, a selective and more conservative approach with routine two-stage repair continues to give good results in the hands of a number of surgeons.[R30]

MORPHOLOGY

The specific morphologic entity of the tetralogy of Fallot encompasses a wide spectrum of morphologic subsets. These vary primarily in the details of the right ventricular outflow obstruction, the ventricular septal defect, and the aortic overriding.

Right Ventricular Outflow Tract

Infundibulum
Infundibular stenosis associated with specific alterations in the position of the infundibular (conal) septum is the hallmark of TF. Specifically, the septal (leftward) end of the infundibular septum is displaced anteriorly, inserting in front of the left anterior division of the septal band (or trabecula septomarginalis),[A17,V3] (Figs. 23-1, 23-2) rather than between its two divisions as in the normal heart (see Chapter 1, Fig. 1-3). In addition, the parietal (rightward) end of the conal septum is rotated anteriorly and passes anteriorly and inferiorly to reach the free wall of the right ventricle (Figs. 23-2, 23-3) so that the infundibular septum and its parietal extension may come to lie almost in a sagittal rather than the usual coronal (frontal) plane. The parietal and septal ends of the conal septum give rise to prominent muscle bands that attach to the right and left sides of the anterior right ventricular free wall.[B23] The anterior free wall may show additional trabeculations or moderate thickening.

There is frequently a localized narrowing or os infundibulum, which usually (72% of cases) lies in a transverse plane at the lower conal septal edge (Fig. 23-3). This siting means that when the conal septum is well developed, there is a large infundibular chamber (Fig. 23-3) (or "third ventricle"), which in older patients occasionally becomes aneurysmal. In older patients, however, the os infundibulum is surrounded by fibrosis, which when the chamber is small or absent, may extend up to and into the pulmonary valve ring. Less commonly (16% of cases), the major stenotic zone at the lower infundibular (conal) septal edge lies almost in a coronal plane, extending inferiorly from the lower infundibular septal edge. This occurs when the hypertrophied muscle bands at the parietal end of the infundibular septum pass more inferiorly to join the free wall nearer to the right ventricular apex, while on the septal (medial or leftward) aspect, there are not only inferiorly directed additional trabeculae, but also often an undue prominence and hypertrophy of the septal band (trabecula septomarginalis). In these circumstances, the inferior boundary of the os infundibulum may be formed by a prominent superiorly displaced moderator band.[A17] (When this type of so-called "low-lying infundibular stenosis" is associated with a small or moderate-sized VSD, it is not termed tetralogy of Fallot—see Section 3 of this chapter). Both transverse and coronal plane stenoses are occasionally present (12% of cases, GLH).

When the infundibular (conal) septum is well developed, an *infundibular chamber* is present. Its walls laterally and

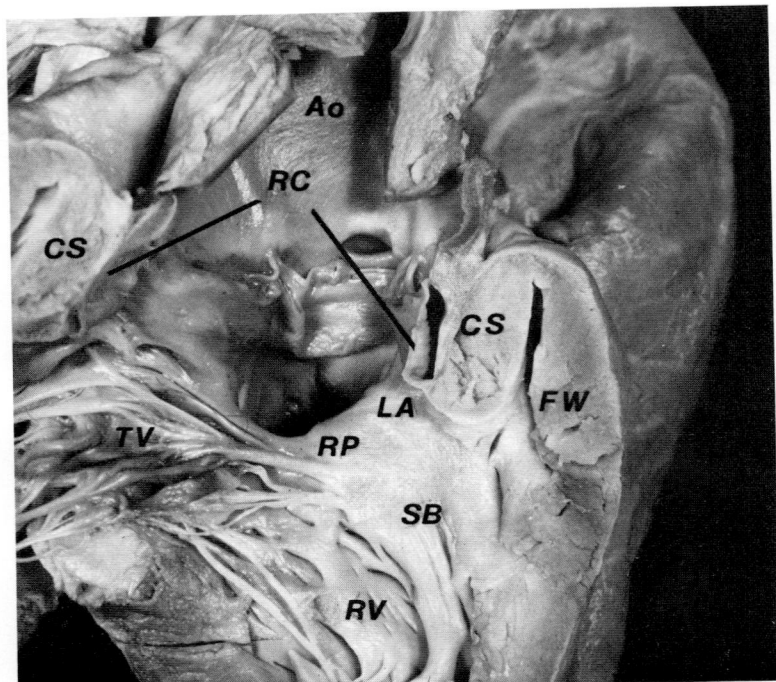

Figure 23-1 Autopsy specimen of tetralogy of Fallot with the right ventricle opened vertically and the incision continued into the overriding ascending aorta, dividing the conal (infundibular) septum and the right aortic cusp transversely (GLH). The right aortic cusp clearly originates within the right ventricle (overrides), its belly attaching to the conal (infundibular) septum and almost reaching its inferior edge. The septal end of the conal (infundibular) septum is displaced anteriorly in front of the left anterior division of the septal band (trabecula septomarginalis). The right posterior division of the septal band gives origin to tricuspid chordae (papillary muscle of the conus or medial papillary muscle). The gap between these two limbs of the septal band, which in a normal heart is occupied by the septal insertion of the conal septum, now forms the inferior and anterior margin of the VSD, which is clearly related to this malalignment of the conal septum with septal band. (In this and the subsequent photographs of autopsied specimens, the orientation is the traditional anatomic one. To view the morphology as the surgeon does at operation, the photograph needs to be rotated 90° counterclockwise.)

Ao, aorta; CS, conal (infundibular) septum; FW, anterior free wall; LA, left anterior division of SB; RP, right posterior division of SB; RC, right coronary cusp; RV, right ventricle; SB, septal band (trabecula septomarginalis); TV, tricuspid valve.

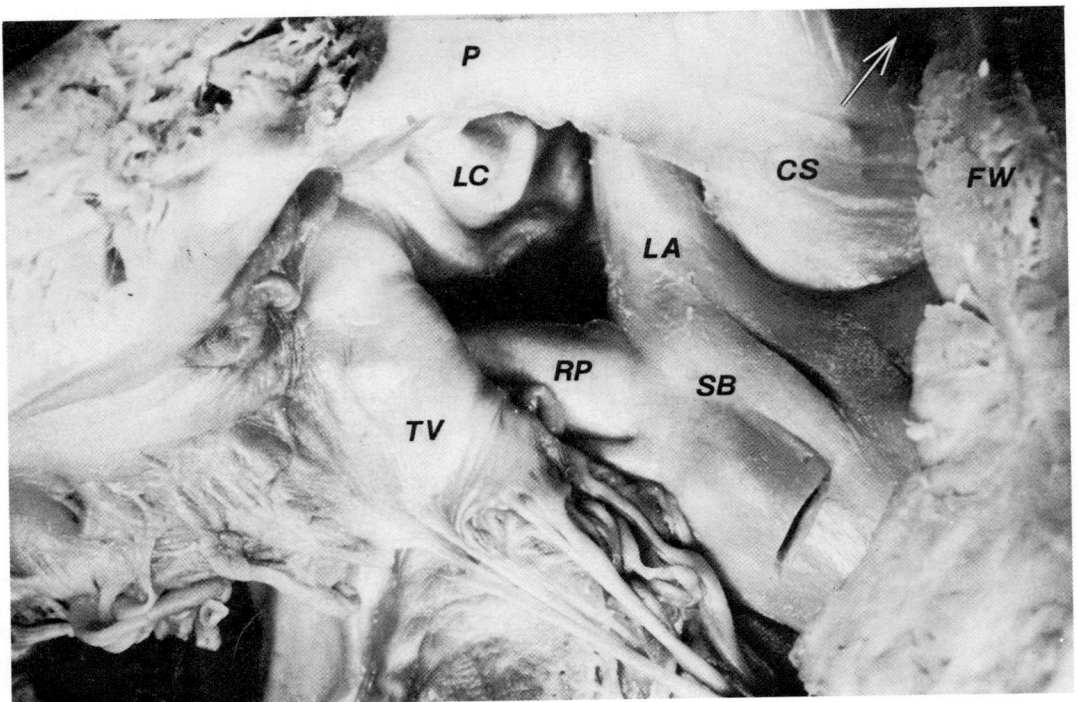

Figure 23-2 Autopsy specimen from a newborn with TF and pulmonary atresia (GLH). The anterior and leftward displacement of the septal end of an unusually bulky conal (infundibular) septum is beautifully shown, inserting in front of the left anterior division of the septal band rather than between the two septal band divisions. The anterior and leftward deviation of the parietal end of the conal septum is also obvious, the septum lying part way between a coronal and sagittal plane. There is a diminutive blind right ventricular outflow tract (arrow) in front of the conal septum.

CS, conal (infundibular) septum; FW, anterior free wall; LA, left anterior division of SB; LC, left coronary cusp; P, parietal end of conal (infundibular) septum; RP, right posterior division of SB; SB, septal band (trabecula septomarginalis); TV, tricuspid valve.

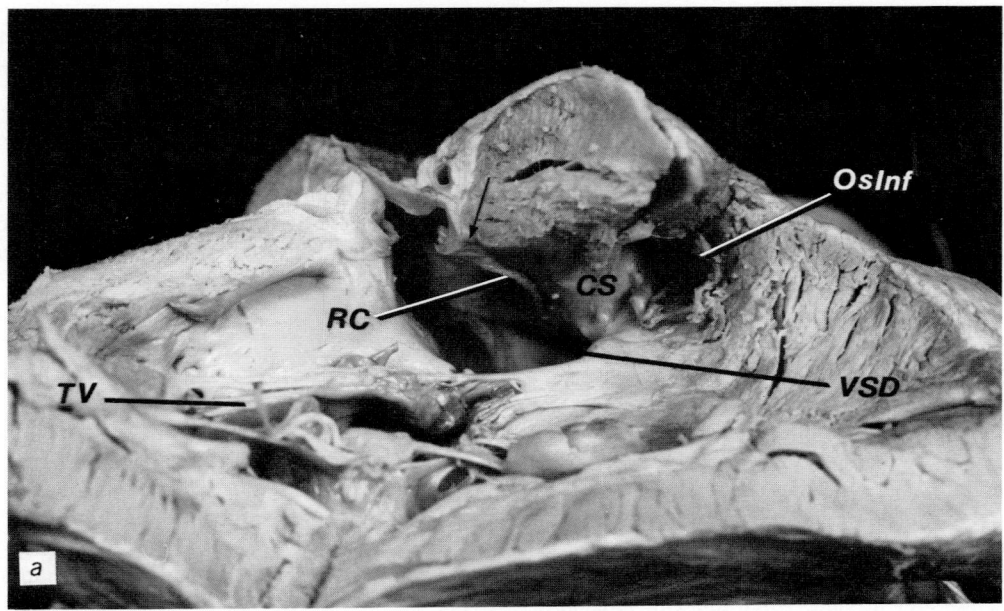

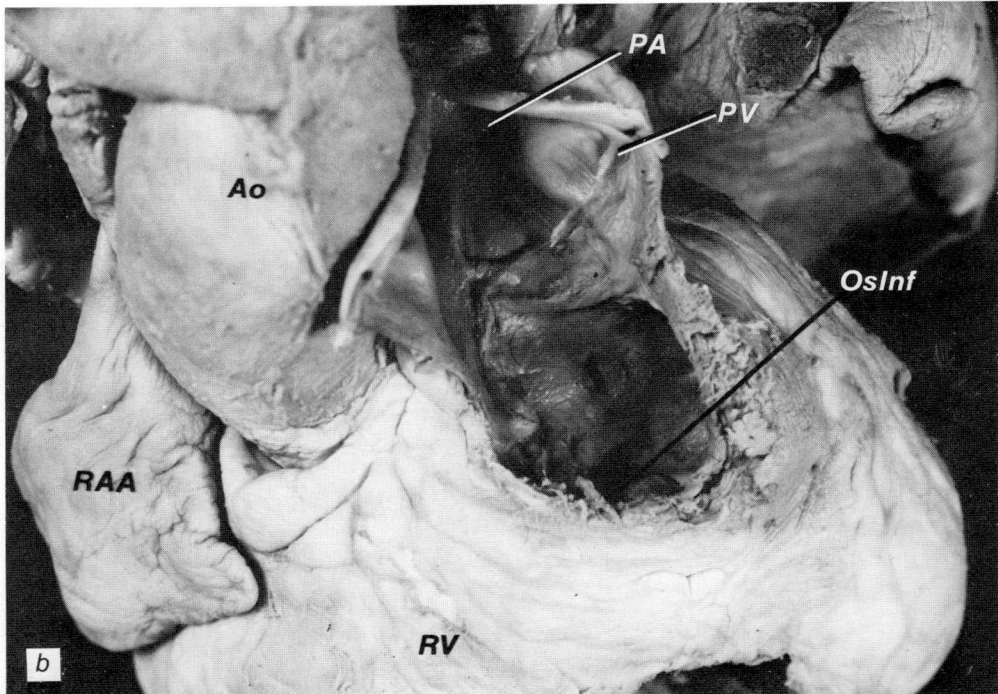

Figure 23-3 Autopsy specimen of TF with low-lying infundibular stenosis (GLH). The isolated infundibular stenosis is viewed (*a*) from below through the opened right ventricle and (*b*) from above after removing the anterior wall of the large infundibular chamber and opening the front of the pulmonary trunk. The infundibular stenosis is localized at the lower border of the conal septum (os infundibulum). Note how the lateral (parietal) end of the conal septum is deviated anteriorly almost into a sagittal plane. The posterosuperior angle of the VSD is well seen (arrow), as is the proximity of the VSD to the right aortic cusp. The infundibular chamber is dilated and thin walled (death occurred without surgical correction at age 3 years) in association with the low, transversely placed infundibular stenosis. The pulmonary valve is tricuspid and not stenotic.

Ao, aorta; CS, conal septum; OsInf, os infundibulum; PA, pulmonary trunk; PV, pulmonary valve; RAA, right atrial appendage; RC, right coronary cusp; RV, right ventricle; TV, tricuspid valve; VSD, ventricular septal defect.

medially consist of numerous trabeculated spaces, some of which may form prominent blind recesses that do not lead directly to the valve ring, or occasionally an accessory opening is present. Endocardial fibrosis is not seen in the first 6–9 months of life and is seldom significant before 2 years of age.[C15] In later years, the fibrosis seems to progress, and this may lead in time to acquired atresia of the infundibulum.

When the infundibular (conal) septum is short (hypoplastic), the infundibular stenosis reaches the pulmonary valve ring without an intervening chamber. When the infundibular septum is absent, the VSD is subpulmonary as well as subaortic and extends superiorly to reach the pulmonary valve. Infundibular stenosis is absent, and the posterior aspect of the right ventricular outflow tract is formed by the VSD itself[N6] (Fig. 23-4). The pulmonary valve and sometimes the annulus are the main sites of the usually moderate stenosis in these hearts. However, once a VSD patch is in position, the hypertrophied right ventricular walls and the dextroposed aorta may combine with the patch to form severe subvalvar stenosis.

Congenital *infundibular atresia,* when present, is usually muscular, the entire conal septum being fused with the anterior free wall (Fig. 23-5), or there may be a small, blind infundibular pouch below a muscular occlusion (Fig. 23-2). Acquired atresia of the infundibulum may develop from a stenosis sited at a low (inferior), medium, or high (superior) level, and an infundibular chamber may therefore remain beyond the atretic site, leading sometimes to a nonstenotic pulmonary valve.

These morphologic changes in the infundibulum produce a variety of *patterns of infundibular stenosis* whose recognition is helpful surgically.

1. *Low:* The stenosis is usually transversely oriented but sometimes is in the coronal plane, and there is a well-formed chamber separating it from the pulmonary valve. Transverse and coronal plane stenoses coexist in hearts with low-lying infundibular stenosis, producing two distinct zones of localized narrowing.

2. *Intermediate:* The stenosis is transversely oriented, and the conal septum is shorter than in the above type. A moderate-sized or small chamber separates the stenotic zone from the pulmonary valve ring.

3. *High:* The stenosis is transverse but reaches the valve, and no infundibular chamber is present. The conal septum is shorter still. A high stenosis may occasionally be entirely fibrous, similar to a membranous subaortic stenosis. (Very rarely, a high fibrous stenosis may occur in a heart with a well-formed conal septum and does not, therefore, correspond in position to the lower conal septal edge.)

4. *Diffuse:* This form is usually associated with infundibular hypoplasia and marked underdevelopment of the entire right ventricular outflow tract. There is no localized os infundibulum (Fig. 23-6); neither is there increased trabeculations nor significant muscular hypertrophy. Nevertheless, the stenosis is usually severe because the narrowing is throughout the outflow tract (Fig. 23-7). This

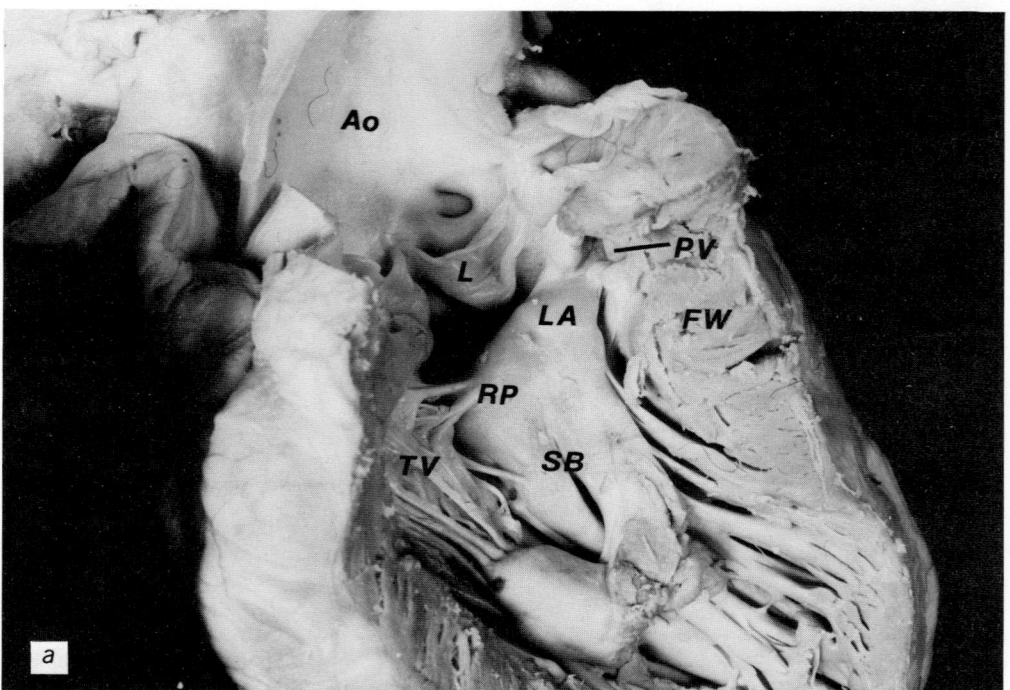

Figure 23-4 Autopsy specimen of TF with subpulmonary (subarterial) ventricular septal defect (GLH).
(a) Viewed from the opened right ventricle with the incision carried across the right cusp of the aortic valve.

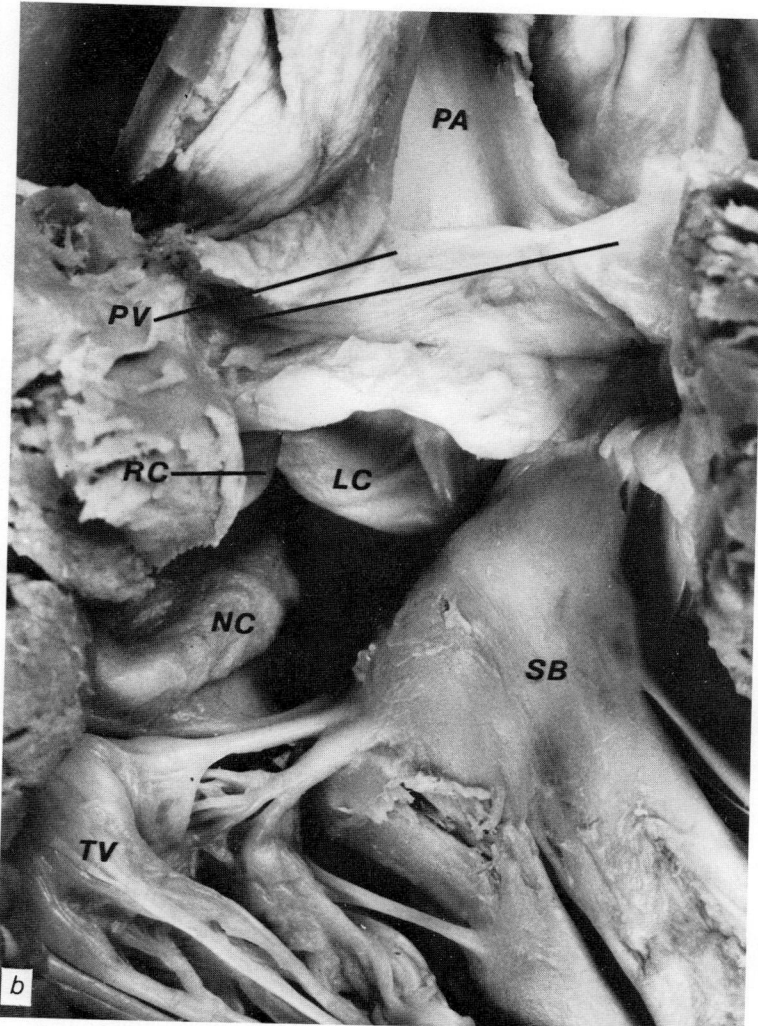

Figure 23-4 *(continued)*

(b) Viewed after opening the right ventricle across the pulmonary valve and pulmonary artery. The infundibular (conal) septum appears to be absent, and the perimembranous ventricular septal defect is bounded superiorly by the fused aortic and pulmonary valve rings. The septal band (trabecula septomarginalis) and right ventricular free wall are severely hypertrophied. There is marked narrowing of the pulmonary anulus and artery and thickening and tethering of the valve leaflets.

Ao, aorta; FW, right ventricular free wall; L, left coronary cusp; LA, left anterior division of SB; LC, left coronary aortic cusp; NC, noncoronary aortic cusp; PA, main pulmonary artery; PV, pulmonary valve; PVC, pulmonary valve cusps; R, fibrous raphe between pulmonary and aortic valve; RC, right coronary aortic cusp; RP, right posterior division of SB; SB, septal band (trabecula septomarginalis); TV, tricuspid valve.

tubular stenosis is usually short but may be of moderate length, depending upon conal septal development (Fig. 23-6).

5. *Absent:* This occurs in TF with so-called subpulmonary VSD (Fig. 23-4), as described above.

Pulmonary Valve

Pulmonary valve is stenotic to a varying degree in 75% of cases of TF. Approximately two-thirds of the stenotic valves are biscuspid[L1,N1] (Table 23-1); a tricuspid configuration oc-

curs more commonly in nonstenotic valves. Even when nonstenotic, the valve area is usually smaller than that of the aortic valve, which is the opposite of normal.

The *leaflets* of a stenotic valve are usually thickened, frequently severely so, a feature that increases the amount of obstruction at valve level (Fig. 23-8). In approximately 10% of cases, the leaflets are replaced by sessile nubbins of fibromyxomatous tissue that themselves offer little obstruction. Such vestigial valves are usually associated with a stenotic pulmonary ring. When the ring is not significantly

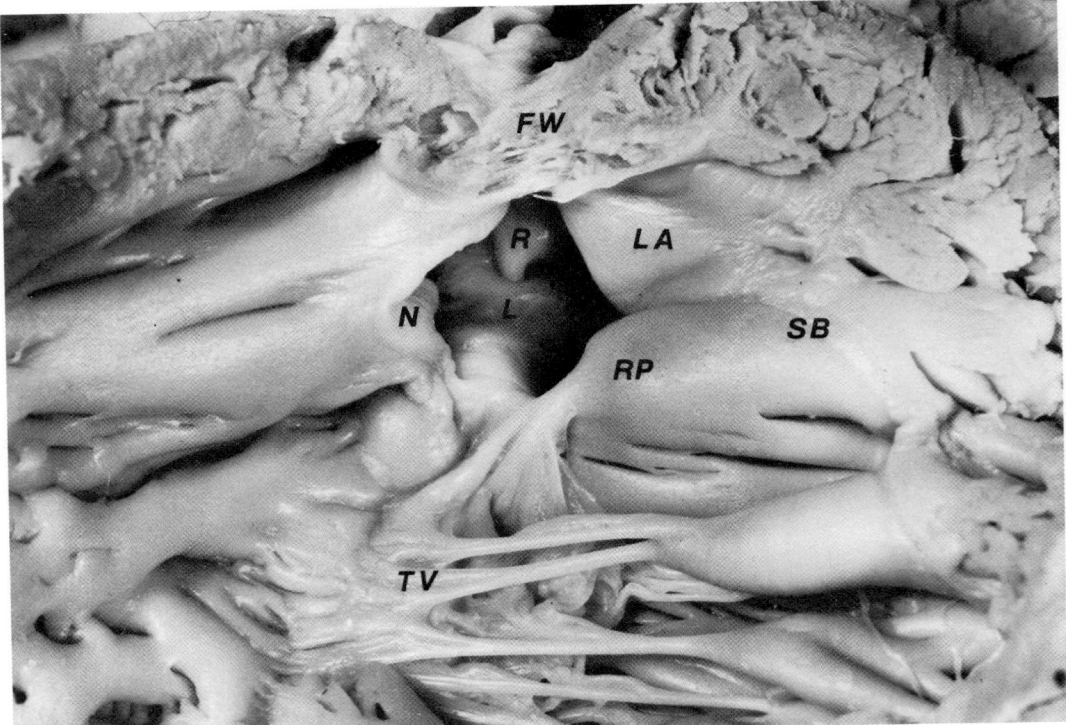

Figure 23-5   A specimen of TF with congenital infundibular atresia (GLH). The conal (infundibular) septum is small. The divisions of the septal band or trabecula septomarginalis are prominent. The ventricular septal defect, as is often the case in this situation, is perimembranous but extends very anteriorly and superiorly almost to the anterior free wall of the ventricle. The danger of inadvertently cutting into the aortic root when making the right ventriculotomy incision is evident. There is marked overriding of the noncoronary aortic cusp.

FW, anterior free wall; L, left coronary cusp; LA, left anterior division of SB; N, noncoronary cusp; R, right coronary cusp of aortic valve; RP, right posterior division of SB; SB, septal band (trabecula septomarginalis); TV, tricuspid valve.

narrowed and the valve is vestigial, pulmonary incompetence results and the condition is called TF with absent pulmonary valve.

The stenosis at the pulmonary valve is usually the result of leaflet tethering rather than commissural fusion (Table 23-1). The length of the free edge of tethered leaflets is considerably shorter than the diameter of the pulmonary artery, so that the valve cannot open adequately and the pulmonary artery is pulled inward at the point of commissural attachment, producing a localized narrowing or waisting of the artery at distal valve level. Thus, both the valve and artery are tethered (Fig. 23-8). In this situation, the sinuses of Valsalva are frequently well formed, but the entry into the sinus (between the leaflet edge and pulmonary artery wall) is often also stenotic, resulting in slow filling of the sinuses with contrast medium on cineangiography. Uncommonly, the leaflets of a tethered valve may be fused for a short distance. Tethering is more common in a biscuspid valve but can occur in a tricuspid one.

Less commonly, thickened leaflets are associated with congenital commissural fusion, resulting in a concentric or eccentric stenotic orifice. An eccentric orifice can also result from a unicuspid configuration.

A fused stenotic pulmonary valve orifice may be beaded with tiny "vegetations" of fibrin. Progressive deposition of fibrin is presumably the mechanism of *acquired valvar atresia. Congenital atresia* may also occasionally be valvar in position; the obstruction then consists of a thick fibrous membrane above a narrow infundibular pouch.

Pulmonary Ring (Anulus)
The pulmonary ring is normally a muscular structure and, like the infundibulum, varies in diameter during the cardiac cycle. In TF, it is almost always smaller in diameter than the aortic ring (the reverse of normal) but may not be obstructive. It is rarely if ever stenotic when the infundibular stenosis is low lying. The ring may become thick from fibrosis, which is usually an extension of endocardial thickening (fibrosis) surrounding an intermediate level or high infundibular stenosis, and is then variably obstructive. The ring is small and obstructive when there is diffuse infundibular hypoplasia, resulting in diffuse right ventricular outflow hypoplasia.

Pulmonary Trunk (Main Pulmonary Artery)

Like the pulmonary valve and ring, the pulmonary trunk is nearly always smaller than the aorta in TF. The reduction in

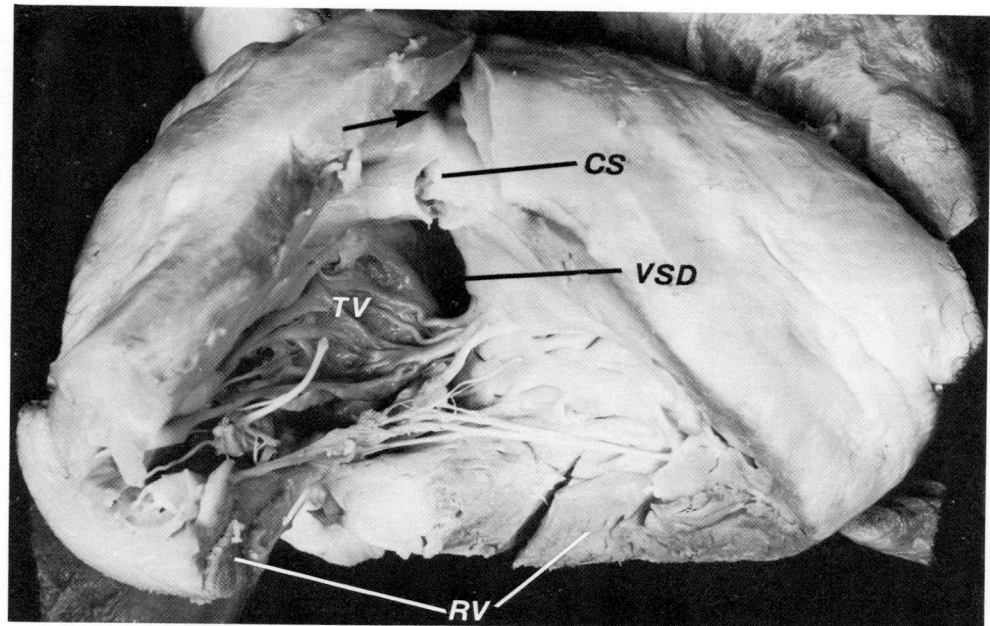

Figure 23-6 Autopsy specimen of TF with diffuse right ventricular outflow hypoplasia (GLH; same specimen as Fig. 23-1). The view is through the opened right ventricle. The stenotic infundibulum (indicated by the arrow) is relatively short with a well-formed anteriorly displaced infundibular (conal) septum. There is no ostium infundibulum but rather a diffuse narrowing of the outflow tract without increased trabeculation or free wall thickening. The ventricular septal defect is perimembranous.

CS, conal septum; RV, right ventricle; TV, tricuspid valve; VSD, ventricular septal defect.

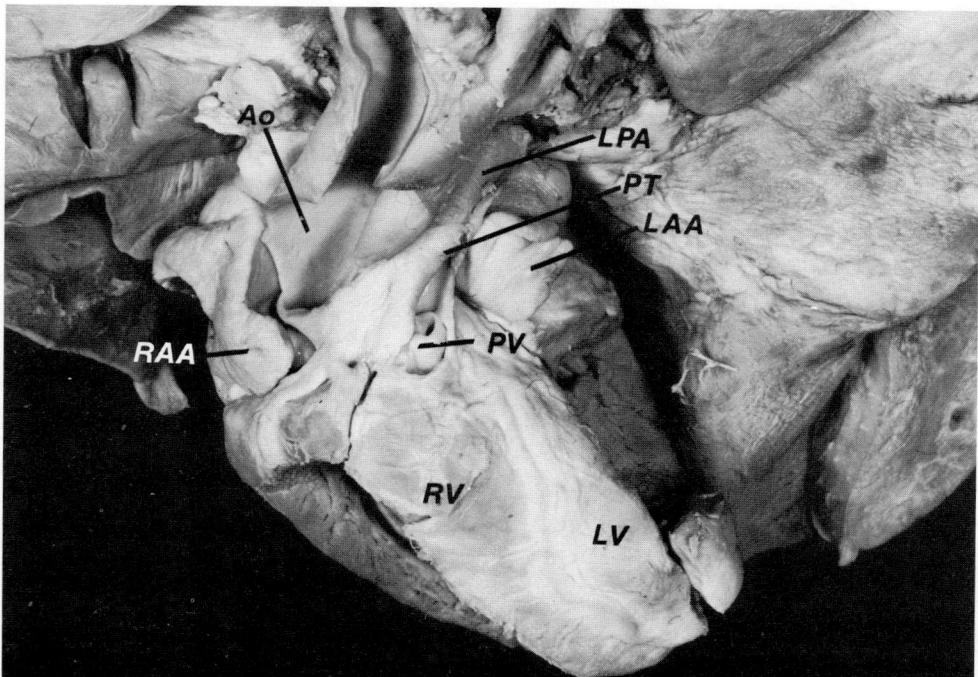

Figure 23-7 Specimen of TF with infundibular, valvular, and supravalvular pulmonary stenosis viewed from in front (GLH). The aorta and main pulmonary artery have been opened. The main pulmonary artery is also diffusely narrowed and continues directly into a left pulmonary artery of satisfactory size without any stenosis at its origin. The right pulmonary artery origin is not visible, passing at right angles directly beneath the aorta.

Ao, aorta; LAA, left atrial appendage; LPA, left pulmonary artery; LV, left ventricle; PT, pulmonary trunk (main pulmonary artery); PV, pulmonary valve; RAA, right atrial appendage; RV, right ventricle.

Table 23-1 Pulmonary valve morphology in 141 surgical patients with stenotic pulmonary valves with or without other types of right ventricular outflow obstruction (GLH; 1968–1978, with exclusions as in Table 23-3).

Valve Configuration	n	%	Valve Lesion	n	%
Bicuspid	93	66%	Tethering alone	89	63%
Tricuspid	21	15%	Fusion alone	20	14%
Vestigial	14	10%	Tethering + fusion	8	6%
Not recorded	13	9%	Vestigial valve	14	10%
			Atretic valve (acquired)	2	1%
			Not recorded	8	6%
Total	141	100%		141	100%

size is most marked when there is diffuse right ventricular outflow hypoplasia. Then, the main pulmonary artery is less than half aortic diameter and is short (Fig. 23-8), passing sharply posteriorly to its bifurcation. The pulmonary trunk is then largely hidden from view at operation by the prominent aorta, which also displaces the origin of the trunk leftward and posteriorly.

When the pulmonary valve is significantly tethered, the main pulmonary artery is also tethered or waisted at the commissural attachment (Fig. 23-8) and may be significantly angulated or kinked at this point. This is the usual mechanism of supravalvar narrowing, and it is not associated with wall thickening. Very rarely there may be a discrete supravalvar narrowing beyond commissural level that is associated with diffuse wall thickening. The main pulmonary artery shows tethering or discrete narrowing in about one-half of surgical patients.

Pulmonary Trunk Bifurcation

The left pulmonary artery (left branch) is usually a direct continuation of the pulmonary trunk, with the right branch arising almost at right angles to it (Fig. 23-9), but there are variations in this pattern (Fig. 23-10). Uncommonly, the distal pulmonary trunk and the origin of the right and left pulmonary arteries are moderately or severely narrowed (*bifurcation stenosis*), and in this situation the bifurcation may have a Y shape.

Right and Left Pulmonary Arteries

Anomalies of the right and left pulmonary arteries are more common in TF with pulmonary atresia (see below) but also occur in patients with pulmonary stenosis (Table 23-2); Fel-

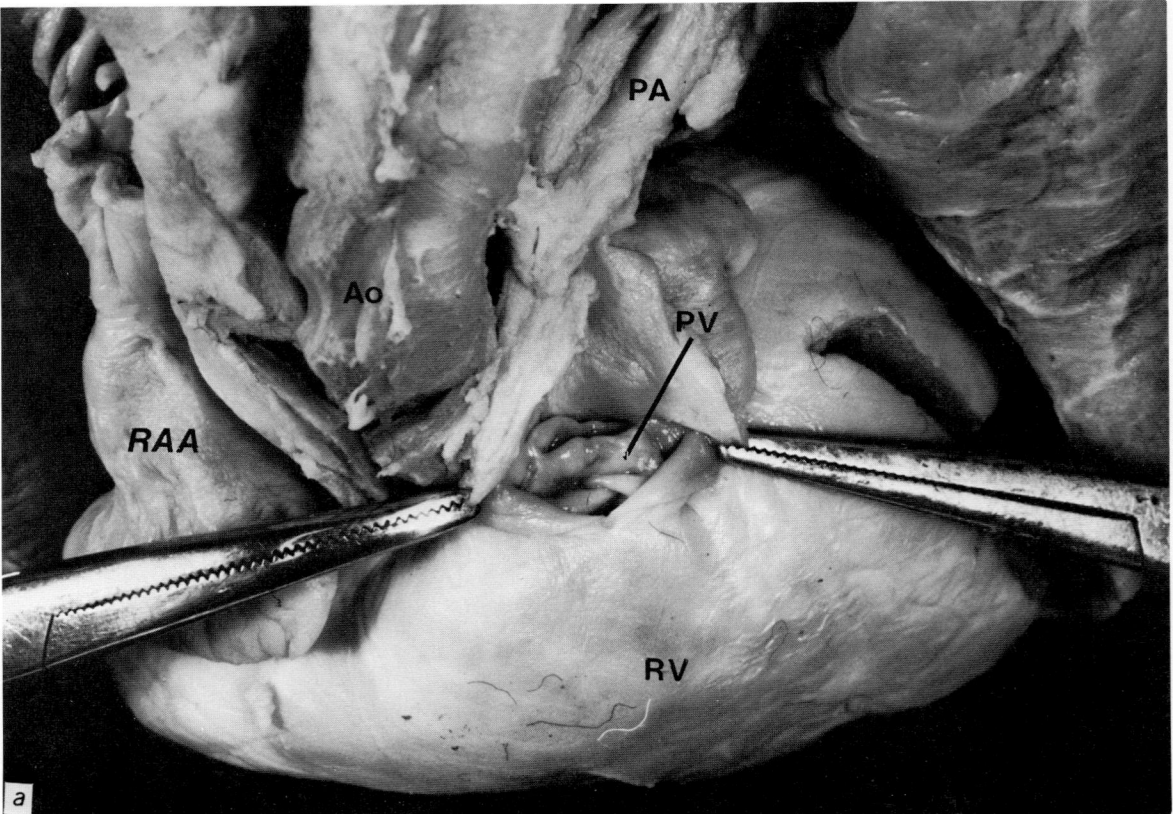

Figure 23-8 Specimen of TF showing thickened stenotic pulmonary valve, and right ventricular cineangiograms in the right anterior oblique projection in an infant with TF showing the same feature (GLH).
(a) Specimen showing the stenotic pulmonary valve viewed through the opened pulmonary artery. There are two thickened leaflets that are not fused, but the pulmonary artery wall is drawn inward where the commissures attach (*tethering*).

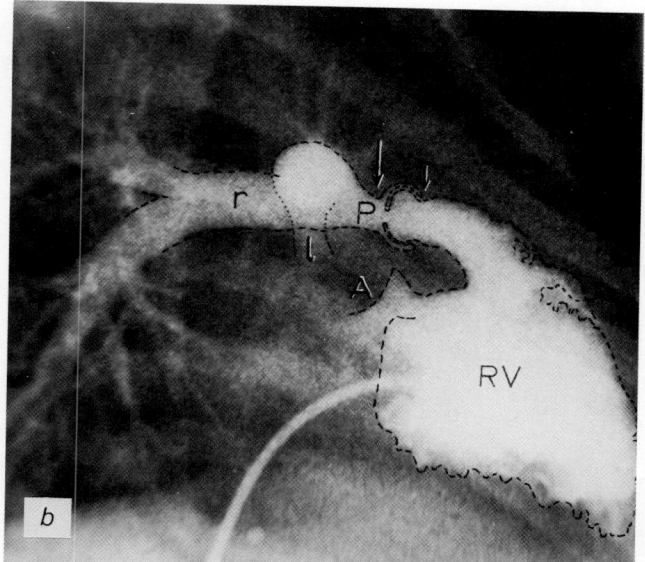
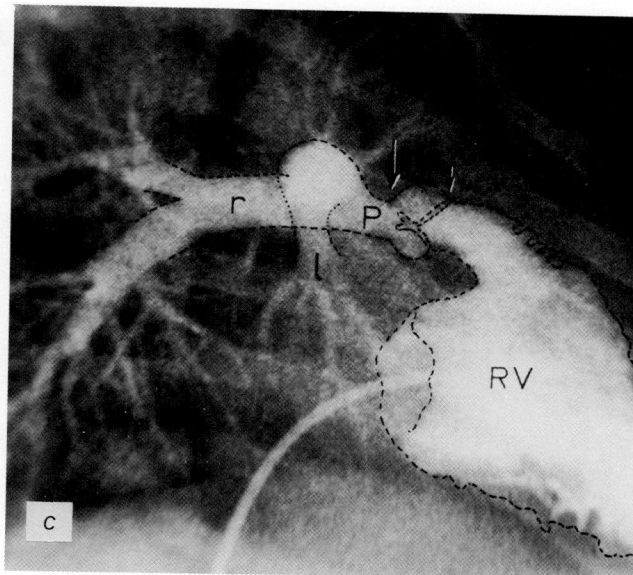

Figure 23-8   *(continued)*

(b) Early systolic frame. The pulmonary valve stenosis is due to valve tethering. The leaflets are thickened and form a dome in systole from their attachments to the pulmonary ring (small arrow). Supravalvular main pulmonary artery narrowing (large arrow) is localized to the region which is junctional between the pulmonary sinuses and the pulmonary artery.

(c) Diastolic frame. The distal edges of the thickened leaflets remain approximated to the narrowed pulmonary artery wall, and the prominent sinuses may be slow to fill with contrast. Note the shortness of the main pulmonary artery.

A, aortic valve; Ao, aorta; l, left pulmonary artery; P, pulmonary artery; PA, main pulmonary artery; PV, pulmonary valve; R, right pulmonary artery; RAA, right atrial appendage; RV, right ventricle.

Reproduced with permission from Calder et al.[C19]

---

lows and colleagues found them in 30% of infants in the latter category presenting for study in the first year of life.[F4]

Hypoplasia

At least mild *generalized* hypoplasia of the central and hilar portions[1] of the right and left pulmonary arteries is nearly always present in TF,[H6] and the hypoplasia is occasionally severe (Fig. 23-11). Hypoplasia of varying degree may also be *localized* and result in localized stenosis. The most common location of a localized area of stenosis is in the left pulmonary artery, adjacent to an open or closed ductus arteriosus (Fig. 23-10). It may also occur at the origin of the left or right pulmonary artery or both. However, single or multiple areas of stenosis may occur anywhere in the right or left pulmonary artery, particularly when there is pulmonary atresia.

Atresia

Atresia may involve the central portion of either pulmonary artery branch but usually of the left. The more distal pulmo-

nary artery is then connected by a fibrous chord to the pulmonary trunk bifurcation.

Absence

The *central portion* of the left and/or right pulmonary artery may be absent, and the phrase *discontinuity of the right and left pulmonary arteries* may be used to describe this situation.[E1] Blood flow to the lung then usually comes from a congenital origin of the hilar portion of its pulmonary artery, from the ductus arteriosus[I2,K9] (Fig. 23-12), the ascending aorta,[K18,R8] or directly from a large aortopulmonary collateral artery (see below). In most cases, a stenosis is present in anomalously originating right or left pulmonary arteries; it is not present when they arise from the ascending aorta. Uncommonly, there is not an anomalous origin of a pulmonary artery whose central portion is absent, but instead numerous small bronchial and intercostal collaterals supply blood flow to the hilar and more distal branches. This uncommon condition (only about 50 reported cases[R4]) is often called *unilateral absence of the pulmonary artery*.[E6] It usually affects the left side.

When the hilar portion is also absent (*absence of central and hilar portions*), the intrapulmonary portions of the pulmonary arteries may be joined end to end by one or more large aortopulmonary (A-P) collateral arteries (Fig. 23-13). Otherwise, only numerous small bronchial anastomotic arteries supply the distal pulmonary arteries.

---

[1] The right and left pulmonary arteries are conveniently divided into a central portion (from origin to within 5 mm of the first branch), a hilar portion (the 5 mm before the first branch and the area of primary branching), an interlobar portion, and an intralobar portion, the latter two being the intrapulmonary portion.

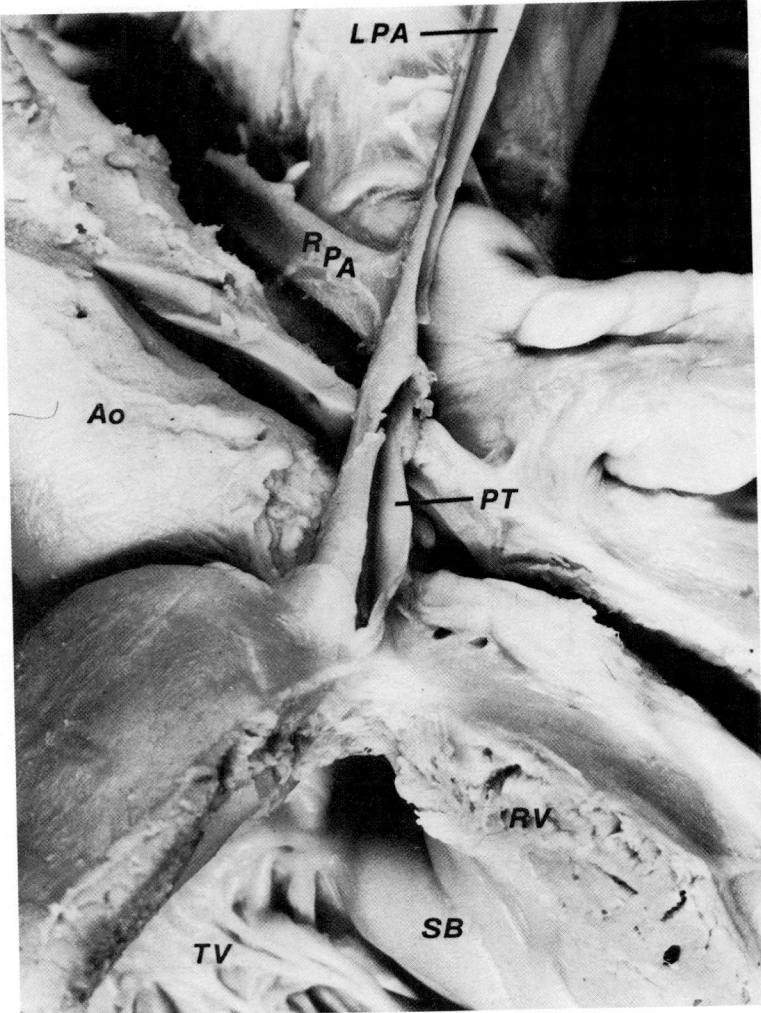

Figure 23-9   Autopsy specimen of TF with congenital pulmonary atresia (GLH; same specimen as Fig. 23-5). The pulmonary trunk ends blindly proximally. Distally, it extends directly into the small left pulmonary artery, whereas in contrast the right pulmonary artery arises almost at right angles from the pulmonary trunk.

Ao, aorta; *LPA*, left pulmonary artery; *PT*, pulmonary trunk (or main pulmonary artery); *RPA*, right pulmonary artery; *RV*, opened right ventricular anterior wall; *SB*, septal band (trabecula septomarginalis); *TV*, tricuspid valve.

Incomplete Distribution

The central and all or part of the hilar portions of the right and/or left pulmonary artery may be present, but the artery may distribute incompletely to the pulmonary lobes and segments. This occurs particularly in patients with large A-P collateral arteries. The one or more lobes and/or segments to which the central or hilar pulmonary arteries do not distribute usually receive their blood supply from the large A-P collateral arteries, which become confluent with the hilar or intrapulmonary arteries in those lobes or segments.

Abnormal Hilar Branching Patterns

Even when the pulmonary arteries distribute to all parts of the right and left lung, the hilar branching patterns may be abnormal, particularly in patients with large A-P collateral arteries coexisting with TF.

Convenient Morphologic Categories of Right Ventricular Outflow Obstruction

The nearly infinitely variable spectrum of right ventricular outflow obstruction in TF can be conveniently categorized in a way that is surgically useful because it relates to the difficulty in obtaining a good relief of the pulmonary stenosis and therefore to surgical techniques and mortality. This supplements the earlier discussion of the patterns of the infundibular portion of the obstruction.

1. *Isolated infundibular stenosis* is encountered in a minority of cases (26%, GLH, Table 23-3). An infundibular chamber is usual when the stenosis is at the intermediate or low level but may be absent when the stenosis is high. The stenosis may lie in a transverse plane (72%) or a coronal plane (16%), or both transverse and coronal plane

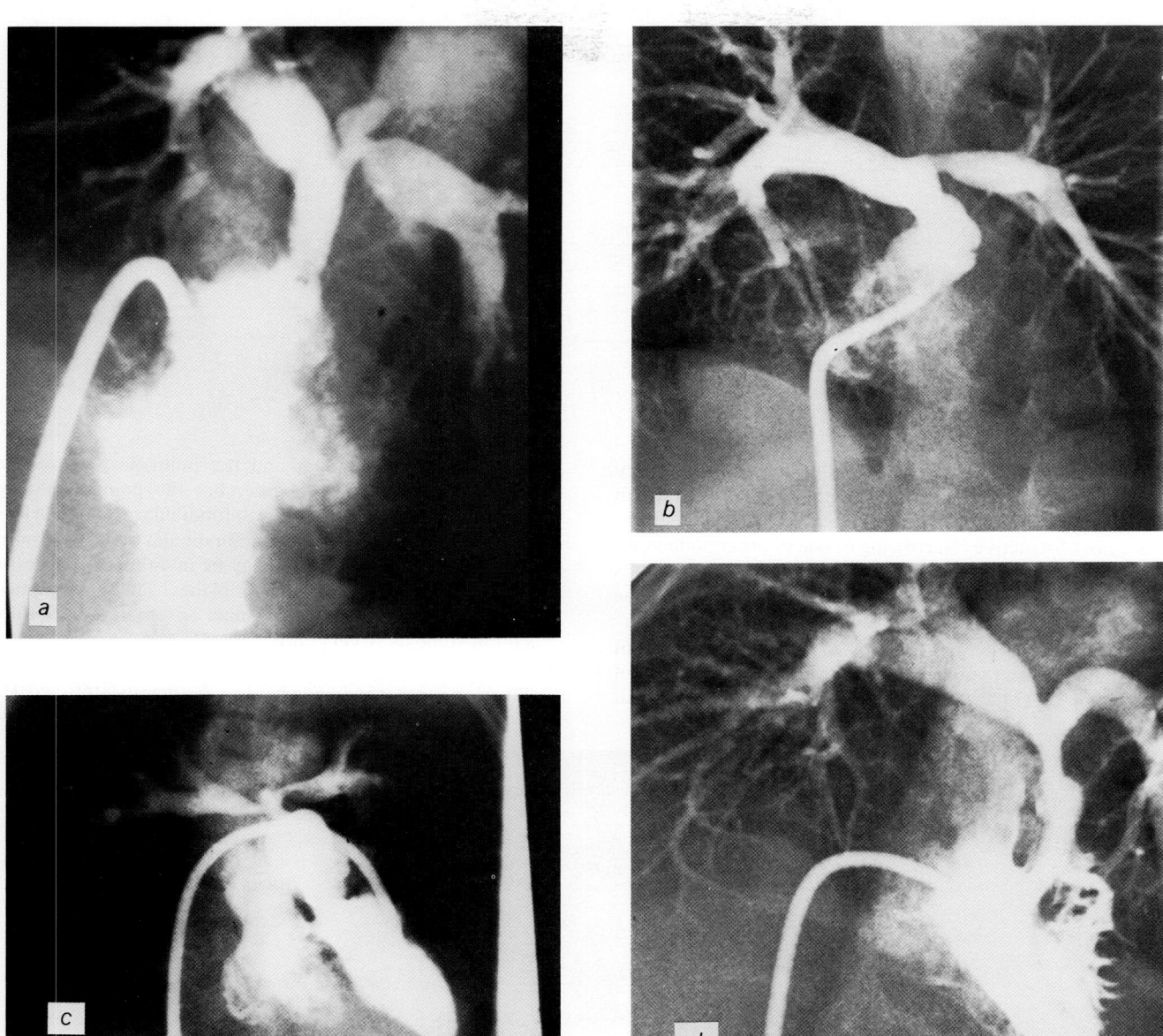

Figure 23-10 Cineangiograms after right ventricular injection showing stenoses of the origins of the pulmonary arteries in patients with TF and pulmonary stenosis (UAB).

(a) Stenosis at the origin of the left pulmonary artery in the region of the ductus arteriosus, which is closed at the aortic end.

(b) Stenosis at the origin of the left pulmonary artery. In this patient, the arrangement is different from usual in that the right pulmonary artery is the continuation of the pulmonary trunk and the left pulmonary artery comes off at right angles.

(c) Bifurcation stenosis. Note that, as usual, the right pulmonary artery comes off at right angles to the pulmonary trunk.

(d) Less severe but probably important bifurcation stenosis.

Table 23-2 Abnormalities of pulmonary trunk bifurcation and of right and/or left pulmonary artery origin in 365 patients with TF and pulmonary stenosis (including those with subpulmonary VSD and absent pulmonary valve syndrome). (GLH; 1960–1978.) Categories are mutually exclusive.

PA Branch Lesion	Degree of Narrowing		Total		Hospital Deaths		
	Severe	Moderate	n	% of 365	No.	%	CL
Congenital							
Left + right origin stenosis[a]	11	8	19	5.2%	3	16%	7%–29%
Left origin stenosis	6	4	10	2.7%	1	10%	1%–30%
Right origin stenosis		1	1	0.3%	0	0%	0%–85%
Left origin atretic or absent			5	1.4%	2	40%	14%–71%
Right origin absent[b]			1	0.3%	1	100%	15%–100%
Diffuse narrowing left + right or left alone	5		5	1.4%	2	40%	14%–71%
Iatrogenic							
Right stenosis or occlusion	3		3	0.8%	0	0%	0%–47%
Total	25	13	44	12.1%	9	20%	14%–29%

KEY: CL, 70% confidence limits; PA, pulmonary artery.

[a] "Bifurcation" stenosis.

[b] Origin right pulmonary artery from ascending aorta.

stenoses may be present (12%). Although the pulmonary valve may be bicuspid, it is by definition not stenotic in this group, and the valve ring and main pulmonary artery are not obstructive. Narrowing of one or other pulmonary artery branch origin is very rare. The risk of operation is low in this group because of the ease with which the pulmonary stenosis is treated.

2. *Infundibular and valvar stenosis.* Some combination of infundibular and valvar stenosis occurs in the majority of cases of TF (74%, GLH, Table 23-3). In 26% of the total cases, the infundibulum and the pulmonary valve are stenotic to a variable degree, but the pulmonary ring (anulus) is of good size. A low infundibular stenosis is less common than in the isolated infundibular stenosis group, but, again, when present it may be in either a transverse plane, a coronal plane, or both planes. The main pulmonary artery may be diffusely small or tethered, but bifurcation stenosis is very rare.

3. *Infundibular plus valvar plus annular stenosis.* This combination is present somewhat less frequently (16%, GLH,

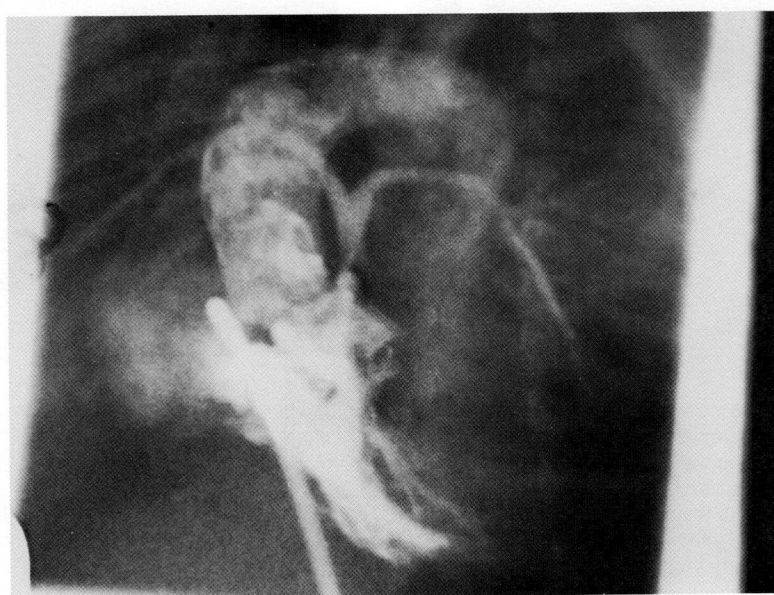

Figure 23-11 Cineangiogram following right ventricular injection in an infant with TF and pulmonary stenosis, without major associated cardiac anomalies (UAB). The striking feature is the diffuse hypoplasia of the right and left pulmonary arteries, which makes them an important obstruction to pulmonary blood flow. The pulmonary trunk and pulmonary anulus and the right ventricular infundibulum are also very narrow. A Gore-Tex interposition shunt between left subclavian and left pulmonary artery was successfully performed, and repair will be accomplished later.

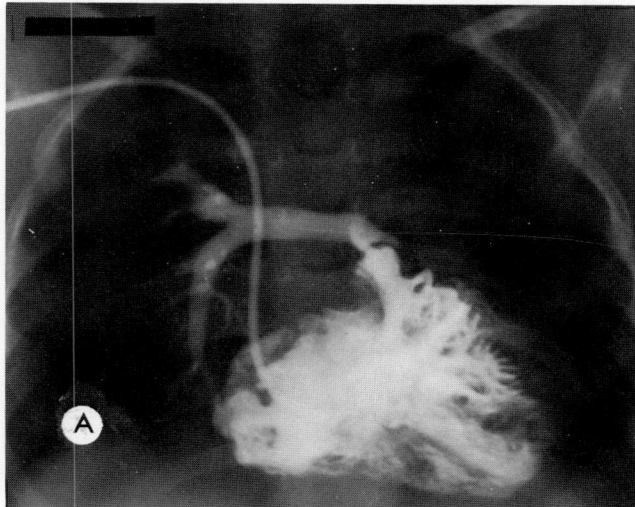

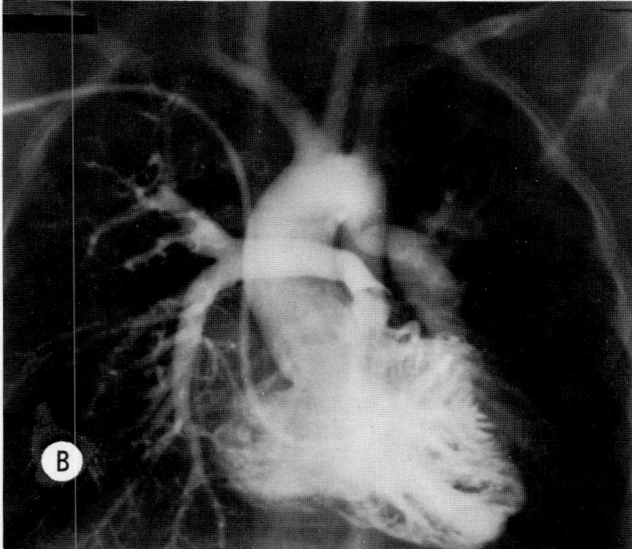

Figure 23-12 Cineangiogram in a patient with TF and absence of the central portion of the left pulmonary artery.
(a) Right ventricular injection shows lack of connection between pulmonary artery and left pulmonary artery.
(b) Later phase shows that the hilar portion of the left pulmonary artery originates from the ductus arteriosus.

Table 23-3). The os infundibulum lies either close to the valve without an intervening chamber (high infundibular stenosis) or at midinfundibular level. The infundibular stenosis is rarely at a low level. Diffuse narrowing or tethering of the main pulmonary artery is rather common, but a significant bifurcation lesion is uncommon.

4. *Diffuse right ventricular outflow hypoplasia*. This morphologic subset (see Table 23-3) is commonly present in infants presenting with severe cyanosis. There is rarely (4%, GLH) an additional proximal coronal stenosis. The pulmonary valve is usually bicuspid, with thickened, tethered, and stenotic leaflets; the pulmonary ring is small and obstructive; and the pulmonary artery diameter is one-half or less of that of the aorta, often with associated

tethering. Branches of the pulmonary artery are involved in 33% of cases (GLH), either at their origins (stenosis or atresia or absence) or more diffusely.

5. *Dominant valvar stenosis* is rare (see Table 23-3). The pulmonary ring is frequently also stenotic, and when the valve stenosis is produced by leaflet tethering the pulmonary artery is also tethered. The infundibular stenosis is mild, but the conal (infundibular) septal deviation characteristic of TF is present. Examples of significant valvar stenosis and a large perimembranous VSD without developmental anomalies of TF type in the infundibulum are uncommon (see Section 5 of this chapter).

6. *Pulmonary atresia. Congenital* pulmonary atresia is less common than pulmonary stenosis in TF, comprising 15%–20% of the total. The main pulmonary artery may be present (Fig. 23-9), widening distally to where it bifurcates, or it may be replaced by a fibrous chord. Occasionally, no fibrous chord is identifiable. Usually there is a confluence between right and left pulmonary artery branches without stenosis of either branch; and usually blood supply to the confluence is via a patent ductus arteriosus (to right or left pulmonary artery depending on the side of the aortic arch and the ductus origin). Alternatively, the blood supply comes from other aortopulmonary collaterals. The confluence may show significant stenoses of either left or right branch origins (usually at the site of the ductus junction and usually on the left side). Uncommonly, both left and right pulmonary artery branches are present but are nonconfluent, and more rarely still, the central and hilar portions of the pulmonary arteries are completely absent.

Acquired pulmonary atresia occurs uncommonly (1.4%, GLH) in the natural history of subjects born with severe stenosis and can be infundibular or valvar. When it is infundibular, a chamber can be present distally and the pulmonary valve can be nonstenotic. When there is acquired valvular atresia, the pulmonary trunk and its bifurcation are usually small. Acquired atresia occurs somewhat more commonly after a large systemic-pulmonary shunt has been made.[F11]

Distal Pulmonary Arteries and Veins

The pulmonary arteries and veins beyond the hilar positions are small in most patients with TF, and the degree of hypoplasia of these vessels is greater than the lung hypoplasia that is also present.[H6] However, the arteries usually enlarge as they pass distally, perhaps reflecting the input of bronchial arterial collateral flow into the distal vessels. The intraacinar arteries are smaller in patients with TF than in normal individuals, and their media is thinner.[J8] In addition, lung volume, alveolar size, and total alveolar number tend to be reduced.[H6,J8]

Pulmonary Artery Thromboses

In severely cyanotic and polycythemic patients with TF, diffuse pulmonary arterial thrombosis can occur. This is initially visible only microscopically,[F1] but rarely it may progress to occlusion of a lobar pulmonary artery or even an

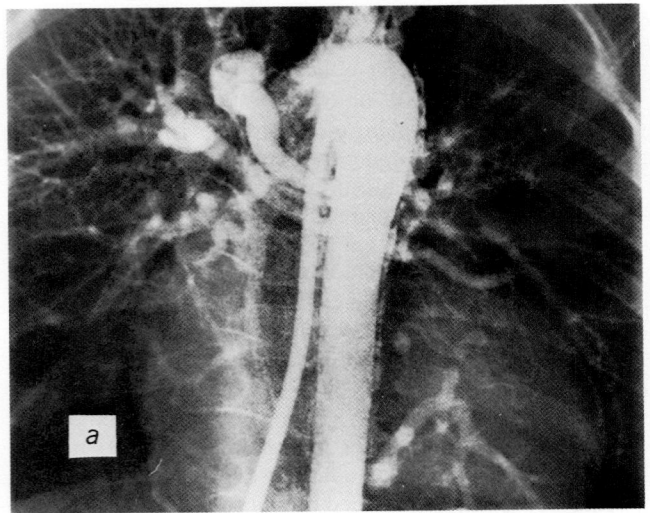

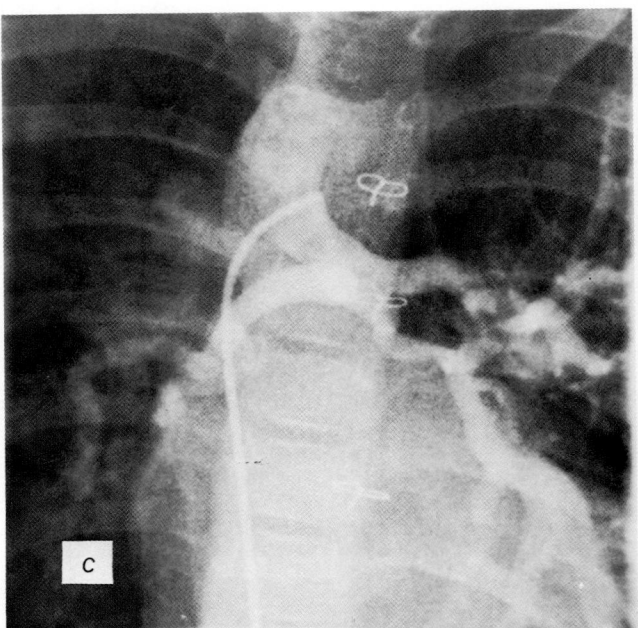

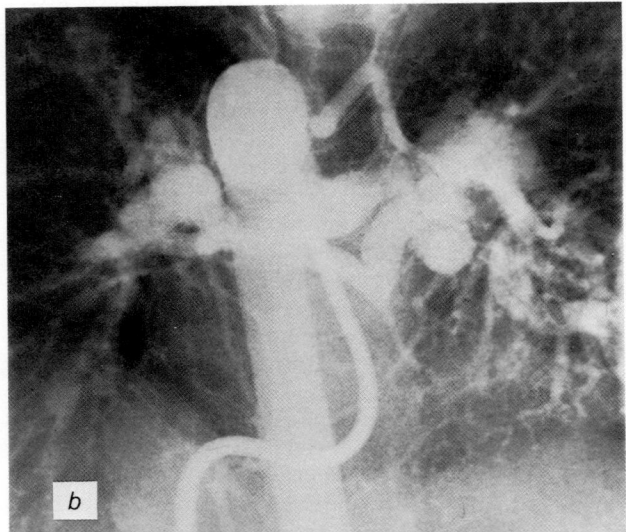

Figure 23-13 Large AP collateral arteries in patients with TF and pulmonary atresia (UAB).

(a) In this patient, two large AP collateral arteries come off the right and anterior aspect of the upper descending thoracic aorta and connect end to end with the hilar arteries of the right upper lobe. A smaller collateral artery supplies part of the lingula of the left lower lobe.

(b) In this patient, a large AP collateral artery passes to the left and joins end to side to the hilar portion of the left pulmonary artery in a manifold. The Y-shaped distal pulmonary trunk and central left and right pulmonary arteries are filled from this manifold. Another large AP collateral passes to the right above the right pulmonary artery.

(c) In this patient, branches of the large AP collateral artery join end to end with hilar branches to the left upper lobe, left lower lobe, and right lower lobe.

Table 23-3 Morphology and sites of right ventricular outflow obstruction in patients undergoing repair of TF with pulmonary stenosis (GLH; 1968–1978; excluding cases with subpulmonary ventricular septal defect, absent pulmonary valve, or congenital pulmonary atresia.) The figures in parentheses indicate the number of patients who had diffuse pulmonary arterial narrowing, pulmonary artery branch origin stenosis or bifurcation stenosis of pulmonary trunk, or absence of the central portion of the right or left pulmonary artery (11% of the total). The percentages in the table indicate percentage of the total group of 190. "High" refers to superiorly placed stenoses and "low" to inferiorly placed stenoses.

| Morphology of RV Outflow Obstruction | Site of Infundibular Stenosis | | | | | | | | Totals | | Hospital Deaths | | | |
| | High | | Inter-mediate | | Low | | Diffuse | | | | | | | |
	No.	%	No.	%	No.	%	No.	%	No.	%	n	No.	%	CL
Infundibular	6	3%	18(1)	9%	25	13%			49(1)	26%	49	0	0%	0%–4%
Infundibular + valvar	9	5%	31(1)	16%	9	5%			49(1)	26%	49	0	0%	0%–4%
Infundibular + valvar + ring	11	6%	20(1)	11%					31(1)	16%	31	3	10%	4%–19%
Diffuse hypoplasia							52(17)	27%	52(17)	27%	52	10	19%	13%–27%
Valvar ± ring									9(1)	5%	9	1	11%	1%–33%
Total	26	14%	69(3)	36%	34	18%	52(17)	27%	190(21)	100%	190	14	7.4%	5.4%–9.9%

KEY: CL, 70% confidence limits.

entire right or left pulmonary artery. Usually pulmonary vascular resistance is not importantly increased by this process, but rarely the thromboses may be so widespread and severe as to be a cause of immediate and sometimes fatal pulmonary hypertension and right ventricular failure following repair.

Pulmonary Vascular Disease

Pulmonary vascular disease rarely develops in surgically untreated patients with TF. It may develop following too large a systemic-pulmonary artery anastomosis (see "Interim Results after Classical Shunting Operations") or in association with nonstenotic, large, naturally occurring aortopulmonary collaterals (usually in patients with TF and pulmonary atresia). When a surgical shunt appears to be the cause, it is possible that preexistent pulmonary arterial thrombosis has compounded the problem.

Iatrogenic Pulmonary Arterial Problems

A functional absence of the central portion of pulmonary artery is produced by a Glenn anastomosis and by end-to-end Blalock-Taussig anastomoses. A palliative transannular patch may later result in severe stenosis at the origin of the left pulmonary artery or, less commonly, of the right one.[F8] An important stenosis or kinking of a right or left pulmonary artery may be produced by an imprecise anastomotic operation, particularly of the Waterston or Potts type, and the distal pulmonary artery may then become relatively hypoplastic because of poor pulmonary blood flow.

Collateral Pulmonary Arterial Blood Flow

A collateral blood flow to the pulmonary circulation is essential to the survival of patients with TF and pulmonary atresia. Patients with TF and pulmonary stenosis usually have less well developed collaterals, but even in some of them the collateral pulmonary blood flow may be greater than that coming directly from the right ventricle. The collateral flow enters into the true pulmonary arteries at some level and thus reaches the capillaries via the very distal branches of the pulmonary arteries.[R22]

Large Aortopulmonary Collateral Arteries
The most dramatic route of collateral flow is through large aortopulmonary (AP) collateral arteries (Fig. 23-13), occurring most commonly in patients with pulmonary atresia, and rarely in patients with TF and pulmonary stenosis. In general, the anatomy of the pulmonary circulation is less complex in the patients with pulmonary stenosis rather than atresia.[R29] The AP collateral arteries are large, discrete arteries, usually from one to three in number, originating from the upper or middescending thoracic aorta.[R6] They generally pursue a somewhat serpiginous course and most commonly terminate by joining an interlobar or intralobar pulmonary artery that then arborizes normally within a pulmonary lobe or segment.[H13,M19]

These large AP collateral arteries arise from the aorta either as elastic vessels with a wide lumen or as muscular arteries with stenotic areas.[H16] In either event, beyond their origins they resemble muscular systemic arteries. Areas of intimal proliferation are frequent, and these result in stenoses. Extensive areas of intimal proliferation (intimal pads) and stenoses are particularly prominent at branching points and at the junction of large AP collateral arteries with pulmonary arteries. This process results in stenoses being present in about 60% of the collateral arteries.[H13,M21,M22] In most patients there are sufficient stenoses to prevent pulmonary overcirculation, but when this is not the case pulmonary overcirculation develops early in life, and pulmonary vascular disease develops in patients surviving past infancy.[H16,T5]

The large AP collateral artery, which joins end to end with an intrapulmonary artery, changes in histologic appearance as it becomes a pulmonary artery; in this process the vessel also changes its positional relation to the bronchi. Thus, peripherally, its histologic appearance and position become typical for "true" pulmonary arteries.[H13] The distal pulmonary arterial branches are then nearly all abnormally small[H13] and fewer in number than in normal patients.[H17]

In about 50% of patients with TF and large AP collateral arteries, the large AP collateral artery enters into a complex manifold in the hilum of the lung. This manifold usually includes the hilar portion of the pulmonary artery, and from this manifold the interlobar and intralobar pulmonary arteries distribute distally, and the central pulmonary arteries may fill in a retrograde fashion.[F12]

Less commonly, a large AP collateral artery may connect end to side to a central pulmonary artery. Rarely, a single large AP artery on each side connects end to end with the hilar portion of the ipsilateral pulmonary artery.[C12,J7,M20] It is this last form that gave origin to the appellation *truncus type IV*.

Large AP collateral arteries are usually associated with abnormal branching patterns and incomplete distribution of the hilar portion of the pulmonary arteries. There may be associated single or multiple, localized or segmental pulmonary arterial stenoses, and/or diffuse hypoplasia of the pulmonary arteries.[O1,H13]

Paramediastinal Collateral Arteries
A large right or left paramediastinal collateral artery occasionally arises from the right or left subclavian artery, most often on the side opposite that of the aortic arch, and cineangiographically closely resembles a surgically created Blalock-Taussig shunt. It usually connects end to side to the right or left central or hilar pulmonary artery, but it may be associated with large AP collateral arteries and distribute end to end to the intrapulmonary arteries of the upper lobe. It may be impossible to distinguish such a collateral from examples of an unusually positioned and tortuous patent ductus arteriosus.

Bronchial Collateral Arteries
Most patients with TF have a diffusely enlarged network of bronchial collateral arteries. These provide a nondiscrete source of pulmonary blood flow, and in some patients, particularly older and deeply cyanotic ones, the collateral blood flow through them is large.

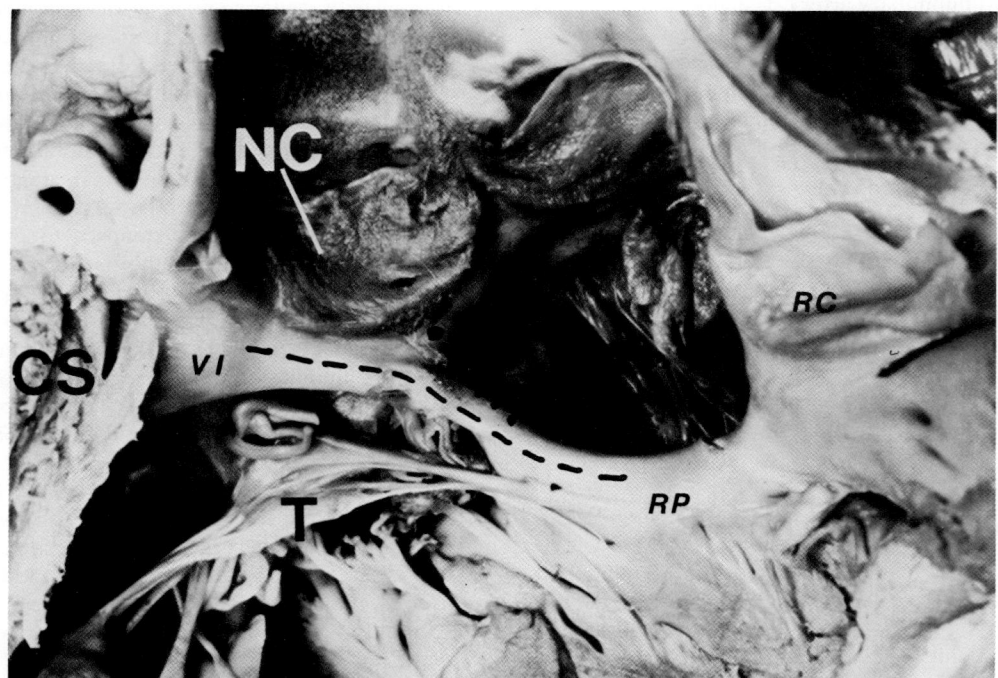

Figure 23-14   Specimen of TF demonstrating the ventricular septal defect and the position of the bundle of His (GLH). In this specimen, there is a narrow muscular bridge separating the VSD from the anterior tricuspid leaflet and tricuspid ring. The right ventricle has been opened, carrying the incision across the conal septum and right coronary cusp out into the ascending aorta as shown in Figure 23-1. The narrow muscular bridge of the septal band (trabecula septomarginalis) consists of the right posterior division of the septal band in continuity with the ventriculo-infundibular fold. The latter can be seen joining the undersurface of the parietal end of the infundibular (conal) septum. Sutures can be passed safely into this ridge along the dashed line (or, alternatively, in the base of the tricuspid leaflet), but the margin for error is small as the course of the bundle of His (dotted line) is not far removed. Note the marked overriding of the right aortic cusp into the right ventricle. CS, conal (infundibular) septum; NC, noncoronary cusp; RC, right coronary cusp; RP, right posterior division of septal band (trabecula septomarginalis); T, tricuspid anterior leaflet; VI, ventriculo-infundibular fold.

Intercostal Collateral Arteries
When pleural adhesions develop spontaneously or because of a previous thoracotomy or poudrage treatment, a very large flow may pass to the lungs through larger collaterals originating from the intercostal arteries, and extensive rib notching then develops. This collateral circulation may be so well developed as to make even the most careful mobilization of the lung hazardous and, on rare occasions, impossible without exsanguinating hemorrhage.

Other Collaterals
Small collateral channels may pass from the coronary arteries to the bronchial arteries.[D5] A *fistula* between the right coronary artery and the pulmonary trunk may rarely be the sole large collateral source of pulmonary blood flow in TF patients with pulmonary atresia.[K24] Even more rarely, an AP window may serve this function.[C2]

Iatrogenically Aggravated Collaterals
After a single Blalock-Taussig shunt, a large collateral arterial supply develops to the arm on the affected side, but parts of it eventually become collateral pulmonary blood flow. Large collateral vessels may develop between the two internal mammary arteries as part of this, and these may produce massive bleeding at sternotomy.

Ventricular Septal Defect

In classical TF, the VSD is subaortic in position and lies adjacent to or involves the membranous septum (perimembranous). It differs from the usual perimembranous defect, however, in that it is associated with malalignment of the conal (infundibular) septum (Fig. 23-2) and is always large.

The VSD is circular and bounded superiorly by the conal (infundibular) septum (Fig. 23-6). The septum may support part or most of the right aortic cusp, depending on the degree of aortic overriding onto the right ventricle (Fig. 23-1). Because of the anterior and leftward deviation of the parietal end (parietal extension) of the conal septum, the postero-superior angle of the defect extends higher than that of the usual isolated perimembranous VSD (Fig. 23-3a) and can be more difficult to expose surgically. When the conal septum is

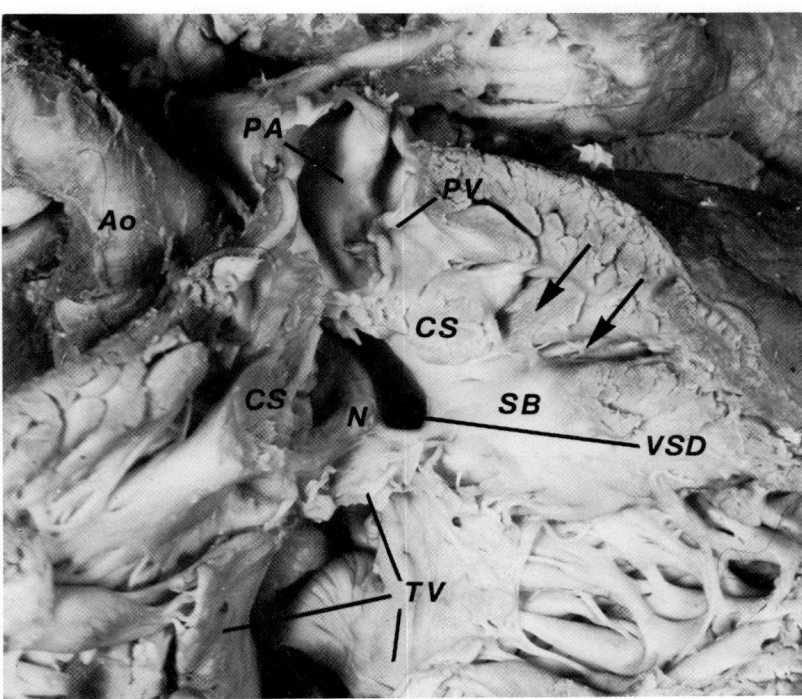

Figure 23-15 Autopsy specimen of TF with the right ventricle and pulmonary trunk opened with an anterior incision and the conal septum divided to expose the ventricular septal defect (GLH). Accessory prominent muscular trabeculations are present in front of the septal attachment of the conal septum (arrows), contributing to the stenosis. The pulmonary valve is bicuspid and tethered with mild leaflet thickening. Marked overriding of the aortic ring is visible, involving the rightward margin of the noncoronary cusp.

Ao, aorta; CS, conal septum; N, noncoronary cusp; PA, main pulmonary artery; PV, pulmonary valve; SB, septal band; TV, tricuspid valve; VSD, ventricular septal defect.

hypoplastic, the defect is larger and extends closer to the pulmonary valve; when the conal septum is absent, the VSD becomes truly subpulmonary.

Posterosuperiorly, the VSD is bounded by muscle (the ventriculo-infundibular fold) adjacent to the rightward edge of the noncoronary aortic cusp (Fig. 23-14). This cusp may override considerably into the right ventricle (Figs. 23-5, 23-15); then the aortic anulus adjacent to the noncoronary cusp forms this boundary.

The posterior margin shows considerable variation. It is related to the base of the tricuspid anteroseptal leaflet commissure and to the right fibrous trigone (central fibrous body) at the nadir of the noncoronary cusp. In most instances, there is tricuspid–aortic–mitral fibrous continuity at this margin and the membranous septum is absent. In some hearts, the VSD may extend inferiorly beneath the tricuspid septal leaflet more than usual. When there is marked clockwise rotation of the overriding aortic root, the right trigone may form the postero-inferior angle of the defect, and the bundle of His (which perforates at this point) is exposed along the edge of the defect (Fig. 23-16). Occasionally, the posterior margin may be formed by a remnant of fibrous tissue (membranous septum) projecting upward from the right trigone region. In at least 20% of hearts, the posterior

margin is formed by a muscular ridge of variable size that separates the right trigone from the base of the anterior tricuspid leaflet.[A16,R9,S9,B13] This ridge is formed by the right posterior division of the septal band (trabecula septomarginalis) as it becomes continuous with the ventriculo-infundibular fold (Figs. 23-14, 23-17). This ridge displaces the right trigone and therefore the bundle of His from the defect edge.

The *inferior* margin of the VSD is formed by the septal band as it cradles the VSD between its limbs. The papillary muscle of the conus (or corresponding chordae only) arises from the right posterior division of the septal band at the *antero-inferior* angle of the defect. Anomalous tricuspid chordal attachments to other margins of the defect are rare, which is in contrast to the situation in the usual perimembranous VSD.

The *anterior* margin of the VSD is formed by the leftward anterior division of the septal band as it becomes continuous with the inferior margin of the conal septum (Fig. 23-2). When the septal band is poorly developed, the defect extends further anteriorly.

Where the infundibular (conal) septum is absent, the VSD is not only subaortic but *subpulmonary* (subarterial or doubly committed) as well.[N6] Posteriorly, this type of VSD is

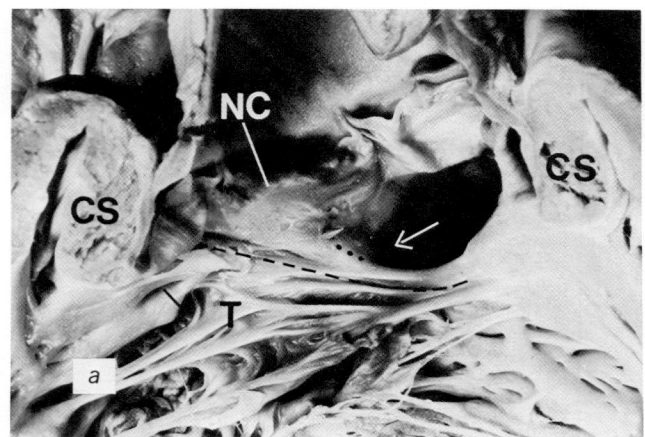
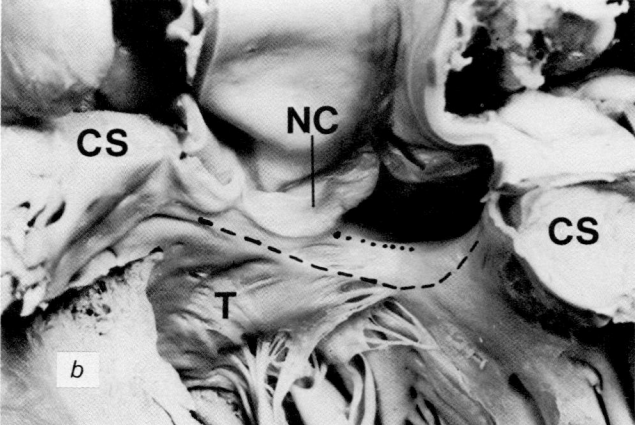

Figure 23-16 Two specimens of TF with perimembranous VSD, opened as in Figure 23-14 (GLH). Although it may not be entirely apparent in the photographs, there is tricuspid–aortic–mitral fibrous continuity at the posterior margin (in the photograph leftward) of the ventricular septal defect.

(*a*) The right fibrous trigone at the nadir of the noncoronary cusp has been perforated by a pin passed from the right atrial side at the point of penetration of the bundle of His; the bundle extends from this point forward and slightly leftward along the margin of the defect (dotted line). The white arrow points to this area. The VSD patch suture line must pass into the base of the anterior tricuspid leaflet (dashed line) and not along the lower defect margin.

(*b*) This photograph shows clearly the position of the right fibrous trigone when there is significant clockwise rotation of the aortic root and overriding of the noncoronary and right aortic cusps into the right ventricle. The bundle position is shown by a dotted line and the position of the VSD suture line (passing into the base of the anterior tricuspid leaflet) by a dashed line.

CS, conal septum; NC, noncoronary cusp; T, tricuspid valve.

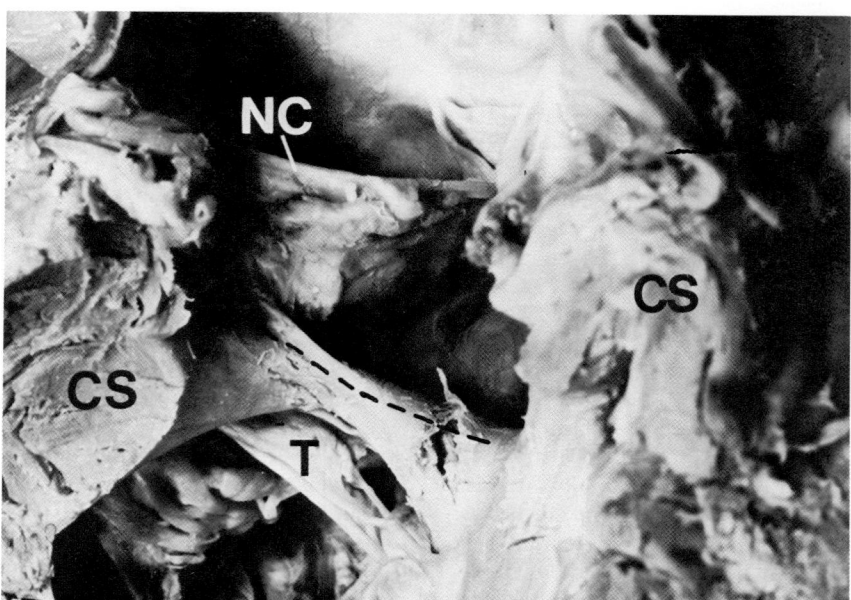

Figure 23-17 In this TF heart the posterior muscular bridge is much bulkier and entirely hides the right trigone that lies several millimeters caudal and leftward of the inferior VSD margin. The bundle will not be damaged by sutures passed into the ridge along the dashed line.

CS, conal septum; NC, noncoronary cusp; T, tricuspid valve.

Table 23-4 Major associated cardiac anomalies and hospital death in patients undergoing repair of TF. Some patients had more than one associated anomaly.

Major Associated Cardiac Anomaly	UAB 1967–1982 (n = 713)				GLH 1968–1978 (n = 205)				Total (n = 918)			
			Hospital Deaths				Hospital Deaths				Hospital Deaths	
	n	% of 713	No.	%	n	% of 205	No.	%	n	% of 918	No.	%
Multiple VSDs	20	2.8%	8	40%	2	1.0%	1	50%	22	2.4%	9	41%
Complete A-V canal defect	20	2.8%	7	35%	0	0%	0	0%	20	2.2%	7	35%
Patent ductus arteriosus	29	4.1%	6	21%	8	3.9%	2	25%	37	4.0%	8	22%
Anomalous origin of LCA from PA	1	0.1%	0	0%	0		0		1	0.1%	0	0%
AP window	2	0.3%	0	0%	0		0		2	0.2%	0	0%
Subaortic stenosis	3	0.4%	2	67%	1	0.5%	0	0%	4	0.4%	2	50%
Moderate or severe aortic incompetence	0		0		1	0.5%	0	0%	1	0.1%	0	0%
PAPVC	7	1.0%	0	0%	2	1.0%	0	0%	9	1.0%	0	0%
TAPVC	1	0.1%	1	100%	0		0		1	0.1%	1	100%
Unroofed coronary sinus	2	0.3%	1	50%	4	2.0%	1	25%	6	0.6%	2	33%
Straddling tricuspid valve	3	0.4	0	0%	0				3	0.3%	0	0%
Small tricuspid valve ring	2	0.3%	0	0%	0				2	0.2%	0	0%
Severe tricuspid incompetence	2	0.3%	1	50%	1	0.5%	0	0%	3	0.3%	1	33%
Mitral stenosis	1	0.1%	0	0%	0				1	0.1%	0	0%
Dextrocardia	6	0.8%	2	33%	3	1.5%	1	33%	9	1.0%	3	33%
Situs ambiguus	2	0.3%	1	50%	0				2	0.2%	1	50%
Situs inversus totalis	2	0.3%	0	0%	3	1.5%	1	33%	5	0.5%	1	20%
Ebstein's malformation	1	0.1%	0	0%	0				1	0.1%	0	0%
Underdeveloped RV	0	NT	NT		3	1.5%	1	33%	3	0.3%	1	33%
RPA origin from asc. ao.	0				1	0.5%	1	100%	1	0.1%	1	100%
Pulmonary vasc. disease	0				2	1.0%	1	50%	2	0.2%	1	50%
Endocarditis RV outflow	0				2	1.0%	0	0%	2	0.2%	0	0%
Total patients	87	12.2%	20	23%	26	13%	6	23%	113	12.3%	26	23%

KEY: AP, aortopulmonary; LCA, left coronary artery; NT, not tabulated; PA, pulmonary artery; PAPVC, partial anomalous pulmonary venous connection; RV, right ventricle; RPA, right pulmonary artery; TAPVC, total anomalous pulmonary venous connection; VSD, ventricular septal defect.

commonly separated from the tricuspid annulus by a 2–5 mm strip of muscle, but it may be truly perimembranous and extend to the tricuspid annulus. Aortic and pulmonary valve rings are contiguous over about one-third of their circumference, being separated at this point by only a thin fibrous ridge (Fig. 23-4). The two valves are often side by side, and the aorta is more than usually dextroposed.[S11] The tetralogy of Fallot with this type of VSD is morphologically similar to double outlet right ventricle with a doubly committed VSD (see Chapter 40).

In 3%–15% of patients with TF (Table 23-4) , one or more *additional VSDs* coexist with the typical subaortic one[F4] (Fig. 23-18). Most commonly, the additional VSD is muscular, and multiple muscular defects sometimes occur. The additional VSD may be in the inlet septum, either as an AV canal type or a muscular defect.

Conduction System

The *sinus and AV nodes* are normal in location (see Chapter 1), and the bundle of His follows the same general course as in patients with isolated perimembranous VSD (see Chapter 20). Thus, it emerges through the right fibrous trigone at the base of the noncoronary cusp and courses forward toward the papillary muscle of the conus along the inferior VSD margin or slightly to the left side of the defect edge.[L14,F13] In hearts showing marked clockwise rotation of the aortic root with overriding, the right trigone (and along with it the penetrating portion of the His bundle) is carried more rightward and superiorly and directly into the VSD margin (Fig. 23-16).

In contrast, the bundle of His does not lie on the VSD margin when there is a muscle ridge present[D12] (Figs. 23-14, 23-17), since the ridge projects superiorly above the right

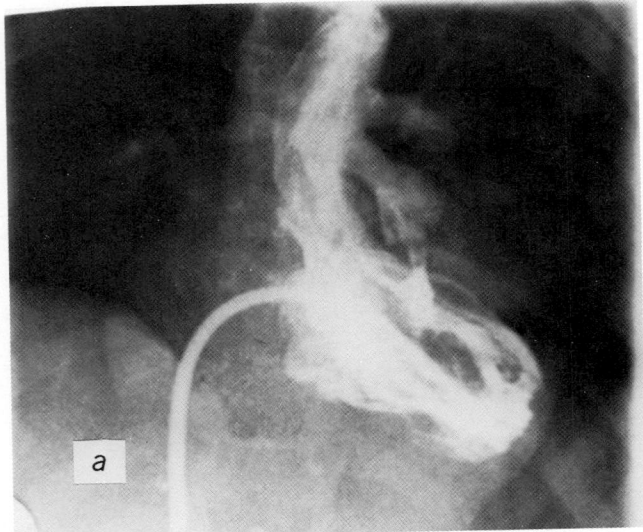

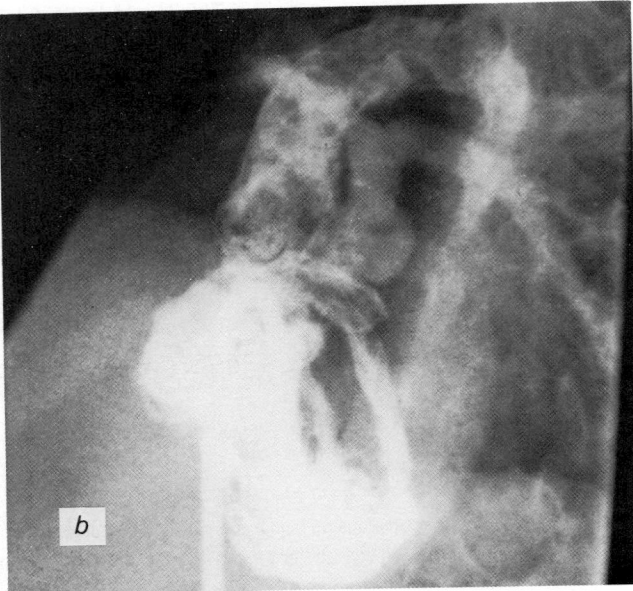

Figure 23-18 Cineangiograms in a patient with TF, pulmonary stenosis, and multiple VSDs (UAB). Note the large trabecular VSD near the apex as well as the usual perimembranous subaortic VSD. (*a*) Systolic frame. (*b*) Diastolic frame.

fibrous trigone and sutures can be safely placed into the muscular tissue.[B13]

Aorta

In TF patients, the aorta is biventricular in origin and is more anteriorly placed than normal, often almost obscuring the smaller pulmonary artery from view at operation. These changes are due to overriding, rotation, and enlargement of the aortic root. Overriding (or dextroposition) of the aorta onto the right ventricle is an almost constant feature. The proportion of the aorta lying above the right ventricle varies

between 30% and 90%.[A17] Generally, about 50% of the aortic orifice is over the right ventricle.

Aortic overriding is associated with a variable degree of clockwise rotation of the aortic root (as viewed from below upward). This rotation moves the base of the noncoronary cusp rightward and superiorly onto the posterosuperior margin of the VSD and away from the base of the anterior mitral leaflet so that in extreme cases it may no longer be continuous with this structure. This cusp may then lie in part just beneath the parietal extension of the infundibular (conal) septum. The rightward rotation of the left aortic cusp results in more of it becoming continuous with the anterior mitral leaflet. Simultaneously, the superiorly positioned right cusp base moves to the left, and in extreme examples it may be just beneath the uppermost extension of the left anterior division of the trabecula septomarginalis (septal band) at the anterosuperior margin of the VSD.

The degree of overriding and clockwise rotation of the aortic root relates to the degree of underdevelopment of the right ventricular outflow tract and to the deviation of the infundibular septum. When these are minimal, as seen with isolated low-lying infundibular stenosis, the aorta is minimally affected, whereas when there is diffuse right ventricular outflow tract hypoplasia in association with a small, markedly deviated infundibular septum and posterior and leftward movement of the origin of the main pulmonary artery, the aorta is markedly rotated and dextroposed. The degree of overriding or dextroposition may be assessed morphologically at operation or autopsy (UAB), and when this is done it may be considered that double outlet right ventricle with pulmonary stenosis, rather than TF, exists when the overriding is more than 90% (UAB). Alternatively, it may be considered that the overriding is best assessed cineangiographically using both left anterior oblique (LAO) and right anterior oblique (RAO) views (Fig. 23-19) and then double outlet right ventricle is diagnosed when the overriding is more than 50% (GLH).

In patients with severe tetralogy, the aortic root is frequently larger than normal, even in infants. Occasionally in adults, it is greatly dilated. This may uncommonly result in aortic valve incompetence.

Aortic Arch and Ductus Arteriosus

The *ductus arteriosus* (or ligamentum arteriosum) is absent in about 30% of hearts with TF patients (GLH autopsy series of 120 cases). Absence of the ductus or ligamentum is about twice as common when there is a right rather than left aortic arch. Patency of the ductus arteriosus is more common in TF with pulmonary atresia than with pulmonary stenosis. In fact, in many patients with TF and pulmonary atresia, the pulmonary circulation at birth is dependent on ductal flow to the site of pulmonary artery confluence. When the ductus is absent, pulmonary blood flow is supplied by large collateral arteries.

A *left aortic arch* is present in about 75% of patients with TF and pulmonary stenosis and in about 70% of those with pulmonary atresia. In patients with TF and pulmonary stenosis and left arch, the arch branching pattern is usually normal (Fig. 23-20). If a patent ductus arteriosus is present, its

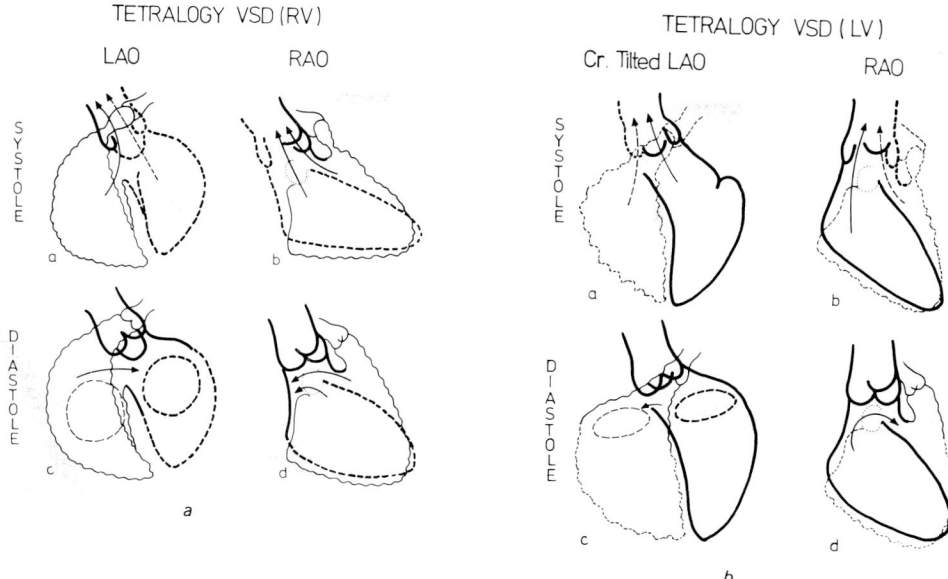

Figure 23-19 Cineangiocardiographic assessment of intracardiac anatomy in TF (GLH). Right ventricle (RV) and pulmonary artery are indicated by thin line; left ventricle (LV) and aorta are indicated by thick line. Continuous line is for structures primarily demonstrated; interrupted line is for those faintly or variably demonstrated.

(a) RV injection in steep (75°–80°) LAO (a,c) and 30°–40° RAO (b,d) in systole (a,b) and diastole (c,d). In *steep LAO projection*, the VSD is profiled beneath the right coronary sinus of the aortic root, adjacent to the upper margin of the tricuspid valve seen in diastole. Any inferior extension of the VSD into the basal sinus septum between the AV valves is accurately shown. In systole contrast medium from RV streams up into the aortic root with relatively nonopaque blood from LV. In diastole contrast medium mixes into the LV showing the left side of the basal septum. This projection shows aortic valve overriding in the region of the noncoronary sinus and adjacent commissure with the right coronary sinus, there being little override in this diagram as is commonly the case. The RV infundibulum, pulmonary valve, and proximal main pulmonary artery are usually superimposed on the aortic root, but distal main pulmonary artery and proximal left pulmonary artery are well seen (not illustrated).

In RAO projection the conal septum is well profiled and the anatomy of the RV infundibulum, pulmonary valve, main pulmonary artery, and proximal right pulmonary artery (not shown) are well displayed. Contrast medium streaming into the anterior part of the aorta through the VSD delineates the VSD margin in relationship to the tricuspid ring. Contrast medium passing beneath the conal septum enters the aortic root directly, since this part overrides. The degree of overriding of the aorta in the region of the right coronary sinus relates to the degree of conal septal displacement into RV from its proper connection to the superior margin of LV. The degree of this displacement and the extent of override, however, are not shown since the LV margin is obscured by RV contrast. In diastole, the aortic valve closes and contrast medium passing beneath the conal septum and through the VSD into LV outlines the atrioventricular septum, usually projected behind the tricuspid valve ring, confirming the LV origin of the posterior part of the noncoronary sinus.

(b) The LV injection in 50°–60° LAO with 30°–40° cranial tilting (a,c), and 30°–40° RAO (b,d). In cranially tilted LAO, the VSD is again profiled beneath the right coronary aortic sinus, although it often looks smaller than in LAO. Aortic override can be assessed in relation to the noncoronary sinus (none illustrated) as in LAO. The extent of VSD inferiorly is less well seen and the tricuspid orifice is foreshortened. The middle and apical parts of the sinus septum are better separated than in LAO, and additional sinus septal defects are therefore more accurately excluded.

In RAO, contrast medium outlines the atrioventricular septum and superior LV margin and streams into the noncoronary and left coronary portions of the aortic root. Initially, the anterior right coronary sinus portion of the aortic root may not outline owing to the nonopaque RV streaming. In diastole, however, contrast medium passing through the VSD shows the right coronary aortic cusp and conal septum in the RV. The degree of displacement of the conal septum from the superior LV margin at the edge of the VSD is accurately shown, indicating the extent of anterior aortic override of the midportion of the right coronary sinus. Additional high anterior muscular VSDs, if present, are profiled in the RAO projection.

RIGHT AORTIC ARCH

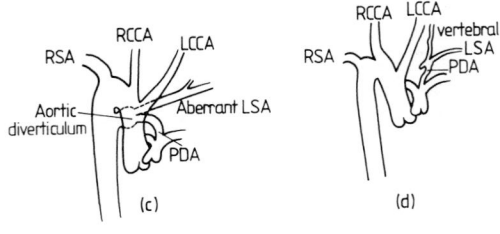

LEFT AORTIC ARCH

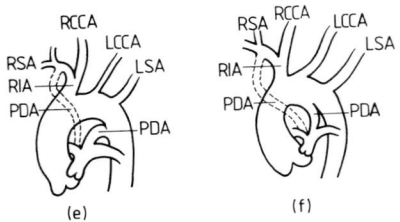

Figure 23-20 Line drawings illustrating the aortic arch branching pattern and ductus origin in hearts with TF. A *right aortic arch* is present in about 25% of hearts with pulmonary stenosis (PS) and 30% with pulmonary atresia. A patent ductus arteriosus is uncommon when there is pulmonary stenosis and common when there is pulmonary atresia.

(a) The usual branching pattern in TF with right aortic arch, present in almost 90% of cases, is the mirror image of normal. The first branch is the left innominate, the second the right common carotid, and the last the right subclavian artery. A left ductus when present arises from the innominate artery. Rarely, there may be a right ductus to the right pulmonary artery, usually from the upper descending aorta (dashed lines).

(b) Less commonly (about 10% of hearts with TF and a right aortic arch), there is an aberrant left subclavian artery. A ductus, if present, may arise near the origin of the left common carotid artery or from the aberrant LSA.

(c) Rarely (about 2% of hearts with TF and a right aortic arch), an aberrant left subclavian artery may arise from an aortic diverticulum, which also gives origin to a left ductus arteriosus. The ductus then passes behind the esophagus. (This is the usual pattern in situs solitus with right aortic arch without TF.)

(d) Least often (in TF and right aortic arch), there is an isolated (sequestered) left subclavian artery. This vessel fills by retrograde flow in the vertebral artery and is connected to the left pulmonary artery by a ductus arteriosus that may or may not be patent.

(e) When a left aortic arch is present in TF with PS, the arch branching pattern is usually normal and if a patent ductus is present its orientation and position is the common one. A right patent ductus

orientation and position on the left side is normal and flow in utero is from pulmonary artery through the ductus arteriosus to the aorta. In patients with TF and pulmonary atresia, the ductus orientation and position are usually abnormal, and it is a downwardly directed branch coming from beneath the left aortic arch.[C20] It is also longer and more tortuous than is otherwise the case (Fig. 23-21) and is often narrowed at its pulmonary end. In the setting of left aortic arch, a right-sided patent ductus arteriosus is rare. When present, it comes off the right subclavian or innominate artery, or, if associated with an aberrant right subclavian artery, it may come from an aortic diverticulum and pass to the right behind the esophagus.

A *right aortic arch* is present in about 25% of patients with pulmonary stenosis and 30% with pulmonary atresia. In 90% of patients with a right arch, there is mirror image branching of the arch (Fig. 23-20). Should a patent ductus arteriosus be present, it usually arises from the innominate or proximal left subclavian artery and joins the left pulmonary artery[S17] (Fig. 23-20). Rarely, there may be a right-sided ductus arteriosus to the right pulmonary artery, usually arising from the upper descending thoracic aorta.

In about 10% of instances, there is an aberrant left subclavian artery, analogous to the aberrant right subclavian artery of dysphasia lusoria in left aortic arch. In right aortic arch with aberrant left subclavian artery, the subclavian artery may arise directly from the descending aorta or from an aortic diverticulum. Thus a ductus arteriosus may arise from the aortic diverticulum and pass to the left behind the esophagus to join the left pulmonary artery.

Rarely, the left subclavian artery is sequestered or isolated from its aortic arch origin but remains connected to the left pulmonary artery by a patent ductus arteriosus (Fig. 23-20). Often in these circumstances there is a vertebral steal present and on arteriography the subclavian artery fills with contrast from the vertebral artery.

Right Ventricle

The external dimensions of the sinus (inflow) portion of the right ventricle are larger than normal due to hypertrophy, so that the interventricular groove is displaced leftward and the left ventricle lies more posteriorly than usual (clockwise rotation of the ventricles). The right ventricular sinus may be clearly separated from the infundibulum during systole by a transverse depression that represents the site of maximal infundibular stenosis inferior to an infundibular chamber.

is rare and would either come off the right subclavian or innominate artery (dashed lines); if arising in conjunction with an aberrant right subclavian via an aortic diverticulum (not shown in diagram), it passes behind the esophagus.

(f) When a left aortic arch is present in TF with pulmonary atresia, the frequently left patent ductus is long and has a downward orientation from the undersurface of the aortic arch, indicating flow in utero from aorta to left pulmonary artery. A right ductus may also be present as in (e) and rarely both left and right ducti may be patent.

LCCA, left common carotid artery; LIA, left innominate artery; LSA, left subclavian artery; PDA, patent ductus arteriosus; RCCA, right common carotid artery; RIA, right innominate artery; RSA, right subclavian artery.

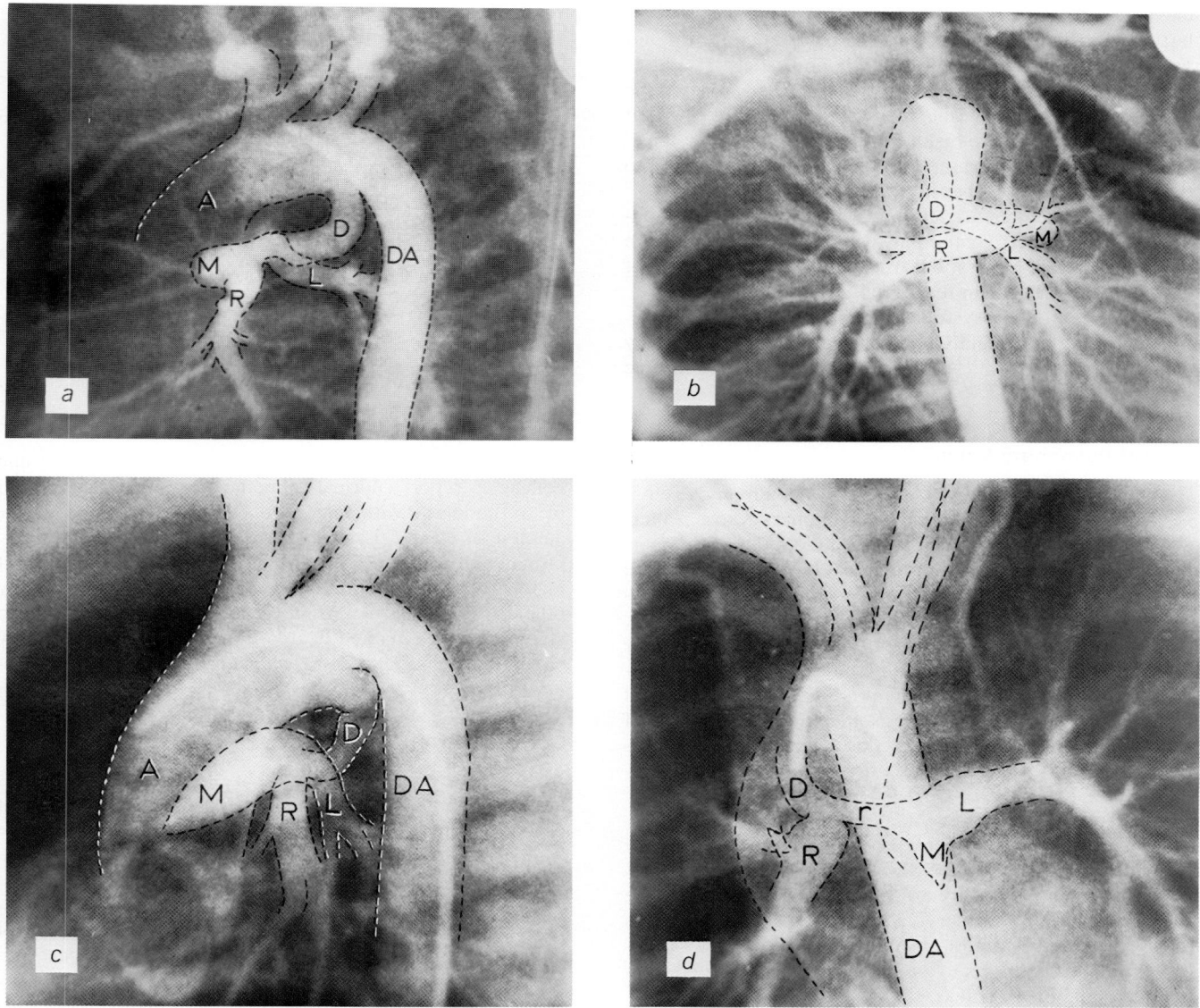

Figure 23-21 Arch aortography in neonate with pulmonary atresia (GLH). Cine frames in (*a*) LAO and (*b*) RAO projections show the typical orientation of a left patent ductus arteriosus in pulmonary atresia with a left aortic arch. The ductus joins the origin of the left pulmonary artery. Contrast medium fills the main and right pulmonary arteries also. The LAO view shows normal (usual) brachiocephalic artery origins.

Cine frames in lateral (*c*) and frontal (*d*) projections show the typical pulmonary atresia orientation of the patent ductus arteriosus when the aortic arch is right-sided. Here the right-sided ductus arises from the distal arch to join the right pulmonary artery. Contrast medium also fills the main and left pulmonary arteries through the narrowed proximal right pulmonary artery.

A, ascending aorta; D, patent ductus arteriosus; DA, descending aorta; L, left pulmonary artery; M, main pulmonary artery; R, right pulmonary artery; r, proximal right pulmonary artery.

The right ventricular wall thickness equals that of the left ventricle and is therefore never excessive unless the large VSD is functionally occluded on its right side by a fibrous flap valve (see Section 2). The normal trabeculations are, however, bulky and prominent. The right ventricular end-diastolic volume may be reduced and the ejection fraction mildly depressed[G1] possibly secondary to the chronic hypoxia. Occasionally (1.5% of cases), the sinus portion of the right ventricle and the tricuspid valve are underdeveloped (Table 23-4).

Left Ventricle

The left ventricle in TF is usually normal in wall thickness[M3] but variable as regards volume. In patients with severe forms of tetralogy and severe cyanosis, the left ventricular end-diastolic volume is normal or somewhat small,[J3,L1,L2,M3,N1] but wall thickness remains normal. Uncommonly, the left ventricle and mitral valve are truly hypoplastic.[G8]

The physiologic contributors to left ventricular size in the tetralogy are complex. The small pulmonary and thus left atrial blood flow tend to result in a small left atrium[M3,N1] and left ventricle. However, the right ventricle ejects blood into the left ventricle as well as into the aorta in this condition,[M3] and this tends to increase left ventricular size. Mild or moderate degrees of left ventricular hypoplasia may result from these physiologic factors, but true hypoplasia is no doubt of morphologic rather than functional origin.

The left ventricular systolic function as estimated by ejection fraction is also mildly reduced, particularly in severely cyanotic patients,[G9,J3,M3] presumably because of the chronic hypoxia.

Absent Pulmonary Valve

About 10% of patients with classic TF and pulmonary stenosis have vestigial nonfunctioning pulmonary valve leaflets (see Table 23-1). When in this situation the stenosis is minimal at both valve and infundibular level, there is severe pulmonary incompetence that is worsened by a modest increase in pulmonary blood flow ($\dot{Q}p/\dot{Q}s$ is generally 1.5–2.0). In this situation, the pulmonary trunk and central and hilar portions of the right and left pulmonary arteries are aneurysmally dilated at birth.[S4] This produces tracheobronchial compression that can be severe, sometimes with collapse of a lobe or a whole lung. There may be extensive tracheobronchitis secondary to the compression and increased pulmonary blood flow.

The cause of the massive dilatation of the pulmonary arteries in utero is unclear, but when there is severe pulmonary incompetence and a large VSD, absence of ductal flow between the main pulmonary artery and the aorta seems to be essential to intrauterine survival.[Z3] Thus, a ductus arteriosus (or ligamentum) is almost always absent at autopsy[E10] (unless the ductus connects to a pulmonary artery isolated from the main pulmonary trunk).

This *absent pulmonary valve syndrome* accounts for only 3%–5% of patients with TF and pulmonary stenosis. The large VSD is a typical malalignment tetralogy defect. In addition to the myxomatous vestigial pulmonary leaflets, there is a mild annular stenosis and conal (infundibular) septal displacement typical of TF but with absent or at most mild stenosis and a tendency toward dilatation and unusual elongation of the right ventricular outflow tract.[Z3] The sinus portion of the right ventricle is markedly enlarged due to dilatation and hypertrophy. Aneurysmal dilatation of the main pulmonary artery is a constant feature, and although both right and left pulmonary arteries may be equally dilated, the right is usually the larger.[L8]

Beyond their hilar portions, the pulmonary arteries are usually normal in size. Rarely, the distal branches are hypoplastic and, rarely also, the hilar branching pattern is abnormal.[R11] There may be origin of the right or left pulmonary artery from the ascending aorta,[C4] or a pulmonary artery may originate from a patent ductus arteriosus.[Z3]

There is controversy as to the histopathology of the di-

Table 23-5 Minor associated cardiac anomalies in patients undergoing repair of the TF with pulmonary stenosis or atresia (UAB; 1967–July 1982).

Minor Associated Cardiac Anomalies	n	% of 836
Atrial septal defect	75	9%
Persistent left superior vena cava	68	8%
Anomalous origin of LAD from RCA	34	4%
Aberrant origin right subclavian artery	2	0.3%
Absent right superior vena cava	1	0.2%
Azygos extension of the inferior vena cava	1	0.2%
Congenital heart block	1	0.2%
Juxtaposition of atrial appendages	1	0.2%
Vascular ring	1	0.2%

KEY: LAD, left anterior descending coronary artery; RCA, right coronary artery.

lated pulmonary arteries in this syndrome. Arensman and colleagues report a normal pulmonary arterial wall in five out of six children, with one child having a reduction in the amount of elastic tissue in the pulmonary arterial wall.[A13] Osman and colleagues have reported similar findings,[O6] but histopathologic abnormalities have been reported by others.[M7,M12,O7,R10,R11] Whatever the histology, physiologic studies indicate marked decrease in right pulmonary artery compliance in sick small babies with TF and absent pulmonary valve.[H8]

Coronary Arteries

As in other cyanotic conditions, in TF the coronary arteries are dilated and tortuous. A large conal branch of the right coronary artery usually courses obliquely across the free wall of the right ventricle. A vertical or transverse ventriculotomy can usually be made downstream to this.

The anterior descending coronary artery arises anomalously from the right coronary artery in about 5% of patients[D5,F4,F5] (Table 23-5). The entire left anterior descending (LAD) artery may originate from the right coronary artery and cross the anterior wall of the infundibulum a variable distance from the pulmonary valve or only the distal part of the LAD may arise anomalously, in this case usually from the large conal branch of the right coronary artery.

Rarely (two cases GLH), the right coronary originates from the left coronary artery, and equally uncommonly (two cases UAB), there is anomalous origin of the left coronary artery from the pulmonary artery.[A14]

Major Associated Cardiac Anomalies

Major associated cardiac anomalies are relatively uncommon in tetralogy (see Table 23-4), particularly in tetralogy with pulmonary atresia (Table 23-6), and are detailed in the tables. *Patent ductus arteriosus, multiple VSDs* (Fig. 23-18), and *complete AV canal defects*[Z1] are the most common.

The *right*[K18] or *left*[M6] *pulmonary artery* may arise anomalously from the ascending aorta[K9] (see Chapter 30). This rare associated anomaly complicates the pathophysiology and the repair, since the lung supplied by the pulmonary artery arising from the aorta usually has overcirculation and the

Table 23-6 Major associated cardiac anomalies other than complete AV canal defects (see Chapter 19) and hospital death in patients undergoing repair for TF with pulmonary atresia (UAB; 1967–July 1982). Some patients had more than one associated anomaly.

| Major Associated Cardiac Anomaly | Pulmonary Atresia (n = 123) | | | |
	n	% of 123	Hospital Deaths No.	%
Multiple VSDs	2	1.6%	0	0%
Coronary-pulmonary artery fistula	4	3%	1	25%
Patent ductus arteriosus	18	15%	4	22%
Moderate or severe aortic incompetence	2	1.6%	1	50%
Partial anomalous pulmonary venous connection	2	1.6%	1	50%
Severe tricuspid incompetence	2	1.6%	0	0%
Total	30	24%	7	23% (CL 15%–34%)

KEY: CL, 70% confidence limits; VSD, ventricular septal defect.

other usually has restriction of flow because of the intracardiac anatomy of TF.

Infrequently, *aortic valve incompetence* may coexist with TF. This may be from typical cusp prolapse in TF with subarterial (subpulmonary and subaortic) ventricular septal defect[M9] (see Chapter 20, Section 2). A bicuspid aortic valve occurs rarely in TF and may result in aortic incompetence.[G11,V2] Occasionally, in patients with TF in the second decade of life or older, aortic incompetence can be from the destructive effects of native aortic valve endocarditis.[B12,C14] Massive dilation of the aortic root with annular ectasia may result in aortic valve incompetence,[C14] particularly in patients with large natural or surgically created AP shunts.

Minor Associated Cardiac Anomalies

Most infants undergoing repair of TF have a patent foramen ovale; when all ages are considered, a true atrial septal defect is found at operation in about 10%. Other minor associated cardiac anomalies may occur (Table 23-5).

Other Convenient Morphologic Categories

Pulmonary Arterial Problems
It is convenient to use the general phrase *pulmonary arterial problems* when important anomalies of the pulmonary arteries complicate the TF. In this text, these include diffuse (Fig. 23-11) or segmental hypoplasia (localized single or multiple stenoses), abnormal hilar branching patterns, incomplete distribution of the hilar portion of the right and/or left pulmonary artery, and absence of portions of the right and left arteries.

Uncomplicated Tetralogy of Fallot
In this text, *uncomplicated TF* is used as a term of convenience to imply absence of pulmonary arterial problems, ma-

jor associated cardiac anomalies, or absent pulmonary valve syndrome and either no previous operation or only a single classical shunt (end-to-side Blalock-Taussig shunt on the side opposite that of the aortic arch or a Gore-Tex interposition shunt).

CLINICAL FEATURES AND DIAGNOSTIC CRITERIA

Clinical Presentation

The usual clinical presentation is with cyanosis, which varies with the severity of the pulmonary stenosis. When there is *pulmonary atresia from birth,* cyanosis is usually evident in the first few days of life and becomes extreme as the ductus narrows and closes. This rapid progression is modified when there are other collaterals of large size supplying the pulmonary bed or when the ductus stays open. Rarely, infants with pulmonary atresia and large AP collaterals have only mild cyanosis and the presentation is with heart failure, which usually develops at 4–6 weeks of age as the neonatal pulmonary vascular resistance falls and pulmonary blood flow becomes large.

Infants with *pulmonary stenosis* and diffuse right ventricular outflow hypoplasia, severe infundibular plus valvar plus annular stenosis or severe infundibular and valvar stenosis (see ''Morphology'') are deeply cyanotic from birth and do not develop heart failure. They are breathless on feeding or other exertion. Hypoxic spells are rare, the cyanosis being constant and gradually worsening. It is seldom lessened by propranolol.

This situation is in contrast to that in infants with dominant infundibular stenosis. In these infants, cyanosis is later in onset, and the infants are subject to hypoxic (cyanotic) spells due to infundibular spasm. These spells are often prevented or lessened in frequency by propranolol. Characteristically, cyanotic spells become less frequent with age, presumably because the stenosis becomes fixed due to acquired endocardial fibrosis and thickening.

In up to 10% of patients with TF who require surgical relief in infancy, presentation is initially as a large VSD with pulmonary plethora and sometimes congestive heart failure at 2–3 months of age, followed at about 6 months of age by gradually increasing cyanosis, frequently with cyanotic spells. In this group, the stenosis is always purely infundibular.

A minority of patients with TF are acyanotic at rest and only mildly cyanotic on exercise because the pulmonary stenosis is mild and right-to-left shunting minimal. In some patients, the shunt may be predominantly left to right. These individuals may remain acyanotic without spells and present at any age within the first and second decades of life, with gradually increasing cyanosis and breathlessness as the pulmonary stenosis slowly increases in severity.

In patients with severe cyanosis and polycythemia, cerebral thrombosis may precipitate a hemiplegia at any age (particularly in association with dehydration from any cause), or hemiplegia may follow paradoxical embolism or a brain abscess. The latter is heralded by fever, headache, and sometimes seizures. Massive hemoptysis may occur in older patients who are severely cyanotic, presumably from rupture of bronchial collateral vessels.

Cyanosis is always accompanied by significant effort dyspnea that is sometimes the dominant symptom, and as the child begins to walk (frequently much later than for a healthy child) cyanosis is often accompanied by squatting that lessens the cyanosis.[K19] There may be an increased incidence of respiratory infection but not to the same extent as in patients with large VSD. Failure to thrive is also less striking than in patients with large VSD.

Physical Examination

Cyanosis of variable degree is generally evident. Deeply cyanotic infants are often quite fat (in contrast to infants with VSD). Severe symmetric clubbing of the fingers and toes is often present in childhood and adult life but not in small infants. Older patients may also have marked acne of the face and anterior chest. The jugular venous pressure is normal and the pulse low volume with a low blood pressure (relative hypotension may persist into the early postoperative period). The heart is not enlarged and is relatively quiet with an unimpressive right ventricular lift. In those few patients with an increased pulmonary blood flow and pulmonary hypertension, there may be a more marked right ventricular lift than usual. It is important to appreciate, however, that when the pulmonary blood flow is very low (as is the case in severely cyanosed patients), it is impossible to detect an elevated pulmonary vascular resistance clinically (or in fact at cardiac catheterization).

A precordial systolic thrill is rare. There is a moderate intensity midsystolic pulmonary (ejection) murmur maximal in the second and third left intercostal spaces, which when the stenosis is very severe becomes less prominent or even disappears. In pulmonary atresia, therefore, a systolic murmur is usually absent. However, there is frequently a continuous murmur in patients with TF and pulmonary atresia (and rarely in patients with TF and pulmonary stenosis) from large AP collateral arteries, a patent ductus arteriosus, or rarely a coronary-pulmonary artery fistula.[O2] This is maximal over the site of the collateral at its point of stenosis and may therefore be heard to the left or right of the sternum or posteriorly.

When there is still a reasonable blood flow in the presence of moderate pulmonary stenoses, the systolic murmur is well heard posteriorly and in the axilla. In the presence of significant cyanosis and low pulmonary blood flow, the second heart sound is single, but in acyanotic patients it may be finely split with a low-intensity pulmonary component. Splitting is also present in modestly cyanosed patients with only a mildly reduced pulmonary blood flow when there are important pulmonary artery origin stenoses.

The signs of congestive heart failure with venous pressure elevation and liver enlargement occur in the rare circumstance of patients with pulmonary atresia with a high pulmonary blood flow or in patients with too large a systemic-pulmonary artery shunt (usually a Waterston or Potts shunt). Congestive heart failure may also appear in untreated severely cyanosed patients in the fourth or fifth decade of life, presumably secondary to myocardial fibrosis, or in association with systemic hypertension or aortic incompetence.

Laboratory Studies

The neonate or very young infant with severe TF with or without pulmonary atresia usually presents with marked reduction of arterial oxygen pressure and saturation and sometimes with metabolic acidosis. Polycythemia is rarely present, and in fact such infants are often anemic.

In older infants and children, the red blood cell count and hematocrit are usually elevated, and the degree of elevation is correlated with the degree of arterial desaturation and thus with the severity of the pulmonary stenosis. In older patients, the hematocrit may reach 90%.

Most cyanotic patients with TF have some depression of their platelet count and prolongation of most of the coagulation tests.

Chest X-Ray

The chest x-ray in children usually shows the typical boot-shaped heart of the TF. In neonates and young infants, the heart may be strikingly small, with an absent pulmonary artery segment along the left upper cardiac border and oligemic lung fields. In older patients, however, there may be a prominence of the left upper cardiac border due to a large infundibular chamber. Large pulmonary arterial collaterals may result in an altered pulmonary blood flow pattern in one or both lungs. Plethora of one lung and oligemia of the other suggest anomalous origin of one pulmonary artery from the ascending aorta (see Chapter 30).

There may be a right aortic arch. Posterior esophageal indentation of the shadow of the barium-filled esophagus results from an aberrant left or right subclavian artery.

Rib notching of the upper ipsilateral ribs may develop in the presence of a long-standing Blalock-Taussig shunt, secondary to the development of a rich collateral blood flow to the arm. Very rarely, collaterals from the pleura to the lung may be sufficiently severe, especially after poudrage or pleural stripping procedures, as to result in bilateral rib notching in the lower half of the thorax. Patients in the second or third decade of life may show progressing kyphoscoliosis.

Electrocardiogram

The electrocardiogram shows moderate right ventricular hypertrophy consistent with a right ventricular pressure that is equal to and not above systemic pressure (in contrast to flap valve VSD; see Section 2, "Tetralogy of Fallot with Flap Valve VSD"). Occasionally there is minimal right ventricular hypertrophy, and in these circumstances right ventricular underdevelopment should be suspected although it may not be present. Left precordial leads are characterized by absent Q waves and low voltage R waves. Occasionally, the frontal plane vectorcardiographic pattern characteristic of atrioventricular canal is found in patients with typical TF.

Echocardiography

The ventricular septal defect, aortic overriding, and narrowing of the right ventricular infundibulum can usually be seen with echocardiography, but details of additional muscular VSDs and of the morphology of the pulmonary trunk and central portions of the left pulmonary arteries may not be reliably visualized. This study is not, therefore, currently considered (UAB and GLH) as providing definitive preoperative information.

Cardiac Catheterization and Angiocardiography

Peak pressure in the cavity of the right ventricle is similar to that in the left, and pulmonary artery pressure is below normal. A systolic pressure gradient can often be demonstrated at infundibular and also valvular level when both zones are stenotic but rarely at a more peripheral site even when severe stenosis is present. When proximal stenoses are severe, however, it may be impossible to enter the pulmonary artery with a catheter.

There is right-to-left shunting at ventricular level and a low pulmonary blood flow, the severity of these changes reflecting the severity of the pulmonary stenosis. In acyanotic patients, there is minimal right-to-left shunting at rest or even a modest increase in pulmonary blood flow, but in most patients right-to-left shunting does occur on exercise. In severely cyanotic patients, the measured pulmonary artery pressure and resistance are not elevated preoperatively, even in the presence of important peripheral pulmonary artery stenoses or thrombosis, because of the low pulmonary blood flow. The pulmonary artery pressure may be elevated when there is a large pulmonary blood flow and an increase in pulmonary vascular resistance.

At the present time, the most important diagnostic study is biplane cineangiography. This demonstrates all the morphologic features of the malformation when performed in an appropriate manner. Oblique[C19] and angled views[B5,S11] are used. The configuration of the right ventricular sinus and the infundibulum and the degree and morphology of the right ventricular outflow obstruction are studied. The morphology of the pulmonary valve and any tethering or narrowing of the main pulmonary artery at the level of the commissural attachment of the valve or beyond are noted. The bifurcation of the pulmonary trunk and the origins of the left and right pulmonary arteries are studied with particular care because the surgeon cannot accurately assess the presence or severity of stenoses in this area at the time of operation. The so-called "sitting-up position" (cranially tilted frontal view) usually offers the best view of this area, although oblique views also usually demonstrate the origins of both arteries. The presence, size, and morphology of the various portions of the right and left pulmonary arteries are studied with care.

With proper profiling of the ventricular septum, the typical large ventricular septal defect and overlying dextroposed aorta are identified (Fig. 23-19). Additional VSDs, if present, are identified on these views.

The coronary arterial anatomy can usually be well seen following the left ventricular injection. Particular search is made for anomalous origin of the LAD artery from the right coronary artery and for the rare but surgically important associated condition of origin of the left coronary artery from the pulmonary artery.

The follow-through frames are searched for evidence of large AP collateral arteries, and an injection is made into the thoracic aorta[R6] and/or selectively into the collateral arteries[C12,P12] if these are present. When the true left or right pulmonary arteries are not visualized following these injections, which must include late filming and sometimes also digital subtraction techniques, a *pulmonary vein wedge injection* is made to fill in a retrograde manner the pulmonary arterial tree[F14,N12,S12,T6] (Fig. 23-22). When all techniques including this one fail to outline a central or hilar portion of a pulmonary artery, it can be safely assumed to be absent.

Any major associated cardiac anomalies are identified by the study. Previously made palliative shunts or transannular patches are visualized, the former if necessary by selective injections. Any iatrogenic pulmonary arterial problems are defined in detail, and particular care is taken to visualize these since this may help the surgeon avoid misidentification of structures at the time of repair.

Careful study of the morphologic category of the right ventricular outflow tract and measurements of these areas in cineangiograms allow a reasonably reliable prediction of the postrepair ratio between peak pressure in right ventricle and that in the left ventricle ($P_{RV/LV}$), with or without a transannular patch or valved extracardiac conduit. (See "Postrepair $P_{RV/LV}$: Its Use and Predictions" in section on Special Situations and Controversies). Such an analysis alerts the surgeon to the probable ease of the relief of the pulmonary stenosis and the techniques that may be needed for this.

CLINICAL FEATURES AND DIAGNOSTIC CRITERIA OF TETRALOGY OF FALLOT WITH ABSENT PULMONARY VALVE

The clinical features of tetralogy of Fallot (TF) with absent pulmonary valve differ strikingly from other forms of TF and must therefore be considered separately.

Clinical Features

It is probable that the age of onset and severity of symptoms are related to the severity of the pulmonary incompetence and the pulmonary blood flow. When pulmonary incompetence is severe and the pulmonary blood flow increased, presentation is early in infancy, often in the first weeks of life, with congestive heart failure and severe intractable tracheobronchitis and respiratory distress responding poorly to routine medical measures. Cyanosis is absent unless hypoxia develops from pulmonary complications. There is marked failure to thrive, and there may be low cardiac output, acidemia, and death.

When pulmonary incompetence is less severe (in association with slightly more pulmonary stenosis, a near normal pulmonary blood flow, and less marked aneurysmal dilatation of the pulmonary arteries), presentation is later in life

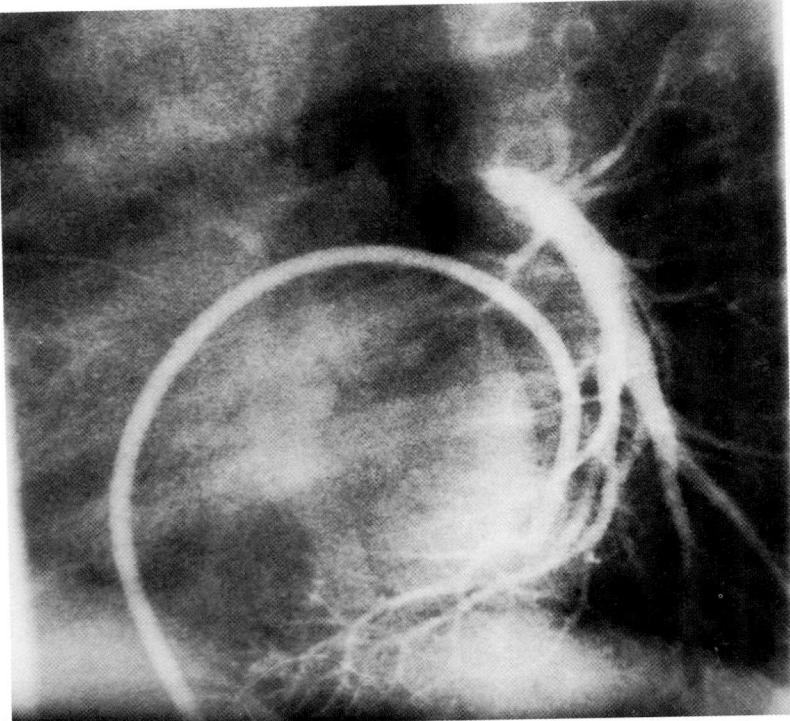

Figure 23-22 Pulmonary vein wedge injection in patients with TF and absent central portion of the left pulmonary artery demonstrating a left hilar pulmonary artery and its normal continuation (GLH). The artery had not been visualized by right ventricular or aortic injection.

and less severe, usually being confined to recurrent respiratory infections or mild heart failure.

Physical Examination

Severely affected infants are in considerable respiratory distress with tachypnea, subcostal retraction, and wheeze with rales and rhonci audible throughout both lung fields. The heart is overactive and the rate is rapid; the pulse of low volume; and there is obvious cardiomegaly, hepatomegaly, and raised venous pressure. There may be a precordial bulge. The infant is frail, cachectic, and febrile. On auscultation, a to and fro murmur is audible along the left sternal edge, with the diastolic component often the more prominent. The second heart sound is single and there may be an apical gallop.

Chest X-Ray

The chest x-ray is distinctive since it shows, from birth, marked supracardiac mediastinal widening due to aneurysmal dilatation of central and hilar pulmonary arteries, usually equal on both sides although sometimes asymmetrical, with relatively oligemic lung fields. Segmental or lobar atelectasis is common, and sometimes an entire lung is collapsed. The aerated portions of lung may appear overinflated. Atelectasis is associated with mediastinal shift, and in cases with partial or complete lung collapse, it is associ-

ated with acquired dextrocardia.[M7] In severe cases, there is considerable cardiomegaly. The left atrium may be pushed downward[M12] and the carina splayed with compression of the lower trachea and both main bronchi.

Other Studies

The electrocardiogram is typical for patients with TF. Cardiac catheterization, including angiography, is required for definitive diagnosis and will demonstrate the pulmonary artery dilatation and the tetralogy-type VSD.

NATURAL HISTORY

The natural history of patients with TF without major associated cardiac anomalies is variable[M5] and is determined primarily by the severity of the right ventricular and pulmonary arterial outflow obstruction.[R16]

Tetralogy of Fallot with Pulmonary Stenosis

Twenty-five percent of surgically untreated infants born with TF and pulmonary stenosis die in the first year of life but uncommonly in the first month of life (Fig. 23-23). These are the patients with the most severe obstruction to pulmonary blood flow. Forty percent are dead by 3 years of age, 70% by 10 years of age, and 95% by 40 years of age. The instanta-

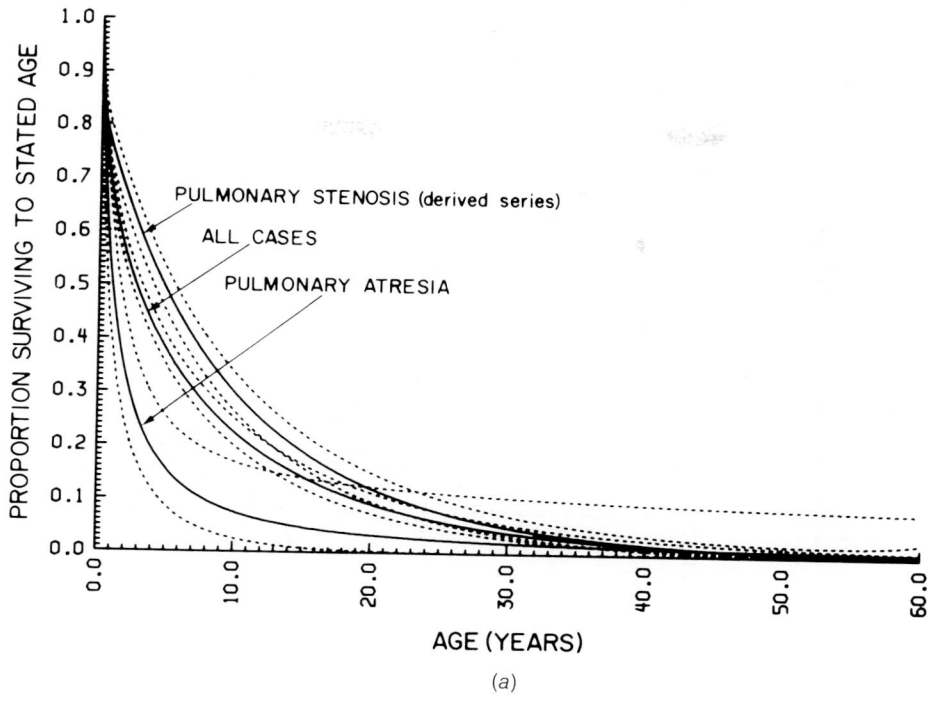

(a)

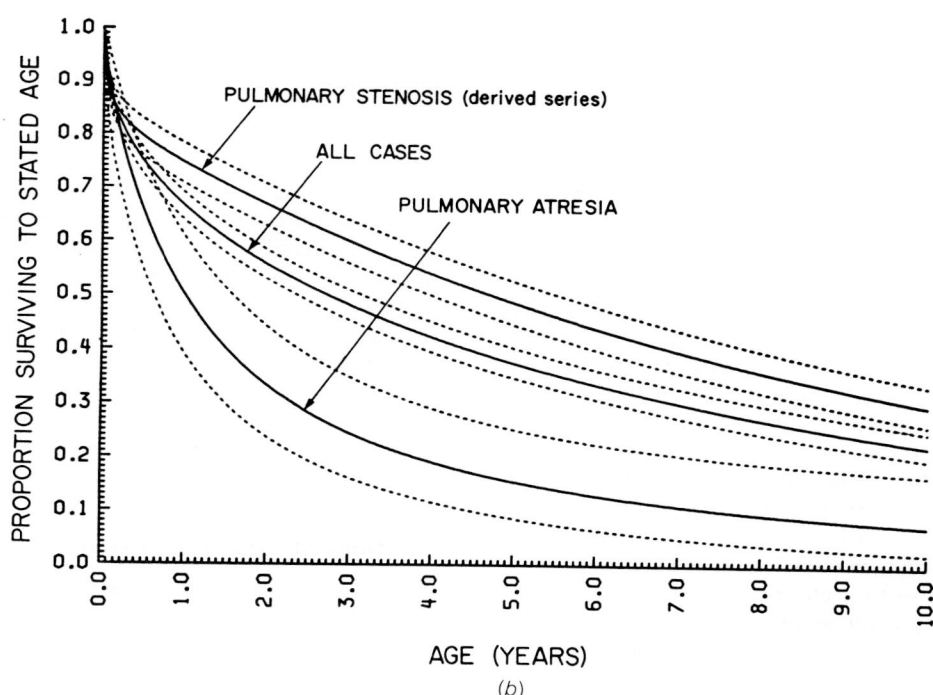

AGE (YEARS)

(b)

Figure 23-23 Nomogram of the survival of surgically untreated patients with TF. The smooth lines represent the survival of the three groups, and the dashed lines enclose the 70% confidence limits around each of these.

(a) Represents survival to age 60 years.

(b) Represents survival to age 10 years on an expanded time scale.

Reproduced with permission from Bertranou et al.[B14]

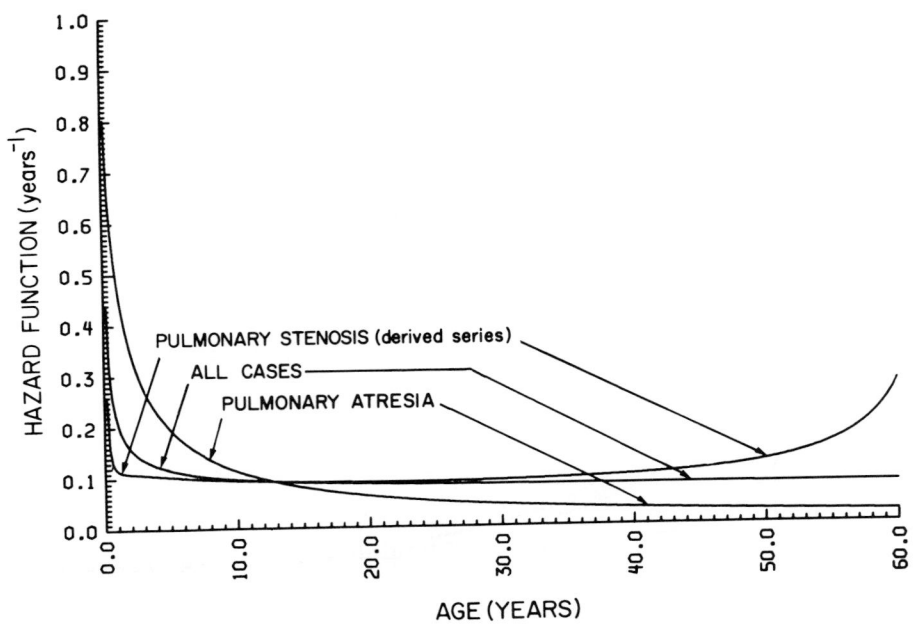

Figure 23-24   Hazard function according to age in three groups of patients with TF.
Reproduced with permission from Bertranou et al.[B14] See reference for equations and statistics.

neous risk of death (hazard function) (see Chapter 6) is greatest in the first year of life (Fig. 23-24). It then stays constant until the age of about 25, when it begins again to rise.

The occurrence of hypoxic spells in the first few years of life is related to the hyperactivity of the infundibulum. This and the fact that the infundibular septum and its parietal extension contract earlier in systole than in normal subjects[G4] produce variable and sometimes severe episodes of right ventricular outflow tract obstruction.

About 25% of patients with the morphology of TF are acyanotic at birth and become cyanotic in the weeks, months, or years that pass, as the pulmonary stenosis increases.[B2,B3,G3,G4] Progression of the arterial desaturation, cyanosis, and polycythemia is variable and is furthered not only by increasing pulmonary stenosis but also by a widespread tendency to thrombosis of the pulmonary arteries, with progressive reduction in pulmonary blood flow.[F1,M4,R2] As part of this same tendency, death may result from cerebral thromboses or abscesses.

In those few surviving into the fourth and fifth decades of life, death is commonly from chronic congestive heart failure due to the secondary cardiomyopathy that results from the right ventricular pressure overload and the chronic hypoxia and polycythemia.

Tetralogy of Fallot with Pulmonary Atresia

Surgically untreated infants born with TF and pulmonary atresia have a poorer prognosis than those with pulmonary stenosis (Fig. 23-23). Fifty percent die of hypoxia by the age of 1 year, and many die in the first month of life. Commonly, early death is caused by spontaneous closure of a ductus arteriosus that has been the sole source of pulmonary blood

flow. Of this group of ductus-dependent patients, 75% are dead by 3 years of age and 92% by 10 years of age. The instantaneous risk of death (hazard function) is high in very early life; and although it falls rapidly as age increases, it remains relatively high throughout the first decade of life (Fig. 23-24).

Many people with TF and pulmonary atresia have large collateral sources of pulmonary blood flow (see "Morphology"). Generally, these are insufficient to maintain near-normal systemic arterial oxygen levels and to increase the pulmonary blood flow during exercise, but they may allow the patient to survive through infancy.[M23] Thereafter, polycythemia gradually develops, which reduces flow through stenoses in the collaterals still further, and a vicious cycle is produced that leads to increasingly severe hypoxia and ultimately death. All of the complications associated with TF and pulmonary stenosis may occur.

Tetralogy of Fallot with Absent Pulmonary Valve

Tetralogy of Fallot with absent pulmonary valve results in a very different natural history. A high percentage of infants born with this syndrome (perhaps 50%) die in the first year of life, and most die in the first few months of life, from respiratory distress caused by the massively dilated right and left pulmonary arteries compressing the tracheobronchial tree.[A13,C4,D7,L8] Such critically ill infants also have heart failure associated with a left-to-right shunt, and the right ventricle is markedly enlarged and systolic function reduced.[H8] Patients who survive infancy, however, generally do well for many years, since the right ventricular outflow obstruction is only moderate and cyanosis is mild or absent. They tend to become symptomatic at about 20–30 years of age and die from intractable right ventricular failure as a result of the chronic right ventricular pressure and volume overload.

Genetic History

Offspring of a parent who has repaired or unrepaired TF are more likely to have TF than offspring of parents without congenital heart disease. It is estimated that about 0.1% of live births will have TF under the latter circumstances and about 1.5% under the former.[S3]

TECHNIQUE OF OPERATION

General Plan and Details Common to All Approaches

Evaluation

The surgeon must come to the operating room with a clear image of the morphology as it has been displayed in the cineangiogram, particularly as it relates to the right ventricular and pulmonary arterial outflow obstruction. After the sternotomy incision is made, the external anatomy of the heart is studied, with particular attention to the right ventricular and pulmonary artery anatomy and the configuration of the coronary arteries crossing the right ventricle. The cineangiogram is mentally reviewed, and with this and the observations of the heart, the morphologic category of the patient's right ventricular outflow obstruction (see "Morphology") is assigned. This in large measure determines the incision that is to be made for the repair and the details of the repair.

Surgical Approach

When there is isolated infundibular stenosis (as described under "Convenient Morphologic Categories of Right Ventricular Outflow Obstruction" in section on Morphology), and particularly if the stenosis is low-lying, a transverse ventriculotomy (GLH) or a right atrial approach (UAB) is optimal, but a vertical ventriculotomy may be used (UAB). When there is diffuse right ventricular outflow hypoplasia or dominant valvar stenosis with a narrow anulus, a transannular patch is almost certainly required, and initially a vertical ventriculotomy is made, limited to the infundibulum. When there is infundibular and valvar stenoses, a transverse ventriculotomy incision may be made (GLH) or a right atrial approach occasionally used (UAB), but a vertical infundibulotomy incision gives maximal flexibility and is most convenient for extension of the incision across the annulus for placement of a transannular patch should measurement of the annular diameter (see later section on "Decision and Technique for Transannular Patching") indicate the need for this. When there is infundibular plus valvar plus annular stenosis, the probability of need for a transannular patch is great, and initially a vertical incision in the infundibulum is generally made.

Preparations for Cardiopulmonary Bypass

Before cardiopulmonary bypass (CPB) is established, the ascending aorta is dissected free from the pulmonary trunk so that when the aortic cross clamp is in position the main and right pulmonary arteries will be undistorted. Unless it is clear from the cineangiogram that the pulmonary trunk bifurcation and the central and hilar portions of the left and right pulmonary arteries are free of stenoses or diffuse hypoplasia, these too must be dissected out. On the left side, this is aided by cutting the pericardium down to the left pulmonary artery, dissecting away and preserving the left phrenic nerve. The ligamentum (or ductus) arteriosum is seen and dissected also. On the right side, the aorta is retracted anterior and to the left, and the right pulmonary artery is dissected completely away from it out to the superior vena cava and beneath it if necessary.

Any surgically created shunts are at least partially dissected before establishing CPB (see later sections on "Repair after Various Shunts").

The Repair

After CPB has been established and the right ventriculotomy or the right atriotomy incision made, the internal anatomy is still further visualized and conceptualized. The plan is to dissect and resect the infundibular stenosis, visualize the pulmonary valve and open it if necessary, measure the outflow tract, valve, and anulus with a Hegar dilator,[D2] and repair the VSD. The pulmonary valvotomy, if needed, may be done through a vertical pulmonary arteriotomy usually closed with a pericardial patch (UAB) or on occasions (UAB) or routinely (GLH) the valvotomy may be done from below via the right ventriculotomy or right atriotomy. When a vertical right ventriculotomy virtually limited to the infundibulum is used, it is closed with a patch of preclotted woven Dacron (UAB), since this particular incision is chosen in large measure because of a narrow infundibulum and because, in any event, direct closure of this incision may narrow the outflow tract. When a transannular patch is needed, a Dacron (UAB) or pericardial[H7] (GLH) one is inserted after extending the infundibular incision across the pulmonary valve ring. The use of a monocusp in the patch[F7,13,M15,Z1] does not appear to result in any less pulmonary incompetence than does a simple patch.[R18]

The repair is basically the same whether a right ventricular (through a vertical or transverse incision) or right atrial approach is chosen and is represented in Figures 23-25 and 23-26, which should be studied in parallel in order to obtain the most complete understanding of the pathologic anatomy and its repair.

Typically, in the *infundibular dissection* the parietal extension of the infundibular (conal) septum is dissected away from the right ventricular free wall and from the ventriculo-infundibular fold and divided transversely 5 mm or so to the right of the attachment of the right coronary cusp to the undersurface of the conal (infundibular) septum. This increases the diameter of the infundibulum at its rightward end and improves exposure of the VSD from a right ventricular approach. Any obstructive trabeculae along the left side of the outflow tract are also incised and partially removed. The aim is to increase the circumference of the infundibulum by enlarging each lateral recess in front of the infundibular (conal) septum. A low-lying (coronal plane) obstruction is relieved by dividing anomalous trabecula above the moderator band and often the moderator band itself while protecting adjacent papillary muscles. When an os infundibulum is present at the level of the inferior edge of the infundibular septum, the *fibrous thickening* all around the ostial orifice is excised, as is any fibrous obstruction extending upstream toward the pulmonary valve.

This type of anatomic dissection is not possible in the presence of diffuse right ventricular outflow hypoplasia and is often not possible when there is infundibular, valvar, and annular stenosis. The structures are all hypoplastic, and patch graft enlargement is often all that can be accomplished.

If a *pulmonary valvotomy* is needed, a vertical incision is made in the pulmonary artery (UAB), taking care to avoid damaging the valve commissures (Fig. 23-27), or (occasionally, UAB; routinely, GLH) the valve is examined from be-

low through the right ventricular or right atrial incision. The pulmonary arteriotomy is not made through a commissure between the leaflets, since placing a patch in such an incision renders the valve incompetent. It is rare to be able to perform an adequate valvotomy by simply dividing one or more sites of commissural fusion, for fusion is present in only 20% of stenotic valves and is almost always associated with important leaflet thickening, particularly at the cusp free edge (see "Morphology"). After valvotomy, therefore, it may be elected to excise the thickened cusp edge to relieve the stenosis adequately, although some pulmonary valve incompetence results (GLH). When there is leaflet tethering only, the most common situation (see "Morphology"), the leaflet edge may be cut from its attachment to the pulmonary artery wall over about 3 mm (GLH). This is done to one leaflet at each commissure. Here, too, excision of thickened leaflet

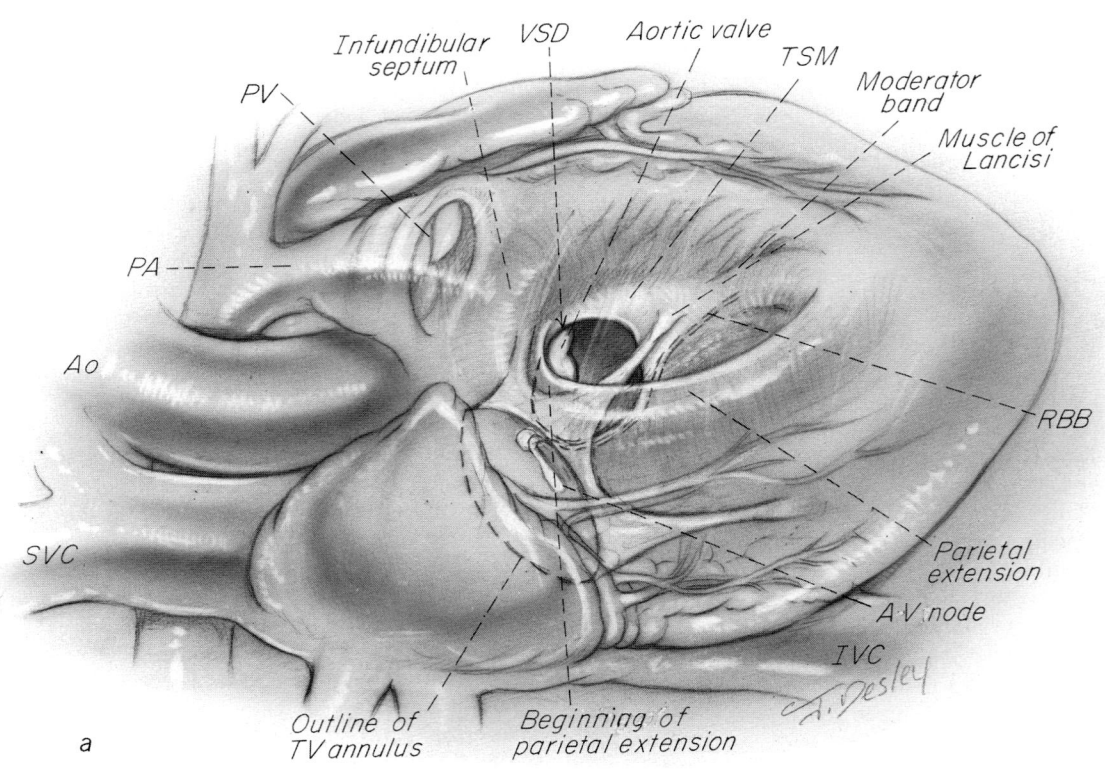

Figure 23-25 the anatomy from the perspective of the right ventricular (RV) approach shown as it the right ventricular free wall were in part translucent.
(a) The separation of the pulmonary valve from the aortic valve by the infundibular septum is evident. The parietal extension arches to the right and over the right ventricular outflow tract, blending in its termination with the free wall of right ventricle. Posteriorly the ventricular septal defect (VSD) abuts the tricuspid anulus. The ventriculo-infundibular fold borders the VSD posterosuperiorly but is unseen because it is overhung by the pariental extension. The VSD comes into relationship anterosuperiorly and anteriorly with the anteriorly displaced infundibular septum. This partially borders the aorta as well in many patients, with an aortic cusp seen on its inferior surface. Anteroinferiorly, a valley-like area may be seen where the infundibular septum merges with the trabecula septomarginalis or septal band that forms the inferior border of the VSD.

Ao, aorta; AV, atrioventricular; IVC, inferior vena cava; PA, pulmonary artery; PV, pulmonary valve; RBB, right bundle branch; SVC, superior vena cava; TSM, trabecula septomarginalis; TV, tricuspid valve; VSD, ventricular septal defect.

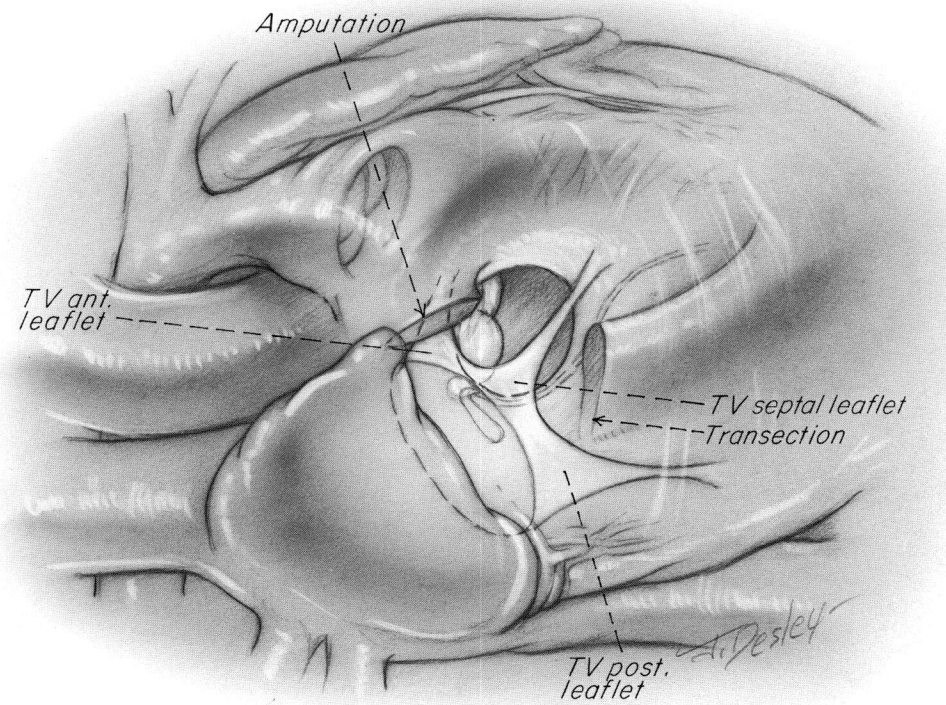

Amputation

*TV ant.
leaflet*

TV septal leaflet
Transection

*TV post.
leaflet*

b

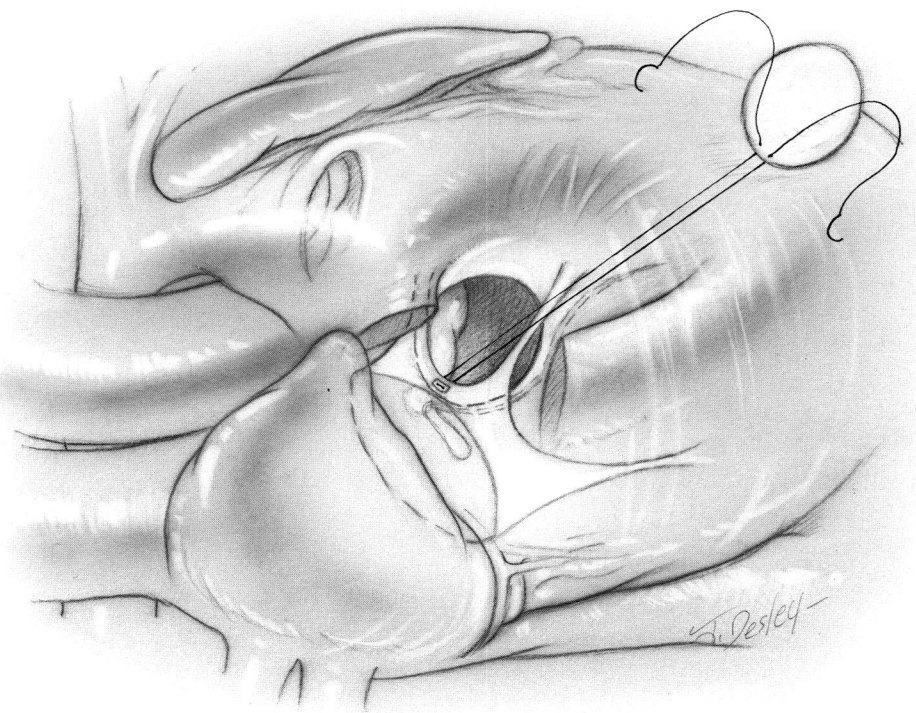

c

Figure 23-25 *(continued)*

(*b*) The parietal extension of the infundibular septum is transected where it begins to fuse with the free wall and is dissected away from the ventriculo-infundibular fold and is then amputated from the infundibular septum. This uncovers the VSD and the tricuspid valve. The ventriculo-infundibular fold remains unseen because it is overhung by the tricuspid valve anterior leaflet.

(*c*) A pledgetted mattress suture is placed from the right atrial side through the base of the commissural tissue between septal and tricuspid leaflets and through the patch. A few more stitches are taken, working superiorly, between the base of anterior leaflet and the patch and then the ventriculoinfundibular fold and the patch.

733

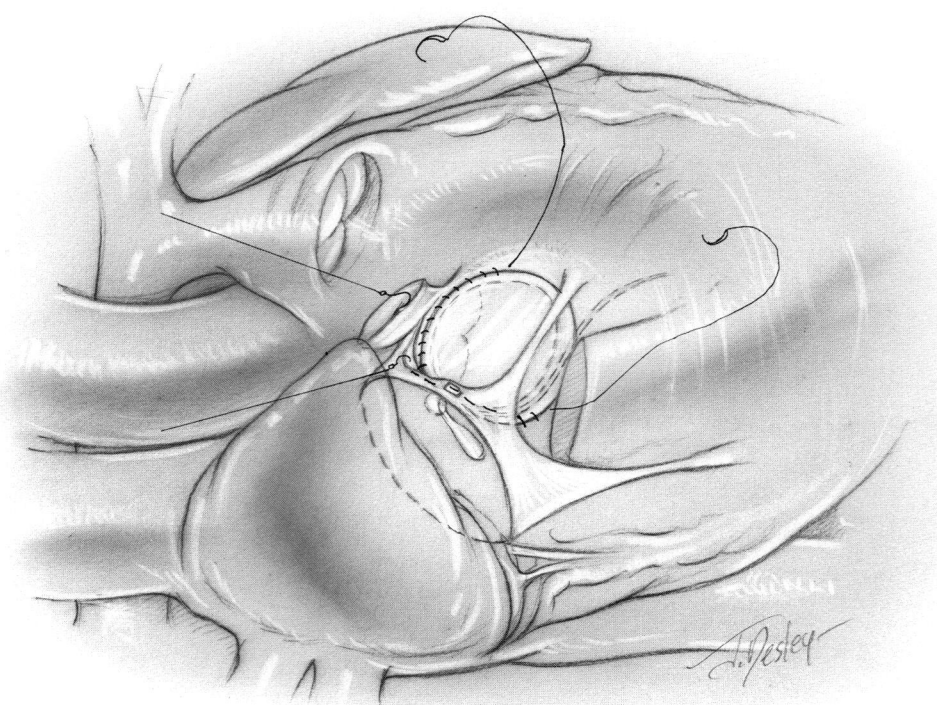

d

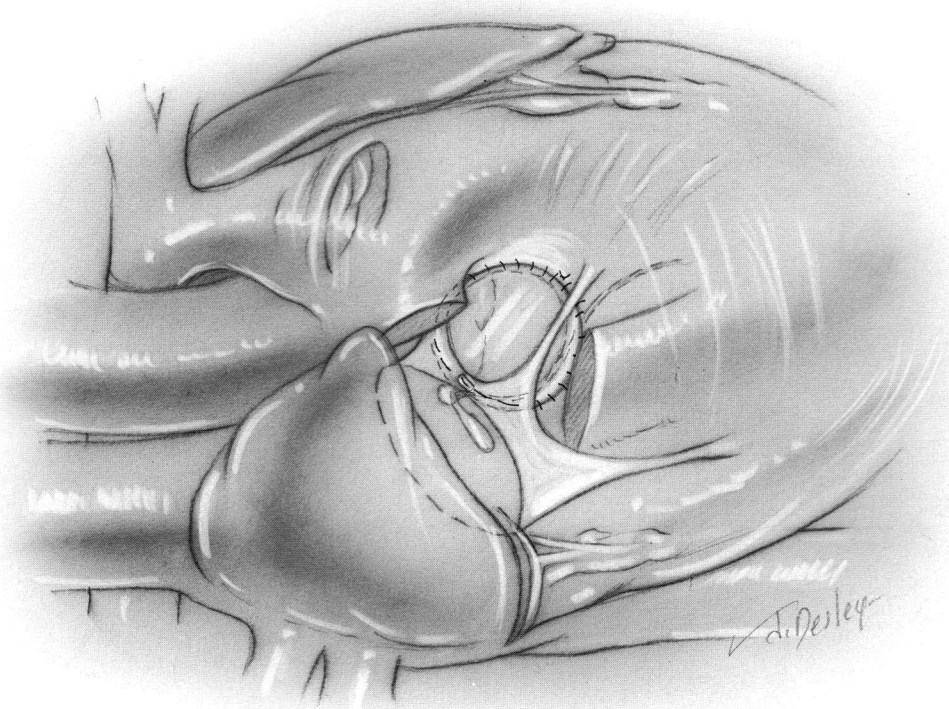

e

Figure 23-25 *(continued)*

(d) The suturing is continued onto the parietal extension and infundibular septum, visualizing and staying close to the aortic valve leaflets so as to avoid leaving a hole between muscular bands. The suture is then held. With the other arm of the suture, a few stitches are taken between septal tricuspid leaflet and patch, weaving beneath any chordae crossing the VSD. When this has taken the suture line about 5 mm inferior to the edge of the VSD, stitches are taken in the septum, well back from the edge of the VSD.

(e) The repair of the VSD is completed. Note that the suture line is away from the bundle of His and its branches, except where it crosses the right bundle branch anteroinferiorly.

tissue may be required. Incompetence from minor detachment of a leaflet may be less than with a transannular patch.[R19] If considerable leaflet incision and detachment are required, incompetence results; if there is also important residual narrowing, it is preferable to excise the leaflets and place a transannular patch after completing the intraventricular part of the repair. If the morphologic assessment and measurements (see later section on "Decision and Technique for Transannular Patching") indicate that a transannular patch is not needed, the pulmonary arteriotomy is closed directly or with a pericardial patch.

The *VSD is closed* with a preclotted knitted Dacron velour patch (UAB) or lightweight woven Dacron patch (GLH); it is trimmed to be slightly larger than the VSD, but not so large as to preclude pulling the infundibular septum down onto the patch in the process of the repair. Exposure for the VSD repair may be obtained entirely with stay sutures (UAB); alternatively (GLH), the VSD is exposed through the right

ventriculotomy by the assistant using two small curved retractors, one beneath each end of the conal (infundibular) septum, which are pulled upward and apart. A third retractor is positioned in the lower margin of the ventriculotomy for gentle inferior traction. The sequencing of the suturing is identical whether the repair is from the right atrium or right ventricle and is similar to that used for isolated VSD (see Figs. 23-25 and 23-26 and Chapter 20, Fig. 20-23). The patch is only partially trimmed before insertion (GLH) and tailored to exact size before placing the last few sutures (see Chapter 20, Fig. 20-24); or final trimming is made before beginning the insertion (UAB).

Decision and Technique for Transannular Patching
After closing the VSD, Hegar dilators are used to estimate the diameter of the narrowest portion of the anulus, pulmonary valve, and pulmonary trunk. If the operating room post-repair $P_{RV/LV}$ is repredicted to be less than 0.85 (see "Post-

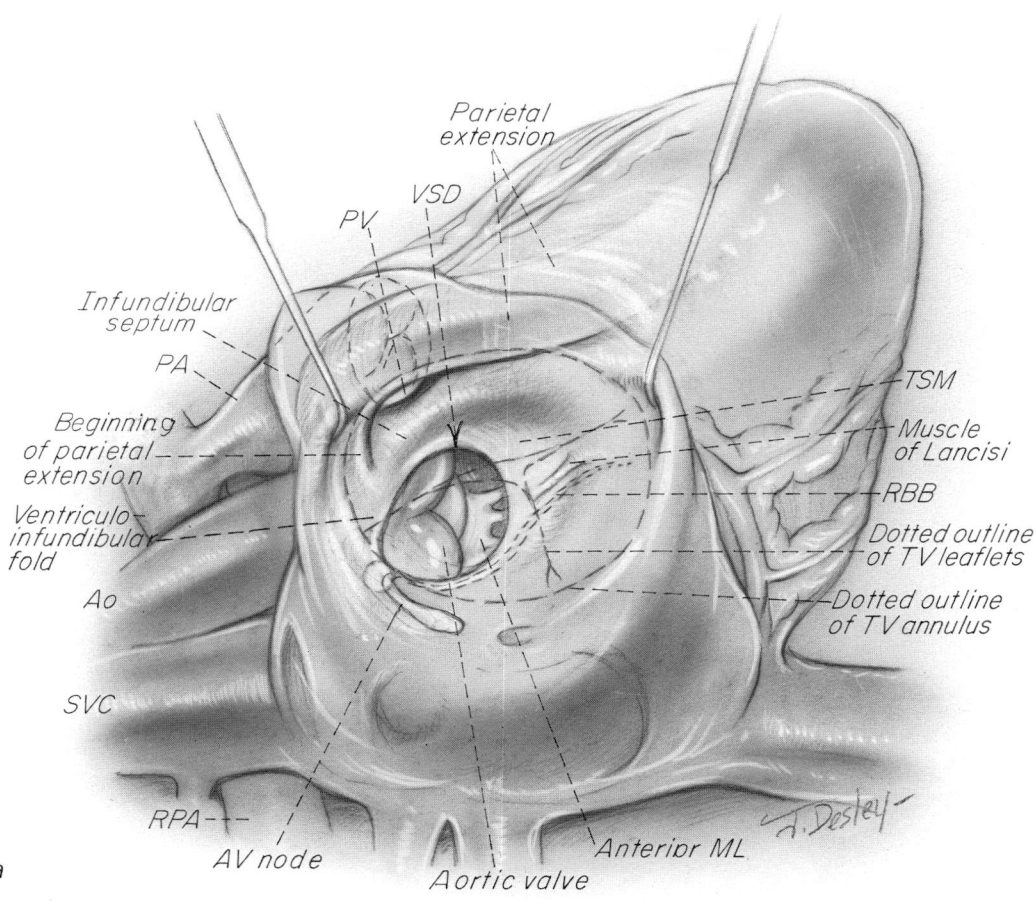

Figure 23-26 The anatomy from the perspective of the right atrial (RA) approach, shown as if the right atrial free wall and tricuspid valve were translucent.
(*a*) The striking difference from the RV perspective (see Fig. 23-25*a*) is in the apparent position of the parietal extension. From the RA perspective, the surgeon is looking *beneath* this, as the parietal extension arches *over* the right ventricular outflow tract. The ventriculo-infundibular fold is easily seen through the tricuspid valve.

Ao, aorta; AV, atrioventricular; ML, mitral leaflet; PA, pulmonary artery; PV, pulmonary valve; RBB, right bundle branch; RPA, right pulmonary artery; SVC, superior vena cava; TSM, trabecula septomarginalis; TV, tricuspid valve; VSO, ventricular septal defect.

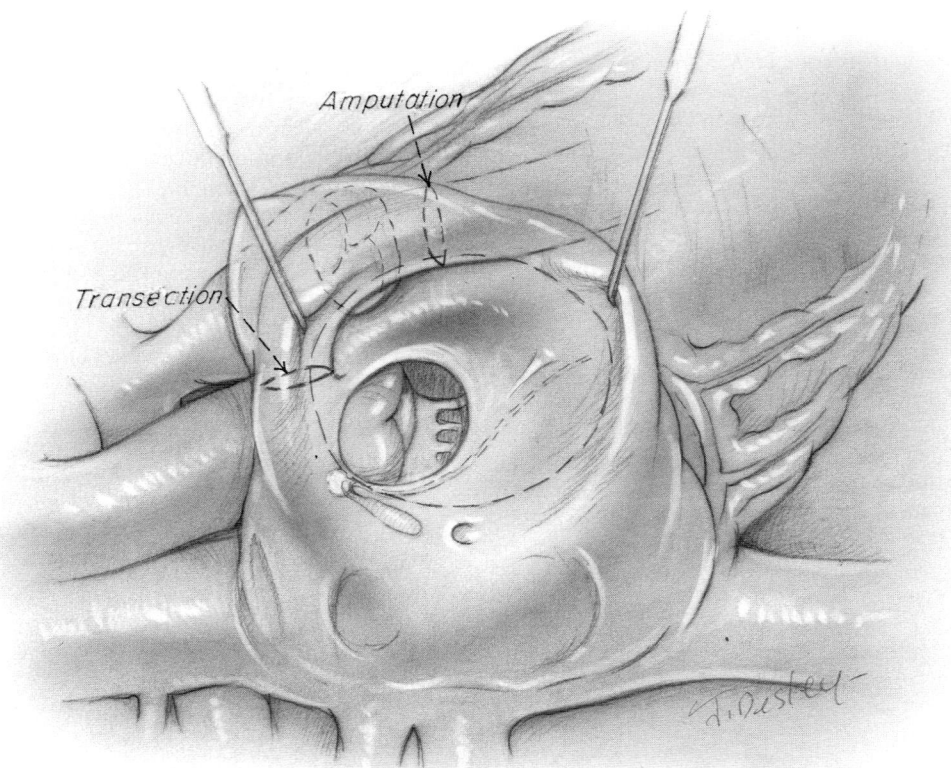

b

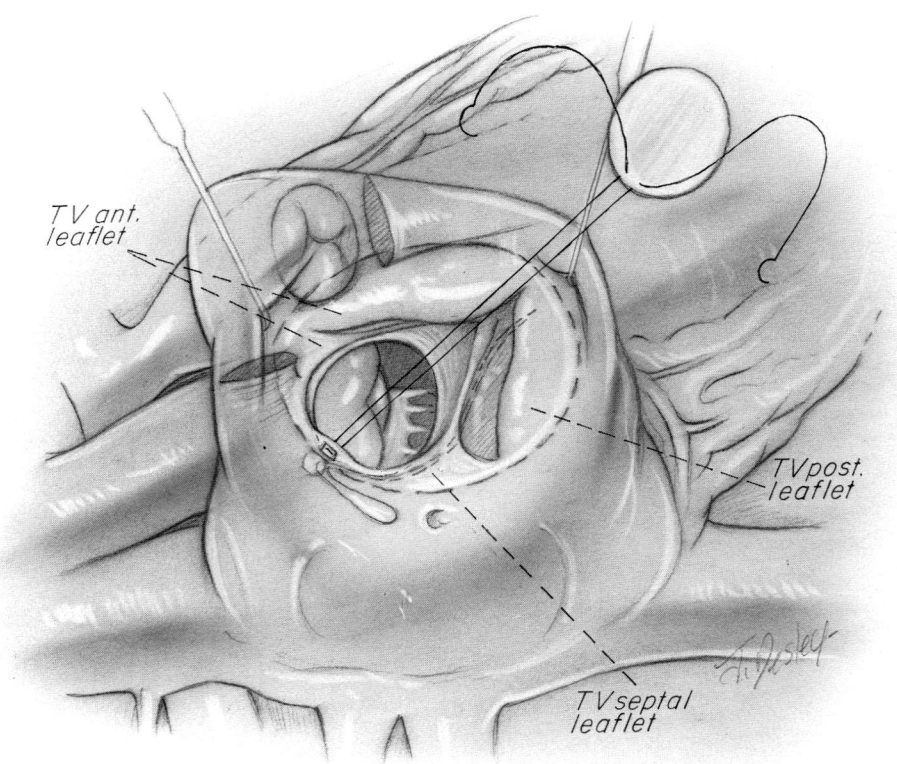

c

Figure 23-26 *(continued)*

(*b*) The same perspective is shown, but without the outline of the tricuspid valve leaflets. The parietal extension is transected at its origin from the infundibular septum, dissected up toward the free wall, and amputated at the free wall. The exposure for an accurate dissection is less good than from the RV approach.

(*c*) For the first time in this series of drawings, the tricuspid valve leaflets are shown. The first step for the repair of the VSD is placed exactly as described in the legend for Figure 23-25(*c*).

736

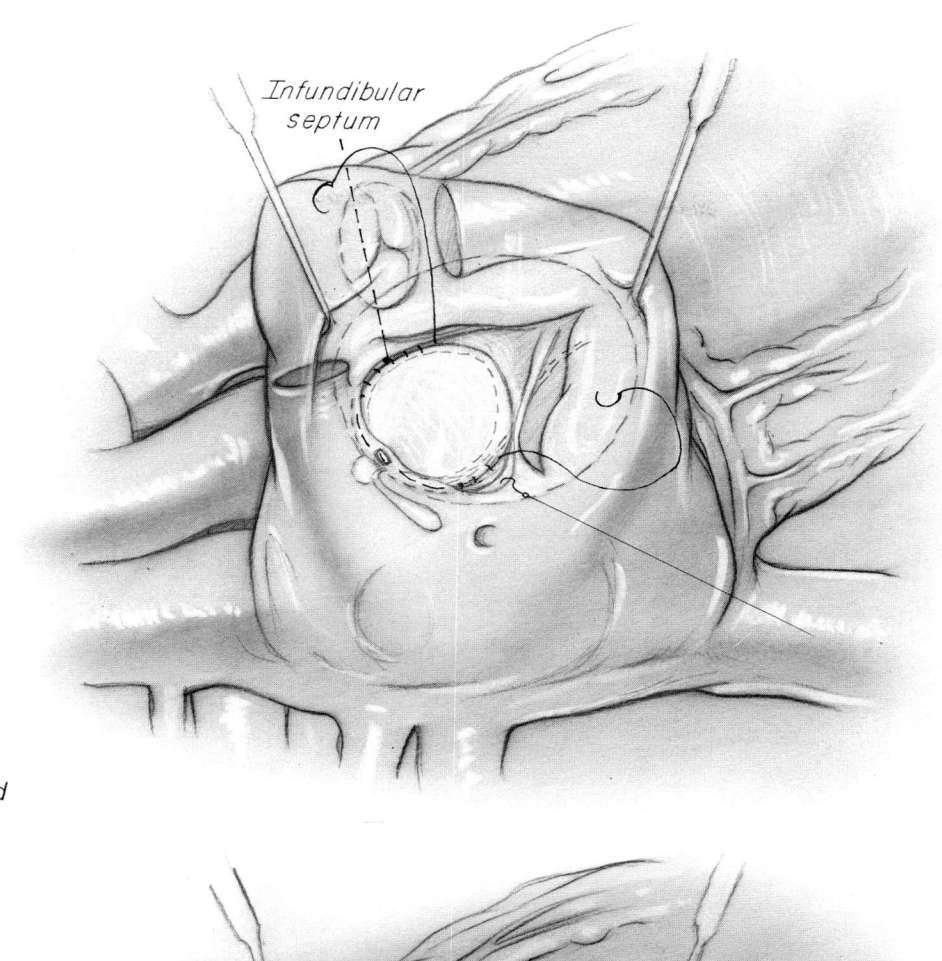

Infundibular septum

d

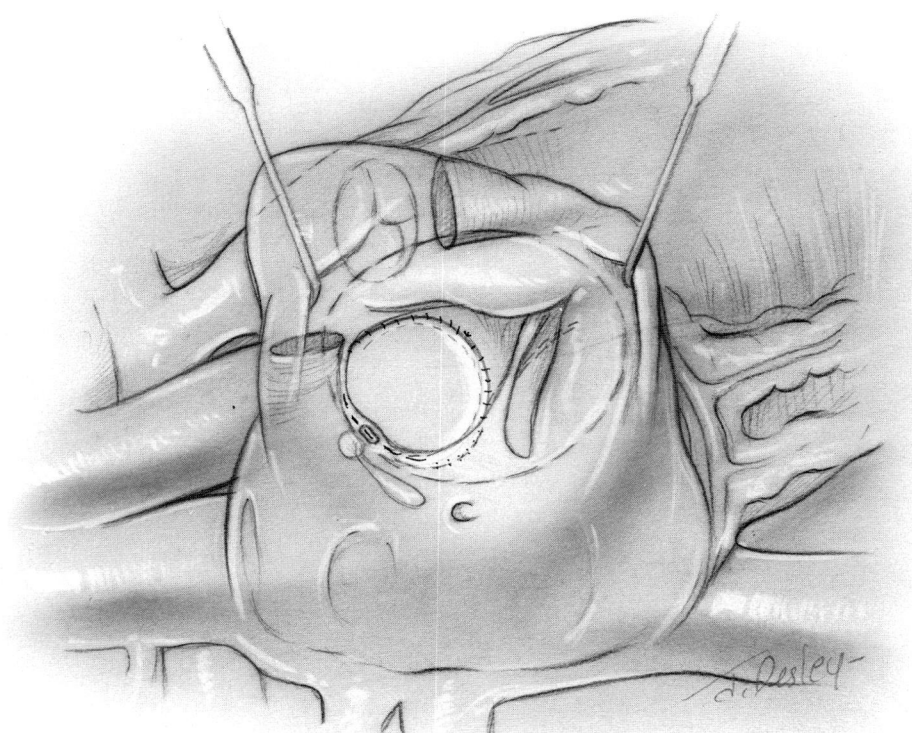

e

Figure 23-26 *(continued)*
(*d*) The suturing continues superiorly exactly as described in the legend for Figure 23-25 (*d*). When working through the RA, it is particularly important to stay close to the aortic valve leaflets and head for the infundibular septum, for it is easy to be misled into going up along the parietal extension, which leads to narrowing or closure of the RV outflow tract.
(*e*) The completed suture line is identical in its appearance to that described in Figure 23-25(*e*).

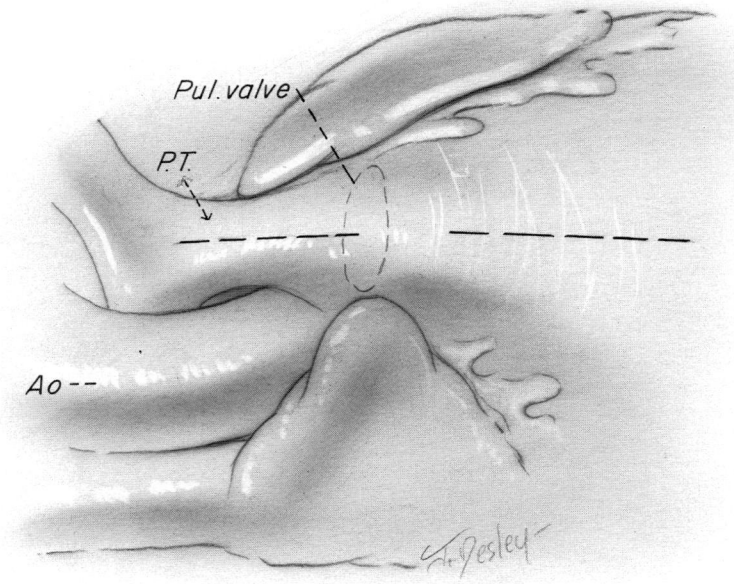

a

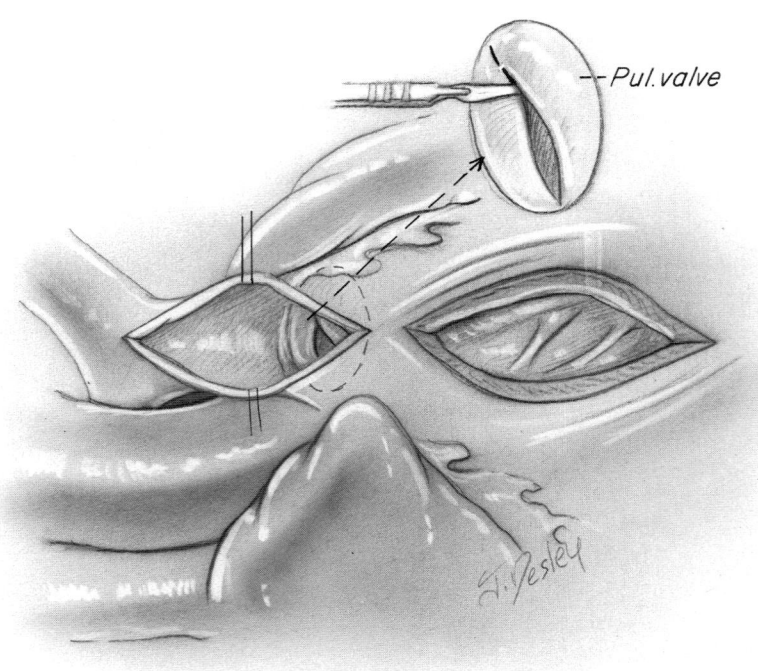

b

Figure 23-27 Repair of TF with separate infundibular and pulmonary artery patches.
(*a*) The proposed pulmonary incision is shown extending to but not into the pulmonary valve ring. The valve ring. The proposed vertical ventriculotomy incision is also shown.
(*b*) Through the pulmonary arteriotomy incision is seen the stenotic pulmonary valve. The fused commissures are incised with a knife to the pulmonary arterial wall. Fine tissue forceps steady the leaflet on each side of the commissure and provide even tension as the incision is being made.

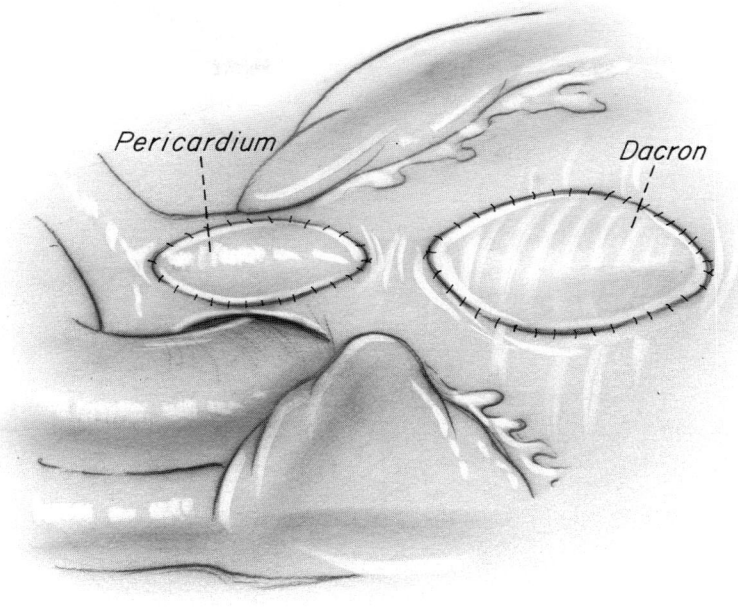

Pericardium   *Dacron*

c

Figure 23-27 *(continued)*
(c) Unless the pulmonary trunk is of normal width, which is uncommon, the incision may be closed with an oval-shaped piece of pericardium (UAB). The ventriculotomy may be closed by sewing into place a segment from a preclotted woven Dacron patch (UAB). The patch is cut in the form shown, and its dimensions (see text) assure that it is convex rather than flat.

repair $P_{RV/LV}$'' in section on Special Situations and Controversies) and particularly if the right ventricular outflow obstruction is infundibular or infundibular and valvar, generally the decision is to proceed without a transannular patch. In this case, if the repair has been made through a transverse ventriculotomy, the incision is closed with interrupted full thickness silk sutures. If the approach has been through a vertical incision (UAB), a preclotted woven Dacron patch is used to close the ventriculotomy (see Fig. 23-27). If the approach has been through a right atriotomy, this is simply closed.

However, if $P_{RV/LV}$ is predicted to be equal to or greater than 0.85 and particularly if the outflow obstruction is diffuse hypoplasia or infundibular plus valvar plus annular, a transannular patch is generally placed (Fig. 23-28), after extending the ventriculotomy incision across the anulus to join the pulmonary arteriotomy and excising the pulmonary valve. The pulmonary arteriotomy should extend distally to the widest part of the pulmonary trunk, which is generally opposite the orifice of the right pulmonary artery. A pericardial transannular patch may be used (GLH), in which case the patch and the underlying gauze are cut together (see Chapter 15, Fig. 15-5) to fashion an outflow gusset of appropriate size. The length can be measured from the length of the incision from right ventricle to pulmonary artery, whereas the maximum width is judged visually by holding the edges of the incision open at valve level and judging the size of the roof required to create a new pulmonary artery anulus whose diameter is no larger than three-fourths of the diameter of the

ascending aorta. Alternatively, in infants a 10-mm Hegar dilator can be placed through the divided anulus and the width of pericardium required to complete the roof over it measured. Usually, the patch is about 50 mm long and 15 mm wide at its center, tapering off sharply at the distal end. The right ventricular end is cut almost transversely. The patch is positioned using continuous 5-0 polypropylene sutures, commencing at the distal end of the incision. The stitch is mattressed at the end and over and over elsewhere, placing the first two or three throws along each side before pulling the pericardial patch (with its underlying gauze) into position as the suture is tightened. The gauze is then removed from beneath the patch and the upstream end of the patch held tight with a curved forcep. Suturing is continued down each side to anulus level, and then the remainder of the right ventriculotomy is closed by incorporating the pericardial patch into it with the continuous sutures. Deep bites of muscle are taken down each side and at the angle.

Alternatively, a Dacron patch for the transannular reconstruction may be cut from a preclotted woven Dacron tube (UAB), the diameter of which corresponds to a patient Z value[2] for the pulmonary anulus of about +2. Too large a patch will increase the pulmonary incompetence.[F7,O4,O5] A

_____

[2] The Z value of the pulmonary anulus is the relative size of that anulus compared to the normal size for the patient's body surface area (or weight), expressed as its standard deviation from the mean normal value of Rowlatt et al (see Fig. 23-60).[R3]

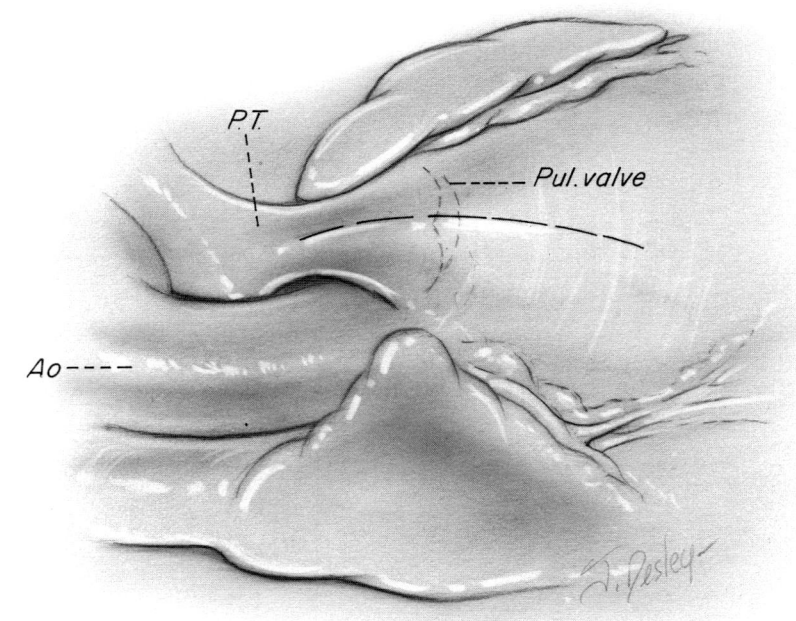

a

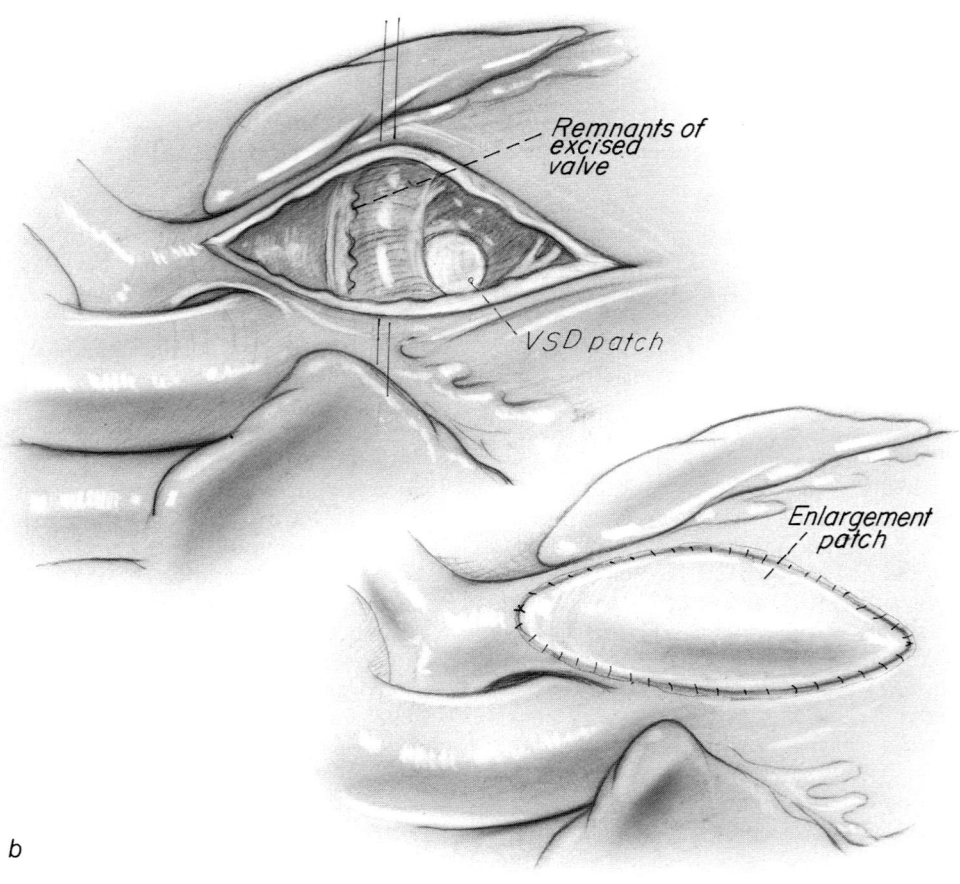

b

Dacron transannular patch is sewed into place as shown in Figure 23-27.

$P_{RV/LV}$ is measured just after discontinuing CPB, before decannulation. Since this preliminary estimate of operating room postrepair $P_{RV/LV}$ may be 10%–20% higher than it will be 30 minutes later, a value up to 0.95 may be accepted in this preliminary estimate if a transannular patch has not been placed and if the hemodynamic state is good. The postrepair $P_{RV/LV}$ is again measured 30 minutes later and a value less than 0.85 accepted if a transannular patch has not been placed. Otherwise, CPB is generally reestablished and a transannular patch placed.

Closure of Foramen Ovale

During the repair a patent foramen ovale (present in about two-thirds of patients[L1,R5]) should be closed. Otherwise, right-to-left shunting at atrial level will occur in the early postoperative period (when right atrial pressure is higher than left atrial pressure), causing hypoxia that will interfere with cardiac performance. Rarely, a persistent atrial communication can be the source of paradoxical cerebral emboli late postoperatively;[L6] or if an atrial septal defect is not closed, there may be significant left-to-right shunting at atrial level.

Repair of Uncomplicated Tetralogy of Fallot with Pulmonary Stenosis via the Right Ventricle

The usual intraoperative preparations are made (see Chapter 2) and a median sternotomy incision employed. Prompt control of major bleeding from collaterals is accomplished with diathermy. The usual dissections are made (see "General Plan"), and purse strings and tapes are placed. A woven Dacron tube (see earlier section on "Decision and Technique of Transannular Patching") may be selected and preclotted under pressure with the patient's blood (UAB), or pericardium may be removed (GLH).

CPB is established using direct (UAB), or indirect (GLH) vena caval cannulation (see Chapter 2). The perfusate is made as cold as possible. The cardioplegic needle is secured into the ascending aorta. By now, because of the cold perfusate, the heart is usually ineffective or fibrillating. After snugging down the caval tapes, a short right atriotomy may be made and a pump-oxygenator sump sucker placed par-

←

Figure 23-28 Enlargement of the right ventricular outflow tract and pulmonary valve ring by a transannular patch.
(a) A primary incision across the valve ring is used when the preoperative cineangiograms and intraoperative observations make it evident that a transannular patch is required. Otherwise, the two separate incisions shown in Figure 23-27(a) are made and joined to form the incision across the pulmonary valve ring only after it has been determined that a transannular patch is needed. (b) After repairing the VSD and performing the infundibular dissection, the pulmonary valve is completely excised. A Dacron (UAB) or pericardial (GLH) patch is used to enlarge the entire area. Its dimensions are such that it is convex in all dimensions (see text for details; the patch may need to be extended farther distally in some cases).

tially across the natural or surgically created foramen ovale (UAB). Alternatively (GLH), the left atrial suction line may be inserted through the base of the right superior pulmonary vein through a purse-string stitch. An efficient system for venting the left heart is essential for precise repair of the TF, since 20% or more of the total flow from the pump oxygenator to the patient passes through collaterals into the pulmonary circulation and then into the left heart.[M1,M2] The aorta is cross clamped, the cold cardioplegic solution injected (the efflux of this from the coronary sinus is aspirated and discarded [UAB] or allowed to escape from the right atrium), and the perfusate temperate is stabilized at 25°C.

The right ventricle is opened through a vertical (longitudinal) or transverse incision (see "General Plan" for the indications for each), and, in any event, large marginal branches of the right coronary artery that cross the right ventricle are spared. The vertical incision is made in the midportion of the right ventricular infundibulum and extended nearly to but not into the pulmonary valve superiorly and just into the sinus portion of the right ventricle. Two pledgetted stay sutures placed through each side of the incision are placed on traction for exposure. A transverse incision is used only when there is adequate lateral width to the infundibulum. The site of the os infundibulum is often indicated by a transverse indentation of the right ventricular free wall over it. Ideally, the transverse incision is made at this level, but a large marginal right coronary branch may overlie this. The incision is then made just downstream to this (if the infundibular chamber is large) or just upstream to it (if there is inadequate infundibular width).

The infundibular resection is performed (see "General Plan," and Fig. 23-25). The pulmonary valve is examined, and if it is stenotic a valvotomy is performed (see earlier discussion in "General Plan"). The diameter of the valve anulus and pulmonary trunk is measured with Hegar dilators. If a transannular patch is considered necessary, the ventriculotomy incision is now carried across the anulus, since this aids exposure of the VSD. If enlargement across the anulus is not considered necessary, the VSD is repaired (see "General Plan").

If the decision has been made earlier not to use a transannular patch, the measurements with the Hegar dilator are now repeated from the right ventricle. If no further narrowing has resulted from the VSD repair, the pulmonary arteriotomy is closed by direct suture or often with a pericardial patch (UAB). The vertical infundibular incision, if made, is closed with a preclotted Dacron patch (UAB) or directly (GLH). When a transverse incision has been used, it is closed by interrupted full thickness 3-0 silk sutures (GLH) or continuous polypropylene (UAB). If the outflow tract is too narrow after the VSD repair, the vertical infundibular incision is carried across the pulmonary valve ring, valve leaflets are excised, and a transannular patch is placed.

Repair of Uncomplicated Tetralogy of Fallot with Pulmonary Stenosis via the Right Atrium

This repair procedure is identical to repair through the right ventricle until CPB has been established. After commencing cooling on CPB, the caval tapes are snugged, a long right atriotomy incision is made that is carried well inferiorly a little anterior to the inferior vena cava (IVC) cannula site, and the pump oxygenator sump sucker is placed partially across the natural or surgically created foramen ovale to keep the left and right atria and pulmonary arterial tree free of blood. The aorta is cross clamped, the cold cardioplegic solution is injected, and the efflux from the coronary sinus is aspirated and discarded. The perfusate temperature is taken to 25°C, and stay sutures are applied to the right atrial wall for exposure. The interior of the right ventricle and its outflow tract are studied through the tricuspid valve (Fig. 23-26).

With properly placed 6-0 polypropylene traction sutures on the septal and anterior leaflets of the tricuspid valve, the edges of the VSD can usually be visualized,[3] although with more difficulty in TF than an isolated perimembranous VSD because of the leftward and anterior displacement of the infundibular septum and its parietal extension. The pathway from sinus to outflow portion of the right ventricle is examined. The obstructive nature of the prominent parietal extension of the infundibular septum (Fig. 23-26) is particularly well appreciated from this approach, and the infundibular chamber, if present, is easily visualized. The pulmonary valve can usually also be well seen.

The parietal extension is deeply incised 2–4 mm beyond (toward the free wall) its origin from the infundibular septum and 4–5 mm above the aortic cusps, which are visualized as the cut is made (Fig. 23-26). The parietal extension is then dissected away from the ventriculo-infundibular fold (inner curvature of the right ventricle) and from the anterior free wall of right ventricle and excised. The free wall of the right ventricle is palpated occasionally from outside during this dissection to avoid perforating it. Any hypertrophied and obstructive trabeculae along the left side of the outflow tract are incised and removed together with the fibrous margins of the infundibulum. The infundibular chamber and areas just upstream to the pulmonary valve are examined to determine (in concert with the preoperative cineangiogram) whether they need widening by an infundibular patch. The pulmonary valve is examined to determine whether a valvotomy should be done through the pulmonary artery. The diameter of the narrowest part of the pulmonary arterial outflow tract is estimated by passage of a Hegar dilator; the probable postrepair $P_{RV/LV}$ without a transannular patch is predicted on the basis of this (see earlier Section on "Decision and Technique for Transannular Patching"). The ventricular septal defect is now repaired by sewing into place a preclotted Dacron velour patch with continuous 4-0 or 5-0 polypropylene (see Fig. 23-26).

---

[3] In about 5% of patients with TF, the aortic dextroposition is sufficiently severe that the cephalad (superior) borders of the VSD cannot be seen except with extreme traction on the tricuspid valve. In such cases, rather than using such strong traction, either the right atrial approach is aborted or a radial incision is made in the anterior and septal tricuspid leaflets, about 2 mm from the anulus, beginning this in the anterior leaflet about 15–20 mm anterior to the commissural leaflet tissue between it and the septal leaflet. Stay sutures of 6-0 polypropylene are applied. (See Chapter 20, Fig. 20-27.)

If a pulmonary valvotomy is needed, it is usually done through a vertical incision in the pulmonary trunk (see Fig. 23-27). After the valvotomy, the postrepair $P_{RV/LV}$ is estimated by sizing the orifice with Hegar dilators, which is usually best done through the right atrium. If need for a transannular patch is not predicted, the pulmonary arteriotomy is closed, usually with a pericardial patch. If there is infundibular and/or subvalvar fibrous narrowing, the pulmonary arteriotomy is left open and a short longitudinal incision is made *limited to* the infundibulum. Care is taken not to damage the pulmonary valve or anulus in making it. Any subvalvar narrowing is excised, and occasionally the anterior free wall can be freed a little more from the parietal extension of the infundibular septum. This incision is closed with a preclotted woven Dacron patch, and the pulmonary arteriotomy is closed with a pericardial patch unless a transannular patch is mandated by predictions from a final measurement with Hegar dilators in which case a transannular patch is placed. (It is recommended [see "General Plan"] that the right atrial approach be restricted to patients thought not to need infundibular or transannular patches, and the steps described in this paragraph, other than the pulmonary valvotomy, should rarely be necessary.)

Returning to the right atrium, the sump sucker is withdrawn from the foramen ovale and positioned in the right atrium; with strong suction on the aortic needle vent, the aortic clamp is released. The foramen ovale is closed, the right atriotomy is closed, and the caval tapes are loosened. The remainder of the operation proceeds as described for repair through the right ventricle.

Repair of Tetralogy of Fallot in Infancy Using Profound Hypothermia and Circulatory Arrest

When the repair of TF is done in infants, CPB at 25°C may be used in most circumstances (UAB), or profound hypothermia with total circulatory arrest may be preferred (GLH). Optical magnification is used as a routine. When CPB is used, the technique is that described in the earlier portions of the section on "Technique of Operation" and in Chapter 2. The general features of the total circulatory arrest technique are described in Chapter 2, Section 4, and the special features in the TF are described here.

Cooling is achieved largely by surface means while pressure monitoring lines are inserted (see Chapter 2, Section 4 for details). A median sternotomy is performed at 25°C and the heart exposed. If the cineangiogram indicates that a transannular patch is required and in borderline cases, the front of the pericardium is removed from where it joins the diaphragm to its most superior reflection from the aorta. This will secure a piece of pericardium at least 6 cm long and 3 cm wide, tapering at both ends. The pericardium is stretched with its epicardial surface downward onto moist gauze and is set aside for later use. The dissection of the pulmonary trunk and right and left pulmonary arteries is easily and rapidly achieved because of the low aortic and pulmonary artery pressures at these low temperatures, which will have reached about 21°C nasopharyngeal by this time.

CPB is established, cooling to a nasopharyngeal temperature of 18°C (14°C rectal) accomplished, and total circulatory arrest established. When the cineangiogram indicates that a transannular patch is not required and when dissection of the main pulmonary artery confirms that it is of adequate diameter, a transverse incision is made into the right ventricle. The infundibular stenosis is completely relieved. The pulmonary valve is examined from below and any stenosis relieved in the manner already described. The VSD is closed.

The tricuspid valve is now retracted and the atrial septum exposed. If a patent foramen ovale is present, it is often possible to close it from this approach; but if not or if there is a more extensive atrial septal defect, the right atrium is opened and the defect closed through this approach, with continuous polypropylene suture. The right atrium is closed. The ventriculotomy is now closed with interrupted silk sutures.

When a transannular patch is indicated and whenever the anterior wall of the right ventricular outflow is too narrow to allow a transverse incision, a vertical ventriculotomy is made. The infundibular stenosis is relieved as completely as possible, and the pulmonary valve and anulus are examined from below. Any pulmonary valve stenosis is opened (see earlier sections). If a transannular patch is not needed, the vertical ventriculotomy incision is closed directly with interrupted silk sutures. Otherwise, the incision is carried across the anulus and out along the main pulmonary artery almost to the origin of the left pulmonary artery and a transannular patch of pericardium is placed. Should there be a left pulmonary artery origin stenosis, the incision passes beyond this to reach the normal diameter left pulmonary artery. When a transannular patch is needed, the VSD repair may be delayed until after inserting the patch into the pulmonary artery.

Should the circulatory arrest period approach 45 minutes before the repair is completed (and this should be uncommon if the procedure has been done precisely and efficiently), CPB is recommended by reinserting the single cannula into the right atrial appendage if only the right ventricular pericardial patch suture line requires completion or otherwise by inserting two small caval cannula via the opened right atrium.

Repair of Uncomplicated Tetralogy of Fallot after a Blalock-Taussig or Gore-Tex Interposition Shunt

The making of the median sternotomy in a patient with TF and a *Blalock-Taussig (B-T) shunt* is usually accompanied by profuse bleeding from the arteries in front of and behind the sternum, which have developed as part of the collateralization that follows ligation of the subclavian artery. As this bleeding is being controlled, rapid volume replacement should not be made with banked blood. This blood passes directly across the VSD into the aorta and coronary arteries. If infused rapidly, because it is cold and has a low calcium content and low pH, the heart may slow and even stop in asystole.

When a right B-T shunt is present in a patient with a left aortic arch, the pericardium is opened, a piece removed if needed, the pericardial stay sutures and the purse-string sutures placed as usual, the lines to the pump oxygenator divided and positioned, and the Dacron tube-graft preclotted if required for the repair. As the assistant elevates and retracts the ascending aorta to the left, the right pulmonary artery is visualized coming from beneath the aorta, and the superior vena cava is dissected off from it and gently retracted rightward[K4] (Fig. 23-29). (In a few cases, exposure of the subclavian artery may be easier with the superior vena cava retracted to the left.) Possible distortions of the right pulmonary artery by the shunt are known from the preoperative cineangiogram, and these are kept in mind as the dissection proceeds. The course of the right subclavian artery coming down to the right pulmonary artery can usually now be suspected from observation and the palpation of a continuous thrill. The entire circumference of the subclavian artery may be freed along a short length of the artery by sharp dissection well superior to the anastomosis, and two heavy ligatures are placed loosely around it. The subclavian artery is then temporarily occluded, and if the vessel identification has been correct the continuous thrill disappears, the systolic and diastolic systemic arterial pressures rise, and pulse pressure narrows. If these things do not occur, the right pulmonary artery has been misidentified as the subclavian artery, or the shunt, is small. The heart is now cannulated and CPB begun. The ligatures around the subclavian artery are tied, and the operation proceeds as usual. An alternative and now preferred method is closure with a sturdy clip, in which case the back wall of the subclavian artery is not dissected and temporary ligatures are not placed (UAB).

When the left B-T shunt is present in a patient with a right aortic arch, the subclavian artery is approached from outside the pericardium. For this, the upper left pericardial stay sutures are placed on strong traction to the patient's right. The level of the left pulmonary artery is noted before this maneuver, and just cephalad (superior) to this level the thymus gland and left phrenic nerve are dissected up from the pericardium, sharply and over a limited area, since excessive dissection in this region can result in major bleeding that is very difficult to control. A narrow Deaver retractor is now slipped under the thymus, and the region of the subclavian artery is located by gentle palpation and sharp dissection. It is dissected out as described for the right side, and the same tests made for accuracy of identification. The operation then proceeds as described above.

If the left subclavian artery cannot be located in this manner or by going over the thymus gland and phrenic nerve, an alternative method is used (Fig. 23-30). The innominate artery is identified beneath the left innominate vein and traced distally to the point when in bifurcates into the left subclavian and left common carotid artery. After identifying the left subclavian artery positively by the maneuvers described and by the fact that the anesthesiologist can feel the left common carotid (or left superficial temporal) pulse when the vessel is temporarily occluded, the operation proceeds as described.

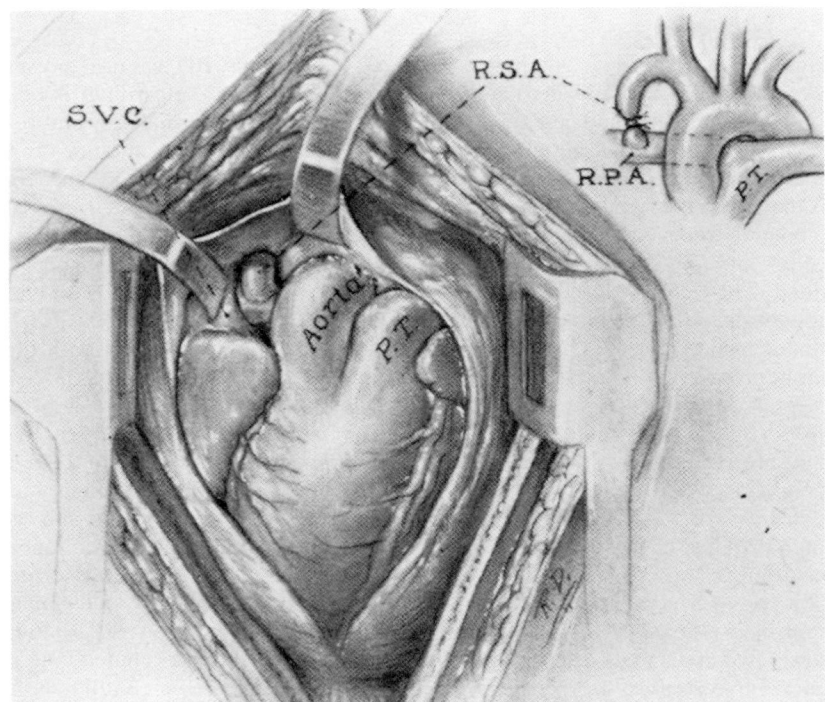

Figure 23-29 Exposure for closure of a right B-T shunt (left aortic arch) at the time of repair of TF. Note that the right subclavian artery is exposed medial to the superior vena cava.

RPA, right pulmonary artery; RSA, right subclavian artery; SVC, superior vena cava.

Reproduced with permission from Kirklin et al.,[K4] and *Surgery, Gynecology and Obstetrics.*

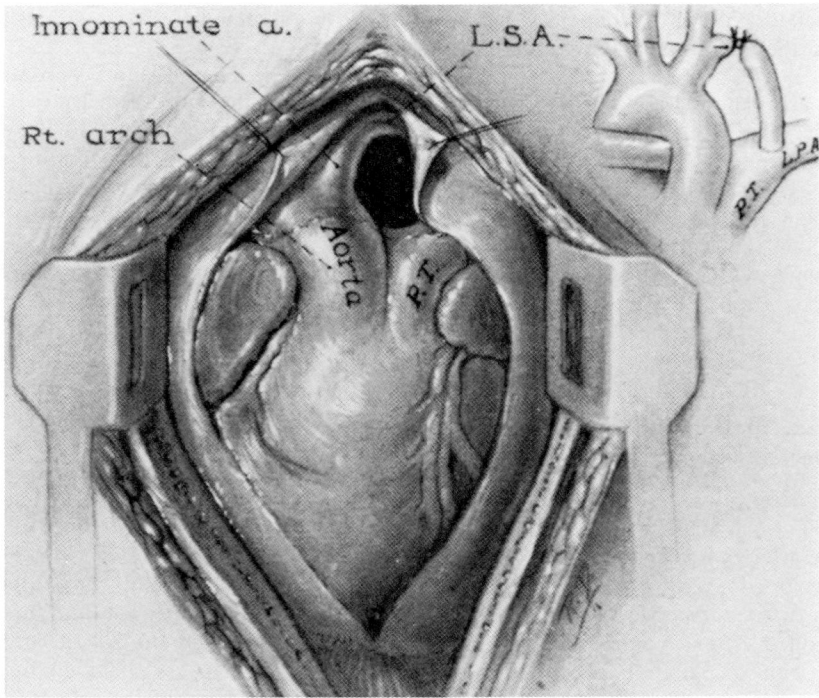

Figure 23-30 An alternative method for approaching the left subclavian artery (right aortic arch) for closure of a B-T shunt at the time of repair of TF. See text for details.

LSA, left subclavian artery.

Reproduced with permission from Kirklin et al.,[K4] and *Surgery, Gynecology and Obstetrics.*

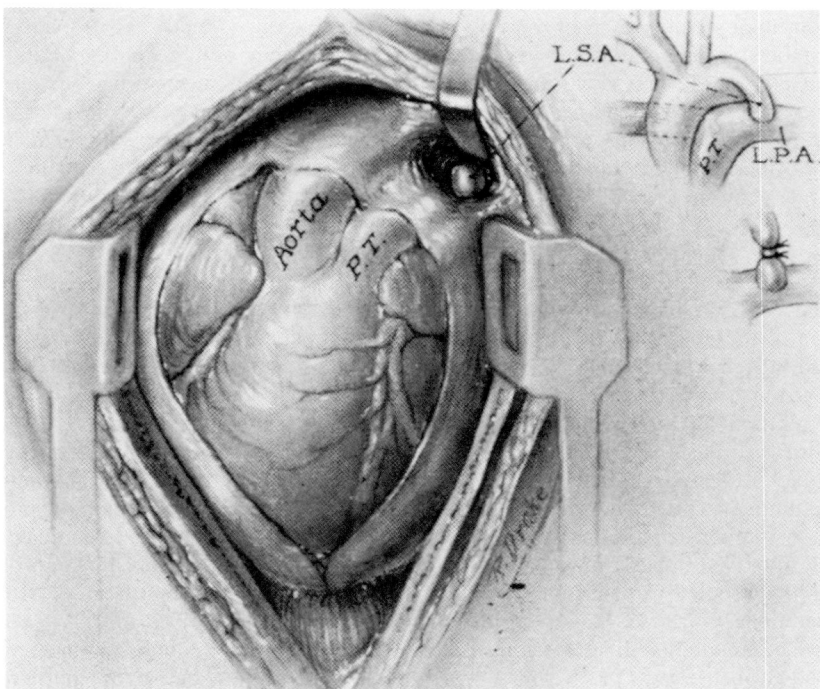

Figure 23-31   Method of extrapericardial approach to the left subclavian artery (right aortic arch) for closure of a B-T shunt at the time of repair of TF. This same approach is used to close a left Gore-Tex interposition shunt (right aortic arch).
LPA, left pulmonary artery; LSA, left subclavian artery; PT, pulmonary trunk.
Reproduced with permission from Kirklin et al.,[K4] and *Surgery, Gynecology and Obstetrics*.

If a left B-T shunt has been made in a patient with a left aortic arch (not recommended) or if a Gore-Tex interposition shunt has been placed between the undivided left subclavian artery and left pulmonary artery, the approach may be started beneath the thymus gland (Fig. 23-31). However, in this circumstance the vessel used for the shunt is farther to the patient's left, and the dissection is usually more easily and quickly accomplished by going outside the thymus gland and into the left pleural space. If a left B-T shunt has been made, its identification may be aided by palpating out along the transverse aortic arch, across which the turned-down subclavian artery passes. Once identified, the artery is dissected sharply, as described earlier. A Gore-Tex interposition graft is felt at reoperation as a hard and rather fixed tube. The dissection is carried down to it, and then by sharp dissection its lateral borders are cleared, but the dissection is not carried completely around it. The operation then proceeds as usual, doubly ligating the subclavian artery, but in the case of the Gore-Tex graft clipping it with a large hemostatic clip.

Repair of Tetralogy of Fallot after a Waterston Shunt

In this situation, the TF repair operation proceeds initially as usual, and the pericardial stay sutures are placed. The superior vena cava is carefully dissected off the right pulmonary artery and retracted laterally, while the right atrial appendage is retracted inferiorly, and the ascending aorta is retracted to the patient's left. Medial to the superior vena cava, the right pulmonary artery is dissected back to its point of anastomosis with the aorta. Then the ascending aorta is retracted to the right, the pulmonary trunk and origin of the right pulmonary artery are dissected away from the left side of the ascending aorta, and a tape is placed around the aorta proximal to the Waterston anastomosis and another one distal to the anastomosis. The purse strings and left atrial line are placed, positioning the aortic purse strings well distally so that there is ample room for the aortic cross clamp between them and the Waterston anastomosis.

When CPB is begun, a soft vascular clamp is placed across the Waterston anastomosis. The perfusate is made as cold as possible, the caval tapes snugged, and the left atrial suction system positioned. The aorta is cross-clamped between the arterial cannula and the Waterston anastomosis, the cold cardioplegic solution infused, the perfusate temperature stabilized at 25°C, and the clamp removed from the Waterston anastomosis when the cardioplegic infusion has been completed. The aorta is rolled to the patient's right by the tapes and medially the right pulmonary artery is freed further from the leftward posterior wall of the aorta. The aorta is next retracted to the patient's left, and an incision is made through the most accessible part of the suture line between the aorta and the right pulmonary artery. This allows a view of the anastomosis from within the aorta; working first from above and then below, the incision through the suture line is extended until the two vessels are completely separated.

A two-row transverse closure of the aorta is made. The first row is placed as a continuous whip stitch of 4-0 polypropylene, brought back to the starting point as an over-and-over adventitial stitch that covers the first row. Occasionally, the right pulmonary artery is quite large, and the opening can be closed transversely without narrowing it. Usually a generous square of pericardium, which is at least one and one-half times larger than the diameter of the right pulmonary artery, is sewn into the opening with continuous 5-0 polypropylene.

(Alternative methods of managing this situation have been described and used at GLH and UAB in the past but are now not recommended. Closure of the anastomosis from within the aorta is a simple method, which works well in the uncommon patient with *no* distortion of a large right pulmonary artery. The more radical method of transection of the ascending aorta at the level of the anastomosis[E4,Y1] gives superb exposure of the entire central portion of the right pulmonary artery and the pulmonary artery bifurcation and certainly facilitates extensive reconstruction in this area. The proximal and distal aortic segments must be well mobilized, or else when reconstructed the ascending aorta will compress the right pulmonary artery. This method is necessary only when simple complete mobilization of all the structures fails to give good exposure.)

Another infusion of the cold cardioplegic solution is given into the ascending aorta, and the remainder of the repair is accomplished as usual.

Repair of Tetralogy of Fallot after a Potts Shunt

The usual preparations for the TF repair operation are made, but a femoral (or external iliac) artery is exposed through a small vertical groin incision (or a transverse iliac fossa incision for retroperitoneal exposure of the iliac artery) before the median sternotomy is made. After the sternotomy is made and the usual stay and purse-string sutures are applied, the anterior aspect of the left pulmonary artery is freed where it exits through the pericardium (see "General Plan"). This dissection is carried as far distally as is possible, which is usually to a point at which the left superior pulmonary vein crosses the artery. The origins of the innominate and left common carotid arteries from the transverse aortic arch are dissected and a single tape placed around them both so that an angled arterial clamp can later be placed across their aortic origins.

The heart is usually grossly enlarged and distorted in the presence of a long-standing Potts anastomosis. The aorta may be very large, and aortic incompetence can be present from annular dilation. Acquired infundibular or valvar atresia is sometimes present.

After placing the arterial cannula in the femoral or iliac artery and cannulating the cavae as usual, CPB is established. A large-bored cold cardioplegic needle is secured in the ascending aorta. The perfusate is made as cold as possible, the caval tapes are left open, the head of the operating table is lowered,[G10] the flow is momentarily reduced to about $1.0 \; l \cdot min^{-1} \cdot m^{-2}$, and a longitudinal incision is made in the left pulmonary artery. The Potts stoma is identified from the blood exiting from it and is digitally occluded.[K8] Full perfusion rate can then be reestablished. When the patient's

nasopharyngeal temperature reaches about 24°C, the perfusion flow rate is reduced to about $0.5 \; l \cdot min^{-1} \cdot m^{-2}$ and the surgeon can relinquish the digital occlusion of the Potts stoma. A small intracardiac sucker placed in the pulmonary artery will return blood escaping from it to the circuit. An angled vascular clamp is now placed across the superior aspect of the aortic arch so that the origins of the innominate and carotid arteries are completely excluded from the aorta. An aortic cross clamp is placed *between* the cardioplegic needle and the heart.

If the stoma is a small one, the repair can be made while perfusion continues at a very low flow. Usually the exposure is inadequate even with the perfusion at a low flow rate and total circulatory arrest is established. The Potts stoma must be securely identified to avoid closing the orifice of a branch of the left pulmonary artery (LPA) because of misidentification. Identification is aided by giving a 1- or 2-second burst of perfusion through the arterial cannula, identifying the Potts stoma as the one from which the blood emerges. Usually the stoma has tough edges and can be closed by a two-row whip stitch of polypropylene and one or two previously placed pledgetted mattress sutures. Very occasionally a pericardial patch is needed for closure.

Often the left pulmonary artery may be closed directly. However, it may be narrow in the region of the Potts stoma. In this case, the incision is made across the stenosis and is reconstructed with a rectangular piece of pericardium that is one and one-half times as long as the incision and one and one-half times as wide as the diameter of the LPA before the stricture.[4] Usually all this can be accomplished within about 20 minutes of circulatory arrest.

Now CPB is reestablished at 28°C at a low flow. Strong suction is placed on the cardioplegic needle, as in the deairing process (see Chapter 2), and full flow is reestablished. Air in the aorta is driven superiorly into the arch by the blood coming up from the femoral cannula and is removed via the needle vent. After determining that all air has been removed, the clamp exteriorizing the innominate and left common carotid arteries is removed as is the aortic cross clamp. The table is straightened. If the heart fibrillates, it is defibrillated. About 5 minutes of a beating heart is now allowed. The perfusate is then made very cold, the left atrial suction system positioned, the aorta cross-clamped, the cold cardioplegic solution given, the perfusate temperature stabilized at 25°C, and the repair performed.

Repair of Tetralogy of Fallot with Stenosis at Origin of Left Pulmonary Artery

In this situation, there is usually sufficient hypoplasia of the pulmonary anulus and trunk that a transannular patch is also required (see "Morphology"). A completely pericardial patch may be used for the entire reconstruction (GLH), which has the advantage of simplifying the procedure as much as possible. Alternatively (UAB), pericardium may be

---

[4]This latter assumes that the pericardium will form the entire anterior half of the circumference of the enlarged LPA. The circumference is roughly three times the diameter and half of this is one and one-half times the diameter.

used for the reconstruction of the delicate left pulmonary artery and a separate Dacron patch used for the transannular reconstruction. Possibly, this makes a perfect geometric reconstruction easier. A right ventricular approach to the intracardiac repair is usually chosen to simplify the procedure as much as possible.

The operation proceeds as usual until the VSD repair is completed. The incision in the right ventricular infundibulum is extended across the anulus and into the pulmonary trunk. This incision is extended to the end of the pulmonary trunk and across the stenosis at the origin of the LPA and into the larger LPA beyond (Fig. 23-32). Even though the preoperative cineangiogram has shown no stenosis at the origin of the *right* pulmonary artery, this orifice is examined from within to be sure this is the case. When two separate patches are used, the pericardial patch is trimmed in a rectangular shape so as to be one and one-half times the length of the incision into the LPA and one and one-half times the estimated diameter of the reconstructed LPA. This patch is sewed into place with continuous 6-0 polypropylene (Fig. 23-32). The preclotted woven Dacron patch is trimmed as described earlier and sewed into place as a transannular patch, attached in part distally to the pericardial patch (Fig. 23-32). When a completely pericardial patch is used, it is trimmed as usual, but an extension for the LPA enlargement is fashioned.

In those uncommon instances in which a transannular patch is not needed, an incision is made across the stenosis in the origin of the LPA. A rectangular patch of pericardium is trimmed and sewed into place as described.

When there is a virtual or total occlusion of the LPA origin, patch graft enlargement is not satisfactory. Instead, after locating the patent portion of the LPA beyond the zone of occlusion by dissecting along the chord of tissue that still connects the LPA to the pulmonary artery bifurcation, the patent LPA is opened longitudinally anteriorly for a short distance. The opened end is then sutured to the adjacent leftward edge of the main pulmonary artery with a running fine polypropylene stitch to create a new posterior wall. The anterior wall is next created by a pericardial patch positioned as for reconstruction of a zone of stenosis (see above). When the LPA is totally disconnected from the main pulmonary artery or is too small for the previously described reconstruction, repair entails locating the LPA in or adjacent to the lung hilum (usually by intrapleural dissection) and disconnecting it from any vessel that supplies it. It is then usually possible to anastomose the LPA end to side to the leftward edge of the distal main pulmonary artery (mobilizing it completely so that it will swing more easily to the left). If the LPA is narrowed proximally, however, a technique similar to that described above is employed.

Repair of Tetralogy of Fallot with Stenosis at the Origin of the Right Pulmonary Artery

This repair occurs uncommonly without associated LPA stenosis. In contrast to the LPA, the right pulmonary artery (RPA) is usually *not* an extension of the pulmonary trunk but comes off its side at a right angle. This makes the simple type of repair utilized for origin stenosis of the LPA less satisfactory, although it may be used when the stenosis is not too severe (GLH).

The operation proceeds as usual until the VSD has been repaired. Then a small longitudinal incision is made in the pulmonary trunk so that the orifice of the right pulmonary artery can be visualized (Fig. 23-33). A button of pulmonary trunk wall containing the orifice is excised, creating a large orifice in the side of the pulmonary trunk. The RPA is incised from its narrow orifice back into its wide portion. A rectangular piece of pericardium is trimmed and sewed to the RPA to make a markedly enlarged proximal RPA. The proximal end of the reconstructed RPA is then sutured to the enlarged orifice in the side of the RPA (Fig. 23-33), taking care to avoid any purse-string effect. Alternatively, the posterior edge of the opened RPA is sutured to the back wall of the opened pulmonary trunk, and then the rectangular piece of pericardium is sewed to the remaining opening to widen it further.

Transection of the ascending aorta improves the exposure but generally is not necessary.

Repair of Tetralogy of Fallot with Bifurcation Stenosis of the Pulmonary Trunk

This condition requires appropriate reconstruction based on a proper understanding of the morphology, although only a few papers discuss the details of this repair.[L11] Both left and right pulmonary artery ostia are usually stenosed to a similar degree and over a short distance (<15 mm), and the distal pulmonary trunk is often similarly narrowed. The pulmonary trunk may be short and the carina between the two branches prominent and unusually proximal, making the bifurcation more Y shaped than usual.

Complete mobilization of aorta, pulmonary trunk, RPA, and LPA is required, preferably before CPB. Before or after repairing the VSD, the vertical ventriculotomy incision is carried across the anulus and into the pulmonary trunk and extended across the narrow origin of the LPA and into the dilated portion. The repair may be made after fashioning a similar anterior incision across the RPA origin stenosis (GLH). The superior edges of both opened arteries are sutured together with 5-0 polypropylene over a distance of about 10 mm (tissue at the original carina may need to be trimmed away to make this area less bulky). This suture line is intended to create a single widely open distal ostium, and a rectangular-shaped pericardial patch of appropriate size is sutured onto its edges to create a new front wall, carrying the patch proximally into the pulmonary trunk and right ventriculotomy. Alternatively (routinely at UAB; only when the RPA comes off at right angles at GLH), the identical repair described earlier is used for the RPA, and the usual steps are used to enlarge the first part of the LPA (Fig. 23-34). The transannular patch is then made from a preclotted woven Dacron tube (UAB), or a pericardial patch may be used (GLH).

Repair of Tetralogy of Fallot with Anomalous Origin of the Left Anterior Descending Coronary Artery from the Right Coronary Artery

In hearts in which there is a large coronary artery crossing the right ventricular outflow tract close to the pulmonary ring (usually an anomalously arising left anterior descending

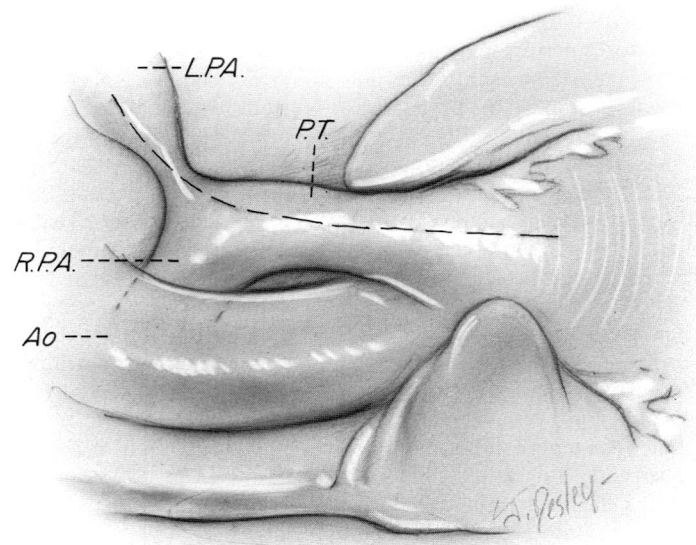

a

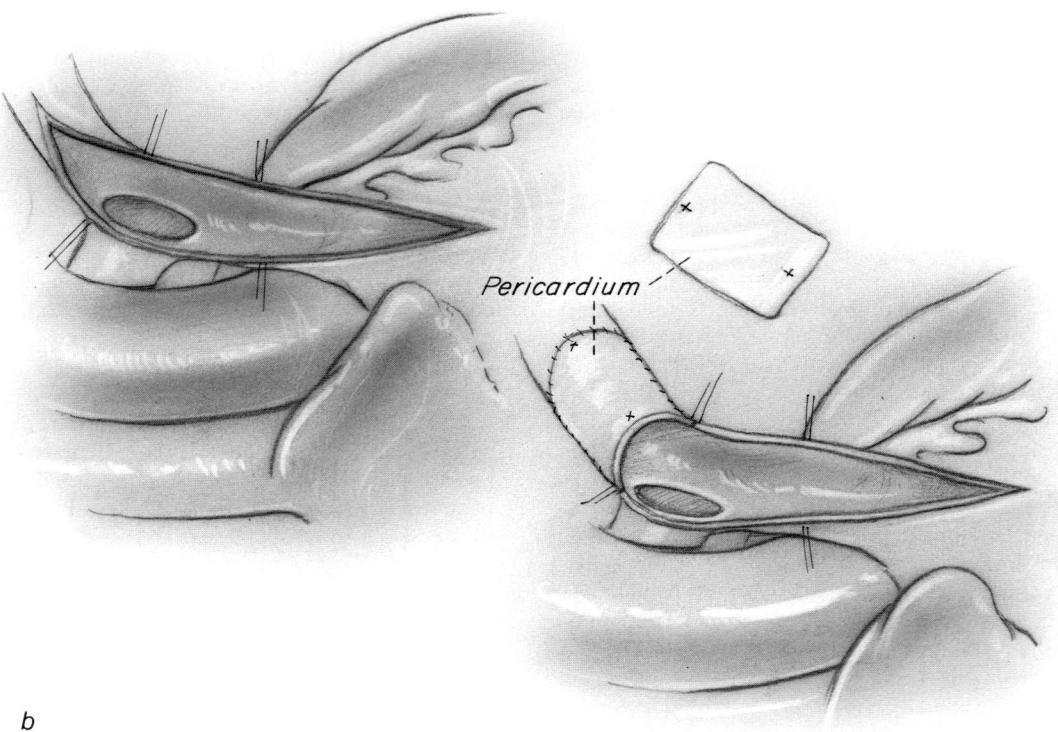

b

Figure 23-32 Repair of stenosis at the origin of the left pulmonary artery. Since the stenosis is usually associated with hypoplasia of the pulmonary valve ring and pulmonary trunk, the repair is shown in this context. Alternatively (GLH), the entire repair may be made with a single pericardial patch.

(*a*) The incision in the pulmonary trunk is carried well across the stenosis in the first part of the left pulmonary artery.

(*b*) A pericardial patch is sewed into place to enlarge the first part of the left pulmonary artery. Note that the pericardial patch is cut in a rectangular shape so as to allow maximum convexity after its insertion (see text for details).

Ao, aorta; LPA, left pulmonary artery; PT, pulmonary trunk; RPA, right pulmonary artery.

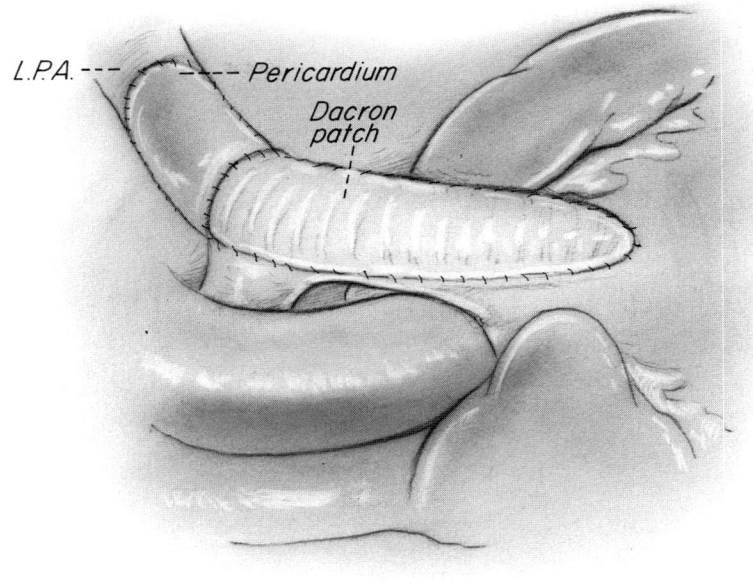

L.P.A. --- --- Pericardium
Dacron patch

c

Figure 23-32 *(continued)*
(c) The preclotted woven Dacron transannular patch is sewed into place, being attached distally in part to the previously placed pericardial patch.

[LAD] artery from the right coronary artery [RCA] but sometimes the entire left coronary artery coming from RCA), the relief of the pulmonary stenosis must not either divide or compromise flow through this vessel. Since such a vessel is occasionally buried in muscle or fat and not apparent on surface inspection at operation, the preoperative cineangiographic study must be of sufficient quality to exclude this anomaly. When there is uncertainty, the usual course of the first part of the LAD artery is inspected, and if the LAD is not there it arises anomalously. When anomalous origin is present, the technique of repair depends on the morphology of the right ventricular outflow obstruction, as usual. When the pulmonary valve ring is of adequate diameter, a transverse right ventriculotomy is made low in the outflow tract and the infundibular stenosis relieved from below. Any valvular stenosis is relieved either from below or via the pulmonary trunk.

When there is a small pulmonary ring and proximal pulmonary trunk, a vertical ventriculotomy may be made after dissecting up the anomalous artery from its bed in the right ventricular wall over almost its entire length from its origin to near the interventricular groove (GLH). The incision is then carried beneath it and across the ring into the pulmonary trunk. The infundibular stenosis is relieved in the usual fashion and a pericardial patch of a size sufficient to relieve the stenosis positioned beneath the artery across the ring. Alternatively (UAB), a homograft valved conduit between right ventricle and pulmonary artery may be used to bypass

the area. If this is done, care is taken to avoid making the native pulmonary valve incompetent by injudicious valvotomy.

Repair of Tetralogy of Fallot with Pulmonary Atresia

Occasionally, and particularly in patients with pulmonary atresia that has developed after a shunting procedure, the atresia is at the level of the infundibulum. The operation described for uncomplicated TF with pulmonary stenosis can then be done, often without a transannular patch. When the atresia is at pulmonary valve level and the infundibulum and pulmonary trunk are separated essentially by a membrane, a transannular patch repair can be used, modifying the shape of the patch (Fig. 23-35). In most cases of TF with pulmonary atresia, these simpler repairs are not feasible and the insertion of a valved conduit is required.

The preparations and initial stages of the operation are as described for TF with pulmonary stenosis. Any patent systemic-pulmonary artery shunt is dissected and later tied and other large collateral arteries dissected and occluded where indicated (see "Tetralogy of Fallot with Large AP Collaterals," under section on Indications for Operation). During the early stages of the procedure, the homograft valve with its ascending aorta is selected, thawed if frozen, and rinsed. In infants, depending on their size, a 14–18-mm homograft valve can be used; in children over 5 years of age, a 22–25-mm valve can be used. These should not be flow limiting.

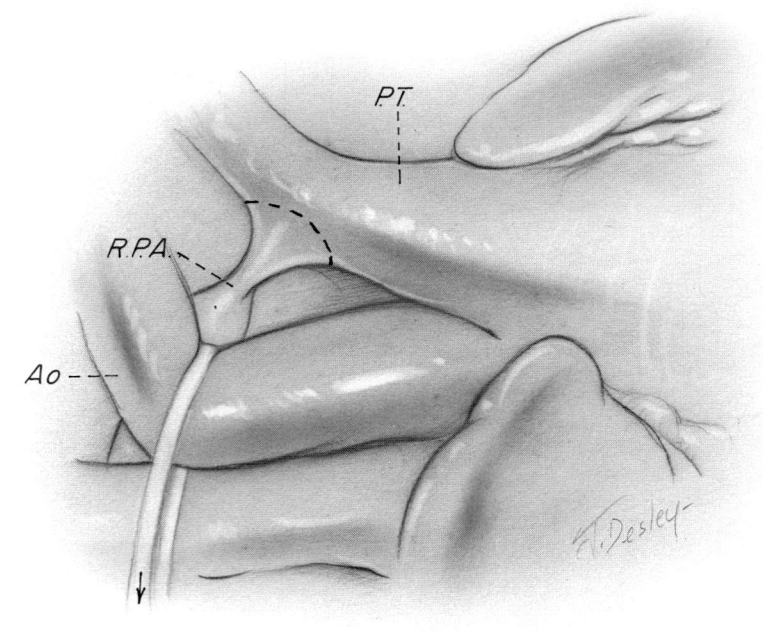

a

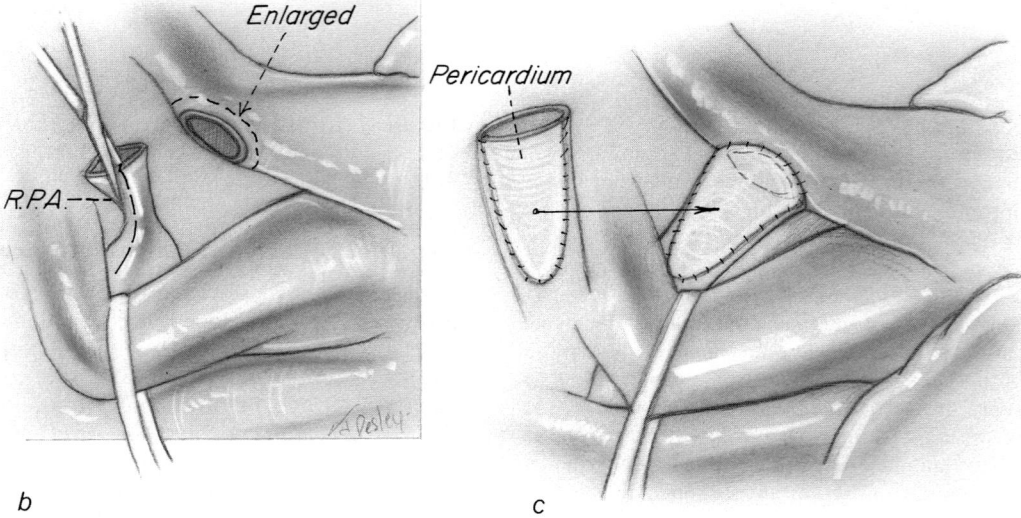

b   *c*

Figure 23-33 One type of repair of stenosis at the origin of the right pulmonary artery (RPA). Initially, a small incision is made in the pulmonary trunk through which the stenotic orifice of the RPA can be viewed from within (not illustrated).

(*a*) The ascending aorta has been mobilized to expose the origin of the RPA. The proposed incision for disconnection of the RPA from the pulmonary trunk is shown.

(*b*) The RPA has been removed from the pulmonary trunk. The resulting orifice in the pulmonary trunk is enlarged as shown. An incision is made down the anterior aspect of the RPA.

(*c*) The RPA is enlarged with a pericardial patch. The enlarged RPA is now reattached to the enlarged aperture in the pulmonary trunk. (At times, it may be easier to suture the posterior wall of the RPA to the posterior aspect of the pulmonary trunk orifice before making the pericardial enlargement of the RPA.)

Ao, aorta; PT, pulmonary trunk; RPA, right pulmonary artery.

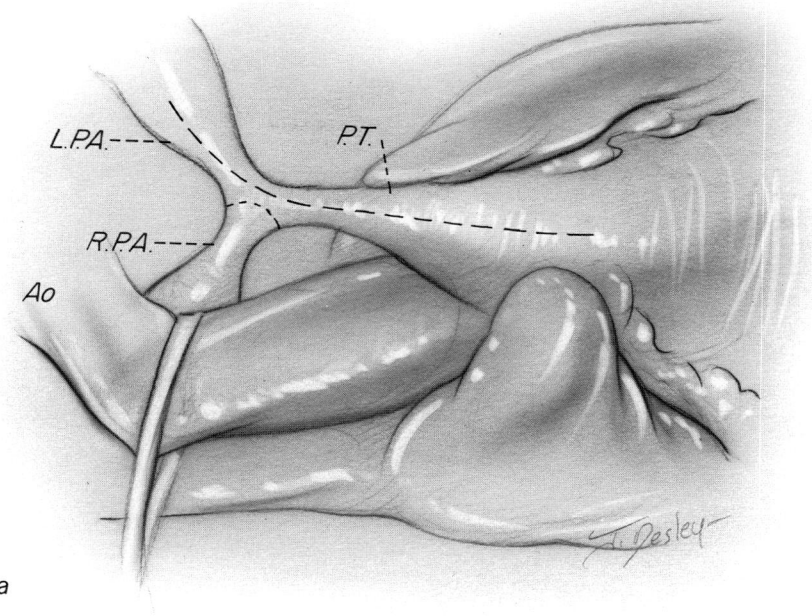

a

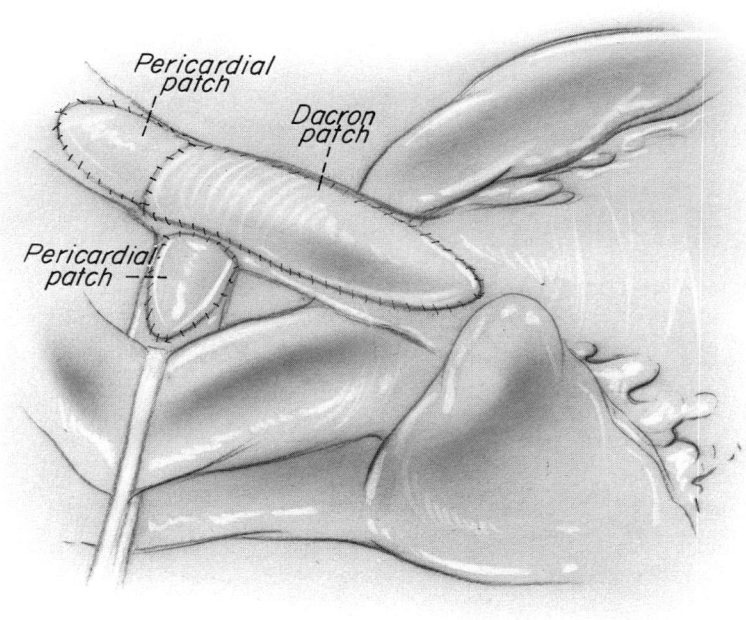

b

Figure 23-34 Repair of bifurcation stenosis of the pulmonary trunk in TF. The illustration is of a situation in which there is marked hypoplasia of the pulmonary trunk and valve ring, as is usually the case.

(*a*) The proposed incisions are shown.

(*b*) After enlarging the proximal portion of the left pulmonary artery as shown in Figure 23-32 and the proximal portion of the right pulmonary artery as shown in Figure 23-33, the repair is completed with the placement of the transannular Dacron patch.

Ao, aorta; LPA, left pulmonary artery; PT, pulmonary trunk; RPA, right pulmonary artery.

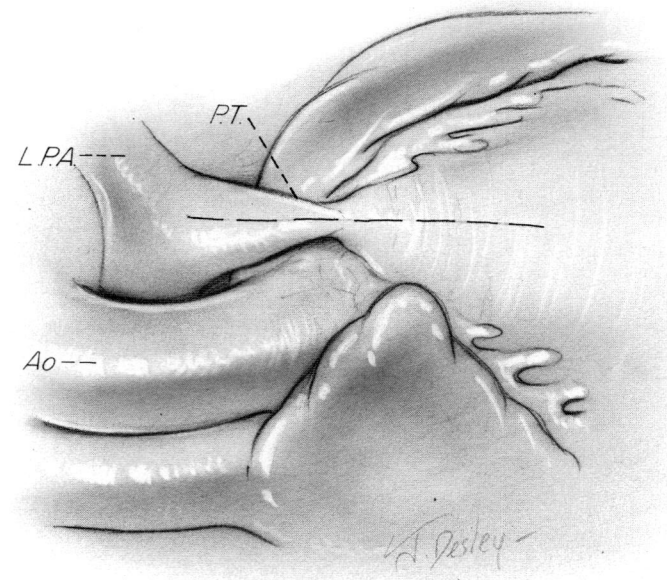

a

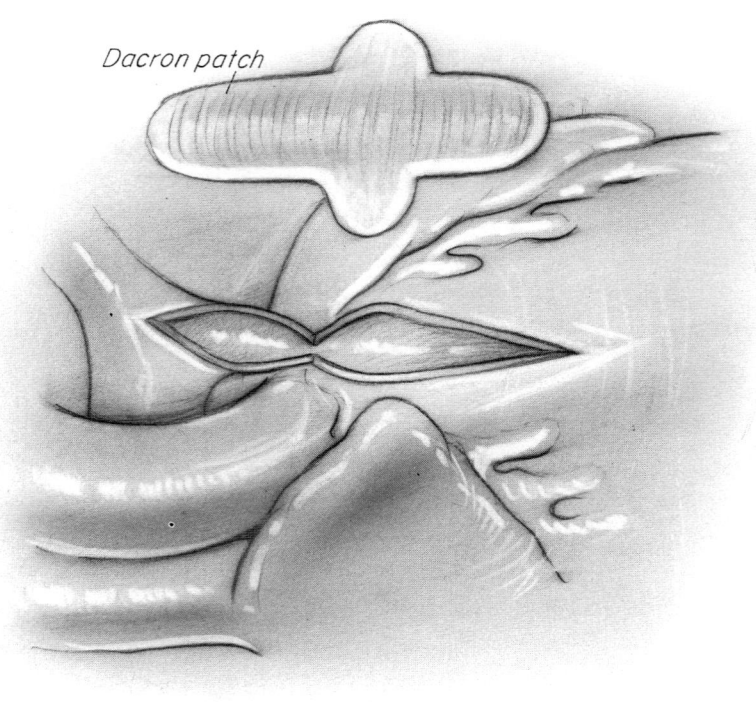

b

Figure 23-35 Modified transannular patch for use in the repair of TF with pulmonary valve atresia.
(a) Proposed incision. Notice that the atresia between the right ventricle and pulmonary trunk is not
evident exteriorly, only a narrowing being visible.
(b) After making the incision, the marked narrowing at the atretic area is again evident. The Dacron
patch is trimmed as shown to compensate for this narrowing.

Ao, aorta; LPA, left pulmonary artery; PT, pulmonary trunk.

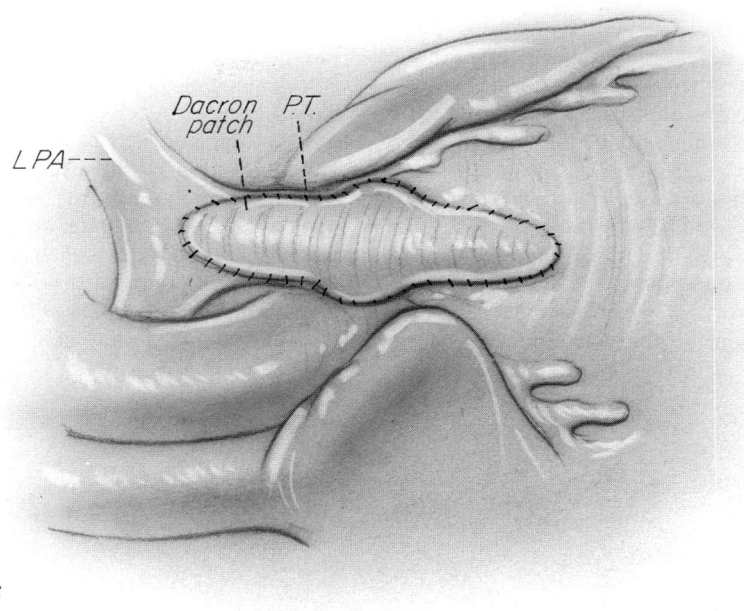

c

Figure 23-35 *(continued)*
(c) After the patch has been inserted, there is a near-uniform widening of the entire area.

(See Chapter 12, Appendix 12C, for a description of the procuring, processing, preservation, and preparation for use of the homograft.)

The pulmonary trunk (if present) and the first portions of the right and left pulmonary arteries may require dissection, and this is done as described earlier. The generally large collateral blood flow through the lungs is collected during the repair by a pump oxygenator sump sucker passed across the atrial septum (UAB) or through the right superior pulmonary vein (GLH).

Two apparently different techniques of inserting the homograft valved conduit are used, which in their end result may not be as different as they may seem to be. In one, that on theoretical grounds is preferable, the proximal end of the homograft is sunk into the right ventricular outflow tract and a piece of pericardium or Dacron is used as a roof over the ventriculotomy incision (Fig. 23-36). The distal end of the homograft is attached to the pulmonary trunk. This method has the advantages of minimal use of foreign material on which a thick neointima may develop and of freedom from sternal compression, but with the method care must be taken that the aortic homograft valve anulus retains its proper circular geometry and that the opening from the right ventricle into the homograft is large. In the second method, a woven preclotted Dacron tube 2–5 mm larger than the diameter of the homograft valve anulus is sutured to the proximal end of the homograft (Fig. 23-37). Before insertion, the proximal Dacron end is cut in a severely beveled fashion so that it serves primarily as a roof on the ventriculotomy incision with only a few millimeters of fully circular Dacron conduit just proximal to the homograft. With care, the conduit can be kept completely away from the sternum. It has the advantage that the perfectly circular geometry of the homograft valve is well maintained and that with it all types of right ventricular and pulmonary trunk morphology can be managed. It has the disadvantage of more Dacron in the conduit than the previous method. There are situations in which one or the other method is mandated, depending on the right ventricular morphology and the availability of the pulmonary trunk, but at times the selection is one of choice.

In either event, the proximal valved end of the homograft is cut transversely about 5 mm below the nadir of the cusps, leaving the muscular remnant at least 4 mm thick (thicker than when the valve is used for aortic valve replacement). In the former method, the aorta at the distal or nonvalved end of the graft is not cut until the exact nature of the pulmonary artery confluence is established by complete dissection and the distance between this and the right ventricular opening has been accurately assessed. When the latter method is used, the same is true but generally a rather short segment of homograft wall is included in the conduit because of the inevitable calcification of this part of the homograft.

With the first method, a limited longitudinal incision is made in the superior right ventricular wall at the position where the pulmonary artery would normally arise. Care is taken in extending the incision distally in order that the anterior margin of the ventricular septal defect and the right coronary cusp of the aortic valve are not damaged. The right ventricular opening is enlarged proximally, and any thick trabeculations arising from the free wall, particularly inferiorly, are excised, along with a limited portion of muscle from both sides of the incision, to convert it into an elliptical opening. The ventricular septal defect is repaired in a fashion similar to that described for TF with pulmonary stenosis. When the infundibular septum is very deficient, the VSD patch may be left unsutured anteriorly (GLH) and this portion of the ventricular septal defect repair incorporated into the proximal conduit suture line. The distal end of the homograft aorta is now cut so that it is the correct shape and the conduit is the correct length. It must not be too long, or else it may kink and possibly compress either branch of the pulmonary artery. The pulmonary artery confluence is opened with an incision that extends out along the right and left branches beyond any zone of proximal narrowing. The opening is made long enough to match exactly the diameter of the homograft aorta (Figs. 23-36, 23-37). Occasionally, it may need to extend further out along one branch to relieve a long

zone of stenosis (usually in the left pulmonary artery). The homograft aorta may be cut with an appropriately shaped flanged extension that extends into and enlarges this new opening (GLH), or the branch may be widened with a separate pericardial patch (UAB) (see earlier section on "Repair of Tetralogy of Fallot with Stenosis at Origin of Left Pulmonary Artery"). After orienting the graft so that the fibrous portion of the aortic ring at the proximal end of the conduit will lie posteriorly, the distal anastomosis is made with continuous 5-0 polypropylene suture. The suture line is commenced superiorly in the midline with a double armed suture, which is carried around each side to meet inferiorly (Fig. 23-36). The suture line must be accurate, and the delicate pulmonary artery wall must not be torn. To facilitate this part of the anastomosis, it may be necessary to have a brief period

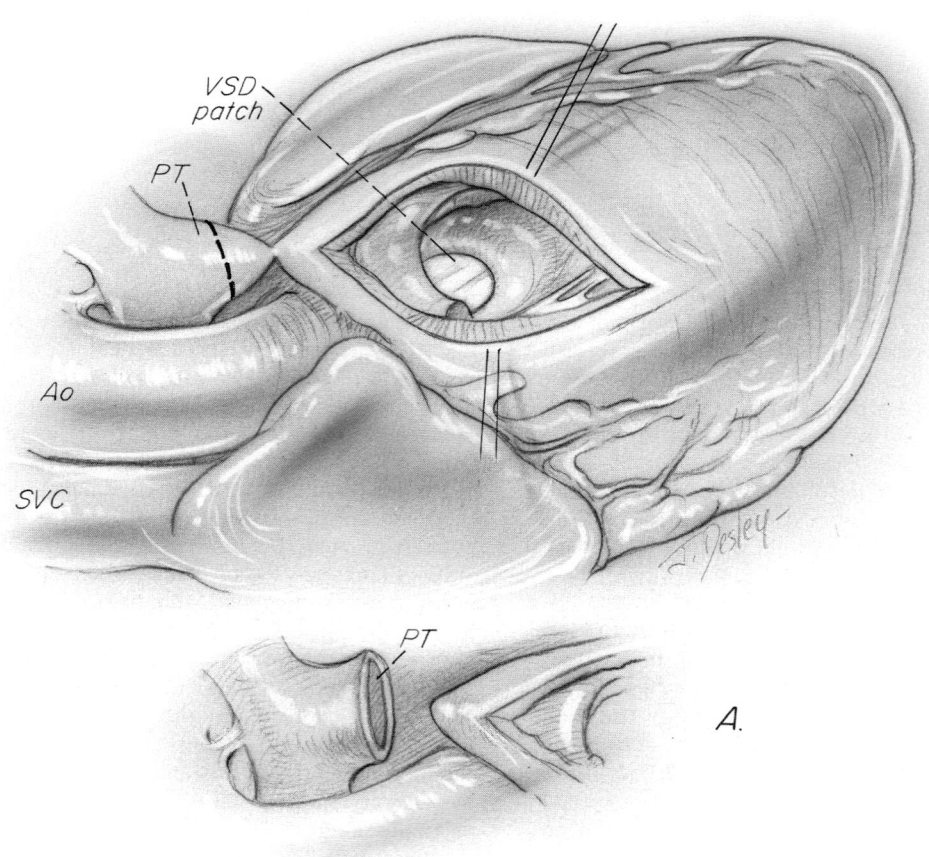

Figure 23-36   Repair of TF with pulmonary atresia (or absent pulmonary valve) using a homograft valve conduit.
(a) A short vertical incision has been made in the right ventricular outflow tract. The ventricular septal defect has been repaired with a patch. In the illustration shown, the infundibular septum is present. When this is severely hypoplastic or virtually absent, the ventricular septal defect repair is nearly to the anterior right ventricular wall superiorly. The sutures for the anterior part of the VSD repair may be left until later and when placed incorporate not only the VSD patch but also the base of the homograft valved conduit (GLH). The pulmonary trunk has been disconnected from any attachment to the right ventricle.
Ao, aorta; PT, pulmonary trunk; SVC, superior vena cava; VSD, ventricular septal defect.

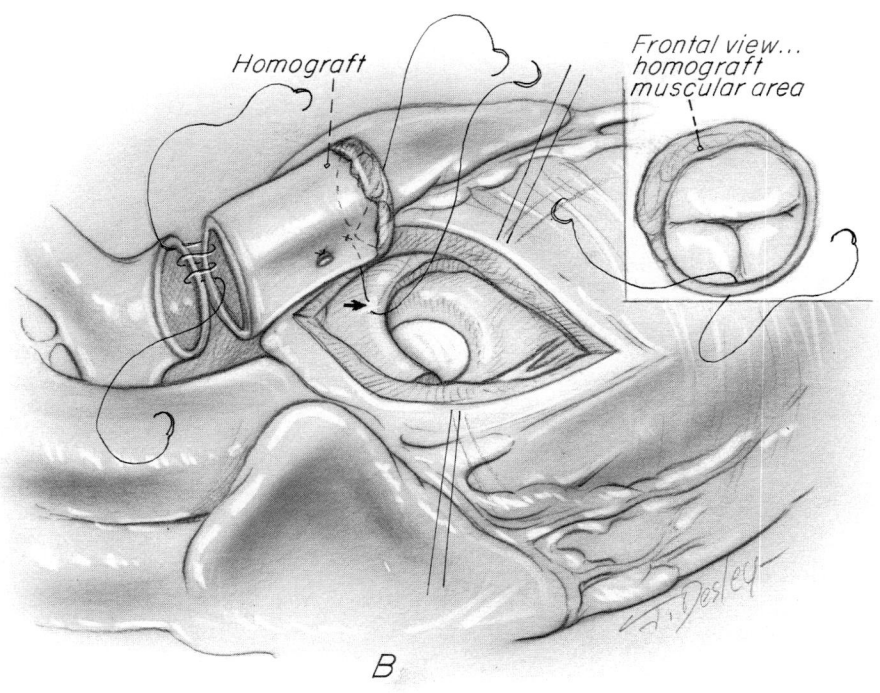

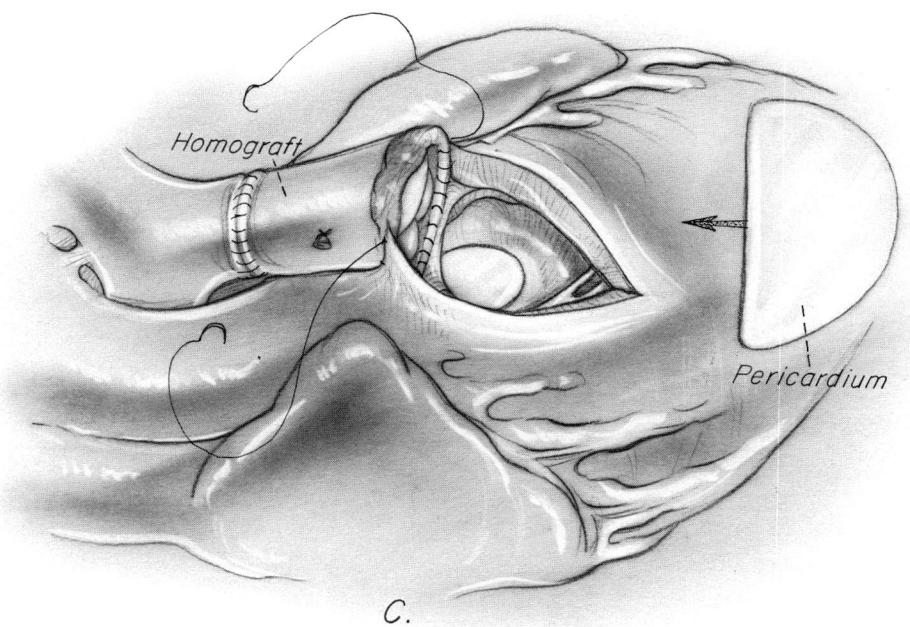

Figure 23-36 *(continued)*

(*b*) The homograft valve has been trimmed appropriately and is oriented so that the muscular portion of its proximal end is anterior. The distal end of the homograft is anastomosed end to side to the pulmonary trunk. One suture method is shown, although others can be used (see text). Anastomosis of the proximal end to the infundibular septum is begun.

(*c*) The suture line between right ventricle and proximal end of the homograft is made and held as shown. A piece of pericardium (or, alternatively UAB, preclotted woven Dacron) is trimmed to an appropriate shape for use as a roof or gusset.

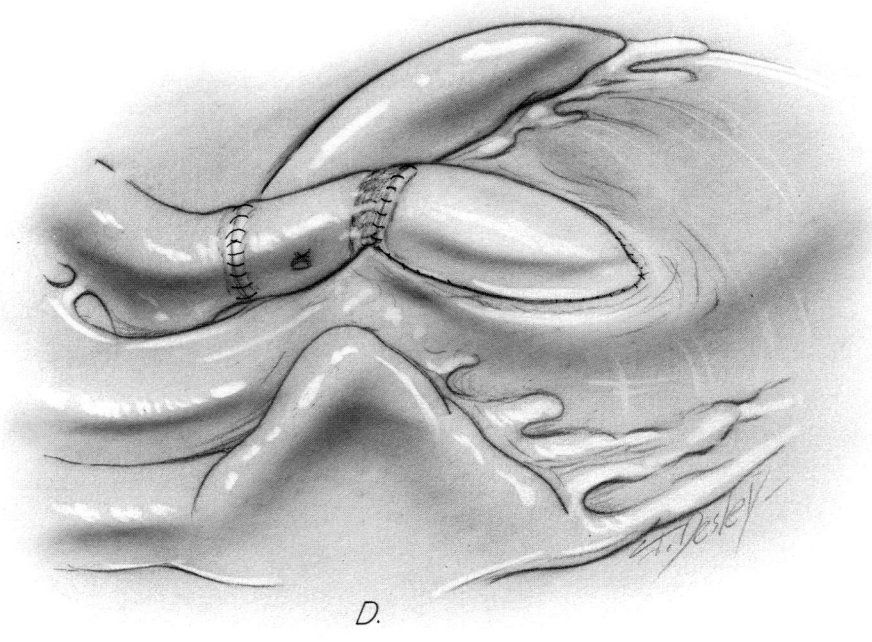

D.

Figure 23-36 *(continued)*
(*d*) The repair is completed by sewing this piece into place. Ordinarily it does not appear quite as long as shown in the illustration.

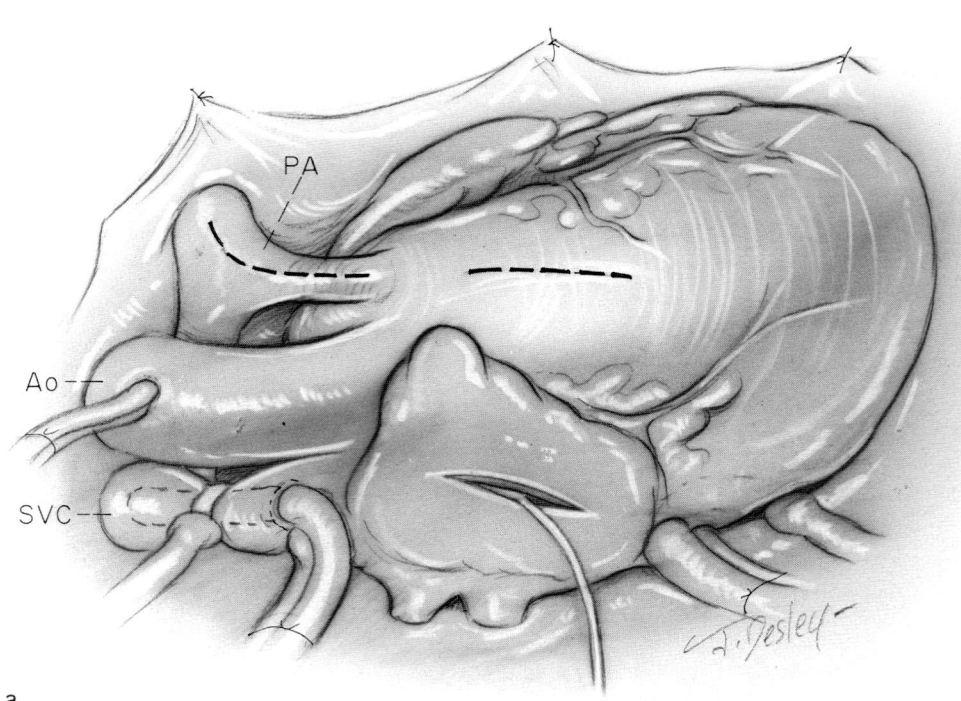

a

Figure 23-37 Repair of TF with pulmonary atresia using a homograft valved conduit and a very short proximal Dacron extension (UAB).
(*a*) The VSD is repaired through a vertical incision in the right ventricle, shown by the dashed line. After the VSD is repaired, a longitudinal incision is made in the pulmonary trunk, which may need to be extended onto the proximal left pulmonary artery to obtain adequate length. If there is little or no pulmonary trunk present, a transverse incision is made across the confluence of the central left and right pulmonary arteries.
(*b*) After the homograft has been rinsed, its coronary arteries doubly ligated, and the woven Dacron

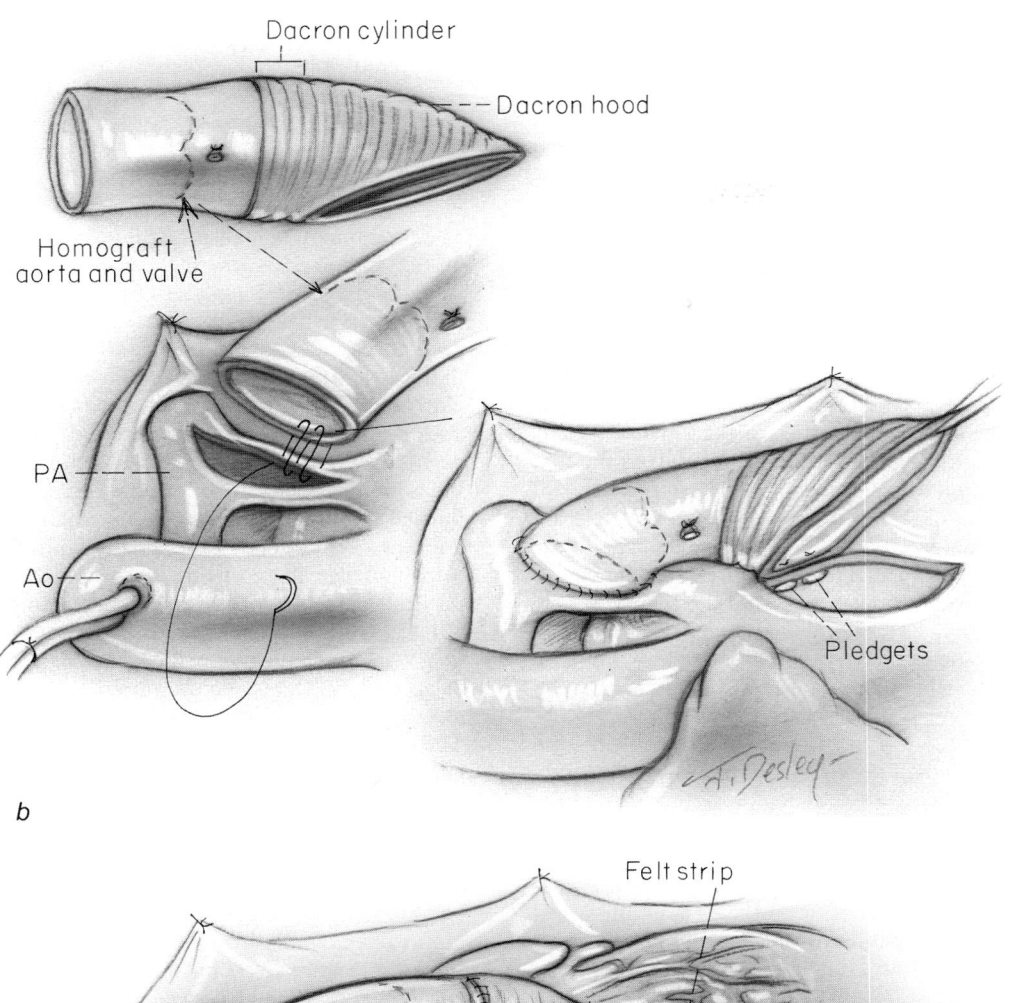

Dacron cylinder

Dacron hood

Homograft
aorta and valve

Pledgets

PA

Ao

b

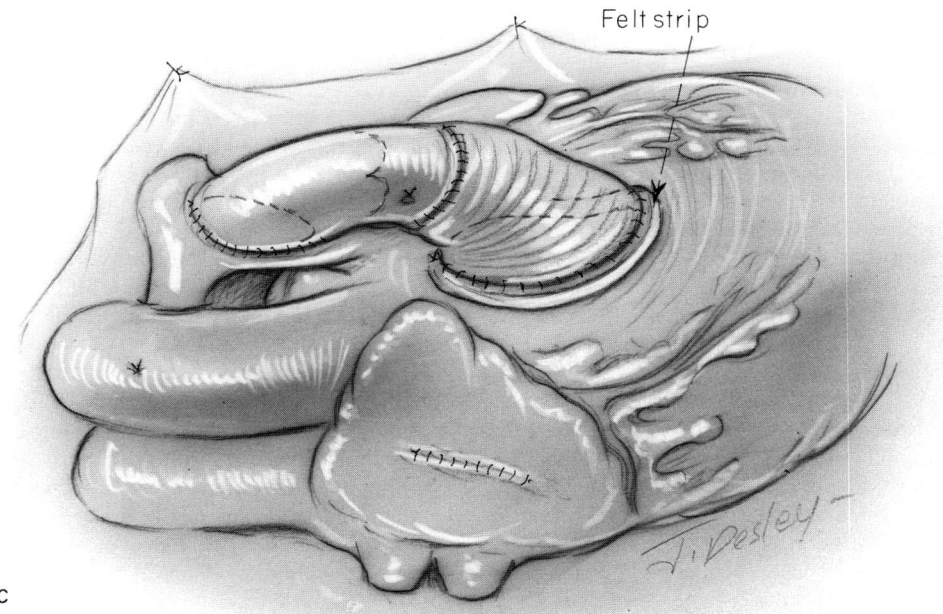

Felt strip

c

Figure 23-37 (*continued*)
tube preclotted, the homograft is trimmed proximally in a manner similar to that for its use in aortic valve replacement (see Chapter 12, "Technique of Operation"), except that the muscle is left 3–4 mm thick and the straight lower margin 3–4 mm below the nadir of the aortic cusp. End-to-end anastomosis is made between the proximal homograft and Dacron tube. The distal end of the homograft is cut square and, if possible, at a level that will allow the proximal end to be trimmed as shown in the insert, leaving a very short piece of Dacron cylinder just beyond the Dacron hood. The entire conduit is trimmed before beginning the insertion. The distal anastomosis is made as shown, placing the initial row from the inside of the vessels.
(*c*) The proximal anastomosis is begun (B) with three or four interrupted felt pledgetted mattress sutures, around the heel, placed from the inside. Just beyond these, on either side an everting mattress suture is placed from the outside through felt strips and continued around as a whip stitch; alternatively interrupted felt pledgetted mattress sutures are used throughout.

Ao, aorta; PA, pulmonary artery; SVC, superior vena cava.

757

of total circulatory arrest, although one of low flow often suffices. The proximal conduit anastomosis is now made by commencing the suturing posteriorly where the fibrous margin of the homograft is opposed to the superior margin of the ventriculotomy and any remnant of infundibular septum. A 4-0 polypropylene suture is used, and usually both the right ventricular wall and the superior edge of the Dacron VSD patch are picked up in the suture line to make it particularly secure posteriorly (GLH). The suture line is continued from the midline along both sides around about half the circumference of the conduit, and the sutures are held. A patch of pericardium (or preclotted Dacron) is now cut to an approximate semilunar shape and sutured into place to complete the anterior half of the anastomosis. Its straight superior edge is anastomosed to the muscular portion of the graft as the first step, and its curved inferior edge is attached to the edges of the right ventriculotomy incision. Good bites of muscle are taken all around and care is used in avoiding damage to the aortic cusps of the graft or the left anterior descending coronary artery. The conduit now arises from the right ventricle in the same position as a normal pulmonary artery and passes superiorly and posteriorly directly to the pulmonary artery bifurcation. It is not in danger of being compressed by the sternum.

In the second method, a longitudinal incision is made in the downstream portion of the right ventricle, and pledgetted stay sutures are applied. If a rudimentary infundibular septum and parietal extension are present, these are dissected away from the right ventricular free wall. The VSD is repaired, as described for TF with pulmonary stenosis. Preparations are now made for insertion of the homograft-valved conduit. The conduit, once in position, should head toward the patient's left shoulder as it comes off the right ventriculotomy (it need not necessarily be oriented parallel to the ventriculotomy) and then curve gently back to the right to approach the pulmonary artery with just a little redundancy and in an undistorted fashion. This is accomplished by cutting the distal end of the homograft exactly transversely (not obliquely). The proximal end of the conduit is cut so that the tubular part of the proximal Dacron extension is only a few millimeters long. The distal and proximal anastomoses are made (Fig. 23-37).

With either method, after the completion of the procedure, the aortic clamp is released with strong suction on the aortic needle vent. Until a good cardiac action is returned, close attention is paid to preventing overdistention of the left ventricle and left atrium by the usually large pulmonary venous return secondary to the large collateral pulmonary blood flow. The remainder of the procedure is completed as described for TF with pulmonary stenosis.

Immediately after discontinuing CPB, the postrepair $P_{RV/LV}$ is measured. (The decision-making implications of the postrepair $P_{RV/LV}$ are discussed in "Postrepair $P_{RV/LV}$" in the section on Special Situations and Controversies.) A polyvinyl catheter is left in the right ventricle (RV) for continuing monitoring of $P_{RV/LV}$, and one is advanced from RV through the conduit for a withdrawal tracing the next morning.

Hemostasis must be patiently secured. Since widespread oozing is common, fresh frozen plasma and platelet concentrates are given routinely after the protamine has been ad-

ministered. When hemostasis is secure, the incision is closed as usual.

Repair of Tetralogy of Fallot with Absent Pulmonary Valve

The preliminaries, incision, and preparations for CPB are as in the previously described procedures. The pulmonary trunk is dissected completely free from the aorta. Since the patients are usually 6–10 years old, a large ($\pm$ 25 mm) homograft aortic valve is chosen (see Chapter 12, Appendix 12C), thawed, and prepared as described earlier. As in tetralogy with pulmonary atresia, either of two very similar techniques may be used. In both procedures, CPB is established, the perfusate cooled, the left atrial suction device positioned, the aorta cross-clamped, and the cold cardioplegic solution infused into the aortic root. In one method (UAB), the conduit has been extended proximally with a Dacron tube (see Repair of Tetralogy of Fallot with Pulmonary Atresia"). A vertical incision is made in the RV infundibulum, and the VSD is repaired. The incision is carried across the anulus and just far enough into the pulmonary trunk so that the orifices of the right and left pulmonary arteries can be visualized. The hypoplastic pulmonary valve leaflets are excised. The pulmonary trunk is then *transected* proximal to the origin of the right pulmonary artery, and the proximal end is dissected back to the right ventricle. The left coronary artery, behind the pulmonary trunk, is preserved. The pulmonary trunk is then amputated from the right ventricle at the level of the pulmonary valve anulus. The distal end of the conduit is transected about 5 mm downstream to the homograft valve commissures, and the proximal end is trimmed as shown in Figure 23-37 but with a shorter hood. End-to-end anastomosis is made between distal pulmonary trunk and homograft. The proximal anastomosis is begun posteriorly, joining the Dacron to the infundibular septum and carrying the suture line up each side until the anterior tongue is sutured into the ventriculotomy. The homograft is now an orthotopic replacement for the pulmonary valve and first part of the pulmonary trunk, much in the manner described by Weldon and colleagues.[W3]

In the other method (GLH), a vertical incision is made into the right ventricular infundibulum and carried across the pulmonary anulus into the dilated main pulmonary artery to a point opposite the inferior edge of the RPA origin. Any obstructive trabeculations are excised from the infundibulum, and the parietal end of the conal (infundibular) septum is divided transversely to improve exposure of the VSD and to allow the septum's deflection backward during patch closure of the VSD to further increase the diameter of the right ventricular outflow tract. The thickened remnants of the pulmonary leaflets are excised. The VSD is closed. The homograft conduit is now inserted inside the opened right ventricular outflow as an internal sleeve, with the muscular portion of its proximal valved end anteriorly. The distal end is cut transversely just beyond the homograft valve commissures. The distal anastomosis is performed within the enormously dilated pulmonary trunk, just proximal to the RPA origin. It is begun posteriorly sewing from inside the graft for the posterior half and outside the graft for the anterior half of the anastomosis. It is simple to perform because of the large diameter of the main pulmonary artery that requires crimping down to match the conduit's diameter. The fibrous portion of the proximal end of the graft is now sutured to the front of the infundibular (conal) septum and to the lateral walls of the outflow tract for about half its circumference. The remaining gap in the right ventriculotomy is filled with a piece of pericardium (or Dacron) positioned with a continuous suture line, exactly as for pulmonary atresia. In either case, the remainder of the operation is completed as usual.

TECHNIQUE OF SHUNTING OPERATIONS

Classical Right Blalock-Taussig Shunt

Generally, an intra-arterial needle is not placed for classical right Blalock-Taussig (B-T) shunt operation. However, in critically ill infants, one is placed in the left radial artery, primarily so that any metabolic acidosis can be identified and treated.

With the patient in the left lateral decubitus position, a right lateral thoracic incision is made. The thorax is entered through the top of the bed of the nonresected fifth rib or through the fourth interspace. A rib spreader is positioned and gradually opened.

The first step in the dissection is the secure identification of the right superior pulmonary vein as it courses obliquely downward (medially and inferiorly) toward the heart to pierce the pericardium posterior to the phrenic nerve. The right pulmonary artery (RPA) is partially overlaid by the vein. The artery, in contrast to the superior pulmonary vein, follows a straight course medially. With the lung retracted toward the surgeon, often best done in the initial stages of the dissection by the surgical nurse (on the surgeon's right) with the left hand, the periarterial sheath over the right pulmonary artery is incised. Usually the superior branch of the artery is first freed, in the process of which the main artery (lying in a slightly different plane of dissection) can be easily overlooked. To find it, the superior surface of the right superior pulmonary vein is cleared, and it and the superior vena cava are elevated (Fig. 23-38). The dissection is carried centrally until the proximal RPA is identified as a single vessel, proximal to the first branch. With lateral traction on a loop of heavy silk placed around the artery, the RPA is dissected in the periarterial tissue plane as far centrally as is possible. The silk loop is now removed so that the artery does not inadvertently become obstructed during the next phase of the operation.

The lung is packed off and retracted inferiorly. An incision is made in the mediastinal pleura over the azygos vein and carried superiorly to the top of the chest, parallel and posterior to the phrenic nerve. The azygos vein is divided between ligatures, and the soft tissue and right paratracheal lymph nodes are divided so as to provide a free pathway for the turned-down right subclavian artery. Any small veins overlying the right subclavian artery are ligated and divided. The vagus and recurrent laryngeal nerves are identified at this time. The periarterial plane over the right subclavian artery is incised. By grasping only the adventitia of the often very delicate subclavian artery, dissection is carried distally in the periarterial plane until the origins of the internal mammary and vertebral arteries are identified. These vessels are divided between ligatures, taking care that the proximal ligature is placed 1–2 mm away from the subclavian artery. Anomalies in the branching of the subclavian artery are of course frequent. The vagus nerve is now gently retracted laterally, and the periarterial plane over the subclavian artery medially is opened and dissected. The subclavian artery is divided between ligatures placed beyond the first two large branches, and a right-angled clamp is passed beneath the vagus nerve from its medial aspect superior to the recurrent laryngeal nerve. The subclavian artery beyond the ligature is grasped with the clamp and pulled out from under the vagus nerve. Holding the artery *beyond* the ligature, the dissection is carried centrally in the periarterial plane until the distal portion of the innominate artery and nearly the entire right common carotid artery are liberated. As this dissection proceeds, a small artery is occasionally found arising from the origin of the subclavian from the innominate artery, and this must be ligated and divided. Now the only thing limiting the turned-down length of the subclavian artery is the common carotid artery itself. Any obstructing bands in the paratracheal soft tissue are divided so that there is nothing in the pathway of the relocated right subclavian artery.

If he is not already using them, the surgeon now puts on magnifying loupes. A light, straight, arterial clamp with a handle long enough to allow easy holding by the first assistant is placed across the subclavian artery about 8 mm proximal to the point of final transection. The artery is now cut squarely across just proximal to its first branch. (Rarely the first branch comes off very proximally and the subclavian artery is unusually large beyond it. In such instances, the artery can be transected beyond this branch.) Double-looped ligatures are placed around the upper branch and main RPA, snugged, and weighted laterally with heavy Kocher clamps. An appropriate-size Baumgartner clamp is placed across the very proximal RPA, the surgeon passing a right-angled clamp beneath the artery for lateral retraction as the first assistant tightens the clamp. A longitudinal incision is now made *in the very superior surface* of the RPA (so that when the occluding devices are removed there will be no torsion of the RPA).

The anastomosis is made with interrupted double-armed 7-0 polypropylene sutures, each stitch being placed from inside to outside in the respective artery (Fig. 23-38). The first assistant holds the two clamps so that the vessels are in perfect opposition and without tension during the anastomosis. Before placing the last few sutures, the lumina are examined and any tiny thrombi or debris irrigated away. After completing the anastomosis, in rather rapid succession the two doubly looped ligatures are cut and removed, the clamp on the subclavian artery is removed, and the Baumgartner clamp is removed. Packing is placed lightly around the anastomosis, any unusual bleeding is controlled digitally, the lung is partially reexpanded, and 5 minutes are allowed to pass. During this time a palpable continuous thrill should be present in the pulmonary artery. When the packs are removed, the field is usually dry. Rarely, an additional adventitial stitch is needed.

A small chest catheter is brought out from the posterior

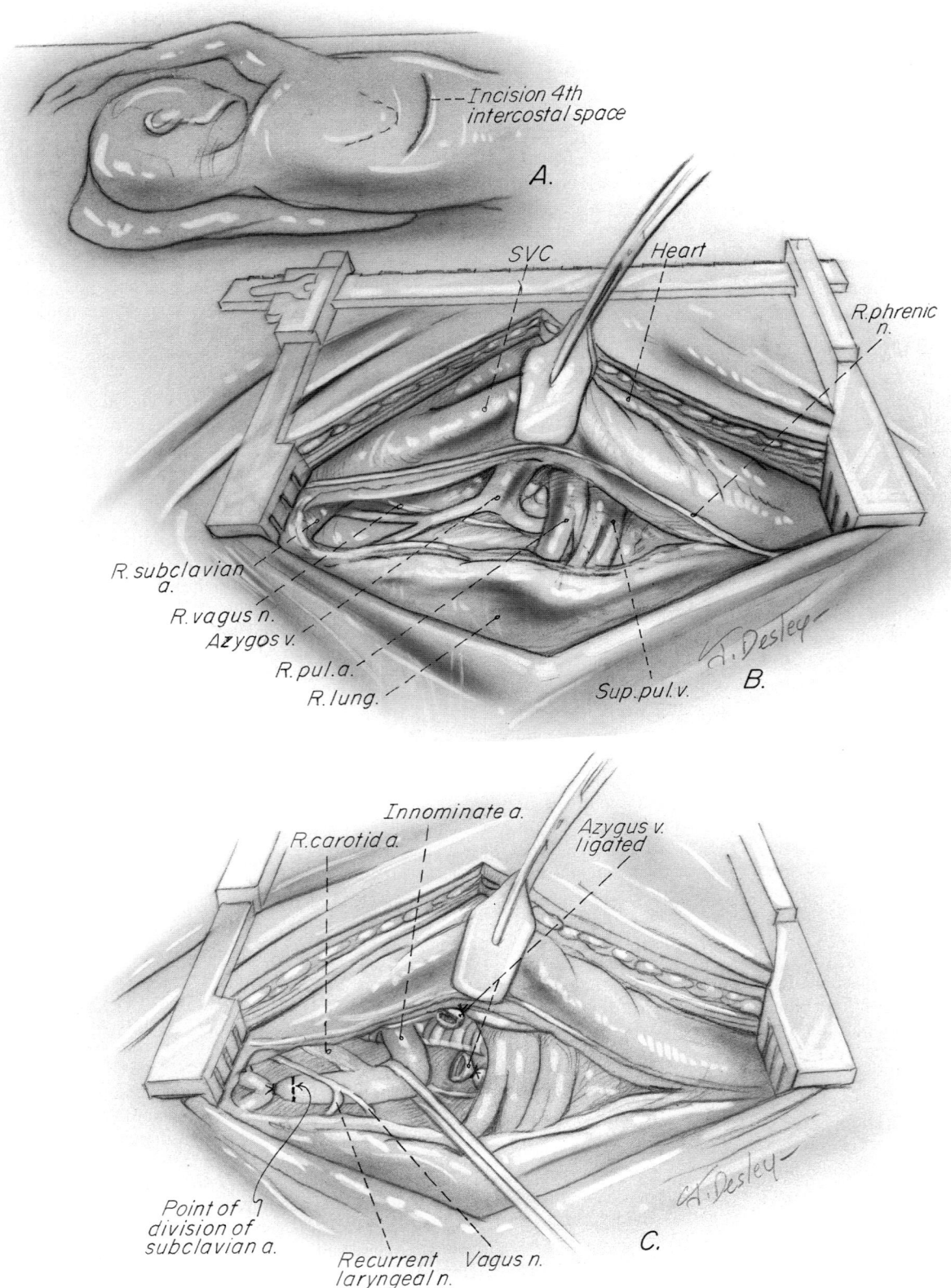

A. — --- Incision 4th intercostal space

SVC   Heart   R.phrenic n.

R. subclavian a.
R. vagus n.
Azygos v.
R. pul. a.
R. lung.
Sup. pul. v.

B.

Innominate a.   Azygus v. ligated
R. carotid a.

Point of division of subclavian a.
Recurrent laryngeal n.   Vagus n.

C.

Figure 23-38 The classical right Blalock-Taussig shunt (left aortic arch).
(a) A right lateral thoracotomy incision is made.
(b) The structures are dissected out.
(c) The right subclavian artery has been completely dissected, mobilized, and ligated just proximal
to its first branch. It will be divided as shown and brought out from beneath the vagus nerve.

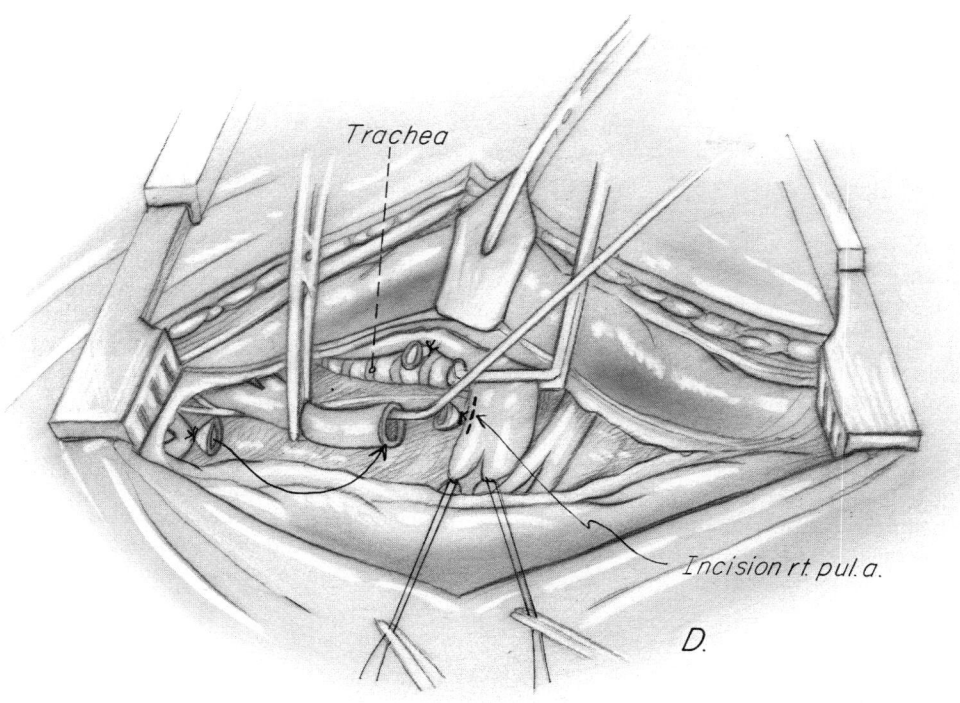

Trachea

Incision rt pul. a.

D.

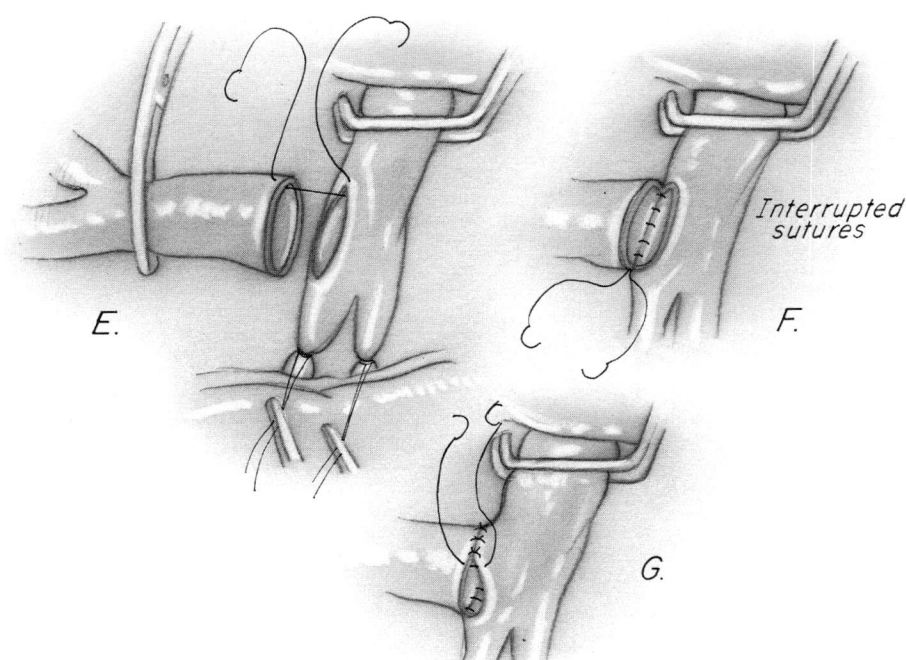

E.

Interrupted
sutures

F.

G.

Figure 23-38 (continued)

(d) The subclavian artery has been divided and appropriate occluding devices placed on the RPA. The proposed incision in the RPA is shown on the very superior aspect of the vessel.

(e,f,g) The anastomosis is made with interrupted 7-0 polypropylene sutures, placing each suture so that the knot lies outside the vessel. The sutures are tied and cut individually after each placement.

gutter through about the seventh interspace and attached to gentle suction. The chest wall is closed, inflating the lung well before bringing the ribs together. The wound is closed in layers with continuous fine Dexon, and the skin is approximated with a continuous subcuticular stitch. With moderate positive pressure on the lung, the chest tube can be removed and the small stab wound closed, generally with a subcuticular stitch. Otherwise, it is removed the next day.

Except in preoperatively acidotic and acutely ill neonates, the anesthesia is managed so that the patient is extubated in the operating room or occasionally an hour or two later.

Gore-Tex Interposition Shunt between Left Subclavian and Left Pulmonary Artery

The monitoring and thoracotomy are as described for the B-T shunt. If necessary, an arterial needle is placed in the right radial artery. The left pulmonary artery is identified and dissected out as described for the right pulmonary artery. The mediastinal pleura is opened over the left subclavian artery and contiguous portion of the aortic arch, and the periarterial

sheath over these structures opened. The subclavian artery is not mobilized.

A 5-mm Gore-Tex tube is generally used. In very small neonates or in the case of a very small LPA, a 4-mm Gore-Tex graft may very occasionally be necessary, but the intermediate (3 years) patency rate is less.[M13] A 6-mm tube is used in older infants. *Before* any occluding devices are placed, the proper length of the Gore-Tex graft is determined. For this, the lung is partially inflated in order to bring the LPA into its usual position. When the anastomosis is completed, the Gore-Tex tube should lie without tension and without redundancy (and thus potential kinking) between the proximal one-half of the subclavian artery and the superior surface of the LPA. One end of the Gore-Tex tube is beveled (Fig. 23-39), the tube is placed in a temporary position, and the other end is cut square at a point that will make the length to the LPA correct.

A delicate side-biting clamp (such as the Castaneda clamp) is placed deeply on the subclavian artery so that the handle lies inferiorly and the clamp occludes the subclavian artery proximally and distally. A longitudinal incision is made in

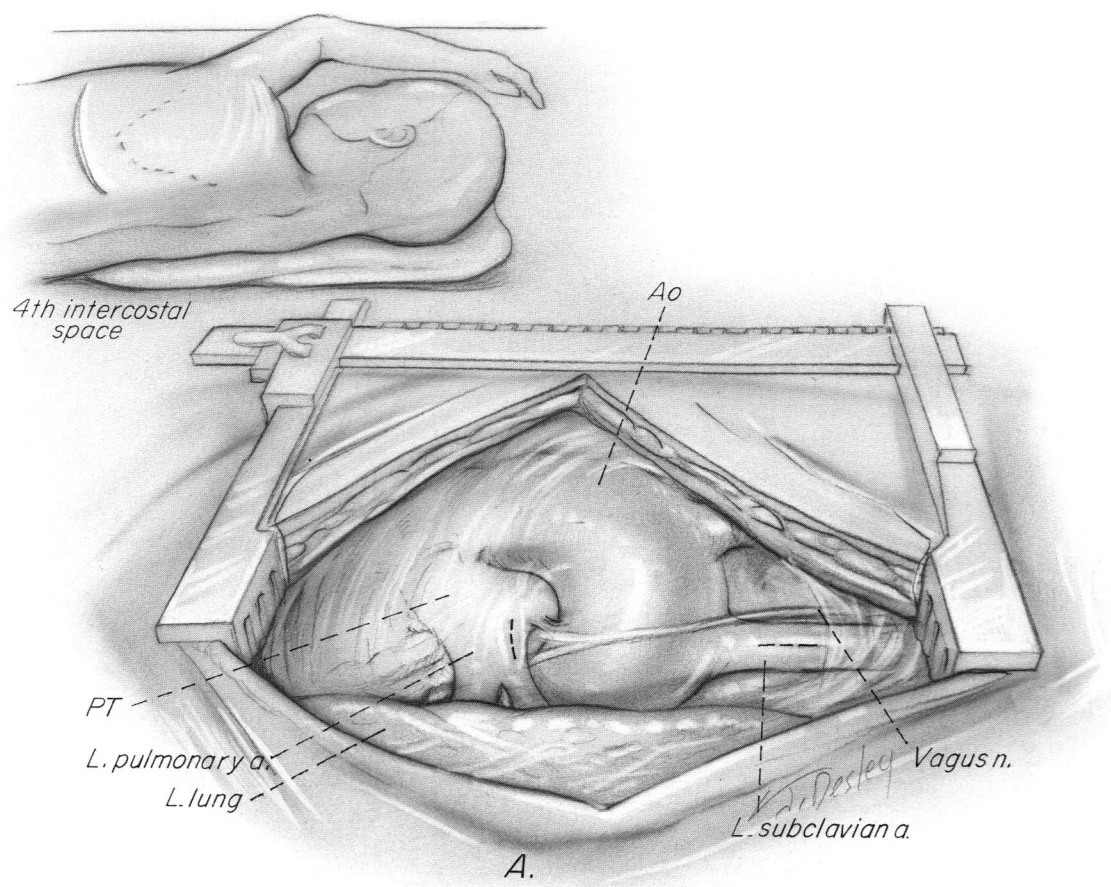

4th intercostal space

Ao

PT

L. pulmonary a.

L. lung

Vagus n.

L. subclavian a.

A.

Figure 23-39   The classical left Gore-Tex interposition shunt (left aortic arch). (a) Exposure and sites of incision (dashed lines) in pulmonary and subclavian arteries.

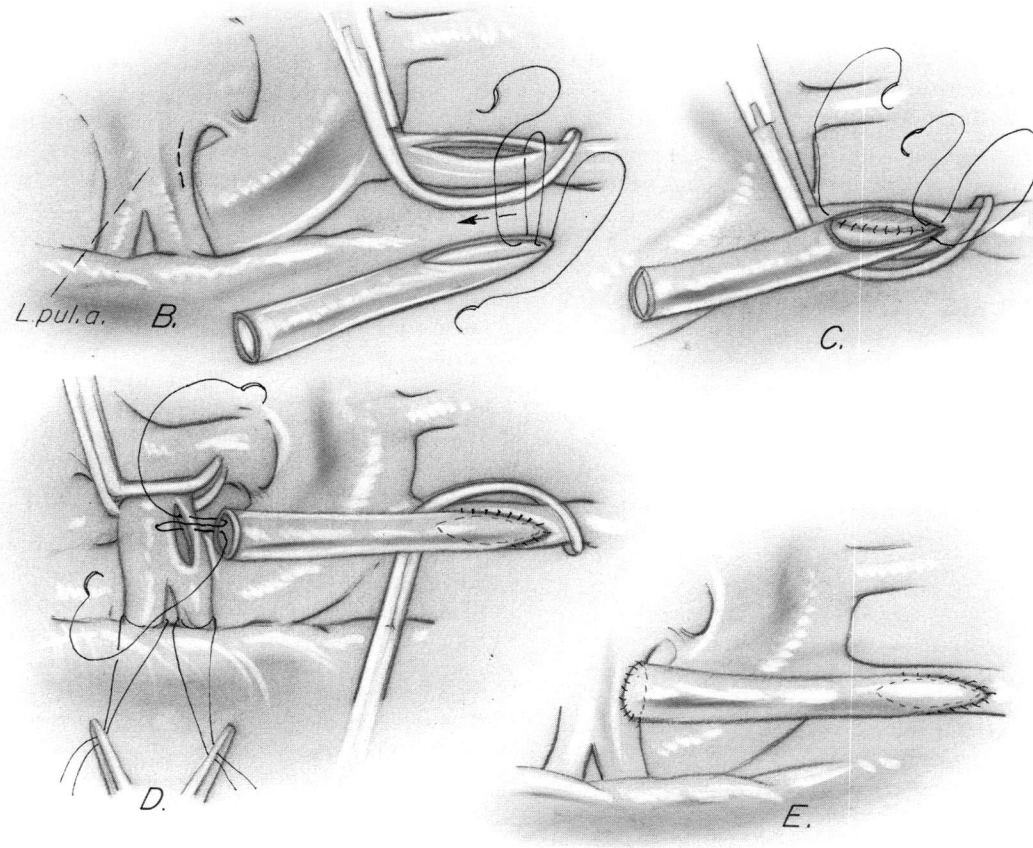

Figure 23-39 (*continued*)

(*b*) The Gore-Tex graft has been trimmed for insertion. End-to-side anastomosis is made between the Gore-Tex and the left subclavian artery. The first portion of the suture line is being made by sewing from within as shown.

(*c*) With the other end of the double-armed suture, the second portion of the suture is begun.

(*d*) The distal anastomosis is made in a similar fashion. The direction of suturing at both anastomoses minimizes the possibility of tearing the delicate subclavian or pulmonary artery.

(*e*) The completed anastomosis.

Ao, aorta; PT, pulmonary trunk (artery).

the excluded portion of the delicate subclavian artery, and an adventitial stay suture is placed on the anterior lip. The proximal anastomosis is made with a continuous stitch of 6-0 polypropylene (Fig. 23-39). The clamp on the subclavian artery is *not* loosened or removed at this time. Heavy silk ligatures are looped twice around the upper branch and the main LPA and snugged, and heavy Kocher clamps are placed on each for lateral traction. A Baumgartner clamp is placed very proximally on the LPA. A longitudinal incision is made in the *superior* surface of the LPA, making this a little shorter than one-half the circumference of the Gore-Tex tube. The distal anastomosis is made with continuous 6-0 polypropylene (Fig. 23-39).

In quick succession, the doubly looped ligatures are cut and removed, the clamp on the subclavian artery is opened and carefully removed from the field, and the Baumgartner clamp opened and removed. A light pack is placed about

each anastomosis, with light digital pressure if needed. A continuous thrill should now be present in the left pulmonary artery. Five minutes are allowed to pass. Nearly always, when the packs are removed the field is dry.

The remainder of the procedure is completed as described for the classical B-T shunt.

Classical Left Blalock-Taussig Shunt (in Patients with Right Aortic Arch)

The monitoring, left thoracotomy incision, and dissection of the left pulmonary artery are as described in the previous two sections. The left subclavian artery is dissected in the cupola of the chest, and the maneuvers for freeing it, bringing it beneath the vagus nerve, and preparing it for the anastomosis are those described for the right side. Occluding devices are placed, the anastomosis performed in the same manner already described, and the operation completed as described.

Right Gore-Tex Interposition Shunt (in Patients with Right Aortic Arch)

This procedure in patients with right aortic arch proceeds exactly as does the procedure on the left side in patients with left aortic arch.

SPECIAL FEATURES OF POSTOPERATIVE CARE

Repair

Management is by the general measures described in Chapter 5. Patients with TF have a particular tendency to increase their interstitial, pleural, and peritoneal fluid early postoperatively. Like other deeply cyanotic people, they probably have abnormal systemic and pulmonary capillary membranes, and this may make them particularly sensitive to the damaging effects of cardiopulmonary bypass (CPB) (see Chapter 2, section 2). Therefore, particular care is taken lest the loss of intravascular plasma to the extravascular spaces produce undesirable hemoconcentration early postoperatively, and attention is given to the possible development of pleural and peritoneal fluid collections. If these do develop, they should be aspirated.

Evaluation is complicated by the fact that in patients convalescing normally after repair of TF, with warm feet and good pedal pulses, the arterial blood pressure tends to be as much as 10% lower than that found in patients who were acyanotic preoperatively. The cardiac index is usually normal for this stage of convalescence, and the tendency to hypotension is related to a relatively low systemic vascular resistance. In the presence of other signs of normal convalescence, treatment of the arterial blood pressure is not indicated.

After repair of TF, the right and left atrial pressures are usually similar or one may be 2–4 mmHg higher than the other. Rarely, the left atrial pressure is 5–10 mmHg higher than the right. When this occurs, a residual left-to-right shunt must be sought (see Chapter 5, "Low Cardiac Output" in Section 2) and if found promptly closed by reoperation. If no shunt is found, the elevated left atrial pressure indicates left ventricular hypoplasia or severe impairment of left ventricular systolic or diastolic function, and the prognosis is not good. Rarely, the right atrial pressure is 5–10 mmHg higher than the left, indicating an important volume or pressure overload of the right ventricle or severe impairment of right ventricular function. If the hemodynamic state is poor and a transannular patch has been used, prompt placement of a homograft valve beneath the patch is considered in this situation; if a transannular patch (or conduit) has not been placed and the $P_{RV/LV}$ is more than 0.70, return to the operating room and placement of a transannular patch is to be considered. If the diagnosis is TF with pulmonary atresia, a valved conduit has been used in the repair, and $P_{RV/LV}$ is more than 0.95, perforation of the VSD patch is considered. (See Chapter 5, Footnote 8, for discussion of the determinants of right and left atrial pressures.)

Although not essential to success, there is an advantage in determining the possible presence and magnitude of any residual shunting, measuring pulmonary artery and right ventricular pressure the morning after the operation, and comparing the latter with radial artery pressure to estimate the $P_{RV/LV}$. This is a more reliable indicator of the late postoperative $P_{RV/LV}$ than is the measurement in the operating room[A6,L10,T1] (see "Postrepair $P_{RV/LV}$" in section on Special Situations and Controversies). Left-to-right shunts of 10%–50% are occasionally present a few hours after operation and absent the next morning; small shunts may still be present the next morning and absent 2 weeks later.[A6] This indicates that some shunting may occur early postoperatively through even a preclotted knitted Dacron patch (or through stitch holes or between sutures), but this does not persist for more than a few hours or days. Even though a shunt of 50% is seen the morning of postoperative day one by dye curve, or doppler, or contrast echocardiography, reoperation should be considered only with great caution since the shunt may be through the patch and temporary.

As regards the $P_{RV/LV}$ measured the morning after the operation, if a transannular patch has not been used and the $P_{RV/LV}$ is more than 0.7, and no more than a small residual shunt is present, the patient should probably be returned to the operating room and a transannular patch placed, although the need for this is rare. This decision may be tempered if the anulus is known to be muscular and the pulmonary valve of good quality, since under these circumstances the $P_{RV/LV}$ may possibly fall more than usual in the months ahead. In the case of TF with pulmonary atresia, a $P_{RV/LV}$ greater than 0.95 is probably an indication to return the patient to the operating room for perforation of the VSD patch (see "Postrepair $P_{RV/LV}$" in section on Special Situations and Controversies).

Particular attention is paid to the possible need for reoperation for bleeding following repair of the TF. The preoperative polycythemia and depletion of many of the clotting factors, the extensive collateral circulation often present, and the damaging effects of CPB often combine to produce a considerable bleeding tendency. The usual criteria for reoperation are followed (Chapter 5), and prompt reoperation is advised as soon as they are violated. This practice was one of the things contributing to the considerable reduction in the risk of operation in the early 1960s. Today, with careful intraoperative hemostasis reoperation is infrequently required.

After the patient leaves the intensive care unit, the body weight is followed closely, since after repair of TF and particularly when a transannular patch has been used transient fluid retention is common. Digoxin is particularly useful in this situation of a volume overloaded right ventricle and if started should be continued for about 6 weeks. Diuretics are used as indicated (see Chapter 5).

Systemic-Pulmonary Arterial Shunting

Except for neonates and occasionally very young infants, care after the creation of a systemic-pulmonary arterial shunt is simple. An arterial needle is generally not placed and the chest tube and endotracheal tube are usually removed in the operating room. The patient is nursed in the

Table 23-7 Hospital mortality after all operations performed for TF (UAB; 1967–July 1982).

| Operation | n | Hospital Deaths | | |
		No.	%	CL
Repair	836	88	10.5%	9.4%–11.7%
Pulmonary stenosis	713	64	9.0%	7.9%–10.2%
Pulmonary atresia	123	24	20%	16%–24%
Palliative operations	186	22	12%	9%–15%
"Manifolding" operations	4	0	0%	0%–38%
Banding of large AP collateral	2	0	0%	0%–61%
Miscellaneous other operations before repair	16	2	12%	4%–27%
Late orthotopic pulmonary valve insertion	14	0	0%	0%–13%
Replacement of valved extracardiac conduit	9	1	11%	1%–33%
Other operations late after repair	36	3	8%	4%–16%
Original repair at UAB	23	2	9%	3%–19%
Original repair elsewhere	13	1	8%	1%–24%
Total	1103	116	10.5%	9.6%–11.6%

KEY: AP, aortopulmonary; CL, 70% confidence limits.

Intensive Care Unit in a humidified oxygen-enriched atmosphere, usually provided by a head box or in older children a mask. Oral intake is resumed 4–6 hours after the operation.

In neonates and young infants, the systemic-pulmonary anastomosis is often done on an emergency or semi-emergency basis because the patient is severely hypoxic and often acidotic. Further, congenital pulmonary arterial problems (see "Morphology") are often present, which increase the risk of shunting procedures. Therefore, careful intra- and postoperative monitoring and control of arterial Po_2 and pH and buffer base are required (see Chapter 5). An intra-arterial needle is placed preoperatively, and the baby is returned to the Intensive Care Unit still intubated. The usual intense postoperative care and protocols are applied (see Chapter 5).

In any event, a chest x-ray is taken as soon as the child reaches the Intensive Care Unit and is repeated about 4 hours later. Infrequently, dense opacification of the ipsilateral lung becomes apparent at this time, and nearly inevitably this localized hemorrhagic pulmonary edema will produce hypoxia and deterioration of the patient. It is an indication for immediately returning the patient to the operating room and narrowing the anastomosis in some way. This complication seems to be the direct effect of the sudden increase in pulmonary blood flow on the abnormal lung of the cyanotic patient with TF and *not* a reflection of elevated pulmonary venous pressure. The reality of this is evident from the report of Ferenz, who found extravasation of red cells and localized but rather extensive areas of hemorrhage and edema in the lung in many patients dying a few days after these anastomotic operations for TF.[F2]

Very infrequently mild renal failure and rarely acute renal failure and anuria develop after a simple shunting procedure. This is related to the renal pathology sometimes present in cyanotic patients with TF and to renal damage by the radiopaque dye that may have been used for the cineangio-gram a few hours or days before the operation. Therefore, urine flow is carefully observed postoperatively.

A surgically created shunt *must* function. Therefore, auscultation is used to assess the patency of the shunt during the entire postoperative hospitalization. If doubt develops concerning the function of the shunt, immediate cineangiographic study is indicated. If it is poorly functioning, prompt reoperation is indicated. In patients with large AP collateral arteries, a continuous murmur is present preoperatively, and therefore simple auscultation is not as useful early postoperatively. In this setting, if the cyanosis is *not* improved, aortography is indicated.

EARLY RESULTS OF OPERATION

Since the TF is morphologically and clinically a highly variable entity, it is difficult to make generalizations about results that are relevant to patient populations other than those that have been studied, and thus to compare the results in one institution with those of another. Even with an institution's total surgical experience available (as an example, see Table 23-7), including all types of operations in all subsets of the tetralogy over a long period extending up to the present, reasonably accurate generalizations require intensive study and analysis. Even then, a comparison of results between centers is seriously hampered by differing indications for operations according to age, morphology, and clinical status and actual differences in the patients coming to various centers.

Hospital Mortality after Repair

The hospital mortality after repair of uncomplicated TF with pulmonary stenosis (see "Morphology") has steadily declined over the last 30 years and in the current era under

Table 23-8 Hospital death after repair of TF and pulmonary stenosis in the first 2 years of life (excluding 3 patients with absent pulmonary valve) (GLH; 1970–1980; n = 89). In 4, a previous shunting operation had been done. Included are patients (n = 11) with pulmonary arterial problems (hospital death in 2, 18%, CL 6%–38%) and patient (n = 6) with other major associated anomalies (1 hospital death, 17%, CL 2%–46%). In patients with uncomplicated TF (n = 72), there were 4 hospital deaths (6%, CL 3%–10%).

Age (mo)		Transannular Patch No				Transannular Patch Yes				Total			
			Hospital Deaths				Hospital Deaths				Hospital Deaths		
≤	<	n	No.	%	CL	n	No.	%	CL	n	No.	%	CL
	1	2	1	50%	7%–93%	1	0	0%	0%–85%	3	1	33%	4%–76%
1	3	2	0	0%	0%–61%	7	2	29%	10%–55%	9	2	22%	8%–45%
3	6	4	0	0%	0% 36%	11	1	9%	1%–28%	15	1	7%	0.9%–21%
6	12	21	0	0%	0%–9%	15	2	13%	4%–29%	36	2	6%	2%–13%
12	23	13	1	8%	1%–24%	13	0	0%	0%–14%	26	1	4%	0.5%–12%
Total		42	2	5%	2%–11%	47	5	11%	6%–17%	89	7	8%	5%–12%

(Brace annotations: No column, rows 1–3: 1/8 12%; CL 2%–36%. Yes column, rows 1–3: 6/34 18%; CL 11%–27%.)

KEY: CL, 70% confidence limits.

proper circumstances is low (1%–5%), whether the repair is done primarily or after a single B-T or Gore-Tex interposition shunt. The risk does not yet approach zero, possibly because the pathophysiology is severe in some patients, the technical demands of the procedure are occasionally great, and cyanotic patients are probably particularly sensitive to the damaging effects of CPB.

As an example of current risks, essentially routine primary repair of uncomplicated TF in the first two years of life has been accompanied by a hospital mortality of 6% (GLH) (CL 3%–10%) (Table 23-8). The safety of this approach has been confirmed by Castaneda and Norwood, who report a hospital mortality of 8% (CL 5%–12%) among 92 patients undergoing repair in the first year of life.[C3] The use of primary repair whenever it was considered safe but a two-stage approach in many very young infants has also allowed a low mortality for repair, which in the current era (UAB) is 2.2% (CL 0.7%–5.3%) (Table 23-9). A low mortality, using basically similar protocols for a selective two-stage approach, has also been reported by others.[A5,A8,B8,B30,B31,O9,R30,S2,S20,V5]

When the TF with pulmonary stenosis is complicated by coexisting diffuse right and left pulmonary artery hypoplasia, other kinds of pulmonary arterial problems (see "Morphology"), major associated cardiac anomalies of various types, or advanced age or severe disability, the risk of hospital death is increased (see Tables 23-8, 23-9). The impact of primary versus two-stage repair and other variations in surgical protocols and techniques on these higher mortalities in complex cases of almost infinite variability is not yet clear. (For further discussions of these matters, see "Incremental Risk Factors for Hospital Death after Repair.")

In uncomplicated cases of TF with pulmonary atresia, the hospital mortality is also low in the current era. For example, it has been 2.4% (CL 0.3%–8%) going back to 1967 (UAB) (Table 23-10). As in TF with pulmonary stenosis, the risk is higher when there are coexisting pulmonary arterial problems (Table 23-10) or other complicating factors. In any event, as reported by Olin and colleagues, overall hospital mortality for repair of TF with pulmonary atresia is less than 10%,[O1] although subsets of patients with a higher mortality can be identified. (See "Incremental Risk Factors for Hospital Death after Repair.")

Table 23-9 Hospital mortality after repair of TF with pulmonary stenosis in the current era (UAB; 1979–July 1982). Only the "uncomplicated" category is a mutually exclusive one.

Category	n	Hospital Deaths No.	%	CL
Uncomplicated	89	2	2.2%	0.7%–5.3%
Pulmonary arterial problems	22	3[a]	14%	6%–26%
Absent pulmonary valve	6	2[b]	33%	12%–62%
Major associated cardiac anomalies	16	5[c]	31%	18%–47%
Multiple VSDs	4	2	50%	18%–82%
Complete AV canal defect	11	3	27%	12%–47%
Others	1	0	0%	0%–85%
More than one previous palliative operation	6	2[d]	33%	12%–62%

KEY: AV, atrioventricular; CL, 70% confidence limits; VSD, ventricular septal defect.

[a]One was 10 months old; two were 30 months old.

[b]Ages were 7 and 15 days.

[c]Ages were 8, 17, 17, 26, 30 months.

[d]Ages were 17 and 69 months.

Modes of Early Death

In about one-half the patients dying in hospital after repair of TF, the mode of death is acute cardiac failure (Table 23-11). The mode is acute or chronic pulmonary insufficiency in about one-fourth of the patients who die, and occasionally death is accompanied by acute pulmonary edema (occasionally with massive tracheobronchial hemorrhage) without elevated left atrial pressure.[K11] The pathologic basis of the pulmonary insufficiency has been described by Harms and colleagues,[H1] who found in their autopsy studies that extensive alveolar and interstitial edema and hemorrhage is characteristic of the lungs of patients dying early after repair of TF. This process is probably caused by the damaging effects of CPB (see Chapter 2),[H1,K6] to which severely cyanotic and polycythemic patients seem particularly sensitive.

Table 23-10 Hospital mortality after repair of TF according to the morphology and type of repair (UAB; 1967–July 1982; n = 836; 88 hospital deaths).

	Uncomplicated Cases				Pulmonary Arterial Problems				Major Associated Cardiac Anomalies				More than One Previous Operation			
		Hospital Deaths				Hospital Deaths				Hospital Deaths				Hospital Deaths		
Category	n	No.	%	CL	n	No.	%	CL	n	No.	%	CL	n	No.	%	CL
Tetralogy of Fallot (Pulmonary stenosis)																
Simple repair	399	15	3.8%	2.8%–5.0%	21	3	14%	6%–27%	26	4	15%	8%–26%	20	3	15%	7%–28%
Transannular patch[a]	126	10	8%	5%–11%	63	13	21%	15%–27%	17	11	65%	49%–78%	11	4	36%	19%–56%
Valved extracardiac conduit[a]	4	0	0%	0%–38%	4	1	25%	3%–63%	5	1	20%	3%–53%				
Orthotopic pulmonary valve[a]	2	0	0%	0%–61%	6	1	17%	2%–46%								
Total	531	25	4.7%	3.8%–5.9%	94	18	19%	15%–24%								
Tetralogy of Fallot (Pulmonary atresia)																
Simple repair	6	0	0%	0%–27%	4	0	0%	0%–38%					2	0	0%	0%–61%
Transannular patch[a]	10	0	0%	0%–17%	18	3	17%	7%–31%	1	0	0%	0%–85%	8	3	38%	17%–62%
Valved extracardiac conduit[a]	24	1	4%	0.5%–13%	35	11	31%	23%–41%	7	2	29%	10%–55%	5	0	0%	0%–32%
Orthotopic pulmonary valve[a]	1	0	0%	0%–85%	3	2	67%	24%–96%								
Total	41	1	2.4%	0.3%–8.1%	60	16	27%	20%–34%					4	2	50%	18%–82%

KEY: CL, 70% confidence limits.

NOTE: Only "uncomplicated cases" (cases exclusive of the other three categories and without absent pulmonary valve) is an exclusive category.

[a] As part of the total repair.

A few patients die with a diffuse hemorrhagic diathesis and a few in other modes.

Heart Block

Permanent heart block has occurred in no cases at UAB from 1967 to July 1, 1983 and in 1.3% of patients at GLH between 1963 and 1978. Clearly the risk currently is negligible. Right bundle branch block and left anterior hemiblock[B20] occur in about the same frequency as after repair of isolated VSD (see Chapter 20, "Conduction Disturbances" in section on Late Results).

Table 23-11 Mode of death following repair of TF in infants (GLH, same cases as in Table 23-8). In the patient 0.4 months of age, toxic serum propranolol levels were present immediately preoperatively on a dose of 10 $\mu g^{-1} \cdot kg^{-1} \cdot day^{-1}$; the patent foramen ovale was not closed in the patient 1.3 months of age; and ruptured polypropylene sutures were found at the pulmonary artery bifurcation suture line in the patient 11 months of age. Preoperative pulmonary arterial problems were present in the patients 0.4 and 11 months of age.

Age (mo)	Mode of Death
0.4	Low cardiac output
1.2	Pulmonary dysfunction
1.3	Pulmonary dysfunction
3	Low cardiac output ($P_{RV/LV}$ = 1.1)
6	Low cardiac output ($P_{RV/LV}$ = 1.2)
11	Hemorrhage
22	Pulmonary dysfunction

Hospital Mortality after Palliative Procedures

Primary B-T and Gore-Tex interposition shunts, referred to as *classical shunts*[5], have a hospital mortality approaching zero when done for TF with pulmonary stenosis[K11] (Tables 23-12, 23-13). Even in the first month of life, the hospital mortality can be expected (UAB) to be 0.6% (CL 0.1%–2.3%) (see later section on "Incremental Risk Factors for Hospital Mortality after Classical Shunting Operations"). Similarly, low risks have been reported by other groups.[A7,A12,G12,I4,K31,L20,S2,T4] When classical shunting operations are done for patients with TF and pulmonary atresia, the hospital mortality has been 12%[K11] (Table 23-12), and most of the deaths are in very small (young) infants with severe hypoplasia of the pulmonary arteries or other kinds of pulmonary arterial anomalies.

Other types of shunting operations have a higher hospital mortality (Table 23-12), in part because with them the shunt rather easily becomes too large or too small. Arciniegas and colleagues found the hospital mortality after the Waterston shunt to be more than twice that after the B-T shunt.[A7]

Palliative transannular patching, with the aid of CPB, has a low hospital mortality in children and young adults,[P3] but the mortality has been high (10%–20%) in infants (Table 23-12).

INCREMENTAL RISK FACTORS FOR HOSPITAL DEATH AFTER REPAIR

Although the risk of repair for TF in the current era is low, there are a number of risk factors for hospital death (Table

---

[5] In this text, a classical shunting procedure is defined as a Blalock-Taussig shunt on the side opposite to that occupied by the aortic arch, or a Gore-Tex interposition shunt on the side of the aortic arch.

Table 23-12 Hospital mortality after primary palliative operations for TF (UAB; 1967–July 1982; $n = 141$).

| | Pulmonary Stenosis | | | | Pulmonary Atresia | | | | Totals | | | |
| | | Hospital Deaths | | | | Hospital Deaths | | | | Hospital Deaths | | |
	n	No.	%	CL	n	No.	%	CL	n	No.	%	CL
Classical B-T shunt	44	0	0%	0%–4%	40	4[a]	10%	5%–17%	84	4	5%	2%–9%
Gore-Tex subclavian–PA shunt	9	0	0%	0%–19%	11	2[b]	18%	6%–38%	20	2	10%	3%–22%
Total	53	0	0%	0%–4%	51	6	12%	7%–18%	104	6	6%	3%–9%
Waterston anastomosis	17	4	24%	12%–39%	6	2	33%	12%–62%	23	6	26%	16%–39%
Palliative RV–PA connection									9	3	33%	15%–56%
Transannular patch	2	1	50%	7%–93%	6	2	33%	12%–62%	8	3	38%	17%–62%
Valved conduit					1	0	0%	0%–85%	1	0	0%	0%–85%
Miscellaneous nonstandard shunts or revisions	1	0	0%	0%–85%	4	0	0%	0%–38%	5	0	0%	0%–32%
Total	73[c]	5	7%	4%–11%	68[c]	10	15%	10%–21%	141	15	11%	8%–14%

KEY: B-T, Blalock–Taussig; CL, 70% confidence limits; PA, pulmonary artery; RV, right ventricle.

[a] Ages 1, 3 days, 1.7, 3 months.

[b] Ages 2, 3 days.

[c] In addition, one patient with pulmonary stenosis survived both inadvertent left subclavian artery anastomosis to left pulmonary *vein* and later complete repair; one patient with pulmonary atresia had Gore-Tex interposition graft inadvertently to AP collateral artery and died after central shunt 1 day later.

23-14). As stated in Chapter 6, these risk factors can, to a greater or lesser degree, be neutralized by skill and experience, but they remain as variables that at least increase the difficulty of obtaining excellent results.

Earlier Date of Operation

Early date of operation is clearly a risk as is evident from a comparison of current results with those of an earlier era or the overall era in almost any institution (see, for example, Table 23-7). Nonetheless, analysis of results over a span of time are useful, since they allow identification of risk factors that may be largely neutralized in the current era in some institutions.

Pulmonary Arterial Problems

Diffuse severe hypoplasia, severe and particularly multiple localized areas of hypoplasia (stenoses), or iatrogenic stenoses of the left and right pulmonary arteries increase the probability of hospital death after repair of TF with either pulmonary stenosis or atresia[K11,S13] (see Tables 23-2, 23-10). Incomplete distribution of the central and hilar portions of the right and left pulmonary arteries also increases the risk of hospital death (see Table 23-2). In patients with pulmonary stenosis, the risk of repair with a transannular patch at 3 years of age is doubled (increased from 4% to 9%) by the presence of pulmonary arterial problems (Fig. 23-40); and in patients with pulmonary atresia, these problems increase the risk of repair with a valved conduit from 6% to 14% (Fig. 23-40).

Table 23-13 Hospital mortality after repair (primary or after a single previous shunt) of uncomplicated TF with pulmonary stenosis (see "Other Convenient Morphologic Categories" in section on Morphology for definition) and after classical shunting operations in the current era (UAB; 1979–July 1982).

	Age (mo)											
	<6		6–12		12–24		>24		Total			
		Hospital Deaths		Hospital Deaths		Hospital Deaths		Hospital Deaths		Hospital Deaths		
	n	No.	n	No.	n	No.	n	No.	n	No.	%	CL
Repair												
Simple			4	0	10	0	55	1	69	1	1.4%	0.2%–4.9%
Transannular patch					4	0	15	1	19	1	5%	0.7%–17%
Other							1	0	1	0	0%	0%–85%
							2	0	23	0	0%	0%–8%
Classical shunts	11	0	4	0	6	0	2	0				
Total	11	0	8	0	20	0	73	2	112	2[a]	1.8%	0.6%–4.2%

KEY: CL, 70% confidence limits.

[a] One was age 28 years, Down's syndrome, institutionalized, NYHA class IV, died on postoperative day 32 with chronic pulmonary insufficiency; one was 3 years of age and died of acute pulmonary insufficiency.

Table 23-14 Incremental risk factors for hospital death after repair of TF (UAB; 1967–July 1982; n = 836; 88 hospital deaths; see reference K11 for variables analyzed and details of the analysis.)

Incremental Risk Factors		Logistic Coefficient ± SD	P Value
Presence of pulmonary arterial problems		1.0 ± 0.32	.002
More than one previous palliative operation		1.6 ± 0.44	.0004
Size of patient			
If pulmonary stenosis	(ln BSA)	− 1.2 ± 0.54	.02
	(ln BSA)^2	1.1 ± 0.52	.04
If pulmonary atresia	(ln BSA)^2	5.3 ± 1.79	.003
If pulmonary stenosis			
High hematocrit (1/hematocrit)		−1.6 ± 0.45	.0003
Use of transannular patch		0.7 ± 0.34	.05
Early date of operation (years since Jan. 1, 1967)		−0.08 ± 0.046	.08
Absent pulmonary valve		1.6 ± 0.81	.04
Presence of major associated cardiac anomaly		2.0 ± 0.43	<.0001
If pulmonary atresia			
Use of valved extracardiac conduit or orthotopic pulmonary valve		2.3 ± 0.82	.006
High postrepair (OR) $P_{RV/LV}(P_{RV/LV})^2$		2.4 ± 0.74	.001
Intercepts		Pulmonary stenosis: −0.25 Pulmonary atresia: −6.5	

KEY: BSA, body surface area (M^2); ln, logarithm; $P_{RV/LV}$ = (Right ventricular systolic pressure)/(left ventricular systolic pressure); OR, operating room; SD, standard deviation.

The mechanisms underlying the increased risk when pulmonary arterial problems are present are several. The operations under these circumstances are often long and complex, which itself tends to increase hospital mortality. Since it is difficult and at times impossible to relieve completely the increased resistance to flow produced by these pulmonary arterial problems, high postrepair $P_{RV/LV}$ with its deleterious effect is often present. Finally, unrelieved pulmonary arterial problems must result in severe underperfusion of some parts of the lung and overperfusion of other parts, leading to important postoperative acute pulmonary dysfunction and sometimes death. In spite of this, in selected cases and under proper circumstances, remarkably good early results are possible, as evidenced by Puga et al.'s report of no deaths (0%, CL 0%–11%) among 16 patients undergoing repair for TF with congenital pulmonary atresia and absence of the central portions of the right and left pulmonary arteries (nonconfluent pulmonary arteries).[P11]

The full impact of pulmonary arterial problems as a risk factor for patients with TF is evident from the fact that they also increase the risk of shunting operations and make some patients unfit for even an attempt at complete repair.

Major Associated Cardiac Anomalies

Major associated cardiac anomalies have increased the risk of operation in the past (see Tables 23-4, 23-6, 23-8, 23-9, 23-10, 23-14) and no doubt continue to be incremental risk fac-

tors. However, their impact has been lessened by more complete preoperative diagnosis and by improved surgical capability for the management of complex lesions such as complete atrioventricular (AV) canal defects.[S8]

Although patent ductus arteriosus is listed as a major associated anomaly and appears to increase the risk of repair, this association may be a spurious one since ductus is uncommon in patients with TF and pulmonary stenosis; and in patients with TF and pulmonary atresia a ductal source of pulmonary blood flow (rather than through some other source) has been considered a favorable feature.

Absent Pulmonary Valve Syndrome

Absent pulmonary valve syndrome has been associated with a very high probability of hospital death after repair in young infants[M27] (see Table 23-14). This is related in part at least to the very poor preoperative condition of these infants and severe respiratory problems.

When operation is undertaken beyond the first year of life, the respiratory problems have usually resolved and the hospital mortality is low.

High Hematocrit

The effect of high hematocrit as a risk factor is illustrated in Table 23-15. An increase of hematocrit from 0.45 to 0.55 nearly doubles the risk of hospital death. The association of a high hematocrit with a higher hospital mortality has also been observed by Richardson and Clarke[R7] and by Kahn.[K13]

The incremental risk of high hematocrit is related to its correlation with and reflection of arterial hypoxia and its widespread chronic effects, including a probably increased capillary permeability and abnormalities of the clotting mechanisms. Perhaps related to this, deeply cyanotic patients have a particularly strong tendency to develop pulmonary hemorrhage and edema early after the construction of a systemic-pulmonary artery shunt.[F2] Also, they have a greater tendency than do acyanotic patients to develop pleural and peritoneal effusions and hemorrhagic pulmonary edema without elevated left atrial pressure after complete repair with CPB. Some surgical groups may elect at times to do a classical shunting operation for even older children with the tetralogy when there is severe polycythemia. From 6 to 12 months later, the hematocrit should be lower and the risk of repair less.

Small Size (Young Age)

In patients with pulmonary stenosis, small size (young age[6]) has increased the probability of hospital death in the past (see Tables 23-8, 23-14). The increased risk became evident[7]

---

[6] Body surface area proves to be a more significant risk factor than young age in the multivariate analysis,[K11] but most groups prefer to use age. Therefore, a regression analysis has been made of the relation of age to body surface area so that the two can be used interchangeably.

[7] See Chapter 6 for the definition of *evident differences*.

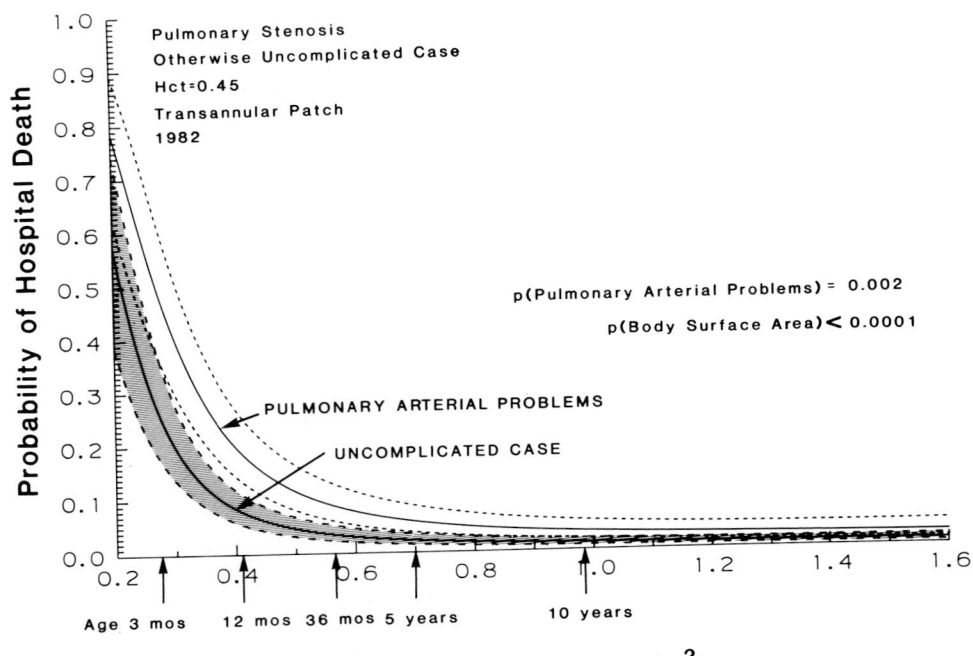

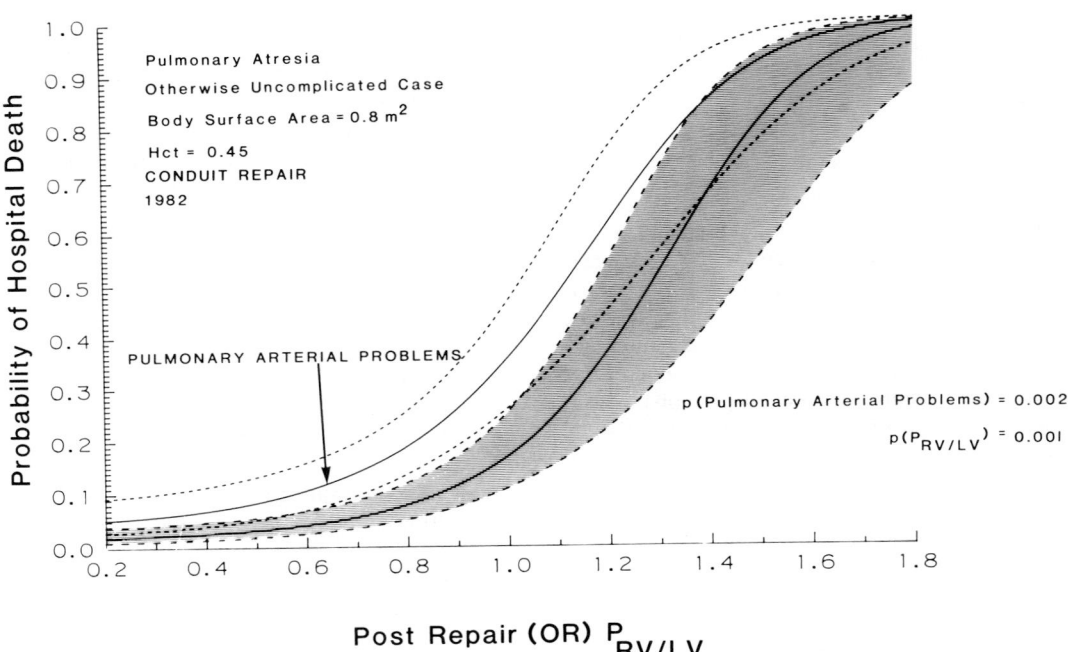

Figure 23-40 Nomograms of the multivariate equation (Table 23-14) showing the effect of pulmonary arterial problems on the hospital mortality after repair of TF. The solid line represents the point estimates, and the dashed lines enclose the 70% confidence limits. The specific conditions for each nomogram are indicated in the upper left-hand corner of the figure; 1982 indicates that the depiction is for an operation done in 1982.

(*a*) Patients with pulmonary stenosis undergoing repair with a transannular patch, showing the risk related to body surface area (or age) as well as to pulmonary arterial problems.

(*b*) Patients with pulmonary atresia, undergoing repair with a valved conduit, showing the risk related to postrepair $P_{RV/LV}$ in the operating room as well as to pulmonary arterial problems.

Hct, hematocrit.

Reproduced with permission from Kirklin et al.[K11]

Table 23-15   Digital nomogram from the multivariate equation (Table 23-14), showing the probability of hospital death after the repair in 1982 of uncomplicated TF and pulmonary stenosis, showing the effect of preoperative hematocrit, a transannular patch, and body surface area of the patient at the time of operation (transformed to age).

		Estimated Probability of Hospital Death									
		3 Months[a]		12 Months[a]		24 Months[a]		36 Months[a]		60 Months[a]	
Hematocrit	Transannular Patch	P	CL	P	CL	P	CL	P	CL	P	CL
0.45	No	16%	10%–24%	4.1%	2.7%–6.3%	2.4%	1.5%–3.8%	1.8%	1.1%–2.9%	1.1%	0.7%–1.9%
	Yes	26%	18%–37%	7.7%	5.3%–11%	4.5%	3.0%–6.7%	3.5%	2.3%–5.3%	2.2%	1.4%–3.5%
0.55	No	26%	17%–38%	7.6%	4.9%–12%	4.5%	2.8%–7.0%	3.4%	2.1%–5.5%	2.2%	1.3%–3.6%
	Yes	41%	29%–53%	14%	9.7%–19%	8.3%	5.7%–12%	6.5%	4.3%–9.6%	4.1%	2.6%–6.4%

KEY: CL. 70% confidence limits; P, probability expressed as percent.

[a]Age at repair, corresponding to median body surface areas (m²) of 0.27, 0.41, 0.50, 0.56, and 0.70, respectively.

(UAB) as the age decreased from 5 years, for example, to 17 months; at 5 years of age, with a hematocrit of 0.45, the probability of hospital death after repair without a transannular patch has been 1.1% (CL 0.7%–1.9%) and at 17 months of age 3.1% (CL 1.9%–4.8%) (Fig. 23-41). The multivariate equation (Table 23-14) yielding these probabilities was derived from an experience going back 16 years,[P8] and the current risks in young infants are probably less. However, similar trends are evident in the GLH experience (Fig. 23-42), but the risk does not appear, on simple contingency table analysis (Table 23-8), to increase until age becomes less than 3 months. Most other experiences support the idea of an increased risk of repair of the TF in the very young.[C9,C10,H14,P7,V5] An exception appears to be that of Cas-

taneda and colleagues,[C1,C3] and their interpretation of their results (Table 23-16) is that an increased risk does not exist.

In TF patients with pulmonary atresia the relations are different in that the risk has been higher both in the very young and in those beyond about 15 years of age (Fig. 23-43). In pulmonary atresia, under the conditions in Figure 23-43, the risk is currently lowest (5%, CL 2%–8%) when the patient size is between 0.65 M² (4½ years of age) and 1.5 M² (< 16 years).

The incremental risk of small size (young age) is probably the result of the increased sensitivity of small cyanotic patients to the damaging effects of CPB[K6] (see Chapter 2) and the fact that the morphology is apt to be more severe in those requiring early operation. Currently, these risks of young

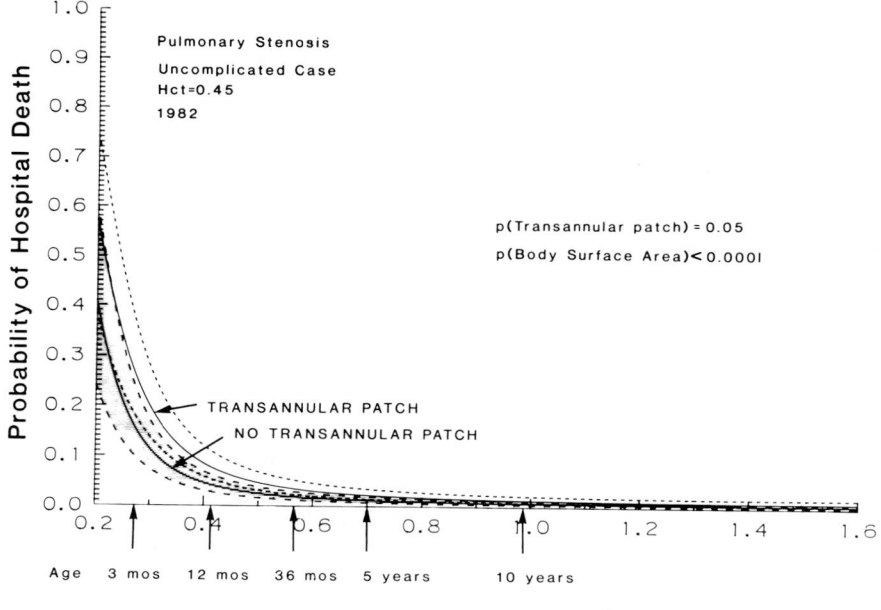

Figure 23-41   Nomogram of the multivariate equation (Table 23-14) showing the effect of size (age) at operation and use of a transannular patch on the hospital mortality after repair of uncomplicated TF with pulmonary stenosis. The presentation is as in Figure 23-40.

Reproduced with permission from Kirklin et al.[K11]

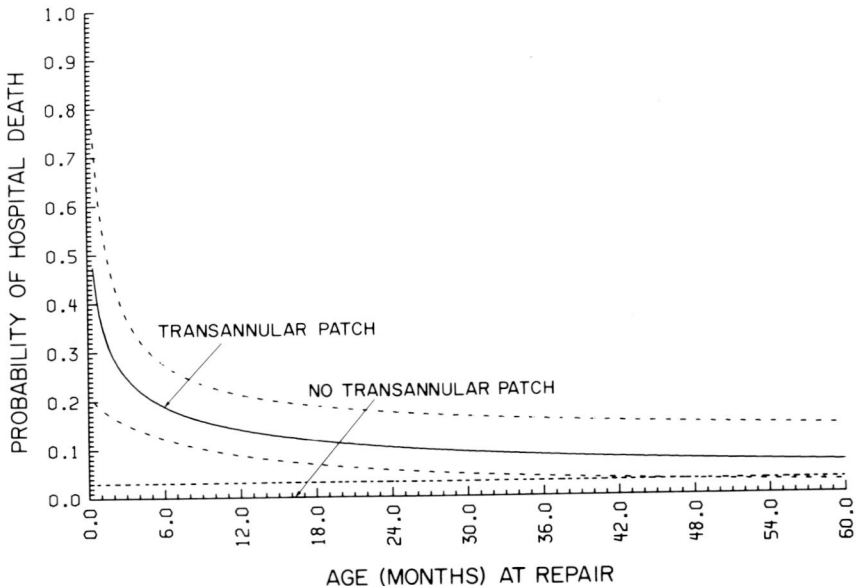

Figure 23-42 Nomogram of a multivariate analysis (equation upon request) of the effect of age at operation and use of a transannular patch on the hospital mortality after repair of TF with pulmonary stenosis. P (age) = .06, P (transannular patch) = 0.001 (The multivariate logistic equation for the nomogram is derived from 125 cases of all ages, GLH, 1970–1978. Included are cases with stenosis of the right and/or left pulmonary arteries, 21 cases with 3 deaths; absent left pulmonary artery, 3 cases with 1 death; patent ductus arteriosus, 8 cases with 2 deaths; and anomalous origin of left anterior descending from right coronary, 11 cases with no deaths. Excluded are cases with multiple VSDs, 7 cases with 1 death; anomalous origin of left or right pulmonary artery, 1 case who died; huge discrete A-P collateral arteries, 2 cases without death; important subaortic stenoses, 1 case without death; and isolated dextrocardia, 2 cases with 1 death. Excluded also are cases in which the aorta arises more than 50% from the right ventricle—see "Assessment of Aortic Overriding" in "Special Situations and Controversies.")

age are being neutralized to a much greater extent than was the case 10 or more years ago but not quite to the extent as in the repair of some acyanotic conditions (see Chapters 19 and 20). In time, with better understanding of the phenomena involved, this should happen in TF as well.

More Than One Previous Palliative Operation

One previous classical palliative operation has not increased the risk of repair (Table 23-17), but more than one has done so (Table 23-14).

Table 23-16 Hospital mortality (Boston Children's Hospital) after primary repair of TF with pulmonary stenosis in the first year of life.[C3]

Age (mo)			Hospital Deaths		
≤	<	n	No.	%	CL
	3	10	1	10%	1%–30%
3---	6	22	2	9%	3%–20%
6---	9	24	2	8%	3%–19%
9---	12	36	2	6%	2%–13%
	Total	92	7	8%	5%–12%

KEY: CL, 70% confidence limits.

Method of Repair of the Pulmonary Stenosis or Atresia

In patients with pulmonary stenosis, the use of a *transannular patch* in the repair has increased the probability of hospital death (Tables 23-14, 23-15, 23-18, and Figs. 23-41, 23-42). Although the confidence limits and P values indicate that this association is not likely due to chance, it is currently a weak risk factor as can be seen from the overlapping confidence limits at any given patient size (age). This incremental risk of transannular patching is evident in the reports from most groups (Table 23-19), including the recent one by Zhao and colleagues.[Z4]

The reasons for transannular patching being a risk factor for hospital mortality may, of course, be complex. One is that cardiac performance after repair is probably somewhat impaired by the sudden diastolic overload imposed on the right ventricle by the free pulmonary valvular incompetence inherent in the repair with a transannular patch. However, it is not possible to dissociate transannular patching completely from the type and severity of the pulmonary stenosis that requires it, and there is an increased mortality when the morphology of the pulmonary stenosis is more extensive[K11] (Table 23-3). This is to be expected since the repair of such lesions is technically more difficult and time consuming and

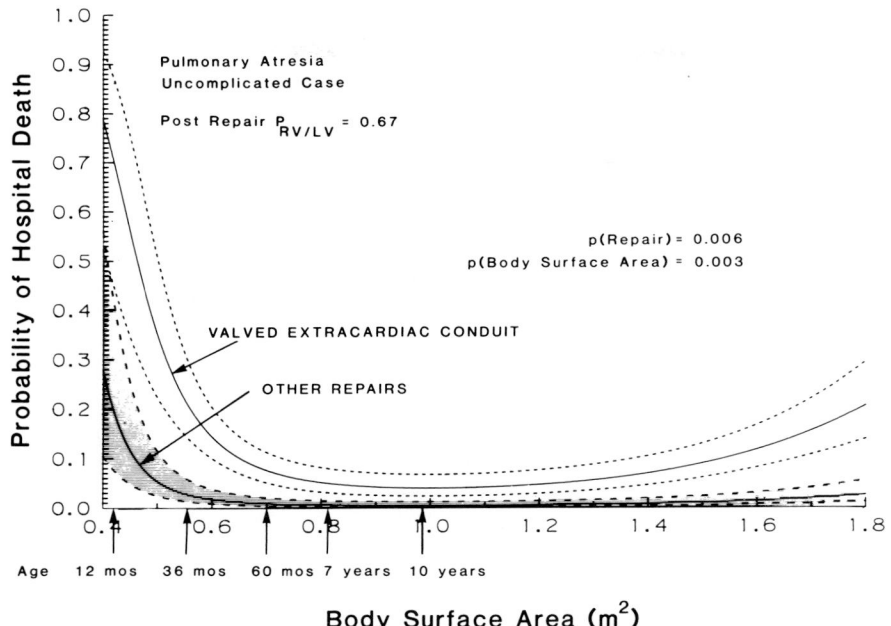

Figure 23-43 Nomogram of the multivariate equation (Table 23-14) showing the effect of the type of repair on the hospital mortality after repair of uncomplicated TF with pulmonary atresia. The presentation is as in Figure 23-40.

Reproduced with permission from Kirklin et al.[K11]

Table 23-17 Hospital mortality after intracardiac repair of TF with pulmonary stenosis, with or without major associated cardiac anomalies (GLH; 1961–1978, *n* = 351; patients with absent pulmonary valves and those with congenital pulmonary atresia are excluded.) Where more than one operation is listed, they were performed sequentially.

		Hospital Deaths		
Previous Palliative Operations	n	*No.*	*%*	*CL*
Single B-T shunt	69[a]	4	6%	3%–10%
Single B-T shunt + pleurectomy	1	1	100%	15%–100%
Right + left B-T shunt	2	0	0%	0%–61%
B-T shunt + Glenn shunt	1	0	0%	0%–85%
B-T + Waterston shunts	2	1	50%	7%–93%
B-T shunt + Brock procedure	1	0	0%	0%–85%
Brock procedure	8	0	0%	0%–21%
Brock procedure + pleurectomy	1	0	0%	0%–85%
Waterston shunt	19	0	0%	0%–10%
Potts shunt	4	0	0%	0%–38%
Central shunt + bilateral pleurectomy	1	1	100%	15%–100%
Subtotal with previous palliative operation	109	7	6%	4%–10%
Subtotal with no previous palliative surgery	242	17	7%	5.3%–9.2%
Total	351	24	7%	5.4%–8.5%

KEY: B-T = Blalock–Taussig; CL, 70% confidence limits.
[a] Five were occluded at the time of repair

Table 23-18 Hospital mortality after primary repair of TF with pulmonary stenosis according to age at operation and the use or not of a transannular patch (GLH; 1970–1978). Details are the same as described for Figure 23-42.

Age		Without Transannular Patch					With Transannular Patch					Total			
			Hospital Deaths					Hospital Deaths					Hospital Deaths		
≤ <	n	No.	%	CL		n	No.	%	CL		n	No.	%	CL
Months														
3	2	0	0%	0%–61%	0/6	10	4	40%	22%–61%		12	4	33%	18%–52%
					0%; CL					5/22				
3---6	4	0	0%	0%–38%	0%; 0%–27%	3	0	0%	9%–47%	23%;CL 13%–36%	7	0	0%	0%–24%
6---12	19	0	0%	0%–10%		9	1	11%	1%–33%		28	1	4%	0.5%–12%
12---24	10	0	0%	0%–17%		8	0	0%	0%–21%		18	0	0%	0%–10%
24---48	12	0	0%	0%–15%		10	1	10%	1%–30%		22	1	5%	0.6%–15%
48---60	10	0	0%	0%–17%		7	2	29%	10%–55%		17	2	12%	4%–26%
Years														
5---10	10	0	0%	0%–17%		3	0	0%	0%–47%		13	0	0%	0%–14%
10---20	2	0	0%	0%–61%		4	0	0%	0%–38%		6	0	0%	0%–11%
20---30						1	0	0%	0%–85%		1	0	0%	0%–86%
30	1	0	0%	0%–85%		—	—				1	0	0%	0%–86%
Total	70	0	0%	0%–3%		55	8	15%	10%–21%		125	8	6%	4%–6%

KEY: CL, 70% confidence limits.

relief of the obstruction is more likely to be incomplete even with transannular patching.

The use of a *valved conduit,* at least when it is a heterograft-valved synthetic conduit used for the repair of pulmonary atresia, is associated with an increased risk of hospital death (Tables 23-14, 23-20, Fig. 23-43). This may in part relate to a splinting effect of the rather rigid heterograft valved conduit, used up until 1982 (UAB), on wall motion of the right ventricle, and consequent impairment of right ventricular systolic function, as well as to the residual gradient usually present with that type of conduit. The incremental risk may be less with homograft conduits.

High Postrepair $P_{RV/LV}$

When the postrepair $P_{RV/LV}$, as measured in the operating room, is greater than about 1.0 and the repair has been made by simple methods (resection or a transannular patch), there is an evident increase in hospital mortality[K11] (Fig. 23-44). When a valved conduit has been used for the repair, the hospital mortality is evidently increased when $P_{RV/LV}$ is greater than about 0.85 (Fig. 23-44, Table 23-20). The effect of postrepair $P_{RV/LV}$ is seen also in the GLH experience (Table 23-21). This effect of a high postrepair $P_{RV/LV}$ was also observed in our early Mayo Clinic experience[K3,K5,K9] and has been reported by others.[H14,L11,R7]

Table 23-19 Hospital mortality after repair of uncomplicated TF (from literature).

Authors	Without Transannular Patch				With Transannular Patch				$P (\chi^2)$ for Difference
			Hospital Deaths				Hospital Deaths		
	n	No.	%	CL	n	No.	%	CL	
Venugopal et al.[V1]	20	0	0%	0%–9%	16	4	25%	13%–41%	P = .12
Jones et al.[J1]	363	58	16%	14%–18%	63	19	30%	24%–37%	P = .007
Azar et al.[A1]	155	13	8%	6%–11%	45	13	29%	21%–37%	P = .0003
Goldman et al.[G2]	150	14	9%	7%–12%	16	8	50%	35%–65%	P = 0.00001
Asano[A2]	79	3	4%	2%–8%	47	8	17%	11%–25%	P = .01
Aigueperse et al.[A3]	50	4	8%	4%–14%	19	5	26%	15%–41%	P = .09
Jaumin et al.[J2]	55	9	16%	11%–23%	36	4	11%	6%–19%	P = .48
Poirier, McGoon, et al.[P1]	216	14	7%	5%–9%	95	12	13%	9%–17%	P = .07
Monties et al.[M1]	34	2	6%	2%–13%	8	5	63%	38%–83%	P = .0001
Castaneda et al.[C1]	12	0	0%	0%–15%	27	2	7%	2%–17%	P = .33
Daily et al.[D1]	144	5	4%	2%–6%	71	3	4%	2%–8%	P = .8
Alfieri et al.[A4]	20	0	0%	0%–9%	41	7	17%	11%–25%	P = .08
Arciniegas et al.[A5]	13	0	0%	0%–14%	36	1	3%	0.4%–9%	P = .5

KEY: CL, 70% confidence limits.

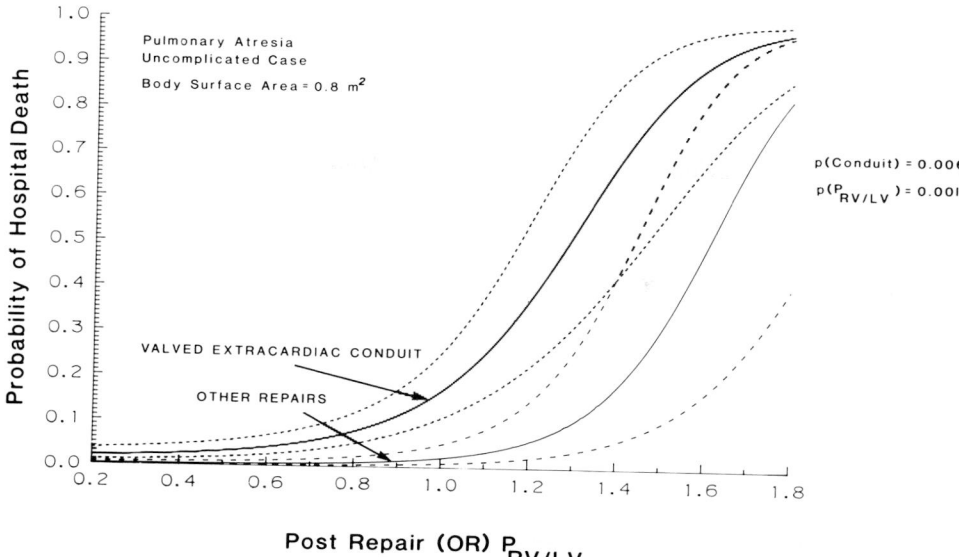

Figure 23-44   Nomogram of the multivariate equation (Table 23-14) showing the effect of postrepair (in the operating room) $P_{RV/LV}$ and the type of repair on hospital mortality after the repair of TF patients with pulmonary atresia. The presentation is as in Figure 23-40.
Reproduced with permission from Kirklin et al.[K11]

Table 23-20   Digital nomogram from the multivariate equation (Table 23-14), showing the probability of hospital death after the repair of "uncomplicated" (without pulmonary arterial problems) TF with pulmonary atresia, showing the effect of postrepair $P_{RV/LV}$, type of repair, and age at operation.

Postrepair $P_{RV/LV}$	Type of Repair	Estimated Probability of Hospital Deaths									
		12 months		36 months[a]		60 months[a]		7 years[a]		10 years[a]	
		P	CL	P	CL	P	CL	P	CL	P	CL
0.5	Simple	15%	5.4%–35%	1.6%	0.7%–3.6%	0.5%	0.2%–1.4%	0.3%	0.1%–0.9%	0.3%	0.1%–0.8%
	Conduit	41%	18%–69%	5.9%	2.8%–12%	2.1%	0.9%–4.7%	1.3%	0.5%–3.2%	1.0%	0.4%–2.7%
0.9	Simple	63%	36%–84%	13%	8.5%–20%	4.9%	3.1%–7.9%	3.1%	1.8%–5.4%	2.5%	1.4%–4.6%
	Conduit	87%	67%–96%	38%	26%–50%	17%	12%–24%	11%	7.3%–17%	9.1%	5.6%–14%

KEY: CL, 70% confidence limits; P, probability expressed as percent.
NOTE: Simple repair indicates repair by resection, valvotomy, or transannular patch.
[a] Age at operation, corresponding to BSA (m²) of 0.41, 0.56, 0.70, 0.81, and 0.98.

The incremental risk of a high postrepair $P_{RV/LV}$ is the result of an increase in right ventricular afterload in the setting of a now-closed VSD. The implications of these findings are discussed in the section on postrepair $P_{RV/LV}$ in "Special Situations and Controversies."

Pulmonary Atresia

Pulmonary atresia per se has not been shown to be an incremental risk factor for hospital death after repair of TF.[K11] However, the rather high incidence of pulmonary arterial problems, conduit repairs, and high postrepair $P_{RV/LV}$ does tend to result in higher hospital mortality in this group as a whole.

Table 23-21   Hospital mortality after primary repair of TF with pulmonary stenosis (GLH; 1970–1978).

Postrepair $P_{RV/LV}$			Hospital Deaths		
≤	<	n	No.	%	CL
	0.40	35	0	0%	0%–6%
0.4	---0.65	47	4	9%	4%–15%
0.65	---0.75	18	0	0%	0%–10%
0.75	---0.85	11	1	9%	1%–28%
0.85	---1.0	6	2	33%	12%–62%
	1.0	1	1	100%	14%–100%
Total		118	8	6.8%	4.4%–10.1%
P (logistic)				.002	

KEY: CL, 70% confidence limits.

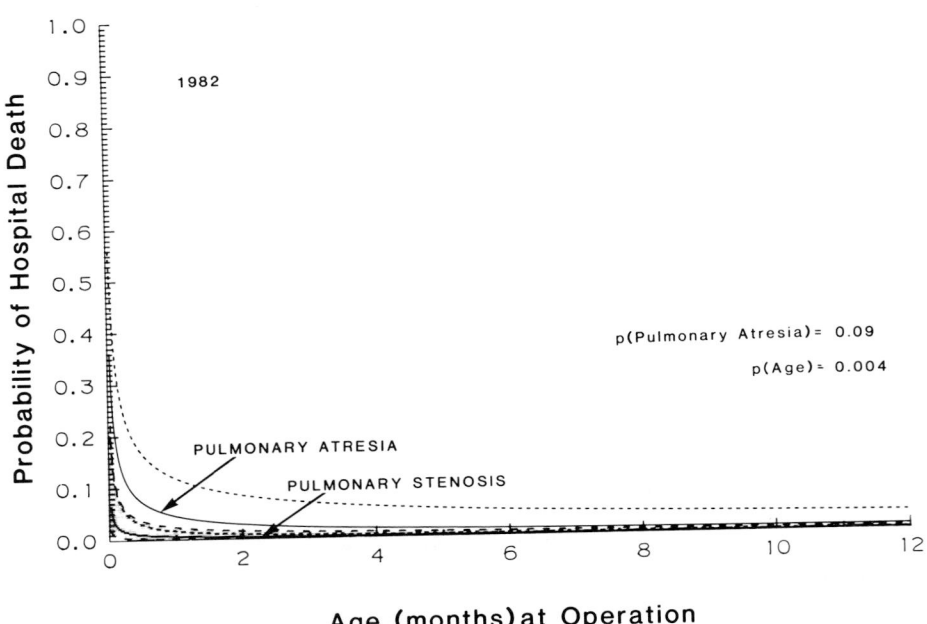

Figure 23-45   Nomogram of the multivariate equation (Table 23-22) showing the effect of age at operation and pulmonary atresia versus pulmonary stenosis on hospital mortality after classical shunting operations for TF. The presentation is as in Figure 23-40.
Reproduced with permission from Kirklin et al.[K11]

Prerepair Left Ventricular Volume

Graham and colleagues proposed that an end-diastolic left ventricular volume less than 55% of normal for age is an important risk factor for hospital death.[G8] Nomoto and colleagues also report that small left ventricular volume is a risk factor, with a demonstrable increase in risk (in their case, an increased need for catecholamine support early postoperatively) when preoperative left ventricular end-diastolic volume is less than about 65% of normal.[N9] Oberhansli and Friedli have reported similar findings.[O8] In addition, in five patients who underwent repair with transannular patching (GLH), left atrial pressure has been more than twice that of right atrial pressure in the early postoperative period, with progressively more severe evidence of pulmonary venous hypertension and pleural effusions. Two patients died, and their left ventricles were at the lowest limit of normal size for age at autopsy.

INCREMENTAL RISK FACTORS FOR HOSPITAL DEATH AFTER CLASSICAL SHUNTING PROCEDURES

As was noted earlier, probably the most important risk factor for hospital death after classical shunting procedures (see Footnote 5) is *pulmonary arterial problems,* an opinion expressed also by Kay and colleagues.[K25] The rather high incidence of these in patients with pulmonary atresia explains why pulmonary atresia is a risk factor (Table 23-22).

Young age has added an increment of risk to shunting

Table 23-22   Incremental risk factors for hospital death after primary classical shunting operations (see footnote 1) for TF (UAB; 1967–July 1982; $n = 127$, seven hospital deaths; see reference K11 for variables analyzed and details of the analysis).

Incremental Risk Factor	Logistic Coefficient ± SD	P Value
TF with pulmonary atresia	2.1 ± 1.22	.09
Young age (ln age)	−0.7 ± 0.25	.024
Earlier date of operation (years since Jan. 1, 1967)	−0.28 ± 0.151	.06
Intercept	1.0	

operations, but a relatively small one (Fig. 23-45). Thus in patients with pulmonary stenosis the current risk of hospital death after a classical shunting procedure is estimated at 0.02% (CL 0.004%–0.09%) at 5 months of age and 0.6% (CL 0.1%–2.3%) at 1 month of age. In patients with pulmonary atresia, the risk is estimated to be 1.8% (CL 0.1%–5.1%) at 5 months of age and 4.5% (CL 1.5%–11.5%) at 1 month of age. If the presence of pulmonary arterial problems were taken into account, the effect of young age might no longer be evident since these are common in patients requiring treatment at a very young age.

Early date of operation has been a risk factor in the multivariate analysis, indicating possible ($P = 0.16$) improvement in results in recent years. The earlier GLH analysis[K1] also indicated that there was need for improvement in the results of shunt operations. The improvement is probably the result of technical improvements in microvascular surgery and of the increased use of the Gore-Tex interposition shunt in very small infants.

Table 23-23   Events other than hospital death after primary classical shunting operations for TF (UAB; 1967–July 1982; $n = 104$).

Events	Pulmonary Stenosis (n = 53)			Pulmonary Atresia (n = 51)			Total (n = 104)		
	No.	%	CL	No.	%	CL	No.	%	CL
Early (< 30 days) shunt closure, with successful reoperation	4	8%	4%–13%	3	6%	3%–11%	7[a]	7%	4%–10%
Premature repair because of shunt closure	2	4%	1%–9%	1	2.0%	0.3%–6.5%	3	2.9%	1.3%–5.7%
Later shunting operations	0	0%	0%–4%	7[b]	14%	9%–21%	7	7%	4%–10%
Sudden death	1[c]	1.9%	0.2%–6.3%	0	0%	0%–4%	1	1.0%	0.1%–3.2%
Brain abscess	1[d]	1.9%	0.2%–6.3%	0	0%	0%–4%	1	1.0%	0.1%–3.2%
Gangrene of the hand	1[e]	1.9%	0.2%–6.3%	0	0%	0%–4%	1	1%	0.1%–3.2%
Planned repair									
Elsewhere	4	8%	4%–13%	1	2.0%	0.3%–6.5%	5	5%	3%–8%
UAB	32	60%	52%–68%	16	31%	24%–39%	48	46%	41%–52%

KEY: CL, 70% confidence limits.

[a] None have occurred since 1979; none had initial Gore-Tex interposition shunts; three were less than 30 days old.

[b] None for shunt closure.

[c] Four months postoperatively, cause entirely unknown; date of operation 1980.

[d] Nonfatal; age 28 months at shunt in 1971; occurred 15 months p.o.

[e] 1971.

INTERIM RESULTS AFTER CLASSICAL SHUNTING OPERATION

Early (< 30 days postoperatively) *nonfatal shunt closure* is uncommon. It has occurred in 7% of patients receiving primary B-T or Gore-Tex interposition shunts for TF (UAB) (Table 23-23). However, in the current era (since January 1979) and with the use of the Gore-Tex interposition shunts in very small babies, this event has not been recognized.

Late shunt closure is likewise infrequent. This occurred in 3 (3%) patients (UAB) and required premature complete repair. Similarly, high early patency rates after Gore-Tex interposition shunts have been reported by Donahoo and colleagues[D4] and by Di Benedetto and colleagues.[D10] The latter group found 95 of 96 such shunts patent 3–36 months postoperatively.[D10] An identical incidence after 5-mm Gore-Tex interposition shunting in infancy was reported by McKay and colleagues.[M13] Kay, Capuani, Franks, and Lincoln have presented particularly useful information on shunt patency after the Gore-Tex interposition shunt.[K25] The actuarial patency rate was 90% at 2 years, with all shunt failures occurring in the first 6 months. The patency rate was 74% when the operation was necessary in the first month of life. There was no demonstrable difference in patency rates between 4-mm grafts and larger ones.

Gangrene of the hand is rare after the ligation of the subclavian artery incident to a B-T shunt. It has occurred in one patient at UAB and one patient at GLH and required digital amputation.

Sudden death, without explanation or autopsy, is uncommon after classical shunting procedures. It occurred 4 months after operation in one patient (UAB) (Table 23-23). Nonfatal brain abscess is also uncommon, occurring in one patient with pulmonary stenosis (UAB). These two irreversible interim events occurred in 1.9% (CL 0.6%–4.5%) of the patients receiving classical shunting operations for TF[K11] (UAB) (see Appendix 23A for use of this in estimating the risk of two-stage repair). A similar low incidence of unfavorable interim events has been reported by others.[A5,S2] Of course, improperly performed classical shunts and Waterston and Potts' anastomoses result in a higher incidence of unsatisfactory interim results, primarily because of iatrogenic pulmonary arterial problems.

Iatrogenic pulmonary arterial problems are uncommon after classical shunts or Gore-Tex interposition shunting operations. For example, none has been identified in the UAB experience. These problems do occur after the Waterston anastomosis, and their incidence varies from 16%[G14,P6,R17] to 64% of cases.[N7]

Ten years after a classical B-T shunt, the arm on the ipsilateral side is a little shorter and smaller than on the opposite side.[H10]

The main *beneficial interim results* of shunting procedures are an increased pulmonary blood flow and consequent reduction in cyanosis and polycythemia and improved functional capacity. The NYHA functional class is usually I or II after shunting. Arterial oxygen saturation at rest is usually 80%–90%, but it always falls with exercise, at times to as low as 50%.[H10,J4]

Another benefit of the classical shunting procedures is diffuse increase in size of the right and left pulmonary arteries in TF patients with pulmonary stenosis[G13,K20] and to some extent of the pulmonary anulus and pulmonary trunk.[R30] These enlargements may very occasionally be enough to allow the subsequent repair to be done without a transannular patch, whereas without the shunting procedure a patch may have been required.[V5] (The enlargement of the annulus and pulmonary trunk is even greater after a Waterston anastomosis,[A15] but the higher incidence of iatrogenic pulmonary arterial problems offsets this advantage.) Somewhat in contrast,

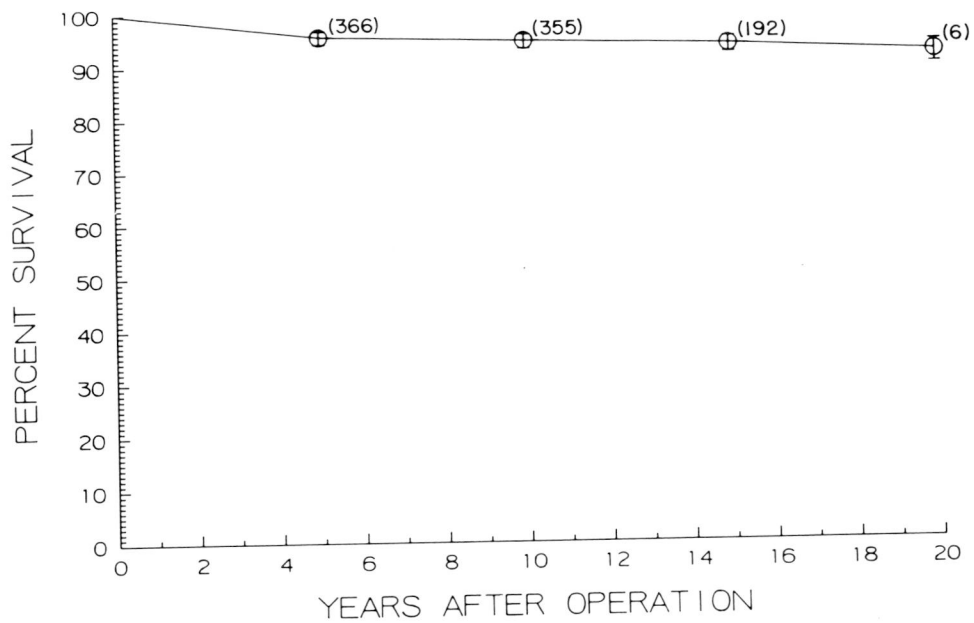

Figure 23-46 Actuarial survival of hospital survivors of repair of TF (Mayo Clinic; 1955–1966; *n* = 396; these patients are also described in the publication by Fuster and colleagues[F3]).

in patients with TF and pulmonary atresia and large A-P collateral arteries, the enlargement is often not diffuse. Instead, the pulmonary trunk and central portions of the right and left pulmonary arteries may enlarge, but scattered short or long narrow segments in the hilar and more peripheral portions may remain as discrete or segmental stenosis.[F8,H15,K21]

Occasionally, severe infundibular or valvar stenoses become complete after a palliative shunting operation.[F11,M14,R15] This, however, does not complicate later complete repair.

Important pulmonary vascular disease may develop after a classical B-T shunt but rarely before 7 years have passed.[H11] Beyond this time, the proportion of patients developing hypertensive pulmonary vascular disease increases with increasing shunt duration[D3,H12,R15] but even up to 23 years remains uncommon.[N11] (The incidence of this complication is greater in patients with Waterston anastomoses[T3] and is still greater after a Potts' anastomosis;[C8,V4] again, however, the incidence is time related, and important pulmonary vascular disease is uncommon before 5 years.[N11])

LATE RESULTS

Survival

The late survival of hospital survivors of the repair of uncomplicated TF with pulmonary stenosis has been good, even in the patients operated upon in the early era of intracardiac repair.[L4] Thus, among the hospital survivors of the repairs done by us at the Mayo Clinic in 1955–1966, 93% survived 10 years and 91% survived 20 years[F3] (Fig. 23-46).

Among the 414 patients who underwent repair at UAB in 1967–1977, the 10-year survival rate was 96% (Fig. 23-47).[K12] Currently, the late results are excellent, survival being 98% (Fig. 23-48) in a selected group who resemble patients being operated on currently. Further evidence as to the excellence of the long-term results comes from the GLH experience, with only eight late deaths (3%) (two of which were noncardiac) amongst 267 hospital survivors of repair between 1963–1978. Similarly good long-term survival has been reported by others.[K29,R28,Z4] However, the operation cannot be considered curative in all patients, since the survival curve at 10 years is slightly but significantly less than that of a matched general population.[F3,K12]

Incremental Risk Factors for Premature Late Death

A *postrepair* $P_{RV/LV}$ in the operating room of 0.85 gives two and one-half times the chance of death within 8 years of the repair as does one of 0.5.[K12] Similar evidence for a high postrepair $P_{RV/LV}$ being a risk factor was found in Fuster and colleagues' analysis of our early Mayo Clinic experience[F3] and McGoon and colleagues' late follow-up of patients receiving valved conduits.[M10]

A *previous Potts anastomosis* (now rarely encountered) also is a risk factor for premature late death.[F3,K12] This is probably related to the damaging effect of the long-standing left ventricular volume overload imposed by the usually large Potts shunt (see Chapter 12) and/or the secondary pulmonary vascular disease.

Older age at operation is a risk factor for premature late death after repair.[K12] This is especially apparent when age is over 20 years at the time of operation. A comparison of the

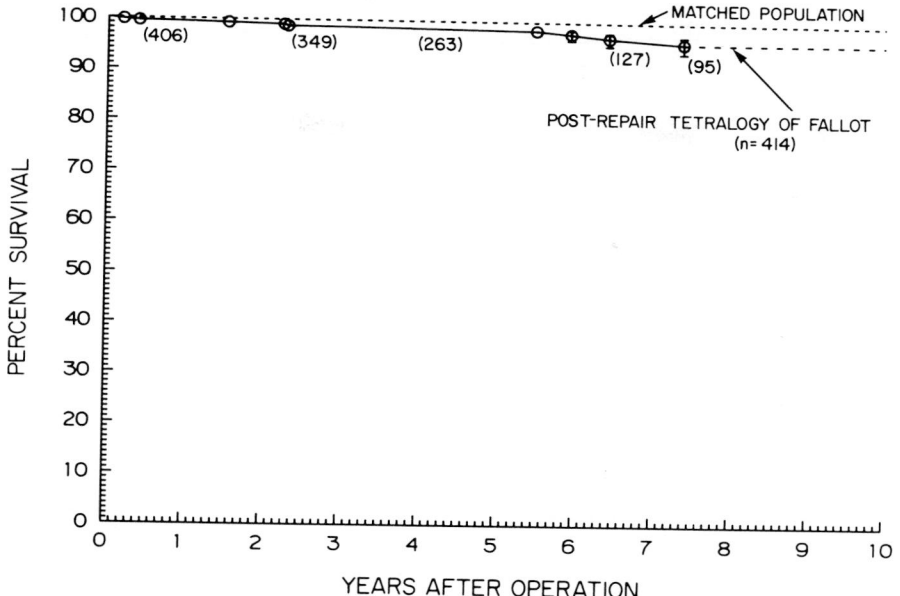

Figure 23-47 Actuarial survival of patients leaving the hospital alive after repair of TF with pulmonary stenosis (UAB; 1967–1977; n = 414). The actuarial 8-year survival is 95.8% (CL 93.9%–97.1%), with the dashed line indicating follow-up beyond this time without any deaths. Each event is indicated by an open circle, and the vertical bars represent the 70% CLs. The dotted line above is the expected survival of the age, race, and sex-matched U.S. population life table.

Reproduced with permission from Katz et al.,[K12] and the American Heart Association, Inc.

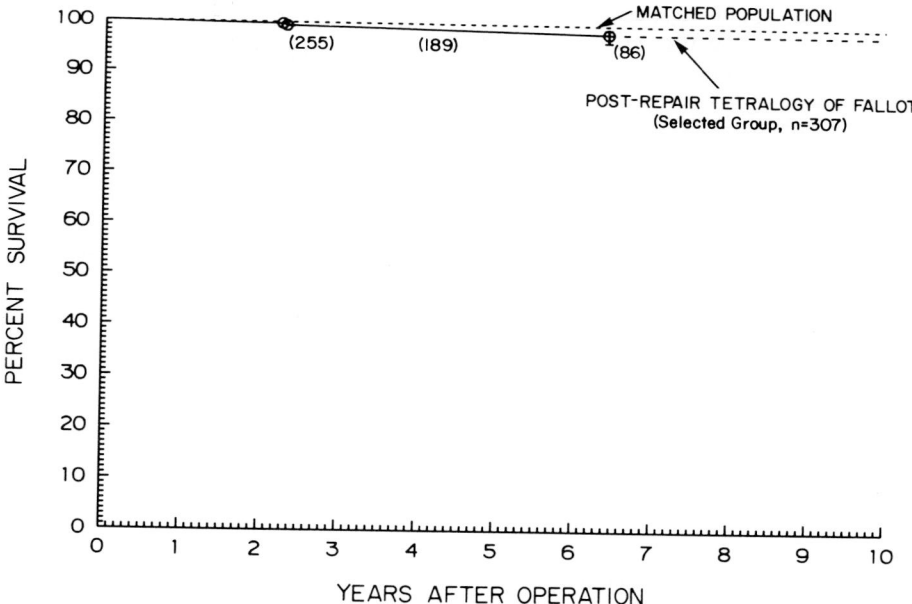

Figure 23-48 Actuarial survival as in Figure 23-47, but including only the 307 patients who were younger than 20 years at repair, had either no previous operation or only a single B-T or Waterston shunt, and had a postrepair $P_{RV/LV}$ (in the operating room) equal to or less than 0.85.

Reproduced with permission from Katz et al.,[K12] and the American Heart Association, Inc.

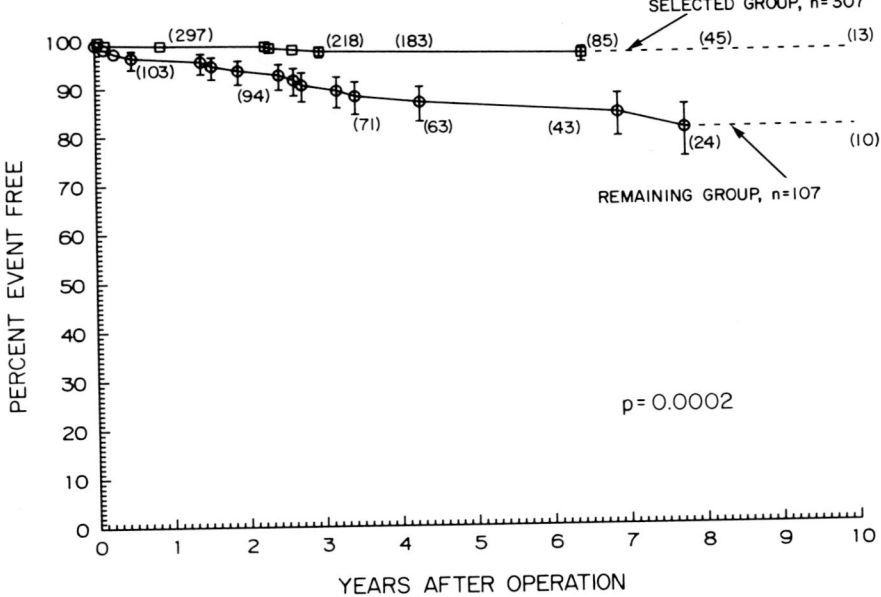

Figure 23-49 Actuarial freedom from premature late death, reoperation, arrhythmic symptoms, or congestive heart failure among patients leaving the hospital alive after repair of TF with pulmonary stenosis. (See text for definition of "selected group.") (UAB; 1967–1978; n = 414.)
Reproduced with permission from Katz et al.,[K12] and the American Heart Association, Inc.

long-term survival of patients over 40 years of age, reported by Hu et al.,[H21] with the survival of patients in the Katz study[K12] supports the inference of older age as a risk factor.

Complete heart block was, in an earlier era, a cause of sudden death late postoperatively. This was no doubt related to the relatively high incidence of temporary postoperative heart block with the early techniques of VSD repair, since late complete heart block is more likely to develop in patients who have had temporary complete heart block present for a number of days after repair, even though sinus rhythm has then resumed. For example, 13 patients operated upon prior to 1964 developed transient complete heart block (GLH), and five of these subsequently reverted to complete heart block late postoperatively, with death in one. None of these five patients had a bifascular block pattern. In fact, no patients has developed late complete heart block without having had transient complete heart block postoperatively (GLH).

Some have found that patients with right bundle branch block plus anterior hemiblock are more apt to develop sudden death, presumably from complete heart block, than are other patients,[W6] but others have not confirmed this[B20,C11,D11,Q1,S9] (see Chapter 20, "Conduction Disturbances" in section on Late Results).

Use of a *transannular patch* in the repair operation has not been identified as a risk factor for premature late death in groups of patients observed during a 10-year period[K12] nor in some groups observed for 20 years.[S3] Klinner and colleagues have identified use of a transannular patch as a risk factor in a group of patients followed for 25 years.[K29]

Symptomatic and Functional Statuses

Over 95% of the patients consider themselves fully active and without symptoms up to 10 years after operation.[K12] In a selected group of patients that resembles those being operated upon in the current era (repair done before the age of 20 years, no previous operation or only a single shunt [exclusive of the Potts], and postrepair [operating room] $P_{RV/LV}$ equal to or less than 0.85), 96% are free from any events, including death, up to 10 years after repair (Fig. 23-49) and considered themselves normal. Wessel and colleagues have found, by standardized exercise testing, that some patients after repair of TF have normal functional capacity (Table 23-24), and an occasional one has the capacity

Table 23-24 Exercise performance under standardized conditions, one or more years after repair of TF.[W2] (Mean values are given for continuous variables.)

Characteristics	10 Highest Performers[a]	10 Lowest Performers[b]	P for Difference
CT Ratio	0.49	0.58	.001
P_{RV}	39 mmHg	76 mmHg	.001
Age at repair	5.83 yr	10.7 yr	.001
Pulmonary valve incompetence	0/10 pts	8/10 pts	.0004
Previous Potts' anastomosis	0/10 pts	4/10 pts	.04

KEY: CT, cardiothoracic; P_{RV}, right ventricular pressure; pts, patients.
[a] Duration of exercise greater than 100% of normal for age.
[b] Duration of exercise 42.8% of normal for age.

Table 23-25 Exercise performance under standardized conditions, one or more years after repair of TF, exclusive of patients with residual ventricular septal defects.[W2]

Subsets	Duration of Exercise (% of Normal Controls) Mean ± SD	P for Difference
P_{RV} < 50 mmHg		
Pulm. V. Incomp. *No*	98.2 ± 20.1	
Pulm. V. Incomp. *Yes*	74.7 ± 8.9	< .05
P_{RV} > 50 mmHg		
Pulm. V. Incomp. *No*	87.7 ± 15.9	
Pulm. V. Incomp. *Yes*	51.0 ± 29.8	< .02

KEY: Incomp., incompetence; P_{RV}, systemic pressure right ventricle; Pulm., pulmonary; SD, standard deviation; V, valve.

of a trained athlete.[W2] Although other investigators have reported similar findings,[D8,F9] it has also been found that some patients have reduced exercise capacity, although to questioning they are without symptoms.[D8,W2]

Incremental Risk Factors for Suboptimal Late Functional Status

Pulmonary Valve Incompetence
Pulmonary valve incompetence resulted in reduced exercise capacity in the study of Wessel and colleagues,[W2] regardless of the right ventricular systolic pressure (Table 23-25). The importance of a competent pulmonary valve has been also demonstrated by exercise testing in patients who have undergone repair of TF with absent pulmonary valve in whom exercise capacity is improved when the repair includes insertion of a valve but otherwise not[I1] (Fig. 23-50). Others have also found that pulmonary valve incompetence late postoperatively, usually the result of a transannular patch, predisposes to impaired exercise capacity.[A16,D8,P9]

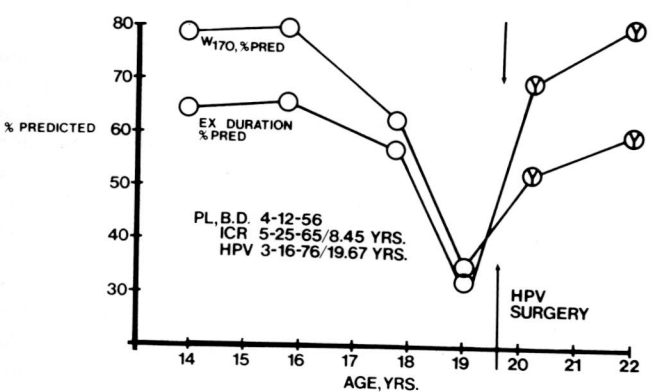

Figure 23-50 The results of serial exercise testing (work capacity above, exercise duration below, expressed as percentage of predicted value for age) in a patient after repair of TF with absent pulmonary valve. Intracardiac repair was performed at 8.45 years of age, and exercise and work capacity steadily decreased. A homograft pulmonary valve was inserted at age 19 years, with subsequent improvement in performance.

Reproduced with permission from Ilbawi et al.[I1]

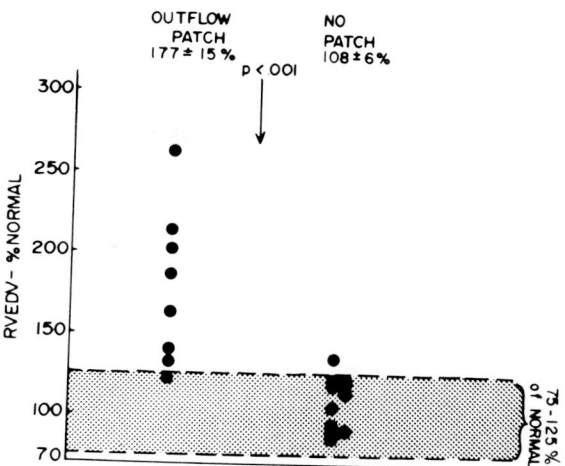

Figure 23-51 Right ventricular end-diastolic volume late postoperatively in patients who have had repair of TF. The patients are separated into those with a transannular patch (called outflow patch in the figure) and those without such a patch. The stippled area represents normal values.

Reproduced with permission from Graham et al.,[G1] and the American Heart Association, Inc.

This, plus the tendency of patients with transannular patches to have larger cardiothoracic ratios[F3] and larger right ventricular volumes (Fig. 23-51) late postoperatively, suggest that eventually a deleterious effect on long-term survival will become evident.[E7]

Residual Right Ventricular Hypertension
Residual right ventricular hypertension, expressed as P_{RV}, or $P_{RV/LV}$, or right ventricle–pulmonary artery (RV–PA) gradient (see "Postrepair $P_{RV/LV}$" in section on Special Situations and Controversies) adversely affects the functional status late after complete repair.[O3,W2] The data of Wessel and colleagues suggest that, in the absence of other problems, a P_{RV} greater than 70 mmHg (corresponding roughly to $P_{RV/LV}$ > 0.7, and a RV–PA gradient greater than 40 mmHg) is likely to exert this effect[W2] (Table 23-25). This is supported by the work of Piccoli and colleagues, who found a greater proportion (36%) of symptomatic patients among those with a postrepair $P_{RV/LV}$ > 0.8 than that (9.8%) among those with a $P_{RV/LV}$ < 0.8 (P = 0.001).[P9] This is compatible with the information concerning risk factors for premature late death and with the natural history of patients with pulmonary stenosis with intact ventricular septum (see Chapter 24).

Fortunately, in patients with TF and pulmonary stenosis, functionally important residual right ventricular (RV) hypertension at rest, secondary to residual right ventricular outflow obstruction, is rare. This is true of both infants (Fig. 23-52) and older patients (Figs. 23-53 23-54). This has been a cause for reoperation in only 0.9% of patients (UAB).[K12] Further, the RV pressure late postoperatively is generally lower and predictable from pressure measurements in the operating room and particularly from those in the intensive care unit the following morning (see "Postrepair $P_{RV/LV}$" in section on Special Situations and Controversies). In fact, the hemodynamic state seems to be remarkably stable after

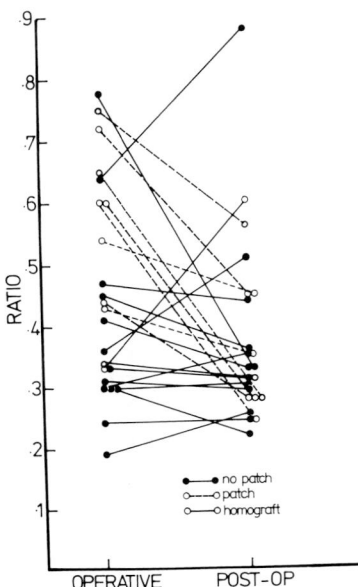

Figure 23-52 The RV/Ao systolic pressure ratios recorded at the end of operation and at postoperative catheterization an average of 30 months later in 23 infants aged 0.7–21 months at the time of operation (GLH). The child with a significant increase in ratio to 0.87 had an inadequately relieved high infundibular and pulmonary anulus (ring) stenosis.

Ao, aorta; patch, transannular patch; ratio, right ventricular/aortic peak pressure ratio; RV, right ventricle.
Reproduced with permission from Calder et al.[C19]

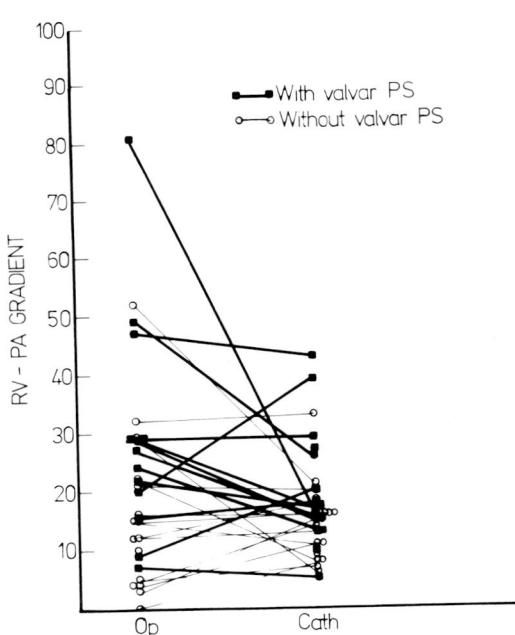

Figure 23-53 The RV–PA peak pressure gradients in 33 patients with TF operated upon between 2 and 8 years of age and restudied an average of 26 months later (GLH). All had a low or midlevel infundibular stenosis. A transannular patch was not used in any patient.

PA, pulmonary artery; PS, pulmonary stenosis; RV, right ventricle.

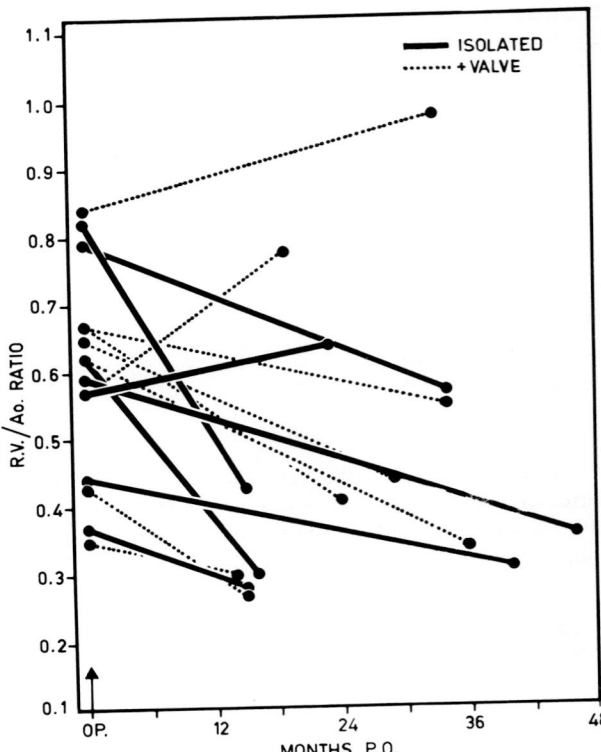

Figure 23-54 The RV/Ao systolic pressure ratio recorded at the end of operation and on follow-up catheterization in 15 patients with either an isolated high-level infundibular stenosis or this plus valve stenosis in whom a transannular patch was not used. The two patients with a significant increase in the ratio both had a borderline residual pulmonary ring stenosis.

Ao, aorta; PO, postoperative; RV, right ventricle.
Reproduced with permission from Barratt-Boyes.[B17]

repair,[F9] and unexpected late postoperative right ventricular hypertension is uncommon.

However, certain morphologic features of the TF may predispose to residual right ventricular outflow obstruction and consequent right ventricular hypertension late postoperatively. Pulmonary trunk bifurcation stenosis is one, and at times in the past this has led to right ventricular hypertension late postoperatively. (It is for this reason that more extensive repairs are currently advised—see section under "Technique of Operation".) Uncommonly, a borderline pulmonary (anulus) ring stenosis that appears to be adequately relieved without transannular patching may appear to be more obstructive on follow-up than was appreciated initially. In fact, there is no evidence that a disproportionate increase in the size of a small pulmonary anulus occurs as the child grows after a repair without transannular patching (Fig. 23-55). (For this reason, reoperation and placement of a transannular patch is considered 24 hours after the repair when $P_{RV/LV}$ is unduly elevated at that time—see "Special Features of Postoperative Care"). Stiffening and eventual calcification of thickened pulmonary valve leaflets left beneath a transannular patch may also result in a rising right ventricular pressure late postoperatively.[H3] (For this reason, thickened pul-

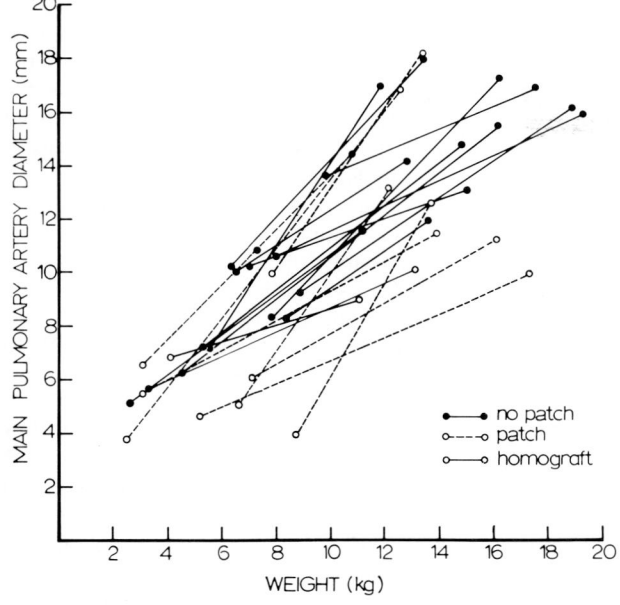

a

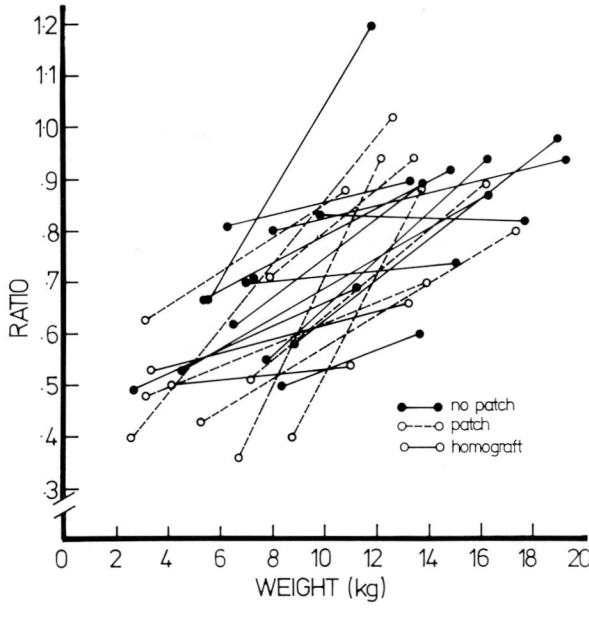

b

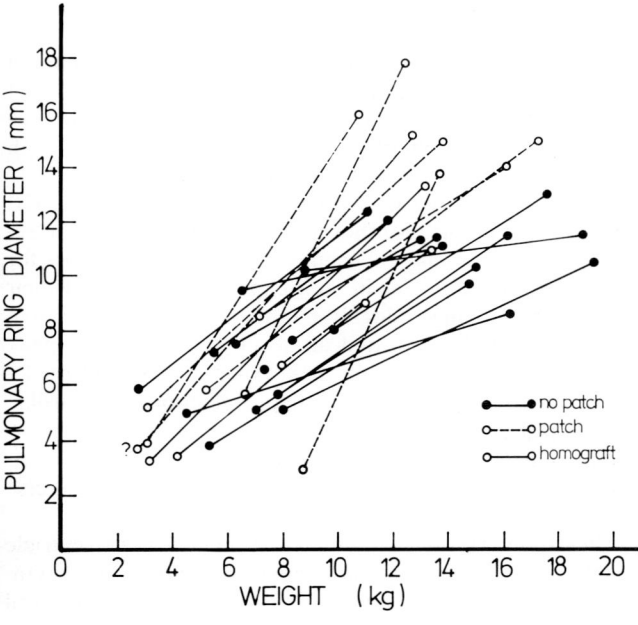

c

Figure 23-55 Pre- and postoperative diameters measured cine-angiographically and corrected for magnification in 23 infants (same series as Fig. 23-52).
(a) Main pulmonary artery diameters.
(b) Ratio of main pulmonary artery to aortic diameters.
(c) Pulmonary anulus (ring) diameters.
Reproduced with permission from Calder et al.[C19]

The greatest interest is in changes in the pulmonary ring diameters in patients *without* a transannular patch or homograft. By converting the measurements to a Z value (exactly as was done for the UAB data[B1]), which expresses the patient's ring diameter in terms of the number of standard deviations it is away from the mean normal value of patients of his size,[R3] it is seen that the pulmonary ring (anulus) enlarged after repair but did not grow disproportionally to the patient's total body growth and remained abnormally small. Thus, we have the following:

| Type of Repair | Pulmonary Anulus (Ring) | | |
	Z (preop) mean ± SD	Z (late postop) mean ± SD	P for difference
No transannular patch or homograft (n = 12)	−2.2 ± 1.54	−2.0 ± 1.25	.7
Transannular patch (n = 8)	−2.4 ± 1.78	1.1 ± 1.77	.004

monary leaflets are excised when a transannular patch is placed.)

As in other types of residual obstructions, any gradient remaining between right ventricle and pulmonary artery after repair of TF is magnified by exercise.[F9,H9,S5] However, the increase is generally considerably less than the increase in cardiac output, indicating that the ability to adapt to increased flow remains. However, large increases in gradients with exercise occur in occasional patients late after complete repair, resulting in right ventricular peak pressure as high as

100–140 mmHg.[E5] According to the studies of Joransen and colleagues,[J6] these marked increases in right ventricular systolic pressure during exercise occur only in patients with resting pressures greater than about 80 mmHg. Other things being equal, the presence of pulmonary incompetence increases the right ventricular peak pressure during exercise. All this again emphasizes the importance of obtaining adequate and appropriate relief of the pulmonary stenosis at the time of repair.

In patients with TF and pulmonary atresia, the proportion

with high P_{RV} late postoperatively is considerably higher but again usually predictable from pressure measurements early after repair. The increased incidence is related to the greater frequency of right and left pulmonary arterial problems in this subset of patients. Also, most of these patients require a valved conduit; and if a heterograft valved conduit has been used, its complications result in a late increase in right ventricular pressure (see "Valved Conduits" in "Special Situations and Controversies").

Residual or Recurrent VSDs
Residual or recurrent VSDs decrease exercise capacity.[W2,Z2] Further, large residual or recurrent VSDs ($\dot{Q}_p/\dot{Q}_s < 2$) strongly predispose to chronic congestive heart failure late postoperatively.[R21]

A single previous B-T shunt does not demonstrably reduce exercise capacity after total repair.[W2]

Age at Repair
Age at total repair affects the late postoperative functional status. Repair in the first 5 years of life appears to result in excellent late postoperative functional status[M18]; James and colleagues found no difference from controls in the exercise capacity of such patients late postoperatively.[J5] Patients averaging 12 years of age at operation had significantly less exercise capacity less postoperatively than did normal controls,[J5] but Wessel and colleagues found no relationship between age at repair and exercise capacity in patients between 1.9 and 15.6 years of age at repair.[W2] However, Bjarke found maximal oxygen uptake during exercise to be only 30%–40% of normal in patients whose total correction was made at an average age of 19.5 years.[B22] When repair is made at a still older age, the functional result is clearly less good than when it is performed in infancy or early childhood.[S6] This is not surprising in view of the effects of chronic pressure overload on the right ventricle, chronic volume overload (if a systemic-pulmonary shunt is in place) on the left ventricle, and chronic hypoxia on the cardiac and other subsystems.

Reoperation

Reoperation is uncommon, occurring in 2.4% (CL 1.7%–3.5%) of the UAB patients 1967–1977.[K12] None has been necessary after the first 5 postoperative years. The importance of performing the initial repair in a complete and precise manner is illustrated by the Stanford experience, which shows that patients requiring rerepair for any reason are considerably more likely to require still another reoperation and suffer premature late death than are patients undergoing their first repair.[M11]

Late Ventricular Arrhythmias

Important ventricular arrhythmias, including multifocal ventricular premature beats, sustained ventricular tachycardia, ventricular fibrillation, and sudden death, occur after repair of TF, and their incidence varies from institution to institution and may in part be related to surgical techniques that allow important residual defects with cardiomegaly.[W5]

The most serious manifestation of late arrhythmic prob-

lems is *sudden death*, which usually seems to be due to ventricular fibrillation and not to the sudden development of complete heart block.[D13,G20,Q1] Sudden death in patients without known complete heart block occurred in 2% of the 396 patients in our early Mayo Clinic experience, followed up to 20 years[F3]; most of these had important cardiomegaly, a finding also reported by Kavey and colleagues,[K28] and half had large residual or recurrent VSDs. In that experience, a transannular patch was also an important contributor to cardiomegaly and thus possibly to sudden death. Only one (0.2%, CL 0.03%–0.9%) of 414 patients at UAB followed up to 10 years died suddenly, and 95% (CL 93.0%–96.8%) were free from any clinical problem related to arrhythmias.[K12] In the select group (age less than 20 years at repair, either primary repair or repair after a single B-T or Waterston shunt, and postrepair $P_{RV/LV} > 0.85$ in the operating room after repair), only two (0.7%, CL 0.4%–1.5%, at 10 years) of 307 patients had any clinical problems related to arrhythmia and none died. Thus, in our early Mayo Clinic experience and at UAB, important late ventricular arrhythmic problems are uncommon and tend to occur in patients who are older than 20 years at operation, have important cardiomegaly preoperatively (as from a previous Potts anastomosis), or have a transannular patch or a high postrepair $P_{RV/LV}$ and cardiomegaly postoperatively.[F3,K12] The data presented by Kavey and colleagues, and by Kobayashi and colleagues, also suggest that serious ventricular arrhythmias are more common in patients whose repair has been delayed beyond the age of 5 years.[K26,K30] Wessel and colleagues also found that important arrhythmic problems occurred only in patients with significant residual hemodynamic abnormalities.[W2]

A higher incidence of sudden death (eight or 3.9%, CL 2.5%–5.9%, among 207 hospital survivors) has been reported by Garson and colleagues,[G6] but the risk factors for sudden death are similar in their experience. Seven of their eight patients dying suddenly had undergone postoperative cardiac catheterization, and all seven had postrepair peak $P_{RV} > 70$ mmHg. In fact, in their experience 33% of the 21 patients with peak $P_{RV} > 70$ mmHg at postoperative cardiac catheterization died suddenly. Patients with important postoperative hemodynamic disturbances also have a strong tendency to develop ventricular arrhythmias during exercise testing.[G7]

Thus the pressure- or volume-overloaded right ventricle has the same tendency toward important ventricular arrhythmias as does the overloaded left ventricle in aortic or mitral valve disease (see Chapters 11 and 12). However, the time course seems slower for the right ventricle, and life-threatening arrhythmias usually develop 8–20 years after repair of TF.

Rarely, the right ventriculotomy scar itself may be arrhythmogenic. This should be considered as a possibility in patients with life-threatening ventricular arrhythmias after repair of TF only when cardiomegaly is absent and there is neither important pressure nor volume overload of the right ventricle. Under these circumstances, electrophysiologic mapping is indicated; when the source of the arrhythmia can be localized to the right ventriculotomy scar, excision of the scar and its replacement with a patch graft have been reported to be beneficial.[H5]

Congestive Heart Failure

Congestive heart failure is a very uncommon late complication of proper repair of the TF. Thus Katz and colleagues found in their select group (those less than 20 years of age at operation, undergoing primary repair or secondary repair after a single B-T or Waterston shunt, and with a postrepair $P_{RV/LV} < 0.85$ in the operating room) an actuarial incidence of congestive heart failure up to 10 years to be 0.7% (CL 0.3%–1.3%).[K12]

Right Ventricular Aneurysms

Right ventricular aneurysms are uncommon. Only 0.9% of patients with TF and pulmonary stenosis (UAB) have undergone reoperation for RV aneurysms, and in all (three patients, two of whom had transannular patches) the $P_{RV/LV}$ in the operating room after the initial repair was greater than 0.79.

The aneurysm may be a false one, but it is usually a true aneurysm that presumably is related to excessive thinning or devascularization of the right ventricular free wall and/or thinning and bulging of pericardium if it has been used as an infundibular or transannular patch.[S7] This latter is rare, since only one patient has developed an aneurysm of a pericardial transannular patch requiring reoperation (GLH) and this in association with a residual high right ventricular pressure due to unrelieved bifurcation stenosis. Rosenthal and colleagues note that most right ventricular aneurysms develop within 6 months of operation, and that the true aneurysms stabilize and rarely progress, whereas false aneurysms may progress rapidly and rupture.[R14]

Right Ventricular Function

Right ventricular systolic and diastolic function is variable late postoperatively and depends on the preoperation status of the ventricle and the type of operative procedure. When a transannular patch has not been used in the repair, right ventricular end-diastolic volume and ejection fraction are usually normal late postoperatively.[B16,G1] However, when a transannular patch has been used, right ventricular end-diastolic volume is increased over normal and in some patients severely so[B16,F7,G1] (Fig. 23-51).

Increased end-diastolic volume is accompanied by a decrease in systolic function in some patients. Thus, when pulmonary regurgitation and the increase in right ventricular end-diastolic volume is severe, right ventricular ejection fraction is usually markedly decreased.[B16,F7]

Even when exercise capacity is normal late postoperatively, a transannular patch is not present, and resting right ventricular systolic function is normal, the right ventricular ejection fraction may not increase normally with exercise[R12] (Fig. 23-56). Subnormal findings such as this, as in the case of the left ventricle, may be related to the myocardial fibrosis that results from the chronic preoperative hypoxia.[L15]

Left Ventricular Function

Variable findings as to left ventricular function late postoperatively have been reported. Some of the variability relates

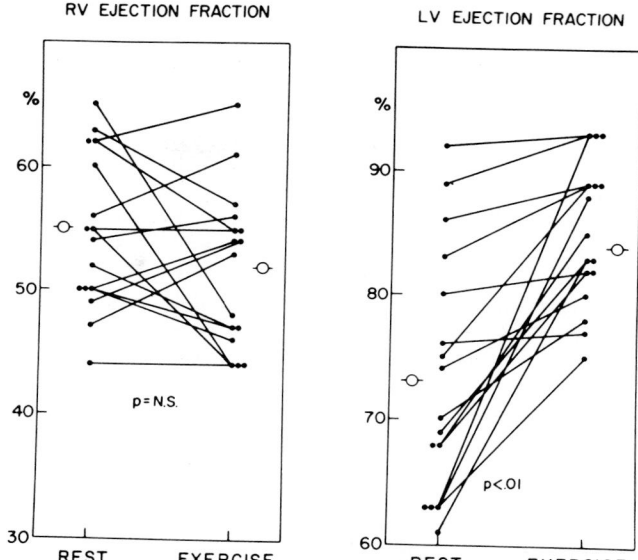

Figure 23-56 The response of right ventricular and left ventricular systolic function to exercise in patients after the repair of the TF. The mean value for each set of data is indicated by the open circle. Reproduced with permission from Reduto et al.[R12]

to the preoperative status of the patient, the age at the time of repair, and the presence or absence of previous palliative operations.

When no residual shunt was present, Jarmakani and colleagues found an increase toward normal in left ventricular mass and end-diastolic volume after repair (as did Oberhansli and colleagues[O8]) and an increase, but not to normal, in left ventricular systolic function.[J3] Findings were similar whether or not a palliative shunt had been done before complete repair. However, Reduto and colleagues found a normal left ventricular response to exercise, with the ejection fraction increasing strikingly, in patients studied an average of 10 years after repair[R12] (Fig. 23-56). Mean age at repair was 10 years. Rosing and colleagues report similar findings.[R13]

The left ventricular function late postoperatively is related to the age of the patient at the time of repair. Although simple tests of left ventricular function at rest may fail to disclose this difference, Borow and colleagues demonstrated that patients undergoing repair in the first 2 years of life have normal or near-normal left ventricular function during stress by afterload increase, whereas those repaired later in childhood have clearly depressed function during stress.[B21] This is consistent with earlier studies; Jarmakani et al. found depressed left ventricular ejection fraction in patients operated upon at an older age,[J3] and Sunderland and colleagues found normal ejection fraction in those undergoing repair when less than 2 years of age.[S10] In part at least, these less favorable results in older children could be due to the myocardial damaging effect of chronic preoperative hypoxia and of long-standing left ventricular overload from the palliative shunting procedure that most of the older patients had undergone.[L15] This study emphasizes the advantages of performing the repair in the early years of life, preferably within the first 3 years.

Lung Function

Patients with an optimal hemodynamic result from repair of TF in infancy or childhood (closed VSD, $P_{RV} < 50$ mmHg, and no pulmonary valve incompetence) have normal lung volumes and capacities late postoperatively.[W7] In general, patients with a good repair of their TF and without pulmonary valve incompetence have only mildly reduced lung function.[W7] Conversely, patients with a less than optimal hemodynamic result and patients operated upon late in the second decade of life[B22] have distinctly subnormal lung function. Wessel and colleagues found that postoperative pulmonary valve incompetence particularly adversely affected late postoperative lung volume and function.[W7]

Recurrent or Residual VSDs

Important recurrent or residual VSDs are uncommon, reoperation for this being necessary (UAB) in less than 1% of cases.[K12] Even small and hemodynamically unimportant leakage is infrequently present under proper circumstances.[B19] Routine left ventriculography an average of 23 months postoperatively in 23 infants showed a tiny residual VSD in only one (GLH).[C19] Others have reported small leakage in up to 10% of patients.[A6]

When important shunts are present, they are usually from inaccurate repair or dehiscence at the posteroinferior angle of the VSD.[C5]

Bacterial Endocarditis

Bacterial endocarditis is rare after repair of patients with TF with pulmonary stenosis. No instances were observed in the 10-year follow-up of 414 cases by Katz et al.[K12]

INDICATIONS FOR OPERATION

The *diagnosis* of TF is an indication for operation in view of the poor prognosis without operation (see "Natural History") and the very good early and late results of repair. However, the morphologic and clinical variants are so numerous that this simple statement requires amplification.

Uncomplicated Tetralogy of Fallot with Pulmonary Stenosis

Intracardiac repair, as a primary procedure or after an initial palliative operation, is advisable and should be performed before the age of 3 years in order to avoid complications such as severe polycythemia, brain abscess, and death, and to ensure a very good long-term result (See "Other Convenient Morphologic Categories" in section on Morphology for definition of uncomplicated TF with pulmonary stenosis or atresia.) Older age, even an adult age, is not, however, a contraindication to operation. Even in infancy, primary repair is theoretically optimal therapy because of its medical, social, and economic advantages; but in some morphologic and clinical subsets of patients and in some treatment situations, initial palliation and later repair (two-stage repair) is safer for the patient.

The decision about primary versus two-stage repair should be made after comparing the risks of the two approaches in the patient at hand, recognizing that a degree of uncertainty must always exist in such comparisons. (See "Primary versus Two-stage Repair" in section on Special Situations and Controversies.) Currently, infants with uncomplicated TF presenting with hypoxia and requiring treatment *in the first 3 months of life* are treated initially by a classical shunting procedure (UAB—see Footnote 5 for description of classical shunting procedures); or propranolol (GLH), with the enthusiasm for the latter tempered by the knowledge that in this setting diffuse right ventricular outflow hypoplasia is common. Nonetheless, particularly when propranolol dosage (usually 2–6 mg $\cdot$ kg^{-1} $\cdot$ day^{-1}) is controlled by intermittent measurements of serum propranolol levels, this has been a satisfactory protocol (GLH). (See "Initial Palliation by Propranolol" in "Special Situations and Controversies.") When palliation is not promptly achieved by propranolol (GLH), a classical shunting procedure is performed (see later discussion of "Indications for the Various Shunting Procedures"). If palliation is successful, the drug is continued but stopped 48 hours prior to the repair.

When any infant with uncomplicated TF is in need of treatment *after the first 3 months of life,* primary repair is advised (GLH). Alternatively (UAB), a shunt may be performed with later repair if the infant is less than 6 months of age and a transannular patch is probably not needed, but primary repair is recommended if the infant is over 6 months of age. In cases in which a transannular patch is probably needed, a shunt is performed with later repair if the infant is less than 8–9 months old (specifically, body surface area less than 0.38 m^2), but otherwise primary repair is done. (For definition and details, see "Primary versus Two-stage Repair," in "Special Situations and Controversies.")

If a shunt is performed for any reason, intracardiac repair is carried out at 2–3 years of age.

Uncomplicated Tetralogy of Fallot with Pulmonary Atresia

Occasionally only infundibular resection or a transannular patch is needed in the repair of patients with TF and pulmonary atresia, in which case the protocols described for patients with TF and pulmonary stenosis apply.

Usually a homograft-valved conduit is needed, and whenever possible one with an internal diameter greater than about 20 mm (adult-sized) is desirable so that it will not be restrictive when the patient is fully grown. Generally, adult-sized homograft-valved conduits can be used in patients over about 5 years of age. Because of this and because the risk of repair with a conduit is lowest between about 5 and 15 years of age (Fig. 23-43 and Table 23-20), a shunting operation is advised for such patients less than about 4 years of age, with repair at some convenient time around 5 years of age. The final repair should generally not be delayed beyond 8–10 years of age because of the risks of increasing hypoxia, polycythemia, and ventricular hypertrophy.

Tetralogy of Fallot with Pulmonary Arterial Problems

Tetralogy of Fallot with Pulmonary Stenosis

When the problem is severe *pulmonary artery hypoplasia* in a patient with TF and pulmonary stenosis (see "Postrepair $P_{RV/LV}$" in "Special Situations and Controversies" for definition of this), an initial shunting operation is performed in anticipation of an eventual good result. Well-performed classical shunts will usually stay open, even when made to very hypoplastic pulmonary arteries. Restudy is carried out a year or two later, and if the pulmonary arteries have increased diffusely and sufficiently in size complete repair is performed. If not, a definitive palliative homograft-valved extracardiac conduit may be placed after about 5 years of age (UAB) and the shunt closed. In a few patients, later repair of the VSD may be possible.

When important *stenosis* is present at the *origins of the right and/or left pulmonary artery* (so-called "bifurcation stenosis" when both are present) in a patient with TF and pulmonary stenosis, the repair can be expected to be more complex and time consuming than in the case of uncomplicated TF. In older patients, the hospital mortality with current techniques can be expected to be low—about 3% (Fig. 23-40), but there is an evident increase in hospital mortality in patients younger than about 3 years of age (BSA < 0.6). Therefore, in patients younger than about 3 years of age with such problems, a preliminary shunting operation may be performed (UAB), reserving the repair to the age of about 3–4 years. Alternatively patients with this type of pulmonary arterial problem are considered acceptable for repair with the same protocols used for uncomplicated TF (GLH).

Tetralogy of Fallot with Pulmonary Atresia

In patients with TF and pulmonary atresia and diffusely hypoplastic left and right pulmonary arteries, the plan is initially the same as in TF patients with pulmonary stenosis. However, at restudy the enlargement may be seen *not* to be diffuse, but instead single- or multiple-segmental or discrete stenoses remain. These can be sufficient to result in an unacceptably high postrepair $P_{RV/LV}$ (see "Postrepair $P_{RV/LV}$" in "Special Situations and Controversies"). *Percutaneous transluminal pulmonary artery angioplasty (PTPA)* has yielded good results in the few cases of this type in which it has been used (UAB) and is advised under these circumstances. Then, if the postrepair $P_{RV/LV}$ predicted from the cineangiogram is acceptable and the patient is 5 years of age or older, repair is performed and usually a homograft-valved conduit is required.

Tetralogy of Fallot with Occlusion of the Origin of One Pulmonary Artery ("Absence of the Central Portion of a Pulmonary Artery")

When, as is usually if not always the case, the more distal pulmonary artery has been determined by appropriate studies to be present (see "Morphology" and "Clinical Features and Diagnostic Criteria") and it is considered possible to join

it to the main pulmonary artery by one of the techniques available (see "Technique of Operation"), primary repair is advisable, with establishment of flow to the involved lung (usually the left). If it is considered that the affected pulmonary artery is too hypoplastic or its proximal portion too distal from the pulmonary trunk to permit establishment of flow to it, primary repair is still considered optimal therapy. When something more than infundibular dissection and pulmonary valvotomy are required, in children over about 5 years of age, a 20 mm or larger homograft-valved conduit is used; in infants and young children a transannular patch seems acceptable. In infants, a classical shunt to the involved lung may be considered within 2 years after the intracardiac repair, hoping that by the time shunt-induced congestive heart failure develops the pulmonary artery will be sufficiently enlarged to connect end to side to the pulmonary trunk via a lateral thoracotomy.

This protocol is recommended, in part because a classical shunting procedure to the single functioning pulmonary artery is hazardous, although with proper precautions (cooling to 33°C, rapid anastomosis, and prompt resuscitative measures should bradycardia or asystole develop while the pulmonary artery is clamped), it can be accomplished with survival of the patient.

Tetralogy of Fallot with Large Aortopulmonary Collateral Arteries

In patients with TF and pulmonary atresia and large aortopulmonary (AP) collateral arteries in addition to the problems already described, there may also be *incomplete distribution* of the right and/or left pulmonary arteries and a direct connection of an AP collateral artery to a lobar or segmental pulmonary artery. Although almost no two cases with this complex pathology are exactly alike, certain general principles have evolved and are the basis for these current protocols:

1. Preoperative evaluation must include cineangiographic visualization of the morphology and distribution of all the large AP collateral arteries and of the pulmonary trunk and right and left pulmonary arteries[M16] (see "Clinical Features and Diagnostic Criteria").

2. As early in life as possible (to give the best chance for enlargement of all portions of the right and left pulmonary arteries), a well-functioning classical B-T or Gore-Tex interposition shunt is established.

3. Soon after operation, a cineangiogram is made, with injection into the shunt. Usually this provides the first clear definition of the morphology and distribution of the right and left pulmonary arteries.[H15,M21] If the shunt is large and working well and the right and left pulmonary arteries distribute to all lobes of both lungs, the large AP collateral arteries are temporarily closed by catheter balloons introduced retrograde into the aorta. If arterial oxygen levels remain good, immediate thrombosis is produced by the catheter introduction of a Gianturco spring with a Dacron fuzz ball[Y2] or, less ideally, with a detachable valved balloon.[G21] This procedure may be done on just one side if the distribution of the other pulmonary artery

is incomplete. (Until recently, the large AP collaterals on the same side as the shunt would have been ligated at the aorta at the time of the shunting operation if the conditions described above seemed to exist, and the appropriateness and accuracy of this would have been verified by arterial oxygen measurement at surgery and immediate postoperative pulmonary arteriogram and aortogram.)

4. Stenoses of the central or more distal parts of the right and left pulmonary arteries are often present in this situation. Although some of the central ones may be well suited to surgical repair (see the description in "Technique of Operation"), some are approached surgically with difficulty. Management of choice for some of these is balloon dilation angioplasty,[L12,L13] and an inoperable situation can sometimes be converted to an operable one by this technique.

5. If the preoperative or immediately postoperative study indicates incomplete distribution of the right and/or left pulmonary arteries, the large AP collateral going to the lobar or segmental arteries that are isolated from the central pulmonary artery is identified. The possible interconnection (manifolding) between that collateral artery and the central and hilar portion of the ipsilateral pulmonary artery is sought by careful study of high-quality cineangiograms. If such a manifold is present, the large AP collateral is occluded with a balloon *proximal* to the interconnection, and after the interconnection is verified by another pulmonary arteriogram via the shunt and by adequate arterial oxygen levels with the collateral occluded, the collateral artery is permanently thrombosed at the site of the balloon, as described.

   If there is *no* intercommunication, that large AP collateral artery must be preserved. Ligation of this collateral in a patient with this situation has in the past resulted in infarction of the lobe, abscess formation and cavitation, and death.[A11] This is analogous to the similar complications that may occur when end-to-end B-T anastomosis is simply ligated at the time of repair of TF.[M8] Surgical attempts to create a manifold have been made (UAB, four cases—direct anastomosis or saphenous vein bypass grafts), but their efficacy has not been proven.

6. Consideration is given to definitive repair, with closure of the VSD and placement of a homograft-valved conduit between right ventricle and pulmonary artery, ideally at 5–10 years of age (see earlier discussion under "Uncomplicated TF with Pulmonary Atresia"). Meanwhile, if palliation is inadequate, a second shunt is created on the opposite side.

7. In some patients, the incompleteness of the distribution of the central and/or hilar portions of the right and left pulmonary arteries may seem to preclude definitive repair. In such cases, at the age of 4–5 years, a palliative homograft-valved conduit is placed between the right ventricle and pulmonary trunk, since this type of repair provides the best palliation and best chance of enlarging the pulmonary arteries,[P3] and the AP shunt is closed. The VSD may be repaired with a slitted patch at that time,[N8] making later complete repair easy via the right atrium should that prove to be possible. The feasibility of this is suggested postoperatively by evidences of a large pulmonary blood flow and an unusually good (> 85%) arterial oxygen saturation.

Tetralogy of Fallot with Absent Pulmonary Valve

Surgical help is urgently needed in small babies with this morphologic variant who present with severe respiratory distress. Some have unrelated congenital hypertrophic lobar emphysema, and a few have severe hypoplasia of the right and left pulmonary arteries, and in either event salvage may be impossible. In the others, complete repair at presentation very early in life with or without inserting a homograft valve has carried a high hospital mortality (see Table 23-9).[A13,11,P5] Several palliative procedures have been used, which likewise have often failed to salvage the infants.[L7]

Therefore, currently an intense medical program is recommended, with the baby continuously in a prone position on a hinged board in the head-up position.[A13] This presumably allows the pulmonary arteries to fall forward and away from the bronchi, particularly the right one.[A13] If, in spite of this, surgical help is needed in the first 6 months of life, the palliative procedure of rather tight *pulmonary banding* is recommended.[O7] If cyanosis is too severe, a classical shunt (see later section on "Indications for Various Shunting Procedures") is added.[B15] If successful, repair with a homograft valve (see below) is performed at about 8–10 years of age or earlier if cyanosis mandates this.

Some patients with this morphology require no special care in early life, and repair can be advised electively. The optimal repair includes orthotopic insertion of a homograft aortic valve (see "Technique of Operation").[11] This operation is advised at age 8–10 years.

Tetralogy of Fallot with Major Associated Cardiac Anomalies

Associated anomalies such as aortopulmonary window,[C2] subaortic stenosis, and total anomalous pulmonary venous connection dictate that total repair be done early in life. However, in the case of others, such as multiple VSDs or complete AV canal defects without important left AV valve incompetence, a shunting procedure gives good palliation and is indicated when patients with TF and these associated cardiac anomalies require surgery in the first year of life (UAB). The definitive repair may then usually be delayed to about age 2–3 years.

Tetralogy of Fallot with Pulmonary Stenosis and Anomalous Origin of the Left Anterior Descending from the Right Coronary Artery

Primary repair may be considered optimal treatment at any age even in the presence of TF with pulmonary stenosis and anomalous origin of the left anterior descending from the right coronary artery when the technique of repair used for this combination obviates the need for a valved conduit (GLH) (see "Technique of Operation"). When there is reluctance to use this technique (UAB) and preoperative studies indicate the possible need for a transannular patch (see "Postrepair $P_{RV/LV}$" in "Special Situations and Controversies"), a shunt is performed when surgical intervention is required in infants and small children, and repair with a valved conduit is performed at 5–10 years of age. When preoperative studies indicate that neither a transannular nor infundibular patch will be required, primary repair via the right atrium or a transverse ventriculotomy is advised in infants over 6 months of age. Still another point of view is that of Castaneda and colleagues, who consider this additional anomaly to be a contraindication to primary repair under any circumstances in infants.[C1]

Indications for the Various Shunting Procedures

When an AP shunt is indicated in infants less than about 2 months of age, a classical (on the side of the aortic arch) Gore-Tex interposition shunt is generally the procedure of choice (see description in "Technique of Operation"). Very hypoplastic pulmonary arteries in neonates do not contraindicate this technique, since high patency rates and lack of pulmonary artery distortion have been achieved in that setting. The interposition shunt may be used on the side opposite that of the aortic arch if special situations make it preferable.

In infants over about 2 months of age and in children, the classical B-T shunt on the side opposite that of the aortic arch is the preferred method for making an AP shunt. However, if the pulmonary arteries are very hypoplastic, a classical Gore-Tex interposition shunt may be advisable in order to avoid pulmonary artery distortion, unless on preoperative study the subclavian artery arising from the innominate is clearly of good size and length.

When for any reason at any age a shunt needs to be made on the side of the aortic arch, the Gore-Tex interposition shunt is preferable to end-to-side use of the subclavian artery by the B-T technique or one of the modifications of that operation.

SPECIAL SITUATIONS AND CONTROVERSIES

Postrepair $P_{RV/LV}$: Its Use and Predictions

In the repair of the TF, the closure of the VSD is usually easily accomplished by a relatively standardized technique. The management of the right ventricular outflow obstruction is more complex, since the morphology is highly variable and there are several surgical techniques for its relief. When the residual right ventricular outflow obstruction is too great after repair, a poor result is obtained. However, unnecessary use of a transannular patch is disadvantageous (see "Incremental Risk Factors for Suboptimal Late Functional Results" in section on Late Results) and so is the unnecessary use of a valved conduit (see "Late Results"), although one or the other is preferable to leaving severe residual right ventricular outflow obstruction. The ratio of the peak pressure in the right ventricle over that in the left ventricle (or aorta) is one way of estimating the residual obstruction. The upper level of *late postoperative $P_{RV/LV}$* that is compatible

with a good result is somewhat controversial, but most would agree that although as low a $P_{RV/LV}$ as possible is desired, one up to *0.70* is acceptable if the only alternative is a transannular patch with its resultant pulmonary valvular incompetence. A postrepair $P_{RV/LV}$ of 0.7 is roughly analogous to a P_{RV} of 70 mmHg, and an RV–PA systolic pressure gradient of 40 mmHg. In patients with TF and pulmonary atresia, there is little certainty as to the upper level of acceptable late postrepair $P_{RV/LV}$. Currently, a figure of 0.85 is used, since usually the only alternative is a purely palliative operation, either a shunting procedure or a transannular patch or valved conduit leaving the VSD open. However, in pulmonary atresia there is little certainty as to the long-term results of repair when the postrepair $P_{RV/LV}$ is high nor of its only alternative, a palliative procedure.

The *ratio between peak pressure in the right ventricle and that in the left ($P_{RV/LV}$)* is easily measured in the operating room after repair of TF, and, therefore, when the pulmonary artery pressure is known to be low, it is a convenient way of assessing the adequacy of the relief of the pulmonary stenosis. It has the disadvantage of being difficult to obtain late postoperatively, and in its place, the ratio of peak right ventricular pressure to peak radial, femoral, or aortic pressure is generally used. The $P_{RV/LV}$ is neither better nor worse for assessing the relief of the pulmonary stenosis than is the theoretically more useful *gradient between right ventricle and pulmonary artery,* this having the disadvantage that measurement of pulmonary artery pressure *distal* to the last stenotic lesion (which may be in the hilar portion of the right or left pulmonary artery) can be difficult in the operating room or early postoperatively[L10] and that interpretation of the gradient requires a measurement of flow through the area, which is not easily available in the operating room. The scanty data available concerning the relationship of the postrepair RV–PA gradient in the operating room to that of the next day or late postoperatively[G18,L10,S1] and concerning the relationship of the gradient to late results are compatible with the information and conclusions drawn from postrepair $P_{RV/LV}$. The *RV pressure alone* is perhaps the least useful measurement, because by itself it conveys no information as to the possible effect of the hemodynamic state of the patient on the measurement.

Postrepair $P_{RV/LV}$ is related to the pulmonary arteriolar resistance, the size of the right and left pulmonary arteries,[M16] the presence and severity of any localized or segmental stenoses or incomplete distributions of the right and left pulmonary arteries, and any residual pulmonary trunk or right ventricular outflow obstructions. It is also related to the flow through the right ventricular outflow tract, and this is increased postoperatively by residual left-to-right shunting across the VSD and by pulmonary valve incompetence.

It is the postrepair $P_{RV/LV}$ *late* after operation that is a determinate of the long-term result of the operation (see "Late Results"), but it is preoperatively and in the operating room that decisions need to be made as to the type of right ventricular outflow tract repair best suited to survival and a good long-term result in the patient at hand. Thus, the relationship between postrepair $P_{RV/LV}$ in the operating room and that late postoperatively is important. Further, the $P_{RV/LV}$ early postoperatively is a determinant of hospital

Table 23-26 The relationship between postrepair $P_{RV/LV}$ in the operating room, 30 minutes after repair, and that late (24 hours) postoperatively in patients with TF and pulmonary stenosis ($n = 82$) or atresia ($n = 18$). The variables affecting the relationship were determined by multivariate linear regression analysis ($n = 100$; UAB 1978–1982), and the postrepair $P_{RV/LV}$ in the operating room was 0.59 ± 0.193 and that late (24 hours) postoperatively was 0.51 ± 0.18 (P for difference $< .0001$).

Variable	Coefficient ± SD	P value
Postrepair $P_{RV/LV}$ (OR)	0.45 ± 0.068	$< .0001$
Body surface area (m²)	-0.07 ± 0.028	.01
Presence of pulmonary atresia	0.10 ± 0.034	.03
Presence of pulmonary arterial problems	0.06 ± 0.032	.05
Intercept	0.27	

mortality. The postrepair $P_{RV/LV}$ in the operating room about 30 minutes after discontinuing CPB is generally 10%–20% lower than that immediately after coming off CPB. Postrepair $P_{RV/LV}$ 24 hours postoperatively is generally lower than that in the operating room[G18,M17,N10] and generally similar to that late postoperatively.[K12] Some of the evidence for the latter statement is indirect and is in the study of Katz et al.[K12] ($P = 0.94$ for the relationship between the time between operation and late $P_{RV/LV}$ measurement and the amount of change in $P_{RV/LV}$); some is in the study of Lang et al.,[L10] who found the RV–PA *gradient* only 8 mmHg ($\pm$ 13.8 SD) higher ($P < 0.0001$) 1 year later than it was 24 hours postoperatively, and in that of Albertal et al.,[A6] who found similar small changes. There is of course some variability, as emphasized by Lang and colleagues.[L10] Some of the variability has been taken into account by a multivariate analysis[K22] (Table 23-26), a digital nomogram of which is in Table 23-27.

In the operating room after repair, the recommended practice in patients with TF and pulmonary stenosis is to accept a postrepair $P_{RV/LV}$ 30 minutes after CPB up to 0.85 before placing a transannular patch or valved conduit, since it is, under these circumstances, usually less than 0.70 the next morning and late postoperatively (Fig. 23-57, Tables 23-28, 23-29). Going to a transannular patch more readily, that is, placing a patch in the face of a lesser operating room postrepair $P_{RV/LV}$ than 0.85, submits unnecessarily many patients to transannular patching who without it would have had a $P_{RV/LV}$ less than 0.7 by the next day and late postoperatively. Thus, if an operating room postrepair $P_{RV/LV}$ only up to 0.8 or 0.75 is accepted, then 79% and 82%, respectively, of patients will receive unnecessary transannular patches, and in fact 49% and 57%, respectively, would have had late postrepair $P_{RV/LV}$ less than 0.6 without one (Table 23-29). True, accepting a postrepair $P_{RV/LV}$ as high as 0.85 without placing a patch means that 32% of individuals with postrepair $P_{RV/LV}$ of exactly 0.85 may have a postrepair $P_{RV/LV}$ less than 0.70 the next morning. Such individuals should usually be returned to the operating room for placement of a transannular patch, but this is infrequently necessary. (See "Special Features of the Postoperative Care.")

There is less certainty as to the postrepair $P_{RV/LV}$ that should be accepted after repair of *TF with pulmonary atre-*

Table 23-27 Digital nomogram of the relationship between postrepair $P_{RV/LV}$ in the operating room, 30 minutes after repair, and that late (24 hours) postoperatively, as it is modified by the other significant variables (the equation and variables are in Table 23-26). The standard deviation for all values is 0.12. (A) Represents TF with pulmonary stenosis and no pulmonary arterial problems (see "Morphology" for definition), and (B) represents TF with pulmonary stenosis and pulmonary arterial problems. (C) represents TF with pulmonary atresia and no pulmonary arterial problems, and (D) represents TF with pulmonary atresia and pulmonary arterial problems.

Postrepair (OR) $P_{RV/LV}$	Postrepair (Late) $P_{RV/LV}$ (mean; SD = 0.12)					
	0.27[a] (3 mo)	0.41[a] (12 mo)	0.50[a] (24 mo)	0.56[a] (36 mo)	0.7[a] (60 mo)	1.0[a]
			(A)			
0.40	0.43	0.42	0.41	0.41	0.40	0.38
0.50	0.48	0.47	0.46	0.45	0.45	0.42
0.60	0.52	0.51	0.50	0.50	0.49	0.47
0.70	0.56	0.55	0.55	0.54	0.53	0.51
0.85	0.63	0.62	0.61	0.61	0.60	0.58
0.90	0.65	0.64	0.64	0.63	0.62	0.60
1.00	0.70	0.69	0.68	0.68	0.67	0.65
			(B)			
0.40	0.49	0.48	0.48	0.47	0.46	0.44
0.50	0.54	0.53	0.52	0.52	0.51	0.49
0.60	0.58	0.57	0.57	0.56	0.55	0.53
0.70	0.63	0.62	0.61	0.61	0.60	0.58
0.85	0.69	0.68	0.68	0.67	0.66	0.64
0.90	0.72	0.71	0.70	0.70	0.69	0.67
1.00	0.76	0.75	0.75	0.74	0.73	0.71
			(C)			
0.40	0.54	0.53	0.52	0.51	0.51	0.48
0.50	0.58	0.57	0.56	0.56	0.55	0.53
0.60	0.62	0.61	0.61	0.60	0.59	0.57
0.70	0.67	0.66	0.65	0.65	0.64	0.62
0.85	0.74	0.73	0.72	0.72	0.71	0.68
0.90	0.76	0.75	0.74	0.74	0.73	0.71
0.95	0.78	0.77	0.76	0.76	0.75	0.73
1.00	0.80	0.79	0.79	0.78	0.77	0.75
			(D)			
0.40	0.60	0.59	0.58	0.58	0.57	0.55
0.50	0.64	0.63	0.63	0.62	0.61	0.59
0.60	0.69	0.68	0.67	0.67	0.66	0.64
0.70	0.73	0.72	0.72	0.71	0.70	0.68
0.85	0.80	0.79	0.78	0.78	0.77	0.75
0.90	0.82	0.81	0.81	0.80	0.79	0.77
0.95	0.84	0.83	0.83	0.82	0.81	0.79
1.00	0.87	0.86	0.85	0.85	0.84	0.81

[a]Body surface area (m²) at repair, age in parentheses.

sia. This is primarily because the alternative of perforating the VSD repair patch and ending up with only a palliative operation is a much less desirable alternative than the simple placement of a transannular patch, which is usually all that is needed when the dilemma arises in patients with TF with pulmonary stenosis. In the absence of any certainty as to its correctness, the recommendation is to accept the complete repair and not perforate the patch unless postrepair $P_{RV/LV}$ is

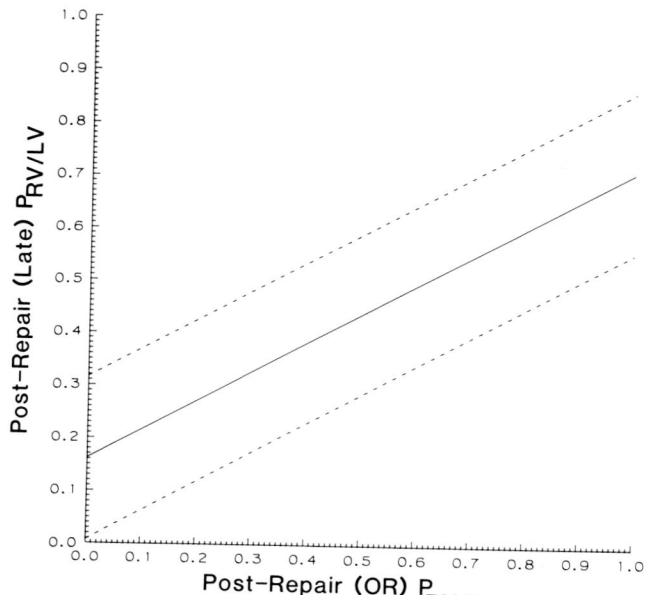

Figure 23-57 Nomogram of the best estimate of the univariate relation between postrepair $P_{RV/LV}$ in the operating room 30 minutes after repair and that late postoperatively. The linear regression equation ($n = 410$) for the nomogram is

$$\text{Late } P_{RV/LV} \text{ (or } P_{RV/Systemic\ arterial})$$
$$= \text{OR } P_{RV/LV} \cdot 0.55 \pm 0.038 + 0.16 \pm 0.023$$

P for the slope of the relationship different from 1 is < .0001. The $n = 410$ is comprised of 33 from Katz et al.[K12]; 82 UAB patients since Katz's study;[K22] and 295 patients from the literature and referenced in Katz et al.[K12] The data in Figures 23-52, 23-53, and 23-54 are included in the 295. Neither these nor the data of Lang et al.[L10] deviate in any significant manner from this best estimate, nor do the data from the three sources deviate from each other or from this best estimate.

greater than 1.2 or the hemodynamic state after repair is unsatisfactory and accompanied by a right atrial pressure that is 50% higher than the left atrial pressure. It is recognized that patients left with a high $P_{RV/LV}$ must be followed very carefully postoperatively and returned to the operating room for patch perforation if the hemodynamic state becomes unsatisfactory or if the $P_{RV/LV}$ is greater than 0.95 the next morning.

It is useful to be able to *predict* the operating room postrepair $P_{RV/LV}$ from cineangiograms before going to the operating room, and this has been demonstrated to be possible.[B1] Such predictions may be considered useful in making decisions in certain infants about one-stage versus two-stage repair (UAB) (see "Indications for Operation") and in deciding about the feasibility of complete correction in patients with TF and pulmonary atresia. An evaluation of the right ventricular outflow morphology is helpful (see "Morphology"), but usually some measurements are of added value. These attempt to quantitate the effect of the pulmonary arteries on the postrepair $P_{RV/LV}$ and, in addition, the effect of any residual right ventricular outflow narrowing.

The first is based in part on[B1] the diameters of the right and left pulmonary arteries, normalizing these by relating them

Table 23-28 Digital nomogram of the relationship of postrepair $P_{RV/LV}$ (ratio of peak pressure in right ventricle (RV) over that in left (LV)) in the OR, about 30 minutes after repair of TF with pulmonary stenosis, to that 24 hours after repair. (The data points are taken from Fig. 23-57.)

Postrepair (OR)	$P_{RV/LV}$ 24 Hours after Repair	
	Point Estimate	CL
0.50	0.44	0.28–0.59
0.55	0.46	0.31–0.62
0.60	0.49	0.34–0.64
0.65	0.52	0.37–0.67
0.70	0.55	0.39–0.70
0.75	0.57	0.42–0.73
0.80	0.60	0.45–0.75
0.85	0.63	0.48–0.78
0.90	0.66	0.50–0.81
0.95	0.68	0.53–0.84
1.00	0.71	0.56–0.87
1.05	0.74	0.59–0.89
1.10	0.77	0.61–0.92

KEY: CL, 70% confidence limits.
NOTE: These univariate relations are refined by the multivariate equation in Table 23-26 and the digital nomogram in Table 23-27.

to the diameter of the descending thoracic aorta (desc th ao) at the diaphragm, as suggested by McGoon and colleagues[M16]:

$$\frac{RPA}{Desc\ Th\ Ao}\ diameter + \frac{LPA}{Desc\ Th\ Ao}\ diameter$$

As can be seen in Figure 23-58, the right and left pulmonary arteries can be considered to be nonrestrictive when the combined diameter ratio is about 2.0 or greater, and they are only mildly restrictive when the ratio is 1.6. When the com-

Table 23-29 The relationship of postrepair $P_{RV/LV}$ in the OR about 30 minutes after repair to the proportion of patients whose late (24 hours or more after operation) postrepair $P_{RV/LV}$ will be greater than 0.7 (and who may need secondary placement of a transannular patch if one is not already in place); and to the proportion whose late postrepair $P_{RV/LV}$ will be less than 0.6 (and who, if they had reestablishment of CPB in the operating room and placement of a transannular patch because of the postrepair $P_{RV/LV}$, would have had it needlessly). (The data points are taken from Fig. 23-57.)

Postrepair (OR) $P_{RV/LV}$	Postrepair (Late) $P_{RV/LV}$	
	% > 0.70	% < 0.6
0.65	12%	70%
0.70	16%	64%
0.75	21%	57%
0.80	26%	49%
0.85	32%	42%
0.90	39%	35%
0.95	46%	29%
1.00	53%	23%

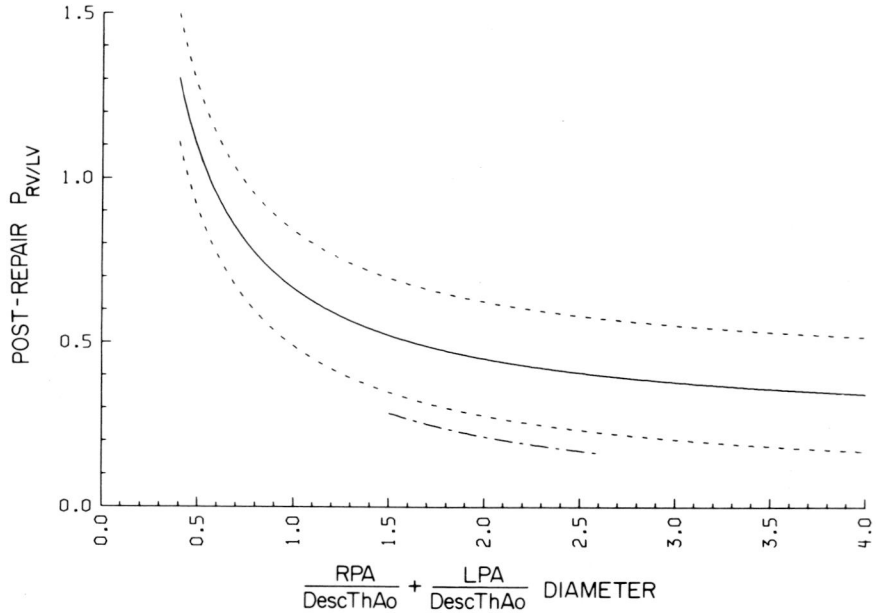

Figure 23-58   The effect of the size of the right and left pulmonary arteries on the postrepair $P_{RV/LV}$ measured in the operating room 30–60 minutes after repair of TF when no residual narrowing is present in the ventricle or in the pulmonary arterial outflow tract and no localized stenosis is present at the origin of right or left pulmonary artery. The relation is expressed by the solid line, the dashed lines enclosing the 70% confidence limits. Note that the right and left pulmonary arteries can be considered to be nonrestrictive when the combined diameter ratio is greater than about 2. The nonlinear regression equation from which this nomogram was derived is

$$P_{RV/LV} = 0.4840/(D_{RPV/Desc\ Th\ Ao} + D_{LPA/Desc\ Th\ Ao}) + 0.2007$$

The standard deviation (the same as the 70% CLs) of the equation, including the incremental factors (see text) is 0.175 $P_{RV/LV}$ units.

  The relations found in normal subjects are shown in the dash-dot line. The difference between them and the tetralogy patients is expressed by the term +0.2007 $P_{RV/LV}$ units. This difference would probably be less if the $P_{RV/LV}$ measurements had been made the morning after operation or later, since $P_{RV/LV}$ is usually 10%–20% lower by then.

Reproduced with permission from Blackstone et al.,[B1] see publication for details.

bined diameter is 1, they are moderately restrictive, but the postrepair $P_{RV/LV}$, when a transannular patch or valved extracardiac conduit is placed as part of the repair, is predicted to be 0.68 (CL 0.51–0.86). When their combined diameters are about 0.8, the postrepair $P_{RV/LV}$ under these circumstances will be 0.81 (CL 0.63–0.98). In addition to taking into account the diameters of the pulmonary arteries, if the cineangiographic study indicates incomplete distribution of the right and left pulmonary arteries and/or peripheral pulmonary arterial stenoses, their effects must be considered. To date, this is quantitated only by three simple terms to be added to the above estimate[B1]:

+0.2569 (if RPA stenosis is present)

+0.1188 (if RPA arborization [distribution] anomaly is present)

+0.7936 (if bilateral arborization anomaly is present)

From this it can be seen that in the current state of knowledge, bilateral incomplete distributions of both the right and left pulmonary arteries predicts a postrepair $P_{RV/LV}$ unacceptably high.

  In assessing the effect of the right ventricular outflow tract on postrepair $P_{RV/LV}$, the assumption is made, based on reasonably good evidence, that infundibular obstruction is virtually completely relieved by dissection and if necessary an infundibular patch. The pulmonary valve anulus seems to grow only in proportion to the child's growth, and if it is small it seems to remain small for the child. Therefore, its size relative to the child's size is expressed as a Z value, which is the number of standard deviations that the patient's pulmonary valve anulus is away from the mean normal value established by Rowlatt, Rimoldi, and Lev.[R3] Thus, the anulus is measured on the cineangiogram, corrected for magnification, and empirically adjusted (Fig. 23-59) to obtain an estimate of the anulus diameter. The anulus diameter is then normalized to the patient's body surface area (or weight in kilograms) (Fig. 23-60). By the equation derived by Blackstone et al.,[B1] the increment in $P_{RV/LV}$ from Z-value sized anulus is determined (Fig. 23-61) and added to the $P_{RV/LV}$

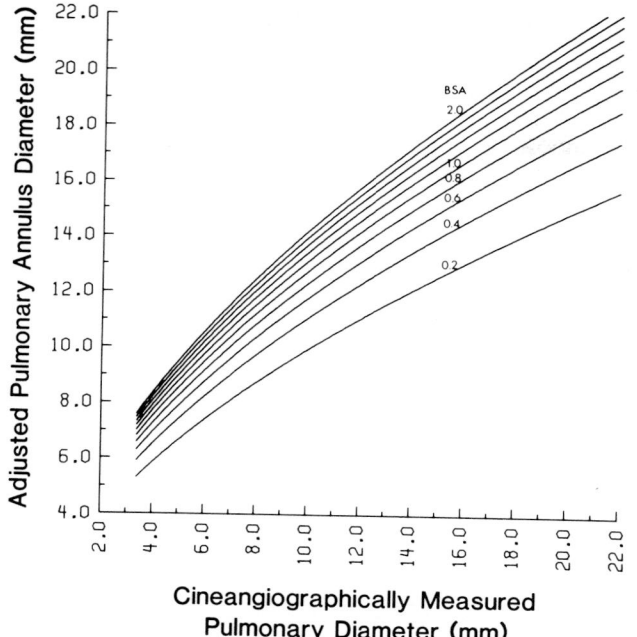

Figure 23-59 Nomogram for obtaining the empirically adjusted pulmonary anulus diameter from the cineangiographic measurements. The equation[B1] is

$$\text{Adjusted pulmonary anulus diameter (mm)} = 3.359 \cdot \text{measured anulus diameter } 0.5789 \cdot \text{body surface area (BSA) } 0.155$$

The standard deviation of the equation is 1.36 mm. The cineangiographically measured anulus diameter has been corrected for magnification.[B1]

related to the size and additional anomalies of the right and left pulmonary arteries described here.

This cineangiographically predicted postrepair $P_{RV/LV}$ and its variability or confidence limits are used in making decisions about operation for primary repair in some small infants (see following section on "Primary versus Two-stage Repair"). The calculations can be accomplished quickly and easily with a programmable handheld calculator.

In the case of patients with TF with pulmonary stenosis, it is possible at operation, after completing the infundibular dissection and pulmonary valvotomy, to refine the prediction of postrepair $P_{RV/LV}$ by measuring directly with Hegar dilators the diameter of the narrowest point in the right ventricular outflow tract, the pulmonary anulus, or the main pulmonary artery. The diameter of the narrowest point is converted to the Z value (Fig. 23-60) and the predicted $P_{RV/LV}$ recalculated (Figs. 23-61 plus 23-58). If from this a postrepair $P_{RV/LV} < 0.85$ is predicted, a transannular patch or valved-extracardiac conduit is not used (see earlier discussion). As a further check, pressures are measured immediately after discontinuing CPB to verify the correctness of the decision. If $P_{RV/LV}$ is higher than expected, it may be necessary to reevaluate the decision (see "Technique of Operation").

Other methods of quantitation of the right ventricular outflow obstruction and prediction of results have been used, some using noninvasive methods.[L19] McGoon used his index finger for this.[H3] Calder and colleagues (GLH),[C19] Naito and colleagues,[N2,N3,N4] Oku,[O4,O5] and Furuse and colleagues[F6] have all presented different methods and equations for this. When the conditions of the measurements and calculations are taken into account, it is apparent that the results of these various methods are comparable.[K14] However, in the future, a method using cross-sectional area of the RPA and LPA, such as that proposed by Nakata and colleagues,[N15] may be the most useful.

Primary versus Two-Stage Repair of Tetralogy of Fallot with Pulmonary Stenosis

Since very few if any institutions perform *routine* primary repair in infants with TF and pulmonary stenosis, some sort of decision-making process is needed. (This would not be the case if shunting were used *routinely* in the first 2 years of life, but currently available information does not support such an approach.) The process may be a simple one (GLH), using primary repair over the age of 3 months except in a few special situations such as patients with TF with complete AV canal, multiple VSDs, or severely hypoplastic pulmonary arteries. Alternatively (UAB), all currently available and regularly updated information can be used in order to arrive rigorously at an individual decision for each patient based upon equations and numerical information, which is not very complicated in an era of handheld calculators and high-speed computers. It may never be possible to prove whether more lives are saved and better long-term results are achieved by the latter method.

In the rigorous method, an estimate is made of the probability of needing a transannular patch from the operating room (OR) postrepair $P_{RV/LV}$ (see previous section). If this is less than or equal to 0.63, a transannular patch will probably not be needed; primary repair is recommended if the patient is over 6 months of age or a shunt and later repair if younger. This is based on the fact that the upper 80% confidence limit of this prediction of 0.63 is 0.85, which means that just 10% of patients with a predicted OR postrepair $P_{RV/LV}$ of 0.63 will have one greater than 0.85. The probable need for a transannular patch in 10% of these patients seems acceptable, with the final decision being made in the operating room as described earlier.

If the predicted OR postrepair $P_{RV/LV}$ is greater than 0.63, there is a greater than 10% chance of the patient needing a transannular patch, and primary repair is recommended only if the BSA is more than 0.38 m^2 (age greater than 8 or 9 months). Otherwise, a shunt is performed initially, with later repair at 2–3 years of age (see "Indications for Operation").

In the rigorous method, the ages below which a two-stage approach is used are derived from a comparison of primary versus two-stage repair. (See Appendix 23A for methodology of the comparisons.) A two-stage approach is recommended at ages (sizes) that are younger (smaller) than that at which there develops separation of the 70% confidence limits of the probability of hospital death after primary and two-stage repair (UAB) (Fig. 23-62). (See Chapter 6 for rationale of using 70% CLs.) Others may wish to use a two-stage repair only below the age at which the 50%, 68%, 90%, or

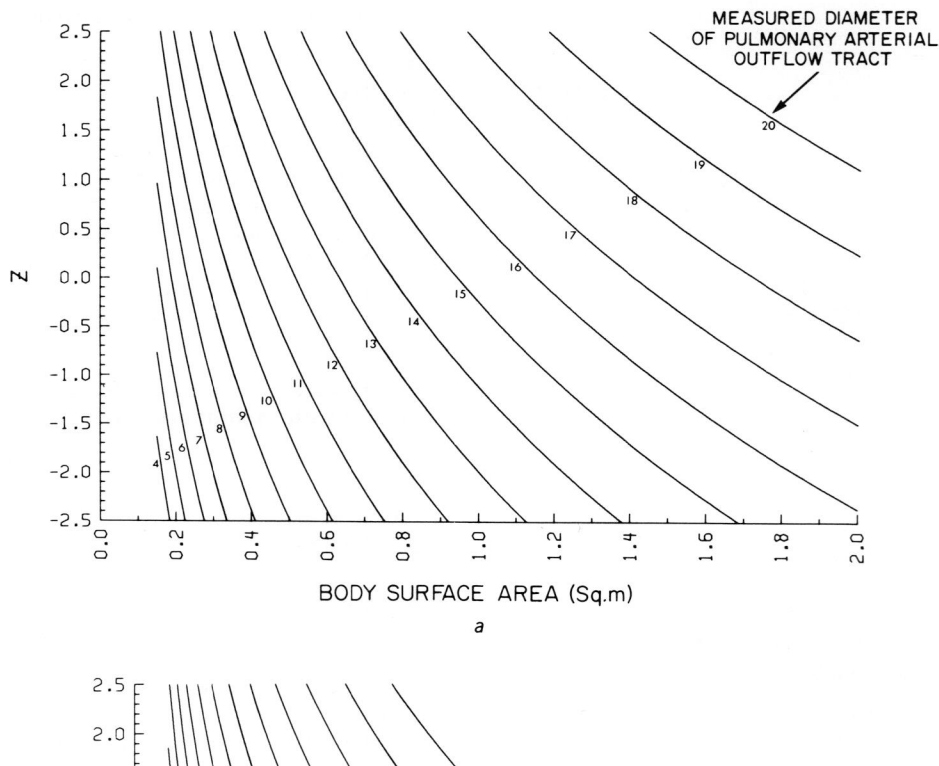

a

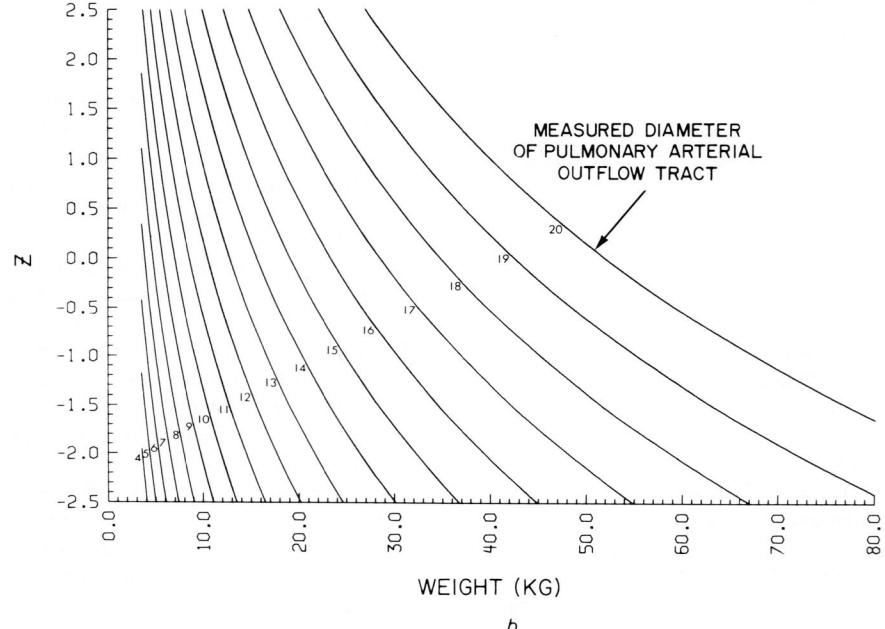

b

Figure 23-60

(*a*) Nomogram, based on BSA, for the determination of the Z value for circumference of the adjusted pulmonary anulus from the cineangiogram (see Fig. 23-59) (or in the case of Hegar dilator measurements in the operating room, the narrowest part of the pulmonary arterial outflow tract) in an individual patient. The nomogram is the solution of the equation for calculating Z value:

$$Z = \frac{\dfrac{\text{Diameter (mm) } \pi}{10} - \text{Mean normal pulmonary anulus circumference}}{\text{SD of normal circumference}}$$

The equation for obtaining mean normal circumference for the patient at hand, based on Rowlatt et al.'s data is:

$$\text{Mean normal (cm)} = 3.5869 \cdot \log_{10}(\text{BSA m}^2 \cdot 10^4) - 9.5431$$

The standard deviation (70% CLs) of the normal value is 0.3624.
(*b*) The same as Figure 23-60*a*, using weight and different constants in the equation.

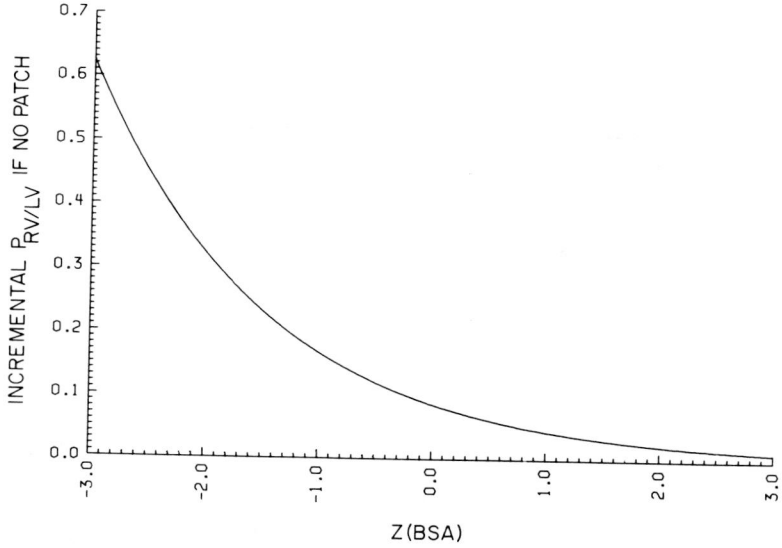

Figure 23-61   Nomogram representing the incremental $P_{RV/LV}$ imposed by the postrepair size of the pulmonary arterial outflow tract, transformed to Z, when a transannular patch is not used. The equation for this nomogram is

$$\text{Incremental } P_{RV/LV} = 0.09437 \cdot \exp(-0.6344 \cdot Z)$$

Reproduced with permission from Blackstone et al.[B1]

95% confidence limit of primary versus two-stage repair separate (Fig. 23-62, Table 23-30) selection of the broader 90% or 95% confidence limits carrying primary repair to a younger age than presented in this text for UAB. Another way of stating the matter is to say that two-stage repair will be performed below an age at which there is the elected *P* value for the difference between the lower hospital mortality of two-stage repair and that of primary repair; *P* values of 0.2, 0.1, 0.05, 0.01, or 0.003 may be elected. The most conservative decision in this setting is the election of 0.2, selection of the smaller *P* values carrying primary repair to a younger age (Table 23-30).

Repair or Palliation in Tetralogy of Fallot and Pulmonary Atresia

Hypoplasia of the right and left pulmonary arteries with or without pulmonary arterial problems may predict a high postrepair $P_{RV/LV}$ even with a transannular patch or a valved conduit. However, in this instance, the alternative is no repair and only a palliative operation. Furthermore, as indicated earlier, an acceptable postrepair $P_{RV/LV}$ in the operating room in patients with pulmonary atresia is not known with assurance. It is, however, reasonable to assume that in patients with TF and pulmonary atresia, *if the cineangiographically predicted OR postrepair $P_{RV/LV}$ is greater than 1.2,* a palliative rather than a corrective operation is to be advised, and if it is less than or equal to 1.2, a repair is advisable. This is based on the fact that if the postrepair $P_{RV/LV}$ in the operating room turns out to be exactly 1.2, the predicted late postrepair $P_{RV/LV}$ in patients without pulmonary arterial anomalies is 0.84 (CL 0.71–0.97) and in patients with pulmonary arterial anomalies is 0.90 (CL 0.78–1.0). (See ''Indications for Operation.'')

Initial Palliation by Propranolol

The advantage of propranolol therapy for severe cyanosis and hypoxic spells in early infancy is that surgery may thereby be deferred and a primary repair done. The disadvantages are that propranolol does not always provide good palliation, and the risk of repair may be higher in patients on propranolol.

Honey and colleagues showed in 1964 that β blockade usually alleviates paroxysmal hypoxic spells from TF,[H4] and this has been confirmed by many others.[C7,K16,P4] When doses of about 2.5 mg $\cdot$ kg^{-1} $\cdot$ day^{-1} of propranolol are used, relief of the hypoxic spells for at least 3 months occurs in 80% of patients.[G5] However, Garson and colleagues found this regimen was more effective in patients older than 1 year, when it could be considered unnecessary (UAB and GLH) and less successful in infants 6 months old.[G5] However, their conclusion was that the drug was effective in the very young patients if the dose was adequate (2–6 mg $\cdot$ kg^{-1} $\cdot$ day^{-1} and serum propranolol levels about 100 ng $\cdot$ ml^{-1}).

Palliative Transannular Patches, or Valved Conduits

Brock suggested in the 1950s that the preliminary palliative operation in TF might be infundibular resection and pulmonary valvotomy, with or without a transannular patch.[B7,B11] Barnard and Schrire in 1961 reported two young children treated palliatively with a transannular patch; one did well but the other developed an apparently false aneurysm from the prosthesis suture line and died suddenly 5 months after operation.[B6] In patients without left and/or right pulmonary arterial problems, this type of palliative operation is probably unwise, for a large left-to-right shunt and heart failure

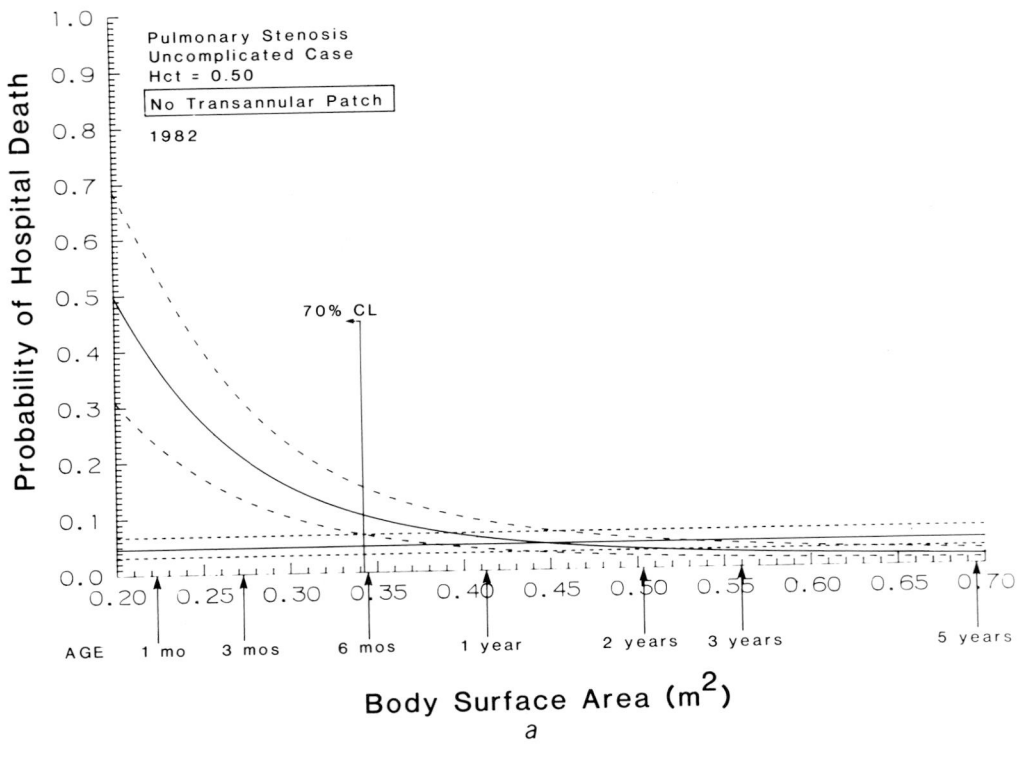

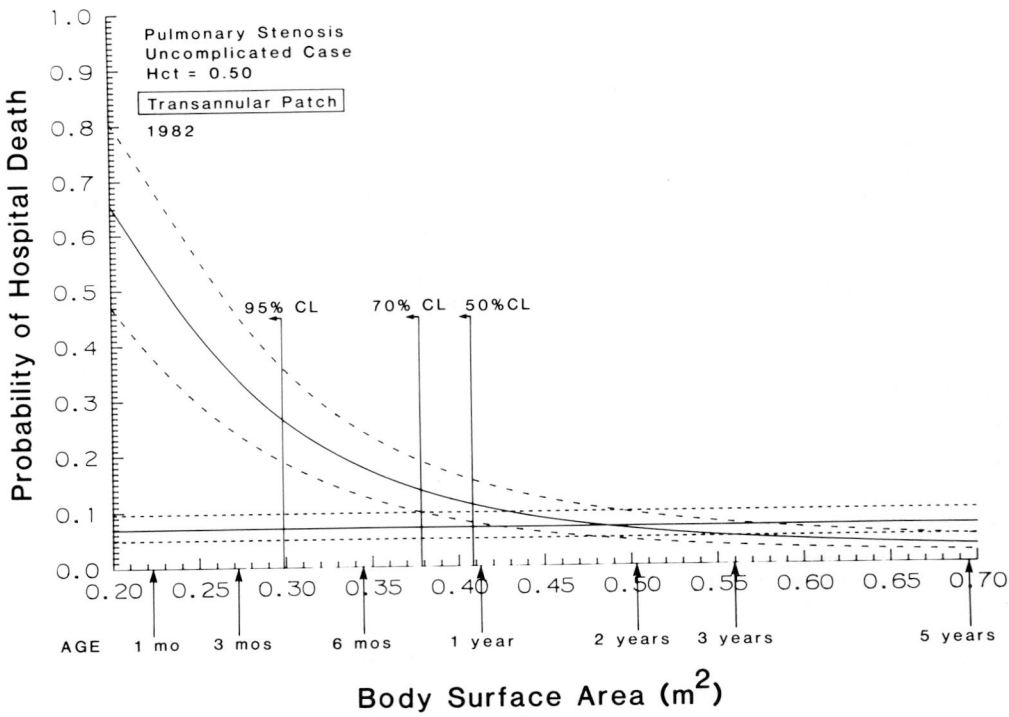

Figure 23-62 A nomogram of the probability of hospital death after primary repair (upper curving line) and two-stage repair (straight line) in TF patients with pulmonary stenosis, according to BSA (or age). Presentation is as in Figure 23-40. The nomograms depict similar information to Table 23-30. (*a*) Repair without a transannular patch. The point of separation of the 70% confidence limits is shown by the vertical line.
(*b*) Repair with a transannular patch. The points of separation of three confidence limits are shown by the vertical lines.
Reproduced with permission from Kirklin et al.[K11]

Table 23-30 Digital nomogram of the degree of uncertainty, at various BSAs and age, that two-stage repair of uncomplicated TF with pulmonary stenosis has in 1982 a lower combined risk (probability of hospital death, interim mortality or important morbidity, and death at secondary repair), than does primary repair. (For details see Appendix 23A.)

Without Transannular Patch				With Transannular Patch	
BSA(m²)	Age (mo)	P value[a]	Confidence Limits[b]	BSA(m²)	Age (mo)
0.38	9	.20	45%	0.42	13
0.37	8	.17	50%	0.41	12
0.35	7	.10	64%	0.39	10
0.341	6.3	.08	68%[c]	0.379	9
0.338	6	.07	70%	0.376	8
0.33	5.5	.05	76%	0.365	8
0.29	3	.01	90%	0.33	6
0.26	2	.003	95%	0.30	4

[a]Single-tailed P-value supporting the null hypothesis that primary repair is as safe as two-stage repair. The smaller the P-value, the greater the likelihood that the null hypothesis is incorrect, and the greater the likelihood that two-stage repair has a lower risk.

[b]The specific confidence limits that separate at the stated BSA (age).

[c]Exactly ± 1 standard deviation of Z, the logistic transformation of the probability of hospital death or morbidity.

frequently develop. For TF patients with pulmonary stenosis and very hypoplastic pulmonary arteries, it may be advised. (See next section.)

Palliative transannular patching has been used particularly in patients with TF and pulmonary atresia and severe underdevelopment of the pulmonary arterial tree.[C13,G15,K20,N8,P10] This was apparently first accomplished by Gerbode in about 1964.[G19] The operation of palliative transannular patching can be done at a low risk in children and young adults,[G15,P3] but the mortality has been appreciable in infants (see Table 23-12). The palliation is often good, and the pulmonary trunk and pulmonary arteries usually enlarge postoperatively.[G15] The response of the more peripheral pulmonary arteries is not uniform and is the same as described after shunting procedures. However, at UAB and in the experience of Freedom and colleagues,[F8] any narrowing present in the proximal left or right pulmonary artery usually becomes very much worse within a year or two of this type of palliative procedure. This may be due to pulmonary regurgitation back into the right ventricle during diastole and the associated collapse of the distal artery. For this reason, current practice is to use a palliative homograft-valved conduit rather than a palliative transannular patch when this type of procedure is indicated (UAB).

A palliative homograft-valved conduit is preferred treatment in patients with TF and pulmonary atresia in whom a definitive repair in the future seems unlikely because of inadequate size and distribution of the right and left pulmonary arteries (UAB).

Choice of the Initial Palliative Operation

The classical B-T shunt, performed with the subclavian artery arising from the innominate artery on the side opposite that of the aortic arch, is the preferred initial palliative procedure except in infants less than 2–3 months of age. In them, the occasionally unsatisfactory shunt resulting from this procedure makes the Gore-Tex interposition graft on the side of the aortic arch the preferred operation. This operation, using Teflon or Dacron rather than Gore-Tex, was reported by Klinner in 1961[K17,K23] and has been more recently emphasized by de Leval and colleagues.[D6] The Gore-Tex shunt, introduced by Gazzaniga and colleagues in 1975,[G16,G17] has been very reliable even in very young infants, with few late occlusions. (See "Interim Results after Classical Shunting Operations.")

Although at one time the Waterston ascending aorta–right pulmonary artery was popular, most groups find with it a higher mortality in infants[A7,D1] (see Table 23-12), a considerably higher proportion of iatrogenic right pulmonary artery problems, and a relatively high incidence of late pulmonary hypertension because of excessive pulmonary blood flow.[G14] The same disadvantages pertain for the Potts descending aorta–left pulmonary artery anastomosis[D3]; in addition it is more difficult to perform in an optimal manner than is the Waterston shunt and is more difficult to close later.

The central Davidson shunt between aorta and pulmonary trunk requires opening the pericardium and usually a median sternotomy. It has no advantages to counteract its disadvantage, namely, that the approach leaves behind adhesions that unnecessarily complicate later intracardiac repair.

Palliative transannular patching is the initial palliative procedure of choice of a few surgical groups, but it has yet to be demonstrated that in small infants it can be done as safely as shunting operations or that the overall results of a two-staged approach with it as the initial procedure are as good as when classical shunts are used. Tucker, Turley, Ullyot, and Ebert report one death (11%; CL 1%–33%) among nine infants receiving this procedure for TF with pulmonary stenosis.[T2] Further, the pulmonary valve is irrevocably destroyed, and the resultant intrapericardial adhesions can complicate the later corrective operation. Palliative transannular patching does usually enlarge the pulmonary arteries.[T2]

Management of the Severely Polycythemic Patient

Severe polycythemia has been an incremental risk factor for hospital death (Tables 23-14, 23-15), and Kahn[K13] and Richardson and Clarke[R7] have reported the same finding. This is probably because the hematocrit reflects the severity of the chronic hypoxia. Chronic hypoxia may damage capillaries, the kidneys, and the myocardium and make the patient more sensitive to the damaging effects of CPB. Therefore, even after the first year of life, severe polycythemia might under these circumstances be considered an indication for a shunting procedure, followed within 6–12 months by complete repair.

Choice of Approach for Repair

Probably, there is a place for all three approaches to the repair of the TF. However, no effect of the type of incision on hospital mortality has been demonstrated in the tetralogy[K7,K11] or in isolated VSD.[R24]

The most generally useful approach is via a *vertical incision* in the *outflow portion of the right ventricle*. The so-called "limited right ventriculotomy" used for placement of a transannular patch when the right atrial approach is used is less than 1 cm shorter than the standard vertical ventriculotomy incision. The advantages of "limiting" the incision in this small way are problematic, and the advantages of the transatrial repair when a transannular patch is needed are slight. When using the vertical ventriculotomy, it need not and should not be carried very far into the sinus portion of the right ventricle. The vertical ventriculotomy incision is closed by suturing into it a preclotted woven Dacron patch (UAB) (see Fig. 23-27), since the infundibulum itself is often narrow, or alternatively it may be closed directly (GLH).

A *transverse ventriculotomy* may be used in those patients in whom the infundibulum and pulmonary valve ring do not require enlargement. Its disadvantage is that if improperly made and an infundibular or transannular patch is unexpectedly required, an inverted T-shaped incision may result. This may be avoided by making the transverse incision low in the outflow tract so that if a subsequent vertical incision is required for transannular patching, there is a bridge of viable muscle between the two incisions. This was the case in 48 (18%) of 277 transverse ventriculotomies (GLH). Among the 48, five (10%; CL 6%–17%) died.

A *right atrial approach* gives very adequate exposure for the infundibular dissection and the repair of the ventricular septal defect.[B10,E2,E3,H2,K15] The pulmonary valve can be seen and assessed through it, and the approach avoids cutting the branches of the right coronary artery and avoids the akinetic or dyskinetic area that results after healing of the right ventriculotomy. Kawashima and colleagues have shown that this may be of some functional advantage since the rise in stroke volume index with isoproterenol infusion is significantly greater when the right atrial approach has been used.[K10] Another advantage of using the approach is that

with it the surgeon acquires an increased understanding of the functional implications of the abnormal right ventricular anatomy of the TF. Its great risk is inadvertent tearing of the tricuspid valve, as pointed out by Ebert in 1976 in his discussion of the paper by Edmond et al.[E11] This has not occurred in the UAB experience, but particular care must be taken to avoid it. In spite of the advantages of not making a ventriculotomy, no improvement in early or late results has yet been demonstrated to result from use of the right atrial approach, although good results have been reported.[E3] Kawashima and colleagues have shown no increase in the frequency or severity of residual pulmonary stenosis at late postoperative cardiac catheterization when the right atrial approach is compared with the conventional approach through the right ventricle.[K10]

The transatrial approach is used when a transannular patch is not needed and the infundibular chamber is wide and an infundibular patch unnecessary (UAB). Alternatively (GLH), a transverse right ventriculotomy incision is made in these circumstances. Unless these conditions pertain, the repair is preferably done through a vertical incision in the right ventricular infundibulum.

Technique of the Infundibular Dissection

Some advocate only an incision in the parietal extension of the infundibular septum (parietal band), rather than dissection and resection as described in this chapter.[C3] Such an approach forces near-routine infundibular or transannular patching and is therefore considered disadvantageous (GLH and UAB).

More "Liberal" Transannular Patching

Several surgical groups currently use transannular patches in most operations for TF. In the past, hospital mortality has been increased in patients in whom transannular patches have been used. Even with a low hospital mortality, the use of transannular patching liberally (that is, in cases in which it may not be necessary) can be considered disadvantageous in view of the unfavorable long-term effects now known to be associated with the resultant free pulmonary valve incompetence (see "Late Results").

Valved Transannular Patches

Periodically, enthusiasm has been expressed for the incorporation of a monocusp valve in the transannular patch (or the use of an opened homograft or heterograft pulmonary artery or aorta with its cusp as the gusset[A10]). There is no evidence that this reduces hospital mortality, and recent studies indicate that there is little valve function postoperatively in most patients.[S14]

Transannular Patching Plus Orthotopic Heterograft Valve Insertion

After carrying a vertical ventriculotomy across the pulmonary valve anulus and onto the pulmonary artery, a stent-mounted heterograft valve may be placed orthotopically be-

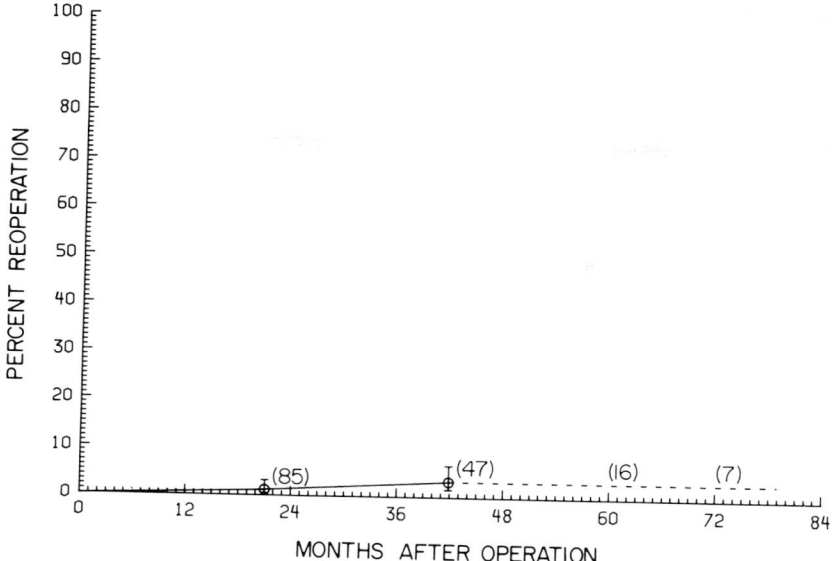

Figure 23-63   Actuarial rate of reoperation after placement of heterograft-valved extracardiac conduit from a ventricle to the pulmonary artery (UAB; September 1972–1979; *n* = 117).[D16] Operations were done in an era in which the importance of positioning the conduit away from the sternum was recognized. Follow-up date was January 1, 1980. The mean follow-up period was 37 months.

neath a transannular patch.[L5] Also, this method may be used in correcting pulmonary valve incompetence late after the repair of TF with a transannular patch[E7] (see Table 23-7). This procedure has been replaced by the technique of using an orthotopically placed homograft aortic valve (UAB and GLH).

Valved Conduits

A number of different types of valved extracardiac conduits have been used in the treatment of patients with TF and pulmonary atresia since they were first introduced by Ross and Somerville in 1966.[R23] These include homografts of the aortic valve and ascending aorta, procured, sterilized, and preserved in many different ways; homograft valves within Dacron tubes; heterograft valves within Dacron tubes; and pericardial and dura mater valves within pericardial tubes.

The most extensively used has been the *heterograft-valved Dacron conduit* of either the Hancock or Carpentier-Edwards type. Complications can occur with this conduit simply because it is improperly routed beneath the sternum. Proper routing to the left of the sternum (or to the *right* when the aorta is in L-malposition) reduces the incidence of reoperation for conduit obstruction within the first five postoperative years.[B27] Thus, even with the limitations of the heterograft-valved extracardiac conduit, 96% of patients can be reoperation free at 6 years (Fig. 23-63).

Even when properly routed, however, gradients may be present across the conduit when first inserted, and these tend to increase with time. Severe conduit stenosis develops with increasing frequency as time passes, independent of any initial gradients. Thus, Bisset and colleagues report a 30% incidence of conduit failure within 6 years,[B18] and Ciaravella and colleagues report that 32% of their patients

developed an increase in the RV–PA gradient across the conduit within 6 years of the insertion and that in some patients the increase was as great as 70 mmHg.[C6] These stenoses may be at the proximal conduit–RV anastomosis, or at the heterograft valve, or very commonly at the conduit–PA anastomosis.[N5]

In part, these stenoses are a result of the type of neointima that forms on the Dacron, a subject that has been carefully studied by Agarwal and colleagues.[A9] In most instances, the neointima begins to develop within 24 hours of operation, when it is a thin layer of platelet-fibrin thrombus into which red blood cells and a few leukocytes become incorporated. Within 2–3 weeks, organization of the thin thrombotic lining begins by fibroplastic migration and proliferation from both proximal and distal anastomoses. The neointima does not develop uniformly, however, and there may be fenestrations in the neointima through which bare areas of Dacron are visible. The neointima appears to be matured by 1 month and normally does not change appreciably thereafter. It is about 3 mm thick, and the luminal surface is shiny gray; the interface between neointima (peel) and conduit usually contains necrotic thrombotic debris. No matter how long the conduit is in place, the peel can be easily stripped away.

When there are many fenestrations in the neointima, there is a greater opportunity for dissection by luminal blood into the loose layer between neointima and the Dacron, a process that is aided by the lack of true adherence between neointima and the Dacron surface. Rapid increase in the thickness of the peel results and obstruction develops. By the same process, the peel can be suddenly dissected away from the Dacron, and its mass within the conduit lumen becomes an obstructing lesion. This is particularly apt to happen at the anastomosis to the ventricle proximally or to the pulmonary artery distally.

Table 23-31 The results of follow-up cardiac catheterization in infants with TF or other anomalies undergoing repair, including the use of an aortic homograft conduit (GLH; 1970–1976).

Age at Repair (Months)	Interval Since Repair (Years)	Pressures (mmHg)					NYHA Class	Interval Since Repair (yr)
		AO	RV	MPA	LPA	RPA		
Tetralogy of Fallot with Pulmonary Atresia								
1	3	95	36	33	—	25	I	10
16	5	130	80	56	—	33	I	5
17	3	130	44	26	15	13	I	9
Complex Tetralogy of Fallot								
3	3	90	48	35	21	33	I	10
14	2	110	37	33	—	25	I	8
Truncus Arteriosus								
1	3	—	50	31	14	29	I	9
2	3	115	42	32	16	—	II	9*
3	3	110	60	29	—	—	I	4
Double Outlet Left Ventricle								
18	2	120	30	26	26	26	I	9
24	3	95	36	28	—	20	I	9
TGA + VSD + PS								
13	2	105	40	26	24	24	I	8
20	10	100	80	18	—	—	II	10

KEY: Ao, aorta; LPA, left pulmonary artery; MPA, main pulmonary artery; NYHA, New York Heart Association; PS, pulmonary stenosis; RPA, right pulmonary artery; RV, right ventricle; TGA, transposition great arteries; VSD, ventricular septal defect.

[a] Severe aortic incompetence.

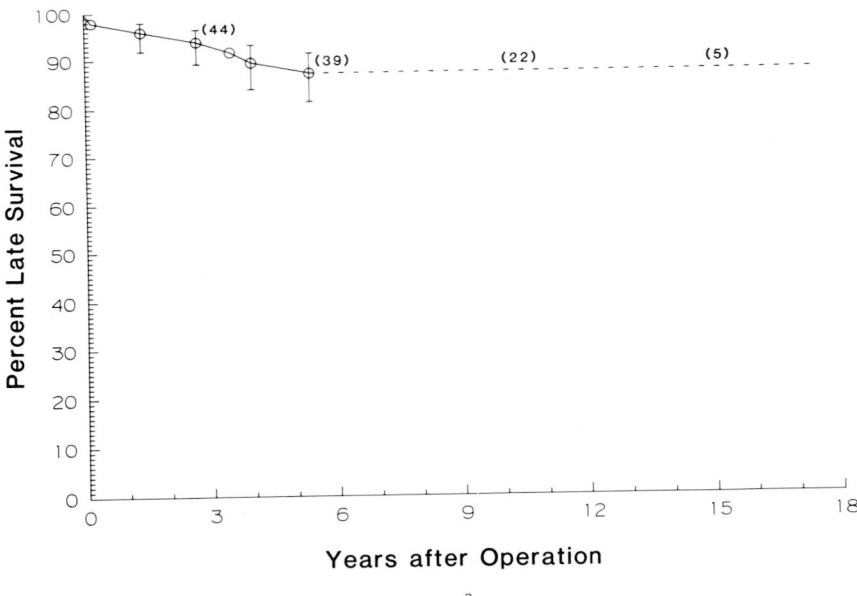

a

Figure 23-64 Actuarial estimates of the long-term results of homograft-valved conduits between right ventricle and pulmonary arteries. (Data supplied by Dr. Jane Somerville and Dr. Donald Ross[R27] and colleagues from the experience of the National Heart Hospital, London, England, 1966–1977; the data concerned 49 hospital survivors.)
(a) Actuarial survival among hospital survivors of homograft-valved conduit to the pulmonary artery in TF. "Death" includes death after reoperation on conduit (two such cases).

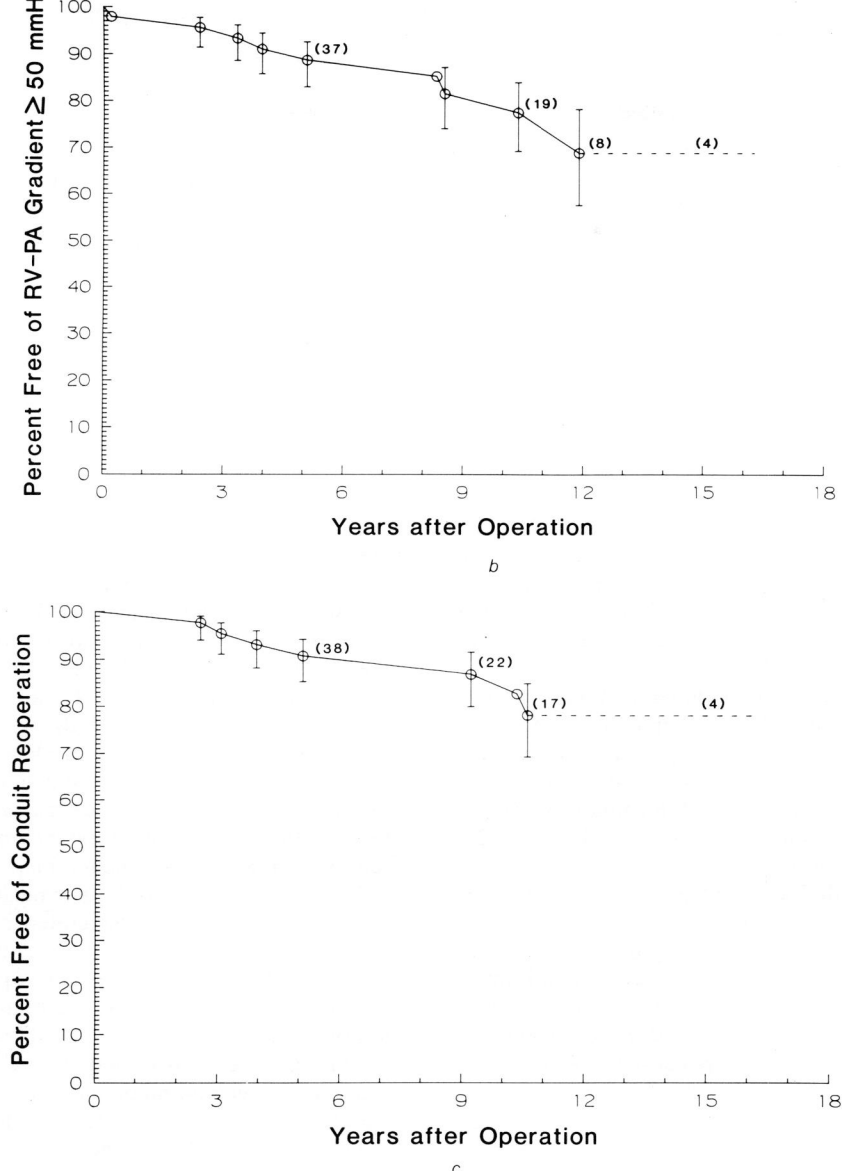

Figure 23-64 *(continued)*
(b) Actuarial estimate of freedom from RV–PA gradient ≥ 50 mmHg among hospital survivors of homograft-valved conduit to the pulmonary artery in TF.
(c) Actuarial estimate of freedom from reoperation on the valved conduit among hospital survivors of homograft-valved conduit to the pulmonary artery in TF.

Heterograft-valved extracardiac conduits can also become obstructive or incompetent because of calcification and degeneration of the heterograft valve itself. This seems to develop in the same manner and at the same rate as it does when the valve is in the mitral, aortic, or tricuspid position (see Chapter 11).

Quite in contrast, *antibiotic sterilized homograft-valved conduits* between right ventricle and pulmonary artery have performed well. The homograft aortic wall usually calcifies within a few years, as was shown experimentally by Rastelli

and colleagues,[R20] but valve function is retained for a very long time and an obstructing neointima does not develop. Thus, among 12 patients followed with such conduits (GLH), only one has required reoperation, and that 10 years later. Five of the patients received their homograft valve in the first year of life, and at recatheterization 3 years later, the gradients across the valved conduits were 8, 10, 13, 19, and 31 mmHg (Table 23-31). There have been no examples of conduit rupture. Fontan and colleagues report no reoperations among 25 patients with variants of the TF who received

Table 23-32 Late events among hospital survivors of homograft-valved conduit to the pulmonary artery in TF (National Heart Hospital, London; n = 49, 1966–1977).[R27] "Death" includes death after reoperation on conduit (two such cases).

PA Extension of Homograft	n	RV → PA Gradient > 50 mmHg[a]			Reoperation on Conduit[b]			Death[c]		
		No	%	CL	No	%	CL	No	%	CL
None	40	5	12%	7%–20%	5	12%	7%–20%	2	5%	2%–11%
Dacron tube	3	3	100%	58%–100%	2	67%	24%–96%	3	100%	58%–100%
Saphenous vein	1	0	0%	0%–85%	0	0%	0%–85%	1	100%	15%–100%
Gusset	5	1	20%	3%–35%	0	0%	0%–32%	0	0%	0%–32%
Dacron	1				0			0		
Pericardium	4	1			0			0		
Total	49	9	18%	12%–26%	7	14%	9%–21%	6	12%	7%–19%

KEY: CL = 70% confidence limits.

[a] Actuarial incidence is 31% at 17 years.

[b] Actuarial incidence is 22% at 17 years.

[c] Actuarial incidence is 13% at 17 years.

either an orthotopically placed homograft replacement of the pulmonary valve or a homograft right ventricular to pulmonary artery conduit, with a mean follow-up of 12 years, and only one patient (gradient 30 mmHg) with a late postoperative gradient over 15 mmHg.[F10]

Somerville and Ross (personal communication)[S19] report an 88% actuarial survival up to 18 years in patients receiving right ventricular to pulmonary artery homograft conduits (Fig. 23-64). Right ventricle to pulmonary artery gradients equal to or greater than 50 mmHg did develop in some patients, and the actuarial incidence at 17 years is 31% (Fig. 23-64). Eighty-one percent of the patients remained free of the need for reoperation on their conduits up to 17 years. In their experience, a proximal extension of the homograft with a Dacron tube between it and the right ventricle did not increase the incidence of important conduit gradient or reoperation; on the other hand, the distal extension of the homograft with a Dacron tube to pulmonary artery did appear to increase the incidence of these complications (Table 23-32).

SECTION 2

TETRALOGY OF FALLOT WITH FLAP VALVE VENTRICULAR SEPTAL DEFECT

DEFINITION

Hearts with tetralogy of Fallot (TF) and flap valve ventricular septal defect (VSD) have the basic morphology of TF but with the constant additional feature of a thick, fibrous flap hinged on the right side of the large VSD that limits right-to-left shunting. The VSD is thus anatomically large but functionally small.

MORPHOLOGY

The large VSD is of malalignment type that is typical for TF. The inferior margin either reaches the tricuspid ring (perimembranous) or is separated from it by a ridge of mus-

cle (see "Morphology" in Section 1). A fibrous flap is attached posteriorly to the aortic margin of the VSD, and its inferior margin may or may not be fused with the base and superior margin of the anterior tricuspid leaflet. Elsewhere, the flap is unattached and it rarely plays any part in tricuspid valve function (Fig. 23-65). It can hinge freely toward the right, but its thickness and bulk prevent movement through the VSD into the left ventricle. Therefore, in the presence of severe pulmonary stenosis and a raised right ventricular pressure, it virtually occludes the defect.[N14] It may be confused with an aneurysm of the membranous ventricular septum but, in fact, is not aneurysmal.

The pulmonary stenosis is typical of TF, but the infundibular component is exaggerated by the severe degree of right ventricular hypertrophy that involves chiefly the sinus portion of the right ventricle, consequent upon the high right ventricular pressure. Thus, there may be a localized high-, intermediate-, or low-level infundibular stenosis or the narrowing may be diffuse, and the valve may or may not be stenotic. Congenital pulmonary atresia is occasionally present and pulmonary artery branch origin stenosis may occur.

This subset of TF is one of the group of conditions in which there is an *accessory fibrous flap or pouch*[C18] *or excrescence* arising in the region of the AV valve apparatus and sometimes from the leaflets themselves. They have sometimes been called, usually erroneously, "aneurysms of the membranous septum."[P15] Such anomalies associated with the tricuspid valve may prolapse into the right ventricular outflow tract and pulmonary valve and cause severe pulmonary stenosis,[C17,F16,P14] and this phenomenon may occur in the absence of a VSD.[E9] A mobile mass of fibrous tissue related to the tricuspid valve may prolapse through a VSD and produce left ventricular outflow obstruction.[N13,S16] This type of subaortic stenosis is easily corrected by operation.[M25] When transposition of the great arteries and VSD coexist, prolapse of accessory tricuspid valve tissue through the VSD results again in left ventricular outflow tract obstruction, which is now subpulmonary.[H21,R26] (See Chapter 39.) In cases with congenitally corrected transposition of the great arteries (see Chapter 42), accessory valvar tissues of

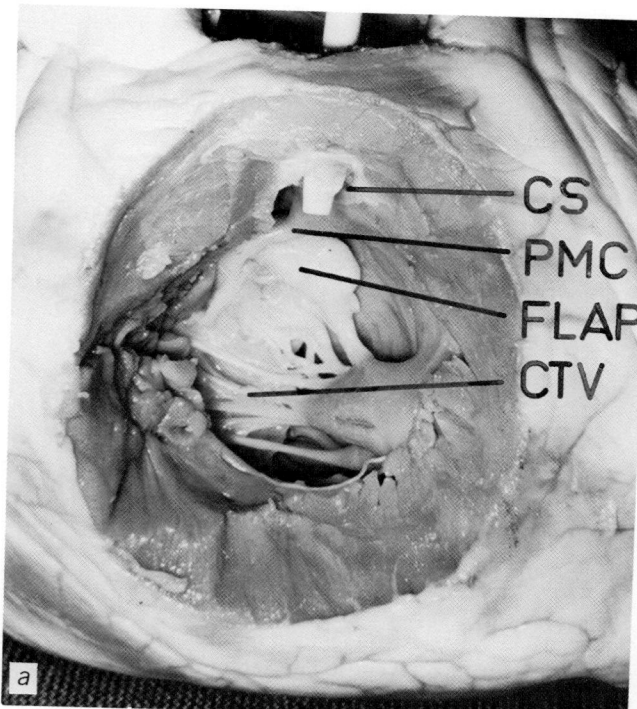

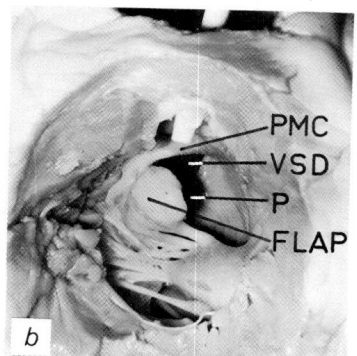

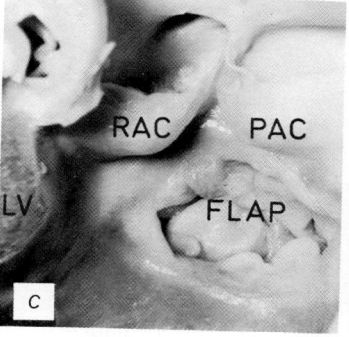

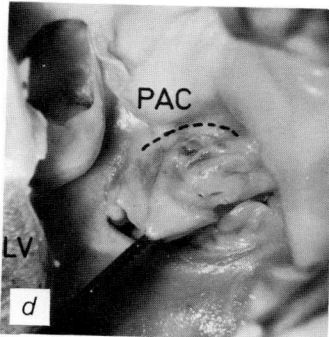

Figure 23-65   A "flap valve" VSD with severe infundibular pulmonary stenosis (GLH). In this heart, the pulmonary valve was normal and the pulmonary artery of near normal size.
(a,b) Viewed from right ventricle. Note the extreme degree of right ventricular hypertrophy and the tight infundibular stenosis (probe). The flap is continuous in this specimen with the anterior tricuspid leaflet. In (b), the flap has been moved rightward to expose the large VSD.
(c,d) Viewed from the left ventricle. The flap is hinged posteriorly (indicated by the dashed line) beneath the noncoronary aortic cusp (PAC) and adjacent right cusp, where it becomes continuous with the membranous septum.

CS, conus (infundibulum) septum; CTV, chordae tricuspid valve; LV, left ventricle; PAC, posterior (noncoronary) aortic cusp; PMC, papillary muscle of the conus; RAC, right aortic cusp; VSD, ventricular septal defect.

the right-sided, morphologically left AV valve may coexist. In this situation, the tendency is for the accessory tissue to prolapse in a ball valve fashion into the morphologically left ventricular outflow tract to produce subpulmonary stenosis.[L18] This may occur with or without an associated VSD Although such prolapsing accessory tissue, uncommon as it is, appears to be more commonly associated with the systemic venous AV valve, it does rarely occur in association with the pulmonary venous (arterial) AV valve. MacLean[M26] and colleagues and Levy and colleagues[L18] each report such a case in which subaortic obstruction resulted. Such a phenomenon may rarely coexist with TF.[V6]

CLINICAL FEATURES AND DIAGNOSTIC CRITERIA

The right-to-left shunt through the restricted VSD may be large enough to produce important cyanosis; but usually it is not, so that when the atrial septum is also intact, the patient is acyanotic or only mildly cyanotic despite severe pulmonary stenosis, and presentation in the first year of life is uncommon. When the pulmonary stenosis is severe, the virtually intact ventricular septum results in severe right ventricular hypertrophy on the electrocardiogram (in contrast to

the moderate right ventricular hypertrophy typical of TF), near normal splitting of the second heart sound (since pulmonary blood flow and pulmonary artery systolic pressure are maintained at a near normal level), and a prominent a wave in the jugular venous pulse. These features and the larger cardiac silhouette on the chest x-ray than in classical TF, make the diagnosis likely. On cardiac catheterization, right ventricular pressure is nearly always suprasystemic. The flap can frequently be visualized on cineangiography.

TECHNIQUE OF OPERATION

The intracardiac repair operation is similar to that for typical TF. However, the severe right ventricular hypertrophy makes relief of the pulmonary stenosis more difficult and may also limit exposure of the VSD. Usually, wide excision of muscle is required. The fibrous flap is identified and excised unless it is atypical and part of the AV valve mechanism. Then, its herniation into the VSD is simply reduced and the VSD repaired in the usual way. It may be necessary to attach the herniated portion to the tricuspid valve to prevent it obstructing the right ventricular outflow tract.

Table 23-33   Hospital death after repair of pulmonary stenosis with VSD but *not* TF.

| | UAB (1967–July 1983) | | | | GLH (1959–1983) | | | |
| | Hospital Deaths | | | | Hospital Deaths | | | |
Category	n	No.	%	CL	n	No.	%	CL
Tetralogy of Fallot with flap valve VSD	5	2	40%	14%–71%	12	2	17%	6%–35%
Low-lying infundibular PS[b]	48	1	2%	0.3%–7%	45	2[c]	4%	1%–10%
With VSD	41	1[a]	2%	0.3%–8%	32	2	6%	2%–14%
Without VSD	7		0%	0%–24%	13	0	0%	0%–14%
Other forms of infundibular PS[b]	22	0	0%	0%–8%				
With VSD	17	0	0%	0%–11%				
Without VSD	5	0	0%	0%–32%				
Valvar PS with VSD	8	0	0%	0%–21%	6	0	0%	0%–27%
Valvar and infundibular PS (or atresia) with VSD	11	2		NA				

KEY: CL, 70% confidence limits; IV, interventricular; NA, not available; PS, pulmonary stenosis; VSD, ventricular septal defect.

[a] Operation in 1971; death with low cardiac output.

[b] In the GLH material these two subsets are combined.

[c] Both deaths in 1960; one in association with underdeveloped right ventricle.

RESULTS

The hospital mortality after repair has, in the past, been relatively high. Four (24%, CL 12%–39%) of 17 patients (GLH and UAB) died in the hospital after repair (Table 23-33). One UAB death occurred in association with anomalous origin of the left main coronary artery from the pulmonary trunk and one GLH death in association with pulmonary atresia and a large fistulous communication between the left coronary artery and the right ventricle.

The late results in hospital survivors have been good.

INDICATIONS FOR OPERATION

Palliative shunting operations are inappropriate since they do not relieve the progressive right ventricular pressure overload. Similarly, blind (or open) pulmonary valvotomy could result in excessive shunting from left to right through the VSD.

Primary repair is the correct treatment and is advisable when the diagnosis is made.

SECTION 3

LOW-LYING INFUNDIBULAR PULMONARY STENOSES WITH OR WITHOUT VENTRICULAR SEPTAL DEFECT

DEFINITION

Low-lying infundibular pulmonary stenosis is a type of intraventricular pulmonary stenosis that clearly separates the sinus (inflow) portion of the right ventricle from a large and thin-walled infundibulum.[H17,L17] It is usually but not always associated with a small or moderate-sized and occasionally large perimembranous ventricular septal defect (VSD), or one with a narrow bar of muscle between it and the anulus of the tricuspid valve. Also included in this section are similar cases with an intact ventricular septum, since such cases may be considered part of this overall spectrum and perhaps with a spontaneously closed VSD (UAB).

Low-lying infundibular pulmonary stenosis may coexist with otherwise typical tetralogy of Fallot.[L16] Such cases are not included in this section but are included in Section I as part of the spectum of TF. The lesion may also coexist with double outlet right ventricle.[G22] (See Chapter 40.)

HISTORICAL NOTE

Like many cardiac anomalies, low-lying infundibular pulmonary stenosis was encountered by the cardiac surgeon in the mid- and late-1950s, before the lesion was recognized by morphologists as a discrete entity.[K27,S15,W8] However, case 1 in the 1933 report by Eakin and Abbot[E8] and cases 1 and 3 in the 1959 report by Blount and colleagues[B26] clearly were examples of the entity, and Grant and colleagues clearly discussed this lesion in their paper of 1961.[G23] However, the credit for the first description of the entity as such is generally given to Tsifutis and colleagues in 1961.[T7]

MORPHOLOGY

The most striking morphologic finding in this subset of cardiac anomalies is the large and thin-walled infundibular chamber, which gives rise to the appellation "two-chambered right ventricle."[H18] The pulmonary valve and anulus are normal sized or large, as is the pulmonary trunk, and the right and left pulmonary arteries are virtually always large and free of stenoses or distributional anomalies.

The stenosis is formed by accessory bulky muscle bundles concentrated at the level of the ring of muscle that separates the sinus portion of the right ventricle from the infundibulum (the infundibular septum and its parietal and septal exten-

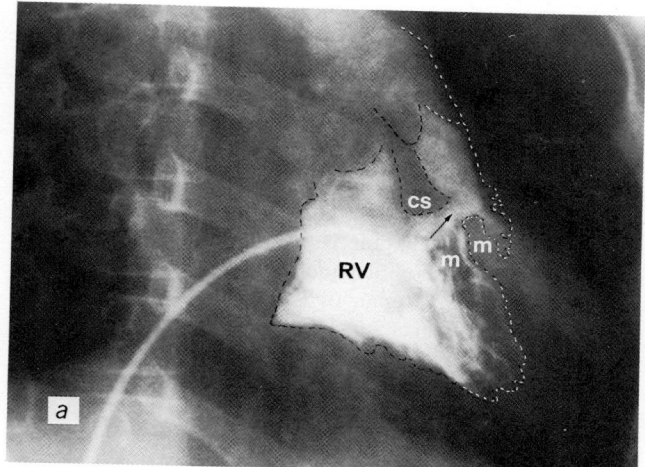

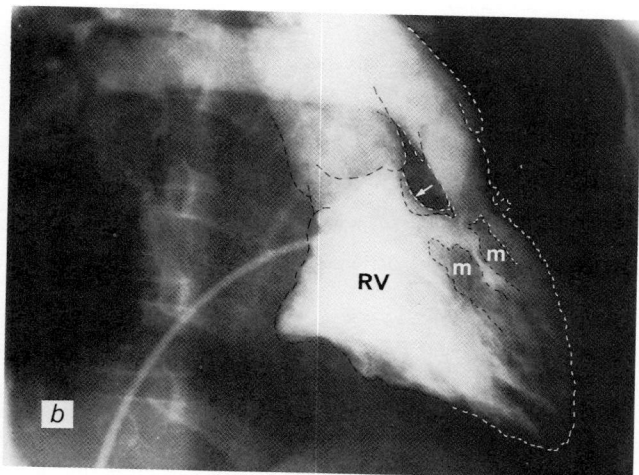

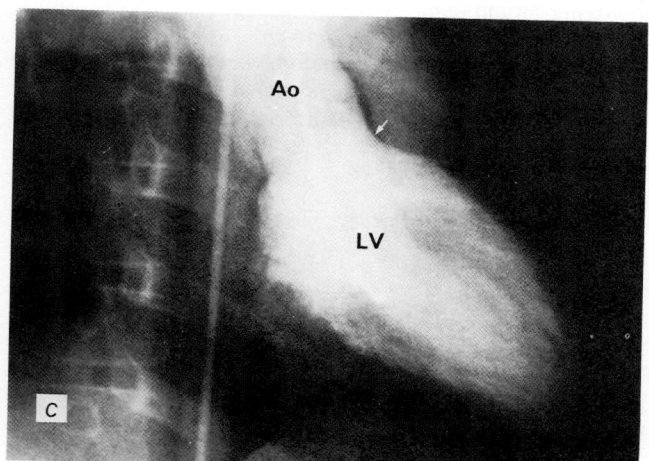

Figure 23-66 Right anterior oblique cineangiograms from a patient with low-lying infundibular pulmonary stenosis and a large ventricular septal defect that has characteristics which tend to distinguish it from TF (GLH).

(*a*) Early frame after right ventricular injection. The anomalous muscle bundles form an extensive coronal plane stenosis between the RV sinus and infundibulum with an ostium (arrow) lying immediately below a normally positioned conal septum.

(*b*) In this later frame, the right-to-left shunting through the ventricular septal defect (not profiled in this view) outlines not only the aorta but also the superior margin of the left ventricle (arrow).

(*c*) Left ventricular injection confirming a normally aligned connection (arrow) between the superior margin of the LV (formed by the conal or infundibular septum) and the aorta. In tetralogy of Fallot this view shows overriding of the aorta onto the RV secondary to conal (infundibular) septal displacement (see Figure 23-19*A*).

Ao, aorta; CS, conal septum; LV, left ventricle; M, muscle bundles; RV, right ventricle.

sions and the moderator bands). In its most florid form, there is a bulky, trabeculated muscular shelf lying almost in a coronal plane that separates a large, relatively thin-walled infundibular chamber from a hypertrophied, thick-walled sinus portion containing the tricuspid valve apparatus and the ventricular septal defect. These are the two chambers of the so-called "two-chambered right ventricle." The shelf is formed by medial and lateral anomalous muscle bundles that join the anterior free wall about halfway between the ventricular apex and base.[B24] The stenotic ostium is usually centrally located, and in older patients it is surrounded by a bulky fibrous collar that further increases the stenosis. There may be more than one ostium. This obstructing muscular diaphragm inserts so far inferiorly on the free wall that it lies nearly in a coronal plane, which predisposes the surgeon's incision to be in the infundibular chamber. The muscular band on the right side usually seems in fact to be the parietal extension of the infundibular septum.

The VSD is usually small or moderate-sized, although it may be large or may have closed and be represented only by a dimple. It is usually perimembranous and overhung by thick tricuspid chordae, but it may have a bar of muscle at its posterior margin rather than abutting against the tricuspid annulus.

In about 5% of cases, important and otherwise typical subaortic *stenosis* (see Chapter 32, Section 2) coexists with low-lying infundibular pulmonary stenosis.[R25] The explanation for the coexistence of these two lesions in this relatively large proportion is not at hand.[B25]

CLINICAL FEATURES AND DIAGNOSTIC CRITERIA

Patients with low-lying infundibular pulmonary stenosis and VSD usually present in the midpart of the first decade of life, but they may present in the second decade or even in adult life. The presentation is often with mild cyanosis.

On examination, the most striking feature is the very loud systolic murmur, which is often grade 6 and heard with the stethoscope off the chest wall. The chest x-ray is not specific, but the pulmonary artery shadow along the upper left cardiac border is usually prominent.

The diagnosis can be made by 2D echocardiography, but cardiac catheterization and cineangiography are performed, particularly to confirm the presence and location of the VSD and the amount of displacement of the infundibular septum and overriding of the aorta (Fig. 23-66).

NATURAL HISTORY

The natural history can only be surmised. Because in some cases only a dimple remains in the perimembranous area at operation, the VSD presumably has a tendency to close spontaneously. Since few patients with this entity present in infancy, it is not surprising that the stenosis has been demonstrated to increase gradually in severity as the child grows.[C16,D15,F15,H19,H20] The progression can lead to complete infundibular atresia.[P13]

TECHNIQUE OF OPERATION

The preparations, median sternotomy incision, and placement of the stay sutures and purse strings are as usual (see Chapter 2, Section 3). The examination of the heart may confirm the presence of a characteristically large and thin-walled infundibular chamber, but this is not always evident externally. Usually a marginal branch of the right coronary artery courses over the underlying infundibular stenosis and should be preserved by making the ventriculotomy incision just downstream to it. A woven Dacron tube about the size of the pulmonary artery is preclotted.

Cardiopulmonary bypass (CPB) is established, employing direct caval cannulation (UAB) or caval cannulation via the right atrium (GLH) (Chapter 2, Fig. 2-19). The perfusate temperature is made as cold as possible; when the heart has become ineffective, a small right atriotomy incision is made and a pump oxygenator sump sucker is passed into the left atrium across a natural or surgically created foramen ovale. The aorta is cross-clamped and the cold cardioplegic solution is infused (see Chapter 3).

A transverse infundibular incision (GLH) or an atrial approach (UAB, see "Repair of Uncomplicated Tetralogy of Fallot with Pulmonary Stenosis via the Right Atrium," in Section 1, Technique of Operation) is made, and stay sutures are inserted (Fig. 23-67). The view is an interesting and unique one from the right ventricular approach, since the interior of the smooth and thin-walled infundibulum is exposed and in its depth inferiorly is seen the ostium of the low-lying infundibular stenosis. A moment of carelessness could lead to the ostium's being misidentified as the VSD,[C15,L17] but further examination confirms it as the ostium infundibulum since the tricuspid valve apparatus, lying entirely in the sinus portion of the right ventricle, cannot be visualized.

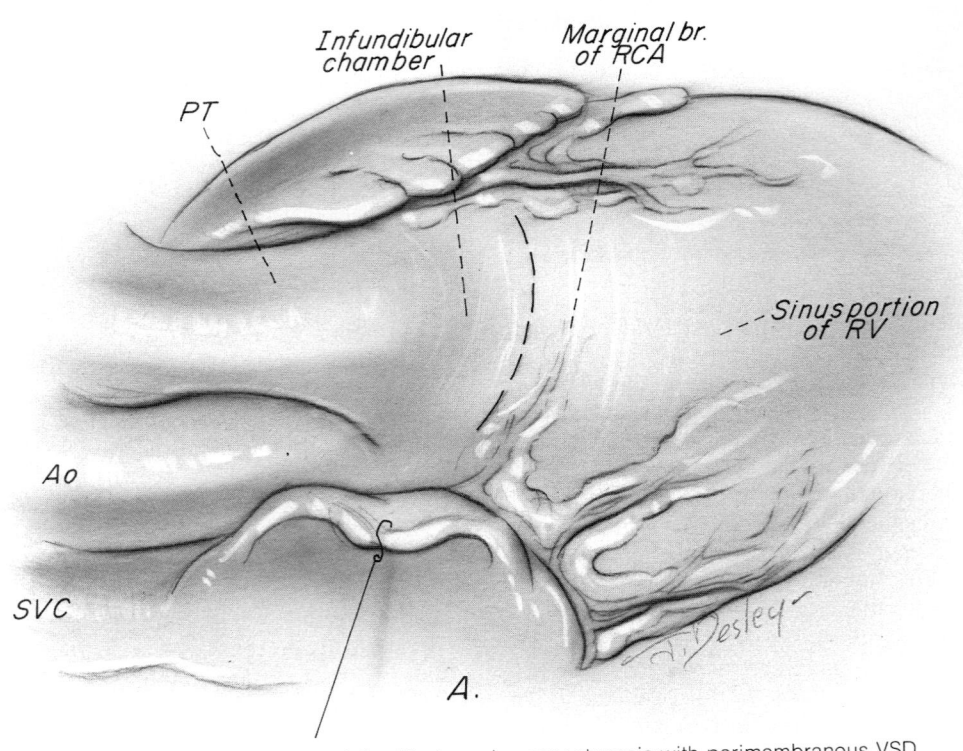

Figure 23-67 Repair of low-lying infundibular pulmonary stenosis with perimembranous VSD.
(a) A transverse right ventricular incision is often well suited for the repair, although at times a vertical incision may be used and closed with a Dacron patch (UAB). A right atrial approach is more frequently used (UAB).
(b) Schematic illustration, made as if the anterior wall of the right ventricle were transparent, of the internal anatomy. The os infundibulum is small in this example; therefore the tricuspid apparatus and ventricular septal defect are not visible from this perspective, which is the same as is achieved by a transverse incision into the infundibular chamber. Note the well-developed infundibular septum and the parietal extension of the infundibular septum that is prominent and contributes importantly to the obstruction, as do anomalous muscle bands.

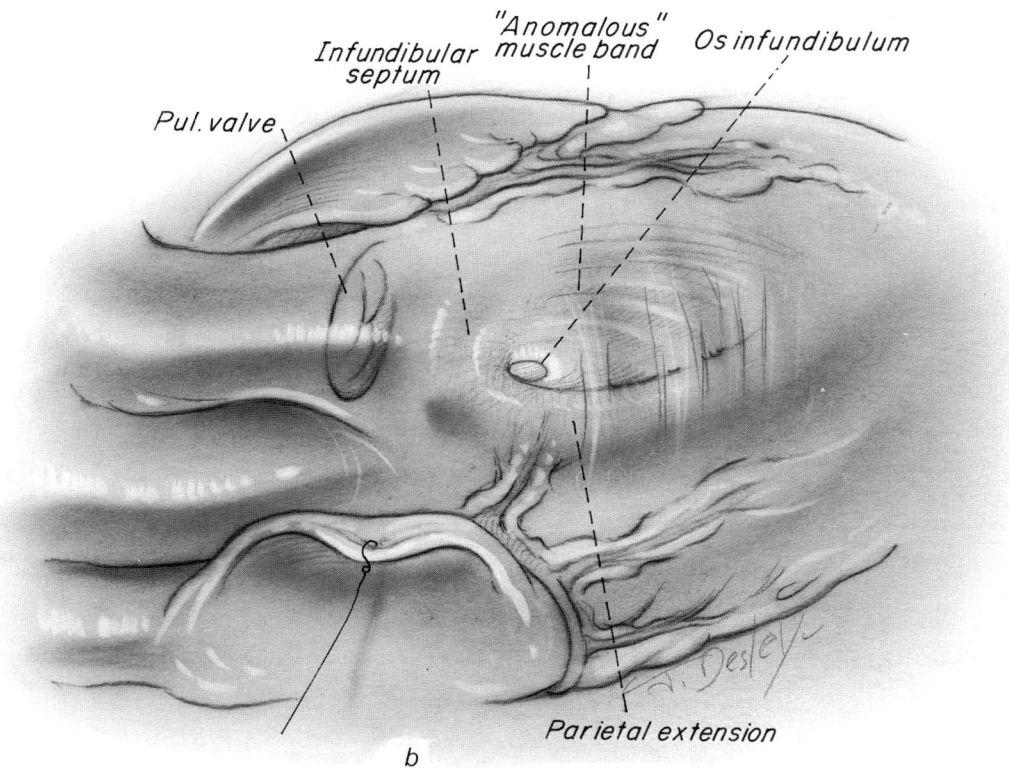

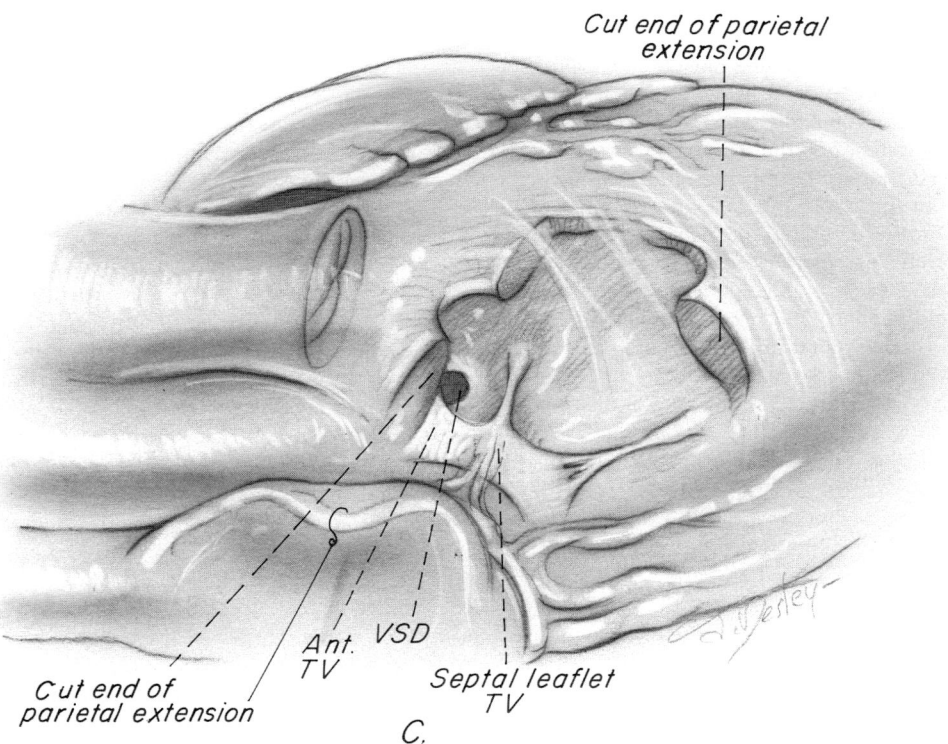

Figure 23-67 *(continued)*

(c) The operation consists of excision of a portion of the parietal extension of the infundibular septum as well as of the anomalous muscle bands. Care is taken not to damage any papillary muscles of the tricuspid valve. After this step has been accomplished, the ventricular septal defect and the tricuspid valve are easily visualized.

Ao, aorta; PT, pulmonary trunk; RCA, right coronary artery; RV, right ventricle; SVC, superior vena cava; TV, tricuspid valve; VSD, ventricular septal defect.

Table 23-34 Hospital death after repair of low-lying infundibular pulmonary stenosis (UAB; 1967–July 1983). Thirty-three of 41 patients had a small or moderate-sized VSD, and among the 33 the infundibular stenosis was severe in 31 and moderate in 2; 8 had a large VSD and moderate stenosis. Among the 7 who had no VSD, 6 had severe and 1 moderate pulmonary stenosis.

VSD	Age at Operation (yr) ≤	<	n	Hospital Deaths No.	%
Yes		1	1	0	
	1---	5	9[a]	0	
	5---	10	9[b]	1	
	10---	20	11[a]	0	
	20---	40	6	0	
	40		5[c]	0	
Total			41	1	2%(CL 0.3%–8%)
No		1			
	1---	5	1	0	
	5---	10	2	0	
	10---	20	4	0	
	20				
Total			7		0%(CL 0%–24%)
All cases			48	1	2%(CL 0.3%–7%)

KEY: CL, 70% confidence limits; VSD, ventricular septal defect.
[a] One patient had associated subaortic stenosis, requiring resection
[b] One patient (surviving) had associated severe tricuspid incompetence
[c] One patient had concomitant coronary artery bypass grafting

An incision is made in the obstructing muscle mass anteriorly and to the left, which allows visualization of the interior of the sinus portion (proximal chamber) of the right ventricle, the tricuspid apparatus, and the VSD. The part of the obstructing muscle mass that arches up and to the right from the infundibular septum (probably the parietal extension of the infundibular septum) is dissected and largely resected. Before resecting the left side of the obstructive muscular collar, which usually is at least in part moderator band, the location of the tricuspid papillary muscles is visualized, and they are protected as the left-sided heavy muscular band is dissected and largely amputated (see Figs. 23-25, 23-26). There is now a wide exposure of the sinus portion of the right ventricle and the VSD. Even though the VSD is small, it is repaired with a patch, just as it is done for other VSDs in this area (see Chapter 20, Fig. 20-24 and Figs. 23-25, 23-26). If the VSD is small and overhung by the thick chordae, a completely interrupted suture technique is preferable.

The right ventriculotomy is closed directly. The sump sucker is removed from the foramen ovale and the left atrium is allowed to fill, the foramen ovale is closed, strong suction is placed on the aortic needle vent, and the aortic cross clamp is released. Rewarming with the perfusate has been started about 5 minutes before this. The right atrium is closed and the rest of the procedure completed as usual.

The morphology is so well suited to repair that usually no gradient is present after repair nor are murmurs present postoperatively.

SPECIAL FEATURES OF POSTOPERATIVE CARE

Postoperative care is performed as usual.

EARLY RESULTS

The hospital mortality after the repair of this cardiac anomaly should approach zero, but the UAB experience (Table 23-34) is marred by an unexplained death in 1971, with low cardiac output and high left atrial pressure.

Neither heart block nor other complications have occurred.

LATE RESULTS

The long-term results are excellent, with no late deaths and all without symptoms.[H20]

INDICATIONS FOR OPERATION

The presence of the malformation is an indication for its repair, and the time of election is the time of diagnosis.

SECTION **4**
OTHER FORMS OF INFUNDIBULAR PULMONARY STENOSIS WITH OR WITHOUT VENTRICULAR SEPTAL DEFECT

There are patients with infundibular pulmonary stenosis, with or without a ventricular septal defect (VSD) whose hearts do not meet the criteria for the diagnosis of tetralogy of Fallot nor for low-lying infundibular stenosis. These are included in this section.

Some of these malformations may be similar in their origin to low-lying infundibular pulmonary stenosis, except that there is mild infundibular hypoplasia and the anomalous muscle bundles arise from the infundibular septum a little more distally (downstream). Others in this subset probably represent instances in which the only discernible lesion at birth is a large VSD. With time, the parietal extension of the infundibular septum hypertrophies out of proportion to the rest of the right ventricle, during which time in some cases the VSD narrows or closes.[C16] In view of this, cases with only mild infundibular pulmonary stenosis associated with an important VSD are included in Chapter 20. (Five of the cases included here in Section 4 were by error included in the 312 cases of VSD published by Rizzoli et al.[R24])

The age distribution at operation of the 22 patients in this subset is similar to that of the patients with low-lying infundibular pulmonary stenosis and, not surprisingly, consists mostly of children and young adults and not infants. In all cases, the surgeon believed the infundibular stenosis sufficiently severe to require resection. Among the 17 patients with associated VSD, the infundibular stenosis was severe in five and moderate in 12. Eight of the VSDs were perimembranous and large, and eight were small; one VSD was subarterial and subpulmonary in position. Among the five patients without VSD, the stenosis was severe in three and moderate in two.

The diagnosis, natural history, and techniques of repair are similar to those for low-lying infundibular pulmonary stenosis, except that a vertical ventriculotomy and infundibular patching should probably be used routinely (UAB). It is important to recognize the infundibular stenosis at the time of repair of the VSD, since otherwise the stenosis can persist or worsen after the repair and reoperation be required for its relief.[D14,M24] The results of complete repair are excellent (Table 23-33). The indications for operation are the same as for low-lying infundibular pulmonary stenosis.

SECTION 5
VALVAR PULMONARY STENOSIS WITH VENTRICULAR SEPTAL DEFECT

With surprising infrequency, isolated valvar pulmonary stenosis coexists with a ventricular septal defect (VSD). Only eight patients with this combination were encountered in the surgical UAB experience 1967–July 1983 (Table 23-33), and their age distribution was similar to that of patients described in Sections 3 and 4. The valvar pulmonary stenosis was anatomic and not "functional" and was severe in five of the 8 patients and moderately severe in three. The VSD was perimembranous and large in four patients and small in two; two patients had small muscular VSDs.

This combination may merely represent coexistence by chance of these two malformations of valvar pulmonary stenosis and VSD. The combination is an indication for operation by techniques described earlier.

SECTION 6
COMBINED VALVAR AND INFUNDIBULAR PULMONARY STENOSIS OR ATRESIA WITH VENTRICULAR SEPTAL DEFECT

Ten patients encountered during the 1967–July 1983 UAB surgical experience had combined valvar and infundibular pulmonary stenosis (or atresia, one additional case) and VSD but were morphologically *not* tetralogy of Fallot (see Table 23-30). In one, situs solitus of the atria, ventricular D-loop, and dextrocardia, as well as a left ventricular diverticulum, coexisted. In one, mesocardia coexisted. In four of the 11, the VSDs were muscular and multiple. In one of these four, who was 10 months old and died after repair, there was also severe stenosis at the origin of the left pulmonary artery. In the other patient who died, there was also severe mitral incompetence and prolapse of tricuspid valve tissue through a perimembranous VSD causing subaortic stenosis (see Section 2).

These seem to be unique cases whose management must be individualized.

APPENDIX

APPENDIX **23A**
COMPARISON OF THE RISK OF PRIMARY VERSUS TWO-STAGE REPAIR OF UNCOMPLICATED TETRALOGY OF FALLOT

1. The estimate of the current probability of *hospital or interim death* (within 3 years of the shunt and including hospital death after both the shunt and the repair) or *morbidity* (specifically brain abscess) *for the two-stage repair* of uncomplicated tetralogy of Fallot with pulmonary stenosis was estimated as follows:

The probability of hospital death after shunting came from the multivariate logistic equation in Table 23-22, solved for TF with pulmonary stenosis, age 5 months (the median age of shunted patients, 1979–July 1982), and year of operation 1982. This probability is 0.02%, CL 0.004%–0.09%. (Had the age of 1 month been used, the probability would be 0.6%, CL 0.1%–2.3%.)

The probability of interim events after shunting was estimated to be 1.9%, CL 0.6%–4.5%. This probability was based on the experience of two such events (brain abscess in one case, sudden death in a second) among 104 patients receiving classical shunts (see Table 23-23). P_{shunt} is the sum of these two probabilities.

The probability of hospital death after secondary repair came from the multivariate equation in Table 23-14, solved for an uncomplicated case with pulmonary stenosis, size of patient 0.56 m^2 (age 36 months), hematocrit 0.50, date of operation 1982. It was solved for transannular patch-no and transannular patch-yes.

These three probabilities were combined to give the total probability of hospital or interim death or brain abscess for two-stage repair without a transannular patch of 4.6%, CL 3.2%–6.8% and with a transannular patch of 6.9%, CL 4.9%–9.6%, as follows:

$$P_{2\text{-stage}} = 1 - (1 - P_{shunt}) \cdot (1 - P_{secondary\ repair})$$

The confidence limits were obtained by first obtaining the variance as follows:

$$Var(P_{2\text{-stage}}) = (1 - P_{2\text{-stage}})^2 \cdot \left[\frac{Var(P_{shunt})}{1 - P_{shunt}} + \frac{Var(P_{interim})}{1 - P_{interim}} + \frac{Var(P_{secondary})}{1 - P_{secondary}} \right]$$

Assuming that the variance of $P_{2\text{-stage}}$ is related to the variance of a logistic Z, where $Z = \ln [(P_{2\text{-stage}}/(1 - P_{2\text{-stage}})]$, the confidence limits were calculated by first solving the following equation for Var(Z):

$$Var(P_{2\text{-stage}}) = (1 - P_{2\text{-stage}})^2 P^2_{2\text{-stage}} \cdot [Var(Z_{2\text{-stage}})]$$

The confidence limits were then calculated as follows:

$$CL(Z) = Z \pm k \sqrt{Var(Z)}$$

For 70% confidence limits, $k = 1.04$; for 95% confidence limits, $k = 1.96$; for 50% confidence limits, $k = 0.6745$.

2. The probability of hospital death after primary repair, with the same stipulations as in (1), were obtained from the multivariate logistic regression equation in Table 23-14.

3. The P value for the difference between the probability of hospital death after primary versus two-stage repair is obtained by solving for t as follows:

$$t = \frac{Z_{2\text{-stage}} - Z_{primary\ repair}}{\sqrt{Var(Z_{2\text{-stage\ repair}}) + Var(Z_{primary\ repair})}}$$

t is then converted to a single-tailed P value using the normal distribution.

4. The equivalent nonoverlapping confidence limits for a given P

value for the difference between primary and two-stage repair was calculated using these relationships:

$$k = \frac{Z_{\text{2-stage repair}} - Z_{\text{primary repair}}}{\sqrt{\text{Var}(Z_{\text{2-stage repair}})} + \sqrt{\text{Var}(Z_{\text{primary repair}})}}$$

which is related to t above by

$$t = k \cdot \frac{(\sqrt{\text{Var}(Z_{\text{2-stage repair}})} + \sqrt{\text{Var}(Z_{\text{primary repair}})})}{\sqrt{\text{Var}(Z_{\text{2-stage repair}})} + \text{Var}(Z_{\text{primary repair}})}$$

where k is converted to a two-tail P value utilizing the normal distribution, and the confidence coefficient is calculated as one minus that P value (e.g., a k of 1.96, $P = 0.05$ converts to 95% confidence limits).

5. The degree of uncertainty (expressed as nonoverlapping confidence limits and P values) in the conclusion that two-stage repair is safer than primary repair for infants with uncomplicated TF can now be calculated for any given patient size (age).

REFERENCES

A

1. Azar H, Hardesty RL, Pontius RG, Zuberbuhler JR, Bahnson HT: A review of total correction in 200 cases of tetralogy of Fallot. *Arch Surg* 99:281, 1969.

2. Asano K: Long-term results of corrective surgery for the tetralogy of Fallot. *Singapore Med J* 14:178, 1973.

3. Aigueperse J, Lemoine G: 140 corrections de tetralogies de Fallot revues avec un recul de la 7 ans. *Coeur Med Interne* 8:709, 1977.

4. Alfieri O, Locatelli G, Bianchi T, Vanini V, Parenzan L: Repair of tetralogy of Fallot after Waterston anastomosis. *J Thorac Cardiovasc Surg* 77:826, 1979.

5. Arciniegas E, Farooki ZQ, Hakimi M, Green EW: Results of two-stage surgical treatment of tetralogy of Fallot. *J Thorac Cardiovasc Surg* 79:876, 1980.

6. Albertal G, Swan HJC, Kirklin JW: Hemodynamic studies two weeks to six years after repair of tetralogy of Fallot. *Circulation* 29:583, 1964.

7. Arciniegas E, Farooki ZQ, Hakimi M, Perry BL, Green EW: Classic shunting operations for congenital cyanotic heart defects. *J Thorac Cardiovasc Surg* 84:88, 1982.

8. Arcienegas E, Farooki ZQ, Hakimi M, Perry BL, Green EW: Early and late results of total correction of tetralogy of Fallot. *J Thorac Cardiovasc Surg* 80:770, 1980.

9. Agarwal KC, Edwards WD, Feldt RH, Danielson GK, Puga FJ, McGoon DC: Pathogenesis of nonobstructive fibrous peels in right-sided porcine-valved extracardiac conduits. *J Thorac Cardiovasc Surg* 83:584, 1982.

10. Asano K, Eguchi S: A new method of right ventricular outflow reconstruction in corrective surgery for tetralogy of Fallot: The application of the valve-retaining pulmonary artery graft as a patch. *J Thorac Cardiovasc Surg* 59:512, 1970.

11. Alfieri O, Blackstone EH, Kirklin JW, Pacifico AD, Bargeron LM Jr: Surgical treatment of tetralogy of Fallot with pulmonary atresia. *J Thorac Cardiovasc Surg* 76:321, 1978.

12. Arciniegas E, Blackstone EH, Pacifico AD, Kirklin JW: Classic shunting operations as part of two-stage repair of tetralogy of Fallot. *Ann Surg* 27:514, 1979.

13. Arensman FW, Francis PD, Helmsworth JA, Benzing III G, Schreiber JT, Schwartz DC, Kaplan S: Early medical and surgical intervention for tetralogy of Fallot with absence of pulmonic valve. *J Thorac Cardiovasc Surg* 84:430, 1982.

14. Akaska T, Itoh K, Ohkawa Y, Nakayama S, Miyamoto H, Nishi T, Satoh H, Takarada M: Surgical treatment of anomalous origin of the left coronary artery from the pulmonary artery associated with tetralogy of Fallot. *Ann Thorac Surg* 31:469, 1981.

15. Alfieri O, Blackstone EH, Parenzan L: Growth of the pulmonary anulus and pulmonary arteries after the Waterston anastomosis. *J Thorac Cardiovasc Surg* 78:440, 1979.

16. d'Allaines C, Soyer R, Rioux C, Blondeau P, Cachera J.-P., Dubost C: Tetralogies de Fallot: Resultats a distance de la correction complete. *Nouv Presse Med* 2:961, 1973.

17. Anderson RH, Allwork SP, Ho SY, Lenox CC, Zuberbuhler JR: Surgical anatomy of tetralogy of Fallot. *J Thorac Cardiovasc Surg* 81:887, 1981.

B

1. Blackstone EH, Kirklin JW, Bertranou EG, Labrosse CJ, Soto B, Bargeron LM Jr: Preoperative prediction from cineangiograms of postrepair right ventricular pressure in tetralogy of Fallot. *J Thorac Cardiovasc Surg* 78:542, 1979.

2. Bonchek LI, Starr A, Sunderland CO, Menashe VD: Natural history of tetralogy of Fallot in infancy. *Circulation* 48:392, 1973.

3. Becu L, Ikkos D, Ljungquist A, Rudhe U: Evolution of ventricular septal defect and pulmonary stenosis with left to right shunt into classic tetralogy of Fallot. *Am J Cardiol* 7:598, 1961.

4. Blalock A, Taussig HB: The surgical treatment of malformations of the heart in which there is pulmonary stenosis or pulmonary atresia. *JAMA* 128:189, 1945.

5. Bargeron LM Jr, Elliott LP, Soto B, Bream PR, Curry G: Axial cineangiography in congenital heart disease. Section I. Concept, Technical and Anatomic Considerations. *Circulation* 56:1075, 1977.

6. Barnard CN, Schrire V: The surgical treatment of the tetralogy of Fallot. *Thorax* 16:346, 1961.

7. Brock RC, Campbell M: Infundibular resection or dilatation for infundibular stenosis. *Br Heart J* 12:403, 1950.

8. Bender HW Jr, Fisher RD, Conkle DM, Martin CE, Graham TP: Selective operative treatment for tetralogy of Fallot. *Ann Surg* 183:685, 1976.

9. Barratt-Boyes BG, Simpson M, Neutze JM: Intracardiac surgery in neonates and infants using deep hypothermia with surface cooling and limited cardiopulmonary bypass. *Circulation* 43:suppl; 1:25, 1971.

10. Binet JP, Hvass U, Bruniaux de J, Langlois J, Planche CL, Dreyfus G, Razafinombana A: Correction complete de la tetralogie de Fallot sans ouverture du ventricle droit. *Arch Mal Coeur* 73:1185, 1980.

11. Brock RC: Direct operations in tetralogy of Fallot. *Am J Cardiol* 3:1, 1959.

12. Beach PM, Bowman FO, Kaiser GA, et al: Total correction of tetralogy of Fallot in adolescents and adults. *Circulation* 43,44:suppl 1:37, 1971.

13. Bharati S, Lev M, Kirklin JW: *Cardiac Surgery and the Conduction System.* New York: John Wiley & Sons, 1983.

14. Bertranou EG, Blackstone EH, Hazelrig JB, Turner ME Jr, Kirklin JW: Life expectancy without surgery in tetralogy of Fallot. *Am J Cardiol* 42:458, 1978.

15. Byrne JP, Hawkins JA, Battiste CE, Khoury GH: Palliative procedures in tetralogy of Fallot with absent pulmonary valve: A new approach. *Ann Thorac Surg* 33:500, 1982.

16. Bove EL, Byrum CJ, Thomas FC, Kavey RW, Sondheimer HM, Blackman MS, Parker FB Jr: The influence of pulmonary insufficiency on ventricular function following repair of tetralogy of Fallot. Evaluation using radionuclide ventriculography. *J Thorac Cardiovasc Surg* 85:691, 1983.

17. Barratt-Boyes BG: The surgery of tetralogy of Fallot, pulmonary atresia with ventricular septal defect and transposition of the great vessels. *Australas Radiol* 12:311, 1968.

18. Bisset III GS, Schwartz DC, Benzing III G, Helmsworth J, Schreiber JT, Kaplan S: Late results of reconstruction of the right ventricular outflow tract with porcine xenografts in children. *Ann Thorac Surg* 31:437, 1981.

19. Blondeau PH, Nottin R, d'Allaines C, Carpentier A, Soyer R, Bouchard F, Durand M, Dubost Ch: Communications interventriculaires residuelles apres reparation complete de la tetralogie de Fallot. *Coeur* 3:31, 1977.

20. Bocala RR, Guller B, Danielson GK, Feldt RH: Left anterior hemiblock and complete repair of tetralogy of Fallot (abstr). *Pediatr Res* 8:347, 1974.

21. Borow KM, Green LH, Castaneda AR, Keane JF: Left ventricular function after repair of tetralogy of Fallot and its relationship to age at surgery. *Circulation* 61:1150, 1980.

22. Bjarke B: Oxygen uptake and cardiac output during submaximal and maximal exercise in adult subjects with totally corrected tetralogy of Fallot. *Acta Med Scand* 197:177, 1975.

23. Bharati S, Paul MH, Idriss FS, Potkin RT, Lev M: The surgical anatomy of pulmonary atresia with ventricular septal defect: Pseudotruncus. *J Thorac Cardiovasc Surg* 69:713, 1975.

24. Barnes RJ, Kwong KH, Cheung ACS: Aberrant muscle bundle of the right ventricle. *Br Heart J* 33:546, 1971.

25. Baumstark A, Fellows KE, Rosenthal A: Combined double chambered right ventricle and discrete subaortic stenosis. *Circulation* 57:299, 1978.

26. Blount SG Jr, Vigoda PS, Swan H: Isolated infundibular stenosis. *Am Heart J* 57:684, 1959.

27. Bailey WW, Kirklin JW, Bargeron LM Jr, Pacifico AD, Kouchoukos NT: Late results with synthetic valved external conduits from venous ventricle to pulmonary arteries. *Circulation* (suppl II):II-56, 1977.

28. Barratt-Boyes BG, Neutze JM: Primary repair of tetralogy of Fallot in infancy using profound hypothermia with circulatory arrest and limited cardiopulmonary bypass: A comparison with conventional two-stage management. *Ann Surg* 178:406, 1973.

29. Brock RC: Pulmonary valvulotomy for relief of congenital pulmonary stenosis. Report of 3 cases. *Br Med J* 1:1121, 1948.

30. Bianchi T, Gamba A, Parenzan L: Two-stage correction for tetralogy of Fallot. *Thorac Cardiovasc Surgeon* 32:229, 1984.

31. Brown JW, Marts B, Gilbert P, Girod D, Hurwitz R, Caldwell R, Mahoney L, King H: Selective two-stage repair of tetralogy of Fallot. *JACC* (Abstract) 5:478, 1985.

32. Blackstone EH, Kirklin JW, Pacifico AD: Decision-making in repair of tetralogy of Fallot based on intraoperative measurements of pulmonary arterial outflow tract. *J Thorac Cardiovasc Surg* 77:526, 1979.

C

1. Castaneda AR, Freed MD, Williams RG, Norwood WI: Repair of tetralogy of Fallot in infancy. Early and late results. *J Thorac Cardiovasc Surg* 74:372, 1977.

2. Castaneda AR, Kirklin JW: Tetralogy of Fallot with aorticopulmonary window. Report of two surgical cases. *J Thorac Cardiovasc Surg* 74:467, 1977.

3. Castaneda AR, Norwood WI: Fallot's tetralogy, in J Stark, M de Leval, (eds): *Surgery for Congenital Heart Defects*. London: Grune & Stratton, 1983.

4. Calder AL, Brandt PWT, Barratt-Boyes BG, Neutze JM: Variant of tetralogy of Fallot with absence pulmonary valve leaflets and origin of one pulmonary artery from the ascending aorta. *Am J Cardiol* 46:106, 1980.

5. Castaneda AR, Sade RM, Lamberti J: Reoperation for residual defects after repair of tetralogy of Fallot. *Surgery* 76:1010, 1974.

6. Ciaravella JM Jr, McGoon DC, Danielson GK, Wallace RB, Mair DD: Experience with the extracardiac conduit. *J Thorac Cardiovasc Surg* 78:920, 1979.

7. Cumming GR, Carr W: Relief of dyspneic attacks in Fallot's tetralogy with propranolol. *Lancet* 1:519, 1966.

8. Cole RB, Muster AJ, Fixler DE, Paul MH: Long-term results of aortopulmonary anastomosis for tetralogy of Fallot. *Circulation* 43:263, 1971.

9. Chiariello L, Meyer J, Wukasch DC, Hallman GL, Cooley DA: Intracardiac repair of tetralogy of Fallot. Five-year review of 403 patients. *J Thorac Cardiovasc Surg* 70:529, 1975.

10. Clayman JA, Ankeney JL, Liebman J: Results of complete repair of tetralogy of Fallot in 156 consecutive patients. *Am J Surg* 130:601, 1975.

11. Cairns JA, Dobell ARC, Gibbons JE, Tessler I: Benign prognosis of right bundle branch block and left anterior hemiblock after intracardiac repair of tetralogy of Fallot. *Am Heart J* 90:549, 1975.

12. Chesler E, Beck W, Schrire V: Selective catheterization of pulmonary or bronchial arteries in the preoperative assessment of pseudotruncus arteriosus and truncus arteriosus type IV. *Am J Cardiol* 26:20, 1970.

13. Crupi G, Locatelli G, Villani M, Tiraboschi R, Parenzan L: Open-heart palliative surgery for pulmonary atresia with ventricular septal defect and hypoplastic pulmonary arteries. *Thorax* 33:625, 1978.

14. Capelli H, Ross D, Somerville J: Aortic regurgitation in tetrad of Fallot and pulmonary atresia. *Am J Cardiol* 49:1979, 1982.

15. Coates JR, McClenathan JE, Scott LW III: The double-chambered right ventricle. A diagnostic and operative pitfall. *Am J Cardiol* 14:561, 1964.

16. Corone P, Doyon F, Gaudeau S, Guerin F, Vernant P, Ducam H, Rumeau-Rouquette C, Gaudeul P: Natural history of ventricular septal defect. A study involving 790 cases. *Circulation* 55:908, 1977.

17. Cosio FG, Wang Y, Nicoloff D: Membranous right ventricular outflow obstruction. *Am J Cardiol* 32:1000, 1973.

18. Chesler K, Korns ME, Edwards JE: Anomalies of the tricuspid valve, including pouches, resembling aneurysms of the membranous ventricular septum. *Am J Cardiol* 21:661, 1968.

19. Calder AL, Barratt-Boyes BG, Brandt PWT, Neutze JM: Postoperative evaluation of patients with tetralogy of Fallot repaired in infancy. *J Thorac Cardiovasc Surg* 77:704, 1979.

20. Calder AL, Kirker JA, Neutze JM, Starling MB: Pathology of the ductus arteriosus treated with prostaglandins. Comparison with untreated cases. *Pediatr Cardiol* 5:85, 1984.

D

1. Daily PO, Stinson EB, Griepp RB, Shumway NE: Tetralogy of Fallot. Choice of surgical procedure. *J Thorac Cardiovasc Surg* 75:338, 1978.

2. Dobell ARC, Charrette EP, Chughtai MS: Correction of tetralogy of Fallot in the young child. *J Thorac Cardiovasc Surg* 55:70, 1968.

3. Daoud G, Kaplan S, Helmsworth JA: Tetralogy of Fallot and pulmonary hypertension. *Am J Dis Child* 3:166, 1966.

4. Donahoo JS, Gardner TJ, Zahka K, Langford Kidd BS: Systemic-pulmonary shunts in neonates and infants using microporous expanded polytetrafluoroethylene: Immediate and late results. *Ann Thorac Surg* 30:146, 1980.

5. Dabizzi RP, Caprioli G, Alazzi L: Distribution and anomalies of coronary arteries in tetralogy of Fallot. *Circulation* 61:84, 1980.

6. de Leval MR, McKay R, Jones M, Stark J, Macartney FJ: Modified Blalock-Taussig shunt. Use of subclavian artery orifice as flow regulator in prosthetic systemic-pulmonary artery shunts. *J Thorac Cardiovasc Surg* 81:112, 1981.

7. D'Cruz I, Lendrum BL, Novak G: Congenital absence of the pulmonary valve. *Am Heart J* 68:728, 1964.

8. Delisle G, Olley PM: Epreuve d'effort sous-maximal chez les enfants atteints de tetralogie de Fallot: Avant et apres correction chirurgicale. *Union Med Can* 103:886, 1974.

9. Davidson JS: Anastomosis between the ascending aorta and the main pulmonary artery in the tetralogy of Fallot. *Thorax* 10:348, 1955.

10. Di Benedetto G, Tiraboschi R, Vanini V, Annecchino P, Aiazzi L, Caprioli C, Parenzan L: Systemic-pulmonary artery shunt using PTFE prosthesis (Gore-Tex). Early results and long-term follow-up on 105 consecutive cases. *Thorac Cardiovasc Surg* 29:143, 1981.

11. Downing JW Jr, Kaplan S, Bore KE: Postsurgical anterior hemiblock and right bundle branch block. *Br Heart J* 34:263, 1972.

12. Dickinson DF, Wilkinson JL, Smith A, Hamilton DI, Anderson RH: Variations in the morphology of the ventricular septal defect and disposition of the atrioventricular conduction tissues in tetralogy of Fallot. *Thorac Cardiovasc Surg* 30:243, 1982.

13. Deanfield JE, Yen Ho S, Anderson RH, McKenna WJ, Allwork SP, Hallidie-Smith KA: Late sudden death after repair of tetralogy of Fallot: A clinicopathologic study. *Circulation* 67:626, 1983.

14. Dolara A, Dellocchio T, Diligenti LM, Manetti A, Vergassola R: Pulmonary infundibular stenosis developing after closure of ventricular septal defect. *Acta Cardiol* (Brux) 30:221, 1975.

15. Danilowicz D, Hoffman JIE, Rudolph AM: Serial studies of pulmonary stenosis in infancy and childhood. *Br Heart J* 37:808, 1975.

16. Del Campo A, Blackstone EH, Kirklin JW: (1979) Unpublished data.

E

1. Edwards JE, McGoon DC: Absence of anatomic origin from heart of pulmonary arterial supply. *Circulation* 47:393, 1973.

2. Edmunds LH, Saxena NC, Friedman S, Rashkind WJ, Dodd PF. Transatrial resection of the obstructed right ventricular infundibulum. *Circulation* 54:117, 1976.

3. Edmunds LH, Saxena NC, Friedman S, Rashkind WJ, Dodd PF. Transatrial repair of tetralogy of Fallot. *Surgery* 80:681, 1976.

4. Ergin MA, Griepp RB: Total correction of tetralogy of Fallot. How to deal with complicated ascending aorta-right pulmonary artery anastomosis. *J Thorac Cardiovasc Surg* 77:469, 1979.

5. Epstein SE, Beiser GD, Goldstein RE, Rosing DR, Redwood DR, Morrow AG: Hemodynamic abnormalities in response to mild and intense upright exercise following operative correction of an atrial septal defect or tetralogy of Fallot. *Circulation* 47:1065, 1973.

6. Emanuel RW, Pattison JN: Absence of the left pulmonary artery in Fallot's tetralogy. *Br Heart J* 18:289, 1956.

7. Ebert PA: Second operations for pulmonary stenosis or insufficiency after repair of tetralogy of Fallot. *Am J Cardiol* 50:637, 1982.

8. Eakin WW, Abbott ME: Stenosis of the pulmonary conus at the lower bulbar orifice (conus a separate chamber) and closed interventricular septum with two illustrative cases. Presented before the Meeting of the American Association of Pathologists and Bacteriologists, Washington, D.C., May 9, 1933.

9. Ehrenhaft JL, Theilen EO, Fisher J: Ectopic tricuspid leaflet producing symptoms of infundibular pulmonic stenosis. *Ann Surg* 150:937, 1959.

10. Emmanouilides GC, Thanopoulos B, Siassi B, Fishbein M: Agenesis of ductus arteriosus associated with the syndrome of tetralogy of Fallot and absent pulmonary valve. *Am J Cardiol* 37:403, 1976.

11. Ebert PA: Discussion of paper by Edmunds et al.[E3]

F

1. Ferencz C: The pulmonary vascular bed in tetralogy of Fallot. I. changes associated with pulmonary stenosis. *Bull Johns Hopkins Hosp* 106:81, 1960.

2. Ferencz C: The pulmonary vascular bed in tetralogy of Fallot. II. changes following a systemic-pulmonary arterial anastomosis. *Bull Johns Hopkins Hosp* 106:100, 1960.

3. Fuster V, McGoon DC, Kennedy MA, Ritter DC, Kirklin JW: Long-term evaluation (12 to 22 years) of open heart surgery for tetralogy of Fallot. *Am J Cardiol* 46:635, 1980.

4. Fellows KE, Smith J, Keane JF: Preoperative angiocardiography in infants with tetrad of Fallot. Review of 36 cases. *Am J Cardiol* 47:1279, 1981.

5. Fellows KE, Freed MK, Keane JR, Van Praagh R, Bernhard WF, Castaneda AR: Results of routine preoperative coronary angiography in tetralogy of Fallot. *Circulation* 51:561, 1975.

6. Furuse A, Mizuno A, Shindo G, Yamaguchi T, Saigusa M: Optimal size of outflow patch in total correction of tetralogy of Fallot. *Jpn Heart J* 18:629, 1977.

7. Furuse A, Mizuno A, Shindo G, Yamaguchi T, Saigusa M: Pulmonary regurgitation following total correction of tetralogy of Fallot. *Jpn Heart J* 18:621, 1977.

8. Freedom RM, Pongiglione G, Williams WG, Trusler GA, Rowe RD: Palliative right ventricular outflow tract construction for patients with pulmonary atresia, ventricular septal defect, and hypoplastic pulmonary arteries. *J Thorac Cardiovasc Surg* 86:24, 1983.

9. Finnegan P, Haider R, Patel RG, Abrams LD, Singh SP: Results of total correction of the tetralogy of Fallot. Long-term haemodynamic evaluation at rest and during exercise. *Br Heart J* 38:934, 1976.

10. Fontan FM, Choussat A, Deville C, Doutremepuich CDC, Coupilland J, Vosa C: Aortic valve homografts in the surgical treatment of complex cardiac malformations. *J Thorac Cardiovasc Surg* 87:649, 1984.

11. Fabricius J, Hansen PF, Lindeneg O: Pulmonary atresia developing after a shunt operation for Fallot's tetralogy. *Br Heart J* 23:556, 1961.

12. Faller K, Haworth SG, Taylor JFN, Macartney FJ: Duplicate sources of pulmonary blood supply in pulmonary atresia with ventricular septal defect. *Br Heart J* 46:263, 1981.

13. Feldt RH, DuShane JW, Titus JL: The anatomy of the atrioventricular conduction system in ventricular septal defect and tetralogy of Fallot: Correlations with the electrocardiogram and vectorcardiogram. *Circulation* 34:774, 1966.

14. Freedom RM, Pongiglione G, Williams WG, Trusler GA, Moes CAF, Rowe RD: Pulmonary vein wedge angiography: Indications, results, and surgical correlates in 25 patients. *Am J Cardiol* 51:936, 1983.

15. Forster JW, Humphries JO: Right ventricular anomalous muscle bundle. Clinical and laboratory presentation and natural history. *Circulation* 43:115, 1971.

16. Flege JB Jr, Vlad P, Ehrenhaft JL: Aneurysm of the tricuspid valve causing infundibular obstruction. *Ann Thorac Surg* 3:446, 1967.

G

1. Graham TP Jr, Cordell D, Atwood GF, Boucek RJ, Boerth RC, Bender HW, Nelson JH, Vaughn WK: Right ventricular volume characteristics before and after palliative and reparative operation in tetralogy of Fallot. *Circulation* 54:417, 1976.

2. Goldman BS, Mustard WT, Trusler GS: Total correction of tetralogy of Fallot. *Br Heart J* 30:563, 1968.

3. Gasul BM, Dillon RF, Urla V: The natural transformation of ventricular septal defects into ventricular septal defects with pulmonary stenosis and/or into tetralogy of Fallot. *Am J Dis Child* 94:424, 1957.

4. Gotsman MS: Increasing obstruction to the outflow tract in Fallot's tetralogy. *Br Heart J* 28:615, 1966.

5. Garson A Jr, Gillette PC, McNamara DG: Propranolol: The preferred palliation for tetralogy of Fallot. *Am J Cardiol* 47:1098, 1981.

6. Garson A Jr, Nihill MR, McNamara DG, Cooley DA: Status of the adult and adolescent after repair of tetralogy of Fallot. *Circulation* 59:1232, 1979.

7. Garson A Jr, Gillette PC, Gutgesell HP, McNamara DG: Stress-induced ventricular arrhythmia after repair of tetralogy of Fallot. *Am J Cardiol* 46:1006, 1980.

8. Graham TP Jr, Faulker Scott, Bender H Jr, Wender CM: Hypoplasia of the left ventricle: Rare cause of postoperative mortality in tetralogy of Fallot. *Am J Cardiol* 40:454, 1977.

9. Graham TP Jr, Erath HG Jr, Boucek RJ Jr, Boerth RC: Left ventricular function in cyanotic congenital heart disease. *Am J Cardiol* 45:1231, 1980.

10. Gross RE, Bernhard WF, Litwin SB: Closure of Potts anastomosis in the total repair of tetralogy of Fallot. *J Thorac Cardiovasc Surg* 57:72, 1969.

11. Glancy DL, Morrow AG, Robert WC: Malformations of the aortic valve in patients with the tetralogy of Fallot. *Am Heart J* 76:755, 1968.

12. Guyton RA, Owens JE, Waumett JD, Dooley KJ, Hatcher CR Jr, Williams WH: The Blalock-Taussig shunt: Low risk, effective palliation, and pulmonary artery growth. *J Thorac Cardiovasc Surg* 85:917, 1983.

13. Gale AW, Arciniegas E, Green EW, Blackstone EH, Kirklin JW: Growth of the pulmonary anulus and pulmonary arteries after the Blalock-Taussig shunt. *J Thorac Cardiovasc Surg* 77:459, 1979.

14. Gay WA Jr, Ebert PA: Aorto-to-right pulmonary artery anastomosis causing obstruction of the right pulmonary artery. *Ann Thorac Surg* 16:402, 1973.

15. Gill CC, Moodie DS, McGoon DC: Staged surgical management of pulmonary atresia with diminutive pulmonary arteries. *J Thorac Cardiovasc Surg* 73:436, 1977.

16. Gazzaniga AB, Elliott MP, Sperling DR, Dietrick WR, Eisenman JI, McRae DM, Bartlett RH: Microporous expanded polytetrafluoroethylene arterial prosthesis for construction of aorto-pulmonary shunts. Experimental and clinical results. *Ann Thorac Surg* 21:322, 1976.

17. Gazzaniga AB, Lamberti JJ, Siewers RD, Sperling DR, Dietrick WR, Arcilla RA, Replogle RL: Arterial prosthesis of microporous expanded polytetrafluoroethylene for construction of aorto-pulmonary shunts. *J Thorac Cardiovasc Surg* 72:357, 1976.

18. Goor DA, Smolinsky A, Mohr R, Caspi J, Shem-Tov A: The 24-hour drop of residual right ventricular pressure after conservative infundibulectomy in repair of tetralogy of Fallot. *J Thorac Cardiovasc Surg* 81:897, 1981.

19. Gerbode, F: In discussion of Pacifico et al.[P10] (1977).

20. Gillette PC, Yeoman MA, Mullins CE, McNamara DG: Sudden death after repair of tetralogy of Fallot. Electrocardiographic and electrophysiologic abnormalities. *Circulation* 56:566, 1977.

21. Grinnell VS, Mehringer CM, Hieshima GB, Stanley P, Lurie PR: Transaortic occlusion of collateral arteries to the lung by detachable valved balloons in a patient with tetralogy of Fallot. *Circulation* 65:1276, 1982.

22. Gallucci V, Scalia D, Thiene G, Mazzucco A, Valfre C: Double-chambered right ventricle: Surgical experience and anatomical considerations. *Thorac Cardiovasc Surgeon* 28:13, 1980.

23. Grant RP, Downey FM, MacMahon H: The architecture of the right ventricular outflow tract in the normal human heart and in the presence of ventricular septal defects. *Circulation* 24:223, 1961.

H

1. Harms D, Hansen P, Fischer K, Bernhard A: Pathology of the "Fallot Lung." *Virchows Arch Abt A Path Anat* 361:77, 1973.

2. Hudspeth AS, Cordell AR, Johnston FR: Transatrial approach to total correction of tetralogy of Fallot. *Circulation* 27:796, 1963.

3. Hawe A, McGoon DC, Kincaid OW, Ritter DG: Fate of outflow tract in tetralogy of Fallot. *Ann Thorac Surg* 13:137, 1972.

4. Honey M, Chamberlain DA, Howard J: The effect of beta-sympathetic blockade on arterial oxygen saturation in Fallot's tetralogy. *Circulation* 30:501, 1964.

5. Harken AH, Horowitz LN, Josephson ME: Surgical correction of recurrent sustained ventricular tachycardia following complete repair of tetralogy of Fallot. *J Thorac Cardiovasc Surg* 80:779, 1980.

6. Hislop A, Reid L: Structural changes in the pulmonary arteries and veins in tetralogy of Fallot. *Br Heart J* 35:1178, 1973.

7. Hjelms E, Pohlner P, Barratt-Boyes BG, Gavin JB: Study of autologous pericardial patch-grafts in the right ventricular outflow tracts in growing and adult dogs. *J Thorac Cardiovasc Surg* 81:120, 1981.

8. Hiraishi S, Bargeron LM, Isabel-Jones JB, Emmanouilides GC, Friedman WF, Jarmakani JM: Ventricular and pulmonary artery volumes in patients with absent pulmonary valve. Factors affecting the natural course. *Circulation* 67:183, 1983.

9. Hirschfeld S, Tuboku-Metzger AJ, Borkat G, Ankeney J, Clayman J, Liebman J: Comparison of exercise and catheterization results following total surgical correction of tetralogy of Fallot. *J Thorac Cardiovasc Surg* 75:446, 1978.

10. Harris AM, Segel N, Bishop JM: Blalock-Taussig anastomosis for tetralogy of Fallot. A ten-to-fifteen year follow-up. *Br Heart J* 26:266, 1964.

11. Hofschire PJ, Rosenquist GC, Ruckerman RN, Moller JH, Edwards JE: Pulmonary vascular disease complicating the Blalock-Taussig anastomosis. *Circulation* 56:124, 1977.

12. Hancock EW, Hultgren HN, March HW: Pulmonary hypertension after Blalock-Taussig anastomosis. *Am Heart J* 67:817, 1964.

13. Haworth SG, Macartney FJ. Growth and development of pulmonary circulation in pulmonary atresia with ventricular septal defect and major aortopulmonary collateral arteries. *Br Heart J* 44:14, 1980.

14. Hamilton DI, Di Eusanio G, Piccoli GP, Dickinson DF: Eight years experience with intracardiac repair of tetralogy of Fallot. Early and late results in 175 consecutive patients. *Br Heart J* 46:144, 1981.

15. Haworth SG, Rees PG, Taylor JFN, Macartney FJ, de Leval M, Stark J: Pulmonary atresia with ventricular septal defect and major aortopulmonary collateral arteries; effect of systemic-pulmonary anastomosis. *Br Heart J* 45:133, 1981.

16. Haworth SG: Collateral arteries in pulmonary atresia with ventricular septal defect. A precarious blood supply. *Br Heart J* 44:5, 1980.

17. Haworth SG, Reid L: Quantitative structural study of pulmonary circulation in the newborn with pulmonary atresia. *Thorax* 32:129, 1977.

18. Hartmann AF Jr, Tsifutis AA, Arvidsson H, Goldring D: The two-chambered right ventricle. Report of nine cases. *Circulation* 26:279, 1962.

19. Hartmann AF Jr, Goldring D, Carlsson E: Development of right ventricular obstruction by aberrant muscular bands. *Circulation* 30:679, 1964.

20. Hartmann AF Jr, Goldring D, Ferguson TB, Burford WH, Smith CH, Kissane JM, Frich RF: The course of children with two chambered RV. *J Thorac Cardiovasc Surg* 60:72, 1970.

21. Hu DCK, Seward JB, Puga FJ, Fuster V, Tajik AJ: Total correction of tetralogy of Fallot at age 40 years and older: Long-term followup. *JACC* 5:40, 1985.

I

1. Ilbawi MN, Idriss FS, Muster AJ, Wessel HU, Paul MH, DeLeon SY: Tetralogy of Fallot with absent pulmonary valve. Should valve insertion be part of the intracardiac repair? *J Thorac Cardiovasc Surg* 81:906, 1981.

2. Imai Y, Nishiya Y, Morikawa T, Kurosawa H, Konno S: Total correction of tetralogy of Fallot associated with an anomalous left pulmonary artery arising from the aortic arch. *J Thorac Cardiovasc Surg* 68:51, 1974.

3. Ionescu MJ, Tandon AP, Macartney FJ: Long-term sequential hemodynamic evaluation of right ventricular outflow tract reconstruction using a valve mechanism. *Ann Thorac Surg* 27:426, 1979.

4. Ilbawi MN, Grieco J, DeLeon SY, Idriss FS, Muster AJ, Berry TE, Klich J: Modified Blalock-Taussig shunt in newborn infants. *J Thorac Cardiovasc Surg* 88:770, 1984.

J

1. Jones EL, Conti R, Neill CA, Gott VL, Brawler RK, Haller JA Jr: Long-term evaluation of tetralogy patients with pulmonary valvular insufficiency resulting from outflow-patch correction across the pulmonic annulus. *Circulation* 47 and 48:(suppl III):III-11, 1973.

2. Jaumin P, Tremouroux-Wattiez M, Vliers A, Stijns J, Kestens-Servaye Y, Ravean A, Goenen M, Tremouroux J, Polour H, Poulet R, Chalant C: Resultats de la chirurgie reparatrice de la tetralogie de Fallot. *Ann Chir Thorac Cardiovasc* 14:221, 1975.

3. Jarmakani JM, Graham TP Jr, Canent RV Jr: Left heart function in children with tetralogy of Fallot before and after palliative or corrective surgery. *Circulation* 46:478, 1972.

4. Jarmakani JM, Nakazawa M, Isabel-Jones J: Right ventricular function in children with tetralogy of Fallot before and after aortic to pulmonary shunt. *Circulation* 53:555, 1976.

5. James FW, Kaplan S, Schwartz DC, Chou TC, Sandker MJ, Naylor V: Response to exercise in patients after total surgical correction of tetralogy of Fallot. *Circulation* 54:671, 1976.

6. Joransen JA, Lucas RV Jr, Moller JH: Postoperative haemodynamics in tetralogy of Fallot. A study of 132 children. *Br Heart J* 41:33, 1979.

7. Jefferson K, Rees S, Somerville J: Systemic arterial supply to the lungs in pulmonary atresia and its relation to pulmonary artery development. *Br Heart J* 34:418, 1972.

8. Johnson RJ, Haworth SG: Pulmonary vascular and alveolar development in tetralogy of Fallot: A recommendation for early correction. *Thorax* 37:893, 1982.

K

1. Kerr AR, Barratt-Boyes BG: Surgery of tetralogy of Fallot in infancy: comparison of shunt palliation and primary intracardiac repair, in BG Barratt-Boyes, JM Neutze, EA Harris (eds): *Heart Disease in Infancy.* Edinburgh: Churchill Livingstone, 1973.

2. Kirklin JW, DuShane JW, Patrick RT, Donald DE, Hetzel PS, Harshbarger HG, Wood EH: Intracardiac surgery with the aid of a mechanical pump-oxygenator system (Gibbon type): Report of eight cases. *Proc Staff Meet Mayo Clin* 30:201, 1955.

3. Kirklin JW, Ellis FH Jr, McGood DC, DuShane JW, Swan HFC: Surgical treatment for the tetralogy of Fallot by open intracardiac repair. *J Thorac Surg* 37:22, 1959.

4. Kirklin JW, Payne WS: Surgical treatment for tetralogy of Fallot after previous anastomosis of systemic to pulmonary artery. *Surg Gynecol Obstet* 110:707, 1960.

5. Kirklin JW, Payne WS, Theye RA, DuShane JW: Factors affecting survival after open operation for tetralogy of Fallot. *Ann Surg* 152:485, 1960.

6. Kirklin JK, Westaby S, Chenoweth D, Blackstone EH, Kirklin JW, Pacifico AD: Complement and the damaging effects of cardiopulmonary bypass. *J Thorac Cardiovasc Surg* 86:845, 1983.

7. Kirklin JW, Blackstone EH, Pacifico AD, Brown RN, Bargeron LM Jr: Routine primary repair vs two-stage repair of tetralogy of Fallot. *Circulation* 60:373, 1979.

8. Kirklin JW, Devloo RA: Hypothermic perfusion and circulatory arrest for surgical correction of tetralogy of Fallot with previously constructed Potts' anastomosis. *Dis Chest* 39:87, 1961.

9. Kirklin JW, Wallace RB, McGoon DC, DuShane JW: Early and late results after intracardiac repair of tetralogy of Fallot: 5-year review of 337 patients. *Ann Surg* 162:578, 1965.

10. Kawashima Y, Kitamura S, Nakano S, Yagihara T: Corrective surgery for tetralogy of Fallot without or with minimal right ventriculotomy and with repair of the pulmonary valve. *Circulation* 64:11–147, 1981.

11. Kirklin JW, Blackstone EH, Kirklin JK, Pacifico AD, Aramendi J, Bargeron LM Jr: Surgical results and protocols in the spectrum of tetralogy of Fallot. *Ann Surg* 198:251, 1983.

12. Katz NM, Blackstone EH, Kirklin JW, Pacifico AD, Bargeron LM Jr: Late survival and symptoms after repair of tetralogy of Fallot. *Circulation* 65:403, 1982.

13. Kahn DR: Discussion of paper by Dobell et al.[D2]

14. Kirklin JW, Blackstone EH: Editorial on papers by Naito, Wessel, and their colleagues. *J Thorac Cardiovasc Surg* 80:594, 1980.

15. Kawashima Y, Mori T, Kitamura S, Hirose H, Nakano S, Yagihara T: Trans-pulmonary arterial, trans-right atrial repair of tetralogy of Fallot. *J Jpn Surg Soc* 80:1259, 1979.

16. Keck EW, Brode P: Beta-receptor blockade in Fallot's tetralogy. *Dtsch Med Wochenschr* 95:766, 1970.

17. Klinner W: Klinische und experimentelle untersuchungen zur operativen korrektur der Fallotschen tetralogie. *Aus der Chirurgischen Klinik der Universitat Munchen*, 1961.

18. Kuers PF, McGoon DC: Tetralogy of Fallot with aortic origin of right pulmonary artery. *J Thorac Cardiovasc Surg* 65:327, 1973.

19. Kirklin JW, Karp RB: *The Tetralogy of Fallot.* Philadelphia: W. B. Saunders Co., 1970.

20. Kirklin JW, Bargeron LM Jr, Pacifico AD: The enlargement of small pulmonary arteries by preliminary palliative operations. *Circulation* 56:612, 1977.

21. Kirklin JW: Reviewer's comment of paper by Freedom et al.[F8] *J Thorac Cardiovasc Surg* 86:24, 1983.

22. Kirklin JK, Blackstone EH, Brown RN, Kirklin JW: Unpublished data.

23. Klinner VW, Pasini M, Schaudig A: Anastomose zwischen system- und lungenarterie mit hilfe von kunststoffprothesen bei cyanotischen herzvitien. *Thoraxchirurgie* 10:68, 1962.

24. Krongrad E, Ritter DG, Hawe A, Kincaid OW, McGoon DC: Pulmonary atresia or severe stenosis and coronary artery-to-pulmonary artery fistula. *Circulation* 46:1005, 1972.

25. Kay PH, Capuani A, Franks R, Lincoln C: Experience with the modified Blalock-Taussig operation using polytetrafluoroethylene (Impra) grafts. *Br Heart J* 49:359, 1983.

26. Kavey REW, Blackman MS, Sondheimer HM: Incidence and severity of chronic ventricular dysrhythmias after repair of tetralogy of Fallot. *Am Heart J* 103:342, 1982.

27. Kirklin JW, Openshaw CR, Tompkins RG: Surgical treatment of infundibular stenosis with intact ventricular septum. *Ann Surg* 137:228, 1953.

28. Kavey REW, Thomas FD, Byrum CJ, Blackman MS, Sondheimer HM, Bove EL: Ventricular arrhythmias and biventricular dysfunction after repair of tetralogy of Fallot. *JACC* 4:126, 1984.

29. Klinner W, Reichart B, Pfaller M, Hatz P: Late results after correction of tetralogy of Fallot necessitating outflow tract reconstruction. Comparison with results after correction without outflow tract patch. *Thorac Cardiovasc Surgeon* 32:244, 1984.

30. Kobayashi J, Hirose H, Nakano S, Matsuda H, Shirakura R, Kawashima Y: Ambulatory electrocardiographic study of the frequency and cause of ventricular arrhythmia after correction of tetralogy of Fallot. *Am J Cardiol* 54:1310, 1984.

31. Kay PH, Capuani A, Franks R, Lincoln C: Experience with the modified Blalock-Taussig operation using polytetrafluoroethylene (Impra) grafts. *Br Heart J* 49:359, 1983.

L

1. Lev M, Eckner FAO: The pathologic anatomy of tetralogy of Fallot and its variations. *Dis Chest* 45:251, 1964.

2. Lev M, Rimoldi HJA, Rowlatt DF: Quantitative anatomy of cyanotic tetralogy of Fallot. *Circulation* 30:531, 1964.

3. Lillehei CW, Cohen M, Warden HE, Read RC, Aust JB, DeWall RA, Varco RL: Direct vision intracardiac surgical correction of the tetralogy of Fallot, pentalogy of Fallot, and pulmonary atresia defects: Report of first ten cases. *Ann Surg* 142:418, 1955.

4. Lillehei CW, Levy MJ, Adams P, Anderson RC: Corrective surgery for tetralogy of Fallot. *J Thorac Cardiovasc Surg* 48:556, 1964.

5. Laks H, Hellenbrand WE, Kleinman CS, Stansel HC Jr, Talner NS: Patch reconstruction of the right ventricular outflow tract with pulmonary valve insertion. *Circulation* 64(suppl II):II-154, 1981.

6. Levine FH, Reis RL, Morrow AG: Incidence and significance of patent foramen ovale after correction of tetralogy of Fallot. *Ann Thorac Surg* 13:464, 1972.

7. Litwin SB, Rosenthal A, Fellows K: Surgical management of young infants with tetralogy of Fallot, absence of the pulmonary valve, and respiratory distress. *J Thorac Cardiovasc Surg* 65:552, 1973.

8. Lakier JB, Stanger P, Heymann MA, Hoffman JIE, Rudolph AM: Tetralogy of Fallot with absent pulmonary valve. Natural history and hemodynamic considerations. *Circulation* 50:167, 1974.

9. Laks H, Castaneda AR: Subclavian arterioplasty for the ipsilateral Blalock-Taussig shunt. *Ann Thorac Surg* 19:319, 1975.

10. Lang P, Chipman CW, Siden H, Williams RG, Norwood WI, Castaneda AR: Early assessment of hemodynamic status after repair of tetralogy of Fallot: A comparison of 24 hour (intensive care unit) and 1 year postoperative data in 98 patients. *Am J Cardiol* 50:795, 1982.

11. Lecompte Y, Hazan E, Baillot F, Jarreau MM, Mathey J: La reparation chirurgicale de la voie pulmonaire dans la tetralogie de Fallot: *Coeur* 3:739, 1977.

12. Lock JE, Niemi T, Einzig S, Amplatz K, Burke B, Bass JL: Transvenous angioplasty of experimental branch pulmonary artery stenosis in newborn lambs. *Circulation* 64:886, 1981.

13. Lock JE, Castaneda-Zuniga WR, Fuhrman BP, Bass JL: Balloon dilation angioplasty of hypoplastic and stenotic pulmonary arteries. *Circulation* 67:962, 1983.

14. Lev M: The architecture of the conduction system in congenital heart disease. II Tetralogy of Fallot. *AMA Arch Pathol* 67:572, 1958.

15. Lange PE, Onnasch DGW, Bernhard A, Heintzen PH: Left and right ventricular adaptation to right ventricular overload before and after surgical repair of tetralogy of Fallot. *Am J Cardiol* 50:786, 1982.

16. Li MD, Coles JC, McDonald AC: Anomalous muscle bundle of the right ventricle. Its recognition and surgical treatment. *Br Heart J* 40:1040, 1978.

17. Lucas RV Jr, Varco RL, Lillehei CW, Adams P Jr, Anderson RC, Edwards JE: Anomalous muscle bundle of the right ventricle. Hemodynamic consequences and surgical considerations. *Circulation* 25:443, 1962.

18. Levy MJ, Lillehei CW, Elliott LP, Carey LS, Adams P Jr, Edwards JE: Accessory valvular tissue causing subpulmonary stenosis in corrected transposition of great vessels. *Circulation* 27:494, 1963.

19. Lappen RS, Riggs TW, Lapin GD, Paul MH, Muster AJ: Two-dimensional echocardiographic measurement of right pulmonary artery diameter in infants and children. *JACC* 2:121, 1983.

20. Lamberti JJ, Carlisle J, Waldman JD, Lodge FA, Kirkpatrick SE, George L, Mathewson JW, Turner SW, Pappelbaum SJ: Systemic-pulmonary shunts in infants and children. *J Thorac Cardiovasc Surg* 88:76, 1984.

M

1. Monties JR, Goudard A, Fogliani J, Bandini A, Blanc-Gauthier T: Correction de la tetralogie de Fallot avant l'age de 5 ans. *Ann Chir Thorac Cardiovasc* 14:229, 1975.

2. Moffitt EA, Kirklin JW, Theye RA: Physiologic studies during whole-body perfusion in tetralogy of Fallot. *J Thorac Cardiovasc Surg* 44:180, 1962.

3. Miller GAH, Kirklin JW, Rahimtoola S, Swan HFC: Volume of the left ventricle in tetralogy of Fallot. *Am J Cardiol* 16:488, 1965.

4. De Matteis A: The vascular pathology of the lung in congenital malformations of the heart with severe pulmonary stenosis or atresia and right-to-left shunt. *Respiration* 26:337, 1969.

5. McCord MC, van Elk J, Blount G Jr: Tetralogy of Fallot clinical and hemodynamic spectrum of combined pulmonary stenosis and ventricular septal defects. *Circulation* 16:736, 1957.

6. Morgan JR: Left pulmonary artery from ascending aorta in tetralogy of Fallot. *Circulation* 45:653, 1972.

7. Miller RA, Lev M, Paul MH: Congenital absence of the pulmonary valve. The clinical syndrome of tetralogy of Fallot with pulmonary regurgitation. *Circulation* 26:266, 1962.

8. Marcelletti C, McGoon DC: Pulmonary infarction following ligation of terminally shunted pulmonary artery. *J Thorac Cardiovasc Surg* 71:746, 1976.

9. Matsuda H, Ihara K, Mori T, Kitamura S, Kawashima Y: Tetralogy of Fallot associated with aortic insufficiency. *Ann Thorac Surg* 29:529, 1980.

10. McGoon DC, Danielson GK, Puga FJ, Ritter DG, Mair DD, Illstrup DM: Late results after extracardiac conduit repair for congenital cardiac defects. *Am J Cardiol* 49:1741, 1982.

11. Miller DC, Rossiter SJ, Stinson EB, Oyer PE, Reitz BA, Shumway NE: Late right heart reconstruction following repair of tetralogy of Fallot. *Ann Thorac Surg* 28:239, 1979.

12. Macartney F, Miller GAH: Congenital absence of the pulmonary valve. *Br Heart J* 32:483, 1970.

13. McKay R, deLeval MR, Rees P, Taylor JFN, Macartney FJ, Stark J: Postoperative angiographic assessment of modified Blalock-Taussig shunts using expanded polytetrafluoroethylene (Gore-Tex). *Ann Thorac Surg* 30:137, 1980.

14. Mizuno A, Sato F, Hasegawa T, Tsuzuki M, Furuse A, Kotoda T, Saigusa M: Acquired obstruction of the right ventricular outflow tract in tetralogy of Fallot after Blalock-Taussig anastomosis. Report of two cases successfully treated with total correction. *Jpn Heart J* 11:113, 1970.

15. Marchand P: The use of a cusp-bearing homograft patch to the outflow tract and pulmonary artery in Fallot's tetralogy and pulmonary valvular stenosis. *Thorax* 22:497, 1967.

16. McGoon DC, Baird DK, Davis GD: Surgical management of large bronchial collateral arteries with pulmonary stenosis or atresia. *Circulation* 52:109, 1975.

17. Muraoka R, Yokota M, Matsuda K, Tabata R, Hikasa Y: Long-term hemodynamic evaluation of primary total correction of tetralogy of Fallot during the first two years of life. *Arch Jpn Chir* 42:315, 1973.

18. Murphy JD, Freed MD, Keane JF, Norwood WI, Castaneda AR, Nadas AS: Hemodynamic results after intracardiac repair of tetralogy of Fallot by deep hypothermia and cardiopulmonary bypass. *Circulation* 62(suppl I):I-168, 1980.

19. Macartney F, Deverall P, Scott O: Haemodynamic characteristics of systemic arterial blood supply to the lungs. *Br Heart J* 35:28, 1973.

20. Macartney FJ, Scott O, Deverall PB: Haemodynamic and anatomical characteristics of pulmonary blood supply in pulmonary atresia with ventricular septal defect-including a case of persistent fifth aortic arch. *Br Heart J* 36:1049, 1974.

21. McGoon MD, Fulton RE, Davis GD, Ritter DG, Neill CA, White RI Jr: Systemic collateral and pulmonary artery stenosis in patients with congenital pulmonary valve atresia and ventricular septal defect. *Circulation* 56:473, 1977.

22. Mocellin R, Krettek M, Sauer U, Buhlmeyer K: Pulmonalatresie mit Ventrikelseptumdefekt. *Z Kardiol* 66:382, 1977.

23. Miller WW, Nadas AS, Bernhard WF, Gross RE: Congenital pulmonary atresia with ventricular septal defect. Review of the clinical course of fifty patients with assessment of the results of palliative surgery. *Am J Cardiol* 21:673, 1968.

24. Maron BJ, Ferrans VJ, White RI Jr: Unusual evolution of acquired infundibular stenosis in patients with ventricular septal defect. Clinical and morphologic observations. *Circulation* 48:1092, 1973.

25. Macedo MEM, Sena Lino JA, Lima M, Salomao CS: Left ventricular outflow tract obstruction due to tricuspid valve prolapse through a high ventricular septal defect. *Thorac Cardiovasc Surg* 31:110, 1983.

26. Maclean LD, Culligan JA, Kane DJ: Subaortic stenosis due to accessory tissue on the mitral valve. *J Thorac Cardiovasc Surg* 45:382, 1963.

27. McCaughan BC, Danielson GK, Driscoll DJ, McGoon DC: Tetralogy of Fallot with absent pulmonary valve. *J Thorac Cardiovasc Surg* 89:280, 1985.

N

1. Nagao GI, Daoud GI, McAdams AJ, Schwartz DC, Kaplan S: Cardiovascular anomalies associated with tetralogy of Fallot. *Am J Cardiol* 20:206, 1967.

2. Naito Y, Kawashima Y, Fujita Y, Miyamoto T, Okamoto S, Mori M, Danno M, Hashimoto S, Kato M, Manabe H: Surgical measures to improve operative results in total correction of severe tetralogy of Fallot. *Journal of Jpn Surg Soc* 72:1484, 1971.

3. Naito Y: Study on total correction of tetralogy of Fallot: Factors affecting operative mortality and surgical measures to improve operative results. *Jpn J Assoc Thorac Surg* 20:131, 1972.

4. Naito Y, Fujita T, Manabe H, Kawashima Y: The criteria for reconstruction of right ventricular outflow tract in total correction of tetralogy of Fallot. *J Thorac Cardiovasc Surg* 80:574, 1980.

5. Norwood WI, Freed MD, Rocchini AP, Bernhard WF, Castaneda AR: Experience with valved conduits for congenital heart disease. *Ann Thorac Surg* 24:223, 1977.

6. Neirotti R, Galindez E, Kreutzer G, et al: Tetralogy of Fallot with subpulmonary ventricular septal defect. *Ann Thorac Surg* 25:51, 1978.

7. Norberg WJ, Tadavarthy M, Knight L, Nicoloff DM, Moller JH: Late hemodynamic and angiographic findings after ascending aorta—pulmonary artery anastomosis. *J Thorac Cardiovasc Surg* 76:345, 1978.

8. Norwood NI, Rosenthal A, Castaneda AR: Tetralogy of Fallot with acquired pulmonary atresia and hypoplasia of pulmonary arteries. Report of surgical management in infancy. *J Thorac Cardiovasc Surg* 72:454, 1976.

9. Nomoto S, Muraoka R, Yokota M, Aoshima M, Kyoku I, Nakano H: Left ventricular volume as a predictor of the postoperative hemodynamics and a criterion for total correction of the tetralogy of Fallot. *J Thorac Cardiovasc Surg* 88:389, 1984.

10. Nottin R, Blondeau Ph, D'Allaines C, Carpentier A, Bouchard F, Dubost Ch: A study of long-term hemodynamic results following complete repair of tetralogy of Fallot. *Thorac Cardiovasc Surgeon* 27:211, 1979.

11. Newfeld EA, Waldman JD, Paul MH, Muster AJ, Cole RB, Idriss F, Riker W: Pulmonary vascular disease after systemic-pulmonary arterial shunt operations. *Am J Cardiol* 39:715, 1977.

12. Nihill MR, Mullins CE, McNamara DG: Visualization of the pulmonary arteries in pseudotruncus by pulmonary vein wedge angiography. *Circulation* 58:140, 1978.

13. Nanton MA, Belcourt CL, Gillis DA, Krause VW, Roy DL: Left ventricular outflow tract obstruction owing to accessory endocardial cushion tissue. *J Thorac Cardiovasc Surg* 78:537, 1979.

14. Neufeld HN, McGoon DC, DuShane JW, Edwards JE: Tetralogy of Fallot with anomalous tricuspid valve simulating pulmonary stenosis with intact septum. *Circulation* 22:1083, 1960.

15. Nakata S, Imai Y, Takanashi Y, Kurosawa H, Tezuka M, Nakazawa M, Ando M, Takao A: A new method for the quantitative standardization of cross sectional areas of the pulmonary arteries in congenital heart diseases with decreased pulmonary blood flow. *J Thorac Cardiovasc Surg* 88:610, 1984.

O

1. Olin CL, Ritter DG, McGoon DC, Wallace RB, Danielson GK: Pulmonary Atresia: Surgical correction and results in 103 patients undergoing definitive repair. *Circulation* 54(suppl III):III-35, 1976.

2. Ongley PA, Rahimtoola SH, Kincaid OW, Kirklin JW: Continuous murmurs in tetralogy of Fallot and pulmonary atresia with ventricular septal defect. *Am J Cardiol* 18:821, 1966.

3. Oku H: Operative results and postoperative hemodynamic results in total correction of tetralogy of Fallot. *Arch Jpn Chir* 45:87, 1976.

4. Oku H, Shirotani H, Yokoyama T, Yokota Y, Kawai J, Makino S, Noguchi K, Setsuie N, Nishioka T, Okamoto F, Shinohara T: Right ventricular outflow tract prosthesis in total correction of tetralogy of Fallot. *Circulation* 62:604, 1980.

5. Oku H, Shirotani H, Yokoyama T, Yokota Y, Kawai J, Mori A, Kanzaki Y, Makino S, Ando F, Setsuie N: Postoperative size of the right ventricular outflow tract and optimal age in complete repair of tetralogy of Fallot. *Ann Thorac Surg* 25:322, 1978.

6. Osman MZ, Meng CCL, Girdany BR: Congenital absence of the pulmonary valve. Report of eight cases with review of the literature. *Amer J Roentgenology* 106:58, 1969.

7. Opie JC, Sandor GGS, Ashmore PG, Patterson MWH: Successful palliation by pulmonary artery banding in absent pulmonary valve syndrome with aneurysmal pulmonary arteries. *J Thorac Cardiovasc Surg* 85:125, 1983.

8. Oberhansli I, Friedli B: Echocardiographic study of left and right ventricular dimension and left ventricular function in patients with tetralogy of Fallot, before and after surgery. *Br Heart J* 41:40, 1979.

9. Oelert H, Hetzer R, Luhmer I, Kalfelz HC, Borst HG: Criteria for and against primary correction of Fallot's tetralogy. *Thorac Cardiovasc Surgeon* 32:215, 1984.

P

1. Poirier RA, McGoon DC, Danielson GK, Wallace RB, Ritter DG, Moodie DS, Wiltse CG: Late results after repair of tetralogy of Fallot. *J Thorac Cardiovasc Surg* 73:900, 1977.

2. Potts WJ, Smith S, Gibson S: Anastomosis of the aorta to a pulmonary artery. *JAMA* 132:627, 1946.

3. Piehler JM, Danielson GK, McGoon DC, Wallace RB, Fulton RE, Mair DD: Management of pulmonary atresia with ventricular septal defect and hypoplastic pulmonary arteries by right ventricular outflow construction. *J Thorac Cardiovasc Surg* 80:552, 1980.

4. Ponce FE, Williams LC, Webb HM, Riopel DA, Hohn AR: Propranolol palliation of tetralogy of Fallot: experience with long-term drug treatment in pediatric patients. *Pediatrics* 52:100, 1973.

5. Pinsky WW, Nihill MR, Mullins CE, McNamara DG: Management of absent pulmonary valve syndrome. *Am J Cardiol* 39:311, 1977.

6. Parenzan L, Alfieri O, Vanini V, Bianchi T, Villani M, Tiraboschi R, Crupi G, Locatelli G: Waterston anastomosis for initial palliation of tetralogy of Fallot. *J Thorac Cardiovasc Surg* 82:176, 1981.

7. Puga FJ, DuShane JW, McGoon DC: Treatment of tetralogy of Fallot in children less than 4 years of age. *J Thorac Cardiovasc Surg* 64:247, 1972.

8. Pacifico AD, Bargeron LM Jr, Kirklin JW: Primary total correction of tetralogy of Fallot in children less than four years of age. *Circulation* 48:1085, 1973.

9. Piccoli GP, Dickinson DF, Musumeci F, Hamilton DI: A changing policy for the surgical treatment of tetralogy of Fallot: Early and late results in 235 consecutive patients. *Ann Thorac Surg* 33:365, 1982.

10. Pacifico AD, Kirklin JW, Blackstone EH: Surgical management of pulmonary stenosis in tetralogy of Fallot. *J Thorac Cardiovasc Surg* 74:382, 1977.

11. Puga FJ, McGoon DC, Julsrud PR, Danielson GK, Mair DD: Complete repair of pulmonary atresia with nonconfluent pulmonary arteries. *Ann Thorac Surg* 35:36, 1983.

12. Pacifico AD, Kirklin JW, Bargeron LM Jr, Soto B: Surgical treatment of common arterial trunk with pseudotruncus arteriosus. *Circulation* 49 and 50(suppl II):II-20, 1974.

13. Perloff JK, Ronan JA Jr, de Leon AC: Ventricular septal defect with the "two-chambered right ventricle." *Am J Cardiol* 16:894, 1965.

14. Pate JW, Richardson RL Jr, Giles HH: Accessory tricuspid leaflet producing right ventricular outflow obstruction. *New Engl J Med* 279:867, 1968.

15. Perasalo O, Halonen PI, Pyorala K, Telivuo L: Aneurysm of the membranous ventricular septum causing obstruction of the right ventricular outflow tract in a case of ventricular septal defect. *Acta Chir Scand* 285(suppl):123, 1961.

Q

1. Quattlebaum TB, Varghese J, Neill CA, Donahue JS: Sudden death among postoperative patients with tetralogy of Fallot. *Circulation* 54:289, 1976.

R

1. Rastelli GC, Ongley PA, Davis GD, Kirklin JW: Surgical repair for pulmonary valve atresia with coronary-pulmonary artery fistula: Report of case. *Mayo Clin Proc* 40:521, 1965.

2. Rich AR: A hitherto unrecognized tendency to the development of widespread pulmonary vascular obstruction in patients with congenital pulmonary stenosis (tetralogy of Fallot). *Bull Johns Hopkins Hosp* 82:389, 1948.

3. Rowlatt JF, Rimoldi HJA, Lev M: The quantitative anatomy of the normal child's heart. *Pediatr Clin North Am* 10:499, 1963.

4. Regis JE, Carvalho W Jr, de Oliveira FM, Araujo JAR, Mont-'Alverne R, Paes JN Jr, de Sousa JR: Tratamento cirurgico da tetralogia de Fallot com agenesia da arteria pulmonar esquerda. Relato de dois casos. *Arq Bras Cardiol* 38/1:39, 1982.

5. Rowe RD, Vlad P, Keith JD: Experiences with 180 cases of tetralogy of Fallot in infants and children. *Can Med Assoc J* 73:23, 1955.

6. Rees S, Somerville J: Aortography in Fallot's tetralogy and variants. *Br Heart J* 31:146, 1969.

7. Richardson JP, Clarke CP: Tetralogy of Fallot. Risk factors associated with complete repair. *Br Heart J* 38:926, 1976.

8. Robin E, Silberberg B, Ganguly SN, Magnisalis K: Aortic origin of the left pulmonary artery. Variant of tetralogy of Fallot. *Am J Cardiol* 35:324, 1975.

9. Rosenquist GC, Sweeney LJ, Stemple DR, Christianson SD, Rowe RD: Ventricular septal defect in tetralogy of Fallot. *Am J Cardiol* 31:749, 1973.

10. Ruttenberg HD, Carey LS, Adams P, Edwards J: Absence of the pulmonary valve in tetralogy of Fallot. *Am J Roentgenology* 91:500, 1964.

11. Rabinovitch M, Grady S, David I, Van Praagh R, Sauer U, Buhlmeyer K, Castaneda AR, Reid L, Silva DK: Compression of intrapulmonary bronchi by abnormally branching pulmonary arteries associated with absent pulmonary valves. *Am J Cardiol* 50:804, 1982.

12. Reduto LA, Berger HJ, Johnstone DE, Hellenbrand W, Wackers F J Th, Whittemore R, Cohen LS, Gottschalk A, Zaret BL: Radionuclide assessment of right and left ventricular exercise reserve after total correction of tetralogy of Fallot. *Am J Cardiol* 45:1013, 1980.

13. Rosing DR, Borer JS, Kent KM, et al. Long-term hemodynamic and electrocardiographic assessment following operative repair of tetralogy of Fallot. *Circulation* 58:(suppl I):I-209, 1978.

14. Rosenthal A, Gross RE, Pasternac A: Aneurysms of right ventricular outflow patches. *J Thorac Cardiovasc Surg* 63:735, 1972.

15. Roberts WC, Freisinger GC, Cohen LS, Mason DT, Ross RS: Acquired pulmonic atresia. Total obstruction to right ventricular outflow after systemic to pulmonary arterial anastomoses for cyanotic congenital cardiac disease. *Am J Cardiol* 24:335, 1969.

16. Rygg IH, Olesen K, Boesen I: The life history of tetralogy of Fallot. *Dan Med Bull* 18:(suppl II):25, 1971.

17. Reitman MJ, Galioto FM Jr, El-Said GM, Cooley DA, Hallman GL, McNamara DG: Ascending aorta to right pulmonary artery anastomosis. Immediate results in 123 patients and one month to six year follow-up in 74 patients. *Circulation* 49:952, 1974.

18. Regensburger D, Sievers HH, Lange PE, Heitzen PH, Bernhard A: Reconstruction of the right ventricular outflow tract in tetralogy of Fallot and pulmonary stenosis with a monocusp patch. *Thorac Cardiovasc Surg* 29:345, 1981.

19. Rohmer J, Van Der Mark F, Zijlstra WG: Pulmonary valve incompetence. II. Application of electromagnetic flow velocity catheters in children. *Cardiovasc Res* 10:46, 1976.

20. Rastelli GC, Titus JL, McGoon DC: Homograft of ascending aorta and aortic valve as a right ventricular outflow: An experimental approach to the repair of truncus arteriosus. *Arch Surg (Chicago)* 95:698, 1967.

21. Rocchini AP, Rosenthal A, Freed M, Castaneda AR, Nadas AS: Chronic congestive heart failure after repair of tetralogy of Fallot. *Circulation* 56:305, 1977.

22. Rabinovitch M, Herrera-DeLeon V, Castaneda AR, Reid L: Growth and development of the pulmonary vascular bed in patients with tetralogy of Fallot with or without pulmonary atresia. *Circulation* 64:1234, 1981.

23. Ross DN, Somerville J: Correction of pulmonary atresia with a homograft aortic valve. *Lancet* 2:1446, 1966.

24. Rizzoli G, Blackstone EH, Kirklin JW, Pacifico AD, Bargeron LM Jr: Incremental risk factors in hospital mortality rate after repair of ventricular septal defect. *J Thorac Cardiovasc Surg* 80:494, 1980.

25. Rowland TW, Rosenthal A, Castaneda AR: Double-chamber right ventricle: Experience with 17 cases. *Am Heart J* 89:455, 1975.

26. Riemenschneider TA, Goldberg SJ, Ruttenberg HD, Gyepes MT: Subpulmonic obstruction in complete (d) transposition produced by redundant tricuspid tissue. *Circulation* 39:603, 1969.

27. Ross DN, Somerville J: (1983) Personal communication.

28. Rosenthal A, Behrendt D, Sloan H, Ferguson P, Snedecor SM, Schork A: Long-term prognosis (15 to 26 years) after repair of tetralogy of Fallot: I. Survival and symptomatic status. *Ann Thorac Surg* 38:151, 1984.

29. Ramsey JM, Macartney FJ, Haworth SG: Tetralogy of Fallot with major aortopulmonary collateral arteries. *Br Heart J* 53:167, 1985.

30. Rittenhouse EA, Mansfield PB, Hall DG, Herndon SP, Jones TK, Kawabor: I, Stevenson JG, French JW, Stamm SJ: Tetralogy of Fallot: Selected staged management. *J Thorac Cardiovasc Surg* 89:772, 1985.

S

1. Starr A, Bonchek LI, Sunderland CO: Total correction of tetralogy of Fallot in infancy. *J Am Cardiovasc Surg* 65:45, 1973.

2. Stephenson LW, Friedman S, Edmunds LH Jr: Staged surgical management of tetralogy of Fallot in infants. *Circulation* 58:837, 1978.

3. Sanchez Cascos, A: Genetics of Fallot's tetralogy. *Br Heart J* 33:899, 1971.

4. Stafford EG, Mair DD, McGoon DC, Danielson GK: Tetralogy of Fallot with absent pulmonary valve. Surgical considerations and results. *Circulation* 47 and 48: suppl.III:III-24, 1973.

5. Shah P, Kidd L: Hemodynamic responses to exercise and to isoproterenol following total correction of Fallot's tetralogy. *J Thorac Cardiovasc Surg* 52:135, 1966.

6. Strieder DJ, Aziz K, Zaver AG, Fellows KE: Exercise tolerance after repair of tetralogy of Fallot. *Ann Thorac Surg* 19:397, 1975.

7. Seybold-Epting W, Chiariello L, Hallman GL, Cooley DA: Aneurysm of pericardial right ventricular outflow tract patches. *Ann Thorac Surg* 24:237, 1977.

8. Studer M, Blackstone EH, Kirklin JW, Pacifico AD, Soto B, Chung GKT, Kirklin JK, Bargeron LM Jr: Determinants of early and late results of repair of atrioventricular septal (canal) defects. *J Thorac Cardiovasc Surg* 84:523, 1982.

9. Steeg CN, Krongrad E, Davazhi F, Bowman FO, Malm JR, Gersony WM: Postoperative left anterior hemiblock and right bundle branch block following repair of tetralogy of Fallot. *Circulation* 51:1026, 1975.

10. Sunderland CO, Rosenberg JA, Menashe VC, Lees MH, Bonchek LI, Starr A: Total correction of tetralogy of Fallot under two years of age. Postoperative hemodynamic evaluation (abstract). *Circulation* 45 and 46:98, 1972.

11. Soto B, Pacifico AD, Ceballos R, Bargeron LM Jr: Tetralogy of Fallot: An angiographic-pathologic correlative study. *Circulation* 64:558, 1981.

12. Singh SP, Rigby ML, Astley R: Demonstration of pulmonary arteries by contrast injection into pulmonary vein. *Br Heart J* 40:55, 1978.

13. Shimazaki Y, Kawashima Y, Hirose H, Nakano S, Matsuda H, Kitamura S, Morimoto S: Operative results in patients with pseudotruncus arteriosus. *Ann Thorac Surg* 35:294, 1983.

14. Sievers HH, Lange PE, Regensburger D, Yankah CA, Onnasch DGW, Bursch J, Heintzen PH, Bernhard A: Short-term hemodynamic results after right ventricular outflow tract reconstruction using a cusp-bearing transannular patch. *J Thorac Cardiovasc Surg* 86:777, 1983.

15. Swan H, Hederman WP, Vigoda PS, Glount SG Jr: The surgical treatment of isolated infundibular stenosis. *J Thorac Cardiovasc Surg* 38:319, 1959.

16. Sellers RD, Lillehei CW, Edwards JE: Subaortic stenosis caused by anomalies of the atrioventricular valves. *J Thorac Cardiovasc Surg* 48:289, 1964.

17. Shuford WH, Sybert RG: *The Aortic Arch and Its Malformations with Emphasis on the Angiographic Features.* Springfield: Charles C. Thomas, 1974.

18. Sellors H: Surgery of pulmonary stenosis. A case in which the pulmonary valve was successfully divided. *Lancet* 1:988, 1948.

19. Somerville J and Ross DN: (1984) Personal communication.

20. Sebening F, Laas J, Meisner H, Struck E, Bühlmeyer K, Zwingers Th: The treatment of tetralogy of Fallot: Early repair or palliation? *Thorac Cardiovasc Surgeon* 32:201, 1984.

T

1. Theye RA, Kirklin JW: Physiologic studies early after repair of tetralogy of Fallot. *Circulation* 28:42, 1963.

2. Tucker WY, Turley K, Ullyot DJ, Ebert PA: Management of symptomatic tetralogy of Fallot in the first year of life. *J Thorac Cardiovasc Surg* 78:494, 1979.

3. Tay DJ, Engle MA, Ehlers KH, Levin AR: Early results and late developments of the Waterston anastomosis. *Circulation* 50:220, 1974.

4. Tyson KRT, Larrieu AJ, Kirchmer JR Jr: The Blalock-Taussig shunt in the first two years of life: A safe and effective procedure. *Ann Thorac Surg* 26:38, 1978.

5. Thiene G, Frescura C, Bini RM, Valente M, Gallucci V: Histology of pulmonary arterial supply in pulmonary atresia with ventricular septal defect. *Circulation* 60:1066, 1979.

6. Takamiya M, Tauge I, Tadokoro M: Retrograde pulmonary arteriography: A new approach to opacification of pulmonary artery in pulmonary atresia (abstr), in *Proceedings of the 13th International Congress of Radiology,* Madrid. Amsterdam: *Excerpta Medica,* 1973:233. (International Congress Series No. 301.)

7. Tsifutis AA, Hartmann AF Jr, Arvidsson H: Two-chambered right ventricle: report on seven patients (abstr). *Circulation* 24:1058, 1961.

V

1. Venugopal P, Subramanian S: Intracardiac repair of tetralogy of Fallot in patients under 5 years of age. *Ann Thorac Surg* 18:228, 1974.

2. Van Praagh R, McNamara JJ: Anatomic types of ventricular septal defect with aortic insufficiency: Diagnostic and surgical considerations. *Am Heart J* 75:604, 1968.

3. Van Praagh R, Van Praagh S, Nebesar RA, Muster AJ, Sinha SN, Paul MH: Tetralogy of Fallot: Underdevelopment of the pulmonary infundibulum and its sequelae. *Am J Cardiol* 26:25, 1970.

4. Von Bernuth G, Ritter DG, Frye RL, Weidman WH, Davis GD, McGoon DC: Evaluation of patients with tetralogy of Fallot and Potts anastomosis. *Am J Cardiol* 27:259, 1971.

5. Villani M, Gamba A, Tiraboschi R, Crupi G, Parenzan L: Surgical treatment of tetralogy of Fallot. Recent experience using a prospective protocol. *Thorac Cardiovasc Surg* 31:151, 1983.

6. Van Praagh R, Corwin RD, Dahlquist EH Jr, Freedom RM, Mattioli L, Nebesar RA: Tetralogy of Fallot with severe left ventricular outflow tract obstruction due to anomalous attachment of the mitral valve to the ventricular septum. *Am J Cardiol* 26:93, 1970.

W

1. Waterston DJ: Treatment of Fallot's tetralogy in children under one year of age. *Rozhl Chir* 41:181, 1962.

2. Wessel HU, Cunningham WJ, Paul MH, Bastanier CK, Muster AJ, Idriss FS: Exercise performance in tetralogy of Fallot after intracardiac repair. *J Thorac Cardiovasc Surg* 80:582, 1980.

3. Weldon CS, Rowe RD, Gott VL: Clinical experience with the use of aortic valve homografts for reconstruction of the pulmonary artery, pulmonary valve, and outflow portion of the right ventricle. *Circulation* 35(Supp II):II-267, 1967.

4. Warden HE, DeWall RA, Choen M, Varco RL, Lillehei CW: A surgical–pathologic classification for isolated ventricular septal defects and for those in Fallot's tetralogy based on observations made on 120 patients during repair under direct vision. *J Thorac Surg* 33:21, 1957.

5. Wessel HU, Bastanier CK, Paul MH, Berry TE, Cole RB, Muster AJ: Prognostic significance of arrhythmia in tetralogy of Fallot after intracardiac repair. *Am J Cardiol* 46:843, 1980.

6. Wolfe GS, Rowland TW, Ellison RC: Surgically induced right bundle branch block with left anterior hemiblock. *Circulation* 46:587, 1972.

7. Wessel HU, Weiner MD, Paul MH, Bastanier CK: Lung function in tetralogy of Fallot after intracardiac repair. *J Thorac Cardiovasc Surg* 82:616, 1981.

8. Williams GR, Richardson WR, Cayler GC, Campbell GC: Infundibular pulmonic stenosis with intact ventricular septum. *Am Surg* 27:307, 1961.

Y

1. Yamamoto N, Reul GJ, Kidd JN, Cooley DA, Hallman GL: A new approach to repair of pulmonary branch stenosis following ascending aorta–right pulmonary artery anastomosis. *Ann Thorac Surg* 21:237, 1976.

2. Yamamoto S, Nozawa T, Aizawa T, Honda M, Mohri M: Transcatheter embolization of bronchial collateral arteries prior to intracardiac operation for tetralogy of Fallot. *J Thorac Cardiovasc Surg* 78:739, 1979.

Z

1. Zavcanella C, Matsuda H, Subramanian S: Successful correction of a complete form of atrioventricular canal associated with tetralogy of Fallot. Case Report. *J Thorac Cardiovasc Surg* 74:195, 1977.

2. Zerbini EJ: The surgical treatment of the complex of Fallot: Late results. *J Thorac Cardiovasc Surg* 58:158, 1977.

3. Zach M, Beitzke A, Singer H, Hofler H, Schellmann B: The syndrome of absent pulmonary valve and ventricular septal defects—anatomical features and embryological indication. *Basic Res Cardiol* 74:54, 1979.

4. Zhao HX, Miller DC, Reitz BA, Shumway NE: Surgical repair of tetralogy of Fallot. *J Thorac Cardiovasc Surg* 89:204, 1985.

24

PULMONARY STENOSIS WITH INTACT VENTRICULAR SEPTUM

DEFINITION

Pulmonary stenosis with intact ventricular septum is a form of right ventricular outflow tract obstruction in which the stenosis is usually valvar or both valvar and infundibular, but it may be only infundibular. This chapter concerns primarily valvar pulmonary stenosis, with or without infundibular stenoses. This condition has been called *simple pulmonary stenosis*,[C1] *pure pulmonary stenosis*,[C1] *isolated pulmonary stenosis*,[B9,F1] and *pulmonary stenosis with normal aortic root*.[A1,K3]

It may be considered that pure infundibular pulmonary stenosis with intact ventricular septum is a part of the spectrum of low-lying infundibular pulmonary stenosis with ventricular septal defect (UAB) and the cases categorized with that entity (see Chapter 23, Section 3). Alternatively, pure infundibular pulmonary stenosis may be considered a subset of pulmonary stenosis with intact ventricular septum (GLH); thus examples of this condition are represented in this chapter.

HISTORICAL NOTE

In 1913, Doyen first attempted to relieve pulmonary stenosis surgically in a 20-year-old woman, thought in retrospect to have infundibular obstruction. This was described by J. Dumont.[D1] Thirty-five years later, in December 1947, Sellors performed a successful closed transventricular instrumental pulmonary valvotomy, following closely the technique of Doyen.[S1] Brock performed three successful closed valvotomies in early 1948.[B1] These patients probably all had tetralogy of Fallot. Blalock and colleagues applied this procedure to patients with pulmonary stenosis and intact ventricular septum soon thereafter, reporting 19 patients with just 2 hospital deaths.[B2] Swan surgically corrected pulmonary stenosis with intact ventricular septum by an open technique in about 1952, approaching the valve via a pulmonary arteriotomy during total circulatory arrest with the patient rendered moderately hypothermic by surface cooling.[S2] Our experiences at the Mayo Clinic during this period with closed valvotomy for this condition led to an appreciation of the importance of acquired obstruction due to hypertrophy[B3,K1] and the need for a pump–oxygenator system that would allow its relief by open operation.[K2] When cardiopulmonary bypass (CPB) became available in 1955, most surgeons began to use it for support of the patient during open valvotomy.

MORPHOLOGY

Valvar pulmonary stenosis with intact ventricular septum consists of a spectrum ranging from critical (pinhole) pulmonary stenosis, at times with right ventricular hypoplasia and presenting in the neonate, through severe pulmonary stenosis with a normal-sized or dilated right ventricle, to mild valvar pulmonary stenosis that remains relatively stable throughout life. Classification of the stenosis as mild, moderate, or severe is somewhat arbitrary, but criteria for this are listed in Table 24-1.

Pulmonary Valve

The pulmonary valve is usually the major and often the only site of stenosis. In severe forms, the valve commonly pre-

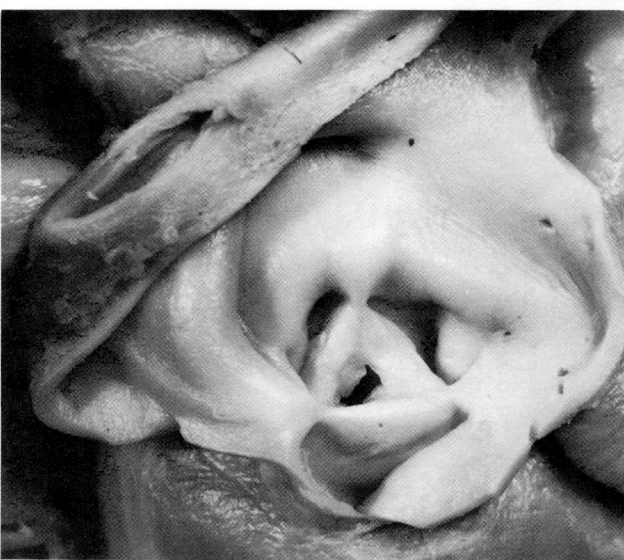

Figure 24-1 Specimen from a neonate with congenital valvar pulmonary stenosis with intact ventricular septum viewed through the open, dilated, pulmonary trunk (GLH). The fibrous cone with its central, very stenotic orifice, the well-formed sinuses of Valsalva, and the potential trileaflet valve structure are typical. There is coexisting moderate right ventricular hypoplasia (see Fig. 24-3).

sents as a uniform fibrous cone with a circular, central, and stenotic orifice and two or three ridges on its pulmonary arterial side (Fig. 24-1). These ridges radiate from the central orifice to the periphery and outline two or three leaflets that correspond to the pulmonary sinuses of Valsalva that are usually well formed. The valvular diaphragm is considerably thicker than normal leaflet tissue, particularly around the ostium, but is mobile. The valve is rarely calcified except in older patients in whom this is particularly likely to follow bacterial endocarditis on the valve.[D2] In milder forms, the two or three or even four pulmonary leaflets are relatively well formed, with only partial commissural fusion and thickening usually confined to the free edge. In infants, the leaflet tissue may have a myxomatous appearance, and occasionally in older patients it may be irregularly deformed and thickened.[G1,S3]

In 1969 Koretzky, Edwards, and colleagues[K4] described a group of patients with congenital pulmonary valvar stenosis, which they labeled *pulmonary valvular dysplasia*. In this condition, the obstruction is due to the thickened, shortened, and rigid cusp tissue alone, since there is no commissural fusion. The pulmonary artery wall is pulled inward or tethered at the site of commissural cusp attachment immediately above the sinuses of Valsalva, and the valve is often bicuspid. The pulmonary anulus is occasionally small, and fibrous bands may occur in the sinuses. This type of morphology occurs in only 5%–15% of patients with intact ventricular septum, but may be more common in infants presenting for surgical treatment.[P3] It is more common in patients with tetralogy of Fallot[M1,S5,W4] (see Chapter 23, Section 1). A dysplastic pulmonary valve is the characteristic cardiac defect in Noonan's syndrome.[N1,R1]

Table 24-1 Numerical and descriptive assessment of the severity of pulmonary stenosis,[K5,N2] assuming that pulmonary blood flow is normal and that the pressure in the distal left and right pulmonary arteries is normal or low.

	Severity of Pulmonary Stenosis		
	Mild	*Moderate*	*Severe*
Peak pressure gradient, RV-distal RPA and LPA (mmHg)	<50	≤50 --- <80	≥80
Peak pressure RV (mmHg)	<75	≤75 --- 100	≥100
Peak pressure ratio RV/LV (or RV/aorta)	<0.5	≤0.5 --- 0.9	≥0.9

KEY: LPA, left pulmonary artery; LV, inlet portion of left ventricle; RPA, right pulmonary artery; RV, inlet portion right ventricle.

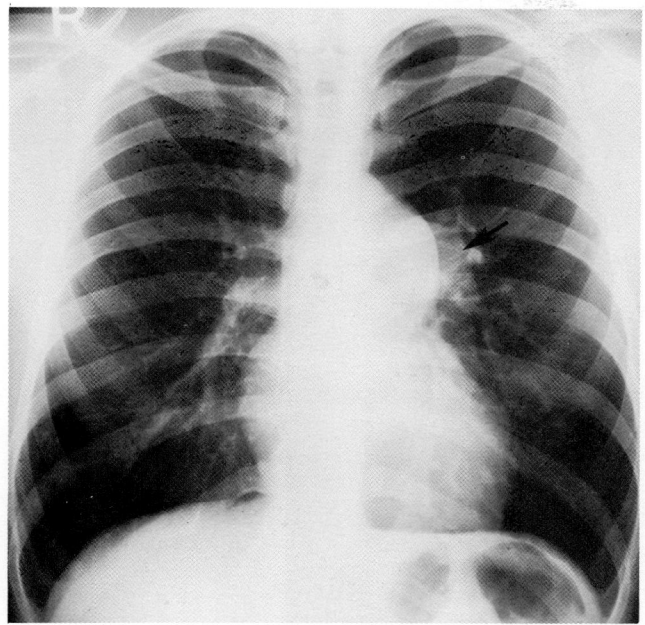

Figure 24-2 Chest x-ray of a patient with valvar pulmonary stenosis, demonstrating poststenotic dilatation of the main pulmonary artery and of the left pulmonary artery (arrow) (UAB). The right pulmonary artery is normal.

Pulmonary Arteries

A poststenotic dilatation of the main and proximal left pulmonary arteries (Fig. 24-2) is present in about 70% of patients with this malformation.[F1,G2] Histologically, the dilated wall may have a thin adventitia and media with destruction of elastic tissue.[P1] The intima becomes hyperplastic.[D3] Cavina[C2] in 1915 demonstrated experimentally that poststenotic dilatation could be acquired and related to mechanical causes, perhaps turbulent flow.[G1] The preferential dilatation of the left pulmonary artery is no doubt related to direction of the jet into this vessel, because it is a more direct continuation of the pulmonary trunk than is the right branch.

Occasionally, the pulmonary trunk or its bifurcation or both may show a localized stenosis, or coarctation, that may add significantly to the obstruction (Table 24-2). Such patients often have a history of intrauterine rubella and may present multiple peripheral pulmonary artery stenoses also.

In about 50% of neonates with critical pulmonary stenosis, the right and left pulmonary arteries appear to be moderately or severely hypoplastic.[C4] This appearance is probably secondary to the very low pulmonary blood flow; in those that survive after surgical treatment, the pulmonary arteries are usually normal in size within a few years.[C4]

Right Ventricle

The obstruction produces concentric hypertrophy of the right ventricle, which, in severe cases, results in *secondary* (functional) *infundibular stenosis* due to progressive thickening of the infundibular septum and its parietal and septal extensions, as well as the free wall.[K1] This is not associated

Table 24-2 Morphologic features of pulmonary stenosis with intact ventricular septum (GLH; 1960–1979; n = 140).

	No.	% of Total Cases
Valve stenosis alone	82	59%
Infundibular stenosis alone[a]	13	9%
Valve + infundibular stenosis[b]	45	32%
Total	140	100%
MPA and/or branch origin stenosis	7	5%
Hypoplastic right ventricle	19	14%

NOTE: The categories in the lower group are not mutually exclusive.

KEY: MPA, main pulmonary artery.

[a] This group is discussed in more detail in Chapter 23, Section 3.

[b] Includes only patients receiving combined valvotomy and infundibular resection.

with endocardial thickening or additional muscle bands and, as pointed out by Engle and colleagues[E1] and others,[G6] usually regresses after relief of the valvar component. In the most extreme examples of right ventricular hypertrophy in hearts with an intact ventricular septum, the right ventricular cavity size is significantly reduced. In the later stages of the disease, the right ventricle may dilate, and tricuspid incompetence may occur.

In occasional cases, infundibular obstruction is contributed to by a low-lying and large moderator band or so-called anomalous muscle bands, and in about 10%–20% of patients with pulmonary stenosis and intact ventricular septum, these are the only sites of obstruction (Table 24-3), the valve being either normal or rarely bicuspid but not stenotic. This type of *infundibular stenosis* occurs more commonly in association with a ventricular septal defect, and is discussed in detail in Chapter 23, Section 3.

The *right ventricle is hypoplastic (underdeveloped)* to a varying degree in about 15% of patients with isolated pulmonary stenosis (Table 24-2, Fig. 24-3). Hypoplasia was present in 50% of the neonates presenting with critical pulmonary

Table 24-3 Morphologic features in patients with pulmonary stenosis and right ventricular hypoplasia (GLH; 1960–1979; 21 surgical cases among an n of 140—see Table 24-2).

Morphology	No.	% of Total Cases
Valve stenosis only	3	14%
Infundibular stenosis only	4	19%
Combined valve and infundibular stenosis	14	67%
Total	21	100%
Atrial communication (PFO or ASD)	18	86%
Small VSD	2[a]	10%
Abnormal myocardial sinusoids	4	19%

NOTE: Nine of 21 patients had severe right ventricular hypoplasia, 10 moderate, and 2 mild. The categories in the lower group are not mutually exclusive.

KEY: ASD, atrial septal defect; PFO, patent foramen ovale; RV, ventricle; VSD, ventricular septal defect.

[a] These two patients are not included in Tables 24-2 and 24-6.

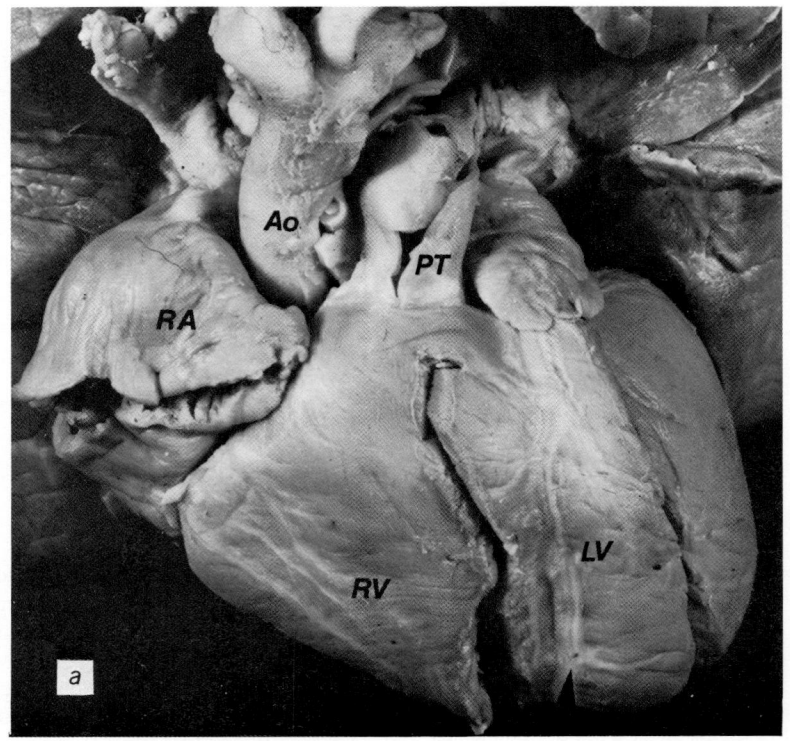

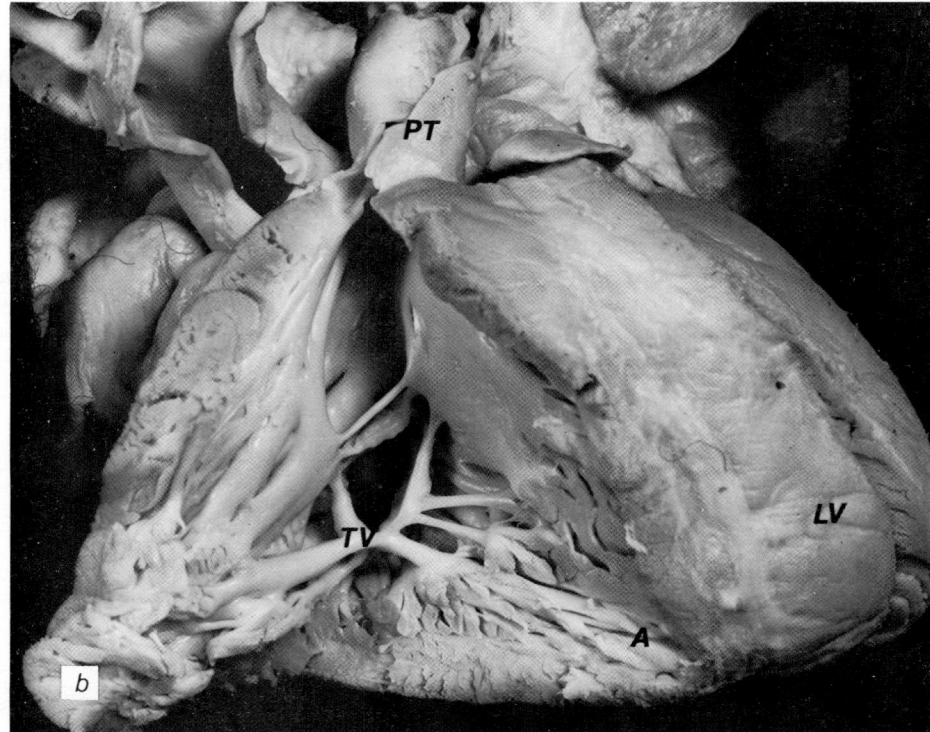

Figure 24-3 Specimen of pulmonary stenosis with intact ventricular septum and moderate right ventricular hypoplasia in a neonate (GLH). (Same specimen as Fig. 24-1.)

(*a*) The external dimensions of the right ventricle are moderately reduced with displacement of the left anterior descending coronary artery (arrow) toward the right.

(*b*) The opened right ventricle shows the almost complete obliteration of the apical half of the sinus portion of the cavity by closely packed muscular trabeculations. These have had to be divided, along with the free wall, to display the potential cavity. Dysplasia of the tricuspid valve is apparent, with leaflet thickening and shortening and abnormally attached and thickened sparse chordae.

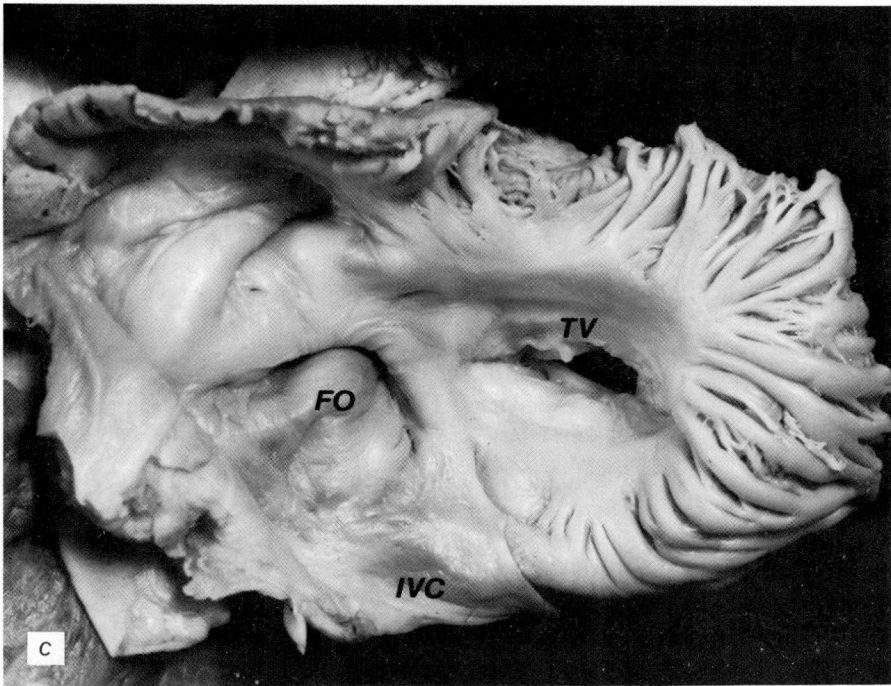

Figure 24-3 (*continued*)
(*c*) The moderately stenotic tricuspid valve viewed from the right atrial aspect. The ring circumference measured 32 mm compared with the mitral ring circumference of 32 mm. This heart is similar in many respects to those with pulmonary atresia and intact ventricular septum (see Chapter 25).

A, heavily trabeculated apical portion of cavity; Ao, aorta; FO, foramen ovale; IVC, inferior vena cava; LV, left ventricle; RA, right atrium; RV, right ventricle; PT, pulmonary trunk (main pulmonary artery); TV, tricuspid valve.

stenosis reported by Coles and associates[C4] (Table 24-4) and in 8 (73%) of the 11 GLH infants operated upon under 3 months of age. Moderate and severe forms of right ventricular hypoplasia can, however, be present in patients presenting for valvotomy beyond 1 year of age (see "Early Results" and Table 24-9). In this event, the pulmonary stenosis is frequently moderate. In right ventricular hypoplasia, the volume of the right ventricular cavity is reduced by heavy fibromuscular trabeculations, particularly at the apex and in

Table 24-4 Hypoplasia and tricuspid insufficiency as shown by cineangiography in 36 consecutive neonates coming to operation for critical pulmonary stenosis with intact ventricular septum (mean age 3.9 days, range 1–14 days). The number in parentheses describes the number of cases. The percent refers to that number divided by 36 (31 in the case of the pulmonary arteries).

		Hypoplasia	
	None	*Mild*	*Moderate–Severe*
Right ventricle	50%(18)	6%(2)	44%(16)
RV infundibulum	42%(15)	14%(5)	44%(16)
Pulmonary arteries (*n* = 31)	29%(9)	6%(2)	65%(20)
	None	*Mild*	*Moderate–Severe*
Tricuspid insufficiency	3%(1)	17%(6)	81%(29)

SOURCE: Modified from Coles et al.[C4]

the infundibulum, where they produce organic obstruction. In the most severe forms, the right ventricular apical cavity is absent, the sinus portion is small, and there is tricuspid stenosis due mainly to a small ring. In many patients with marked hypoplasia of the sinus portion of the right ventricle, there is also infundibular hypoplasia (Table 24-4), which may be fixed and persist after valvotomy.[C4]

When severe right ventricular hypoplasia occurs in the neonate who presents with extreme or so-called critical valvar stenosis (pinhole orifice), it may be associated, as in pulmonary atresia, with abnormal myocardial sinusoids connecting with the coronary arteries (Table 24-3). Morphologically and functionally, some of these severe forms resemble pulmonary atresia with intact ventricular septum (see Chapter 25), but in most neonates with critical pulmonary stenosis the sinus portion of the right ventricle has the capability of growth after valvotomy.

A small ventricular septal defect (VSD) may occasionally be present in cases that are otherwise similar to the condition of pulmonary stenosis with intact ventricular septum.

The *histologic appearance* of the right ventricle varies. Concentric right ventricular hypertrophy is characterized by increase in muscle cell size and diffuse fibrosis.[A2] The former is greater in the fibers near the endocardial surface, and in some areas muscle fibers can be seen to be disintegrating. Fibrosis is diffuse or patchy, but the papillary muscles are always the most severely affected. The fibrosis increases *pari passu* with the hypertrophy and is probably the result of imbalance in the myocardial oxygen supply–demand ratio.[A2,F1] Fibrosis of both the endocardium and the trabeculations is a marked feature when the right ventricle is hypoplastic and contributes to the poor compliance in this condition.

Tricuspid Valve

In infants and older children, the tricuspid valve is usually morphologically normal although mild tricuspid incompetence or, in the face of right ventricular failure, moderate or severe incompetence may develop. In neonates with critical pulmonary stenosis, marked tricuspid incompetence is usually present (Table 24-4). The tricuspid valve, although small, is often morphologically normal, allowing disappearance of the incompetence after successful treatment.[C4] However, the tricuspid valve is occasionally grossly abnormal in the neonates with critical pulmonary stenosis and marked right ventricular hypoplasia, with abnormal chordal attachments and abnormal fused leaflets. When this is present, critical pulmonary stenosis closely resembles pulmonary atresia with intact ventricular septum.

Right Atrium

The right atrial wall is hypertrophied secondary to the increased right atrial pressure. In about one-quarter of infants and adults with valvar pulmonary stenosis, the atrial septum is intact; but in most, the foramen ovale is patent or there is a small fossa ovalis atrial septal defect (ASD).[F2,K1] When a left-to-right shunt is present, there is usually a large ASD and mild or moderate pulmonary stenosis.[R3]

There is nearly always at least a patent foramen ovale in neonates who present with critical pulmonary stenosis. Because of the right ventricular hypertension and low compliance, a large right-to-left shunt occurs at this level.

Left Ventricle

Alterations in the left ventricle such as myocardial infarction, myocardial dysplasia, obstructive changes in the coronary arteries, and abnormal media of the ascending aorta have been shown occasionally to complicate pulmonary stenosis with intact ventricular septum.[B4,S4] According to Harinck, Becker, and colleagues,[H1] some of these changes could be related to a direct effect of massive right ventricular hypertrophy on the left ventricle. In other cases, muscular subaortic stenosis, histologically of the variety seen in idiopathic hypertrophic subaortic stenosis, is present. A combination of muscular subaortic and subpulmonary obstruction may be associated with abnormal facies and is a possible variant in Noonan's syndrome.[N1]

Associated Anomalies

Pulmonary stenosis is a very common anomaly in most varieties of congenital heart disease; but in this text when it occurs with another defect it is considered under that heading. (See Chapters 20, 23 and 15.)

Associated anomalies present in patients included in this chapter are partial anomalous pulmonary venous connection (present in 3 of 137 patients at GLH); left superior vena cava (in 3 of 137 patients); patent ductus arteriosus (in 8 of 137 patients); and supravalvar aortic stenosis (in 1 of 137 patients). Congenital valvar aortic stenosis and muscular subaortic stenosis can but rarely does coexist with pulmonary stenosis.

Pulmonary stenosis with intact ventricular septum occurs frequently in Noonan's syndrome[N1] (small stature, hypertelorism, mild mental retardation, and at times ptosis, undescended testes, and skeletal malformations). It is also associated with intrauterine rubella. One patient in the series with isolated infundibular stenosis had neurofibromatosis (GLH). The stenosis was unusually distal in the right ventricle and fibrous and may have been etiologically related to the neurofibromatosis.

CLINICAL FEATURES AND DIAGNOSTIC CRITERIA

Symptoms

Neonates presenting with this malformation are usually critically ill, irritable, tachypneic, and severely hypoxic from right-to-left shunting at atrial level. The chest x-ray shows a large heart. Less often, when the atrial septum is closed, cyanosis is absent. *Infants* who present later in the first year of life have similar but usually less severe symptoms. *After the first year of life,* patients often present because of a murmur only, produced by a mild or moderate stenosis. *In the second, third, and fourth decades,* the presentation may be in chronic right ventricular failure.

In all, 30%–40% of patients with severe pulmonary stenosis and intact ventricular septum are asymptomatic when first examined.[F1,K5] When symptoms occur, the first is often effort dyspnea,[A3,F1] which results from inability to increase pulmonary (and thus systemic) blood flow with exercise because of the relatively fixed resistance of the pulmonary valve. Cyanosis appears when, in the presence of an atrial communication, the right ventricle becomes less compliant than the left or the pressure becomes severely elevated. With a normally developed right ventricle, this occurs only when the right ventricular pressure is suprasystemic, and it is associated with the electrocardiographic evidence of considerable right ventricular hypertrophy. When cyanosis is marked in older patients, polycythemia becomes severe, and all the complications associated with this (see Chapter 23 "Clinical Presentation" in Section 1, Clinical Features and Diagnostic Criteria) can develop.[M2] Interestingly, however, these patients rarely squat for symptomatic relief as do those with tetralogy of Fallot.[A3,F1]

Effort-related precordial pain is not uncommon in patients with severe stenosis and is presumably right ventricular angina. Sudden death can occur in cyanotic and acyanotic children and young adults with this malformation.[M2,W1]

Patients in the second and third decades of life with severe and long-neglected pulmonary stenosis with intact ventricular septum develop and die from right heart failure with elevated jugular venous pressure, hepatomegaly, and ascites.

Signs

Except in young infants presenting with severe heart failure, a systolic murmur (best heard in the second left interspace) is present, often with a thrill. The peak intensity of the murmur occurs later in systole in those with severe rather than mild stenosis.[G3] The pulmonary component of the second sound may be normal, decreased, or inaudible, whereas the aortic component is usually obscured by the murmur. The tighter the pulmonary stenosis, the longer the right ventricular ejection time and the greater the delay in pulmonary valve closure.[G3,V1] In early systole, an ejection click often is heard and the Q-ejection click interval has a significant reversed relationship to peak pressure.[G3] In severe stenosis, the click is absent since the dome of the pulmonary valve is pushed upward into the pulmonary artery by the vigorous right atrial contraction before ventricular systole occurs. In some patients with mild stenosis, the abnormality of cusp movement may be insufficient to produce a click, although in other patients it may be quite prominent, the sound being magnified by a dilated pulmonary trunk. The hypertrophied right ventricle can often be appreciated as a right ventricular heave palpable to the left of the sternum. The jugular venous *a* wave increases in amplitude[W1] as the pulmonary stenosis increases in severity and is made more obvious by a noncompliant right ventricle.

Neonates with critical pulmonary stenosis and intact ventricular septum, half of whom have moderate or severe right ventricular hypoplasia,[C4] present seriously ill and usually with both marked cyanosis and heart failure. The chest x-ray shows a large heart, and tricuspid incompetence is usually marked.

When the *right ventricle is significantly hypoplastic,* symptoms and signs are importantly altered. Important symptoms are not necessarily present in infancy, but when they appear they tend to be more rapidly progressive. Classically, there are a markedly prominent *a* wave and reversed (expiratory) splitting of the second heart sound.[W2]

In older children, the diagnosis of associated right ventricular hypoplasia is suspected when the signs of pulmonary stenosis are combined with heart failure and cyanosis in the absence of severe right ventricular hypertrophy in the electrocardiogram. Thus, in contrast to pulmonary stenosis with a normally developed right ventricle, cyanosis may occur when the right ventricular pressure is less than systemic and the electrocardiogram unremarkable.[S5,W2]

Electrocardiogram

Right atrial enlargement of moderate or severe pulmonary stenosis is reflected in prominent P waves in the electrocardiogram.[S6] When pulmonary stenosis is mild or moderate, the R wave height in V_1 is less than 10 mm, or there is a pattern of incomplete right bundle branch block. When it is severe, the R or R' in V_1 becomes greater than 10 mm and corresponding in its height to the degree of right ventricular hypertension.[E2] In fact, a high correlation exists between the height of the R wave in V_1 and systolic pressure in right ventricle ($r = .88$),[E3] and pulmonary valve resistance ($r = .74$) and area ($r = .79$).[B5] An even better correlation is produced by relating right maximal spatial vector of the vectorcardiogram to right ventricular systolic pressure.[E4] Right axis deviation in the frontal plane is present, usually less than $+150°$.[S7] With increasing severity of the pulmonary stenosis, additional abnormalities appear, including steep inversion of T waves in right precordial leads.[S6] Bassingthwaighte and colleagues found good correlation of the average angle of the QRS and angle of the T waves with pulmonary valve area ($r = .72$) and with right ventricular–pulmonary artery (RV–PA) peak pressure gradient.[B5]

Pulmonary stenosis with hypoplastic right ventricle is associated with less than the expected degree of right ventricular hypertrophy, and in severe hypoplasia, left ventricular forces are dominant despite severe stenosis.[E2] The diminished right ventricular potentials are due to the smallness of the right ventricular cavity rather than to a diminution in muscle mass.[B6]

Echocardiography

In a critically ill neonate with clear lung fields and a large cardiac silhouette, 2D echocardiography provides a near-certain diagnosis. The thick stenotic pulmonary valve is visualized, the right ventricular cavity is seen, and the size and leaflet thickness of the tricuspid valve can be determined. Likewise, in older children 2D echocardiography can often provide a near-certain diagnosis. Currently (UAB and GLH), cardiac catheterization and cineangiography are added in patients for whom treatment is being considered in order to measure the peak systolic gradient and to study in more detail the morphology of the right ventricle and pulmonary arteries.

Cardiac Catheterization and Cineangiography

The cardiac catheterization and cineangiography study provides information on the peak systolic pressure in the right ventricle and pulmonary artery and the pressure gradient between the two. Detection of possible left-to-right shunting at atrial level is made by saturation data and of right-to-left shunting by indicator dilution curves or cineangiocardiography. Studies during exercise are valuable in assessing the magnitude of rise in right ventricular systolic and diastolic pressures under these circumstances.

Cineangiography (Fig. 24-4) provides precise information regarding the site of stenosis, the size of the right ventricular cavity and infundibulum, the presence or absence of tricuspid incompetence, and the morphology of the pulmonary trunk and the right and left pulmonary arteries.

NATURAL HISTORY

Frequency

Pulmonary stenosis with intact ventricular septum accounts for about 10% of congenital heart disease and is thus a common anomaly. Most surgical series show a predominance of females. (At GLH the male-to-female ratio is 3 to 4.)

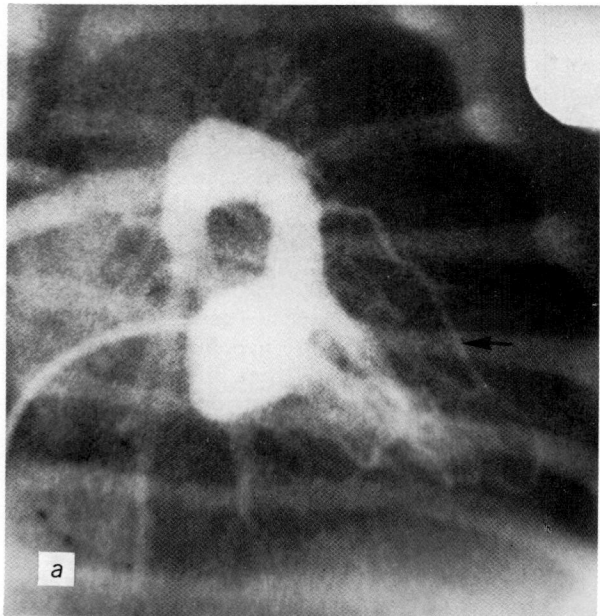

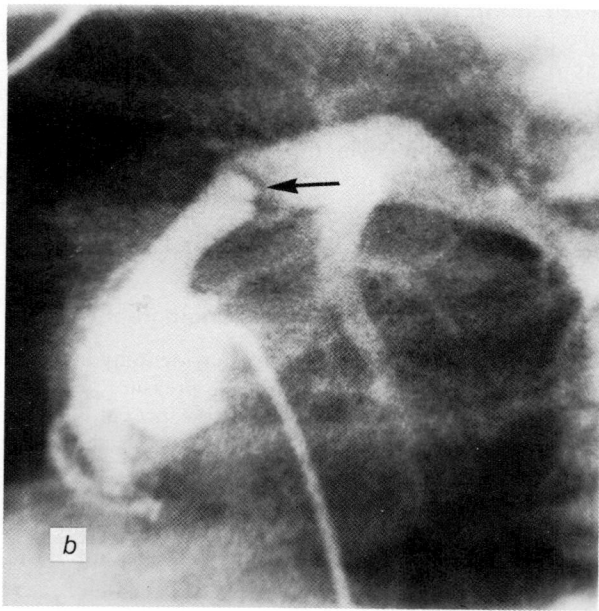

Figure 24-4 Cineangiocardiogram of a neonate with extreme (pinhole) pulmonary stenosis and severe right ventricular hypoplasia (GLH).

(a) Right anterior oblique view in diastole to show the maximal degree of filling of the apical half of the sinus portion that is mainly occupied by thick muscular trabeculations. The infundibulum, main pulmonary artery, and branches are of good size. The left anterior descending artery (arrow) is filling retrogradely from the right ventricle. There is no tricuspid incompetence.

(b) Left anterior oblique view in systole demonstrates the thickened, domed pulmonary valve. The tiny central jet (arrow) is barely visible, but the flow through it is sufficient to fill the pulmonary arteries well after several cardiac cycles.

Patients Presenting as Neonates

Symptoms in neonates are not common, but when they do develop the prognosis without treatment is very poor. Related to this is the fact that 5 (14%, CL 8%–22%) of the 36 newborns known to have valvar pulmonary stenosis with intact ventricular septum who were followed prospectively by Mitchell and colleagues[M3] died before 28 days of age, whereas none of those who remained reasonably well in this period died during the following period (mean follow-up 3–7 years).

The presentation is nearly always within the first 2 weeks of life, with the mean age at operation in the Toronto Sick Children's series being 3.9 days.[C4] The neonates developing severe hypoxia, with or without heart failure, essentially all die without treatment.[G5] Autopsy reports indicate that death from the malformation in neonates is always associated with very severe (critical) pulmonary stenosis and often (50% of cases[C4]) with right ventricular hypoplasia.[F3,N2]

Patients Presenting in Infancy

Those patients who survive the neonatal period to present later in infancy have a wide variation in the degree of pulmonary valve narrowing. As determined from the reported studies[D4,M4,W3] (n = 58), 40%(CL 32%–47%) have *mild obstruction,* 47%(CL 39%–54%) *moderate,* and only 14%(CL 9%–20%) *severe.* However, these percentages probably underestimate the proportion of patients in this age group with severe obstruction, since Nugent and colleagues found that 58%(CL 51%–64%) of an unselected group of infants presenting in the first 2 years of life (n = 81) with this entity had severe right ventricular outflow obstruction.[N2] Even in early life, and probably more so as time passes, infundibular (muscular) narrowing adds to the right ventricular output resistance.

When the *right ventricular outflow obstruction* is *severe* in the first 2 years of life, congestive heart failure and/or cyanosis are common (more so than in older patients who have developed the same degree of obstruction[L1,N2]). The prognosis of this group is probably poor, since Levine and Blumenthal found that 56% of patients with this complication of congestive heart failure died during their follow-up.[L1] Even when the *obstruction is moderate* in this young age group, an important proportion have congestive heart failure, with its same poor prognostic implication. It is probable that a degree of right ventricular hypoplasia is often implicated in the heart failure under these circumstances. According to the studies of Mody,[M4] of 17 patients with moderate right ventricular outflow tract obstruction in the first year of life, 53%(CL 38%–68%) experienced progression to a severe lesion in the next several years (average time 4.5 years). Similar conclusions can be obtained from the data of Wennevold and colleague[W3] and Danilowicz and colleagues.[D4]

Patients Presenting after Two Years of Age

When patients are over about 2 years of age, *severe pulmonary stenosis* is prone eventually to produce chronic congestive heart failure (and thus premature death), the tendency being greater the older the patient. According to the Joint Study of the Natural History of Congenital Heart Disease sponsored by the U.S. National Institute of Health,[N2] 19%(CL 5%–23%) of patients with severe stenosis aged 2–11 years had symptoms, whereas 37%(27%–48%) aged 12–21 had symptoms ($P = .03$). Probably secondary changes in the severely stenotic valve make it more obstructive as time passes, the outflow tract becomes more hypertrophied and stenotic, and the right ventricle in this situation becomes thicker, more fibrotic, less contractile, and less compliant.

Patients over the age of about 2 with *moderate pulmonary stenosis* have much less tendency toward progressive increase of their outflow tract obstruction than do infants. However, such increases can occur.

Patients with *mild pulmonary stenosis* at 2 or more years of age rarely have symptoms or develop increasing obstruction. Indeed, 89%(CL 76%–96%) of patients in this category stayed in it during a 4.5 year mean follow-up in one study,[M4] and other studies report similar findings.[M5,M6]

Effect of Right Ventricular Hypoplasia

The incidence and effect of right ventricular hypoplasia on natural history has been unclear in the literature. The GLH surgical series from 1960 to 1979 includes 14% of patients with varying degrees of right ventricular hypoplasia. Thus, it seems to affect natural history unfavorably. However, some patients with hypoplasia do not die in infancy but present later in life, usually with progressive cyanosis from a right-to-left shunt at atrial level. Untreated, progressive right heart failure develops and causes death.

TECHNIQUE OF OPERATION

Infants, Children, and Adults

The preparation and initial phases of the operation are those used for most cardiac operations (see Chapter 2, Section 3). The pulmonary trunk and aorta are separated from each other by sharp dissection so that the aorta may be cross-clamped without impinging on the pulmonary trunk. The usual support techniques for cardiopulmonary bypass (CPB) or profound hypothermia and total circulatory arrest (see Chapter 2) are used for these patients. When CPB is used, the right atrium may be opened and a left atrial pump sump sucker placed across the naturally present or iatrogenic foramen ovale (UAB). Alternatively, no vent may be used and the intracardiac sucker inserted distally into the opened pulmonary artery to provide a clear field.

After the aorta is cross-clamped and the cold cardioplegic solution infused (see Chapter 3), an anterior vertical incision is made in the proximal main pulmonary artery (pulmonary trunk). The incision is carried into the anterior sinus of Valsalva once the position of the valve commissures is visualized. A valvotomy is performed (Fig. 24-5). When the edges of the cusps are bulky and obstructive, and particularly when the valve is bicuspid, valvectomy may be necessary since a taut bicuspid valve cannot open properly even after incising the two fused commissures.

When infundibular resection and patch graft enlargement are not required (see "Indications for Operation" and "Indications for Infundibular Resection" in "Special Situations and Controversies"), the pulmonary arteriotomy is usually closed directly with 5-0 polypropylene sutures. If there is concern about its size, a patch of pericardium may be used in the closure. If a left atrial sucker has been placed across the foramen ovale, it is then removed. In any event, the foramen ovale or atrial septal defect is closed after filling the left atrium with saline. The right atrium is closed. Air is aspirated from the apex of the left ventricle with a needle. With strong suction on the aortic needle vent, the aortic clamp is released, 5 minutes before which rewarming by the pump oxygenator has commenced. The remainder of the operative procedure is carried out as usual (see Chapter 2, Section 3).

Right ventricular, left ventricular, and pulmonary artery pressures are measured at this point, but they are of little value in decision making (see "Indications for Operation" and "Indications for Infundibular Resection" in "Special Situations and Controversies"). A polyvinyl catheter is brought from the pulmonary artery out the low right ventricle in any case in which an infundibular resection has not been done (UAB), since pressure measurements made the following morning may indicate the need for return to the operating room and relief of infundibular or annular stenosis.

When an *infundibular resection* is felt to be indicated (Fig. 24-6), it may be performed through a transverse ventriculotomy (GLH), sited proximally in the infundibulum, and closed with full-thickness interrupted silk sutures placed 5 mm apart (Fig. 24-6). Alternatively (UAB), a vertical infundibular incision is made; after the resection, the incision is closed using an oval-shaped patch of preclotted woven Dacron (see Chapter 23, Fig. 23-27).

In a few patients (6% of the combined UAB and GLH series), a *transannular patch* is required because of a small pulmonary valve ring. Patients requiring this often have dysplastic pulmonary valves. The cineangiogram may suggest the need for the transannular patch, but the final decision is usually made in the operating room. At the time of valvotomy through the pulmonary arteriotomy, the anulus is sized with Hegar dilators. If it is small (a diameter with a Z-value of −2 or less; see Chapter 23, Figs. 23-60 and 23-61), the arteriotomy incision is carried across the anulus and down the infundibular free wall. If there is doubt about need for transannular patching, the pulmonary arteriotomy is left open and the vertical incision made in the infundibulum. After muscle resection has been accomplished, the anulus is again sized by Hegar dilators passed through the valve from below. If it is too small, the two incisions are joined by cutting across the anulus, and a transannular patch is inserted (see Chapter 23, Fig. 23-28).

In the occasional patient with a *stenosis of the main pulmonary artery or its branches,* the latter are dissected to a point beyond the stenosis and an enlarging repair made (see Chapter 23, Figs. 23-32, 23-33, and 23-34). The preliminary dissection of these branches is best made during CPB cooling. These stenoses must be identified at preoperative cineangiography, since they may be difficult to detect at operation.

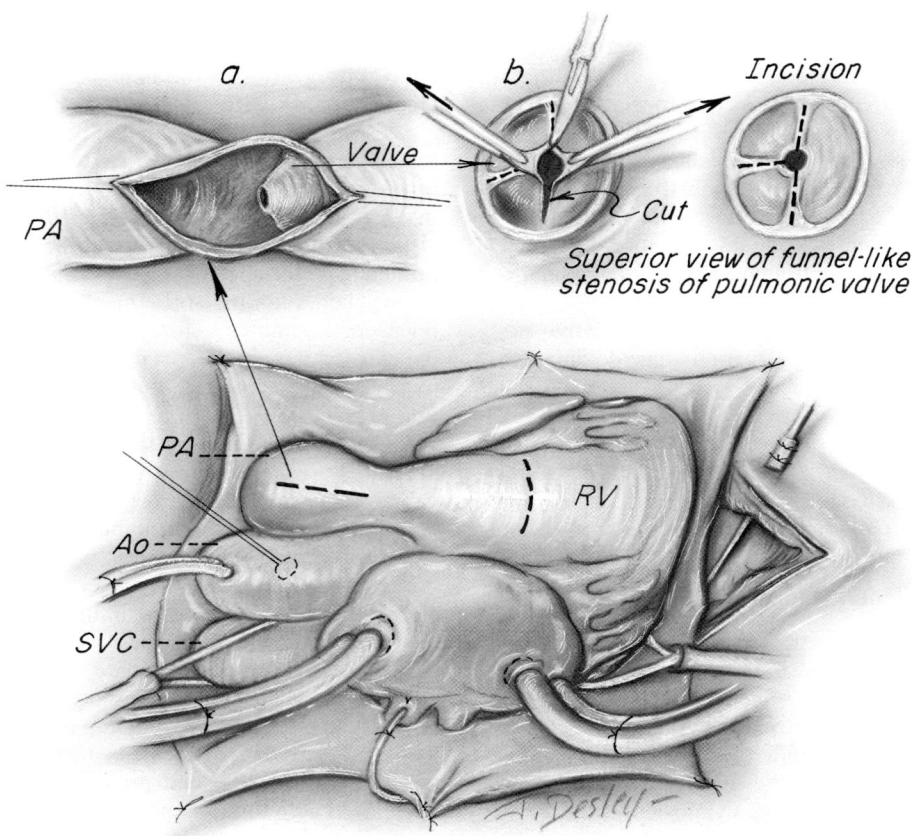

Figure 24-5   Pulmonary valvotomy through the pulmonary artery during cardiopulmonary bypass.
(a) Detailed illustrations of the pulmonary arteriotomy incision, which must be made with care to avoid damaging the pulmonary valve.
(b) The commissures are being incised sharply with the knife. As this is done, the surgeon and an assistant must carefully stabilize the cusp on either side in order to avoid inaccuracy in the incision. If necessary, thickened valve tissue around the orifice may be resected or a cusp may be partially detached; but this is done only if the opening is otherwise unacceptable, since some degree of incompetence results.

When an infundibular dissection and resection are also required but a transannular patch is unnecessary, the right ventricle may be opened through a transverse incision low in the infundibulum (GLH). After performing the dissection and resection (see Fig. 24-6), the transverse ventriculotomy is closed with simple, full-thickness interrupted sutures.

Ao, aorta; PA, pulmonary artery; RV, right ventricle; SVC, superior vena cava.

Neonates

Without a Concomitant Shunt Procedure
Inflow stasis at more or less normothermia is generally used for the valvotomy[M1,V2] *when a concomitant shunt procedure is not contemplated* (see "Type of Operation in Neonates" in "Special Situations and Controversies"). Generally, this is in the subset without severe infundibular hypoplasia, comprising about half the cases (see Table 24-4).

For this procedure, the usual devices for open intracardiac operations are placed, the usual room temperature is maintained, and before the circulatory arrest no effort is made either to cool or warm the patient. Thus, the baby's nasopharyngeal temperature usually drifts down to about 34.5°C by the time of the arrest period.

A median sternotomy is made, and pericardial stay sutures are inserted as usual. Superior and inferior vena caval tapes are placed (see Chapter 2, Section 3). The aorta and pulmonary arteries are dissected apart so that a clamp can subsequently be placed across the very distal end of the pulmonary artery. Stay sutures are applied at four quadrants in the pulmonary artery, and a fine-bladed side-biting clamp is placed, taking care to exteriorize enough of the artery to allow a longitudinal incision of about 1 cm in length, which is now made. A light vascular clamp is nestled into place across the very distal end of the pulmonary trunk and held by an assistant in such a way that he can close it.

Preparations are then made for total circulatory arrest. The anesthesiologist hyperventilates the patient with 100% oxygen, is certain that the baby is paralyzed (to prevent

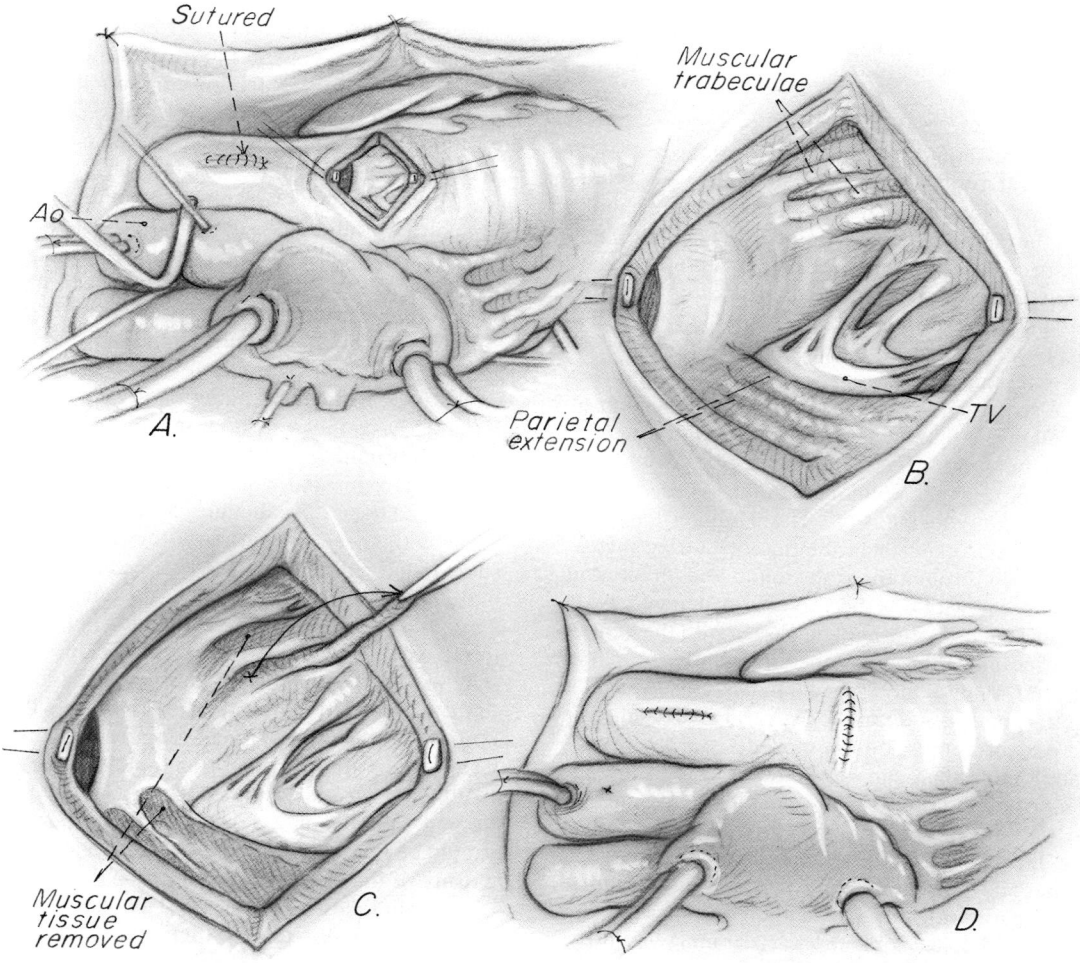

Figure 24-6 Infundibular resection in operations for pulmonary stenosis with intact ventricular septum. In contrast to the situation in TF, this is a resection of muscle from the entire circumference of the severely hypertrophied outflow tract.

(*a*) The approach is through a transverse incision (GLH), or alternatively through a vertical incision that is closed with a Dacron patch as in tetralogy of Fallot (UAB).

(*b*) and (*c*) Working from below upward, muscle is cored out with a knife up to valve level. More muscle can be excised from recesses in front of either end of the infundibular septum than elsewhere. The excision is often also necessary from the walls (anterior, medial, and lateral) for a short distance below the ventriculotomy.

(*d*) When a transverse incision is used, it is closed with a whip stitch, as is the pulmonary arteriotomy.

Ao, aorta; TV, tricuspid valve.

respiratory movements during the total circulatory arrest period), and gives sodium bicarbonate (to counteract the metabolic acidosis that develops during circulatory arrest; see Chapter 4). The surgeon rehearses the surgical team members on their roles during circulatory arrest, and the few needed instruments are set aside. The procedure should be completed during 1 minute of total circulatory arrest, but 2 minutes (temperature is usually 34.5°C) are allowable. The anesthesiologist calls out the arrest time at 30-second intervals.

First the inferior and then the superior vena caval tapes are snugged; and after 2 or 3 heart beats, and the assistant closes the pulmonary artery cross-clamp, the surgeon re-

moves the side-biting clamp, and the first assistant clears the field with the sucker while holding the stay suture on his or her side. While the surgical nurse holds the stay suture on the surgeon's side, the valvotomy is performed using fine thumb forceps and knife or scissors. The valve is opened as widely as possible, even if violent stretching with a hemostat is required. The caval tapes are then released. The first assistant holds both lateral stay sutures, the nurse uses the suction, and the surgeon replaces the side-biting clamp. The pulmonary artery cross clamp is released. If necessary, the usual resuscitative measures are followed (see Chapter 4). The pulmonary arteriotomy is closed with continuous 6-0 polypropylene sutures.

The remainder of the operation is completed as usual. A right atrial polyvinyl catheter is placed. A single 16 F catheter is used to drain the pericardium.

With a Concomitant Shunt Procedure

When a concomitant shunt procedure is to be done, a closed transventricular valvotomy may be accomplished. Unless the baby is severely hypoxic, this is done before the shunt.

A left lateral thoracotomy incision is made usually through the fifth interspace and extending rather far anteriorly beneath the nipple. The pericardium is opened anterior to the phrenic nerve, and stay sutures are placed on the pericardial edge. The exposure should permit a palpating finger to be placed on the pulmonary artery just beyond the pulmonary valve. A purse-string suture is placed on the midportion of the anterior wall of the right ventricle. A small stab wound is made and a 3- or 4-mm Hegar dilator is passed into the ventricle and up through the pulmonary valve in order to find the pathway to the valve easily. The Himmelstein valvulotome,[H2] or some other small dilating or cutting instrument, is then passed through the stab wound and up into the pulmonary valve, and with this the valve is opened widely. If desired, a larger Hegar dilator may be passed into the ventricle to confirm the enlarged valve opening. While the purse string is snugged mildly, the stab wound is closed with a single pledgetted mattress suture or several over-and-over sutures. The pericardium is loosely closed.

The operating table then can be rotated a little to the patient's right side and a Gore-Tex interposition shunt carried out between the left subclavian and left pulmonary artery (see Chapter 23, "Gore-Tex Interposition Shunt Between Left Subclavian and Left Pulmonary Artery" in Section 1, Technique of Operation). A small catheter is brought out from the left pleural space for temporary drainage, and the incision is closed in the usual manner.

SPECIAL FEATURES OF POSTOPERATIVE CARE

General

The postoperative care is accomplished as described in Chapter 5. One special feature (UAB) is that a withdrawal pressure tracing is made across the right ventricular outflow when the pulmonary artery pressure-monitoring catheter is removed 24 hours after operation. These pressures are more reliable in predicting the late results from operation than those taken in the operating room. However, provided the patient's hemodynamic state is good, reoperation within a few days of the initial procedure is rarely necessary, even when the right ventricular pressure is high, because of the known tendency for infundibular hypertrophy to regress with time.

Critical Pulmonary Stenosis in Neonates

The proper perioperative management of neonates is essential for success. Generally these deeply cyanotic and critically ill babies have been started on prostaglandin E_1 (PGE_1) intravenously in doses of $0.05-0.4$ μg · kg · min even before any studies were done and the resultant enlargement of the ductus arteriosus has increased pulmonary blood flow and arterial oxygen levels by the time of operation.

When pulmonary valvotomy is done without a concomitant shunt, PGE_1 is continued intra- and postoperatively, and the infant is left intubated and ventilated. The arterial oxygen pressure (PaO_2) is measured frequently. If after 24 hours, PaO_2 remains well above 30 mmHg, the PGE_1 can be gradually withdrawn. Then, if PaO_2 stays well above 30 mmHg and the hemodynamic state is good, the baby is gradually weaned from the ventilator and extubated. Even though some arterial desaturation persists, as long as the PaO_2 stays above 30 mmHg and the clinical condition is good, the infant is patiently followed in anticipation of continued improvement as pulmonary vascular resistance falls. If the PGE_1 cannot be withdrawn or if after withdrawal PaO_2 falls to 30 mmHg or below, the patient is returned to the operating room and a left Gore-Tex interposition shunt is performed (see "Technique of Operation," Chapter 23). Even with these precautions, the Toronto experience has shown that pulmonary valvotomy alone, with or without *preoperative* PGE_1, has a higher hospital mortality than does valvotomy plus proper provision for pulmonary blood flow in the early postoperative period[C4] (Table 24-5).

When both a valvotomy and shunt have been done, the PGE_1 is stopped in the operating room or within a few hours after operation if PaO_2 remains above 30 mmHg. The baby is weaned from the ventilator as rapidly as possible.

When a systemic-pulmonary artery shunt has been performed initially or a few days after operation, the infant should be restudied at about 1 year of age and plans made for closure of the shunt and repair of the pulmonary stenosis by open techniques if necessary. This plan should be followed because Blalock's early experience[B2] and that reported by Freed[F3] indicate that a systemic-pulmonary artery shunt tends to result in severe congestive heart failure within a few years in this group of patients.

The postoperative care does not end after the first few postoperative weeks. The babies are closely followed, since

Table 24-5 Hospital mortality after operation for critical pulmonary stenosis in neonates at the Toronto Sick Children's Hospital. In the $n = 5$ group, the prostaglandin E_1 was continued after the valvotomy, usually for 24–48 hours.

Procedure	n	No.	%	CL	
		Hospital Death			
Pulmonary valvotomy	22	12	55%[a]	41%–67%	
Shunt alone	1	1	100%	15%–100%	
Pulmonary valvotomy plus shunt[b]	8	2	25%	9%–50%	15%[a]
Pulmonary valvotomy + continued PGE_1	5	0	0%	0%–32%	CL 5%–33%
Total	36	15	42%	32%–52%	

SOURCE: Modified from Coles et al.[C4]

KEY: CL, 70% confidence limits; PGE_1, prostaglandin E_1.

[a] P(Fisher) for difference = 0.02.

[b] Concomitant or within 24 hours.

Table 24-6 Hospital mortality after the repair of pulmonary stenosis with intact ventricular septum (UAB; January 1967–1979 and GLH; 1960–1979).

| Age at Operation (yr) | | UAB | | | | GLH | | | | Combined Series | | | |
| | | | Hospital Deaths | | | | Hospital Deaths | | | | Hospital Deaths | | |
≤	<	n	No.	%	CL	n	No.	%	CL	n	No.	%	CL
	1/12	8	6	75%	50%–91%	6	2	33%	11%–62%	14	8	57%	40%–73%
1/12 ---	3/12	5	0	0%	0%–32%	5	1	20%	3%–53%	10	1	10%	1%–30%
3/12 ---	6/12	7	1	14%	2%–41%	1	0	0%	0%–86%	8	1	12%	2%–36%
6/12 ---	1	8	0	0%	0%–21%	4	0	0%	0%–38%	12	0	0%	0%–15%
1 ---	2	9	0	0%	0%–19%	3	0	0%	0%–47%	12	0	0%	0%–15%
2 ---	5	16	0	0%	0%–11%	25	2	8%	3%–18%	41	2	5%	2%–11%
5 ---	10	15	0	0%	0%–12%	27	0	0%	0%–7%	42	0	0%	0%–5%
10 ---	20	29	0	0%	0%–6%	40	1	2.5%	0.3%–8%	69	1	1%	0.2%–5%
20 ---	30	13	0	0%	0%–14%	12	0	0%	0%–15%	25	0	0%	0%–7%
30		16	0	0%	0%–11%	17	0	0%	0%–11%	33	0	0%	0%–6%
	Subtotal[a]	118	1	0.8%	0.1%–3.0%	134	4	3.0%	1.5%–5.4%	252	5	2.0%	1.1%–3.4%

KEY: CL, 70% confidence limits.

[a] The subtotal reflects the experience with all patients except neonates (those less than 1 month [1/12 year] of age).

about 25% will require another operation within 5 years and 50% within 10 years[C4] (see "Late Results").

EARLY RESULTS

Infants, Children, and Adults

The hospital mortality after repair of pulmonary stenosis with intact ventricular septum is very low (Table 24-6) and, in general, has been so for many years,[D5] including in our earlier Mayo Clinic experience.[M7] This fact is also evident in the overall GLH experience going back to 1960 (Table 24-7). It approaches zero when patients with severe right ventricular hypoplasia or advanced chronic congestive heart failure are excluded.

In this subset, young age (down to 1 month) is not a risk factor, the apparently higher risk in reports from some institutions (Table 24-8) likely resulting from the indiscriminate inclusion of neonates in whom the problem and the risks are clearly different (see below).

The few deaths that occur in the infant, children, and adult age group are associated either with *severe right ventricular hypoplasia* (Table 24-9) or, particularly in adults, advanced chronic congestive heart failure.

No difference in hospital mortality can be shown between the patients operated upon with a closed transventricular valvotomy, mild hypothermia (induced by surface cooling), and inflow stasis, and those operated with CPB or profound hypothermia and total circulatory arrest (see Table 24-7). However, the greater convenience and flexibility and more complete repair with CPB support the current preference for it in this age group.

Neonates

In the past, and with the exception of the Boston Children's Hospital report of no deaths in 12 cases in 1973,[F3] the hospital mortality has been high (±50%) after operation for

"critical" pulmonary stenosis in neonates[L2,M8] (see Table 24-6). This is also evident in the overall results reported by Coles et al.[C4] (see Table 24-5). The hospital mortality has in the past been thought to be related to the severity of the right ventricular hypoplasia, but a multivariate analysis by Coles and colleagues has failed to confirm this.[C4] Probably the high mortality was related to the very poor condition of the neonate when brought to the operating room before the days of PGE_1 and to the general lack of appreciation of the need for a shunt or continuation postoperatively of the PGE_1 in many patients. However, this latter was recognized in the early

Table 24-7 Surgical results in patients with pulmonary stenosis and intact ventricular septum in two eras (GLH; 1960–1979). Figures in parentheses represent the number of patients dying within 30 days of operation.

| Age at Operation (yr) | | 1960–1966 | | 1967–1979 | | | Totals |
≤	<	H	CPB	PH	CPB	B[a]	
	1/12	1	0	1(1)	1	3(1)	6(2)
1/12 ---	3/12	1(1)	0	2	0	2	5(1)
3/12 ---	6/12	0	0	1	0	0	1
6/12 ---	1	0	0	4	0	0	4
1 ---	2	0	0	0	3	0	3
2 ---	5	4	7(1)	0	14(1)	0	25(2)
5 ---	10	9	5	0	13	0	27
10 ---	20	17	7(1)	0	16	0	40(1)
20 ---	30	3	7	0	2	0	12
30		0	10	0	7	0	17
Total		35(1)	36(2)	8(1)	56(1)	5(1)	140(6)
		71(3), 4%, CL 2%–8%		69(3), 4%, CL 2%–9%			

KEY: B, Brock (closed transventricular) valvotomy; CPB, cardiopulmonary bypass (at normothermia or mild hypothermia); PH, profound hypothermia (18–22°C) with circulatory arrest and limited CPB; H, mild hypothermia (30–32°C) combined with inflow stasis.

[a] Three of these patients also had a Waterston shunt.

Table 24-8 Results of pulmonary valvotomy in infants with pulmonary stenosis and intact ventricular septum.

Author	Oldest Age (mo)	Method	Hospital Deaths			
			n	No.	%	CL
Gersony et al.[G5] (1967)	12	Closed	19	4	21%	11%–35%
Langlois et al.[L2] (1972)	24	Closed	21	5	24%	14%–37%
Leca-Chetochine[L4] (1976)	4	Inflow stasis	12	3	25%	11%–44%
Mustard[M10] (1968)	12	Inflow stasis	26	1	4%	0%–12%
Dobell et al.[D7] (1971)	12	CPB	63	1	2%	0%–5%
Langlois et al.[L2] (1972)	24	CPB	18	9	50%	36%–64%

KEY: CL, 70% confidence limits; CPB, cardiopulmonary bypass.

1970s by a few groups[B10,B11,L5] and by Murphy and colleagues in the case of pulmonary atresia with intact ventricular septum.[M11]

Currently, using the intra- and postoperative techniques recommended in this text and based upon the above information, a lower hospital mortality is anticipated, judging from the Toronto experience (Table 24-5) and current UAB–GLH experiences.

LATE RESULTS

Infants, Children, and Adults

Survival

Long-term *survival* is the rule after surgical treatment of valvar pulmonary stenosis with intact ventricular septum. There are only 3 (1.2%, CL 0.5%–2.4%) known late cardiac

Table 24-9 Age and mortality in 21 patients with pulmonary stenosis, intact ventricular septum (except for two with a small VSD), and right ventricular hypoplasia (GLH; 1960–1979).

Age at Operation (yr) ≤	<	Degree of Hypoplasia Severe	Moderate	Mild	Hospital Deaths	Late Deaths
	1/12	3	1		2	1
1/12 ---	3/12	1	3		1	
3/12 ---	1			1		
1 ---	2					
2 ---	10	2	1	1	1[b]	
10 ---	20		2			
20 ---	30	1	1			1[c]
30 ---	40	1[a]				
40 ---	50	1[a]	1		1[b]	
50 ---	60		1			
Total		9	10	2	5 (26% CL 15%–41%)[d]	2

KEY: CL, 70% confidence limits.

[a] Blalock-Taussig shunt performed at an earlier age.

[b] These two patients had a small VSD and severe hypoplasia. They are, therefore, not included in Table 24-2.

[c] Glenn procedure.

[d] Five of 19.

deaths among 247 hospital survivors of valvotomy in this age group (GLH, 20-year experience; UAB, 14-year experience). One was in a patient with severe right ventricular hypoplasia. The other two were related to severe chronic heart failure in patients without right ventricular hypoplasia. One of these two was a 63-year-old man with long-standing severe organic infundibular stenosis, as well as valvar stenosis, well relieved by operation. The other was a 19-year-old girl with Noonan's syndrome and a dysplastic pulmonary valve and small anulus. The repair included placement of a transannular patch, and restudy failed to show any residual stenosis.

Completeness of Relief of Pulmonary Stenosis

The ultimate completeness of the relief of the pulmonary stenosis can only be determined by late postoperative cardiac catheterization because of the known tendency for the right ventricular peak pressure to drop as time passes after the valvotomy.[E1] Presumably, this drop is due primarily to regression of right ventricular hypertrophy and lessening of the infundibular narrowing.[B7,G4,K1,L3,M8,N2,R2,T1] The final hemodynamic result after an adequate operative procedure in a wide spectrum of cases is not known in a precise way, but the experience indicates that important residual pulmonary stenosis is uncommon.

It is known, however, that adequate, isolated pulmonary valvotomy does not routinely provide excellent relief of the pulmonary stenosis in this entity, even in infants. Thus, among Steinbicker, Swan, and colleagues' 37 patients undergoing isolated open valvotomy with surface cooling and inflow occlusion who were later restudied, six (16%; CL 10%–25%) had important residual pulmonary stenosis (peak pressure gradient between right ventricle and pulmonary artery of 30 mmHg or more).[S8] One patient (3%; CL 0.3%–9%) had sufficiently severe residual stenosis to require reoperation. Tandon and colleagues have reported that when open pulmonary valvotomy is done without infundibular resection, about 10% of patients have important residual pulmonary stenosis late postoperatively.[T2] These late residual pulmonary stenoses can be due primarily to important secondary infundibular pulmonary stenosis that has not regressed postvalvotomy,[B8,J1,K1,M7] and this is the reason for the use of concurrent infundibular resection when indicated. Late residual stenosis can also be due to residual valvar stenosis or a narrow pulmonary valve ring.

Table 24-10 Reoperations in patients with pulmonary stenosis and intact ventricular septum following an initial open operation (GLH; 1960–1979). In addition, two infants required reoperation following a Brock procedure.

Site of Residual Defect	Technique at First Operation	Associated RVA	Age		Final Result
			Operation 1	2	
Valve stenosis	H	No	2 yr	7 yr	Good
Valve stenosis	H	No	7 yr	14 yr	Good
Valve stenosis	CPB	Yes	4 yr	10 yr	Good
Anulus stenosis	CPB	No	2 yr	8 yr	Good
Anulus stenosis	CPB	Yes	1 yr	8 yr	Good
ASD[a]	CPB	No	53 yr	54 yr	Good
Right atrium[b]	PH	No	2 mo	2 mo	Good

KEY: ASD, atrial septal defect; CPB, cardiopulmonary bypass; H, mild hypothermia and inflow stasis; PH, profound hypothermia, limited CPB, and total circulatory arrest; RVA, right ventricular aneurysm.

[a] Also RV hypoplasia.

[b] Misdirection of IVC to LA by pericardial patch at first repair plus partial anomalous pulmonary venous connection of right lung to right atrium.

Reoperation

The conclusion that residual pulmonary stenosis is uncommon following a properly performed operation is supported by an analysis of reoperations (Table 24-10). There have been five reoperations (4% of cases exclusive of neonates) for residual stenosis at valve or anulus level following an initial open valvotomy (GLH). In all three with valve stenosis, the initial valvotomy was probably incomplete (the valvotomy performed using CPB was unwisely carried out through a right ventriculotomy), although valve restenosis can occur. In the two with a narrow anulus, misjudging the need for a transannular patch at the first operation was the cause of a need for reoperation. In two of the three patients with a ventriculotomy scar, the high residual pressure had produced a right ventricular aneurysm that required excision. The lack of reoperations for residual infundibular stenosis is a consequence of a policy of infundibular resection at the initial operation, when indicated.

Cyanosis

Cyanosis may persist late postoperatively when the foramen ovale or atrial septal defect is not closed, even when the stenosis has been relieved, due to impaired right ventricular compliance.[D6,M9,O1] This can occur occasionally with a normally developed severely hypertrophied right ventricle presumably secondary to diffuse fibrosis, but it is the rule in the hypoplastic right ventricle. The data from Freed et al.[F3] suggest that the reversed atrial shunt may lessen as a neonate grows and as the right ventricle increases in size, and later surgical closure of the atrial septal defect thus may not be required. This favorable sequence cannot be expected in infants and older patients with hypoplastic right ventricle (see Table 24-9), and it is well known that significant anoxia can occur from a right-to-left shunt through a small atrial communication. For this reason, great care is taken at operation to close the atrial communication securely.

Pulmonary Incompetence

The incidence of late postoperative pulmonary incompetence has been reported to be as low as 10% by Engle and colleagues[E5] and as high as 50% by the group at the Boston Children's Hospital.[T2] Talbert and colleagues concluded from cardiac catheterization data that some degree of pulmonary incompetence was nearly always present, even when a diastolic murmur could not be heard.[T3] Rhomer and colleagues, using a semiquantitative method, found the incompetence mild or moderate after pulmonary valvotomy for this condition and less than that resulting from a transannular patch.[R4]

Functional Capacity

Knowledge of the late functional capacity of these patients after an adequate operation is also incomplete, in part because of the wide variability of the clinical spectrum and of the operations that have been done. Certainly, however, many patients have an excellent late functional result. Stone and colleagues have shown that children who have undergone pulmonary valvotomy for this condition have during exercise a normal relationship between cardiac output and oxygen consumption, no increase in right ventricular end-diastolic pressure after exercise (preoperatively it increased), and less increase than preoperatively in right ventricular peak systolic pressure after exercise.[S9]

The late result in patients with a *hypoplastic right ventricle* is inferior to that in patients with a normally developed ventricle. The late mortality is higher, there may be a reversed shunt through an unclosed atrial communication, and there may be residual infundibular obstruction. Finally, there may be persistent or recurrent right heart failure despite complete relief of the stenosis. It may be inferred that late congestive heart failure can be prevented in this group (GLH), particularly in those who are young, by a complete valvotomy combined with enlargement of the right ventricular cavity by excision of trabeculations.

Neonates

Survival

The late survival rates in neonates have been good, but less so than in infants and older patients, and reoperations have been more frequent. This is well demonstrated in the data from the Toronto Sick Children's Hospital. Of 21 hospital survivors 2 (10%; CL 3%–21%) *died late postoperatively* (average follow-up was 61 months), both in the first year after the initial operation.[C4]

Reoperation

Reoperation was required within 5 years in 28% and within 10 years in 58% of the hospital survivors in the Toronto experience.[C4] The need for another operation occurred more frequently in those with a hypoplastic infundibulum than in those with a normal infundibulum (Fig. 24-7). Among the 8 reoperations, 5 were for placement of a transannular patch and 2 for repeat pulmonary valvotomy. An atrial septal defect alone was repaired in 1, and as part of the procedure in 6 of the other 7 patients.

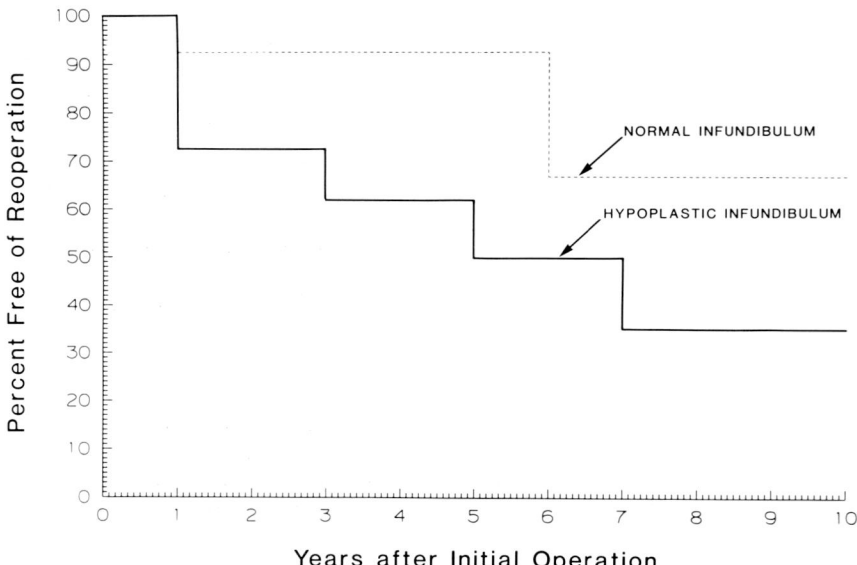

Figure 24-7 Actuarial freedom from reoperation after initial valvotomy for critical pulmonary stenosis in the neonate. The dashed line represents patients with a preoperatively normal-sized infundibulum. The solid line represents those with a hypoplastic infundibulum. The *P* value for the difference between the two is .07. These variables are also significant in a Cox multivariate analysis. (Slightly modified from the report of Coles et al.[C4] of 20 hospital survivors of the initial operation at Toronto Sick Children's Hospital.)

Functional Capacity and Morphologic and Functional Changes

The functional capacity of surviving patients is generally good. The patients are usually active and without symptoms. This is not surprising in view of the favorable morphologic and functional changes that occur after the initial operation (Table 24-11). The sinus portion of the right ventricle enlarges and becomes normal in size in most patients. This is in contrast to the situation in patients with pulmonary atresia with intact ventricular septum (see Chapter 25). The infundibulum enlarges in many patients; but as in tetralogy of Fallot (see Chapter 23, Fig. 23-55), a narrow pulmonary anulus (ring) may fail to enlarge disproportionately as the

child grows. This is evident in the overall GLH experience as well (see Table 24-10). The apparent size of the pulmonary arteries increases, and in most patients the arteries become normal sized. Of great significance, and again in contrast to pulmonary atresia with intact ventricular septum, the preoperatively severe tricuspid incompetence is usually absent late postoperatively (Table 24-11).

INDICATIONS FOR OPERATION

Neonates

Patients with critical pulmonary stenosis with intact ventricular septum, presenting in the first few weeks of life, demand emergency treatment (see "Natural History"). As soon as these deeply cyanotic babies present and the diagnosis has been made presumptively, an intravenous infusion of PGE$_1$ is begun.[F4,N3,O2] At a dose of 0.1–0.4 µg · kg · min, arterial Po$_2$ can be expected to rise about 10 mmHg. The diagnosis is established forthwith by cardiac catheterization and cineangiography. Operation is undertaken promptly, although not as an emergency, since a continuation of PGE$_1$ therapy for a few more hours often improves the clinical and metabolic state of the neonate.

When there is associated severe infundibular hypoplasia, a closed transventricular valvotomy and left Gore-Tex interposition graft are indicated, followed by cessation of the PGE$_1$ infusion. When there is no or mild infundibular hypoplasia, pulmonary valvotomy through a median sternotomy incision is indicated, recognizing that closed pulmonary valvotomy also can provide good initial results.[G4,M12] The PGE$_1$

Table 24-11 Hypoplasia and tricuspid insufficiency remaining late after the initial pulmonary valvotomy for critical pulmonary stenosis in neonates (20 hospital survivors). The percent is the number of cases in the category divided by the *n* of 20. The percent in parentheses is that present preoperatively.

	Hypoplasia		
	None	*Mild*	*Moderate–Severe*
Right ventricle	88%(vs. 50%)	12%	0%(vs. 44%)
Right ventricular infundibulum	75%(vs. 42%)	19	6%(vs. 44%)
Pulmonary arteries	94%(vs. 29%)	6%	0%(vs. 65%)
	None	*Mild*	*Moderate–Severe*
Tricuspid insufficiency	81%(vs. 3%)		19%(vs. 81%)

SOURCE: Adapted from Coles et al.[C4]

NOTE: All percentages are different from preoperative ones with $P \leq 0.03$ (Fisher).

infusion is continued for 1–4 days, and if PaO$_2$ does not remain above 30 mmHg with its discontinuance, a left Gore-Tex interposition shunt is performed promptly.

Since the need for reoperation—usually for further relief of the right ventricular outflow obstruction, closure of the ASD, or both—is frequent late postoperatively, close follow-up and frequent restudy are required to determine whether the indications for these are present. Temporary balloon occlusion of the ASD may be helpful in determining whether right ventricular competence is sufficient to allow the defect to be closed.[B11]

Infants

When patients first develop signs and symptoms at 1 or more months of age, they are nearly always less critically ill than when the presentation is in the first few weeks of life. Nonetheless, when the diagnosis is made, operation is advisable without undue delay, using CPB and an open technique. Operation is similarly advised in asymptomatic infants who are shown to have severe stenosis (see Table 24-1). Operation is usually postponed until preschool age in those with moderate stenosis and is not recommended when the stenosis is mild.

Children and Young Adults

In older patients, management differs only in the group with moderate stenosis. In this subset, the older the age at diagnosis the less likely is there to be significant progression and therefore the less the need for operation. Generally, however, operation is advisable even for asymptomatic patients with moderate stenosis.

The presence and degree of *right ventricular hypoplasia* are taken into account when deciding upon operation. Because of its effect in increasing cyanosis and heart failure, severe right ventricular hypoplasia makes operation more urgent in infants. In older children and adults presenting with this lesion, the indications for operation do not differ unless there is severe heart failure unresponsive to medical measures. Under these circumstances, the risk of operation is increased, and a percutaneous balloon pulmonary valvuloplasty (see section in "Special Situations and Controversies") is probably preferable.

SPECIAL SITUATIONS AND CONTROVERSIES

Technique of Valvotomy

Pulmonary valvotomy has been performed by a simple, closed transventricular technique;[B1,M12,S10] a more sophisticated transventricular technique using special instruments such as the Himmelstein valvulotome;[D8,G6,H2] an open technique through the pulmonary artery during simple inflow stasis; an open technique with surface cooling and inflow stasis; and an open technique with profound hypothermia and total circulatory arrest, or cardiopulmonary bypass (CPB) approaching the pulmonary valve from the pulmonary artery or right ventricle.

However, in critical pulmonary stenosis in neonates, a simple, atraumatic method is required, and either a closed transventricular procedure or an open valvotomy through the pulmonary artery with a brief period of inflow stasis is generally used. The accuracy of the valvotomy is of lower priority here than is the obtaining of the widest opening possible with the simplest and least traumatic method.

In infants, children, and adults, occasionally a well-formed three-leaflet valve is present with commissural fusion. Then a precise opening of the valve through the fused commissures has a reasonable chance of resulting in a competent but widely opened valve. In other instances, some tailoring or partial excision of the valve is needed, and the capability for infundibular resection or placement of a trans-annular patch is also desirable. For all of these reasons, an open technique is clearly desirable, and this requires CPB or, alternatively (GLH), in small infants profound hypothermia and total circulatory arrest (see Chapter 2, Section 4).

Percutaneous Balloon Pulmonary Valvuloplasty

It has been shown that the pulmonary valve can be enlarged by percutaneous balloon pulmonary valvuloplasty.[C3,K6,L6,P2] The efficacy of this compared with surgical valvotomy remains to be assessed, but a small experience with six patients indicates a good immediate relief of the right ventricular-pulmonary artery gradient (UAB).[B12] In patients with pulmonary valve dysplasia and those in whom the valve is a uniform fibrous cone, probably the incompetence is similar either after balloon valvuloplasty or surgical enlargement of the valve. Possibly, however, the incompetence will be less after surgical valvotomy than after balloon valvuloplasty when the pulmonary valve has three leaflets and is reasonably well formed albeit stenotic (see "Technique of Valvotomy"). This is suggested by the report of Lababidi and colleagues in which at open operation after balloon valvuloplasty, it was seen that the valvuloplasty had torn the cusp alongside but not through the fused raphe.[L6]

Indications for Infundibular Resection

An associated and presumably secondary infundibular narrowing during systole is often present in association with valvular pulmonary stenosis, particularly in patients with suprasystemic right ventricular pressure. It is arguable whether this is all a functional narrowing or in part at least morphologic, but the latter is likely.[K1] Regression of morphologic changes certainly occurs in many patients after valvotomy but not in all (see "Late Results"). Thus, the management of the infundibulum is highly controversial, with some recent studies suggesting that the secondary infundibular narrowing need never be approached directly.[G6] The late results of pulmonary valvotomy have been discussed earlier (see "Late Results") and do not support such a conclusion.

In view of the data presented earlier (see "Early Results" and "Late Results"), infundibular resection (UAB and GLH) and patch graft enlargement (UAB) are advised in addition to valvotomy when preoperatively there is suprasystemic right ventricular systolic pressure or when particularly marked systolic narrowing of the infundibulum is seen cineangiographically in patients with lesser degrees of right ventricular hypertension.

Certainly, pressure measurements immediately after repair in the operating room are of no value in deciding which cases require infundibular resection. Frequently, the right ventricular pressure and the gradient are greater at this time than preoperatively. This may be due to the high catecholamine levels prevailing at that time. Thus the decision for or against infundibular resection is best made preoperatively.

The presence of significant *hypoplasia of the right ventricle* is considered an indication for right ventriculotomy in infants and older patients, because in this condition abnormal muscle bands contribute to the infundibular obstruction, and should be excised.

Closure of the Foramen Ovale

If the catheterization data fail to show a shunt in either direction, the right atrium is left unopened and any possible small foramen ovale defect ignored (GLH). Alternatively it may be elected routinely to open the atrium and vent through the foramen ovale (UAB). Following this, the foramen ovale is closed.

When there is a right-to-left shunt at atrial level, even though it is through a patent foramen ovale, closure is wise. Otherwise, severe right ventricular hypertrophy may continue to compromise right ventricular compliance, despite complete relief of the stenosis, so that right-to-left shunting at atrial level and cyanosis persist.

When there is severe right ventricular hypoplasia, the decision concerning closure of the interatrial communication may be difficult. Occlusion of the defect by catheter balloon at the time of preoperative study is an effective means of judging whether or not closure can be tolerated.[B11] Unless it indicates that closure cannot be tolerated, the near-routine closure of the interatrial communication is recommended.

Type of Operation in Neonates

Critical pulmonary stenosis presenting with symptoms in the neonate is a special problem because of the severity of the disease, its profound effects, and its relative infrequency. Some might disagree with the surgical protocols presented for this group and would support an alternative method.[W5]

Another view is that, should there be associated severe right ventricular hypoplasia, the enlargement of the right ventricular cavity and relief of any organic infundibular stenosis with the use of the profound hypothermia-circulatory arrest technique may possibly be superior to techniques that allow valvotomy only (GLH). Such an approach may obviate the need for a systemic-pulmonary artery shunt in this condition.

Type of Operation in Children and Adults with Right Ventricular Hypoplasia and Severe Congestive Heart Failure

Management in this rare group of patients is at present unclear, since even after complete valvotomy, infundibular resection, and cavity enlargement by excision of apical right ventricular trabeculations, they may succumb in persistent heart failure. It is likely that if there is severe right ventricular hypoplasia and particularly some tricuspid stenosis and a reversed shunt at atrial level, a Fontan-type procedure should be performed (see Chapter 26).

REFERENCES

A

1. Abrahams DG, Wood P: Pulmonary stenosis with normal aortic root. *Br Heart J* 13:519, 1951.
2. Allanby KD, Campbell M: Congenital pulmonary stenosis with closed ventricular septum. *Guy's Hosp Rep* 98:18, 1949.
3. Anderson IM, Nouri-Moghaddam S: Severe pulmonary stenosis in infancy and early childhood. *Thorax* 24:312, 1969.

B

1. Brock RC: Pulmonary valvulotomy for the relief of congenital pulmonary stenosis. *Br Med J* 1:1121, 1948.
2. Blalock A, Kieffer RF Jr: Valvulotomy for the relief of congenital valvular pulmonary stenosis with intact ventricular septum. Report of nineteen operations by the Brock method. *Ann Surg* 132:496, 1950.
3. Brock RC: *The Anatomy of Congenital Pulmonary Stenosis.* London: Cassell, 1957.
4. Becu L, Somerville J, Gallo A: "Isolated" pulmonary valve stenosis as part of more widespread cardiovascular disease. *Br Heart J* 38:472, 1976.
5. Bassingthwaighte JB, Parkin TW, DuShane JW, Wood EH, Burchell HB: The electrocardiographic and hemodynamic findings in pulmonary stenosis with intact ventricular septum. *Circulation* 28:893, 1963.
6. Brody DA: A theoretical analysis of intracavitary blood mass influence on the heart-lead relationship. *Circ Res* 4:731, 1956.
7. Blumenthal S, Jesse MJ, Hayes C: The natural history of pulmonary stenosis, in BSL Kidd, JD Keith (eds): *Congenital Heart Defects.* Springfield: Charles C Thomas, 1971, pp 61–80.
8. Blount SG Jr, van Elk J, Balchum OJ, Swan H: Valvular pulmonary stenosis with intact ventricular septum. Clinical and physiologic response to open valvuloplasty. *Circulation* 15:814, 1957.
9. Blount SG Jr, McCord MC, Mueller H, Swan H: Isolated valvular pulmonic stenosis. *Circulation* 10:161, 1954.
10. Bianchi T, Locatelli G, Vanini V, Parenzan L, Alfieri O, Branchini B, Tiraboschi R: Correzione chirurgica della stenosi serrata e atresia valvolare polmonare nel primo anno di vita. *Ateneo Parmense (Acta Biomed)* 42:3, 1971.
11. Bass JL, Fuhrman BP, Lock JE: Balloon occlusion of atrial septal defect to assess right ventricular capability in hypoplastic right heart syndrome. *Circulation* 68:1081, 1983.
12. Bargeron LM: (1985) Personal communication.

C

1. Campbell M: Simple pulmonary stenosis. *Br Heart J* 16:273, 1954.

2. Cavina G: Stenosi sperimentale dellarteria polmonare. *Arch Sci Med (Torino)* 39:112, 1915.

3. Cooper R, Ritter S, Golinko R: Percutaneous balloon valvuloplasty (PBV): Initial and long term results. *JACC* 5:405, 1982.

4. Coles JG, Freedom RM, Olley PM, Coceani F, Williams WG, Trusler GA: Surgical management of critical pulmonary stenosis in the neonate. *Ann Thorac Surg* 38:458, 1984.

D

1. Dumont J: Chirurgie des malformations congenitales ou acquises du coeur. *Presse Med* 21:860, 1913.

2. Dinsmore RE, Sanders CA, Hawthorne JW, Austen WG: Calcification of the congenitally stenotic pulmonary valve. *N Engl J Med* 275:99, 1966.

3. Dow JW, Levine HD, Elkin M, Haynes FW, Helems HK, Whittenberger JW, Ferris BG, Godale WT, Harvey WP, Eppinger EC, Dexter L: Studies of congenital heart disease. IV. Uncomplicated pulmonic stenosis. *Circulation* 1:267, 1950.

4. Danilowicz D, Hoffman JIE, Rudolph AM: Serial studies of pulmonary stenosis in infancy and childhood. *Br Heart J* 37:808, 1975.

5. Danielson GK, Exarhos ND, Weidman WH, McGoon DC: Pulmonic stenosis with intact ventricular septum. *J Thorac Cardiovasc Surg* 61:228, 1971.

6. deCastro CM, Nelson WP, Jones RC, Hall RJ, Hopeman AR, Jahnke EJ: Pulmonary stenosis: Cyanosis, interatrial communication and inadequate right ventricular distensibility following pulmonary valvotomy. *Am J Cardiol* 26:540, 1970.

7. Dobell ARC, Fagan JE, Sheverini M, Collins GF, Murphy DR, Gibbons JE: Results of pulmonary valvotomy—early and late, in BSL Kidd, JD Keith (eds): *Congenital Heart Defects.* Springfield: Charles C Thomas, 1971, pp 68–80.

8. Daskalopoulos DA, Pieroni DR, Gingell RL, Roland JA, Subramanian S: Closed transventricular pulmonary valvotomy in infants. *J Thorac Cardiovasc Surg* 84:187, 1982.

E

1. Engle MA, Holswade GR, Goldberg HP, Lukas DS, Glenn F: Regression after open valvulotomy of infundibular stenosis accompanying severe valvular pulmonary stenosis. *Circulation* 17:862, 1958.

2. Engle MA, Ito T, Goldberg HP: The fate of the patient with pulmonic stenosis. *Circulation* 30:554, 1964.

3. Engle MA, Ito T, Lukas DS, Goldberg HP: Electrocardiographic evaluation of pulmonic stenosis. *J Pediatr* 57:171, 1960.

4. Ellison RC, Restieaux NJ: Vectorcardiography, in *Congenital Heart Disease.* Philadelphia: WB Saunders, 1972.

5. Engle MA, Redo SF, Stewart HJ: Pulmonic stenosis: Direct surgical approach. *Surg Clin North Am* 41:377, 1961.

F

1. Fabricius J: *Isolated Pulmonary Stenosis.* Munksgaard. Copenhagen, 1959.

2. Farber S, Hubbard J: Fetal endomyocarditis—intrauterine infection as the cause of congenital cardiac anomalies. *Am J Med Sci* 186:705, 1933.

3. Freed MD, Rosenthal A, Bernhard WF, Litwin SB, Nadas AS: Critical pulmonary stenosis with a diminutive right ventricle in neonates. *Circulation* 48:875, 1973.

4. Freed MD, Heymann MA, Lewis AB, Reischer S, Kensey RC: Prostaglandin E₁ in infants with ductus arteriosus-dependent cyanotic congenital heart disease. *Circulation* 64:899, 1981.

G

1. Greene DG, Baldwin ED, Baldwin JS, Himmelstein A, Roh CE, Cournand A: Pure congenital pulmonary stenosis and idiopathic congenital dilatation of the pulmonary artery. *Am J Med* 6:24, 1949.

2. Gibson S, Clifton WM: Congenital heart disease. *Am J Dis Child* 55:761, 1938.

3. Gamboa R, Hugenholtz PG, Nadas AS: Accuracy of the phonocardiogram in assessing severity of aortic and pulmonic stenosis. *Circulation* 30:35, 1964.

4. Gomez-Engler HE, Grunkemeier GL, Starr A: Critical pulmonary valve stenosis with intact ventricular septum. *Thorac Cardiovasc Surg* 27:160, 1979.

5. Gersony WM, Bernhard WF, Nadas AS, Gross RE: Diagnosis and surgical treatment of infants with critical pulmonary outflow obstruction. *Circulation* 35:765, 1967.

6. Griffith BP, Hardesty RL, Siewers RD, Lerberg DB, Ferson PF, Bahnson HT: Pulmonary valvulotomy alone for pulmonary stenosis: Results in children with and without muscular infundibular hypertrophy. *J Thorac Cardiovasc Surg* 83:577, 1982.

H

1. Harinck E, Becker AE, Groot ACG, Oppenheimer-Dekker A, Versprille A: The left ventricle in congenital isolated pulmonary valve stenosis. *Br Heart J* 39:429, 1977.

2. Himmelstein A, Jameson AG, Fishman AP, Humphreys GH II: Closed transventricular valvulotomy for pulmonic stenosis. Description of a new valvulotome and results based on pressures during operation. *Surgery* 42:121, 1957.

J

1. Johnson AM: Hypertrophic infundibular stenosis complicating simple pulmonary valve stenosis. *Br Heart J* 21:429, 1959.

K

1. Kirklin JW, Connolly DC, Ellis FE Jr, Burchell HB, Edwards JE, Wood EH: Problems in the diagnosis and surgical treatment of pulmonic stenosis with intact ventricular septum. *Circulation* 8:849, 1953.

2. Kirklin JW: Open-heart surgery at the Mayo Clinic. The 25th Anniversary. *Mayo Clin Proc* 55:339, 1980.

3. Kjellberg SR, Mannheimer E, Rudhe J, Jonsson B: Pulmonary stenosis with normal aortic root, in *Diagnosis of Congenital Heart Disease.* Chicago: Book Publishers, 1959, p 136.

4. Koretzky ED, Moller JH, Korns ME, Schwartz CJ, Edwards JE: Congenital pulmonary stenosis resulting from dysplasia of valve. *Circulation* 40:43, 1969.

5. Keith JD, Rowe RD, Vlad P: *Heart Disease in Infancy and Childhood.* New York: Macmillan, 1967.

6. Kan JS, White RI Jr, Mitchell SE, Gardner TJ: Percutaneous balloon valvuloplasty: A new method for treating congenital pulmonary-valve stenosis. *N Engl J Med* 9:540, 1982.

L

1. Levine OR, Blumenthal S: Pulmonic stenosis. *Circulation* 31–32 (suppl III):III–33, 1965.

2. Langlois J, Binet JP: La place de la valvulotomie de Brock dans le traitement des stenoses pulmonaires a septum interven-

triculaire intact chez l'enfant de moins de 2 ans. *Ann Chir Infant* 13:45, 1972.

3. Lillehei CW, Simmons RL, Tood DB: Late hemodynamic response to correction of isolated pulmonary stenosis by open operation during pulmonary bypass. *Circulation* 32:258, 1965.

4. Leca-Chetochine F, Thibert M, Neveux JY, Louville Y, Fiemeyer A, Mathey J: Aspects anatomiques et traitment chirurgical des stenoses et atresies pulmonaires a septum interventriculaire intact du nouveune et du nourrisson de moins de 6 mois. *Arch Mal Coeur* 69:639, 1976.

5. Linde RM, Turner SW, Sparker RS: Pulmonary valvular dysplasia: A cardiofacial syndrome. *Am Heart J* 35:301, 1973.

6. Lababidi Z and Wu J: Percutaneous balloon pulmonary valvuloplasty. *Am J Cardiol* 52:560, 1983.

M

1. Mistrot J, Neal W, Lyons G, Moller J, Lucas R, Castaneda A, Varco R, Nicoloff D: Pulmonary valvulotomy under inflow stasis for isolated pulmonary stenosis. *Ann Thorac Surg* 21:30, 1976.

2. Moss AJ, Adams FH, Emmanoulides GC, Editors: *Heart Disease in Infants, Children, and Adolescents* (ed 2). Baltimore: Williams and Wilkins, 1977.

3. Mitchell SC, Korones SB, Berendes HW: Congenital heart disease in 56,109 births. Incidence and natural history. *Circulation* 43:323, 1971.

4. Mody MR: The natural history of uncomplicated valvular pulmonic stenosis. *Am Heart J* 90:317, 1975.

5. Moller I, Wennevold A, Lyngborg KE: The natural history of pulmonary stenosis. *Cardiology* 58:193, 1973.

6. Moller JH, Adams P Jr: The natural history of pulmonary valvular stenosis. *Am J Cardiol* 16:654, 1965.

7. McGoon DC, Kirklin JW: Pulmonic stenosis with intact ventricular septum. Treatment utilizing extracorporeal circulation. *Circulation* 17:180, 1958.

8. Miller GAH, Restifo M, Shinebourne EA, Paneth M, Joseph MC, Lennox SC, Kerr IH: Pulmonary atresia with intact ventricular septum and critical pulmonary stenosis presenting in first month of life. Investigation and surgical results. *Br Heart J* 35:9, 1973.

9. Mirowski M, Shah KD, Neill CA, Taussig HB: Long-term (10 to 13 years) follow-up study after transventricular pulmonary valvotomy for pulmonary stenosis with intact ventricular septum. *Circulation* 28:906, 1963.

10. Mustard WT, Jain SC, Trusler GA: Pulmonary stenosis in the first year of life. *Br Heart J* 30:255, 1968.

11. Murphy DA, Murphy RD, Gibbons JE, Dobell RC: Surgical treatment of pulmonary atresia with intact ventricular septum. *J Thorac Cardiovasc Surg* 62:213, 1971.

12. Milo S, Yellin A, Smolinsky A, Blieden LC, Neufeld HN, Goor DA: Closed pulmonary valvotomy in infants under 6 months of age: Report of 14 consecutive cases without mortality. *Thorax* 35:814, 1980.

N

1. Noonan JA, Ehmke DA: Associated noncardiac malformations in children with congenital heart disease. *J Pediatr* 63:468, 1963.

2. Nugent EW, Freedom RM, Nora JJ, Ellison RC, Rowe RD, Nadas AS: Clinical course in pulmonary stenosis. *Circulation* 56:(suppl I):I-38, 1977.

3. Neutze JM, Starling MB, Elliott RB, Barratt-Boyes BG: Pallia-tion of cyanotic congenital heart disease in infancy with E-type prostaglandins. *Circulation* 55:238, 1977.

O

1. Oakley CM, Braimbridge MV, Bentall HH, Cleland WP: Reversed interatrial shunt following complete relief of pulmonary valve stenosis. *Br Heart J* 26:662, 1964.

2. Olley PH, Coceani F, Bodach E: E-type prostaglandins: A new emergency O_2 therapy for certain cyanotic congenital heart malformations. *Circulation* 53:728, 1976.

P

1. Provenzale L: Contribution to the understanding of a not infrequent heart malformation amenable to surgery: Congenital "isolated" pulmonary stenosis. *Sci Med Ital* 3:233, 1954.

2. Pepine CJ, Gessner IH, Feldman RL: Percutaneous balloon valvuloplasty for pulmonic valve stenosis in the adult. *Am J Cardiol* 50:1442, 1982.

3. Polansky DB, Clark EB, Doty DB: Pulmonary stenosis in infants and young children. *Ann Thorac Surg* 39:159, 1985.

R

1. Rodriquez-Fernandez HZ, Char F, Kelly D, Rowe RD: The dysplastic pulmonic valve and the Noonan's syndrome. *Circulation* 45 and 46:(suppl II):II–98, 1972 (abstr).

2. Rao PS, Liebman J, Borkat G: Right ventricular growth in a case of pulmonic stenosis with intact ventricular septum and hypoplastic right ventricle. *Circulation* 53:389, 1976.

3. Roberts WC, Shemin RJ, Kent KM: Frequency and direction of interatrial shunting in valvular pulmonic stenosis with intact ventricular septum and without left ventricular inflow or outflow obstruction. *Am Heart J* 99:142, 1980.

4. Rhomer J, Van Der Mark F, Zijlstra WG: Pulmonary valve incompetence. II. Application of electromagnetic flow velocity catheters in children. *Cardiovasc Res* 10:46, 1976.

S

1. Sellors TH: The surgery of pulmonary stenosis. *Lancet* 1:988, 1948.

2. Swan H, Zeavin L, Blount SG Jr, Virtue RW: Surgery by direct vision in the open heart during hypothermia. *J Am Med Assoc* 153:1081, 1953.

3. Selzer A, Carnes WH, Noble CA Jr, Higgins WH Jr, Holmes RO: The syndrome of pulmonary stenosis with patent foramen ovale. *Am J Med* 6:3, 1949.

4. Somerville J, Becu L: "Isolated" pulmonary valve stenosis: A possible misnomer. *Br Heart J* 38:316, 1976 (abstr).

5. Schieken RM, Friedman S, Pierce WS: Severe congenital pulmonary stenosis with pulmonary valvular dysplasia syndrome. *Ann Thorac Surg* 15:570, 1973.

6. Silverman BK, Nadas AS, Wittenborg MH, Goodale WT, Gross RE: Pulmonary stenosis with intact ventricular septum. *Am J Med* 20:53, 1956.

7. Scherlis L, Koenker RJ, Lee Y-C: Pulmonary stenosis. *Circulation* 28:288, 1963.

8. Steinbicker PG Jr, Pryor R, Swan H, Blount SG Jr: Valvular pulmonary stenosis. *Am J Cardiol* 17:310, 1966.

9. Stone FM, Bessinger FB Jr, Lucas RV Jr, Moller JH: Pre- and postoperative rest and exercise hemodynamics in children with pulmonary stenosis. *Circulation* 49:1102, 1974.

10. Srinivasan V, Konyer A, Broda JJ, Subramanian S: Critical pulmonary stenosis in infants less than three months of age: A reappraisal of closed transventricular pulmonary valvotomy. *Ann Thorac Surg* 34:46, 1982.

T

1. Taussig HB: Pulmonary stenosis, in *Congenital Malformations of the Heart* (ed 2), vol. 2. Cambridge: Harvard University Press, 1960, p 380.

2. Tandon R, Nadas AS, Gross RE: Results of open-heart surgery in patients with pulmonic stenosis and intact ventricular septum. *Circulation* 31:190, 1965.

3. Talbert JL, Morrow AG, Collins NP, Gilbert JW: The incidence and significance of pulmonic regurgitation after pulmonary valvulotomy. *Am Heart J* 65:590, 1963.

V

1. Vogelpoel L, Schrire V: Auscultatory and phonocardiographic assessment of pulmonary stenosis with intact ventricular septum. *Circulation* 22:55, 1960.

2. Varco RL (in discussion of Muller WH Jr, Longmire WP Jr): Surgical treatment of cardiac valvular stenosis. *Surgery* 30:41, 1951.

W

1. Wood P: Pulmonary stenosis with normal aortic root, in *Disease of the Heart and Circulation* (ed 2). Philadelphia: JB Lippincott, 1956, p 408.

2. Williams JCP, Barratt-Boyes BG, Lowe JB: Underdeveloped right ventricle and pulmonary stenosis. *Am J Cardiol* 11:458, 1963.

3. Wennevold A, Jacobsen JR: Natural history of valvular pulmonary stenosis in children below the age of two years. *Eur J Cardiol* 8:371, 1978.

4. Watkins L, Donahoo JS, Harrington D, Haller JA Jr, Neill CA: Surgical management of congenital pulmonary valve dysplasia. *Ann Thorac Surg* 24:498, 1977.

5. Weldon CS, Harmann AF Jr, McKnight RC: Surgical management of hypoplastic right ventricle with pulmonary atresia or critical pulmonary stenosis and intact ventricular septum. *Ann Thorac Surg* 37:12, 1984.

25

PULMONARY ATRESIA WITH INTACT VENTRICULAR SEPTUM

DEFINITION

Pulmonary atresia with intact ventricular septum is a congenital malformation in which the pulmonary valve and sometimes the infundibulum are atretic, the right ventricle including its inlet portion and the tricuspid valve apparatus is present although usually small, and the ventricular septum is intact. Atrioventricular and ventriculoarterial connections are concordant.

HISTORICAL NOTE

In 1839, Peacock collected 7 patients with pulmonary atresia with intact ventricular septum from his records and gave credit to John Hunter for reporting the first case in 1783.[P1] Hunter described a premature male child who died on the thirteenth day of life. The right ventricle had ''scarcely any cavity'' and the tricuspid valve was ''especially small.''

In 1955, Greenwold and colleagues at the Mayo Clinic suggested that pulmonary valvotomy was appropriate treatment when the right ventricle was near normal in size.[G3,G4] In 1961, Davignon and colleagues at the same institution suggested that an aortopulmonary (AP) shunt be done for patients in whom the right ventricle was small.[D1] Reports of successful surgery from the University of Minnesota, the Mayo Clinic, and Henry Ford Hospital appeared in 1961.[B2,D1,Z1]

MORPHOLOGY

The two surgically important morphologic features of the malformation are the wide *variability* in the atretic portion and in the size of the right ventricle and the nearly constant association of important *tricuspid valve malformations* resulting in stenosis, incompetence, or both.

Pulmonary Valve

The pulmonary valve is usually replaced by an imperforate fibrous membrane[E1] (membranous type of pulmonary atresia[C1]). Commissural ridges may be prominent and converge to meet in the center of the valve,[Z2] an appearance similar to that in congenital pulmonary stenosis. In some patients, commissural ridges are present only in the periphery, the center being a smooth fibrous membrane. This type of valve, which can be seen to be domed on cineangiography, is usually associated with lesser degrees of right ventricular hypoplasia and with an open infundibulum.[B9] Occasionally, when the pulmonary trunk is small, there is only poorly structured, imperforate fibrous tissue present within the pulmonary anulus.

Right Ventricle

There is now general agreement that right ventricular cavity size and configuration in pulmonary atresia with intact ventricular septum comprise a spectrum, although originally Greenwold and colleagues described only two types of right ventricle (small and normal or large sized.[G4] At one extreme are the very small (diminutive) right ventricles with a tiny cavity and very hypertrophied walls with heavy trabeculations.[C1,E1] The right ventricle was of this type in 27% (CL 23%–32%) of 121 cases collected from the literature.[C2,D2,E3,F1] The small cavity size of the right ventricle in this situation results mainly from the massive wall hypertrophy extending into the cavity, as also occurs in some cases of critical pulmonary stenosis with intact ventricular septum (see Chapter 24, Fig. 24-3b). At the other extreme are the significantly dilated and often thin-walled right ventricles (which are usually associated with Ebstein's malformation) and severe incompetence of the tricuspid valve.[A1,B1,C3,F5,M1,V1,Z2] These form less than 5% of the total. Rarely, the wall may be very thin (Uhl's anomaly or parchment right ventricle[C3]). In the majority, the cavity is nontrabeculated adjacent to the tricuspid valve and heavily trabeculated in its apical half.

The same general spectrum of right ventricular pathology occurs in pulmonary atresia with intact ventricular septum as occurs in critical pulmonary stenosis with intact ventricular septum presenting in neonates, but in the former there is a higher proportion of severe hypoplasia. Bull and colleagues, on the basis of the early concepts of Goor and Lillehei,[G8] modified the usual division of the right ventricle into sinus and outlet (infundibular) portions (see Chapter 1) by further subdividing the sinus portion into inlet and trabecular portions.[B8] This corresponds to one of the systems used to describe the parts of the right ventricular side of the ventricular septum (UAB) (see Chapter 1, "Right Ventricle" in section on Cardiac Chambers and Major Vessels). Bull and colleagues as well as Coles and colleagues found that in examples of critical pulmonary stenosis the inflow, trabecular, and infundibular portions of even a severely hypoplastic right ventricle were nearly always present; in contrast, in only 53%(CL 43%–65%) of 32 autopsied cases of pulmonary atresia with intact ventricular septum were all three portions present (tripartite right ventricle), albeit with more-or-less severe generalized hypoplasia.[B8,C4] Since the tricuspid

valve, although abnormal, is not atretic in any cases, by definition the inflow portion of the right ventricle is present in all cases. In 19%(CL 11%–29%) of the examples reported by Bull and colleagues, the trabecular portion was so ingrown by hypertrophied myocardium as to be effectively absent, and in 28%(CL 19%–39%) this was true of both trabecular and infundibular portions. This latter type may be considered to have muscular as well as valvar atresia,[C1,M2] and in some series has included the majority of cases.[P4]

There is associated diffuse fibrosis of the hypertrophied muscle and, especially when the right ventricular cavity is small, a modest degree of right ventricular endocardial fibroelastosis.[C1,E3,P2,Z2] Bulkley and colleagues found typical myocardial fiber disarray in 69% of the right ventricular free wall and in 73% of the ventricular septum in this condition.[B7] The potential for impaired left as well as right ventricular dysfunction is evident.

Intramyocardial Sinusoids

As a part of the right ventricular malformation, communications may be present between the right ventricular cavity and the coronary arteries and through them with the aorta.[E3,G5] They particularly occur when the right ventricular cavity is small and the tricuspid valve is largely competent.[F1,P4] Grant and others[G5,L1,W1] have suggested that they represent persistent primitive communications secondary to severe fetal right ventricular hypertension. These so-called intramyocardial sinusoids occasionally end blindly in the myocardium,[L1] but usually they have either multiple communications with the coronary arteries or converge to a single vessel[L1,W1] that joins either the left anterior descending coronary artery or the right coronary artery. The coronary artery participating in the communication is dilated and tortuous. Considered originally as a pathologic curiosity, it is now apparent that the desaturated blood these sinusoids carry from right ventricle to the vessel to which they connect compromises myocardial oxygen supply. The left anterior descending coronary artery, for example, may be seen on cineangiography to fill from the right ventricle during systole and from the aorta in diastole, or it may remain filled from the right ventricle throughout the cycle and constitute a circular right-sided shunt.[F2] Left ventricular myocardial ischemia, necrosis, and fibrosis, which have been amply documented in pulmonary atresia with intact ventricular septum, are no doubt related to this phenomenon.[E3,V2]

Tricuspid Valve

The frequency and importance of the associated tricuspid valve abnormalities are apparent from the early work by Davignon and colleagues[D1] and from Lev's considering this entity as a subset of tricuspid valve malformations.[P2] Freedom's study of 60 hearts with congenital pulmonary atresia and intact ventricular septum included *no* specimen with a strictly normal tricuspid valve[F1] nor did the 32 specimens examined by Bull and colleagues.[B8] The size of the tricuspid anulus has generally been considered to be directly related to the size of the right ventricular cavity;[E2,E3,F1] Zuberbuhler and Anderson have confirmed this correlation ($r = .84$).[Z2] The size of the tricuspid valve is also related to the degree of cavity obliteration, the smallest valves being found in examples of pulmonary atresia with no trabecular or infundibular cavity, larger ones when only the trabecular cavity is obliterated, and still larger ones (although still smaller than normal) when all three portions are present.[B8]

The changes in the leaflets are variable. Occasionally, in association with a hypoplastic right ventricle with all 3 cavity components, they have no significant abnormality other than their small size (a miniature valve). Usually, however, the leaflets contribute to the stenosis by virtue of thickening, which includes the chordae (these are also reduced in number and abnormally attached) and sometimes by commissural fusion (a failure of development). Local agenesis of leaflet tissue and incomplete separation of the septal leaflet from the right ventricular wall so that its origin appears to be displaced have been described[C1,E3,F1] but are uncommon when the orifice is smaller than normal.

In the rare cases in which the right ventricular cavity is enlarged, the leaflets almost always show the features of Ebstein's anomaly, with enlargement of the anterior leaflet and downward displacement onto the ventricle of the origin of a dysplastic septal leaflet. The posterior leaflet may or may not be abnormal.[B6] These valves are usually severely incompetent[B3] and might more appropriately be considered under Ebstein's anomaly (see Chapter 27).

Pulmonary Arteries

The main pulmonary artery (pulmonary trunk) is usually near normal in size.[C1,C2,E1,E2,Z2] The right and left pulmonary arteries are variable in size but are usually near normal. Uncommonly, one or the other is quite hypoplastic.[E3,V2]

Right Atrium

The right atrium is always enlarged, particularly so when there is severe tricuspid incompetence. An interatrial communication is present in all cases, usually in the form of a patent foramen ovale of adequate size.[E1]

The eustachian valve is frequently prominent. This was the case in 7 of 18 autopsied hearts with this anomaly (GLH). Kauffman and Anderson[K1] postulated that this directs the caval return preferentially through the foramen ovale into the left atrium and results in poor development of the right ventricle.

Left-Sided Chambers

The *left atrium* is almost always hypertrophied and somewhat enlarged, the *mitral orifice* is usually larger than normal, and the *left ventricle* shows some hypertrophy and may show endocardial fibroelastosis.[C1] A convex bulging of the ventricular septum into the left ventricular cavity has been noted, with speculation that this might produce subaortic obstruction.[Z2]

Aorta

The aorta usually has adult morphology without isthmal narrowing[M1] and is almost always left sided.

Ductus Arteriosus

The ductus arteriosus is, as usual, patent at birth, but its tendency to close is lethal for the patient with this malformation. Usually, the bronchial arteries are normal and important AP collateral arteries are absent.[E1] However, one of 18 autopsied specimens shows an absent ductus and large mediastinal collaterals (GLH).

CLINICAL FEATURES AND DIAGNOSTIC CRITERIA

Symptoms and Signs

Fetal distress before birth is usually not evident, and deliveries are typically uncomplicated and at term.[E2] The infants are generally well developed and are likely initially to appear healthy except for cyanosis.[B2] Cyanosis is usually obvious on the first day of life and becomes rapidly more severe as the ductus closes and there is respiratory distress and progressing metabolic acidosis.[D2,G6] In the New England series,[B5] 81% of the infants presented in the first week of life. Only 11% had low birth weight, and none had severe extracardiac anomalies.

Absence of a right ventricular impulse in a cyanotic infant with a palpable left ventricle should arouse suspicion of pulmonary atresia with intact ventricular septum, tricuspid atresia, Ebstein's anomaly, or critical pulmonic stenosis with hypoplastic right ventricle.[B4,P3] Typically, no murmur[B2,E1] or a systolic murmur of tricuspid incompetence can be heard,[B2,B4] sometimes with a thrill. Despite the presence of a patent ductus arteriosus, a continuous murmur is seldom heard.[C2,E1] The second heart sound is always single.[P3]

The classical findings on chest x-ray include clear lung fields with diminished (or normal) vascular markings and a flat or concave pulmonary artery segment. The heart size is variable and may be large, even when the right ventricular cavity is small.

Electrocardiogram

The P waves can be normal at birth, but evidence of right atrial enlargement develops quickly, and within a few weeks prominent right atrial P waves are uniformly present.[B2,C1,P3,S2] The means QRS axis in the frontal plane is usually normal or shows a rightward deviation,[C1,G7,M3,S1] and there is absence of the usual right ventricular hypertrophy pattern present in the neonate. However, electrocardiographic evidence of right ventricular hypertrophy may be present even though the right ventricular cavity is small, and this must not, therefore, be used to predict right ventricular cavity size.

Echocardiography

Echocardiography shows normal left-sided echoes. The right ventricle may not be found, and the pulmonary valve is absent.

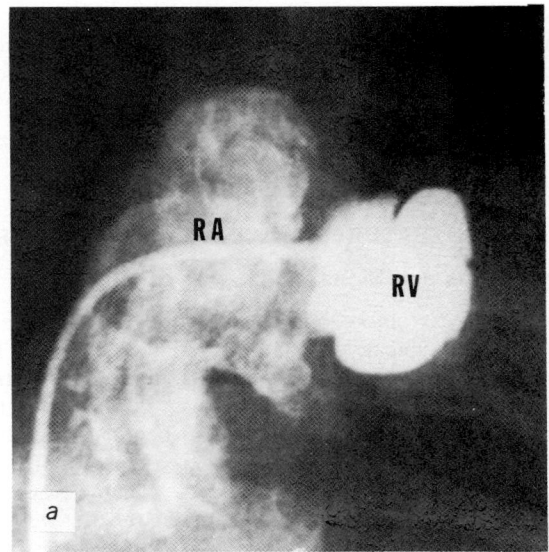

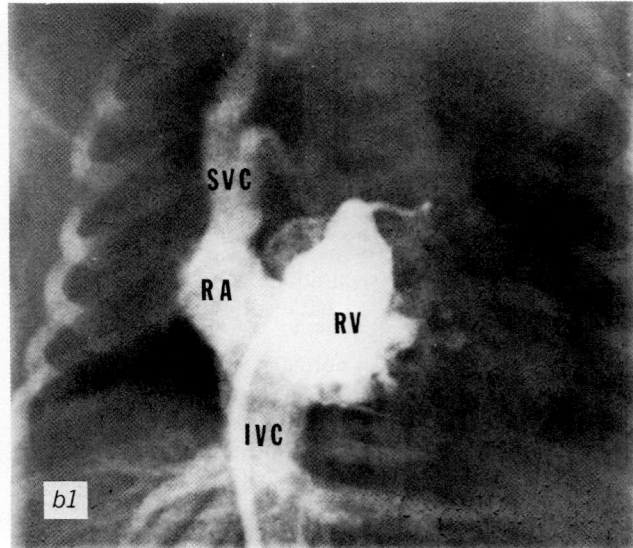

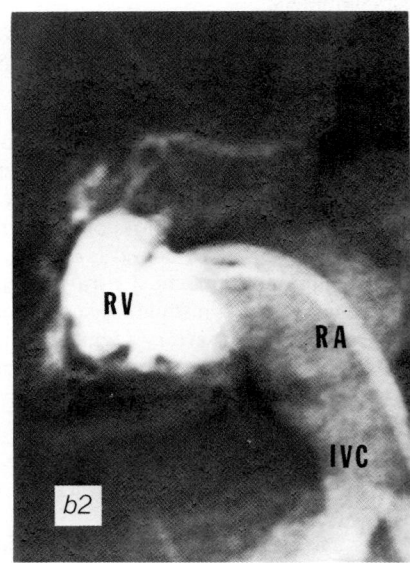

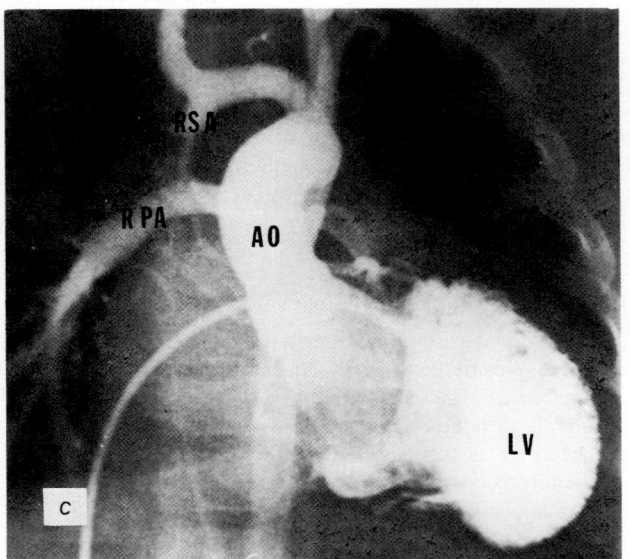

Figure 25-1 Cineangiograms in neonates with pulmonary atresia and intact ventricular septum (UAB).

(a) Right ventriculogram, frontal view: The small right ventricle has smooth borders. The infundibulum is atretic. The tricuspid valve shows severe insufficiency.

(b) Right ventriculogram from another patient in (1) frontal and (2) lateral views. The right ventricle is very small, but its walls are trabeculated. Sinusoid channels are seen, which are connected with the coronary circulation.

(c) Left ventriculogram in frontal view in another patient. The LV has the usual appearance and supports the aorta. A right Blalock-Taussig shunt has been made.

AO, aorta; IVC, inferior vena cava; LV, left ventricle; RA, right atrium; RPA, right pulmonary artery; RSA, right subclavian artery; RV, right ventricle; SVC, superior vena cava.

Cardiac Catheterization and Cineangiography

When pulmonary atresia with intact ventricular septum is suspected, cardiac catheterization and angiography are indicated to confirm the diagnosis and to delineate the intracardiac anatomy.

The right atrial mean pressure is usually higher than the left and a prominent a wave can be seen in the pressure tracing.[C1,C2] The right ventricular peak pressure is usually higher than or equal to systemic, although it may be less in association with severe tricuspid incompetence and a thin-walled right ventricle.[C2,D2,G2,J1,S1] The systemic arterial saturation is always low but varies according to the flow through the patent ductus arteriosus.

Angiocardiography is essential in establishing the diagnosis and planning treatment[E2] (Fig. 25-1). The degree of separation of the pulmonary trunk from the patent infundibulum can be exactly determined when, in the same frame, there is filling of both the infundibulum (via a right ventricular injection) and the pulmonary trunk (filled via the ductus from an aortic injection).[F3] High-quality angiography is required, since in Ebstein's anomaly with severe tricuspid incompetence presenting in the neonatal period in association with a high pulmonary vascular resistance, right ventricular systole may fail to open a normal pulmonary valve.[N1]

NATURAL HISTORY

Pulmonary atresia with intact ventricular septum, a rather rare malformation, occurs in 1%–1.5% of individuals born with congenital heart disease.[F4,M4] It comprises 3% of the critically ill infants with congenital heart disease in the New England Series.[B5]

Pulmonary atresia with intact ventricular septum is a highly lethal malformation, about 50% of patients dying within 2 weeks of birth and about 85% being dead by the age of 6 months (Fig. 25-2). Death is caused by severe hypoxia and metabolic acidosis and usually coincides with the spontaneous closure of the ductus arteriosus.

Rarely, patients survive into young adult life. McArthur and colleagues[M5] described a 21-year-old patient whose pulmonary blood flow came from a right coronary–pulmonary arterial fistula, and Robicsek[R1] described another patient of similar age who survived because of a congenital AP window.

TECHNIQUE OF OPERATION

Initial Operation of Pulmonary Valvotomy and Shunting

The neonate is brought to the operating room with a prostaglandin E_1 (PGE_1) infusion continuing. A radial (or brachial) artery needle is inserted (see Chapter 2) and anesthesia is induced and maintained with consideration for the serious nature of the condition and the tendency to acidosis (see Chapter 4).

A left lateral incision is made similar to that for an isolated left-sided Gore-Tex interposition shunt (see Chapter 23, "Gore-Tex Interposition Shunt between Left Subclavian and Left Pulmonary Arteries" in Section 1, Technique of Shunting Operations) except that the skin incision is carried anteriorly beneath the nipple nearly to the midline. The interspace is also opened well anteriorly. The Gore-Tex interposition shunt is made and the occluding devices released (see Chapter 23). The pericardium is opened longitudinally, anterior to the phrenic nerve, in preparation for the transpulmonary valvotomy. No caval tapes are used. A clamp is

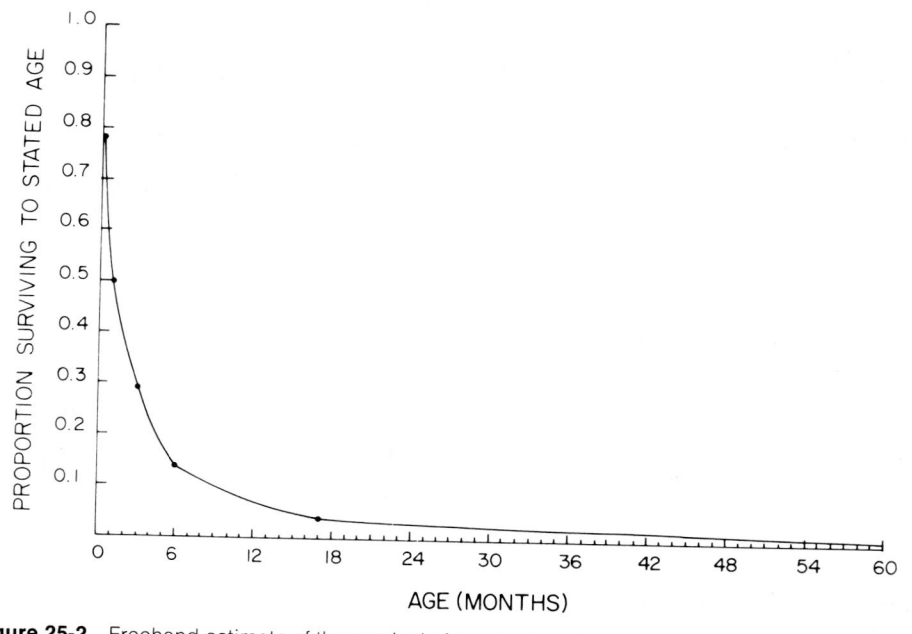

Figure 25-2 Freehand estimate of the survival of surgically untreated patients with pulmonary atresia and intact ventricular septum based upon reports in the literature.[B5,D1,D2,D3,F3,F4,L2,M1,M4,M9,S4,W2]

placed across the distal pulmonary artery, and a longitudinal arteriotomy made. The field is dry because of the atretic pulmonary valve. A stay suture is placed on each lip of the arteriotomy. With a small sharp knife, a stab incision is made in the valve. A small curved hemostat is then used to enlarge the opening forcefully in two directions. A side-biting clamp is placed on the lips of the arteriotomy, and the pulmonary arteriotomy closed with a whip stitch and the clamp removed. Pharmacologic support (see Chapter 4) may be necessary for a time. The pericardium is irrigated and loosely closed. The incision is closed, leaving a small catheter for pleural drainage.

Initial Shunting Operation Only

With the same precautions and preparations as described above, a left Gore-Tex interposition shunt is performed (see Chapter 23, "Gore-Tex Interposition Shunt between Left Subclavian and Left Pulmonary Arteries" in Section 1, Technique of Shunting Operations).

Later Right Ventricular Outflow Operations

When further increase in pulmonary blood flow is required in the first few months of life, a closed transventricular pulmonary valvotomy (see Chapter 24, "Neonates" in section on Technique of Operation) may be performed if the initial operation did not include this procedure. However, there is often severe infundibular narrowing or atresia and an open operation with transannular patching is then required. The technique is similar to the placement of a transannular patch in the repair of tetralogy of Fallot with congenital pulmonary atresia (see Chapter 23, Figure 23-35), using cardiopulmonary bypass (UAB) or profoundly hypothermic total circulatory arrest (GLH).

When the initial operation was only a valvotomy and severe cyanosis persists, a classical Blalock-Taussig or Gore-Tex interposition shunt may be chosen (see Chapter 23, Section 1, "Technique of Shunting Operations").

When a more or less definitive right ventricular outflow operation is indicated (see "Indications for Operation"), it is done with cardiopulmonary bypass (CPB) (see Chapter 2) and cold cardioplegic myocardial protection (see Chapter 3) in the usual manner. The previously constructed shunt is usually closed as part of the procedure (see Chapter 23, "Repair of Uncomplicated Tetralogy of Fallot after a Blalock-Taussig or Gore-Tex Interposition Shunt" in Section 1, Technique of Operation). A transannular patch is generally placed. As a part of this procedure, muscle and fibrous tissue are excised from all four walls of the outflow tract and pulmonary ring. Prior to this, the sinus portion of the ventricle is examined and enlarged as much as possible by excising trabeculations passing from the septum to the free wall (including the moderator band). The tricuspid valve attachments must not be damaged. The foramen ovale is closed surgically.

Later Orthotopic Pulmonary Valve Insertion and Tricuspid Valve Replacement

These procedures are described in Chapters 23 and 14. They may be performed simultaneously as the third procedure in patients who have undergone initial valvotomy and shunting and subsequently an open repair with a transannular patch.

Later Fontan-type Procedure

The details of the Fontan-type procedure are in the section on Technique of Operation in Chapter 26. The direct right atrial to pulmonary artery anastomosis is used. The only special feature of the operation, when it is done for pulmonary atresia with intact ventricular septum, is that the hypoplastic tricuspid valve is excised in its entirety. The right ventricle is very hypoplastic and the cavity nearly nonexistent in the patients with pulmonary atresia and intact ventricular septum in whom the Fontan-type procedure is chosen, and its presence in communication with the right atrium has had no unfavorable effect. The other alternatives for the management of the right ventricle (plication,[W3] closure of the tricuspid orifice) have been considered less desirable.

SPECIAL FEATURES OF POSTOPERATIVE CARE

After the initial operative procedure, the postoperative care is the same as described in Chapter 24 for the care after operation for critical pulmonary stenosis in neonates except that PGE_1 is not generally continued into the postoperative period unless the shunt is poorly functioning.

The care after later right ventricular outflow tract operations is the same as after repair of tetralogy of Fallot (see Chapter 23). Care after the Fontan-type procedure is described in Chapter 26.

EARLY RESULTS

Hospital Mortality

With current indications and methods, an overall hospital mortality after the initial operation of about 10% is possible. In the combined UAB and GLH experience (Table 25-1), there was one hospital death (9%, CL 1%–28%) among 11 patients undergoing a systemic-pulmonary artery shunt alone or a shunt plus closed pulmonary valvotomy. De Leval and colleagues have had a similar experience since 1977, with a protocol of shunting or shunting plus transpulmonary valvotomy, depending on the morphology.[D4] Only 1 (7%, CL 0.9%–21%) of their 15 patients died in the hospital.

Other protocols for initial treatment have resulted in a high mortality (Tables 25-1, 25-2). Both de Leval's and the UAB and GLH data (Table 25-1) illustrate the poor results in this entity with valvotomy alone by any technique.

De Leval and colleagues also report disappointing overall results in an earlier era, 17 hospital deaths (55%, CL 44%–65%) occurring among 31 patients undergoing initial operations.[D4]

Early Reoperation

About 25% (3 of 10 at GLH and UAB; 7 of 28 in the report by de Leval et al.[D4]) of the patients require a second operation

Table 25-1 Initial surgical treatment of pulmonary atresia with intact ventricular septum (GLH and UAB; 1965–July 1980).

Age at Initial Operation	RV Hypoplasia	Other Operations	Result
Primary Brock valvotomy	7 Patients, hospital death in 6 (86%, CL 59%–98%)		
1 d	Severe	—	HD
2 d	Moderate	Shunt (3 d)	
		OV (5 mo)	D (5 mo)
2 d	NA	—	HD
3 d	Moderate	—	HD
4 d	Mild	—	HD
5 d	Mild	—	HD
Primary shunt:	8 Patients, hospital death in 1 (12%, CL 2%–36%)		
1 d	Moderate	—	Alive
1 d	Severe	OV (1 mo)	Alive
1 d	Moderate	—	Alive
2 d	Severe	—	Alive
3 d	Severe	—	Alive (cerebral abscess)
3 d	Severe	OV (13d)	HD
8 d	Severe	—	Alive (CHF,PVR)
8 mo	Severe	Shunt (2 mo)	D (2 mo)
	Large RV	—	Alive
Primary Brock valvotomy + Waterston shunt	3 Patients, hospital death in 0 (0%, CL 0%–47%)		
2 d	Moderate	PDAB (21 d)	Alive
2 d	Moderate	TAP (28 d)	Alive
3 d	Moderate	—	Alive
Primary Glenn Procedure			
9 mo	Severe	Fontan (5 yr)	(5 yr)
Primary open valvotomy (profound hypothermia)	6 Patients, hospital death in 5 (83%, CL 54%–98%)		
		(Additional Operative Steps)	
1 d		TAP	HD
3 d	Large RV[b]	TAP,PDAC,PFOC	HD
5 d	Mild	TAP,PDAC,PFOC	HD
11 d	Mild	IR,PDAC,PFOC	Alive
3 wk	Mild	IR	HD
4 wk	Large RV[b]	TVR,PDAC,TAP	HD

KEY: CHF, congestive heart failure; CL, 70% confidence limits; d, day; D, later death; HD, hospital death; IR, infundibular resection; mo, month; NA, not available; OV, open valvotomy; PDAB, patent ductus arteriosus banded; PDAC, patent ductus arteriosus closed; PVR, high pulmonary vascular resistance; TAP, transannular patch; TVR, tricuspid valve replacement; yr, year.

[a] Formalin injection patent ductus arteriosus instead of shunt.

[b] Associated Ebstein's anomaly with severe tricuspid incompetence.

within 1 month of the original procedure because of continuing hypoxia from low pulmonary blood flow. Another shunt, closed pulmonary valvotomy, or open repair with placement of transannular patch was done. Usually good additional palliation was provided.

LATE RESULTS

Interim Reoperations

Additional palliative operations to increase pulmonary blood flow are required in the first few years of life in 25%–50% of cases (Fig. 25-3). The hospital mortality of these procedures is less than 10%.

Right Ventricular and Tricuspid Valve Growth

Even a very small right ventricular cavity can increase in size as the patient grows,[G1,L2,M8,M9,S4] and right ventricular ejection fraction may increase.[G1] However, in most cases the cavity remains smaller than normal.[P4] The increase in size incorporates the area of extensive myocardial sinusoidal trabecular spaces, and with this process, the connections of these spaces with the coronary arteries may disappear.[P4]

Table 25-2   Reports of initial surgical treatment of pulmonary atresia with intact ventricular septum, 1970–1980.

Institution	Age (years)	Shunt			Shunt + Atrial Septostomy[a]			Valvotomy			Shunt + Valvotomy			Shunt + Valvotomy + Atrial Septostomy		
			Hospital Deaths			Hospital Deaths			Hospital Deaths			Hospital Deaths			Hospital Deaths	
		n	No.	%	n	No.	%	n	No.	%	n	No.	%	n	No.	%
Montreal Children's Hosp. (1977)[D3]	0–8/12	2	2	100%				19	9	47%	1	1	0%			
Toronto Sick Children's Hosp. (1976)[T2]	0–17/12	10	7	70%				17	13	76%				10	2	20%
New England Infant Cardiac Program (1976)[B5]		36	27	75%				11	7	64%	12	10	83%			
Texas Children's Hosp. (1970)[D2]	1/365–11/12	14	4	29%	1	0	0%	2	2	100%						
Univ. of Kansas Hosp. (1972)[L2]	1/365–5/12	6	2	33%	5	0	0%	2	0	0%						
Univ. of Minn. Hosp. (1970)[M9]	1/365–10/12							19	15	79%						
Brompton Hosp. (1973)[M1]	1/365–8/365	6	3	50%	4	0	0%	4	3	75%	1	1	100%			
Buffalo Children's Hosp. (1972)[S3]		1	1	100%				11	5	45%	4	3	75%			
Long Island Med. Ctr. (1977)[W2]	1/52	8	2	25%				3	1	33%	4	3	75%			
Babies Hosp., NYC (1979)[M7]	1/52	6	3	50%				6	6	100%	17	3	18%			
Children's Med. Ctr. (1979)[M8]	2–4/365				4	1	25%				3	0	0%			
Total		89	51	57%	30	7	23%	94	61	65%	42	20	48%	10	2	20%

[a] Some had Blalock-Hanlon operation instead.

Much of the growth occurs within a relatively short time postoperatively.[G1]

Knowledge of the factors that stimulate right ventricular growth is incomplete, but the two most important are the presence of severe tricuspid incompetence and of continuity between the right ventricle and pulmonary artery.[L3] However, growth can occur with severe tricuspid incompetence alone despite persistent pulmonary atresia (see Fig. 25-4). Even when the right ventricular cavity has grown, there usually remain significant abnormalities in right ventricular compliance,[G1] probably related to the fibrous endocardium and myocardium.

In view of the difficulty of quantitating changes in right ventricular size in this condition, it is reasonable instead to measure *changes in tricuspid valve diameter*. The tricuspid valve may show a normal rate of growth in patients in whom right ventricle-to-pulmonary artery continuity is present and very occasionally may become of normal size (Fig. 25-5).

When this continuity does not exist, little or no growth occurs.[D4,L3]

Pulmonary Vascular Resistance

Pulmonary vascular resistance is occasionally considerably elevated after the palliative operations. This occurred in one child at GLH and in 2 of the 8 patients described by Patel and colleagues.[P4] The elevated pulmonary vascular resistance may be contributed to by polycythemia and spontaneous pulmonary vascular thrombosis, but a large Waterston or Potts' shunt can also produce it.

Brain Abscess

Right-to-left shunting persists until a definitive repair is done. Brain abscess is therefore an ever-present risk and has occurred in 1 child at GLH.

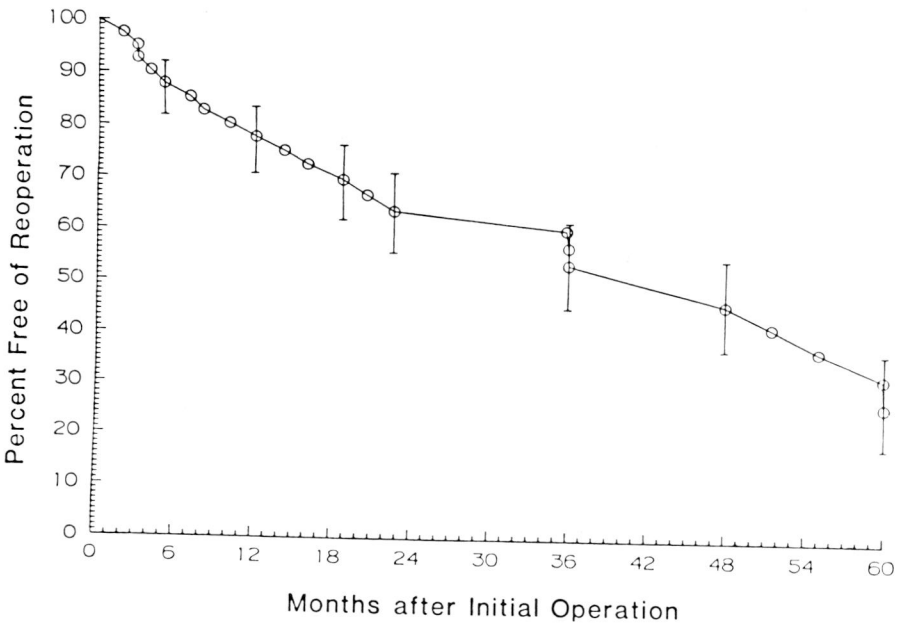

Figure 25-3 Proportion of 42 patients (collected from the literature)[D3,L2,W2] not reoperated upon at various intervals after surviving the initial operative procedure (shunting in 23, valvotomy in 9, shunting plus valvotomy in 10). Note that only 50% have not undergone a second operation within 36 months.

Definitive Repairs

Definitive repairs at a later age have carried an appreciable mortality to date, 25% (CL 3%–63%) after a right ventricular outflow repair (Table 25-3) with or without a procedure on the tricuspid valve, and 40% (CL 14%–71%) (see Chapter 26, Table 26-1) after the Fontan-type procedure. The considerable degree of left ventricular fibrosis that is usually present, the impaired left ventricular compliance that is apt to be present when creation of a right ventricular-pulmonary artery pathway was not possible,[S5] and the occasionally small left and right pulmonary arteries have no doubt contributed to these deaths. However, surviving patients after either procedure generally are in New York Heart Association (NYHA) class I or II.

Summary

Although actuarial survival after surgical treatment falls steeply during the first 6 months of life (Fig. 25-6), the additional actuarial mortality is about 15% over the next 4–5 years. Most surviving children are leading an active life.

INDICATIONS FOR OPERATION

The presence of the malformation is generally an indication for operation, and because of the highly lethal nature of the condition (see "Natural History"), a decision usually must be made during the first few weeks of life (see "Appropriateness of Surgical Treatment" in section on Special Situations and Controversies).

As soon as the diagnosis is suspected, an infusion of PGE_1 is begun in order to reverse spontaneous ductal closure.[C5,C6,E4,F6,H1,N2,O1] The full dose is $0.1 \text{ mg} \cdot \text{kg}^{-1} \cdot \text{min}^{-1}$, but if this dose is used from the outset, a period of apnea is usual. Therefore, one-fourth to one-tenth of this dose is recommended initially. Usually, the response is favorable, with lessening of cyanosis and decrease or disappearance of acidosis. Once the diagnosis is established (see earlier section), operation is undertaken within a few hours; but in view of the favorable effect of PGE_1, it is not done as an emergency. Prostaglandin E_1 is continued until a systemic-pulmonary artery shunt has been constructed. (For further discussion of preoperative PGE_1, see Chapter 24 "Neonates" in section on Indications for Operation.)

When a tripartite right ventricle has been shown to be present, which can be anticipated in no more than half the cases (see "Morphology"), a combined transpulmonary valvotomy and left Gore-Tex interposition graft insertion are performed. When there is infundibular atresia, only the Gore-Tex interposition graft operation is performed. A systemic-pulmonary shunt is always included because it is the most certain method of promptly increasing pulmonary blood flow.[D3,D4,M1,M6,T1]

If it has been possible to open the right ventricular outflow tract at the initial operation, and if the tricuspid valve has no more than mild incompetence and a diameter within the 70% confidence limits of normal as established by Rowlatt et al.[D4,R3] (see Chapter 19, Figure 19-21a, for the nomogram of these normal valves), and if the patient has reached the age of 1 or 2 years or more, then closure of the shunt, right ventricular outflow tract reconstruction usually with a transannular patch, and closure of the atrial septal defect are

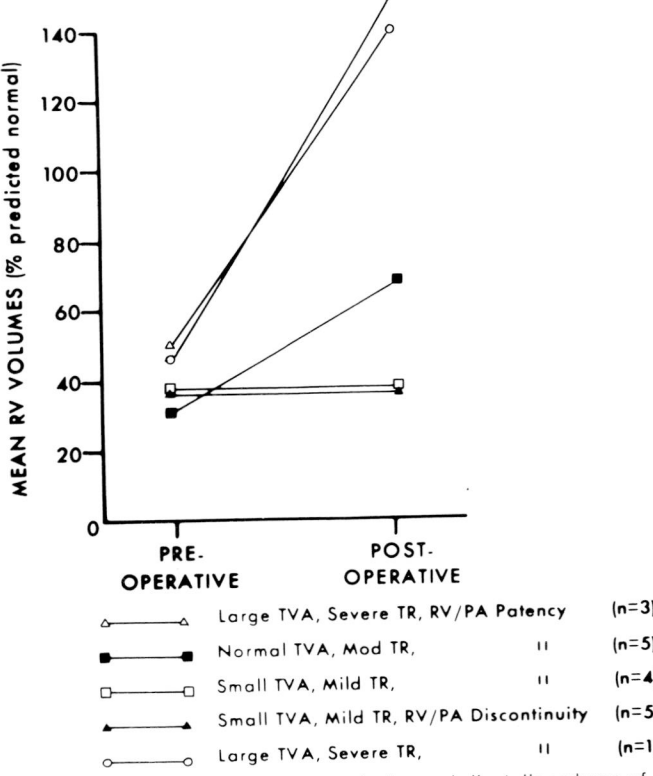

Large TVA, Severe TR, RV/PA Patency   (n=3)

Normal TVA, Mod TR,   "   (n=5)

Small TVA, Mild TR,   "   (n=4)

Small TVA, Mild TR, RV/PA Discontinuity   (n=5)

Large TVA, Severe TR,   "   (n=1)

Figure 25-4   Change in right ventricular end-diastolic volume after palliative operations for pulmonary atresia with intact ventricular septum. The mean right ventricular end-diastolic volumes are expressed as a percentage of expected volume both before operation and at the time of last assessment.

PA, pulmonary artery; RV, right ventricle; TR, tricuspid regurgitation; TVA, tricuspid valve anulus.

Reproduced with permission from Patel et al.,[P4] and the American Heart Association, Inc.

Table 25-3   Results of subsequent operations in patients surviving an initial procedure for pulmonary atresia and intact ventricular septum (UAB; 1967–1979).

Age (yr)	Previous Procedure	Procedure	Outcome
5	Potts anastomosis (neonate)	Transannular patch, closure of Potts, tricuspid annuloplasty	Alive[a]
3	Balloon septostomy (1/365)	Valved external conduit	Alive[b]
30/12	Balloon septostomy Waterston shunt (2/365)	Transannular patch	Death from hypoxia
23	Blalock-Taussig shunt	Fontan operation	Alive and in good condition
8	Potts shunt (3/365)	Valved external conduit	Alive and in good condition

[a] At 9 years, a third operation (insertion of tricuspid valve) was done with good result to date.

[b] At 6 years, a third operation (closure of Waterston shunt and atrial septal defect) was done, with death.

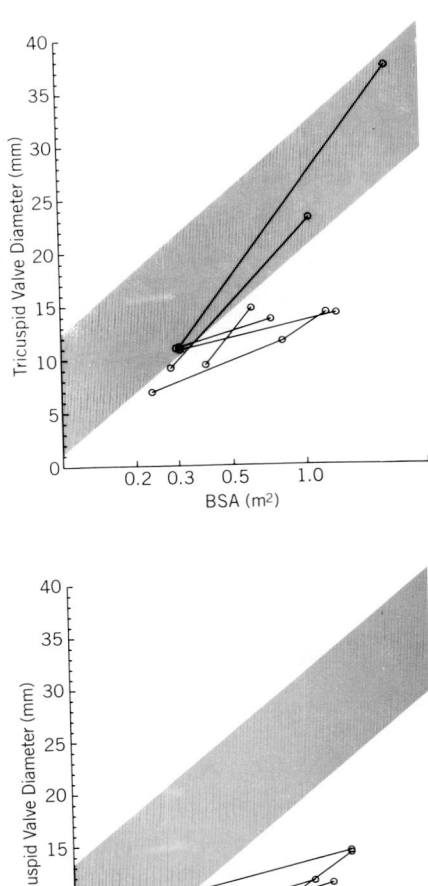

Figure 25-5   Tricuspid valve diameter related to body surface area (BSA) during growth of infants surviving an initial operation for pulmonary atresia with intact ventricular septum. In the top panel are patients in whom there was created a pathway from right ventricle to pulmonary artery; in the bottom panel are those without such a pathway. The horizontal axis, representing body surface area (m²), is on a logarithmic scale.

Modified from de Leval et al.,[D4] and the American Heart Association, Inc.

probably indicated as a definitive repair. (All this occurs infrequently and implies an originally tripartite right ventricle.) When there is concern that closure of the atrial septal defect may not be tolerated for any reason, the response at catheterization to temporary balloon closure should be determined before operation.[B10] If hypoxia develops at a younger age, a second shunt (or possibly a closed transventricular valvotomy) is indicated as a temporizing measure. In the years after the repair described, insertion of a homograft valve between right ventricle and pulmonary artery may become necessary, as well as replacement of the tricuspid valve.

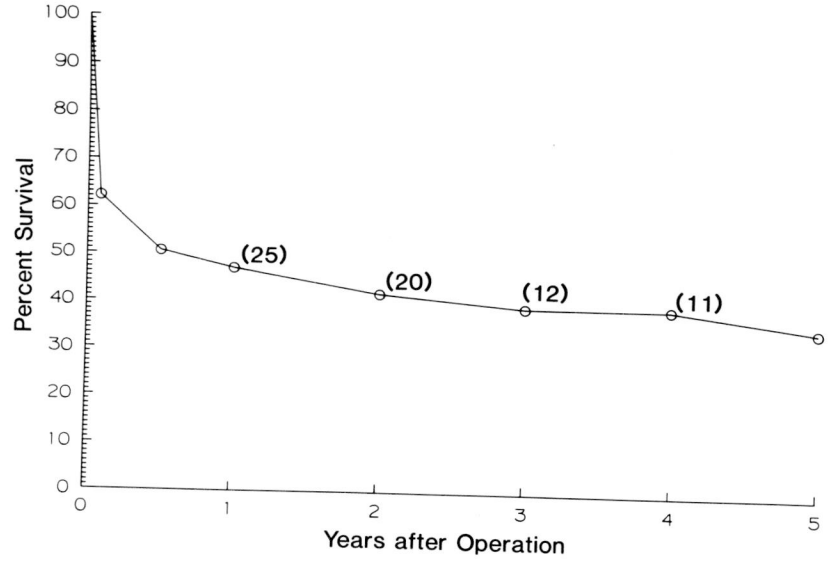

Figure 25-6 Actuarial survival after initial palliative operations for pulmonary atresia with intact ventricular septum. Hospital deaths are included.
Modified from de Leval et al.[D4]

More commonly, the criteria necessary for establishing a good right ventricular to pulmonary artery pathway are not present, in contrast to the situation in critical pulmonary stenosis with intact septum. Then a Fontan-type repair at an appropriate age is indicated if the right and left pulmonary arteries are of an adequate size (see Chapter 26, section on Indications for Operation). This may prove to be optimal surgical treatment for this malformation under most conditions. A temporizing additional shunt may be indicated in the interim.

SPECIAL SITUATIONS AND CONTROVERSIES

Appropriateness of Surgical Treatment

The current hospital mortality of 10% for the initial operation, the incidence of reoperation during the same hospitalization of 25% (albeit with a low risk), the need for additional palliative operations in 25%–50% of patients over the next few years, and the current hospital mortality of 25%–50% for the later definitive repairs could raise a question as to the appropriateness of embarking on a program of surgical treatment in the neonate with pulmonary atresia and intact ventricular septum. On the other hand, the considerable lowering in the current era of the risk of the initial operation suggests that overall risks in the future may also be lower. Also, the fact that the infants with this cardiac anomaly are otherwise usually well developed and without other anomalies argues in favor of strenuous cardiac surgical efforts.

On balance, intense surgical efforts seem clearly indicated unless limitation in resources make it necessary to curtail surgical procedures that have a relatively low probability of long-term success (see Chapter 6, Section 5). Part of the obligation in treating these infants surgically is a full discussion with the parents preoperatively, in which the risks and imponderables of surgical treatment are described.

Formalin Infiltration of the Wall of the Patent Ductus Arteriosus

Rudolph and colleagues in 1975 introduced formalin infiltration of the wall of the ductus via a left thoracotomy as a means of maintaining patency and avoiding the need for an artificial shunt.[R2] In one such patient (GLH) in whom this was done, the ductus required banding at 21 days of age because of an excessive shunt. Others (including UAB) have observed ductal closure within a few weeks or months of the procedures,[D4,M7] and its use is not currently recommended.[D5]

Surgical Obliteration of Right Ventricular Myocardial Sinusoids

The myocardial sinusoids present in some infants with pulmonary atresia and intact ventricular septum, particularly those with small right ventricular cavities and high intracavitary pressure, are physiologically active. As indicated in the section on Morphology, the sinusoids connect with coronary vessels and deliver deoxygenated blood to the myocardium.[F2] Deoxygenated blood may also pass via the left coronary artery to the aorta.[D6] Waldman and colleagues and de Leval propose surgical obliteration of the large fistulae or of the right ventricular cavity iself.[D6,W3] Since even the natural history of these sinusoids is uncertain,[P4] as well as the efficacy of these surgical measures, these procedures have not been used (UAB, GLH).

REFERENCES

A

1. Azcarate AO, Gonzalez LF, Alarcon AV: Atresia pulmonar con tabique interventricular integro. *Arch Inst Cardiol Mex* 44:388, 1974.

B

1. Bowman FO Jr, Malm JR, Hayes CJ, Gersony WM, Ellis K: Pulmonary atresia with intact ventricular septum. *J Thorac Cardiovasc Surg* 61:85, 1971.
2. Benton JW Jr, Elliott LP, Adams P Jr, Anderson RC, Hong CY, Lester RG: Pulmonary atresia and stenosis with intact ventricular septum. *Am J Dis Child* 104:83, 1962.
3. Becker AE, Becker MJ, Edwards JE: Pathologic spectrum of dysplasia of the tricuspid valve. *Arch Pathol* 91:167, 1971.
4. Bialostozky D, Attie F, Lupi E, Contreras R, Velo JE: Atresia pulmonar con septum interventricular intacto. I. *Arch Inst Cardiol Mex* 44:195, 1974.
5. Buckley LP, Dooley KJ, Fyler DC: Pulmonary atresia and intact ventricular septum in New England. *Am J Cardiol* 37:124, 1976 (abstr).
6. Bharati S, McAllister HA, Chiemmongkeltip P, Lev M: Congenital pulmonary atresia with tricuspid insufficiency: morphologic study. *Am J Cardiol* 40:70, 1977.
7. Bulkley BH, D'Amico B, Taylor AL: Extensive myocardial fiber disarray in aortic and pulmonary atresia. Relevance to hypertrophic cardiomyopathy. *Circulation* 67:191, 1983.
8. Bull C, de Leval MR, Mercanti C, Macartney FJ, Anderson RH: Pulmonary atresia and intact ventricular septum: A revised classification. *Circulation* 66:266, 1982.
9. Braunlin EA, Formanek AG, Moller JH, Edwards JE: Angiopathological appearances of pulmonary valve in pulmonary atresia with intact ventricular septum. Interpretation of nature of right ventricle from pulmonary angiography. *Br Heart J* 47:281, 1982.
10. Bass JL, Fuhrman BP, Lock JE: Balloon occlusion of atrial septal defect to assess right ventricular capability in hypoplastic right heart syndrome. *Circulation* 68:1081, 1983.

C

1. Cole RB, Muster AJ, Lev M, Paul MH: Pulmonary atresia with intact ventricular septum. *Am J Cardiol* 21:23, 1968.
2. Celermajer JM, Bowdler JD, Gengos DC, Cohen DH, Stuckey DS: Pulmonary valve rusion with intact ventricular septum. *Am Heart J* 76:452, 1968.
3. Cote M, Davignon A, Fouron JC: Congenital hypoplasia of right ventricular myocardium (Uhl's anomaly) associated with pulmonary atresia in a newborn. *Am J Cardiol* 31:658, 1973.
4. Coles JG, Freedom RM, Olley PM, Coceani F, Williams WG, Trusler GA: Surgical management of critical pulmonary stenosis in the neonate. *Ann Thorac Surg* 38:458, 1984.
5. Coceani F, Olley PM: The response of the ductus arteriosus to prostaglandins. *Can J Physiol Pharmacol* 51:220, 1973.
6. Christansen NC, Fabricus J: Medical manipulation of the ductus arteriosus. *Lancet* 2:24, 1975.

D

1. Davignon AL, Greenwold WE, DuShane JW, Edwards JE: Congenital pulmonary atresia with intact ventricular septum—Clinicopathologic correlation of two anatomic types. *Am Heart J* 62:591, 1961.
2. Dhanavaravibul S, Nora JJ, McNamara DG: Pulmonary valvular atresia with intact ventricular septum: Problems in diagnosis and results of treatment. *J Pediatr* 77:1010, 1970.
3. Dobell ARC, Grignon A: Early and late results in pulmonary atresia. *Ann Thorac Surg* 24:264, 1977.
4. de Leval M, Bull C, Stark J, Anderson RH, Taylor JFN, Macartney JF: Pulmonary atresia and intact ventricular septum: Surgical management based on a revised classification. *Circulation* 66:272, 1982.
5. Deanfield JE, Rees PG, Bull CM, de Leval M, Stark J, Macartney FJ, Taylor JFN: Formalin infiltration of ductus arteriosus in cyanotic congenital heart disease. *Br Heart J* 45:573, 1981.
6. de Leval M: (1984) Personal communication.

E

1. Edwards JE, Carey LS, Neufeld HN, Lester RG: Pulmonary atresia with intact ventricular septum, in *Congenital Heart Disease*. Philadelphia: W.B. Saunders, 1965, pp 576–598.
2. Ellis K, Casarella WJ, Hayes CJ, Gersony WM, Bowman FO Jr, Malm JR: Pulmonary atresia with intact ventricular septum. *Am J Roentgenol* 116:501, 1972.
3. Elliott LP, Adams P Jr, Edwards JE: Pulmonary atresia with intact ventricular septum. *Br Heart J* 25:489, 1963.
4. Elliott RB, Starling MB, Neutze JM: Medical manipulation of the ductus arteriosus. *Lancet* 1:140, 1975.

F

1. Freedom RM, Dische MR, Rowe RD: The tricuspid valve in pulmonary atresia and intact ventricular septum. *Arch Pathol Lab Med* 102:28, 1978.
2. Freedom RM, Harrington DP: Contributions of intramyocardial sinusoids in pulmonary atresia and intact ventricular septum to a right-sided circular shunt. *Br Heart J* 36:1061, 1974.
3. Freedom RM, White RI Jr, Ho CS, Gingell RL, Hawker RE, Rowe RD: Evaluation of patients with pulmonary atresia and intact ventricular septum by double catheter technique. *Pediatr Cardiol* 33:892, 1974.
4. Freedom RM, Keith JD: Pulmonary atresia with normal aortic root, in Keith JD, Rowe RD, Vlad P (eds): *Heart Disease in Infancy and Childhood* (ed 3). New York: Macmillan, 1978, pp 506–517.
5. Freedom RM, Wilson G, Trusler GA, Williams WG, Rowe RD: Pulmonary atresia and intact ventricular septum. *Scand J Thorac Cardiovasc Surg* 17:1, 1983.
6. Freed MD, Heymann MA, Lewis AB, Roehl SL, Kensey RC: Prostaglandin E₁ in infants with ductus arteriosus-dependent congenital heart disease. *Circulation* 64:899, 1981.

G

1. Graham TP, Bender HW, Atwood GF, Page DL, Sell CGR: Increase in right ventricular volume following valvulotomy for pulmonary atresia or stenosis with intact ventricular septum. *Circulation* 49, 50:(suppl II):II-69, 1974.
2. Gersony WM, Bernhard WF, Nadas AS, Gross RE: Diagnosis and surgical treatment of infants with critical pulmonary outflow obstruction. *Circulation* 35:765, 1967.

3. Greenwold WE: *A clinico-pathologic study of congenital tricuspid atresia and of pulmonary stenosis or pulmonary atresia with intact ventricular septum,* thesis. University of Minnesota, November 1955.

4. Greenwold WE, DuShane JW, Burchell HB, Bruwer A, Edwards JE: Congenital pulmonary atresia with intact ventricular septum: Two anatomic types. *Circulation* 14:945, 1956 (abstr).

5. Grant RT: An unusual anomaly of the coronary vessels in the malformed heart of a child. *Heart* 13:273, 1926.

6. Gootman NL, Scarpelli EM, Rudolph AM: Metabolic acidosis in children with severe cyanotic congenital heart disease. *Pediatrics* pp 251–254, February 1963.

7. Gamboa R, Gersony WM, Nadas AS: The electrocardiogram in tricuspid atresia and pulmonary atresia with intact ventricular septum. *Circulation* 34:24, 1966.

8. Goor DA, Lillehei CW: *Congenital Malformations of the Heart.* New York: Grune & Stratton, 1975, p 11.

H

1. Heymann MA, Rudolph AM: Ductus arteriosus dilatation by prostaglandin E$_1$ in infants with pulmonary atresia. *Pediatrics* 53:325, 1977.

J

1. Jimenez MQ, Sarachaga IH, Granados FM, Martul EV, Fanjul IT, Dieguez CG, Diaz FA: Atresia pulmonary con tabique interventricular integro. *Arch Inst Cardiol Mex* 46:182, 1976.

K

1. Kauffman SL, Anderson DH: Persistent venous valves, maldevelopment of the right heart, and coronary artery-ventricular communications. *Am Heart J* 66:664, 1963.

L

1. Lauer RM, Fink HP, Petry EL, Dunn MI, Diehl AM: Angiographic demonstration of intramyocardial sinusoids in pulmonary-valve atresia with intact ventricular septum and hypoplastic right ventricle. *N Engl J Med* 271:68, 1964.

2. Luckstead EF, Mattioli L, Crosby IK, Reed WA, Diehl AM: Two-stage palliative surgical approach for pulmonary atresia with intact ventricular septum (Type I). *Am J Cardiol* 29:490, 1972.

3. Lewis AB, Wells W, Lindesmith GG: Evaluation and surgical treatment of pulmonary atresia and intact ventricular septum in infancy. *Circulation* 67:1318, 1983.

M

1. Miller GAH, Restifo M, Shinebourne EA, Paneth M, Joseph MC, Lennox SC, Kerr IH: Pulmonary atresia with intact ventricular septum and critical pulmonary stenosis presenting in first month of life. *Br Heart J* 35:9, 1973.

2. Morgan BC, Stacy GS, Dillard DH: Pulmonary valvular and infundibular atresia with intact ventricular septum. *Am J Cardiol* 16:746, 1965.

3. Mangiardi JL, Sullivan JJ, Bifulco E, Lukash L: Congenital tricuspid stenosis with pulmonary atresia. *Am J Cardiol* 11:726, 1963.

4. Mitchell SC, Korones SB, Berends HW: Congenital heart disease in 56,109 births. *Circulation* 43:323, 1971.

5. McArthur JD, Munsi SC, Sukumar IP, Cherian G: Pulmonary valve atresia with intact ventricular septum. *Circulation* 44:740, 1971.

6. Murphy DA, Murphy DR, Gibbons JE, Dobell ARC: Surgical treatment of pulmonary atresia with intact ventricular septum. *J Thorac Cardiovasc Surg* 62:213, 1971.

7. Moulton AL, Bowman FO Jr, Edie RN, Hayes C, Ellis K, Malm JR: Pulmonary atresia with intact ventricular septum—A 16 year experience. *J Thorac Cardiovasc Surg* 78:527, 1979.

8. Mansfield PB, Hall DG, Rittenhouse EA, Sauvage LR, Herndon PS, Stamm SJ: Surgical treatment of pulmonary atresia with right ventricular hypoplasia and intact septum. *Mod Prob Pediatr* 22:167, 1983.

9. Moller JH, Girod D, Amplatz K, Varco RL: Pulmonary valvotomy in pulmonary atresia with hypoplastic right ventricle. *Surgery* 68:630, 1970.

N

1. Newfeld EA, Cole RB, Paul MH: Ebstein's malformation of the tricuspid valve in the neonate with functional or anatomic pulmonary outflow obstruction. *Am J Cardiol* 19:727, 1967.

2. Neutze JM, Starling MB, Elliott RB, Barratt-Boyes BG: Palliation of cyanotic congenital heart disease in infants with E type prostaglandins. *Circulation* 55:238, 1977.

O

1. Olley PM, Coceani F, Bodach E: E-type prostaglandins. A new emergency therapy for certain cyanotic congenital heart malformations. *Circulation* 53:728, 1976.

P

1. Peacock TB: Malformation of the heart: Atresia of the orifice of the pulmonary artery. *Trans Pathol Soc London* 20:61, 1869.

2. Paul MH, Lev M: Tricuspid stenosis with pulmonary atresia. *Circulation* 12:198, 1960.

3. Perloff JK: Pulmonary atresia with intact ventricular septum, in *The Clinical Recognition of Congenital Heart Disease.* Philadelphia: WB Saunders, 1978, pp 604–618.

4. Patel RG, Freedom RM, Moes CAF, Bloom KR, Olley PM, Williams WG, Trusler GA, Rowe RD: Right ventricular volume determinations in 18 patients with pulmonary atresia and intact ventricular septum. Analysis of factors influencing right ventricular growth. *Circulation* 61:428, 1980.

R

1. Robicsek F, Bostoen H, Sander PW: Atresia of the pulmonary valve with normal pulmonary artery and intact ventricular septum in a 21-year-old woman. *Angiology* 17:896, 1966.

2. Rudolph AM, Hemann MA, Fishman N, Lakier JB: Formalin infiltration of the ductus arteriosus. A method for palliation of infants with selected congenital cardiac lesions. *N Engl J Med* 292:1263, 1975.

3. Rowlatt UF, Rimoldi JHA, Lev M: The quantitative anatomy of the normal child's heart. *Pediatr Clin North Am* 10:499, 1963.

S

1. Shams A, Fowler RS, Trusler GA, Keith JD, Mustard WT: Pulmonary atresia with intact ventricular septum. Report of 50 cases. *Pediatrics* 47:370, 1971.

2. Schrire V, Sutin GJ, Barnard CN: Organic and functional pulmonary atresia with intact ventricular septum. *Am J Cardiol* 8:100, 1961.

3. Subramanian S, Wagner H, Tsehai G, Menon VA: Pulmonary atresia with intact ventricular septum. *Ann Chir Infantile* 13:225, 1972.

4. Subramanian S: Surgical treatment of complex cyanotic anomalies in infants: Pulmonary atresia with intact ventricular septum, in JC Davila (ed): *Second Henry Ford Hospital International Symposium on Cardiac Surgery*. New York: Appleton-Century-Crofts, 1977, p 316.

5. Sideris EB, Olley PM, Spooner E, Farina M, Foster E, Trusler G, Shaher R: Left ventricular function and compliance in pulmonary atresia with intact ventricular septum. *J Thorac Cardiovasc Surg* 84:192, 1982.

6. St. Cyr J, Braunlin E, Moller J, Ring WS, Molina JE, Foker J: Management of pulmonary atresia and intact ventricular septum. *JACC* 5:477, 1985 (abstr).

T

1. Trusler GA, Fowler RS: The surgical management of pulmonary atresia with intact ventricular septum and hypoplastic right ventricle. *J Thorac Cardiovasc Surg* 59:740, 1970.

2. Trusler GA, Yamamoto N, Williams WG, Izukawa T, Rowe RD, Mustard WT: Surgical treatment of pulmonary atresia with intact ventricular septum. *Br Heart J* 38:957, 1976.

V

1. Vlad P: Pulmonary atresia with intact ventricular septum, in BG Barratt-Boyes, JM Neutze, EA Harris (eds): *Heart Disease in Infancy*. Baltimore, Md: Williams & Wilkins, 1973, pp 245–249.

2. Van Praagh R, Ando M, Van Praagh S, Senno A, Hougen TJ, Novak G, Hastreiter AR: Pulmonary atresia: Anatomic considerations, in BSL Kidd, RD Rowe (eds): *The Child with Congenital Heart Disease after Surgery*. New York: Futura, 1976, p 103.

W

1. Williams RR, Kent GB Jr, Edwards JE: Anomalous cardiac blood vessel communicating with the right ventricle. *Arch Pathol* 52:480, 1951.

2. Weisz D, Gootman N, Silbert D, Voleti C, Wisoff BG: Pulmonary atresia with intact ventricular septum. *NY State J Med*, pp 2068–2072, 1977.

3. Waldman JD, Lamberti JJ, Mathewson JW, George L: Surgical closure of the tricuspid valve for pulmonary atresia, intact ventricular septum, and right ventricle to coronary artery communications. *Pediatr Cardiol* 5:221, 1984.

Z

1. Ziegler RF, Taber RE: Diagnostic criteria and successful surgery in an operable form of complete pulmonary valve atresia. *Circulation* 26:807, 1962.

2. Zuberbuhler JR, Anderson RH: Morphological variations in pulmonary atresia with intact ventricular septum. *Br Heart J* 41:281, 1979.

26

TRICUSPID ATRESIA

DEFINITION

Tricuspid atresia is a congenital cardiac malformation in which the right atrium fails to open into a ventricle through an atrioventricular (AV) valve. There is thus a univentricular AV connection consisting of a left-sided mitral valve between the morphologically left atrium and left ventricle. The atrial situs is almost invariably solitus (normal) in association with a ventricular D-loop, and the right ventricle is hypoplastic. There is almost always a ventricular septal defect. The ventriculoarterial connection may be concordant or discordant (transposition). Tricuspid atresia occurs in situs inversus with L-ventricular loop (mirror image pattern), but this is very rare.

Hearts with situs solitus of the atria and ventricular L-loop in which the left-sided left atrium is separated from a left-sided hypoplastic right ventricle by an atretic tricuspid valve are excluded from this chapter.

HISTORICAL NOTE

In 1906, Kuhne apparently recognized the entity of congenital tricuspid atresia and described the two basic types, those with ventriculoarterial concordant connections and those with discordant (transposed) connections.[K1] In 1949, Edwards and Burchell further emphasized these two subgroups and added the presence or absence of pulmonary stenosis as a categorizing feature of tricuspid atresia.[E1] Tandon and Edwards added further descriptive features in 1974.[T1] The clinical features of tricuspid atresia were described by Bellet and colleagues in 1933[B9] and by Taussig[T2] and Brown[B5] in 1936. Controversy arose early and continues as to whether tricuspid atresia should be considered as a subset of single ventricle (see section on Historical Note in Chapter 43). From a surgical point of view, it is best considered as such, but its frequency supports presenting it as a separate entity.

The systemic-pulmonary arterial shunts developed in 1945 by Blalock and Taussig and later by Potts and by Waterston (see section on Historical Notes, Chapter 23) soon were applied to cyanotic patients with tricuspid atresia; and in 1958 the superior vena caval–right pulmonary artery anastomosis was applied specifically to tricuspid atresia by Glenn.[G1] The basis for the Glenn procedure was provided by the experimental studies reported by Carlon and colleagues in 1951,[C1] by Glenn and co-workers,[G2,N1,P1] and by Robicsek and colleagues,[R3] which showed that systemic venous pressure was an adequate driving force for pulmonary blood flow. In Moscow, Bakuljev and Kolesnikov independently developed these same concepts.[B8]

Successful repair of tricuspid atresia with separation of the right and left circulations was accomplished in 1968 by Fontan and colleagues and was reported in 1971.[F1,F2] This was preceded by experimental studies in 1943 by Isaac Starr and colleagues, showing that destruction of the dog's right ventricle did not result in systemic venous hypertension,[S1] in 1949 by Rodbard and Wagner, showing that the right ventricle could be bypassed,[R1] and in 1954 by Warden, DeWall, and Varco, showing the feasibility of bypassing the right ventricle by a right atrial–pulmonary artery anastomosis.[W1] Based on these studies, Hurwitt and colleagues reported an unsuccessful attempt to correct tricuspid atresia by a right atrial to pulmonary artery anastomosis in 1955.[H1] Fontan's procedure involved the construction of a cavopulmonary (Glenn) anastomosis with, in the first patient, a direct anastomosis between the right atrial appendage and the proximal end of the divided right pulmonary artery. In the subsequent two patients, one of whom had ventriculoarterial discordance (transposition), an aortic homograft-valved conduit was placed between the right atrium and the right pulmonary artery. In all three patients, a second homograft valve was inserted into the inferior vena caval ostium, the foramen ovale was closed, and the main pulmonary artery was ligated or divided. In 1973, Kreutzer and colleagues reported a modification of Fontan's operation in which the patient's main pulmonary artery with its intact pulmonary valve was dislocated from the right ventricle and anastomosed to the right atrial appendage after closing the ventricular septal defect (VSD) and atrial septal defect (ASD). A Glenn procedure was not performed, and no inferior vena caval valve was used.[K2,K4]

Other early reports of successful repairs are those of Ross and Somerville[R7] and Stanford and colleagues.[S7] Fontan has subsequently modified the operation originally done by himself and Baudet,[F3,F4] as have many others.[B4,B11,D1,H2,N2] Perhaps the most important of these was the report by Bjork[B4] describing a direct anastomosis between the right atrial appendage and the right ventricular outflow in patients with a normal pulmonary valve, using a roof of pericardium in order to avoid a synthetic tube graft. The direct right atrial–pulmonary artery connection used by Fontan in his first case has been modified and subsequently widely used.[D1,G4,G6,K3]

MORPHOLOGY

In tricuspid atresia there is no direct connection between the right atrium and right ventricle, but the left atrium connects through the mitral valve to the left ventricle. The atresia (or absent right atrioventricular connection) is usually muscular (75% of cases), but it may also be membranous. In the *muscular* type, the presence of a tiny dimple in the floor of the right atrium may or may not represent the atretic valve. The dimple has been said to lie above the left ventricle[A1,B3,W2] or ventricular septum in most cases and may then transilluminate from the left ventricle.[R6,R8] In such instances, it may in fact be a remnant of the membranous atrioventricular septum.[A3] In an autopsy collection of 26 hearts with tricuspid atresia, however, a dimple was present in only 13 hearts, and it transilluminated from the left ventricle in only 4 (15%) (GLH). The *membranous* type has three variants. In one, a fibrous diaphragm blocks the atrioventricular orifice, and remnants of the valvular apparatus are occasionally found beneath the membrane in the right ventricle. This type is often associated with left-sided juxtaposition of the atrial appendages and transposition.[D7] In the second variant, there is a classical Ebstein malformation of the tricuspid valve (see Chapter 27), which is imperforate because the leaflets are completely fused to each other, as well as to the wall of a small right ventricle[A1,R2,W2] (Fig. 26-1). In the rarest variant, there is an AV canal defect in which the right-sided valve is imperforate and blocks the opening between the right atrium and right ventricle (Fig. 26-2).

Two morphologic subsets of tricuspid atresia exist. In one, the origins of the great arteries are normal (a concordant ventriculoarterial connection) (60%–70% of cases); in the other there is transposition of the great arteries (a discordant ventriculoarterial connection) (about 30%–40% of cases).[A1,E1] Rarely, the ventriculoarterial connection is double outlet right or left ventricle or single outlet with truncus arteriosus.[A1]

Tricuspid Atresia with Normal Origin of the Great Arteries (Concordant Ventriculoarterial Connection)

This form of tricuspid atresia was referred to as type 1 by Edwards and Burchell[E1] and also by Vlad.[V1] The atria are nearly always in situs solitus.

The *right atrium* and its appendage are enlarged and thick walled, and an interatrial communication is always present, usually through a fossa ovalis type of ASD (Fig. 26-3). The valve of the fossa ovalis may be redundant and bulge into the left atrium and may contain multiple fenestrations. The ASD is generally large; Dick and colleagues found by hemodynamic studies that only 4% of patients had a *restrictive ASD*.[D4] Uncommonly, the defect is an ostium primum ASD in association with a cleft in the left atrioventricular valve (Fig. 23-2b), and rarely there is a common atrium (see Chapter 19).

The *eustachian valve* is often prominent, and in about 5% of cases it may extend superiorly to form a veil or partition across the right atrium, the so-called cor triatriatum dexter.[B3] At operation, this may be confusing to the unprepared surgeon.

The *left atrium* is morphologically normal but is also enlarged due to the obligatory shunt of systemic venous blood across the ASD. The *mitral valve* is usually larger than normal, which is related to the fact that both systemic and pulmonary venous return pass through it. The *left ventricle* is

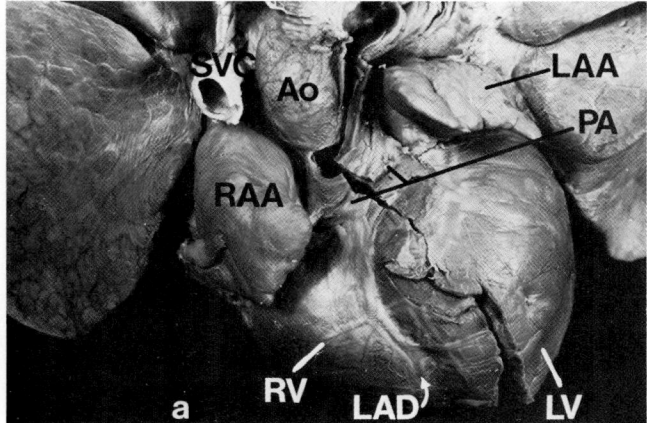

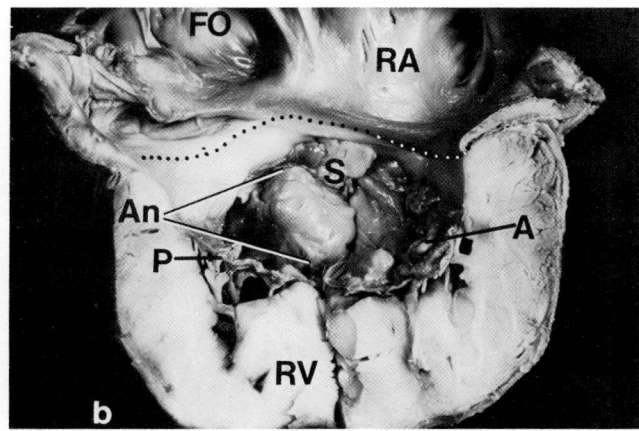

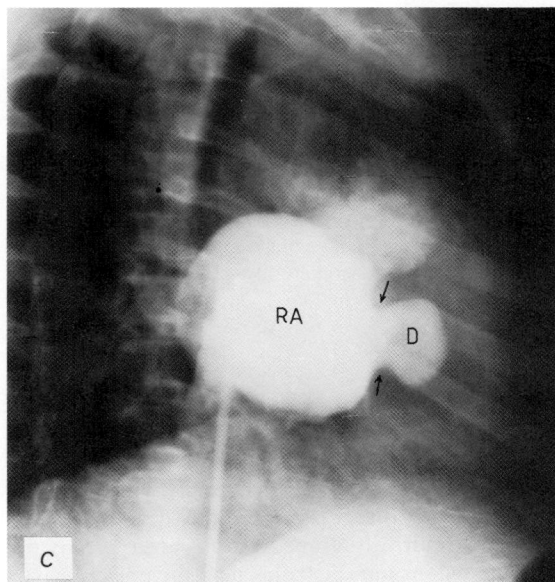

Figure 26-1 Specimen and cineangiogram of tricuspid atresia of Ebstein type (GLH).

(a) Exterior view of heart clearly shows the displaced left anterior descending coronary artery and the small right ventricle to its right. There was also pulmonary atresia, the cordlike pulmonary artery remnant wrapping around the proximal aorta where it arises from the left ventricle.

(b) Interior of RV and right atrium. The septal and posterior leaflets are downwardly displaced from the tricuspid anulus (dotted line). All three leaflets are loosely adherent to the RV wall and join to form an imperforate membrane. The aneurysmal bulge of the septal leaflet covers a potential ventricular septal defect. The blind RV is markedly hypertrophied.

(c) A cineangiogram frame from a similar patient in RAO projection shows the site of the tricuspid ring (arrow) and the blind diverticulum formed by the fused leaflets.

A, anterior leaflet; An, aneurysm septal leaflet; Ao, aorta; D, diverticulum; FO, fossa ovalis; LAA, left atrial appendage; LAD, left anterior descending coronary artery; LV, left ventricle; P, posterior tricuspid leaflet; PA, pulmonary artery; RA, right atrium; RAA, right atrial appendage; RV, right ventricle; S, septal tricuspid leaflet; SVC, superior vena cava.

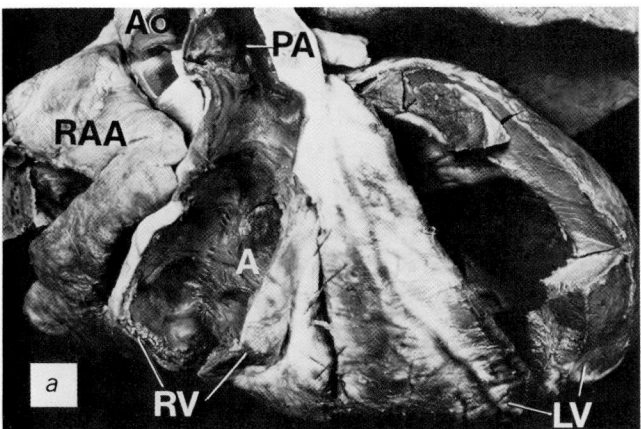

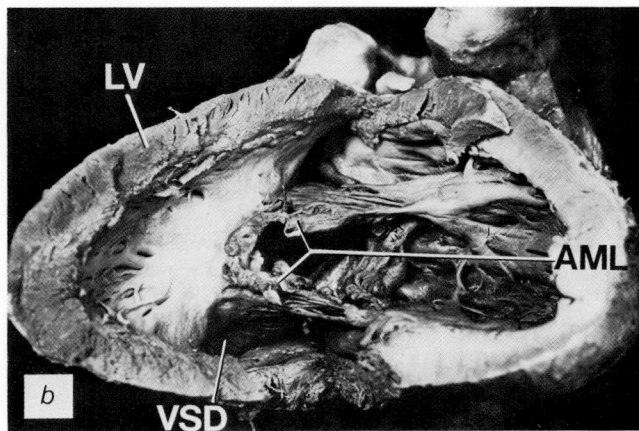

Figure 26-2 Specimen of tricuspid atresia with an AV canal defect (GLH).

(a) Frontal view with the thin-walled small right ventricle and pulmonary artery open. The rightward portions of the AV valve are fused to form an imperforate fibrous membrane. Note the large thick-walled left ventricle. The pulmonary valve is normal. The VSD is not visible in this view.

(b) View of opened left ventricle to show the typical scooped-out ventricular septal crest and the superior and inferior leaflets of the left side of the AV valve. The VSD is adjacent to the inferior leaflet.

A, imperforate membrane; AML, left AV valve leaflets; Ao, aorta; LV, left ventricle; PA, pulmonary artery; RAA, right atrial appendage; RV, right ventricle; VSD, ventricular septal defect.

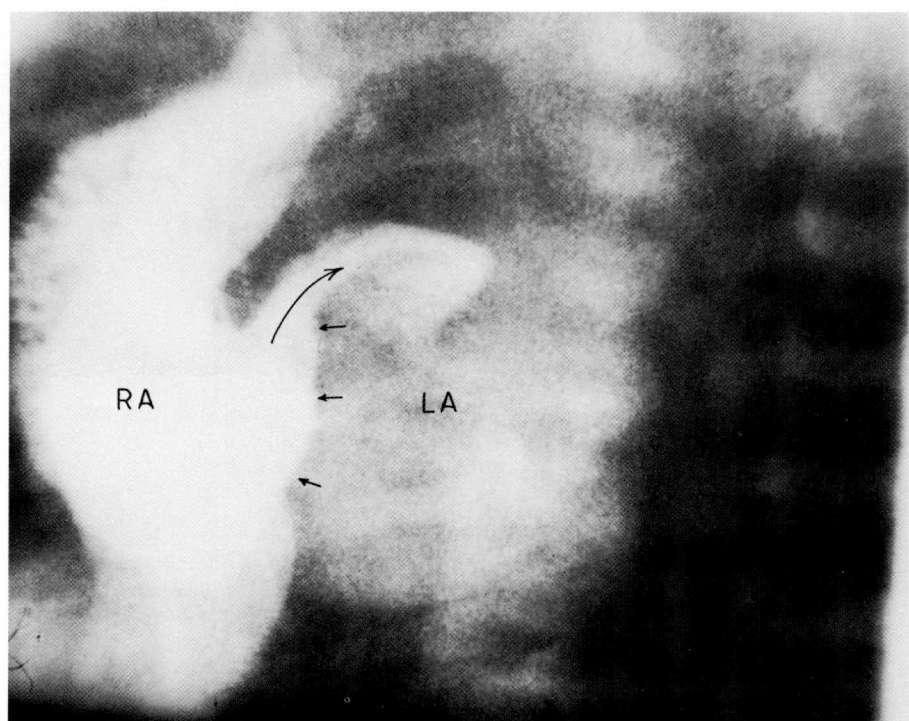

Figure 26-3 Cineangiogram frame in tilted LAO projection in a patient with tricuspid atresia that shows the right-to-left atrial shunt through a stretched patent foramen ovale (large arrow) (GLH). The valve of the fossa ovalis is outlined by the small arrows. There is no right ventricular filling.

RA, right atrium; LA, left atrium.

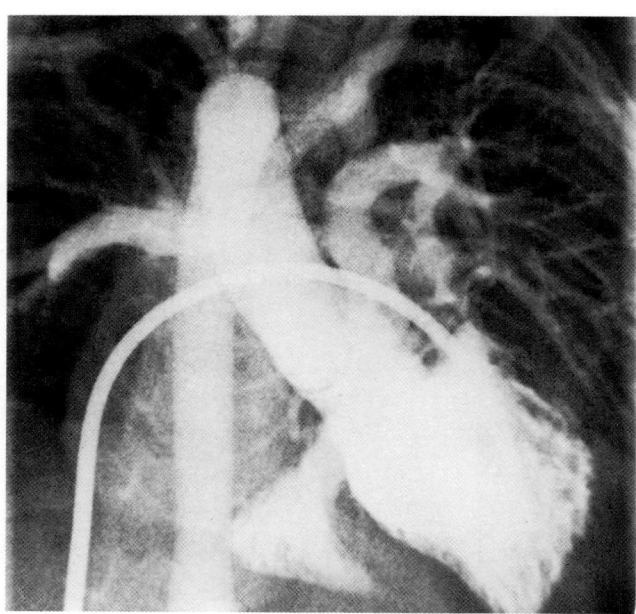

Figure 26-4 Cineangiogram in a patient with tricuspid atresia and normally positioned great arteries (ventriculoarterial concordant connection) in the four-chambered view (UAB). The injection is into the left ventricle. The left ventricle is mildly enlarged. The severely hypoplastic sinus portion of the right ventricle is evident, as is the infundibular portion. The pulmonary valve ring and pulmonary arteries are slightly small but are not restrictive. The bifurcation of the pulmonary artery is normal.

hypertrophied and larger than normal, which is no doubt related to the fact that it receives both systemic and pulmonary venous return. Its trabeculations are typically fine, although anomalous muscle bands near the posterior papillary muscle are occasionally present.

The normally positioned *right ventricle* (RV) is highly abnormal and similar in most instances to the small right ventricle of double inlet left ventricle[D2] (see Chapter 44, section on Morphology). Thus, in the majority of hearts it comprises a distal tubular smooth-walled portion with a thin free wall and a smaller proximal trabeculated pouch into which a VSD opens (Fig. 26-4). The VSD is variable in size and position and sometimes multiple. In general, the larger the VSD, the larger the right ventricle. The VSD usually lies below the conal (infundibular) septum and from the left ventricular side is separated from the noncoronary aortic cusp by conal muscle. In two autopsy hearts (GLH), there was deviation of the conal septum into the left ventricular outflow tract producing potential obstruction. When the VSD is large, it may extend inferiorly to the membranous septum, or it may be entirely muscular, lower in the septum, and sometimes slitlike. The VSD and trabeculated portion of the right ventricle into which it opens are frequently separated from the smooth-walled distal portion by a narrow opening that looks like an os infundibulum (see Chapter 23, "Infundibulum" in Section 1, Morphology). Like other VSDs, it frequently narrows spontaneously and is therefore often small and may close completely. In a minority of hearts, the right ventricle is large and has a true sinus portion (Fig. 26-5). Usually this has

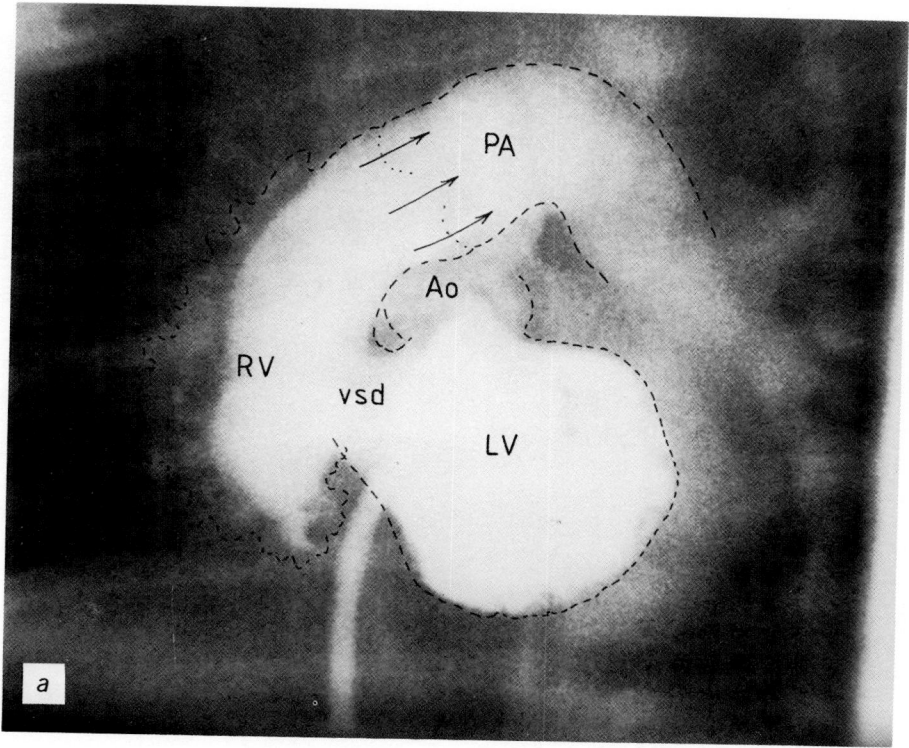

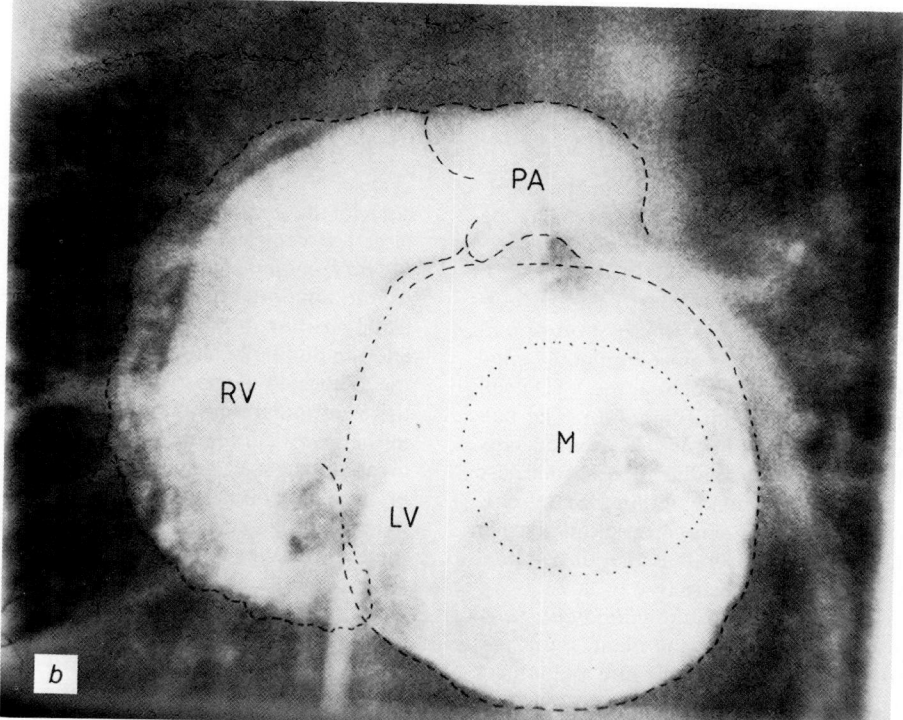

Figure 26-5 Cineangiogram in LAO projection of a patient with tricuspid atresia and a reasonably large right ventricle (GLH).

(*a*) Systolic frame shows a large ventricular septal defect entering the right ventricle and a wide channel to the pulmonary artery.

(*b*) Shows enlargement of both right and left ventricles in diastole and the large mitral valve orifice.

Ao, aorta; LV, left ventricle; PA, pulmonary artery; RV, right ventricle; VSD, ventricular septal defect.

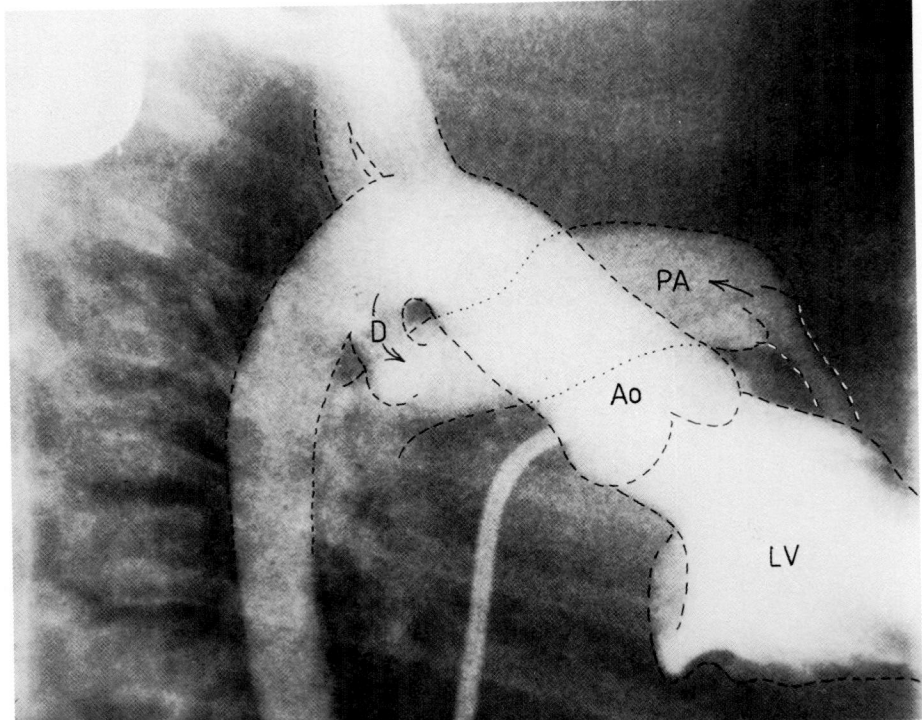

Figure 26-6   Cineangiogram in RAO in a patient with tricuspid atresia showing severe infundibular pulmonary stenosis beneath a normal, although small, pulmonary valve (GLH). There is also a patent ductus arteriosus.

Ao, aorta; D, patent ductus arteriosus; LV, left ventricle; PA, pulmonary artery.

no tricuspid valve remnants, but occasionally in the membranous varieties of tricuspid valve atresia there may be chordal remnants or in the Ebstein variety an atrialized portion beneath the adherent leaflets (Fig. 26-1*b*) (see Chapter 27).

In about 75% of patients with tricuspid atresia and normally positioned great arteries, there is *obstruction to pulmonary blood flow.* The obstruction is most commonly sited at the ostium infundibulum, or it may occur at the VSD itself or throughout the entire infundibulum (Fig. 26-6). The pulmonary valve is bicuspid in about 20% of cases, but usually it and the anulus, although a little smaller than normal, are not obstructive (the diameter is usually within 1 SD of normal). The main, right, and left pulmonary arteries are usually a little small, but only uncommonly (about 5% of patients) are they severely hypoplastic and restrictive to flow.[B3,C3]

In about 10% of cases in this subset, the *pulmonary valve is atretic.* Under these circumstances, the main, right, and left pulmonary arteries are usually small, and pulmonary blood flow is via a patent ductus arteriosus or aortopulmonary collateral artery; the right ventricle is usually extremely small, represented only by a miniscule endothelium-lined slit that is often inapparent to gross examination.[B3] The same is usually true when the VSD is absent.

About 15% of cases have no pulmonary stenosis and a normal or increased pulmonary blood flow. The VSD is larger than usual, and there is no infundibular stenosis.

The *coronary arteries* are normally distributed, and the system is usually a right dominant one. The well-formed anterior descending artery is displaced to the right by the large left ventricle.

The *conduction system* is basically normal but is affected by the abnormalities present. Thus, the AV node is in the usual position in the AV septum between the coronary sinus and the dimple of the atretic tricuspid valve.[B1] It penetrates the abnormally formed central fibrous body to the left side of the ventricular septum and becomes the branching bundle in the lower confines of the pars membranacea.[B2,G3] Here it gives off most of the posterior radiation of the left bundle branch. The bifurcation of the bundle and the formation of the right bundle branch occurs at the posteroinferior angle of the VSD on the left ventricular side. The right bundle branch proceeds here on the left ventricular side and then intramyocardially along the inferior (caudal) border of the VSD. Then it emerges on the right ventricular side and proceeds along the hypoplastic septal band (Fig. 26-7).

Associated defects in this subset of tricuspid atresia are uncommon, but a persistent left superior vena cava entering the coronary sinus occurs in about 15% of cases. Partially unroofed coronary sinus, with coronary sinus–left atrial communication (see Chapter 18), occurs in 1%–5% of patients. This is important, since after a Fontan repair the high right atrial pressure will produce a significant right-to-left shunt through it, even though a shunt was not apparent preoperatively.

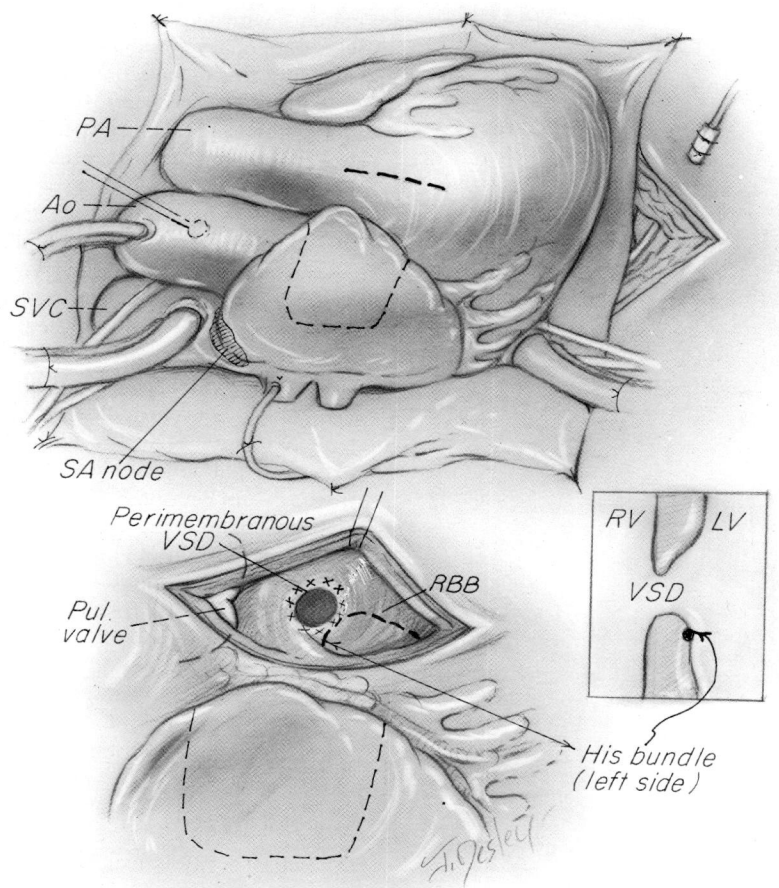

Figure 26-7 The conduction system in tricuspid atresia with normally positioned great arteries. Note the course of the His bundle and its protection from the surgeon by the thickness of the ventricular septum.

Ao, aorta; LV, left ventricle; PA, pulmonary artery; RBB, right bundle branch; RV, right ventricle; SVC, superior vena cava; VSD, ventricular septal defect.

Reproduced with permission from Bharati, Lev, and Kirklin.[B2]

Tricuspid Atresia with Transposition of the Great Arteries (Ventriculoarterial Discordant Connection)

In this tricuspid atresia subset (called type 2 by Edwards and Burchell[E1]), which includes 30%–40% of cases, the aorta arises from the right ventricle and the pulmonary artery from the left ventricle (Fig. 26-8). Generally, the aorta is anterior and to the right of the pulmonary artery (D malposition), in the position generally occupied in transposition of the great arteries, but uncommonly there is L-malposition.[T1,T5]

The atrial anatomy is generally similar to that described above. However, left juxtaposition of the atrial appendages occurs in about 10% of these cases,[B3] and in about half the ASD is small.[W2]

The *right ventricle* is larger in this subset and thicker walled. It is usually a single smooth-walled cavity without a proximal trabeculated extension. The VSD is usually large and may be nearly subaortic in position. In about 65% of cases, there is no subpulmonary left ventricular outflow obstruction, and the pulmonary valve and anulus are normal or

as large as the pulmonary artery. Thus, infants born with this malformation usually have a large or near-normal pulmonary blood flow.

The *left ventricle* is normal although enlarged. Subpulmonary stenosis in the left ventricle does occur in about 35% of cases, and very occasionally pulmonary atresia is present. These conditions result in a low pulmonary blood flow and hypoxia after birth.

The *coronary arteries* usually arise from the posterior aortic sinuses of Valsalva.

Associated cardiac anomalies in this subset usually involve the aortic arch. Coarctation of the aorta coexists in about 30% of cases and interrupted aortic arch less frequently.

CLINICAL FEATURES AND DIAGNOSTIC CRITERIA

Symptoms and Signs

Patients with tricuspid atresia with normal origin of the great arteries (ventriculoarterial concordant connection) are usu-

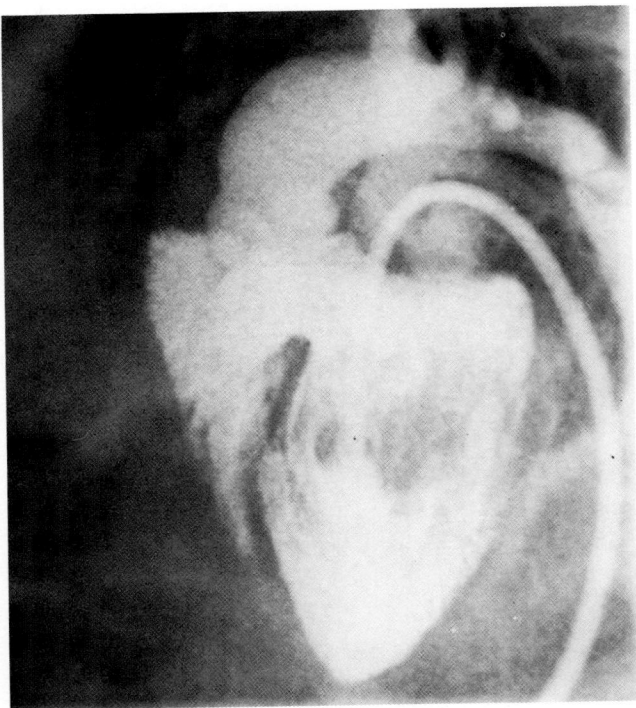

Figure 26-8   Tricuspid atresia with transposition of the great arteries (ventriculoarterial discordant connection) (UAB). The injection is into the left ventricle. In this long axial view, the aorta is seen to arise from the right ventricle, which is usually larger than when the aorta arises from left ventricle. The single ventricular septal defect is large and subaortic in position. There is moderate subpulmonary stenosis, poorly seen in this view, in the left ventricular outflow tract. The left ventricle is typically larger than normal.

ally cyanotic from birth because of the small pulmonary blood flow secondary to the right ventricular outflow obstruction. Dick and colleagues report that 50% of patients with tricuspid atresia are recognized to have congenital heart disease on their first day of life.[D4] The cyanosis is severe and progressive and is often accompanied by hypoxic spells characterized by increased cyanosis, dyspnea, and occasional syncope. These spells may occur in the first 6 months of life, and they are a grave prognostic sign. In patients with increasing obstruction to pulmonary blood flow resulting from progressive infundibular stenosis or closure of the ventricular septal defect, the degree of cyanosis becomes rapidly more severe, and patients who were previously acyanotic may become cyanotic in a matter of a few months. Clubbing of the fingers is commonly seen in children who survive beyond the first 2 years of life, but it may occasionally develop as early as 3 or 4 months of age. Squatting is uncommon. Dyspnea is often apparent with crying or feeding.

Most patients have loud, harsh, ejection systolic murmurs maximal over the lower left sternal border, which may be associated with an apical middiastolic rumble from the large mitral valve flow. In cases of progressive obstruction to pulmonary flow as the result of infundibular stenosis or closure of the VSD, the murmurs decrease or disappear. A continu-

ous murmur from a ductus arteriosus may also be heard in patients with pulmonary atresia and occasionally in babies with pulmonary stenosis.

A minority of patients with tricuspid atresia and normal origin of the great arteries has no obstruction to pulmonary blood flow and a nonrestrictive VSD. Such patients may present in infancy with all the signs and symptoms of excessive pulmonary blood flow or they may have more or less normal pulmonary blood flow and only mild cyanosis. In this latter instance, the physical findings, chest x-ray, and electrocardiogram are similar to those of other patients with normal origin of the great arteries. The vectorcardiogram, however, is similar to that in patients with tricuspid atresia with transposition of the great arteries.

Patients with *tricuspid atresia and transposition of the great arteries* (ventriculoarterial discordant connection) often present in early life with the symptoms and signs of excessive pulmonary blood flow (see Chapter 20, "Clinical Features" in Section 1, Clinical Features and Diagnostic Criteria). Usually an apical middiastolic rumble is present, and there is fixed splitting of the second heart sound at the base. However, occasionally moderate subvalvar pulmonary stenosis is present and results in either mildly increased or normal pulmonary blood flow. Such patients usually present after the neonatal period and sometimes after infancy, with mild cyanosis and few if any symptoms. The physical findings are similar to those in patients with tricuspid atresia and concordant ventriculoarterial connection.

Chest X-Ray

The chest x-ray is usually characteristic of reduced pulmonary blood flow and hypoplasia of the right ventricular chamber in patients with *tricuspid atresia* and *concordant ventriculoarterial connection*. Pulmonary vascular markings are reduced, and hilar shadows are diminutive. The left apical heart border may be rounded, forming a high, arched contour. The vascular pedicle is narrow, and the left border in the area of the main pulmonary artery is usually concave. However, the radiographic appearance of the heart in tricuspid atresia in this subset is variable and may resemble that of tetralogy of Fallot or occasionally appear normal. The chest x-ray in patients with this anomaly and discordant ventriculoarterial connection usually shows pulmonary plethora and cardiomegaly, and the narrow supracardiac waist and left ventricular contour make the x-ray resemble that of ordinary complete transposition.

Electrocardiogram

The electrocardiogram in patients with tricuspid atresia *and concordant ventriculoarterial connection* typically demonstrates left axis deviation (0° to −90°),[O1] left ventricular hypertrophy, and abnormalities of the P wave.[D4] Leftward deviation of the QRS axis is found in about 90% of cases, whereas left ventricular hypertrophy is noted in virtually all. The P wave is frequently tall (greater than 2.5 mV) and notched. Vectorcardiographic analysis reveals a narrow loop in the horizontal plane, often with a figure-of-eight contour, and with small QRS forces. The electrocardiogram may show left axis deviation in patients with tricuspid atresia and discordant ventriculoarterial connection, but a normal QRS axis between 0° and +90° is present in more than half the patients. In contrast to most patients with tricuspid atresia and normal origin of the great arteries, the QRS loop in the vectorcardiogram is usually wide, and large vector forces are directed posteriorly and to the left.

Two-Dimensional Echocardiography

Echocardiography confirms the clinical impression of tricuspid atresia and identifies the position of the great arteries, as well as the diminutive right ventricle and large left ventricle. Contractility of the left ventricle can be assessed.

Cardiac Catheterization and Cineangiography

Cardiac catheterization and cineangiography are performed prior to operation to determine the right ventricular and pulmonary arterial morphology and the arterial connections and to identify any major associated cardiac anomalies.

NATURAL HISTORY

Tricuspid atresia occurs more commonly than other types of univentricular atrioventricular connection and accounts for 1%–3% of congenital heart disease.

The natural history is determined primarily and early by the presence and severity of obstruction to pulmonary blood flow and secondarily and later by the left ventricular cardiomyopathy that develops in response to the volume overload.

Patients with tricuspid atresia and normal origin of the great arteries most commonly have important right ventricular outflow obstruction and are cyanotic at birth. In most of these the VSD narrows rapidly[R4] (in common with the general tendency of muscular VSDs to close spontaneously), pulmonary blood flow diminishes still further, cyanosis worsens, and increasing hypoxia causes the death of 90% of surgically untreated patients by the age of 1 year (Fig. 26-9).

When patients with tricuspid atresia and normal origin of the great arteries have a normal or increased pulmonary blood flow, the life history is more favorable than in any other subset (Fig. 26-9). Some die in early infancy of congestive heart failure secondary to the large pulmonary blood flow, but the spontaneous narrowing of the VSD and progression of infundibular narrowing usually produces a more balanced flow and better hemodynamic state within a few months of birth. Mild cyanosis and mild-to-moderate exercise intolerance persist at a plateau level for several years. The spontaneous narrowing of most VSDs continues,[R4,R5] however, and approximately 90% of the patients are dead by the age of 10 years. A few survive into the second and third decade of life and even beyond, presumably because neither the VSD nor the right ventricular outflow tract continue to narrow.

In patients surviving into the second decade of life and

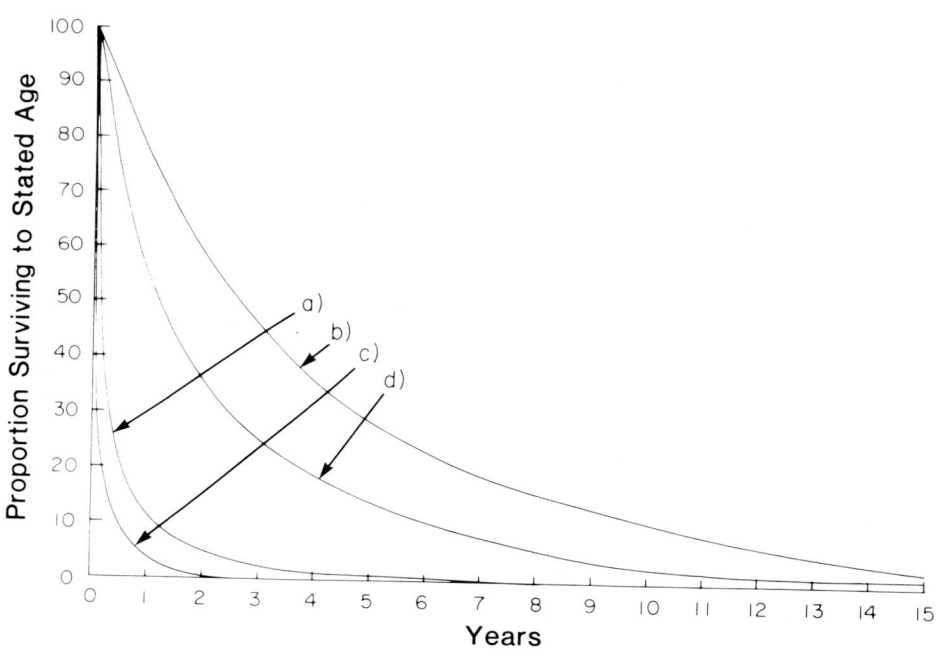

Figure 26-9 Free-hand representation of the left expectancy of surgically untreated patients with tricuspid atresia (based in part on Vlad[V1] and Dick et al.[D4]). (*a*) Represents patients with ventriculoarterial concordant connection and reduced pulmonary blood flow at birth. (*b*) Represents patients with ventriculoarterial concordant connection and normal or increased pulmonary blood flow at birth. (*c*) Represents patients with ventriculoarterial discordant connection and increased pulmonary blood flow at birth. (*d*) Represents patients with ventriculoarterial discordant connection and decreased or normal pulmonary blood flow at birth.

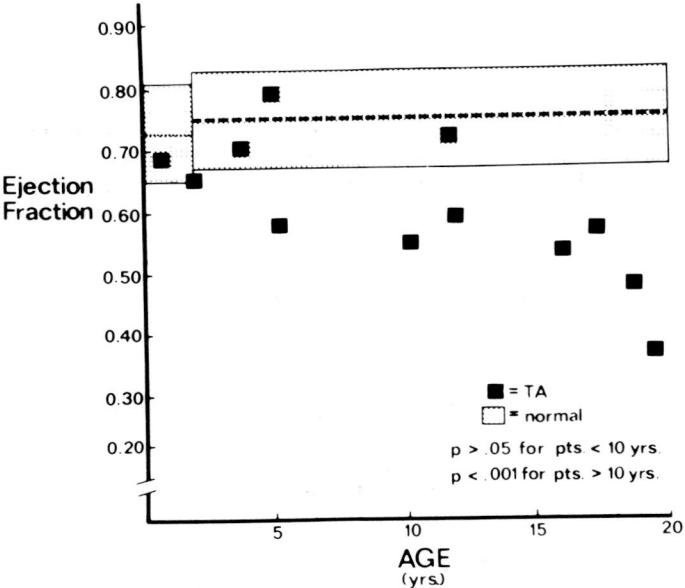

Figure 26-10 Left ventricular ejection fraction in patients with tricuspid atresia and surgically created systemic-pulmonary arterial shunts (solid squares) compared with normal subjects (stippled area). Note that ejection fraction becomes progressively more depressed as the patients become older.

TA, tricuspid atresia; normal, normal subjects.

Reproduced with permission from LaCorte et al.,[L2] and the American Heart Association, Inc.

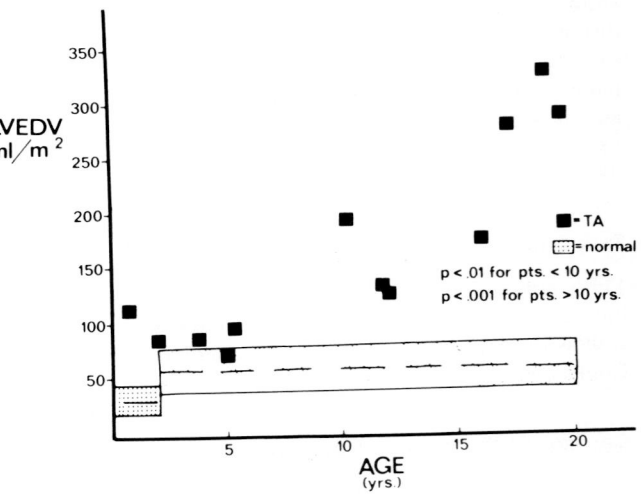

Figure 26-11 Left ventricular end-diastolic volume in patients with tricuspid atresia and systemic-pulmonary arterial shunts. (Presentation is as in Fig. 26-10.) Note the progressive increase with time in the left ventricular size.

LVED, left ventricular end diastolic volume; TA, tricuspid atresia.

Reproduced with permission from LaCorte et al.,[L2] and the American Heart Association, Inc.

longer, the chronic volume overload of the left ventricle usually produces a secondary left ventricular cardiomyopathy and reduced systolic function (Fig. 26-10). On this basis, mitral incompetence may develop. These factors produce a lower left ventricular output and consequent increasing cyanosis and congestive heart failure.

Surgically untreated patients with tricuspid atresia and transposed great arteries usually have a severely increased pulmonary blood flow, because the left ventricle ejects directly and without restriction into the pulmonary artery. Any tendency to closure of the VSD worsens the pulmonary plethora and reduces systemic blood flow. This unfavorable situation results in most of the babies with this type of tricuspid atresia being dead by the age of 1 year (Fig. 26-9).

A few such patients have associated mild or moderate left ventricular (subpulmonary) outflow narrowing at birth and a decreased pulmonary blood flow. The progression of the VSD and right ventricular outflow narrowing is slower in this subset, so that about 50% of these patients survive to about 2 years of age (Fig. 26-9). The hypoxia does, however, worsen with time, and about 90% of surgically untreated patients are dead by the age of 6 or 7 years.

The volume-overloaded left ventricle, receiving both pulmonary and systemic venous return in patients with tricuspid atresia, plays an important role in the natural life history. Surgically untreated infants with diminished pulmonary blood flow have depressed left ventricular systolic function (reduced ejection fraction) and end-diastolic volume larger than normal.[L2,N3] The reduced ejection fraction at this young age may be related to hypoxia. As these patients become

older, usually surviving because of a palliative systemic-pulmonary arterial shunt, ejection fraction becomes progressively more depressed (Fig. 26-10) and left ventricular volume progressively larger[L2] (Fig. 26-11). This is related to the progression of the left ventricular cardiomyopathy secondary to the chronic volume overload.[N3] In some patients, this leads to the gradual development of mitral incompetence in the second, third, and fourth decades of life.

TECHNIQUE OF OPERATION

Fontan-Type Procedure

Various technical options are available for the repair itself. These include (1) a nonvalved connection between right atrium and right ventricle with exclusion of any trabecular (sinus) portion of the ventricle, (2) a homograft-valved conduit between right atrium and right ventricle with preservation of the trabecular portion of the right ventricle (these two are applicable only when there is a concordant ventriculoarterial connection), and (3) a nonvalved connection between right atrium and pulmonary artery. (See "Indications for Operation" for discussion on selection of the most appropriate procedure.)

When the Fontan-type procedure is used for conditions other than tricuspid atresia, some additional steps are required. Patients with double inlet left ventricle require either closure of the right AV valve[D9] or a complex atrial baffle to divert pulmonary venous blood through both valves.[A4] These procedures are discussed in Chapter 44, "Fontan-type Procedure" in section on Technique of Operation. Patients with mitral atresia require a similar type of baffle.

In all, the preparations for operation, the incision, and the preparations for cardiopulmonary bypass (CPB) are generally those described in Chapter 2, including those for profound hypothermia and total circulatory arrest. The latter may be used in infants less than 8 kg in weight (GLH). The aortic cannulation and cardioplegia pursestrings are placed as usual, as are those for direct superior vena cava (SVC) and inferior vena cava (IVC) cannulation (see Chapter 2, Fig. 2-19). Any previously made systemic-pulmonary artery anastomosis is dissected (see Chapter 23, ''Repair of Uncomplicated Tetralogy of Fallot after a Blalock-Taussig or Gore-Tex Interposition Shunt'' in Section 1, Technique of Operation) and closed immediately after the start of CPB. If Dacron is to be used, an appropriate-sized woven tube graft is preclotted. CPB is established, the aorta cross-clamped, and the cold cardioplegic infusion given. The perfusate temperature is rapidly lowered by taking the heat exchanger water bath to 4°C so that the heart cools profoundly and soon becomes quiescent, the aorta is cross-clamped, and the cold cardioplegic solution is infused. Body temperature is stabilized at 25°C. During cooling, a left atrial suction line may be inserted through the base of the right superior pulmonary vein (GLH), or the field may be freed of blood after the right atrium is opened by a pump oxygenator sump sucker across the ASD (UAB).

Nonvalved Right Atrial–Right Ventricular Connection (GLH)

This procedure, which is essentially the Bjork modification[B4] of the Fontan procedure, may be performed when the trabecular portion of the right ventricle is vestigial and when the pulmonary valve and ring are nonrestrictive. The atrial appendage is opened at its tip along its longest axis and internal trabeculations excised to make certain there is no narrowing at the appendage waist (Fig. 26-12). The atrial septum is carefully studied through this opening, with knowledge of the frequency with which cor triatriatum dexter occurs to confuse the morphology. If this is present, the proliferation of eustachian valve tissue is cut away so that the atrial septum is seen clearly. The coronary sinus is explored with a fine right-angled clamp to be certain it is not unroofed in its midportion (see Chapter 18). The fossa ovalis type of ASD and the entire fossa ovalis are examined to determine whether additional defects are present. The ASD is then closed, usually with a patch of either pericardium or knitted Dacron velour. When the atrial suction line has been placed across the defect, the last few stitches of the ASD repair are placed but left on rubber shod clamps and set aside to be tied later.

A vertical incision is made in the right ventricular infundibulum (Fig. 26-12). Particular care is taken to keep it proximal to the pulmonary valve, which often extends further into the infundibulum than is apparent externally. The incision is then extended distally just to the pulmonary valve and far enough proximally to make the opening nonrestrictive. It is often necessary to excise a portion of the thin anterior wall of the infundibulum so that the rightward side of the opening lies fairly close to the atrioventricular (AV) groove. The VSD is closed off from the infundibulum with a knitted Dacron velour patch, which also excludes any trabecular portion of the ventricle.[N2]

The leftward edge of the opened appendage is sutured to the rightward edge of the ventriculotomy with a continuous whip stitch. A previously tailored piece of pericardium (GLH) or dacron (UAB) is now used to make a convex roof over the entire area (Fig. 26-12).[B4,S4] Before this is finished, the left atrial suction line is removed from the foramen ovale, the left atrium is filled with saline, and the atrial septal patch sutures are pulled up and tied. With strong suction on the aortic needle vent, the aortic clamp is released. Rewarming by the perfusate has been initiated about 5 minutes before this point is reached. After the ''roof'' has been completely sutured into place, the caval tapes are loosened.

After a good cardiac action has returned, the usual de-airing procedures are followed (Chapter 2). Two right atrial and one ventricular temporary myocardial wires are placed. After assuring hemostasis in the cardiac suture lines, CPB is discontinued. Pressure is measured in right atrium and pulmonary artery to assure that there is no pressure gradient. Should a gradient be found, the anastomosis must be undone and refashioned. When the operation has been properly done, the ratio between the mean right atrial and mean left atrial pressures (P_{RA}/P_{LA}) at this time should be less than 2.

The operation is completed as usual, but in addition both pleural spaces are opened and a chest tube brought from each. This is done because of the tendency to develop pleural effusion early after a Fontan operation.

Nonvalved Right Atrial–Right Ventricular Connection (UAB)

This operation is no longer employed as a routine but may still be indicated in a few special situations. Before cardiopulmonary bypass (CPB), fine 5-0 silk stitches are placed, tied, and cut to serve as markers for the cardiac incisions (Fig. 26-13). An appropriate-sized woven Dacron tube graft (often 20 mm) is selected and preclotted properly (see Chapter 23). After CPB is established, the aorta cross-clamped, and cold cardioplegia given, the right atrium is opened through one limb of the proposed trapdoor incision, and a pump oxygenator sump sucker is inserted across the foramen ovale.

A trapdoor opening is made into the right atrium (Fig. 26-13).[S4] After the usual careful examination of the interior of the RA, the ASD is closed with a patch of knitted Dacron velour. The repair is not completed at this time; instead, the last few stitches of the ASD repair are placed but let on rubber-shod clamps and set aside so that the left atrial sump sucker can remain in place across the defect.

A vertical incision is made in the right ventricular infundibulum (Fig. 26-13). Again, particular care is taken to keep it *proximal* to the pulmonary valve, which often is deeper in the infundibulum than is apparent externally. The incision is then extended distally just to the pulmonary valve and proximally far enough into the underdeveloped trabecular portion of the right ventricle to make the opening nonrestrictive. The trabecular portion of the ventricle, with the VSD, is closed off from the infundibulum with a knitted Dacron velour patch (Fig. 26-13).

The right atrial trapdoor flap is turned anteriorly, and its leading edge is sutured to the right side of the infundibular incision (Fig. 26-13). The previously tailored segment of the preclotted Dacron tube is now used to roof the entire area

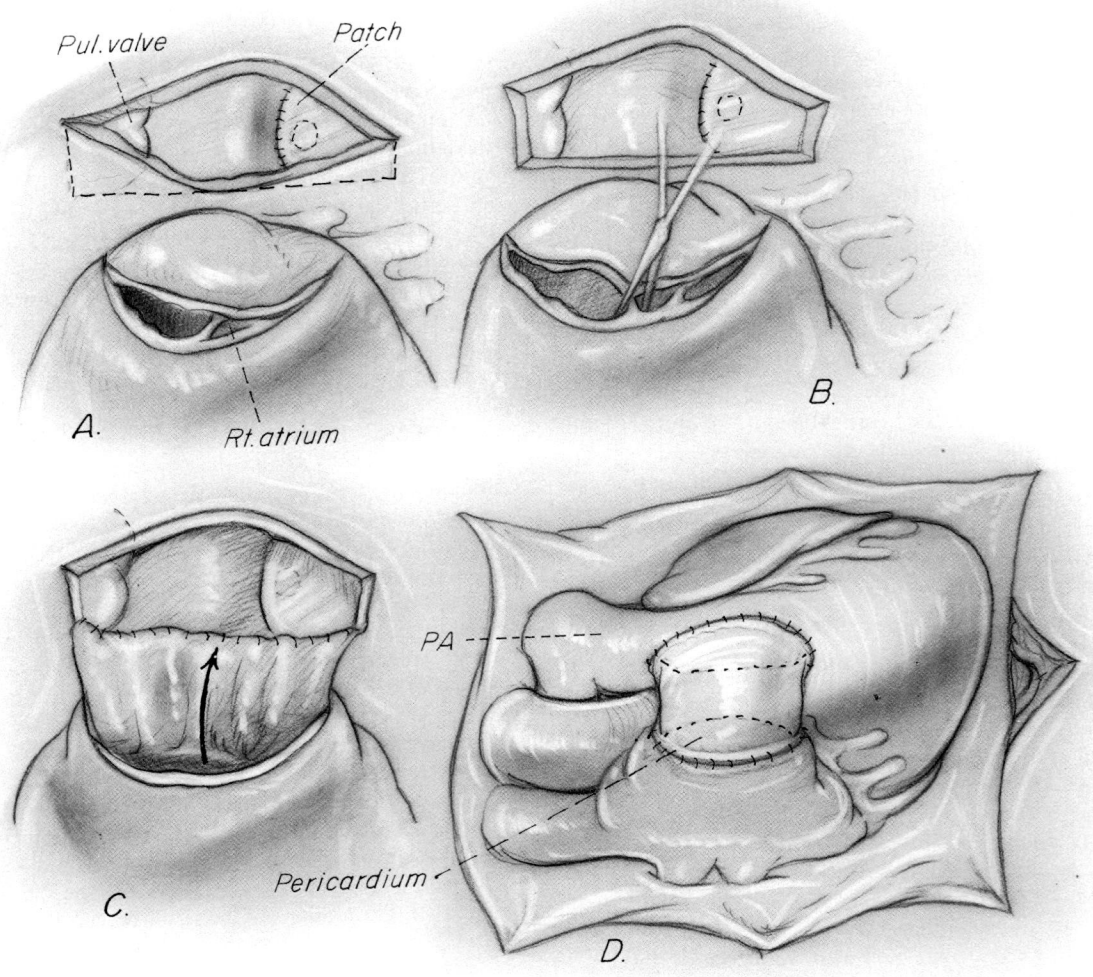

Figure 26-12 Fontan-type procedure using a nonvalved right atrial–right ventricular connection by the Bjork method.

(a) The hypoplastic right ventricle has been opened vertically, and a patch has been placed to isolate the infundibulum from the ventricular septal defect and the sinus portion of the ventricle. The right atrial appendage has been opened along its tip.

(b) The trabeculations are cut away to ensure a wide opening. A portion of the rightward side of the ventriculotomy has been incised to enlarge the opening.

(c) The posterior wall of the pathway is created by suturing together the contiguous edges of the right atrium and the right ventricular infundibulum.

(d) A concave roof of pericardium is used to complete the pathway.

PA, pulmonary artery.

(Fig. 26-22).[S4] Before this is finished, the sump sucker is removed from the foramen ovale, the left atrium is filled with saline, and the atrial septal patch sutures pulled up and tied. The suturing of the roof is completed, and with strong suction on the aortic needle vent, the aortic clamp is released. The caval tapes are loosened, and the remainder of the procedure is completed as usual.

Valved Right Atrial–Right Ventricular Connection (GLH)
When this technique is selected, the right atrial appendage is opened at its tip and an ellipse of atrial wall excised from the leftward aspect of the appendage, almost to the AV groove, creating an opening of sufficient size to accommodate a 22–

24-mm diameter homograft in a child and a 26–28-mm graft in an adult (Fig. 26-14). The adjacent rightward edge of the right ventricle (where it projects in front of the AV groove) is opened in similar fashion, excising an ellipse of tissue and extending the opening if necessary into the anterior right ventricular wall in a V-shaped fashion (Fig. 26-14). The VSD and ASD are both closed with a Dacron velour patch, working through these incisions, and any muscular restriction in the right ventricular infundibulum is excised. Since the distance between the appendage and right ventricular incisions is short, the homograft is trimmed transversely 2 mm below the aortic leaflets, and its aortic end is cut obliquely just above the leaflets. The valved end is sewn into the appendage opening with continuous 4-0 polypropylene and the aortic end into the right ventricular opening in similar fashion, with the longer flange of the obliquely cut aortic wall lying anteriorly (Fig. 26-15).

With suction on the aortic needle vent, the aortic clamp is released and rewarming begun. The operation is completed in the usual fashion.

Direct Right Atrial–Pulmonary Artery Connection

The direct right atrial–pulmonary artery (RA–PA) connection may be used as a routine (UAB) or in the Fontan-type

procedure only in selected cases (GLH). Before CPB, the main pulmonary artery is completely dissected away from the ascending aorta, and the right and left pulmonary arteries are mobilized beyond the bifurcation (Fig. 26-16). This procedure is done so the pulmonary trunk can be pulled beneath the aorta and to the right into a new position if this is required for a proper right atrial–pulmonary artery anastomosis. The ligamentum arteriosum is usually seen and can be simply ligated or ligated and divided. Meticulous hemostasis must be obtained with the electrocautery as the dissection is being done to prevent serious bleeding after CPB.

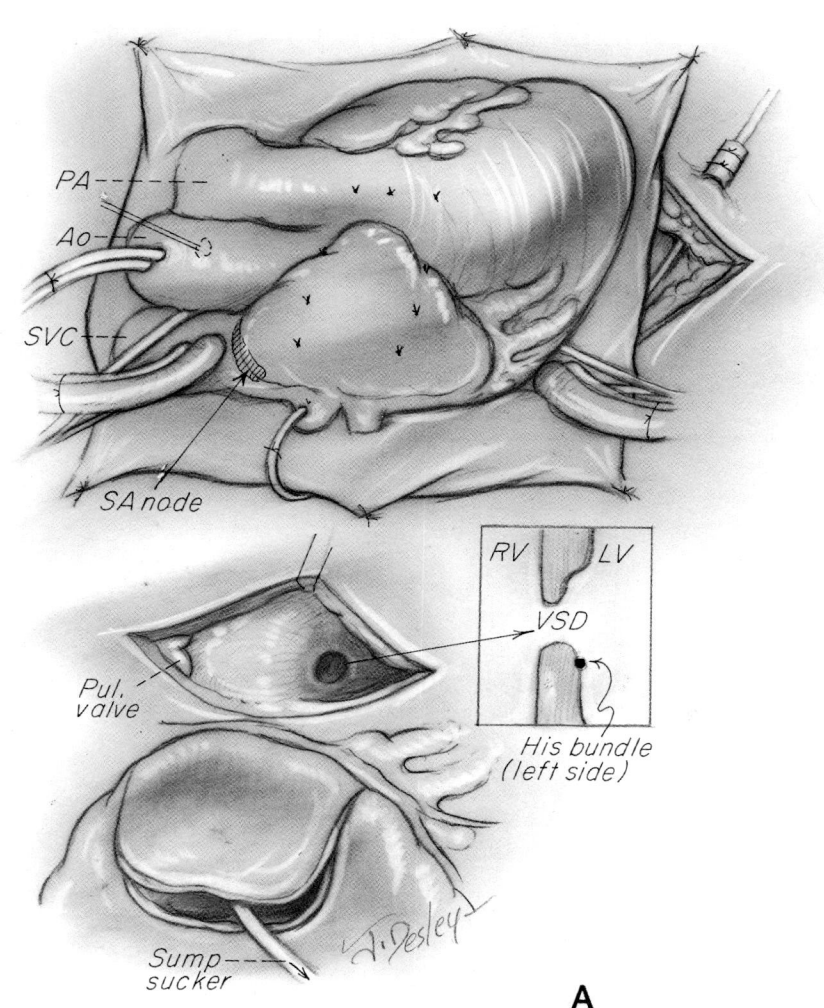

A

Figure 26-13 Fontan-type procedure using nonvalved right atrial–right ventricular connection (UAB).

(a) The tied 5-0 silk sutures outline the proposed right atrial trap door incision and the incision into the right ventricular infundibulum. Cardiopulmonary bypass (CPB) is established, cannulating the vena cavae directly. The right atrial trapdoor incision is made before the right ventricle is opened. Through it the atrial septal defect is nearly closed with a patch (not illustrated, but described in the text), and the sump sucker is left through the defect and into the left atrium. A longitudinal incision is made in the right ventricular infundibulum, extending it just far enough into the sinus portion of the right ventricle to make an adequate-sized opening (see text). The VSD is seen, and the insert shows the His bundle on the left ventricular side of the defect.

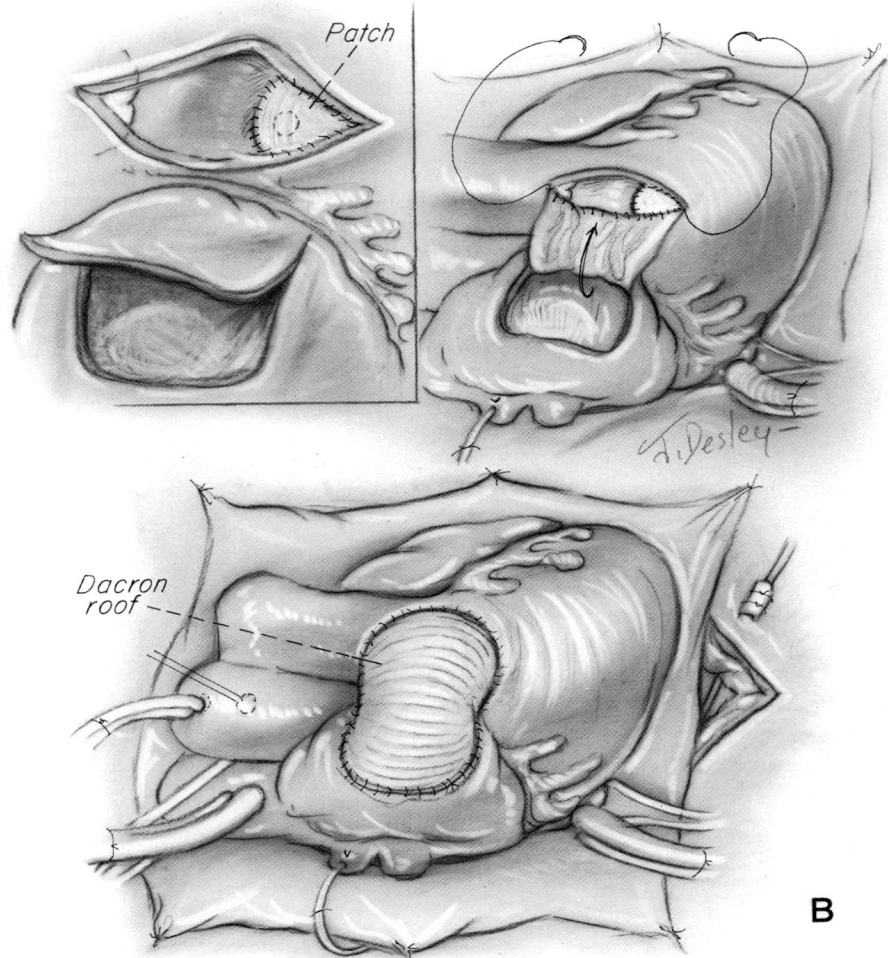

Figure 26-13 *(continued)*
(b) The sinus portion of the hypoplastic right ventricle and the VSD are excluded from the pulmonary blood flow pathway by a patch. The right atrial trapdoor is rotated forward, and its leading edge is sutured to the rightward edge of the ventriculotomy incision with continuous 4-0 polypropylene suture. The Dacron convex "roof," which has been made before CPB by trimming a preclotted woven Dacron tube to just the right dimensions, is sutured into place, beginning anteriorly. Not illustrated is the pulling up and tying of the atrial septal defect closure sutures (see text) before completing this.

Ao, aorta; LV, left ventricle; PA, pulmonary artery; RV, right ventricle; SVC, superior vena cava; VSD, ventricular septal defect.

Reproduced with permission from Bharati et al.[B2]

After CPB is established, the aorta is cross-clamped, taking care to leave the pulmonary arteries undisturbed, the cold cardioplegic solution is injected, the right atrium is opened through an oblique incision, and the pump oxygenator sump sucker is inserted across the foramen ovale. If the pulmonary trunk and its bifurcation and the first 1–2 cm of the right and left pulmonary arteries have not been fully mobilized, this is now completed. The pulmonary trunk is transected as close to the pulmonary valve as possible, and the proximal end is closed with two rows of continuous 4-0 polypropylene sutures supplemented with a few pledgetted mattress sutures. The distal well-mobilized end of the pulmonary trunk is pulled beneath the aorta to the right side

(Fig. 26-16). If the distal pulmonary trunk is very large, the opening is suitable for the anastomosis, but usually it must be extended onto the right pulmonary artery (Fig. 26-16).

The roof of the atria, just inferior to the right pulmonary artery, is visualized both externally and from within the right atrium. A right-angle clamp within the right atrium tents up the roof of the right atrium so that an incision can be made in it from outside. Now every consideration is given to making the largest possible opening between the right atrium and in the pulmonary artery. This requires extension of the opening in the atrial roof rightward to the superior vena cava and leftward well beneath the great arteries. An incision is made anteriorly from the midportion of this incision, and usually

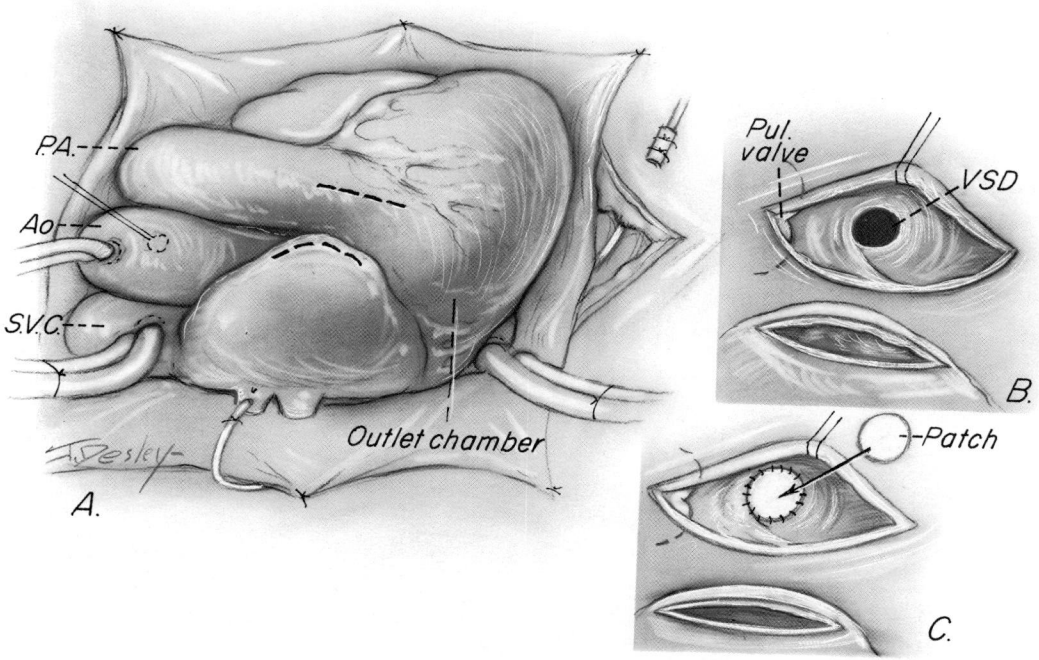

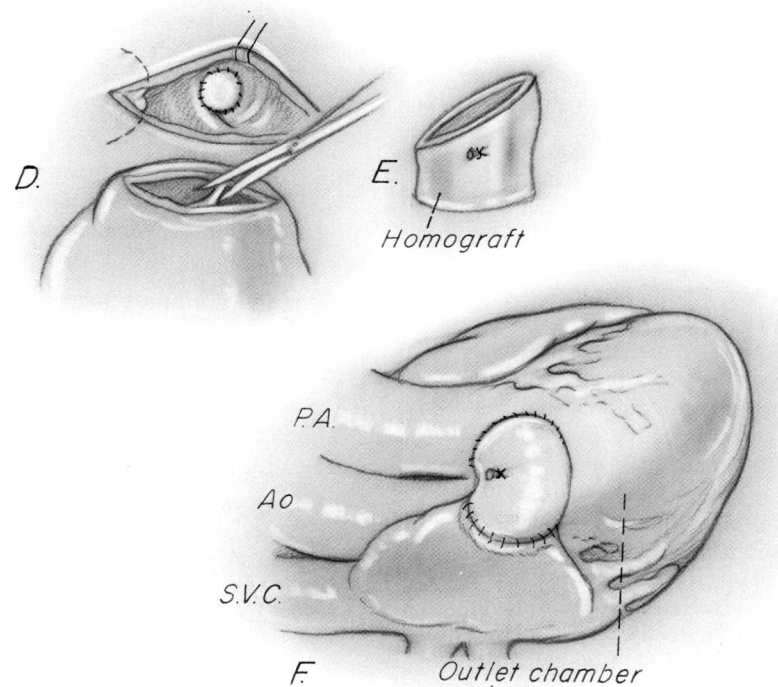

Figure 26-14 The Fontan-type repair using a valved right atrial–right ventricular connection.
(a) Incisions are made in the right atrial appendage and in the infundibulum of the very hypoplastic right ventricle.
(b) The incision in the ventricle is extended a short distance into the sinus portion of the ventricle to expose the ventricular septal defect and to provide the sinus portion free access to the pathway. This is to encourage later growth of the sinus portion.
(c) The ventricular septal defect *itself* is closed with the patch.
(d) Any muscular bands within the right atrial appendage are cut in order to ensure a free pathway from the right atrium into the conduit.
(e) A homograft-valved conduit is prepared and trimmed in an appropriate shape.
(f) The conduit is sutured into place between the right atrium and right ventricle (see text for details).
Ao, aorta; PA, pulmonary artery; SVC, superior vena cava; VSD, ventricular septal defect.

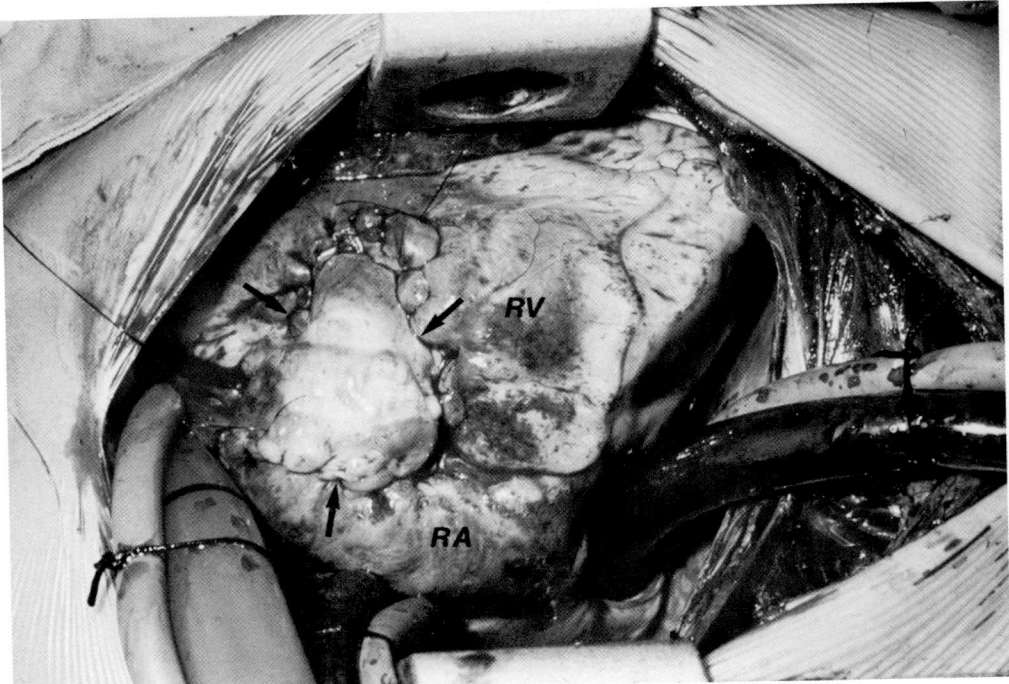

Figure 26-15   Aortic homograft-valved conduit between the right atrial appendage and the right ventricle, as viewed by the surgeon standing on the patient's right (GLH). The graft has been inset into the heart and does not project forward. The three arrows mark the visible portion of the suture line.

RA, right atrium; RV, right ventricle.

the angles are excised to create a large and essentially circular opening into the right atrium. (In anomalies such as single ventricle in which a complex atrial baffle is required, the atrial septum is excised and the opening in the atrial roof may be over both right and left atria.)

Usually a direct large anastomosis between the atrial roof incision and the distal end of the pulmonary artery is possible. The posterior row is made with a continuous suture of 4-0 or 5-0 polypropylene and the anterior row with interrupted 4-0 or 5-0 sutures. Occasionally, a convex roof is required to keep the RA–PA connection large, and this is made by sewing into place an appropriately shaped piece cut from the preclotted Dacron tube (Fig. 26-16). From within the right atrium, the ASD is simply closed, usually with a knitted Dacron velour patch. In some complex cases, most of the atrial septum must be excised and a new septum or right atrial wall flap used (see Chapter 44, "Fontan-type Procedure" in Section on Technique of Operation) to insure that the pulmonary veins drain to the mitral valve and access from the right atrium to the pulmonary artery is unobstructed. A polyvinyl catheter is placed through the anastomosis into the pulmonary artery, and the other end is brought out through the right atrial wall and later brought out through the skin.

The right atriotomy incision is closed. With strong suction on the aortic needle, the aortic clamp is released. The remainder of the operation is completed as usual. The usual left atrial polyvinyl catheter has been inserted before CPB, and a right atrial catheter and the usual temporary pacing wires are placed. A large window is made between the

pericardial and right pleural spaces by excising a large piece of pericardium anterior to the phrenic nerve. The remainder of the operation is completed as described above.

Systemic-Pulmonary Arterial Shunting

The types and techniques of shunting procedures and the circumstances leading to the choice of one over the other are exactly the same as in the tetralogy of Fallot (see Chap-

Figure 26-16   Fontan-type procedure, with direct right atrial–pulmonary artery connection. The pulmonary trunk is dissected free of the aorta before cardiopulmonary bypass, and the right and left pulmonary arteries are completely mobilized.

(a) After establishing cardiopulmonary bypass (see text), cross-clamping the aorta, and infusing the cold cardioplegic solution, the right atrium is opened through an oblique incision. The pulmonary trunk is transected just above the pulmonary valve commissure.

(b) The proximal end is closed (see text), and the distal end is brought rightward beneath the aorta.

(c) The opening into the pulmonary arteries is enlarged as shown by the dashed line. After incising and then excising the atrial septum if a complex atrial septal baffle is required, a circular button of the atrial roof is removed. (In classical tricuspid atresia, only the roof of the *right* atrium need be opened and partially excised.)

(d) The posterior wall of the openings into the pulmonary artery and the atria are brought together with a continuous whip stitch. The atrial septum has been excised as shown in the dashed line (a procedure necessary only when a complex atrial baffle is required and not in cases of classical tricuspid atresia).

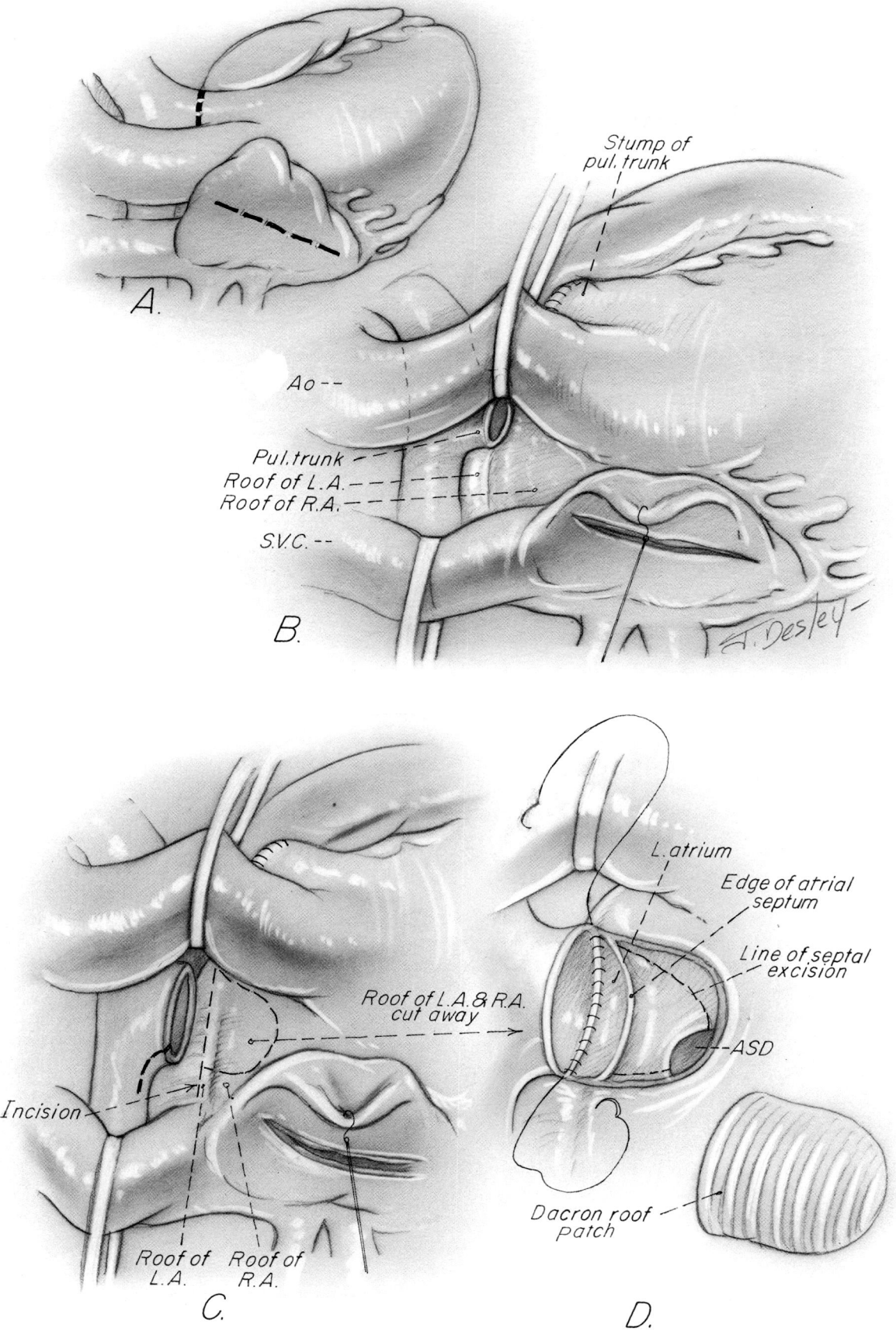

A.

B.

Stump of pul. trunk

Ao --

Pul. trunk -
Roof of L.A. --
Roof of R.A. --

S.V.C. --

J. Desley

C.

Roof of L.A. & R.A.
cut away

Incision -

Roof of   Roof of
L.A.   R.A.

D.

L. atrium

Edge of atrial
septum

Line of septal
excision

--- ASD

Dacron roof
patch

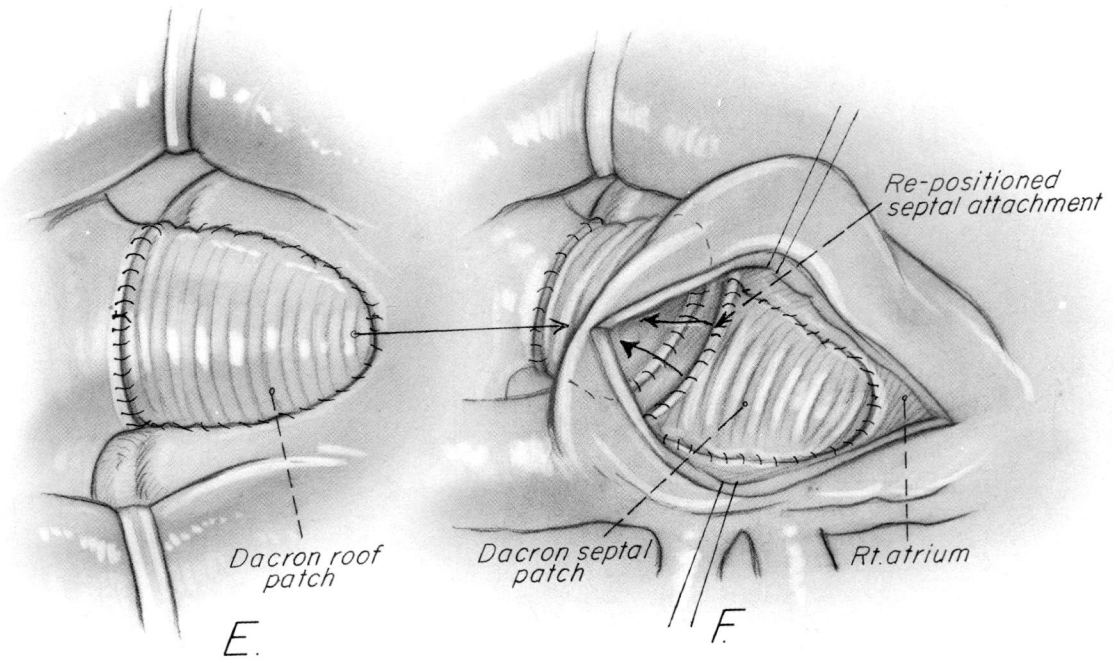

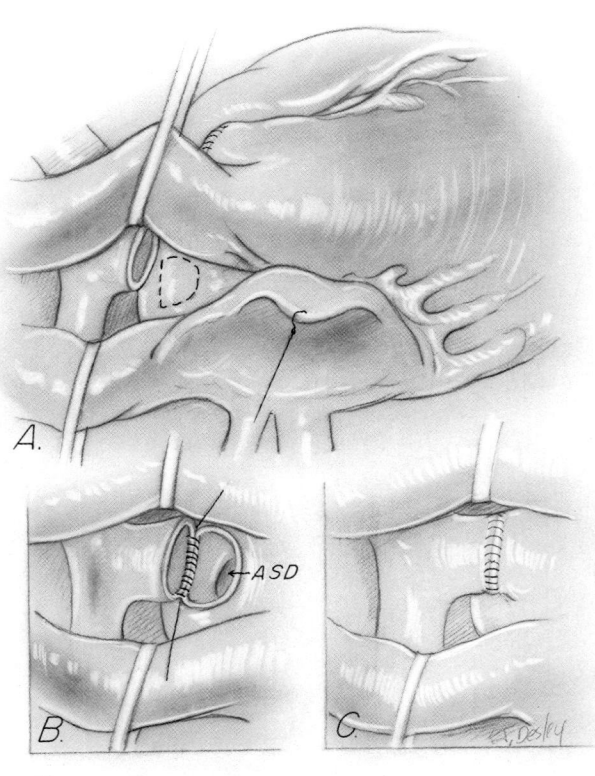

Re-positioned
septal attachment

Dacron roof
patch

Dacron septal
patch

Rt. atrium

E.

F.

A.

B.

C.

g

Figure 26-16 (*continued*)

(*e*) In most cases, the anterior wall of the right atrium and pulmonary artery can be brought together with interrupted sutures to complete a direct anastomosis (illustrated in Fig. 26-16*g*). Occasionally, it may seem that this would narrow the anastomosis, in which case a convex roof is placed over the opening to maintain a large aperture.

(*f*) The atrial septal defect is closed with a patch of knitted Dacron velour repositioned so as to provide a wide orifice from right atrium to pulmonary artery and free access of pulmonary venous blood to the left-sided AV valve. The repositioning is not necessary in tricuspid atresia.

(*g*) Alternatively, at least in tricuspid atresia, the repair may be done through a single incision in the roof of the right atrium. This approach, however, is not entirely desirable because it is nearly impossible to search the entire atrial septum and the coronary sinus carefully for any perforations allowing right atrial–left atrial communication postoperatively. The atrial septal defect (ASD) can usually be visualized through this incision and closed after placing the posterior row of the direct atriopulmonary artery anastomosis. If the anastomosis can be made as a wide circle rather than oval and narrow by a direct anastomosis of the distal end of the main pulmonary artery to the right atrium, this is done.

Ao, aorta; ASD, atrial septal defect; LA, left atrium; RA, right atrium; SVC, superior vena cava.

ter 23, Section 1, "Technique of Operation" and "Indications for Operation").

Pulmonary Artery Banding

The operation is done through a left anterolateral incision through the fourth or fifth interspace so as to allow the later median sternotomy for repair to be a primary one and, after the banding the pericardium is closed, to minimize intrapericardial adhesions.

The technique of banding is the same as described for VSD (see Chapter 20, "Pulmonary Artery Banding" in Section 1, Technique of Operation). The same procedure is used whether the ventriculoarterial connection is discordant or concordant, and the "transposition" rules apply.

SPECIAL FEATURES OF POSTOPERATIVE CARE

Fontan-Type Procedure

These patients are managed generally by the methods described in Chapter 5, but some modifications are used because of the absence of a pumping chamber for the pulmonary circulation and consequently higher pressure in the right atrium than in the left atrium.

Right atrial (RA) and left atrial (LA) pressures are monitored. Whenever possible, pulmonary artery pressure is also monitored by a fine polyvinyl catheter that enters the right atrium and passes across the anastomosis and into the pulmonary artery. A pressure tracing is made from this catheter as it is pulled back through the anastomosis and removed about 24 hours after operation.

There is a tendency for fluid to leave the intravascular compartment and pass into the interstitial space and into the pleural and peritoneal cavities. Thus, 5% albumin or stable plasma protein solution (SPPS) (see Chapter 5) is administered to keep the right atrial pressure at about 10–15 mmHg. Pleural effusions drain through the tubes placed at operation. On rare occasion, a peritoneal catheter may be required to drain a rapidly developing ascites.

If mean RA pressure must be kept above 16 mmHg to maintain an adequate hemodynamic state in the early postoperative hours, an explanation must be sought. As a first step, RA and LA pressures are compared. If LA pressure is also elevated, ventricular or AV valve dysfunction (incompetence or stenosis) is responsible for the right atrial hypertension. If the RA pressure is more than 5 mmHg higher than the LA pressure, the pathway from the right atrium through the lungs is probably restrictive at some point. If PA pressure is being recorded and is also elevated, either small size of the pulmonary arteries or pulmonary vascular disease are the likely explanation for the RA hypertension. Nothing definitive can be done about this, although pulmonary vascular resistance is sometimes transiently elevated for 12–36 hours after CPB and then returns to normal. Most importantly, if PA pressure is low and the difference between it and the mean RA pressure is greater than 1–2 mmHg, important stenosis exists somewhere in the RA–PA pathway. Under these circumstances, if the RA pressure is greater

than 18 mmHg and/or the hemodynamic state of the patient is suboptimal, consideration is given to prompt reoperation with revision of the pathway. The addition of a Glenn anastomosis may be advantageous.[D5]

The patient is nursed in semi-Fowler's position, and positive end-expiratory pressure (PEEP) is not used. As usual, spontaneous breathing is encouraged as early as possible (see Chapter 5). Extubation is usually accomplished within 6–24 hours of operation. The stay in the Intensive Care Unit is usually 48–72 hours, rather than the usual 24 hours, because of the slightly less robust performance of the cardiac subsystem than usually pertains when the energy for pulmonary blood flow is generated by a ventricle committed to this purpose. Likewise, the hospital stay is usually 14–28 days.

Careful follow-up is required for at least 3–6 weeks. A tendency to fluid retention, hepatomegaly, and ascites usually persists for most of this time, making sodium and fluid restriction and diuretic therapy usually necessary during this period. Close attention must be given to the possibility that fluid may accumulate in the pleural or pericardial space late postoperatively, producing important pulmonary or cardiac dysfunction. Prompt and, if necessary, repeated aspirations may be required. Chylothorax is always suspected under these circumstances.

Chylothorax is occasionally a serious problem after the Fontan-type of repair. An effusion that early postoperatively seems clearly not chylous may gradually over a period of days assume all of the characteristics of chyle. Chylous fluid may accumulate in either pleural space or in the pericardium if the pericardium does not communicate with the pleural spaces. The chyle very likely escapes from the vascular system at multiple points, rather than simply through an area of trauma to the thoracic duct. Although at times chylous effusions after the Fontan-type procedure gradually subside, they may persist and eventually become a fatal complication. The risk factors for the development of chylothorax after the Fontan-type procedure are still not clear, but at least on occasions this complication may develop in patients without inordinately elevated caval pressures. Special measures for the management of chylothorax are discussed in Chapter 5, "Chylothorax" in Section 3, Special Problems and Controversies.

Other Operations

Patients who have received *shunting operations* or *pulmonary artery banding* are managed as are patients who have received these operations for other malformations (see Chapters 20 for the latter and 23 for the former).

EARLY RESULTS

Hospital Mortality after the Fontan-Type Procedure

In most institutions, the early experience with the Fontan-type procedure for tricuspid atresia had an appreciable mortality (15%–30%).[T3,V2] Thus, at UAB, between 1967 and November 1, 1983 (first Fontan procedure in 1975), 40 patients with tricuspid atresia underwent the Fontan proce-

Table 26-1 Hospital and late deaths after Fontan-type procedure for congenital heart disease (UAB; 1967–Nov. 1, 1983; $n = 73$, first operation was in 1975).

		Deaths								
		Hospital			Late			Total		
Diagnosis	n	No.	%	CL	No.	%[a]	CL	No.	%	CL
Tricuspid atresia	46	7	15%	10%–23%	2	5%	2%–12%	9	20%	13%–27%
Severe TV hypoplasia	1	0	0%	0%–85%	0	0%	0%–85%	0	0%	0%–85%
Single ventricle	14	4	29%	15%–46%	1	10%	1%–30%	5	36%	21%–53%
Pulmonary atresia or near atresia with intact ventricular septum	5	2	40%	14%–71%	0	0%	0%–47%	2	40%	14%–71%
VSD with severe RV hypoplasia and PA band	1	0	0%	0%–85%	0	0%	0%–85%	0	0%	0%–85%
Complex double outlet RV	4	2	50%	18%–82%	0	0%	0%–61%	2	50%	18%–82%
Complex congenital heart disease with situs ambiguus	1	1	100%	15%–100%	—			1	100%	15%–100%
Complex corrected transposition	1	0	0%	0%–85%	0	0%	0%–85%	0	0%	0%–85%
Total	73	16	22%	17%–28%	3	5%	2%–10%	19	26%	20%–32%
$P(\chi^2)$		.3								

KEY: CL, 70% confidence limits; PA, pulmonary artery; RV, right ventricle; TV, tricuspid valve; VSD, ventricular septal defect.

[a] Percent of hospital survivors.

dure, with seven hospital deaths (15%; CL 10%–23%) (Table 26-1), and at GLH the mortality in this period in patients over 12 months of age was also 15% (2 out of 13). The Mayo Clinic experience between 1973 and 1979, reported by Gale and colleagues, included 29 patients with 4 hospital deaths (14%);[G4] the hospital mortality was 17% for about the same time frame at the Boston Children's Hospital;[S2] and it was 17% at the hospitals Marie-Lennelonge and Laennec.[B13] Since the operation is now applied to other types of single ventricle and other congenital anomalies,[L3,M3,Y1] the results of the Fontan-type procedure in general will be discussed from this point on since the large numbers provide more reliable information.

Current risks of hospital death after the Fontan-type procedure are certainly lower than those obtained earlier[K3] and may be 5%–10% or even less. This is suggested by the experience of Fontan and colleagues, in which the overall mortality in 100 patients with tricuspid atresia was 12% but in their most recent experience was 8.7% (CL 6%–13%)[F3]; by the UAB experience, in which the mortality for all Fontan-type procedures for the year 1983 was 7% (CL 1%–22%) (Table 26-2); and by the report of Ashraf and colleagues in the recent era of no deaths (0%, CL 0%–24%) among 7 children with double inlet left ventricle in whom a Fontan-type of repair was done.[A4] The lower current risks are primarily the result of technical improvements resulting in a higher proportion of patients with a completely nonrestrictive pathway between RA and PA and, to a lesser extent, of avoiding this type of operation when the pulmonary arteries are restrictive because of their small size. An important and not yet completely answered question is whether or not the hospital

mortality would approach zero if routinely adequate pathways were created, the pulmonary arteries were not restrictive, and the main ventricular chamber and its AV valve were well functioning. It may not, because of the sensitivity of the patient after the Fontan-type procedure to any transient rise in pulmonary vascular resistance secondary to the damaging effects of CPB.

Complete Heart Block

Heart block is rare after the Fontan-type procedure; there was only one instance in the combined UAB and GLH experiences, although it has been reported by others.[G4]

Table 26-2 Hospital deaths among the 65 patients undergoing the Fontan-type procedure without concomitant AV valve repair or extensive reconstruction of the right and left pulmonary arteries or proximal pulmonary trunk to aorta anastomosis (UAB; 1967–Nov. 1, 1983).

Date of Operation	n	Hospital Deaths		
		No.	%	CL
Before 1983	51	11[a]	22%	15%–29%
1983	14	1[b]	7%	1%–22%
Total	65	12	18%	13%–25%
P(Fisher)		.20		

KEY: CL, 70% confidence limits.

[a] Two late deaths; thus 12 total deaths (24%, CL 17%–31%).

[b] One late death; thus two total deaths (14%, CL 5%–31%).

Table 26-3 Incremental risk factors for hospital death after the Fontan-type procedure for all cardiac anomalies (UAB; 1967–November 1983; n = 73).

Incremental Risk Factor	Logistic Coefficient ± SD	P Value
Young age at repair (ln years)	−1.7 ± 0.47	.0003
Tricuspid atresia = no	1.6 ± 0.75	.03
Complex *additional* procedures	2.5 ± 1.08	.02
Intercept	−0.64	

KEY: ln, logarithm; SD, standard deviation.

NOTE: "Complex *additional* procedures" includes AV valve replacement (two cases, two deaths); anastomosis of proximal pulmonary trunk to ascending aorta (one case, one death); and extensive reconstruction of the right and left pulmonary artery (five cases, one death).

Incremental Risk Factors for Hospital Death after the Fontan-Type Repair

The larger number of patients in the overall group of patients receiving the Fontan-type of repair (Table 26-1) makes it more suitable for examination of risk factors (Table 26-3).

Although no difference that could not be due to chance exists in hospital mortality after the Fontan-type procedure according to the individual cardiac anomaly for which it was done (Table 26-1), *tricuspid atresia* was associated with a lower risk than the other malformations combined into one group (Table 26-3). In other words, all lesions other than tricuspid atresia, as a group, were a risk factor. Whether this difference is an inherent one and will continue in the future or whether it will disappear as the operative procedures become more perfect is problematic. Although it is possible that inherent problems exist with a complex atrial baffle plus a Fontan-type repair as suggested by Di Carlo, Marcelletti, et al.,[D6] there is no firm evidence for this. If the pathways, including the approach to the AV valve, are nonrestrictive, the complex baffle should not affect the flow of systemic venous blood into the pulmonary artery. However, a small and noncompliant *pulmonary* venous atrium could result in elevated pulmonary venous (left) atrial pressure (as it does after the Mustard or Senning operation or repair of total anomalous pulmonary venous connection; see Chapters 39 and 16) and thus secondarily in elevated right atrial pressures.

Young age appears to be an incremental risk factor for hospital death after the Fontan-type procedure[F3,G4] (Table 26-3). It is not certain, as one moves toward infants and neonates, at what age the increased risk is evident, but it seems to be somewhere between 1 and 4 years of age (Tables 26-4, 26-5, Fig. 26-17).

When *AV valve replacement* has been combined with the Fontan-type procedure, the mortality has been high (Tables 26-3, 26-6). This may be related to the gradient usually present across a valve replacement device and the consequently increased left atrial pressure. *Complex additional procedures* have also been risk factors (Tables 26-3, 26-7).

A *significant elevation of pulmonary vascular resistance* did not appear in the UAB analysis as a risk factor, because it is known to be a contraindication to a Fontan-type re-

Table 26-4 Hospital mortality according to age after Fontan-type operation for tricuspid atresia with ventriculoarterial concordant connection (GLH; 1975–1984).

Age (months)			Hospital Deaths		
≤	<	n	No.	%	CL
	6	5	3	60%	29%–85%
6 ---	12	2	1	50%	7%–93%
12 ---	24	4	1	25%	3%–63%
24 ---	48				
48		10	2	20%	7%–41%
	Total	21	7	33%	22%–47%
	P(χ²)			.4	

KEY: CL, 70% confidence limits.
[a] One additional patient died 5 months after operation.

pair,[C7] and patients with a known increase have been excluded. However, it may be a significant factor in some patients in whom it cannot be measured preoperatively, in small infants, particularly when there has been a low pulmonary blood flow from birth, and in whom the pulmonary vessels are probably less compliant in the early postoperative period.

Hospital Mortality after the Systemic-Pulmonary Arterial Shunting

The hospital mortality in earlier times was high (25%–50%) for shunting procedures in the sick small baby with tricuspid atresia and reduced pulmonary blood flow.[D3,D4] Since about 1970 in centers prepared for infant cardiac surgery, it has been about 5% (Table 26-8). Crupi and colleagues report four (7%, CL 4%–13%) hospital deaths among 56 patients treated in Bergamo, Italy.[C3]

The hospital mortality and the incremental risk factors for hospital death after systemic-pulmonary artery shunting are currently the same as in tetralogy of Fallot. (See Chapter 23, "Hospital Mortality after Palliative Procedures" in Section 1, Early Results.)

Table 26-5 Hospital mortality after Fontan-type procedure, without valve replacement, or proximal pulmonary artery to aorta conduit, or extensive left and right pulmonary artery reconstruction for congenital heart disease (UAB; 1967–Nov. 1, 1983).

Age (yr)			Hospital Deaths		
≤	<	n	No.	%	CL
	2	6	4	67%	38%–88%
2 ---	4	7	2	29%	10%–55%
4 ---	8	20	5	25%	14%–39%
8 ---	16	21	1	5%	0.6%–15%
16		11	0	0%	0%–16%
	Total	65	12	18%	13%–25%
	P(logistic)			.008	

KEY: CL, 70% confidence limits.

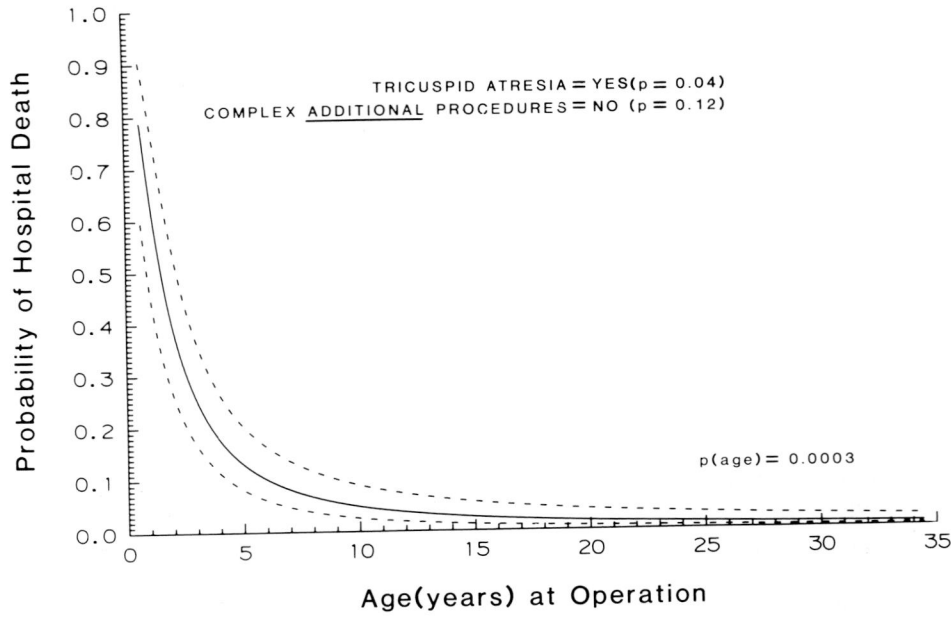

Figure 26-17 Nomogram from the multivariate equation (Table 26-4), showing hospital mortality after the Fontan-type procedure for tricuspid atresia as a function of age at operation. The dashed lines enclose the 70% confidence limits.

Hospital Mortality after the Glenn Operation

As demonstrated earlier by Edwards and Bargeron[E2] and by others,[C4,M1,T4] the hospital mortality is also reasonably low after the Glenn operation (Table 26-8).

LATE RESULTS

Fontan-Type Procedure

Premature Late Death
Premature late death, at least up to 15 years postoperatively, is uncommon after the Fontan-type repair, Fontan and colleagues reporting an actuarial 14-year survival rate of 80%, including deaths in the hospital[F3] (Fig. 26-18). When hospital deaths are excluded, the actuarial survival was over 90%, with all deaths but one occurring within 1 year of operation. The overall late survival after the Fontan-type procedure for all types of congenital heart disease at UAB are indistinguishable from these (Fig. 26-19).

Reoperation
Reoperation has occasionally been necessary in the past, but with current techniques it should rarely be necessary (Fig. 26-20).

Early Stenosis of Porcine Valves
An important incidence of early stenosis of porcine valves used either in a conduit or at the entrance of the inferior vena cava has been reported by most groups who have used this type of valve;[B14,G4,S3,S5,S8] and Gale and colleagues[G4] note that a peel inside the Dacron conduit may also narrow this (see Chapter 23, section on ''Special Situations and Controversies''). These complications may require reoperation often within a year or so of implantation, indicating that porcine valves should not be used. Homograft valves have so far not required replacement.[B12,F3]

Table 26-6 Hospital mortality after Fontan-type procedure for congenital heart disease (UAB; 1967–Nov. 1, 1983; $n = 73$).

AV Valve Replacement	n	Hospital Deaths		
		No.	%	CL
No	71	14	20%	15%–26%
Yes	2	2	100%	39%–100%
Total	73	16	22%	17%–28%

KEY: AV, atrioventricular; CL, 70% confidence limits.

Table 26-7 Circumstances of hospital death among 73 patients undergoing the Fontan-type procedure (UAB; 1967–Nov. 1, 1983).

Associations and Modes of Death	No.	Proportion of 73	
		%	CL
Right atrial hypertension[a]	9	12%	8%–18%
Complex surgical procedure or complex situs ambiguus	6	8%	5%–13%
Neurologic death	1	1%	0.1%–5%
Total	16	22%	17%–28%

KEY: CL, 70% confidence limits; PA, pulmonary artery; RA, right atrium.
[a]In two cases, this is known to have resulted from an inadequate RA–PA pathway.

Table 26-8 Hospital mortality after surgical procedures ($n = 146$) for tricuspid atresia in 92 patients (UAB; 1967–September 1982).

Operation (All UAB Operations)	No.	Hospital Deaths n	%	CL	
Fontan	37	6	16%	10%–25%	
Fontan take down	1	0	0%	0%–86%	
Systemic-pulmonary artery shunting	69	5	7%	4%–12%	
Blalock-Taussig	31	2	6%	2%–15%	3/44, 7%, CL 3%–13%
Gore-Tex interposition	13	1	8%	1%–24%	
Others	25	2	8%	3%–18%	
Glenn operation	11	2	18%	6%–38%	
Revisions of shunts	8	2	25%	9%–50%	
Open palliative procedures	7	1	14%	2%–41%	
Pulmonary artery banding	6	0	0%	0%–27%	
Coarctation repair and pulmonary artery banding	1	0	0%	0%–86%	
Miscellaneous other palliative procedures	6	1	17%	2%–46%	
Total	146	17	12%	9%–15%	
(Total patients)	92	14	15%	11%–20%	

KEY: CL, 70% confidence limits.

SOURCE: Reproduced with permission from Cleveland et al.[C6]

Functional Status

The functional status is generally good, Fontan and colleagues reporting that 94% of surviving patients with tricuspid atresia and a Fontan-type repair are in N.Y. Heart Association (NYHA) functional class I or II.[F3] At UAB, this proportion is similar in patients with various anomalies (Table 26-9), and there is no difference in late results among the various anomalies. Late deterioration has not yet been seen in either the Bordeaux, UAB, or GLH experience (Table 26-10) except in patients who required reoperation for conduit obstruction, all of whom are now in NYHA class I.

It is important to remember that the follow-up remains relatively short after the Fontan-type procedure. Fontan has followed only five patients for longer than 7 years,[F3] and

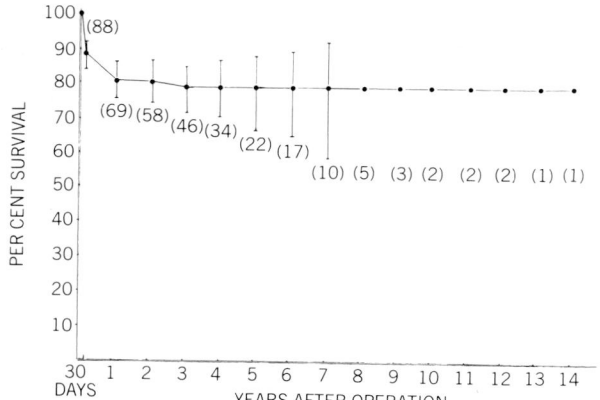

Figure 26-18 Actuarial survival after the Fontan repair for tricuspid atresia. Note that 93% of the hospital survivors are alive up to 14 years after the repair, with the few premature late deaths having occurred in the first preoperative year.

Reproduced with permission from Fontan et al.[F3]

these patients have not all had exactly the same operation. Many of the procedures performed to date may prove imperfect because of the known tendency of Dacron conduits and porcine valves to obstruct when used in the right heart. It seems theoretically desirable to augment flow into the pulmonary artery by making use of the right ventricle if this is possible and not in other ways detrimental. This presupposes that only a homograft conduit will be used, and the need for subsequent reoperation is accepted.

Hemodynamic Status

The good clinical results suggest a satisfactory hemodynamic state on intermediate follow-up in spite of the absence of a right ventricular pumping chamber. This has been documented by Peterson and colleagues in 16 patients, 11 of whom had no valve used in the Fontan-type repair done an average of 25 months earlier. They found that resting and exercise cardiac indexes were not different in these patients from those of healthy children.[P3] The mechanisms used by the patients in achieving high cardiac outputs during exercise included an increase in heart rate. However, ventricular ejection fraction was low, being 0.45 ± 0.11 at rest and 0.51 ± 0.13 at peak exercise; and ventricular end-diastolic volumes were considerably greater than those of controls. Laks and colleagues have shown that right atrial pressure also rises during exercise.[L4] The findings by Shachar and associates[S5] were similar, indicating a reduced ejection fraction and an increased left ventricular end-diastolic volume at rest and on exercise. Their study, performed 4–25 months postoperatively on eight patients with a heterograft-valved conduit placed between right atrium and pulmonary artery, also showed a lower cardiac index at rest and on exercise than in a control group ($P < .05$), with a corresponding fall in mixed venous saturation. At rest there was a significant conduit gradient in only one patient, whereas on exercise all

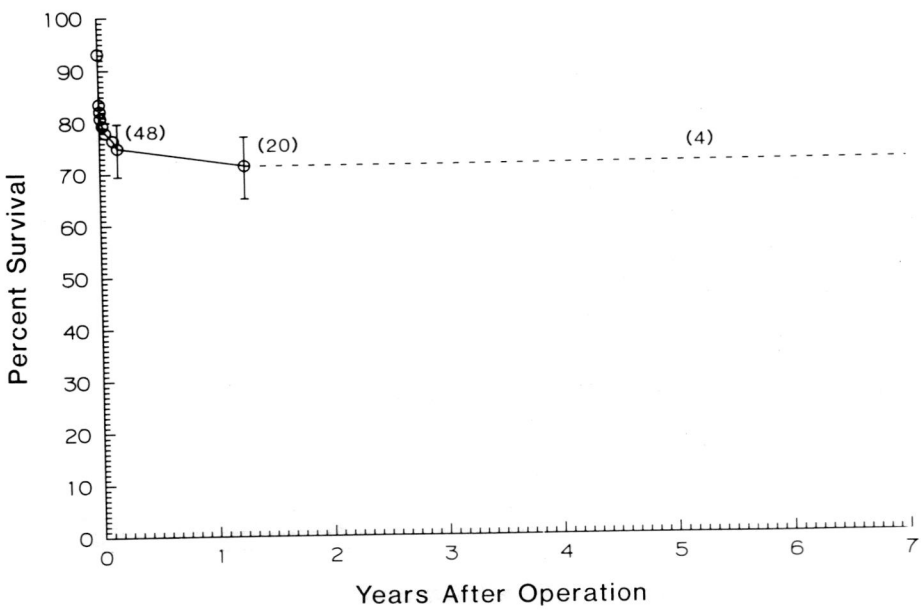

Figure 26-19 Actuarial survival, including hospital deaths, after Fontan-type repair for congenital heart disease (UAB; 1967–Nov. 1, 1983, *n* = 73).

Reproduced with permission from Stefanelli et al.[S6]

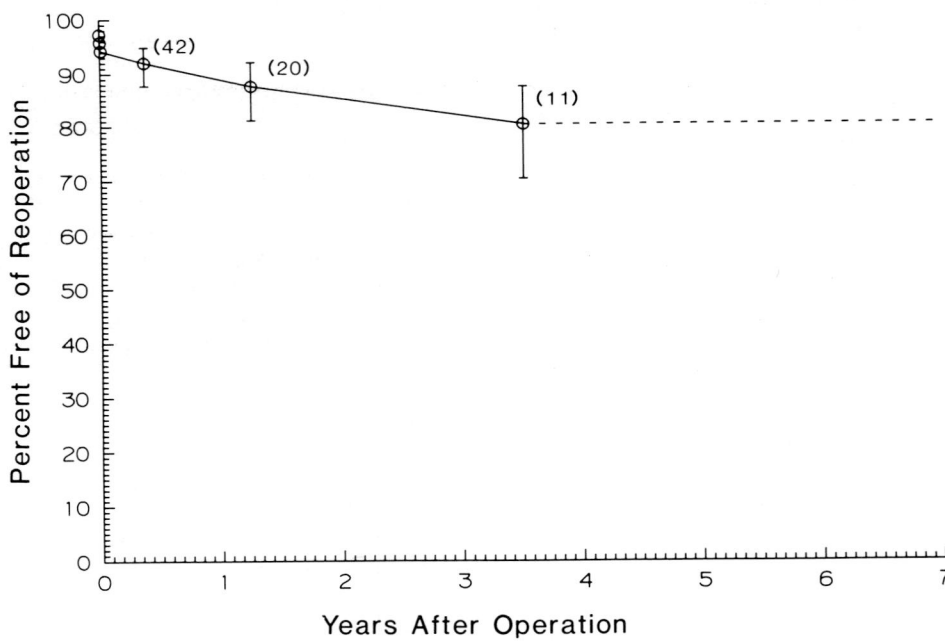

Figure 26-20 Actuarial freedom from reoperation, including very early postrepair Glenn operations, after the Fontan-type procedure for congenital heart disease (UAB; 1967–Nov. 1, 1983; *n* = 73).

Table 26-9 Functional status of surviving patients ($n = 54$) after the Fontan-type procedure (UAB).

NYHA Class	n	% of Surviving Patients (n = 47[a])		
		%	CL	
I	36	77%	69%–83% }	96%, CL 90%–99%
II	9	19%	13%–27% }	
III	0	0%	0%–4%	
IV	2[b]	4%	1%–10%	
Total	47			

KEY: CL, 70% confidence limits.

NOTE: Three patients are untraced as to NYHA functional class, and four additional patients are too recently operated upon to evaluate. (Date of inquiry for tricuspid atresia Nov. 1, 1982; for all others Nov. 15, 1983.)

[a]The functional status is not known in seven additional living patients.

[b]Previous Potts anastomosis in one patient; in the other, combined Glenn and Fontan procedure done electively, and recatheterization showed no gradient across Hancock RA–PA valved conduit.

patients developed a significant gradient (maximum 14 mmHg, mean 8 mmHg) despite the fact that they were in NYHA class 1.

There is, of course, a right atrial mean pressure greater than normal and at least in some cases reflux into caval and hepatic veins during atrial systole (Fig. 26-21).[D8] When this is extreme, it could be detrimental to long-term results.

Pulmonary artery flow is bi-phasic after the Fontan-type repair, with both right atrial relaxation and contraction as well as left atrial emptying into the ventricle influencing pulmonary arterial flow.[D8,H3,L4,M5] The type of connection made

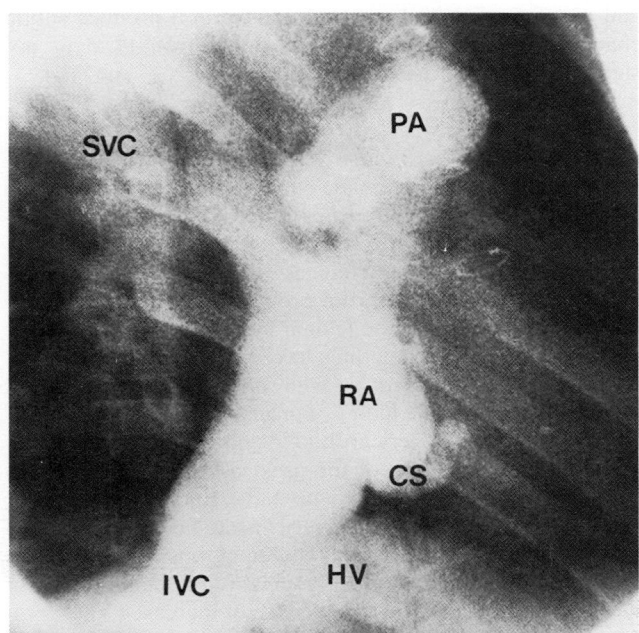

Figure 26-21 Right atrial cineangiogram during atrial systole in RAO projection 7 years after a Kreutzer procedure (GLH). Right atrial mean pressure is 14 mmHg. There is no gradient across the pulmonary valve. The pulmonary trunk is seen on. During atrial diastole there is no reflux from the pulmonary artery, but during systole there are contrast refluxes into the superior vena cava, inferior vena cava, hepatic veins, and coronary sinus.

CS, coronary sinus; HV, hepatic veins; IVC, inferior vena cava; PA, pulmonary trunk; RA, right atrial; SVC, superior vena cava.

Table 26-10 Fontan-type operations in patients under 4 years of age with ventriculoarterial concordance (GLH; 1975–1984). In the 2 month old, the RA was stretched over the large aneurysm of the AV septum (which was excised) and was atonic. In the 11 month old, death was probably due to an anastomotic gradient.

Age (months)	RV Size	Other Anomaly	Modification of Fontan Procedure	Outcome
1.75	Moderate		Bjork	Hospital death
2	Small	Aneurysm AV septum	Kreutzer	Hospital death
3	Small		Kreutzer	Good (7 yr)
3	Moderate		Homograft(18 mm) RA-RV	Death (5 mo)
5	Moderate		Homograft(20 mm) RA-RV	Hospital death[a]
7	Small		Bjork	Good (1 yr)
11	Small		Kreutzer	Hospital death
12	Small		Kreutzer	Good (5 yr)
12	Small	Pulmonary incompetence No ventricular septal defect, Right Blalock-Taussig shunt	Homograft(20 mm) RA-MPA	Hospital death
18	Small		Kreutzer	Good (4 yr)
18	Small		Bjork	Good (1 mo)
24	Small		Bjork	Good (3 yr)

[a]Complete heart block present.

and the presence or absence of a valve in it produce subtle changes in pulmonary artery flow,[B12] but may not significantly affect these flow patterns.[L4,N5]

Protein-Losing Enteropathy

Some relatively asymptomatic patients after the Fontan-type procedure have a protein-losing enteropathy. Routine laboratory examinations are generally normal except for depressed serum albumin concentrations.[H4] Special studies show excessive loss of serum proteins from the gut and dilated lymph vessels in the jejunal mucosa.

Protein-losing enteropathies have been reported in almost all situations in which there is chronically elevated central venous pressure, including congestive heart failure,[D10] chronic constrictive pericarditis,[W4] and venous switch operations for transposition of the great arteries.[M5] It has also been observed in patients who have undergone superior vena cava–right pulmonary artery anastomoses[G7] and in patients with isolated superior vena caval obstruction after a venous switch operation.[H4] Presumably the combination of increased lymph production because of increased IVC pressure and impaired lymph drainage because of increased SVC pressure contribute to this complication. However, there is no easily discernible difference in right atrial pressure after the Fontan-type procedure between those patients with and without a protein-losing enteropathy.

When severe, the protein-losing enteropathy may be relieved by insertion of a valve in the inferior vena caval orifice.[C8]

Risk Factors for a Poor Late Result

The risk factors for a poor postoperative functional status have not been clearly defined. Certainly persisting elevation of right atrial pressure (above about 18 mmHg) is one, but this should not occur when the indications for operation are appropriate and a pathway without obstruction is present between the right atrium and pulmonary arteries.

The evidence for the need for a valve (or valves) in the circuit is at present incomplete. Fontan and colleagues report data from standardized exercise testing that support the idea that a homograft valve in the connection between right atrium and right ventricle provides a better late functional result than a nonvalved connection.[F3] However, no patients with nonvalved direct connections between right atrium and pulmonary artery are included in their study.

When a homograft-valved conduit is placed between right atrium and right ventricle with preservation of function of a trabecular (sinus) portion, this sinus portion can enlarge late postoperatively and its pumping action can then contribute to pulmonary blood flow and reduction of right atrial mean pressure.[B12] Moreover, pulmonary artery systolic and pulse pressures increase almost to normal. Ottenkamp and colleagues have also reported physiologic evidence than an enlarged right ventricular sinus provides a hemodynamically significant pumping action late postoperatively when a valved right atrial to right ventricular conduit is placed.[O2] Bowman and colleagues were the first to demonstrate pro-

gressive enlargement of the right ventricle when a valved right atrial to right ventricular conduit was used.[B11] Whether the magnitude of this contribution is sufficient to affect the long-term functional results favorably is as yet uncertain.

Studies (GLH) suggest that a valve does not function when the right ventricle is totally excluded, as in the Kreutzer modification of the Fontan procedure, despite the fact that the valve remains structurally perfect.[I1] Bull and colleagues also showed, using echo studies, that the valve in a valved-homograft conduit between right atrium and pulmonary artery closed momentarily or not at all.[B12] In similar circumstances, Sharratt and colleagues found the conduit valve showed delayed opening and slow closure, suggesting that its presence in the pulmonary circuit may not contribute much to the hemodynamic state.[S9] Finally, in acute animal experiments, Shemin and colleagues[S3] showed that flow through a right atrial to pulmonary artery conduit was similar whether or not a valve was present. This is not the case, however, if an inferior vena caval valve is added,[Y1,Y2] for then the conduit valve does function and the right atrium may act as a true pump.

Considerable enlargement of the trabecular portion of the right ventricle late postoperatively in a patient without a valve in a right atrial to right ventricular connection can result in a poor late functional result. Crupi and colleagues have reported such a case, with complete remission of the peripheral edema, ascites, and protein-losing enteropathy after placing a valve in the connection.[C2] When the sinus portion of the right ventricle is excluded, as in the modification of the Fontan-type procedure described in this chapter, this complication cannot occur.

The importance of *sinus rhythm postoperatively* is also unclear. The acute animal experiments of Matsuda and colleagues[M4] and Shemin and colleagues[S3] indicated that loss of sinus rhythm did not alter flow through a right atrial to pulmonary artery conduit whether or not it contained a valve. It would appear that in these circumstances the right atrium is not acting as an effective pump and that conduit flow is influenced more by left atrial pressure, which is a function of left ventricular behavior. The long-term detrimental effects of atrial fibrillation (or junctional rhythm) are likely to be the result of its effect on the left ventricle. This presumption ignores the importance of sinus rhythm in providing a pulsatile pulmonary flow. Bull and colleagues using Doppler techniques confirmed that pulmonary flow accelerates during atrial systole,[B12] and this was confirmed by Ishikawa and colleagues using low-pressure contrast injection into the pulmonary artery.[I1]

Systemic-Pulmonary Arterial Shunting Procedures

The systemic-pulmonary arterial shunt serves well for palliation and maintenance of life for 18 months to 3 years, by which time a Fontan-type repair can be done electively. Crupi and colleagues found the actuarial survival of hospital survivors to be 93% at 4 years;[C3] and in 95% of the survivors, the pulmonary arterial tree was deemed adequate for repair by the Fontan method.

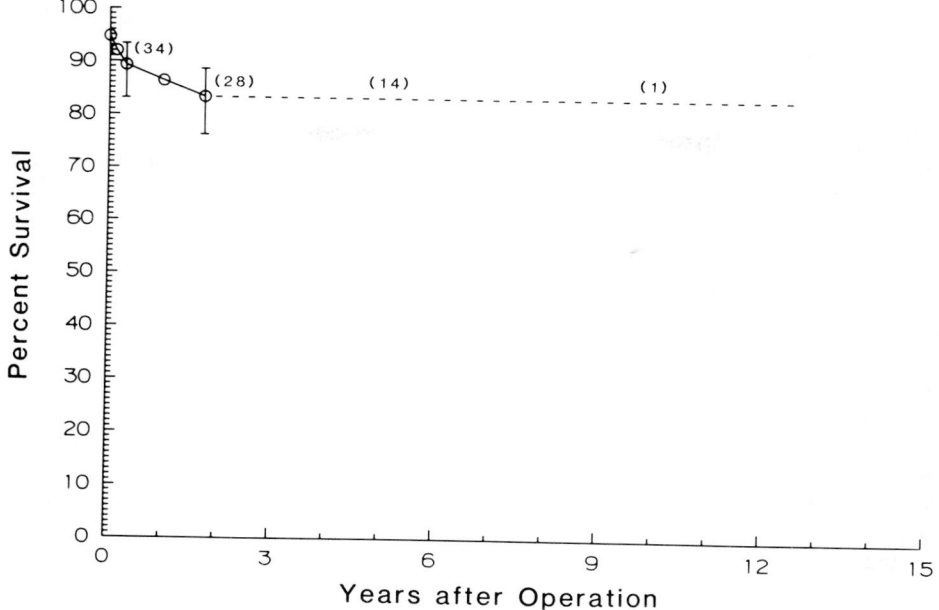

Figure 26-22   Actuarial survival including hospital deaths of patients who have received classical shunting procedures (UAB). Patients were not censored from follow-up if they subsequently received a Fontan-type repair.

The long-term (±15 years) results of systemic-pulmonary artery shunting operations in the management of tricuspid atresia are surprisingly satisfactory, with 50%–70% of patients surviving and remaining reasonably well for 15 years.[B13,D4,K4,T4,T6,W3] However, the good 12-year actuarial survival of 80% (Fig. 26-22) is accomplished only because the shunting operation was later followed by Fontan-type procedures, electively or when deterioration commenced (UAB). The deterioration in patients who do not undergo a secondary Fontan-type procedure is related to the narrowing of the VSD and the relative narrowing of the Blalock-Taussig shunt as the patient grows, as well as to the left ventricular cardiomyopathy secondary to the chronic volume overload, which worsens with time (see "Natural History").

Glenn Operation

The long-term results of the Glenn anastomosis per se are generally satisfactory.[E2] About 85% of patients survive 10 or more years after the creation of such a shunt,[C4] and the UAB experience and that of others[C4,M1,T4] indicate that the Glenn anastomosis nearly always remains patent.[B7] When symptoms do recur, they are almost never caused by shunt closure but rather to rising hematocrit (with consequent decrease in right lung pulmonary blood flow), or decreasing left lung pulmonary blood flow because of progressive narrowing of the VSD or of the pulmonary valve or subvalvar area, or increasing flow through the venous collaterals developing around the ligated superior vena cava.[B6,B7,C4,L1] There have been a few reports of the development of right-sided pulmonary arteriovenous fistulae late after the Glenn procedure,

usually confined to the right lower lobe.[C5,M1,M2,V3] Although this occurrence is apparently rare and has not been recognized at UAB or by many others, the Mayo Clinic group considers it can be confidently diagnosed using contrast M-mode echocardiography at a stage when the pulmonary angiogram is still normal.[M2] Although lung scans show there is a redistribution of pulmonary blood flow, most of which goes to the lower lobe, studies by Laks and colleagues have shown no deterioration in right lung gas exchange with time.[L1] This information relative to the long-term results of the Glenn anastomosis is reassuring as to the long-term results of a similar hemodynamic state in *both* lungs produced by the Fontan procedure.

INDICATIONS FOR OPERATION

When patients are born with tricuspid atresia and *reduced pulmonary blood flow* (usually in this setting the great arteries are normal in origin but occasionally are transposed), severe cyanosis usually is present and operation is required in the first 6–12 months of life. A *systemic-pulmonary artery anastomosis* is indicated, usually by a Gore-Tex interposition graft between the left subclavian and left pulmonary artery or alternatively if the child is more than about 2 months old by a classical Blalock-Taussig shunt on the side opposite that of the aortic arch (see Chapter 23). The Fontan-type procedure is currently indicated as a primary procedure if surgical intervention is first required after about 6 (GLH) to 12 (UAB) months of age. If a palliative shunt has been done in infancy, the Fontan-type procedure is indicated before the age of about 2–3 years, to avoid a longer period of left ventricular overload with its tendency to promote the development of a secondary left ventricular cardiomyopathy. The current practice of performing the Fontan-type repair within the first few years of life may seem to ignore the incremental risk of young age (see Fig. 26-17). The practice is based on the more favorable current experiences (GLH and UAB) with the operation. It is also based on the unproven assumption that the direct RA-PA connection will enlarge as the child grows.

When the neonate has tricuspid atresia with a *large pulmonary blood flow* (usually patients with discordant ventriculoarterial connection) and heart failure in the first few weeks or months of life that does not respond to vigorous medical management, *pulmonary artery banding* is indicated. The Fontan-type procedure is carried out between 1–5 years of age. Narrowing of the VSD during the interval is to be expected, producing functional subaortic stenosis if the ventriculoarterial connection is discordant or reduction in pulmonary blood flow and worsening cyanosis if it is concordant. Thus close follow-up is necessary in the interval between banding and repair.

There are *contraindications* to the Fontan-type repair. These include pulmonary arteries so narrow as to restrict blood flow (the ratio of the diameter of the right pulmonary artery and left pulmonary artery divided by that of the descending thoracic aorta should be 2.0 or greater to assure nonrestrictiveness—see Chapter 23, Fig. 23-58). Pulmonary vascular resistance above four units · m^2 is probably a contraindication to a Fontan-type repair, although the exact level remains unclear, particularly in patients in whom pulmonary blood flow is increased preoperatively[J1] or who are severely polycythemic.[N4] Elevated pulmonary artery pressure per se is not a contraindication. An elevated left atrial pressure secondary to mitral valve abnormalities (unless correctable) or left ventricular dysfunction is likely to result in a high (> 18 mmHg) postrepair right atrial pressure and thus an unfavorable result after the Fontan procedure. The apparent contraindication in the past of young age (< 4 years according to Choussat and Fontan and colleagues[C7,F3]) probably does not apply currently (see "Incremental Risk Factors for Hospital Death after the Fontan-type Repair"). Right atrial hypertrophy and an atrium of normal volume are not essential prerequisites. Chronic atrial fibrillation preoperatively is an unfavorable finding and may constitute a contraindication if there is also left ventricular dysfunction or other unfavorable features.[C7]

The indications for the various types of operation remain somewhat controversial. The *direct nonvalved connection* between right atrium and pulmonary artery may be considered indicated whenever the Fontan-type procedure is done (UAB) or, alternatively, only when the great arteries are transposed or when they arise normally but the pulmonary valve is abnormal (GLH). In this latter view, the *right atrial–right ventricular connection* is preferred when the great arteries arise normally and the pulmonary valve is normal (GLH), using a homograft conduit when the sinus portion of the right ventricle is likely to be capable of enlarging (except in infants) and otherwise using a nonvalved connection.

SPECIAL SITUATIONS AND CONTROVERSIES

Palliation by Direct Relief of the Obstruction to Pulmonary Blood Flow

This palliation procedure was first suggested by Brock in 1964.[B15] Experience with one case at UAB, the report of five cases by Annechino, Fontan, and colleagues,[A2] and of seven by Gersbach, Friedli, and Hahn indicate that, just as in the tetralogy of Fallot, palliation is possible by a direct approach to the anatomic obstruction to pulmonary blood flow, at least in patients with tricuspid atresia and ventriculoarterial concordant connections.[G5] This consists of enlargement of a restrictive VSD anterosuperiorly or resection of an obstructive ostium infundibulum, with or without patch graft enlargement of the right ventricular infundibulum. When the pulmonary valve anulus is small, the patch graft enlargement can be carried across the anulus. CPB is used for these repairs, but the right atrial appendage must not be cannulated since it may be needed at a later repair.

The use of the definitive Fontan-type procedure itself in young patients and preference for the extrapericardial systemic-pulmonary shunt for younger infants whose cyanosis requires palliation have largely eliminated the need for this direct type of operation. It may be appropriate in some unusual circumstances.

Glenn Operation

Side-to-side anastomosis of the SVC to the distal end of the divided right pulmonary artery, with closure of the SVC–right atrial junction, has been demonstrated to give good palliation in patients with tricuspid atresia. However, the operation results in right–left pulmonary arterial discontinuity. Even though continuity can be reestablished by a major reconstruction,[P2] this aspect of the Glenn anastomosis must be considered a serious disadvantage. Therefore, the current recommendation is that it not be used as a planned procedure. It may still be indicated in some situations when the Fontan-procedure results in an inadequate right atrial to pulmonary artery pathway.

Management of Subaortic Stenosis Following Pulmonary Artery Banding

Pulmonary artery banding is most often required when transposition of the great arteries is associated with tricuspid atresia, and the subsequently appearing subaortic stenosis is usually in the form of an infundibular muscular narrowing associated with narrowing of the VSD. It can be relieved at the time of the Fontan operation by opening the right ventricular outflow chamber anteriorly and excising the hypertrophied muscle beneath the aortic valve. The VSD may also require enlargement by excising muscle from its anterosuperior margins. Alternatively, the proximal end of the divided main pulmonary artery is anastomosed either directly or with an intervening Dacron conduit end to side to the adjacent ascending aorta (provided there is no pulmonary stenosis) as suggested by Yacoub.[Y1] The risk of hospital death after this procedure is high (53% in the Mayo Clinic experience[C7]), and it may be less desirable than to attempt a direct relief of the obstruction first.

Occasionally, the VSD alone may be restrictive in patients with tricuspid atresia and transposition who have not undergone prior pulmonary artery banding. If a pressure gradient is demonstrated across it at preoperative catheterization, the VSD must be enlarged at the time of the repair.

Leftward Juxtaposition of the Atrial Appendages

Left juxtaposition of the appendages is more common in patients with tricuspid atresia and ventriculoarterial discordance than in those with normally originating great arteries. It is not a contraindication to a Fontan-type repair.[R7] It does not prevent a direct right atrial to pulmonary artery anasto-

mosis using the superior right atrial–left atrial wall. The left atrial appendage may occasionally be conveniently anastomosed side to side to the left pulmonary artery.[D1]

Right Atrial to Pulmonary Ring Connection

In the right atrial to pulmonary ring connection[K2] (a Kreutzer modification of the Fontan-type procedure), the pulmonary trunk, anulus, and valve are dissected away from the right ventricular infundibulum, and the connection is made between the right atrial appendage and the pulmonary valve ring. This procedure is no longer used (GLH), despite the fact that the dislocated pulmonary ring and valve grow with the child and are then nonobstructive,[11] because it is technically more difficult and there is usually a significant gradient across the anastomosis at the conclusion of the operation.

REFERENCES

A

1. Anderson RH, Wilkins JL, Gerlis LM, Smith A, Becker AE: Atresia of the right atrioventricular orifice. *Br Heart J* 39:414, 1977.

2. Annecchino FP, Fontan F, Chauve A, Quaegebeur J: Palliative reconstruction of the right ventricular outflow tract in tricuspid atresia: A report of 5 patients. *Ann Thorac Surg* 29:317, 1980.

3. Ando M, Satami G, Takao A: Atresia of tricuspid or mitral orifice: Anatomic spectrum and morphogenetic hypothesis, in Van Praagh R, Takao A (eds): *Etiology and Morphogenesis of Congenital Heart Disease*. New York: Futura Publishing, 1980, p 421.

4. Ashraf H, Cotroneo J, Han S, Dhar N, Pieroni D, Subramanian S: Right atrial to pulmonary artery diversion for double inlet ventricle. *JACC* 5:478, 1985 (abstr).

B

1. Bharati S, Lev M: The conduction system in tricuspid atresia with and without regular (D-) transposition. *Circulation* 56:423, 1977.

2. Bharati S, Lev M, Kirklin JW: *Cardiac Surgery and the Conduction System.* New York: John Wiley, 1983.

3. Bharati S, McAllister HA Jr, Tatooles CJ, Miller RA, Weinberg M Jr, Bucheleres G, Lev M: Anatomic variations in underdeveloped right ventricle related to tricuspid atresia and stenosis. *J Thorac Cardiovasc Surg* 72:383, 1976.

4. Bjork VO, Olin CL, Bjarke BB, Thoren CA: Right atrial-right ventricular anastomosis for correction of tricuspid atresia. *J Thorac Cardiovasc Surg* 77:452, 1979.

5. Brown JW: Congenital tricuspid atresia. *Arch Dis Child* 11:275, 1936.

6. Boruchow IB, Swenson EW, Elliott LP, Bartley TD, Wheat MW, Schiebler GL: Study of the mechanisms of shunt failure after superior vena cava—right pulmonary artery anastomosis. *J Thorac Cardiovasc Surg* 80:531, 1970.

7. Bargeron LM Jr, Karp RB, Barcia A, Kirklin JW, Hunt D, Deverall PB: Late deterioration of patients after superior vena cava to right pulmonary artery anastomosis. *Am J Cardiol* 30:211, 1972.

8. Bakuljev AN, Kolesnikov SA: Anastomosis of the superior vena cava and pulmonary artery in the surgical treatment of certain congenital defects of the heart. *J Thorac Cardiovasc Surg* 37:693, 1959.

9. Bellet S, Stewart HL: Congenital heart disease, atresia of tricuspid orifice. *Am J Dis Child* 45:1247, 1933.

10. Blackstone EH, Kirklin JW, Bertranou EG, Labrosse CJ, Soto B, Bargeron LM Jr: Preoperative prediction from cineangiograms of postrepair right ventricular pressure in tetralogy of Fallot. *J Thorac Cardiovasc Surg* 78:542, 1979.

11. Bowman FO, Malm JR, Hayes CJ, Gersony WM: Physiological approach to surgery for tricuspid atresia. *Circulation* 58(suppl I):I-83, 1978.

12. Bull C, de Leval MR, Stark J, Taylor JFN, Macartney FJ, McGoon DC: Use of a subpulmonary ventricular chamber in the Fontan circulation. *J Thorac Cardiovasc Surg* 85:21, 1983.

13. Brux JL, Zannini L, Binet JP, Neveux JY, Langlois J, Hazan E, Planche C, Leca F, Marchand M: Tricuspid atresia. Results of treatment in 115 children. *J Thorac Cardiovasc Surg* 85:440, 1983.

14. Behrendt DM, Rosenthal A: Cardiovascular Status after repair by Fontan procedure. *Ann Thorac Surg* 29:322, 1980.

15. Brock R: Tricuspid atresia: a step toward corrective treatment. *J Thorac Cardiovasc Surg* 47:17, 1964.

C

1. Carlon CA, Mondini PG, de Marchi R: Surgical treatment of some cardiovascular diseases. *J Intern Coll Surgeons* 16:1, 1951.

2. Crupi G, Locatelli G, Tiraboschi R, Villani M, Tommasi M De, Parenzan L: Protein-losing enteropathy after Fontan operation for tricuspid atresia (imperforate tricuspid valve). *Thorac Cardiovasc Surg* 28:359, 1980.

3. Crupi G, Alfieri O, Locatelli G, Villani M, Parenzan L: Results of systemic-to-pulmonary artery anastomosis for tricuspid atresia with reduced pulmonary blood flow. *Thorax* 34:290, 1979.

4. di Carlo D, Williams WG, Freedom RM, Trusler GA, Rowe RD: The role of cava-pulmonary (Glenn) anastomosis in the palliative treatment of congenital heart disease. *J Thorac Cardiovasc Surg* 83:437, 1982.

5. Calabrese CT, Carrington CB, Harley RA, Rojas RH, Glenn WWL: The long-term functional and morphological changes in the pulmonary circulation following cava-pulmonary artery shunt. *J Surg Res* 8:593, 1968.

6. Cleveland DC, Kirklin JK, Naftel DC, Kirklin JW, Blackstone EH, Pacifico AD, Bargeron LM Jr: Surgical Treatment of Tricuspid Atresia. *Ann Thorac Surg* 38:447, 1984.

7. Choussat A, Fontan I, Besse P, Vallot F, Chauve A, Bricand H: Selection criteria for Fontan's procedure, in RH Anderson, EA Shinebourne (eds): *Pediatric Cardiology 1977.* Edinburgh: Churchill Livingstone 1978, Chap. 64.

8. Crupi G, Locatelli G, Tiraboschi R, Villani M, De Tommasi M, Parenzan L: Protein-losing enteropathy after Fontan operation for tricuspid atresia (imperforate tricuspid valve). *Thorac Cardiovasc Surg* 28:359, 1980.

D

1. Doty DB, Marvin WJ Jr, Lauer RM: Modified Fontan procedure. *J Thorac Cardiovasc Surg* 81:470, 1981.

2. Deanfield JE, Tommasini G, Anderson RH, Macartney FJ: Tricuspid atresia: Analysis of coronary artery distribution and ventricular morphology. *Br Heart J* 48:485, 1982.

3. Deverall PB, Lincoln JCR, Aberdeen E, Bonham-Carter RE, Waterston DJ: Surgical management of tricuspid atresia. *Thorax* 24:239, 1969.

4. Dick M, Gyler DC, Nadas AS: Tricuspid atresia. Clinical course in 101 patients. *Am J Cardiol* 36:327, 1975.

5. DeLeon SY, Idriss FS, Ilbawi MN, Muster AJ, Paul MH, Cole RB, Riggs TW, Berry TE: The role of the Glenn shunt in patients undergoing the Fontan operation. *J Thorac Cardiovasc Surg* 85:669, 1983.

6. Di Carlo D, Marcelletti C, Nijveld A, Lubbers LJ, Becker AE: The Fontan procedure in the absence of the interatrial septum. *J Thorac Cardiovasc Surg* 85:923, 1983.

7. Dickinson DF, Wilkinson JL, Smith A, Anderson RH: Atresia of the right atrioventricular orifice with atrioventricular concordance. *Br Heart J* 42:9, 1979.

8. DiSessa TG, Child JS, Perloff JK, Wu L, Williams RG, Laks H, Friedman WF: Systemic venous and pulmonary arterial flow patterns after Fontan's procedure for tricuspid atresia or single ventricle. *Circulation* 70:898, 1984.

9. di Donato R, Becker AE, Nijveld A, Lam J, Bulterijs A, Squitieri C, Marcelletti C: Ventricular exclusion during Fontan Operation: An evolving technique. *Ann Thorac Surg* 39:283, 1985.

10. Davidson JD, Waldmann TA, Goodman DS, Gordon RS: Protein-losing enteropathy in congestive heart failure. *Lancet* 1:899, 1961.

E

1. Edwards JE, Burchell HB: Congenital tricuspid atresia: A classification. *Med Clin North Am* (1949):1177, 1949.

2. Edwards WS, Bargeron LM Jr: The superiority of the Glenn operation for tricuspid atresia in infancy and childhood. *J Thorac Cardiovasc Surg* 55:60, 1968.

F

1. Fontan F, Mounicot F-B, Baudet E, Simonneau J, Gordo J, Gouffrant J-M: "Correction" de l'atresie tricuspidienne. Rapport de deux cas "corriges" par l'utilisation d'une technique chirurgicale nouvelle. *Ann Chir Thorac Cardiovasc* 10:39, 1971.

2. Fontan F, Baudet E: Surgical repair of tricuspid atresia. *Thorax* 26:240, 1971.

3. Fontan F, Deville C, Quaegebeur J, Ottenkamp J, Sourdille N, Choussat A, Brom GA: Repair of tricuspid atresia in 100 patients. *J Thorac Cardiovasc Surg* 85:647, 1983.

4. Fontan F, Choussat A, Brom AG, Chauve A, Deville C, Castro-Cels A: Repair of tricuspid atresia—surgical considerations and results, in RH Anderson, EA Shinebourne (eds): *Pediatric Cardiology 1977.* Edinburgh: Churchill Livingstone 1978, Chap. 65.

G

1. Glenn WWL: Circulatory bypass of the right side of the heart. IV. Shunt between superior vena cava and distal right pulmonary artery—report of clinical application. *N Engl J Med* 259:117, 1958.

2. Glenn WWL, Patino JF: Circulatory by-pass of the right heart. I. Preliminary observations on the direct delivery of vena caval blood into the pulmonary arterial circulation. Azygous vein-pulmonary artery shunt. *Yale J Biol Med* 27:147, 1954.

3. Guller B, DuShane JW, Titus JL: The atrioventricular conduction system in two cases of tricuspid atresia. *Circulation* 40:217, 1969.

4. Gale AW, Danielson GK, McGoon DC, Wallace RB, Mair DD: Fontan procedure for tricuspid atresia. *Circulation* 62:91, 1980.

5. Gersbach PH, Friedli B, Hahn C: Treatment of tricuspid atresia with small pulmonary flow (type 1b) by surgical enlargement of the ventricular septal defect. *Thorac Cardiovasc Surg* 29:82, 1981.

6. Gale AW, Danielson GK, McGoon DC, Mair DD: Modified Fontan operation for univentricular heart and complicated congenital lesions. *J Thorac Cardiovasc Surg* 78:831, 1979.

7. Gleason WA Jr, Roodman ST, Laks H: Protein-losing enteropathy and intestinal lymphangiectasia after superior vena cava–right pulmonary artery (Glenn) shunt. *J Thorac Cardiovasc Surg* 77:843, 1979.

H

1. Hurwitt ES, Young D, Escher DJW: The rationale of anastomosis of the right auricular appendage to the pulmonary artery in the treatment of tricuspid atresia. *J Thorac Surg* 30:503, 1955.

2. Henry JH, Devloo RAE, Ritter DG, Mair DO, Davis GD, Danielson GK: Tricuspid atresia. Successful surgical "correction" in two patients using porcine xenograft valves. *Mayo Clin Proc* 49:803, 1974.

3. Hagler DJ, Seward JB, Tajik AJ, Ritter DG: Functional assessment of the Fontan operation: Combined M-Mode, Two-Dimensional and Doppler Echocardiographic Studies. *JACC* 4:756, 1984.

4. Hess J, Kruizinga K, Bijleveld C-A, Hardjowijono R, Eygelaar A: Protein–losing enteropathy after Fontan operation. *J Thorac Cardiovasc Surg* 88:606, 1984.

I

1. Ishikawa T, Neutze JM, Brandt PWT, Barratt-Boyes BG: Hemodynamics following the Kreutzer procedure for tricuspid atresia in patients under 2 years of age. *J Thorac Cardiovasc Surg* 88:373, 1984.

J

1. Juaneda E, Haworth SG: Pulmonary vascular structure in patients dying after a Fontan procedure. The lung as a risk factor. *Br Heart J* 52:575, 1984.

K

1. Kuhne M: Uber zwei Falle kongenitaler atresie des ostium venosum dextrum. *Jahrbuch Kinderheildkunde Physiche Erziehung* 63:235, 1906.
2. Kreutzer G, Galindez E, Bono H, de Palma C, Laura JP: An operation for the correction of tricuspid atresia. *J Thorac Cardiovasc Surg* 66:613, 1973.
3. Kreutzer GO, Vargas FJ, Schlichter AJ, Laura JP, Suarez JC, Coronel AR, Kreutzer EA: Atriopulmonary anastomosis. *J Thorac Cardiovasc Surg* 83:427, 1982.
4. Kyger ER III, Reul GJ Jr, Sandiford FM, Wukasch DC, Hallman GL, Cooley DA: Surgical palliation of tricuspid atresia. *Circulation* 52:685, 1975.

L

1. Laks H, Mudd JG, Standeven JW, Fagan L, Willman VL: Long term effect of the superior vena cava-pulmonary artery anastomosis on pulmonary blood flow. *J Thorac Cardiovasc Surg* 74:253, 1977.
2. LaCorte MA, Dick M, Scheer G, LaFarge CG, Flyer DC: Left ventricular function in tricuspid atresia. Angiographic analysis in 28 patients. *Circulation* 52:996, 1975.
3. Laks H, Williams WG, Hellenbrand WE, Freedom RM, Talner NS, Rowe RD, Trusler GA: Results of right atrial to right ventricular and right atrial to pulmonary artery conduits for complex congenital heart disease. *Ann Surg* 192:382, 1980.
4. Laks H, Milliken JC, Perloff JK, Hellenbrand WE, George BL, Chin A, DiSessa TG, Williams RG: Experience with the Fontan procedure. *J Thorac Cardiothorac Surg* 88:939, 1984.

M

1. Mathur M, Glenn WWL: Long-term evaluation of cava-pulmonary artery anastomosis. *Surgery* 74:899, 1973.
2. McFaul RC, Tajik AJ, Mair DD, Danielson GK, Seward JB: Development of pulmonary arteriovenous shunt after superior vena cava-right pulmonary artery (Glenn) anastomosis. *Circulation* 55:212, 1977.
3. Marcelletti C, Mazzera E, Olthof H, Sebel PS, Duren DR, Losekoot TG, Becker AE: Fontan's operation: An expanded horizon. *J Thorac Cardiovasc Surg* 80:764, 1980.
4. Matsuda H, Kawashima Y, Takano H, Miyamoto K, Mori T: Experimental evaluation of atrial function in right atrium-pulmonary artery conduit operation for tricuspid atresia. *J Thorac Cardiovasc Surg* 81:762, 1981.
5. Moodie DS, Feldt RH, Wallace RB: Transient protein-losing enteropathy secondary to elevated caval pressures and caval obstruction after the Mustard procedure. *J Thorac Cardiovasc Surg* 72:379, 1976.

N

1. Nuland SB, Glenn WWL, Guilfoil PH: Circulatory bypass of the right heart. III. Some observations on long-term survivors. *Surgery* 43:184, 1958.
2. Neveux J-Y, Dreyfus G, Leca F, Marchand M, Bex J-P: Modified technique for correction of tricuspid atresia. *J Thorac Cardiovasc Surg* 82:457, 1981.
3. Nishioka K, Kamiya T, Ueda T, Hayashidera T, Mori C, Konishi Y, Tatsuta N, Jarmakani JM: Left ventricular volume characteristics in children with tricuspid atresia before and after surgery. *Am J Cardiol* 47:1105, 1981.
4. Nihill MR, McNamara DG, Vick RL: The effects of increased blood viscosity on pulmonary vascular resistance. *Am Heart J* 92:65, 1976.
5. Nakazawa M, Nakanishi T, Okuda H, Satomi G, Nakae S, Imai Y, Takao A: Dynamics of right heart flow in patients after Fontan procedure. *Circulation* 69:306, 1984.

O

1. O'Neill CA: Left axis deviation in tricuspid atresia and single ventricle. *Circulation* 12:612, 1955.
2. Ottenkamp J, Rohmer J, Quaegebeur JM, Brom AG, Fontan F: Nine years' experience of physiological correction of tricuspid atresia: long-term results and current surgical approach. *Thorax* 37:718, 1982.

P

1. Patino JF, Glenn WWL, Guilfoil PH, Hume M, Fenn J: Circulatory bypass of the right heart. II. Further observations on vena caval pulmonary artery shunts. *Surg Forum* 6:189, 1957.
2. Pacifico AD, Kirklin JW: Take-down of cava-pulmonary artery anastomosis (Glenn) during repair of congenital cardiac malformations. Report of 5 cases. *J Thorac Cardiovasc Surg* 70:272, 1975.
3. Peterson RJ, Franch RH, Fajman WA, Jennings JG, Jones RG: Noninvasive determination of exercise cardiac function following Fontan operation. *J Thorac Cardiovasc Surg* 88:263, 1984.

R

1. Rodbard S, Wagner D: Bypassing the right ventricle. *Proc Soc Exp Biol Med* 71:69, 1949.
2. Rao PS, Jue KL, Isabel-Jones J, Ruttenberg HD: Ebstein's malformation of the tricuspid valve with atresia. Differentiation from isolated tricuspid atresia. *Am J Cardiol* 32:1004, 1973.
3. Robicsek F, Temesvari A, Kadar RL: A new method for the treatment of congenital heart disease associated with impaired pulmonary circulation. *Acta Med Scandinav* 154:151, 1956.
4. Rao PS: Natural history of the ventricular septal defect in tricuspid atresia and its surgical implications. *Br Heart J* 39:276, 1977.
5. Rao PS: Further observations on the spontaneous closure of physiologically advantageous ventricular septal defects in tricuspid atresia: surgical implications. *Ann Thorac Surg* 35:121, 1983.
6. Rigby ML, Gibson DG, Joseph MC, Lincoln JCR, Shinebourne EA, Shore DF, Anderson RH: Recognition of imperforate atrioventricular valves by two dimensional echocardiography. *Br Heart J* 47:329, 1982.
7. Ross DN, Somerville J: Surgical correction of tricuspid atresia. *Lancet* 1:845, 1973.
8. Rosenquist GC, Levy RJ, Rowe RD: Right atrial-left ventricular relationships in tricuspid atresia: position of the presumed site of the atretic valve as determined by transillumination. *Am Heart J* 80:493, 1970.

S

1. Starr I, Jeffers WA, Meade RH: The absence of conspicuous increments of venous pressure after severe damage to the right ventricle of the dog, with a discussion of the relation between clinical congestive failure and heart disease. *Am Heart J* 26:291, 1943.
2. Sanders SP, Wright GB, Keane JF, Norwood WI, Castaneda AR: Clinical and hemodynamic results of the Fontan operation for tricuspid atresia. *Am J Cardiol* 49:1733, 1982.

3. Shemin RJ, Merrill WH, Pfeifer JS, Conkle DM, Morrow AG: Evaluation of right atrial-pulmonary artery conduits for tricuspid atresia. *J Thorac Cardiovasc Surg* 77:685, 1979.

4. Stanton RE, Lurie PR, Lindesmith GG, Meyer BW: The Fontan procedure for tricuspid atresia. *Circulation* 64(suppl II):II–140, 1981.

5. Shachar GB, Fuhrman BP, Wang Y, Lucas R Jr, Lock JE: Rest and exercise hemodynamics after the Fontan procedure. *Circulation* 65:1043, 1982.

6. Stefanelli G, Kirklin JW, Naftel DC, Blackstone EH, Pacifico AD, Kirklin JK, Soto B, Bargeron LM Jr: Early and intermediate-term (10-year) results of surgery for single ventricle. *Am J Cardiol* 54:811, 1984.

7. Stanford W, Armstrong RG, Cline RE, King TD: Right atrium–pulmonary artery allograft for correction of tricuspid atresia. *J Thorac Cardiovasc Surg* 66:105, 1973.

8. Serratto M, Miller RA, Tatooles C, Ardekani R: Hemodynamic evaluation of Fontan operation in tricuspid atresia. *Circulation* 54(suppl III):III–99, 1976.

9. Sharratt GP, Johnson AM, Monro R: Persistence and effect of sinus rhythm after Fontan procedure for tricuspid atresia. *Br Heart J* 42:78, 1979.

T

1. Tandon R, Edwards JE: Tricuspid atresia. A re-evaluation and classification. *J Thorac Cardiovasc Surg* 67:530, 1974.

2. Taussig HB: The clinical and pathological findings in congenital malformations of the heart due to defective development of the right ventricle associated with tricuspid atresia or hypoplasia. *Bull Johns Hopkins Hosp* 59:435, 1936.

3. Tatooles CJ, Ardekani RG, Miller RA, Serratto M: Operative repair for tricuspid atresia. *Ann Thorac Surg* 21:499, 1976.

4. Trusler GA, Williams WG: Long-term results of shunt procedures for tricuspid atresia. *Ann Thorac Surg* 29:312, 1980.

5. Tandon R, Marin-Garcia J, Moller JM, Edwards JE: Tricuspid atresia with l-transposition. *Am Heart J* 88:417, 1974.

6. Taussig HB, Keinonen R, Momberger N, Kirk H: Long-time observations on the Blalock-Taussig operation. IV: Tricuspid atresia. *Johns Hopkins Med J* 132:135, 1973.

V

1. Vlad P: Tricuspid atresia, in Keith JD, Rowe RD, Vlad P (eds): *Heart Disease in Infancy and Childhood* (ed 3) New York: Macmillan, 1978, pp 518–541.

2. de Vivie ER, Ruschewski W, Koveker G, Risch D, Weber H, Beuren AJ: Fontan procedure—indication and clinical results. *Thorac Cardiovasc Surg* 29:348, 1981.

3. Van Den Bogaert-Van Heesvelde AM, Derom F, Kunnen M, Van Egmond H, Devloo-Blancquaert A: Surgery for arteriovenous fistulas and dilated vessels in the right lung after the Glenn procedure. *J Thorac Cardiovasc Surg* 76:1953, 1978.

W

1. Warden HE, DeWall RA, Varco RL: Use of the right auricle as a pump for the pulmonary circuit. *Surg Forum* 5:16, 1954.

2. Weinberg PM: Anatomy of tricuspid atresia in its relevance to current forms of surgical therapy. *Ann Thorac Surg* 29:306, 1980.

3. Williams WG, Rubis L, Fowler RS, Rao MK, Trusler GA, Mustard WT: Tricuspid atresia: Results of treatment in 160 children. *Am J Cardiol* 38:225, 1976.

4. Wilkinson P, Pinto B, Senior JR: Reversible protein–losing enteropathy with intestinal lymphangiectasia secondary to chronic constrictive pericarditis. *N Engl J Med* 273:1178, 1965.

Y

1. Yacoub MH, Radley-Smith R: Use of a valved conduit from right atrium to pulmonary artery for "correction" of a single ventricle. *Circulation* 54(suppl III):III-63, 1976.

2. Yacoub MH. Fontan's operation—are caval valves necessary? in RH Anderson, EA Shinebourne (eds): *Pediatric Cardiology, 1977.* Edinburgh: Churchill Livingstone, 1978, Chap. 66.

27

EBSTEIN'S MALFORMATION

DEFINITION

Ebstein's malformation (anomaly) is a congenital defect of the tricuspid valve in which the origins of the septal or posterior tricuspid leaflets or both are displaced downward into the right ventricle and the leaflets are variably deformed. Characteristically, the anterior leaflet is enlarged and sail-like. There is a wide spectrum of severity, so that in the mildest asymptomatic forms the valve may, at first sight, appear normal[S9] and classification as Ebstein's anomaly be debatable.

In this chapter, Ebstein's malformation in hearts with atrioventricular corcordant connection and without another major cardiac anomaly is discussed. Patients with an Ebstein type of tricuspid atresia and those with Ebstein's anomaly associated with pulmonary atresia are discussed elsewhere (see Chapters 25 and 26), as are those associated with atrioventricular discordant connections (see Chapters 42 and 43). Details of the Wolff-Parkinson-White syndrome, occasionally associated with Ebstein's anomaly, are presented in Chapter 48.

HISTORICAL NOTE

Ebstein's scholarly description of the tricuspid valve abnormality that bears his name was published in 1866.[E1] The report describes a single autopsy specimen and includes Ebstein's hypothesis of the pathophysiology based on a correlation of the morphology and the clinical notes supplied by a colleague (since Ebstein did not apparently see the patient alive[S3]). According to the historical review by Mann and Lie,[M1] the second case was not described until 20 years later, and the first description in the English literature was by MacCallum in 1900. The eponym "Ebstein's disease" was first suggested by Arnstein in 1927[A5] and was used by Yater and Shapiro in their 1937 review article that reported the 16th case and the first to be examined by both roentgenography and electrocardiography.[Y1] These authors commented that "it would appear impossible to make the diagnosis during life." In 1950, Engle and colleagues[E2] and also Reynolds[R1] suggested that the disease was associated with a clinical syndrome that should make diagnosis possible. In 1951, Van Lingen and colleagues[V1] and Soloff and colleagues[S6] made the diagnosis during life, using cardiac catheterization and, in the case of the latter group, angiocardiography. In 1955 Lev[L2] and colleagues described a patient with associated Wolff-Parkinson-White (WPW) syndrome and provided histologic details of the course of the conducting tissue in this disease.

Palliative surgery was attempted unsuccessfully using a Blalock-Taussig shunt in 1950.[E3] A superior vena cava (SVC) to right pulmonary artery anastomosis (Glenn proce-

Table 27-1 Summary of autopsy findings in 16 hearts with Ebstein's anomaly (GLH).
(One or other detail was missing in 2 hearts.)

Tricuspid Leaflet	Totally Absent	Leaflet Origin			Leaflet Size		
		Normal	Displaced	Adherent	Normal	Small	Elongated
Septal	1	0	10	8[a]	2	11[b]	1
Posterior	1	3	5	7	1	1	12
Anterior	0	14	1	0	0	0	15[c]

NOTE: Dilatation of the functional right ventricle was present in 15; of the atrialized chamber in 4; and the tricuspid anulus in 12. There was an atrial communication in all specimens (small, probe patent, foramen ovale in 2, an enlarged foramen ovale in 7, fossa ovalis atrial septal defect in 7).

[a] In two the whole cusp was adherent.

[b] In three up to half the leaflet was missing.

[c] In three the elongation was slight.

dure[G5]) was used successfully by Gasul and colleagues in 1959[G3,G6] and subsequently by McCredie and colleagues[M4] and Scott and colleagues.[S7] Barnard and Schrire[B5] were the first to report the use of prosthetic valve replacement in 1962 followed by Cartwright and colleagues[C2] and Lillehei and colleagues.[L3] Hardy and colleagues[H3] reported the first successful "valvuloplasty" in 1964 based on the concepts of Hunter and Lillehei.[H2] A similar technique was used by Bahnson in 1965.[B2]

MORPHOLOGY

Tricuspid Valve

Both the origin of the tricuspid valve from the atrioventricular (AV) ring and its chordal attachments with the ventricle are malpositioned, and the leaflets are malformed.[A1,A4,B3,L1,Z1] The leaflets are either enlarged or reduced in size and frequently dysplastic (thickened and distorted). These deformities vary widely in severity (Table 27-1). In the mildest forms, the valve is functionally near normal,[P1] whereas in the fully developed syndrome function is severely compromised. The displacement of the origin of the leaflets from the AV ring is reasonably constant. The septal leaflet appears always to be affected, the posterior leaflet nearly always, and the anterior leaflet seldom (Fig. 27-1). As noted by Anderson and colleagues,[A1] when both septal and posterior leaflets are displaced, the point of maximum displacement is usually at the commissure between these two leaflets. In the few cases in which the anterior leaflet is displaced, the commissural area between anterior and septal leaflet, attached to the right trigone at the point of penetration of the bundle of His, remains in normal position[L2] (Fig. 27-1). In a significant proportion of patients, the apparent displacement is in fact due to adherence of the base of the leaflet to the right ventricular wall (Table 27-1, Fig. 27-1). When adherence is incomplete, there is a potential or obvious pocket beneath the leaflet.

The septal or posterior leaflet may be partially absent (Fig. 27-1b), in which event the belly of the leaflet is small or may be totally absent (Fig. 27-1c). The posterior leaflet is more often elongated than reduced in size (Table 27-1) due in part to lack of a commissure between posterior and anterior

cusps. This was the case in 8 of 15 hearts (GLH) (Fig. 27-1c and d). The septal-posterior leaflet commissure may also occasionally be absent. Leaflet enlargement and elongation are characteristic of the anterior leaflet that has been described as saillike. The leaflet is usually diffusely thickened or ridged and occasionally consists partly of muscle (Fig. 27-1d). All the leaflets are frequently dysplastic (Fig. 27-1b), and isolated accessory leaflets may occur.[L1]

The distal leaflet attachments are variable and usually abnormal. The displaced and dysplastic posterior and septal leaflets frequently have multiple, short chordae connecting to multiple, small papillary muscles. The saillike anterior leaflet may also have multiple, short chordae arising around most of its free edge, which bind it relatively closely to the septum and occasionally to the free wall (Fig. 27-1d); or the leaflet edge may be directly adherent to the anterior papillary muscle and moderator band or the posterior edge of the septal band.[Z1]

Should the entire free margin of the leaflets be adherent and imperforate, one variety of tricuspid atresia is produced[R2,Z1] (see Chapter 26). When the adherence is partial, the large anterior leaflet produces a variable degree of stenosis between the portion of ventricle proximal to it (atrialized ventricle) and that distal to it (functional or ventricularized ventricle) since the blood can pass only between the openings that remain between the leaflet margin and the ventricular wall (or through the commissures when these are present) (Fig. 27-2). The stiffness of the anterior leaflet contributes to stenosis.

Although important stenosis is uncommon, most Ebstein valves are incompetent, often severely so (Fig. 27-3). This is contributed to by marked dilatation of the true tricuspid anulus and the right ventricle, as well as the morphologic abnormalities of the tricuspid valve.

Right Ventricle

The downward displacement of the valve divides the right ventricle into a proximal (atrialized) and distal functional (ventricularized) portion. The proximal portion lies between the true tricuspid ring and the valve attachment and comprises a variable portion of the posterior and inferior (diaphragmatic) aspects of the ventricular cavity (Figs. 27-2, 27-3).

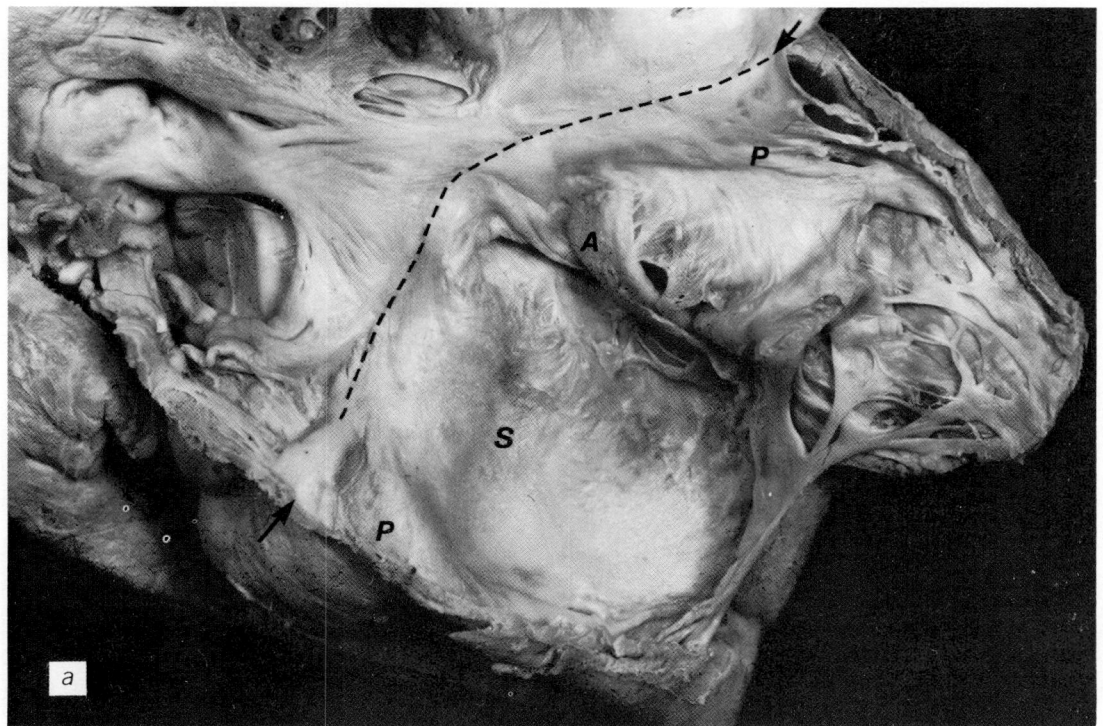

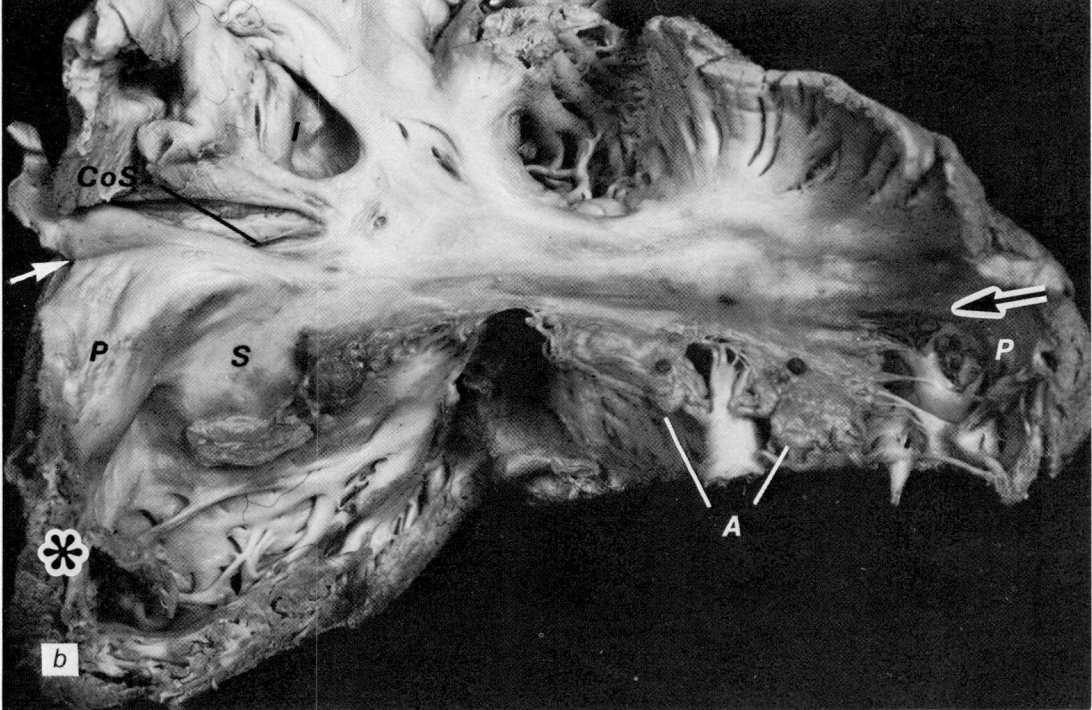

Figure 27-1 Autopsy specimens of Ebstein's anomaly with varying degrees of deformity of the tricuspid valve (GLH). The right atrium and right ventricle have been opened. The site of the true AV ring is marked by the dashed line between the arrows.

(a) All three leaflets are enlarged and elongated (the anterior leafflet is poorly displayed). The septal leaflet is completely adherent to the ventricular septal surface and has abnormal distal chordal attachments as does the posterior leaflet. Note the normal leaflet origin at the right trigone (anteroseptal commissure).

(b) The septal leaflet origin is displaced well downward into the ventricle and the leaflet tissue is diminutive and dysplastic. The posterior leaflet is adherent from the ring to the point marked *. The anterior leaflet origin is normal, the belly is mildly elongated and cleft, and there are multiple short chordal attachments.

A, anterior leaflet of the tricuspid valve; CoS, coronary sinus; P, posterior leaflet of the tricuspid valve; S, septal leaflet of the tricuspid valve.

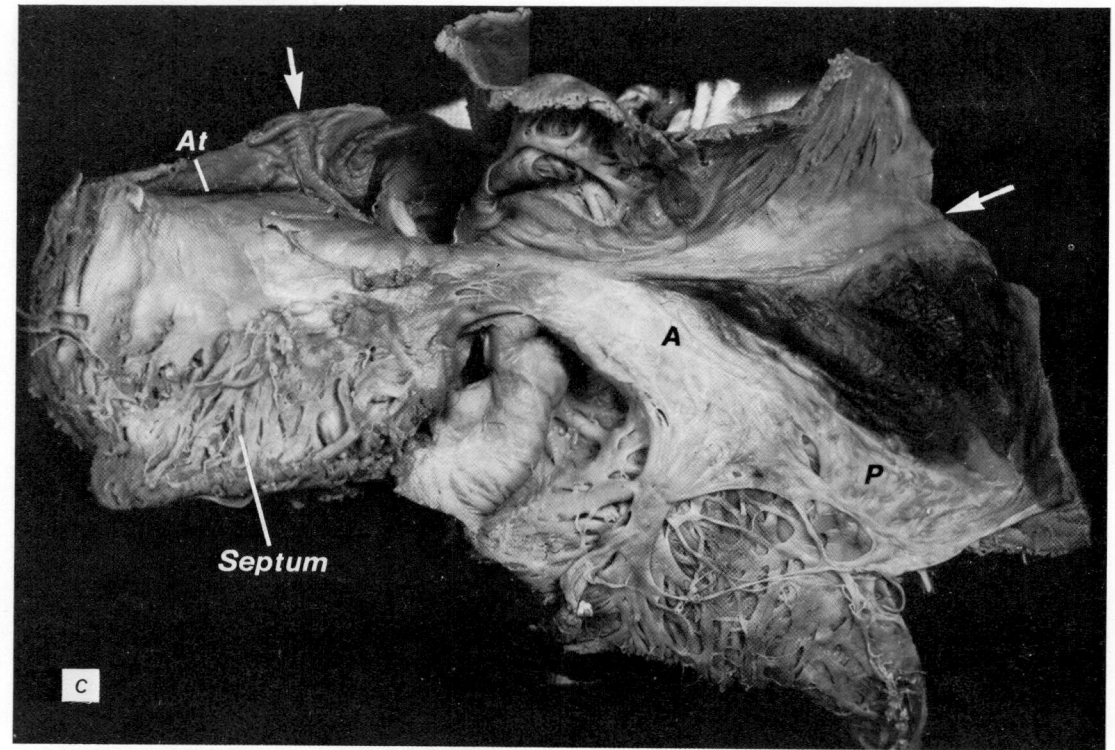

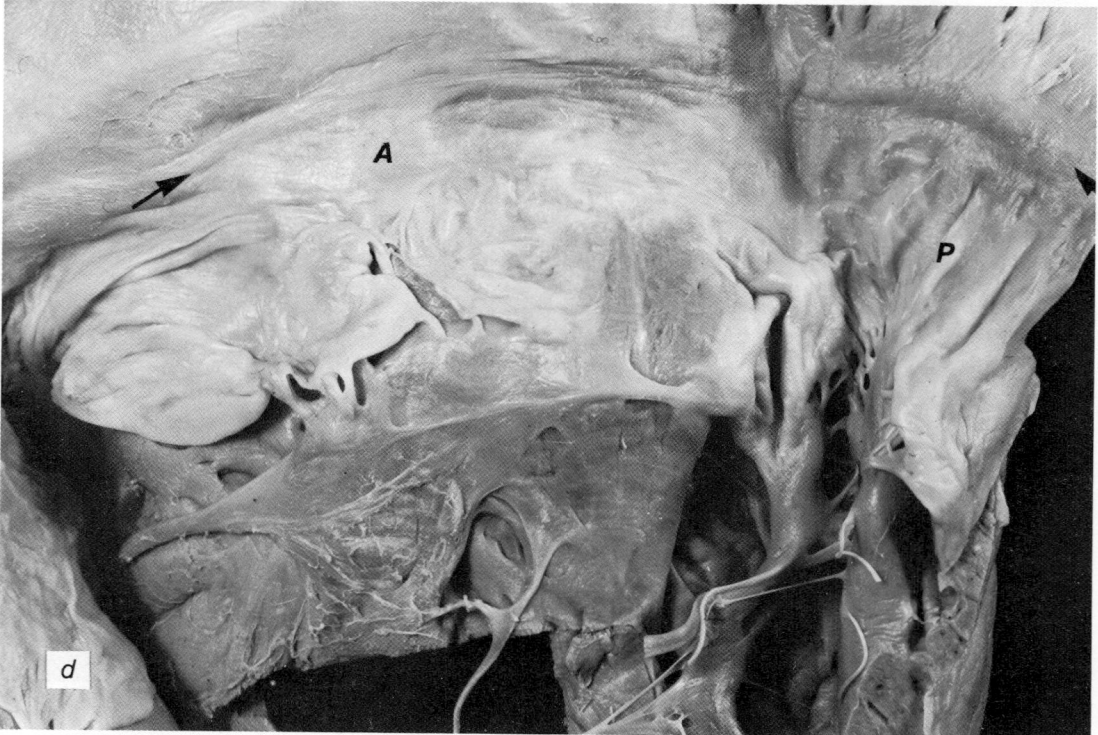

Figure 27-1 *(continued)*
(c) The septal leaflet is absent except for a strand of fibrous tissue. The anterior leaflet origin is downwardly displaced (except at the right trigone) as is the posterior leaflet origin. The darkened bruised portion of ventricular wall is thinned, atrialized ventricle.
(d) Elongated anterior and posterior leaflets originating normally from the ring but with poor commissural development. The central part of the distal anterior leaflet edge is completely fused to a broad muscle group on the right ventricular free wall, and adjacent to this are thickened short chordae. The septal leaflet is not visible.

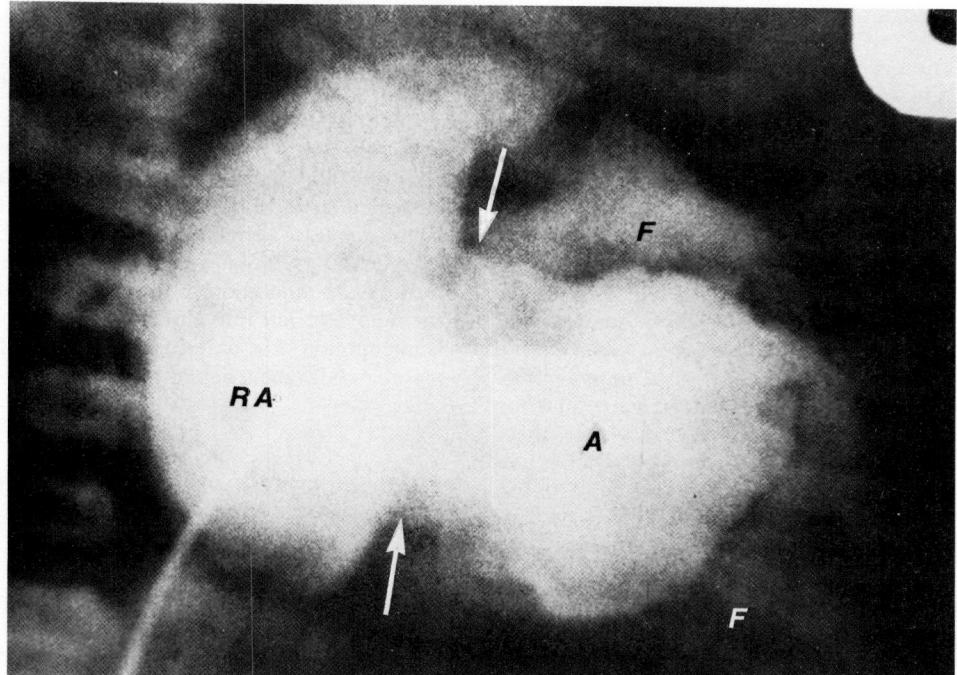

Figure 27-2 Cineangiogram in RAO position in a patient with Ebstein's anomaly, with injection into a large atrialized ventricle, which well demonstrates the dome formed by the fused leaflets (GLH). Free reflux is present into the right atrium through the atrioventricular ring (arrow). The relatively small functional (ventricularized) ventricle is poorly outlined because the displaced valve is stenotic (the specimen showed virtual tricuspid atresia).

A, atrialized portion of right ventricle; F, functional portion; RA, right atrium.

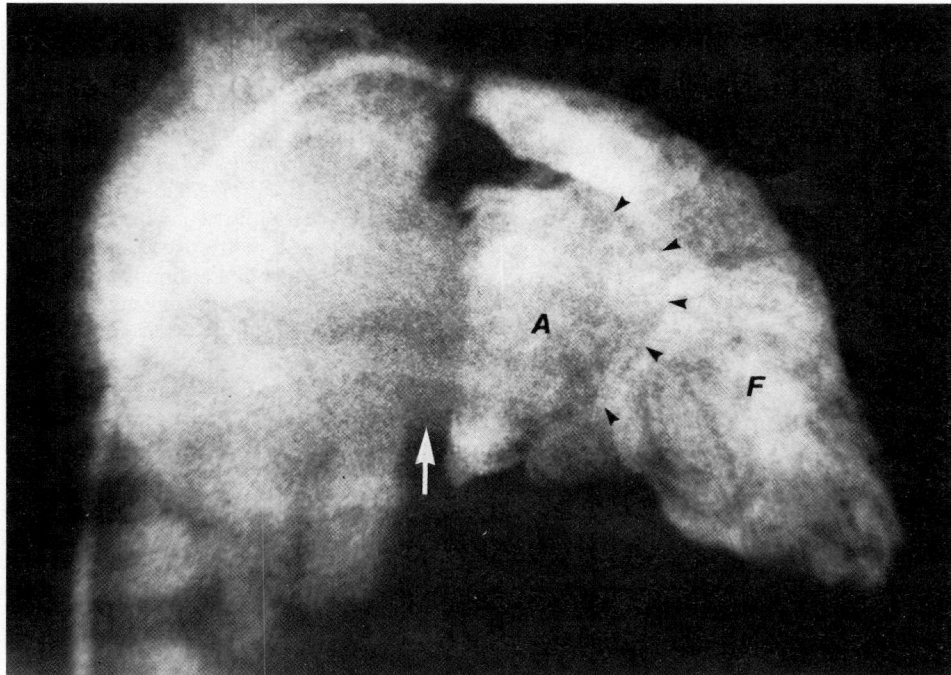

Figure 27-3 Cineangiogram in RAO position of neonate with pulmonary atresia and Ebstein's anomaly (GLH). The injection was made into right ventricle, but the catheter has recoiled into right atrium. The curved margin (arrows) represents a dome formed by the abnormally tethered distal edge of the tricuspid leaflets. This margin separates the atrialized ventricle from the functional ventricle. There is severe tricuspid incompetence. The normally positioned atrioventricular ring is readily identified (thick arrow).

A, atrialized portion of right ventricle; F, functional portion.

The proximal portion is obviously *atrialized* in about one-quarter of the hearts in which the posterior and septal leaflets are severely displaced. This atrialized portion of ventricular wall is dilated. Uncommonly, it is so thin walled as to seem aneurysmal, in which case the wall is largely fibrous tissue and the endocardium is smooth. When very thin, it moves paradoxically during ventricular systole and may also expand during atrial systole. Its electrical potentials are ventricular, but its pressure pulse has an atrial contour. More commonly, the wall of the atrialized portion is thicker and contains variable amounts of muscle.

The *functional* (ventricularized) *portion* of the right ventricle lies distal (downstream) to the displaced valve and is therefore smaller than the normal ventricle. However, this feature is modified by right ventricular dilatation, which is an almost constant finding. The functional portion consists of the infundibulum (conus), the trabeculated apex, and that portion of the ventricle beneath the large anterior cusp (the anterolateral recess)[A4] (Figs. 27-4, 27-5). The dilated functional ventricle is usually thinner walled than normal and contains fewer than the normal number of muscle fibers. Anderson and Lie[A2] have suggested that there may be a congenital paucity of myocardial cells in the right ventricle in this disease, so that the dilatation of both portions of the ventricle is a part of the developmental anomaly rather than entirely its hemodynamic consequence.

Right Atrium

The right atrium is enormously dilated in advanced cases. There is usually an interatrial communication (present in necropsy specimens in 60% and at catheterization in 42% according to Watson,[W1] and in 21 of 22 surgical cases [UAB]), most commonly a patent foramen ovale, although an atrial septal defect (ASD) of any type may be present.[W1] Rarely, an ostium primum defect ASD co-exists (UAB).

The bundle of His and AV node lie in their usual locations, although the right bundle and node may be compressed by the thickened endocardium[L1,L2] (a possible explanation of the frequent right bundle branch block pattern in the electrocardiogram). There are anomalous (Kent) bundles and a Wolff-Parkinson-White (WPW) syndrome present in about 5% of individuals with Ebstein's anomaly.

Left Ventricle

Monibi and colleagues[M3] and Ng and colleagues[N3] report that left ventricular abnormalities, consisting of abnormal left ventricular contraction and contour and mitral valve prolapse, are frequently present. Mitral valve prolapse has been noted by others.[R4] The mitral valve is frequently nodular and thickened.[C3,L2]

Associated Defects

The most common associated defect is *pulmonary atresia or stenosis,* which may be present in up to one-third of autopsied hearts.[B3] Other associated anomalies include ventricular septal defect, tetralogy of Fallot, patent ductus arteriosus, transposition of the great arteries, coarctation of the aorta, and congenital mitral stenosis.[B3,K1,L1,W1]

In congenitally *corrected transposition* with visceroatrial situs solitus, the tricuspid valve lies within a left-sided systemic morphologically right ventricle. Although 30% of these left-sided tricuspid valves are incompetent,[A1,A3] this is frequently, but by no means always, due to Ebstein's anomaly. The Ebstein's anomaly differs from the usual right-sided form in that dilatation of the AV ring and the separation of the right ventricle into atrialized and ventricularized portions is uncommon. The anterior leaflet is also less prominent and may be cleft (see Chapter 42).

CLINICAL FEATURES AND DIAGNOSTIC CRITERIA

Mechanisms of Symptoms and Signs

Several mechanisms are involved in the production of the variable symptoms and signs of Ebstein's anomaly. One is right ventricular dysfunction of a variable degree, related to the variable decrease in the number of muscle fibers in the right ventricle[A2] and to the variable extent of the cardiomyopathy secondary to tricuspid valve incompetence. In addition, an aneurysmal atrialized portion of the right ventricle may move paradoxically. The functional or ventricularized right ventricular chamber may be of small size and also contribute importantly to right ventricular dysfunction in some patients.

A variable degree of malfunction of the tricuspid valve is another mechanism for symptoms, as well as for the production of a secondary right ventricular cardiomyopathy. When incompetence is present but mild and right ventricular dysfunction is mild, symptoms and signs may be few or even absent. When tricuspid incompetence is severe, right atrial and systemic venous hypertension often develop, as do ascites and peripheral edema. Right ventricular dysfunction often coexists with tricuspid incompetence in this setting. A variable degree of tricuspid stenosis may also occur in patients with Ebstein's anomaly, usually with incompetence.

Another mechanism for symptoms and signs is the right-to-left shunting that is often present. With this is the potential for paradoxic emboli and cerebral embolism. Occasionally, the right-to-left shunt is large (secondary to the right ventricular and tricuspid dysfunction described above), and severe hypoxia and polycythemia may develop with their untoward sequelae.

Large left-to-right shunts occur uncommonly, but when they are present (because of minimal right ventricular and tricuspid valve dysfunction), they provide a mechanism for developing heart failure, as in the case of any atrial septal defect (see Chapter 15).

Symptoms and Signs

Symptoms may appear in the first week of life and then consist of breathlessness in association with cyanosis, severe cardiomegaly, and often congestive heart failure. However, many patients do not have sufficient symptoms in the first week of life to bring them to medical attention and pre-

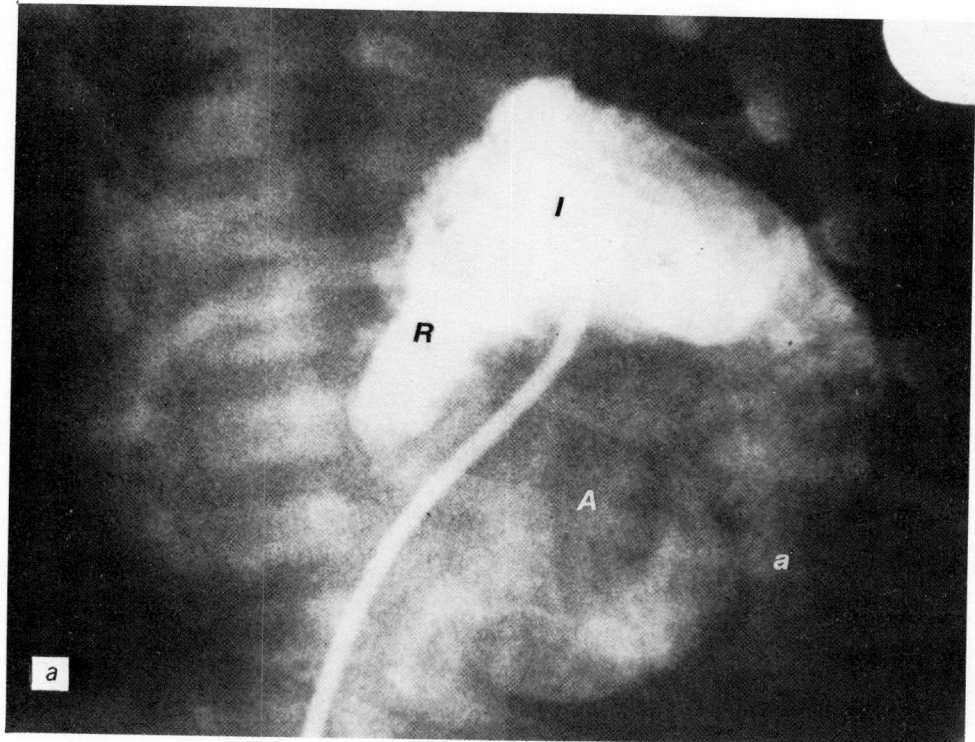

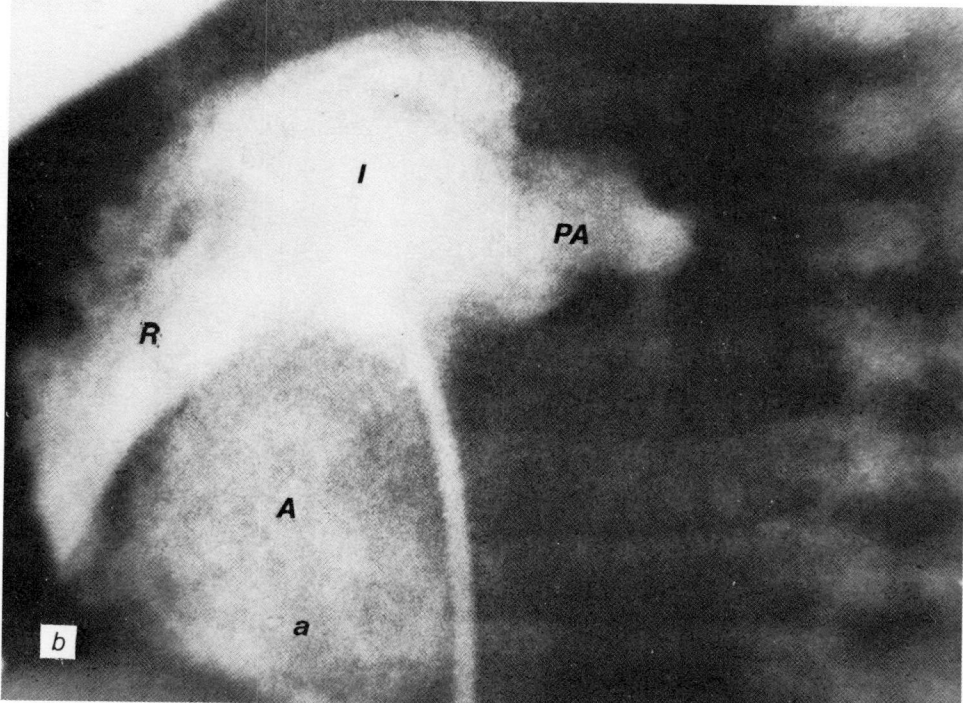

Figure 27-4 Right anterior oblique (*a*) and left anterior oblique (*b*) cineangiogram frames of a patient with Ebstein's anomaly (GLH). The injection was made into the outflow portion of the functional (ventricularized) right ventricle which also extends around the anterior and rightward free wall aspects of the atrialized portion to form the anterolateral recess. The apical portion of the functional ventricle fills poorly and is superimposed on the atrialized portion in the LAO view.

a, apical portion of functional right ventricle; A, atrialized portion of right ventricle; I, outflow portion of the functional right ventricle; PA, pulmonary artery; R, anterolateral recess.

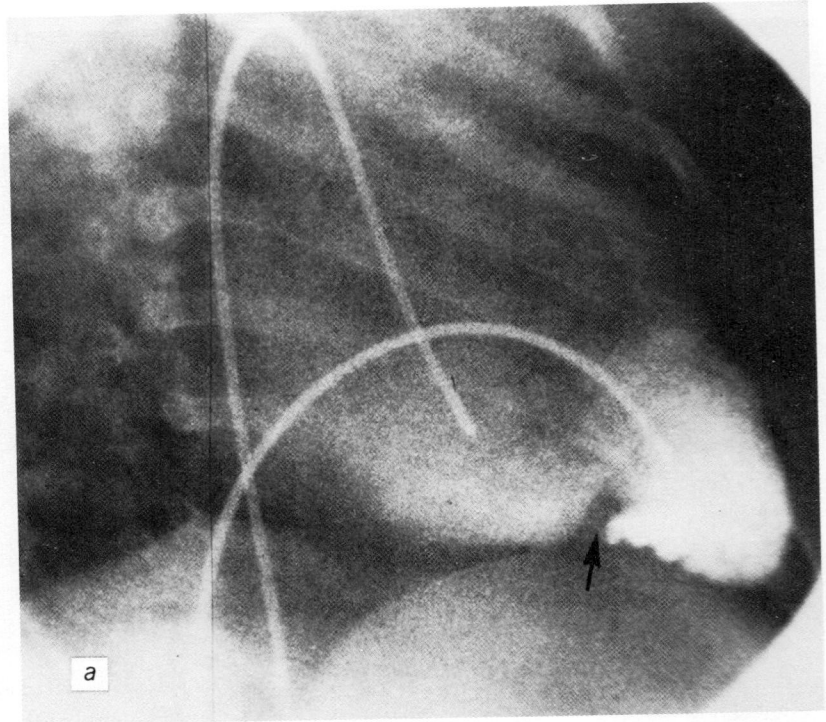

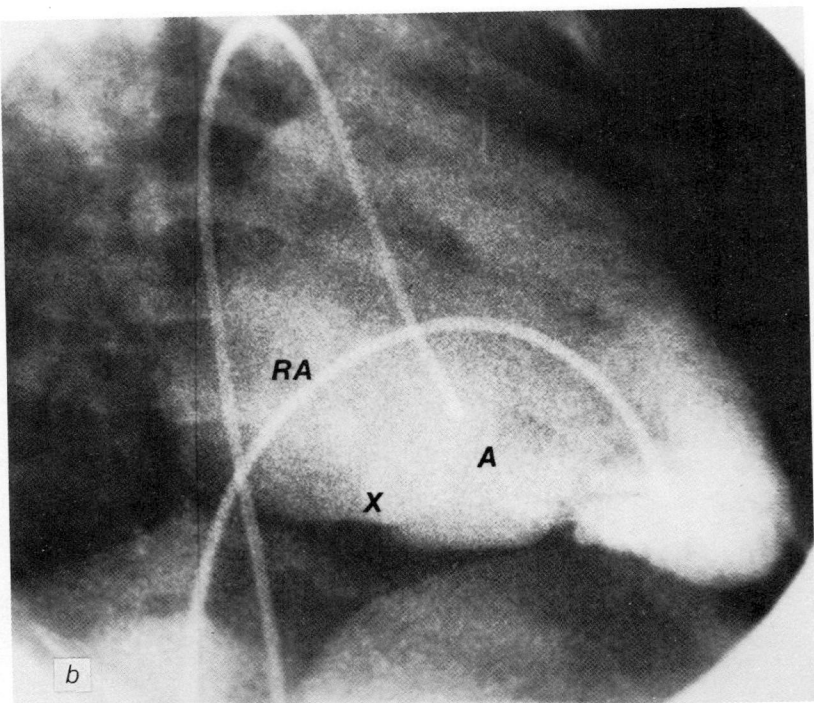

Figure 27-5 Right anterior oblique cineangiogram frames of a patient with Ebstein's anomaly with injection into right ventricular apex (GLH).
(a) Early frame showing reflux through displaced leaflets into the atrialized ventricle. The deep notch (arrow) represents the attachment of a dysplastic posterior leaflet to the inferior wall.
(b) Later frame showing more extensive filling of atrialized ventricle and right atrium. The X marks the position of the true AV ring.

A, atrialized ventricle; RA, right atrium.

Table 27-2 Clinical features of 19 patients with Ebstein's disease who were referred *after* the first week of life (from 29 days to 55 years) (GLH).

	No. of Patients	% of Total
Cyanosis	11	58
Arrhythmia	11	58
L → R atrial shunt (ASD closure)	3	16
CHF during course	6	32
Deaths	6	32
CHF	2	11
Sudden	2	11
Surgery[a]	2	11
Asymptomatic[b]	7	37
Mild symptoms[b]	6	32
Total	19	100

KEY: ASD, atrial septal defect; CHF, congestive heart failure; WPW, Wolff-Parkinson-White.

NOTE: The mean follow-up in the 13 survivors is 13 years (5–23 years) (see Fig. 27-7).

[a] One surgical death followed a Glenn operation in 1963. The other was a late death 3.9 years after valve replacement.

[b] Status at last assessment.

sent later in life. In these patients, mild dyspnea and fatigue may become evident in childhood or early adult life, or more severe symptoms and signs of various types may develop. Should congestive heart failure appear, the patient becomes severely limited by breathlessness and fatigue.

Cyanosis is a common sign of Ebstein's malformation, occurring in more than half the patients (Table 27-2), and is severe in about a third.[K1] It may appear at birth; but in most, the onset is in infancy and early childhood. Palpitations due to various types of dysrhythmia are common.[B4] More severe arrhythmic symptoms are frequent in patients with Ebstein's malformation of all ages and may be severe and disabling. The WPW syndrome is the best known type of arrhythmia, but less specific types of supraventricular tachycardias are much more common. Numerous electrophysiologic abnormalities have been identified,[K2] which no doubt account for the frequent occurrence and persistence of arrhythmic symptoms even after operation. Symptoms are more severe when there are significant associated cardiac anomalies.

A malar flush, similar to the so-called "mitral facies," was noted by Ebstein and occurs in about one-third of the patients.[S5] It is unrelated to cyanosis or polycythemia or the cardiac output.[K1]

The left anterior chest is often prominent in association with marked cardiomegaly, and there may be a systolic thrill along the left sternal edge originating from the tricuspid valve. Characteristically, the precordium and apex remain quiet despite marked cardiomegaly. The jugular venous pressure is generally unremarkable[W3] and rarely suggests tricuspid incompetence or stenosis, despite the fact that free tricuspid incompetence is present on an angiogram. This is related to the large size and compliance of both the right atrium and the atrialized right ventricle, as well as the low right ventricular and pulmonary artery pressures.

On auscultation the most constant finding is wide splitting of the first sound with accentuation of the delayed component that is caused by closing (or termination of motion[C1,F1]) of the large anterior tricuspid leaflet. The delayed tricuspid valve closure is probably mechanical[G1] rather than related to right bundle branch block, although Crews and colleagues[C1] considered it correlated with the latter. The large anterior leaflet is also responsible for an opening snap in diastole, and in addition there may be an atrial fourth sound. The pulmonary component of the second sound is delayed and soft (in relation to the right bundle branch block) or absent when pulmonary artery pressure is very low. A pansystolic murmur maximal at the lower left sternal edge is due to tricuspid incompetence and is heard in about one-third of patients. Finally, there is usually a diastolic murmur often low pitched and sometimes scratchy in quality, commencing with the opening snap and sometimes augmented by the fourth sound. The diastolic murmur is presumably due to movement of blood across the malformed tricuspid orifice.

Chest X-Ray

In classical Ebstein's disease, the chest x-ray shows marked cardiomegaly with a rounded or boxlike cardiac contour beneath a narrow pedicle (Fig. 27-6). In the pulmonary artery view, the whole of the silhouette is then formed by right atrium and right ventricle, and because of their minimal excursion and the normal or oligemic lung fields, the silhouette has a peculiarly sharp edge. However, as with other features of the disease, there is a wide variation in heart size.[S5] In a few it remains normal, and in most it is only moderately enlarged.[K1]

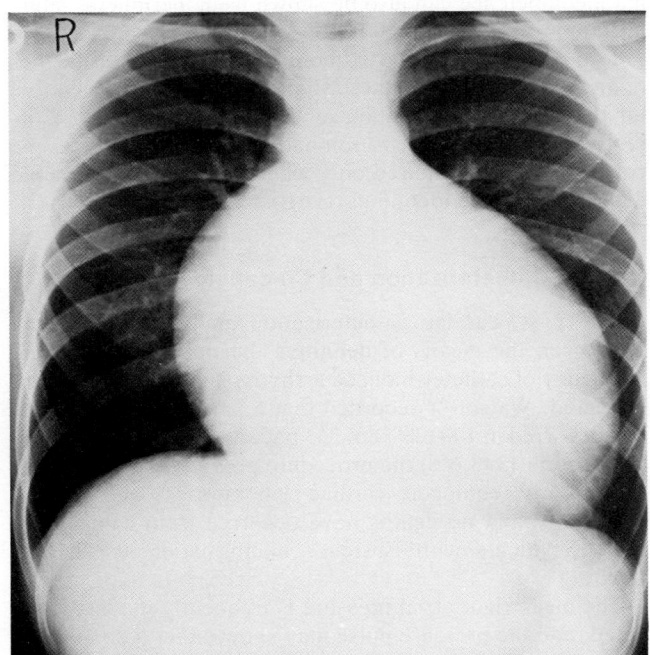

Figure 27-6 Chest x-ray of a 12-year-old girl with classical Ebstein's anomaly (UAB).

Electrocardiogram

A right bundle branch pattern together with relatively low amplitude R wave in right-sided chest leads and right atrial hypertrophy are characteristic of the anomaly. According to Kumar and associates,[K1] the height of the P wave varies inversely with the arterial oxygen saturation ($r = .82$, $P < .001$). In addition, the taller the P wave, the shorter the survival time ($P < .001$). Right ventricular hypertrophy does not occur in uncomplicated Ebstein's, and inverted T waves in leads V_1–V_4 are fairly common. Using intralumenal electrode catheters, Kastor and colleagues[K2] have demonstrated prolonged intraright atrial and infranodal conduction in patients with a large right atrium and well-defined atrialized ventricle.

In approximately 5% of patients the electrocardiogram (ECG) shows a type B (right-sided) WPW syndrome. In any cyanotic patient with this type of preexcitation, Ebstein's anomaly should always be considered. Supraventricular arrhythmias occur in more than half the patients, and they may be paroxysmal and recurrent. Paroxysmal atrial tachycardia, atrial fibrillation and nodal rhythm can all occur, as can first-degree heart block.

Echocardiography

M-mode echocardiography is a useful screening test. It will usually demonstrate delayed tricuspid valve closure and displacement of the tricuspid valve to the left. According to Giuliani,[G1] the greater the delay in tricuspid valve closure, the more severe the disease. Wide excursion of the anterior tricuspid valve leaflet, a decreased E-F slope, increased right ventricular dimensions, and paradoxic septal motion can also be demonstrated. A right-to-left atrial shunt and tricuspid incompetence can also be shown using peripheral saline injections.

Two-dimensional echo is more helpful, and with further refinement of technique these studies have become definitive for the anatomic evaluation of Ebstein's anomaly.[S12] Currently, cardiac catheterization and cineangiography may be considered to be required only when specific hemodynamic details need to be identified (UAB).[S12]

Cardiac Catheterization and Cineangiography

In the past, cardiac catheterization and cineangiography have been the means of definitive diagnosis, although the frequency of catheter-induced arrhythmias has long been appreciated. Watson[W1] recorded that a paroxysmal dysrhythmia occurred in 100 (28%) of 363 patients during catheterization, and in 13 (3.6%) the procedure proved fatal. However, in properly equipped cardiac laboratories, the risk is minimal,[K1] and no deaths have occurred from catheterization of patients with Ebstein's malformation at GLH or UAB.

The mean right atrial pressure is frequently modestly elevated, and the pressure pulse may show either a dominant a or v wave. These correlate poorly with the degree of tricuspid incompetence or stenosis. An additional "s" wave, which precedes the v wave and interrupts the c wave, is said to indicate tricuspid incompetence.[G,K1,S5] The right atrial waveform is also recorded in the atrialized portion of the right ventricle so that the tricuspid valve is noted to be displaced well toward the left of the spine. An *electrode catheter* may define the position and size of the atrialized right ventricular chamber.[M4,Y2] Right ventricular systolic pressure is normal or low, and right ventricular end-diastolic pressure is frequently raised, more so when there is the syndrome of chronic congestive heart failure. It is uncommon to record a significant gradient across the tricuspid valve,[K1] although Takayasu and colleagues noted this in 8 of their 26 cases and considered that stenosis could still be significant in its absence.[T1]

When there is an interatrial communication, the shunt through it is usually right to left in association with systemic arterial desaturation and a reduced $\dot{Q}p$. The right-to-left shunt can be quantitated using indicator dilution curves. The shunt may occasionally be left to right[M2] and the resultant increase in $\dot{Q}p$ may be associated with congestive heart failure. The direction of shunting is no doubt influenced by the right ventricular compliance.

In the newborn with Ebstein's anomaly, a functional pulmonary outflow obstruction can occur.[N1] Thus, a normal pulmonary valve may fail to open following a right-sided injection of contrast due to a combination of massive tricuspid incompetence, poor right ventricular contraction, and a high neonatal pulmonary vascular resistance with or without a large shunt at ductal level. High-quality cineangiocardiography is therefore necessary to distinguish this not uncommon situation from true pulmonary atresia.

Cineangiocardiography (see Figs. 27-2–27-5) is usually diagnostic,[D2] provided there is significant displacement and dysplasia of septal or posterior leaflets. In the right anterior oblique projection, the conjoined posterior and anterior cusps, and therefore the distal limit of the atrialized ventricle, can frequently be identified. Contrast trapped beneath the posterior leaflet can indicate the degree of its adherence to and level of its origin from the diaphragmatic border of the right ventricle, which may be notched at this point.[S6] The site of the true anulus is also visible more proximally. An injection into the functional right ventricle enables tricuspid incompetence to be assessed together with the size and behavior of the functional ventricle. Angiography in left anterior oblique projection also allows the right-to-left shunt at atrial level to be visualized, and any ventricular septal defects can be localized by left ventriculography.

NATURAL HISTORY

Ebstein's malformation is uncommon, occurring in less than 1% of subjects with congenital heart disease. The incidence is equal in the two sexes. Familial Ebstein's has been reported rarely[E3,G4,S4] but was present in one of the UAB surgical cases.

In keeping with the wide morphologic spectrum of this disease, the subject may be asymptomatic throughout a normal life span or symptoms may not develop until very late in

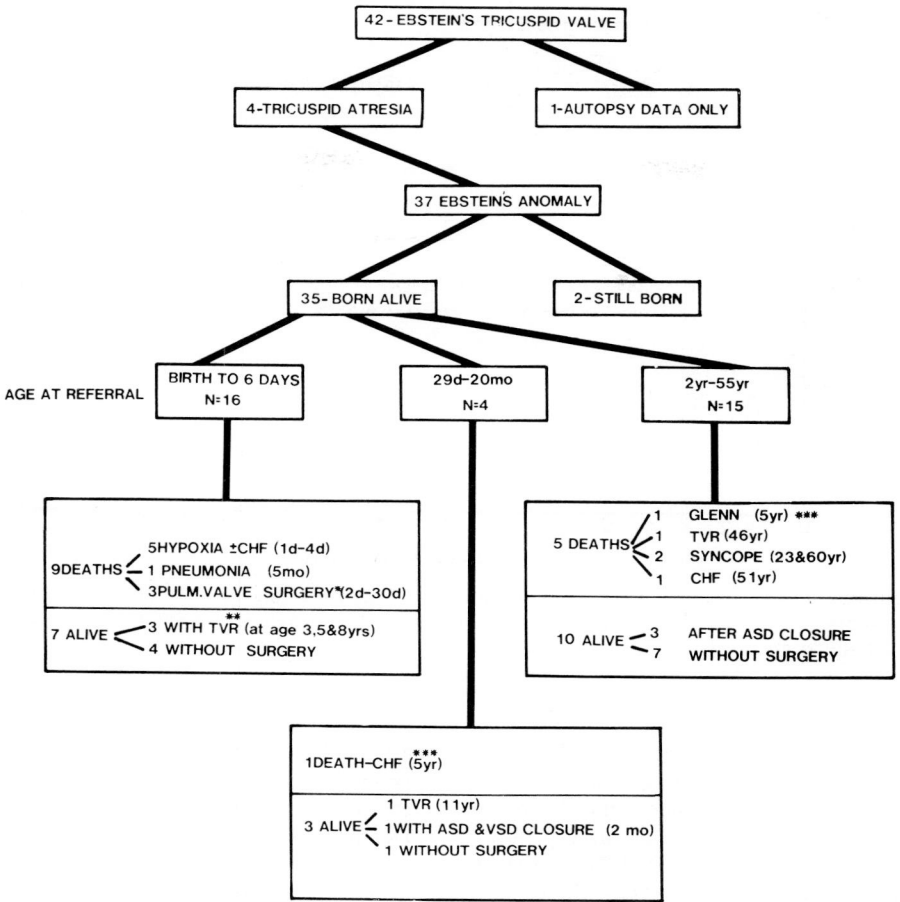

Figure 27-7 A flowchart depicting the fate of patients with Ebstein's anomaly seen between 1958 and 1980 (GLH). In all patients but one the diagnosis was confirmed by cardiac catheterization or autopsy, and all patients have been followed for a mean of 6.2 years. Patients are divided into three groups according to their age at first referral to the hospital. Ages in parentheses are ages at death or operation.

* One had a normal pulmonary valve (presumed pulmonary atresia) and two had pulmonary atresia. One also had tricuspid valve replacement with a stented aortic homograft at 30 days of age; **, one also had a blind valvotomy for pulmonary stenosis at 19 days of age; ***, both deaths occurred in 1963 and are not representative of recent management.

ASD, atrial septal defect; CHF, congestive heart failure; TVR, tricuspid valve replacement; VSD, ventricular septal defect.

life.[H4] In contrast, severe symptoms may appear in the first week of life. Many patients are in the middle of the spectrum.

Natural History Related to Age at Referral

The disease is a recognized cause of death in utero,[G2] and the babies may be stillborn (two at GLH). A surprising number of patients, slightly less than half (16/35 = 46%, CL 36%–56%) are referred with cyanosis and often congestive heart failure within the *first week of life,* most in the first 48 hours and all before the fifth day (Fig. 27-7). About half of these die (9/16 = 56%, CL 40%–71%), usually within days of being seen. Those who survive this period tend to remain alive, some with the aid of surgery at a later age. In most of them,

the cyanosis disappears spontaneously, sometimes to reappear later. It would therefore seem that provided a symptomatic neonate with Ebstein's anomaly survives the neonatal period, there is a good chance of long-term survival, and that this can be further improved, where appropriate, by surgery on the tricuspid valve.

Obstruction to pulmonary blood flow is uncommon in patients presenting at an older age (none at GLH). However, 6 (38%) of the 16 babies presenting in the first week of life had infundibular or pulmonary valve obstruction (GLH), and thus had Ebstein's anomaly with a major associated lesion. As is usual when major associated lesions complicate a congenital cardiac lesion in infancy, mortality is high.[K1] The 3 with pulmonary atresia succumbed (GLH), despite valvotomy in 2 of them, whereas the 3 with pulmonary stenosis

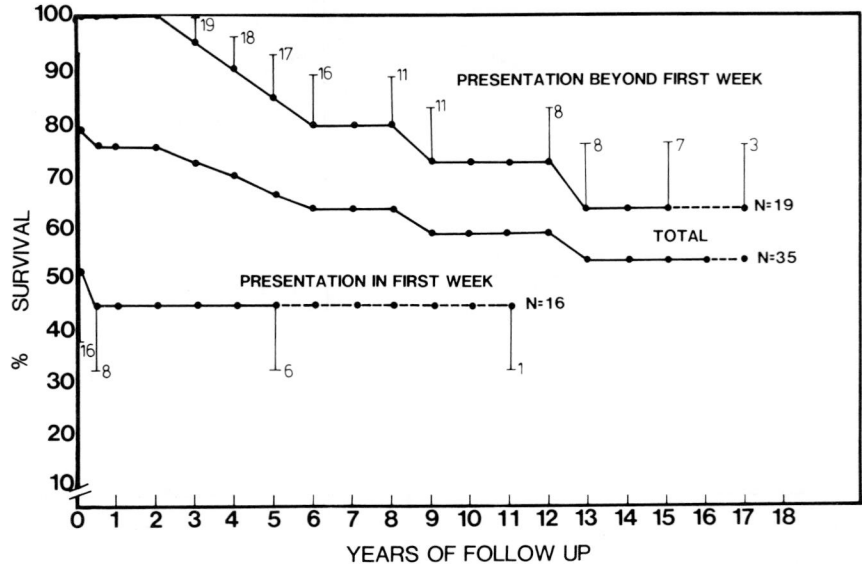

Figure 27-8 Actuarial survival curves of patients with Ebstein's anomaly, stratified according to age at presentation (GLH). The numbers at risk are noted. The *P* value for the difference between the two stratified curves is .01.

survived (1 required early valvotomy). Importantly, transient cyanosis may occur (6 of the 35 GLH patients) in the first week of life, which rapidly subsides and is never significant enough to require early referral to surgery.

Many studies have probably underestimated the incidence and the severity of this entity in *neonates*. Thus, the review by Vacca and colleagues of 108 clinical or autopsy cases reported between 1866 and 1957[V2] recorded only 2 patients less than 1 month of age. In Watson's collected review of 505 cases[W1] only 35 (7%) were less than 1 year old (half of them were under 1 month). In Bialostozky's review of 65 patients[B4] the authors comment that neonates are not included. In the current Mayo Clinic series[G1] only 10 of the 67 patients were diagnosed in infancy. The Boston Children's Hospital series[K1] also probably underestimates the frequency of serious symptoms in neonates. Twelve of their 55 patients (22%) were seen in the first week of life, and 34 (64%) were under 2 years of age. Eleven of the 34 died early. These series must have been in some way selective and, therefore, not useful in assessing natural history. In contrast, Schiebler and colleagues'[S5] earlier study from the Mayo Clinic found that 12 of the 23 patients presented in the neonatal period, and 5 of these 12 died—figures similar to those from GLH.

Presentation in infancy but beyond the first month of life is not associated with a high risk of death or of severe symptoms (Fig. 27-7 and Table 27-2). Other studies do suggest an increased mortality in the infant group,[G1,K1] at least until 6 months of age.[W1] Beyond this age Watson's series[W1] indicates a prognosis similar to that of older children. He states that "whereas 72% of those under 1 year of age were in heart failure, 71% of the children and adolescents had little or no disability." Between the ages of 1 and 25 years, 15% (50/346) of the patients died from natural causes.

Many patients with this disease are only mildly symptom-

atic and do not present until *late in life*.[S1] Genton and Blount[G2] point out that only about half of those over 50 years of age are cyanotic, and their hearts are often normal in size. Death in this age group is more often due to paroxysmal embolus or paroxysmal atrial tachycardia with congestive heart failure appearing only very late in the course.

Actuarial analysis (Fig. 27-8) confirms the improved survival in patients who present beyond the first week of life compared with those presenting in the first week.

Incremental Risk Factors for Premature Death

Cyanosis, when present, tends to be slowly progressive and survival can be related to its severity.[G1] Kumar and colleagues[K1] found that with severe cyanosis the 8-year survival was 20% and with mild cyanosis, 94%. Between 15% and 20% of patients remain acyanotic throughout their course. This does not necessarily mean that the atrial septum is intact, since there are patients with left-to-right shunting at atrial level[M2,V2] (see "Symptoms and Signs").

A similar, but probably less marked, association has been demonstrated with *increasing cardiomegaly.*[G1,K1] However, marked cardiomegaly may be present without significant symptoms and with a surprisingly stable course.

The *onset of congestive heart failure* is a grave prognostic sign, death usually following within 2 years.[K1,W1] Heart failure may be precipitated by prolonged tachycardia or by acute infections, and with few exceptions such patients also have gross cardiomegaly.[W1] After the age of 6 months, about half the deaths occur in association with congestive heart failure.[W1]

As would be anticipated, NYHA classes III and IV patients have a much poorer prognosis,[G1,W1] and death from any cause is much less common in patients with few symptoms (classes I and II). It is important to note that about 70% of patients between 1 and 25 years of age and 60% of those greater than 25 years are in classes I and II.[W1]

Other Events

Sudden death occurs in about 3% of patients, and about 20% of all the deaths are of this nature,[G2,W1] presumably from arrhythmia with or without WPW. *Cerebral abscess* or *paradoxical emboli and stroke*[M7] occur at all ages but are said to be a more common cause of death in patients over 50 years.[G2] Bacterial endocarditis does not occur.

TECHNIQUE OF OPERATION

Tricuspid Valve Replacement and Atrial Septal Defect Closure

The usual preparations are made for operation, anesthetic management (see Chapter 4), and preparation for cardiopulmonary bypass (CPB) using two venous cannulae (see Chapter 2). Prior to commencing CPB, the atrialized portion of the right ventricle is assessed noting particularly whether it moves paradoxically, and an exploring finger is inserted into the right atrium through the appendage to confirm the presence and degree of tricuspid incompetence. Care must be taken with this, since very gross incompetence (such as would occur were the tricuspid valve absent) produces no jet and only gross turbulence may be felt.

After establishing CPB (see Chapter 2) and cold cardioplegia (Chapter 3), the lateral right atrial wall is incised obliquely, and the pump oxygenator sump sucker is placed across the atrial septal defect.

The tricuspid leaflet tissue is excised, leaving a more generous portion of the base of the anterior and septal cusps where they attach to the membranous septum and right trigone at the point of penetration of the bundle of His. The general suture technique for insertion of the valve replacement device is that described in Chapters 11 and 14. When the septal and posterior tricuspid leaflets are displaced into the right ventricle, or the septal leaflet is absent, sutures may be passed through the usual location of the tricuspid ring (GLH). Alternatively, the suture line in this area can be placed well posterior to the AV node area and coronary sinus (UAB), as described by Barnard and Schrire[B5] (Fig. 27-9). In Ebstein's malformation, the replacement valve of choice is a stented, antibiotically treated semilunar valve homograft (GLH; see Chapter 14, Appendix) or, alternatively, in young adults a large-sized mechanical prosthesis and in older adults a 34-mm diameter heterograft valve (UAB).

As an alternative to cold cardioplegia, electrical fibrillation without aortic cross-clamping may be used and the heart defibrillated before placing the valve replacement sutures (GLH). Should heart block occur, the offending stitch is removed and repositioned.

When the atrialized ventricle is thin walled and fibrous and moves paradoxically, it is plicated by passing the sutures used to position the valve first through the tissue that forms the margin of the atrialized ventricle (corresponding to the attachment of the displaced septal and posterior leaflets) and then through the true tricuspid ring (GLH). The valve is seated and the sutures tied and cut. If the atrialized ventricle has been plicated, this portion is further obliterated by a running polypropylene suture, placed from outside the heart, taking care not to compromise the arterial supply of the remainder of the right ventricle by occluding significant-sized coronary arteries. Plication is unnecessary in most cases.[W5]

The interatrial communication is closed. In many instances, the septal tissue is stretched and the fossa ovalis tissue thinned. A patch must then be used (pericardium is ideal, although knitted Dacron velour serves well) and positioned without tension using a continuous 4-0 polypropylene suture (Fig. 27-9). Direct suture is avoided unless the tissues are strong and the hole is small, because even stitch holes can result in significant residual right-to-left shunting. The left atrium is deliberately not emptied of blood, and the patch suture line is completed at the highest point (superiorly) to avoid air entrapment on the left side of the septum.

The right atriotomy is now closed. When the atrium is very large, its size may be reduced by first excising an ellipse from the lateral wall (GLH). With strong suction on the aortic needle vent, the aortic clamp is released. The procedure is completed in the usual fashion, including atrial and ventricular pacing wires and left-and-right atrial pressure lines (see Chapter 2).

When a WPW syndrome is present and there is a history of life-threatening paroxysmal arrhythmia,[S8] the accessory conduction pathways should be divided at the same operation, after proper electrophysiologic study (see Chapter 48, "Division of Accessory AV Conduction Pathways" in section on Technique of Operation). This is generally done before the valve replacement.

Simple Atrial Septal Defect Closure

Simple ASD closure is done as described for closure in conjunction with valve replacement.

SPECIAL FEATURES OF POSTOPERATIVE CARE

Postoperative care is as usual (see Chapter 5). Convalescence is generally rapid and normal.

EARLY RESULTS

Valve Replacement and Atrial Septal Defect Closure

The early results of valve replacement and closure of the ASD are good, but hospital mortality does not yet approach zero even for patients in NYHA classes II and III. Thus, in the combined UAB and GLH series, hospital mortality was about 5% in patients preoperatively in NYHA class II or III (one death, 6%, CL 1%–19% in 16 patients, Table 27-3). This is similar to the results reported by Danielson and colleagues.[D3] The mortality is very much higher when the patients are in advanced heart failure (Table 27-3). These facts account for the overall mortality of 20% in the combined UAB and GLH experience (Table 27-3). All deaths

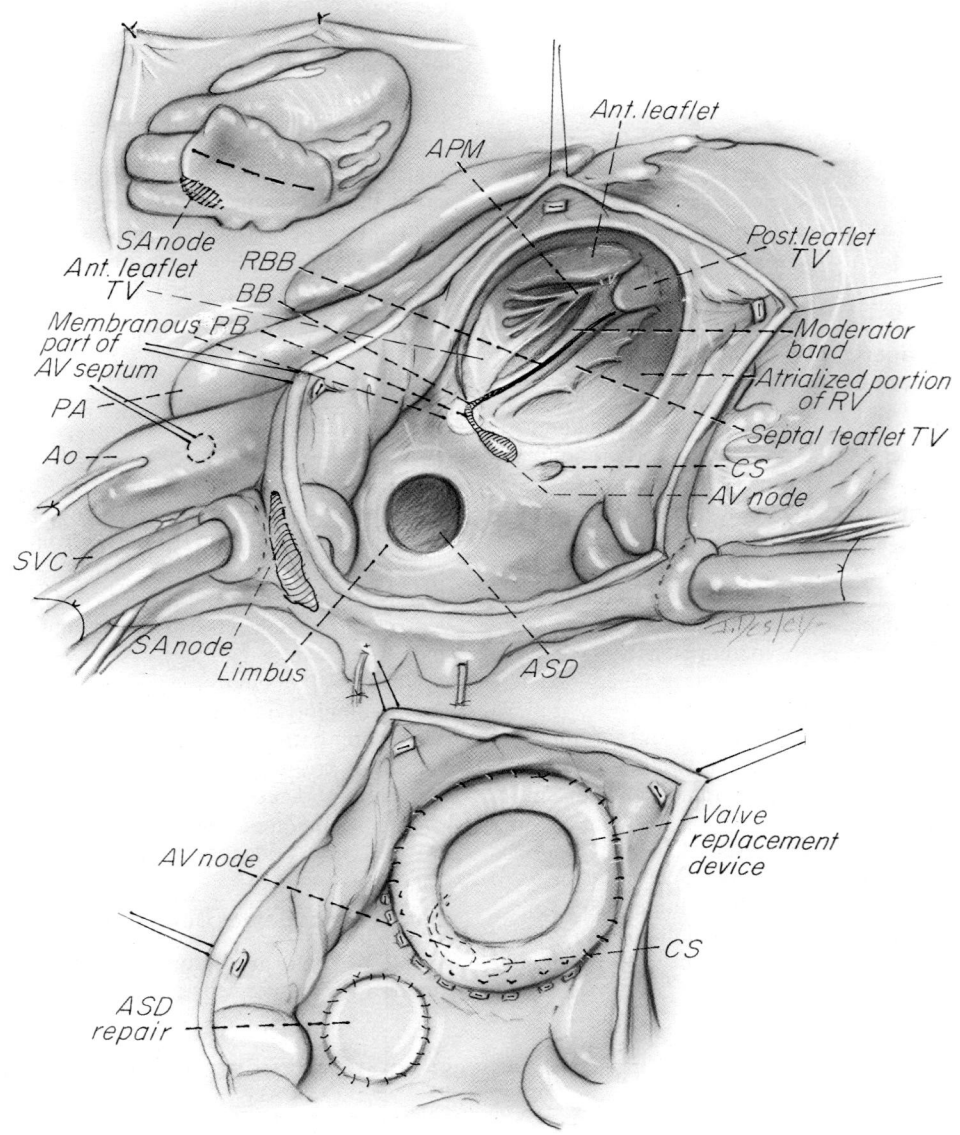

Figure 27-9 Replacement of the tricuspid valve and closure of the atrial septal defect in Ebstein's malformation. The upper left insert shows the siting of the atriotomy incision well anterior to the sinoatrial node. The upper drawing shows the anatomic details seen by the surgeon and indicates the position of the conduction tissue and its vulnerability to damage. The lower drawing shows closure of the ASD and one method (UAB) of insertion of the tricuspid prosthesis when the septal leaflet is absent or severely displaced into the right ventricle. Even then, the suture can be placed in the actual tricuspid ring in that area (GLH) (see text). Interrupted sutures may be used throughout (GLH). When septal leaflet remnants are present, the posterior sutures are passed through them and the valve replacement device is positioned in the true anulus (see text for details).

APM, anterior papillary muscle; AV node, atrioventricular node; BB, branching bundle; Cos, coronary sinus; PA, pulmonary artery; PB, penetrating bundle; RBB, right bundle branch; SA, sinoatrial.

Reproduced with permission from Bharati et al.[B1]

Table 27-3 Preoperative NYHA functional class and hospital mortality after tricuspid valve replacement and ASD closure for Ebstein's anomaly (UAB and GLH combined series; GLH 1958–Apr. 1981, UAB 1967–1980).

| Preoperative NYHA Class | n | Hospital Deaths | | |
		No.	%	CL
I	—			
II	4	1[a]	25%	3%–63%
III	12		0%	0%–15%
IV	4	3[b]	75%	37%–97%
Total	20	4	20%	10%–33%

KEY: CL, 70% confidence limits.

[a] Associated partial AV canal defect.

[b] One was a neonate with pulmonary atresia.

were associated with acute cardiac failure. This is similar to the mortality of 12 deaths (18%, CL 13%–24%) among the 68 patients reported in the literature prior to 1981.[B6,B7,J1,K3,M5,P2,R3,S2,S9]

Complete heart block occurred in one patient in the combined series. It should not occur with the methods currently used (see "Technique of Operation"). With the exception of the series of Judgutt et al.,[J1] in which all 4 patients developed complete heart block, this complication has been reported in only 2 (3%) of 64 patients in the literature prior to 1981.

Repair of Atrial Septal Defect Alone

The risk of simple ASD closure is low in properly selected cases. Nine patients with either left-to-right or right-to-left shunts and competent although abnormal tricuspid valves underwent simple closure of the ASD (GLH and UAB) with no hospital deaths (0%, CL 0%–19%). It is a little surprising that closure of the ASD was so well tolerated in the face of right-to-left shunting, but that was the early experience at the Mayo Clinic[W2] and has been the experience in pulmonary stenosis with intact ventricular septum (see Chapter 24).

Other Procedures

Danielson and colleagues have reported a low hospital mortality (9%, CL 4%–17%) among 34 patients undergoing *tricuspid annuloplasty*, usually in conjunction with repair of the ASD and right ventricular plication.

Pulmonary valvotomy can have a low hospital mortality in patients with Ebstein's anomaly when indications are appropriate (Tables 27-4, 27-5). This procedure may be lifesaving in the neonate, since it decreases the degree of tricuspid incompetence.

Tricuspid valvotomy for severe stenosis of the displaced tricuspid valve plus closure of the ASD may be successful,[P2] but important tricuspid incompetence may result. One 3-year-old child underwent tricuspid valvotomy and died 2 weeks after hospital dismissal with severe tricuspid valve incompetence (UAB).

The sectioning of accessory AV conduction pathways does not increase the early risk of repair[S8] (see Chapter 48).

Table 27-4 Surgery for Ebstein's anomaly without tricuspid valve surgery or right ventricular plication. (GLH, 1958–Apr., 1981; UAB 1967–1981). No hospital deaths occurred.

Operation	Indication	No. of Patients
Repair of ASD	L → R shunt	3[a]
	R → L shunt	3
	Bidirectional	2
Repair of ASD and VSD	L → R shunt	1
Repair of ASD and pulmonary valvotomy	RV outflow obstruction, L → R shunt	1
Repair of ASD and tricuspid valvotomy	R → L shunt, obstruction at tricuspid V	1[b]
Repair of ASD	L → R shunt, suspected atrial myxoma	1
Total		12

KEY: ASD, atrial septal defect; RV, right ventricular; V, valve; VSD, ventricular septal defect; WPW, Wolff-Parkinson-White.

[a] Two patients had WPW syndrome, and Kent bundles were divided at operation; in another, the bundles were not divided.

[b] Patient (3 yr old) had severe tricuspid incompetence after the operation and died 2 weeks after hospital dismissal.

LATE RESULTS

Tricuspid Valve Replacement and Closure of Atrial Septal Defect

Although the surviving patients are generally in NYHA functional class I or II[B6,M6,S10,S13] (Table 27-7), the operation is not curative. A late mortality of 10%–15% is usual[B8,D3,W5] (Table 27-6) and is reported in the literature (4 late deaths among 56 hospital survivors). From 10% to 20% of patients have troublesome supraventricular tachycardia not WPW.[W5] Late results appear to be as good without as with plication of the atrialized portion of the right ventricle.[S2]

The usual late complications of tricuspid valve replacement also occur (see Chapter 14).

Closure of Atrial Septal Defect Alone

When a left-to-right shunt is present preoperatively, the late results are good (Table 27-7). Thus, 3 patients in this category were hospital survivors and 2 of the 3 have an excellent long-term result (UAB and GLH). One of the 3 has WPW syndrome, with episodic dysrhythmias.

If the indication is appropriate, the late results of simple ASD closure are also good in patients with right-to-left shunting preoperatively and important cyanosis. Four of 5 such patients are alive at late postoperative follow-up and are acyanotic (GLH and UAB), but all have episodic dysrhythmias, which are severe in 3 of them. Two consider themselves functionally normal (NYHA class I), whereas 2 are in NYHA class II (Table 27-7). One patient had an initially good result, and then cyanosis and severe disability recurred. Three years after his initial operation he died after reoperation elsewhere for reclosure of the septal defect and tricuspid valve replacement.

Table 27-5 Total surgical experience in Ebstein's disease (GLH; 1958–1980).

	Preoperative Features				Postoperative Features			
Age	NYHA Class	CTR	Cyanosis	Other Surgery	Follow-Up	NYHA Class	CTR	Comments
Valve replacement + ASD closure								
30 d	IV	85	Severe	Pulm valve PDA closed	Hospital death			Pulmonary atresia
3.7 yr	II	77	Severe	Plication atrialized RV	5.9 yr	I	61	Reop. at age[a] 9.3 yr
5.5 yr	III	68	Severe	Pulm valve	6 mo	I	61	
8 yr	II	79	Mild	Brock valve at 19 days	5 yr	I	?	
11 yr	III	71	Severe	Nil	9 yr	I	53	
43 yr	IV	62	Moderate	Nil	3.9 yr	I	?	Dextrocardia late death[b]
ASD closure alone								
2.7 mo	IV	69	Nil	Mod. VSD closed	6 yr	I	50	$\dot{Q}p/\dot{Q}s = 3.5$
11 yr	II	67	Nil	Nil	18 yr	II	?	WPW, $\dot{Q}p/\dot{Q}s = 1.9$
14 yr	I	66	Nil	Nil	4 yr	I	64	RA myxoma suspected $\dot{Q}p/\dot{Q}s = 1$
59 yr	II	72	Nil	Nil	1 yr	I	61	$\dot{Q}p/\dot{Q}s = 3.7$
Glenn shunt								
5 yr	III	68	Severe	Nil	Hospital death			Operation 1963

KEY: ASD, atrial septal defect; CTR, cardiothoracic ratio; NYHA, New York Heart Association; Pulm, pulmonary; $\dot{Q}p/\dot{Q}s$, pulmonary to systemic blood flow ratio; RA, right atrial; Reop, reoperation; RV, right ventricle; VSD, ventricular septal defect; WPW, Wolff-Parkinson-White.

NOTE: Not included are two neonates who had surgery for correction of an associated anomaly only. One had a blind valvotomy for presumed pulmonary atresia and the other a transannular patch for true pulmonary atresia.

[a] Reoperation for homograft valve stenosis and incompetence. Second homograft inserted.

[b] Late death from bronchopneumonia complicating surgically produced cerebral damage.

Table 27-6 Late results of tricuspid valve replacement and atrial septal defect closure (GLH and UAB; $n = 16$).

Institution	Age at Operation (yr)	Preop NYHA	Length of Follow-up (yr)	Postop NYHA Class	Comments
GLH	3.7	II	6	I	Reop age 9 yr for homograft replacement
GLH	5.5	III	½	I	
GLH	8	II	5	I	
GLH	11	III	9	I	
UAB	12	III	5	I	Occasional SV tachycardia
UAB	18	III	½	I	Died suddenly 6 mo postop from ruptured intracranial aneurysm
UAB	18	II	5	I	Occasional SV tachycardia
UAB	18	III	½	I	
UAB	19	IV	3	I	
UAB	20	IV	3	II	Mild fluid retention, fatigue
UAB	21	II	5	I	Occasional SV tachycardia
UAB	21	III	3	I	
UAB	29	III	½	I	
GLH	43	IV	4	I	Death 4 yr postop of complications of surgically produced cerebral damage
UAB	46	III	1½	II	Severe SV tachycardia
UAB	50	III	9	I	

KEY: NYHA, New York Heart Association; Postop, postoperative; Preop, preoperative; Reop, reoperation; SV, supraventricular.

Table 27-7 Late results of atrial septal defect closure without tricuspid valve repair or replacement (GLH and UAB).

Institution	Age at Operation (yr)	Shunt	Preop NYHA	Length Follow-up (yr)	Postop NYHA	Comments
GLH	2.7 mo	L → R	IV	6	I	Moderate-sized VSD also closed
UAB	8	L → R	II	3.2	I	Kent bundle cut; pulmonary valvotomy performed; SV tachycardia PO
GLH	11	L → R	II	18	II	WPW, with episodic dysrhythmia PO
UAB	13	R → L	III	10	I	Episodic SV tachycardia postoperatively
GLH	14	0	I	4	I	Operation for suspected RA myxoma
UAB	17	R → L[a]	I	3	I	Operation for peripheral embolism; episodic SV tachycardia PO
UAB	20	R → L	II	14	II	Episodic severe dysrhythmia PO
UAB	26	L → R	III	6	II	Kent bundles cut; severe dysrhythmias PO
UAB	32	R → L	IV	3		Late death at operation elsewhere for TVR
UAB	40	R → L	III	12	II	Episodic severe SV tachycardia PO
GLH	59	L → R	II	1	I	

KEY: NYHA, New York Heart Association; Preop, Postop/PO, preoperative, postoperative; RA, right atrial; SV, supraventricular; TVR, tricuspid valve replacement; VSD, ventricular septal defect; WPW, Wolff-Parkinson-White

NOTE: ASD repair alone in eight; ASD and VSD repair in one; ASD repair and pulmonary valvotomy in one; ASD repair in patient with suspected myxoma one. One patient with ASD repair and tricuspid valvotomy not included in this table died 2 weeks after hospital dismissal.

[a] bidirectional but dominantly R → L.

Sectioning of the Accessory Atrioventricular Conduction Pathways

Two patients (UAB) who had sectioning of electrophysiologically demonstrated accessory conduction pathways in the right AV groove have episodic dysrhythmias late postoperatively but not WPW (see Chapter 48 for more details).

INDICATIONS FOR OPERATION

Valve replacement (or repair) and closure of the ASD are indicated in patients with important tricuspid incompetence and moderate or severe cyanosis or symptoms of congestive heart failure. Severe limitations and severe hypoxia are not contraindications to repair, although the increased hospital mortality in patients in functional NYHA class IV argue strongly in favor of advising operation before disability is this advanced. Contrary to the advice of Watson,[W1] an age under 15 years is not a contraindication to this procedure. In the very young, however, tricuspid valve replacement is disadvantageous and usually can be avoided by intensive medical management.

Simple repair of the ASD is indicated when there is a large left-to-right shunt and symptoms of heart failure. When there is significant left-to-right shunting at atrial level ($\dot{Q}p/\dot{Q}s > 2$),

the ASD should be closed even in the absence of significant symptoms.

In patients with WPW syndrome that is producing life-threatening arrhythmia, the accessory conduction pathways should be divided[S9] and the valve defect should be treated concomitantly on its merits. Atrial communications should be closed at the time of the accessory pathways division. Other arrhythmias are not an indication for operation, since their incidence is not altered by correction of the valve defect. However, they are undoubtedly less well tolerated in the presence of severe tricuspid incompetence, cardiomegaly, and cyanosis and can then be an added indication for operation on the valve.

SPECIAL SITUATIONS AND CONTROVERSIES

Morphology

Confusion as to morphologic classification has arisen in some infants who have pulmonary atresia and minor downward displacement (or adherence) of the septal tricuspid leaflet origin (see Chapter 25). When this is the only Ebstein-like leaflet abnormality present, the defect is not classified as Ebstein's disease. In a number of infants with pulmonary atresia, however, the tricuspid valve shows additional typical and often florid features of Ebstein's anomaly in association with gross tricuspid incompetence. Such patients form one variety of complex Ebstein's disease.

Tricuspid Valve Repair

Most surgical groups advise replacement rather than repair when tricuspid valve surgery is indicated in patients with Ebstein's malformation.[W1] However, there is controversy concerning this,[B2,D1,H1,M5] and Danielson and colleagues have reported satisfactory results with valve repair.[D1,D3,D4] Most groups have found that patients who have morphology that is suitable for repair are uncommon, and that when there is important tricuspid incompetence, valve replacement is indicated. Danielson and colleagues report tricuspid valve repair rather than replacement in 34 (81%) of 42 patients undergoing operation between 1972 and 1982, with two hospital deaths and two further deaths 6 weeks and 4 months postoperatively from arrhythmias.[D3,D4] The functional results in the survivors were satisfactory, with a majority being in NYHA class I or II.[D4] However, some patients in this series, as well as in the earlier series of Hardy and colleagues,[H1] have residual tricuspid incompetence. Schmidt-Habelmann and colleagues also report residual tricuspid incompetence, although they, like Danielson, believe that when the anterior leaflet is of adequate size, tricuspid valvuloplasty can be done.[S11]

Type of Prosthesis for Tricuspid Valve Replacement

A stent-mounted glutaraldehyde porcine bioprosthesis may be considered optimal in most patients in Ebstein's malformation (UAB), but it is subject to the usual problems of a bioprosthesis.[W4] Mechanical prostheses may also be used.[C5] Melo and colleagues report excellent long-term results in Ebstein's anomaly using a Starr-Edwards ball valve prosthesis for the tricuspid replacement,[M6] as do Najafi and associates.[N2] A stented antibiotic-treated homograft may be favored (GLH), since it has a favorable orifice size and no thromboembolic risk, nor is there significant risk of endocarditis. It may, however, become stenotic or incompetent long term, albeit with a benign course leading to reoperation. (See Chapter 14 for a full discussion of valve replacement devices for the tricuspid position.)

Indications for Plication of the Atrialized Ventricle

Indications for plication of the atrialized ventricle are controversial. In the literature, there is the suggestion that omission of plication compromises right ventricular function postoperatively.[H1,T2] This has not been the experience at GLH and UAB, and plication may be considered indicated only when the atrialized portion of ventricle is very thin walled and aneurysmal (GLH) (probably about 10%–15% of cases).[B6,K3,N4,P2] It may be considered unnecessary in even these cases (UAB),[W5] since good function has been shown to result even when plication is not done.[C1,C4]

Excision or Plication of the Right Atrial Wall

Excision or plication of the right atrial wall was suggested by Timmis, Hardy, and Watson,[T2] who considered it important "to promote atrial emptying and lessen the likelihood of clot formation" when a prosthetic valve was used for valve replacement. Danielson incorporates excision of the right atrial wall in his repair.[D1,M5] The simplicity of this maneuver in the operation of valve replacement makes it an attractive step when the right atrium is markedly enlarged. However, this may be omitted (UAB).

REFERENCES

A

1. Anderson KR, Zuberbuhler JR, Anderson RH, Becker AE, Lie JT: Morphologic spectrum of Ebstein's anomaly of the heart. A review. *Mayo Clin Proc* 54:174, 1979.

2. Anderson KR, Lie JT: The right ventricular myocardium in Ebstein's anomaly. A morphometric histopathologic study. *Mayo Clin Proc* 54:181, 1979.

3. Anderson KR, Danielson GK, McGoon DC, Lie JT: Ebstein's anomaly of the left-sided tricuspid valve. Pathological anatomy of the valvular malformation. *Circulation* 58(suppl I):I-87, 1977.

4. Anderson KR, Lie JT: Pathologic anatomy of Ebstein's anomaly of the heart revisited. *Am J Cardiol* 71:739, 1978.

5. Arnstein A: Eine Seltene Missbildung der Trikuspikalklappe ("Ebsteinsche Krankheit"). *Virchows Arch* (Pathol Anat) 266:274, 1927.

B

1. Bharati S, Lev M, Kirklin JW: *Cardiac Surgery and the Conduction System*. New York: John Wiley, 1983.

2. Bahnson HT, Bauersfeld SR, Smith JR: Pathological anatomy and surgical correction of Ebstein's anomaly. *Circulation* 31–32 (suppl I):I-3, 1965.

3. Becker AE, Becker MJ, Edwards JE: Pathologic spectrum of dysplasia of the tricuspid valve: features in common with Ebstein's malformation. *Arch Pathol* 91:167, 1971.

4. Bialostozky D, Horwitz S, Espino-Verla J: Ebstein's malformation of the tricuspid valve. A review of 65 cases. *Am J Cardiol* 29:826, 1972.

5. Barnard CN, Schrire Y: Surgical correction of Ebstein's malformation with a prosthetic tricuspid valve. *Surgery* 54:302, 1963.

6. Barbero-Marcial M, Verginelli G, Awad M, Ferreira S, Ebaid M, Zerbini EJ: Surgical treatment of Ebstein's anomaly. Early and late results in 20 patients subjected to valve replacement. *J Thorac Cardiovasc Surg* 78:416, 1979.

7. Bove EL, Kirsh MM: Valve replacement for Ebstein's anomaly of the tricuspid valve. *J Thorac Cardiovasc Surg* 78:229, 1979.

8. Behl PR, Blesovsky A: Ebstein's anomaly: sixteen years' experience with valve replacement without plication of the right ventricle. *Thorax* 39:8, 1984.

C

1. Crews TL, Pridie RB, Benham R, Leatham A: Auscultatory and phonocardiographic findings in Ebstein's anomaly. Correlation of first heart sound with ultrasonic records of tricuspid valve movement. *Br Heart J* 34:681, 1972.

2. Cartwright RS, Smeloff EA, Cayler GG, Fong W, Huntley AC, Blake JR, McFall RA: Total correction of Ebstein's anomaly by means of tricuspid replacement. *J Thorac Cardiovasc Surg* 47:755, 1964.

3. Cabin HS, Roberts WC: Ebstein's anomaly of the tricuspid valve and prolapse of the mitral valve. *Am Heart J* 101:177, 1981.

4. Caralps JM, Aris A, Bonnin JO, Solanes H, Torner M: Ebstein's Anomaly: Surgical treatment with tricuspid replacement without right ventricular plication. *Ann Thorac Surg* 31:277, 1981.

5. Charles RG, Barnard CN, Beck W: Tricuspid valve replacement for Ebstein's anomaly: A 19 year review of the first case. *Br Heart J* 46:578, 1981.

D

1. Danielson GK, Maloney JD, Devloo RAE: Surgical repair of Ebstein's anomaly. *Mayo Clin Proc* 54:185, 1979.

2. Deutsch V, Wexler L, Blieden LC, Yahini JH, Neufeld HN: Ebstein's anomaly of tricuspid valve: Critical review of roentgenological features and additional angiographic signs. *Am J Roentgenol* 125:395, 1975.

3. Danielson GK, Fuster V: Surgical repair of Ebstein's anomaly. *Ann Surg* 196:499, 1982.

4. Danielson GK: Ebstein's anomaly: Editorial comments and personal observations. *Ann Thorac Surg* 34:396, 1982.

E

1. Ebstein W: Ueber einen sehr seltenen Fall von Insufficient der valvula tricuspidalis, bedingt durch eine angedorene hochgradige missbjldung derselben. *Arch Anat Physiol* 328, 1866.

2. Engle MA, Payne TPB, Bruins C, Taussig HB: Ebstein's anomaly of the tricuspid valve. Report of 3 cases and analysis of clinical syndrome. *Circulation* 1:1246, 1950.

3. Emanuel R, O'Brien K, Ng R: Ebstein's anomaly: genetic study of 26 families. *Br Heart J* 38:5, 1976.

F

1. Fontana ME, Wooley CF: Sail sound in Ebstein's anomaly of the tricuspid valve. *Circulation* 46:155, 1972.

G

1. Giuliani ER, Fuster V, Brandenberg RO, Mair DD: The clinical features and natural history of Ebstein's anomaly of the tricuspid valve. *Mayo Clin Proc* 54:163, 1979.

2. Genton E, Blount G: The spectrum of Ebstein's anomaly. *Am Heart J* 73:395, 1967.

3. Gasul BM, Weinberg M Jr, Luan LL, Fell EH, Bicoff J, Steiger Z: Superior vena cava-right main pulmonary artery anastomosis. *J Am Med Assoc* 171:1979, 1959.

4. Gueron M, Hirsch M, Stern J, Cohen W, Levy MJ: Familial Ebstein's anomaly with emphasis on the surgical treatment. *Am J Cardiol* 18:105, 1966.

5. Glenn WL: Circulatory bypass of the right side of the heart: Shunt between superior vena cava and right pulmonary artery. Report of clinical application. *N Engl J Med* 259:117, 1958.

6. Gasul BM, Weinberg MJV, Lendrum BL, Fell EH: Indications for and evaluation of surgical therapy in congenital heart disease. *Prog Cardiovasc Dis* 3:763, 1960.

H

1. Hardy KL, Roe BB: Ebstein's anomaly: Further experiences with definitive repair. *J Thorac Cardiovasc Surg* 58:553, 1969.

2. Hunter SW, Lillehei CW: Ebstein's malformation of the tricuspid valve with suggestions of a new form of surgical therapy. *Dis Chest* 33:297, 1958.

3. Hardy KL, May IA, Webster CA, Kimball KG: Ebstein's anomaly: A functional concept and successful definitive repair. *J Thorac Cardiovasc Surg* 48:927, 1964.

4. Hansen JF, Leth A, Dorph S, Wennevold A: The prognosis in Ebstein's disease of the heart. Long-term follow-up of 22 patients. *Acta Med Scand* 201:331, 1977.

J

1. Judgutt BI, Brooks CH, Sterns LP, Callaghan JC, Rossall RE: Surgical treatment of Ebstein's anomaly. *J Thorac Cardiovasc Surg* 73:114, 1977.

K

1. Kumar AJ, Fyler DC, Miettinen OS, Nadas AS: Ebstein's anomaly. Clinical profile and natural history. *Am J Cardiol* 28:84, 1971.

2. Kastor JA, Goldreyer BN, Josephson ME, Perloff JK, Scharf DL, Manchester JH, Shelburne JC, Hirschfeld JW Jr: Electrophysiologic characteristics of Ebstein's anomaly of the tricuspid valve. *Circulation* 52:987, 1975.

3. Kitamura S, Johnson JL, Redington JR, Mendez A, Zubiate P, Kay JH: Surgery for Ebstein's anomaly. *Ann Thorac Surg* 11:320, 1971.

L

1. Lev M, Liberthson RR, Joseph RH, Seten CE, Junske D, Miller RA, Eckner FA: The pathologic anatomy of Ebstein's disease. *Arch Pathol* 90:334, 1970.

2. Lev M, Gibson S, Millar RA: Ebstein's disease with Wolff-Parkinson-White syndrome: Report of a case with histopathologic study of possible conduction pathways. *Am Heart J* 49:724, 1955.

3. Lillehei CW, Kalke BR, Carlson RG: Evolution of corrective surgery for Ebstein's anomaly. *Circulation* 35 (suppl I):I-111, 1967.

M

1. Mann RJ, Lie JT: The life story of Wilhelm Ebstein (1836–1912) and his almost overlooked description of a congenital heart disease. *Mayo Clin Proc* 54:197, 1979.

2. Mayer FE, Nadas AS, Ongley PA: Ebstein's anomaly. Presentation of 10 cases. *Circulation* 16:1057, 1957.

3. Monibi AA, Neches WH, Lenox CC, Park SC, Mathews RA, Zuberbuhler JR: Left ventricular anomalies associated with Ebstein's malformation of the tricuspid valve. *Circulation* 57:303, 1978.

4. McCredie RM, Oakley C, Mahoney EB, Yu PN: Ebstein's disease: Diagnosis by electrode catheter and treatment by partial bypass of the right side of the heart. *N Engl J Med* 267:174, 1962.

5. McFaul RC, Davis Z, Giuliani ER, Ritter DG, Danielson GK: Ebstein's malformation. *J Thorac Cardiovasc Surg* 72:910, 1976.

6. Melo J, Saylam A, Knight R, Starr A: Long-term results after surgical correction of Ebstein's anomaly. Report of 2 cases. *J Thorac Cardiovasc Surg* 78:233, 1979.

7. Mathews JL, Pennington WS, Isobe JH, Gaskin TA, Dumas JH, Kahn DR: Paradoxical embolization with Ebstein's anomaly. *Arch Surg* 118:1101, 1983.

N

1. Newfeld EA, Cole RB, Paul MH: Ebstein's malformation of the tricuspid valve in the neonate. Functional and anatomic pulmonary outflow tract obstruction. *Am J Cardiol* 19:727, 1967.

2. Najafi H, Hunter JA, Dye WS, Javid H, Julian OC: Ebstein's malformation of the tricuspid valve. *Ann Thorac Surg* 4:334, 1967.

3. Ng R, Sommerville J, Ross D: Ebstein's anomaly: Surgical results of late correction. *Eur J Cardiol* 9:39, 1979.

4. Nawa S, Kioka Y, Sano S, Shirakawa K, Ozaki K, Beika M, Nagase H, Nakayama Y, Mondori E, Shigenobu M, Murakami T, Uchida H, Senoo Y, Teramoto S: Surgical correction of Ebstein's anomaly by tricuspid valve replacement and its late problems. *J Cardiovasc Surg* 25:142, 1984.

P

1. Pocock WA, Tucker RBK, Barlow JB: Mild Ebstein's anomaly. *Br Heart J* 31:327, 1969.

2. Peterfly A, Bjork VO: Surgical treatment of Ebstein's anomaly. Early and late results in 7 consecutive cases. *Scand J Thorac Cardiovasc Surg* 13:1, 1979.

R

1. Reynolds G: Ebstein's disease. A case diagnosed clinically. *Guys Hosp Rep* 99:276, 1950.

2. Rao PS, Jue KL, Isabel-Jones J, Ruttenberg H: Ebstein's malformation of the tricuspid valve with atresia. *Am J Cardiol* 32:1004, 1973.

3. Ross D, Sommerville J: Surgical correction of Ebstein's anomaly. *Lancet* 2:280, 1970.

4. Roberts WC, Glancy DL, Seningen RP, Maron BJ, Epstein SE: Prolapse of the mitral valve (floppy valve) associated with Ebstein's anomaly of the tricuspid valve. *Am J Cardiol* 38:377, 1976.

S

1. Seward JB, Tajik AJ, Feist DJ, Smith HC: Ebstein's anomaly in an 85-year-old man. *Mayo Clin Proc* 54:193, 1979.

2. Seno Y, Ohishi K, Nawa S, Teramoto S, Sunada T: Total correction of Ebstein's anomaly by replacement with a biological aortic valve without plication of the atrialized ventricle. *J Thorac Cardiovasc Surg* 72:243, 1976.

3. Schiebler GL, Grauvenstein JS, Van Mierop LH: Ebstein's anomaly of the tricuspid valve. Translation of original description with comments. *Am J Cardiol* 22:867, 1968.

4. Simcha A, Bonham-Carter RE: Ebstein's anomaly. Clinical study of 32 patients in childhood. *Br Heart J* 33:46, 1971.

5. Schiebler GL, Adams P Jr, Anderson RC, Amplatz K, Lester RG: Clinical study of 23 cases of Ebstein's anomaly of the tricuspid valve. *Circulation* 19:165, 1959.

6. Soloff LA, Stauffer HM, Zatuchni J: Ebstein's disease: report of the first case diagnosed during life. *Am J Med Sci* 222:554, 1951.

7. Scott LP III, Dempsey JJ, Timmis HH, McClenathan JE: Surgical approach to Ebstein's disease. *Circulation* 27:574, 1963.

8. Sealy WC, Gallaher JJ, Pritchett ELC, Wallace AG: Surgical treatment of tachyarrhythmias in patients with both an Ebstein's anomaly and a Kent bundle. *J Thorac Cardiovasc Surg* 75:847, 1978.

9. Sealy WC: The cause of the hemodynamic disturbances in Ebstein's anomaly based on observations at operation. *Ann Thorac Surg* 27:536, 1979.

10. Shigenobu M, Mendez MA, Zubiate P, Kay JH: Thirteen years experience with Kay-Shiley disc valve for tricuspid replacement in Ebstein's anomaly. *Ann Thorac Surg* 29:423, 1979.

11. Schmidt-Habelmann P, Meisner H, Struck E, Sebening F: Results of valvuloplasty for Ebstein's anomaly. *Thorac Cardiovasc Surgeon* 29:155, 1981.

12. Shina A, Seward JB, Edwards WD, Hagler DJ, Tajik AJ: Two-dimensional echocardiographic spectrum of Ebstein's anomaly: Detailed anatomic assessment. *JACC* 3:356, 1984.

13. Silver MA, Cohen SR, McIntosh CL, Cannon RO III, Roberts WC: Late (5 to 132 months) clinical and hemodynamic results after either tricuspid valve replacement or anuloplasty for Ebstein's anomaly of the tricuspid valve. *Am J Cardiol* 54:627, 1984.

T

1. Takayasu S, Obunai Y, Konno S: Clinical classification of Ebstein's anomaly. *Am Heart J* 95:154, 1978.

2. Timmis HH, Hardy JD, Watson DG: The surgical management of Ebstein's anomaly. The combined use of tricuspid valve replacement, atrioventricular plication and atrioplasty. *J Thorac Cardiovasc Surg* 53:385, 1967.

V

1. Van Lingen B, McGregor M, Kaye J, Meyer MJ, Jacobs HD, Braudo JL, Bothwell TH, Elliott GA: Clinical and cardiac catheterization. Findings compatible with Ebstein's anomaly of the tricuspid valve. A report of 2 cases. *Am Heart J* 43:77, 1952.

2. Vacca JB, Bussman DW, Mudd JG: Ebstein's anomaly. Complete review of 108 cases. *Am J Cardiol* 1:210, 1958.

W

1. Watson H: Natural history of Ebstein's anomaly of the tricuspid valve in childhood and adolescence: An international co-operative study of 505 cases. *Br Heart J* 36:417, 1974.

2. Wright JL, Burchell HB, Kirklin JW, Wood EH: Congenital displacement of the tricuspid valve (Ebstein's malformation). Report of a case with closure of the associated foramen ovale for correction of the right to left shunt. *Proc Mayo Clin* 29:278, 1954.

3. Wood P: *Diseases of the Heart and Circulation* (ed 3). London: Eyre and Spottiswoode, 1968, p 412.

4. Williams JB, Karp RB, Kirklin JW, Kouchoukos NT, Pacifico AD, Zorn GL Jr, Blackstone EH, Brown RN, Piantadosi S, Bradley EL: Considerations in selection and management of

patients undergoing valve replacement with glutaraldehyde-fixed porcine bioprostheses. *Ann Thorac Surg* 30:247, 1980.

5. Westaby S, Karp RB, Kirklin JW, Waldo AL, Blackstone EH: Surgical treatment in Ebstein's malformation. *Ann Thorac Surg* 34:388, 1982.

Y

1. Yater WM, Shapiro MJ: Congenital displacement of a tricuspid valve (Ebstein's disease): Review and report of a case with electrocardiographic abnormalities and detailed histological study of the conduction system. *Ann Int Med* 11:1043, 1937.

2. Yim BJB, Yu PN: Value of an electrode catheter in diagnosis of Ebstein's disease. *Circulation* 17:543, 1958.

Z

1. Zuberbuhler JR, Allwork SP, Anderson RH: The spectrum of Ebstein's anomaly of the tricuspid valve. *J Thorac Cardiovasc Surg* 77:202, 1979.

28

TRUNCUS ARTERIOSUS

DEFINITION

Truncus arteriosus (persistent truncus arteriosus, truncus arteriosus communis, common aorticopulmonary trunk) is a congenital cardiovascular malformation in which one great artery arises from the base of the heart by way of a single semilunar (truncal) valve. This artery gives origin to the coronary, the systemic, and one or two pulmonary arteries proximal to the origin of the brachiocephalic branches. Beneath the truncal valve is a ventricular septal defect.

This definition excludes those hearts wherein there are no true pulmonary arteries and the lungs are supplied only by large aortopulmonary arteries (Collett and Edwards type IV[C1]), which are considered to be tetralogy of Fallot and pulmonary atresia with absence of the pulmonary trunk and of the central and hilar portions of the right and left pulmonary arteries (see Chapter 23, "Absence" under Right and Left Pulmonary Arteries in Section 1, Morphology). Also excluded are hearts with a common arterial trunk but two semilunar valves or an intact ventricular septum.[C4,D2,S10,V1]

HISTORICAL NOTE

The first well-documented case of truncus arteriosus was reported by Wilson in 1798,[W2] and the existence of the entity was confirmed in the accurate clinical and autopsy report of the disease in a 6-month-old infant by Buchanan in 1864.[B7] In the early literature, there was frequent confusion with single arterial trunk, and although Vievordt clarified this aspect in 1898 (quoted by Victoria et al.[V3]), there was still confusion as late as 1930 when Shapiro[S12] distinguished it from hearts with aortic and pulmonary atresia. Lev and Saphir proposed the basic morphologic criteria necessary for the disease in 1942,[L3] and in 1949 Collett and Edwards[C1] reviewed previously published cases and proposed a classification. An alternative classification was suggested by the Van Praaghs in 1965.[V1]

Surgical treatment was initially confined to banding of one or both pulmonary arteries.[A7,H2,S9] Intracardiac repair was first successfully accomplished in 1962 at the University of Michigan utilizing a nonvalved Teflon conduit; this patient

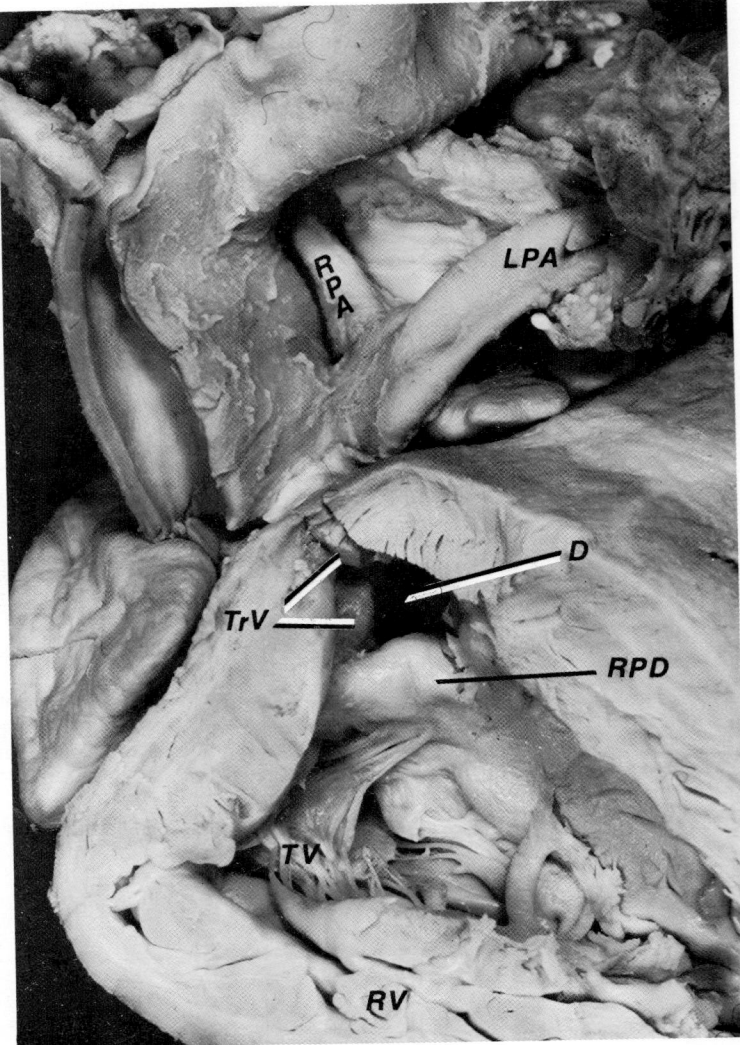

Figure 28-1   Autopsy specimen from 12-day-old neonate with type I truncus arteriosus (GLH). There is a distinct, although short, main pulmonary artery arising from the left lateral aspect of the truncal artery. The right ventricle has been opened, revealing its thick wall. The ventricular septal defect lies immediately beneath the truncal valve. Note that the defect's lower margin is separated from the tricuspid valve by a prominent right posterior division of the septal band, or trabecula septomarginalis.

D, ventricular septal defect; LPA, RPA, left and right pulmonary arteries; RPD, right posterior division of the septal band; RV, right ventricle; TrV, truncal valve; TV, tricuspid valve.

was alive and well 11 years later.[B1] Experimental work using aortic homograft-valved conduits was reported from Japan by Arai and colleagues in 1965[A5] and by Rastelli and colleagues at the Mayo Clinic in 1967.[R2,S11] Prior to this, in 1966 Ross had successfully used a homograft-valved conduit in the reconstruction of tetralogy of Fallot with pulmonary atresia.[R1] McGoon was the first to repair truncus arteriosus successfully using a homograft-valved conduit in September 1967.[M1,W1] The first homograft conduit to be used by GLH for repair of truncus arteriosus was in April 1967, but this patient did not survive. Weldon and Cameron reported a successful case in 1968.[W3] Binet used a heterograft valve incorporated in a Dacron tube in 1971 (see discussion of

paper by Moore et al.[M7]), and Bowman, Hancock, and Malm reported the use of a glutaraldehyde-treated porcine aortic valve in a Dacron conduit in 1973.[B6]

The first successful conduit repair in infancy was carried out at GLH in 1971 in a 6-week old baby.[G4]

Morphology

Truncus arteriosus has been classified on the basis of the arrangement of the origins of the pulmonary arteries from the truncal artery by Collett and Edwards[C1] and also by taking account of those cases with a single pulmonary artery

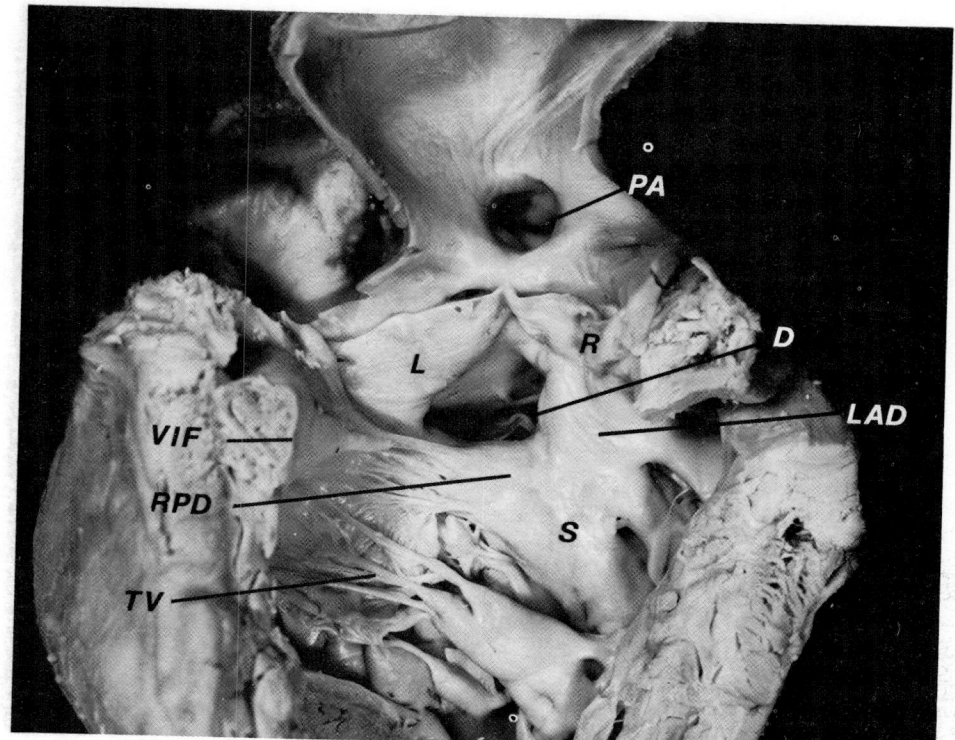

Figure 28-2 Autopsy specimen from 6-week-old infant with type I truncus arteriosus viewed from the opened right ventricle and truncal artery (GLH). The truncal valve has three leaflets of normal appearance. The orifice of the main pulmonary artery arises from the truncal artery close to the commissure between the right and left leaflets of the truncal valve. There is lack of continuity between the right posterior division of the septal band, or trabecula septomarginalis, and the ventriculo-infundibular fold, allowing tricuspid-truncal valve fibrous continuity at the posteroinferior margin of the ventricular septal defect (VSD). The bundle of His therefore lies along this edge of the VSD.

D, ventricular septal defect; LAD, left anterior division, septal band; PA, pulmonary artery; R, L, right and left leaflets of truncal valve; RPD, right posterior division of the septal band; S, septal band; TV, tricuspid valve; VIF, ventriculo-infundibular fold.

Truncus Artery

The arterial trunk (truncus artery) is larger than a normal aorta and is the only vessel arising from the base of the heart. The trunk originates in part from both ventricles but usually is more over the right than the left ventricle.[B2,C3,T1] From the truncal artery arise the coronary arteries and one or two pulmonary arteries.

Pulmonary Arteries

The pulmonary arteries usually originate just downstream from the truncal valve on the left posterolateral aspect of the truncus artery, although the origin may lie truly laterally or truly posteriorly[A3] or rarely anterolaterally. There is frequently a single orifice leading into a *short main pulmonary artery* (type I of Collett and Edwards), which then divides into left and right pulmonary arteries that follow a normal course (Figs. 28-1 and 28-2). Alternatively and less commonly, the orifice is double, the *left and right branches arising separately* side by side (Fig. 28-3) or occasionally with the left ostium superior (anterior) to the right rather than left (type II Collett and Edwards). Types I and II merge into each other and are best considered together. They comprise the great majority of cases[B2,C1,C2,C3] (43 of 50 [86%] in the GLH autopsy series).

Rarely, the ostia of left and right pulmonary arteries may be widely separated and arise from opposite lateral walls of the truncal artery either at the same or different levels above the valve (type III Collett and Edwards). The GLH autopsy series contains one example (2%). This arrangement poses special problems at the time of repair.[S4]

Occasionally, *only one pulmonary artery* originates from the truncal artery. Rarely, the central and hilar portions of the other pulmonary artery may be absent, and the normally branching intrapulmonary pulmonary arteries of the affected lung are then supplied only by bronchial or mediastinal collaterals. Much more commonly, the hilar portion of the nonconfluent pulmonary artery, usually the left, is present and

and the varying degree of development of the ascending aorta and ductus arteriosus by the Van Praaghs.[V1]

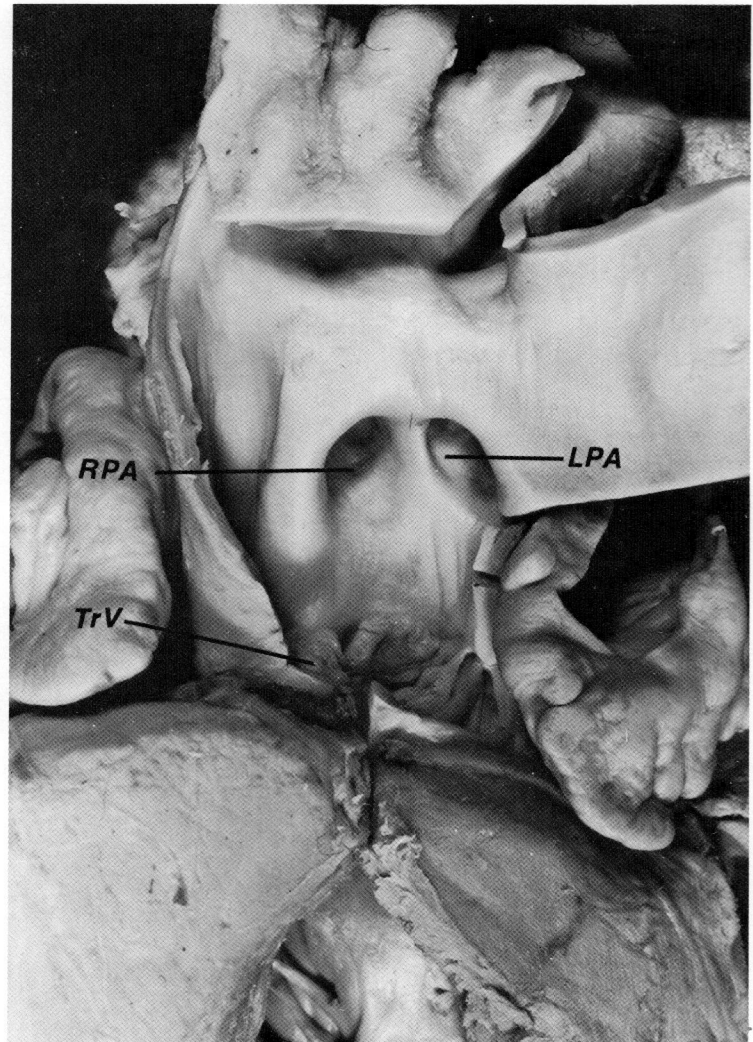

Figure 28-3 Autopsy specimen from a 4-week-old infant with type II truncus arteriosus (GLH). The proximal carina between the left and right pulmonary arteries is well seen lying flush with the posterolateral wall of the widely opened truncal artery. The truncal valve is quadricuspid with moderately abnormal leaflets, which, clinically, were considered to be both stenotic and incompetent. LPA, RPA, left and right pulmonary arteries; TrV, truncal valve.

arises from a left-sided patent ductus arteriosus (or in the case of a nonconfluent right pulmonary artery, from a right-sided ductus.[V2])

The Van Praaghs, who classify cases with a single pulmonary artery arising from the truncus artery separately,[C2,V1] point out that when the left pulmonary artery is absent, the right often continues to arise from the *left* posterolateral surface of the proximal truncal artery. In their more recent autopsy series, 8% of truncus hearts had only one pulmonary artery arising from the truncal artery. In the GLH series, there is one example only (2%).

Stenosis of the origin of one or both branch pulmonary arteries is more frequent than absence; it is probably underestimated in autopsy compared with cineangiocardiographic studies. Thus, it was noted in five clinical cases (10%) but in only 2% of the autopsy cases (GLH).[C2]

Ascending Aorta and Ductus Arteriosus

In truncus arteriosus, there is reciprocal development between the ascending and transverse aortic arch (arising from the fourth aortic arch) and the ductus arteriosus (arising from the sixth aortic arch).[V1] Thus, in the majority of cases the ascending aorta is a direct continuation of the truncus artery and of about the same diameter (Fig. 28-1), whereas the ductus arteriosus is usually entirely absent. This was the case in all but one of the GLH autopsy cases [3%] in this category. In contrast, when the ductus arteriosus is widely

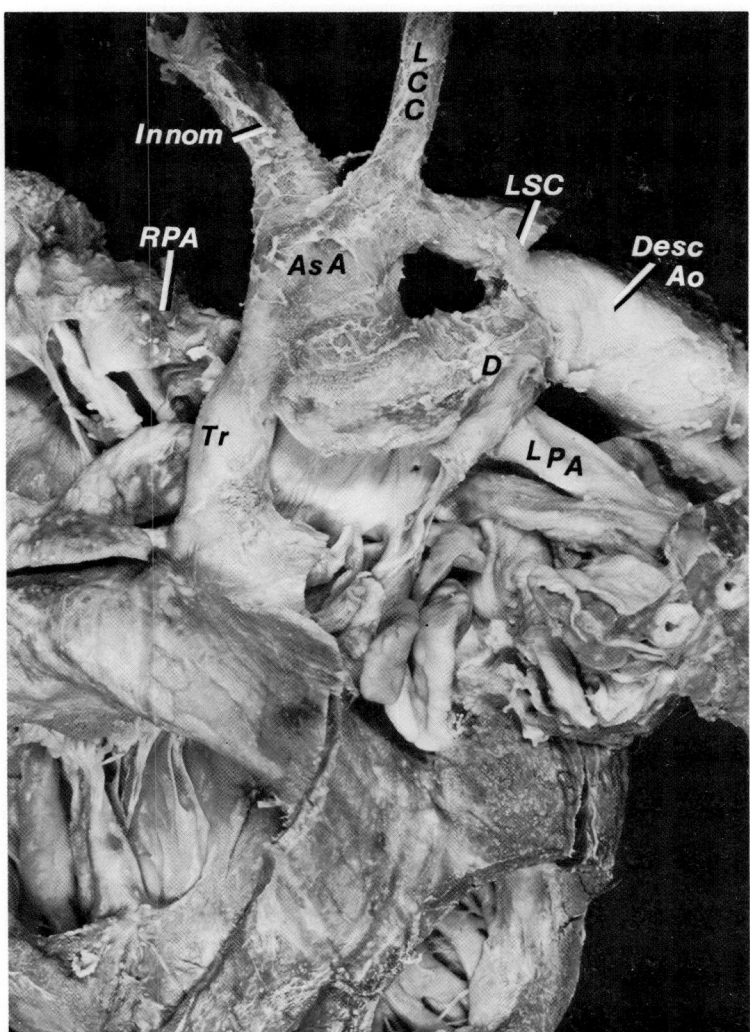

Figure 28-4 Autopsy specimen from 7-day-old neonate with truncus arteriosus (Van Praagh's type 4) (GLH). There is a large patent ductus arteriosus similar in diameter to the descending aorta. There is also severe coarctation of the aorta consisting of a short, totally atretic segment and a hypoplastic arch between the left common carotid and left subclavian arteries. The truncal artery (opened anteriorly) is wider than is usual with this arrangement. The origins of the left and right pulmonary arteries, although not visible in the photograph, are widely separated.

D, patent ductus arteriosus; Des. Ao, descending aorta; Innom, innominate artery; LCC, left common carotid artery; LPA, RPA, left and right pulmonary arteries; LSC, left subclavian artery; Tr, truncal artery.

patent, the transverse arch and usually the ascending aorta are underdeveloped. The ductus is a direct continuation of the truncus artery arching leftward to join the descending aorta (Fig. 28-4). In this situation, the left and right branches of the pulmonary arteries usually arise separately from superior and inferior (leftward and rightward) walls of the truncal artery (Collett and Edwards type III arrangement). The ascending aorta now arises from the superior rightward aspect of the truncus artery as the relatively smaller branch. Usually the transverse aorta is interrupted beyond the origin of the left common carotid artery (type B interrupted aortic arch; see Chapter 34, Section 2), or there is a severe coarcta-tion including tubular hypoplasia of the aortic isthmus and arch[T4] (Fig. 28-4). This arrangement (Van Praaghs' type A4) was present in 12% of the GLH autopsy series (6/50) and in 12% of Van Praaghs' cases also.[C2]

Coronary Arteries

The coronary arteries usually arise from the sinuses of Valsalva above the truncal leaflets. In about two-thirds of cases, the left coronary artery arises from the left posterior aspect of the truncal artery and the right coronary artery from the right anterior aspect in a position similar to the normal.[A1]

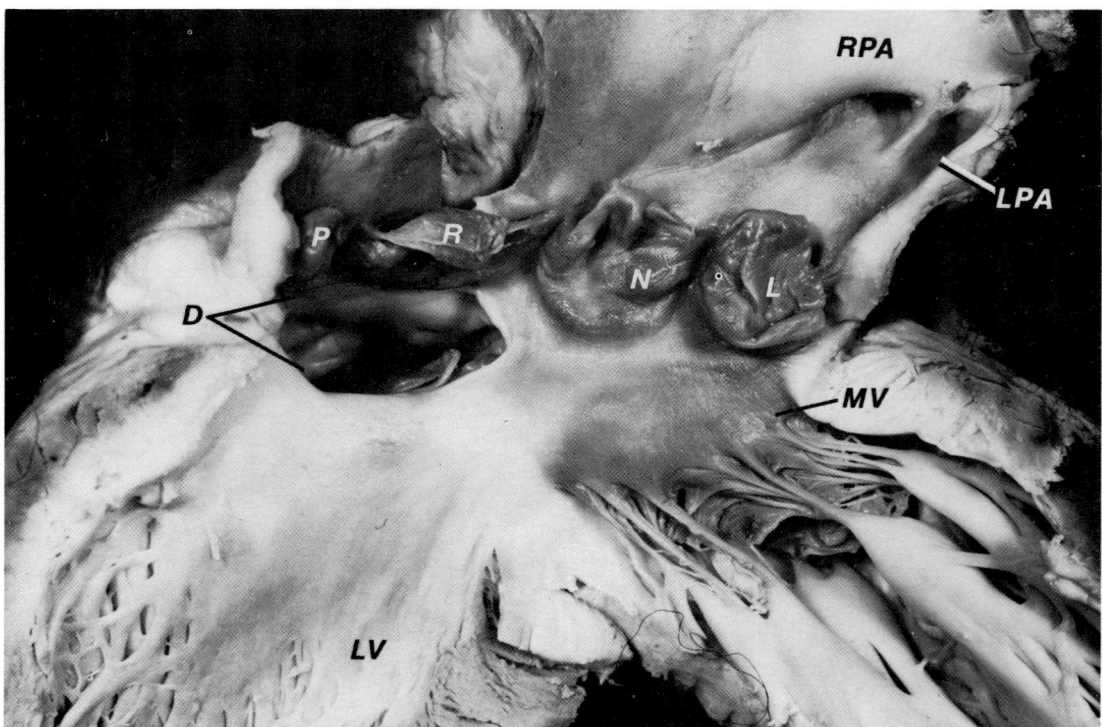

Figure 28-5 Autopsy specimen from a 3-day-old neonate with type II truncus arteriosus (GLH), in which the truncus artery and the left ventricle have been opened to demonstrate the fibrous continuity between the anterior leaflet of the mitral valve and the noncoronary and left coronary truncal valve leaflets, as in the normal heart. The truncal valve is quadricuspid with the ventricular septal defect lying directly beneath the right and pulmonary leaflets of the truncal valve.

D, ventricular septal defect; LPA and RPA, left and right pulmonary arteries; LV, left ventricle; MV, mitral valve; N, L, non-coronary and left coronary truncal valve leaflets; R, P, right and pulmonary leaflets of the truncal valve.

Variations from this pattern occur in the remainder of cases and include a single ostium, closely approximated right and left ostia, and a high origin of the left ostium and less frequently the right.[A1,B2,C3,S3,V1] Rarely, a coronary artery may arise from a pulmonary artery rather than the truncal artery; Daskalopoulos and colleagues report the circumflex artery's origin from the right pulmonary artery in a case in which pulmonary artery banding was not tolerated.[D3]

The proximal part of the left anterior descending coronary artery is frequently displaced to the left of the interventricular sulcus and does not reach it until about halfway down the front of the heart. This artery tends to be small. Larger than normal diagonal branches from the right coronary artery cross the anterior right ventricle inferior to the conal branches and contribute to the blood supply of the upper interventricular septum and occasionally part of the left ventricle.[A1,B2] Damage to these vessels at the time of surgical repair can seriously compromise the myocardium.[A1]

Semilunar Valve

The single truncal valve is posterior and inferior in position, similar to the normal aortic valve, although it points more anteriorly.[C2] There is fibrous continuity between its poste-

rior leaflets and the anterior mitral leaflet, as in the normal heart[C2] (Fig. 28-5). The valve is tricuspid in half to two-thirds of cases, and in most of the remainder there are four cusps. Rarely (5% in GLH autopsy cases), the valve is bicuspid. Not infrequently a raphe is present partially dividing a cusp into two, but it is doubtful if there are ever more than four well-formed cusps.[V1] There may be variations in length and width of individual leaflets, but in the majority of patients who survive infancy the leaflets are well formed (Fig. 28-2 and 28-5).

However, in autopsy material, obvious severe myxomatous thickening of the leaflets is present in one-third of all cases and is much more common in those dying as neonates (Table 28-1 and Fig. 28-6). These same changes in less severe form are present in two-thirds of older infants (Fig. 28-7), and microscopic increase in thickness of the distal portions of the leaflets is apparent in many more.[B3] Severe myxomatous changes often are associated with severe truncal valve incompetence, and their frequency in autopsy specimens from neonates and very young infants corresponds to the high incidence of truncal incompetence in neonates and very young infants who develop severe congestive heart failure or die. These morphologic changes are also reminiscent of those seen in congenital valvar aortic stenosis in the neonate (see Chapter 32), and may make the valve stenotic.[B4,G5,L1,P3]

Table 28-1 The incidence of abnormal truncal valve leaflets in an autopsy series of cases with truncus arteriosus (GLH).

| | Truncal Valve Leaflets | | | | |
| | | Abnormal | | | |
Age	Normal	Mild	Moderate	Severe	Total
Stillborn to 28 d	3	3	3	10	19
1–10 mo	4	4	4	1	13
> 2 yr	0	1	2	1	4
Totals	7 (19%)	8 (22%)	9 (25%)	12 (33%)	36

The pathologic findings suggest a significant stenosis in nine hearts (18%) in the GLH series, and this has been confirmed in some by withdrawal gradients. Rarely, stenosis is contributed to by commissural fusion.[B3]

A redundant truncal valve leaflet may obstruct the pulmonary artery ostium during ventricular ejection when the ostium is proximally placed[C2] causing obstruction to pulmonary blood flow.

Ventricular Septal Defect

The ventricular septal defect (VSD) is high and anterior and usually large. It lies immediately beneath the truncal valve, which forms its superior margin (Figs. 28-2 and 28-5). In-feriorly and anteriorly it is bounded by the two divisions of the septal band (trabecula septomarginalis) and posteriorly by the free wall muscle band that separates the semilunar from the tricuspid valve (the ventriculo-infundibular fold) (Fig. 28-2). Usually, the junction of right posterior division of the septal band and the ventriculo-infundibular fold forms a muscle bridge that separates the defect from the tricuspid valve and right trigone (Fig. 28-1) and therefore the bundle of His.[B2,C3,C6,V1] Occasionally, this muscle bridge is absent (Fig. 28-2) or poorly formed (Fig. 28-7), and the lower margin of the defect then approaches the tricuspid ring in which case the His bundle is at risk of damage when repair is performed. Part of the membranous ventricular septum may still be present at the posteroinferior margin of the VSD. In these hearts there may be fibrous truncal-tricuspid-mitral valve continuity.

Right Ventricle

The infundibular (conal) septum is absent from the right ventricular outflow tract.[C3,V1] It can sometimes be recognized, however, fused to the distal anterior (free) right ventricular wall, and, rarely, there is a persistent blind right ventricular outflow pouch in front of it. The morphology of the VSD and right ventricular outflow tract is thus very similar to that present in tetralogy of Fallot with pulmonary atresia[V1] (see Chapter 23). In both, the infundibular septum is malaligned (it normally inserts between the two divisions of the septal band).

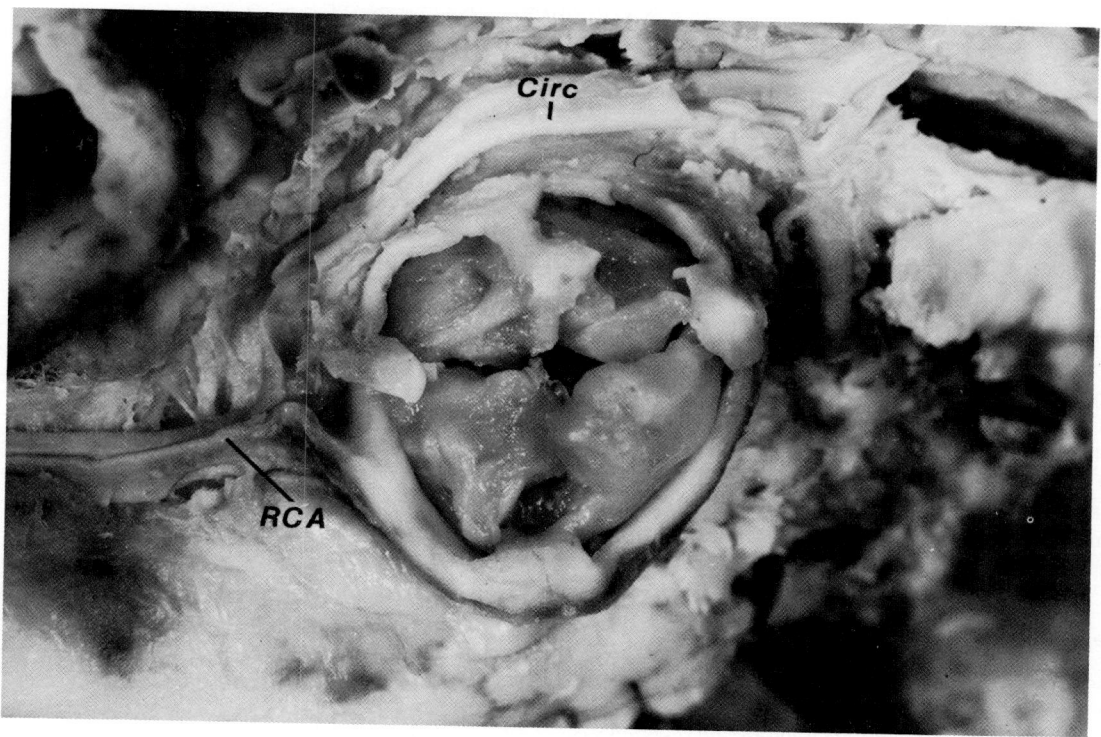

Figure 28-6 Autopsy specimen from 3-week-old neonate with truncus arteriosus to show a severely abnormal truncal valve viewed from above (GLH). The four cusps are thickened, nodular, myxomatous, and stiff. Clinically the valve was considered to be stenotic.
Circ, circumflex coronary artery; RCA, right coronary artery.

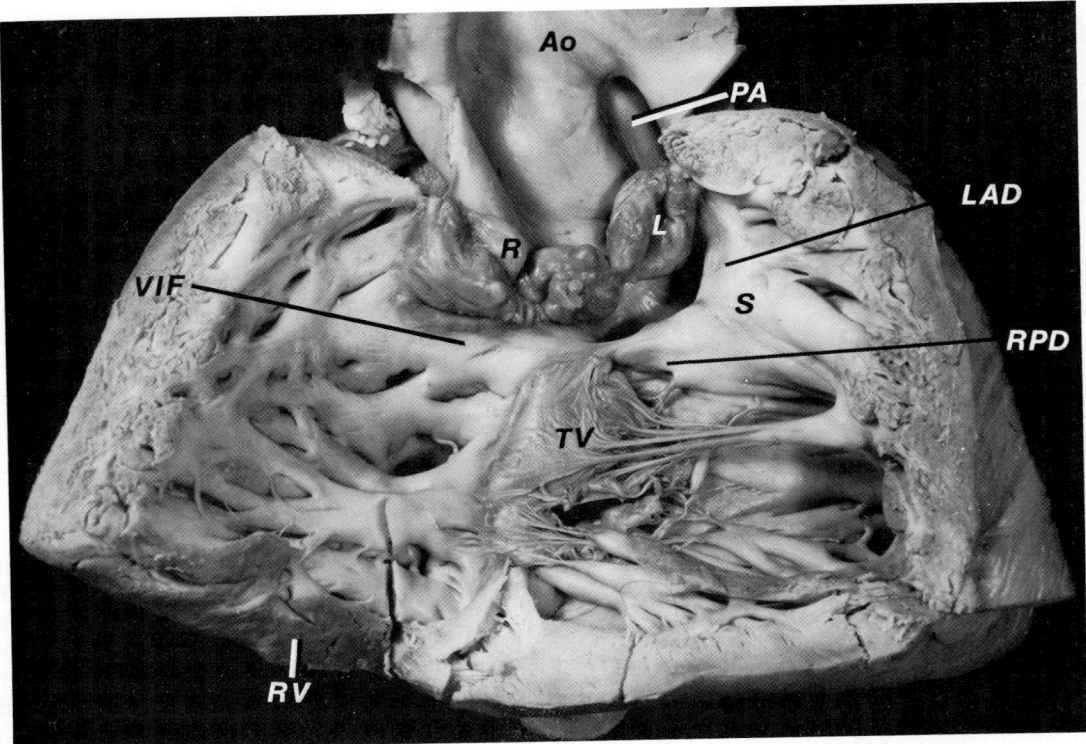

Figure 28-7 Autopsy specimen from 3-week-old neonate with type I truncus arteriosus (GLH). The truncal artery and right ventricle have been opened. The tricuspid truncal valve has severely abnormal leaflets. There is a diminutive muscular ridge separating truncal and tricuspid valves at the posteroinferior margin of the ventricular septal defect.

Ao, aorta (in fact, the truncal artery beyond the takeoff of the pulmonary arteries); LAD, left anterior division of septal band; L, R, left, right truncal valve leaflets; PA, main pulmonary artery origin; RPD, right posterior division of septal band; RV, right ventricle; S, septal band (or trabecula septomarginalis); TV, tricuspid valve; VIF, ventriculo-infundibular fold; VSD, ventricular septal defect.

Left Ventricle

In contrast to the right ventricular outflow tract, the left ventricular outflow tract is relatively normal in hearts with truncus arteriosus (Fig. 28-5), and flow from this chamber into the truncal artery is restricted only when the truncal artery originates mainly from the right ventricle and the VSD is small. A pressure gradient demonstrable on catheter withdrawal from left ventricle to aorta in such rare instances will lie at VSD level rather than at the truncal valve. Although a moderate-sized VSD will not be restrictive prior to surgical repair, it may prove so afterward and may therefore need to be enlarged at operation (see "Technique of Operation").

Associated Anomalies

Truncus arteriosus is rarely associated with other complex congenital cardiac defects. For example, atrioventricular discordance, situs inversus, and asplenia or polysplenia are all very rarely seen and dextrocardia is most uncommon. Single ventricle is also very rare,[V1] although mitral stenosis or atresia with left ventricular hypoplasia does occur (Table 28-2).

Table 28-2 Associated anomalies in an autopsy series of 50 patients with truncus arteriosus (GLH).

Associated Anomalies	No.		%
R aortic arch	8		16
Anomalous origin R and L subclavian artery	4		8
Anomalous origin R innominate artery	1		2
Persistent LSVC to coronary sinus	3		6
Moderate-sized or large ASD	5		10
Partial anomalous pulmonary venous connection	2		4
Additional muscular VSD	2		4
Mitral valve anomalies	5		10
Severe stenosis + LV hypoplasia		1	
Atresia + LV hypoplasia		1	
Mild stenosis		2	
Double orifice		1	
Complete AV canal defect	1		2
Extracardiac defects[a]	5		10

KEY: ASD, atrial septal defect; AV, atrioventricular, L, left; LSVC, left superior vena cava; LV, left ventricle; R, right; VSD, ventricular septal defect.

[a] The Di George syndrome was present in one infant.

The frequent total absence of the ductus arteriosus has already been mentioned together with the association of a widely patent ductus arteriosus in the 12% of patients in whom there is also aortic arch interruption or less often aortic coarctation or atresia. When hearts with aortic arch interruption are excluded, right aortic arch is as common in truncus arteriosus as in tetralogy of Fallot (25%–35%).[C2,V1] Anomalous branch origins occur frequently, usually of the subclavian arteries (10%). A persistent left superior vena cava draining to coronary sinus occurs in about 10% of patients, and occasionally there is partial anomalous pulmonary venous connection (Table 28-2). A patent foramen ovale is very common, and a significant-sized atrial septal defect is found in about 10% of patients. Mitral valve anomalies of various types are present with similar frequency. Other rare lesions include AV canal defects, double aortic arch,[C1] and according to Bharati et al.[B2] tricuspid stenosis and, rarely, atresia.

Extracardiac congenital defects are not uncommon and may occasionally contribute to death. The Di George syndrome (thymic and parathyroid aplasia or hypoplasia) is known to be associated with truncus arteriosus (and tetralogy of Fallot).[F2]

CLINICAL FEATURES AND DIAGNOSTIC CRITERIA

Symptoms

The presenting symptoms are almost always tachypnea, tachycardia, irritability, and unwillingness to take either breast or bottle feedings in the early weeks of life, all manifestations of heart failure.[A4] Rarely, respiratory distress is aggravated by compression of the left upper lobe bronchus between an anteriorly placed left pulmonary artery and the posterior aortic arch.[C2,H1] Even more rarely (one 2-day-old infant at GLH), an aneurysmal truncal artery associated with interrupted aortic arch may severely compress the right main bronchus and produce total right lung collapse. Mild cyanosis accompanies these symptoms in about one-third of cases and rarely is the presenting feature. On the other hand, in those infants who survive for longer periods, recurrent respiratory infections, dyspnea, and failure to thrive are usually present and cyanosis is more apparent, secondary to a rising pulmonary vascular resistance. Older children may occasionally present with increasing cyanosis (Eisenmenger's syndrome) and fail to give a history of heart failure in infancy.

Physical Examination

On examination, the signs of congestive heart failure are accompanied by a jerky to collapsing arterial pulse, produced by the rapid runoff from the truncal artery into the pulmonary arteries. The heart is overactive, and a prominent left parasternal systolic murmur and often thrill are appreciated. There is frequently an ejection click coinciding with full opening of the truncal valve,[A6] and an apical gallop rhythm may be present although it is surprisingly rare in neonates. An aortic early diastolic murmur (from truncal valve incompetence) is highly suggestive of truncus ar-

teriosus, particularly when it is accompanied by pulmonary plethora on the chest x-ray and a right aortic arch. The second heart sound is usually single but is split (impure or multiple) in about one-third of cases. A continuous murmur is noted occasionally and is most often due to stenosis at the origin of one or both pulmonary arteries. Significant truncal valve stenosis is a confusing feature and usually results in diminished peripheral pulses accompanied by a harsh ejection systolic murmur and thrill maximal in the right upper intercostal spaces.[B4,L2]

Chest X-Ray

Chest x-ray shows marked cardiomegaly in the neonate and infant as well as plethora. The main pulmonary artery segment is deficient (as in transposition), but a high origin or arching of the left pulmonary artery may be evident in older children as a "comma" sign on the left upper mediastinal border.[C2] A solitary right pulmonary artery arising from the left side of the truncus artery may give a similar appearance. The hemithorax may be smaller and the vascularity less on the side of the "absent" pulmonary artery (when this lung is supplied by bronchial collaterals or by a relatively small patent ductus arteriosus). In truncus arteriosus with aortic arch interruption, the descending aorta is often prominent in the chest x-ray.[C2] In those few infants who survive without treatment, plethora becomes less, as does the cardiomegaly, in association with increasing pulmonary vascular disease.

Electrocardiogram

Electrocardiogram (ECG) usually shows combined ventricular hypertrophy and a normal or slightly rightward axis, although left ventricular hypertrophy is usually dominant in the tracing and occasionally ventricular hypertrophy is absent.[C2] P-pulmonale can occur.[V3]

Echocardiography

Echocardiography is useful since it demonstrates a single vessel overriding the ventricular septum and will show abnormalities in the truncal valve leaflets.[A6,H4,P3] With currently available technology, 2D echocardiography can be diagnostic of the entity truncus arteriosus.

Cardiac Catheterization and Angiocardiography

Cardiac catheterization and angiocardiography are still performed to define the pulmonary arteries, the aortic arch, and the hemodynamic state.

In infants, there is left-to-right shunting at ventricular level with a high pulmonary-to-systemic blood flow ratio ($\dot{Q}p/\dot{Q}s$) and systemic pressures in the right ventricle and pulmonary artery. The high pulmonary blood flow keeps the aortic oxygen saturation up to 85% or more.[M2] The pulmonary vascular resistance is mildly raised (2–4 units · m^2). Rarely, when the VSD is restrictive and the truncal origin is mainly from the right ventricle, left ventricular pressure may exceed right ventricular pressure; when there is truncal valve stenosis, there is a withdrawal gradient across this valve. It may prove difficult to identify the site of stenosis preoperatively. Pulmonary artery pressure is frequently slightly below systemic pressure, but it is significantly reduced when there is a stenosis at the origin of one or other artery.

The progressive rise in pulmonary vascular resistance that occurs in virtually all the children who survive infancy is associated with a fall in Q̇p and therefore in arterial oxygen saturation. Arterial oxygen saturations less than 80% are usually an indication that the pulmonary vascular resistance is beyond the operable range.[M2]

Cineangiocardiography with contrast injections into both ventricles and ascending aorta demonstrates the exact site of origin of the pulmonary arteries and differentiates this lesion from a patent ductus arteriosus. Special views are required to demonstrate the origin of right and left pulmonary artery branches in order to assess any proximal stenosis. Should one pulmonary artery fail to outline after routine contrast injections, the origin and distribution of the blood supply to the other lung must be identified. This is usually possible by injections into the upper descending thoracic aorta. In addition, a pulmonary vein wedge injection can be used to fill retrogradely true pulmonary arteries that fill inadequately or not at all from an aortic injection.

These studies also provide information on the alignment of the truncal artery and truncal valve with the two ventricles, truncal valve leaflet thickening, and truncal valve stenosis or incompetence. A bicuspid or quadricuspid valve may show doming in systole without stenosis being present. The site of the VSD is demonstrated, as are the two ventricles.

NATURAL HISTORY

Truncus arteriosus is relatively rare, occurring in 2.8% of the cases of congenital heart disease in the cardiac registry of the Children's Hospital Medical Center, Boston,[C2] and in 1.7% of Tandon's autopsy series.[T2] In the GLH autopsy series of congenital heart disease, the incidence is 4.6% (36/780).

The natural history of patients with truncus arteriosus is unfavorable. Only about 50% of infants born with this condition survive beyond the first month of life (Table 28-3), 30% beyond the age of 3 months, 18% beyond 6 months, and 12% beyond 1 year (Fig. 28-8). There is little further mortality beyond this age until pulmonary vascular disease becomes severe and death occurs with the Eisenmenger's syndrome in about the third decade of life.

Death in infancy is invariably due to congestive heart failure, and when it occurs in the neonatal period it is usually contributed to by severe truncal valve incompetence as well as the large left-to-right shunt. The situation may be compounded by severe respiratory infection, as in other malformations with large left-to-right shunts in early life. Longer term survivors may occasionally succumb from bacterial endocarditis or cerebral abscess,[C1] but most die eventually from the consequences of severe pulmonary vascular disease (see Chapter 20, "Pulmonary Vascular Disease" in Section 1, Natural History). When pulmonary vascular disease develops in the first year of life (and it may develop more rapidly than in patients with isolated VSD[M5]) or later, the patient has a good chance of surviving at least into the

Table 28-3 The natural history of truncus arteriosus as shown by analysis of a consecutive series of cases (New Zealand born) admitted for diagnosis and treatment (GLH; 1958–1981). The median age of death was 1 month.

Onset of Symptoms	n	Age at Death (mo)			Alive (yr)
		< 1	1 < 3	3 < 12	2–20
< 1 wk	17	13 (76%)	2 (12%)	1	1[a]
1 < 4 wk	15	6 (40%)	5 (33%)	4	0
1 mo	7	0	5 (71%)	2	0
2 mo–9 mo	6	0	0	2	4[b]
Total	45	19 (42%)	12 (27%)	9 (20%)	5 (11%)

NOTE: ( ) encloses the percent of n.

NOTE: Sixteen of the 45 had surgery; all were in severe (usually critical) congestive heart failure preoperatively and for the purpose of this analysis are considered to have died at the time of operation. Two additional infants not in heart failure at the time of operation and three stillborn subjects have been excluded.

[a] LPA stenosis present.

[b] Two with and 2 without pulmonary vascular disease.

teens, as is usually the case with Eisenmenger's syndrome. Thus, 7 of 10 of the Mayo Clinic patients with a pulmonary vascular resistance greater than 8 units · m² at diagnosis under 1 year of age were alive (without treatment) 1–15 years (average 8.3 years) later.[M5]

Rather remarkably, a few patients survive infancy and early childhood without the development of severe pulmonary vascular disease and with large left-to-right shunts. These patients probably represent less than half of those surviving beyond 1 year of age and less than 5% of all infants born with truncus arteriosus.

This concept of natural history, based on the GLH experience (Table 28-3), is compatible with the meager information from other sources, primarily reports of autopsied cases by the Van Praaghs and Calder,[C2,V1] Edwards and associates,[C1,F1] and Lev and associates.[B2] In two reports, the median age of death was 5 weeks,[C2,F1] in another, two-thirds were noted to be dead before reaching 6 months of age,[C1] and similar statistics are available from the studies of Fontana and Edwards.[F1] Bharati and associates give a mean age of death at 6 months in 177 cases.[B2] Other isolated case reports[C5,H5] confirm that some subjects, perhaps 10%, survive into adolescence or young adult life but usually with severe pulmonary vascular disease.

Survival is adversely affected by severe truncal valve incompetence,[E4] as noted earlier, or by truncal valve stenosis.[G1] As an example, of 10 infants with severe myxomatous nodular leaflets (GLH autopsy series), 9 presented with congestive heart failure in the first 3 weeks of life and 9 died between 2 days and 3 months of age (median age at death 12 days). Even in older patients, truncal valve incompetence can be shown to be present in 60%–70% of cases.[H3] The regurgitation may be predominantly into the right ventricle.

Survival is also adversely affected by coexisting interrupted aortic arch or coarctation.[V1] The median age of death in such patients has been 7 days (GLH). Survival is also less good when there are other associated severe lesions, such as left ventricular hypoplasia and a small or atretic mitral valve,

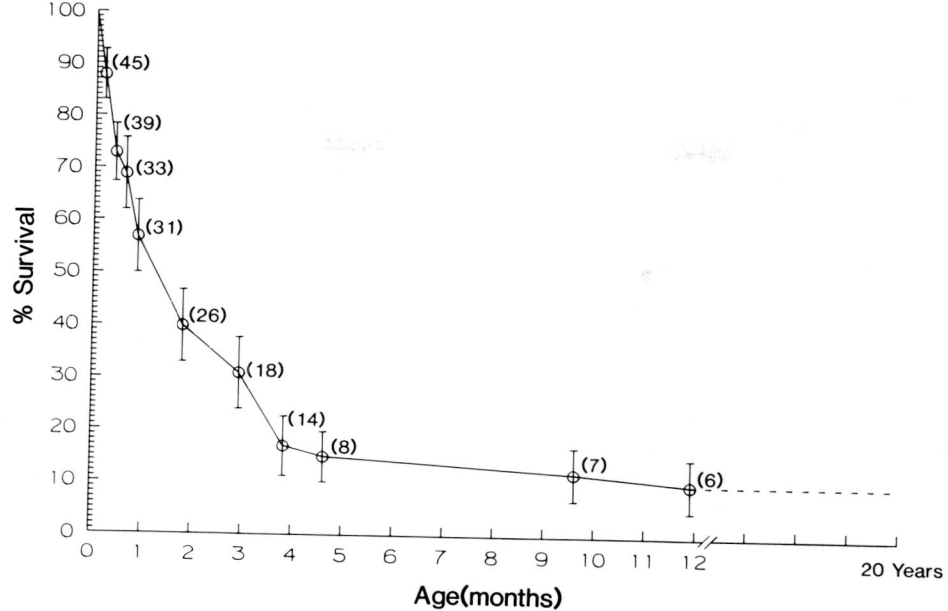

Figure 28-8 Actuarial survival of truncus arteriosus patients (GLH; same patients and conditions as in Table 28-3). The numbers at risk at each time interval are noted. The bars represent one standard error (approximately 70% confidence limits). The actuarial curve may be considered a representation of the survival of surgically untreated patients.

complete AV canal defect, or serious extracardiac anomalies.

Survival is favorably affected by pulmonary stenosis (narrowing at the origins of right or left or main pulmonary artery). Thus, of the 5 GLH patients with this feature, only 1 died in the neonatal period and 3 remained alive at 9 months, 2 years, and 5 years without surgical treatment or significant pulmonary vascular disease; and 4 of the first 28 (14%) truncus patients repaired beyond infancy at the Mayo Clinic had naturally occurring pulmonary artery stenosis.[M8]

TECHNIQUE OF OPERATION

Repair of Truncus Arteriosus Type I or II

The usual preparations (see Chapter 2, Section 3) and anesthetic managements (see Chapter 4) are currently used. The operation now is nearly always performed in infancy, and profound hypothermia and total circulatory arrest may be used routinely (GLH) or only in patients weighing less than 2–3 kg (UAB) (see Chapter 2, Section 4). Otherwise, cardiopulmonary bypass (CPB) is used (see Chapter 2, Section 3), with venting through the opened right atrium and across a natural or surgically occurring foramen ovale (UAB) or a directly inserted left atrial vent (GLH). Cold cardioplegia may be used routinely (UAB) or omitted (GLH) when profound hypothermia and total circulatory arrest are used. (See ''Support Techniques during the Repair of Truncus Arteriosus in Infants,'' in section on Special Situations and Controversies.)

After making a primary median sternotomy incision, a piece of pericardium may be taken and laid aside in a moist sponge for use with the conduit (GLH). The left and right pulmonary arteries are dissected and a snare placed loosely around each of them. The usual purse strings are placed (see Chapter 2), positioning that for the aortic cannulation as far downstream as possible in order that the aortic cross-clamp (placed proximal or upstream to the cannula) will be as far distal as possible on the ascending aorta. No purse string is placed for the cardioplegic needle site. A segment of a 14- or 16-mm woven Dacron tube is preclotted (UAB). The steps of the operation are carefully organized so as to conserve CPB or total circulatory arrest time, as well as the aortic cross-clamp time, as much as possible.

When CPB is used, the aorta is cross-clamped immediately after beginning the bypass, the pulmonary artery snares tightened, the right atrium opened, a pump oxygenator sump sucker placed across a natural or surgically created foramen ovale, and the cold cardioplegic solution infused while the effluent from the coronary sinus is aspirated and the needle withdrawn (UAB). The snares on the pulmonary arteries are loosened and the repair is begun. As usual, the perfusate is kept as cold as possible until the patient's temperature is 27°C. Then it is stabilized at 25°C and a flow rate of $1.6 \ 1 \cdot \min^{-1} \cdot m^{-2}$, and periods of low flow ($0.5 \ 1 \cdot \min \cdot m^2$) or occasional short ($< 5$ min) periods of total circulatory arrest are used whenever needed to improve exposure.

The pulmonary artery origin is detached from the truncal artery (Fig. 28-9), including an appropriate ellipse of truncal wall in truncus type II. The incision for detachment is begun on the left side, 6 mm or so distal to the truncal valve anulus. It is carried across anteriorly far enough so that the interior of the truncal artery and valve, the ostia of the coronary arteries, and the orifices of the right and left pulmonary ar-

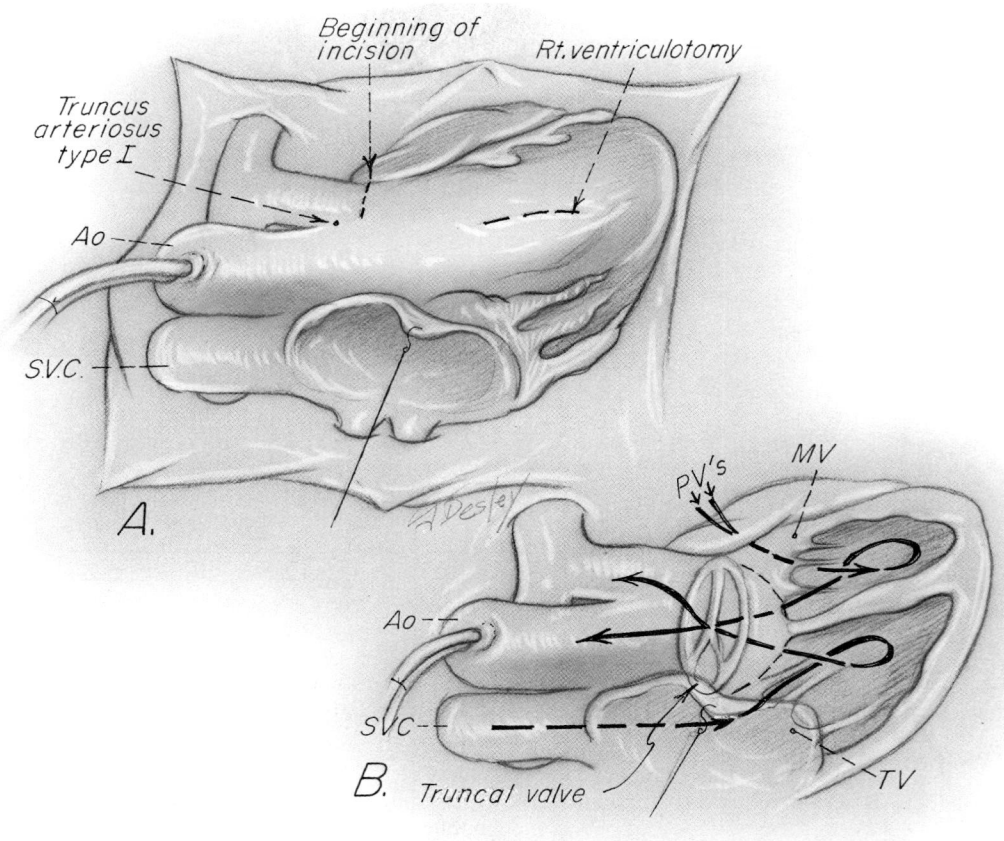

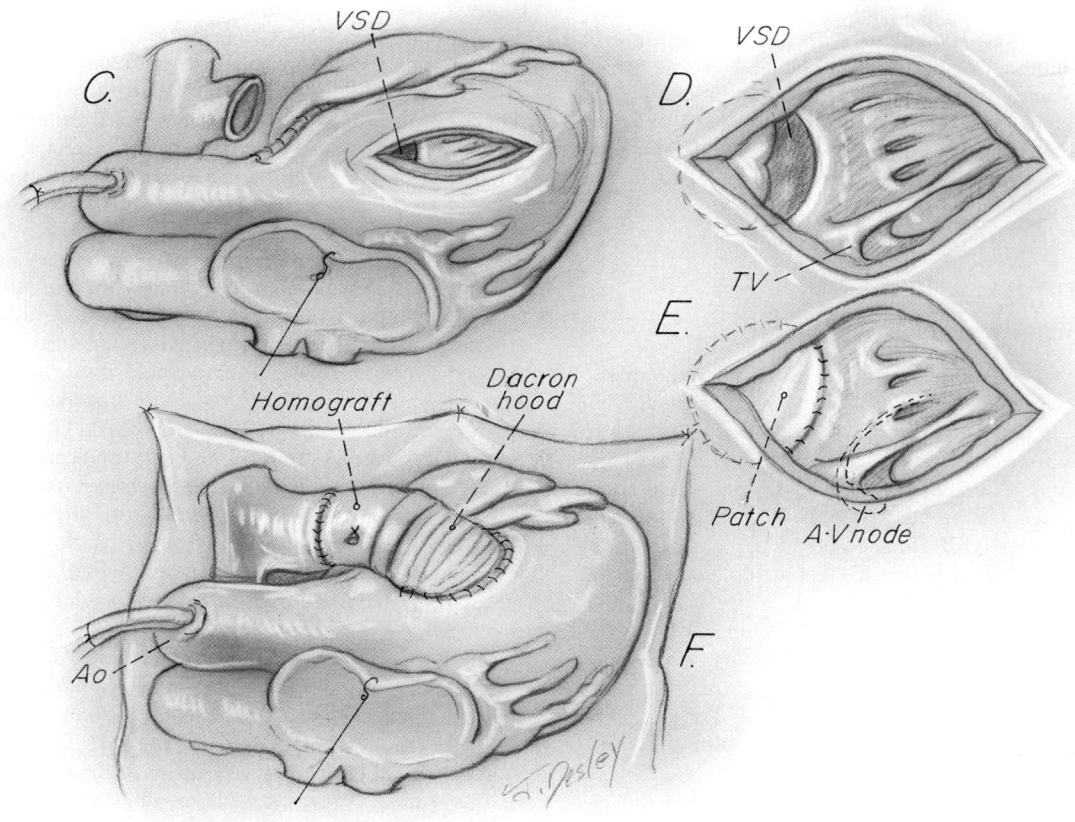

teries begin to be exposed. The detachment is then completed while viewing from within all these structures. The deficiency in what is now the aorta is closed with two rows of continuous 4-0 or 5-0 polypropylene sutures, using the second row to bring adventitia over the first row.

A vertical ventriculotomy about 2 cm in length is made just proximal to the truncal valve, and stay sutures may be placed for exposure (UAB). Alternatively, the opening may be enlarged to an oval shape by excising muscle from the anterior wall, leaving adequate tissue to the right and left for subsequent suturing so that neither the anterior descending nor right coronary arteries will be compromised (GLH). The ventricular septal defect (VSD) is repaired just as described in the repair of tetralogy of Fallot (see Chapter 23, Fig. 23-25), remembering that in truncus arteriosus there is usually a rim of muscle between the VSD and the tricuspid anulus (see ''Morphology''). As in the repair of tetralogy of Fallot with pulmonary atresia (see Chapter 23, Fig. 23-36), the superior sutures may pass into the anterior right ventricular wall where it forms the distal margin of the circular opening just proximal to the truncal valve ring (GLH), and they may not be positioned until the stage at which the conduit is attached to the right ventricular opening. If the lower margin of the VSD lies so close to the truncal valve that following patch closure the left ventricular outflow tract would be narrowed, the VSD may be enlarged by excising a wedge of muscle from its anteroinferior margin. The defect is then closed with a Dacron patch in a manner similar to that used in the repair of double outlet right ventricle (see Chapter 40, Fig. 40-12), and the truncal valve is incorporated into the left ventricular outflow tract.

The aortic homograft valve conduit is then trimmed to an appropriate length. The conduit may have been made as described under tetralogy of Fallot (UAB) (see Chapter 23, Fig. 23-37), except that the distal aorta trimmed from the homograft may at times be used for the proximal extension in

place of the segment of preclotted Dacron tube. Alternatively (GLH), a pericardial skirt has been attached with a running 5-0 polypropylene suture to the muscular half of the circumference of the valved end of the homograft conduit. The muscular half is chosen since it is the more bulky portion and will produce a posterior shelf with angulation of the conduit if it is positioned posteriorly. It is usually necessary to trim off transversely the redundant distal aorta just above the valve commissures. Too long a conduit tends to kink the pulmonary artery bifurcation. A 14–18-mm conduit diameter will usually match the pulmonary artery in a neonate or small infant. If there is narrowing at the origins of right or left pulmonary artery, the offending branch is opened longitudinally across the stenosis and a tongue of aorta is left on the distal conduit end to widen this point. If the carina of the pulmonary artery bifurcation is too proximal and prominent, making the branch pulmonary artery origins borderline in diameter, the origins can be widened by dividing the carina longitudinally and suturing the walls of the arteries together along the edges of this incision (GLH). The end-to-end distal conduit to pulmonary artery anastomosis is constructed with continuous 5-0 polypropylene after orienting the conduit so that the heavy muscular base lies anteriorly and the homograft portion curves gently posteriorly as it passes superiorly. The proximal end of the conduit is anastomosed to the right ventriculotomy as described in tetralogy of Fallot (see Chapter 23, Fig. 23-37). When an anterior pericardial skirt is used, the proximal valved end of the conduit is sutured to oval right ventriculotomy with continuous polypropylene, commencing with the distal right ventricular edge (GLH). Each bite of posterior portion of the conduit suture line picks up the adjacent edges of the VSD patch, right ventricular wall, and fibrous conduit margin. When the free right ventricular wall is reached on either side, the sutures pass into the pericardial skirt of the homograft, which is trimmed to an appropriate shape for incorporation into the right ventriculotomy so that the conduit valve lies in a transverse plane, just as it does when a tubular proximal extension is used.

As the proximal conduit–right ventricle suture line is being made, rewarming is begun. The sump-type sucker is removed, the foramen ovale is closed, the aortic cross-clamp is removed, and free egress of blood (and air) are allowed by enlarging, if necessary, the tract made by the cardioplegia needle. The procedure is completed as described for conduit repair of tetralogy of Fallot (see Chapter 23).

When profound hypothermia and total circulatory arrest are used (GLH), the techniques are in general those described in Chapter 2. The aorta is cross-clamped distal to the arterial cannula (GLH). The repair then proceeds until the distal conduit anastomosis is completed. About 30 minutes of circulatory arrest time will generally have elapsed by then. To avoid too long a period of arrest before completing the repair, the right atrium is now opened with an oblique incision commencing at the appendage; both cavae are then cannulated directly from within the atrium, using a 5 mm cannula for the superior vena cava and a 6 mm one for the inferior vena cava. These cannulae are joined with a Y connector to the venous pump line and CPB recommenced at

---

◀

Figure 28-9 Repair of truncus arteriosus.

(a) After establishing CPB and cross-clamping the aorta, the incision for separation of the pulmonary trunk from the truncus artery is begun. After looking through the incision and determining the precise origin of the coronary arteries and the pulmonary arteries, the excision of the pulmonary trunk is completed. The proposed vertical right ventriculotomy is shown with a dashed line.

(b) Schematic representation of the ventricular outflow in truncus arteriosus. Both ventricles eject through the truncal valve into the base of the truncus artery. There is some preferential flow of left ventricular blood into the systemic arteries.

(c) The suture line in the truncal artery has been completed, and the distal end of the pulmonary trunk is prepared for the conduit. The vertical ventriculotomy has been made.

(d) The VSD illustrated is the typical one for truncus arteriosus, with a band of muscle (see Fig 28-1) separating it from the tricuspid anulus.

(e) The VSD is closed by suturing the patch to the edges of the ventricular septal defect, the AV node and bundle of His being away from this edge.

(f) The operation is completed by suturing into place the homograft-valved conduit (see text for details).

16°C and 80 ml · kg^{-1} · min^{-1} flow. Since the aorta has been cross-clamped distal to the arterial line, as flow through the arterial cannula commences the aorta proximal to the clamp is de-aired by flooding the field with electrolyte solution and making the aortic valve incompetent with a curved forceps introduced through the valve via the still open anterosuperior portion of the VSD repair. The aortic clamp is then released. Coronary sinus return is aspirated from the atrium with the open heart sucker, and the atrial septal defect or patent foramen ovale is closed with a running 5-0 polypropylene suture followed by closure of the atriotomy, bringing the cannulae to the atrial appendage as this is done. Rewarming is commenced soon after CPB is restarted. The left heart is de-aired before closure of the VSD is completed since the heart by this stage is beating. Rewarming CPB is continued after the right ventricular suture lines are completed and discontinued at 36°C.

Repair of Truncus Arteriosus Type III

Left and right pulmonary artery branches that arise posteriorly from the right and left lateral aortic walls are kept in continuity by excising a large button of aorta that includes these origins. The aorta is reconstructed as described earlier. When the right and left pulmonary arteries come off the lateral truncal walls, it may be necessary to excise that segment of the truncal artery. The front of the segment is then excised to create an elliptical opening for anastomosis to the conduit.[G2,S4] The aorta is reconstituted by end-to-end anastomosis, or if the ends are too widely separated for this, by the undesirable alternative of interposing a short segment of Dacron graft.[G2]

Repair of Other Types of Truncus Arteriosus

When only one pulmonary artery takes origin from the truncus artery, the aortic connection may be closed from within the truncus artery and an end-to-side anastomosis made between conduit and pulmonary artery; alternatively, if the pulmonary artery is of good size, it may be managed by excision from the truncal artery and usual end-to-end conduit pulmonary anastomosis.[W1]

When the left pulmonary artery arises from the ductus arteriosus, the ductus can be ligated (or oversewn) very close to the aorta, and the end of the pulmonary artery attached end to side to the homograft conduit or to the right pulmonary artery; or the end of the right pulmonary artery may be anastomosed to the left. In older children, it may be necessary to use a bifurcated Dacron graft with end-to-end or end-to-side anastomosis to each pulmonary artery, although this technique is less satisfactory.

Repair of Truncus Arteriosus with Interrupted Aortic Arch or Coarctation

In this setting, it is not necessary to reconstruct the aortic arch since the ductus remains widely patent and can be used as the permanent conduit to the descending aorta. The pulmonary artery branches are detached from the truncus artery and the repair proceeds as usual.[G3]

Repair of Truncus Arteriosus with Truncal Valve Incompetence

Important truncal valve incompetence greatly complicates the repair of truncus arteriosus, particularly when an operation is required in the very young. The decision to replace the truncal valve (with a homograft, accomplished successfully in one 2-month-old infant [UAB]) is difficult and in general should be made only when the incompetence is gross.

Lesser degrees of truncal valve incompetence complicate the perfusion, myocardial protection, and myocardial reperfusion. One of the advantages of Ebert's technique of aortic cross-clamping immediately after beginning CPB and releasing the cross clamp and maintaining a beating heart after disconnecting the pulmonary arteries and repairing the opening left in the truncal artery is that the disadvantages of some degree of truncal valve incompetence are minimized (see "Support Techniques during the Repair of Truncus Arteriosus in Infants" in section on Special Situations and Controversies). With the methods described earlier, less than severe truncal valve incompetence is generally manageable. When CPB is used for the repair (UAB), the aorta is cross-clamped proximal to the perfusion cannula just after establishing CPB, and if the cold cardioplegia infusion cannot distend the truncal root because of truncal valve incompetence, the infusion is given directly into one or both coronary ostia after partially disconnecting the pulmonary arteries. This is possible because the ostium of at least the left coronary artery is usually large. The truncal closure is made around a Frater pull-out stitch (see Chapter 20, "Technique of Operation" in Section 2, Ventricular Septal Defect and Aortic Incompetence), which keeps the truncal valve competent when the cross-clamp is later removed. It is not necessary to use a more formal whip stitch for temporary valve approximation as described by De Leval et al.[D1]

When the technique of profound hypothermia and total circulatory arrest has been used (GLH), truncal valve incompetence rarely poses problems.

Repair of Truncus Arteriosus with Truncal Valve Stenosis

True severe stenosis of the truncal valve is rare. The preoperative left-ventricular-to-truncus-artery gradient overestimates the amount of anatomic narrowing, because both systemic and pulmonary blood flows are passing through the truncal valve. When valvotomy is required, the principles used in the surgical treatment of congenital aortic stenosis are followed (see Chapter 32).

SPECIAL FEATURES OF POSTOPERATIVE CARE

Management is accomplished with the concepts and techniques described in Chapter 5. Following the repair of truncus arteriosus in infants, pulmonary artery or right ventricular pressure is continuously monitored through a polyvinyl catheter placed through the right ventricular wall after the repair (UAB). When important residual hypertension is present, muscle paralysis or continuous intravenous anesthesia for 24–48 hours is helpful in preventing paroxysms of severely elevated pulmonary arterial pressure (see Chapter 2, "Low Cardiac Output" in Section 2, "Cardiovascular Subsystem").

EARLY RESULTS

Hospital Mortality

The hospital mortality after the correction of truncus arteriosus is higher than that after the repair of most congenital cardiac malformations.[A2,B2,B9,M4] Thus, even in the large Mayo Clinic experience, there were 18 deaths (21%, CL 16%–26%) among 86 patients over 2 years of age reported in 1977[M4] and 48 hospital deaths (29%, CL 25%–33%) among the overall group of 167 patients reported in 1985.[D4]

More pertinent to current management problems is the mortality after repair in the first year of life, since only about 10% of patients born with truncus arteriosus survive beyond 1 year, and many of these have severe pulmonary vascular disease (see "Natural History"). The hospital mortality for repair of truncus arteriosus in the first 6 months of life can be as low as 16% (CL 12%–21%), as has been shown by Ebert and colleagues[E4,E5] (Table 28-4; since the six babies dying under medical treatment might elsewhere have been submitted to operation in NYHA class V, they are included in the mortality). Few other groups have been able to present such a satisfactory experience, although many have reported successful operations in infants.[S1,S6,S8] The GLH and UAB experiences (Tables 28-5 and 28-6), both of which go back to 1967, with a combined mortality of 13 deaths among 21 patients operated upon in the first 6 months of life (62%, 48%–74%), may be more representative of what most other groups have experienced in this period. Current hospital mortality rates are no doubt lower.

Incremental Risk Factors for Hospital Death after Repair

The most lethal risk factor is a very *poor preoperative clinical status* of the patient as is evident in both the UAB (Table 28-7) and GLH (Table 28-5) results. Eight of 9 patients in NYHA class V preoperatively died after repair in the combined UAB (Table 28-8) and GLH (Table 28-5) experiences, both of which go back to 1967. Not surprisingly, the patients

Table 28-4 Hospital deaths in 106 patients less than 7 months of age presenting with truncus arteriosus. In addition, three deaths occurred after hospital dismissal.

| Category | n | Hospital Deaths | | |
		No.	%	CL
Medical treatment	6	6	—	—
Repaired	100	11	11%	8%–15%
Total	106	17	16%	12%–21%

KEY: CL, 70% confidence limits.

SOURCE: Adapted from Ebert et al.[E5]

Table 28-5 Hospital deaths after repair of truncus arteriosus with and without major associated cardiac anomalies (GLH; 1967–1981).

| Age | | | Hospital Deaths | | |
≤ <		n	No.	%	CL
Months					
1		3	3	100%	53%–100%
1 --- 3		6	2	33%	12%–62%
3 --- 6		4	2	50%	18%–82%
6 --- 12		1	1	100%	15%–100%
Years					
1 --- 10		6	4	67%	38%–88%
Total		20	12	60%	46%–73%

KEY: CL, 70% confidence limits.

NOTE: Four of the patients less than 3 months of age were in preoperative NYHA class V; three died after repair.

Table 28-6 Hospital deaths after repair of truncus arteriosus with or without major associated cardiac anomalies (UAB; 1967–1984).

| Age | | | Hospital Deaths | | |
≤ <		n	No.	%	CL
Months					
1		5	5	100%	68%–100%
1 --- 3		4	4	100%	62%–100%
3 --- 6		8	6	75%	50%–91%
6 --- 12		13	8	62%	43%–77%
12 --- 24		12	7	58%	40%–75%
24 --- 48		10	5	50%	30%–70%
Years					
4 --- 10		9	3	33%	15%–56%
10		7	1	14%	2%–41%
Total		68	39	57%	50%–64%
P(logistic)			.0008		

KEY: CL, 70% confidence limits.

NOTE: Major associated cardiac anomalies include origin of left pulmonary artery from ductus arteriosus (1 case, 0 death); absent left pulmonary artery (4 cases, 1 death); absent right pulmonary artery (1 case, 0 death); obstruction of RPA by previously placed band (1 case, 1 death); interrupted aortic arch (3 cases, 3 deaths).

Table 28-7 Incremental risk factors for hospital death after the repair of truncus arteriosus, with and without major associated cardiac anomalies (UAB; 1967–1984; n = 68, 39 events).

Incremental Risk Factor	Coefficient ± SD	P Value
NYHA class (I–V)	1.1 ± 0.53	0.03
Truncal valve incompetence (0–3)	1.2 ± 0.50	0.01
PA band	2.1 ± 0.96	0.03
(Young) age (months)	−0.7 ± 0.37	0.05
(Early) date of operation (years)	−0.15 ± 0.098	0.12
Female	1.6 ± 0.78	0.04
Intercept	−1.3	

KEY: SD, standard deviation.

NOTE: There are no hypotheses as to why being female is a risk factor, and this may well be a spurious association.

Table 28-8 Hospital mortality after repair of truncus arteriosus with and without major associated cardiac anomalies (UAB; 1967–1984).

NYHA Class	n	No.	%	CL
I	—	—		
II	24	7	29%	19%–42%
III	23	14	61%	48%–73%
IV	16	13	81%	66%–92%
V	5	5	100%	68%–100%
Total	68	39	57%	50%–64%
$P(x^2)$			.002	

Hospital Deaths columns: No., %, CL

KEY: CL, 70% confidence limits.

Table 28-10 Hospital mortality after repair of truncus arteriosus in the first 6 months of life (Ebert; 1974–1980).

Clinical Features	n	No.	%	CL
High $\dot{Q}p/\dot{Q}s$	41	1	2%	0.3%–8%
$\dot{Q}p/\dot{Q}s \pm 1$	13	3	23%	10%–41%
Cyanotic	2	2	100%	39%–100%
Total	56	6	11%	6%–17%

Hospital Deaths columns: No., %, CL

SOURCE: Adapted from publication by Ebert.[E4]

KEY: CL, 70% confidence limits.

NOTE: In this series, 4 were less than 1 month old, 30 were 1–3 months old, and 22 were 3–6 months old; 16 weighed 2–3 kg, 31 weighed 3–4 kg, and 9 weighed 4–5 kg; 46 were in heart failure; 14 had some degree of truncal incompetence; and 8 had increased pulmonary resistance.

with the most advanced symptoms were generally the youngest (Table 28-9).

Important truncal valve incompetence is also an important risk factor for hospital death (Table 28-7), as has been noted by Ebert and colleagues.[E5] All 4 infants with preoperatively severe truncal valve incompetence died after repair, including 2 who underwent simultaneous truncal valve replacement (UAB). Severe truncal valve incompetence has not been any more common among the very young neonates than among other infants.

A previously placed *pulmonary artery* band has increased the risk of repair (Table 28-7), which is no doubt related to distortions of the pulmonary arteries produced by the band or its migration.[M3] However, in older patients the incremental risk of a previously placed band is less evident.[M4,P1]

Young age has increased the risk,[D4] in part because of the probably increased sensitivity of the young to the damaging effects of cardiopulmonary bypass (see Chapter 2). However, the relatively high mortality among infants undergoing repair in the first few months of life is related primarily to the fact that, in most experiences, the infants are in NYHA functional class IV or V. Survivors of repair have been obtained in the first month of life,[E3,S4] however, although not commonly. As age becomes even a month or two older, survivors become more common.[E1,P4,S4,S7]

Pulmonary vascular disease is a risk factor. In the Mayo Clinic series, for example, the hospital mortality was 14% when the pulmonary vascular resistance was 8 units · m^2 or less and 39% when it was greater than 8 units · m^2 ($P < .01$).[M4] Although this is more relevant when an operation is being considered in older patients rather than infants, infants

occasionally do have high pulmonary vascular resistance. Thus, infants with a large pulmonary blood flow (and thus low pulmonary vascular resistance) have a lower hospital mortality than do those with smaller pulmonary blood flows (Table 28-10).

Earlier date of operation has been a risk factor in most experiences, with the improvements in time relating to general improvements in cardiac surgery.

Major coexisting cardiac anomalies must be an incremental risk factor for hospital death, although they were not identified as such in the multivariate analysis (Table 28-7). Absence of one pulmonary artery increased the risk in the Mayo Clinic experience, in part as a consequence of the associated pulmonary vascular disease.[M10] Success has been reported in the face of coexisting aortic arch interruption.[D5,G3]

The *type of conduit* would seem likely to affect the hospital mortality, but it has not been demonstrated to do so. Success has been reported using nonvalved conduits.[B1] A nonvalved pericardial tube has the disadvantage that the thickening that occurs with this material may lead to stenosis at the pulmonary artery bifurcation when the branch origins are small.[S13] Although it would seem that the well-fitting homograft-valved conduit should provide optimal results, the lowest hospital mortality (Ebert) has been obtained with the heterograft-valved Dacron conduit.

A *previous pericardiotomy* may increase the risk of repair because of adhesions that may increase the risk of damage to coronary arteries.[A1]

LATE RESULTS

Survival

As in most cardiac operations, a few deaths occur in the early months after hospital dismissal[B8,M9,P4] (Tables 28-4 and 28-5) and are properly considered part of the early risks.

Thereafter, premature late deaths in the intermediate term (10 years) are few when the operation is done with a properly preserved and prepared homograft-valved conduit in a young patient with little or no preoperative elevation of pulmonary vascular resistance. There have been no intermediate term deaths in the GLH experience (Table 28-11),

Table 28-9 Some correlations in patients undergoing repair of truncus arteriosus (UAB; 1967–1984; n = 68).

Variables	R Value	P Value
Age (months) and NYHA class (I–V)[a]	−.7	<.0001
Age (months) and truncal valve incompetence (0–3)[a]	−.2	.18
NYHA and truncal valve incompetence	.03	.8

[a] Age is age at operation.

Table 28-11 Postoperative cardiac catheterization and other relevant data in survivors of conduit repair of truncus arteriosus (GLH; 1967–1981).

| Age at Operation | Conduit | Time Interval | Postoperative Catheterization | | | | | | | Preop AI | Length of Follow-Up |
| | | | Systolic Pressures (mmHg) | | | | | Q̇p/Q̇s | AI | | |
			Ao	Rv	MPA	LPA	RPA				
1 mo	Homo (14 mm)	3 yr		50	31	14	29	1	Mod[b]	Mild	9 yr
2 mo	Pericardium	7 wk	85	85	85	—[a]	—[a]	1.5	None	None	2 mo (death after reoperation)
2 mo	Homo (19 mm)	3 yr	115	42	32	16		1	Severe	Trivial	9 yr
2 mo	Homo (18 mm)	4 wk	105	48	48	35		1[c]	NA	None	4 yr (faint EDM)
3 mo	Homo (18 mm)	3 yr	110	60	20			1	Severe	Trivial	4 yr
3 mo	Homo (18 mm)	7 wk	55	80	65	65[d]	16	1[c]	NA	None	2 mo (death)
5 yr	Homo (22 mm)	5 yr		44			44	1	Mild	None	5 yr
9 yr	Homo (20 mm)								—	None	4 yr (faint EDM)

KEY: AI, aortic incompetence; Ao, aorta; EDM, early diastolic aortic or pulmonary murmur; Homo, homograft valved; LPA, MPA, RPA, left, main, and right pulmonary arteries; NA, not assessed; Q̇p/Q̇s, pulmonary to systemic blood flow ratio; RV, right ventricle.

[a] Severe bifurcation stenosis on angio and at reoperation.

[b] Clinical assessment.

[c] Tiny jet visible through VSD repair on angio.

[d] PVR 9 units • m² using LPA pressure.

which has been accomplished under these conditions. Similarly, in the Mayo Clinic experience there have been no late deaths out to 13 years in patients operated upon when they were less than 2 years old; increasing age at operation was associated with shorter long-term survival ($P = .004$).[D4] In the Mayo Clinic experience, unilateral pulmonary artery, something less than a large pulmonary blood flow, and moderate or severe truncal valve incompetence were also risk factors for premature late death.[D4]

Truncal Valve Incompetence

Important truncal valve incompetence may develop in some survivors as time passes, even though preoperatively and early postoperatively it was not prominent. This has developed in 3 of 6 long-term survivors at GLH (50%; CL 24%–76%) (Table 28-11).

Conduit Complications

False aneurysms have developed at the proximal suture line in a few patients, and reoperation has been required for this. Otherwise, no patients in whom a homograft-valved conduit has been used has as yet required reoperation (GLH and UAB) (Table 28-11). This is similar to the experiences with homograft-valved conduits between right ventricle and pulmonary artery for other conditions.[B5] (See Chapter 23, "Valved Conduits" in Section 1, Special Situations and Controversies) for a detailed discussion of late results with homograft-valved conduits.)

When a heterograft-valved synthetic conduit is used, heterograft-valve degeneration and neointimal proliferation within the Dacron tube make ultimate reoperation nearly inevitable (see Chapter 23). Also, the small size of a heterograft-valved conduit that must be used in an infant necessi-

tates relatively early reoperation, earlier with the 12-mm conduit than the 14-mm conduit.[E5] When the operation is done with such a conduit in the first 6 months of life, over half of the hospital survivors require conduit replacement within 5 years; thus in the experience of Ebert and colleagues, 55 (64%, CL 58%–70%) of 86 cases required reoperation at a median time after insertion of 4 years.[E5] Replacement of the heterograft-valved conduit in patients in whom it has been used as part of the repair of truncus arteriosus can be done at a low risk[M6] (0 deaths in 9 cases, UAB; 0 deaths in 55 cases, Ebert and colleagues[E5]), although still further reoperations may be necessary when nonvalved or heterograft-valved conduits are inserted at reoperation.

Progression of Pulmonary Vascular Disease

Progression of pulmonary vascular disease has not been observed in patients operated upon in the first 6 months of life,[E5] as would be predicted from the larger and longer followed experience with repair of isolated VSD (see Chapter 20, "Pulmonary Hypertension" in Section on Late Results). As the VSD experience would also predict, when repair of truncus arteriosus is done at an older age and/or with preoperatively elevated pulmonary vascular resistance, the pulmonary vascular disease may persist or progress after repair. In the Mayo Clinic experience with children 6 to 9 years of age, the 13-year survival was only 68% and many of the late deaths were related to pulmonary vascular disease.[D4] The patient may die suddenly or with chronic right heart failure.

INDICATIONS FOR OPERATION

The diagnosis of truncus arteriosus is an indication for its repair. This should, when possible, be carried out before the development of advanced functional disability (NYHA class IV or V), this being more important than reaching some age of election before repair. However, when the left-to-right shunt is large and heart failure well controlled out of the hospital by medication, repair may be deferred until 3 or possibly 6 months of age but not beyond that time.[J1] During the period of deferral, the infant is closely observed and repair undertaken at the first suggestion of worsening heart failure or increasing pulmonary vascular resistance.

If severe and intractable heart failure is present when the patient is first seen, especially if this is in the first few months of life, the problem is a difficult one. Repair under these circumstances can result in some survivors and should be carried out, albeit at an increased risk. Consideration may be given to a palliative operation to reduce pulmonary blood flow (see "Special Situations and Controversies") and perhaps even to concomitant homograft replacement of the truncal valve if it is severely incompetent and later complete repair at 6–12 months of age.

When pulmonary vascular resistance is already elevated when the patient is first seen, the indications for repair are the same as in isolated VSD (see Chapter 20). When there is only one pulmonary artery, the criteria are possibly altered.[M10]

SPECIAL SITUATIONS AND CONTROVERSIES

Support Techniques during the Repair of Truncus Arteriosus in Infants

The techniques used by Ebert and colleagues for the repair of truncus arteriosus have given the best reported results in infants,[E5] and serious consideration should be given to their adoption by others, particularly in very young infants.

The operating room time is reduced to a minimum by streamlining the anesthesia induction and placement of devices, much as described in Chapter 2. After making the median sternotomy, the aortic purse-string suture for arterial cannulation is placed and a purse-string suture is placed on the atrial appendage through which the single venous cannula is placed (see Chapter 2). Ebert has demonstrated that CPB can be maintained during a right ventriculotomy with a single venous cannula whose tip is positioned in the inferior vena cava and in which there is an extra hole that lies in the right atrium. The tricuspid valve remains closed, allowing the perfusion to be nicely maintained even with a right ventriculotomy. This is facilitated by the perfusionists maintaining just enough suction on the venous line so that the perfusion is satisfactory and blood does not well up into the right ventricle but not so much as to suck air into the right atrium. The right and left pulmonary arteries are not dissected, but a snare is passed behind the aorta distal to the takeoff of the pulmonary trunk and then through the transverse sinus. The snare is then effectively around the pulmonary trunk or the origin of the right and left pulmonary arteries.

Cardiopulmonary bypass is established with the perfusate as cold as possible, the snare previously passed around the pulmonary trunk is snugged, and the aorta is clamped after the heart is cooled or if ventricular ejections cease. At that point, the perfusate temperature is stabilized at 26°C. The pulmonary trunk or arteries are excised from the truncus artery as described earlier, and the defect in what is now the aorta is closed. The aortic clamp is released, and rewarming with the perfusate is begun. Any important leakage in the aortic suture line is closed with a stitch or two. The right ventricle is opened as described earlier, and the VSD is closed with a patch, placing the sutures a little farther apart than usual and all from the right ventricular side. If exposure is difficult for the VSD repair, the aorta may be cross-clamped a second time. The homograft-valved conduit would be sewed into place as described earlier (a departure from Ebert's method) and perfusion discontinued and decannulation accomplished.

The very short aortic cross-clamp time with this technique and the avoidance of the use of cold cardioplegia may be of particular advantage in the repair of truncus arteriosus in small infants. Dissection and temporary occlusion of the pulmonary arteries are unnecessary. The short aortic cross-clamp time neutralizes any potential advantage of cold cardioplegia (see Chapter 3, Fig. 3-10). The frequently present truncal valve incompetence complicates proper use of cold cardioplegia in any event but usually does not prevent prompt restarting of the heart by aortic declamping with Ebert's method. The rather anterior position of the VSD in most patients with truncus arteriosus makes it particularly suitable for repair with these perfusion techniques. With the VSD in this position, no sutures need be placed in the base of the tricuspid leaflet, which might distort the valve and complicate the CPB.

Other Methods of Separating the Pulmonary Arteries from the Truncal Artery

Instead of detaching the pulmonary arteries, a transverse incision may be made anteriorly in the truncus artery. From within the truncus, a patch of pericardium or Dacron may then be sewn into place over the truncal aperture leading to the pulmonary arteries, to separate the pulmonary arteries

Table 28-12 Results of pulmonary artery banding (GLH; 1965–1970). A single band was placed around the main pulmonary trunk or the closely approximated origins of the two arteries in all except the 2-year-old child.

Age	Associated Anomalies	Result
3 wk	Aortic incompetence	Died at operation
6 wk	Nil	Died 4 h p.o.
6 wk	Nil	CHF persisted
		Conduit repair (pericardial tube) at 2 mo; died age 4 mo
2 mo	Nil	Died at operation
3 mo	Aortic stenosis	Died 18 h p.o.
3 mo	Nil	Alive; conduit repair age 9 yr
2 yr	Interrupted arch (B)	Alive until after 9 yr then died at cardiac repair
	LPA stenosis[a]	
	Muscular VSD	

[a] Right pulmonary artery only banded.

from the truncus.[S8] When this method is used, care must be taken so that the patch does not interrupt the confluence between the left and right pulmonary arteries. The conduit is then anastomosed end to side to the pulmonary trunk or left pulmonary artery.

Use of a Valveless Conduit

Success was achieved in the past with the use of a valveless conduit,[B1] and Spicer and colleagues and Oelert currently are using these with success at the primary operation in infants.[O1,S14] Ebert and colleagues have inserted valveless conduits in about one-half the patients in whom they have replaced the original conduit, without mortality.[E5] However, with the known late effects of pulmonary valve incompe-

tence and the excellent long-term results of properly prepared homograft conduits (see Chapter 23 and Table 28-11), there seems little reason to recommend valveless conduits.

Pulmonary Artery Banding

Theoretically, narrowing of the pulmonary artery by external banding or internal constriction[L4,M11] should be a good palliative procedure for truncus arteriosus, especially when there is little or no truncal valve incompetence. However, the hospital mortality in the past has been 30%–50%[A2,B1,E2,H6,K1,M3,M12,P2,S5,T3] (Table 28-12). Whether it could be made less by excluding those cases with important truncal valve incompetence (or replacing the valve) and providing better intra- and postoperative care is problematic.

REFERENCES

A

1. Anderson KR, McGoon DC, Lie JT: Surgical significance of the coronary arterial anatomy in truncus arteriosus communis. *Am J Cardiol* 41:76, 1978.

2. Appelbaum A, Bargeron LM Jr, Pacifico AD, Kirklin JW: Surgical treatment of truncus arteriosus with emphasis on infants and small children. *J Thorac Cardiovasc Surg* 71:436, 1976.

3. Angelini P, Vrdugo AL, Illera JP, Leachman RD: Truncus arteriosus communis. Unusual case associated with transposition. *Circulation* 56:1167, 1977.

4. Anderson RC, Obata W, Lillehei CW: Truncus arteriosus. Clinical study of 14 cases. *Circulation* 26:586, 1957.

5. Arai T, Tsuzuki Y, Nazi M, Kurashize K, Kayanazi H, Nishida H: Experimental study on bypass between the right and left ventricle and aorta by means of homograft with valve. *Bull Heart Inst Jpn* 9:49, 1965.

6. Assad-Morell JL, Seward JB, Tajik AJ, Hagler DJ, Giuliani ER, Ritter DG: Echo-phonocardiographic and contrast studies in conditions associated systemic arterial trunk over-riding the ventricular septum. Truncus arteriosus, tetralogy of Fallot and pulmonary atresia with ventricular septal defect. *Circulation* 53:663, 1976.

7. Armer RM, De Oliveira PF, Lurie PR: True truncus arteriosus: Review of 17 cases and report of surgery in 7 patients. *Circulation* 24:878, 1961 (abstr).

B

1. Behrendt DM, Kirsch MM, Stern A, Sigmann J, Perry B, Sloan HB: The surgical therapy for pulmonary artery-right ventricular discontinuity. *Ann Thorac Surg* 18:122, 1974.

2. Bharati S, McAllister HA, Rosenquist GC, Miller RA, Tatooles CJ, Lev M: The surgical anatomy of truncus arteriosus communis. *J Thorac Cardiovasc Surg* 67:501, 1974.

3. Becker AE, Becker MJ, Edwards JE: Pathology of the semilunar valve in persistent truncus arteriosus. *J Thorac Cardiovasc Surg* 62:16, 1971.

4. Burnell RH, McEnery G, Miller GAH: Truncal valve stenosis. *Br Heart J* 33:423, 1971.

5. Barratt-Boyes BG: Corrective surgery for congenital heart disease in infants with the use of profound hypothermia and circulatory arrest techniques. *Aust NZ J Surg* 47:737, 1977.

6. Bowman FOG, Hancock WD, Malm JR: A valve-containing dacron prosthesis: its use in restoring pulmonary artery-right ventricular continuity. *Arch Surg* 107:724, 1973.

7. Buchanan A: Malformation of the heart. Undivided truncus arteriosus. Heart otherwise double. *Trans Path Soc London* 15:89, 1864.

8. Brawley RK, Gardner TJ, Donahoo JS, Neill CA, Rowe RD, Gott VL: Late results after right ventricular outflow tract reconstruction with aortic root homografts. *J Thorac Cardiovasc Surg* 64:314, 1972.

9. Burakovsky VI, Falkovsky GE, Ivanitsky AV: Surgical repair of truncus arteriosus. *Pediatr Cardiol* 5:111, 1984.

C

1. Collett RW, Edwards JE: Persistent truncus arteriosus: A classification according to anatomic types. *Surg Clin North Am* 29:1245, 1949.

2. Calder L, Van Praagh R, Van Praagh S, Sears WP, Corwin R, Levy A, Keith JD, Paul MH: Truncus arteriosus communis. Clinical angiocardiographic and pathologic findings in 100 patients. *Am Heart J* 92:23, 1976.

3. Crupi G, Macartney FJ, Anderson RH: Persistent truncus arteriosus. A study of 66 autopsy cases with special reference to definition and morphogenesis. *Am J Cardiol* 40:569, 1977.

4. Carr I, Bharati S, Kusnoor VS, Lev M: Truncus arteriosus communis with intact ventricular septum. *Br Heart J* 42:97, 1979.

5. Carr FB, Goodale RH, Rockwell AEP: Persistent truncus arteriosus in a man aged 36 years. *Arch Pathol* 19:833, 1935.

6. Ceballos R, Soto B, Kirklin JW, Bargeron LM Jr: Truncus arteriosus. An anatomical-angiographic study. *Br Heart J* 49:589, 1983.

D

1. de Leval MR, McGoon DC, Wallace RB, Danielson GK, Mair DD: Management of truncal valvular regurgitation. *Ann Surg* 180:427, 1974.

2. Deely WJ, Hagstrom JWC, Engle MA: Truncus insufficiency. Common truncus arteriosus with regurgitant truncal valve: Report of 4 cases. *Am Heart J* 65:542, 1963.

3. Daskalopoulos DA, Edwards WD, Driscoll DJ, Schaff HV, Danielson GK: Fatal pulmonary artery banding in truncus ar-

teriosus with anomalous origin of circumflex coronary artery from right pulmonary artery. *Am J Cardiol* 52:1363, 1983.

4. DiDonato RM, Fyfe DA, Puga FJ, Danielson GK, Ritter DG, Edwards WD, McGoon DC: Fifteen-year experience with surgical repair of truncus arteriosus. *J Thorac Cardiovasc Surg* 89:414, 1985.

5. Davis JT, Ehrlich R, Blakemore WS, Lev M, Bharati S: Truncus arteriosus with interrupted aortic arch: Report of a successful surgical repair. *Ann Thorac Surg* 39:82, 1985.

E

1. Ebert P, Robinson S, Stanger P, Engle M: Pulmonary artery conduits in infants younger than 6 months of age. *J Thorac Cardiovasc Surg* 72:351, 1976.

2. Edmunds LH Jr, Fishman NH, Gregory GA, Heymann MA, Hoffman JIE, Robinson SJ, Roe RB, Rudolph AM, Stanger P: Cardiac surgery in infants less than six weeks of age. *Circulation* 46:250, 1972.

3. Ebert P: (1981) Personal communication.

4. Ebert PA: Truncus arteriosus, in L. Parenzan, G. Crupi, G. Graham (eds): *Congenital Heart Disease in the First 3 Months of Life*. Bologna, Italy: Patron Editore, 1981.

5. Ebert PA, Turley K, Stanger P, Hoffman JIE, Heymann MA, Rudolph AM: Surgical treatment of truncus arteriosus in the first six months of life. *Ann Surg* 200:451, 1984.

F

1. Fontana RS, Edwards JE: Congenital cardiac disease: *A Review of 357 Cases Studied Pathologically*. Philadelphia and London: WB Saunders, 1962, p 95.

2. Freedom RM, Rosen FS, Nadas AS: Congenital cardiovascular disease and anomalies of the third and fourth pharyngeal pouch. *Circulation* 46:165, 1972.

G

1. Gelband H, Van Meter S, Gersony WM: Truncal valve abnormalities in infants with persistent truncus arteriosus. A clinicopathological study. *Circulation* 45:397, 1972.

2. Griepp RB, Stinson EB, Shumway NE: Surgical correction of types II and III truncus arteriosus. *J Thorac Cardiovasc Surg* 73:345, 1977.

3. Gomes MMR, McGoon DC: Truncus arteriosus with interrupted aortic arch: report of a case successfully repaired. *Mayo Clin Proc* 46:40, 1971.

4. Girinath MR: Case presentation: Truncus arteriosus: Repair with homograft reconstruction in infancy, in BG Barratt-Boyes, JM Neutze, EA Harris (eds): *Heart Disease in Infancy. Diagnosis and Surgical Treatment*. Edinburgh: Churchill Livingstone 1973, p 234.

5. Gerlis LM, Wilson N, Dickinson DF, Scott O: Valvar stenosis in truncus arteriosus. *Br Heart J* 52:440, 1984.

H

1. Habbema L, Losekoot TG, Becker AE: Respiratory distress due to bronchial compression in persistent truncus arteriosus. *Chest* 77:230, 1980.

2. Heilbrunn A, Kittle CF, Diehl AM: Pulmonary arterial banding in the treatment of truncus arteriosus. *Circulation* 29:1, 102, 1964.

3. Hallermann FJ, Kincaid OW, Tsakiris AG, Ritter DG, Titus JL: Persistent truncus arteriosus: A radiographic and angiocardiographic study. *Am J Roentgen* 107:827, 1969.

4. Hagler DJ, Tajik AJ, Seward JB, Mair DD, Ritter DG: Wide-angle two-dimensional echocardiographic profiles of conotruncal abnormalities. *Mayo Clin Proc* 55:73, 1980.

5. Hicken P, Evans D, Heath D: Persistent truncus arteriosus with survival to the age of 38 years. *Br Heart J* 28:284, 1966.

6. Hunt CE, Formanek G, Levine MA, Castaneda A, Moller JH: Banding of the pulmonary artery. Results in 111 children. *Circulation* 43:395, 1970.

J

1. Juaneda E, Haworth SG: Pulmonary vascular disease in children with truncus arteriosus. *Am J Cardiol* 54:1314, 1984.

K

1. Kreidberg MB, Fisher JH, De Luca FG, Chernoff HL: Pulmonary artery banding for persistent truncus arteriosus. Report of a case. *J Pediatr* 64:557, 1964.

L

1. Lee MH, Bellon EM, Liebman J, Perrin EV: Truncal valve stenosis. *Am Heart J* 85:397, 1973.

2. Ledbetter MK, Tandon R, Titus JL, Edwards JE: Stenotic semilunar valve in persistent truncus arteriosus. *Chest* 69:182, 1976.

3. Lev M, Saphir O: Truncus arteriosus communis persistens. *J Pediatr* 20:74, 1943.

4. Litwin SB, Friedbert DZ: Pulmonary artery plication: A new surgical procedure for small infants with Type I truncus arteriosus. *Ann Thorac Surg* 35:193, 1983.

M

1. McGoon DC, Rastelli GC, Ongley PA: An operation for the correction of truncus arteriosus. *J Am Med Assoc* 205:59, 1968.

2. Mair DD, Ritter DG, Davis GD, Wallace RB, Danielson GK, McGoon DC: Selection of patients with truncus arteriosus for surgical correction: anatomic and hemodynamic considerations. *Circulation* 49:144, 1974.

3. McFaul RC, Mair DD, Feldt RH, Ritter DG, McGoon DC: Truncus arteriosus and previous pulmonary arterial banding: Clinical and hemodynamic assessment. *Am J Cardiol* 38:626, 1976.

4. Marcelleti C, McGoon DC, Danielson GK, Wallace RB, Mair DD: Early and late results of surgical repair of truncus arteriosus. *Circulation* 55:636, 1977.

5. Marcelleti C, McGoon DC, Mair DD: The natural history of truncus arteriosus. *Circulation* 54:108, 1976.

6. Moodie DS, Mair DD, Fulton RE, Wallace RB, Danielson GK, McGoon DC: Aortic homograft obstruction. *J Thorac Cardiovasc Surg* 72:553, 1976.

7. Moore CH, Martelli V, Ross DN: Reconstruction of right ventricular outflow tract with a valved conduit in 75 cases of congenital heart disease. *J Thorac Cardiovasc Surg* 71:11, 1976.

8. McGoon DC, Rastelli GC, Wallace RB: Discontinuity between right ventricle and pulmonary artery: Surgical treatment. *Ann Surg* 172:680, 1970.

9. Moseley PW, Ochsner JL, Mills NL, Chapman J: Management of an infected Hancock prosthesis after repair of truncus arteriosus. *J Thorac Cardiovasc Surg* 73:306, 1977.

10. Mair DD, Ritter DG, Danielson GK, Wallace RB, McGoon DC: Truncus arteriosus with unilateral absence of a pulmonary artery. Criteria for operability and surgical results. *Circulation* 55:641, 1977.

11. Mistrot JJ, Varco RL, Nicoloff DM: Palliation of infants with truncus arteriosus through creation of a pulmonary artery ostial stenosis. *Ann Thorac Surg* 22:495, 1976.

12. Musumeci F, Piccoli GP, Dickinson DF, Hamilton DI: Surgical experience with persistent truncus arteriosus in symptomatic infants under 1 year of age. Report of 13 consecutive cases. *Br Heart J* 46:179, 1981.

O

1. Oelert I: (1984) Personal communication.

P

1. Parker RK, McGoon DC, Danielson GK, Wallace RB, Mair DD: Repair of truncus arteriosus in patients with prior banding of the pulmonary artery. *Surgery* 78:761, 1975.

2. Poirier RA, Berman MA, Stansel HC Jr: Current status of the surgical treatment of truncus arteriosus. *J Thorac Cardiovasc Surg* 69:169, 1975.

3. Patel RG, Freedom RM, Bloom KR, Rowe RD: Truncal or aortic valve stenosis in functionally single arterial trunk. A clinical hemodynamic and pathologic study of six cases. *Am J Cardiol* 42:800, 1978.

4. Parenzan L, Alfieri O: Surgical repair of persistent truncus arteriosus in infancy, in RH Anderson, EA Shinebourne (eds): *Pediatric Cardiology, 1977.* Edinburgh: Churchill Livingstone 1978, p 551.

R

1. Ross DN, Somerville J: Correction of pulmonary atresia with a homograft aortic valve. *Lancet* 2:1446, 1966.

2. Rastelli GC, Titus JL, McGoon DC: Homograft of ascending aorta and aortic valve as a right ventricular outflow. *Arch Surg* 95:698, 1967.

S

1. Singh A, de Leval M, Stark J: Total correction of type I truncus arteriosus in a 6-month-old infant. *Br Heart J* 37:1314, 1975.

2. Stark J, Aberdeen E, Waterston DJ, Bonham-Carter RE, Tynan M: Pulmonary artery constriction (banding): A report of 146 cases. *Surgery* 65:808, 1969.

3. Shrivastava S, Edwards JE: Coronary arterial origin in persistent truncus arteriosus. *Circulation* 55:551, 1977.

4. Stark J, Gandhi D, de Leval M, Macartney F, Taylor JFN: Surgical treatment of persistent truncus arteriosus in the first year of life. *Br Heart J* 40:1280, 1978.

5. Singh AL, de Leval MR, Pincott JR, Stark J: Pulmonary artery banding for truncus arteriosus in the first year of life. *Circulation* 53, 54(suppl 3):17, 1976.

6. Stanger P, Robinson SJ, Engle MA, Ebert PA: "Corrective" surgery for truncus arteriosus in the first year of life. *Am J Cardiol* 39:393, 1977 (abstr).

7. Sullivan H, Sulayman R, Replogle R, Arcilla RA: Surgical correction of truncus arteriosus in infancy. *Am J Cardiol* 38:113, 1976.

8. Smith JM, Cooley DA: Modified procedure for correction of truncus arteriosus types II and III. *Ann Thorac Surg* 29:387, 1980.

9. Smith GW, Thompson WM, Damman JF, Muller WH: Use of the pulmonary artery banding procedure in treating type II truncus arteriosus. *Circulation* 29(suppl):1–108, 1964.

10. Swift LH, Shimomura A, Ryan SF, Van Praagh R: New type of truncus arteriosus communis with two semilunar valves, aortic valvular atresia and no ventricular septal defect. *Circulation* 40:111, 1969.

11. Seki S, Rastelli GC, McGoon DC, Titus JL: Replacement of the pulmonary artery with a pulmonary arterial homograft. *J Thorac Cardiovasc Surg* 60:853, 1970.

12. Shapiro PF: Truncus solitarus pulmonalis. A rare type of congenital cardiac anomaly. *Arch Pathol* 10:671, 1930.

13. Smith HJ: Case presentation: Truncus arteriosus: Two-stage repair, in BG Barratt-Boyes, JM Neutze, EA Harris (eds): *Heart Disease in Infancy. Diagnosis and Surgical Treatment.* Edinburgh: Churchill Livingstone, 1973, p 232.

14. Spicer RL, Behrendt D, Crowley DC, Dick M, Rocchini AP, Uzark K, Rosenthal A, Sloan H: Repair of truncus arteriosus in neonates with the use of a valveless conduit. *Circulation* 70(suppl I):I-26, 1984.

T

1. Thiene G, Bortolotti A, Gallucci V, Terribile V, Pellegrino PA: Anatomical study of truncus arteriosus communis with embryological and surgical considerations. *Br Heart J* 38:1109, 1976.

2. Tandon R, Hanck AJ, Nadas AS: Persistent truncus arteriosus: A clinical, hemodynamic and autopsy study of 19 cases. *Circulation* 28:1050, 1963.

3. Tatooles CJ, Miller RA: Palliative surgery in infants with congenital heart disease. *Prog Cardiovasc Dis* 15:331, 1973.

4. Thiene G, Cucchini F, Pellegrino PA: Truncus arteriosus communis associated with underdevelopment of the aortic arch. *Br Heart J* 37:1268, 1975.

V

1. Van Praagh R, Van Praagh S: The anatomy of common aorticopulmonary trunk (truncus arteriosus communis) and its embryonic implications. A study of 57 necropsy cases. *Am J Cardiol* 16:406, 1965.

2. Van der Horst RL, Gotsman MS: Type 3C truncus arteriosus. Case report with clinical and surgical implications. *Br Heart J* 36:1046, 1974.

3. Victoria BE, Krovetz LJ, Elliott CP, Van Mierop LHS, Bartley TD, Gessner IH, Schiebler GZ: Persistent truncus arteriosus in infancy. *Am Heart J* 77:13, 1969.

W

1. Wallace RB, Rastelli GC, Ongley PA, Titus JL, McGoon DC: Complete repair of truncus arteriosus defects. *J Thorac Cardiovasc Surg* 57:95, 1969.

2. Wilson J: A description of a very unusual malformation of the human heart. *Philos Trans R Soc Lond [Biol]* 18:346, 1798.

3. Weldon CS, Cameron JL: Correction of persistent truncus arteriosus. *J Cardiovasc Surg* 9:463, 1968.

29

AORTOPULMONARY WINDOW

DEFINITION

Aortopulmonary window is a round or oval opening between the ascending aorta and the pulmonary artery occurring as a congenital anomaly in hearts with separated aortic and pulmonary valves. This malformation has also been termed aortic septal defect, aortopulmonary fistula or fenestration or septal defect, and aorticopulmonary window or fistula or fenestration or septal defect.[R2]

HISTORICAL NOTE

The first report of an aortopulmonary window was by Elliotson in 1830[E1] and in the American literature by Cotton about 70 years later.[C6] The first reported correct clinical diagnoses are attributed to Dodds and Hoyle in 1949[D3] and to Gasul and colleagues in 1951.[G3]

In 1952, Gross[G1] reported the successful ligation of an aortopulmonary (AP) window using a closed technique. In 1953, Scott and Sabiston reported the successful division of an AP window by a closed technique,[S1] as did we in 1954 at the Mayo Clinic.[F1] The operation was, however, difficult and hazardous by closed techniques.

The advent of open operation with cardiopulmonary bypass (CPB) in 1954–1955 brought the capability of more easily correcting this malformation. Division of the connection between aorta and pulmonary artery was used in our early cases done at the Mayo Clinic with CPB, and Cooley and colleagues in 1957 reported three successful cases by this method.[C2] Bjork[B4] advised closure of the defect by the simple method of patching it from within the pulmonary artery. This was later also suggested by Putnam and Gross.[P1] In 1968, Wright and colleagues reported the transaortic ap-

proach to the intraluminal closure of an AP window by direct suture.[W1] A year later Deverall and colleagues also reported the use of a transaortic approach but with Dacron patch closure of the defect.[D1]

MORPHOLOGY

An aortopulmonary (AP) window is usually a large, oval defect between the aorta and pulmonary trunk (main pulmonary artery), although in about 10% of patients the defect is small. As the term *window* implies, there is little or no length to the communication. Nearly always it is a single orifice, although it may be fenestrated. The window is in the left lateral wall of the ascending aorta, usually close to the orifice of the left coronary artery, and in the contiguous right wall of the main pulmonary artery inferior to the origin of the right pulmonary artery.[N1] It is not surprising, therefore, that occasionally the right coronary artery[B1,B3,L1] and rarely the left[D2] may be transposed onto the pulmonary trunk close to the edge of the defect. When viewed from within the pulmonary artery, the AP window can be confused with the orifice of the right pulmonary artery.

Rarely, the orifice is more downstream in the ascending aorta.[M1,M3] Doty has encountered four such patients in his group of 25.[D2] It may then lie between the aorta and right pulmonary artery.[B2,D2]

Since the defect is usually a large one, pulmonary vascular disease develops with at least the same rapidity as it does in patients with ventricular septal defect (VSD) (see Chapter 20, "Pulmonary Vascular Disease" in Section 1, Morphology).

There is an association between AP window (particularly distally located ones) and anomalous origin of the right pulmonary artery from the ascending aorta (see Chapter 30). The AP window may open between the right pulmonary artery and aorta.[D2,M3] The right pulmonary artery may straddle the AP window ("unroofing" of the right pulmonary artery) or may originate completely from the aorta while maintaining continuity with the left pulmonary artery by way of the AP window.[B2] Finally, the two conditions may simply coexist.[G2] Rarely, there is a complex syndrome of AP window usually in the downstream portion of the ascending aorta,[T2] aortic origin of the right pulmonary artery, intact ventricular septum, patent ductus arteriosus, and interrupted aortic arch or severe coarctation.[B1,C5,J2,T2] This is a particularly lethal combination, most infants with it dying a short time after birth. Interrupted aortic arch may also occur as the only associated anomaly or it may coexist along with a VSD.

Other major associated cardiac anomalies may occasionally coexist with AP window, including VSD,[F2,T1] tetralogy of Fallot,[C1,T1] and subaortic stenosis. In all, from one-third to one-half of all patients with AP window have a major associated cardiac anomaly,[B1,N1,T2] From 5% to 10% of patients with the malformation have less severe associated cardiac anomalies, such as right aortic arch (7%),[F2] ostium secundum atrial septal defects, or patent ductus arteriosus.[B1,C4,D1]

CLINICAL FEATURES AND DIAGNOSTIC CRITERIA

Infants with AP window usually develop symptoms and signs of congestive heart failure early in life, and their presentation is similar to that of infants with large VSD (see Chapter 20, "Clinical Features" in Section 1). Thus, they generally are small, underdeveloped, tachypneic infants who tend to have repeated respiratory infections.

On examination, the left precordium is prominent because of marked cardiomegaly. The second heart sound at the base is usually accentuated. The murmur is usually only systolic and of variable intensity.[D1,M2,N1] In about 15% of patients it is continuous,[M2,N1] in which event the AP window is smaller and the pulmonary hypertension less than usual. When the left-to-right shunt through the defect is large, there are peripheral signs of a rapid aortic runoff, such as jerky or collapsing peripheral pulses, but these signs are not evident when heart failure is marked or pulmonary vascular resistance is severely elevated.

The chest x-ray and electrocardiogram are similar to those of infants and young children with VSD or large patent ductus arteriosus, giving evidence of left and right ventricular enlargement and large pulmonary blood flow.[B1] Left atrial enlargement (as a result of the large pulmonary blood flow) is usually prominent.

The differential diagnoses before special study include large patent ductus arteriosus, truncus arteriosus, and in patients beyond the infant age group, VSD with aortic incompetence and ruptured aneurysm of the sinus of Valsalva.

The diagnosis can be made using two-dimensional echocardiography,[S2] but cardiac catheterization and cineangiography currently provide the definitive diagnosis and identify associated cardiac anomalies. Blood oxygen saturation in the pulmonary artery is elevated over that in the right ventricle and right atrium in most cases. Occasionally, blood oxygen saturation in right ventricle is increased over that in

right atrium, which may suggest VSD or truncus arteriosus until cineangiography shows this to be from pulmonary valve incompetence associated with AP window. The definitive study is ascending aortic angiography, which shows rapid filling of the pulmonary artery through the AP window, and separate aortic and pulmonary valves. Because of the variability in location of the AP window and because coronary arteries may arise from the pulmonary artery, the angiographic visualization of all defects must be precise.

NATURAL HISTORY

Aortopulmonary window is a rare malformation. For example, at the Hospital for Sick Children in Toronto, only 23 (0.15%) of the 15,104 patients with congenital heart disease seen over a 20-year period had AP window.[R1]

There is no known tendency for AP windows to close spontaneously. The natural history of infants with large AP windows is at least as unfavorable as that of infants with persistently large VSDs. In fact, patients with large AP windows are rarely seen in childhood or adult life, and those who do survive beyond early life have important pulmonary vascular disease.[M1] This natural history is, therefore, similar to that of surgically untreated older patients with large VSD (see Chapter 20).

TECHNIQUE OF OPERATION

After proper preparation (Chapters 2 and 4), a median sternotomy incision is made and pericardial stay sutures applied. A left atrial monitoring line may be inserted at this time (UAB) or, alternatively, after the repair (GLH). The diagnosis can usually be verified at operation from outside the heart. The first portion of the aorta and pulmonary artery form a large confluence at the level of the AP window, which suggests truncus arteriosus. However, separate semilunar valve rings can usually be verified by the finding of a dimple between the two great arteries where they arise from the heart. Even in very young infants, the left ventricle is enlarged, usually about grade 3 (1–6), as are the left atrium and right ventricle. In older children, the ventricular enlargement and hypertrophy are grotesquely severe.

The operation may be done with cardiopulmonary bypass (CPB) unless the infant weighs less than about 2.5 kg (see Chapter 2, Section 3), in which case it would be done with profoundly hypothermic total circulatory arrest (UAB); or profoundly hypothermic total circulatory arrest may be used as a routine in infants weighing less than 8 kg (GLH) (see Chapter 2, Section 4). For CPB, particular care must be taken in selecting the site for aortic cannulation. In order to have room for the aortic cross-clamp between the AP window and the aortic cannula, the latter must be as far downstream as possible. Also, before establishing CPB, a narrow dissection is made between aorta and pulmonary artery, downstream to the AP window but still proximal to the aortic cannulation site. Care is taken to identify and protect the right pulmonary artery during this dissection and during placement of the aortic cross clamp. A single venous cannula may be used; or the cavae may be cannulated directly, the

Table 29-1 Hospital mortality after repair of AP window (UAB; 1967–July 1, 1983).

Age (mo) ≤	<	n	Hospital Deaths No.	%	CL
	3	2		0%	
3 ---	6	5		0%	
6 ---	12	1		0%	
12 ---	24	1		0%	
24 ---	48	1		o%	
48		—		0%	
Total		10 .		0%	0%–17%

KEY: CL, 70% confidence limits.

NOTE: In addition, an AP window was repaired along with tetralogy of Fallot in a 26-month-old infant, who lived.[C1] One patient 5 years of age died at reoperation for recurrence of an AP window after attempted closure elsewhere.

right atrium opened, and a pump oxygenator sump sucker placed across the foramen ovale into left atrium (see Chapter 2, Section 3).

When profoundly hypothermic total circulatory arrest is used, the arterial cannula is inserted proximal to the site of cross-clamping (GLH; see Chapter 2, Section 4). Surface cooling to low temperature has a particular advantage in conditions such as this in which there is severe aortic runoff, since when the chest is opened the arterial pressure is low so that aortic cannulation and dissection are simplified and there is no danger of overdistention of the pulmonary vascular bed.

With either technique, as soon as CPB has been initiated and core cooling begun, a side-biting clamp (such as a Satinsky clamp or small Cooley clamp) is placed across the window from the pulmonary artery side to occlude it. The aortic cross-clamp is positioned exactly at the place provided by the prior dissection. The cold cardioplegic solution is injected into the ascending aorta unless total circulatory arrest is to be used (GLH; see Chapter 3). When the repair is to be done during CPB, the perfusate temperature is stabilized at 25°C.

The aorta is opened, usually transversely, at the level of the AP window. The ostium of the left coronary artery, often close to the window, is noted. Small or moderate-sized AP windows may be closed transversely by direct suture, using one or two rows of continuous 4-0 polypropylene sutures. A large window is closed with a patch of Dacron or pericardium sewn into place with continuous 4-0 polypropylene sutures. The aortotomy incision is then closed with one row of continuous polypropylene sutures. The remainder of the operation, including the de-airing procedure and rewarming where circulatory arrest has been used, is carried out as usual (see Chapter 2).

In the event that the AP window involves the front wall of the proximal right pulmonary artery, the approach may be best made through a vertical aortotomy and the defect closed with a teardrop-shaped patch that extends out along the right pulmonary artery.

SPECIAL FEATURES OF POSTOPERATIVE CARE

The postoperative care is usual, as described in Chapter 5. The hemodynamic state is generally excellent because the left ventricle is large, no ventriculotomy has been made, and the operation is short.

EARLY RESULTS

The *hospital mortality* is low after the repair of AP window unless unusual circumstances are present, no deaths having occurred among 12 patients (UAB and GLH) undergoing primary repair (Tables 29-1, 29-2). Even when major associated lesions coexist, the risk of total repair may also be low.[C1,C3]

One patient first seen with recurrent AP window and severe pectus excavatum died of hemorrhage at the secondary sternotomy in 1971 (UAB). Another patient undergoing reoperation died from low cardiac output related to severe pulmonary vascular disease (GLH).

Table 29-2 Results of surgical treatment of AP window (GLH; 1958–1983).

Year of Operation	Age at Operation	Associated Anomalies	Operation	Outcome
1961	8 yr	Subaortic stenosis	CPB; AP window closed via MPA Excision subaortic membrane	Hospital death grade 4 PVD[a]
1961	4 yr		AP window divided (no CPB)	Excellent
1968	6 mo	Moderate VSD	AP window suture closure (no CPB)	Closure incomplete PVR 17 units • m² at restudy
1976	6 mo		PH-CA AP window closed via aorta	Excellent

KEY: CPB, cardiopulmonary bypass; MPA, main pulmonary artery; PH-CA, profound hypothermia circulatory arrest; PVD, pulmonary vascular disease; PVR, pulmonary vascular resistance; VSD, ventricular septal defect.

NOTE: In addition, AP window has been diagnosed at autopsy in three neonates, two with interrupted aortic arch (one with a ventricular septal defect also) and one with atresia of the aortic isthmus.

[a] Heath Edwards classification.

Among the 11 patients (10 isolated, one with tetralogy of Fallot) operated upon (UAB), the transaortic approach was used in 10 and the transpulmonary in 1; suture closure was done in 6 and patch closure in 5.

LATE RESULTS

The late results are excellent when the operation is performed in infancy. There have been no late deaths among the patients operated on. One patient, whose AP window seemed to be an isolated lesion when it was repaired at age 18 months, at age 9 was successfully reoperated upon for supravalvar and subvalvar aortic stenosis and valvar and subvalvar pulmonary stenosis (UAB).

In those rare circumstances in which repair of a large AP window is done in older children, the late result may be compromised by pulmonary vascular disease. The probability of "surgical cure" will be dependent upon age at operation and level of pulmonary vascular resistance at the time of operation (see Chapter 20, Figs. 20-35 through 20-39).

INDICATIONS FOR OPERATION

Symptomatic infants with AP window should be operated on promptly when the diagnosis is made. Electively, repair is advised at 3 months of age.

Older children should be operated on unless high pulmonary vascular resistance renders them inoperable. The criteria of operability described for patients with VSD are directly applicable to those with large AP windows (see Chapter 20, Section 1, "Indications for Operation").

SPECIAL SITUATIONS AND CONTROVERSIES

Diagnosis

When AP window coexists with other malformations, the diagnosis may be difficult. This is because of the hemodynamic similarity, for example, between AP window with VSD and truncus arteriosus.

Patch Closure versus Direct Suture

Clarke and colleagues have stated that patch closure is preferable to direct suture.[C3] Narrowing of the aorta or pulmonary artery has not resulted from transverse direct closure (UAB).

Alternative Surgical Technique

Recently, a somewhat different technique of repair has been reported by Johansson and colleagues.[J1] A vertical incision is made in the anterior wall of the AP window itself, more or less transecting its anterior one-half. After carefully identifying the orifice of the right pulmonary artery and the left coronary artery, the patch for closure is sutured to the posterior, superior, and inferior walls of the window. The incision into the window is then closed by incorporating the front edge of the patch, with each stitch passing through the aortic wall, the patch, and the pulmonary artery wall. This technique allows visualization of the left coronary ostium and orifice of the right pulmonary artery and provides a secure partitioning of the ascending aorta from pulmonary artery. Unless there is aneurysmal thinning of the window, this technique seems ideal and is recommended.

A modification of this technique is required when the right coronary artery arises from the pulmonary trunk just to the left of the anterior wall of the AP window. Then the anterior incision into the window curves to the left into the pulmonary trunk to create a flap of anterior pulmonary artery wall that includes the origin of the right coronary artery. The flap should be large enough to cover the entire window.[L1] It is sewn into position over the window with a continuous polypropylene stitch. The repair is completed by closing the deficiency in the pulmonary artery with a pericardial patch.

Surgical Treatment when Associated Lesions Are Present

Patients with AP window and associated cardiac malformations can undergo successful surgical correction. Their management must be individualized. Examples are AP window associated with tetralogy of Fallot,[C1,C3] anomalous origin of right pulmonary artery from aorta,[G2] and transposition of the great arteries.[V1] A special problem is the coexistence of AP window, aortic isthmic hypoplasia or interrupted arch, and patent ductus arteriosus (see "Morphology"). Neonates with this anomaly usually are critically ill, and under these circumstances a two-staged procedure may be advisable. At the first stage, the interrupted arch is repaired (see Chapter 34) and partial closure of the AP window is obtained by a plication technique; 6 months or so later, the AP window is closed definitively by standard methods.[T2]

REFERENCES

B

1. Blieden LC, Moller JH: Aorticopulmonary septal defect. An experience with 17 patients. *Br Heart J* 36:630, 1974.
2. Berry TE, Bharati S, Muster AJ, Idriss FS, Santucci B, Lev M, Paul MH: Distal aortopulmonary septal defect, aortic origin of the right pulmonary artery, intact ventricular septum, patent ductus arteriosus and hypoplasia of the aortic isthmus: A newly recognized syndrome. *Am J Cardiol* 49:108, 1982.
3. Burroughs JT, Schumutzer KJ, Linder F, Neuhans G: Anomalous origin of the right coronary artery with aortico-pulmonary window and ventricular septal defect. *J Cardiovasc Surg* 3:142, 1968.
4. Bjork VO: (1964) Personal communication.

C

1. Castaneda AR, Kirklin JW: Tetralogy of Fallot with aorticopulmonary window. Report of two surgical cases. *J Thorac Cardiovasc Surg* 74:467, 1977.

2. Cooley DA, McNamara DG, Latson JR: Aorticopulmonary septal defect: Diagnosis and surgical treatment. *Surgery* 42:101, 1957.

3. Clarke CP, Richardson JP: The management of aorticopulmonary window. Advantages of transaortic closure with a Dacron patch. *J Thorac Cardiovasc Surg* 72:48, 1976.

4. Coleman EN, Barclay RS, Reid JM, Stevenson JG: Congenital aortopulmonary fistula combined with persistent ductus arteriosus. *Br Heart J* 29:571, 1967.

5. Chiemmongkoltip P, Moulder PV, Cassels DE: Interruption of the aortic arch with aorticopulmonary septal defect and intact ventricular septum in a teenage girl. *Chest* 60:324, 1971.

6. Cotton AC: Report of a case of anuria. *Arch Pediatr* 16:774, 1899.

D

1. Deverall PB, Lincoln JCR, Aberdeen E, Bonham-Carter RE, Waterston DJ: Aortopulmonary window. *J Thorac Cardiovasc Surg* 57:479, 1969.

2. Doty DB, Richardson JV, Falkovsky GE, Gordonova MI, Burakovsky VI: Aortopulmonary septal defect: Hemodynamics, angiography, and operation. *Ann Thorac Surg* 32:244, 1981.

3. Dodds JH, Hoyle C: Congenital aortic septal defect. *Br Heart J* 11:390, 1949.

E

1. Elliotson J: Case of malformation of the pulmonary artery and aorta. *Lancet* 1:247, 1830.

F

1. Fletcher G, DuShane JW, Kirklin JW, Wood EH: Aorticopulmonary septal defect. Report of a case with surgical division along with successful resuscitation from ventricular fibrillation. *Mayo Clin Proc* 29:285, 1954.

2. Faulkner SL, Oldham RR, Atwood GF, Graham TP: Aortopulmonary window, ventricular septal defect, and membranous pulmonary atresia with a diagnosis of truncus arteriosus. *Chest* 65:3, 1974.

G

1. Gross RE: Surgical closure of an aortic septal defect. *Circulation* 5:858, 1952.

2. Gula G, Chew C, Radley-Smith R, Yacoub M: Anomalous origin of the right pulmonary artery from the ascending aorta associated with aortopulmonary window. *Thorax* 33:265, 1978.

3. Gasul BM, Fell EH, Casas R: The diagnosis of aortic septal defect by retrograde aortography: Report of a case. *Circulation* 4:251, 1951.

J

1. Johansson L, Michaelsson M, Westerholm CJ, Abert T: Aortopulmonary window: A new operative approach. *Ann Thorac Surg* 25:564, 1978.

2. Jacobson JG, Trusler GA, Izukawa T: Repair of interrupted aortic arch and aortopulmonary window in an infant. *Ann Thorac Surg* 28:290, 1979.

L

1. Luisi SV, Ashraf MH, Gula G, Radley-Smith R, Yacoub M: Anomalous origin of the right coronary artery with aortopulmonary window: Functional and surgical considerations. *Thorax* 35:446, 1980.

M

1. Meisner H, Schmidt-Habelmann P, Sebening F, Klinner W: Surgical correction of aorto-pulmonary septal defects. A review of the literature and report of eight cases. *Dis Chest* 53:750, 1968.

2. Morrow AG, Greenfield LJ, Braunwald E: Congenital aortopulmonary septal defect. Clinical and hemodynamic findings, surgical technique, and results of operative correction. *Circulation* 25:463, 1962.

3. Mori K, Ando M, Takao A, Ishikawa S, Imai Y: Distal type of aortopulmonary window. Report of 4 cases. *Br Heart J* 40:681, 1978.

N

1. Neufeld HN, Lester RG, Adams P Jr, Anderson RC, Lillehei CW, Edwards JE: Aorticopulmonary septal defect. *Am J Cardiol* 9:12, 1962.

P

1. Putnam TC, Gross RE: Surgical management of aortopulmonary fenestration. *Surgery* 59:727, 1966.

R

1. Rowe RD: Aortopulmonary septal defect, in JD Keith, RD Rowe, P Vlad (eds): *Heart Disease in Infancy and Childhood* (ed 3). New York: Macmillan, 1978.

2. Richardson JV, Doty DB, Rossi NP, Ehrenhaft JL: The spectrum of anomalies of aortopulmonary septation. *J Thorac Cardiovasc Surg* 78:21, 1979.

S

1. Scott HW Jr, Sabiston DC Jr: Surgical treatment for congenital aorticopulmonary fistula. Experimental and clinical aspects. *J Thorac Surg* 25:26, 1953.

2. Satomi G, Kakamus K, Imai Y, Takao A: Two-dimensional echocardiographic diagnosis of aorticopulmonary window. *Br Heart J* 43:351, 1980.

T

1. Tandon R, DaSilva CL, Moller JH, Edwards JE: Aorticopulmonary septal defect coexisting with ventricular septal defect. *Circulation* 50:188, 1974.

2. Tabak C, Moskowitz W, Wagner H, Weinberg P, Edmunds LH Jr: Aortopulmonary window and aortic isthmic hypoplasia. *J Thorac Cardiovasc Surg* 86:273, 1983.

V

1. Vanini V: (1980) Personal communication.

W

1. Wright JS, Freeman R, Johnston JB: Aortopulmonary fenestration. A technique of surgical management. *J Thorac Cardiovasc Surg* 55:280, 1968.

30

ORIGIN OF THE RIGHT OR LEFT PULMONARY ARTERY FROM THE ASCENDING AORTA

DEFINITION

In patients with origin of the right or left pulmonary artery from the ascending aorta, the right pulmonary artery or, much less commonly, the left pulmonary artery arises from the *ascending* aorta in the presence of separate aortic and pulmonary valves and without the interposition of ductal tissue. Rarely, both right and left pulmonary arteries arise from the ascending aorta in the presence of two separate semilunar valves.

Origins of one or both pulmonary arteries from the transverse aortic arch via a ductus arteriosus or collateral arteries and from the descending thoracic aorta via collateral arteries are not included. These conditions are almost always part of the tetralogy of Fallot and are discussed in Chapter 23. When both right and left pulmonary arteries arise from the ascending aorta with a common semilunar valve, the condition is truncus arteriosus, which is discussed in Chapter 28.

HISTORICAL NOTE

Apparently, the first description of this entity was by Fraentzel,[F1] who in 1868 reported the case of a 25-year-old woman dying in congestive heart failure with the right pulmonary artery (RPA) arising from the ascending aorta and an aortopulmonary (AP) window. Doering reported aortic origin of the RPA in an infant dying at age 8 months, whose only associated anomaly was a patent ductus arteriosus.[D1] Bopp, in 1949, gave a detailed report of this condition,[B1] and since

then and with the development of cardiac catheterization and angiocardiography other cases have been reported.

Caro and colleagues, in 1957, corrected the malformation by disconnecting the RPA from the ascending aorta and connecting it with an interposition graft to the main pulmonary artery.[C1] The patient, a 23-year-old man, died a short time after operation. The first successful repair, which was in a 12-month-old infant, was reported by Armer, Shumacker, and Klatte in 1961.[A1] They interposed a graft between the pulmonary trunk and the distal end of the divided RPA and closed a coexisting patent ductus arteriosus. Kirkpatrick and colleagues, in 1967, reported the first successful cases of retroaortic direct anastomosis of the divided RPA to the pulmonary trunk.[K1]

The first report of successful surgical treatment of aortic origin of the *left* pulmonary artery (LPA), which was in a 6-week-old child, was by Herbert and colleagues in 1973.[H1]

MORPHOLOGY

The *right pulmonary artery* (RPA) usually arises from the right or posterior aspect of the ascending aorta in this condition, but occasionally it arises from the leftward posterior aspect.[C6] Its origin is within 1–3 cm of the aortic valve.[B4,G1,K2,W1,W3] The RPA origin is rarely stenosed, and the vessel is usually as large or larger than the normally connected LPA[G1,K2] and is normal as regards its structure, course, and distribution.

When the RPA arises anomalously from the ascending aorta and no other anomalies are present, the pulmonary vascular beds of the two lungs may be similar despite the differences in the origin of the pulmonary arteries.[C2,H1,M1,P1,R1,R2] Surprisingly, Keane and colleagues report no significant obstructive vascular changes in either lung in the majority of patients dying in the first 6 months of life.[K3] Among older patients, hypertensive pulmonary vascular disease is usually present, often to a similar extent in the two lungs, sometimes greater in the right lung, and sometimes greater in the left.

Occasionally, the *pulmonary* and *tricuspid* valves are dilated secondary to right heart failure, and the tricuspid leaflets may be thickened and the edges rolled.[G1]

Aortic origin of the RPA is an isolated lesion in about 20% of cases.[C6,R4] In the remainder, the most common coexisting lesion is patent ductus arteriosus, which is present in about 50% of cases.[C6,P3] Other much less common associations are with tetralogy of Fallot,[C3,C6,K4,M2] ventricular septal defect,[F2,M4] aortopulmonary window[G2] (see Chapter 29), coarctation of the aorta, interrupted aortic arch, and atrial septal defect.

Severe contralateral (left) *pulmonary vein stenosis* coexisted with aortic origin of the RPA in two out of four cases (UAB). The stenoses were typically tubular, and there was dilation of the left pulmonary veins proximal to the stenoses. Also, Sievers and colleagues report anomalous origin of the right pulmonary artery coexisting with subtotal obstruction of the left pulmonary vein orifices by a membrane which could be excised at operation.[S5]

Origin of the *left pulmonary artery* (LPA) from the ascending aorta is an even more rare condition,[C2,H1,R5,S2] and when it occurs as an isolated lesion it may be limited to patients with right aortic arch. It occurs as an isolated lesion in about 40% of cases;[C6] and in contrast to aortic origin of the RPA, the most common associated anomaly is tetralogy of Fallot.[P3] Then the aortic arch may be left sided.[C6,R5] Two cases had tetralogy of Fallot with absent pulmonary valve syndrome (GLH)[C6] (Fig. 30-1).

Origin of *both RPA and LPA from the ascending aorta* has been reported in one patient[B2] who had no other cardiac anomaly. The origin was by way of a short single trunk coming off the posterior aspect of the ascending aorta, with the main pulmonary artery arising normally from the right ventricle and connected only to a patent ductus arteriosus. Operation was attempted unsuccessfully at 11 days of age.

CLINICAL FEATURES AND DIAGNOSTIC CRITERIA

When the condition is isolated except for a patent ductus arteriosus, the patient characteristically presents early in infancy with respiratory distress and congestive heart failure.[C2,G1,K1,K3,O1,R3,S1] The infant is frequently acutely ill. There may be cyanosis due either to venous admixture in the lungs or to reversed shunting through a patent foramen ovale secondary to right heart failure or through a patent ductus arteriosus.

There are no typical auscultatory findings, and murmurs may or may not be present.[C4,G1,K3,O1,S1] When present, the

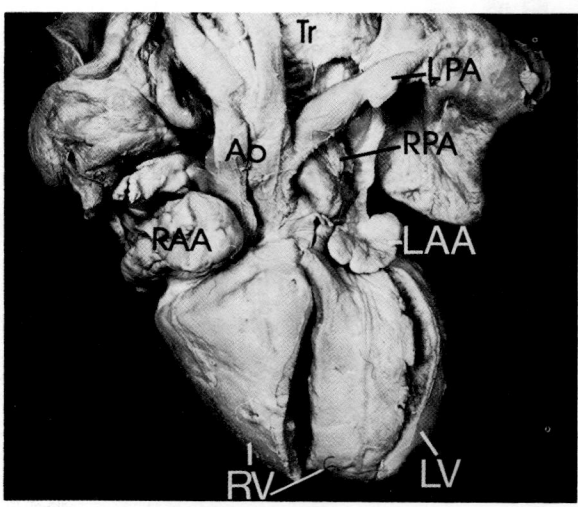

Figure 30-1 Heart specimen from 1-month-old infant viewed from in front (GLH). The left pulmonary artery arises from the ascending aorta and crosses in front of the dilated right pulmonary artery that arises normally from the main pulmonary artery. This infant had tetralogy of Fallot with absent pulmonary valve and pulmonary incompetence.

Ao, aorta; *LAA,* left atrial appendage; *LPA,* left pulmonary artery; *LV,* left ventricle; *RAA,* right atrial appendage; *RPA,* right pulmonary artery; *RV,* right ventricle; *Tr,* trachea.

Reproduced with permission from Calder et al.[C6]

murmur is usually systolic and heard along the left sternal border. Rarely, it may be continuous due to kinking or stenosis of the artery. The peripheral pulses are jerky or bounding secondary to the rapid runoff from the aorta into the lung and the consequent left-to-right shunting.

The electrocardiographic findings are not diagnostic and usually indicate biventricular and right atrial enlargement. Cardiomegaly is usually severe on the chest x-ray, with the heart assuming a globular shape.[G1,W1] Pulmonary plethora is usually of similar degree bilaterally.[C2,K2,S1]

When tetralogy of Fallot is present with severe pulmonary stenosis, the clinical features are dominated by the tetralogy. The condition may be suspected, however, because the lung supplied by the anomalously arising artery is usually plethoric, whereas the other lung is oligemic.[C6,M2,R5]

The diagnosis can be made by two-dimensional echocardiography.[D2,K7] However, cardiac catheterization and cineangiography provide additional information. The pressure in the pulmonary artery arising from the aorta is systemic in almost all cases since ostial stenosis is rare.[S1] As has already been indicated, pressure in the pulmonary artery that arises normally is usually also elevated to systemic or suprasystemic levels.[S4] The precise measurement of pulmonary and systemic blood flows is difficult in this situation, but it is not critical since the infants usually present with clear clinical evidence of increased pulmonary blood flow. The pulmonary vascular resistance in the normally connected lung can be readily calculated and is a useful guide to operability and an essential one in older patients. Cineangiography is diagnostic, and a right ventriculogram or pulmonary arteriogram opacifies only the normally connected pul-

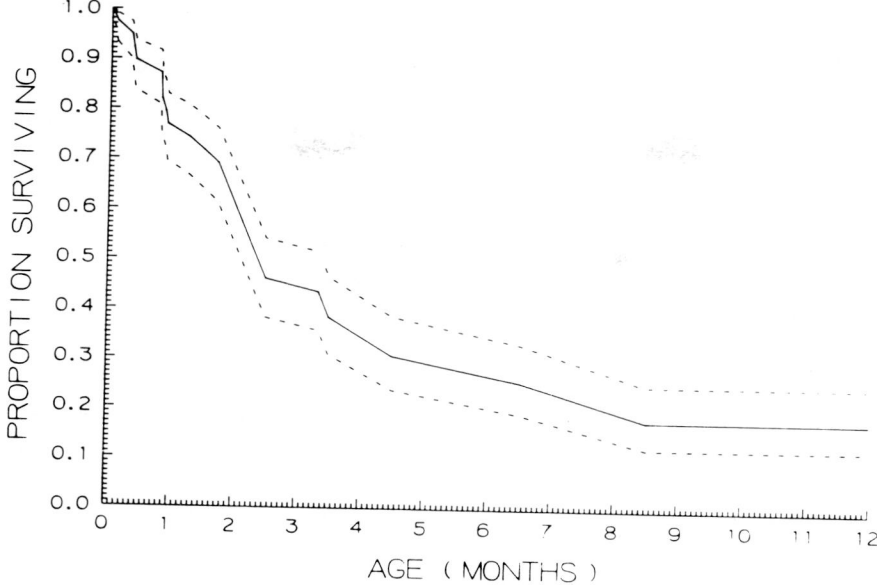

Figure 30-2 Natural history of isolated aortic origin of right pulmonary artery, with or without patent ductus arteriosus, *n* = 39. Autopsied nonsurgical cases reported in the literature[B1,C5,D1,F2,G1,K2, K3,K5,K6,K8,K9,M3,O1,P1,R1,S1,S3,T1,T2,V1,V2,W1] have been tabulated and an actuarial analysis made of the proportion alive (vertical axis) at any stated age (horizontal axis).[W2] Some cases and reports may be missing from this analysis, but the general shape of the relationship is probably correct.

monary arteries. Antegrade or retrograde aortography visualizes the pulmonary artery that arises from the ascending aorta. Cineangiography is also used to define other cardiac anomalies that may be present.[G1,R1]

NATURAL HISTORY

This anomaly is rare, only 56 cases being reported by 1980; by far, the majority involved the right pulmonary artery.[C6,P3]

Anomalous origin of the RPA from the ascending aorta is a lethal condition. Wideman and colleagues found reports in the literature of 39 unoperated patients, among whom patent ductus arteriosus was present in 26 (67%).[W2] Actuarial analysis indicates that about 70% of surgically untreated patients born with this condition are dead by 6 months of age and 80% are dead by 1 year (Fig. 30-2). Intractable heart failure is the usual mode of death.

Those patients living beyond the first few months of life develop pulmonary hypertension in both the right lung and the normally connected left lung. The development of pulmonary hypertension and pulmonary vascular disease in the normally connected left lung is related to the observation of Pool and colleagues that 19% of infants born with unilateral absence of a pulmonary artery and no associated malformations develop pulmonary hypertension[P2] and to the observation of these workers that ligation of one pulmonary artery within 24 hours of birth in 5 calves resulted in severe pulmonary hypertension in the opposite lung within 2 months.

It is likely that the natural history of origin of the LPA

from the ascending aorta is similar, but too few patients have been observed to establish this.

TECHNIQUE OF OPERATION

The preparations for operation, median sternotomy incision, and preparation for cardiopulmonary bypass (CPB) are those normally used (see Chapter 2). In infants smaller than about 2.5 kg, profound hypothermia and total circulatory arrest are used (see Chapter 2, Section 4). For infants larger than about 2.5 kg, CPB with two venous cannulae may be used (UAB) (see Chapter 2, Section 3) or, alternatively, the technique of profound hypothermia and total circulatory arrest is used in infants up to about 8 kg in weight (GLH). The procedure is described for anomalously arising RPA; it is similar when the LPA is affected.

Once the pericardium has been opened, the anomalously originating RPA is visualized coming from either the posterior or right lateral aspect of the ascending aorta. It passes into the right hemithorax beneath the superior vena cava.

The aorta is completely dissected from the main pulmonary artery, and if convenient the ductus arteriosus may be dissected out at this point or after establishing CPB (see Chapter 20, Fig. 20-28). The purse-string sutures and preparation for CPB are made as usual, except that care is taken to place the aortic purse string suture and the aortic cannula far enough downstream so that the cross-clamp can be placed distal to the aortic origin of the RPA.

CPB is established as usual, and as soon as it has begun a

temporary arterial clamp is placed across the RPA. The ligamentum arteriosum or ductus arteriosum is dissected out and ligated. The perfusate may now be made as cold as possible, the aorta cross-clamped well distal to the RPA, and the cold cardioplegic infusion given. (If the repair is made during total circulatory arrest, the cardioplegic infusion is omitted [GLH]). The right atrium is opened through a small incision, and a pump oxygenator sump sucker placed across the naturally occurring or surgically created foramen ovale since the collateral circulation is usually large.

The clamp is now removed from the RPA, which has been thoroughly mobilized beneath the superior vena cava either before CPB or just after establishing it. The pulmonary artery is then disconnected from the ascending aorta. The defect left in the ascending aorta may be closed transversely by direct suture, but in one case this narrowed the aorta to such an extent that it had to be taken down and a patch graft used for closure (UAB). Thus, if there is any uncertainty on this point, a piece of pericardium is sewn into the defect to close the aortic aperture.

The aorta is now rotated up anteriorly and leftward and the right side of the main pulmonary artery pulled out from beneath it. A longitudinal incision is made in this and an end-to-side anastomosis made between the well mobilized RPA and the side of the main pulmonary artery. A 6-0 polypropylene suture can conveniently be used to make the posterior suture line, sewing from within the vessels and carrying this suture line around anteriorly to complete the repair.

Rewarming is begun, the sump sucker removed from the foramen ovale, the foramen ovale closed, and the right atrium closed. Suction may be placed upon the cardioplegic needle if left ventricular distention occurs from the large aortopulmonary collateral flow. Air is aspirated from the apex of the left ventricle, and with strong suction on the aortic needle vent the aortic clamp is released. After an effective cardiac action has returned, the usual de-airing procedures are carried out (see Chapter 2). After rewarming is complete, CPB is discontinued and the remainder of the procedure completed as usual.

It is advisable to place not only the usual left and right atrial pressure catheters but also to insert an additional catheter into the lower right ventricle and pass it to the main pulmonary artery for the monitoring of pulmonary artery pressure for the first 24 postoperative hours.

SPECIAL FEATURES OF POSTOPERATIVE CARE

The management usually given to infants after open intracardiac surgery, described in Chapter 5, is used. In some cases, pulmonary pressure is severely elevated and cardiac output reduced early postoperatively, and special methods of management of the infant are indicated (see Chapter 5, ''Low Cardiac Output'' in Section 2, Cardiovascular Subsystem).

EARLY RESULTS

When origin of RPA or LPA from ascending aorta is an isolated condition (apart from patent ductus arteriosus), operation can be a low-risk procedure even in very small infants (Table 30-1). This is confirmed by the Boston Children's Hospital experience with three infants aged 15, 18, and 56 days who have survived repair.[P3]

When there are important associated anomalies, such as

Table 30-1 Outcome in 7 infants with anomalous origin of right or left pulmonary arteries from the ascending aorta. (UAB; 1967–1980 and GLH; 1960–1980. The GLH patients have been reported in detail by Calder and colleagues.[C6])

Age (mo)	Institution	Anomalous Vessel	Associated Lesions	Surgical Procedure	Result
3	UAB	RPA	PDA	Closure PDA Anast RPA to MPA	Excellent
12	UAB	RPA	PDA	Closure PDA; anast RPA to MPA	Excellent
3/4	UAB	RPA	LPV Stenosis	Anast RPA to MPA	Died
3	UAB	RPA	LPV Stenosis	Anast RPA to MPA	Died
1	GLH	LPA	TF (absent pulm. valve syndrome)	None	Died
8	GLH	LPA	TF (absent pulm. valve syndrome)	None	Died
4	GLH	RPA	TF (absent pulm. valve syndrome)	Repair tetralogy (valved homograft conduit) anast RPA to MPA	Died

KEY: LPA, left pulmonary artery; LPV, left pulmonary vein; MPA, main pulmonary artery; PDA, patent ductus arteriosus; RPA, right pulmonary artery; TF, tetralogy of Fallot.

tetralogy of Fallot with absence of the pulmonary valve or pulmonary vein stenosis, the results have in the past been less good (Table 30-1). These may improve as techniques for managing coexisting lesions improve.

LATE RESULTS

Survivors of repair of isolated aortic origin of RPA in infancy, with or without patent ductus arteriosus, have generally done well and have normal pulmonary artery pressure late postoperatively and presumably a normal life expectancy.[B3,K3,P3] Thus, both infants surviving operation (Table 30-1) are well (UAB). One was catheterized 5 years postoperatively and had normal right ventricular and pulmonary artery pressures and a small gradient between main pulmonary artery (26/15 mmHg) and RPA (13/9). At least an intermediate term good result can be obtained even in some older patients, Juca and colleagues reporting a satisfactory fall in right and left pulmonary artery pressure in a patient who was 20 years of age at operation.

INDICATIONS FOR OPERATION

The diagnosis of aortic origin of the right or left pulmonary artery from ascending aorta in infancy is an indication for urgent operation. This is true regardless of the pulmonary vascular resistance in the two lungs, since at least in infants operated upon under 12 months of age, these changes are almost always reversible. In those rare examples of presentation beyond infancy, excessive elevation of pulmonary vascular resistance in the normally connected lung is a contraindication to operation.[P3] Unfortunately, the experience is inadequate to allow a confident statement of the exact level of pulmonary vascular resistance in the normally connected lung that makes the patient inoperable; it may be in the vicinity of 20 units $\cdot$ m^2.

REFERENCES

A

1. Armer RM, Shumacker HB, Klatte EC: Origin of right pulmonary artery from the aorta: Report of a surgically corrected case. *Circulation* 24:662, 1961.

B

1. Bopp VF: Anormale arterielle Gefassversorgung der Rechten Lunge. *Zentralbl Allg Pathol* 85:155, 1949.
2. Beitzke A, Shinebourne EA: Single origin of right and left pulmonary arteries from ascending aorta, with main pulmonary artery from right ventricle. *Br Heart J* 43:363, 1980.
3. Binet JP, Ribierre M, Daggonet Y, Le Loch H, Loth P, Planch CL, Lortat-Jacob S: Artere pulmonaire droite naissant de l'aorte ascendante. *Arch Mal Coeur* 68:415, 1975.
4. Björk VO, Rudhe U, Zetterqvist P: Aortic origin of the right pulmonary artery and wide patent ductus arteriosus. *Scand J Thor Cardiovasc Surg* 4:87, 1970.

C

1. Caro C, Lermanda VC, Lyons HA: Aortic origin of right pulmonary artery. *Br Heart J* 19:345, 1957.
2. Caudill DR, Helmsworth JA, Daoud G, Kaplan S: Anomalous origin of left pulmonary artery from ascending aorta. *J Thorac Cardiovasc Surg* 57:493, 1969.
3. Czarnecki SW, Hopeman AR, Child PL: Tetralogy of Fallot with aortic origin of the left pulmonary artery: Radiographic and angiocardiographic considerations. *Dis Chest* 46:97, 1964.
4. Cumming GR, Ferguson CC, Sanchez J: Aortic origin of the right pulmonary artery. *Am J Cardiol* 30:674, 1972.
5. Calazel P, Martinez J: Naissance anormale à partir de l'aorta ascendante de l'une des deux arteres pulmonaires. *Arch Mal Coeur* 68:397, 1975.
6. Calder AL, Barndt PWT, Barratt-Boyes BG, Neutze JM: Variants of tetralogy of Fallot with absent pulmonary valve leaflets and origin of one pulmonary artery from the ascending aorta. *Am J Cardiol* 46:106, 1980.

D

1. Doering H: Angeborener defekt der rechten lungenarterie. *Stud Pathol Entwick* 2:41, 1914.
2. Duncan WJ, Freedom RM, Olley PM, Rowe RD: Two dimensional echocardiographic identification of hemitruncus: Anomalous origin of one pulmonary artery from ascending aorta with the other pulmonary artery arising normally from the right ventricle. *Am Heart J* 102:892, 1981.

F

1. Fraentzel O: Ein fall von abnormer communication der aorta mit der arteria pulmonalis. *Virchows Arch [Pathol Anat]* 43:420, 1868.
2. Findlay CW, Maier HC: Anomalies of the pulmonary vessels and their surgical significance: With a review of the literature. *Surgery* 29:604, 1951.

G

1. Griffiths SP, Levine OR, Andersen DH: Aortic origin of right pulmonary artery. *Circulation* 25:73, 1962.
2. Gula G, Chew C, Radley-Smith R, Yacoub H: Anomalous origin of the right pulmonary artery from the ascending aorta associated with aortopulmonary window. *Thorax* 33:265, 1978.

H

1. Herbert WH, Hohman M, Farnsworth P, Swamy S: Anomalous origin of the left pulmonary artery from ascending aorta, right aortic arch, and right patent ductus arteriosus. *Chest* 63:459, 1973.

J

1. Jucá ER, Carvalho W Jr, deSousa JR, Araujo JA, Maia F, Karbage JM, Silva F: Origem anômala da artéria pulmonar direita na aorta ascendente. *Arq Bras Cardiol* 33:347, 1979.
2. Jucá ER: Origin of right pulmonary artery from ascending aorta (Letter to the Editor). *J Thorac Cardiovasc Surg* 88:458, 1984.

K

1. Kirkpatrick SE, Girod DA, King H: Aortic origin of the right pulmonary artery: Surgical repair without a graft. *Circulation* 36:777, 1967.

2. Kauffman SL, Yao AC, Webber CB, Lynfield J: Origin of the right pulmonary artery from the aorta: A clinical-pathologic study of two types based on caliber of the pulmonary artery. *Am J Cardiol* 19:741, 1967.

3. Keane JF, Maltz D, Bernhard WF, Corwin RD, Nadas AS: Anomalous origin of one pulmonary artery from the aorta: Diagnostic, physiologic and surgical considerations. *Circulation* 50:588, 1974.

4. Kuers PFW, McGoon DC: Tetralogy of Fallot with aortic origin of the right pulmonary artery. *J Thorac Cardiovasc Surg* 65:327, 1973.

5. Kuetel J, Kampmann A, Kyrieleis C: Abnormer Ursphrung der rechten lungernarterie aus der aszendierenden aorta. *Z Kardiol* 62:567, 1972.

6. Kleinschmidt HJ, Lignitz E: Ursphrung der rechten arteria pulmonalis aus der aorta ascendens. *Zentralbl Allg Pathol* 115:547, 1972.

7. King DH, Huhta JC, Gutgesell HP, Ott DA: Two-dimensional echocardiographic diagnosis of anomalous origin of the right pulmonary artery from the aorta: Differentiation from aortopulmonary window. *JACC* 4:351, 1984.

8. Kondo M, et al: Origin of the right pulmonary artery from the ascending aorta associated with patent left ductus arteriosus. *Resp Circ* 23:637, 1975.

9. Kadoma K, Sugiura S, Saito M, Takao T: Anomalous origin of right pulmonary artery from ascending aorta. *Heart* 3:786, 1971.

M

1. Mudd JG, Willman VL, Riberi A: Origin of one pulmonary artery from the aorta. *Am Rev Resp Dis* 89:255, 1964.

2. Morgan JR: Left pulmonary artery from ascending aorta in tetralogy of Fallot. *Circulation* 45:653, 1972.

3. Maier HC: Absence of hypoplasia of a pulmonary artery with anomalous systemic arteries to the lung. *J Thorac Surg* 28:145, 1954.

4. Morgan J, Pitman R, Goodwin JF, Steiner RE, Hollman A: Anomalies of the aorta and pulmonary arteries complicating ventricular septal defect. *Br Heart J* 24:279, 1964.

O

1. Odell JE, Smith JC: Right pulmonary artery arising from ascending aorta. *Am J Dis Child* 105:87, 1963.

P

1. Porter DD, Canent, Jr RV, Spach MS, Baylin GJ: Origin of the right pulmonary artery from the ascending aorta: Unusual cineangiocardiographic and pathologic findings. *Circulation* 27:589, 1963.

2. Pool PE, Averill KH, Vogel JHK: Effect of ligation of left pulmonary artery at birth on maturation of pulmonary vascular bed. *Med Thorac* 19:362, 1962.

3. Penkoske PA, Castaneda AR, Fyler DC, Van Praagh R: Origin of pulmonary artery branch from ascending aorta. *J Thorac Cardiovasc Surg* 85:537, 1983.

R

1. Rosenberg HS, Hallman GL, Wolfe RR, Latson JR: Origin of the right pulmonary artery from the aorta. *Am Heart J* 72:106, 1966.

2. Rosenburg HS, McNamara DG, Leachman RA, Buzzi RM: The pulmonary vascular structure of children with ventricular septal defect. *Arch Pathol* 70:141, 1960.

3. Redo SF, Foster Jr HR, Engle MA, Ehler KH: Anomalous origin of the right pulmonary artery from the ascending aorta. *J Thorac Cardiovasc Surg* 50:726, 1965.

4. Richardson JV, Doty DB, Rossi NP, Ehrenhaft JL: The spectrum of anomalies of aortopulmonary septation. *J Thorac Cardiovasc Surg* 78:21, 1979.

5. Robin E, Silberg B, Ganguley S, Magnisalis K: Aortic origin of the left pulmonary artery. Variant of tetralogy of Fallot. *Am J Cardiol* 35:324, 1975.

S

1. Stanton RE, Durnin RE, Fyler DC, Lindesmith GG, Meyer BW: Right pulmonary artery originating from ascending aorta. *Am J Dis Child* 115:403, 1968.

2. Schillar M, Williams TE Jr, Craenen J, Hosier DM, Sirak HD: Anomalous origin of the left pulmonary artery from the ascending aorta. *Vasc Surg* 5:126, 1971.

3. Sikl H: Neobvykla malformace arteriosniho trunku: Odstup jedne halvni vetve plicnice z aorty. *Cas Lek Cesk* 91:1366, 1952.

4. Semb BKH, Björnstad PG: Correction of isolated anomalous origin of the right pulmonary artery from the ascending aorta. *Thorac Cardiovasc Surg* 29:255, 1981.

5. Sievers HH, Lange PE, Radtcke W, Hahne HJ, Heintzen P, Bernhard A: Repair of anomalous origin of the right pulmonary artery from the ascending aorta associated with subtotal left cor triatriatum. *Ann Thor Surg* 39:80, 1985.

T

1. Turpin R, Cruveiller J, Bocquet L, Gorin R, Malafosse M: Artere pulmonaire droite branch de l'aorta ascendante (un cas d'hemitruncus). *Ann Pediatr (Par)* 9:429, 1962.

2. Tobise K, Kobayashi T, Tateda K, Kishi F, Onodera K: Origin of right pulmonary artery from ascending aorta. A case report. *Jpn J Intern Med* 62:154, 1973.

V

1. Vasquez-Perez J, Pereda-Perez A, Frontera-Izquierdo: Origin aortico de la arteria pulmonar derecha: A proposito de dos casos. *Am Esp Pediatr* 9:584, 1976.

2. Vasquez SF, Trevino CP, Angulo O: Naciemiento de arteria pulmonar derecha de la aorta y fibroelastosis endocardica derecha. *Arch Dis Cardiol Mex* 36:184, 1966.

W

1. Weintraub RA, Fabian CE, Adams DF: Ectopic origin of one pulmonary artery from ascending aorta. *Radiology* 86:666, 1966.

2. Wideman FE, Blackstone EH, Kirklin JW: Natural history of aortic origin of the right pulmonary artery (unpublished study, 1980).

3. Wagenvoort CA, Neufeld HN, Birge RF, Caffrey JA, Edwards JE: Origin of right pulmonary artery from ascending aorta. *Circulation* 23:84, 1961.

31

CONGENITAL ANOMALIES OF THE CORONARY ARTERIES

SECTION 1

CORONARY ARTERIOVENOUS FISTULA

DEFINITION

A congenital coronary arteriovenous fistula is a direct communication between a coronary artery and the lumen of any one of the four cardiac chambers or the coronary sinus or its tributary veins or the superior vena cava, pulmonary artery, or pulmonary veins close to the heart. Fistulous coronary connections that occur in congenital pulmonary or aortic atresia (see Chapter 25 or 35), in which blood flow is from the ventricle to the aorta, are excluded.

HISTORICAL NOTE

A congenital coronary arteriovenous (AV) fistula was first described by Krause in 1865.[K1] The first report in the English literature was that of Trevor in 1912 who described the autopsy findings in a case with a fistula from the right coronary artery opening into the right ventricle, the patient dying from associated endocarditis.[T4] Autopsy reports from Blakeway[B8] and from Halpert[H3] followed. The first report of surgical correction was in 1947 by G. Biorck and Crafoord[B3] in which a fistulous connection to the main pulmonary artery was discovered at thoracotomy in a patient presumed to have a patent ductus arteriosus. It was closed with sutures. Probably the first reported case of a fistula that was correctly

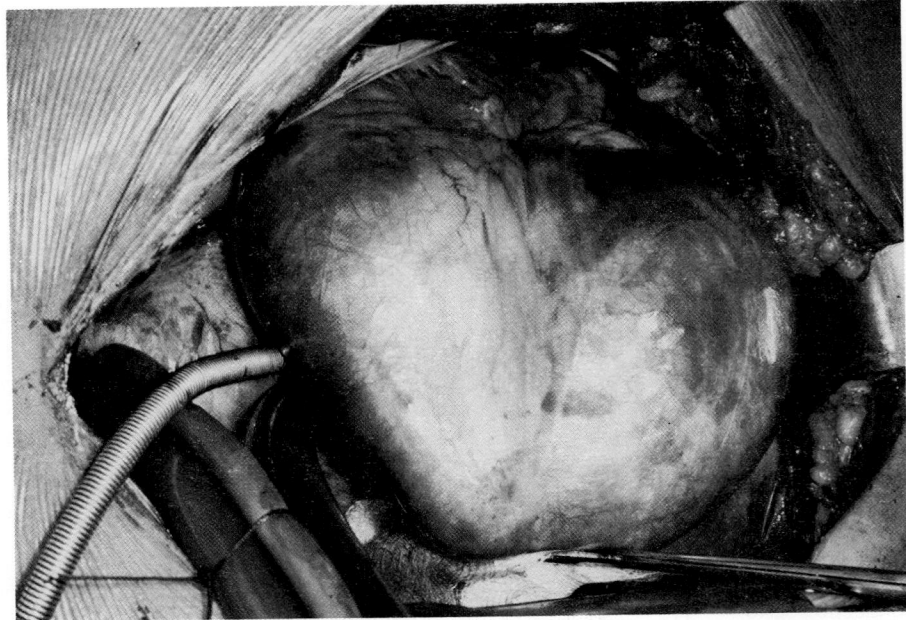

Figure 31-1   Photograph taken during operation in a 43-year-old man with a coronary arteriovenous fistula and a giant aneurysm of the right coronary artery that occupies the entire surgical field (GLH). The fistula was of moderate-to-large diameter and entered the left ventricle posteriorly close to the interventricular groove and apex.

diagnosed preoperatively is that of Fell and associates in 1958,[F1] and the first report of repair of the lesion using cardiopulmonary bypass (CPB) is that of Swan and colleagues in 1959.[S4] Currarino and colleagues described the use of angiography in diagnosis also in 1959.[C3] The first GLH patient with this lesion was operated upon in 1960 and our first Mayo Clinic patient in 1961.[E1] About 350 surgical cases have now been reported in the literature, and several times this number are no doubt unreported.

MORPHOLOGY

Coronary Artery Site

The right coronary artery or its branches are the site of the fistula in 50%–55% of cases.[L2,L3] The left coronary artery is the involved vessel in about 35%, and both coronary arteries in 5%.[B2] The fistulous artery is almost invariably part of a normally distributed coronary artery with a normal branching pattern. The fistula is either in the main vessel that continues beyond the fistula (a side-to-side pattern) or occurs at the termination of the main vessel itself or a branch (an end artery).[S5] Occasionally, the involved artery is anomalous.[U1] It is always dilated and elongated and may be serpiginous, the degree of these changes being roughly proportional to the size of the shunt through the fistula. Usually the dilatation is uniform throughout, but it may become aneurysmal opposite the fistula and sometimes elsewhere along its course. Rarely, a giant aneurysm occurs involving the whole artery. This is

particularly prone to occur in fistulae from the right main coronary artery entering either the posterior wall of the left ventricle[L7,O3,W4] or the right ventricle (Fig. 31-1).[M6] Although such aneurysms have been shown to enlarge progressively,[L7] rupture is rare. Should the artery continue beyond the fistula, it reduces abruptly to a diameter smaller than expected. It is probable that in such cases a coronary steal phenomenon occurs.[H5] There is no convincing evidence that these "feeding arteries" are prone to develop atheroma.[J1]

Site of the Fistulous Connection

The fistulous connection between the coronary artery and the heart may enter any of the four cardiac chambers, the coronary sinus or its tributary veins, or the great arteries or veins adjacent to the heart (main pulmonary artery, proximal pulmonary veins or proximal superior vena cava, or left superior vena cava). There are, however, certain predilections. Over 90% of the fistulae open into the right heart chambers or its connecting vessels, true AV fistulae to the veins themselves (coronary sinus or its major branches or the cavae) being quite uncommon. Thus, about 40% drain to the right ventricle, 25% to the right atrium, 15%–20% to the pulmonary artery, 7% to the coronary sinus, and only 1% to the superior vena cava.[L1,L3] Fistulae entering the right side of the circulation result in a rapid systolic and diastolic runoff from the aorta and a left-to-right shunt. The $\dot{Q}p/\dot{Q}s$ is seldom larger than 1.8 and is often less than this, and the arterial pulse pressure is seldom greatly widened.

About 8% of the fistulae drain into the left heart chambers

Table 31-1 An institutional experience with coronary arteriovenous fistulae (GLH; 1957–1984).

Fistula Drainage Site	Fistula Size		Total	
	Large	Small	n	% of 21
Right atrium	3 (3)	1	4	19%
Right ventricle	3 (3)	—	3	14%
Pulmonary artery	1 (1)	8 (3)[a]	9	43%
Left atrium	—	1	1	5%
Left ventricle	1 (1)[b]	3[c]	4	19%
Total	8 (8)	13 (3)	21 (11)	100%

NOTE: Number of patients undergoing surgical closure is in parentheses.
[a] Closure undertaken during operation for associated lesions.
[b] Giant right coronary artery aneurysm. Hospital death.
[c] Includes one patient with diffuse fistulation (Fig. 31-5).

or their tributaries, usually the left atrium, less often the left ventricle (about 3%), and, rarely, the proximal pulmonary veins. The left heart fistulae are of course not AV fistulae, but arterioarterial (arteriocameral,[A6] arteriosystemic) and do not therefore produce a left-to-right shunt. There may be significant runoff from the aorta during both systole and diastole when they enter the left atrium or only during diastole when they enter the left ventricle, the fistula usually closing off during systole. The volume overload on the left ventricle is therefore similar to that produced by aortic incompetence.

The information on sites of fistulous connections comes in large part from the numerous collective reviews of this subject,[H4,L1,L2,L3] and most of the patients were surgically treated. When all cases, large and small, discovered on coronary angiography are the source of the data (Table 31-1), the site of fistulous connection is most commonly in the pulmonary artery (Fig. 31-2) and lower in the right ventricle (14%) and in the right atrium and its connecting veins (Fig. 31-3). Fistulae (localized and diffuse) to the left heart are more common in coronary arteriographic series than in surgical series.

Size and Multiplicity of the Fistulae

In surgically treated cases, the fistulous opening, when single, is seldom larger than 2–5 mm (Fig. 31-4) and usually has fibrous margins, although uncommonly it may itself be aneurysmal[U1] as in the first reported case.[B3] Occasionally, there may be several openings or a localized angiomatous network of vessels. Among the 58 patients reported from the Texas Heart Institute, multiple fistulae were identified in 16%, an angiomatous lesion in 10%, and the fistula was stated to be aneurysmal in 19%.[U1] In a number of instances (no doubt many times the number of surgically reported cases), the fistula is small, these lesions being recognized only as a result of the development of high-quality cineangiography.

As in other sites, most left ventricular fistulae are single, but there is a separate small group of patients in whom there is a diffuse sponge work of tiny connections from a number of, if not most, branches of the left coronary and sometimes the right coronary artery also (Fig. 31-5).[A6,C4,R4] These pre-sumably represent persistence of embryonic trabecular spaces.

Cardiac Chambers

The chamber or vessel into which the fistula drains is variably affected. When the right atrium receives the fistula, it tends to become considerably dilated, whereas the right ventricle and main pulmonary artery show little change apart from that to be expected from an increase in pulmonary blood flow or until congestive heart failure occurs when they participate in the cardiomegaly. Similarly, the left ventricle tends to remain normal in size despite a fistulous connection to it, probably because the runoff that occurs only in diastole is seldom very large and is seldom comparable to that which occurs in severe aortic regurgitation. Left ventricular hypertrophy may be present. The left atrium rarely may become aneurysmally dilated.[F2] The coronary sinus may also dilate to aneurysmal proportions (one case, UAB) and has been the site of rupture. This is the only reported site of preoperative rupture in this condition.[H1] It is possible that runoff through the coronary sinus is limited by the coronary sinus ostium. Arterialization of the coronary sinus occurs, and possibly in relation to this, there is an unusually high incidence of congestive heart failure in such patients.[O4]

Bacterial Endocarditis

The fistula is the site of endocarditis in about 5% of cases, no doubt because of the turbulence it produces.

Associated Lesions

Most coronary arteriovenous fistulae occur as isolated lesions. There may, however, be coincidental congenital or acquired lesions of almost any type. Among 21 patients, 13 had no other lesions, 4 had acquired valvular disease, 2 atrial septal defect, 1 a ventricular septal defect, and 1 associated coronary artery disease (GLH). In the series reported by Urrutia-S and colleagues, 21 among 58 patients had somewhat similar associated lesions.[U1]

CLINICAL FEATURES AND DIAGNOSTIC CRITERIA

Age at Presentation

Most patients present for treatment late in life, 15 of 27 patients being over 20 years old (UAB and GLH). The presentation may be in childhood and rarely in infancy.

Symptoms

The majority of patients who are considered for operation are asymptomatic and present either because of a continuous murmur[O1,R1] or mild cardiomegaly and plethora on the chest x-ray. Eighty percent of patients under 20 years at the time of consideration are asymptomatic whereas only 40% of those over this age are without symptoms.[L1]

More patients are now being detected with small fistulae because of the frequency of coronary angiography for unre-

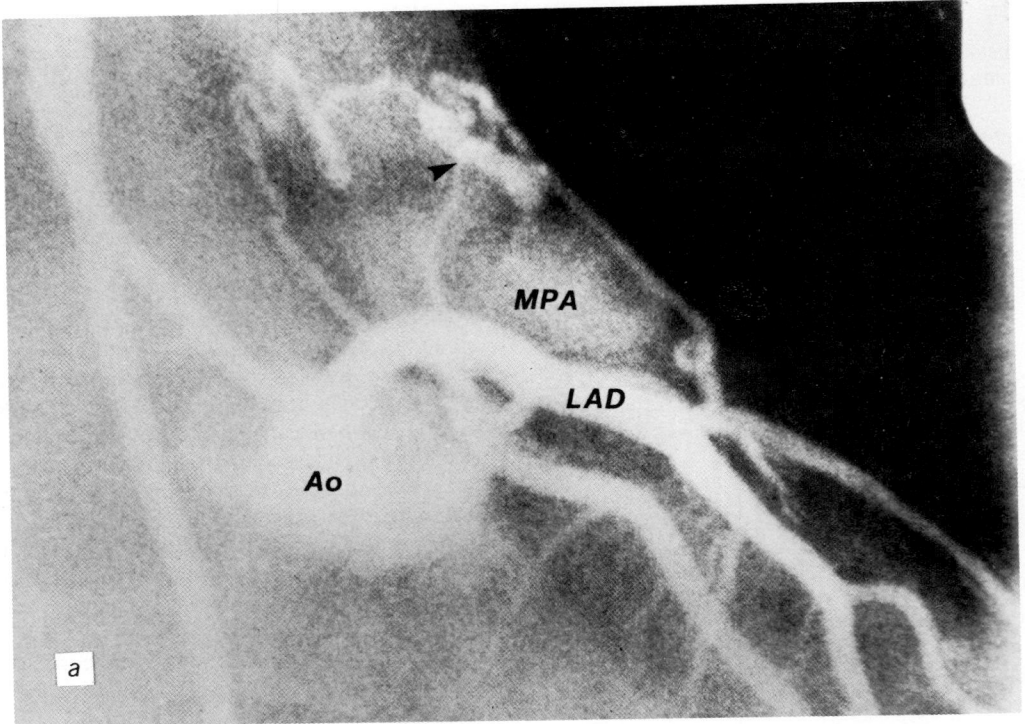

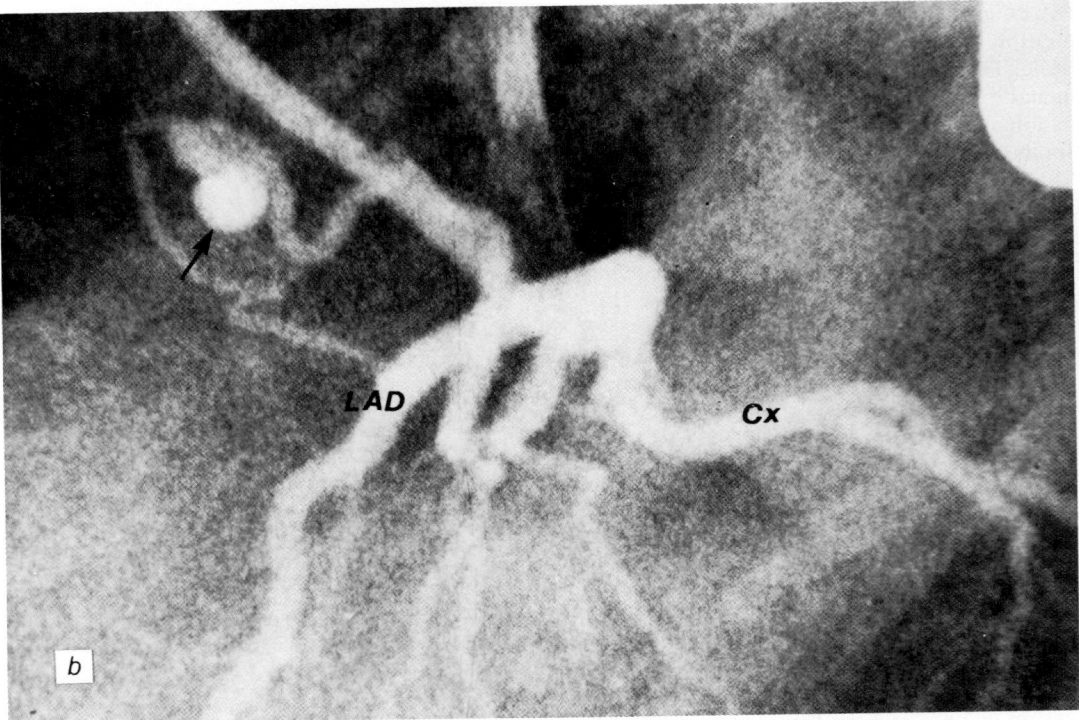

Figure 31-2 Cineangiograms in two patients with small fistulae to the main pulmonary artery (GLH). (a) Right anterior oblique projection. The fistula (arrow) is supplied by small branches from the second diagonal and proximal anterior descending arteries. The pulmonary artery opacifies faintly during part of each cardiac cycle. Operation is not indicated.

(b) Left anterior oblique projection. The fistula (arrow) is supplied by two branches from the proximal anterior descending artery (the origin of the superior one is overlapped by the shadow of the cardiac catheter). The pulmonary artery opacified faintly. This lesion was closed at the time of atrial septal defect repair.

Ao, aorta; Cx, circumflex artery; LAD, left anterior descending artery; LCA, left coronary artery; MPA, main pulmonary artery.

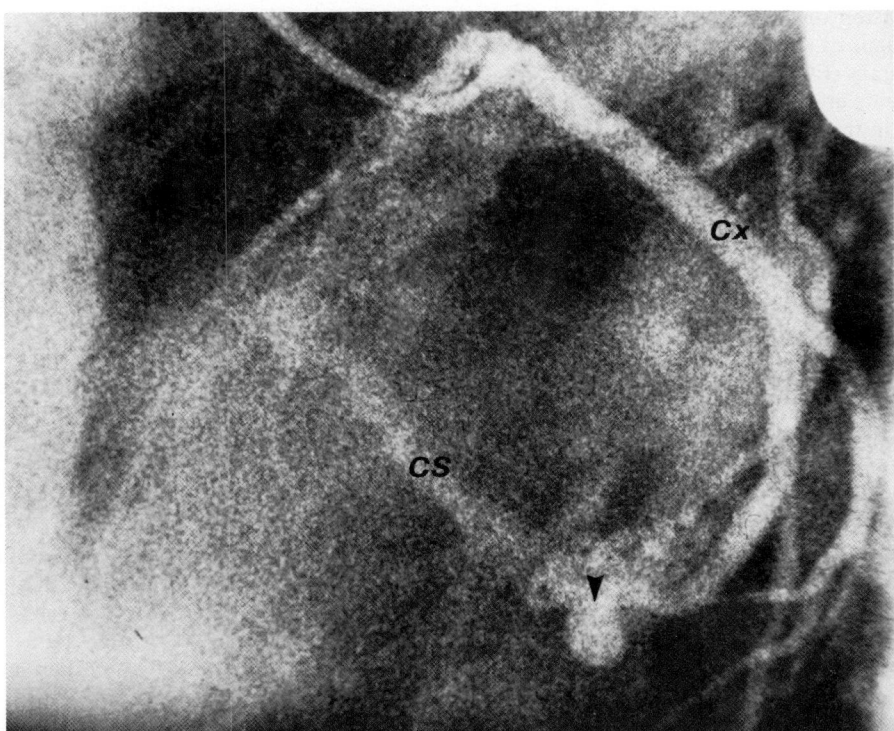

Figure 31-3 Cineangiogram frame in LAO projection showing a small fistula (arrow) entering the coronary sinus (GLH). The feeding left circumflex artery is a large vessel and forms a small aneurysm at the site of the fistulous connection. An atrial branch joins with the terminal circumflex artery in this area. The shunt is small.

Cs, coronary sinus; Cx, circumflex artery.

lated conditions.[G1] Those with small fistulae are asymptomatic and presumably will continue to be so, as was the case in 10 of the 21 GLH patients detected at coronary arteriography, although 3 of them had symptoms from other lesions requiring operation.

The most common symptom is effort *dyspnea* and *fatigue* from the left-to-right shunt. *Angina* is uncommon (about 7%) and myocardial infarction rare (about 3%).[R1] It is postulated that these ischemic symptoms are due to coronary artery steal.

Congestive heart failure occurs in 12%–15% of all surgically treated patients[D7,L1] but is much more common in older patients (the same is true for angina).[L1] Thus, in the review by Liberthson and colleagues, only 6% of patients under 20 years had congestive heart failure, whereas 19% of those 20 years or older had it.[L1] Heart failure may occasionally occur in infancy in patients with large shunts, including in an occasional child with a large right-coronary–left-ventricular fistula comparable to an aortic–left-ventricular tunnel.[D2] In older patients, the likelihood of having heart failure is not directly related to shunt size. Presumably it is related to a long-standing modest left-to-right shunt, as in the case of atrial septal defect. Ogden and Stansel noted that congestive heart failure was more common in patients with a fistulous connection to the coronary sinus (50% versus 14% in overall group).[O4] It may also be more common with the onset of

atrial fibrillation, which is said to occur more often when the connection is to the right atrium.[S5]

When bacterial endocarditis occurs, presentation may be with chills and fever.

Diagnosis

The diagnosis can frequently be strongly suspected from the physical signs,[D1] but it may be difficult on this basis to distinguish coronary AV fistula from other lesions with rapid aortic runoff and continuous murmurs, such as patent ductus arteriosus, ventricular septal defect with aortic incompetence, ruptured sinus of Valsalva aneurysm, and, in infancy, aorta–left-ventricular tunnel. In coronary AV fistula there is usually a continuous murmur that is maximal to the right of the sternum when the fistula enters the right atrium and usually at the lower left sternal edge when it enters the right ventricle or left ventricle. However, when the pulmonary artery is involved, the murmur is sited as for a patent ductus arteriosus. When the fistula enters the left ventricle, the murmur is usually only diastolic (the fistula closing during systole), but it may also have a systolic component.

A systolic thrill is occasionally palpable when the fistula lies anteriorly (entry into right atrium or right ventricle). When the shunt and the aortic diastolic runoff are large, there is a wide pulse pressure and a jerky pulse. Rarely, infants with a connection to the left ventricle may present with the full-blown signs of severe aortic incompetence.[D2]

The electrocardiogram (ECG) is entirely normal in about half the surgical patients and shows evidence of right or left ventricular overload in the remainder.[M5]

The chest x-ray may also be normal or may show mild cardiomegaly and plethora. Cardiomegaly is more marked when congestive heart failure appears. There may be evidence of right or left atrial enlargement, and occasionally the dilated and tortuous or aneurysmal coronary artery or fistulous site may distort the cardiac silhouette. This is most obvious when there is a giant aneurysm of the right coronary artery draining usually to the left ventricle (Fig. 31-6),[L7,O3,W4] although this is a rare occurrence.

Two-dimensional echocardiography can detect significantly enlarged coronary arteries and may also confirm specific chamber enlargement.[R5] The actual diagnosis of a coronary arteriovenous fistula can be made in some circumstances by two-dimensional and Doppler echocardiography.[A8]

Cardiac catheterization, aortography, and selective coronary angiography are necessary for definitive diagnosis and the planning of the surgical repair (see Figs. 31-2, 31-3, 31-4).[L2,W3] The left-to-right shunts are calculated and right heart pressures measured.

NATURAL HISTORY

The natural history of coronary arteriovenous fistula is not precisely known, but its general outlines are clear. The fistula, if not present at birth, develops early in life. It is likely that small fistulae remain small permanently and that the moderate fistulae slowly increase in size, although there may be little change over a 10–15-year period.[J1] The onset of dyspnea, congestive heart failure, and angina can occur in young patients with large fistulae. However, as the fistula shunt is usually only moderate, symptoms usually do not appear until later in life as a result of the long-standing moderate left ventricular volume overload. Daniel and colleagues found from a review of the literature that if congestive heart failure did not occur early in infancy it was virtually unknown until 20 years of age.[D7] The maximum incidence of congestive heart failure occurs in the fifth and sixth decades.[D7]

The only other event that may precipitate symptoms and cause premature death is bacterial endocarditis, which occurs in about 5% of patients and may develop at any age.[D7]

Spontaneous rupture is very rare[H1] despite the fact that the feeding coronary artery or the fistula itself may become aneurysmal and that, as with other aneurysms, there is progressive dilatation of the sac.[L7]

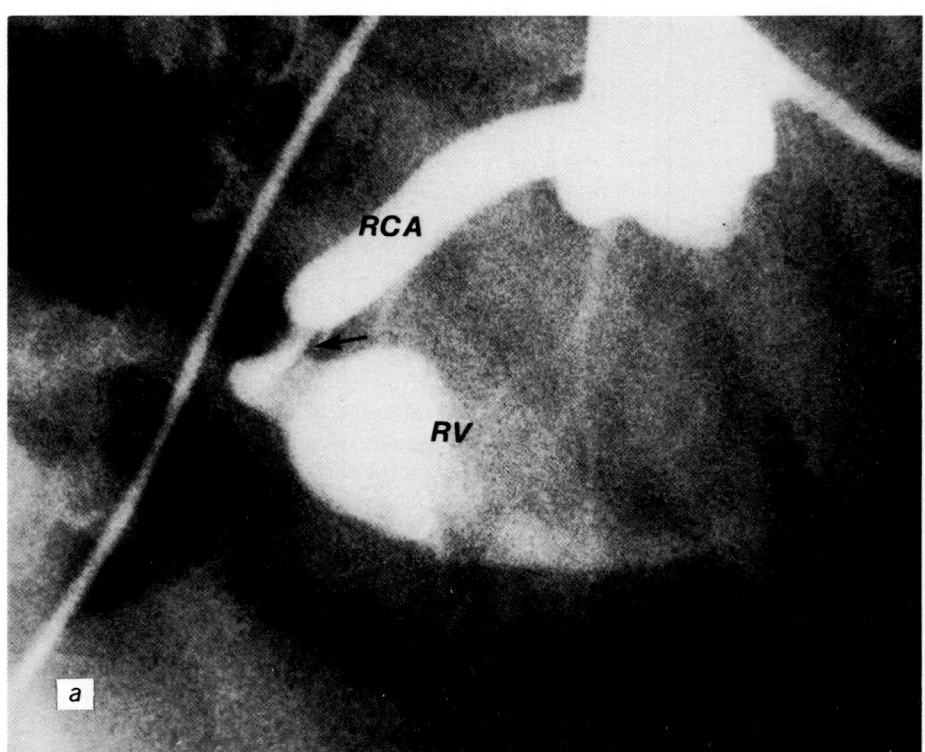

Figure 31-4 Cineangiogram frames in right anterior oblique projection in two patients with coronary arteriovenous fistulae from the main right coronary artery to the right ventricle (GLH).
(a) The dilated right coronary artery runs in its usual position in the AV groove and beyond the fistula (arrow) continues around the acute margin to divide into posterior descending and inferior left ventricular (posterolateral segment) branches (not seen).

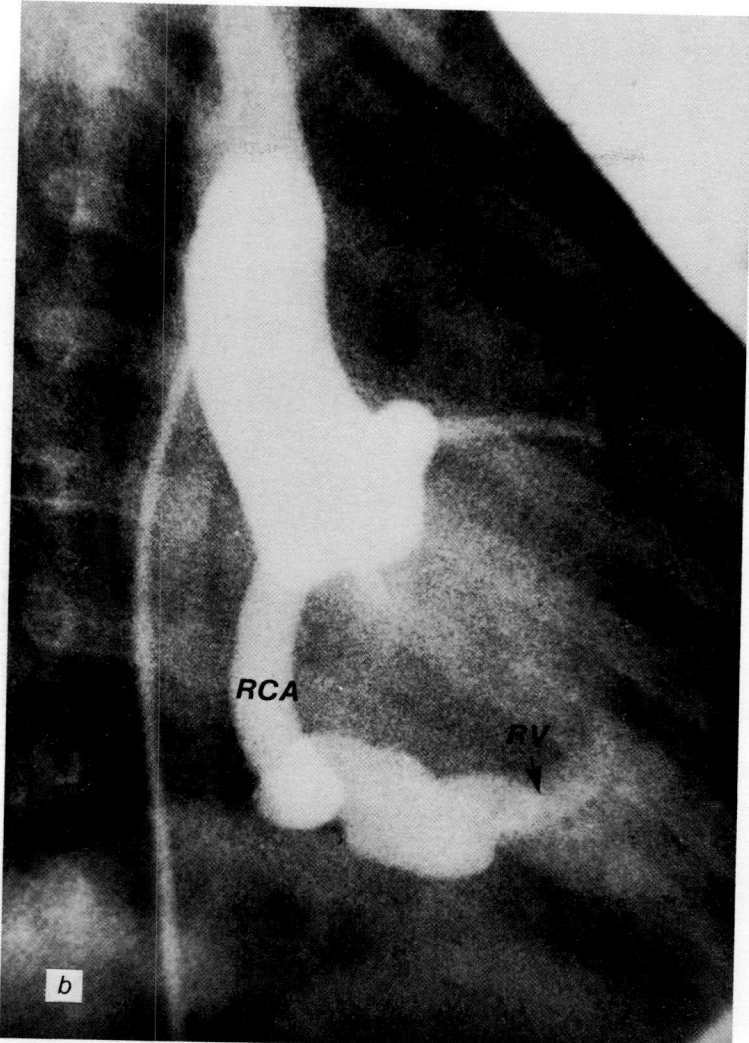

Figure 31-4   (*continued*)
(*b*) The right coronary artery is again normally positioned and very dilated and tortuous. The fistula (arrow) arises from the posterior descending branch about halfway along the posterior interventricular groove and lies therefore at the termination of this vessel.
RCA, right coronary artery; RV, right ventricle.

Liberthson and colleagues found that among 173 reported cases with a mean age of 24 years, death was due to the fistula in 6% of cases; the incidence falling to 1% in those presenting under 20 years and rising to 14% in those presenting over 20 years (mean age 43 years).[L1]

Spontaneous closure of a fistula has been recorded[G4,J1,S1] but is rare.

TECHNIQUE OF OPERATION

The approach in all patients is through a median sternotomy with preparations made for the use of cardiopulmonary bypass (CPB) (see Chapter 2, Section 3). After opening the pericardium, the site of the fistula and the location, size, and pathology of the coronary artery leading to it are carefully noted. *CPB is indicated* when the artery is dilated and tortuous in order to prevent catastrophic hemorrhage during closure of the fistula and when the fistula is relatively inaccessible, such as when it is in the left atrioventricular groove or in the distribution of the circumflex or distal right coronary artery. It is also indicated when the fistula is in the course of the coronary artery rather than at its termination in order that the fistula itself can be closed without ligation of the coronary artery (Table 31-2) and in those instances where an aneurysm requires excision.

The fistulous connection may be safely *closed without CPB* when it represents the termination of a major coronary artery branch into an easily accessible site and the other factors mentioned above are absent. In such instances, a

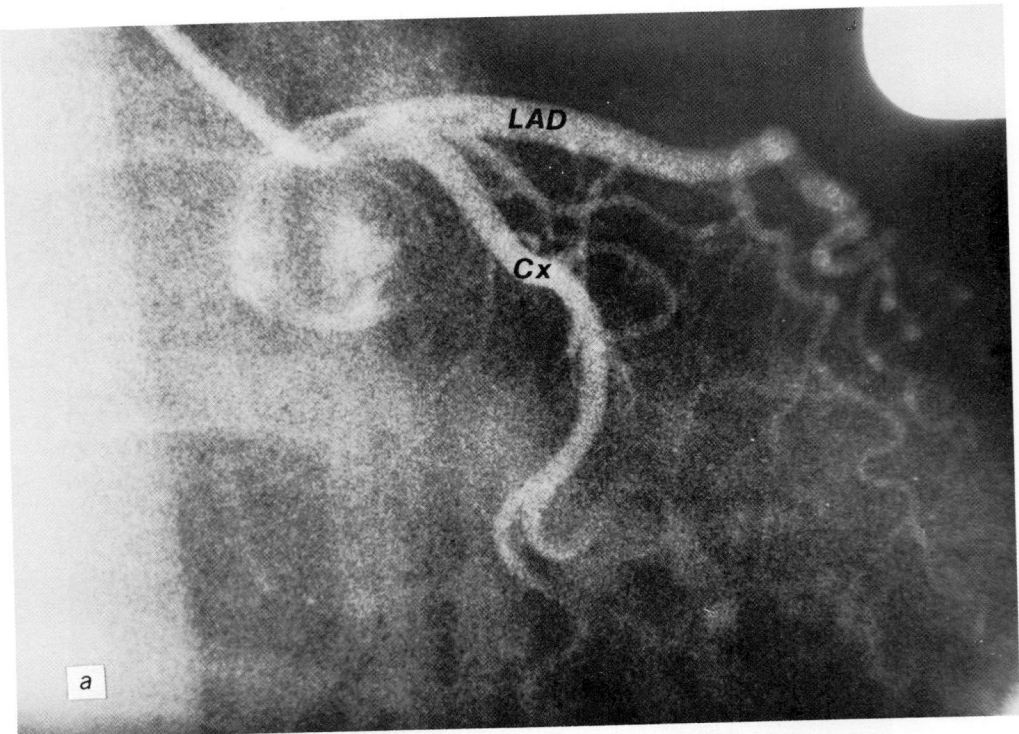

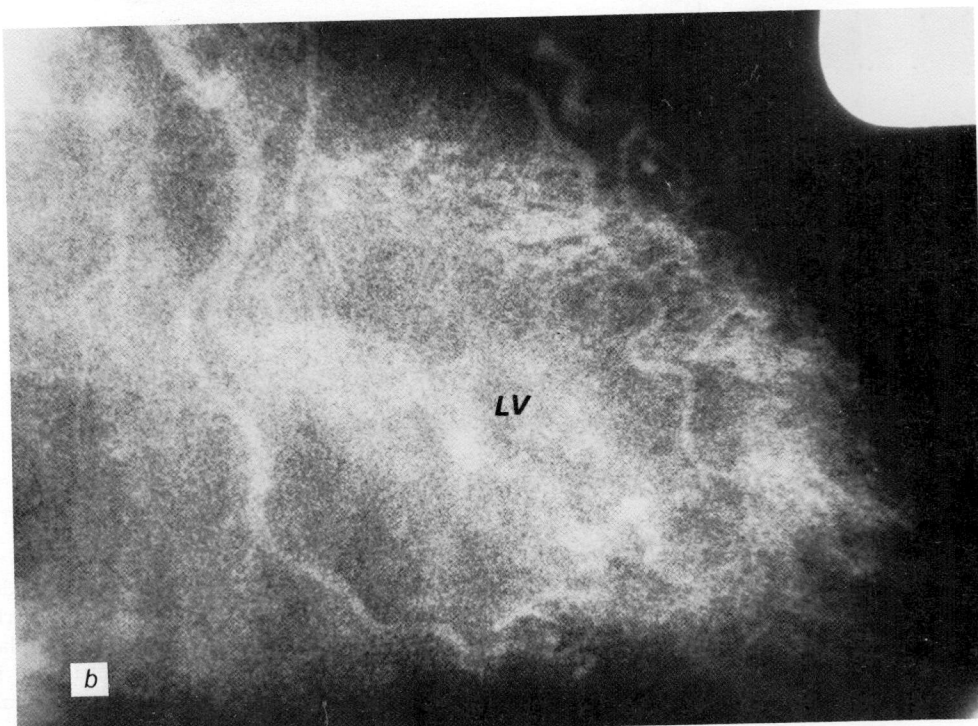

Figure 31-5 Four cineangiogram frames in right anterior oblique projection to demonstrate diffuse fistulation from both left and right coronary arteries to the cavity of the left ventricle (GLH). (*a*), (*b*) are diastolic frames, (*b*) being later in the sequence, whereas (*c*) is a systolic frame that indicates a significant shunt to the left ventricle. (*d*) shows similar shunting from branches of the right coronary artery. This 41-year-old woman complained of angina.

Cx, circumflex; LAD, left anterior descending; LV, left ventricle; RCA, right coronary artery.

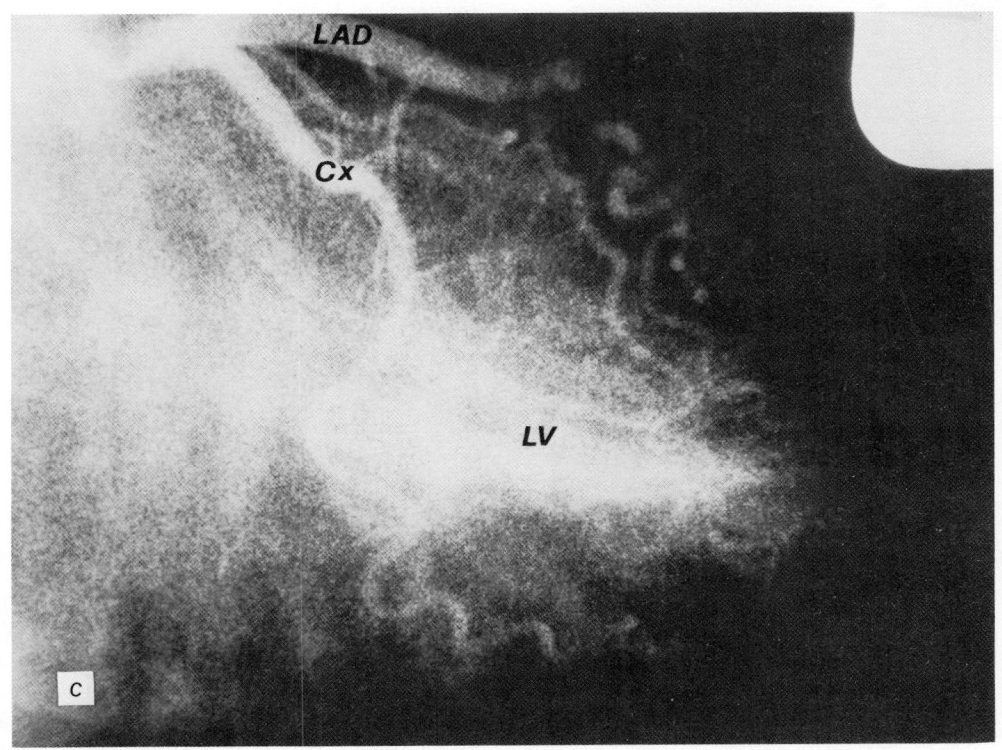

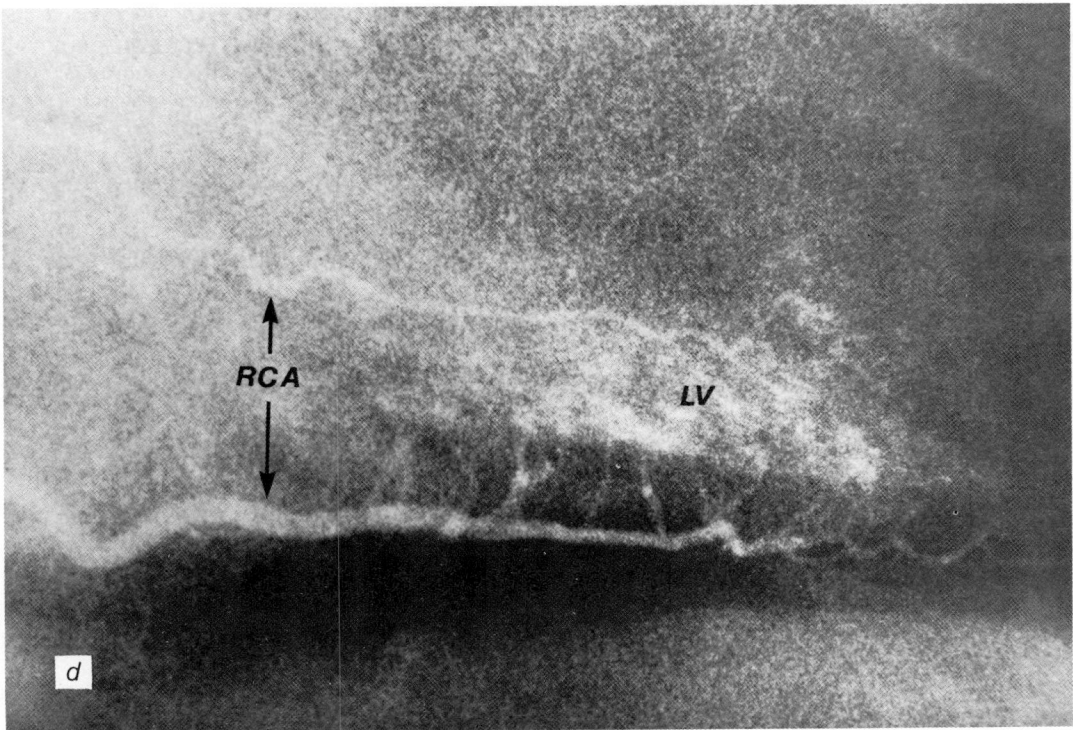

Figure 31-5 (continued)

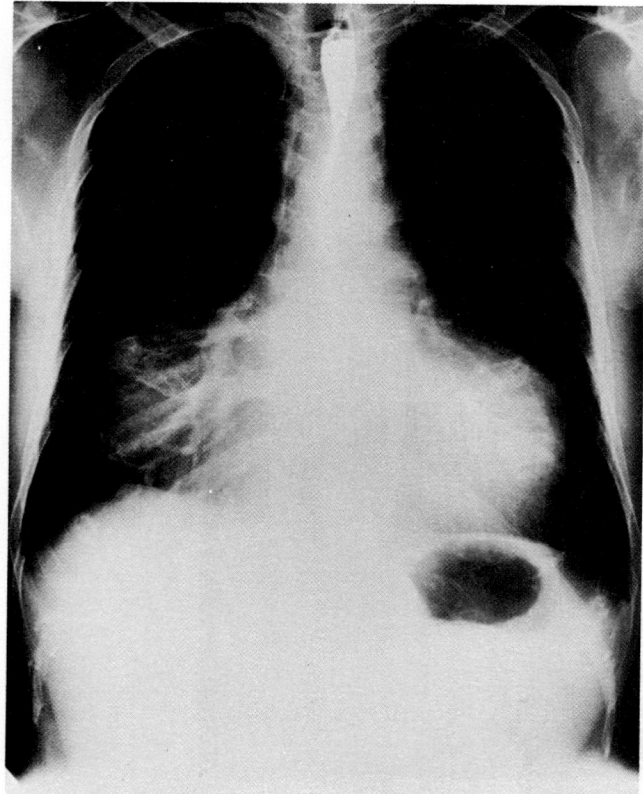

Figure 31-6 Chest x-ray of patient with the aneurysm demonstrated in Figure 31-5 (GLH).

Table 31-2 Method of repair of coronary AV fistulae (UAB; 1967–August 1, 1983; $n = 15$).

Method of Obliteration of Coronary AV Fistula	CPB	No. of Cases
Ligation of coronary artery just proximal to fistula	No	3
	Yes	1
Closure of fistula		
Transarterial	Yes	2
Transchamber		
Right atrium	Yes	3
Coronary sinus	Yes	1
Right ventricle	Yes	2
Pulmonary artery	Yes	1
Left atrial appendage	Yes	1
Total		15

NOTE: No deaths occurred.

suture ligature is placed around the "feeding" coronary artery very close to the fistulous connection. With this, the fistula is temporarily completely closed (as evidenced by complete ablation of the thrill) and the electrocardiogram is monitored for several minutes. If there is no ECG change, the ligature is tied down and a suture ligature placed for additional security. When the fistula is less clearly localized and consists of a leash of vessels, secure closure requires a running suture that encloses all the involved vessels and the underlying walls.

When CPB is used, the precise location of the coronary AV fistula is determined and marked with a stitch before establishing CPB, since this is difficult to do later. After establishing CPB (see Chapter 2, Section 3) and reducing the perfusate temperature, the aorta is cross-clamped; while the fistula is digitally closed, the cold cardioplegic solution is administered. When the chamber into which the fistula opens is an atrium or the pulmonary artery, the chamber is opened and the fistula closed from within with over-and-over sutures supplemented with a pledgetted mattress suture. The cold cardioplegic solution can again be infused to test the security of the closure. When the fistula enters a ventricle or when the coronary artery is large and continuing beyond the fistula, the coronary artery itself is opened and the fistula closed with a running suture, followed by closure of the arteriotomy with 6-0 polypropylene sutures. (The use of a

running mattress suture beneath the artery through the fistulous site[U1] is not recommended, since this may lead to fistula recurrence.)

When a large aneurysm is present (Fig. 31-1), it requires excision. If the aneurysm is localized over the fistula site, it entails trimming away the edges of the dilated vessel and resuture of its walls to create an artery of near normal size. This is possible since the posterior wall invariably consists of strong tissue. This is necessary, however, only when the artery continues beyond the site of the fistula. When it is an end artery, the aneurysm is totally excised and the vessel remnants oversewn. When the aneurysm involves most of the feeding coronary artery as in Figure 31-1, there is usually no option but to deroof it completely and close the coronary artery proximal and distal to the sac, the latter closure including the fistula site. In such circumstances, it is always appropriate to consider the use of coronary artery bypass vein or internal mammary artery grafting to the vessel beyond the fistula,[L3] but this may not be possible when it is too small.

After completing the repair, if a left-sided chamber has been opened it is aspirated for air; with strong suction on the aortic vent needle, the aortic clamp is released and rewarming begun. The remainder of the operation is completed as usual.

SPECIAL FEATURES OF POSTOPERATIVE CARE

Patients are managed as described in Chapter 5.

EARLY RESULTS

The hospital mortality for repair of coronary AV fistula in the absence of giant aneurysm formation approaches zero, no deaths (0%, CL 0%–7%) having occurred among 25 such patients (UAB and GLH). The same is true of other series.[L3,U1] In fact, the review of the literature by Liberthson and colleagues indicates a mortality of 4% (CL 2.5%–6.2%) in 173 patients.[L1] When there is a giant aneurysm, almost always of the right coronary artery, which necessitates its complete excision and usually regrafting of the remaining right coronary system, there is an increased danger of ischemia and arrhythmia. This was the cause of death in one patient with this pathology (GLH). It may be significant that 3 of the 10 reported cases of right-coronary-artery–left-ventricular fistula have died postoperatively.[D2,L7,M7,W4]

Complications of the operation are rare. Myocardial ischemia, either temporary or with infarction, has been reported in 3% of cases and fistula recurrence in 4%.[A1,R1] Using the techniques described here, these complications have been uncommon.

LATE RESULTS

Late results of repair are excellent. Twenty-four of 25 patients have been traced and all are in NYHA class 1 (UAB and GLH), although one of the early patients required early reoperation using CPB for a recurrence that followed ligation. Identical results are reported by Edis and colleagues.[E1] Lowe and colleagues at Duke University found no late deaths and no recurrent fistulas among 22 survivors of repair, with a mean follow-up time of 10 years.[L3] Although involution of the greatly dilated leading artery can occur when repair is performed in early life,[O1] this is not the case in adults.[J1]

INDICATIONS FOR OPERATION

Some believe that the prognosis of a surgically untreated coronary AV fistula is excellent and that operation is indicated only if symptoms are present. However, in view of the probability that at least some of these fistulae increase in size and therefore eventually produce symptoms and heart failure, the tendency of patients with them to develop bacterial endocarditis, the very low probability of spontaneous closure, plus the safety and efficacy of the operation, it is recommended that the diagnosis of a coronary AV fistula is an indication for operation unless the shunt is small ($\dot{Q}p/\dot{Q}s <$ 1.3).

SECTION 2

ANOMALOUS ORIGIN OF THE LEFT CORONARY ARTERY FROM THE PULMONARY ARTERY

DEFINITION

In anomalous origin of the left coronary artery from the pulmonary artery, the whole of the left main coronary artery or only the left anterior descending or circumflex branch arises anomalously from the proximal main pulmonary artery or very rarely from the proximal right pulmonary artery. The branching pattern of the anomalously arising left coronary artery remains normal. The right coronary artery arises normally from the aorta and has a normal branching pattern.

Collaterals from it feed the left coronary artery, in which flow is reversed, so that the left coronary artery drains into the pulmonary artery. In the strictest sense, therefore, the condition is one variety of coronary AV fistula. Very rarely, both coronary arteries arise from the pulmonary artery by a single trunk.[G5]

HISTORICAL NOTE

In 1886, Brooks in Dublin described, apparently for the first time, the anomalous origin of a coronary artery from the pulmonary trunk,[B4] and in 1908, Abbott described anomalous origin of the left coronary artery from the pulmonary trunk.[A1]

Bland, White, and Garland in 1933 described the clinical syndrome associated with anomalous origin of the left coronary artery from the pulmonary trunk on the basis of their experience with a 3-month-old infant who died from the condition.[B5] The pathophysiology, impoverishment of left ventricular myocardial blood flow in spite of good collaterals between right and left coronary arteries because of retrograde flow from the left coronary artery to pulmonary trunk, was suggested by Brooks in his original paper.[B4] Edwards supported this hypothesis[E2] as did Case, Morrow, Stainsby, and Nestor in 1958.[C1] Case and colleagues also reported the postmortem observation that radiopaque dye injected into the ascending aorta passed out through the normal right coronary artery and by collaterals filled in retrograde fashion the left coronary artery.[C1]

Sabiston and colleagues verified the retrograde flow at the first successful operation for the condition in 1959 by measuring a striking increase in the left coronary artery pressure when its anomalous connection from the pulmonary trunk was occluded.[S2] The actual demonstration of left-to-right shunt into the pulmonary trunk was by Augustasson and colleagues in 1961[A2] and by Rudolph, Gootman, and colleagues in 1963.[R2]

The earliest surgical attempts to ameliorate the condition were indirect. The first was apparently that of Potts, who created an aortopulmonary (AP) fistula to increase the saturation in the main pulmonary artery.[P2] Kittle and associates banded the pulmonary artery,[K3] and Paul and Robbins used pericardial poudrage.[P3] These procedures are, of course, now obsolete. The successful ligation of the anomalous left coronary artery origin by Sabiston and colleagues in 1959 was followed by a similar report from Rowe and Young in 1960.[R6] As early as 1953, Mustard reported attempts to anastomose the turned-down left common carotid artery to the anomalous left coronary artery that he detached from the pulmonary artery together with a button of pulmonary artery wall[M8]; Apley and colleagues attempted a similar procedure using the left subclavian artery in 1957.[A7] Meyer and colleagues first used this latter procedure successfully to create a two-coronary artery system in 1968,[M1] and others have reported such a repair.[P1] In 1966, Cooley and associates reported the use of coronary artery bypass vein grafting from the aorta to the left main or proximal left anterior descending artery, after closing the left coronary ostium from within the pulmonary artery.[C5] The next procedure to evolve was direct transplantation of the anomalous coronary artery from the pulmonary artery to the ascending aorta. Such a procedure was performed unsuccessfully at GLH in 1972 using profoundly hypothermic circulatory arrest techniques.[B10] This was first performed successfully for the rare condition of right coronary artery origin from the pulmonary trunk (where the artery lies anteriorly and is more readily transposed) by Tingelstad and colleagues in 1971[T3] and for the left coronary artery by Neches and colleagues in 1974.[N1] In their report, Neches and associates also described the successful interposition of a free left subclavian artery segment between the left coronary artery and the back of the ascending aorta. The last modification, in 1979, was the use of a tunnel within the main pulmonary artery to connect the ostium of the anomalous coronary artery to the aorta via an AP window, created either of pericardium by Hamilton and colleagues[H2] or of pulmonary artery wall by Takeuchi and colleagues.[T2] Arciniegas modified this concept by placing a free subclavian artery graft inside the pulmonary artery.[A4]

At GLH, the aneurysmal left ventricular wall was excised unsuccessfully in 1960.[B9] This procedure was subsequently performed successfully by Turina and colleagues in 1973 combined with ligation of the left coronary artery[T5] and by Fleming and colleagues in 1975.[F3]

MORPHOLOGY

The anomalous left main coronary artery arises most commonly from the sinus of Valsalva immediately above the left or posterior cusps and rarely from that above the right cusp.[W1] The left main coronary artery is of variable length but usually divides into anterior descending and circumflex branches within 5 or 6 mm of its origin. Anastomoses between the right and left coronary arteries are always present but vary in extent and are grossly visible in only a minority of cases and mainly in adults. Uncommonly, only the circumflex branch arises anomalously from the pulmonary trunk, and rarely (8 patients reported in the literature) only the left anterior descending branch arises anomalously.[R8]

Very rarely, the left main coronary artery or only the circumflex artery (two cases, GLH) arises from the right pulmonary artery near its origin rather than the pulmonary trunk.[D5,O2] Even more rarely, both the left and right coronary arteries arise from the pulmonary trunk.[K2,R3]

The left ventricle is always hypertrophied and usually greatly dilated, with the dilatation often involving primarily the left ventricular apex. Diffuse left ventricular fibrosis is virtually always present, and patients dying in infancy usually also have evidence of recent and old anterolateral myocardial infarction. The fibrosis is most marked in the subendocardial layer. Focal calcification may be present in the fibrotic areas. Secondary subendocardial fibroelastosis of variable degree is usually present.

Several pathologic features may result in *mitral valve incompetence.*[W1] There may be extensive fibrosis and sometimes calcification in the papillary muscles, leading to papillary muscle dysfunction. Endocardial fibroelastosis may involve the mitral apparatus with fusion and shortening of chordae tendinae. Also, the papillary muscles may be abnormally positioned, which may lead to mitral incompe-

tence.[M2,N2] Extensive left ventricular fibrosis can produce left ventricular and mitral annular dilatation and mitral incompetence.[B6,T1]

CLINICAL FEATURES AND DIAGNOSTIC CRITERIA

Infant Presentation

Symptoms may be recognized within a week or so of birth. When there are no other anomalies, these are very seldom severe enough to warrant referral before 2 months of age. Presumably the high postnatal pulmonary artery pressure limits runoff into the pulmonary artery so that there is less coronary steal and infarction is gradual in onset rather than sudden.

There is often circumoral pallor and blueness. The cardinal symptom is poor feeding. The baby takes the first 2–3 ounces well but then stops; there is breathlessness and sweating and the baby may draw up the knees, arch the back, and uncommonly cry or scream. The presumed cause is angina. As a result of the feeding problem, weight gains are poor. Very few infants with these symptoms improve spontaneously. Usually by 2–3 months of age there is frank congestive heart failure with persistent tachypnea and tachycardia, the infant by then being seriously ill and occasionally moribund.

The clinical signs are difficult to distinguish from those of a cardiomyopathy or endocardial fibroelastosis. There may be a nonspecific systolic murmur at the base or a more definite apical pansystolic murmur due to mitral regurgitation and an apical gallop rhythm. A continuous murmur is not audible in infants. A precordial lift is common in association with marked and frequently gross cardiomegaly, and there is hepatomegaly and rales throughout the lungs.

The electrocardiogram (ECG) is frequently helpful in diagnosis, since it usually shows anterolateral infarction with Q waves and ST segment elevation in lateral chest lead[A5] and evidence of left ventricular hypertrophy. However, left ventricular hypertrophy alone may be reflected in the ECG. Myocardial enzymes may be elevated. The horizontal plane vectorcardiogram is uniformly characteristic of anterolateral myocardial infarction with clockwise rotation, the initial vector pointing anteriorly and rightward and the loops then progressing posteriorly.[A5]

The chest x-ray in addition to cardiomegaly shows interstitial pulmonary edema. Echocardiography shows a dilated, poorly contracting left ventricle. Two-dimensional and pulsed Doppler echocardiography may detect the anomalous origin of the left coronary artery from the pulmonary trunk in infants otherwise thought to have a dilated cardiomyopathy.[C6,K4] This technique can also identify an anomalously originating right coronary artery.[W5]

Definitive diagnosis currently requires *cardiac catheterization and cineangiography.* An aortogram demonstrates the single right coronary artery arising from the aorta and retrograde filling of the left coronary artery that produces a varying degree of opacification of the main pulmonary artery (Fig. 31-7). A left ventriculogram is also required to assess left ventricular function and the degree of mitral regurgitation. It may also demonstrate the coronary anatomy, making an aortogram unnecessary. Right heart catheterization may show an increase in blood oxygen content at pulmonary artery level.

Adult Presentation

In patients who present later in life, the collateral circulation from the right coronary artery is apparently adequate enough to prevent massive infarction since very few adults give a history of hospitalization in infancy, although there may have been feeding difficulties. When severe symptoms do not occur in infancy, presentation is often delayed to beyond 20 years of age.[M3,R7,W2] Some adult patients remain asymptomatic or complain only of fatigue, dyspnea, or palpitations. About half have effort angina.

On examination, there is usually a nonspecific systolic murmur, sometimes an apical pansystolic murmur from mitral regurgitation, and occasionally a continuous murmur over the upper left sternal edge. Occasionally, mitral regurgitation dominates the clinical picture, producing congestive heart failure. In an earlier era, some such patients were operated upon or died without the diagnosis of anomalous left coronary artery being made.[B6,D3,G2,U2]

The resting ECG is virtually always abnormal, with ST-T segment changes or frank evidence of old anterolateral infarction. The exercise ECG usually shows an abnormal ischemic response, and stress thallium myocardial imaging is usually abnormal.[M3] The chest x-ray may be normal or show cardiac enlargement.

Cineangiography shows more prominent collaterals from the right coronary artery in adults than in infants and usually a near normal left ventricular ejection fraction but with anterolateral hypokinesia. Mitral regurgitation is occasionally severe.

NATURAL HISTORY

This is a rare congenital anomaly occurring in 0.26% of patients with congenital heart disease catheterized at the Children's Hospital in Boston.[A5]

About 65% of infants born with anomalous origin of the left coronary artery from the pulmonary artery die in the first year of life from intractable left ventricular failure (Fig. 31-8).[W1] However, as noted earlier, they uncommonly do so in the first 2 months of life. The explanation for this symptom-free interval is not entirely clear, since extensive left ventricular scarring, particularly of the subendocardium, and evidence of old and recent infarction are usually present by 3 months of age.

If death does not occur in the first year, the hazard to the patient is considerably less and the more chronic phase of the natural history is reached. Survival to this stage may be related to rich interarterial collaterals present in some patients, possibly associated with a slightly restrictive opening between the left coronary artery and the pulmonary trunk. In support of this is the fact that about 5% of patients with anomalous origin of the left coronary artery have continuous murmurs, and many of these patients are in good health and a few have normal ECGs.[W1] Survival beyond the first year may also relate to a marked right coronary dominance, with this vessel supplying not only the diaphragmatic portion of

the left ventricle but a good deal of the septum and lateral wall as well.[W1] Patients with this arrangement may occasionally only have papillary muscle ischemia and fibrosis, and mitral incompetence may dominate the clinical picture.

Having survived infancy, most patients continue to be at risk of death from chronic congestive heart failure secondary to the ischemic left ventricular cardiomyopathy. This hazard apparently lessens by the fourth decade of life (Fig. 31-8), and those few patients living to the fifth and sixth decades occasionally die suddenly, as do older patients with long-standing ischemic heart disease (see Chapter 7). In patients in adult life, myocardial ischemia and fibrosis are prominent, and occasionally extensive myocardial calcification develops. However, left ventricular ejection fraction is only moderately depressed or normal in most of these patients.[M3]

TECHNIQUE OF OPERATION

Construction of a Two-Coronary System

Tunnel Operation

These seriously ill infants are liable to develop ventricular fibrillation before the heart can be cannulated and CPB commenced (this occurred in 5 of 10 such infants at UAB, in three of them as the sternotomy was being made). For this reason, surface cooling prior to the sternotomy is preferred (GLH), followed by profound hypothermia-circulatory arrest techniques (see Chapter 2, Section 4). In any event, great vigilance is required to maintain an optimal hemodynamic state during the preparations for operation and cannulation of the heart.

After opening the sternum, the pericardium is opened and stay sutures are placed without touching the heart, since the least trauma may induce fibrillation in the very ischemic left ventricle. An aortic purse-string suture is placed for cannulation, heparin is administered, and the aorta is cannulated. When the technique of profoundly hypothermic total circulatory arrest is to be used, a purse-string stitch is placed around the right atrial appendage, a single venous cannula is inserted, and CPB is begun. The patient is cooled to 18°C and the repair done after establishing the profoundly hypothermic total circulatory arrest. Alternatively (UAB), after inserting the venous cannula and commencing CPB the tip of the single venous cannula is advanced a short distance into the inferior vena cava and the repair done during CPB at 25°C with periods of low perfusion flow rate when improved visibility is required (see Chapter 2, Section 3). Instead of using a single venous cannula during CPB, initially a superior vena caval purse-string stitch may be placed, the cannula inserted, and CPB established at a flow of about 1.2 $l \cdot min^{-1} \cdot m^{-2}$, and then the inferior vena caval purse-string stitch placed and the cannula inserted (UAB). The aorta is cross-clamped, and the cold cardioplegic solution is infused (UAB), digitally occluding the origin of the left coronary artery from the pulmonary trunk. If left heart decompression is necessary, the tip of the left atrial appendage may be amputated and later ligated or oversewn.

A transverse incision is made in the left pulmonary artery just downstream to the commissure of the pulmonary valve (Fig. 31-9). When, as is usually the case, the opening of the anomalously originating left coronary artery arises from the

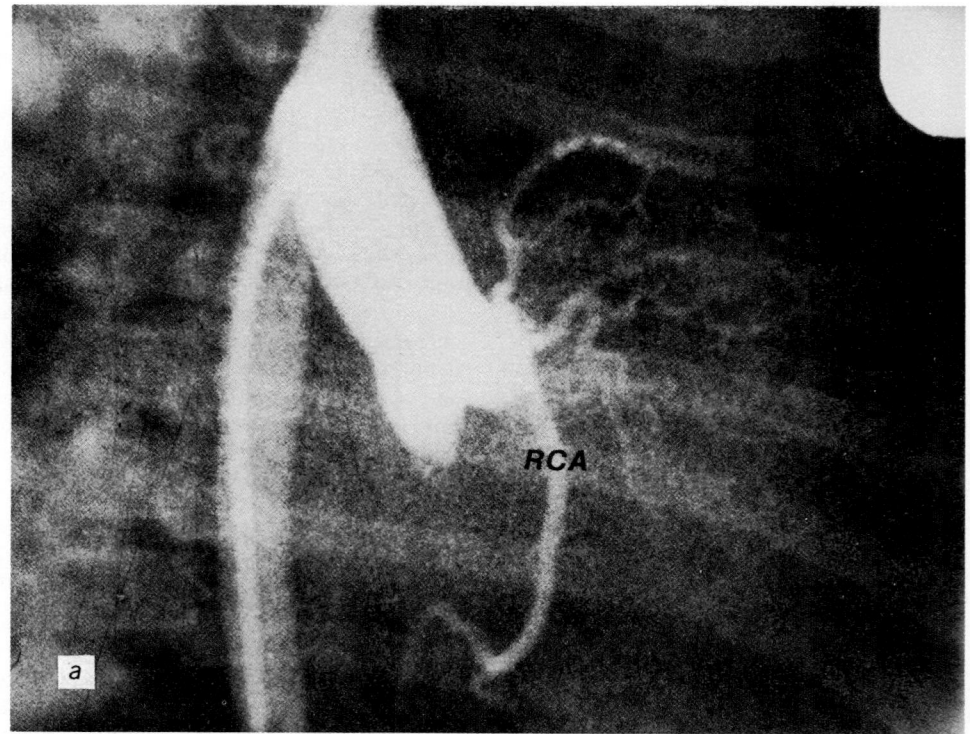

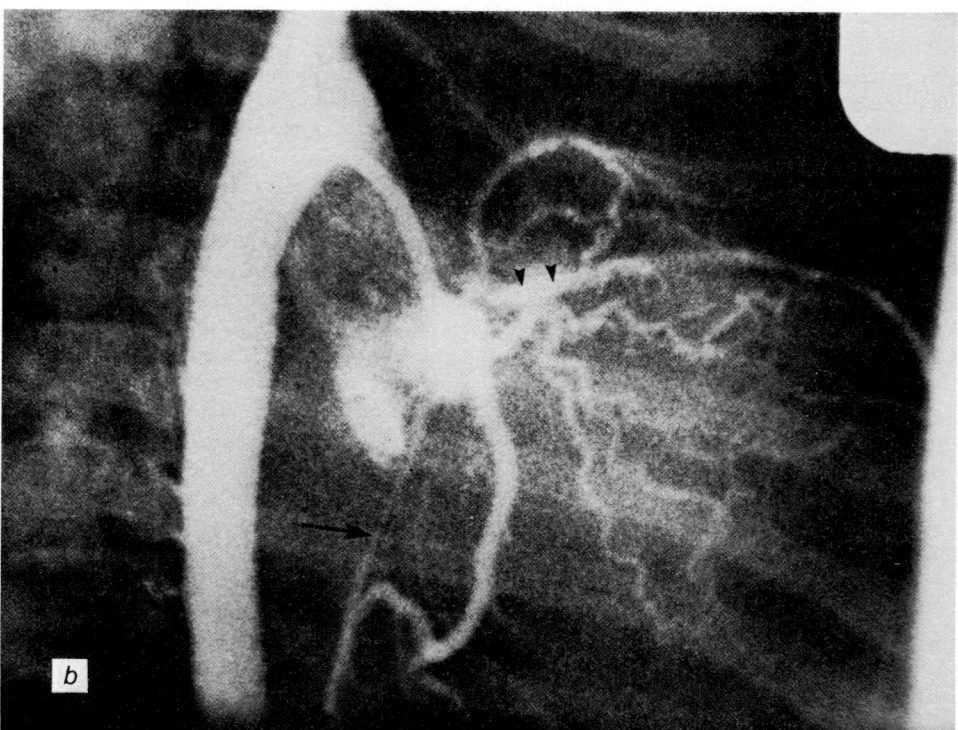

Figure 31-7 Biplane cineangiographic frames in a 3-month-old infant with anomalous origin of the left coronary artery from the pulmonary artery (GLH). (*a*) and (*b*) In right anterior oblique projection; (*c*) and (*d*) in left anterior oblique projection. In (*a*) and (*c*), the right coronary artery fills directly from the aorta and the prominent conal branch collaterals are visible. In (*b*) and (*d*), there is delayed retrograde filling of the left anterior descending (double arrows) and circumflex arteries (single arrow). A whiff of contrast can be seen in the main pulmonary artery (cross) in (*d*).

RCA, right coronary artery.

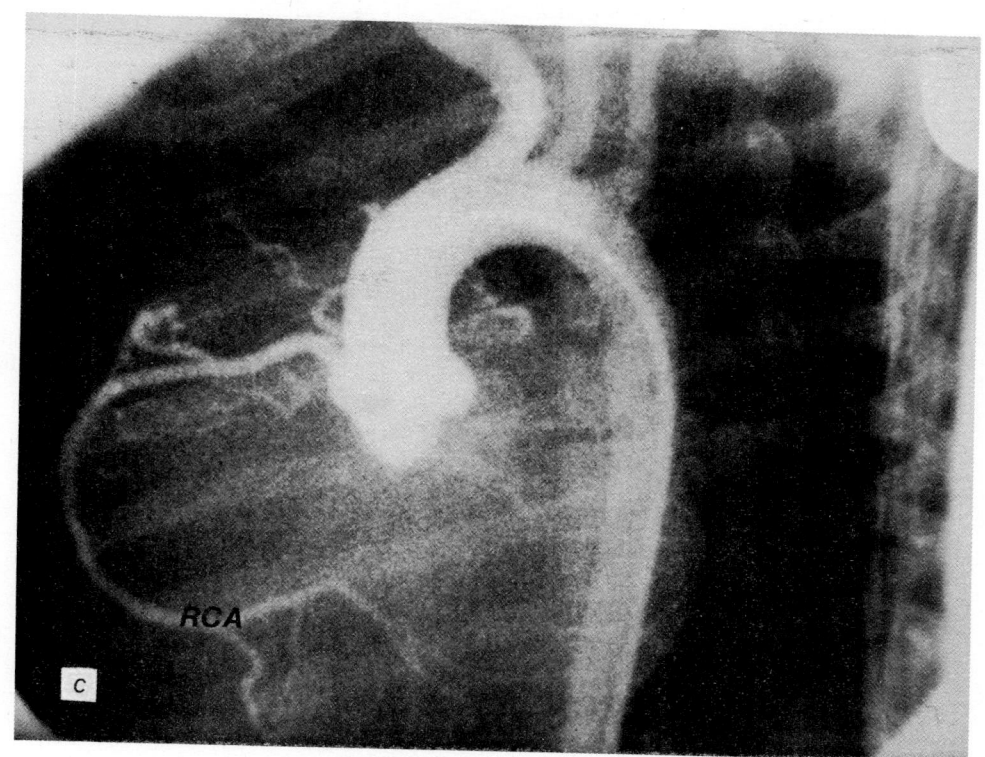

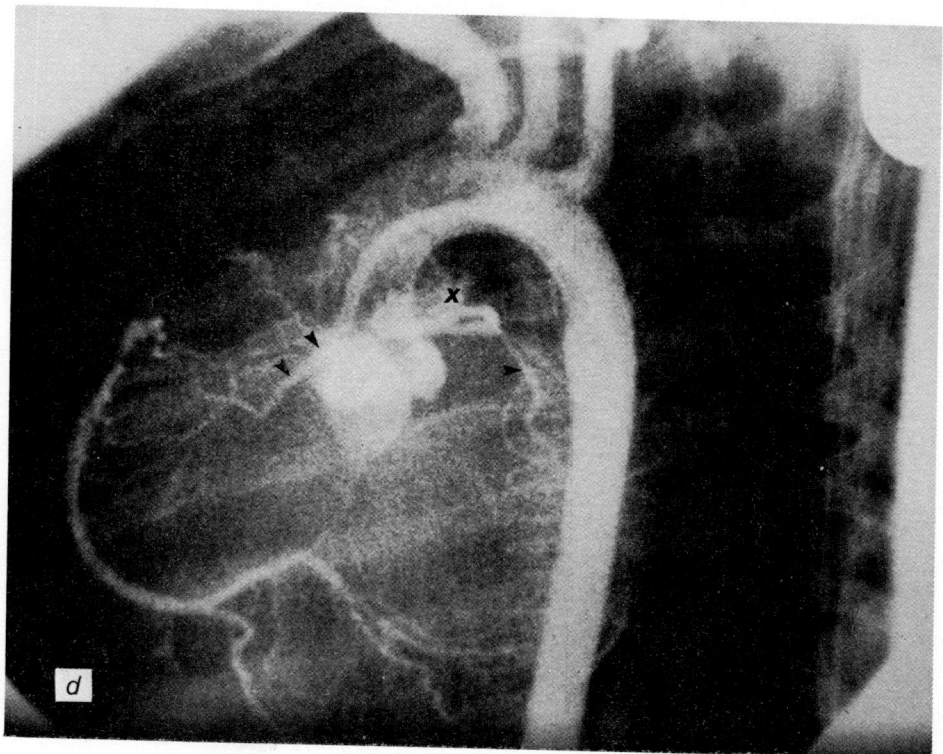

Figure 31-7 *(continued)*

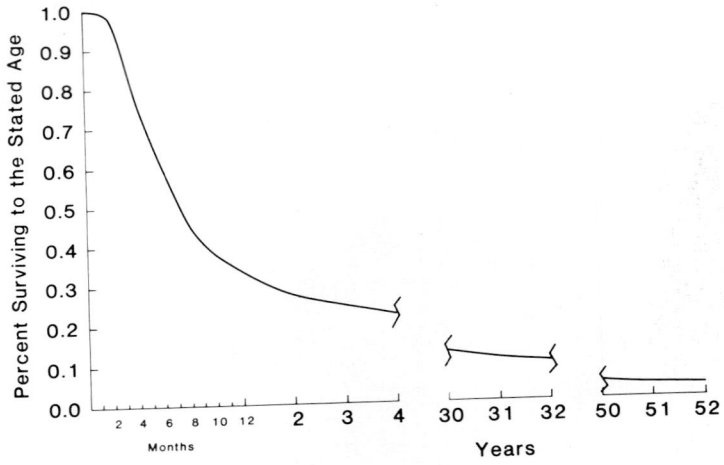

Figure 31-8 Freehand depiction of actuarial survival without surgical treatment of patients with anomalous origin of the left coronary artery from the pulmonary trunk. (This is based primarily on the collective review of 140 cases by Wesselhoeft and colleagues.[W1])

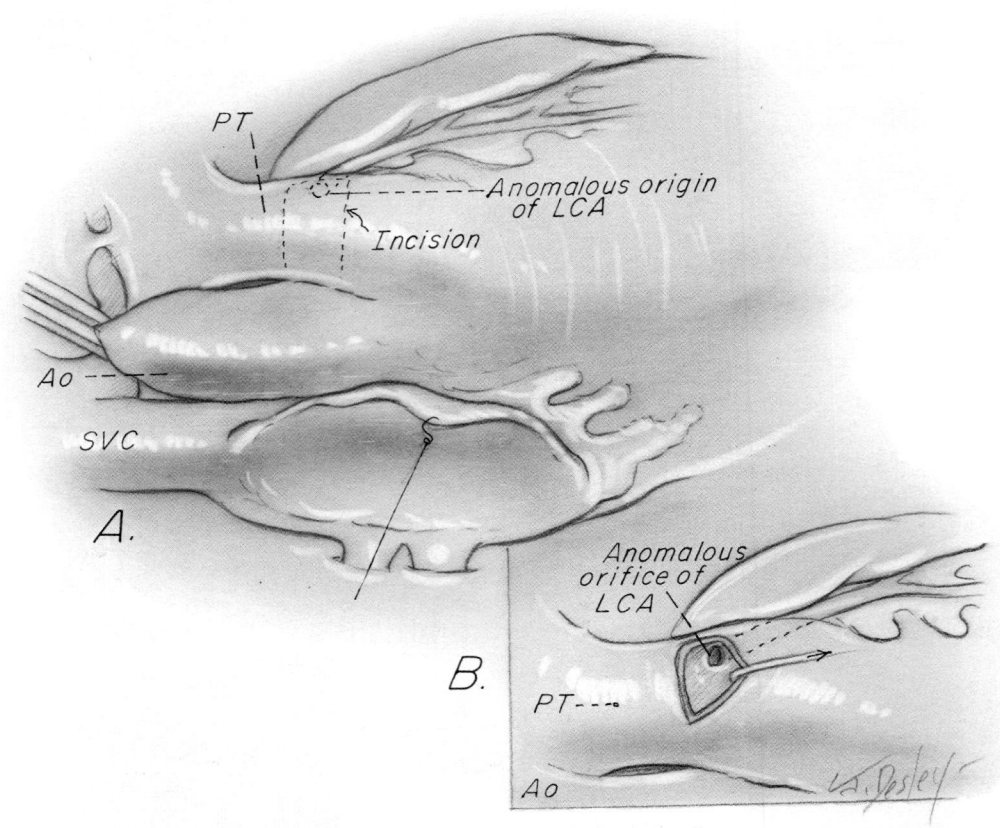

Figure 31-9 Intrapulmonary artery tunnel repair for anomalous origin of the left coronary artery.

(a) Depiction in dashed circle of the usual position within the left pulmonary artery of the anomalous origin of the left coronary artery. Not illustrated is the fact that the origin within the sinus of Valsalva is close to the pulmonary valve. The dashed lines indicate the proposed incisions for the pulmonary artery flap.

(b) The initial incision in the pulmonary trunk is made to determine the exact location of the anomalous orifice. After verifying that the position eliminates the possibility of reimplantation of the orifice directly into the aorta, the tunnel operation proceeds.

(c) The dashed circles show the proposed circular opening to be made in the contiguous wall of aorta and pulmonary trunk. These are made with a punch, exactly as in coronary artery bypass grafting (see Chapter 7, Fig. 7-10).

(d) The aortopulmonary window is being made by suturing together these two openings.

(e) The initial incision has been extended to create the flap of pulmonary trunk wall.

(f) The flap has been sutured into place to form the convex roof of a tunnel through which aortic blood passes to the anomalous orifice of the left coronary artery.

(g) A piece of pericardium is used to close the opening that remains in the anterior wall of the pulmonary trunk.

Ao, aorta; LCA, left coronary artery; PT, pulmonary trunk; SVC, superior vena cava.

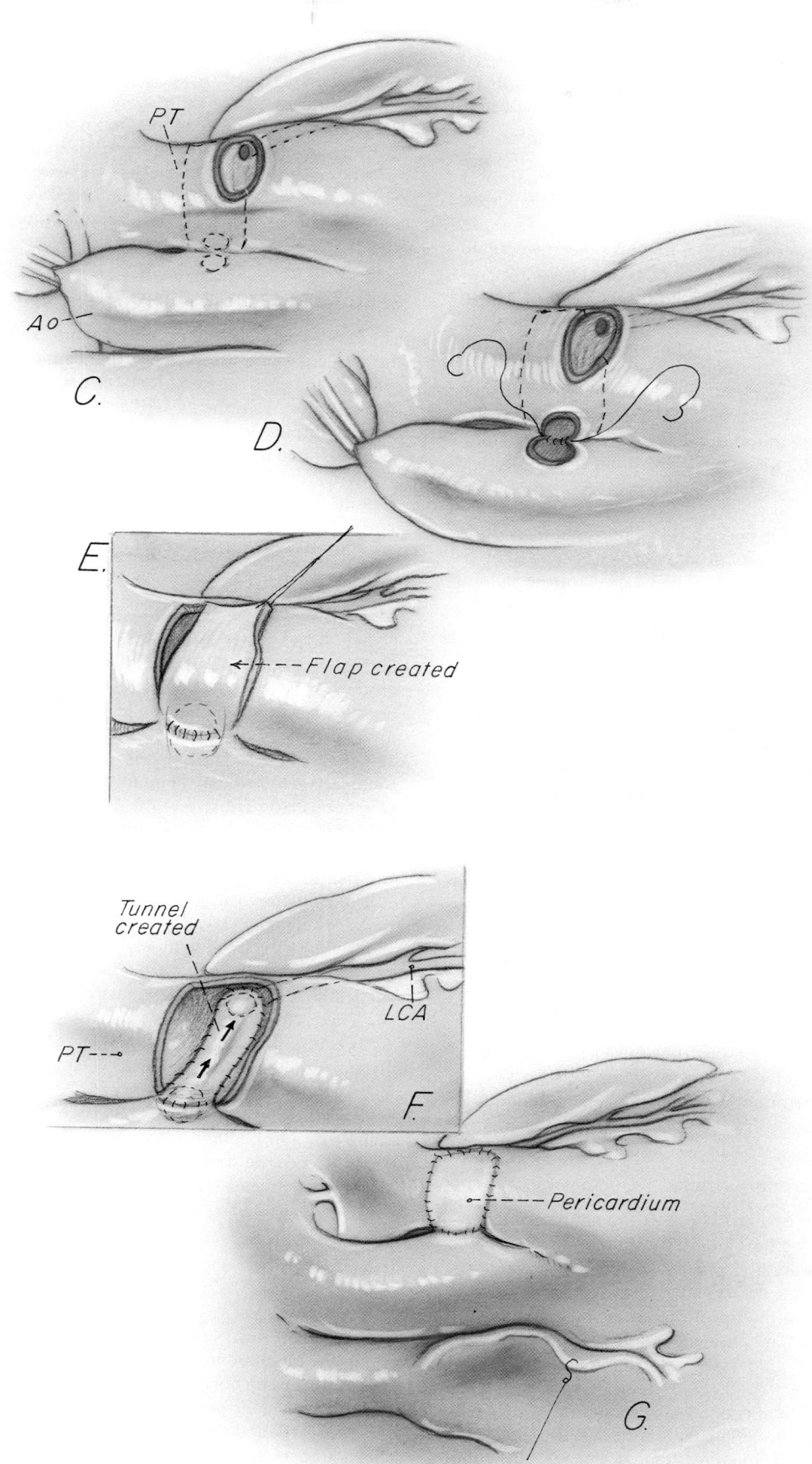

C.

PT

Ao

D.

E.

Flap created

F.

Tunnel
created

LCA

PT

Pericardium

G.

left-sided rather than the posterior or right-sided aspect of the main pulmonary artery the *tunnel operation*[T2] is selected (UAB).

A button of aortic wall about 5 to 6 mm in diameter is excised at a point at which the aorta is in contact with the left side of the pulmonary trunk. Directly opposite this a button is excised from the pulmonary trunk. These openings are sewn together with continuous 5-0 polypropylene to create an AP window (Figs. 31-9c and 31-9d). Using either a flap of anterior pulmonary trunk wall hinged on the right or a strip of anterior pulmonary trunk wall made by a parallel incision downstream to the original transverse one, the anterior wall of the tunnel is created, the tunnel conveying blood from the AP window across the back of the pulmonary trunk to the anomalously originating left coronary artery (Fig. 31-9f) The large defect in the anterior wall of the pulmonary trunk is reconstructed with a piece of pericardium (Fig. 31-9g).

Reimplantation
Alternatively, when after making the transverse incision in the pulmonary trunk the left coronary artery is seen to originate from the posterior or right-sided aspect of the pulmonary trunk, the incision is continued until the trunk is completely divided.[G3,L6] The incision is arranged so that a sizable button of pulmonary artery wall around the coronary ostium may be excised in preparation for its reimplantation into the aorta (UAB). The left coronary artery may be carefully mobilized for a short distance. An opening is made in the adjacent posterolateral portion of the aorta, taking care to avoid valve leaflet damage. The button around the coronary ostium is anastomosed to the aorta with 7-0 polypropylene sutures, and the pulmonary trunk is reconstructed by end-to-end anastomosis.

Rewarming is begun, and with strong suction on the aortic needle vent the aortic clamp is released. The remainder of the operation is completed in the usual fashion. Weaning the patient from CPB may require patience, intravenous nitroglycerine, Neo-Synephrine, and care as to left and right atrial pressures.

Coronary Artery Bypass Grafting
The techniques are the same as those used for the surgical treatment of arteriosclerotic coronary artery disease (see "Indications for Operation" and Chapter 7, "Technique of Operation").

Ligation of Left Coronary Artery

This procedure may be carried out in the simplest manner, through a limited left anterolateral fourth interspace incision (GLH). The pericardium is opened in front of the phrenic nerve after mobilizing the thymus from its upper part. A ligature is tied around the tip of the left atrial appendage to retract it superiorly. The anomalous left coronary artery is immediately obvious and is rapidly dissected and ligated close to the pulmonary artery wall with a single transfixing suture of 3-0 silk. Venous collaterals around the artery may require diathermy control. The pericardium is loosely closed and the chest closed with or without drainage. The entire procedure can be complete within 30–45 minutes.

CPB may be used, especially if the anomalous coronary artery attaches to the pulmonary trunk posteriorly (UAB). Using a single venous cannula and perfusion at 37°C and no aortic cross-clamping, the pulmonary trunk is opened transversely and the origin of the left coronary artery oversewn with a few simple sutures reinforced with a pledgetted mattress suture. The CPB time is approximately 15 minutes.

SPECIAL FEATURES OF POSTOPERATIVE CARE

The care of patients undergoing repair of anomalous origin of the left coronary artery from the pulmonary artery is the same as that for other patients undergoing cardiac surgery (see Chapter 5). In the case of critically ill small infants, low cardiac output can be anticipated in the first few postoperative days, and appropriate measures applied (see Chapter 5, "Low Cardiac Output" in section on Cardiovascular Subsystem).

EARLY RESULTS

The hospital mortality following *operation in infancy* has been high in most reported series.[A5,D6,L4] Ten hospital deaths (59%, CL 43%–73%) occurred among 17 patients in this age group (GLH and UAB; Tables 31-3, 31-4). The series reported by Arciniegas and colleagues is the only one with a low mortality, 2 deaths (17%, CL 6%–35%) occurring among 12 patients (Table 31-5).[A4] It is noteworthy, however, that in their series, 6 seriously ill infants were not operated upon, all of whom died. Thus, 8 (40%, CL 27%–54%) among 20 patients seen by Arciniegas and colleagues died. It is the preoperative condition of the patient, not age per se, that is the risk factor (Table 31-6).

The safest operation in the infant group has yet to be established (Table 31-7). Arciniegas and colleagues had 2 deaths among 3 infants undergoing ligation and no death in 9 undergoing anastomotic procedures,[A4] whereas there were no deaths with ligation regardless of age (GLH; see Table 31-3). Thus it may be that the risk of simple ligation without CPB is less than that for occlusion of the anomalous ostium from within the pulmonary artery using CPB, but this has not been established with certainty.

Operation beyond infancy has been associated with a mortality rate approaching zero (see Tables 31-3, 31-4).[A4,C2] This seems to be true whatever operation is used, including coronary artery bypass vein grafting.[C2]

LATE RESULTS

Survival

The survival rate is generally high, and dependent primarily upon the hospital mortality rate. Premature late death is uncommon among hospital survivors,[C2,M3,W2] only 1 having occurred among 19 patients after a maximum follow-up of 19 years (UAB and GLH). It is apparent that late death has been uncommon even when the left coronary artery occludes late after the various procedures that establish a two-

Table 31-3 A surgical experience with anomalous origin of the left coronary artery from the pulmonary artery (GLH; 1957–1984).

Year at Operation	Age	CHF	CTR	Infarct	Operation	Outcome[a]
1960	7 mo	None	>70%	Yes	Excision infarct	HD
1963	2 yr	None	58%	No	Ligation	1982 NYHA I
1966[b]	47 yr	None	52%	Yes	Ligation	Died 1971
1966[b]	23 yr	None	52%	No	Ligation	1979 NYHA I
1972	4 mo	Yes	69%	Yes	LCA-Ao	HD
1973	4 mo	Yes	69%	Yes	LCA-Ao	HD
1974	8 mo[c]	Yes	76%	Yes	Ligation	1980 NYHA I[e]
1974	4 mo	Yes	>70%	Yes	Ligation	1980 NYHA I
1978	1 mo[d]	Yes	75%	No	Ligation	1983 NYHA I
1979	4 mo	Yes	>70%	Yes	Ligation	1980 NYHA I

KEY: CHF, congestive heart failure; CTR, cardiothoracic ratio; HD, hospital death; LCA-Ao, reimplantation operation.

NOTE: Ligation was performed without CPB. During this period, only one additional patient (aged 2 months) was seen and not operated upon, death occurring before investigation could be carried out.

[a] Includes year of follow-up and NYHA class.
[b] Previously reported.[R7]
[c] Circumflex from RPA + origin LAD from RCA.
[d] Circumflex from RPA + severe coarctation of aorta.
[e] Residual severe mitral regurgitation.

Table 31-4 Hospital mortality, according to the age of the patient, after repair of origin of left coronary artery from the pulmonary trunk (UAB; 1967–July, 1983).

Age (mo)			Hospital Deaths		
≤	<	n	No.	%	CL
	6	8	5	63%	38%–83%
6	12	2	2	100%	39%–100%
12	24				
24	48	3	0	0%	0%–47%
48		6	0	0%	0%–27%
	Total	19	7	37%	24%–51%

KEY: CL, 70% confidence limits.

NOTE: No infants were seen and not operated upon. Patients older than 48 months were 5, 11, 13, 17, 19, and 52 years old.

Table 31-5 Hospital mortality after surgery for anomalous origin of the left coronary artery from the pulmonary trunk, in the experience of Arciniegas and colleagues.[A4]

Age (mo)			Hospital Deaths		
≤	<	n	No.	%	CL
	3	1		0%	0%–85%
3	6	7	2	29%	10%–55%
6	12	4		0%	0%–38%
12	24	5		0%	0%–32%
24		2		0%	0%–61%
	Total	19	2	11%	4%–23%

KEY: CL, 70% confidence limits.

coronary system.[C2,M3,W2] (See below for the instance of saphenous vein bypass grafting.)

Functional Status

The functional status is generally good late postoperatively. In a group of 18 long-term survivors, 17 are in NYHA class I and the other in NYHA class II (GLH and UAB). The size of the left ventricle (including the cardiothoracic ratio) is nearly always markedly reduced by operation,[L4] and signs of myocardial ischemia are reduced.[D4,M3] The type of operation has not been shown to be related to the late postoperative

Table 31-6 Hospital mortality, according to NYHA preoperative functional class, after surgical treatment of anomalous origin of left coronary artery from the pulmonary trunk (UAB; 1967–July, 1983).

NYHA Class	Hospital Deaths						
	n	No.	%	CL			
I	1	0	0%	0%–85%			
II	3	0	0%	0%–47%	0/9	0%	0%–19%
III	5	0	0%	0%–38%			
IV	6	3	50%	18%–82%	7/10	70%	49%–86%
V	4	4	100%	62%–100%			
Total	19	7	37%	24%–51%			
P(logistic)		.002					

KEY: CL, 70% confidence limits.

NOTE: NYHA class V indicates emergency operation for acute hemodynamic deterioration.

Table 31-7 Hospital mortality, according to type of procedure used for repair of origin of left coronary artery from pulmonary trunk (UAB; 1967–July 1983).

Procedure	n	No.	%	CL
			Hospital Deaths	
Occlusion of origin of LCA	7	2	29%	10%–55%
Reimplantation in aorta				
Coronary artery anastomosis	12	5	42%	25%–60%
Tunnel anastomosis	4	2	50%	18%–22%
Left subclavian–left coronary anastomosis	4	3[a]	75%	37%–97%
Saphenous vein bypass grafting	4[b]		0%	0%–38%
Total	19	7	37%	24%–51%

KEY: CL, 70% confidence limits.

[a] One death was a 7-month-old infant in whom concomitant mitral valve replacement was performed.

[b] Ages 2½, 11, 17, 52 years.

results,[M3] although there is a suggestion in the report by Wilson and colleagues that in adult patients closure of the anomalous origin of the left coronary artery and saphenous vein bypass grafting is superior to simple closure of the origin.[W2] The late postoperative functional status in patients operated upon in infancy or in adult life appears to depend primarily on the status of the left ventricle before operation,[M3] just as it does in arteriosclerotic ischemic heart disease (see Chapter 7).

Conduit Patency and Hemodynamic State

When saphenous vein bypass grafts are used in adults, *graft patency rates* may be higher than in arteriosclerotic coronary artery disease. Donaldson and colleagues report 4 of 5 grafts patent 14 years postoperatively[D4]; when the reports of Moodie et al. and Chiariello and colleagues are combined, 11 out of 15 grafts were patent.[C2,M3] However, concern exists about the potentially lethal effect of vein graft closure should it occur, particularly in view of the demonstrated regression of the right coronary artery collaterals that follows successful revascularization.[D4,M3] Indeed, Anthony and colleagues have reported sudden death in a 9-year-old girl 5 months after closure of the anomalous origin of the left coronary artery from the pulmonary trunk and saphenous vein bypass grafting; at autopsy the graft was shown to be occluded and to have extensive intimal fibrous hyperplasia.[A3] Similar obliterative changes have been observed in these vein grafts by El-Said and colleagues.[E3]

Few studies of patency of the tunnel repair have been reported. However, Midgley and colleagues reported a patent tunnel conduit in an infant studied 14 months after repair.[M9] Objective evidence of improved left ventricular function has been obtained after all types of operations (Figs. 31-10, 31-11).[A4,S3] There is no certainty that one type of operation is better than another in this regard, although exercise testing in a small number of patients has supported the superiority of a two-vessel system after operation.[M4]

Ischemic mitral incompetence of moderate degree appears to persist late postoperatively in many cases. Thus, among 12 long-term survivors 6 (50%) have a mild-to-moderate intensity apical systolic murmur (UAB), which probably results from mitral incompetence, and one other patient has persistent severe mitral incompetence (GLH).

INDICATIONS FOR OPERATION

The diagnosis of anomalous origin of the left coronary artery from the pulmonary artery in an infant, usually seriously ill, is an indication for urgent operation. The recommendation that operation be delayed until an older age[D6] is no longer tenable.

The optimal operation in infancy remains controversial, as is evident from the hospital mortality rates after the various operations. In the critically ill infant, simple ligation by a closed (GLH) or open (UAB) technique is currently the procedure of choice. It is possible that simple ligation should be followed by an elective bypass procedure later to avoid the potential risk of late sudden death.[W3] Theoretically, the creation of a two-vessel coronary artery system is desirable, provided this can be done at low risk and with a good chance of permanent patency. The tunnel operation, using pulmonary artery wall[T2] or, alternatively, reimplantation when this can be accomplished without tension or kinking can be recommended for infants who are not critically ill (UAB).

Beyond infancy, the optimal operation would seem to be a tunnel procedure (or reimplantation), avoiding coronary artery bypass vein grafting because of the virtual certainty of ultimate late vein graft occlusion. Internal mammary artery grafting is, however, a reasonable alternative when the size of the mammary artery allows this procedure (see Chapter 7, "The Internal Mammary Artery for the CABG Operation" in section on Special Situations and Controversies).

SPECIAL SITUATIONS AND CONTROVERSIES
Analogy with Arteriosclerotic Ischemic Heart Disease

Infants who are seriously ill because of anomalous origin of the left coronary artery from the pulmonary trunk present

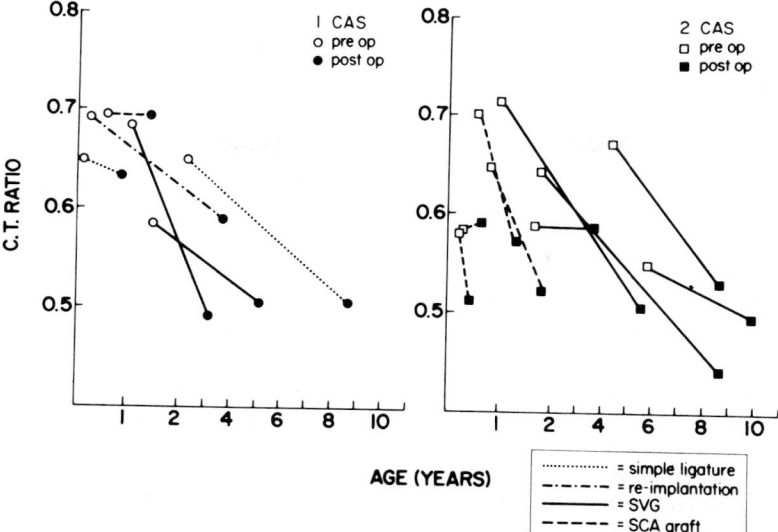

Figure 31-10 Change in cardiothoracic ratio after surgery for anomalous origin of left coronary artery from pulmonary trunk. Along the horizontal axis is age in years at the time of the observation. "1 CAS" (in the leftward frame) indicates patients with one coronary arterial system postoperatively; "2 CAS" (in the rightward frame) indicates patients with two coronary arterial systems postoperatively.

Reproduced with permission from Arciniegas et al.,[A4] and the American Heart Association, Inc.

because of myocardial ischemia, usually having suffered several silent myocardial infarctions and occasionally presenting with acute myocardial infarction. The evolving experience with adult acute myocardial infarction (see Chapter 7, "CABG for Acute Myocardial Infarction" in section on Special Situations and Controversies) indicates that such infants should be operated upon as emergencies.

Such infants rarely have true left ventricular aneurysms, so that aneurysmectomy is rarely if ever required. The assumption can be made that there are viable myocardial cells scattered throughout the scarred ventricle and that improvement of coronary blood flow to the left ventricle should improve left ventricular function. The good functional state of patients after repair and the reduction in left ventricular

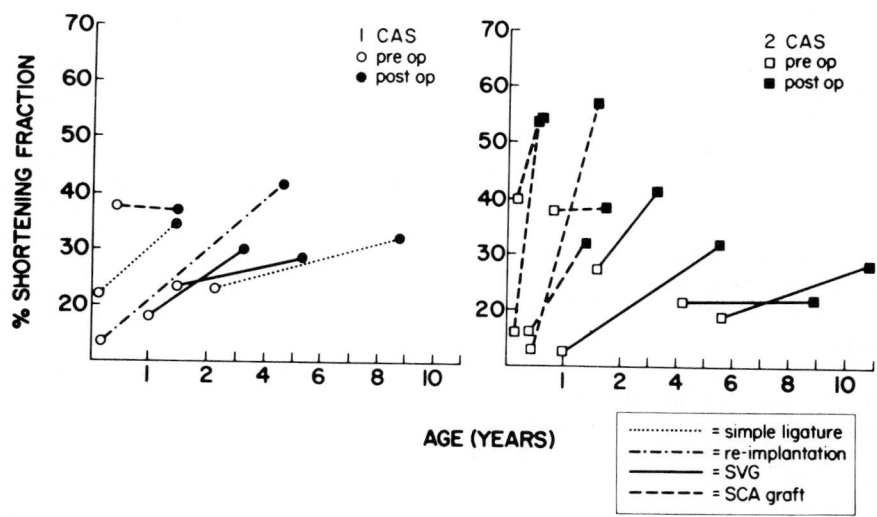

Figure 31-11 Change in left ventricular shortening fraction after surgery for anomalous origin of left coronary artery from the pulmonary trunk. Depiction as in Figure 31-10.

Reproduced with permission from Arciniegas et al.,[A4] and the American Heart Association, Inc.

size that usually occurs supports this belief. This reasoning also supports increasing the amount of revascularization obtained, not only by occluding the anomalous origin of the left coronary artery (and thus stopping the coronary steal), but also by constructing an aorta–left coronary artery connection when this can be done at a low risk.

Mitral Incompetence

Recognition of the analogies between the congenital malformation of anomalous origin of the left coronary artery from the pulmonary trunk and adult arteriosclerotic coronary artery disease helps in the management of the mitral incompetence that may coexist with the former condition. In fact, the principles described for managing adult ischemic mitral incompetence (see Chapter 10, "Indications for Operation") apply directly. However, it is probable that the mitral valve should not be interfered with when operation is performed in infancy even when regurgitation is judged moderate or severe, since it almost always lessens postoperatively.[S3] Un-

commonly severe incompetence does not regress, however, and then valve replacement is necessary.[B11]

Anomalous Origin of the Right Coronary Artery from the Pulmonary Trunk

An anomaly even more rare than anomalous origin of the left coronary artery from the pulmonary trunk is the similarly anomalous origin of the right coronary artery. In 1975, only 11 cases were recorded in the world literature.[B7] This anomaly is a much less lethal one than is anomalous origin of the left coronary artery, and the diagnosis is usually made at autopsy or incidentally in asymptomatic adults. Occasionally, the anomaly is associated with symptoms in an older child or adult or with sudden death.[L5] Surgical correction consists of excising the anomalous origin of the right coronary artery from the anterior aspect of the pulmonary trunk, along with a button of pulmonary arterial wall, and reimplanting it into the anterior aspect of the ascending aorta.[T3] Probably operation is advisable when the diagnosis is made.

REFERENCES

A

1. Abbott ME: *Congenital Heart Disease, Osler's Mod. Med.* Philadelphia, 1927, vol IV.

2. Augustasson MN, Gasul BM, Lundquist R: Anomalous origin of the left coronary artery from the pulmonary artery (adult type). *Pediatrics* 29:274, 1962.

3. Anthony CL, McAllister HJA, Cheitlin MD: Spontaneous graft closure in anomalous origin of the left coronary artery. *Chest* 68:4, 1975.

4. Arciniegas E, Farooki ZQ, Hakimi M, Green EW: Management of anomalous left coronary artery from the pulmonary artery. *Circulation* 62(suppl I):I-180, 1980.

5. Askenazi J, Nadas AS: Anomalous left coronary artery originating from the pulmonary artery. Report on 15 cases. *Circulation* 51:976, 1975.

6. Ahmed SS, Haider B, Regan TJ: Silent left coronary—cameral fistula: probable cause of myocardial ischemia. *Am Heart J* 104:869, 1982.

7. Apley J, Horton RE, Wilson MG: The possible role of surgery in the treatment of anomalous left coronary artery. *Thorax* 12:23, 1957.

8. Agatston AS, Chapman E, Hildner FJ, Samet P: Diagnosis of a right coronary artery—right atrial fistula using two-dimensional and Doppler echocardiography. *Am J Cardiol* 54:238, 1984.

B

1. Barcia A, Kincaid OW, Swan HJC, Weidman WH, Kirklin JW: Coronary artery-to-right ventricle communication: Report of two cases studied by selective angiocardiography. Staff Meetings of the Mayo Clinic 37 (No. 24):623, 1962.

2. Baim DS, Kline H, Silverman JF: Bilateral coronary artery—pulmonary artery fistulas. Report of five cases and review of the literature. *Circulation* 65:810, 1982.

3. Biorck G and Crafoord C: Arteriovenous aneurysm on the pulmonary artery simulating patent ductus arteriosus botalli. *Thorax* 2:65, 1947.

4. Brooks SJ: Two cases of an abnormal coronary artery of the heart arising from the pulmonary artery: With some remarks upon the effect of this anomaly in producing cirsoid dilatation of the vessels. *J Anat Phys* 20:26, 1886.

5. Bland EF, White PD, Garland J: Congenital anomalies of the coronary arteries: Report of an unusual case associated with cardiac hypertrophy. *Am Heart J* 787, 1933.

6. Burchell HB, Brown AL: Anomalous origin of the coronary artery from pulmonary artery masquerading as mitral insufficiency. *Am Heart J* 63:388, 1962.

7. Bregman D, Brennan FJ, Singer A, Vinci J, Parodi EN, Cassarella WJ, Edie RN: Anomalous origin of the right coronary artery from the pulmonary artery. *J Thorac Cardiovasc Surg* 72:626, 1976.

8. Blakeway HA: A hitherto undescribed malformation of the heart. *J Anat Physiol* 52:354, 1918.

9. Barratt-Boyes BG: Cardiac surgery in infancy. *NZ Med J* 64(suppl):17, 1965.

10. Barratt-Boyes BG: The technique of intracardiac repair in infancy using deep hypothermic with circulatory arrest and limited cardiopulmonary bypass, in MI Ionescu, GH Wosler (eds): *Current Techniques in Extracorporeal Circulation.* London: Butterworth 1976, p 219.

11. Bojar RM, Ilbawi MN, DeLeon SY, Riggs TW, Idriss FS: Surgical management of anomalous left coronary artery with mitral insufficiency in infancy: Contribution of echocardiography. *Pediatr Cardiol* 5:35, 1984.

C

1. Case RB, Morrow AG, Stainsby W, Nestor JO: Anomalous origin of the left coronary artery: The physiologic defect and suggested surgical treatment. *Circulation* 17:1062, 1958.

2. Chiariello L, Meyer J, Reul G, Hallman GL, Cooley DA: Surgical treatment for anomalous origin of left coronary artery from pulmonary artery. *Ann Thorac Surg* 19:443, 1975.

3. Currarino G, Silverman FN, Landing BH: Abnormal congenital

fistulous communications of the coronary arteries. *Am J Roentgenol* 82:392, 1959.

4. Cha SD, Singer E, Maranhao V, Goldberg H: Silent coronary artery-left ventricular fistula: A disorder of the Thebesian system? *Angiology* 29:169, 1978.

5. Cooley DA, Hallman GL, Bloodwell RD: Definitive qualified treatment of anomalous origin of left coronary artery from pulmonary artery. *J Thorac Cardiovasc Surg* 59:789, 1966.

6. Caldwell RL, Hurwitz RA, Girod DA, Weyman AF, Feigenbaum H: Two-dimensional echocardiographic differentiation of anomalous left coronary artery from congestive cardiomyopathy. *Am Heart J* 106:710, 1983.

D

1. de Nef JJE, Varghese PJ, Losekoot G: Congenital coronary artery fistula. Analysis of 17 cases. *Br Heart J* 33:857, 1971.

2. Dobell ARC, Long RW: Right coronary–left ventricular fistula mimicking aortic valve insufficiency in infancy. *J Thorac Cardiovasc Surg* 82:785, 1981.

3. Dietrich W: Ursprungder vorderen Kranz-arterie aus der Lungenschlagader mit ungewohnlichen Veranderungen des Herz muskels und der Gefasswande. *Virchows Arch [Pathol Anat]* 303:436, 1939.

4. Donaldson RM, Raphael MJ, Yacoub MH, Ross DN: Hemodynamically significant anomalies of the coronary arteries: Surgical aspects. *Thorac Cardiovasc Surg* 30:7, 1982.

5. Doty DB, Chandramouli B, Schieken RE, Lauer RM, Ehrenhaft JL: Anomalous origin of the left coronary artery from the right pulmonary artery. *J Thorac Cardiovasc Surg* 71:787, 1976.

6. Driscoll DJ, Nihill MR, Mullins CE, Cooley DA, McNamara DG: Management of symptomatic infants with anomalous origin of the left coronary artery from the pulmonary artery. *Am J Cardiol* 47:640, 1981.

7. Daniel TM, Graham TP, Sabiston DC Jr: Coronary artery-right ventricular fistula aorto congestive heart failure: Surgical correction in the neonatal period. *Surgery* 67:985, 1970.

E

1. Edis AJ, Schattenberg TT, Feldt RH, Danielson GK: Congenital coronary artery fistula. Surgical considerations and results of operation. *Mayo Clin Proc* 47:567, 1972.

2. Edwards JE: Functional pathology of congenital cardiac disease. *Pediat Clin North Am* 1:13, 1954.

3. El-Said GM, Ruzyllo W, Williams RL, Mullins CE, Hallman GL, Cooley DA, McNamara DG: Early and late result of saphenous vein graft for anomalous origin of left coronary artery from pulmonary artery. *Circulation* (suppl. III)47, 48:III-2, 1973.

F

1. Fell EH, Weinberg J, Gordon AS, Gasul BM, Johnson FR: Surgery for congenital arteriovenous fistulas. *Arch Surg* 77:331, 1958.

2. Floyd WL, Young WG, Johnsrude IS: Coronary arterial–left atrial fistula. Case with obstruction of the inferior vena cava by a giant left atrium. *Am J Cardiol* 25:716, 1970.

3. Fleming RJ, Marx L, Litwin SB, Gallen WL: Left ventricular aneurysmectomy in a child. *Ann Thorac Surg* 19:457, 1975.

G

1. Goebel N, Gander MP, Steinbrunn W: Small coronary artery fistulae. *Ann Radiol* 22:277, 1979.

2. George JM, Knowlan DM: Anomalous origin of the left coronary artery from the pulmonary artery in an adult. *N Engl J Med* 261:993, 1959.

3. Grace RR, Angelini P, Cooley DA: Aortic implantation of anomalous left coronary artery arising from pulmonary artery. *Am J Cardiol* 39:608, 1977.

4. Griffiths SP, Ellis K, Hordof AJ, Martin E, Levine OR, Gersony WM: Spontaneous complete closure of a congenital coronary artery fistula. *JACC* 2:1169, 1983.

5. Goldblatt E, Adams APS, Ross IK, Savage JP, Morris LL: Single-trunk anomalous origin of both coronary arteries from the pulmonary artery. *J Thorac Cardiovasc Surg* 87:59, 1984.

H

1. Habermann JH, Howard ML, Johnson ES: Rupture of the coronary sinus with hemopericardium. *Circulation* 28:1143, 1963.

2. Hamilton DI, Ghosh PK, Donnelly RJ: An operation for anomalous origin of left coronary artery. *Br Heart J* 41:121, 1979.

3. Halpert B: Arteriovenous communication between the right coronary artery and the coronary sinus. *Heart* 15:129, 1930.

4. Horiuchi T, Abe T, Tanake S, Koyamada K: Congenital coronary arteriovenous fistulas. *Ann Thorac Surg* 11:102, 1971.

5. Hudspeth AS, Linder JH: Congenital coronary arteriovenous fistula. *Arch Surg* 96:832, 1968.

J

1. Jaffe RB, Glancy DL, Epstein SE, Brown BG, Morrow AG: Coronary arterial–right heart fistulae. *Circulation* 47:133, 1973.

K

1. Krause W: Ueber den Ursprung einer accessorischen A. coronaria cordis aus der A. pulmonalis. *Z Ratl Med* 24:225, 1865.

2. Keeton BR, Keenan DJM, Monro JL: Anomalous origin of both coronary arteries from the pulmonary trunk. *Br Heart J* 49:397, 1983.

3. Kittle CF, Diehl AM, Heilbruun A: Anomalous left coronary artery arising from pulmonary artery. *J Pediatr* 47:198, 1955.

4. King DH, Danford DA, Huhta JC, Gutgesell HP: Noninvasive detection of anomalous origin of the left main coronary artery from the pulmonary trunk by pulsed Doppler echocardiography. *Am J Cardiol* 55:608, 1985.

L

1. Liberthson RR, Sagar K, Berkoben JP, Weintraub RM, Levine FH: Congenital coronary arteriovenous fistula. Report of 13 patients, review of the literature and delineation of management. *Circulation* 59:849, 1979.

2. Levin DC, Fellows KE, Abrams HL: Hemodynamically significant primary anomalies of the coronary arteries. Angiographic aspects. *Circulation* 58:25, 1978.

3. Lowe JE, Oldham HN, Sabiston DC: Surgical management of congenital coronary artery fistulas. *Ann Surg* 194:373, 1981.

4. Laborde F, Marchand M, Leca F, Jarreau MM, Dequirot A, Hazan E: Surgical treatment of anomalous origin of the left coronary artery in infancy and childhood. *J Thorac Cardiovasc Surg* 82:423, 1981.

5. Lerberg DB, Ogden JA, Zuberbuhler JR, Bahnson HT: Anomalous origin of the right coronary artery from the pulmonary artery. *Ann Thorac Surg* 27:87, 1979.

6. Levitsky S, van der Horst RL, Hastreiter AR, Fisher EA: Anomalous left coronary artery in the infant. Recovery of ventricular function following early direct aortic implantation. *J Thorac Cardiovasc Surg* 79:598, 1980.

7. Lien CH, Tan NC, Tan L, Seah CS, Tan D: Congenital aneurysm of right coronary artery. *Am J Cardiol* 39:751, 1977.

M

1. Meyer BW, Stefanik G, Stiles QR, Lindesmith GG, Jones JC: A method of definitive surgical treatment of anomalous origin of left coronary artery—a case report. *J Thorac Cardiovasc Surg* 56:104, 1968.

2. Moller JH, Lucas RV, Adams P, Anderson RC, Jorgens J, Edwards JE: Endocardial fibroelastosis: Clinical and anatomic study of 47 patients with emphasis on its relationship to mitral insufficiency. *Circulation* 30:759, 1964.

3. Moodie DS, Fyfe D, Gill CG, Cook SA, Lytle BW, Taylor PC, Fitzgerald R, Sheldon WC: Anomalous origin of the left coronary artery from the pulmonary artery (Bland-White-Garland syndrome) in adult patients: Long-term follow-up after surgery. *Am Heart J* 106:381, 1983.

4. McNamara DG, El-Said G: Treatment of anomalous origin of the left coronary artery from the pulmonary artery. *Eur J Cardiol* 1:497, 1973.

5. McNamara JJ, Gross RE: Congenital coronary artery fistula. *Surgery* 65:59, 1969.

6. Meyer MH, Stephenson HE Jr, Keats TE, Martt JM: Coronary artery resection for giant aneurysmal enlargement and arteriovenous fistula. *Am Heart J* 74:603, 1967.

7. Masuya K, Kusunoki N, Hara S, Funatsu T, Takegosh N, Marakami E, Ueyama T, Takeda R: Congenital right coronary artery fistula communicating with the left ventricle. *South Med J* 68:1007, 1975.

8. Mustard WT: Anomalies of the coronary arteries, in *Pediatric Surgery*. Chicago: Year Book, 1953, vol 1, p 433.

9. Midgley FM, Watson DC Jr, Scott LP III, Kuehl KS, Perry LW, Galioto FM Sr, Ruckman RN, Shapiro SR: Repair of anomalous origin of the left coronary artery in the infant and small child. *JACC* 4:1231, 1984.

N

1. Neches WH, Mathews RA, Park SC, Lenox CC, Zuberbuhler JR, Siewers RD, Bahnson HT: Anomalous origin of the left coronary artery from the pulmonary artery. *Circulation* 50:582, 1974.

2. Noren GR, Raghib G, Moller JH, Amplatz K, Adams P, Edwards JE: Anomalous origin of the left coronary artery from the pulmonary trunk with special reference to the occurrence of mitral insufficiency. *Circulation* 30:171, 1964.

O

1. Oldham HN, Ebert PA, Young WG, Sabiston DC: Surgical management of congenital coronary artery fistula. *Ann Thorac Surg* 12:503, 1971.

2. Ott DA, Cooley DA, Pinsky WW, Mullins CE: Anomalous origin of circumflex coronary artery from right pulmonary artery. *J Thorac Cardiovasc Surg* 76:190, 1978.

3. Okuda Y, Tsuneda T, Morishima A, Matsumoto S, Ito Y, Isuzaki M: Right coronary artery to left ventricle fistula. The sixth case in the literature and discussion. *Jpn Heart J* 14:184, 1973.

4. Ogden JA, Stansel HC Jr: Coronary arterial fistulas terminating in the coronary venous system. *J Thorac Cardiovasc Surg* 63:172, 1972.

P

1. Pinsky WW, Fagan LR, Mudd JFG, Willman VL: Subclavian-coronary artery anastomosis in infancy for the Bland-White-Garland syndrome. *J Thorac Cardiovasc Surg* 72:15, 1976.

2. Potts WJ: (1955) Personal communication.

3. Paul RN, Robbins SG: A surgical treatment prognosed for either endocardial fibroelastosis or anomalous left coronary artery. *Pediatrics* 47:196, 1955.

R

1. Rittenhouse EA, Doty DB, Ehrenhaft JL: Congenital coronary artery–cardiac chamber fistula. *Ann Thorac Surg* 20:468, 1975.

2. Rudolph AM, Gootman NL, Kaplan N, Rohman M: Anomalous left coronary artery arising from the pulmonary artery with large left-to-right shunt in infancy. *J Pediatr* 63:543, 1963.

3. Roberts WC: Anomalous origin of both coronary arteries from the pulmonary artery. *Am J Cardiol* 68:595, 1962.

4. Reddy K, Gupta M, Hamby RI: Multiple coronary arteriosystemic fistulas. *Am J Cardiol* 33:304, 1974.

5. Rodgers DM, Wolf NM, Barrett MJ, Zuckerman GL, Meister SG: Two-dimensional echocardiographic features of coronary arteriovenous fistula. *Am Heart J* 104:872, 1982.

6. Rowe GG, Young WP: Anomalous origin of the coronary arteries with special reference to surgical treatment. *J Thorac Cardiovasc Surg* 39:777, 1960.

7. Roche AHG: Anomalous origin of the left coronary artery from the pulmonary artery in the adult. Report of uneventful ligation in two cases. *Am J Cardiol* 20:561, 1967.

8. Roberts WC, Robinowitz M: Anomalous origin of the left anterior descending coronary artery from the pulmonary trunk with origin of the right and left circumflex coronary arteries from the aorta. *Am J Cardiol* 54:1381, 1984.

S

1. Shubrooks SJ, Naggar CZ: Spontaneous near closure of coronary artery fistula. *Circulation* 57:197, 1978.

2. Sabiston DC, Neill CA, Taussig HB: The direction of blood flow in anomalous left coronary artery arising from the pulmonary artery. *Circulation* 22:591, 1960.

3. Shrivastava S, Castaneda AR, Moller JH: Anomalous left coronary artery from the pulmonary trunk. *J Thorac Cardiovasc Surg* 76:130, 1978.

4. Swan H, Wilson JH, Woodwark G, Blount SG: Surgical obliteration of a coronary artery fistula to right ventricle. *Arch Surg* 79:820, 1959.

5. Sakakibara S, Yokoyama M, Takao A, Nogi M, Gomi H: Coronary arteriovenous fistula. *Am Heart J* 72:307, 1966.

T

1. Talner NS, Halloran KH, Mahdavy M, Gardner TH, Hipona F: Anomalous origin of the left coronary artery from the pulmonary artery: Clinical spectrum. *Am J Cardiol* 15:689, 1965.

2. Takeuchi S, Imamura H, Katsumoto J, Hayashi I, Katohgi T, Yozu R, Ohkura M, Inoue T: New surgical method for repair of anomalous left coronary artery from the pulmonary artery. *J Thorac Cardiovasc Surg* 78:7, 1979.

3. Tingelstad JB, Lower RR, Eldredge WJ: Anomalous origin of the right coronary artery from the main pulmonary artery. *Am J Cardiol* 30:670, 1972.

4. Trevor RS: Aneurysm of the descending branch of the right coronary artery situated in the wall of the right ventricle and opening into the cavity of the ventricle, associated with great dilatation of the right coronary artery and non-valvular infective endocarditis. *Proc R Soc Med* 5:20, 1912.

5. Turina M, Real F, Neier W, Senning A: Left ventricular aneurysmectomy in a 4-month-old infant. *J Thorac Cardiovasc Surg* 67:915, 1974.

U

1. Urrutia-S CO, Falaschi G, Ott DA, Cooley DA: Surgical management of 56 patients with congenital coronary artery fistulas. *Ann Thorac Surg* 35:300, 1983.

2. Usman A, Fernandez B, Uricchio JF, Nichols HT: Aberrant origin of left coronary artery combined with mitral regurgitation in an adult. *Am J Cardiol* 8:130, 1961.

W

1. Wesselhoeft H, Fawcett JS, Johnson AL: Anomalous origin of the left coronary artery from the pulmonary trunk. *Circulation* 38:403, 1968.

2. Wilson CL, Dlabal PW, McGuire SA: Surgical treatment of anomalous left coronary artery from pulmonary artery: Follow-up in teenagers and adults. *Am Heart J* 98:440, 1979.

3. Wilde P, Watt I: Congenital coronary artery fistulae: Six new cases with a collective review. *Clin Radiol* 31:301, 1980.

4. White H, Wilde P, Wattie J, Barratt-Boyes BG: Aneurysmal right coronary artery with a fistula into the left ventricle (1985) Personal communication.

5. Worsham C, Sanders SP, Burger BM: Origin of the right coronary artery from the pulmonary trunk: Diagnosis by two-dimensional echocardiography. *Am J Cardiol* 55:233, 1985.

CONGENITAL AORTIC STENOSIS

Congenital aortic stenosis is a cardiac anomaly in which narrowing at valvar, subvalvar, supravalvar, or combined (multiple) levels results in a systolic pressure gradient between the inflow portion of the left ventricle and the aorta beyond the obstruction.

SECTION 1
CONGENITAL VALVAR AORTIC STENOSIS

DEFINITION

Congenital valvar aortic stenosis is an obstruction at valve level due to imperfect cusp development with leaflet thickening. In this chapter, congenital valvar aortic stenosis is discussed only in the age group from birth to 25 years (GLH) or to 20 years (UAB). The leaflet abnormalities may or may not be severe in early life; in the latter instance significant obstruction may not develop until later in life when calcification occurs.[R1,R2]

HISTORICAL NOTE

Congenital valvar aortic stenosis has been long recognized by morphologists. Initial efforts to find a surgical solution to this malformation were made by Carrel and Jeger, who independently attempted experimentally to place conduits between the left ventricular apex and the aorta.[C17,J4] In 1955, Marquis and colleagues reported the surgical treatment of congenital valvar aortic stenosis by dilators introduced through the apex of the left ventricle, as did Downing in 1956.[D7,M21] Also in 1956, valvotomy was done by an open technique during inflow stasis and with moderate hypothermia induced by surface cooling.[L9,S16,S19] The first report of its treatment by accurate valvotomy during cardiopulmonary bypass was by Spencer and colleagues in 1958,[S1] although we at the Mayo Clinic had performed the procedure in 1956.[E2,E6]

MORPHOLOGY

Aortic Valve

In patients with stenosis severe enough to require operation in infancy or childhood, the valve is bicuspid in about 70% of cases (Table 32-1) and usually consists of thickened right and left leaflets in association with an anterior and a posterior commissure and a slitlike orifice with its long axis in the sagittal plane (Fig. 32-1). The left cusp is frequently the larger and may contain a transversely placed central thickened ridge (or buttress), representing a rudimentary commissure between the normal right and left cusps. Less commonly, the two cusps are anterior and posterior, and the orifice is then oriented in a coronal plane. There is usually fusion peripherally of one or, occasionally, both commissures. However, severe stenosis can occur without this feature, purely as a result of thickened leaflets and a bicuspid configuration. If the free edges of both thickened bicuspid leaflets are taut, they are then equal in length to the diameter of the aortic root and cannot open (Fig. 32-1b).[E4]

Table 32-1 Morphology of congenital valvar aortic stenosis in a surgical series of patients operated on at age 1–25 years (GLH; 1958–1977).

	No.	% of 39
Bicuspid valve	17	44%
Bicuspid valve with rudimentary commissure in one cusp	9	23%
Tricuspid valve	12	30%
Unicuspid valve	1	3%
Total	39	100%

NOTE: The frequency of the unicuspid variety has possibly been underestimated, since a bicuspid valve in which the commissures are very rudimentary might better be termed "unicuspid."

In about 30% of cases (Table 32-1), the valve is tricuspid, with three thickened leaflets of approximately equal size and three recognizable commissures that are fused peripherally to varying degrees, creating a dome with a central stenotic orifice. This type of valve is the more favorable for valvotomy since all three commissures can usually be opened.

Rarely, the valve may have a unicuspid configuration (Fig. 32-2) with only one commissure. This variety is more common in infants presenting with severe stenosis,[M18] but occasionally the stenosis is not severe and signs and symptoms develop in later life as the valve thickens and calcifies.[F8] A thickened unicuspid valve is inherently stenotic, whether or not the commissure is fused, unless the leaflets are particularly redundant.

Diffuse leaflet thickening, most marked at the free leaflet edges, contributes importantly to the valvar stenosis. This process is more extreme in neonates and infants, and the cusps may be very irregular and myxomatous or dysplastic in appearance.[C2] In addition, particularly in infants, the aortic anulus may be small and itself stenotic, frequently in association with endocardial fibroelastosis of a hypoplastic left ventricle (Fig. 32-3), coarctation of the aorta, patent ductus arteriosus, and mitral incompetence or stenosis.[H3,L2]

Left Ventricle

The left ventricle is always concentrically hypertrophied in children with severe aortic stenosis, but in infants the hypertrophy is occasionally extreme (Fig. 32-4) with a tiny cavity and extensive fibrosis in the wall. The fibrosis is primarily in the subendocardial region.[C16] Extensive endocardial fibroelastosis may also be present, and it is possibly the result of ischemia of the subendocardial layers. In these hearts, the ventricle may be dilated (Fig. 32-5).

Coexisting Cardiac Anomalies

Congenital valvar aortic stenosis may be associated with a fibrous subvalvar or a supravalvar stenosis. Hastreiter and associates have noted that in severe aortic stenosis presenting in infancy, the valvar stenosis and hypoplasia of the aortic anulus may be associated with a subvalvar stenosis as well as coarctation of the aorta.[H5] Many other congenital cardiac anomalies such as ventricular septal defect, atrial septal defect, and pulmonary stenosis may coexist (Table 32-2).

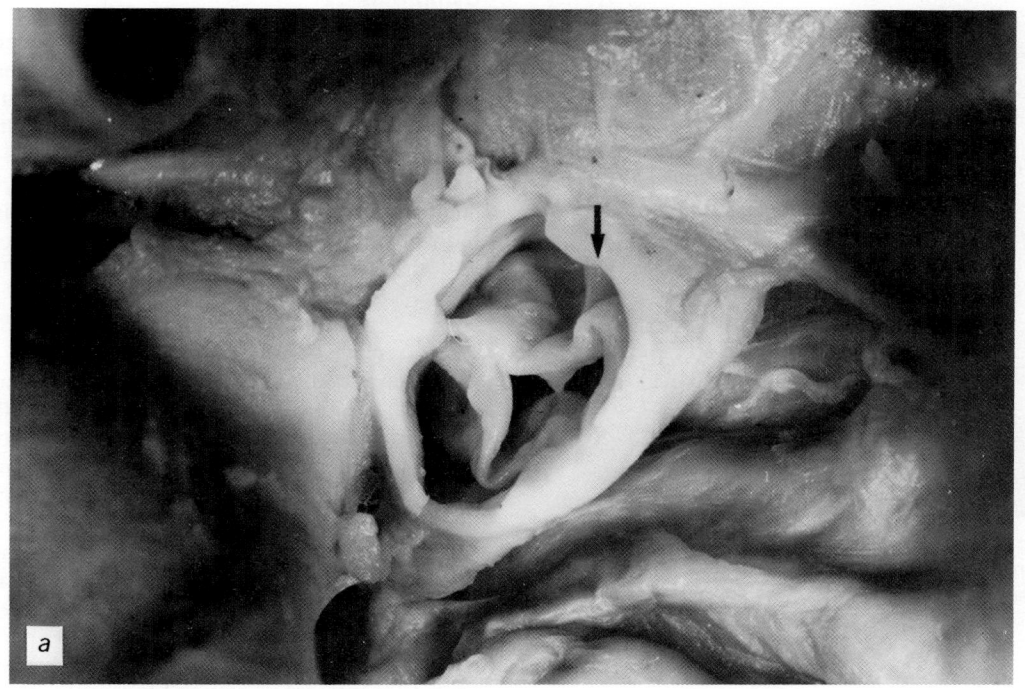

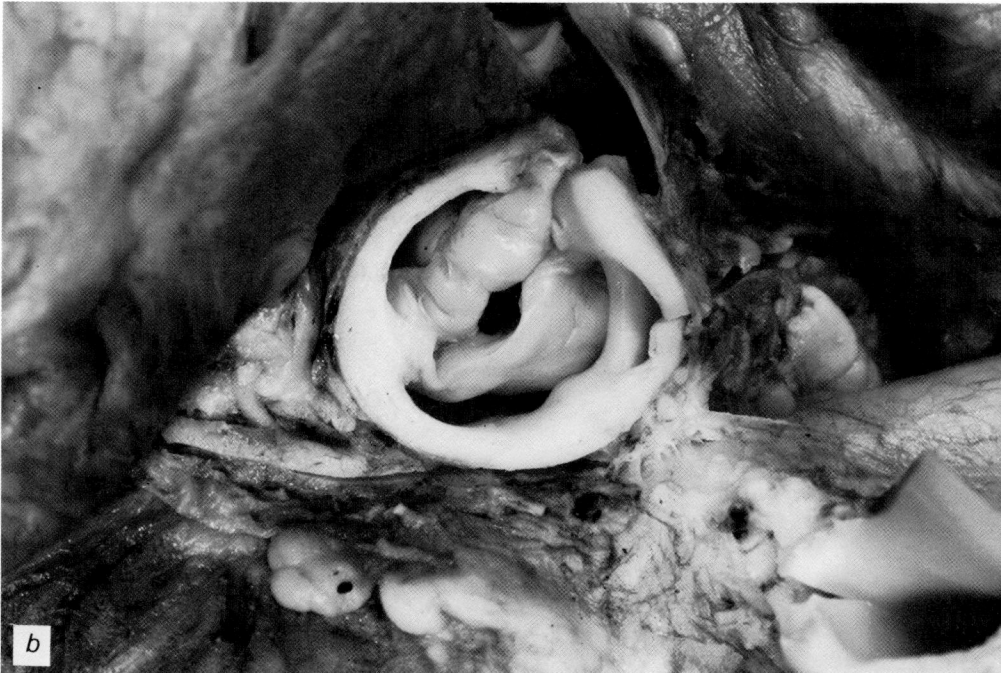

Figure 32-1 Specimens of congenital aortic stenosis with a bicuspid valve (GLH).
(a) Bicuspid valve with mild leaflet thickening, moderately redundant leaflets, and fusion of one commissure. There is a diminutive buttress in the anterior leaflet (arrow).
(b) Bicuspid valve from a neonate with severe aortic stenosis. The leaflets are very thickened and obstructive, but there is no commissural fusion and no buttress formation.

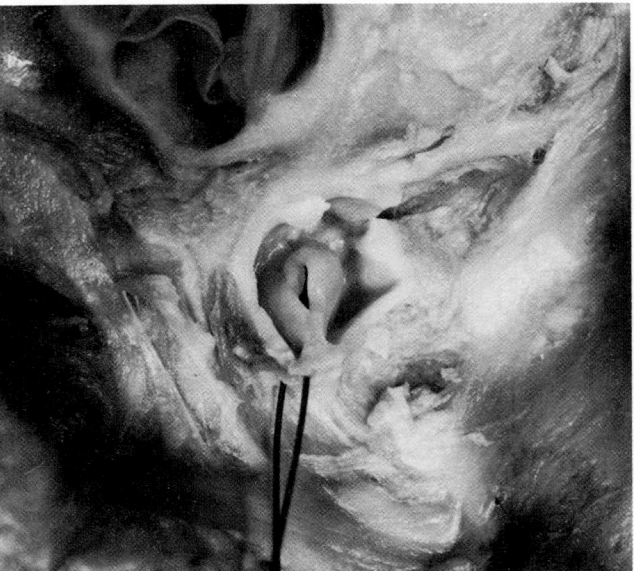

Figure 32-2 Specimen of a unicuspid aortic valve (GLH). The single fused commissure is suitable for valvotomy, but the cusps cannot be divided elsewhere without producing incompetence.

CLINICAL FEATURES AND DIAGNOSTIC CRITERIA

Symptoms

In neonates and infants presenting with severe valvar aortic stenosis, the presentation is usually with pallor, perspiration, and inability to feed. Shortness of breath and cyanosis may be present. In children and young adults, even important congenital valvar aortic stenosis may be without symptoms. However, the presence of effort dyspnea, effort angina, or effort syncope, singly or in combination, usually indicates a severe lesion.[D1,G1,H1] Dyspnea may be present with moderate stenosis.

Signs

In neonates and infants presenting with severe valvar aortic stenosis, the most striking feature is the small pulse volume, pallor, dyspnea, and sometimes cyanosis. Both the murmur and the gradient across the valve may be unimpressive because of a low cardiac output. There also may be a hyperactive right ventricular impulse.

Clinical signs in children and young adults include an ejection systolic murmur (and thrill) at the base radiating to the carotid vessels accompanied by a systolic ejection click. An aortic diastolic murmur is uncommon, particularly when compared to patients with discrete subvalvar stenosis. A severe lesion is characterized by a pulse that is palpably of low volume and slow upstroke, single or reversed splitting of

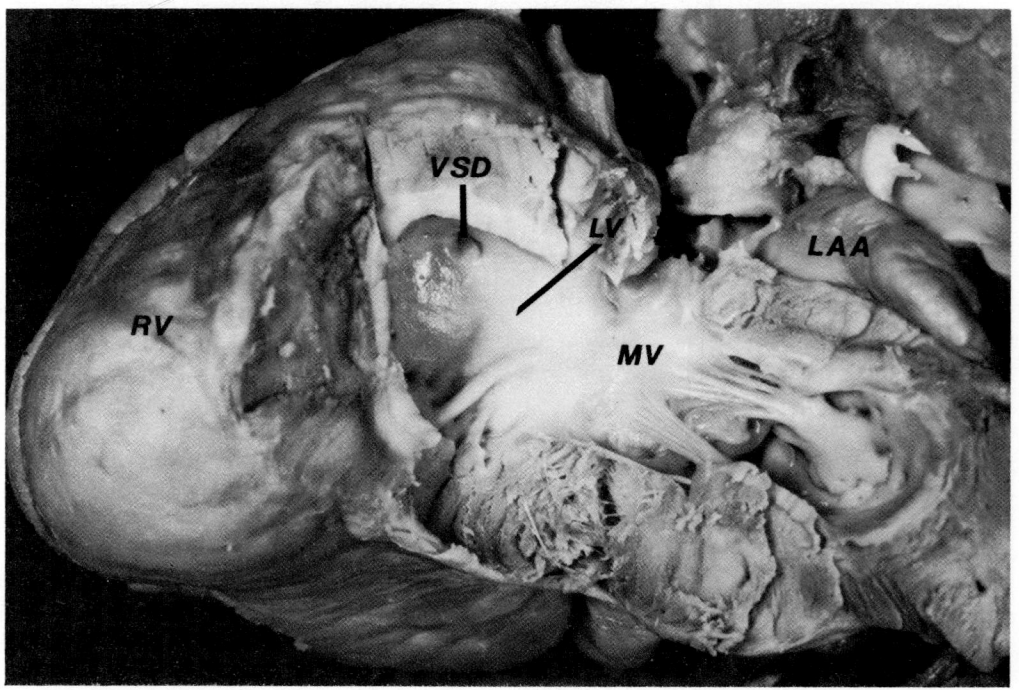

Figure 32-3 Specimen from a 10-day-old infant with severe aortic valvar stenosis (GLH). The opened left ventricle is relatively hypoplastic compared to the enlarged right ventricle, with thick walls and marked endocardial fibroelastosis. A small anterior, midmuscular ventricular septal defect is present.

AoV, aortic valve; LAA, left atrial appendage; LV, left ventricle; MV, mitral valve; RV, right ventricle; VSD, ventricular septal defect.

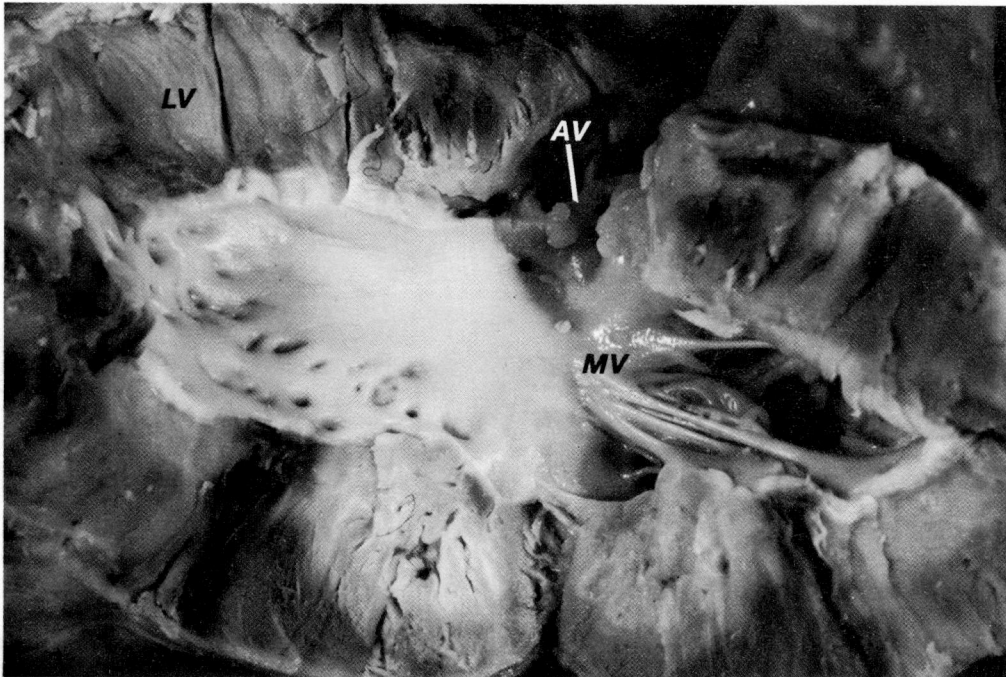

Figure 32-4 Specimen of congenital aortic stenosis from a 9-month-old infant (GLH). The aortic valve leaflets are thickened, nodular, and myxomatous. The opened left ventricle is small and has extreme hypertrophy and moderate endocardial fibroelastosis, which also involves the papillary muscles of the mitral valve.

AV, aortic valve; LV, left ventricle; MV, mitral valve.

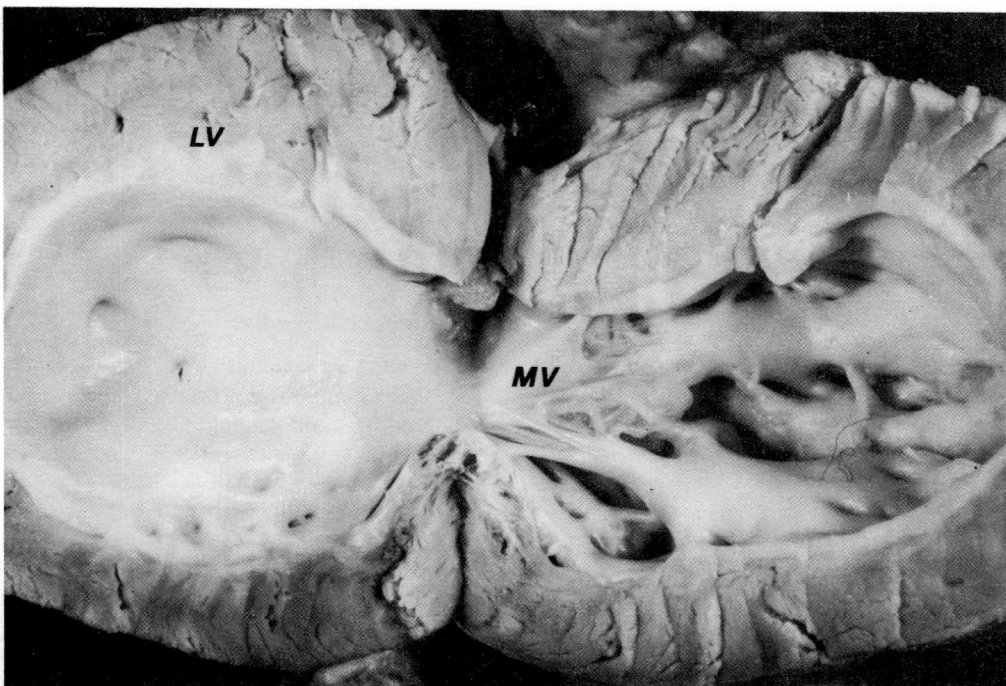

Figure 32-5 Specimen of congenital aortic stenosis from a 12-day-old infant (GLH). The opened left ventricle is hypertrophied and dilated. The septal surface is smooth because of the endocardial fibroelastosis that measures 1.5 mm in thickness. There is associated congenital mitral valve disease, with thickened leaflets and chordae and obliteration of interchordal spaces (see Chapter 36 for details concerning congenital mitral valve disease).

LV, left ventricle; MV, mitral valve.

Table 32-2 Coexisting cardiac anomalies (previously or concurrently repaired or left unrepaired) in patients coming to operation for congenital aortic stenosis (UAB; 1967–1982; $n = 142$).

Type of Congenital Aortic Stenosis	Associated Anomaly	No. of Cases
Valvar ($n = 78$)	Isolated PDA	8
	PDA + ASD	3
	PDA + coarctation	3
	Isolated coarctation	3
	Isolated VSD	1
	PDA + coarctation + VSD	1
	Left SVC	1
		20 (26%)
Subvalvar ($n = 41$)	Isolated PDA	2
	PDA + coarctation	1
	Coarctation + congenital mitral stenosis	1
	VSD + important PS	3
	Unroofed coronary sinus syndrome	1
	Left SVC + single coronary orifice	1
	AI (3 mild, 2 important)	5
	VSD	4
		18 (44%)
Supravalvar ($n = 10$)	Pulmonary artery stenosis	1
	Left SVC	1
		2 (12%)
Combined ($n = 7$)	PDA + coarctation	1
	Congenital mitral stenosis	1
	VSD	1
		3 (43%)

KEY: AI, aortic incompetence; ASD, atrial septal defect; PDA, patent ductus arteriosus; PS, pulmonary stenosis; SVC, superior vena cava; VSD, ventricular septal defect.

NOTE: ( ) is % of n. The categories are mutually exclusive.

the second heart sound, an apical fourth and sometimes a third heart sound, and a thrusting left ventricular impulse.

Many investigators have concluded that physical signs are unreliable in assessing the severity of valvar stenosis in children.[C1,E1,F1,G1,J1,W1] However, it is possible to differentiate on the basis of physical signs among mild, moderate, and severe lesions in most instances, and severe lesions can always be distinguished from those that are only mild.[H1]

Electrocardiogram

The electrocardiogram usually shows severe left ventricular hypertrophy but can be near normal.[H2] There may be right ventricular hypertrophy in the electrocardiogram in association with a left-to-right shunt at atrial level through a stretched patent foramen ovale and sometimes a reversed shunt at ductus level.[S2]

Chest X-Ray

The ascending aorta frequently is prominent. Increase in heart size is seldom seen except in neonates and infants in congestive heart failure, where it may be very marked.

Radiologically demonstrable valvar calcification is rare in patients under 25 years of age.

Noninvasive Studies

Noninvasive techniques used to assess the severity of stenosis include analysis of the carotid upstroke with phonocardiography[B1] and echocardiography, which is helpful in assessing left ventricular size, wall thickness and ejection fraction, and possibly orifice size.[B15,G2,W2] The estimation of subendocardial oxygen requirements has also been said to be helpful in assessing severity of the stenosis.[K1,L4]

Currently, noninvasive methods of estimating the pressure gradient across the congenitally stenotic aortic valve are being perfected, and these play an increasingly important role in the necessary continuous reevaluation of patients with this anomaly. Although two-dimensional echocardiography has been limited in its ability to measure aortic valve area, Doppler ultrasound is capable of measuring the velocity of flow across stenotic valves,[H9] and this can be used to quantify the transvalvar pressure gradient. Stamm and colleagues have found, in patients with aortic stenosis, a correlation coefficient (r) of .94 (with the standard error of the estimate

12.8 mmHg) between peak aortic gradients determined at cardiac catheterization and those by Doppler ultrasound.[S12]

Cardiac Catheterization and Angiography

The definitive diagnosis currently depends on the demonstration of a systolic gradient across the aortic valve at cardiac catheterization, usually through a retrograde aortic approach but, if this is not possible, by a transeptal approach. Cardiac output is also measured so that a valve area can be calculated. A gradient greater than 75 mmHg or a valve area less than 0.5 cm^2 · m^{-2} is indicative of severe stenosis (see below). A raised left ventricular end-diastolic pressure indicates left ventricular failure unless it is merely a function of an augmented a wave.

Angiocardiography demonstrates thickened leaflets that form a dome in systole with a localized jet of contrast entering the aorta (Fig. 32-6), but this type of study is not reliable in assessing the severity of stenosis. It will, however, assess the size of the aortic ring and left ventricle, and an aortic root injection allows quantitation of aortic regurgitation when this is present.

Summary

By a combination of clinical and hemodynamic assessments, patients with congenital valvar aortic stenosis can be categorized as having mild, moderate, or severe obstruction.[H1] *Mild* implies that pulse volume and contour are normal, as is the second heart sound. Patients with these findings have a left ventricular–aortic (LV-Ao) systolic pressure difference less than 40 mmHg at rest, and the mean value for a group of such patients is 20 mmHg. Patients considered to have *moderate* stenosis have an abnormally small pulse volume to palpation and by contour, and narrow inspiratory splitting of the second heart sound may be present. Such patients generally have gradients less than 75 mmHg, and the mean value is 50 mmHg. Patients with *severe* stenosis have a gradient in excess of 75 mmHg and an abnormal pulse volume and contour, as well as a single second heart sound or reverse splitting. These patients have a mean calculated aortic valve area index of 0.38 ± 0.15 cm^2 · m^{-2}.[H1]

NATURAL HISTORY

Congenital valvar aortic stenosis is three to four times more common in males than in females and occurs in about 5% of patients with congenital heart disease.

Presentation in Infancy

When valvar stenosis presents in infancy, the lesion is almost always severe as evidenced by rapidly progressive congestive heart failure and death within a few days to a few weeks of birth. This accounts for the fact that most neonates and young infants come to operation critically ill and in NYHA class IV or V (Table 32-3). Many have other associated left heart lesions. Over a 10-year period, 17 infants pre-

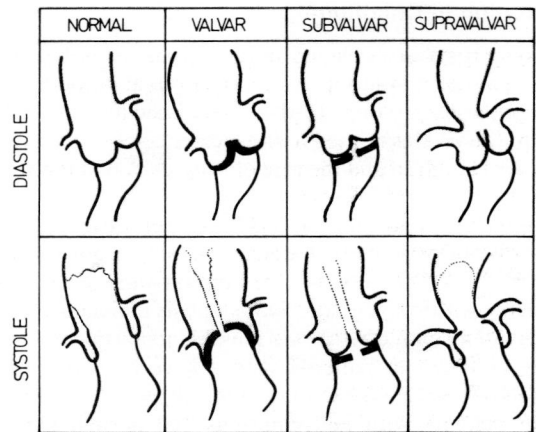

Figure 32-6 Diagrammatic representation of angiocardiographic signs of aortic stenosis (GLH). In *valvar stenosis*, there is systolic doming and a jet between the thickened leaflets. Poststenotic dilatation of the aorta is visible. In fibrous *subvalvar* stenosis, a jet may be seen and the leaflets may not open fully but doming is absent. The membrane should be visible and there is often mild aortic incompetence. In *supravalvar* stenosis, the narrowing commencing above the aortic leaflets is visible. The sinuses of Valsalva are prominent, and the coronary arteries are often dilated.

sented in heart failure with severe valvar stenosis, 15 in the first 2 weeks of life and the oldest at 6 weeks, but only 4 did not have significant associated lesions (GLH, 1967–1977). All died, except 3 of those who had valvotomy.

The various coexisting left heart anomalies are left ventricular hypoplasia of varying degrees (5 in the 17 GLH patients), extreme left ventricular hypertrophy with small cavity size (2), endocardial fibroelastosis (9), congenital mitral stenosis (6) or incompetence (1), patent ductus arteriosus (7), severe coarctation (2), and subaortic stenosis due to mitral valve abnormalities (2). In addition, a ventricular septal defect (4), as well as pulmonary atresia (1), may be present.

Table 32-3 NYHA functional class according to age at the time of the first repair of congenital aortic stenosis (UAB; 1967–1982; n = 142).

Age at Operation ≤ <	NYHA Functional Class (mean ± SD)			
	Valvar (n = 78)	Subvalvar (n = 41)	Supravalvar (n = 16)	Combined (n = 7)
Weeks				
1	4.8 ± 0.45			
1 --- 4	4.1 ± 0.94			4.0
Months				
1 --- 3	4.5 ± 0.71			
3 --- 12	3.0 ± 1.26			
12 --- 48	2.2 ± 0.98	3.2 ± 0.96	1.0 ± 0.00	3.0
Years				
4 --- 12	1.7 ± 0.76	1.8 ± 0.94	1.7 ± 0.52	2.0 ± 1.00
12 --- 20	1.7 ± 0.73	1.8 ± 1.19	1.7 ± 0.58	2.5 ± 0.71
20		1.9 ± 0.74	2.8 ± 0.84	

NOTE: The patients were categorized into NYHA classes I–V, class V indicating those operated upon as an emergency because of shock or metabolic acidosis.

Presentation in Childhood

When symptoms are delayed until the patient is beyond 1 year of age, heart failure is rare and survival without treatment is generally prolonged. Also, associated lesions are less common. Survival is related to the incidence of sudden death in untreated children and the rate of progression of the stenosis.

The reported incidence of *sudden death* varies between 1% and 19% of patients with congenital valvar aortic stenosis.[B2,C3,G1,M1,O1,P1] Analysis of the literature and of a series of 218 patients with congenital valvar stenosis indicates that the risk of sudden death directly attributable to aortic stenosis is virtually confined to patients with a severe lesion (GLH; mean follow-up 13 years, maximum 20 years).[H1] Sudden death in patients with no symptoms and normal physical findings apart from the murmur of aortic stenosis has not been documented. Sudden death may occur in patients with a normal electrocardiogram,[H1] but this finding is not incompatible with severe stenosis. Thus, the true incidence of sudden death in children and adolescents in whom surgery is deferred until the lesion is considered severe on clinical grounds is probably in the vicinity of 1%.

When congenital aortic valvar deformities are nonobstructive in infancy and childhood, less than 10% *progress* to mild obstruction within about 10 years. Mills and colleagues have obtained information on a group of 26 patients who were aged 1 week to 29 years when first seen and in whom the diagnosis of nonobstructive aortic valve deformity was made on the basis of an isolated aortic ejection sound.[L1] During a 5–16-year follow-up, 2 (7%, CL 2%–16%) developed signs of mild stenosis after 7 and 15 years.[M2] As many more years pass, an undetermined time-related proportion of people with deformed (usually congenitally bicuspid) aortic valve develop progressive thickening and calcification and ultimately important stenosis.

When mild stenosis is present at the first evaluation in childhood, progression is somewhat more rapid. Within 10 years, about 20% of such patients have developed moderate or severe stenosis; within about 20 years, 45% have done so (Fig. 32-7). Even after this long interval, therefore, 55% of the mild lesions remained mild.

When moderate stenosis is present initially, the lesion had become severe within 10 years in about 60% of cases (Fig. 32-8).

Spontaneously occurring bacterial endocarditis appears in fewer than 1% of cases. The incidence was 2.7 episodes per 1,000 patient years (GLH),[H1] and in a series reported by Gersony and colleagues it was 1.8 per 1,000 patient years.[G3] Bacterial endocarditis may produce aortic incompetence and be a cause of death.

TECHNIQUE OF OPERATION

Valvotomy in Neonates and Critically Ill Infants

The technique of surface cooling and profoundly hypothermic total circulatory arrest may be used (GLH). The technique as described earlier is followed (see Chapter 2, Section 4). By the time the heart is exposed and preparations are completed, including the insertion of a single venous cannula into the right atrial appendage but not of the arterial cannula, the temperature is at 21–22°C. The circulation is then arrested by snugging down the caval tapes and cross-clamping the aorta. The ascending aorta is opened with an

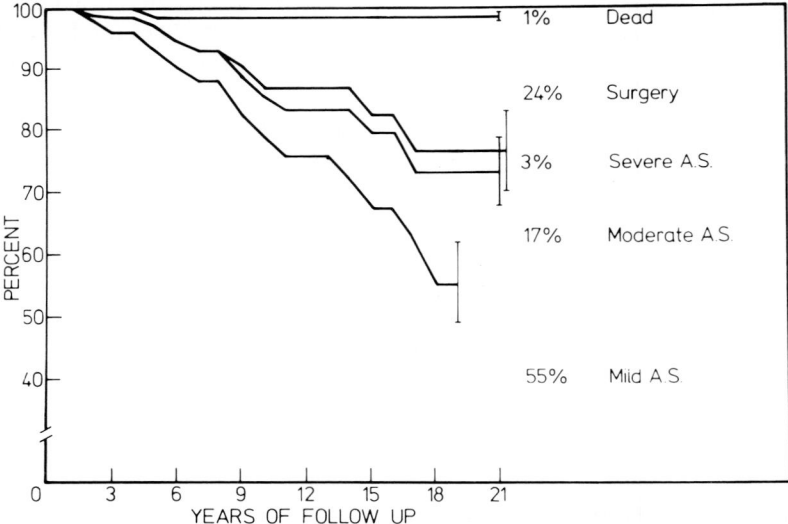

Figure 32-7 Cumulative actuarial curves for 153 patients presenting with originally mild congenital valvar aortic stenosis (GLH). The vertical bars represent 70% confidence limits. Mean age at presentation was 6.5 years (1–25 years) and mean follow-up time 8.8 years (1–26 years). The one death in this group was due to bacterial endocarditis. The patients underwent operation when the stenosis was considered severe.

Reproduced with permission from Hossack et al.[H1]

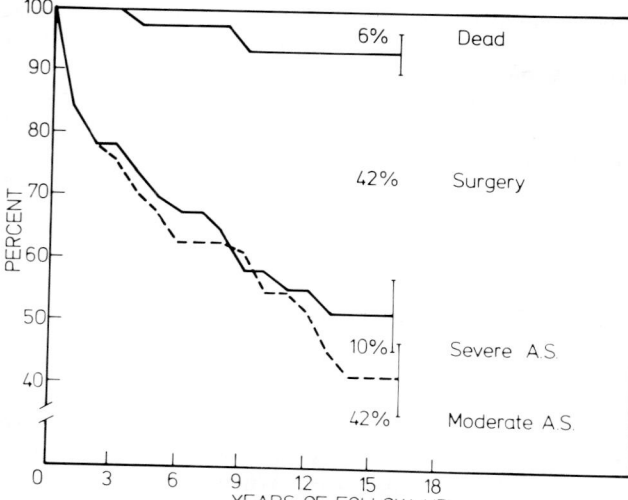

Figure 32-8 Cumulative actuarial curves for 54 patients presenting with originally moderate congenital valvar aortic stenosis (GLH). The vertical bars represent 70% confidence limits. Mean age at presentation was 11.8 years (1–25 years) and mean follow-up time 8.5 years (1–24 years). The two deaths in this group were both sudden, 4 and 9 years after presentation, in association with progression to severe stenosis.

Reproduced with permission from Hossack et al.[H1]

oblique incision that passes into the noncoronary sinus of Valsalva.

The valvotomy is performed by dividing fused commissures with a knife to within 1 mm of the aortic wall. In this, it is important that even tension be placed on the two adjoining cusps so that the incision is precise. Only those commissures with adequate leaflet attachment to the aortic wall are opened because division of rudimentary commissures produces incompetence. The incisions are deepened in stages, and the cusps on each side are evaluated as to their competence and lack of prolapse before each further incision.[E6] If it is sensed that a further incising of the commissure will cause cusp prolapse, the incision is carried no further. Very occasionally, myxomatous nodules can be excised from the cusp-free edge or fibrous thickening can be shaved off the ventricular aspect of one or more cusps. The aortotomy is then closed with a running suture. The arterial cannula is inserted proximal to the aortic cross-clamp, the left heart is de-aired, and rewarming CPB is begun after releasing the aortic cross-clamp (see Chapter 2, Section 4).

Alternatively, the technique of CPB at 37°C, with simple aortic cross-clamping and no cardioplegia, may be used (UAB). The anesthetic and supportive management must be precise and delicate (see Chapter 4). The preparation and median sternotomy are as described earlier (see Chapter 2). As the pericardium is being opened, care is taken to touch the heart as little as possible, since ventricular fibrillation is easily provoked. The purse-string suture is placed for the aortic cannula, the patient heparinized, and the cannula inserted and connected to the arterial line. Only then is a purse-string suture placed around the right atrial appendage,

for if the heart then fibrillates, CPB can be established in less than a minute. A single venous cannula is inserted (see Chapter 2 for details), CPB is begun at 25°C, the aorta is cross-clamped, and the perfusate temperature is taken to 37°C.

The usual transverse aortotomy incision is made (see Chapter 12, Fig. 12-2), and the ventricular cavity is cleaned of blood with a small high-power sucker. Two stay sutures are placed on the upstream side of the aortotomy for exposure. Aortic valvotomy is performed as described above. The aortotomy is closed with a simple whip stitch. A small stab wound is made in the aorta proximal to the clamp for de-airing, and the clamp is removed. The remainder of the procedure is completed as usual, closing the stab wound with a simple stitch after de-airing. A pulmonary artery pressure-monitoring catheter may be placed through the right ventricle when insertion of a left atrial catheter in this circumstance is deemed hazardous.

Valvotomy in Older Infants, Children, and Adults

The preparation for operation, the incision, and the preparations for CPB are those described earlier (see Chapter 2, Section 3). Using a single venous cannula (UAB) or caval cannulation (GLH), CPB is established at 28°C. No left atrial or left ventricular vent is used. External cardiac cooling is applied. The aorta is cross-clamped, and the cold cardioplegic solution is infused (see Chapter 3). The transverse aortotomy is made (see Chapter 12, Fig. 12-2), and stay sutures are applied to the edges of the incision for exposure. The commissurotomy is performed as described earlier. The aortotomy is closed with a simple whip stitch.

With strong suction on the aortic needle vent and after aspirating air from the apex of the left ventricle, the aortic clamp is released and rewarming is begun. The remainder of the operation is completed as usual. Left ventricular and aortic pressures are measured and recorded before closing the chest.

Aortic Valve Replacement in Children

When the congenitally stenotic aortic valve is viewed at operation, it may be apparent that it is too extensively deformed to allow its being opened and remaining reasonably competent. However, this situation is rare in primary operations in patients less than 10 years old and uncommon in those less than 20 years of age. It is more common when a second or third valvotomy is being done for a patient receiving an original valvotomy in early life.

A homograft valve or, if this is not feasible, a St. Jude valve is preferred. The techniques for these operations, including when necessary enlargement of the aortic root, are described in Chapter 12.

SPECIAL FEATURES OF POSTOPERATIVE CARE

The postoperative care after aortic valvotomy or the other procedures discussed in this section are conducted in the manner generally used after open cardiac operations (see Chapter 5).

Whenever valvotomy is performed for congenital valvar aortic stenosis, long-term follow-up is indicated because of the possible occurrence of restenosis and need for reoperation.

EARLY RESULTS

Hospital Mortality

The overall hospital mortality for the surgical treatment of congenital valvar aortic stenosis in patients less than 20–25 years of age is a nearly meaningless figure, since it is so heavily affected by the age of the patients. This mortality has been 18% (CL 14%–22%) in the combined UAB-GLH experience (23 deaths among 128 patients) (Tables 32-4 and 32-5). The very differing mortality among the subsets is illustrated by the fact that both at GLH and UAB there have been no deaths after valvotomy in children and young adults, and mortality was also low in this age group in an earlier era,[E2] whereas in neonates the mortality has been 62%–100% (Tables 32-5 and 32-6). However, the potential safety of an open approach in neonates with severe congenital aortic stenosis has been demonstrated by Messina, Ebert, and colleagues who report one hospital death (9%; CL 1%–28%) among 11 neonates in this category and no late deaths.[M22]

In contrast to many situations in cardiac surgery, nearly all deaths after surgery for congenital valvar aortic stenosis occur early postoperatively (Figure 32-9) and most within 48 hours of operation.

INCREMENTAL RISK FACTORS FOR HOSPITAL DEATH

Poor Preoperative Functional Class

Advanced symptoms, that is being in NYHA class IV and particularly class V, are associated with a considerable increased risk of hospital death. When this is taken into account in a multivariate way, no other risk factors are apparent (Table 32-7). The risk in patients (nearly always neonates and young infants) in NYHA class V is extraordinarily high (Table 32-8).

Table 32-4 Types of operation and hospital deaths after primary operations for congenital aortic stenosis (UAB; 1967–1982; $n = 142$).

Site of Stenosis	Procedure	n	Hospital Deaths
Valvar	Aortic valvotomy	75	14
	Aortic valve replacement	2	0
	Sternotomy (intended valvotomy)	1	1
		78	15 (19%, CL 14%–25%)
Subvalvar	Excision, and	26	0
	Septal myotomy	11	0
	Modified Konno repair	2	0
	LV-Ao Conduit	2	0
		41	0 (0%, CL 0%–5%)
Supravalvar	Patch widening of ascending aorta	16	2 (12%, CL 4%–27%)
Valvar + supravalvar	AVR and patch widening	1	0
	Aortic valvotomy and patch widening	1	0
		2	0
Valvar + subvalvar	Aortic valvotomy, and		
	Excision of subvalvar stenosis at early reoperation	1	0
	Excision	2	0
	Modified Konno repair after ineffective myotomy	1	1
		4	1
Valvar + subvalvar + supravalvar	Excision of subvalvar stenosis, with later reoperation	1	0

KEY: AVR, aortic valve replacement; CL, 70% confidence limits; LV-Ao, left ventricular to aortic.

NOTE: In the subvalvar group, two patients also had aortic valve replacement for preoperatively severe incompetence as did one adult patient with supravalvar stenosis. The 16-year-old patient with stenosis at all three levels had early reoperation with patch graft enlargement ascending aorta, mitral valve replacement and resection of hypertrophied, obstructing papillary muscles for coexisting congenital aortic stenosis, and left-ventricular–aortic conduit.

Table 32-5 Results of surgery for congenital valvar aortic stenosis (GLH; 1958–1977).

Procedure	n	Age Presentation	Age Surgery	Hospital Deaths No.	Hospital Deaths %	Hospital Deaths CL	Late Deaths	Reoperation	SBE
Valvotomy	30	8.8(1–25)yr	12.1(2–30)yr	0	0%	0%–6%	4	10	2
Primary valve replacement	9	12.5(6–23)yr	23.6(14–35)yr	0	0%	0%–19%	1	1	1
Valvotomy in infancy	11[a]	(0.3–3)wk	(0.4–38)wk	8	72%	53%–88%	0	0	0
Total	50			8	16%	11%–23%	5	11	3

KEY: CL, 70% confidence limits.

[a] Includes five neonates with five (100%, CL 68%–100%) deaths and six infants older than 30 days with three (50%, CL 24%–76%) deaths.

Table 32-6 Hospital deaths after surgery for congenital aortic stenosis (UAB; 1967–1982; $n = 142$, 18 deaths).

Age at Operation ≤ <	Valvar n	No.	%	CL	Subvalvar n	No.	%	CL	Supravalvar n	No.	%	CL	Combined n	No.	%	CL
Weeks																
1	5	4	80%	47%–97%												
1 --- 4	11	6[a]	55%	35%–73%									1	0	0%	0%–85%
Months																
1 --- 3	2	2	100%	39%–100%												
3 --- 12	11	3	27%	12%–47%												
12 --- 48	6	0	0%	0%–27%	4	0	0%	0%–38%	2	1	50%	7%–93%	1	1	100%	15%–100%
Years																
4 --- 12	23	0	0%	0%–8%	5	0	0%	0%–12%	6	1	17%	2%–46%	3	0	0%	0%–47%
12 --- 20	20	0	0%	0%–9%	12	0	0%	0%–15%	3	0	0%	0%–47%	2	0	0%	0%–61%
20					10	0	0%	0%–17%	5	0	0%	0%–32%				
Total	78	15	19%	14%–25%	41	0	0%	0%–5%	16	2[b]	12%	4%–27%	7	1	14%	2%–41%

KEY: CL, 70% confidence limits.

[a] Includes one patient dying at sternotomy before repair.

[b] Diffuse type.

Young Age

Very young age at operation is associated with a high risk of early death postoperatively[L3] (Tables 32-5, 32-6). However, most patients coming to operation in very early life have been in NYHA functional class IV or V (see Table 32-3). The poor functional status preoperatively better explains the deaths, statistically (Table 32-7) and intuitively, than does the young age. It is important to recall, however, that survival after operation is possible in critically ill neonates and young infants (Table 32-5 and 32-6).[B3,C6,K7,T2]

The hospital mortality after operations for congenital valvar aortic stenosis in patients over 1 year of age approaches zero (0 deaths [0%, CL 0%–2%] in 88 cases in the combined UAB-GLH experience). Even in an earlier era, the mortality was low under these circumstances (Table 32-9).

Coexisting Major Cardiac Anomalies

Coexisting severe left-sided cardiac defects (severe endocardial fibroelastosis, congenital mitral valve disease, left ventricular hypoplasia, extreme left ventricular hypertrophy with small cavity size[K7]) are associated with a high mortality rate after operation.[C7,H3] Again, coexisting major cardiac anomalies, poor preoperative functional class, and young age tend to occur together, but the coexisting cardiac anomalies along with the severity of the valvar aortic stenosis are probably the basic incremental risk factors.

Type of Congenital Valvar Aortic Stenosis

In a few patients, a unicusp or severely dysplastic bicuspid valve may be essentially uncorrectable,[C2] and in a few patients the very small aortic anulus may prevent a satisfactory outcome.

LATE RESULTS

Survival

Overall survival up to 15 years is good after the primary operation for congenital valvar aortic stenosis and is marred primarily by the high early risks in the very ill neonates and young infants (Fig. 32-10 and see Table 32-5).[L3]

Thus, for patients preoperatively in NYHA class I or II (and this means for most older infants and children), the 15-year survival (taking into account all deaths including those in hospital) after the primary valve operation is about 90% (Fig. 32-11).[A1,B3] In patients preoperatively in NYHA class

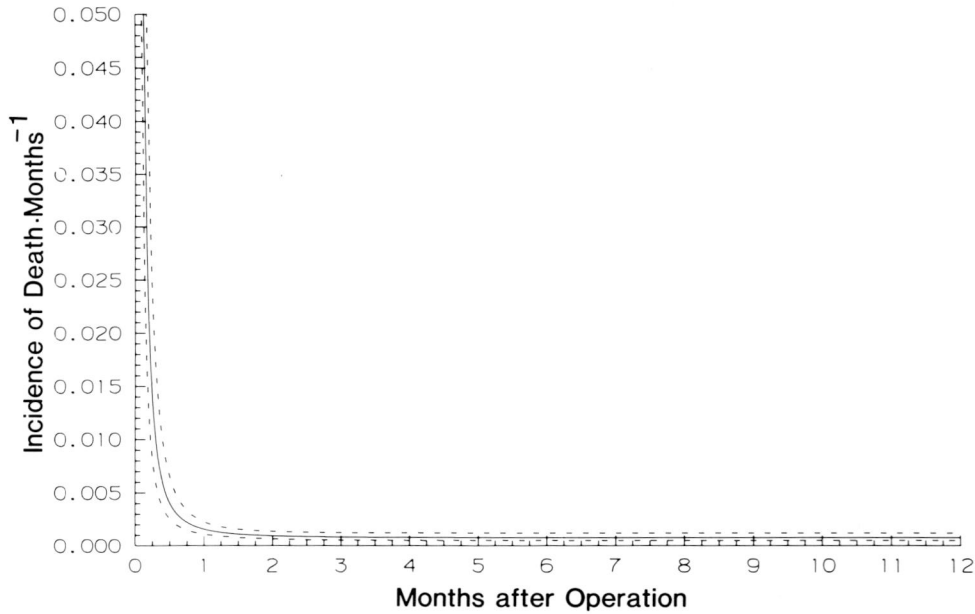

Figure 32-9 Nomogram of the hazard function (instantaneous risk of death at any time after one operation, depicted along the vertical axis) after the primary valve operation for congenital valvar aortic stenosis (UAB; 1967–1982; *n* = 78, all patients traced). Time zero is at the end of cardiopulmonary bypass. Patients were not censored at reoperation. The solid line is the point estimate, and the dashed lines enclose the 70% confidence limits. There is an early phase, which lasts about 5 weeks after operation, and a low constant late phase. (For discussion of the hazard function, see Chapter 6, "Parametric Methods" in Analysis of Time-Related Events in Section 4.)

IV or V (nearly all of whom are very ill neonates and young infants), the 15-year survival is 27%. However, the risk of death in the late phase (that is, after about 5 weeks postoperatively) is no greater in this group than in those preoperatively in NYHA class I or II.

Reoperation

About 35% of patients undergo a repeat aortic valve operation within 15–20 years of the original valve operation for congenital valvar aortic stenosis (Figs. 32-12 and 32-13). Recurrent or persistent stenosis is usually the indication (see later section, "Residual or Recurrent Left Ventricular–

Table 32-7 Incremental risk factors for death after original operation for congenital valvar aortic stenosis using hazard function analysis (see Fig. 32-9) (UAB; 1967–1982; *n* = 77, one neonate dying at sternotomy being omitted).

| | Hazard Phases | | |
| | Early | | |
Incremental Risk Factor	Coefficient ± SD	P value	Constant
NYHA class (I–V)	2.5 ± 0.72	.0004	
Intercepts	− 10.5		− 4.7

NOTE: The variables included in the analysis are NYHA classes I–V; age (months) at operation; sex; race; left atrial pressure at catheterization; LV size (surgical estimate); LV hypertrophy (surgical and autopsy estimate); cardioplegia, yes–no; aortic cross-clamp time in cardioplegia groups. Patients were not censored at reoperation. No risk factors were found for death in the late constant phase.

Aortic Pressure Gradients").[D6,K9,P5] The likelihood of having to undergo reoperation appears to be constant across time after the valvotomy (Fig. 32-14). Young age at valvotomy is not an incremental risk factor for reoperation in the early or intermediate length follow-up (Table 32-10).

The procedures done at reoperation are generally more varied than at the initial operation (Table 32-11). A satisfactory repeat valvotomy is sometimes possible, especially when the initial operation has been done in infancy.[F9,K7] At times, an overlooked second level of obstruction is found and requires treatment, such as patch graft supravalvar enlargement or a Konno procedure (see "Repair of Tunnel Stenosis by Atrioventriculoplasty (Konno Operation)" in Technique of Operation in Section 2). Since a small aortic anulus may be present, when aortic valve replacement is carried out, a Manouguian type of annular enlargement may be required (see Chapter 12). These procedures can be carried out at low risk at reoperation, no deaths having occurred in 10 reoperations (UAB) (Table 32-10), but no doubt at a somewhat greater risk than at the primary operation.[S14,S15]

In spite of efforts to save the native aortic valve, only 70% of patients surviving an initial aortic valvotomy have not required aortic valve replacement within 10 years of the valvotomy (Fig. 32-15).

Functional Status

Most surviving patients, including those who have had reoperations, are in NYHA class I or II (Table 32-12). Objective evidence of the improvement in functional capacity is pro-

Table 32-8 Digital nomogram of probability of death after valve surgery for congenital valvar aortic stenosis taken from the multivariate analysis (Table 32-7) of the hazard function (UAB; 1967–1982; $n = 78$, 15 deaths).

Preoperative NYHA Class	Probability of Death					
	48 Hours PO		2 Weeks PO		Early Phase of Hazard	
	%	CL	%	CL	%	CL
I	0.04%	0.005%–0.27%	0.08%	0.03%–0.22%	0.04%	0.004%–0.34%
II	0.4%	0.08%–1.9%	0.5%	0.12%–2.0%	0.4%	0.09%–2.1%
III	5%	1.9%–11%	5%	2.1%–12%	5%	2.1%–12%
IV	37%	27%–49%	40%	29%–52%	41%	30%–52%
V	87%	76%–93%	89%	79%–95%	89%	79%–95%

KEY: CL, 70% confidence limits.

NOTE: The probability of death within 48 hours of the end of cardiopulmonary bypass (PO) and within 2 weeks of it are shown, as well as within the entire early hazard phase (see Fig. 32-9).

Table 32-9 Composite results of aortic valvotomy for congenital valvar aortic stenosis in patients older than 1 year at operation. Noncardiac deaths have been excluded from the late mortality.

Reference	Number of Patients	Length of follow-up Mean (Range)	Early Mortality (%)	Late Mortality (%)	Reoperation Rate (%)	Significant AI (%)	Significant AS (%)	Endo-carditis (%)	Good Results (%)
Spencer (1958)[S1]	8	NS (1–6 mo)	0%	0%	NS	25%	12%		NS
Lees (1961)[L3]	26	17 mo (9 mo–3.5 yr)	4%	0%	NS	4%	2 of 7%	0%	
Ellis (1962)[E6]	33	18 mo (6–39 mo)	6%	6%	NS	18%	NS	3%	67%
Morrow (1963)[M7]	30	NS (2.5–17 mo)	10%	0%	NS	13%	7%	NS	NS
Cooley (1965)[C4]	39	NS (1–8 yr)	2.5%	NS	NS	NS	NS	NS	NS
Thomson (1965)[T1]	23	3.4 yr (1–6 yr)	0%	4%	4%	22%	4%	NS	74%
Fisher (1970)[F2]	26	18 mo (6 mo–5 yr)	0%	4%	NS	8%	20%	NS	68%
Shackleton (1972)[S2]	25	7.5 yr (3–10 yr)	4%	8%	8%	20%	NS	NS	NS
Bernhard (1973)[B3]	116	NS (1–15 yr)	2.5%	5%	9%	43%	14%	1%	NS
Conkle (1973)[C5]	38	10 yr (5–14 yr)	0%	2.5%	8%	10%	16%	10%	69%
Jack (1976)[J2]	47 (5 lost to follow-up)	10.6 yr (10–16.3 yr)	0%	8%	11%	25%	6 of 15 studied preop and postop	6%	56%
Wagner (1977)[W1]	162 (> 2 years of age)	6.5 yr (3–9 yr)	1.2%	2%	NS	3%	NS	NS	35 (45 of 12-7)
Hossack (1980)[H1]	30	13 yr (1–17 yr)	0%	13%	33%	27%	40%	7%	30%

KEY: NS, not stated.

NOTE: Significant aortic incompetence (AI) is defined as a pulse pressure >50 mmHg. Significant aortic stenosis is defined as a peak left ventricular–aortic (LV-Ao) pressure difference >75 mmHg. A good result is an asymptomatic patient who has no more than mild aortic stenosis (AS).

SOURCE: Modified from Hossack, Neutze, Barratt-Boyes.[H1]

vided by Whitmer and colleagues, who demonstrated marked regression of exercise-induced ST depression one year after operation, and increase in mean total work and in peak exercise systolic blood pressure.[W7]

Aortic Valve Incompetence

Important aortic valve incompetence is not common after valvotomy when the operation has been performed as described in the section on "Technique of Operation." Thus, moderate-to-severe incompetence without residual stenosis is present at late follow-up in about 10% of cases; but some incompetence is combined with moderate or severe continu-

ing or restenosis in an additional 15%–20% of cases.[H1] Postoperative incompetence occurs more frequently when the valvotomy is radical[S2,T1] and particularly when an attempt is made to convert a bicuspid into a tricuspid valve.[L5]

Residual or Recurrent Left-Ventricular–Aortic Pressure Gradients

There is usually a significant reduction in the pressure gradient after valvotomy, which persists for 5–10 years.[F2,J2,L5,M23] Thereafter, the gradient tends to rise steadily. It has been stated that the rise occurs earlier and more frequently when

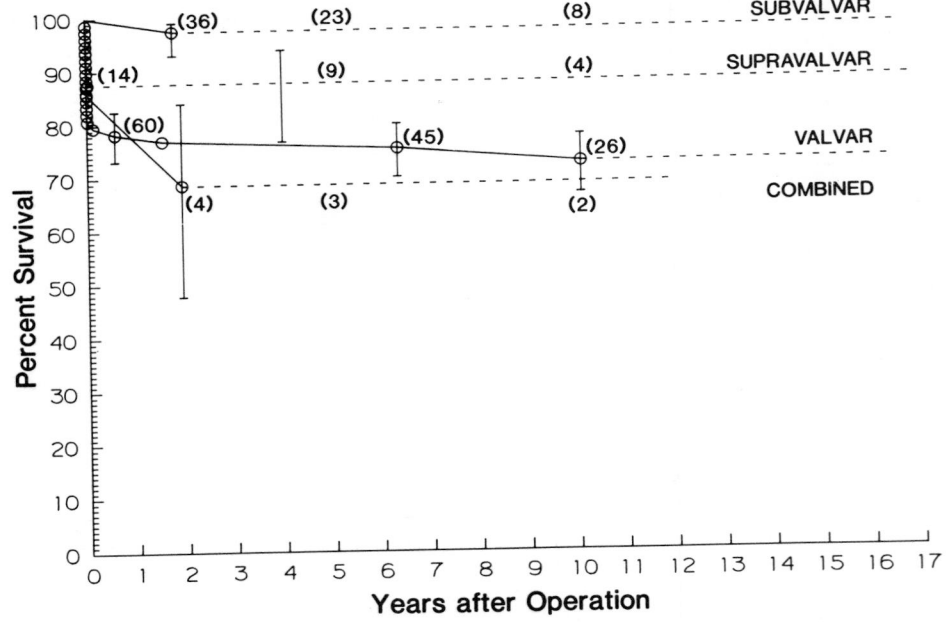

Figure 32-10   Actuarial survival after surgery for congenital aortic stenosis (UAB; 1967–1982; *n* = 142). All patients are traced, and patients were not censored at reoperation.

the valvotomy has been done in infancy.[K7] But this is not necessarily true, since as stated earlier, age at original operation is not a risk factor for the event reoperation (Table 32-10). In cases with a good initial result, the later rise in gradient is mainly the result of progressive cusp immobility and calcification.[R1] It is the recurrence and progression of the left ventricular–aortic (LV-Ao) pressure gradient that is usually the indication for reoperation.

Electrocardiographic Changes

There may be persistent left ventricular hypertrophy (LVH) after valvotomy or valve replacement either because of residual stenosis or incompetence or a progressive secondary cardiomyopathy. This can be contributed to or produced either by intraoperative damage to the ventricle or by preexistent ischemic myocardial fibrosis[E3,M4] made worse by de-

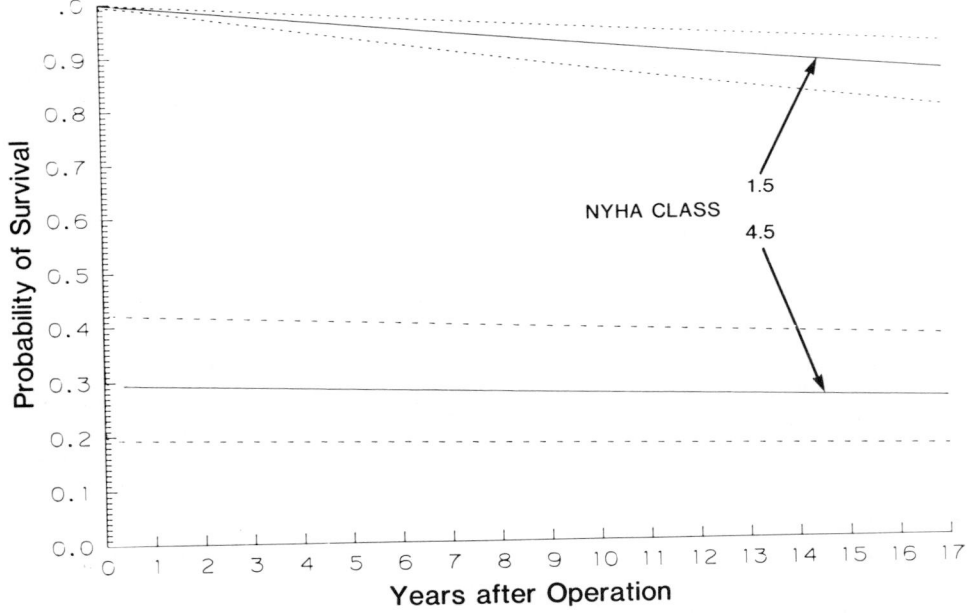

Figure 32-11   Nomogram of the parametric survival estimate from the hazard function analysis (see Fig. 32-9 and Table 32-7), after surgery for congenital valvar aortic stenosis according to preoperative clinical status. NYHA class "1.5" depicts patients in NYHA class I or II; "4.5" depicts those in NYHA class IV or V.

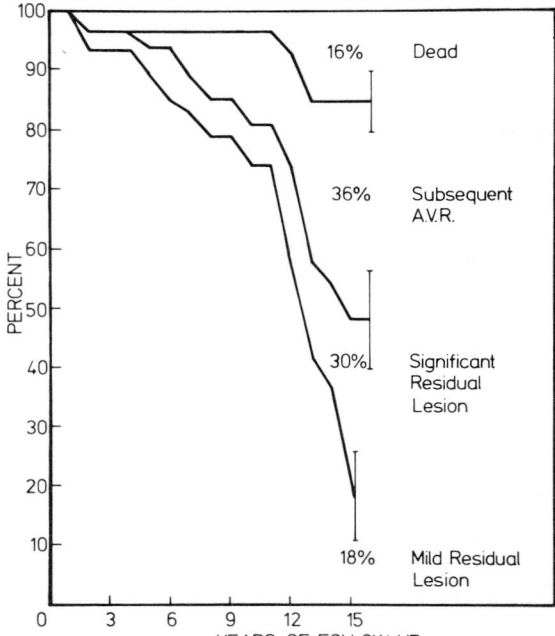

Figure 32-12 Cumulative actuarial curves for 30 children and young adults (infants excluded) undergoing valvotomy for congenital valvar aortic stenosis (GLH). The vertical bars represent 70% confidence limits. Mean follow-up time was 13 years (1–17 years).

Reproduced with permission from Hossack et al.[H1]

laying the operation for too long. Among 22 patients who had only mild residual stenosis or incompetence, LVH was absent or mild in 13 (59%) and severe in only three, an indication that the changes were usually reversible (GLH; Table 32-13).

Bacterial Endocarditis

The incidence of endocarditis is not lessened by valvotomy,[G3,H1,R9] and actually it may be somewhat higher than in the natural history.[H1]

INDICATIONS FOR OPERATION

Original Valvotomy

In neonates with severe congenital valvar aortic stenosis, operation is indicated on an emergency basis as soon as the diagnosis is made. Delay results in worsening of the clinical condition and a higher operative risk.[K7] When the diagnosis is suspected before transport to a cardiac surgical center of a neonate in the first week or two of life, or when such a patient is moribund or in metabolic acidosis on admission, prostaglandin E_1 is begun (see Chapter 25, section on "Indications and Strategy for Operation"). This usually opens the ductus arteriosus, particularly if the neonate is just a few days old, and improves the systemic circulation and relieves metabolic acidosis, thereby improving the patient's tolerance to operation.[J5] As soon as is possible operation is undertaken.[M24] The circumstances under which the risk of postoperative hospital death is high could be considered indications of inoperability (see "Incremental Risk Factors for Hospital Death"), but the good late results in surviving patients contradict this.

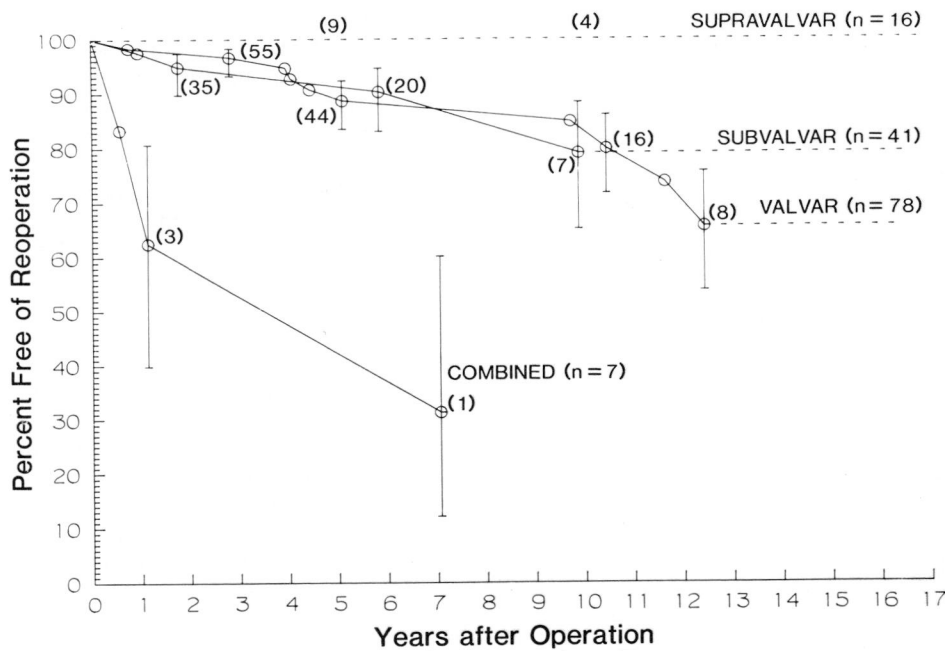

Figure 32-13 Actuarial percent of patients free of *reoperation* on the left ventricular or aortic outflow tracts after a primary operation for congenital aortic stenosis (UAB; 1967–1982; *n* = 142).

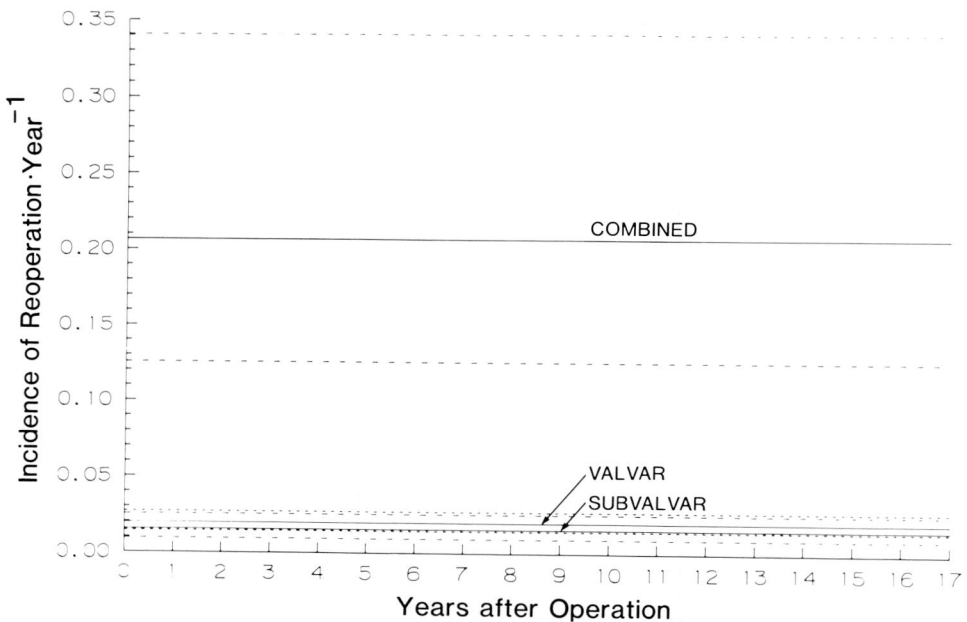

Figure 32-14   Hazard function for the event ''reoperation'' after surgery for congenital aortic stenosis (UAB; 1967–1982; $n = 142$). There were no reoperations after repair of supravalvar stenosis. (Presentation is as in Fig. 32-9.)

In young infants severe congenital valvar aortic stenosis is an indication for urgent but usually not emergent operation.

In older infants and children, severe congenital valvar aortic stenosis is an indication for operation (see summary in ''Clinical Features and Diagnostic Criteria'' for definitions of severity). Symptoms of angina or syncope in this age group always indicate severe stenosis and thus are indications for operation.[D1] Conversely, severe stenosis requiring operation frequently occurs without symptoms, but in such circumstances there will usually be physical signs,[H1] particularly in the pulse and the behavior of the second heart sound. Also, the electrocardiogram will usually show left ventricular hy-

pertrophy. An electrocardiogram that shows severe hypertrophy (that is, significant ST-T depression) is an indication for operation even though the gradient may be less than 50 mmHg.

Mild congenital valvar aortic stenosis is not an indication for operation. Because of the natural history, patients with mild congenital aortic stenosis require long-term periodic noninvasive reevaluation (see ''Clinical Features and Diagnostic Criteria'') and invasive study and operation if they become indicated.

Older infants and children with moderate stenosis are a controversial group, although it has been recommended by many that an operation be advised for them.[B3,C4,C5,E2,M3] Others have recommended periodic reevaluation with repeated measurements of LV-Ao gradients,[C1,E1,F1,W1] or subendocardial oxygen requirements,[K1,L4] or calculations of valve area. Factors arguing against prematurely advising operation in this group are that sudden death related to congenital aortic stenosis is rare in children whose LV-Ao gradient is between 50 and 75 mmHg, that reoperation and probable valve replacement will someday be necessary in any event, and that the latter cannot be delayed by early reoperation. Therefore, in most circumstances operation is not advised in this group but is advised when and if the patient moves into the severe group. In this regard, the central importance of the LV-Ao pressure gradient in deciding upon the need for operation is no longer a problem, since it can be assessed noninvasively and repeatedly (see earlier statements) in children being followed because of mild or moderate congenital valvar aortic stenosis.

Reoperation

When restenosis becomes severe (see summary in ''Clinical Features and Diagnostic Criteria'') or when symptoms de-

Table 32-10   Incidence of reoperation at UAB or elsewhere in patients who are hospital survivors of a primary valvotomy (UAB; 1967–1982; $n = 61$) for congenital valvar aortic stenosis, according to age at initial valvotomy.

Age at Valvotomy			Reoperation		
≤ <		n	No.	%	CL
Weeks					
1		1	0	0	0%–85%
1 --- 4		5	0	0	0%–32%
Months					
1 --- 3		0	0		
3 --- 12		8	2	25%	9%–50%
12 --- 48		6	2	33%	12%–62%
Years					
4 --- 12		22	4	18%	9%–31%
12 --- 20		19	2	11%	4%–23%
Total		61	10	16%	11%–23%
P (parametric)				.9	

KEY: CL, 70% confidence limits.

NOTE: P value obtained in the hazard function domain.

Table 32-11 First reoperation for congenital aortic stenosis (UAB; 1967–1982), categorized according to the morphologic category and procedure at the first operation. The numbers in parentheses indicate the patients whose first operations were also at UAB.

Category	Procedure	Prior Procedure	n	(UAB)	Hospital Death
Valvar	Aortic valvotomy	Aortic valvotomy	2	(1)	0
	AVR	Aortic valvotomy	2	(0)	0
	AVR + patch ascending aorta	Aortic valvotomy	3	(0)	0
	AVR + Konno	Aortic valvotomy	1	(0)	0
	AVR + Manougian aortic root enlargement	Aortic valvotomy	2	(1)	0
			10		0
Subvalvar	Excision	Excision	1	(0)	0
	Excision + myototomy + modified Konno	Excision	1	(0)	0
	Myototomy + modified Konno	Excision	1	(0)	0
	Excision + patch ascending aorta	Excision	1	(0)	0
	AVR + excision + patch ascending aorta	Excision	1	(0)	0
	LV-Ao conduit	Excision	1	(1)	0
			6		0
Supravalvar	Excision of subvalvar stenosis	Ascending aortic patch	1	(0)	0
	Aortic valvotomy + myotomy + ascending aortic patch	Ascending aortic patch	1	(0)	0
			2		0
Combined valvar + supravalvar	Excision of subvalvar stenosis AVR + ascending aortic patch	Valvotomy + ascending aortic patch	1	(0)	1
	AVR + ascending aortic patch	Valvotomy + ascending aortic patch	1	(0)	0
			2		1
Combined valvar + subvalvar	Valvotomy + excision of accessory mitral tissue	Valvotomy	1	(1)	0
	AVR + Konno	Valvotomy + excision of subaortic stenosis	1	(1)	0
	AVR + excision of fibromuscular stenosis and accessory mitral tissue + Konno	Valvotomy + excision of subaortic stenosis	1	(1)	0
			3		0
Combined valvar + subvalvar + supravalvar	Patch ascending aorta + LV-Ao conduit	Excision of subaortic stenosis	1	(1)	0

KEY: AVR, aortic valve replacement; LV-Ao, left ventricular to aortic.

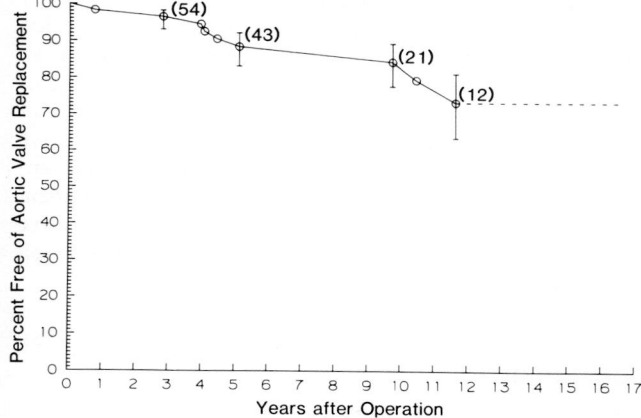

Figure 32-15 Actuarial incidence of freedom from aortic valve *replacement* after initial aortic valvotomy (UAB; 1967–1982; *n* = 75). The aortic valve replacement may have been late after a repeat valvotomy.

Table 32-12 Preoperative functional class and functional class when last traced postoperatively in patients undergoing a primary operation for congenital valvar aortic stenosis (UAB; 1969–1982).

Follow-up NYHA Class	Preoperative NYHA Class					Total
	I	II	III	IV	V	
I	22	20	5	6	0	53
II	0	2	1	1	0	4
III	0	0	0	0	0	0
IV	0	0	0	0	0	0
Dead	0	2	3	5	10	20
Uncertain	0	1	0	0	0	1
Total	22	25	9	12	10	78

Table 32-13 Comparison of evidences of left ventricular hypertrophy in the pre- and postoperative ECGs in patients with a good hemodynamic result (only mild stenosis or incompetence) after valvotomy or valve replacement for congenital aortic stenosis (GLH; 1958–1977).

Preoperative Grade	n	Postoperative Grade			
		1	2	3	4
5	3			2	1
4	8	3	1	2	2
3	7	3	2	2	
2	4	1	3		
Total	22	7	6	6	3

NOTE: The follow-up ranged from 13 to 201 months. The criteria for the degrees of LVH are: 1, none; 2, mild; 3, moderate; 4, severe (ST-T inverted 0–3 mm); 5, extreme (ST-T inverted > 3 mm).

velop with moderate restenosis, reoperation is indicated. Although repeat valvotomy or valve replacement is the operation usually required, the possibility that important subvalvar stenosis has also developed must not be overlooked. When this is present, there is often a small anulus, as well as some supravalvar narrowing. If this is the case, a Konno operation rather than simple valvotomy or valve replacement is indicated.

SPECIAL SITUATIONS AND CONTROVERSIES

Technique of Operation

There is periodic enthusiasm for the use of a closed transventricular approach in critically ill neonates and young infants, which has been motivated by the high early mortality in this group.[T3] Williams, Trusler, and colleagues at Toronto Sick Childrens Hospital have reduced the hospital mortality in neonates from 11 deaths (69%, CL 53%–82%) among 16 patients done with CPB to seven deaths (39%, CL 25%–54%) among 18 patients done by a closed transventricular approach (*P* for difference = .08).[W9] However, there is no convincing evidence that, considering both early mortality and the amount of valvar incompetence produced, the method is either superior to or as good as the techniques described here.

A few groups have preferred to do the operation under inflow stasis at normothermia or mild hypothermia.[C6] The operation under these circumstances is a semiopen one, and forceful stretching or tearing of the valve may result if exposure is not ideal. In children, the method can be used safely, but 7 (26%, CL 17%–37%) of 27 patients followed-up to 15 years by Stewart and colleagues had moderate or severe aortic valve incompetence.[S18] Sink and colleagues have reported 2 (25%, CL 9%–50%) hospital deaths among 8 infants, 6 of whom were neonates.[S17]

Anecdotal reports of percutaneous balloon valvuloplasty for congenital valvar aortic stenosis indicate that severe aortic valvar incompetence sometimes results. However, Walls and colleagues report only one instance of more than mild aortic regurgitation after percutaneous balloon aortic valvuloplasty in 14 patients.[W11] No neonates were treated by

them in this manner. Thus, the evidence is not complete that semiopen techniques and balloon angioplasty represent improvements over the methods described under "Technique of Operation."

CONGENITAL DISCRETE SUBVALVAR AORTIC STENOSIS

DEFINITION

Congenital discrete subvalvar aortic stenosis is an obstruction beneath the aortic valve due either to a short, localized fibrous or fibromuscular ridge or a longer (diffuse) fibrous tunnel. "Diffuse subvalvar aortic stenosis" is a phrase best avoided as being currently confusing, since it was originally used[K3] to contrast what is now termed *hypertrophic obstructive cardiomyopathy* (see Chapter 33) from the subject of this chapter.

Subvalvar aortic stenosis may also be a part of other cardiac anomalies. In these situations, the obstruction may be fibromuscular or may consist of a localized muscular bar or shelf (such as in coarctation or aortic arch interruption with ventricular septal defect) or of abnormalities of the mitral valve (see Chapter 36).

HISTORICAL NOTE

The first description of discrete subvalvar stenosis is attributed to Chevers in 1842.[C13] Brock and Fleming[B5] from Guys Hospital in London published an early report of the diagnosis of the condition during life, using transventricular puncture to measure left ventricular pressure. The catheter was then advanced across the aortic valve from below and the level of obstruction demonstrated.

Brock[B6] reported the results of transventricular dilatation as treatment in 1956. Spencer and colleagues[S5] published the first substantial report of treatment using cardiopulmonary bypass in 1960. We at the Mayo Clinic illustrated the lesion clearly in 1961, referring to cases operated upon between 1956 and 1960. The long fibrous tunnel form of the stenosis was described by Spencer in 1960[S5] and was later reemphasized by Reis, Morrow, and colleagues.[R3] Its effective treatment became possible with the introduction of aortoventriculoplasty by Rastan and Koncz[R7,R8] and independently by Konno and colleagues,[K8] in 1975. An alternative form of treatment, left ventricular-aortic conduit, was developed at about the same time.[C12,N3]

MORPHOLOGY

Left Ventricular Outflow Tract

Localized Subvalvar Aortic Stenosis
The localized form of discrete subvalvar aortic stenosis described here may be fibrous or fibromuscular. The *fibrous* form involves a spectrum of pathology varying between a discrete short fibrous ridge, a thicker but still discrete

fibromuscular shelf and a long fibrous tunnel. The situation in which a fibrous ridge is firmly adherent to a hypertrophied septum anteriorly and to the left is termed *discrete fibromuscular stenosis*.[K2,M7,N1] Whether or not isolated, localized, and purely muscular subvalvar stenosis occurs as an entity separate from obstructive hypertrophic cardiomyopathy is controversial (see Chapter 33).

An obstructing localized circumferential fibrous shelf or ridge can be situated at any level between the nadir of the aortic cusps and the free edge of the anterior mitral leaflets posteriorly (that is, anywhere at the level of the aortic-mitral anulus). An immediately subvalvar fibrous ridge may be adherent to the base of the aortic leaflets[F10] (either the right only or all three), but more often it is separated from the cusps by several millimeters. Such a high ridge tends to be relatively narrow, and unless there is very severe left ventricular hypertrophy, the remainder of the outflow beneath it remains relatively normal.[K2] A low fibrous ridge may be attached almost at the hinge line of the anterior mitral leaflet, but most frequently it occupies an intermediate position well above this and several millimeters below the aortic valve (Fig. 32-16). Usually the ridge is 2–3-mm thick and is more prominent anteriorly and laterally than posteriorly on the mitral-aortic anulus, but it may be present as a complete fibrous diaphragm, and the stenotic orifice may be central and circular or eccentric and slitlike. The mitral-aortic anulus is longer than normal in hearts with discrete subvalvar aortic stenosis, and the diameter of the aortic valve anulus, on the average, is smaller than normal.[R4] The muscular ventricular septum beneath the right aortic cusp shows a variable degree of hypertrophy and prominence and in severe cases may contribute importantly to the stenosis.

Tunnel Subvalvar Aortic Stenosis
The much less common tunnel stenosis presents as a circumferential irregular zone of fibrosis commencing at, or close to, the valve ring and extending downward for 10–30 mm.[M5,R3,S5] Tunnel stenosis has varying degrees of severity, and its spectrum blends into localized subvalvar aortic stenosis. In the most severe form and the form that requires a special surgical procedure, the stenotic tunnel is long and the diameter of aortic anulus is small even though the aortic valve cusps are normally formed. In patients with less severe examples, the tunnel may be shorter and the aortic anulus normal sized; then the morphology resembles that of the localized fibromuscular form of discrete subvalvar aortic stenosis.[K2] These gradations no doubt explain the differing incidences in various series. Fibrous stenosis is sufficiently long to justify the term *tunnel* in about one-fifth of cases of congenital subvalvar aortic stenosis (GLH, 6 patients [16%] out of 37), and the full-blown entity with annular hypoplasia is rare (GLH, 1 case [3%]).

Aortic Valve

The aortic valve is usually tricuspid and either entirely normal or with some diffuse leaflet thickening in patients with congenital subvalvar aortic stenosis. Nonetheless, trivial or mild aortic incompetence is present in about two-thirds of the cases. The aortic valve may, however, be bicuspid and there may be congenital commissural fusion producing a varying degree of valvar stenosis (Table 32-14). The valve may have been damaged by endocarditis, a not uncommon complication of subvalvar stenosis,[M10,M11] and this can result in severe incompetence. The base of the valve cusps are thick when a high-lying fibrous ridge is continuous with them.

Very occasionally supravalvar as well as valvar stenosis coexists with the subvalvar narrowing.

Left Ventricle

The left ventricle is usually concentrically hypertrophied. Subendocardial ischemia and probably fibrosis are known to occur here as well as in congenital valvar stenosis.[C11] Rarely, there may be excessive hypertrophy of the septum (in comparison with the thickening of the posterior left ventricular wall) and muscle fiber disorientation histologically.[B4,M5] It is this that complicates the distinction, in a few patients, between discrete subvalvar aortic stenosis and obstructive hypertrophic cardiomyopathy (see Chapter 33).

Roberts and associates[M5,M11] have noted the presence of lumenal narrowing due to structural wall changes in the intramural coronary arteries of both humans and dogs with fibrous subvalvar aortic stenosis. These changes have not been observed in valvar aortic stenosis.

Coexisting Cardiac Anomalies

Discrete subvalvar aortic stenosis occurs as an isolated anomaly in only about one-half to two-thirds of patients coming to operation (Table 32-15, and see Table 32-2).[C8,H4,K2] Coexisting anomalies include a ventricular septal defect (VSD) that is frequently large,[L7,M8,N1] and the fibromuscular obstruction is then often located immediately below (upstream to) the VSD. When there is aortic arch interruption and patent ductus arteriosus (and also occasionally coarctation) there may be localized muscular subvalvar stenosis in association with a subpulmonary VSD.[F3,V1] Valvar or infundibular pulmonary stenosis[N2] and occasionally tetralogy of Fallot, atrial septal defect, aortopulmonary (AP) window, sinus of Valsalva aneurysm, and aneurysm of the membranous ventricular septum may also coexist (Table 32-15). These are more frequent in patients undergoing operation in childhood (Table 32-16).

The complexity of the relation between VSD and discrete subvalvar aortic stenosis is further evident from the fact that discrete subvalvar aortic stenosis may develop after spontaneous closure or narrowing of the VSD.[C15] Typical discrete subvalvar aortic stenosis may also develop after repair of a complete atrioventricular (AV) canal defect or may be present and progress before repair (see Chapter 19).[B17,G8]

Other Types of Discrete Subvalvar Aortic Stenosis

Localized subaortic stenosis may be caused by morphology and mechanisms other than those just described. In fact, in an autopsy series that included complex congenital heart disease, Freedom and associates[F3] found the typical fibrous or fibromuscular variety to be the least common in infancy.

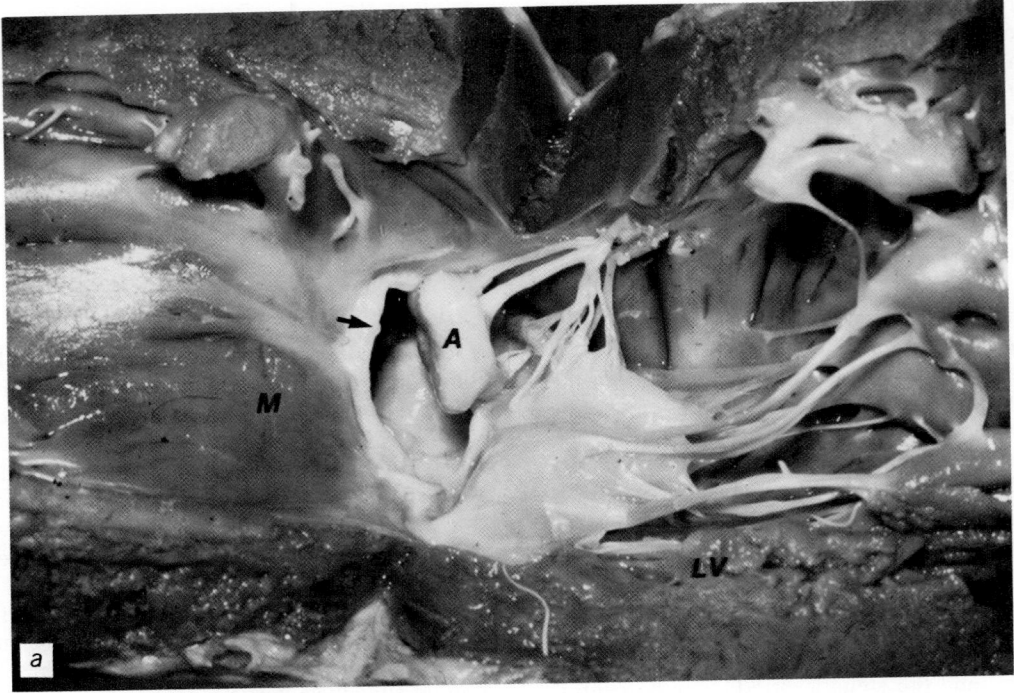

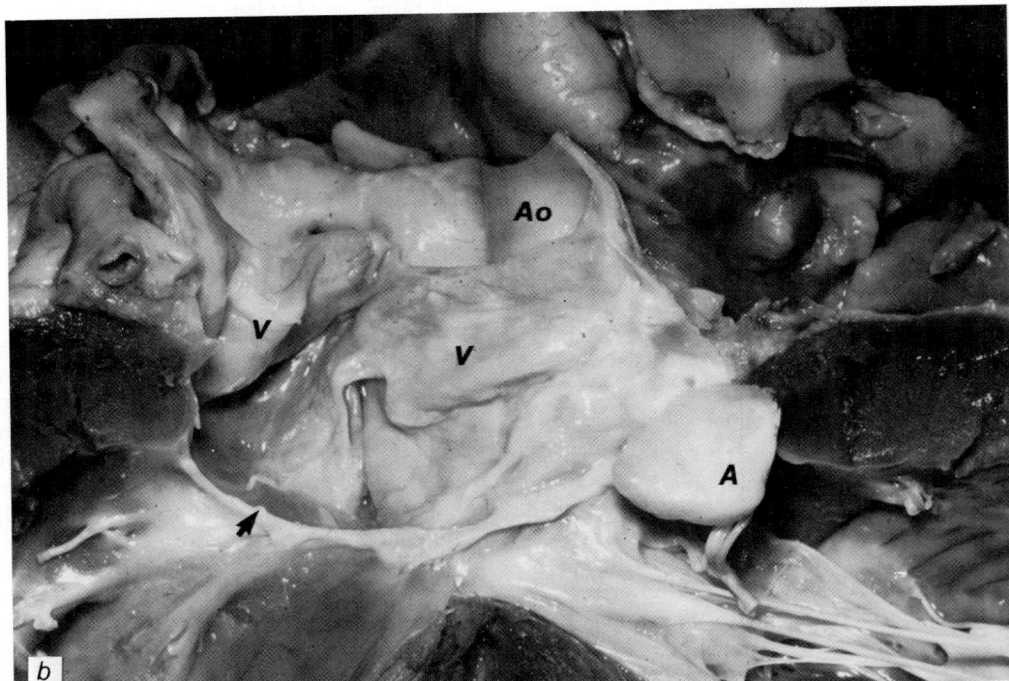

Figure 32-16 Autopsy specimen with medium-level discrete fibrous subvalvar aortic stenosis (GLH).

(a) The stenosis is viewed intact from below. Note the thickness of the left ventricular wall and the associated muscular hypertrophy anteriorly beneath the localized fibrous ridge (arrow).

(b) The stenotic zone has been opened out into the ascending aorta to show its relationship to the aortic valve. Accessory mitral leaflet tissue contributes to the stenosis.

A, accessory mitral leaflet tissue; Ao, ascending aorta; LV, left ventricular wall; M, muscular hypertrophy, V, aortic valve.

Table 32-14 Aortic valve anomalies in patients with discrete subaortic stenosis (GLH; 1958–1979; n = 37). The categories are not mutually exclusive.

Category	No.	
Membrane adherent to tricuspid aortic valve	6	
Bicuspid aortic valve	4	
With leaflet fusion		2
Without leaflet fusion		2
Tricuspid valve	7	
With leaflet fusion		2
With leaflet thickening		5
Aortic incompetence	24	
Trivial or mild		23
Severe (active endocarditis)		1
Total	41	

Table 32-15 Associated lesions and age at operation for discrete subvalvar aortic stenosis (GLH; 1960–1979; n = 34). The categories are mutually exclusive.

Category	Number of Patients	Ages (yr)	Hospital Deaths	Late Deaths
VSD	3	4, 15, 48	0	2
VSD + PS	2[a]	7, 8	0	
VSD + coarctation	2[b]	5, 8	0	
Coarctation (±PDA)	2[b]	5, 9	0	
AP window	1	8	1[c]	
PS (infundibular)	1	9	0	
IHSS	1	9	0	
Situs inversus	1	50	0	
Total	13		1	2

KEY: IHSS, hypertrophic obstructive cardiomyopathy; PDA, patent ductus arteriosus; PS, pulmonary stenosis; VSD, ventricular septal defect.

[a] One patient had classical tetralogy of Fallot.

[b] The associated lesions were corrected in infancy.

[c] Grade 4 pulmonary vascular disease present at autopsy (operation 1961).

Table 32-16 Age at operation and associated anomalies in patients with discrete subaortic stenosis (GLH; 1960–1979; n = 37).

Age at Operation (yr) ≤ <	n	Patients with Associated Anomalies No.	%	Hospital Deaths	Late Deaths
5	1	1	90%	0	
5 --- 10	10	9		1	2
10 --- 20	12	1		0	
20 --- 30	8	0		0	1
30 --- 40	2	0	12%	1	
40 --- 50	2	1		0	1
50	2	1		0	
Total	37	13	35%	2(5%; CL 2%–12%)	4

KEY: CL, 70% confidence limits.

Mitral valve anomalies involving accessory tissue or leaflet malposition (including that found in AV canal defects) may be a cause of obstruction,[E5,G10,K10] and these may occur in the absence of functional abnormality of the mitral valve or other cardiac anomalies.[M20] Localized muscular obstructions related to abnormal infundibular development or malalignment are relatively frequent and often associated with a VSD and aortic coarctation or interruption. A developmental complex described by Shone and associates[S4] (see Chapter 36) consists of a parachute mitral valve and left ventricular outflow obstruction that usually includes a localized fibromuscular subaortic stenosis. Discrete muscular subvalvar aortic stenosis may develop after pulmonary artery banding for VSD (see Chapter 26).[F4]

CLINICAL FEATURES AND DIAGNOSTIC CRITERIA

Symptoms

The symptoms of congenital subvalvar aortic stenosis are similar to those of the valvar variety. About 25% of patients requiring operation are asymptomatic despite the presence of significant obstruction.

Signs

A systolic ejection murmur is heard, but a click is rare. There is an unimpressive aortic diastolic murmur in 65% of patients. It is either secondary to leaflet thickening with or without adherence of the fibrous ridge to the cusps or to the effects of the eddy currents produced by the subvalvar stenosis on aortic valve closure.

When severe stenosis is present, the pulse is slow rising, the second heart sound is single or paradoxically split, a third and occasionally a fourth heart sound are audible, and a middiastolic murmur may be heard at the apex in association, usually with a fibrotic obstruction that limits movement of the anterior mitral leaflet.[K2] It is important to recognize, particularly in children, that one or more of these signs may be minimal or absent despite severe obstruction.

Occasionally important aortic incompetence may be secondary to severe congenital cusp deformities or endocarditis. When endocarditis does occur on the aortic valve, the signs of incompetence produced by leaflet destruction may be less than expected, since a tight fibrous stenosis beneath the valve may limit aortic runoff. Moreover, vegetations on the fibrous shelf itself may increase the subaortic obstruction.[M11]

Chest X-Ray

The ascending aorta is not usually dilated in the chest x-ray, and valvar calcification is absent.

Electrocardiogram

The electrocardiogram usually shows severe left ventricular hypertrophy.

Echocardiography

Two-dimensional echocardiography can be particularly useful in diagnosis and can demonstrate the obstructing shelf.[C15,M5,W3] M-mode echocardiography is helpful in differentiating this lesion from obstructive hypertrophic cardiomyopathy.[B4,M5]

Cardiac Catheterization and Cineangiography

On cardiac catheterization, there is a systolic pressure gradient below the valve on withdrawal of the catheter across the left ventricular outflow area. When the fibrous ridge is immediately beneath the valve, the gradient may be apparently at valve level. The postectopic pressure pulse response is normal, and the aortic pulse contour does not show an accessory wave; these are features that distinguish the lesion from obstructive hypertrophic cardiomyopathy.

Angiocardiography provides a definitive diagnosis.[H4,K2,M5,N1] The tilted left anterior oblique (LAO) view provides good visualization of the fibrous ridge since it overcomes the foreshortening of the left ventricular outflow region present in the conventional LAO projection (Figs. 32-17, 32-18, 32-19). The level and thickness of the obstruction can be accurately defined in this manner, and additional valvar stenosis and incompetence can be evaluated also.

Summary

In discrete subvalvar aortic stenosis, features characteristic of obstructive hypertrophic cardiomyopathy are usually absent. It would appear, however, that rarely, particularly in severe forms of fibrous subvalvar aortic stenosis,[B4] including the tunnel variety,[M5] there may be abnormal systolic anterior mitral leaflet motion and an abnormal postectopic response. These indicate either a particularly prominent anterior muscular shelf or, in those patients who also show an abnormal septal-posterior wall thickness ratio on echocardiography (with disorientation of the muscular pattern of hypertrophy histologically), associated obstructive hypertrophic cardiomyopathy.

NATURAL HISTORY

Discrete subaortic stenosis comprises between 8% and 30% of cases with congenital left ventricular outflow tract obstruction (see Table 32-6).[B14,K4,K5,M6,N1]

The striking absence of operations for discrete subvalvar aortic stenosis in the first year of life (see Tables 32-6 and 32-16) clearly indicates the difference in life history of patients with congenital subvalvar aortic stenosis, compared with that of patients with valvar stenosis. Thus, it would appear that typical discrete subvalvar aortic stenosis is rarely a cause of important obstruction in infancy.[F3,H5,N1,S13] Rather, the obstruction begins to be evident after the first year of life, in a few patients by 3–5 years of age, but in most in early childhood or young adult life. Also, the lesion appears uncommonly beyond 30 years of age, suggesting that if surgery has not been performed, survival beyond this time is infre-

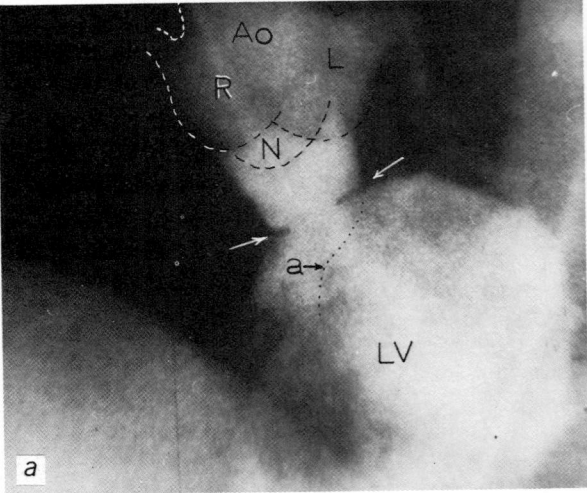

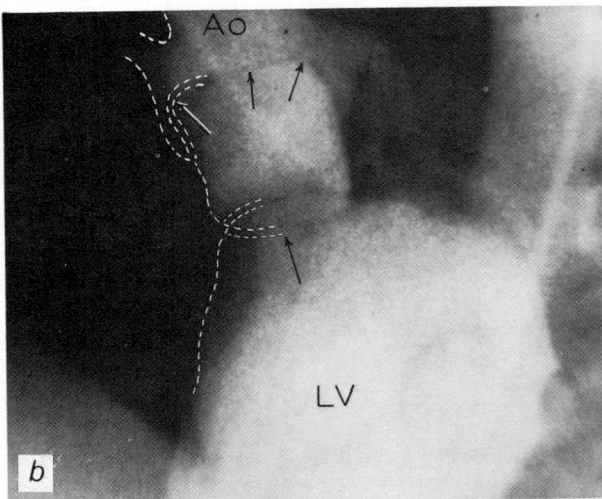

Figure 32-17 Left ventricular cineangiocardiogram in a cranially tilted left anterior oblique projection, in a patient with localized fibrous subvalvar aortic stenosis (GLH). Cineangiogram frames in diastole (a) and early systole (b). A thin ridge obstructing the left ventricular outflow tract about 1 cm below the aortic valve is well profiled and indicated by the white arrows. In systole, the aortic valve is domed (arrows), indicating a valvular abnormality in addition to the subaortic ridge.

a, anterior mitral leaflet; Ao, aorta; L, left; LV, left ventricle; N, noncoronary cusps; R, right.

quent or that the lesion gradually merges with obstructive hypertrophic cardiomyopathy.[K1]

Further support for these concepts is provided by the interesting study of Pyle and associates[P2] of fibrous subaortic stenosis in Newfoundland dogs. In these animals, subaortic stenosis was never present at birth but was significant by 12 weeks of age. There was also evidence of an inherited trait. A familial incidence has also been reported in humans.[G4,L7,M5]

Reports of serial cardiac catheterizations indicate that discrete subvalvar aortic stenosis progresses relatively rapidly,[H4,M9,N1] probably more rapidly than valvar stenosis. There

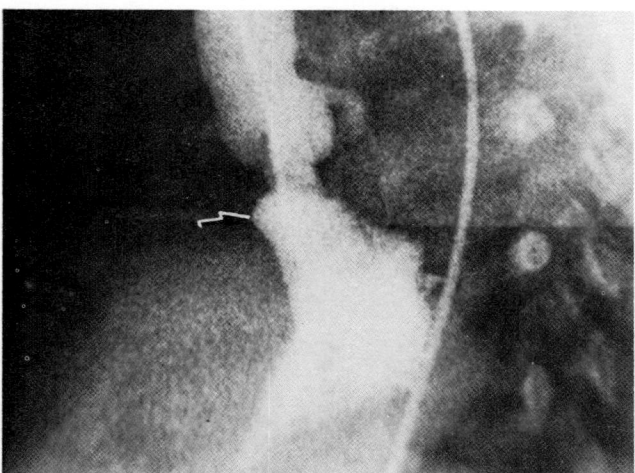

Figure 32-18 Left ventricular cineangiocardiogram in a cranially tilted left anterior oblique projection in a patient with fibromuscular subvalvar aortic stenosis (GLH). Cineangiogram frame in systole shows a thick fibromuscular outflow obstruction commencing just beneath the aortic valve. The aortic leaflets fail to open completely but show no doming. Just below obstructing shelf on the septal aspect of the outflow tract there is a diverticulum (arrow) representing a surgically closed ventricular septal defect.

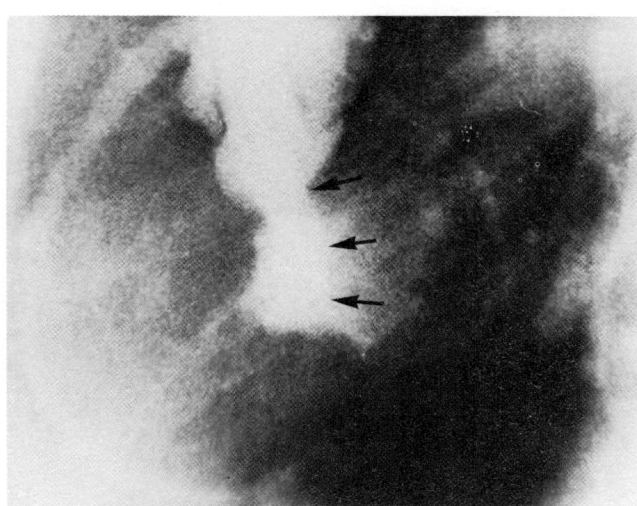

Figure 32-19 Left ventricular cineangiocardiogram in lateral projection in a patient with tunnel subvalvar aortic stenosis (GLH). Cineangiogram frame in late systole shows the outflow tract narrowing 1 cm below the aortic ring and extending down into the base of the left ventricle. The anterior mitral valve leaflet forms the posterior margin of the stenotic zone (arrows) and is prevented from moving back to its normal systolic position. The anterior (septal) margin of the outflow tract shows irregular encroachment by the obstructing fibromuscular tissue.

are two proven examples of the first appearance of the subvalvar gradient several years after an earlier study in infancy, performed prior to VSD and coarctation repair (GLH).

These features are the probable explanation of the fact that in published surgical series in which the ages of all patients are listed (Table 32-17, and see Table 32-6), the youngest patients operated upon were between 3 and 6 years and surgery was uncommon beyond 20 years of age.[C8,H4,K2,K5,L6,M5,S5]

It has been suggested that the aortic incompetence that is commonly associated with discrete subvalvar aortic stenosis is a progressive lesion secondary to leaflet thickening from the poststenotic turbulence.[N1] The leaflet thickening is the probable explanation for the frequency of endocarditis that can occur before or after surgical excision of the membrane.[M10,S6] In the autopsy series reported by Fontana and Edwards, 13 of 29 patients with subvalvar aortic stenosis had evidence of endocarditis.[F5] Muna and associates suggest that endocarditis may be more common here than in any other congenital cardiac anomaly.[M11]

TECHNIQUE OF OPERATION

Resection of Localized Subvalvar Aortic Stenosis

The operation proceeds just as described in Section 1 for valvotomy for congenital valvar aortic stenosis in children. The aortotomy may be a reversed hockey-stick incision extending into the noncoronary sinus of Valsalva (GLH) or a transverse one directed posteriorly toward the commissure between left and noncoronary cusp (UAB; see Chapter 12, Fig. 12-2).

The aortic cusps are retracted and the subvalvar fibrous ridge exposed. Beginning beneath the nadir of the right coronary cusp, a vertical incision is made through the ridge and into the underlying muscle, the depth of the incision being proportional to the estimated thickness of the septum (Fig. 32-20). The fibromuscular ridge to the patient's left of this is grasped either with toothed dissecting forceps or by passing stay sutures into it. The resection of the fibromuscular ridge begins by carrying the vertical incision circumferentially toward the patient's left, removing fibrous tissue and muscle until the mitral apparatus is encountered at the leftward extremity of the left ventricular outflow tract. In this process care is taken not to penetrate the ventricular septum and produce a ventricular septal defect. As the dissection is carried down over the anterior mitral leaflet, only the fibrous ridge is removed, shaving it off the leaflet or mitral-aortic anulus with the knife. This is carried rightward as far as the mitral leaflet and mitral-aortic anulus extend.

Returning anteriorly, only the fibrous ridge is shaved off the muscular septum to the right of the nadir of the right coronary cusp (Fig. 32-20). The ridge excision is carried rightward over the membranous septum. This technique preserves the integrity of the underlying bundle of His and cores out the entire subvalvar stenosis as a single mass. When the fibromuscular ridge is attached to the undersurface of the belly of one or more of the aortic cusps, it is carefully shaved away from the cusp tissue.

The procedure is not considered complete unless a generous amount of muscle has been removed leftward of the nadir of the right coronary cusp. If this has not occurred, for example if only the fibrous component has been enucleated,[G9] a deep trough of muscle is cut from the ventricular

Table 32-17 Composite results following excision of discrete subaortic stenosis (compiled 1979). Reoperations were for residual or recurrent stenosis.

Reference (Years of Study)	n	Age (yr)	Tunnel Stenosis	Hospital Deaths		Surgical CHB	Complications		Reoperation	Late Death
				No.	%		VSD	MI		
Spencer[S5] (1956–1960)	12	6–18	2	3	25%	0	1	0	NA	NA
Cooley[C4] (1956–1964)	21[a]	NA	NA	0	0%	NA	NA	NA	NA	NA
Lillehei[L6] (1956–1966)	15	4–58	NA	1	7%	0	0	0	2	1
McGoon[M6] (1956–1966)	30	NA	NA	2	7%	0	0	1	NA	2
Reis[R3] (1960–1969)	30	5–44	9	2	7%	0	0	0	0	2
Kelly[K2] (1957–1970)	20[a]	3–18	2	0	0%	1	0	0	3	NA
Katz[K5] (1958–1970)	26	3–54	NA	1	4%	0	1	1	2	1
Shariatzadeh[S3]	20	6–28	0	0	0%	1	0	0	0	1
Champsaur[C8] (1960–1971)	20	4–14	Excluded	0	0%	1	0	0	2	1
Chiariello[C9] (1967–1974)	11[a]	>1	NA	0	0%	0	0	0	2	0
Newfeld[N1] (1959–1975)	40	NA	NA	2	5%	4	2	0	3	2
Hardesty[H4] (1962–1976)	35	3–16	1	2	6%	1	0	2	2	3
Bernhard[B3] (1956–1972)	30	NA	4	2	6%	1	0	2	3	2
GLH (1960–1979)	37	4–15	6	2	5%	0	0	0	0	4
Total	347			17	4.8%		4	6	19	19

KEY: CHB, complete heart block; NA, information not available; MI, mitral incompetence; VSD, production of a ventricular septal defect.

[a] Patients with associated valvar stenosis excluded.

septum anteriorly. The trough is centered beneath the commissure between right and left cusps as in the operation for obstructive hypertrophic cardiomyopathy (see Chapter 33). This step is of value even when the fibrous ridge is immediately subvalvar, since the ventricular septum is always hypertrophied.

In those instances in which adequate relief of the anterior portion of the obstruction is not possible from above, and this may be the case when there is excessive muscular hypertrophy or extensive fibrous (tunnel) stenosis, the excision may be completed from below through the left ventricle (GLH; see details in Chapter 33, "Technique of Operation").

After determining that the ventricular septum has not been perforated and the valve cusps have not been damaged, the aortotomy is closed and the remainder of the procedure accomplished as described in Section 1 for valvotomy.

Aortic valve replacement may also be required in those rare instances in older children or adults in which there is important incompetence. It is performed in conventional fashion after excising the subvalvar obstruction (see Chapter 12, "Technique of Operation").

Repair of Tunnel Stenosis by Aortoventriculoplasty (Konno Operation)

When a tunnel-type of subaortic stenosis coexists with hypoplasia of the aortic valve anulus, aortoventriculoplasty is indicated[K8,R7,R8] using the modification described by Misbach, Ebert, and colleagues.[M19]

The preliminaries and the preparations for cardiopulmonary bypass (CPB) are identical to those described earlier for the operation for congenital valvar aortic stenosis. CPB is established using two caval cannulae and caval taping since the right ventricle will be opened. The aorta is cross-clamped, the cold cardioplegic infusion is given, and the perfusate temperature is stabilized at 25°C. Through a small oblique right atriotomy incision, the pump oxygenator sump sucker is placed across a naturally occurring or surgically created foramen ovale.

Prior to establishing CPB, the position of the right coronary artery has been accurately noted and a silk stitch placed leftward from this to indicate the siting of the incision. A vertical aortotomy is made, beginning about 10-mm downstream to the level of the right coronary artery (Fig. 32-21a).

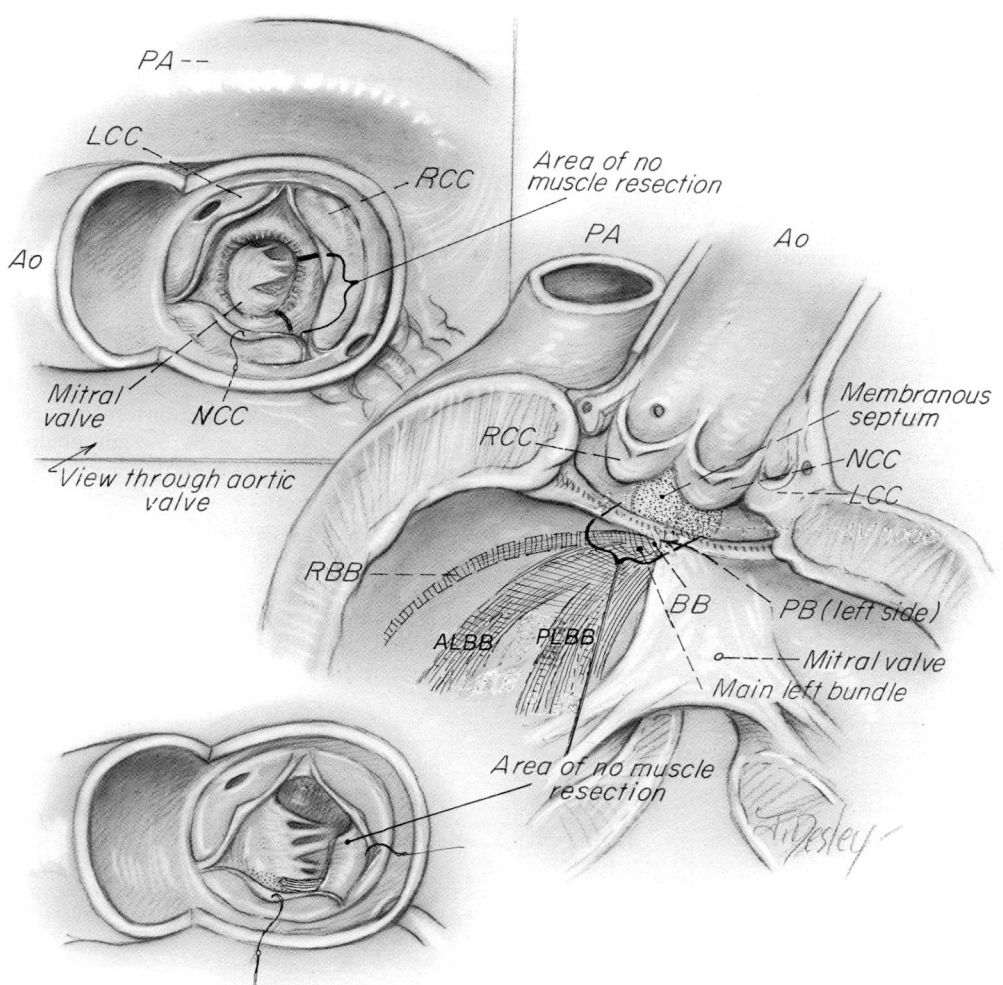

Figure 32-20 The surgical repair of discrete fibromuscular subvalvar aortic stenosis. Above and to the left is the exposure of the stenosis after retracting the cusps. The initial incision beneath the nadir of the right coronary cusp is shown. The resection proceeds as described in the text. The muscle and membranous septum over the bundle of His are left intact, shaving off only the fibrous ridge in this area.

ALBB, anterior left bundle branch; Ao, aorta; BB, bundle branch; LCC, left coronary cusp; NCC, noncoronary cusp; PA, pulmonary artery; PLBB, posterior left bundle branch; RBB, right bundle branch; RCC, right coronary cusp.

Reproduced with permission from Bharati et al.[B19]

The incision is carried well to the left of the right coronary artery and onto the right ventricle over the junction of the contiguous portions of the right and left coronary cusps.[D2] The right ventriculotomy may be made first, so as to visualize the pulmonary valve leaflets. In any event, care is necessary to avoid damaging the pulmonary valve cusps while the right ventricle is being opened, because these lie very near the point of entry of the incision into the right ventricle. After the right ventricle is opened (Fig. 32-21b), the scissors are positioned with one blade in the left ventricle through the aortotomy and one in the right through the ventriculotomy; with them a cut is made to the left side of the nadir of the right coronary cusp. This incision is carried far enough into the two ventricles to get below (or upstream to) the tunnel stenosis. The newly created and enlarged anulus is sized, and an appropriately sized prosthesis, usually a St. Jude type, is chosen and sutured into place posteriorly (Fig. 32-21c). A double velour woven Dacron graft, whose diameter is somewhat larger than that of the ascending aorta, has been preclotted prior to CPB, and from this an oval-shaped patch is trimmed whose width is about two-fifths of the tube graft's circumference. Beginning at the inferior angle of the incision through the ventricular septum, this patch is sewn into place from the right ventricular side out to beyond the aortic anulus (Fig. 32-21c). Then the horizontal mattress sutures in the anterior aspect of the prosthesis are passed through the patch and tied (Fig. 32-21d). The remainder of the Dacron patch is sutured into place to enlarge and close the aortotomy (Fig. 32-21d).

The piece of pericardium which had been taken and set aside as the incision was being made is now trimmed to an appropriate size and is sutured into place to cover the aortic portion of the previous Dacron patch and at the same time close the opening into the right ventricle (Fig. 32-21e). Particular care is taken to anchor the patch with several interrupted pledgetted mattress sutures at the junction of right ventricle and aorta so that hemostasis is particularly secure in that area.

The left atrial suction line is removed from across the foramen ovale and the foramen closed. With strong suction on the aortic needle vent, the aortic clamp is released and rewarming is begun. The right atrium is closed. The remainder of the operation including the de-airing procedure is carried out in the usual manner (see Chapter 2, Section 3).

Modified Konno Operation

The modified Konno operation may be effective in some patients with difficult and complex localized subaortic stenosis or tunnel stenosis when the aortic anulus and valve are normal.

The preparations for operation and the establishment of CPB are exactly as described for the Konno operation. The aorta is cross-clamped, the cold cardioplegic infusion is given, and the pump oxygenator sump sucker is placed across the foramen ovale. Since the Konno operation usually would not be done with a normal-sized anulus and normal valves, a transverse aortotomy is made just as for the operation for aortic valvotomy or resection of discrete subaortic stenosis (see "Technique of Operation" in Section 1 and "Resection of Localized Subvalvar Aortic Stenosis" in Section 2). When it has been determined that the usual procedures will not enlarge the left ventricular outflow tract sufficiently, the right ventricle is opened through a transverse incision about 2 cm inferior (upstream) to the level of the pulmonary valve cusps. A right-angled clamp is passed into the left ventricular outflow tract through the aortic valve and positioned 1 cm or so upstream to the valve (Fig. 32-22). This then can be palpated through the ventricular septum, and at this point an incision is made in the septum from the right ventricular side. The incision is extended inferiorly for about 1 cm, making it parallel to the left ventricular outflow tract and thus at an angle to the right ventricular outflow tract. The incision through the ventricular septum is now

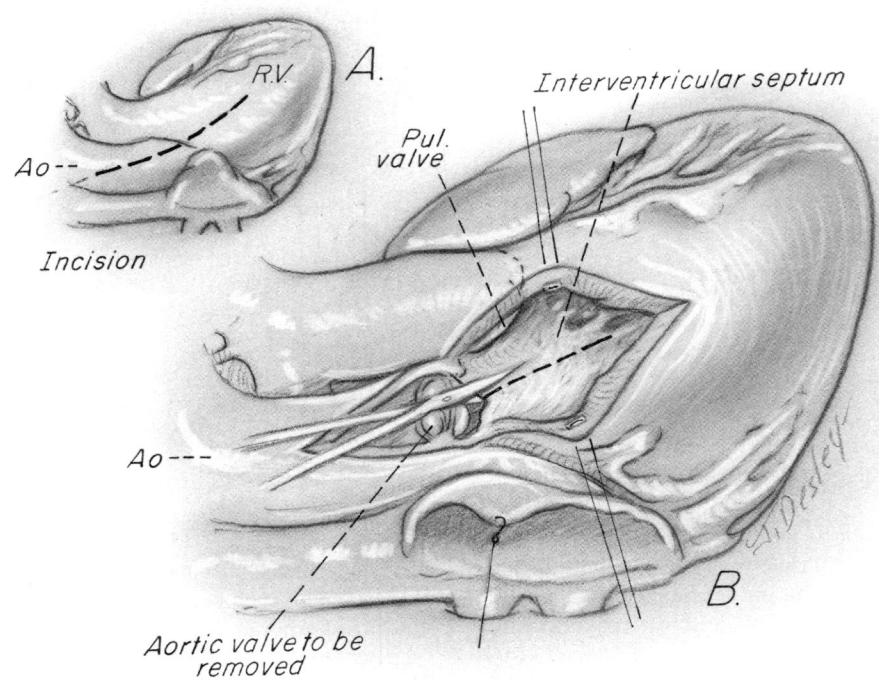

Figure 32-21 Aortoventriculoplasty (Konno operation) and aortic valve replacement.
(a) A vertical aortotomy is made, which heads a little rightward of the commissure between left and right coronary cusps of the aortic valve. As the incision is being made, the orifice of the right coronary artery is visualized and the incision passes clearly leftward of this. The right ventricle is opened with an oblique incision, the pulmonary valve is located, and the two incisions are joined.
(b) Before or after excising the aortic valve, an incision is made into the base of the right coronary cusp just to the left of its nadir. This incision is extended into the ventricular septum and toward the apex of the left ventricle. It is leftward of the conduction system (see Fig. 32-20).

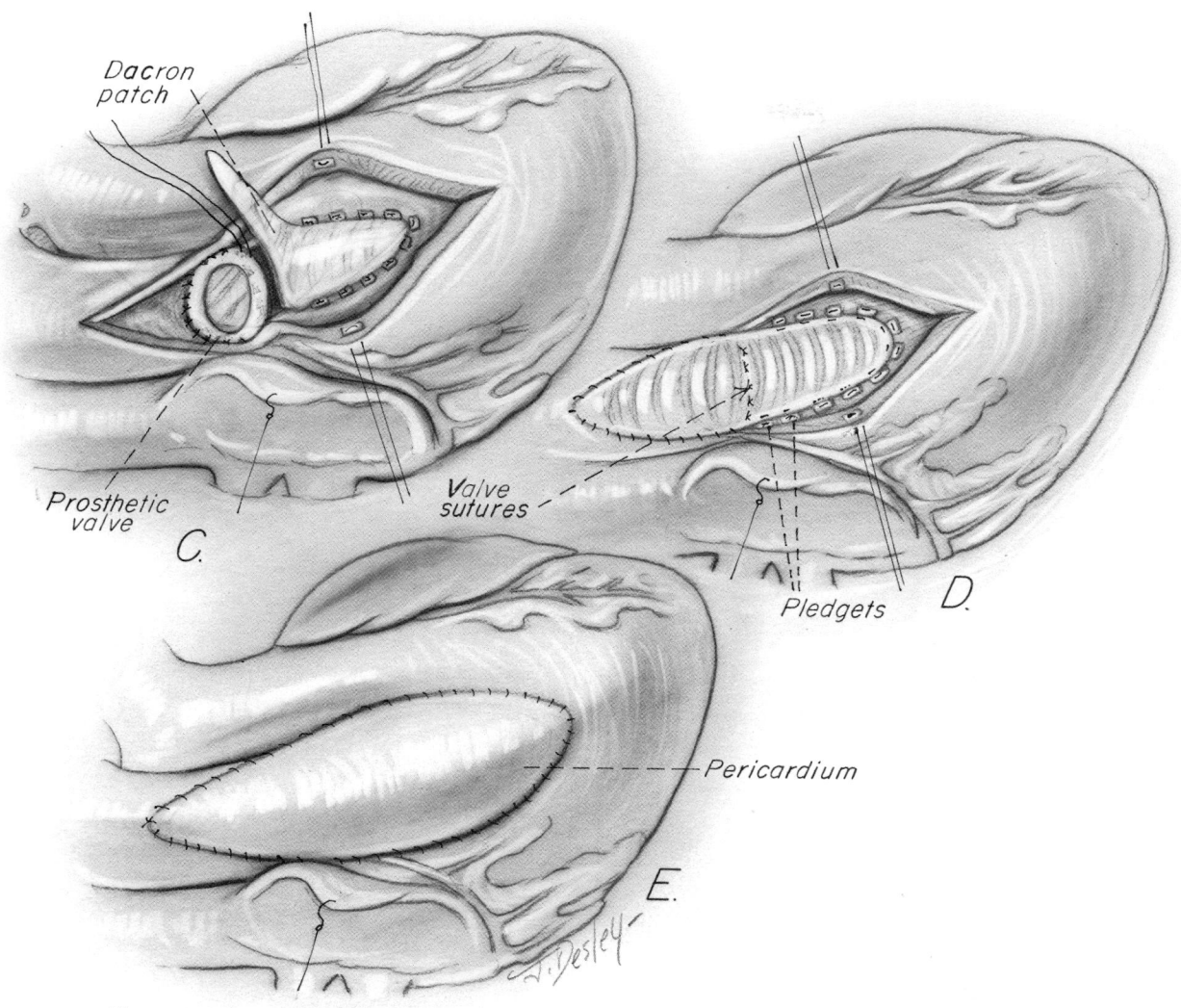

Figure 32-21 *(continued)*

(c) After excising the aortic valve, the valve replacement device (prosthetic valve) is sutured into place posteriorly by the usual interrupted technique. Anteriorly double-armed mattress sutures may be placed through the sewing ring and set aside for the moment. A preclotted woven velour Dacron patch is sutured into the left ventricular outflow tract, often with interrupted pledgetted mattress sutures.

(d) The sutures previously placed in the anterior aspect of the prosthesis are passed through the Dacron patch and tied. The remainder of the patch is sutured into place so as to close the aortotomy.

(e) A pericardial patch is now used to close the right ventriculotomy and is sewn onto the aorta just outside the previous suture line.

Ao, aorta; Pul. valve, pulmonary valve; RV, right ventricle.

extended superiorly with great care in order that it be kept clearly upstream to the aortic valve. As described for the Konno operation, an oval patch is trimmed from a preclotted woven Dacron tube. This is sewn into place so as to enlarge the left ventricular outflow tract. The septum is always thick in this circumstance, and four or five pledgetted mattress sutures with the pledgetts on the left ventricular side are placed initially to obtain a secure attachment of the patch; a whip stitch is used around the entire circumference.

The right ventriculotomy and the aortotomy are closed with continuous sutures. The remainder of the operation is carried out exactly as described for the Konno procedure.

EARLY RESULTS

Hospital Mortality

The hospital mortality for repair of *localized* subvalvar aortic stenosis is low but has not quite approached zero. In the combined GLH-UAB series (see Tables 32-4, 32-6 and 32-

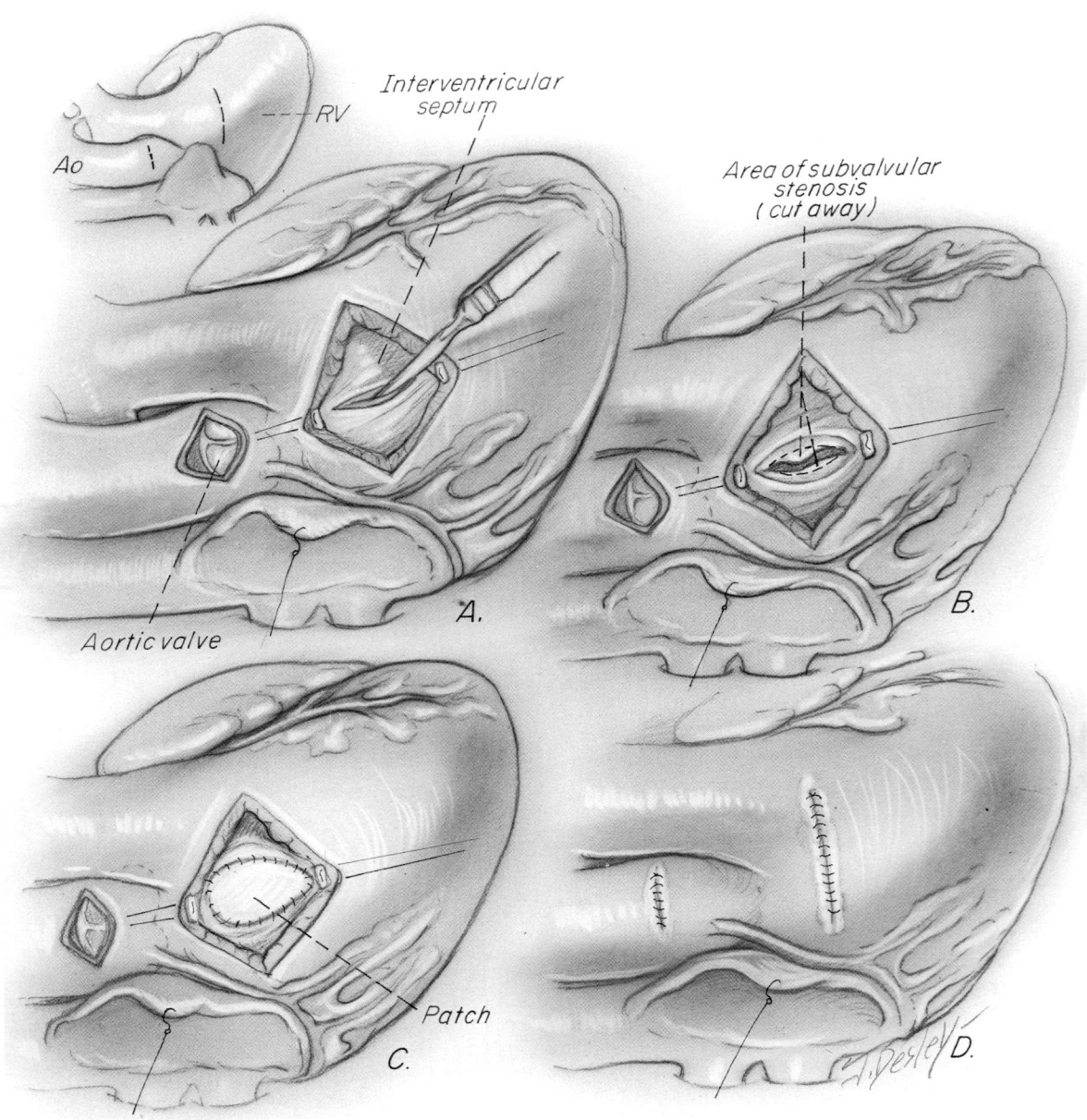

Figure 32-22 Modified Konno operation used only for complex or recurrent discrete subaortic stenosis or tunnel stenosis without a small aortic anulus. The ascending aorta is opened through a small transverse incision, to inspect the valve and guide the incision into the ventricular septum. A transverse incision is made in the infundibulum of the right ventricle (insert).

(a) After the transverse right ventriculotomy has been made, an incision is made through the ventricular septum parallel with the direction of the left ventricular outflow tract, keeping the incision well anterior to the level of the muscle of Lancisi in order to avoid the production of heart block. Usually a finger or instrument is passed through the aortic valve to protect it during the making of this incision.

(b) The fibromuscular components of the subvalvar stenosis are excised as much as is possible. The incision in the septum is carried to within 1 or 2 mm of the aortic valve anulus.

(c) The left ventricular outflow tract is widened by insertion of a patch. Widely spaced interrupted pledgetted mattress sutures, with the pledgets on the left ventricular side, may be placed through the patch and tied before the continuous suture line shown is placed.

(d) The ventriculotomy and aortotomy are closed with continuous sutures.

Ao, aorta; RV, right ventricle.

Table 32-18 Results of primary repair in the various types of congenital aortic stenosis according to morphology (UAB; 1967–1982).

Morphology of Stenosis	n^a	Hospital Deaths		
		No.	%	CL
Valvar	78(55%)	15	19%	14%–25%
Discrete subvalvar	41(29%)	0		
Localized	39	0		
Tunnel type	2	0		
Supravalvar	16(11%)	2	12%	4%–27%
Diffuse	5	2		
Localized	11	0		
Combined levels of stenosis	7(5%)	1	14%	2%–41%
Valvar + subvalvar	4	1		
Valvar + supravalvar	2	0		
Annular + subvalvar + supravalvar	1	0		
Total	142	18	13%	10%–16%

KEY: CL, 70% confidence limits.
^{a}( ) is percent of 142.

16), two deaths (2.6%, CL 0.8%–6%) occurred among 78 patients. In a combined series of 314 patients from the literature, mostly in an earlier era, the mortality was 4.8% (see Table 32-17).

Incremental Risk Factors for Hospital Death

Although it is not evident in the UAB-GLH combined series (Table 32-18), no doubt the early risks are greater in patients with *tunnel stenosis*. Thus, in the earlier report by Spencer and colleagues[S5] both patients with tunnel subvalvar aortic stenosis and severe infundibular pulmonary stenosis died; four of the 10 patients with tunnel stenosis, frequently in association with hypoplasia of the aortic anulus, died in the series of Maron and associates.[M5] Death was due to inadequate relief of the stenosis using an aortic approach.

No doubt also, the association of localized subvalvar aortic stenosis with *obstruction at other levels* (valvar, supravalvar, aortic, coarctation) and with the rather frequent *coexisting cardiac anomalies* such as ventricular septal defect (VSD), or pulmonary stenosis increase the early risks of death. This is all difficult to quantify, in part because the coexisting lesions may receive surgical treatment in early infancy before the discrete subaortic stenosis has become evident (for example, all four patients with associated VSD and coarctation or coarctation alone had these repaired in infancy [GLH]) and in part because in some patients the multiplicity of levels of obstruction may not be evident until after the first operation for valvar stenosis (Table 32-10).

The risk of the surgical treatment of localized subvalvar stenosis also depends in part on the procedure used. The mortality nearly approaches zero for the *resection technique* described. The *modified Konno operation* has been used in five primary operations and reoperations for complex varieties of localized subvalvar stenosis (UAB), with one death. The *Konno procedure* has been used in four primary operations and reoperations for complex subvalvar stenosis (UAB), with no deaths. With Ebert's modification, it is con-

sidered a low-risk operation. Thus, Misbach, Ebert, and colleagues report only 1 hospital death (6%, CL 0.7%–18%) among 18 patients.[M19] de Vivie and colleagues report 7 deaths (12%, CL 8%–18%) among 57 patients undergoing the Konno procedure,[D2] and others have reported similar results.[B16,R6] There have been no deaths (UAB, GLH) after five *left-ventricular–aortic conduit operations*. Norwood and colleagues reported two hospital deaths (22%, CL 8%–45%) among nine infants age 3 days to 13 months at operation; the conduit was placed between the left ventricle and the thoracic aorta.[N5]

Complications

Complications of the resection procedure are rare with current techniques. Only 1 case of surgically related complete heart block has occurred in the combined UAB-GLH series of 78 patients (and that in a complex case in a young child associated with congenital mitral stenosis and requiring a Konno operation and mitral valve replacement [UAB]); one instance of a small iatrogenic VSD has occurred (GLH); and no instance of iatrogenic mitral incompetence has developed. These are all potential complications of the resection of discrete subvalvar aortic stenosis. In an earlier era, these complications did occur (see Table 32-17).

LATE RESULTS

Survival

About 80% of patients coming to operation for discrete subvalvar aortic stenosis are alive 15 years later (Fig. 32-10 and 32-23). The early and late deaths are virtually all related to residual left ventricular outflow obstruction or subsequent efforts to relieve it, except for the few patients who die with bacterial endocarditis. This is illustrated by the experience with patients whose postrepair operating room gradients between left ventricle and aorta were greater than 20 mmHg (Table 32-19). Norwood and colleagues experienced two late deaths (29%, CL 10%–55%) among seven hospital survivors.

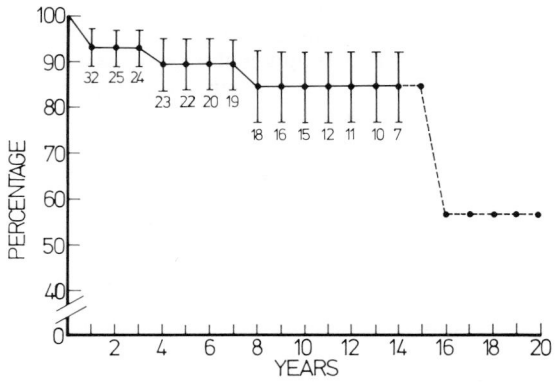

Figure 32-23 Actuarial survival, excluding hospital mortality, in patients operated on for discrete subaortic stenosis (GLH). The vertical bars represent 70% confidence limits. The data are not significant beyond 14 years. The patient dying within the first postoperative year had tunnel stenosis and annular hypoplasia, with incomplete relief of the obstruction by a subvalvar operation.

Table 32-19   Details of patients with a gradient >20 mmHg at the end of operation for discrete subvalvar aortic stenosis (GLH; 1960–1979, *n* = 37).

Case Number	LV-Ao Gradient (mmHg)			Type of Obstruction	Other Anomalies	Muscle Excised	Outcome
	Preoperatively	Operation	Recatheterization				
1	110	22	20	High	MN	Yes	Asymptomatic (5 yr)
2	35	35	—	High	AVA	Yes	Asymptomatic (3 mo)
3	140	72	—	High	AVA	Partial	Asymptomatic (7 yr)
4	116	26	25	Low	None	No	Late death SBE (8 yr)
5	90	28	—	Low	BAV	Yes	Asymptomatic (3 mo)
6	85	35	0	Low	None	Yes	Asymptomatic (5 yr)
7	78	56	—	Low	VSD	No	Late death (5 wk)
8	125	48	—	Tunnel	BAV; small anulus	Yes	Late death (6 wk)

KEY: AVA, extensive adherence of membrane to aortic valve cusps; BAV, bicuspid aortic valve; LV-Ao, left ventricular to aortic; MV, hypertrophied anterior papillary muscle adherent to mitral leaflet edge; SBE, subacute bacterial endocarditis; VSD, ventricular septal defect.

NOTE: In cases 1, 2, 5, and 8 there were congenital valvar aortic stenoses as components of the residual gradient.

Functional Status

The functional status of surviving patients operated upon for subvalvar aortic stenosis is generally good.[B8] Thus, 31 (82%, CL 73%–88%) of 38 surviving and traced patients are in NYHA functional class I and 6 (16%, CL 6%–24%) are in NYHA class II (UAB). Whitmer and colleagues have shown objective evidence of improvement by exercise testing.[W7]

Hemodynamic State

Most patients, including those with the less severe forms of tunnel stenosis, have an excellent hemodynamic result late (10 years) postoperatively. The operation usually results in a dramatic immediate gradient reduction, which is sustained or improved over the subsequent 10 years (Fig. 32-24). In a few patients, the gradient is mildly increased 5–10 years postoperatively, compared to measurements in the operating room, but this is difficult to interpret because of the variability of the postrepair operating room measurements.

The results from simple resection are less good in patients with severe tunnel stenosis.[M25] This is illustrated by the finding of Wright and colleagues that in six patients in this category the mean LV-Ao gradient was reduced from 102 to only 72 mmHg.[W8] This was a significantly smaller reduction in gradient (30 ± 17 mmHg) than was achieved in patients with discrete subvalvar aortic stenosis (52 ± 40 mmHg) (*P* for difference < .05). The advantages of the Konno procedure in this setting are clear.

Recurrence of Discrete Subvalvar Stenosis

This is a controversial matter. Several authors have reported an increase in the residual stenosis at the time of late postoperative catheterization, particularly in the fibromuscular and tunnel stenoses,[C8,K2,K5,N1,R8] and some have suggested that this is caused by a recurrence of the stenosis either from failure of growth of the stenotic zone in children or regrowth of fibrous tissue.[K5,N1] Reoperation has been undertaken in a

number of these patients and has not always been effective in relieving the obstruction.[C18]

However, to date no reoperations have been required in the GLH group; and the overall actuarial incidence of freedom from reoperation at 17 years is 78% (UAB; see Fig. 32-13). In only one case was there really a recurrence in a patient with only discrete subvalvar stenosis, and it was treatable by another resection. In the other three, the stenosis originally was over a long area, the original procedure was inadequate, and at reoperation a left-ventricular–aortic conduit (two) or a Konno operation (one) was required. Fortunately, the risk of reoperation has been low in patients whose first operation was for isolated or combined discrete

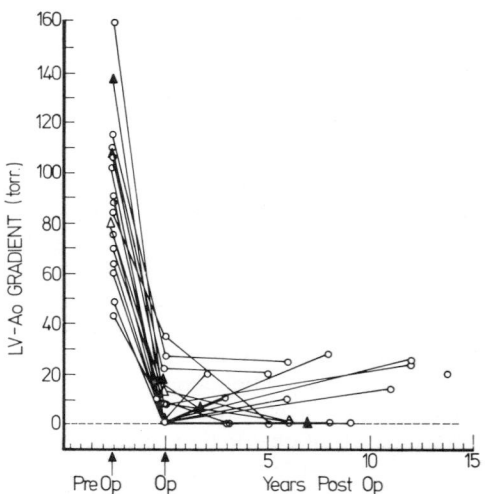

Figure 32-24   The results of cardiac catheterization in 19 patients operated upon for discrete subaortic stenosis and restudied an average of 6.6 years (1.5–14 years) later (GLH). A zero gradient was recorded at the completion of operation (Op) in 10 of 18 patients and at late follow-up in 8 of 19 patients. No patient had a gradient 30 mmHg or more at late study. The three patients with tunnel stenosis are shown as triangles: A closed triangle indicates treatment by a combined excision via aorta and left ventricle.

subvalvar stenosis, no deaths (0%, CL 0%–19%) having occurred among the nine patients (UAB) in which this has been performed (Table 32-10; only five of the nine had their first operation at UAB).

Aortic Incompetence

Some have suggested that aortic incompetence may progress after a satisfactory operation,[C9] but in the GLH-UAB experiences and that reported by others,[H4,K2] although the aortic incompetence persists, it remains trivial or mild unless endocarditis occurs.

INDICATIONS FOR OPERATION

Since the obstruction from localized congenital subvalvar aortic stenosis tends to progress rather rapidly (see "Natural History") and since the tendency to develop sudden death when it becomes severe is presumably the same as in the case of severe congenital valvar aortic stenosis, operation is advisable whenever the stenosis is moderate (LV-Ao gradient > 50 mmHg). When the stenosis (gradient > 100 mmHg) is severe, operation without delay is indicated. Resection of the subvalvar obstruction is the procedure of choice (see "Technique of Operation").

When the discrete subvalvar stenosis is long (tunnel stenosis), particularly when it is associated with annular hypoplasia, a simple repair by resection is often not effective. In these circumstances, an initial Konno operation is indicated.

When there are multiple levels of left ventricular outflow obstruction or major associated cardiac anomalies, the general indications described above pertain, but each patient must be considered in the light of his or her particular morphology and circumstances. The Konno procedure is the most generally applicable one, but the required aortic valve replacement is disadvantageous for the very young patient.

SPECIAL SITUATIONS AND CONTROVERSIES

Aortoseptal Approach for Tunnel Stenosis

The modified Konno procedure provides only a limited exposure of the subvalvar area (see "Technique of Operation"). Vouhe and colleagues have used an approach more like the Konno operation but without the need for replacement of the aortic valve.[V2] Although not yet used (UAB, GLH), the approach appears to have merit. A longitudinal incision in the aorta is carried obliquely down toward the top of the adjacent portions of the right and left aortic cusps. A more-or-less transverse incision is made in the right ventricular infundibulum, beginning at a point just over this. The aortic and right ventricular incisions come together just over the top of the left anterior fibrous trigone. The aortic ring is now divided through the trigone, going exactly between the adjacent extremities of the left and right cusps. It is said that this can be done without damage to the cusps. This incision is now carried well into the ventricular septum, as in the

Konno procedure, opening the left ventricular outflow tract widely. After resecting the obstructing tissue, the septal incision is closed, the left anterior fibrous trigone reconstructed, and the right ventricular and aortic incisions closed. It would seem a widening Dacron patch could be used in closing the septal incision, as in the modified Konno procedure.

Left Ventricular–Aortic Conduit

This operation has enjoyed some popularity in the past.[B7,C10,E7] Complications both early and late postoperatively are frequent with this procedure, and 4 (24%, CL 12%–39%) of 17 hospital survivors reported by Brown and colleagues have required reoperation, as have 7 (78%, CL 55%–92%) of 9 hospital survivors reported by Di Donato and colleagues.[B18,D8] Currently (GLH and UAB), there are no indications for the procedure in cases of congenital aortic stenosis.

SECTION 3
CONGENITAL SUPRAVALVAR AORTIC STENOSIS

DEFINITION

Congenital supravalvar aortic stenosis is an obstruction caused by localized or diffuse narrowing of the aortic lumen commencing immediately above the aortic valve.

HISTORICAL NOTE

The first description of supravalvar aortic stenosis is attributed to Mencarelli in 1930.[M16] It was seldom recognized, however, until Denie and Verheugt emphasized in 1958 that supravalvar stenosis could be differentiated from other varieties of aortic stenosis by retrograde arterial catheterization.[D5] In 1959, Morrow and associates pointed out the usefulness of angiography in diagnosis.[M12] In 1961, the GLH group of Williams, Barratt-Boyes, and Lowe described the association of supravalvar aortic stenosis with unusual "elfin" facies and mental retardation,[W4] a syndrome that was soon confirmed by others.[B11,F6]

In 1964, Beuren and colleagues reported that their 10 cases of the GLH syndrome all suffered from multiple peripheral pulmonary artery stenoses.[B12] Watson and Bourassa and Campeau had also noted this association 1 year before.[B13,W6] The similarity between the facies of patients with supravalvar aortic stenosis and severe infantile hypercalcemia was noted in 1963 by Hooft and colleagues and Black and Bonham Carter[B9,H7]; 1 year later, Garcia and colleagues reported the first patient with the GLH syndrome and a documented history of infantile hypercalcemia.[G5] The occurrence of a familial form of supravalvar stenosis without elfin facies was reported first from Johns Hopkins in 1959.[S10]

Successful surgery for supravalvar stenosis using patch graft enlargement of the noncoronary sinus of Valsalva was reported by us from the Mayo Clinic in 1961,[M14] the first patient being operated upon in 1956. Prior to this publication, successful procedures using a similar technique had been carried out in 1959 at GLH[W4] and elsewhere.[G6,S7] In 1960, Hara and associates successfully performed an excision and end-to-end anastomosis in a patient with supravalvar aortic stenosis,[H6] and Hancock satisfactorily relieved the stenosis by excision of the intimal ridge without patch enlargement.[H8] Neither of these procedures is currently recommended.

MORPHOLOGY

Supravalvar Stenosis

The stenosis may be localized or diffuse.[P3] Most commonly, it is *localized* to the supravalvar area of the aorta just above or at the level of the attachments of the valve commissures.[D5,W4] There is usually an external waisting of the aorta at this point, which produces, in association with some dilatation of the sinuses of Valsalva and absence of poststenotic dilatation, an hourglass appearance. In addition, there is a variable amount of intimal thickening in the form of an internal shelf, which increases the stenosis significantly.

Less often, the narrowing is *diffuse,* extending throughout the length of the ascending aorta and even beyond into the transverse arch and the origins of the arch vessels.[N4]

Associated Other Aortic Stenoses

In about a third of the patients, the aortic valve leaflets are thickened,[D3] but true valvar stenosis due to leaflet fusion is rare as is a bicuspid valve.[R5] Occasionally, the aortic anulus may be hypoplastic.[K6] Subvalvar stenosis is uncommon but can coexist.[K6]

Coronary Arteries

The aortic valve leaflet edges may be adherent to the intimal shelf, producing a stenosis at the entry into the sinus of Valsalva and obstructing the coronary flow. This is more common in the left cusp[D5,P3,R5] but can occur in the right.[W4] In the absence of obstruction to inflow into the sinus of Valsalva or of ostial stenosis, which may also occur,[N4] the coronary arteries are exposed to a high pressure and show dilatation, tortuosity and medial hypertrophy,[N4] and the early onset of atherosclerosis.

Associated Cardiac Anomalies

The most common associated anomaly consists of multiple stenoses in the peripheral pulmonary arteries,[B12] which may be severe enough to produce right ventricular hypertension and hypertrophy. Pulmonary valve stenosis occurs uncommonly.[B13] Diffuse hypoplasia of the main pulmonary artery may be associated with diffuse hypoplasia of the aorta,[M17,S9,S11] both arteries showing marked wall thickening and fibromuscular dysplasia histologically in association with disorganization and replacement of the elastic tissue of

the media. These patients usually give a familial history, and sudden death in infancy is common.

Less common anomalies include stenosis of the origins of subclavian and carotid and rarely other major systemic arteries, coarctation of the aorta (with or without patent ductus arteriosus), and ventricular septal defect. Mitral incompetence occurs rarely, and the mitral valve may be thickened and redundant.[B10] The patient reported by Denie and Verheugt in 1958 had Marfan's syndrome,[D5] and this has been noted subsequently in about 5% of patients with supravalvar aortic stenosis.[P3]

CLINICAL FEATURES AND DIAGNOSTIC CRITERIA

Symptoms

Symptoms rarely develop in infancy and frequently do so in childhood, but in some patients they may appear as late as the second or third decade. They are similar to those in other types of congenital aortic stenosis, although angina may be more frequent because of the increased incidence of early onset coronary atherosclerosis.

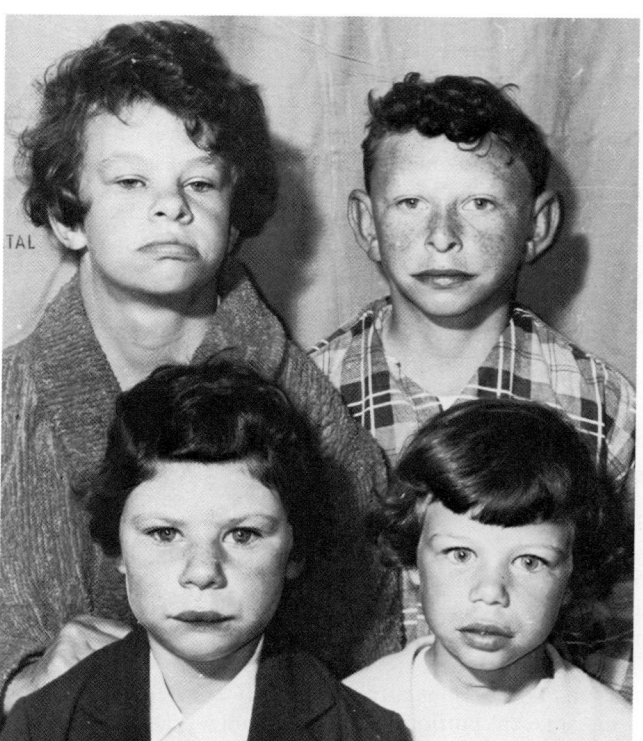

Figure 32-25 Photograph of the four children with elfin facies and supravalvar congenital aortic stenosis reported in 1961 (GLH).[W4] The appearance is characterized by a depressed nasal bridge with anteverted nares, thick lips, mandibular recession, short palpebral fissures, and medial eyebrow flare. Dental malocclusion is also present.

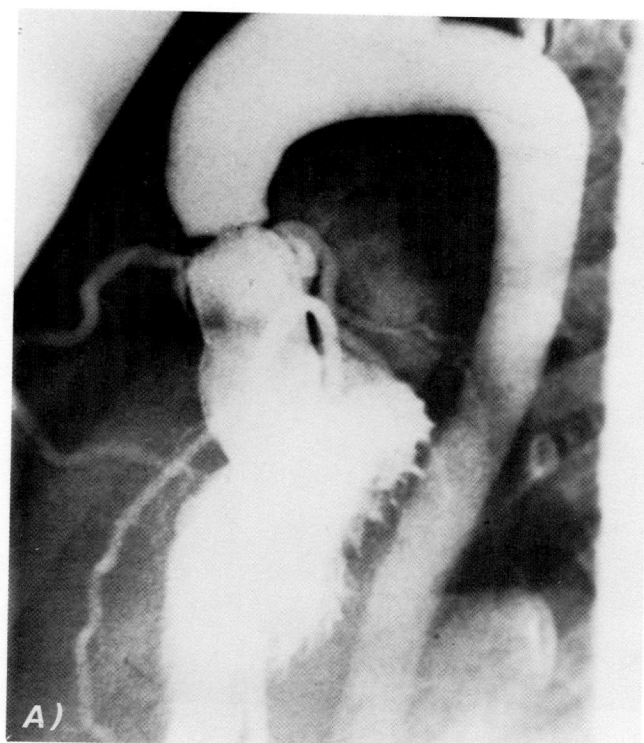

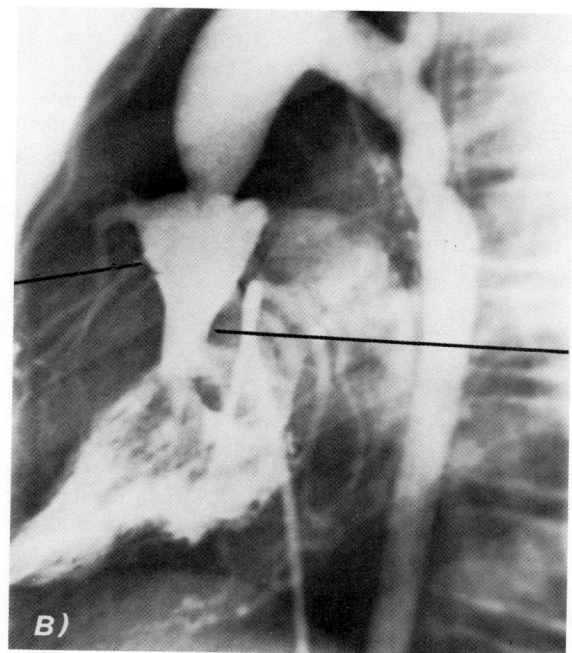

Figure 32-26 Left ventriculogram and aortogram in the long axial position in a patient with localized congenital supravalvar stenosis (UAB).
(*a*) In the lateral view the subvalvar area is seen to be widely open. The hourglass deformity and supravalvar ridge are evident and produce severe obstruction.
(*b*) In the regular lateral view, the base of the right aortic cusp is seen well below the supravalvar narrowing. The anterior mitral leaflet is open.

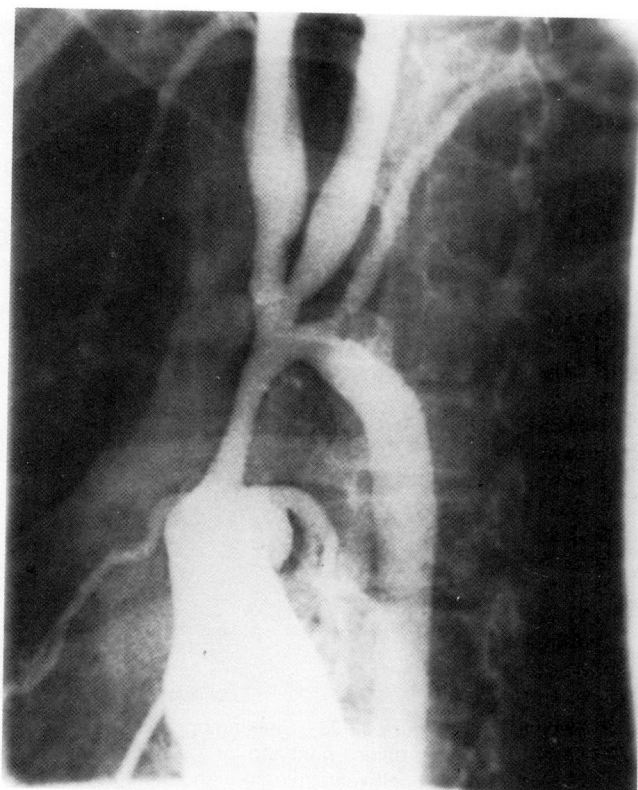

Figure 32-27 Left ventriculogram and aortogram in lateral projection in the long axial position in a patient with diffuse supravalvar aortic stenosis, which was successfully repaired (UAB). The ascending aorta becomes diffusely narrow at the level of the aortic valve commissures, just beyond the takeoff of the right and left coronary arteries. The narrowing extends into the transverse arch.

Signs

The auscultatory findings are similar to those in valvar aortic stenosis so that the correct diagnosis may not be possible from the physical signs. However, an ejection click is absent, and the murmur and thrill tend to be sited higher than in valvar stenosis. An aortic diastolic murmur is uncommon.[L8] The blood pressure may be lower in the left arm than the right.[C14,K6,W4] This is due in some cases to stenosis at the origin of the left subclavian artery and in others to a jet effect.[F7,G7] Similarly, the left carotid pulse may be diminished.[L8]

A diagnostic clinical feature in some cases are elfin facies (Fig. 32-25), combined with a reduced intelligence quotient and failure to thrive.[W4] These retarded children are characteristically small, friendly, and loquacious. Each component of the syndrome varies in severity, however, and the supravalvar stenosis may in fact be mild or occasionally absent in patients with the typical facies.[J3] The disease in this form is always sporadic, and the facies are identical to those present in severe infantile hypercalcemia. Hypercalcemia has been documented in less than 5% of these infants,[M3] al-

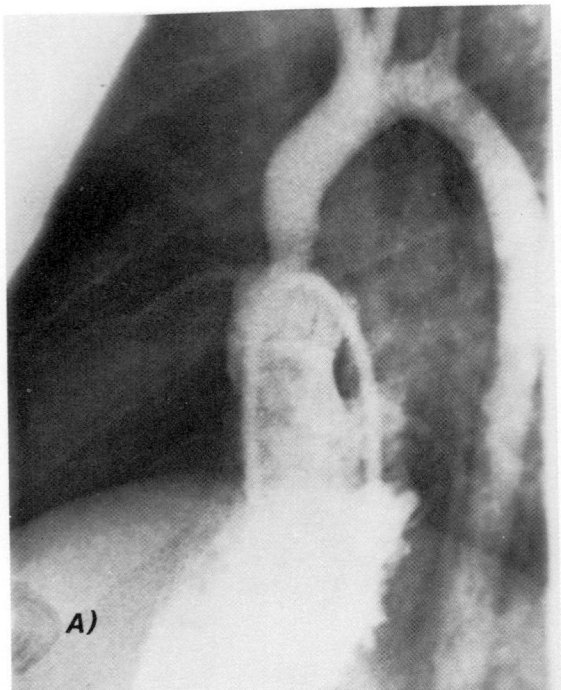
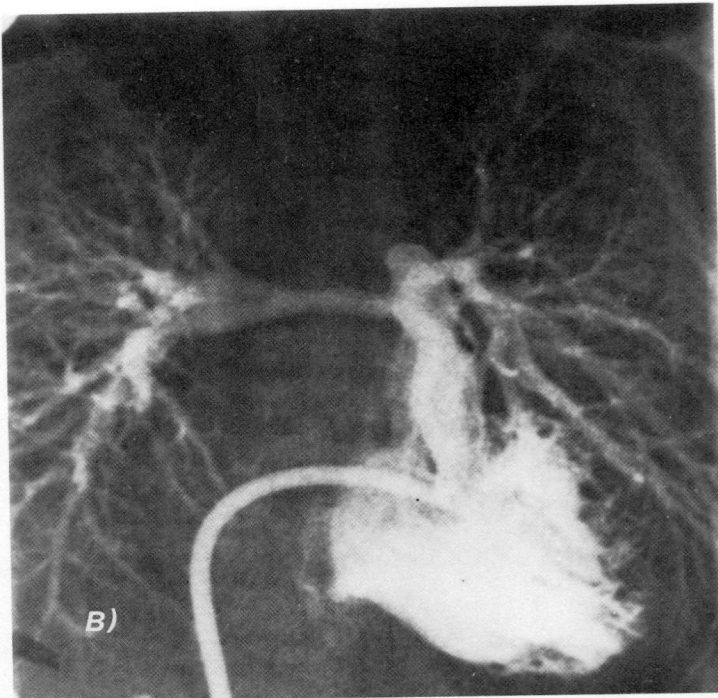

Figure 32-28 Cineangiograms in a patient with localized supravalvar aortic stenosis with coexisting diffuse right and left pulmonary artery narrowing (UAB).
(a) Left ventriculogram and aortogram in the lateral projection in the long axial position.
(b) Right ventriculogram in the PA projection.

though it is more common when the elfin facies is not present.^M13

Somewhat fewer than half the patients with congenital supravalvar aortic stenosis have elfin facies and mental retardation. Of the remainder, some are familial and some sporadic.

Cardiac Catheterization and Angiocardiography

The site of pressure change can be localized on withdrawal of a catheter from left ventricle to aorta. The morphology of the supravalvar stenosis can be outlined on angiography (Figs. 32-26 and 32-27), and coexisting anomalies can be identified (Fig. 32-28).

NATURAL HISTORY

This is the least common type of congenital aortic stenosis. The sexes are equally affected.

In infants with elfin facies and mental retardation and combined congenital supravalvar aortic stenosis and pulmonary stenoses of the diffuse variety, sudden death is common early in life.^S9 Also, sudden death can occur in all age groups, presumably in part from severe left ventricular outflow obstruction and in part from coronary artery disease.

Progression of the stenosis has been documented occasionally; the time course is probably comparable to that of valvar stenosis. It is probable that most untreated patients with supravalvar stenosis die before reaching adult life, since the lesion is uncommon in adults.^P4 Death before adult life is particularly likely to occur in those with elfin facies, since they comprise only 11% of adults with the anomaly and 60% of the children with it. Some of the children with elfin facies and the severe form of infantile hypercalcemia die from complications of hypercalcemia.

TECHNIQUE OF OPERATION

Localized Type

The operation is begun exactly as described for the procedure of valvotomy for congenital valvar aortic stenosis. After cross-clamping the aorta and infusing the cold cardioplegic solution, the aortotomy is made (Fig. 32-29).

The aorta is opened above the valve and the incision carried into the right (GLH) or noncoronary (UAB) sinus of Valsalva. If the former is used, the right coronary artery origin must first be dissected and the incision placed between it and the commissure between right and noncoronary cusps. The aortic valve and subvalvar areas are examined to exclude obstruction at those levels. The intimal shelf is now resected, in part to ensure adequate inflow into the sinuses of Valsalva. A diamond-shaped patch of pericardium (or if not available, preclotted woven Dacron) is then incorporated into the incision with a running polypropylene suture; it must be of sufficient size to enlarge the aortic diameter to normal. With strong suction on the aortic needle vent, the aortic clamp is released and rewarming is begun. The remainder of the procedure is completed as usual (see Chapter 2, Section 3), including measurement of pressure in left ventricle and ascending aorta.

Diffuse Type

The operation proceeds as described for the localized type, except that the skin incision is carried about 2 cm more superiorly than usual. The femoral artery is exposed for arterial cannulation. The origins of the innominate, left common carotid, and left subclavian arteries and the transverse portion of the aortic arch are dissected below and above the left innominate vein.

Cardiopulmonary bypass (CPB) is established with arterial inflow to the patient through the femoral artery, and the body temperature is taken to 20°C. The operating table is placed in moderate Trendelenburg position. The aorta is cross-clamped, usually just proximal to the left subclavian artery (which is usually not reconstructed), the origins of the left common carotid and innominate arteries are clamped, and the cold cardioplegic solution is infused. Total circulatory arrest is usually established.

A longitudinal incision is made in the ascending aorta, and it is carried well down into the noncoronary sinus of Valsalva, as in the case of the repair of the localized form. Any intimal ridge above each sinus of Valsalva is excised as described earlier. The incision is carried up the ascending aorta, which is usually thick walled and has a small lumen, and around onto the transverse portion of the aortic arch and, if necessary, into the upper descending thoracic aorta after establishing total circulatory arrest and removing the cross-clamp that is there. Incisions are made across any stenosis present at the origin of the innominate and left common carotid artery, and any intimal proliferations at these orifices are dissected away. A patch of preclotted woven double

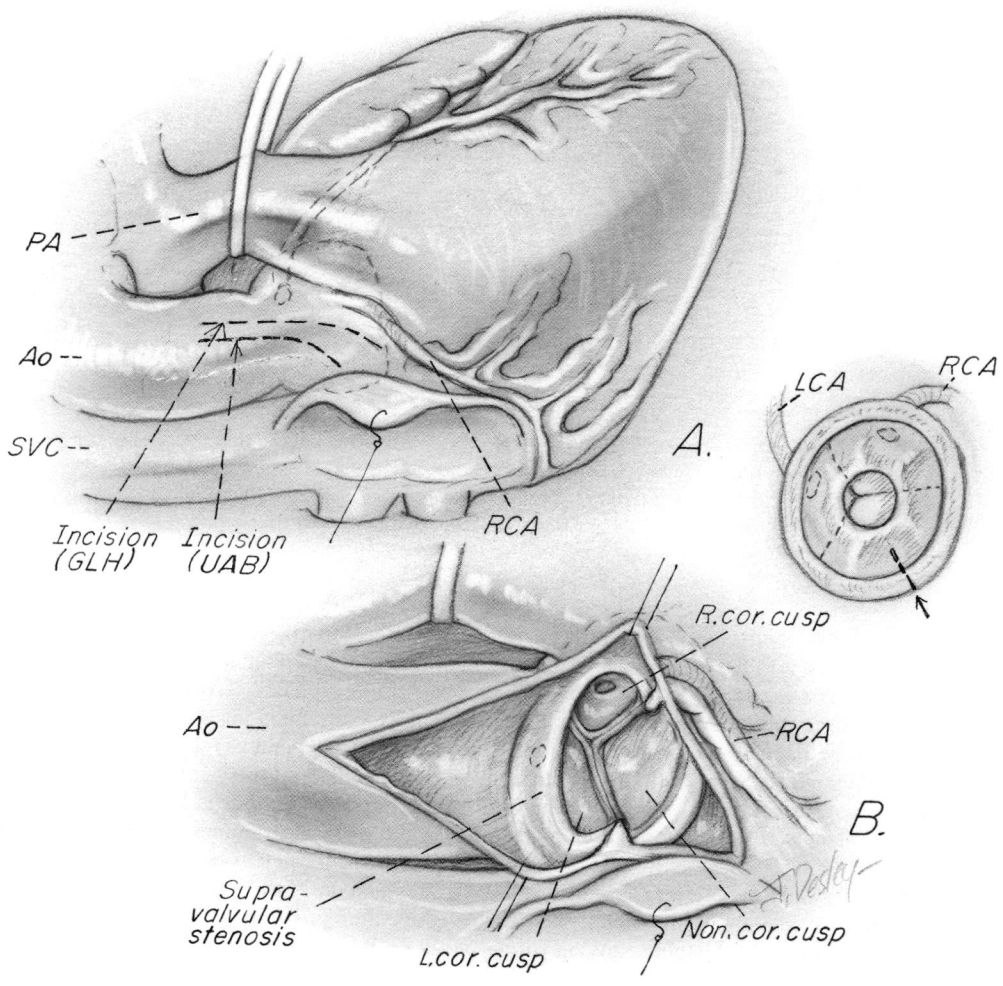

Figure 32-29 Repair of congenital supravalvar aortic stenosis.
(a) The aortotomy is directed into the right coronary sinus of Valsalva, to the right of the right coronary artery origin (GLH) or is extended down into the noncoronary sinus (UAB).
(b) After obtaining exposure with stay sutures, the fibrous intimal ridge is visible. The insert illustrates the added severity of stenosis imparted by the ridge.

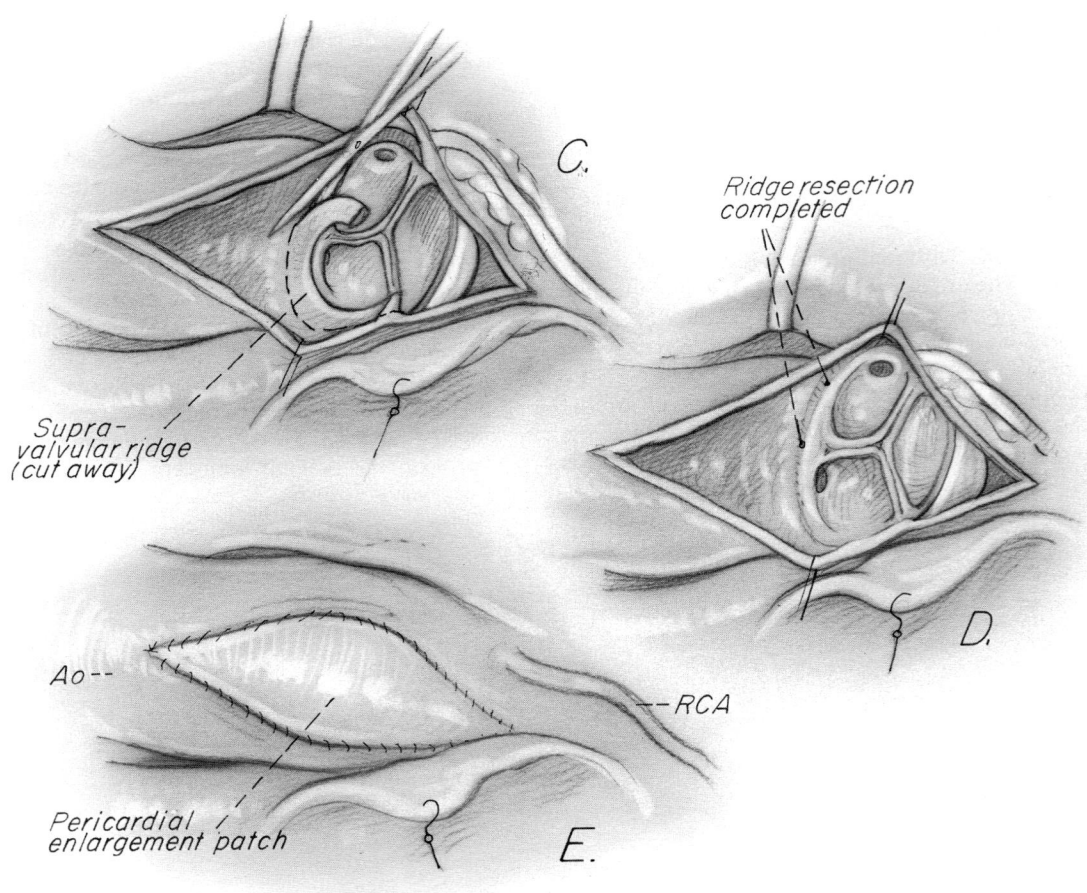

Figure 32-29 (continued)
(c) When this ridge is prominent (as is usually the case), it is excised.
(d) The excision opens up entrance into the sinuses of Valsalva, particularly the left.
(e) The supravalvar narrowing is eliminated by incorporating an enlarging patch of pericardium (or Dacron) into the closure of the incision.

Ao, aorta; LCA, left coronary artery; L.cor.cusp, left coronary cusp; Non.cor.cusp, noncoronary cusp; PA, pulmonary artery; RCA, right coronary artery; R.cor.cusp, right coronary cusp; SVC, superior vena cava.

velour Dacron cut from a tube graft or of pericardium if enough is available is fashioned to an appropriate size and shape. Beginning distally, it is sutured into place with continuous 4-0 or 5-0 polypropylene suture. An ear or projection is fashioned into the patch to go across the orifice of the left common carotid and innominate arteries. The most proximal angle of the suture line is not completed at this moment. If circulatory arrest has been used, CPB is now recommenced at $0.5-1.0 \; l \cdot min^{-1} \cdot m^{-2}$ at 25°C, releasing the distal aortic clamp to allow free bleeding out the proximal angle. The clamps on the left common carotid and innominate artery are then removed and the vessels jiggled to displace any air into the arch and out the proximal angle of the suture line. Then the aortic cross-clamp is repositioned just proximal (upstream) to the innominate artery, full perfusion flow is established, and rewarming is begun. The proximal angle of the patch is then sutured into place, and the aortic clamp is removed. The operation is completed as described earlier.

Alternatively, if there is uncertainty about air after jiggling the brachiocephalic vessels to remove the air, the distal clamp is replaced, CPB is again discontinued, and a right-angled cannula is inserted through a purse-string suture into the superior vena cava. The vena cava is occluded between the cannula and the right atrium, the cannula attached to the arterial line, and perfusion of the cerebral circulation begun in a retrograde manner. Then when air and blood have been flushed out, perfusion through the regular arterial line is reestablished, air extruded from beneath the patch graft, and the clamp positioned on the ascending aorta just proximal to the innominate artery.

EARLY RESULTS

The primary repair of isolated *localized* congenital supravalvar aortic stenosis has a low hospital mortality. Thus, in the combined GLH-UAB series of 19 patients, there were no hospital deaths (0%, CL 0%–10%) (Tables 32-18 and 32-20). An additional 6-year-old patient with peripheral pulmonary artery stenosis and aortic native valve endocarditis with a large aneurysm of the ascending and transverse aortic arch died 11 days postoperatively (GLH).

The early risks are greater in patients with *diffuse* congenital supravalvar aortic stenosis. Two (40%, CL 14%–71%) of five patients died in hospital after repair (UAB). Although allegedly the high risk is related to inadequate relief of the obstruction,[K6] the gradient had been abolished in these five cases.

LATE RESULTS

The late *survival* is good. Thus, there have been two late deaths in the GLH series and none to date in the UAB series. The actuarial survival is 87% (UAB) (see Fig. 32-13); the two deaths are in patients with diffuse supravalvar narrowing who died in hospital.

Table 32-20 Surgical series of repair of congenital localized supravalvar aortic stenosis (GLH; 1959–1984). One patient with the diffuse form has undergone repair.

Age (yr)		GLH Syndrome	Hospital Deaths	
≤ <	n	No.	No.	%
5				
5 --- 10	3	3		
10 --- 20	4	3		
20	1			
Total	8	6		0% (CL 0%–24%)

KEY: CL, 70% confidence limits.

NOTE: There are two late deaths (age 11 and 9 years at operation) and no reoperations. In addition to the patients in the table, one patient aged 6 years died 1 month after repair of supravalvar aortic stenosis complicated by bacterial endocarditis and large mycotic aneurysm of ascending and transverse aorta; he also had peripheral pulmonary artery stenosis, a familial history, and no elfin facies.

Most patients are without symptoms.[M15,S8] Thus, 10 (77%) of 13 traced cases are in NYHA class I and 3 are in NYHA class II (UAB).

There have been no *reoperations* at UAB or GLH.

Residual left ventricular-aortic *gradients* are rare[K6,R5,W5] and were present in only one patient (UAB, GLH). A residual gradient is usually caused by an overlooked coexisting valvar or subvalvar stenosis.[R5]

INDICATIONS FOR OPERATION

Operation is advisable in patients with localized or diffuse congenital supravalvar aortic stenosis when the peak pressure gradient across the stenosis is 50 mmHg or more. The operation should be performed at whatever age the criteria for surgery are met. Coexisting diffuse right and left pulmonary artery stenoses are uncorrectable by current techniques, and their presence may make surgery inadvisable.

SPECIAL SITUATIONS AND CONTROVERSIES

Type of Repair

The insertion of a diamond-shaped patch of prosthetic material or pericardium to enlarge the aortic diameter[M14] combined with resection of the intimal shelf[R5] is a safe and effective procedure. There is the theoretical danger of a false aneurysm developing at the edge of a Dacron onlay patch, similar to that which occurs when a Dacron patch is used in the repair of coarctation (see Chapter 34). Pericardium is a more desirable material for this reason.

Most surgeons have placed the patch into the noncoronary sinus of Valsalva,[C14,D4,M14,S7] but it has always (GLH) been placed into the right sinus since this maneuver relieves any narrowing between the right cusp and aortic wall.[W4] More recently, Doty and colleagues have recommended using a double-flanged patch that extends separately into both noncoronary and right sinuses.[D3,H10] There is no evidence that the double-flanged patch produces superior results.

REFERENCES

A

1. Ankeney JL, Tzeng TS, Liebman J: Surgical therapy for congenital aortic valvular stenosis. *J Thorac Cardiovasc Surg* 85:41, 1983.

B

1. Bonner AJ, Sacks HN, Tavel ME: Assessing the severity of aortic stenosis by phonocardiography and carotid pulse recordings. *Circulation* 48:247, 1973.
2. Braverman IB, Gibson S: The outlook for children with congenital aortic stenosis. *Am Heart J* 53:487, 1957.
3. Bernhard WF, Keane JF, Fellows KE, Litwin SB, Gross RE: Progress and problems in surgical management of congenital aortic stenosis. *J Thorac Cardiovasc Surg* 66:404, 1973.

4. Bloom KR, Meyer RA, Bove KE, Kaplan S: The association of fixed and dynamic left ventricular outflow obstruction. *Am Heart J* 89:586, 1975.
5. Brock R, Felming PR: Aortic subvalvar stenosis. A report of 5 cases diagnosed during life. *Guy's Hosp Rep* 105:391, 1956.
6. Brock R: Aortic subvalvar stenosis with surgical treatment. *Guy's Hosp Rep* 108:144, 1959.
7. Bernhard WF, Porier V, La Farge CG: Relief of congenital obstruction to left ventricular outflow with a ventricular-aortic prosthesis. *J Thorac Cardiovasc Surg* 69:223, 1975.
8. Binet JP, Losay J, Demontoux S, Planche C, Langlois J: Subvalvar aortic stenosis. Long-term surgical results. *Thorac Cardiovasc Surg* 31:96, 1983.
9. Black JA, Bonham Carter RE: Association between aortic ste-

nosis and facies of severe infantile hypercalcemia. *Lancet* 2:745, 1963.

10. Becker AE, Becker MJ, Edwards JE: Mitral valvular abnormalities associated with supravalvular aortic stenosis. *Am J Cardiol* 29:90, 1972.

11. Beuren AJ, Apitz J, Harmjanz E: Supravalvular aortic stenosis in association with mental retardation and a certain facial appearance. *Circulation* 26:1235, 1962.

12. Beuren AJ, Schulze C, Eberle P, Harmjanz E, Apitz J: The syndrome of supravalvular aortic stenosis, peripheral pulmonary stenosis, mental retardation and similar facial appearance. *Am J Cardiol* 13:471, 1964.

13. Bourassa MG, Campeau L: Combined supravalvular aortic and pulmonic stenosis. *Circulation* 28:572, 1963.

14. Braunwald E, Goldblatt A, Aygen MM, Rockoff SD, Morrow AG: Congenital aortic stenosis. 1. Clinical and hemodynamic findings in 100 patients. *Circulation* 27:426, 1963.

15. Blackwood RA, Bloom KR, Williams SN: Aortic stenosis in children. Experience with echocardiographic prediction of severity. *Circulation* 57:263, 1978.

16. Bjornstad PB, Rastan H, Keutel J, Beuren AJ, Koncz J: Aortoventriculoplasty for tunnel subaortic stenosis and other obstructions of the left ventricular outflow tract. Clinical and hemodynamic results. *Circulation* 60:59, 1979.

17. Ben-Shachar G, Moiler JH, Castaneda-Zuniga W, Edwards JE: Signs of membranous subaortic stenosis appearing after correction of persistent common atrioventricular canal. *Am J Cardiol* 48:340, 1981.

18. Brown JW, Girod DA, Hurwitz RA, Caldwell RL, Rocchini AP, Behrendt DM, Kirsh MM: Apicoaortic valved conduits for complex left ventricular outflow obstruction: Technical considerations and current status. *Ann Thorac Surg* 38:162, 1984.

19. Bharati S, Lev M, Kirklin JW: *Cardiac Surgery and the Conduction System.* John Wiley & Sons, New York, 1983.

C

1. Cohen LS, Friedman WF, Braunwald E: Natural history of mild congenital aortic stenosis elucidated by serial hemodynamic studies. *Am J Cardiol* 30:1, 1972.

2. Cheitlin MD, Fenoglio JJ Jr, McAllister HA Jr, Davia JE, De Castro CM: Congenital aortic stenosis secondary to dysplasia of congenital bicuspid aortic valves without commissural fusion. *Am J Cardiol* 42:102, 1978.

3. Campbell M: The natural history of congenital aortic stenosis. *Br Heart J* 30:514, 1968.

4. Cooley DA, Beall AC, Hallman GC, Bucker DL: Obstructive lesions of the left ventricular outflow tract. Surgical treatment. *Circulation* 31:612, 1965.

5. Conkle DM, Jones M, Morrow AG: Treatment of congenital aortic stenosis. An evaluation of the late results of aortic valvotomy. *Arch Surg* 107:649, 1973.

6. Coran AG, Bernhard WF: The surgical management of valvular aortic stenosis during infancy. *J Thorac Cardiovasc Surg* 58:401, 1969.

7. Chiariello L, Vlad P, Subramanian S: Surgical treatment of congenital valvular aortic stenosis. *Thorax* 31:398, 1976.

8. Champsaur G, Trusler GA, Mustard WT: Congenital discrete subvalvar aortic stenosis. Surgical experience and long-term follow-up in 20 pediatric patients. *Br Heart J* 35:443, 1973.

9. Chiariello L, Agosti J, Vlad P, Subramanian S: Congenital aortic stenosis. Experience with 43 patients. *J Thorac Cardiovasc Surg* 72:182, 1976.

10. Cooley DA, Norman JC, Reul GJ, Kidd JN, Nihill MR: Surgical treatment of left ventricular outflow tract obstruction with apicoaortic valved conduit. *Surgery* 80:674, 1976.

11. Cassels GA, Benjamin JD, Lakier JB: Subendocardial ischemia in patients with discrete subvalvar aortic stenosis. *Br Heart J* 40:388, 1978.

12. Cooley DA, Norman JC, Mullins CE, Grace RR: Left ventricle to abdominal aorta conduit for relief of aortic stenosis. *Cardiovasc Dis* 2:376, 1975.

13. Chevers N: Observations on the diseases of the orifice and valves of the aorta. *Guy's Hosp Rep* 387, 1842.

14. Cornell WP, Elkins RC, Criley M, Sabiston DC Jr: Supravalvar aortic stenosis. *J Thorac Cardiovasc Surg* 51:484, 1966.

15. Chung KJ, Fulton DR, Kriedberg MB, Payne DD, Cleveland RJ: Combined discrete subaortic stenosis and ventricular septal defect in infants and children. *Am J Cardiol* 53:1429, 1984.

16. Chietlin MD, Robinowitz M, McAllister H, Hoffman JIE, Bharati S, Lev M: The distribution of fibrosis in the left ventricle in congenital aortic stenosis and coarctation of the aorta. *Circulation* 62:823, 1980.

17. Carrel A: On the experimental surgery of the thoracic aorta and the heart. *Ann Surg* 52:83, 1910.

18. Cain T, Campbell A, Paton B, Clarke D: Operation for discrete subvalvular aortic stenosis. *J Thorac Cardiovasc Surg* 87:366, 1984.

D

1. Doyle EF, Arumugham P, Lara E, Ruthowsky MR, Kiely B: Sudden death in young patients with congenital aortic stenosis. *Pediatrics* 53:481, 1974.

2. de Vivie ER, Hellberg K, Heisig B, Rupprath G, Vogt J, Beuren AJ: Surgical treatment of various types of left ventricular outflow tract stenosis by aortoventriculoplasty—Clinical results. *Thorac Cardiovasc Surg* 29:266, 1981.

3. Doty DB, Polansky DB, Jenson CB: Supravalvular aortic stenosis. Repair by extended aortoplasty. *J Thorac Cardiovasc Surg* 74:362, 1977.

4. De Bakey ME, Beall AC Jr: Successful surgical correction of supravalvular aortic stenosis. *Circulation* 27:858, 1963.

5. Denie JJ, Verheugt AP: Supravalvular aortic stenosis. *Circulation* 18:902, 1958.

6. Dobell ARC, Bloss RS, Gibbons JE, Collins GF: Congenital valvular aortic stenosis. *J Thorac Cardiovasc Surg* 81:916, 1981.

7. Downing BF: Congenital aortic stenosis: Clinical aspects and surgical treatment. *Circulation* 14:188, 1956.

8. Di Donato RM, Danielson GK, McGoon DC, Driscoll DJ, Julsrud PR, Edwards WD: Left ventricle-aortic conduits in pediatric patients. *J Thorac Cardiovasc Surg* 88:82, 1984.

E

1. El-Said G, Galioto FM, Mullins CE, McNamara DG: Natural hemodynamic history of congenital aortic stenosis in childhood. *Am J Cardiol* 30:6, 1972.

2. Ellis FH, Ongley PA, Kirklin JW: Results of surgical treatment for congenital aortic stenosis. *Circulation* 25:29, 1962.

3. Esterly JR, Oppenheimer EH: Some aspects of cardiac pathology in infancy and childhood: Part 4. Myocardial and coronary lesions in cardiac malformations. *Pediatrics* 39:896, 1967.

4. Edwards JE: The congenital bicuspid aortic valve. *Circulation* 23:485, 1961.

5. Edwards JE: Pathology of left ventricular outflow tract obstruction. *Circulation* 31:586, 1965.

6. Ellis FH Jr, Kirklin JW: Congenital valvular aortic stenosis: Anatomic findings and surgical techniques. *J Thorac Cardiovasc Surg* 43:199, 1962.

7. Ergin MA, Cooper R, La Corte M, Golinko R, Griepp RB: Experience with left ventricular apico-aortic conduits for complicated left ventricular outflow obstruction in children and young adults. *Ann Thorac Surg* 32:369, 1981.

F

1. Friedman WF, Modlinger J, Morgan JR: Serial hemodynamic observations in asymptomatic children with valvar aortic stenosis. *Circulation* 43:91, 1971.

2. Fisher RD, Mason DT, Morrow AG: Results of operative treatment in congenital aortic stenosis. Pre- and postoperative hemodynamic evaluations. *J Thorac Cardiovasc Surg* 59:218, 1970.

3. Freedom RM, Dische MR, Rowe RD: Pathologic anatomy of subaortic stenosis and atresia in the first year of life. *Am J Cardiol* 39:1035, 1977.

4. Freed MD, Rosenthal A, Plauth WH Jr, Nadas AS: Development of subaortic stenosis after pulmonary artery banding. *Circulation* 47 & 48(Suppl III):III-7, 1973.

5. Fontana RS, Edwards JE: *Congenital Cardiac Disease: A Review of 357 Cases Studied Pathologically.* Philadelphia: W.B. Saunders, 1962.

6. Farrehi C, Dotter CT, Griswold HE: Supravalvular aortic stenosis. *Am J Dis Child* 108:335, 1964.

7. French JW, Guntheroth WG: An explanation of asymmetric upper extremity blood pressures in supravalvular aortic stenosis. The Coanda effect. *Circulation* 42:31, 1970.

8. Falcone MW, Roberts WC, Morrow AG, Perloff JK: Congenital aortic stenosis resulting from a unicommissural valve. *Circulation* 44:272, 1971.

9. Fulton DR, Hougen TJ, Keane JF, Rosenthal AR, Norwood WI, Bernhard WF: Repeat aortic valvotomy in children. *Am Heart J* 1067:60, 1983.

10. Feigl A, Feigl D, Lucas RV Jr, Edwards JE: Involvement of the aortic valve cusps in discrete subaortic stenosis. *Pediatr Cardiol* 5:185, 1984.

G

1. Glew RH, Varghese PJ, Krovetz LG, Dorst JP, Rowe RD: Sudden death in congenital aortic stenosis. A review of 8 cases with an evaluation of premonitory clinical features. *Am Heart J* 78:615, 1969.

2. Glanz S, Hellenbrand WE, Berman MA, Talner NS: Echocardiographic assessment of the severity of aortic stenosis in children and adolescents. *Am J Cardiol* 38:620, 1976.

3. Gersony WM, Hayes CG: Bacterial endocarditis in patients with pulmonary stenosis, aortic stenosis or ventricular septal defect. *Circulation* 56:(suppl I), I-84, 1977.

4. Gale AW, Cartmill TB, Bernstein L: Familial subaortic membranous stenosis. *Aust NZ J Med* 4:576, 1974.

5. Garcia RE, Friedman WF, Kaback MM, Rowe RD: Idiopathic hypercalcaemia and supravalvular aortic stenosis. Documentation of a new syndrome. *N Engl J Med* 271:117, 1964.

6. Gordon AS: The surgical management of congenital supravalvular, valvular and subvalvular aortic stenosis using deep hypothermia. *J Thorac Cardiovasc Surg* 43:141, 1962.

7. Goldstein RE, Epstein SE: Mechanism of elevated innominate

artery pressure in supravalvular aortic stenosis. *Circulation* 42:23, 1970.

8. Gow RM, Freedom RM, Williams WG, Trusler GA, Rowe RD: Coarctation of the aorta or subaortic stenosis with atrioventricular septal defect. *Am J Cardiol* 53:1421, 1984.

9. Gallotti R, Wain WH, Ross DN: Surgical enucleation of discrete sub-aortic stenosis. *Thorac Cardiovasc Surg* 29:312, 1981.

10. Gomes AS, Nath PH, Singh A, Lucas RV Jr, Amplatz K, Nicoloff DM, Edwards JE: Accessory flaplike tissue causing ventricular outflow obstruction. *J Thorac Cardiovasc Surg* 80:211, 1980.

H

1. Hossack KF, Neutze JM, Lowe JB, Barratt-Boyes BG: Congenital valvar aortic stenosis. Natural history and assessment for operation. *Br Heart J* 43:561, 1980.

2. Hohn AR, Van Praagh S, Moore D, Vlad P, Lambert EC: Aortic stenosis. *Circulation* 32:(suppl III):III-4, 1965.

3. Hastreiter AR, Oshima M, Miller RA, Lev M, Paul MH: Congenital aortic stenosis syndrome in infancy. *Circulation* 28:1084, 1963.

4. Hardesty RL, Griffith BP, Mathews RA, Siewers RD, Neches WH, Park SC, Bahnson HT: Discrete subvalvular aortic stenosis. An evaluation of operative therapy. *J Thorac Cardiovasc Surg* 74:352, 1977.

5. Hastreiter AR, Oshima M, Miller RA, Lev M, Paul MH: Congenital aortic stenosis syndrome in infancy. *Circulation* 28:1084, 1963.

6. Hara M, Dungan T, Lincoln B: Supravalvular aortic stenosis. Report of successful excision and aortic re-anastomosis. *J Thorac Cardiovasc Surg* 43:212, 1962.

7. Hooft C, Vermassen A, Blancquaert A: Observation concerning the evolution of the chronic form of idiopathic hypercalcaemia in children. *Helv Paediatr Acta* 18:138, 1963.

8. Hancock E: Differentiation of valvular, subvalvular and supravalvular aortic stenosis. *Guy's Hosp Rep* 110:1, 1961.

9. Hatle L, Angelsen BA, Tromsdol A: Noninvasive assessment of aortic stenosis by Doppler ultrasound. *Br Heart J* 43:284, 1980.

10. Harlan JL, Clark EB, Doty DB: Congenital aortic stenosis with hypoplasia of the left sinus of Valsalva. Anatomic reconstruction of the aortic root. *J Thorac Cardiovasc Surg* 89:288, 1985.

J

1. Jones RC, Walker WJ, Jahnke EJ, Winn DF: Congenital aortic stenosis: correlation of clinical severity with haemodynamic and surgical findings in 43 cases. *Ann Intern Med* 58:486, 1963.

2. Jack WD, Kelly DT: Long term follow-up of valvulotomy for congenital aortic stenosis. *Am J Cardiol* 38:231, 1976.

3. Jones KL, Smith DW: The Williams elfin facies syndrome. A new perspective. *J Pediatr* 86:718, 1975.

4. Jeger E: *Die Chirurgie der Blutgafassen und des Herzens.* Berlin: August Hirchwald, 1913.

5. Jonas RA, Lang P, Mayer JE, Castaneda AR: The importance of prostaglandin E$_1$ in resuscitation of the neonate with critical aortic stenosis. *J Thorac Cardiovasc Surg* 89:314, 1985.

K

1. Krovetz LG, Kurlinski JP: Subendocardial blood flow in children with congenital aortic stenosis. *Circulation* 54:961, 1976.

2. Kelly DT, Wulfsberg BA, Rowe RD: Discrete subaortic stenosis. *Circulation* 46:309, 1972.

3. Kirklin JW, Ellis FH Jr: Surgical relief of diffuse subvalvular aortic stenosis. *Circulation* 24:739, 1961.

4. Keith JD, Rowe RD, Vlad P: *Heart Disease in Infancy and Childhood* (ed 2). New York: Macmillan 1967, p 250.

5. Katz NM, Buckley MJ, Liberthson RR: Discrete membranous subaortic stenosis. Report of 31 patients, review of the literature, and delineation of management. *Circulation* 56:1034, 1977.

6. Keane JF, Fellows KE, La Farge G, Nadas AS, Bernhard WF: The surgical management of discrete and diffuse supravalvar aortic stenosis. *Circulation* 54:112, 1976.

7. Keane JF, Bernhard WF, Nadas AS: Aortic stenosis in infancy. *Circulation* 52:1138, 1975.

8. Konno S, Imai Y, Iida Y, Nakajima M, Tatsuno K: A new method for prosthetic valve replacement in congenital aortic stenosis associated with hypoplasia of the aortic valve ring. *J Thorac Cardiovasc Surg* 70:909, 1975.

9. Kugelmeier J, Egloff L, Real F, Rothlin M, Tarina M, Senning A: Congenital aortic stenosis. Early and late results of aortic valvotomy. *Thorac Cardiovasc Surg* 30:91, 1982.

10. Kuribayashi R, Imai T, Yagi Y, Gomi H: Subaortic stenosis caused by an accessory tissue of the mitral valve. *J Cardiovasc Surg (Torino)* 20:591, 1979.

L

1. Leech G, Mills P, Leatham A: The diagnosis of a non-stenotic bicuspid aortic valve. *Br Heart J* 40:941, 1978.

2. Lakier JB, Lewis AB, Heymann MA, Stanger P, Hoffman JIE, Rudolph AM: Isolated aortic stenosis in the neonate. Natural history and hemodynamic considerations. *Circulation* 50:801, 1974.

3. Lees MH, Hauck AJ, Starkey GWB, Nadas AS, Gross RE: Congenital aortic stenosis: Operative indications and surgical results. *Br Heart J* 24:31, 1961.

4. Lewis AB, Heymann MA, Stanger P, Hoffman JIE, Rudolph AM: Evaluation of subendocardial ischemia in valvar aortic stenosis in children. *Circulation* 49:978, 1974.

5. Lawson RM, Bonchek LI, Menashe V, Starr A: Late results of surgery for left ventricular outflow tract obstruction in children. *J Thorac Cardiovasc Surg* 71:334, 1976.

6. Lillehei CW, Bonnabeau RC Jr, Sellers RD: Subaortic stenosis. Diagnostic criteria, surgical approach and late follow-up in 25 patients. *J Thorac Cardiovasc Surg* 55:94, 1968.

7. Lauer RM, Du Shane JW, Edwards JE: Obstruction of left ventricular outlet in association with ventricular septal defect. *Circulation* 22:110, 1960.

8. Logan WF, Wyn Jones E, Walker E, Coulshed N, Epstein EJ: Familial supravalvar aortic stenosis. *Br Heart J* 27:547, 1965.

9. Lewis FJ, Shumway NE, Niazi SA: Aortic valvulotomy under direct vision during hypothermia. *J Thorac Cardiovasc Surg* 32:481, 1956.

M

1. Marquis RM, Logan R: Congenital aortic stenosis and its surgical treatment. *Br Heart J* 17:373, 1955.

2. Mills P, Leech G, Davies M, Leatham A: The natural history of a non-stenotic bicuspid aortic valve. *Br Heart J* 40:951, 1978.

3. Morrow AG, Goldblatt A, Braunwald E: Congenital aortic stenosis 11. Surgical treatment and the results of operation. *Circulation* 27:450, 1963.

4. Moller JH, Nakib A, Edwards JE: Infarction of papillary muscles and mitral insufficiency associated with congenital aortic stenosis. *Circulation* 34:87, 1966.

5. Maron BJ, Redwood DR, Roberts WL, Henry WL, Morrow AG, Epstein SE: Tunnel subaortic stenosis. Left ventricular outflow tract obstruction produced by fibromuscular tubular narrowing. *Circulation* 54:404, 1976.

6. McGoon DC, Geha AS, Scofield EL, Du Shane JW: Surgical treatment of congenital aortic stenosis. *Dis Chest* 55:388, 1969.

7. Morrow AG, Goldblatt A, Braunwald E: Congenital aortic stenosis 11. Surgical treatment and the results of operation. *Circulation* 27:426, 1963.

8. Manouguian S, Kirckhoff PG, Koncz J, Corovic D, Dahn D: Ventricular septal defect associated with fibrous subvalvar aortic stenosis: Diagnostic problems and surgical management. *Thoraxchirurgie* 23:444, 1975.

9. Mody MR, Mody GT: Serial hemodynamic observations in congenital valvular and subvalvular aortic stenosis. *Am Heart J* 89:137, 1975.

10. Morrow AG, Fort L III, Roberts WL, Braunwald E: Discrete subaortic stenosis complicated by aortic valvular regurgitation. Clinical, hemodynamic and pathologic studies and the results of operative treatment. *Circulation* 31:163, 1965.

11. Muna WFT, Ferrans VJ, Pierce JE, Roberts WL: Discrete subaortic stenosis in Newfoundland dogs: Association of infective endocarditis. *Am J Cardiol* 41:746, 1978.

12. Morrow AG, Waldhausen JA, Peters RL, Bloodwell RD, Braunwald E: Supravalvular aortic stenosis. Clinical, hemodynamic and pathologic observations. *Circulation* 20:1003, 1959.

13. Martin EC, Moseley IF: Supravalvar aortic stenosis. *Br Heart J* 35:758, 1973.

14. McGoon DC, Mankin HT, Vlad P, Kirklin JW: The surgical treatment of supravalvular aortic stenosis. *J Thorac Cardiovasc Surg* 41:125, 1961.

15. Merin G, Copperman IJ, Borman JB: Surgical correction of diffuse supravalvar aortic stenosis involving the branches of the aortic arch. *Chest* 70:546, 1976.

16. Mencarelli L: Stenosis sopravalvolare aortica e anello. *Arch Ital Anat Istol Pat* 1:829, 1930.

17. McDonald AH, Gerlis LM, Somerville J: Familial arteriopathy with associated pulmonary and systemic arterial stenoses. *Br Heart J* 31:375, 1969.

18. Moller JH, Nakib A, Eliot RS, Edwards JE: Symptomatic congenital aortic stenosis in the first year of life. *J Pediatr* 69:728, 1966.

19. Misbach GA, Turley K, Ullyot DJ, Ebert PA: Left ventricular outflow enlargement by the Konno procedure. *J Thorac Cardiovasc Surg* 84:696, 1982.

20. Matthewson JW, Riemenschneider TA, McGough EC, Concon VR: Left ventricular outflow tract obstruction produced by redundant mitral valve tissue in a neonate. Clinical, angiographic, and operative findings. *Circulation* 53:198, 1976.

21. Marquis RM, Logan A: Congenital aortic stenosis and its surgical treatment. *Br Heart J* 17:373, 1955.

22. Messina LM, Turley K, Stanger P, Hoffman JIE, Ebert PA: Successful aortic valvotomy for severe congenital valvular aortic stenosis in the newborn infant. *J Thorac Cardiovasc Surg* 88:92, 1984.

23. Mavroudis C, Rees A, Solinger R, Elbl F: The prognostic value of intraoperative pressure gradients with congenital aortic stenosis. *Ann Thorac Surg* 38:237, 1984.

24. Messina L, Turley K, Stanger P, Hoffman JIE, Ebert A: Reply

to Jonas' et al Letter to the Editor. *J Thorac Cardiovasc Surg* 89:315, 1985.

25. Moses RD, Barnhart GR, Jones M: The late prognosis after localized resection for fixed (discrete and tunnel) left ventricular outflow tract obstruction. *J Thorac Cardiovasc Surg* 87:410, 1984.

N

1. Newfeld EA, Muster AJ, Paul MH, Idriss PS, Riker WL: Discrete subvalvular aortic stenosis in childhood. Study of 51 patients. *Am J Cardiol* 38:53, 1976.
2. Neufeld HN, Ongley PA, Edwards JE: Combined congenital subaortic stenosis and infundibular pulmonary stenosis. *Br Heart J* 22:686, 1960.
3. Norman JC, Cooley DA, Hallaran GL, Nihill MR: Left ventricular apical-abdominal aortic conduits for left ventricular outflow tract obstructions. *Circulation* 56(suppl II):II-62, 1977.
4. Neufeld HN, Wagenvoort CA, Ongley PA, Edwards JE: Hypoplasia of ascending aorta. An unusual form of supravalvular aortic stenosis with special reference to localized coronary arterial hypertension. *Am J Cardiol* 10:746, 1962.
5. Norwood WI, Lang P, Castaneda AR, Murphy JD: Management of infants with left ventricular outflow obstruction by conduit interposition between the ventricular apex and thoracic aorta. *J Thorac Cardiovasc Surg* 86:771, 1983.

O

1. Ongley PA, Nadas AS, Paul MY, Rudolph AM, Starkey GWB: Aortic stenosis in infants and children. *Pediatrics* 21:207, 1958.

P

1. Peckham GB, Keith JD, Evans JR: Congenital aortic stenosis: Some observations on the natural history and clinical assessment. *Can Med Assoc J* 91:639, 1964.
2. Pyle RL, Patterson DF, Chacko S: Genetics and pathology of discrete subaortic stenosis in the Newfoundland dog. *Am Heart J* 92:324, 1976.
3. Peterson TA, Todd DB, Edwards JE: Supravalvular aortic stenosis. *J Thorac Cardiovasc Surg* 50:734, 1965.
4. Pasengrau DG, Kioshos JM, Durnin RE, Kroetz FW: Supravalvular aortic stenosis in adults. *Am J Cardiol* 31:635, 1973.
5. Presbitero P, Somerville J, Revel-Chion R, Ross D: Open aortic valvotomy for congenital aortic stenosis. Late results. *Br Heart J* 47:26, 1982.

R

1. Roberts WC: The structure of the aortic valve in clinically isolated aortic stenosis. An autopsy study of 162 patients over 15 years of age. *Circulation* 42:91, 1970.
2. Roberts WC: The congenitally bicuspid aortic valve. A study of 85 autopsy cases. *Am J Cardiol* 26:72, 1970.
3. Reis RL, Peterson LM, Mason DT, Simon AL, Morrow AG: Congenital fixed subvalvar aortic stenosis. An anatomical classification and correlations with operative results. *Circulation* 43:(suppl I)I-11, 1971.
4. Rosenquist GC, Clark EB, McAllister HA, Bharati S, Edwards JE: Increased mitral-aortic separation in discrete subaortic stenosis. *Circulation* 60:70, 1979.
5. Rastelli GC, McGoon DC, Ongley PA, Mankin HT, Kirklin JW: Surgical treatment of supravalvular aortic stenosis. Report of 16

cases and review of literature. *J Thorac Cardiovasc Surg* 51:873, 1966.

6. Rastan H, Abu-Aishah N, Rastan D, Heisig B, Koncz J, Bjoornstad PG, Beuren AJ: Results of aortoventriculoplasty in 21 consecutive patients with left ventricular outflow tract obstruction. *J Thorac Cardiovasc Surg* 75:659, 1978.
7. Rastan H, Koncz J: Plastische Erweiterung der linken Ausflubahn. Eine neue Operationsmethode. *Thoraxchirurgie* 23:169, 1975.
8. Rastan H, Koncz J: Aortoventriculoplasty. A new technique for the treatment of left ventricular outflow tract obstruction. *J Thorac Cardiovasc Surg* 71:920, 1976.
9. Reid JM, Coleman EN: The management of congenital aortic stenosis. *Thorax* 37:902, 1982.

S

1. Spencer FC, Neill CA, Bahnson HT: The treatment of congenital aortic stenosis with valvotomy during cardiopulmonary bypass. *Surgery* 44:109, 1958.
2. Shackleton J, Edwards FR, Bickford BJ, Jones RS: Long term follow-up of congenital aortic stenosis after surgery. *Br Heart J* 34:47, 1972.
3. Shariatzadeh AN, King H, Girod D, Schumacker HB Jr: Discrete subaortic stenosis. A report of 20 cases. *J Thorac Cardiovasc Surg* 63:258, 1972.
4. Shone JD, Sellers RD, Anderson RL, Adams P, Lillehei CW, Edwards JE: The developmental complex of parachute mitral valve, supravalvular ring of left atrium, subaortic stenosis and coarctation of aorta. *Am J Cardiol* 11:714, 1963.
5. Spencer FC, Neill CA, Sank L, Bahnson HT: Anatomical variations in 46 patients with congenital aortic stenosis. *Am Surg* 26:204, 1960.
6. Sung C, Price EC, Cooley DA: Discrete subaortic stenosis in adults. *Am J Cardiol* 42:283, 1978.
7. Starr A, Dotter C, Griswold H: Supravalvular aortic stenosis: Diagnosis and treatment. *J Thorac Cardiovasc Surg* 41:134, 1961.
8. Schumacker HB Jr, Mandelbaum I: Surgical considerations in the management of supravalvular aortic stenosis. *Circulation* 31 & 32 (suppl I)I-36, 1965.
9. Strong WB, Perrin E, Liebman J, Silbert DR: Systemic and pulmonary artery dysplasia associated with unexpected death in infancy. *J Pediatr* 77:233, 1970.
10. Sissman NJ, Neill CA, Spencer FC, Taussig HB: Congenital aortic stenosis. *Circulation* 19:458, 1959.
11. Schmidt RE, Gilbert EF, Amend TC, Chamberlain CR, Lucas RV Jr: Generalized arterial fibromuscular dysplasia and myocardial infarction in familial supravalvular aortic stenosis syndrome. *J Pediatr* 74:576, 1969.
12. Stamm RB, Martin RP: Quantification of pressure gradients across stenotic valves by Doppler ultrasound. *JACC* 2:707, 1983.
13. Somerville J, Stone S, Ross D: Fate of patients with fixed subaortic stenosis after surgical removal. *Br Heart J* 43:629, 1980.
14. Salomon NW, Stinson EB, Oyer P, Copeland JG, Shumway NE: Operative treatment of congenital aortic stenosis. *Ann Thorac Surg* 26:452, 1978.
15. Sandor GGS, Olley PM, Trusler GA, Williams WG, Rowe RD, Morch JE: Long-term follow-up of patients after valvotomy for congenital valvular aortic stenosis in children. *J Thorac Cardiovasc Surg* 80:171, 1980.

16. Swan H, Blount SG, Wilkinson RH: Visual repair of congenital aortic stenosis during hypothermia. *J Thorac Cardiovasc Surg* 35:139, 1958.

17. Sink JD, Smallhorn JF, Macartney FJ, Taylor JFN, Stark J, de Leval MR: Management of critical aortic stenosis in infancy. *J Thorac Cardiovasc Surg* 87:82, 1984.

18. Stewart JR, Paton BC, Blount Jr SG, Swan H: Congenital aortic stenosis. Ten to 22 years after valvulotomy. *Arch Surg* 113:1248, 1978.

19. Swan H, Kortz A: Direct vision trans-aortic approach to the aortic valve during hypothermia: Experimental observations and report of a successful clinical case. *Ann Surg* 144:205, 1956.

T

1. Thomson NB, Fisher FC: Long term postoperative follow-up in surgery for congenital valvular stenosis. *Circulation* 32:732, 1965.

2. Trinkle JK, Grover FL, Arom KV: Closed aortic valvotomy in infants. Late results. *J Thorac Cardiovasc Surg* 76:198, 1978.

3. Trinkle JK, Norton JB, Richardson JD, Grover FL, Noonan JA: Closed aortic valvotomy and simultaneous correction of associated anomalies in infants. *J Thorac Cardiovasc Surg* 69:758, 1975.

V

1. Van Praagh R, Bernhard WF, Rosenthal A, Parisi LF, Fyler DC: Interrupted aortic arch: Surgical treatment. *Am J Cardiol* 27:200, 1971.

2. Vouhe PR, Poulain H, Bloch G, Loisance DY, Gamain J, Lombaert M, Quiret J, Lesbre J, Bernasconi P, Pietri J, Cachera J: Aortoseptal approach for optimal resection of diffuse subvalvular aortic stenosis. *J Thorac Cardiovasc Surg* 87:887, 1984.

W

1. Wagner HR, Ellison RC, Keane JF, Humphries JO, Nadas AS: Clinical course in aortic stenosis. *Circulation* 56(suppl I):I-47, 1977.

2. Weyman AE, Fergenbaum H, Hurwitz RA, Girod DA, Dillon JC: Cross-sectional echocardiographic assessment of the severity of aortic stenosis in children. *Circulation* 55:773, 1977.

3. Weyman AE, Feigenbaum H, Hurwitz RA, Girod DA, Dillon JC, Chang S: Cross sectional echocardiography in evaluating patients with discrete subaortic stenosis. *Am J Cardiol* 37:358, 1976.

4. Williams JCP, Barratt-Boyes BG, Lowe JB: Supravalvar aortic stenosis. *Circulation* 24:1311, 1961.

5. Weisz D, Hartmann AF Jr, Weldon CS: Results of surgery for congenital supravalvular aortic stenosis. *Am J Cardiol* 37:73, 1976.

6. Watson GH: Supravalvular pulmonary and aortic stenosis coexisting. *Br Heart J* 25:817, 1963.

7. Whitmer JT, James FW, Kaplan S, Schwartz DC, Knight MJ: Exercise testing in children before and after surgical treatment of aortic stenosis. *Circulation* 63:254, 1981.

8. Wright GB, Keane JF, Nadas AS, Bernhard WF, Castaneda AR: Fixed subaortic stenosis in the young: medical and surgical course in 83 patients. *Am J Cardiol* 52:830, 1983.

9. Williams WG, Trusler GA: (1983) Personal communication.

10. Walls JT, Lababidi Z, Curtis JJ, Silver D: Assessment of percutaneous balloon pulmonary and aortic valvuloplasty. *J Thorac Cardiovasc Surg* 88:352, 1984.

33

HYPERTROPHIC OBSTRUCTIVE CARDIOMYOPATHY

DEFINITION

Hypertrophic cardiomyopathy (HCM) is a primary hypertrophy of cardiac muscle associated with a small left ventricular cavity, increased systolic function, and impaired diastolic function. It is of unknown etiology but has a genetic basis. The obstructive forms, so-called hypertrophic obstructive cardiomyopathy or idiopathic hypertrophic subaortic stenosis, are of surgical significance and are characterized by massive ventricular hypertrophy and myocardial fiber disarray that are concentrated in the ventricular septum and a variable, dynamic obstruction that is usually subaortic and is then associated with abnormal systolic anterior motion of the anterior mitral leaflet. The more common nonobstructed forms are not considered for operation.

HISTORICAL NOTE

Pathologic findings compatible with hypertrophic obstructive cardiomyopathy (HOCM) were described by two nineteenth-century French pathologists[H7,L2] and an early twentieth-century German pathologist, Schmincke.[S11] Davies, in 1952, described a family from Cardiff with five of nine siblings affected and three dying suddenly[D1] who probably suffered from this disease. Although each of these reports and the surgical report of Brock in 1957[B5] describe a diffuse form of muscular subaortic stenosis, the disease was first accurately categorized by Teare, a London pathologist, in 1958.[T3] Teare described both the disproportionate thickening of the ventricular septum in comparison with the free wall and the presence of myocardial fiber disarray in a group of young people who died suddenly. These pathologic findings were rapidly confirmed,[B6,M11] and the clinical features were further elucidated by Braunwald[B7,B8,B10] and others.[G5,M10,V1,W3] To distinguish it from other cardiomyopathies, the term *hypertrophic obstructive cardiomyopathy* was applied by Goodwin, Hollman, Cleland, and Teare,[G4,G5] whereas Braunwald and associates called it *idiopathic hypertrophic subaortic stenosis* (IHSS),[B8] and Wigle and associates called it *muscular subaortic stenosis.*[W3] At this time, left ventricular outflow tract obstruction was thought to be distinctive for the disease. That the anterior mitral leaflet contributed to the obstruction was first documented in 1964 in Stockholm,[F3] and its abnormal systolic anterior motion (SAM) was subsequently demonstrated angiocardiographically.[A4,D5,S13] By the mid-1960s, HOCM was a well-defined clinical entity,[B7] and it was realized that some patients had a form of the disease in which there was no, or minimal, obstruction.[B4,M17] Particular attention was paid to this group by Goodwin and Oakley,[G4,G6] who emphasized the importance of reduced left ventricular compliance as the major determinant of cardiac dysfunction ("inflow" obstruction) rather than outflow obstruction. The knowledge that the nonobstructive group was by far the more common had to await the introduction of echocardiography, since with this noninvasive technique it was possible to detect asymmetric septal hypertrophy (ASH),[A2,H6] one of the hallmarks of the disease, as well as the presence or absence of SAM of the anterior mitral leaflet.[P2,S10] In the early 1970s, ASH and SAM were thought to be specific for the disease,[H6] but this is now known to be incorrect. Echocardiography not only established that the disease is relatively common but also that it is usually genetically transmitted rather than sporadic.[C5]

Surgical awareness of the obstructive form of the disease began with Brock's reports in 1957 and 1959.[B5,B9] However, in Brock's patients and in our first patient operated on at the Mayo Clinic in February 1958,[K3] nothing was done surgically since the nature of the disease was not understood. Credit for the first myotomy, consisting of a simple incision of the prominent anterior muscular ridge in the septum, probably belongs to Cleland.[G5] Myotomy was used by a number of others at about this same time,[K2,M9,M12,W3] although beginning with our very earliest Mayo Clinic cases we used myectomy.[K2,K3] A left ventriculotomy was devised to allow adequate excision of muscle under direct vision,[K3] and this approach has been subsequently favored (GLH).[A3,B2,K2] Over the next few years, the surgical approach to septectomy (myectomy) was modified by others in a number of ways. Dobell and Scott[D3] used a left atrial approach, exposing the hypertrophied septum by dividing the anterior mitral leaflet across its center, whereas Lillehei used a similar approach but with detachment of the base of the mitral leaflet near the ring.[L3] Swan[S8] described the use of a corkscrew to excise septal muscle from a limited left ventricular approach, and Julian et al.[J1] used a fishmouth left ventricular incision

that detached the lower part of the free wall from the septum and gave an excellent exposure of the subaortic septal bulge that was then excised. Cooley[C4] developed an approach through the right ventricle used first by Harken[H5] in which septal muscle was shaved off the right ventricular side, judging septal thickness by means of a finger inserted into the left ventricle through the aortic valve. None of these techniques is in use currently. Simple myotomy via an aortic approach was persisted with for a considerable time by the Toronto group[B3,T2] but more recently modified to include excision of muscle (myectomy) as advocated by Morrow.[M1,M5] More recently, two further procedures have been suggested, namely, mitral valve replacement by Cooley[C1,C2] and the use of a left ventricular–aortic (LV-Ao) valved conduit to bypass the obstruction.[D4]

MORPHOLOGY

The idiopathic muscular hypertrophy present in hypertrophic obstructive cardiomyopathy (HOCM) involves the left ventricle and is variable in site and severity.

Ventricular Septum

In the classical obstructive form of the disease, the hypertrophy is maximal in the cephalad portion of the ventricular septum. A longitudinal section of the septum shows that it bulges into both left and right ventricles and that the point of maximal thickening lies just apical (caudad) to the free edge of the anterior mitral leaflet in its open position. This diffuse muscular prominence or mound tapers off gradually toward the aortic anulus and toward the apex. At the point opposite the free edge of the anterior mitral leaflet, the left ventricular endocardium is thickened by a localized plaque of fibrous tissue that lies at right angles to the long axis of the outflow tract. Since this plaque is usually present in nonobstructive as well as obstructive forms of the disease, it is presumably related to contact between the anterior mitral leaflet and the septal bulge in diastole rather than systole, the leaflet snapping open rapidly at the onset of diastole (in part because of high left atrial pressure) and hitting the ventricular septal prominence.[E1]

Hypertrophy of the ventricular septum is not always maximal in its anterior basal parts. Occasionally, it may be maximal at a site below the anterior mitral leaflet adjacent to the papillary muscles, producing a so-called midcavity obstruction[F4] in which papillary muscle and free-wall hypertrophy contribute and there is no systolic anterior motion (SAM), or it may be confined to the posterior or apical septum.[S16] Occasionally, the entire septum may be of equal thickness.[M22,S15]

Dynamic Morphology of the Septum and Mitral Valve

When the septal hypertrophy is of this usual classic type, the obstruction is sited low in the left ventricular outflow tract between the hypertrophied ventricular septum and the free edge of the anterior mitral leaflet. In systole, the posterior mitral leaflet closes against the body of the anterior leaflet at about the junction of its mid- and free-edge third (rather than at its free edge as in the normal heart), and the free-edge portion of the anterior mitral leaflet beyond the point of coaptation hinges (angulates) on the remainder of the leaflet in a cephalad direction toward the aortic anulus. This brings the free edge of the anterior mitral leaflet close to the ventricular septal bulge. This so-called SAM of the anterior leaflet is a constant feature of classic HOCM, and the degree of movement correlates with the severity of the obstruction,[H8] as does the diameter of the left ventricular outflow tract at this point.[S13] Ventricular ejection is rapid and early, mostly occurring within the first half of ventricular systole.

The mechanism of SAM is disputed. Most probably it is secondary to forward (anterior) displacement of the mitral valve relative to the septum,[S13] so that in association with the marked septal hypertrophy opposite the mitral leaflet and rapid and early ventricular ejection and Venturi effect of the high velocity stream carries the protruding edge of the anterior mitral leaflet toward the aortic anulus in early systole. As a secondary event, the higher pressure below the anterior leaflet then forces it further into the outflow tract.[H2] There are other less convincing explanations of the mechanism of SAM.[P1,R2] It is absent in nonobstructive forms of HOCM and when the obstruction is sited at a lower level. It can occur also in transposition of the great arteries with intact ventricular septum (see Chapter 39) and rarely in other disease states.[M20,M21]

Left Ventricular Free Wall

In the obstructive forms of the disease, free-wall hypertrophy is more marked than in nonobstructive forms[H4] and is fairly uniform, particularly in the anterolateral and apical portions. There is, however, less thickening of the posterior free wall in almost all varieties of HOCM.[M28] Thus, the ratio between the thick upper anterior part of the ventricular septum and the thinner posterior wall beneath the posterior mitral leaflet (that portion through which the beam passes in M-mode echocardiography) is 1.3 or more in almost all cases of HOCM whether or not there is obstruction. This so-called asymmetric septal hypertrophy (ASH) may be absent when the septal hypertrophy is unusually located, and it may occasionally be present in diseases other than HOCM so that it is not pathognomonic of the disease.[C3,M13,M20,M22] In fact, it has been demonstrated in numerous varieties of congenital heart disease, particularly in neonates and infants.[L1,M15,M16,S4] Also, it has been demonstrated in association with lesions that produce long-standing right ventricular hypertension,[M20] in discrete subvalvar and valvar aortic stenosis, and even occasionally in normal hearts.[L1] Larter and colleagues have pointed out that when ASH is present in early life in association with congenital heart disease, it tends to lessen or disappear with growth.[L1] ASH (and SAM) has recently been described in infants of diabetic mothers. This is a transient nonfamilial condition and not a true hypertrophic cardiomyopathy.[G9]

Unusual combinations and sites of septal and free-wall thickening in HOCM result in a variable pattern. Not only can there be midcavity obstruction,[F4] but more often in these varieties, obstruction is absent and hypertrophy is symmetric rather than asymmetric or involves a portion of septum or free wall in the sinus portion of the ventricle rather than the outflow region.[M22,M23,S15] Extreme hypertrophy of the apical portion of the septum and free wall can result in obliteration of the apical portion of the left ventricular cavity without either SAM or ASH being present.[S16,Y1]

Left Ventricular Cavity

In association with the unusual shape of the ventricular septum, the left ventricular cavity is small, even when heart failure occurs in the later stages of the disease, and has an S or sigmoid shape in systole when viewed in its longitudinal axis (Fig. 33-1). When ventricular hypertrophy is located in the midportion of the ventricle, a dumbbell-shaped cavity results[F4]; when it is confined to the apex, there may be complete obliteration of the lower half of the cavity and a spade-shaped basal portion.[S16,Y1]

Very rarely, the left ventricle may become dilated in the late stages of the disease. This can be the result of transmural myocardial infarction[W5] or of severe long-standing congestive heart failure.[G8]

Histopathology of the Left Ventricle

The microscopic findings in the hypertrophied ventricular septum are distinctive.[H9] In addition to focal areas of increased fibrosis and to an increase in muscle cell diameter,[H8] there are numerous foci of muscle cell disarray interspersed among areas of hypertrophied but normally arranged parallel cells.[F1,T3] In the areas of disarray, the muscle cells are wider and shorter than in the case of hypertrophy from other causes, and there is increased cellular branching, extensive side-to-side intercellular junctions, widened Z bands, and evidence of formation of new sarcomeres. There are also less specific abnormalities in the orientation of the myofibrils.[F1] In obstructive forms, the disarray is confined to the ventricular septum, whereas in nonobstructive forms, it may occur also in the left ventricular free wall.[M3,W1] It is present also, but to a much less-marked degree, in many other conditions.[B1] Using a quantitative histologic method to determine the extent of myocardial fiber disarray, Maron and Roberts found that the average degree of ventricular septum involved in HOCM was 30% compared with 1.5% in control hearts (those with congenital or acquired cardiac disease or normal hearts) and that when more than 5% of the relevant areas of the tissue section were involved it was both highly sensitive (90%) and specific (93%) for HOCM.[M18,M20] In contrast, Bulkley and colleagues considered that myocardial fiber disarray found in HOCM was qualitatively and quantitatively similar in the left ventricle of hearts with aortic atresia and a patent mitral valve and in the right ventricle of hearts with pulmonary atresia and intact ventricular septum.[B13] Thus, it is unlikely that fiber disarray is a morphologic manifestation of a genetically transmitted myocardial defect present in HOCM[H3,M3]; rather, it is likely to be the result of the incoordinate type of muscular contraction present in these various conditions.[B13,H1]

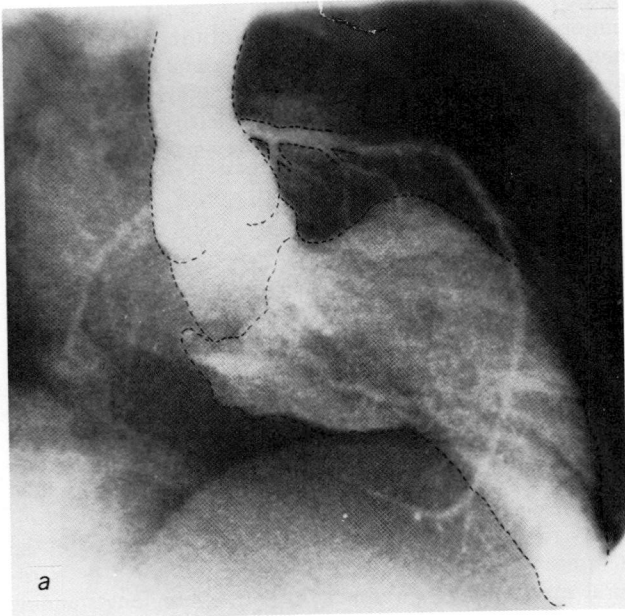

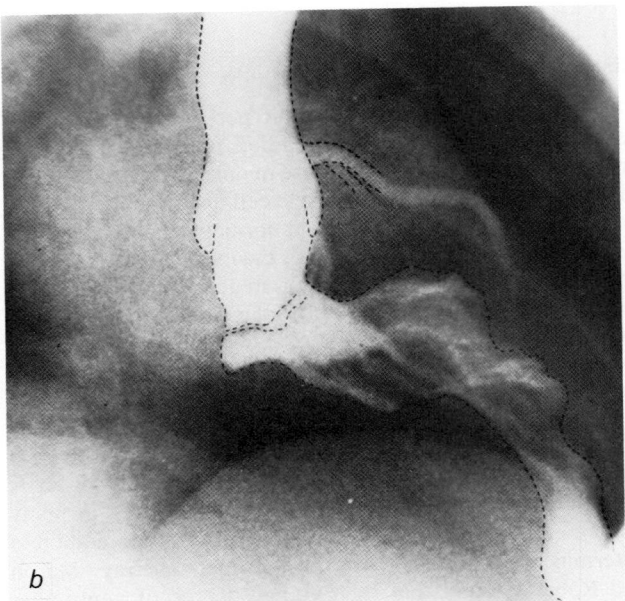

Figure 33-1 Left ventricular cineangiogram in right anterior oblique projection in a patient with HOCM (GLH).
(a) Diastole.
(b) Systole.
Note the characteristic deformity of the left ventricular (LV) cavity shape with septal muscle encroaching upon the anterior margin of the outflow tract and the grossly hypertrophied papillary muscles contributing to virtual obliteration of the mid-LV cavity in systole. The interrupted line crossing low LV outflow in (a) represents the free wall portion of the mitral ring delineated by contrast medium trapped behind the opened posterior leaflet. The interrupted lines in (b) indicate a radiolucent filling defect caused by contact between mitral leaflet and septum in systole, a feature infrequently observed in this projection.

Left Atrium

The left atrium is often dilated and thick walled, secondary to the decreased compliance of the left ventricle. These changes may be contributed to by mitral incompetence.

Mitral Valve

As already noted, in obstructive forms of the disease the mitral valve is positioned closer to the ventricular septum than in the normal heart.[M7] The anterior leaflet is diffusely thickened, particularly at its leading edge, presumably secondary to SAM. A further consequence of SAM is the production of mitral incompetence in mid- or late systole as the anterior leaflet moves forward[S14] (Fig. 33-2). The studies by Wigle and colleagues suggest that its severity correlates with the left ventricular outflow gradient (and therefore with the degree of SAM).[W2] However, 18 of 42 (43%, CL 34%–52%) patients with important obstruction had no mitral incompetence preoperatively and it was moderate or severe in 24% (CL 17%–32%; GLH).[A3] Occasionally, mitral regurgitation in HOCM can be due to chordal rupture,[A3] congenital abnormalities,[W2] or rheumatic disease. Calcification of the mitral anulus is not uncommon in older patients with HOCM.[K1,T4]

Right Ventricle

The right ventricular chamber is distorted by the hypertrophied ventricular septum that projects into the right ven-

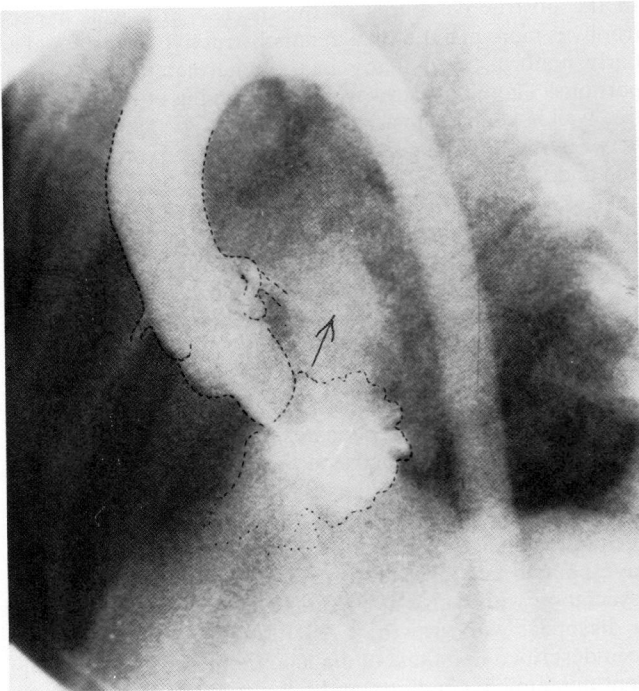

Figure 33-2 Left ventricular (LV) cineangiocardiogram in lateral projection in a patient with HOCM and mild mitral regurgitation (GLH). Maximal LV outflow tract obstruction toward the end of systolic ejection is illustrated. The arrow indicates the site of the regurgitant jet emerging beneath the anterior mitral leaflet during abnormal systolic anterior motion.

tricular outflow tract and may cause a significant gradient and, in long-standing cases, hypertrophy of the free wall secondary to this. Right ventricular hypertrophy may also occur secondary to pulmonary hypertension from long-standing left heart failure and elevated left atrial pressure.

Coronary Arteries

The coronary arteries are larger in diameter than normal. Significant coronary atherosclerosis is present in about 5% of cases.[G3,M14,T1] Spray and colleagues have noted the presence of wall thickening and luminal narrowing of intramural branches located primarily in the ventricular septum and also occasionally in the left and right ventricular free walls in about half the patients with HOCM.[S3] These lesions are not seen in other forms of aortic stenosis. Muscular bridging of the left anterior descending coronary artery during part of its course is more common in HOCM than in normal hearts. The artery may become totally occluded during systole at these points[K4] or may show an irregular sawtooth appearance.[B16] Septal perforating arteries and other epicardial vessels may also be obliterated or severely narrowed during systole. The hemodynamic effect of these changes is not known, although Maron and colleagues have reported that transmural myocardial infarction does occur in HOCM in the absence of atheromatous coronary artery disease.[M24,W5]

Associated Lesions

There is a specific association between HOCM and diffuse lentiginosis.[S9] There is no evidence that this condition is inherited.[S17] The association with essential hypertension noted in Brock's original report[B5] is probably coincidental, although Wei and colleagues[W4] suggest that a hypertrophic cardiomyopathy with features indistinguishable from HOCM can occur in a number of other disease states, including severe long-standing hypertension and severe aortic valvar stenosis. Similarly, there may be a coincidental association with any other congenital or acquired cardiac disease such as atrial septal defect and rheumatic heart disease.

CLINICAL FEATURES AND DIAGNOSTIC CRITERIA

In obstructive forms of the disease, usually the symptoms and signs are such as to make a confident diagnosis on clinical grounds possible. This is in contrast to nonobstructive types, in mild forms of which there may be no symptoms or clinical signs. In severe forms, when there is no murmur, it may be impossible to distinguish this clinically from other causes of congestive heart failure.[G7,G8]

Symptoms

Presentation can occur at any age from infancy to beyond 70 years. The symptoms are those of aortic stenosis, namely, effort dyspnea, effort syncope or dizziness, and effort angina, singly or in combination. Palpitation may occur and is most often due to atrial fibrillation that may initially be paroxysmal but is permanent in about 10% of patients in the later stages of the disease. The onset of atrial fibrillation is usually heralded by a sudden increase in dyspnea and sometimes by heart failure[G1] and hypotension due in part to the rapid rate and in part to loss of the atrial component of ventricular filling that is important to the noncompliant ventricle present in this disease. Arrhythmia may also be due to ventricular premature beats or bouts of ventricular tachycardia and is then an important cause of sudden death.[M25,S18]

Almost half the patients with atrial fibrillation give a history of systemic embolism.

The later stages of the disease are associated with severe and progressive congestive heart failure with paroxysmal nocturnal dyspnea, orthopnea, and pulmonary edema. Rarely, there is ascites and peripheral edema secondary to tricuspid incompetence.

Signs

The physical signs in classic cases with obstruction differ in important respects from other forms of aortic stenosis. Thus, the pulse is jerky with a rapid upstroke and with prominent pulsation of the abdominal aorta (in contrast to the anacrotic pulse of valvar aortic stenosis). An abnormal jugular a wave is frequently present. The thrusting, overactive left ventricular impulse is frequently double due to transmission of the forceful atrial contraction that may also be audible as a fourth heart sound. Frequently, there is also a third sound at the apex. Splitting of the second heart sound may be paradoxic, but this feature, as well as the gallop rhythm, is characteristically variable in line with the dynamic and variable obstruction. A midsystolic murmur, roughly proportional in intensity to the degree of obstruction, is maximal between the left sternal edge and apex rather than in the aortic area, although it radiates to the base and a thrill may be present. The murmur increases in intensity following a Valsalva maneuver (or inhalation of amyl nitrite), since both of these increase the obstruction. When there is significant mitral incompetence present, the murmur is maximal at the apex and pansystolic. There is no aortic ejection click or dilatation of the ascending aorta. Valvar calcification and an aortic diastolic murmur are also absent (except in the rare instances in which the valve is abnormal).

The three cardinal signs are the late onset systolic ejection murmur between the left sternal edge and apex, the jerky arterial pulse, and the palpable left atrial contraction.[G7]

Electrocardiogram

In obstructive forms of the disease, the electrocardiogram (ECG) characteristically shows a left ventricular strain pattern, although Q waves may be present, and there are rarely minimal changes of left ventricular hypertrophy despite a significant gradient.[K2,M26,M27] Occasionally, the ECG shows a complete right or left bundle branch block and more often a left anterior hemiblock.[M5,S2] Left atrial enlargement is often noted and right atrial enlargement less often.

Chest X-Ray

The chest x-ray shows mild-to-moderate cardiomegaly more often than in other forms of aortic stenosis. The raised left atrial pressure may be reflected in the lung fields by evidence of pulmonary venous hypertension or frank interstitial edema.[K2]

Echocardiography

The diagnosis can usually be made by M-mode echocardiography, since with rare exceptions, patients with familial hypertrophic obstructive cardiomyopathy (HOCM) have asymmetric septal hypertrophy (ASH) (ratio of thickness of basal ventricular septum to posterior left ventricular wall of 1.3 or more measured at end diastole), and all those with obstruction should show systolic anterior motion (SAM), although this may appear only on provocation, for example, after a Valsalva maneuver. The degree of obstruction can be quantitated by M-mode echocardiography using an obstruction index that correlates well with the gradient measured at catheterization.[H6] The diagnosis of classical familial HOCM is confirmed by demonstrating ASH (with M-mode echo) in a first-degree relative (the likelihood that five first-degree relatives will fail to show ASH is about 3%).[M20] However, when classic findings are present, a firm diagnosis is appropriate in the absence of a proven genetic link. Other M-mode echocardiographic findings are the demonstration of early (midsystolic) aortic valve closure (this is nonspecific since it occurs in any situation in which almost all ejection of blood occurs in early systole),[T5] decreased systolic thickening, decreased excursion of the hypertrophied septum,[C6,R3] a small left ventricular cavity, and a large left atrial cavity.

Wide-angle two-dimensional echocardiography displays more of the left ventricle than M mode and can identify left ventricular hypertrophy of unusual distribution, for example, when it involves mainly the posterior or apical septum and apical free wall.[M22,M23,Y1] In these circumstances, ASH and SAM are absent and there is no obstruction.

Cardiac Catheterization and Cineangiocardiography

Cardiac catheterization and cineangiocardiography continue to be used for diagnosis when operation is considered, since the echocardiographic findings can be misleading.[G8,W4] Right heart catheterization will show any infundibular stenosis (occasionally this is severe) or any elevation of pulmonary artery pressure, which may also be marked because of high left atrial pressures.[F2] Retrograde left heart catheterization will quantitate and localize the obstruction. The catheter tip should be positioned near the base of the ventricle to avoid apical entrapment that can produce a falsely high left ventricular pressure.[C7] The left ventricular end-diastolic pressure is usually raised, often markedly, due to transmission of a large left atrial a wave (Fig. 33-3). The central and peripheral arterial pulse contours show a rapid ascending limb with a short upstroke time (0.06–0.08 second) but a total ejection time that is >0.33. A secondary systolic tidal wave results in the characteristic "spike-and-dome" pulse contour initially described by Benchimol and associates (Fig. 33-3).[B11] The beat following a ventricular ectopic beat shows an abnormal response, namely, a reduced arterial pulse pressure (and an exaggerated spike and dome contour) secondary to the increased obstruction generated by the overfilled left ventricle (Fig. 33-3).[B12] In fact, the obstruction is increased by any maneuver that increases left ventricular contractility or that decreases left ventricular preload or afterload. Whenever the obstruction increases, the pulse pressure decreases and the total left ventricular ejection time increases. It is useful at catheterization to confirm this dynamic characteristic of the obstruction by various provocative maneuvers,[B10] such as isoproterenol administration, exercise, and the Valsalva maneuver that increase the gradient and methoxamine administration that decreases it.

Left ventricular cineangiography is best performed in the left lateral view if the vertical x-ray beam is used, since in

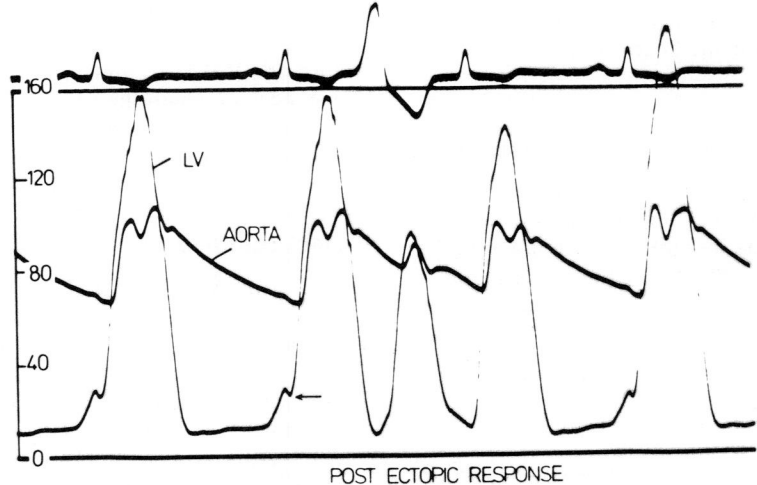

Figure 33-3 Left ventricular (LV) and aortic pressure tracings from a patient with HOCM and a peak systolic gradient of 60 mmHg (GLH). The aortic pressure pulse shows the typical double contour ("spike and dome") and the LV tracing an elevated end-diastolic pressure in association with transmission of an a wave from the left atrium (arrow). The beat following an ectopic beat demonstrates the reduction in aortic pulse pressure characteristic of hypertrophic obstructive cardiomyopathy.

this position the cardiac apex moves caudally and does not overshadow the mitral area. The mitral valve is profiled rather nearer the posterior than the anterior commissure. The prominent septal bulge can be seen to form the anterior boundary of the outflow tract and the anterior mitral leaflet to form its posterior boundary. SAM can usually be demonstrated when obstruction is present (Fig. 33-4). The abnormal sigmoid shape of the left ventricular cavity, the prominent papillary muscles, and the small end systolic volume are variable features well shown in the right anterior oblique projection (Fig. 33-1). The abnormal shape of the ventricular septum can be further demonstrated in a left anterior oblique projection with simultaneous injection into both right and left ventricles.[D2] In patients with concentric left ventricular hypertrophy, both sides of the septum are parallel, whereas in HOCM, the superior part of the septum is thicker and bulges into both ventricles and the inferior part near the apex is thinner. The degree of mitral incompetence is assessed from the left ventricular cineangiogram. Multiple ectopic beats can make quantitation difficult.[M5] Coronary angiography should be added to the procedure in patients over 30 years of age in whom occlusive disease may be present.

NATURAL HISTORY

Hypertrophic obstructive cardiomyopathy (HOCM) is a genetically determined disorder of cardiac muscle transmitted as an autosomal dominant trait,[C5] although nonfamilial cases probably also occur. In familial HOCM, isolated asymmetrical septal hypertrophy (ASH) identified by M-mode echocardiography is an important part of the clinical spectrum and has the same genetic implications as HOCM. It is uncertain whether isolated ASH, an asymptomatic disease, develops into clinical HOCM; if so, this sequence is uncommon after 20 years of age.[E2]

HOCM can present at any age, from early infancy[M8] to the sixth or even seventh decade, but it most commonly presents in the second or third decade of life.[E1,S7] Early studies using cardiac catheterization and angiocardiography for diagnosis suggested that about 80% of patients with HOCM developed outflow tract obstruction, but more recent studies using echocardiography and including those with isolated ASH suggest that obstruction is present in only about 20% of the entire spectrum. How often obstruction is present de novo or develops as a new feature in patients who present first without it is unclear. Serial cardiac catheterizations in a few patients (GLH) would suggest that once obstruction occurs, the gradient may increase, but the lability of the obstruction makes this assessment difficult.

Older patients with obstruction (either at rest or on provocation only) generally have been more symptomatic than younger ones, suggesting that symptoms progress in severity with age.[A1,E1,F2,S7] Thus, the incidence of severe symptoms (NYHA classes III and IV) increases from 9% of the patients for the first decade to 70% for the sixth to eighth decades. The data from the National Heart and Lung Institute (NHLI) suggest that there are two populations: a younger group of patients who are asymptomatic or only mildly disabled and an older group in whom the clinical manifestations develop later in life and who become progressively more disabled.[F2] However, in some patients the symptomatic course is extremely variable, fluctuating from prolonged stability to progressive deterioration, and there is no way to predict when it will change. The sudden onset of congestive heart failure is frequently precipitated by atrial fibrillation, and this may be associated with systemic embolism. It is probable that the longer the follow-up, the higher the incidence of heart failure, atrial fibrillation, and embolism. In the studies reported by Oakley, the incidence of heart failure was approximately 12%, of stable atrial fibrillation 10%, and of embolism 6%.[O1]

The correlation between symptomatic class and degree of obstruction has in general been poor, although in the multicenter trial reported by Shah and colleagues there were no asymptomatic patients once the gradient exceeded 100 mmHg.[S7] Also, the study by Frank and Braunwald indicated a significantly higher gradient in NYHA classes III and IV compared with those without symptoms.[F2] Studies by Goodwin and Oakley suggest that progressive symptomatic deterioration is associated with loss of outflow tract obstruction,[G2,O1,S12] but this has been documented only rarely and most often in association with congestive heart failure and a falling cardiac output.

The mortality of the disease without surgery (but not necessarily without propranolol) appears to be about 15% at 5 years and 25% at 10 years, with an annual attrition rate of 3.5%. This figure excludes death from causes unrelated to HOCM.[G2,M16,S7,S12]

Most cardiac deaths are *sudden*, only about 10% being due to congestive heart failure.[M16] In Shah's study, sudden death was unrelated to symptomatic class or the type of symptoms including a history of effort syncope, and there was no correlation of sudden death with age, sex, length of follow-up, or degree of obstruction.[S7] However, the report by Maron and colleagues of ASH presenting in patients under 15 years of age indicates that of 35 children who were referred because of overt symptoms of the disease and were followed for an average of 7.4 years, 11 (31%) died suddenly and 10 (29%) deteriorated clinically.[M4] Excluding 4 surgically treated cases, 8 (40%) of 20 with obstruction died suddenly, and only 1 (9%) of 11 without obstruction died suddenly. In those with obstruction, the incidence of sudden death was not, however, related to the degree of obstruction or symptoms, electrocardiographic changes, heart size, left ventricular end-diastolic pressure, left ventricular ejection, or upstroke time.[M4] Maron and colleagues were also able to review 26 *asymptomatic* patients who had died suddenly from the disease.[M2] In this group, there was no correlation with obstruction (some had no obstruction), but 23 of the 36 were under 25 years of age at the time of death and all 26 had a distinctly abnormal ECG and moderate-to-severe ventricular septal thickening on echocardiogram. Finally, one-third of them gave a family history of sudden death in a first-degree relative.

Many of the above features are confirmed by the study of the natural history of HOCM undertaken by McKenna and colleagues[M16] who examined 254 patients retrospectively over a mean follow-up period of 6 years (1–23 years). The average age at death (30 years) was significantly less than that of the survivors ($P < .03$). Cardiac deaths attributed to

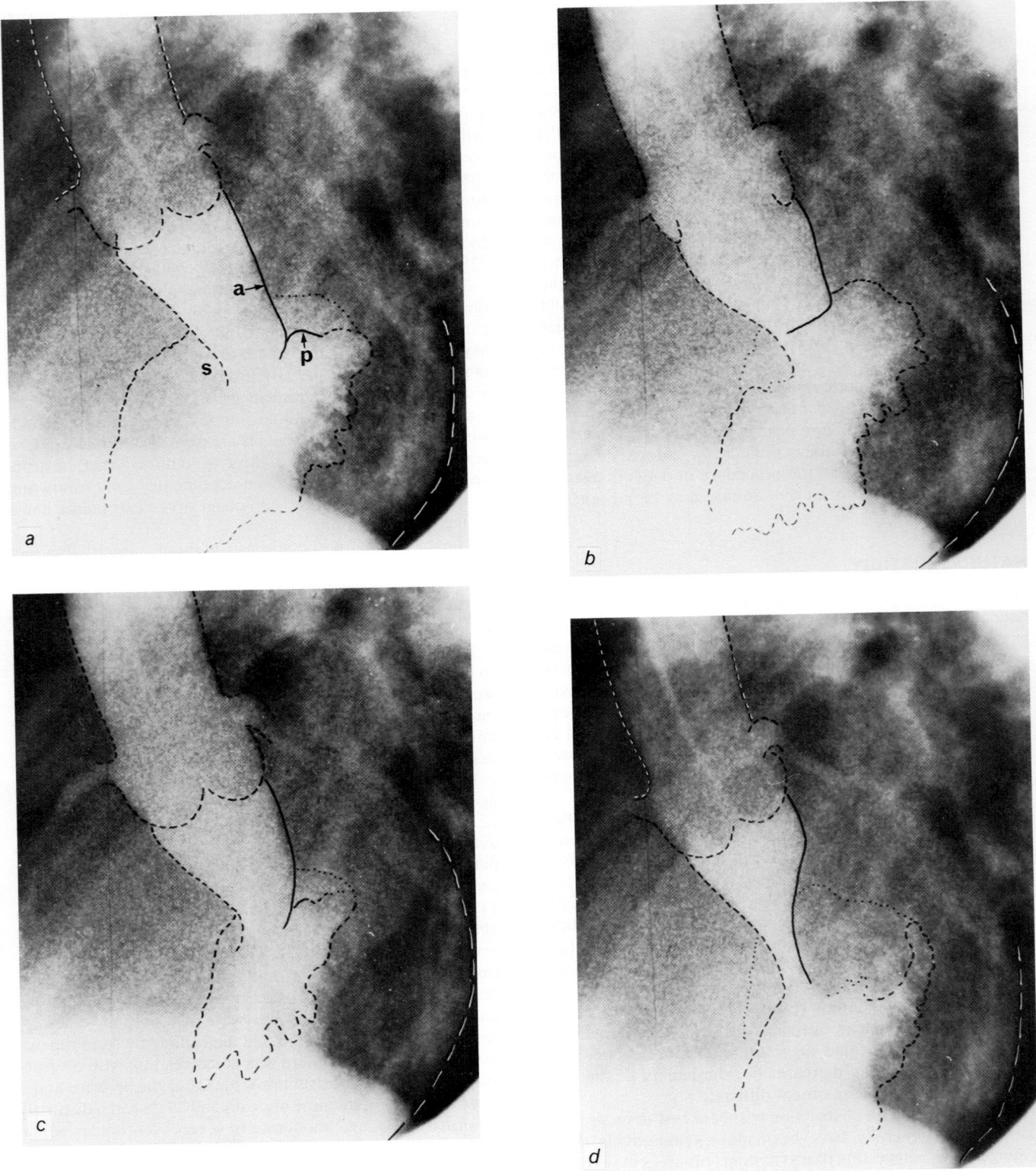

Figure 33-4 Left ventricular (LV) cineangiocardiogram in left lateral projection showing systolic anterior motion of the anterior mitral leaflet (GLH).

(a) Isovolumetric contraction: The anterior and posterior mitral leaflets are apposed in relatively normal systolic position giving only slight narrowing low in the left ventricular outflow tract in spite of prominent septal muscle anteriorly. Aortic valve is still closed.

(b) Systolic ejection phase: The apposed free edges of the mitral leaflets have risen to the maximal level of radiologic obstruction, the leaflet shelf almost meeting the septal muscle. In spite of severe

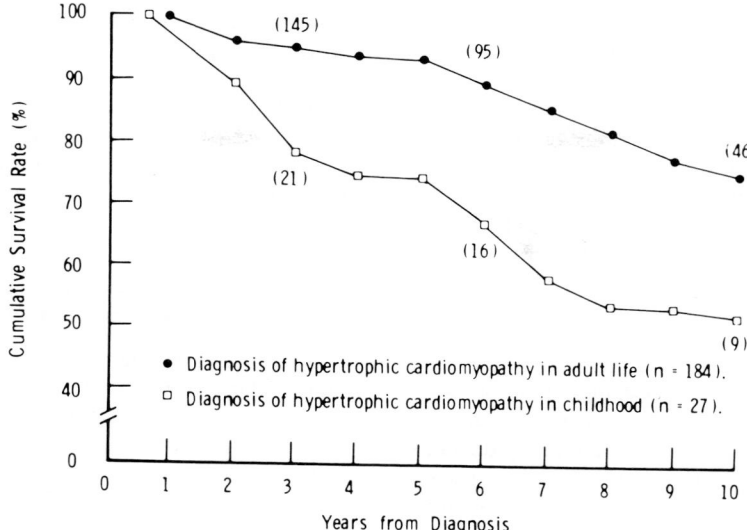

Figure 33-5 Actuarial survival of 211 medically treated patients with hypertrophic cardiomyopathy (with or without obstruction) considering only those deaths that were sudden or due to congestive heart failure. The 10-year survival for those in whom the diagnosis was made in adult life (15 years and over) was 74%, compared with 52% in those in whom the diagnosis was made in childhood ($\leqslant$14 years).

Reproduced with permission from McKenna et al.[M16]

HOCM (sudden or from cardiac failure) were found on discriminant analysis to be more common in patients diagnosed in childhood (<15 years of age) (Fig. 33-5), in those with a strong family history of sudden death, especially if it was known to be due to HOCM, in those with a history of syncope at diagnosis, and in those in whom there was severe dyspnea present at the last follow-up examination. Cardiac death was unrelated to the presence or severity of obstruction or to any other hemodynamic or ECG findings.

Ventricular arrhythmia is thought to be the antecedent of sudden death.[M25,S18] Treatment with β blockage (propranolol) or calcium antagonists (verapamil) is ineffective against ventricular arrhythmia in HOCM and these drugs have no effect on the incidence of sudden death.

Death can be caused by cerebral embolism in patients with stable or paroxysmal atrial fibrillation or uncommonly from bacterial endocarditis on aortic or mitral valves (a 2%–4% incidence). In the multicenter study by Shah and colleagues in patients not operated upon and followed for an average of 5.2 years, all of whom had obstruction, there was only 1 death from heart failure and 2 from bacterial endocarditis compared with 23 that were sudden.[S7]

---

obstruction (systolic gradient 100 mm), note the absence of mitral regurgitation in this patient.

(c) Isovolumetric relaxation: The mitral leaflets have returned to a more normal systolic position, and the aortic leaflets have closed.

(d) Diastole: The mitral valve is open, the anterior leaflet showing normal forward convexity from its hinge beneath the aortic root in contrast to the appearance during abnormal systolic anterior motion shown in (b) .

a, anterior mitral leaflet; p, posterior mitral leaflet; s, septal muscle.

TECHNIQUE OF OPERATION

Although a combined aortic and left ventricular approach is necessary in at least some cases (UAB, GLH), it may be used as a routine (GLH) or only under specific conditions (UAB).

Myectomy by a Combined Aortic and Left Ventricular Approach (GLH)

A median sternotomy is used and cardiopulmonary bypass (CPB) is established in standard fashion (see Chapter 2, Section 3). During cooling, a left atrial suction line to the pump oxygenator is inserted through the base of the right superior pulmonary vein. The aorta is cross-clamped, and the cold cardioplegic solution is infused through the aortic needle. The aorta is then opened with an incision extending into the noncoronary sinus of Valsalva (see Chapter 12, Fig. 12-2 b). Both coronary ostia are now cannulated with cuffed-tip metal cannulae that are held in position with stay sutures passed through the aortic wall.[B17] (The technique is described in detail in Chapter 3, "Technique of Myocardial Protection in Patients with Aortic Valve Incompetence.") The coronary perfusion system is maintained intact throughout the operation to prevent air entering the coronary ostia, which will otherwise occur when the heart is subsequently dislocated from the pericardium, particularly in hearts with extreme left ventricular hypertrophy and particularly into the coronary branches on the front of the heart.

The right aortic cusp is retracted forward with a cloth-covered retractor, and removal of hypertrophied muscle is commenced from above using a no. 15 (small rounded) scalpel blade. A deep U of muscle is excised from the septum anteriorly, beginning beneath the nadir of the right coronary cusp and extending to the left to the commissure between right and left cusps. The trough must not extend further toward the right since this will inevitably produce complete left bundle branch block or even complete heart block from damage to the main bundle of His (Fig. 33-6). The trough extends directly inferiorly rather than inferiorly and toward the right (remembering that the hypertrophied septum occupies the anterior as well as the right wall of the outflow tract). It extends inferiorly only as far as the surgeon can see. Blind extension of the incision into the depths of the ventricle is avoided.

The left ventricle is now dislocated and a pack placed behind it. It is opened through a 4-cm-long oblique incision in the lower anterior wall approximately at the junction of mid- and lower third (Fig. 33-6). Exact positioning depends upon the lowermost diagonal artery. The incision lies inferior and roughly parallel to this (if present) and far enough away so that the artery will not be damaged with the sutures used to close it. The incision enters the ventricle below the origin of the anterior papillary muscle. Exposure of the interior of the ventricle is obtained by careful retraction of both edges of the incision. The anterior mitral leaflet is identified and moved away from and to the left of the ventricular septum. Muscle is now excised from the *anterior* portion of the ventricular septum, working from below upward using a no. 10 (regular) scalpel blade. A wide, deep U is created, extending from opposite the ventriculotomy into the ventricular outflow tract, to become continuous with the anterior block already cut out from above. Excision of the block of muscle from the floor of the trough is completed with scissors. The depth of the trough depends upon the degree of septal hypertrophy but is at least 15 mm and often 20 mm. The trough extends superiorly and toward the left from its lowermost point. When the trough is partly completed, the surgeon's left index finger is passed into the outflow tract via the aortotomy to define better the area of excision superiorly and to protect the anterior mitral leaflet (which is displaced behind the finger). Final muscle removal in the depths of the trough (the most cephalad superior portion in front of the finger) is accomplished using medium-sized bone rongeurs. Great care is taken not to leave loose fragments of muscle that could embolize.

When the trough is deemed adequate, the heart is returned to the pericardium and the trough is examined again through the aortotomy. Further muscle fragments can often be removed to align the aortic excision site with that completed from below. The ventricle is again dislocated (the coronary cannulae are still in position), and the ventriculotomy is closed with a single row of interrupted 0 silk sutures placed with a large, curved needle. Each stitch must be full thickness, and all are placed before any are tied. Five sutures usually suffice. The heart is returned to the pericardium, and the aortotomy is closed with a continuous running 3-0 silk suture. The coronary cannulae are removed after the posterior half of the closure is completed. The left ventricle will have filled with blood during this stage. Aortic closure is completed and the left ventricle needled for air (without dislocating it).

Rewarming with CPB is begun as the ventriculotomy is being closed. When the aortic closure is completed, the aortic cross clamp is released while suction is applied to the aortic vent needle. The heart is defibrillated and de-aired (see Chapter 2, Section 3). Before reducing CPB flows, the heart is dislocated to examine the ventriculotomy and any bleeding sites are controlled with additional sutures. The remainder of the operation is completed in the usual manner.

Myectomy and Myotomy Primarily by an Aortic Approach (UAB)

The operation proceeds as described above through the infusion of the cold cardioplegic solution into the aortic root. A transverse aortotomy is made (see Chapter 12, Fig. 12-2b), extending it a little further than usual in both directions to improve exposure. Stay sutures are applied to the lips of the aortotomy for retraction. The right coronary cusp is collapsed against the sinus wall where it will then usually stay. When the hypertrophied septum can be seen bulging down into the anterior aspect of the left ventricular outflow tract (as is usually the case), the operation proceeds through the aortic root.

As described in the previous section ("Myectomy by a Combined Aortic and Left Ventricular Approach [GLH]"), a deep incision is made in the septum, exactly beneath the nadir of the right coronary cusp. A no. 10 (regular) scalpel blade is used, passing it into position with care to avoid aortic valve cusp damage. A second parallel deep incision is made as far leftward as possible without damaging the mitral apparatus. As suggested by Morrow,[M1] a sponge stick is now pressed against the right ventricular free wall, which depresses the ventricular septum and brings it into better view through the aortotomy. Both incisions are now deepened and carried inferiorly as far as possible and indeed beyond the point of visibility, since there are no structures there that can be damaged. Now, using a no. 15 (small curved) blade on the scalpel, the depths of the two incisions are connected by a transverse incision beneath the right coronary cusp. With continuing pressure by the sponge stick, this transverse incision is extended downwards into the ventricle, first with the knife and then with scissors, until a thick, rectangular piece of septum has been excised. Care is taken not to lose any small bits of muscle. If the finger passed through the valve into the left ventricular cavity confirms by palpation that the excision has traversed the entire length of the muscular obstruction, the decision is made to forego left ventriculotomy. By blunt dissection with the finger, at times working against the counterpressure of the sponge stick, the trough is considerably deepened and widened. The aortotomy is closed; with strong suction to the aortic needle vent, the aortic clamp is released and rewarming begun. The remainder of the operation is completed as usual. (See Chapter 2, Section 3.)

When the initial examination through the aortic valve shows the muscular obstruction to be deeper (more inferior or more upstream) in the left ventricular outflow tract than usual or when the trough excision leaves a residual muscular obstruction inferiorly, the left ventricular approach is added. This is carried out exactly as described in the previous section, with the exception that the left ventriculotomy is closed

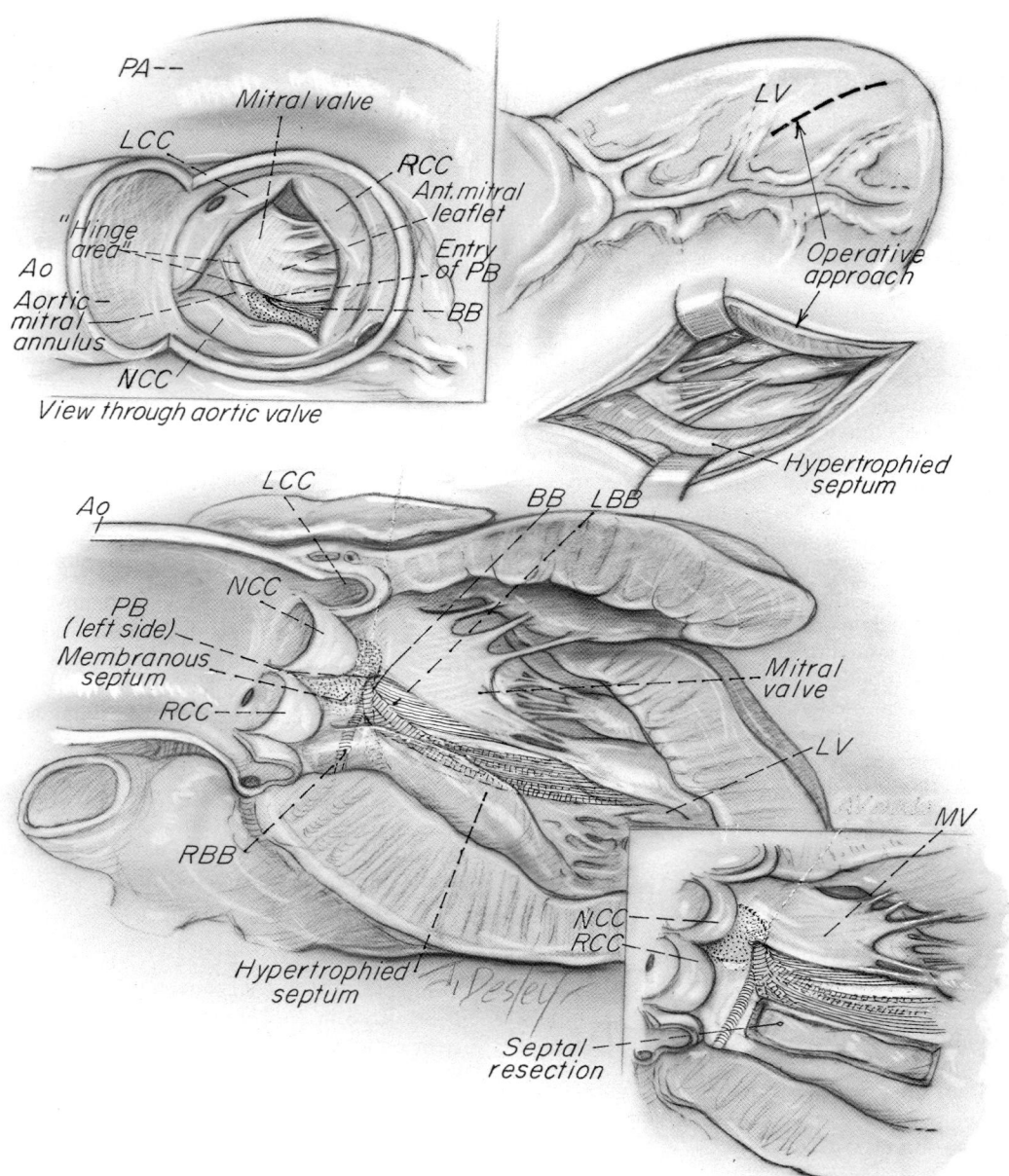

Figure 33-6 The conduction system and surgery for hypertrophic obstructive cardiomyopathy. The upper left insert shows the anatomic details as viewed through the aortic valve. The muscular left ventricular outflow obstruction is not evident in this view. The upper right drawing shows the location of the left ventriculotomy (see text for details). The relationship of the trough of septal resection to the conduction system is shown in the lower right insert.

Ao, aorta; AV, atrioventricular; BB, bundle branch; LBB, left bundle branch; LCC, left coronary cusp; LV, left ventricle; NCC, noncoronary cusp; PA, pulmonary artery; PB, penetrating bundle; RBB, right bundle branch; RCC, right coronary cusp.

Reproduced with permission from Bharati et al.[B18]

with interrupted mattress sutures over felt strips supplemented by a continuous whip stitch.

SPECIAL FEATURES OF POSTOPERATIVE CARE

The patient is cared for with the principles and protocols described in Chapter 5. The marked left ventricular hypertrophy of patients with HOCM reduces the compliance of the ventricle to such an extent that left atrial pressures of 16–18 mmHg may be required in the early postoperative period for adequate preload (see Chapter 5, footnote 9).

EARLY RESULTS

Hospital Mortality

The hospital mortality for surgical procedures directed against hypertrophic obstructive cardiomyopathy is low but does not yet approach zero (see Chapter 6 for definition). Thus, 5 hospital deaths (6%, CL 3%–10%) have occurred after 84 operations (GLH, Table 33-1), although no deaths (0%, CL 0%–8%) have occurred among 22 patients undergoing operation since 1976; 5 such deaths (7%, CL 4%–11%) have occurred after 76 operations (UAB; Table 33-2), although only 1 death (2%, CL 0.2%–6%) occurred, and that in 1971, among 55 patients undergoing myectomy and myotomy alone, with or without coronary artery bypass grafting. This is similar to the mortality achieved in other centers in which there is experience in the surgery of this condition.[R1,S1] Thus, Maron and colleagues report 19 hospital deaths (8%, CL 6%–10%) among 233 patients[M19] and Beahrs and colleagues 4 deaths (10%, CL 5%–17%) among 40 patients.[B14]

Modes of Death

Among the 10 deaths occurring in hospital in the combined GLH and UAB experience, 5 were in acute cardiac failure (low cardiac output) (Tables 33-3 and 33-4). All had some procedure in addition to the myectomy. Two deaths were neurologic (both operated upon before 1977), and these as well as those associated with ventriculotomy dehiscence (1966) and ventricular rupture appear to be prevented by the techniques of operation now used.

Table 33-1 Myectomy and myotomy for hypertrophic obstructive cardiomyopathy (GLH; 1960–1984). The aortic approach was used between 1960 and 1963 and the combined aortic and left ventricular approach from 1963 to the present.

| Technique of Operation | n | Hospital Deaths | | | Late Reoperations |
		No.	%	CL	No.
Aortic approach	9	0	0%	0%–19%	4
Aortic and LV approach	75[a]	5	7%	4%–11%	0
Total	84	5	6%	3%–10%	4

KEY: CL, 70% confidence limits; LV, left ventricular.

[a] The 75 operations were performed on 71 patients, four reoperations after an initial aortic approach being required for unrelieved obstruction with severe persistent symptoms.[K2]

Table 33-2 Cardiac surgical procedures in addition to myectomy and myotomy in patients with hypertrophic obstructive cardiomyopathy (UAB; 1967–1984; n = 76).

| Procedures | n | Hospital Deaths | | |
		No.	%	CL
None	41	1[a]	2%	.3%–8%
CABG	14		0%	0%–13%
MVR	9[b]	4	44%	24%–66%
AVR	7[c]		0%	0%–24%
MVR + AVR	2		0%	0%–61%
TVA	1		0%	0%–85%
MVR (no myectomy)	2[d]		0%	0%–61%
Total	76	5	7%	4%–11%

MVR through TVA bracketed: 21%; CL 11%–35%

KEY: AVR, aortic valve replacement; CABG, coronary artery bypass grafting; CL, 70% confidence limits; MVR, mitral valve replacement; TVA, tricuspid valve annuloplasty.

[a] Neurologic death after operation in 1971.
[b] One (who died) had also CABG.
[c] Without and with (three, zero deaths) CABG.
[d] One had also CABG.

Incremental Risk Factors for Hospital Death

Multivariate analysis did not identify any risk factors (GLH), but this would in any event be difficult because of the relatively small number of cases and deaths. However, associated cardiac conditions leading to concomitant procedures as a group increased the risk of hospital death (GLH, Table 33-5; UAB, see Table 33-2). This is not surprising in view of the incremental risk of severe left ventricular hypertrophy, which all patients with HOCM have, in any cardiac operation. Age at operation (Table 33-6) and preoperative NYHA functional class (Table 33-7) have not been demonstrated to be risk factors for hospital death.

Conduction Disturbances

Complete heart block is uncommonly produced at operation. It occurred in 2 (3%) patients (GLH), both of whom had a right bundle branch block preoperatively and in 5% of the series reported by Maron and colleagues in 1978.[M6] When a preoperative complete right bundle branch block is present, creation of a left bundle branch block (LBBB) at the time of operation results in a complete block. A complete LBBB occurred in 57% of the GLH patients and had no effect on mortality.[M5] In the series reported by Reis and colleagues, complete LBBB occurred in only 1 of the 30 patients postoperatively; in 12 the ECG was essentially unchanged and in 16 only a left anterior hemiblock occurred. This low incidence was attributed to positioning the myectomy more to the left.[R1]

Perioperative Myocardial Infarction

Perioperative myocardial infarction occurs occasionally at sites removed from the myotomy and can occur without associated coronary atheroma.[M24] It was detected electrocardiologically in 3 (4%) of the patients (GLH). Most of the operations were performed prior to the advent of cold

Table 33-3 Modes of hospital death in patients undergoing operation for hypertrophic obstructive cardiomyopathy using a combined aortic–left ventricular approach (GLH; 1963–1984; $n = 75$).

Mode of Death	Preoperative NYHA Class	Resting Gradient (mmHg)	Age (yr)	Date of Operation
Dehiscence ventriculotomy	I	118	35	1966
Acute cardiac failure (myocardial infarction) (CAD)	III	150	67	1972
Acute cardiac failure (TR)	V	40	56	1973
Acute cardiac failure (CABG × 3)	IV	50	59	1974
Neurologic death (CABG × 3)	III	126	73	1976

KEY: CABG, coronary artery bypass grafts; CAD, coronary artery disease; TR, gross tricuspid regurgitation.

cardioplegia. The current use of this technique should lessen the incidence.

Iatrogenic Ventricular Septal Defect

A ventricular septal defect (VSD) has been reported to have been produced in 3% of patients operated on by transaortic myectomy,[M6] but it has not occurred with this approach (UAB). It may not be recognized until some weeks after operation and could then be the result of septal infarction rather than surgical perforation.[S3] It may contribute to hospital mortality and may be large enough to require subsequent repair.[M6] It has not occurred during an open approach through the left ventricle (GLH, UAB).[A3]

Iatrogenic Aortic and Mitral Incompetence

Iatrogenic aortic and mitral incompetence have been reported by others but have been avoidable (GLH, UAB).

LATE RESULTS
Survival

Actuarial survival including all late deaths from whatever cause but excluding hospital mortality has been 76% 10 years postoperatively and 53% 17 years (204 months) postoperatively, by which time there were only 8 patients at risk

(GLH) (Fig. 33-7). When the hospital mortality is added, these figures became 70% and 49%, respectively. Four of the 16 deaths occurred in the first 14 postoperative months, but thereafter there continued to be a significant late mortality due to the progressive nature of the disease.

Deaths directly attributable to the cardiomyopathy are those from congestive heart failure or arrhythmia (sudden). Those less directly related but still cardiac in origin are the result of cerebral embolism (in association with atrial fibrillation) or myocardial infarction (Table 33-8). When only deaths from congestive heart failure and sudden death are examined, 10-year survival is 87% (1.3%/year) and 17-year (204 months) survival is 61% (2.3%/year) (Fig. 33-8).

Only 25% of the deaths were sudden. This is in contrast to late deaths with purely medical management where sudden death is the most common mode.[M16,S7] Thus, the 10-year mortality from syncope (sudden death) and congestive heart failure in the study by McKenna and colleagues of medically treated patients was 65%, and 55% of these deaths were due to syncope[M16]; in the study by Shah and colleagues, in which all patients had obstruction, 26 (53%) of the 49 deaths in patients on medical treatment were sudden.[S2] Shah's study also suggested that sudden death was less frequent in surgically treated patients.

Table 33-4 Modes of hospital death in patients undergoing operations for hypertrophic obstructive cardiomyopathy (UAB; 1967–1984; $n = 76$).

Mode of Death	No.	Procedure in Addition to Myectomy	No. of Cases
Acute cardiac failure	3	MVR	2
		MVR + CABG	1
Hemorrhage (ventricular rupture)	1	MVR	1
Neurologic	1[a]	None	1
Total	5		5

KEY: CABG, coronary artery bypass grafts; MVR, mitral valve replacement.
[a]Operation in 1971.

Table 33-5 Cardiac surgical procedures in addition to myectomy and myotomy in patients with hypertrophic obstructive cardiomyopathy (GLH; 1963–1984; $n = 75$).

Procedures	n	Hospital Deaths No.	%	CL
None	68	3	4%	4%–9%
CABG	3	2	67%	24%–96%
Mitral valve repair (chordal rupture)	1	0	0%	0%–85%
AVR (congenital stenosis)	1	0	0%	0%–85%
Mitral valvotomy + aortic valvotomy (rheumatic)	1	0	0%	0%–85%
Repair ASD	1	0	0%	0%–85%
Total	75	5	7%	4%–11%

KEY: ASD, atrial septal defect; AVR, aortic valve replacement; CABG, coronary artery bypass graft; CL, 70% confidence limits.

Table 33-6   Age at operation and hospital (< 30 days) and late mortality in patients undergoing surgery for hypertrophic obstructive cardiomyopathy (GLH; 1963–1984; *n* = 75).

Age at Operation (yr) ≤ <	n	Hospital Deaths No.	Late Deaths No.	Total Deaths No.	%	
5 --- 10	2	0	0	0	0%	⎫
10 --- 20	6	0	2	2	33%	⎪
20 --- 30	14	0	2	2	14%	⎬ 14/63
30 --- 40	17	1	3	4	24%	22%; CL 17%–29%
40 --- 50	8	0	2	2	25%	⎪
50 --- 60	16	2	2	4	25%	⎭
60 --- 70	10	1	4	5	50%	⎫ 7/12
70	2	1	1	2	100%	⎬ 58%; CL 40%–75%
Total	75	5(7%)	16(21%)	21	28%	(CL 22%–34%)
$P(\chi^2)$		.24			.19	

KEY: CL, 70% confidence limits.

These surgical late results are virtually identical to those of Maron and colleagues, where the overall 10-year actuarial survival was 70%; when late mortality from deaths due to syncope and congestive heart failure only were considered, 10-year survival was 82% (1.8% per year).[M6] The late mortality for surgically treated patients reported by McKenna and colleagues was also 1.8% per year[M16] and for those reported by Beahrs and colleagues with a mean 13-year follow-up, 1.6% per year (86% 10-year survival).[B14]

Incremental Risk Factors for Death after Hospital Dismissal

History of Congestive Heart Failure
A history preoperatively of congestive heart failure was a risk factor for late death in the multivariate analysis (Table 33-9), but preoperative NYHA functional class was not (Table 33-7). This finding is similar to that from the study of McKenna et al., which showed that the presence of congestive heart failure and syncope at diagnosis increased the risk of subsequent death in patients medically treated.[M16] Fighali and colleagues have also reported similar findings.[F5]

Age
Older age (over 60 years) was a risk factor for late death (see Tables 33-6 and 33-9). However, a more detailed analysis (Table 33-10) shows that the mean follow-up time is 7 years

Table 33-7   Preoperative NYHA class and mortality in patients undergoing surgery for hypertrophic obstructive cardiomyopathy (GLH; 1963–1984; *n* = 75).

NYHA Class	n	Hospital Deaths	Late Deaths	Total Deaths n	%	CL
I	9	1	1	2	22%	8%–50%
II	22	0	5	5	23%	13%–36%
III	32	2	7	9	28%	19%–39%
IV	9	1	2	3	33%	15%–56%
V	3	1	1	2	67%	24%–96%
Total	75	5	16	21	28%	22%–34%
P(logistic)		.21			.19	

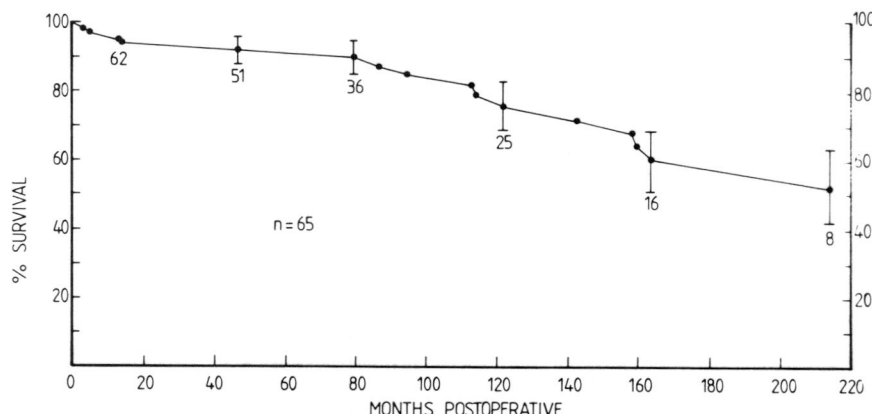

Figure 33-7   Actuarial survival of hospital survivors (*n* = 70) of myectomy and myotomy for HOCM (GLH; 1963–1984). Five patients are untraced, and the analysis is of the remaining 65. The bars enclose the 70% confidence limits; the number at risk at various intervals are indicated.

Table 33-8 Modes of late death in 65 traced patients following surgery for hypertrophic obstructive cardiomyopathy (GLH; 1963–1984).

Mode of Death	No.	Age at Operation (yr)
Sudden (arrhythmia)	4	14, 31, 51, 56
Congestive heart failure	6	11, 25, 34, 63, 66, 67
Cerebrovascular episode[a]	3	38, 46, 47
Bronchopneumonia	1	72
Myocardial infarction	1	64
Probable carcinoma	1	21
Total	16	11–72 (mean 44)

[a] Two from cerebral emboli in association with atrial fibrillation.

Table 33-9 Incremental risk factors for death after hospital dismissal after surgery for hypertrophic obstructive cardiomyopathy (GLH; 1963–1984; *n* = 75).

Variable	Coefficient	SD	P value
CHF history	1.77	±0.66	.008
(High) LVEDP (if age <60 yr)	0.09	±0.04	.015
Age >60 yr	3.15	±0.96	.001

KEY: CHF, congestive heart failure; LVEDP, left ventricular end-diastolic pressure.

NOTE: The analysis was of 61 patients (75 operations in 71 patients, with 5 hospital deaths and 5 untraced patients) with 16 late deaths; LVEDP values were missing in 4 patients. Variables examined in assessing incremental risk factors for posthospital death using Cox's proportional hazards model included age at operation ≥ 60 years yes/no; dyspnea (grades 1–5); angina (grades 1–5); congestive heart failure yes/no; NYHA class (grades I–V); mitral incompetence (grades 0–5); other valve lesions yes/no; other cardiac lesions (chiefly coronary artery disease) yes/no; left ventricular end diastolic pressure (continuous); outflow tract resting gradient (continuous); cardioplegia yes/no; complete left bundle branch block (pre- or postop) yes/no; atrial fibrillation (pre- or postop) yes/no.

and that the five late deaths occurred from 6.6 to 13.2 years postoperatively, at which time the patients were between 69 and 81 years old (average 75.2 years). Symptomatic deterioration prior to death was rapid, so that the patients experienced long periods of improved functional class. This was also true of the patient who had deteriorated to NYHA class III on assessment 5 years postoperatively, since she was in class I for the first 3 years. These findings are not inconsistent with the report of Koch and colleagues of superior results in a group of 20 patients 65 years of age or older, since the duration of follow-up is shorter in their series.[K5]

Left Ventricular End-Diastolic Pressure
Marked elevation of left ventricular end-diastolic pressure (LVEDP) was the only preoperative hemodynamic measurement that related to late death, and this was true only in patients <60 years of age (Table 33-9). The preoperative pressure gradient across the left ventricular outflow tract was not a risk factor.

Postoperative Pressure Gradients

The preoperative gradients are virtually always relieved by operation,[A3,M6] although on provocation a mild gradient can be demonstrated in about 25% of cases (Fig. 33-9). In patients in whom a gradient was present preoperatively only on provocation, these maneuvers do not produce a gradient postoperatively.[A3,M6] In addition, operation almost always abolishes the abnormal postectopic response and the abnormal arterial pulse contour. In patients with several postoperative catheterizations extending over many years, the residual gradient either remains the same or is further reduced (Fig. 33-10).[A3,M6] Both echocardiography and cineangiography show reduction or abolition of systolic anterior motion of the mitral valve in most patients postoperatively.[A3,M5] In addition, the surgical grooves created by myectomy and reduction in thickness of the myectomy site are demonstrable by these techniques,[A3,S6] and have been shown to result in enlargement of the left ventricular outflow tract.[S5]

Mitral Incompetence

Mitral incompetence is usually abolished or significantly reduced following adequate myectomy (Fig. 33-11).[A3] Persis-

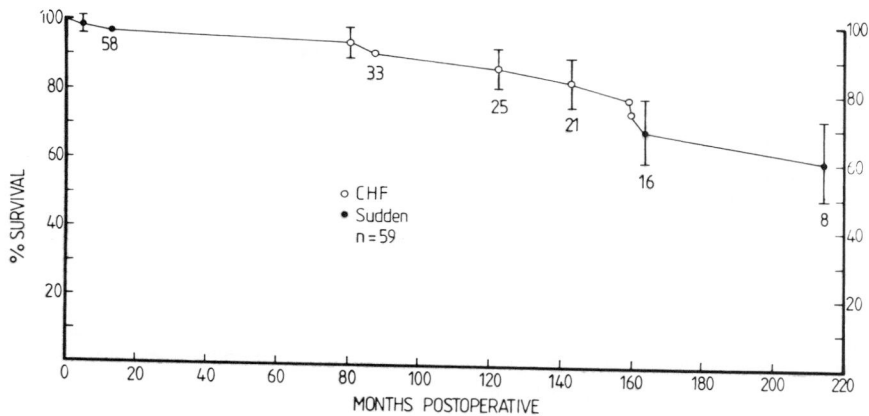

Figure 33-8 Actuarial survival of hospital survivors of myectomy and myotomy for HOCM, considering only deaths that were sudden or due to congestive heart failure (GLH; 1963–1984; combined aortic–left ventricular approach). The presentation is as in Figure 33-7.

Table 33-10 Characteristics and results in patients over 60 years of age undergoing surgery for hypertrophic obstructive cardiomyopathy using a combined approach (GLH; 1963–1984).

Preoperative				Follow-Up			
Age (yr)	NYHA Class	LVEDP (mmHg)	Resting Gradient	Duration (yr)	Age (yr)	Rhythm	Status
61	III	12	80	2.2	63	SR	NYHA I
61	III	10	150	5.3	67	SR	NYHA III
61	IV	22	0(50)[a]	9.2	71	SR	NYHA II
63	II	1	80	6.6	69	AF	LD (CHF)
63	II	11	83	7.0	70	CHB[c]	NYHA I
64	III	22	20(115)	7.8	72	SR	LD (infarct)
66	III	24	89	13.2	80	AF	LD (CHF)
67	III	20	150	HD			
67	III	14	110	7.2	74	CHB[c]	LD (CHF)
68	III	13	90	2.3	70	SR	NYHA I
72	II	24	66	9.4	81	AF	LD (pneumonia)
73	III	26	126	HD[b]			
Mean 65		17	87	7.0	72		

KEY: AF, atrial fibrillation; CHB, complete heart block; HD, hospital death; LD, late death; LVEDP, left ventricular end-diastolic pressure; NYHA, New York Heart Association; SR, sinus rhythm.

[a] ( ) gradient on provocation with isoproterenol.

[b] Plus coronary artery bypass grafts × 3.

[c] Complete heart block of late onset paced.

tent significant mitral regurgitation usually suggests a coexisting mitral lesion, such as spontaneous chordal rupture or damage from bacterial endocarditis.

Left Ventricular Aneurysm

The ventriculotomy is potentially a cause of aneurysm. A false aneurysm can occur at the ventriculotomy site because of insecure closure, and reoperation may be required to repair it.[A3] This complication is avoidable since it has not occurred at GLH since 1968 and prior to that occurred only once. A true left ventricular aneurysm occurred in one GLH patient secondary to an anterior myocardial infarction.

Symptomatic Status

When the obstruction is not relieved by operation, symptoms persist.[K2] In contrast, following an adequate myectomy all recent reports indicate striking symptomatic improvement.[A3,M6,M19,R1,S1] Most patients promptly become either totally asymptomatic or complain of mild effort dyspnea only, and syncope is almost always abolished (Table

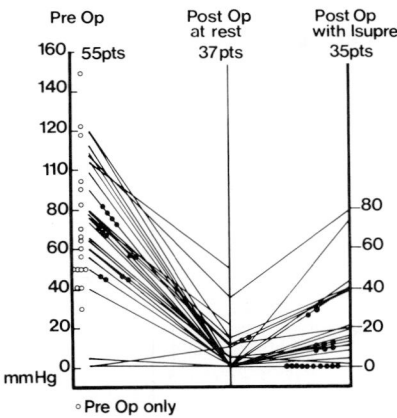

Figure 33-9 Preoperative resting peak systolic left ventricular outflow tract gradients in 55 patients operated upon for HOCM, and postoperative gradients measured at rest (37 patients), and after provocation with isoproterenol (35 patients) (GLH; 1963–1978; combined aortic–left ventricular approach). Three patients in the series had no resting gradient preoperatively but did develop gradients of 50–60 mmHg on provocation (one of these had mild valvar stenosis from a bicuspid valve, and one had severe mitral regurgitation from chordal rupture).

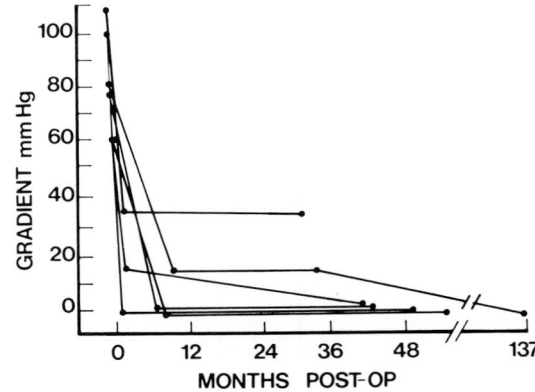

Figure 33-10 Pre- and postoperative resting peak systolic left ventricular outflow tract gradients in six patients operated upon for HOCM who have had two or more postoperative studies (GLH).

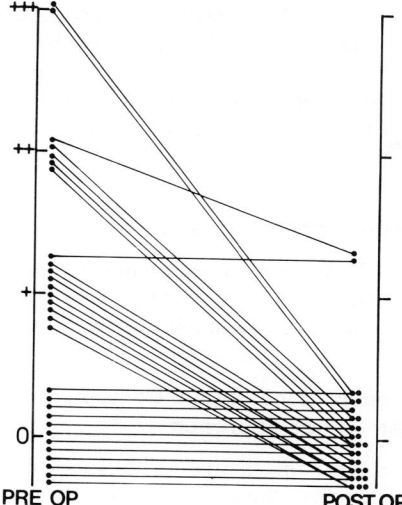

Figure 33-11 Degree of mitral regurgitation assessed cineangiocardiographically in 29 patients with pre- and postoperative studies (GLH; 1963–1975).

0, none; +, mild; + +, moderate; + + +, severe.

Reproduced with permission from Agnew et al.[A3]

33-11).[A3,M5,R1] Eighty-nine percent of patients are in class I or II after a follow-up of 9.4 years (1–21 years; GLH). Only 2 patients showed marked deterioration (from class II to IV), both in association with atrial fibrillation. There is no evidence that late recurrence of symptoms is related to recurrence of obstruction. The NYHA class was known at an interval reasonably close to the time of late death in 10 of the 16 patients who died; 5 were in class I, 4 were in class II, and 1 (a class V patient preoperatively) was in class IV. A few patients do show subsequent deterioration on longer-term follow-up.[M6]

Atrial fibrillation undoubtedly has an adverse effect on symptoms,[A3,B13] although it is not associated with an increased risk of late death. Surgical relief of the obstruction in

Table 33-11 NYHA class pre- and postoperatively in 48 surviving patients (five other patients are lost to follow-up, and in three others NYHA class postoperatively is uncertain) (GLH; 1963–1984).

Preop NYHA	Postoperative NYHA				
	I	II	III	IV	V
I	6				
II	15			2[a]	
III	11	5	1		
IV	2	3	1		
V			1		
Total	34	8	3[b]	2	

KEY: NYHA, New York Heart Association functional class.

[a] One deteriorated 16 years postop with onset of atrial fibrillation and now has a dilated cardiomyopathy; one is in long-standing atrial fibrillation and has obesity and alcoholism.

[b] One of three in chronic atrial fibrillation.

HOCM does not abolish chronic atrial fibrillation or permit successful cardioversion, and when this rhythm occurs as a new feature in the later stages of the disease there is further symptomatic deterioration (and if anticoagulants are not given a 50% chance of embolism). Atrial fibrillation is present in approximately 50% of the patients at the time of late death (GLH).

Left Ventricular Function

The preoperatively markedly increased resting ejection fraction characteristic of HOCM (76 ± 2%) is reduced postoperatively ($P < .001$) to 67 ± 2%, a figure that lies well within the range of normal.[B15] On exercise, preoperatively the ejection fraction falls to within the normal range (71 ± 3%) and postoperatively it also falls slightly (66 ± 4%). These figures do not give any evidence of significant damage to the left ventricle from a transaortic myectomy; similar data are not available in patients who have also had a ventriculotomy, but the similarity in the symptomatic relief obtained with either technique strongly suggests that the findings would be the same in the latter group.[B15]

Left ventricular diastolic function is probably not affected by the operation, although left ventricular cavity size is increased. There is no significant change in LVEDP in the late postoperative studies when these are compared with preoperative studies.[A3]

INDICATIONS FOR OPERATION

Surgery may be considered (GLH, UAB) in any patient with an important gradient at rest (>50 mmHg) who has significant limitations (NYHA class III or more) that have not been relieved by β blockade (propranolol) or the administration of a calcium antagonist (verapamil[A5,R4,S20] or nifedipine) in adequate dosage. A properly performed myectomy currently is associated with a very low risk and with about a 90% chance of providing long-term and almost complete symptomatic relief, particularly in patients in sinus rhythm. Neither age nor severity of symptoms is a contraindication.

Similar indications may be considered to exist when there is no resting gradient but a gradient >50 mmHg is present on provocation (isoproterenol) or after an ectopic beat (GLH). The symptomatic relief obtained by operation is less certain in this circumstance in patients in chronic atrial fibrillation, since operation does not alter this rhythm.

These indications may be widened to include less symptomatic patients with severe gradients, particularly in the presence of significant mitral regurgitation or with a history of syncope (without insisting upon a trial of propranolol therapy),[M24] although this is controversial. It is considered justified because of the likely effect of an operation in reducing the incidence of sudden death and the low risk of operation.

Since additional procedures seem to increase the risk of hospital death after the repair of HOCM and particularly since mitral incompetence regresses after adequate repair (see "Late Results"), mitral valve replacement for mitral incompetence should be limited to situations in which the incompetence is either very severe or due to mitral structural abnormalities unsuitable for repair or valvotomy. Since coronary artery bypass grafting alone does not relieve symptoms in patients with HOCM and coronary artery disease,[G10,S19] myectomy plus coronary artery bypass grafting is indicated when the two conditions coexist.

SPECIAL SITUATIONS AND CONTROVERSIES

Mitral Valve Replacement

Mitral valve replacement has been recommended as surgical treatment for HOCM by Cooley and colleagues.[C1,C2] Excision of the anterior mitral leaflet is said to relieve the obstruction entirely so that myectomy is not a necessary part of the operation; this did not prove to be true in at least one case (UAB). This approach may now be considered contraindicated because it substitutes a prosthesis with its long-term hazards for a mitral valve that is structurally essentially normal and that usually becomes competent after myectomy alone, because there may be an increased risk of periprosthetic leakage because of the lack of thickening in the mitral leaflets and the occasional ring calcification, and because exposing the valve may be difficult in the presence of extreme left ventricular hypertrophy and a relatively small left atrium (GLH, UAB). The small left ventricular cavity and bizarre shape make a low profile valve mandatory and, even then, disk movement can be compromised. Finally, few patients fail to obtain relief of obstruction by myectomy, which is a more satisfactory operation with more predictable long-term results.

Left Ventricular–Aortic Conduit

The use of a LV-Ao conduit device in patients with HOCM is not indicated because myectomy, properly performed, makes it an unnecessarily complex alternative.

Aortic Approach Alone versus Combined Aortic and Left Ventricular Approach

The results of these alternative techniques are comparable, and firm recommendations are therefore not appropriate. The combined operation may be preferred as a routine because myectomy can be more accurately performed under direct vision and because a left ventriculotomy does not add additional mortality or morbidity to the procedure (GLH). Moreover, an iatrogenic VSD is more confidently avoided. However, iatrogenic VSD has not occurred using primarily an aortic approach, and this approach may be preferred when applicable because of its simplicity (UAB).

REFERENCES

A

1. Adelman AG, Wigle ED, Ranganathan N, Webb GD, Kidd BSL, Bigelow WG, Silver MD. The clinical course in muscular subaortic stenosis. A retrospective and prospective study of 60 hemodynamically proved cases. *Ann Intern Med* 77:515, 1972.

2. Abasi AS, MacAlpin RN, Eber LM, Pearce ML. Echocardiographic diagnosis of idiopathic hypertrophic cardiomyopathy without outflow obstruction. *Circulation* 46:897, 1972.

3. Agnew TM, Barratt-Boyes BG, Brandt PWT, Roche AHG, Lowe JB, O'Brien KP. Surgical resection in idiopathic hypertrophic subaortic stenosis using a combined approach through aorta and left ventricle. A long-term follow-up study of 49 patients. *J Thorac Cardiovasc Surg* 74:307, 1977.

4. Adelman AG, McLoughlin MJ, Marquis Y, Auger P, Wigle ED: Left ventricular cineangiographic observations in muscular subaortic stenosis. *Am J Cardiol* 24:689, 1969.

5. Anderson DM, Raff GL, Ports TA, Brundage BH, Parmley WW, Chatterjee K: Hypertrophic obstructive cardiomyopathy. Effects of acute and chronic verapamil treatment on left ventricular systolic and diastolic function. *Br Heart J* 51:523, 1984.

B

1. Bjork VL, Radegran K: Obstructive cardiomyopathy. *J Cardiovasc Surg (Torino)* 17:376, 1976.

2. Barratt-Boyes BG, O'Brien KP: Surgical treatment of idiopathic hypertrophic subaortic stenosis using a combined left ventricular aortic approach in hypertrophic obstructive cardiomyopathy. Ciba Foudation Study Group No. 37. GEW Wolstenholme, M O'Connor (eds). London: J and A Churchill, 1971, p 150.

3. Bigelow WG, Trimble AS, Auger P, Marquis Y, Wigle ED: The ventriculomyotomy operation for muscular subaortic stenosis. A reappraisal. *J Thorac Cardiovasc Surg* 52:514, 1966.

4. Braunwald E: Editorial. Hypertrophic subaortic stenosis—a broadened concept. *Circulation* 26:161, 1962.

5. Brock RC: Functional obstruction of the left ventricle. *Guy's Hosp Rep* 106:221, 1957.

6. Bercu BA, Diettert GA, Danforth WH, Pund EE Jr, Ahlvin RC, Belliveau RR: Pseudoaortic stenosis produced by ventricular hypertrophy. *Am J Med* 25:814, 1958.

7. Braunwald E, Lambrew CT, Rockoff SD, Ross J Jr, Morrow AG: Idiopathic hypertrophic subaortic stenosis. 1. A description of the disease based upon an analysis of 64 patients. *Circulation* 29 and 30 (suppl IV):IV-1, 1964.

8. Braunwald E, Morrow AG, Cornell WP, Aygeu MM, Hilbish TF: Idiopathic hypertrophic subaortic stenosis: Clinical hemodynamic and angiographic manifestations. *Am J Med* 29:924, 1960.

9. Brock R: Aortic subvalvar stenosis: Surgical treatment. *Guy's Hosp Rep* 108:126, 1959.

10. Braunwald E, Ebert PA: Hemodynamic alterations in idiopathic hypertrophic subaortic stenosis induced by sympatho-mimetic drugs. *Am J Cardiol* 10:489, 1962.

11. Benchimol A, Legler JF, Dimond EG: The carotid tracing and apexcardiogram in subaortic stenosis and idiopathic myocardial hypertrophy. *Am J Cardiol* 11:427, 1963.

12. Brockenbrough EC, Braunwald E, Morrow AG: A hemodynamic technique for the detection of hypertrophic subaortic stenosis. *Circulation* 23:189, 1961.

13. Bulkley BH, D'Amico B, Taylor A: Extensive myocardial fiber

disarray in aortic and pulmonary atresia. Relevance to hypertrophic cardiomyopathy. *Circulation* 67:191, 1983.

14. Beahrs MM, Tajik AJ, Seward JB, Giuliani ER, McGoon DC: Hypertrophic obstructive cardiomyopathy: 10 to 21 year follow-up after partial septal myotomy. *Am J Cardiol* 51:1160, 1983.

15. Borer JS, Bacharach SL, Green MV, Kent KM, Rosing DR, Seides SF, Morrow AG, Epstein SE, Mack B, Farkas S: Effect of septal myotomy and myectomy on left ventricular systolic function at rest and during exercise in patients with IHSS. *Circulation* 60(suppl I):1–82, 1979.

16. Brugada P, Blar FW, de Zwaan C, Roy D, Green M, Wellens JH: "Saw-fish" systolic narrowing of the left anterior descending coronary artery—an angiographic sign of hypertrophic cardiomyopathy. *Circulation* 66:800, 1982.

17. Barratt-Boyes BG: A method of preserving and inserting a homograft valve. *Br J Surg* 52:11, 1965.

18. Bharati S, Lev M, Kirklin JW: *Cardiac Surgery and the Conduction System.* John Wiley & Sons, 1983.

C

1. Cooley DA, Wukasch DC, Leachman RD: Mitral valve replacement for idiopathic hypertrophic subaortic stenosis—results in 27 patients. *J Cardiovasc Surg (Torino)* 17:380, 1976.

2. Cooley DA, Leachman RD, Wukasch DC: Diffuse muscular subaortic stenosis: Surgical treatment. *Am J Cardiol* 31:1, 1973.

3. Come PC, Balkley BH, Goodman ZD, Hutchins GM, Pitt B, Fortuin NJ: Hypercontractile cardiac states simulating hypertrophic cardiomyopathy. *Circulation* 55:901, 1977.

4. Cooley DA, Bloodwell RD, Hallman G, La Sorte AF, Leachman RD, Chapman DW: Surgical treatment of muscular subaortic stenosis. Results from septectomy in 26 patients. *Circulation* 35 and 36(suppl I):I-124, 1967.

5. Clark CE, Henry WL, Epstein SE: Familial prevalence and genetic transmission of idiopathic hypertrophic subaortic stenosis. *N Engl J Med* 289:709, 1973.

6. Cooperman LB, Rosenblum R, Cohen MV: Abnormal septal contraction in idiopathic hypertrophic subaortic stenosis. *Circulation* 50(suppl III):III-29, 1974.

7. Criley MJ, Lewis KB, White RI, Ross RS: Pressure gradients without obstruction: A new concept of hypertrophic subaortic stenosis. *Circulation* 32:881, 1965.

D

1. Davies LG: A familial heart disease. *Br Heart J* 14:206, 1952.

2. Desilets DT, Kadell BM, Buttenberg HD, Goldbert SJ, MacAlpin RN: Angiographic demonstration of the ventricular septum. A new technique. *Radiology* 91:329, 1968.

3. Dobell ARC, Scott HJ: Hypertrophic subaortic stenosis: Evolution of a surgical technique. *J Thorac Cardiovasc Surg* 47:26, 1964.

4. Dembitsky WP, Weldon CS: Clinical experience with the use of a valve-bearing conduit to construct a second left ventricular outflow tract in cases of unresectable intra-ventricular obstruction. *Ann Surg* 184:317, 1976.

5. Dinsmore RE, Sanders CA, Hawthorne JW: Mitral regurgitation in idiopathic hypertrophic subaortic stenosis. *New Engl J Med* 275:1225, 1966.

E

1. Epstein SE, Henry WL, Clark CE, Roberts WC, Maron BJ, Ferrans VJ, Redwood DR, Morrow AG: NIH Conference: Asymmetric septal hypertrophy. *Anat Intern Med* 81:650, 1974.

2. Emanuel R, Marcomichelakis J, Withers R, O'Brien K: Asymmetric septal hypertrophy and hypertrophic cardiomyopathy. *Br Heart J* 49:309, 1983.

F

1. Ferrans VJ, Morrow AG, Roberts WC: Myocardial ultrastructure in idiopathic hypertrophic subaortic stenosis. A study of operatively excised left ventricular outflow tract muscle in 14 patients. *Circulation* 45:769, 1972.

2. Frank S, Braunwald E: Idiopathic hypertrophic subaortic stenosis. Clinical analysis of 126 patients with emphasis on the natural history. *Circulation* 37:759, 1968.

3. Fix P, Moberg A, Soderberg H, Karnell J: Muscular subvalvular aortic stenosis. Abnormal anterior mitral leaflet possibly the primary factor. *Acta Radiol (Diagn) (Stockh)* 2:177, 1964.

4. Falicov RE, Resnekov L: Mid-ventricular obstruction in hypertrophic obstructive cardiomyopathy. New diagnostic and therapeutic challenge. *Br Heart J* 39:701, 1977.

5. Fighali S, Krajcer Z, Leachman RD: Septal myomectomy and mitral valve replacement for idiopathic hypertrophic subaortic stenosis: Short- and long-term follow-up. *JACC* 3:1127, 1984.

G

1. Glancy DL, O'Brien KP, Gold HK, Epstein SE: Atrial fibrillation in patients with idiopathic hypertrophic subaortic stenosis. *Br Heart J* 32:652, 1970.

2. Goodwin JF: ? IHSS. ? HOCM. ? ASH. A plea for unity. *Am Heart J* 89:269, 1975 (editorial).

3. Gulotta SJ, Hamby RI, Aronson AL, Ewing K: Coexistent idiopathic hypertrophic subaortic stenosis and coronary artery disease. *Circulation* 46:890, 1972.

4. Goodwin FJ: Cardiac function in primary myocardial disorders. Part 1. *Br Med J* 1:1527, 1964.

5. Goodwin JF, Hollman A, Cleland WP, Teare D: Obstructive cardiomyopathy simulating aortic stenosis. *Br Heart J* 22:403, 1960.

6. Goodwin JF, Oakley CM: The cardiomyopathies. *Br Heart J* 34:545, 1972 (editorial).

7. Goodwin JF: Editorial. Hypertrophic cardiomyopathy: A disease in search of its own identity. *Am J Cardiol* 45:177, 1980.

8. Goodwin JF: The frontiers of cardiomyopathy. *Br Heart J* 48:1, 1982.

9. Gutgesell HP, Mullins CE, Gillette PC, Speer M, Rudolph AJ, McNamara DG: Transient hypertrophic subaortic stenosis in infants of diabetic mothers. *J Pediatr* 89:120, 1976.

10. Gill CC, Duda AM, Kitazume H, Kramer JR, Loop FD: Idiopathic hypertrophic subaortic stenosis and coronary atherosclerosis. Results of coronary artery bypass alone and myectomy combined with coronary artery bypass. *J Thorac Cardiovasc Surg* 84:856, 1982.

H

1. Hutchins GM, Bulkley BH: Catenoid shape of the interventricular septum: Possible cause of idiopathic hypertrophic subaortic stenosis. *Circulation* 58:392, 1978.

2. Henry WL, Clark CE, Griffith JM, Epstein SE: Mechanism of left ventricular outflow obstruction in patients with obstructive asymmetric septal hypertrophy (idiopathic hypertrophic subaortic stenosis). *Am J Cardiol* 35:337, 1975.

3. Henry WL, Clark CE, Epstein SE: Asymmetric septal hypertrophy (ASH): The unifying link in the IHSS disease spectrum.

Observations regarding its pathogenesis, pathophysiology and course. *Circulation* 47:827, 1973.

4. Henry WL, Clark CE, Roberts WC, Morrow AG, Epstein SE: Differences in distribution of myocardial abnormalities in patients with obstructive and non-obstructive asymmetric septal hypertrophy (ASH). Echocardiographic and gross anatomic findings. *Circulation* 50:447, 1974.

5. Harken DE: Discussion. *J Thorac Cardiovasc Surg* 47:33, 1964.

6. Henry WI, Clark CE, Epstein SE: Asymmetric septal hypertrophy. Echocardiographic identification of the pathognomonic anatomic abnormality of IHSS. *Circulation* 47:225, 1973.

7. Hallopeau. Retrecissement ventriculo-aortique. *Gaz Med Paris* 24:683, 1869.

8. Hoshino T, Fujiwara H, Kawai C, Hamashima Y: Myocardial fiber diameter and regional distribution in the ventricular wall of normal adult hearts, hypertensive hearts and hearts with hypertrophic cardiomyopathy. *Circulation* 67:1109, 1983.

9. Hoshino T, Fujiwara H, Kawai C, Hamashima Y: Diagnostic value of disarray in endomyocardial biopsy specimens in hypertrophic cardiomyopathy: A critical report based on distribution of disarray in the subendocardial region of autopsied hearts. *Jpn Circ J* 46:1281, 1982.

J

1. Julian OC, Dye WS, Javid H, Hunter JA, Muenster JJ, Najafi H: Apical left ventriculotomy in subaortic stenosis due to a fibromuscular hypertrophy. *Circulation* 31 and 32 (suppl I):I-44, 1965.

K

1. Krauss KR, Weisinger B, Glassman E: Mitral annular calcification and subaortic stenosis. *Circulation* 46(suppl II):II-178, 1972.

2. Kelly DT, Barratt-Boyes BG, Lowe JB: Results of surgery and hemodynamic observations in muscular subaortic stenosis. *J Thorac Cardiovasc Surg* 51:353, 1966.

3. Kirklin JW, Ellis FH Jr: Surgical relief of diffuse subvalvular aortic stenosis. *Circulation* 24:739, 1961.

4. Kitazume H, Kramer JR, Kruthamer D, Tobgi SE, Proudfit WL, Sones FM: Myocardial bridges in obstructive hypertrophic cardiomyopathy. *Am Heart J* 106:131, 1983.

5. Koch JP, Maron BJ, Epstein SE, Morrow AG: Results of operation for obstructive hypertrophic cardiomyopathy in the elderly. Septal myotomy and myectomy in 20 patients 65 years of age or older. *Am J Cardiol* 46:963, 1980.

L

1. Larter WE, Allen HD, Sahn DJ, Goldbert SJ: The asymmetrically hypertrophied septum. Further differentiation of its causes. *Circulation* 53:19, 1976.

2. Liouiville: Retrecissement cardiaque sous mortique. *Gaz Med Paris* 24:161, 1869.

3. Lillehei CW, Levy MJ: Transatrial exposure for correction of subaortic stenosis. A new approach. *JAMA* 186:8, 1963.

M

1. Morrow AG: Hypertrophic subaortic stenosis. Operative methods utilized to relieve left ventricular outflow obstruction. *J Thorac Cardiovasc Surg* 76:423, 1978.

2. Maron BJ, Roberts WC, Edwards JE, McAllister HA Jr, Foley DD, Epstein SE: Sudden death in patients with hypertrophic cardiomyopathy: Characterization of 26 patients without functional limitation. *Am J Cardiol* 41:803, 1978.

3. Maron BJ, Ferrans VJ, Henry WL, Clark CE, Redwood DR, Roberts WC, Morrow AG, Epstein SE: Differences in distribution of myocardial abnormalities in patients with obstructive and nonobstructive asymmetric septal hypertrophy (ASH). Light and electron microscopic findings. *Circulation* 50:436, 1974.

4. Maron BJ, Henry WL, Clark CE, Redwood DR, Roberts WC, Epstein SE: Asymmetric septal hypertrophy in childhood. *Circulation* 53:9, 1976.

5. Morrow AG, Reitz BA, Epstein SE, Henry WL, Conkle DM, Itscoitz SB, Redwood DR: Operative treatment in hypertrophic subaortic stenosis. Techniques and the results of pre- and postoperative assessments in 83 patients. *Circulation* 52:88, 1975.

6. Maron BJ, Merrill WH, Freier PA, Kent KM, Epstein SE, Morrow AG: Long-term clinical course and symptomatic status of patients after operation for hypertrophic subaortic stenosis. *Circulation* 57:1205, 1978.

7. Maron BJ, Gottdiener JS, Roberts WC, Henry WL, Savage DD, Epstein SE: Left ventricular outflow tract obstruction due to systolic anterior motion of the anterior mitral leaflet in patients with concentric left ventricular hypertrophy. *Circulation* 57:527, 1978.

8. Maron BJ, Edwards JE, Henry WL, Clark CE, Bingle GJ, Epstein SE: Asymmetric septal hypertrophy (ASH) in infancy. *Circulation* 50:809, 1974.

9. Morrow AG, Brockenbrough EC: Surgical treatment of idiopathic hypertrophic subaortic stenosis: Technique and hemodynamic results of subaortic ventriculomyotomy. *Ann Surg* 154:181, 1961.

10. Menges H Jr, Brandenberg RO, Brown AL Jr: The clinical, hemodynamic, and pathologic diagnosis of muscular subvalvular aortic stenosis. *Circulation* 24:1126, 1961.

11. Morrow AG, Braunwald E: Functional aortic stenosis. A malformation characterized by resistance to left ventricular outflow without anatomic obstruction. *Circulation* 20:181, 1959.

12. Morrow AG, Lambrew CT, Braunwald E: Idiopathic hypertrophic subaortic stenosis. 11. Operative treatment and the results of pre and postoperative hemodynamic evaluations. *Circulation* 29 and 30(suppl IV):IV-120, 1964.

13. Mintz GS, Kotler MN, Segal BL, Parry WR: Systolic anterior motion of the mitral valve in the absence of asymmetric septal hypertrophy. *Circulation* 57:256, 1978.

14. Maron BJ, Savage DD, Clark CE, Henry WL, Vlodaver Z, Edwards JE, Epstein SE: Prevalence and characteristics of disproportionate ventricular septal thickening in patients with coronary artery disease. *Circulation* 57:250, 1978.

15. Maron BJ, Edwards JE, Ferrans VJ, Clark CE, Lebowitz EA, Henry WL, Epstein SE: Congenital heart malformations associated with disproportionate ventricular septal thickening. *Circulation* 52:926, 1975.

16. McKenna W, Deanfield J, Farugui A, England D, Oakley C, Goodwin J: Prognosis in hypertrophic cardiomyopathy: Role of age and clinical electrocardiographic and hemodynamic features. *Am J Cardiol* 47:532, 1981.

17. Maron BJ, Epstein SE: Hypertrophic cardiomyopathy: A discussion of nomenclature. *Am J Cardiol* 43:1242, 1979.

18. Maron BJ, Roberts WC: Quantitative analysis of cardiac muscle cell disorganization in the ventricular septum of patients with hypertrophic cardiomyopathy. *Circulation* 59:689, 1979.

19. Maron BJ, Koch JP, Kent KM, Epstein SE, Morrow AG: Re-

sults of surgery for idiopathic hypertrophic subaortic stenosis. *J Cardiovasc Med* Feb:145, 1980.

20. Maron BJ, Epstein SE: Hypertrophic cardiomyopathy: Recent observations regarding the specificity of the three hallmarks of the disease: Asymmetric septal hypertrophy, septal disorganization and systolic anterior motion of the anterior mitral leaflet. *Am J Cardiol* 45:141, 1980.

21. Maron BJ, Gottdiener JS, Perry LW: Specificity of systolic anterior motion of anterior mitral leaflet for hypertrophic cardiomyopathy. Prevalence in large population of patients with other cardiac diseases. *Br Heart J* 45:206, 1981.

22. Maron BJ, Gottdiener JS, Epstein SE: Patterns and significance of distribution of left ventricular hypertrophy in hypertrophic cardiomyopathy. A wide angle, two dimensional echocardiographic study of 125 patients. *Am J Cardiol* 48:418, 1981.

23. Maron BJ, Gottdiener JS, Bonow RO, Epstein SE: Hypertrophic cardiomyopathy with unusual locations of left ventricular hypertrophy undetectable by M-mode echocardiography. Identification by wide-angle two-dimensional echocardiography. *Circulation* 63:409, 1981.

24. Morrow AG, Koch JP, Maron BJ, Kent KM, Epstein SE: Left ventricular myotomy and myectomy in patients with obstructive hypertrophic cardiomyopathy and previous cardiac arrest. *Am J Cardiol* 46:313, 1980.

25. Maron BJ, Epstein SE, Roberts WC: Hypertrophic cardiomyopathy and transmural myocardial infarction without significant atherosclerosis of the extramural coronary arteries. *Am J Cardiol* 43:1086, 1979.

26. McKenna WJ, Chetty S, Oakley CM, Goodwin JF: Arrhythmias in hypertrophic cardiomyopathy: Exercise and 48-hour non-ambulatory electrocardiographic assessment with and without eta adrenergic blocking therapy. *Am J Cardiol* 45:1, 1980.

27. Maron BJ, Wolfson JK, Cirjo E, Spirito P: Relation of electrocardiographic abnormalities and patterns of left ventricular hypertrophy identified by 2-dimensional echocardiography in patients with hypertrophic cardiomyopathy. *Am J Cardiol* 51:189, 1983.

28. Maron BJ: Asymmetry in hypertrophic cardiomyopathy: The septal to free wall thickness ratio revisited. *Am J Cardiol* 55:835, 1985 (editorial).

O

1. Oakley CM: Hypertrophic obstructive cardiomyopathy. Patterns of progression in hypertrophic obstructive cardiomyopathy. Ciba Foundation Study Group No. 37. GEW Wolstenholme, M O'Conner (eds). London: J and A Churchill 1971, p 9.

P

1. Pridie RB, Oakley CM: Mechanism of mitral regurgitation in hypertrophic obstructive cardiomyopathy. *Br Heart J* 32:203, 1970.

2. Popp RL, Harrison DC: Ultrasound in the diagnosis and evaluation of therapy in idiopathic hypertrophic subaortic stenosis. *Circulation* 40:905, 1969.

R

1. Reis RL, Hannah H III, Carley JE, Pugh DM: Surgical treatment of idiopathic hypertrophic subaortic stenosis (IHSS). Postoperative result in 30 patients following ventricular septal myotomy and myectomy (Morrow procedure). *Circulation* 56(suppl II):II-128, 1977.

2. Rodger JC: Motion of mitral apparatus in hypertrophic cardiomyopathy with obstruction. *Br Heart J* 38:732, 1976.

3. Rossen RM, Goodman DJ, Ingham RE, Popp RL: Ventricular septal thickening and excursion in idiopathic hypertrophic subaortic stenosis. *Circulation* 50(suppl III):III-29, 1974.

4. Rosing DR, Idänpään-Heikkilä U, Maron BJ, Bonow RO, Epstein SE: Use of calcium-channel blocking drugs in hypertrophic cardiomyopathy. *Am J Cardiol* 55:185B, 1985.

S

1. Senning A, Transventricular relief of idiopathic hypertrophic subaortic stenosis. *J Cardiovasc Surg (Torino)* 17:371, 1976.

2. Savage DD, Seides SF, Clark CE, Henry WL, Maron BJ, Robinson FC, Epstein SE: Electrocardiographic findings in patients with obstructive and non-obstructive hypertrophic cardiomyopathy. *Circulation* 58:402, 1978.

3. Spray TL, Maron BJ, Morrow AG, Epstein SE, Roberts WC: Clinical pathologic conference. A discussion on hypertrophic cardiomyopathy. *Am Heart J* 95:511, 1978.

4. Somerville J, Becu L: Congenital heart disease associated with hypertrophic cardiomyopathy. *Br Heart J* 40:1034, 1978.

5. Spirito P, Maron BJ, Rosing DR: Morphologic determinants of hemodynamic state after ventricular septal myotomy-myectomy in patients with obstructive hypertrophic cardiomyotomy: M mode and two-dimensional echocardiographic assessment. *Circulation* 70:984, 1984.

6. Shapira JN, Stemple DR, Martin RP, Rakowski H, Stinson EB, Popp RL: Single and two-dimensional echocardiographic visualization of the effects of septal myectomy in idiopathic hypertrophic subaortic stenosis. *Circulation* 58:850, 1978.

7. Shah PM, Adelman AG, Wigle ED, Gobel FL, Burchell HB, Hardarson T, Curiel R, de la Calzada C, Oakley CM, Goodwin JF: The natural (and unnatural) history of hypertrophic obstructive cardiomyopathy. A multicenter study. *Circ Res* 34–35(suppl II):179, 1974.

8. Swan H: Subaortic muscular stenosis: A new surgical technique for repair. *J Thorac Cardiovasc Surg* 47:681, 1964.

9. Somerville J, Bonham Carter RE: The heart in lentiginosis. *Br Heart J* 34:58, 1972.

10. Shah PM, Gramiak R, Kramer DH: Ultrasound location of left ventricular outflow obstruction in hypertrophic obstructive cardiomyopathy. *Circulation* 40:3, 1969.

11. Schmincke A: Ueber linksseitige muskulose conusstenosen. *Dtsch Med Wochenschr* 2:2082, 1907.

12. Swan DA, Bell B, Oakley CM, Goodwin J: Analysis of symptomatic course and prognosis and treatment of hypertrophic obstructive cardiomyopathy. *Br Heart J* 33:671, 1971.

13. Spirito P, Maron BJ: Significance of left ventricular outflow tract cross-sectional area in hypertrophic cardiomyopathy: A two-dimensional echocardiographic assessment. *Circulation* 67:1100, 1983.

14. Shah PM, Taylor RD, Wong M: Abnormal mitral valve coaptation in hypertrophic obstructive cardiomyopathy: Proposed role in systolic anterior motion of mitral valve. *Am J Cardiol* 48:258, 1981.

15. Shapiro LM, McKenna WJ: Distribution of left ventricular hypertrophy in hypertrophic cardiomyopathy: A two-dimensional echocardiographic study. *JACC* 2:437, 1983.

16. Sheikhzadeh A, Ghabussi P: A case of asymmetrical apical hypertrophy which is a form of hypertrophic nonobstructive cardiomyopathy with giant negative T waves. *Jpn Heart J* 23:843, 1982.

17. St. John Sutton MG, Tajik AJ, Giuliani ER, Gordon H, Su WP: Hypertrophic obstructive cardiomyopathy and lentiginosis: A little known neural ectodermal syndrome. *Am J Cardiol* 47:214, 1981.

18. Savage DD, Seides SF, Maron BJ, Myers DJ, Epstein SE: Prevalence of arrhythmias during 24-hour electrocardiographic monitoring and exercise testing in patients with obstructive and nonobstructive hypertrophied cardiomyopathy. *Circulation* 59: 866, 1979.

19. Stewart S, Schreiner B: Coexisting idiopathic hypertrophic subaortic stenosis and coronary artery disease. Clinical implications and operative management. *J Thorac Cardiovasc Surg* 82:278, 1981.

20. Spicer RL, Rocchini AP, Crowley DC, Rosenthal A: Chronic verapamil therapy in pediatric and young adult patients with hypertrophic cardiomyopathy. *Am J Cardiol* 53:1614, 1984.

T

1. Tajik AJ, Giuliani ER, Weidman WH, Brandenberg RO, McGoon DC: Idiopathic hypertrophic subaortic stenosis. Long-term surgical follow-up. *Am J Cardiol* 34:815, 1974.

2. Trimble AS, Bigelow WG, Wigle ED, Chrysohon A: Simple and effective surgical approach to muscular subaortic stenosis. *Circulation* 29(suppl):125, 1964.

3. Teare RD: Asymmetrical hypertrophy of the heart in young adults. *Br Heart J* 20:1, 1958.

4. Tajik AJ, Giuliani ER, Frye RL, Davis GD, McGoon DC, Brandenberg RO: Mitral valve and/or annulus calcification associated with idiopathic hypertrophic subaortic stenosis (IHSS). *Circulation* 46(suppl II):II-228, 1972 (abstr).

5. Tajik AJ, Giuliani ER: Electrocardiographic observations in idiopathic hypertrophic subaortic stenosis. *Mayo Clin Proc* 49:89, 1974.

V

1. Van Der Bel-Kahn J: Muscle fiber disarray in common heart diseases. *Am J Cardiol* 40:355, 1977.

W

1. Wigle ED, Silver MD: Editorial. Myocardial fiber disarray and ventricular septal hypertrophy in asymmetrical hypertrophy of the heart. *Circulation* 58:398, 1978.

2. Wigle ED, Adelman AG, Auger P, Marquis Y: Mitral regurgitation in muscular subaortic stenosis. *Am J Cardiol* 24:698, 1969.

3. Wigle ED, Heimbecker RO, Gunton EW: Idiopathic ventricular septal hypertrophy causing muscular subaortic stenosis. *Circulation* 26:325, 1962.

4. Wei JY, Weiss JL, Bulkley BH: The heterogenicity of hypertrophic cardiomyopathy: An autopsy and one dimensional echocardiographic study. *Am J Cardiol* 45:24, 1980.

5. Waller BF, Maron BJ, Epstein SE, Roberts WC: Transmural myocardial infarction in hypertrophic cardiomyopathy: A cause of conversion from left ventricular asymmetry to symmetry and from normal-sized to dilated left ventricular cavity. *Chest* 79:461, 1981.

Y

1. Yamaguchi H, Ishimura T, Nishiyama S, Nakanishi S, Takatsu F, Nishijo T, Ameda T, Machi K: Hypertrophic unobstructive cardiomyopathy with giant negative T waves (apical hypertrophy): Ventriculographic and echocardiographic features in 30 patients. *Am J Cardiol* 44:401, 1979.

34

COARCTATION OF THE AORTA AND AORTIC ARCH INTERRUPTIONS

SECTION 1

COARCTATION OF THE AORTA

DEFINITION

Coarctation of the aorta is classically a congenital narrowing of the upper descending thoracic aorta adjacent to the site of attachment of the ductus arteriosus which is sufficiently severe that there is a pressure gradient across the area. Sometimes it is combined with more proximal aortic narrowing. Uncommonly, coarctation occurs more proximally, between the left common carotid and subclavian arteries. The aortic lumen may be atretic, but in coarctation the aortic walls above and below the atresia are in continuity, as distinguished from the situation in aortic arch interruption, in which a short distance separates the aortic ends (see Section 2). The occasional examples of coarctation of the lower thoracic and abdominal aorta are not considered in this chapter.

Coarctation with or without patent ductus arteriosus but without other major associated cardiac anomalies is termed *primary*, or *pure, coarctation*.

HISTORICAL NOTE

Morgagni is credited in 1760 with the first description of an aortic coarctation that was found at autopsy, whereas Paris some 30 years later was the first to describe the pathologic features fully.[C1] In 1903, Bonnett suggested dividing the lesion into adult (postductal) and infantile (preductal) types,[B1] a classification that has tended to persist ever since. By 1928, Maude Abbott was able to review 200 autopsy cases in subjects over 2 years of age.[A1] The natural history of this age group was further elucidated by review of the 104 autopsy cases reported subsequently between 1928 and 1946 and collected by Reifenstein, Levine, and Gross.[R1] The fact that coarctation was frequently a cause of death in infancy was not appreciated in these earlier reports. Indeed, it was not until the 1950s that this aspect was adequately documented.[B7,C2]

Animal experiments designed to develop surgical treatment were published in 1944 by Blalock and Park.[B2] Their procedure involved turndown of the divided left subclavian artery onto the aorta, a technique that they recognized would not provide complete relief. Experiments involving excision and end-to-end anastomosis were commenced in

1938 by Gross and Hufnagel.[G1] In their classic article published in 1945, they described in detail the technique of end-to-end anastomosis, including the method of suturing and the design of appropriate clamps. They also noted that the hindquarter paralysis that occurred in some of their experimental animals was unlikely to be a problem in humans with coarctation because of the presence of a collateral circulation and that it seemed to be prevented "by packing the entire back of the animal in ice." They predicted the use of homograft aorta where end-to-end anastomosis was not practicable.

The first coarctation repair in a patient was performed by Crafoord in October 1944.[C3] Gross's first patient was operated upon in June 1945.[G2] The procedure was rapidly adopted worldwide. Thus, Clagett in 1948 was able to report the first 21 patients operated upon at the Mayo Clinic.[C4] In 8 of them end-to-end anastomosis was not considered wise, and Blalock's left subclavian turndown operation was performed instead. The first coarctectomy at GLH was performed in 1949. Extension of the operation into the infant group began in 1950 when Burford attempted unsuccessfully to reconstruct an infant aorta using an arterial graft.[C2] A successful end-to-end anastomosis in an infant was reported by Lynxwiler and associates in 1951[L1] and by us at the Mayo Clinic in a 10-week-old infant in 1952.[K1] Mustard reported a successful result in a 12-day-old infant in 1953.[M1]

Subsequent modifications in surgical technique include the use of prosthetic onlay grafts across the coarctation site or of a simple vertical incision and its transverse closure by Vorsschulte in 1957[V1] and the subclavian patch aortoplasty by Waldhausen in 1966.[W1] The use of a prosthetic tube graft as an alternative to the homograft, which was preferred by Gross,[G3] was reported by Morris, Cooley, DeBakey, and Crawford in 1960.[M2]

MORPHOLOGY

Coarctation

Coarctations vary in severity. When the stenosis is localized, the lumen must be reduced in cross-sectional area by more than about 50% before there is a pressure gradient across it, but longer tubular coarctations may be hemodynamically significant with lesser narrowing.[G4] Thirty-three percent of autopsy specimens show moderate luminal narrowing, 42% severe (pinhole) stenosis, and 25% luminal atre-

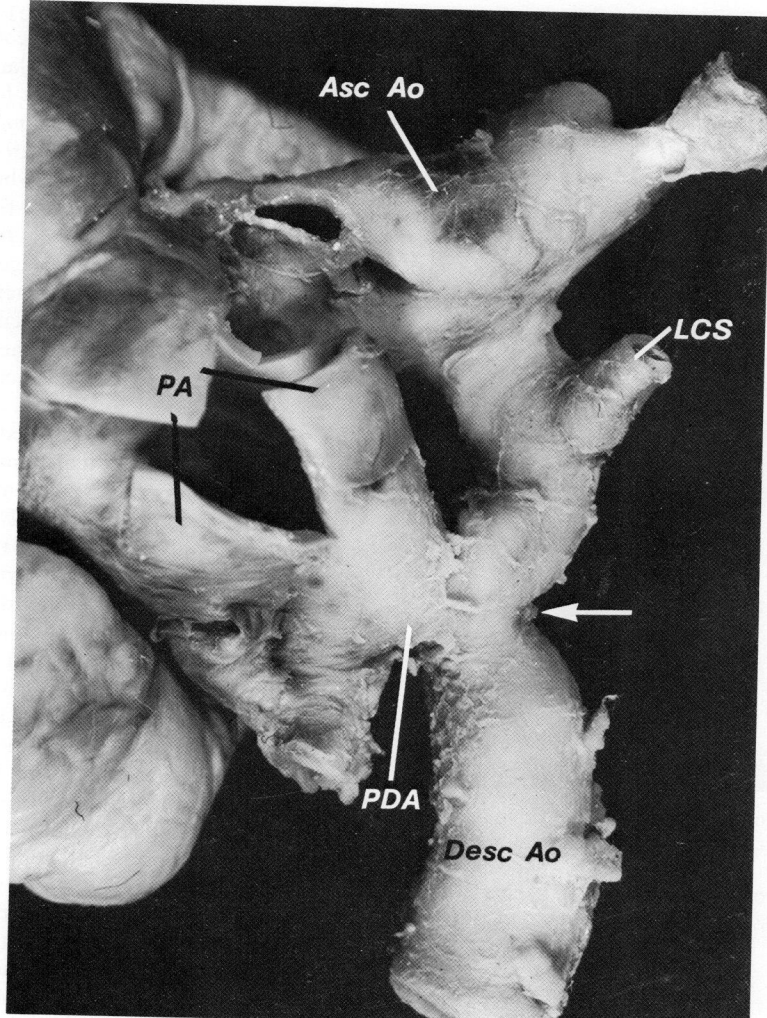

Figure 34-1 Autopsy specimen from 6-week-old girl showing a juxtaductal coarctation due to a localized shelf with a typical external deformity of the aorta at the site of narrowing (arrow) (GLH). Asc Ao, ascending aorta; Desc Ao, descending aorta; LSC, left subclavian artery; PA, main pulmonary artery; PDA, patent ductus arteriosus.

sia.[R1] Occasionally, the adult aorta may be redundant and severely kinked opposite the ligamentum arteriosum without any pressure gradient, the so-called pseudocoarctation lesion.[W2]

The localized lesion of classic coarctation is a *shelf*, or projection, or infolding of the aortic media into the lumen, which is most prominent in that portion of the circumference opposite the ductus arteriosus (the superior or leftward wall). This inward projection of the media is present also on the anterior and posterior walls but absent on the ductal side (inferior or rightward wall). The shelf is usually marked externally by a localized indentation or waisting of the left aortic wall as if a string had been tied around it, pulling the aorta toward the mediastinum[E1,P8] (Figs. 34-1 and 34-2). The external narrowing may be absent in the young infant.[H1] The aorta beyond the narrowing usually shows poststenotic dilatation, and paradoxically the wall beyond the stricture is usually thicker than that just proximal to it where the pres-

sure is higher. The localized shelf or curtain of media and intima lies adjacent to the ductus arteriosus in utero and to the ligamentum arteriosum should the ductus close. The shelf may be pre- or postductal but is usually juxtaductal.[R2] Hutchins has pointed out that the histologic features of this aortic media infolding are identical to those seen at a branch point of the normal aorta.[H2]

In addition to the infolding of aortic media, there is usually a localized ridge of *intimal hypertrophy* (so-called intimal veil) that extends the shelf circumferentially and further narrows the lumen. Pellegrino and colleagues have considered this to resemble ductal tissue.[P8] This intimal change is believed to be secondary and progressive.[E2,K2] Rodbard has presented experimental and theoretical evidence that would indicate that the lowering of lateral pressure on the aortic wall secondary to the increase in velocity that occurs across a site of narrowing (according to the Bernoulli principle) allows the endothelial cells to multiply until probe patency is

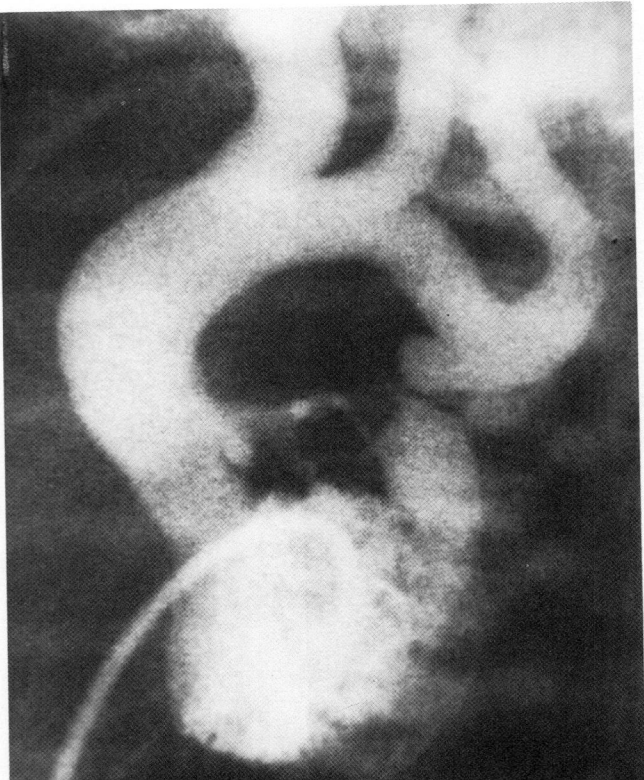

Figure 34-2 Cineangiocardiogram in left anterior oblique view with injection into left ventricle, showing severe coarctation due to a localized shelf opposite an obliterated ductus arteriosus in a 5-day-old infant (GLH). No other cardiovascular anomaly was demonstrated. Note the marked angulation of the aorta toward the mediastinum.

reached.[R3,R4] The resistance to flow across this stenosis then lowers the velocity so that ingrowth usually stops.

Many specimens of aortic coarctation show, in addition to the localized shelf, a more diffuse narrowing due to hypoplasia of the aortic isthmus between the left subclavian artery and the coarctation, or between the left subclavian artery and the left common carotid artery, or both (Fig. 34-3). This lesion is conveniently called *tubular hypoplasia*. Since there may occasionally be severe tubular hypoplasia without a localized shelf, particularly in infants, the term *coarctation* should not be confined to a localized infolding of the aortic media as originally suggested by Edwards.[E2] DeBoer, Lev, and associates have postulated that in some specimens with tubular hypoplasia a localized narrowing may be entirely acquired;[D1] Allan and colleagues, however, have studied the evolution of coarctation in intrauterine life by echocardiography and consider the isthmal hypoplasia to be secondary to the coarctation.[A6] In so-called preductal coarctation, the aortic isthmus is invariably narrowed. This lesion nearly always presents in infancy in association with a still patent ductus arteriosus and usually in combination with other congenital cardiac defects. In 78 infants under 6 months of age, Sinha et al. found that 16 had a localized shelf only, 7 a tubular hypoplasia only, and 55 had both lesions.[S2]

Rudolph postulates that the type of coarctation is related to fetal flow patterns through the ductus and the aorta.[R2] He has shown in the normal fetal lamb, that flow through the aortic isthmus is approximately half that across the ductus (25% compared to 42%), explaining the smaller diameter of the aortic isthmus compared with ascending and descending aorta in the normal human newborn.[R2] The localized shelf opposite the ductus may result from a reorientation of the angle at which the ductus meets the aorta. The tendency for a shelf to develop could be exaggerated in those instances in which ductal flow is further increased relative to isthmal flow, for example, with a ventricular septal defect (VSD).[H2] In addition, the isthmus becomes more hypoplastic when ascending aortic flow is diminished by lesions that impair left ventricular output in utero (e.g., aortic and mitral stenosis). In contrast, the diameter of the isthmus (and flow through it) is increased by those malformations that decrease flow through the ductus (e.g., pulmonary stenosis), and in these conditions coarctation is virtually unknown.[H2,S1]

Rudolph has also pointed out that a localized juxtaductal aortic shelf may be present at birth without producing aortic obstruction, provided the ductus remains widely patent.[R2] The ductus closes first at its pulmonary end, and obliteration of its aortic end may be delayed for several days; it is only then that a gradient occurs.[T1] The earlier suggestion that the process indicating ductal closure could extend to involve and narrow the juxtaductal aorta (the Skodaic theory)[B3] is supported by the recent report from Ho and Anderson.[H1] Using serial sectioning techniques, these authors have confirmed that there is a sling of ductal tissue completely surrounding the juxtaductal aorta so that "the ductus and descending aorta form a common channel of structural continuity, and the isthmus enters this channel rather than the reverse."

Tubular hypoplasia between the left subclavian and left common carotid arteries in young infants is common, but usually there is no pressure gradient across the area. The explanation for the frequently found hypoplasia of this segment of aortic arch is uncertain. Hutchins has suggested that in those cases in which ductal flow exceeds that in the ascending aorta, flow in the isthmus may be reversed so that the left subclavian artery is supplied via the ductus arteriosus.[H2] Under such circumstances, flow in the arch between the left subclavian and common carotid arteries would be low and its diameter reduced.

Collateral Circulation

The collateral circulation between aorta proximal to the coarctation and that distal to it is one of the striking features of coarctation. When well developed, it is responsible for some of the classic signs of the malformation, such as parascapular pulsations and rib notching. It is usually present to some extent in newborns but increases in size and extensiveness as the patient ages (Fig. 34-4).

Inflow into the collateral circulation is widespread but is primarily from the branches of both subclavian arteries, particularly the internal mammary, vertebral, costocervical, and thyrocervical trunks. *Outflow* from the collateral system

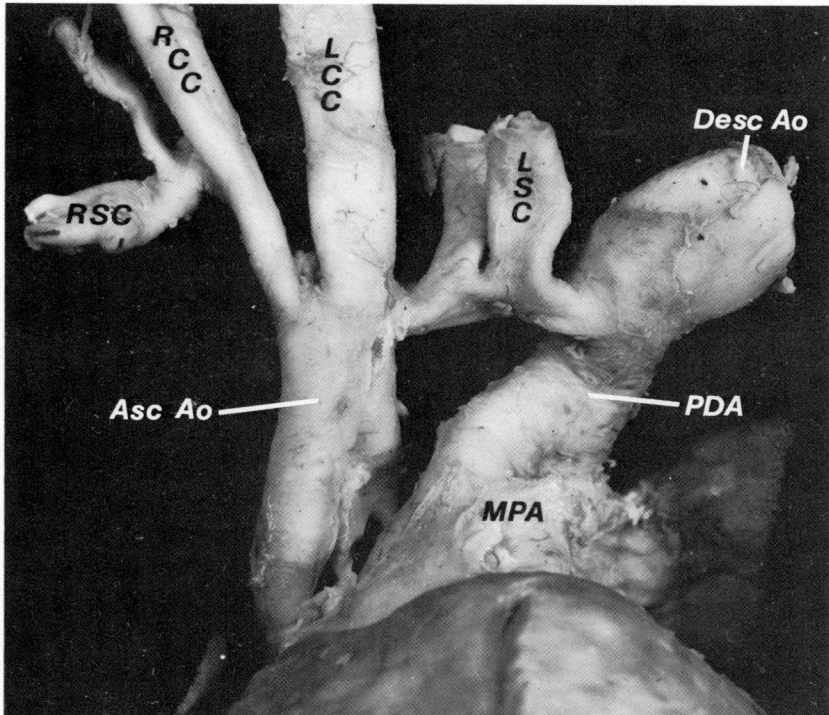

Figure 34-3 Autopsy specimen from 5-day-old infant with coarctation demonstrating tubular hypoplasia of the aortic arch between the left common carotid artery and the patent ductus arteriosus (a variety of so-called preductal coarctation) (GLH). A large left vertebral artery arises separately from the arch proximal to the left subclavian artery. This infant also had perimembranous and muscular ventricular septal defects and mild mitral valve hypoplasia.

Asc Ao, ascending aorta; Desc Ao, descending aorta; LCC, left common carotid artery; LSC, left subclavian artery; LSC, left subclavian artery; MPA, main pulmonary artery; PDA, patent ductus arteriosus; RCC, right common carotid; RSC, right subclavian artery.

to the lower body is more limited and is primarily into the descending thoracic aorta. The largest *vessels* participating in this outflow are usually the first two pairs of intercostal arteries distal to the coarctation. These are the third and fourth intercostal arteries, and they are greatly enlarged by the large reversed collateral flow. This reversed flow into the aorta has been demonstrated at operation by directional Doppler velocity detector probes; the flow returns to a normal direction immediately after coarctation repair.[B4] (Only the intercostals carrying this large reversed flow are sufficiently enlarged to produce rib notching, which explains the lack of notching of the first and second ribs.) The lower intercostal arteries also provide outflow pathways from the collateral circulation, as do the inferior epigastric artery and other branches of the abdominal aorta.

The collateral circulation and its clinical manifestations are altered by anatomic variations around a classic coarctation. Associated stenosis at the origin of the left subclavian artery excludes this artery as an important source of inflow into the collateral circulation, and thus rib notching occurs only on the *right* side. When the right subclavian artery arises as the fourth aortic branch (see Chapter 38) and distal to the coarctation, it does not serve as a source of inflow, and rib notching occurs only on the *left* side.

Aneurysm Formation

The enlarged, tortuous third and fourth intercostal arteries may become aneurysmal,[E2] but this is rare before about 10 years of age. These thin-walled *aneurysms* are usually saccular and are prone to occur at the aortic origin of the intercostals. That this is a weak point is a fact of surgical significance; if an enlarged intercostal artery in coarctation must be ligated, the ligature should be a few millimeters *beyond* its aortic origin.

The aorta itself may become aneurysmal adjacent to the site of maximal narrowing as a result of hemodynamic effects, aortic dissection, or a mycotic aneurysm. These also are uncommon in young children. The overall incidence of aneurysm is about 10% by the end of the second decade of life, 20% by the end of the third decade, and probably even higher in older patients[S3] (Table 34-1).

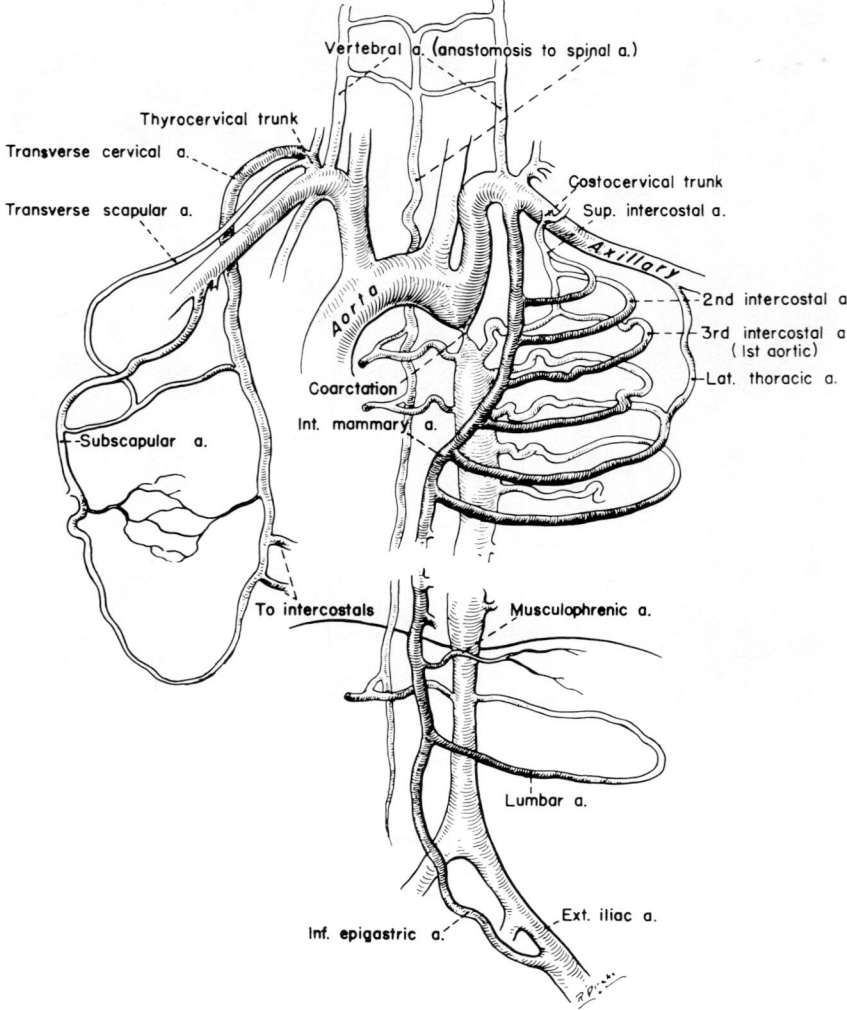

Figure 34-4   The major collateral channels in coarctation of the aorta. Reproduced with permission from Edwards et al.[E2]

Coronary Arteries

The left ventricular hypertrophy that occurs in untreated cases is accompanied by histologic changes in the coronary arteries.[V2] In the young patients, nonatherosclerotic lesions are conspicuous in the intimal layer. These consist of degenerative and proliferative changes of the elastic fibers and excess collagenous tissue. There is medial thickening to about twice normal with a rich elastic fiber network and often hyaline changes. The mean total area of the coronary arteries is increased so that they have a greater than normal capacity, presumably in response to the increased metabolic requirements of the left ventricle. As a result of prolonged hypertension, atheromatous changes are prone to occur more often and at a younger age.

Left Ventricle

Left ventricular hypertrophy without volume increase is present in most patients with coarctation within a few days of birth. This progresses as the patient ages and may be aggravated by associated cardiac anomalies.

Aortic Valve

A bicuspid aortic valve has long been known to be common in patients with coarctation. The exact incidence of bicuspid aortic valves in coarctation remains speculative. In two autopsy series it was 46%[B5] and 27%,[T2] with an additional 6% and 7%, respectively, with congenital valvar stenosis. Tawes and associates note in their report[T2] that among 250 living

Table 34-1 Aneurysms present at operation in patients age 1–64 years (GLH; *n* = 224).

Site of Aneurysm	No. of Cases	Age at Operation (yr)	
		Mean	Range
Aortic isthmus	4	27	(7–35)
Postcoarctation aortic segment	5	28	(5–64)
Intercostal arteries			
Single	6	27	(10–45)
Multiple	5	46	(31–54)
Subclavian artery	1	5	
Total	21	31	(5–64)

children with long-term follow-up, 32 (13%) had clinical evidence of aortic valve disease (mainly stenosis but also incompetence). When aortic incompetence appears in coarctation, it is usually on the basis of a bicuspid aortic valve combined with persistent hypertension.

Intracranial Aneurysm

There appears to be a coexistence of coarctation and berry-type intracranial aneurysm in some patients. Some instances of sudden death in untreated (and also treated) patients with coarctation have been shown to be from rupture of the intracranial aneurysm.

Associated Cardiac Anomalies

When coarctation presents in older children and young adults (as it generally did in the early years after surgical treatment began), the frequency of associated cardiac anomalies is not evident. When it presents in younger children and infants, and particularly in neonates, this frequency becomes clearly evident. Forty percent of patients coming to operation after the first year of life have an associated cardiac lesion (other than bicuspid aortic valve), compared with about 80% of infants (GLH; Tables 34-2 and 34-3). About 60% of those undergoing coarctation repair in the first 3 months of life have a major associated cardiac lesion, compared with 25% of those between 6 and 12 months of age (GLH). This high incidence in the very young is corroborated by Shinebourne and colleagues, who reported that 85% of neonates presenting with coarctation have major associated cardiac defects, compared with 52% of those aged 1–11 months.[S4]

A patent ductus arteriosus is present in almost 100% of neonates and in most infants with a preductal type of coarctation.[T3] This is considered as part of the coarctation complex rather than an additional anomaly. Tubular hypoplasia is also included as part of the anomaly rather than as an associated defect. Atrial septal defect is not considered as an additional anomaly unless large enough to need closure. This excludes the fairly numerous examples of infants presenting with a left-to-right shunt through a stretched patent foramen ovale that may subsequently close.

As previously mentioned, it is postulated that in many

instances it is the disturbance in the flow pattern that the associated lesions produce that influences the formation of the juxtaductal shelf of coarctation, or a tubular hypoplasia, or both.[R2] Thus, the association of coarctation with left-sided obstructive lesions, which divert flow away from the ascending aorta, such as aortic stenosis in its various forms, mitral valve lesions producing stenosis or incompetence, and those varieties of truncus arteriosus with a large patent ductus arteriosus and a hypoplastic ascending aorta, is well documented.[B5,F1,R2,S1,T3,V3] Conversely, malformations in which pulmonary (and ductal) flow is reduced in utero and isthmal flow is correspondingly increased are generally *not* associated with coarctation.[H2,S1] Examples are pulmonary stenosis and atresia, tetralogy of Fallot, and tricuspid atresia with normally positioned great arteries. The cause of the frequent association of coarctation with lesions producing a *left-to-right shunt postpartum* (VSD, atrial septal defect, atrioventricular canal, common ventricle, total anomalous pulmonary venous connection, double outlet right ventricle, transposition of the great arteries with a large ventricular septal defect) is less clear, although in some instances these lesions may be associated with subaortic obstruction.[R2] Coarctation is rare in *right-sided aortic arch*,[H3] presumably because of altered flow patterns in ductus and isthmus with this arrangement of great vessels.[R2]

CLINICAL FEATURES AND DIAGNOSTIC CRITERIA

The diagnostic criteria and mode of presentation vary according to age.

Infancy

The signs and symptoms of coarctation presenting in the neonate are those of heart failure. After a variable period of well being, the infant develops tachypnea, feeding problems, and sweating. On examination, there is a gallop rhythm and a systolic murmur along the left sternal edge and usually posteriorly over the coarctation site. The femoral pulse is absent or reduced in volume and delayed in comparison with the radial or brachial pulse, although in small, sick infants with tachycardia pulse delay may be difficult to detect. There is a higher blood pressure in the arms than the legs (>20 mmHg). The delay in onset of heart failure is probably related, at least in primary or pure coarctation, to the variable time it may take for the ductus to close. Closure usually commences at the pulmonary end, and it is not until the aortic end is occluding that the juxtaductal aortic shelf produces severe obstruction (see "Morphology").[F3,R2,T1] Thus, femoral pulses can be normal at birth but absent at 1 week.[T1]

When the ductus arteriosus remains widely patent and a severe coarctation lies proximal to it (preductal coarctation), there may be a right-to-left shunt into the descending aorta and, classically, cyanosis of the toes and sometimes the left hand while the right hand and lips remain pink (differential cyanosis). The femoral pulse under these circumstances is normal, and there is no ductus murmur. In fact, differential

Table 34-2 Associated congenital cardiac anomalies in patients undergoing repair of coarctation (GLH; 1949–1978).

Associated Cardiac Anomaly		< 1 Year (1960–1979) No.	% of 94	1–64 Years (1949–1977) No.	% of 224
No associated lesion		18	19% } 36%	135	60% } 69%
Patent ductus arteriosus only		16	17%	21	9%
Patent ductus arteriosus^a		53(53)^c	56%	33(33)	15%
Large	21			3	
Moderate	10			4	
Small	22			26	
Ventricular septal defect		32(11)	34%	13(5)	6%
Large	16(10)			6(4)	
Moderate	10(1)			1	
Small	6			6(1)	
Mitral stenosis^a		0	0%	2(1)	0.9%
Mitral stenosis + other lesions^a		2(1)	2%		
Mitral incompetence^a		4	4%	6	3%
Aortic stenosis^b		6(5)	6%	13(7)	6%
Aortic incompetence^a		2	2%	26(8)	12%
Pulmonary stenosis^a		0	0%	2	0.9%
Peripheral pulmonary arterial stenosis		0	0%	1	0.4%
Atrial septal defect^a		1(1)	1%	1(1)	0.4%
Partial AV canal^a		1(1)	1%	0	0%
PAPVC^a		1	1%	1	0.4%
TAPVC^a		0	0%	1(1)	0.4%
Single ventricle		3	3%		
TGA + VSD ± PDA		8(6)	9%		
DORV ± PDA		5(1)	5%		
Congenitally corrected TGA		0	0%	1(1)	0.4%
Origin LCC from RPA		1(1)	1%	0	0%
Total		94	100%	224	100%

KEY: AV, atrioventricular; DORV, double outlet right ventricle; LCC, left circumflex coronary artery; PAPVC, partial anomalous pulmonary venous connection; PDA, patent ductus arteriosus; RPA, right pulmonary artery; TAPVC, total anomalous pulmonary venous connection; TGA, transposition of the great arteries; VSD, ventricular septal defect.

^a These anomalies did not preclude categorization of the patient as "primary, pure coarctation."

^b Five of the 19 had discrete subvalvar aortic stenosis.

^c ( ) Indicates operations for correction of the associated cardiac lesions.

cyanosis is uncommon either because flow through the coarctation is significant or because the Po_2 of the pulmonary artery blood is high from an additional intracardiac shunt through a ventricular septal defect (VSD), or an atrial communication, or both. Moreover, despite the presence of a severe coarctation proximal to a patent ductus arteriosus, the systemic vascular resistance in the lower compartment usually exceeds pulmonary vascular resistance so that the ductal shunt is left to right.[K3]

In infancy, hypertension may be present but is seldom severe, and a collateral circulation is not palpable although it is usually present angiographically[11] (Fig. 34-5). Marked cardiomegaly is almost invariable on the chest x-ray. The electrocardiogram usually shows right ventricular hypertrophy in the first few months of life even with isolated coarctation.[S2] About two-thirds of the infants operated upon in the first year of life have right ventricular hypertrophy or combined hypertrophy, and fewer than 25% have pure left ventricular hypertrophy.[H4,P1]

When associated intracardiac defects are present, heart failure tends to be more severe, even earlier in onset, and responds less well to decongestive measures. Thus, a complicating lesion should be suspected when the baby does not respond promptly to medical management.[F4]

Coarctation may be unsuspected in complex lesions when the baby is in extremis, since even when the ductus is closed, a large left-to-right shunt proximal to the aorta can decrease the manifestation of hypertension in the arms. Severe proximal obstructing lesions (aortic or mitral stenosis) can have a similar effect.[F4] Control of the heart failure and tachycardia in these situations frequently make the differential pressures in upper and lower extremities apparent as cardiac output improves.[M3]

It should be noted that a left-to-right shunt through a stretched patent foramen ovale is not uncommon in infants with severe coarctation in heart failure. When the heart failure disappears, so does the atrial shunt. Congenital aortic stenosis may not be evident clinically (or on catheter with-

Table 34-3 Associated cardiac anomalies in patients undergoing repair of coarctation in infancy (UAB; 1967–1981; n = 55).

	All Cases	
Associated Cardiac Anomaly	n	% of 55
None or only PDA	16	29%
VSD	20	36%
Congenital mitral stenosis	4	7%
Congenital aortic stenosis	1	2%
Congenital mitral stenosis + VSD	1	2%
Congenital aortic stenosis + VSD	1	2%
Complete AV canal defect	1	2%
Single ventricle	4	7%
TGA + VSD	4	7%
DORV	2	4%
DOLV	1	2%
Total	55[a]	100%

SOURCE: Modified from Bergdahl et al.[B8]

KEY: AV, atrioventricular; DOLV, double outlet left ventricle; DORV, double outlet right ventricle; PDA, patent ductus arteriosus; TGA, transposition of the great arteries; VSD, ventricular septal defect.

[a]45 of the 55 patients were less than 3 months old.

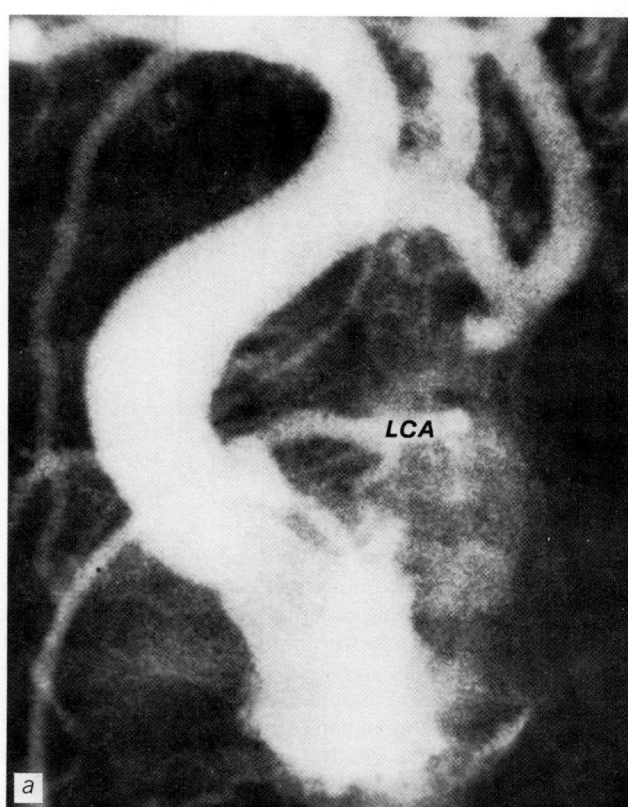

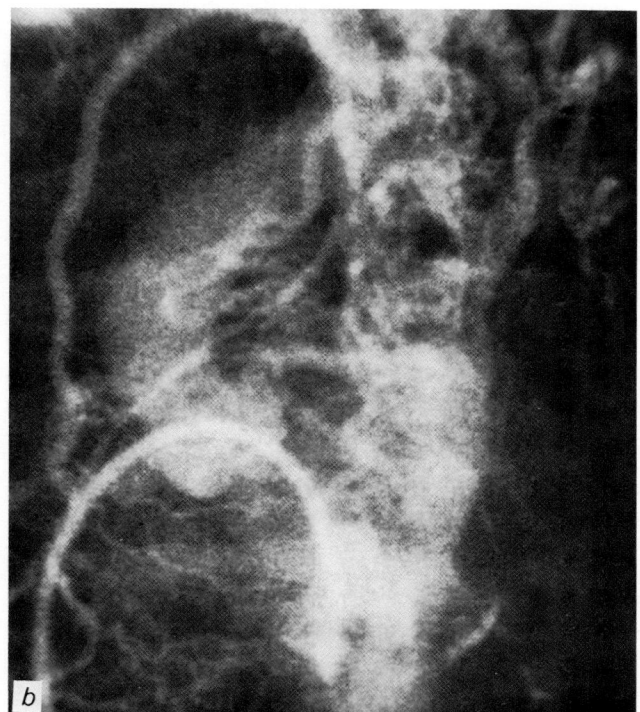

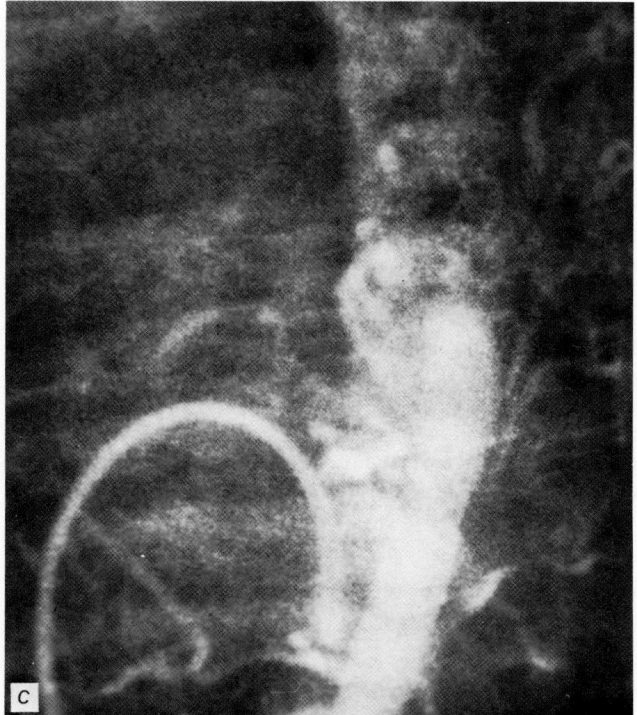

Figure 34-5 Cineangiocardiograms in left anterior oblique view with injection into left ventricle of a severe coarctation 5 mm in length in a 7-week-old infant without other associated anomalies (GLH). (a) The aortic arch and branches are outlined proximal to the coarctation, but the distal aorta is not opacified. Collateral vessels are visible. (b) A dense collateral network is visible in this later frame with contrast in the descending aorta below the coarctation. (c) The descending aorta is well outlined, most of its filling coming from the collaterals although a tiny lumen about 5 mm long could be identified connecting the two ends. LCA, left coronary artery.

drawal pressures) in infancy and yet be severe enough to require surgical relief at 2–5 years of age, particularly when the stenosis is subvalvar (see Chapter 32, Section 2).

Childhood (Aged 1–14 Years)

Almost all patients aged 1–14 years are asymptomatic unless they have significant associated lesions. Tawes and colleagues noted that children with associated lesions can continue to present in heart failure up to 3 years of age,[T3] and Patel et al.[P1] noted heart failure in 7 of 65 children (11%) aged 1–14 years. Subarachnoid hemorrhage from rupture of a berry aneurysm occurs occasionally but is rare in children under 7 years of age,[S5] and spontaneous paresis or paraplegia due to dilated intercostal arteries compressing the anterior spinal artery or to epidural hemorrhage is even less common.[B6] Hypertension occurs in almost 90% of patients.

The chest x-ray shows cardiomegaly in 33% and rib notching in about 15% (Fig. 34-6), but this feature does not occur before 3 years of age.[P1,T3] The electrocardiogram shows predominantly left ventricular hypertrophy with right ventricular hypertrophy present only when there is pulmonary hypertension with an elevated pulmonary vascular resistance. The electrocardiogram is normal in about one-third of the children.

Adolescence (beyond 14 Years) and Adult Life

Many adolescent and young adult patients remain asymptomatic and are diagnosed at routine examination because the femoral pulses are noted to be absent or reduced and delayed in the presence of a cardiac murmur, hypertension, or an abnormal chest x-ray. Hypertension is very common and more severe than in younger patients, and heart failure reappears at about 30 years of age. It is preceded by effort dyspnea, cardiomegaly, and significant left ventricular hypertrophy on the electrocardiogram. Headache, nose bleeds, fatigue, and calf claudication all occur occasionally. Collaterals are usually palpable or audible posteriorly. The radiographic findings include a figure 3 sign in the left upper mediastinal shadow (Fig. 34-7) and, almost always, rib notching. Absence of rib notching in the right chest suggests an anomalous right subclavian artery and in the left chest a stenosis of the left subclavian artery origin.

Associated Syndromes

There is a known association between *Turner's syndrome* and coarctation of the aorta[A2] (noted in six, or 2%, of the GLH cases) and of *Von Recklinghausen's disease* (present in one GLH case). Rarely, patients with coarctation have *Noonan's syndrome* or congenital rubella.

Special Diagnostic Methods

Two-dimensional echocardiography can visualize a coarctation in infancy, and high-quality studies are of value in excluding such a lesion in doubtful cases with complex disease.

Cardiac catheterization and particularly *aortography* are required for exact diagnosis. A withdrawal gradient is pres-

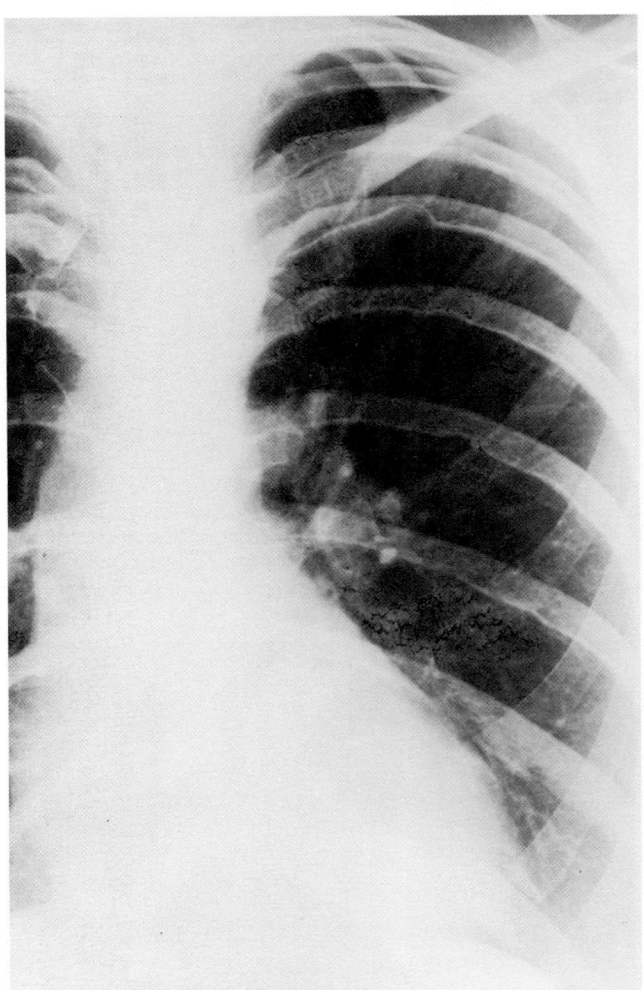

Figure 34-6 A portion of the chest x-ray showing severe rib notching in a patient with coarctation of the aorta (UAB). Note that the changes are not present in the first two ribs and are typically less severe below the fifth rib.

ent at rest across the coarctation, and in borderline cases measurement of cardiac output and the gradient during exercise will help in assessing severity. When there is preductal coarctation in association with pulmonary hypertension and a widely patent ductus arteriosus, a gradient is absent and aortography is required to demonstrate the coarctation. The severity of the coarctation can be better assessed on aortography than on catheter withdrawal pressures, particularly in infancy when the aorta is relatively small and the ductus patent. Aortography will also reveal any hypoplasia of the isthmus or transverse arch which may be present, the arrangement of the aortic arch branches, the degree of collateral circulation, and the presence of an aneurysm, and it will help in assessing the status of the ductus arteriosus. Demonstration of ductus patency may, however, require intracardiac contrast injections.

These investigations are indicated whenever associated cardiac anomalies are suspected clinically and as a routine in infancy where associated anomalies are common. These

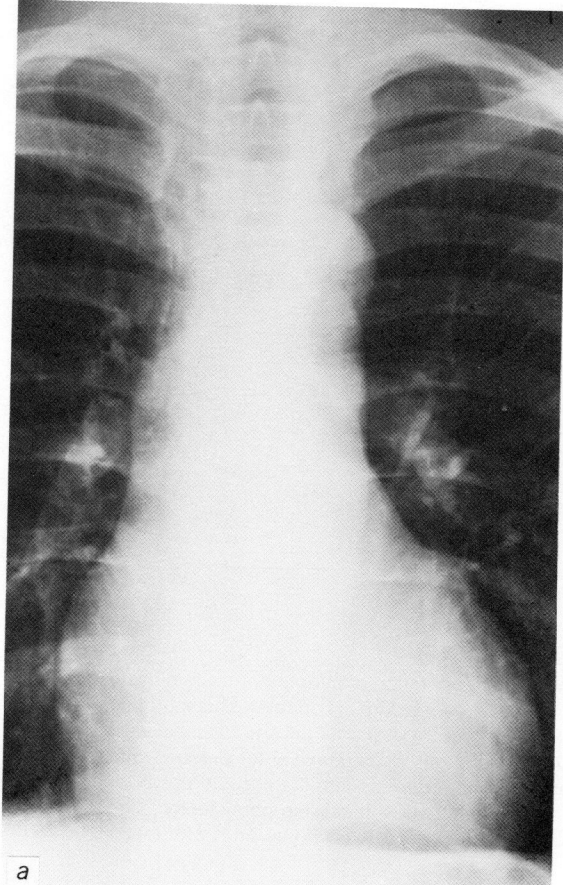
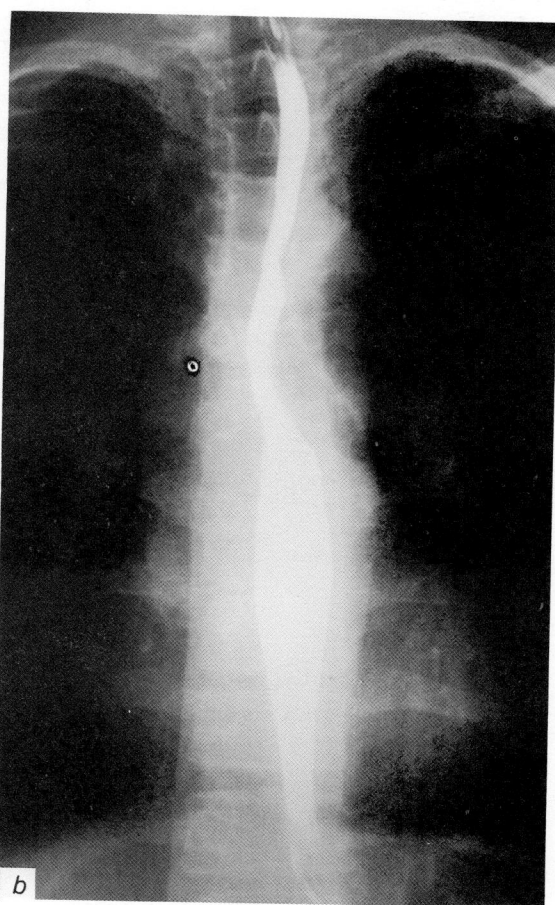

Figure 34-7 Radiographic studies in a patient with coarctation, demonstrating the classical figure 3 sign present in some patients with coarctation of the aorta (GLH).
(a) Chest x-ray. The upper convexity of the sign is formed by the aortic isthmus and left subclavian artery, the lower convexity by the upper descending aorta at the site of poststenotic dilatation.
(b) Barium esophagogram. Note how the two shadows overlap. The isthmus and descending aorta produce the upper and lower indentations on the leftward margin of the barium-filled esophagus.

should be accurately defined prior to operation so that appropriate treatment can be planned for them. Investigation is also probably indicated routinely in patients over 20 years of age because of the higher incidence of aneurysm. Special investigations are not considered necessary in children and adolescents with classic features of isolated coarctation, including equal pressures in both arms and palpable collaterals. Unequal arm pressures usually indicate involvement of the left subclavian artery origin or an anomalous right subclavian artery arising below the coarctation, and the absence of palpable collaterals and rib notching usually means an inadequate collateral circulation. Each of these variants requires preliminary aortography.

NATURAL HISTORY

Coarctation accounts for 5%–8% of congenital heart disease.[F2] Isolated coarctation is slightly more than twice as common in males as it is in females, but there is no sex difference in complex coarctation.[S4]

Primary or Pure Coarctation

This category includes patients with an associated patent ductus arteriosus.

Survival

Among infants born with primary or pure coarctation, about 5% (13 of the 268) develop intractable congestive heart failure in the first few weeks of life and would probably die without an operation[1] (Fig. 34-8). Another 10% (23 patients were operated upon 1–6 months of age) develop less severe congestive heart failure and might survive into early childhood without an operation. The other 85% live at least into late childhood or young adult life according to available

---

[1] These inferences concerning the natural history of primary coarctation are in large part derived by assuming that the 268 GLH referrals are representative of the complete population of New Zealand, that most patients with coarctation were identified and operated upon eventually, and that all 224 cases operated upon over the age of 1 year had pure coarctation (GLH).

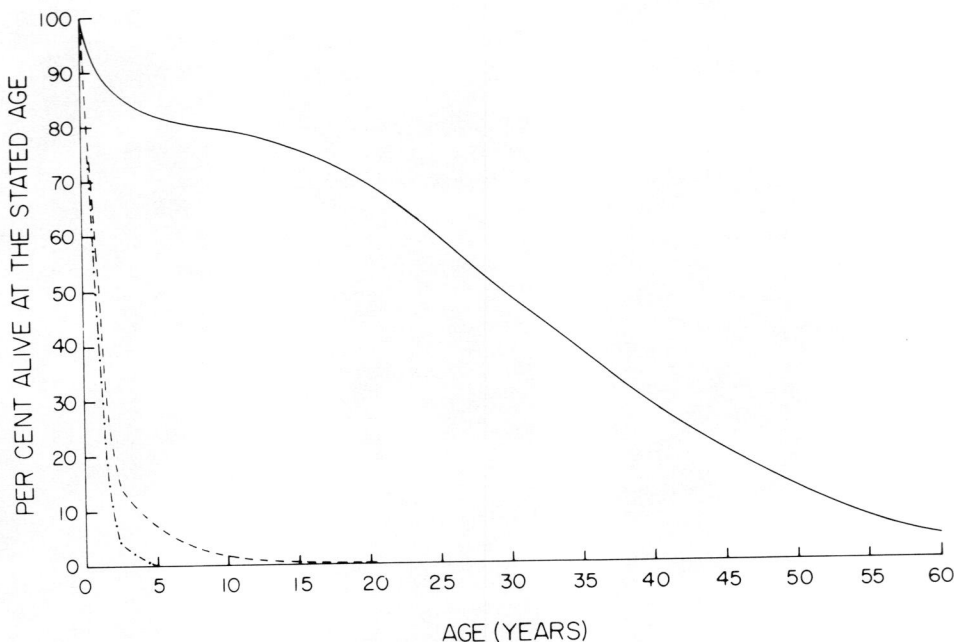

Figure 34-8   Freehand depiction of the survival curve without operation of people born with classic coarctation and interrupted aortic arch based upon material presented in this chapter. The solid line depicts survival of those with coarctation either isolated or only with patent ductus arteriosus. In view of the high spontaneous closure rate of moderate-sized and small VSDs, survival for persons with these coexisting anomalies is probably similar. The dashed line depicts that the survival curve for people born with coarctation and major associated cardiac anomalies, including persistently large or multiple ventricular septal defects. The dash-dot line depicts interrupted aortic arch with major associated cardiac anomalies.

data.[A1,C5,R1] Probably about one-quarter of this group die before reaching age 20, leaving 65% entering the third decade of life (Fig. 34-8). Another 25% die during both the fourth and fifth decades, and 98% die by the age of 60 years. The few survivors to age 60 are probably women, who tend to develop hypertensive and atherosclerotic complications more slowly than men.

Heart Failure in Infancy

There are a number of factors that act singly or in combination to produce heart failure in infancy: (1) Ductal closure, as it progresses from the pulmonary to the aortic end during the first 7–10 days of life, increases the degree of aortic narrowing,[R2,T1] which prior to this event may have been mild and of no functional significance. The relatively sudden appearance of severe coarctation precipitates left ventricular failure at 1–2 weeks of age. Should the coarctation not become severe, heart failure does not occur. (2) The degree to which the collateral circulation has developed at birth may also be important, although information on this point is incomplete. Mathew and colleagues found that all infants with isolated coarctation had collaterals on angiography performed at 8 days to 15 months of age, indicating that they developed either during fetal life or soon after.[M4] The site of the coarctation, be it preductal, juxtaductal, or postductal, is not per

se a factor, except as it relates to collateral development. Presumably collateral development is absent or inadequate in preductal coarctation as long as the ductus is widely patent and there is pulmonary hypertension.[B7] (3) The presence of major noncardiac anomalies also contributes. Thus, in the 46 autopsied infants with coarctation reported by Malm et al. in 1963,[M3] 12 died in the first week of life from major noncardiac anomalies (prematurity, tracheoesophageal fistula, etc.). In the New England Regional Study,[F2] 26% of the infants had extracardiac anomalies that, when severe, contributed to mortality.

The sequence of pathophysiologic events leading to severe heart failure in the 5% of patients with pure coarctation who develop this in the first few weeks of life has been further elucidated by Graham and colleagues.[G5] They found in this subset that left ventricular wall mass was normal and left ventricular stroke volume and ejection fraction severely depressed. Since left ventricular systolic function as reflected in stroke volume and ejection fraction returned to normal after coarctation repair, the mechanism of its preoperative reduction is clearly the *afterload mismatch* (see Chapter 12, "Natural History") brought about by sudden increase in left ventricular afterload from the rapidly developing coarctation as the ductus closes in the presence of a nonhypertrophied left ventricle. Severe cardiomegaly is present, but it is the result of markedly increased *right* ventricular end-diastolic volume; left ventricular end-diastolic volume is normal. The right ventricular enlargement usually is associated with left-to-right shunting through the stretched foramen ovale.

Graham and colleagues report somewhat different findings in the 10% of patients with pure (or primary) coarctation presenting with mild or moderate heart failure at 1–6 months of age. Left ventricular wall mass was significantly increased in this group (as it is in older children with coarctation[G6]) and left ventricular ejection fraction and stroke volume only *mildly* decreased. The increased left ventricular thickness had by this time significantly reduced left ventricular after-load (see Chapter 5, footnote 10); that is "afterload mis-match" had largely been overcome.

Death after infancy in patients with primary or pure coarctation is generally due (apart from incidental causes) to heart failure, bacterial endocarditis, aortic rupture or dissection (each in about 20% of cases), and rupture of an intracranial aneurysm in about 10%.[A1,R1]

Heart Failure in Childhood and Adult Life
Heart failure causes death in surgically untreated older patients at an average age of 39 years. In Reifenstein's series, there was only one death from heart failure below 20 years of age, most occurring in the fourth and fifth decades.[R1] In most instances, there was associated valvular heart disease, usually aortic but occasionally mitral, that combined with the hypertension to produce heart failure. A contribution from a patent ductus arteriosus, VSD, or more complex congenital malformation was uncommon, no doubt because most such subjects had died in infancy. A congenitally abnormal aortic valve (bicuspid valves were present in 42% of the hearts in Reifenstein's series[R1]) was the usual cause of the aortic stenosis or incompetence. Clearly, heart failure has a bimodal distribution in coarctation. It occurs in about two-thirds of the infants, is uncommon between 1 and about 30 years of age, and reappears in about two-thirds of the patients who have survived beyond 40 years.[L2]

Bacterial Endocarditis or Endarteritis
Bacterial endocarditis or endarteritis causes death at an average age of 29 years and was equally common in the first five decades of life. Infection usually occurred on a bicuspid aortic valve and rarely on a mitral valve or in relationship to a VSD. Endarteritis is less common and usually occurred in the poststenotic segment in relation to the jet lesion on the aortic wall. Mycotic aneurysms can result. Bacterial endocarditis occurred prior to operation in 6 of the 224 patients (3%) over 1 year of age (GLH).

Aortic Rupture
Rupture occurs at an average age of 27 years and is most common in the second and third decades.[A1,R1] It usually involved the ascending aorta when rupture often occurred into the pericardium with tamponade; less often the aorta immediately beyond the coarctation ruptured at the site of poststenotic dilatation where the wall was dilated and thin.

Many of these ruptures are probably true dissecting aneurysms, but pathologic details of the aortic wall are scarce.

Intracranial Lesions
Intracranial lesions caused death at an average age of 28 years in Reifenstein's series and 30 years in Abbott's series.[A1,R1] Among the 35 patients less than 21 years of age with coarctation and cerebrovascular disease reported in the literature and reviewed by Shearer and colleagues only 3 were less than 7 years old at the time and in most the incident was fatal.[S5] In the great majority there is a subarachnoid hemorrhage from rupture of a congenital berry aneurysm on the circle of Willis arteries. These lesions are considerably more common in coarctation than in the general population and are more likely to rupture because of the associated hypertension.[S5] Other causes of cerebrovascular accidents are atherosclerosis, particularly in older patients, and emboli, particularly in the presence of bacterial endocarditis. In the treated series reported by Liberthson and colleagues a cerebrovascular accident had occurred in only 1 of 91 patients less than 11 years old at the time of diagnosis and in 12 of 143 (8%) aged 11–39 years.[L2] However, in those over 40 years, 21% (5/24) had had a cerebrovascular accident. A documented subarachnoid hemorrhage occurred preoperatively in only 2% of patients (GLH) beyond infancy.

Coarctation Associated with Ventricular Septal Defect

Most infants born with large VSD and coarctation develop severe congestive heart failure in the first month of life. In contrast, presentation so early is uncommon in patients with isolated large VSD (see Chapter 20, "Natural History"). Unless the VSD rapidly diminishes in size, most of these babies die within a few months without surgical treatment (Fig. 34-8). In many of these infants, the VSD does become small quite rapidly (see Chapter 20), and the natural history then becomes that of primary, isolated coarctation.

Coarctation Associated with Other Major Cardiac Anomalies

The combination of coarctation with other major cardiac anomalies nearly always produces severe heart failure in the early weeks of life. From 80% to 100% of such babies die in their first year of life without surgical treatment (Fig. 34-8).[F4,L3,S2]

All reported series show a high proportion of associated cardiovascular lesions in those patients with coarctation presenting in infancy (Table 34-2).[C6,F4,G7,T3] In such infants, isthmal hypoplasia is almost constant as a consequence of the disturbed fetal blood flow patterns (see "Morphology").[R2] In many of these infants, particularly those with complex and severe intracardiac defects, the natural history is primarily that of the associated defect. However, the associated severe coarctation undoubtedly precipitates early heart failure in such infants.

TECHNIQUE OF OPERATION

Subclavian Flap Aortoplasty in Neonates and Infants

In critically ill neonates with coarctation, intravenous prostaglandin E_1 (PGE$_1$) (0.1 mg · kg^{-1} · min^{-1}) is begun immediately and continued until the situation is remedied at operation.[N1,W4] (For more details about the use of PGE$_1$, see Chapter 25, section on "Indications for Operation.") The response is dramatic in about 80% of such infants,[F5] with reappearance of femoral pulses and disappearance of the metabolic acidosis from hypoperfusion of the lower body. Operation is then delayed 6–12 hours until the baby has stabilized in this improved condition. When an immediate response is *not* obtained, immediate operation is indicated since a later response will not occur.

Since there is always uncertainty about the collateral circulation in a young infant with coarctation, after anesthetic induction the body temperature is allowed to drift down to a nasopharyngeal temperature of about 33°C. This downward drift is helped by reducing the operating room temperature to about 18°C (65°F), and by use of the cooling mode in the heating–cooling pad under the child. The blood pressure in the right arm is monitored either by the usual cuff method or by Doppler techniques, but an indwelling radial or brachial catheter is used in particularly critical situations.

The approach is made through a left posterolateral thoracotomy with the patient in a full lateral position, secured with strapping across the hip and onto the operating table and a sandbag tucked against the front of the chest. The chest is entered through the fourth intercostal space (Fig. 34-9). For this, the intercostal muscles may be incised in the center of the interspace or entry made via the fifth rib bed, elevating the periosteum from the superior half of this rib and incising the rib bed rather than the intercostal muscles. Care is required posteriorly, since careless elevation of the periosteum too far in this direction or attempts to dislocate the costotransverse joint will result in excessive bleeding from collaterals. The rib spreader is inserted and opened in stages to avoid rib fractures. The lung is retracted anteriorly, and the mediastinal pleura opened over the aorta downward for about 4 cm below the coarctation site and upward across the entire left subclavian artery. Numerous rather closely placed stay sutures are placed along each side of the pleural incision, and the ends are gathered into clamps for exposure. No other retractors are then required. The left superior intercostal vein is ligated and divided.

Keeping the dissection in the areolar tissue just superficial to the adventitial aortic coat, the proximal left subclavian artery and the distal transverse arch and aortic isthmus are dissected and tapes may be placed around them (Fig. 34-9). All dissection is kept close to the aorta, in part because this is the best plane of dissection and in part to minimize the possibility of damage to the thoracic duct. "Abbott's artery," which occasionally arises from the medial aspect of the isthmus, should be remembered and, when present, ligated and divided. Next, with great care to avoid damage to intercostals and bronchial arteries, the aorta beyond the coarctation is dissected. It is occasionally necessary to divide one or more bronchial arteries medially. A tape may be

placed around the aorta beyond the coarctation. Finally, the ductus arteriosus or ligamentum arteriosum is dissected.

If by now the nasopharyngeal temperature has not dropped to 33°C, the left pleural space is lavaged with ice cold saline for the few minutes that are required to accomplish this (see Chapter 53, "Paraplegia" in section on Special Situations and Controversies). To begin the subclavian flap aortoplasty,[W1] the dissection of the subclavian artery is carried distally to expose the branches. The vertebral artery may be ligated and divided together with any more proximal branches (GLH); alternatively (UAB), in order to preserve all the collateral circulation to the arm, the subclavian artery may be ligated and divided proximal to all branches, none of which are ligated. A light clamp, such as a Potts fine-toothed clamp or an angled light Castaneda infant clamp, is placed across the transverse arch between the left common carotid artery and left subclavian artery, and a second clamp is placed well distal to the coarctation but proximal to the intercostal arteries. Uncommonly, it must be placed beyond the third pair of intercostal arteries (the first set beyond the coarctation), which are then controlled with a single bulldog clamp. The ligamentum arteriosum or a small patent ductus arteriosus is ligated; or, if there is a large patent ductus arteriosus, this is clamped at its pulmonary end and the divided ends oversewn with a running polypropylene stitch.

The subclavian artery is split open longitudinally along its posterior margin, carrying this incision across the coarctation into the dilated distal aorta for at least 1 cm (Fig. 34-9). Stay sutures are placed on either side at the level of the coarctation. The intimal shelf is excised as completely as possible but care is taken not to damage the aortic wall. The subclavian artery is now divided 3 or 4 mm proximal to the ligature. The sharp corners at the end of the opened subclavian artery are trimmed off; if the subclavian flap is unusually wide, the lateral edge is trimmed so that its width is about one and one-half times the diameter of the aorta (GLH). The turned-down subclavian flap may be tacked to the distal opened aorta using a double-ended 5-0 or 6-0 polypropylene suture that is then carried proximally as a continuous whip stitch (GLH). Alternatively, the suture line may be started proximally on the medial side and carried just beyond the inferior angle of the aortic incision (UAB); another suture line is then started proximally on the lateral side and carried down to the previous one. Five-0 or 6-0 absorbable suture[2] may be used (see "Late Results"), or alternatively 6-0 or 7-0 interrupted sutures. The angles at either end of the turned-down subclavian flap must lie beyond the level of the coarctation, achieving this when necessary by sliding the flap distally in the process of the suturing. In this manner, a proper "cobra-head" appearance to the flap repair is achieved.

The anesthesiologist has given a dose of sodium bicarbonate during the cross-clamping, and an infusion of a pure peripheral vasoconstrictor is begun just before the cross-clamps are removed (see Chapter 4). The distal clamp is removed. After the proximal clamp has been *slowly* opened, great care is taken to maintain proper ventilation and slight

---

[2] Ethicon polydioxanone suture (PDS) is currently preferred.[R10]

arterial hypertension for at least the next 5 minutes as a precaution against the sudden development of intractable ventricular fibrillation 3–4 minutes after release of the clamp (the declamping syndrome[T3]).

After the subclavian flap operation (or any other type of operation), pressures are measured proximal and distal to the repair with fine needles. If there is a systolic gradient of > 10 mmHg (a rare occurrence), the clamps are reapplied, the sutures removed, and the repair refashioned. The usual problem is inadequate excision of the intimal shelf combined with failure to carry the incision in the aorta far enough distally.

After the clamps are removed, the heating blanket, warming lamps, a warmed operating room, and warmed and humidified inspired gases are used to warm the infant. Usually the suture line is hemostatic, and the mediastinal pleura can soon be closed over it. A small chest tube is placed through a lateral and inferior stab wound. The incision through the interspace is closed with a few interrupted sutures. The muscles and subcuticular layers are closed with a continuous suture.

The chest tube may be removed in the operating room in neonates and infants after closing the incision (UAB). Unless the baby is critically ill, the relaxants are reversed, and the baby is extubated in the operating room.

Subclavian Flap Aortoplasty or End-to-End Anastomosis in Children (up to 10 Years of Age)

The operation is technically more demanding than in infants because the collateral circulation is much larger. The appropriate operation is also controversial.

The subclavian flap operation may be used in children up to 10 years of age unless the anatomy is perfect for resection and end-to-end anastomosis (very discrete coarctation without any isthmus hypoplasia) or the subclavian artery is involved and too small (UAB). End-to-end anastomosis may be preferred as a routine in this age group, reserving the subclavian flap repair for cases with marked isthmus hypoplasia (GLH) (see ''Special Situations and Controversies'').

A radial artery pressure catheter is not required. A long posterolateral thoracotomy incision is made, cutting 1–4 cm of the trapezius muscle posteriorly and carrying the incision to the nipple line anteriorly. The pleural space is entered through the top of the bed of the nonresected fifth rib. The rib spreader is opened gradually until a wide exposure is obtained.

The mediastinal pleura is opened widely over the upper one-half of the descending thoracic aorta and the subclavian artery. Numerous stay sutures are applied as described for the infants.

The aortic and subclavian dissection then proceeds as described for infants. However, it must be done with particular precision because of the large intercostal arteries. Even the smallest subadventitial dissection must be scrupulously avoided by keeping the dissection in the areolar tissue just superficial to the adventitia. Usually, after incising the pleura over the aorta and subclavian artery and dividing the superior intercostal vein, the dissection is carried around the aorta just proximal to the coarctation and a tape placed

around it. A similar sharp dissection is made just distal to the coarctation, taking care to avoid damage to a hidden Abbott's artery above or an enlarged intercostal artery below. Further dissection is facilitated by gentle traction on the tapes.

The ligamentum arteriosum, the third and sometimes fourth pair of intercostal arteries, Abbott's artery if present, and the left subclavian artery are now completely dissected. Abbott's artery requires ligation and division, as may a bronchial (or esophageal) artery beyond the stricture. All the dissection details described for infants are important here as well.

If *the subclavian flap operation* is elected, it is carried out as described for infants. More often than in infants, the distal clamp must be placed downstream to the third or fourth pair of intercostal arteries, in which instances these are temporarily controlled by special small bulldog clamps. When the suturing is completed, one of these is loosened to test for hemostasis. If it is satisfactory, the clamp is replaced, the distal clamp is removed, the bulldog clamps are carefully removed, and the proximal clamp is slowly opened over a 30–60-second period.

The remainder of the operation is completed as in infants, except that chest tubes (one with the tip positioned posteroinferiorly in the paravertebral gutter and the other anteriorly and superiorly) are routinely left for 24 hours.

If *end-to-end anastomosis* is elected, the dissection is identical (Fig. 34-10). The proximal clamp is usually placed across the aorta close to the origin of the left subclavian artery, but if more length is required in the isthmus area it is positioned between the subclavian and left common carotid, controlling the subclavian with a separate clamp or using a single curved or angled clamp across both vessels. The distal clamp is placed as for the subclavian flap operation. The ligamentum arteriosum, which has been tied at its pulmonary end, is transected at its aortic insertion. The aorta is transected proximal to the coarctation, sometimes extending the opening obliquely onto the under surface of the transverse arch in order to obtain a wide diameter. A similar transection is made beyond the coarctation, where the aortic diameter is usually ample. With the aortic clamps held by the assistant to the surgeon's right, the end-to-end anastomosis is begun at the deep angle with an interrupted horizontal mattress suture of 5-0 or 6-0 silk (Fig. 34-10b). The clamps are brought together, the suture tied, and the medial half of the anastomosis made with interrupted simple (UAB) or horizontal mattress (GLH) sutures. Then the surgeon steadies the clamps as they are rotated over to the first assistant across the table to hold. The lateral half of the suture line is similarly completed.

Finally, the clamps are removed as described above and the operation completed similarly.

End-to-End Anastomosis in Adolescents and Adults

The operation is carried out in the same steps as in younger patients. However, the vessels are much more friable, the intercostal arteries larger and more easily damaged, and the dissection potentially more hazardous. The use of controlled hypotension by the anesthesiologist (see Chapter 4) during

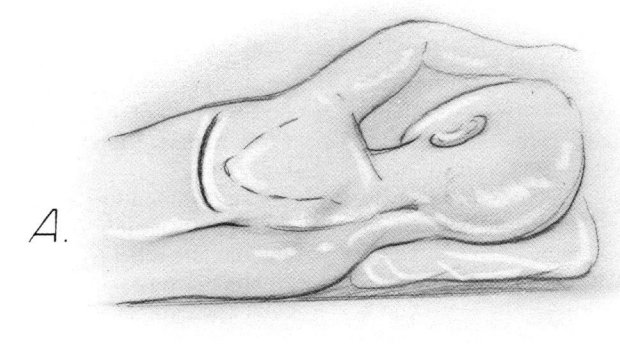

A.

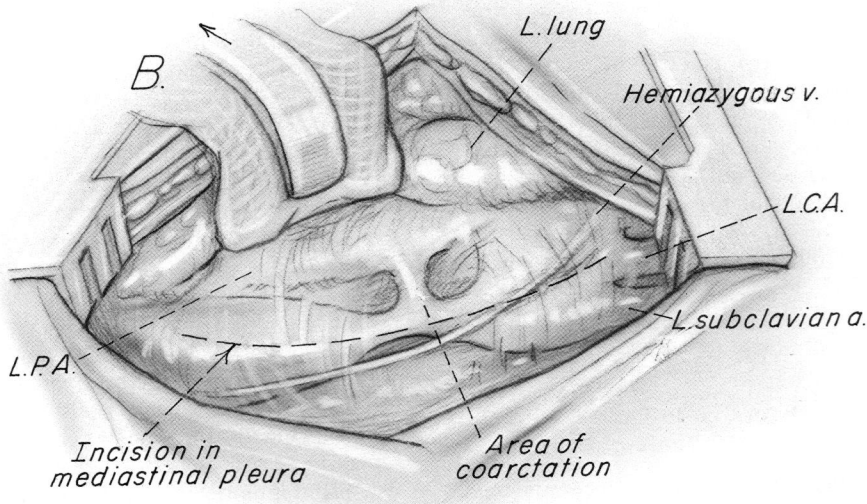

B.

L. lung

Hemiazygous v.

L.C.A.

L. subclavian a.

L.P.A.

Incision in
mediastinal pleura

Area of
coarctation

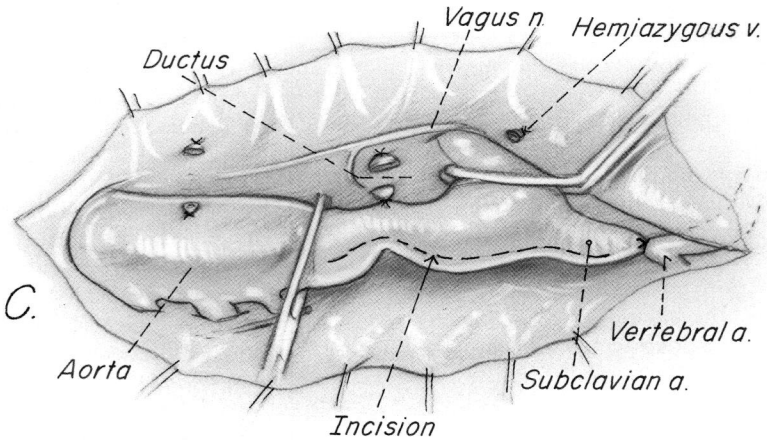

C.

Ductus

Vagus n.

Hemiazygous v.

Aorta

Incision

Vertebral a.

Subclavian a.

Figure 34-9 Subclavian flap repair for coarctation.

(a) The patient, often an infant, is positioned in the right lateral decubitus position, and a curving incision is made around the angle of the scapula. In infants it is usually not necessary to incise the trapezius muscle.

(b) The rib spreader is in place, and the lung is retracted anteriorly to expose the area of the coarctation. The proposed incision in the mediastinal pleura is shown by the dashed line.

(c) The mediastinal pleura has been opened and stay sutures have been placed on the edges for exposure. After the dissection has been completed (see text) and after the left subclavian artery has been ligated just proximal to the vertebral artery (UAB) or beyond this with individual ligation of the branches (GLH), a vascular clamp is placed across the aortic arch between the left common carotid and left subclavian arteries. The distal clamp nearly always can be placed just upstream to the third pair of intercostal arteries and yet well below the coarctation (see text). The dashed line indicates the proposed incision.

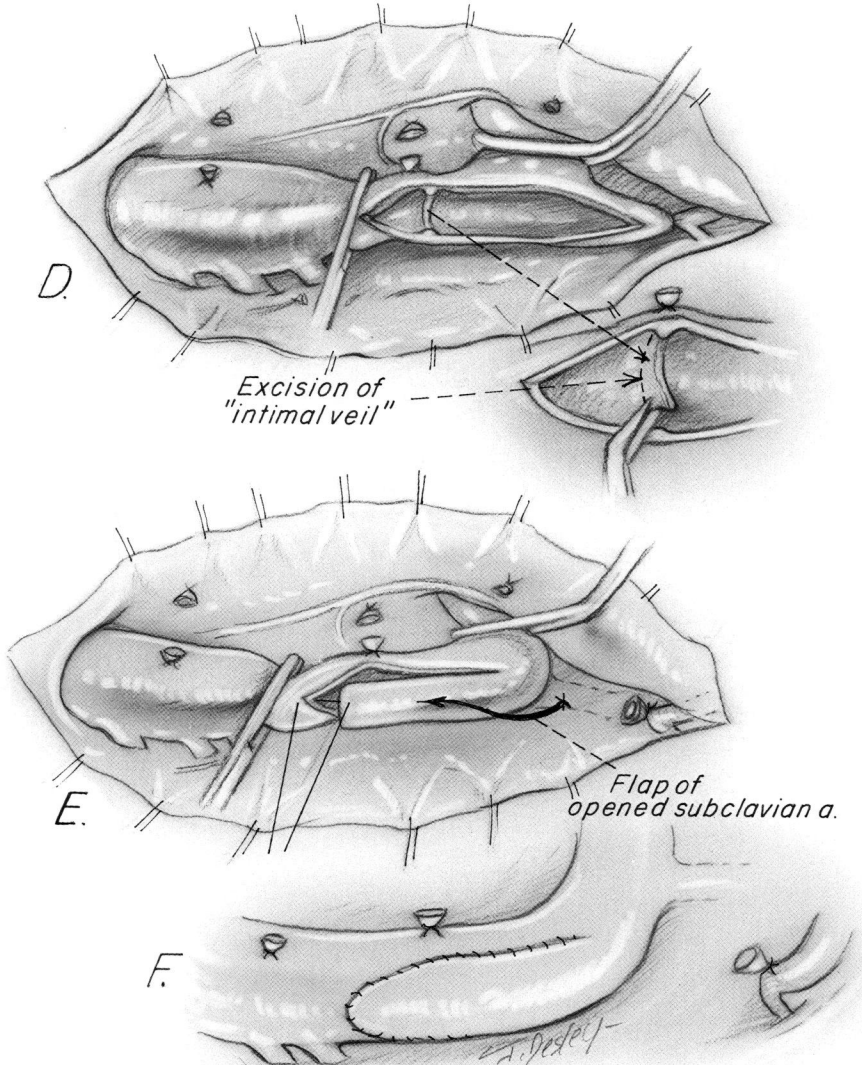

Figure 34-9 *(continued)*
(d) After the aorta and subclavian artery have been opened, the intimal veil is dissected away if it is present.
(e) The subclavian artery has been divided distally and turned down for the flap.
(f) The flap has been sewn into place (see text).
LCA, left coronary artery; LPA, left pulmonary artery.

the dissection is very important since it allows the dissection to be done more safely and expeditiously. Once the aortic clamps are in place, the upper body blood pressure is allowed to rise to moderately hypertensive levels (to promote collateral blood flow, see Chapter 53, ''Paraplegia'' in section on Special Situations and Controversies). The hypotensive agents must be withdrawn before the clamps are removed.

Hemorrhage from the intercostal arteries or from Abbott's artery can be massive and difficult to control, especially if one of these vessels is damaged early in the dissection before

adequate exposure is obtained. Therefore, no effort is made to dissect these until tapes are around the aorta just above and below the coarctation, the left subclavian artery, and in these older patients the aorta distal to the fourth, or if it is large, the fifth intercostal artery. With traction on the pleural stay sutures in one direction and on the aortic tapes in the other, the structures can be liberated gradually by precise sharp dissection. The most inaccessible structures are the right third and fourth intercostal arteries, and they must be approached and dissected with particular care. The junction of the enlarged intercostal artery with aorta is the most

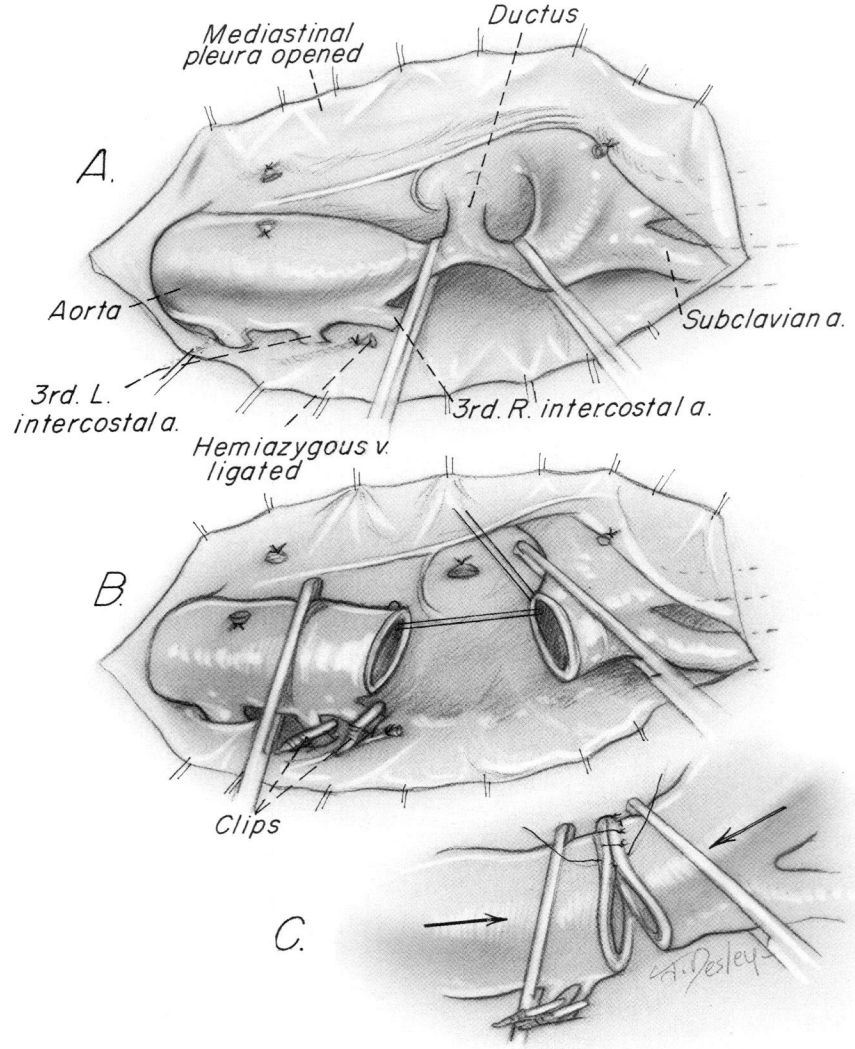

Figure 34-10 Resection and end-to-end anastomosis for the repair of coarctation.

(a) The patient has been positioned in the right lateral decubitus position, a curving incision made around the angle of the scapula, the chest opened, and stay sutures placed on the cut edges of the mediastinal pleura and held under tension to aid exposure. After sharply dissecting out the coarctation and contiguous structures, tapes are placed around the aorta just above and below the coarctation. Traction on the tapes elevates the aorta anteriorly or posteriorly to provide an exposure that facilitates the dissection.

(b) The ligamentum arteriosum has been ligated and divided, and small bull-dog clamps (clips) have been placed on the third pair of intercostal arteries. The proximal clamp is positioned across the aorta and base of the subclavian artery so as to leave ample length for the proximal cuff. The coarctation is excised, getting back to a wide orifice proximally and distally. A horizontal mattress suture has been placed between the two ends of aorta at the deep angle anteriorly.

(c) The mattress suture has been tied, and several additional simple sutures have been placed to begin the anterior part of the anastomosis (see text).

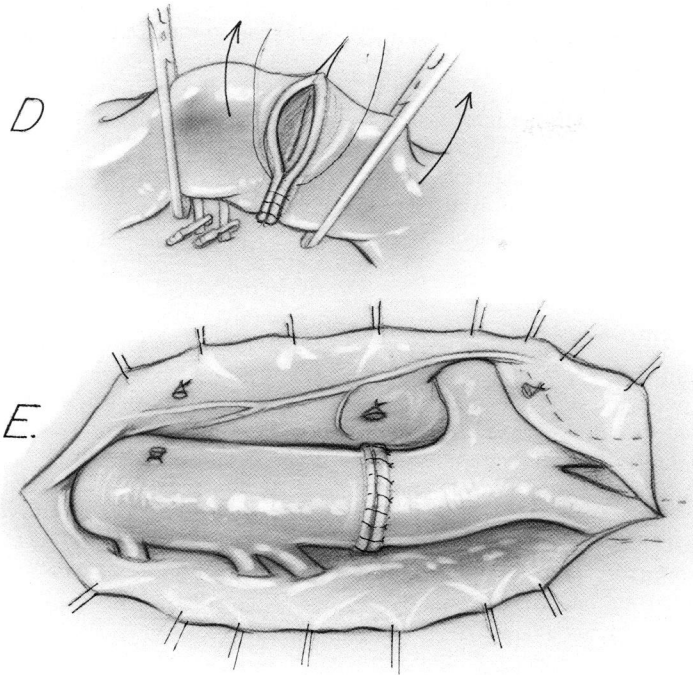

Figure 34-10 (*continued*)
(*d*) The clamps have been rotated to the first assistant across the table from the surgeon, and the posterior row of interrupted sutures are being placed.
(*e*) The completed anastomosis is shown after removal of the clamps.

fragile and easily damaged point. After dissecting from one side for a time, a sponge can be tucked against the aorta, the tapes swung to the other side, and the dissection continued.

It is safer to control the intercostals temporarily with special small metal bulldog clamps during the resection and anastomosis than it is to ligate and divide them, since delayed hemorrhage can occur from slippage of such a ligature.

Rarely, end-to-end anastomosis is not possible and an interposed Dacron tube graft is necessary.

Repair of Coarctation Proximal to Left Subclavian Artery

When severe coarctation occurs proximal to the left subclavian artery, the usual methods of repair can be unsatisfactory. When the situation is encountered in infants, a *reversed subclavian flap aortoplasty* may be used.[H14,T9] Since a collateral circulation is usually poorly developed in the setting of coarctation in this area, the infant should be surface cooled to 30°C to lessen the risk of paraplegia and the aortic cross clamp time kept as short as possible. After the usual exposure and dissection, the left common carotid artery and the aortic arch between this and the subclavian artery are completely dissected. Clamps are placed on the left common carotid artery and on the aorta just proximal to this vessel and on the aorta distal to the left subclavian artery. The subclavian artery is ligated and divided distally. The subclavian artery is split down its *medial side* and the incision extended proximally onto the arch and the origin of the left

common carotid artery. The subclavian artery is turned down, in reverse to the classic subclavian flap operation, and sewn into place.

In older patients, *replacement of the coarcted area* with an interposed tube graft may be done when the lesion is severe, but the techniques for aneurysms of the distal portion of the transverse aortic arch may be necessary (see Chapter 55) or a temporary shunt placed from ascending to descending aorta. The simpler palliative placement of a bypassing Dacron tube graft between the ascending aorta and lower descending thoracic aorta via a right thoracotomy may be used but is less satisfactory[A5,E3] (see "Special Situations and Controversies" for further discussion).

Repair when Aneurysm is Present

When an aneurysm is present, either of the intercostal arteries (single or multiple) or of the aorta (see discussion under "Morphology"), resection of the segment of aorta involved along with the coarctation is required, and continuity is reestablished with an interposed tubular woven Dacron graft. This procedure can be hazardous, particularly as regards hemostatic control of the large intercostal artery feeding into the aneurysm. Pharmacologically induced hypotension is helpful to the dissection. Early placement of the proximal aortic clamp and then ligation and division of the ligamentum arteriosus and placement of a clamp across the coarctation itself allows transection of the aorta proximal to the coarctation. Then gentle forward traction on the clamp across the coarctation allows the distal aorta and the posteriorly placed intercostal artery aneurysm to be brought into better view for dissection and management.

Postrepair paraplegia is a greater than usual hazard in these situations because of the need to sacrifice intercostal arteries (see Chapter 53, "Paraplegia" in section on Special Situations and Controversies). The special precautions required for all aneurysm surgery in this area are used (see Chapter 55, "Repair of Aneurysms of the Descending Thoracic Aorta" in section on Technique of Operation).

Repair of Persistent or Recurrent Coarctation

Whenever possible, the operation consists of either a standard subclavian flap repair or, under some circumstances, of resecting the recurrent or residual stricture, performing end-to-end reanastomosis of the posterior one-half or two-thirds of the circumference and completing the anterior part as a subclavian flap or patch-graft repair. When the subclavian artery is unsuitable in diameter or length and end-to-end anastomosis is clearly not appropriate, an interposed Dacron graft is required for the reconstruction. In particularly difficult technical situations in older patients, a bypassing Dacron tube graft on the left or right side may be all that is possible,[A5,E3] but is not ideal (see "Late Aneurysm Formation" in section on Late Results).

SPECIAL FEATURES OF POSTOPERATIVE CARE

General

Generally, the care of patients after coarctation repair is that accorded any patient after simple thoracotomy. In most very young infants, especially those in whom a subsequent intracardiac operation may be required, an arterial needle is avoided. The infant is extubated and the chest tube is removed in the operating room. This simplifies postoperative care, which then consists only of humidified and oxygen-enriched inspired air, feeding after 6 hours, and antibiotics for 4 days.

In critically ill babies, this accelerated convalescence may not be possible and more elaborate postoperative care is necessary. Most of the measures used after other cardiac surgical procedures in seriously ill neonates and infants are then required (see Chapter 5). In older patients with their enormous collateral arteries, more than the usual bleeding may occur, and retention of the chest tube for 24 hours or longer is indicated.

Management of Systemic Arterial Hypertension

Systemic arterial hypertension is usually present after operation, and its management is controversial. In older patients, the mean arterial blood pressure is lowered to about 110 mmHg with nitroprusside for the first 24 hours, and the drug is then rapidly tapered and discontinued (see Chapter 5). Aldomet is then substituted in doses of 250–500 mg every 6 hours unless systolic blood pressure is below 150 mmHg.

In infants and young children, no treatment is given routinely for postoperative hypertension. This practice differs from the recommendations of Ho and Moss,[H5] who reported that routine treatment with antihypertensive drugs resulted in fewer (no) instances of laparotomy for abdominal pain than did nontreatment ($P < .001$; see "Early Postoperative Morbidity").

Abdominal Pain

Careful interrogation and observation of patients postoperatively indicate that most have mild abdominal discomfort for a few postoperative days. In 5%–10% of cases this is prominent, and abdominal distension with hypoactive bowel sounds may develop.

Treatment consists of bowel decompression via a nasogastric tube and antihypertensive drugs. Reserpine 0.07 mg · kg^{-1} is almost magical in relieving these symptoms within 12–24 hours. Hydralazine HCL 0.15 mg · kg^{-1} intramuscularly every 12 hours, or intravenous sodium nitroprusside 1–5 $\mu g \cdot kg^{-1} \cdot min^{-1}$ may be used. Intravenous fluids may be required for a day or two.

Chylothorax

The nature of the chest tube drainage should be observed. Copious serous or milky drainage is probably *chyle,* a finding in about 5% of patients. The chest tube should be left in place until this stops. If it continues profusely until the sixth or seventh postoperative day, reoperation is indicated.

A chest x-ray is made about 7 days after coarctation repair, since chylothorax may develop late and be initially manifest as an unexpected pleural effusion. If present, it should be aspirated. Occasionally, repeated aspirations are required; if the chyle reaccumulates after the third aspiration, reoperation is indicated (see Chapter 5, "Chylothorax" in Section 3, for this and other aspects of chylothorax).

EARLY RESULTS

Hospital Mortality in Neonates and Infants

Currently, the hospital mortality after repair of coarctation in infants approaches zero, except when operation is required in patients with complex major associated cardiac anomalies at a very young age. Indeed, the hospital mortality after repair of primary, or pure, coarctation with or without associated patent ductus arteriosus (PDA) in the first year of life has been 3% in the entire GLH and UAB experience (Table 34-4).

However, in an earlier era (combined overall GLH and UAB experience) and including complex cases, 36 of 149 patients (24%; CL 20%–28%) less than 1 year of age died in the hospital. This is similar to the results in 252 cases in the same age group reported in the literature (81 deaths, 32%, CL 29%–35%).[A3,C7,C8,C9,F2,F3,F6,G7,H4,H6,H7,K4,L4,M5,M6,S4,T3,W3]

Most hospital deaths are associated with postoperative acute cardiac failure (Table 34-5), and occasionally this mode of death may occur in the operating room 5–15 minutes after removing the aortic cross-clamp. Tawes and col-

Table 34-4 The effect of associated cardiac anomalies on hospital mortality after repair of coarctation (UAB and GLH).

	GLH (1960–1979)				UAB (1967–1981)				Total			
		Hospital Deaths				Hospital Deaths				Hospital Deaths		
Category	n	No.	%	CL	n	No.	%	CL	n	No.	%	CL
Primary ("pure") coarctation[a]	44	1	2%	0.3%–8%	16	1	6%	0.8%–20%	60	2	3%	1%–8%
Coarctation with VSD	32	8	25%	17%–35%	20	4	20%	10%–33%	52	12	23%	17%–31%
Coarctation with other major associated cardiac anomalies	18	11	61%	46%–75%	19	11	58%	43%–71%	37	22	59%	50%–69%
Total	94	20	21%	17%–27%	55	16	29%	22%–37%	149	36	24%	20%–28%
$P(\chi^2)$	≤ .0001				.002				≤ .0001			

KEY: CL, 70% confidence limits; VSD, ventricular septal defect.

[a] Includes patients with patent ductus arteriosus as only associated malformation (UAB) or as indicated in Table 34-2.

leagues have referred to this as the *acute declamping syndrome*.[T3] Next most commonly (5 of 16 deaths, UAB experience), the death occurs after prolonged ventilatory support for severe pulmonary insufficiency. This is particularly common in neonates and infants with associated complex cardiac anomalies.

Incremental Risk Factors for Hospital Death in Neonates and Infants

The hospital mortality after repair of coarctation in neonates and infants is related to a number of risk factors.

Associated major cardiac anomalies other than ventricular septal defect (VSD)[B8] are an incremental risk factor (Tables 34-6, 34-7, and 34-8; see also Table 34-4), and their effects are not exerted entirely by their predilection to be present in very young (and thus very small) infants.

Very young age (small size) is an incremental risk factor (Fig. 34-11), although not a very strong one in the primary coarctation group and in those with only an associated VSD. It is a strong incremental risk factor in those with other major associated cardiac anomalies (see Fig. 34-11 and Table 34-8),[T3] but this may be because of the severity of the associ-

ated anomalies in infants who require operation at an early age.

The *preoperative functional status* of the patient before operation probably relates to the risk of operation and may also explain the incremental risk of young age since many neonates and infants are critically ill before coarctation repair. However, it has not been possible to document this.[B8]

Date of operation is an incremental risk factor, hospital mortality being higher in the earlier experiences (UAB, GLH; see Table 34-6).

The *adoption of the subclavian flap repair* has apparently been a factor in the reduction of hospital mortality in recent years (UAB). This is suggested by simple comparison of the results of the two methods (Table 34-9) and supported by the results of multivariate analysis (see Table 34-6). With the subclavian flap method in infants with primary coarctation or coarctation with VSD, hospital mortality approaches zero (CL 0%–5%) except in tiny babies whose body surface area is less than 0.2 m² (see Fig. 34-11). Even in these infants, the risk is less than 10%. Similar results in 27 infants are reported by Penkoske and colleagues.[P9] The reason for the improved results with the subclavian flap operation is probably the high proportion of patients who have complete or nearly complete relief of the aortic obstruction and thus an immediate improvement in left ventricular systolic function because of the sudden fall in afterload.[B8]

However, the improvement in hospital mortality with time (GLH; see Table 34-7) deemphasizes the importance of the

Table 34-5 Mode of death in infants (< 1 year of age) after repair of coarctation in relation to associated cardiac anomalies (UAB; 1967–1981).[B8]

Mode of Death	Coarctation (n = 16)	Coarctation with VSD (n = 20)	Coarctation with Other Major Associated Lesions (n = 19)
Acute cardiac failure[a]	0	2	7
Severe pulmonary dysfunction	1	1	3
Bleeding from suture line[b]	0	1	0
Indeterminate (sudden death)	0	0	1

KEY: VSD, ventricular septal defect.

[a] One death was with acute declamping syndrome.

[b] Dacron patch graft repair.

Table 34-6 Multivariate analysis for risk factors for hospital death after coarctation repair in infants (UAB; 1967–1981).

Incremental Risk Factors	Logistic Coefficient ± SD	P Value
Type of repair[a]	2.6 ± 0.89	.004
Small size (ln[BSA])	−11 ± 5.2	.04
Associated major cardiac anomalies (*not* VSD)	5.1 ± 1.80	.005
Intercept	−22 ± 9.0	

SOURCE: Reproduced from Bergdahl et al.[B8] See publication for variables analyzed.

KEY: BSA, body surface area; SD, standard deviation; VSD, ventricular septal defect.

[a] Repair: 0, subclavian flap; 1, patch graft; 2, end-to-end anastomosis.

Table 34-7 Hospital mortality for repair of coarctation in infants (< 1 year of age) in two time periods (GLH).

Category	1960–1970			1971–1978			P for Difference (Fisher)
	n	No.	%	n	No.	%	
		Hospital Deaths			Hospital Deaths		
Primary ("pure") coarctation	26	0	0%	18	1	6%	.4
Coarctation with VSD	15	7	47%	17	1	6%	.01
Coarctation with other major associated cardiac anomalies	8	7	88%	10	4	40%	.06
Total	49	14	29%	45	6	13%	.06

KEY: VSD, ventricular septal defect.

Table 34-8 Relationship of age at coarctation repair in infants and associated lesions to hospital death (GLH; 1960–1978).

Age (Months) ≤ <	Coarctation			Coarctation with VSD			Coarctation with Other Major Associated Cardiac Anomalies			P(χ^2) for Difference
	n	Hospital Deaths No.	%	n	Hospital Deaths No.	%	n	Hospital Deaths No.	%	
1	13	1	8%	14	4	29%	9	6	67%	.01
1 --- 3	15	0	0%	13	4	31%	5	3	60%	.01
3 --- 6	8	0	0%	3	0	0%	4	2	50%	.04
6 --- 12	8	0	0%	2	0	0%	0	0	—	—
Total	44	1	2%	32[a]	8	25%	18	11	61%	
P(χ^2)	.05			.6			.8			

KEY: VSD, ventricular septal defect.

[a] In six patients, the VSD was small, and all survived.

subclavian flap technique (versus end-to-end anastomosis) in achieving excellent results in infants since the subclavian flap was not adopted routinely at GLH until after this time. Probably the routine postrepair operating room measurement of pressures above and below the anastomosis (GLH) and the selective use of the subclavian flap in cases with difficult anatomy for resection and anastomosis account for this.

Hospital Mortality in Children and Adults

The hospital mortality for repair of coarctation in children and adults approaches zero. Among 224 such patients, 3 (1.3%, CL 0.6%–2.7%) died in the hospital (GLH; Table 34-10). Two of these deaths occurred in 1949, and one of them was associated with important aortic incompetence. The third death, which occurred in 1961, was a patient with a high pulmonary vascular resistance (patent ductus arteriosus and VSD). The associated lesions present in these patients are listed in Table 34-2.

Among 174 patients, 2 (1.1%, CL 0.4%–2.7%) died in the hospital (UAB). One operated upon in 1967 was 11 years old and had an associated large PDA and VSD and severe pulmonary vascular disease and died suddenly 24 hours postoperatively. The other, 22 years old and operated upon in 1971,

died 6 hours postoperatively from sudden suture line hemorrhage related to a technical error of subadventitial dissection at operation.

Both of these mortality rates are a little lower than that reported in the literature,[B3,B9,L5,M2,S3,S6] (1,658 patients, 52 deaths or 3.1%, CL 2.7%–3.6%), but probably can be considered representative of current risks.

Incremental Risk Factors for Hospital Mortality in Children and Adults

In children and adults, the type of operation is not a risk factor (Table 34-11) nor is the age of the patient (Table 34-10). Aneurysm formation must increase the surgical risk, but this cannot be demonstrated in this material. In any event, incremental risk factors are hard to demonstrate when surgical advances have reduced hospital mortality to such a low level.

Early Postoperative Morbidity

Paraplegia
Two (0.6%, CL 0.2%–1.5%) among 318 surgically treated patients (GLH, 1949–1978) developed paraplegia. The incidence in the combined series (UAB and GLH) is 2 (0.4%, CL 0.1%–0.9%) among 547 such patients, which is not different

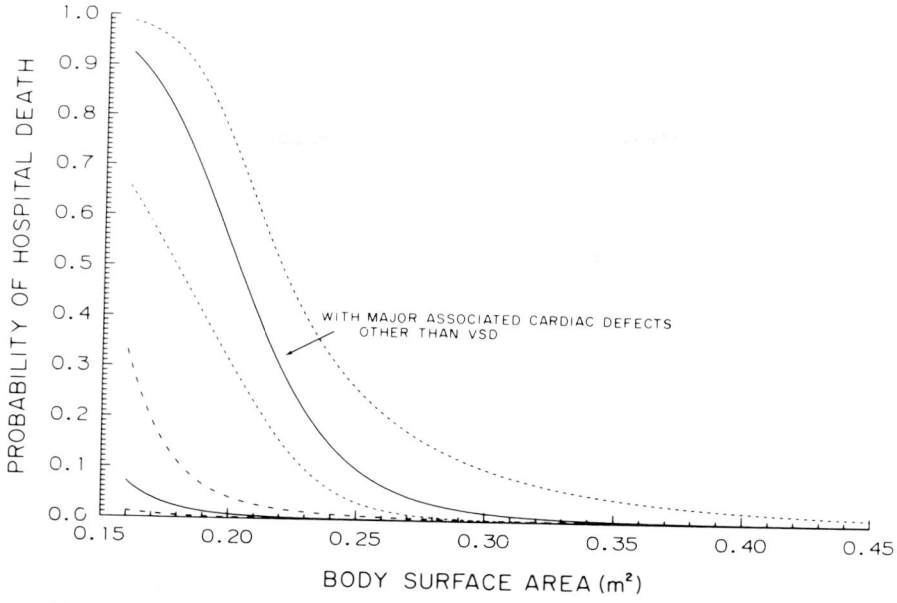

Figure 34-11 Nomogram of the logistic equation (Table 34-6) for the incremental risk factors for hospital death after repair of coarctation, presented for the subclavian flap repair. The unlabeled line represents primary (pure) coarctation and coarctation with ventricular septal defect, which were not different as regards hospital mortality. The labeled line represents those with major associated cardiac anomalies other than ventricular septal defect. The dashed lines enclose the 70% confidence limits. P(body surface area) = .04, and P(major associated cardiac defects other than VSD) = .005.

Reproduced with permission from Bergdahl et al.[B8]

from that reported in a collective review by Brewer[B6] of 51 instances (0.41%, CL 0.35%–0.48%) among 12,532 coarctectomies.

Incremental Risk Factors for Paraplegia

Enough knowledge of the incremental risk factors for paraplegia and their neutralization (see Chapter 53, "Paraplegia" in section on Special Situations and Controversies) is now available to make it possible that the incidence of paraplegia after coarctectomy approaches zero. Wherever the collateral circulation typical of coarctation has not developed, the risk of paraplegia is increased. This is probably because the blood pressure in the distal aorta is lower during aortic clamping when the collaterals are poorly developed.[K9] Thus, neither of the patients with this complication had developed

the typical collateral circulation of coarctation (GLH). One was operated upon for aortic aneurysm developing at a mild coarctation; the other was a 4-year-old child with preductal coarctation and a large PDA supplying the descending thoracic aorta. Situations that may fail to stimulate the development of the usual collateral circulation of coarctation include coarctations in infants, coarctations proximal to the left subclavian artery, coarctation with PDA supplying the descending thoracic aorta, coarctation associated with stenosis at the origin of the left subclavian artery or with the right subclavian artery arising as the fourth branch distal to the coarctation, and something less than severe narrowing at the coarcted area. These situations increase the risk of para-

Table 34-9 Hospital mortality in relation to method of coarctation repair in infants (UAB; 1967–1981).[B8]

Method of Repair	No.	Hospital Deaths		
		No.	%	CL
Resection and end-to-end anastomosis	21	13	62%	48%–74%
Subclavian flap	30	2	7%	2%–15%
Total	51[a]	15		
P		< .0001		

KEY: CL, 70% confidence limits.

[a] In 1972–1977, four additional patients had Dacron patch graft aortoplasty, one died.

Table 34-10 Absence of relationship of age at coarctation repair beyond infancy to hospital death (GLH; 1949–1977).

Age (yr)			n	Hospital Deaths	
≤		<		No.	%
1	---	4	17	0	0%
5	---	10	48	1	2%
10	---	20	82	2	2%
20	---	30	32	0	0%
30	---	40	22	0	0%
40	---	50	13	0	0%
50	---	64	10	0	0%
	Total		224	3	1.3%

Table 34-11   Type of operation used for repair of coarctation in patients aged 1–64 years (GLH; 1949–1977).

Type of Operation	No.	% of 224	Hospital Deaths	Poor Results
Resection + end-to-end anastomosis	147	66%	2	4
Resection + end-to-end anastomosis + patch graft	7	3%	0	0
Tube graft (end-to-end)	22	10%	0	4[c]
Dacron patch graft (onlay)	31	14%	0	2
Bypass tube graft (LSC − Desc. Ao)	1	0.5%	0	1[c]
Aortoplasty[a]	6	3%	0	0
LSC − Desc. Ao. anastomosis[b]	4	2%	1	2
Subclavian flap aortoplasty	6	3%	0	0
Total	224	100%	3(1.3%)	13(5.8%)

[a] Vertical incision with transverse closure in four; excision portion of circumference in one; excision diaphragm only in one.

[b] The left common carotid artery was used in one patient.

[c] Two of these five patients required reoperation for aneurysm, the other three had recoarctation.

plegia as a complication of operation. The risk is also increased at re-repair.[B6]

Postoperative Hypertension and Abdominal Pain
Nearly all patients, including infants, have some systolic and diastolic hypertension for a variable period after the repair of coarctation. Many patients, if observed carefully, have mild abdominal discomfort and distension during the first 5 or 6 postoperative days.[H5,R5] Uncommonly (10%–20% of cases), this becomes sufficient to produce important discomfort and distension. Then there may be abdominal tenderness, fever, ileus, and leukocytosis. In a 30-year experience with coarctation at the Mayo Clinic and UAB, during which routine treatment of postoperative hypertension was not practiced, no instance of the syndrome severe enough to require laparotomy or prolonged special treatment has been seen; at GLH, 2 patients underwent laparotomy, but in retrospect it is not certain if it was required. Thus, management should be nonsurgical in virtually all cases. (See "Special Features of Postoperative Care" for treatment.)

Further discussion of this syndrome is difficult, because in the early years of coarctation surgery many complications which are now rarely observed were reported as examples of the syndrome. Also, so-called paradoxic hypertension is really the rule after coarctation repair rather than the hallmark of a special syndrome. The syndrome was first described in a single case by Sealy in 1953.[S7] At laparotomy on the tenth postoperative day, the jejunum and proximal ileum were "edematous and cyanotic but the superior mesenteric arteries and veins were patent." At autopsy there was "inflammation of small arteries and arterioles confined to the body area below the coarctation" and infarcts in liver, spleen, kidney, and intestines. Lober and Lillehei added two cases in 1954[L6] and Perez-Alvarez and Oudkerk another in 1956.[P2] Ring and Lewis in 1956[R6] considered that the lesion justified the term "syndrome" and that it was due to sudden increase in pulsatile pressures in vessels distal to the coarctation with acute overdistension of these vessels. In 1957, Sealy[S8] linked the onset of abdominal pain with the presence of paradoxic hypertension, which he described in detail. He

noted that following successful coarctectomy, the patient could develop an early systolic hypertension within the first 36 postoperative hours or a more delayed mainly diastolic hypertension after 48 hours that lasted for 7–14 days. This delayed phase was associated with abdominal pain in 6 of 14 of his patients. This observation has been confirmed by many others.[H5,V4] Sealy suggested that the hypertension might be due to an altered baroreceptor response plus an increased excretion of epinephrine or norepinephrine.[G8,S8] The study by Rocchini and colleagues[R7] suggests that the sympathetic nervous system is responsible for the early phase and that the renin–angiotensin system plays a major role in the later phase, although more recent information would indicate the renin–angiotensin system also plays a role in the early phase.[P3]

Pathologic findings have been described in the small arteries and arterioles in vessels below the repaired coarctation[S7] in these patients, and they probably are present to some degree routinely after coarctation repair. They include thrombosis, inflammatory cell infiltration of the entire wall, fragmentation of the internal elastic lamina, and fibroblastic proliferation, as well as marked mesenteric lymphadenitis in the jejunum and proximal ileum.[D2] Rarely there may be infarcts in liver, spleen and kidneys, and rupture of aneurysms that may have formed on large intraabdominal arteries.[L6]

In a review of the literature up to 1970, Ho and Moss[H5] found the syndrome was reported in 9% (107 of 1,193) of patients surviving coarctectomy. The fully developed syndrome was present in 6% of patients (GLH), but as noted earlier it occurs to some degree in most patients. It is said to be rare below 2 years of age,[G9,R6,T4,V4] but since in young infants it is difficult to be sure of its presence or absence, this is questionable.

LATE RESULTS

Survival

Actuarial survival of all hospital survivors of coarctation *repair in infancy* is 83% at 15 years (Fig. 34-12). The survival is

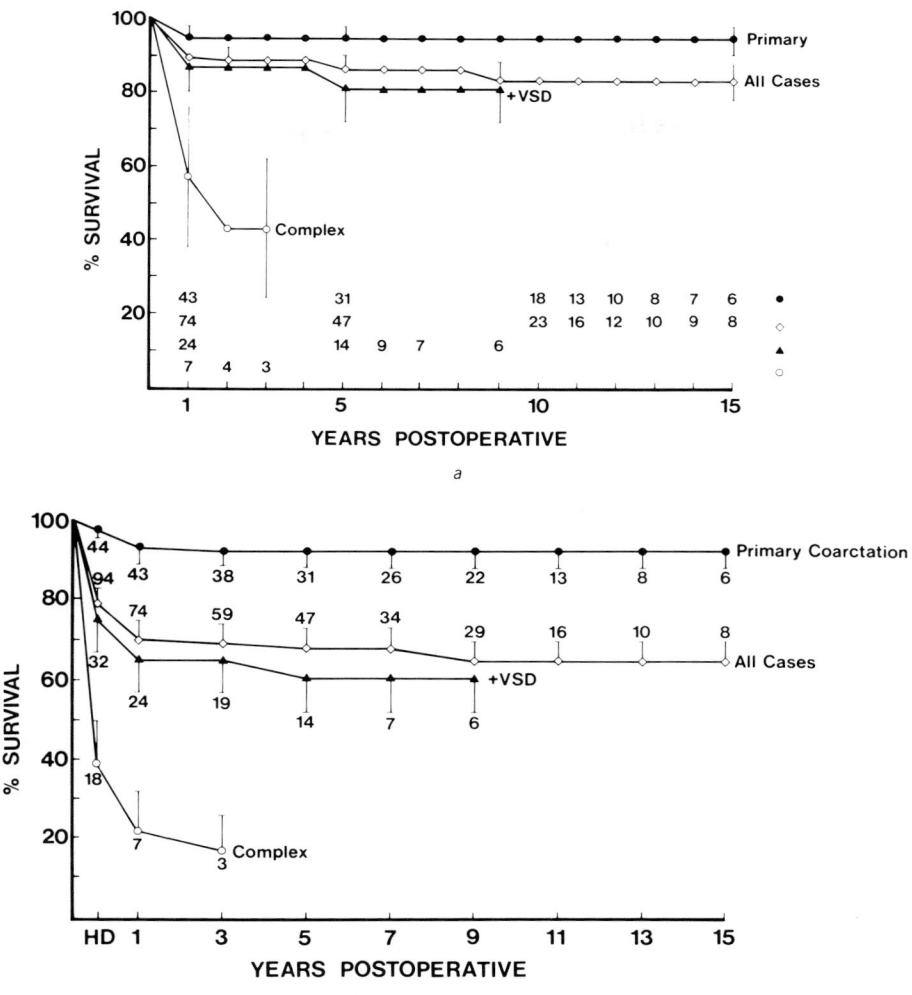

Figure 34-12 Patient survival expressed actuarially following repair of coarctation *in infancy*, including those with primary (pure) coarctation, coarctation with VSD, and coarctation with other major (complex) associated cardiac anomalies (GLH, 1960–1978). The numbers at risk in each category are noted.
(*a*) Hospital survivors.
(*b*) All cases coming to operation, including those dying in hospital. Primary versus VSD, *P* = .008; VSD versus complex, *P* ≤ .0001.
HD, hospital deaths; VSD, ventricular septal defect.

best for those with primary (pure) coarctation (92%), less good for those with coarctation and ventricular septal defect (VSD) (81%), and relatively poor for those with coarctation and other major associated cardiac anomalies (41% at 3 years). It is noteworthy that almost all the late deaths occur within 1 year of operation, and this probably represents the extension of the early phase of high hazard function so frequently seen after other kinds of cardiac surgery (see for example Chapter 7, "Incremental Risk Factors for Hospital and Early-Phase Death" in section on Early Results).

Actuarial survival of hospital survivors of coarctation *repair after infancy*, most of whom had pure coarctation, is 89% at 15 years and 83% at 25 years (Fig. 34-13). By 25 years after operation, about 90% of hospital survivors of coarcta-

tion repair after infancy are still living (GLH, 197 late survivors among 221 hospital survivors).

Mode of Late Death

When the repair of coarctation of the aorta is done *in infancy*, late death is usually related to recoarctation or to the associated lesions and their need for treatment (Table 34-12). In all, over a 25-year follow-up period, late death occurs in 15% of hospital survivors following coarctation repair in infancy (GLH). Data reported by McManus and colleagues support this idea.[M6]

When the coarctation *repair* is performed *after infancy*,

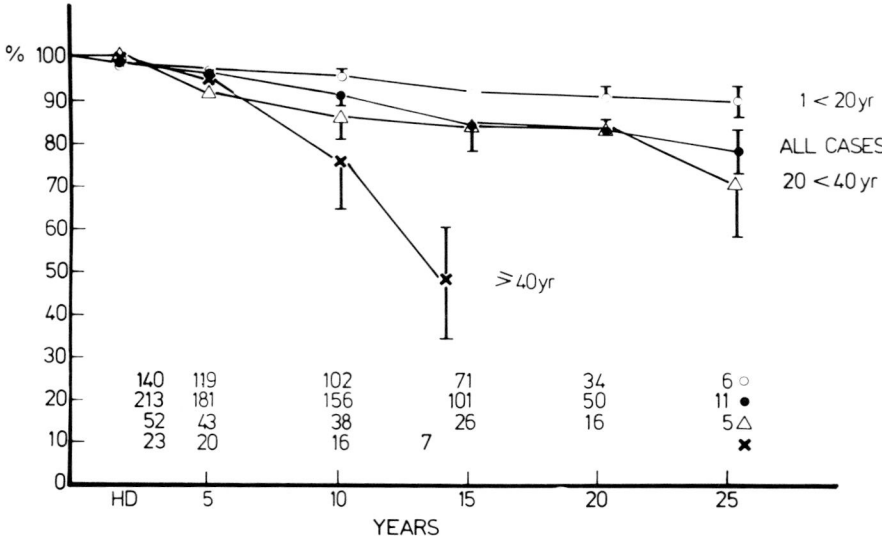

Figure 34-13 Survival following repair of coarctation in *1–64 year-old-age group* (GLH, 1949–1977). Hospital mortality is included. The ages to the right of the lines refer to age at operation. The numbers at risk are noted. 1–20 years versus 20–39 years, *P* = .07; 20–39 years versus 40 + years, *P* = .006.

HD, hospital deaths.

late death is associated with acute myocardial infarction in about 30% of cases (GLH; Table 34-13). About 20% of late deaths are related to the aortic valve disease that commonly coexists with coarctation (Table 34-13)[B9] and about 15% to aortic disease, either secondary to the coarctation repair or to aortic wall abnormalities probably related to the coarctation. Ruptured congenital intracranial aneurysms account for about 15% of late deaths,[M7] as do other forms of con-

genital heart disease (Table 34-13). Heart failure without mechanical cause is rare.

Incremental Risk Factors for Premature Late Death

Incremental risk factors for premature late death have not been rigorously defined, but some are apparent.

Major Associated Cardiac Anomalies
Other than VSD, major associated cardiac anomalies impose an incremental risk because of interim risks before the second repair, the risks of a second major cardiac operation, and the late risks after the second repair. As might be expected from the excellent late survival rate of VSD repaired in the first 2 years of life (see Chapter 20), an associated VSD

Table 34-12 Postcoarctectomy late deaths in patients undergoing repair in infancy (GLH; 1960–1978).

Age at Operation	Age at Death	Mode of Death	Recoarctation
		Coarctation	
21 d	3 mo	At repair ASD (1967)	None
3 mo	11 mo	Bronchopneumonia	Moderate
		Coarctation + VSD	
28 d	4 mo	Sudden	None
21 d	11 mo	Heart failure from recoarctation	Severe
7 wk	4 yr	At repair VSD[a] (+ debanding)	Mild
5 wk	6 mo	At repair VSD (+ debanding)	Severe
		Coarctation + Complex CHD	
4 d	12 mo	At re-repair[b] TGA + VSD	Mild
6 d	3 mo	At repair TGA + VSD	None
5 mo	8 yr	At repair TGA + VSD	Mild
3 mo	9 mo	At repair TGA + VSD	None
12 d	7 mo	Untreated single ventricle	Unknown

KEY: ASD, atrial septal defect; CHD, congenital heart disease; TGA, transposition of the great arteries; VSD, ventricular septal defect.

[a] Swiss cheese defects.

[b] For pulmonary vein stenosis.

Table 34-13 Postcoarctectomy late deaths in 1–64-year-old age group (GLH; 1949–1977).

Mode of Death	No.	Autopsied	Comments
Myocardial infarction	8	6	3 less than 40 yr old at death
Aortic valve disease	5	4	4 had aortic valve surgery
Heart failure	1	0	Normotensive
Aortic disease	3	3	1 ruptured false aneurysm after Dacron patch repair
			1 ruptured intercostal artery
			1 dissecting aneurysm
Associated CHD	3	2	1 high PVR (PDA + VSD)
			1 congenital mitral stenosis
			1 fibrous subaortic stenosis
Unrelated	3	2	
Unknown	1	0	
Total	24	17	

KEY: CHD, congenital heart disease; PDA, patent ductus arteriosus; PVR, pulmonary vascular resistance; VSD, ventricular septal defect.

is only a weak incremental risk factor for premature late death. Other more complex anomalies are stronger risk factors.

Older Age at Operation

Older age at operation seems clearly a risk factor. Thus, age over 20 years seems to provide less likelihood of survival for 15 postoperative years than does operation at a younger age (Fig. 34-13). There have been no deaths after the first postoperative year among patients having coarctation repair in the first year of life (GLH).

Type of Operation

It is not yet apparent whether end-to-end anastomosis, rather than the subclavian flap repair, is an incremental risk for premature late death. There is, however, a suggestion in the study of Cobanoglu and colleagues that this is the case.[C18]

Persistent or Recurrent Coarctation

Persistent or recurrent coarctation must increase the risk of premature late death, as must late postoperative upper body hypertension.

Persistent or Recurrent Coarctation

General Features

Persistent or recurrent coarctation is a postoperative condition characterized by a resting peak pressure gradient exceeding 20 mmHg across the repair area. This discussion is limited to situations in which there is a true luminal narrowing rather than simply a stiff segment of aorta. The latter can result in a pressure gradient, and the important physiologic consequence of either cause of the gradient is upper body hypertension. Assessment of the incidence and severity of persistent or recurrent coarctation is difficult, because many patients are not studied in a way that can establish the gradient, and in still fewer patients is the gradient during exercise known. Substitution of the freedom from reoperation rate for known absence of the resting gradient is unsatisfactory and must underestimate the incidence of persistent or recurrent coarctation.

Clinically, the diagnosis is established when femoral pulsation is diminished and delayed compared with the radial or brachial pulse. The pressure gradient can be measured by arm and leg cuff pressures, but more optimally by intra-arterial or intra-aortic pressure measurements. Usually, a narrowing can be visualized at the site of repair when an important gradient is present, but not unexpectedly the correlation between the gradient and angiographically determined narrowing is not great.[H8]

It is probable that many early "recoarctations" are in fact persistent coarctations.[H10,N2,P5] True recurrent recoarctations probably occur, although their demonstration by serial aortography has been infrequent. *True recoarctation* after end-to-end anastomosis has been attributed to lack of growth of the suture line and the presence of abnormal mesodermal tissue that proliferates and produces marked intimal and medial hypertrophy.[I1,K5,M8,P5,P6,P7,T6] Remnants of ductal tissue could behave in this way.[B3] Damage to the aorta from the

vascular clamps used at repair has also been implicated.[F3] Also, the mucopolyssacharides in the aortic wall in coarctation show a relative increase in the chondroitin sulfate fraction, more marked in recoarctation specimens,[B11] a change that leads to an increase in wall rigidity (a decrease in distensibility) that could predispose to restenosis.[R4] Technical factors are no doubt responsible for *persistent coarctation*, for example, insufficient resection of a long, narrow segment followed by end-to-end anastomosis or excessive tension on the suture line because of inadequate mobilization of the aorta above and below the coarctation. Other technical causes include incorrect fashioning of a subclavian flap or Dacron onlay patch, failure to resect an obstructing intimal ridge, the use of too small a tube graft in a child, or kinking of such a graft particularly when used as a bypass. A residual hypoplastic segment of transverse aortic arch, usually between the left subclavian and common carotid arteries (tubular hypoplasia), can possibly contribute to a residual gradient. However, serial aortograms have shown progressive growth of this segment after coarctectomy (GLH),[C10] no doubt secondary to restoration of normal arch blood flow.

The experimental animal data showing that normal growth of an artery can occur after end-to-end anastomosis[B10,S10] are not necessarily relevant to the situation after coarctectomy if indeed the tissue left behind is abnormal and has a tendency to proliferate and produce excessive scar tissue. The experimental data do not conclusively demonstrate the superiority of one particular suture technique for end-to-end anastomosis, although interrupted sutures are generally thought to be less likely to impede growth.[J1]

It is important to note that recoarctation in children and adults is considerably more common when the anatomy of the coarctation is unsuitable for direct end-to-end anastomosis because of a long narrowing or aneurysm formation, necessitating some other type of repair (see Table 34-11). The indications for and results of reoperation in patients with persistent or recurrent coarctation are discussed in "Special Situations and Controversies."

Incidence after End-to-End Anastomosis

The incidence of persisting coarctation or recoarctation is strongly related to the age at operation when the operation is end-to-end anastomosis (Table 34-14, and Fig. 34-14). The incidence is about 50% when the operation is performed in neonates, and it decreases from about 15% at 6 months of age (GLH) to less than 5% after infancy. Cobanoglu and colleagues have suggested that their incidence of persistent or recurrent coarctation after end-to-end anastomosis is much lower, but they have used the reoperation free rate as evidence for this.[C18] Harlan and colleagues interpret their data to indicate a lower incidence of these complications when 7-0 polypropylene rather than silk sutures are used, but they also used the reoperation free rate rather than measurement of gradient as their criterion.[H16]

Incidence after Subclavian Flap Aortoplasty

The subclavian flap operation appears to have reduced the incidence of persistent coarctation in neonates and infants (Table 34-15).[H7,P4,T5] Thus, Hamilton and colleagues report that of 34 infants less than 6 months of age treated by the

Table 34-14 Incidence of persisting coarctation or recoarctation (resting systolic pressure difference across coarctation [or upper extremity vs. lower extremity] ≥ 20 mmHg) after end-to-end anastomosis (GLH; 1949–1978).

Age at Operation		Traced Hospital Survivors[a]	Persistent or Recurrent Coarctation		
≤	<	n	No.	%	CL
(Months)					
	1	18	10	56%	41%–70%
1 ---	3	16	1	6%	0.8%–20%
3 ---	6	9	3	33%	15%–56%
6 ---	12	9	1	11%	1%–32%
1 to 54	(years)	147	4	3%	1%–5%
	Total	199	19	10%	7%–12%
	P (logistic)			<.0001	

KEY: CL, 70% confidence limits.

NOTE: There were an additional 15 examples of recoarctation seen following various other types of operation. Expressed actuarially, the incidence among all cases was 5% at 10 years, 7% at 15 years, and 9% at 25 years.

[a] Infant follow-up 7 years (range 2 months–19 years). Child and adult follow-up average 17.5 years (range 10–28 years).

subclavian flap operation, 0 (0%, CL 0%–6%) had residual or recurrent coarctation when followed up to 6 years postoperatively.[H7] The recent report of Waldhausen and colleagues also indicates a zero incidence (0%, CL 0%–8%) within 6 or more months of operation in 23 infants less than 14 months of age so treated.[W4] Both percentages are lower than that for end-to-end anastomosis (see Table 34-14 and Fig. 34-14), and the nonoverlapping confidence limits make it unlikely that the differences are due to chance. Campbell, Waldhausen, and colleagues report small gradients (15 and 20 mmHg) in 2 of 4 patients studied an average of 42 months after repair in infancy using continuous nonabsorbable suture, and no gradients in 7 in whom a subclavian flap aortoplasty was made using interrupted or absorbable sutures (see "Subclavian Flap Repair in Infants" in section of Technique of Operation).[C16] Penkoske and colleagues at Toronto Sick Children's Hospital found persisting or recoarctation in 6% (CL 3%–10%) of 81 infants repaired by the subclavian flap, in contrast to 27% using end-to-end anastomosis.[P9] Furthermore, in a group of 8 patients studied 4 years after subclavian flap aortoplasty, Fripp and colleagues found a normal arm–leg blood pressure response to exercise.[F12] Growth of the subclavian flap has been demonstrated by Moulton and colleagues.[M15]

The favorable experience reported by Campbell and colleagues included a considerable number (45) of neonates and infants less than 8 weeks of age, as did that of Hamilton and colleagues.[C16,H7] This is also true of the UAB and GLH experiences. In contrast, Metzdorff and colleagues infer from their experience that the incidence of persistent or recurrent coarctation is excessive when subclavian flap angioplasty is performed when the patient is less than 8 weeks old.[M17] They report a 75% 2-year actuarial freedom from reoperation rate after subclavian flap aortoplasty in infants less than 8 weeks of age and one of 100% in older patients. The differences in results in the various series cannot currently be reconciled, but possibly differences in surgical technique and methods of study of clinical experiences contribute to the dilemma.

The subclavian flap method does have the disadvantage that late postoperatively the left upper arm is mildly shortened and the left arm slightly less strong.[T10] Handedness is not affected.

Incidence after Patch Aortoplasty
The late results of Dacron or Gore-Tex patch aortoplasty in this regard have been variable. Sade and colleagues report persisting coarctation (mean arm–leg systolic blood pressure difference 33 ± 7.5 mmHg) after end-to-end anastomosis in infants but not after Gore-Tex patch aortoplasty (difference was 5.1 ± 2.3 mmHg).[S9] They also report growth of both the preoperatively hypoplastic isthmus and the intact posterior aortic wall at the site of repair.[S14] Similar findings were reported by Connor and Baker.[C13] Smith and colleagues found the arm–leg pressure gradient during exercise to be only mildly increased over the minimal resting gradient when patch aortoplasty had been used, but a large increase when end-to-end anastomosis had been used.[S15] However, Hesslein and colleagues from Houston report an incidence of persistent or recoarctation (by the criteria used in this chapter) of 18% with *no* difference for end-to-end anastomosis versus patch aortoplasty.[H9] Younger patients had a higher incidence with either operation.

Upper Body Arterial Hypertension without Resting Gradients

There remains some uncertainty, in patients with upper body hypertension after the repair of coarctation, as to the frequency with which the hypertension is associated with a pressure gradient across the repair at rest or during exercise but not at rest (Fig. 34-15). Exercise gradients develop in most patients whose repair has been made by resection and end-to-end anastomosis, even if gradients at rest are minimal or absent.[F2,V4] In any event, the mechanism of upper body hypertension late after coarctation repair is probably multifactorial and not in all cases simply a residual aortic narrowing. For example, Gidding and colleagues have shown increased vascular reactivity in the forearm of patients who are hypertensive after coarctation repair.[G10]

Many, but not all, patients leave the hospital with upper body arterial hypertension. Thus, in patients over 5 years of age at operation, only about 40% have normal systolic and diastolic blood pressures at hospital dismissal (GLH). During the next 5 years there is a steady increase in the percent of normotensive patients (Fig. 34-16), so that 90% of those observed 5 years postoperatively are normotensive at rest (GLH). However, by 20 years after operation, only 50% of patients treated by end-to-end anastomosis are without hypertension (normotensive), and by 25 years only 25% remain without this complication (Fig. 34-17). The significance of the incidence of hypertension after coarctation repair is better appreciated when this subset of patients is compared with the general population. In the 20–39 and 40–59 year age groups, the incidence of hypertension in the general population is 4% and 17%, respectively,[C14] whereas in the post-coarctectomy population the incidence is 36% and 78%, respectively. Clearly, those studies in which the mean fol-

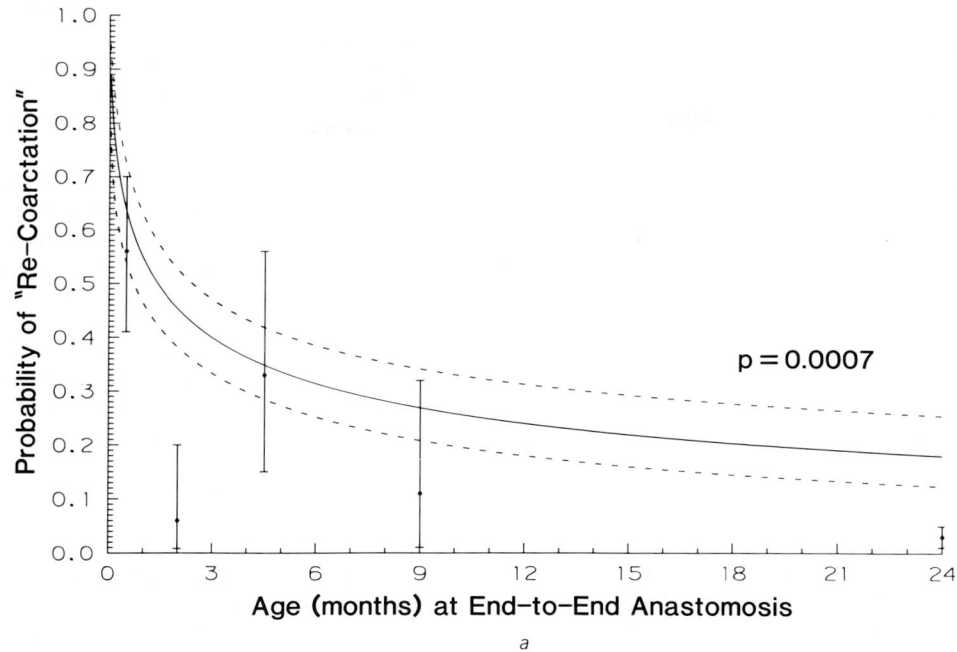

a

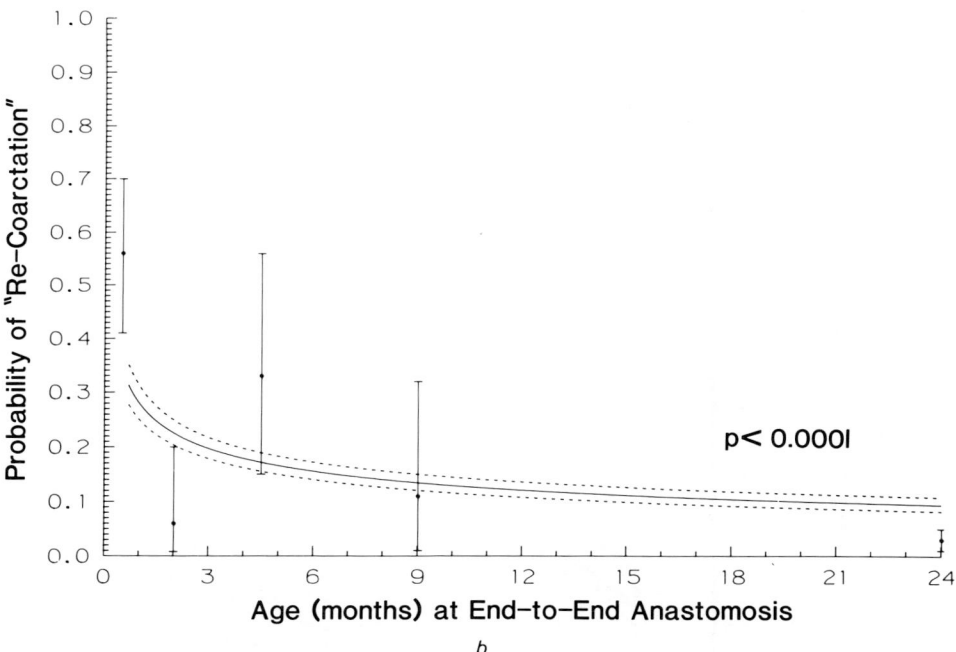

b

Figure 34-14   Probability of persistent or recurrent coarctation (criteria given in text) according to age at which coarctation was repaired by end-to-end anastomosis. Also shown by the solid circles with their 70% confidence limits is the GLH experience (Table 34-14).

(*a*) Logistic single-variable analysis from 69 cases *reported as individuals* in the literature.

(*b*) The same analysis and depiction from 161 cases *reported in groups* in the literature. The GLH data suggest that the relationship obtained from analysis of the grouped cases is probably close to the truth except in the very young patients, where the truth was probably often hidden by the grouping of 0–3 months or 0–6 months. In these two youngest age groups, the $n = 69$ analysis is probably closer to the truth.

See Appendix 34A for details and equations.

Table 34-15 Quality of femoral pulses early after coarctation repair in relation to type of operation in infants (UAB; 1967–1981).

| Type of Operation | n | PO Femoral Pulses Grade 3 or 4 | | |
		No.	%	CL
End-to-end anastomosis	12[a]	9	75%	56%–89%
Subclavian flap	30	29[b]	97%	89%–99.6%
P (Fisher)			.06	

KEY: CL, 70% confidence limits; No., number; PO, postoperative.
[a] PO pulses unknown in nine others (six of whom died in operating room).
[b] 28 grade 4 (full), one grade 3.

low-up period is less than 5 years[H6,L2,N2,P6,R5,S4] cannot be used as predictors of the risk of hypertension later in life.

Some of the *incremental risk factors* (other than persistent or recurrent coarctation) for upper body arterial hypertension late postoperatively are known. Age at operation is one. Late hypertension is more common in patients operated upon $\geq$ 20 years than 5–19 years (P = .007), although younger patients are not exempt (GLH; Fig. 34-17). Liberthson and colleagues, in the late follow-up of 234 patients with coarctation operated upon at the Massachusetts General Hospital, also noted an increasing incidence of postoperative hypertension as age at operation increased.[L2] Both the group 5–9 years old at operation and the 10–19 year-old group (GLH) have a significantly lower incidence of late hypertension than the group of patients 30 years of age at the time of operation (P = .02 and .001).

The late incidence of hypertension in infants and children less than 5 years old at the time of coarctectomy is less well known, although several publications indicate that hypertension can persist postoperatively in the absence of a residual anastomotic gradient.[N2,P1,R5,S4] However, in a 7-year follow-up of 118 patients having coarctation repair in the first year of life, Williams and colleagues found *no* instances of hypertension without persistent or recurrent coarctation.[W5] The actuarial incidence of hypertension in 18 patients aged 0–4 years at operation, without residual coarctation and followed for at least 10 years is no different from that in the 5–9 year olds (GLH), but it is at present assumed that hypertension will be less common in the 0–4 year olds when the follow-up period is longer.

Systemic arterial hypertension at hospital dismissal is an incremental risk factor in the GLH experience. Thus, patients who are normotensive at hospital discharge are more likely to remain normotensive 20 years later than those who are hypertensive at hospital discharge (P = .01).

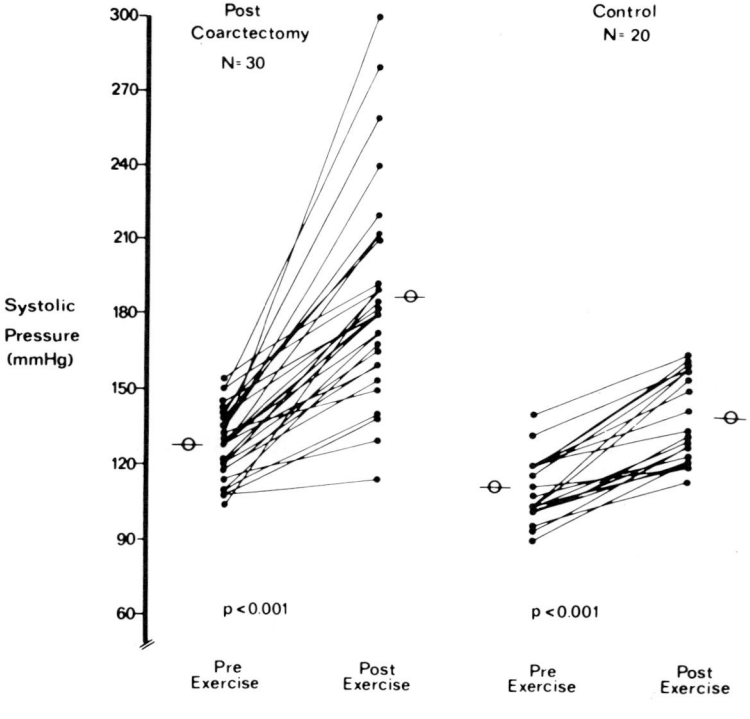

a

Figure 34-15 (*a*) Systolic blood pressure in the arm before and after exercise in patients after coarctectomy and end-to-end anastomosis and in 20 control subjects. The systolic pressure increased in both groups but was higher in the coarctectomy patients.

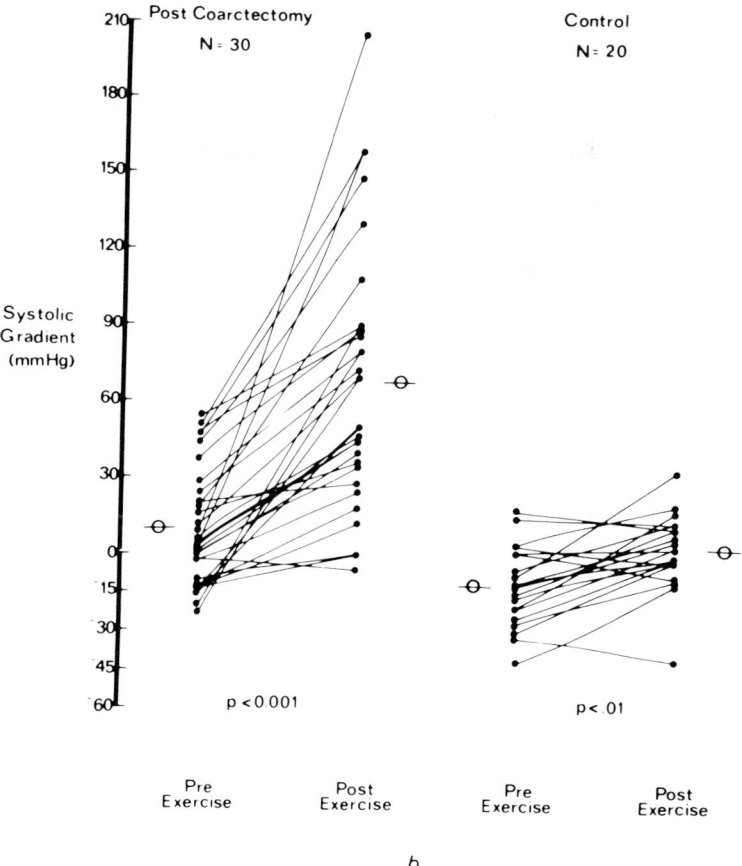

b

Figure 34-15 (*continued*)

(*b*) Systolic blood pressure difference between the arm and leg before and after exercise in the coarctectomy patients and the control subjects. The difference increased significantly, often to very high levels, in the coarctectomy group.

ɵ, average values; N, number of patients; p, probability.

Reproduced with permission from Freed et al.[F7]

Late Aneurysm Formation

A true or false aneurysm may occur late postoperatively. A *true aneurysm* from progressive deterioration of the aortic wall opposite a prosthetic onlay patch has been reported on long follow-up by Vorsschulte,[V1] Bergdahl and colleagues,[B12] Olsson and colleagues,[O2] and Rheuban and colleagues.[R12] Ala-Kulju and colleagues found this to develop in 27% (CL 21%–34%) of 62 patients followed 2–14 years.[A4] Presumably, the stiff patch transmits additional tension to the adjacent elastic aortic wall, which thus bears the total burden of the pulse wave and dilates.[O2,B12] This makes the Dacron onlay patch technique undesirable in most circumstances. A true aneurysm after a Dacron onlay patch repair has always (GLH) been associated with a false (suture line) aneurysm (see below). The incidence was 10% but increased to 25% in the 8 patients followed 15 years or more (GLH; Table 34-16). Aneurysms have not occurred in patients operated upon below 10 years of age (GLH; Table 34-17),

although the follow-up in the younger age group does not yet extend to 15 years.

An interposed aortic *homograft* tube may become aneurysmal (this has occurred in one of the four cases, GLH), but this is not common even with long follow-up.[F10,S3]

A *dissection* may occur occasionally either in the ascending or descending aorta, proximal or distal to the coarctation repair site (2 cases, GLH). This may lead to late aneurysm formation.

False (suture line) *aneurysms* can be mycotic when they occur early in the postoperative period[B12,K6] but they are usually uninfected and have a similar etiology to the false femoral aneurysm that occurs at the distal anastomosis of an aortofemoral prosthetic graft. They may complicate prosthetic tubular grafts as well as prosthetic onlay patches. In the former instance they are said to be more common at the proximal anastomosis of a bypass tube graft where the suture line is more oblique in relationship to the transverse forces in the aortic lumen.[O2] They are rare with end-to-end tubular grafts unless mycotic.

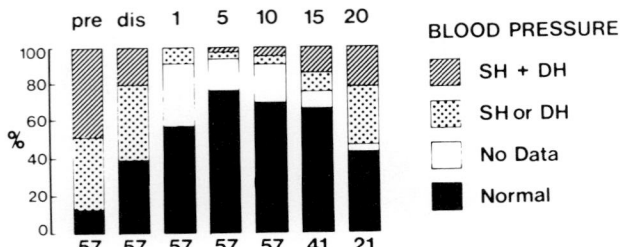

Figure 34-16 Histogram depicting the frequency of hypertension (excluding patients with persistent or recurrent coarctation) in 10–19-year age group preoperatively (pre), at hospital discharge (dis), and at 1–20 years postoperatively (GLH; operations in 1949–1968). The numbers beneath the bars are the number of patients at risk. The time intervals are noted in years at the top of the bars. The exact intervals were 1–2, 5 ± 1, 10 ± 1, 15 ± 1 and 20 ± 1 years. The analysis is based upon 10–28-year follow-up (mean 17.5 years). Note that the percent of patients with hypertension decreases in the first 5 postoperative years and then increases. This pattern occurred in all age groups.

DH, diastolic hypertension; SH, systolic hypertension.

Valvar Disease

Valvar disease may complicate long-term management of patients who have undergone coarctation repair and occasionally prevents a good result.[B16] Surgery for *aortic stenosis* (4 subvalvar, 1 valvar) has been required at 3–7 years of age in 7% of patients whose coarctation was repaired in infancy, excluding those with complex lesions (GLH). In patients beyond their first birthday at coarctation repair, 46 (21%) of 224 have definitive signs of aortic valve disease at last follow-up. To date, 14 (6%) of these have required surgery for stenosis or incompetence and 2 additional patients died before surgery was performed. No doubt a significantly larger number will require surgery for calcific aortic stenosis when more of those patients with bicuspid valves reach their fifth

and sixth decades of life. Thus, among the 23 patients in Crafoord's original series, followed by Bjork et al. for more than 26 years, 11 (48%) had developed definite aortic valve disease, although in four operation had not been required.[B9]

Congenital mitral valve disease has been thought to be infrequent in this setting. It was known to be present in only 8 patients (4%) in the GLH series; six remain well without valvular surgery, and 2 with congenital mitral stenosis died. It is probable that a number of additional infants had significant congenital mitral valve disease. Celano and colleagues found coexisting mitral valve anomalies in 12 (21%) of 56 patients with coarctation studied by two-dimensional echocardiography.[C17]

Other Late Events

Congestive heart failure may occasionally persist postoperatively in older patients who have it preoperatively,[L2] and coronary artery disease with myocardial infarction or angina also occurs but is not common.[M7] Bacterial endocarditis occasionally occurs on the aortic or mitral valve. Cerebrovascular accidents are more common in patients with persistent hypertension. Maron and colleagues noted a high incidence of conduction defects in the electrocardiograms (ECG) of their patients.[M7] Finally, Bjork and colleagues found degenerative disease of the hip joints present in 20% of their 25 patients who had been followed for 27–32 years and who were 7–31 years at the time of coarctectomy.[B9]

Summary

The late results following coarctectomy and end-to-end anastomosis in patients 1 year and over at the time of surgery include a small 1.3% hospital mortality (GLH; Fig. 34-18). The mortality increases as the follow-up lengthens. In the 84% of patients alive 25 years postoperatively, 4% had a recoarctation (or an aneurysm) that had either been

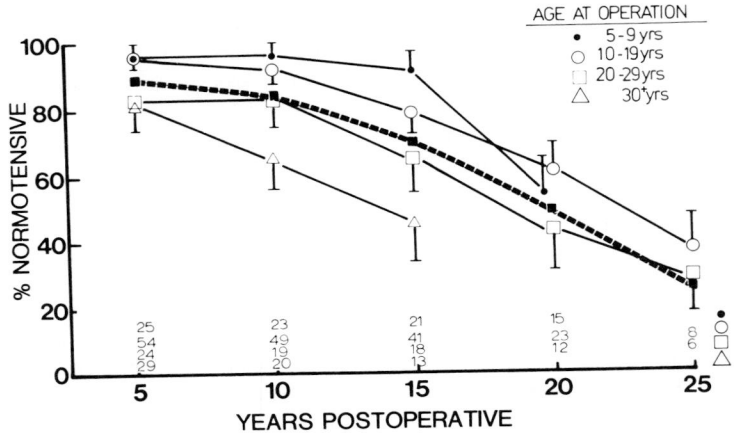

Figure 34-17 Actuarial incidence of patients free of hypertension after coarctectomy, excluding those with persistent or recurrent coarctation (GLH; operations in 1949–1968). The numbers at risk are shown. The dashed line represents the incidence for all cases combined. Age 5–9 versus age ≥ 30, P = .02; age 10–19 versus age ≥ 30, P = .001; age 5–19 versus age ≥ 20, P = .007.

Table 34-16 Incidence of late aneurysm formation following Dacron onlay patch grafting as primary repair or for re-repair of coarctation of the aorta (GLH; 1949–1979).

Duration of Follow-up (yr) ≤ / <	Primary Repair									Rerepair With Patch Alone			Total		
	Patch Alone			Patch + End-to-End Anastomosis			Patch Plus Subclavian Flap								
	n	Aneurysms No.	%	n	Aneurysms No.	%	n	Aneurysms No.	%	n	Aneurysms No.	%	n	Aneurysms No.	%
5	2		0%	1									3		
5 --- 10	12		0%	1			2			3	1	33%	18	1	6%
10 --- 15	15	2	13%	6						1		0%	22	2	9%
15 --- 20	4	2	50%	4									8	2	25%
Total	33	4 (CL 6%–20%)	12%	12		0% (CL 0%–15%)	2		0% (CL 0%–61%)	4	1 (CL 3%–63%)	25%	51	5 (CL 6%–16%)	10%

KEY: CL, 70% confidence limits.

NOTE: Screening of the patients was initially by plain chest x-ray, and only if this suggested an aneurysm was an aortogram performed. The incidence is thus probably underestimated.

reoperated upon or was producing significant obstruction; and a further 13% had one or another miscellaneous event of importance, such as symptomatic aortic valve disease usually treated by operation, angina, congestive heart failure, or a cerebrovascular accident. Finally, an increasing number of patients developed hypertension so that by 25 years postoperatively 47% of the living patients, excluding those with recoarctation or other miscellaneous events, had hypertension of varying degree. No one in this subset of patients had significant symptoms. Looked at in this fashion, 67% of the patients operated upon beyond infancy remain alive 25 years later, but only 20% are well and normotensive. The incremental risk factors for this accumulation of events may be similar to those already described in "Incremental Risk Factors for Premature Late Death" and in "Upper Body Arterial Hypertension without Resting Gradients."

INDICATIONS FOR OPERATION

Primary or Pure Coarctation

The presence of isolated, classic, severe coarctation of the aorta (diminished or delayed femoral pulses, reduction of luminal diameter at the coarcted area greater than 50%, and

Table 34-17 Incidence of late aneurysm in patients having a Dacron onlay patch alone as primary repair for coarctation in relation to age at operation (GLH; 1949–1979).

Age at Operation (yr) ≤ / <	Duration Follow-Up (yr)				
	<5	5–9	10–14	15–19	Total
5	1	4	2		7
5 --- 10		2	4		6
10 --- 20		4	3	2(1)	9(1)
20 --- 30	1	1	4(1)a	1	7(1)
30		1	2(1)	1(1)	4(2)
Total	2	12	15(2)	4(2)	33(4)

a ( ) Number with aneurysm.

enlarged collateral vessels) is an indication for operation. When the patient is first seen at age 3–4 years, operation should be advised forthwith. When the patient is first seen at an older age including in adult life, operation is still advisable, although as seen earlier the long-term results are less good. Even the presence of congestive heart failure is not a contraindication to operation,[L2] but preoperatively this should be controlled medically.

When the patient with isolated severe coarctation is seen in the first few weeks of life with congestive heart failure, intense medical treatment is indicated. Should the heart failure resolve completely so that decongestive therapy can be reduced and then discontinued, operation is delayed until the optimum age. Should the heart failure not resolve completely, operation is performed promptly.

Occasionally, young infants not in heart failure and with pure coarctation have severe upper body hypertension with systolic blood pressure over 150 mmHg. This is an indication for prompt operation.

The *optimum age* for repair and the type of repair both remain controversial. When end-to-end anastomosis is used, elective operation should be advised at age 3–4 years, since late hypertension is less common when it is done while the patient is young. Advising operation in the first year of life when end-to-end anastomosis is used, as advocated by some,[P1,S4] is unwise because of the high incidence of persistent or recoarctation that occurs in this age group. In contrast, when a subclavian flap operation is used, the optimum age for repair is considered to be between 6 and 12 months (UAB, GLH).[C18]

A subclavian flap repair is advisable in infants and may also be preferred between 1 and about 10 years of age (UAB) because of the 5% incidence of residual coarctation or recoarctation and the exercise gradients that occur following end-to-end anastomosis.[H11] However, when the anatomy is ideal for end-to-end anastomosis, this technique can be used and it remains the technique of choice in patients over about 10 years of age. This could change if long-term follow-up of the subclavian flap procedure shows that it is less likely to be associated with late hypertension.

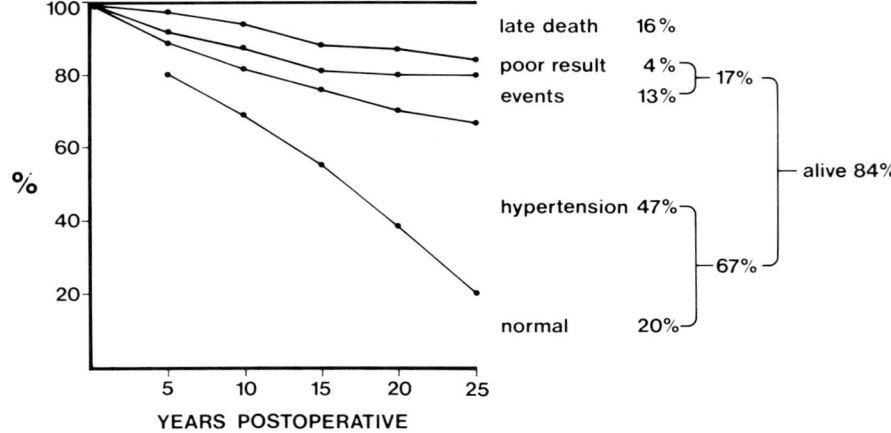

Figure 34-18 Cumulative actuarial portrayal of late events after repair with end-to-end anastomosis of coarctation in patients aged 1 year and over at the time of operation (GLH; operations in 1949–1968).

A Dacron or Gore-Tex patch graft enlargement, although advocated by some,[F6,S9] is not advised for routine use because of the incidence of late aneurysm formation. It should be reserved for special circumstances when other procedures are inappropriate. An example would be a long, tubular narrowing with hypoplasia of the subclavian artery in a young patient.

Resection and interposition of a tube graft of Dacron is rarely followed by late aneurysm formation and is therefore a superior operation to patch grafting when subsequent growth of the site of repair is not a consideration. It is the operation required when aneurysm is present either on the proximal segment of the intercostal arteries or on the adjacent aorta and may be required in adults for coarctations proximal to the left subclavian artery.

A bypassing Dacron tube graft may be all that is possible without undue risk very occasionally in older children and adults with complex forms of coarctation. These grafts are not recommended because of the increased risk of anastomotic aneurysms.

Coarctation and Ventricular Septal Defect

When infants present in heart failure with severe coarctation and ventricular septal defect (VSD), urgent repair of the coarctation is indicated (see above). This is particularly the case when the VSD is large, the patient very young and small, and the blood urea elevated.[L8] If the VSD is small or moderately sized, only coarctation repair is needed.

When the VSD is large or multiple, the situation is controversial. A policy of coarctation repair and pulmonary artery banding and later repair of the VSD has provided good results (GLH; Table 34-18), and this continues to be the policy in neonates (GLH). In infants over 1 month of age, simultaneous repair is preferred (GLH). Alternatively only the coarctation is repaired in neonates and young infants; if the neonate or infant is not extubated and progressing well 48 hours after this operation, the VSD is then repaired (UAB). Among 12 patients treated in this manner by Penkoske and colleagues, spontaneous VSD closure has occurred in 5, and

spontaneous narrowing in 6.[P9] They did not find cineangiographic estimation of VSD size helpful in predicting the tendency of the defect to narrow or close. (See Chapter 20 for more details.)

Coarctation and Other Coexisting Cardiac Anomalies

When neonates and young infants present in heart failure with severe coarctation and a major associated cardiac anomaly other than VSD, the situation is a hazardous one (see Fig. 34-11). When the associated anomaly is correctable, the coarctation is repaired and the infant is followed closely medically. If the child is not doing well within 2 or 3 days of the repair, then the associated lesion should be repaired also. In some patients, repair of the coarctation through a left thoracotomy and concomitant repair of the associated cardiac anomaly through a median sternotomy is

Table 34-18 Results of surgical treatment in patients with coarctation and ventricular septal defect (GLH; 1974–1984; 4 patients await VSD repair).

		Deaths	
Categories	No.	Hospital	Late
Moderate coarctation + large VSD			
VSD closure only	3	0	0
Severe coarctation + moderate VSD			
Coarctectomy only	3	0	1[a]
Severe Coarctation + large VSD			
Stage 1: coarctectomy + banding	16	1	1[b]
Stage 2: VSD closure + debanding	10	3[c]	0
Severe coarctation + large VSD			
Simultaneous repair	3[d]	0	0
Total	25	4	2

KEY: VSD, ventricular septal defect.

[a] Recoarctation.

[b] Noncardiac.

[c] Recoarctation two, Swiss cheese in one.

[d] Ages 3, 5, and 9 months.

appropriate. Satisfactory results with this one-stage approach have been reported by Tiraboschi and colleagues.[T7]

SPECIAL SITUATIONS AND CONTROVERSIES

Coarctation Proximal to the Left Subclavian Artery

Coarctation proximal to the left subclavian artery is rare (about 1% of all cases). The stenosis is localized, and femoral pulses are usually only slightly decreased and the systolic pressure gradient across the coarctation mild (< 20 mmHg) or moderate. The coarctation is often not detected until young adult life, at which time upper body hypertension is often present. A well-developed collateral circulation is generally not present.

The natural history of this lesion and its prognosis with antihypertensive medication is not clear, and thus neither are the indications for operation. However, when upper body systolic and diastolic hypertension are severe during moderate exercise, operation is advised.

A reverse subclavian flap is optimal treatment in infants and young children (see "Technique of Operation"). When a resection and anastomosis is used in older children and adults, either directly or with interposition of a tubular Dacron graft, the risk of hospital death or a major complication is probably 5%–10%. When a right-sided bypass Dacron graft (ascending aorta to descending thoracic aorta) is used, the risk is lower and the hemodynamic result is good on intermediate term follow-up (up to 11 years),[E3] but there is an increased risk of anastomotic aneurysm and of upper body hypertension during exercise.

When an operation is performed in this subset of patients, particular attention must be paid to preventing paraplegia (see "Repair of Coarctation Proximal to the Left Subclavian Artery" in section on Technique of Operation).

Mild and Moderate Coarctation in the Classic Position

Uncommonly, in infants and older patients *moderate* coarctation is present in the classic position. Collateral vessels are absent. The natural history of this entity is not clear and thus neither are the indications for operation. Degenerative changes are, however, prone to occur in the region of the coarctation, and when calcification is apparent, resection and replacement of this area with a tube graft may be recommended (UAB). The surgical techniques are the same as for thoracic aneurysms in this area (see Chapter 55).

When the coarctation is so *mild* that there is no gradient across the area, in which case the lesion is usually found because of the buckled appearance of the aorta on chest x-ray (pseudocoarctation),[N3] operation is advised only when degenerative changes and thus an increased risk of aneurysm formation have developed.

Prevention of Paraplegia as a Complication of the Repair

In the combined experiences (GLH 1949 to the present, Mayo Clinic 1950–1966, and UAB 1966–1982), paraplegia has not occurred as an operative complication in classic coarctation of the aorta with well-developed collateral circulation. Thus, in preventing paraplegia after the repair of coarctation great importance attaches to the *preoperative* identification of patients with potentially inadequate collateral circulation. In children and adults with juxtaductal coarctation, the absence of rib notching on the chest x-ray or of palpable parascapular pulsations suggest that the collateral circulation is not well developed. Only mildly diminished femoral pulsations in such patients are often associated with a poorly developed collateral circulation, as are a diminished left radial pulse (usually due to involvement of the origin of the left subclavian artery in the coarctation) or a diminished right radial pulse (present when the right subclavian artery arises distal to the coarctation). Aortography is indicated under these circumstances, and when adequate collateral arteries are not present, special measures are taken at operation (see Chapter 53, "Paraplegia" in section on Special Situations and Controversies). If uncertainty remains, pressure is measured at thoracotomy in the descending aorta with the proximal aortic cross-clamp temporarily in place (GLH); if this is less than 50 mmHg, special measures are used.

Many infants with coarctation have a good collateral circulation around the coarctation but some do not, and the routine use of mild hypothermia to about 33°C when the aorta is cross-clamped probably allows 45 minutes of safe cross-clamping in all cases (see "Subclavian Flap Aortoplasty in Infants" in section on Technique of Operation for details). This degree of hypothermia is as protective in older patients as in infants and a similar technique may be used when the collateral circulation is not well developed. The ice cold saline lavage may need to be prolonged to 10 minutes or so. Instead, a temporary bypass shunt, usually from the left subclavian to the descending thoracic aorta or femorofemoral cardiopulmonary bypass may be used during the period of aortic cross-clamping (see Chapter 53, "Paraplegia," in section on Special Situations and Controversies). Another alternative is the placement of a large bypass graft as a permanent method of repair.

Indication for and Results of Operation for Persistent or Recurrent Coarctation

The current indications for reoperation are the demonstration of a resting gradient across the coarctation of > 20 mmHg and angiographic demonstration of reduction of luminal diameter of greater than 50% at the anastomosis. Under these circumstances, heart failure or upper body hypertension (systolic pressure > 140 mmHg in infants and children) is an indication for prompt reoperation. However, of 21 infants with persistent or recurrent coarctation, only 3 (14%) died late postoperatively, all without reoperation (GLH); and none of the children or adults with these problems have died from them.

Hospital mortality has been low, since no deaths have occurred in the combined GLH-UAB experience with reoperation, although reports in the literature indicate a potential mortality of 10%–20%.[E4,11]

The physiologic results are reasonably good, but the aortic scarring or residual narrowing often prevent an ideal result.

Balloon Angioplasty for Coarctation

Percutaneous balloon angioplasty is being used in some cardiac centers for the treatment of coarctation of the aorta. It has been found to be useful in patients with persistent or recurrent coarctation after operation.[A7,K10] In patients who have not undergone repair, the situation remains highly controversial. The aortic gradients have usually been reduced, but they may remain greater than 20 mmHg.[C19,D5,M18] Marvin and colleagues found a mean peak systolic pressure gradient of 23 mmHg after balloon angioplasty in 10 young children;[M16] a further decrease of 12 mmHg occurred in the subsequent 6 months. De Lezo and colleagues have reported some good results in neonates and young infants, but they have encountered early recoarctation and in another patient death soon after the dilation.[L9] Lock, from his considerable experience, has warned against premature enthusiasm for the use of balloon angioplasty as a primary method of treatment for aortic coarctation.[L11] More experience and intermediate and long-term follow-up evaluation will be required before this technique can be considered an acceptable alternative to surgical treatment for primary coarctation.

SECTION **2**

INTERRUPTED AORTIC ARCH

DEFINITION

Interrupted aortic arch is complete luminal and anatomic discontinuity between two segments of the aortic arch. Also those rare specimens that exhibit a fibrous strand connecting the two widely separated ends are included under aortic arch interruption rather than coarctation.

HISTORICAL NOTE

The first description of interrupted aortic arch is attributed to Steidele in 1778.[S12] In this case the aortic isthmus was absent so that the morphology was similar to preductal coarctation. The description of the absence of more proximal portions of the arch occurred later; for the segment between the left subclavian and left common carotid they occurred in 1818 by Siedel[S13] and for that between the left common carotid and innominate arteries by Weisman and Kesten not until 1948.[W7] By 1959, Celoria and Patton were able to collect 28 cases that they classified according to the site of obstruction into types A, B, and C.[C11]

The first patient to have successful surgical treatment was a 3-year-old girl operated upon by Samson in 1955.[M9] The aortic isthmus was absent between the left subclavian artery and a widely patent ductus arteriosus, but both structures were adjacent and it was possible to join the divided ductus to the under surface of the proximal left subclavian artery. The two ventricular septal defects (VSDs) were closed 4 years later. Mustard apparently performed a similar successful procedure in a similar patient aged 7 months in 1957.[V6] Villalobos and colleagues[V7] and Blake and colleagues[B15] each reported a successful case in the early 1960s using a prosthetic graft to bridge the gap. Sirak et al.[S11] were the first to use the turned-down arch branches successfully (left subclavian or left common carotid artery or both) for end-to-end anastomosis to the descending aorta (combined with pulmonary artery banding for the VSD), although this type of operation was attempted as early as 1959.[V6] Sirak's patient was also the first neonate to survive operation, followed by an 18-hour-old boy reported by Norton et al.[N4] and an 11-day-old infant operated upon in Houston in 1970.[V5] In 1970, a palliative operation consisting of a Dacron graft between the main pulmonary artery and the descending aorta combined with pulmonary artery banding was used successfully by Litwin et al.[L7] in an 11-day-old infant, but this procedure is no longer advocated.

The first simultaneous repair of both the interrupted arch and all intracardiac lesions was performed successfully at GLH in 1970[B13] in an 8-day-old infant with an interruption distal to the left subclavian artery, a VSD, and total anomalous pulmonary venous connection. A 12-mm Dacron conduit was used first, with a left thoracotomy to join its distal end to descending aorta and then with a median sternotomy to join the proximal end to ascending aorta and to repair both intracardiac lesions. The procedure demonstrated that circulatory arrest techniques made an anastomosis to the ascending aorta feasible. In 1973, Murphy and colleagues reported a successful complete repair in a 3-day-old infant with interruption proximal to the left subclavian artery, and a VSD, using profound hypothermia-circulatory arrest techniques.[M10] They used a segment of the father's basilic vein as the graft between descending and ascending aorta and approached the heart and descending aorta through a median sternotomy with an extension into the third left intercostal space. In 1975, Trusler demonstrated that a median sternotomy alone provided adequate exposure for this procedure in small infants, and, again using circulatory arrest techniques, he was able to anastomose the descending aorta successfully, after excising ductus tissue, end-to-side to the ascending and transverse aortic arch without interposing a graft.[T8] The VSD was also closed. In 1976, the remarkable immediate preoperative improvement produced by the ductus-opening effect of prostaglandin E_1[E5,N1] was reported in the preoperative treatment of interrupted aortic arch.[H12,R8]

MORPHOLOGY

Types

The aortic arch may be interrupted at one of three sites. It may be interrupted just distal to the left subclavian artery (type A of Celoria and Patton[C11]), and flow into the descending aorta is from the ductus arteriosus. All forms of interrupted aortic arch display this latter feature with the rare exception of those cases in which the ductus is absent or closes during fetal life. About 40% of cases are of this type.[V6] The most common site of interruption (55% of cases) is proximal to the left subclavian artery, between it and the left common carotid artery (type B). In only about 5% of cases is the interruption proximal to the left common carotid artery, between it and the innominate artery[V6] (type C).

Aortic Arch

Anomalies of the origins of the brachiocephalic vessels are frequent in association with interrupted arch.[R9] Thus, an aberrant right subclavian artery is not uncommon in type B but can also occur in type A;[B13] the right subclavian may in fact arise high in the neck from the right common carotid artery (cervical origin of the right subclavian artery).[K7] A right-sided ductus may also persist from the right pulmonary artery and give origin to the right subclavian artery, and the right pulmonary artery may arise from the ascending aorta. Rarely, interrupted arch occurs with a right aortic arch, and in this instance both left and right ducti may remain patent and give origin to the subclavian arteries.[R9]

Characteristically, the ascending aorta is about half the normal diameter and is straight, dividing into two branches of about equal size (the V sign), whereas the main pulmonary artery is huge. The descending aorta is a direct continuation of the ductus arteriosus, as in the fetus, and is usually a little larger than the ascending aorta.

In the newborn, there is usually a wide gap between the aortic ends, although when the interruption is beyond the left subclavian artery the gap may be short. Rarely, there is a fibrous strand connecting the two ends.

Since the ductus arteriosus is almost always widely patent at birth, a collateral circulation does not develop and death occurs when the ductus closes soon after birth. When the ductus is obliterated in fetal life, a collateral circulation is already present at birth[D3] and survival is usual.

Left Ventricular Outflow Anomalies

The aortic valve is bicuspid in 30%–50% of patients, analogous to the situation in coarctation. Congenital valvar aortic stenosis may be present occasionally and subaortic stenosis may be present or develop (see below).[F8,12,V6] The aortic ring is frequently small, compared to the diameter of the ascending aorta.

Coexisting Cardiac Anomalies

A large ventricular septal defect (VSD) is nearly always present. The majority of these (about 60%) are subpulmonary, and most lie within the substance of the conal (infundibular) septum so that muscle persists between pulmonary and aortic leaflets. This portion of the conal septum is often displaced leftward beneath the aortic valve to produce a subaortic stenosis,[F8,V6] either initially or after repair (see "Late Results"); Ho and colleagues found significant left ventricular outflow tract obstruction by this mechanism in 9 (41%, CL 29%–54%) of 22 autopsy specimens of interrupted aortic arch and VSD (see Chapter 32).[H15] Less commonly, the VSD is subaortic and immediately subpulmonary with contiguous aortic and pulmonary leaflets. In about 25% of cases, the VSD is perimembranous or in the muscular septum. The VSDs may be multiple.

As in coarctation of the aorta, a wide variety of other often complex associated cardiac anomalies can occur[D4,F11,V6] with the exception of those associated with pulmonary stenosis. There is, however, a particular association with *truncus arteriosus* and *aortopulmonary (AP) window*.

Associated Syndromes

Absence of thymic tissue (Di George's syndrome) is a rather frequently associated syndrome[C12,F9,V6] and should be looked for routinely. Van Mierop and Kutsche found this association only in type B interrupted arch, and believe this finding has pathogenetic significance.[V8] When Di George's syndrome is present, hypocalcemia will require treatment,[N4] as will immunologic problems.

CLINICAL FEATURES AND DIAGNOSTIC CRITERIA

Almost all patients with interrupted aortic arch present as critically ill neonates in severe congestive heart failure due to the combined effects of volume overload from the left-to-right intracardiac shunting and the high afterload imposed by the closing ductus in the presence of total aortic interruption. Metabolic acidosis and anuria develop rapidly. Femoral pulses become diminished and then impalpable as the ductus closes and may vary in volume from hour to hour.[H13] It is of interest that when the ductus closes flow reverses in the vessels distal to the interruption (left subclavian and left common carotid) without recognizable neurologic symptoms developing.[H13] With the ductus still shunting, the expected differential cyanosis between arms and legs is usually not visible, in part because the intracardiac bidirectional shunt minimizes the oxygen saturation differences between ascending and descending aorta. Reversed differential cyanosis (blue arms and pink legs) can be obvious, however, when there is associated transposition of the great arteries.

Cardiac murmurs are not specific, nor is the electrocardiogram. The chest x-ray shows gross cardiomegaly and pulmonary plethora.

In those occasional instances in which the ductus remains widely patent and the intracardiac lesions are not complex, presentation is delayed for several weeks and heart failure and cardiomegaly are less severe. In the few patients who survive unrecognized into childhood, an Eisenmenger syndrome with cyanosis commonly develops. Rarely, interrupted aortic arch presents as an entirely isolated lesion in childhood or young adult life, in a manner similar to that of classic coarctation and in association with an obvious collateral circulation.[D3,R11]

Cardiac catheterization with cineangiocardiography is required for diagnosis and should be proceeded with promptly. A prostaglandin E_1 infusion is commenced prior to the study or during it. The study must include multiple contrast injections in both ventricles to outline not only the ascending and descending aorta, including when possible the size of the aortic outflow region beneath and at valve level, but also any other cardiac anomaly.[B13] Calculations of pulmonary vascular resistance are particularly important beyond the first year of life.

NATURAL HISTORY

Interrupted aortic arch comprised 1%–4% of autopsy cases of congenital heart disease and 1.3% of infants presenting with critical congenital heart disease at the Boston Children's Hospital.[C12,V6] The estimated incidence is 0.003 per 1,000 births.

This uncommon anomaly is highly lethal since the median age of death is 4–10 days and 75% of such babies are dead within 1 month of birth.[F8,R9,V6] If the ductus arteriosus stays open, longer survival is possible, but even then 90% are dead by 1 year of age (see Fig. 34-8). In those unusual circumstances in which major associated cardiac anomalies are absent, the natural history is similar to that of coarctation without major associated cardiac anomalies (see Fig. 32-8).

TECHNIQUE OF OPERATION

In the absence of a generally applicable method of surgical treatment, the methods that have been used are described briefly. In any event, a prostaglandin E_1 infusion is in place when the patient comes to the operating room (see "Indications for Operation").

Direct Anastomosis

Direct anastomosis is applicable primarily to aortic arch interruptions below the left subclavian artery. It can be done through a left thoracotomy or, with more difficulty, through a median sternotomy when profound hypothermia and total circulatory arrest are used. The technique is advantageous because of its simplicity, but the anastomosis may be under enough tension to compromise the lumen (see "Early Results" and "Late Results"). After division of the ductus arteriosus and closure of the pulmonary end, friable ductal tissue must be removed from the descending aorta before making the anastomosis.

Direct anastomosis has been used by Turley and colleagues for aortic arch interruption between the left common carotid and left subclavian arteries.[T12] The patients were nearly all neonates, and an anterior approach was used and simultaneous repair of the associated ventricular septal defect.

Interposed Gore-Tex or Other Grafts

Grafts may be used for interruptions distal to the left subclavian artery and for some that are between the left common carotid and subclavian arteries. The approaches include those used for direct anastomosis; alternatively, the distal anastomosis may be performed through a left thoracotomy and then the proximal anastomosis and intracardiac repair through a median sternotomy.[B13,V4]

Pulmonary Artery Banding

When pulmonary artery banding is to be done for an associated anomaly, a left thoracotomy is made for the repair and banding (see the rules for banding in Chapter 20, "Pulmonary Artery Banding" in Section 1, Technique of Operation).

One-Stage Repair

A median sternotomy approach and profound hypothermia and total circulatory arrest are optimal. (See Chapter 2, Section 4.) As noted, a left thoracotomy may be made first for distal anastomosis of a tube graft to the descending aorta.

The ice bags are removed from the front of the chest at 24°C and a median sternotomy approach made. After opening the pericardium and the ascending aorta and its branches, the distal pulmonary artery, the ductus, and its continuation into the descending aorta are dissected fully extrapleurally. This is a relatively simple matter since the aortic pressure is about 40 mmHg at these low temperatures. Presuming that the heart has continued to beat effectively throughout, circulatory arrest is established at 20–22°C without cannulating the small ascending aorta at this stage and, therefore, without any period of additional core cooling. A single venous cannula is, however, inserted into the right atrial appendage and connected to the cardiopulmonary bypass (CPB) circuit, and blood is drained off the infant through this line into the machine. The arch branches are occluded with a single clamp. The ductus is detached from the descending aorta removing all the friable and often heaped-up ductal tissue.[C15] In situations in which the interruption is between the left common carotid and subclavian arteries, this opening can be enlarged upward into the origin of the left subclavian artery. An appropriate length incision is made into the ascending aorta posteriorly, if necessary carrying this upward onto the left subclavian artery or left common carotid origin as the case may be. An end-to-side anastomosis may be made between the lower and upper aortic segments using interrupted simple or everting 6-0 polypropylene or Dacron sutures. Alternative measures for establishing aortic continuity may be used.

The anterior ascending aorta is next cannulated for arterial return opposite or proximal to the anastomosis and CPB commenced, cooling the infant to 18°C. During this perfusion, which is now equally effective in upper and lower body compartments, the anastomosis is checked for leaks and additional sutures applied to control any bleeding. The pulmonary artery end of the ductus that has been clamped earlier is now closed with a suture. The circulation is again arrested to repair the intracardiac anomaly. With the repair completed and the heart closed, CPB is reestablished and the operation completed as usual (see Chapter 2).

The sequence described may need to be altered if the circulation is inadequate during surface cooling or while dissecting the arch vessels and ductus. In this event, the ascending aorta is cannulated for a short period of core cooling prior to establishing circulatory arrest for the anastomosis; if this is accomplished expeditiously, a VSD can be repaired during the same arrest period.

SPECIAL FEATURES OF POSTOPERATIVE CARE

Care is as usual (see Chapter 5). Special attention is paid to the possible occurrence of hypocalcemia, should Di George's syndrome be present.

EARLY RESULTS

The early risks are higher after repair of interrupted aortic arch then after most other operations for congenital heart disease.

One-Stage Repair

When the interrupted arch (usually between the left common carotid and subclavian artery but sometimes beyond the left subclavian artery) and a coexisting VSD are repaired at one stage, the mortality can be as low as 20% but is frequently 80%–100%. Thus, Norwood and colleagues report 3 hospital deaths (23%, CL 10%–41%) among 13 neonates treated in this manner.[N5] In most of their cases, a tube graft was anastomosed to the descending thoracic aorta via a left thoracotomy and then through a median sternotomy anastomosed to the ascending aorta; the ductus was then ligated and the VSD closed during profoundly hypothermic total circulatory arrest. Turley and colleagues report 2 deaths (20%, CL 7%–41%) among 10 neonates and young infants in whom a direct anastomosis and repair of the VSD were used.[T12] Moulton and Bowman, performing the entire procedure through a median sternotomy, reported 2 deaths (33%, CL 12%–62%) in 6 infants aged 7 days to 5 months.[M12] One of their 2 neonates survived. In a collected review of five series,[B14,M10,M12,M14,T8] these authors noted 6 hospital deaths (32%, CL 20%–26%) among 19 patients undergoing complete repair of a type B interruption and VSD. Less favorably, 4 (100%, CL 62%–100%) of 4 (UAB; Table 34-19) one-stage repairs have died as have 6 (86%, CL 59%–98%) of 7(GLH; Table 32-20).

Repair of Interrupted Arch and Secondary Repair of Intracardiac Defects

When only the aortic arch interruption is repaired in neonates with coexisting VSD[M13] and in some a pulmonary artery band placed, the initial hospital mortality can be as low as 30% or as high as 80%–100%. Thus, Norwood and colleagues report 3 deaths (27%, CL 12%–47%) among 11 neo-

nates managed in this way.[N5] Zahka and colleagues report 7 infants, all less than 4 days old, treated with prostaglandin E₁ infusion, Gore-Tex grafting between upper and lower aortic segments combined with ductal division and pulmonary artery banding, with zero hospital mortality (CL 0%–24%);[Z1] using a comparable management protocol, Higgins and colleagues[H13] reported 4 deaths (50%, CL 27%–73%) among 8 infants. However, in the Norwood series there were 1 late death and 3 deaths after subsequent repair of the VSD 5 days to 16 months later for an overall mortality of 7 (67%, CL 44%–81%) among 11 patients.

LATE RESULTS

Survival

In Moulton and Bowman's experience with four hospital survivors of one-stage primary repair using direct anastomosis of the upper-to-lower aortic segments (all had type B interruption), three (75%, CL 37%–97%) were intermediate term survivors up to 6 years.[M5] They seemed healthy and active.

In the collected review of the 19 patients undergoing primary one-stage repair discussed under hospital mortality, 11 of the 13 hospital survivors (85%, CL 67%–95%) were alive 1–9 years later. The overall intermediate term survival rate was 11 of 19 or 58% (CL 43%–71%).

Zahka et al. report only fair intermediate results in their series of seven neonates successfully treated by the first stage of a two-stage repair.[Z1] Only one has had complete repair and is alive, although two others await complete repair. One graft has had to be replaced with a larger one. Braunlin and colleagues report seven patients, all of whom survived the initial repair and pulmonary artery banding; four (57%, CL 32%–80%) are alive after completion of both stages.[B17] Fowler and colleagues have also reported their results in 14 children undergoing an initial palliative repair of the interrupted arch and pulmonary artery banding in most cases. Ten (71%, CL 54%–85%) survived the initial palliation and six (43%, CL 27%–60%) are currently surviving, three with a now complete repair.[F13]

Aortic Anastomotic Narrowing

Date are available in three of Moulton and Bowman's hospital survivors with a direct aortic anastomosis.[M12] Of the two who were 3 months of age at operation, no anastomotic narrowing was seen at autopsy 8 months later in one and none was apparent by pressure measurements or aortography 2½ years later in the other. The baby who was 7 days old at operation had a 30-mmHg systolic pressure difference between upper and lower extremities 3 years postoperatively. Norwood and colleagues reported important gradients late postoperatively in their patients in whom the left subclavian or left common carotid arteries were used for anastomosis to the descending thoracic aorta.[N5] When a tube graft is used for aortic reconstruction, gradients are insignificant 1–3 years later. However, the development of gradients with growth of the child is inevitable. The single GLH survivor (Table 32-18) developed calcification in the

Table 34-19 Hospital mortality after repair of aortic arch interruption (UAB; 1967–Aug. 1, 1981).

		Hospital Deaths		
Procedure	n	*No.*	%	*CL*
Repair of aortic interruption only[a]	5	4	80%	47%–97%
Repair plus PA band[b]	3	1[c]	33%	4%–76%
One-stage repair of aortic interruption and intracardiac defect[d]	4	4	100%	62%–100%
Total	12	9	75%	56%–88%

KEY: CL, 70% confidence limits; PA, pulmonary artery; TGA, transposition of the great arteries; VSD, ventricular septal defect.

[a] Direct anastomosis in one, subclavian artery graft in one, Gore-Tex graft in three.

[b] Direct anastomosis in two, Gore-Tex graft in one.

[c] One other died after repair of multiple VSDs 6 weeks later.

[d] VSD in one, truncus arteriosus type III in one, TGA + VSD in one (arterial swtich repair).

Table 34-20   Results of repair of interrupted arch (GLH; 1970–1981).

Age at Operation	Type of Interruption	Associated Defects	Repair of Interruption	Result
8 days	A	VSD, TAPVC	Tube graft	Satis (12 yr)
8 days	B	VSD, ASD	Direct anastomosis	Died (OR)
10 days	B	VSD, ASD, AS	Direct anastomosis	Died (12 hr)
17 days	B	VSD, ASD	Direct anastomosis	Died (OR)
24 days	B	TGA, VSD	Direct anastomosis	Died (12 hr) LCO
6 months	A	VSD	Direct anastomosis	Died (31 hr) LCO
6 years	A	VSD, MS, PVR 12 units · m²	Tube graft	Died (OR)
9 years	B	TA; Banded RPA (aged 2)	Homograft-valved conduit	Died (OR) bleeding
15 years	A	TGA, VSD PVR 12 units · m²		Died (6 hr) LCO

KEY: AS, aortic stenosis; ASD, atrial septal defect; CR, complete repair; DA, direct anastomosis; DG, Dacron graft; LCO, low cardiac output; MPA, RPA, main and right pulmonary artery; MS, mitral stenosis; TA, truncus arteriosus; TAPVC, total anomalous pulmonary venous connection; VSD, ventricular septal defect.

NOTE: All had complete one-stage repair except the 24-day-old infant who had repair of the interruption and pulmonary artery banding and the 15-year-old who had only a palliative venous switch operation.

Teflon conduit, and at restudy 12 years postoperatively the conduit is occluded; where the graft passes in front of the pulmonary artery, it has distorted but not narrowed the left pulmonary artery origin.

Development of Subvalvar Aortic Stenosis

Six (67%, CL 44%–85%) of nine children studied 1–3 years after primary or staged repair (the second stage of the repair was performed at about 6 months of age) had developed subaortic stenosis in the experience of Norwood and colleagues.[N5] In four it was severe and required a left ventricular-thoracic aortic conduit in three and resection in one.

INDICATIONS FOR OPERATION

With an overall intermediate term survival rate of 50%–75%, and the likelihood that important subaortic stenosis will develop in at least one-half of these and require further extensive surgery, a case could be made for allowing the very poor natural history to unfold. However, as long as resources permit it, operation is advisable, preferably by a one-stage approach. If the intracardiac lesion is uncorrectable (which is rare), operation is contraindicated.

As soon as the baby is seen, an infusion of prostaglandin E_1 (PGE$_1$) is begun, the baby is intubated, and cardiac catheterization and cineangiocardiography are performed. About 4–8 hours are allowed for the PGE$_1$ infusion to have a maximum effect before operation is performed.[L10]

SPECIAL SITUATIONS AND CONTROVERSIES

Technique of Repair

Several techniques have been described for repair. The standard ones include techniques for bypass of the surgically interrupted arch, such as the use of tube grafts,[B13,M10,T11] left subclavian artery,[B14] venous homograft,[B18] and direct anastomosis of descending aorta to ascending aorta.[K8,T8,V5] In patients in whom the ductus is not stenotic and presumably not prone to close (probably most of the cases), methods have been devised to use the ductus as part of the conduit in reconstruction, such as with Dacron grafts,[M14] flaps of pulmonary artery,[M11] or conduits fashioned from the pulmonary artery.[F3,V6] Also, Utley and colleagues have described the making of a large window between ascending aorta and proximal pulmonary trunk and placing an internal baffle within the pulmonary trunk connecting this window with the pulmonary orifice of the ductus arteriosus to provide blood flow around the interruption.[U1] A technique such as this may ultimately prove superior to the use of an interposed tube graft.

APPENDIX

APPENDIX 34A
ANALYSES OF THE PROBABILITY OF RECOARCTATION

The data used in obtaining the equations for Figure 34-14 came from all reports found in the literature in which adequate follow-up data were given for individual patients (Fig. 34-14a) or for groups of patients (Fig. 34-14b). The data considered adequate include age at operation (varied from 1 day to 41 years in the 69 individual cases), resection and end-to-end anastomosis specified as the type of operation, and blood pressure recordings in arm and leg at least 6 months after operation. A difference of 15 mmHg between arm and leg (arm higher) was taken as evidence of persisting or recurrent coarctation, as was "absent or markedly diminished femoral pulses," or the statement that "reoperation was done for recoarctation," or that "angiography showed recurrent coarctation."

1. Sixty-nine individually reported cases were analyzed. The results are

Probability of persisting or recoarctation =
$$1/(1 + \exp[-0.18 \pm 0.334 + 0.54 \pm 0.159 \cdot \ln(\text{age})])$$

where exp is the base of the natural logarithm (ln), $P(\text{slope}) = .0007$. Individual cases came from references C1,C2,H4, M9,W6.

2. Six hundred sixty-one cases reported as group data in nonover-lapping age group were analyzed. The 69 individual cases were also included. The results are

Probability of recurrent or residual recoarctation =
$$1/(1 + \exp[0.95 \pm 0.155 + 0.42 \pm 0.060 \cdot \ln(\text{age})])$$

$P < .0001$

Cases came from references C1,C2,E1,F1,G1,H4,H6,T1,K1,L2, L4,M1,M9,N1,N2,O1,P1,P3,R2,S1,S3,S4,T1,T4,W3, and W6.

REFERENCES

A

1. Abbott ME: Coarctation of the aorta of the adult type. II. A statistical study and historical retrospect of 200 recorded cases with autopsy of stenosis or obliteration of the descending aorta in subjects over the age of two years. *Am Heart J* 3:574, 1928.
2. Albright F, Smith PH, Fraser R: A syndrome characterized by primary ovarian insufficiency and decreased stature. Report of 11 cases with a digression on hormonal control of axillary and pubic hair. *Am J Med Sci* 204:625, 1942.
3. Adam M, Johnson A, Davis M, Mitchel B: Surgical management of coarctation of the aorta in infancy. *Ann Thorac Surg* 2:188, 1966.
4. Ala-Kulju K, Jarvinen A, Maamies T, Mattila S, Merikallio E: Late aneurysms after patch aortoplasty for coarctation of the aorta in adults. *Thorac Cardiovasc Surg* 31:301, 1983.
5. Akl BF: Ascending-Distal Aorta Bypass. Letter to the Editor. *Ann Thorac Surg* 39:196, 1985.
6. Allan LD, Crawford DC, Tynan M: Evolution of coarctation of the aorta in intrauterine life. *Br Heart J* 52:471, 1984.
7. Allen HD, Marx GR, Ovitt TW: Balloon angioplasty for coarctation: Serial evaluation. *JACC* 5:405, 1985.

B

1. Bonnett LM: Sur la lesion dite stenose congenitale de l'aorte dans la region de l'isthme. *Rev de Med* 23:108, 1903.
2. Blalock A, Park EA: Surgical treatment of experimental coarctation (atresia) of aorta. *Ann Surg* 119:445, 1944.
3. Brom AG: Narrowing of the aortic isthmus and enlargement of the mind. *J Thorac Cardiovasc Surg* 50:166, 1965.
4. Barnes RW, Rittenhouse EA, Kongtahworn C, Doty DB, Rossi NP, Ehrenhaft JL: Reversed intercostal arterial flow in coarctation of the aorta. *Ann Thorac Surg* 19:27, 1975.
5. Becker AE, Becker MJ, Edwards JE: Anomalies associated with coarctation of aorta. Particular reference to infancy. *Circulation* 41:1067, 1970.
6. Brewer LA, Fosburg RA, Mulder GA, Verska JJ: Spinal cord complications following surgery for coarctation of the aorta. *J Thorac Cardiovasc Surg* 64:368, 1972.
7. Bahn RC, Edwards JE, DuShane JW: Coarctation of the aorta as a cause of death in early infancy. *Pediatrics* 8:192, 1952.
8. Bergdahl LAL, Blackstone EH, Kirklin JW, Pacifico AD, Bargeron LM Jr: Determinants of early success in repair of aortic coarctation in infants. *J Thorac Cardiovasc Surg* 83:736, 1982.
9. Bjork VO, Bergdahl L, Jonasson R: Coarctation of the aorta. The world's longest follow-up. *Adv Cardiol* 22:205, 1978.
10. Bull C, Hoeksema T, Duckworth JA, Mustard WT: An experimental study of the growth of arterial anastomoses. *Can J Surg* 6:383, 1963.
11. Berry CL, Tawes RL: Mucopolysaccharides of the aortic wall in coarctation and recoarctation. *Cardiovasc Res* 4:244, 1970.
12. Bergdahl L, Ljungqvist A: Long-term results after repair of coarctation of the aorta by patch grafting. *J Thorac Cardiovasc Surg* 80:177, 1980.
13. Barratt-Boyes BG, Nicholls TT, Brandt PWT, Neutze JM: Aortic arch interruption associated with patent ductus arteriosus, ventricular septal defect, and total anomalous pulmonary venous connection. *J Thorac Cardiovasc Surg* 63:367, 1972.
14. Bailey LL, Jacobson JG, Vyhmeister E, Petry E: Interrupted aortic arch complex. Successful total correction in the neonate. *Ann Thorac Surg* 25:66, 1978.
15. Blake HA, Manion WC, Spencer FC: Atresia or absence of the aortic isthmus. *J Thorac Cardiovasc Surg* 43:607, 1962.
16. Bergdahl L, Bjork VO, Jonasson R: Surgical correction of coarctation of the aorta. Influence of age on late results. *J Thorac Cardiovasc Surg* 85:532, 1983.
17. Braunlin EA, Lock JE, Foker JE: Repair of type B interruption of the aortic arch. Results and follow-up. *J Thorac Cardiovasc Surg* 86:920, 1983.
18. Bailey LL, Jacobson JG, Doroshow RW, Merritt WH, Petry EL: Anatomic correction of interrupted aortic arch complex in neonates. *Surgery* 89:553, 1981.

C

1. Christensen NA: Coarctation of the aorta: Historical review. *Proc Staff Meet Mayo Clin* 23:322, 1948.
2. Colodney NM, Carson MJ: Coarctation of the aorta in early infancy. *J Pediatr* 37:46, 1950.
3. Crafoord C, Nylin G: Congenital coarctation of the aorta and its surgical treatment. *J Thorac Surg* 14:347, 1945.
4. Clagett OT: The surgical treatment of coarctation of the aorta. *Proc Staff Meet Mayo Clin* 23:359, 1948.
5. Campbell M: Natural history of coarctation of the aorta. *Br Heart J* 32:633, 1970.
6. Chang JT, Barrington JD: Coarctation of the aorta in infants and children. *J Pediatr Surg* 7:127, 1972.
7. Chen S, Fagan LF, Mudd GJF, Willman VL: Prognosis of infants with coarctation of aorta. *Am Heart J* 94:557, 1977.
8. Connors JP, Harmann AF Jr, Weldon CS: Considerations in the surgical management of infantile coarctation of aorta. *Am J Cardiol* 36:489, 1975.

9. Campbell J, Delorenzi R, Brown J, Girod D, Hurwitz R, Caldwell R, King H: Improved results in newborns undergoing coarctation repair. *Ann Thorac Surg* 30:273, 1980.

10. Clarkson PM, Nicholson MR, Barratt-Boyes BG, Neutze JM, Whitlock RM: Results after repair of coarctation of the aorta beyond infancy: A 10 to 28 year follow-up with particular reference to late systemic hypertension. *Am J Cardiol* 51:1481, 1983.

11. Celoria GC, Patton RB: Congenital absence of the aortic arch. *Am Heart J* 58:407, 1959.

12. Collins-Nakai RL, Dick M, Parisi-Buckley L, Fyler D, Castaneda AR: Interrupted aortic arch in infancy. *J Pediatr* 88:959, 1976.

13. Connor TM, Baker WP: A comparison of coarctation resection and patch angioplasty using postexercise blood pressure measurements. *Circulation* 64:567, 1981.

14. Christmas BW, Turner AS: Prevalence of high blood pressure treated and untreated in an urban adult New Zealand population. Napier 1973. *NZ Med J* 86:419, 1977.

15. Calder AL, Kirker JA, Neutze JM, Starling MB: Pathology of the ductus arteriosus treated with prostaglandins: Comparison with untreated cases. *Pediatr Cardiol* (in press).

16. Campbell DB, Waldhausen JA, Pierce WS, Fripp R, Whitman V: Should elective repair of coarctation of the aorta be done in infancy? *J Thorac Cardiovasc Surg* 88:929, 1984.

17. Celano V, Pieroni DR, Morera JA, Roland JMA, Gingell RL: Two-dimensional echocardiographic examination of mitral valve abnormalities associated with coarctation of the aorta. *Circulation* 69:924, 1984.

18. Cobanoglu A, Teply JF, Grunkemeier GL, Sunderland CO, Starr A: Coarctation of the aorta in patients younger than three months. *J Thorac Cardiovasc Surg* 89:128, 1985.

19. Cooper RS, Ritter SB, Golinko RJ: Balloon dilatation angioplasty: nonsurgical management of coarctation of the aorta. *Circulation* 70:903, 1984.

D

1. DeBoer A, Grana L, Potts WJ, Lev M: Coarctation of the aorta. *Arch Surg* 82:801, 1961.

2. Downing DF, Grotzinger PJ, Weller RW: Coarctation of the aorta. The syndrome of necrotizing arteritis of the small intestine following surgical therapy. *Am J Dis Child* 96:711, 1958.

3. Dische MR, Tsai M, Baltaze HA: Solitary interruption of the arch of the aorta. *Am J Cardiol* 35:271, 1975.

4. DeLeon SY, Idriss FS, Ilbawi MN, Tin N, Berry T: Transmediastinal repair of complex coarctation and interrupted aortic arch. *J Thorac Cardiovasc Surg* 82:98, 1981.

5. D'Souza VJ, Velasquez G, Weesner KM, Prabhu S: Transluminal angioplasty of aortic coarctation with a two-balloon technique. *Am J Cardiol* 54:457, 1984.

E

1. Edwards JE, Christensen NA, Clagett OT, McDonald JR: Pathologic considerations in coarctation of the aorta. *Proc Staff Meet Mayo Clin* 23:324, 1948.

2. Edwards JE, Clagett OT, Drake RL, Christensen NA: The collateral circulation in coarctation of the aorta. *Proc Staff Meet Mayo Clin* 23:333, 1948.

3. Edie RN, Janani J, Attai LA, Malm JR, Robinson G: Bypass grafts for recurrent or complex coarctations of the aorta. *Ann Thorac Surg* 20:558, 1975.

4. Eshagpour E, Olley PM: Recoarctation of the aorta following

coarctectomy in the first year of life: A follow-up study. *J Pediatr Surg* 80:809, 1972.

5. Elliott RB, Starling MB, Neutze JM: Medical management of the ductus. *Lancet* 1:140, 1975.

F

1. Freed MD, Keane JF, Van Praagh R, Castaneda AR, Bernhard WF, Nadas AS: Coarctation of the aorta with congenital mitral regurgitation. *Circulation* 49:1175, 1974.

2. Fyler DC: Report of the New England regional infant cardiac program. *Pediatrics* 64:(suppl):432, 1980.

3. Fishman NH, Bronstein MH, Berman W Jr, Roe BB, Edmunds LH Jr, Robinson ST, Rudolph AM: Surgical management of severe aortic coarctation and interrupted aortic arch in neonates. *J Thorac Cardiovasc Surg* 71:35, 1976.

4. Freundlich E, Engle MA, Goldberg HP: Coarctation of aorta in infancy (analysis of 10 year experience) with medical management. *Pediatrics* 27:427, 1961.

5. Freed MD, Hemann MA, Lewis AB, Roehl SL, Kensey RC: Prostaglandin E₁ in infants with ductus arteriosus-dependent congenital heart disease. *Circulation* 64:899, 1981.

6. Fleming WH, Sarafian LB, Clarke ED, Dooley KJ, Hofshire PJ, Hopeman AR, Ruckman PK, Mooring PK: Critical aortic coarctation: Patch aortoplasty in infants less than age 3 months. *Am J Cardiol* 44:687, 1979.

7. Freed M, Rocchini A, Rosenthal A, Nadas AS, Castaneda AR: Exercise-induced hypertension after surgical repair of coarctation of the aorta. *Am J Cardiol* 43:253, 1979.

8. Freedom RM, Bain HH, Esplugas E, Dische R, Rowe RD: Ventricular septal defect in interruption of aortic arch. *Am J Cardiol* 39:572, 1977.

9. Freedom RM, Rosen FS, Nadas AS: Congenital cardiovascular disease and anomalies of the third and fourth pharyngeal pouch. *Circulation* 46:165, 1972.

10. Foster JH, Collins HA, Jacobs JK, Scott HW: Long-term follow-up of homografts used in the treatment of coarctation of the aorta. *J Cardiovasc Surg* 6:111, 1965.

11. Freed MD, Rosenthal A, Plauth WH Jr, Nadas AS: Development of subaortic stenosis after pulmonary artery banding. *Circulation* 47, 48(suppl III):III-7, 1973.

12. Fripp RR, Whitman V, Werner JC, Nicholas GC, Waldhausen JA: Blood pressure response to exercise in children following the subclavian flap procedure for coarctation of the aorta. *J Thorac Cardiovasc Surg* 85:682, 1983.

13. Fowler BN, Lucas SK, Razook JD, Thompson WM Jr, Williams GR, Elkins RC: Interruption of the aortic arch: Experience in 17 infants. *Ann Thorac Surg* 37:25, 1984.

G

1. Gross RE, Hufnagel CA: Coarctation of the aorta. Experimental studies regarding its surgical correction. *N Engl J Med* 233:287, 1945.

2. Gross RE: Surgical correction for coarctation of the aorta. *Surgery* 18:673, 1945.

3. Gross RE: Treatment of certain aortic coarctations by homologous grafts. *Ann Surg* 134:753, 1951.

4. Gupta TC, Wiggens CJ: Basic hemodynamic changes produced by aortic coarctation of different degrees. *Circulation* 3:17, 1951.

5. Graham TP Jr, Atwood GF, Boerth RC, Boucek RJ Jr, Smith

CW: Right and left heart size and function in infants with symptomatic coarctation. *Circulation* 56:641, 1977.

6. Graham P Jr, Lewis BW, Jarmakani JM, Canent RV Jr, Capp MP: Left heart volume and mass quantification in children with left ventricular pressure overload. *Circulation* 41:203, 1970.

7. Goodall M, Sealey WC: Increased sympathetic nerve activity following resection of coarctation of the thoracic aorta. *Circulation* 39:345, 1969.

8. Grunkemeier GL, Lambert MS, Bonchek LI, Starr A: An unproven statistical method for assessing the results of operation. *Ann Thorac Surg* 20:289, 1975.

9. Groves LK, Effler DB: Problems in the management of coarctation of the aorta. *J Thorac Cardiovasc Surg* 39:60, 1960.

10. Gidding SS, Rocchini AP, Moorehead C, Schork MA, Rosenthal A: Increased forearm vascular reactivity in patients with hypertension after repair of coarctation. *Circulation* 71:495, 1985.

H

1. Ho SY, Anderson RH: Coarctation, tubular hypoplasia and the ductus arteriosus. Histological study of 35 specimens. *Br Heart J* 41:268, 1979.

2. Hutchins GM: Coarctation of the aorta explained as a branch point of the ductus arteriosus. *Am J Pathol* 63:203, 1971.

3. Honey M, Lincoln JCR, Osborne MP, deBono DP: Coarctation of aorta with right aortic arch. Report of surgical correction in 2 cases: One with associated anomalous origin of left circumflex coronary artery from the right pulmonary artery. *Br Heart J* 37:937, 1975.

4. Hallman GL, Yasher JJ, Bloodwell RD, Cooley DA: Surgical correction of coarctation of the aorta in the first year of life. *Ann Thorac Surg* 4:106, 1969.

5. Ho ECK, Moss AJ: The syndrome of mesenteric arteritis following surgical repair of aortic coarctation. *Pediatrics* 49:40, 1972.

6. Herrmann VM, Laks H, Fagan L, Terschluse D, Willman VL: Repair of aortic coarctation in the first year of life. *Ann Thorac Surg* 25:57, 1978.

7. Hamilton DJ, Eusanio GD, Sandrasagra FA, Donnelly RJ: Early and late results of aortoplasty with a left subclavian flap for coarctation of the aorta in infancy. *J Thorac Cardiovasc Surg* 75:699, 1978.

8. Hanson E, Eriksson BO, Sorensen SE: Intra-arterial blood pressures at rest and during exercise after surgery for coarctation of the aorta. *Eur J Cardiol* 11:245, 1980.

9. Hesslein PS, McNamara DG, Morriss MJH, Hallman GL, Cooley DA: Comparison of resection versus patch aortoplasty for repair of coarctation in infants and children. *Circulation* 64:164, 1981.

10. Hartmann AF Jr, Goldring D, Hernaulez A, Behrer MR, Schad N, Ferguson T, Burford T: Recurrent coarctation of the aorta after successful repair in infancy. *Am J Cardiol* 25:405, 1970.

11. Hamilton DI, Medici D, Oyonarte M, Dickinson DF: Aortoplasty with the left subclavian flap in older children. *J Thorac Cardiovasc Surg* 82:103, 1981.

12. Heyman MA, Berman WB, Rudolph AM, Whitman V: Dilation of the ductus arteriosus by prostaglandin E$_1$ in aortic arch abnormalities. *Circulation* 59:169, 1976.

13. Higgins CB, French JW, Silverman JF, Wexler L: Interruption of the aortic arch: Preoperative and postoperative clinical, hemodynamic and angiographic features. *Am J Cardiol* 39:563, 1977.

14. Hart JC, Waldhausen JA: Reversed subclavian flap angioplasty for arch coarctation of the aorta. *Ann Thorac Surg* 36:715, 1983.

15. Ho SY, Wilcox BR, Anderson RH, Lincoln JCR: Interrupted aortic arch—anatomical features of surgical significance. *Thorac Cardiovasc Surg* 31:199, 1983.

16. Harlan JL, Doty DB, Brandt B III, Ehrenhaft JL: Coarctation of the aorta in infants. *J Thorac Cardiovasc Surg* 88:1012, 1984.

I

1. Ibarra-Perez C, Castaneda AR, Varco RL, Lillehei CW: Recoarctation of the aorta. Nineteen year clinical experience. *Am J Cardiol* 23:778, 1969.

2. Immagoulou A, Anderson RC, Moller JH: Interruption of the aortic arch. *Circulation* 26:39, 1962.

J

1. Johnson J, Kirby CK: The relationship of the method of suture to the growth of end-to-end arterial anastomosis. *Surgery* 27:17, 1950.

K

1. Kirklin JW, Burchell HB, Pugh DG, Burke EC, Mills SD: Surgical treatment of coarctation of the aorta in a ten-week-old infant. Report of a case. *Circulation* 6:411, 1952.

2. Kennedy A, Taylor DG, Durrant TE: Pathology of the intima in coarctation of the aorta: A study using light and scanning electron microscopy. *Thorax* 34:366, 1979.

3. Keith JD, Rowe RD, Vlad P: *Heart Disease in Infancy and Childhood.* New York: Macmillan, 1978, p 738.

4. Kamau P, Miles V, Toews W, Kelminson L, Friesen R, Lockhart C, Butterfield J, Hernandez J, Hawes CR, Pappas G: Surgical repair of coarctation of the aorta in infants less than six months of age. *J Thorac Cardiovasc Surg* 81:171, 1981.

5. Khoury GH, Hawes CR: Recurrent coarctation of the aorta in infancy and childhood. *J Pediatr* 72:801, 1968.

6. Kirsh MM, Perry B, Spooner E: Management of pseudoaneurysm following patch grafting for coarctation of the aorta. *J Thorac Cardiovasc Surg* 74:636, 1977.

7. Kutsche LM, Van Mierop LHS: Cervical origin of the right subclavian artery in aortic arch interruption: pathogenesis and significance. *Am J Cardiol* 53:892, 1984.

8. Kawashima Y, Oyama C, Mori T, Manabe H: Interruption of the aortic arch associated with patent ductus arteriosus and ventricular septal defect. Proposal of a new surgical technique for total correction. *J Cardiovasc Surg* 16:426, 1975.

9. Kreiger KH, Spencer FC: Is paraplegia after repair of coarctation of the aorta due principally to distal hypotension during aortic cross-clamping? *Surgery* 97:2, 1985.

10. Kan JS, White RI, Mitchell SE, Farmlett EJ, Donahoo JS, Gardner TJ: Treatment of restenosis of coarctation by percutaneous transluminal angioplasty. *Circulation* 68:1087, 1983.

L

1. Lynxwiler CP, Smith S, Babich J: Coarctation of the aorta; report of a case. *Arch Pediatr* 68:203, 1951.

2. Liberthson RR, Pennington DG, Jacobs MC, Daggett WM: Coarctation of the aorta: Review of 234 patients and clarification of management problems. *Am J Cardiol* 43:835, 1979.

3. Lang HT Jr, Nadas AS: Coarctation of the aorta with congestive heart failure in infancy—medical treatment. *Pediatrics* 17:45, 1956.

4. Litwin SB, Bernhard WF, Rosenthal A, Gross RE: Surgical resection of coarctation of the aorta in infancy. *J Pediatr Surg* 6:307, 1971.

5. Lindesmith GG, Stanton RE, Stiles QR, Meyer BW, Jones JC: Coarctation of the thoracic aorta. *Ann Thorac Surg* 11:482, 1971.

6. Lobert PH, Lillehei CW: Necrotizing panarteritis following repair of coarctation. *Surgery* 35:950, 1954.

7. Litwin SB, Van Praagh R, Bernhard WF: A palliative operation for certain infants with aortic arch interruption. *Ann Thorac Surg* 14:369, 1972.

8. Leanage R, Taylor JFN, de Leval MR, Stark J, Macartney FJ: Surgical management of coarctation of aorta with ventricular septal defect. Multivariate analysis. *Br Heart J* 46:269, 1981.

9. de Lezo JS, Fernandez R, Sancho M, Concha M, Arizon J, Franco M, Alemany F, Barcones F, Lopez-Rubio F, Valles. Percutaneous transluminal angioplasty for aortic isthmic coarctation in infancy. *Am J Cardiol* 54:1147, 1984.

10. Leoni F, Huhta JC, Douglas J, Mackay R, de Leval MR, Macartney FJ, Stark J: Effect of prostaglandin on early surgical mortality in obstructive lesions of the systemic circulation. *Br Heart J* 52:654, 1984.

11. Lock JE: Now that we can dilate, should we? *Am J Cardiol* 54:1358, 1984.

M

1. Mustard WT, Rower RD, Keith JD, Sirek A: Coarctation of the aorta with special reference to the first year of life. *Ann Surg* 141:249, 1955.

2. Morris GC, Cooley DA, DeBakey ME, Crawford ES: Coarctation of the aorta with particular emphasis upon improved techniques of surgical repair. *J Thorac Cardiovasc Surg* 40:705, 1960.

3. Malm JR, Blumenthal S, Jameson AG, Humphreys GH: Observations on coarctation of the aorta in infants. *Arch Surg* 86:96, 1963.

4. Mathew R, Simon G, Joseph M: Collateral circulation in coarctation of aorta in infancy and childhood. *Arch Dis Child* 47:950, 1972.

5. Midgley FM, Scott LP, Perry CW, Shapiro SR, McClenathan JE: Subclavian flap aortoplasty for treatment of coarctation in early infancy. *J Pediatr Surg* 13:265, 1978.

6. McManus Q, Starr A, Lambert LE, Grunkemeier G: Correction of aortic coarctation in neonates: Mortality and late results. *Ann Thorac Surg* 24:544, 1977.

7. Maron BJ, Humphries JO, Rowe RD, Mellits ED: Prognosis of surgically corrected coarctation of the aorta: A 20-year postoperative appraisal. *Circulation* 47:119, 1973.

8. Mulder DG, Linde LM: Recurrent coarctation of the aorta in infancy. *Am Surg* 25:908, 1959.

9. Merrill DL, Webster CA, Samson PC: Congenital absence of the aortic isthmus. *J Thorac Surg* 33:311, 1957.

10. Murphy DA, Lemire GG, Tessler I, Dunn GL: Correction of type B aortic arch interruption with ventricular and atrial septal defects in a three-day-old infant. *J Thorac Cardiovasc Surg* 65:882, 1973.

11. Moller JH, Edwards JE: Interruption of the aortic arch. Anatomic patterns and associated cardiac malformations. *Am J Roentgenol Rad Theror Nucl Med* 95:557, 1965.

12. Moulton AL, Bowman FO Jr: Primary definitive repair of type B interrupted aortic arch, ventricular septal defect, and patent ductus arteriosus. *J Thorac Cardiovasc Surg* 82:501, 1981.

13. Muraoka R, Yokota M, Aoshima M, Nomoto S, Osaragi M, Kyoku I, Nakano H, Ueda K, Saito A: Simplified method for total correction of interrupted aortic arch with ventricular septal defect in infancy. *J Thorac Cardiovasc Surg* 78:744, 1979.

14. Monro JL, Brown W, Conway N: Correction of type B interrupted aortic arch with ventricular septal defect in infancy. *J Thorac Cardiovasc Surg* 74:618, 1977.

15. Moulton AL, Brenner JI, Roberts G, Tavares S, Ali S, Nordenbert A, Burns JE, Ringel R, Berman MA: Subclavian flap repair of coarctation of the aorta in neonates. Realization of growth potential. *J Thorac Cardiovasc Surg* 87:220, 1984.

16. Marvin WJ, Mahoney LT: Balloon angioplasty of unoperated coarctation in young children. *JACC* 5:405, 1985 (abstr).

17. Metzdorff MT, Cobanoglu A, Grunkemeier GL, Sunderland CO, Starr A: Influence of age at operation on late results with subclavian flap aortoplasty. *J Thorac Cardiovasc Surg* 89:235, 1985.

18. McCredie RM, Allan RM, Swinburn MJ, Wright JS: Percutaneous transluminal balloon angioplasty in coarctation re-stenosis in infancy. *The Cardiac Society of Australia and New Zealand.* 580, 1984 (abstr).

N

1. Neutze JM, Starling MB, Elliott RB, Barratt-Boyes BG: Palliation of cyanotic congenital heart disease in infancy with E-type prostaglandins. *Circulation* 55:238, 1977.

2. Nanton MA, Olley PM: Residual hypertension after coarctectomy in children. *Am J Cardiol* 37:769, 1976.

3. Nasser WK, Helmen C: Kinking of the aortic arch (pseudocoarctation). *Ann Intern Med* 64:971, 1966.

4. Norton JB, Ullyot DJ, Stewart ET, Rudolph AM, Edwards LH: Aortic arch atresia with transposition of the great vessels: Physiological considerations and surgical management. *Surgery* 67:1011, 1970.

5. Norwood WI, Lang P, Castaneda AR, Hougen TJ: Reparative operations for interrupted aortic arch with ventricular septal defect. *J Thorac Cardiovasc Surg* 86:837, 1983.

O

1. Ostermiller WE Jr, Somerndike JM, Hunter JA, Dye WS, Javid H, Najafi H, Julian OC: Coarctation of the aorta in adult patients. *J Thorac Cardiovasc Surg* 61:125, 1971.

2. Olsson P, Sonderlund S, Dubiel WT, Ovenfors CO: Patch graft or tubular grafts in the repair of coarctation of the aorta. A follow-up study. *Scand J Thorac Cardiovasc Surg* 10:139, 1976.

P

1. Patel R, Singh SP, Abrams L, Roberts KD: Coarctation of the aorta with special reference to infants. Long-term results of operation in 126 cases. *Br Heart J* 39:1246, 1977.

2. Perez-Alvarez JJ, Oudkerk S: Necrotizing arteritis of the abdominal organs as a postoperative complication following correction of coarctation of the aorta. A case report. *Surgery* 37:833, 1955.

3. Parker FB, Farrell B, Streeten DHP, Blackman MS, Sondheimer HM, Anderson GH: Hypertensive mechanisms in coarctation of the aorta. Further studies of the renin-angiotensin system. *J Thorac Cardiovasc Surg* 80:568, 1980.

4. Pierce WS, Waldhausen JA, Berman W Jr, Whitman V: Late results of the subclavian flap procedure in infants with coarctation of the thoracic aorta. *Circulation* 58:(suppl I):I-78, 1978.

5. Parsons CG, Astley R: Recurrence of aortic coarctation after operation in childhood. *Br Med J* 1:573, 1966.

6. Pelletier C, Davignon A, Ethier MF, Stanley P: Coarctation of the aorta in infancy. *J Thorac Cardiovasc Surg* 57:171, 1969.

7. Parsons CG: Recurrent coarctation of the aorta. *Am Heart J* 73:1, 1967 (editorial).

8. Pellegrino A, Deverall PB, Anderson RH, Smith A, Wilkinson JL, Russo P, Tynan M: Aortic coarctation in the first three months of life. An anatomopathological study with respect to treatment. *J Thorac Cardiovasc Surg* 89:121, 1985.

9. Penkoske PA, Williams WG, Olley PM, LeBlanc J, Trusler GA, Moes CAF, Judakin R, Rowe RD: Subclavian arterioplasty. Repair of coarctation of the aorta in the first year of life. *J Thorac Cardiovasc Surg* 87:894, 1984.

R

1. Reifenstein GH, Levine SA, Gross RE: Coarctation of the aorta. A review of 104 autopsied cases of the "adult type" 2 years of age or older. *Am Heart J* 33:146, 1947.

2. Rudolph AM, Hemann MA, Spitznas U: Haemodynamic considerations in the development of narrowing of the aorta. *Am J Cardiol* 30:514, 1972.

3. Rodbard S: Vascular modifications induced by flow. *Am Heart J* 51:926, 1956.

4. Rodbard S: Physical factors in the progression of stenotic vascular lesions. *Circulation* 17:410, 1958.

5. Rathi L, Keith JD: Postoperative blood pressures in coarctation of the aorta. *Br Heart J* 26:671, 1964.

6. Ring DM, Lewis FJ: Abdominal pain following surgical correction of coarctation of the aorta. A syndrome. *J Thorac Surg* 31:718, 1956.

7. Rocchini AP, Rosenthal A, Barger AC, Castaneda AR, Nadas AS: Pathogenesis of paradoxical hypertension after coarctation resection. *Circulation* 54:382, 1976.

8. Radford DT, Blook KR, Coceani F, Fariello R, Olleg PM: Prostaglandin E₁ for interrupted aortic arch in the neonate. *Lancet* 2:95, 1976.

9. Roberts WC, Morrow AG, Braunwald E: Complete interruption of the aortic arch. *Circulation* 26:39, 1962.

10. Ray JA, Doddi N, Regula D, Williams JA, Melveger A: Polydioxanone (PDS), a novel monofilament synthetic absorbable suture. *Surg Gynecol Obstet* 153:497, 1981.

11. Reardon MJ, Hallman GL, Cooley DA: Interrupted aortic arch: Brief review and summary of an eighteen-year experience. *Texas Heart Institute Journal* 11:250, 1984.

12. Rheuban K, Carpenter M, Jedeikin R, Dammann F, Kron I, Wellons J, Nolan SP: Aortic aneurysm after patch angioplasty for coarctation in childhood. *JACC* 5:476, 1985 (abstr).

S

1. Shinebourne EA, Elseed AM: Relation between fetal flow patterns, coarctation of the aorta and pulmonary blood flow. *Br Heart J* 36:498, 1974.

2. Sinha SN, Kardatzke MF, Cole RB, Muster AJ, Wessel HV, Paul MH: Coarctation of the aorta in infancy. *Circulation* 40:385, 1969.

3. Schuster SR, Gross RE: Surgery for coarctation of the aorta: A review of 500 cases. *J Thorac Cardiovasc Surg* 43:54, 1962.

4. Shinebourne EA, Tam ASY, Elseed AM, Paneth M, Lennox SC, Cleland WP, Lincoln C, Joseph MC, Anderson RH: Coarc-

tation of the aorta in infancy and childhood. *Br Heart J* 38:375, 1976.

5. Shearer WT, Turman JY, Weinberg WA, Godring D: Coarctation of the aorta and cerebrovascular accident. A proposal for early corrective surgery. *J Pediatr* 77:1004, 1970.

6. Sellors TH, Hobsley M: Coarctation of the aorta: Effect of operation on blood pressure. *Lancet* 1:1387, 1963.

7. Sealy WC: Indications for surgical treatment of coarctation of the aorta. *Surg Gynecol Obstet* 97:301, 1953.

8. Sealy WC, Harris JS, Young WG Jr, Calloway HA Jr: Paradoxical hypertension following resection of coarctation of the aorta. *Surgery* 42:135, 1957.

9. Sade RM, Taylor AB, Chariker EP: Aortoplasty compared with resection for coarctation of the aorta in young children. *Ann Thorac Surg* 28:346, 1979.

10. Shumaker HB Jr, Freeman LW, Hutchings IM, Radigan L: Studies in vascular repair; further observations on growth of anastomosis and free vascular transplants in growing animals. *Angiology* 2:263, 1951.

11. Sirak HD, Ressahat M, Hosier DM, deLorimier AA: A new operation for repairing aortic arch atresia in infancy: Report of 3 cases. *Circulation* 37(suppl II):II-43, 1968.

12. Steidele RJ: Samml *Chir Med Beob Vienna* 1778, Vol 2, p 114.

13. Seidel JF: *Index Musei Anatomici Kiliensis.* Kiel, CF Mohr, 1818, p 61.

14. Sade RM, Crawford FA, Hohn AR, Riopel DA, Taylor AB: Growth of the aorta after prosthetic patch aortoplasty for coarctation in infants. *Ann Thorac Surg* 38:21, 1984.

15. Smith RT Jr, Sade RM, Riopel DA, Taylor AB, Crawford FA Jr, Hohn AR: Stress testing for comparison of synthetic patch aortoplasty with resection and end to end anastomosis for repair of coarctation in childhood. *JACC* 4:765, 1984.

T

1. Talner NS, Berman MA: Postnatal development of obstruction in coarctation of the aorta: Role of the ductus arteriosus. *Pediatrics* 56:562, 1975.

2. Tawes RL, Berry CL, Aberdeen E: Congenital bicuspid aortic valves associated with coarctation of the aorta in children. *Br Heart J* 31:127, 1969.

3. Tawes RL, Aberdeen E, Waterston DJ, Bonhan-Carter RE: Coarctation of the aorta in infants and children. A review of 333 operative cases including 170 infants. *Circulation* 39, 40:(suppl I):I-173, 1969.

4. Tawes RL, Bull JC, Rowe BB: Hypertension and abdominal pain after resection of aortic coarctation. *Ann Surg* 171:409, 1970.

5. Thibault WN, Sperling DR, Gazzaniga AB: Subclavian artery patch angioplasty. *Arch Surg* 110:1095, 1975.

6. Tucker BL, Stanton RE, Lindesmith GG, Stiles QR, Meyer BW, Jones JC: Recurrent coarctation of the thoracic aorta. *Arch Surg* 102:556, 1971.

7. Tiraboschi R, Alfieri O, Carpentier A, Parenzan L: One stage correction of coarctation of the aorta associated with intracardiac defects in infancy. *J Cardiovasc Surg* 19:11, 1978.

8. Trusler GA, Izukawa T: Interrupted aortic arch and ventricular septal defect. Direct repair through a median sternotomy incision in a 13-day-old infant. *J Thorac Cardiovasc Surg* 69:126, 1975.

9. Tiraboschi R, Locatelli G, Bianchi T, Parenzan L: Correction of coarctation of the aorta during the first year of life by means of

the subclavian flap technique. 8 cases operated on successfully. *Surg Italy* 5:244, 1975.

10. Todd PJ, Dangerfield PH, Hamilton DI, Wilkinson JL: Late effects on the left upper limb of subclavian flap aortoplasty. *J Thorac Cardiovasc Surg* 85:681, 1983.

11. Tyson KRT, Harris LC, Nghiem QX: Repair of aortic arch interruption in the neonate. *Surgery* 67:1006, 1970.

12. Turley K, Yee ES, Ebert PA: The total repair of interrupted arch complex in infants: the anterior approach. *Circulation* 79(suppl I)I-16, 1984.

U

1. Utley JR, Swain JA, Higgins CB, Kashani IA: Pulmonary artery partition: New method for correction of interrupted aortic arch. *J Thorac Cardiovasc Surg* 86:309, 1983.

V

1. Vorsschulte K: Surgical correction of the aorta by an "isthmus plastic" operation. *Thorax* 16:338, 1961.

2. Vlodaver Z, Neufeld HN: Coronary arteries in coarctation of the aorta. *Circulation* 37:449, 1968.

3. Van Praagh R, Van Praagh S: The anatomy of common aorto-pulmonary trunk (truncus arteriosus communis) and its embryological implications. *Am J Cardiol* 16:406, 1965.

4. Verska JJ, DeQuattro V, Woolley MM: Coarctation of the aorta. The abdominal pain syndrome and paradoxical hypertension. *J Thorac Cardiovasc Surg* 58:746, 1969.

5. Ventemiglia R, Oglietti J, Wukasch DC, Hallman GL, Cooley DA: Interruption of the aortic arch. *J Thorac Cardiovasc Surg* 72:235, 1976.

6. Van Praagh R, Bernhard WF, Rosenthal A, Parisi LF, Fyler DC: Interrupted aortic arch: Surgical treatment. *Am J Cardiol* 27:200, 1971.

7. Villalobos MCR, Balderrama DP, Lopez JL, Castellanos M: Complete interruption of the aorta. *Am J Cardiol* 8:664, 1961.

8. Van Mierop LHS, Kutsche LM: Interruption of the aortic arch and coarctation of the aorta: Pathogenetic relations. *Am J Cardiol* 54:829, 1984.

W

1. Waldhausen JA, Nahrwold DL: Repair of coarctation of the aorta with a subclavian flap. *J Thorac Cardiovasc Surg* 51:532, 1966.

2. Winer HE, Kronzon I, Glassman E, Cunningham JN Jr, Madayag M: Pseudocoarctation and mid-arch aortic coarctation. *Chest* 72:519, 1977.

3. Waldhausen JA, King H, Nahrwold DL, Lurie PR, Shumaker HB Jr: Management of coarctation in infancy. *JAMA* 187:270, 1964.

4. Waldhausen J, Whitman V, Pierce W: Coarctation in infants: Management with prostaglandin E_1 and the subclavian flap procedure. World Congress of Pediatric Cardiology, London, 1980 (abstr).

5. Williams WG, Shindo G, Trusler GA, Dische MR, Olley PM: Results of repair of coarctation of the aorta during infancy. *J Thorac Cardiovasc Surg* 79:603, 1980.

6. Wright L, Burchell HB, Wood EH, Hines EA, Clagett OT: Hemodynamic and clinical appraisal of coarctation four to seven years after resection and end-to-end anastomosis. *Circulation* 14:806, 1956.

7. Weisman D, Kesten HD: Absence of transverse aortic arch with defects of cardiac septums. Report of a case simulating acute abdominal disease in a newborn infant. *Am J Dis Child* 76:326, 1948.

Z

1. Zahka KG, Roland JMA, Cutilletta AF, Gardner TJ, Donahoo JS, Kidd L: Management of aortic arch interruption with prostaglandin E_1 infusion and microporous expanded polytetrafluoroethylene grafts. *Am J Cardiol* 46:1001, 1980.

35

AORTIC ATRESIA

DEFINITION

Aortic atresia is a developmental anomaly in which the aortic valve is atretic and the ascending aorta is hypoplastic. With few exceptions there is in addition mitral atresia or mitral valve hypoplasia, severe left ventricular hypoplasia, and an intact ventricular septum, a condition called the hypoplastic left heart syndrome. The exceptions are those few examples of aortic atresia with a large ventricular septal defect and a left ventricle which is not hypoplastic; in this setting the mitral valve may be near normal, hypoplastic, or atretic. Hypoplastic left heart syndrome is, along with other forms of mitral atresia, an example of a univentricular atrioventricular connection (see Chapter 44), but because of its special clinical and surgical significance, it is discussed separately. Mitral atresia in the absence of aortic atresia is also one of the forms of univentricular atrioventricular connection considered in Chapter 44.

This chapter discusses primarily aortic atresia with hypoplastic left heart syndrome.

HISTORICAL NOTE

The first description of aortic atresia was apparently by Canton in 1850.[C1] Although Abbott had recognized congenital aortic and mitral atresia,[A1] Brockman in 1950 first emphasized that in about 50% of cases of mitral atresia there was coexisting aortic atresia and severe underdevelopment of the left side of the heart.[B1] Lev, in 1952, further emphasized the group of congenital cardiac malformations associated with underdevelopment of the left-sided cardiac chambers and a small ascending aorta and arch.[L4] Noonan and Nadas in 1958 brought together the morphological features of combined aortic and mitral atresia and introduced the phrase "hypo-

plastic left heart syndrome."[N1] Roberts and colleagues in 1976 organized still further the knowledge about aortic atresia by emphasizing the differing morphology depending on whether a ventricular septal defect was present.[R2]

Palliative surgical treatment was of temporary benefit in a neonate with a ventricular septal defect and a normal-sized left ventricle reported by Freedom and colleagues in 1976.[F1] A Potts anastomosis was performed together with separate banding of the left and right pulmonary arteries. Litwin and colleagues suggested that the difficulties of individually banding the left and right pulmonary arteries might be overcome by banding the pulmonary trunk distal to a conduit placed from the pulmonary trunk to the descending aorta and ligating the patent ductus arteriosus.[L5] This was practiced by Levitsky and colleagues[L2] and Mohri and colleagues.[M2] Doty and colleagues reported somewhat similar palliative treatment[D2] which included placement of a perforated patch inside the pulmonary trunk to restrict pulmonary flow. Behrendt and Rocchini described an alternative palliative approach in one infant in 1981.[B2] Successful two-stage correction of the hypoplastic left heart syndrome was reported in 1983 by Norwood, Lang, and Hansen.[N3] Successful correction of aortic atresia without mitral atresia was first reported by Norwood and Stellin in 1981[N2] and again in 1983 by Duffy and colleagues.[D3]

MORPHOLOGY

The heart is significantly enlarged and about twice normal weight for age. Its shape is determined by the large right and small left heart chambers (Fig. 35-1a).[V2] In 95% of cases the morphology is remarkably constant, the only variable being the presence of either mitral atresia or severe mitral valve

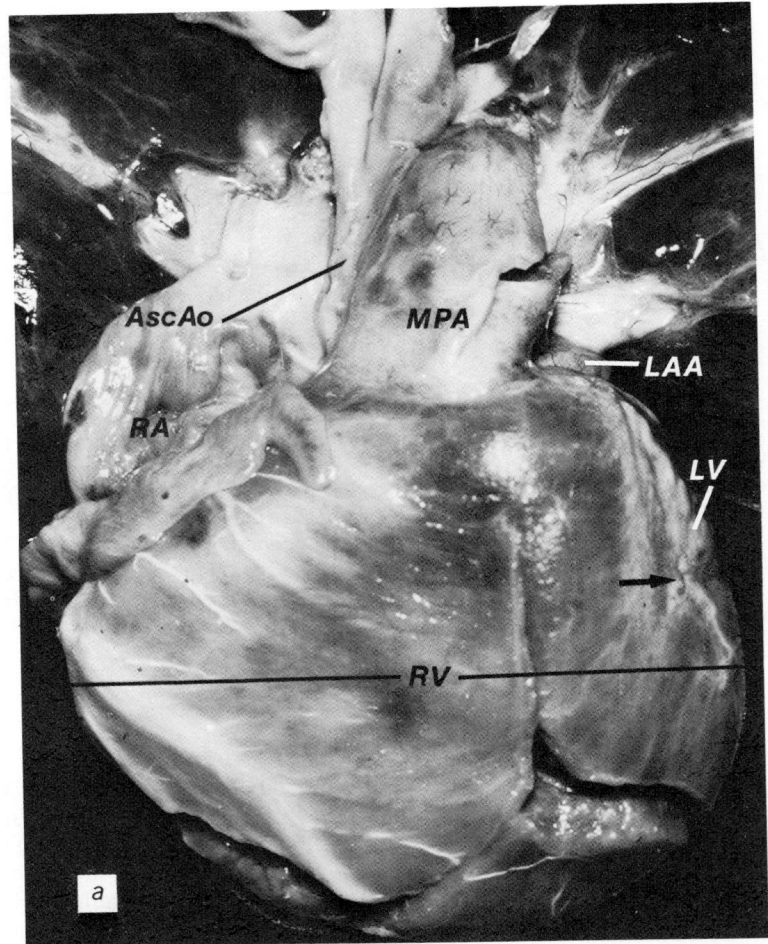

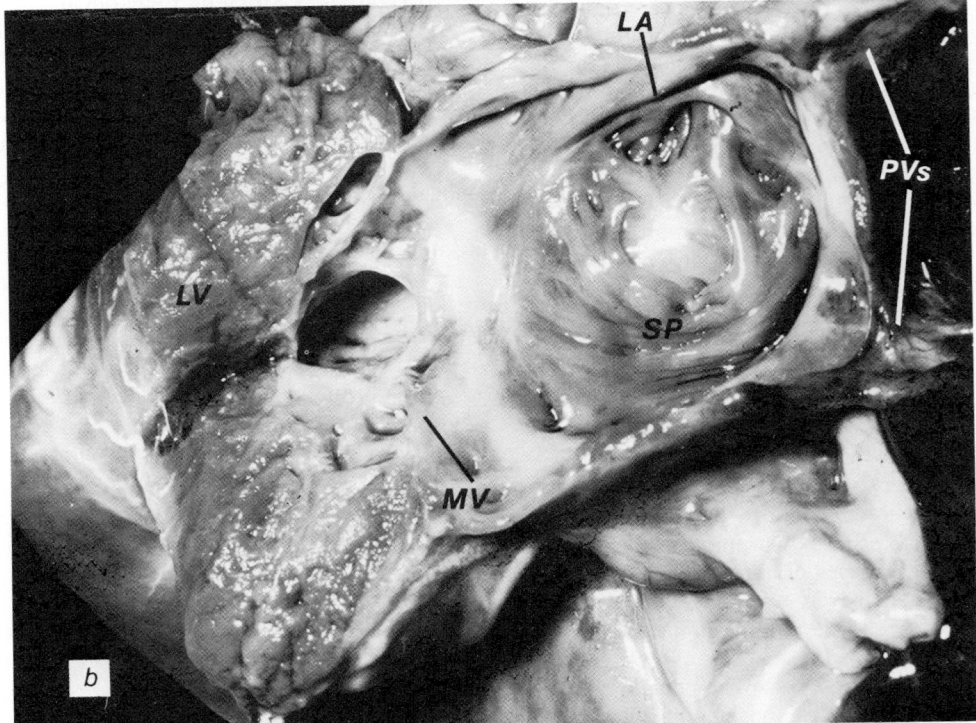

Figure 35-1 Autopsy specimen of aortic atresia and hypoplastic left heart syndrome from a 4-day-old neonate (GLH).

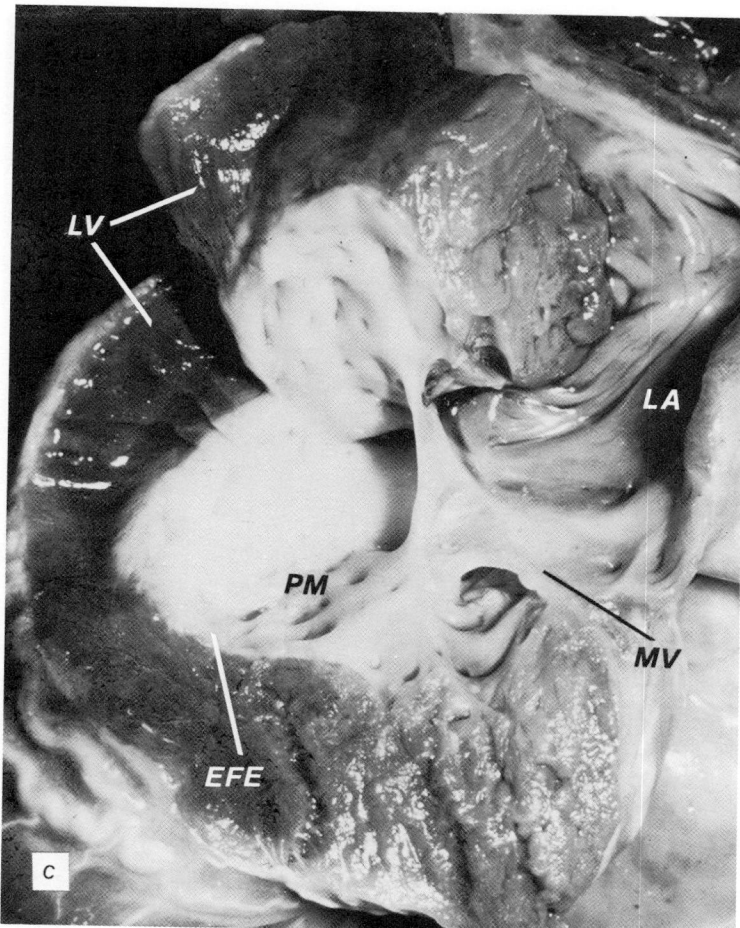

Figure 35-1 *(continued)*
(a) The globular external shape of the heart results from the massive right ventricular hypertrophy and enlargement. The main pulmonary artery is large and the ascending aorta small. The left ventricle is small and displaced posteriorly and does not reach the cardiac apex. The arrow points to the left anterior descending coronary artery.
(b) Interior of the left atrium and partly opened left ventricle. The septum primum (fossa ovalis) is thickened and protrudes into the right atrium. The mitral valve is very hypoplastic and stenotic and the left ventricular wall grossly thickened.
(c) Interior of the fully opened left ventricle. The cavity is small and there is marked endocardial fibroelastosis, which also involves the rudimentary papillary muscles of the small mitral valve.

AscAo, ascending aorta; EFE, endocardial fibroelastosis; LA, left atrium; LAA, left atrial appendage; LV, left ventricle; MPA, main pulmonary artery; MV, mitral valve; PM, papillary muscles; PVs, pulmonary veins; RA, right atrium; RV, right ventricle; SP, septum primum (fossa ovalis).

hypoplasia. Fetal pulmonary vasculature is present, resulting in a high pulmonary vascular resistance.[H1]

Aortic Valve and Ascending Aorta

The aortic valve is totally absent, but diminutive aortic sinuses of Valsalva are frequently present, giving origin to relatively normally positioned right and left coronary arteries which have a normal distribution pattern. The ascending aorta is narrow (Fig. 35-1*a*), the portion between the innominate artery and the atretic valve serving only as a conduit to supply coronary blood flow (Fig. 35-2). Distally, the transverse arch gradually widens and is joined beyond the origin of the left subclavian by a large, downwardly directed patent ductus arteriosus which is of larger diameter than the aortic isthmus and carries blood from the right ventricle into the descending aorta and retrogradely up the transverse and ascending arch. There is frequently a forme fruste coarctation at or proximal to the ductus, consisting of a mild infolding of the aortic media on the wall opposite the ductus. In 15–20% of cases a significant coarctation coexists.[M1,V1]

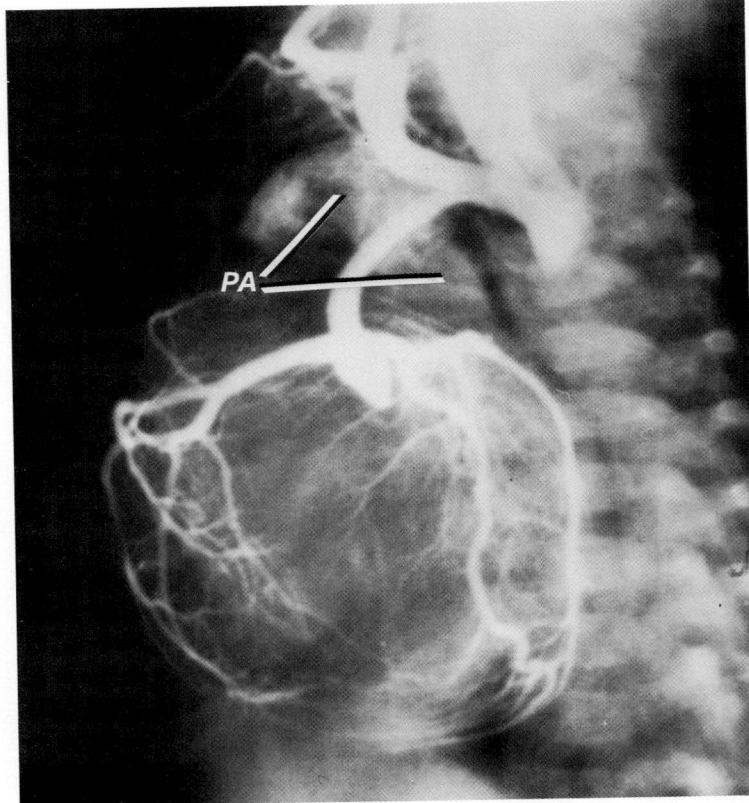

Figure 35-2   Lateral cineangiocardiogram obtained after a pressure injection of contrast medium into a brachial artery cannula in a neonate with hypoplastic left heart syndrome (GLH). (This resulted in marked bradycardia and hypotension and is not a recommended technique.) The size of the blind ascending aorta, which supplies the large coronary arteries, and the larger transverse arch and its branches are displayed. The main pulmonary artery is faintly outlined by contrast medium reaching it through the ductus arteriosus.

PA, pulmonary artery.

Left Ventricle and Mitral Valve

In 95% of cases the left ventricle is severely hypoplastic and the ventricular septum intact. The left ventricular cavity is slitlike and tiny and its wall is very thick. Rarely, however, the left ventricle is normal in size when the ventricular septum is intact.[E1] The inlet mitral valve is either atretic (about one-third of patients) or patent but severely hypoplastic (about two-thirds) (Figs. 35-1b and 35-1c).[R2]

When the valve is patent, there may be ventriculocoronary connections (Fig. 35-3) similar to those present in the right ventricle in pulmonary atresia with intact ventricular septum (see Chapter 25, "Right Ventricle" in section on Morphology).[O1] It is postulated that these serve to decompress the blind left ventricular chamber.[O1] Localized thickening of the coronary arteries occurs adjacent to these connections and there is also a variable degree of endocardial thickening (endocardial fibroelastosis). Rarely, there is focal calcification and scarring limited to the left ventricular subendocardium.[O1] The hypoplastic left ventricle shows myocardial fiber disarray quantitatively and qualitatively similar to that present in the left ventricle in hypertrophic obstructive cardiomyopathy (see Chapter 33, "Histopathology of the Left Ventricle" in section on Morphology) and in the right ventricle in pulmonary atresia with intact ventricular septum (see Chapter 25, "Right Ventricle" in section on Morphology).[B3]

In 5% of cases the left ventricular cavity is near normal in size in association with a large ventricular septal defect and either a relatively normal mitral valve or mitral valve atresia.[R2] There is left ventricular hypertrophy but no fibroelastosis and no ventriculocoronary connections or myocardial fiber disarray.

Right Ventricle

The right ventricle is enlarged, and the diffuse hypertrophy and marked increase in cavity size (to about three times normal) worsen with increasing age.[H2,V2] Both the tricuspid

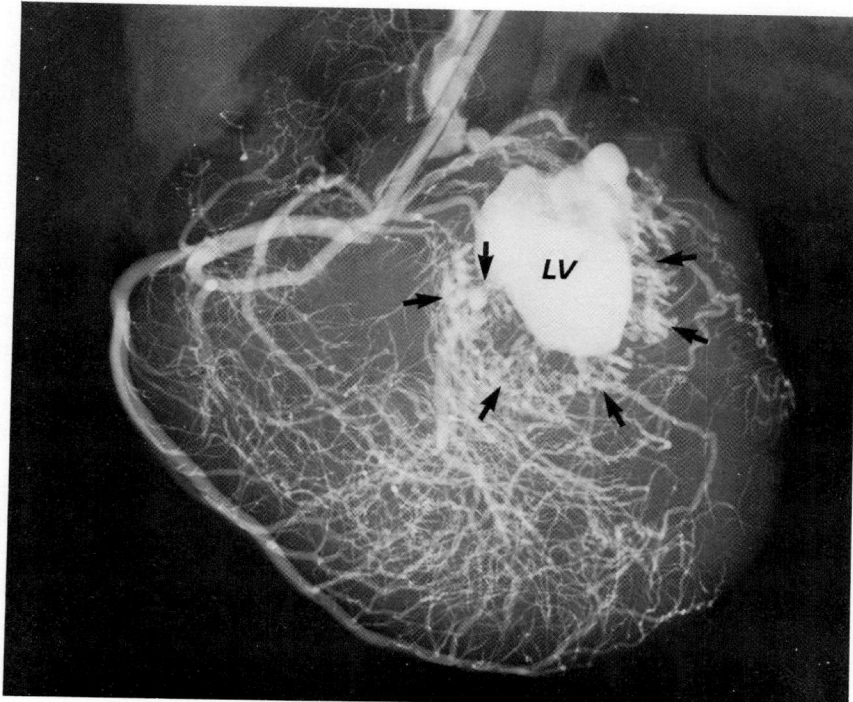

Figure 35-3 Postmortem coronary angiogram obtained by cannulation and injection of contrast medium into a coronary artery ostium in a heart with aortic atresia and hypoplastic left heart syndrome (GLH). The small left ventricular cavity was filled rapidly by the contrast medium's reaching it through numerous coronary–LV fistulous connections. These form a prominent network within the thickened LV myocardium (arrows). The large arrow marks the site of a particularly large connection which was the first to fill.

LV, left ventricle.

and pulmonary valves are larger than normal and there is sometimes tricuspid incompetence.

Pulmonary Artery

The main pulmonary artery is large and continues directly into a large patent ductus arteriosus. The right and then the left branches arise at right angles from the short parent trunk.

Atria and Atrial Septum

The *left atrium* is relatively small and thick-walled (except in those rare instances where the left ventricle and mitral valve are of normal size) with its long axis directed transversely toward the right atrium. The *atrial septum* is also thick, making balloon atrial septostomy generally unsatisfactory.[B4,L3] There is virtually always an atrial communication, which in the great majority of cases is a stretched patent foramen ovale. The valve of the fossa ovalis is thickened and stretched so that it herniates into the right atrium and allows left-to-right shunting (Fig. 35-1*b*). There may be a frank aneurysm of the atrial septum projecting to the right. Occasionally, the valve of the fossa ovalis has multiple perforations and there is a common atrium or there is an ostium primum–

type defect in association with a complete AV canal.[F1,N4,R2] The *right atrium* is larger than normal with hypertrophy of its walls.

Other Associated Anomalies

Other associated anomalies are uncommon.[F2,M4] Juxtaposed atrial appendages and a double tricuspid orifice have been reported, as has the coexistence of complete transposition of the great arteries.[M5,N4]

CLINICAL FEATURES AND DIAGNOSTIC CRITERIA

Presentation is in the newborn period with mild cyanosis and respiratory distress and tachycardia. There is usually rapid deterioration with signs of congestive heart failure and death within a week of birth.

On examination there is a hyperactive right ventricular precordial impulse and a moderate-intensity midsystolic murmur along the left sternal border. The second heart sound is accentuated and single. Congestive heart failure is associated with rales and liver enlargement. In most instances, peripheral pulses are of poor volume and the arm blood pressure is low.

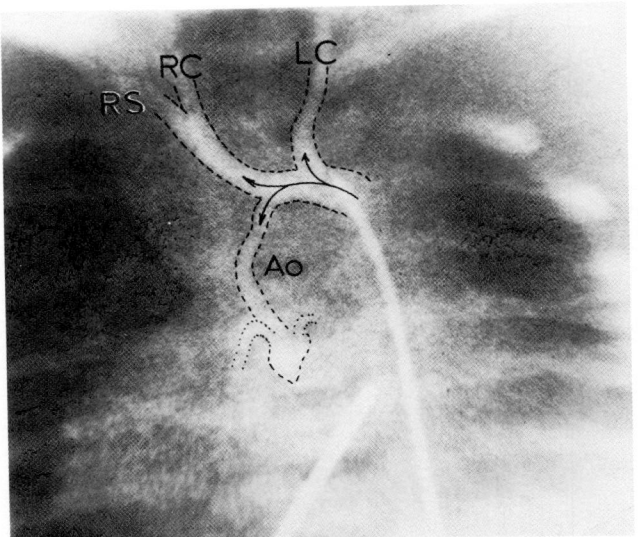

Figure 35-4 A shallow left anterior oblique cineangiogram frame obtained after a hand injection of contrast medium into the aorta adjacent to the ductus origin (GLH). The retrograde flow present in this condition results in adequate definition of the atretic aortic valve and small ascending aorta.

Ao, aorta; LC, left carotid artery; RC, right carotid artery; RS, right subclavian artery.

The chest x-ray shows moderate cardiomegaly and significant pulmonary plethora secondary to the increased pulmonary blood flow. The electrocardiogram demonstrates right axis deviation and right ventricular hypertrophy, and usually no left ventricular forces. However, good ventricular voltages can be present and do not necessarily signify an adequate left ventricular cavity.[F1]

Two-dimensional echocardiography is diagnostic. It demonstrates the large right ventricle and tricuspid valve and the small or absent left ventricle, mitral valve, and ascending aorta.[M3]

Cardiac catheterization and cineangiography are indicated in infants being considered for operation. The entire ascending aorta can be clearly outlined with contrast by a hand injection at the aortic end of the patent ductus arteriosus via a catheter advanced from the right heart or from the femoral artery, since flow into the aorta is both retrograde and antegrade from this site (Fig. 35-4). A right ventriculogram is performed to assess right ventricular function and exclude significant tricuspid incompetence.

NATURAL HISTORY

Aortic atresia with the hypoplastic left heart syndrome is the fourth most common congenital cardiac defect.[F2] Almost all afflicted babies are otherwise well developed and have normal birth weights. About 70% are males.[N4,R2]

Severe heart failure usually develops in the first week of life. Many infants with the syndrome die within 1–2 weeks of birth, only 40% survive the neonatal period, and survival beyond 6 weeks of age is uncommon.[B1,F2,L1,R1] The hypo-

plastic left heart syndrome accounts for 25% of cardiac deaths during the first week of life and 15% of those in the first month of life.[F2,N1]

The ductus arteriosus may remain patent, and perinatal survival is dependent upon this. Death can be the result of a progressive increase in pulmonary blood flow as the neonatal pulmonary vascular resistance falls. However, coronary perfusion in this anomaly is clearly abnormal, particularly to the left ventricle but also to the right ventricle, for it occurs in systole rather than diastole. Also, it is dependent on continuing patency of the ascending aorta and adequate systemic arterial blood flow. As pulmonary blood flow increases, systemic arterial flow decreases, as does coronary blood flow. The ductus arteriosus does begin to close shortly after birth, functionally at least, in some infants with the hypoplastic left heart syndrome, and this leads to impoverishment of systemic blood flow, metabolic acidosis, and death. The occasional patient surviving the neonatal period has continuing patency of the ductus and pulmonary blood flow limited either by a restricted atrial communication or pulmonary arteriolar constriction with or without organic vascular disease.

TECHNIQUE OF OPERATION

The ability to maintain patency of the ductus arteriosus and thereby an adequate blood flow to the systemic circulation by means of a continuous infusion of prostaglandin E_1 (PGE_1) makes it possible to plan an initial palliative procedure with a view to proceeding with a Fontan-type second-stage operation at an age when the pulmonary vascular resistance has fallen to normal.[D1,D2,Y1] PGE_1 may exert its temporarily favorable effect by other mechanisms as well.

First-Stage Palliative Procedure

The aims of the initial palliative operation are to provide an unobstructed pathway from the right ventricle to the aorta, and ideally to enlarge the ascending aorta also; to maintain but limit pulmonary blood flow and thus prevent progression of congestive heart failure and later pulmonary vascular disease; and to ensure an adequate interatrial communication.[N3] The connection of the right ventricle to aorta has been accomplished with prosthetic or homograft conduits from right ventricle or pulmonary trunk to the descending aorta,[D2,L2,M2,N4,N5] but a direct connection between the proximal pulmonary trunk and ascending aorta that also enlarges the ascending aorta has seemed preferable but more difficult to accomplish.[B2] Pulmonary blood flow seems best maintained in a controlled manner by using a Gore-Tex tube between right ventricle and pulmonary artery; a 3 mm hole in a pulmonary artery flap interposed between proximal and distal pulmonary artery;[B2] a classic Blalock-Taussig shunt; or a Gore-Tex interposition shunt between innominate artery and right pulmonary artery. The patent ductus arteriosus is interrupted. The atrial septum is excised so that pulmonary venous blood has free access to the tricuspid valve.[B2]

Currently the initial operation is performed during profound hypothermia and total circulatory arrest, with surface cooling to about 28°C before the sternotomy (see Chapter 2, Section 4), after the usual preparations are made for cardiac surgery (UAB). Prostaglandin E_1 has been started immediately upon suspicion of the diagnosis and is continued until cardiopulmonary bypass (CPB) is begun. (See Chapter 25, "Indications and Strategy of Operation," for more details about the use of prostaglandin E_1.) After the median sternotomy incision has been made, a piece of pericardium is set aside on a moist gauze for later use. (See Fig. 15-15 in Chapter 15 for the technique.) The main and central portions of the right and left pulmonary arteries as well as the ascending aorta are dissected, and silastic loops are placed around the left and right pulmonary arteries.

Using a single venous cannula in the right atrium and the arterial cannula in the pulmonary trunk, cardiopulmonary bypass (CPB) is begun, and the loops on the left and right pulmonary arteries are snugged. When nasopharyngeal temperature reaches 18°C, total circulatory arrest is established. Both the venous and arterial cannulae are removed. The ductus arteriosus is divided and the ends oversewn. The pulmonary trunk is divided proximal to its bifurcation, and the distal opening is closed with a pericardial patch in order to preserve a widely patent confluence between the left and right pulmonary arteries.

Formerly, the proximal opening in the pulmonary trunk was extended downward toward the pulmonary valve on the right side to form a large flap. An incision was made in the left side of the narrow ascending aorta, extending it distally across the coarctation if one was present. The flap of pulmonary trunk was sutured over this opening in the aorta (and as a patch graft enlargement across the associated coarctation if this was present) to create a large pathway between the right ventricle and the systemic and coronary arteries. Because this suture line is sometimes under tension, serious bleeding has been a problem. Thus, in the last three cases, following the suggestion of Castaneda,[C2] only the pulmonary end of the ductus is closed after ductal division. Ductal tissue is trimmed away from the opening in the aorta, and the opening is enlarged across any coarctation that may be present. After dividing the pulmonary trunk and closing the distal end with pericardium as described earlier, a cylinder of descending aortic homograft is interposed between the proximal end of the pulmonary trunk and the aortic arch after excising the ductal remnant.

A 4 mm Gore-Tex interposition shunt is then placed between the innominate artery (or the homograft) and the right pulmonary artery. Biologic glue (if available) is placed on all suture lines. The atrial septum is excised either through the opening in the atrial appendage or an extension of it, so that there is free access of pulmonary venous blood to the tricuspid valve.

The cannulae are replaced, CPB is reestablished, and rewarming is begun after a total circulatory arrest period that is usually about 60 minutes. The remainder of the procedure is completed in the usual fashion. Fresh frozen plasma and platelet concentrates are given immediately after discontinuing CPB.

Second-Stage Definitive Procedure

The second stage is performed at 6–24 months of age in surviving infants. At this procedure, the surgically created shunt is closed, a direct anastomosis is made between the right atrium and pulmonary artery (see Chapter 26, "Direct Right Atrial-Pulmonary Artery Connection" in section on Technique of Operation), and an atrial baffle is inserted to direct caval flow to the right atrial-pulmonary artery anastomosis and pulmonary venous blood to the tricuspid valve.

EARLY RESULTS

The mortality of the first stage repair has been high, even in experienced hands. Lang and Norwood experienced 22 (63%, CL 53%–72%) hospital deaths among 35 neonates and infants undergoing a first-stage repair, although in many a technique now known not to be optimal was used.[L3] Among 8 patients undergoing the first-stage repair of the hypoplastic left heart syndrome, 6 (75%, CL 50%–91%) died in the hospital (UAB). Four died in the operating room of acute cardiac failure complicated by a bleeding diathesis. A fifth patient died on the eighth postoperative day with sepsis, after an initially satisfactory postoperative course. The last three patients were operated on with the current technique, and two survived to leave the hospital in good condition. Both subsequently died.

Lang and Norwood report four patients undergoing the second and final stage of repair. Two (50%, CL 18%–82%) hospital deaths occurred, one related to pulmonary vascular disease and the other to presumed acute cardiac failure.

LATE RESULTS

The 2 patients (6%, CL 2%–13% of an original group of 35 neonates and infants with hypoplastic left heart syndrome) who survived two-stage repair are reported by Lang and Norwood to be doing well 1 year after the second stage.[L3]

Late postoperative hemodynamic studies of 10 infants surviving the first stage of repair of the hypoplastic left heart showed regression of pulmonary vascular resistance to normal in all.[L3] The studies also demonstrated the long-term ineffectiveness of balloon septostomy in this setting, which is probably related to the very thick and abnormal atrial septum found in the hypoplastic left heart.[B4] One patient developed severe tricuspid incompetence, which is probably related to the marked right ventricular enlargement that develops in this situation.[H3,V2]

INDICATIONS FOR OPERATION

The presence of the anomaly may be considered an indication for operation (UAB), or the surgical survival rates may be considered too low and the achieved and potential benefits of the repairs too small to justify the considerable human and material resources required (GLH). However, insufficient information is available to allow the latter conclusion to be made with confidence, and a continuation of this clinical trial is appropriate in order to obtain this information.

SPECIAL SITUATIONS AND CONTROVERSIES

Aortic Atresia, Large Ventricular Septal Defect, and Normal-sized Left Ventricle

One success has been reported by Duffy and colleagues from a two-stage procedure in a patient with aortic atresia and large left ventricle and VSD.[D3] An earlier success in a more complex situation with coexisting interrupted aortic arch was reported by Norwood and Stellin in 1981.[N2] The operative procedures have been similar to those used when the left ventricle is severely hypoplastic. The ductus arteriosus is closed, a conduit or a direct side-to-side anastomosis is placed between the undivided pulmonary artery and aorta, and the right and left pulmonary arteries are banded separately. The definitive procedure has consisted of closing the VSD, releasing the right and left pulmonary artery bands with dilation or patch graft enlargement if needed, taking down the pulmonary artery–aortic connection, and placing a valved conduit between the apex of the left ventricle and the descending thoracic or infradiaphragmatic aorta.[D3,S1]

REFERENCES

A

1. Abbott ME: Aortic, mitral, and tricuspid atresia, in *Atlas of Congenital Cardiac Disease*. New York: American Heart Association, p 48, 1936.

B

1. Brockman JL: Congenital mitral atresia. *Am Heart J* 40:301, 1950.
2. Behrendt DM, Rocchini A: An operation for the hypoplastic left heart syndrome: Preliminary report. *Ann Thorac Surg* 32:284, 1981.
3. Bulkley BH, D'Amico B, Taylor AL: Extensive myocardial fiber disarray in aortic and pulmonary atresia. Relevance to hypertrophic cardiomyopathy. *Circulation* 67:191, 1983.
4. Bharati S, Lev M: The surgical anatomy of hypoplasia of aortic tract complex. *J Thorac Cardiovasc Surg* 88:97, 1984.

C

1. Canton M: Congenital obliteration of origin of the aorta. *Trans Pathol Soc (Lond)* 2:38, 1850.
2. Castaneda AR: (1984) Personal communication.

D

1. Doty DB, Knott HW: Hypoplastic left heart syndrome. *J Thorac Cardiovasc Surg* 74:624, 1977.
2. Doty DB, Marvin WJ Jr, Schieken RM, Lauer RM: Hypoplastic left heart syndrome: Successful palliation with a new operation. *J Thorac Cardiovasc Surg* 80:148, 1980.
3. Duffy CE, Muster AJ, De Leon SY, Idriss FS, Ilbawi M, Riggs TW, Paul MH: Successful surgical repair of aortic atresia associated with normal left ventricle. *JACC* 6:1503, 1983.

E

1. Esteban I, Cabrara A: Aortic atresia with normal left ventricle and intact ventricular septum. *Chest* 73:883, 1978.

F

1. Freedom RM, Williams WG, Dische MR, Rowe RD: Anatomical variants in aortic atresia—potential candidates for ventriculo-aortic reconstruction. *Br Heart J* 38:821, 1976.
2. Fyler DC: Report of the New England Regional Infant Cardiac Program. *Pediatrics* 65:376, 1980.

H

1. Heidelberger KP, Newman MS, Dick M, Rosenthal A: Fetal pulmonary vascular changes associated with hypoplastic left ventricle syndrome. *Am J Cardiol* 43:364, 1979 (abstr).
2. Hastreiter AR, Van der Horst RL, Dubrow IW, Eckner FO: Quantitative angiographic and morphologic aspects of aortic valve atresia. *Am J Cardiol* 51:1705, 1983.
3. Hawkins JA, Doty DB: Aortic atresia: Morphologic characteristics affecting survival and operative palliation. *J Thorac Cardiovasc Surg* 88:620, 1984.

L

1. Lambert EC, Canet RV, Hohn AR: Congenital cardiac anomalies in the newborn. A review of condition causing death or severe distress in the first month of life. *Pediatrics* 37:343, 1966.
2. Levitsky S, van der Horst RL, Hastreiter AR: Surgical palliation in aortic atresia. *J Thorac Cardiovasc Surg* 79:456, 1980.
3. Lang P, Norwood WI: Hemodynamic assessment after palliative surgery for hypoplastic left heart syndrome. *Circulation* 68:104, 1983.
4. Lev M: Pathologic anatomy and interrelationship of hypoplasia of the aortic tract complexes. *Lab Invest* 1:61, 1952.
5. Litwin SB, Van Praagh R, Bernhard WF: A palliative operation for certain infants with aortic arch interruption. *Ann Thorac Surg* 14:369, 1972.

M

1. Milo S, Ho SY, Anderson RH: Hypoplastic left heart syndrome: Can this malformation be treated surgically? *Thorax* 35:351, 1980.
2. Mohri H, Horiuchi T, Haneda K, Sato S, Kahata O, Ohmi M, Ishizawa E, Kagawa Y, Fukuda M, Yoshida Y, Shima T: Surgical treatment of hypoplastic left heart syndrome. *J Thorac Cardiovasc Surg* 78:223, 1979.
3. Meyer RA, Kaplan S: Echocardiography in the diagnosis of hypoplasia of the right and left ventricle in the neonate. *Circulation* 46:55, 1972.
4. Mahowald JM, Lucas RV Jr, Edwards JE: Aortic valvular atresia. Associated cardiovascular anomalies. *Pediatr Cardiol* 2:99, 1982.
5. McGarry KN, Taylor JF, Macartney FJ: Aortic atresia occurring with complete transposition of the great arteries. *B Heart J* 44:711, 1980.

N

1. Noonan JA, Nadas AS: The hypoplastic left heart syndrome: An analysis of 101 cases. *Pediatr Clin North Am* 5:1029, 1958.

2. Norwood WI, Stellin GJ: Aortic atresia with interrupted aortic arch. *J Thorac Cardiovasc Surg* 81:239, 1981.

3. Norwood WI, Lang P, Hansen D: Physiologic repair of aortic atresia-hypoplastic left heart syndrome. *N Engl J Med* 308:23, 1983.

4. Norwood WI, Lang P, Castaneda AR, Campbell DN: Experience with operations for hypoplastic left heart syndrome. *J Thorac Cardiovasc Surg* 82:511, 1981.

5. Norwood WI, Kirklin JK, Sanders SP: Hypoplastic left heart syndrome. Experience with palliative surgery. *Am J Cardiol* 45:87, 1980.

O

1. O'Connor WN, Cash JB, Cottrill CM, Johnson GL, Noonan JA: Ventriculocoronary connections in hypoplastic left hearts: An autopsy microscopic study. *Circulation* 66:1078, 1982.

R

1. Redo SF, Engle MA, Ehlers KH, Farnworth PB: Palliative surgery for mitral atresia. *Arch Surg* 95:717, 1967.

S

1. Sarnoff S, Donovan TJ, Case RB: The surgical relief of aortic stenosis by means of apical-aortic valvular anastomosis. *Circulation* 11:564, 1955.

2. Roberts WC, Perry LW, Chandra RS, Myers GE, Shapiro SR, Scott LP: Aortic valve atresia. A new classification based on necropsy study of 73 cases. *Am J Cardiol* 37:753, 1976.

V

1. von Rueden TJ, Knight L, Moller JH, Edwards JE: Coarctation of the aorta associated with aortic valvular atresia. *Circulation* 52:951, 1975.

2. van der Horst RL, Hastreiter AR, DuBrow IW, Eckner FAO: Pathologic measurements in aortic atresia. *Am Heart J* 106:1411, 1983.

Y

1. Yabek SM, Mann JS: Prostaglandin E_1 infusion in the hypoplastic left heart syndrome. *Chest* 76:330, 1979.

36

CONGENITAL MITRAL VALVE DISEASE

DEFINITION

Congenital mitral valve disease is a developmental malformation of one or more of the components of the mitral valve apparatus, including that portion of left atrial wall immediately adjacent to the mitral anulus, which produces stenosis or incompetence or, occasionally, a combined lesion. It often coexists with other cardiac anomalies, particularly those involving the left-sided cardiac chambers and aorta.

Left atrioventricular valve anomalies associated with atrioventricular canal defects (Chapter 19), aortic atresia with left ventricular hypoplasia (Chapter 35), various forms of atrioventricular discordant connection (Chapter 43), or transposition of the great arteries (Chapter 39) are special situations that are discussed in the chapters describing these conditions. The mitral valve anomalies associated with straddling mitral valves or univentricular atrioventricular connections are described in Chapter 44. Mitral incompetence related to mitral valve prolapse as part of the syndrome of myxomatous degeneration in patients 20 years of age or older and that associated with atrial septal defect in older patients without demonstrable congenital anomalies of the valvar apparatus are described in Chapters 11 and 15, respectively.

HISTORICAL NOTE

The heterogeneity of congenital mitral valve disease and the frequency of its association with other cardiac anomalies make it difficult to trace the historical evolution of knowledge about this entity. However, as early as 1902 Fisher described "2 cases of congenital disease of the left side of the heart," one of which was a stenotic supravalvar ring.[F1] "Parachute mitral valve," another entity in this spectrum, was not described until 1961[S3] and was not fully documented until 1963.[S1]

One of the first reports of the surgical treatment of congenital mitral valve disease was that by Starkey in 1959.[S5] In 1962, Creech and colleagues reported a well-documented case of repair of congenital mitral incompetence resulting from a cleft in the posterior leaflet in a 2-year-old girl. Although the child was improved by suturing the cleft, moderate mitral incompetence persisted.[C1]

MORPHOLOGY

The congenital abnormality may involve any component of the mitral apparatus and may result in stenosis with or without incompetence or in pure incompetence. Although only one component may be involved, more often the entire valve is affected, as emphasized by Carpentier and colleagues.[C2]

Supravalvar Ring

A tough fibrous ring may be situated just on the left atrial side of the mitral anulus.[A2] A supravalvar ring is distinguished from the "diaphragm" or fibrous ridge of cor triatriatum (see Chapter 17) by the fact that in the former the pulmonary veins and left atrial appendage enter the same chamber (the left atrium) above or proximal to the ring. The supravalvar ring may be nonobstructive and an incidental finding, or it may protrude into the orifice and provide a variable degree of obstruction in the left atrioventricular (AV) pathway.[A2,D1] Occasionally, an isolated ring may be severely stenotic and contribute importantly to death in the first year of life (Fig. 36-1).[D1] More commonly, it coexists with other cardiac anomalies and particularly with other mitral valve anomalies and with left ventricular outflow obstruction.[S1]

Mitral Anulus

The mitral anulus uncommonly is small and obstructive in the absence of severe left ventricular hypoplasia or other abnormalities of the valve.[C5] It may be small but not obstructive, particularly in hearts with coarctation of the aorta.[R1]

The anulus may be enlarged, usually secondary to mitral incompetence resulting from some other deformity of the mitral valve. However, the basic valvar anomaly leading to incompetence may be subtle and difficult to identify. Carpentier and colleagues found essentially isolated annular dilatation in 8 (17%) of 47 cases with congenital mitral valve disease, although some deficiency of commissural tissue is implied by their description.[C2]

Leaflet Anomalies

The orifice through the mitral valve is frequently narrowed by a congenital absence of one or both commissures, which are replaced by a continuous sheet of leaflet tissue. Small perforations may be present at what is usually a commissure. The leaflets often then take the form of an inverted cone, and in these circumstances the chordae are usually short and intermixed and the orifice obstructed further by abnormal and hypertrophied papillary muscles beneath it (the so-called hammock valve).[C3] In other cases, there may be congenital leaflet thickening and immobility and consequent orifice narrowing, even though commissures are present (Fig. 36-2).

When congenital mitral regurgitation without important stenosis is the functional lesion, a variety of mitral leaflet anomalies may be responsible. The posterior leaflet may be severely hypoplastic and represented only by tags of fibrous tissue.[C2] In other cases the anterior leaflet may be long and billowing and the chordae thin and elongated and occasion-

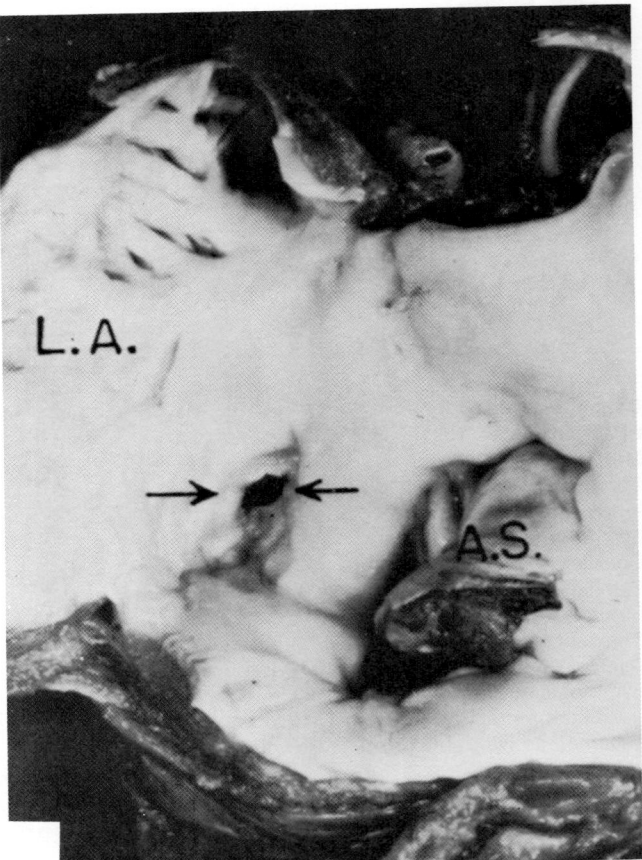

Figure 36-1 Supravalvar ring producing severe obstruction above the mitral orifice in an infant dying of heart failure at age 9 months. Arrows indicate the small (3 mm) orifice produced by the stenosing ring.

AS, fossa ovalis atrial septal defect; LA, left atrium.

Reproduced with permission from Davichi et al.,[D1] and the American Heart Association.

ally ruptured.[D1,F2] This has been observed as a cause of severe mitral incompetence in patients as young as 2 years of age (UAB). (This may represent prolapse, or myxomatous degeneration, of the mitral valve appearing in the very young. In this chapter, only those requiring operation before age 20 are considered. For a consideration of this entity in older patients, see Chapter 11.)

In still other patients, without any of the stigmata of an AV canal defect, the anterior leaflet or, less commonly, the posterior leaflet[C1] of the mitral valve may be separated into two leaflets by an accessory commissure (or cleft), with resultant regurgitation through that area.[D3] Chordae tendinae may pass from the edges of the cleft to the ventricular septum or rudimentary papillary muscles (as was the case in two of five such cases reported by Carpentier and colleagues[C2]), or the cleft may simply represent leaflet deficiency in that area (Fig. 36-3) without chordal support.[B1,F2] Rarely, there may be a hole in the belly of the anterior cusp.[F2]

Commissural leaflet tissue may be absent at one or the other commissures, resulting in an accessory orifice and mitral incompetence.[S2]

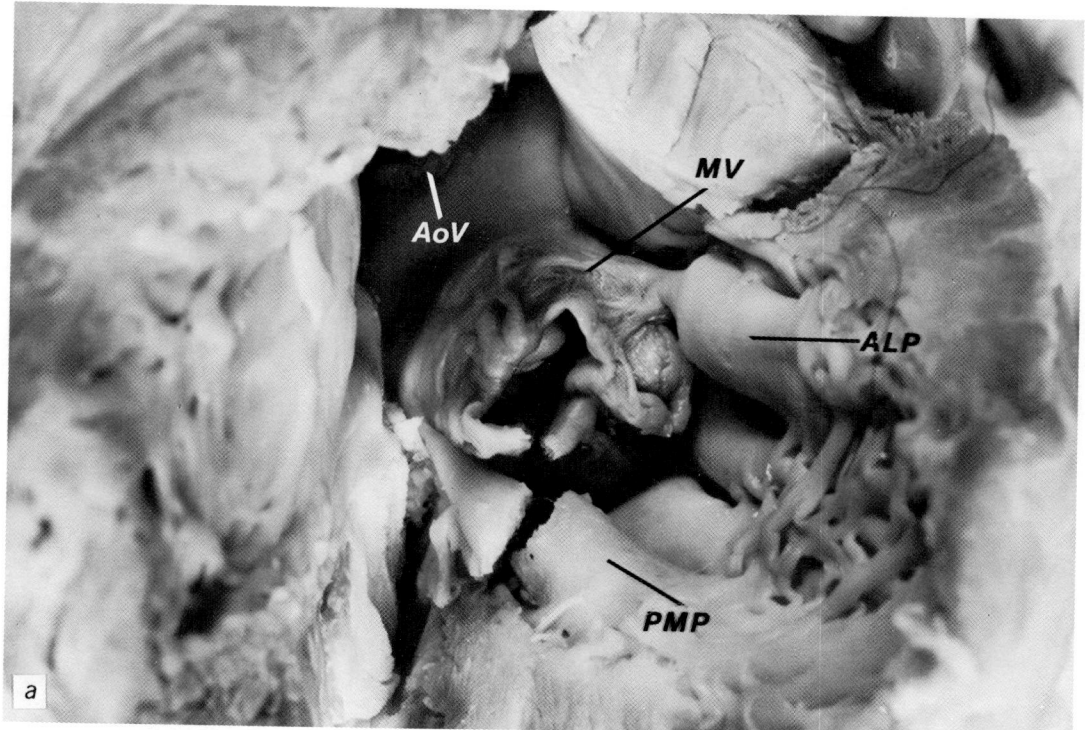

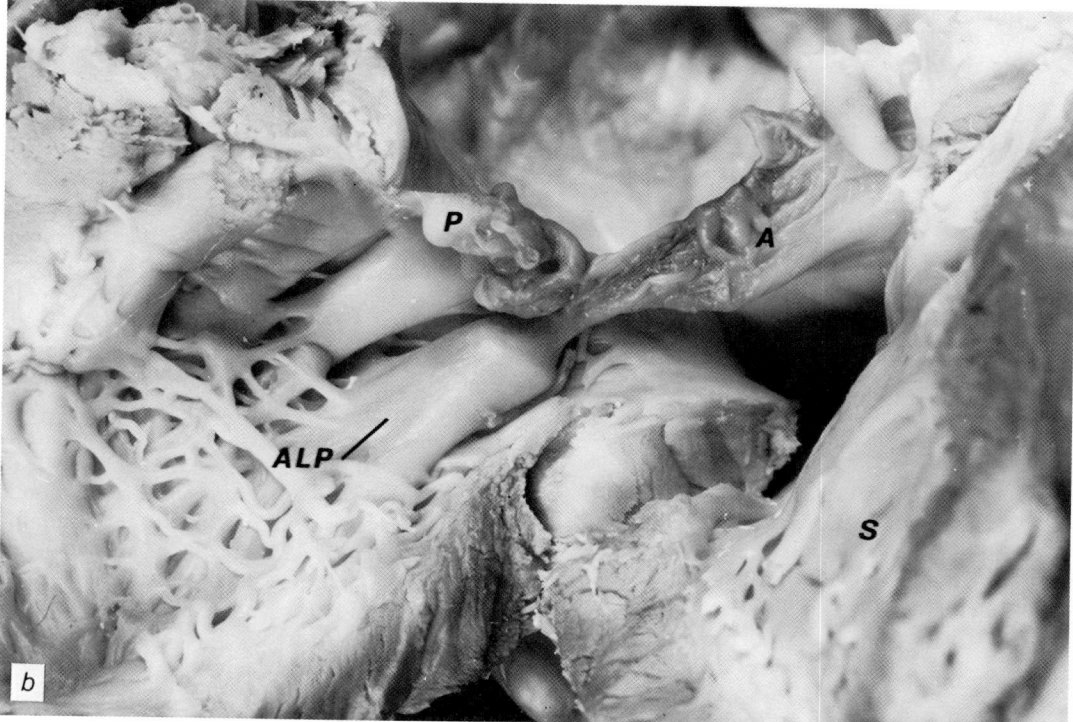

Figure 36-2 Specimen with severe congenital mitral stenosis from an infant dying at 10 weeks of age with an associated ventricular septal defect (GLH). All components of the valve are very abnormal and contribute to the stenosis.

(a) Viewed from the left ventricle with the mitral valve essentially intact. The leaflets are diffusely thickened without commissures, the papillary muscles are bulky and almost reach the leaflets, and the chordae are thick, fused, and short.

(b) Viewed from the left ventricle with the mitral ring divided.

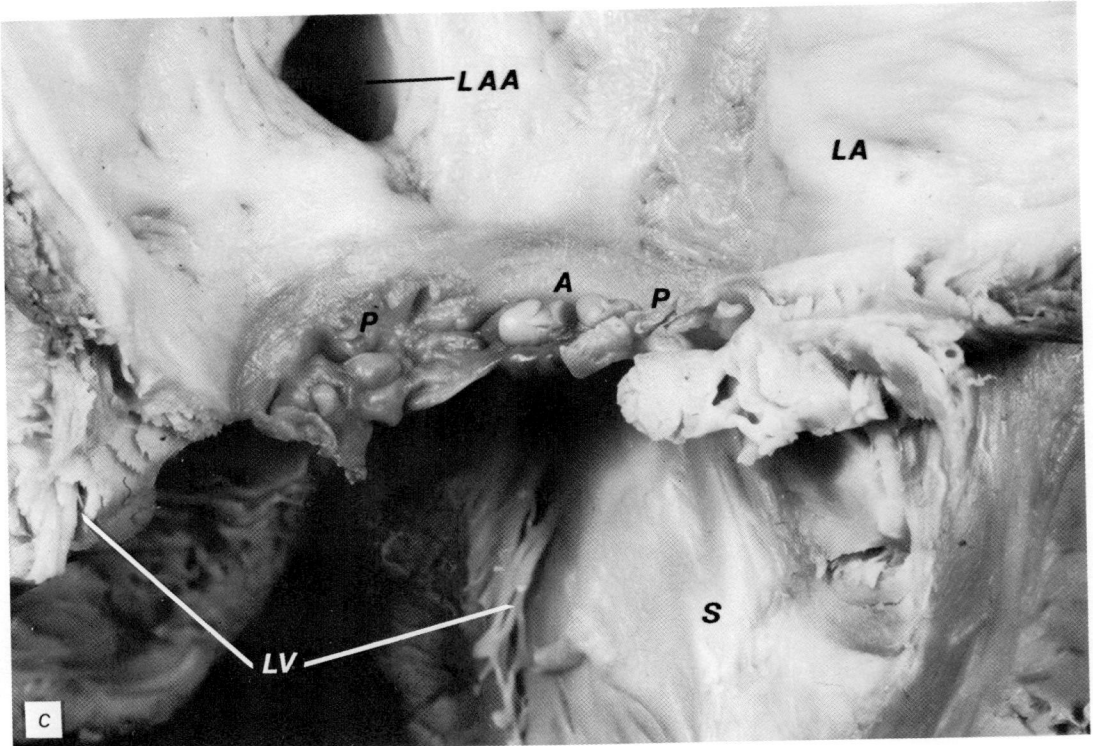

Figure 36-2 (*continued*)
(c) Viewed from the left atrium. It is not possible to distinguish the anterior from the posterior leaflet except by their attachments to the ring.

A, anterior mitral leaflet; ALP, anterolateral papillary muscle; AoV, aortic valve; LA, left atrium; LAA, left atrial appendage; LV, left ventricle; MV, mitral valve; PMP, posteromedial papillary muscle; P, posterior mitral leaflet; S, muscular interventricular septum.

Chordal Anomalies

Very short chordae, which are often thick and fused, can produce severe orifice narrowing. This, or complete chordal absence, brings the leaflet tissue down onto the papillary muscle(s) and results in a thick and narrow orifice. Accessory chordae that attach along the entire free edge of the anterior leaflet rather than leaving its central third free[R1] are a cause of restricted leaflet movement and, therefore, stenosis.

Chordal abnormalities can also result in congenital mitral incompetence. Most commonly these are chordal elongation, sometimes with lengthened papillary muscles, the tips of which actually prolapse along with the leaflet into the left atrium during ventricular systole.[C2]

Papillary Muscle Anomalies

There may be a single large papillary muscle, with all chordae attaching to it, the so-called parachute valve described first by Schiebler and colleagues[S3] and emphasized by Shone and colleagues (Fig. 36-4).[S1] Usually the chordae are short and thick and limit leaflet movement. This restricts the primary orifice through the opened valve as well as the secondary orifices between the chordae and results in mitral stenosis. In other cases, there is a single large papillary muscle, whereas near it is a hypoplastic one with only a few chordae attached to it, and the valve orifice is small by the same mechanisms. A parachute valve usually produces only severe stenosis, but it may also result in mitral regurgitation.[G4]

Two hypertrophied and abnormally placed, contiguous, papillary muscles, usually situated posteriorly,[C2] are also a cause of subvalvar obstruction.[C3,D1] The obstruction in this situation is often aggravated by the coexistence of short thick chordae and anomalous thick muscular bands.[R2] In still other cases, there are three or more closely placed and hypoplastic or bulky papillary muscles, a situation in which short thick chordae are often also present and contribute to the congenital mitral stenosis. In all of these, absence of the normal wide interpapillary distance contributes to the obstruction in the mitral pathway.

In still other situations, an *anomalous papillary muscle arcade* is formed by a bridge of fibrous tissue that runs through the free aspect of the anterior mitral leaflet between the anterolateral and posteromedial papillary muscles (Fig. 36-5).[D1,L1]

Summary

Congenital mitral *stenosis* without or with incompetence may result from supravalvar, annular, or valvar narrowing

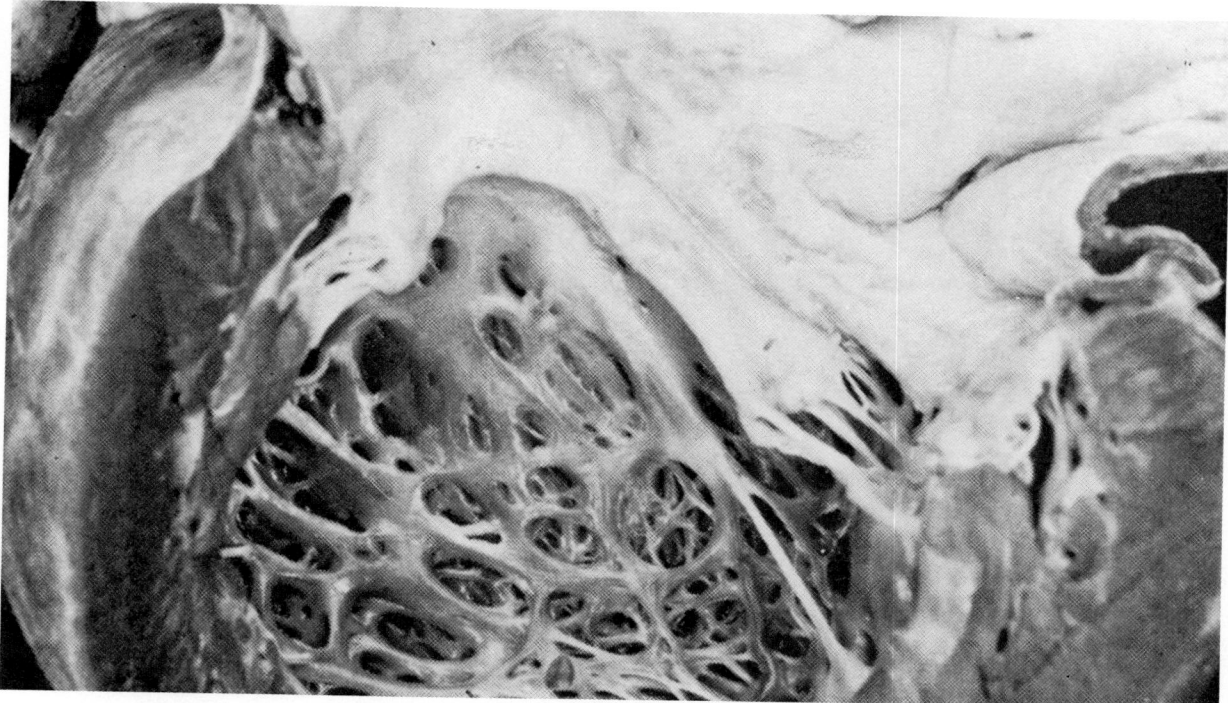

Figure 36-3 Specimen from a 9-year-old boy who died with congestive heart failure from severe mitral incompetence. There is a large cleft, or gap, without chordae in the anterior mitral leaflet. Reproduced with permission from Edwards.[E1]

and may be accentuated by subvalvar obstruction produced by hypertrophied and misplaced papillary muscles or sheets of fused chordae. Frequently the stenosis is a result of abnormalities at multiple levels (see Fig. 36-2). Congenital mitral *incompetence* may result from annular dilation secondary to anterior or posterior leaflet prolapse or to hypoplasia of the posterior leaflet with chordal shortening. Chordal elongation and valve prolapse may be so severe that chordal rupture can develop, even in young children, and produce severe incompetence. Congenital mitral incompetence may also be produced by clefts or gaps or perforations in the anterior mitral leaflet, accessory commissures, or leaflet hypoplasia at the medial or lateral commissures.

Coexisting Cardiac Anomalies

Patients with congenital mitral incompetence often have coexisting cardiac anomalies, but they tend to be less severe than in the case of congenital mitral stenosis (Table 36-1).

Congenital mitral stenosis is an isolated malformation in only about 25% of cases (6 of the 26 in the combined UAB and GLH surgical series). In another 30%, congenital mitral stenosis coexists with a ventricular septal defect. In about 40% of cases (11 of 26 in the UAB and GLH combined surgical series), congenital mitral stenosis coexists with one or another form of left ventricular (LV) outflow obstruction, a situation quite properly termed "Shone's syndrome."[S1] This may consist only of coarctation or some hypoplasia of the distal aortic arch, with or without patent ductus arteriosus. The left ventricular outflow obstruction may be in

the form of valvar or discrete subvalvar or combined valvar and subvalvar aortic stenosis, with or without coarctation. Rarely, there is diffuse or "tunnel" subvalvar stenosis, with or without the other forms of LV outflow obstruction. The frequency of the association of LV outflow obstruction with congenital mitral valve disease is evidenced by Rosenquist's finding of 31 instances of coexisting important congenital mitral valve anomalies among specimens from 53 patients whose primary diagnosis in life was coarctation of the aorta.[R1] However, when a large surgical series of coarctation repair is considered and includes adults as well as infants and children, only 2% of patients with coarctation severe enough to require repair have demonstrable congenital mitral valve disease.[F2]

The rare coexistence of a stenosing supravalvar ring with tetralogy of Fallot is noteworthy, since if undetected it may cause death after the repair of the tetralogy.[B2,C5] Congenital mitral valve disease and subaortic stenosis may rarely coexist with subpulmonary stenosis and an intact ventricular septum,[B4] or with subpulmonary stenosis and a VSD,[G4] or with valvar pulmonary stenosis.[G4]

CLINICAL FEATURES AND DIAGNOSTIC CRITERIA

Symptoms and Signs

Isolated Mitral Valve Disease
The symptoms and clinical signs are identical to those present in acquired mitral valve disease, the congenital etiology

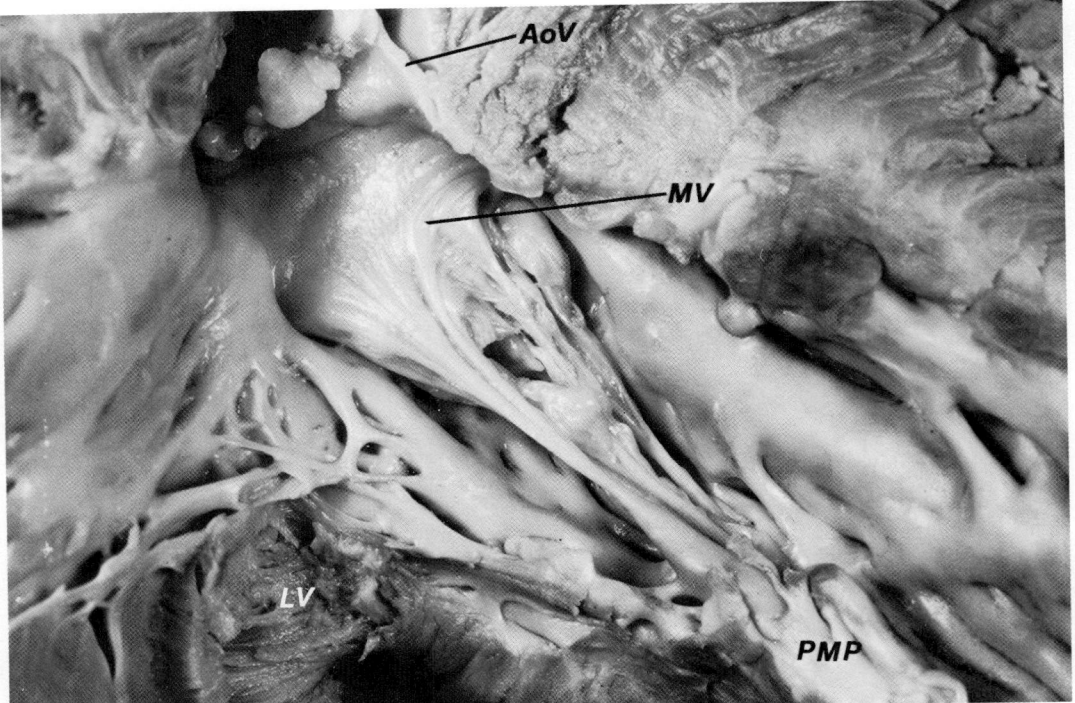

Figure 36-4 Specimen of a heart with congenital mitral stenosis from parachute mitral valve, viewed from left ventricular aspect (GLH). The chordae are thickened, and all of them attach to a single posteromedial papillary muscle. The anterolateral papillary muscle is absent.

AoV, aortic valve; LV, left ventricle; MV, mitral valve; PMP, posteromedial papillary muscle.

being apparent only when presentation is in infancy or early childhood and there is no rheumatic history. Symptoms of pulmonary venous hypertension include dyspnea, orthopnea or paroxysmal nocturnal dyspnea, and recurrent pulmonary infection.[C5] Pulmonary hypertension is nearly always present in severe lesions, terminating in frank congestive heart failure often with peripheral and central cyanosis.[C5]

Mitral stenosis is associated with a prominent apical mid-diastolic murmur sometimes with presystolic accentuation, and there may be an opening snap,[D2] although the morphologic features that commonly result in a limitation of leaflet movement make this less common than in acquired mitral stenosis.[A2] Mitral incompetence is evidenced by an apical pansystolic murmur radiating to the axilla, frequently with a third heart sound or a short, middiastolic murmur and left ventricular overactivity. When there is pulmonary hypertension, the second heart sound is accentuated and there is a right ventricular lift.

Combined with Left Ventricular Outflow Tract Obstruction
Unless a ventricular septal defect or patent ductus arteriosus is also present, the mitral signs are usually clinically diagnostic, particularly when the only additional significant site of obstruction is a coarctation. When there is severe congenital aortic stenosis, the mitral lesion, unless also severe, may not be clinically obvious. Again, the mitral lesions worsen the clinical presentation.

Electrocardiogram

Evidence of left atrial hypertrophy of greater degree than usually found in the coexisting cardiac anomaly suggests associated congenital mitral valve disease. Right ventricular hypertrophy is evident when there is the usual raised pulmonary vascular resistance and there is also right atrial enlargement, whereas left ventricular hypertrophy is present when there is severe mitral regurgitation or associated left ventricular outflow tract obstruction. Atrial fibrillation is rare.

Chest X-Ray

Left atrial enlargement out of proportion to that usually present in any coexisting cardiac anomaly that the patient may have is the most important clue in the chest x-ray of the possible presence of congenital mitral valve disease. There is always cardiac enlargement, whether the lesion is isolated or complex. Signs of pulmonary venous hypertension and occasionally overt pulmonary edema may be present in severe cases, but pulmonary plethora from a coexisting left-to-right shunt may confuse these signs.

Two-Dimensional Echocardiography

Two-dimensional echocardiography is ideally combined with Doppler interrogation studies and can provide a nearly com-

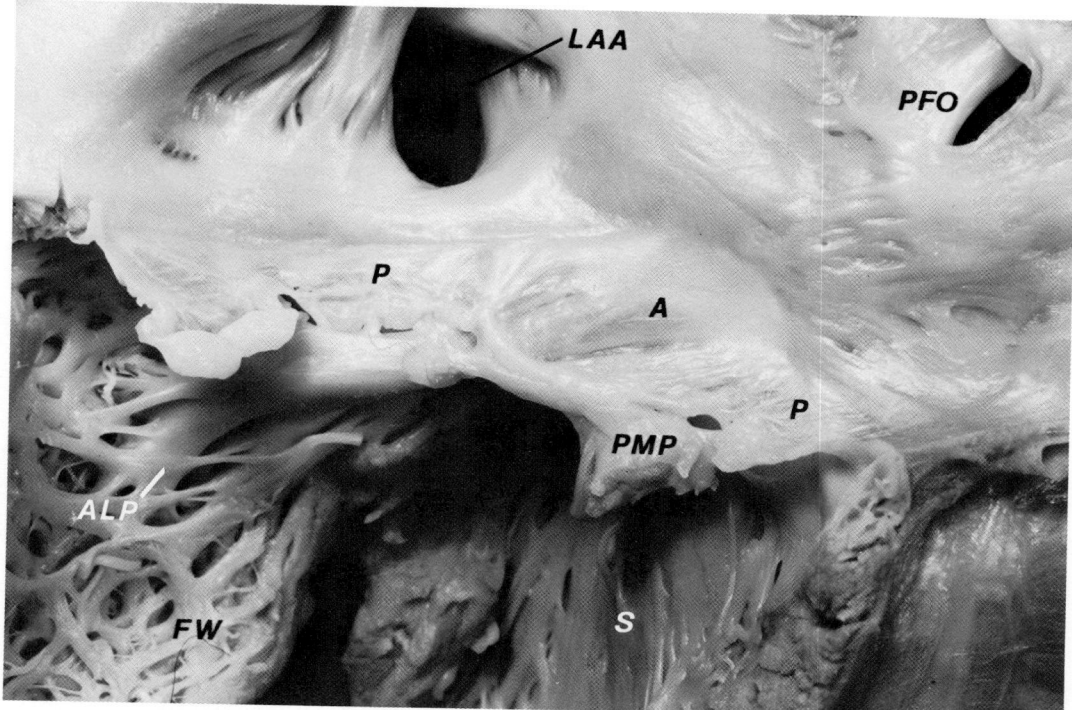

Figure 36-5   Specimen of a heart with mitral arcade producing mitral incompetence (GLH). There is a thick fibrous band stretching between the tips of the two papillary muscles along the edge of the anterior leaflet.

A, anterior mitral leaflet; ALP, anterolateral papillary muscle; LAA, left atrial appendage; FW, left ventricular free wall; P, posterior mitral leaflet; PFO, patent foramen ovale; PMP, portion of posteromedial papillary muscle; S, muscular septum.

Table 36-1   Coexisting cardiac anomalies in patients coming to operation primarily for congenital mitral incompetence (UAB and GLH; 1967–1984; *n* = 22). The categories are mutually exclusive.

Coexisting Cardiac Anomaly	No. of Patients
ASD	6
ASD + malformed pulmonary valve	1
Absent coronary sinus syndrome	1
ASD + left SVC + WPW syndrome	1
Hypoplastic left pulmonary artery	1
Moderate tricuspid incompetence	1
PDA + pulmonary AV fistula	1
PDA + coarctation	1
VSD	2
SVD + severe infundibular PS	1
Total	16

KEY: ASD, atrial septal defect; PA, pulmonary artery; PDA, patent ductus arteriosus; SVC, superior vena cava; VSD, ventricular septal defect; WPW, Wolff-Parkinson-White.

NOTE: Congenital mitral valve incompetence occurred in some other patients primarily operated upon for another congenital cardiac anomaly, and these are not accounted for in this table.

plete analysis of the morphology and function of congenitally abnormal mitral valves.[G3,S6] It may be the only method of study that can securely identify isolated cleft mitral valve.[D4] Routine echocardiographic study is required in all forms of congenital heart disease that may coexist with congenital mitral valve disease, since otherwise the presence of the mitral lesion may be overlooked.

Cardiac Catheterization and Cineangiographic Studies

Cardiac catheterization and cineangiographic studies are usually also necessary, primarily for the evaluation of possible associated lesions and for definition of the degree of pulmonary vascular disease.[C4] Also, the morphology of the congenitally abnormal valve can be further evaluated by its cineangiographic appearance.[M1]

NATURAL HISTORY

Congenital mitral valve disease is a rare congenital cardiac anomaly, occurring in 0.6% of autopsied patients with congenital heart disease and in 0.21%–0.42% of clinical cases of congenital heart disease.[C5]

As implied in the foregoing section, the natural history of these patients is highly variable and depends on the severity

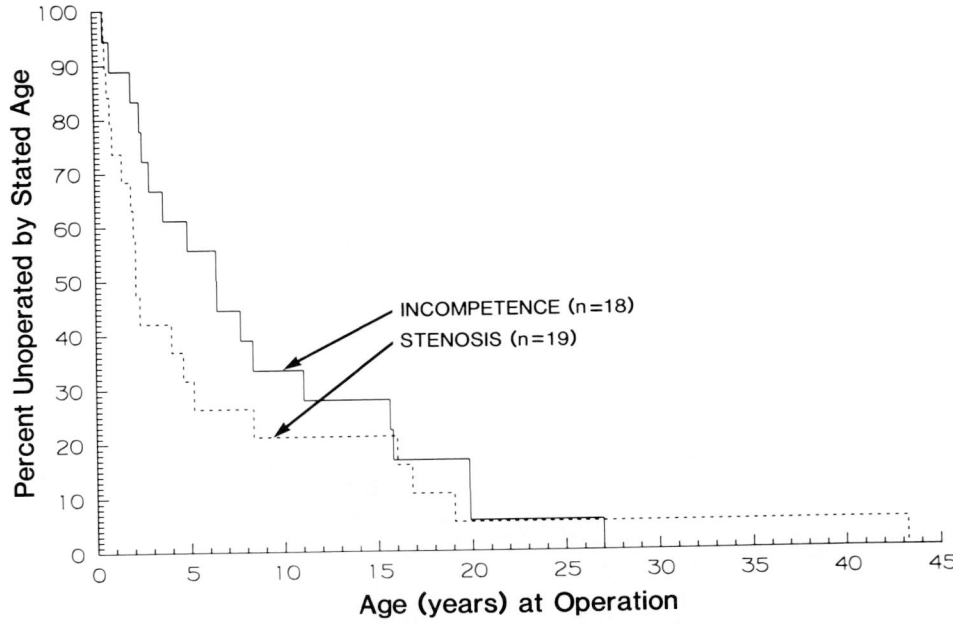

Figure 36-6 Percent of surgical patients with congenital mitral valve disease who have not yet come to operation at any given age (UAB; 1967–1984; *n* = 37). The hypothesis is that to some extent this mirrors natural history.

of the resultant stenosis or incompetence and the type and severity of coexisting lesions.

Congenital mitral valve disease often causes symptoms in very early life, van der Horst and Hastreiter observing the onset of symptoms in the first month of life in one-third of their cases and in the first year in three-fourths of them.[V1] Symptoms are particularly likely to appear early when other cardiac anomalies coexist. With the onset of symptoms, the patient's condition tends to deteriorate rapidly, and one-half die within 6 months. In patients referred for surgery, the presentation is not so early in childhood as in van der Horst and Hastreiter's series (Figs. 36-6 and 36-7). Collins-Nakai and colleagues at the Boston Children's Hospital found the average age of onset of symptoms to be 1.6 years, and presentation and diagnosis was complete by 4.5 years in 50% of their cases.[C5] This corresponds to the finding that 39% of the patients coming to surgery for congenital mitral incompetence and 62% of those coming with mitral stenosis do so by 4 years of age (Fig. 36-6). The still earlier age at which patients with congenital mitral stenosis and left ventricular outflow obstruction come to operation (86% by 4 years) emphasizes the serious nature of this combination (Fig. 36-7).

Symptoms of pulmonary venous hypertension (dyspnea, orthopnea, paroxysmal nocturnal dyspnea, and frank pulmonary edema) and recurrent pulmonary infection tend to dominate in the early years. However, pulmonary vascular disease usually develops in childhood, and symptoms of right ventricular failure then begin to develop.

The patients who fail to develop symptoms in the first year of life usually have no or mild coexisting cardiac anomalies and only mild or moderate functional impairment from the congenital anomalies of the mitral valve. Such individuals may remain relatively well for 10–30 years, but symptoms usually develop and progress at some time.

TECHNIQUE OF OPERATION

Repair of Isolated Congenital Mitral Incompetence

The preparations for operation, the sternotomy incision, cannulation, and establishment of cardiopulmonary bypass (CPB) are the same in the infant and child with isolated congenital mitral incompetence as in adults with mitral incompetence (see Chapter 11). The aorta is cross-clamped, and the cold cardioplegic solution is infused (see Chapter 3). The left atrium is opened from the right side and the exposure obtained as in other operations on the mitral valve.

The mitral valve is now carefully examined, with the possible pathologic bases for congenital mitral incompetence clearly in mind since these determine the type of operation that is most appropriate. A repair based on the pathology is performed whenever possible (see below). After repair, the left atrium is allowed to fill with blood as it is closed. Rewarming of the perfusate and the patient is begun, the apex of the left ventricle is aspirated for air, and with strong suction on the aortic needle vent, the aortic clamp is released. The remainder of the procedure, including the de-airing, is carried out as usual (see Chapter 22).

Annuloplasty
Occasionally annular dilation is the dominant pathology at operation, even in young children, but it is usually associ-

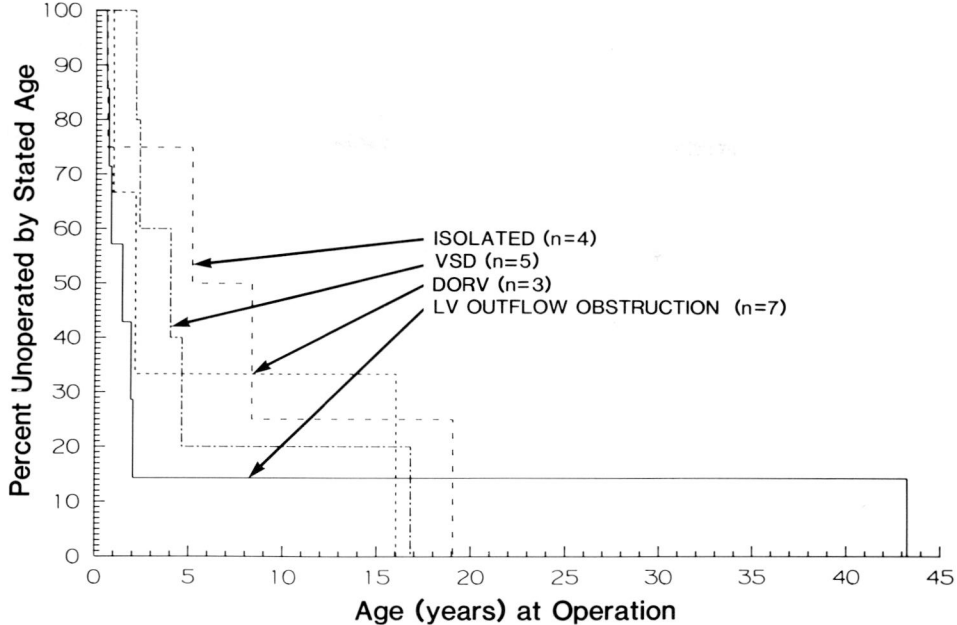

Figure 36-7 Percent of surgical patients with congenital mitral stenosis who have not yet come to operation at any given age (UAB; 1967–1984; *n* = 19).

ated with some abnormal thickening and prolapse of a billowing anterior leaflet.[1,2] If a reasonable anterior leaflet without ruptured chordae is present, annuloplasty is indicated. This is also an appropriate operation when there is marked hypoplasia or near absence of the posterior leaflet, which probably initially was responsible for the incompetence and subsequent annular dilation.

Although the use of the Carpentier ring for mitral annuloplasty is optimal in adults, it is not used in infants and children since with it, growth of the anulus is not possible. Thus, a technique such as the Reed asymmetric measured annuloplasty is chosen (see Chapter 11, Fig. 11-5).

Repair for Ruptured Chordae
When ruptured chordae to less than one-half of the posterior leaflet is the cause of the incompetence, a rectangular excision and leaflet repair, usually combined with annuloplasty, is indicated (see Chapter 11, Fig. 11-4).

Repair of Cleft Mitral Leaflet
When sufficient anterior or posterior mitral leaflet tissue is present on both sides of a cleft of the leaflet, the cleft is sutured closed to achieve competence. A posteromedial (Wooler type) annuloplasty may be helpful.

Repair of Congenital Mitral Stenosis

After placing the patient on CPB, cross-clamping the aorta, infusing the cold cardioplegic solution, and opening the left atrium from the right side, the valve pathology is carefully examined. When the valve leaflets are fused into one and are stenotic, leaflet incisions may be made in the areas in which

commissures would be expected to have developed. At times, fused papillary muscles or chordae may be split or partly excised in an attempt to enlarge the orifice.

Since these maneuvers may result in incompetence of the valve, immediately after discontinuing CPB a regurgitant mitral jet is sought by palpation of the posterior left atrial wall and then the superior left atrial wall beneath the aorta. If a prominent thrill is found and is accompanied by a high left atrial pressure and a suboptimal hemodynamic state, CPB is reestablished and the valve replaced, since otherwise the early and late results are unsatisfactory (see later sections on "Early Results" and "Late Results").

Mitral Valve Replacement

When repair is not possible, mitral valve replacement is performed (see Chapter 11 for the techniques of this procedure). Stent-mounted glutaraldehyde porcine heterografts are not appropriate in infants and children because of their rapid degeneration in the young (see "Late Results," and Chapter 11, "Choice of the Replacement Device" in section on Special Situations and Controversies); however, as an alternative to this, a stent-mounted aortic homograft is used (GLH). The favorable orifice-to-anulus ratio of the St. Jude Medical valve (see Chapter 11, "Choice of the Replacement Device") makes it the mitral valve replacement device of choice in infants and children (UAB).

SPECIAL FEATURES OF POSTOPERATIVE CARE

The usual practices and protocols are used (see Chapter 5).

EARLY RESULTS

Hospital Mortality

The overall hospital mortality after the treatment of congenital mitral stenosis is higher than that after operations for most kinds of congenital heart disease. In an earlier era, prior to 1967, a hospital mortality of 50% or more was frequently reported,[V1] and even since 1967 the mortality has not approached zero.[K2] Thus, 10 (21%; CL 15%–29%) of 48 patients (UAB and GLH combined series) have died after the initial operation for congenital mitral valve disease (Table 36-2). Collins-Nakai and colleagues report 5 hospital deaths (38%, CL 23%–57%) among 13 patients undergoing valvotomy for congenital mitral stenosis at the Boston Children's Hospital. The overall hospital mortality at initial valve operation was 13% (CL 8%–20%) in a group of 47 patients reported by Carpentier and colleagues.[C2]

Mode of Death

Almost all patients die with the sequelae of left atrial hypertension as a direct result of incomplete relief of the mitral valve lesion or of associated obstructive left-sided lesions.

Incremental Risk Factors for Hospital Death

The risk of hospital death does not seem to be influenced by whether the operation has been done for *stenosis or incompetence* (Table 36-2) nor by whether the mitral valve was *repaired or replaced* (Tables 36-3 and 36-4). The frequent coexistence of *major associated cardiac anomalies* probably affects hospital mortality after the operation on the mitral valve for congenital mitral stenosis, but the available information does not document this (Tables 36-5 and 36-6). *Young age* at operation is associated with an increased risk of hospital death (Table 36-7).

An important risk factor has been the *functional state* of the patient at the time of operation (Table 36-8). This is similar to the findings after surgery for other types of congenital heart disease and in the surgical treatment of acquired mitral valve disease (see Chapter 11). It may be this which explains the increased risk of operation in very young patients.

LATE RESULTS

Survival

Ten-year survival has been 63% in patients undergoing an initial repair and 30% in those undergoing valve replacement, the difference between the two being likely due to chance (UAB; Fig. 36-8). Nearly identical figures have been reported from the Boston Children's Hospital.[C5] This rather low intermediate-term survival relates largely to the high early mortality rate.

Functional Status

Most survivors of valve repair or replacement are in NYHA class I or II, in spite of the usual presence of some residual

Table 36-2 Hospital deaths after initial surgical treatment for congenital mitral valve disease with or without associated cardiac anomalies (UAB and GLH; 1967–1984).

	UAB				GLH				Total			
		Hospital Deaths				Hospital Deaths				Hospital Deaths		
Category	n	No.	%	CL	n	No.	%	CL	n	No.	%	CL
Mitral stenosis	19[a]	4	21%	11%–35%	7	2[b]	29%	10%–55%	26	6	23%	14%–35%
Mitral incompetence	18	3	17%	7%–31%	4	1	25%	3%–63%	22	4	18%	9%–31%
Total	37	7	19%	12%–28%	11	3	27%	12%–47%	48	10	21%	15%–29%

KEY: CL, 70% confidence limits.
[a] One patient had only a successful Blalock-Hanlon operation and pulmonary artery banding.
[b] One patient aged 9 months had also severe congenital aortic stenosis and endocardial fibroelastosis of the left ventricle.

Table 36-3 Hospital deaths after the surgical treatment of congenital mitral valve disease with incompetence and no stenosis (UAB and GLH; 1967–1984). Only one patient undergoing valve repair had an associated cardiac anomaly (ASD).

	UAB				GLH				Total			
		Hospital Deaths				Hospital Deaths				Hospital Deaths		
Method of Treatment	n	No.	%	CL	n	No.	%	CL	n	No.	%	CL
Repair	10	1[a]	10%	1%–30%	2	1	50%	7%–93%	12	2	17%	6%–35%
Replacement	8	2[b]	25%	9%–50%	2	0	0%	0%–61%	10	2	20%	7%–41%
Total	18	3	17%	7%–31%	4	1	25%	3%–63%	22	4	18%	9%–31%

KEY: CL, 70% confidence limits.
NOTE: Ages at operation (UAB) ranged from 6 months to 27 years, median 6.4 years; the ages of the GLH patients were 2, 3, 6, and 8 years.
[a] Operation in 1969, preoperative NYHA class IV.
[b] Operations in 1972 and 1974, preoperative NYHA classes V and IV, respectively.

Table 36-4 Hospital deaths after surgical treatment of congenital mitral stenosis (UAB and GLH; 1967–1984).

Method of Treatment	UAB				GLH				Total			
		Hospital Deaths				Hospital Deaths				Hospital Deaths		
	n	No.	%	CL	n	No.	%	CL	n	No.	%	CL
Repair	12	3	25%	11%–44%	6	2	33%	12%–62%	18	5	28%	16%–43%
Replacement	6	1	17%	2%–46%	1	0	0%	0%–85%	7	1	14%	2%–41%
Total	18	4	22%	12%–37%	7	2	29%	10%–55%	25	6	24%	15%–36%

KEY: CL, 70% confidence limits.

Table 36-5 Surgical treatment for congenital mitral valve stenosis (UAB and GLH; 1967–1984).

Morphologic Category	UAB				GLH				Total			
		Hospital Deaths				Hospital Deaths				Hospital Deaths		
	n	No.	%	CL	n	No.	%	CL	n	No.	%	CL
Isolated	4	0	0%	0%–38%	2	0	0%	0%–61%	6[a]	0	0%	0%–27%
Coexisting VSD	5	1	20%	3%–53%	2	0	0%	0%–61%	6[b]	1	17%	2%–46%
Coexisting DORV and VSD	3	0	0%	0%–47%	NI				3	0	0%	0%–47%
Coexisting LV outflow obstruction	7	3	43%	20%–68%	3	2	67%	24%–96%	11[c]	5	45%	27%–65%
Total	19	4	21%	11%–35%	7	2	29%	10%–55%	26	6	23%	14%–35%

KEY: CL, 70% confidence limits; DORV, double outlet right ventricle; LV, left ventricle; NI, not included in the GLH tabulation; VSD, ventricular septal defect.
NOTE: One patient (UAB) included in this table, with coexisting DORV and VSD, had only a Blalock-Hanlon operation and is not included in Table 36-4.
[a] One had associated patent ductus arteriosus (PDA).
[b] Three also had PDA; all had mitral valve repair.
[c] Includes coarctation and valvar and subvalvar aortic stenosis; two patients had also a significant VSD.

stenosis or incompetence.[C2] This good functional status of surviving patients results in part from the practice of advising reoperation for patients in a poor functional status.

Hemodynamic Result

Most but not all patients who have had a reparative operation for congenital mitral stenosis have a lessened diastolic gradient after repair but continue to have a residual gradient up to about 10 mmHg.[C5] Exceptions are the rare case of

Table 36-6 Further details of the surgical treatment for congenital mitral stenosis coexisting with left ventricular outflow obstruction (UAB; 1967–1984).

Details of Coexisting Cardiac Anomalies	Hospital Deaths	
	n	No.
Hypoplasia of aortic arch or coarctation only	3	1
Coarctation plus PDA	1	
Coarctation plus valvar and subvalvar AS	1	0
Coarctation plus PDA plus valvar AS plus VSD	1	1
Valvar AS plus tunnel subvalvar AS	1	1
Total	7	3 (43%, CL 20%–68%)

KEY: AS, aortic stenosis; CL, 70% confidence limits; PDA, patent ductus arteriosus.

isolated supravalvar ring in which a complete relief of the diastolic gradient may be obtained.[C5,M1,N1]

Most patients with either congenital mitral stenosis or incompetence have at least some incompetence after reparative operations. Carpentier and colleagues report that in 22 of the 34 such patients there was an apical systolic murmur late postoperatively, and only 7 of the 34 showed significant decrease in heart size.[C2] Of 12 patients recatheterized 7 had moderate or severe mitral regurgitation. Flege and colleagues reported a virtually complete repair in only 4 of 13 patients with congenital mitral incompetence.[F3] One of 4 patients treated for mitral stenosis (GLH; 2 with a supravalvar ring and 2 with valvar stenosis) had severe mitral regurgitation after repair, requiring valve replacement 1 month later.

The hemodynamic state after *replacement* of a congenitally abnormal mitral valve depends on the type and size of the replacement device used (see Chapter 11). In general, the hemodynamic state and valve function are satisfactory unless a device complication develops.

Reoperation

Among patients undergoing *repair* of congenital mitral valve disease, 79% are free of reoperation on the valve up to 10 years postoperatively (Fig. 36-9). This indicates that function at the repaired valve is reasonably good, although most patients have some residual stenosis or incompetence (see above).

Table 36-7   Hospital mortality after operations for congenital mitral valve disease, according to whether there was stenosis or incompetence at the valve and to the age of the patient (UAB and GLH; 1967–1984).

Age	Incompetence (n = 22)				Stenosis (n = 26)			
		Hospital Deaths				Hospital Deaths		
≤ <	n	No.	%	CL	n	No.	%	CL
Months								
6	0				2	1	50%	7%–93%
6---12	2	1	50%	7%–93%	7	3	43%	20%–68%
12---24	1	0	0%	0%–85%	3	0	0%	0%–47%
24---48	6	1	17%	2%–46%	6	2	33%	12%–62%
Years								
4---10	7	2	29%	10%–55%	4	0	0%	0%–38%
10---20	5	0	0%	0%–32%	3	0	0%	0%–47%
20	1	0	0%	0%–85%	1	0	0%	0%–85%
Total	22	4	18%	9%–31%	26	6	23%	14%–35%

KEY: CL, 70% confidence limits.

NOTE: P (logistic) for the effect of age when n = 22 and n = 26 are combined is .03.

Table 36-8   Hospital deaths after operation for congenital mitral valve disease, according to preoperative functional class (UAB and GLH; 1967–1984).

NYHA Functional Class	UAB				GLH				Total			
		Hospital Deaths				Hospital Deaths				Hospital Deaths		
	n	No.	%	CL	n	No.	%	CL	n	No.	%	CL
I	7		0%	0%–24%	0				7	0	0%	0%–24%
II	12	1	8%	1%–26%	1	0	0%	0%–85%	13	1	8%	1%–24%
III	7	1	14%	2%–41%	0				7	1	14%	2%–41%
IV	10	4	40%	22%–61%	8	2	25%	9%–50%	18	6	33%	21%–48%
V	1	1	100%	15%–100%	2	1	50%	7%–93%	3	2	67%	24%–96%
Total	37	7	19%	12%–28%	11	3	27%	12%–47%	48	10	21%	15%–29%
P (logistic)												.01

KEY: CL, 70% confidence limits; NYHA, New York Heart Association.

NOTE: NYHA class V indicates emergency operation for shock or metabolic acidoses.

Among patients undergoing mitral valve *replacement* for congenital mitral valve disease, reoperations are frequent and early when a porcine heterograft has been used (Figs. 36-9 and 36-10). This is in accord with the known inverse relationship between the age of the patient and the rate of degeneration of this bioprosthesis[A1,B3,G2,K1,S4,T1] (see Chapter 11, Fig. 11-29). The one surviving patient with a stented aortic homograft valve remains well without signs of mitral valve dysfunction 11 years postoperatively (GLH; operation at age 2 years).

When a prosthetic valve has been used initially, reoperation has been required mainly for outgrowth of the device and has always allowed the insertion of a larger valve. In one patient with a 17-mm Bjork-Shiley valve inserted at 7 months of age, a fibrous pannus obstructed the atrial side of the device 12 months postoperatively and again 24 months postoperatively, when it caused death (GLH). Prosthetic valves in children have resulted in no higher incidence of thromboembolism and complications from anticoagulation with coumadin than in adults.[A1,G1]

INDICATIONS FOR OPERATION

Severe symptoms and signs of important pulmonary venous hypertension are an indication for prompt operation in infants with congenital mitral valve anomalies in view of the natural history of this disease. A reparative operation is indicated if at all feasible. These same indications prevail in children and young adults. When symptoms are mild or even moderate, operation is delayed in the hope that when it becomes necessary and if valve replacement is required, an adult-sized device can be used. Operation is indicated, even in the absence of marked symptoms, when pulmonary hypertension is severe, in which situation there may be right-to-left shunting across a patent ductus arteriosus or a foramen ovale.

When a reparative operation is performed, long-term follow-up is indicated because of the need in some patients for reoperation. When valve replacement is performed in infants, children, and young adults, a porcine bioprosthesis is contraindicated because of its rapid degeneration in this age

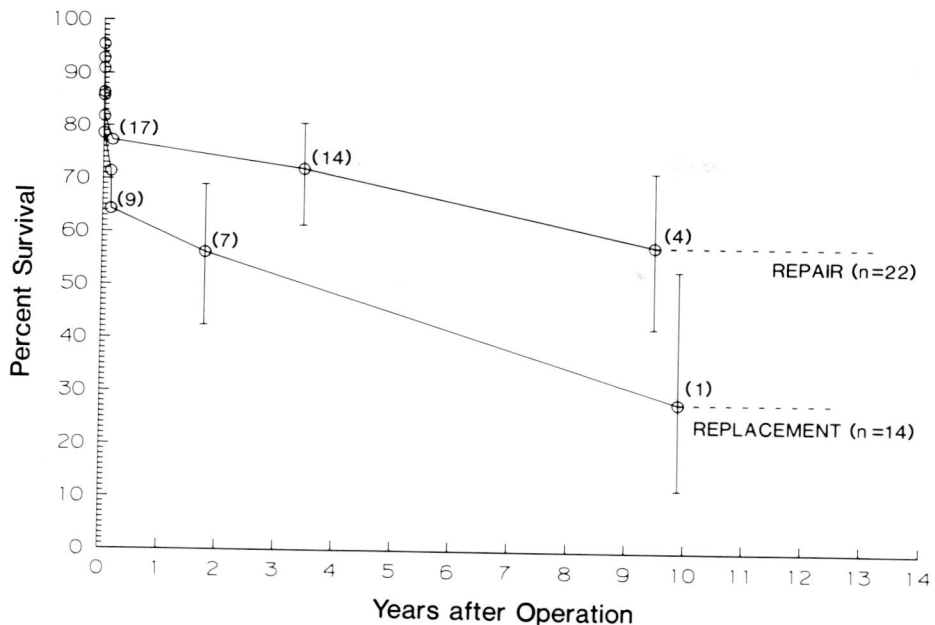

Figure 36-8 Actuarial survival after initial valve repair or replacement for congenital mitral valve disease (UAB; 1967–1984; $n = 36$). All patients are traced, with a median follow-up among survivors of 71 months (5.9 years). Seventy-five percent are followed 43 or more months and 25% 98 or more months. Patients were not censored at reoperation. Each circle represents a death. The numbers of patients traced to a time period are indicated in parentheses. The vertical bars indicate 70% confidence limits (1 SD).

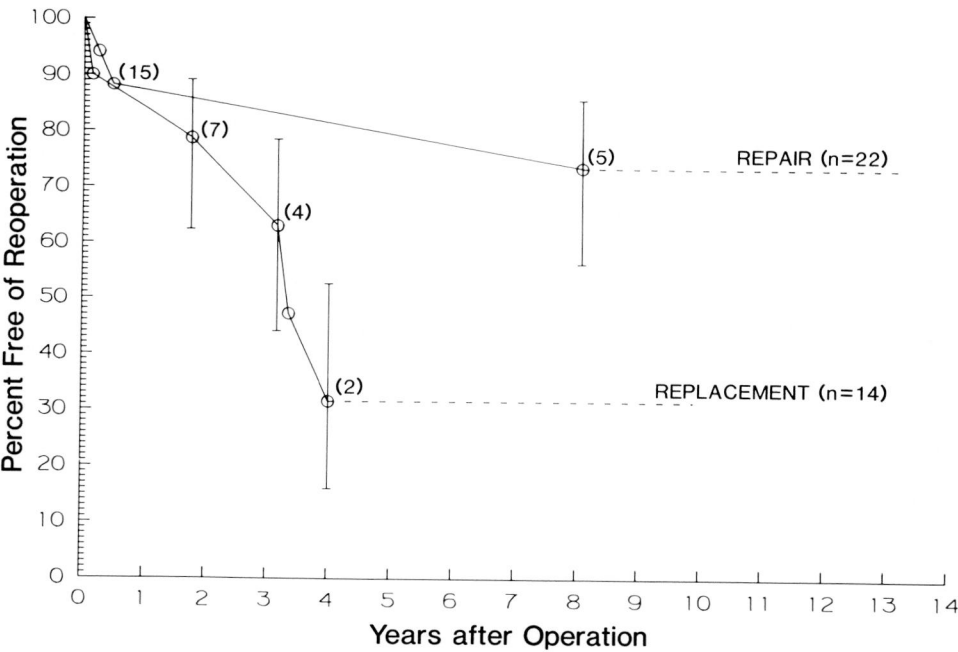

Figure 36-9 Actuarial freedom from reoperation after an initial valve operation for congenital mitral valve disease (UAB; details are as in Fig. 36-8). Patients were censored at death.

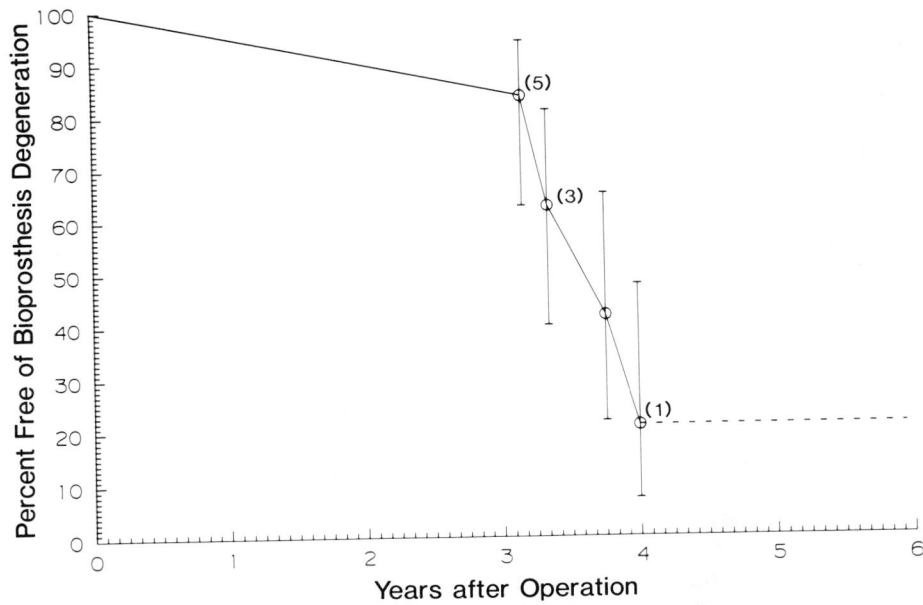

Figure 36-10   Actuarial incidence of important degeneration (causing reoperation or death) of porcine heterograft bioprosthesis placed at initial operation or reoperation for congenital mitral valve disease (UAB; 1967–1984; *n* = 18). Presentation is as in Figure 36-8.

group (Fig. 36-10). A stented aortic homograft valve may be preferred in infants and children because of its large orifice and despite the fact that there is risk of late buttress detachment from the stent and leaflet rupture (GLH; see Chapter 11). However, a St. Jude medical prosthesis is currently the device of choice (UAB), with long-term anticoagulation with warfarin.

It is important to identify coexisting congenital mitral valve disease in patients being considered for surgical repair of left ventricular outflow obstruction, ventricular septal defect, tetralogy of Fallot, or double outlet right ventricle. When present and moderate or severe, the mitral disease must also be treated surgically.

SPECIAL SITUATIONS AND CONTROVERSIES

Use of St. Jude Valve without Anticoagulation

Pass, Sade, and colleagues have reported no thromboembolic episodes in 12 infants and children followed 1–50 months in whom the mitral valve has been replaced with a St. Jude valve and warfarin not given.[P1] Although this is an attractive protocol, it requires confirmation before being generally adopted.

Other Reparative Operations

Procedures have been described for the repair of congenital mitral valve anomalies that are not currently used because of lack of evidence as to their efficacy (UAB, GLH). A *sliding plasty* has been used by Carpentier and colleagues to correct congenital elongation of chordae to part of a papillary muscle.[C2] The papillary muscle is incised longitudinally and reconstructed by suturing the halves together asymmetrically, with the part attached to the elongated chordae fixed at a lower level. Elongation of all chordae to a papillary muscle may be treated by *chordal shortening*.[C2] The extremity of the papillary muscle is incised longitudinally, and the redundant chordae are buried in the trench so created and the papillary muscle closed firmly around them by sutures.

When the mitral anulus is very small, a *valved conduit* (similar to that used for right ventricular–pulmonary artery reconstruction) may be placed between left atrium and left ventricle. Laks and colleagues reported such a procedure, which was unsuccessful in 1980,[L3] and Lansing and colleagues reported a successful case in a 10-year-old girl in 1983.[L4] Late results are not available.

REFERENCES

A

1. Attie F, Kuri J, Zononiani C, Renteria V, Buendia A, Ovseyevitz J, Lopez-Soriano F, Garcia-Cornejo M, Martinez-Rios MA: Mitral valve replacement in children with rheumatic heart disease. *Circulation* 64:812, 1981.

2. Anabtawi IN, Ellison RG: Congenital stenosing ring of the left atrioventricular canal (supravalvular mitral stenosis). *J Thorac Cardiovasc Surg* 49:994, 1965.

B

1. Berghuis J, Kirklin JW, Edwards JE, Titus JL: The surgical anatomy of isolated congenital mitral insufficiency. *J Thorac Cardiovasc Surg* 47:791, 1964.

2. Benrey J, Leachman RD, Cooley DA, Klima T, Lufschanowski R: Supravalvular mitral stenosis associated with tetralogy of Fallot. *Am J Cardiol* 37:111, 1976.

3. Barros MM, Sato YMC: Alteracoes morfologicas de duramater empregada em proteses valvulares. Consideracoes etiopatologicas. *Arq Bras Cardiol* 33(suppl I):I-314, 1979.

4. Billig DM, Kreidberg MB, Chernoff HL, Khan MAA: Mitral stenosis and insufficiency with subaortic and subpulmonic stenosis. *J Thorac Cardiovasc Surg* 61:121, 1971.

C

1. Creech O, Ledbetter MK, Reemtsma K: Congenital insufficiency with a cleft in the posterior leaflet. *Circulation* 25:390, 1962.

2. Carpentier A, Branchini B, Cour JC, Asfaou E, Villani M, Deloche A, Relland J, D'Allaines C, Blondeau P, Piwnica A, Parenzan L, Brom G: Congenital malformations of the mitral valve in children. Pathology and surgical treatment. *J Thorac Cardiovasc Surg* 72:854, 1976.

3. Castaneda AR, Anderson RC, Edwards JE: Congenital mitral stenosis resulting from anomalous arcade and obstructing papillary muscles. Report of correction by use of ball valve prosthesis. *Am J Cardiol* 24:237, 1969.

4. Carney EK, Braunwald E, Rogerts WC, Aygen M, Morrow AG: Congenital mitral regurgitation. *Am J Med* 33:223, 1962.

5. Collins-Nakai RL, Rosenthal A, Castaneda AR, Bernhard WF, Nadas AS: Congenital mitral stenosis. A review of 20 years' experience. *Circulation* 56:1039, 1977.

D

1. Davichi F, Moller JH, Edwards JE: Diseases of the mitral valve in infancy. *Circulation* 43:565, 1971.

2. Daoud G, Kaplan S, Perrin EV, Dorst JP, Edwards FK: Congenital mitral stenosis. *Circulation* 27:185, 1963.

3. Di Segni E, Edwards JE: Cleft anterior leaflet of the mitral valve with intact septa. A study of twenty cases. *Am J Cardiol* 51:915, 1983.

4. Di Segni E, Bass JL, Lucas RV Jr., Einzig S: Isolated cleft mitral valve: A variety of congenital mitral regurgitation identified by 2-dimensional echocardiography. *Am J Cardiol* 51:927, 1983.

E

1. Edwards JS: In *An Atlas of Congenital Anomalies of the Heart and Great Vessels*. Springfield, Ill: Charles C Thomas, 1954, p 41.

F

1. Fisher T: Two cases of congenital disease of the left side of the heart. *Br Med J* 1:639, 1902.

2. Freed MD, Keane JF, Van Praagh R, Castaneda AR, Bernhard WF, Nadas AS: Coarctation of the aorta with congenital mitral regurgitation. *Circulation* 49:1175, 1974.

3. Flege JB, Vlad P, Ehrenhaft JL: Congenital mitral incompetence. *J Thorac Cardiovasc Surg* 53:138, 1967.

G

1. Gardner TJ, Roland JM, Neill CA, Donahoo JS: Valve replacement in children. A fifteen-year perspective. *J Thorac Cardiovasc Surg* 83:178, 1982.

2. Geha AS, Laks H, Stansel HC, Cornhill JF, Kilman JW, Buckley MJ, Roberts WC: Late failure of porcine valve heterografts in children. *J Thorac Cardiovasc Surg* 78:351, 1979.

3. Grenadier E, Sahn DJ, Valdes-Cruz LM, Allen HD, Lima CO, Goldbert SJ: Two-dimensional echo Doppler study of congenital disorders of the mitral valve. *Am Heart J* 107:319, 1984.

4. Glancy DL, Chang MY, Dorney ER, Roberts WC: Parachute mitral valve. Further observations and associated lesions. *Am J Cardiol* 27:309, 1971.

K

1. Kutsche L, Oyer PE, Shumway NE, Baum D: An important complication of Hancock mitral valve replacement in children. Cardiovascular Surgery. *Circulation* 60(suppl I):I-98, 1979.

2. Khalil KG, Shapiro I, Kilman JW: Congenital mitral stenosis. *J Thorac Cardiovasc Surg* 70:40, 1975.

L

1. Layman TE, Edwards JE: Anomalous mitral arcade. A type of congenital mitral insufficiency. *Circulation* 35:389, 1967.

2. Levy MJ, Varco RL, Lillehei CW, Edwards JE: Mitral insufficiency in infants, children, and adolescents. *J Thorac Cardiovasc Surg* 45:434, 1963.

3. Laks H, Hellenbrand WE, Kleinman C, Talner NS: Left atrial-left ventricular conduit for relief of congenital mitral stenosis in infancy. *J Thorac Cardiovasc Surg* 80:782, 1980.

4. Lansing AM, Elbl F, Solinger RE, Rees AH: Left atrial-left ventricular bypass for congenital mitral stenosis. *Ann Thorac Surg* 35:667, 1983.

M

1. Macartney FJ, Scott O, Ionescu MI, Deverall PB: Diagnosis and management of parachute mitral valve and supravalvar mitral ring. *Br Heart J* 36:641, 1974.

N

1. Neirotti R, Kreutzer G, Galindez E, Becu L, Ross D: Supravalvular mitral stenosis associated with ventricular septal defect. *Am J Dis Child* 131:862, 1977.

P

1. Pass HI, Sade RM, Crawford FA, Hohn AR: Cardiac valve prostheses in children without anticoagulation. *J Thorac Cardiovasc Surg* 87:832, 1984.

R

1. Rosenquist GC: Congenital mitral valve disease associated with coarctation of the aorta. A spectrum that includes parachute deformity of the mitral valve. *Circulation* 49:985, 1974.

2. Ruckman RN, Van Praagh R: Anatomic types of congenital mitral stenosis: Report of 49 autopsy cases with consideration of diagnosis and surgical implications. *Am J Cardiol* 42:592, 1978.

S

1. Shone JD, Sellers RD, Anderson RC, Adams P Jr, Lillehei CW, Edwards JE: The developmental complex of "parachute mitral valve," supravalvular ring of left atrium, suboaortic stenosis, and coarctation of aorta. *Am J Cardiol* 11:714, 1963.

2. Schraft WC, Lisa JR: Duplication of the mitral valve: Case report and a review of the literature. *Am Heart J* 39:136, 1950.

3. Schiebler GL, Edwards JE, Burchell HB, DuShane JW, Ongley PA and Wood EH: Congenital corrected transposition of the great vessels. A study of 33 cases. *Pediatrics* (suppl)27:851, 1961.

4. Silver MM, Pollock J, Silver MD, Williams WG, Trusler GA; Calcification in porcine xenograft valves in children. *Am J Cardiol* 45:685, 1980.

5. Starkey GWB: Surgical experiences in the treatment of congenital mitral stenosis and mitral insufficiency. *J Thorac Surg* 38:336, 1959.

6. Smallhorn J, Tommasini G, Deanfield J, Douglas J, Gibson D, Macartney F: Congenital mitral stenosis. Anatomical and functional assessment by echocardiography. *Br Heart J* 45:527, 1981.

T

1. Thandroyen FT, Whitton IN, Pirie D, Rogers MA, Mitha AS: Severe calcification of glutaraldehyde-preserved porcine xenografts in children. *Am J Cardiol* 45:690, 1980.

V

1. van der Horst RL, Hastreiter AR: Congenital mitral stenosis. *Am J Cardiol* 20:773, 1967.

37

CONGENITAL PULMONARY VEIN STENOSIS

DEFINITION

Congenital pulmonary vein stenosis is an important morphologic and functional narrowing of the junctional area between the pulmonary veins and left atrium.

HISTORICAL NOTE

In 1951, Reye reported severe stenosis of three pulmonary veins and obliteration of the orifice of the fourth in an 8-year-old girl who died from these findings,[R1] and Edwards and Burchell at the Mayo Clinic described what is probably a similar case in the same year.[E3] In the subsequent 10 years, a few other groups reported similar cases.[B3,E1,E2,L1,S1,S2] Successful surgical treatment, with a 2-year follow-up, has been reported by Kawashima and colleagues.[K1]

MORPHOLOGY

The basic pathologic process of this poorly understood condition seems to be a nonspecific fibrous intimal thickening, which may progress to a complete obliteration of the lumen between one or more of the four pulmonary veins and the left atrium.[E1] The morphologic abnormality may be localized to the pulmonary vein ostium[M1] or may involve the adjacent extrapulmonary venous segment in a tubular fashion.[B1,C2] In addition to the morphologic narrowing, there may be a functional narrowing of the ostium and adjacent vein, which is very apparent cineangiographically and manometrically but is not apparent on inspection during surgery.

The lesion is usually not evident at birth but may appear after a few weeks or months of life. Usually all four pulmonary veins are involved, and progression in the severity of the stenosis is the rule.

As a result of this lesion, pulmonary vascular disease rapidly develops.[C1,N1,S3] Even though pulmonary vein stenosis involves only three of the four pulmonary veins, the pulmonary vascular disease can be found in all four lobes[G1] and may be so severe that the pulmonary capillary wedge pressure is normal. Numerous thrombi may be found in the pulmonary arteries.[B4] Ultimately, interstitial fibrosis of the lung can develop.[A1]

Congenital pulmonary vein stenosis is often an isolated lesion, but it may coexist with total anomalous pulmonary venous connection,[W1] complete transposition of the great arteries, anomalous origin of the right pulmonary artery, patent ductus arteriosus, ventricular septal defect, and no doubt other anomalies.

CLINICAL FEATURES AND DIAGNOSTIC CRITERIA

The presenting symptoms in patients with pulmonary vein stenosis usually develop in infancy, infrequently in the first month of life, and infrequently in childhood. They consist of failure to thrive and respiratory distress. There may be recurrent hemoptysis. When such symptoms persist and then worsen, the diagnosis of pulmonary venous hypertension is usually suspected and confirmed by chest x-ray. Then pulmonary venous stenosis must be differentiated from other causes of pulmonary venous hypertension such as congenital mitral stenosis, cor triatriatum, and total anomalous pulmonary venous connection.

The presence of congenital pulmonary vein stenosis may not be suspected in infants presenting with coexisting defects such as large ventricular septal defect, patent ductus arteriosus, or anomalous origin of a pulmonary artery from the ascending aorta. The clue in such patients may then be the very slow passage of dye through the pulmonary arteries in a pulmonary angiogram.

Two-dimensional echocardiography may visualize the pulmonary vein stenoses directly.[B1]

Cardiac catheterization and cineangiography are diagnostic. If precise details of the pulmonary vein–left atrial junction are not obtained, selective injections in the right and left pulmonary artery branches or pulmonary artery wedge injections can usually provide diagnostic data.[B2] It usually is not possible to pass even a small catheter retrograde across the stenosis. If, however, a small catheter can be passed, the finding of a pressure gradient between pulmonary vein and left atrium is diagnostic.

NATURAL HISTORY

Symptoms are rarely present in the first month of life and more commonly appear in the first year. This makes it likely that the condition of congenital pulmonary vein stenosis is either not present at birth or is mild and that it either develops or rapidly worsens after birth. An early onset of severe symptoms suggests that all four pulmonary veins are involved. In these circumstances, severe and usually suprasystemic pulmonary artery hypertension quickly develops. Once symptoms appear, they usually rapidly worsen and death occurs within 3–12 months.

Occasionally, symptoms do not develop until later in the first decade of life[E1] or even early in the second decade.[K1] Such patients usually have fewer than four veins involved. It is noteworthy that involvement of the pulmonary veins on just one side can result in severe and bilateral pulmonary hypertension. Progression to death is usually the rule, even in these initially less severe cases.

TECHNIQUE OF OPERATION

No surgical procedure has been demonstrated as yet to be of long-term benefit for patients with congenital pulmonary vein stenosis. The operation described here has been used and appears to be the one most likely to provide an adequate repair (GLH,UAB).

The preliminaries to the operation are as described in Chapter 2, with the use of cardiopulmonary bypass and cardioplegia or profound hypothermia and total circulatory arrest. When other lesions (ventricular septal defect, total anomalous pulmonary venous connection, transposition of the great arteries) require correction, the sequencing of the procedure for correction of the vein stenosis and of the associated anomaly requires individual planning.

The right upper and middle lobe, right lower lobe, left upper lobe, and left lower lobe veins are individually dissected outside the atrium to define the length of the stenosis and to locate the point at which each of the four veins returns to normal diameter and wall consistency. The left atrium is now entered from the right side for complete inspection of the ostia of all four veins. When the stenosis is localized to the ostium and is due to localized intimal thickening, this material is completely excised working from within. This is the only maneuver possible for the stenosed left lower lobe vein, but it should form a part of the operation for each of the

other ostia if there is material suitable for excision and this can be done without breaching the vein wall.

After now opening the right atrium, the atrial septum is opened with a small incision between the superior limbus and the fossa ovalis, and the tissue of the fossa ovalis then detached from the atrial wall laterally with a vertical extension of the original incision. The posterior portion of the limbus in front of the right pulmonary veins requires excision. A longitudinal incision is made in the anterior wall of the right upper venous trunk where it has returned to normal diameter (usually within 5 mm of its ostium) and carried across the stenosis into the adjacent right atrial wall with the intention of performing a V–Y atrioplasty to enlarge the anterior wall of the stenotic portion of vein. The vertical limb of the Y is that portion of the incision in the vein itself, whereas the two limbs of the Y comprise a V incision that encloses a portion of right atrial wall immediately in front of the stenotic ostium. The angle of the V is made as obtuse as possible. The V of atrial wall is now advanced laterally into the pulmonary vein to create a new and wide anterior wall, suturing it accurately with continuous 5-0 or 6-0 polypropylene. Should the flap of right atrial wall be too thick at the site of the crista terminalis, the excess tissue is removed from the endocardial surface with scissors before suturing commences. The size of the new ostium should be confirmed as adequate with Hegar dilators (8–10 mm diameter is ideal).

The right lower pulmonary vein lies more posteriorly as well as inferiorly and is more difficult to correct. However, relief may be practicable by advancing the detached atrial septum as a V flap into a longitudinal incision in the anterior vein wall that crosses the stenosis and extends onto the adjacent left atrial wall. The tissue of the fossa ovalis, previously detached as described, is used for the repair, leaving it intact inferiorly so that it remains viable. If this type of procedure seems practicable, it is performed as the first step before the V–Y atrioplasty to the right upper vein.

The procedure is completed by closing the interatrial communication with a pericardial patch so that both pulmonary veins continue to drain correctly into the left atrium. The pericardial suture line must pass well in front of the enlarged right upper lobe venous ostium.

Repair of the left upper pulmonary vein is accomplished from outside the atrium. The heart is retracted inferiorly and to the right to expose the left upper lobe vein, which is dissected beyond its point of narrowing. The vein passes almost vertically and lies adjacent to the left atrial appendage base. A vertical incision is made in the superior wall of the vein *distal* to the stenosis, leaving the stenosis undisturbed. A similar length opening is made in the adjacent wall of the left atrial appendage, excising an ellipse of tissue to create an elliptical opening. The two incisions are anastomosed together with continuous 5-0 polypropylene with knots at the angles to prevent purse-stringing.

Alternatively, if a left superior vena cava of adequate size (which drains to the coronary sinus) is present, the side-to-side anastomosis can be conveniently made between it and the left upper lobe vein. The left superior vena cava is then ligated distal to the anastomosis and the coronary sinus ostium directed into the left atrium by creating a coronary sinus–left atrial window and closing the coronary sinus ostium by direct suture, taking care to avoid the atrioventricular nodal tissue. (See the description of repair of total anomalous pulmonary venous connection to the coronary sinus in Chapter 16.)

The operation is completed in the usual fashion.

SPECIAL FEATURES OF POSTOPERATIVE CARE

The usual postcardiac surgery care is appropriate (see Chapter 5). At operation, a polyvinyl catheter is brought from the pulmonary artery out the right ventricle; with this, pulmonary artery pressure is monitored for at least 24 hours postoperatively. Persistent severe pulmonary artery hypertension strongly suggests that the pulmonary vein stenosis has not been completely relieved.

EARLY RESULTS

Three (33%, CL 15%–56%) of nine patients undergoing surgical treatment (UAB, 1967–1984) died in the hospital; death was from pulmonary edema in all UAB cases. Among four patients operated upon (GLH, 1967–1984), one died in the hospital, and two died within 1 year after operation.

Most reports of success in the literature are of individual cases.[B3,K1]

LATE RESULTS

Five of six hospital survivors died within 6 months of operation (UAB), and autopsy showed recurrence of pulmonary venous stenosis in each case; one case (GLH) is clinically well 12 months postoperatively and one case (UAB) is progressing well 6 months after operation. Thus, the combined early and intermediate mortality to date is 11 deaths (85%, CL 67%–95%) among 13 patients in whom operation was done (UAB, GLH). Many of the operations were done by techniques now known to be ineffective, and with the techniques described, results may improve. Kawashima and colleagues report a 2-year good result in a 15-year-old boy with three pulmonary veins involved in whom the localized intimal hyperplasia was excised at operation.[K1]

Even when early postoperative study has shown improvement in the stenosis, early recurrence of the stenosis and death have occurred.[P1]

Transvenous balloon dilation has also only afforded temporary relief.[D1]

INDICATIONS FOR OPERATION

The diagnosis of the condition is an indication for an attempt at surgical correction, and in view of the uniformly fatal natural history even a suspicion of the presence of congenital pulmonary vein stenosis should lead to an intensive effort to prove or disprove its presence.

Optimal surgical techniques remain to be defined.

REFERENCES

A

1. Andrews EC Jr: Five cases of an undescribed form of pulmonary interstitial fibrosis caused by obstruction of the pulmonary veins. *Bull Johns Hopkins* 100:28, 1975.

B

1. Bini RM, Cleveland D, Ceballos R, Bargeron LM Jr, Pacifico AD, Kirklin JW: Congenital pulmonary venous stenosis. *Am J Cardiol* 54:369, 1984.

2. Bini RM, Bargeron LM Jr: Visualization of pulmonary vein obstruction by pulmonary artery wedge injection. *Pediatr Cardiol* 2:161, 1982.

3. Binet JP, Bouchard F, Langlois J, Chetochine F, Conso JF, Pottemain M: Unilateral congenital stenosis of the pulmonary veins. A very rare cause of pulmonary hypertension. *J Thorac Cardiovasc Surg* 63:397, 1972.

4. Bernstein J, Nolke AC, Reed JO: Extrapulmonic stenosis of the pulmonary veins. *Circulation* 19:891, 1959.

C

1. Contis G, Fung RH, Vawter GF, Nadas AS: Stenosis and obstruction of the pulmonary veins associated with pulmonary artery hypertension. *Am J Cardiol* 20:718, 1967.

2. Cabrera A, Nazquez C, Lekuona I: Isolated atresia of the left pulmonary veins. *Int J Cardiol* 7:298, 1985.

D

1. Driscoll DJ, Hesslein PS, Mullins CE: Congenital stenosis of individual pulmonary veins: Clinical spectrum and unsuccessful treatment by transvenous balloon dilation. *Am J Cardiol* 49:1767, 1982.

E

1. Emslie-Smith D, Hill IGW, Lowe KG: Unilateral membranous pulmonary venous occlusion, pulmonary hypertension, and patent ductus arteriosus. *Br Heart J* 17:79, 1955.

2. Edwards J: Congenital stenosis of pulmonary veins. *Lab Invest* 9:46–66, 1960.

3. Edwards JE, Burchell HB: Multilobar pulmonary venous obstruction with pulmonary hypertension. *Arch Intern Med* 87:372, 1951.

G

1. Geggel RL, Fried R, Tuuri DT, Gyler DC, Reid LM: Congenital pulmonary vein stenosis: Structural changes in a patient with normal pulmonary artery wedge pressure. *JACC* 3:193, 1984.

K

1. Kawashima Y, Ueda T, Naito Y, Morikawa E, Manabe H: Stenosis of pulmonary veins. *Ann Thorac Surg* 12:196, 1971.

L

1. Lucas R, Anderson R, Amplatz K, Adams P, Edwards J: Congenital causes of pulmonary venous obstruction. *Pediatr Clin North Am* 10:781, 1963.

M

1. Mortensson W, Lundstrum N: Congenital obstruction of the pulmonary veins at their atrial junction. *Am Heart J* 87:359, 1974.

N

1. Nasrallah AT, Mullins CE, Singer D, Harrison G, McNamara DG: Unilateral pulmonary vein atresia: Diagnosis and treatment. *Am J Cardiol* 36:969, 1975.

P

1. Park SC, Neches WH, Lenox CC, Zuberbuhler JR, Siewers RD, Bahnson HT: Diagnosis and surgical treatment of bilateral pulmonary vein stenosis. *J Thorac Cardiovasc Surg* 67:755, 1974.

R

1. Reye RDK: Congenital stenosis of the pulmonary veins in their extrapulmonary course. *Med J Aust* 1:801, 1951.

S

1. Sherman F, Stengel W, Bauersfeld S: Congenital stenosis of pulmonary veins at their atrial junctions. *Am Heart J* 56:908, 1958.

2. Shone J, Amplatz K, Anderson R, Adams P, Edwards J: Congenital stenosis of individual pulmonary veins. *Circulation* 26:574, 1962.

3. Sade RM, Freed MD, Matthews EC, Castaneda AR: Stenosis of individual pulmonary veins. *J Thorac Cardiovasc Surg* 67:953, 1974.

W

1. Whight CM, Barratt-Boyes BG, Calder AL, Neutze JM, Brandt PWT: Total anomalous pulmonary venous connection. Long-term results following repair in infancy. *J Thorac Cardiovasc Surg* 75:52, 1978.

38

VASCULAR RINGS AND SLINGS

SECTION 1

AORTIC ARCH ANOMALIES (VASCULAR RINGS)

DEFINITION

Vascular rings are anomalies of the great arteries (aortic arch and its branches) that compress the trachea and/or esophagus.

HISTORICAL NOTE

The condition of double aortic arch was apparently first described by Hommel in 1737 (cited by Turner[T1]) and a century later by Von Siebold.[V1] Wolman is credited with describing the syndrome of tracheal and esophageal compression produced by a double arch in 1939.[W6] A description of a patient with dysphagia thought to be due to an aberrant right subclavian artery was published in 1794 by Bayford,[B1] although the vessel is illustrated to pass between the esophagus and trachea rather than in its actual position posterior to the trachea.[B7]

The first surgical correction of a double aortic arch was performed by Gross in 1945,[G5] and this was the stimulus for the modern interest in these anomalies. Subsequently, he pioneered the surgical treatment of most of the other forms of vascular rings.[G3,G6,G7] The basis for the radiologic diagnosis of these anomalies was initially described by Neuhauser.[N2]

The complex development of the human aortic arches in the embryo had been placed on a secure basis by the observations of Congdon in 1922,[C2] but until Gross's pioneering surgical work, this information had been little used by clinicians. Edwards in 1948 introduced the hypothetical double aortic arch scheme to conceptualize the numerous anomalies of the arch complex,[E3] and this was further elaborated by us in 1950[K2] and by Stewart, Kincaid, and Edwards in 1967.[S2] Meantime, Barry in 1951 had provided a clear summary and review of Congdon's basic work.[B5]

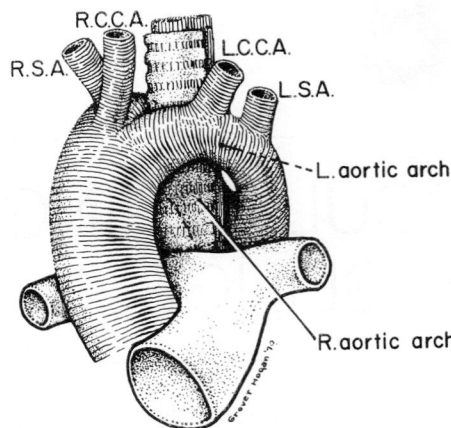

Figure 38-1   Drawing of a complete double aortic arch taken from a frontal angiocardiogram. The descending aorta is on the left.
LCCA, left common carotid artery; LSA, left subclavian artery; RCCA, right common carotid artery; RSA, right subclavian artery.
Reproduced with permission from Shuford and Sybers.[S5]

MORPHOLOGY

Variations in the arrangement of the ascending, transverse, and descending aorta and its branches are numerous. Several categories of these variations may produce compression of the trachea or esophagus or both and are of surgical significance.

Double Aortic Arch

In patients with double aortic arch, the ascending aorta arises normally but as it leaves the pericardium divides into two branches, a left and a right aortic arch that join posteriorly to form the descending aorta. The left arch passes anteriorly and to the left of the trachea in the usual position and is joined where it becomes the descending aorta by the ductus arteriosus (or more usually a ligamentum arteriosum). The right aortic arch passes to the right and then posterior to the esophagus to join the left-sided descending aorta, thus completing the vascular ring (Fig. 38-1).[E1] Occasionally the descending aorta is right sided, in which case the left arch (or its remnant) passes behind the esophagus. This was the case in 13 of the 19 cases reported by Lincoln and colleagues.[L2] Alternatively, the descending aorta may be essentially a midline structure.

The right arch gives origin to two arch vessels, the right common carotid and the right subclavian, whereas the left arch gives origin to the left common carotid and left subclavian arteries in that order. The left arch is often narrower than the right, either throughout its course or in its distal part, usually beyond the origin of the left subclavian artery (Fig. 38-2). This portion may remain patent or be represented by a fibrous chord that joins the descending aorta, often at the site of a diverticulum.[S3] This fibrous chord, at its origin from the base of the left subclavian artery, lies close to the ligamentum arteriosum. The latter structure passes from this point to the adjacent proximal part of the left pulmonary artery (Fig. 38-3). Uncommonly, the right arch may be smaller in its distal part (Fig. 38-4) but is rarely atretic.

Associated cardiovascular anomalies are not common but include tetralogy of Fallot and transposition of the great arteries.[H2,S2]

Right Aortic Arch

Without Retroesophageal Component
In the common situation of a right aortic arch without a retroesophageal segment, there is no vascular ring. The arch branches arise in mirror image of the normal (Fig. 38-5). This arrangement of the aortic arch branches is the result of interruption of the embryonic left arch distal to the ductus arteriosus (Fig. 38-6, type 1, right aortic arch) and is particularly common in tetralogy of Fallot (see Chapter 23) and truncus arteriosus (see Chapter 28).

With Retroesophageal Component
In the situation of a right aortic arch with a retroesophageal component, a vascular ring is usually present, but the anatomic details vary depending upon the site of interruption of the embryonic left arch.

WITH MIRROR-IMAGE BRANCHING AND A RETROESOPHAGEAL LIGAMENTUM ARTERIOSUM. Here the interruption of the left arch is proximal (upstream) to the ductus arteriosus (type 2 right aortic arch in Fig. 38-6). The left-sided ligamentum arteriosum extends from a diverticulum on the upper descending thoracic aorta, behind the esophagus, forward to the left pulmonary artery. A vascular ring is present, formed by the ascending portion of the right arch and innominate artery anteriorly, the aortic diverticulum posteriorly, and the ligamentum arteriosum laterally; it may be symptomatic.[A2,M3,W7] This anomaly is rare.[S5]

WITH RETROESOPHAGEAL ANOMALOUS LEFT SUBCLAVIAN ARTERY AND LIGAMENTUM (DUCTUS) ARTERIOSUM. Here the interruption of the left arch occurs between the left subclavian artery and the left common carotid artery (type 3 right aortic arch in Fig. 38-6). The first branch of the right arch becomes the left common carotid artery, and the de-

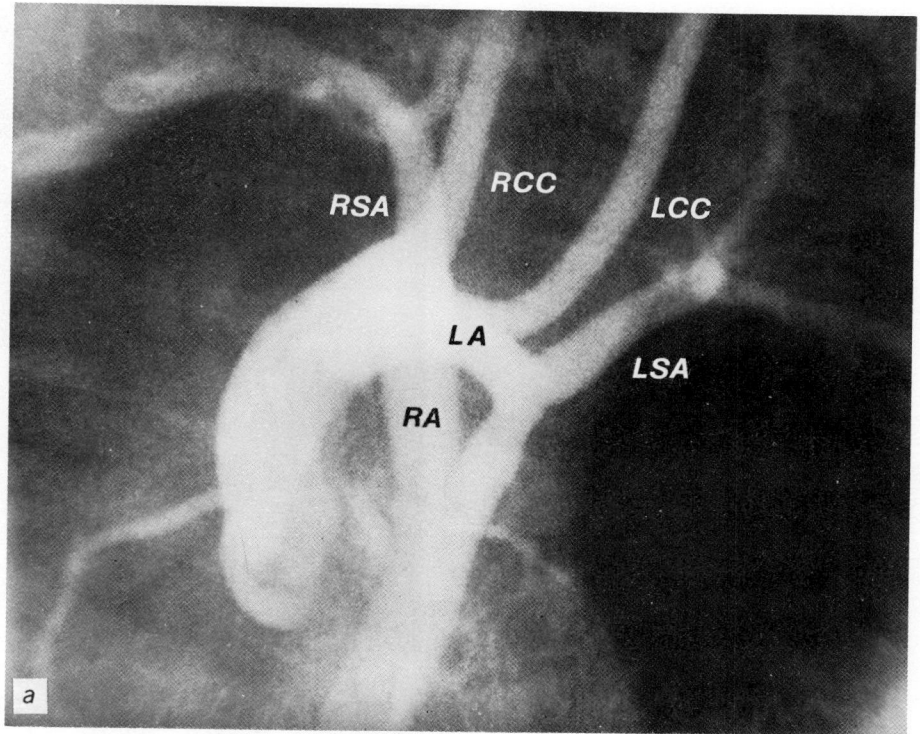

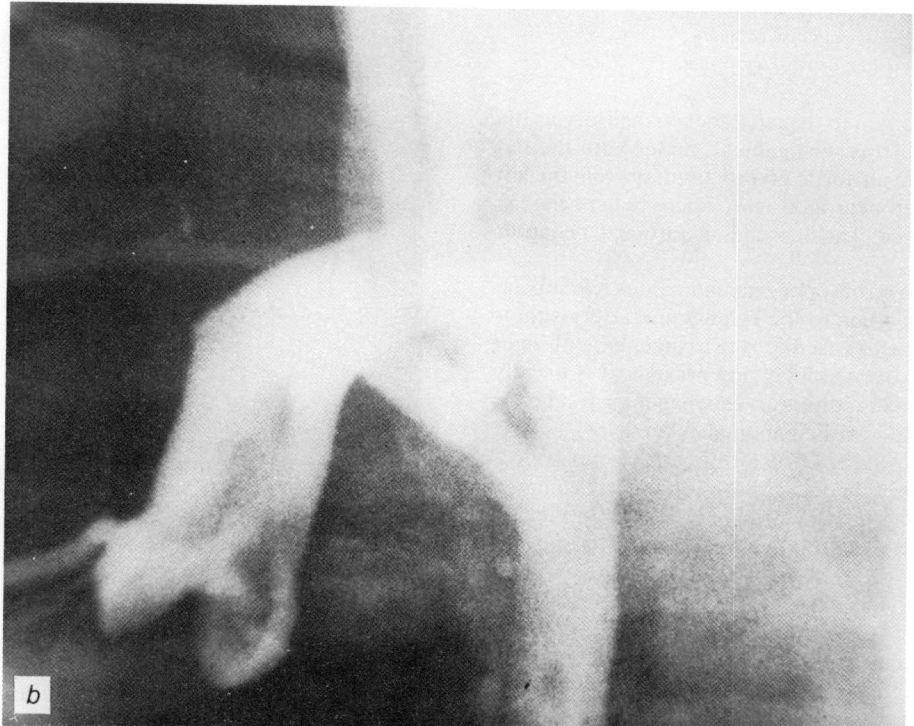

Figure 38-2 Aortogram in a patient with double aortic arch in (*a*) frontal view and (*b*) lateral view with cranial tilt (GLH). The left aortic arch is distinctly narrowed beyond the origin of the left subclavian artery.

LA, left arch; LCC, left common carotid artery; LSA, left subclavian artery; RA, right aortic arch; RCA, right common carotid artery; RSA, right subclavian artery.

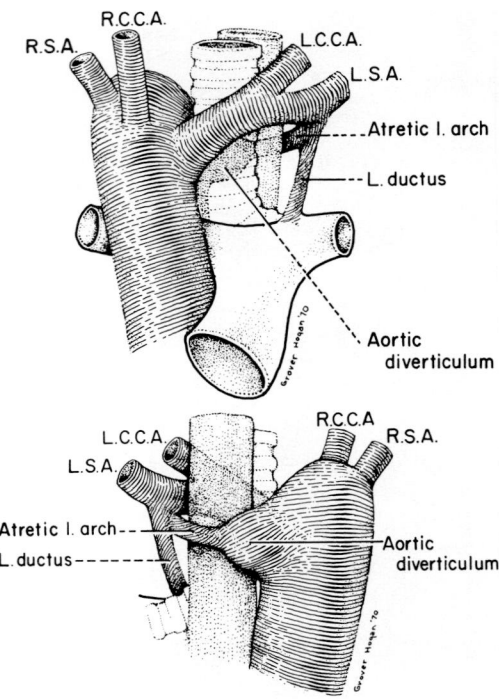

Figure 38-3 Drawings of a double aortic arch with left arch atresia forming a vascular ring. Above frontal view; below posterior view. LCCA, left common carotid artery; LSA, left subclavian artery; RCCA, right common carotid artery; RSA, right subclavian artery.
Reproduced with permission from Shuford and Sybers.[S5]

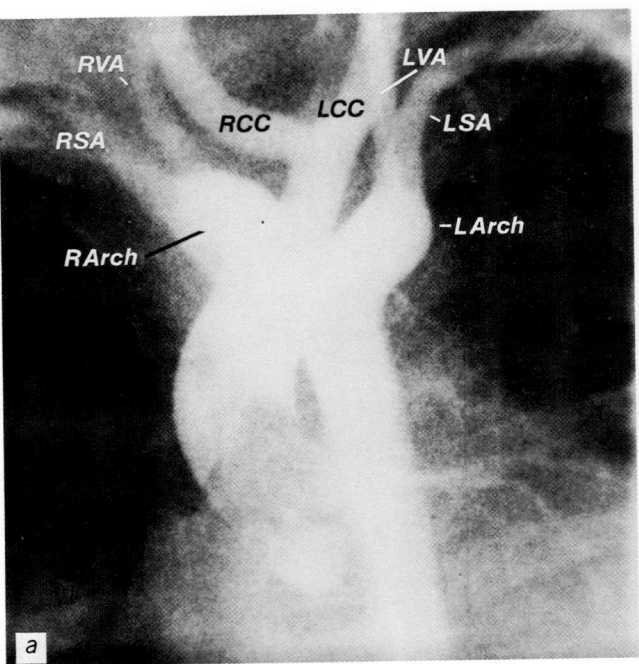

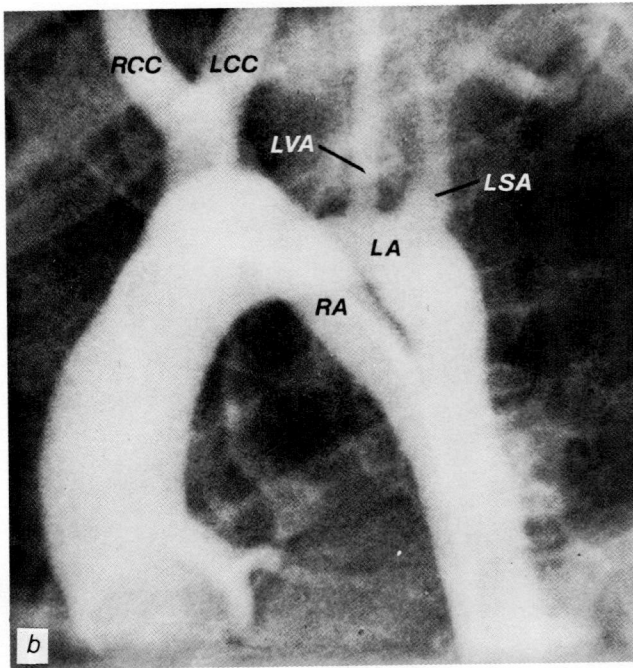

Figure 38-4 Aortogram in a patient with double aortic arch in (a) frontal and (b) lateral views (GLH). The right aortic arch is slightly smaller than the left arch where it joins the left-sided descending aorta. (The right arch was divided via a right thoracotomy.) The right and left common carotid arteries arise from a large common trunk.

LA, left arch; LCC, left common carotid artery; LSA, left subclavian artery; LVA, left vertical artery; RA, right arch; RCC, right common carotid artery; RSA, right subclavian artery; RVA, right vertebral artery.

scending aorta gives origin to the left subclavian artery as the fourth branch. The ductus, or ligament, arises with the left subclavian artery from an aortic diverticulum or from the left subclavian artery itself near its origin, where the subclavian artery may be narrowed. The descending aorta can be left or right sided.

A right arch with a retroesophageal anomalous left subclavian artery that gives origin to the ligamentum arteriosum is the most common type of vascular ring associated with right arch. Although there is a vascular ring present, it is usually loose so that compression of either esophagus or trachea is uncommon. Associated cardiac anomalies are rare.

WITH RETROESOPHAGEAL ANOMALOUS LEFT INNOMINATE ARTERY. Here interruption occurs between the left common carotid and the right arch (type 4 right aortic arch in Fig. 38-6). A vascular ring is present, but the anomaly is rare.

Left Aortic Arch

A vascular ring is associated with a left aortic arch much less commonly than with a right aortic arch.

Anomalous Right Subclavian Artery
In the past, the relatively common aberrant right subclavian artery arising as the fourth branch of an otherwise normal aortic arch and passing upward and to the right behind the esophagus was thought to be a cause of dysphagia (dysphagia lusorium).[L2,M3] Rarely, a right ligamentum arteriosum

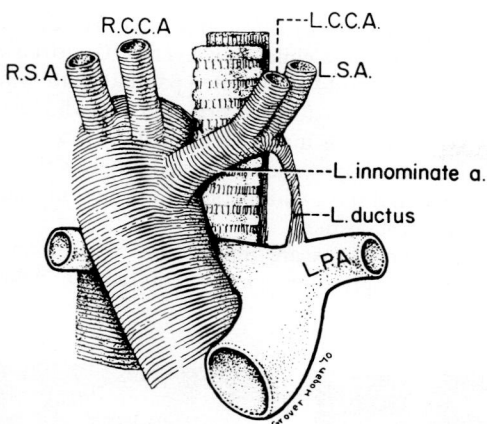

Figure 38-5 Drawing of the common type of right aortic arch with mirror-image branching. There is no retroesophageal component and no vascular ring. Abbreviations are as for Figure 38-3. Reproduced with permission from Shuford and Sybers.[S5]

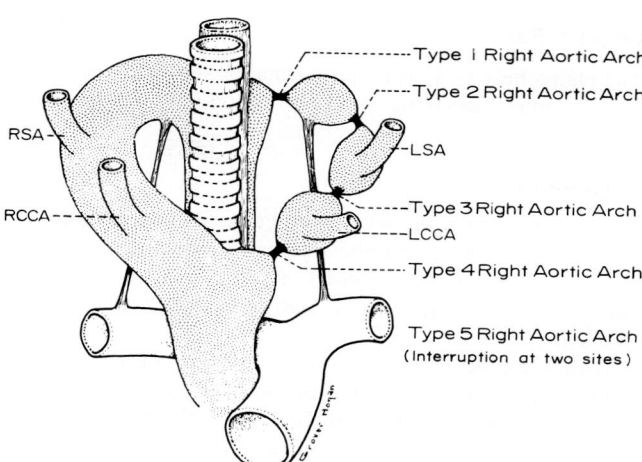

Figure 38-6 Drawing showing sites of interruption in the hypothetical double aortic arch. See text for descriptions of the various types of right aortic arch that result. When there is interruption of the arch at two sites, a sequestered subclavian artery results (see Chapter 23, "Aortic Arch and Ductus Arteriosus" in Section 1, Morphology and Fig. 23-20d). Abbreviations are as in Figure 38-1. Reproduced with permission from Shuford and Sybers.[S5]

passing from the aberrant right subclavian artery to the right pulmonary artery may form a vascular ring that is symptomatic.

Left Aortic Arch and Right Descending Aorta

Vascular rings are likely in the uncommon combination of a left aortic arch and right descending aorta. The left arch crosses behind the esophagus. In combination with a right patent ductus arteriosus or ligamentum arteriosum, a vascular ring is formed.[B6,M6] When the right arch gives origin to the aberrant left subclavian artery via an aortic diverticulum, a ring also is formed.[P2] Often, such cases are associated with a cervical position of the apex of the aortic arch[W8] as a part of the cervical aortic arch complex.[M7] In this, there is a retroesophageal descending aorta on the side opposite that of the aortic arch, and the retroesophageal segment of the aorta may be tortuous and severely narrowed.[H5]

Associated congenital heart disease is said to be more common in this situation than in the other types of vascular ring.[D3]

Ductus Arteriosus Sling

Binet and colleagues[B3] have described an infant with respiratory obstruction in which an anomalous vessel from the right pulmonary artery origin crossed to the left between the esophagus and trachea to join the descending aorta adjacent to the origin of an anomalous right subclavian artery.

Abnormal Course of the Innominate or Left Common Carotid Artery

These arteries may be drawn taut across the anterior wall of the trachea and are a potential but very rare cause of respiratory obstruction.[E2,F1,L2,M2]

Severe Malrotation of the Heart

Compression of the lower trachea can occur with a normal left arch when there is severe malrotation of the heart into the right chest in association with agenesis or hypoplasia of the right lung.[M5,V2,W4] (See Fig. 38-9 in Section 2.) Also, Scherer and Westcott describe a case with dextrocardia and normal lungs in which the main pulmonary artery lay anterior to the trachea and somewhat to the right and the patent ductus arteriosus connecting with a normally positioned descending aorta pulled the main pulmonary artery backward, compressing the front of the trachea. Compression was relieved by dividing the patent ductus arteriosus.[S7]

CLINICAL FEATURES AND DIAGNOSTIC CRITERIA

Symptoms and Signs

Presentation is usually within the first 6 months of life. Inspiratory stridor may be present at birth, often in association with an expiratory wheeze and tachypnea. The stridor may be worse in various positions, for example, when the baby is lying on its back rather than its side. Often, the stridor is relieved by extending the neck. The baby's cry may be hoarse and in the absence of frank stridor the breathing noisy. A persistent barking cough is frequently present. There may be episodes of apnea, severe cyanosis, and unconsciousness. When obstruction is severe, there is obvious subcostal retraction. Recurrent respiratory infections are common and aggravate the respiratory obstruction; when obstruction is less severe, obstructive symptoms may be apparent only at such times.

The baby often feeds poorly, and there may be obvious difficulty in swallowing liquids with episodes of choking and increased respiratory obstruction at these times. Dysphagia for solids is common (most severe cases are operated upon before they are old enough to be offered solid food), the infant refusing to swallow them or choking and regurgitating.

Chest X-Ray

The plain chest x-ray is either normal or shows a right aortic arch. Tracheal deviation or compression may be evident.

Esophagram

The esophagram is the most useful diagnostic measure.[A2,L2] The recording of the esophagogram on cine film at the time of cineangiography is optimal, since it allows a detailed study that shows the pulsatile nature of the obstruction and trachea.

With a double aortic arch, the esophagus shows left- and right-sided indentations, that for the right arch usually being higher and deeper (Fig. 38-7a). In addition, the retroesophageal component produces a prominent posterior esophageal indentation that courses downward and to the left. In contrast, an aberrant left subclavian artery arising from the right arch produces a narrower esophageal impression that courses upward and leftward. A right arch and a left ligamentum arteriosum show a more marked right-sided than left-sided indentation (Fig. 38-7b).

Bronchoscopy

Bronchoscopy is rarely done, although it does identify sites of tracheal compression and show its pulsatile nature.[M3]

Aortography

Aortography is now performed routinely via a catheter positioned in the ascending aorta and is usually combined with cineangiocardiography to assess associated congenital cardiac defects. Using biplane techniques, the first injection depicts both lateral and anteroposterior (AP) views and the second both left and right oblique views. A degree of cranial tilt may separate the arches better in the oblique views.[T2] Only aortography (or contrast computed tomography [CT] scan) will establish that the anomaly is a complete double aortic arch, and it will show sites of narrowing in the left or rarely the right arch (see Figs. 38-2 and 38-4). It cannot distinguish between a double arch with an atretic segment and a right aortic arch with a retroesophageal component. A sharp angulation of one of the brachiocephalic arteries may indicate the site of an atretic segment in a double arch or a constricting ligamentum arteriosum in a right arch with a retroesophageal component (Fig. 38-8).

NATURAL HISTORY

Vascular rings of aortic arch origin comprise only about 1%–2% of cases of congenital heart disease.[N1]

Only fragmentary information exists concerning the natural history of these anomalies. Untreated severe respiratory obstruction present in the first 6 months of life is presumably fatal before 1 year, particularly when symptoms are present from birth. Symptoms that first appear after 6 months are less severe and rarely if ever progressive, except at times of respiratory infection or regurgitation and choking.

When symptoms are of borderline severity, they almost always disappear as the child grows. Thus, Godtfredsen and colleagues[G4] followed 11 unoperated patients with symptoms not severe enough to justify surgery. Of the 6 who had either a double aortic arch or a right arch with a retroesophageal component producing a vascular ring, 4 outgrew their symptoms by age 4, and the 2 with persistent symptoms had other anomalies to explain them.

Generally, symptoms are milder and of later onset and dysphagia is less prominent in patients with a right aortic

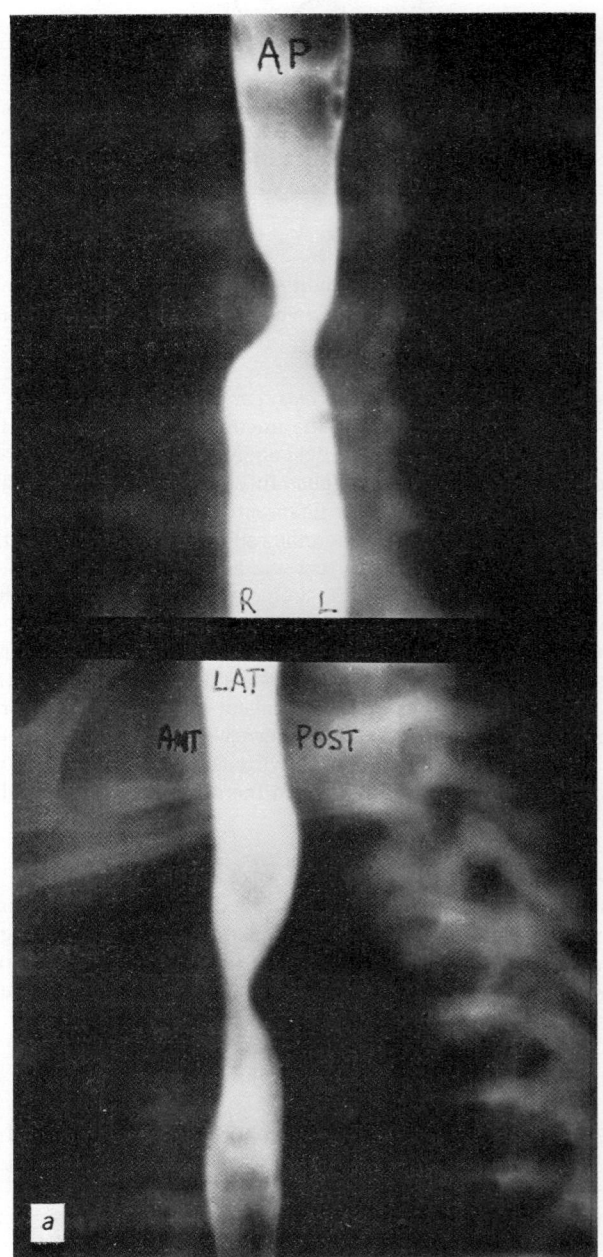

Figure 38-7 Esophagograms in anteroposterior and lateral projections (GLH).
(a) A double aortic arch.

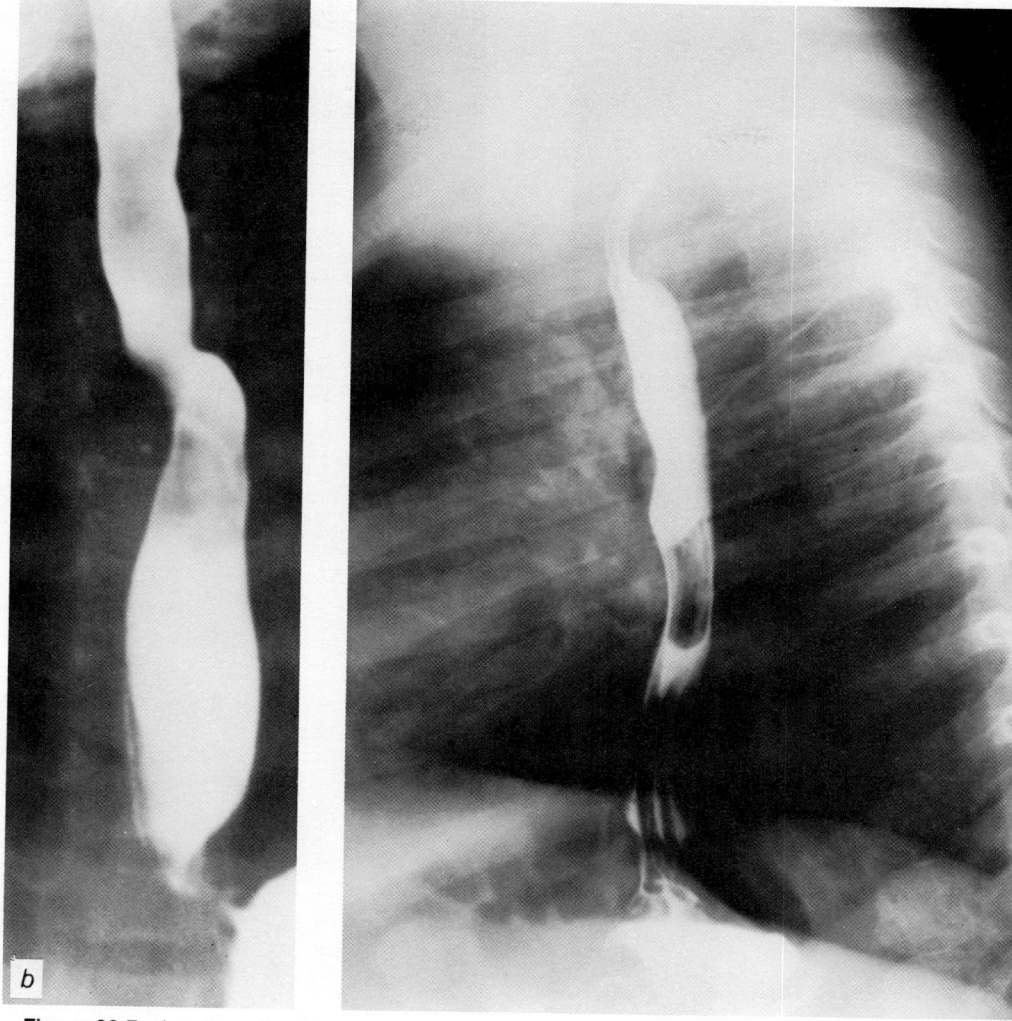

Figure 38-7 (*continued*)

(*b*) A right aortic arch and a retroesophageal aortic diverticulum giving origin to an aberrant left subclavian artery and the ligamentum arteriosum. The anteroposterior views show the typical bilateral indentations and the lateral views a posterior indentation.

AP, anteroposterior view; L, left side of patient; LAT, lateral view; POST, posterior aspect of patient; R, right side of patient.

arch and retroesophageal component than in those with a double aortic arch.[A2]

TECHNIQUE OF OPERATION

Double Aortic Arch

When *both arches* are of *equal size,* the vascular ring may be approached through the fourth interspace or bed of the non-resected fifth rib from the left side, as in the operation for patent ductus arteriosus (see Chapter 22 and Fig. 22-3) or coarctation (see Chapter 34 and Fig. 34-9). However, a similar approach from the right side is preferred in this situation. (GLH,UAB). The right arch is dissected out completely, including the part passing behind the esophagus. The right

arch is divided between clamps close to its junction with the descending aorta. The ends are oversewn with two rows of 4-0 or 5-0 polypropylene sutures. The mediastinal surface of the right arch is then dissected further to free it and allow the divided ends to separate. The descending aorta is also mobilized and sometimes sutured to rib periostium to keep it away from the esophagus. In this and other operations for the relief of vascular rings "all strands or bands of tissue which form a part of the constricting mechanism" must be dissected away from the trachea or esophagus.[G8] The operation is completed by closing the chest wound in layers after inserting a single intercostal tube for drainage.

More often, the *distal left arch is narrowed,* and the approach is made from the left side. The vascular structures and the ligamentum arteriosum are dissected out and separated thoroughly from the surrounding structures. The liga-

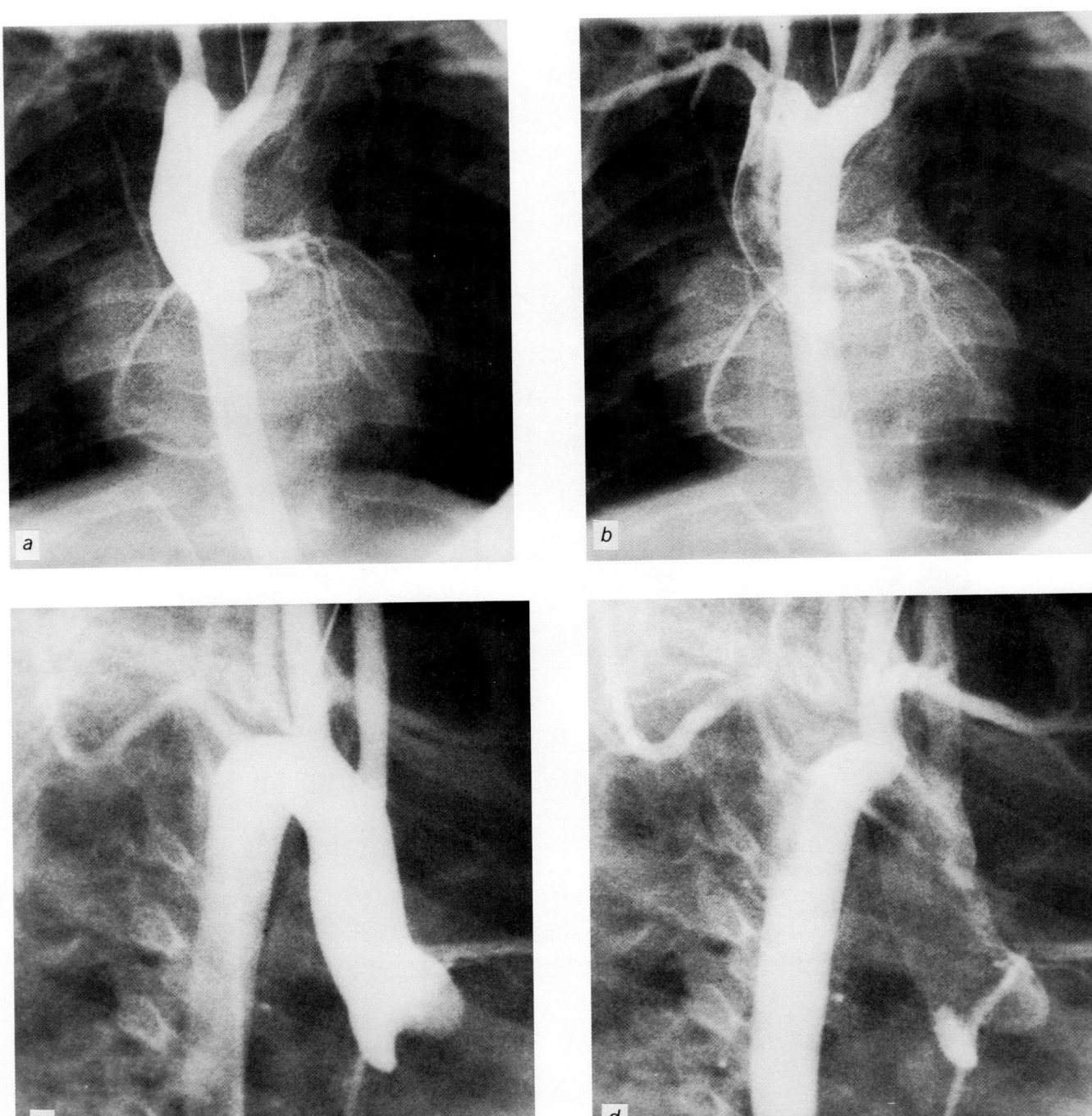

Figure 38-8 Aortogram of a patient with a right aortic arch with an anomalous left subclavian artery and a ligamentum arteriosum arising from a retroesophageal aortic diverticulum (GLH). The frontal views, (a) and (b) and right anterior oblique views. (c) and (d), are both at different phases in the cardiac cycle. The angulation at the origin of the left subclavian artery from the diverticulum suggests the presence of a ligamentum arteriosum under tension passing forward to the left pulmonary artery (as was the case at operation). The angulation is downward in the frontal view and anterior in the right anterior oblique view. The absence of a similar angulation along the course of the left common carotid artery suggests that this artery is not connected to the diverticulum by an atretic ligament that forms part of a complete left aortic arch.

mentum arteriosum is divided, and the junction of the left arch with the descending aorta is divided between vascular clamps and the ends oversewn. The end of the left arch is now further dissected from the underlying mediastinal tissues to allow it to retract forward. The medial surface of the descending aorta and the distal divided end are also dissected away from the esophagus. The adventitia over the lateral wall of the aorta may be stitched to the adjacent rib periosteum to pull it laterally and posteriorly away from the esophagus.

Right Aortic Arch

When there is a *right arch with a retroesophageal component*, it is generally approached from the left side. After the dissection is completed, the ligamentum arteriosum is divided. The descending aorta is dissected away from the esophagus and is sutured to the periosteum of the rib if necessary.

Left Aortic Arch

A right-sided thoracotomy is used in the rare patients with a *left aortic arch and right-sided ligamentum arteriosum* producing a vascular ring.[P6,W8] The ligamentum is dissected and divided in the same fashion for a right arch with retroesophageal component.

When there is compression of the lower trachea by an anomalous innominate artery or by a malrotated left aortic arch associated with severe rightward malrotation of the heart, the approach is through a *median sternotomy*. The anomalous vessel is fully dissected and then suspended from the posterior aspect of the sternum or adjacent ribs with strong sutures that pick up the adventitia of the vessel.

SPECIAL FEATURES OF POSTOPERATIVE CARE

Few patients obtain immediate relief of stridor,[L2] and, in fact, symptoms may be worse in the first postoperative week. Special respiratory care is therefore required, particularly in small infants. Occasionally, intubation is necessary for several days in order to allow adequate tracheal aspiration toilet and, if necessary, ventilation. The use of continuous positive airway pressure with the infant breathing spontaneously (see Chapter 5, "Pulmonary Subsystem" in Section 2) is often advantageous in this setting.[S9] After extubation, positive pressure is maintained, if necessary, for some days by using nasal prongs with an appropriate flow of humidified gas. Full humidification and meticulous suctioning techniques are required to keep the airway clear and to avoid damage to the mucosa.

RESULTS

Hospital mortality is low but does not approach zero (Table 38-1).[A2,L2,W7]

Late survival and relief of symptoms are both excellent unless prevented by complications from associated con-

Table 38-1 Surgical cases of vascular ring (GLH; 1958–1984 and UAB; 1967–1984, but includes only three cases, all with double aortic arch, because the other cases were cared for by the pediatric general surgery service.)

Category	n	Hospital Deaths No.	%	CL
Double aortic arch	10	0	0%	0%–17%
Right aortic arch	6	1	17%	2%–46%
Retroesophageal ligamentum arteriosum	2	0	0%	0%–61%
Retroesophageal left subclavian artery	4	1	25%	3%–63%
Left aortic arch, with anterior tracheal compression and right lung hypoplasia	2	0	0%	0%–61%
Total	18	1	6%	1%–18%

KEY: CL, 70% confidence limits.

NOTE: The one death was in a 7-week-old baby who died 2 weeks postoperatively from cerebral symptoms present preoperatively.

genital heart disease or congenital extracardiac anomalies.[R3] Rarely, an arteriosclerotic aneurysm may occur at the site of an aortic diverticulum and require excision.[R2]

INDICATIONS FOR OPERATION

Operation is indicated in all patients with significant obstructive symptoms. It is not indicated if symptoms are mild or absent.

Section 2
ANOMALOUS LEFT PULMONARY ARTERY (VASCULAR SLING)

DEFINITION

Vascular sling is a congenital condition in which the left pulmonary artery arises anomalously from the right pulmonary artery extrapericardially and courses to the left behind the tracheal bifurcation and in front of the esophagus to reach the left lung hilum and form a sling around the trachea.

HISTORICAL NOTE

Aberrant left pulmonary artery was first recognized by Glaevecke and Doehle in 1897[G1] during an autopsy performed on a 7-month-old child who died from asphyxia. The next report was that of Scheid, again in the German literature in 1938[S1] and again from autopsy findings, this time in a 7-month-old child who died from respiratory obstruction. The description of the anomalous course of the artery is exact in both reports, whereas Scheid also described in detail an associated diffuse tracheal stenosis due to the presence of complete cartilaginous rings. This latter condition was again accurately described by Wolman 3 years later.[W5]

Quist-Hanssen from Norway detailed the clinical findings of pulmonary artery sling premortem in 1949,[Q1] although the exact diagnosis was not made until the autopsy was performed. Welsh and Munro first suggested, on the basis of their autopsy findings, that in this anomaly the barium swallow should show an anterior esophageal indentation,[W1] whereas Wittenborg soon after accurately defined these features on the esophagram.[W2] In 1958, Contro and colleagues coined the term *vascular sling* to distinguish the condition from vascular ring.[C1]

Potts and colleagues in 1954 were the first to report a successful operation for this anomaly in a patient in whom the anatomy of the malformation was not established prior to the operation. Potts divided the left pulmonary artery at its origin from the right pulmonary artery, transferred the vessel in front of the trachea, and reanastomosed it to the proximal stump.[P1] Soon after, Morse and Gladding reported a case diagnosed at right thoracotomy and confirmed at autopsy[M1] in whom the anomalously arising left pulmonary artery was dissected away from the trachea in an attempt to relieve compression but not divided.

Hiller and Maclean operated successfully upon a patient correctly diagnosed by barium swallow and angiography in 1955; after mobilizing and dividing the anomalously arising left pulmonary artery, they anastomosed it to the side of the main pulmonary artery (the operation currently practiced). Moreover, they performed a postoperative angiogram 3 weeks later that showed that the left pulmonary artery was occluded, although the patient's stridor had been relieved completely and the chest x-ray remained normal.[H1] In 1962, Mustard and colleagues reported relief of respiratory obstruction following division of the ligamentum arteriosum only,[M3] and a year later Lochard and colleagues reported a case in which the right main stem bronchus was successfully relocated in front of the anomalous left pulmonary artery.[L3] Neither of these latter two procedures is practiced currently.

MORPHOLOGY

Anomalous Left Pulmonary Artery

The left pulmonary artery arises extrapericardially from the posterosuperior wall of a normally positioned right pulmonary artery lying in front of the proximal right main bronchus. The right pulmonary artery in these circumstances is a direct continuation of the main pulmonary artery, the junction between them being marked by the attachment of the ligamentum arteriosum (or ductus arteriosus). From its point of origin, the left pulmonary artery curves upward and backward over the proximal right main bronchus and then to the left behind the lower trachea and its bifurcation at or slightly above the carina[J1] (Fig. 38-9). It courses slightly inferior to lie behind the proximal left main stem bronchus and then appears immediately superior to it to enter the left lung and then divides. The left lung hilum is lower than normal in relation to the main pulmonary artery.[C6] The left pulmonary artery (LPA) usually indents the posterior wall of the trachea and left main bronchus as it passes behind them and displaces (bows) the distal trachea and carina toward the left. The right main bronchus is bowed anteriorly.[C6] The LPA

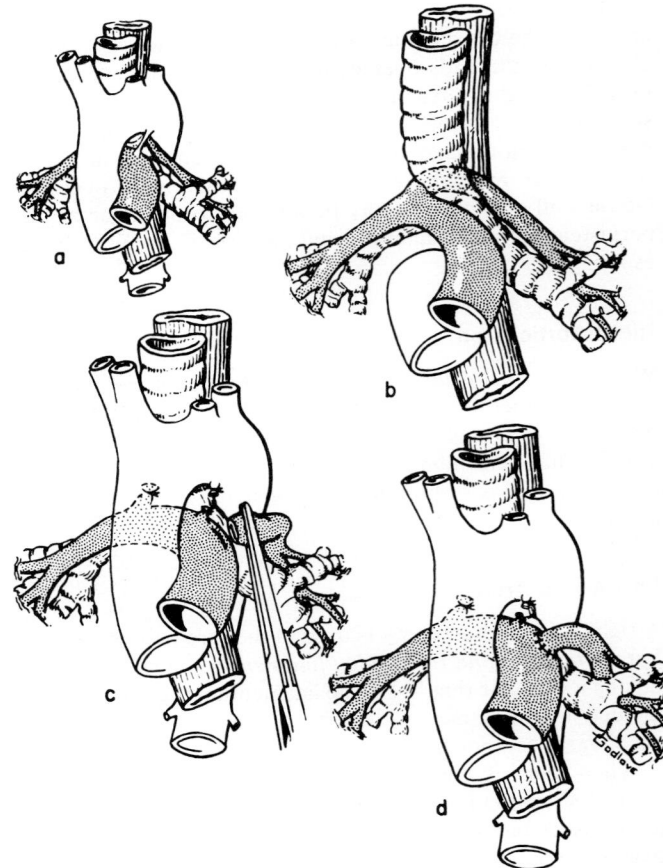

Figure 38-9 Drawings to show an anomalous left pulmonary artery arising from the right pulmonary artery. (a) is the complete depiction. In (b), the aortic arch has been removed in order to display the anatomy better. (c) and (d) indicate the surgical technique used for correction of the anomaly.
Reproduced with permission from Clarkson et al.[C7]

passes in front of the esophagus, which is usually indented across its entire anterior aspect or less often on its leftward anterior surface only.

The anomalous LPA is frequently slightly smaller than normal in comparison with the right pulmonary artery. Rarely, the *right* upper lobe artery may come off the LPA near its origin.[T3] Bamman and colleagues describe one case in which the left lung was partly supplied by a left pulmonary artery in normal position; the anomalous LPA supplied only the left lower lobe and crossed behind the left atrium rather than behind the tracheal bifurcation.[B2]

The ligamentum arteriosum (or ductus arteriosus) follows a normal course from the junction of the main pulmonary artery and right pulmonary artery, passing backward directly superior to the left main bronchus and the anomalous LPA (not between them as depicted by Williams and colleagues[W3]) to join the descending aorta.

Tracheobronchial and Pulmonary Abnormalities

The trachea near the bifurcation is usually narrowed as a result of posterior compression by the anomalous LPA. This mainly affects the origin of the right main bronchus and trachea just above the main carina.[J1] Rarely, the left main bronchus may be narrowed by a similar mechanism.

In about 50% of patients with this vascular anomaly, narrowing of the trachea and/or proximal main bronchi is secondary to the presence of complete ring cartilages,[S6] which are also often more numerous than normal.[S1] In these areas, the pars membranacea is absent and the lumen is usually severely narrowed. This process may involve the entire length of the trachea or only its proximal or distal portions. The major bronchi may be similarly involved or their cartilaginous rings may be wide and irregular and the bronchi variable in diameter and length.[C5]

The so-called bronchus suis, consisting of separate high origin from the trachea of the eparterial bronchus to the right upper lobe, is more frequent than normal.[A1] It is not a cause of obstruction per se.

When the right main bronchus is selectively narrowed, there is hyperinflation of the right lung (not affecting the right upper lobe when there is a bronchus suis present); when the left main bronchus is the narrower, there is hyperinflation of the left lung.[A1] More complete obstruction leads to atelectasis. When obstruction to the right main bronchus is significant in utero, there may be retention of fetal fluid in the right lung at birth.

Either the left or right lung may be unilobar.[S6] Rarely, the right lung may be hypoplastic.[H3] In a case in the GLH series (Table 38-2), the lung hypoplasia was part of the scimitar syndrome.

Other Cardiovascular Anomalies

Other cardiovascular anomalies are associated with half the cases of anomalous LPA.[S6] The more common are left superior vena cava, atrial septal defect, patent ductus arteriosus, and ventricular septal defect, but there may be tetralogy of Fallot, single ventricle, transposition of the great arteries, tricuspid atresia, or aortic arch anomalies (see Table 38-2).

Noncardiovascular Development Anomalies

A wide variety of noncardiovascular developmental anomalies occur relatively frequently.[C7]

CLINICAL FEATURES AND DIAGNOSTIC CRITERIA

Symptoms and Signs

The majority of patients with anomalous left pulmonary artery (LPA), possibly as many as 90%,[C7,S6] have significant and usually severe symptoms, and in the majority these are present at birth or soon after.[C7]

The most common presentation is with wheezing and stridor, often with prolongation of the expiratory phase suggesting asthma and with a harsh cough and intercostal indrawing. In addition, there may be choking and rapid breathing or apneic spells and associated episodes of cyanosis. The symptoms are episodic, but acute episodes of dyspnea and cyanosis or severe exacerbations of respiratory obstruction are common and may result in unconsciousness, convulsions, or even death.

Symptoms may be precipitated by respiratory infections and are occasionally altered by changes in posture of the infant. They may be made worse by feeding,[Q1,W2] with or without regurgitation and choking. Dysphagia, however, is very uncommon.

Table 38-2 Patients with anomalous left pulmonary artery (GLH; 1956–1984).

Age at Diagnosis	Symptoms	Complete Tracheal Rings	Other Anomalies	Surgery for Anomalous LPA (Age)	Outcome (Age)
5 mo	Severe	Yes	None	None	Mild dyspnea
1 wk	Severe	No	Scimitar syndrome Hypoplastic lung PDA	None	Died (30 d)
1 mo	Severe (NYHA IV)	Yes	VSD (large)	Yes (2 mo)	Hospital death
Not diagnosed (autopsy)	Severe	Yes	Tricuspid atresia Aberrant RSA LSVC Cong IVC occlusion	None	Died (7 mo)
3 mo	Severe (NYHA IV)	Yes	Aplasia RUL	Yes (3 mo)	Late death (8 mo)
6 yr	Mild	No	VSD (small) Aberrant RSA	Division ligamentum Division aberrant RSA (operation 1956)	Mild dyspnea (30 yr)
14 yr	Nil	No	None	None	Asymptomatic
2 mo	Nil[a]	No	TGA	None	Asymptomatic

KEY: IVC, inferior vena cava; LPA, left pulmonary artery; LSVC, left superior vena cava; PDA, patent ductus arteriosus; RSA, right subclavian artery; TGA, transposition of the great arteries; VSD, ventricular septal defect.

NOTE: Complete tracheal rings were always associated with severe diffuse tracheal stenosis.

[a] The LPA supplied only the left lower lobe.

Chest X-Ray

The plain chest x-ray gives important clues to the correct diagnosis.[C6] It shows anterior bowing of the right main bronchus and deviation of the lower trachea and carina to the left. In addition, the left lung hilum is lower than normal in relation to the position of the main pulmonary artery, and there is frequently unequal aeration of the lungs. Usually, the right lung is overinflated, but sometimes the left may be.[A1] When obstruction is more complete, there may be areas of atelectasis. There is a mediastinal density between the trachea and esophagus on the lateral view (Fig. 38-10) and, in older patients in particular, a right-sided mediastinal density opposite the carina in the posteroanterior view (Fig. 38-11).[H1,K1,M4]

In the newborn, the initial chest x-ray may show retention of fetal fluid in the right lung, evidenced by a uniform opacity of the right lung without loss of volume (this is, in fact, increased) and without an air bronchogram. Once the fetal fluid has been resorbed or suctioned off, the right lung will appear hyperinflated.[Z1]

Esophagram

Barium swallow usually shows an anterior indentation of the esophagus in the *lateral* view just above the level of the carina (Fig. 38-11). On the anteroposterior view there may be no abnormality or a leftward lateral indentation.[G2,S4] The only other conditions known to produce an anterior esophageal indentation at this level are the ductus arteriosus sling[B3] (see "Ductus Arteriosus Sling" in Section 1, Morphology) and a long, tortuous patent ductus arteriosus.[B4]

In patients with anomalous LPA, these findings are by no means always present[D1,W2] and are variable in their appearance during the esophagram, since they are in part dependent upon the phase of the cardiac and respiratory cycles.[B4] High-quality cine film recordings of the barium swallows are therefore required. The esophagram can be more difficult to interpret when there is also an aberrant subclavian artery passing posterior to the esophagus at a slightly higher level than the LPA.[W2]

Other Investigations

A *tracheogram* with or without *bronchoscopy* is an important part of the assessment,[C4,C6] and it is made to evaluate the additional zones of narrowing that are frequently present and that influence surgical management. It is best done in conjunction with esophageal studies and recorded on cine film. The diagnosis can be confirmed by computed tomography with or without contrast enhancement, since this will show the LPA arising from the right pulmonary artery and passing leftward between the trachea and esophagus.[R1,S8]

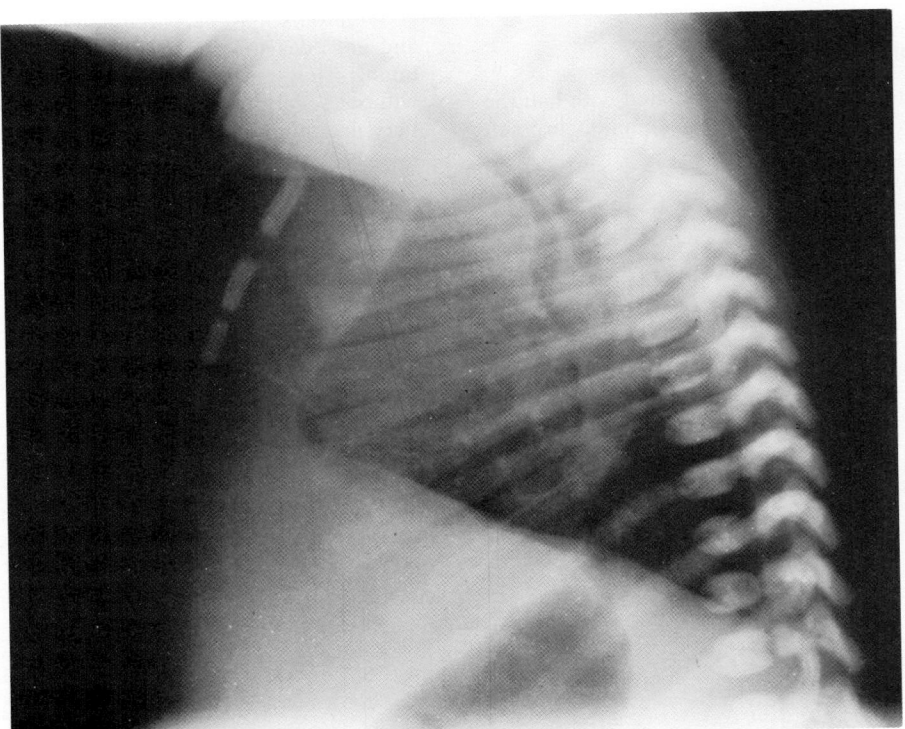

Figure 38-10   Lateral chest x-ray in infant with a scimitar syndrome and an anomalous left pulmonary artery forming a vascular sling (GLH). The separation of the lower trachea from the esophagus (which is also air filled) by a rounded mass is typical of the condition. Also in this infant, the acquired dextrocardia, resulting from the hypoplasia of the right lung that was part of the scimitar syndrome, has caused the ascending aorta to compress the trachea (arrow) at a high level.

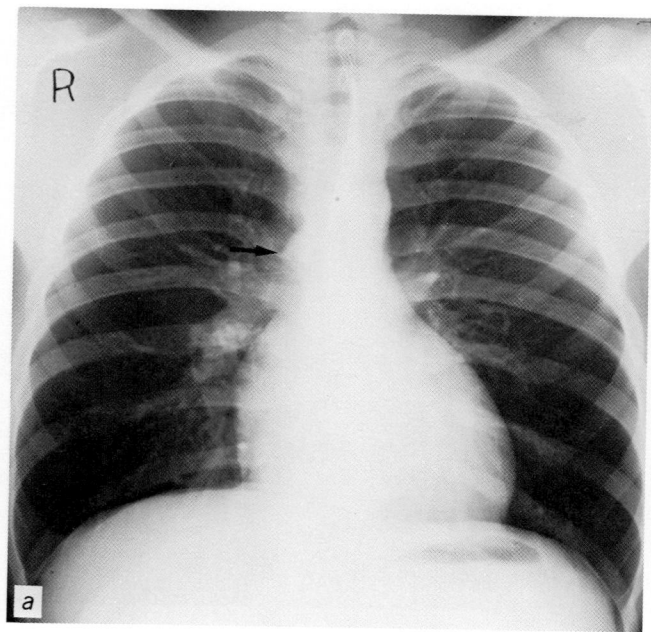

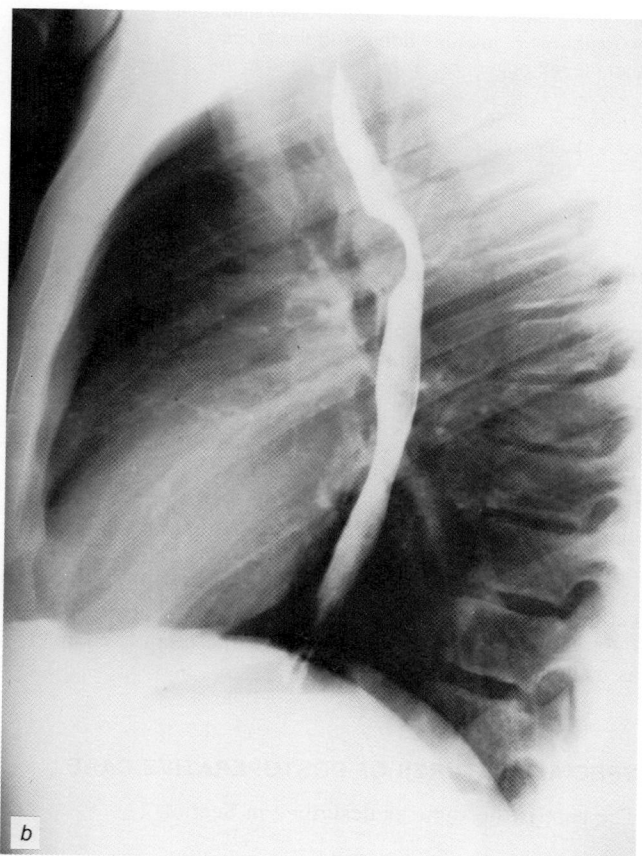

Figure 38-11 Chest x-ray (a) and lateral esophagogram (b) in a 14-year-old asymptomatic youth with an anomalous left pulmonary artery (LPA) (GLH). The LPA is visible as a curved density along the right mediastinal border and as a prominent indentation in the anterior wall of the esophagus immediately above the tracheal bifurcation.

Cardiac Catheterization and Angiocardiography

Cardiac catheterization and angiocardiography are usually required to confirm the diagnosis (Fig. 38-12) and to assess associated cardiovascular anomalies. The LPA is visualized best in a cranially tilted frontal view.

NATURAL HISTORY

Knowledge of the natural history of this uncommon anomaly is fragmentary.

When significant respiratory obstruction is present in the neonate, most are dead before 1 year of age.[C7] It is probable that when presentation is a little later in life, survival is possible without surgical intervention (provided the trachea does not show more diffuse narrowing) and obstruction may become less severe with growth.[K3,P4] It is now apparent that a number of patients in whom anomalously originating LPA is an isolated anomaly are asymptomatic throughout their lives.[H4,K2,M4]

TECHNIQUE OF OPERATION

The repair may be done through a left posterolateral thoracotomy without cardiopulmonary bypass (CPB)[G9] (GLH) or through a median sternotomy with CPB (UAB).

Left Posterolateral Thoracotomy Approach

A left posterolateral thoracotomy is made, entering the chest via the fourth interspace or fifth rib bed, as described in Section 1. The anomalous left pulmonary artery (LPA) is identified by dissection of the superior part of the left lung hilum. The ligamentum arteriosum is divided, since this improves exposure and may possibly relieve compression on the left main bronchus.[M3] The dissection of the left pulmonary artery is continued medially (centrally) and behind the proximal left main bronchus and tracheal bifurcation. The artery is freed completely from the posterior wall of these structures and followed as far as possible into the mediastinum to gain adequate length. Care is taken not to obstruct flow into the right pulmonary artery by undue tension on the LPA. The patient is given heparin in a dose of $1.5 \text{ mg} \cdot \text{kg}^{-1}$ to obtain partial systemic heparinization. The LPA is then divided between vascular clamps and its distal end oversewn with continuous polypropylene suture and the clamp removed.

The pericardium is opened with a vertical incision anterior to the phrenic nerve to expose the main pulmonary artery, and a second similar incision is made posterior to this structure through which the distal end of the anomalous LPA is passed. The tip of the left atrial appendage is retracted by a ligature tied to it, and the left wall of the main pulmonary artery is excluded in a curved vascular clamp. The clamp is positioned to allow the LPA to reach the main pulmonary artery without kinking or tension. The excluded portion of the main pulmonary artery is opened, excising an ellipse of the wall, and an end-to-side anastomosis performed between

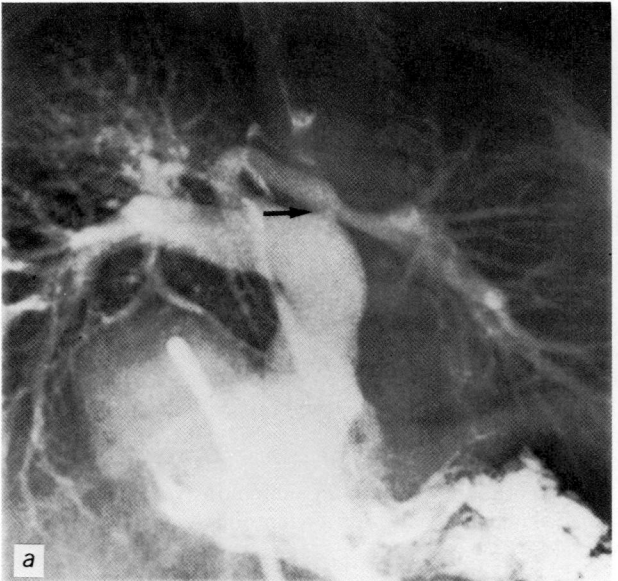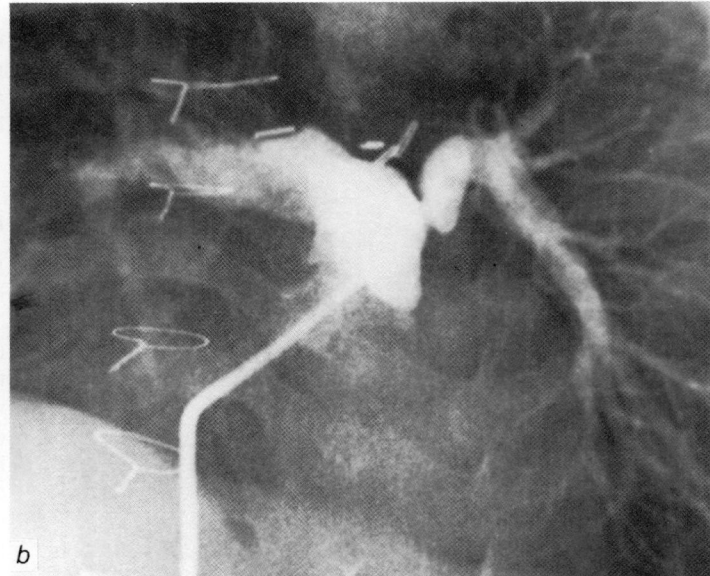

Figure 38-12 Cineangiogram in an infant with anomalous left pulmonary artery (vascular sling) (UAB).
(*a*) Preoperative study showing the left pulmonary artery originating from the right. A very small patent ductus arteriosus (arrow) is present between the distal left pulmonary artery and the pulmonary trunk. The concavity apparent in the upper surface of the left pulmonary artery just lateral to the ductus is the impression of the descending aorta.
(*b*) Late postoperative study showing stenosis at the anastomosis of left pulmonary artery to pulmonary trunk. This was successfully treated by percutaneous balloon dilation.

the left and main pulmonary artery (Fig. 38-9), refashioning the left pulmonary artery end obliquely to increase the diameter of the anastomosis. The posterior layer of the anastomosis is performed from within using continuous 5-0 polypropylene and the anterior from outside using interrupted sutures. The clamps are then removed. The heparin is not reversed.

The pericardium is left open and the chest closed, leaving one intercostal tube for drainage.

Median Sternotomy Approach with Cardiopulmonary Bypass

After the usual preparations (see Chapter 2, Section 3), the median sternotomy is made. The pericardium is opened and stay sutures are applied. The aorta is dissected completely away from the pulmonary artery. The ligamentum arteriosum is dissected and divided between ligatures.

CPB is established, using a single venous cannula, and with it the patient is cooled to 25°C so that periods of very low CPB flow may be used if needed. The left pleural space is opened widely, either now or later. The left pulmonary artery is usually easily identified coming off the right pulmonary artery. It is dissected out well distally, completely separating it from the surrounding structures including the trachea anteriorly and the esophagus posteriorly.

The LPA is cut away from the right pulmonary artery, and

the defect in the latter is closed with two rows of 5-0 or 6-0 polypropylene sutures. The left pulmonary artery is then pulled out into the left pleural space. A large window is made in the pericardium behind the phrenic nerve and along side the main pulmonary artery, and the left pulmonary artery is brought into the pericardial space through it. An incision is made in the left lateral aspect of the main pulmonary artery. Taking care that the LPA lies nicely and without kinking or rotation, its proximal end is anastomosed to the side of the main pulmonary artery with interrupted 6-0 or 7-0 sutures.

After rewarming the patient, CPB is discontinued and decannulation is effected. A polyvinyl pressure-recording catheter is brought out from the pulmonary artery via the right ventricle. The remainder of the operation is completed as usual (see Chapter 2, Section 3).

SPECIAL FEATURES OF POSTOPERATIVE CARE

The care is the same as described in Section 1.

RESULTS

Survival

Only 50%–60% of patients have survived the operation and the postoperative period of hospitalization[S6] (Table 38-3).

Table 38-3 Surgical cases of anomalous left pulmonary artery (vascular sling) (UAB; 1967–1984 and GLH; 1958–1984).

Age at Operation	Associated Anomalies	Complete Tracheal Rings	Surgical Approach	Outcome
2	VSD	Yes	Left thoracotomy	Hospital death
2	L superior vena cava		Median sternotomy[a]	Hospital death 48 hours
2.5	PDA		Median sternotomy[a]	Asymptomatic
3	Aplasia RUL	Yes	Left thoracotomy	Death 8 months PO
8		Stenosis L main bronchus	Median sternotomy	Asymptomatic

KEY: L, left; PDA, patent ductus arteriosus; PO, postoperatively; RUL, right upper lobe; VSD, ventricular septal defect.

[a]With cardiopulmonary bypass.

Coexisting anatomic tracheal narrowing is often present in patients who fail to survive (see Table 38-3).[S6] When no coexisting anomalies are present, the chances for early survival are good.[D2]

Most of the patients who survive the early postoperative period become long-term survivors.[S6] Two asymptomatic patients (Table 38-3) are alive 1.5 and 8 years postoperatively.

Relief of Respiratory Obstruction

Relief of respiratory obstruction is virtually always complete when it is due only to compression by the anomalous LPA. However, relief of symptoms has been obtained in a few patients in whom only the ligamentum arteriosum or a patent ductus arteriosus has been divided.[M3,P4,P5] When there is diffuse anatomic tracheal stenosis associated with complete cartilaginous rings, the prognosis is usually poor, with recurrent episodes of acute respiratory stridor and ultimately death. Occasionally, however, this is not the case. One non-surgical case in whom a severe diffuse stenosis has become less marked (repeat tracheograms) over a 10-year period is doing well (GLH; Table 38-2).

When the tracheal stenosis is localized, resection of the stenotic zone is a possible second-stage procedure.

Left Pulmonary Artery Patency

The left pulmonary artery anastomosis has frequently occluded,[P5,S6] but this may not be the case currently, with more meticulous techniques and the use of heparin.[D2,L1] In two surviving cases, restudy early postoperatively showed patent anastomoses (UAB). Dunn and colleagues have reported all anastomoses (100%, CL 62%–100%) in their 4 patients to be patent by radioisotope perfusion studies 9–21 months postoperatively.[D2] Earlier, Sade and associates reported a patent left pulmonary artery in only 2 (18%, CL 6%–38%) of 11 patients with late studies.

Despite left pulmonary artery occlusion, the symptomatic result is good in most patients, and no changes in the chest x-ray seem to develop at the time of occlusion. Thus, the first patient to be operated upon by Potts is reported to be asymptomatic 24 years later but with an occluded left pulmonary artery.[C3] Late development of pulmonary hypertension in the right lung is a possibility in such circumstances. Attempts to reestablish left pulmonary artery patency by reoperation have not been successful.[S6]

INDICATIONS FOR OPERATION

When anomalously arising left pulmonary artery (LPA) is an isolated anomaly and there are symptoms and radiologic signs of important respiratory obstruction, operation is indicated. When symptoms are absent or mild, surgery is not recommended.[P3]

When there is severe diffuse tracheal stenosis with complete cartilaginous rings, relief of the stenosis due to anomalous LPA is indicated only when this stenosis is more severe than the former.

Associated cardiac defects also complicate matters. They are usually best corrected or palliated first, with the anomalously arising LPA then operated upon if respiratory obstruction persists.

REFERENCES

A

1. Aytac A, Ozme S, Sarikayalar F, Saylam A: Pulmonary artery sling. *Ann Thorac Surg* 22:596, 1976.

2. Arciniegas E, Hakimi M, Hertzler JH, Farooki ZQ, Green EW: Surgical management of congenital vascular rings. *J Thorac Cardiovasc Surg* 77:721, 1979.

B

1. Bayford D: An account of a singular case of obstructed deglutition. *Mem Med Soc London* 2:275, 1794.

2. Bamman JL, Ward BH, Woodrum DE: Aberrant left pulmonary artery. Clinical and embryologic factors. *Chest* 72:67, 1977.

3. Binet JP, Conso JF, Losay J, Narcy Ph, Raynaud EJ, Beaufils Fr, Dor C, Bruniaux J: Ductus arteriosus sling: Report of a newly recognized anomaly and its surgical correction. *Thorax* 33:72, 1978.

4. Brandt PWT, Clarkson PM, Barratt-Boyes BG, Neutze JM: An unusual esophageal indentation caused by a long tortuous patent ductus arteriosus. *Australas Radiol* 17:394, 1973.

5. Barry A: The aortic derivatives in the human adult. *Anat Rec* 111:221, 1951.

6. Berman W Jr, Yabek SM, Dillon I, Neal JF, Ake B, Burnstein J: Vascular ring due to left aortic arch and right descending aorta. *Circulation* 63:458, 1981.

7. Beabout JW, Stewart JR, Kincaid OW: Aberrant right subclavian artery. Dispute of commonly accepted concepts. *Am J Roentgenol* 92:855, 1964.

C

1. Contro S, Miller RA, White H, Potts WJ: Bronchial obstruction due to pulmonary artery anomalies: 1. Vascular sling. *Circulation* tion 17:418, 1958.

2. Congdon ED: Transformation of the aortic arch system during the development of the human embryo. Carnegie Trust. Washington. Publ 277. *Contrib Embryol* 1(68):47, 1922.

3. Campbell CD, Wernly JA, Koltip PC, Vitullo D, Replogle RL: Aberrant left pulmonary artery (pulmonary artery sling): Successful repair and 24-year follow-up report. *Am J Cardiol* 45:316, 1980.

4. Castaneda AR: Pulmonary artery sling (editorial). *Ann Thorac Surg* 28:210, 1979.

5. Cohen SR, Landing BH: Tracheostenosis and bronchial abnormalities associated with pulmonary artery sling. *Ann Otol Rhinol Laryngol* 85:582, 1976.

6. Capitanio MA, Ramos R, Kirkpatrick JA: Pulmonary sling. Roentgen Observations. *Am J Roentgenol* 112:28, 1971.

7. Clarkson PM, Ritter DG, Rahimtaoola SH, Hallermann FJ, McGoon DC: Aberrant left pulmonary artery. *Am J Dis Child* 113:373, 1967.

D

1. Derrick JR, Stoeckle H: Bronchial obstruction secondary to an aberrant pulmonary artery. *Am J Dis Child* 99:830, 1960.

2. Dunn JM, Gordon I, Chrispin AR, de Leval MR, Stark J: Early and late results of surgical correction of pulmonary artery sling. *Ann Thorac Surg* 28:230, 1979.

3. D'Cruz IA, Cautez T, Namin EP, Licata R, Hastreiter A: Right-sided aorta. Part II. Right aortic arch, right descending aorta and associated anomalies. *Br Heart J* 28:725, 1966.

E

1. Ekstrom G, Sandblom P: Double aortic arch. *Acta Chir Scand* 102:183, 1951.

2. Ericsson NO, Soderland S: Compression of the trachea by an anomalous innominate artery. *J Pediatr Surg* 4:424, 1969.

3. Edwards JE: Anomalies of the derivatives of the aortic arch system. *Med Clin North Am* (July) 925, 1948.

F

1. Fineberg C, Stofman HC: Tracheal compression caused by an anomalous innominate artery arising from a brachiocephalic trunk. *J Thorac Surg* 37:214, 1959.

G

1. Glaevecke H, Doehle H: Ueber eine seltene Angeborene. Anomalie der Pulmonalarterie. *Munchen Med Wschr* 44:950, 1897.

2. Gumbiner, CH, Mullins CE, McNamara DG: Pulmonary artery sling. *Am J Cardiol* 45:311, 1980.

3. Gross RE, Neuhauser EBD: Compression of the trachea or esophagus by vascular anomalies. Surgical therapy in 40 cases. *Pediatrics* 7:69, 1951.

4. Godtfredsen J, Wennerold A, Efsen F, Lauridsen P: Natural history of vascular ring with clinical manifestations. A follow-up study of 11 unoperated cases. *Scand J Thorac Cardiovasc Surg* 11:75, 1977.

5. Gross RE: Surgical relief for tracheal obstruction from a vascular ring. *N Engl J Med* 233:586, 1945.

6. Gross RE: Surgical treatment for dysphagia lusoria. *Ann Surg* 124:532, 1946.

7. Gross RE, Ware PF: The surgical significance of aortic arch anomalies. *Surg Gynecol Obstet* 83:435, 1946.

8. Gross RE: Arterial malformations which cause compression of the trachea or esophagus. *Circulation* XI:124, 1955.

9. Grover FL, Norton JB, Webb GE, Trinkle JK: Pulmonary sling. *J Thorac Cardiovasc Surg* 69:295, 1975.

H

1. Hiller HG, Maclean AD: Pulmonary artery ring. *Acta Radiol* 48:434, 1957.

2. Higashino SM, Ruttenberg HD: Double aortic arch associated with complete transposition of the great vessels. *Br Heart J* 30:579, 1968.

3. Han BD, Dunbar JS, Bove K, Rosenkrantz JG: Pulmonary vascular sling with tracheobronchial stenosis and hypoplasia of the right pulmonary artery. *Pediatr Radiol* 9:113, 1980.

4. Hatten HP Jr, Lorman JG, Rosenbaum HD: Pulmonary sling in the adult. *Am J Roentgen* 128:919, 1977.

5. Hellenbrand WE, Kelley MJ, Talner NS, Stansel HC Jr, Berman MA: Cervical aortic arch with retroesophageal aortic obstruction: Report of a case with successful surgical intervention. *Ann Thorac Surg* 26:86, 1978.

J

1. Jue KL, Raghib G, Amplatz K, Adams P Jr, Edwards JE: Anomalous origin of the left pulmonary artery from the right pulmonary artery. Report of 2 cases and review of the literature. *Am J Roentgen* 95:598, 1965.

K

1. Kale MK, Rafferty RE, Carton RW: Aberrant left pulmonary artery presenting as a mediastinal mass. Report of a case in an adult. *Arch Intern Med* 125:121, 1970.

2. Kirklin JW, Clagett OT: Vascular "rings" producing respiratory obstruction in infants. *Proc Mayo Clin* 25:360, 1950.

3. King HA, Walker D: Pulmonary artery sling. *Thorax* 39:462, 1984.

L

1. Lenox CC, Crisler C, Zuberbuhler JR, Park SC, Neches WH, Mathews RA, Fricker FJ, Golding LA: Anomalous left pulmonary artery: Successful management. *J Thorac Cardiovasc Surg* 77:748, 1979.

2. Lincoln JCR, Deverall PB, Stark J, Aberdeen E, Waterston DJ: Vascular anomalies compressing the esophagus and trachea. *Thorax* 24:295, 1969.

3. Lochard J, Vert P, Chalnot P: Trajet aberrant de l'artere pul-

monaire gauche compriment l'origine de la bronche souche droite. *Ann Chir Thorac Cardiovasc* 17:458, 1963.

M

1. Morse HR, Gladding S: Bronchial obstruction due to misplaced left pulmonary artery. *Am J Dis Child* 89:351, 1955.

2. Mustard WT, Baylis CE, Fearon B, Pelton D, Trusler GA: Tracheal compression by the innominate artery in children. *Ann Thorac Surg* 8:312, 1969.

3. Mustard WT, Trimble AW, Trusler GA: Mediastinal vascular anomalies causing tracheal and esophageal compression and obstruction in childhood. *Can Med Assoc J* 87:1301, 1962.

4. Mayer JE Jr, Joyce LD, Reinke D, McGeachie R, Humphrey EW, Varco RL: Aberrant left pulmonary artery presenting as a right paratracheal mass in an adult. *J Thorac Cardiovasc Surg* 72:571, 1976.

5. McCormick TL, Kuhns LR: Tracheal compression by a normal aorta associated with right lung agenesis. *Radiology* 130:659, 1979.

6. Murthy K, Mattioli L, Diehl AM, Holder TM: Vascular ring due to left aortic arch, right descending aorta, and right patent ductus arteriosus. *J Pediatr Surg* 5:550, 1970.

7. Mullins CE, Gillette PC, McNamara DG: The complex of cervical aortic arch. *Pediatrics* 51:210, 1973.

N

1. Nadas AS, Fyler DC: *Pediatric Cardiology*. Philadelphia: Saunders, 1972, p. 497.

2. Neuhauser EBD: The roentgen diagnosis of double aortic arch and other anomalies of the great vessels. *Am J Roentgen* 56:1, 1946.

P

1. Potts WJ, Holinger PH, Rosenblum AH: Anomalous left pulmonary artery causing obstruction to right main bronchus: Report of a case. *JAMA* 155:1409, 1954.

2. Park SC, Siewers RD, Neches WH, Lenox CC, Zuberbuhler JR: Left aortic arch with right descending aorta and right ligamentum arteriosum. A rare form of vascular ring. *J Thorac Cardiovasc Surg* 71:779, 1976.

3. Phelan PD: Management of anomalous left pulmonary artery (letter). *J Thorac Cardiovasc Surg* 79:639, 1980.

4. Phelan PD, Venables AW: Management of pulmonary artery sling (anomalous left pulmonary artery arising from right pulmonary artery): A conservative approach. *Thorax* 33:67, 1978.

5. Philp T, Sumerling MD, Fleming J, Grainger RG: Aberrant left pulmonary artery. *Clin Radiol* 23:153, 1972.

6. Price DA, Slaughter RE, Fraser DKB: Abnormalities of the aortic arch system compressing the esophagus and trachea. *Aust Pediatr J* 18:46, 1982.

Q

1. Quist-Hanssen S: Mutual compression of the right main bronchus and an abnormal left pulmonary artery as causes of the death of a 7 week old child. *Acta Paediat* 37:87, 1949.

R

1. Rheuban KS, Ayres N, Still JG, Alford B: Pulmonary artery sling: A new diagnostic tool and clinical review. *Pediatrics* 69:472, 1982.

2. Rowe LE, Lowry LD, Keane WM, Fallenjad M: Aortic arch anomalies in adult disorders of deglutition. *Ann Otol* 87:498, 1978.

3. Roesler M, de Leval M, Chrispin A, Stark J: Surgical management of vascular ring. *Ann Surg* 197:139, 1983.

S

1. Scheid P: Missbildung des Trachealskelettes und der linken Arteria pulmonalis mit Erstickungstod bei 7 Monate Altem Kind. *Z Path* 52:114, 1938.

2. Stewart JR, Kincaid OW, Edwards JE: *An Atlas of Vascular Rings and Related Malformations of the Aortic Arch System*. Springfield, Ill.: Charles C Thomas, 1964.

3. Symbas PN, Shuford WH, Edwards FK, Sehdera JS: Vascular ring. *J Thorac Cardiovasc Surg* 61:149, 1971.

4. Sprague PL, Kennedy JC: Anomalous left pulmonary artery with an unusual barium swallow. *Pediatr Radiol* 4:188, 1976.

5. Shuford WH, Sybers RG: *The Aortic Arch and Its Malformations with Emphasis on the Angiographic Features*. Springfield, Ill.: Charles C Thomas, 1974.

6. Sade RM, Rosenthal A, Fellows K, Castaneda AR: Pulmonary artery sling. *J Thorac Cardiovasc Surg* 69:333, 1975.

7. Scherer D, Westcott JL: Dextrocardia, left aortic arch and tracheal compression. An unusual type of vascular ring. *Radiology* 103:383, 1972.

8. Stone DN, Bein ME, Garris JB: Anomalous left pulmonary artery: Two new adult cases. *Am J Roentgenol* 135:1259, 1980.

9. Stewart S III, Edmunds LH Jr, Kirklin JW, Allarde RR: Spontaneous breathing with continuous positive airway pressure after open intracardiac operations in infants. *J Thorac Cardiovasc Surg* 65:37, 1973.

T

1. Turner W: *Br Foreign Med Chir Rev* 30:173, 1962.

2. Tonkin CL, Elliott LP, Bargeron LM Jr: Concomitant axial cineangiography and barium esophagoscopy in the evaluation of vascular rings. *Radiology* 135:69, 1980.

3. Turner AF, Pacuilli JR, Lau FY, Mikity VG, Johnson JL: Partial tracheal obstruction due to anomalous origin of the left pulmonary artery. *Calif Med* 114:59, 1971.

V

1. Von Siebold CT: Ringfermiger aorten-bogen bei einem neugeboraen blansuchtigen. *Kinde J Geburtsch Faruenzimmer-Kinderkrank* 16:294, 1837.

2. Van Praagh R, Van Praagh S, Vlad P, Keith JD: Diagnosis of the anatomic types of congenital dextrocardia. *Am J Cardiol* 15:234, 1965.

W

1. Welsh TM, Munro IB: Congenital stridor caused by an aberrant pulmonary artery. *Arch Dis Child* 29:101, 1954.

2. Wittenborg MH, Tantiwongse T, Rosenberg BF: Anomalous course of left pulmonary artery with respiratory obstruction. *Radiology* 67:339, 1956.

3. Williams RG, Jaffe RB, Condon VR, Nixon GW: Unusual features of pulmonary sling. *Am J Roentgenol* 133:1065, 1979.

4. Wheeler PC, Wolff LJ, Stevens EM: Pseudovascular ring resulting from right lung agenesis, normal aortic arch and patent ductus arteriosus. *Am J Roentgenol* 98:365, 1966.

5. Wolman IJ: Congenital stenosis of the trachea. *Am J Dis Child* 61:1263, 1941.

6. Wolman IJ: Syndrome of constricting double aortic arch in infancy. Report of case. *J Pediatr* 14:527, 1939.

7. Wychulis AR, Kincaid OW, Danielson GK: Congenital vascular ring: surgical considerations and results of operation. *Mayo Clin Proc* 46:182, 1971.

8. Whitman G, Stephenson LW, Weinberg P: Vascular ring: Left cervical aortic arch, right descending aorta, and right ligamentum arteriosum. *J Thorac Cardiovasc Surg* 83:311, 1982.

Z

1. Zumbro GI, Treasure RL, Geiger JP: Respiratory obstruction in the newborn associated with increased volume and opacification of the hemithorax. *Ann Thorac Surg* 18:622, 1974.

39

COMPLETE TRANSPOSITION OF THE GREAT ARTERIES

DEFINITION

Complete transposition of the great arteries is a congenital cardiac anomaly in which the aorta arises entirely or in large part from the right ventricle,[1] and the pulmonary artery arises entirely or in large part from the left ventricle (ventriculoarterial discordant connection).

Although the phrase *complete transposition of the great arteries* may properly be applied whenever this situation exists no matter what the other aspects of the cardiac anomaly may be, in this chapter it is used to imply a cardiac anomaly with atrioventricular concordant connection and ventriculoarterial discordant connection. The phrase *complete*

transposition of the great arteries most appropriately describes this group, and the only reason that it is not used throughout in this chapter, rather than simply transposition of the great arteries (TGA), is simplification of expression. Thus, this chapter describes complete transposition of the great arteries, a phrase that is not applicable to patients with transposed great arteries and tricuspid or mitral atresia or double inlet left or right ventricle (see Chapters 26 and 44), or atrioventricular discordant connection (congenitally corrected transposition of the great arteries; see Chapter 43, Fig. 43-1).

HISTORICAL NOTE

The first morphologic description of transposition of the great arteries (TGA) is attributed to Baillie in 1797.[B1] The

---

[1] As in other chapters (see Chapters 40–46), the adjectives right or left modifying an atrium or ventricle refer to their morphology; the phrases right sided and left sided refer to position.

term *transposition of the aorta and pulmonary artery* was coined by Farre when he described the third known case of this anomaly in 1814, transposition (trans = across, ponere = to place), meaning that the aorta and pulmonary artery are displaced across the ventricular septum.[F1] In subsequent pathologic descriptions that included attempts to explain its embryologic basis, the word transposition was used to describe an anterior position of the aorta relative to the pulmonary artery, and by the early 1900s, it had become accepted practice to include any abnormal position of the aorta, regardless of its ventricular origin, under this heading.[A1] This broad confusing definition was clarified by Van Praagh and colleagues as recently as 1971, when they strongly advocated a return to Farre's original definition of transposition, and introduced the useful term *malposition* for those abnormal positions of the aorta in which both great arteries failed to be displaced across the ventricular septum.[V1] This literal meaning of transposition is now accepted by most pathologists and surgeons.

The recognition of TGA during life resulted from the observations of Fanconi in 1932 and Taussig in 1938.[T9] The importance of the early appearance of pulmonary vascular disease, even when the ventricular septum was intact, was described by Ferguson and colleagues in 1960[F2] and Ferencz in 1966.[F3]

The surgery of TGA commenced in 1950 when Blalock and Hanlon at the Johns Hopkins Hospital described a closed method of atrial septectomy[B2] designed to provide mixing of pulmonary and systemic venous return at atrial level. Edwards and Bargeron modified the Blalock-Hanlon procedure in 1964 by resuturing the septum so as to connect the right pulmonary veins to the right atrium (UAB).[E1]

In 1953, Lillehei and Varco described a partial physiologic correction (or atrial switch), consisting of the anastomosis of the right pulmonary veins to the right atrium and the inferior vena cava (IVC) to the left atrium,[L1] a technique that became known as the Baffes operation. Baffes operation incorporated the use of a homograft aortic tube to connect the IVC to the left atrium.[B3]

The palliation of TGA was revolutionized when Rashkind and Miller in Philadelphia introduced balloon atrial septostomy (BAS) in 1966.[R1,R2] However, in 1971 at Great Ormond Street Hospital in London, Tynan showed that BAS did not allow all babies with TGA to survive until repair.[T2] A modification of this procedure was introduced in 1975 by Park and colleagues with their substitution of a blade rather than a balloon at the end of the catheter.[P1]

Throughout the 1950s there were surgical attempts to correct TGA either at the atrial or great artery levels. The concept of a physiologic correction at the atrial level by switching the atrial septum so that caval return was directed to the left ventricle and pulmonary venous return to the right was first proposed by Albert at a meeting of the American College of Surgeons in 1954.[A2] This concept was amplified by Merendino and colleagues in 1957.[M1] The first successful operation of this type was accomplished by Senning in 1959 by refashioning the walls of the right atrium and the atrial septum.[S1,S3] Modifications were suggested by many, including Barnard and colleagues in 1962[B4] and Schumaker in 1961.[S2] We at the Mayo Clinic used the Senning procedure between 1960 and 1964 with some successes (a few of whom

are still alive and well today) but with many disappointing results, related in part to the fact that most of the infants and children had a large ventricular septal defect (VSD) and varying degrees of pulmonary vascular disease.[B24,K1] Mustard's procedure, in which the atrial septum is excised and a pericardial baffle is used to redirect caval flow, was devised in an attempt to create larger atria than were produced by the Senning procedure[T8] and was successfully introduced at the Toronto Sick Childrens Hospital in 1963 and reported in 1964.[M2] (Actually Wilson and colleagues described essentially the same operation in 1962.[W9]) Mustard's initial results were better than had been achieved by anyone using the Senning procedure, in part at least because Mustard had available to him at Toronto Sick Childrens Hospital a reservoir of young children with TGA and intact ventricular septum who had been well palliated by a Blalock-Hanlon operation. The Mustard technique soon was adopted in nearly all cardiac surgical centers. However, a slightly modified Senning repair was reintroduced by Quaegebeur, Rohmer, and Brom in 1977,[Q1] mainly because of persisting problems with baffle obstruction[B6,S5] and arrhythmia[A3,E2,Z1] following the Mustard procedure.

Soon after successful atrial swtich operations began, it became conventional to delay this definitive procedure for 12–24 months after BAS. In occasional patients, the Mustard procedure was extended to smaller infants by Dillard and colleagues in 1969,[D1] by Bonchek and Starr,[B5] and Subramanian and Wagner.[S4] The first substantiated proposal that repair was necessary and possible in the first 3 months in order to avoid a considerable prerepair mortality was from us (GLH).[B14]

TGA with large VSD remained a difficult problem throughout this early era because of a relatively high hospital mortality after repair and the rapid development of pulmonary vascular disease in many patients. However, enough successes were obtained with the atrial switch procedures to indicate the value of continuing to treat patients surgically in this subset. In 1972, Lindesmith and colleagues introduced the use of a palliative Mustard procedure, in which the VSD was left unclosed, for patients with a high pulmonary vascular resistance.[L2] The modification in which a large VSD is created in TGA with intact ventricular septum was used by Stark and colleagues in 1976.[S25]

Successes were few in patients with TGA, VSD, and important left ventricular outflow tract obstruction (LVOTO) in this early period of intracardiac surgery for TGA. Daicoff and colleagues in 1969 reported a few successful repairs by direct relief of the LVOTO associated with a venous switch by Mustard's technique.[D2] Later, in 1969, Rastelli and colleagues combined the intraventricular tunnel repair (left ventricle → aorta) of the double outlet right ventricle operation (see Chapter 40) with a rerouting valved extracardiac conduit (right ventricle → pulmonary artery) and closure of the origin of the pulmonary artery from the left ventricle to produce an anatomic repair of TGA, VSD, and LVOTO.[R3,R4]

The somewhat disappointing results of the atrial switch operation for TGA and large VSD continued to be a stimulus for the development of an arterial switch operation, particularly since the right (systemic) ventricle sometimes failed late postoperatively in these patients. Very early (1954) Mustard had described unsuccessful attempts to perform an arterial switch operation in seven patients, with transfer of the left coronary ostium to the pulmonary artery and use of a monkey lung as the oxygenator.[M3] Other reports of unsuccessful operations of this general type were those of Bailey and colleagues[B7] and Kay and Cross.[K2] Idriss and colleagues attempted such a procedure in two patients with an intact ventricular septum in 1961 using cardiopulmonary bypass (CPB), transferring the great vessels and a ring of aorta carrying the coronary arteries.[I1] Interest then lagged in this development in many centers, but a few groups persisted with efforts to perfect this approach. Jatene and colleagues in Brazil achieved a major breakthrough in 1975, with the first successful use of the arterial switch procedure, applying it in infants with TGA and VSD.[J1,J2] Soon after, Yacoub reported successful cases.[Y1] An important technical modification of the original Jatene procedure has been the demonstration by Lecompte and colleagues that direct anastomosis of both great arteries without the interposition of a tube graft is possible when the pulmonary artery bifurcation is transferred in front of the distal ascending aortic arch.[L3]

Yacoub's attempts in London to perform the same procedure in three infants with TGA and an intact ventricular septum were unsuccessful in 1972, but reports by Abe and colleagues[A4] in 1977 and Mauck and colleagues[M4] in 1978 indicated that such a repair was possible in infancy. However, most infants with intact ventricular septum did not survive arterial switching. Yacoub approached this problem of the low-pressure left ventricle's not being prepared for sustaining systemic pressure by performing pulmonary artery banding as a first stage.[Y2] However, the idea of performing the arterial switch operation for patients with TGA and intact ventricular septum in the neonatal period before left ventricular pressure falls rapidly developed, and Quaegebeur and Brom in Holland[Q3] and Castaneda in Boston[C1] have now demonstrated the feasibility of this approach.

As the arterial switch operation was evolving, the use of a valved extracardiac conduit to effect the anatomic repair was also developed. This was described simultaneously by Kaye[K7] and Stansel[S6] and earlier by Damus and colleagues[D3,D4] and consists of division of the pulmonary trunk and anastomosis of its proximal end to the posterior aspect of the ascending aorta. A valved conduit is placed between the right ventricle and distal pulmonary artery. The left ventricle thus becomes the systemic ventricle, the aortic valve remaining closed because of the higher upstream pressure. If a VSD is present, it is closed.

MORPHOLOGY

Right Ventricle

The right ventricle (RV) is normally positioned, hypertrophied, and large. Its inflow and sinus portions are essentially normal in their architecture. In about 90% of cases, there is a subaortic conus (infundibulum), and the aorta is rightward and anterior and ascends parallel to the posterior and leftward pulmonary trunk (artery) (Fig. 39-1). In such hearts there is also an infundibular (conal) septum, which in the absence of a ventricular septal defect (VSD), joins nor-

mally with the ventricular septum between the limbs of the septal band (trabecula septomarginalis, TSM). The infundibulum does not deviate to the left as in the normal heart but projects directly superiorly from the sinus portion of the ventricle (Fig. 39-2).

According to Anderson and colleagues, there is less wedging of the pulmonary artery between mitral and tricuspid valves in TGA than of the aorta in normal hearts.[A5] As a result, there is a larger area of contiguity between mitral and tricuspid valves than normally.[A5] These atrioventricular (AV) valves may be at virtually the same level, and the AV septum and the membranous interventricular septum are then smaller than usual or, rarely, even absent. The right fibrous trigone of the central fibrous body is abnormally shaped and attenuated.

In about 10% of hearts with TGA and intact ventricular septum,[V1,W1] the subaortic conus in the RV is absent or very hypoplastic. Then the aorta is either directly anterior or anterior and to the left of the pulmonary artery origin, or rarely posterior.[V1] In a few instances, however, a posteriorly placed aorta is associated with a subaortic conus.[B32] This combination may make the arterial switch operation difficult.

Left Ventricle

The left ventricle (LV) rarely contains an infundibulum (conus), there usually being pulmonary–mitral fibrous continuity comparable to the aortic–mitral continuity present in the normal heart (Fig. 39-3). In about 8% of hearts with TGA and most commonly in those with a VSD, a subpulmonary conus is present in the left ventricle.[V6,V1] The subpulmonary conus is frequently stenotic.[G6] In the majority of these cases, the aorta still lies anteriorly and to the right[S7] but it may be leftward or posterior.

Ventricular Wall Thickness, Cavity Shape, and Function

In the normal heart the left ventricular wall is thicker than the right ventricular wall in utero. After birth, the left ventricular wall thickness increases progressively, whereas the right ventricular wall becomes relatively thinner.[H2,S11]

In TGA, the right ventricular wall is considerably thicker than normal at birth and increases in thickness with age. The left ventricular wall thickness varies depending upon the presence or absence of a VSD and pulmonary stenosis. When the ventricular septum is intact and there is no significant pulmonary stenosis, the left ventricular wall is of normal thickness at birth and remains static as regards its wall thickness. It thus begins to be of less than normal thickness within a few weeks of birth and by 2–4 months of age is relatively thin walled.[B23,C14,D13,M26] When a VSD is present, left ventricular wall thickness increases slightly less than in the normal heart but remains well within the normal range during the first year of life.[H2,S11] When there is left ventricular outflow tract obstruction (LVOTO) (pulmonary stenosis), the evolution is similar, although when the obstruction is severe and the ventricular septum is intact, left ventricular

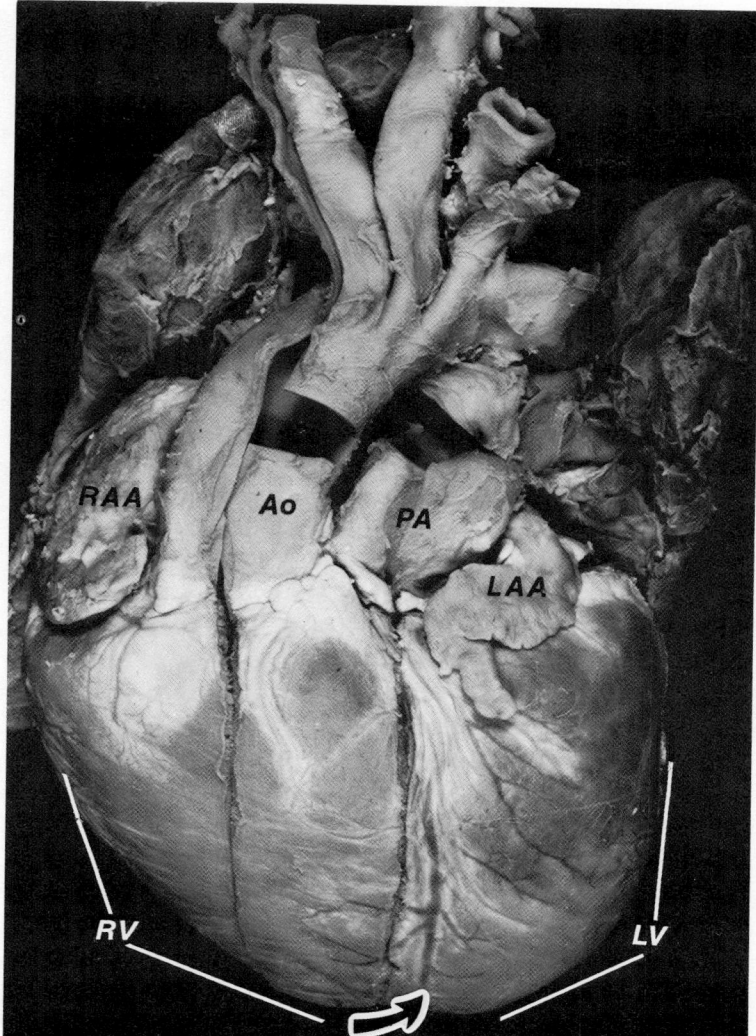

Figure 39-1 Specimen showing the external appearance of a heart with TGA (GLH). The infundibulum of the morphologically right ventricle extends directly superiorly from the sinus portion to give rise to a rightward anterior aorta. The pulmonary trunk lies parallel to the aorta in a posterior leftward position and arises from the morphologically left ventricle. The arrow points to the left anterior descending coronary artery.

Ao, aorta; LAA, left atrial appendage; LV, left ventricle; PA, pulmonary trunk; RAA, right atrial appendage; RV, right ventricle.

wall thickness eventually exceeds right ventricular wall thickness.[K3] Although left ventricular wall thickness is not equivalent to left ventricular work potential, it does reflect the functional capacity.

In infants with TGA, the left ventricular cavity is ellipsoid in shape at birth, as is the normal, but soon becomes banana shaped.[B6] Alterations in left ventricular function no doubt occur with this geometric change.

Right ventricular function is usually normal in TGA in the perinatal period. Thereafter, when the ventricular septum is intact, the right ventricular end-diastolic volume is increased, and the right ventricular ejection fraction is decreased.[G2,J3] The depressed right ventricular ejection fraction is unlikely to be due to increased afterload or decreased preload and is probably due to depressed right ventricular function from relative myocardial hypoxia or the geometry of the chamber itself.[G2]

The left ventricular end-diastolic volume is increased, and the left ventricular ejection fraction is normal. The ratio of right ventricular end-diastolic and left ventricular end-diastolic volumes (normally 1), is increased to 1.46 ± 0.33.

Atria

The atria are normally formed. Right atrial size is usually increased above normal, particularly when the ventricular septum is intact.

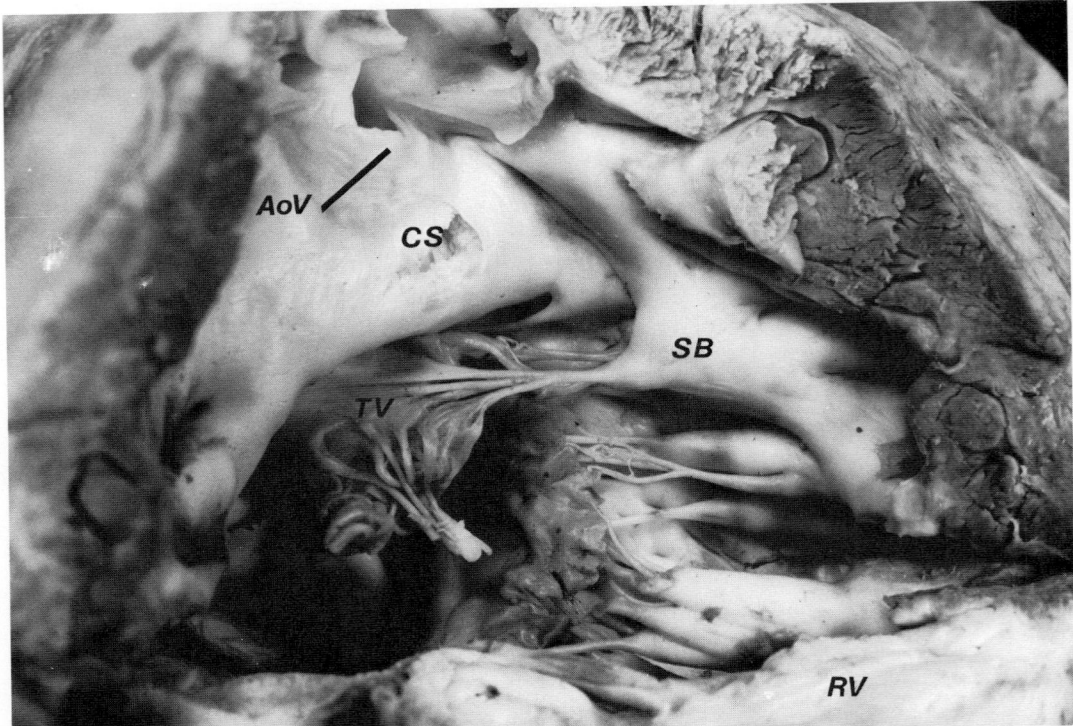

Figure 39-2   Specimen showing the interior of the right ventricle in a heart with TGA with an intact ventricular septum (GLH). The conal (infundibular) septum inserts in a normal way between the two divisions of the septal band (trabecula septomarginalis). These structures and the right ventricular free wall are hypertrophied. The infundibulum projects directly superiorly from the sinus portion of the ventricle rather than superiorly, anteriorly, and leftward, as in the normal heart, and gives origin to the aorta and aortic valve.

AoV, aortic valve; CS, conal septum; RV, right ventricle; SB, septal band; TV, tricuspid valve (one of the chordae has been cut).

Conduction System

The AV node and His bundle lie in a normal position although the AV node is abnormally shaped and may be partly engulfed in the right trigone.[B8] The left bundle branch originates more distally than usual from the bundle of His and as a single cord rather than a sheath; damage to the bifurcation of the bundle at the time of VSD closure is therefore more likely to produce a complete heart block than in the normally structured heart.[B8]

Coronary Arteries

The coronary arteries in TGA arise from the aortic sinuses that face the pulmonary artery, irrespective of the interrelationships of the great arteries.[G10] Thus, the noncoronary sinus is usually the anterior one.

The right coronary usually arises from the rightward posterior sinus and the left coronary from the leftward posterior sinus. Both usually have a normal branching pattern, although not infrequently the right coronary gives origin to the circumflex artery that passes to the left behind the pulmonary artery[E3,R6] (Fig. 39-4).

The variations of coronary artery anatomy in hearts with TGA are considerable and important to the surgeon when doing the arterial switch operation (Fig. 39-4).[Y3] The right coronary artery arises from the right sinus in 90% and from the left sinus in 10% of cases. The usual pattern of origin and distribution (Fig. 39-4[a]) is present in over 60% of cases. Both coronary arteries arise from the right sinus (from a single or double ostium) in 10% of cases. Shaher and Puddu[S28] reported two cases in which a single coronary artery arose from the left sinus and one case in which both right and left coronary arteries arose from the anterior, noncoronary sinus.

Of considerable potential significance in the atrial switch (Mustard or Senning) operation is the course of the sinus node artery in hearts with TGA. This artery usually arises from the right coronary close to its origin and passes superiorly and rightward, usually partly embedded in the most superior portion of the limbus of the atrial septum where it can be damaged if this portion of the atrial septum is widely excised.[T6] It then usually passes behind or branches to form an arterial circle around the caval-atrial junction.[A5]

Pulmonary Vascular Disease

The frequent occurrence of pulmonary vascular disease in patients with TGA has been well documented.[C2,F2,F3,F6,N1,V10]

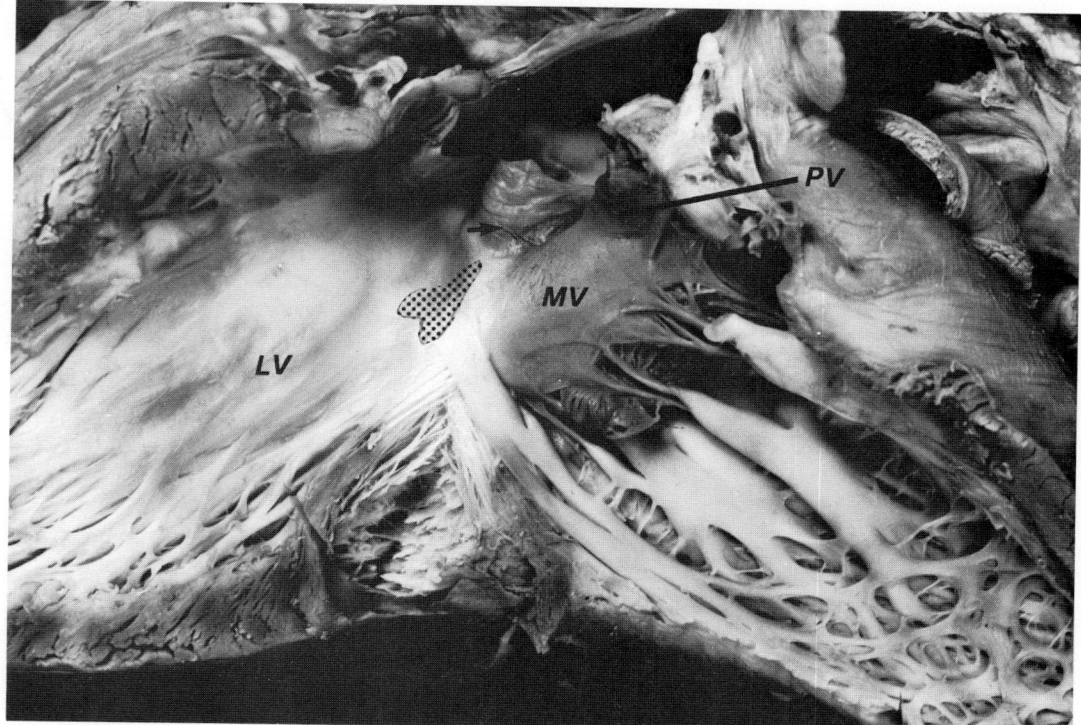

Figure 39-3 Specimen showing the interior of the left ventricle in a heart with TGA (GLH). There is fibrous continuity between the mitral valve and pulmonary valve analogous to the aortic–mitral continuity present in the normal heart. The bundle of His penetrates the right fibrous trigone (arrow). The approximate course of the left bundle branch is shown by the cross-hatched area.
LV, left ventricle; MV, mitral valve; PV, pulmonary valve.

The histologic changes in the pulmonary arteries are comparable to those found in isolated large VSD and can be graded in a similar fashion according to the criteria described by Heath and Edwards or by Reid and colleagues (see Chapter 20, "Pulmonary Vascular Disease" in Section 1, Morphology).

In addition, however, pulmonary microthrombi are present in about 25% of the lungs examined at autopsy[N3] or on lung biopsy.[W7] Pulmonary microthrombi produce a variety of intimal lesions, including eccentric cushion lesions and occlusion with recanalization of nonlaminar intimal fibrosis that can result in irregular fibrous septa within the vessel lumen.[N3] These changes occur with and without the laminar and circumferential changes secondary to hypertensive pulmonary vascular disease and are of uncertain etiology and significance. They are seldom severe enough per se to cause an increase in pulmonary vascular resistance and occur with equal frequency in TGA with intact ventricular septum, large VSD, and large VSD and LVOTO.[N3]

Using lung biopsy specimens, Wagenvoort and colleagues have also described wall thinning and dilatation of pulmonary arteries and, to a lesser extent, pulmonary veins in TGA with intact ventricular septum, particularly when the hematocrit is high.[W7] Yamaki and Tezuka[Y5] also noted that medial hypertrophy was retarded in TGA in the first 5 months of life compared with isolated large VSD and postu-

lated that this weakened the arterial wall and might be a reason for the accelerated hypertensive changes that appear mainly after this age in TGA. The frequency and time of appearance of pulmonary vascular disease varies according to whether or not there is a large VSD, patent ductus arteriosus (PDA), or LVOTO.

When the *ventricular septum is essentially intact*, the incidence of pulmonary vascular disease at autopsy in infants is little different from patients with TGA and a large VSD (Table 39-1). However, this is misleading, and in clinical series only 10%–15% of such infants have significant pulmonary vascular disease. The incidence rises significantly, however, beyond 1 year of age, when 14 of 30 (47%) are known to have significant pulmonary vascular disease[E7,N3] (Fig. 39-5). It is likely that a large patent ductus arteriosus (PDA) has an effect similar to that of a large VSD.

When a *moderate or large VSD* is present, about 25% of infants coming to autopsy at an average age of about 6 months have severe pulmonary vascular disease (grade 3 changes or more), and the incidence rises to 80% or more beyond 12 months of age (Table 39-1). In patients coming to operation, the incidence is lower, although in some patients important pulmonary vascular disease previously unrecognized is present late postoperatively (Fig. 39-6). The severity and rapidity of onset of pulmonary vascular disease is greater in patients with TGA and VSD than in those with

Single Coronary Artery Origin

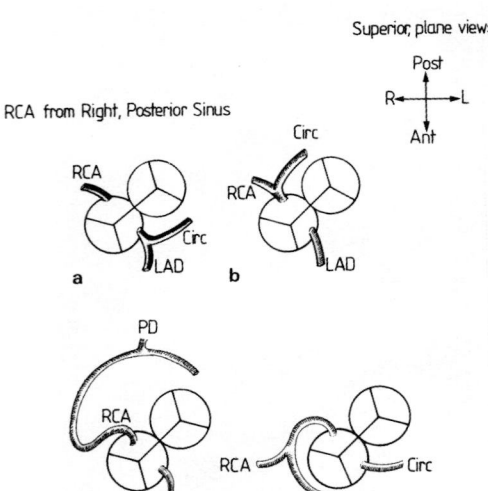

RCA from Right, Posterior Sinus

Superior, plane views

```
        Post
    R ——+—— L
        Ant
```

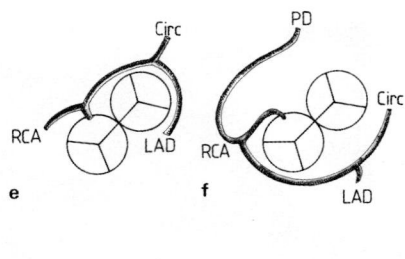

e   f

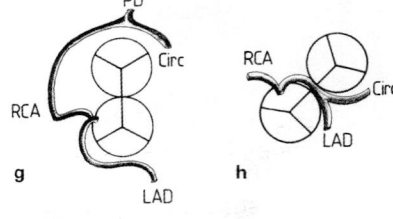

g   h

Aorta in Right, Posterior Position

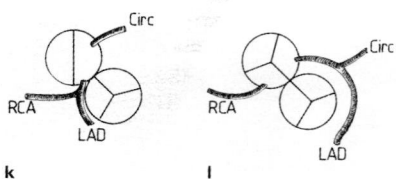

k   l

Aorta in Left, Anterior Position

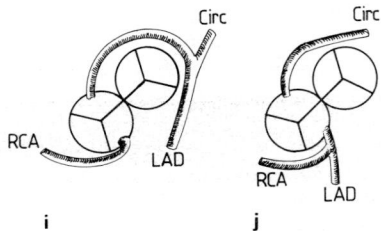

RCA from Left, Anterior Sinus

i   j

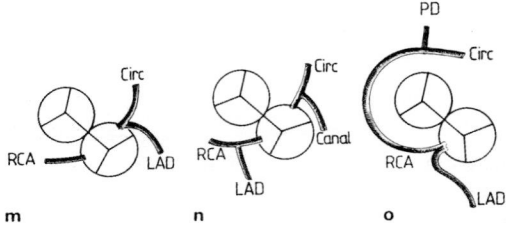

m   n   o

Figure 39-4 Superior views of the coronary arterial patterns as seen in 141 autopsy cases (GLH). In *a–j, the aorta was situated to the right of the pulmonary artery,* either in a side-by-side, oblique, or anterior position. Cases with one or two coronary ostia from the same sinus have been grouped together.

In (*a*), the right coronary artery (RCA) arises from the posterior sinus and the left coronary artery from the left sinus (present in 62% of specimens). In (*b*), the circumflex coronary artery (Circ) arises from the right coronary artery (10%). In (*c*), the right coronary artery supplies the posterior descending (PD) and left atrioventricular groove arteries (5%), and in (*d*), the left anterior descending coronary artery (LAD), which arises from the right coronary artery, passes anteriorly to the aorta (1%).

Origins of the coronary arteries from a single sinus are illustrated in (*e*)–(*h*) and (*o*). In all cases, the single coronary arterial origin was from the right or posterior sinus (GLH). In (*e*), the left coronary artery passes posteriorly to the pulmonary artery, (4%), whereas in (*f*), the left coronary artery passes anteriorly to the aorta (2%). In (*g*), the LAD passes anteriorly to the aorta, and the circumflex arises as a continuation of the RCA (1%). In (*h*), the left coronary artery passes between the aorta and pulmonary artery (3%).

The right coronary artery arises from the left, anterior sinus in 10% of specimens. In (*i*), the left coronary artery arises from the right posterior sinus (6%), and in (*j*) the LAD arises from the RCA and the circumflex coronary artery from the right posterior sinus (4%).

In (*k, l*), two cases are illustrated with *the aorta in a right, posterior position* in which the coronary artery origins are similar to those in normally connected great arteries, with variations in the origin of LAD.

In (*m*) to (*o*), three cases are illustrated with *the aorta in a left, anterior position.* In (*m*), the RCA arises from the right posterior sinus and the left coronary artery from the left posterior sinus. In (*n*), the LAD arises from RCA, and an additional conal branch arises from the circumflex coronary artery. In (*o*), a single coronary artery arises from the right, posterior sinus.

Table 39-1 Incidence of significant (≥ grade 3 Heath-Edwards) pulmonary vascular disease at autopsy in patients with TGA aged 3 months and older.

| | Intact Ventricular Septum | | | | | | Large VSD | | | | | |
| | 3–12 Months[a] | | | >12 Months[a] | | | 3–12 Months[a] | | | >12 Months[a] | | |
Author	n	No.	%	n	No.	%	n	No.	%	n	No.	%
Ferencz[F3]	13[b]	3	23%	12	7	58%	14	1	7%	18	10	56%
Viles et al.[V10]	4	1	25%	3	2	67%	6	3	50%	9	9	100%
Newfeld et al.[N1]	12	0	0%	26	4	15%	17	5	29%	28	26	93%
Clarkson et al.[C2]	6[b]	2	33%	9	4	44%	7	2	29%	5	2	40%
Total	35	6	17%	50	17	34%	44	11	25%	60	47	78%

KEY: VSD, ventricular septal defect; No., number with pulmonary vascular disease.
[a] Age at death.
[b] Includes patients with small ventricular septal defect.

isolated VSD.[F7,L7,N1,V10,W7] The mechanisms for this are multiple and complex but may include hypoxemia and a prominent bronchopulmonary collateral circulation.[A10]

When there is LVOTO, pulmonary vascular disease is less common[V10] (Fig. 39-7). When the ventricular septum was intact, 2 (14%) of 14 patients (one of whom had dynamic and one fibrous LVOTO) developed significant pulmonary vascular disease (GLH). It occurs somewhat more commonly when there is a VSD associated with LVOTO. Thus, in 12 such patients studied pre- or postoperatively between 3 and 11 months of age, 4 had moderate pulmonary vascular disease, whereas in those 1 year or older the incidence was higher (GLH; Fig. 39-7).

Coexisting Anomalies

About half (51%) the hearts with TGA have no other anomaly except for a naturally occurring atrial septal defect (ASD) or patent foramen ovale or PDA.[F5] Left ventricular outflow tract obstruction is present in about 5%–10%, a VSD (all sizes) in about 30% (about one-third of which are small), and a combination of VSD and LVOTO (pulmonary stenosis or atresia) in 10%.[C9,F5] These coexisting anomalies are an integral part of the complex morphology of TGA.

Ventricular Septal Defect

PERIMEMBRANOUS. About one-third of the VSDs in hearts with TGA are typical perimembranous defects (Table 39-2). These lie adjacent to the membranous ventricular septum and the tricuspid anulus at the anteroseptal tricuspid valve commissure and inferior to the normally positioned conal (infundibulum) septum (Fig. 39-8). They may extend in any direction, just as do isolated perimembranous VSDs (see Chapter 20, Figs. 20-2 through 20-5). Viewed from the left ventricular side, the VSD is separated from the pulmonary valve by a muscular ridge so that it is not immediately subpulmonary (Fig. 39-8).

MALALIGNMENT. A little less than a third of the VSDs in hearts with TGA are cradled within the limbs of the septal band, or TSM, and associated with malalignment of the infundibular septum and ventricular outflow obstruction. The VSD may or may not extend back to the tricuspid anulus. These are termed *malalignment VSDs*, since in them the conal (infundibular) septum fails to insert within the Y of the septal band and is frequently less bulky than normal.

Often the infundibular septum is displaced to the left of the anterior division of the septal band and is associated with varying degrees of subpulmonary LVOTO[V1] (Figs. 39-9 and 39-10). In other cases, the infundibular septum is displaced to the right (Fig. 39-11), with the result that the VSD may be subpulmonary and the pulmonary artery may override onto the right ventricle. This type of TGA may be associated with subaortic stenosis.[M5,S8] It may also be associated with aortic arch obstruction (arch hypoplasia, coarctation, or interruption)[M5,S8] and is related to and merges with double outlet right ventricle with subpulmonary VSD[G1,T1,V3] (see Chapter 40, "Taussig-Bing Heart" in section on Morphology).

SUBAORTIC. There is a smaller group of malalignment VSDs in which there is no outflow tract obstruction. In them, the VSD is immediately subaortic and the aorta is usually leftward and anterior.

SUBARTERIAL. This type of VSD, with absence or near absence of the infundibular (conal) septum, occurs rarely[H1,V2] (Table 39-2). Because of the absence of the conal septum, the upper defect margin is formed by the confluent aortic and pulmonary valves[L4] (Fig. 39-12).

MUSCULAR. About a quarter of the VSDs are muscular in hearts with TGA, as in isolated VSD (see Chapter 20). These may occur in any part of the septum and occasionally are multiple (Table 39-2, Fig. 39-13). Most muscular defects are in the midseptum.

ATRIOVENTRICULAR CANAL TYPE. A type of perimembranous VSD, which extends inferiorly beneath the tricuspid leaflet, is a little more common in TGA than in otherwise normal hearts (see Chapter 20, "Ventricular Septal Defect beneath Tricuspid Septal Leaflet" in Section 1, Morphology). The bundle of His ascends from the AV node along the posteroinferior margin[M6] (see Chapter 20, Fig. 20-5). Rarely, a VSD lying inferiorly in the inlet septum is associated with overriding of the tricuspid valve, and this unusual variant also occurs more commonly in hearts with TGA than in otherwise normal hearts. The ventricular septum fails to reach the crux cordis, and the conduction tissue is grossly abnormal, arising from an anomalously positioned posterolateral node sited where the malaligned ventricular septum makes contact with the AV junction.

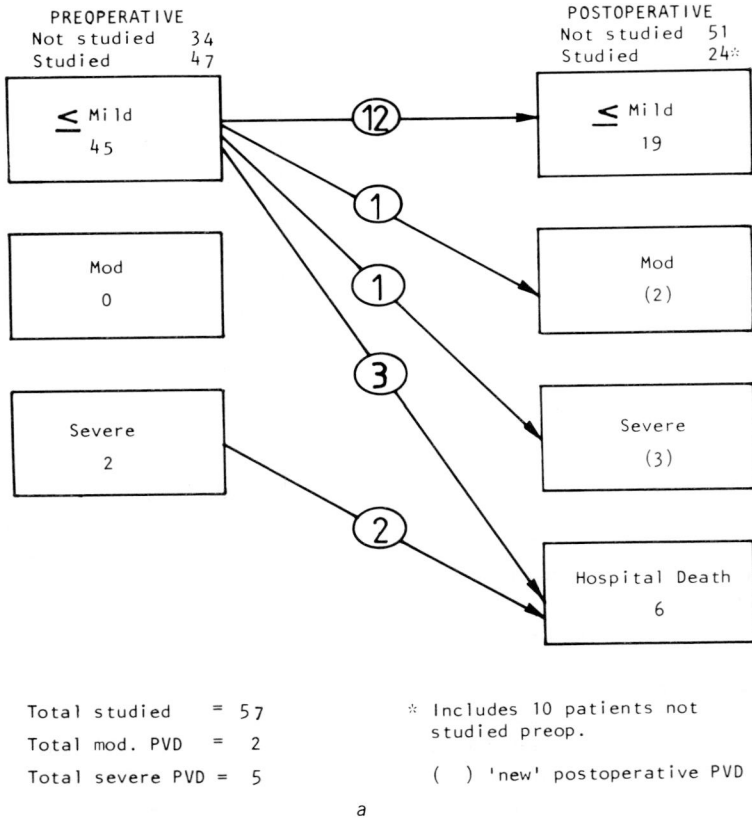

PREOPERATIVE
Not studied   34
Studied   47

POSTOPERATIVE
Not studied   51
Studied   24※

≤ Mild
45

⑫ → ≤ Mild
19

Mod
0

① → Mod
(2)

① → Severe
(3)

Severe
2

③

② → Hospital Death
6

Total studied   = 57
Total mod. PVD   = 2
Total severe PVD   = 5

※ Includes 10 patients not
studied preop.

( ) 'new' postoperative PVD

a

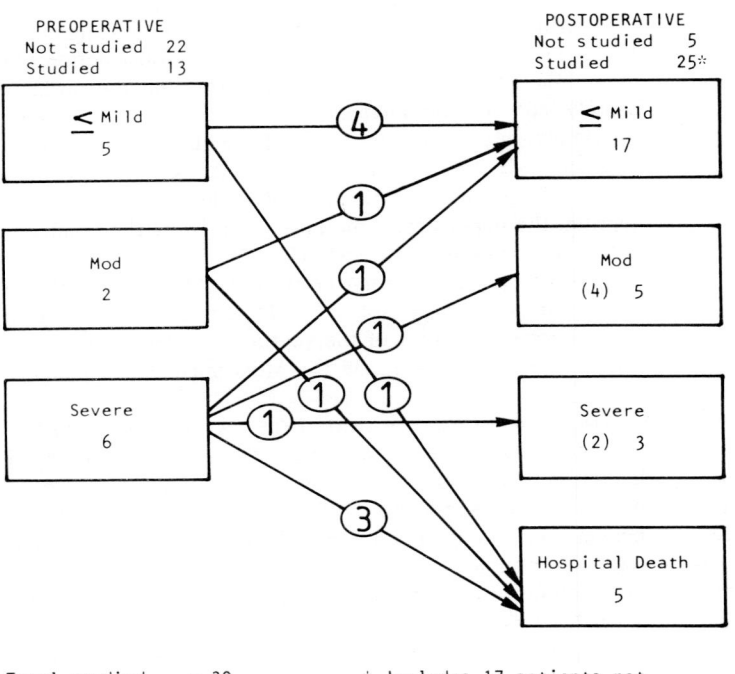

PREOPERATIVE
Not studied   22
Studied   13

POSTOPERATIVE
Not studied   5
Studied   25※

≤ Mild
5

④ → ≤ Mild
17

Mod
2

①

①

Severe
6

① ①

① ①

① → Severe
(2) 3

③

Mod
(4) 5

Hospital Death
5

Total studied   = 30
Total mod. PVD   = 6
Total severe PVD   = 8

※ Includes 17 patients not
studied preop.

( ) 'new' postoperative PVD.

b

Figure 39-5 Assessment of pulmonary vascular disease (PVD) in simple TGA (see footnote 3 for definition), but excluding those with left ventricular outflow tract obstruction (GLH; 1964–1984).

(*a*) Aged 3–11 months at operation.
(*b*) Aged 1 year or older at operation.

"Studied" means an accurate assessment of PVD made close to the time of operation (preoperative) and on follow-up (postoperative) either by calculation of pulmonary vascular resistance or by histologic assessment of the pulmonary vessels at autopsy. In situations in which the two criteria were discrepant (rare), histologic grading (Gr.) was used. The following grades were used: Mild, pulmonary vascular resistance (PVR) < 4 units·m² and/or lung histology Heath-Edwards Gr. < 2; Moderate, PVR 4–8 units·m² or Heath-Edwards Gr. 2; Severe, PVR > 8 units·m² or Heath-Edwards Gr. 3–6.

Mod, moderate; PVD, pulmonary vascular disease.

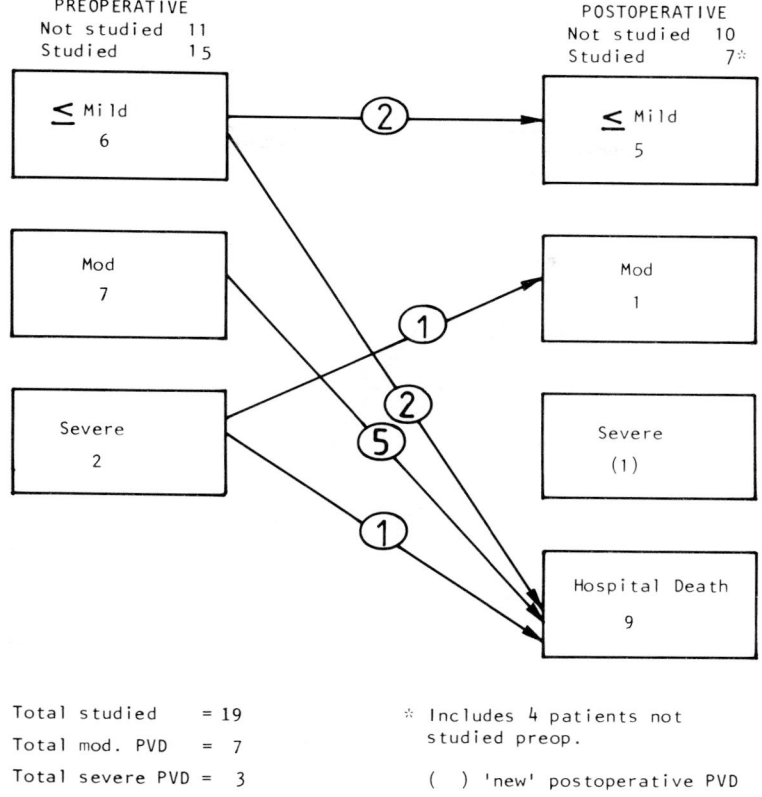

Figure 39-6 Assessment of pulmonary vascular disease in patients with TGA and moderate-sized or large VSD aged 3–11 months at atrial switch repair (GLH; 1964–1984). (See Fig. 39-5 for details.) PVD, pulmonary vascular disease.

Left Ventricular Outflow Tract Obstruction (Pulmonary Stenosis)

LVOTO is a rather common coexisting anomaly in hearts with TGA (Table 39-3). The incidence and morphology vary according to whether a VSD is present.[R3,S7,S9,S10,V5]

INTACT VENTRICULAR SEPTUM. LVOTO is present in about 20% of surgical cases of TGA with intact ventricular septum. In the majority, it is the result of leftward bulging of the muscular ventricular septum secondary to the higher right ventricular pressure (*dynamic obstruction*).[N4,S10] This may be particularly likely to occur if the aorta lies anterior and more to the left than usual with increased wedging of the subpulmonary area.[C12] The septum impinges against the anterior mitral leaflet in combination with abnormal systolic anterior leaflet motion. Thus, the mechanism is similar to that present in hypertrophic obstructive cardiomyopathy (see Chapter 33, "Dynamic Morphology of the Septum and Mitral Valve" in section on Morphology), but there is no asymmetric septal hypertrophy. The gradient may be contributed to by the high velocity of blood flow produced by the usually large pulmonary–systemic blood flow ratio and the deformation of the left ventricular outflow tract.[A9] When this dynamic type of obstruction is severe, a ridge of endocardial thickening is produced on the septum at its point of contact with the mitral leaflet[C6] (Fig. 39-14). Dynamic obstruction is not present at birth, but in untreated children or

those having a balloon septostomy it may develop and progress in severity thereafter.

Less commonly, the subpulmonary stenosis is due to a *subvalvar fibrous ridge* that extends onto the anterior mitral leaflet near its hinge. This lesion is analogous to discrete subvalvar aortic stenosis occurring in otherwise normal hearts with ventriculoarterial concordant connection (see Chapter 32, "Morphology" in Section 2) and is usually localized but may be the tunnel type. At times, there may be difficulty in distinguishing this from the secondary fibrous ridge that develops in the dynamic type of obstruction.

Rarely, the LVOTO may be due to *fibrous tags* arising from the mitral apparatus or the membranous septum. *Valvar stenosis* is quite uncommon in this situation and annular hypoplasia even less common. However, Shaher and colleagues found 4 of 12 autopsy specimens of TGA with intact septum and pulmonary stenosis with valvar stenosis and 3 with a small pulmonary ring. There were also 3 examples of a bicuspid pulmonary valve.[S9] In an angiographic study only 2 of 176 children with TGA and intact septum had valvar pulmonary stenosis (UAB).[S10]

VENTRICULAR SEPTAL DEFECT. In hearts with TGA and a VSD, LVOTO (pulmonary stenosis) coexists in 30%–35% of cases.[R3,S7,S9,S10,V5] The stenosis is often more severe and more complex than in hearts with TGA and intact ventricular septum. The stenosis is usually subvalvar, either in the form

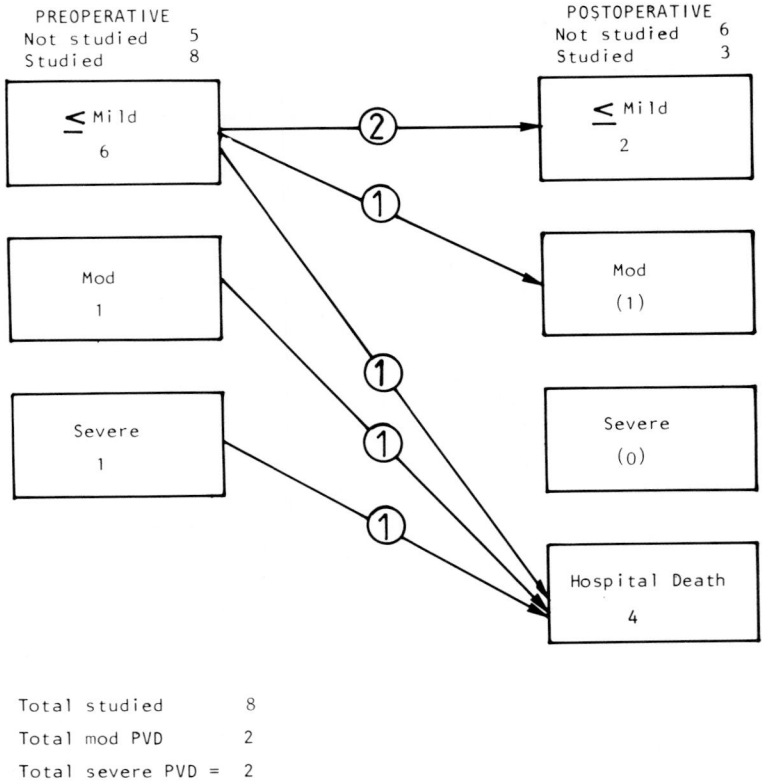

Total studied   8
Total mod PVD   2
Total severe PVD =   2

Figure 39-7 Assessment of pulmonary vascular disease in TGA, moderate or large VSD, and left ventricular outflow tract obstruction in patients 1 year or older at operation (GLH; 1964–1984). (See legend for Fig. 39-5 for details.)
PVD, pulmonary vascular disease.

Table 39-2 Types of VSD present in autopsy series of hearts with TGA (GLH; *n* = 81).

Type of VSD	n		% of Total
Perimembranous	27		33%
Conal septal malalignment	24		30%
Displaced to left		10	
Displaced to right		10	
Subaortic[a]		4	
Subarterial (conal septal deficiency)	4		5%
Muscular	22[b]		27%
Basal (posterior, inflow)		6	
Mid septum		12	
Apical septum		1	
High anterior septum		3	
AV canal (inlet)[c]	4		5%
Total	81		100%

NOTE: See Chapter 1 for GLH subdivisions of the right ventricular side of the ventricular septum used here in the classification of muscular VSD. See text for definition of malalignment VSD.

[a] In two, the aorta was anterior and to the left, in one it was rightward and posterior.

[b] Multiple VSDs present in six.

[c] In this group, an inlet VSD was up against the right tricuspid anulus; in one patient the tricuspid valve was overriding.

of a localized fibrous ring, a long, tunnel type of fibromuscular narrowing, or a muscular obstruction related to protrusion of the infundibular septum into the medial or anterior aspect of the left ventricular outflow tract.[V5] When the septal displacement is severe, it may not only narrow the left ventricular outflow tract but also displace it posteriorly, so that it no longer lies in its normal position anterior to the mitral leaflet (Figs. 39-15 and 39-16).

An important but fortunately rare form of subvalvar stenosis is attachment of the anterior mitral leaflet to the muscular outflow septum by anomalous fibrous or chordal tissue[R3,R7,S7] (Fig. 39-17). Sometimes this occurs in combination with a cleft anterior mitral leaflet with or without mitral valve overriding or straddling.[M7] Other rare causes of subvalvar pulmonary stenosis associated with TGA and VSD are parachute mitral valve[R3,S7] and accessory mitral leaflet tissue.

Subvalvar LVOTO can also be caused by an aneurysm of the membranous ventricular septum, which bulges as a windsock into the left ventricular outflow tract due to the higher right ventricular pressure. Its walls are thick and usually immobile, at least by the time operation is performed, and the VSD is either below the aneurysm or within its sac.[S10,V4] However, some, or perhaps most of these so-called aneurysms are examples of redundant fibrous tissue prolaps-

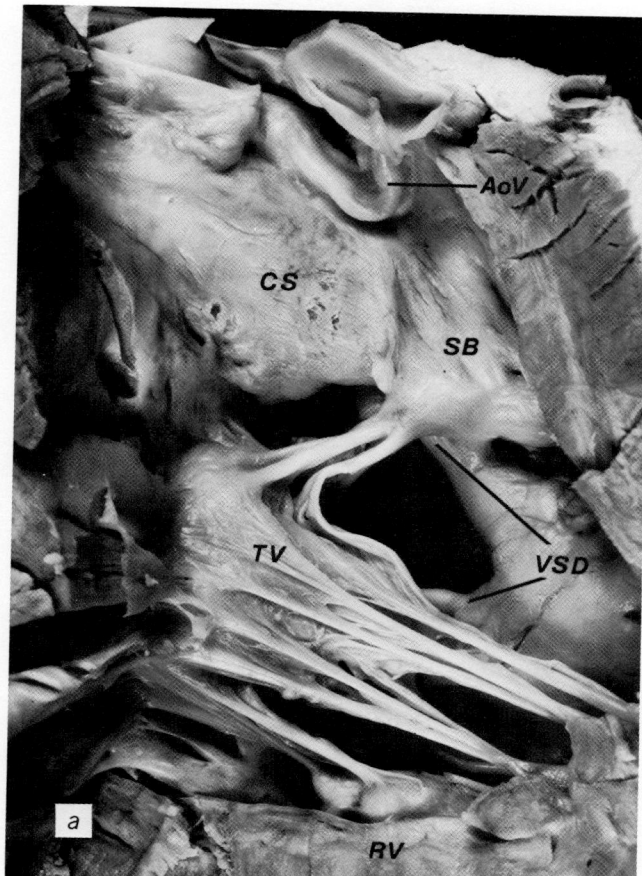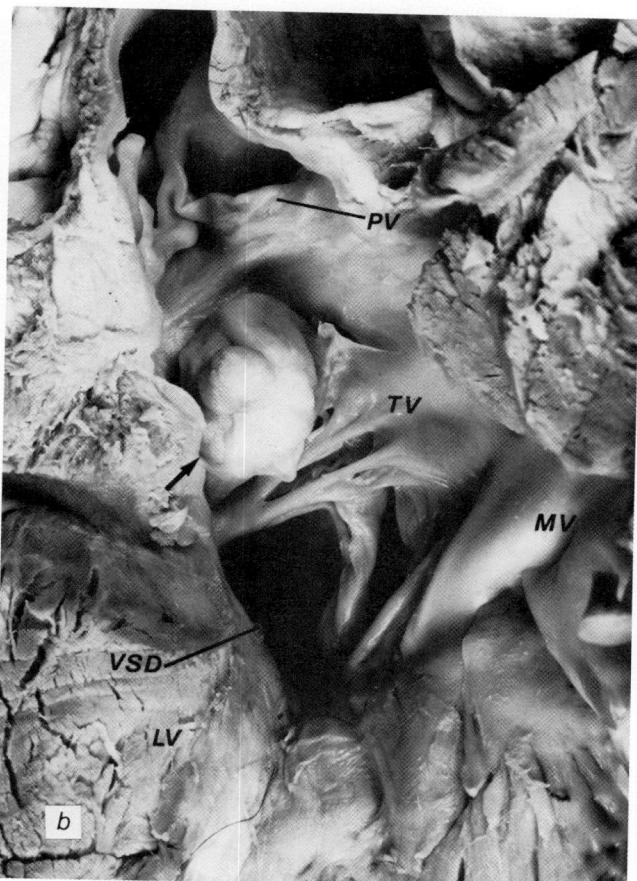

Figure 39-8   Specimen of TGA with large perimembranous ventricular septal defect (GLH).
(a) From the right ventricular side, the defect can be seen to be adjacent to the tricuspid valve anulus and to extend inferiorly beneath it. The conal (infundibular) septum is normally aligned with the trabecula septomarginalis or septal band.
(b) From the left ventricular side, the VSD is separated from the pulmonary valve in part by an anomalous bulky fibrous pouch (arrow) that originates from the left side of the septal tricuspid leaflet and is a cause of left ventricular outflow tract obstruction. There is mitral–tricuspid continuity across the floor of the defect.

AoV, aortic valve; CS, conal septum; LV, left ventricle; MV, mitral valve; PV, pulmonary valve; RV, right ventricle; SB, septal band; TV, tricuspid valve; VSD, ventricular septal defect.

ing through the VSD from the tricuspid valve[H1,L5,R8] (Fig. 39-8) or accessory fibrous tags (Fig. 39-10), possibly in association with a closing perimembranous VSD (see Chapter 23, Section 2) or with the anterior mitral valve leaflet.

Valvar stenosis is rare and when present is nearly always associated with subvalvar lesions. The pulmonary valve may be bicuspid.

Rarely, there is a stenotic muscular subpulmonary (infundibulum) conus.[S7,S10]

Patent Ductus Arteriosus
Patent ductus arteriosus is more common in hearts with TGA than in hearts with ventriculoarterial concordant connection. At the time of initial cardiac catheterization (at an average of 2 weeks of age), it is present in almost half[W2] but is usually functionally (although not necessarily anatomically) closed at 1 month. Thus, in 65 neonates undergoing balloon septostomy (UAB; 1970–1981), 20 (31%) had a large

PDA, 20 (31%) a small PDA, and 25 (38%) no demonstrable PDA. By the time of surgical repair, a PDA is present in 10%–15% of patients, but less than half are of significant size (Table 39-3).

Persistence of a large PDA for more than a few months is associated with an increased incidence of pulmonary vascular disease.[N1,W2]

Other Associated Anomalies

Tricuspid Valve Anomalies
In hearts with TGA, the ratio of the circumference of the tricuspid to mitral anulus is <1 in 46% of cases (in normal hearts this ratio is always >1).[C10] The reduction in this ratio is most marked in hearts with associated coarctation (Fig. 39-18).

Functionally important tricuspid valve anomalies are present in only about 4% of surgical patients (Table 39-3). How-

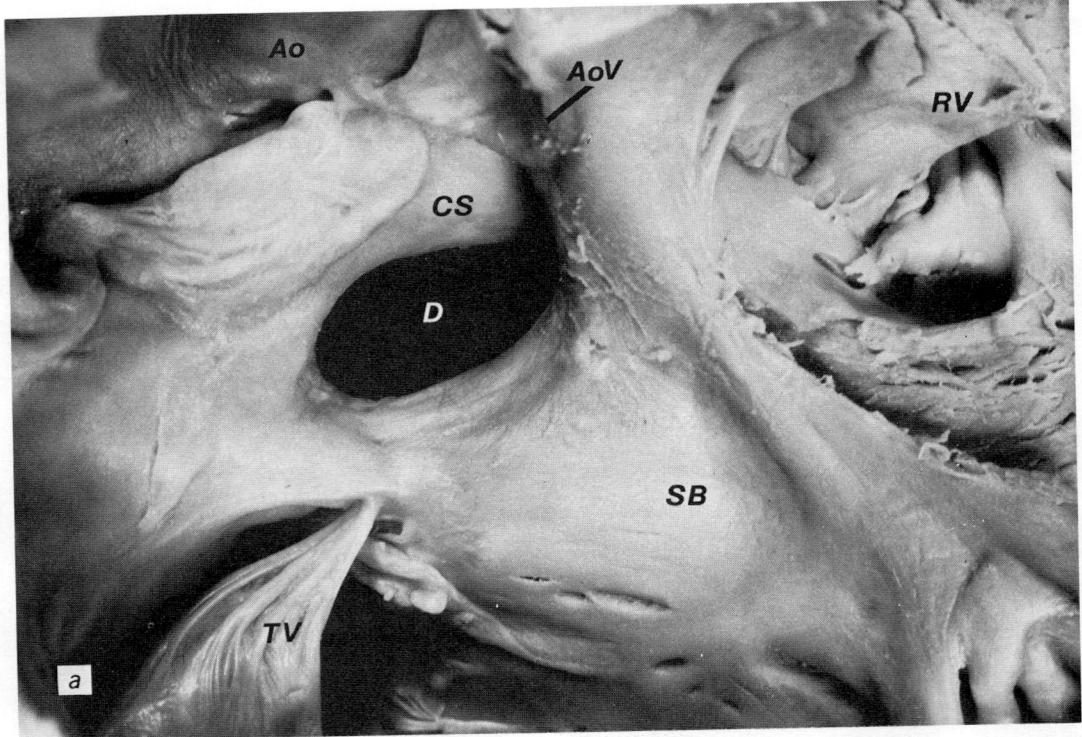

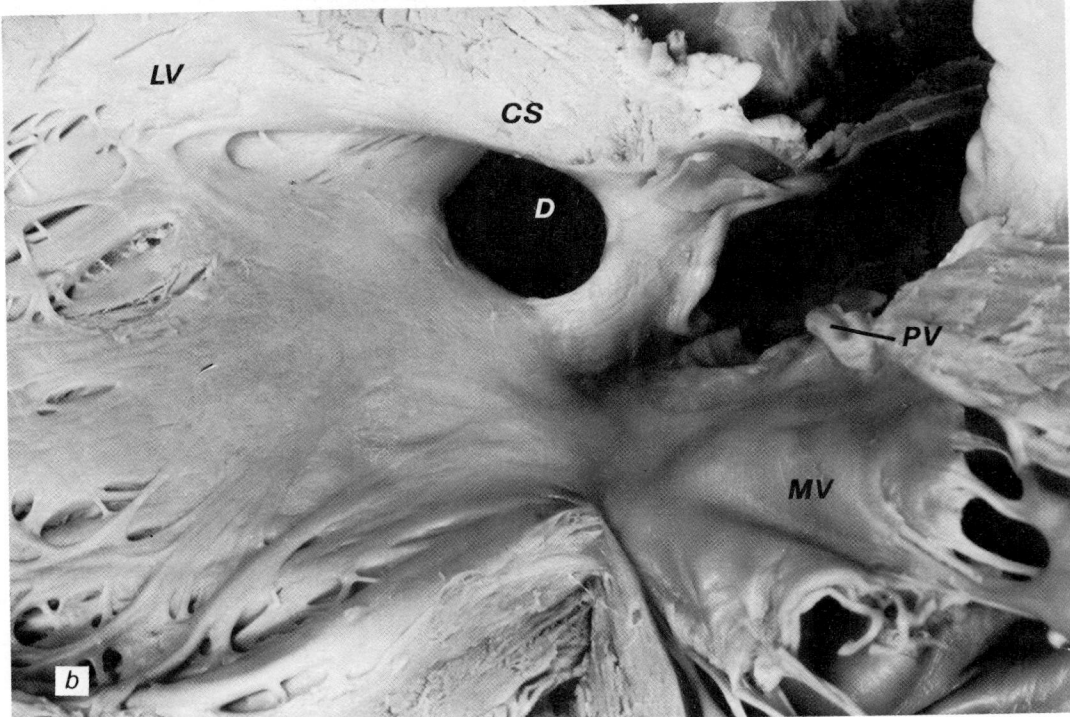

Figure 39-9 Specimen of TGA with large malalignment ventricular septal defect with leftward displacement of the conal (infundibular) septum (GLH).

(a) From right ventricular side.

(b) From left ventricular side. The conal septum is fused with the left ventricular anterior free wall, left ventricular outflow tract obstruction being only moderate.

AoV, aortic valve; CS, conal septum; D, ventricular septal defect; LV, left ventricle; MV, mitral valve; PV, pulmonary valve; RV, right ventricle; SB, septal band; TV, tricuspid valve.

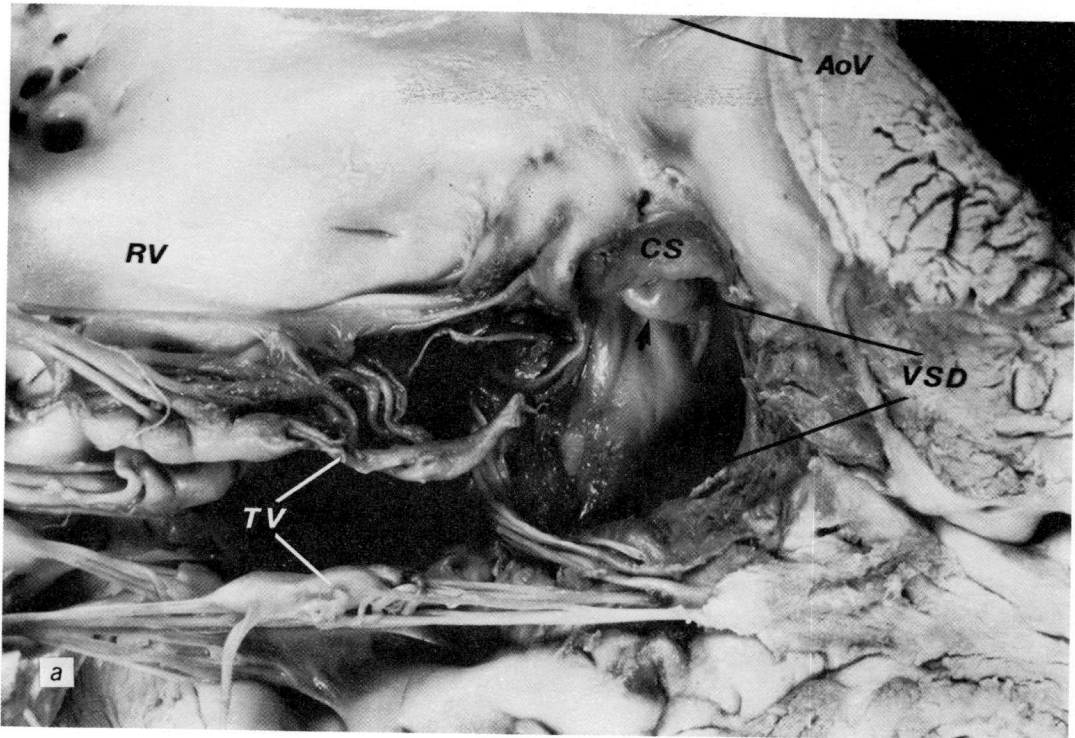

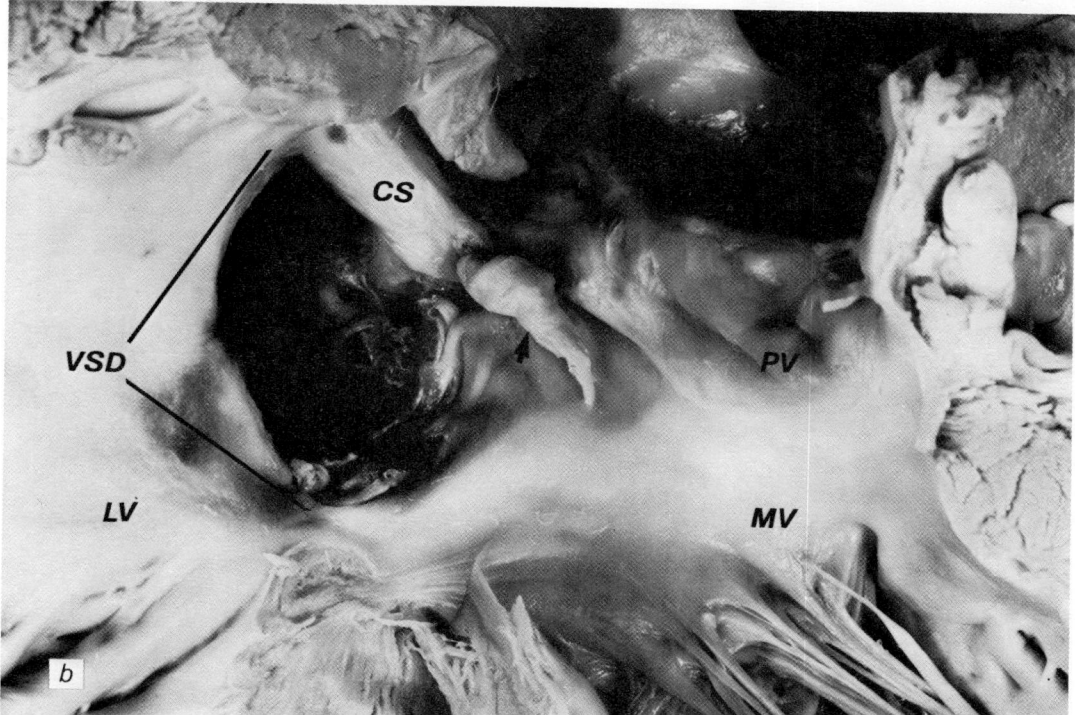

Figure 39-10 Specimen of TGA with large malalignment ventricular septal defect and leftward displacement of the conal septum that is relatively small (GLH).
(a) From right ventricular side. The fibrous tag (arrow), which also contributes to the left ventricular outflow tract obstruction can be seen through the VSD.
(b) From left ventricular side.

AoV, aortic valve; CS, conal septum; LV, left ventricle; MV, mitral valve; PV, pulmonary valve; RV, right ventricle; VSD, ventricular septal defect.

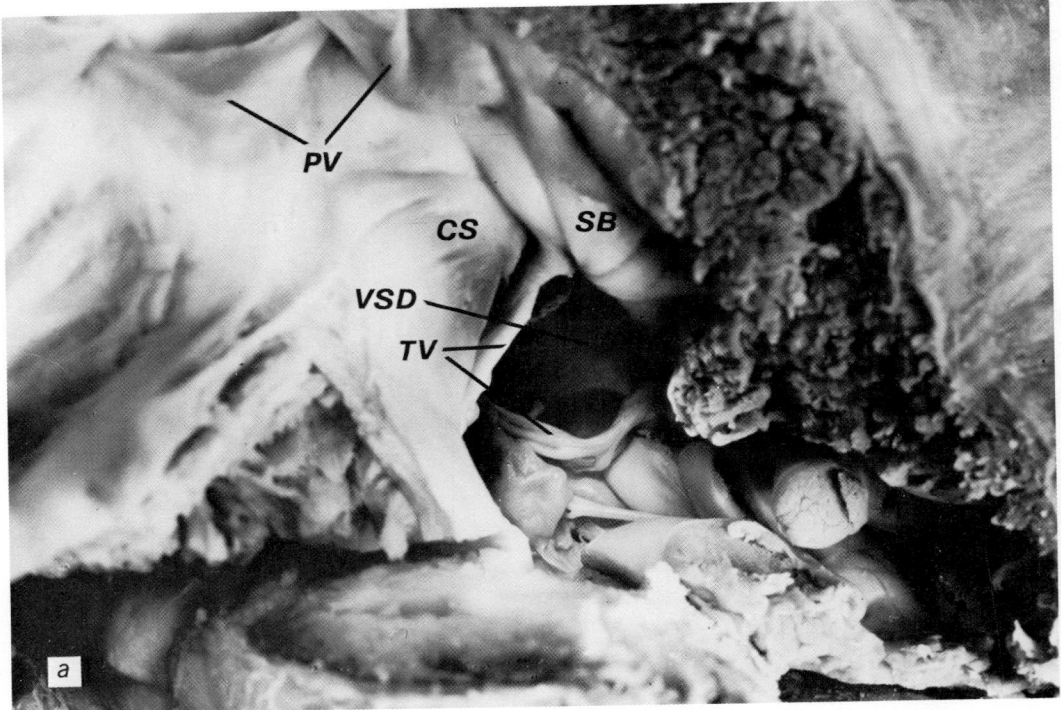

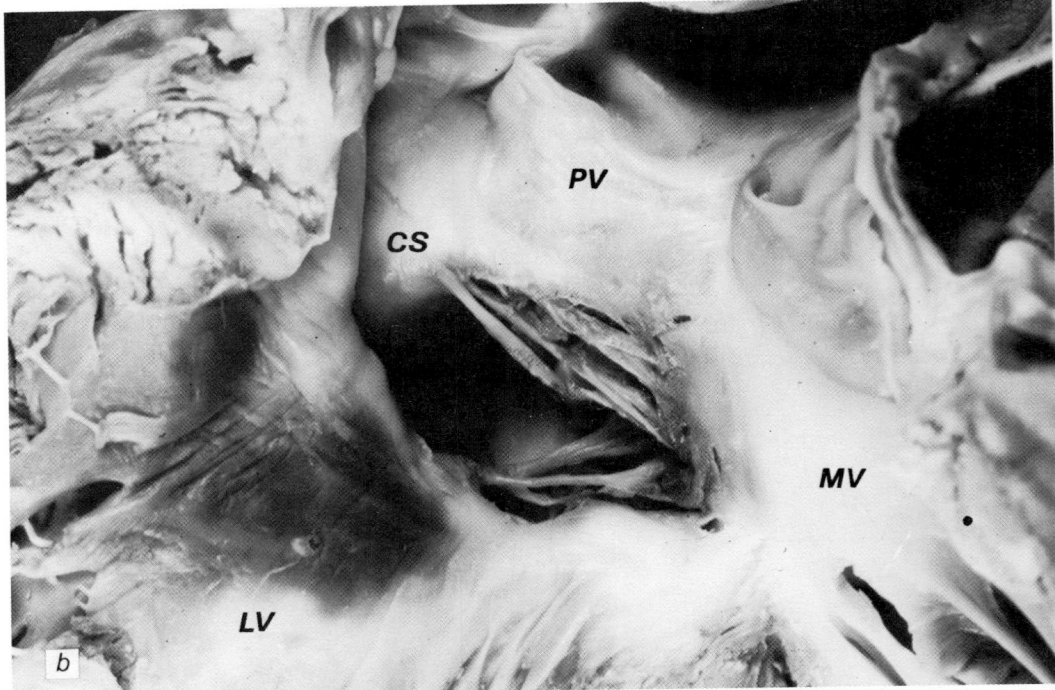

Figure 39-11 Specimen of TGA with a malalignment ventricular septal defect and rightward deviation of the conal (infundibular) septum that tends to produce subaortic obstruction (GLH).
(*a*) From right ventricular side. The deviation is best appreciated by noting the deep position of the tricuspid valve relative to the conal septum. (Compare to Fig. 39-8*a*.)
(*b*) From the left ventricular side. The gap between the conal septum and the ventricular septum is obvious. There are anomalous tricuspid chordae attaching to the edge of the ventricular septal defect.

CS, conal septum; LV, left ventricle; MV, mitral valve; PV, pulmonary valve; SB, septal band; TV, tricuspid valve; VSD, ventricular septal defect.

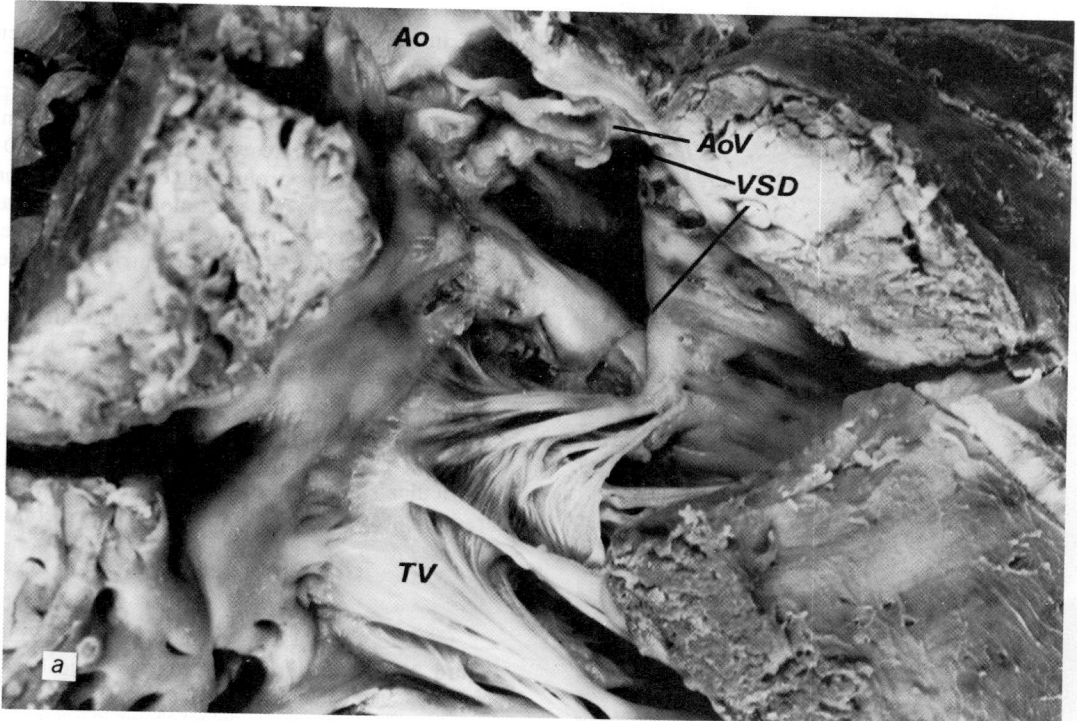

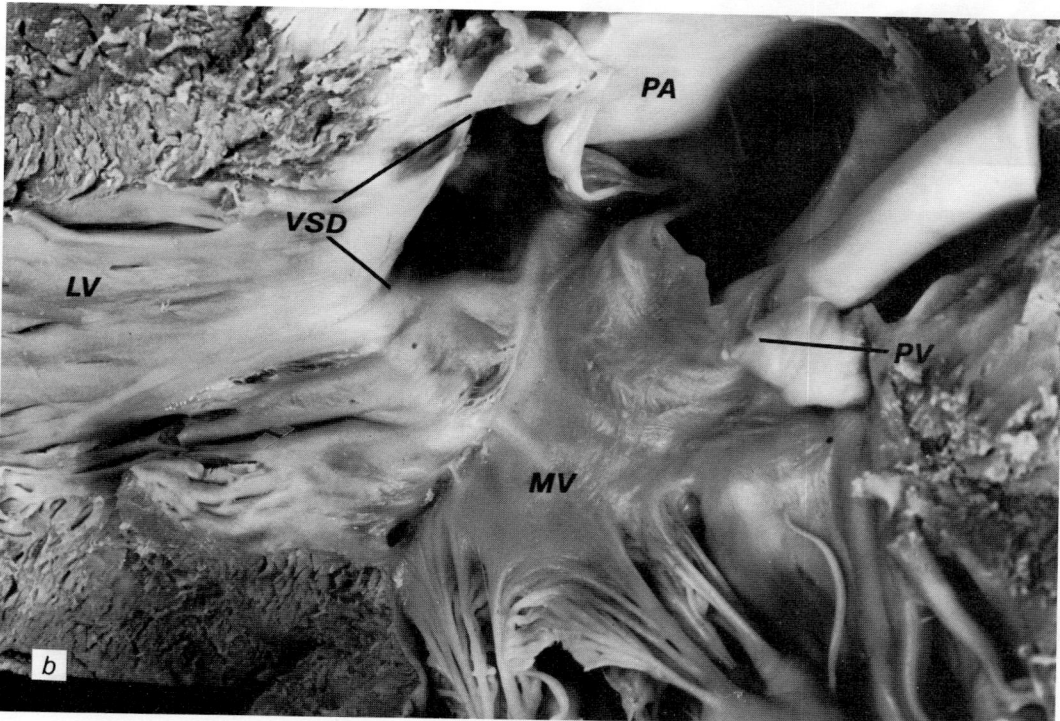

Figure 39-12 Specimen of TGA with large subarterial (conal) ventricular septal defect (GLH). The conal (infundibular) septum is absent, and the upper defect margin is formed by the confluent aortic and pulmonary valve rings. The defect is thus doubly committed and subarterial. There is mild overriding of the pulmonary artery and valve into the right ventricle.

(*a*) From right ventricular side.

(*b*) From left ventricular side. There is pulmonary-mitral continuity.

Ao, aorta; AoV, aortic valve; LV, left ventricle; MV, mitral valve; PA, pulmonary artery; PV, pulmonary valve; RV, right ventricle; TV, tricuspid valve; VSD, ventricular septal defect.

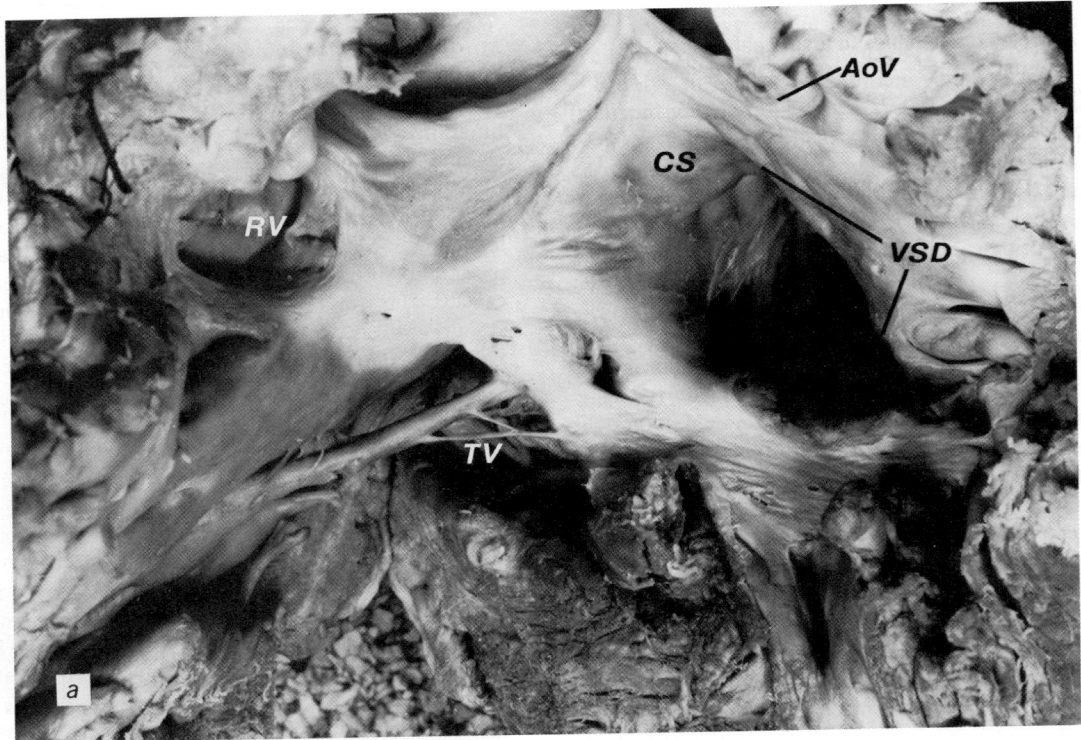

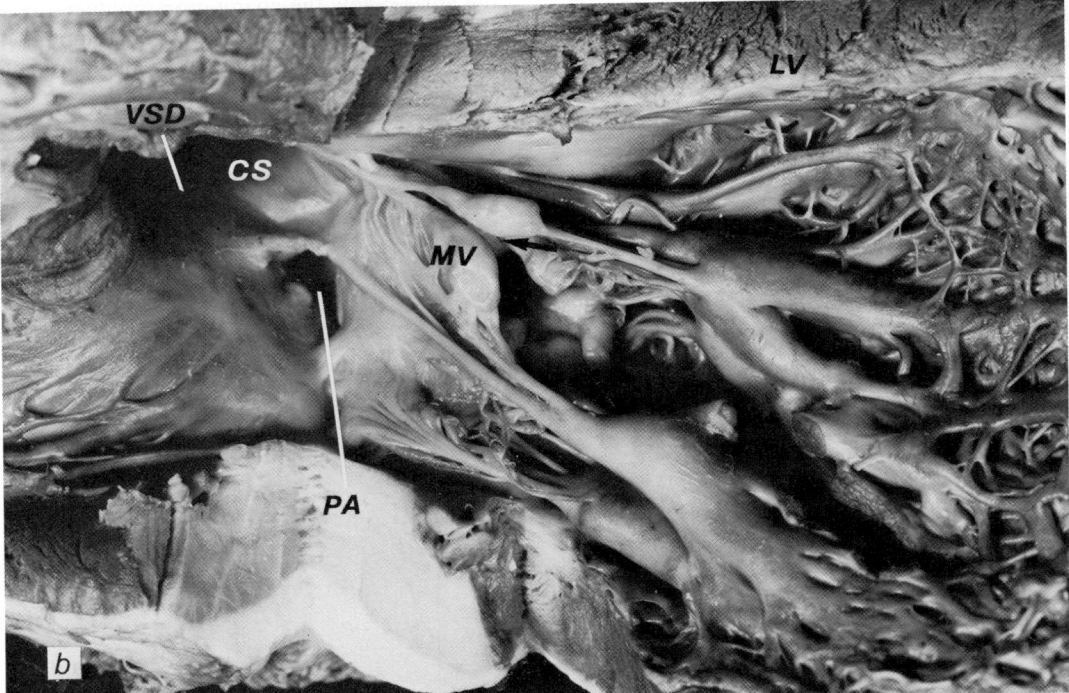

Figure 39-15 Specimen of TGA, VSD, and LVOTO (GLH). The VSD is associated with conal (infundibular) septal malalignment and leftward displacement into the left ventricular outflow tract.
(a) From right ventricular side.
(b) From left ventricular side. The conal septum has fused with the base of the anterior mitral valve leaflet, which is cleft (arrow). The pulmonary valve ostium is displaced posteriorly and is severely stenotic.

AoV, aortic valve; CS, conal septum; LV, left ventricle; MV, mitral valve; PA, pulmonary valve ostium; RV, right ventricle; TV, tricuspid valve; VSD, ventricular septal defect.

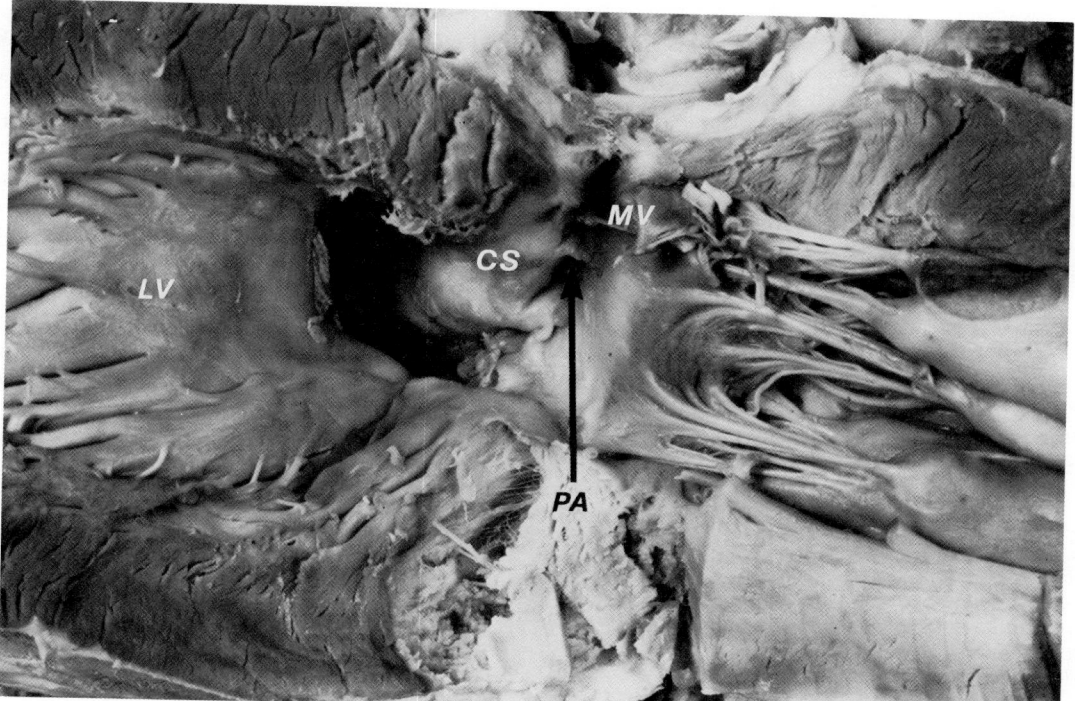

Figure 39-16 Specimen of TGA, VSD, and LVOTO (GLH), viewed from left ventricular side. There is severe conal septal malalignment and severe left ventricular outflow tract stenosis in the form of a muscular tunnel that is displaced posteriorly together with the left ventricular outflow tract.

CS, conal septum; LV, left ventricle; MV, mitral valve; PA, pulmonary artery.

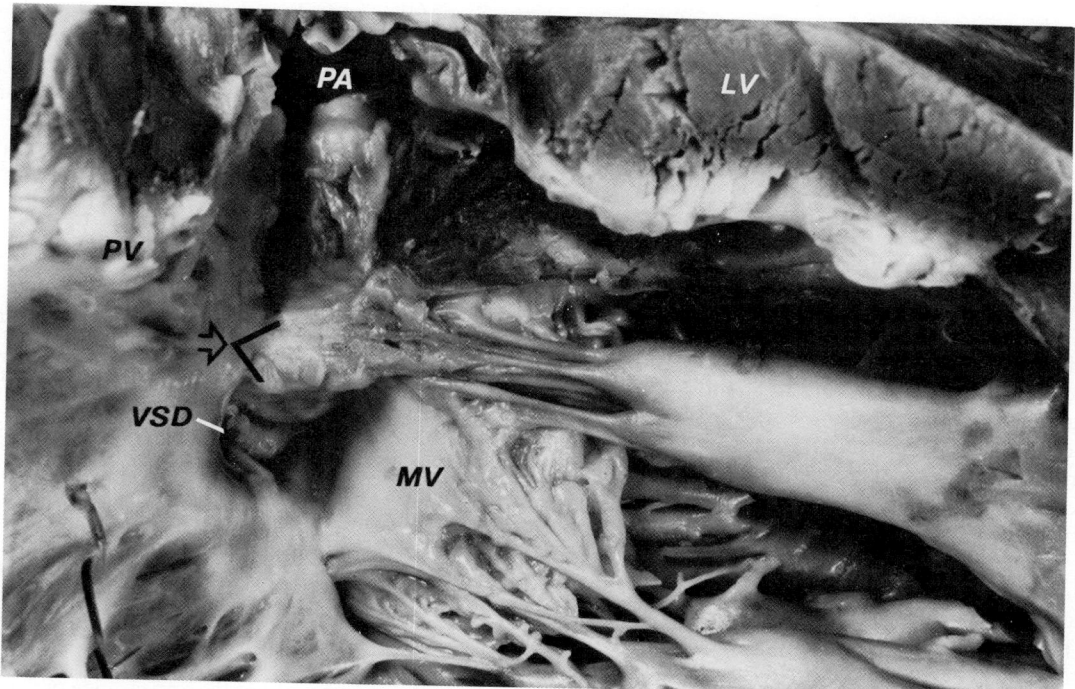

Figure 39-17 Specimen of TGA, VSD, and LVOTO (GLH), viewed from the left ventricle. Left ventricular outflow tract is a stenotic fibrous tunnel formed by bulky fibrous tissue (arrow) extending from the mitral leaflet to the septal surface superior to the VSD. The pulmonary valve is in its normal position.

LV, left ventricle; MV, mitral valve leaflet; PA, pulmonary artery; PV, pulmonary valve; VSD, ventricular septal defect.

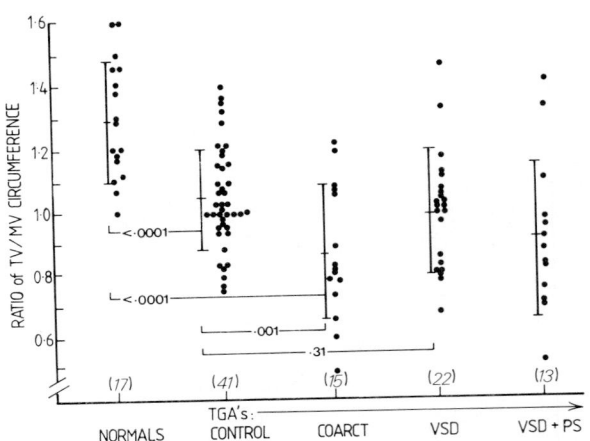

Figure 39-18 The ratio of tricuspid to mitral valve circumferences in a series of autopsy hearts (GLH), with TGA compared with 17 normal hearts.[C10] The control TGA specimens were those with a completely intact ventricular septum with or without a small patent ductus arteriosus, and/or atrial septal defect and/or patent foramen ovale. Only unoperated specimens and those obtained within 30 days of an intracardiac repair are included. The vertical bars indicate the standard deviations. Individual *P* values are noted.

Coarct, coarctation; PS, pulmonary stenosis; TV/MV, tricuspid to mitral; VSD, ventricular septal defect.

noted above, the tricuspid/mitral anulus circumference is less than in other TGA subsets.

Right Aortic Arch
Right aortic arch occurs in about 5% of cases.[M9] It is more common when there is an associated VSD than when the ventricular septum is essentially intact and when there is an associated leftward juxtaposition of the atrial appendages.[M10]

Leftward Juxtaposition of the Atrial Appendages
Leftward juxtaposition of the atrial appendages is more commonly associated with TGA than with any other variety of congenital heart disease.[M10] It occurs in about 2.5% of patients coming to intracardiac repair.[U1,W3] It is associated with a higher than usual incidence of significant underdevelopment of the right ventricular sinus. Bilateral conus and dextrocardia seem more common in TGA associated with leftward juxtaposition than in TGA generally.

Right Ventricular Hypoplasia
Right ventricular hypoplasia was found to some degree in 17% of the necropsy series of TGA reported by Riemenschneider and colleagues.[R9] This is highly relevant to the choice of operation.

Others
Rarely, TGA coexists with congenital valvar aortic stenosis[L5] and very rarely with total anomalous pulmonary venous connection.[S12] It can also coexist with complete AV canal defects (see Chapter 19).

CLINICAL FEATURES AND DIAGNOSTIC CRITERIA

Pathophysiology

When the great arteries are transposed in hearts with atrioventricular (AV) concordant connection, the systemic and pulmonary circulation are in parallel. Unless there is shunting between the two, this is incompatible with life for more than a short period. With this arrangement, pulmonary and systemic blood flow can vary independently, and shunting between the two circulations over more than very short periods of time must be equal in both directions lest all the blood eventually be in one or the other circulation. The magnitude of the bidirectional shunt is highly variable and is referred to as *the degree of mixing.*

The symptoms and clinical presentation in patients with TGA depend in large part upon the degree of mixing between the two parallel circulatory circuits. When there is a high degree of mixing and a large pulmonary blood flow, the arterial oxygen saturation may be near normal and, unless there is pulmonary venous hypertension, symptoms are minimal. When there is little mixing, the arterial oxygen saturation is low and the symptoms of hypoxia severe.

Adequate mixing can occur only when there are communications of reasonable size at the atrial, ventricular, or ductus level. With adequate-sized communications, mixing tends to be directly related to pulmonary blood flow. Factors that reduce pulmonary blood flow, such as left ventricular outflow tract obstruction (LVOTO) or pulmonary vascular disease, reduce mixing and increase cyanosis.

Symptoms and clinical presentation also depend in part upon left atrial and pulmonary venous pressure. When pulmonary blood flow is even moderately elevated, these pressures tend to become elevated and produce symptoms. Both left and right ventricular failure usually result.

The clinical features and diagnostic criteria of patients with TGA fall into three groups on the basis of these criteria.[N5]

Presentation, Symptoms, and Signs

Transposition of the Great Arteries with Essentially Intact Ventricular Septum (Poor Mixing)
Included in this group are infants without a ventricular septal defect (VSD) or with one of 3 mm or less in diameter. A patent foramen ovale or naturally occurring atrial septal defect (ASD) is usually present.

Cyanosis is apparent in half of such infants within the first hour of life and in 90% within the first day[L8] and is rapidly progressive. Pulmonary blood flow is usually increased to a pulmonary-systemic blood flow ratio ($\dot{Q}p/\dot{Q}s$) of about 2; but because of the poor mixing across the small communication, this does not alleviate the hypoxia. The baby becomes critically ill with tachypnea and tachycardia and dies from hypoxia and acidosis without the appearance of frank congestive heart failure. This rapidly downhill course is usually obviated when there is a naturally occurring ASD of significant size, since cyanosis is then less severe. In surviving infants, the appearance of moderate or severe dynamic LVOTO is associated with increasing cyanosis and hypoxic spells, even following an adequate septostomy.[A7,T3,Y4]

The *clinical signs* in most newborns with this subset of TGA are unimpressive. Generally, they are of average birth weight and in good general condition although with severe cyanosis. Clubbing of the fingers and toes is absent and generally does not appear unless the infant survives to about 6 months of age. There is a mild increase in heart and respiratory rates. The heart is not hyperactive and the liver barely palpable. A faint midsystolic ejection-type murmur is present along the midleft sternal edge in less than half the infants. This murmur is more prominent when there is organic or dynamic LVOTO, and in the latter instance it first appears at 1 or 2 months of age and then gradually increases in intensity. The second heart sound is unremarkable (it is often apparently single or very narrowly split), and the third heart sound and an apical middiastolic flow murmur are both rare.

The *chest x-ray* has three characteristic features, which are an oval or egg-shaped cardiac silhouette with a narrow superior mediastinum, mild cardiac enlargement, and moderate pulmonary plethora (Fig. 39-19). In the first week of life, however, the chest x-ray may be normal, or occasionally cardiac enlargement may be more marked. The narrow mediastinum is due in part to the great artery positions and in part to shrinkage of the thymus usually associated with stress[N2] and the plethora is due to the increase in pulmonary blood flow. Plethora is less marked when there is significant LVOTO.

The *electrocardiogram* (ECG) in this subset is often normal at birth, with the usual neonatal right ventricular pattern. By the end of the first week, persistence of an upright T wave in right precordial leads indicates abnormal right ventricular hypertrophy, and right axis deviation predominates.

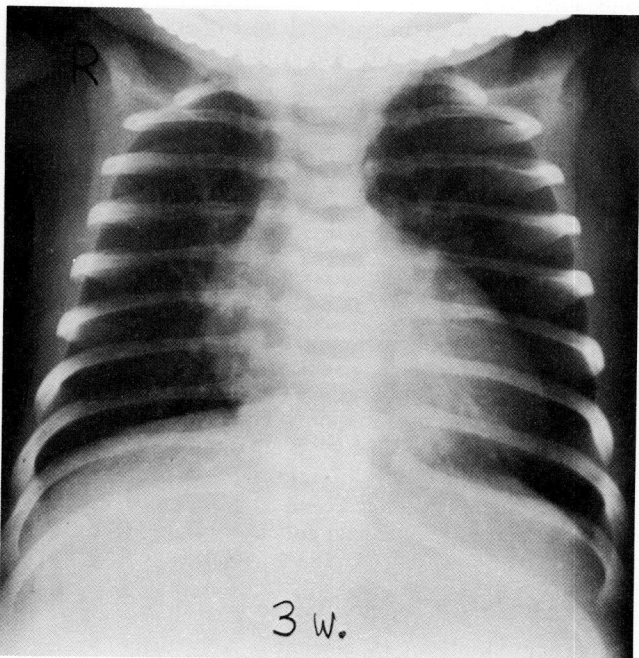

Figure 39-19 Chest x-ray of an infant with TGA and essentially intact ventricular septum showing the typical egg-shaped cardiac silhouette with a narrow superior mediastinum and mild pulmonary plethora (GLH).

The *vectorcardiogram* shows a clockwise horizontal plane loop that is indicative of a near normal left ventricular systolic pressure and a dominant right ventricular mass.[M13] When significant LVOTO is present or the pulmonary vascular resistance is raised, there is ECG evidence of biventricular hypertrophy.

Transposition of the Great Arteries with Large Ventricular Septal Defect or Large Patent Ductus Arteriosus or Both (Good Mixing)

Presentation in this group generally occurs in the latter half of the first month of life, with mild cyanosis and the signs of congestive heart failure resulting from pulmonary venous hypertension and myocardial failure.[C3] There is tachycardia, tachypnea, significant liver enlargement, and moist lung bases. The heart is more active and usually larger than in the poor mixing group.

A large VSD is associated with a moderate intensity pansystolic murmur along the lower left sternal edge, which may not be present initially. There is usually an apical middiastolic murmur or gallop rhythm and narrow splitting of the second heart sound with accentuation of the pulmonary component.

When there is a large patent ductus arteriosus (PDA), a continuous murmur, bounding pulses, and an apical middiastolic murmur are present in less than half even when the ventricular septum is intact.[W2] Sudden spontaneous closure of a large PDA when there is no VSD results in increase in cyanosis (see "Natural History").

The *chest x-ray* in the good mixing group may show more cardiomegaly, more plethora, and a wider superior mediastinum than in the poor mixing group. The *ECG* shows biventricular hypertrophy and when there is a persistent large VSD, a Q wave in V_6. Isolated left ventricular hypertrophy is rare and suggests right ventricular hypoplasia with tricuspid valve overriding.[R9]

The development of pulmonary vascular disease is associated with a reduction in pulmonary blood flow and less plethora, particularly in the peripheral lung fields, and a reduction in heart size, but these features generally appear after the neonatal period.

When *coarctation* of the aorta is present in addition to VSD and PDA, the femoral pulses are usually normal, since the coarctation is preductal and the ductus arteriosus large. Rarely, there may be differential cyanosis with cyanosis confined to the upper torso. All patients with this combination present early in life in congestive heart failure and respond poorly to decongestive treatment. Isolated left ventricular hypertrophy may be present on the ECG because of the frequent association of coarctation with right ventricular hypoplasia.[M8]

Transposition of the Great Arteries with Large Ventricular Septal Defect and Left Ventricular Outflow Tract Obstruction (Poor Mixing without Large Pulmonary Blood Flow)

This group is the least common. The LVOTO is associated with a decreased pulmonary blood flow and poor mixing, but pulmonary venous hypertension and symptoms and signs related to it do not develop because of the lack of increase in pulmonary blood flow. Congestive heart failure is therefore not present. The clinical findings are similar to those of tetralogy of Fallot with severe pulmonary stenosis or pulmonary atresia (see Chapter 23), and cyanosis is severe from birth. The heart is not overactive, and there is a pulmonary ejection murmur and often a single heart sound without an apical gallop or middiastolic murmur. The chest x-ray shows a near-normal-sized heart with normal or ischemic lung fields and the ECG shows biventricular hypertrophy.

Additional Investigations

Echocardiography
The definitive diagnosis can be made using 2D[B10] or, with less confidence, M mode[B9] echocardiography. Two-dimensional echocardiography is also particularly valuable in detecting tricuspid valve abnormalities, including overriding and straddling[L9] and the various varieties of subpulmonary stenosis, including dynamic obstruction.[C15,R11] Echocardiographic features of dynamic LVOTO include leftward deviation of the ventricular septum, abnormal fluttering and premature closure of the pulmonary valve, systolic anterior motion of the mitral leaflet (present in about 50%), and prolonged diastolic apposition of the anterior mitral valve leaflet to the septum.[A9,Y4]

Cardiac Catheterization
Currently, cardiac catheterization (and cineangiocardiographic) studies are performed prior to surgical intervention (although not necessarily prior to balloon septostomy) (UAB, GLH). A full study includes calculation of systemic and pulmonary blood flows and pressures, including those across the left ventricular outflow tract (GLH). Because of the presence of intracardiac communications in patients with TGA, the Fick method is usually the only practical way of measuring pulmonary and systemic flows. Despite the complexity of the circulation, standard calculations apply. Meticulous care is required in measuring oxygen consumption. This is done in infants using a closed box technique (GLH). Equations are as follows:

$$\dot{Q}p = \frac{\dot{V}o_2}{Cpvo_2 - Cpao_2}$$

$$\dot{Q}s = \frac{\dot{V}o_2}{Cao_2 - C\bar{v}o_2}$$

$$\dot{Q}ep = \frac{\dot{V}o_2}{Cpvo_2 - C\bar{v}o_2}$$

where Cao_2 = systemic arterial oxygen content ml · l^{-1}
$Cpao_2$ = pulmonary arterial oxygen content ml · l^{-1}
$Cpvo_2$ = pulmonary venous oxygen content ml · l^{-1}
$C\bar{v}o_2$ = mixed venous oxygen content ml · l^{-1}
$\dot{V}o_2$ = oxygen consumption ml · min^{-1}
$\dot{Q}p$ = pulmonary blood flow
$\dot{Q}ep$ = effective pulmonary blood flow
$\dot{Q}s$ = systemic blood flow

$\dot{Q}ep$ represents the flow of blood from the systemic to the pulmonary circuit at atrial, ventricular, and/or great arterial level. Clearly, there must be equal flow in the opposite direction (anatomic left-to-right shunt or effective systemic blood flow) or, in time, one circuit would be deprived of blood.

There are inherent errors in measurement of these flows. Where $\dot{Q}p$ is high and pulmonary arterial saturation therefore high, the Fick calculation is apt to be inaccurate. This error may be compounded by difficulties in recovering a truly mixed pulmonary venous saturation. Fortunately, these errors are greatest in those patients in whom there is a very high pulmonary flow and thus little concern about a high pulmonary vascular resistance. Calculations are more accurate when the pulmonary blood flow is low and the resistance correspondingly high. There is a potential error if pulmonary arterial sampling is made proximal to the site of entry of sizeable systemic (bronchial) collaterals. The true mixed pulmonary arterial saturation would then be lower than that measured and the pulmonary flow correspondingly lower,[L7] but in practice this situation is uncommon.

Thus, with careful technique, pulmonary vascular resistance in patients with TGA can be calculated with reasonable accuracy. A specific problem arises, however, if the hematocrit is particularly high, since when it is above 60 the viscosity of the blood increases sharply. The effect of the viscosity on pulmonary blood flow may then become important and the calculated resistance higher than that dictated by the pulmonary vascular bed alone.[M9] The only solution to this is to repeat the measurements after lowering the hematocrit by venesection.

$\dot{Q}ep$ is the flow on which life depends. In an individual with TGA, this flow is relatively fixed. Since it is commonly only about 1–1.5 l · min · m^{-2}, this places a major constraint on oxygen supply to the patient. These relationships become evident in rewriting the Fick equation:

$$\dot{V}o_2 = \dot{Q}ep (Ppvo_2 - C\bar{v}o_2)$$
$$= \dot{Q}ep (Spvo_2 - S\bar{v}o_2) \times Hb \times CAP$$

where $Spvo_2$ = pulmonary venous oxygen saturation
$S\bar{v}o_2$ = mixed venous oxygen saturation
CAP = oxygen capacity per gram of Hb
Hb = hemoglobin concentration in g · l^{-1}
$\dot{V}o_2$ = oxygen consumption
$\dot{Q}ep$ = effective pulmonary blood flow

Clearly, on this basis any reduction in hemoglobin will reduce oxygen uptake, and in patients with TGA compensation for this is not possible.[M15] If stress or exercise increases oxygen requirement, the difference in oxygen content of pulmonary venous and mixed venous blood must widen, and since pulmonary venous content cannot increase, mixed venous content (and hence tissue Po_2) must fall.

Cineangiography
Using appropriate views, cineangiography demonstrates the cardiac connections and great artery positions (Fig. 39-20), the position and number of VSDs (Fig. 39-21), the site of any LVOTO (Figs. 39-20, 39-22), the size and function of the AV

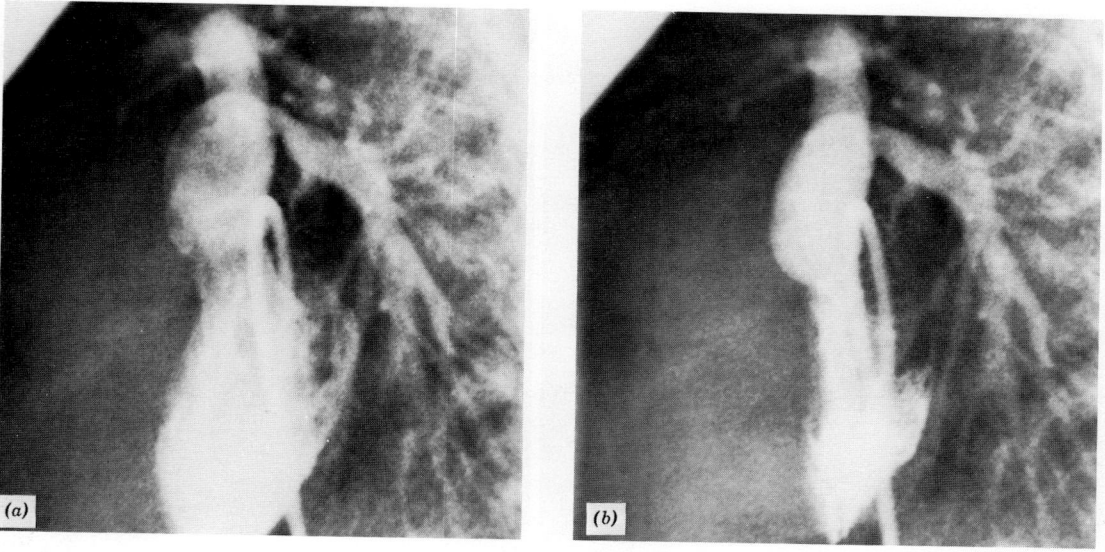

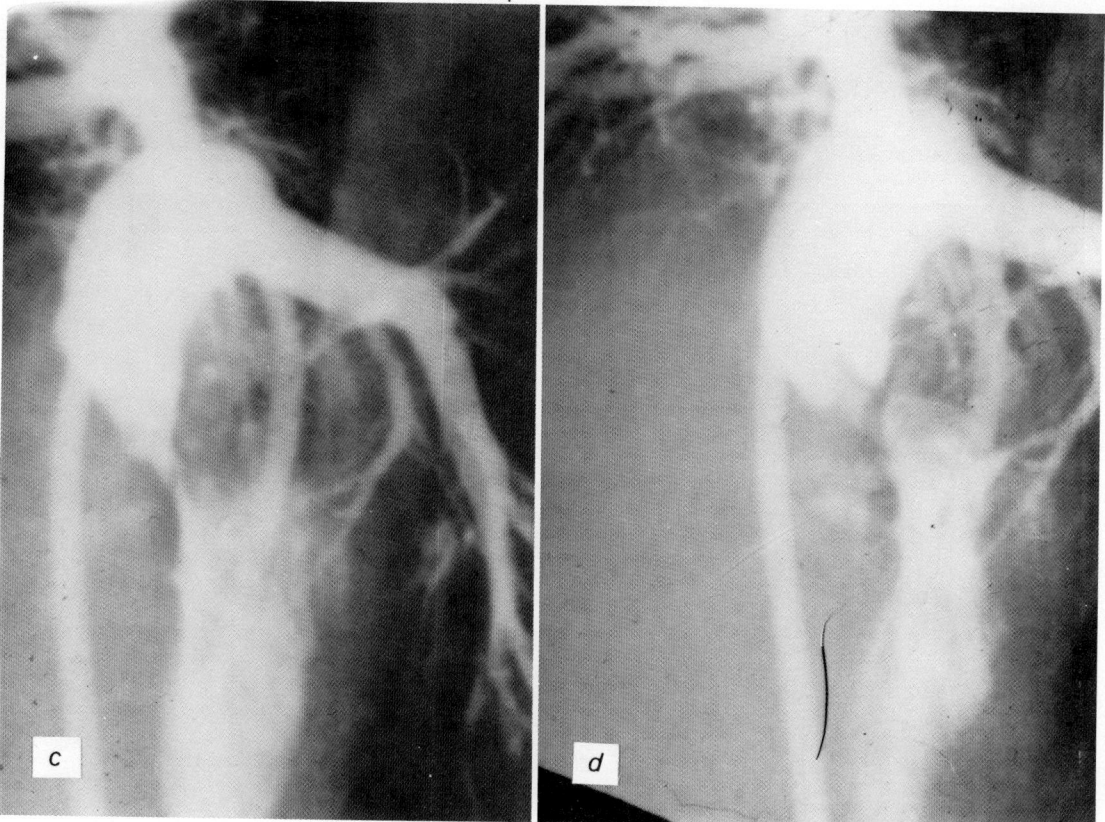

Figure 39-20 Cineangiograms in infants with simple TGA (UAB).
(*a* and *b*) Left ventricular injection, long axial view, in diastole (to the left) and systole. The left ventricular outflow tract is widely open. The apparent narrowing at the origin of the left pulmonary artery is frequently seen, and, as here, usually disappears during systole.
(*c* and *d*) Left ventricular injection, similar views and position, in another infant. The left ventricle gives origin to the pulmonary artery, and there is a long area of subpulmonary left ventricular outflow tract obstruction.

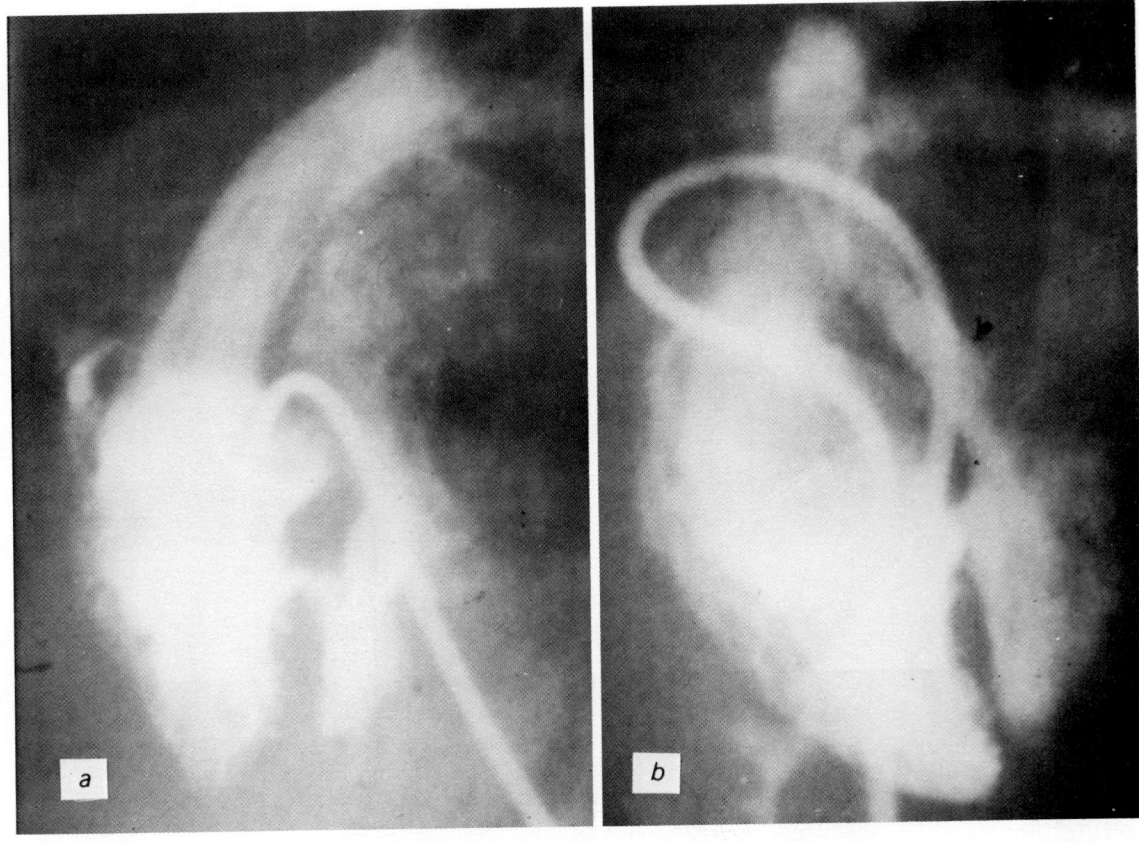

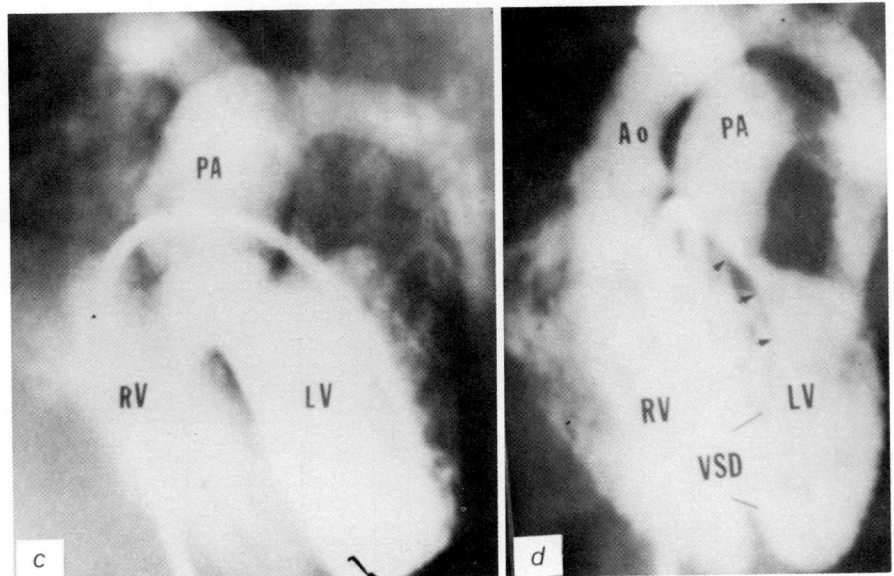

Figure 39-21 Cineangiograms of infants with TGA and VSD (UAB).
(a) A small midmuscular VSD is demonstrated by right ventricular injection in the long axial view.
(b) A large VSD in the inflow portion of the septum is demonstrated by right ventricular injection in the four-chamber position.
(c) A large perimembranous VSD is shown with left ventricular ejection in the long axial view.
(d) Multiple muscular VSDs are demonstrated with a right ventricular injection in the long axial view.

Ao, aorta; LV, left ventricle; PA, pulmonary artery; RV, right ventricle; VSD, ventricular septal defect.

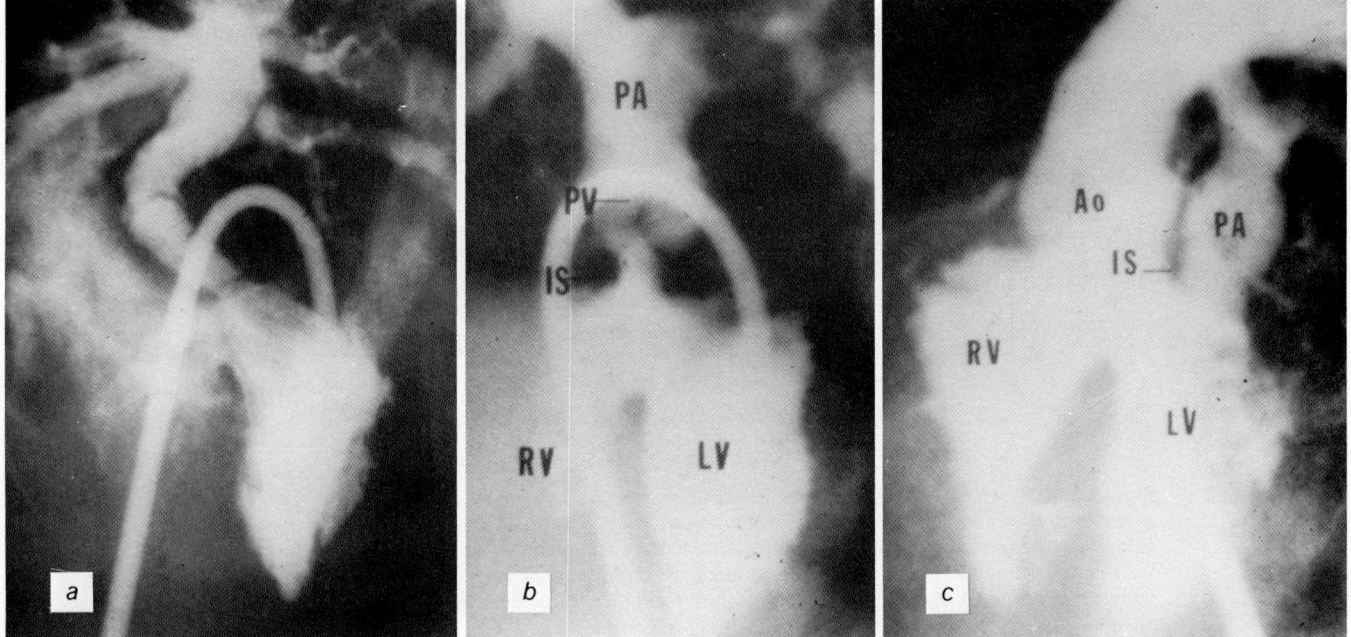

Figure 39-22 Cineangiograms in patients with TGA, VSD, and LVOTO (UAB).
(a) Subvalvar LVOTO is associated with a large perimembranous VSD, as shown by left ventricular injection and the four-chamber view.
(b) Long subvalvar LVOTO is associated with a large perimembranous VSD, as shown by LV injection and the four-chamber view.
(c) Discrete subvalvar LVOTO with large VSD and mild overriding of the aorta onto the left ventricle. LV injection, four-chamber view.
Ao, aorta; IS, infundibular septum; LV, left ventricle; PA, pulmonary artery; RV, right ventricle.

valves, the size and function of both ventricles, and the presence of any other cardiac anomalies.

NATURAL HISTORY

Incidence

Transposition of the great arteries (TGA) is a common form of congenital heart disease, occurring in between 1:2,100 and 1:4,500 births,[G3,L6] and accounting for 7%–8% of all congenital heart disease. In the Auckland area of New Zealand, the incidence over a 10-year period was 1:2,400, whereas in the New England (US) study it was 1:4,000[F5] ($P < .005$). Prior to the advent of effective treatment, at least 16% of deaths due to congenital heart disease at all ages in childhood were due to TGA.[L6]

There is a 2:1 male to female ratio. This male predominance increases to 3.3:1 when the ventricular septum is essentially intact and disappears in complex forms.[L6]

Survival

When patients with all varieties of TGA are considered, 55% survive 1 month, 15% survive 6 months, and only 10% survive 1 year[A6,K4,K5,L6,M12] (Fig. 39-23). The mean life expectancy at birth is 0.65 year, rising to 4 years for those who survive to 12 months and to 6 years for the very few who

survive for 10 years. Thereafter, life expectancy again declines rapidly (Fig. 39-23).

Survival without treatment is different among the various subsets of patients. Survival is particularly poor in untreated patients with *TGA and essentially intact ventricular septum,* 80% being alive at 1 week but only 17% at 2 months and 4% at 1 year.[L6] Survival in this group is better when there is a true atrial septal defect (ASD) (Fig. 39-24).

In patients with *TGA and an important ventricular septal defect (VSD)* the early survival rate is higher, 91% at 1 month, 43% at 5 months, and 32% at 1 year.[L6] Early survival is less good in this morphologic subset when there is a very large pulmonary blood flow (see Fig. 39-24). The combination of *large VSD and coarctation* of the aorta is particularly lethal. All die within a few months of birth, with severe congestive heart failure. Paradoxically, obstructive pulmonary vascular disease in patients with TGA and VSD improves early survival to 40% at 1 year, but there is a rapid decline thereafter so that none are alive by age 5 years.

In patients with *TGA, VSD, and left ventricular outflow obstruction (LVOTO),* early survival is still better, reaching 70% at 1 year and 29% at 5 years, because in many the LVOTO is only moderate initially.

Leibman and colleagues found that a *patent ductus arteriosus (PDA)* increased the risk of early death in all subsets of patients.[L6] This is particularly the case when the ductus is large.

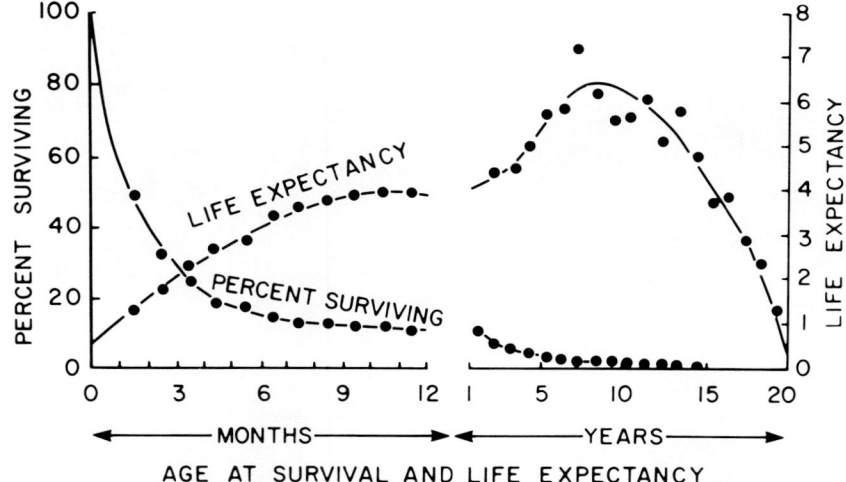

Figure 39-23 Actuarial survival and life expectancy of 655 children with TGA of all types, all of whom died between 1957 and 1964. Seventy-three living children and 14 miscellaneous deaths are excluded. The group is impure in that about 15% of the total had either single ventricle, hypoplasia of the left ventricle with mitral stenosis or atresia, or hypoplasia of the right ventricle with tricuspid stenosis or atresia. However, the trends are representative of patients with TGA.

Reproduced with permission from Liebman et al.,[L6] and the American Heart Association, Inc.

Modes of Death

The poor survival in patients with TGA and *essentially intact ventricular septum* is related primarily to anoxia. Intercurrent pulmonary infections may develop and are particularly lethal because they reduce effective pulmonary blood flow and lead rapidly to increasing hypoxia, acidemia, and death. Death in this group may also result from cerebrovascular events. These are usually due to the polycythemia and increased blood viscosity secondary to severe cyanosis, par-

ticularly in association with dehydration. However, hypoxia plus hypochromic microcytic anemia have also been implicated in the etiology of these events.[P3] Nonfatal cerebrovascular events also occur in about 6% of patients treated by balloon atrial septostomy[P4] and include cerebral abscess.

Patients with *TGA and important ventricular septal defects* (VSDs) usually die with congestive heart failure. The modes of death described for patients with simple transposition sometimes pertain in this group as well and include frequent intercurrent pulmonary infections.

Hypoxia is the primary cause of morbidity and mortality in

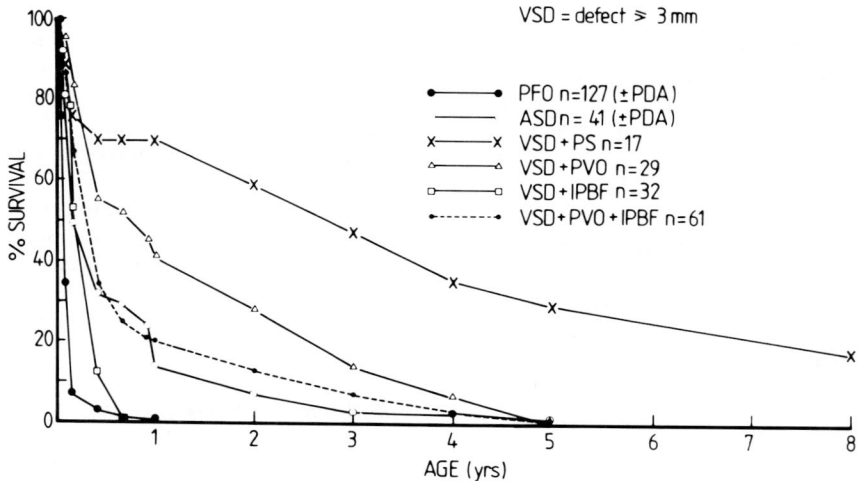

Figure 39-24 Actuarial survival of various subsets of patients with TGA.

ASD, atrial septal defect; IPBF, increased pulmonary blood flow; PFO, patent foramen ovale; PS, pulmonary stenosis; PVD, pulmonary vascular disease; VSD, ventricular septal defect.

Plotted from data presented by Liebman et al.[L6]

patients with *TGA, VSD, and important left ventricular outflow tract obstruction* (LVOTO).

Other Dynamic Events

Patent Ductus Arteriosus

A patent ductus arteriosus (PDA) is present at 1 week of age in about half the patients with TGA, but thereafter the incidence falls fairly rapidly.[P2] When patent, the ductus is small (less than 3 mm in diameter) in about two-thirds of the cases and seems to have little influence on natural history.[L6] When the ductus is large, left ventricular output is increased and hypoxia lessens, but heart failure becomes more severe. Under these circumstances, the acute and often early closure of the ductus results in sudden increase in hypoxia and clinical deterioration.[P2,W2] This is related not only to the decreased mixing at ductus level but also to decreased mixing at atrial level because of the fall in left atrial pressure that results from decreased pulmonary venous return.[W2]

Atrial Septal Defects

In patients with TGA, the patent foramen ovale tends to close at the usual rate. This is the major cause of the time-related increase in hypoxia and death in patients with TGA and essentially intact ventricular septum without an important PDA. A true atrial septal defect (ASD), on the other hand, remains unchanged in size and palliates the patient for a longer time.[P2] The same is true for those rare examples of coexisting partial anomalous pulmonary venous connections.

Ventricular Septal Defects

Large VSDs close or narrow in what is probably a smaller proportion (about 20%) of patients with TGA than is the case in patients with isolated VSD (see Chapter 20, "Spontaneous Closure" in Section 1, Natural History). However, in most instances, the VSD is initially small and often muscular, and spontaneous closure has been documented to occur as late as the last part of the first decade of life.[P2] This process was rarely documented prior to the era of balloon atrial septostomy (BAS), as so few patients survived beyond the first few months of life.[S13]

Left Ventricular Outflow Tract Obstruction

LVOTO of the dynamic type is not present at birth but can appear within several weeks thereafter. It gradually progresses in severity. It develops uncommonly in patients with TGA and important VSD. The awareness of this process has increased since the era of BAS, following which it frequently develops. When LVOTO of the dynamic type becomes important, hypoxia returns and life expectancy is shortened.

Pulmonary Vascular Disease

Pulmonary vascular disease develops more commonly in patients with TGA than in other forms of cyanotic congenital heart disease. It can occur when the ventricular septum is intact[F1,F2] or when there is pulmonary stenosis.[C2] Lakier and colleagues found that 5 (17%, CL 10%–28%) of 29 neonates with simple TGA and a closed ductus arteriosus subsequently developed an increased pulmonary vascular resis-

tance between 7 months and 2.5 years of age.[L7] Its development reduces pulmonary blood flow, increases hypoxia, and shortens life.

Pulmonary vascular disease develops more frequently when there is a large VSD or a large PDA. It appears particularly early in life under these circumstances and can be quite marked by age 3 months. Its development temporarily improves the hemodynamic state by reducing pulmonary blood flow and left atrial pressure, and survival through the first year or two of life is improved. The progression of the pulmonary vascular disease thereafter decreases survival.

Right versus Left Lung Blood Flow

Several groups have documented a relative increase in the blood flow to the right lung compared with that to the left in patients with TGA, using cineangiography and radionuclide lung imaging.[M11,R10,V7] The degree of increase is influenced by the degree of angulation between the main pulmonary artery and right pulmonary artery. If these are at right angles there is a minimal effect, whereas when the angle is increased to 135° so that the pulmonary trunk is directed toward the right pulmonary artery, about 75% of patients are affected. The data suggest that the disparity between right and left lung blood flows is not present at birth and increases with age.

The tendency of infants with intact ventricular septum to develop dynamic LVOTO after the first few months increases the velocity of flow, which increases the momentum effect toward the more directly aligned vessel. Once right lung flow increases, the right vascular bed grows more and there is a relative increase in vascular resistance and reduced compliance in the left lung, which further reduces left lung flow.

It is unlikely that this phenomenon has any significant effect on the natural history of untreated TGA.

TECHNIQUE OF OPERATION

Atrial Switch Operation (Senning Technique)

The preparations for operation and the median sternotomy incision are performed as usual (see Chapter 2). The operation is performed either routinely (GLH) or only in infants less than about 3 kg in weight (UAB), during profound hypothermia to about 18°C and total circulatory arrest (see Chapter 2, Section 4). In infants weighing about 3 kg or more the operation is performed using cardiopulmonary bypass (CPB) and direct caval cannulation (UAB) (see Chapter 2, Section 3). When CPB is used, the patient is cooled to 25°C, the flow is then stabilized at $1.6 \; l \cdot m^{-1} \cdot m^{-2}$, and if necessary a period of 10–15 minutes of low flow or total circulatory arrest may be employed; cold cardioplegic myocardial protection is used.

Before CPB is established, marking sutures are placed to identify points that are critical in the subsequent incisions (UAB) (Fig. 39-25a). First, the circumferences of the superior and inferior vena cavae are determined (by compressing them with a clamp, measuring the length of clamp occupied by the compressed cava, and multiplying by 2).

The superior and inferior extent of the proposed left atriotomy are defined by marking sutures, placed superiorly and inferiorly at the point of junction of the left atrial and right pulmonary vein wall with the most rightward aspect of the right atrial wall surface. The incision must not be extended further superiorly or inferiorly, which would necessitate its being carried leftward and behind the cavae. Marking sutures are then placed to define the superior and inferior extent of the right atriotomy. The superior extent is 3 or 4 mm anteriorly to the sulcus terminalis and thus anterior to the sinus node, and is anterior to the corresponding marking suture at the superior end of the proposed left atriotomy by a distance that is about two-thirds of the circumference of the superior vena cava. The inferior extent of the right atriotomy is placed anterior to the corresponding marking suture at the inferior end of the proposed left atriotomy by a distance that is a minimum of 15 mm but equal to two-thirds of the circumference of the inferior vena cava. With direct caval cannulation, the eustachian valve rarely can be used in the repair, and a marking suture is placed for an anterior extension of the inferior end of the incision. A marking suture for an anterior extension is placed superiorly as well, so that later a right atrial flap can be created (UAB) (Fig. 39-25b).

CPB is established, either with a simple venous cannula for the profoundly hypothermic technique (GLH) or with direct caval cannulation (UAB). Initially, during cooling the interatrial groove on the right side is dissected (Fig. 39-25b). Care is taken to keep the dissection shallow and not to enter the atria. The aorta is cross-clamped, and the cold cardioplegic solution is infused. (When total circulatory arrest is used [GLH], the aortic cross-clamping is delayed until just before its establishment, and cardioplegia is not used.)

The left atriotomy is made and the pump-oxygenator sump sucker is inserted if the patient is on CPB. The right atriotomy and anterior extensions are made (UAB) (Fig. 39-25b). Alternatively, a longitudinal incision is made with a slight

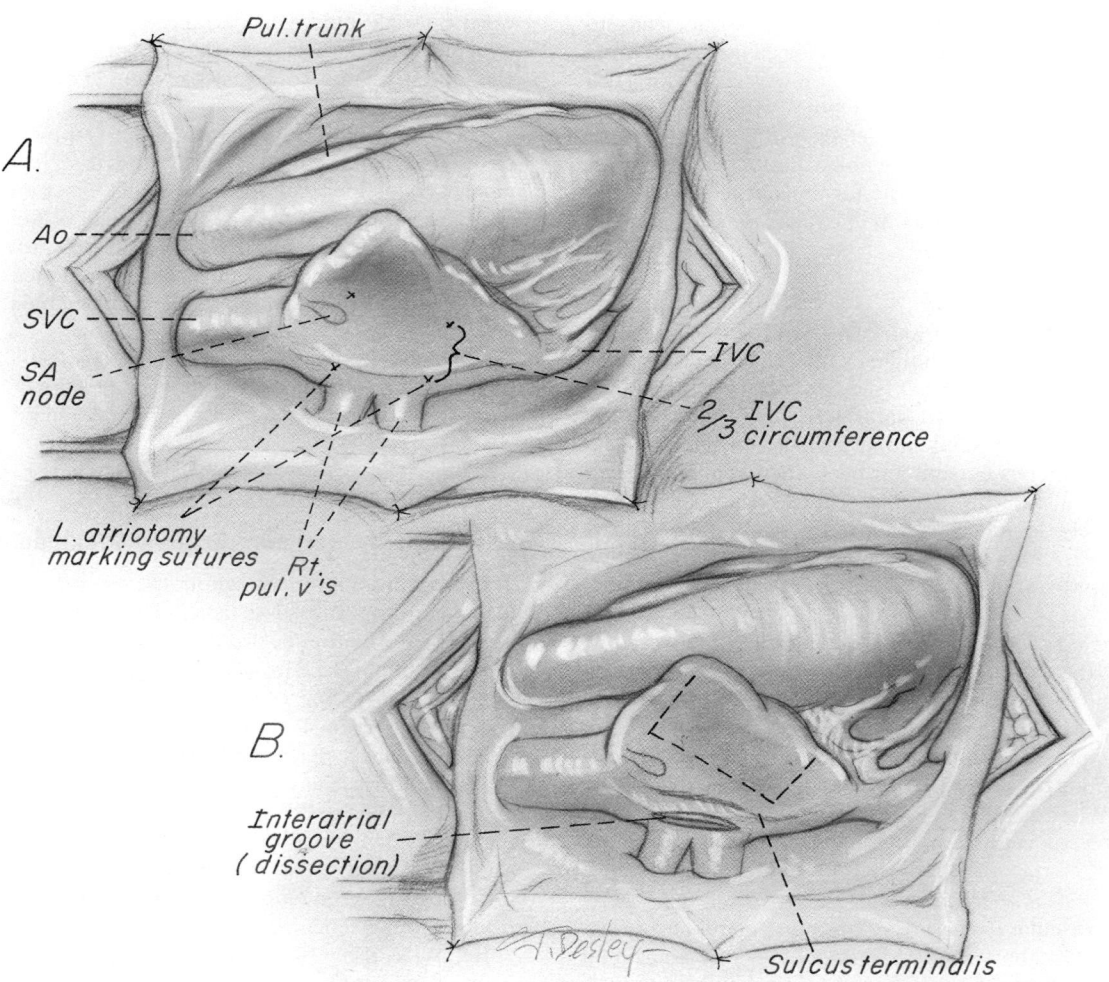

Figure 39-25 The atrial switch operation (modified Senning technique) for patients with TGA.
(a) The placement of initial marking sutures (see text).
(b) The proposed right atriotomy (UAB) is indicated by the dashed lines. The dissection of the interatrial groove, performed after commencing CPB, is also shown.

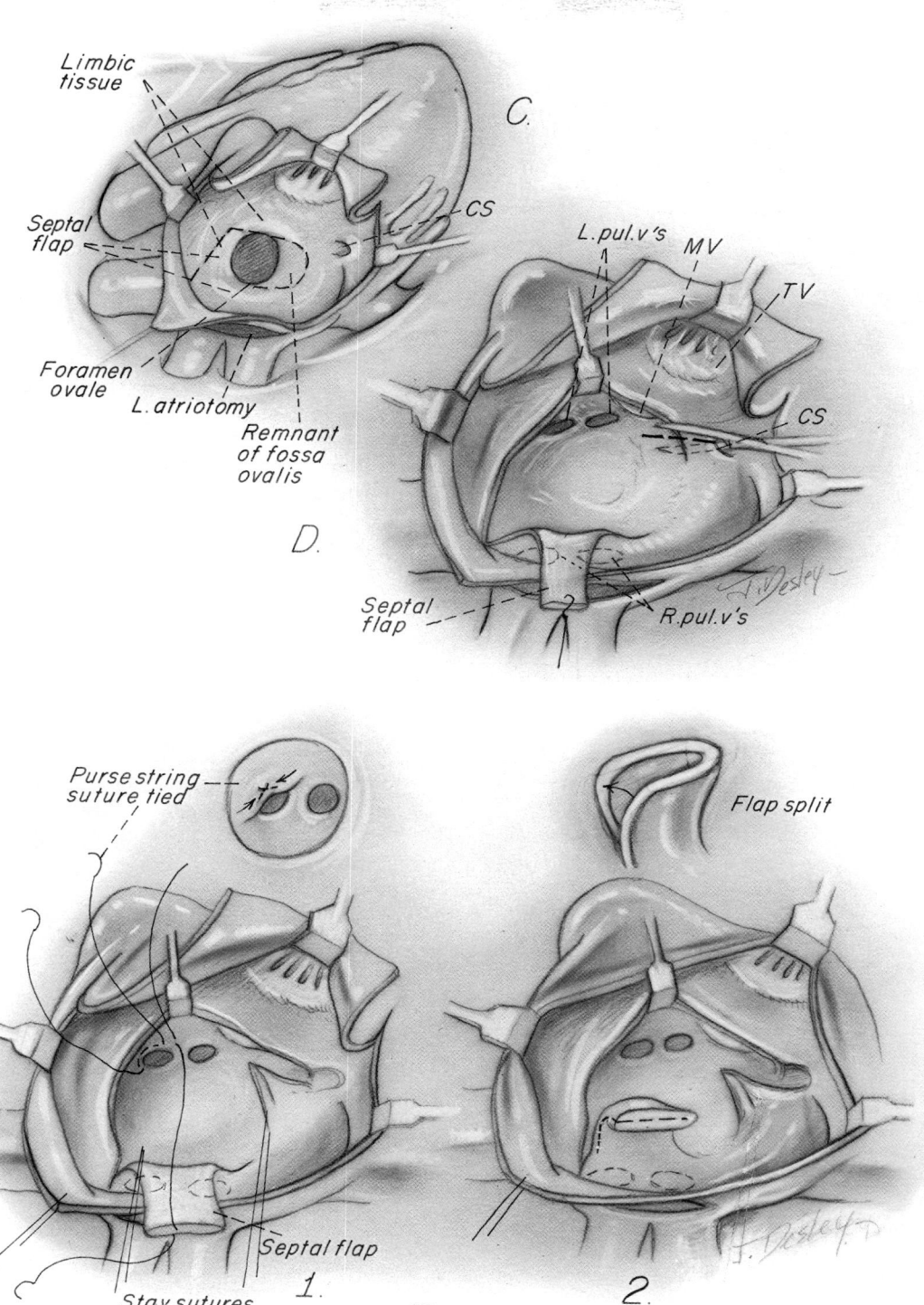

Figure 39-25 *(continued)*

(c) The left atriotomy has been made and the right atrium opened. When the foramen ovale is large, the small inferior remnant of the fossa ovalis is excised and the septal flap fashioned by incisions shown.

(d) The wall between coronary sinus and left atrium is cut down with scissors in such a manner as to leave as wide a posterior-wall remnant (flap) as possible.

(e) (1-UAB) Stay sutures are placed as shown to guide the suturing of the septal flap into position. If necessary, a semi-purse-string suture is placed at the base of the left atrial appendage (insert), which when tied advances this tissue.

(2-GLH) Alternatively, the limbus after its detachment may be split superiorly so that it opens like the leaves of a book.

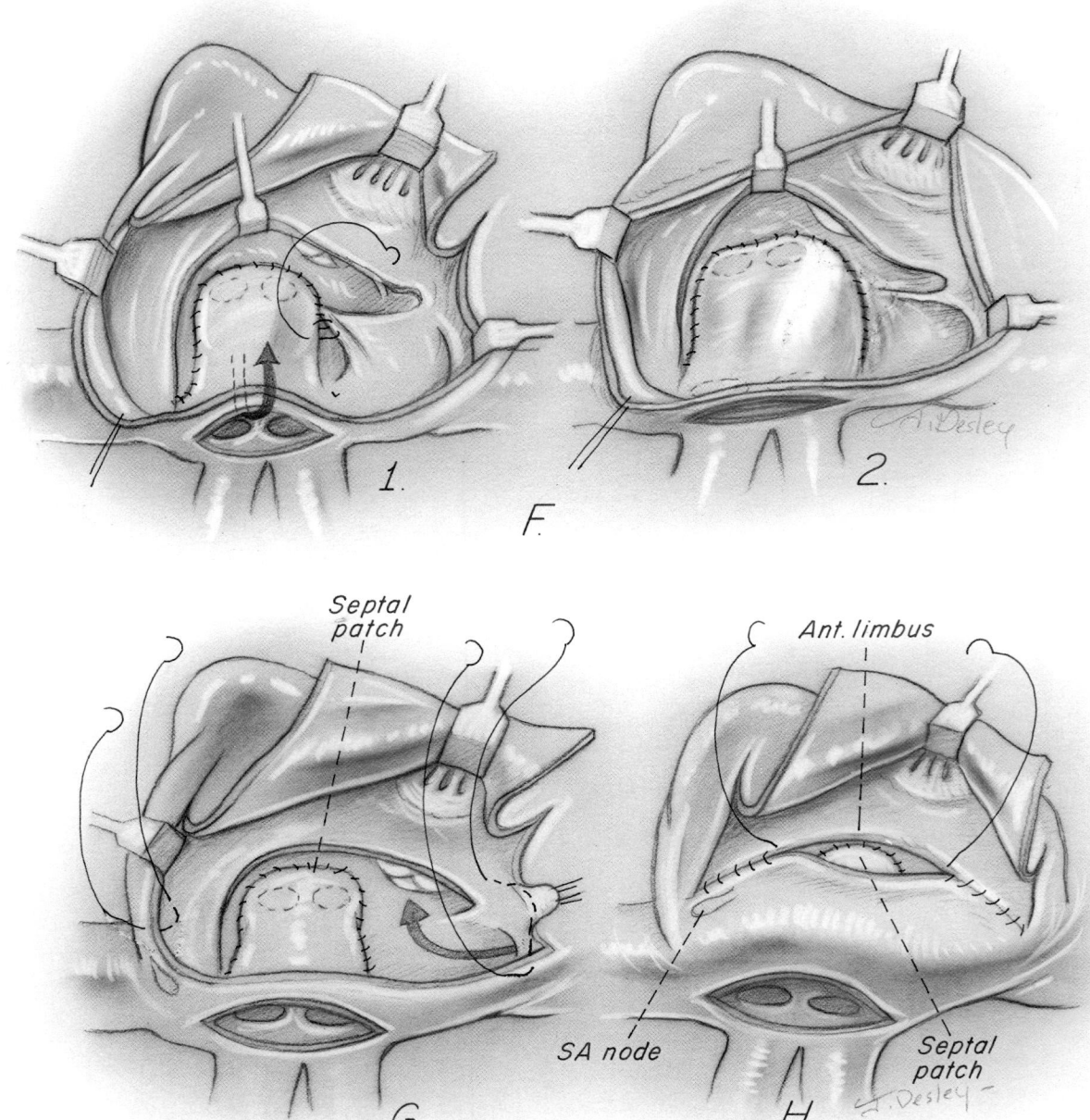

Figure 39-25 (*continued*)

(*f*) (1-UAB) The septal flap has been sewn into place, widened inferiorly by sewing to the large posterior lip or flap created by the cutting down of the coronary sinus. Note the wide pathway now available to the inferior caval blood and the large pathway (indicated by the arrow), anterior to the right pulmonary veins, between the posterior pulmonary venous chamber and that anterior to the septal flap now that the suturing of the septal flap has pulled the posterior atrial wall forward. At this stage, the posterior pulmonary venous pathway can be inspected through the aperture for appropriate width.

(2-GLH) The split septal flap has been opened and sewn into place. Similarly wide pathways result.

(*g*) The wide pathway from inferior vena cava to mitral valve is indicated by the arrow. As the first step in completing this caval pathway to the mitral valve, an inferiorly placed purse-string suture gathers together the right atrial wall and the inferior aspect of the posterior atrial flap. Later, a similar suture is placed superiorly.

(*h*) The inferior suture line between the posterior right atrial flap and the limbus anteriorly is carried to the midpoint of the limbus. The superior purse-string suture is placed, and this suture line is carried toward the first one.

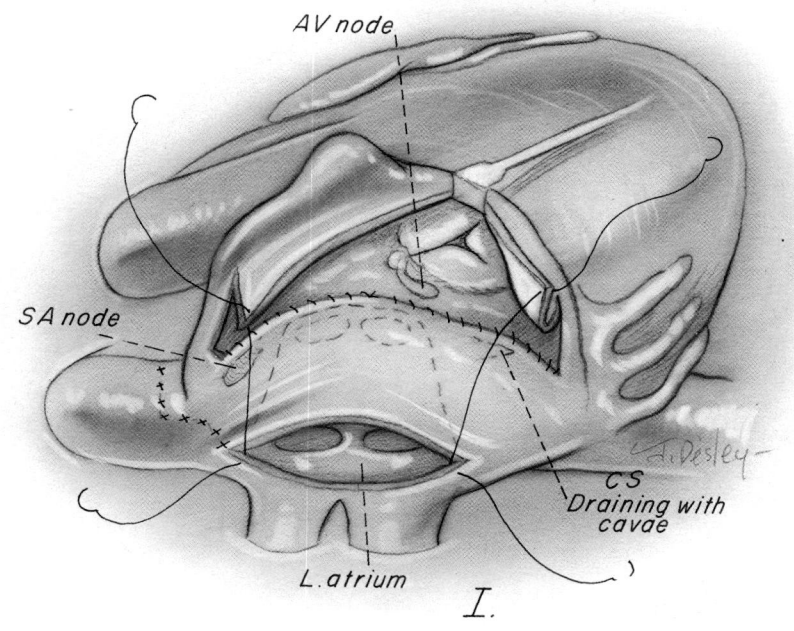

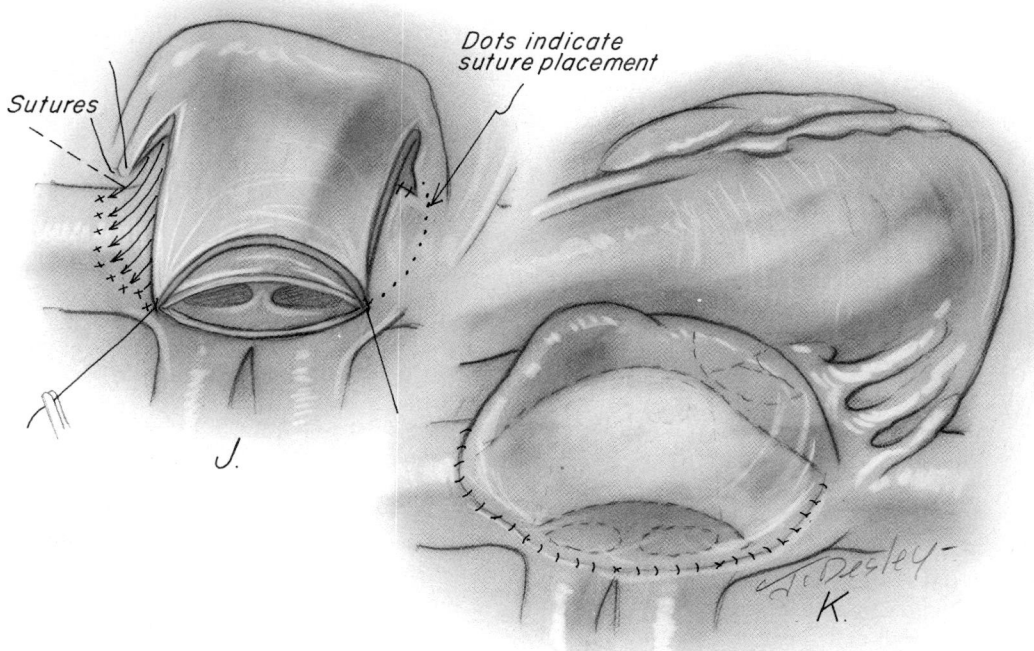

Figure 39-25 *(continued)*

(*i*) The pulmonary venous pathway to the tricuspid valve remains to be completed. In one technique (UAB), the angle of the anterior right atrial flap (see Fig. 39-25*b*) is brought to the upper angle of the incision into the left atrium as shown and the suture tied. The x x x line indicates the proposed line of attachment of the flap.

(*j*) With one arm, the flap is sewn to the lateral aspect of the atrium and the superior vena cava along the x x x line, which is posterior and then superior to the sinoatrial node. This suture line is facilitated by placing a traction suture just above the most superior x. Interrupted sutures may be used. With the other arm of the suture, the anterior right atrial flap is attached to the left atrium over the superior pulmonary vein, and the suture is then held.

(*k*) An entirely similar suture line is placed inferiorly to complete the repair.

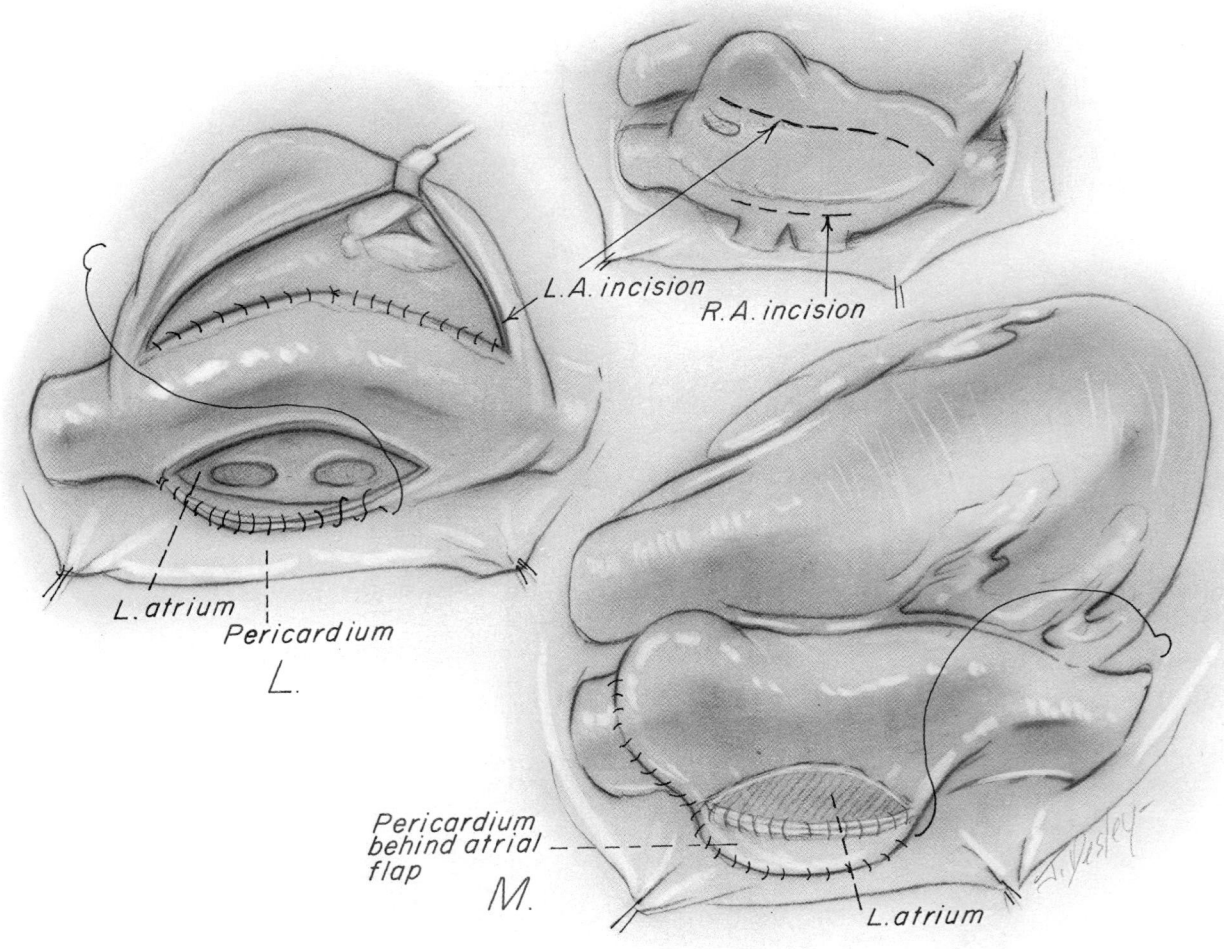

Figure 39-25 *(continued)*
(*l*) In the other technique (GLH), a linear right atriotomy incision has been made initially (insert). The right atrial flap then may not easily come to the left atrial wall over the pulmonary veins (about 30% of cases). In this case, the in situ pericardium is sutured to the lateral side of the left atriotomy.
(*m*) The anterior right atrial flap is sutured superiorly and inferiorly as just described, but the suture lines are joined by suturing the flap to the pericardium as shown, resulting in a large opening between the posterior and anterior pulmonary venous compartments.

Ao, aorta; AV node, atrioventricular node; CS, conal septum; IVC, inferior vena cava; LA incision, left anterior incision; L. atrium, left atrium; L. pul. v's, left pulmonary veins; MV, mitral valve; Pul. trunk, pulmonary trunk; RA, right anterior incision; SA node, sinoatrial node; SVC, superior vena cava; TV, tricuspid valve.

anterior convexity (GLH) (see later Fig. 39-25*l*), which extends inferiorly to the junction of the eustachian valve with the lateral right atrial wall and superiorly to a point 3 mm anterior to the right atrial–superior vena caval junction just in front of the sinus node. Appropriate stay sutures are placed for exposure.

The atrial septal flap, which will form the anterior wall of the posterior pulmonary venous compartment, is fashioned (Fig. 39-25*c*). When the foramen ovale is small, it is closed transversely with a few interrupted sutures and the flap created. When the foramen ovale is large, the flap consists solely of the superior and posterior aspects of the limbus (Fig. 39-25*d*), but this is quite adequate when the maneuvers described below are used.

After making the septal flap, the coronary sinus is cut down precisely so as to leave a large posterior lip to be used in making the inferior septal flap suture line (Figs. 39-25*d* and 39-25*e*). If the septal flap is particularly small, a half purse-string suture is placed and tied at the base of the left atrial appendage (UAB; Fig. 39-25*e*1), which advances this corner of the left atrium toward the right. The septal flap may be split and opened like the leaves of a book (GLH; Fig. 39-25*e*2). Then either the simple septal flap (Fig. 39-25*f*1) or the split flap (Fig. 39-25*f*2) is sewn into place.

The caval pathway to the mitral valve is formed posteriorly by the repositioned septal flap (Fig. 39-25*f*1) and is now completed by suturing the posterior right atrial flap anteriorly to the limbus. Half purse-string sutures are used at each end to begin this (Fig. 39-25*g*), placing these with great care so that these extensions of the cavae will be undistorted. Each suture line is carried toward the midportion of the posterior margin of anterior limbus (Fig. 39-25*h*). The sutures are placed along the cut edge of the limbus anteriorly, visualizing and avoiding the position of the AV node (Fig. 39-25*i*).

The pulmonary venous pathway to the tricuspid valve is now completed. The anterior extensions of each end of the right atriotomy incision allow the right atrial flap to come to the right and posteriorly with ease (UAB). The suturing is begun superiorly (Fig. 39-25*i*), and this suture line is completed before beginning the inferior one. After tying the first stitch, the suture line is carried anteriorly (Fig. 39-25*j*). A traction suture at the most anterior end of the proposed suture line facilitates the suturing, which may be done with 5-0 or 6-0 interrupted or continuous polypropylene sutures. This suture line passes posterior and then superior to the location of the sinus node. With the other arm of the suture, the right atrial flap is sutured to a portion of the anterior lip of the left atriotomy, over the right superior pulmonary vein. A similar suture line is made inferiorly to complete this last step of the operation (Fig. 39-25*k*).

Alternatively (GLH), when a near linear right atriotomy is made and the right atrial flap does not always come easily to the anterior lip of left atrium, the posterior wall of the left atriotomy incision is sutured to the adjacent in situ pericardium (Fig. 39-25*l*). The flap is then sutured to the pericardium at a convenient distance from the suture line to produce a wide opening between the posterior and anterior portions of the pulmonary venous compartment (Fig. 39-25*m*).

When CPB is used, rewarming is begun about 5 minutes before the completion of the suturing of the right atrial flap; when the suturing is completed, and with strong suction on the aortic needle vent, the aortic clamp is released and rewarming is begun. The remainder of the procedure, including the de-airing, is completed as usual (see Chapter 2, Section 3).

When profoundly hypothermic total circulatory arrest is used with a single venous cannula, the venous cannula is reinserted through the right atrial appendage into the pulmonary venous atrium, CPB is reestablished, and rewarming is begun after removing the aortic clamp (see Chapter 2, Section 4). A stab wound is made in the most anterior part of the right ventricle just below the aortic valve to allow the escape of any entrapped air as the heart begins to contract (GLH). When a single venous cannula is used in this manner, pulmonary venous blood is returned to the pump oxygenator and the circuit is in reality a systemic (right) ventricular bypass only. Thus, it is necessary to massage the heart gently in order to push blood through the lungs until an adequate pulmonary (left) ventricular beat returns. This is required for only a few minutes as a rule. The single venous cannula tip often partially obstructs the caval tunnels beneath the baffle so that caval pressures of 10–20 mmHg are usual during rewarming, usually falling to that in the pulmonary venous atrium after the cannula has been removed. The remainder of the procedure is completed as usual.

With either technique, it may be useful to leave a polyvinyl catheter through the right atrial appendage into the pulmonary venous atrium and one through the left atrial appendage into the systemic venous atrium. These plus an internal jugular catheter and a radial artery catheter placed at the beginning of the operation allow complete monitoring of the hemodynamic state in the early postoperative period.

In the unusual event that the procedure cannot be completed within 45 minutes of total circulatory arrest, after completing the creation of the systemic venous atrium the single venous return cannula is inserted into the left atrial appendage (which is first opened and snared with a purse-string stitch) or, if this is too small, into the apex of the left ventricle through a stab incision also controlled with a purse-string stitch (GLH). CPB is then commenced at a relatively low flow and the pulmonary venous return collected from the posterior portion of the new pulmonary venous atrium with the pump-oxygenator sucker system. When the repair has been completed and normal venous cannulation and flow rates achieved, rewarming is begun.

Atrial Switch Operation (Mustard Technique)

Preparations for the operation and the support techniques are the same as when the Senning technique is used.

After establishing CPB and aortic cross-clamping with cold cardioplegia, or establishing profoundly hypothermic total circulatory arrest, the right atrium is opened through the usual oblique incision (Fig. 39-26*a*1) (UAB) or so that a V–Y plasty can be used as a part of the operation (GLH) (Fig. 39-26*a*2). In the latter instance, the incision's posterior extension between the pulmonary veins, which converts the incision into a Y, is not made until later. Atrial stay sutures are placed for exposure.

The atrial septal remnants are excised, beginning this by dividing the limbus superiorly with scissors, centering the cut just to the left of the midpoint of the superior limbus (Fig. 39-26*b*). The incision is carried nearly into the roof of the atrium and then posteriorly beneath the superior vena cava (SVC) and then inferiorly, removing the thick tissue from behind the SVC and in front of the right pulmonary veins. Occasionally, the incision goes outside the atria, and if so, the opening is closed with fine interrupted sutures. Any remnant of the fossa ovalis is completely excised.

The center of the free wall of the coronary sinus is divided downward with scissors for 7–10 mm, exactly as described for the Senning procedure (Fig. 39-26*b*). This transfers the coronary sinus opening into the left atrium and widens the area that will be the extension of the inferior vena cava (IVC) toward the mitral valve.

The most appropriate material, configuration, and size of the atrial baffle that is to be inserted has been confusing and controversial through the years. Pericardium is considered the material of choice because of the higher proportion of baffle complications when Dacron is used (GLH, UAB). However, if at a secondary operation pericardium is not available, very thin knitted Dacron may be used. One concept is to use a relatively small pericardial baffle and sew it snugly in place away from the caval orifices in such a manner that as much of the caval pathways as is possible is atrial wall rather than baffle (GLH). A different concept, based upon the Toronto technique,[T6] uses a larger baffle that is

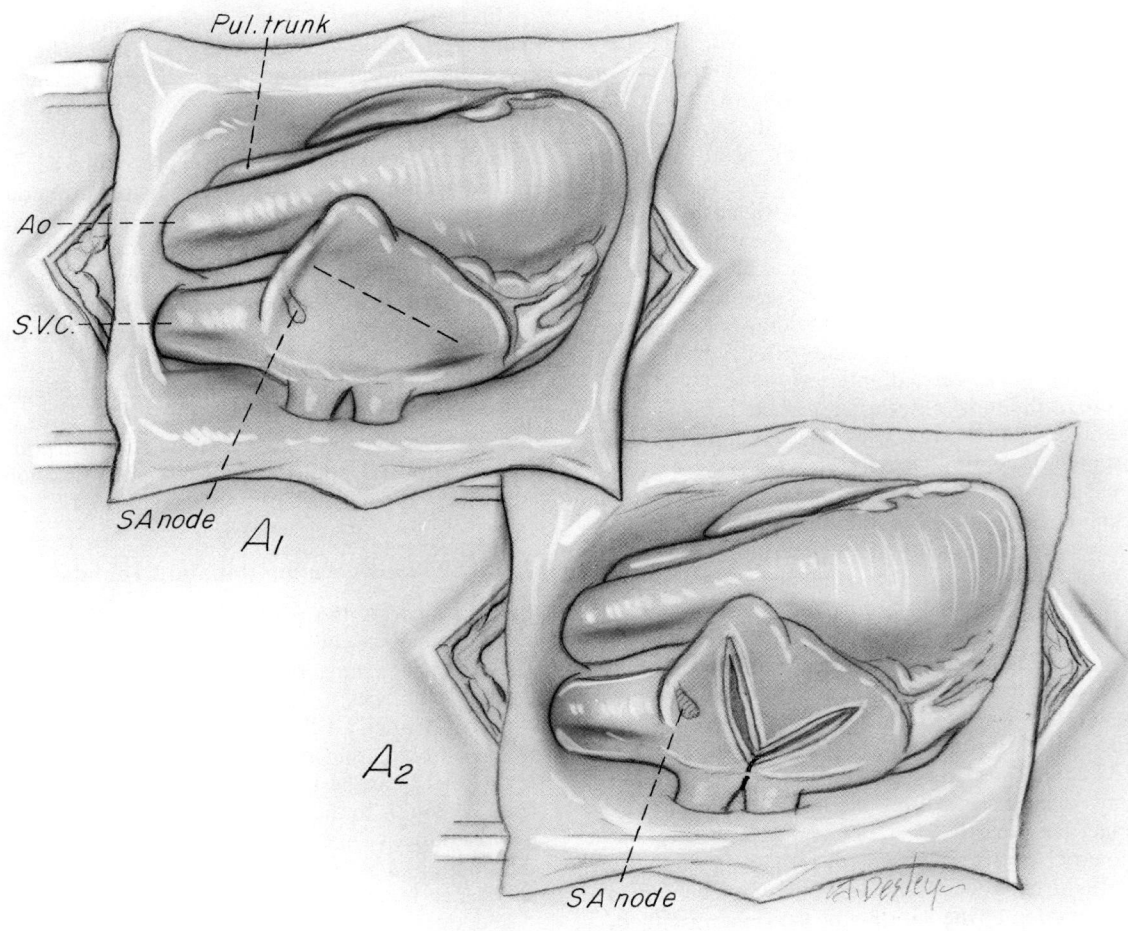

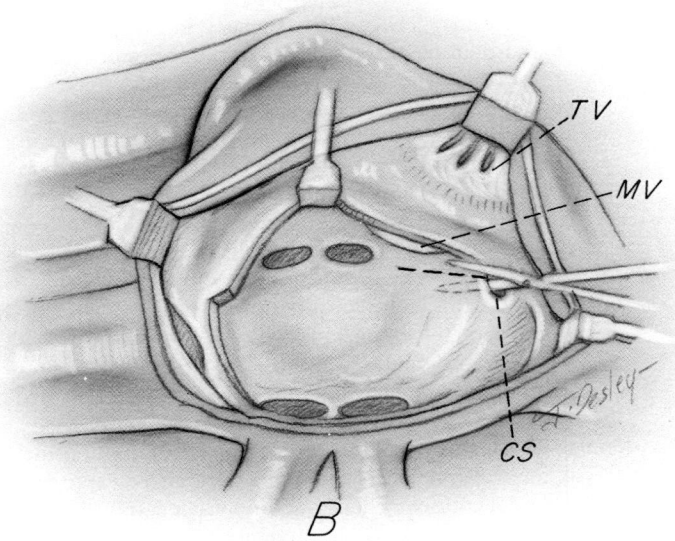

Figure 39-26 Atrial switch operation by the Mustard technique.

(*a*) (1-UAB) The usual oblique atriotomy is made.

(2-GLH) A V–Y incision is used.

(*b*) After excising the atrial septum (see text), the coronary sinus is cut down, just as in the Senning procedure.

(*c*) The pericardial baffle is made from pericardium. In one technique (UAB), the Toronto-type baffle is used and is sewn around the caval orifices. The dimensions in the large diagram and in (c1) are for a 5-kg. infant. Dimensions of 7 × 4 cm are used for a 10-kg child, and proportionately larger ones for larger children. The main drawing represents the shape and dimensions of this pericardial baffle as it is initially excised. In the other technique (GLH), the patch does not reach to the orifices of the cavae but rather to the atrial wall and proximal to the cavae and thus can be smaller (c2).

(1-UAB) The Toronto baffle for a 5-kg child.

(2-GLH) The baffle for a 5-kg child.

(*d*) The baffle is first sutured over the left pulmonary veins. The small circles show the suture line (UAB), and the dashed lines show an alternative one (GLH). Stay sutures may be inserted to aid in placement of the suture line (see text).

(*e*) Continuation of the baffle suture line (see text).

(1-UAB) With the larger patch, the suture line is continued around the orifices of the superior and inferior vena cavae.

(2-GLH) With the smaller patch, the suture line is kept well away from the caval orifices (see text). Each stitch in the atrial wall penetrates the wall completely and gathers the wall down onto the pericardial patch.

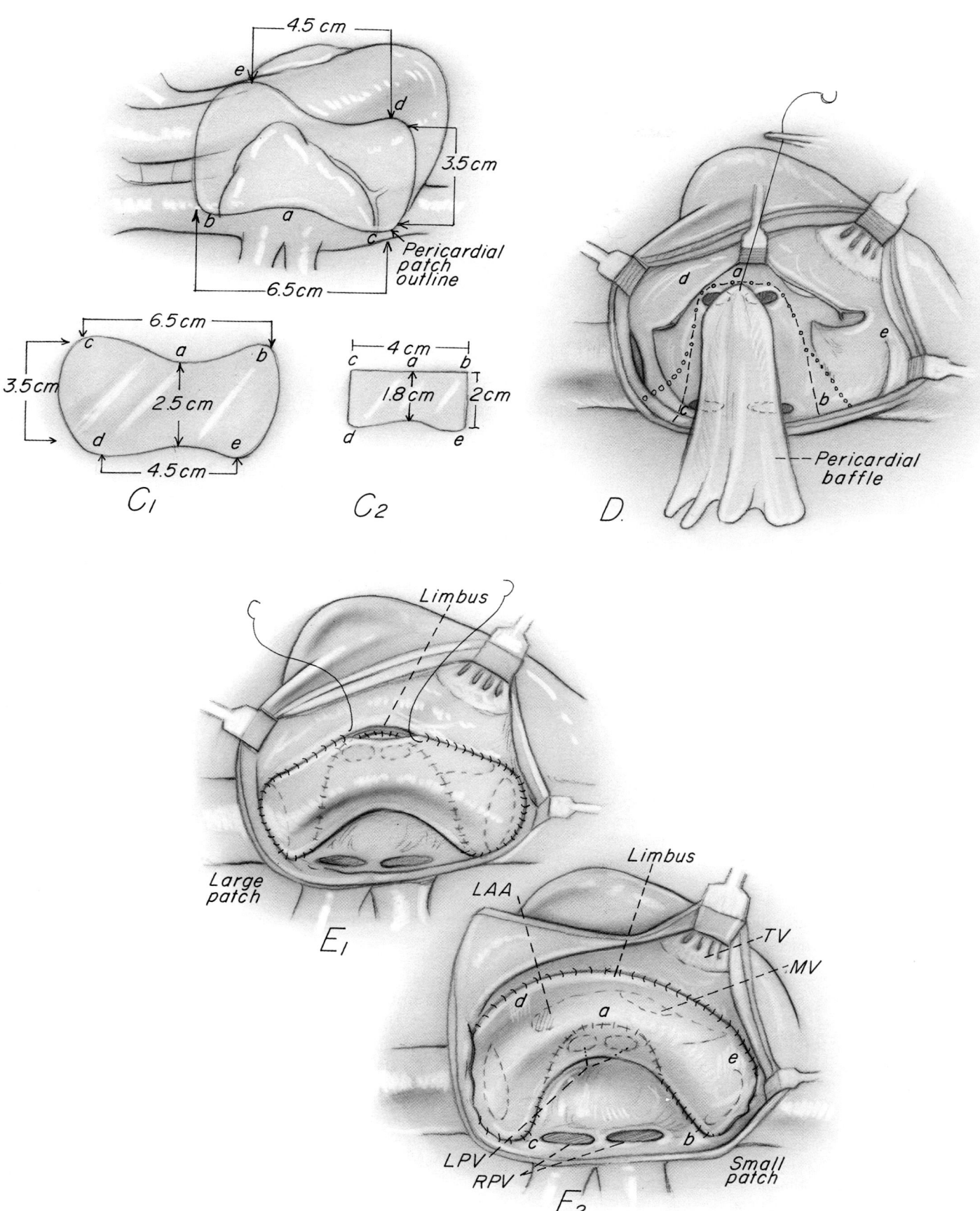

C_1

C_2

$D.$ — Pericardial baffle

E_1 — Large patch — Limbus

E_2 — Small patch — Limbus — LAA — TV — MV — LPV — RPV

Pericardial patch outline

4.5 cm
3.5 cm
6.5 cm
6.5 cm
3.5 cm
2.5 cm
4.5 cm
4 cm
1.8 cm
2 cm

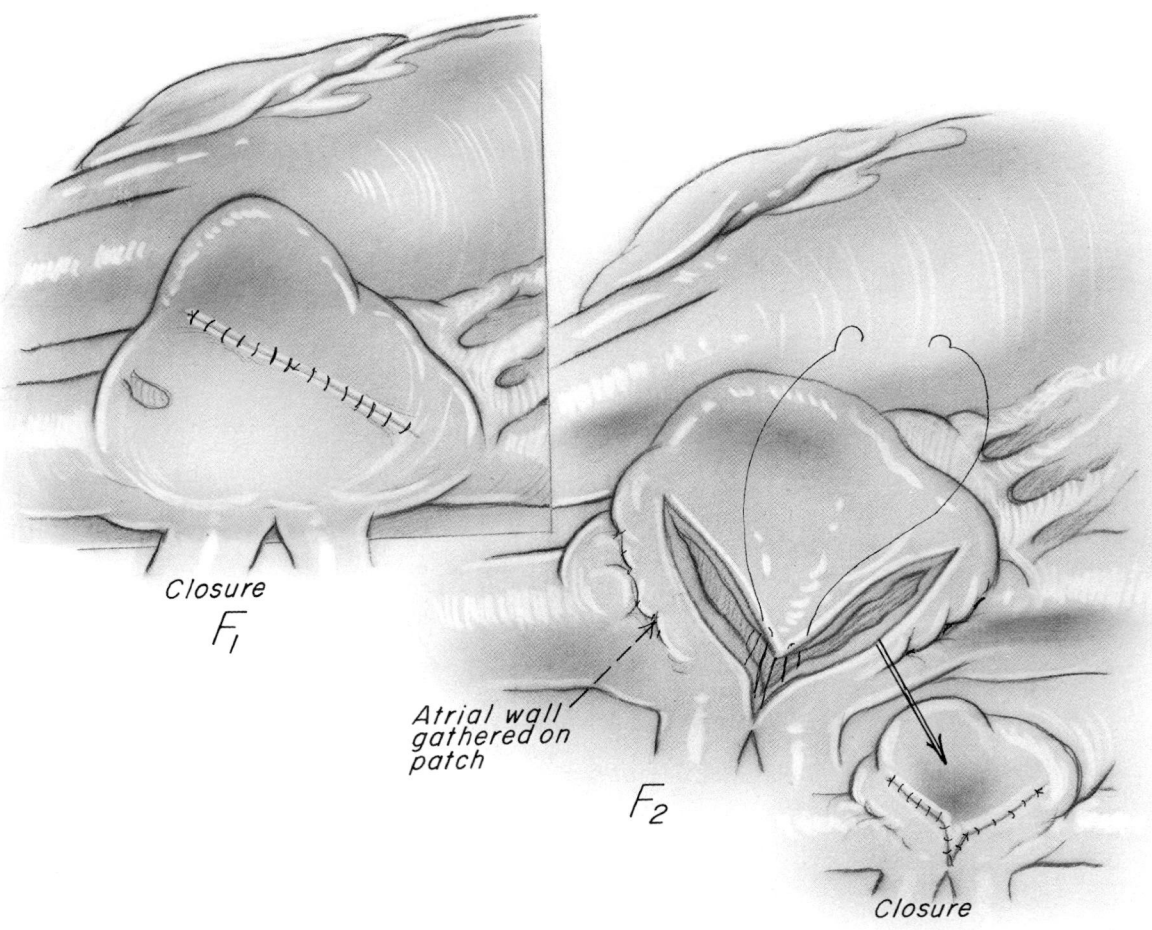

Closure

F_1

Atrial wall gathered on patch

F_2

Closure

Figure 39-26   *(continued)*
(*f*) (1-UAB) Simple closure of the right atriotomy (see text for details).
(2-GLH) Closure of the V–Y plasty to enlarge the pulmonary venous atrium. Note the desired purse-string effect of the baffle suture line in the atrial wall near the superior and inferior vena cava (GLH method).

Ao, aorta; CS, conal septum; LAA, left atrial appendage; LPV, left pulmonary vein; MV, mitral valve; RPV, right pulmonary vein; SA node, sinoatrial node; SVC, superior vena cava; TB, tricuspid valve.

sewn into place around the caval orifices, with a redundancy of the baffle around the cavae to minimize the chance of narrowing the superior or inferior vena cava pathway (UAB).

GLH Method
The pericardial baffle is cut to a generally rectangular shape with a curving posterior edge (Fig. 39-26c2). The dimensions shown in the figure are appropriate for the average 5-kg infant.

Alternatively, the distance *a–b* (from in front of the left pulmonary veins to the crista terminalis just superior and anterior to the IVC orifice) is measured and reduced by two-thirds, since left pulmonary veins are to be pulled somewhat rightward by the suture line. The long dimension of the patch is twice this reduced length. The baffle width is made half the

length of the patch, and the baffle waist is 2–3 mm less than the width.

The pericardial baffle is sewn into place by commencing a double-armed 5-0 polypropylene suture line between baffle and atrium at *a* (Fig. 39-26*d*) and continuing it to *b* (Fig. 39-26*e2*). The two appropriate corners of the patch are held taut as the edge of the pericardium is sutured across the back wall of the left atrium, using a whip stitch that is held tightly by the assistant. Since the pericardial length is one-third shorter than the distance on the heart, the stitches pick up larger bites of atrium than of pericardium and pull the atrium onto the patch. If when point *b* is reached on the heart there is excess pericardium, this is trimmed, while retaining a 90° angle on the patch at *b*. The suture line from *a–b* follows a gentle curve that lies about 10 mm from the apex of the incision that has opened the coronary sinus. Point *b* lies 5 mm superior to the IVC ostium at the junction of the posterior and lateral right atrial (RA) walls just behind the crista terminalis and in front of the plane of the right pulmonary vein.

The other arm of the polypropylene suture is used to attach the baffle to the back wall of left atrium (LA) along the curved line *a–c* (Fig. 39-26*e*2) in a similar manner, pulling the excess atrial wall onto the patch. This suture line passes at least 10 mm below and behind the excised limbus to reach *c*, which lies 5 mm inferior to the SVC ostium and bears the same relationship to the crista terminalis as *b*. If, when the suture line is completed, the patch is too long, it is trimmed back appropriately.

The suture line is continued superiorly and anteriorly, staying well clear of the orifice of the SVC. The distance *c–d* on the heart is almost twice as long as on the patch edge, and the bites of atrial wall are therefore much more widely spread than those on the patch. Moreover, because of the heavily trabeculated atrial wall, each stitch is passed completely through the atrial wall. Suture line *c–d* curves first below and then in front of the SVC, halfway between the sinus node and the atrial appendage purse string, to reach point *d* (Fig. 39-26*e*2). The midportion of this suture line lies close to the edge of the atriotomy. Point *d* lies where the trabeculated free wall joins the smooth atrial wall, which becomes continuous with the anterior remnant of the limbus.

The inferior suture line around the IVC orifice is now made in a similar manner. The suture line *b–e* (Fig. 39-26*e*2) passes through the right atrial free wall, initially near the edge of the atriotomy and then well in front of the inferior caval orifice. The bites on the atrium are larger than those on the patch but less so than around the SVC. The aim both superiorly and inferiorly is to fashion the caval tunnels in an oval or even a D shape, the straight edge of the D being made of pericardium and the curved longer edge of atrial wall.

Finally, the anterior long dimension of the pericardial rectangle is sutured to the anterior limbus in a manner entirely analogous to the suturing of the posterior atrial flap to the limbus in the Senning procedure (Fig. 39-26*e*2).

The right atrium having been opened by the V–Y plasty incision, the atriotomy is now extended posteriorly between the orifices of the right superior and inferior pulmonary veins to convert the V atriotomy into a Y-shaped incision. This releases the potentially narrow waist of the pathway between posterior and anterior pulmonary venous compartments. The atriotomy is closed by advancing the apex of the V-shaped atrial wall flap into the posterior angle of the newly made incision between the pulmonary veins (Fig. 39-26*f*2). Three or four throws of the suture are placed in the angle before snugging them, and then the suture line is completed in the usual manner.

After closing the atrium, the remainder of the operation is completed as described for the Senning-type repair.

UAB Method

Just after making the sternotomy and before opening the pericardium, the pericardium is cleared laterally to within 4 or 5 mm of each phrenic nerve, generally a distance of 5 or 6 cm in a 5-kg infant. Superiorly, the pericardium is cleared nearly to the level of the innominate vein after reflecting and

partially excising the thymus gland. A longitudinal incision is made in the pericardium a few millimeters anterior to the right phrenic nerve (Fig. 39-26*c*). In a 5-kg infant, the length of this incision is about 6.5 cm. Next, a transverse incision is made in the pericardium, along the diaphragm, extending to within 4 or 5 mm of the left phrenic nerve, a distance of about 3.5 cm in a 5-kg child but proportionately longer in a larger patient. Superiorly, a similar but convex incision is made. A left-sided longitudinal incision is made parallel to the left phrenic nerve but with a mild concavity in its midportion. After the patch is removed, a similar concavity is made in the midportion of the other long dimension of the rectangle (Fig. 39-26*c*1).

A double-armed 4-0 or 5-0 polypropylene suture is passed through point *a* on the baffle and through the left atrial wall just above the spur between left superior and inferior pulmonary veins (Fig. 39-26*d*), just as in the GLH method. The superior suture line between *a* and more or less *c* (see Fig. 39-26*e*1) is made as described in the GLH method, but as the point just superior to the left superior pulmonary vein is reached, the suture line is carried superiorly to the posterolateral border of the orifice of the SVC and then up around the lateral margin of the caval orifice (Fig. 39-26*e*1). A larger distance is left between the bites on the patch than between those around the caval orifice so as to avoid purse stringing this orifice and to bring a redundant amount of pericardial patch into the area. The inferior suture line between *a* and more or less *b* is made, using the lip of the coronary sinus cut down as described in the Senning repair (Fig. 39-26*e*1). The remainder of the suturing of the baffle to the limbus anteriorly is accomplished in a fashion similar to that described for the Senning method.

The right atriotomy incision is closed primarily (Fig. 39-26*f*1). With strong suction on the aortic needle vent, the aortic clamp is released and rewarming is begun. The remainder of the operation is completed as described for the Senning procedure.

Atrial Switch Operation Plus Repair of Ventricular Septal Defect

Nearly all ventricular septal defects (VSDs) in TGA can be repaired through the tricuspid valve,[12] using the techniques described for the transatrial repair of isolated VSDs (see Chapter 20, Figs. 20-23, 20-26, and 20-27). This may be done at any point in the procedure, but with the Senning technique it is convenient to do it either just before or just after creating the anterior wall of the posterior pulmonary venous compartment with the septal flap; with the Mustard technique it is generally most convenient to repair the VSD before beginning insertion of the baffle.

Atrial Switch Operation Plus Repair of Left Ventricular Outflow Tract Obstruction

This discussion refers primarily to transposition with essentially intact ventricular septum, since it is uncommon for direct relief of left ventricular outflow obstruction (LVOTO) to be possible in TGA, VSD, and LVOTO.

When the obstruction is dynamic and the systolic pressure

in the left ventricle similar to or less than that in the right (systemic) ventricle, nothing is done directly to the LVOTO. When the left ventricular systolic pressure is considerably higher, surgical relief of the LVOTO is generally required. This may be in the form of resection of muscle, but in extreme cases a valved extracardiac conduit may be needed (see below).

When the LVOTO is in the form of localized or diffuse fibromuscular obstruction, the obstructive tissue is resected. One approach is through the mitral valve (UAB),[O1,O2,W5] after creation of the septal flap (Senning repair) or excision of the atrial septum (Mustard repair). Alternatively, the resection is performed through the pulmonary artery and valve (GLH). In the uncommon circumstances in which the obstruction is valvar, valvotomy through the pulmonary artery is performed.

When the LVOTO is severe and cannot be relieved by resection, the placement of a homograft valved conduit between left ventricle and pulmonary artery is required. The conduit is prepared as described earlier (see Chapter 12, Appendix 12C for a description of the preservation of the homograft and its preparation for use at operation; and see Chapter 23, "Tetralogy of Fallot with Pulmonary Atresia" in Section 1, Technique of Operation, and Figure 23-37 for a description of the preparation of the conduit). After the first part of the atrial switch procedure has been completed, a longitudinal incision is made along the left side of the pulmonary artery; if necessary, the incision is carried on to the left pulmonary artery. The proposed left ventriculotomy, between or beyond the diagonal branches of the left anterior descending coronary artery and along the anterolateral aspect of the ventricle near the apex, is marked with 5-0 silk sutures. The heart is allowed to fall back against the pericardium, and the position on the pericardium of the proposed ventriculotomy is noted. Then, with the heart retracted upward and to the right, the proper length of the conduit can be estimated from the curving course between the pulmonary arteriotomy and the designated points on the pericardium. The conduit is trimmed to a proper length. It is cut short (about 5 mm beyond the aortic valve commissures) distally and beveled proximally (see Chapter 23, Fig. 23-37). The conduit is sewn into position exactly as is done for other ventricular-pulmonary artery conduits (see "Rastelli Operation for TGA, VSD, and LVOTO" and Chapter 23, Fig. 23-37).

After completing this, the last stages of the atrial switch operation are carried out, during which, if necessary, the aortic cross-clamp is released and rewarming begun.

Arterial Switch Operation

The preparations for operation, the median sternotomy, and the opening of the pericardium and placement of pericardial stay sutures proceed as usual. The pulmonary trunk is dissected as completely as possible before establishing cardiopulmonary bypass (CPB). This includes the sharp dissection of the trunk away from the ascending aorta, the dissection of the ligamentum arteriosum, and the complete dissection of the left and right pulmonary arteries beyond the point at which they penetrate the pericardium to become

extrapericardial. The purse string suture for the aortic cannulation is placed as far downstream as possible (Fig. 39-27a), and preparations are made for direct vena caval cannulation.

The coronary arteries are now examined as to their suitability for transfer to the pulmonary trunk. Currently, it is considered that only when there is a *single* coronary artery (particularly with patterns illustrated in *h* and *o*, Fig. 39-4) is there a considerably increased probability of problems from the coronary artery transfer; however, it is controversial whether this arrangement is an indication for using a procedure other than an arterial switch operation.

The arterial switch operation may be done during profoundly hypothermic total circulatory arrest (GLH). It may be done with CPB, except in infants less than 3 kg in weight, when total circulatory arrest is preferred (UAB). When CPB is used, this is established using direct caval cannulation (see Chapter 2) and the perfusate temperature made as cold as possible. After establishing CPB and during cooling, the final dissection of the pulmonary arteries is done. The ligamentum arteriosum is divided between ligatures (Fig. 39-27b). The aorta is cross-clamped, the cold cardioplegic solution is injected, the right atrium is opened, and the pump-oxygenator sump sucker is placed across the foramen ovale. The perfusate temperature is stabilized at 18°–25°C and the flow at 1.2–1.6 $l \cdot min^{-1} \cdot m^{-2}$. When a VSD is present, it is repaired through the tricuspid valve at this time.

The aorta is transected in about its midportion, well downstream to the level of the aortic valve commissures. The pulmonary artery is divided more distally, near its bifurcation (Fig. 39-27c). Marking sutures are placed on the outside of the pulmonary trunk to mark the location of the three pulmonary valve commissures. The distal segment of the divided aorta is passed behind the pulmonary artery bifurcation (the Lecompte maneuver) and anastomosed to the proximal end of the pulmonary trunk with continuous sutures (Fig. 39-27d). These are 5-0 or 6-0 monofilament absorbable sutures throughout (see Chapter 34, footnote 2). When there is a large VSD, the distal aortic segment is smaller than the pulmonary trunk and the aorta is enlarged by a vertical cut prior to the anastomosis (Fig. 39-27d).

The left and right coronary arteries along with a generous button of aortic wall are removed from the proximal aorta (Fig. 39-27e). The button of aorta seems to allow normal growth of the transplanted coronary ostia.[D11] The aortic cross-clamp is momentarily released, and marking sutures placed at the two points at which the coronary arteries can be implanted without tension or distortion. The aortic clamp is replaced, and buttons of tissue are removed from these points[2] using the sutures previously placed as guides in avoiding damage to the valve commissures (Fig. 39-27e). First the right and then the left coronary artery button is sutured into place with interrupted or continuous 6-0 or 7-0 sutures (Figs. 39-27f, 39-27g).

Quaegebeur now recommends an alternative protocol of

---

[2] A convenient way of accomplishing this is with an initial stab wound and punch removal of the button. (Goosen Aortic Punch made by Deknatal, 1018 Jerico Turnpike, Flora Park, New York.)

removing the coronary artery buttons just after dividing the great arteries. Then, while the valve leaflets of the neoaorta are in view, the buttons of tissue are removed and the coronary arteries implanted.[Q3] Then the anastomosis to create the neoaorta is made.

In patients with TGA and VSD, the defects created by excision of the coronary arteries need not be filled in. A vertical cut is made in the distal pulmonary artery to adapt it to the shape of the proximal neopulmonary trunk segment (Fig. 39-27g), and end-to-end anastomosis then creates the new pulmonary trunk. However, in neonates, failure to fill in these defects puts excess tension on the suture line of the neopulmonary artery; in addition, the aorta and pulmonary artery are of similar size in neonates with simple TGA. Thus, a disk of pericardium is sutured into the defects (Fig. 39-27h). Then a simple end-to-end anastomosis is made between the distal pulmonary artery and the proximal neopulmonary trunk segment (Fig. 39-27i).

Returning now to the right atrium, the sump sucker is removed and the foramen ovale closed. A small de-airing stab wound is made in the ascending aorta, the aortic cross-clamp is released, and rewarming is begun. The right atriotomy is closed. The remainder of the procedure is completed in the usual manner. Since bleeding can be troublesome, the suture lines are made as hemostatic as possible before discontinuing CPB, and fibrin glue is applied if available.

Intraventricular Repair

In hearts with TGA and large VSD, occasionally a completely intraventricular repair can be done by the intraven-

tricular tunnel technique.[C13,M25] Its applicability depends on the relation of the VSD to the great arteries and the tricuspid valve. The techniques for doing this are variable and may require enlargement of the VSD, but the operation is essentially the same as the intraventricular repair that may occasionally be possible in the Taussig-Bing heart (see Chapter 40, Fig. 40-12). In some cases, the tunnel may be made superior to the pathway to the pulmonary artery rather than inferior to it.[M25]

A partially intraventricular repair, associated with the placement of a valved extracardiac conduit between right ventricle and pulmonary artery, has been described, but in the largest reported series the hospital mortality was high.[P13]

Rastelli Operation for TGA, VSD, and LVOTO

The usual preparations for the operation are made. An estimate is made of the largest size of extracardiac conduit that can comfortably be placed within the patient's thorax, and the appropriate cryopreserved homograft valve and ascending aorta are removed from the graft bank and brought to the operating room. This is nearly always an 18 mm or larger homograft and most commonly one that is 22–25 mm; these sizes would be expected to function well after the child has reached adult life. A woven double velour Dacron tube 3–5 mm larger than the base of the homograft valve is selected and later preclotted. (See Chapter 12, Appendix 12C for a description of the preservation of the homograft and its preparation for use at operation; and Chapter 23, ''Tetralogy of Fallot with Pulmonary Atresia'' in Section 1, Technique of Operation, and Fig. 23-37 for a description of the preparation of the conduit.)

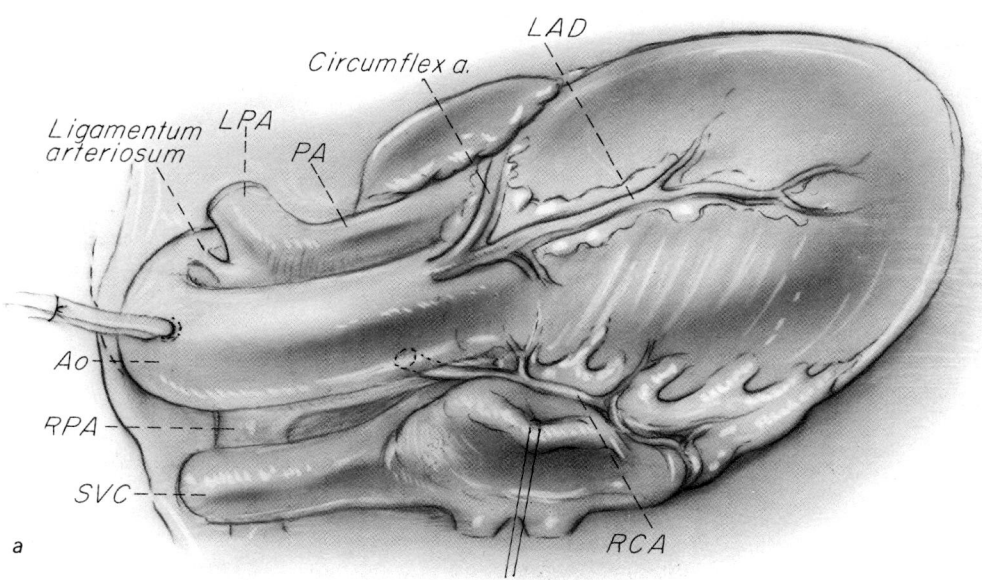

Figure 39-27 Arterial switch operation.
(a) The pulmonary artery (PA) is dissected completely away from the ascending aorta. The ligamentum arteriosum has been dissected out and the PA bifurcation and the left (LPA) and right (RPA) pulmonary arteries completely mobilized.

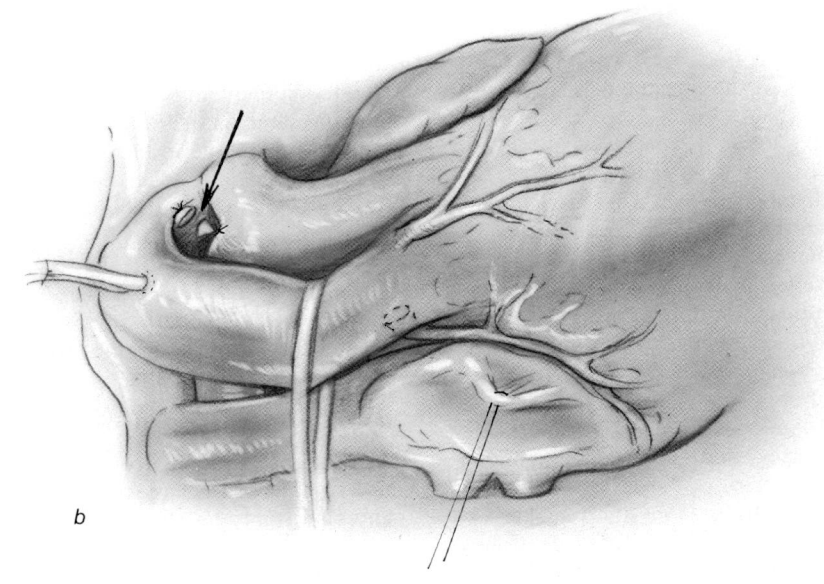

b

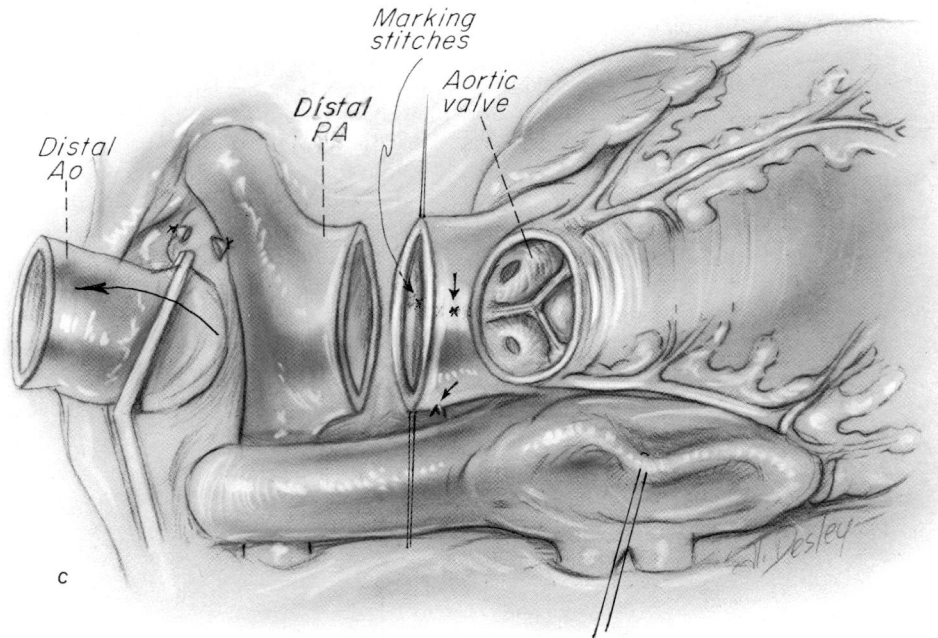

c

Figure 39-27 (*continued*)

(*b*) After establishing CPB, the dissection of the LPA and RPA is completed and the ligamentum arteriosum divided between ligatures.

(c) The aorta (Ao) has been divided well downstream to the valve commissures, the PA has been divided above its midsection, and marking sutures have been placed on the outside of the pulmonary artery to mark the location of the pulmonary valve commissures.

(d) End-to-end anastomosis is made between the proximal neoaorta and the distal aortic segment, after bringing this segment behind the PA bifurcation. The illustration is for patients with TGA and large VSD, in which the pulmonary artery is apt to be considerably larger than the aorta, and therefore the aorta is enlarged by the cut shown.

(e) The coronary arteries, with as large a button of aorta as possible, are cut out from the proximal aortic segment. A small stab incision is made in the neoaorta at the site of the marking sutures, and usually with a small punch, a segment of wall is removed. The commissural attachment of the valve cusps can be visualized from the previously placed three marking sutures.

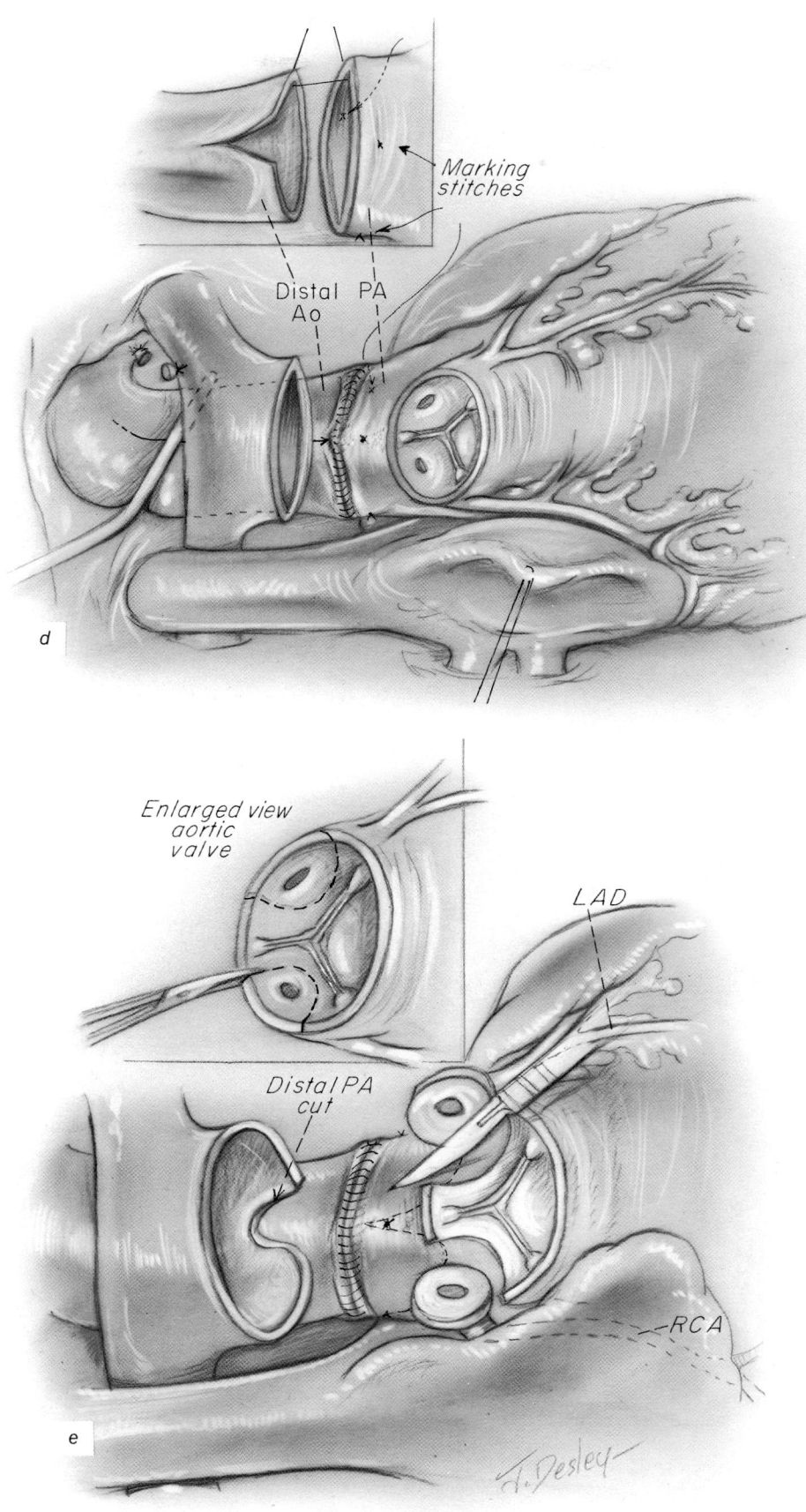

Marking stitches

Distal Ao   PA

d

Enlarged view aortic valve

Distal PA cut

LAD

RCA

e

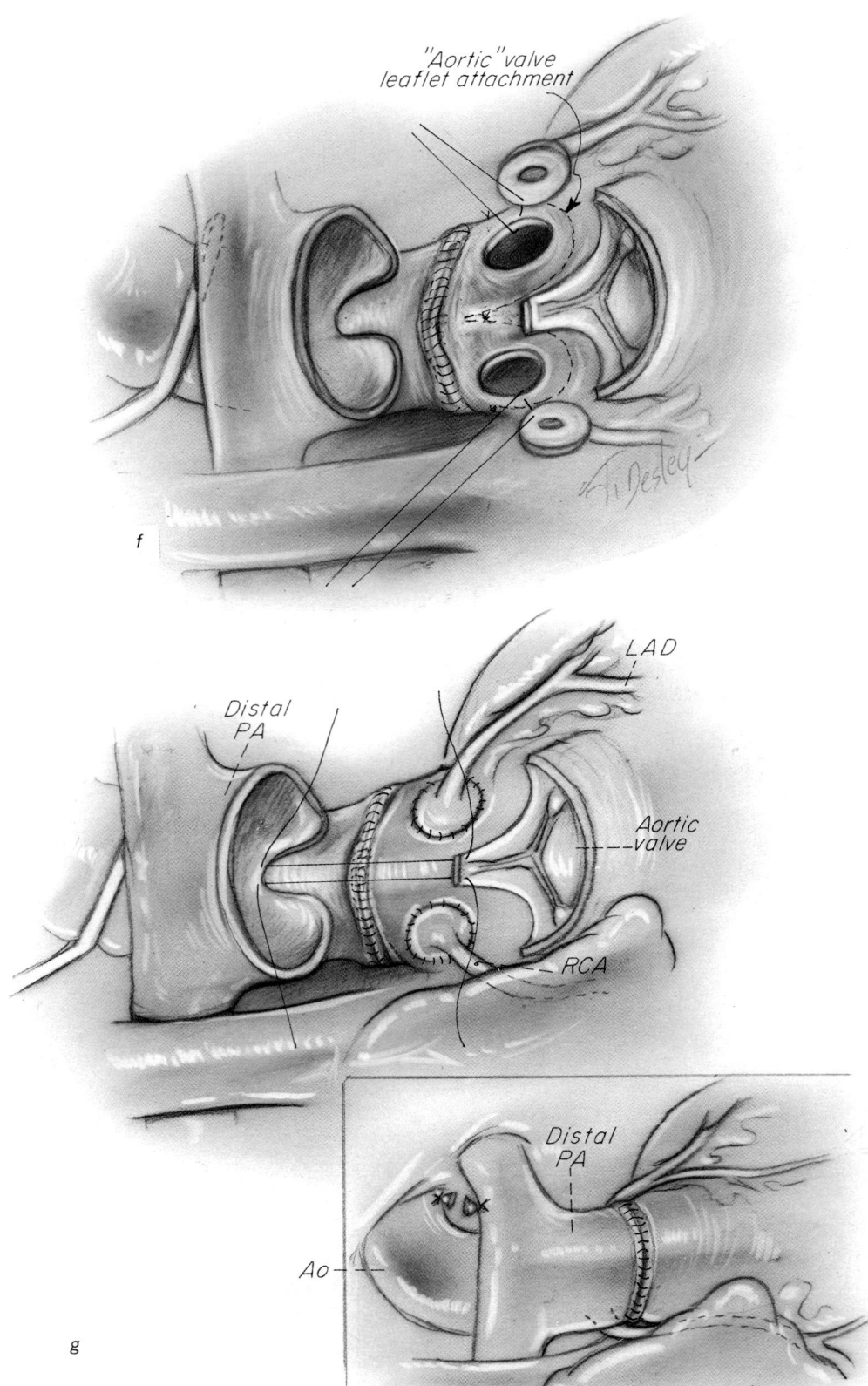

Figure 39-27 (*continued*)

(*f*) The buttons of aorta around the coronary arteries are anastomosed to the opening in the neoaortic root, generally with interrupted 7-0 sutures. (See text for alternative protocol.)

(*g*) In patients with TGA and large VSD, the pulmonary artery is large, and a direct anastomosis can be made between the proximal neopulmonary artery segment and the distal pulmonary artery, after contouring the pulmonary artery as shown.

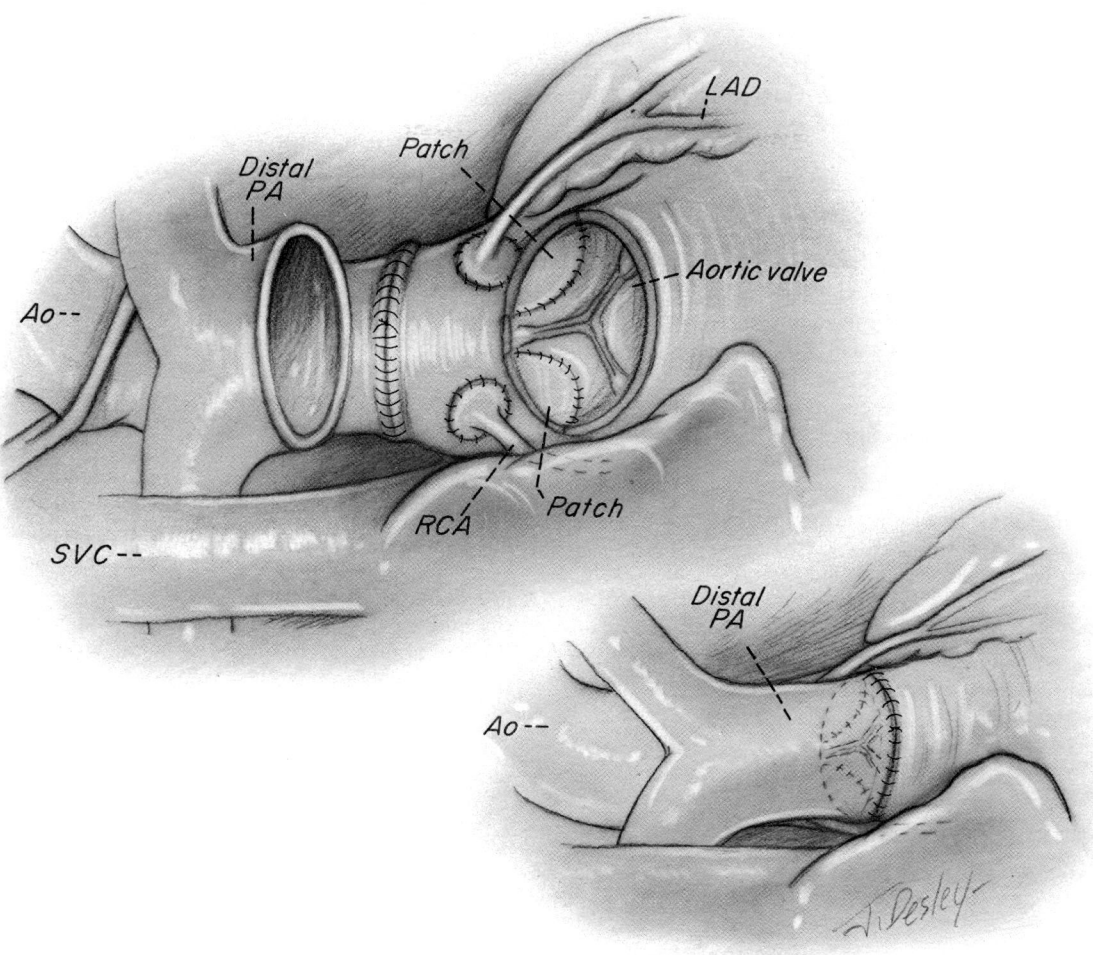

Figure 39-27   *(continued)*

(h) When the arterial switch operation is done in neonates and young infants, the aorta and pulmonary artery are of about the same size and it becomes particularly important to avoid tension on the pulmonary artery suture line. Therefore, the defects left by excision of the coronary arteries are filled in by suturing into place small patches of pericardium.

(I) End-to-end anastomosis is then made between the proximal neopulmonary artery segment and the distal pulmonary artery. The pulmonary arteries lie nicely only if they have been thoroughly mobilized earlier in the procedure.

Ao, aorta; LAD, left anterior descending; LPA, left pulmonary artery; PA, pulmonary artery; RCA, right coronary artery; RPA, right pulmonary artery; SVC, superior vena cava.

Some of these figures are reproduced with permission from Pacifico et al.,[P12] and the American Heart Association, Inc.

A median sternotomy incision is made, and if stenoses are present at the pulmonary trunk bifurcation or in the proximal portions of the right and left pulmonary arteries, a piece of pericardium is removed and set aside. Pericardial stay sutures are placed. The pulmonary trunk in most patients with this anomaly is posterior and to the left of the ascending aorta. Therefore, in order to avoid conduit compression between the right-sided and anterior ascending aorta and the sternum, preparations are made for the routing of the homograft so that it approaches the pulmonary trunk from the patient's *left* side. The pulmonary artery and its bufurcation are dissected completely free of the ascending aorta, and the first portion of the left and right pulmonary arteries are also mobilized. Purse-string sutures are placed appropriately (see Chapter 2, Section 3). Any previously made anastomotic operations are dissected and are closed just after establishing CPB (see Chapter 23, appropriate sections in "Technique of Operation" Section 1).

After the homograft-Dacron conduit has been prepared, CPB is established and the perfusate temperature is made as cold as possible; as soon as the heart has become ineffective a small right atriotomy is made, the pump-oxygenator sump sucker placed across a naturally occurring or surgically created foramen ovale, the aorta cross-clamped, and the cold cardioplegic infusion given. The perfusate temperature is stabilized at 25°C.

The midportion of the free wall of the right ventricle is opened by a moderate-sized vertical ventriculotomy which avoids major coronary artery branches (Fig. 39-28*a*). Appropriate stay sutures are placed on the ventriculotomy edge (Fig. 39-28*b*) and on the septal and anterior leaflets of the tricuspid valve. The origins of the aorta from the right ventricle and of the pulmonary trunk from the left ventricle are confirmed. It has already been determined by preoperative cineangiographic study that the VSD is a perimembranous or malalignment type in the outflow portion of the ventricular septum, but this is now confirmed visually. The tricuspid valve and its tensor apparatus are usually well away from the pathway between the VSD and aorta, but if not special measures are required. Unless the VSD is clearly large and non-restrictive, it is enlarged by an incision into the septum anterior to the defect (Fig. 39-28*b*). Care is taken that the incision is in the septum and not in the ventricular free wall. Generally, this provides considerable enlargement of the VSD, and actual excision of muscle with increased risk to septal coronary artery branches is unnecessary.

The generally subvalvar pulmonary stenosis is sought from within the ventricles. It is usually just superior to the common area of mitral and tricuspid anuli. Usually this can easily be closed, working through the VSD, with a whip stitch of polypropylene suture, supplemented by interrupted

pledgetted mattress sutures (Fig. 39-28*c*). If this is not convenient, after opening the pulmonary trunk a thickened and stenotic pulmonary valve can be similarly closed. Generally, the pulmonary trunk is not divided, since the conduit lies in an ideal position when end-to-side rather than end-to-end anastomosis is made to the pulmonary artery.

An intraventricular tunnel repair is now done, just as described for simple double outlet right ventricle (see Chapter 40, "Intraventricular Tunnel Repair for Simple DORV without Pulmonary Stenosis" in section on Technique of Operation and Fig. 40-12). The left ventricle now ejects into the aorta through this tunnel (Figs. 39-28*d*, 39-28*e*).

The pulmonary trunk is opened with a longitudinal incision along its left side, carrying this if necessary on to the proximal portion of the left pulmonary artery. The previously prepared homograft-valved conduit is now trimmed so that it will lie smoothly in an arc shape with the convexity to the left. Distally, the conduit is cut transversely and generally about 4 or 5 mm beyond the valve cusp commissures; proximally, it is trimmed obliquely (see Chapter 23, Fig. 23-37). Usually the tubular segment that is entirely Dacron is no more than 0.5–1 cm in length, the rest of the Dacron being the hood over the ventriculotomy. End-to-side anastomosis is made of the graft to the pulmonary trunk (Fig. 39-28*f*), and the proximal end is then anastomosed to the right ven-

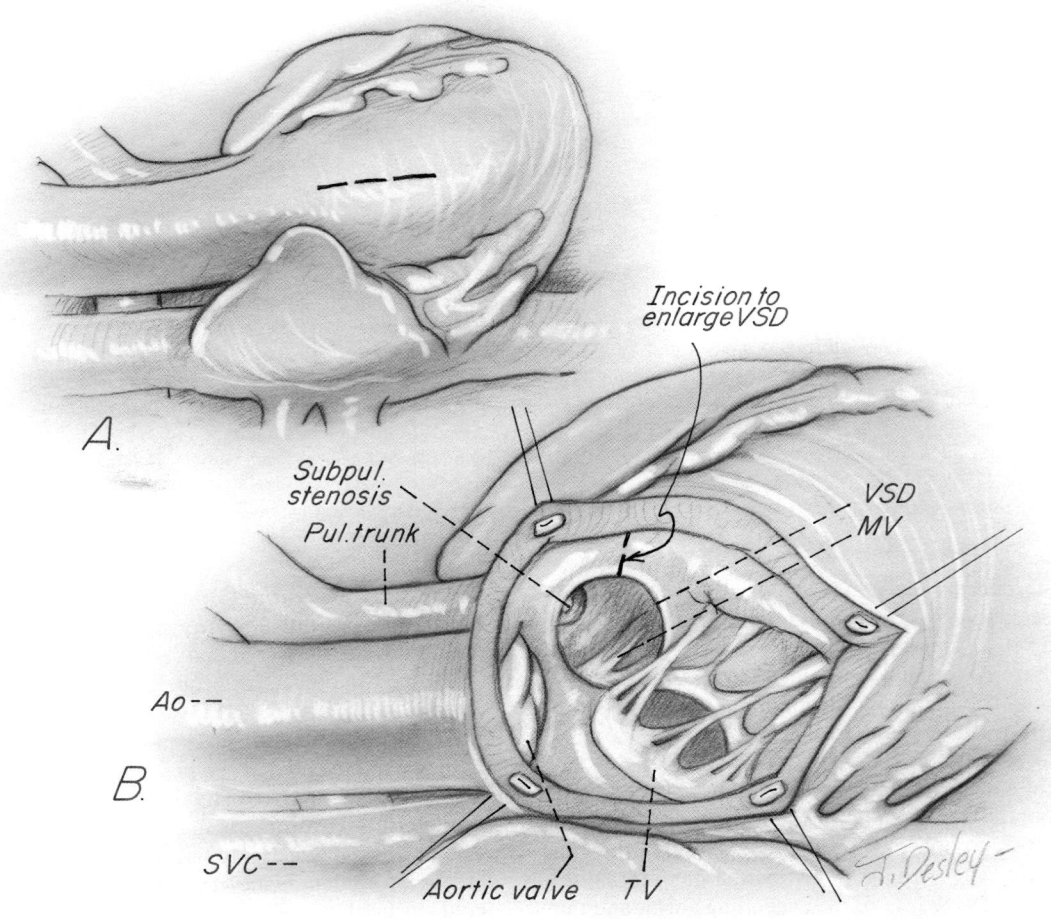

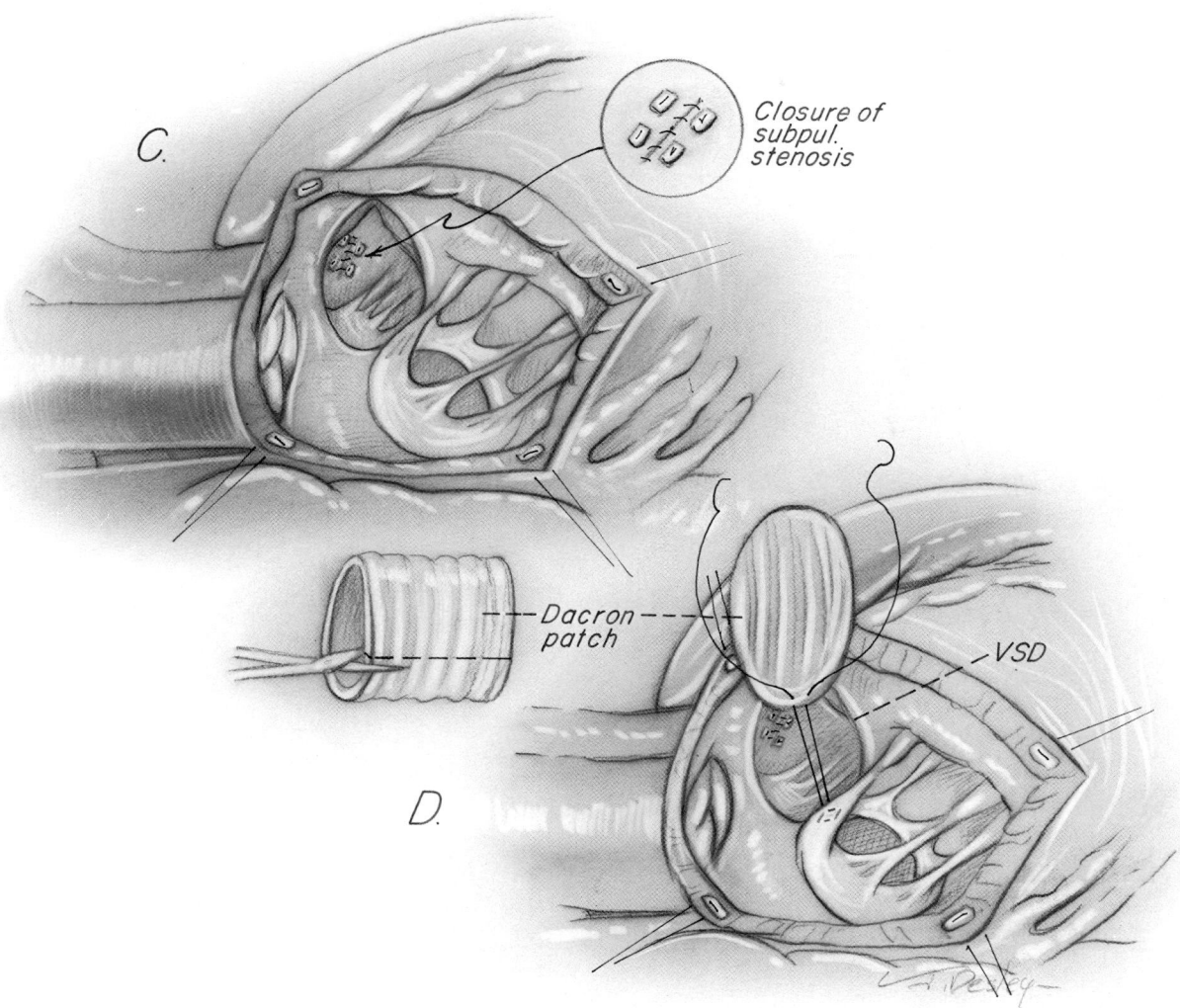

Figure 39-28 The Rastelli repair for TGA, VSD, and LVOTO, combining an intraventricular tunnel repair and a rerouting valved extracardiac conduit.

(a) After the median sternotomy incision has been made, the pulmonary trunk and the left and right pulmonary arteries are completely dissected away from the aorta and surrounding structures. The proposed vertical incision in the right ventricle is shown.

(b) After cross-clamping the aorta and establishing cold cardioplegia and after opening the right atrium and inserting a pump-oxygenator sump sucker through a natural or surgically created foramen ovale, the right ventricle is opened through a vertical incision. Stay sutures are applied. After examining the interior of the right ventricle, the VSD is usually enlarged by an incision as shown. Generally, this considerably increases the orifice size and excision of septal tissue is not necessary.

(c) Generally, the entrance into the pulmonary artery is closed from within the ventricles as shown.

(d) To create the patch used in making the intraventricular tunnel, a segment taken from the preclotted woven double velour Dacron graft is trimmed appropriately. The patch, carefully oriented is sewn into position, with all the precautions described in the intracardiac tunnel repair for simple double outlet right ventricle (see Chapter 40).

Ao, aorta; MV, mitral valve; Subpul. stenosis, subpulmonary stenosis; SVC, superior vena cava; TV, tricuspid valve; VSD, ventricular septal defect.

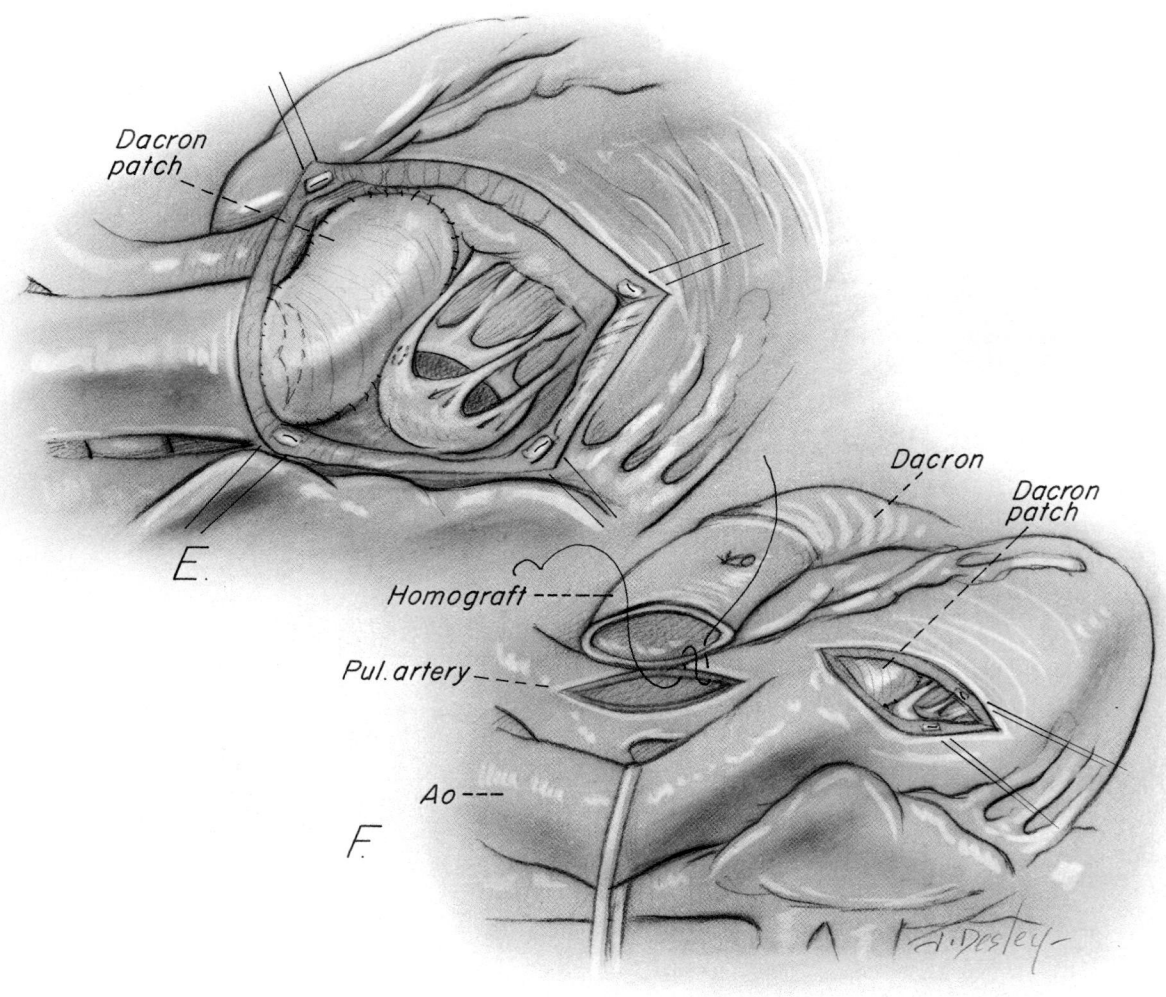

Labels on illustration:
Dacron patch

E.

Dacron

Dacron patch

Homograft

Pul. artery

Ao

F.

Figure 39-28 (*continued*)
(*e*) After the completion of the intraventricular tunnel, left ventricular blood passes freely through the tunnel into ascending aorta.
(*f*) The homograft-valved extracardiac conduit is prepared (see Chapter 23, Fig. 23-37). The distal anastomosis of homograft to pulmonary artery is constructed. With the graft pushed off into the left side of the pericardium, the first portion of the anastomosis is made by sewing from within the structures. After completing this, the rest of the anastomosis is made sewing from outside the structures. Exposure for this is facilitated by traction inferiorly on the ventriculotomy stay sutures.

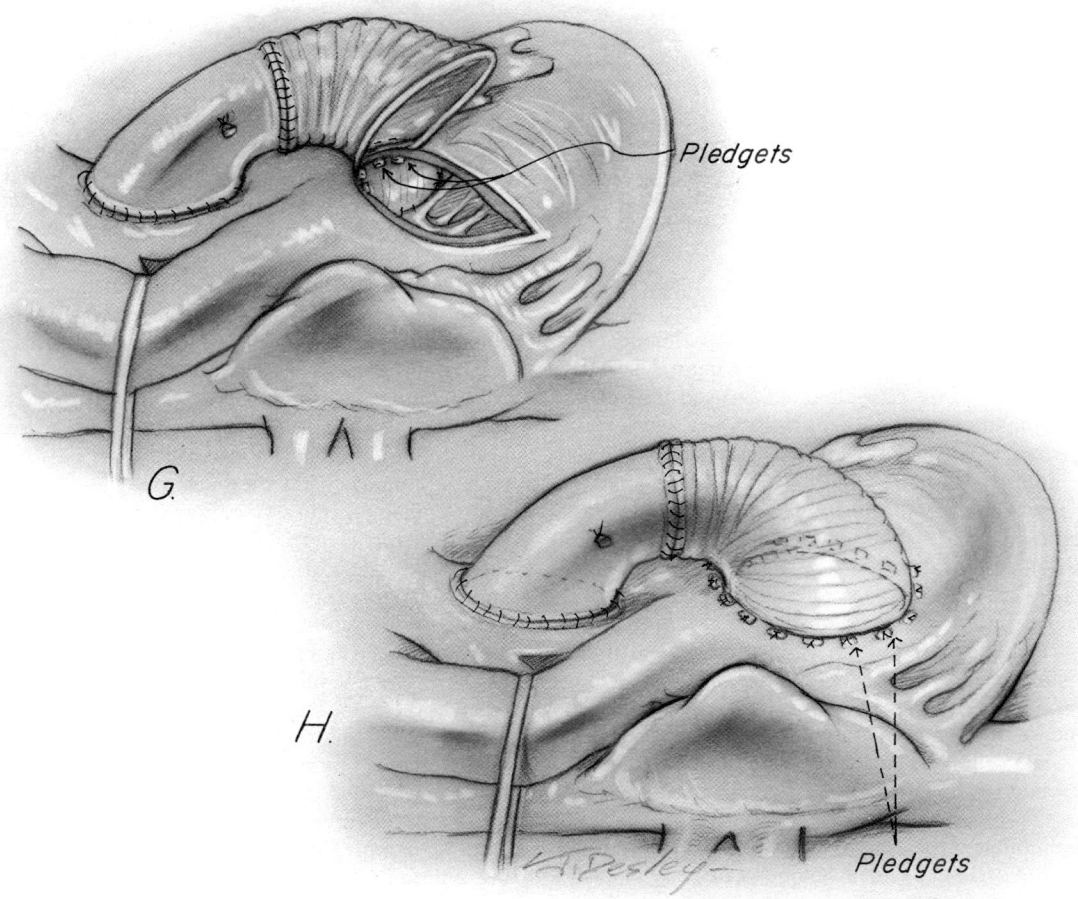

Pledgets

G.

H.

Pledgets

Figure 39-28 (*continued*)

(*g*) The proximal anastomosis is being made. Interrupted pledgetted mattress sutures of Dacron are placed from within around the heel of the graft. The remainder of the suture line is made by placing similar sutures from without so as to evert this part of the anastomosis.

(*h*) When the anastomosis is complete, the conduit lies in a smooth curve, well away from the sternum and off to the patient's left side. This is less evident in the drawing than in actuality.

Note that this technique and configuration of the conduit are deemed necessary in order that there be a smooth pathway between the right ventricle and the often posteriorly placed pulmonary trunk, which is well to the left of the sternum (UAB). An alternative concept dictates the making of the right ventriculotomy as far superior as is possible and attaching the base of the homograft proximally to the superior part of the ventriculotomy (GLH). A pericardial roof then completes the proximal anastomosis (see Chapter 23, Fig. 23-36).

triculotomy (Figs. 39-28g, 39-28h). When inserted in this manner, the conduit lies in a gentle, and smoothly curved shape and well away from the sternum and anterior chest wall.

The sump sucker is removed from across the foramen ovale and the foramen is closed. With strong suction on the aortic needle vent, the aortic clamp is released and rewarming of the patient with the perfusate is begun. The right atrium is closed. After a good cardiac action has been established, the usual de-airing procedures are carried out and the remainder of the operation completed in the usual manner.

In addition to the usual polyvinyl recording catheters in left and right atrium, an additional one may be brought from the pulmonary artery through the conduit and out the low right ventricle.

Blalock-Hanlon Atrial Septectomy

The operation is usually performed in seriously ill neonates or infants with complex types of congenital heart disease, including complex types of TGA, and is not used for failed balloon atrial septostomies in patients with TGA and intact ventricular septum or with VSD (UAB, GLH) (see "Indications for Operation").

Because the patients are seriously ill, a catheter for pressure recording is inserted in the left radial artery. With the patient in the left lateral decubitus position, a right lateral thoracotomy is made and the chest entered through the fifth interspace or the inferior aspect of the bed of the nonresected fifth rib. The pericardium is opened with a long incision *behind* the phrenic nerve, taking care to avoid damaging the nerve. It may, however, be necessary to mobilize the nerve in the midportion of the field and displace it anteriorly. The cautery is not used near the nerve. Stay sutures are applied to the edges of the pericardium for traction.

The right pulmonary artery is dissected just lateral to the superior vena cava (SVC), and a heavy ligature is placed doubly and loosely around it. The pericardial reflection behind the inferior vena cava (IVC) is cut and the posterior pericardium incised transversely between the intrapericardial portion of the right pulmonary artery and the roof of the left atrium; this incision is carried rightward beneath the superior vena cava (SVC). This allows an instrument to be passed behind the IVC and left atrium to emerge superior to the right pulmonary vein and posterior to the SVC. Double ligatures are placed loosely around the superior and inferior pulmonary veins, usually within the pericardium.

Since placement of the occluding devices may be associated with severe hemodynamic deterioration of the sick small infant, the steps of the operation to be done are carefully reviewed at this point with the anesthesiologist and the surgical nurse. A somewhat U-shaped clamp (Derra clamp or small modification of the Satinsky clamp) of proper size is selected. Two good quality small curved clamps are selected for later grasping of the atrial wall. The anesthesiologist is asked to give an appropriate amount of sodium bicarbonate since acidosis will probably develop, the patient is paralyzed, and gentle ventilation established; it is agreed that neither resuscitative measures nor vigorous ventilation will

be begun until the clamps are off. Since the infant's body temperature has usually by now dropped to about 33°C, 3–5 minutes of very low cardiac output is well tolerated.

The operation proceeds in an expeditious but controlled manner. The double ligature on the right pulmonary artery and then those on the right and left pulmonary veins are made snug. The U-shaped clamp is placed, usually from below but sometimes from above (depending upon which fits better), so that one blade is behind the left atrium and emerging from above beneath the SVC and below from beneath the IVC, and the other is closed onto the free right atrial wall. Some temporary SVC obstruction may be produced. The clamp now encompasses the right atrial wall anteriorly, the left atrial wall posteriorly, and the atrial septum in between. A longitudinal incision is made into the left atrium just in front of the confluence of the right superior and inferior pulmonary veins. An incision parallel to this is made in the right atrial wall anterior to the interatrial sulcus. Care is taken that these incisions enter the atrial cavities. The two especially selected small curved clamps are used to grasp the external aspect of the now isolated interatrial groove between the two parallel incisions. With scissors, a cut is made centrally into the atrial septum at the lower end of the groove and at the upper end, although the latter must not be so superior as to chance going outside the heart. With traction on the small curved clamps, these two incisions are extended with scissors into the atrial septum. The occluding clamp may be loosened slightly to pull out still more septum toward the surgeon. While these incisions are being extended centrally, the posterior septal fragment usually tears away as the region of the foramen ovale is approached. If after this the cardiac remnant of the septum does not spontaneously retract, the clamp is again slightly loosened until this occurs. Usually with this the hemodynamic state improves. A few widely placed continuous whip stitches of 5-0 polypropylene suture are placed to bring the anterior right atrial wall to the lip of the posterior left atrial wall before removing the occluding clamp. Then the double ligatures are removed from the pulmonary veins and finally from the right pulmonary artery. A few additional stitches may be needed in the atriotomy for hemostasis.

The pericardium is irrigated and closed with rather widely spaced interrupted 5-0 or 6-0 sutures. A drainage catheter is brought out from the pleural space through a stab wound. The thoracotomy incision is closed in the usual manner.

Pulmonary Artery Banding

Pulmonary artery banding is discussed in detail in Chapter 20 (see "Pulmonary Artery Banding" in Section 1, Technique of Operation), including the Trusler rules for patients with transposition and large VSDs.

Systemic-Pulmonary Artery Shunting Procedures

These procedures are described in detail in Chapter 23 (see "Technique of Shunting Operations" in Section 1). The same guidelines are followed concerning the type of shunt as in the tetralogy of Fallot.

Repair of Post-Mustard Caval Obstruction

The usual preparations for operations through a median sternotomy are made, although others have preferred a right anterolateral thoracotomy.[S18] The oscillating saw is used for the secondary sternotomy, and the usual limited dissection is made (see Chapter 2, Section 3), without freeing the front and leftward aspect of the heart.

Tapes are passed around the cavae beyond the caval-atrial junctions and the cavae are cannulated directly (see Chapter 2, Section 3). Cardiopulmonary bypass (CPB) is commenced and conducted in the usual fashion. The aorta is cross-clamped and cold cardioplegic solution infused into the aortic root. Alternatively (GLH), in infants less than 8 kg the profound hypothermia-circulatory arrest technique is employed (see Chapter 2, Section 4) but with double caval cannulation as above; however, if caval dissection should prove hazardous, a single cannula can be inserted into the left ventricle through an apical purse string and stab wound for venous return. The right atrium is opened with a centrally placed transverse (GLH) or oblique (UAB) incision.

When the obstruction involves only the pathway from the superior vena cava (SVC), this portion of the baffle may be enlarged. The baffle is incised vertically at its midpoint with a knife and the incision carried upward to lay open the pathway from the SVC. When this is totally occluded, the SVC–right atrial (RA) junction, which is always still patent beneath the baffle, is defined by inserting the tip of a curved forcep through a stab wound in the SVC (avoiding the sinus node area) and cutting down onto the tip of the instrument as it tents the baffle toward the right atrial cavity (pulmonary venous compartment). Alternatively, it may be possible to use the tip of the curved forcep to dissect bluntly the area of obstruction from above downward so that the tip appears below it. The baffle is opened at the point at which it joins the RA wall in front of the SVC junction, and fibrous thickening is excised to recontour the baffle and the floor of the new tunnel. An elliptical Dacron patch is now sewn into the baffle incision with continuous 4-0 polypropylene suture to create a new roof to the pathway. An opened, preclotted, knitted or woven double velour Dacron graft of appropriate diameter is used for the patch since this contours toward the pulmonary venous atrium. The patch must not compromise the pulmonary venous channel.

Alternatively, the baffle can be removed entirely. When the entire baffle is grossly thickened and distorted and particularly if it contains folded Dacron and the pathway from the IVC is obstructed, the entire baffle must be excised.[S18] A new baffle is inserted using pericardium if enough is available or otherwise Dacron.

The remainder of the operation is completed in the usual fashion.

Repair of Post-Mustard Pulmonary Venous Obstruction

The initial stages of the operation and the establishment of cardiopulmonary bypass (CPB) and cold cardioplegia are as described above. A transverse incision is made through the right atrial wall and into the anterior pulmonary venous compartment. The incision is carried posteriorly through the waist between the anterior and posterior pulmonary venous compartments and directly between the right upper and right lower pulmonary veins. Excess fibrous tissue surrounding the open stenosis is excised without breaching the baffle. One technique for repair involves closure of the transverse atriotomy with continuous 4-0 polypropylene suture to create a vertical atrial suture line (GLH) in much the same manner as described by Dillard and colleagues as part of the Mustard baffle technique in 1969.[D1] Instead (GLH), a V-atrial flap may be fashioned from the lateral right atrial wall anterior to the stenotic site and the apex of the V advanced posteriorly as a V–Y atrioplasty (see ''Atrial Switch Operation [Mustard Technique]''). Alternatively, a properly sized and shaped preclotted double velour woven Dacron gusset, cut from a tube so as to have convex contour, is sutured into the atriotomy (UAB). This has the potential disadvantage that the stenosis may recur as the patch thickens,[D6] but this has not as yet occured. The remainder of the operation is completed as usual.

Palliative Atrial Switch Operation

Transposition of the Great Arteries with Large Ventricular Septal Defect
When a large VSD is present, the Senning (or Mustard) procedure is performed in the usual manner, leaving the VSD open.

Transposition of the Great Arteries with Intact Ventricular Septum
When the ventricular septum is essentially intact (in association with a high pulmonary vascular resistance), along with the palliative atrial switch operation a large VSD is created in the apex of the ventricular septum through a limited apical left ventriculotomy. The right atrium is opened in preparation for the atrial switch operation. After the ventriculotomy is made, a finger is inserted through the tricuspid valve to tent the ventricular septum toward the left, and a limited opening is made with a knife onto the finger. The opening is then progressively enlarged to a 20 mm size using the knife, avoiding damage to the inferior papillary muscle. Hegar dilators are used to measure the size of the created defect. The ventriculotomy is closed and the atrial switch procedure is completed.

SPECIAL FEATURES OF POSTOPERATIVE CARE

Postoperative care after operations for TGA is as usual for patients undergoing all types of intracardiac operations (see Chapter 5), with special considerations after some types of procedures. When an atrial switch operation has been done, positive end-expiratory pressure (PEEP) is not used since it tends to obstruct the superior vena cava. The infants are nursed in a slightly head-up position. The atrial pressures are kept as low as is compatible with an adequate cardiac output, and if necessary a low dose (2.5 mg · kg^{-1} · min^{-1}) of dopamine during the early postoperative hours is helpful in this regard.

When an arterial switch operation has been performed, particularly in a neonate, left atrial (or pulmonary artery diastolic) pressure should remain low, less than about 12 mmHg. Since restlessness or agitation increases metabolic demands and cardiac output, neonates and infants are usually kept intubated and sedated for 24 to 48 hours after operation (see Chapter 5). If cardiac output is less than optimal, and particularly when 2-D echocardiographic study indicates poor left ventricular function, catecholamine support is used, rather than further increase in left ventricular filling pressure.[C17,Q3]

RESULTS

Although in most chapters the in-hospital deaths and other events are presented in a traditional manner under "Early Results" and those occurring later under "Late Results," they are here presented in a single section on "Results." A single presentation was also used in Chapter 7, "Incremental Risk Factors for Hospital and Early-Phase Death" in section on Early Results. The traditional method usually underestimates the incidence of early events and cannot take advantage of a comprehensive analysis of time-related events after cardiac surgery (see Chapter 6).

Atrial Switch Procedure for Simple Transposition of the Great Arteries[3]

Survival to Atrial Switch Repair
Somewhat in contrast to the situation in which an arterial switch operation is done for simple TGA in the first few days or weeks of life, when the atrial switch operation is used the mortality before the definitive repair must be considered along with the early and late mortality after the repair.

A few neonates with simple TGA are so severely hypoxic

---

[3]Throughout the discussions from this point on, the phrase *simple TGA* applied to a group of patients means that they had either an intact ventricular septum or a ventricular septal defect ≤3 mm in diameter, that they were with or without (±) a patent ductus arteriosus of any size, and that they were with or without (±) left ventricular outflow tract obstruction.

a short time after birth, that they die before balloon atrial septostomy (BAS). This has been the case in three (2%, CL 0.7%–3%) of 188 patients (GLH; 1970–1984) admitted to hospital with simple TGA.

After hospital admission and BAS and in spite of the infrequency of complications of BAS compared with earlier years,[R15] some infants (5%–20%) die before their atrial switch operation. This was initially documented by Tynan and colleagues,[T2] who found that by 3 months of age only about 81% survived without repair. Furthermore, early in the experience with BAS, surgical septectomy was often considered necessary in the interval between BAS and a definitive atrial switch operation.[B20,D8,G3,T6]

The survival after BAS and before repair is 89% (GLH) at 3 months of age (Fig. 39-29) and 81% (UAB) (CL 76%–86%) (Fig. 39-30). Most of the deaths are in the first few days after BAS, the instantaneous risk of dying falling to a low level by the age of 45 days (Fig. 39-31). Most deaths are in neonates who are severely ill with acidosis and hypoxia on admission (Table 39-4). However, occasional deaths can occur several months after septostomy from cerebral thrombosis[C3,P11] and intercurrent respiratory infections.

The presence or absence of left ventricular outflow tract obstruction (LVOTO) in patients with simple TGA seems not to affect survival after septostomy and before repair, but associated patent ductus arteriosus (PDA) decreases it (Tables 39-4 and 39-5). The effect on survival is particularly important when the PDA is large (Fig. 39-32). The 3-month survival (it is the same at 6 months) before an atrial switch operation in the current era in patients with no (25 of 65, UAB) or a small (20) PDA is 95% (CL 90%–98%), whereas it is 85% (CL 71%–93%) in those with large PDA (Fig. 39-32). This unfavorable effect of PDA was also evident in the experience of Powell and colleagues.[P14]

Repeat balloon septostomy seems to have little effect in improving these results.[P11,T2] Surgical septectomy may result in a better survival until repair[G3,L13,T2,T6] but for many reasons is undesirable.

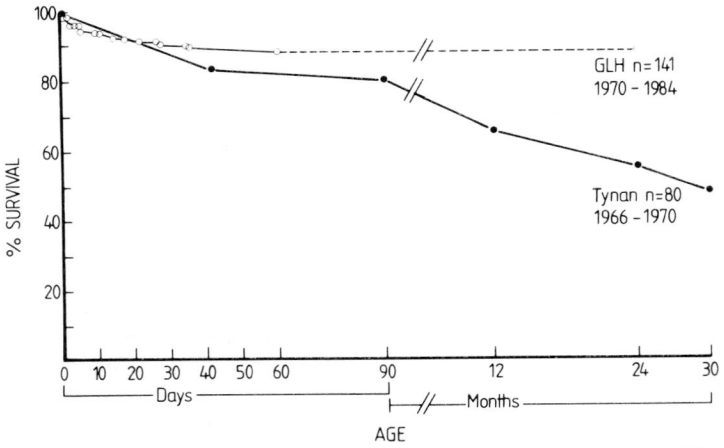

Figure 39-29 Actuarial survival up to the time of atrial baffle repair following initial palliation by balloon atrial septostomy (BAS). Patients were not censored if other palliative procedures were done. Initial palliation in the GLH series was BAS (except for five septectomies) and for Tynan's series,[T2] BAS only. The GLH series includes only patients with simple TGA (see footnote 3 for definition). Tynan's series also includes those with large VSD, but there was no difference in survival prior to repair between these two subsets.

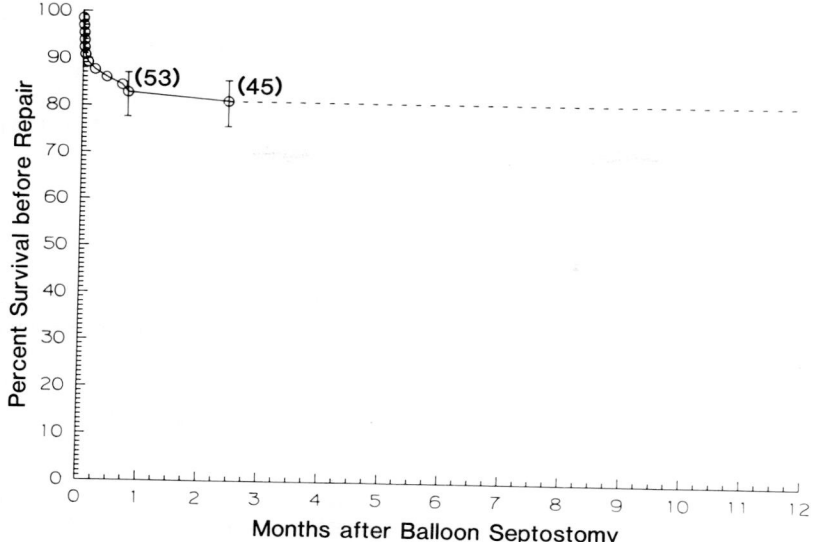

Figure 39-30 Actuarial survival before repair of patients with simple TGA (see footnote 3 for definition) (UAB; 1970–1981; *n* = 65, 12 deaths). Patients were not censored when procedure other than repair was performed but were censored when an atrial switch repair was done (1 had repair 3 days after septostomy, 10 others had repair before 90 days of age).

Survival after Atrial Switch Repair

Hospital mortality after the atrial switch repair for simple TGA varies between 0% and 15% (Tables 39-6–39-8). The variability is in part related to lower survival in earlier eras, considerable morphologic variability even within this subset, different criteria for operation and inclusion of cases within a given data set, and variability of incremental risk factors from one experience to another. Five-year survival, including hospital deaths, varies between 82% (Fig. 39-33) and 90% (Fig. 39-34). The 10- and 20-year survivals are probably less by 5% and 10%, respectively. The instantaneous risk of death is highest early after repair, falls to very low levels about 6 weeks after repair, and continues thereafter at a very low constant level for as long as patients have been followed (Fig. 39-35).

The modes of early death are variable, but early in most experiences include baffle obstruction (Table 39-9). In this regard, it must be remembered that the patient population may be complex even in patients with simple TGA since this group includes patients with large patent ductus arteriosus (PDA) and/or left ventricular outflow tract obstruction (LVOTO) (Tables 39-7 and 39-10).

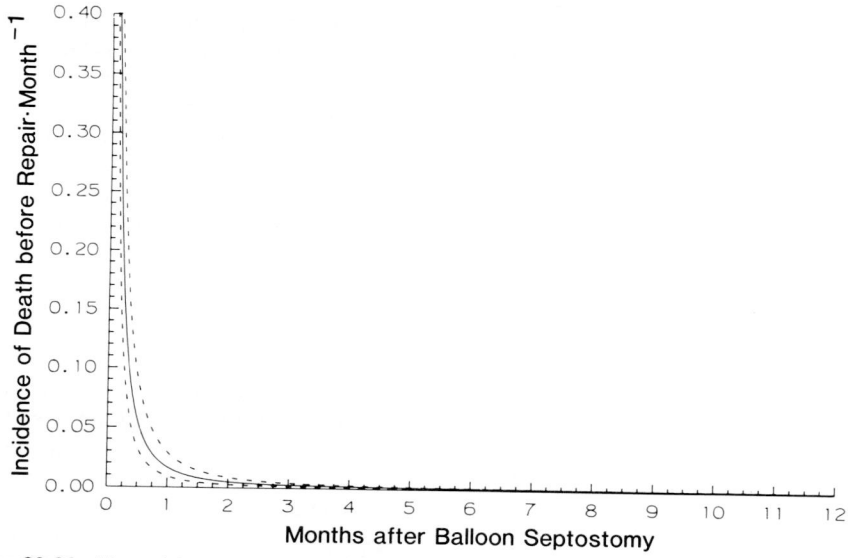

Figure 39-31 Hazard function (instantaneous risk of death) after balloon atrial septostomy before atrial switch repair in patients with simple TGA (see footnote 3 for definition) (UAB; 1970–1981; *n* = 65, 12 deaths). The data set is the same as in Fig. 39-30. The dashed lines enclose the 70% confidence limits. Only one phase is present in the hazard function.

Table 39-4 Category of death in infants with simple TGA (see footnote 3 for definition) who died prior to atrial switch repair (GLH; 1970–1984; n = 188 patients admitted to hospital).

Category	No. of Patients
NYHA class V on admission and death in continuing hypoxia	4
Cerebral death after late (>12 d old) referral in NYHA class V	6
Associated large PDA and NYHA class IV	3
Intercurrent respiratory infection	1
E. Coli sepsis	1
Necrotizing enterocolitis	1
Accident at balloon septostomy	1
Total	17

NOTE: 3 of the 17 patients died before balloon septostomy could be done. The accident at balloon septostomy was avulsion of a pulmonary vein. In addition to these 17 patients, 6 await repair and 165 have undergone repair.

Overall Survival

An estimate of overall survival of patients with simple TGA committed in the current era to a protocol of BAS and atrial switch repair 1–3 months later is of great importance but can only be made informally. Using data representing the most current era (based on Tables 39-7 and 39-11 and Fig. 39-36) (UAB), the overall 5-year survival, including deaths after septostomy before repair as well as early and late deaths after repair, is 85% (CL 80%–89%) and projected to be 77% (CL 68%–84%) at 20 years (Table 39-12). (This assumes no deaths between hospital admissions and septostomy, which is not quite accurate; see above.) The survival would be about 5%–10% lower at these time periods were a large PDA present because of its adverse effect on survival after septostomy and before atrial switch repair (see Fig. 39-32). Comparing these data with the other portion (GLH) of the combined UAB-GLH experience (see Table 39-6 and Fig. 39-34) suggests that these informally combined data are representative of current results. These figures will be important in comparisons with the results of the *arterial* switch operation in the various subsets of TGA.

Table 39-5 Incremental risk factors (in the hazard function domain, see Fig. 39-31) for death before atrial switch repair after balloon septostomy for simple TGA (see footnote 3 for definition) (UAB; 1970–1981; n = 65, 12 events[a]). Risk factors examined were age at septostomy, PDA (presence of large PDA; presence of small PDA; presence of any size PDA; size of PDA [0 = none, 1 = small, 2 = large]), presence of left ventricular outflow tract obstruction, presence of small (unimportant) VSD, date of septostomy (years since 1/1/1970).

Incremental Risk Factor	Early Phase Hazard	
	Coefficient ± SD	P value
PDA size (0 = none, 1 = small, 2 = large)	0.8 ± 0.43	.06
(Earlier) date of septostomy (years since 1/1/70)	−0.17 ± 0.108	.12
Intercept	−1.49	

[a] Patient who died at 6.9 years was censored at death.

Incremental Risk Factors for Premature Death

Certain risk factors for premature death (in hospital or later) after the atrial switch procedures for simple TGA have been identified, both informally and by separate multivariate analyses of the experiences (GLH, UAB) with the atrial switch procedures for all types of TGA (see Table 39-11, and Tables 39-13, and 39-14).

THE ERA. The early or hospital survival has been steadily increasing (mortality has been decreasing) in recent years in most cardiac surgical centers, as evidenced in the overall GLH experience (see Table 39-6) and in the overall (Table 39-15) and recent (see Table 39-7) UAB experiences. (A possible reason for the later appearance of improved results [UAB vs. GLH] is the use of Dacron baffles [UAB] in the early 1970s.) These trends must be taken into account in making comparisons with other types of operations recently introduced.

AGE AT REPAIR. Age less than 1 month has been an incremental risk factor for hospital death when earlier experiences are included (see Table 39-13). When the analysis of all early and late deaths is limited to the current era, this is no longer the case (see Table 39-11). This is also the experience of DeLeon and colleagues from the Boston Children's Hospital, where 2 (11%, CL 4%–23%) of 19 neonates died in hospital after a Senning atrial switch procedure, a mortality no different from that of older patients.[D10] However, 2 of the 17 hospital survivors developed important pulmonary venous obstruction. The feasibility and safety of performing the atrial switch operation in very early life, in the current era, is also illustrated by the reports of several other groups.[B11,F9] These trends are less evident in contingency table analysis (Table 39-16), but in this combined GLH-UAB series, operation at less than 1 month of age was done only for critically ill patients. *Routinely* performing the atrial switch operation in neonates would no doubt carry a lower risk than shown here.

PATENT DUCTUS ARTERIOSUS. As in the natural history and after BAS (see earlier sections), the presence of a PDA increases the risk of premature death after an atrial switch repair for simple TGA (see Table 39-13). The reasons for this are not evident, but it has been noted by others.[L15,R17]

TYPE OF ATRIAL SWITCH OPERATION. The standard Mustard repair (rather than the V–Y Mustard or the Senning repair) has been a risk factor for premature death after hospital dismissal (see Table 39-14). This is consistent with the somewhat increased incidence of baffle obstruction with the standard Mustard-type repair.

POSTREPAIR CAVAL AND PULMONARY VENOUS OBSTRUCTIONS. When these complications develop late postoperatively, the risk of premature death is increased (see Table 39-14). In part, this is related to the risk of reoperation (see later section in "Special Situations and Controversies").

OTHER POSSIBLE RISK FACTORS. In patients with simple TGA, coexisting *LVOTO* has not been identified as a risk factor in the UAB and GLH experiences, either in the multivariate analyses (see Tables 39-11, 39-13, and 39-14) or in contingency table study (see Tables 39-6 and 39-7). The favorable results in patients with simple TGA and LVOTO are also evident in the actuarial survival curve (Fig. 39-37). Even when an LV → pulmonary artery valved conduit has been used, the risks have not been increased.[S27]

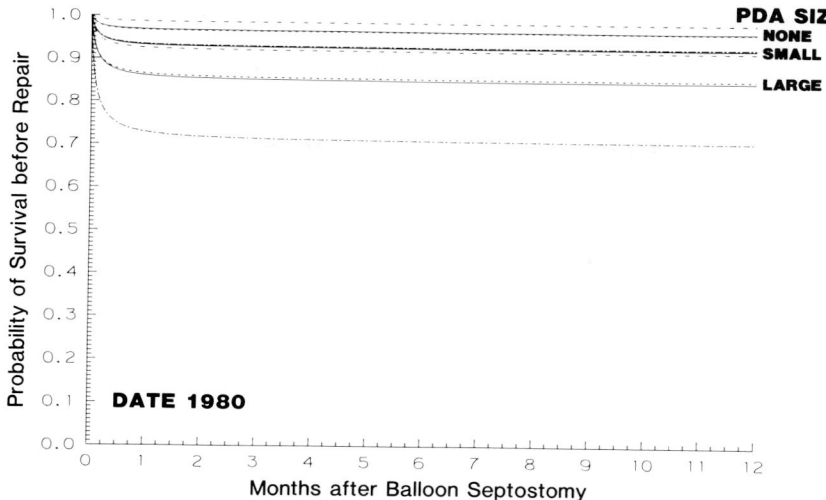

Figure 39-32 Stratified parametric estimate of survival after balloon atrial septostomy and before repair in patients with simple TGA (see footnote 3 for definition) (UAB; 1970–1981; $n = 65$). For this nomogram, the date of septostomy was set at 1980. The dotted and dot-dashed lines enclose the 70% confidence limits. (The multivariate equation used for the nomogram is in Table 39-5.) The survival is higher than that in the actuarial (Fig. 39-30) because the effect of date of septostomy is taken into account (the effect is probably more related to better care during and after septostomy and very early repair in sick babies in the current era than it is to changes in septostomy technique).

Severe hypoxia and acidosis preoperatively would seem to be incremental risk factors for hospital death after atrial switch operations in infants with simple TGA (Tables 39-17 and 39-18), although this has not been demonstrated to be the case in either the GLH or UAB multivariate analyses.

A *high pulmonary vascular resistance* (above 8–10 units · m²) greatly increases the risk of atrial switch repair when the ventricular septum is intact (Table 39-9). In these circumstances, simultaneous creation of a ventricular septal defect (VSD) virtually abolishes the risk.[S25]

Growth and Functional Status

Most patients appear to be asymptomatic after an atrial switch procedure[T3] (Table 39-19). However, graded exercise testing has shown that about 50% of them have a reduced exercise capacity associated with lower maximal oyxgen consumption values, compared with normal. These abnormalities are more prominent in patients operated upon at an older age[M21] and are often accompanied by abnormal cardiac

rhythms (see section on "Electrophysiologic Disturbances"). Those patients found to have normal or near normal exercise capacity tend to have a normal response of right ventricular systolic function to exercise.[M22] Functional capacity may be better in patients receiving the Senning rather than the Mustard type of atrial switch procedure, since Bjornstad and colleagues found atrial function to be superior with the former operation.[B26]

There is a considerable increase in height and weight after an atrial switch repair, particularly in those in whom these are importantly depressed preoperatively.[L16] A return of these parameters to normal may be achieved within 2 years of operation.

Venous Pathway Obstruction

Venous pathway obstruction is a potentially serious complication of an atrial switch operation. However, superior vena caval obstruction (SVCO) may exist in asymptomatic patients. All varieties of venous pathway obstruction predis-

Table 39-6 Hospital mortality after operations which included an atrial switch procedure with or without other procedures, in patients with simple TGA (see footnote 3 for definition) (144 Mustard procedures and 20 more recent Senning procedures).

| Year of Operation | NO LVOTO | | | | LVOTO | | | | Total | | | |
| | | Hospital Deaths | | | | Hospital Deaths | | | | Hospital Deaths | | |
	n	No.	%	CL	n	No.	%	CL	n	No.	%	CL
1964–1970	21	5	24%	14%–37%	2	0	0%	0%–61%	23	5	22%	12%–34%
1970–1984	116	10	9%	6%–12%	25	0	0%	0%–7%	141	10	7%	5%–10%
Total	137	15	11%	8%–14%	27	0	0%	0%–7%	164	15	9%	7%–12%
$P (\chi^2)$												0.02

KEY: CL, 70% confidence limits; LVOTO, left ventricular outflow tract obstruction.

NOTE: Direct relief of LVOTO was undertaken in 20 (8 severe, 9 moderate, 3 mild), whereas in 7 (2 moderate, 5 mild) nothing was done. The table excludes one patient with situs inversus and LVOTO who died.

Table 39-7 Hospital mortality after Senning-type atrial switch operation for simple TGA (see footnote 3 for definition) (UAB; 1977–1984).

Associated Procedures	n	Hospital Deaths		
		No.	%	CL
None	68	9	13%	9%–19%
Closure PDA	14	1	7%	1%–22%
Repair TV	1	1	100%	85%–100%
Resection LVOTO obstruction	7	0	0%	0%–24%
LV → PA Conduit	2	0	0%	0%–61%
VSD Repair	3	0	0%	0%–47%
VSD repair + other procedures for LVOTO	4	1	25%	3%–63%
VSD repair plus closure large PDA	2	2	100%	39%–100%
Total	101	14	14%	10%–18%

KEY: CL, 70% confidence limits; LV, left ventricle; LVOTO, left ventricular outflow tract obstruction; PA, pulmonary artery; PDA, patent ductus arteriosus; TV, tricuspid valve.

NOTE: The VSDs were small and closed with one stitch.

pose to premature late death[S5,V8] (Table 39-14), and acute postoperative obstruction can occur, particularly early in an experience with atrial switch procedures, and predispose to hospital death (Table 39-18).

CAVAL OBSTRUCTION. *Superior vena caval* pathway obstruction appears late postoperatively in 5%–10% of survivors of the *Mustard-type* of atrial switch procedure (Table 39-20). The incidence appears to be higher when the operation is performed in infants[K8]; the reoperation-free rate was 59% in patients less than seven months of age at operation, compared with 95% in those over one year of age, in the experience of Cobanoglu and colleagues.[C16] Although a significant incidence of *inferior vena caval* pathway obstruction was reported in the early series of Stark and associates[S5] and Venables and associates[V8] using Dacron baffles, the current incidence is very low (1%–2%).[A8,G4,M17,P6,T6] Its incidence is particularly low (GLH; 1 instance [0.6%, CL 0.1%–2%] among 166 patients) when at the atrial switch procedure the coronary sinus is opened down into the left atrium (see description in "Technique of Operation").

SVCO is maximal at the site of excision of the superior remnant (limbus) of the atrial septum beneath the upper baffle compartment and thus lies within the right atrium rather than at the SVC–RA junction. It was first described

by Mazzei and Mulder in 1971.[M18] The venous pathway may be totally occluded for over 1 cm or more in this area, or there may be only a localized zone of narrowing. Baffle shape, size, and composition are each important in its production as is the position of the suture lines within the atrium. It need not be more common when operation is performed in very early life (Table 39-20). The fact that it has proven impossible to eliminate SVCO after the Mustard procedure, despite intense study of the problem, indicates that the exact mechanism is not understood.

The incidence of late SVCO following a *Senning operation* is probably lower than following a Mustard operation[B12,F4,P7,W8] (Table 39-21). This is because the geometry of the pathway is, on average, better with the Senning-type repair, and the entire compartment is composed of viable atrial wall. Chin and colleagues, however, found SVCO present in 2 of 28 (7%) recatheterized patients after the Senning repair.[C5]

PULMONARY VENOUS OBSTRUCTION. Pulmonary venous obstruction is a less common but more lethal type of venous pathway obstruction. Severe obstruction has been recognized in 4 (2%, CL 1%–4%) of 166 patients (GLH) undergoing the Mustard-type atrial switch operation and has been identified in no case in which the V–Y angioplasty technique has been used (GLH). Pulmonary venous obstruction is more common when a Dacron baffle is used in the Mustard-type repair.[D5,R14] This complication has been reported after the Senning-type repair as well,[C5,S17] although no instances of pulmonary venous obstruction have been recognized in the recent UAB experience (1977–1984) with the Senning procedure. (See "Special Situations and Controversies" for further discussions of venous obstruction after atrial switch procedures.)

Reoperations

Reoperation may be required after the atrial switch repair, most commonly because of caval (see Table 39-20) or pulmonary venous obstruction after the Mustard repair but occasionally for other reasons. Dacron baffles require reoperation more frequently than do pericardial ones. Reoperation is particularly uncommon after the Senning-type atrial switch procedure, only one late reoperation (for tricuspid valve repair) being required among patients operated upon in the 1977–1984 era (UAB; n = 132) (see Table 39-21). Two acute reoperations (one Glenn anastomosis and one revision) were

Table 39-8 Results of atrial switch repair in simple TGA (see footnote 3 for definition), as reported in the literature.

Author	Years	n	Hospital Deaths			Age Range
			No.	%	CL	
Arcienegas et al.[A8]	1971–1979	90	4	4%	2%–8%	3 mo–17 yr
Mahony et al.[M17]	1975–1981	52	0	0%	0%–4%	< 100 d
Trusler et al.[T6]	1973–1979	100	2	2%	0.7%–5%	2 mo–4 yr
Locatelli et al.[L14a]	1977–1978	32	0	0%	0%–6%	3 mo–3 yr
Egloff et al.[E8]	1973–1977	63	5	8%	4%–13%	2 d–24 mo
Ullal et al.[U2]	1973–1978	95	10	11%	7%–15%	14 d–28 yr

KEY: CL, 70% confidence limits.

[a] Senning repair.

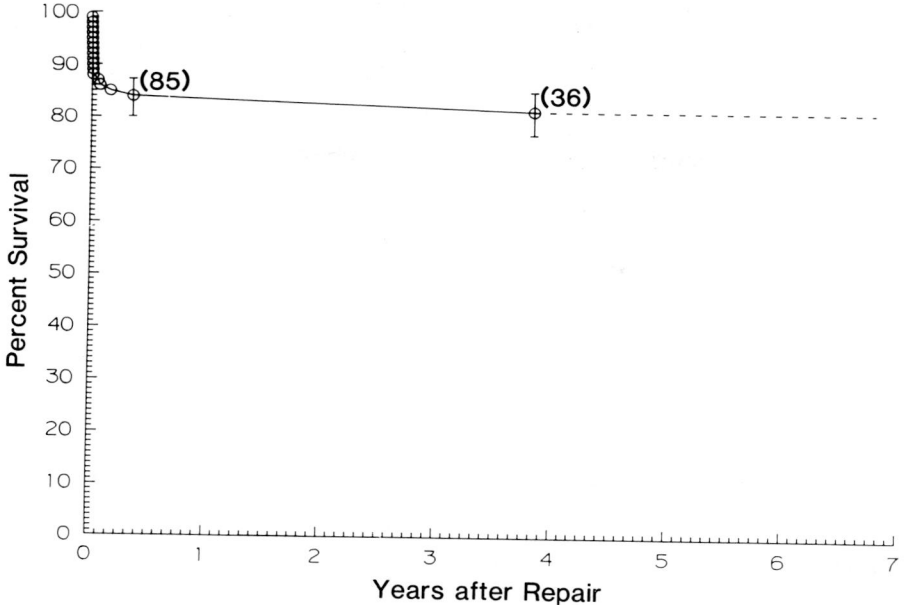

Figure 39-33   Actuarial survival, including hospital deaths, after Senning-type atrial switch operation for simple TGA (see footnote 3 for definition) (UAB; 1977–1984; *n* = 101, 14 hospital deaths and 3 late deaths). See Table 39-7 for details of the data base. Survival at specific intervals:

Time after Repair	Survival	
	%	CL
1 week	88%	85%–91%
1 month	86%	82%–89%
1 year	84%	80%–87%
5 years	82%	77%–86%

required in the early (1977) Senning experience (UAB), both for superior caval obstruction.

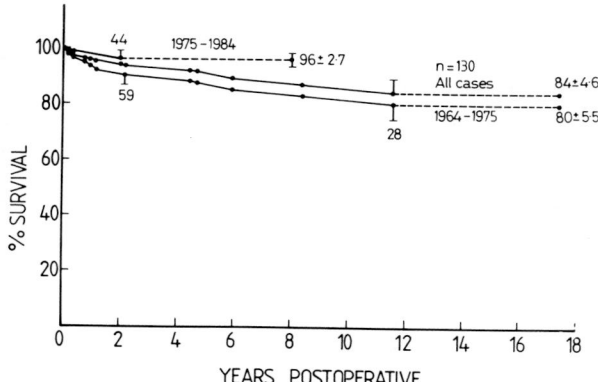

Figure 39-34   Actuarial survival of patients with simple TGA (see footnote 3 for definition) following an atrial switch procedure and direct relief when necessary of the left ventricular outflow tract obstruction (GLH; 1967–1984). Hospital deaths are excluded. The depiction is for the total group, and an early and current era. The numbers of patients at risk are noted. The bars depict the standard error (approximately the 70% confidence limits). When hospital deaths are included, the 8-year survival (operation in the current era of 1975–1984) is 90%.

When reoperation is done for caval or pulmonary venous obstruction, the results are generally good, although the symptoms and signs of inferior caval obstruction may require several months to regress. Recurrence of obstruction is uncommon after reoperation, having been recognized in only 1 of 8 (GLH) hospital survivors of reoperation and suspected but unproven in 1 of 15 (UAB). Reoperations are, however, not without risk when delayed until the patient is very ill (see Table 39-21).

Electrophysiologic Disturbances
Electrophysiologic disturbances occur in some patients after atrial switch operations. Their analysis is complex, in part because the frequency with which arrhythmias are detected on follow-up depends on whether only surface ECGs or 24-hour ECG ambulatory monitoring are used and upon the definition of abnormal. The 24-hour monitoring of *normal* infants and children has established that many apparently abnormal rhythms can occur (Table 39-22) and that abrupt changes in heart rate over a 24-hour monitoring period are relatively common.[D7,S21,S22]

Changes in *P-wave amplitude and contour* are virtually constant following a Mustard repair.[C7,E2] Postoperatively, the P wave is markedly diminished in amplitude and is frequently bifid in shape. The mean frontal plane P-wave axis is, however, unchanged.

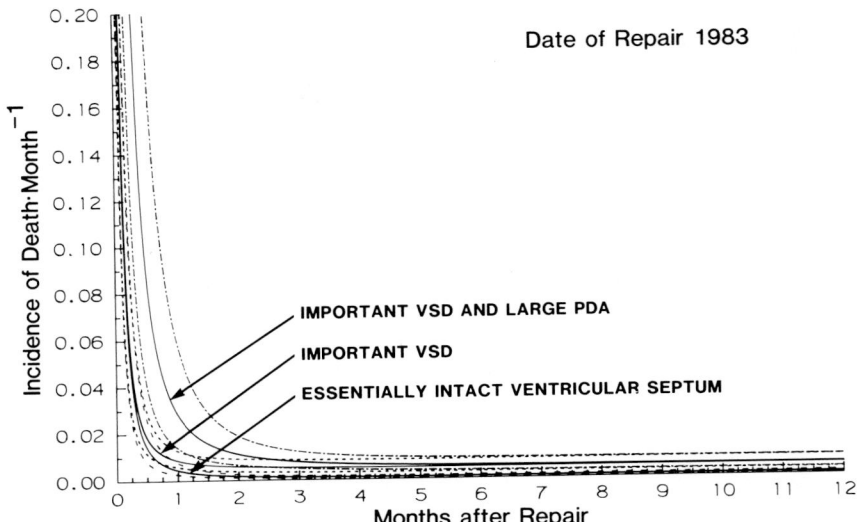

Figure 39-35 Stratified hazard function (instantaneous risk of death) from the multivariate analysis (Table 39-11) of death after the Senning-type atrial switch repair of all types of TGA (UAB; 1977–1984; *n* = 132). The dashed lines enclose the 70% confidence limits for the estimate. There is an early phase, merging with a constant late phase at 4–8 weeks after operation, but there is no phase of rising late risk within the follow-up period. In this analysis, neither left ventricular outflow tract obstruction nor patent ductus arteriosus were risk factors in patients with essentially intact ventricular septum, so-called simple TGA (see footnote 3 for definition).

PDA, patent ductus arteriosus; VSD, ventricular septal defect.

Usually *sinus rhythm* is present on standard ECG tracings at the time of hospital discharge following an atrial switch operation for simple TGA.[C7] About 10% of such patients are in a varying sinus-junctional rhythm, and only a few show a pure, benign-type junctional rhythm (Table 39-23). Thereafter there is a gradual decrease in the incidence of sinus rhythm after the Mustard-type repair as follow-up lengthens,[B17,F8] so that the probability of being alive and in sinus rhythm at 1 year is 72%, at 5 years 56%, at 10 years 50%, and at 13 years 43% (Fig. 39-38). Thus, at 13 years, half the GLH patients have persistent sinus rhythm and half a benign junctional rhythm without a conduction anomaly. Apart from the apparent slight increase in the risk of sudden death when a benign junctional rhythm is present, this rhythm appears to have no other significance. In this regard,

Table 39-10 Simultaneous procedure performed at the time of atrial switch repair in simple TGA (see footnote 3 for definition) (GLH; 1970–1984; *n* = 141; 10 hospital deaths).

Associated Procedure	n	Hospital Deaths
Ligation large collaterals	1	0
Ligation PDA		
Small or doubtful	31	3
Moderate	2	1
Large	4	1
Closure small VSD	7	0
Relief LVOTO	20	0
Excision RA ball thrombus	1	0

KEY: LVOTO, left ventricular outflow tract obstruction; PDA, patent ductus arteriosus; VSD, ventricular septal defect.

Table 39-9 Modes of hospital death in simple TGA (see footnote 3 for definition) (GLH; 1970–1984; *n* = 141; 10 hospital deaths; see Table 39-6).

Major Association with Death	Age at Operation	Other Factors
High pulmonary vascular resistance[a]	6, 7, 21 mo	
Low cardiac output	3, 3, 2 mo	NYHA class V in two *E. coli* enteritis in one
Baffle obstruction	19 d	
Respiratory complications	11 d	NYHA class V CHF (large PDA)
Arrhythmia (at 27 days PO)	5 mo[b]	
Chylopericardium (at 26 days PO) and tamponade	10 mo[b]	

KEY: CHF, congestive heart failure; PDA, patent ductus arteriosus; NYHA, New York Heart Association.

[a] Preop 8.3, 14.0, 22.0 units · m². All showed Gr 4 Heath-Edwards changes at autopsy.

[b] Senning repair.

Table 39-11 Incremental risk factors for death (hazard function domain) early and late after the Senning type of atrial switch operation for all subsets of patients with TGA. (UAB; 1977–1984; $n = 132$, 28 deaths throughout the follow-up period, including 22 hospital deaths; data set is that shown for Senning repair, 1977–1984, in Table 39-15.)

Incremental Risk Factor	Early Phase Hazard		Constant Phase Hazard	
	Coefficient ± SD	P value	Coefficient ± SD	P value
(Earlier) date of operation (years since 1977)	−0.28 ± 0.137	.04		
Presence of important VSD			2.1 ± 0.99	.03
Important VSD with PDA	2.1 ± 0.92	.02		
Intercepts	2.1		−7.5	

NOTE: The variables entered into the analysis are in Appendix 39A.

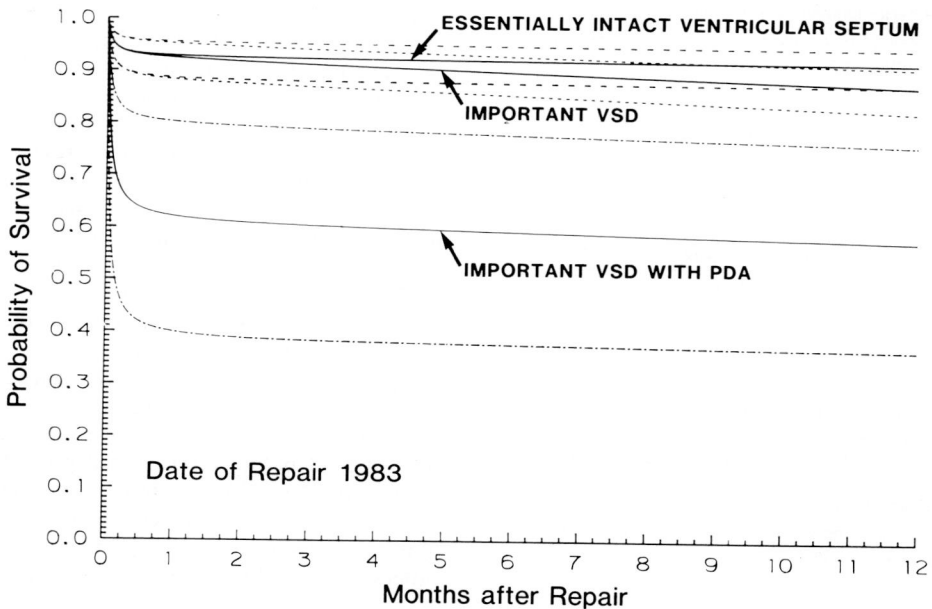

Figure 39-36 Stratified parametric survival estimates, including hospital deaths, for patients undergoing Senning atrial switch repair of all types of TGA (UAB; 1977–1984; $n = 132$; 28 deaths including 22 hospital deaths). See Table 39-15 for details; the multivariate equation is in Table 39-11). The dashed lines enclose the 70% confidence limits. The estimated late survival for the group with essentially intact ventricular septum (simple transposition—see footnote 3 for definition) at 5, 15, and 20 years are 89% (CL 85%–93%); 84% (CL 75%–90%) and 81% (CL 70%–88%), respectively.

PDA, patent ductus arteriosus; VSD, ventricular septal defect.

Table 39-12 Informal estimate of the survival of patients after treatment for simple TGA (see footnote 3 for definition) but without large patent ductus arteriosus, including the risks at and after balloon septostomy (BAS) and after the Senning repair in the current era (1983) (UAB).

Time after Repair (Survival)		Senning Survival		BAS Survival to 1–6 Months without Large PDA	Combined Survival	
		%	CL		%	CL
Days	7	94%	90%–96%		90%	85%–93%
	14	93%	89%–96%		89%	84%–92%
	30	93%	89%–96%		89%	84%–92%
				95%(CL 90%–98%)		
Months	6	92%	88%–95%		88%	83%–91%
	12	92%	88%–95%		88%	83%–91%
Years	5	89%	85%–93%		85%	80%–89%
	20	81%	70%–88%		77%	68%–84%

KEY: BAS, balloon atrial septostomy; CL, 70% confidence limits; PDA, patent ductus arteriosus.

NOTE: The BAS estimate is from the multivariate equation (Table 39-5, represented in Fig. 39-32), including only patients with no or small PDA. The Senning estimates are from the multivariate equation in Table 39-11, the nomogram for which is Figure 39-36.

Table 39-13 Incremental risk factors for hospital death after atrial switch operation for all types of TGA, with or without associated procedure (GLH; 1970–1984; $n = 203$, 38 hospital deaths).

Incremental Risk Factor	Coefficient ± SD	P value
Moderate or large VSD	2.25 ± 0.44	<.001
PDA[a]	0.96 ± 0.49	.05
Age ≤ 30 d	2.33 ± 0.79	.003
Intercept	2.89	

[a] Small, moderate, or large, regardless of time or method of closure.

NOTE: These have been obtained by multivariate logistic regression analysis (see Appendix 39B for variables analyzed).

Table 39-14 Incremental risk factors for premature late death after hospital dismissal among all subsets of patients undergoing an atrial switch procedure (GLH; 1970–1984).

Incremental Risk Factor	Coefficient ± SD	P value
Moderate or large VSD	1.85 ± 0.46	.0001
SVC obstruction[a]	1.35 ± 0.62	.003
PV obstruction[a]	1.89 ± 0.45	.002
Standard Mustard[b]	1.29 ± 0.53	.01

KEY: PV, pulmonary venous; SVC, superior vena caval.

NOTE: The multivariate analysis was done with the Cox proportional hazards model. Variables analyzed are described in Appendix 39B. Since inferior caval obstruction occurred only once in the GLH experience (in association with SVC obstruction), it does not appear as a risk factor.

[a] Mild, moderate, or severe versus none, assuming that in noncatheterized, asymptomatic patients these factors were absent.

[b] Compared with V-Y Mustard or Senning repair.

it should be noted that in some normal subjects in sinus rhythm the heart rate can fall below 40 beats per minute during sleep and the rhythm is then usually junctional.[D7,S21,S22]

In those in *slow junctional rhythm* there is a relatively normal rate response to exercise, often with reversion to sinus rhythm.[H5] Occasionally, rapid (accelerated) junctional rhythm can occur. This rhythm, and occasionally also supraventricular tachycardias or atrial flutter, can lead to a so-called malignant (active) arrhythmia, which reduces cardiac output and requires active measures for control.[E2] The sinus node recovery time after an atrial switch operation may be abnormal,[E6,G8,H5] and even when in sinus rhythm the maximal exercise heart rate response and the recovery rate following exercise may be abnormal.[H5]

Twenty-four-hour Holter monitoring following both Mustard and Senning operations may reveal dysrhythmias that are infrequent enough to be missed on standard ECGs, even when these are repeated on many occasions.[B12,M20] This technique allows the frequency of the rhythm disturbances to be assessed, as well as their categorization as a normal or probably abnormal variant. Holter studies that fail to make this latter differentiation overstate the arrhythmia incidence.[B17] Before a postoperative arrhythmia can be categorized as due to the surgical procedure, it is necessary to know that it was not present on a preoperative Holter monitor recording.[S23] Using these criteria, dysrhythmias are not frequent before atrial switch procedures. Thus, 24 patients (GLH) with TGA, aged 1–10 months, had preoperative monitoring; using the criteria in Table 39-22, only 1 was abnormal (frequent atrial premature beats), although 5 others showed abnormalities within the normal range.

Table 39-15 Hospital mortality after repair of TGA of all types with an atrial switch operation (UAB; 1967–1984; $n = 339$).

Associated Procedures	1967–1977 Mustard				1977–1984 Mustard				1977–1984 Senning				1977–1984 Total			
		Hospital Deaths				Hospital Deaths				Hospital Deaths				Hospital Deaths		
	n[a]	No.	%	CL	n	No.	%	CL	n	No.	%	CL	n	No.	%	CL
None	98	17	17%	13%–22%	15	2	13%	4%–29%	68	9	13%	9%–19%	83	11	13%	9%–18%
Closure PDA					1	0	0%	0%–85%	14	1	7%	1%–22%	15	1	7%	1%–21%
Repair TV									1	1	100%	85%–100%	1	1	100%	15%–85%
Resection subpulmonary stenosis	13	6	46%	29%–64%	3	1	33%	4%–76%	7	0	0%	0%–24%	10	1	10%	1%–30%
LV → PA conduit					2	2[a]	100%	39%–100%	2	0	0%	0%–61%	4	2	50%	18%–82%
VSD repair	44	25	57%	48%–65%	4	0	0%	0%–38%	21	4	19%	10%–32%	25	4	16%	8%–27%
VSD repair + other procedures for PS					5	0	0%	0%	8	2	25%	9%–50%	13[b]	2	15%	5%–33%
VSD repair plus other procedures					4	3	75%	37%–97%	11	5	45%	27%–65%	15[c]	8	53%	37%–69%
Total	155	48	31%	27%–35%	34	8	24%	16%–33%	132	22	18%	14%–22%	166	30	18%	15%–22%

KEY: CL, 70% confidence limits.

NOTE: In the 1967–1977 data, patients with major associated lesions or VSD and PS are not included.

[a] One also had closure PDA.

[b] Other procedures: repair AV valve (1, 1 death); close PDA (9, 5 deaths); PA debanding (5, 2 deaths).

[c] Other procedures: LV → PA conduits (5, 1 death); pulmonary valvotomy (4, 0 deaths); resection subpulmonary stenosis (3, 0 deaths); resection subpulmonary stenosis + LV → PA conduit (1, died).

Table 39-16 Hospital mortality following atrial switch procedure in patients with simple TGA (see footnote 3 for definition) (GLH; 1970–1984 and UAB; 1977–1984, Senning repair only).

| Age at Operation (months) | | GLH | | | | UAB | | | | Combined Series | | | |
| | | | Hospital Deaths | | | | Hospital Deaths | | | | Hospital Deaths | | |
≤	<	n	No.	%	CL	n	No.	%	CL	n	No.	%	CL
	1	4	2[a]	50%	18%–82%	9	4	44%	24%–66%	13	6	46%	29%–64%
1 ---	3	22	2	9%	3%–20%	18	1	6%	1%–18%	40	3	8%	3%–15%
3 ---	6	48	3	6%	3%–12%	32	4	12%	6%–22%	80	7	9%	5%–13%
6 ---	12	41	0	0%	0%–5%	31	4	13%	7%–22%	74	6	8%	5%–13%
12 ---	24	12	0	0%	0%–15%	8	1	12%	2%–36%	21	2	10%	3%–21%
24		11	0	0%	0%–16%	3	0	0%	0%–47%	14	0	0%	0%–13%
Total		138[b]	7	5%	3%–8%	101	14	14%	10%–18%	242	24	10%	8%–12%

KEY: CL, 70% confidence limits.

NOTE: These tables do not include deaths in the early phase (see Fig. 39-35) *after* hospital dismissal.

[a]One death from baffle obstruction (operation 1973) and one from low cardiac output (large patent ductus arteriosus in severe heart failure).

[b]Excludes three patients aged 6, 7, and 21 months operated upon knowing of their severe pulmonary vascular disease who died. They are included in the total combined series.

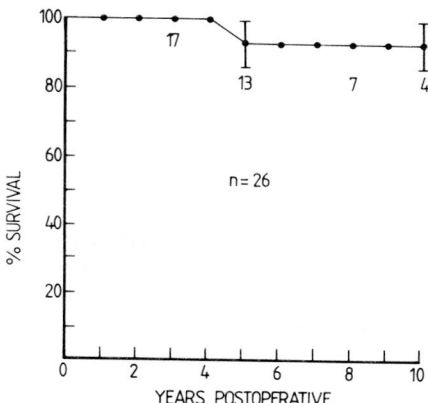

Figure 39-37 Actuarial survival of patients with simple TGA (see footnote 3 for definition) and left ventricular outflow obstruction following an atrial switch procedure and direct relief of left ventricular outflow tract obstruction (GLH; 1964–1984). No hospital deaths occurred in this subset.

Table 39-17 Hospital mortality after atrial switch procedure in patients with simple TGA (see footnote 3 for definition), according to the patients preoperative status (GLH; 1970–1984).

| Preoperative Status | | n | Hospital Deaths | | |
			No.	%	
Urgent operation	"NYHA class V"	6	2	33%	24%; 5/21 CI 14%–37%
Semiurgent operation		15	3	20%	
Elective Operation					
NYHA class IV		33	0	0%	4%; 5/20 CL 2%–7%
NYHA class III		87	5	6%	
Total		141	10	7%	CL 5%–10%
$P(\chi^2)$				.08	

KEY: CL, 70% confidence limits.

Table 39-18 Characteristics (not mutually exclusive) of hospital deaths after atrial switch operation for TGA, without other procedures (UAB; 1977–1984; the analysis is of the $n = 83$ in Table 39-15).

Characteristics	No. of Patients	
NYHA class V	2	
NYHA class IV	2	
Age < 30 d	4	
Preoperatively simple uncomplicated TGA	7	(5 Operated upon before 1980)
SVC obstruction	2	All redone
IVC obstruction	1	
Pulmonary venous pathway obstruction	1	
Typical syndrome of protamine reaction	1	

Table 39-19 Functional status among 103 living patients following the Senning-type atrial switch repair of TGA with or without large VSD (UAB; 1977–1984; $n = 132$).

NYHA Functional Status	n	% of 103 Survivors
I	99	96%
II	1	1%
III	0	
IV	0	
Unclassified	3	3%

NOTE: The one patient in class II had repair of TGA with large muscular VSD at age 2 months and subsequently underwent tricuspid valve replacement for severe tricuspid valve incompetence. She still tires easily.

Table 39-20 Incidence of superior vena caval (upper systemic venous compartment) obstruction (SVCO) in hospital survivors after the Mustard operation for all subsets of TGA (GLH; 1964–July 1981).

Age at Operation (months)		Hospital Survivors	SVCO (Mod-Severe)		Reoperation	Late Death
≤	<	n	No.	%	No.	No.
	1	3	—	0%		
1 ---	3	26	3[a]	12%	3	1
3 ---	6	57	4	7%	2	3[b]
6 ---	12	48	3	6%	2	0
12 ---	24	14	0			
24		18	2	11%	2	0
Total		166	12	7%	9	4 (2%)

NOTE: Ninety-four late postoperative cardiac catheterizations were performed in the 166 hospital survivors. In the patients with SVCO, the pressure gradients ranged between 9 and 22 mmHg.

[a] One had associated significant lower venous compartment obstruction.

[b] Two of these three deaths occurred without reoperation (one from associated severe pulmonary venous compartment obstruction, the other from noncardiac causes).

Postoperative Holter monitoring does reveal additional dysrhythmias (Table 39-24), particularly when the patient is in junctional rhythm. However, if the standard ECG always shows sinus rhythm, in about two-thirds of cases the Holter monitor study is normal. Rarely is an important abnormality in rhythm disclosed for the first time in Holter monitoring. As yet the dysrhythmias that predispose to sudden death in this context are not known.

Rhythm monitoring *during maximal exercise* testing may provide additional information, although at present its prognostic implications are also unknown. Mathews and associates noted that of 15 patients in sinus rhythm at rest who underwent exercise testing a mean of 9 years post-Mustard,

9 developed either premature atrial or ventricular contractions or junctional rhythm during exercise.[M21] This contrasted with a control group of whom none developed an arrhythmia.[M21]

The event of *sudden death* may well be related to some of these dysrhythmias. Sudden death occurs in about 5% of hospital survivors over a period of 10–20 years (4 sudden deaths have occurred [GLH] among 112 hospital survivors [see Fig. 39-38]; 1 sudden death [UAB] occurred 3½ years after the Senning repair, [see Fig. 39-33]). This complication was emphasized early by Aberdeen.[A11] Sudden death is rare in patients who remain in sinus rhythm postoperatively and when pacemaker recovery times are normal.[E6,G8,H5] The risk

Table 39-21 Reoperations (UAB; 1977–1984) after atrial switch operations done in any era or elsewhere. All cases have been followed after reoperation as of July 1, 1984.

Original Operation		Obstructed Pathway	No.	Hospital Deaths	Recurrence
Type	Site				
Mustard	UAB	SVC	3	1	
	UAB	SVC, IVC	5		Suspected IVC
	UAB	SVC, PV	1		
	UAB	SVC, IVC, PV	1		
	EW	SVC, IVC	3		
	EW	PV	2		
	EW	SVC, IVC, PV	1	1	
Senning	UAB[a]	SVC	2	2	
	UAB[b]	PV	1	1	
	UAB[b]	SVC	1		
Total			18	3 (17%; CL 7%–31%)	

KEY: EW, = elsewhere; IVC, inferior vena caval; PV, pulmonary venous; SVC, superior vena caval.

NOTE: All the original UAB Mustard operations were done prior to 1977. No late reoperations for pathway obstruction have been required in patients receiving the Senning operation in 1977–1984; one late reoperation was required for tricuspid valve replacement in a patient who had preoperative tricuspid incompetence.

[a] Operations in 1977 and reoperations (one Glenn anastomosis, and one revision) same day.

[b] Original operations in 1976.

Table 39-22 Definition of arrhythmia present on 24-hour ambulatory ECG monitoring in normal infants and children (normal criteria) and the criteria that can be considered to lie outside this normal range (abnormal criteria).

Arrhythmia	Normal Criteria	Abnormal Criteria
Junctional (nodal)	Rare, unsustained	Frequent, sustained
Accelerated junctional (> 100/min)	Unsustained (< 6 beats)	Prolonged, repetitive
Tachy/bradycardias	Occasional	Frequent episodes
Sinus pauses	50%–99% duration[a] infrequent (< 10/h)	50%–99% duration[a] when ≥ 10/h ≥ 100% duration[a] Total pause ≥ 1,800 msec
Premature AV beats	Infrequent (< 10/h)	≥ 10/h
Atrial bi/trigemini	Infrequent (< 3 episodes) Unsustained	Repetitive Sustained
Supraventricular tachycardia[b]	Unsustained (< 6 beats)	Sustained Chaotic, repetitive

[a] P–P (or R–R) interval length of sinus pause beat compared with preceding normal beat.

[b] Some are due to atrial flutter.

of sudden death in patients in junctional rhythm is 7% (GLH). No other risk factors for sudden death could be identified in a collaborative study of 372 patients.[F8]

Episodes of *supraventricular tachycardia* occur in 3%–5% of hospital survivors of the Mustard-type atrial switch procedure.

Risk factors for both conduction and rhythm disturbances are incompletely defined. The Mustard-type and Senning-type atrial switch procedures are not known to be different in this regard.[M20,M27] Patients in whom a VSD is repaired along with the atrial switch procedure appear to be at greater risk, although this has not been established with certainty.

The morphologic basis of the conduction and rhythm disturbances provides only an imperfect understanding of the reasons for their occurrence. Histologic examination of the sinus node region has revealed that the sinus node itself, the sinus node artery, and the paranodal tissues are frequently abnormal following the Mustard operation.[B16,E2,E4] Acute changes include compression of the sinus node artery by sutures or less often intimal thickening or thrombus for-

mation and suture compression, necrosis, or infarction of the sinus node itself with interstitial hemorrhage and edema of nodal tissue and the adjacent myocardium. Edwards and Edwards found that in nine cases with sinus node artery compression the sinus node showed acute infarction in seven.[E4] Chronic changes include marked fibrosis in the node and paranodal tissue, such that in some cases the sinus node can no longer be identified. The surgical maneuvers responsible for this damage include incorrect techniques for SVC cannulation (siting too close to the node so that the purse-string suture damages it and the use of excluding crushing clamps in this region), overzealous excision of the limbus and reendothelialization of the bare area so created that may damage the sinus node artery, and siting of suture lines too close to the sinus node. Although these abnormalities are associated with dysrhythmias and are present in a significant number of individuals with late sudden death, it is not certain that they are the explanation for all late benign arrhythmias after the Mustard or Senning operation. The extensive suture lines within the atria, combined with excision of virtually the

Table 39-23 Cardiac rhythm in 112 hospital survivors following a Mustard type atrial switch repair in patients with simple TGA (see footnote 3 for definition) (GLH; 1964–1982). Follow-up extends to 17 years.

Rhythm	Incidence at Hospital Dismissal		Rhythm at Last Review					
			Sinus		Junctional		CHB	
	No.	%	No.	%	No.	%	No.	%
Sinus	88	79%	59	53%	28	25%	1	1%[c]
Junctional	9[a]	8%	2	2%	6[b]	5%	1	1%
Sinus/junctional	12	11%	2	2%	10	9%	0	
Uncertain	3	3%	3	3%	0		0	
Total	112	100%	66	59%	44	39%	2	2%

KEY: CHB, complete heart block.

NOTE: Among the 88 patients in sinus rhythm only at discharge, 28 (32%) later converted to junctional rhythm, whereas of 28 patients who showed junctional rhythm, only 4 (19%) later converted to sinus rhythm.

[a] One known to be present preop.

[b] One with P–R 0.27.

[c] Temporary CHB postop.

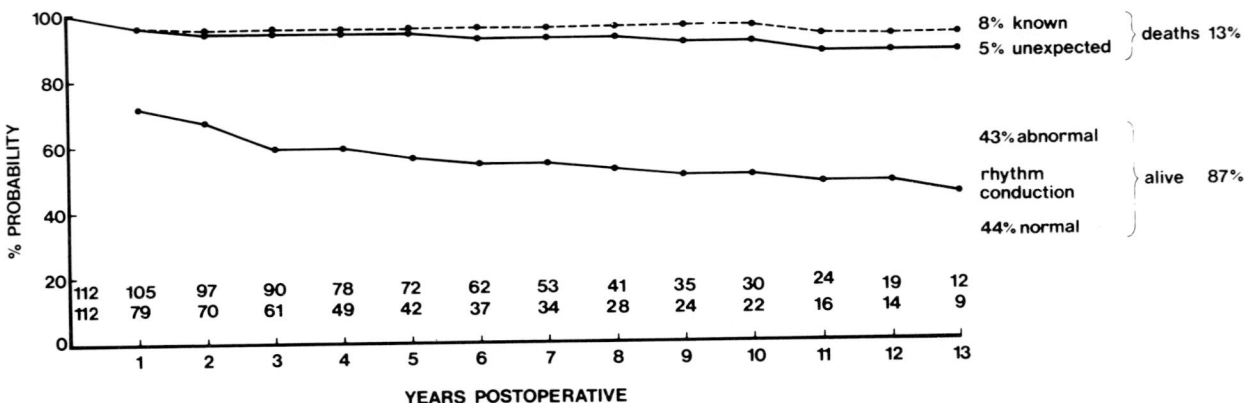

Figure 39-38 Actuarial cumulative arrhythmic risks in hospital survivors of a Mustard-type atrial switch procedure (GLH; 1964–1982; n = 112). All had simple TGA (see footnote 3 for definition). Follow-up extends to 17 years, but numbers are small beyond 13 years. The numbers at risk are shown. The 5% incidence of unexpected (sudden) late death represents four patients (one was in complete heart block and unpaced; one had first-degree heart block and junctional rhythm; one had junctional rhythm and episodes of supraventricular tachycardia; one had junctional rhythm that was also present preoperatively).

whole of the atrial septum, may also be related.[G7,W6] Although it is no longer believed that atrial conduction occurs through discrete, well-defined internodal tracts (see Chapter 1, "Internodal Pathways" in section on the Conduction System),[J4] it is possible that preservation of the anterosuperior portion of the limbus decreases the incidence of dysrhythmia.[C7,T6] In contrast, division of the free wall of the coronary sinus is not detrimental.[C7,T6]

A number of reports indicate that the incidence of dysrhythmia has decreased in operations performed in more recent years.[E5,L12,T6] The most important reason for this improvement may be that surgeons have taken greater care to preserve the sinus node and its artery.

Right Ventricular Function

Right ventricular systolic function (usually studied by measurement of ejection fraction at rest or during exercise or another form of stress) is usually reduced after an atrial switch operation in patients with simple TGA.[B12,G9,H6,M22] However, at least some of these patients have a reduced

Table 39-24 Arrhythmias disclosed on Holter monitoring of patients following a Mustard atrial switch procedure (GLH). The definitions used to denote whether the Holter monitor arrhythmia was a normal or abnormal variant are given in Table 39-22.

Rhythm on Holter Monitor	Persistent Sinus Rhythm[a] (n = 19)			Persistent Junctional Rhythm[a] (n = 17)		
		Abnormal			Abnormal	
	Normal	No.	% of 19	Normal	No.	% of 17
Sinus rhythm	16	0	0%	3	0	0%
Junctional rhythm	0	3	16%	1	14	82%
Accelerated JR	1	0	0%	1	2	12%
Tachy/bradycardias	0	0	0%	1	1	6%
Sinus pauses[b]						
50%–99%	5	6	32%	4	6	35%
≥ 100%	0	3	16%	0	2	12%
≥ 1,800 msec	0	0	0%	0	2	12%
Atrial premature beats	9	2	11%	2	7	41%
Ventricular premature beats	3	1	5%	0	3	18%
Bitrigemini	0	0	0%	2	2	12%
SVT	0	1	5%	2	2	12%
Total arrhythmias[c]	18	13		16	27	
Total patients	11	8	42%,CL 29%–57%	0	17	100%,CL 89%–100%

KEY: CL, 70% confidence limits; SVT, supraventricular tachycardia; JR, junctional rhythm.

[a] On surface ECGs.

[b] See Table 39-22.

[c] Excluding junctional rhythm (JR).

ejection fraction preoperatively, and it is not certain that a further reduction postoperatively is common.[G9] When there is a decrease in right ventricular systolic function after an atrial switch procedure, it is usually associated with increased right ventricular end-diastolic volume.[H6]

During exercise, the right ventricular ejection fraction may increase, remain unchanged, or decrease; patient age at operation, time of study, and the postoperative interval are not predictive of the change.[B18,M22,P10,R5]

Further evidence as to the possible decrease in right ventricular function after an atrial switch operation was obtained by Borow and colleagues.[B19] The systemic right ventricles in patients in whom the procedure was performed in the first year of life responded to afterload stress (methoxamine infusion) with a smaller increase in minute work index than did those in normal patients or patients after repair of isolated VSD or tetralogy of Fallot. Parrish and colleagues found a similar impairment of systemic right ventricular response in patients with congenitally corrected transposition.[P10] Thus, the morphologic right ventricle may be incapable of functioning normally as a systemic ventricle. The reasons for this are not entirely evident. Possibly the myocardial fiber arrangement in the right ventricle differs from that in the left, and this may render the right ventricle less able to function systemically.[S24] Possibly the right ventricle cannot benefit from the septal component of ejection because of the bellowslike action of the ventricular free wall.[B18] Benson and colleagues suggest that there may be a mismatch between the right ventricular blood supply and demand.[B18]

In any event, progressive deterioration of right ventricular function is uncommon after the atrial switch procedure in patients with simple TGA. Thus, obvious right ventricular failure, with marked hypokinesis and increased end-diastolic volume and signs and symptoms of congestive heart failure,[B12] is rare.[C4,P6] It is more common in patients in whom a large VSD also required repair (see later section on "Atrial Switch Operation for TGA and VSD").[G9,P10]

Left Ventricular Function

Left ventricular function at rest is often normal late after atrial switch operations.[H6] However, in some patients left ventricular ejection fraction fails to increase with exercise.[M22]

Tricuspid Valve Incompetence

Important (moderate or severe) tricuspid incompetence occurs uncommonly after the atrial switch procedure for simple TGA (it has occurred in only one patient in the GLH experience). Exceptional patient groups with an incidence up to 15% have been reported[H4]; the reasons for this variability are not evident. Trivial and mild incompetence occasionally occur.[C4,G5,M17,M19]

Left Ventricular Outflow Tract Obstruction

When an atrial switch procedure is performed for patients with simple TGA and the dynamic type of LVOTO (see "Morphology"), the obstruction rarely progresses after the atrial switch procedure.[P6] In fact, it usually regresses to some degree, whether or not a myotomy–myectomy is performed (Fig. 39-39).

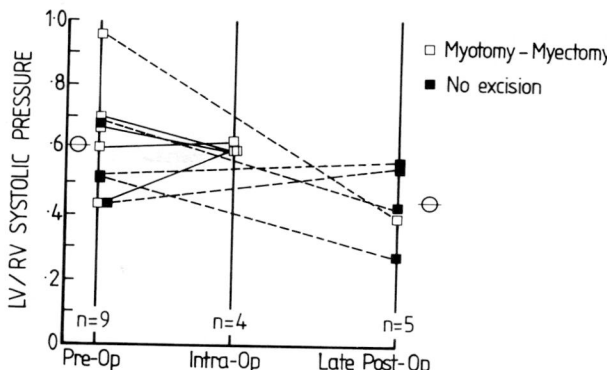

Figure 39-39 Preoperative, intraoperative, and late postoperative (mean 35 months) pressure measurements in patients with simple TGA and the dynamic type of left ventricular outflow obstruction undergoing an atrial switch procedure (GLH; 1964–1984). The follow-up time is 23–134 months (mean 56 months). When myotomy–myectomy was performed, the approach was through the pulmonary artery.

LV, left ventricle; RV, right ventricle.

The results of direct relief of the other types of LVOTO are also reasonably good (Fig. 39-40). When direct relief has not been possible, bypassing the obstruction with a left ventricular–pulmonary artery valved conduit gives good relief.[C6]

Residual Atrial Shunting

Trivial leaking at the baffle suture line occurs in a small proportion of patients (15%, GLH[C4]; 26%, CL 24%–29% in 390 collected cases[A8,G4,G5,H4,M17,M19,P6,S19,T4,T6]). Severe leaks, requiring reoperation, are uncommon (3 [2%, CL 0.8%–4%] of 166 patients, GLH; 12 [3%, CL 2%–4%] of the

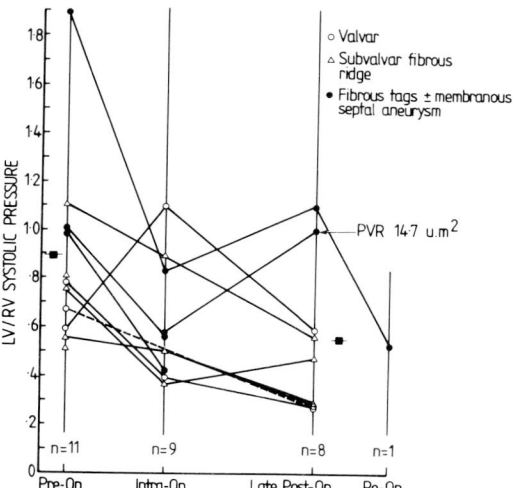

Figure 39-40 Depiction and patients as in Figure 39-37, except that the left ventricular outflow obstruction was morphologic rather than dynamic (GLH; 1964–1984). The obstruction was relieved through a pulmonary artery approach. The follow-up time is 16–55 months (mean 35 months).

PVR, pulmonary vascular resistance; $u \cdot m^2$, units $\cdot m^2$.

Table 39-25   Patients with simple TGA (see footnote 3 for definition) with presumably normal pulmonary vascular resistance preoperatively and an elevated pulmonary vascular resistance after an atrial switch operation performed at 3 or more months of age (GLH; 1964–1984).

| Preoperative Study | | Operation | Postoperative Study | | |
Age (months)	PVR (units · m^2)	Age (months)	Age (months)	PVR (units · m^2)	Comment
3	2.0	4	57	35	
		3[a]	21	14.7	
		5	45	9.2	
		35	103	8.9	(LD) small PDA; Gr 4 PVD
		24	44	8.1	
		43	102	7.7	Large PDA
4	1.6	4	49	6.7	Large baffle leak (reop)
		45	98	7.2	
		38	47	6.2	
		26	45	4.2	
		46[b]	78	4.0	

KEY: LD, late death; PDA, patent ductus arteriosus; PVR, pulmonary vascular resistance; PVD, pulmonary vascular disease.

NOTE: Two patients who died from pulmonary venous compartment obstruction and showed Gr 2 and 3 pulmonary vascular disease at autopsy have been excluded. Patients in whom no data are available preoperatively are presumed to have then had a normal resistance.

[a] Mild fibrous left ventricular outflow tract obstruction.

[b] Mild dynamic left ventricular outflow tract obstruction.

390 collected cases referenced above). Leaks are most common in the trabeculated upper portion of the atrium.

Pulmonary Vascular Disease
When an atrial switch operation is performed in the first 3 months of life for patients with TGA and essentially intact ventricular septum, new and progressive pulmonary vascular disease is uncommon; Mahoney and colleagues found no instances (0%, CL 0%–7%) among 28 patients in whom the operation was performed in the first 100 days of life.[M17] However, when the repair is done in older infants in this morphologic category, some patients (5%–10%) with a normal pulmonary vascular resistance preoperatively do develop pulmonary vascular disease postoperatively[N3,R16] (Table 39-25; and see Fig. 39-5). This often progresses and causes death.[B21]

Infants with simple TGA who evidence elevation of pulmonary vascular resistance preoperatively to levels less than about 12 units · m^2 may experience a satisfactory fall in resistance by the time of the late postoperative follow-up study[C2] (Table 39-26). Some of this fall is related to the reduction in hematocrit that occurs postoperatively.[C2,D9,H8] In some instances, however, the already present pulmonary vascular disease may progress postoperatively and be a cause of late mortality.[M23]

Atrial Switch Operation for Transposition of the Great Arteries with Ventricular Septal Defect

The results of the atrial switch operation are somewhat different for patients with TGA and important (moderate or large) VSD, although less so in the current era.

Survival to Atrial Switch Repair
As in the case of simple TGA and even with a policy of definitive repair within the first 6 months of life, not all pa-

tients with TGA and VSD survive to the time of repair. As noted earlier, Tynan found the survival in this group no different from that in simple TGA[T2] (see Fig. 39-29), and this is also the case in the UAB and GLH experience. However, the shape of the survival curve is different (Fig. 39-41), with fewer deaths in the early days of life and relatively more after the neonatal period. The patients usually die with pulmonary complications and congestive heart failure, rather than with hypoxia as is generally the case in simple TGA.

Thus, unless the repair is done in the first few months of life, only about 85% of patients entering the hospital with TGA and VSD can be expected to survive until repair.

Survival after Atrial Switch Repair
Hospital survival after the atrial switch operation and repair of the VSD has been lower (mortality higher) than when the atrial switch operation has been done for simple TGA, but the difference has become less in recent years. Thus, in 234 cases collected from the literature, there have been 54 deaths (mortality 23%, CL 20%–26%).[A8,E8,P9,S26,T7,V2] The hospital mortality in this subset (GLH; 1964–1972) was 68% (CL 55%–79%) (Table 39-27) and at UAB (1967–1977) 57% (CL 48%–65%) (see Table 39-15). More recently, the mortality has been less, the improvement being evident in the GLH (1972–1984) experience in which it was 38% (CL 30%–46%) (see Table 39-27) and the UAB (1977–1984) experience in which it was 26% (CL 17%–36%). However, in cases with just TGA and VSD, the mortality is 17% (CL 9%–28%) (Table 39-28).

In part as a result of this improved early survival, the combined early and late survival of patients after the atrial switch operation and repair of important VSD is better than in earlier eras (see multivariate analysis in Table 39-11), although the presence of such a VSD remains an incremental risk factor for premature death after repair (Table 39-13), especially when combined with a large PDA (Table 39-11).

Table 39-26   Postoperative pulmonary vascular resistance in patients with simple TGA (see footnote 3 for definition) 3 months of age or older at atrial switch operation and with preoperatively moderate or severe pulmonary vascular disease (GLH; 1964–1984).

Preoperative Study		Operation	Postoperative Study (or Autopsy)	
Age (months)	PVR (units · m²)	Age (months)		PVR (units · m²)
5[a]	22.0	5	(HD)	Gr 4 PVD
6[b]	14.0	7	(HD)	Gr 4 PVD
10	10.8	12		3.6
57	10.1	58		4.2
19	8.3	20	(HD)	Gr 4 PVD
		20	(HD)	Gr 4 PVD
		40	(HD)	Gr 4 PVD
		37	(HD)	Gr 4 PVD
30	7.8	32		3.1
		32	(HD)	Gr 2 PVD

KEY: HD, hospital death; PVD, pulmonary vascular disease; PVR, pulmonary vascular resistance.

NOTE: The cardiac output used in the resistance calculations in this table and in Table 39-25 has been obtained either by using a measured oxygen uptake (Fick) or from indicator dilution curves.

[a] Small PDA.

[b] Moderate PDA.

The unfavorable effect of the VSD (and its repair) is evident late postoperatively (see Table 39-11, late phase, and Table 39-14 and Figs. 39-35, 39-36; Fig. 39-42) as well as early.

Overall Survival

An estimate of the overall survival to be expected in patients operated upon in the current era can only be made informally as in the case of simple TGA. This informal estimate (UAB; Table 39-29) suggests a 5-year survival of 67% (53%–78%) for patients operated upon in the current era. This is less than the 85% (CL 80%–89%) predicted in simple TGA (see Table 39-12).

Incremental Risk Factors for Premature Death

THE ERA. As has already been seen, the risk of premature death after the atrial switch procedure and closure of the VSD is less in the current era.

AGE AT REPAIR. Young age has been a risk factor for premature death (see Table 39-13), but this is not apparent in the current era (see Tables 39-11 and 39-28).

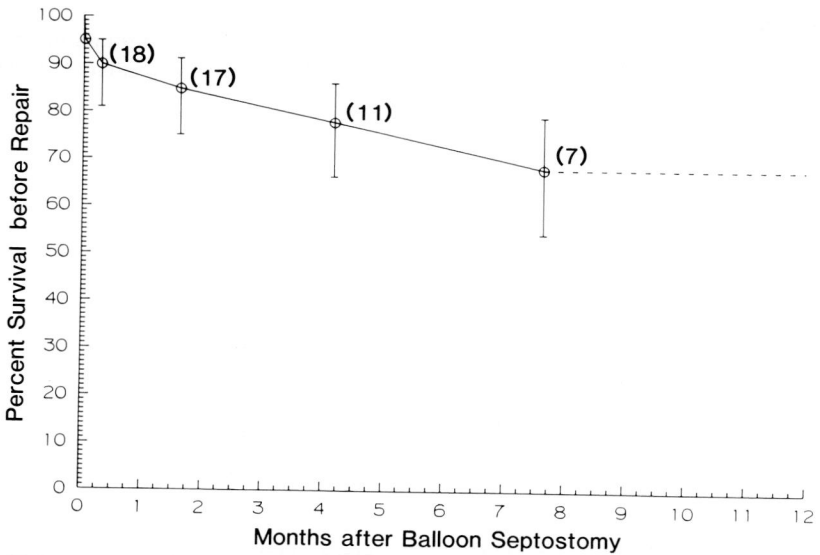

Figure 39-41   Actuarial survival before repair of patients with TGA and important (moderate-sized or large) VSD and without left ventricular outflow tract obstruction, submitted to balloon atrial septostomy (UAB; 1970–1981, *n* = 20, five deaths). The actuarial survival at 1 month is 90% (CL 81%–95%); 2 months, 85% (CL 75%–91%); 6 months 78% (CL 66%–86%).

Table 39-27 Hospital mortality in patients with TGA and moderate-sized or large VSD, following atrial switch procedure and repair of ventricular septal defect with or without repair of patent ductus arteriosus and/or left ventricular outflow tract obstruction but excluding patients receiving the Rastelli repair (GLH; 1964–1972).

Age at Operation (months)		1964–1972				1972–1984				Total			
			Hospital Deaths				Hospital Deaths				Hospital Deaths		
≤	<	n	No.	%	CL	n	No.	%	CL	n	No.	%	CL
	1	7	6	86%	59%–98%	2	2	100%	39%–60%	9	8	89%	67%–99%
1 ---	3	2	1	50%	7%–93%	8	3	38%	17%–62%	10	4	40%	22%–61%
3 ---	6	4	2	50%	18%–82%	23	10	43%	31%–56%	27	12	44%	33%–56%
6 ---	12	0				11	4	36%	19%–56%	11	4	36%	19%–56%
12 ---	24	3	2	66%	24%–96%	2	0	0%	0%–61%	5	2	40%	14%–71%
24		6	4	66%	38%–88%	4	0	0%	0%–38%	10	4	40%	22%–61%
Total		22	15	68%	55%–79%	50	19	38%	30%–46%	72	34	47%	41%–54%
P(logistic)			0.6				0.04				0.09		

CL, 70% confidence limits.

PATENT DUCTUS ARTERIOSUS. In this setting, associated PDA is a risk factor for premature death after repair (see Tables 39-11, 39-13). This may be related to the increment in the left ventricular volume overload and the pulmonary vascular disease imposed preoperatively by this additional anomaly.

ADDITIONAL RISK FACTORS. The other risk factors described for premature death after atrial switch procedure for simple TGA apply also to those with TGA and important VSD.

Growth and Functional Statuses
The growth and functional status is good at least up to 5 years in most surviving patients (see Table 39-19).

Venous Pathway Obstruction
This is similar to that described for simple TGA.

Electrophysiologic Disturbances
These are similar to those described for simple TGA but perhaps more common.

Table 39-28 Hospital mortality after Senning-type atrial switch repair in patients with transposition of the great arteries and moderate-sized or large VSD (UAB; 1977–1984; n = 24).

Age at Operation (months)				Hospital Deaths	
≤	<	n	No.	%	CL
	1	0		0%	0%–85%
1 ---	3	2	0	0%	0%–61%
3 ---	6	7	2	29%	10%–55%
6 ---	12	7	1	14%	2%–41%
12 ---	24	5	0	0%	0%–32%
24		3	1	33%	4%–76%
Total		24	4	17%	9%–28%

KEY: CL, 70% confidence limits.

NOTE: Not included are patients with co-existing large patent ductus arteriosus (n = 6, all < 6 months old, with 3 hospital deaths) or severe LVOTO (n = 1, age 10 months, who died). Thus, hospital mortality after the Senning repair in the entire group of TGA with important VSD is 8 deaths (26%; CL 17%–36%) among 31 patients. This, plus Table 39-7, reconciles with Table 39-15.

Right Ventricular Function
Right ventricular dysfunction is more common in patients in whom a large VSD required repair than in those with simple TGA, and it is particularly apt to occur when the VSD is repaired via a right ventriculotomy.[C4,H4,P6] In these circumstances, it may be accompanied or precipitated by tricuspid incompetence (see below).

Left Ventricular Function
This appears to be similar to that described for simple TGA.

Tricuspid Valve Incompetence
The incidence of important tricuspid incompetence late postoperatively is higher in this subset than after repair in simple TGA.[C4,C5,G4,H4,P6,T5] Four (24%) of 17 patients with a large VSD had on late postoperative cineangiography moderate or severe tricuspid incompetence, 7 (41%) had mild tricuspid incompetence, and only 6 (35%) had no incompetence (GLH). This complication is more common when the VSD closure is performed through the right ventricle (rather than the right atrium), presumably because of the higher inci-

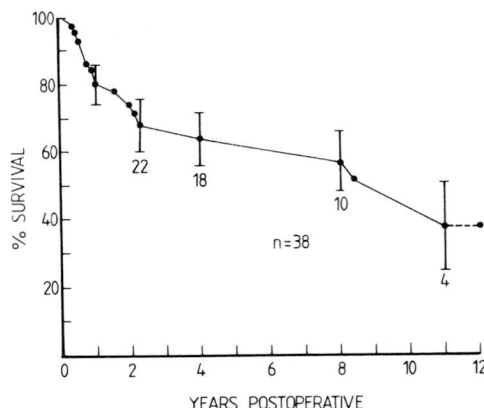

Figure 39-42 Actuarial survival of patients with TGA and a moderate or large VSD ± PDA ± LVOTO following an atrial switch procedure, repair of VSD, and direct relief where necessary of LVOTO (GLH; 1964–1984). Hospital deaths are excluded. Depiction is as in Figure 39-34.

Table 39-29 Informal estimate of the over-all survival of patients after treatment in the current era (1983) for TGA with important ventricular septal defect but without large patent ductus arteriosus, including the risks at and after balloon septostomy (BAS) and after the Senning repair (UAB).

Time after Repair (Survival)		Senning Survival		BAS Survival to 1–3 Months	Combined Survival	
		%	CL		%	CL
Days	7	94%	90%–96%			
	14	93%	89%–96%		89%	84%–93%
	30	92%	88%–95%		88%	83%–92%
					88%	83%–92%
Months	6	90%	86%–93%	95% (CL 87%–98%)		
	12	88%	83%–91%		86%	81%–90%
Years	5	70%	58%–80%		83%	77%–87%
					67%	53%–78%

KEY: BAS, balloon atrial septostomy; CL, 70% confidence limits.

NOTE: The BAS estimate is from the actuarial analysis, assuming a similar trend of improvement in the current era as for patients undergoing BAS with essentially intact ventricular septum (Fig. 39-41). The Senning estimates are from a solution of the multivariate equation in Table 39-11, represented in Figure 39-36.

dence of right ventricular dysfunction following this former approach, but it also occurs when a right atrial approach has been used.[C5,T5]

Left Ventricular Outflow Tract Obstruction

In those patients with TGA and important VSD in whom LVOTO can be effectively relieved directly, the long-term results are satisfactory[14] (Fig. 39-43).

Residual Ventricular Shunting

This is uncommon and can be the result of overlooked multiple VSDs or of incomplete or dehisced repair of a large VSD. Two (6%, CL 2%–13%) of 34 patients (GLH) surviving an atrial switch procedure and repair of a large VSD had a large residual shunt at the repair site, and 4 others (12%, CL 6%–20%) had small shunts through unclosed additional small VSDs.

Pulmonary Vascular Disease

When an atrial switch operation and closure of a large VSD are performed in the first 6 months of life in patients with

TGA whose pulmonary vascular resistance is less than about 10 units · m², the resistance usually falls to satisfactory levels late postoperatively.[C2] As with simple TGA, however, the resistance may progress or apparently new disease may appear; this is more common when repair is performed beyond 1 year of age. Ten (53%) of 19 patients in this subset had moderate or severe pulmonary vascular disease at some stage in their course (see Fig. 39-6).

Arterial Switch Operation for Simple Transposition of the Great Arteries

When the arterial switch operation has been done in the first month of life, the early (in-hospital) survival has been good. Castaneda and colleagues report that 19 (86%, CL 74%–94%) of 22 neonates have left the hospital alive[C11]; Radley-Smith and Yacoub report 10 survivors (91%, CL 72%–99%) among 11 neonates[R13]; Quaegebeur reports 18 survivors (100%, CL 90%–100%) among 18 neonates[Q3]; Idriss and colleagues report 6 survivors among 6 neonates (100%, CL 73%–100%).[15] It remains to be determined whether these results can be reproduced generally. Reoperation has been necessary in 2 among 17 survivors (Castaneda) because of pulmonary artery stenosis.

Little is yet known concerning the late results, except that they may be similar to those following the arterial switch operation for TGA and large VSD (see below).

Arterial Switch Operation for Transposition of the Great Arteries and Ventricular Septal Defect

Survival

The hospital mortality has been variable but in general in the range of 25%–40%. Thus early survival rate in the category of TGA and important VSD has been 67% (CL 44%–85%) (UAB) (Table 39-30). To date, there have been no late deaths (Fig. 39-44), and the clinical status of all surviving patients is good.

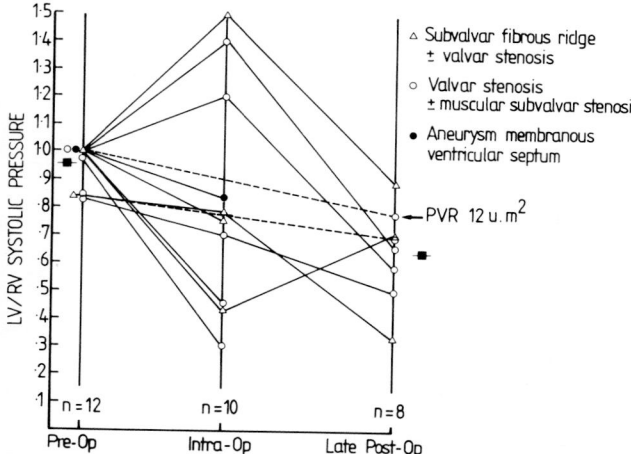

Figure 39-43 Hemodynamic results of direct relief of LVOTO (with an atrial switch procedure and VSD repair) in patients with TGA, VSD, and LVOTO (GLH). Follow-up time is 1–50 months (mean 20 months).

Table 39-30 Hospital mortality after repair of TGA by arterial switch operation (UAB; 1977–1984; first operation 1981).

Arterial Switch Operation	n	Hospital Deaths		
		No.	%	CL
With closure of large PDA	2	2	100%	39%–100%
With closure VSD	9[a]	3	33%	15%–56%
Total	11	5	45%	27%–65%

KEY: CL, 70% confidence limits.

NOTE: Nine arterial switch operations have been performed in infants with TGA and large VSD (GLH). Five hospital deaths occurred among the first six patients (1976–1979); no early or late deaths have occurred in the last 3 patients (operations in 1983).

[a] Two also had small PDA.

Electrophysiologic Disturbances

Granting the relatively short follow-up periods to date, patients with TGA and either intact ventricular septum or VSD treated by the arterial switch operation have been free of the supraventricular rhythm disturbances that many patients have after the atrial switch procedures. Arensman and colleagues report that this is true whether or not a right ventriculotomy has been made for repair of the VSD.[A13]

This casts some doubt on the supposition that such rhythm disturbances are an inherent part of the malformation of TGA.

Left Ventricular Function

Left ventricular function is usually normal after the arterial switch operation. In a study of 12 patients, Borow and colleagues found normal contractility and normal dimensions and wall thickness in 10 of 12 patients studied between 2 and 7 years postoperatively.[B28] However, Hausdorf and colleagues identified one patient among 14 studied late after the arterial switch operation, in whom left ventricular stiffness was severely increased,[H10] and Okuda and colleagues three patients with reduced ejection fractions associated with neoaortic valve incompetence.[O3]

Of great interest is the fact that dynamic LVOTO, even with a gradient up to 120 mmHg, disappears after the arterial switch procedure.[Y4]

Right Ventricular Outflow Obstruction

Residual or new right ventricular outflow obstruction has complicated the early and intermediate term course of some patients after the arterial switch operation. Castaneda and colleagues have experienced two examples of pulmonary artery stenosis requiring reoperation among 13 hospital survivors.[C1] Bical and colleagues have reoperated upon 5 (16%, CL 9%–26%) of 31 hospital survivors of the arterial switch operation for stenosis of the right ventricular outflow tract.[B31]

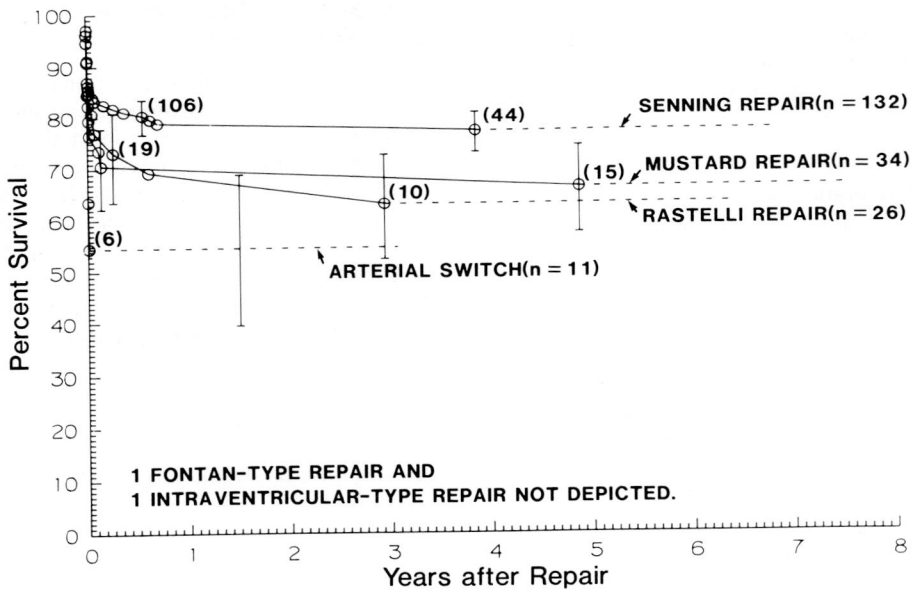

Figure 39-44 Actuarial survival including hospital deaths for all patients undergoing repair of all morphologic subsets of transposition of the great arteries (UAB; 1977–1984; n = 205). The actuarial curves are stratified according to the type of repair. Patients with simple TGA and with TGA plus important VSD (with or without PDA and/or LVOTO) are included in the Senning and Mustard group. For the best estimate of the survival of the morphologic subsets, see Fig. 39-36. Each death is represented by a circle, and the vertical bars represent 70% confidence limits of the estimates. The dashed lines represent traced living patients. The numbers in parentheses represent the number of patients traced beyond that point. All patients have been traced as of July 1984. The patient with the Fontan-type repair is alive and in NYHA functional class I 1 year after repair; the one with the intraventricular repair is alive and in class I 2.5 years after repair.

Table 39-31 Hospital mortality after the Rastelli operation for TGA, VSD, and LVOTO (UAB; 1967–1984; n = 57).

| Years of Operation | n | Hospital Deaths | | |
		No.	%	CL
1969–1973	11	4	36%	19%–56%
1973–1977	20	6	30%	19%–44%
1977–1981	16	6	38%	23%–54%
1981–1984	10	0	0%	0%–17%
Total	57	16	28%	22%–36%

KEY: CL, 70% confidence limits.

Rastelli Operation for TGA, VSD, and LVOTO

Survival

Although the in-hospital mortality has been high in earlier years, it is currently much lower. Thus, among 57 patients (UAB; 1967–1984) undergoing the Rastelli operation (Table 39-31), 16 patients (28%, CL 22%–36%) have died and the other part (GLH) of the combined (UAB and GLH) experience has been similar, 4 deaths (44%, CL 24%–66%) having occurred among 9 patients (1967–1979). The recent experience is much improved, no deaths (0%, CL 0%–17%) having occurred among 10 patients undergoing the operation since 1980 (UAB; see Table 39-31).

Late death is uncommon after the Rastelli repair in patients with TGA, VSD, and LVOTO, but in series going back into an earlier era the relatively high hospital mortality has limited the long-term survival. Thus, survival up to 16 years (UAB; 1967–1984) is only 60% (Fig. 39-45). Most of the deaths occurred within 2 weeks of the operation; only 2 later deaths occurred among the 37 patients (UAB) alive at 10 months after operation. This is reflected in the finding of only an early phase in the hazard function (Fig. 39-46), which falls to a very low level within 6 months of operation, indicating

that late survival should be much better in patients undergoing operations in the current era.

Incremental Risk Factors for Premature Death

Only an earlier date of operation and preoperative functional class are identified as incremental risk factors for premature late death (Table 39-32). The era (date of operation) effect is also illustrated by the fact that the hospital mortality has been much lower since 1980 (see Table 39-31). The cryopreserved homograft-valved conduit (see "Technique of Operation") has been used in the current era (Table 39-33).

It is of interest that enlargement of the VSD as part of the repair was not found to be a risk factor (see Table 39-32), presumably because proper precautions were taken in performing this (see "Technique of Operation"). Between 1978 and 1984 (UAB), the VSD was not enlarged in 16 patients, among whom 2 died (12%, CL 4%–27%), and was enlarged in 10, among whom 4 died (40%, CL 22%–61%).

Functional Status

Most survivors of the Rastelli operation are in good health. Thus, among 35 hospital survivors (UAB; 1967–1984), 77% are in NYHA functional class I, 14% are in NYHA class II; in 3 (9%) the functional status is unknown.

Conduit Obstruction

Both the Dacron conduits containing irradiated homografts and those (Hancock) containing porcine heterograft valves have been subject to late conduit obstruction (see Chapter 23, "Special Situations and Controversies") and thus the need for reoperation (Fig. 39-47). The incidence of reoperation, even with the heterograft-valved conduits, has been low for the first 5 years, probably related to the fact that the conduit has always been placed to the patient's *left* side. The technically easier maneuver, in patients with D-malposition of the aorta, of placing it to the right (as in the original

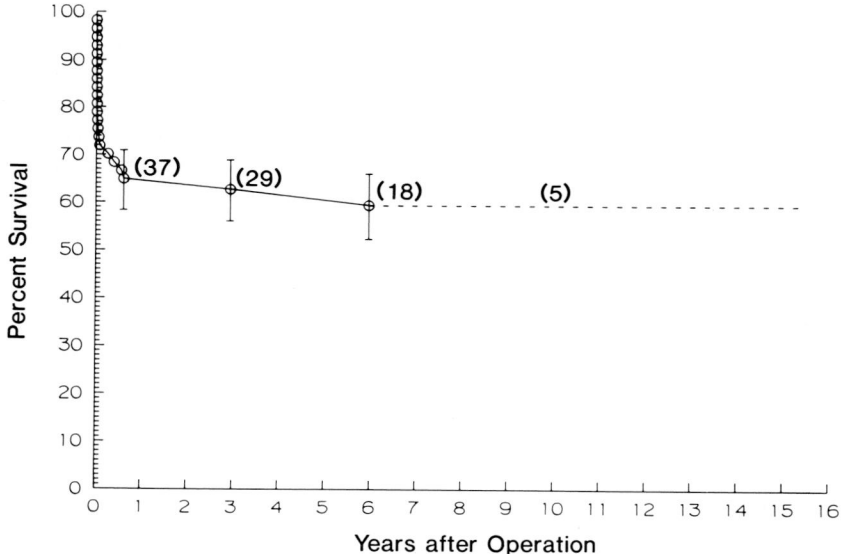

Figure 39-45 Actuarial survival, including hospital deaths, after the Rastelli operation for TGA, VSD, and LVOTO (UAB; 1967–1984; n = 57). All patients are traced as of July 1984. (Note that Fig. 39-44 includes only patients operated on in 1977–1984.)

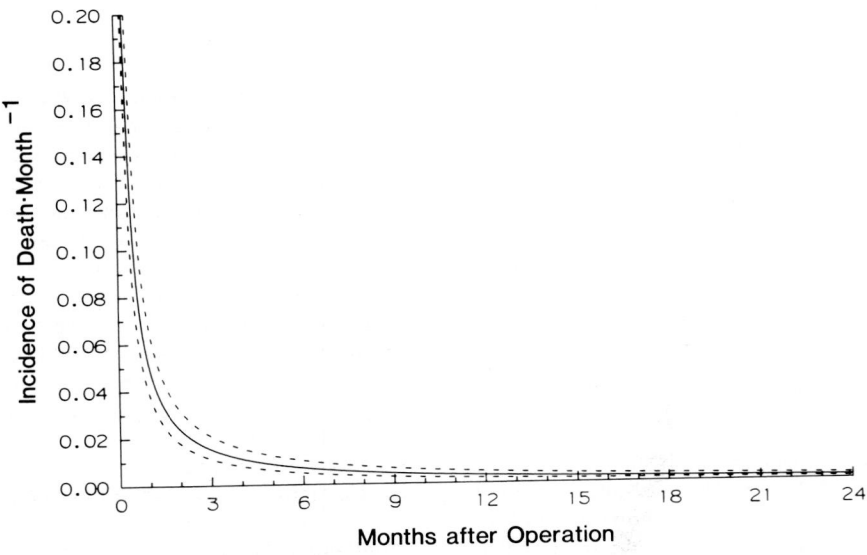

Figure 39-46   Hazard function for death (incidence of death · month^{-1}) after the Rastelli operation for TGA, VSD, and LVOTO (UAB; 1967–1984; $n = 57$, 22 events).

Rastelli description[R3]) results in a higher incidence because the conduit is compressed by the sternum. The need for reoperation is considerably less when the cryopreserved homograft valved conduit is used (see Fig. 39-47, and Chapter 23, "Valved Conduits" in Section 1, Special Situations and Controversies).

Conduit replacement, although undesirable, can be done safely. Thus, no deaths have occurred among 6 patients requiring it (UAB).

Table 39-32   Incremental risk factors for premature death, including hospital deaths, after the Rastelli operation for TGA, VSD, and LVOTO (UAB; 1967–1984; $n = 57$, 22 events). There is no late constant hazard phase (see Fig. 39-46). (See Appendix 39C for variables entered.)

Incremental Risk Factor	Early Phase Hazard	
	Coefficient ± SD	P value
Earlier date of operation (months since 1/1/67)	−0.14 ± 0.085	.10
NYHA functional class	0.6 ± 0.42	.14
Intercept	0.112	

Electrophysiologic Disturbances

Complete heart block has occurred as a result of repair (UAB, 4 instances [13%, CL 7%–22%] among 31 patients operated upon prior to 1977). The incidence may be less in the current era (UAB, 1 instance [4%, CL 0.5%–12%] among 26 patients operated upon 1977–1984).

The development of heart block or other arrhythmia late postoperatively is uncommon, no instances having occurred (UAB or GLH).

INDICATIONS FOR OPERATION

The indications for operation in any condition, always the product of comparisons between the natural history of the disease and the early and late results of the various surgical interventions, are continuously subject to change with the development of new information and new procedures. This is particularly true for the various subsets of transposition of the great arteries (TGA), because of the relatively recent advent of the arterial switch operation and the lack of information concerning its intermediate (5–10 years) and long-

Table 39-33   Hospital mortality after the Rastelli operation for TGA, VSD, and LVOTO (UAB; 1967–1984).

Type of Conduit	n	Hospital Deaths			
		No.	%	CL	
Dacron conduit containing irradiated homograft valve	12	4	33%	18%–52%	16/51; 31% (CL 24%–39%)
Hancock heterograft-valved conduit	39	12	31%	23%–40%	
Cryopreserved homograft-valved conduit	6	0	0%	0%–27%	
Total	57	16	28%	22%–36%	

KEY: CL, 70% confidence limit.

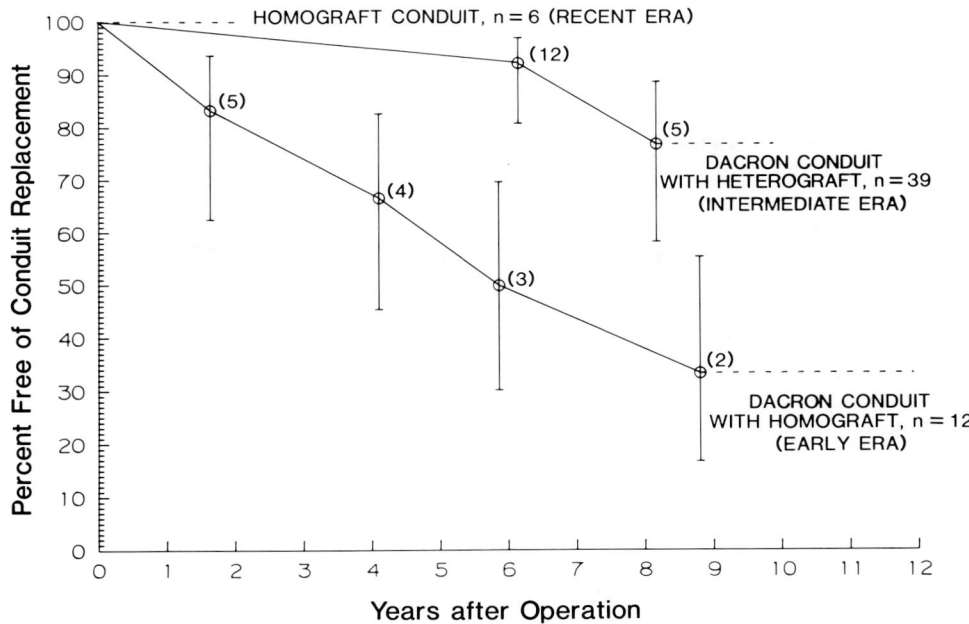

Figure 39-47 Actuarial incidence of freedom from reoperation for conduit obstruction after the Rastelli operation for TGA, VSD, and LVOTO (UAB; 1967–1984; *n* = 57). (Patients were censored when death occurred before reoperation.) There were no deaths at reoperation. The early era homografts were sterilized by irradiation.

term (20 or more years) results. Thus, current indications are subject to modification in a particular institution for study purposes or generally as new information becomes available.

Simple Transposition of the Great Arteries without Associated Cardiac Anomalies

(See footnote 3 for definition of simple TGA.) Currently, a protocol of balloon atrial septostomy (BAS) and later atrial switch repair is used (GLH and UAB). The BAS is performed a short time after birth, and careful medical management is used for the first several weeks after this. If hypoxia is extreme, an infusion of prostaglandin is occasionally given before the procedure.[B15,H9,L11] This decreases cyanosis by dilating the ductus arteriosus, but its effect on lowering pulmonary vascular resistance may also be beneficial since this further increases pulmonary blood flow. Continued support with prostaglandin infusion may rarely be required postseptostomy for a few days, when there is concern about persistent marked hypoxia.[L11] In the uncommon circumstances of persisting, severe cyanosis and symptoms, an atrial switch procedure of the Senning type is performed at the initial hospitalization or later in the first month of life. Repeat balloon septostomy or a Blalock atrial septectomy are not used. Generally, the Senning procedure can be done electively at 3 months of age, avoiding further delay in order to reduce the waiting morbidity and mortality to as low a level as possible and to lessen the likelihood of irreversible pulmonary vascular disease and impairment of cognitive function.[N6] Cardiac catheterization is repeated immediately preoperatively to assess the pulmonary vascular resistance and any LVOTO.

Generally, when the atrial switch procedure is indicated, the Senning technique is used. When there is leftward juxtaposition of the atrial appendages, however, this type of atrial switch is more difficult because of the smaller right atrial wall, and a Mustard-type repair is done. Also, in referred cases in which a large posterior type of ASD has already been created by the Blalock-Hanlon technique, the Mustard-type repair is often selected.

An *arterial* switch procedure may be considered the procedure of choice in simple TGA, although information concerning the results in this subset are incomplete. When this procedure is used, the repair is done in the neonatal period as soon after the diagnosis is made as is possible and generally after balloon septostomy.

Simple Transposition of the Great Arteries with Patent Ductus Arteriosus

In view of the high incidence of early death when a moderate-sized or large patent ductus arteriosus (PDA) is present, an aggressive surgical approach is indicated. When pulmonary blood flow is excessive and heart failure cannot be medically controlled in the first 2–3 weeks of life, the PDA is divided via a left thoracotomy (GLH). The infant is closely observed in the days following this procedure, and if cyanosis is too severe an atrial switch repair is carried out. Otherwise, the repair is delayed until 3 months of age.

Alternatively, an atrial or an arterial switch operation and ductal closure are performed in the neonatal period (UAB).

Simple Transposition of the Great Arteries with Left Ventricular Outflow Tract Obstruction

When the left ventricular outflow tract obstruction (LVOTO) is dynamic and particularly when left ventricular pressure is not suprasystemic, the protocol used for patients with simple TGA alone is appropriate. When the obstruction is discrete and correctable by a direct operation (as judged by cineangiographic appearance), an atrial switch procedure plus direct relief of the LVOTO within the first 3 months of life is indicated.

When the pressure in the left ventricle is suprasystemic and the LVOTO seems not amenable to direct relief, an atrial switch operation plus a left ventricle-to-pulmonary artery homograft-valved conduit is indicated (UAB). Alternatively (GLH), a simple atrial switch operation is done initially with direct relief of the stenosis as far as possible, followed later by the conduit operation if suprasystemic left ventricular systolic pressure persists.

Transposition of the Great Arteries with Important Ventricular Septal Defect

Currently, an arterial switch operation is indicated in the first 3 months of life, although complete information on the results of this protocol is not available. If symptoms become severe in the first month of life, the arterial switch operation is indicated forthwith. In view of the improved results of the *atrial* switch operation in patients with TGA and important VSD in the current era, this procedure (and transatrial closure of the VSD) may be used in place of the arterial switch procedure if coronary anatomy is considered at operation to be unfavorable for the arterial switch procedure. In a few cases, the position of the VSD and its relations to the great arteries make a completely intraventricular tunnel repair advisable. Pulmonary artery banding is no longer performed (UAB, GLH).

When pulmonary vascular resistance is severely elevated (>10 units · m²), a palliative atrial or arterial switch procedure is indicated. Close follow-up is needed, since pulmonary vascular resistance may fall postoperatively, and even in older patients later repair of the VSD may be possible. In situations in which the ventricular septum is intact, a similar procedure is performed combined with the creation of a large VSD in the apex of the septum via a left ventriculotomy.

Transposition of the Great Arteries with Important Ventricular Septal Defect and Left Ventricular Outflow Tract Obstruction

The Rastelli operation is the indicated definitive procedure when the VSD is in an appropriate position and of an appropriate size. When the VSD is less than moderate-sized, the surrounding structures often limit the amount of surgical enlargement of the VSD that is possible, and make the Rastelli operation inadvisable.[V11] If the LVOTO is amenable to direct repair, this and an atrial switch operation with VSD repair may be used. Otherwise, a left ventricular pulmonary artery conduit is added.

Because a valved extracardiac conduit is needed for the Rastelli procedure, the repair is deferred when possible to the age of 3–5 years, at which time a relatively large homograft-valved extracardiac conduit can be used. Usually severe cyanosis indicates the need for an initial shunting operation, which may be a Gore-Tex interposition shunt (particularly if palliation is required in the first 3 months of life) or a classic Blalock-Taussig shunt on the side opposite to the aortic arch.

Transposition of the Great Arteries Plus Severe Right Ventricular Hypoplasia

Fortunately, severe forms of right ventricular hypoplasia are rare when the ventricular septum is intact.[R9] It is more common when the VSD is large, particularly when there is coarctation of the aorta.[M8] In these patients, provided the pulmonary vascular resistance is normal, a Fontan-type procedure with right atrial-pulmonary artery anastomosis is indicated (see Chapter 26, "Fontan-type Procedure" in section on Technique of Operation).

SPECIAL SITUATIONS AND CONTROVERSIES

Superior Vena Caval Obstruction after Atrial Switch Procedures

As was noted earlier (see "Results"), the obstruction is not in the cava itself but lies within the right atrium at the site of the excision of a portion of the superior limbus. The mechanism of the obstruction is variable. When a redundant Dacron baffle has been used, folding of the cloth upon itself can frequently be identified (in association with an increase in baffle thickness by neointima), and the same probably occurs with redundant pericardium. Primary adherence of the baffle to the bare area created by excision of the limbus is a possibility, but if so this is not entirely prevented by reendothelializing this area with interrupted sutures.

Clinical Features
The patients may be asymptomatic. Venables and colleagues found that although symptoms could be present with a superior vena cava (SVC) mean pressure as low as 10 mmHg, they were not constant until it rose above 16 mmHg.[V8]

The least conspicuous clinical feature but one that suggests the diagnosis is ruddiness of the cheeks, and there may also be puffiness of the eyelids, face, and neck, which can mask fixed distention of the jugular veins. Tortuous subcutaneous venous collaterals can occur[P6] but are uncommon. A bilateral or right-sided pleural effusion may be present, sometimes chylous. With SVC obstruction there may be bilateral cervical and axillary lymphadenopathy and paramediastinal densities (due to tortuous collaterals) on the chest x-ray.[M18]

Less common features are an increasing head circumference and hydrocephalus associated with widening of the cranial sutures, which is a response to an increase in intracranial venous pressure in children less than 18 months of age (the upper age limit for normal closure of the cranial sutures).[M17,R12,S14,S16,V8] Children over 3 years of age may de-

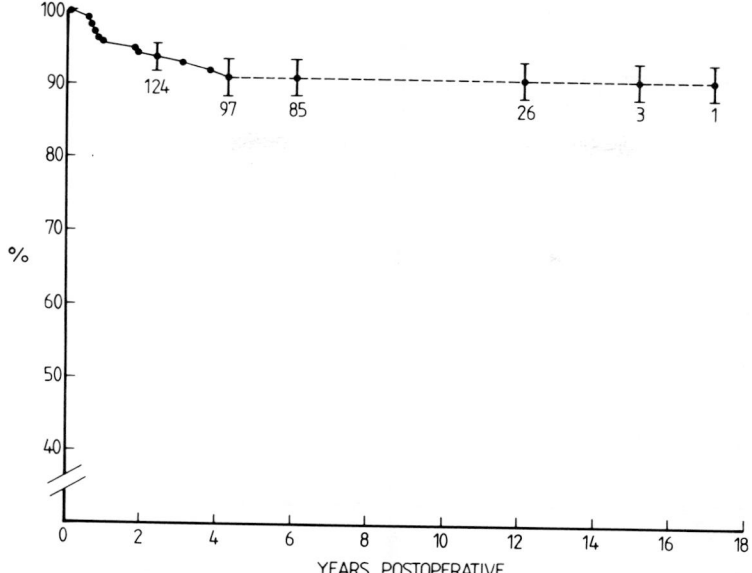

Figure 39-48 Actuarial freedom from SVC obstruction in hospital survivors of the Mustard-type atrial switch operation (GLH; 1964–1981). The time of appearance of obstruction is taken as the time of postoperative cardiac catheterization (n = 10) or of recognition of increase in head circumference to > 2 SD of the expected mean for age at 6 and 9 months postoperatively. Those documented as appearing beyond 1 year postoperatively were either without symptoms at an earlier stage or, in one patient, had serial cardiac catheterization showing progression of a mild stenosis. Of the 166 patients 94 had late postoperative cardiac catheterization.

velop pseudotumor cerebri.[R12] There may also be a protein-losing enteropathy,[K6,M16] presumably due to interference with the normal return of intestinal lymph to the venous system, secondary to a high venous pressure. (This is more common with inferior vena caval obstruction.[M16])

Time of Onset
SVC obstruction is usually apparent within 12 months of operation, although asymptomatic patients may not be discovered until they are later investigated. The appearance between 12 and 18 months of a new stenosis has not been convincingly documented, although slow progression of a mild-to-severe stenosis has been (GLH). The actuarial incidence is 9% at 4 years, with no further events up to 17 years postoperatively (GLH) (Fig. 39-48).

Diagnosis
The diagnosis can be made noninvasively, using two-dimensional echocardiography,[C5,S14] Doppler ultrasound,[W4] pulse Doppler echocardiography,[S20] and radionuclide angiography.[H3] However, cardiac catheterization and cineangiography are advisable before reoperation. In severe cases, this demonstrates a striking difference in wave form between the SVC and the systemic venous atrium (SVA), similar to a situation that may be present at the end of operation,[P5] and a high mean pressure in the SVC (Fig. 39-49). The large amplitudes of phasic pressure in the SVA are considered due to its small volume, which can cause a rapid rise in pressure as the chamber fills, followed by a rapid fall when it empties into a more compliant left ventricle.[P5,V8] These abnormal

wave forms are not necessarily present late postoperatively (Fig. 39-50) nor is there necessarily a gradient,[C4] but they are common.[S13,V8] When the SVC obstruction is mild, the striking feature is the damped wave form in the SVC tracing (Fig. 39-51).

Obstruction severe enough to become apparent clinically is associated with an SVC mean pressure above about 15 mmHg and an SVC–SVA gradient of ⩾10 mmHg.[P6,M17,V8] In 19 patients with severe obstruction, Silove and Taylor recorded a mean gradient of 16.9 ± 9.0.[S13] The SVC pressure tends to be higher when there is also an inferior vena caval obstruction.[V8] Occasionally, the SVC tracing may show tall *a* waves due to contraction of the right atrial appendage (when it lies above the site of stenosis); in this circumstance blood refluxes up the SVC[S13] (Fig. 39-49*a*).

Angiography shows either a complete obstruction or a severe stenosis (Fig. 39-49*b*).

Treatment
When symptoms are present, reoperation is indicated. It is also indicated in any child who shows progressive increase in head size beyond the normal range. (For the technique of reoperation, see "Technique of Operation.")

Inferior Vena Caval Obstruction after Atrial Switch Procedures

Postoperative inferior vena caval (IVC) obstruction, like SVC obstruction, occurs within the heart at about the midpoint of the lower portion of the systemic venous compart-

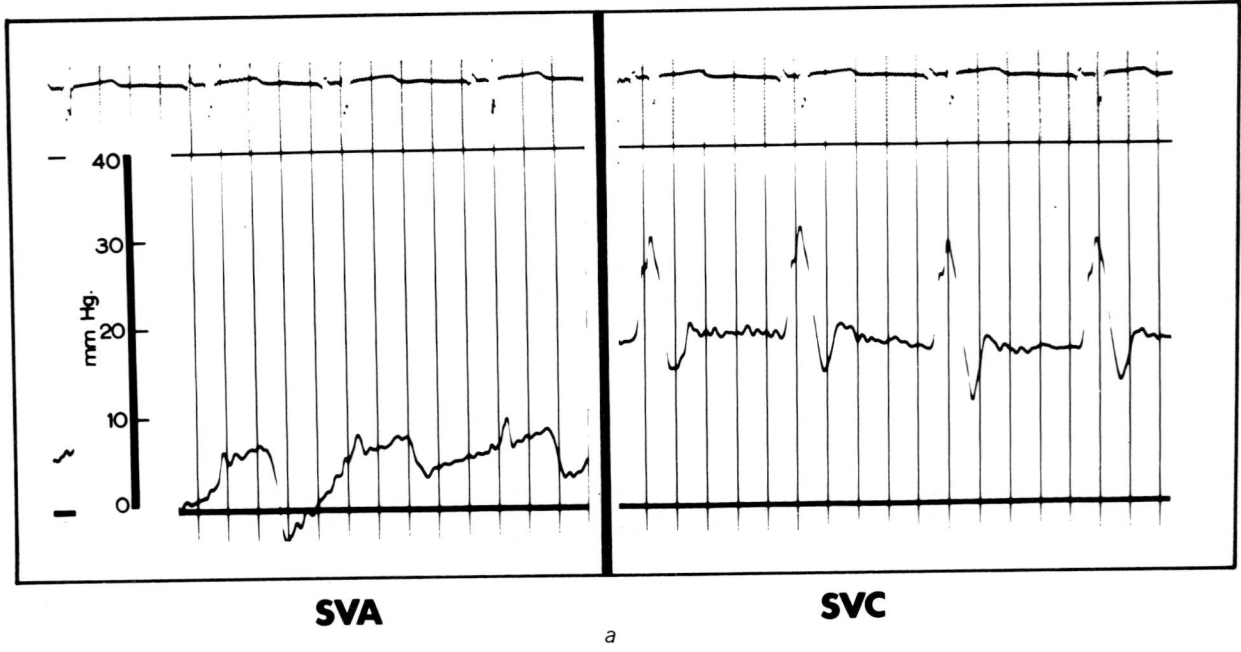

SVA   **SVC**

a

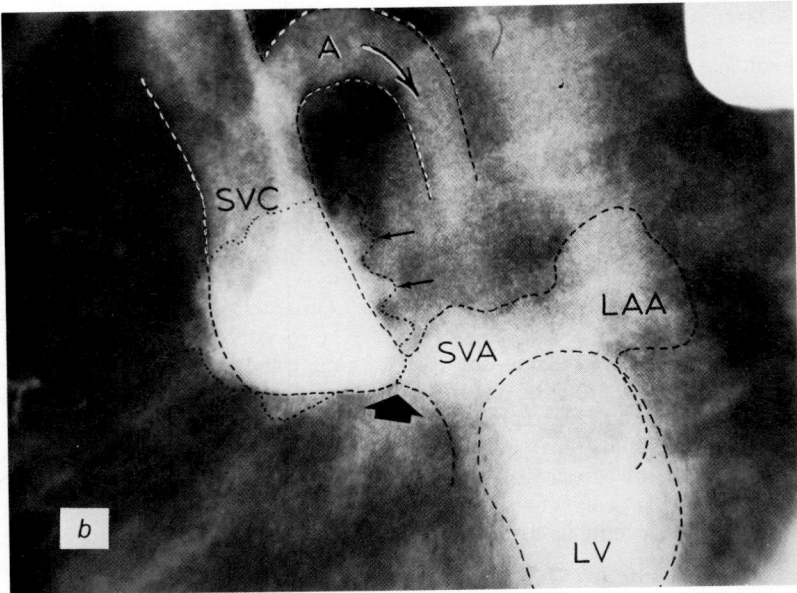

b

Figure 39-49 Data from postoperative cardiac catheterization in a patient who had undergone a Mustard repair and developed severe obstruction to superior vena caval (SVC) flow into the systemic venous atrium (GLH).

(*a*) Phasic withdrawal pressures from systemic venous atrium (SVA) to SVC. Mean pressures were 5 and 20 mmHg, respectively. Note the dominant a wave in the SVC tracing. This is due to contraction of the portion of right atrial appendage that lies above the site of obstruction.

(*b*) Cineangiogram after injection into the superior vena cava, in 20° left anterior oblique projection. The heavy arrow marks the site of obstruction. The fine dotted lines (small arrows) outline that portion of the original right atrial appendage that lies in the upper venous compartment beneath the baffle and above the site of obstruction. There is retrograde flow into the azygous vein.

A, azygous vein; LAA, left atrial appendage; LV, left ventricle; SVA, systemic venous atrium; SVC, superior vena cava.

Reproduced with permission from Clarkson et al.,[C4] and the American Heart Association, Inc.

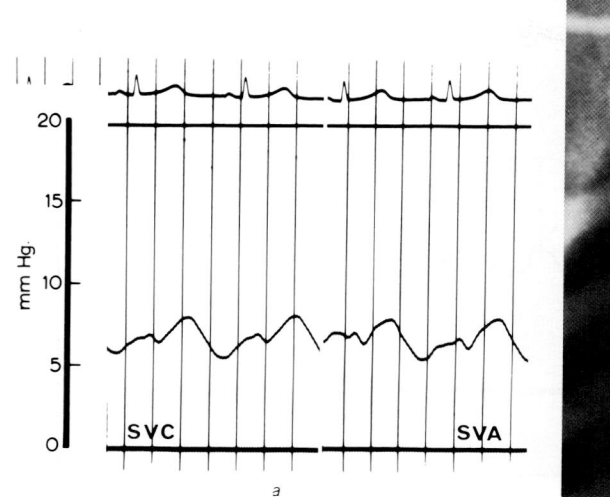
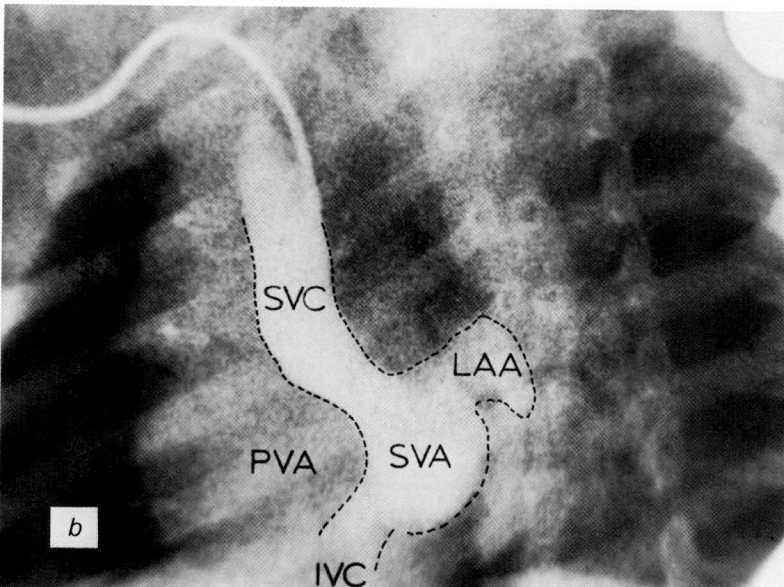

Figure 39-50   Data from postoperative cardiac catheterization in a patient who had undergone a Mustard-type atrial switch operation and has unrestricted systemic venous drainage (GLH).
(a) Phasic withdrawal pressures.
(b) Cineangiogram as in Fig. 39-49.

IVC, inferior vena cava; LAA, left atrial appendage; PVA, pulmonary venous atrium; SVA, systemic venous atrium; SVC, superior vena cava.

Reproduced with permission from Clarkson et al.,[C4] and the American Heart Association, Inc.

ment, adjacent to the coronary sinus ostium. It is, when significant, almost always symptomatic with liver enlargement, ascites, and leg edema. A protein-losing enteropathy may occur more frequently than with SVC obstruction,[M16] and particularly when combined with some degree of SVC obstruction, there may be low cardiac output and premature late death.

The diagnostic techniques used are similar to those for SVC obstruction; pressure gradients are also similar, averaging 17.8 ± 8.8 mmHg in the series reported by Silove and associates.[S15]

Reoperation with insertion of a new baffle is always indicated for IVC obstruction (see details in ''Technique of Operation'').

Pulmonary Venous Obstruction after Atrial Switch Procedures

Pulmonary venous obstruction usually occurs at the waist of the pulmonary venous atrium (PVA), which lies just anterior to the entry of the right pulmonary veins, between the crista terminalis on the lateral right atrial wall and the center of the baffle in the Mustard operation. In severe stenosis there is a circular fibrotic ostium at this point, which is less than 10 mm in diameter and which divides the PVA into two almost equal compartments of adequate size. The right pulmonary vein ostia are usually not stenotic. Rare examples of isolated left pulmonary vein stenosis or occlusion have been reported, presumably secondary to placement of the baffle suture line too close to these ostia,[L10,T6] although rarely congenital pulmonary vein stenosis coexists with TGA (see Chapter 37).

Symptoms

Pulmonary venous obstruction produces pulmonary venous hypertension and symptoms of progressive dyspnea with cough, fatigue, and sometimes cyanosis. Pulmonary venous congestion is visible on the plain chest x-ray. This may progress to interstitial pulmonary edema. These signs are unilateral when only the left pulmonary veins are stenotic. There may be a continuous murmur with diastolic accentuation heard along the lower left sternal edge.[B13,D5,P8]

Time of Onset

The time of onset is similar to that of caval obstruction, and is usually within 6–12 months of operation. However, occasional cases of late onset up to 10 years postoperatively have been documented by serial cardiac catheterizations.[B13,D5] However, mild early pulmonary venous obstruction does not necessarily progress, since none of the six patients with documented mild pulmonary venous obstruction (GLH; 1964–1971) have subsequently been recognized to develop more severe obstruction.

Diagnosis

The diagnosis is confirmed by cardiac catheterization at which, ideally, the catheter is passed retrogradely across the stenosis to the posterior pulmonary venous compartment to obtain a withdrawal gradient. If this is impossible, a comparison is made between a pulmonary artery wedge pressure

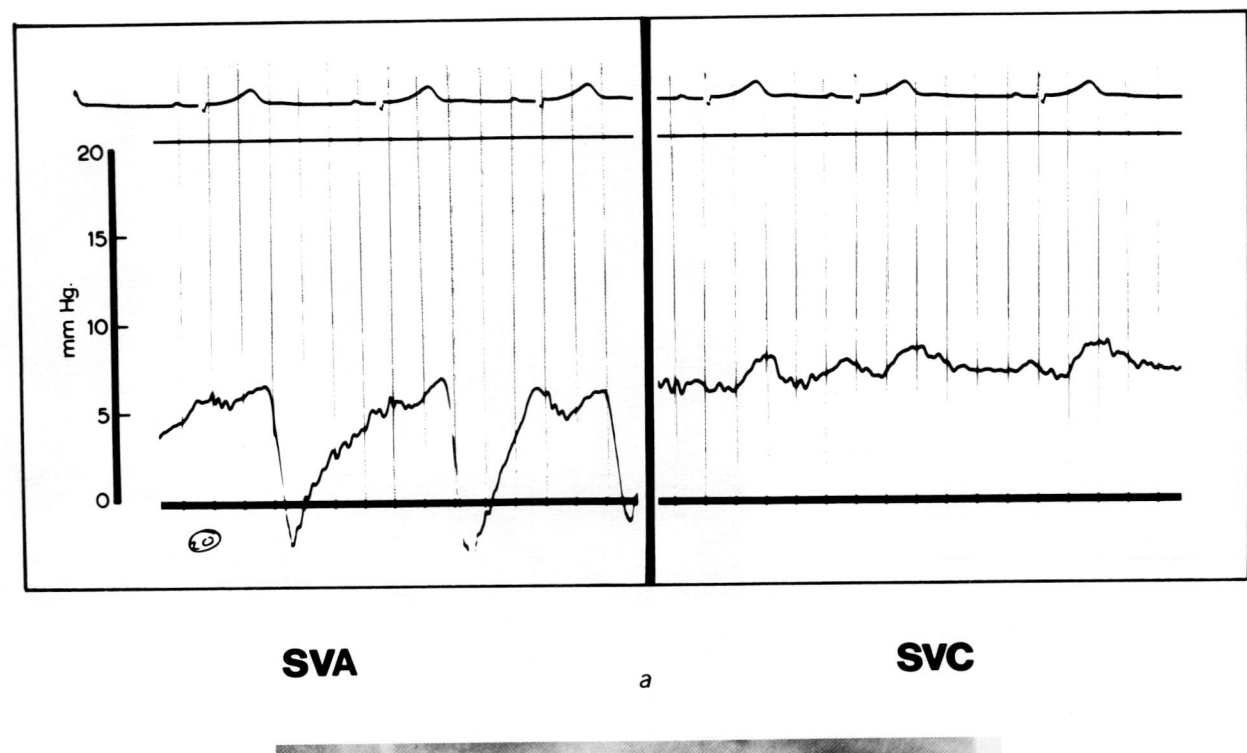

SVA   *a*   **SVC**

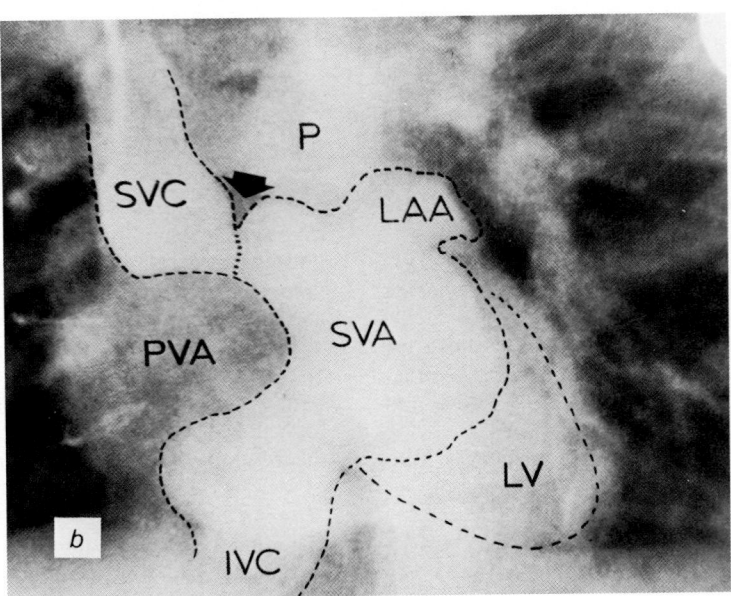

Figure 39-51 Data from postoperative cardiac catheterization in a patient who had undergone a Mustard-type atrial switch procedure and developed mild superior vena caval (SVC) obstruction (GLH).

(*a*) Phasic withdrawal pressures from systemic venous atrium (SVA) to SVC. Mean pressures were 4 and 7 mm, respectively.

(*b*) SVC cineangiogram in 20° left anterior oblique projection in the same patient. The site of restriction is arrowed. The dotted line crossing the upper venous channel marks the site of a faint radiolucent band representing continuation of the stenosing ridge profiled superiorly. Reflux shows a good caliber lower venous compartment.

IVC, inferior vena cava; LAA, left atrial appendage; LV, left ventricle; PVA, pulmonary venous atrium.

Reproduced with permission from Clarkson et al.,[C4] and the American Heart Association, Inc.

and right ventricular diastolic pressure. A gradient of >10 mmHg is certainly significant, although it is frequently higher than this.[D5] Pulmonary hypertension and usually an elevation of the calculated pulmonary vascular resistance are present. Normal pulmonary artery and left ventricular systolic pressures argue against significant stenosis. On cineangiography, narrowing of the PVA waist can be seen best in a lateral projection.[C4] Diagnosis is also possible using two-dimensional echocardiography.[C5,S17]

Treatment

Urgent reoperation is indicated (see "Technique of Operation").

Surgical Atrial Septectomy

Prior to the advent of balloon atrial septostomy (BAS) in 1966,[R1,R2] surgical atrial septectomy carried a high mortality, particularly in neonates with intact ventricular septum where it was needed most. In this early era, the mortality using open atrial septectomy with inflow stasis and mild hypothermia was 29% (GLH),[C3] at Boston Children's Hospital using inflow stasis under hyperbaric conditions 21%, and in institutions using the Blalock-Hanlon technique somewhat higher but variable.[D8,H7,V9] In some institutions, surgical atrial septectomy continues to be used in patients in whom BAS has failed, and since 1970 the hospital mortality of the procedure has been considerably lower. Currently (GLH, UAB), however, surgical atrial septectomy is essentially never done for patients with TGA, although it is still used on occasions for patients with certain types of univentricular atrioventricular connections, such as mitral atresia (see Chapter 44).

Palliative Mustard or Senning Operation

This operation is indicated when there is an elevation of pulmonary vascular resistance beyond about 10 units · m².[M24] It consists of an atrial switch procedure without closure of an existing VSD or of the creation of a VSD when one is not present. Alternatively, in the latter circumstances a Potts anastomosis can be considered,[L17] since it has the theoretical advantage that the right-to-left shunting occurs distal to the arch vessels and there is no danger of cerebral abscess or emboli. It remains to be shown, however, whether mixing through this is adequate, and it has not been used (GLH, UAB).

The hemodynamic consequences of a high pulmonary vascular resistance in TGA include a reduction in pulmonary blood flow and in intercirculatory mixing and thus increasing cyanosis and polycythemia (see "Pathophysiology" in section on Clinical Features and Diagnostic Criteria).[M14] Arterial oxygen saturation in TGA depends upon the relative proportions of systemic venous and pulmonary venous blood reaching the aorta and the saturation of the systemic venous blood. Thus, as pointed out by Mair and Ritter,[M14] if the total systemic flow is 6 l · min⁻¹ · m⁻² and the effective systemic flow (amount of pulmonary venous blood reaching the aorta) is 1.5 l · min⁻¹ · m⁻², the proportions of blood reaching the aorta are 1 part of fully saturated pulmonary venous blood to 3 parts of markedly desaturated systemic venous blood. After palliative atrial switch repair, the effective systemic flow is markedly increased, the ratio usually

changing from 1:3 to approximately 2:1. The decrease in the proportion of systemic venous blood entering the aorta is also influenced by the rise in systemic arteriolar resistance that follows the rise in arterial oxygen saturation, since the increase in systemic vascular resistance decreases the right-to-left shunting of systemic venous blood through the open VSD. Finally, the doubling of effective systemic flow results in a significant increase in systemic venous saturation despite the concomitant reduction in hemoglobin concentration. As a result of these complex interactions, there is an absolute increase in arterial oxygen saturation of approximately 20% in most patients following a palliative switch operation[M14]; the increase varies between 6%–48% (mean 24%) in the report by Byrne and colleagues.[B22] The only preoperative variable that correlated with the postoperative systemic arterial oxygen saturation was the pulmonary arteriovenous oxygen difference. Thus, a higher arteriovenous oxygen difference was associated with a higher postoperative arterial oxygen saturation.[B22]

The hospital mortality of this procedure has been surprisingly low. Thus, Lindesmith and colleagues report no deaths in 10 patients with a VSD[L18]; Byrne and colleagues report no deaths in 23 patients (20 with a VSD and 3 with an intact ventricular septum[B22]); and Bernhard and colleagues report 1 death among 8 patients.[B25] At GLH, 6 such procedures have been performed with 2 hospital deaths and at UAB (1977–1984) 3 with no deaths.

The intermediate term results are good, with no late deaths in the combined GLH and UAB group of hospital survivors, marked lessening of cyanosis, and improvement in exercise capacity. Occasionally (2 cases, UAB), pulmonary vascular resistance falls, and successful repair of the VSD is later possible.

Other Types of Arterial Switch Operations

The current surgical techniques (see "Arterial Switch Procedure" under "Technique of Operation") for the arterial switch operation have evolved from the original descriptions of Jatene and of Yacoub, in which a synthetic tube was used to aid in reconstruction of the neopulmonary artery. This is now rarely necessary.

An ingenious technique for arterial switching was described by Bex and colleagues[B29,B30] in which the subaortic conus is divided so that the whole aortic root, together with a muscular subvalvular rim and the coronary arteries, is switched to lie over the left ventricle. To provide maximal length to the neopulmonary artery, the pulmonary artery is transected through the pulmonary artery–ventricular junction, sacrificing the pulmonary valve leaflets. The pulmonary artery is then switched and anastomosed to the right ventricular outflow tract, often with the aid of a patch in the anterior portion of the suture line.

The Damus-Kaye-Stansel type of arterial switch procedure has also been used in patients with TGA and large VSD.[D3,D4,D12,K7,S6] In this operation, the main pulmonary artery is transected near its bifurcation and the proximal end anastomosed end to side to the ascending aorta. A valved extracardiac conduit is placed between the right ventricle and distal pulmonary artery. The VSD is closed. The right ventricular (pulmonary) systolic pressure falls to about 30 mmHg, and aortic pressure, which is above 100 mmHg, keeps the aortic valve closed. Some have recommended suturing the aortic valve closed. The mortality in this relatively simple and theoretically attractive operation has been considerable; Ceithaml and colleagues from the Mayo Clinic report 10 deaths (53%; CL 38%–66%) among 19 patients.[C8] However, if patients less than 1 year of age or those with severe pulmonary vascular disease or left ventricular systolic pressure less than two-thirds systemic are excluded, the hospital mortality consists of 1 patient (14%; CL 2%–41%) among 7. The patients have been clinically well after the repair. Thus, in complex situations in which the usual type of arterial switch operation seems to be contraindicated, this procedure can be considered. It is not recommended in simple TGA.

Two-stage Arterial Switch Operation for Simple Transposition of the Great Arteries and Intact Ventricular Septum

This procedure was introduced by Yacoub and colleagues[Y2] to prepare the left ventricle to withstand systemic pressure (produced after arterial switching) in infants with intact ventricular septum in whom the postnatal fall in pulmonary artery pressure has reduced left ventricular wall thickness (see "Morphology").

The first stage of the operation consisted of banding of the pulmonary artery; in about 15% of patients, a subsequent Blalock-Taussig shunt was required because of severe cyanosis.[B27] The arterial switch operation was performed as a second-stage procedure an average of 15 weeks later.

Bernhard, Yacoub and colleagues have reported 3 early deaths (9%, CL 4%–17%) among 33 patients undergoing the first stage operation and 5 early deaths (20%, CL 11%–32%) among 24 patients undergoing the second-stage arterial switch procedure.[B27] Thus, the overall mortality, beginning with the first-stage procedure and considering only the early deaths after the second stage, is 27%.

Although the postoperative assessment of surviving patients indicates a good hemodynamic state,[B27] with evidence of growth of the anastomoses, the overall mortality rate and the generally cumbersome nature of the approach suggest that it will give way to primary arterial switch operations in the first week of life in simple TGA.

APPENDIXES

APPENDIX **39A**
MULTIVARIATE ANALYSIS OF RISK FACTORS FOR DEATH AFTER ATRIAL SWITCH OPERATION (UAB)

Variables entered into the multivariate analysis in the hazard function domain of all deaths (early and late) after atrial switch operations for TGA (UAB; 1977–1984) are as follows:

Age at repair

Patent ductus arteriosus (yes/no)

Important pulmonary stenosis (yes/no)

Important VSD (yes/no)

Date of repair

APPENDIX **39B**
MULTIVARIATE ANALYSIS OF RISK FACTORS FOR DEATH AFTER ATRIAL SWITCH OPERATION (GLH)

Variables entered into the multivariate logistic regression analysis of hospital deaths in TGA (GLH; 1970–1984) following atrial switch repair are as follows:

Age at operation

Date of operation

Atrial septal defect creation (none, septostomy, repeat septostomy, septectomy)

Other palliation (Blalock-Taussig, Waterston, banding, ductus ligation, coarctation repair)

Atrial septal defect size at repair (none, small, moderate, large)

Ventricular septal defect size (small, moderate, large)

Additional ventricular septal defects (yes/no)

Left ventricular outflow tract obstruction (yes/no) and type (valve, fibrous, muscular)

Coarctation (yes/no)

Right ventricular size (moderate or severe hypoplasia; yes/no)

Urgency of operation (elective, NYHA class IV, semiurgent, urgent)

Type of operation (standard Mustard, V-Y Mustard, Senning)

Technique of cardiopulmonary bypass (standard/profound hypothermia; circulatory arrest)

Preoperative pulmonary vascular resistance (or lung histology) in patients ≥3 months of age

Early reoperation (for bleeding, baffle obstruction, baffle leak, infection)

Discharge ECG (sinus, junctional, complete heart block)

Patent ductus arteriosus (absent/small, moderate, large in various combinations)

Operation (baffle repair) ≤30 days of age (yes/no)

Early operation (repair or palliation) ≤30 days (yes/no)

Growth preop (normal, the third percentile, well below the third percentile, always below the third percentile but steady, always below the third percentile but declining and various combinations)

Additional variables considered in Cox's proportional hazard's model for late mortality in same data set are as follows:

Upper systemic venous compartment obstruction (none/mild, moderate, severe)

Lower systemic venous compartment obstruction (same criteria)

Pulmonary venous compartment obstruction (same criteria)

Baffle leak (same criteria)

Residual left ventricular outflow tract obstruction

Residual ventricular septal defect (yes/no)

MULTIVARIATE ANALYSIS OF RISK FACTORS FOR DEATH AFTER RASTELLI OPERATION (UAB)

Risk factors entered into the multivariate analysis of death, in the hazard function domain, after the Rastelli operation (UAB) are as follows:

Demographic: sex, age at operation, body surface area

Clinical: NYHA functional class, hematocrit

Morphology: juxtaposition of atrial appendages

Surgical: cardioplegia; aortic cross-clamp time in cardioplegic group; type of valved conduit; enlargement of VSD

REFERENCES

A

1. Abbott ME: Congenital cardiac diseases, in W Osler, T McCrae (eds): *Modern Medicine* (ed 3). Philadelphia: Lea & Febiger, 1927, Vol 4, Chap 21.

2. Albert HM: Surgical correction of transposition of the great vessels. *Surg Forum* 5:74, 1954.

3. Aberdeen E, Waterston DJ, Carr I, Graham G, Bonham-Carter RE, Subramanian S: Successful "correction" of transposed great arteries by Mustard's operation. *Lancet* 1:1233, 1965.

4. Abe T, Kuribayashi R, Sato M, Nieda S, Takahashi M, Okubo T: Successful Jatene operation for transposition of the great arteries with intact ventricular septum. A case report. *J Thorac Cardiovasc Surg* 75:64, 1978.

5. Anderson RH, Becker AE, Lucchese FE, Meier MA, Rigby ML, Soto B: *Morphology of Congenital Heart Disease.* Maryland: University Park Press, 1983, Chap 6.

6. Abrams HL, Kaplan HS, Purdy A: Diagnosis of complete transposition of the great vessels. *Radiology* 57:500, 1951.

7. Aziz KU, Paul MH, Idriss FS, Wilson AD, Muster AJ: Clinical manifestations of dynamic left ventricular outflow tract stenosis in infants with d-transposition of the great arteries with intact ventricular septum. *Am J Cardiol* 44:290, 1979.

8. Arcienegas E, Farooki ZQ, Hakimi M, Perry BL, Green EW: Results of the Mustard operation for dextro-transposition of the great arteries. *J Thorac Cardiovasc Surg* 81:580, 1981.

9. Aziz PU, Paul MH, Muster AJ: Echocardiographic assessment of left ventricular outflow tract in D-transposition of the great arteries. *Am J Cardiol* 41:543, 1978.

10. Aziz KU, Paul MH, Rowe RD: Bronchopulmonary circulation in d-transposition of the great arteries: Possible role in genesis of accelerated pulmonary vascular disease. *Am J Cardiol* 39:432, 1977.

11. Aberdeen E: Correction of uncomplicated cases of transposition of the great arteries. *Br Heart J* 33(suppl):66, 1971.

12. Aziz KU, Paul MH, Muster AJ, Idriss FS: Positional abnormalities of atrioventricular valves in transposition of the great arteries including double outlet right ventricle, atrioventricular valve straddling and malattachment. *Am J Cardiol* 44:1135, 1979.

13. Arensman FW, Bostock J, Radley-Smith R, Yacoub MH: Cardiac rhythm and conduction before and after anatomic correction of transposition of the great arteries. *Am J Cardiol* 52:836, 1983.

B

1. Baillie M: *The Morbid Anatomy of Some of the More Important Parts of the Human Body.* London: Johnson and Nichol, 1797, p 38.

2. Blalock A, Hanlon CR: The surgical treatment of complete transposition of the aorta and the pulmonary artery. *Surg Gynecol Obstet* 90:1, 1950.

3. Baffes TG: A new method for surgical correction of transposition of the aorta and pulmonary artery. *Surg Gynecol Obstet* 102:227, 1956.

4. Barnard CN, Schrire V, Beck W: Complete transposition of the great vessels: Successful complete correction. *J Thorac Cardiovasc Surg* 43:768, 1962.

5. Bonchek LI, Starr A: Total correction of transposition of the great arteries in infancy as initial surgical management. *Ann Thorac Surg* 14:376, 1972.

6. Berman MA, Taylor JF, Talner NS, Stansel HC Jr: Successful repair of pericardial patch stenosis after Mustard procedure. Diagnostic and therapeutic considerations in two patients. *J Thorac Cardiovasc Surg* 65:276, 1973.

7. Bailey CP, Cookson BA, Downing DF, Neptune WB: Cardiac surgery under hypothermia. *J Thorac Cardiovasc Surg* 28:229, 1954.

8. Bharati S, Lev M: The conduction system in simple, regular (D), complete transposition with ventricular septal defect. *J Thorac Cardiovasc Surg* 72:194, 1976.

9. Bass NM, Roche AHG, Brandt PWT, Neutze JM: Echocardiography in assessment of infants with complete d-transposition of great arteries. *Br Heart J* 40:1165, 1978.

10. Bierman FZ, Williams RG: Prospective diagnosis of D-transposition of the great arteries in neonates by subxiphoid two-dimensional echocardiography. *Circulation* 60:1496, 1979.

11. Bailey LL, Jacobson JG, Merritt WH, Doroshow RW, Petry EL: Mustard operation in the 1st month of life. *Am J Cardiol* 49:766, 1982.

12. Bender HW Jr, Graham TP Jr, Boncek RJ Jr, Walker WE, Boerth RC: Comparative operative results of the Senning and Mustard procedures for transposition of the great arteries. *Circulation* 61:(suppl II)II-2, 1980.

13. Berman MA, Barash PS, Hellenbrand WE, Stansel HC Jr, Talner NS: Late development of severe pulmonary venous obstruction following the Mustard operation. *Circulation* 56(suppl II):II-1191, 1977.

14. Barratt-Boyes BG, Simpson M, Neutze JM: Intracardiac surgery in neonates and infants using deep hypothermia with surface cooling and limited cardiopulmonary bypass. *Circulation* 43–44(suppl I):I-25, 1971.

15. Beitzke A, Suppan CH: Use of prostaglandin E₂ in management of transposition of great arteries before balloon atrial septostomy. *Br Heart J* 49:341, 1983.

16. Bharati S, Molthan WE, Veasy LG, Lev M: Conduction system in two cases of sudden death two years after the Mustard procedure. *J Thorac Cardiovasc Surg* 77:101, 1979.

17. Beerman LB, Neches WH, Fricker FJ, Mathews RA, Fischer DR, Park SC, Lenox CC, Zuberbuhler JR: Arrhythmias in transposition of the great arteries after the Mustard operation. *Am J Cardiol* 51:1530, 1983.

18. Benson LN, Bonet J, McLaughlin P, Olley PM, Feiglin D, Druck M, Trusler G, Rowe RD, Morch J: Assessment of right ventricular function during supine bicycle exercise after Mustard's operation. *Circulation* 65:1052, 1982.

19. Borow KM, Keane JF, Castaneda AR, Freed MD: Systemic ventricular function in patients with tetralogy of Fallot, ventricular septal defect and transposition of the great arteries repaired during infancy. *Circulation* 64:878, 1981.

20. Baker F, Baker L, Zoltun R, Zuberbuhler JR: Effectiveness of the Rashkind procedure in transposition of the great arteries in infants. *Circulation* 43(suppl I):I-1, 1971.

21. Berman W Jr, Whitman V, Pierce WS, Waldhausen JA: The development of pulmonary vascular obstructive disease after successful Mustard operation in early infancy. *Circulation* 58:181, 1978.

22. Byrne J, Clarke D, Taylor JF, Macartney FJ, de Leval M, Stark J: Treatment of patients with transposition of great arteries and pulmonary vascular obstructive disease. *Br Heart J* 40:221, 1978.

23. Bano-Rodrigo A, Quero-Jimenez M, Moreno-Granado F, Gamallo-Amat C: Wall thickness of ventricular chambers in transposition of the great arteries. *J Thorac Cardiovasc Surg* 79:592, 1980.

24. Barcio A, Kincaid OW, Davis GD, Kirklin JW, Ongley PA: Transposition of the great arteries. An angiocardiographic study. *Am J Roentgenol* C:249:1967.

25. Bernhard WF, Dick M, Sloss LJ, Castaneda AR, Nadas AS: The palliative mustard operation for double outlet right ventricle or transposition of the great arteries associated with ventricular septal defect, pulmonary arteries hypertension, and pulmonary vascular obstructive disease. A report of 8 patients. *Circulation* 54:810, 1976.

26. Bjornstad PG, Tjonneland S, Semb BKH: Echocardiographic evaluation of atrial function after Senning and Mustard correction for transposition of the great arteries. *Thorax* 39:114, 1984.

27. Bernhard A, Yacoub M, Regensburger D, Sievers HH, Smith RR, Stephan E, Lange PE, Keck EW, Heintzen PH: Further experience with the two-stage anatomic correction of simple transposition of the great arteries. *Thorac Cardiovasc Surg* 29:138, 1981.

28. Borow KM, Arensman FW, Webb C, Radley-Smith R, Yacoub M: Assessment of left ventricular contractile state after anatomic correction of transposition of the great arteries. *Circulation* 69:106, 1984.

29. Bex JP, Lecompte Y, Baillot F, Hazan E: Anatomical correction of transposition of the great arteries. *Ann Thorac Surg* 29:86, 1980.

30. Bex JP, Lecompte Y: New surgical approaches for complete correction of transposition of the great arteries. *Ped Cardiol* 4(suppl. 1):67, 1983.

31. Bical O, Hazan E, Lecompte Y, Fermont L, Karam J, Jarreau MM, Tran Viet T, Sidi D, Leca K, Neveux JY: Anatomic correction of transposition of the great arteries associated with ventricular septal defect: midterm results in 50 patients. *Circulation* 70:891, 1984.

32. Buchler JR, Bembon JC, Buchler RD: Transposition of the great arteries with posterior aorta and subaortic conus: anatomical and surgical correlation. *Int J Cardiol* 5:13, 1984.

C

1. Castaneda AR, Norwood WI, Lang P, Sanders SP: Transposition of the great arteries and intact ventricular septum: Anatomical repair in the neonate. *Ann Thorac Surg* 38:438, 1984.

2. Clarkson PM, Neutze JM, Wardill JC, Barratt-Boyes BG: The pulmonary vascular bed in patients with complete transposition of the great arteries. *Circulation* 53:539, 1976.

3. Clarkson PM, Barratt-Boyes BG, Neutze JM, Lowe JB: Results over a 10-year period of palliation followed by corrective surgery for complete transposition of the great arteries. *Circulation* 45:1251, 1972.

4. Clarkson PM, Neutze JM, Barratt-Boyes BG, Brandt PWT: Late postoperative hemodynamic results and cineangiocardiographic findings after Mustard atrial baffle repair for transposition of the great arteries. *Circulation* 53:525, 1976.

5. Chin AJ, Sanders SP, Williams RG, Lang P, Norwood WI, Castaneda AR: Two-dimensional echocardiographic assessment of caval and pulmonary venous pathways after the Senning operation. *Am J Cardiol* 52:118, 1983.

6. Crupi G, Anderson RH, Ho SY, Lincoln C: Complete transposition of the great arteries with intact ventricular septum and left ventricular outflow tract obstruction. Surgical management and anatomic considerations. *J Thorac Cardiovasc Surg* 78:730, 1979.

7. Clarkson PM, Barratt-Boyes BG, Neutze JM: Late dysrhythmias and disturbances of conduction following Mustard operation for complete transposition of the great arteries. *Circulation* 53:519, 1976.

8. Ceithaml EL, Puga FJ, Danielson GK, McGoon DC, Ritter DG: Results of the Damus-Stansel-Kaye procedure for transposition of the great arteries and for double-outlet right ventricle with subpulmonary ventricular septal defect. *Ann Thorac Surg* 38:433, 1984.

9. Clarkson PM: A study of 143,222 live births, Auckland, NZ (1971–1981) (1984) unpublished study.

10. Calder, L: (1984) Unpublished study.

11. Castaneda AR: (1984) Personal communication.

12. Chiu I, Anderson RH, Macartney FJ, de Leval MR, Stark J: Morphologic features of an intact ventricular septum susceptible to subpulmonary obstruction in complete transposition. *Am J Cardiol* 53:1633, 1984.

13. Cooley DA, Angelini P, Leachman RD, Kyger ER: Intraventricular repair of transposition complexes with ventricular septal defect. *J Thorac Cardiovasc Surg* 3:461, 1976.

14. Carbonera-Giani P: Wall thickness and chamber volume of right and left ventricles in transposition of the great arteries: An anatomic study. *Ped Cardiol* 4:9, 1983.

15. Chin AJ, Yeager SB, Sanders SP, Williams RG, Bierman FL, Burger BM, Norwood WI, Castaneda AR: Accuracy of two-dimensional echocardiographic evaluation of left ventricular outflow tract in complete transposition of the great arteries. *Am J Cardiol* 55:759, 1985.

16. Cobanoglu A, Abbruzzese PA, Freimanis I, Garcia CE, Grunkemeier G, Starr A: Pericardial baffle complications following the Mustard operation. Age-related incidence and ease of management. *J Thorac Cardiovasc Surg* 87:371, 1984.

17. Copeland JG, Emery RW, Marx GR, Allen HD: Evaluation of the vessel switch operation in infants with transposition of the great vessels. *JACC* 5:479, 1985 (abstr).

18. Coto EO, Jimenez MQ, Deverall PB, Bain H: Anomalous mitral 'cleft' with abnormal ventriculo-arterial connection: Anatomical findings and surgical implications. *Pediatr Cardiol* 5:1, 1984.

D

1. Dillard DH, Mohri H, Merendino KA, Morgan BC, Baum D, Crawford EW: Total surgical correction of transposition of the great arteries in children less than six months of age. *Surg Gynecol Obstet* 129:1258, 1969.

2. Daicoff GR, Schiebler GL, Elliott LP, Van Mierop LH, Bartley TD, Gessner IH, Wheat MW Jr: Surgical repair of complete transposition of the great arteries with pulmonary stenosis. *Ann Thorac Surg* 7:529, 1969.

3. Damus R: Correspondence. *Ann Thorac Surg* 20:724, 1975.

4. Damus PS, Thomson NB Jr, McLoughlin TG: Arterial repair without coronary relocation for complete transposition of the great vessels with ventricular septal defect. Report of a case. *J Thorac Cardiovasc Surg* 83:316, 1982.

5. Driscoll DJ, Nihill MR, Vargo TA, Mullins CE, McNamara DG: Late development of pulmonary venous obstruction following Mustard's operation using a dacron baffle. *Circulation* 55:484, 1977.

6. Driscoll DJ, Nihill MR, Cooley DA: Failure of pulmonary venous atrioplasty to relieve pulmonary venous obstruction following Mustard's operation. (1977) Personal communication.

7. Dickinson DF, Scott O: Ambulatory electrocardiographic monitoring in 100 healthy teenage boys. *Br Heart J* 51:179, 1984.

8. Deverall PB, Tynan MJ, Carr I, Panagopoulos P, Aberdeen E, Bonham-Carter RE, Waterston DJ: Palliative surgery in children with transposition of the great arteries. *J Thorac Cardiovasc Surg* 58:721, 1969.

9. Drakeley MJ: Case presentation: Transposition of the great arteries with elevated pulmonary vascular resistance, in BG Barratt-Boyes, JM Neutze, EA Harris (eds): *Heart Disease in Infancy*. Edinburgh: Churchill Livingstone, 1973, p 284.

10. DeLeon VH, Hougen TJ, Norwood WI, Lang P, Marx GR, Castaneda A: Results of the Senning operation for transposition of the great arteries with intact ventricular septum in neonates. *Circulation* 70(suppl I):I-21, 1984.

11. de la Riviere AB, Quaegebeur JM, Hennis PJ, de la Riviere GB, Huysmans HA, Brom AG: Growth of an aorto-coronary anastomosis: An experimental study in pigs. *J Thorac Cardiovasc Surg* 86:393, 1983.

12. Danielson GK, Tabry IF, Mair DD, Fulton RE: Great-vessel switch operation without coronary relocation for transposition of great arteries. *Mayo Clin Proc* 53:675, 1978.

13. Danford DA, Huhta JC, Gutgesell HP: Left ventricular wall stress and thickness in complete transposition of the great arteries. *J Thorac Cardiovasc Surg* 89:610, 1985.

E

1. Edwards WS, Bargeron LM, Lyons C: Reposition of right pulmonary vein in transposition of the great vessels. *JAMA* 188:522, 1964.

2. El-Said G, Rosenberg HS, Mullins CE, Hallman GL, Cooley DA, McNamara DG: Dysrhythmias after Mustard's operation for transposition of the great arteries. *Am J Cardiol* 30:526, 1972.

3. Elliott LP, Amplatz K, Edwards JE: Coronary arterial patterns in transposition complexes. Anatomic and angiocardiographic studies. *Am J Cardiol* 17:362, 1966.

4. Edwards WD, Edwards JE: Pathology of the sinus node in d-transposition following the Mustard operation. *J Thorac Cardiovasc Surg* 75:213, 1978.

5. El-Said GM, Gillette PC, Cooley DA, Mullins CE, McNamara DG: Protection of the sinus node in Mustard's operation. *Circulation* 53:788, 1976.

6. El-Said GM, Gillette PC, Mullins CE, Nihill MR, McNamara DG: Significance of pacemaker recovery time after the Mustard operation for transposition of the great arteries. *Am J Cardiol* 38:448, 1976.

7. Edwards WD, Edwards JE: Hypertensive pulmonary vascular disease in alpha-transposition of the great arteries. *Am J Cardiol* 41:921, 1978.

8. Egloff LP, Freed MD, Dick M, Norwood WI, Castaneda AR: Early and late results with the Mustard operation in infancy. *Ann Thorac Surg* 26:474, 1978.

F

1. Farre JR: Pathological researches. Essay 1: *On Malformation of the Human Heart*. London: Longman, Hurst, Rees, Orme, Brown, 1814, p 28.

2. Ferguson DJ, Adams P, Watson D: Pulmonary arteriosclerosis in transposition of the great vessels. *Am J Dis Child* 99:653, 1960.

3. Ferencz C: Transposition of the great vessels. Pathophysiologic considerations based upon a study of the lungs. *Circulation* 33:232, 1966.

4. Feder E, Meisner H, Buhlmeyer K, Struck E, Sebening F: Operative treatment of TGA: Comparison of Senning's and Mustard's operation in patients under 2 years of age. *Thorac Cardiovasc Surg* 28:7, 1980.

5. Fyler DC: Report of the New England regional infant cardiac program. *Pediatrics* 65:375, 1980.

6. Forenz C, Greco JM, Libi-Sylora M: Variability of pulmonary vascular disease in certain malformations of the heart, in BSL Kidd, JD Keith (eds): *The Natural History and Progressive Treatment of Congenital Heart Defects*. Springfield: Charles C. Thomas, 1971, p 300.

7. Ferencz C: Transposition of the great vessels. Pathophysiologic considerations based upon a study of the lungs. *Circulation* 33:232, 1966.

8. Flinn CJ, Wolff GS, Dick M, Campbell RM, Borkat G, Casta A, Hordof A, Hougen TJ, Kavey RE, Kugler J, Liebman J, Greenhouse J, Hees P: Cardiac rhythm after the Mustard operation for complete transposition of the great arteries. *N Engl J Med* 310:1635, 1984.

9. Fortune RL, Paquet M, Collins-Nakai RL, Duncan NF: Intracardiac repair of dextro-transposition of the great arteries in the newborn period. *J Thorac Cardiovasc Surg* 85:371, 1983.

G

1. Goor DA, Lillehei CW: In *Congenital Malformations of the Heart*. New York: Grune and Stratton, 1975, p 210.

2. Graham TP Jr, Atwood GF, Boucek RJ Jr, Boerth RC, Nelson JH: Right heart volume characteristics in transposition of the great arteries. *Circulation* 51:881, 1975.

3. Gutgesell HP, Garson A, McNamara DG: Prognosis for the newborn with transposition of the great arteries. *Am J Cardiol* 44:96, 1979.

4. Graham TP Jr: Hemodynamic residua and sequelae following interatrial repair of transposition of the great arteries. A review. *Pediatr Cardiol* 2:203, 1982.

5. Godman MJ, Friedli B, Pasternac A, Kidd BS, Trusler GA, Mustard WT: Hemodynamic studies in children four to ten years after the Mustard operation for transposition of the great arteries. *Circulation* 53:532, 1976.

6. Goor DA, Lillehei CW: In *Congenital Malformations of the Heart.* New York: Grune & Stratton, 1975, p 215.

7. Gillette PC, Kugler JD, Garson A Jr, Gutgesell HP, Duff DF, McNamara DG: Mechanisms of cardiac arrhythmias after the Mustard operation for transposition of the great arteries. *Am J Cardiol* 45:1225, 1980.

8. Gillette PC, El-Said GM, Sivarajan N, Mullins CE, Williams RL, McNamara DG: Electrophysiologic abnormalities after Mustard's operation for transposition of the great arteries. *Br Heart J* 36:186, 1974.

9. Graham TP Jr, Atwood GF, Boucek RJ Jr, Boerth RC, Bender HW Jr: Abnormalities of right ventricular function following Mustard's operation for transposition of the great arteries. *Circulation* 52:678, 1975.

10. Gittenberger-de Groot AC, Sauer U, Oppenheimer-Dekker A, Quaegebeur J: Coronary arterial anatomy in transposition of the great arteries: A morphologic study. *Ped Cardiol* 4:15, 1983.

H

1. Huhta JC, Edwards WD, Danielson GK, Feldt RH: Abnormalities of the tricuspid valve in complete transposition of the great arteries with ventricular septal defect. *J Thorac Cardiovasc Surg* 83:569, 1982.

2. Huhta JC, Edwards WD, Feldt RH, Puga FJ: Left ventricular wall thickness in complete transposition of the great arteries. *J Thorac Cardiovasc Surg* 84:97, 1982.

3. Hurwitz RA, Papanicolaou N, Treves S, Keane JF, Castaneda A: Radionuclide angiocardiography in evaluation of patients after repair of transposition of the great arteries. *Am J Cardiol* 49:761, 1982.

4. Hagler DJ, Ritter DG, Mair DD, Davis GD, McGoon DC: Clinical, angiographic, and hemodynamic assessment of late results after Mustard operation. *Circulation* 57:1214, 1978.

5. Hesslein PS, Gutgesell HP, Gillette PC, NcNamara DG: Exercise assessment of sinoatrial node function following the Mustard operation. *Am Heart J* 103:351, 1982.

6. Hagler DJ, Ritter DG, Mair DD, Tajik AJ, Seward JB, Fulton RE, Ritman EL: Right and left ventricular function after the Mustard procedure in transposition of the great arteries. *Am J Cardiol* 44:276, 1979.

7. Herrmann V, Laks H, Kaiser GC, Barner HB, Willman VL: The Blalock-Hanlon procedure. Simple transposition of the great arteries. *Arch Surg* 110:1387, 1975.

8. Hoffman JE: Diagnosis and treatment of pulmonary vascular disease. Birth defect: Original article series 8:9, 1972.

9. Henry CG, Goldring D, Hartmann AF, Weldon CS, Strauss AW: Treatment of d-transposition of the great arteries: Management of hypoxemia after balloon atrial septostomy. *Am J Cardiol* 47:299, 1981.

10. Hausdorf G, Gravinghoff L, Sieg K, Keck EW, Radley-Smith R, Yacoub MH: Left ventricular performance after anatomic correction of d-transposition of the great arteries. *JACC* 5:479, 1985.

I

1. Idriss FS, Goldstein IR, Grana L, French D, Potts WJ: A new technic for complete correction of transposition of the great vessels: An experimental study with a preliminary clinical report. *Circulation* 24:5, 1961.

2. Idriss FS, Aubert J, Paul M, Nikaidoh H, Lev M, Newfeld EA: Transposition of the great vessels with ventricular septal defect. Surgical and anatomic considerations. *J Thorac Cardiovasc Surg* 68:732, 1974.

3. Indeglia RA, Moller JH, Lucas RV Jr, Castaneda AR: Treatment of transposition of the great vessels with an intra-atrial baffle (Mustard procedure). *Arch Surg* 101:797, 1970.

4. Idriss FS, deLeon SY, Nikaidoh H, Muster AJ, Paul MA, Newfeld EA, Albers W: Resection of left ventricular outflow obstruction in d-transposition of the great arteries. *J Thorac Cardiovasc Surg* 74:343, 1977.

5. Idriss FS, Albanic MN, DeLeon SY, Berry TE, Muster AJ, Paul MH, Duffy CE: Transposition of the great arteries with intact ventricular septum: Arterial switches in the first month of life. *JACC* 5:477, 1985 (abstr).

J

1. Jatene AD, Fontes VF, Paulista PP, Souza LCB, Neger F, Galantier M, Sousa JE: Successful anatomic correction of transposition of the great vessels. A preliminary report. *Arg Braz Cardiol* 28:461, 1975.

2. Jatene AD, Fontes VF, Paulista PP, Souza LCB, Neger F, Galantier M, Sousa JE: Anatomic correction of transposition of the great vessels. *J Thorac Cardiovasc Surg* 72:364, 1976.

3. Jarmakani JM, Canent RV Jr: Preoperative and postoperative right ventricular function in children with transposition of the great vessels. *Circulation* 50(suppl II):II-39, 1974.

4. Janse MJ, Anderson RH: Specialized internodal atrial pathway: Fact or fiction. *Am J Cardiol* 2:117, 1974.

K

1. Kirklin JW, Devloo RA, Weidman WH: Open intra-cardiac repair for transposition of the great vessels: 11 cases. *Surgery* 50:58, 1961.

2. Kay EB, Cross FS: Surgical treatment of transposition of the great vessels. *Surgery* 38:712, 1955.

3. Keane JF, Ellison RC, Rudd M, Nadas AS: Pulmonary blood flow and left ventricular volumes in transposition of the great arteries and intact ventricular septum. *Br Heart J* 35:521, 1973.

4. Keith JD, Neill CA, Vlad P, Rowe RD, Chute AL: Transposition of the great vessels. *Circulation* 7:830, 1953.

5. Kidd BSL: The fate of children with transposition of the great arteries following balloon atrial septostomy, in BS Kidd, RD Rowe (eds): *The Child with Congenital Heart Disease after Surgery.* Mt. Kisco, NY: Futura Publishing, 1976.

6. Krueger SK, Burney DW, Ferlic RM: Protein-losing enteropathy complicating the Mustard procedure. *Surgery* 81:305, 1977.

7. Kaye MP: Anatomic correction of transposition of great arteries. *Mayo Clin Proc* 50:638, 1975.

8. Kron IL, Rheuban KS, Joob AW, Jedeiken R, Mentzer RM, Carpenter MA, Nolan SP: Baffle obstruction following the Mustard operation: Cause and treatment. *Ann Thorac Surg* 39:112, 1985.

L

1. Lillehei CW, Varco RL: Certain physiologic, pathologic and surgical features of complete transposition of the great vessels. *Surgery* 34:376, 1953.

2. Lindesmith GG, Stiles QR, Tucker BL, Gallaher ME, Stanton RE, Meyer BW: The mustard operation as a palliative procedure. *J Thorac Cardiovasc Surg* 63:75, 1972.

3. Lecompte Y, Zannini L, Hazan E, Jarreau MM, Bex JP, Tu TV, Neveus JY: Anatomic correction of transposition of the great arteries. *J Thorac Cardiovasc Surg* 82:629, 1981.

4. Lincoln C, Hasse J, Anderson RH, Shinebourne E: Surgical correction in complete levotransposition of the great arteries

with an unusual subaortic ventricular septal defect. *Am J Cardiol* 38:344, 1976.

5. Layman TE, Edwards JE: Anomalies of the cardiac valves associated with complete transposition of the great vessels. *Am J Cardiol* 19:247, 1967.

6. Liebman J, Cullum L, Belloc NB: Natural history of transposition of the great arteries. Anatomy and birth and death characteristics. *Circulation* 40:237, 1969.

7. Lakier JB, Stanger P, Heymann MA, Hoffman JI, Rudolph AM: Early onset of pulmonary vascular obstruction in patients with aortopulmonary transposition and intact ventricular septum. *Circulation* 51:875, 1975.

8. Levin DL, Paul MH, Muster AJ, Newfeld EA, Waldman JD: The clinical diagnosis of D-transposition of the great vessels in the neonate. *Arch Intern Med* 137:1421, 1977.

9. La Corte ME, Fellows KE, Williams RG: Over-riding tricuspid valve: Echocardiographic and angiographic features. *Am J Cardiol* 37:911, 1976.

10. Lock JE, Lucas RV Jr, Amplatz K, Bessinger FB Jr: Silent unilateral pulmonary venous obstruction. Occurrence after surgical correction of transposition of the great arteries. *Chest* 73:224, 1978.

11. Lang P, Freed MD, Bierman FZ, Norwood WI Jr, Nadas AS: Use of prostaglandin E$_1$ in infants with d-transposition of the great arteries and intact ventricular septum. *Am J Cardiol* 44:76, 1979.

12. Lewis AB, Lindesmith GG, Takahashi M, Stanton RE, Tucker BL, Stiles QR, Meyer BW: Cardiac rhythm following the Mustard procedure for transposition of the great vessels. *J Thorac Cardiovasc Surg* 73:919, 1977.

13. Litwin SB, Plauth WH Jr, Jones JE, Bernhard WF: Appraisal of surgical atrial septectomy for transposition of the great arteries. *Circulation* 43(suppl I):I-7, 1971.

14. Locatelli G, Benedetto GD, Villani M, Vanini V, Bianchi T, Parenzan L: Transposition of the great arteries. Successful Senning's operation in 35 consecutive patients. *J Thorac Cardiovasc Surg* 27:120, 1979.

15. Leanage R, Agnetti A, Graham G, Taylor J, Macartney FJ: Factors influencing survival after balloon atrial septostomy for complete transposition of the great arteries. *Br Heart J* 45:559, 1981.

16. Levy RJ, Rosenthal A, Castaneda AR, Nadas AS: Growth after surgical repair of simple D-transposition of the great arteries. *Ann Thorac Surg* 25:225, 1978.

17. Levinsky L, Srinivasan V, Gingell RL, Choh JH, Peironi DR, Fisher J, Subramanian S: Senning repair with ductal decompression: Palliative approach to d-TGA and irreversible pulmonary vascular disease. *Ann Heart J* 106:409, 1983.

18. Lindesmith GG, Stanton RE, Lurie PR, Takahashi M, Tucker BL, Stiles QR, Meyer BW: An assessment of Mustard's operation as a palliative procedure for transposition of the great vessels. *Ann Thorac Surg* 19:514, 1975.

M

1. Merendino EA, Jesseph JE, Herron PW, Thomas GI, Vetto RR: Interatrial venous transposition. A one-stage intracardiac operation for the conversion of complete transposition of the aorta and pulmonary artery to corrected transposition. *Surgery* 42:898, 1957.

2. Mustard WT: Successful two-stage correction of transposition of the great vessels. *Surgery* 55:469, 1964.

3. Mustard WT, Chute AL, Keith JD, Sivek A, Rowe RD, Vlad P:

A surgical approach to transposition of the great vessels with extracorporeal circuit. *Surgery* 36:39, 1954.

4. Mauck HP Jr, Robertson LW, Parr EL, Lower RR: Anatomic correction of transposition of the great arteries without significant ventricular septal defect or patent ductus arteriosus. *J Thorac Cardiovasc Surg* 74:631, 1977.

5. Moene RJ, Oppenheimer-Dekker A, Bartelings MM: Anatomic obstruction of the right ventricular outflow tract in transposition of the great arteries. *Am J Cardiol* 51:1701, 1983.

6. Milo S, Ho SY, Macartney FJ, Wilkinson JL, Becker AE, Wenink AC, Gittenberg de Groot A, Anderson RH: Straddling and over-riding atrioventricular valves: Morphology and classification. *Am J Cardiol* 44:1122, 1979.

7. Moene RJ, Oppenheimer-Dekker A: Congenital mitral valve anomalies in transposition of the great arteries. *Am J Cardiol* 49:1972, 1982.

8. Milanesi O, Thiene G, Bini RM, Pellegrino PA: Complete transposition of great arteries with coarctation of aorta. *Br Heart J* 48:566, 1982.

9. Mair DD: Effect of markedly elevated hematocrit level on blood viscosity and assessment of pulmonary vascular resistance. *J Thorac Cardiovasc Surg* 77:682, 1979.

10. Melhuish BP, Van Praagh R: Juxtaposition of the atrial appendages. A sign of severe cyanotic congenital heart disease. *Br Heart J* 30:269, 1968.

11. Muster AJ, Paul MH, Van Grondelle A, Conway JJ: Asymmetric distribution of the pulmonary blood flow between the right and left lungs in d-transposition of the great arteries. *Am J Cardiol* 38:352, 1976.

12. Miller RA: Complete transposition of the great arteries, in DP Morse (ed): *Congenital Heart Disease. Pathogenetic Factors, Natural History, Diagnosis, and Surgical Treatment.* Philadelphia: F. A. Davis, 1962, p 74.

13. Mair DD, Macartney FJ, Weidman WH, Ritter DG, Ongley PA, Smith RE: The vectorcardiogram in complete transposition of the great arteries: correlation with anatomic and hemodynamic findings and calculated left ventricular mass. *J Electrocardiol* 3:217, 1970.

14. Mair DD, Ritter DG: Factors influencing intercirculatory mixing in patients with complete transposition of the great arteries. *Am J Cardiol* 30:653, 1972.

15. Mair DD, Ritter DR, Ongley PA, Helmholz HF: Hemodynamics and evaluation for surgery of patients with complete transposition of the great arteries and ventricular septal defect. *Am J Cardiol* 28:632, 1971.

16. Moodie DS, Feldt RH, Wallace RB: Transient protein-losing enteropathy secondary to elevated caval pressures and caval obstruction after the Mustard procedure. *J Thorac Cardiovasc Surg* 72:379, 1976.

17. Mahony L, Turley K, Ebert P, Heymann MA: Long-term results after atrial repair of transposition of the great arteries in early infancy. *Circulation* 66:253, 1982.

18. Mazzei EA, Mulder DG: Superior vena cava syndrome following complete correction (Mustard repair) of transposition of the great vessels. *Ann Thorac Surg* 11:243, 1971.

19. Morgan JR, Miller BL, Daicoff GR, Andrews EJ: Hemodynamic and angiocardiographic evaluation after Mustard procedure for transposition of the great arteries. *J Thorac Cardiovasc Surg* 64:878, 1972.

20. Martin TC, Smith L, Hernandez A, Weldon CS: Dysrhythmias following the Senning operation for dextro-transposition of the great arteries. *J Thorac Cardiovasc Surg* 85:928, 1983.

21. Mathews RA, Fricker FJ, Beerman LB, Stephenson RJ, Fischer DR, Neches WH, Park SC, Lenox CC, Zuberbuhler JR: Exer-

cise studies after the Mustard operation in transposition of the great arteries. *Am J Cardiol* 52:1526, 1983.

22. Murphy JH, Barlai-Kovach MM, Mathews RA, Beerman LB, Park SC, Neches WH, Zuberbuhler JR: Rest and exercise right and left ventricular function late after the Mustard operation: Assessment by radionuclide ventriculography. *Am J Cardiol* 51:1520, 1983.

23. Mair DD, Danielson GK, Wallace RB, McGoon DC: Long-term follow-up of Mustard operation survivors. *Circulation* 50(suppl II):II-46, 1974.

24. Mair DD, Ritter DG, Danielson GK, Wallace RB, McGoon DC: The palliative Mustard operation: rationale and results. *Am J Cardiol* 37:762, 1976.

25. McGoon DC: Intraventricular repair of transposition of the great arteries. *J Thorac Cardiovasc Surg* 64:430, 1972.

26. Maroto E, Fouron JC, Douste-Blazy MY, Carceller AM, van Doesburg N, Kratz C, Davignon A: Influence of age on wall thickness, cavity dimensions and myocardial contractility of the left ventricle in simple transposition of the great arteries. *Circulation* 67:1311, 1983.

27. Marx GR, Hougen TJ, Norwood WI, Fyler DC, Castaneda AR, Nadas AS: Transposition of the great arteries with intact ventricular septum: Results of Mustard and Senning operations in 123 consecutive patients. *JACC* 2:476, 1983.

N

1. Newfeld EA, Paul MM, Muster AJ, Idriss FS: Pulmonary vascular disease in complete transposition of the great arteries: A study of 200 patients. *Am J Cardiol* 34:75, 1974.

2. Nogrady MB, Dunbar JS: Complete transposition of the great vessels; re-evaluation of the so-called "typical configuration" on plain films of the chest. *J Can Assoc Radiol* 20:124, 1969.

3. Newfeld EA, Paul MH, Muster AJ, Idriss FS: Pulmonary vascular disease in transposition of the great vessels and intact ventricular septum. *Circulation* 59:525, 1979.

4. Nanda NC, Gramiak R, Manning JA, Lipchik EO: Echocardiographic features of subpulmonic obstruction in dextro-position of the great vessels. *Circulation* 51:515, 1975.

5. Neutze JM: Transposition of the great arteries in infancy. *NZ Med J* 64(suppl):13, 1965.

6. Newburger JW, Silbert AR, Buckley LP, Tyler DC: Cognitive function and age at repair of transposition of the great arteries in children. *New Engl J Med* 310:1495, 1984.

O

1. Oelert H, Stegmann Th, Leitz KH, Luhmer I, Reichelt W, Borst HG: Transposition of the great arteries, ventricular septal defect, and left ventricular outflow obstruction: Results of conservative correction. *Thorac Cardiovasc Surg* 27:219, 1979.

2. Oelert H, Borst HG: Transmitral resection of subpulmonary stenosis in transposition of the great arteries. *Thorac Cardiovasc Surg* 27:58, 1979.

3. Okuda H, Nakazawa M, Imai Y, Kurosawa H, Takanashi Y, Hoshino S, Takao A: Comparison of ventricular function after Senning and Jatene procedures for complete transposition of the great arteries. *Am J Cardiol* 55:530, 1985.

P

1. Park SC, Zuberbuhler JR, Neches WH, Lenox CC, Zoltan RA: A new atrial septostomy technique. *Cathet Cardiovasc Diagn* 1:195, 1975.

2. Plauth WH Jr, Nadas AS, Bernhard WF, Fyler DC: Changing hemodynamics in patients with transposition of the great arteries. *Circulation* 42:131, 1970.

3. Phornphutkul C, Rosenthal A, Nadas AS: Cerebrovascular accidents in infants and children with cyanotic congenital heart disease. *Am J Cardiol* 32:329, 1973.

4. Paul MH: Transposition of the great arteries, in FH Adams, GC Emmanouilides (eds): *Heart Disease in Infants, Children and Adolescents* (ed 3). Baltimore: Williams and Wilkins, 1983, chap 21.

5. Parr GV, Blackstone EH, Kirklin JW, Pacifico AD, Lauridsen P: Cardiac performance early after interatrial transposition of venous return in infants and small children. *Circulation* 50(suppl II):II-2, 1974.

6. Park SC, Neches WH, Mathews RA, Fricker FJ, Beerman LB, Fischer DR, Lenox CC, Zuberbuhler JR: Hemodynamic function after the Mustard operation for transposition of the great arteries. *Am J Cardiol* 51:1514, 1983.

7. Parenzan L, Locatelli G, Alfieri O, Villani M, Invernizzi G: The Senning operation for transposition of the great arteries. *J Thorac Cardiovasc Surg* 76:305, 1978.

8. Park SC, Weiss FH, Siewers RD, Neches WH, Zuberbuhler JR, Lennox CC: Continuous murmur following Mustard operation for transposition of the great arteries. A sign of pulmonary venous obstruction. *Circulation* 54:684, 1976.

9. Penkoske PA, Westerman GR, Marx GR, Rabinovitch M, Freed MD, Norwood WI, Castaneda AR: Transposition of the great arteries and ventricular septal defect: results with the Senning operation and closure of the ventricular septal defect in infants. *Ann Thorac Surg* 36:281, 1983.

10. Parrish MD, Graham TP Jr, Bender HW, Jones JP, Patton J, Partain CL: Radionuclide angiographic evaluation of right and left ventricular function during exercise after repair of transposition of the great arteries. Comparison with normal subjects and patients with congenitally corrected transposition. *Circulation* 67:178, 1983.

11. Parsons CG, Astley R, Burrows FG, Singh SP: Transposition of great arteries. A study of 65 infants followed for 1 to 4 years after balloon septostomy. *Br Heart J* 33:725, 1971.

12. Pacifico AD, Stewart RW, Bargeron LM Jr: Repair of transposition of the great arteries with ventricular septal defect by an arterial switch operation. *Circulation* 68 (suppl II)II-49, 1983.

13. Pitlick P, French J, Guthaner D, Shumway N, Baum D: Results of intraventricular baffle procedure for ventricular septal defect and double outlet right ventricle or d-transposition of the great arteries. *Am J Cardiol* 47:307, 1981.

14. Powell TG, Dewey M, West CR, Arnold R: Fate of infants with transposition of the great arteries in relation to balloon atrial septostomy. *Br Heart J* 51:371, 1984.

Q

1. Quaegebeur JM, Rohmer J, Brom AG: Revival of the Senning operation in the treatment of transposition of the great arteries. Preliminary report on recent experience. *Thorax* 32:517, 1977.

2. Quaegebeur JM, Brom AG: The trouser-shaped baffle for use in the Mustard operation. *Ann Thorac Surg* 25:240, 1978.

3. Quaegebeur JM: (1985) Personal communication.

R

1. Rashkind WJ, Miller WW: Creation of an atrial septal defect without thoracotomy: A palliative approach to complete transposition of the great arteries. *JAMA* 196:991, 1966.

2. Rashkind WJ, Miller WW: Transposition of the great arteries. Results of palliation by balloon atrioseptostomy in thirty-one infants. *Circulation* 38:453, 1968.

3. Rastelli GC, Wallace RB, Ongley PA: Complete repair of transposition of the great arteries with pulmonary stenosis. A review and report of a case corrected by using a new surgical technique. *Circulation* 39:83, 1969.

4. Rastelli GC: A new approach to "anatomic" repair of transposition of the great arteries. *Mayo Clin Proc* 44:1, 1969.

5. Ramsay JM, Venables AW, Kelly MJ, Kalff V: Right and left ventricular function at rest and with exercise after the Mustard operation for transposition of the great arteries. *Br Heart J* 51:364, 1984.

6. Rowlatt UF: Coronary artery distribution in complete transposition. *JAMA* 179:269, 1962.

7. Rosenquist GC, Stark J, Taylor JF: Congenital mitral valve disease in transposition of the great arteries. *Circulation* 51:731, 1975.

8. Riemenschneider TA, Goldberg SJ, Ruttenberg HD, Gyepes MT: Subpulmonic obstruction in complete (d) transposition produced by redundant tricuspid tissue. *Circulation* 39:603, 1969.

9. Riemenschneider TA, Vincent WR, Ruttenberg HD, Desilets DT: Transposition of the great vessels with hypoplasia of the right ventricle. *Circulation* 38:386, 1968.

10. Rabinovitch M, Rosenthal A, Sade RM, Castaneda AR, Treves S, Nadas AS: Regional lung function studies and radionuclide angiography in D-transposition of the great arteries: *Pediatr Res* 11:1117, 1977.

11. Riggs TW, Muster AJ, Aziz KU, Paul MH, Ilbawi M, Idriss FS: Two-dimensional echocardiographic and angiocardiographic diagnosis of subpulmonary stenosis due to tricuspid valve pouch in complete transposition of the great arteries. *JACC* 1:484, 1983.

12. Rosman NP, Shands KN: Hydrocephalus caused by increased intracranial venous pressure: A clinicopathologic study. *Ann Neurol* 3:445, 1978.

13. Radley-Smith R, Yacoub MH: One stage anatomic correction of simple complete transposition of the great arteries in neonates. *Br Heart J* 51:685, 1984.

14. Reul GJ, Cooley DA, Sandiford FM, Hallman GL: Complications following the contoured dacron baffle in correction of transposition of the great arteries. *Surgery* 76:946, 1974.

15. Rashkind WJ: The complications of balloon atrioseptostomy. *J Pediatr* 76:649, 1970.

16. Rosengart R, Fishbein M, Emmanouilides GC: Progressive pulmonary vascular disease after surgical correction (Mustard procedure) of transposition of the great arteries with intact ventricular septum. *Am J Cardiol* 35:107, 1975.

17. Rashkind WJ: Balloon atrioseptostomy. *Adv Cardiol* 11:2, 1974.

S

1. Senning A: Surgical correction of transposition of the great vessels. *Surgery* 45:966, 1959.

2. Schumaker HB Jr: A new operation for transposition of the great vessels. *Surgery* 50:773, 1961.

3. Senning A: Surgical correction of transposition of the great vessels. *Surgery* 59:334, 1966.

4. Subramanian S, Wagner H: Correction of transposition of the great arteries in infants under surface-induced deep hypothermia. *Ann Thorac Surg* 16:391, 1973.

5. Stark J, Silove ED, Taylor JF, Graham GR: Obstruction to

systemic venous return following the Mustard operation for transposition of the great arteries. *J Thorac Cardiovasc Surg* 68:742, 1974.

6. Stansel HC Jr: A new operation for d-loop transposition of the great vessels. *Ann Thorac Surg* 19:565, 1975.

7. Shrivastava S, Tadavarthy SM, Fukuda T, Edwards JE: Anatomic causes of pulmonary stenosis in complete transposition. *Circulation* 54:154, 1976.

8. Schneeweiss A, Motro M, Shem-Tov A, Neufeld HN: Subaortic stenosis: An unrecognized problem in transposition of the great arteries. *Am J Cardiol* 48:336, 1981.

9. Shaher RM, Puddu GC, Khoury G, Moes CA, Mustard WT: Complete transposition of the great vessels with anatomic obstruction of the outflow tract of the left ventricle. Surgical implications of anatomic findings. *Am J Cardiol* 19:658, 1967.

10. Sansa M, Tonkin IL, Bargeron LM Jr, Elliott LP: Left ventricular outflow tract obstruction in transposition of the great arteries: An angiographic study of 74 cases. *Am J Cardiol* 44:88, 1979.

11. Smith A, Wilkinson JL, Arnold R, Dickinson DF, Anderson RH: Growth and development of ventricular walls in complete transposition of the great arteries with intact septum (simple transposition). *Am J Cardiol* 49:362, 1982.

12. Sapsford RN, Aberdeen E, Watson DA, Crew AD: Transposed great arteries combined with totally anomalous pulmonary veins. A report of a successful correction. *J Thorac Cardiovasc Surg* 63:360, 1972.

13. Shaher RM, Fowler RS, Kidd BS, Moes CA, Keith JD: Spontaneous closure of a ventricular septal defect in a case of complete transposition of the great vessels. *Can Med Assoc J* 93:1037, 1965.

14. Silverman NH, Snider AR, Colo J, Ebert PA, Turley K: Superior venal obstruction after Mustard's operation: detection by two-dimensional contrast echocardiography. *Circulation* 64:392, 1981.

15. Silove ED, Taylor JF: Haemodynamics after Mustard's operation for transposition of the great arteries. *Br Heart J* 38:1037, 1976.

16. Sweeney MF, Bell WE, Doty DB, Schieken RM: Communicating hydrocephalus secondary to venous complications following intra-atrial baffle operation (Mustard procedure) for d-transposition of the great arteries. *Pediatr Cardiol* 3:237, 1982.

17. Satomi G, Nakamura K, Takao A, Imai Y: Two-dimensional echocardiographic detection of pulmonary venous channel stenosis after Senning's operation. *Circulation* 68:545, 1983.

18. Szarnicki RJ, Stark J, de Leval M: Reoperation for complications after inflow correction of transposition of the great arteries: Technical considerations. *Ann Thorac Surg* 25:150, 1978.

19. Sunderland CO, Henken DP, Nichols GM, Dhindsa DS, Bonchek LI, Menashe VD, Rahimtoola SH, Starr A, Lees MH: Postoperative hemodynamic and electrophysiologic evaluation of the interatrial baffle procedure. *Am J Cardiol* 35:660, 1975.

20. Stevenson JG, Kawabori I, Guntheroth WG, Dooley TK, Dillard D: Pulsed Doppler echocardiographic detection of obstruction of systemic venous return after repair of transposition of the great arteries. *Circulation* 60:1091, 1979.

21. Southall DP, Johnston F, Shinebourne EA, Johnston PGB: 24-hour electrocardiographic study of heart rate and rhythm patterns in population of healthy children. *Br Heart J* 45:281, 1981.

22. Scott O, Williams GJ, Fiddler GI: Results of 24-hour ambulatory monitoring of electrocardiogram in 131 healthy boys aged 10 to 13 years. *Br Heart J* 44:304, 1980.

23. Southall DP, Keeton BR, Leanage R, Lam L, Joseph MC, Anderson RH, Lincoln CR, Shinebourne EA: Cardiac rhythm and conduction before and after Mustard's operation for complete transposition of the great arteries. *Br Heart J* 43:21, 1980.

24. Streeter DD Jr, Spotitz HM, Patel D, Ross J Jr, Sonnenblick EH: Fiber orientation in the canine left ventricle during diastole and systole. *Circ Res* 24:339, 1969.

25. Stark J, de Leval MR, Taylor JF: Mustard operation and creation of ventricular septal defect in two patients with transposition of the great arteries, intact ventricular septum and pulmonary vascular disease. *Am J Cardiol* 38:524, 1976.

26. Stark J, Weller P, Leanage R, Cunningham K, de Leval M, Macartney F, Taylor JFN: Late results of surgical treatment of transposition of the great arteries. *Adv Cardiol* 27:254, 1980.

27. Singh AK, Stark J, Taylor JF: Left ventricle to pulmonary artery conduit in treatment of transposition of great arteries, restrictive ventricular septal defect and acquired pulmonary atresia. *Br Heart J* 38:1213, 1976.

28. Shaher RM, Puddu CG: Coronary artery arterial anatomy in complete transposition of the great vessels. *Am J Cardiol* 17:355, 1966.

T

1. Taussig HB, Bing RJ: Complete transposition of aorta and levoposition of pulmonary artery. *Am Heart J* 37:551, 1949.

2. Tynan M: Survival of infants with transposition of great arteries after balloon atrial septostomy. *Lancet* 1:621, 1971.

3. Tonkin IL, Sansa M, Elliott LP, Bargeron LM Jr: Recognition of developing left ventricular outflow tract obstruction in complete transposition of the great arteries. *Radiology* 134:53, 1980.

4. Takahashi M, Lindesmith GG, Lewis AB, Stiles QR, Stanton RE, Meyer BW, Lurie PR: Long-term results of the Mustard procedure. *Circulation* 56(suppl II):II-11, 1977.

5. Tynan M, Aberdeen E, Stark J: Tricuspid incompetence after the Mustard operation for transposition of the great arteries. *Circulation* 45(suppl I):I-1, 1972.

6. Trusler GA, Williams WG, Izukawa T, Olley PM: Current results with the Mustard operation in isolated transposition of the great arteries. *J Thorac Cardiovasc Surg* 80:381, 1980.

7. Turley K, Ebert PA: Total correction of transposition of the great arteries. Conduction disturbances in infants younger than three months of age. *J Thorac Cardiovasc Surg* 76:312, 1978.

8. Trusler GA, Bull RC, Hoeksema F, Mustard WT: The effect on cardiac output of a reduction in atrial volume. *J Thorac Cardiovasc Surg* 46:109, 1963.

9. Taussig HB: Complete transposition of the great vessels; clinical and pathologic features. *Am Heart J* 16:728, 1938.

U

1. Urban AE, Stark J, Waterston DJ: Mustard's operation for transposition of the great arteries complicated by juxtaposition of the atrial appendages. *Ann Thorac Surg* 21:304, 1976.

2. Ullal RR, Anderson RH, Lincoln C: Mustard's operation modified to avoid dysrhythmias and pulmonary and systemic venous obstruction. *J Thorac Cardiovasc Surg* 78:431, 1979.

V

1. Van Praagh R, Perez-Trevino C, Lopez-Cuellar M, Baker FW, Zuberbuhler JR, Quero M, Perez VM, Moreno F, Van Praagh S: Transposition of the great arteries with posterior aorta, anterior pulmonary artery, subpulmonary conus and fibrous continuity between aortic and atrioventricular valves. *Am J Cardiol* 28:621, 1971.

2. Van Praagh R, Weinberg PM, Calder L, Buckley LF, Van Praagh S: The transposition complexes: how many are there? in JC Davila (ed): *Second Henry Ford Hospital International Symposium on Cardiac Surgery*. New York: Appleton-Century-Crofts 1977, chap 35.

3. Van Praagh R: What is the Taussig-Bing malformation? *Circulation* 38:445, 1968.

4. Vidne BA, Subramanian S, Wagner HR: Aneurysm of the membranous ventricular septum in transposition of the great arteries. *Circulation* 53:157, 1976.

5. Van Gils FA, Moulaert AJ, Oppenheimer-Dekker A, Wenink CG: Transposition of the great arteries with ventricular septal defect and pulmonary stenosis. *Br Heart J* 40:494, 1978.

6. Van Doesburg NH, Bierman FZ, Williams RG: Left ventricular geometry in infants with d-transposition of the great arteries and intact interventricular septum. *Circulation* 68:733, 1983.

7. Vidne BA, Duszynski D, Subramanian S: Pulmonary blood flow distribution in transposition of the great arteries. *Am J Cardiol* 38:62, 1976.

8. Venables AW, Edis B, Clarke CP: Vena caval obstruction complicating the Mustard operation for complete transposition of the great arteries. *Eur J Cardiol* 1:401, 1974.

9. Venables AW: Complete transposition of the great vessels in infancy with reference to palliative surgery. *Br Heart J* 28:335, 1966.

10. Viles PH, Ongley PA, Titus JL: The spectrum of pulmonary vascular disease in transposition of the great arteries. *Circulation* 40:31, 1969.

11. Villagra F, Quero-Jimenez M, Maitre-Azcarate MJ, Guitierrez J, Brito JM: Transposition of the great arteries with ventricular septal defects. Surgical considerations concerning the Rastelli operation. *J Thorac Cardiovasc Surg* 88:1004, 1984.

W

1. Wilkinson JL, Arnold R, Anderson RH, Acerete F: "Posterior" transposition reconsidered. *Br Heart J* 37:757, 1975.

2. Waldman JD, Paul MH, Newfeld EA, Muster AJ, Idriss FS: Transposition of the great arteries with intact ventricular septum and patent ductus arteriosus. *Am J Cardiol* 39:232, 1977.

3. Wood AE, Freedom RM, Williams WG, Trusler GA: The Mustard procedure in transposition of the great arteries associated with juxtaposition of the atrial appendages with and without dextrocardia. *J Thorac Cardiovasc Surg* 84:451, 1983.

4. Wyse RK, Haworth SG, Taylor JF, Macartney FJ: Obstruction of superior vena caval pathway after Mustard's repair. Reliable diagnosis by transcutaneous Doppler ultrasound. *Br Heart J* 42:162, 1979.

5. Wilcox BR, Henry GW, Anderson RH: The transmitral approach to left ventricular outflow tract obstruction. *Ann Thorac Surg* 35:288, 1983.

6. Wittig JH, Stark J: Intraoperative mapping of atrial activation before, during and after the Mustard operation. *J Thorac Cardiovasc Surg* 73:1, 1977.

7. Wagenvoort CA, Nauta J, Schaar PJ van der, Weeda HW, Wagenvoort N: The pulmonary vasculature in complete transposition of the great vessels, judged from lung biopsies. *Circulation* 38:746, 1968.

8. Wyse RK, Macartney FJ, Rohmer J, Ottenkamp J, Brom AG, Wyse RK: Differential atrial filling after Mustard and Senning

repairs. Detection by transcutaneous Doppler ultrasound. *Br Heart J* 44:692, 1980.

9. Wilson HE, Nafrawi AG, Cardozo RH, Aguillon A: Rational approach to surgery for complete transposition of the great vessels: Analysis of the basic hemodynamics and critical appraisal of previously proposed corrective procedures with a suggested approach based on laboratory and clinical studies. *Ann Surg* 155:258, 1962.

Y

1. Yacoub MH, Radley-Smith R, Hilton CJ: Anatomical correction of complete transposition of the great arteries and ventricular septal defect in infancy. *Br Med J* 1:1112, 1976.

2. Yacoub MH, Radley-Smith R, Maclaurin R: Two-stage operation for anatomical correction of transposition of the great arteries with intact ventricular septum. *Lancet* 1:1275, 1977.

3. Yacoub MH, Radley-Smith R: Anatomy of the coronary arteries in transposition of the great arteries and methods for their transfer in anatomical correction. *Thorax* 33:418, 1978.

4. Yacoub MH, Arensman FW, Keck E, Radley-Smith R: Fate of dynamic left ventricular outflow tract obstruction after anatomic correction of transposition of the great arteries. *Circulation* 68 (suppl II):II-11, 1983.

5. Yamaki S, Tezuka F: Quantitative analysis of pulmonary vascular disease in complete transposition of the great arteries. *Circulation* 54:805, 1976.

Z

1. Zuberbuhler JR, Bauersfeld SR: Unusual arrhythmias after corrective surgery for transposition of the great vessels. *Am Heart J* 73:752, 1967.

40

DOUBLE OUTLET RIGHT VENTRICLE

DEFINITION

Double outlet right ventricle (DORV) is a congenital cardiac anomaly in which both great arteries arise wholly or in large part from the right ventricle.[1] It is, then, a type of ven-

triculoarterial connection (see Chapter 1, "Cardiac Connections" in section on Terminology and Classification of Heart Disease).

In this chapter, DORV with atrioventricular (AV) concordant connection is discussed in detail. It can be held that DORV is a basic entity (Fig. 40-1) and that patients with AV discordant connection should be considered along with those with AV concordant connection (GLH); thus they are included in some tables in this chapter (GLH). Alternatively, it

---

[1] The adjectives left and right used to modify atrium or ventricle always mean morphologic left and morphologic right, respectively. The position of the chamber is referred to as right sided or left sided.

DOUBLE OUTLET RIGHT VENTRICLE

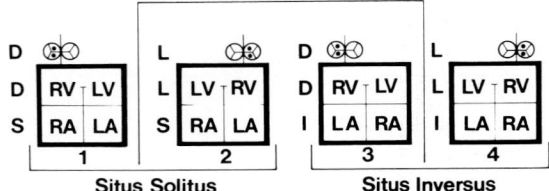

Figure 40-1 Model of the four basic hearts as they occur in DORV, with the usual great vessel positions (aorta lateral to pulmonary artery) (GLH). Models 2 and 3 show AV discordance. The Van Praagh symbolic convention is used (see Chapter 1, "Symbolic Convention of Van Praagh," in section on Terminology and Classification of Heart Disease).

LA, left atrium; LV, left ventricle; RA, right atrium; RV, right ventricle.

can be held that when the AV connection is discordant, it becomes the surgically more important feature of the malformation (UAB) and that patients with this combination are better considered along with others with AV discordant connection. (A detailed discussion of this matter, and the UAB data concerned with it, are presented in Chapter 43.) There are precedents for both points of view.

DORV may also occur in patients with univentricular AV connections (see Chapter 44). It is frequent in patients with atrial isomerism (UAB cases with atrial isomerism are included in Chapter 46).

One or both great arteries may overlie the ventricular septal defect (VSD) in hearts with DORV. When one great artery arises biventricularly, it is assigned to the ventricle that by morphologic examination it overlies by more than 50%; thus when one great artery arises wholly or nearly so from the right ventricle and the other more than 50% from it, the condition is termed *DORV*. Rarely, both great arteries arise biventricularly in association with a doubly committed VSD. One convention is arbitrarily to assign each great artery to the ventricle above which more than 50% arises and categorize the condition accordingly (UAB); the alternative method, and probably a preferable one, is to term the malformation *double outlet both ventricles* (GLH).

Within this scheme, a few additional rules may be used (UAB). (1) The tetralogy of Fallot is an entity with a variable amount of dextroposition of the aorta. Cases in which the aorta arises more than 50% from the right ventricle are kept in the category of tetralogy of Fallot unless on morphologic examination the aorta arises nearly wholly (90% or more) from the right ventricle, in which case they are categorized as DORV with pulmonary stenosis (UAB). Alternatively (GLH), such cases in which the aorta arises more than 50% from the right ventricle may be considered DORV (see Chapter 23, "Definitions"). Edwards uses still different criteria for distinguishing between these two conditions.[E5] (2) The Taussig-Bing heart (see below for description) is an entity with variability in the origin of the pulmonary artery. This diagnosis may be made when the pulmonary artery arises wholly or nearly so from the right ventricle, equally from the right and left ventricle, or more than 50% but not

more than 90% from the left ventricle (LV) (UAB). When it arises more than 90% from the LV, the categorization is to "transposition of the great arteries with ventricular septal defect (VSD)." Alternatively, when in this situation the pulmonary artery arises more than 50% from the left ventricle, the diagnosis can be transposition of the great arteries with VSD (GLH).

HISTORICAL NOTE

When the first repair of DORV (which was of the simple type, with a subaortic VSD) was performed in May 1957 by us at the Mayo Clinic,[K2] the entity was virtually unknown and the preoperative diagnosis was large VSD with a high pulmonary blood flow. The diagnosis was correctly made at operation, the term *double outlet right ventricle* or *origin of both great vessels from the right ventricle* was coined in the operating room, the position of the His bundle deduced, and an intraventricular tunnel repair performed in much the same manner as is done today.[K2] An identical sequence occurred at GLH in September 1958.[B11] Earlier, in 1952, Braun and colleagues reported what is clearly a case of DORV with pulmonary stenosis and used the phrase *double outlet ventricle*, but the title of the paper was confusing and it escaped notice.[B5] At about the time of the first repair, the first morphologic paper with the title "Double Outlet Right Ventricle" was published by Witham,[W3] and subsequently other early descriptions of the morphology appeared.[C1,E1,E2,N1,N2] Redo, Engle, and colleagues, in 1963, also reported repair of this entity.[R1]

The Taussig-Bing heart was described in 1949,[T1] but its place in the spectrum of DORV was recognized only later.[H4,N3,V2] Many early papers understandably referred to it under "transposition."[A5,B7,C4] Lev and colleagues recognized it as a form of DORV in which the VSD was subpulmonary.[L1] They and earlier workers did not clearly state, however, that the Taussig-Bing heart is different from the heart with classical DORV with subaortic VSD, not only as regards the relationships of the VSD, but also as regards the position and interrelations of the great arteries[A3] and the position of the infundibular (outlet) septum.[A2,W1] Early reports of successful surgical treatment, were our own in 1967[D3] and 1969,[H1] that of Patrick and McGoon in 1968,[P1] and that of Kawashima and colleagues in 1971.[K1]

The other types of DORV with AV concordant connection began to be clarified in Lev and colleagues classical paper in 1972.[L1] Only in very recent years has successful correction of the unusual forms been reported.[K3,P2,S3]

MORPHOLOGY

Within the spectrum of DORV and concordant atrioventricular (AV) connection, an enormous variability exists.[W1] Therefore, all attempts to group the cases into subsets are difficult and controversial. Likewise, definitions of the relations of the ventricular septal defect (VSD) to the great arteries (subaortic, subpulmonary, doubly committed, and noncommitted) are arbitrary and controversial and at times difficult to apply. Although a conus (or infundibulum) is easy to define as the presence of muscle between a semilunar and AV valve, the muscle strip may be a few millimeters or a few centimeters wide. An aorta that is to the right and side by side with the pulmonary trunk may seem essentially normal in position to one observer or in D-malposition to another. These matters complicate gathering diverse information and data into a cohesive whole.

The surgical treatment depends primarily upon the feasibility of an intraventricular tunnel repair, fashioned so that left ventricular blood passes across the VSD and through the tunnel to the aorta. It is the assessment of this, not the naming of the malformation, that is of practical morphologic importance.

Ventricular Septal Defect

The VSD is usually large, but in about 10% of cases it is smaller than the aortic root and flow restrictive.[E3,L4,M2,M3,S6] The VSD may be multiple. Rarely, it is absent.[A6,M6,S7,Z1]

Since the relation of the VSD to the aorta is of great surgical significance, the position of the VSD and this relation are of central morphologic importance. In most hearts with DORV, the VSD lies between the limbs of the septal band (trabecula septomarginalis, or TSM), which therefore form its inferior and anterior (leftward) boundaries.[T1] Only when the VSD is remote (noncommitted) to the great arteries is this not the case. Thus, the differences in position among subaortic, subpulmonary, and doubly committed VSDs relate primarily to the variability in the position of the septal band (TSM) and in the superior and rightward (posterior) boundaries of the VSD.

Subaortic Ventricular Septal Defect

When the VSD is subaortic, it and the septal band lie more posteriorly in the ventricular septum than in the case of subpulmonary and doubly committed VSDs and are tucked beneath the infundibular septum (Fig. 40-2). The distance between the VSD and the aortic valve varies, depending upon the presence and length of the subaortic conus (infundibulum).

When there is aortic-mitral fibrous continuity and absence of a subaortic conus, the posterosuperior margin of the VSD is formed by the left aortic cusp or the base of the anterior mitral leaflet, depending upon the degree of overriding. The ventriculo-infundibular fold and the rightward posterior division of the TSM may form the posterior margin of the VSD; or the defect may reach the tricuspid ring (opposite the anteroseptal leaflet commissure), in which case it can be called perimembranous (see Chapter 20, "Perimembranous Ventricular Septal Defect" in Section 1, Morphology). In this event the rightward posterior division of the septal band is deficient, and the bundle of His lies along the posterior border of the VSD and is at risk during surgical repair (Fig. 40-3).[A2] Occasionally, the VSD may extend further inferiorly beneath the septal leaflet of the tricuspid valve.[S3] Inferiorly, the VSD is bordered by the TSM and anteriorly by the infundibular septum.

The chordal attachments of the anterior and septal tricuspid leaflets are variable, and they may be anomalously at-

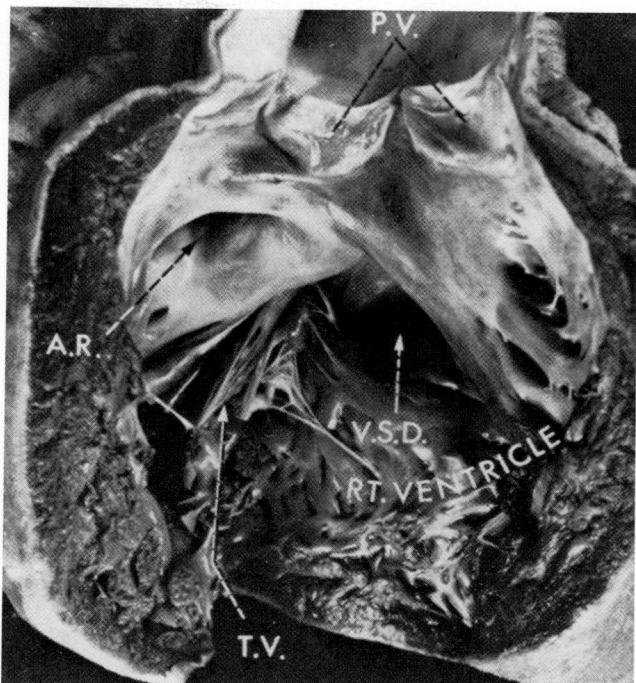

Figure 40-2 Autopsy specimen of simple DORV with subaortic ventricular septal defect. There is a prominent subaortic conus, and a well-developed infundibular (outlet) septum separates the pulmonary valve from the aorta, tricuspid valve, and the VSD.

AR, aortic root (conus); PV, pulmonary valve; TV, tricuspid valve; VSD, ventricular septal defect.

Reproduced with permission from Kirklin et al.[K2]

tached around the edge of the VSD and seriously interfere with placement of the tunnel patch (Fig. 40-4).[B8]

The VSD is also frequently subaortic when there is DORV associated with L-malposition of the aorta. The VSD and the TSM (septal band), within whose limbs the VSD is cradled,[V1] lie more anteriorly and superiorly than when the aorta is to the right. The septal band and its limbs form the inferior and posterior margins of the defect and the aortic valve superiorly. The VSD may occasionally extend to the tricuspid anulus and be perimembranous.

Subpulmonary Ventricular Septal Defect

The VSD and septal band lie more superiorly and anteriorly in the ventricular septum, directly beneath the pulmonary conus or valve, than they do in subaortic VSD with right-sided aorta but in a position similar to that of subaortic VSD with aortic L-malposition. If there is a subpulmonary conus lying entirely over the right ventricle, conal (infundibular) muscle forms the superior margin of the defect. If there is no subpulmonary conus, there is pulmonary-mitral and occasionally pulmonary-tricuspid continuity (Fig. 40-5); then the posterosuperior margin of the VSD is formed by the zone of the fibrous continuity or by the pulmonary cusps, depending on the degree of overriding of the pulmonary valve. The posteroinferior margin is formed by the zone of tricuspid-mitral continuity or by the ventricular septum (Fig. 40-5). As with the subaortic VSD, the defect may extend to the tricus-

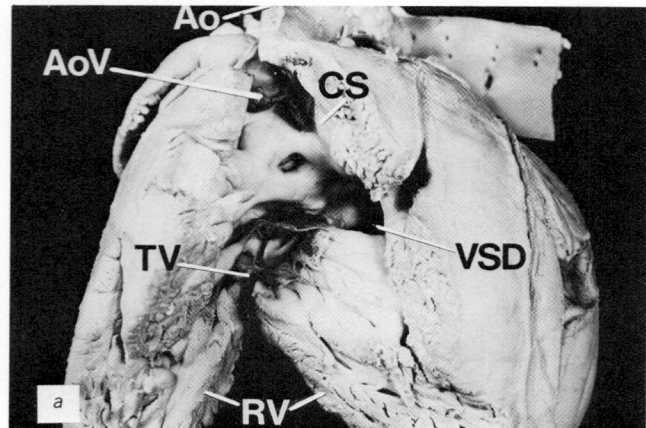

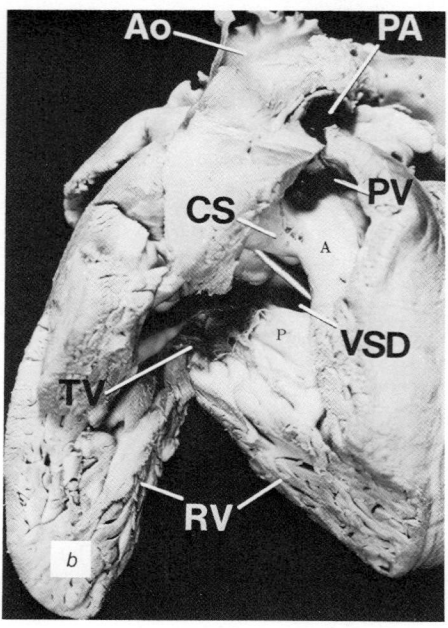

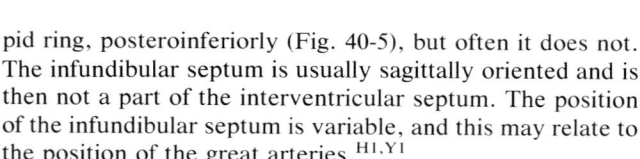

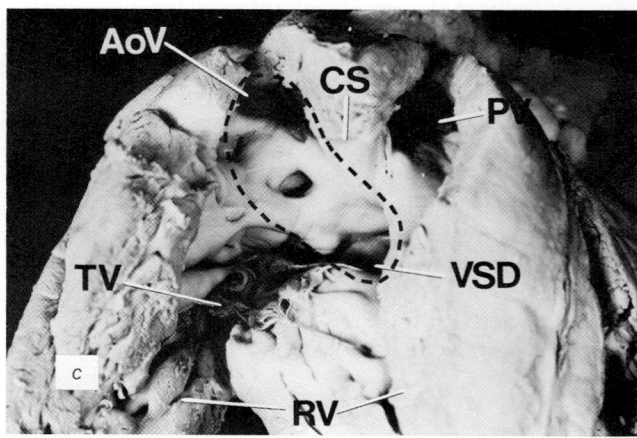

Figure 40-3 Three specimens of DORV with subaortic VSD (GLH). The right ventricle has been opened.

(a) The conal septum has been displaced to the left to reveal the aortic valve and the aorta. A broad band of subaortic conal muscle separates the aortic from the tricuspid valve.

(b) The conal septum and the adjacent portion of anterior wall to which it attaches have been swung to the right to reveal the pulmonary outflow, pulmonary valve, and pulmonary artery. The VSD lies between the two limbs of the septal band and reaches the tricuspid ring inferiorly (probe through VSD passes out to the aorta). The infundibular septum inserts behind the left anterior division of the septal band, and its leftward end contributes to the interventricular septum in front of the VSD.

(c) Close-up view of right ventricular outflow to both great arteries. The posterior and leftward insertions of the conal septum are clearly seen. The dashed line shows the position of the suture line for the patch used in an intraventricular tunnel repair.

A, left anterior division of septal band; Ao, aorta; AoV, aortic valve; CS, conal septum; P, right posterior division of septal band; PA, pulmonary artery; PV, pulmonary valve; RV, right ventricle; TV, tricuspid valve; VSD, ventricular septal defect.

Reproduced with permission from Barratt-Boyes and Calder.[B8]

pid ring, posteroinferiorly (Fig. 40-5), but often it does not. The infundibular septum is usually sagittally oriented and is then not a part of the interventricular septum. The position of the infundibular septum is variable, and this may relate to the position of the great arteries.[H1,Y1]

The Taussig-Bing heart characteristically has this type of VSD.

Doubly Committed Ventricular Septal Defect
In this uncommon variant, the VSD as well as the septal band lie more superiorly in the septum than in the case of subaortic or subpulmonary VSDs. This plus the absence (or severe hypoplasia) of the infundibular septum and consequent confluence of the aortic and pulmonary valve ring place the defect in a subarterial position.[A2,B8] The semilunar valves are related to the posterior and superior boundaries of the defect. The anterior and inferior borders of the VSD are formed by the septal band (TSM) and its left anterior division and the posteroinferior border by the posterior division. This

muscle band usually but not always separates the VSD from the tricuspid valve ring. There is usually no conus; if present, it is very narrow, and there may be aortic-tricuspid and pulmonary-mitral continuity (Fig. 40-6).

In this entity, the VSD and its relations resemble those of isolated subarterial VSD (see Chapter 20), of tetralogy of Fallot with subarterial (subpulmonary) VSD (see Chapter 23), and of some types of double outlet left ventricle (see Chapter 41). In this setting, both semilunar valves usually lie over the right ventricle, but it can be difficult to decide whether this is the case or whether they lie mostly over the left ventricle. At times, they may arise equally over both ventricles, a condition that can properly be called ''double outlet both ventricles.''[B2]

Noncommitted or Remote Ventricular Septal Defect
Trabecular VSDs are not related to the septal band and its divisions in the manner described earlier and are clearly away from the semilunar valves.[L1,Z1] Occasionally, an AV

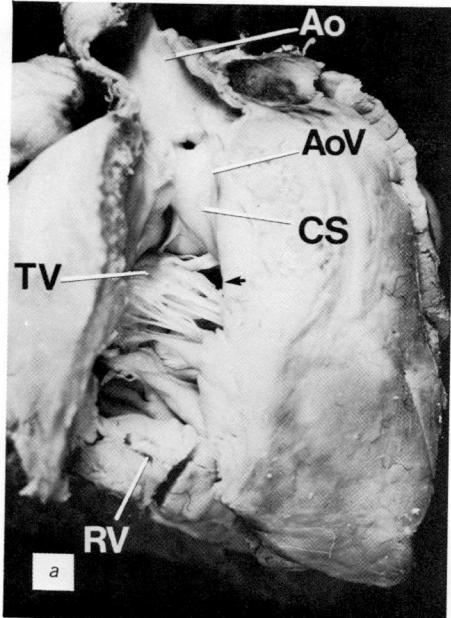

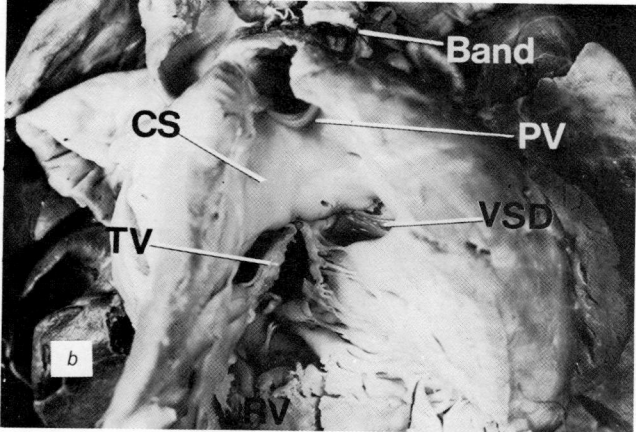

Figure 40-4 Specimen of DORV with bilateral conus and subaortic VSD (GLH) in a patient with a pulmonary artery band.
(a) Right ventricular outflow tract has been opened as has the aortic valve and aorta. The VSD (arrow) is only just visible since it is partly overlaid by anomalously attached chordae from the tricuspid valve, which may interfere with placement of an intraventricular tunnel patch.
(b) Conal septum displaced to right to reveal the pulmonary valve and extensive subpulmonary conus. The conal septum inserts posteriorly and is unrelated to the interventricular septum. In some respects, this ventricular septal defect is intermediate between a subaortic and a subpulmonary defect and illustrates the difficulties of precise categorization.

Ao, aorta; AoV, aortic valve; CS, conal septum; PV, pulmonary valve; RV, right ventricle; TV, tricuspid valve.

Reproduced with permission from Barratt-Boyes and Calder.[B8]

canal-type VSD is sufficiently remote from the great arteries as to be considered noncommitted (Fig. 40-7).[L7]

Conus (Infundibulum) and Infundibular Septum

There may be bilateral conuses,[2] one beneath both the aortic and mitral valves.[V3] Rarely, neither aortic nor mitral valve is separated from the AV valves, and there is no conus. Rather commonly in hearts with DORV, there is just one conus.

The infundibular (conal) septum in DORV is not an integral part of the interventricular septum, as in the normal heart, but is to a variable degree malaligned.[3] In certain hearts with DORV, notably the Taussig-Bing heart, the infundibular septum lies in a sagittal plane and is not at all a part of the interventricular septum. The infundibular septum may be entirely absent in some examples of DORV.

Great Arteries

Both of the great arteries may lie over the right ventricle in their entirety, such as in the rare instance of DORV with intact ventricular septum and in hearts with a noncommitted VSD. This is usually the situation as well when the VSD is subaortic. When the VSD is doubly committed or subpulmonary, there is usually a variable degree of overriding of one or both great arteries over the VSD.

The positional interrelations of the great arteries are variable in hearts with DORV. Occasionally, they are normal, with the aorta to the right and slightly posterior to the anteriorly placed pulmonary trunk and then the aorta tends to twist around the pulmonary artery as in the normal heart.[A2,P2] Frequently, the great arteries are side by side, with the aorta to the right. This may be difficult to distinguish from a normal relation. D-malposition is often present in hearts with DORV, with the aorta anterior and to the right or at times directly anterior. Rarely, it is anterior and to the left. Occasionally, there is L-malposition and the aorta is to the left but side by side with the pulmonary arteries.

Interrelations among Ventricular Septal Defect, Great Artery Position, and Conal Pattern

Although the position of VSD relative to the great arteries (subaortic, subpulmonary, doubly committed, noncommitted) may occasionally be difficult to categorize in an individual heart before operation, from a surgical viewpoint, it remains the most useful morphologic feature in patients with DORV. Since the position of the great arteries is variable, not all subaortic VSDs, for example, are in the same position in the ventricular septum (see "Ventricular Septal Defect").

This has led to attempts to organize the classification of DORV around the position of the great arteries.[S3] This has been less useful surgically than had been hoped. Although typically subaortic VSDs are associated with *more-or-less normally related great arteries* (simple DORV), only hearts

---

[2]The infundibulum, or conus, is a muscular structure of variable length, separating a semilunar valve from an AV valve.

[3]The infundibular, or outlet, septum is a muscular structure separating the aortic and pulmonary valves.

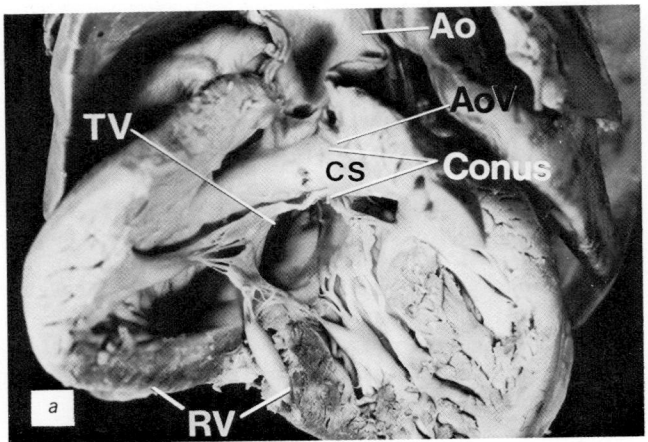

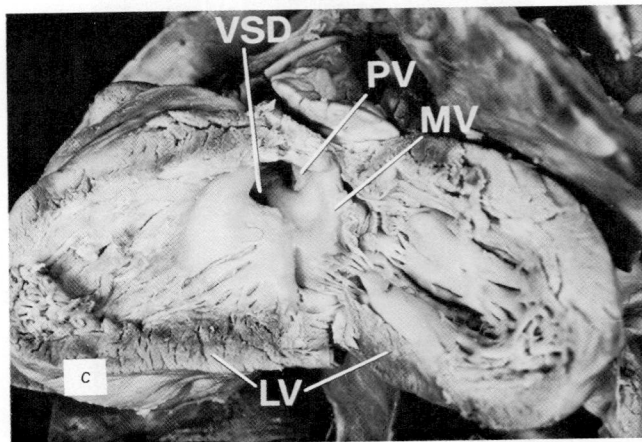

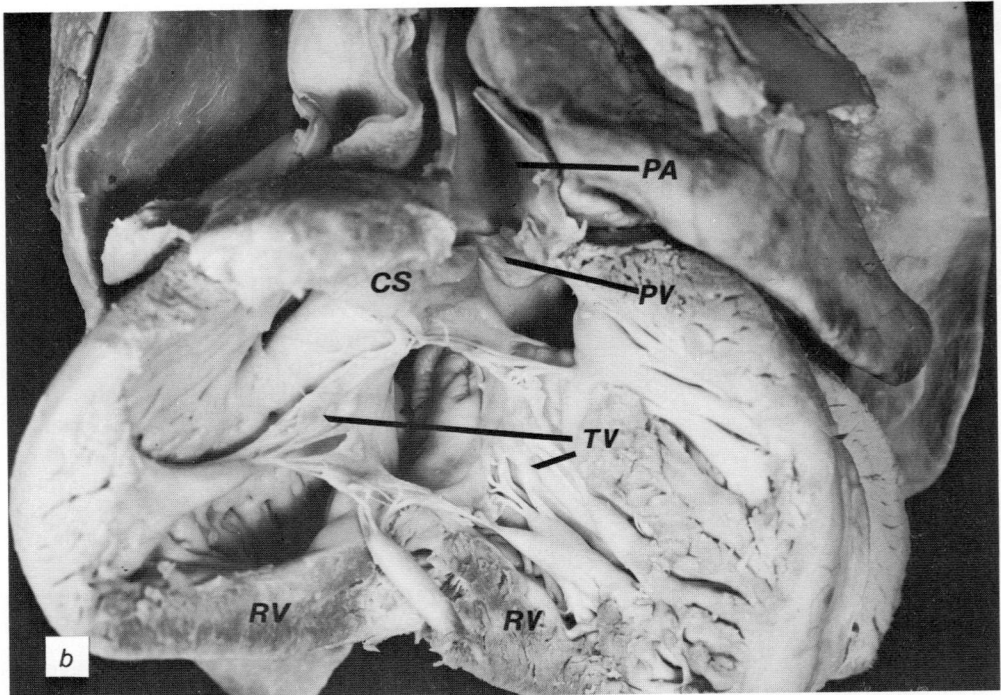

Figure 40-5 Specimen of DORV with subpulmonary VSD (Taussig-Bing heart) (GLH).
(a) Right ventricular outflow tract, aortic valve, and aorta have been opened. The subaortic conus separates the aortic from the tricuspid valve. The rightward aspect of the conal septum is visible.
(b) The conal septum and adjacent portion of free wall are displaced toward the aorta to reveal the opened pulmonary outflow, pulmonary valve, and pulmonary artery. The conal septum lies in a sagittal plane and has no attachment to the ventricular septum. Moreover, it separates the ventricular septal defect from the aortic valve. The VSD lies directly above the septal band, but because the rightward posterior division of the septal band is deficient it reaches the tricuspid ring (and can be called perimembranous). The pulmonary valve overrides the VSD onto the left ventricle. There is no subpulmonary conus. The aorta is to the right and slightly anterior to the pulmonary artery.
(c) View from opened left ventricle. The overriding pulmonary valve is in direct fibrous continuity with the anterior leaflet of the mitral valve.

Ao, aorta; AoV, aortic valve; CS, conal septum; LV, left ventricle; MV, mitral valve; PA, pulmonary artery; PV, pulmonary valve; RV, right ventricle; TV, tricuspid valve; VSD, ventricular septal defect.

Reproduced with permission from Barratt-Boyes and Calder.[B8]

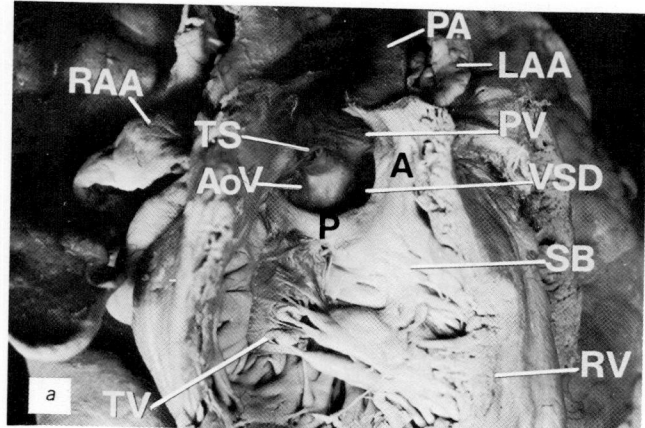

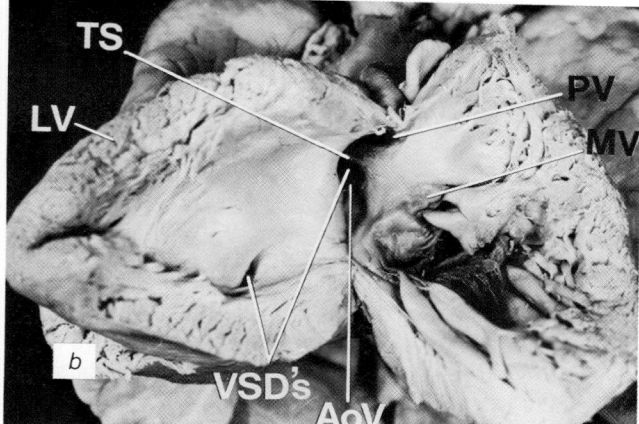

Figure 40-6 Specimen of DORV with doubly committed VSD (GLH).

(*a*) Right ventricular outflow tract. Both great arteries override the ventricular septum. Aortic and pulmonary valves are in fibrous continuity, since there is no conal septum. The aortic valve lies rightward and posterior to the pulmonary valve, making a tunnel repair to create a series circulation (Ao → LV) satisfactory. If the aorta lies to the right and anterior to the pulmonary valve, this becomes more difficult. The VSD lies between the two divisions of the septal band. Persistence of the right posterior division of the septal band prevents aortic-tricuspid valve continuity.

(*b*) View from opened left ventricle. The pulmonary and aortic valves are in tenuous fibrous continuity with the mitral valve, since there is no conus. There is an additional slitlike VSD in the sinus septum.

A, left anterior division of septal band; AoV, aortic valve; LAA, left atrial appendage; LV, left ventricle; MV, mitral valve; P, right posterior division of septal band; PA, pulmonary artery; PV, pulmonary valve; RAA, right atrial appendage; RV, right ventricle; SB, septal band (trabecula septomarginalis); VSD, ventricular septal defect; TV, tricuspid valve.

Reproduced from Brandt et al.[B2]

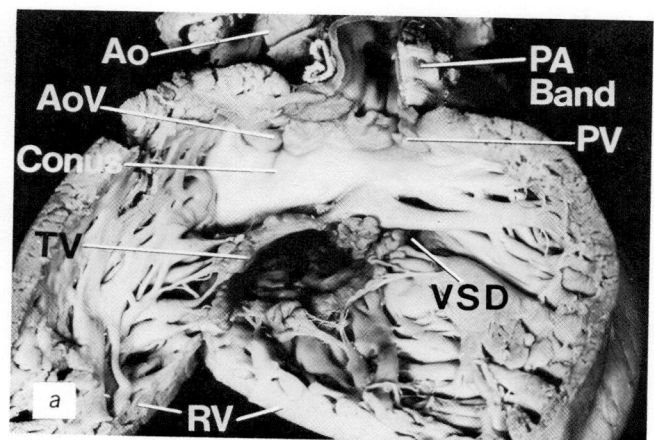

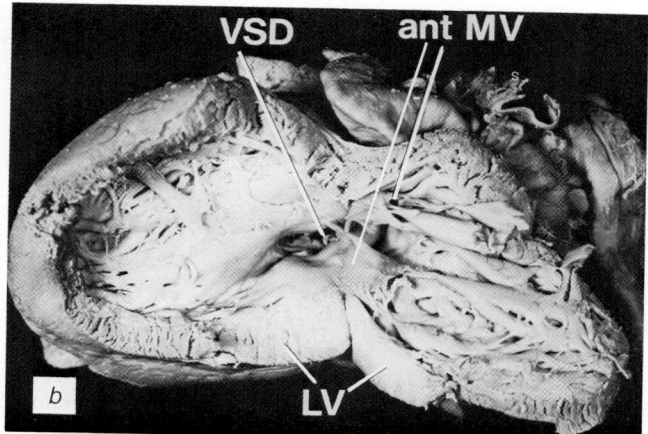

Figure 40-7 Specimen of DORV with noncommitted VSD (GLH).

(*a*) Right ventricular outflow to opened pulmonary valve and banded main pulmonary artery and to aortic valve. A well developed subsemilunar conus separates the aortic and pulmonary valves from the tricuspid valve and from the VSD, which is partly obscured by the tricuspid valve. The aortic and pulmonary valves are joined (i.e., the conal septum is absent). The aorta and pulmonary artery lie side by side, with the valves at the same level.

(*b*) View from opened left ventricle. The only exit is via the VSD (which is of AV canal type) through which tricuspid valve tissue can be seen. The anterior mitral valve leaflet is cleft.

Ant MV, anterior mitral leaflet; Ao, aorta; AoV, aortic valve; LV, left ventricle; PA, pulmonary artery; PV, pulmonary valve; RV, right ventricle; TV, tricuspid valve; VSD, ventricular septal defect.

Reproduced with permission from Barratt-Boyes and Calder.[B8]

with noncommitted VSDs have a distribution of great artery positions different from all others (Table 40-1). Although in 77% of hearts with subaortic VSD the aorta is to the right and either side by side or posterior to the pulmonary trunk (more-or-less normally related), it is anterior (D-malposition) in 23% (Table 40-1). Further, more-or-less normally related great arteries are not unique to hearts with subaortic VSD,

those with subpulmonary VSD having it in the same frequency. Only in hearts with noncommitted VSD is the frequency of more-or-less normally related great arteries less (33%) (*P* for difference = .06; Table 40-1). Although *D-malposition of the aorta* may be considered characteristic of ordinary transposition (see Chapter 39) and by implication the Taussig-Bing heart, hearts with DORV and subpulmonary VSD are associated with typical D-malposition in a minority of cases (Table 40-1). In fact, the incidence is no greater than when the VSD is subaortic (*P* for difference = .8). Hearts with doubly committed VSD tend to have more-or-less normally related great arteries (Table 40-1).

Thus, observing the great artery position at cineangiocar-

Table 40-1 The position of the VSD and the great arteries in DORV in patients with AV concordant connection (autopsy series; GLH; *n* = 42). Specimens (nine) with atrial isomerism (all with noncommitted AV canal-type VSD) are excluded, as are those with L-malposition.

		Aortic Position Relative to PA							
		Side by side or Posterior[a]			Anterior[b]				P for Difference
Position of VSD	n	No.	% of n	CL	No.	% of n	CL		
Subaortic	22	17	77%	64%–87%	5	23%	13%–36%	P = .8[c]	.23
			(59%	47%–69%)		(38%	23%–57%)		
Subpulmonary	11	8	73%	53%–88%	3	27%	12%–47%		.8
			(28%	18%–39%)		(23%	10%–41%)		
Doubly committed	3	2	67%	24%–96%	1	33%	4%–76%		.7
			(7%	2%–16%)		(8%	1%–24%)		
Noncommitted	6	2	33%	12%–62%	4	67%	38%–88%		.06
			(7%	2%–16%)		(31%	16%–49%)		
Total	42	29	69%	60%–77%	13	31%	23%–40%		
			(100%)			(100%)			

KEY: CL, 70% confidence limits; PA, pulmonary artery; VSD, ventricular septal defect percent of 42.

NOTE: In parentheses are the percentages of the various VSD locations within each great artery position. The *P* value column refers to the differences in the incidence of the given VSD position in the two great artery positions.

[a]Side by side or posterior refers to the aorta being to the right and beside or slightly posterior to the pulmonary trunk (artery), with the great arteries being more or less normally interrelated.

[b]Anterior refers to D-malposition, with the aorta being anterior and more or less to the right.

[c]Refers to the difference in incidence of subaortic and subpulmonary VSDs in DORV with anteriorly placed aorta.

diography or operation does not permit a reasonably accurate inference as to the position of the VSD and the category of DORV. There is no greater certainty that the VSD is subaortic when the great arteries are more-or-less normally interrelated than when in D-malposition (*P* for difference = .23). When the aorta is in D-malposition, there is no greater certainty that the VSD will be subpulmonary (*P* for difference = .8) than subaortic (Table 40-1).

There is greater specificity in the relationship of the position of the VSD to the conal pattern (Table 40-2), but this is of limited help at operation because conal patterns cannot be determined from external examination of the heart. The distribution of conal patterns is different from all others in the case of subaortic (*P* = .008), subpulmonary (*P* = .01), and

doubly committed (*P* = .003) VSDs but not in the case of noncommitted VSD (*P* = .3). Also, distribution of conal patterns is different in subaortic and subpulmonary VSD (*P* = .0004); most hearts with a subaortic VSD have bilateral conuses, but in hearts with DORV and subpulmonary VSD, there is a solitary subaortic conus in 23% of cases (a situation not found with subaortic VSD) and a bilateral conus in 45%. Thus, bilateral conus is not unique to subaortic VSD or any other type (*P* = .3) and occurred frequently in hearts with doubly committed and noncommitted VSDs as well. Only subpulmonary and noncommitted VSDs were associated with a solitary subaortic conus (*P* = .0007), suggesting a fundamental relation.

There is a pattern of relations between the conus and the

Table 40-2 The position of the VSD and the conus pattern in DORV (autopsy series; GLH; *n* = 42).

		Type of Conus (Infundibulum)												
		Bilateral			Subpulmonary Only			Subaortic Only			Absent			P fo
Position of VSD	n	No.	% of n	CL	No.	% of n	CL	No.	% of n	CL	No.	% of n	CL	Differe
Subaortic	22	17	77%	64%–87%	5	23%	13%–36%	0	0%	0%–8%	0	0%	0%–8%	.000
			(63%	51%–74%)		(100%	68%–100%)		(0%	0%–19%)		(0%	0%–85%)	
Subpulmonary	11	5	45%	27%–65%	0	0%	0%–16%	6	55%	35%–73%	0	0%	0%–16%	.01
			(19%	11%–29%)		(0%	0%–32%)		(67%	44%–85%)		(0%	0%–85%)	
Doubly committed	3	2	67%	24%–96%	0	0%	0%–47%	0	0%	0%–47%	1	33%	4%–76%	.003
			(7%	2%–17%)		(0%	0%–32%)		(0%	0%–19%)		(100%	15%–100%)	
Noncommitted	6	3	50%	24%–76%	0	0%	0%–27%	3	50%	24%–76%	0	0%	0%–27%	.3
			(11%	5%–21%)		(0%	0%–32%)		(33%	15%–56%)		(0%	15%–100%)	
Total	42	27	64%	55%–73%	5	12%	7%–19%	9	21%	15%–30%	1	2%	0.3%–8%	
P(χ²)			.3			.16			.0007					

KEY: CL, 70% confidence limits.

NOTE: See Table 40-1 for details of the presentation and analysis. In addition, the *P*-values along the bottom of the table refer to the difference in incidence of the ty conus of the column in the various positions of the VSD.

Table 40-3   The type of conus and position of the great arteries in DORV (autopsy series; GLH; $n = 42$).

Type of Conus	n	Side by side or Posterior			Anterior			P for Difference
		No.	% of n	CL	No.	% of n	CL	
Bilateral	27	20	74% (69%	63%–83% 58%–79%)	7	26% (54%	17%–37% 36%–71%)	.3
Subpulmonary only	5	5	100% (17%	68%–100% 10%–28%)	0	0% (0%	0%–32% 0%–14%)	.14
Subaortic only	9	3	33% (10%	15%–56% 5%–20%)	6	67% (46%	44%–85% 29%–64%)	.009
Absent	1	1	100% (3%	15%–85% 0.4%–11%)	0	0% (0%	0%–85% 0%–14%)	.7
Total	42	29	69%	60%–77%	13	31%	23%–40%	
$P(\chi^2)$			.04				.4	

KEY: CL, 70% confidence limits; PA, pulmonary artery.

NOTE: See Tables 40-1 and 40-2 for details of the presentation.

position of the great arteries (Table 40-3), as has long been known. An anterior position (D-malposition) of the aorta is uncommon (26%) when there are bilateral conuses; but when there is only a subaortic conus, this position occurs commonly (67%). An anterior position has not been observed to occur with only subpulmonary conus or no conus. An aorta side by side or posterior to the pulmonary artery occurs in all conal patterns.

Pulmonary Stenosis

Pulmonary stenosis is common in hearts with a subaortic VSD. The stenosis is most often infundibular (Fig. 40-8), but there may also be valvar and annular stenosis and stenosis at the origin of the right or left pulmonary arteries, as in the tetralogy of Fallot. Rarely, the infundibular stenosis may be of the isolated, low-lying variety, producing a two-chambered right ventricle and DORV.[J2,M3]

Pulmonary stenosis is also common in hearts with doubly committed VSD (five of five; GLH). Pulmonary stenosis is uncommon in association with the Taussig-Bing heart[L5] and hearts with a noncommitted VSD.[L1]

Conduction System

In DORV with concordant AV connection, the AV node is in its normal position in the AV septum and the bundle of His penetrates the right fibrous trigone in the usual way. Thus, the course of the bundle of His relative to the VSD is the same as in primary VSD and in tetralogy of Fallot (see Chapters 20 and 23). The bundle is at risk of damage during the repair only when the defect reaches the tricuspid anulus (and becomes perimembranous). This is true whether the defect is subaortic or subpulmonary[B4] and whether the ascending aorta is right or left sided.[L2] However, as in other conditions with clockwise rotation and dextroposition of the aorta, the bundle is more on the left ventricular side of the septum than is usual.[B4] Further, the trigone is often attenuated in DORV when there is a subaortic conus, which removes the aortic anulus from the central fibrous skeleton of the heart.

When a complete AV canal defect coexists, the node and bundle course are altered accordingly (see Chapter 19).

Coronary Arteries

The coronary artery pattern depends upon the position of the great arteries. Thus, in most varieties of DORV it is similar to normal except that the aortic sinuses are rotated in a clockwise direction (viewed from below) so that the right coronary arises anteriorly and the left coronary posteriorly.[E4] When the aorta is anterior and rightward, the pattern is usually similar to that in transposition of the great arteries, with the right coronary artery arising from a rightward posterior sinus.[L9] In 15% there may be a single coronary ostium supplying the left and right sides of the heart arising either anteriorly or posteriorly.[G1,W1] The branching pattern is also usually normal, except for the occasional origin of the left anterior descending from the right coronary artery, this vessel crossing the right ventricular outflow from right to left as in tetralogy of Fallot. This anomaly was found in 25% of the DORV hearts reported in the early Mayo Clinic series[G1,G2] but has not been encountered in the 43 GLH surgical cases.

When the aorta is to the left in L-malposition, the right coronary artery passes to the right from the anterior sinus of the leftward anterior aorta to reach the AV groove in front of the main pulmonary artery. Its position prohibits extensive anterior patching across the pulmonary ring.

Associated Anomalies

Major associated cardiac anomalies, in addition to pulmonary stenosis of the tetralogy of Fallot type, may coexist. Coarctation of the aorta may be present and require repair in the neonatal period,[S1] and rarely discrete subvalvar aortic stenosis may coexist with DORV.[G4] Various other cardiac anomalies coexisted in about 30% of the patients coming to intracardiac repair of DORV with a subaortic or doubly committed VSD (Tables 40-4 and 40-5).[P2]

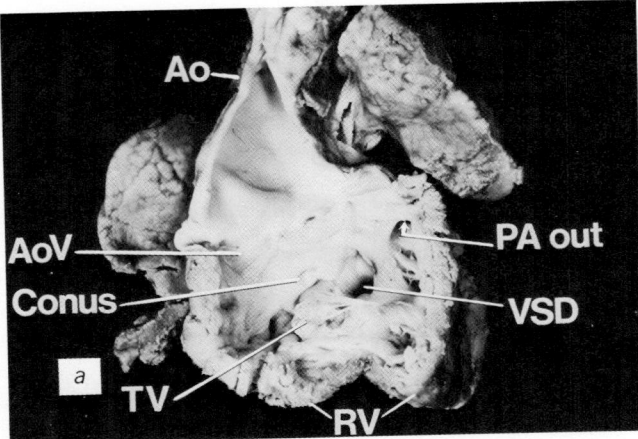

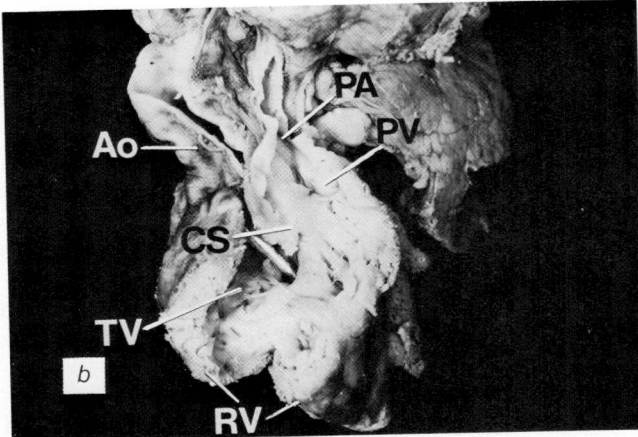

Figure 40-8 Specimen of DORV with subaortic VSD and infundibular pulmonary stenosis (GLH).
(a) Right ventricular outflow is opened to aortic valve and aorta. A subaortic conus separates the aortic and tricuspid valves. Poorly expanded subpulmonary conus narrows the pulmonary outflow.
(b) Conal septum displaced to reveal the opened pulmonary outflow. The pulmonary valve is bicuspid, and it and the pulmonary artery are smaller than normal. The aorta is slightly anterior to the pulmonary artery. A probe passes through the VSD and into the aorta.
Ao, aorta; AoV, aortic valve; PA, pulmonary artery; PA out, pulmonary outflow; PV, pulmonary valve; RV, right ventricular outflow; TV, tricuspid valve; VSD, ventricular septal defect.
Reproduced with permission from Barratt-Boyes and Calder.[B8]

Morphologic Syndromes of Double Outlet Right Ventricle

Simple Double Outlet Right Ventricle

The phrase simple DORV connotes the rather commonly occurring and easily repaired type of DORV in which the VSD is subaortic and the aorta is to the right, usually by the side of the pulmonary trunk or slightly posterior to it but in about 20% of the cases somewhat anterior to the pulmonary trunk (see Table 40-1). The aorta may spiral around the pulmonary trunk as it leaves the heart,[A2] or the great arteries may course parallel one to the other. The internal architecture of the heart has been described in "Subaortic Ventricu-

Table 40-4 Associated cardiac anomalies (exclusive of pulmonary stenosis and ASD) in patients undergoing surgical correction of DORV with subaortic or doubly committed VSD (UAB; 1967–1982; n = 42 and GLH; 1958–1984; n = 28). Since some patients had multiple anomalies, the total is not cumulative, nor is the list mutually exclusive.

Associated Cardiac Anomalies	No.	Percent of Total (N = 70)	Hospital Deaths
Multiple VSDs	9	13%	1[a]
Patent ductus arteriosus	8	11%	3[a]
Pulmonary artery distribution deficiencies or postshunt stenoses	9	13%	1
Pulmonary atresia	2	3%	1[a]
LV hypoplasia + MV hypoplasia or incompetence	2	3%	2
Congenital mitral stenosis	1	1.4%	
Subaortic stenosis	2	3%	
Tricuspid incompetence (severe)	2	3%	1
Unroofed coronary sinus syndrome	3	4%	
Azygous continuation IVC	1	1.4%	
Right aortic arch	1	1.4%	
Aberrant right subclavian artery	1	1.4%	
Origin right coronary from left coronary artery	1	1.4%	
Juxtaposed atrial appendages	1	1.4%	1
Situs inversus totalis (Van Praagh's ILL)	2	3%	
No associated anomalies	41	59%	12

KEY: IVC, inferior vena cava; LV, left ventricular; MV, mitral valve; VSD, ventricular septal defect.
[a] All but one of these five patients had LV hypoplasia.

lar Septal Defect." Usually there is a conus (infundibulum) beneath both the aorta and pulmonary valve, but in some cases there may be no subaortic conus (see Table 40-2).

This type of DORV, in borderline cases, merges with the type of DORV in which a noncommitted perimembranous VSD is of the AV canal type and, on the other hand, with the type in which the VSD is doubly committed.

Taussig-Bing Heart

In the most representative cases, the Taussig-Bing anomaly is very similar from heart to heart. The VSD is anterior and superior and subpulmonary. The pulmonary artery arises biventricularly over the VSD, and the aorta is to the right and slightly anterior to or along side the pulmonary trunk (see Table 40-1). The first portions of the aorta and pulmonary artery are parallel[A2,A3,D2] rather than tending to spiral as do the normally positioned great arteries. The infundibular septum is in the sagittal plane and is not part of the interventricular septum. Lev and colleagues are able to use specific morphologic features within the right ventricle as the hallmark of the Taussig-Bing heart,[L3] but this is rarely possible clinically or surgically.

Subaortic stenosis, from narrowing of the subaortic infundibulum[T2] may develop with the Taussig-Bing heart.[Y1] Pulmonary stenosis is uncommon but does occur.[L5] The mitral valve may straddle across the subpulmonary VSD,[K4,M5] and

Table 40-5 Associated cardiac anomalies in patients with varieties of DORV other than those with subaortic or doubly committed VSDs (GLH; 1964–1984). Five of the 15 patients (33%) died in the hospital, and all but 1 of these had major associated anomalies. Since most patients had multiple anomalies, the total is not cumulative.

Associated Cardiac Anomalies	n	Percent of Total (n = 15)	Hospital Deaths
Hypoplasia LV and MV	1	7%	1
Congenital mitral stenosis	1	7%	1
Two-storied heart	2	13%	1
Dextrocardia	2	13%	0
Juxtaposed atrial appendages	3	20%	1
LSVC → CS	3	20%	1
Coarctation aorta	1	7%	0
MV override and/or straddling	1	7%	1
TV override and/or straddling	1	7%	0
Hypoplastic RV and TV	1	7%	0
AV discordance (Van Praagh's SLL)	3	20%	0
Multiple VSDs	2	13%	2
ASD (moderate or large)	6	40%	2
No associated anomalies (apart from PS and/or ASD)	5	33%	1

KEY: CS, coronary sinus; LSVC, left superior vena cava; LV, left ventricle; MV, mitral valve; RV, right ventricle; TV, tricuspid valve.

in such cases the left ventricle may be hypoplastic.[K4] Associated coarctation of the aorta is common[N3,S1,Y1] and is said by Parr and colleagues to be present in 50% of cases.[P3] This is very much in contrast to the 6% incidence in transposition with VSD.[P3]

This type of DORV, in borderline cases, merges with transposition of the great arteries and large VSD and, on the other hand, may merge with DORV and noncommitted VSD of the trabecular type.

Double Outlet Right Ventricle with Doubly Committed Ventricular Septal Defect

In this uncommon syndrome, the VSD is immediately beneath both aorta and pulmonary artery.

Double Outlet Right Ventricle with Noncommitted Ventricular Septal Defect

When the VSD is in the trabecular septum and clearly far removed from the great arteries, the anomaly is easily categorized into this subset. When the VSD is in the inlet septum and up against the tricuspid valve, the so-called AV canal type of VSD, categorization as DORV with noncommitted VSD can always be questioned, but at least the defect is further removed from the aorta than in most hearts with DORV and subaortic VSD.

Double Outlet Right Ventricle with L-Malposition

DORV with L-malposition usually has a subaortic VSD (rarely extending back to the tricuspid anulus) and pulmonary stenosis and presents a rare but distinctive clinical and surgical syndrome.[D1,L2,L6,P4,V1] Rarely, the VSD may be

perimembranous and extend up toward the pulmonary artery,[Y2] or it may be truly subpulmonary.[S4,W2] The VSD may, contrariwise, extend into the inlet septum[A4] and be noncommitted. Mehrizi has reported DORV with L-malposition and doubly committed VSD.[M1]

Double Outlet Right Ventricle with Complete Atrioventricular Canal Defect

In the cases of DORV with complete AV canal defect, the interventricular communication is large and usually extends deeply beneath a bridging left superior leaflet (see Chapter 19, "AV Valves" in section on Morphology) to be subaortic in position.[S8] Occasionally, however, the interventricular communication does not extend in this manner, and is noncommitted.[B6]

Double Outlet Right Ventricle with Superior–Inferior Ventricles

Uncommonly, in DORV with situs solitus of the atria, AV concordant connection, and D-ventricular loop, there is a positional anomaly termed *superior-inferior ventricles* (*over-and-under ventricles, upstairs-downstairs ventricles*) (see Chapter 1, "Cardiac and Arterial Positions" in section on Terminology and Classification of Heart Disease). In most hearts with this ventricular position, there is a ventricular L-loop, atrial situs solitus, and AV discordant connection; these are discussed in Chapters 42 and 43. When the AV connection is concordant, the right ventricle is superior (and sometimes a little posterior) and the left ventricle inferior. There may be D- or L-malposition of the aorta. The VSD is usually perimembranous and in the inlet portion of the septum. The right AV valve is usually more superiorly placed than usual, relative to the left AV valve, and either AV valve may straddle. Severe left ventricular hypoplasia may be present. Pulmonary stenosis is common.

CLINICAL FEATURES AND DIAGNOSTIC CRITERIA

Pathophysiology

The clinical features of patients with the morphologically highly variable group of cardiac anomalies with double outlet right ventricle (DORV) and atrioventricular (AV) concordant connection are of necessity also highly variable. In general, however, such patients who have a large ventricular septal defect (VSD) and are without pulmonary stenosis or severe pulmonary vascular disease are not cyanotic because pulmonary blood flow is high and the resultant mixture of blood in the right ventricle has a high enough oxygen saturation to prevent clinically evident cyanosis. However, there is always some arterial desaturation.

Streamlining of Blood Flow

Arterial saturation is also affected by the streaming within the right ventricle, which is determined by the relationship of the semilunar valves to the VSD and the position and presence of the infundibular septum.[N3,S7] Thus, in simple DORV, flow of highly oxygen-saturated left ventricular blood through the VSD is directed preferentially beneath the infundibular septum into the adjacent aorta (particularly when the subaortic conus is short or absent), whereas systemic venous blood passes largely out the pulmonary artery. Patients with this arrangement, therefore, present with a high pulmonary blood flow in congestive heart failure without cyanosis in infancy and cannot be clinically distinguished from those with a large VSD (see Chapter 20).

When the VSD is subpulmonary, as in the Taussig-Bing heart, the flow of highly saturated left ventricular blood through it is directed into the adjacent pulmonary artery by the vertically positioned infundibular septum. The pulmonary artery oxygen saturation is then higher than aortic saturation, systemic venous blood from the right ventricle tending to flow more into the aorta.[W4] This situation is aggravated when there is overriding of the pulmonary artery onto the LV. Thus, these infants present in a similar fashion to transposition of the great arteries with large VSD and are in congestive heart failure with mild cyanosis (see Chapter 39).

Pulmonary Vascular Disease

Pulmonary vascular disease may be of somewhat more rapid onset in patients with DORV without pulmonary stenosis than in patients with simple large VSD, particularly in the Taussig-Bing heart.[S3] The resultant reduction in pulmonary blood flow has a more marked influence on arterial saturation than in simple VSD since it reduces the amount of highly saturated blood in a common mixing chamber.

Pulmonary Stenosis

When there is important pulmonary stenosis in patients with any type of DORV, cyanosis becomes severe and the clinical features and presentation are similar to those with tetralogy of Fallot (see Chapter 23).

Examination

On physical examination there are no clinical signs that distinguish patients with DORV with and without pulmonary stenosis from the conditions that they simulate. The electrocardiogram (ECG) is not diagnostic nor is the chest x-ray. However, in those uncommon instances in which there is L-malposition of the aorta, this vessel may be evident on the posteroanterior chest x-ray as it ascends vertically from the cardiac silhouette in the left upper mediastinum.[L2,V1] This finding is not specific, however, to DORV with L-malposition of the aorta (see discussion in Chapter 45, "Clinical Features and Diagnostic Criteria").

Two-dimensional echocardiography provides a considerable amount of information, particularly with regard to AV valve abnormalities.[H2,S2,S7] The VSD and its relation to the AV valves and the aorta and pulmonary artery can also be defined.[M7]

Cardiac Catheterization and Cineangiography

Cardiac catheterization and cineangiography are necessary preoperatively for definition of the hemodynamic state (as described in Chapters 20 and 23) and for identification and characterization of the morphologic details, including those of any associated anomalies. Biplane cineangiography using appropriate views is the critical diagnostic procedure (Fig. 40-9). The whole of the ventricular septum must be profiled so that its upper part can be projected cranially to assess the great vessel positions relative to the two ventricles and the location of the VSDs determined (this is discussed in more detail in Chapter 23, Fig. 23-19).[B3,B8] The size of the VSD can be judged (Fig. 40-10). Subsets such as the Taussig-Bing heart can be identified (Fig. 40-11). Cineangiography is of particular value in assessing the complex interrelationships present in DORV with superior-inferior ventricles and crisscross hearts.[B9]

NATURAL HISTORY

The natural history of patients with double outlet right ventricle (DORV) and atrioventricular (AV) concordant connection is also highly variable, but some general trends can be identified.

When there is a large subaortic VSD without pulmonary stenosis, the natural history is similar to that of simple VSD (see Chapter 20), and this is probably also true for patients with DORV whose VSDs are doubly committed or noncommitted. The exception is that spontaneous closure of the VSD, although occurring,[M4] is rare in DORV. Further, in the setting of DORV, spontaneous closure is fatal rather than curative.

When the VSD is subpulmonary as in the Taussig-Bing heart, the natural history is similar to that for transposition and large VSD but even more unfavorable. This is in part because severe pulmonary vascular disease occurs early in the life history of these patients. The poor prognosis in these patients may also be related to the frequent occurrence of left-sided cardiac lesions, such as coarctation of the aorta and left ventricular and mitral valve hypoplasia.

When pulmonary stenosis or atresia is present in patients with subaortic VSD and probably in those with doubly committed or noncommitted VSDs, the natural history is indistinguishable from that of patients with tetralogy of Fallot and pulmonary atresia (see Chapter 23).

The natural history in some patients is dominated by an associated cardiac anomaly such as a complete AV canal defect (see Chapter 19).

TECHNIQUE OF OPERATION

The preparation for operation, draping, arrangement of the lines for cardiopulmonary bypass (CPB), the median sternotomy incision, and placement of stay sutures and sutures for cannulation are as usual (see Chapter 2, Section 3). The pericardium is cleared in case it is needed, and a woven Dacron tube whose diameter is about 20% larger than that of the aorta is preclotted. The intrapericardial anatomy is carefully evaluated. A final decision is then made concerning the support technique to be used. Cardiopulmonary bypass (CPB) with direct caval cannulation at 25°C may be used routinely (UAB) (see Chapter 2, Section 3) and brief periods of low flow or total circulatory arrest added when needed to improve exposure; alternatively (GLH), this technique may

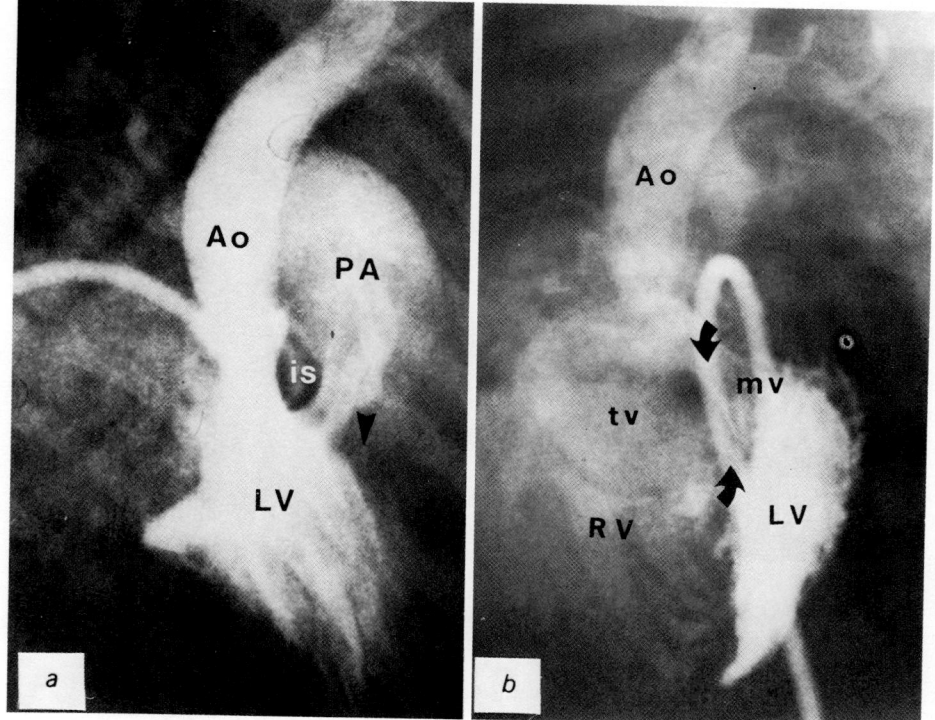

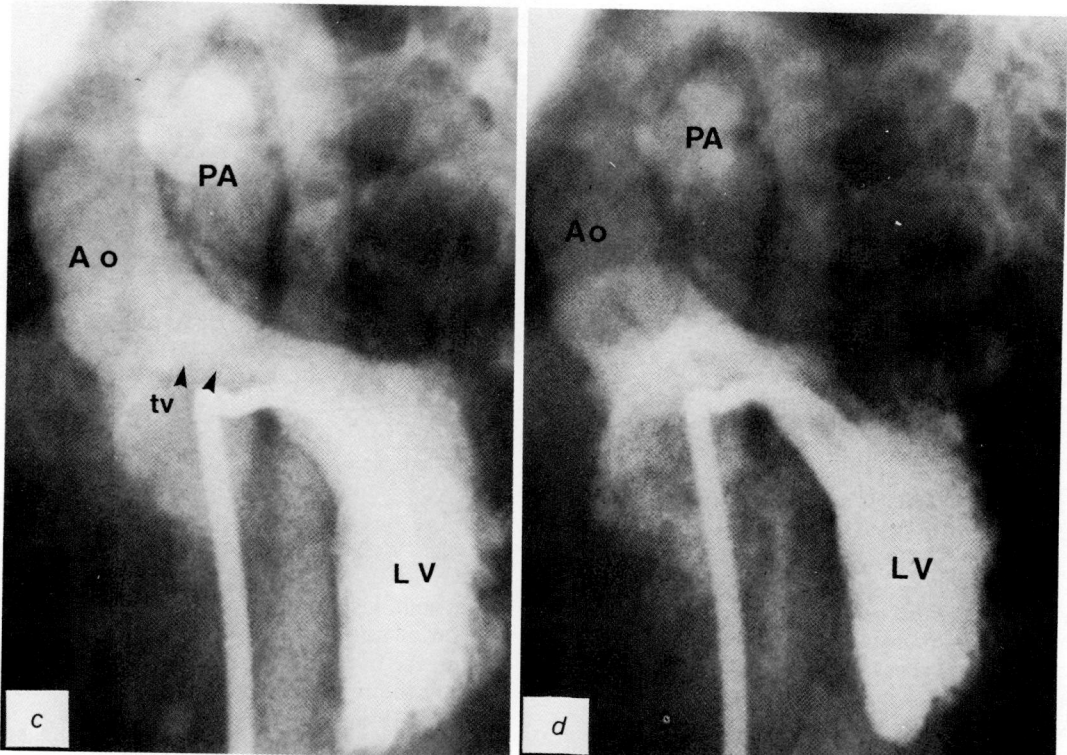

Figure 40-9 Cineangiograms in a patient with simple DORV with a perimembranous VSD (UAB).
(a) Left ventriculogram in an elongated RAO view. The infundibular septum is well shown.
(b) Four-chambered view. The VSD is perimembranous, and abuts the tricuspid valve.
(c) Left ventriculogram in the four-chambered view of another patient in whom the VSD is separated from the tricuspid valve (indicated by arrows) by a bar of muscle (UAB).
(d) This is from the same cineangiogram a few frames later.

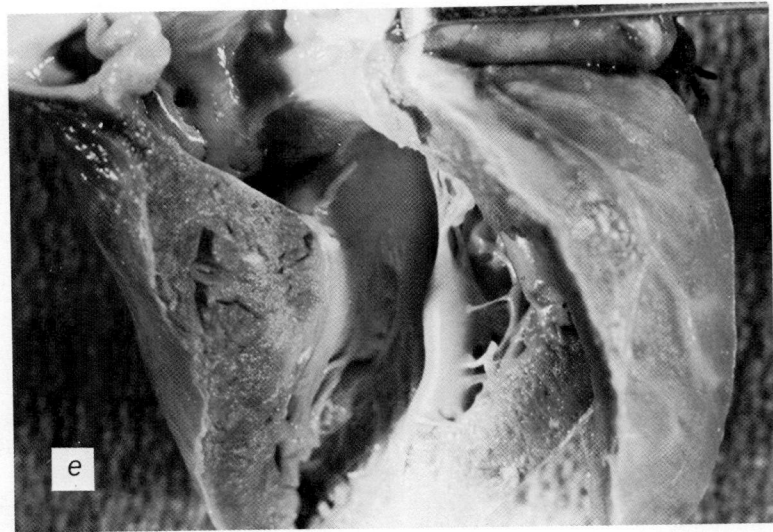

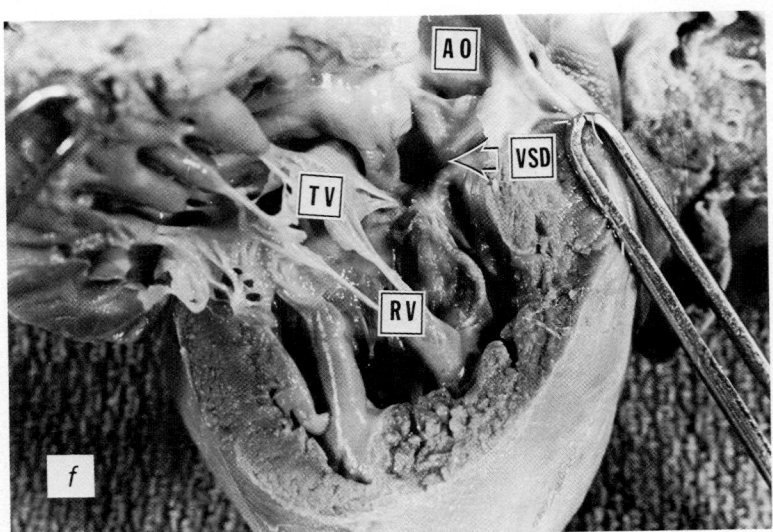

Figure 40-9 *(continued)*
(e) Specimen illustrating DORV of the same type as shown in *c* and *d* (UAB), viewed from the left ventricular aspect.
(f) The same specimen viewed from the right ventricular aspect. Note the rim of muscle between the VSD and the tricuspid valve.

Ao, aorta; AV, aortic valve; IS, infundibular (conal) septum; LV, left ventricular; MV, mitral valve; PA, pulmonary artery; RV, right ventricle; TV, tricuspid valve; VSD, ventricular septal defect.

be replaced with limited CPB and profoundly hypothermic total circulatory arrest in infants less than 8 kg in weight (see Chapter 2, Section 4). Cold cardioplegia (see Chapter 3) may be used routinely (UAB), or omitted in favor of simple cold ischemic arrest in infants less than 8 kg in weight (GLH).

After CPB has been established and cooling begun, the perfusate temperature is made as cold as possible. Later, when the patient's temperature is 26°C, the perfusate is taken to 25°C. Soon the cardiac action becomes ineffective and the caval tapes are snugged, the right atrium is opened (in a special manner if a venous switch operation is a possibility), and a pump oxygenator sump sucker line is placed across a natural or surgically created foramen ovale into the

left atrium. Usually a thorough examination of the intraventricular anatomy can be made through the tricuspid valve, and on the basis of this the repair is planned (UAB). Occasionally the repair is performed through this approach (see "Special Situations and Controversies"). Alternatively (GLH), the right atrium is not opened early in the procedure unless the intraventricular repair is to be done through it or the intraventricular anatomy examined from this route, because a right atriotomy prevents effective external cardiac cooling by irrigation of the pericardial space with cold electrolyte solution during aortic cross-clamping. Therefore, the left atrial suction line is normally positioned through a purse-string stitch placed in the base of the right superior pulmo-

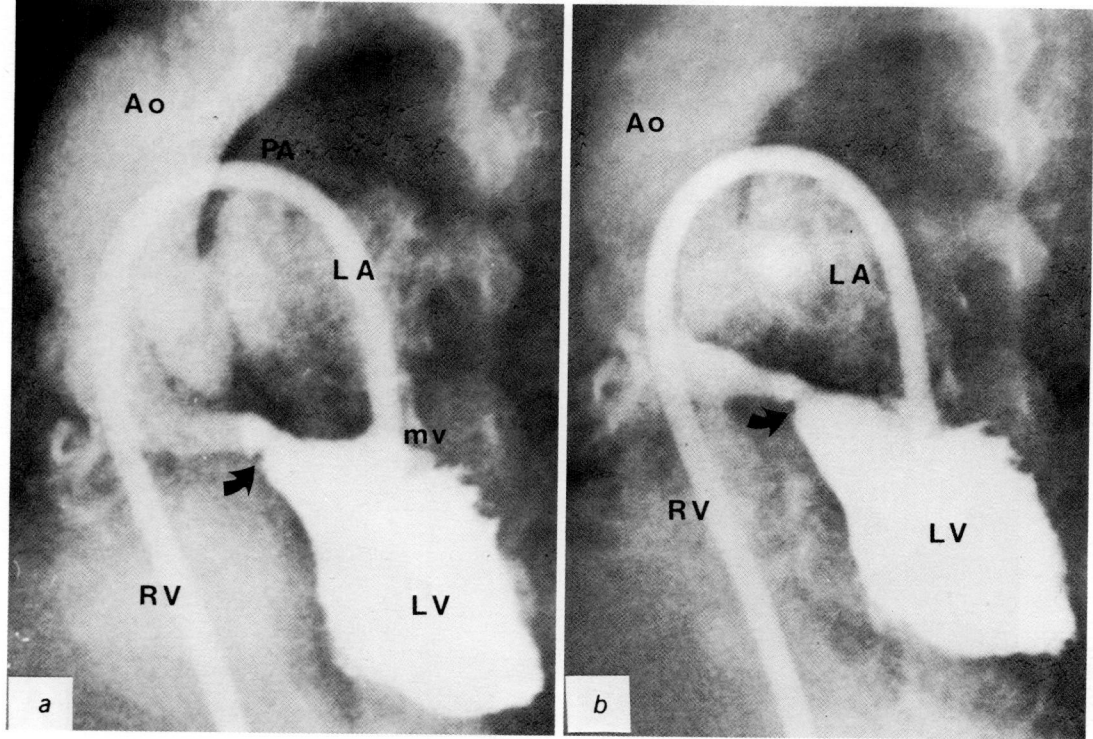

Figure 40-10   Cineangiogram in a patient with simple DORV and a restrictive subaortic VSD (UAB). (a) An early phase and (b) a late phase of a cineangiogram made in the long axial projection after injection into the left ventricle.

Ao, aorta; LA, left atrium; LV, left ventricle; MV, mitral valve; PA, pulmonary artery; RV, right ventricle.

nary vein. The aorta is cross-clamped, and the cold cardioplegic solution is infused if it is to be used.

Intraventricular Tunnel Repair of Simple Double Outlet Right Ventricle without Pulmonary Stenosis

For the repair of simple DORV with subaortic VSD, an intraventricular tunnel is created within the right ventricle which conducts left ventricular blood from the ventricular septal defect (VSD) to the aorta. For this, a transverse ventriculotomy is made low in the right ventricular (RV) outflow tract, unless the distance between the anterior descending coronary artery on the left and the right coronary artery on the right is not adequate in which case a vertical infundibular incision is used. Special care is required if there is an anomalous origin of the left anterior descending from the right coronary artery. Stay sutures are placed on the ventriculotomy for exposure.

The anatomy is carefully assessed, verifying the anatomic details of the diagnosis. The location and size of the VSD are noted, as well as whether it abuts the tricuspid valve or has a rim of muscle for its posterior border. The latter determines the relationship of the bundle of His to the posterior margin of the VSD. Note is made as to the subaortic and subpulmonary conuses and the position of the infundibular septum.

If the VSD is not clearly large and nonrestrictive, it is enlarged anteriorly. Before this is done, the area of the proposed enlargement is carefully examined to be certain that it

is interventricular septum and not hypertrophied and trabeculated anterior ventricular wall. Cutting into the latter places the left anterior descending coronary artery at risk of damage and risks the development of a false aneurysm of the left ventricle.[E3] Generally, a simple incision made anteriorly from the VSD suffices to enlarge the defect, but occasionally some muscle must be excised.

The VSD patch is then cut from a knitted or woven double velour Dacron tube. The geometry of the patch is critically important in preventing subaortic stenosis after the repair (Fig. 40-12). The patch will form the anterior half of the tunnel connecting the VSD to the aortic orifice; the posterior half of the tunnel will be the heart tissue itself, and experience indicates that this provides adequately for the growth of the tunnel. Thus, the initial trimming is made to retain about one-half to two-thirds of the circumference of the tube graft, which was selected so as to have a diameter about 20% greater than of the ascending aorta. The patch is then trimmed so that its *length* is the distance from the anterior angle of the VSD to the anterior edge of the subaortic conus (or if this is hypoplastic the aortic valve anulus).

The technique for insertion of the patch for the intraventricular tunnel is analogous to that for inserting the VSD repair patch in isolated VSD (see Chapter 20, Figs. 20-23 and 20-24) or tetralogy of Fallot (see Chapter 23, Figs. 23-25 and 23-26). Since the correct orientation of the patch is essential to the creation of a geometrically correct tunnel between left ventricle and aorta, a marking stitch is placed at the most

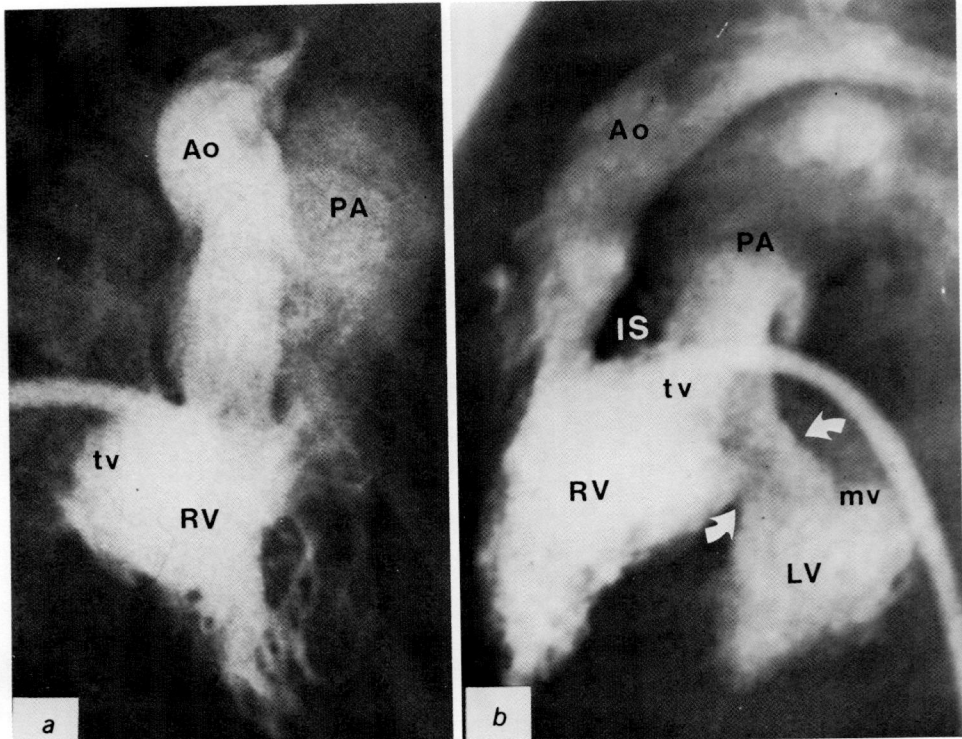

Figure 40-11 Cineangiogram made in an elongated RAO view (a) and in a long axial view (b) in a patient with the Taussig-Bing heart (UAB). The prominent infundibular septum is seen between the aorta and the pulmonary artery, but it is clearly not interventricular in position. The VSD is between the arrows. The pulmonary artery somewhat overrides the VSD.

Ao, aorta; IS, infundibular (conal) septum; LV, left ventricle; MV, mitral valve; PA, pulmonary artery; RV, right ventricle; TV, tricuspid valve.

anterior part of the repair, and one is placed through the patch at a similar point. A similar marking stitch is placed over the midportion of the aorta and in the patch. The first pledgetted mattress stitch is passed from atrial to ventricular side through the base of the tricuspid commissural tissue between anterior and septal leaflets (Fig. 40-12). (If a bar of muscle separates the VSD from the tricuspid anulus, the sutures may be placed just on the right side of the edge of this muscle, as in a similar anatomic situation in tetralogy of Fallot; see Chapter 23, Fig. 23-17). The suturing is carried to the left for a short distance between patch and tricuspid leaflet tissue and after a few stitches between patch and ventriculo-infundibular fold and up along the right side of the subaortic infundibulum. When the marking stitch is reached, the suture is held. With the other arm of the suture, the patch is sewn to the right ventricular side of the septum, 5–7 mm back from the edge of the VSD, proceeding anteriorly and then superiorly (Fig. 40-12). When the repair is completed, the contoured Dacron patch forms the anterior portion of an unobstructed intraventricular tunnel between VSD and the aorta.

As the right ventriculotomy incision is being closed, rewarming of the patient by the perfusate is begun. The left atrial sucker is removed from across the foramen ovale, and the interatrial communication is closed with a few sutures. With strong suction on the aortic needle vent, the aortic

clamp is removed and the intracardiac sucker is used to remove blood from the right atrium. The right atriotomy is closed, and the caval tapes are loosened.

The remainder of the operation is carried out as usual (see Chapter 2, Section 3). In addition to the usual measurements, left ventricular and aortic pressures are measured to exclude any gradient across the baffle; when the repair is done as described, none is present.

Repair of Simple Double Outlet Right Ventricle with Pulmonary Stenosis

The repair of the pulmonary stenosis is entirely similar to that described for the tetralogy of Fallot (see Chapter 23, "Technique of Operation"). The initial steps of the operation are the same as described for simple DORV without pulmonary stenosis, except that the woven Dacron tube is preclotted (UAB) or a pericardial patch is prepared (GLH). In this setting, a vertical right ventriculotomy may be made routinely (UAB), or a transverse ventriculotomy may be used if preliminary angiographic assessment shows a pulmonary valve and ring of adequate size (GLH).

An infundibular dissection and resection are performed (see Chapter 23, Figs. 23-25 and 23-26). If valvar pulmonary stenosis is present, valvotomy is done through a pulmonary arteriotomy (UAB) or from below (GLH,UAB) (see Chapter

23, Fig. 23-27). The pulmonary valve ring is sized with Hegar dilators, and the decision as to a valved extracardiac conduit or a transannular patch is made according to the tetralogy rules (see Chapter 23, ''General Plan and Details Common to All Approaches,'' in Section 1, Technique of Operation). If a transannular patch is elected, the incision is carried across the anulus now, since this improves the intraventricular exposure. The intraventricular tunnel repair is then made as described above.

If a conduit or transannular patch is not required, a vertical ventriculotomy is closed with a Dacron patch, tailored and sewed into place as in the tetralogy (UAB) (see Chapter 23, Fig. 23-27); or a transverse incision is closed by direct suture (GLH). Rewarming is begun as this suturing is completed, and the remainder of the operation is completed as in simple DORV without pulmonary stenosis. After discontinuing CPB, measurements are made to be certain the post-repair $P_{RV/LV}$ is satisfactory (see Chapter 23, ''General Plan and Details Common to All Approaches'' in Section 1, Tech-

nique of Operation). If a transannular patch is used, it is placed as in the tetralogy of Fallot (see Chapter 23, Fig. 23-28). If there is pulmonary atresia or for other reasons a conduit is elected, a homograft valved extracardiac conduit is placed (see Chapter 23, Figs. 23-36 and 23-37).

Intraventricular Repair of the Taussig-Bing Heart

When repair by the ideal completely intraventricular technique is contemplated,[A1,K1,P1,S9,Y1] the caval tapes are snugged after CPB has been established and the heart made ineffective by the cooling, the right atrium opened, and a pump oxygenator sump sucker placed across a patent or surgically created foramen ovale. The aorta is cross-clamped and the cold cardioplegic solution injected. The morphology within the right ventricle is assessed through the tricuspid valve. Although the limits to the intraventricular repair of the Taussig-Bing heart have not been established, it is made

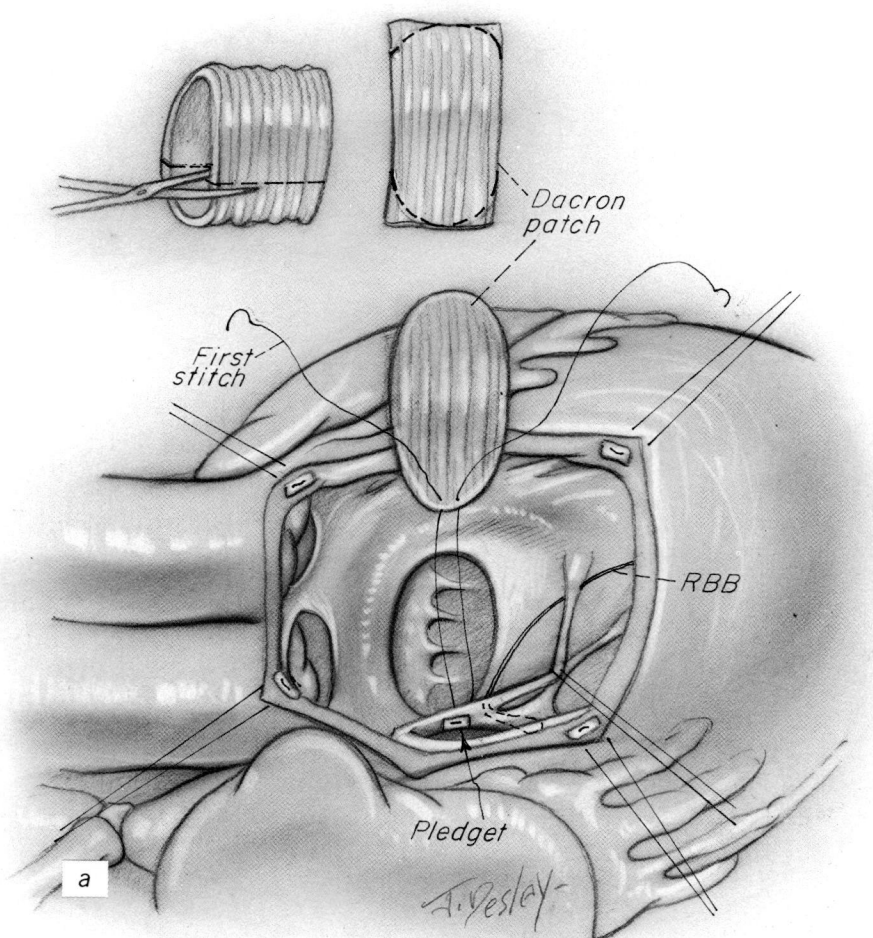

Figure 40-12 Intraventricular tunnel repair for simple DORV with subaortic VSD. (a) The perimembranous VSD has been exposed through a right ventriculotomy. A Dacron tube of a diameter about 20% larger than that of the aortic root has been cut to a length that is the same as the distance from the anterior border of the VSD to the aortic valve. It is contoured as shown in the drawing. A pledgetted mattress suture is placed through the base of the commissure between septal and anterior leaflet to begin the tunnel repair.

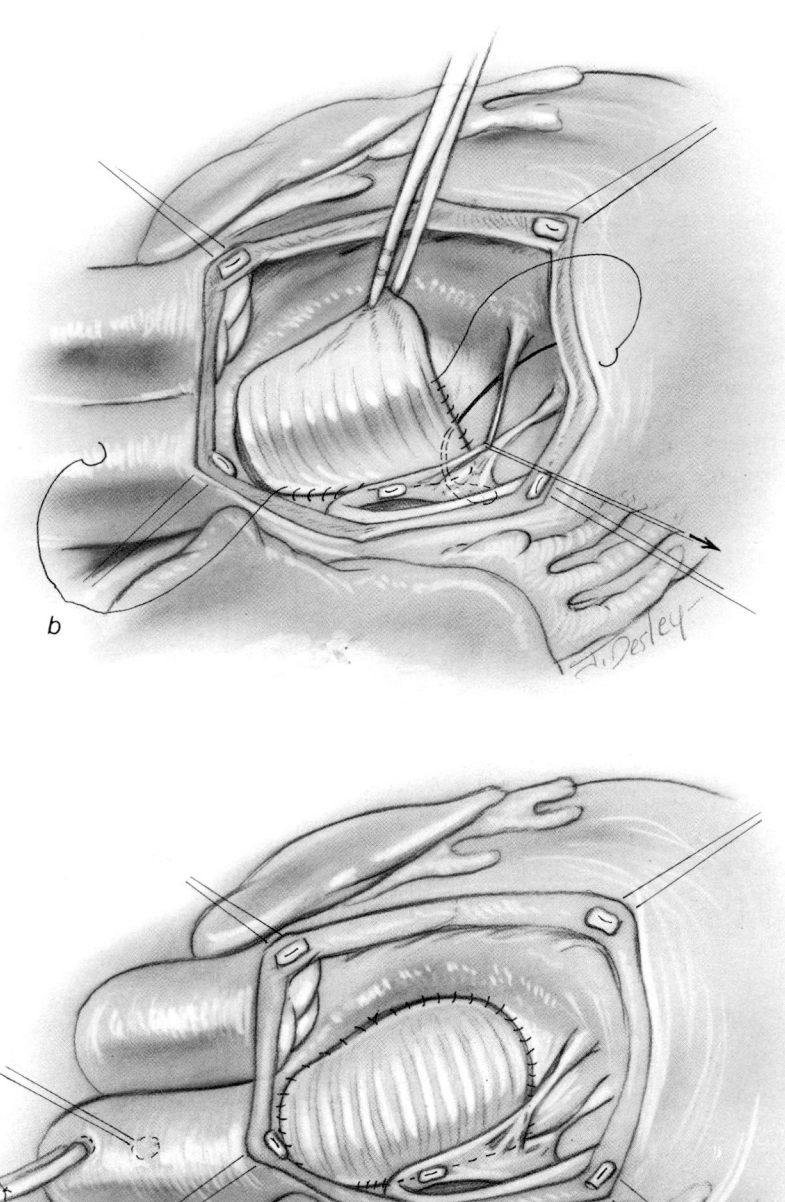

Figure 40-12 (*continued*)
(*b*) The suturing has been carried to the left along the ventriculo-infundibular fold and up over the subaortic conus.
(*c*) With the other arm of the suture, the inferior and superior portions of the repair are completed (see text for details). The contoured tunnel offers no obstruction to flow from left ventricle to aorta.
RBB, right bundle branch.

at least difficult in some by tricuspid chordal attachment to the infundibular septum.[Q2] If an intraventricular repair is deemed feasible, it may be done from the right atrium but is generally carried out through a right ventriculotomy.

The right ventricle is opened longitudinally in part to allow the placement of a patch in the ventriculotomy should this be necessary to enlarge the right ventricular access to the pulmonary valve. At least when the great arteries are side by side, the infundibular septum is in the sagittal plane between aorta and pulmonary artery and directly obstructs the pathway between the VSD and the aorta. As noted earlier, the infundibular septum is *not* interventricular in position nor does it contain conduction tissue, and it is excised as the first step in the repair. Additional muscle along the pathway may also need to be resected.[P1] An intraventricular tunnel conducting blood from the VSD to the aorta is then created in a fashion similar to the procedure used in simple DORV, but the Dacron patch is contoured slightly differently (Fig. 40-13). The precautions with regard to avoidance of damage to the bundle of His are identical to those in creating the intraventricular tunnel in simple DORV, but usually in the Taussig-Bing heart a bar of muscle does separate the VSD from the tricuspid valve.

The details of the creation of the intraventricular tunnel vary from patient to patient because of the variations in the intraventricular anatomy. Occasionally the intraventricular tunnel repair is made anteriorly to the subpulmonary area.[M8,P1]

In absence of pulmonary stenosis, right ventricular access to the pulmonary valve can often be maintained after the tunnel has been completed and the right ventricular incision closed with or without a patch. Otherwise, a valved extracardiac conduit is placed between right ventricle and pulmonary artery (see Chapter 23).

With strong suction on the aortic needle vent, the aortic clamp is released and rewarming is begun. The remainder of the operation is completed as in simple DORV.

Repair of the Taussig-Bing Heart by an Arterial Switch Procedure

When the operation is likely to be either repair of the VSD so that the left ventricle ejects into the pulmonary artery plus an arterial switch or a completely intraventricular tunnel repair, the required dissections of the aorta, pulmonary artery and bifurcation, and ductus arteriosus are made before CPB. A right atriotomy is made, and the position of the infundibular septum and the interrelations between it, the VSD, the aortic valve, the pulmonary valve, and particularly the tricuspid tensor apparatus are carefully evaluated through the tricuspid valve. If a completely intraventricular repair is not elected, the VSD is closed so that the LV ejects into the pulmonary artery. An arterial switch procedure is then performed[B1,Q1,S5] (see Chapter 39, "Arterial Switch Operation" in section on Technique of Operation).

Repair of the Taussig-Bing Heart by an Atrial Switch Procedure

There are situations, particularly in older children, in which an atrial switch procedure may still be useful for the repair of the Taussig-Bing heart. Such situations include left ventricular hypoplasia with or without a straddling mitral valve and important left ventricular outflow obstruction (see "Morphology"). These situations should be identified preoperatively or by examination of the interior of the right ventricle through the right atrium and tricuspid valve and a right ventriculotomy *avoided*. The VSD repair, or septation procedure if needed because of mitral valve straddling, can be performed through the right atrium or, occasionally, in the case of the VSD repair, through the large pulmonary artery.[O1]

The operation is begun through the incision mandated by the venous switch procedure to be used (see Chapter 39, "Atrial Switch Operation (Senning Technique)" in section on Technique of Operation). Working through the tricuspid valve, the VSD is repaired so that the left ventricle (LV) ejects into the pulmonary artery (PA). An atrial switch procedure is done (see Chapter 39). When important left ventricular outflow obstruction is present, a homograft-valved extracardiac conduit is also placed between the LV and PA (see Chapter 39, "Atrial Switch Operation Plus Repair of Left Ventricular Outflow Tract Obstruction" in section on Technique of Operation).

With strong suction on the aortic needle vent, the aortic clamp is released and rewarming is begun. The remainder of the procedure is carried out in the usual manner.

Repair of Double Outlet Right Ventricle with Doubly Committed Ventricular Septal Defect

After establishing CPB and cold cardioplegia, a transverse right ventriculotomy is made; when pulmonary stenosis coexists a vertical ventriculotomy is used (UAB). A slightly modified tunnel repair is usually done, very much as described in "Intraventricular Tunnel Repair for Simple Double Outlet Right Ventricle." However, when the two semilunar valves lie side by side and the pulmonary ring is the larger, contouring the patch to achieve this may be difficult without obstructing flow into the pulmonary artery. This problem can be minimized by enlarging the VSD anteriorly as much as possible before placing the patch. When there is pulmonary stenosis that cannot be relieved directly, the outflow to the pulmonary artery is enlarged with a transannular patch. If this is inadequate, or electively (UAB), a bypassing homograft-valved conduit is placed from pulmonary artery to right ventricle (see Chapter 23, Figs. 23-36 and 23-37).

Repair of Double Outlet Right Ventricle with Noncommitted Ventricular Septal Defect

The operation proceeds as described for simple DORV. In most patients the operative procedure can be decided upon only after the right ventricle has been opened.

When the noncommitted VSD is of the so-called "AV canal type" of perimembranous VSD (see Chapter 20, "Ventricular Septal Defect beneath Tricuspid Septal Leaflet" in Section 1, Morphology), it extends beneath the tricuspid septal leaflet rather than anteriorly or superiorly. Often, it is possible to enlarge this defect anteriorly and superiorly (Fig. 40-14) so that a tunnel repair can be per-

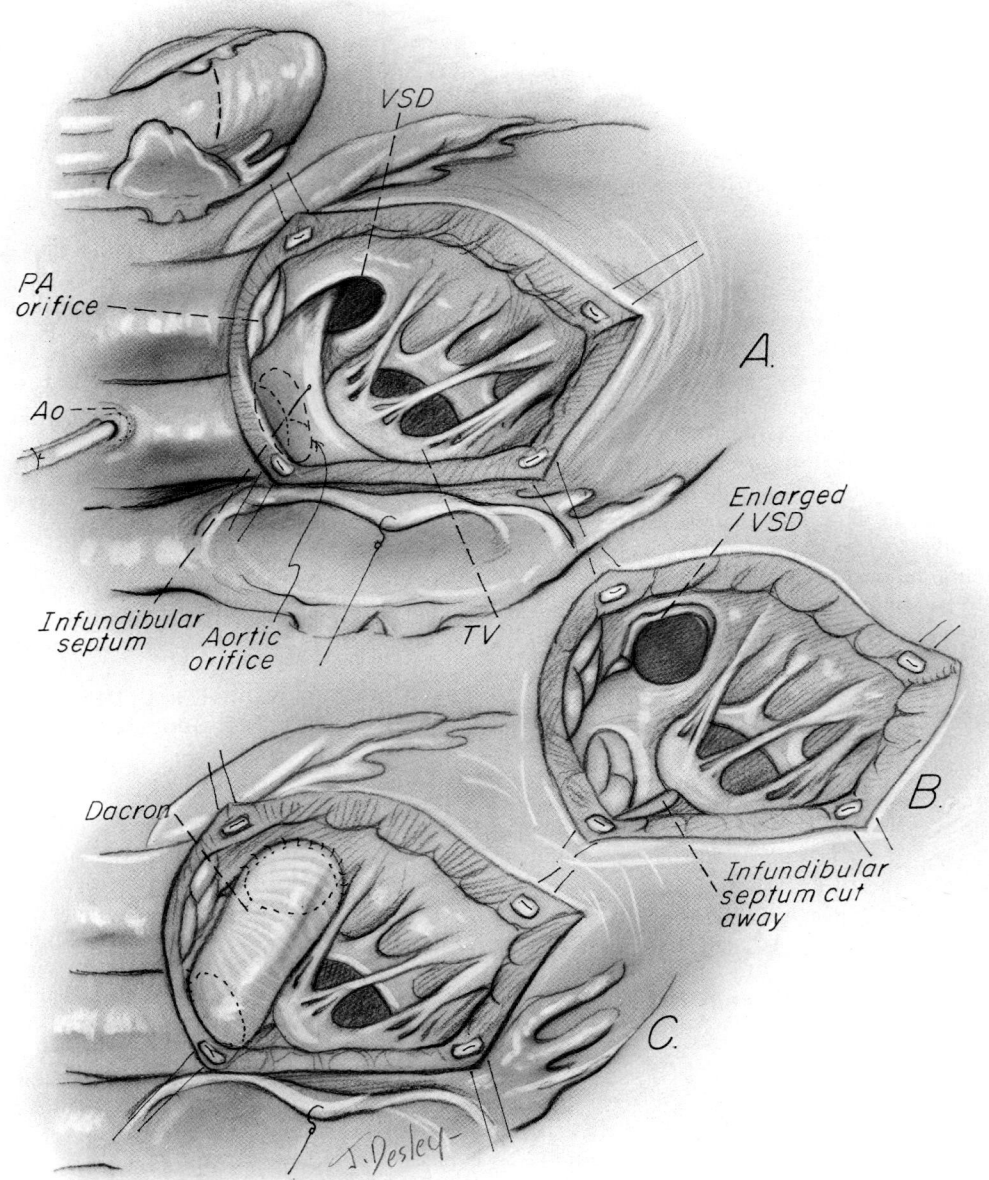

Figure 40-13 Intraventricular tunnel repair of the Taussig-Bing heart. In the case illustrated, the great arteries are side by side, with the aorta to the right of the pulmonary artery.

(a) The right ventricle is opened through a transverse incision, sited as is shown in the upper inset. In the case illustrated, the tricuspid valve apparatus is away from the infundibular septum and VSD, which facilitates the intraventricular repair.

(b) The VSD is enlarged by excising the ventricular septum anteriorly, and the infundibular septum is partially cut away to provide better access of the intraventricular tunnel to the aortic orifice.

(c) The intraventricular tunnel repair is complete, an appropriately sized and shaped patch (made from a Dacron tube—see Fig. 40-12) having been sewn in place. The tunnel conducts blood from left ventricle to aorta.

Ao, aorta; PA, pulmonary artery; TV, tricuspid valve; VSD, ventricular septal defect.

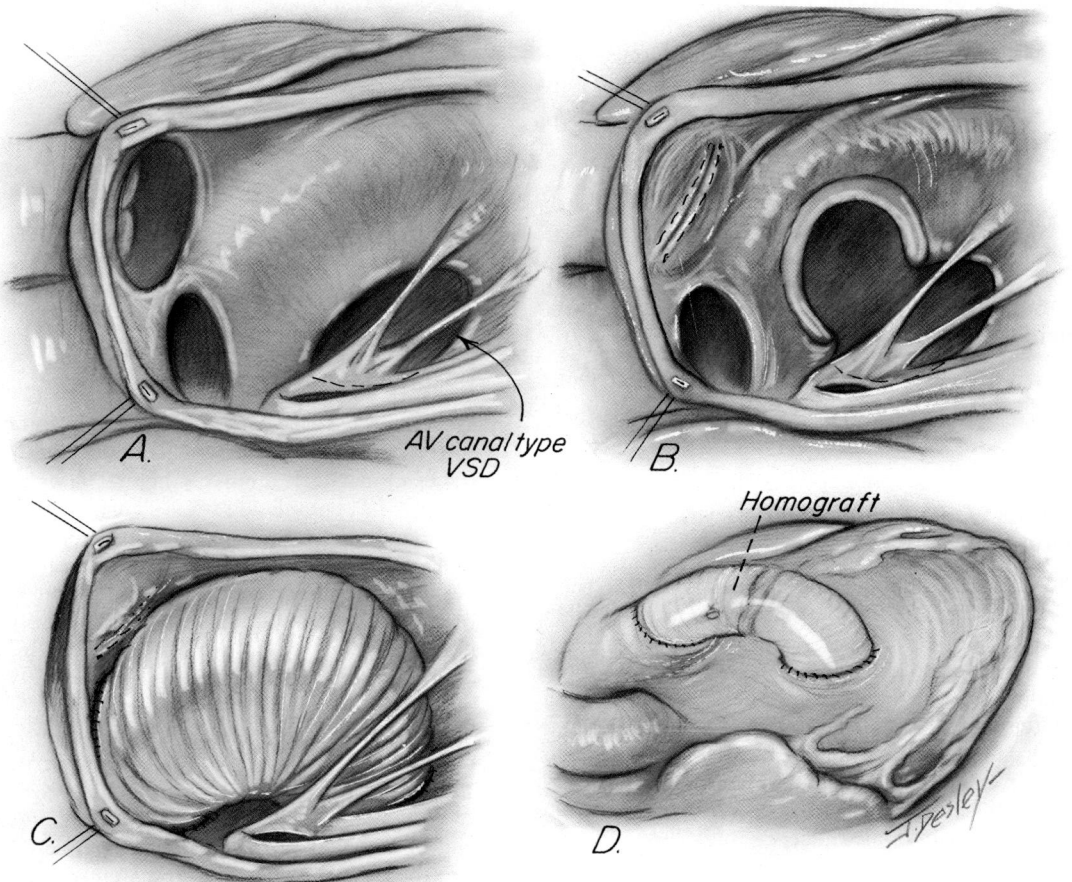

Figure 40-14 Repair of DORV with noncommitted AV canal-type VSD.
(a) The VSD is noncommitted, but typically is not far from being either subaortic or subpulmonary.
(b) The VSD has been enlarged anteriorly, after visualizing the mitral apparatus and being certain not to damage the anterior free wall and the anterior descending coronary artery with the enlargement.
(c) An intraventricular tunnel repair is made. In the case illustrated, the pulmonary artery is left on the right ventricular side, but the tunnel partially obstructs the approach to it. In some others, an appropriate tunnel cannot be made except by leaving the pulmonary artery on the left ventricular side of the tunnel; in such cases, the entry into the pulmonary artery is closed off before making the tunnel repair, or the pulmonary trunk is divided when the conduit is placed.
(d) Right ventricular–pulmonary artery continuity is established with a homograft-valved extracardiac conduit.

AV, atrioventricular; VSD, ventricular septal defect.

formed, which connects the LV to the aorta. The precautions used against damage to the conduction system are those used for the repair of AV canal-type VSD (see Chapter 20, Fig. 20-26). If the tunnel obstructs access to the pulmonary valve, a homograft-valved conduit is placed from RV to pulmonary artery.

In some patients with an AV canal type of noncommitted VSD, tricuspid valve chordae may overhang the defect so that its enlargement as described is not possible, and then a tunnel repair cannot be carried out. The same situation may exist when there is a large single or multiple muscular VSD in the trabecular septum. *When pulmonary stenosis is present,* a Fontan-type repair is carried out. The pulmonary

trunk is disconnected from the RV and the proximal end closed. The distal end is brought beneath the aorta to the right side and anastomosed to a wide opening in the roof of the atrial septum. The atrial septum is repositioned and closed so that the cavae drain through this anastomosis and the pulmonary veins drain through the mitral valve. The tricuspid valve is closed. (For details of this surgical procedure, see Chapter 26, ''Direct Right Atrial to Pulmonary Artery Connection'' in section on Technique of Operation and Chapter 44, ''Fontan-Type Procedure'' in section on Technique of Operation.) If the noncommitted VSD is not completely nonrestrictive, it is enlarged.

When the tunnel repair cannot be made, *and pulmonary*

stenosis is absent the Fontan-type repair is not feasible. Instead, the VSD is closed and either (1) the pulmonary valve is surgically closed, a homograft-valved extracardiac conduit placed between left ventricle and pulmonary artery (see Chapter 39, "Atrial Switch Operation Plus Repair of Left Ventricular Outflow Tract Obstruction" in section on Technique of Operation), and an atrial switch operation performed, or (2) the VSD is closed, the aortic valve is closed, and a valved conduit is placed between the LV and the ascending or descending thoracic aorta.

Repair of Double Outlet Right Ventricle with Complete Atrioventricular Canal

This operation is discussed in Chapter 19, "Repair with Double Outlet Right Ventricle" in section on Technique of Operation.

Repair of Double Outlet Right Ventricle with L-Malposition of the Aorta

In nearly all surgical patients in this subset, the VSD is subaortic. The heart is opened by a vertical incision in the right ventricle. Usually, the VSD is easily visualized anterosuperiorly in the ventricular septum and well away from the tricuspid anulus. An intraventricular tunnel repair with a contoured patch may not be necessary, and a simple knitted Dacron velour patch may be used to close the VSD in such a way that the left ventricle ejects into the aorta. Stitches may be placed along the edge of the VSD posteriorly unless the defect abuts the tricuspid valve (see Chapter 23). A homograft-valved extracardiac conduit is nearly always placed between right ventricle and pulmonary artery, because of associated severe pulmonary and subpulmonary stenosis (see Chapter 23, Figs. 23-36 and 23-37).

Palliative Operations

Shunting operations are described in Chapter 23 (see "Technique of Shunting Operations" in Section 1, Technique of Operation) and atrial septectomy in Chapter 39 (see "Blalock-Hanlon Operation" in section on Technique of Operation).

SPECIAL FEATURES OF POSTOPERATIVE CARE

The care after corrective or palliative operations is that described in Chapter 5.

EARLY RESULTS

Hospital Mortality

Over the past 30 years, the overall hospital mortality after the repair of the various types of double outlet right ventricle (DORV) has been relatively high. Thus, among 139 patients (UAB-GLH combined series, Tables 40-6 and 40-7) undergoing repair for DORV and AV concordant connection, 42 patients (30%, CL 26%–35%) died in the hospital. Our earlier Mayo Clinic experience was similar and is included in the report by Gomes and associates[G1,G2] and in other publications.[H1,K2,K3,K5] In almost all cases, death has been associated with acute or subacute heart failure with low cardiac output.

In the recent era and particularly in certain subsets of patients, the mortality is low. Thus, in the era 1978–July 1982, 2 hospital deaths (9%, CL 3%–19%) occurred among 23 patients undergoing repair of DORV and subaortic VSD, and one of these had coexisting complete AV canal defect and the other severe subaortic stenosis (UAB; Table 40-6). All those without pulmonary stenosis in the subaortic VSD group were under 2 years of age at operation (Table 40-8). The experience in this subset from GLH (1967–1984) is similar, the hospital mortality being 6% (Table 40-9). A low mortality in similar patients has also been reported from Toronto (1 death in 17 patients),[H3] although the youngest patient in their series was 1.7 years.

Throughout the 1967–1982 era, when an atrial switch oper-

Table 40-6   Hospital mortality after repair of DORV (UAB; 1967–July 1982; $n = 98$).

| | | 1967–1978 | | | | 1978–July 1982 | | | | Total | | |
| | | Hospital Deaths | | | | Hospital Deaths | | | | Hospital Deaths | | |
Position of VSD	n	No.	%	CL	n	No.	%	CL	n	No.	%	CL
Subaortic	28	12	43%	32%–54%	23	2[a]	9%	3%–19%	51	14	27%	21%–35%
Subpulmonary	20	6	30%	19%–44%	7	5[b]	71%	45%–90%	27	11	41%	30%–53%
Doubly committed	7	0	0%	0%–24%	1	0	0%	0%–85%	8	0	0%	0%–21%
Noncommitted	6	4	67%	38%–88%	6	0	0%	0%–27%	12	4	33%	18%–52%
Total	61	22	36%	29%–43%	37	7	19%	12%–28%	98	29	30%	25%–35%
$P(\chi^2)$			.06				.001				.16	

KEY: CL, 70% confidence limits; VSD, ventricular septal defect.

NOTE: The discrepancy between this table and those in the paper by Piccoli et al.[P2] results from recent deletion of one patient (who lived) from the DORV group because he is now considered to have tetralogy and the recent discovery in the files of an additional patient (who died) with DORV.

[a]One, age 30, had coexisting complete AV canal with common atrium and pulmonary stenosis; repair included a valved extracardiac conduit and left AV valve replacement. The other, age 8 months, had coexisting subaortic stenosis, and died with hemorrhagic pulmonary edema with low left atrial pressures.

[b]Ages 1, 1.8, 2.5, 8, and 13 months at VSD repair and atrial switch operation.

Table 40-7 Hospital death after the repair of DORV in patients with AV concordant (top four columns) or discordant connection (GLH; 1958–1984). There were no examples of L-malposition in patients with AV concordant connection.

Type of VSD	n	No.	%	CL
		Hospital Deaths		
Subaortic	23	6	26%	16%–39%
Doubly committed	6	2	33%	12%–62%
Subpulmonary (Taussig-Bing)	6	3	50%	24%–76%
Noncommitted	6	2	33%	12%–62%
Total	41	13	32%	24%–41%
$P(\chi^2)$			.7	
AV discordant connection (SLL)	3[a]	0	0%	0%–47%

KEY: AV, atrioventricular; CL, 70% confidence limits; VSD, ventricular septal defect.

[a] VSD closure and extracardiac conduit (LV → PA) in all three; two of the three had dextrocardia.

Table 40-9 Hospital mortality after surgical correction of simple DORV with subaortic VSD in the current era (GLH; 1967–1984). Thirteen of the patients had pulmonary stenosis (with one Waterston shunt performed elsewhere) and one had pulmonary atresia (with a previously performed Gore-Tex shunt).

Age (mo) ≤ <	n	No.	%	CL
		Hospital Deaths		
6	3[a]	0	0%	0%–47%
6 --- 12	3	0	0%	0%–47%
12 --- 24	7	1	14%	2%–41%
24	4	0	0%	0%–38%
Total	17	1	6%	0.8%–19%

KEY: CL, 70% confidence limits.

NOTE: This table excludes two patients with left ventricular hypoplasia and mitral valve hypoplasia or incompetence (aged 3 months and 7 years) who died.

[a] Aged 2, 3, and 4 months.

ation has been included in the repair, the hospital mortality has been high (Table 40-10), as it has been in experiences of others.[H3,P2,S3] This experience plus the reports of Yacoub and Radley-Smith,[Y1] suggest that currently the hospital mortality is lowest when the repair leaves left (rather than the right) ventricle ejecting into aorta. This may be accomplished by an intraventricular tunnel repair with or without an associated procedure for pulmonary stenosis (UAB; 1978–July 1982, 1 death [5%, CL 0.6%–15%] in 22 patients, Table 40-10) or by closure of the VSD and an arterial switch

Table 40-8 Hospital mortality after surgical correction of uncomplicated simple DORV with subaortic VSD in the current era (UAB; 1978–July, 1982; n = 17).

Pulmonary Stenosis	Age (mo) ≤ <	n	No.	%	
			Hospital Deaths		
No	6	5	0		
	6 --- 12	3	1		
	12 --- 24	2	0		
Total		10	1	10%	(CL 1%–30%)
Yes	12	0	0		
	12 --- 24	3	0		
	24 --- 48	1	0		
	48 --- 120	1	0		
	120	2	0		
Total		7	0	0%	(CL 0%–24%)
Total		17	1	6%	(CL 0.8%–19%)

KEY: CL, 70% confidence limits.

NOTE: In cases with pulmonary stenosis, the repair was by resection ± right ventricular outflow tract patch (3), transannular patch (2), transannular patch with orthotopic valve (1), or valved extracardiac conduit (1). This table excludes 3 patients with subaortic VSD and complete AV canal (1 death), 1 (who lived) with subaortic DORV and aortic L-malposition and 1 (who lived) with subaortic VSD and D-malposition (anterior) of the aorta, and 1 (who lived) with subaortic VSD, superior-inferior ventricle, and D-malposition of the aorta. (See Table 40-6 for the total of the 23 patients with subaortic VSD including those just enumerated.)

operation (Yacoub and colleagues report no deaths [0%, CL 0%–38%] among 4 patients treated in this manner; Quaegebeur reports 1 death [10%, CL 1%–30%] among 10 patients).[Q3] Others have reported similarly favorable results with the arterial switch operation (see Chapter 39 for discussion of the results of the arterial switch operation).

The Fontan procedure may be used in selected patients with complex forms of DORV with good results. Three such patients have been treated in this manner, with no deaths (GLH). (See also Chapters 26 and 44 for UAB results.)

Palliative systemic-pulmonary artery shunts, either as a preliminary-to-definitive repair or as permanent palliation for uncorrectable situations, have carried a low hospital risk. One death (5%, CL 0.0%–15%) has occurred after 21 such operations for various types of DORV with pulmonary stenosis (UAB; 1967–July 1982), and the death was in a 4-day-old baby with severe origin stenosis of the left pulmonary artery and hypoplasia of the right ventricle.

Incremental Risk Factors for Hospital Death

Location of the Ventricular Septal Defect
The location of the VSD (subaortic, subpulmonary, doubly committed, noncommitted) is a risk factor currently for hospital death after repair (Table 40-11). The very low risk of repair of uncomplicated simple DORV with subaortic VSD is evident even in infants (see Table 40-8 and 40-9), and repair of DORV with doubly committed VSD is also accomplished at low risk. Even in the case of subpulmonary VSD, a similarly low mortality is predicted when the same operation is done as in the case of simple DORV (intraventricular tunnel repair conducting left ventricular blood to aorta with or without a transannular patch or valved conduit) (Table 40-12), and this is reflected in the contingency table analysis for the entire period (Table 40-13). The increased risk in patients with noncommitted VSD has been apparent no matter what repair was done (Tables 40-14 and 40-15) but seems to be less in the current era (see Table 40-6).

Table 40-10 Hospital mortality according to the type of repair of DORV (UAB; 1967–July 1982; n = 98).

Type of Repair	1967–1978				1978–July 1982				Total			
		Hospital Deaths				Hospital Deaths				Hospital Deaths		
	n	No.	%	CL	n	No.	%	CL	n	No.	%	CL
Intraventricular tunnel repair	9	2	22%	8%–45%	10[a]	1[d]	10%	1%–30%	19	3	16%	7%–29%
Intraventricular tunnel repair with pulmonary valvotomy or infundibular resection	6[a]	0	0%	0%–27%	3	0	0%	0%–47%	9	0	0%	0%–19%
Intraventricular tunnel repair with transannular patch	6	5[a]	83%	54%–98%	3[b]	0	0%	0%–47%	9	5	56%	34%–76%
Intraventricular tunnel repair with RV → PA valved extracardiac conduit	22	6	27%	17%–40%	5	0	0%	0%–32%	27	6	22%	14%–33%
Intraventricular tunnel repair with orthotopic pulmonary valve insertion	1	0	0%	0%–85%	1	0	0%	0%–85%	2	0	0%	0%–61%
Closure of VSD (leaving LV → PA) and atrial switch with or without LV → PA conduit	12	5	42%	25%–60%	7	4[d]	57%	32%–80%	19	9	47%	34%–62%
Closure of VSD, closure of PA, and LV → PA valved extracardiac conduit and atrial switch					5[c]	1	20%	3%–53%	5	1	20%	3%–53%
Closure of VSD and double conduit	1	1	100%	15%–100%	—	—			1	1	100%	15%–100%
Repair complete AV canal and DORV	4	3	75%	37%–97%	3	1[e]	33%	4%–76%	7	4	57%	32%–80%
Total	61	22	36%	29%–43%	37	7	19%	12%–28%	98	29	30%	25%–35%

KEY: AV, atrioventricular; CL, 70% confidence limits; LV, left ventricle; PA, pulmonary artery; RV, right ventricle; VSD, ventricular septal defect.

[a] One (who lived) had tricuspid valve annuloplasty.

[b] One (who lived) had repair of partial anomalous pulmonary venous connection.

[c] One (who survived) had also resection of supravalvar mitral stenosis.

[d] One had subvalvar aortic stenosis.

[e] One (who died) had left AV valve replacement.

Table 40-11 Incremental risk factors for hospital death after repair of DORV with concordant AV connection (UAB; 1967–July 1982; n = 98). The cases are those described in Table 40-6. The risk factors were obtained by multivariate logistic analysis.

Incremental Risk Factor	Logistic Coefficient ± SD	P Value
Noncommitted VSD	−1.9 ± 0.95	.05
Complete AV canal defect	3.3 ± 1.19	.006
Age (months) at operation younger age (In months)	−1.9 ± 0.56	.0005
Age	0.019 ± 0.0075	.01
Use of transannular patch	4.6 ± 1.42	.001
Use of valved extracardiac conduit (RV → PA)	2.2 ± 1.02	.03
Closure of VSD and atrial switch (with or without LV → PA conduit)	2.1 ± 0.94	.02
Aortic cross-clamp time[a]	0.05 ± 0.021	.02
Earlier date of operation (months since January 1967)	−0.026 ± 0.0118	.03
Intercept	5.3	

KEY: AV, atrioventricular; In, logarithm; SD, standard deviation; VSD, ventricular septal defect.

[a] Intercept if cardioplegia used: 0.86.

Associated Cardiac Anomalies

The incremental risk of an associated complete AV canal defect has been considerable (Tables 40-11, 40-15). Also, left ventricular hypoplasia, particularly when combined with mitral valve hypoplasia, increases the risk of repair (GLH).[B10] Significant right ventricular hypoplasia is likely to be a risk factor also.

Young Age

In the past, young age has increased the risk of repair of DORV (Table 40-11). This has been particularly striking in patients (generally with subpulmonary VSD) undergoing repair such that the aorta remained over the RV and pulmonary artery (PA) over the LV, with or without an LV to PA extracardiac conduit (Fig. 40-15); the predicted mortality at 2 months of age has been about 50%, but at 5 years of age about 1%.

An increased risk associated with young age is not present currently in patients with simple DORV (see Tables 40-8, 40-9); and Quaegebeur has demonstrated that it is not present in patients with the Taussig-Bing heart treated by an arterial switch operation.[Q3]

Technique of Repair

The *intraventricular tunnel repair* is associated with the lowest risk (Table 40-16). In patients with subaortic VSD, the

Table 40-12 Probability of hospital death after an intraventricular tunnel repair for DORV with subaortic, subpulmonary, or doubly committed VSD (UAB; 1967–July 1982; $n = 98$) obtained by solving the multivariate logistic equation (Table 40-11).

	Predicted Probability of Hospital Death after Intraventricular Tunnel Repair					
	Alone		Plus Transannular Patch		Plus Valved Extracardiac Conduit	
Age at Operation	%	CL	%	CL	%	CL
6 mo	2.3%	0.9%–5.9%	70%	40%–89%	18%	8%–36%
12 mo	0.7%	0.2%–2.1%	40%	16%–70%	6%	2%–15%
24 mo	0.2%	0.05%–0.9%	18%	6%–45%	2%	0.6%–6%
48 mo	0.09%	0.02%–0.4%	8%	2%–27%	2%	0.2%–3.0%
8 yr	0.06%	0.01%–0.3%	6%	1%–20%	0.8%	0.2%–3.0%
16 yr	0.1%	0.02%–0.5%	9%	2%–29%	0.5%	0.1%–2.1%

KEY: CL, 70% confidence limits.

NOTE: Date of operation was entered as mid-1982, aortic cross-clamp time with cardioplegia as 75 minutes, complete AV canal—no, and noncommitted VSD—no.

Table 40-13 Hospital mortality after repair of Taussig-Bing type of DORV (UAB; 1967–July 1982; $n = 28$).

		Hospital Deaths		
Type of Repair	n	No.	%	CL
Intraventricular tunnel,[a] LV → aorta	1		0%	0%–86%
Intraventricular tunnel,[a] LV → aorta plus PA closure and RV → PA VEC	8	1	12%	2%–36%
Close VSD so LV → PA, plus atrial switch	18	9	50%	36%–64%
Close VSD, plus closure PA and LV → PA VEC, and atrial switch	1	1	100%	14%–100%
Total	28	11	39%	29%–51%

(Intraventricular tunnel rows bracketed: 11%; CL 1%–33%)

KEY: CL, confidence limits; LV, left ventricle; PA, pulmonary artery; RV, right ventricle; VEC, valved extracardiac conduit; VSD, ventricular septal defect.

[a] With or without VSD enlargement.

Table 40-14 Hospital mortality after repair of DORV with noncommitted VSD (UAB; 1967–July 1982; $n = 12$).

	1967–1978				1978–July 1982				Total			
		Hospital Deaths				Hospital Deaths				Hospital Deaths		
Type of Repair	n	No.	%	CL	n	No.	%	CL	n	No.	%	CL
Intraventricular tunnel and RV → PA valved extracardiac conduit[a] (VSD enlarged in 4, PA closed in 5)	5	3	60%	29%–86%	1	0	0%	0%–85%	6	3	50%	24%–76%
Closure of VSD[b] leaving LV → PA and atrial switch (VSD enlarged)					1	0	0%	0%–85%	1	0	0%	0%–85%
Closure of VSD, closure of PA, LV → PA valved extracardiac conduit, and atrial switch					4[c]	0	0%	0%–38%	4	0	0%	0%–38%
Closure of VSD and double conduit	1	1	100%	15%–100%					1	1	100%	15%–100%
Total	6	4	67%[d]	38%–88%	6	0	0%[d]	0%–27%	12	4	33%	15%–100%

KEY: CL, 70% confidence limits.

[a] VSD enlarged in four, PA closed in five.

[b] VSD enlarged.

[c] Ages 2, 5, 6, and 7 years.

[d] P(Fisher) for difference = .03.

Table 40-15 Probability of hospital death after intraventricular tunnel repair (conducting left ventricular blood to aorta) and a right ventricle to pulmonary artery valved extracardiac conduit in patients with DORV (UAB; 1967–July 1982; *n* = 98), according to the type of VSD.

	Predicted Probability of Hospital Death According to Age at Operation					
	24 Months		4 Years		8 Years	
Type of VSD	%	CL	%	CL	%	CL
Noncommitted VSD	12%	5%–26%	5.1%	1.9%–13%	3.4%	1.2%–9.5%
Complete AV canal	34%	14%–64%	18%	6%–43%	12%	4%–34%
Others	2%	0.6%–6%	0.8%	0.2%–3.0%	0.5%	0.1%–2.1%

KEY: CL, 70% confidence limits.

NOTE: The digital nomogram is obtained from a solution of the multivariate logistic equation (Table 40-11). Date of operation was entered as mid-1982, aortic cross-clamp time 75 minutes with cardioplegia, transannular patch—no, and atrial switch—no.

only death in the current era was in an 8-month-old infant with associated subaortic stenosis (UAB) (see Table 40-8). In the UAB and GLH experience, this repair has been done only rarely in patients with the Taussig-Bing heart (subpulmonary VSD), but even when combined with an RV-to-PA-valved conduit in such patients, the risk has been about 10% (see Table 40-13).

The addition to the repair of a *valved extracardiac conduit* between right ventricle and pulmonary trunk increased the risk but less so than use of a transannular patch (see Table 40-12). However, the difference in risk between simple tun-

nel repair and tunnel repair plus valved conduit is not apparent except in infants (see Table 40-12).

Yacoub and Quaegebeur have each demonstrated that the risk is not increased when an *arterial switch* operation is used.[Q3,Y1]

Repair by closing the VSD so as to leave the aorta above the right ventricle, and either the pulmonary trunk above the left ventricle or a valved conduit between left ventricle and pulmonary trunk is of necessity accompanied by an *atrial switch procedure*. This combination has increased the risk of hospital mortality. This is particularly evident in the young; in older children the effect is less (see Fig. 40-15).

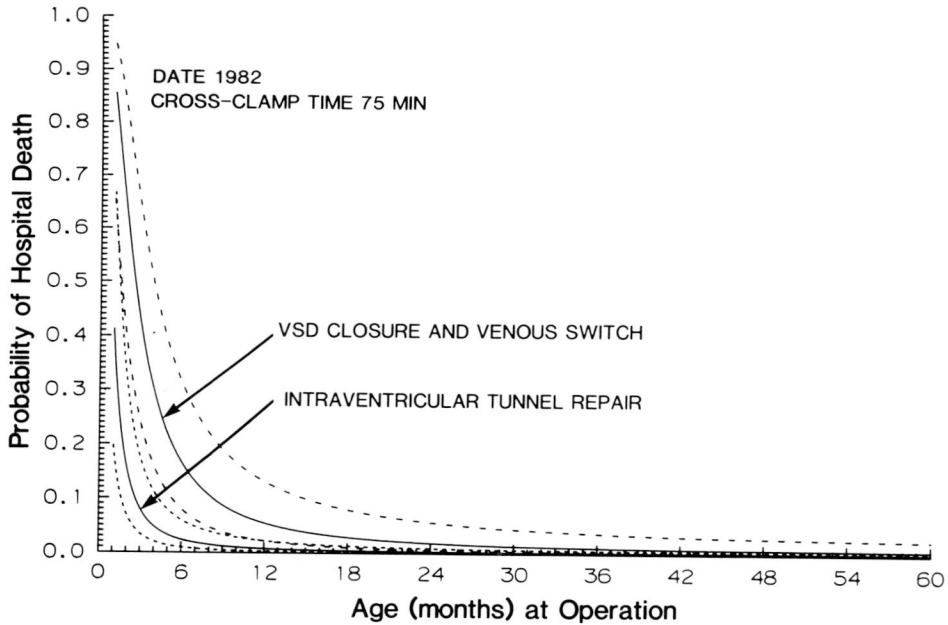

Figure 40-15 Nomogram of the probability of hospital death after repair of DORV without pulmonary stenosis, related to age at repair and to two types of repair (intraventricular tunnel repair versus VSD repair and venous [atrial] switch operation) (UAB; 1967–July 1982; *n* = 98). The dashed lines enclose the 70% confidence limits of the point estimates. The nomogram is a solution of the multivariate logistic analysis (Table 40-11). The other variables in the model were entered as follows: noncommitted VSD—no, complete AV canal defect—no, use of transannular patch—no, use of valved extracardiac RV → PA conduit—no.

Table 40-16 Probability of hospital death after repair of DORV according to type of repair and date of operation.

Type of Repair and Date of Operation	Predicted Probability of Hospital Death According to Age at Operation							
	6 Months		24 Months		4 Years		8 Years	
	%	CL	%	CL	%	CL	%	CL
Intraventricular tunnel repair								
1967	73%	28%–95%	20%	4%–62%	9%	2%–40%	6%	1%–30%
1972	36%	12%–68%	5%	1%–18%	2%	0.5%–9%	1.4%	0.3%–6%
1977	10%	4%–23%	1.1%	0.3%–3.5%	0.4%	0.1%–1.7%	0.3%	0.07%–1.2%
1982	2%	0.9%–6%	0.2%	0.05%–0.9%	0.09%	0.02%–0.4%	0.06%	0.01%–0.3%
Intraventricular tunnel repair and valved extracardiac conduit								
1967	96%	75%–99.5%	70%	26%–94%	49%	13%–86%	38%	9%–79%
1972	84%	53%–96%	32%	11%–65%	16%	5%–44%	11%	3%–32%
1977	51%	27%–75%	9%	3%–22%	4%	1.3%–11%	3%	0.8%–8%
1982	18%	8%–36%	2%	0.6%–6%	0.8%	0.2%–3.0%	0.5%	0.1%–2.1%
VSD closure and venous switch								
1967	96%	79%–99%	68%	31%–91%	47%	16%–81%	36%	11%–72%
1972	82%	59%–94%	30%	13%–56%	15%	6%–35%	10%	4%–27%
1977	49%	32%–66%	8%	4%–18%	4%	1%–9%	2%	0.8%–7%
1982	16%	8%–31%	2%	0.6%–6%	0.8%	0.2–2.9%	0.5%	0.1%–2.1%

KEY: CL, 70% confidence imits.

NOTE: The nomogram was obtained by solving the multivariate logistic equation (Table 40-11). Aortic cross-clamp time with cardioplegia was entered as 75 minutes, complete AV canal defect—no, and noncommitted VSD—no.

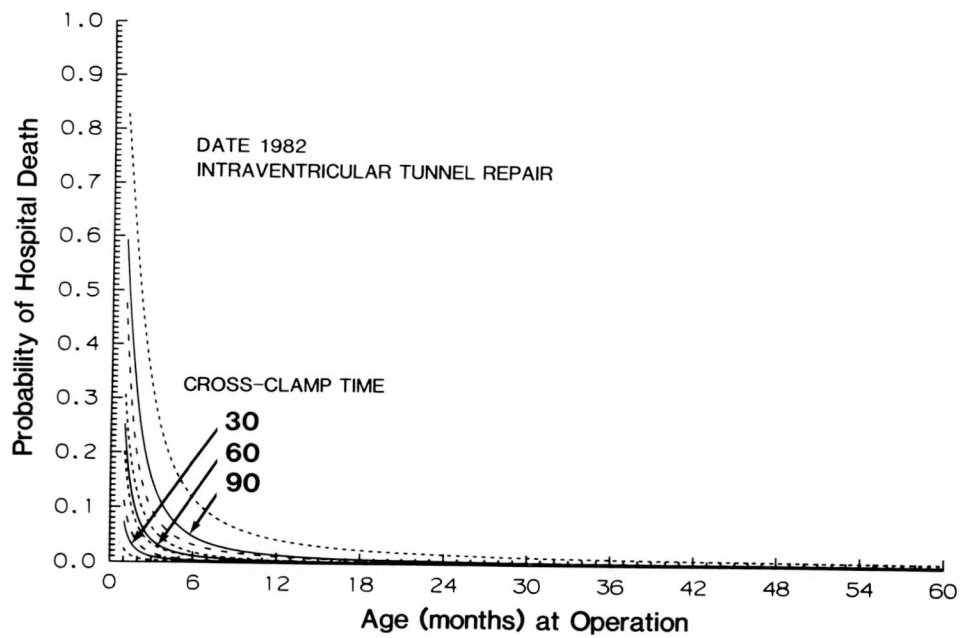

Figure 40-16 Nomogram of the probability of hospital death after repair of DORV (same types as in Fig. 40-15) related to age at repair and the aortic cross-clamp time. The presentation is as in Figure 40-15; the variables in the equation were also the same as in Figure 40-15, except that closure of VSD and atrial switch repair was entered as no, and the equation was solved for three aortic cross-clamp times.

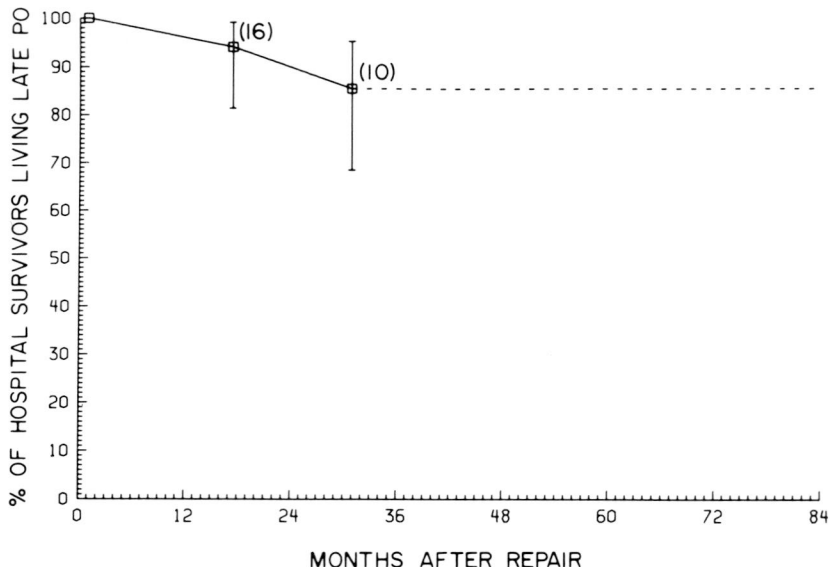

Figure 40-17   Actuarial survival of hospital survivors of repair of DORV with subaortic or doubly committed VSD. The two deaths were in patients with preoperatively severe pulmonary vascular disease.

Reproduced with permission from Stewart et al.[S3]

Time of Myocardial Ischemia (Aortic Cross-Clamp Time)
At least when cold cardioplegia has been used, longer cross-clamp times increase the risk of death. This is not a very powerful effect, but it is more evident in very young infants (Fig. 40-16).

Date of Operation
The date of operation has been a powerful risk factor, so that hospital mortalities are much lower in the current era (Tables 40-6 and 40-14). In 1985, for example, the risk of repair of simple DORV in infants and children approaches zero.[K6] Specific advances during the past 15 years that may account for the improvements include more precise and complete preoperative diagnoses, these leading to better repair with shorter operative and aortic cross-clamp times, cold cardioplegic myocardial protection, and improved surgical understandings of complex cardiac anomalies and their repair.

LATE RESULTS

Survival

The survival to date in patients after repair of *DORV with either subaortic or doubly committed VSD* has been good, although the follow-up is still relatively short and the numbers small (Fig. 40-17).[S3] Arrhythmias were an important cause of late death in the series reported by Judson and colleagues,[J1] but this has not been the GLH and UAB experience. Exercise tolerance in these patients is good, and most can lead a normal life.[H3]

In contrast, survival is much less satisfactory after repair of *DORV with subpulmonary VSD* (Taussig-Bing heart) (Fig. 40-18), all five late deaths being in patients who had an atrial switch procedure as part of the repair. In four of the five,

there was at least moderate elevation of pulmonary vascular resistance preoperatively. With earlier repair and the use of the arterial switch operation or of intraventricular tunnel repairs and of homograft-valved conduits rather than Dacron porcine conduits when these are required, long-term survival rates should improve.

Morbidity and Reoperations

Reoperation for recurrent VSD at the site of the tunnel repair has been required late postoperatively in 2 (6%) of 35 hospital survivors and in a further patient in whom multiple apical VSDs were overlooked at the time of the initial repair (GLH). Judson and colleagues have reported a reoperation incidence for VSD at the site of tunnel repair of 17%.[J1]

Infrequently, residual pulmonary stenosis requires reoperation. This was the case in 3 (9%) of 35 hospital survivors (GLH). In one, the stenosis was valvar, in another it was at the site of a Waterston shunt, and in a third reoperation was required to join a proximally occluded left pulmonary artery onto the main pulmonary artery; all these procedures were successful. Reoperation may be required for replacement of a porcine-valved conduit.[J1]

Other problems that have been reported but not recognized in the UAB and GLH series are obstruction beneath the intraventricular Dacron baffle,[C2,L8,R2] development of a false right ventricular aneurysm at the site of VSD enlargement,[E3] and nonfatal atrial and ventricular arrhythmias.[J1]

When an atrial or arterial switch operation is required, the late results are affected by complications peculiar to these procedures (see Chapter 39, "Results"). The late results and complications following the Fontan-type procedure are described in Chapter 26, section on "Late Results."

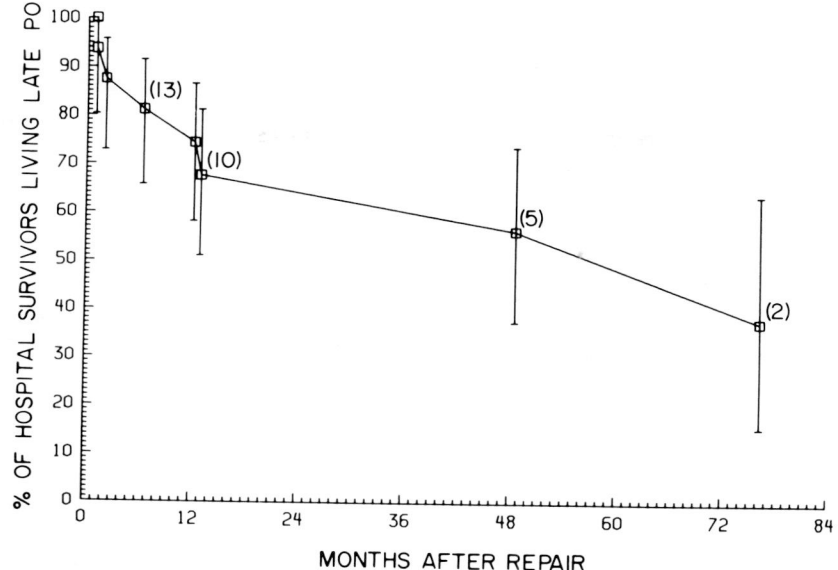

Figure 40-18 Actuarial survival of hospital survivors of repair of the Taussig-Bing heart. The late deaths were all in patients who had an atrial switch as part of the repair, and four of the five had preoperative evidence of at least moderate pulmonary vascular disease.
Reproduced with permission from Stewart et al.[S3]

Late Results of Palliative Operations

The late results after shunting procedures are the same as described for the tetralogy of Fallot (see Chapter 23) and for single ventricle (see Chapter 44). The late results of atrial septectomy depend upon the pulmonary blood flow and ventricular performance in the individual patient.[S3]

INDICATIONS FOR OPERATION

Early repair is indicated for uncomplicated simple DORV with subaortic VSD, and for DORV with doubly committed VSD, just as in the case of isolated ventricular septal defect (see Chapter 20). In the current era, operation should electively be done at about 6 months of age. If symptoms of intractable heart failure develop before this, prompt primary repair is indicated.

When simple DORV and important pulmonary stenosis coexist, the protocol is similar to that for tetralogy of Fallot, with initial shunting being reserved only for patients less than about 3 months (GLH) to 9–12 (UAB) months of age (see Chapter 23).

Patients with DORV and subpulmonary VSD (the Taussig-Bing heart) should have repair in the first 6 months of life whenever possible. An operation in which the atrial switch procedure is part of the repair should be avoided. Either an arterial switch operation or, if it is feasible, an intraventricular tunnel repair may be chosen.

In the uncommon circumstance of a patient with the Taussig-Bing heart in whom a pulmonary artery band was placed in early life and there is opportunity for surgical repair in childhood rather than infancy, in addition to the above pro-

cedures repair of the VSD so that the left ventricle ejects into the pulmonary artery and an atrial switch procedure may be used.

Patients with DORV and noncommitted VSDs are apt to require a complex operation. In view of the poor prognosis without operation, this is indicated; when possible, it is deferred until about 2 years of age.

In patients with DORV and L-malposition, pulmonary stenosis and the need for a valved extracardiac conduit are frequent (see "Coronary Arteries" in "Morphology") and the protocols used for the tetralogy of Fallot apply (see Chapter 23, "Indications for Operation" in Section 1). Patients with DORV and complete AV canal are managed by the protocols described for complete AV canal in general (see Chapter 19).

SPECIAL SITUATIONS AND CONTROVERSIES

Right Atrial Approach to Repair of Simple Double Outlet Right Ventricle

The repair of simple DORV can be accomplished through the right atrium,[C3,G3,11] although the most superior part of the repair must sometimes be made through the additional exposure afforded by a radial incision along the base of the tricuspid anterior and septal leaflets (see Chapter 20, Fig. 20-26). It is considered more difficult through the atrial approach to be certain that the geometry of the intraventricular tunnel is exactly correct. In view of this and the lack of any firm evidence of the increased safety of the atrial approach to the repair of isolated VSD (see Chapter 20) or tetralogy of Fallot (see Chapter 23), the right ventricular approach is generally used (GLH,UAB).

REFERENCES

A

1. Agarwala B, Doyle EF, Danilowicz D, Spencer FC, Mills NM: Double outlet right ventricle with pulmonic stenosis and anteriorly positioned aorta (Taussig-Bing variant). *Am J Cardiol* 32:850, 1973.

2. Anderson RH, Becker AE, Wilcox BR, Macartney FJ, Wilkinson JL: Surgical anatomy of double-outlet right ventricle—a reappraisal. *Am J Cardiol* 52:555, 1983.

3. Angelini P, Leachman RD: Spectrum of double outlet right ventricle: an embryologic interpretation. *Card Dis Bull Texas H Inst* 3:127, 1976.

4. Anderson RH, Pickering D, Brown R: Double outlet right ventricle with l-malposition and uncommitted ventricular septal defect. *Eur J Cardiol* 3/2:133, 1975.

5. Azevedo A deC, Toledo AN, deCarvalho AA, Rowbach R: Transposition of the aorta and levoposition of the pulmonary artery (Taussig-Bing syndrome). *Am Heart J* 52:249, 1956.

6. Ainger LE: Double outlet right ventricle, intact ventricular septum, mitral stenosis and blind left ventricle. *Am Heart J* 70:521, 1965.

B

1. Binet JP, Lacour-Gayet F, Conso JF, Dupuis CL, Bruntiaux J: Complete repair of the Taussig-Bing type of double-outlet right ventricle using the arterial switch operation without coronary translocation—report of one successful case. *J Thorac Cardiovasc Surg* 85:272, 1983.

2. Brandt PST, Calder AL, Barratt-Boyes BG, Neutze JM: Double outlet left ventricle: Morphology, cineangiography, diagnosis, and surgical treatment. *Am J Cardiol* 38:897, 1976.

3. Baron MG: Radiologic notes in cardiology: Angiographic differentiation between tetralogy of Fallot and double outlet right ventricle. *Circulation* 43:451, 1971.

4. Bharati S, Lev M: The conduction system in double outlet right ventricle with subpulmonic ventricular septal defect and related hearts (the Taussig-Bing group). *Circulation* 54:459, 1976.

5. Braun K, De Vries A, Feingold DS, Ehrenfeld NE, Feldman J, Schorr S: Complete dextroposition of the aorta, pulmonary stenosis, interventricular septal defect, and patent foramen ovale. *Am Heart J* 43:773, 1952.

6. Bharati S, Kirklin JW, McAllister HA, Jr., Lev M: The surgical anatomy of common atrioventricular orifice associated with tetralogy of Fallot, double outlet right ventricle and complete regular transposition. *Circulation* 61:1142, 1980.

7. Beuren A: Differential diagnosis of the Taussig-Bing heart from complete transposition of the great vessels with a posterior overriding pulmonary artery. *Circulation* 21:1071, 1960.

8. Barratt-Boyes BG, Calder AL: Double outlet ventricle: Classification and surgical management, in JC Davila (ed): *Second Henry Ford Hospital International Symposium on Cardiac Surgery*. New York: Appleton-Century-Crofts, 1977, p. 49.

9. Brandt PWT: Cineangiography of atrioventricular and ventriculo-arterial connections, in *Pediatric Cardiology*, Volume 4. London: Churchill Livingstone, 1981, p 191.

10. Barratt-Boyes BG, Kirklin JW: Surgical management of double outlet right and left ventricle, in MJ Godman (ed): *Pediatric Cardiology*, Volume 4. London: Churchill Livingstone, 1981, p 492.

11. Barratt-Boyes BG, Lowe JB, Watt WJ, Cole DS, Williams JCP: Initial experiences with extracorporeal circulation in intracardiac surgery. *Br Med J* 2:1826, 1960.

C

1. Cheng TO: Double outlet right ventricle: Diagnosis during life. *Am J Med* 32:637, 1962.

2. Chaitman BR, Grondin CM, Theroux P, Bourassa MG: Late development of left ventricular outflow tract obstruction after repair of double-outlet right ventricle. *J Thorac Cardiovasc Surg* 72:265, 1976.

3. Cherian KM, John TA, Abraham KA: Transatrial correction of origin of both great vessels from right ventricle with pulmonary hypertension. *J Thorac Cardiovasc Surg* 84:783, 1982.

4. Chiechi MA: Incomplete transposition of the great vessels with biventricular origin of the pulmonary artery (Taussig-Bing complex): Report of 4 cases and review of the literature. *Am J Med* 22:234, 1957.

D

1. Danielson GK, Ritter DG, Coleman HN III, DuShane JW: Successful repair of double-outlet right ventricle with transposition of the great arteries (aorta anterior and to the left), pulmonary stenosis, and subaortic ventricular septal defect. *J Thorac Cardiovasc Surg* 63:741, 1972.

2. de la Cruz MV, Berrazueta JR, Artega M, Attie F, Soni J: Rules for diagnosis of atrioventricular discordance and spatial identification of ventricles. *Br Heart J* 38:341, 1976.

3. Daicoff GR, Kirklin JW: Surgical correction of Taussig-Bing malformation. Report of three cases. *Am J Cardiol* 19:125, 1967 (abstr).

E

1. Engle MA, Holswade GR, Campbell WG, Goldberg HP: Ventricular septal defect with transposition of aorta masquerading as acyanotic ventricular septal defect. *Circulation* 22:745, 1960 (abstr).

2. Engle MA, Steinberg I: Angiocardiography in diagnosis of transposition of aorta with subaortic ventricular septal defect (origin of both great vessels from right ventricle). *Circulation* 24:927, 1961 (abstr).

3. Edwards WD, Wilcox WD, Danielson GK, Feldt RH: Postoperative false aneurysm of left ventricle and obstruction of left circumflex coronary artery complicating enlargement of restrictive ventricular septal defect in double-outlet right ventricle. *J Thorac Cardiovasc Surg* 80:141, 1980.

4. Elliott LP, Amplatz K, Edwards JE: Coronary arterial patterns in transposition complexes: Anatomic and angiocardiographic studies. *Am J Cardiol* 17:362, 1966.

5. Edwards WD: Double-outlet right ventricle and tetralogy of Fallot. Two distinct but not mutually exclusive entities. *J Thorac Cardiovasc Surg* 82:418, 1981 (editorial).

G

1. Gomes MMR, Weidman WH, McGoon DC, Danielson GK: Double-outlet right ventricle without pulmonic stenosis: Surgical considerations and results of operation. *Circulation* 43(suppl I):I-31, 1971.

2. Gomes MMR, Weidman WH, McGoon DC, Danielson GK: Double-outlet right ventricle with pulmonic stenosis. Surgical considerations and results of operation. *Circulation* 43:889, 1971.

3. Goor DA, Massini C, Shem-Tov A, Neufeld HN: Transatrial repair of double-outlet right ventricle in infants. *Thorax* 37:371, 1982.

4. Golan M, Hegesh J, Massini C, Goor DA: Double-outlet right ventricle associated with discrete subaortic stenosis. *Ped Cardiol* 5:157, 1984.

H

1. Hightower BM, Barcia A, Bargeron LM Jr., Kirklin JW: Double-outlet right ventricle with transposed great arteries and subpulmonary ventricular septal defect; The Taussig-Bing malformation. *Circulation* 49,50(suppl I):I-207, 1969.

2. Hagler DJ, Tajik AJ, Seward JB, Mair DD, Ritter DQ: Double outlet right ventricle. Wide angle two-dimensional echocardiographic observations. *Circulation* 63:419, 1983.

3. Harvey JC, Sondheimer HM, Williams WG, Olley PM, Trusler GA: Repair of double-outlet right ventricle. *J Thorac Cardiovasc Surg* 73:611, 1977.

4. Hinkes P, Rosenquist GC, White RI, Jr: Roentgenographic reexamination of the internal anatomy of the Taussig-Bing heart. *Am Heart J* 81:335, 1971.

I

1. Ionescu MI, Scott O, Wooler GH: Surgical treatment of acyanotic double-outlet right ventricle. *Thorax* 22:336, 1976.

J

1. Judson JP, Danielson GK, Puga FJ, Mair DD, McGoon DC: Double-outlet right ventricle. *J Thorac Cardiovasc Surg* 85:32, 1983.

2. Judson JP, Danielson GK, Ritter DG, Hagler DJ: Successful repair of coexisting double-outlet right ventricle and two-chambered right ventricle. *J Thorac Cardiovasc Surg* 84:113, 1982.

K

1. Kawashima Y, Fujita T, Miyamoto T, Manabe H: Intraventricular rerouting of blood for the correction of Taussig-Bing malformation. *J Thorac Cardiovasc Surg* 62:825, 1971.

2. Kirklin JW, Harp RA, McGoon DC: Surgical treatment of origin of both vessels from right ventricle, including cases of pulmonary stenosis. *J Thorac Cardiovasc Surg* 48:1026, 1964.

3. Kirklin JK, Castaneda AR: Surgical correction of double-outlet right ventricle with noncommitted ventricular septal defect. *J Thorac Cardiovasc Surg* 73:399, 1977.

4. Kitamura N, Takao A, Ando M, Imai Y, Konno S: Taussig-Bing heart with mitral valve straddling. *Circulation* 49:761, 1974.

5. Kiser JC, Ongley PA, Kirklin JW, Clarkson PM, McGoon DC: Surgical treatment of dextrocardia with inversion of ventricles and double-outlet right ventricle. *J Thorac Cardiovasc Surg* 55:6, 1968.

6. Kirklin JW, Blackstone EH: (1985) Unpublished data.

L

1. Lev M, Bharati S, Meng CCL, Liberthson RR, Paul MH, Idriss F: A concept of double-outlet right ventricle. *J Thorac Cardiovasc Surg* 64:271, 1972.

2. Lincoln C, Anderson RH, Shinebourne EA, English TAH, Wilkinson JL: Double outlet right ventricle with L-malposition of the aorta. *Br Heart J* 37:453, 1975.

3. Lev M, Rimoldi HJA, Eckner FAO, Melhuish BP, Meng L, Paul MH: The Taussig-Bing heart: Qualitative and quantitative anatomy. *Arch Pathol* 81:24, 1966.

4. Lavoie R, Sestier F, Gilbert G, Chameides L, Van Praagh R, Grondin P: Double outlet right ventricle with left ventricular outflow tract obstruction due to small ventricular septal defect. *Am Heart J* 82:290, 1971.

5. Lopez FN, Dobben GC, Rabinowitz M, Ferguson LA, Reisler H, Cassels DE, Lev M: Taussig-Bing complex with pulmonary stenosis. *Dis Chest* 50:1, 1966.

6. Lincoln C: Total correction of d-loop double-outlet right ventricle with bilateral conus, l-transposition, and pulmonic stenosis. *J Thorac Cardiovasc Surg* 64:435, 1972.

7. Luisi VS, Verunelli F, Eufrate S: Double outlet right ventricle, non-committed ventricular septal defect and pulmonic stenosis. Anatomical and surgical considerations. *Thorac Cardiovasc Surg* 28:368, 1980.

8. Luber JM, Castaneda AR, Lang P, Norwood WI: Repair of double-outlet right ventricle: early and late results. *Circulation* 68(suppl II):II-144, 1983.

9. Lev M, Bharati S: Transposition of the arterial trunks in levocardia, in SC Sommers (ed): *Cardiovascular Pathology Decennial 1966–1975.* New York: Appleton-Century-Crofts, 1975, p 30.

M

1. Mehrizi A: The origin of both great vessels from the right ventricle I with pulmonic stenosis. Clinico-pathological correlation in 18 autopsied cases; 11 without pulmonic stenosis. Clinico-pathological correlation in 13 autopsied cases. *Bull Johns Hop Hosp* 117:75, 1965.

2. Marin-Garcia J, Neches WH, Park SC, Lenox CC, Zuberbuhler JR, Bahnson HT: Double-outlet right ventricle with restrictive ventricular septal defect. *J Thorac Cardiovasc Surg* 76:853, 1978.

3. Mason DT, Morrow AG, Elkins RC, Friedman WF: Origin of both great vessels from the right ventricle associated with severe obstruction to left ventricular outflow. *Am J Cardiol* 24:118, 1969.

4. Marino B, Loperfido F, Sardi CS: Spontaneous closure of ventricular septal defect in a case of double outlet right ventricle. *Br Heart J* 49:608, 1983.

5. Muster AJ, Bharati S, Aziz KU, Idriss FS, Paul MH, Lev M, Carr I, DeBoer A, Anagnostopoulos C: Taussig-Bing anomaly with straddling mitral valve. *J Thorac Cardiovasc Surg* 77:832, 1979.

6. McMahon JE, Lips M: Double outlet right ventricle with intact ventricular septum. *Circulation* 30:745, 1964.

7. Macartney FJ, Rigby ML, Anderson RH, Stark J, Silverman NH: Double outlet right ventricle. Cross sectional echocardiographic findings, their anatomical explanation, and surgical relevance. *Br Heart J* 52:164, 1984.

8. Metras D, Coulibaly AO, Ouattara K: Successful intraventricular repair of Taussig-Bing anomaly in infancy. Report of a case. *J Thorac Cardiovasc Surg* 88:311, 1984.

N

1. Neufeld HN, DuShane JW, Wood EH, Kirklin JW, Edwards JE: Origin of both great vessels from the right ventricle. I. Without pulmonary stenosis. *Circulation* 23:399, 1961.

2. Neufeld HN, DuShane JW, Edwards JE: Origin of both great vessels from the right ventricle. II. With pulmonary stenosis. *Circulation* 23:603, 1961.

3. Neufeld HN, Lucas RV, Lester RG, Adams P, Anderson RC, Edwards JE: Origin of both great vessels from the right ventricle without pulmonary stenosis. *Br Heart J* 24:393, 1962.

O

1. Ottino G, Kugler JD, McNamara DG, Hallman GL: Taussig-Bing anomaly: Total repair with closure of ventricular septal defect through the pulmonary artery. *Ann Thorac Surg* 29:170, 1980.

P

1. Patrick DL, McGoon DC: Operation for double-outlet right ventricle with transposition of the great arteries. *J Cardiovasc Surg* 9:537, 1968.

2. Piccoli G, Pacifico AD, Kirklin JW, Blackstone EH, Kirklin JK, Bargeron LM Jr: Changing results and concepts in the surgical treatment of double-outlet right ventricle: Analysis of 137 operations in 126 patients. *Am J Cardiol* 52:549, 1983.

3. Parr GVS, Bharati S, Lev M, Waldhausen JA: Fetal coarctation in complete transposition of the great arteries with ventricular septal defect vs. Taussig-Bing group of hearts. Surgical significance. *Circulation* 66(suppl II):II-195, 1982 (abstr).

4. Paul MH, Van Praagh S, Van Praagh R: Transposition of the great arteries, in H Watson (ed): *Paediatric Cardiology*. London: Lloyd-Luke, 1968, p 576.

Q

1. Quaegebeur JM: The optimal repair for the Taussig-Bing heart. *J Thorac Cardiovasc Surg* 85:276, 1983 (editorial).

2. Quaegebeur JM, Bartelings M, Gittenberger-DeGroot AC: Double outlet right ventricle with sub-pulmonary ventricular septal defect: an anatomical basis for surgical repair. *Pediatr Cardiol* 5:234, 1984.

3. Quaegebeur JM: (1985) Personal communication.

R

1. Redo SF, Engle MA, Holswade GR, Goldbert HP: Operative correction of ventricular septal defect with origin of both great vessels from the right ventricle. *J Thorac Cardiovasc Surg* 45:526, 1963.

2. Rocchini AP, Rosenthal A, Castaneda AR, Keane JF, Jeresaty R: Subaortic obstruction after the use of an intracardiac baffle to tunnel the left ventricle to the aorta. *Circulation* 54:957, 1976.

S

1. Sondheimer HM, Freedom RM, Olley PM: Double outlet right ventricle: Clinical spectrum and prognosis. *Am J Cardiol* 39:709, 1977.

2. Sanders SP, Bierman FZ, Williams RG: Conotruncal malformations: Diagnosis in infancy using subxiphoid two-dimensional echocardiography. *Am J Cardiol* 50:1361, 1982.

3. Stewart RW, Kirklin JW, Pacifico AD, Blackstone EH, Bargeron LM Jr: Repair of double outlet right ventricle. An analysis of 62 cases. *J Thorac Cardiovasc Surg* 78:502, 1979.

4. Shafer AB, Lopez JF, Kline IK, Lev M: Truncal inversion with biventricular pulmonary trunk and aorta from right ventricle (variant of Taussig-Bing complex). *Circulation* 36:783, 1967.

5. Smith EEJ, Pucci JJ, Walesby RK, Oakley CM, Sapsford RN: A new technique for correction of the Taussig-Bing anomaly. *J Thorac Cardiovasc Surg* 83:901, 1982.

6. Serratto M, Arevalo F, Goldman EJ, Hastreiter A, Miller RA: Obstructive ventricular septal defect in double outlet right ventricle. *Am J Cardiol* 19:457, 1967.

7. Sridaromont S, Ritter DG, Feldt RH, Davis GD, Edwards JE: Double-outlet right ventricle. Anatomic and angiocardiographic correlations. *Mayo Clin Proc* 53:555, 1978.

8. Stridaromont S, Feldt RH, Ritter DG, Davis GD, McGoon DC, Edwards JE: Double-outlet right ventricle associated with persistent common atrioventricular canal. *Circulation* 52:933, 1975.

9. Stewart S: Double-outlet right ventricle (S,D,D), VSD related to pulmonary artery, and pulmonic stenosis absent. Correction with an intraventricular conduit in infancy. *J Thorac Cardiovasc Surg* 74:70, 1977.

T

1. Taussig HB, Bing RJ: Complete transposition of the aorta and a levoposition of the pulmonary artery. *Am Heart J* 37:551, 1949.

2. Thanopoulos BD, Dubrow IW, Fisher EA, Hastreiter AR: Double outlet right ventricle with subvalvular aortic stenosis. *Br Heart J* 41:241, 1979.

V

1. Van Praagh R, Perez-Trevino C, Reynolds JL, Moes CAF, Keith JD, Roy DL, Belcourt C, Weinberg PM, Parisi LF: Double outlet right ventricle (S,D,L) with subaortic ventricular septal defect and pulmonary stenosis. *Pediatr Cardiol* 35:42, 1975.

2. Van Praagh R: What is the Taussig-Bing malformation? *Circulation* 38:445, 1968 (editorial).

3. Van Praagh R: Conotruncal malformation, in BG Barratt-Boyes, JM Neutze, EA Harris (eds): *Heart Disease in Infancy. Diagnosis and Surgical Management*. London: Churchill Livingstone, 1973, p 145.

W

1. Wilcox BR, Ho SY, Macartney FJ, Becker AE, Gelis LM, Anderson RH: Surgical anatomy of double-outlet right ventricle with situs solitus and atrioventricular concordance. *J Thorac Cardiovasc Surg* 82:405, 1981.

2. Wesselhoeft H, Beuren AJ, Stoermer J, Kyrielis C: Ursprung beider grossen Gefasse aus dem rechten Ventrikel. *Arch Kreisl-Forsch* 66:80, 1971.

3. Witham AC: Double outlet right ventricle: A partial transposition complex. *Am Heart J* 53:928, 1957.

4. Wedemeyer AL, Lucas RV, Castaneda AR: Taussig-Bing malformation, coarctation of the aorta, and reversed patent ductus arteriosus. *Circulation* 42:1021, 1970.

Y

1. Yacoub MH, Radley-Smith R: Anatomic correction of the Taussig-Bing anomaly. *J Thorac Cardiovasc Surg* 88:380, 1984.

2. Yamaguchi M, Horikoshi K, Toriyama A, Kimura K, Mito H, Tei G, Kaneda H, Ogawa K, Asada S: Successful repair of double-outlet right ventricle with bilateral conus, 1-transposition of great arteries (S,D,L), and subpulmonary ventricular septal defect. *J Thorac Cardiovasc Surg* 71:366, 1976.

Z

1. Zamora R, Moller JH, Edwards JE: Double-outlet right ventricle. Anatomic types and associated anomalies. *Chest* 68:672, 1975.

41

DOUBLE OUTLET LEFT VENTRICLE

DEFINITION

Double outlet left ventricle (DOLV) is a cardiac anomaly in which both great arteries arise from the left ventricle (LV).[1] The great arteries are assigned to one or another ventricle by the rules described in Chapter 40, "Definition."

DOLV may occur with atrioventricular (AV) concordant or discordant connection, as does double outlet right ventricle (DORV). The same controversy exists as to the categorization of patients primarily by the ventriculoarterial connection (DOLV) or the AV connection as exists in the case of DORV (see Chapter 40, "Definition"). Because of its rarity, DOLV with AV discordant connection and DOLV with AV concordant connection are both discussed in this chapter. DOLV with AV discordant connection is discussed further in Chapter 43 (which is concerned with AV discordant connection in general).

DOLV, like DORV, may also occur in patients with univentricular AV connections (see Chapter 44) and in those with atrial isomerism (see Chapter 46).

HISTORICAL NOTE

Marechal is credited with describing the first case of DOLV in 1819,[M1] but this was in a heart with double inlet left ventricle with an infundibular outlet chamber. The first reported case in a heart with two ventricles and without pulmonary stenosis is that of Sakakibara and colleagues in 1967 in which they performed a successful intraventricular repair.[S1] DOLV is another congenital cardiac anomaly, therefore, that remained for all practical purposes undescribed until the advent of intracardiac surgery. In this regard, it is of interest that the first case reported by Potts and colleagues as tetralogy of Fallot and receiving a side-to-side aortopulmonary artery anastomosis[P3] underwent subsequent repair for well-documented DOLV with pulmonary stenosis (UAB). A unique case of DOLV with an intact ventricular septum was

---

[1] The adjectives left and right used to modify atrium or ventricle always mean morphologic right or morphologic left. The position of the chamber is referred to as right sided or left sided.

DOUBLE OUTLET LEFT VENTRICLE

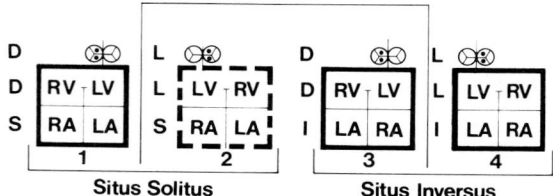

Figure 41-1 Model of the four basic hearts as they occur in DOLV with the usual positions of the great arteries (aorta medial to the pulmonary artery) (GLH). Models 2 and 3 are in AV discordant connection.

LA, left atrium; LV, left ventricle; RA, right atrium; RV, right ventricle.

Table 41-1 Surgical cases of DOLV (UAB; 1967–Nov. 15, 1983 and GLH; 1966–1983).

Segmental Arrangement	n	Hospital Deaths		
		No.	%	CL
AV concordant connection	22	5	23%	13%–36%
SDD	17	4	24%	12%–39%
SDL	4	1	25%	3%–63%
ILD	1		0%	0%–85%
AV discordant connection	4	1	25%	3%–63%
SLL	3	1	33%	4%–76%
IDD	1		0%	0%–85%
Total	26	6	23%	14%–35%

KEY: CL, 70% confidence limits.

reported by Paul and colleagues in 1970,[P1] and this established with certainty the existence of the entity.

Our publications (UAB) in 1971[K1] and 1973[P2] expanded the surgical possibilities by reporting the reconstruction of the pulmonary pathway in cases in which a completely intraventricular repair was not possible, preferably by a valved extracardiac conduit from right ventricle to pulmonary artery.[K1,P1] Anderson and colleagues reported the sixth case of DOLV in 1974.[A1] Five cases were added to the literature by our publication in 1976 (GLH).[B1] The first GLH patient was completely repaired in September 1966 using a valved aortic homograft conduit but died in low cardiac output postoperatively. Sharratt and colleagues in 1976[S2] reported the use of a Fontan-type procedure in hearts with DOLV and severe right ventricular hypoplasia. Additional cases have been reported by Urban and colleagues[U1] and Stegmann and colleagues.[S3]

MORPHOLOGY

As in the case of hearts with DORV, there is great variability among hearts with DOLV and AV concordant connection. Because of the rarity of DOLV, generalizations are even more difficult than in the case of DORV.

As in all complex cardiac anomalies, a segmental approach[B1,V1] is necessary for the complete understanding of this malformation (see Chapter 1, "Terminology and Classification of Heart Disease"). DOLV occurs in each of the four basic hearts (Fig. 41-1) but is most common in hearts with atrial situs solitus and ventricular right handedness or D-loop (SDD).[2] Examples of each of the four basic types are found in the combined GLH and UAB surgical experience (Table 41-1).

Atrial Situs Solitus and Ventricular Right Handedness (D-Loop) (Atrioventricular Concordant Connection)

In this subset, the aorta is usually in D-malposition (SDD, by the Van Praagh convention), but examples are seen with the

aorta in L-malposition (SDL). In the former, the great vessels may appear in relatively normal position (aorta to the right and somewhat posterior to the pulmonary artery), or they may be side to side, or the aorta may be somewhat anterior to the pulmonary artery.[B2]

Ventricular Septal Defect
Although the ventricular septum is rarely intact,[P1] nearly always a large ventricular septal defect (VSD) is present and lies between the limbs of the septal band (trabecula septomarginalis).

Most commonly, the VSD is *subaortic* in position (Fig. 41-2). As in other types of VSDs in this area, the defect may extend back to the tricuspid ring or be separated from it by a muscular bridge.[B2] When the aorta overrides the VSD, and arises in part from the right ventricle, this entity begins to merge with transposition of the great arteries.

When the VSD is *subpulmonary*, it is usually more anterior and well separated from the tricuspid valve by a rather wide band of muscle. In some cases, the pulmonary artery origin overrides the VSD and lies in part over the right ventricle. As the overriding becomes more severe, this entity merges with tetralogy of Fallot and subpulmonary VSD.

Occasionally, the VSD lies immediately below both great arteries (*doubly committed*). (For an example of a defect of this type, see Chapter 40, Fig. 40-6.) It is frequently difficult to decide whether DOLV or DORV is present, in which case the term *double outlet both ventricles* is appropriate.[B1]

Conal Pattern
Most often there is an absent subaortic conus (infundibulum) with aortic-mitral fibrous continuity and a subpulmonary conus that is displaced into the left ventricle (Fig. 41-3). Rarely, a bilaterally absent conus permits aortic-mitral-tricuspid and pulmonary-tricuspid fibrous continuity (see Fig. 41-2). In this event, both semilunar valves arise at the same level. Very rarely, only a subaortic conus is present.

Pulmonary Stenosis
Pulmonary stenosis is present in the majority of cases and is either valvar (sometimes with annular stenosis) or subvalvar, when it is due to a restrictive subpulmonary infundibulum (conus) with secondary fibrosis of the ostium. When the VSD is subaortic and there is infundibular pulmonary

---

[2]See Chapter 1, "Symbolic Convention of Van Praagh" in section on Terminology and Classification of Heart Disease, for explanation of this and the other symbols used by Van Praagh.

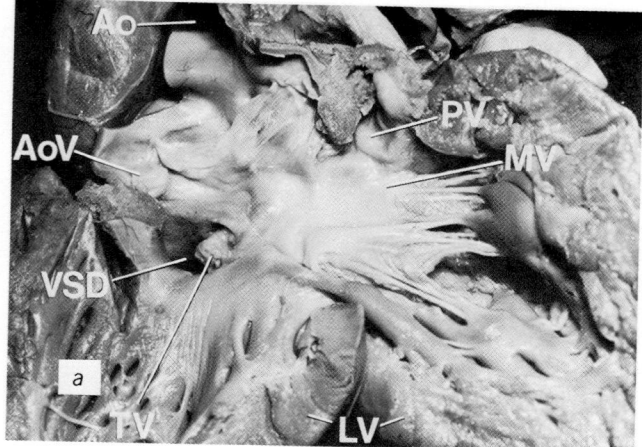

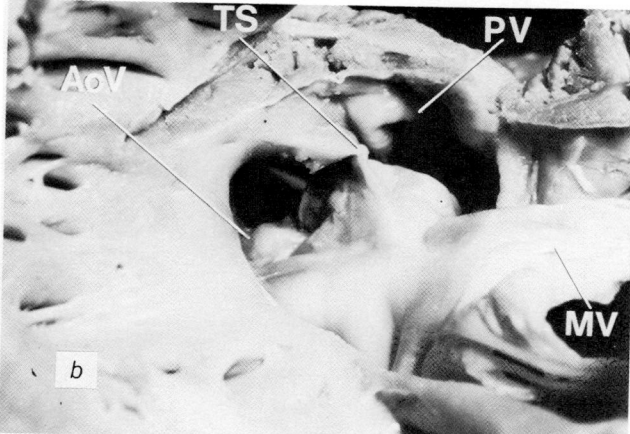

Figure 41-2 Specimen of DOLV and AV concordant connection (GLH).

(a) Viewed from the opened left ventricle and aorta. The aortic valve is bicuspid but otherwise normal. The ventricular septal defect (VSD) is subaortic, its upper margin being separated from the aortic valve by 4 mm. The tricuspid valve is visible through the VSD (there is an Ebstein's anomaly of the tricuspid valve).

(b) Close-up view of the left ventricular outflow tract before the aorta was opened. The pulmonary valve is not stenotic. The aortic and pulmonary valves are in continuity, being separated only by a thin fibrous ridge that has been called the truncal septum. There is pulmonary-mitral valve fibrous continuity and aortic-mitral valve fibrous continuity; that is, the conus is absent bilaterally.

Ao, aorta; AoV, aortic valve; LV, left ventricle; MV, mitral valve; PV, pulmonary valve; TS, truncal septum; TV, tricuspid valve; VSD, ventricular septal defect.

Reproduced with permission from Brandt et al.[B1]

stenosis, the great vessels are usually relatively normally interrelated.[B2] This type of DOLV has been called the tetralogy type.

Right Ventricular Hypoplasia
There is an increased tendency in hearts with DOLV for the right ventricular sinus and the tricuspid valve to be hypoplastic.[B2] The extreme example of this is the occurrence of tricuspid atresia, the two reported cases both having had

classic tricuspid atresia with ventricular right-handedness (SDD).[V1,V2] Also, the tricuspid valve may rarely show an Ebstein anomaly.[B1]

Left Ventricle
The left ventricle is nearly always well formed. One case of mitral atresia with a large left ventricle and an infundibular outlet chamber (SDD segmental arrangement) has been reported.[V1]

Conduction System
The position of the AV node and bundle of His is normal. Thus, the bundle penetrates from a normally positioned posterior AV node through the right trigone in the region of the commissure between tricuspid septal and anterior leaflet and at the base of the noncoronary aortic cusps, and its two branches are distributed in normal fashion. Whether or not it is at risk during the repair depends on the relationship of the lower VSD margin to the tricuspid ring (see Chapter 23).

Atrial Situs Inversus and Ventricular Left-Handedness (L-Loop) (Atrioventricular Concordant Connection)

Both the ILL and the ILD arrangements have been reported (that is, the aorta to the left or to the right), although both are rare. Usually the VSD is subaortic in position and there is coexisting pulmonary stenosis.

Atrial Situs Solitus and Ventricular Left-Handedness (L-Loop) (Atrioventricular Discordant Connection)

In this subset, the aorta is usually to the left (SLL). Usually the VSD is subaortic, the conus absent bilaterally, and pulmonary stenosis present.

In hearts with this arrangement and in those with the IDD arrangement (see below), the position of the *conduction system* is similar to that in other subsets of AV discordant connection (see Chapter 43, "Atrioventricular Node and Bundle of His" in section on Morphology). The AV node is usually anterior, but there may be a normally positioned posterior AV node as well. The penetrating bundle usually arises from the anterior node and passes around the superior and anterior margins of the VSD.

Atrial Situs Inversus and Ventricular Right-Handedness (D-Loop) (Atrioventricular Discordant Connection)

In this subset (IDD), the VSD is usually subaortic, the conuses absent bilaterally, and pulmonary stenosis present.

CLINICAL FEATURES AND DIAGNOSTIC CRITERIA
Pathophysiology

In hearts with double outlet left ventricle (DOLV), the left ventricle is a common mixing chamber. In those with atrioventricular (AV) concordant connections, the left ventricle receives pulmonary venous blood through the mitral valve

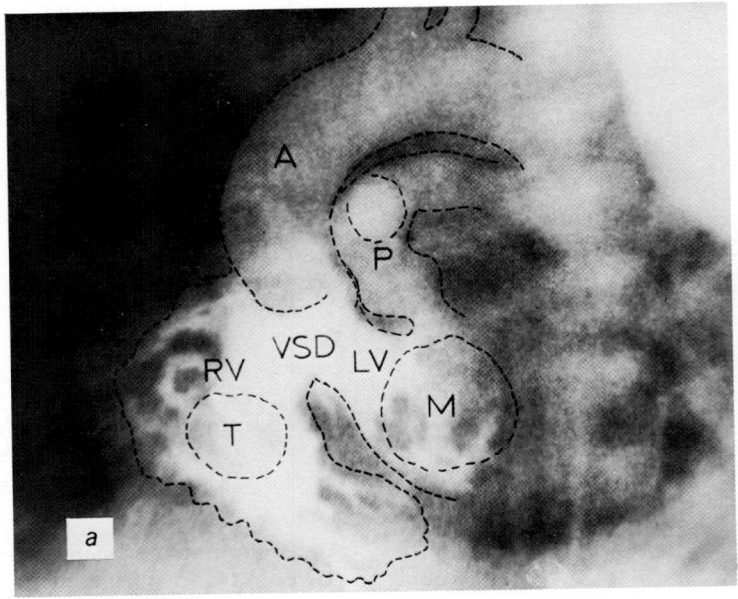

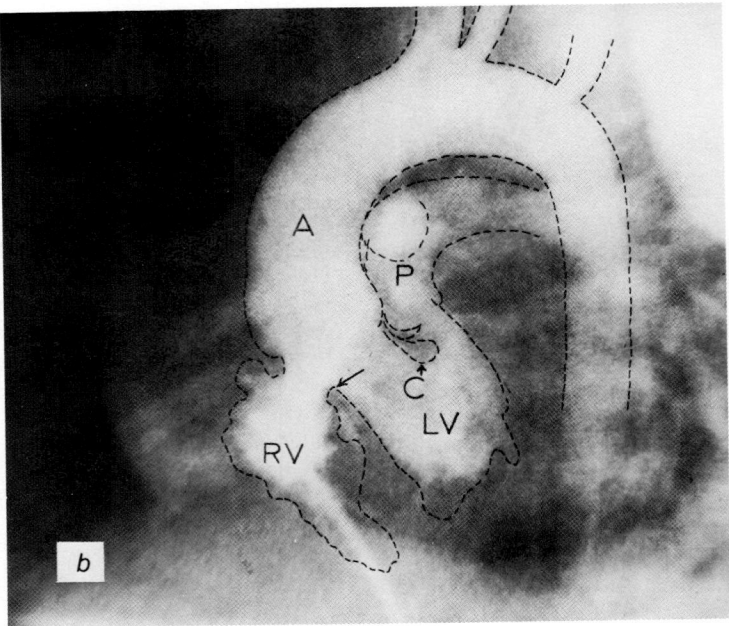

Figure 41-3 Cineangiograms in a patient with a normally positioned heart with AV concordant connection and DOLV and a subaortic ventricular septal defect (VSD) and pulmonary stenosis (GLH). (a) Diastolic frame in left anterior oblique (LAO) projection. Nonopaque flow outlines the tricuspid and mitral valves opening into their respective ventricles. The tricuspid ring is smaller than the mitral ring, but the right ventricle is not hypoplastic compared with the left ventricle (LV). The distance between aortic and mitral valves in this view is within the normal range and is consistent with aortic to mitral fibrous continuity.

(b) Systolic frame in LAO confirms the subaortic position of the VSD. The position of the upper margin of the basal septum, that is, the lower margin of the VSD (large arrow), indicates that the aorta arises from the LV except for the rightward anterior sinus, which arises from the right ventricular free wall. The conal (infundibular) septum is entirely within the LV.

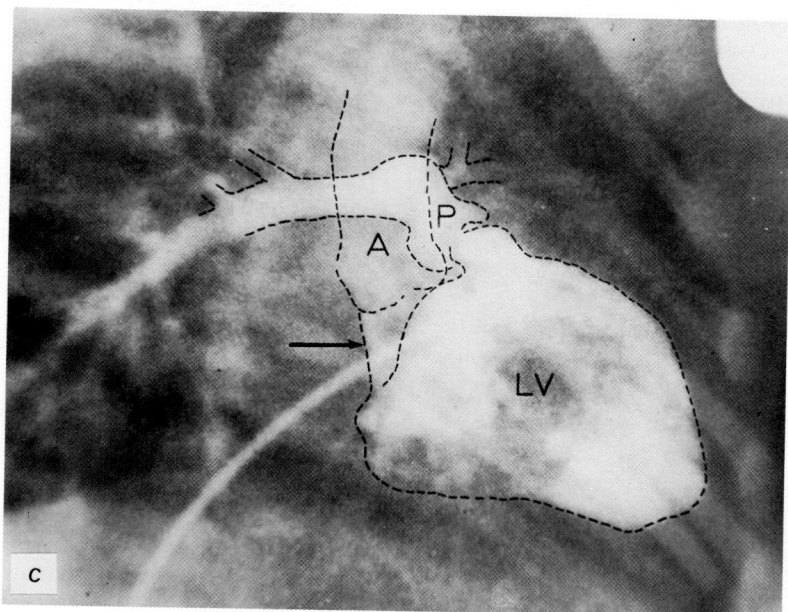

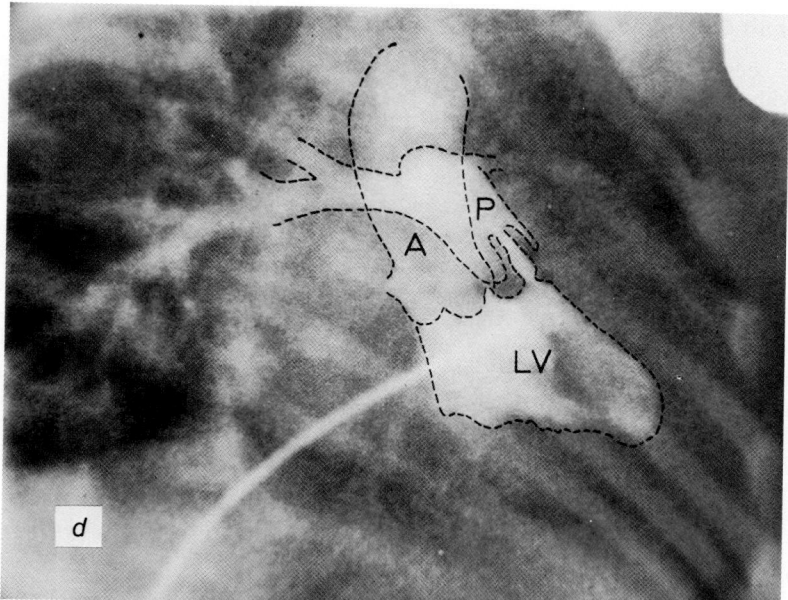

Figure 41-3 (continued)

(c) Diastolic frame in right anterior oblique (RAO) projection with LV injection of contrast. The low position of the aortic root showing a normal relationship to the intact AV septum (arrow) suggests a normal deficiency of the subaortic conus. Overlap of the aorta indicates (by correlating with the LAO views) that it is to the right and slightly anterior to the pulmonary artery.

(d) Systolic frame in RAO shows severe narrowing of the subpulmonary conus, indicating its muscular nature.

A, aorta; C, conal septum; LV, left ventricle; M, mitral valve; P, pulmonary artery; RV, right ventricle; T, tricuspid valve; VSD, ventricular septal defect.

Reproduced with permission from Brandt et al.[B1]

and caval blood by way of the right ventricle and ventricular septal defect (VSD). The clinical presentation, however, is dominated by the very frequent occurrence of pulmonary stenosis, which results in severe cyanosis. Thus, 7 of 11 patients with pulmonary stenosis had undergone a shunting operation in early life (UAB). In the absence of pulmonary stenosis, pulmonary blood flow is large and congestive heart failure often develops early in life. Thus, 3 of the 6 surgical patients in the combined GLH and UAB series had undergone pulmonary artery banding in very early life. Streaming of desaturated right ventricular blood into the aorta may occur when the VSD is subaortic, leading to unexpectedly severe cyanosis.

In hearts with DOLV and AV discordant connection, the left ventricle receives caval blood through the mitral valve and pulmonary venous blood by way of the right ventricle and VSD. The tendency to cyanosis is more severe than in the previous group.

Examination

The physical findings, chest x-ray, and electrocardiogram (ECG) are not diagnostic, and echocardiography has not been entirely reliable for definitive diagnosis to date.

Cardiac Catheterization and Cineangiography

Biplane cineangiography, selecting injection sites and projections suited to the individual problem, are diagnostic.[B1] Both left[K1] and right ventricular injections[B1] are desirable. It is essential to profile the sinus septum so that the plane of the septum can be projected cranially and its relation to the great vessel origins, including the degree of override of the aorta or pulmonary artery, can be defined exactly. When the ventricles are in normal position, this can be achieved with a left anterior oblique projection, but in other circumstances a frontal or a lateral view may be more appropriate. Angiography must also accurately define the position and number of VSDs, the presence and site of pulmonary and aortic stenosis, and the size of the right ventricle and tricuspid valve relative to the left ventricle and mitral valve (Fig. 41-3).

NATURAL HISTORY

The natural history of patients with double outlet left ventricle (DOLV) without pulmonary stenosis appears to be similar to that of patients with isolated large ventricular septal defect (VSD) (see Chapter 20), except that the tendency for the VSD to narrow and close spontaneously is less when DOLV coexists. Progressive narrowing of the VSD has not, in fact, been documented in DOLV. Mild cyanosis may occur because of the common mixing chamber beneath the great arteries, but considerable streamlining of flow is often present and accounts for the considerable variability in the arterial oxygen levels.

The natural history of patients with DOLV and pulmonary stenosis is similar to that of patients with tetralogy of Fallot (see Chapter 23), and in both entities the degree of hypoxia and the clinical course are directly related to the severity of the pulmonary stenosis.

TECHNIQUE OF OPERATION

Identification of Morphology

There are no clues to the specific diagnosis of double outlet left ventricle (DOLV) from external examination of the heart as it is exposed at operation. Generally, only the preoperative identification of the AV connection as being concordant or discordant can be confirmed by external observation. It is for this reason that a detailed and complete preoperative study must be made to identify all aspects of the cardiac anomaly. Even when this has been done, the relation of the great arteries to the ventricular septal defect (VSD), and of the VSD to the atrioventricular (AV) valves may be different from that visualized preoperatively. For this reason, after the heart is opened, an accurate evaluation must be made of all aspects of the morphology but particularly of these.

When the AV connection is concordant, the finding of a large VSD located far downstream (distally) and anterosuperiorly in the ventricular septum mandates a thorough consideration of all the diagnostic possibilities associated with a VSD in this position, including not only DOLV but also ordinary subpulmonary VSD with ventriculo-arterial concordant connection, tetralogy of Fallot with subpulmonary VSD (if pulmonary stenosis coexists), anterosuperior VSD with complete transposition of the great arteries, DORV with doubly committed VSD, and DORV of the Taussig-Bing type (which has its VSD in this same position but the aorta far removed from the VSD and originating quite clearly from the right ventricle alone). A similar appearance may also be given by cases in which both of the great arteries seem to arise from a smooth-walled muscular chamber (infundibulum) that communicates freely with the right ventricle and, via the VSD, with the left ventricle.

When the AV connection is discordant, the same detailed observations must be made. This evaluation generally reveals findings quite similar to those in congenitally corrected transposition of the great arteries (see Chapter 42), but in DOLV the aorta as well as the pulmonary artery arise entirely or in large part from the right-sided (in atrial situs solitus) left ventricle. (For more details see Chapters 42 and 43.)

Repair of Double Outlet Left Ventricle and Atrioventricular Concordant Connection

The preparations for operation, the sternotomy, and the placement of the purse-string sutures are those generally used (see Chapter 2, Section 3). Cardiopulmonary bypass (CPB) is established, the perfusate temperature taken to 25°C, the aorta cross-clamped, and the cold cardioplegic infusion given. The usual oblique right atriotomy is made (see Chapter 15, Fig. 15-12), and the interior of the right ventricle is inspected through the tricuspid valve. It can usually be confirmed through this that neither great artery arises from the right ventricle and that the VSD is in the outlet portion of the ventricular septum.

Usually the repair is made through a vertical incision in the distal portion of the right ventricle. After placing stay sutures, the position of the VSD, the origin of the aorta and pulmonary artery from the left ventricle and their relationships to the VSD, and the nature of any pulmonary stenosis are verified.

When *pulmonary stenosis is present* in a tetralogy-type DOLV, it is usually not possible to relieve the pulmonary stenosis directly and do a completely intraventricular repair, as is described for patients with no coexisting pulmonary stenosis. However, if examination of the pulmonary valve through a vertical anterior incision in the pulmonary artery or from the ventricle shows it to be widely patent and the subvalvar fibromuscular obstructing ring is localized, the ring may satisfactorily be excised and then a completely intraventricular repair may be possible. Usually, the pulmonary ring is small and the subvalvar stenosis too long and narrow for this to be effective. It is not possible to place a transannular patch because the left anterior descending coronary artery is immediately in front of the pulmonary ring, and a valved extracardiac conduit is necessary. Thus usually, by working through the VSD, the subvalvar stenosis is completely closed by placing two rows of continuous polypropylene sutures supplemented by one or two pledgetted mattress sutures. Then the VSD is closed by suturing into place a preclotted knitted Dacron patch, taking the usual precautions for avoiding damage to the bundle of His (Fig. 41-4). A homograft-valved extracardiac conduit is prepared (see Chapter 23, Figs. 23-36 and 23-37) and sutured distally to a longitudinal incision in the pulmonary trunk and proximally to the right ventriculotomy. Returning to the right atrium, the foramen ovale is closed, and with strong suction on the aortic needle vent, the aortic clamp is released and rewarming begun. The remainder of the operation is completed in the usual manner.

When *pulmonary stenosis is not present*, the arrangement in a particular case may allow an intraventricular tunnel repair in which a contoured patch is placed into the VSD so that the right ventricle now ejects into the pulmonary artery while the left ventricle continues to eject into aorta. The VSD may need to be enlarged anteriorly and superiorly before this is done. When this is not possible, the pulmonary orifice is closed off from within the ventricle or from within the pulmonary trunk or the pulmonary trunk is divided; the VSD is closed, leaving the aorta coming off left ventricle; and a homograft-valved extracardiac conduit is placed between the right ventricle and pulmonary artery.

Rarely, in the absence of pulmonary stenosis, this type of repair is not possible. It may then be possible to close the VSD with a contoured patch so that right ventricle ejects into the aorta and the left ventricle into the pulmonary artery and complete the operation by performing an arterial switch or an atrial switch procedure (see Chapter 39).

When there is *atrial situs inversus,* there is a mirror image of the relations and the operation.

Repair of Double Outlet Left Ventricle with Atrioventricular Discordant Connection

In this setting of DOLV, it is surgically helpful to remember that the operative procedure is in some ways similar to that for the repair of a VSD in patients with congenitally corrected transposition of the great arteries. Thus, the precautions for minimizing the incidence of heart block are the same as those used in congenitally corrected transposition

(see Chapter 42, Fig. 42-9). At the end of the operation, the aorta should emerge from the left-sided (in atrial situs solitus) right ventricle, just as it does in congenitally corrected transposition. When a valved extracardiac conduit is used as a pulmonary pathway, it is positioned in a manner similar to that used in congenitally corrected transposition (see Chapter 42, Fig. 42-11).

The preparations for operation, the median sternotomy, the placement of purse-string sutures, and the commencement of CPB are accomplished in the usual manner (see Chapter 2, Section 3). The perfusate temperature is taken to 25°C, the aorta cross-clamped, the cold cardioplegic infusion given (see Chapter 3), and the right atrium opened in the usual oblique manner. The diagnosis of DOLV is confirmed by examination of the interior of the right-sided (atrial situs solitus) left ventricle through the right atrium. If at all possible, an intraventricular tunnel repair is made, contouring the patch so that right ventricle ejects into the aorta and left ventricle into the pulmonary artery. Generally, this repair can be made from the right atrium through the mitral valve, although exposure may have to be obtained by a radial incision through the base of the superior aspect of the anterior and posterior mitral leaflets (see Chapter 42, Fig. 42-10). If this is not possible, the repair is made through a left ventriculotomy.

When pulmonary stenosis coexists or if the intraventricular tunnel repair obstructs access to the pulmonary artery, a homograft-valved extracardiac conduit is placed between the right-sided left ventricle and the pulmonary trunk.

When there is *atrial situs inversus,* there is a mirror image of the relationships and the operation.

Double Outlet Left Ventricle with Atrioventricular Concordant Connection and Important Hypoplasia of the Right Ventricle and Tricuspid Valve

A significant degree of hypoplasia of the right ventricle and tricuspid valve makes the type of repair described above inadvisable. A Fontan-type operation is then indicated. The tricuspid valve is closed, the pulmonary artery divided and its proximal end closed, and an anastomosis made between right atrium and pulmonary artery (see Chapter 26, "Direct Right Atrial-Pulmonary Artery Connection" in section on Technique of Operation).

SPECIAL FEATURES OF POSTOPERATIVE CARE

The care of the patient after repair is given in accordance with the usual protocols (see Chapter 5).

EARLY RESULTS

Hospital Mortality

The hospital mortality has been relatively high, 6 (23%, CL 13%–36%) of 26 patients dying in the combined GLH and UAB experience (Table 41-1). This experience dates back nearly 20 years, and in the current era the risk of repair is no doubt lower.

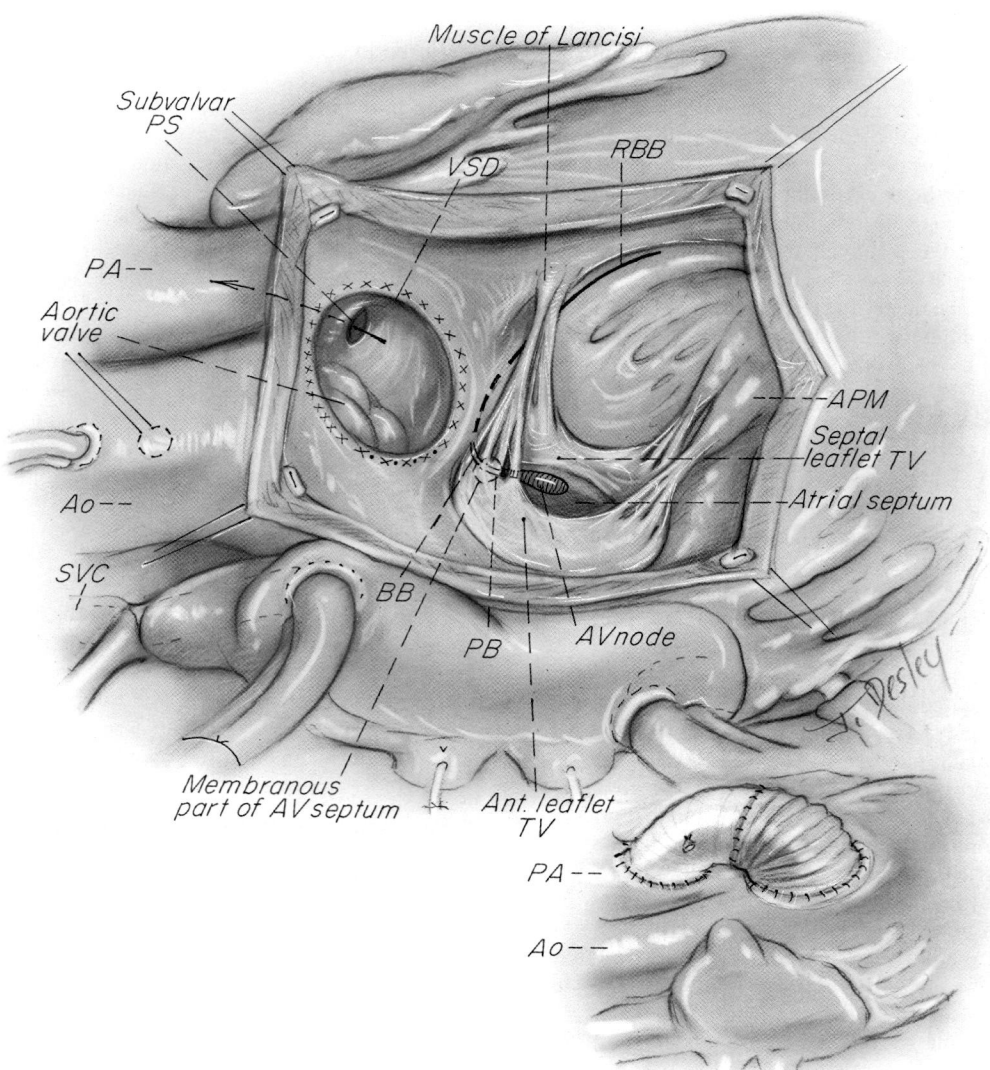

Figure 41-4 Repair of DOLV, and pulmonary stenosis. The aorta is to the right and slightly posterior to the pulmonary artery. The right ventricle has been opened by a vertical incision. The subvalvar stenotic pathway to the pulmonary artery is closed (see text for details). The ventricular septal defect (VSD) is then closed with a patch. Since in this example a band of muscle lies between the VSD and the tricuspid valve, the bundle of His is away from the posterior border of the VSD and sutures for the patch closure can be placed in the muscular border as shown. Suture siting in trabecular (septal band) and infundibular septa and right ventricular musculature is indicated by ×'s; alternating dots and ×'s represent suture siting in the posterior muscular border (ventriculo-infundibular fold). The repair is completed by placing a homograft-valved conduit between the right ventricle and pulmonary artery (lower right insert).

Ao, aorta; APM, anterior papillary muscle; AV, atrioventricular; PA, pulmonary artery; PB, BB, penetrating and branching portions of bundle of His; PS, pulmonary stenosis; RBB, right bundle branch; SVC, superior vena cava; TV, tricuspid valve; VSD, ventricular septal defect.

Table 41-2   Type of repair of DOLV with AV concordant connection (UAB; 1967–Nov. 15, 1983 and GLH; 1966–1983).

| Type of Repair | UAB | | | | GLH | | | | Combined UAB and GLH | | | |
| | | Hospital Deaths | | | | Hospital Deaths | | | | Hospital Deaths | | |
	n	No.	%	CL	n	No.	%	CL	n	No.	%	CL
Intraventricular repair (LV → aorta; RV → PA)	3	0	0%	0%–47%	0				3	0	0%	0%–47%
Intraventricular repair (LV → aorta) plus valved extracardiac conduit (RV → PA)	13	3	23%	10%–41%	5	2	40%	14%–71%	18	5	28%	16%–43%
Intraventricular repair (LV → PA; RV → aorta) plus arterial switch	1	0	0%	0%–85%	0				1	0	0%	0%–85%
Total	17	3	18%	8%–32%	5	2	40%	14%–71%	22	5	23%	13%–36%

KEY: CL, 70% confidence limits; LV, left ventricle; RV, right ventricle; PA, pulmonary artery.

No risk factors for hospital death can be identified with any reasonable certainty, which is probably related to the small number of heterogeneous cases (Table 41-1). When the patients with *AV concordant connection* are looked at separately, in neither the individual nor combined experiences is there an evident effect on mortality of the type of repair (Table 41-2) or age at operation (Table 41-3). The status of the pulmonary outflow tract in this group of patients likewise did not seem to be related to hospital mortality (Table 41-4). When the patients with *AV discordant connection* are looked at separately, the type of operation is not evidently related to hospital mortality (Table 41-5). (For further details in this last subset, see Chapter 43, ''Incremental Risk Factors for Hospital Death'' in section on Early Results.)

Heart Block

Heart block, occurring in one patient with AV concordant connection who died after operation early in the experience (UAB), should be rare in the current era in patients with AV concordant connection. Although in the small number of patients (four) with AV discordant connection in the combined

series heart block did not occur, in a larger group of patients its incidence would probably be similar to that after the repair of congenitally corrected transposition (see Chapter 43, ''Incremental Risk Factors for the Development of Complete Heart Block'' in section on Early Results).

LATE RESULTS

Survival

When the repair can be made without a valved extracardiac conduit, the late results are good and entirely comparable to those obtained with isolated large VSD (see Chapter 20) or tetralogy of Fallot when a transannular patch or valved extracardiac conduit is not used (see Chapter 23). No late deaths have occurred in patients with AV concordant connection in this category in the combined UAB and GLH experience. One 26-year-old patient with AV discordant connection had complete heart block preoperatively and died suddenly 2 years postoperatively (GLH).

In the group in whom a valved extracardiac conduit was

Table 41-3   Age distribution of patients undergoing repair of DOLV and AV concordant connection (UAB; 1967–Nov. 15, 1983 and GLH; 1966–1983).

| Age (yr) ≤   < | UAB | | GLH | | Total | | | |
| | | Hospital Deaths | | Hospital Deaths | | Hospital Deaths | | |
	n	No.	n	No.	n	No.	%	CL
2	4[a]	1	2	1[b]	6	2	33%	12%–62%
2 --- 4	5	2	3	1[c]	8	3	38%	17%–62%
4 --- 8	3				3		0%	0%–47%
8 --- 16	2				2		0%	0%–61%
16	3				3		0%	0%–47%
Total	17	3 (18%; CL 8%–32%)	5	2 (40%; CL 14%–71%)	22	5	23%	13%–36%

(Age 4–8, 8–16, 16 rows: 0% (CL 0%–21%))

KEY: CL, 70% confidence limits.

NOTE: The 4-month-old infant who died after repair had repair of coarctation and pulmonary artery banding at age 3 weeks.

[a] Ages 4 (died), 5, 6, and 8 months.

[b] Moderate right ventricular hypoplasia, death with right heart failure.

[c] Operation—1966.

Table 41-4 Status of the pulmonary outflow tract in patients undergoing repair of DOLV and AV concordant connection (UAB; 1967–Nov. 15, 1983 and GLH; 1966–1983).

Pulmonary Stenosis	n	Hospital Deaths		
		No.	%	CL
No—unbanded	4	2	50%	18%–82%
No—banded	3	0	0%	0%–47%
Yes	8	3	38%	17%–62%
Yes plus anastomotic operation	7	0	0%	0%–24%
Total	22	5	23%	13%–36%

KEY: CL, 70% confidence limits.

Table 41-5 Hospital deaths after intracardiac repair in patients with DOLV and AV discordant connection (UAB; 1967–Nov. 15, 1983; n = 3 and GLH; 1966–1983; n = 1).

Operation	n	Hospital Deaths		
		No.	%	CL
Intraventricular tunnel repair (RV → aorta)	2[a]	1	50%	7%–93%
Intraventricular tunnel repair plus valved extracardiac conduit (LV → PA)	2	0	0%	0%–61%
Total	4	1	25%	3%–63%

KEY: CL, 70% confidence limits; LV, left ventricle; PA, pulmonary artery; RV, right ventricle.
[a]One patient who lived also had pulmonary valvotomy (GLH).

used, one late sudden death occurred 4 years postoperatively.

Reoperation

The incidence and timing of reoperation are determined by the nature of the conduit. With a heterograft-valved Dacron conduit, reoperation within 10 years for conduit replacement can be expected in 10%–20% of cases (see Chapters 23 and 42), and among 13 patients in whom these conduits were used as part of the repair of DOLV, 2 have undergone this type of reoperation (UAB). When a properly preserved and prepared homograft-valved conduit is used, over a period of 20 years less than 20% of patients can be expected to require reoperation on the conduit (see Chapter 23, ''Valved Conduits'' in Section 1, Special Situations and Controversies).

INDICATIONS FOR OPERATION

The diagnosis of DOLV is an indication for operation. When pulmonary stenosis coexists, a homograft-valved conduit is almost always a necessary part of the repair. Because of this and the safety and efficacy of shunting procedures, a classic shunting operation (see Chapter 23) is performed if the patient presents before the age of 2 years, and complete repair is deferred until the age of 3–5 years if possible.

When there is no pulmonary stenosis, the timing of intracardiac repair depends upon whether or not a valved extracardiac conduit will likely be required. Management will thus depend upon the accuracy of the preoperative diagnosis and whether it is possible to predict from the cineangiocardiograms whether or not repair can be accomplished by an intraventricular baffle alone. If an external conduit can be avoided, repair can be carried out at an early age, preferably before 12 months, in order to prevent the development of pulmonary vascular disease. If a conduit is required, pulmonary artery banding should be performed if there is congestive heart failure or if the pulmonary vascular resistance is rising and repair be delayed until 3–5 years of age.

When there is moderate or severe right ventricular hypoplasia, a Fontan-type procedure is required, although, at present, it is difficult to predict the degree of right ventricular hypoplasia that makes a Fontan-type procedure mandatory. This operation can be done only when the pulmonary vascular resistance is near normal and is feasible beyond 6 months of age (see Chapter 26).

SPECIAL SITUATIONS AND CONTROVERSIES

Morphology

Some pathologists consider DOLV to be an exceedingly rare condition, whereas clinically it has seemed to be an uncommon but not rare malformation. This paradox results from the fact that the ventricular septal defect (VSD) in this condition is always subarterial, and thus the assignment of a great artery to one or the other ventricle is made by projecting the plane of the septum anterosuperiorly through the VSD.[B1,C1] Clinically, the projection is made on echocardiographic images and on cineangiography but primarily by observations made at the time of operation. The result may be different when the projection is made in the isolated autopsy heart.

REFERENCES

A

1. Anderson R, Galbraith R, Gibson R, Miller G: Double outlet left ventricle. *Br Heart J* 36:554, 1974.

B

1. Brandt PWT, Calder AL, Barratt-Boyes BG, Neutze JM: Double outlet left ventricle. Morphology, cineangiocardiographic diagnosis and surgical treatment. *Am J Cardiol* 38:897, 1976.

2. Bharati S, Lev M, Stewart R, McAllister HA Jr, Kirklin JW: The morphologic spectrum of double outlet left ventricle and its surgical significance. *Circulation* 58:558, 1978.

C

1. Coto EO, Jimenez MQ, Castaneda AR, Rufilanchas JJ, Deverall PB: Double outlet from chambers of left ventricular morphology. *Br Heart J* 42:15, 1979.

K

1. Kerr AR, Barcia A, Bargeron LM, Kirklin JW: Double-outlet left ventricle with ventricular septal defect and pulmonary stenosis: Report of surgical repair. *Am Heart J* 81:688, 1971.

M

1. Marechal: Confirmation vicieuse du Coeur d'un infant affecté de la maladie bleue. *J Gen de Med* 69:354, 1819.

P

1. Paul MH, Muster AJ, Sinha SN, Cole RB, Van Praagh R: Double-outlet left ventricle with an intact ventricular septum: Clinical and autopsy diagnosis and developmental implications. *Circulation* 41:129, 1970.
2. Pacifico AD, Kirklin JW, Bargeron LM Jr, Soto B: Surgical treatment of double-outlet left ventricle. Report of four cases. *Circulation* 47 and 48 (suppl III):III-19, 1973.
3. Potts WJ, Smith S, Gibson S: Anastomosis of the aorta to a pulmonary artery. *JAMA* 132:627, 1946.

S

1. Sakakibara S, Takao A, Arai T, Hashimoto A, Nogi M: Both great vessels arising from the left ventricle. *Bull Heart Inst Jpn* 66, 1967.
2. Sharratt GP, Sbokos CG, Johnson AM, Anderson RH, Monro JL: Surgical "correction" of solitus-concordant, double-outlet left ventricle with L-malposition and tricuspid stenosis with hypoplastic right ventricle. *J Thorac Cardiovasc Surg* 71:853, 1976.
3. Stegmann T, Oster H, Bissenden J, Kallfelz HC, Oelert H: Surgical treatment of double-outlet left ventricle in 2 patients with D-position and L-position of the aorta. *Ann Thorac Surg* 27:121, 1979.

U

1. Urban AE, Anderson RH, Stark J: Double outlet left ventricle associated with situs inversus and atrioventricular concordance. *Am Heart J* 94:91, 1977.

V

1. Van Praagh R, Weinberg PM: Double outlet left ventricle, in FH Adams, GC Emmanouilides (eds): *Heart Disease in Infants, Children, and Adolescents* (ed 3). Baltimore: Williams and Wilkins, 1983, chap 24.
2. Vaseenon I, Diehl AM, Mattioli L: Tricuspid atresia with double outlet left ventricle and bilateral conus. *Chest* 74:676, 1978.

42

CONGENITALLY CORRECTED TRANSPOSITION OF THE GREAT ARTERIES

DEFINITION

Congenitally corrected transposition of the great arteries is a congenital cardiac anomaly with ventriculoarterial discordant connection (transposition of the great arteries) and atrioventricular discordant connection, the right atrium connecting to the left ventricle and the left atrium connecting to the right ventricle.[1] The circulatory pathways are, therefore, in series. The condition can occur in atrial situs solitus or in atrial situs inversus. The ventricles may lie in any position.[2]

HISTORICAL NOTE

Probably, Rokitansky was the first to describe a case of congenitally corrected transposition of the great arteries (CTGA) in 1875.[R1] After that, pathologists recognized the condition easily but considered it rare.[L1] With the advent of cardiac surgery, interest and knowledge expanded rapidly and the papers by Anderson and colleagues from the University of Minnesota in 1957[A2] and by Schiebler and colleagues from the Mayo Clinic in 1961[S1] established the clinical syndromes associated with it.

In 1913, Monckenberg[M1] and again in 1936, Uher[U1] described the anterior position of the atrioventricular (AV) node usually present in corrected transposition. In 1931, Walmsley recognized that there were fundamental differences in the cardiac structure in hearts with corrected transposition, including a different coronary arterial pattern and altered morphology in the central fibrous body and in the conduction system.[W1] In 1963, Lev and colleagues again described the anomalous position of the AV node and bundle.[L5] Clinicians, however, remained generally unaware of these observations until Anderson and colleagues again confirmed the unusual position of the AV node and extended the knowledge of the pathway of the bundle of His.[A1,A3]

The first repairs of a cardiac anomaly associated with CTGA were reported in 1957 by Anderson, Lillehei, and Lester from the University of Minnesota.[A2] Our experience began at the Mayo Clinic in 1958 and was reported as part of the overall Mayo Clinic report in 1974[B7] and again in 1980.[M2] The first patient was operated upon in 1960 (GLH).

---

[1] The adjectives left and right used to modify atrium or ventricle always mean morphologic right or morphologic left. The position of the chamber is referred to as right sided or left sided.

[2] Because many of the bibliographic references in this Chapter and Chapter 43 are the same, one bibliography has been used for the two chapters, and included in Chapter 43. The reference symbols in this chapter refer to that bibliography.

TRANSPOSITION OF GREAT ARTERIES

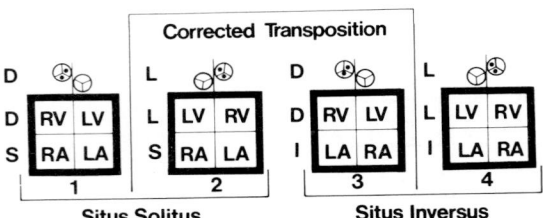

Figure 42-1 Diagrammatic models of the four basic hearts (see Chapter 1) as they occur in transposition of the great arteries (ventriculoarterial discordance), with the most common great arterial positions indicated (GLH). The degree of elevation of the great arteries above their respective ventricles corresponds to the usual type of conal development. Models 1 and 4 are complete transposition of the great arteries, and models 2 and 3 are CTGA.

LA, left atrium; LV, left ventricle; RA, right atrium; RV, right ventricle.

MORPHOLOGY

In atrial situs solitus, the most common arrangement in patients with congenitally corrected transposition of the great arteries (CTGA) is a ventricular L-loop and L-malposition of the aorta (SLL in the Van Praagh convention; see Chapter 1, "Symbolic Convention of Van Praagh," in section on Terminology and Classification of Heart Disease) (Fig. 42-1). The left ventricle usually lies to the right and the right ventricle to the left. The left ventricle is usually slightly posterior and inferior to the right ventricle. Mirror-image relations pertain when there is atrial situs inversus (IDD).

Ventricles

Usually there is fibrous continuity in the left ventricle between the right-sided mitral and pulmonary valves and a well-developed right ventricular infundibulum separating the left-sided tricuspid and aortic valves. However, rare cases have been described with bilateral conus or bilaterally deficient conus.[V6]

The left ventricular outflow tract beneath the pulmonary valve lies between the septal (pulmonary) leaflet of the mitral valve on the right and the muscular ventricular septum on the left (Fig. 42-2). In its anterior part, there is often a promi-

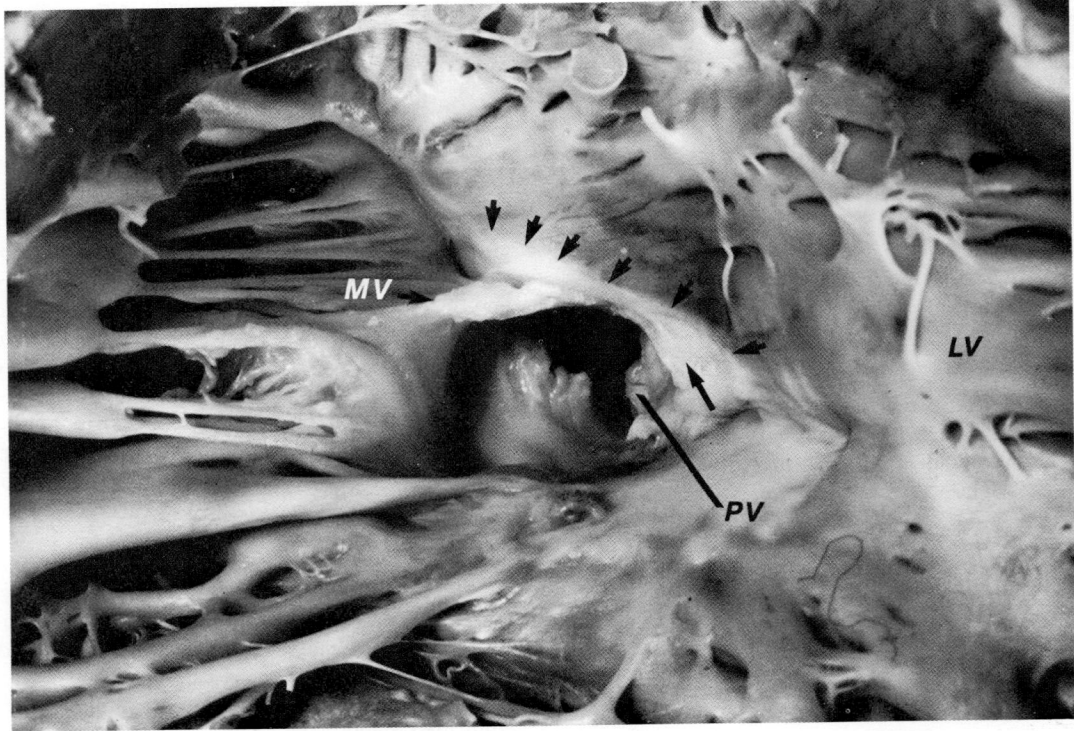

Figure 42-2 Specimen of a heart with CTGA and atrial situs solitus viewed from below, showing the outflow tract of the right-sided left ventricle (GLH). The septal leaflet of the mitral valve has been swung to the right. A fibrous subvalvar membrane is visible (large arrows) and is continuous with the anterior part of the pulmonary ring. Part of the membrane was removed at operation and the fused, thickened pulmonary valve leaflets were also divided. The bundle of His is visible as a raised pale ridge crossing the anterior wall of the outflow tract just beneath the valve ring (small arrows). This heart had a large AV canal-type ventricular septal defect (not shown).

LV, left ventricle; MV, mitral valve; PV, pulmonary valve.

nent recess.[A3] The ventricular outflow tracts do not cross, and the aorta and pulmonary artery lie parallel one to the other.

In CTGA with atrial situs solitus, the apex of the heart is usually to the left and is formed by the right ventricle. There is dextrocardia in about 25% of cases, however, and there is occasionally mesocardia.[C1] In CTGA with atrial situs inversus, there is nearly always dextrocardia.

More bizarre rotational anomalies may occur in this and other hearts with AV discordant connections (see Chapter 43, "Morphology").

Pulmonary Outflow Tract

The pulmonary valve lies in a transverse plane and arises from the left ventricle to the right and posterior to the aortic valve in a wedged position between the mitral and tricuspid valves. The axis of the AV valves is part way between a transverse and sagittal plane as in the normal heart. The wedging of the pulmonary valve is said to be more marked in CTGA than in complete transposition (see Chapter 39), and more marked than that of the aorta in the normal heart (see Chapter 1).[L1]

The long axis of the pulmonary outflow from the left ventricle is obliquely oriented[A5] and is potentially restrictive, particularly when there is left ventricular hypertrophy. There is, however, organic obstruction present in about half the hearts,[A4,A5] and in at least 25% of hearts it is surgically significant.[L1] The pulmonary valve leaflets may be thickened and fused or occasionally bicuspid or even unicuspid; occasionally, there is pulmonary atresia. In the last event there may or may not be a pulmonary artery confluence between right and left pulmonary arteries. When valve stenosis is present, the main pulmonary artery may be narrowed by valve tethering, as in the tetralogy of Fallot (see Chapter 23, "Pulmonary Valve" in Section 1, Morphology). In most cases, there is additional subvalvar pathology, or this may be the only site of obstruction. The subvalvar narrowing is due either to a subvalvar membrane that is adherent to its right (laterally) with the anterior mitral leaflet (Fig. 42-2) or to a frank aneurysmal bulging of the membranous septum into the posterior part of the outflow tract[K2] with or without a ventricular septal defect (VSD; Fig. 42-3).[A4] Less severe obstruction is usually due to fibrous tags (valvar excrescences) attached to the pulmonary anulus or membranous septum or the right-sided mitral valve or to valvar excrescences projecting through a VSD from the tricuspid valve leaflet.[L4,W3]

Atrial Septa

There is malalignment of the atrial and ventricular septa except where the pulmonary, mitral, and tricuspid valves lie in close proximity and are joined by the right fibrous trigone. Elsewhere, the atrial septal attachment to the fibrous skeleton of the heart is moved to the right of the ventricular septal attachment.[A3,B10] These changes in alignment are usually severe enough in hearts with atrial situs solitus to prevent the normally positioned (regular) AV node (so-called "posterior," "inferior," or "lateral node") from reaching the underlying ventricular septum.

Mitral Valve

The mitral valve lies at the entrance to the right-sided left ventricle. Because of the wedged position of the pulmonary valve, the mitral ring extends anterior to the pulmonary ring so that the pulmonary valve is tucked beneath (to the left of) the septal mitral valve leaflet (Fig. 42-2). The mitral valve is rotated so that its usual septal (aortic) leaflet, which is in fibrous continuity with the pulmonary valve and can therefore be called the pulmonary leaflet, is posterior and its mural leaflet anterior (see Fig. 42-3). The smaller papillary muscle arises from the anterolateral free wall of the ventricle, where it can be damaged by a left ventriculotomy. Its position is frequently marked by direct branches crossing the front of the left ventricle from the anterior descending coronary artery.[A4] The larger papillary muscle arises from the posterolateral left ventricular free wall (Fig. 42-4).

Aortic Valve

The aortic valve, usually normal, is over the right ventricular infundibulum, and it and the aorta are usually in a leftward and anterior position (SLL by the Van Praagh convention). Occasionally, the aorta may lie to the right and anterior to the pulmonary artery (SLD), associated with rotation of the infundibulum in this direction.[A4] In CTGA with atrial situs inversus, the aorta is virtually always to the right (IDD).

Subaortic obstruction rarely occurs in the right ventricular outflow tract.

Tricuspid Valve

The tricuspid valve lies at the entrance to the left-sided right ventricle, which has the usual coarse trabeculations, a septal band, and an infundibular septum. The valve is positioned almost in a sagittal plane and has the usual three leaflets but with the septal leaflet more medial and anterior than normal. It is nearly always structurally abnormal (90% of cases according to Allwork and colleagues[A4]). In most instances, there is leaflet dysplasia with abnormal, thickened chordal attachments of septal and posterior leaflets,[B2,B3,T1] and in a minority there is a true Ebstein's anomaly with downward displacement of the origins of the septal and posterior cusps. The Ebstein's anomaly of CTGA often but not always differs from that in a heart with normal connections in three respects. The anterior leaflet is normal in size rather than large and saillike, the valve ring is not dilated, and the right ventricular sinus is not enlarged.[A6] In about 30% of hearts, the morphologic changes make the tricuspid valve incompetent or, rarely, stenotic.

There may be a thinned dilated atrialized portion of the right ventricle.[A6,L1] For this reason and occasionally without this feature, the right ventricle may be mildly or more severely hypoplastic.[E1]

Atrioventricular Node and Bundle of His

The AV node and bundle of His in CTGA (and in most if not all hearts with AV discordant connection) differs from the normal. Although a regular (posterior) AV node is present in

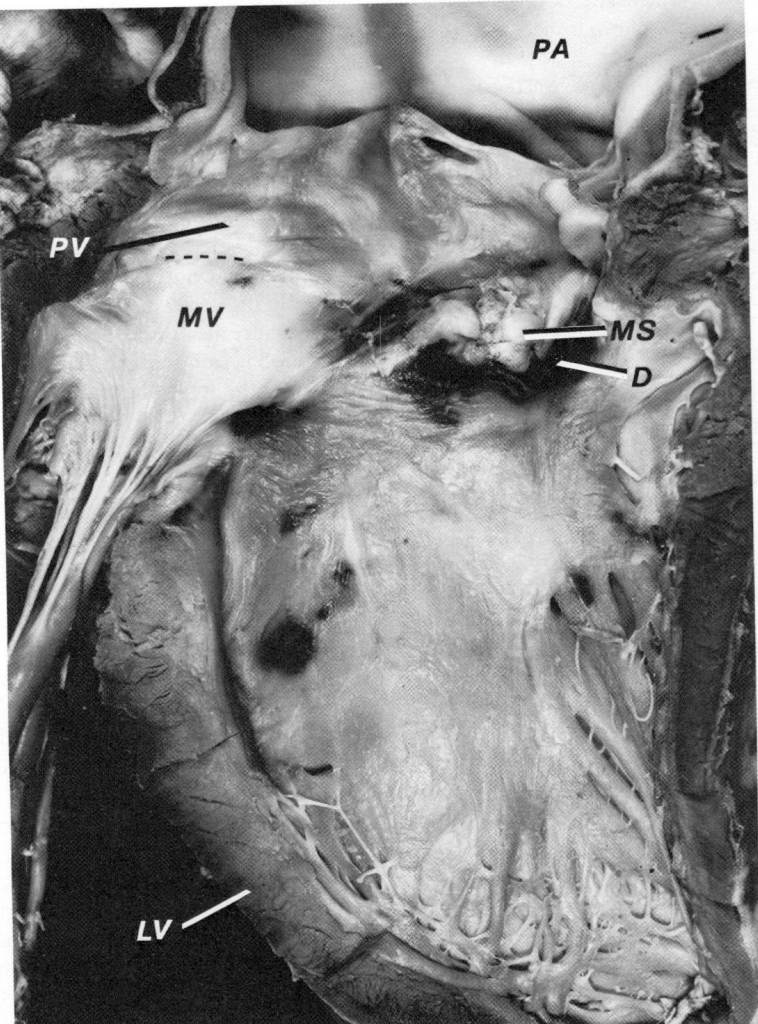

Figure 42-3 Specimen of a heart with CTGA with the opened right-sided left ventricle (LV) and pulmonary artery (GLH). The exposed ventricular septal surface is smooth and has fine apical trabeculations. There is a moderate-sized aneurysm of the membranous ventricular septum bulging into the LV outflow tract, associated with a perimembranous ventricular septal defect. There is pulmonary-mitral valve fibrous continuity, the pulmonary leaflet reaching to the dashed line.

D, ventricular septal defect; LV, left ventricle; MS, membranous ventricular septum; MV, mitral valve; PA, pulmonary artery; PV, pulmonary valve.

front of the coronary sinus ostium in the apex of the triangle of Koch, the penetrating bundle of His rarely extends from it because of the septal malalignment at this point. However, when there is atrial situs inversus, the penetrating bundle of His nearly always extends from the regular or posterior node.[D2,M2,T1,W2] The bundle of His arising from the regular AV node then lies adjacent to the posteroinferior margin of the VSD.[D2] An anterior AV node is generally also present but without a connection to a bundle of His.

In all hearts with atrial situs solitus, there is a second anterior (superior) node located adjacent to the right AV orifice beneath the ostium of the right atrial appendage at its junction with the anterior atrial wall where the anterior horn of the limbus of the atrial septum joins the AV ring (see Fig. 42-4). Immediately beneath this point is the right fibrous

trigone through which the penetrating bundle passes to lie immediately inferior (caudad) to the pulmonary anulus in the anterior right ventricular free wall (Fig. 42-2). It then passes over the anulus and descends away from it onto the anterior part of the infundibular septum.[A1,A3] The bundle descends for some distance before branching, lying between the membranous and muscular portions of the septum. It is subendocardial in position and frequently visible as a pale ridge of tissue (Fig. 42-2). A cordlike right branch penetrates across the crest of the muscular septum to reach the left-sided right ventricular septal surface near the origin of the papillary muscle of the conus and passes downward on the surface of the septal band to reach the moderator band. The sheetlike left bundle branch continues downward on the left ventricular septal surface from the branching bundle.

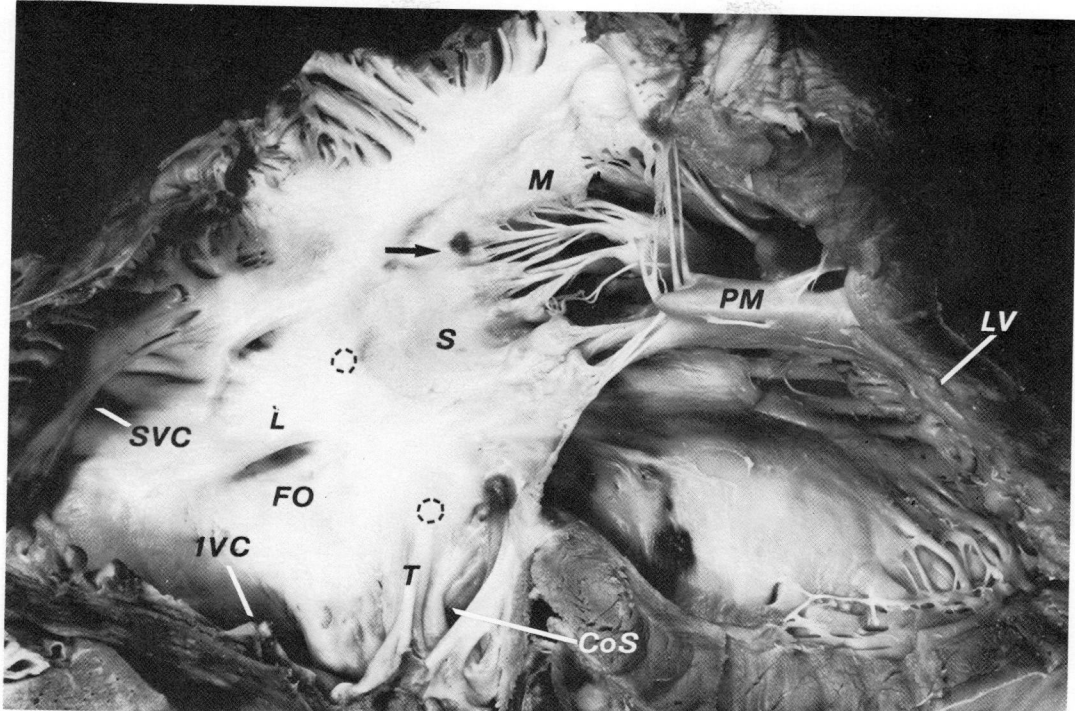

Figure 42-4 Specimen with CTGA in which the right atrium and right-sided left ventricle have been opened, the incision passing across the inferior mitral valve commissure (GLH). The superior commissure between the septal (pulmonary) mitral leaflet and mural leaflet is marked with an arrow. The likely position of the two AV nodes are shown with dotted lines. The larger posterolateral papillary muscle is well seen.

CoS, coronary sinus; FO, fossa ovalis; IVC, inferior vena cava; L, limbus; LV, left ventricle; M, mural leaflet; PM, papillary muscle; S, septal mitral leaflet; SVC, superior vena cava; T, tendon of Todaro.

Occasionally, penetrating bundles pass from both the regular and the anterior AV nodes to form a complete sling of conducting tissue surrounding the pulmonary ring.[A3,B1,S2]

The encircling portion of the AV bundle is prone to fibrosis in older people,[A3] a feature that may explain the spontaneous occurrence of complete heart block. Occasionally, when there is congenital complete heart block, anatomic discontinuity has been demonstrated between the node and bundle of His[B4,L5] or a sling of conduction tissue in the ventricular septum.[B6,W4] In cases with Wolff-Parkinson-White (WPW) syndrome, accessory pathways are present (see Chapter 48, Section 1).[B6,S2]

Ventricular Septum

In the absence of positional anomalies, most of the muscular sinus septum lies in a sagittal plane and is therefore profiled in the anteroposterior view (rather than the left anterior oblique) on cineangiography.[L1] However, the right ventricular cavity is circular in cross section and the lower pressure left ventricle wraps around it.

The septal malalignment and separation result in enlargement of the membranous septum and a filling of the gap created between atrial, ventricular, and conal septa. The AV part of the membranous septum lies between the left atrium and left ventricle (rather than the right atrium and left ventricle as

in the normal heart), and its interventricular portion lies beneath the posterior part of the pulmonary anulus. An aneurysm of this portion of the septum is relatively common with or without a VSD (Fig. 42-3) and can be a cause of left ventricular outflow tract obstruction.[A4,A6,K2] When a VSD is present, the aneurysm lies along its superior margin.

Ventricular Septal Defect

A VSD is the most common additional anomaly and is present in about 80% of hearts with CTGA.[A4] Usually, it is large and subpulmonary and associated with virtual absence of the membranous septum (perimembranous). The pulmonary valve commonly overrides the VSD to arise in part from the right ventricle. As viewed from the right (left ventricular) side (Fig. 42-5), the VSD is bounded superiorly by the pulmonary ring or the pulmonary valve itself depending on the degree of overriding. There may be membranous septal remnants along this margin (Fig. 42-3). Posteriorly, it is bounded by that part of the mitral ring from which the septal leaflet arises and anteriorly and inferiorly by the infundibular and muscular interventricular septa, respectively. Its postero-inferior margin may extend to the mitral ring with a zone of mitral-pulmonary-tricuspid fibrous continuity. The VSD is not infrequently narrowed or nearly closed by an aneurysm of the membranous septum (Fig. 42-3) or valvar excres-

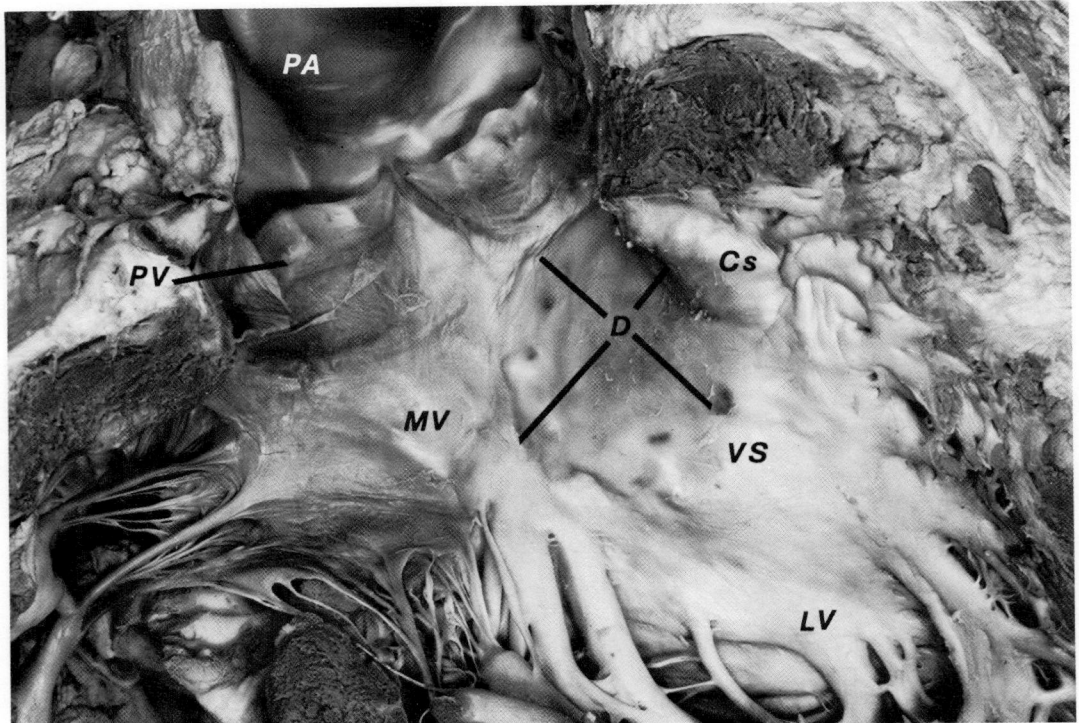

Figure 42-5 Specimen of a heart with CTGA in which a large perimembranous ventricular septal defect has been closed with a Dacron patch 4 years prior to death (GLH). The left ventricle and pulmonary artery have been opened. The limits of the patch are easily discernible. The defect is bounded superiorly by the pulmonary ring, posteriorly by the mitral ring, anteriorly by the infundibular (conal) septum, and inferiorly by the muscular ventricular septum.

Cs, infundibular (conal) septum; D, ventricular septal defect closed by a patch; LV, left ventricle; MV, septal mitral valve leaflet; PA, pulmonary artery; PV, normal pulmonary valve; VS, ventricular septum.

cences from the left-sided tricuspid valve (see Chapter 23, Section 4).[A4]

Viewed from the right ventricular (left) side, this perimembranous VSD lies, as usual, within the Y of the septal band and beneath the conal septum. The bundle of His courses along its anterior margin on the left ventricular (right) side in a subendocardial position and bifurcates at its anteroinferior angle with the right bundle branch crossing this angle of the defect to reach the right ventricle.

In about 10% of cases (more often in Japan),[O1] the VSD lies within the conal septum (subaortic); when it completely replaces it, it is immediately below both great arteries (doubly committed, subarterial) (Fig. 42-6). Uncommonly, the VSD may be muscular, lying in the sinus (trabecular) septum.

A large, typical AV canal-type VSD may uncommonly occur. Also, there may be more than one VSD present.

Coronary Arteries

The coronary arteries demonstrate the anatomy appropriate to their ventricles. Thus, the left coronary artery with its left anterior descending and circumflex branches supplies the left ventricle, and the right coronary artery and its conal and posterior descending branches supplies the right ventricle.

The aortic origins are, however, peculiar to the malformation, bearing in mind that the anterior sinus is the noncoronary one. The right-sided left coronary artery arises from the right posterior sinus and passes directly in front of the pulmonary ring to divide into left anterior descending and circumflex branches, the latter passing in front of the right atrial appendage in the atrioventricular groove. The left-sided right coronary artery arises from the left posterior sinus and runs in the AV groove and in front of the left atrial appendage, terminating posteriorly as the posterior descending artery. Lev and Rowlatt used the terms "right sided" and "left sided" to describe these vessels.[L6] The most common variation from this arrangement is for a single coronary artery to arise from the right sinus and divide into right and left main branches.

Associated Anomalies

VSD, pulmonary stenosis, and left-sided tricuspid valve anomalies have been discussed, although 1%–2% of hearts with CTGA have no coexistent anomalies.[A4,A8,L1,L2] Other coexisting anomalies include a supravalvar left atrial ring, which may be a cause of left-sided (tricuspid valve) stenosis,[A4] and coarctation of the aorta in association with a VSD. A patent ductus arteriosus is sometimes present, as is a true

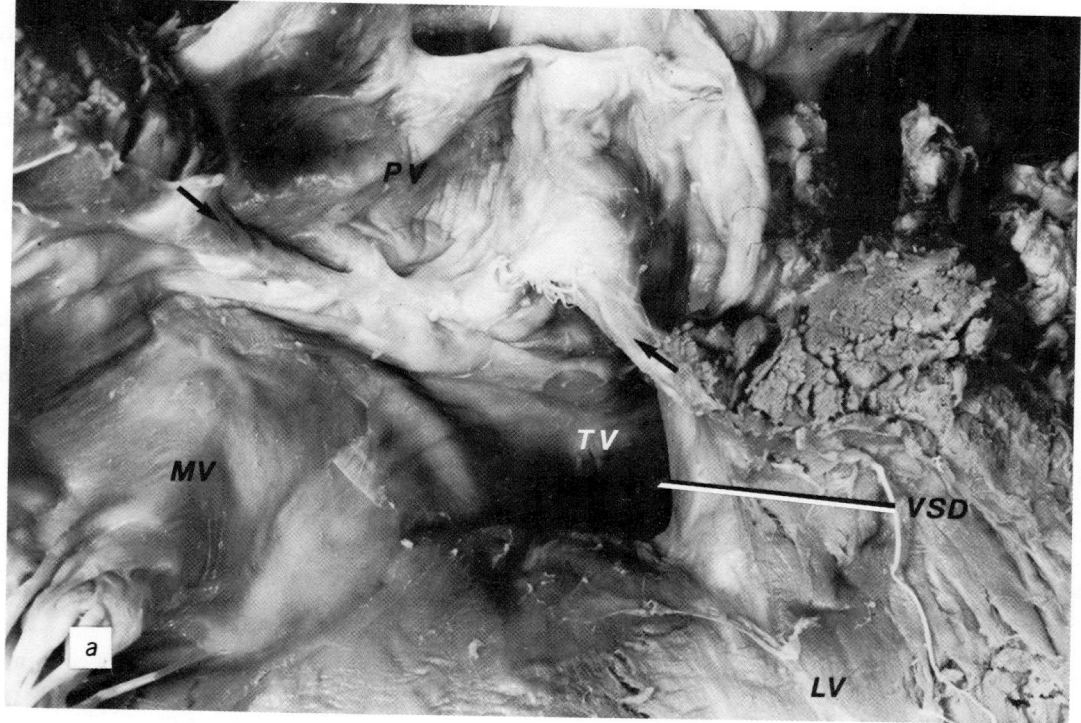

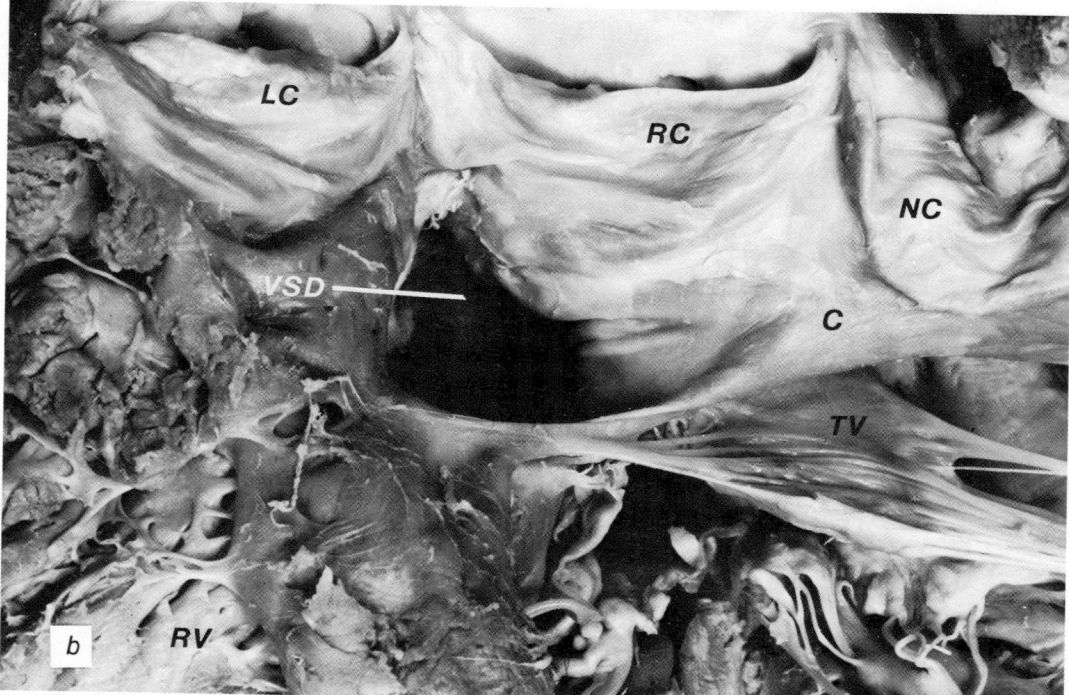

Figure 42-6 Specimen of a heart with CTGA and doubly committed subarterial ventricular septal defect (GLH).

(a) Viewed from the right-sided left ventricle. There is also a partially obstructed subpulmonary fibrous membrane present (arrows).

(b) Viewed from the left-sided right ventricle. The conal septum is absent, but there is a relatively short subaortic conus. There is tricuspid-mitral-pulmonary fibrous continuity through the VSD.

C, subaortic conus; LC, left coronary (right-sided) aortic leaflet; LV, left ventricle; MV, mitral valve; NC, noncoronary (anterior) aortic leaflet; PV, pulmonary valve; RC, right coronary (left-sided) aortic leaflet; RV, right ventricle; TV, tricuspid valve; VSD, ventricular septal defect.

atrial septal defect in about 20% of cases. One patient with pulmonary atresia and atrial situs inversus also had an unroofed coronary sinus (right superior vena cava draining to left atrium) (GLH).

Overriding or straddling of AV valves is more common when there are positional anomalies, as is hypoplasia of one or other ventricle.[E1] A left-sided tricuspid valve may override and straddle a VSD,[L7] which is at times associated with hypoplasia of the left-sided right ventricle and at times with superior-inferior ventricles (see Chapter 43, "Positional Anomalies" and Chapter 1, "Cardiac and Arterial Positions" in section on Terminology and Classification of Heart Disease). The left-sided tricuspid valve straddles the posterior part of the ventricular septum, which is then prevented from reaching the crux, and the conduction tissue passes anterior to the pulmonary ring.[M6] More rarely, the right-sided mitral valve may behave similarly (as it does at times in AV discordant connection with double outlet right ventricle); invariably this is associated with left ventricular hypoplasia and superior-inferior ventricles.[B8,S4] The mitral valve straddles the anterior part of the septum so that the ventricular septum does extend to the crux, and a regular posterior node only may be present with the bundle passing posterior to the pulmonary anulus.[B8]

CLINICAL FEATURES AND DIAGNOSTIC CRITERIA

In congenitally corrected transposition of the great arteries (CTGA), despite the usually large ventricular septal defect (VSD) and even though there is no organic obstruction, there is usually some restriction of pulmonary blood flow due to the morphology of the subpulmonary left ventricular outflow tract. Therefore, symptoms from the sequelae of a large pulmonary blood flow are not common in the first year of life. Friedberg and Nadas estimate such symptoms to occur in about 30% of their cases,[F4] and the UAB experience is similar (Fig. 42-7). This is in contrast to the situation in primary large VSD (see Chapter 20).

Also, it is uncommon for the pulmonary stenosis to be severe enough to require a shunting procedure in the first year of life (UAB; Fig. 42-7). Friedberg and Nadas found only 30% of their patients presented in the first year of life as a result of cyanosis, although cyanosis was present at some time during the course of the disease in two-thirds. Most often, the presentation is in childhood or in the second decade (see Fig. 42-7) because of growth failure and exercise intolerance from a left-to-right shunt or, if there is important pulmonary stenosis, mild or moderate cyanosis or effort intolerance. Left-sided tricuspid valve incompetence may complicate the other anomalies present, or it may occur as an isolated finding. The incompetence seems to worsen with time, and therefore patients with it may occasionally not present until the third, fourth, or fifth decade of life.

The clinical feature bringing some patients with CTGA to medical attention is bradycardia from congenitally complete heart block (present from birth or soon after), a complication occurring in 10%–30% of cases.[C2,F4,L2] The complete heart block at times is episodic and induced temporarily by cardiac catheterization, anesthesia, exercise, or thoracotomy.[S1] First- or second-degree heart block is found in an additional 20%–30% of cases,[B7,S1] many of whom earlier had normal AV conduction,[F4] and this degree of heart block may be a prelude to the development of complete heart block (see

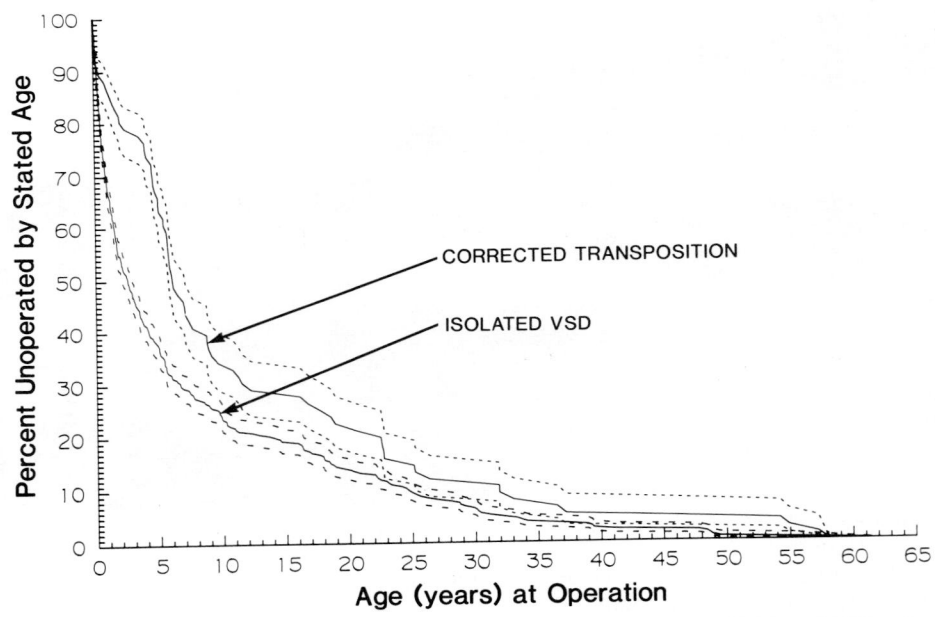

Figure 42-7 Cumulative distribution of age at operation of patients with CTGA and VSD with or without pulmonary stenosis (UAB; 1967–1983) compared with patients with concordant AV connection having isolated VSD repair (Rizzoli et al.[R4]). The dashed lines enclose the 70% confidence limits. Note that only 67% of the VSD patients are without operation by age 1 year, whereas 88% of those with CTGA remain without operation by that age.

"Natural History"). Wolff-Parkinson-White syndrome (WPW), either type A or B, coexists with some frequency in patients with CTGA.[B4,G1,S1,S3]

The physical findings are generally not diagnostic,[F4] but the finding of a loud second heart sound at the second left intercostal space is said to be suggestive of the diagnosis since it may represent closure of the leftward and anterior aortic valve.[H2,S1]

Although the chest x-ray may suggest that a congenital cardiac malformation has AV discordant connection by the finding of the shadow of the ascending aorta along the left upper cardiac silhouette, this is not diagnostic since there are many other anomalies in which the aorta is in L-malposition (see Chapter 45, "Clinical Features and Diagnostic Criteria"). The electrocardiogram (ECG) may suggest a correct diagnosis when there is reversal of the precordial Q wave pattern with deep Q waves in leads V_2 and AVR and QS complexes in leads V_3 and AVF and right precordial leads. The presence of congenital or developing complete heart block is also suggestive of the diagnosis of CTGA.[L1]

The echocardiogram can provide the diagnosis of CTGA with reasonable accuracy.[H3,S5] When the spatial orientation of the ventricular septum is abnormal, the left-sided AV valve inserts more toward the apex than the right-sided one and has direct chordal attachments to the inlet septum. There is also continuity between the right-sided AV valve and the posterior (pulmonary) semilunar valve.[L1]

Currently, however, cardiac catheterization and biplane cineangiography provide the definitive diagnostic data in this group of cardiac malformations (Fig. 42-8). Pressure and flows are measured to quantitate the severity of pulmonary stenosis and any intracardiac shunt. As with other complex cardiac anomalies, the angiographic views must profile the ventricular septum and establish the morphology of the various chambers and the site of systemic and pulmonary venous return and thus the cardiac connections present. They must define the site and number of VSDs, the nature of the pulmonary stenosis and of tricuspid valve function, and any other associated anomalies.[B9,L1,S6]

NATURAL HISTORY

The only specific and certain contribution of the discordant atrioventricular (AV) connection to the natural history is the tendency to the development of AV conduction abnormalities and, ultimately, complete heart block. About 5%–10% of infants with congenital transposition of the great arteries or other types of AV discordant connection have complete heart block at birth,[C2,F4,L2] and this proportion slowly increases at a rate of about 2% a year to reach about 30%.[H5]

At least 40%–50% of patients with AV discordant connection are born with first-degree or second-degree AV block.[B7] As time passes, a prolongation of PR interval sometimes develops in those with originally normal intervals.[F4] Thus, Gillette and colleagues found normal AV conduction at 6–7 years of age in only 38% (CL 29%–47%) of 40 patients with CTGA.[G2] Prolongation of the PR interval, when present, slowly increases and this may eventuate in episodic or per-

manent complete heart block.[S1] However, about 40% of patients with AV discordant connection retain throughout their lives normal PR intervals and QRS durations.

The site of first degree AV block may be in the AV node, the bundle of His, or the bundle branch system.[G2] These same sites may be responsible for higher degrees of heart block, although multiple and diffuse sites of block may be involved. Further, in some infants born with complete heart block. bundle of His potentials cannot be recorded,[G2] and morphologic evidence of a connection between an AV node and the more distal parts of the bundle of His cannot be found.

It is difficult to prove that the systemic right ventricle present in CTGA and in other forms of AV discordant connection is detrimental to cardiac performance or life expectancy. Graham and colleagues have shown that the right ventricle's ejection fraction tends to be normal in childhood in this setting but depressed after the second decade of life.[G3] However, most patients have associated cardiac anomalies that could have caused the deterioration. Kishon and colleagues followed six healthy infants with CTGA without any associated anomaly and found functional deterioration over 10–15 years in none of them.[K5]

The natural history of patients with CTGA and *large VSD* tends to be a little better than that of patients with isolated large VSDs (Fig. 42-7). This is not as apparent as it might be in the report of Friedberg and Nadas,[F4] and this may relate to their inclusion of patients with univentricular AV connection (single ventricle) in their study. However, chronic symptoms of effort intolerance and growth failure are common in such patients in the first two decades of life, but death during this period of life is infrequent. Although an actuarial estimate of survival in patients with corrected transposition and large VSD is not available, presumably death from chronic congestive heart failure occurs with increasing frequency in the third, fourth, and fifth decades of life.

When *important pulmonary stenosis coexists with VSD*, cyanosis is produced in early life and the natural history of the patient is presumably similar to that of tetralogy of Fallot (see Chapter 23).

The natural history of the *left AV valve* in patients with CTGA and other types of AV discordance is unclear. Presumably, this valve is nearly always competent in the first few years of life, but the incidence and magnitude of incompetence progressively increases during the second through fifth decades.

TECHNIQUE OF OPERATION

Repair of the Ventricular Septal Defect

The preparations for operation and the median sternotomy and placement of pericardial stay sutures are as usual (see Chapter 2, Section 3). Placement of the purse-string sutures for aortic cannulation and the cannulation itself are more difficult than usual because of the aortic L-malposition. These procedures are facilitated by grasping the aortic adventitia with one or two small curved hemostats and retracting these inferiorly. The usual purse-string sutures are

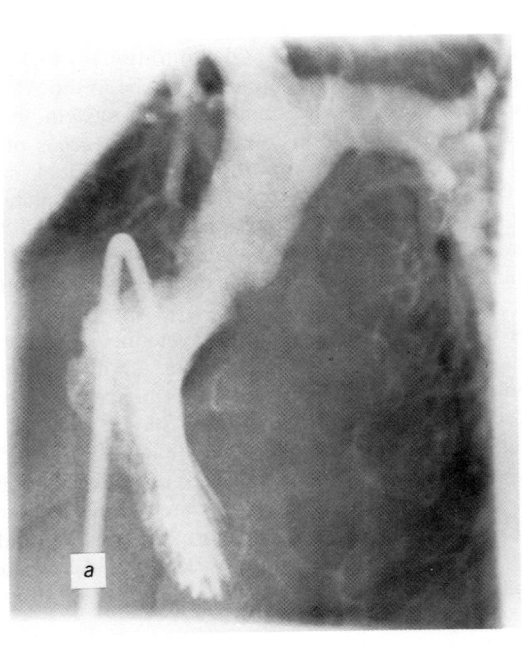
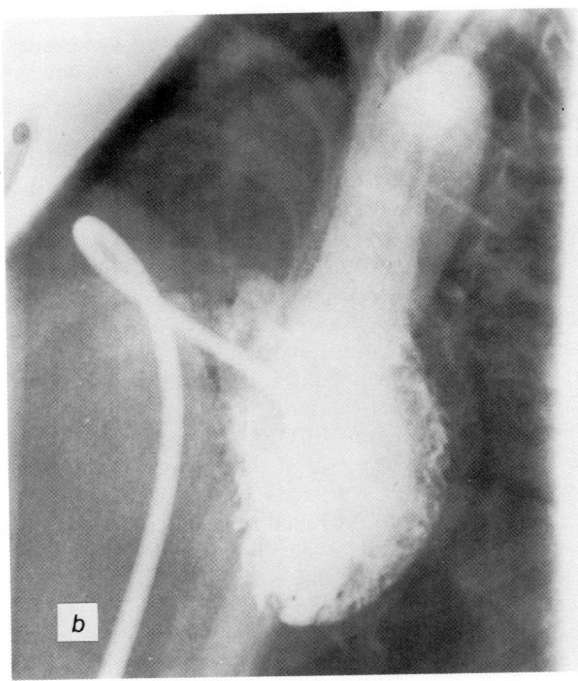
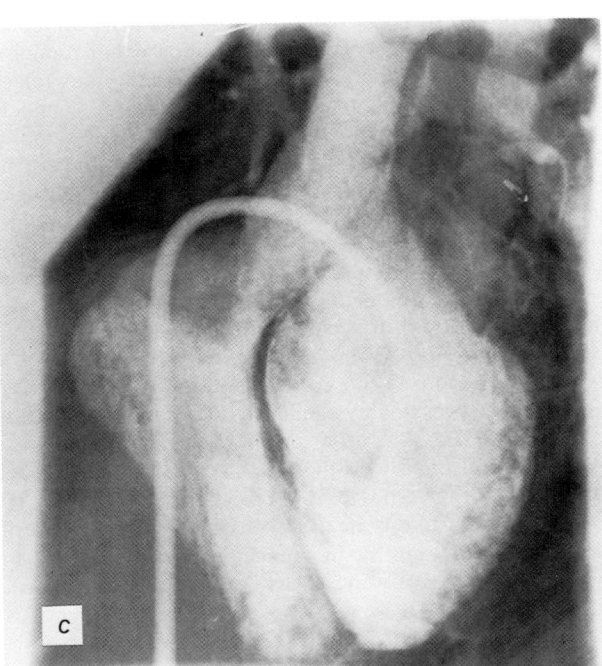
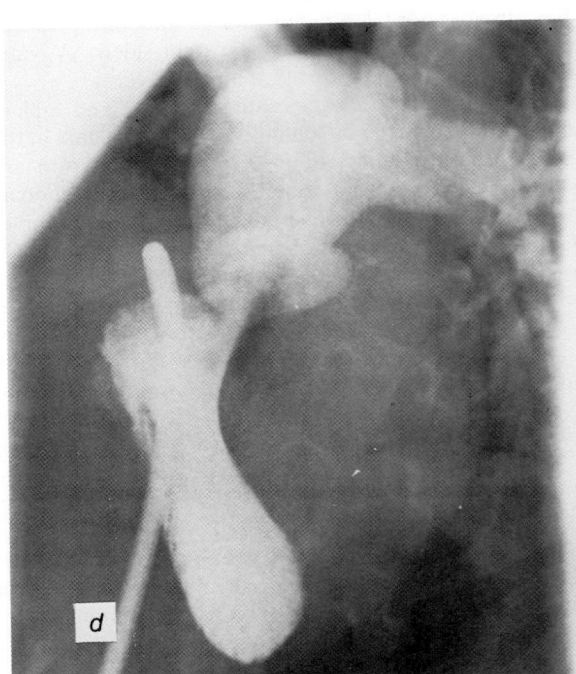

Figure 42-8 Cineangiograms in patients with CTGA (UAB).

(a) Left ventricular injection in the four-chamber position, AP projection. The pulmonary artery arises from the right-sided left ventricle. Note the concavity into the low-pressure left ventricle produced by the nonopacified high-pressure right ventricle.

(b) In the same patient, right ventricular injection in the four-chamber position, AP projection. The aorta arises from the left-sided right ventricle.

(c) In another patient, right ventricular injection in the four-chamber position, AP projection. In this patient, in contrast to the first one, a ventricular septal defect allows dye to pass into the left ventricle and out the pulmonary artery. The pulmonary artery and ascending aorta are superimposed.

(d) In a patient with coexisting subvalvar pulmonary stenosis, left ventricular injection in the four-chamber position, AP projection. The severe subvalvar narrowing is evident, as well as the post-stenotic dilation of the pulmonary artery.

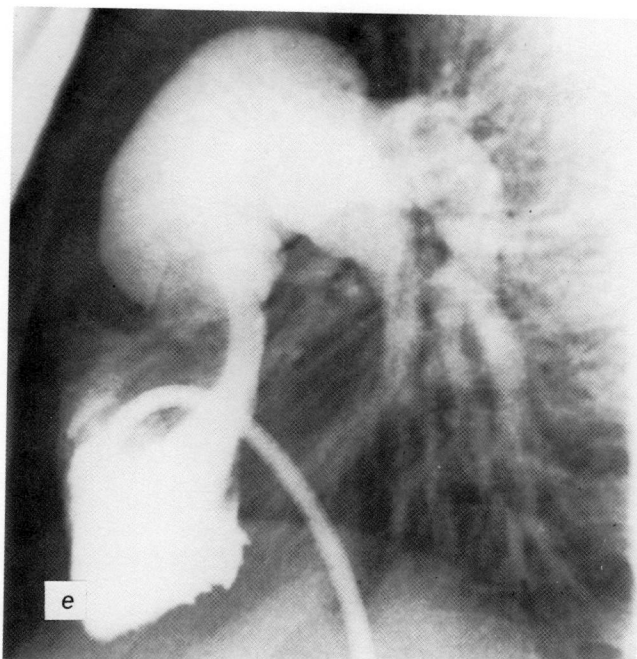

Figure 42-8 *(continued)*
(e) In the same patient, left ventricular injection, lateral projection. The long severe subvalvar narrowing is again evident.

placed for aortic cannulation and for the cardioplegic needle, and caval tapes and purse-string sutures are also placed. When there is atrial situs solitus and dextrocardia, the right atrium and cavae are hidden behind the ventricle making right atrial cannulation difficult (GLH), although the difficulty of direct caval cannulation is not increased (UAB). It may be best to cannulate only the right atrial appendage prior to commencing cardiopulmonary bypass (CPB), then when the heart has been emptied it is dislocated and a second cannula positioned (GLH).

The exterior of the heart is examined, and palpation behind the left atrium and then along its roof is carried out to detect any regurgitant jet from the left-sided tricuspid valve.

CPB is established in the usual manner. The perfusate is made as cold as possible, and as soon as the heart becomes ineffective the right atrium is opened through an oblique incision (see Chapter 15, Fig. 15-12). A pump-oxygenator sump sucker is placed across the foramen ovale (UAB) or introduced through the right superior pulmonary vein (GLH). The aorta is cross-clamped and the cold cardioplegic solution infused. Stay sutures are placed to provide a wide atrial exposure.

The ventricular septal defect (VSD) is examined through the right-sided mitral valve. This valve does not permit quite as free access to the interior of the ventricle as the normal right-sided tricuspid valve. However, in about two-thirds of the cases, the VSD can be repaired through the intact mitral valve. In about one-third of cases, the exposure is suboptimal. Then, a circumferential incision is made in the base of the septal (pulmonary) leaflet of the mitral valve near the superior commissural tissue and carried forward, if necessary, through the commissural tissue into the mural leaflet.

The technique is similar to that used occasionally for AV canal type of VSD (see Chapter 20, Fig. 20-26). Working through the aperture that is created, the repair of the VSD can be accomplished nicely.

The subpulmonary (left ventricular outflow) tract is examined. Unless the pulmonary valve itself is stenotic or there are valvar excrescences obstructing the subvalvar area, little can be done to improve the variable degree of narrowing that is usually present (see "Results"). Only the placement of a bypassing valved extracardiac conduit will provide good relief. However, if the pulmonary blood flow has been large ($\dot{Q}p/\dot{Q}s > 2.0$ preoperatively), even a 50 mmHg gradient does not necessarily indicate the need for a conduit. With ablation of the left-to-right shunt by closure of the large VSD, the right-sided left ventricular pressure will usually fall to half systemic pressure.

The margins of the VSD are studied (Fig. 42-9). The location of the anterior node and the bundle of His arching over the subpulmonary outflow tract and passing anterior to the VSD are conceptualized, and in fact the bundle often can be seen as a thin, pale line. Electrophysiologic mapping is not necessary (see "Results"). The left-sided tricuspid valve can usually be seen through the VSD, and some of its chordae often attach to the inferior VSD border.

The repair is made by sewing into place a proper sized Dacron velour patch, keeping the sutures on the left (right ventricular) side of the defect anterosuperiorly, anteriorly, and as much as possible inferiorly (Fig. 42-10). The chordae from the tricuspid valve, often attaching to the inferior edge of the VSD, limit this possibility inferiorly. A continuous 4-0 polypropylene suture may usually be used, although interrupted pledgetted mattress sutures are used if the exposure is difficult. After the repair is complete and if a circumferential incision has been made in the mitral leaflets, this incision is closed with continuous 6-0 polypropylene suture, using the previously placed fine stay sutures to keep the closure properly orientated so that valve distortion is avoided.

The left atrial suction line is removed from across the foramen ovale (UAB) and the left atrium filled, the foramen ovale closed, and the apex of the left-sided right ventricle aspirated for air; with strong suction on the aortic needle vent, the aortic clamp is released. Rewarming with the pump oxygenator has been started about 5 minutes before. The right atriotomy is closed, the caval tapes released, and the usual de-airing procedures are carried out. The remainder of the procedure, including the placing of temporary atrial and ventricular pacing wires, is carried out in the usual manner (see Chapter 2, Section 3). The matter of permanent pacing electrodes is discussed in "Special Situations and Controversies."

Pulmonary Valvotomy for Pulmonary Stenosis

When the pulmonary valve is stenotic, it is approached through a pulmonary arteriotomy during moderately hypothermic CPB and cold cardioplegia. The pulmonary valvotomy is done as described for isolated pulmonary valve stenosis (see Chapter 24, Fig. 24-5). When there are obstructing fibrous subvalvar tags, these are excised bearing in mind the bundle position (Fig. 42-2). A subvalvar fibrous

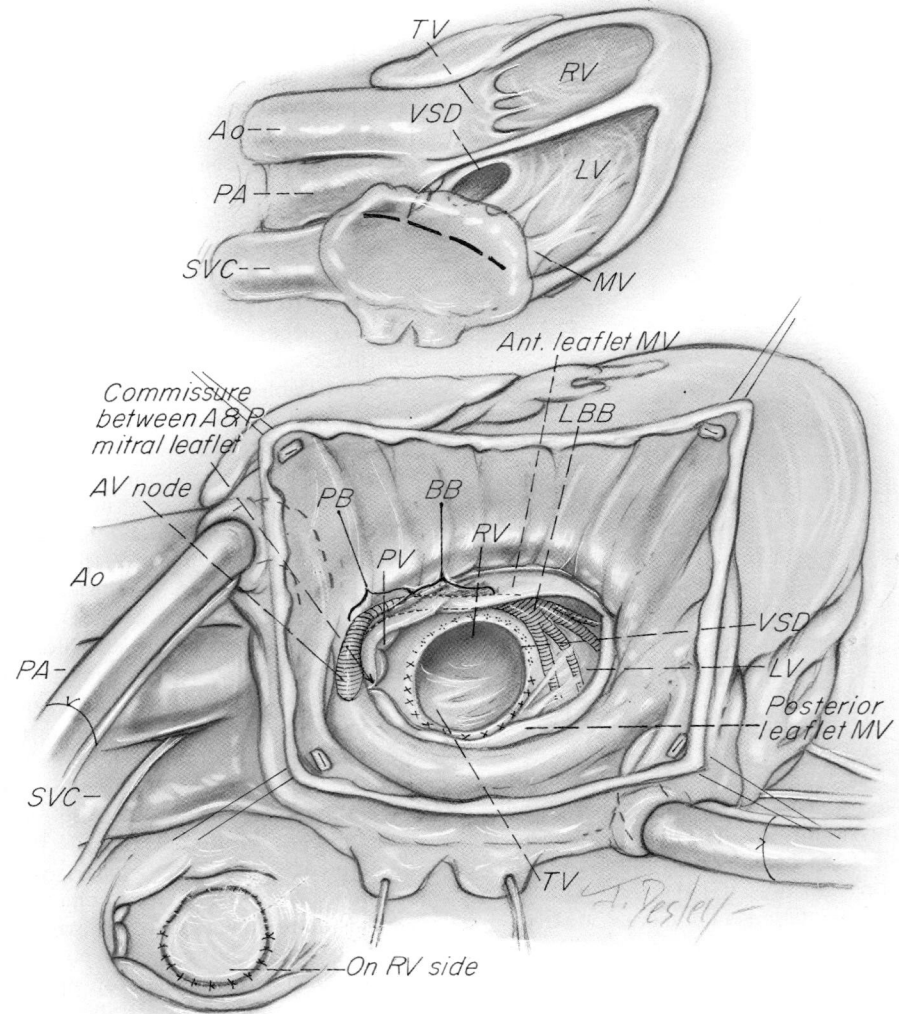

Figure 42-9   Anatomy, conduction system, and suture siting for repair of the ventricular septal defect in patients with atrial situs solitus and CTGA. A dashed line represents the atrial incision. Suture siting on the right-sided left ventricular aspect of ventricular septum is indicated by ×'s. Suture siting on the left-sided right ventricular aspect of the ventricular septum is indicated by a double row of dots.

A, anterior; Ao, aorta; AV, atrioventricular; LBB, left bundle branch; LV, right-sided left ventricle; MV, right-sided mitral valve; P, posterior; PA, pulmonary artery; PB, BB, penetrating and branching portions of bundle of His; PV, pulmonary valve; RV, left-sided right ventricle; SVC, superior vena cava; TV, left-sided tricuspid valve; VSD, ventricular septal defect.

Reproduced with permission from Bharati et al.[B11]

membrane can also be excised except for that portion at the anteroinferior angle. Aneurysms of the membranous ventricular septum are similarly excised. When there is a VSD, the resultant deficiency is closed as part of the VSD repair. When the ventricular septum is intact, the VSD so created is closed with a running polypropylene suture. Muscle must never be removed from the rightward (medial) aspect of the left ventricular outflow tract nor from the anterior part adjacent to the pulmonary ring, since the bundle of His lies in these positions.

Hegar dilators are used to measure the resulting orifice and the Z value estimated (see Chapter 23, "General Plan and Details Common to All Approaches" in Section 1, Technique of Operation). Usually the results of valvotomy are disappointing in the setting of CTGA, because of a bicuspid valve, supravalvar pulmonary trunk narrowing (tethering) at the level of commissural attachment, or a narrow subpulmonary left ventricular outflow tract. However, if the Z value is > −1 after the valvotomy, the pulmonary artery is closed, the usual de-airing and other procedures are carried out, and CPB is discontinued.

Pressures are measured before removing the cannulae. The relationship between the postvalvotomy $P_{RV/LV}$ in the operating room and that the next morning and late postop-

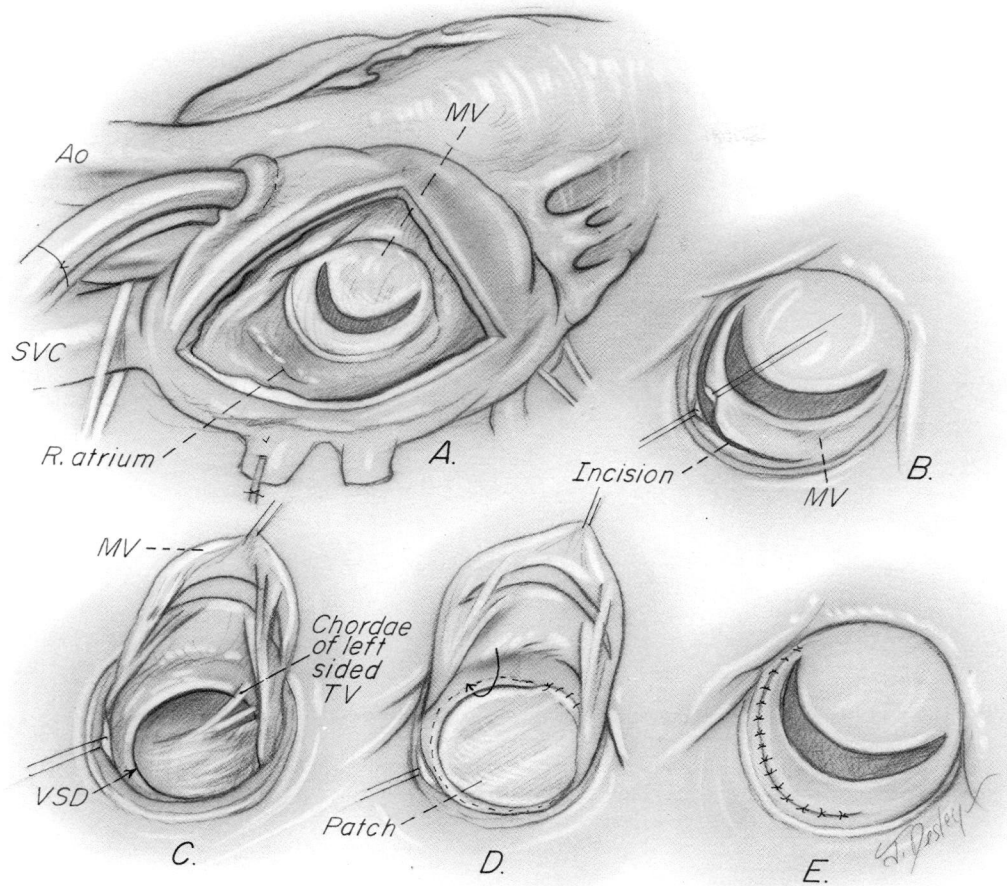

Figure 42-10   Steps in the repair of the ventricular septal defect (VSD) in CTGA.
(*a*) The initial approach through the right atrium. Frequently, the repair can be carried out through the intact right-sided mitral valve.
(*b*) If exposure is not good, a radial incision is made in the leaflets as shown. Stay sutures are placed opposite each other to aid in proper reconstruction of the leaflet.
(*c*) With the leaflet elevated by stay sutures, excellent exposure of the VSD is obtained. In this case, as is frequent, chordae from the left-sided tricuspid valve attach along the inferior edge of the ventricular septum. This prevents keeping the patch on the right ventricular left side for the entire repair.
(*d*) The patch has been sewn into place, keeping the sutures well on the right ventricular side throughout except where prevented by chordae. An alternative is to cut a slot in the patch so that the chordae come through the patch that has been placed on the right ventricular side (see Chapter 44, "Straddling and Overriding AV Valves"). However, this risks an incomplete closure of the VSD.
(*e*) The right-sided mitral valve is reconstructed with continuous 6-0 polypropylene sutures.
Ao, aorta; MV, mitral valve; SVC, superior vena cava; TV, tricuspid valve; VSD, ventricular septal defect.

eratively is not known in CTGA. However, it has seemed reasonable to go back on CPB and place a valved extracardiac conduit if the $P_{RV/LV}$ is > 0.85.

In any event, a polyvinyl catheter is placed in the right-sided left ventricle, and if possible this is threaded into the pulmonary artery. The left ventricular pressure is remeasured the next morning in the intensive care unit with this catheter, and if the calculated $P_{RV/LV}$ is > 0.7, the patient is returned to the operating room and a valved extracardiac conduit is placed (UAB).

Placement of Valved Extracardiac Conduit to the Pulmonary Trunk

When pulmonary stenosis coexists with a VSD and is of sufficient severity to result in important cyanosis, a valved extracardiac conduit is usually a necessary part of the repair. Doty and colleagues have proposed using a transannular patch instead, the patch going across the pulmonary valve ring posteriorly, with or without an orthotopically placed valve replacement. However, this method has not been well

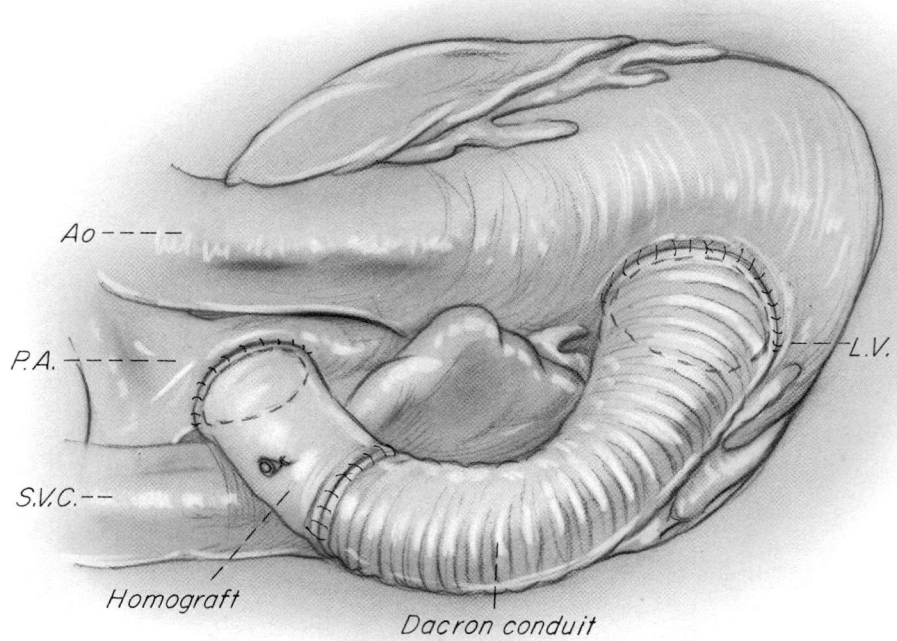

Ao ----

P.A. ----

S.V.C. --

Homograft

Dacron conduit

---- L.V.

Figure 42-11 Final position of the homograft-valved extracardiac conduit used for repair in patients with CTGA, ventricular septal defect, and pulmonary stenosis. This routing of the conduit, which is virtually routine in patients with AV discordant connection and atrial situs solitus, allows it to lie away from the sternum and prevents its compression.

Ao, aorta; LV, left ventricle; PA, pulmonary artery; SVC, superior vena cava.

tested, and the average gradient after repair in their report was 40 mmHg.[D3]

After the VSD has been repaired by working through the right atrium, the site is chosen for the left ventriculotomy by examination of the interior of the left ventricle through the mitral valve. A site is chosen that is on the anterior left ventricular wall but rather inferior and away from any papillary muscles. This incision is then made. An incision in the

right side of the pulmonary trunk is made for the distal end of the conduit and is extended if necessary onto the right pulmonary artery.

The homograft-valved conduit has previously been prepared by extending it proximally with a woven Dacron tube (see Chapter 23, Fig. 23-37 for details). This is necessary in this situation, in contrast to tetralogy of Fallot and complete transposition, because the conduit must be of sufficient

Table 42-1 Hospital and late mortality after primary cardiac operations in patients with CTGA (GLH; 1958–1983).

Operation	n	Hospital Deaths			Late Deaths		
		No.	%	CL	No.	%[b]	CL
VSD repair	4	0	0%	0%–38%	3	75%	
VSD + PS repair	4[a]	0	0%	0%–38%	1	25%	
VSD + LV–PA conduit	4	2	50%	18%–82%	1	50%	
TV replacement							
Isolated	1	0	0%	0%–85%	1	100%	
With VSD repair	2	0	0%	0%–61%	1	50%	
With VSD + PS repair	1	1	100%	15%–100%			
PS repair	3	0	0%	0%–47%	0	0%	
Total	19	3	16%	7%–29%	7	44%	29%–60%

KEY: ASD, atrial septal defect; CABG, coronary artery bypass grafting; CL, 70% confidence limits; LV, left ventricle; PA, pulmonary artery; PS, pulmonary stenosis; TV, tricuspid valve; VSD, ventricular septal defect.

NOTE: Six patients (no deaths) with atrial situs solitus had dextrocardia. Three patients (no deaths) had atrial situs inversus.

[a] One with banded PA.

[b] Percentage of hospital survivors.

Table 42-2 Hospital and late mortality after primary cardiac operations in patients with corrected CTGA (UAB; 1967–1983).

Operation	n	Hospital Deaths			Late Deaths		
		No.	%	CL	No.	%[d]	CL
Repair VSD	16	1	6%	1%–20%	5	33%	
Repair VSD + PS	15[a]	2	13%	4%–29%	2	15%	
Repair VSD + valved extracardiac conduit to PA	26[b,c]	2	8%	3%–17%	2	8%	
Tricuspid valve repair	1		0%	0%–85%			
Tricuspid valve replacement							
Isolated	5[a]	1	20%	3%–53%			
With VSD Repair	8	1	12%	2%–36%	1	14%	
With VSD + PS repair	1		0%	0%–85%			
With PS repair + CABG	1[a]		0%	0%–85%			
Repair ASD	1[a]		0%	0%–85%			
Fontan-type operation	1		0%	0%–85%			
Total	75	7	9%	6%–14%	10	15%	10%–21%

KEY: ASD, atrial septal defect; CABG, coronary artery bypass grafting; CL, 70% confidence limits; PA, pulmonary artery; PS, pulmonary stenosis; VSD, ventricular septal defect.

NOTE: Seventeen (24%, CL 18%–30%) of the 71 patients with atrial situs solitus had dextrocardia, and 2 (12%, CL 4%–26%) of the 17 died. In the years 1967–1978, 4 (11%, CL 6%–19%) of 37 patients died; in the years 1978–1983, 3 (8%, CL 3%–15%) of 38 died.

[a] One patient who lived had atrial situs inversus.

[b] Three patients who lived had atrial situs inversus.

[c] One patient also had aortic valvotomy.

[d] Percentage of hospital survivors.

length to prevent kinking, and the valve must lie away from the left ventricle so that it is not distorted. The estimation of the length and lie of the conduit is particularly important in order to avoid conduit compression by the sternum. The conduit is trimmed to size, cutting the distal end square but leaving more of the ascending aorta beyond the aortic valve than in the case of tetralogy, because this facilitates a smooth conduit contour and limits the length of the Dacron part of the conduit. The proximal Dacron end of the conduit is trimmed to make a cobra head (see Chapter 23, Fig. 23-37). The distal aortic end is anastomosed end to side to the

Table 42-3 Complete heart block after repairs in patients with CTGA (GLH; 1958–1983).

Operation	n[a]	PO Permanent CHB		
		No.	%	CL
VSD repair	4	1	25%	
VSD + PS repair	3	1	33%	
VSD + PA–LV conduit	3[b]	0	0%	
TV replacement				
Isolated	1	0	0%	
With VSD repair	1	0	0%	
With VSD + PS repair	1	0	0%	
PS repair	3	0	0%	
Total	16[b]	2	12%	4%–27%

KEY: CHB, complete heart block; CL, 70% confidence limits; LV, left ventricle; PA, pulmonary artery; PO, postoperative; PS, pulmonary stenosis; TV, tricuspid valve; VSD, ventricular septal defect.

NOTE: Among 7 patients undergoing VSD repair since 1969, none (0%, CL 0%–24%) has developed complete heart block.

[a] Number without preoperative complete heart block.

[b] Excludes one patient who died in the operating room.

incision in the pulmonary trunk, and the proximal Dacron end is anastomosed to the ventriculotomy. The conduit curves to the right, around the right atrium and atrial appendage (Fig. 42-11). The remainder of the operation is completed as usual.

Correction for an Incompetent Left-Sided Tricuspid Valve

When important left-sided tricuspid valve incompetence coexists, repair of the valve by annuloplasty is rarely successful but should be attempted if the situation for it seems favorable. If replacement is required, the same considerations apply to the replacement device as in ordinary left-sided mitral valve replacement (see Chapter 11, "Choice of the Replacement Device").

The valve replacement proceeds in the same manner as in the usual case of left-sided mitral valve replacement, including the choice of venous cannulae and the approach through the right side of the left atrium (see Chapter 11, "Mitral Valve Replacement" in section on Technique of Operation, and Fig. 11-6). The replacement device is either sewn in with interrupted pledgetted mattress sutures (UAB) or simple interrupted sutures (GLH). A continuous suture technique is not desirable when there is absence of a well-defined anulus in some areas, occasioned by downward displacement into the ventricle of some of the left-sided tricuspid leaflets.

Placement of Epicardial Pacemaker Leads

When complete heart block has been present intermittently or permanently preoperatively or developed intraoperatively, permanent epicardial atrial and ventricular pacemaking leads are placed. Atrioventricular sequential pacing is

Table 42-4 Heart block after operation in patients with CTGA (UAB; 1967–1983).

Operation	n	Preoperative Complete Heart Block	PO Permanent Complete Heart Block		
			No.	% of (n − Preop Block)	CL
Repair VSD	16	2	2	14%	5%–31%
Repair VSD + PS	15	1	3	21%	10%–38%
Repair VSD + valved extracardiac conduit to PA	26	3[a]	6	26%	16%–39%
Tricuspid valve repair	1			0%	0%–85%
Tricuspid valve replacement					
Isolated	5	1		0%	0%–38%
With VSD repair	8	2		17%	2%–46%
With VSD + PS repair	1	1			
With VSD repair + CABG	1			0%	0%–85%
Repair ASD	1			0%	0%–85%
Fontan-type operation	1			0%	0%–85%
Total	75	10	12	18%	13%–25%
		13% (CL 9%–19%)			

KEY: ASD, atrial septal defect; CABG, coronary artery bypass grafting; CL, 70% confidence limits; PA, pulmonary artery; PO, postoperative; PS, pulmonary stenosis; VSD, ventricular septal defect.

NOTE: Heart block developed in 0 (0%, CL 0%–24%) of 7 patients whose repair did not include closure of a VSD and in 12 (21%, CL 15%–28%) of 58 who had a VSD closed as part of the procedure (P (Fisher) = .22).

[a] In one, complete heart block preoperatively was episodic and was permanent after repair.

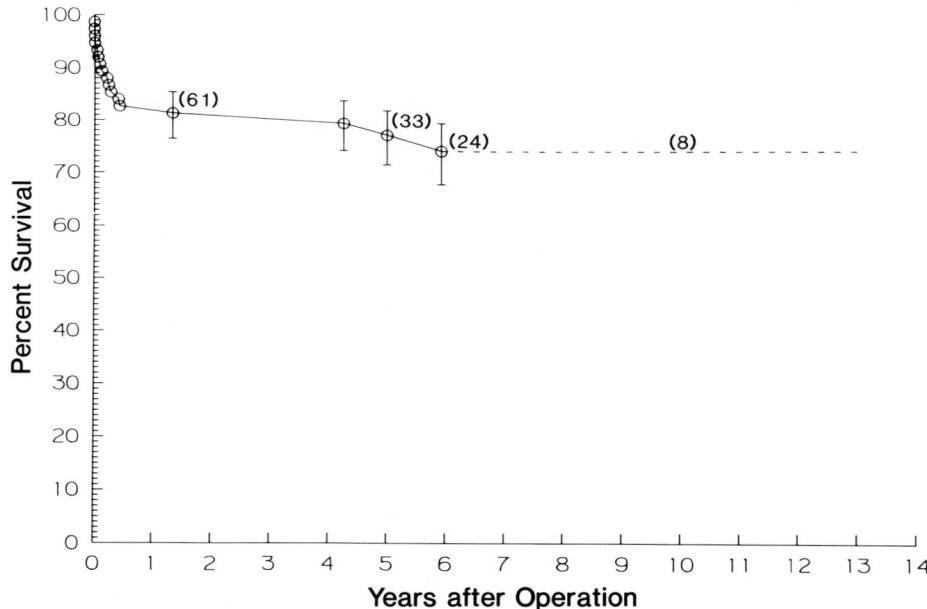

Figure 42-12 Actuarial survival after intracardiac repair in patients with congenitally corrected transposition (UAB; 1967–1983; $n = 75$). Hospital deaths are included. Each circle represents a death. The vertical bars enclose the 70% confidence limits of the actuarial estimates. The number of patients alive at specific intervals is shown in parentheses. A dashed line is drawn beyond the last event, indicating that living patients are traced beyond this point, but no actuarial estimate is possible.

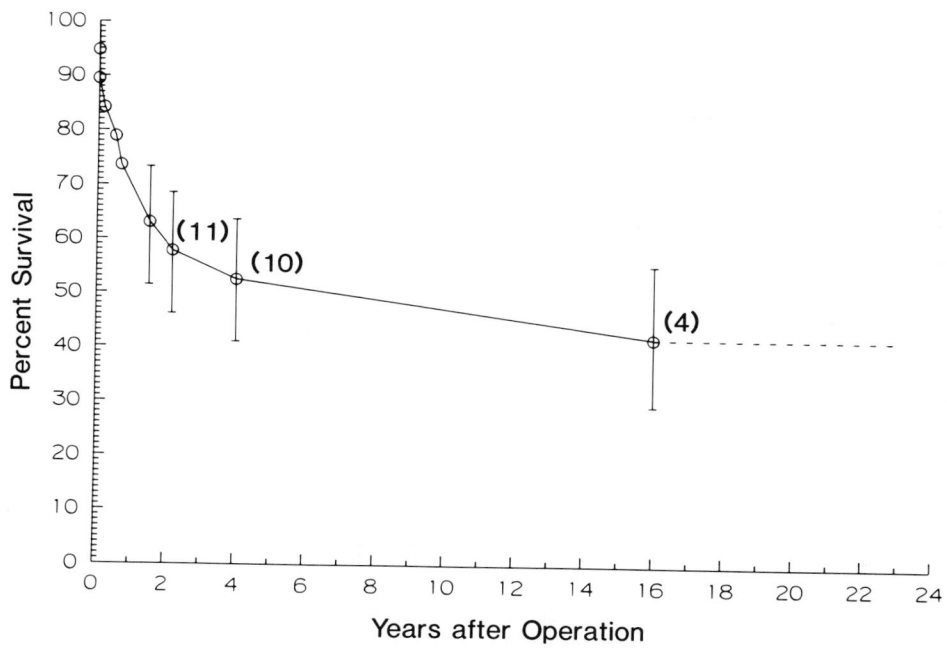

Figure 42-13 Actuarial survival after intracardiac repair in patients with congenitally corrected transposition (GLH; 1958–1983; $n = 19$). Presentation is as in Figure 42-12.

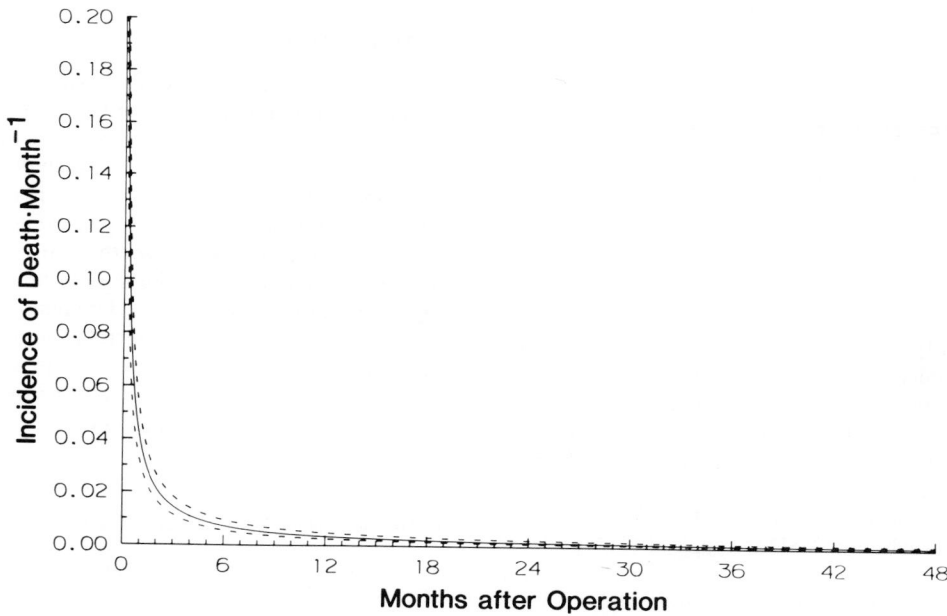

Figure 42-14 Hazard function (instanteous death rate) for death after intracardiac repair in patients with congenitally corrected transposition (UAB; 1967–1983; $n = 75$). The dashed lines enclose the 70% confidence limits. Only one phase of hazard was identified.

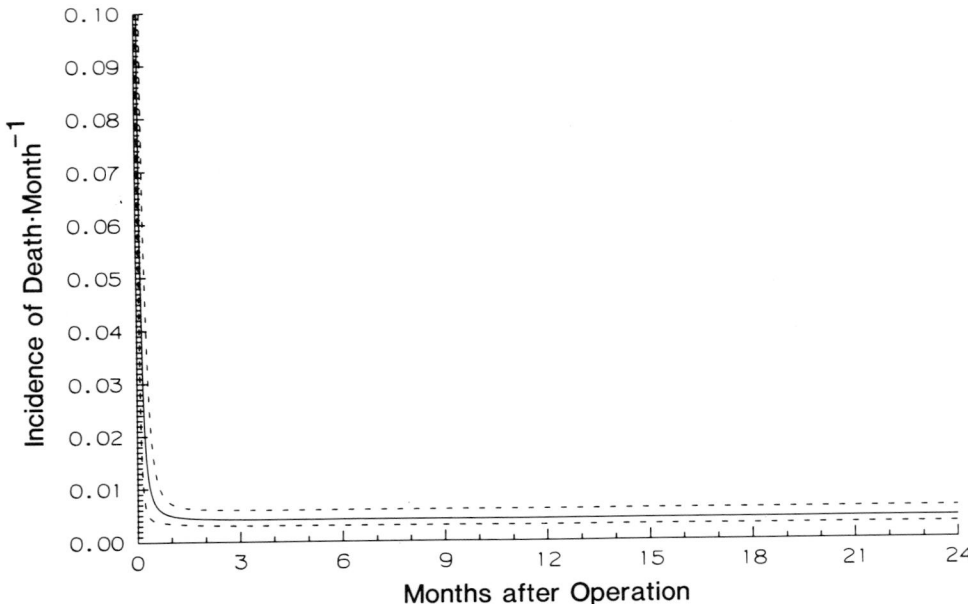

Figure 42-15 Hazard function (instantaneous death rate) for death after intracardiac repair in patients with congenitally corrected transposition (GLH; 1958–1983; $n = 19$). Presentation is as in Figure 42-14. Both early and late phases of hazard were identified.

carried out for 24–48 hours via the usual temporary epicardial wires, and then a permanent pacemaker pulse generator is placed subcutaneously (see Chapter 47 for details). Alternatively, the pulse generator can be placed at the end of the intracardiac repair, but there seems greater risk of hemorrhage into the pocket with this plan.

SPECIAL FEATURES OF POSTOPERATIVE CARE

The special features of postoperative care are discussed in Chapter 43.

EARLY RESULTS

The hospital mortality after repairs of cardiac defects in patients with congenitally corrected transposition of the great arteries (CTGA) is about 10% (Tables 42-1 and 42-2); this is probably higher than the hospital mortality after similar repairs in patients with AV concordant connections (see Chapter 43, "Early Results").

Complete heart block develops in about 10%–20% of patients with CTGA in whom a VSD is repaired (Tables 42-3 and 42-4).

These and other early results and the incremental risk factors for death and for complete heart block are further discussed in Chapter 43. Also discussed are the interrelations in these and other matters between CTGA and the other subsets of AV discordant connection.

LATE RESULTS

Late deaths probably occur somewhat more frequently after cardiac repairs in patients with CTGA than in patients with AV concordant connections (Tables 42-1 and 42-2). Actuarial survival (freedom from death including hospital deaths) up to about 10 years is only 50%–75% in patients with CTGA who have undergone cardiac repairs (Figs. 42-12 and 42-13). The instantaneous risk of death across time (hazard function; see Chapter 6) may have only an early phase (UAB; Fig. 42-14) or both an early and late phase (GLH; Fig. 42-15).

The late results and the interrelation between those in patients with CTGA and those in patients with other subsets of AV discordant connection, as well as incremental risk factors, are discussed in Chapter 43.

INDICATIONS FOR OPERATION

The indications for operation are included in the discussion of indications for patients with AV discordant connection in general in Chapter 43.

43

ATRIOVENTRICULAR DISCORDANT CONNECTION

DEFINITION

Atrioventricular (AV) discordant connection is a congenital cardiac anomaly in which the right atrium connects to the left ventricle and the left atrium connects to the right ventricle.[1] (See Chapter 1 for definitions and morphology of right and left atria and ventricles and of the other types of AV connections.) Atrioventricular discordant connection may occur in atrial situs solitus, in which case there is a ventricular L-loop (left handedness of the ventricular internal architecture[A10,V4,V5]); or it may occur in atrial situs inversus, in which case there is a ventricular D-loop (right handedness).

Conditions with AV discordant connection are discussed together in this chapter, because it may be held that their special morphologic features separate them in a fundamental and surgically important way from conditions with other types of AV connections (UAB) and that in view of the infrequency of some of the subsets within this group, surgi-

---

[1]The adjectives left and right used to modify atrium or ventricle always mean morphologic right or morphologic left. The position of the chamber is referred to as right sided or left sided.

cally relevant information can best be obtained by considering them together. A contrary view is that categorization of cardiac anomalies by their ventriculoarterial connection is more relevant to cardiac surgical procedures than is one by the AV connection (GLH). Material concerning patients with AV discordant connection (UAB) is concentrated in this chapter; that concerning patients with univentricular AV connections is concentrated in Chapter 44. Material on patients with AV discordant connections (GLH), although reported in these chapters, is also recorded in the chapters on double outlet right ventricle (DORV) (Chapter 40) and double outlet left ventricle (DOLV) (Chapter 41). Each approach has been advocated by others in the past.

HISTORICAL NOTE

The history of the development of knowledge and surgical treatment of congenitally corrected transposition of the great arteries (CTGA) is discussed in Chapter 42.

The time of first recognition of atrioventricular (AV) discordant connection associated with double outlet right ventricle (DORV) is not clear, but as late as 1960 the entity was not clearly distinguished from DORV with concordant AV connection. Ruttenberg and colleagues described DORV coexisting with AV discordant connection in 1964.[R2] In 1965 at the Mayo Clinic, we recognized and repaired this type of DORV (with ventricular septal defect [VSD] and pulmonary stenosis) associated with AV discordant connection. In this repair, an extracardiac conduit was used for rerouting pulmonary blood flow, perhaps for the first time. Double outlet left ventricle associated with AV discordant connection has been rare and the first surgical case was reported by us from GLH in 1976.[B5]

Isolated ventricular inversion was named by Van Praagh in 1966 when he described one such case.[V1] A similar malformation had, however, been reported by Ratner, Abbott, and Beattie in 1921[R5] and by Lev and Rowlatt in 1961.[L6] In 1975, Quero-Jimenez and associates reviewed six reported cases, including two of their own.[Q1] Isolated atrial inversion was named when the first such case was reported at GLH in 1972.[C3]

MORPHOLOGY

Among hearts with atrioventricular (AV) discordant connection there is a great variability, not only in ventriculoarterial connections but also in many other morphologic details.[A11]

Ventricular Architecture

The ventricles are said to be inverted in this entity. However, because of the many ventricular positional anomalies that occur, the phrase *ventricular inversion* is not very useful, and it is necessary to describe the internal architecture of each ventricle more specifically in a given case. A convenient way of doing this is with Van Praagh's phrases *ventricular D-loop* and *ventricular L-loop,* defined as in Chapter 1

(see "Situs of the Ventricles"), or the phrases *right handedness* and *left handedness,*[A10,V4,V5] also defined in Chapter 1. Thus, in patients with AV discordant connection and situs solitus, there is a ventricular L-loop, or left-handed internal architecture. With atrial situs inversus, there is a D-loop, or right handedness.

Ventricular Position and Rotation

In patients with atrial situs solitus and AV discordant connection, the right ventricle is generally left sided and the left ventricle lies side by side to it and to the right. Related to this is the fact that the entire length of the ventricular septum is usually visualized in profile in an anteroposterior view during angiocardiography. However, there may be variations in the anterosuperior orientation of the ventricles and variations in their rotation (see Chapter 1, "Cardiac and Arterial Positions").

Positional Anomalies
An extreme variation in anterosuperior position is the so-called superior-inferior ventricles ("over-and-under," "upstairs-downstairs," "two-story," or "parking deck" ventricles). In this, the septum is not vertically oriented as is usual in AV discordant connection but is horizontal, and the left ventricle lies inferiorly and the right ventricle superiorly. This may first have been described by Kinsley, McGoon, and Danielson.[K4] Most commonly, when the ventricles are positioned in this manner, there is AV discordant connection, an inlet ventricular septal defect (VSD), and DORV. One chamber may be hypoplastic, and there may be AV valve straddling. Rarely, a superior-inferior position of the ventricle may be associated with AV concordant connection and DORV (see Chapter 40, "Double Outlet Right Ventricle with Superior-Inferior Ventricles" in section on Morphology).

Rotational Anomalies
When rotational anomalies are present in patients with AV discordant connection, even more bizarre situations occur. Although the left ventricular inlet portion generally remains on the right side in patients with atrial situs solitus, the trabecular and outlet portions may be left sided and present a confusing picture.[S2] Generally, however, the ventricular septum is in the coronal plane, the left ventricle is posterior, and the right ventricle is anterior.[K4] It is in the domain of these extreme rotational anomalies that so-called crisscross hearts occur[A9,F2,F5,S2,T2] in which the inflow pathways of the two ventricles appear to cross rather than being parallel. It is also here that the question arises as to whether an AV discordant connection necessarily implies a ventricular L-loop, or left-handedness, in atrial situs solitus and D-loop, or right handedness, in atrial situs inversus. In this text, the assumption is made that it does.

Ventricular Size

Varying degrees of hypoplasia of the left-sided right ventricle may be present.[E1] When the ventricles are in a superior-inferior position, the morphologic left ventricle may be hypoplastic. Ventricular hypoplasia is frequently associated with straddling and overriding of the AV valve of the hypoplastic ventricle.

Cardiac Position

It is estimated that about 25% of cases with atrial situs solitus and AV discordant connection have dextrocardia,[C1] and rarely there is levocardia when the atrial situs is inverted.

Ventriculoarterial Connection

Ventriculoarterial Discordant Connection
The morphology of congenitally corrected transposition of the great arteries (AV discordant connection and ventriculoarterial discordant connection) is described in Chapter 42.

Double Outlet Right Ventricle
Double outlet right ventricle (DORV) may coexist with AV discordant connection and ventricular left handedness (L-loop), and in nearly all cases VSD and pulmonary stenosis also coexist. Since the right ventricle in this situation is the systemic ventricle (receives pulmonary venous blood from the atrium to which pulmonary veins are connected), cyanosis is not a necessary result of the malformation, but it is usually produced by the associated pulmonary stenosis. The apex of the heart may point to the right (dextrocardia with atrial situs solitus and ventricular D-loop)[K1]; this occurred in 5 (33%, CL 19%–50%) of 15 cases (UAB), an incidence not significantly different from that in corrected transposition (25%, CL 19%–32%). The aorta is usually in L-malposition, but it may be in any position. The VSD is usually very distal in the septum and beneath the adjacent great arteries (usually the pulmonary artery), but it can be anywhere in the septum.

In this entity, the pulmonary artery is not in a wedged position. Probably related to this, the location of the conduction system tends to be different from that in corrected transposition (see "Atrioventricular Node and Bundle of His").[L1]

This entity is, of course, closely related to the subset of corrected transposition with VSD in which the pulmonary artery somewhat overrides the VSD and in part arises over the left-sided right ventricle. When this overriding is so severe that more than 50% of the pulmonary artery overlies the left-sided right ventricle, the case is assigned the diagnosis of AV discordant connection with DORV. (See Chapter 40, "Definition.") However, in most cases of DORV, the pulmonary artery is nearly completely over the left-sided right ventricle.

Double Outlet Left Ventricle
Double outlet left ventricle (DOLV) may coexist with AV discordant connection.[B5,V7] Since the left ventricle in this setting is the pulmonary ventricle (receives systemic venous blood from the atrium to which the cavae are connected), cyanosis is a necessary result of this cardiac anomaly. The VSD is in a similar position as in DORV with AV discordant connection, but the aorta overrides the VSD to such an extent that it emerges wholly or in large part from the right-sided left ventricle. This subset may occur in patients with atrial situs inversus.[A12]

Ventriculoarterial Concordant Connection
Ventriculoarterial concordant connection is even more unusual in patients with AV discordant connection and is of two types, *isolated ventricular inversion*[Q1,V1] and *isolated atrial inversion*.[C3] The systemic and pulmonary circulations are parallel in this setting, the physiology is that of ordinary transposition of the great arteries (see Chapter 39, "Pathophysiology" in section on Clinical Features and Diagnostic Criteria), and cyanosis results.

In isolated ventricular inversion with atrial situs solitus, as originally defined,[V1] the aortic origin lies to the right and posterior to the pulmonary artery origin and there is aortic-mitral fibrous continuity and a muscular subpulmonary infundibulum (conus) as in the normal heart. The condition differs from normal, however, in that there is AV discordant connection and the aorta arises from a right-sided morphologically left ventricle and, for this reason, both great arteries are parallel. Usually there is a large VSD, and pulmonary stenosis is generally absent.[Q1] When there is situs inversus, a mirror image pattern occurs.[A7,L8]

As in corrected transposition of the great arteries (CTGA), the inverted ventricles in patients with isolated atrial or ventricular inversion usually lie side by side with the ventricular septum in a sagittal plane and with a similar coronary artery distribution pattern to that in CTGA. However, it is important surgically to note that in isolated ventricular inversion, the right-sided left coronary artery does not cross in front of the pulmonary outflow so that enlargement of the outflow anteriorly is feasible, if required. Although Losekoot and colleagues have suggested that the conduction tissue will be as for CTGA,[L1] the position of the cardiac conduction tissue in this condition is, at present, uncertain.

In the case of isolated atrial inversion reported from GLH[C3] and that reported subsequently by Leijala and associates,[L8] there was atrial situs inversus with a ventricular D-loop and dextrocardia with fibrous aortic-mitral continuity and a subpulmonary conus (model 3, Fig. 43-1*a*). However, in the GLH case (Fig. 43-2), the great arteries crossed in a virtually normal fashion with the morphologically right ventricle lying to the right and posterior to the morphologically left ventricle. The unusual feature about this heart was the presence of visceroatrial discordance, since the abdominal organs were in a situs solitus position, whereas the atria (and their venous connections) were inverted. This rare additional feature did not, however, alter the circulatory pathways from those present in isolated ventricular inversion.

In addition to the heart just described, there are others with identical connections (AV discordant connection and ventriculoarterial concordant connection) but with conal development that is the reverse of that described in isolated ventricular inversion (Fig. 43-1*b*, models 2 and 3). That is, the aorta arises from the morphologically left ventricle and lies, in a situs solitus heart, to the right of the pulmonary artery but is separated from the mitral valve by a muscular subaortic conus. Usually in these circumstances there is pul-

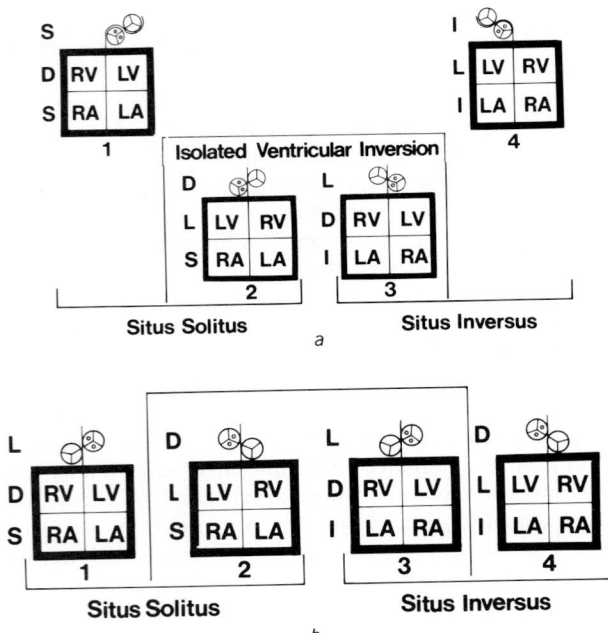

Figure 43-1 Models illustrating isolated ventricular inversion and anatomically corrected malposition of the great arteries (GLH).[V3] (*a*) Models of isolated ventricular inversion (2,3) (models 1 and 4 are the normal heart, with the origin of the pulmonary artery indicated by the spiraled vertical extension of the partition line). The similarities between models 2 and 3 here and in (*b*) are apparent. Isolated ventricular inversion is a cyanotic condition because of the AV discordant connection.

(*b*) Models of anatomically corrected malposition of the great arteries. In this text, it is considered that only models 1 and 4 represent anatomically corrected malposition of the great arteries.

LA, left atrium; LV, left ventricle; RA, right atrium; RV, right ventricle.

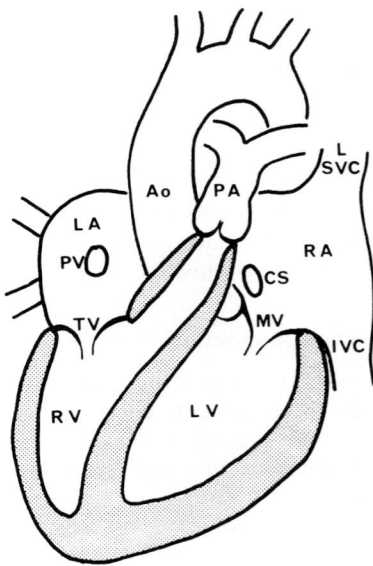

Figure 43-2 Line drawing of exact relationships of cardiac chambers and great arteries in isolated atrial inversion (GLH). The right superior vena cava and left pulmonary veins are not shown.

Ao, aorta; CS, coronary sinus; IVC, inferior vena cava; LA, left atrium; LSVC, left superior vena cava; LV, left ventricle; MV, mitral valve; PA, pulmonary artery; PV, pulmonary valve; RA, right atrium; RV, right ventricle; TV, tricuspid valve.

Reproduced with permission from Clarkson et al.[C3]

When there is DOLV, the AV node giving rise to the penetrating bundle is usually the anterior one.

The position of the conduction tissue is uncertain in patients with isolated ventricular or atrial inversion.

Accessory Conduction Pathways

Kent's bundles may occur in patients with AV discordant connections, particularly in those with corrected transposition, and may give rise to preexcitation and the Wolff-Parkinson-White (WPW) syndrome (see Chapter 48, Section 1, for a detailed discussion of WPW syndrome).[B6,S2] Kent's bundle may be in the posterior wall of the left-sided right ventricle or in the posterolateral wall of the right-sided morphologic left ventricle.[B6] It is presumed by Bharati and colleagues that the relative frequency of these findings in hearts with AV discordant connection is associated with the high incidence of Ebstein's anomaly of the left-sided tricuspid valve in these cases.[B6]

Coronary Arteries

The coronary arteries are expectedly abnormal in hearts with AV discordant connection, but the appropriate terminology for describing them is controversial. The simple terms *right sided* and *left sided* seem the best.[L6] The right-sided coronary artery, arising from the right posterior coronary sinus and analogous to the normal left coronary artery, gives rise to the anterior descending coronary artery coursing from right to left and to the circumflex artery. The left-sided coronary artery arises from the left posterior aortic sinus and passes around the left-sided tricuspid orifice usu-

monary-tricuspid fibrous continuity, but a subpulmonary conus may also, rarely, be present. These hearts can be considered to have anatomically corrected malposition of the great arteries[V8] or contrariwise (as in this text), a variant within the general category of AV discordant connection and ventriculoarterial concordant connection.

Atrioventricular Node and Bundle of His

The AV conduction tissue is abnormal in most patients with AV discordant connection and typically so in the subset of corrected transposition with atrial situs solitus, where an anterior AV node gives rise to the bundle of His (see Chapter 42, "Atrioventricular Node and Bundle of His" in section on Morphology for details concerning this).

When a left-sided DORV coexists with an AV discordant connection, wedging of the pulmonary trunk is not present, and usually both the anterior and posterior AV nodes persist, connected by a sling of conduction tissue around the VSD, which continues on as the branching bundle.[L1] However, only the anterior AV node or the regular posterior one may give rise to the penetrating bundle.[L1] This variability may predispose to surgically induced complete heart block.

ally to become the posterior descending artery on the back of the heart.[L1]

Atrioventricular Valves

The right-sided *mitral valve* typically has two leaflets and usually is in fibrous continuity with the pulmonary valve. As in the normal heart, it has no septal attachments but rather has typically paired papillary muscles.

The left-sided *tricuspid valve* consists of three leaflets. The septal leaflet, and often the posterior (inferior) leaflet, is displaced more than normally into the ventricle, but the deformity in most such hearts is not typically an Ebstein malformation (see Chapter 42, "Tricuspid Valve" in section on Morphology for more details).

The AV valves may, uncommonly, *straddle* and *override* the ventricular septum in hearts with AV discordant connection. When the overriding is greater than 50%, by convention the diagnosis is made of univentricular AV connection (single ventricle) with straddling and overriding AV valve (see Chapter 44). When the overriding is less than this, the diagnosis is AV discordant connection with straddling AV valve. A left-sided tricuspid valve may override and straddle a VSD,[L7] which is at times associated with hypoplasia of the left-sided right ventricle and at times with a superior-inferior position of the ventricles. More rarely, the right-sided mitral valve may straddle and override a VSD,[B8,S4] invariably associated with hypoplasia of the left ventricle and superior-inferior position of the two ventricles.[B8] When an AV valve straddles, the ventriculoarterial connection may be discordant, in which case the AV node is still anterior but is even farther anteriorly along the superior aspect of the right-sided mitral valve.[B8] The penetrating bundle descends directly onto the ventricular septum without passing anterior to the pulmonary outflow tract. The ventriculoarterial connection may also be DORV.

CLINICAL FEATURES AND DIAGNOSTIC CRITERIA

The clinical features of patients with AV discordant connection vary widely, depending upon the ventriculoarterial connection and on the associated cardiac anomalies.

Corrected Transposition of the Great Arteries

In this condition, the pulmonary and systemic circulations are in series. A large VSD is common, but usually some degree of subpulmonary stenosis is produced by the morphology of the subpulmonary left ventricular outflow tract, even though it is not apparent. Therefore, it is not common for the presentation to be in the first year of life from the sequelae of a large pulmonary blood flow.

The clinical features and diagnostic criteria of this subset are fully discussed in Chapter 42.

Double Outlet Right Ventricle and Double Outlet Left Ventricle

There are no characteristic presentations of either double outlet right ventricle (DORV) or double outlet left ventricle (DOLV) coexisting with AV discordant connection. However, since in patients with AV discordant connection and DORV there is usually coexisting pulmonary stenosis, cyanosis is usually evident; and since in this setting with DOLV the aorta arises from the ventricle receiving systemic venous blood (see "Morphology"), cyanosis is usually evident here as well. The diagnosis is made by the same methods as described for corrected transposition (see Chapter 42).

Isolated Ventricular or Atrial Inversion

Patients with these anomalies present in a similar fashion to patients with complete transposition of the great arteries. When the ventricular septum is intact, there is severe cyanosis in infancy[C1]; when there is a large VSD, moderate cyanosis is accompanied by congestive heart failure and cardiomegaly.[Q1] Pulmonary stenosis adds to the degree of cyanosis. The diagnosis is made by the same methods as described for corrected transposition (see Chapter 42). Cineangiography is particularly important for definitive diagnosis (Fig. 43-3).

NATURAL HISTORY

Most of the information concerned with the natural history of patients having AV discordant connection is drawn from patients with congenitally corrected transposition of the great arteries. This is discussed in Chapter 42.

TECHNIQUE OF OPERATION

Repairs in Corrected Transposition of the Great Arteries

See Chapter 42.

Repair of Atrioventricular Discordant Connection with Double Outlet Right Ventricle and Pulmonary Stenosis

Since in this setting the right ventricle receives pulmonary venous blood (see "Morphology"), the origin of the aorta from it is appropriate; the pulmonary trunk must be repositioned so as to receive blood from the left ventricle.

The proper approach to repair in this subset is less certain than it is in corrected transposition because information about the conduction system is less complete. Further, there has been controversy as to whether a completely intraventricular repair is usually adequate or the use of a valved extracardiac conduit between left ventricle and the pulmonary artery is usually necessary.[K1,V2] In part because of the data presented by Tabry and colleagues[T3] and in part because important subpulmonary stenosis is usually present, the use of a valved extracardiac conduit is preferred (UAB, GLH).

The details of the initial stages of the operation are the same as those for corrected transposition, including the opening of the right atrium and the infusion of the cold car-

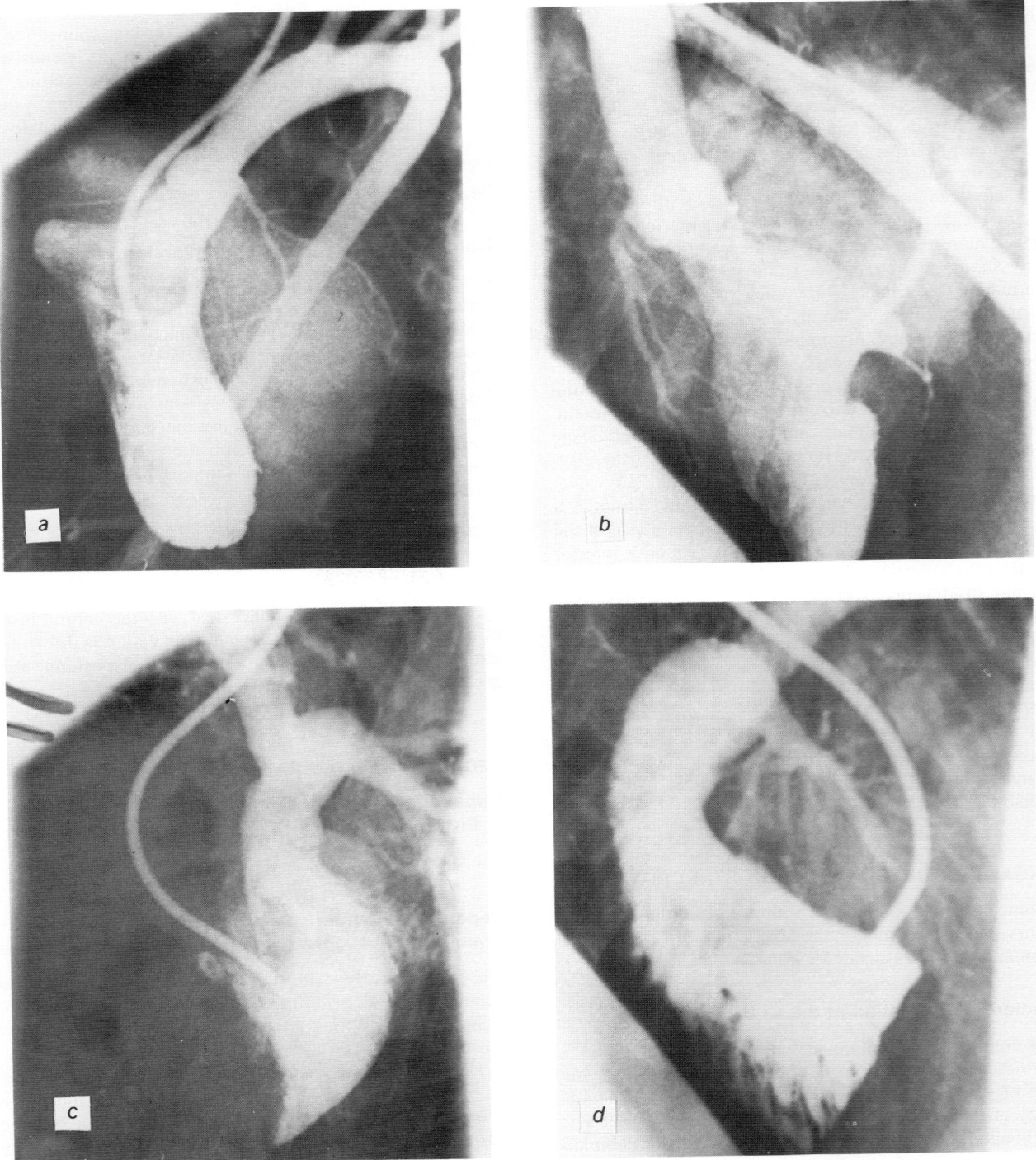

Figure 43-3 Cineangiogram in a patient with isolated ventricular inversion (AV discordant connection and ventriculoarterial concordant connection) (UAB).
(a) Left ventricular injection, four-chamber position, AP projection. The aorta arises from the right-sided left ventricle.
(b) Lateral projection.
(c) Right ventricular injection, four-chamber position, AP projection. The pulmonary artery arises from the left-sided right ventricle.
(d) Lateral projection.

dioplegic solution. The interior of the right-sided left ventricle (in atrial situs solitus) is examined through the right-sided mitral valve, and inasmuch as is possible, the interior of the left-sided right ventricle including the subaortic and subpulmonary areas is examined through the VSD. The planning is then made for closing off the origin of the pulmonary trunk from the left-sided right ventricle and repairing the VSD from the right atrial approach, and placing a valved conduit from left ventricle to pulmonary trunk. Matsuda and colleagues prefer transaortic closure of the VSD.[M7]

Through the right atrial approach and working first through the VSD, the usually narrow subpulmonary pathway is generally closed with two rows of continuous polypropylene sutures supplemented with interrupted pledgetted mattress sutures. If this is difficult, the pulmonary trunk can later be opened longitudinally (see below) and the thickened valve leaflets closed by a similar suture technique. In view of what is known about the location of the conduction system, sutures for closure of the VSD are placed entirely on the patient's left (right ventricular) side of the defect. Posteriorly, if possible they are placed in the base of the septal leaflet of the left-sided tricuspid leaflet.

After completing this part of the operation through the right atrium, the pulmonary trunk is opened from the right side. The incision may need to be extended somewhat onto the right pulmonary artery. The left ventricular incision and the routing and steps of insertion of the homograft-valved extracardiac conduit are those described for corrected transposition. (See Chapter 42, "Technique of Operation" and Fig. 42-11.)

Repair of Atrioventricular Discordant Connection and Double Outlet Left Ventricle

Since the left ventricle receives sytemic venous blood (see "Morphology"), the aorta must be repositioned so as to receive blood from the right ventricle. An alternative surgical option consists of leaving the aorta with the right-sided left ventricle, connecting the left ventricle to the pulmonary artery with a conduit, and performing an atrial switch operation[S7]; this seems more complicated and less desirable.

This entity is so rare as to make reliable surgical recommendations difficult. In any event, an intraventricular tunnel repair must be used (see Chapter 40, "Intraventricular Tunnel Repair of Simple Double Outlet Right Ventricle without Pulmonary Stenosis") and constructed so as to conduct blood from the left-sided right ventricle (in atrial situs solitus) through the VSD and then to the aorta. The sutures between the Dacron patch for the tunnel and the ventricular septum are placed with due regard for the location of the conducting tissue (see "Repair of Atrioventricular Discordant Connection with Double Outlet Right Ventricle and Pulmonary Stenosis"). On occasions, it may be possible to do this repair without obstructing the left ventricular access to the pulmonary trunk. However, if access is compromised or if pulmonary stenosis is present, a homograft-valved extracardiac conduit is placed between left ventricle and pulmonary trunk (Chapter 42, Fig. 42-11). Further details of the operations are discussed in Chapter 41.

Repair of Isolated Ventricular or Atrial Inversion

When the ventricular septum is intact, balloon septostomy is required in infancy followed by an atrial switch operation. This returns the circulation functionally and anatomically to normal, since the left ventricle is the systemic ventricle.[C3]

When there is a large VSD, it is closed via the right ventricle (pulmonary ventricle) in a fashion similar to that for primary VSD, the bundle being presumed to lie on the left ventricular side; an atrial switch operation is then performed.

Placement of Epicardial Pacemaker Leads

When complete heart block has been present preoperatively or develops intraoperatively and when in sinus rhythm the P-R interval is very long, permanent epicardial atrial and ventricular pacemaking leads are placed. (See Chapter 47 for the details of the technique.) Atrioventricular pacing is carried out for 24–48 hours via the usual temporary epicardial wires, and then a permanent pacemaker pulse generator is placed subcutaneously (see Chapter 47 for the details). Alternatively, the pulse generator can be placed immediately after repair, but there seems greater risk of hemorrhage into the pocket with this plan.

SPECIAL FEATURES OF POSTOPERATIVE CARE

Patients with atrioventricular (AV) discordant connection undergoing cardiac repair are managed with protocols generally used after cardiac surgery (see Chapter 5). In patients with AV discordant connection, particular attention is paid to the cardiac rhythm. When complete heart block is present, AV sequential pacing is advantageous to cardiac output and therefore is used routinely.

EARLY RESULTS

Hospital Mortality after Repairs

The hospital mortality for the repair of the cardiac malformations in patients with atrioventricular (AV) discordant connections has not yet approached zero. Thus, in the combined overall UAB and GLH experience with 122 such patients, there have been 18 (15%, CL 11%–19%) hospital deaths (Tables 43-1, 43-2).

The reasons for the risk of hospital death not yet approaching zero are not clear (see Chapter 6 for definition of this). One may be that the operations are more complex than those for similar defects in patients with AV concordant connections. Another may be the infrequency with which repairs are made in patients with AV discordant connections and thus the relative unfamiliarity of the surgeon with the procedure. Most importantly, perhaps, the cardiac morphology associated with AV discordant connection and the complexity of the malformation in many of the patients may themselves present risks that have not yet been neutralized.

Table 43-1 Hospital and late deaths after intracardiac repair in patients with AV discordant connection (UAB; 1967–1983).

Ventriculoarterial Connection	Hospital Deaths				Late Deaths			
	n	No.	%	CL	n	No.	%	CL
Discordant[a]	75	7	9%	6%–14%	68	10	15%	10%–21%
DORV	16	6	38%	23%–54%	10	3	30%	14%–51%
DOLV	3	1	33%	4%–76%	2	0	0%	0%–61%
Concordant[b]	4	1	25%	3%–63%	3	0	0%	0%–47%
Total	98	15	15%	11%–20%	83	13	16%	11%–21%

KEY: CL, 70% confidence imits; DOLV, double outlet left ventricle; DORV, double outlet right ventricle.

[a] Corrected transposition of the great arteries.

[b] Isolated ventricular inversion.

(See "Incremental Risk Factors for Premature Death" under "Late Results" for further discussion of this.)

The hospital mortality after the repair of defects associated with *corrected transposition of the great arteries* (CTGA) is about 10% (see Tables 43-1 and 43-2, and see Chapter 42, Tables 42-1 and 42-2). Similar hospital mortalities are reported by Williams and colleagues (9%, CL 4%–17%),[W3] Marcelletti and colleagues, 1971–1980 (18%, CL 11%–27%),[M2] de Leval and colleagues (15%, CL 5%–33%),[D1] and Westerman and colleagues (9%, CL 3%–19%).[W5] In earlier times, the hospital mortality was higher.[F1,M5] Thus, in the Mayo Clinic experience, 1958–1971, including our cases 1958–1967, the hospital mortality was 50% (CL 33%–67%).[M2] Risks in the current era for most subsets with corrected transposition are probably about 5% (see "Incremental Risk Factors for Premature Death").

The repair of *double outlet right ventricle* (DORV) and AV discordant connection is associated with a higher risk of hospital death than are the repairs in patients with CTGA (Tables 43-1 and 43-2). Thus, 6 deaths (38%, CL 23%–54%) occurred among 16 cases (UAB), although no deaths (0%, CL 0%–47%) occurred among 3 (GLH; see Chapter 40, Table 40-7). In the Mayo Clinic experience, the mortality has been 15% (CL 7%–28%).[T3] There is no convincing evidence that the type of repair influences hospital mortality in these patients (Table 43-3).

The repair of *double outlet left ventricle* (DOLV) and of *ventriculoarterial concordant connection* with AV discordant connection has been done infrequently[A12] and this pre-

Table 43-2 Hospital mortality after intracardiac repair in patients with AV discordant connection (GLH; 1958–1983).

Ventriculoarterial Connection	Hospital Deaths			
	n	No.	%	CL
Discordant[a]	19	3	16%	7%–29%
DORV	3	0	0%	0%–47%
DOLV	1	0	0%	0%–85%
Concordant[b]	1	0	0%	0%–85%
Total	24	3	12%	6%–24%

KEY: CL, 70% confidence limits; DOLV, double outlet left ventricle; DORV, double outlet right ventricle.

[a] Corrected transposition of the great arteries.

[b] Isolated atrial inversion.

cludes a useful prediction of a current hospital mortality rate, but it is probably similar to that for the repair of DORV with AV discordant connection (Tables 43-1, 43-2, 43-4, and 43-5; see Chapter 41, Tables 41-1 and 41-5 for details of GLH case).

Incremental Risk Factors for Hospital Death

These risks are described under "Late Results," in which death is considered as a time-related event across the entire spectrum of time, beginning with the end of the operation.

Conduction Disturbances

It is disappointing that reasonably secure knowledge of the location of the bundle of His has not allowed complete heart block to disappear as a postoperative complication of the repair of a ventricular septal defect (VSD) or of an intraventricular tunnel repair in patients with AV discordant connection, including those with CTGA. Currently, such patients have about a 20% risk of developing complete heart block after repair of a VSD (Table 43-6 and see Chapter 42, Table 42-3), considerably greater than the risk in patients with AV concordant connection who undergo VSD repair (see Chapters 20 and 23). de Leval's recent experience with 11 patients is encouraging in that none (0%, 0%–16%) developed heart block,[D1] as is the GLH recent experience (see Chapter 42, Table 42-3), but the data indicate that these improved results could be due to chance. Hwang et al. report an incidence (17%, CL 6%–35%) similar to that at UAB.[H4] The unusually high incidence of complete heart block of 46% (CL 29%–64%) for the current era experienced by Westerman and colleagues may be explained by their frequent use of resection in the treatment of subpulmonary stenoses.[W5]

Abandoning electrocardiographic (ECG) monitoring of each stitch[F1] in favor of a repair[D1] based on knowledge of morphology during cold cardioplegic cardiac arrest has not increased the risk of heart block.[M4] Also, the incidence of surgically induced heart block has not been demonstrated to have been reduced by electrophysiologic mapping at the time of surgery (Table 43-7).[F1,M2] Among all of the patients with AV discordant connection (UAB, GLH), only those with VSD repair appear to be at risk of developing complete heart block at operation (see Chapter 42, Table 42-4).

The development of complete heart block has not adversely affected hospital mortality (Table 43-8). This matter

Table 43-3 Hospital and late death after intracardiac operation in patients with AV discordant connection and DORV and VSD (UAB; 1967–1983). Five (33%, CL 19%–50%) of the 15 patients who had atrial situs solitus had dextrocardia, and 3 (60%, CL 29%–86%) of the 5 died.

Operation	n	Hospital Deaths			Late Deaths	
		No.	%	CL	No.	%[a]
VSD closure + valved extracardiac conduit to PA	12[b,c]	5	42%	25%–60%	2	29%
Intraventricular repair	3	1[d]	33%	4%–76%	1	50%
Cardiac transplantation	1[e]	0	0%	0%–85%		
Total	16	6	38%	23%–54%	3	30%
						(CL 14%–51%)

KEY: CL, 70% confidence limits; PA, pulmonary artery; VSD, ventricular septal defect.

NOTE: In these patients, the valved extracardiac conduit is placed from the left ventricle (which receives caval blood) to the pulmonary artery, the VSD closure leaving the aorta arising from the right ventricle. When an intraventricular repair is used, a spiral patch leaves the right ventricle in communication with the aorta but baffles left ventricular blood to the pulmonary artery.

[a]Percentage of hospital survivors.

[b]One patient who lived had atrial situs inversus.

[c]Four had superior-inferior ventricles, and two died.

[d]Patient had superior-inferior ventricles.

[e]Patient had superior-inferior ventricles, a shunting operation in infancy, and severely depressed ventricular function.

is controversial, however, in view of different experiences by others.

When complete heart block is not produced by the repair, the P-R interval is generally not lengthened over that present preoperatively.[C4] Delayed intraventricular conduction is present in about one-half of the cases, the delay usually being in activation of the left-sided right ventricle and less often of the left ventricle. This delay appears to result from damage to the proximal bundle branches near the VSD. However, no patients who did not have complete heart block at the time of hospital dismissal have developed it late postoperatively (UAB, GLH).

Incremental Risk Factors for the Development of Complete Heart Block

When chordae straddle across the VSD or insert on the crest of the ventricular septum, the risk of developing complete heart block is increased (Table 43-9). This is probably because this arrangement has necessitated sutures being placed on the left ventricular side of the septum anteroinferiorly,

thus putting the bundle of His at risk. Probably complete heart block is more likely to develop in patients with DORV than in other subsets of AV discordant connection (Tables 43-9 and 43-10). Tabry and colleagues report this complication to have followed repair in 30% (19%–44%) of patients with AV discordant connection and DORV.[T3] Under some circumstances, older age at repair may predispose to surgical heart block (Table 43-9).

Left Atrioventricular Valve Repair or Replacement

Valve repair or replacement does not increase the hospital mortality in patients with AV discordant connection undergoing cardiac repair (Table 43-11, and see Chapter 42, Tables 42-1 and 42-2).

Table 43-5 Hospital deaths after repair in patients with AV discordant connection and ventriculoarterial concordant connection, so-called isolated ventricular inversion (UAB; 1967–1983). There were no late deaths.

Operation	n	Hospital Deaths		
		No.	%	CL
Intraventricular tunnel repair + valved extracardiac conduit to PA	2[a]	0	0%	0%–61%
VSD closure + venous switch	2[b]	1[c]	50%	7%–93%
Total	4	1	25%	3%–63%

KEY: CL, 70% confidence limits; PA, pulmonary artery; VSD, ventricular septal defect.

NOTE: In this group of patients, an intraventricular (left) tunnel repair is made to conduct blood from the right ventricle to the aorta; the pulmonary artery is closed off from the right ventricle and a valved extracardiac conduit connects the left ventricle to the pulmonary artery.

[a]One patient had atrial situs solitus and dextrocardia.

[b]One patient who lived had superior-inferior ventricles with dextrocardia.

[c]Patient had atrial situs inversus.

Table 43-4 Hospital deaths after intracardiac repair in patients with AV discordant connection and DOLV and VSD (UAB; 1967–1983). There were no late deaths.

Operation	n	Hospital Deaths		
		No.	%	CL
Intraventricular tunnel repair	1[a]	1	100%	15%–100%
Intraventricular tunnel repair + valved extracardiac conduit, LV → PA	2	0	0%	0%–61%
Total	3	1	33%	4%–76%

KEY: CL, 70% confidence limits; LV, left ventricle; PA, pulmonary artery.

NOTE: The intraventricular (left) tunnel conducts right ventricular blood to the aorta.

[a]Patient had superior-inferior ventricles.

Table 43-6 Development of postoperative complete heart block after intracardiac repair in patients with AV discordant connection (UAB; 1967–1983).

| Ventriculoarterial Connection | n | Preoperative Complete Heart Block | | | n | Developed Postoperative Complete Heart Block | | |
		No.	%	CL		No.	%	CL
Discordant[a]	75	10	13%	9%–19%	65	12	18%	13%–25%
DORV	16	0	0%	0%–11%	15[c]	7	47%	31%–63%
DOLV	3	1	33%	4%–76%	2	1	50%	7%–93%
Concordant[b]	4	0	0%	0%–38%	4	0	0%	0%–38%
Total	98	11	11%	8%–16%	86	20	23%	18%–29%
$P(\chi^2)$			.23				.06	

KEY: CL, 70% confidence limits; DOLV, double outlet left ventricle; DORV, double outlet right ventricle.

[a] Corrected transposition of the great arteries.

[b] Isolated ventricular inversion.

[c] Heart transplant patient not considered at risk.

Table 43-7 The relationship of intraoperative electrophysiologic mapping to the development of complete heart block after the repair of VSD ($n = 78$) in patients with AV discordant connection (UAB; 1967–1983).

| Ventriculoarterial Connection | No Electrophysiologic Mapping | | | | | Electrophysiologic Mapping | | | |
| | | Developed Heart Block | | | | | Developed Heart Block | | |
	n	No.	%	CL	n	No.	%	CL
Discordant[a]	44	11	25%	18%–34%	13	1	8%	1%–24%
DORV	12	6	50%	32%–68%	3	1	33%	4%–76%
DOLV	1	0	0%	0%–85%	1	1	100%	15%–100%
Concordant[b]	4	0	0%	0%–38%	0			
Total	61	17	28%	22%–35%	17	3	18%	8%–32%

KEY: CL, 70% confidence limits; DOLV, double outlet left ventricle; DORV, double outlet right ventricle; VSD, ventricular septal defect.

NOTE: $P(\chi^2)$ for difference in incidence of heart block among those with no electrophysiologic mapping and those with it is .4.

[a] Corrected transposition of the great arteries.

[b] Isolated ventricular inversion.

Table 43-8 Heart block and hospital mortality after intracardiac repair in patients with AV discordant connection (UAB; 1967–1983).

| Ventriculoarterial Connection | No Complete Heart Block | | | | Preop Complete Heart Block | | | | PO Development of Complete Heart Block | | | | Total[d] |
| | | Hospital Deaths | | | | Hospital Deaths | | | | Hospital Deaths | | | |
	n	No.	%	CL	n	No.	%	CL	n	No.	%	CL	
Discordant[a]	53	5	9%	5%–16%	10	1	10%	1%–30%	12	1	8%	1%–26%	75 (7)
DORV[b]	8	4	50%	27%–73%					7	2	29%	10%–55%	15 (6)
DOLV	1	0	0%	0%–85%	1	0	0%	0%–85%	1	1	100%	15%–100%	3 (1)
Concordant[c]	4	1	25%	3%–63%									4 (1)
Total	66	10	15%	10%–21%	11	1	9%	1%–28%	20	4	20%	10%–33%	97 (15)

KEY: CL, 70% confidence limits; DOLV, double outlet left ventricle; DORV, double outlet right ventricle; PO, postoperative.

[a] Corrected transposition of the great arteries.

[b] Not included is one patient who received heart transplantation.

[c] Isolated ventricular inversion.

[d] Numbers in parentheses refer to hospital deaths; see table 43-1.

Table 43-9 Incremental risk factors for repair-related complete heart block in patients with AV discordant connection without preoperative heart block and with VSD closure as part of the repair (UAB; 1967–1983). These were determined by a multivariate logistic analysis initially entering a large number of demographic and morphologic variables.

Incremental Risk Factor	Logistic Coefficient ± SD	P value
Chordae straddling or inserting on crest of septum	2.6 ± 0.84	.002
DORV	1.3 ± 0.73	.08
If no chordae straddling (older) age at repair (years)	0.05 ± 0.030	.09
Intercept	−2.7	

KEY: DORV, double outlet right ventricle; SD, standard deviation.

Development of Left-Sided Tricuspid Valve Incompetence

Immediately after the repair of a VSD in patients with CTGA, left-sided tricuspid valve incompetence sometimes appears. Fox and colleagues reported this to have been apparent immediately after the repair in 6 (43%, CL 27%–60%) of 14 patients in whom left-sided AV valve incompetence was not present prior to operation.[F1] Westerman and colleagues have observed the same phenomenon.[W5] The mecha-

nism for this is unknown, but as best as can be determined the incompetence does not result from direct damage to the valvar tissue or chordae. It may be associated with the development of complete heart block.[W5] In any event, the incompetence may be sufficiently severe to require later valve replacement.

Hospital Mortality after Palliative or Staged Operations

As usual (see for example Chapter 23, "Hospital Mortality after Palliative Procedures" in Section 1, Early Results of Operation), hospital mortality is low after classical Blalock-Taussig shunting operations (Table 43-12). Palliative or staged operations are otherwise uncommonly performed.

LATE RESULTS

Premature Late Death

The actuarial survival of the entire group of patients undergoing repairs for anomalies associated with atrioventricular (AV) discordant connection is 69% at 10 years, including hospital mortality (Fig. 43-4). The survival of the various subsets are different only in the case of DORV (Fig. 43-5).

The instantaneous risk of death (hazard function) in the group as a whole has a single phase (Fig. 43-6) of rapidly

Table 43-10 Heart block after intracardiac operation in patients with AV discordant connection and DORV and VSD (UAB; 1967–1983). (See footnote in Table 43-3 for description of the operations.)

Operation	n	Preoperative Complete Heart Block	PO Permanent Complete Heart Block		
			No.	% of (n-Preop Block)	CL
VSD closure + valved extracardiac conduit to PA	12		6	50%	32%–68%
Intraventricular Repair	3		1	33%	4%–76%
Total[a]	15	0	7	47%	31%–63%

KEY: CL, 70% confidence limits; PA, pulmonary artery; PO, postoperative; VSD, ventricular septal defect.
[a] In addition, one patient who has survived had cardiac transplantation.

Table 43-11 Tricuspid (systemic AV) valve repair or replacement as part of the intracardiac operation in patients with AV discordant connection (UAB; 1967–1983).

Ventriculoarterial Connection	Valve Repair				Valve Replacement			No Valve Surgery		
	n	n	Hospital Deaths No.	%	n	Hospital Deaths No.	%	n	Hospital Deaths No.	%
Discordant	75	1	0	0%	15[a]	2	13% (CL 4%–29%)	59	5	8% (CL 5%–14%)
DORV	16	0			0 ⎱			16	6	38%
DOLV	3	0			0 ⎰ [a]			3	1	33%
Concordant	4	0			0			4	1	25%
Total	98	1	0	0%	15	2	13%	82	13	16%

KEY: CL, 70% confidence limits; DOLV, double outlet left ventricle; DORV, double outlet right ventricle.
[a] P(Fisher) = .01 for 15/75 (20%; CL 15%–26%) versus 0/23 (0%, CL 0%–8%) valve replacements.

Table 43-12 Hospital and late deaths after palliative operations in patients with AV discordant connection (UAB; 1967–1983).

Other Patients	n	Hospital Deaths				n	Late Deaths		
		No.	%	CL			No.	%	CL
Shunts	4[a]	1	25%	3%–63%		3	2	67%	24%–96%
PDA + Coarctation	2[b]	2	100%	39%–100%					
Other	2	1	50%	7%–93%		1	0	0%	0%–85%
Total	8	4	50%	27%–73%		4	2	50%	18%–82%

KEY: CL, 70% confidence limits; DOLV, double outlet left ventricle; DORV, double outlet right ventricle; PDA, patent ductus arteriosus.

[a] Ages 21 days and 2.0, 2.5, and 8.0 years.

[b] Ages 1.6 and 1.8 months.

falling risks tending to level off after 6 months. There is no late phase of hazard.

Incremental Risk Factors for Premature Death

The ventriculoarterial connection of double outlet right ventricle (DORV) is the only morphologic feature that appears to be a risk factor for death early or late after cardiac repair in patients with AV discordant connection (Table 43-13, Fig. 43-7). The effect of this risk factor is primarily on hospital mortality.

The mechanism of the increased risk produced by high hematocrit is no doubt the same as in tetralogy of Fallot (see Chapter 23, "High Hematocrit" in Section 1, Incremental Risk Factors for Hospital Death after Repair).

Both very young and very old age have increased the risk of operation during this experience (see Table 43-13). Repair

has been accomplished with the lowest risk between the ages of about 5 and 15 years (Fig. 43-8).

As time has passed, the risk of intracardiac repairs in patients with AV discordant connection has decreased, as indicated by the incremental risk of an earlier date of operation (Table 43-13). The decline was particularly striking in the years prior to 1976 (Fig. 43-9). Thus, currently, in subsets other than DORV, the risk of early death after repair is about 7%. The improvement has probably resulted from improved precision and completeness of the preoperative diagnosis and advances in surgical techniques and the techniques of myocardial protection.

Functional Status

The functional status of most surviving patients with AV discordant connection who have undergone the repair of as-

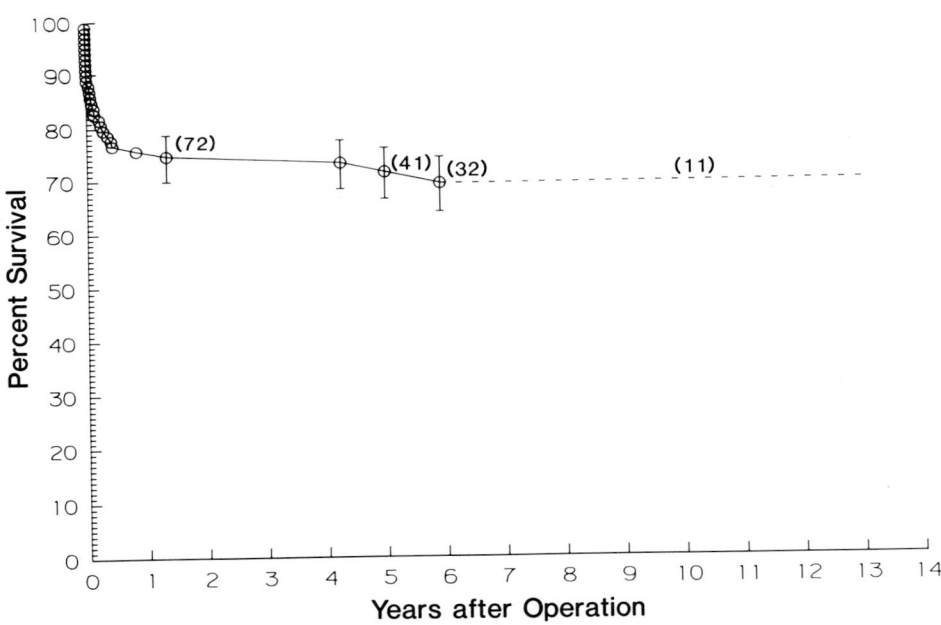

Figure 43-4 Actuarial survival after intracardiac repair in patients with AV discordant connection (UAB; 1967–1983; n = 98). Time 0 is the end of cardiopulmonary bypass. Each circle represents a death. The vertical bars enclose the 70% confidence limits (1 SD) of the actuarial estimates. The dashed lines represent follow-up beyond the last event. The numbers of patients followed to a given time point are enclosed in parentheses. All patients are traced.

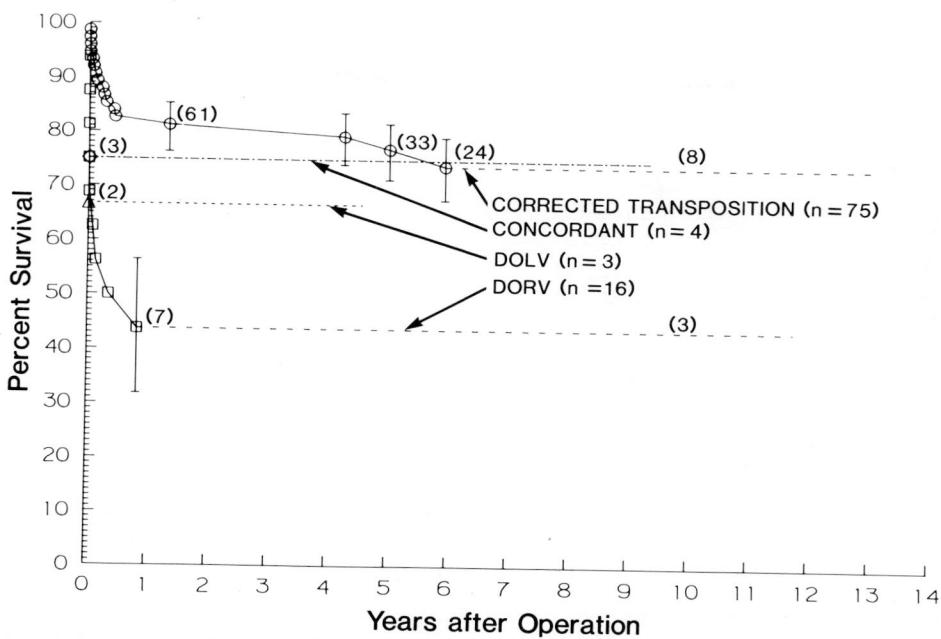

Figure 43-5 Actuarial survival after intracardiac repair in patients with AV discordant connection (UAB; 1967–1983) stratified according to the type of ventriculoarterial connection. Presentation is as in Figure 43-4.

DOLV, double outlet left ventricle; DORV, double outlet right ventricle.

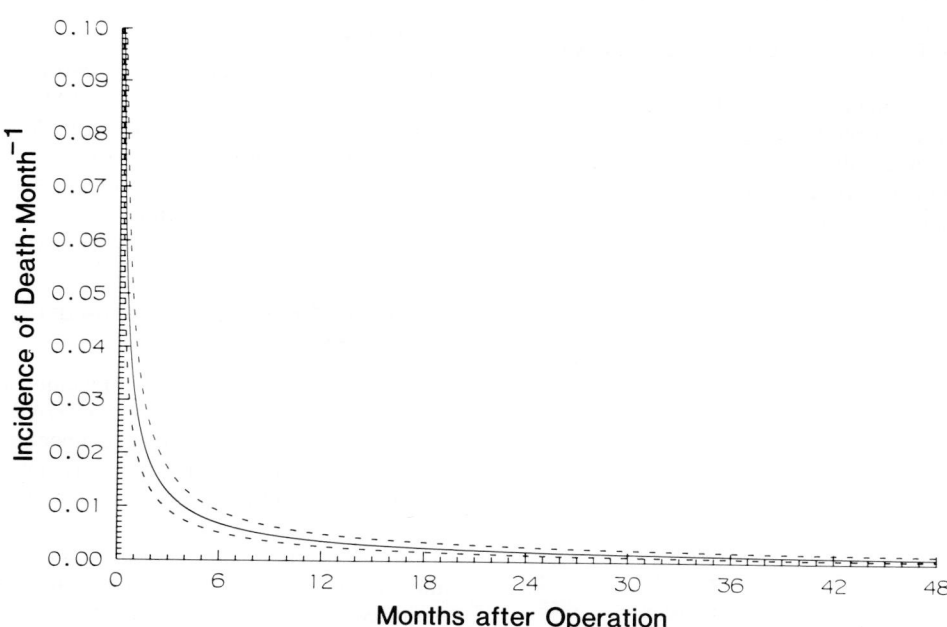

Figure 43-6 Hazard function for death (instantaneous risk of death per month) across time after intracardiac repair in patients with AV discordant connection (UAB; 1967–1983; n = 98). The dashed lines enclose the 70% confidence limits (1 SD) of the estimates. Only one hazard phase was identified.

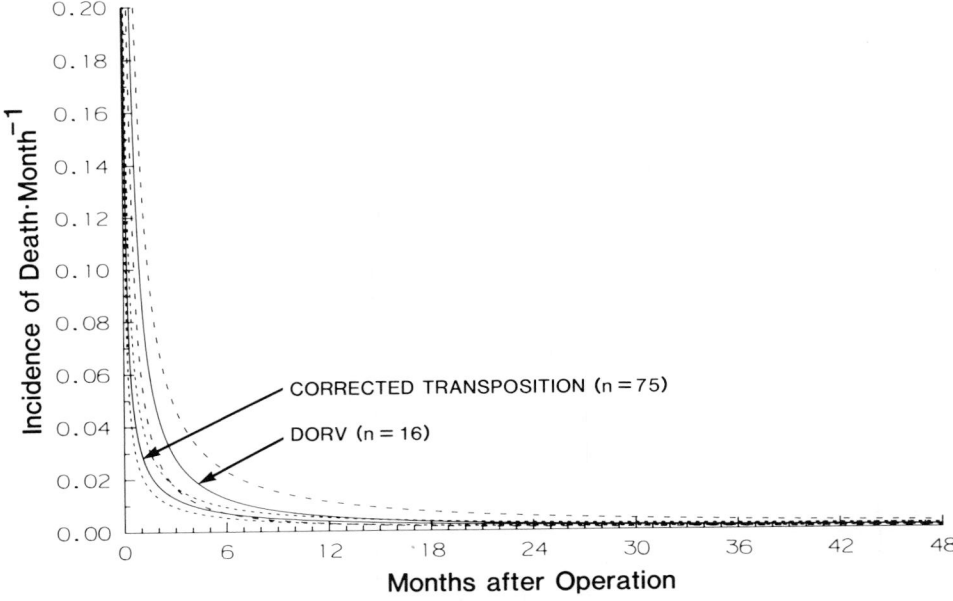

Figure 43-7 Hazard function for death (instantaneous risk of death per month) across time after intracardiac repair by separate analysis in patients with corrected transposition of the great arteries and in patients with AV discordant connection with DORV (UAB; 1967–1983).
DORV, double outlet right ventricle.

sociated anomalies is good in all subsets. Among 69 traced and surviving patients, 83% are in NYHA class I and 17% in NYHA class II (UAB, 1967–1983); in the corrected transposition group, among 9 living and traced patients, 7 (78%) are in NYHA class I and the remainder (22%) in NYHA class II (GLH).

There was no suggestion in the study of late results by Fox and colleagues that the morphologic right ventricle's systolic or diastolic function gradually fails under the pressure load of being the systemic ventricle. In fact, Hwang and colleagues found normal right ventricular systolic function late postoperatively in their patients except in one who had severe left-sided tricuspid valve incompetence.[H4]

Sudden Death

Sudden death has occurred late postoperatively in a few patients,[M5,W3] just as has happened after the septation operation for single ventricle (see Chapter 44, "Septation Operation" under Late Results). Whether this is due to the sudden appearance of unidentified complete heart block with ventricular asystole or of ventricular fibrillation, or of pacemaker failure in those with such a device, is problematic.

Tricuspid (Systemic Atrioventricular) Valve Incompetence

Tricuspid valve incompetence develops late after the repair of a VSD in some patients (15%; UAB, actuarially determined) with AV discordant connection.[F1,M5] The exact mechanism is uncertain, but it has not been due to direct surgical damage to the valve. In four patients, this has led to reoperation and replacement of the tricuspid valve (UAB; Table 43-14); two additional patients have died with severe incompetence but without reoperation. One patient (GLH) required a late tricuspid valve replacement and another died with severe incompetence.

Reoperation seems common after repair (rather than replacement) of left-sided tricuspid valve incompetence. Williams and colleagues report using valvuloplasty of an unspecified type in six children with AV discordance and tricuspid valve incompetence, and three (50%, CL 24%–

Table 43-13 Incremental risk factors for death at any time, including hospital deaths, after intracardiac repair in patients with AV discordant connection (UAB; 1967–1983; n = 98; 28 deaths). Only one hazard phase was identified.

Incremental Risk Factor	Early Phase Hazard	
	Coefficient ± SD	P value
DORV	1.5 ± 0.70	.03
(Higher) hematocrit (%)	0.10 ± 0.034	.004
Age (years) at operation		
Age	0.09 ± 0.041	.02
ln(age)	−1.1 ± 0.53	.03
Date of operation (years since 1967)		
Date	0.5 ± 0.31	.09
ln(date)	−6 ± 2.6	.03
Intercept	2.9	

KEY: DORV, double outlet right ventricle; ln, logarithm; SD, standard deviation; VA, ventriculoarterial.

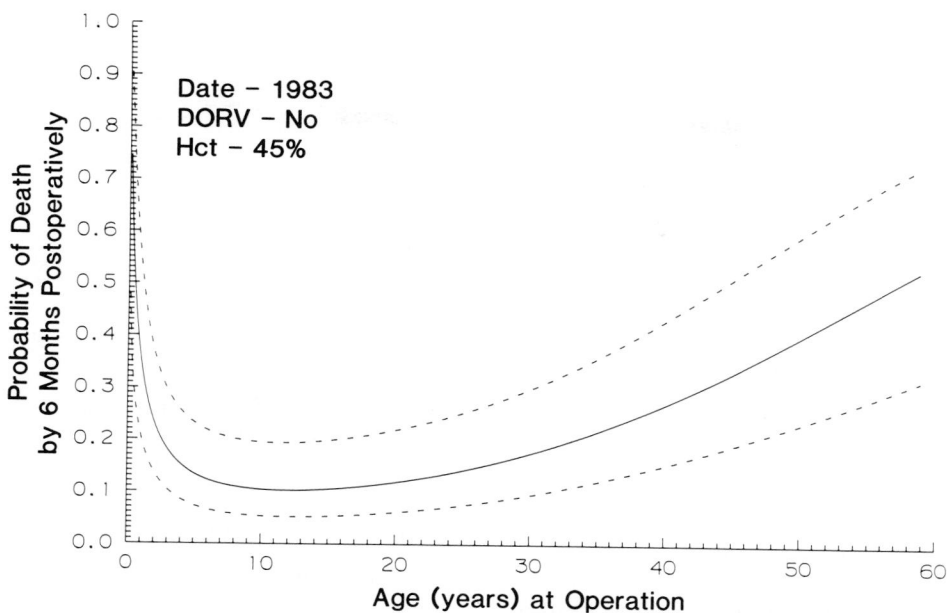

Figure 43-8 Nomogram of the relation of age at operation to probability of death within 6 months of intracardiac repair of congenitally corrected transposition of the great arteries and other ventriculoarterial connections except DORV. The dashed lines enclose the 70% confidence limits (1 SD) of the estimates. This nomogram is a solution of the equation in Table 43-13.

DORV, double outlet right ventricle; Hct, hematocrit.

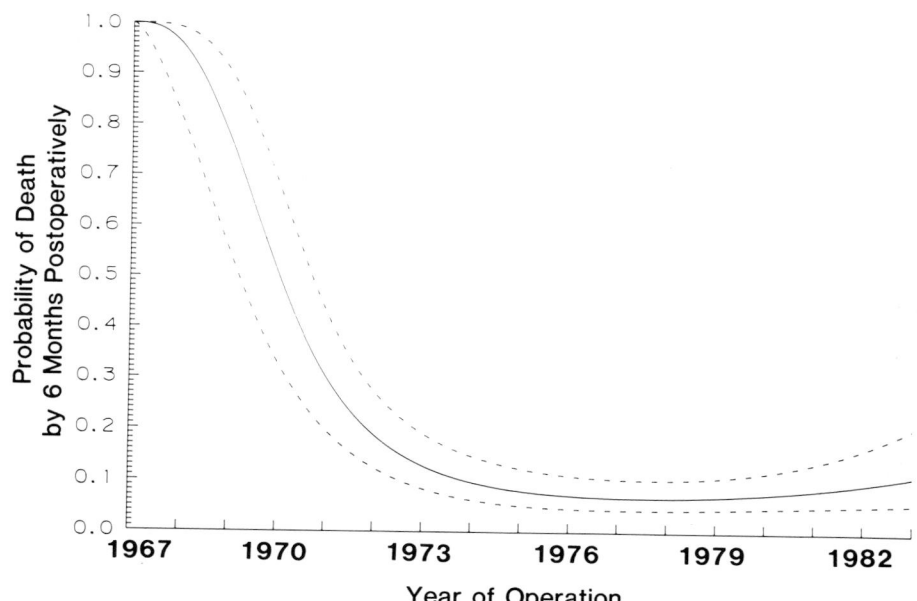

Figure 43-9 Relation of date of operation to probability of death within 6 months of intracardiac repair in patients with AV discordant connection. Depiction is as in Figure 43-7. The equation in Table 43-13 was solved with hematocrit entered as 0.4, age as 7.5 years, and DORV as no.

Table 43-14 Hospital and late deaths after reoperations following initial intracardiac repair in patients with AV discordant connection (UAB; 1967–1983).

		Hospital Deaths			Late Deaths		
Reoperation	n	No.	%	CL	No.	%[a]	CL
Tricuspid valve replacement	4	1	25%	3%–63%	2	67%	24%–96%
Mitral valve replacement	1	0	0%	0%–85%	0	0%	0%–85%
Tricuspid valve re-replacement	2	0	0%	0%–61%	0	0%	0%–61%
Valved extracardiac conduit	1	1	100%	15%–100%			
Replacement of valved extracardiac conduit	3	0	0%	0%–47%	0	0%	0%–47%
VSD patch repair	2	1	50%	7%–93%	1	100%	15%–100%

KEY: CL, 70% confidence limits; AV, atrioventricular; VSD, ventricular septal defect.

[a] Percentage of hospital survivors.

76%) underwent reoperation in a follow-up period averaging 4.9 years, one of whom died at reoperation.[W3]

Relief of Pulmonary Stenosis

Unless the subpulmonary and/or pulmonary valve stenoses are mild, the relief of the pulmonary stenosis in corrected transposition by measures short of a valved extracardiac conduit is apt to be disappointing.[E3] Among seven patients so treated by Westerman and colleagues and restudied later, five had gradients greater than 50 mmHg and two greater than 100 mmHg.[W5]

Reoperations for Valved Extracardiac Conduit Complications

Up to 10 years, 86% of patients with AV discordant connection are free of reoperation for conduit obstruction (UAB; Fig. 43-10). This indicates that the special positioning of the

conduit used in these patients has prevented an increased risk of conduit obstruction.

INDICATIONS FOR OPERATION

The indications for operation are not specific for the atrioventricular (AV) discordant connection but rather are specific for the coexisting anomalies.

Thus, when only a ventricular septal defect (VSD) coexists with corrected transposition of the great arteries (CTGA), the indications and contraindications are those for VSD in otherwise normal hearts (see Chapter 20). When VSD and important pulmonary stenosis coexist, the repair will usually require a homograft-valved extracardiac conduit; the surgical indications and staging are therefore the same as described for tetralogy of Fallot with pulmonary atresia (see Chapter 23, "Uncomplicated Tetralogy of Fallot with Pulmonary Atresia" in Section 1, Indications for Oper-

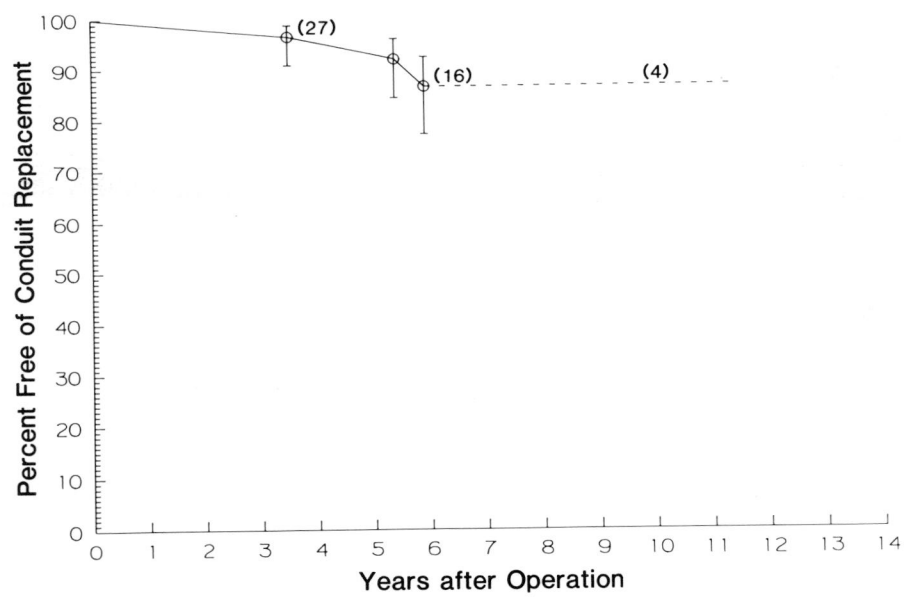

Figure 43-10 Replacement of a valved extracardiac conduit used in the intracardiac repair in 42 patients with AV discordant connection (UAB; 1967–1983). Patients were censored at death. Presentation is as in Figure 43-4.

ation), with the repair generally being advised between about 5 and 15 years of age. When important left-sided tricuspid incompetence coexists with AV discordant connections, the indications for operation are the same as those described for ordinary mitral incompetence in Chapter 11. When complete heart block develops, the indications and techniques for pacemaker intervention are those described in Chapter 47.

When double outlet right ventricle (DORV) coexists with AV discordant connection, there is usually a large VSD and pulmonary stenosis, and a valved extracardiac conduit is required in the repair. The surgical indications and staging are therefore the same as described above for CTGA corrected transposition with important pulmonary stenosis.

Double outlet left ventricle is a rare condition, and decisions are made individually in such situations. Since a valved extracardiac conduit is apt to be required, the definitive operation is postponed to the age of 5–10 years when possible.

When the ventriculoarterial connection is concordant (isolated ventricular or atrial inversion), the indications and techniques of operation are those for ordinary transposition (see Chapter 39, "Atrial Switch Operation" in section on Technique of Operation). However, the venous switch operation, rather than the arterial switch operation, is mandated by isolated ventricular inversion.

When the indications for cardiac transplantation are present, the procedure should be carried out (UAB, one case). As emphasized by Reitz and colleagues, the abnormal position of the great arteries does not prevent technically satisfactory cardiac transplantation.[R3]

SPECIAL SITUATIONS AND CONTROVERSIES

Intraoperative Electrophysiologic Mapping

It has been demonstrated that the bundle of His can often be identified during cardiac operations by electrophysiologic mapping techniques,[F3,K3,M3] and this technique has been used (UAB and GLH). Mapping usually, but not always, allows localization of the bundle of His, and by implication the locus of the AV node can also be determined. However, the procedure is cumbersome surgically because the heart must be open but perfused and beating during the mapping, which means that the patient must be on cardiopulmonary bypass (CPB) at a normal or near-normal temperature and the aorta may not be clamped for more than a few minutes. A risk of air embolization exists, and the CPB time is pro-

longed by 5–20 minutes. Also, in the Mayo Clinic[M2] and UAB experiences,[F1] mapping did not significantly reduce the incidence of complete heart block in the repair of the VSD in patients with corrected transposition (see "Early Results"). Thus, currently, mapping is not used as a routine in these operations.

Approach to the Repair of the Ventricular Septal Defect

Although the right atrial approach is generally preferred, an approach through the *morphologic left ventricle* is reasonable, except in those unusual cases of isolated ventricular inversion where it remains the ventricle supporting the systemic circulation after the repair. Often, however, the exposure for the repair is less good through the left ventricle than through the right atrium. An approach through the right ventricle may be advantageous as regards the avoidance of heart block,[N1] but it is not an approach to be recommended since the right ventricle remains the systemic ventricle after the repair in most cases. Olinger and Maloney described performing the VSD repair through the pulmonary trunk,[O2] but this would seem to have no advantage to repair via the right atrium. Even repair through the aorta has been advocated, but it has little to recommend it.

Routine Placement of Permanent Epicardial Pacemaker Leads

A selective approach to the placement of permanent epicardial pacemaking leads is followed (UAB, GLH; see earlier section on "Technique of Operation"), but some prefer the routine placement of such leads. The GLH and UAB protocol is based on the finding that no patients who have been in sinus rhythm after the operation have developed complete heart block late postoperatively (GLH, UAB). Should it develop, the transvenous route of placement (usually through the subclavian vein[H1]) is simple, and there has not been difficulty with stability of the intraventricular endocardial pacemaker lead in spite of the relatively smooth interior of the right-sided morphologic left ventricle.[E2] Further, it seems irrational to place prophylactic epicardial myocardial leads at operation without connecting them to a pacemaker pulse generator, and unless a clear indication of need exists this appears to be unwise.

REFERENCES

A

1. Anderson RH, Arnold R, Wilkinson JL: The conducting tissue in congenitally corrected transposition. *Lancet* 1:1286, 1973.

2. Anderson RC, Lillehei CW, Lester RG: Corrected transposition of the great vessels of the heart. *Pediatrics* 20:626, 1957.

3. Anderson RH, Becker AE, Arnold R, Wilkinson JL: The conducting tissues in congenitally corrected transposition. *Circulation* 50:911, 1974.

4. Allwork SP, Bentall HH, Becker AE, Cameron H, Gerlis LM, Wilkinson JL, Anderson RH: Congenitally corrected transposition of the great arteries: Morphologic study of 32 cases. *Am J Cardiol* 38:910, 1976.

5. Anderson RH, Becker AE, Gerlis LM: The pulmonary outflow tract in classically corrected transposition. *J Thorac Cardiovasc Surg* 69:747, 1975.

6. Anderson KR, Danielson GK, McGoon DC, Lie JT: Ebstein's

anomaly of the left-sided tricuspid valve. Pathological anatomy of the valvular malformations. *Circulation* 58(suppl I):I-87, 1978.

7. Anderson RH, Arnold MB, Jones RS: D-bulboventricular loop with L transposition in situs inversus. *Circulation* 46:173, 1972.

8. Anselmi G, Munoz S, Machado I, Blanco P, Espino-Vela J: Complex cardiovascular malformations associated with the corrected type of transposition of the great vessels. *Am Heart J* 66:614, 1963.

9. Anderson RH, Shinebourne EA, Gerlis LM: Criss-cross atrioventricular relationships producing paradoxical atrioventricular concordance or discordance. *Circulation* 50:176, 1974.

10. Anderson RH: Criss-cross hearts revisited: A question of definition. *Pediatr Cardiol* 3:305, 1982.

11. Albuquerque de AT, Rigby ML, Anderson RH, Lincoln C, Shinebourne EA: The spectrum of atrioventricular discordance. A clinical study. *Br Heart J* 51:498, 1984.

12. Akagawa H, Yoshioka F, Isomura T, Ohishi K, Hirata K, Kato H, Koga M: Surgical treatment of double-outlet left ventricle in situs inversus {I,D,D}. *Ann Thorac Surg* 37:337, 1984.

B

1. Bharati S, Lev M: The course of the conduction system in dextrocardia. *Circulation* 57:163, 1978.

2. Becu LM, Swan HFC, Du Shane JW, Edwards JE: Ebstein malformation of the left atrioventricular valve in corrected transposition of the great vessels with ventricular septal defect. *Staff Mtg Mayo Clin* 30:483, 1955.

3. Brenner JI, Bharati S, Winn WC, Lev M: Absent tricuspid valve with aortic atresia in mixed levocardia (atria situs solitus, L-loop). A hitherto undescribed entity. *Circulation* 57:836, 1978.

4. Bharati S, McCue C, Tingelstad JB, Mantakas M, Shiel F, Lev M: Lack of connection between the atria and the peripheral conduction system in a case of corrected transposition with congenital atrioventricular block. *Am J Cardiol* 42:147, 1978.

5. Brandt PWT, Calder AL, Barratt-Boyes BG, Neutze JM: Double outlet left ventricle. Morphology, cineangiocardiographic diagnosis and surgical treatment. *Am J Cardiol* 38:897, 1976.

6. Bharati S, Rosen K, Steinfield L, Miller RA, Lev M: The anatomic substrate for preexcitation in corrected transposition. *Circulation* 62:831, 1980.

7. Bonfils-Roberts EA, Guller B, McGoon DC, Danielson GK: Corrected transposition—surgical treatment of associated anomalies. *Ann Thorac Surg* 17:200, 1974.

8. Becker AE, Ho SY, Caruso G, Milo S, Anderson RH: Straddling right atrioventricular valves in atrioventricular discordance. *Circulation* 61:1133, 1980.

9. Brandt PWT: Cineangiography of atrioventricular and ventriculo-arterial connections, in MJ Godman (ed): *Pediatric Cardiology*. London: Churchill Livingstone 1981, vol 4, p 191.

10. Becker AE, Anderson RH: Conditions with discordant atrioventricular convexions—anatomy and conductive tissues, in RH Anderson, EA Shinebourne (eds): *Pediatric Cardiology, 1977*. London: Churchill Livingstone, 1978, p 184.

11. Bharati S, Lev M, Kirklin JW: *Cardiac Surgery and the Conduction System*. New York: John Wiley and Sons, 1983.

C

1. Carey LS, Ruttenberg HD: Roentgenographic features of congenital corrected transposition of the great vessels. *Am J Roentgenol* 92:623, 1964.

2. Cardell BS: Corrected transposition of the great vessels. *Br Heart J* 18:186, 1956.

3. Clarkson PM, Brandt PWT, Barratt-Boyes BG, Neutze JM: Isolated atrial inversion. Visceral situs solitus, viscero-atrial discordance, discordant ventricular d-loop without transposition, dextrocardia: Diagnosis and surgical correction. *Am J Cardiol* 29:877, 1972.

4. Castagna RC, Bastos P, de Leval M, Stark J, Taylor JFN, Anderson RH, Macartney FJ: Changes in ventricular depolarization in patients in sinus rhythm following closure of ventricular septal defect associated with atrioventricular discordance. *Thorac Cardiovasc Surg* 29:148, 1981.

D

1. de Leval MR, Bastos P, Stark J, Taylor JFN, Macartney FJ, Anderson RH: Surgical technique to reduce the risks of heart block following closure of ventricular septal defect in atrioventricular discordance. *J Thorac Cardiovasc Surg* 78:515, 1979.

2. Dick M, Van Praagh R, Rudd M, Folkerth T, Castaneda AR: Electrophysiological delineation of the specialized atrioventricular conduction system in two patients with corrected transposition of the great arteries with situs inversus (I,D,D). *Circulation* 55:896, 1977.

3. Doty DB, Truesdell SC, Marvin WJ Jr: Techniques to avoid injury of the conduction tissue during the surgical treatment of corrected transposition. *Circulation* 68(suppl II):II-63, 1983.

E

1. Erath HG Jr, Graham TP Jr, Hammon JW Jr, Smith CW: Hypoplasia of the systemic ventricle in congenitally corrected transposition of the great arteries. Preoperative documentation and possible implications of operation. *J Thorac Cardiovasc Surg* 79:770, 1980.

2. Estes NAM III, Salem DN, Isner JM, Gamble WJ: Permanent pacemaker therapy in corrected transposition of the great arteries: Analysis of site of lead placement in 40 patients. *Am J Cardiol* 52:1091, 1983.

3. Egloff L, Rothlin M, Schneider J, Arbenz U, Schonbeck M, Senning A, Turina M: Congenitally corrected transposition of the great arteries: A clinical and surgical study. *Thorac Cardiovasc Surg* 28:228, 1980.

F

1. Fox LS, Kirklin JW, Pacifico AD, Waldo AL, Bargeron LM Jr: Intracardiac repair of cardiac malformations with atrioventricular discordance. *Circulation* 54:123, 1976.

2. Freedom RM, Culham G, Rowe RD: The criss-cross heart and superoinferior ventricular heart, an angiocardiographic study. *Am J Cardiol* 42:620, 1978.

3. Fiddler GI, Maloney JD, Danielson GK, McGoon DC, Ritter DG: Intraoperative identification of the conduction system in dextrocardia with complex congenital heart disease. *Am J Cardiol* 39:301, 1977.

4. Friedberg DZ, Nadas AS: Clinical profile of patients with congenital corrected transposition of the great arteries. A study of 60 cases. *N Engl J Med* 282:1053, 1970.

5. Franco-Vazquez JS, Perez-Trevino G, Gaxiola A: Corrected transposition of the great arteries with extreme counterclockwise torsion of the heart. *Acta Cardiol (Bruxelles)* 28:636, 1973.

G

1. Grolleau R, Baissus C, Puech P: Transposition corrigee des gros vaisseaux et syndrome de preexcitation. A propos de deux observations. *Arch Mal Coeur* 70:69, 1977.
2. Gillette PC, Busch U, Mullins CE, McNamara DG: Electrophysiologic studies in patients with ventricular inversion and "corrected transposition." *Circulation* 60:939, 1979.
3. Graham TP Jr, Parrish MD, Boucek RJ Jr, Boerth RC, Breitweser JA, Thompson S, Robertson RM, Morgan JR, Griesinger GC: Assessment of ventricular size and function in congenitally corrected transposition of the great arteries. *Am J Cardiol* 51:245, 1983.

H

1. Holmes DR, Maloney JP, Feldt RH: The use of percutaneous subclavian technique for permanent cardiac pacing. *Mayo Clin Proc* 55:579, 1980.
2. Honey M: The diagnosis of corrected transposition of the great vessels. *Br Heart J* 25:313, 1963.
3. Hagler DJ, Tajik AJ, Seward JB, Edwards WD, Mair DD, Ritter DG: Atrioventricular and ventriculoarterial discordance (corrected transposition of the great arteries). *Mayo Clin Proc* 56:591, 1981.
4. Hwang B, Bowman F, Malm J, Krongrad E: Surgical repair of congenitally corrected transposition of the great arteries: Results and follow-up. *Am J Cardiol* 50:781, 1982.
5. Huhta JC, Maloney JD, Ritter DG, Ilstrup DM, Feldt RH: Complete atrioventricular block in patients with atrioventricular discordance. *Circulation* 67:1374, 1983.

K

1. Kiser JC, Ongley PA, Kirklin JW, Clarkson PM, McGoon DC: Surgical treatment of dextrocardia with inversion of ventricles and double outlet right ventricle. *J Thorac Cardiovasc Surg* 55:6, 1968.
2. Krongrad E, Ellis K, Steeg CN, Bowman FO, Malm JR, Gersony WM: Subpulmonary obstruction in congenitally corrected transposition of the great arteries due to ventricular membranous septal aneurysms. *Circulation* 54:679, 1976.
3. Kupersmith J, Krongrad E, Gersony WM, Bowman FO Jr: Electrophysiologic identification of the specialized conducting system in corrected transposition of the great arteries. *Circulation* 50:795, 1974.
4. Kinsley RH, McGoon DC, Danielson GK: Corrected transposition of the great arteries. Associated ventricular rotation. *Circulation* 49:574, 1974.
5. Kishon Y, Shem-Tov AA, Schneeweiss A, Neufeld HN: Corrected transposition of the great arteries without associated defects—study of 10 patients. *Int J Cardiol* 3:112, 1983.

L

1. Losekoot TG, Anderson RH, Becker AE, Danielson GK, Soto B: *Congenitally Corrected Transposition.* New York: Churchill Livingstone, 1983.
2. Losekoot G: Gecorrigeerde transposities. Thesis. Scheltema en Holkema, Amsterdam, 1967.
3. Lev M, Licata RH, May RC: The conduction system in mixed levocardia with ventricular inversion (corrected transposition). *Circulation* 28:232, 1963.
4. Levy MJ, Lillehei CW, Elliott LP, Carey LS, Adams P, Edwards JE: Accessory valvular tissue causing subpulmonary ste-

nosis in corrected transposition of great vessels. *Circulation* 27:494, 1963.
5. Lev M, Fielding RT, Zaeske D: Mixed levocardia with ventricular inversion (corrected transposition) with complete A-V block. *Am J Cardiol* 12:875, 1963.
6. Lev M, Rowlatt UF: The pathologic anatomy of mixed levocardia. A review of thirteen cases of atrial or ventricular inversion with or without corrected transposition. *Am J Cardiol* 216, 1961.
7. Liberthson RR, Paul MH, Muster AJ, Arcilla RA, Eckner FAO, Lev M: Straddling and displaced atrioventricular orifices and valves with primitive ventricles. *Circulation* 43:213, 1971.
8. Leijala MA, Lincoln CR, Shinebourne EA, Nellen M: A rare congenital cardiac malformation with situs inversus and discordant atrio-ventricular and concordant ventriculo-arterial connections. *Am Heart J* 101:355, 1981.

M

1. Monckeberg JG: Zur Entwicklungsgeschichte des Atrioventrikularsystems. *Verh Dtsch Pathol* 16:228, 1913. (In *Centralblatt Allg Path Path Anat* 24).
2. Marcelletti C, Maloney JD, Ritter DG, Danielson GK, McGoon DC, Wallace RB: Corrected transposition and ventricular septal defect: Surgical experience. *Ann Surg* 191:751, 1980.
3. Maloney JD, Ritter DG, McGoon DC, Danielson GK: Identification of the conduction system in corrected transposition and common ventricle at operation. *Mayo Clin Proc* 50:387, 1975.
4. McGrath L, Kirklin JW, Blackstone EH, Pacifico AD, Kirklin JK, Bargeron LM Jr: Early and intermediate term results of surgery in atrioventricular discordant connection. *J Thorac Cardiovasc Surg,* in press.
5. Metcalfe J, Somerville J: Surgical repair of lesions associated with corrected transposition. *Br Heart J* 50:476, 1983.
6. Milo S, Ho SY, Macartney FJ, Wilkinson JL, Becker AE, Wenink ACG, Gittenberger De Groot AC, Anderson RH: Straddling and over-riding atrioventricular valves—morphology and classification. *Am J Cardiol* 44:1122, 1979.
7. Matsuda H, Kawashima Y, Hirose H, Nakano S, Shirakura R, Shimazaki Y, Nagai I: Transaortic closure of ventricular septal defect in atrioventricular discordance with pulmonary stenosis or atresia. *J Thorac Cardiovasc Surg* 88:776, 1984.

N

1. Nagai I, Kawashima Y, Fujita T, Mori T, Manabe H: Successful closure of ventricular septal defect through a left-sided ventriculotomy in corrected transposition of the great vessels. *Ann Thorac Surg* 21:6, 1976.

O

1. Okamura K, Donno S: Two types of ventricular septal defect in corrected transposition of the great arteries: Reference to surgical approaches. *Am Heart J* 85:483, 1973.
2. Olinger GN, Maloney JV Jr: Trans-pulmonary artery repair of ventricular septal defect associated with congenitally corrected transposition of the great arteries. *J Thorac Cardiovasc Surg* 73:353, 1977.

Q

1. Quero-Jimenez M, Raposo-Sonnefeld I: Isolated ventricular inversion with situs solitus. *Br Heart J* 37:293, 1975.

R

1. Rokitansky CF von: *Die Defecte der Scheidewande des Herzens.* Vienna: Wilhelm Braumuller, 1875.

2. Ruttenberg HD, Anderson RC, Elliott LP, Edwards JE: Origin of both great vessels from the arterial ventricle: A complex with ventricular inversion. *Br Heart J* 26:631, 1964.

3. Reitz BA, Jamieson SW, Gaudiani VA, Oyer PE, Stinson EB: Method for cardiac transplantation in corrected transposition of the great arteries. *J Cardiovasc Surg (Torino)* 23, 1982.

4. Rizzoli G, Blackstone EHB, Kirklin JW, Pacifico AD, Bargeron LM Jr: Incremental risk factors in hospital mortality rate after repair of ventricular septal defect. *J Thorac Cardiovasc Surg* 80:494, 1980.

5. Ratner B, Abbott ME, Beattie WW: Rare cardiac anomaly. Cor triloculare biventriculare in mirror-picture dextrocardia with persistent omphalomesenteric bay, right aortic arch and pulmonary artery forming descending aorta. *Am J Dis Child* 22:508, 1921.

S

1. Schiebler GL, Edwards JE, Burchell HB, Dushane JW, Ongley PA, Wood EH: Congenital corrected transposition of the great vessels: A study of 33 cases. *Pediatrics* 27(suppl II):II-849, 1961.

2. Symons JC, Shinebourne EA, Joseph MC, Lincoln C, Ho SY, Anderson RH: Criss-cross heart with congenitally corrected transposition: report of a case with d-transposed aorta and ventricular preexcitation. *Eur J Cardiol* 5:493, 1977.

3. Swiderski J, Lees MH, Nadas AS: The Wolff-Parkinson-White syndrome in infancy and childhood. *Br Heart J* 24:561, 1962.

4. Sieg K, Hagler DG, Ritter DG, McGoon DC, Maloney JD, Seward JB, Davis GD: Straddling right atrioventricular valve in criss-cross atrioventricular relationships. *Mayo Clin Proc* 52:561, 1977.

5. Sutherland GR, Smallhorn JF, Anderson RH, Rigby ML, Hunter S: Atrioventricular discordance. Cross-sectional echocardiographic-morphological correlative study. *Br Heart J* 50:8, 1983.

6. Soto B, Bargeron LM Jr, Bream PR, Elliott LP: Conditions with atrioventricular discordance—angiographic study, in RH Anderson, EA Shinebourne (eds): *Pediatric Cardiology 1977.* London: Churchill Livingstone, 1978, p 207.

7. Subirana MT, de Leval M, Somerville J: Double-outlet left ventricle with atrioventricular discordance. *Am J Cardiol* 54:1385, 1984.

T

1. Thiene C, Nava A, Rossi L: The conduction system in corrected transposition with situs inversus. *Eur J Cardiol* 6:57, 1977.

2. Todd DB, Anderson RC, Edwards JE: Inverted malformations in corrected transposition of the great vessels. *Circulation* 32:298, 1965.

3. Tabry IF, McGoon DC, Danielson GK, Wallace RB, Davis Z, Maloney JD: Surgical management of double-outlet right ventricle associated with atrioventricular discordance. *J Thorac Cardiovasc Surg* 76:336, 1978.

U

1. Uher V: Zur Pathologie des Reizleitungssystems bei kongenitalen Herzanomalien. *Frankfurter Z Pathol* 49:347, 1936.

V

1. Van Praagh R, Van Praagh S: Isolated ventricular inversion. *Am J Cardiol* 17:395, 1966.

2. Villani M, Ross DN: Successful surgical repair of solitus, dextrocardia, atrioventricular discordance, and double outlet right ventricle with l-malposition of the aorta. *Europ J Cardiol* 7/2-3:105, 1978.

3. Van Praagh R, Van Praagh S: Anatomically corrected transposition of the great arteries. *Br Heart J* 29:112, 1967.

4. Van Praagh R, David I, Gordon D, Wright GB, Van Praagh S: Ventricular diagnosis and designation, in MJ Godman (ed): *Pediatric Cardiology.* London: Churchill Livingstone 1981, vol 4, p 153.

5. Van Praagh S, La Corte M, Fellows KE, Bossina K, Busch JH, Beck EW, Weinberg P, Van Praagh R: Superior-inferior ventricles: Anatomic and angiocardiographic findings in 10 postmortem cases, in R. Van Praagh (ed): *Etiology and Morphology of Congenital Heart Disease.* Mt. Kisco, NY: Futura, 1980, p 317.

6. Van Praagh R, Layton WM, Van Praagh S: The morphogenesis of normal and abnormal relationships between the great arteries and the ventricles: Pathologic and experimental data, in R Van Praagh, A Takao (eds): *Etiology and Morphogenesis of Congenital Heart Disease.* Mt. Kisco, NY: Futura, 1980, p 282.

7. Van Praagh R, Weinberg PM: Double outlet left ventricle, in AJ Moss, FH Adams, GC Emmanouilides (eds): *Heart Disease in Infants, Children and Adolescents* (ed 2). Baltimore: Williams and Wilkins, 1977, p 367.

8. Van Praagh R, Durnin RE, Jockin H, Wagner HR, Korn SM, Garabedian H, Ando M, Calder AL: Anatomically corrected malposition of the great arteries (S,D,L). *Circulation* 51:20, 1975.

W

1. Walmsley T: Transposition of the ventricles and the arterial stems. *J Anat* 65:528, 1931.

2. Wilkinson JL, Smith A, Lincoln C, Anderson RH: The conducting tissues in congenitally corrected transposition with situs inversus. *Br Heart J* 40:41, 1978.

3. Williams WG, Suri R, Shindo G, Freedom RM, Morch JE, Trusler GA: Repair of major intracardiac anomalies associated with atrioventricular discordance. *Ann Thorac Surg* 31:527, 1981.

4. Wenink ACG: Congenitally complete heart block with an interrupted Monckeberg sling. *Eur J Cardiol* 9:89, 1979.

5. Westerman GR, Lang P, Castaneda AR, Norwood WI: Corrected transposition and repair of associated intracardiac defects. *Circulation* 66:I-197, 1982.

44

UNIVENTRICULAR ATRIOVENTRICULAR CONNECTION (SINGLE VENTRICLE)

DEFINITION

Hearts with univentricular atrioventricular (AV) connection comprise a diverse group of cardiac malformations characterized by both AV valves or a common AV valve opening into the same ventricle, or the presence of only a solitary AV valve. Although *single ventricle* is an imprecise and inaccurate phrase, its frequent use in the past and its simplicity recommend it as shorthand for univentricular AV connection. Univentricular AV connection is one type of AV connection (the others being AV concordant connection, AV discordant connection, and ambiguus AV connection, see Chapter 1, ''Cardiac Connections''). This chapter does not discuss classic tricuspid atresia (univentricular AV connection with atrial situs solitus, ventricular D-loop, single inlet left ventricular main chamber, absence of the right-sided AV valve,[1] and either concordant or discordant AV connection[E1,A1]), which because of its frequency and its special surgical considerations is considered by itself in Chapter 26. Neither does this chapter discuss aortic atresia, which in many of its forms is a subset of univentricular AV connection. Because of the special considerations of this anomaly and the hypoplastic left heart syndrome, they are discussed in Chapter 35.

The same need for arbitrary decisions exists in regard to the AV connections as it does in regard to the ventriculoarterial connections in double outlet ventricle, and the same rules are applied to both. Thus, if one AV valve opens into a given ventricle and the other AV valve overrides so severely that half or more is over that given ventricle, the case is considered as having univentricular AV connection and is included under single ventricle; that valve is noted as being overriding. If less than half is overriding, the AV connection is considered to be concordant or discordant as the case may be, and that AV valve is noted as being overriding (see "Special Situations and Controversies").

HISTORICAL NOTE

Because of the morphologic diversity of this group of malformations and the many changes in terminology, it is difficult to trace the historical development of present knowledge and surgical techniques concerned with what is now known as single ventricle. Rokitansky certainly described and illustrated a case of single ventricle in 1875,[R1] as did Mann in 1907,[M1] although they used different terms. Lev and colleagues list a number of other descriptions of certain types of single ventricle published a hundred years ago.[L2] Taussig described "single ventricle with a diminutive outlet chamber" in 1939.[T1] As time passed, a dilemma in terminology became more and more apparent, since the phrase *single ventricle* was being used for a condition in which in many instances there obviously were two muscular chambers.

The clear definition of the entity as one in which both AV valves empty into the same ventricle, by Van Praagh, Ongley, and Swan[V1] in 1964 at the Mayo Clinic, was an important event. At about the same time, Elliott and colleagues expressed the view, now accepted,[R4] that hearts with atresia of one AV valve and thus a single AV valve had morphologically much in common with hearts with a double inlet ventricle,[E1] but Lev and colleagues and others preferred not to include tricuspid atresia in the general category of single ventricle.[L2] Lev clearly established the *exclusion* from the single ventricle category cases with a huge VSD (common ventricle) in which one side of the common chamber was morphologically right ventricle and the other left ventricle.[L2]

There followed a confusing period in which the term *ventricle* was redefined in order to escape from the paradox that there were two muscular chambers, or ventricles. Currently a unifying concept has emerged from the work of Anderson and colleagues[A1,A3] that is both rational and useful, namely, that this group of malformations has as its least common denominator the fact, as Van Praagh and colleagues stated in 1964,[V1] that just one ventricle has an AV connection. This has led to the practice adopted in this text of defining single ventricle as a spectrum of malformations that have in common a univentricular AV connection.[A1]

The surgical palliation of single ventricle without pulmonary stenosis began with the original description of pulmonary artery banding by Muller and Damman in 1952.[M2] The palliation of single ventricle with pulmonary stenosis has as its genesis the original description of the Blalock-Taussig shunt,[B4] and its application to patients with single ventricle and pulmonary stenosis was only a matter of time.

The concept of septating the main chamber to establish two circulations in series emerged from our experience of encountering unexpectedly a patient with single ventricle at the Mayo Clinic in 1956.[M5] The preoperative diagnosis was corrected transposition with ventricular septal defect (VSD), but the correct diagnosis was made after opening the ventricle. A septation was done, but the patient died about 6 months after operation, probably in a Stokes-Adams episode. This concept lay dormant for some years, but in 1972 it was further developed by Sakakibara and colleagues[S3] and in 1973 by Edie, Malm, and colleagues, who reported four successful septation repairs.[E2] Three long-term survivors of septation also were reported in 1973 by Arai, Sakakibara, and colleagues,[A4] and one by Ionescu and colleagues.[I1] McGoon, Danielson, and colleagues began to report successful results from the Mayo Clinic at about this same time.[M5] The right atrial approach to septation was suggested and applied by Doty in 1979.[D1]

A different surgical concept, namely that of using the main (or large, or dominant) ventricular chamber for generating systemic blood flow and allowing the vis a tergo of the systemic venous system to generate pulmonary blood flow was stimulated by the work of Fontan and colleagues, published in 1971,[F4] and of Kreutzer and colleagues.[K4,K5] The application of this concept to the surgical treatment of single ventricle was reported by Yacoub and Radley-Smith in 1976.[Y1]

MORPHOLOGY

Hearts with single ventricle are described by detailing the situs of the atria (solitus, inversus, or ambiguus), situs of the ventricles (which can be done in terms of D-loop and L-loop, see Chapter 1, "Situs of the Ventricles"), presence and degree of development (size) of each when two ventricles are present, details of the univentricular AV connection (double inlet with or without straddling, single AV valve with atretic or imperforate other valve, common AV valve), and the details of the ventriculoarterial connections (ventriculoarterial concordance, ventriculoarterial discordance or transposition, double outlet ventricle, common or single arterial trunk). The ventricles are referred to as left or right ventricles, depending on their internal architecture, recognizing that in hearts with univentricular AV connections, the *main ventricular chamber* (larger of the two ventricles) and the *minor, or accessory, or rudimentary, or hypoplastic ventri-*

---

[1] The adjectives left and right used to modify atrium or ventricle always mean morphologic right or morphologic left. The position of a chamber or valve is referred to as right-sided or left-sided.

Table 44-1 Ventricular architectural pattern and atrial situs in surgical cases of univentricular AV connection (single ventricle), (UAB; 1967–July 1982). Cases of classic tricuspid atresia ($n = 89$) are included and underlined.

Atrial Situs	n	Solitary Ventricle — Indeterminate	Two Ventricles Right-Handed (D-Loop)	Left-Handed (L-Loop)	Undetermined Loop
Solitus	101(87%) + 89	15	32 + 89	50	4
Inversus	2(2%)	0	2	0	0
Ambiguus	12(10%)	7	5	0	0
Bilateral right-sidedness	8(7%)	5	3		
Bilateral left-sidedness	4(3%)	2	2		
Unknown	1(1%)	1	0	0	0
Total	116 + 89 = 205	23(20%)	39(34%) + 89	50(43%)	4

KEY: ( ), percent of 116.

NOTE: All solitary ventricles in this era are of indeterminate morphology. Two additional ones with right ventricular morphology on one side and left ventricular on the other were in the group septated between July 1, 1982 and November 1, 1983.

cle (if present) may not, in precise terms, be identical with the usual morphologic left or right ventricle.

Most surgical patients (87%) with single ventricle have situs solitus of the atria (Table 44-1), only 2% have situs inversus, and about 10% have atrial isomerism.

Generalizations

The essence of hearts with a univentricular AV connection to a *large left ventricle*, recognized as such by its trabecular pattern,[L1,V2,V3] is that the atria connect with the ventricle that lies posterior to an interventricular septum that does not extend to the crux cordis. The small or minor ventricle is always positioned anterosuperiorly within the ventricular mass[A1] and can be left sided (most commonly) or right sided; that is, a ventricular L-loop or D-loop may be present. When the univentricular AV connection is to a *large right ventricle*, recognized by its trabecular pattern, the atria connect with the ventricle which lies anterior to an interventricular septum that usually does not extend to the crux. The small or minor left ventricle may be left sided or right sided (rare, Table 44-2) but is always positioned posteroinferiorly. In a third type, the ventricular chamber is solitary and of *indeterminate trabecular pattern* (primitive ventricle).

The volume of the main chamber is largest when there is no pulmonary stenosis and is considerably smaller when pulmonary stenosis is present.[K3] The increase in pulmonary blood flow ($\dot{Q}p/\dot{Q}s$) from creation of a systemic-pulmonary artery shunt increases the volume of the main chamber, whose size is correlated positively with the $\dot{Q}p/\dot{Q}s$;[S7] pulmonary artery banding often results in increase in wall thickness and decrease in volume of the main chamber, which is

Table 44-2 Ventricular architectural pattern and dominance and the status of the pulmonary outflow tract in surgical cases of univentricular AV connection (UAB; 1967–July 1982). Cases with classic tricuspid atresia are excluded.

Ventricular Architectural Pattern	Main (Dominant) Ventricular Chamber	n	Pulmonary Outflow Stenosis	Atresia	Open
Solitary ventricle	NA	23	19	3	1
Two ventricles					
Right handed (D-loop)		37	25	2	10
	LV	24	15	2	7
	RV	13	10	0	3
Left handed (L-loop)		50	27	0	23
	LV	47	24	0	23
	RV	3	3	0	0
Undetermined		4	2	1	1
	LV	3	2	1	0
	RV	1	0	0	1
Total		114	73(64%)	6(5%)	35(31%)

NOTE: "Open" indicates that no pulmonary stenosis is present. The (%) refers to percentage of 114. Not included are two patients with atrial situs inversus (see legend for Table 44-3 for details).

associated with reduction in size of the ventricular septal defect (VSD).

The morphology of the AV node and conduction system is abnormal in single ventricle and varies from one type to another. It is the inlet septum and its relation to the atrial septum at the AV junction that primarily determines the location of the AV node. This is so, except that when the right ventricle is the main chamber, the right ventricular architecture also plays a role. From the surgeon's standpoint, it is important to know that the AV node in single ventricle collectively can be anywhere around the perimeter of the right-sided AV valve, and in order to avoid heart block when closing off this valve or placing an intra-atrial baffle near it sutures must be placed 9 or 10 mm *away from* the anulus *anywhere* around the valve.

The terminology of the coronary arteries is disputed, primarily because the criteria for naming a vessel the *anterior descending coronary artery* are applicable with difficulty in single ventricle. Certainly, one characteristic of many types of single ventricles is the presence of right and left delimiting coronary arteries, which often demarcate the small ventricle (outlet chamber).[L2,R2]

An almost infinite number of morphologic subsets of single ventricle occurs.[A6] Those most apt to be encountered surgically are described here.

Double Inlet Left Ventricular Main Chamber, Subaortic Small Left-Sided Right Ventricle (Outlet Chamber), and Ventriculoarterial Discordant Connection

This is the most common type of single ventricle, occurring in about half the surgical cases (Table 44-1), and is characterized by both the left and right AV valves opening into a right-sided large left ventricular main chamber (double inlet LV), the small right ventricle lying anterosuperiorly and to the left. Presumably the internal ventricular architecture is left-handed. The ventriculoarterial connection is discordant,

with the pulmonary artery to the right and usually posterior, arising from the right-sided left ventricular main chamber, and the aorta arising from the small right ventricle (outlet chamber).

The internal architecture of this type of single ventricle is similar to that of corrected transposition, as is the position of the great arteries. The right-sided AV valve resembles a mitral valve, the left a tricuspid valve, and a heavy trabeculum often separates the papillary muscles of the two AV valves as they insert into the diaphragmatic free wall of the left ventricle. Not infrequently, both AV valves have mitral valve characteristics. Six of 48 examples of this subset have left-sided AV valve mitral atresia (Table 44-3).

The pulmonary artery arises just anterior and superior to the right-sided AV valve, and this is the anatomic feature that facilitates surgical septation. The left-sided AV valve, through which pulmonary venous blood enters the left ventricular main chamber, is to the left of and somewhat inferior to the right AV valve.

A large and usually nonrestrictive VSD (outlet foramen, bulboventricular foramen) connects the right-sided, dominant, left ventricular chamber with the small smooth-walled and rudimentary right ventricle (bulboventricular chamber, outlet chamber, infundibulum), which lies to the left and anterosuperiorly. From this chamber arises the aorta.

The AV node is anterior and away from the atrial septum and lies in the right atrial wall adjacent to the superior commissural tissue between anterior and posterior leaflets of the right-sided AV valve.[A5,B3,E3] (This arrangement also pertains in ventricular D-loop when the left ventricle is the main chamber, because here again there is no interventricular septum extending to the crux in the usual inlet position.) The bundle of His passes anterior to the pulmonary valve to reach the interventricular septum, where it descends anterior to the VSD.[A5,B2,B3]

The configuration of the coronary arteries is similar to that in corrected transposition.

Table 44-3 Ventricular architectural pattern and dominance and the nature of the univentricular AV connection in surgical cases of univentricular AV connection (UAB; 1967–July 1982).

Ventricular Architectural Pattern	Main (Dominant) Ventricular Chamber	n	AV Valves			
			Common	Double Inlet	Left-Sided AV Valve Atresia	Right-Sided AV Valve Atresia
Solitary ventricle	NA	23(20%)	13	10	0	0
Two ventricles						
Right handed		37 + <u>89</u>	6	24	6	1 + <u>89</u>
(D-loop)	LV	24	4	19	1	0 + <u>89</u>
	RV	13	2	5	5	1
Left handed		50	0	43	6	1
(L-loop)	LV	47	0	41	6	0
	RV	3	0	2	0	1
Undetermined		4	1	2	1	0
	LV	3	1	2	0	
	RV	1	0	0	1	
Total		114 + <u>89</u>	20(18%)	79(69%)	13(11%)	2 + <u>89</u>(2%)

NOTE: The underlined number refers to classic tricuspid atresia. The (%) refers to the percentage of 114. Not included are the two patients with atrial situs inversus, both of whom had two ventricles in D-loop. One of these had a dominant left ventricle with common AV valve, ventriculoarterial concordant connection, and pulmonary stenosis; the other had dominant right ventricle, common AV valve, double outlet right ventricle, and pulmonary stenosis.

Subvalvar or valvar pulmonary stenosis is present in over one-half the surgical cases (Table 44-2).

Double Inlet Left Ventricular Main Chamber, Subpulmonary Right-Sided Right Ventricle, and Ventriculoarterial Concordant Connection

This type of single ventricle occurs in less than 10% of cases, and pulmonary stenosis commonly coexists (Table 44-2). The large, left ventricular main chamber, lying posteriorly and to the left, usually receives two AV valves (double inlet left ventricle), although single or common AV valve may be present instead (see Table 44-3). The small right ventricle lies to the right and anterosuperiorly and gives origin to the pulmonary trunk. Presumably the internal ventricular architecture is right-handed. The aorta arises from the large left ventricle (Table 44-4). This has been called the *Holmes heart*.[A2,H1]

When the small right ventricle is right sided, as it is in this particular subset, the AV node is again anterior at about the 11 o'clock position relative to the right AV valve as seen by the surgeon from the exposure shown in Figure 44-1. The bundle of His descends from the anteriorly positioned AV node directly onto the interventricular septum without coming into relation with the ventricular outflow tract.[E4,W1] Rarely, the AV node and bundle may encircle the anterior aspect of the right AV valve orifice in this subset of single ventricle.[A2]

Right-Sided Right Ventricular Main Chamber

In this rather uncommon subset, the small rudimentary left ventricle (ventricular pouch) lies posteriorly and often has neither an AV nor a ventriculoarterial connection.[K2,S9] Pulmonary stenosis may coexist, and the presentation is often because of hypoxia in early life.[S8]

The AV node has its usual posterior position in the atrial septum, with its normal relation to the ostium of the coronary sinus.[W3] From the node, the perforating bundle of His passes through the AV valve anulus onto ventricular myocardium, either on the interventricular septum or on a trabeculum in the posterior ventricular wall.

Although AV valve atresia may coexist with any type of single ventricle, single ventricle with ventricular D-loop and right ventricular main chamber is that most frequently associated with left-sided AV valve atresia (see Table 44-3).[R4] This is the entity commonly called *mitral atresia*; in the absence of aortic atresia, it is included in this chapter. (With aortic atresia, it is considered in Chapter 35.) The left-sided AV valve may be absent or simply imperforate.[S10]

Left-Sided Right Ventricular Main Chamber

In this uncommon subset, the right-sided small left ventricle may be extremely hypoplastic (vestigial ventricle, vestigial pouch) and be visible only in the wall of the main chamber. Both great arteries originate from the right ventricular main chamber. Presumably there is a ventricular L-loop.

The conduction system is variable, but in a given case, both a conventionally located AV node may be present as well as a more rudimentary one nearby but more anteriorly and superiorly along the right-sided AV valve anulus[E3]; the nonbranching bundle then descends onto a free-running trabecula in the main chamber.

Indeterminate (Primitive) Ventricle

This form of single ventricle, which is common in atrial isomerism (see Table 44-1) and which often has a common AV valve (Table 44-3) and pulmonary stenosis (see Table 44-2), has only a single (solitary) ventricular chamber that is of primitive (nonspecific) architecture. The great arteries are often more-or-less normally interrelated. It comprises about 20% of the surgical cases of single ventricle (10% if tricuspid atresia is included).

The AV node is usually in a posterior position when there

Table 44-4 Ventricular architectural pattern and dominance and the nature of the ventriculoarterial connection in surgical cases of univentricular AV connection (UAB; 1967–July 1982).

Ventricular Architectural Pattern	Main (Dominant) Ventricular Chamber	n	Ventriculoarterial Connection		
			Concordant	Discordant	Double Outlet
Solitary ventricle	NA	23	NA	NA	23
Two ventricles					
Right handed		37	12	11	14
(D-loop)	LV	24	12	10	2
	RV	13	0	1	12
Left handed		50	0	47	3
(L-loop)	LV	47	0	46	1
	RV	3	0	1	2
Undetermined		4	1	1	2
	LV	3	1	0	2
	RV	1	0	1	0
Total		114	13	59	42

NOTE: There were no patients with common arterial trunk. Not included are the two patients with atrial situs inversus (see legend to Table 44-3).

is a rudimentary posterior ridge in the ventricle and distinct papillary muscles to both AV valves[W2] and passes down a free-running trabecula. When the ridge is absent, the AV node is usually situated laterally (away from the atrial septum) and anteriorly, and the nonbranching bundle descends into the right parietal wall of the primitive ventricle.[W2]

So-Called Common Ventricle

Rare examples of an apparently single ventricle have no discernible ventricular septum but one side of the solitary ventricle is morphologically right ventricle and the other is morphologically left ventricle. Some have named this condition common ventricle, while Lev has considered this to be an example of a huge VSD.[L2]

Associated Cardiac Anomalies

Excluding VSD, associated cardiac anomalies occur in at least a third of patients with univentricular AV connections. Straddling AV valves are the most common (Table 44-5).

CLINICAL FEATURES AND DIAGNOSTIC CRITERIA

The clinical manifestations of single ventricles vary with the morphology. Cases without pulmonary stenosis or atresia, which comprise about one-third of the cases, have a presentation similar to that of large VSD (see Chapter 20) except that since the main chamber acts as a common mixing chamber mild cyanosis may also be present. Cardiomegaly, pulmonary plethora on the chest x-ray, and congestive heart failure in the early months of life result from the high pulmonary blood flow and usually result in presentation at a young age.

Contrariwise, when mild or moderate pulmonary stenosis coexists, the early years of life may be without important symptoms. A pulmonary/systemic blood flow ratio of 1.75 to 2, in this setting, results in only moderate cardiomegaly and mild pulmonary overcirculation on the chest x-ray and a good functional status, albeit with mild cyanosis. Presentation in early or midchildhood rather than in infancy is common and usually occasioned by the cyanosis, a cardiac murmur, or the chest x-ray. This is in contrast to tricuspid atresia, where the pulmonary stenosis is more commonly severe and presentation is usually very early in life (Fig. 44-1).

When the pulmonary stenosis is severe or pulmonary atresia is present, important cyanosis usually results in presentation in the early days or weeks of life.

The clinical presentation is considerably altered by coexisting anomalies. Atresia of the AV valve draining the left atrium, which receives pulmonary venous blood when combined with a very restrictive foramen ovale, results in severe pulmonary venous hypertension with its typical chest x-ray and severe respiratory distress in early life. This situation may be masked initially by pulmonary stenosis and a small pulmonary blood flow, only to become apparent after a systemic-pulmonary artery shunt is created. Severe incompetence of an AV valve results in elevated atrial pressure and the early appearance of congestive heart failure. Pulmonary vascular disease may become prominent in early life in patients without pulmonary stenosis and result in marked alteration in the clinical presentation (see Chapter 20, ''Pulmonary Vascular Disease'' in Section 1, Morphology).

The electrocardiogram (ECG) and the chest x-ray may raise suspicion of the presence of single ventricle, but echocardiography usually is the first definitive diagnostic procedure. Absence of the posterior (inlet) septum between the AV valves, one of the hallmarks of single ventricle, can usually be diagnosed from the echocardiogram,[C1,F1] particularly when associated with apposition of the unsupported septal cusps of the two AV valves.[B1]

Table 44-5   Associated cardiac anomalies in surgical cases of univentricular AV connection, according to atrial situs (UAB; 1967–July 1982; n = 116).

Associated Cardiac Anomaly		Number[a]			
		Situs Solitus (n = 101)	Situs Inversus (n = 2)	Situs Ambiguus (n = 12)	Total (n = 116)
Straddling AV valves	Straddling + overriding	6	0	0	6
	Straddling only	8	0	0	8
	Overriding only	1	0	0	1
ASD—fossa ovalis type		23	0	1	24
ASD—sinus venous type		1	0	0	1
ASD—ostium primum type		1	0	1	2
ASD—common atrium		5	2	10	17
PDA		15	0	4	19
TAPVC		1	0	2	3
LSVC		7	2	3	12
Other anomalies of venous return		5	2	11	18
Multiple VSDs		9	0	0	9
Dextrocardia		3	0	5	8
Over-Under Ventricle: RV superior		2	0	0	2
Others		9	0	1	10

[a] One patient has unknown situs without other associated cardiac anomaly.

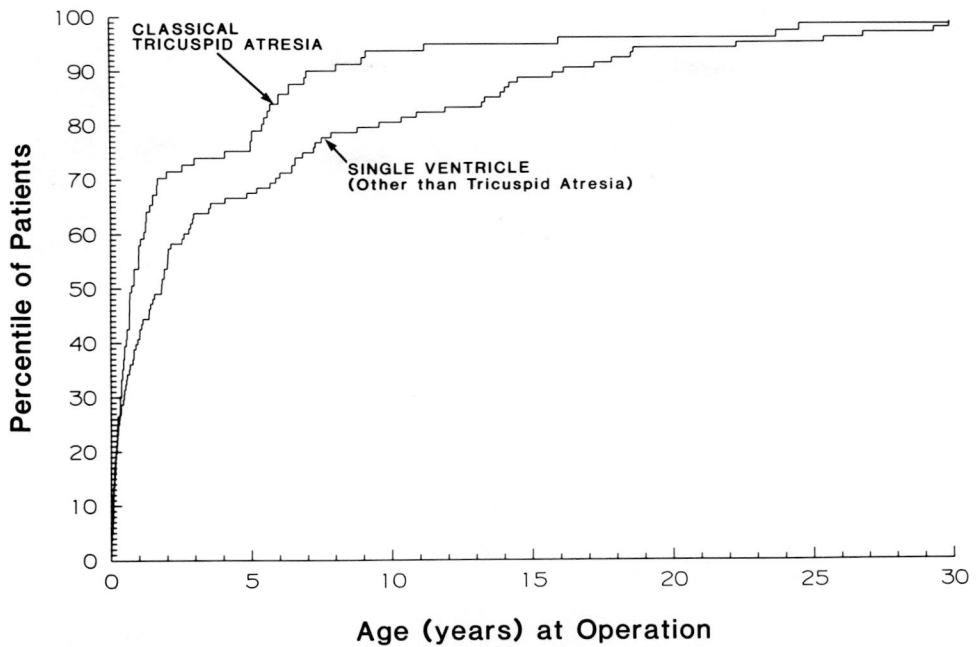

Figure 44-1 Cumulative frequency plot of age at first operation, anywhere, of surgical patients with univentricular AV connection (UAB first operation 1967–July 1982; *n* = 116 + 89 with tricuspid atresia). Not shown in the plot is the oldest patient with single ventricle, who was 46 years old at first operation and the oldest with tricuspid atresia, who was 34 years old at operation.

Reproduced with permission from Stefanelli et al.[S14]

Cineangiography is currently carried out in all cases in which surgical treatment is being considered (Fig. 44-2). In this regard, it must be recalled that the Holmes heart is easily misdiagnosed as tetralogy of Fallot if cineangiography is not precise.[S2]

NATURAL HISTORY

Generalizations

The natural history of patients with univentricular atrioventricular (AV) connections is almost as varied as the morphology, but certain generalizations may be made. Taken as a group, patients with single ventricle seem to be at less risk of death during the neonatal and infant periods than patients with total anomalous pulmonary venous connection, pulmonary atresia with intact septum, hypoplastic left heart, or severe tetralogy of Fallot. Thus, at least among the UAB surgical group, only about 15% of the patients have required a surgical procedure in the first month of life, about 33% in the first 6 months of life, and about 40% by the end of the first year of life (Fig. 44-1). By the end of the second year of life, only about 50% of surgical patients with a univentricular AV connection have had their surgical procedure. However, only 50% of the patients remain alive after 4 years of age.[M9]

Thus, a univentricular AV connection itself, with a resulting lack of separateness of pulmonary and systemic venous return and the potential for systemic ventricular ejection directly into the pulmonary circulation, does not usually pre-

dispose to rapidly progressing disability and early death. Inherently, it is a more lethal lesion than a very large atrial septal defect or common atrium, in which there is a common atrial mixing chamber, because the systemic ventricle ejects into the pulmonary artery.

Double Inlet Left Ventricle

The natural history of patients with double inlet left ventricle resembles that of large VSD except that spontaneous cure does not occur (see Chapter 20). However, either because of congenital anomalies of the valvar apparatus inherent in the internal architecture of a heart with a univentricular AV connection or because such a ventricle is nearly always volume overloaded and susceptible to a secondary cardiomyopathy and thus to secondary AV valve incompetence, one or both AV valves usually begin to be incompetent during the second decade of life, which usually leads to progressive deterioration and death by the beginning of the third decade. The stage may be set for this by the disturbances in myocardial function that appear to be present from early life in patients with single ventricle.[G1] Although global ejection fraction is often normal in early life, there is usually impairment in systolic wall motion anteroapically.

With Mild or Moderate Pulmonary Stenosis

When the single ventricle is associated with mild or moderate pulmonary stenosis, the natural history is ameliorated, just as it is in the case of large VSD. The volume overload of

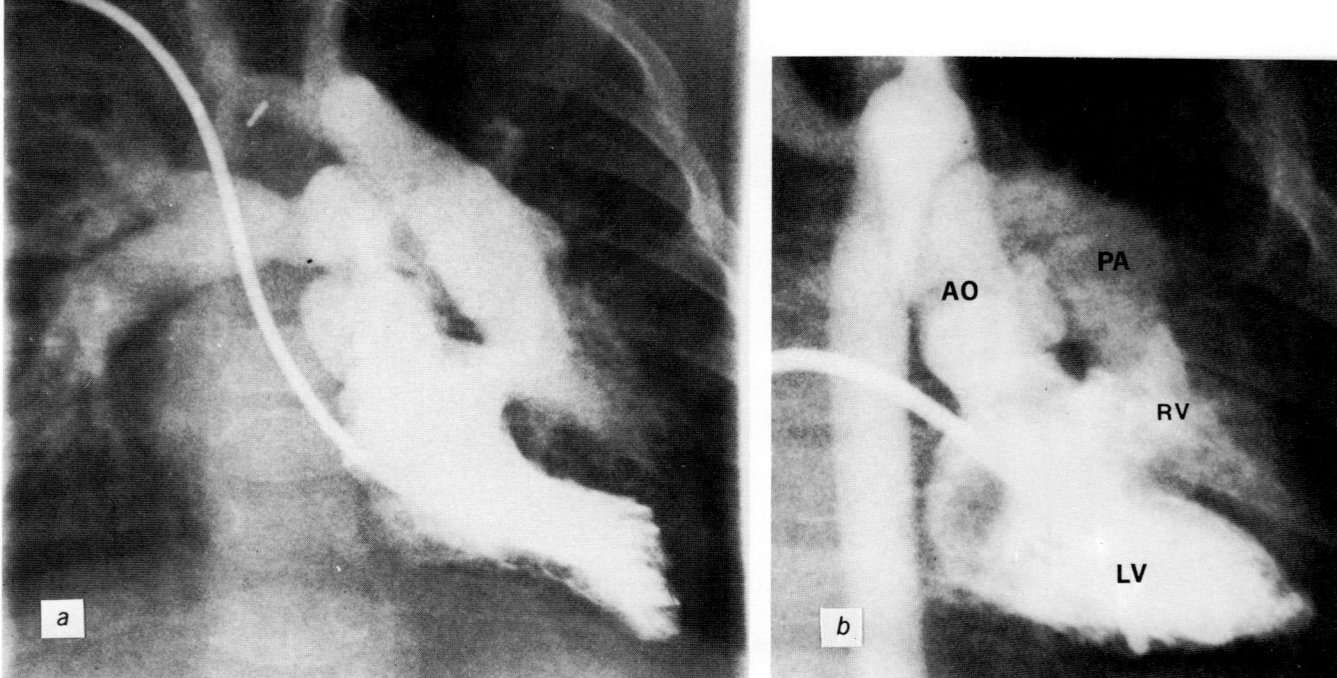

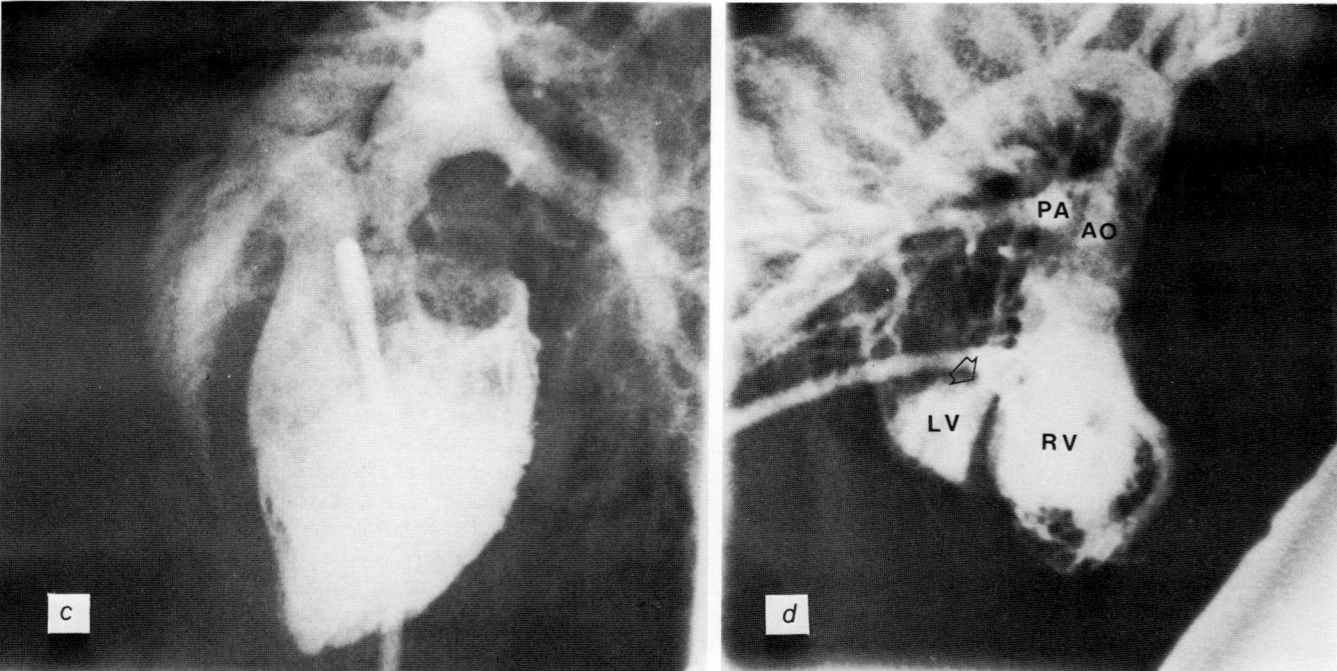

Figure 44-2 Cineangiograms in patients with single ventricle (UAB).

(a) Ventriculogram (frontal projection) in a patient with atrial situs solitus, ventricular L-loop, double inlet left ventricular main chamber, subaortic small right ventricle (outlet chamber) on the left side, and ventriculoarterial discordant connection.

(b) Ventriculogram (frontal projection) in a patient with atrial situs solitus, ventricular L-loop, double inlet left ventricular main chamber, subpulmonary small right ventricle (outlet chamber), and ventriculoarterial concordant connection.

(c) Ventriculogram (long axial view) in a patient with atrial situs solitus, ventricular D-loop, double inlet left ventricular main chamber, and ventriculoarterial discordant connection.

(d) Ventriculogram (elongated right anterior oblique view) in a patient with atrial situs solitus, ventricular L-loop, double inlet right ventricular main chamber, rudimentary left ventricle (or trabecular pouch), and double outlet right ventricle. Other projections clearly demonstrate the coarse trabeculations in the main chamber.

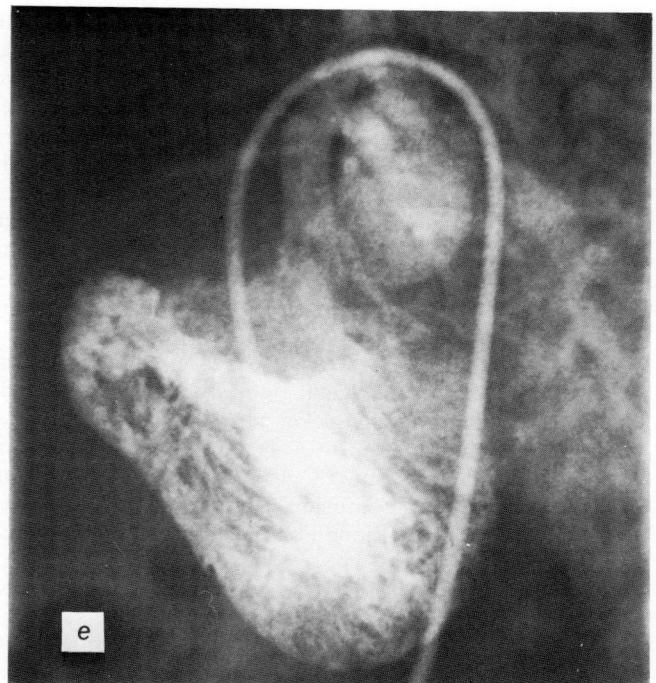

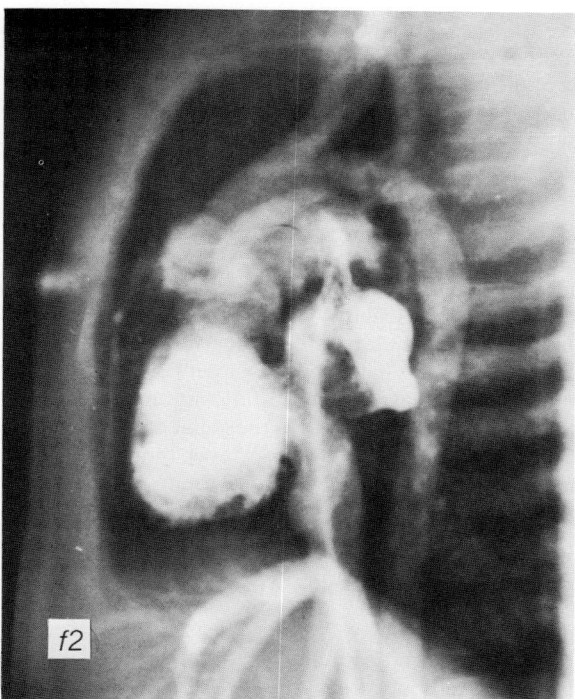

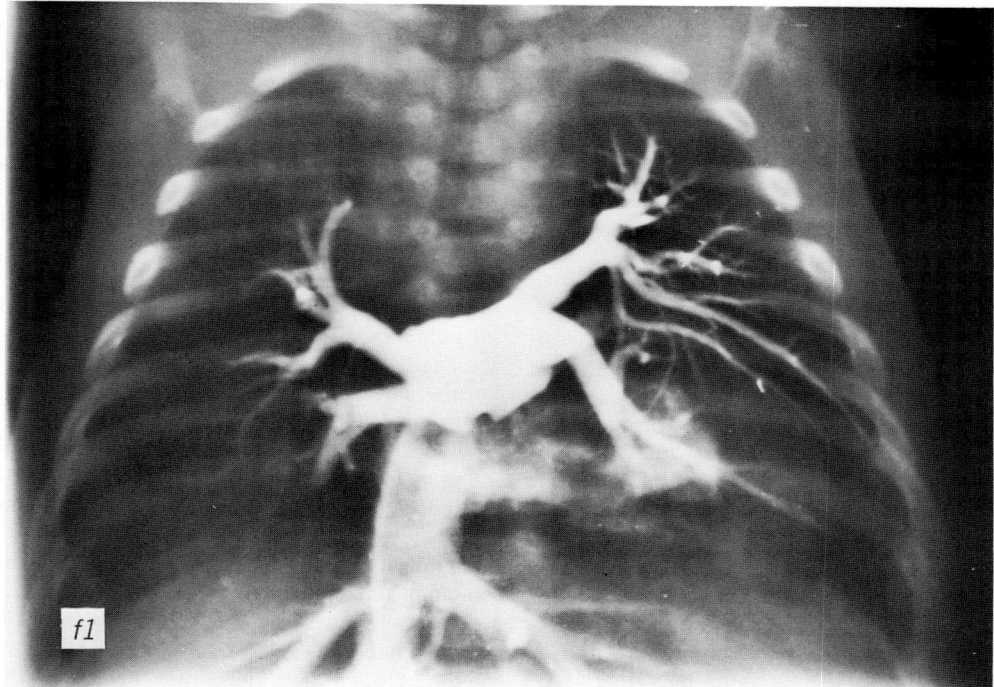

Figure 44-2 *(continued)*

(e) Ventriculogram (long axial view) in a patient with azygos extension of the inferior vena cava (see catheter course) and double-inlet and double outlet indeterminate (primitive) ventricle. There is associated severe subpulmonary stenosis.

(f) Cineangiograms in a patient with atrial situs solitus, ventricular D-loop, left AV valve atresia, and double outlet right ventricle.

(f1) Frontal projection, showing left-sided AV valve atresia.

(f2) Later phase, lateral projection, shows both aorta and pulmonary artery arising from the right ventricle.

Ao, aorta; LV, left ventricle; PA, pulmonary artery; RV, right ventricle.

Reproduced, in part, with permission from Soto et al.[S13]

the ventricle is less and thus the tendency for the development of AV valve incompetence is less, whereas the ill effects of the mild cyanosis and polycythemia are generally not severe. Such patients often live into their 30s or 40s or occasionally even longer before they succumb to myocardial failure.

With Severe Pulmonary Stenosis

When severe pulmonary stenosis or pulmonary atresia coexists with a univentricular AV connection, this dominates the natural history, which then becomes very similar to that of severe tetralogy of Fallot (see Chapter 23). Thus, it is evident that the arterial oxygen saturation is an important determinate of the natural history of these patients. This, in turn, is primarily related to the $\dot{Q}p/\dot{Q}s$,[M4] even though streamlining of flow through the single ventricle occurs in about 65% of patients.[M4,R3]

With Atrioventricular Valve Atresia

When atresia of one AV valve coexists with a restrictive opening in the atrial septum, the situation is rapidly lethal and death usually occurs within the first few months of life. Thus, in patients with so-called "mitral atresia" (atrial situs solitus, ventricular D-loop, right ventricular main chamber, and absent or imperforate left AV valve), most of whom do not have pulmonary stenosis, death often occurs in the first few months of life. The prognosis is the same in patients with ventricular L-loop and left-sided AV valve atresia (i.e., left-sided tricuspid atresia).

TECHNIQUE OF OPERATION

Septation

Although septation can be applied under proper circumstances to several types of single ventricle with double inlet left ventricular main chamber and anterior outlet chamber (and possibly a few with double inlet right ventricle), it is most commonly applied to single ventricle without pulmonary stenosis and with atrial situs solitus, double inlet left ventricular main chamber, and small left-sided subaortic right ventricle. Thus, it is described for this situation.

The preparations, draping, incision, and preliminaries to cardiopulmonary bypass (CPB) are the same as for most operations (see Chapter 2, Section 3). The aortic purse-string suture may be awkward to place and is most easily done as described for corrected transposition (see Chapter 42).

The cardiac morphology is examined, looking particularly for any anomalies of pulmonary or systemic venous return or of atrioventricular (AV) valve incompetence. The ventricular mass is usually enlarged (at least grade 3 on the basis of 1–6). The left atrium is usually enlarged. Interestingly, the right atrium does not usually appear to be as large as it is in patients with isolated ventricular septal defect (VSD), atrial septal defect, or tetralogy of Fallot, but this should not be discouraging to the use of the atrial approach.

The approximate size of the septation patch is now deter-

mined. This is done by noting the external dimensions of the ventricular mass and estimating the wall thickness. An appropriate-sized piece of knitted Dacron velour is backed with pericardium to create an impervious patch, or it is cut from a large double velour woven Dacron tube that has been preclotted. The patch will usually seem too small, but this relatively small size is appropriate[S5] since if it is made too large, it bulges into the right ventricle with each systole and impairs cardiac function. However, if it is made too small there is an increased tendency to dehiscence.

Cardiopulmonary bypass (CPB) is established by the usual techniques (see Chapter 2, Section 3), the perfusate made as cold as possible, the caval tapes snugged as soon as the heart becomes ineffective, a small right atriotomy made, and a pump-oxygenator sump sucker passed across a natural or surgically created foramen ovale. Then the perfusate temperature is stabilized at 25°C, the aorta cross-clamped, and the cold cardioplegic infusion given. The atriotomy is extended into the usual long oblique atriotomy, and stay sutures are applied (Fig. 44-3).

The interior of the left ventricular main chamber is now examined through the right-sided AV valve. The subpulmonary area is visualized, as is the VSD, the left-sided AV valve, and the relation among these structures. A determination is made as to whether the repair can be made through the intact right AV valve or whether a radial incision needs to be made in its base. Working through the aperture created by such an incision (see Chapter 20, Fig. 20-26, and Chapter 42, Fig. 42-10) facilitates the exposure and gives a direct approach to the area in which the sutures for septation must be placed between the tension apparatus of the left-sided and right-sided AV valves but this incision is not necessary in all cases.

A few stay sutures are placed to outline the proposed septation suture line (Fig. 44-3). The goal is to partition the two ventricles about equally, provide unobstructed pathways from the right atrium through the right-sided AV valve to the pulmonary artery and from the left atrium through the left-sided AV valve to the VSD, outlet chamber (right ventricle), and aorta, and to avoid damage to the coronary arteries by placing all sutures from within the ventricle. As McGoon and colleagues have emphasized, the position of the suture line is predetermined by the anatomy of the tension apparatuses of the AV valves posteriorly and inferiorly and by the location of the semilunar valves and VSD superiorly. Therefore, only anteriorly can the surgeon select the suture siting in an attempt to partition the ventricle equally.[M5]

Pledgetted 2-0 Dacron mattress sutures are placed and held individually by small hemostatic forceps. The most difficult area is the heavily trabeculated diaphragmatic surface. The suturing is begun here, if necessary invaginating the ventricular wall with a finger outside the heart as the stitches are placed. The suture placement is then carried posteriorly and superiorly between the tension apparatus of the right-sided AV valve and that of the left-sided AV valve. Starting again at the diaphragmatic surface, the suture placement is carried to the left and anteriorly and then superiorly along the anterior left ventricular wall in the previously determined line. The suture line passes over the VSD and then swings posteriorly and to the right beneath the subpulmo-

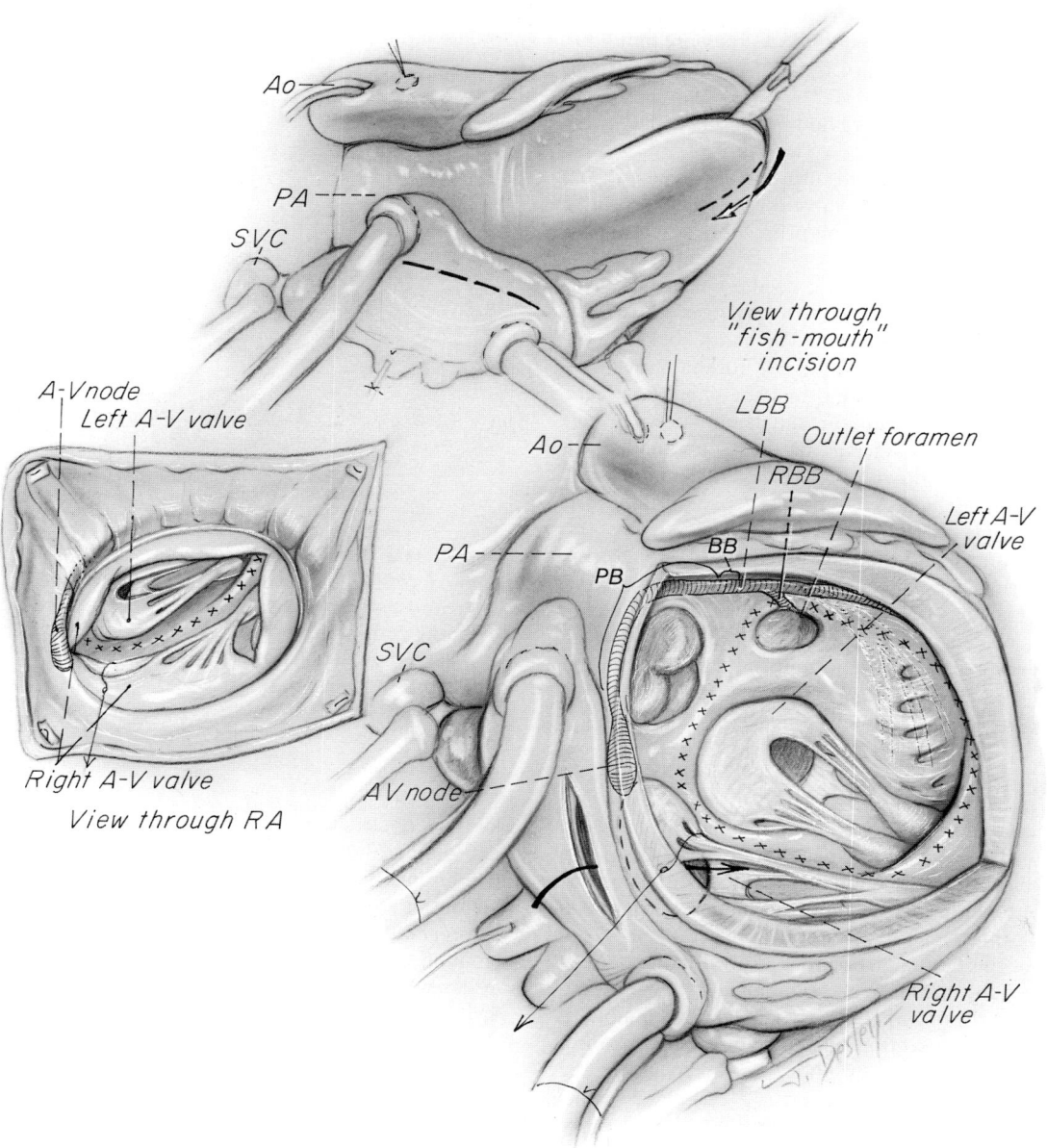

Labels in figure:

Ao
PA
SVC

View through "fish-mouth" incision

A-V node
Left A-V valve

Ao
PA
SVC

LBB
RBB
BB
PB

Outlet foramen
Left A-V valve

AV node

Right A-V valve

View through RA

Right A-V valve

J. Desley

Figure 44-3 The septation operation is performed through a right atrial approach, but it is best illustrated through the alternative fish-mouth incision in the ventricular main chamber. The illustration is of septation for single ventricle with atrial situs solitus, double inlet left ventricular main chamber, and left-sided, small subaortic right ventricle. The positions of the AV node and bundle of His are shown. Also shown are incisions and suture placement for the septation operation. Note that the AV node is in an anterior position, in the right atrial wall at about the junction of the right atrial roof and atrial septum. The bundle of His penetrates the junction of the right AV valve and pulmonary valve to pass over the subpulmonary area along the anterior left ventricular free wall. As it passes along the interventricular septum, it courses anterior to the VSD (or outlet foramen) and divides into left and right bundle branches. The septation operation usually results in heart block. The ×'s indicate suture siting for inserting the septation patch.

Ao, aorta; AV, atrioventricular; LBB, left bundle branch; PA, pulmonary artery; PB,BB, penetrating and branching portions of bundle of His; PM, papillary muscle; RA, right atrium; RBB, right bundle branch; SVC, superior vena cava.

Reproduced from Bharati et al.[B5]

nary area (Fig. 44-3). The sutures must be placed together, and 20–30 are usually required. As they are individually clamped and set aside, care is taken to maintain their
proper order.

The size and shape of the previously trimmed patch are
inspected and altered if needed. The sutures are passed
through the patch, the patch slid into position, and the sutures tied. If the right-sided AV valve has been incised, it is
repaired with continuous 6-0 polypropylene sutures (see
Chapter 20, Fig. 20-26).

With strong suction on the aortic needle vent, the aortic
clamp is released. Rewarming with the perfusate has been
started about 5 minutes before this. The sump sucker is removed from the right atrium, and the foramen ovale is
closed. The right atrium is closed, and the caval tapes are
loosened. A groove, or indentation, can usually now be seen
in the ventricular wall along part of the suture line. Two
temporary right atrial and two temporary ventricular epicardial wires are placed, and AV sequential pacing is begun.
The usual de-airing procedures are then carried out (see
Chapter 2, Section 3), and the remainder of the operation is
completed as usual.

After hemostasis has been secured, two permanent pacing
electrodes are placed on the right atrium and two on the
ventricle. The ends of these are brought subcutaneously into
the right upper quadrant, and an appropriate pacemaker is
inserted a day or two later (see Chapter 45).

Fontan-Type Procedure

Connection of the right atrium to the pulmonary arteries with
maintenance of the ventricular main chamber as the pump
for systemic blood flow is another technique that may be
used for patients with various types of single ventricle and
more or less normal pulmonary vascular resistance.

The details of the Fontan-type procedure with direct anastomosis of the right atrium to the pulmonary artery are described in Chapter 26 (see ''Direct Right Atrial-Pulmonary
Artery Connection'' in section on Technique of Operation).
A roof of Dacron or Gore-Tex may be used to widen the
anastomosis, but is usually not necessary.[M10] When a double
inlet ventricle is part of the malformation, the right-sided AV
valve may be closed surgically (Fig. 44-4), producing an
anatomic situation similar to that in tricuspid atresia. This
option must be used if the right AV valve is incompetent.
Alternatively, both AV valves (if present) may be left draining into the ventricle, and the pathway from the cavae to the
pulmonary artery separated from the pulmonary venous
pathway to the AV valve(s). This option is mandatory if the
left-sided AV valve is atretic or stenotic. The technique of
the separation is critically important, since an improper
method obstructs one or the other pathway and particularly
that to a large right-sided AV valve.[D4] At times a right atrial
wall flap can be improvised and used for the partition after
the atrial septum is excised completely. The wall between
the coronary sinus and left atrium is usually cut down from
the coronary ostium to open the area widely. More commonly, a taut pericardial baffle is sewed into place so as to
divert caval blood to the anastomosis to the pulmonary artery and pulmonary venous blood to both AV valves.

A special problem can exist in single ventricle with aortic

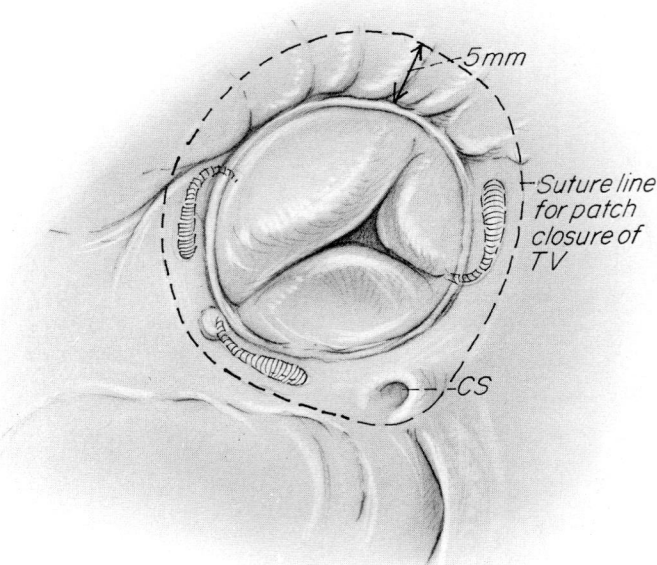

Figure 44-4 The right AV valve may be closed as part of the
surgical procedure in which a Fontan-type repair is performed in
patients with double inlet left ventricle. Several possible locations
of the AV node and proximal bundle of His are shown in the drawing. Since the location in a given patient is not known precisely, the
suture line for patch closure of the right-sided AV valve is 5 mm
outside the anulus all the way around.

CS, coronary sinus; TV, right-sided AV valve.

outflow obstruction. One example of this is a restrictive VSD
(or outlet foramen, or bulboventricular foramen) between
the double inlet left ventricular main chamber and a subaortic outlet chamber. When a nonobstructed pulmonary artery
is present, the proximal end may be connected by a Dacron
conduit to the side of the ascending aorta[D3,Y1] rather than
oversewing it as usually done when the distal end is to be
used for atriopulmonary anastomosis.

Other Operations

Pulmonary artery banding is described in Chapter 20 (see
''Pulmonary Artery Banding'' in Section 1, Technique of
Operation). *Atrial septectomy* is described in Chapter 39
(see ''Blalock-Hanlon Atrial Septectomy'' in section on
Technique of Operation). The *shunting operations* are described in Chapter 23 (see ''Technique of Shunting Operations'' in Section 1).

Repair of Ventricular Septal Defect with Straddling
or Overriding Atrioventricular Valves

A VSD may be complicated by straddling or overriding AV
valves in patients with either AV concordant connection or
discordant connection. Surgical treatment for VSD complicated by straddling AV valves may consist simply of making a slot in the VSD patch, which permits the passage of the
chordae into the other ventricle. Alternatively, a minor septation of the other ventricle can be produced by attaching a
part of the VSD closure patch to the other side of the septum
(rather than to the septal edge) so that the straddling chordae

are now on the appropriate side of the VSD patch (Fig. 44-5). A more major septation[D2,P1] of the opposite (or large) ventricle may be appropriate when there is also overriding of the anulus and some hypoplasia of the ventricle to which the overriding valve normally relates (Fig. 44-6).[P1,T4] Valve replacement, the most direct solution, should be limited to situations in which either the AV valve is importantly incompetent or no other surgical solution is possible. Alternatively, when pulmonary vascular resistance is low, a Fontan-type procedure can be used, in which an intra-atrial baffle is also placed to divert pulmonary venous blood to both AV valves (see ''Fontan-Type Procedure'' in Technique of Operation).

SPECIAL FEATURES OF POSTOPERATIVE CARE

Septation Operation

The usual protocols are followed postoperatively (see Chapter 5). Following septation, the right atrial pressure is usually a few millimeters of mercury higher than the left and should be maintained at about 12–14 mmHg in the early hours after operation.

Fontan-Type Procedure

The care after a Fontan-type procedure is discussed in Chapter 26.

Other Operations

The special features of the postoperative care after pulmonary artery banding, atrial septectomy, and shunting operations are described in the chapters dealing with these procedures (see above).

EARLY RESULTS

Septation Operation

Since the technical details and indications for the septation operation continue to evolve, the current early results may not pertain in the future.

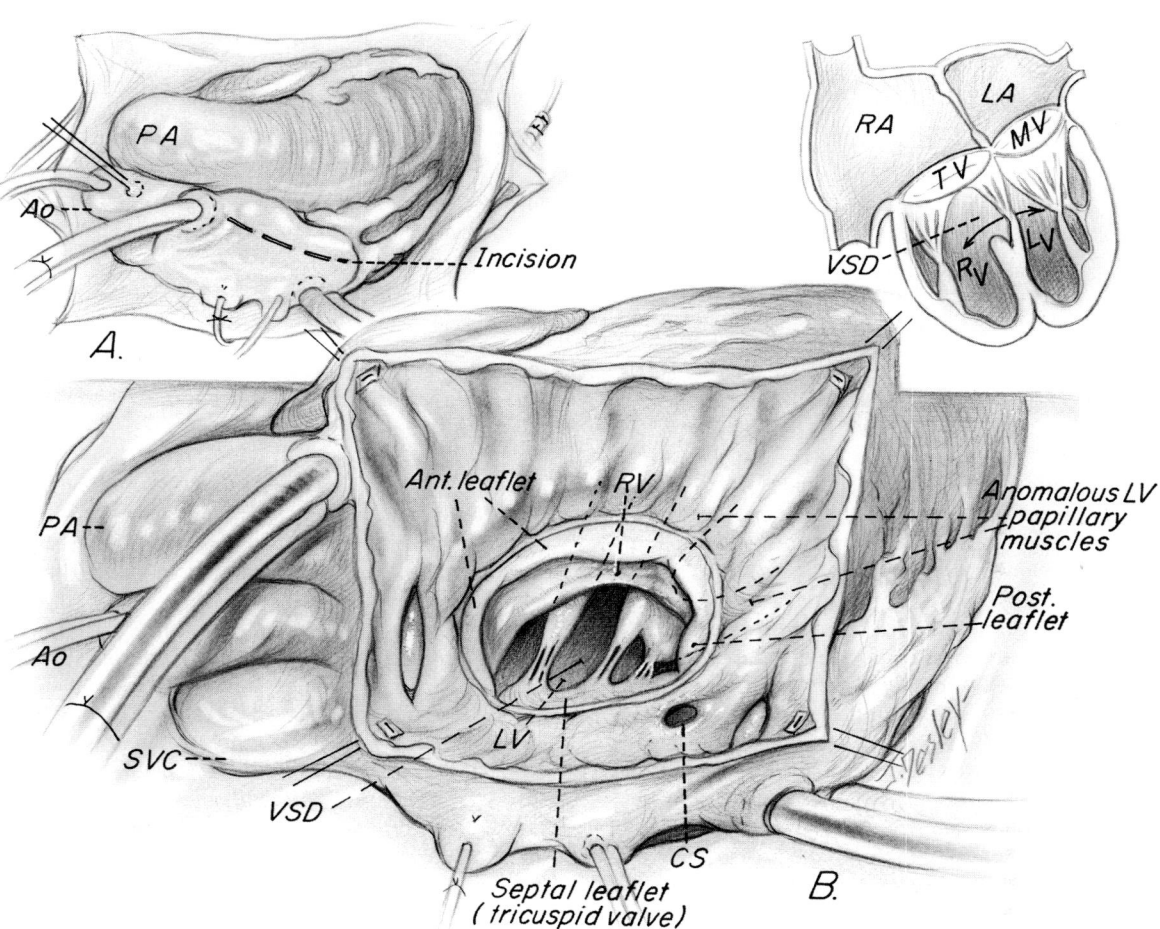

Figure 44-5 Minor septation for inlet VSD associated with straddling and overriding tricuspid valve.
(*a*) Approach through the usual oblique right atrial incision.
(*b*) The anatomy is examined through the right atrial approach and through the tricuspid valve. The chordal straddling on to the anomalous left ventricular papillary muscles is shown, with the origins of the papillary muscles from within the left ventricle outlined by the dashed lines. The AV node is adjacent to the tricuspid anulus at about the 4 o'clock position as viewed by the surgeon.

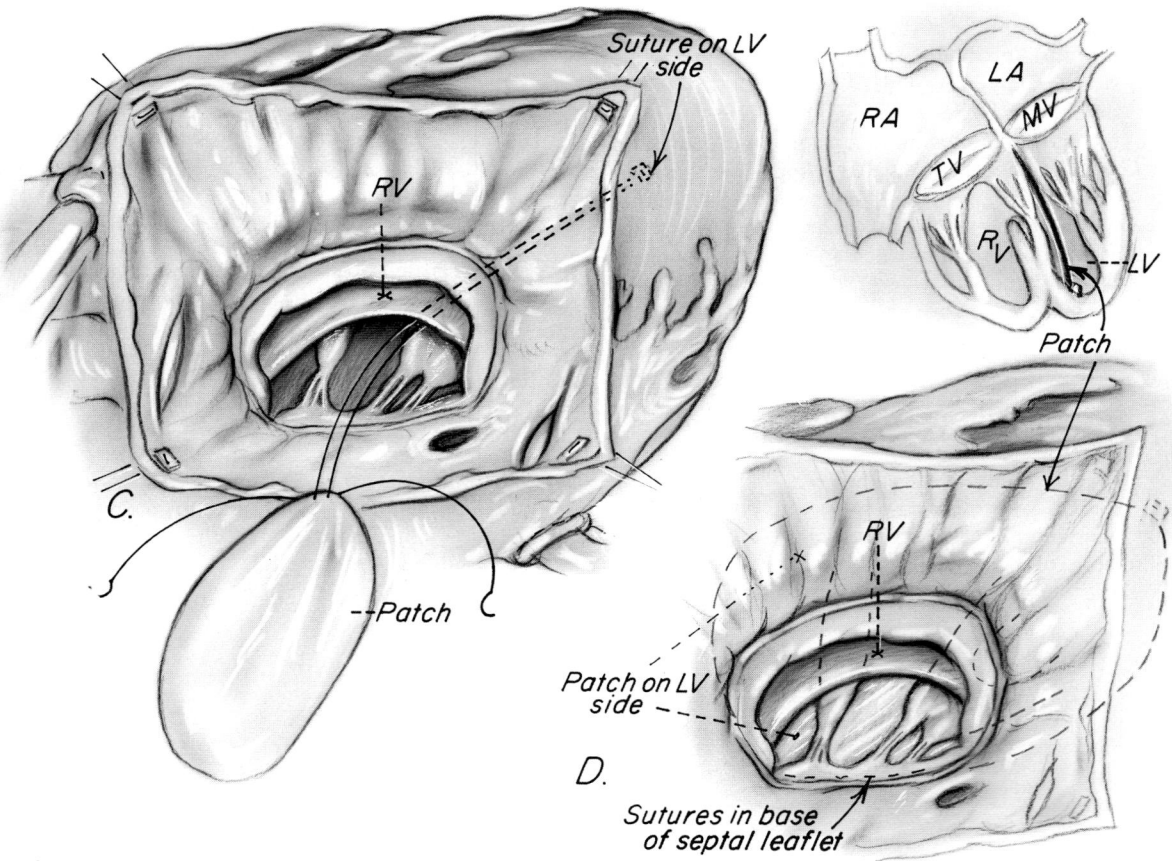

Figure 44-5 *(continued)*
(c) The patch for the minor septation is anchored on the *left* ventricular side of the septum.
(d) In the completed repair, the straddling chordae are now on the right ventricular side of the patch.

Ao, aorta; CS, coronary sinus; LA, left atrium; LV, left ventricle; MV, mitral valve; PA, pulmonary artery; RA, right atrium; RV, right ventricle; SVC, superior vena cava; TV, tricuspid valve; VSD, ventricular septal defect.

Reproduced with permission from Pacifico et al.,[P1] and the American Heart Association, Inc.

Current information (Table 44-6) indicates the hospital mortality under proper circumstances (no concomitant valve replacement or valved extracardiac conduit in patients with main chamber enlargement grade 3 or more) is 6% (CL 1%–20%, 1 death in 16 cases; UAB, 1967–Oct. 1983). This is similar to the Mayo Clinic experience in which 11 patients were operated upon under similar circumstances, among whom only 2 (18%, CL 6%–38%) died early *or* late (within an average of 3¼ years) after septation.[F2] The total hospital mortality has been 36% (UAB; Table 44-7).

The incremental risk factors for hospital death after septation include *indeterminate (primitive) ventricular morphology* (Table 44-7); this has also been true in the Mayo Clinic experience.[F2] Too little experience has been had with the rare double inlet right ventricular main chamber types to know if this morphology is also a risk factor. A *small main chamber* (enlargement grade 2 or less on the basis of 1–6) is an important risk factor (see Table 44-6). *Concomitant AV valve replacement* may also be a risk factor (Table 44-8), although its deleterious effects are more apparent in the late results (see below). Finally, the use of a *valved extracardiac conduit* between a ventricle and the pulmonary artery (or orthotopic pulmonary valve replacement) has been an incremental risk factor for hospital death (Table 44-9). *Age at repair* has not been demonstrated to be a risk factor (Table 44-10).

Complete heart block has developed after septation in 25 of the 28 traced patients known to be at risk (UAB). Three of the 32 patients had congenital heart block; in one other patient the postoperative cardiac rhythm is not known. Three of the patients who escaped heart block had ventricular L-loop, double inlet left ventricular main chamber, and ventriculoarterial discordant connection. The other had ventricular D-loop, double inlet left ventricular main chamber, and ventriculoarterial concordant connection.

Fontan-Type Procedure

Overall, *hospital mortality* has been relatively high (22%, CL 17%–28%) among the 73 patients undergoing Fontan-type procedures for various congenital anomalies (UAB; see Chapter 26, Table 26-1). Among the 14 patients with single ventricle, there have been 4 deaths (29%). Similar mortalities have been reported by Gale and colleagues and Marcelletti and colleagues.[G2,G3,M3]

It is difficult to surmise *risks in the current era* from these overall experiences. Possibly, they are represented by the somewhat lower hospital mortality during January–November 1, 1983, 1 patient (7%, CL 1%–22%) having died among 14 without concomitant AV valve replacement or other major associated procedures (UAB; see Chapter 26, Table 26-2). This is similar to the risks predicted from the experience of Fontan and colleagues,[F4,F5] Kreutzer and colleagues,[K6] and Ashraf and colleagues.[A7]

Further details of the early results after Fontan-type procedures are discussed in Chapter 26.

Classical Shunting Operations

The hospital mortality for classical shunting procedures for single ventricle is low, 2% (Table 44-11), just as it is when they are performed for tetralogy of Fallot and other types of cyanotic congenital heart disease (see Chapter 23, Table 23-12).

Pulmonary Artery Banding

No hospital deaths occurred among the four patients subjected to this procedure (Table 44-12).

Atrial Septectomy

Atrial septectomy was performed without mortality either as an isolated procedure or combined with pulmonary artery banding or a systemic-pulmonary artery shunting procedure (Table 44-13). Shore and colleagues report a higher mortality (23%, CL 10%–41%),[S10] which is perhaps related to their performing the septectomy by open techniques (with inflow occlusion or CPB) rather than by the Blalock-Hanlon technique.

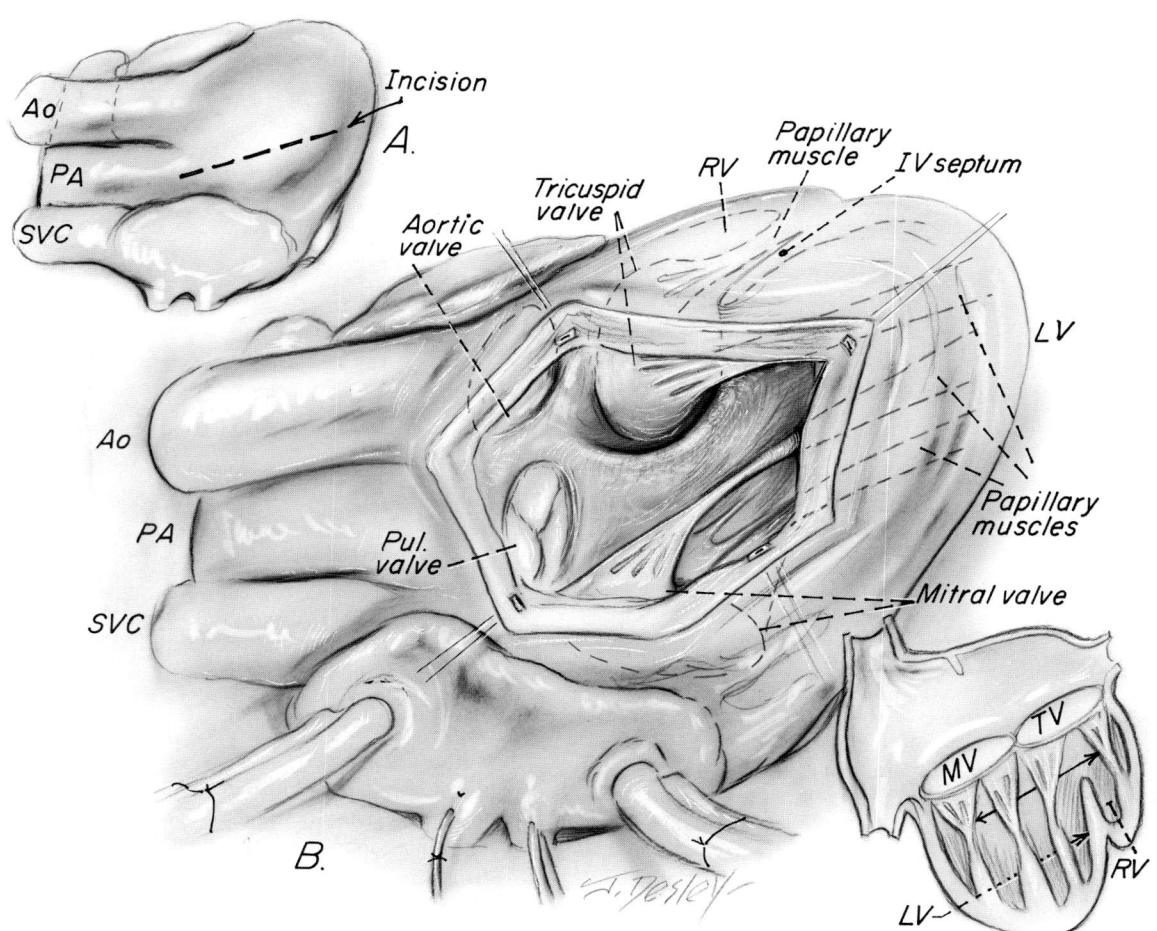

Figure 44-6 Major septation for corrected transposition of the great arteries (ventricular L-loop), large VSD and straddling and overriding, left-sided tricuspid valve. The approach through the right-sided left ventricle is illustrated, but currently an approach through the right-sided AV valve is preferred.
(*a*) Ventriculotomy incision.
(*b*) Details of the anatomic arrangement.

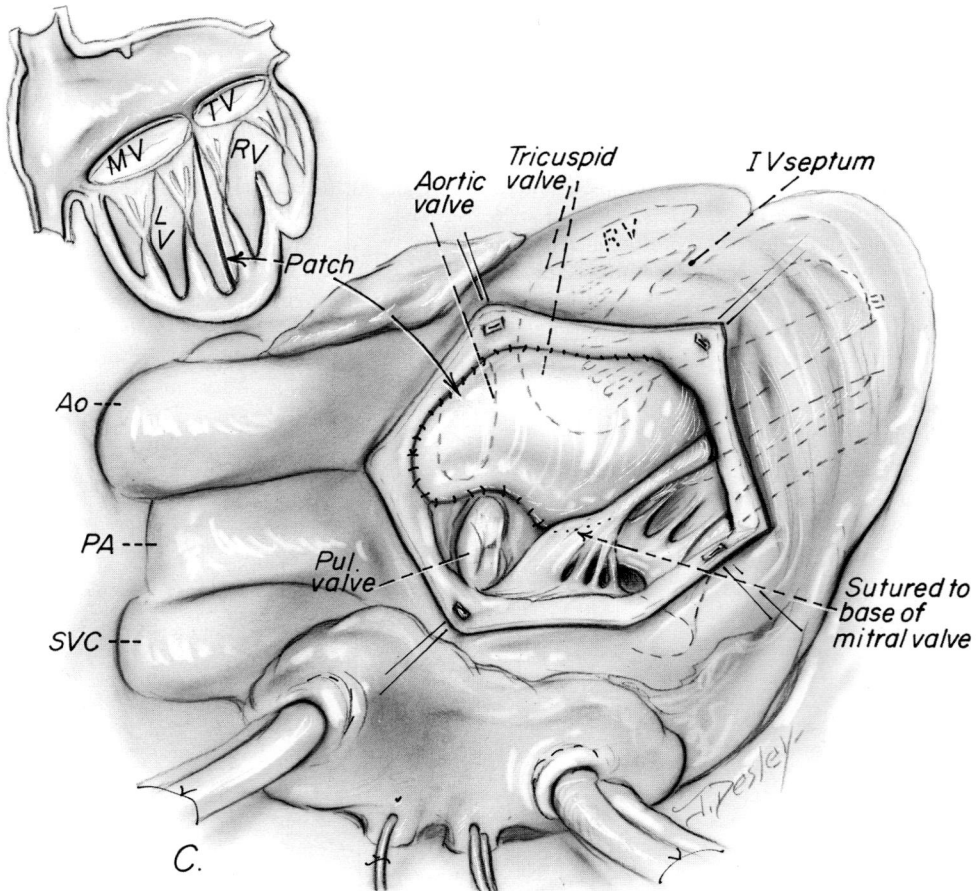

Figure 44-6 (continued)
(c) The repair is by placement of a septation patch leaving the left AV valve and its tension apparatus completely on the left side of the patch.

Ao, aorta; IV, interventricular; LV, left ventricle; MV, mitral valve; PA, pulmonary artery; Pul, pulmonary; RV, right ventricle; SVC, superior vena cava; TV, tricuspid valve.

Reproduced from Pacifico et al.,[P1] and the American Heart Association, Inc.

LATE RESULTS

Septation Operation

Survival

Late survival after the septation operation, even in selected groups, has to date been suboptimal. Thus, among a group of 16 patients with main chamber enlargement grade 3 or more undergoing septation without AV valve replacement or use of a valved extracardiac conduit, the 2-year survival (including hospital death) has been 57% (CL 41%–71%) (Fig. 44-7). Feldt and colleagues from the Mayo Clinic in a study of a somewhat similar group of 11 patients (age at operation 5–15 years, no previous surgery, and in something other than NYHA class IV), found 9 (82%, CL 62%–94%) were alive and reasonably well 3¼ years after coming to septation.[F2]

When the entire septation group (*n* = 36) is considered, the 5-year survival is 47% (CL 37%–57%) (UAB; Fig. 44-8). This is because of the much higher proportion of early deaths in the overall group. Thus, the survival at 6 months (including all 36 patients) was only 58% (CL 49%–66%), in contrast to 79% (67%–88%) in the group of 16.

Reoperation

Several patients also have required reoperation (other than pacemaker change) during the late postoperative period. Thus, of the group of 16 at UAB, freedom from death (early or late) or reoperation at 5 years was 57% (41%–72%) (Fig. 44-9), with 1 of the 5 events being secondary AV valve replacement (and thus 1 or 7%, CL 1%–21%, of 15 hospital survivors have undergone secondary AV valve replacement). In the group as a whole (*n* = 36) and in part related to the high early mortality, the freedom from death or reoperation at 5 years was only 34% (CL 24%–46%), with 5 of the 23 hospital survivors having reoperation as their event and 1 of those having undergone 2 reoperations. In 4 of these 5 patients (17%, CL 9%–29%, of the 23 hospital survivors), the

Table 44-6 Hospital mortality after septation operation for univentricular AV connection with double inlet ventricle, without AV or semilunar valve replacement and without a valved extracardiac conduit (UAB; 1967–Nov. 1, 1983). The one death among the n = 16 group was in a 1-month-old baby undergoing one-stage coarctation repair and septation.

Main Chamber Enlargement (Grade[a])		n	Hospital Deaths		
≤	<		No.	%	CL
	2	4	3	75%	37%–97%
2	--- 6	16	1	6%	1%–20%
Total		20	4	20%	10%–33%
P(Fisher)					.01

KEY: CL, 70% confidence limits.
[a]On the basis of 0–6.

Table 44-7 Hospital mortality after septation operation for univentricular AV connection with double inlet ventricle (UAB; 1967–Nov. 1, 1983).

Morphology[a]	n	Hospital Deaths		
		No.	%	CL
Ventricular L-loop, 2 ventricles with dominant and double inlet LV and rudimentary and leftward RV, VA discordant connection, L-malposition of the aorta	28	10	36%	25%–47%
Solitary ventricle[b]	5	2	40%	14%–71%
Ventricular L-loop, 2 ventricles with dominant and double inlet and double outlet RV, superior-inferior ventricles, D-malposition of the aorta[c]	1	1	100%	15%–100%
Ventricular D-loop, 2 ventricles with dominant and double inlet LV, concordant VA connection, more-or-less normally positioned great arteries	1		0%	0%–85%
Ventricular D-loop, 2 ventricles with dominant and double inlet and double outlet LV, more-or-less normally positioned great arteries[d]	1		0%	0%–85%
Total	36	13	36%	27%–46%

KEY: CL, 70% confidence limits; LV, left ventricle; RV, right ventricle; VA, ventriculoarterial.
[a]No patients with atrial situs inversus had septation; the cases are with or without pulmonary stenoses.
[b]One patient, who lived after operation in 1983, had ventricular L-loop, essentially AV and VA discordant connections with essentially 2 ventricles, an absent septum, right-sided LV morphology, and left-sided RV morphology; another patient, who also lived after operation in 1983, had ventricular D-loop, essentially AV and VA concordant connections with essentially 2 ventricles, an absent septum, right-sided RV morphology, and left-sided LV morphology; the other 3 patients had an indeterminate, primitive ventricle.
[c]Severely overriding right-sided left ventricular AV valve.
[d]Severely overriding right-sided right ventricular AV valve with right ventricular hypoplasia.

Table 44-8 Hospital mortality after septation operation for single ventricle (UAB; 1967–Nov. 1, 1983).

AV Valve Replacement	n	Hospital Deaths		
		No.	%	CL
No	29	10	34%	24%–46%
Yes	7	3	43%	20%–68%
Total	36	13	36%	27%–46%

KEY: AV, atrioventricular; CL, 70% confidence limits.

Table 44-9 Hospital mortality after septation operation for single ventricle without AV valve replacement (UAB; 1967–Nov. 1, 1983).

Valved Extracardiac Conduit to PA	n	Hospital Deaths		
		No.	%	CL
No	20	4	20%	10%–33%
Yes	9[a]	6	67%	44%–85%
Total	29	10	34%	24%–46%
P(Fisher)				.02

KEY: CL, 70% confidence limits; PA, pulmonary artery.
[a]One, who lived, in fact had an orthotopic pulmonary valve replacement.

Table 44-10 Hospital mortality and age distribution in septation for single ventricle with main chamber enlarged grade 3 or more, without concomitant AV valve replacement or use of a valved extracardiac conduit (UAB; 1967–Nov. 1, 1983).

Age (yr)		n	Hospital Deaths
≤	<		No.
	2	1[a]	1
2	--- 4	1	
4	--- 8	4	
8	--- 16	7	
16		3	
Total		16	1

[a]One-month-old infant, undergoing one-stage repair of coarctation and single ventricle.

Table 44-11 Hospital mortality after classic shunting operation for single ventricle done as the first operation (UAB; 1967–July, 1982).

Age (mo)		n	Hospital Deaths		
≤	<		No.	%	CL
	1	6	0	0%	0%–27%
1	--- 3	2	1[a]	50%	7%–93%
3	--- 6	1	0	0%	0%–86%
6	--- 12	4	0	0%	0%–38%
12	--- 24	5	0	0%	0%–32%
24	--- 48	6	0	0%	0%–27%
48		21	0	0%	0%–9%
Total		45	1	2%	0%–7%

KEY: CL, 70% confidence limits.
[a]Operation in 1969 at age 2.7 months.

Table 44-12 Hospital mortality after initial and subsequent operation at UAB for single ventricle (UAB; 1967–July, 1982; *n* = 116, 21 hospital deaths).

Operation (UAB Only)	n	Hospital Deaths			
		No.	%	CL	
Septation	27	11	41%	30%–53%	
Fontan-type procedure	8	2	25%	9%–50%	
Systemic-pulmonary artery shunting	73	6	8%	5%–13%	
Blalock-Taussig	41	1	2%	0.3%–8%	1/55
Gore-Tex interposition	14	0	0%	0%–13%	(2%; CL 0.2%–6%)
Other shunts	18	5	28%	16%–43%	
Pulmonary artery banding	4	0	28%	16%–43%	
Atrial septectomy	9	0		9%–38%	
Repair only of associated cardiac anomaly	7	2	29%	10%–55%	
Combined closed palliative procedures	9	0	0%	0%–19%	
Others	9	2	20%	7%–41%	
Total	147	23	16%	12%–19%	

KEY: CL, 70% confidence limits.

NOTE: The nine other procedures included seven exploratory cardiotomies, including or not pulmonary valvotomy or a valved extracardiac conduit (seven cases, one hospital death), and two revision of previous procedures (one hospital death).

reoperation included AV valve replacement or re-replacement (for thrombosis). In this regard, it is interesting to recall that in an experimental study, Seki and colleagues found that ventricular septal excision and insertion of a prosthetic septum plus tricuspid valve repair resulted in a high incidence of mitral incompetence.[S12]

Residual Shunting
Residual shunting has occurred in some cases,[F2] but in the current era double indicator-dilution dye curves (see Chapter 5) 24 hours after operation (UAB) have routinely demonstrated no residual shunting. Thus, secure repairs are possible.

Functional Status
The functional status of patients surviving septation is generally good, most patients being in NYHA class I or II (Table 44-14). This might be expected from the experimental study

Table 44-13 Hospital mortality after isolated or combined atrial septectomy for single ventricle (1967–July 1982).

Category	n	With or Without Previous Operation UAB or Elsewhere		
		Hospital Deaths		
		No.	%	
Isolated atrial septectomy	9	0	0%	
Atrial septectomy plus PA band	7	0	0%	
Atrial septectomy plus SP shunt	1	0	0%	
Total	17	0	0%	CL 0%–11%

KEY: CL, 70% confidence limits; PA, pulmonary artery; SP, systemic-pulmonary.

NOTE: Eleven of the 17 patients had coexisting left AV valve atresia; 5 others had coexisting severe left AV valve narrowing (hypoplasia); 1 of the 17 had only left atrial hypertension because of large pulmonary blood flow.

by Seki, Tsakiris, and McGoon, which showed no demonstrable detrimental hemodynamic effect of replacing the dog's ventricular septum (and tricuspid valve) with prostheses.[S4] This possibility of good functional status after septation is also supported by a detailed hemodynamic study of two patients late after septation made by Shimazaki and colleagues[S6]; in one patient, who was 8 years postseptation, both right and left ventricular ejection fractions were normal and the hemodynamic response to exercise was normal.

Fontan-Type Procedure

Survival
Death after hospital dismissal is uncommon after this operation, and actuarial late survival of hospital survivors is 92% (CL 85%–96%). This corresponds closely to the longer follow-up in a larger series of patients by Fontan and colleagues.[F5] When hospital deaths are included, the actuarial survival at 5 years has been 71% (CL 65%–77%; Fig. 44-10), and with current techniques this is anticipated to be about 90%. (See "Late Results" in Chapter 26 for further details.) Sixty-five percent of patients are alive and free of reoperation at 3½ years after the procedure (Fig. 44-11).

Functional Status
The functional status is good in most patients. A few are participating in strenuous athletic games, and 93% of survivors are in NYHA class I or II. However, abnormalities of ventricular systolic function are often evident at rest and on exercise.[D5] (See "Late Results" in Chapter 26 for further details.)

Pulmonary Artery Banding

Although death in hospital or during intermediate-term follow-up is infrequent after pulmonary artery banding, the late results are marred by the not infrequent development, at

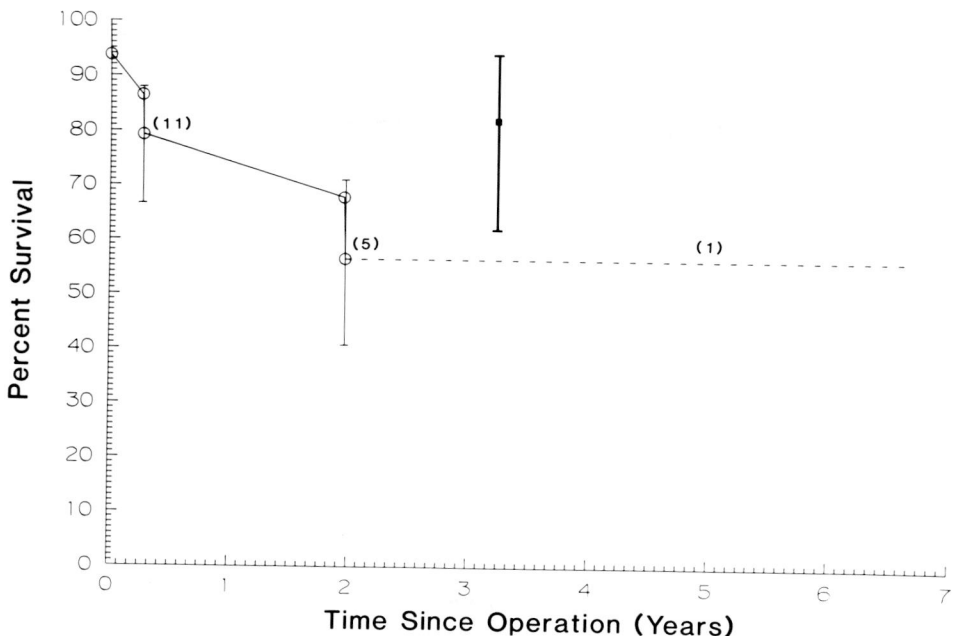

Figure 44-7 Actuarial survival, including hospital deaths, with its 70% confidence limits, after septation operation for single ventricle, without AV valve replacement and without valved extracardiac conduit, in patients with main chamber enlargement greater than grade II (see Table 43-6) (UAB; 1967–Oct. 1983; n = 16). The solid circle represents similar information from the Mayo Clinic experience (n = 11).[F2]

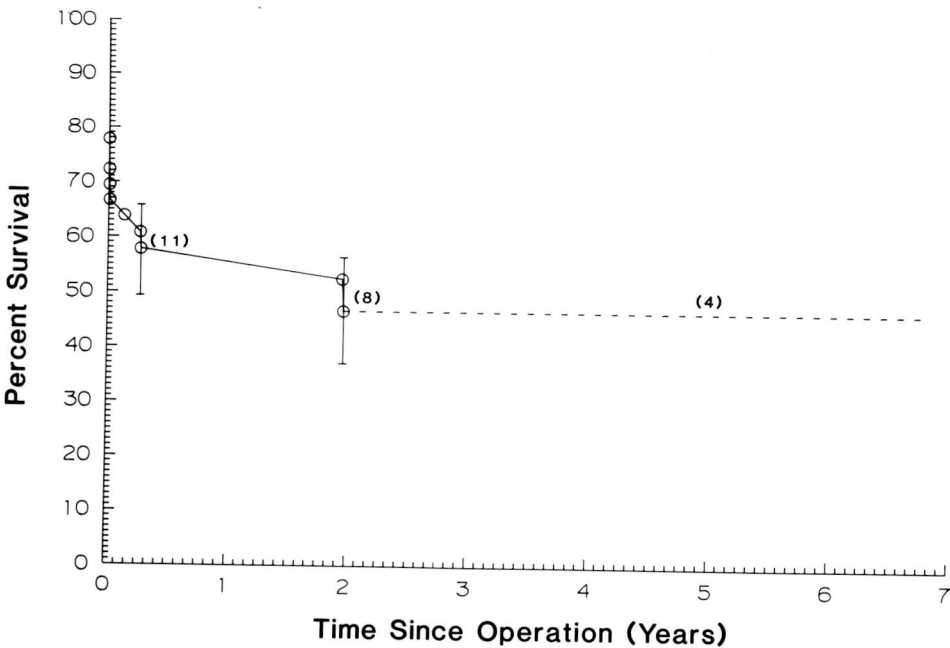

Figure 44-8 Actuarial survival, including hospital deaths, after all septation operations for single ventricle (UAB; 1967–Nov. 1983; n = 36).

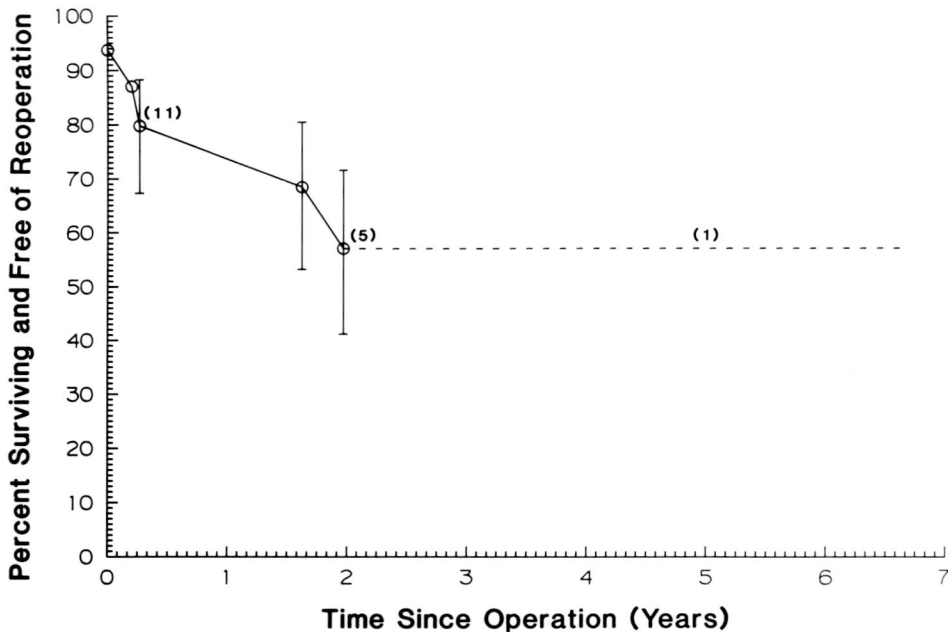

Figure 44-9 Actuarial freedom from death, including hospital deaths, or reoperation, after septation operation without AV valve replacement and without valved extracardiac conduit, in patients with main chamber enlargement greater than grade 2 (see Table 44-6) (UAB; 1967–Oct. 1983; n = 16).

least in patients with ventricular L-loop, double inlet left ventricular main chamber, and ventriculoarterial discordance of severe and progressive subaortic stenosis due partly to narrowing of the VSD.[F3,S1] This is accompanied by massive hypertrophy of the wall of the left ventricular main chamber and decrease in its end-diastole volume. Although ingenious surgical procedures have been devised to overcome this problem, they are not often successful. Penkoske and colleagues have reported 10 deaths (59%, CL 43%–73%) among 17 patients after these complex procedures.[P2]

Shunting Procedures

Including all in-hospital and late deaths, the actuarial 5-year survival following a classic shunting procedure is 85% (Fig. 44-12). Slightly less favorable results have been reported by

Table 44-14 Functional status of surviving patients (n = 36) after the septation operation. (Date of inquiry Nov. 1, 1983.)

NYHA Class	n	% of Traced Survivors[a]		
		%	CL	
I	10	62%	46%–77%	100%
II	6	38%	23%–54%	CL 89%–100%
III	0			
IV	0			
Total	16	100%		

KEY: CL, 70% confidence limits.

[a]The functional status is not known in three additional living patients.

Moodie and colleagues.[M8] Taussig in 1976 provided up to 27 years of follow-up in patients with single ventricle treated by a Blalock-Taussig shunt; among her group, the 10-year survival of hospital survivors was only 72%,[T3] presumably because the patients were older at the time the shunting procedure was performed. Nonetheless, the 20-year-survival rate was 50% (Fig. 44-13).

Atrial Septectomy

Actuarial 10-year survival was 76% after atrial septectomy with or without an associated procedure.

Summary

Including all surgical procedures and hospital as well as late deaths, the actuarial 10-year survival is 66% (Fig. 44-14), and 90% of traced survivors whose statuses are known are in NYHA class I or II. Similarly encouraging results, although with shorter follow-up, have been reported by Villani and colleagues.[V4] Thus, surgical efforts do improve both life expectancy and functional status of patients with most types of single ventricle.

INDICATIONS FOR OPERATION

In view of the reasonably good intermediate term (10-year) results of surgical treatment for single ventricle and the high probability that these are better than the natural history, a univentricular AV connection is not an indication to give up aggressive measures to improve and prolong the patient's

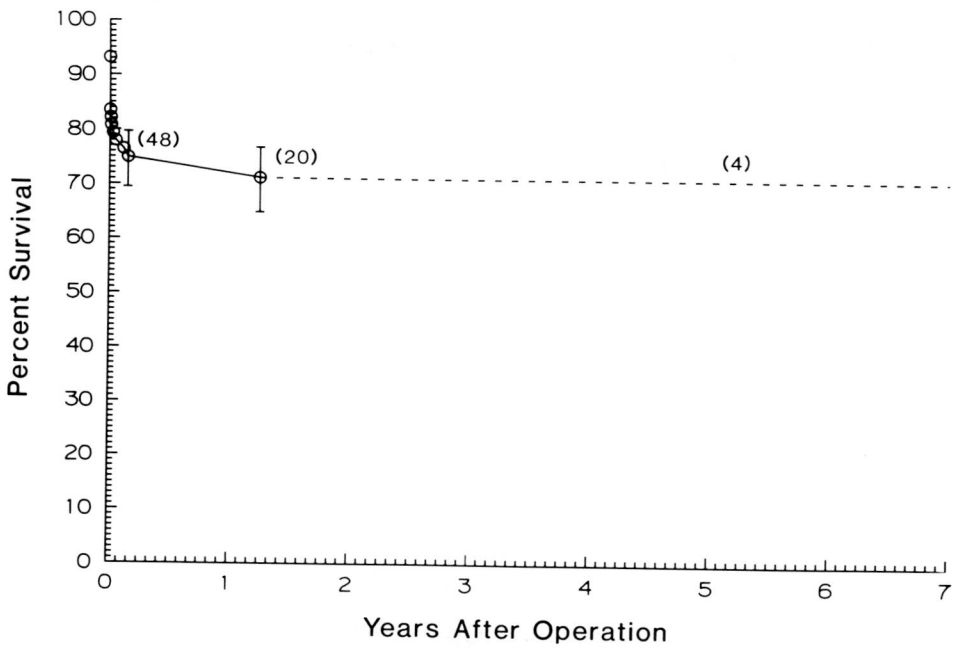

Figure 44-10 Actuarial survival, including hospital deaths, after Fontan-type repair for congenital heart disease (UAB; 1967–Nov. 1, 1983; *n* = 73).
Reproduced with permission from Stefanelli et al.[S14]

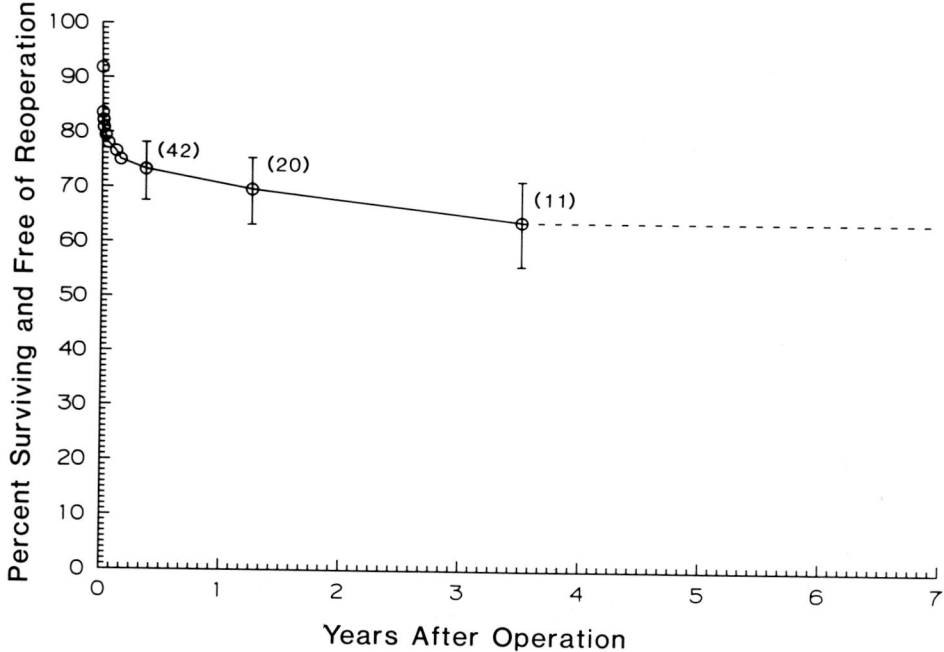

Figure 44-11 Actuarial freedom from death, including hospital death, and reoperation after Fontan-type procedure for congenital heart disease (UAB; 1967–Nov. 1, 1983; *n* = 73).

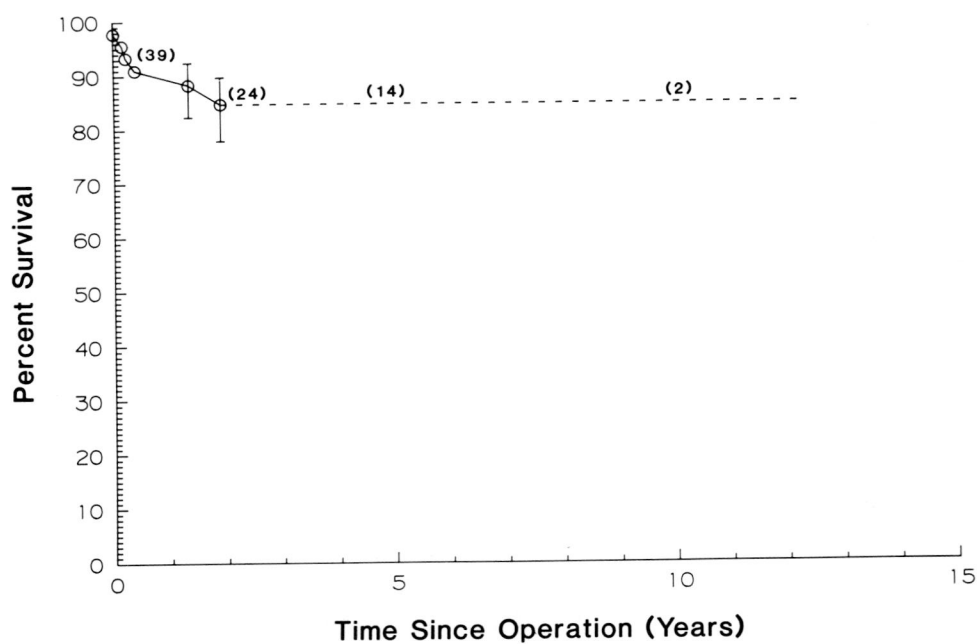

Figure 44-12 Actuarial survival, including hospital deaths, after a classical shunting operation, done as the primary operation at UAB for single ventricle (UAB; 1967–July 1982; n = 45).
Reproduced with permission from Stefanelli et al.[S14]

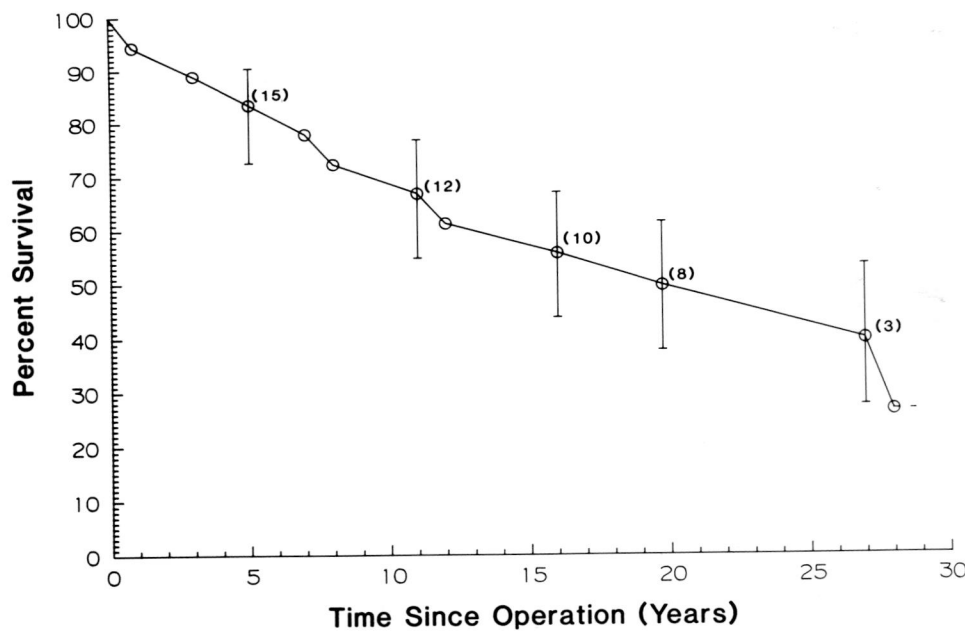

Figure 44-13 Actuarial survival of hospital survivors of the Blalock-Taussig shunt in patients with single ventricle.
Calculated from the data of Taussig.[T3]

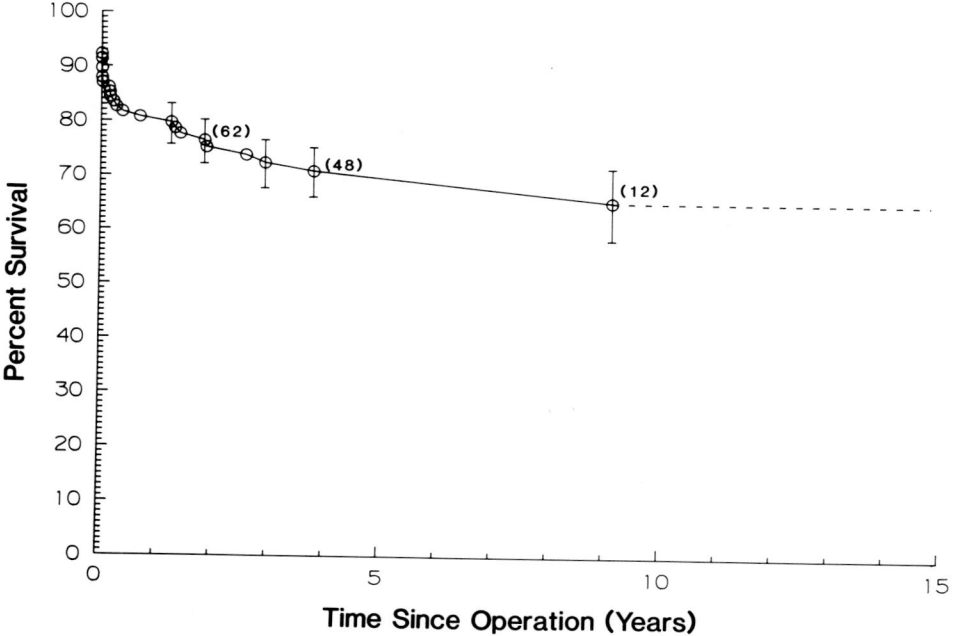

Figure 44-14 Actuarial survival, including hospital deaths, after surgical procedures of any kind at UAB for single ventricle (UAB; 1967–July 1982; *n* = 116).
Reproduced with permission from Stefanelli et al.[S14]

life. Either ventricular septation or a Fontan-type procedure are possible, and there is no certainty that, with current techniques, the overall intermediate or long-term results of one are superior to those of the other. However, in view of the increased early risks when a valved extracardiac conduit is added to septation and the increased early and late risks when concomitant AV valve replacement is done, septation should usually not be chosen when these additional procedures are required. The Fontan-type procedure should not be chosen when pulmonary vascular resistance is elevated, when the right and left pulmonary arteries are restrictive (D_{RPA} + D_{LPA} < 1.6, see Chapter 23, Fig. 23-58), or when main chamber systolic function is poor. In view of the potential for cardiac transplantation in the future, all operative procedures must be planned to avoid both pulmonary vascular disease and any pulmonary artery bifurcation or right or left pulmonary arterial problems.

The identification of this form of congenital heart disease and its detailed diagnosis should be made as early in life as possible, so that early planning can be accomplished for the later repair.

If in infancy pulmonary blood flow is so small, because of pulmonary stenosis or atresia, that arterial desaturation and cyanosis are prominent, a classic shunting procedure is indicated. (See Chapter 23 for details of the type to be chosen.) A commitment is made to ultimate reconstruction by the Fontan-type procedure, which probably can be done as early as 6 months of age but which is usually deferred until about 2–4 years of age if the clinical condition allows.

If in early infancy pulmonary blood flow is large, as it usually is in single ventricle without pulmonary stenoses or atresia, management is more complex and difficult because

the best treatment has not yet been identified. This is particularly true in the common circumstance of atrial situs solitus, ventricular L-loop, double inlet left ventricular main chamber and discordant ventriculoarterial connection as most examples of this subset have the morphologic potential for later septation.[G4] Pulmonary artery banding in this setting is disadvantageous because it frequently results in progressive narrowing of the VSD (and thus subaortic stenoses) plus main chamber wall thickening, volume reduction, and histologic changes of chronic ischemia. These are all disadvantageous to a final repair by septation or a Fontan-type repair.[B6] Thus, patients in this situation should be managed medically if possible and septation done electively at about 2 years of age or as young as 6 months of age if congestive heart failure is intractable or pulmonary vascular resistance is rising rapidly. If in the first few months of life the heart failure becomes life threatening, pulmonary artery banding must be done, but septation or a Fontan-type repair and band removal should then be carried out at 6–12 months of age. This same plan is applicable to all types of single ventricle with a double inlet main chamber and an anteriorly placed outlet chamber giving rise to a great artery. When subaortic stenosis has already developed in infancy, a procedure similar to the first stage of the operation for hypoplastic left heart may be advised (see Chapter 35, "First Stage Palliative Procedure").[J1] In this procedure the proximal pulmonary artery is anastomosed to the ascending aorta, and a controlled pulmonary blood flow is established. Later, a Fontan-type repair is performed.

When the single ventricle is without pulmonary stenosis and is of the indeterminate (primitive) type or when there is a common or single AV valve, the Fontan-type procedure is the only definitive option and pulmonary artery banding should be done in the first few months of life and the Fontan-type procedure at 3–5 years of age or as young as 6 months of age if necessary. (This same protocol can be followed routinely if septation is never used.)

The pulmonary artery banding should probably be done through a median sternotomy incision, using a narrow band anchored proximally so as to preserve the distal segment of pulmonary trunk for later use in the Fontan-type procedure. The band should result in a pulmonary artery peak pressure about 50% of main chamber pressure. The pericardium should be carefully closed without drainage.

In any event, if the atrial septum is intact or has only a restrictive opening and there is left-sided AV valve atresia or severe stenoses (atrial situs solitus), an atrial septectomy by the Blalock-Hanlon technique is indicated (see Chapter 39).

When important AV valve incompetence is present, ventricular septation should usually not be done; instead, the incompetent AV valve should be closed off as a part of a planned Fontan-type procedure if circumstances are appropriate for this procedure. When the incompetent AV valve is a single one, such as in the case of a common AV valve or in tricuspid atresia, the decision is particularly difficult. Probably valve repair or replacement is indicated, along with the Fontan-type procedure, but the risks and imponderables are greater than usual.

SPECIAL SITUATIONS AND CONTROVERSIES

Straddling and Overriding Atrioventricular Valves

Although straddling AV valves may complicate single ventricle (in which case all of one AV valve and at least half the straddling and overriding valve open into or override onto the same ventricle), they may also coexist with a VSD in hearts with concordant or discordant AV connections.[L4,T2]

Rastelli and colleagues called attention to straddling AV valves in 1968.[R5] Pacifico and colleagues and Danielson and colleagues described the management of at least some cases by a septation procedure within the larger of the two ventricular chambers.[P1,D2]

An AV valve may be said to *straddle* when its tension apparatus is attached to both sides of the ventricular septum. An AV valve *overrides* when its anulus in part overlies or opens into the ventricle opposite to the one over which the valve normally lies. The ventricular chamber into which the overriding AV valve normally empties is often somewhat smaller than usual. When the straddling valve is morphologically a tricuspid one, it extends across a posteriorly placed VSD in a septum that does not extend to the crux, whether it

is in a heart with ventricular D-loop (see Chapter 20) or ventricular L-loop; when the straddling valve is morphologically a mitral valve, it straddles an anteriorly placed VSD (as in the Taussig-Bing heart) in a septum that does extend to the crux cordis.[M6]

An unusual position of the AV node and bundle of His coexists with VSD and straddling tricuspid valve, which is related to the fact that the inlet septum does not extend to the crux cordis. The AV node is thus lateral to (away from) the atrial septum. When the right AV valve override is severe, the AV node is next to the tricuspid valve anulus at about the 3 o'clock position as seen by the surgeon through a right atriotomy incision, a position dictated by the position of the inlet septum. When the override is less severe, the node is at the 5 o'clock or 6 o'clock position.[M6] When the VSD is repaired, this and the corresponding position of the bundle of His must be borne in mind during suture placement, but avoidance of heart block may be difficult.

The diagnosis of straddling and overriding AV valves can be made preoperatively with considerable accuracy by echocardiography and by angiocardiography.[L3,S11] The details need to be confirmed at operation by the surgeon.

The surgical treatment of VSD complicated by straddling or overriding AV valves is described under "Technique of Operation."

Ventricular Approach for Septation

A ventricular approach to septation was used originally and is still used by some. Whereas this approach may occasionally be indicated, the right atrial approach and placement of sutures entirely from within the ventricular cavity are preferred. One important reason is that with the atrial approach, the otherwise frequent damage to major coronary arterial branches is avoided.[K1] If a ventricular approach is used, the fish-mouth incision is recommended.[M7]

Staged Septation

Ebert has reported a two-stage approach to septation in a selected subset of single ventricle with a presumably so-called common ventricle (see "Morphology"). At the first stage, performed in infancy, a partially septating patch is placed at the apex of the ventricle and a second one at the superior portion between the AV valves.[E5] Only widely spaced interrupted sutures are used. A pulmonary artery band is placed. In Ebert's cases, septation was completed with a third patch 6 to 18 months later. The other patches were by then completely sealed into position. The band was removed. All patients survived, all in sinus rhythm.

REFERENCES

A

1. Anderson RH, Macartney FJ, Tynan M, Becker AE, Freedom RM, Godman MJ, Hunter S, Quero-Jimenez M, Rigby ML, Shinebourne EA, Sutherland G, Smallhorn JG, Soto B, Thiene G, Wilkinson JL, Wilcox BL, Zuberbuhler JR: Univentricular Atrioventricular Connection: Single ventricle trap unsprung. *Pediatr Cardiol* 4:273, 1983.

2. Anderson RH, Lenox CC, Zuberbuhler JR, Ho SY, Smith A, Wilkinson JL: Double-inlet left ventricle with rudimentary right ventricle and ventriculoarterial concordance. *Am J Cardiol* 52:573, 1983.

3. Anderson RA: Weasel words in paediatric cardiology; Single ventricle. *Intern J Cardiol* 2:425, 1983.

4. Arai T, Sakakibara S, Ando M, Takao A: Intracardiac repair for single or common ventricle, creation of a straight artificial septum. *Singapore Med J* 14:187, 1973.

5. Anderson RH, Arnold R, Thapar MK, Jones RS, Hamilton DI: Cardiac specialized tissues in hearts with an apparently single ventricular chamber (double inlet left ventricle). *Am J Cardiol* 33:95, 1974.

6. Anderson RH, Tynan M, Freedom RM, Quero-Jimenez M, Macartney FJ, Shinebourne EA, Wilkinson JL, Becker AE: Ventricular morphology in the univentricular heart. *Herz* 4:184, 1979.

7. Ashraf H, Cotroneo J, Han S, Dhar N, Pieroni D, Subramanian S: Right atrial to pulmonary artery diversion for double inlet ventricle. *JACC* 5:478, 1985 (abstr).

B

1. Beardshaw JA, Gibson DG, Peason MC, Upton MT, Anderson RH: Echocardiographic diagnosis of primitive ventricle with two atrioventricular valves. *Br Heart J* 39:266, 1977.

2. Becker AE, Wilkinson JL, Anderson RH: Atrioventricular conduction tissues in univentricular hearts of left ventricular type. *Herz* 4:166, 1979.

3. Bharati S, Lev M: The course of the conduction system in single ventricle with inverted (L-) loop and inverted (L-) transposition. *Circulation* 51:723, 1975.

4. Blalock A, Taussig HB: The surgical treatment of malformations of the heart in which there is pulmonary stenosis or pulmonary atresia. *JAMA* 128:189, 1945.

5. Bharati S, Lev M, Kirklin JW: *Cardiac Surgery and the Conduction System.* New York: John Wiley and Sons, 1983.

6. Barber G, Hagler DJ, Edwards WD, Puga FJ, Danielson GK, McGoon DC, Driscoll DJ: Surgical repair of univentricular heart (double inlet left ventricle) with obstructed anterior subaortic outlet chamber. *JACC* 4:771, 1984.

C

1. Chesler E, Joffe HS, Beck W, Shrire V: Echocardiography in the diagnosis of congenital heart disease. *Pediatr Clin North Am* 18:1163, 1971.

D

1. Doty DB, Schieken RM, Lauer RM: Septation of the univentricular heart; Transatrial approach. *J Thorac Cardiovasc Surg* 78:423, 1979.

2. Danielson GK, Tabary IF, Fulton RE, Hagler DJ, Ritter DG:

Successful repair of straddling atrioventricular valve by technique used for septation of univentricular heart. *Ann Thorac Surg* 28:554, 1979.

3. Doty DB, Marvin WJ Jr, Lauer RM: Single ventricle with aortic outflow obstruction. *J Thorac Cardiovasc Surg* 81:636, 1981.

4. diDonato R, Becker AE, Nijveld A, Lam J, Bulterijs A, Squitiera C, Marcelletti C: Ventricular exclusion during Fontan operation: An evolving technique. *Ann Thorac Surg* 39:283, 1985.

5. Del Torso S, Kelly MJ, Kalff V, Venables AW: Radionuclide assessment of ventricular contraction at rest and during exercise following the Fontan procedure for either tricuspid atresia or single ventricle. *Am J Cardiol* 55:1127, 1985.

E

1. Elliott LP, Anderson RC, Edwards JE: The common cardiac ventricle with transposition of the great vessels. *Br Heart J* 26:289, 1964.

2. Edie RN, Ellis K, Gersony WM, Krongrad E, Bowman FO, Malm JR: Surgical repair of single ventricle. *J Thorac Cardiovasc Surg* 66:350, 1973.

3. Essed CE, Ho SY, Hunter S, Anderson RH: Atrioventricular conduction system in univentricular heart of right ventricular type with right-sided rudimentary chamber. *Thorax* 35:123, 1980.

4. Essed CE, Ho SY, Shinebourne EA, Joseph MC, Anderson RH: Further observations on conduction tissues in univentricular hearts—surgical implications. *Eur Heart J* 2:87, 1981.

5. Ebert PA: Staged partitioning of single ventricle. *J Thorac Cardiovasc Surg* 88:908, 1984.

F

1. Felner JM, Brewer DB, Franch RH: Echocardiographic manifestations of single ventricle. *Am J Cardiol* 38:80, 1976.

2. Feldt RH, Mair DD, Danielson GK, Wallace RB, McGoon DC: Current status of the septation procedure for univentricular heart. *J Thorac Cardiovasc Surg* 82:93, 1981.

3. Freedom RM, Sondheimer H, Dische R, Rowe RD: Development of "subaortic stenosis" after pulmonary arterial banding for common ventricle. *Am J Cardiol* 39:78, 1977.

4. Fontan F, Baudet E: Surgical repair of tricuspid atresia. *Thorax* 26:240, 1971.

5. Fontan F, Deville C, Quaegebeur J, Ottenkamp J, Sourdille N, Choussat A, Brom GA: Repair of tricuspid atresia in 100 patients. *J Thorac Cardiovasc Surg* 85:647, 1983.

G

1. Gibson DG, Traill TA, Brown DJ: Abnormal ventricular function in patients with univentricular heart. *Herz* 4:226, 1979.

2. Gale AW, Danielson GK, McGoon DC, Mair DD: Modified Fontan operation for univentricular heart and complicated congenital lesions. *J Thorac Cardiovasc Surg* 78:831, 1979.

3. Gale AW, Danielson GK, McGoon DC, Wallace RB, Mair DD: Fontan procedure for tricuspid atresia. *Circulation* 62:91, 1980.

4. Girod DA, Lima RC, Anderson RH, Ho SY, Rigby ML, Quaegebeur JM: Double-inlet ventricle: Morphologic analysis and surgical implications in 32 cases. *J Thorac Cardiovasc Surg* 88:590, 1984.

H

1. Holmes AF: Case of malformation of the heart. *Trans Med Chir Soc Edinb* 1:252, 1824.

I

1. Ionescu MI, Macartney FJ, Wooler GH: Intracardiac repair of single ventricle with pulmonary stenosis. *J Thorac Cardiovasc Surg* 65:603, 1973.

J

1. Jonas RA, Castaneda AR, Lang P: Single ventricle (single- or double-inlet) complicated by subaortic stenosis: surgical options in infancy. *Ann Thorac Surg* 39:362, 1985.

K

1. Keeton BR, Lie JT, McGoon DC, Danielson GK, Ritter DG, Wallace RB: Anatomy of coronary arteries in univentricular hearts and its surgical implications. *Am J Cardiol* 43:569, 1979.

2. Keeton BR, Macartney FJ, Hunter S, Mortera C, Rees P, Shinebourne EA, Tynan M, Wilkinson JL, Anderson RH: Univentricular heart of right ventricular type with double or common inlet. *Circulation* 59:403, 1979.

3. Kitamura S, Kawashima Y, Shimazaki Y, Mori T, Nakano S, Beppu S, Kozuka T: Characteristics of ventricular function in single ventricle. *Circulation* 60:849, 1979.

4. Kreutzer G, Galindez E, Bono H, de Palma C, Laura JP: An operation for the correction of Tricuspid Atresia. *J Thorac Cardiovasc Surg* 66:613, 1973.

5. Kreutzer G, Schlichter A, Laura JP, Suarez JC, Vargas JF: Univentricular heart with low pulmonary vascular resistances: septation vs. atriopulmonary anastomosis. *Arq Bras Cardiol* 37:301, 1981.

6. Kreutzer GO, Vargas FJ, Schlichter AJ, Laura JP, Suarez JC, Coronel AR, Kreutzer EA: Atriopulmonary anastomosis. *J Thorac Cardiovasc Surg* 83:427, 1982.

L

1. Lev M: Pathologic diagnosis of positional variations in cardiac chambers in congenital heart disease. *Lab Invest* 3:71, 1954.

2. Lev M, Liberthson RR, Kirkpatrick JR, Eckner EAO, Arcilla RA: Single (primitive) ventricle. *Circulation* 39:577, 1969.

3. LaCorte MA, Fellows KE, Williams RG: Overriding tricuspid valve: echocardiographic and angiocardiographic features. *Am J Cardiol* 37:911, 1976.

4. Liberthson RR, Paul MH, Muster AJ, Arcilla RA, Eckner FAO, Lev M: Straddling and displaced atrioventricular orifices and valves with primitive ventricles. *Circulation* 43:213, 1971.

M

1. Mann JD: Cor triloculare biatriatum. *Br Med J* 1:614, 1907.

2. Muller WH Jr, Damman JF Jr: Treatment of certain congenital malformations of the heart by the creation of pulmonic stenosis to reduce pulmonary hypertension and excessive pulmonary blood flow (a preliminary report). *Surg Gynecol Obstet* 95:213, 1952.

3. Marcelletti C, Mazzera E, Olthof H, Sebel PS, Duren DR, Losekoot TG, Becker AE: Fontan's operation: an expanded horizon. *J Thorac Cardiovasc Surg* 80:764, 1980.

4. Macartney FJ, Partridge JB, Scott O, Deverall PB: Common or single ventricle. An angiocardiographic and hemodynamic study of 42 patients. *Circulation* 53:543, 1976.

5. McGoon DC, Danielson GK, Ritter DG, Wallace RB, Maloney JD, Marcelletti C: Correction of the univentricular heart having two atrioventricular valves. *J Thorac Cardiovasc Surg* 74:218, 1977.

6. Mico S, Ho SY, Macartney FJ, Wilkinson JL, Becker AE, Wenink ACG, Groot ACG, Anderson RH: Straddling and overriding atrioventricular valves: Morphology and classification. *Am J Cardiol* 44:1122, 1979.

7. McKay R, Pacifico AD, Blackstone EH, Kirklin JW, Bargeron LM Jr: Septation of the univentricular heart with left anterior subaortic outlet chamber. *J Thorac Cardiovasc Surg* 84:77, 1982.

8. Moodie DS, Ritter DG, Tajik AH, McGoon DC, Danielson GK, O'Fallon WM: Long-term follow-up after palliative operation for univentricular heart. *Am J Cardiol* 53:1648, 1984.

9. Moodie DS, Ritter DG, Tajik AJ, O'Fallon WM: Long-term follow-up in the unoperated univentricular heart. *Am J Cardiol* 53:1124, 1984.

10. Molina JE, Wang Y, Lucas R, Moller J: The technique of the Fontan procedure with posterior right atrium-pulmonary artery connection. *Ann Thorac Surg* 39:371, 1985.

P

1. Pacifico AD, Soto B, Bargeron LM Jr: Surgical treatment of straddling tricuspid valves. *Circulation* 60:655, 1979.

2. Penkoske PA, Freedom RM, Williams WG, Trusler GA, Rowe RD: Surgical palliation of subaortic stenosis in the univentricular heart. *J Thorac Cardiovasc Surg* 87:767, 1984.

R

1. Rokitansky CF von: *Die Defecte der Scheidewande des Herzens*. Vienna: Wilhelm Braumuller, 1875, pp 27–29.

2. Rowlatt WF: Coronary artery distribution in complete transposition. *JAMA* 179:269, 1972.

3. Rahimtoola SH, Ongley DA, Swan HJC: The hemodynamics of common (or single) ventricle. *Circulation* 34:14, 1966.

4. Restivo A, Ho SY, Anderson RH, Cameron H, Wilkinson JL: Absent left atrioventricular connection with right atrium connected to morphologically left ventricular chamber, rudimentary right ventricular chamber, and ventriculoarterial discordance. Problem of mitral versus tricuspid atresia. *Br Heart J* 48:240, 1982.

5. Rastelli GC, Ongley PA, Titus JL: Ventricular septal defect of atrioventricular canal type with straddling right atrioventricular valve and mitral valve deformity. *Circulation* 37:816, 1968.

S

1. Somerville J, Becu L, Ross D: Common ventricle with acquired subaortic obstruction. *Am J Cardiol* 34:206, 1974.

2. Saalouke MG, Perry LW, Okoroma EO, Shapiro SR, Scott LP: Primitive ventricle with normally related great vessels and stenotic subpulmonary outlet chamber. Angiographic differentiation from tetralogy of Fallot. *Br Heart J* 40:49, 1978.

3. Sakakibara S, Tominaga S, Imai Y, Uehara K, Matsumuro M: Successful total correction of common ventricle. *Chest* 61:192, 1972.

4. Seki C, Tsakiris A, McGoon DC: The effect of a prosthetic ventricular septum on canine cardiac function. *Surgery* 71:241, 1972.

5. Seki C, McGoon DC: Surgical techniques for replacement of the interventricular septum. *J Thorac Cardiovasc Surg* 6:919, 1971.

6. Shimazaki Y, Kawashima Y, Mori T, Matsuda H, Kitamura S, Yokota K: Ventricular function of single ventricle after ventricular septation. *Circulation* 61:653, 1980.

7. Shimazaki Y, Kawashima Y, Mori T, Kitamura S, Matsuda H, Yokota K: Ventricular volume characteristics of single ventricle before corrective surgery. *Am J Cardiol* 45:806, 1980.

8. Shinebourne EA, Lau K, Calcaterra G, Anderson RH: Univentricular heart of right ventricular type: Clinical, angiographic and electrocardiographic features. *Am J Cardiol* 46:439, 1980.

9. Soto B, Bertranou EG, Bream PR, Souza J Jr, Bargeron LM Jr: Angiographic study of univentricular heart of right ventricular type. *Circulation* 60:1325, 1979.

10. Shore D, Jones O, Rigby ML, Anderson RH, Lincoln C: Atresia of left atrioventricular connection. *Br Heart J* 47:35, 1982.

11. Seward JB, Tajik AJ, Ritter DG: Echocardiographic features of straddling tricuspid valve. *Mayo Clin Proc* 50:427, 1975.

12. Seki S, Tsakiris AG, Mair DD, McGoon DC: Radical correction of single ventricle in experimental model: Experimental and clinical results. *Ann Surg* 6:748, 1972.

13. Soto B, Pacifico AD, Di Sciascio G: Univentricular Heart: An Angiographic Study. *Am J Cardiol* 49:787, 1982.

14. Stefanelli G, Kirklin JW, Naftel DC, Blackstone EH, Pacifico AD, Kirklin JK, Soto B, Bargeron LM Jr: Early and intermediate-term (10-year) results of surgery for univentricular atrioventricular connection ("single ventricle"). *Am J Cardiol* 54:811, 1984.

T

1. Taussig HB: A single ventricle with a diminutive outlet chamber. *J Tech Meth* 19:120, 1939.

2. Tandon R, Becker AE, Moller JH, Edwards JE: Double inlet left ventricle. Straddling tricuspid valve. *Br Heart J* 36:747, 1974.

3. Taussig HB: Long-time observations on the Blalock-Taussig operation IX. Single ventricle (with apex to the left). *Johns Hopkins Med J* 139:69, 1976.

4. Tabry IF, McGoon DC, Danielson GK, Wallace RB, Tajik AJ, Seward JB: Surgical management of straddling atrioventricular valve. *J Thorac Cardiovasc Surg* 77:191, 1979.

V

1. Van Praagh R, Ongley PA, Swam HJC: Anatomic types of single or common ventricle in man. Morphologic and geometric aspects of 60 necropsied cases. *Am J Cardiol* 13:367, 1964.

2. Van Praagh R, David I, Gordon D, Wright GB, Van Praagh S: Ventricular diagnosis and designation, in MJ Godman (ed): *Paediatric Cardiology*. Edinburgh: Churchill Livingstone, 1982, vol 4, pp 153–181.

3. Van Praagh R, Plet JA, Van Praagh S: Single ventricle. *Herz* 4:113, 1979.

4. Villani M, Crupi G, Locatelli G, Tiraboschi R, Vanini V, Parenzan L: Experience in palliative treatment of univentricular heart including tricuspid atresia. *Herz* 4:256, 1979.

W

1. Wenink ACG: The conduction tissues in primitive ventricle with outlet chamber: two different possibilities. *J Thorac Cardiovasc Surg* 75:747, 1978.

2. Wilkinson JL, Anderson RH, Arnold R, Hamilton DI, Smith A: The conducting tissues in primitive ventricular hearts without an outlet chamber. *Circulation* 53:930, 1976.

3. Wilkinson JL, Dickinson D, Smith A, Anderson RH: Conducting tissues in univentricular heart of right ventricular type with double or common inlet. *J Thorac Cardiovasc Surg* 77:691, 1979.

Y

1. Yacoub MH, Radley-Smith R: Use of a valved conduit from right atrium to pulmonary artery for "correction" of single ventricle. *Circulation* 54(suppl III):III-63, 1976.

45

ANATOMICALLY CORRECTED MALPOSITION OF THE GREAT ARTERIES

DEFINITION

In this text, anatomically corrected malposition is considered an anomaly in the position of the great arteries and not in cardiac connections. Thus, there is atrioventricular (AV) and ventriculoarterial concordant connection, as in the normal heart, but the aortic origin lies to the left and usually anterior to the pulmonary artery origin when there is situs solitus (SDL) and to the right of the pulmonary origin when there is situs inversus (ILD). The circulatory pathways remain in series.

HISTORICAL NOTE

Anatomically corrected malposition of the great arteries was first reported by Theveanin in 1895 (cited by Van Praagh and associates[V1]) and was first termed *anatomically corrected transposition of the great arteries* by Harris and Faber[H1] in 1939. It is possible that similar cases were described earlier under a variety of names. This confusion is exemplified by the case of Raghib and associates described in 1966 with the phrase *isolated bulbar inversion in corrected transposition*.[R1] The Van Praaghs, who had doubted its existence, described three cases in 1967 using the term *anatomically corrected transposition of the great arteries*.[V1] At that time, Abbott's influential definition of transposition, published in 1927, according to which any abnormality in the relationship of the great arteries or between the great arteries and ventricles was called *transposition,* was still accepted.[A2] This confusion was clarified when Van Praagh and colleagues redefined *transposition* in 1971 as the origin of the aorta from the morphologically right ventricle and the pulmonary artery from the morphologically left ventricle[V2] (i.e., ventriculo-

arterial discordant connection) and proposed that other positional and connection abnormalities be included in the definition of *malposition*. The present condition was thus renamed *anatomically corrected malposition of the great arteries*.[V1,V2]

MORPHOLOGY

In anatomically corrected malposition, when there is situs solitus of the atria, usually the right atrium is connected to the morphologically right ventricle (D-loop), which lies to the right, and the left atrium is connected to the morphologically left ventricle, which lies to the left (SDL arrangement). The structure of the sinus portions of both ventricles is normal. However, although the aorta arises from the left ventricle and the pulmonary artery from the right ventricle, there are abnormalities of the outlet, or infundibulum, in both ventricles. The left ventricle probably always exhibits a subaortic conus (infundibulum) with a well-formed conal septum and muscle between the aortic and mitral valve rings. The aortic origin is accordingly displaced superiorly and anteriorly. The right ventricle may also have an infundibulum, but it may be less well developed than normal and in some cases is absent.[V1] In that case, there is pulmonary-tricuspid fibrous continuity. The aorta lies to the left and usually anterior to the pulmonary artery, and both vessels are parallel. Rarely, there may be situs inversus with an ILD arrangement.[A1]

Hearts with similar types of infundibular development but with atrioventricular discordant connection, although originally included in this category by both the Van Praaghs[V1] and Anderson,[A1] are not called *anatomically corrected*

1329

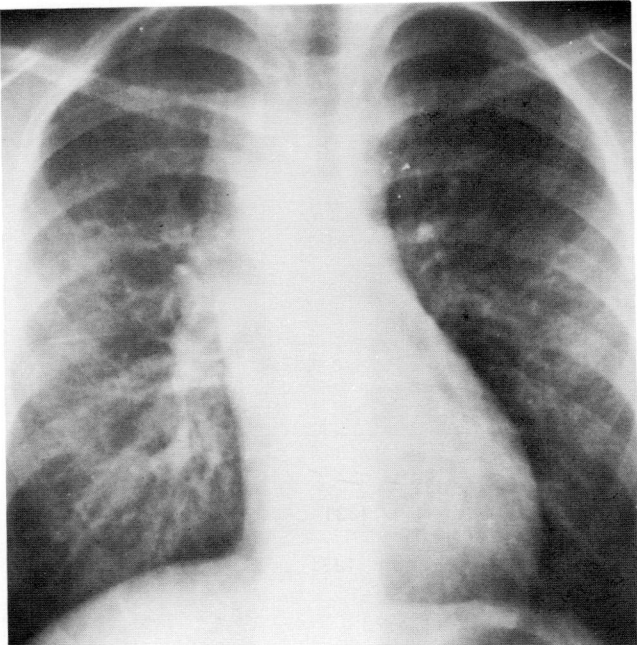

Figure 45-1 Posteroanterior roentgenogram of the chest of a patient with anatomically corrected malposition of the great arteries and a ventricular septal defect (UAB). The ascending aorta is the border-forming structure in the upper left cardiac silhouette.

Reproduced with permission from Kirklin et al.,[K1] and the American Heart Association, Inc.

malposition in this text but are included as variants of isolated ventricular inversion (see Chapter 43).

Associated Anomalies

All reported cases of anatomically corrected malposition have been associated with other congenital cardiac anomalies.[F1] A large ventricular septal defect (VSD) has always been present, usually in the perimembranous area, but occasionally elsewhere, and the VSDs may be multiple. When the VSD is subpulmonary, the pulmonary artery may override onto the left ventricle such that the condition merges with double-outlet left ventricle[K1] (see Chapter 41). When the VSD is subaortic, the aorta may override onto the right ventricle such that the condition merges with double-outlet right ventricle (see Chapter 40).[K1] The aorta was overriding less than 50% in the single GLH patient, in whom there was virtual absence of the ventricular septum but two well-formed ventricles.

Pulmonary stenosis is usual and often infundibular in association with the subpulmonary conus, but there may be valvular stenosis as well. Subaortic stenosis may occur due to a narrowing of the muscular subaortic conus. Tricuspid atresia or tricuspid valve hypoplasia have been noted in half the reported cases, along with associated hypoplasia of the right ventricle. A right aortic arch is relatively common, as is leftward juxtaposition of the atrial appendages and dextrocardia.

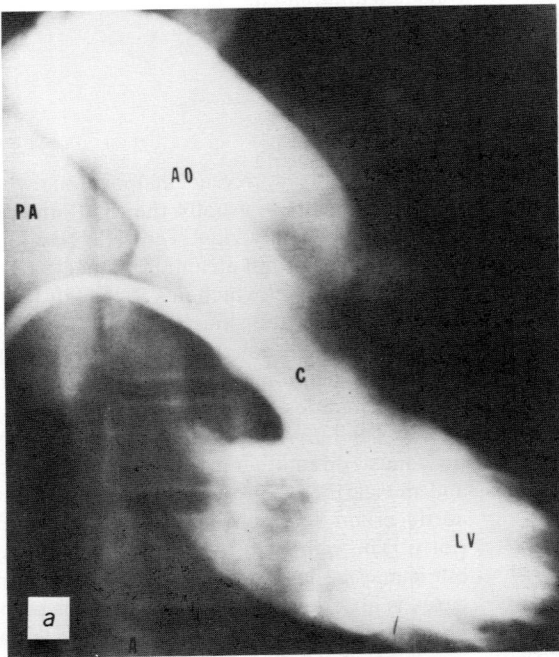
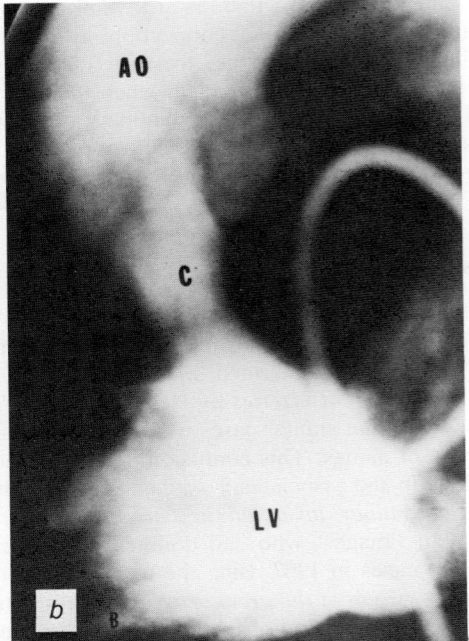

Figure 45-2 Left ventriculograms of a patient with anatomically corrected malposition of the great arteries, a ventricular septal defect, and atrioventricular and ventriculoarterial concordant connections (UAB). There is an infundibulum beneath both the aorta and the pulmonary artery. The aorta is to the left of the pulmonary artery, and the great arteries are parallel with each other. There is also subvalvar pulmonary stenosis.
(*a*) Anteroposterior projection.
(*b*) Lateral projection.

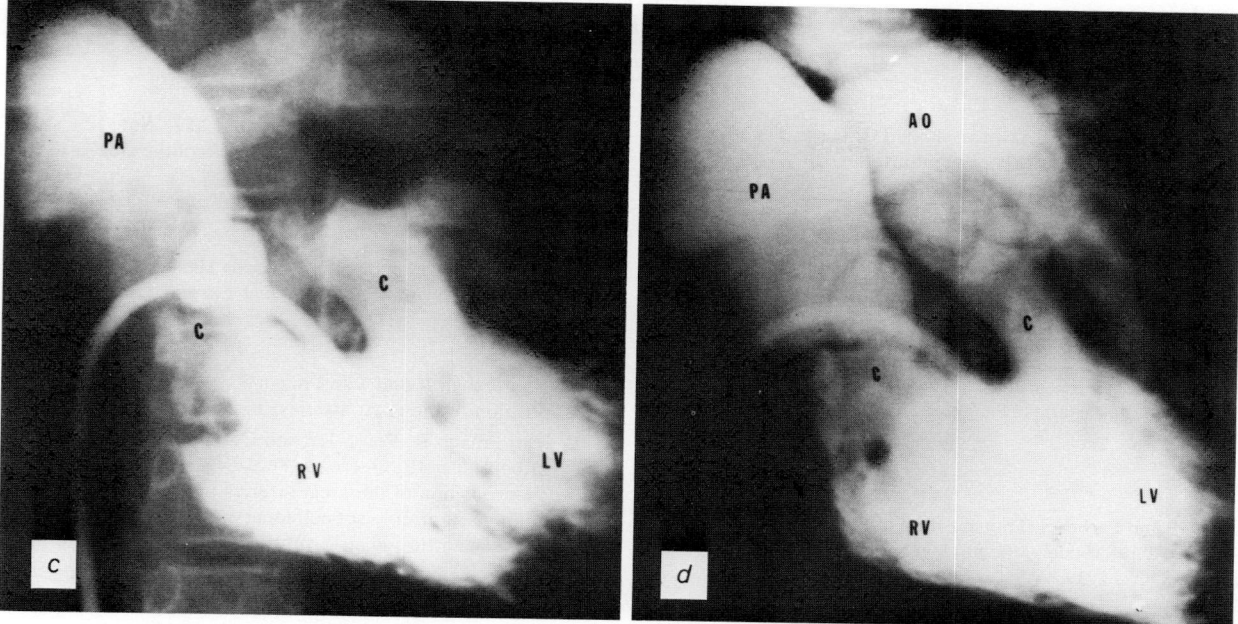

Figure 45-2 *(continued)*
(c, d) Later sequences.

AO, aorta; C, infundibulum (conus); LV, left ventricle; PA, pulmonary artery; RV, right ventricle.
Reproduced with permission from Kirklin et al.,[K1] and the American Heart Association, Inc.

CLINICAL FEATURES AND DIAGNOSTIC CRITERIA

The clinical features of anatomically corrected malposition of the great arteries depend on the associated anomalies, such as VSD.

The correct diagnosis may first be suspected from the characteristic appearance of L-malposition in the chest x-ray (Fig. 45-1). Additional studies, including cineangiograms, are required to establish the presence of atrial situs solitus, atrioventricular and ventricular arterial concordant connections, and the ventricular and great artery position (Fig. 45-2).

Possible diagnoses other than anatomically corrected malposition in the presence of atrial situs solitus and L-malposition of the aorta include complete transposition with L-malposition; AV concordant connection with double-outlet right ventricle and L-malposition (see Chapter 40); AV concordant connection with double-outlet left ventricle (see Chapter 41); congenitally corrected transposition of the great arteries (see Chapter 42); AV discordant connection with double-outlet right or left ventricle (see Chapter 43); and several forms of univentricular atrioventricular connection, most commonly that associated with double-inlet left ventricle, rudimentary left-sided right ventricle, and ventriculoarterial discordant connection (see Chapter 44).

NATURAL HISTORY

The simple positional anomaly of anatomically corrected malposition per se has no impact on the natural history of

patients. However, the presence of associated cardiac anomalies may affect natural history.

TECHNIQUE OF OPERATION

The surgical treatment of anatomically corrected malposition is determined by the associated cardiac anomalies.[K1] The few special problems imposed on aortic cannulation by the L-malposition are discussed under the surgical treatment of corrected transposition (see Chapter 42, ''Technique of Operation'').

When there is tricuspid atresia or significant right ventricular hypoplasia, a Fontan-type procedure is performed. When both ventricles are of adequate size, the VSD is closed, and the pulmonary stenosis is treated by valvotomy and infundibular resection with, when necessary, a transannular patch or a homograft valved extracardiac conduit.

RESULTS

Two patients (UAB) and one patient (GLH) survived repair, although one patient (GLH) died 3 years later. Autopsy then confirmed the morphology.

INDICATIONS FOR OPERATION

Anatomically corrected malposition of the great arteries is not an indication for operation. Coexisting cardiac anomalies may present an indication for operation.

REFERENCES

A

1. Anderson RH, Becker AE, Losekoot TG, Gerlis LM: Anatomically corrected malposition of great arteries. *Br Heart J* 37:993, 1975.

2. Abbott ME: Congenital cardiac disease, in W Osler, T McCrae (eds): *Modern Medicine*, vol 4 (ed 3). Philadelphia: Lea & Febiger, 1927, p 162.

F

1. Freedom RM, Harrington DP: Anatomically corrected malposition of the great arteries. *Br Heart J* 36:207, 1974.

H

1. Harris JS and Farber S: Transposition of the great cardiac vessels with special reference to the phylogenetic theory of Spitzer. *Arch Pathol* 28:427, 1939.

K

1. Kirklin JW, Pacifico AD, Bargeron LM Jr, Soto B: Cardiac repair in anatomically corrected malposition of the great arteries. *Circulation* 48:153, 1973.

R

1. Raghib G, Anderson RC, Edwards JE: Isolated bulbar inversion in corrected transposition. *Am J Cardiol* 17:407, 1966.

V

1. Van Praagh R and Van Praagh S: Anatomically corrected transposition of the great arteries. *Br Heart J* 29:112, 1967.

2. Van Praagh R, Perez-Trevino C, Lopez-Cuellar M, Baker FW, Zuberbuhler JR, Quero M, Perez VM, Moreno F, Van Praagh S: Transposition of the great arteries with posterior aorta, anterior pulmonary artery, subpulmonary conus, and fibrous continuity between aortic and atrio-ventricular valves. *Am J Cardiol* 28:621, 1971.

46

ATRIAL ISOMERISM

DEFINITION

Atrial isomerism is a condition in which the right-sided and left-sided atria, normally morphologically different, are morphologically similar.[1] Atrial isomerism is a subset of situs ambiguus, a condition in which usually asymmetric structures tend to be symmetric.[V1]

This chapter presents clinical information on all surgical patients with atrial isomerism (UAB). In the analysis of the experience with double-outlet right ventricle presented in Chapter 40, cases with atrial isomerism (UAB) are excluded, but the few cases of atrioventricular (AV) canal defects and single ventricle with atrial isomerism are included in their respective chapters as well as in this one. Cases of atrial isomerism (GLH) are included, not here, but in chapters concerning their coexisting cardiac anomalies.

MORPHOLOGY

Atrial Isomerism

In atrial isomerism, both atria have similar internal and external configuration and appendage morphology. They are considered either bilaterally right atria[R2,V1] or bilaterally left

atria.[M3,V1] Atrial situs is most usefully determined by the morphology of the atrial appendages,[C1] since all other studies provide indirect information. Right atrial appendage morphology may be said to be present when the appendage is blunt and has a broad junction with a smooth-walled atrium. This type of junction is accompanied by the protrusion of the crista terminalis into the atrial cavity.[M1] Left atrial appendage morphology may be said to be present when the left atrial appendage is long and thin with constrictions along its length. Such appendages have a rather constricted junction with a smooth atrium, within which a crista terminalis is not identifiable.[M1] However, it is important to note that rarely the atria and their appendages may have mixed right and left atrial morphology.

While the atrial isomerism (right or left) nearly always corresponds to thoracic isomerism, this is not invariably the case.[C1] Atrial and thoracic isomerism (i.e., bilateral atrial and thoracic right- or left-sidedness) usually corresponds to bilateral right-sidedness (asplenia) or left-sidedness (polysplenia) of the abdominal viscera, but exceptions to this correspondence are not infrequent.[L1] Also, abdominal asplenia or polysplenia may exist occasionally without atrial isomerism. Thus, the splenic state does not always predict the atrial morphology.[S1]

In patients coming to surgery, left atrial isomerism is more common than right (UAB; Table 46-1). However, in an autopsy series of 23 hearts with atrial isomerism, only 6 had left atrial isomerism, whereas 17 had right atrial isomerism (GLH).

---

[1]The adjectives left and right used to modify atrium or ventricle always mean morphologic right or morphologic left. The position of a chamber or valve is referred to as right-sided or left-sided.

Table 46-1 Systemic venous connections in surgical patients with atrial isomerism (UAB; 1967–1984; $n = 51$).

	Isomeric Type			
	Left (n = 34)	Right (n = 17)	P(χ²) for Difference	Total (n = 51)
Inferior Vena Caval Connection				
Direct atrial connection from below	5 (15%)	14 (82%)	< .0001	19 (37%)
Right side	4 (12%)	7 (41%)		11 (22%)
Left side	1 (3%)	6 (35%)		7 (14%)
Midline	0 (0%)	1 (6%)		1 (2%)
Connection to SVC	29 (85%)	3 (18%)	< .0001	32 (63%)
Right-sided SVC	17 (50%)	1 (6%)		18 (35%)
Left-sided SVC	12 (35%)	2 (12%)		14 (27%)
Superior Vena Caval Connection				
Bilateral	15 (44%)	3 (18%)	.06	18 (35%)
Right	13 (38%)	6 (35%)		19 (37%)
Left	4 (12%)	4 (24%)		8 (16%)
Unknown	2	4		6 (12%)

KEY: SVC, superior vena cava.

NOTE: In this and subsequent tables, the value in parentheses is percent of *n*.

The Conduction System

In cases of atrial isomerism, the conduction system may be abnormal. Right atrial isomerism is usually accompanied by the presence of bilateral sinus nodes.[B1,D1,V1] Two AV nodes may be present, with a sling of conduction tissue between them. In left atrial isomerism, the sinus node is unusually positioned and often hypoplastic.

The AV node may be normally situated when the ventricular architecture is right-handed (D-loop); when it is left-handed (L-loop), two AV nodes and a sling may be present.[D1] Other more severe abnormalities of the conduction system must occasionally be present, since neonatal complete heart block occurs in some patients with atrial isomerism.[G1,M4]

Anomalies of Systemic Venous Return

In patients with atrial isomerism, anomalies of systemic venous return are common. The inferior vena cava often does not connect directly to the atrium from below but instead passes superiorly along the right-sided paravertebral gutter (azygos extension of the inferior vena cava) or the left-sided gutter (hemiazygos extension of the inferior vena cava) to empty into a right-sided or left-sided superior vena cava (see Table 46-1). The so-called *azygos extension* of the inferior vena cava is much more common in patients with left atrial isomerism, in whom it occurs in about 85% of surgical cases, than in those with right atrial isomerism (UAB; see Table 46-1).

Bilateral superior vena cavae occur in about one-third of cases, but they are more likely to occur in patients with left atrial isomerism (see Table 46-1). When present, each connects to the corresponding top corner of the atria.[M1]

When the inferior vena cava connects directly to the atria from below, it most commonly connects to the right side and rarely in the midline (see Table 46-1).

The hepatic veins most commonly connect directly and separately to the atria from below (Table 46-2), usually to one atrium but sometimes to both or to both sides of a common atrium (Table 46-2).[M1] Such a direct hepatic vein connection is present in all patients with an azygos extension of the inferior vena cava, but it also occurs in patients (in 8 of 19) whose inferior vena cava connects to the atria from below. The coronary sinus orifice is absent in about one-third of cases (Table 46-2).

Anomalies of systemic venous return do not occur exclusively in patients with atrial isomerism (Table 46-3).

Anomalies of Pulmonary Venous Return

In surgical patients with atrial isomerism, extracardiac total anomalous pulmonary venous connection has been uncommon and limited to those with right atrial isomerism (Table 46-3). When the pulmonary veins are connected to an atrium, there is a variable pattern of connection (Table 46-4). Of importance is the fact that there is nearly always the normal wide area of posterior atrial wall between the pulmonary veins when the heart is viewed from behind.[M1]

An abortive cor triatriatum (see Chapter 17) was considered present in 8 (16%) of the 51 patients (UAB). In this regard, the association between cor triatriatum and persistence of the superior vena cava on the left side is to be kept in mind (see Chapters 17, 18). When abortive cor triatriatum was present, it was to the morphologically left atrium that a left-sided superior vena cava was also connected. However, in the two cases of abortive cor triatriatum in the presence of right isomerism, the pulmonary venous chamber (or confluence) was connected to the left-sided superior vena cava at its junction with the left-sided, morphologically right atrium; these might be considered examples of total anomalous pulmonary venous connection.

Atrioventricular Connections

Most patients with atrial isomerism have biventricular atrioventricular connections, which are ambiguus (Table 46-5).[T1] However, there is a univentricular atrioventricular connec-

Table 46-2 Hepatic vein and coronary sinus connections in surgical patients with atrial isomerism (UAB; 1967–1984; *n* = 51).

	Isomeric Type				
	Left (n = 34)		Right (n = 17)		Total (n = 51)
Hepatic Venous Connection					
Via IVC	3 (9%)		8 (47%)		11 (22%)
Direct connections to atrium from below	26 (76%)		3 (18%)		29 (57%)
Right side[a]		15 (44%)		2 (12%)	17 (33%)
Midline[b]		5 (15%)		0 (0%)	5 (10%)
Left side[a]		6 (18%)		1 (6%)	7 (14%)
Unknown	5 (15%)		6 (35%)		11 (22%)
Coronary Sinus Orifice					
Right-sided	12 (35%)		2 (12%)		14 (27%)
Absent	14 (41%)		5 (29%)		19 (37%)
Unknown	8 (24%)		10 (59%)		18 (35%)

KEY: IVC, inferior vena cava.

[a] Direct atrial hepatic venous connections via single or multiple orifices; includes one patient with connection to both right atrium and IVC.

[b] Includes three patients, each with two orifices, one on either side of the midline and one with direct connection to a common atrium (unspecified location).

Table 46-3 Surgical patients with atrial situs solitus, interruption of the inferior vena cava, and azygos extension into the right superior vena cava or hemiazygos extension into the left superior vena cava (UAB; 1967–1984).

Case No.	Atrioventricular Connection	Ventriculo-arterial Connection	Anomaly
1	Discordant	Discordant	VSD, ASD
2	Discordant	Discordant	VSD, PA, about RPA, dextrocardia
3	Discordant	DORV	VSD, PA
4	Discordant	Discordant	ASD
5, 6	Concordant	Concordant	ASD
7	Concordant	Concordant	VSD, TAPVC

KEY: ASD, atrial septal defect; DORV, double-outlet right ventricle; PA, pulmonary atresia; RPA, right pulmonary artery; TAPVC, total anomalous pulmonary venous connection; VSD, ventricular septal defect.

tion (see Chapter 44) in about 25% of the patients, a considerably higher percentage than in any other type of atrial situs; and most of these patients have a solitary ventricular chamber.

Ventriculoarterial Connections

In the surgical series (UAB; Table 46-6), ventriculoarterial connections were most commonly concordant, but an unusually high proportion (33%) of the patients had double-outlet right ventricle.[R1] In autopsy material (GLH), 85% of the specimens with right atrial isomerism had ventriculoarterial discordance (transposition) or double-outlet right ventricle; in left atrial isomerism, this was true in 43% of the specimens.

Atrioventricular Canal and Other Atrial Septal Defects

The complexities of pulmonary and systemic venous return, the variability in the position and nature of the atrioventricu-

Table 46-4 Pulmonary venous connections in surgical patients with atrial isomerism (UAB; 1967–1984; *n* = 51).

	Isomeric Type				
Pulmonary Venous Connection	Left (n = 34)		Right (n = 17)		Total (n = 51)
Extracardiac TAPVC	0 (0%)		4 (24%)		4 (8%)
Atrial connection	34 (100%)		13 (76%)		47 (92%)
Right side of atrium		5 (15%)		5 (29%)	9 (18%)
Midline		8 (24%)		1 (6%)	9 (18%)
Left side of atrium		20 (59%)		3 (18%)	24 (47%)
Laterally unknown		1 (3%)		4 (24%)	5 (10%)
Abortive cor triatriatum	6 (18%)		2 (12%)		8 (16%)

KEY: TAPVC, total anomalous pulmonary venous connection.

Table 46-5   Atrioventricular connections and ventricular morphology in surgical patients with atrial isomerism (UAB; 1967–1984; $n = 51$).

Atrioventricular Connections	Isomeric Type		P(χ^2) for Difference	Total ($n = 51$)
	Left ($n = 34$)	Right ($n = 17$)		
Ambiguus (biventricular)	29 (85%)	8 (47%)		37 (73%)
D-loop	21 (62%)	5 (29%)		26 (51%)
L-loop	8 (24%)	3 (18%)		11 (22%)
Univentricular	5 (15%)	9 (53%)	.004	14 (27%)
Two ventricular chambers	3 (9%)	2 (12%)		5 (10%)
D-loop	3	2		5
L-loop	0	0		0
Solitary ventricular chamber	2 (6%)	7 (41%)		9 (17%)

NOTE: *Loop* refers to ventricular loop.

Table 46-6   Ventriculoarterial connections in surgical patients with atrial isomerism (UAB; 1967–1984; $n = 51$).

Ventriculoarterial Connection	Isomeric Type		Total ($n = 51$)
	Left ($n = 34$)	Right ($n = 17$)	
Concordant	18 (53%)	2 (12%)	20 (39%)
Discordant	3 (9%)	6 (35%)	9 (18%)
DORV	12 (35%)	5 (29%)	17 (33%)
DOIV	1 (3%)	4 (24%)	5 (10%)

KEY: DOIV, double-outlet indeterminate (solitary) ventricle; DORV, double-outlet right ventricle.

lar valves through which the atria empty, and the anomalous muscle bands that sometimes transverse the atria often make it difficult to apply the conventional terms describing atrial septal defects (ASDs) to atrial isomerism. However, a common atrium (see Chapter 19) is present in a high proportion of cases (43%; UAB; see Table 46-7), and an ostium primum ASD (associated with a partial or complete AV canal defect) is present in an additional 18%. This high incidence of AV canal defects (common atrium and ostium primum ASDs) in surgical patients corresponds to the autopsy finding (GLH) that 20 (83%) of 23 cases had some type of AV canal defect. Most patients with atrial isomerism and AV canal defects have a common AV orifice (complete AV canal; see Chapter 19) rather than two AV orifices (Table 46-8).

Rarely (6% in surgical cases; see Table 46-7) in patients with atrial isomerism, the atrial septum is well formed and intact or has only a probe-patent foramen ovale.

Ventricular Morphology and Ventricular Septal Defects

The complexities of the AV valves and the AV connections and the frequency of solitary ventricular chambers in atrial isomerism again make it difficult to apply the conventional terms. Clearly, however, it is rare for surgical patients with atrial isomerism to have an intact ventricular septum; this condition existed in 9 (13%) of the patients (UAB; Table 46-9), one of whom had an interventricular communication located centrally beneath the leaflets of an AV canal defect.

Pulmonary Outflow

Unobstructed pulmonary outflow is rare in right atrial isomerism but common in left atrial isomerism (Table 46-10). In right atrial isomerism, pulmonary stenosis is present in slightly more than half the patients and pulmonary atresia in about one-third.

Other Coexisting Cardiac Anomalies

Anomalies other than those inherent in the atrial isomerism syndrome are surprisingly infrequent in surgically treated

Table 46-7   Atrial septal defects in surgical patients with atrial isomerism (UAB; 1967–1984; $n = 51$).

Description of ASD	Isomeric Type					
	Left ($n = 36$)		Right ($n = 17$)		Total ($n = 51$)	
	No.	% of 34	No.	% of 17	No.	% of 51
Common atrium ⎫ AV canal defects	13[a]	38%	9	53%	22	43%
Ostium primum ⎭	3	9%	6	35%	9	18%
Fossa ovalis type	10[a]	29%	1	6%	11	22%
Coronary sinus type	1	3%	0	0%	1	2%
Posteroinferior (inferior caval) type	0	0%	1	6%	1	2%
Unspecified (not primum)	3	9%	0	0%	3	6%
None or probe-patent foramen ovale only	4	9%	0	0%	4	6%

KEY: AV, atrioventricular.

[a] Or with vestigial ventricle without inlet or outlet.

Table 46-8 Details of AV canal defects in surgical patients with atrial isomerism (UAB; 1967–1984; n = 51).

AV Canal Defect	Number of AV Orifices	Interventricular Communication	AV Connection	Isomeric Type Left (n = 34)	Right (n = 17)	Total (n = 51)
Yes (n = 31)				16 (47%)	15 (88%)	31 (61%)
	2			7	1	8
		None		2	1	3
		Beneath superior or inferior leaflets		4	0	4
		Centrally only		1[a]	0	1
	Common orifice			9	14	23
			Biventricular (ambiguus)	7	6	13
			Univentricular	2	8	10
			Severe straddling[b]	0	1	1
			Solitary ventricular chamber[c]	2	7	9
No (n = 20)				18 (53%)	2 (12%	20 (39%)

KEY: AV, atrioventricular; V, ventricular.

[a] Not counted as a VSD in Table 46-7.

[b] In this case, a common AV orifice lay 90% over one ventricle and 10% over a hypoplastic ventricle; the severity of the straddling (overriding) of the common AV valve orifice and the severity of the ventricular hypoplasia distinguished it from the cases with common orifice listed as *biventricular, ambiguus AV connections.*

[c] Or with rudimentary ventricle without inlet or outlet.

patients (Table 46-11). In autopsy series, obstructive lesions on the left side of the heart, excluding left ventricular hypoplasia and mitral stenosis, are common.[P4]

Summary

In the surgically more common left atrial isomerism, anomalies of systemic venous return are common, as are abortive forms of cor triatriatum, but extracardiac total anomalous venous connections are rare. Common atrium and other types of AV canal defects occur in about one-half of the cases. Univentricular atrioventricular connections are un-

common, as are solitary ventricular chambers, but double-outlet right ventricle is common. Pulmonary stenosis or atresia is present in about one-half of the cases.

In patients with right atrial isomerism coming to surgery, anomalies of systemic venous return occur in only about 20% of cases, as does the abortive form of cor triatriatum, but extracardiac forms of total anomalous pulmonary venous connection also occur in about 20% of cases. Common atrium and other forms of AV canal defects occur in 95% of the patients, and solitary ventricular chamber occurs in nearly one-half of the patients. The fact that cardiac anomalies are more complex and numerous in hearts with right

Table 46-9 Ventricular septal defects in surgical patients with atrial isomerism (UAB; 1967–1984; n = 51).

Description of VSD	Isomeric Type Left (n = 34)	Right (n = 17)	Total (n = 51)
Patients with AV canal defects	16 (47%)	15 (88%)	31 (61%)
Interventricular communication	11[a]	7[b]	18
NA (solitary ventricular chamber)	2	7	9
Intact ventricular septum	3[c]	1	4
Patients without AV canal defects	18 (53%)	2 (12%)	20 (39%)
NA (solitary ventricular chamber)	1 (3%)	1 (6%)	2 (4%)
Applicable cases	17 (50%)	1 (6%)	18 (35%)
Perimembranous	8[b]	1[b]	9
Muscular (only entrance to outlet chamber)	2	0	2
Outlet (subarterial)	2[b]	0	2
Intact ventricular septum	5	0	5

KEY: AV, atrioventricular; NA, not applicable.

[a] Two with multiple VSDs.

[b] One with multiple VSDs.

[c] One with a central bare area of septum (the case with AV canal defect and central interventricular communication).

Table 46-10 Status of the pulmonary outflow tract in surgical patients with atrial isomerism (UAB; 1967–1984; n = 51).

Pulmonary Outflow	Isomeric Type			Total (n = 51)
	Left (n = 34)	Right (n = 17)	P (χ²) for Difference	
Stenosis	16 (47%)	10 (59%)		26 (51%)
Atresia	1 (3%)	6 (35%)		7 (14%)
Unobstructed	17 (50%)	1 (6%)	.002	18 (35%)

Table 46-11 Coexisting cardiac anomalies in surgical patients with atrial isomerism (UAB; 1967–1984; n = 51).

Coexisting Anomalies	Isomeric Type		Total
	Left (n = 34)	Right (n = 17)	
Subaortic stenosis	4	0	4 (8%)
Congenital valvar and supravalvar AS	1	0	1 (2%)
Aortic coarctation	1	0	1 (2%)
Patent ductus arteriosus	5	3	8 (16%)
Nonconfluent pulmonary arteries	1	1	2 (4%)
Stenosis of the RPA	1	0	1 (2%)
Coronary artery anomalies	1	1	2 (4%)
Aortic insufficiency (mild)	1	0	1 (2%)
Congenital heart block	1	0	1 (2%)

KEY: AS, aortic stenosis; RPA, right pulmonary artery.

atrial isomerism than in those with left atrial isomerism probably explains the higher incidence of the latter in surgical series than in autopsy series.

CLINICAL FEATURES AND DIAGNOSTIC CRITERIA

The finding of an increased number of Howell-Jolly bodies in the routine blood smear in newborns or persistent Howell-Jolly bodies in older infants is associated with asplenia. There are no other specific clinical features of atrial isomerism, as there is no specific functional derangement. The clinical features depend, therefore, on the other cardiac anomalies that may be present.

Atrial situs (solitus, inversus, or isomeric, with either bilateral right-sidedness or bilateral left-sidedness) is best diagnosed preoperatively by determining the thoracic situs, since atrial and thoracic situs are nearly always the same.[P1,S2,V2] Thoracic situs is best indicated by the bronchial anatomy,[L1,V2] which does not always correspond to lung lobulation.[L1,L2] The length of each main stem bronchus and the relationship to its respective pulmonary artery provide the most reliable clinical prediction of thoracic situs.[L3,P1,S1] The right main stem bronchus is relatively short and the right pulmonary artery is anterior and inferior to the bronchus; the left main stem bronchus is relatively long and the left pulmonary artery is posterior and superior to the bronchus.

The determination of these relationships, and thus the diagnosis of the thoracic situs, are reliably accomplished from the plain frontal and lateral chest radiograms,[P1,S2] although meticulous attention must be paid to radiologic technique. If the ratio of the length of the shorter (normally right)

bronchus divided by that of the longer (normally the left) one is 2 or greater, there is thoracic lateralization; if the ratio is 1.5 or less, thoracic, and thus usually atrial, isomerism is nearly always present. Also, right isomerism is usually present when each pulmonary artery is anterior to its respective bronchus; and left isomerism is usually present when on both sides the pulmonary artery is superior and posterior to its respective bronchus (Fig. 46-1). The use of special radiologic techniques[D2] and two-dimensional echocardiography[H1] may contribute to the clinical diagnosis of thoracic and thus atrial isomerism, but such techniques are not necessary in most cases.

At operation, the surgeon must make additional direct observations of the atrial appendages and atrial walls to confirm or deny the preoperative diagnosis of right or left atrial isomerism.

NATURAL HISTORY

The natural history of patients with atrial isomerism is determined primarily by the details of the cardiac structures and the nature of the coexisting cardiac anomalies. However, atrial isomerism itself may contribute to the natural history of the patient because of its association with neonatal complete heart block and sometimes neonatal death.[G1,M4]

Right atrial isomerism is often accompanied by asplenia, a condition believed to render the patient susceptible to infection, particularly pneumococcal infections, and thus unfavorable to long-term survival. Left atrial isomerism is often accompanied by polysplenia and a high incidence of extrahepatic biliary atresia.[C2,D3]

TECHNIQUE OF OPERATION

Cardiopulmonary Bypass

In patients with atrial isomerism, cardiopulmonary bypass (CPB) presents no special problems of arterial cannulation, but because of the frequency of systemic venous anomalies, CPB often presents problems of venous cannulation. The basic venous cannulation techniques already described (see Chapter 2, ''Venous Cannulation'' in Section 3) are used, as well as those described for situations involving three vena cavae (see Chapter 2, ''Left Superior Vena Cava'' in Section 3, Special Situations and Controversies). Direct caval cannulation is particularly advantageous in patients with atrial isomerism cases because of the complex intra-atrial repairs often required. In patients with atrial isomerism and two superior vena cavae it must be remembered in selecting the venous cannula size that one of the superior cavae is probably returning the entire inferior vena caval flow as well as its usual flow and that a larger than usual cannula is required (see Chapter 2, Table 2-4). In such situations, the blood returning from the hepatic veins connected directly to an atrium is picked up by a pump-oxygenator sump sucker placed in the depths of the atrium.

One solution to the venous cannulation problem and the

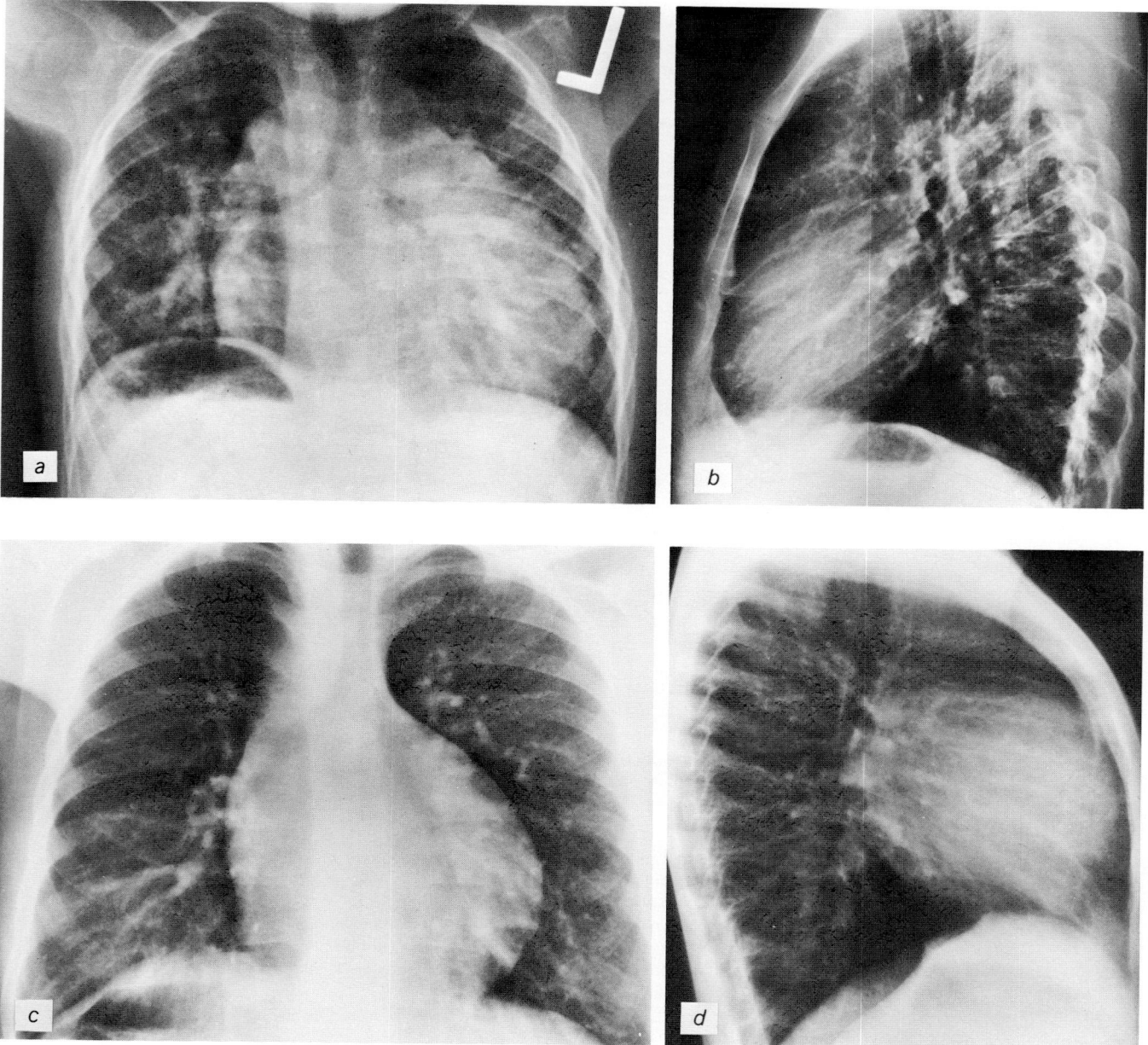

Figure 46-1 Chest roentgenograms of patients with atrial isomerism (UAB).
(a) Left isomerism, frontal chest film. Each bronchus has a similar length.
(b) Lateral view. The pulmonary arteries are superior and posterior to the tracheobronchial tree.
(c) Right isomerism, frontal chest film. Each bronchus has a similar length.
(d) Lateral view. The pulmonary arteries are anterior and inferior to the bronchi.

complexities of the repair is to use the technique of profound hypothermia and total circulatory arrest, cooling and rewarming with a single venous cannula through an atrial appendage. The advantages and disadvantages of this technique have been described (see Chapter 2, Section 4) and generally, this is the method chosen for infants (GLH). Another solution is cardiopulmonary bypass at 25°C and cannulation as described (see Chapter 2, Section 3), with periods of very low perfusion flow rate ($0.5 \; l \cdot min^{-1} \cdot m^{-2}$) when

needed for exposure of complicated parts of the repair (UAB).[P3]

Since the repairs are often complex, they must be carefully planned so that they can be done efficiently. Otherwise, unduly long CPB times themselves become an added risk. Since aortic cross-clamp times may in some cases be as long as 100–120 minutes, the cold cardioplegic technique is always used (see Chapter 3), and the temperature during CPB may be reduced to 20°C.

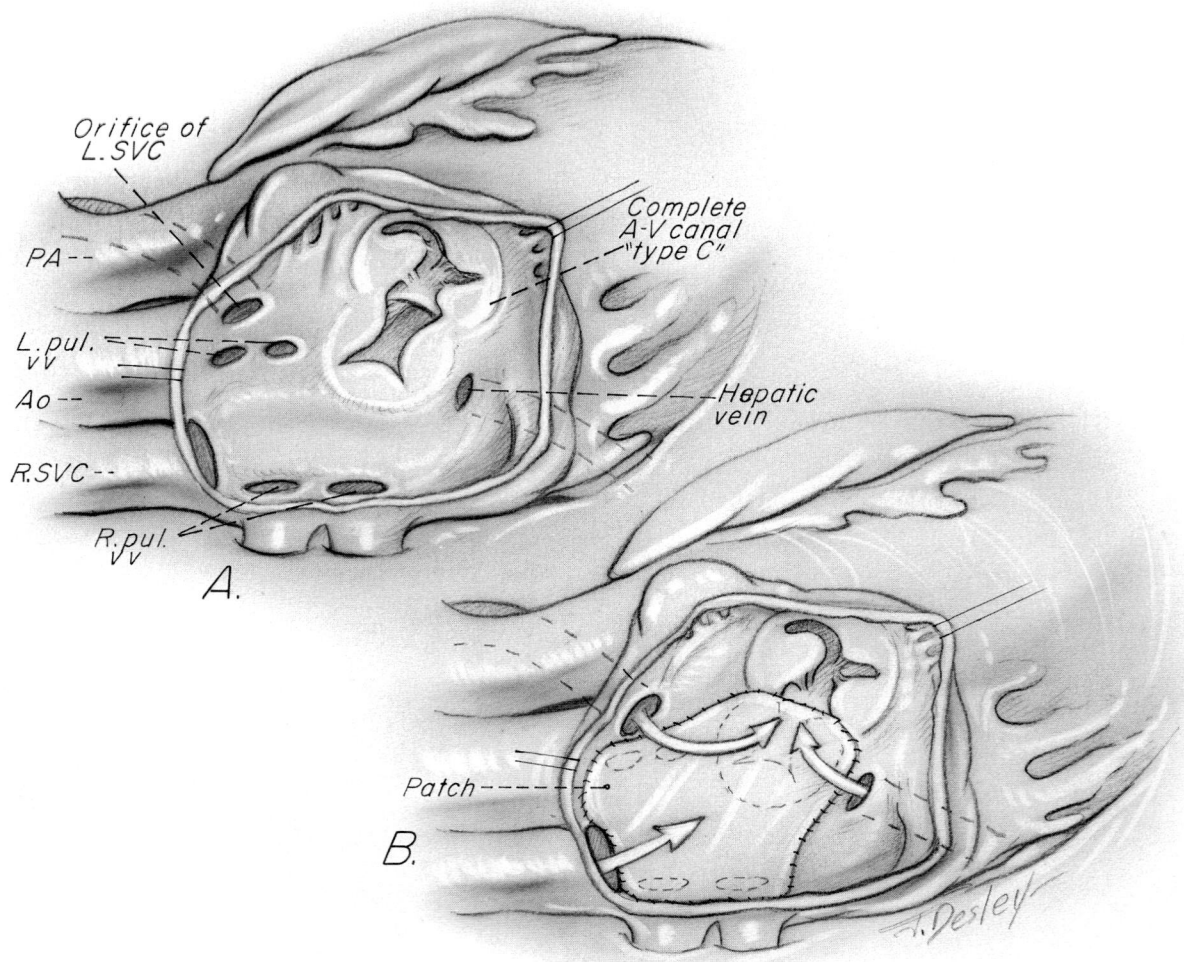

Figure 46-2 Use of a complex atrial baffle in intracardiac repair in a patient with atrial isomerism, bilateral superior vena cavae, and common AV valve orifice (complete AV canal defect).
(*a*) Appearance of the atria after complete excision of the atrial septum.
(*b*) The pericardial baffle has been sewn into place so as to divert pulmonary venous blood to the left side of the partitioned, once common AV valve orifice and systemic venous blood from multiple sources to the right side. The baffle should not be redundant but taut, and care is taken to ensure that it does not restrict any of the pathways.

Ao, aorta; L.SVC, left superior vena cava; L.pul.vv, left pulmonary veins; PA, pulmonary artery; R.pul.vv, right pulmonary veins; R.SVC, right superior vena cava.

Intracardiac Repair

A wide variety of intracardiac repairs are required in patients with atrial isomerism, and in individual patients the repair may incorporate two or three procedures. These procedures are described in chapters on the specific anomaly encountered. The procedures used in the repair of AV canal defects, including common atrium (see Chapter 19) are particularly needed.

Complex Atrial Baffle

In the repairs of the anomalies of pulmonary or systemic venous connections that are frequently part of the cardiac anomaly in patients with atrial isomerism, a complex atrial baffle is often required. The first step is usually excision of the remnants of atrial septum, except for the anterior limbus which, if present, may contain the AV node or bundle of His. The temptation to retain part of the septum as a flap should generally be resisted in such complex repairs because it tends to increase the complexity. When a coronary sinus is present, it is usually cut down, as in the Senning or Mustard repair (see Chapter 39, Fig. 39-25).

Then the complex spatial arrangements involving the orifices of the pulmonary veins, the orifice of the left-sided superior vena cava in the upper left corner of the atrium, the orifice of the right-sided superior vena cava in the upper right atrial corner, and the orifices of the hepatic veins lying inferiorly must be visualized in three dimensions and clearly understood (Fig. 46-2*a*). Also, the superior vena cava receiving the venous drainage from the lower body must be recognized as requiring a larger pathway to the AV valve than is usual if flow is to be unimpeded. The relationship of these arrangements to the orifices of the left-sided and right-sided AV valves is clarified, for the proper positioning of the atrial baffle depends on this knowledge.

In planning the baffle and the potential drainage pathways to the AV valves, the ventriculoarterial connections that will exist at the end of the repair must also be clearly visualized. In this regard, the ventricular situs (or handedness or loop) per se is not important, since, in what will ultimately be a two-ventricle system, the pulmonary venous return must be routed to the ventricle that does or will connect to the aorta regardless of whether it is a morphologically right or left ventricle; similarly, the systemic venous return must be routed to the ventricle connected to the pulmonary artery.

After these structures and relationships have been visualized clearly, the proposed suture line of the baffle is marked with four to six interrupted suture markers, the pericardium that was taken initially and set aside (see Chapter 15, footnote 2) is trimmed to a proper shape and size, and then this pericardium is sutured into place (Fig. 46-2b). This complex atrial baffle is similar to that used for the repair of the simple unroofed coronary sinus syndrome (see Chapter 18, Fig. 18-1) and to that used for the Fontan type of repair in single ventricle (see Chapter 44).

The frequent association of such anomalies of venous connection with AV canal defects in patients with atrial isomerism often necessitates combining the baffle repair with repair of a complete AV canal defect. In such a procedure, the extension of the atrial baffle toward the AV valves is best thought of as simply the pericardial portion of the two-patch technique used in the repair of complete AV canal defects (see Chapter 19, "Technique of Operation").

Fontan Type of Repair

The frequent occurrence of pulmonary stenosis or atresia in patients with atrial isomerism associated with other complex cardiac anomalies means that a Fontan type of repair must sometimes be used (2 cases among 28 at UAB). Under such circumstances, a complex atrial baffle is usually necessary to divert the venous blood from the lungs to one or both AV valves and to create a chamber or pathway into which all systemic venous blood drains and that can be anastomosed to the pulmonary trunk. Thus, it is again of great importance to avoid obstruction in any of the venous pathways created by the complex baffle (see Chapter 44, "Fontan-Type Procedure" in section on Technique of Operation").

Total Cavopulmonary Shunt Operation

Although not used to date (UAB, GLH), the operation of total cavopulmonary shunting may be useful for some patients with atrial isomerism. The pulmonary trunk is divided from the heart, and the ends are closed; the end of the superior vena cava receiving inferior vena cava drainage is then anastomosed end to side to a confluent left or right pulmonary artery, as is the opposite superior vena cava if two are present.[K1] Only hepatic blood and coronary venous

Table 46-12 Hospital mortality after all operations (n = 62) for cardiac anomalies in patients (n = 51) with atrial isomerism (UAB; 1967–1984).

| Operation | n | Hospital Deaths | | |
		No.	%	CL
Corrective procedures	28	9	32%	22%–44%
Palliative procedures	28	6	21%	13%–32%
First procedure	22	4	18%	9%–31%
Second procedure	6	2	33%	12%–62%
Revisions[b]	6	2	33%	12%–62%
First revision	5	1	20%	3%–53%
Second revision	1[c]	1	100%	15%–100%

KEY: CL, 70% confidence limits.

[a] Among the first-time noncorrective procedures were 15 classic Blalock-Taussig shunts, with two (13%, CL 4%–29%) hospital deaths.

[b] Revisions of previous corrective procedure.

[c] In the same hospitalization; the death was counted only after the second revision.

blood now contaminate the pulmonary venous blood entering the heart and passing to the systemic circulation.

Palliative Operations

Standard techniques are used for shunting procedures (see Chapter 23, "Technique of Shunting Operations" in Section 1) and pulmonary artery banding (Chapter 20, "Pulmonary Artery Banding" in Section 1).

SPECIAL FEATURES OF POSTOPERATIVE CARE

The usual measures of postoperative care are employed after repair of cardiac anomalies in patients with atrial isomerism. The special measures employed after the Fontan type of procedure are described in Chapter 26.

EARLY RESULTS

Hospital Mortality

The hospital mortality has been high after repair of cardiac anomalies in patients with atrial isomerism. Thus, in a study including an earlier era as well as the current one, it was 32%

Table 46-13 Hospital mortality with the use of certain repair techniques in the correction of cardiac anomalies in patients with atrial isomerism (UAB; 1967–1984; n = 28, 9 hospital deaths). More than one technique was used in nearly all patients.

| Repair Technique | n | Hospital Deaths | | |
		No.	%	CL
Repair of AV canal defect	15	4	27%	14%–43%
Complex atrial baffle	12	4	33%	18%–52%
Atrial switch	5	0	0%	0%–32%
Valved conduit to PA	6	4	67%	38%–88%
Repair of extracardiac TAPVC	3	1	33%	4%–76%

KEY: AV, atrioventricular; CL, 70% confidence limits; PA, pulmonary artery; TAPVC, total anomalous pulmonary venous connection.

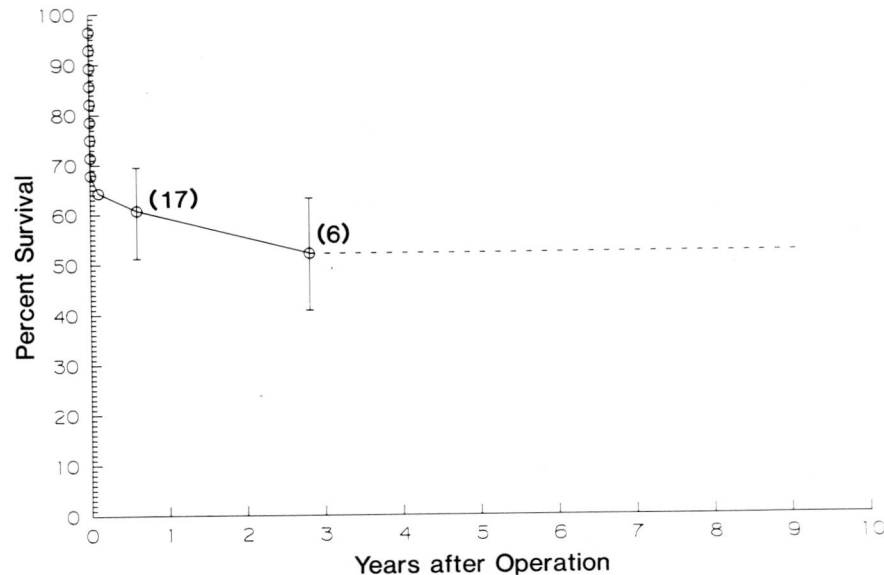

Figure 46-3 Actuarial survival, including hospital deaths, after repair of cardiac anomalies in patients with atrial isomerism (UAB; 1967–1984; *n* = 28; 13 deaths, including 9 hospital deaths). All patients have been traced. The vertical bars enclose the 70% confidence limits. The dashed line indicates patients followed beyond the time of any event.

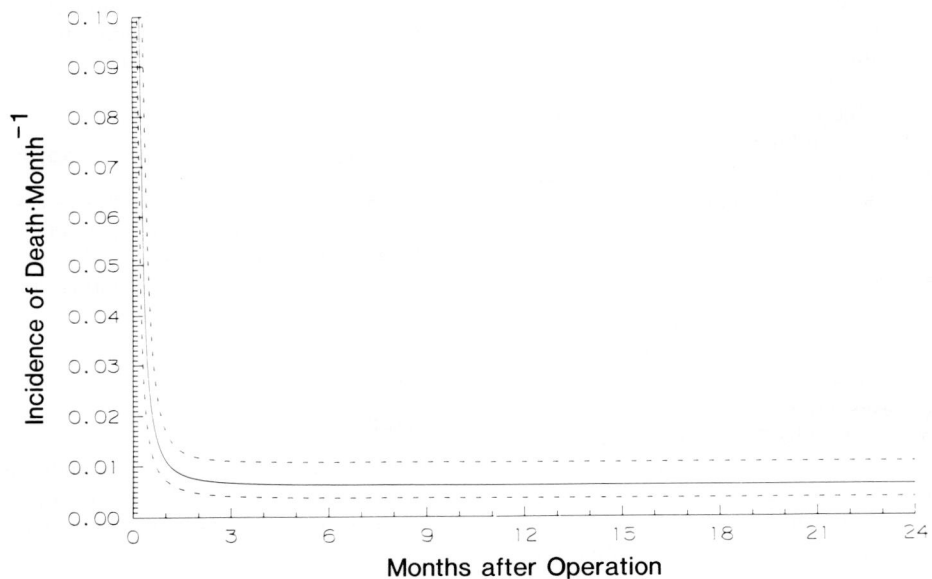

Figure 46-4 Instantaneous risk of death across time by hazard function analysis (see Chapter 6, "Parametric Methods" in Section 4, Analysis of Time–Related Events) after repair of cardiac defects in patients with atrial isomerism (details are as in Fig. 46-3). There is an early phase and a late constant phase.

(CL 22%–44%) (UAB; Table 46-12). However, the risk of repair of these complex procedures is lower in the current era—with more complete preoperative diagnosis, better understanding of the repair techniques required, and better myocardial protection—so that satisfactory results are now being reported.[A1,M2,P2,T2]

The types of repair techniques used have not seemed to be related to hospital mortality (Table 46-13).

In patients with atrial isomerism undergoing palliative operations, the hospital mortality has also been higher than in less complex situations (see Table 46-12).

Heart Block

The development of heart block has not occurred after any reparative procedures in patients with cardiac anomalies and atrial isomerism.

Table 46-14 Incremental risk factors for death as a time-related event after cardiac repair in patients with atrial isomerism (UAB; 1967–1984; *n* = 28; 13 deaths, including 9 hospital deaths).

Incremental Risk Factor	Early Coefficient ± SD	Early P value	Late (constant) Coefficient ± SD	Late (constant) P value
NYHA class (I–V)			2.3 ± 1.35	.09
Discordant ventriculoarterial connection			3.3 ± 1.30	.01
Aortic cross-clamp time (min)	0.041 ± 0.0190	.03		
Intercept	−3.94		−12.4	

KEY: AV, atrioventricular; NYHA, New York Heart Association; SD, standard deviation; VA, ventriculoarterial; VSD, ventricular septal defect.

NOTE: See Chapter 6 for methodology of the parametric method. Factors analyzed were age at repair and its logarithm, hematocrit level, date of operation, preoperative NYHA class, number of systemic venous pathways, nonclosure of a VSD, use of a complex baffle, ventriculotomy, the conduit used in repair, whether the right ventricle was made the systemic ventricle, aortic cross-clamp time, and the presence of a common atrium, any form of AV canal defect, interventricular communication in an AV canal defect, right isomerism, discordant VA connection, concordant VA connection, and a VSD.

Table 46-15 Functional status of survivors late after corrective or palliative cardiac procedures in patients with atrial isomerism. All surviving patients were traced (UAB; 1967–1984).

Procedure	n	No. in Postoperative NYHA Functional Class I	II	III	IV
Corrective	15	14 (93%)	1 (7%)	0	0
Palliative	12	5 (42%)	7 (58%)	0	0

KEY: NYHA, New York Heart Association.

functional classes and a discordant ventriculoarterial connection are risk factors for death in the late constant phase.

Functional Status

The functional status of all surviving patients with atrial isomerism is good after both corrective and palliative operations, but the percentage of patients in NYHA class I is higher for those who have undergone a corrective procedure than for those who have had a palliative operation (Table 46-15).

INDICATIONS FOR OPERATION

The need for surgical treatment is dictated by the associated cardiac anomalies, not by the atrial isomerism. Atrial isomerism, particularly right atrial isomerism and asplenia, strongly suggests the presence of complex cardiac anomalies and a higher than usual surgical risk, but the coexisting anomalies are usually severe and the natural history unfavorable. Therefore, the indications for operation are usually clear.

The complex repairs often require more than the usual amount of cardiopulmonary bypass or total circulatory arrest time. Thus, when possible, repairative procedures should be deferred to the age of 6–12 months or older, since at these ages longer cardiopulmonary times seem to be accompanied by less morbidity and mortality than in younger infants (see Chapter 2, "Damaging Effects of Cardiopulmonary Bypass" in Section 2).

LATE RESULTS

Survival

The actuarial 3-year survival rate after repair of cardiac anomalies associated with atrial isomerism is 52%, with no further deaths occurring in a follow-up period of 9 years (Fig. 46-3). Most deaths have occurred within 6 weeks of repair (Fig. 46-4), although there is a continuing late phase of constant risk.

Incremental Risk Factors for Premature Death

Only long aortic cross-clamp time has been a risk factor for deaths in the early phase, including hospital deaths (Table 46-14). The higher New York Heart Association (NYHA)

REFERENCES

A

1. Ando F, Shirotani H, Kawai J, Kanzaki Y, Setsuie N, Yamaguchi K, Okamoto F, Yokoyama T, Makino S, Tateishi K, Nishi K: Successful total repair of complicated cardiac anomalies with asplenia syndrome. *J Thorac Cardiovasc Surg* 72:33, 1976.

B

1. Bharati S, Lev M: The course of the conduction system in dextrocardia. *Circulation* 57:163, 1978.
2. Brandt HM, Liebow AA: Right pulmonary isomerism associated with venous, splenic, and other anomalies. *Lab Invest* 7:469, 1958.

C

1. Caruso G, Becker AE: How to determine atrial situs? Considerations initiated by 3 cases of absent spleen with a discordant anatomy between bronchi and atria. *Br Heart J* 41:559, 1979.
2. Chandra RS: Biliary atresia and other structural anomalies in the congenital polysplenia syndrome. *J Pediatr* 85:649, 1974.

3. Coles J, Kirklin JW, Blackstone EH, Pacifico ADP, Kirklin JK, Bargeron LM Jr: Cardiac surgery in patients with atrial isomerism. Unpublished data, 1985.

D

1. Dickinson DF, Wilkinson JL, Anderson KR, Smith A, Ho SY, Anderson RH: The cardiac conduction system in situs ambiguus. *Circulation* 59:879, 1979.
2. Deanfield J, Leanage R, Stroobant J, Chrispin AR, Taylor JFN, Macartney FJ: Use of high kilovoltage filtered beam radiographs for detection of bronchial situs in infants and young children. *Br Heart J* 44:577, 1980.
3. Dimmick JE, Bove KE, McAdams AJ: Extrahepatic biliary atresia and the polysplenia syndrome. *J Pediatr* 86:644, 1975.

G

1. Garcia OL, Mehta AV, Pickoff AS, Tamer DF, Ferrer PL, Wolff GS, Gelband H: Left isomerism and complete atrio-ventricular block: a report of 6 cases. *Am J Cardiol* 48:1103, 1981.

H

1. Huhta JC, Smallhorn JF, Macartney FJ: Two-dimensional echocardiographic diagnosis of situs. *Br Heart J* 48:97, 1982.

K

1. Kawashima Y, Kitamura S, Matsuda H, Shimazaki Y, Nakano S, Hirose H: Total cavopulmonary shunt operation in complex cardiac anomalies. *J Thorac Cardiovasc Surg* 87:74, 1984.

L

1. Lev M, Liberthson RR, Eckner FAO, Arcille RA: Pathologic anatomy of dextrocardia and its clinical implications. *Circulation* 37:979, 1968.
2. Liberthson RR, Hastreiter AR, Sinha SN, Bharati S, Novak GM, Lev M: Levocardia with visceral hetrotaxy-isolated levocardia: Pathologic anatomy and its clinical implications. *Am Heart J* 85:40, 1973.
3. Landing BH, Lawrence TK, Payne VC, Wells TR: Bronchial anatomy in syndromes with abnormal visceral situs, abnormal spleen and congenital heart disease. *Am J Cardiol* 128:456, 1971.

M

1. Macartney FJ, Zuberbuhler JR, Anderson RH: Morphological considerations pertaining to recognition of atrial isomerism: Consequences for sequential chamber localization. *Br Heart J* 44:657, 1980.
2. Marcelletti C, Di Donato R, Nijveld A, Squitieri C, Bulterijs AH, Naeff M, Schuller J, Becker AE: Right and left isomerism: The cardiac surgeon's view. *Ann Thorac Surg* 35:400, 1983.
3. Moller JH, Nakib A, Anderson RC, Edwards JE: Congenital cardiac disease associated with polysplenia: A developmental complex of bilateral "left-sidedness." *Circulation* 36:789, 1967.

4. Mehta AV, Sanchez GR: Left isomerism (polysplenia syndrome) and complete atrioventricular block (letter to editor). *Am J Cardiol* 52:429, 1983.

P

1. Partridge MC, Scott O, Deverall PB, Macartney FJ: Visualization and measurement of the main bronchi by tomography as an objective indicator of thoracic situs in congenital heart disease. *Circulation* 51:188, 1975.
2. Pillai R, Lima R, Anderson RH, Shinebourne EA, Lincoln C: Surgical correction in mirror-image atrial arrangement or left atrial isomerism with systemic venous return to the left-sided atrium. *J Thorac Cardiovasc Surg* 86:288, 1983.
3. Pacifico AD, Fox LS, Kirklin JW, Bargeron LM: Surgical treatment of atrial isomerism, in RH Anderson, FJ Macartney, EA Shinebourne, M Tynan (eds): *Paediatric Cardiology* (ed 5). London: Churchill Livingstone, 1983, p 223.
4. Peoples WM, Moller JH, Edwards JE: Polysplenia: A review of 146 cases. *Pediatr Cardiol* 4:129, 1983.

R

1. Rose V, Izukawa T, Moes CAF: Syndromes of asplenia and polysplenia: A review of cardiac and non-cardiac malformations in 60 cases with special reference to diagnosis and prognosis. *Br Heart J* 37:840, 1975.
2. Ruttenberg HD, Neufeld HN, Lucas RV Jr, Carey LS, Adams P Jr, Anderson RC, Edwards JE: Syndrome of congenital cardiac disease with asplenia: Distinction from other forms of congenital cyanotic cardiac disease. *Am J Cardiol* 13:387, 1964.

S

1. Shinebourne EA, Macartney FJ, Anderson RH: Sequential chamber localization: Logical approach to diagnosis in congenital heart disease. *Br Heart J* 38:327, 1976.
2. Soto B, Pacifico AD, Souza AS Jr, Bargeron LM, Ermocilla R, Tonkin IL: Identification of thoracic isomerism from the plain chest radiograph. *Am J Roentgenol* 131:995, 1978.
3. Stanger P, Rudolph AM, Edwards JE: Cardiac malpositions. *Circulation* 56:159, 1977.

T

1. de Tommasi SM, Daliento L, Ho SY, Macartney FJ, Anderson RH: Analysis of atrioventricular junction, ventricular mass, and ventriculoarterial junction in 43 specimens with atrial isomerism. *Br Heart J* 45:236, 1981.
2. Turley K, Tarnoff H, Snider R, Ebert P: Repair of combined total anomalous pulmonary venous connection and anomalous systemic venous connection. *Ann Thorac Surg* 31:70, 1981.

V

1. Van Mierop LHS, Wiglesworth FW: Isomerism of the cardiac atria in the asplenia syndrome. *Lab Invest* 11:1303, 1962.
2. Van Mierop LHS, Eisen S, Schiebler GL: The radiographic appearance of the tracheobronchial tree as an indicator of visceral situs. *Am J Cardiol* 26:432, 1970.

CARDIAC RHYTHM
DISTURBANCES

PART V

47

BRADYCARDIAS

DEFINITION

Abnormal bradycardia is a slow cardiac rate that results chronically or episodically in an inadequate cardiac output.

HISTORICAL NOTE

In the early 1700s, the peripheral pulsations of the circulation began to be timed, and in 1719 Gerbezius recognized bradycardia as a deviation from the usual pulse rate. Morgagni is believed to have surmised the relationship between bradycardia and syncope in 1761, but he attributed both to melancholy. In 1827, Adams accurately described the syndrome now known as the Adams-Stokes syndrome and proposed that it had a cardiac origin. This idea was not well accepted until Stokes, in 1846, collected reports of seven patients with the condition and agreed with Adams's con-

cepts. The phrase *maladie de Adams-Stokes* was originated in 1899 by Huchard.

Understanding of the morphologic basis of the Adams-Stokes syndrome began after Harvey's description of the cardiac cycle. Cardiac conduction tissues were first described by Purkinje in 1830. The atrioventricular (AV) conduction bundle was described by His in 1893. In 1896, Aschoff and Tawara described the AV node and its connection to the bundle of His. Then, in 1907, Keith and Flack described the sinoatrial (SA), or sinus, node. Its function was actually demonstrated in 1906 by Einthoven.

It has long been known that the heart is capable of responding to external electrical stimulation. As long ago as 1804, Aldini successfully stimulated systole in the hearts of decapitated criminals. Apparently it was known in the late 1800s that direct puncture of the heart with or without the installation of drugs would occasionally produce effective cardiac contractions. It is said by Mond[M2] that Lidwill, in

1347

Australia, in 1929 successfully paced the heart of a stillborn infant for a time by direct ventricular puncture. In 1932, Hyman[H3] atrially paced several patients with what he termed an *artificial pacemaker,* and Bigelow and Callaghan,[B2] in Toronto, paced canine hearts by esophageal and precordial electrodes in 1950.

In 1952, Zoll, in Boston, reported the successful pacing, with external cutaneous electrodes and a large and relatively nonmobile pulse generator, of the hearts of patients with complete heart block.[Z1] This method was the only one available when open cardiac surgery came into existence in the mid-1950s, and although the stimulation of each heartbeat was accompanied by skeletal muscle contractions and the skin under the electrodes quickly became excoriated, this method kept some cardiac surgical patients alive until sinus rhythm returned. However, as the days passed in patients in whom sinus rhythm did not return, the agony of the skeletal muscle contractions and skin excoriations increased. Sheer terror developed with the approach of the surgeon, who would each day provoke an Adams-Stokes episode by turning off the pacer to see if an adequate idioventricular rhythm, let alone sinus rhythm, would replace the electrocardiographic image of P waves without any QRS complex.

The change began when Lillehei in Minneapolis, Minnesota enlisted the help of a television engineer named Earl Bakken (later founder of the Medtronics Corporation) in developing a small portable pacemaker. More important, he devised the technique of leaving at operation a wire attached to the ventricular epicardium and brought out externally and used it and an external electrode to pace the heart with minimal discomfort to the patient.[W1] Later, Thevenet, Hodges, and Lillehei devised a method of inserting the wire into the ventricle through a needle passed through the skin of the precordium without an operation.[T2] These systems used the small portable pacemaker system devised by Bakken.

In 1959, Elmquist and Senning, in Stockholm, reported the placement of the first totally implantable pacemaker system, using epicardial electrodes.[E3] This development was made possible by the development of transistors in the 1950s. In 1960, Chardack, Gage, and Greatbatch described a self-contained, mercury cell battery–driven, implantable pulse generator for use with implanted epicardial leads.[C1]

In the previous year, Furman and Robinson had reported the use of endocardial electrodes introduced transvenously rather than epicardial electrodes placed at thoracotomy.[F5] Their paper reported data supporting the idea that endocardial and epicardial electrodes perform in an entirely similar manner. These developments led to the widespread availability by 1961 of both transvenously inserted endocardial electrodes and epicardial electrodes inserted by thoracotomy. These early pacemakers paced at a factory-set rate only and did not sense. They were crude by present standards but did make the difference between less than 50% 1-year survival and 85% 1-year survival for patients having Adams-Stokes episodes.

Rapid developments followed, and pulse generators that sensed the QRS and fired only when no spontaneous QRS occurred within the specified time period became available in the mid-1960s. Much work in the late 1960s and early 1970s to improve the cells (batteries), led by Greatbatch, resulted in the commercial availability of lithium-cell–powered pulse generators in the early 1970s. The lithium cells were much more reliable, and with hydrogen gas no longer being liberated in the pulse generator, hermetic sealing of the entire device became possible. To allow programming of rate and stimulus duration and to allow better QRS sensing, more complicated electronic circuits were developed, with an evolution from transistorized circuits with a few components to hybrid circuits with more components to integrated circuits and finally to implantable pulse generators containing microprocessors.

Further improvements have permitted atrial sensing and pacing as well as ventricular sensing and pacing (i.e., universal pacing) and ventricular pacing synchronized with the patient's atrial contractions as well as sequential atrioventricular pacing. Finally, the combination of multiprogrammability with diagnostic radio transmission has permitted precise evaluation of pacemaker function and improved treatment.

Improvements in the wires and electrodes have also been made through the years, in the form of improved alloys, antifracture characteristics, electrode pacing threshold properties, and lead insulation. These improvements have diminished the incidence of high pacing thresholds and lead fracture.

MORPHOLOGY

Abnormal bradycardia may be the result of complete heart block, a condition in which the P waves have a constant interval but are unrelated to less frequently occurring and often broad QRS complexes, or absent QRS complexes. Important bradycardia may result from abnormal or absent sinoatrial (sinus) node function.

Heart Block

Complete heart block may be present at birth or develop in later life.

Congenital Complete Heart Block
The musculature of the atrial septum may be congenitally deficient near the atrioventricular valves so that there is a diminished or absent connection between the atria and the AV node.[L1] Lev described morphologic discontinuity between the AV node and bundle of His as another basis for congenital complete heart block in otherwise normal hearts.[L2] In hearts with atrioventricular discordant connections, complete heart block may be present at birth, presumably related to these same mechanisms.

Spontaneously Developing Complete Heart Block
Some congenital anomalies of the bundle of His may predispose the patient to the development of complete heart block. Thus, in hearts with AV discordant connection, the unusually long length of the bundle of His is believed to predispose it to fibrosis and loss of function.

Certain disease processes may damage the conduction system. Calcification of the aortic valve may extend into the underlying ventricular septum and damage the bundle of His by a shearing effect during certain phases of the cardiac cycle. Mitral calcification less commonly does the same. Acute posteroinferior myocardial infarctions may be associated with temporary AV node ischemia and heart block.

An increase in the fibrous tissue of the bundle of His and its branches, accompanied by a decrease in the number of conduction fibers present, seems to be part of the aging process. Progressive fibrosis and fiber loss in the left and right bundle branches and resultant heart block (Lev's disease, Lenegre's disease) may be an abnormal acceleration of this process. Anteroseptal myocardial infarctions produce ischemic necrosis in and around the right and left bundle branches and may result in permanent heart block, and chronic ischemic heart disease may gradually result in septal fibrosis, with loss of function in both bundle branches. Dilated cardiomyopathy (see Chapter 51) may be associated with long-standing left ventricular fibrosis that may involve the bundle branches and produce complete heart block.

During surgical procedures for the repair of ventricular septal defects (isolated or as part of the tetralogy of Fallot and other complexes; see Chapters 20, 23, 39–44) or AV canal defects (see Chapter 19), the resection of discrete subvalvar aortic stenosis (see Chapter 32), and the replacement of the mitral or aortic or tricuspid valves (see Chapters 11–14), the bundle of His and/or the contiguous AV node may be severed, sutured, or even, in the absence of such direct injuries, functionally damaged by hemorrhage, with resultant complete heart block. Interestingly, in spite of the fibrosis that must develop in these surgical areas late postoperatively, late postoperative development of complete heart block is rare.

Other Bradycardias

Sinus Node Dysfunction

Important sinus node dysfunction may develop without any identifiable morphologic change in the node.[D1] However, the normal loss of sinus node cells with aging may accelerate and cause dysfunction, or this process in patients with a subnormal nodal cell population at birth may cause it.

Amyloid deposition may occur within the sinus node and produce dysfunction.

Direct damage to the sinus node by surgical procedures occurs but is uncommon. Damage to the sinus node can result in a junctional rhythm that becomes slower as time passes. In the absence of direct injury, surgical procedures in the region of the sinus node (such as the atrial switch operation; see Chapter 39) may result in late perinodal fibrosis, with consequent loss of sinus node function.

Dysfunction of Pathways between Sinus and Atrioventricular Nodes

Preferential conduction pathways between the sinus and AV nodes (see Chapter 1) may be interrupted by congenital absence of electrical continuity in these areas.[L2]

Surgical procedures, especially atrial switch operations (see Chapter 39) and the Fontan-type procedure (see Chapter 26), may rarely immediately damage the preferential conduction pathways. More commonly, late postoperative fibrosis develops and interferes with conduction along these pathways, and a slow junctional rhythm results.

CLINICAL FEATURES AND DIAGNOSTIC CRITERIA

Pathophysiology

Hemodynamic Effects

Although blood flow into the aorta and large arteries is intermittent (pulsatile), the combined effects of the aortic valve, the elasticity of the aorta and great arteries, and the characteristics of the arterial distributing system make the flow relatively constant in capillaries. Thus, the cells of the brain and other organs receive a continuous nutrient flow. The magnitude of this flow is related to, among other things, the net forward flow across the aortic valve with each ventricular systole, and the heart rate. When the stroke volume is large and the heart rate slow, as in trained athletes at rest, the elasticity of the aorta and its filling during systole are sufficient to maintain an adequate volume of runoff during a long diastolic period and thus an adequate nutrient flow to the cells of the brain and other organs.

When stroke volume is not large, the runoff during the late part of chronically long diastolic periods may be inadequate to maintain the proper internal milieu of cells of the brain and other organs. Since the brain is particularly sensitive to hypoxia, cerebral symptoms usually develop before those from dysfunction of other organs.

Cardiac Electrophysiologic Effects

The longer the intervals between the periodic depolarizations of heart muscle, the greater the degree of QT prolongation and the likelihood of the development of ventricular extrasystoles and/or tachycardia, especially of the torsades de pointe variety.[M4] Thus, bradycardia predisposes the patient to life-threatening ventricular arrhythmias. Further, at least with complete heart block, there always remains the possibility of prolonged ventricular asystole.

Heart Block

Clinical manifestations of first-degree heart block (PR interval > 0.2 seconds in adults) are rare. Second-degree heart block (intermittent lack of AV conduction[1]) may be manifested by bradycardia and symptoms. In third-degree (complete) heart block (all atrial impulses fail to be conducted to the ventricle), bradycardia is present, and symptoms are frequent.

The proportion of patients with spontaneously developing complete heart block who remain asymptomatic is not known. The most common clinical manifestation is an Adams-Stokes episode, which is part of the history in 60%–70% of patients presenting with complete heart block.[P1,S3]

---

[1]The two types of second-degree heart block are Mobitz I, in which AV conduction time is progressively prolonged (Wenckebach period) until one atrial impulse is not conducted to the ventricle; and Mobitz II, in which AV conduction times are constant, but episodically an atrial impulse is not conducted to the ventricles.

Palpitations and angina occur infrequently. Symptoms of chronic cardiac failure occur in about half the patients presenting with spontaneously developing complete heart block.

Sinus Node Dysfunction

Patients presenting with bradycardia from spontaneous sinus node dysfunction (or failure of conduction from the sinus to the AV node) may be without other signs of cardiac disease. However, 25% have associated ischemic heart disease.[O1,S3]

Many patients are without symptoms when first seen, but about 20% are symptomatic.[L3,S2] Most patients eventually become symptomatic. Syncope is the predominant symptom,[R1,S3] but palpitations, dyspnea, and angina also occur.

Diagnostic Criteria

Bradycardias are diagnosed largely by electrocardiographic criteria (Table 47-1).

Atrioventricular Block

Established complete (third-degree) AV block and symptomatic incomplete AV block (e.g., 2:1 second-degree AV block) are diagnosed in the standard electrocardiogram (ECG). When paroxysmal AV block is suspected as the cause of symptoms, prolonged ambulatory ECG monitoring may provide confirmation of the diagnosis. In a minority of patients with chronic bundle-branch block of their resting ECG, unexplained transient neurologic symptoms, and negative ambulatory monitoring, electrophysiologic study is indicated. Among such symptomatic patients, the finding of prolongation of the HV interval $\geq$ 70 milliseconds supports a diagnosis of paroxysmal AV block as the cause of symptoms and justifies elective pacemaker implantation.[S7] It must be emphasized, however, that in the absence of neurologic symptoms, the finding of such HV prolongation rarely, if ever, warrants prophylactic pacemaker implantation.[D3]

Sick Sinus Syndrome

Symptomatic arrhythmias in the sick sinus syndrome include profound sinus bradycardia, junctional bradycardia, sinus arrest and/or sinus node exit block, and the so-called *bradycardia-tachycardia syndrome,* in which paroxysmal atrial tachycardia, flutter, or fibrillation is often followed by symptomatic pauses due to overdrive suppression of the sinus node and subsidiary pacemakers. Unfortunately, in most patients the resting ECG is nondiagnostic, and prolonged ambulatory ECG monitoring is required to document the symptomatic rhythm. When symptoms are relatively infrequent, the decision to advise permanent pacing may rest on the demonstration of asymptomatic sinus pauses and/or sinoatrial exit block. At present, electrophysiologic study is of limited help, since abnormal sinus node recovery times or sinoatrial conduction times are demonstrable in only a small minority of symptomatic patients. Ongoing research to refine the sensitivity of these tests and the direct recording of sinus node potentials may, however, change this in the future.[T4]

Carotid Sinus Syndrome

A hyperactive carotid sinus reflex is said to be present when digital stimulation of the carotid sinus results in cardiac asystole lasting 3 or more seconds.[T3] The carotid sinus syndrome is diagnosed when, in addition to the presence of a hyperactive reflex, the patient's spontaneous symptom complex can be reproduced by stimulation of one or both (not simultaneously) carotid sinuses. In patients with only a cardioinhibitory response, pacemaker therapy may completely relieve symptoms. However, the presence of a simultaneous vasodepressor response should also be sought by repetition of massage after intravenous atropine and measurements of the blood pressure. In such patients, preservation of the heart rate may not prevent symptoms due to hypotension.

NATURAL HISTORY

Bradycardia from both spontaneous heart block and spontaneous sinus node dysfunction tends to occur in elderly patients. The mean age of patients at the time of diagnosis of spontaneously occurring heart block is 70 years.[A1,S3]

Spontaneously Developing Complete Heart Block

Probably the majority of patients with complete heart block eventually develop symptoms, the exact proportion in part determined by the functional status of the heart as a whole. Likewise, the tendency toward premature death is related to the functional status of the rest of the heart as well as other risk factors.

Patients who develop Adams-Stokes episodes as a manifestation of complete heart block and who are not paced have a 1-year survival rate of 50%–75%,[E1,F2,P1] less than that of an age-, race-, and sex-matched general population. The 1-year survival rate is said to be 70%–80% in patients with complete heart block but without a history of syncope.

Table 47-1 Electrocardiographic indications in patients undergoing the implantation of permanent pacemakers (GLH; 1981; *n* = 120).

ECG Indications	No. of Patients	% of 120
Second-degree AVB		
Mobitz II	1	0.8%
2:1 AVB	7	6%
High-grade AVB	14	12%
Alternating bundle-branch block	2	2%
Complete AVB	47	39%
Sick sinus syndrome (including transient asystole three patients)	29	24%
None[a]	20	17%
Totally normal ECG	4	
1° AVB only	1	
Unifasicular block or ICD	3	
Bifasicular block	12	
Total	120	

KEY: AVB, atrioventricular block; ICD, intraventricular conduction defect.
[a]Eighteen of these 20 patients had syncope.

These differences persist over a follow-up period of 15 years and appear to be related to the considerably higher incidence of sudden death in the patients who have syncopal attacks.[P1] Syncopal attacks as well as sudden death in patients with complete heart block (who are surviving with an idioventricular or bundle of His rhythm) usually result from sudden asystole but may be precipitated by a sudden reduction in stroke volume or increased metabolic demands.

Congenital Complete Heart Block

For infants born with congenital complete heart block and hearts that are otherwise normal, the prognosis may be somewhat better than that for patients with spontaneously developing complete heart block.[E2,M1,P2] The 10-year survival rate is said to be about 85%,[E2,P2] with most of the deaths occurring in the first month of life. Deaths that occur after this time are related to Adams-Stokes episodes.

About two-thirds of surviving patients with congenital complete heart block and otherwise normal hearts are asymptomatic during their first 10 years. When symptoms develop, they usually do so in the first month of life and consist of symptoms of heart failure or Adams-Stokes episodes. The probability of survival is lessened considerably when symptoms are present.

Surgically Induced Complete Heart Block

In the first few years of cardiac surgery, when epicardial and transvenous pacing was not possible, hospital mortality was greatly increased in patients in whom complete heart block developed perioperatively. Unpaced hospital survivors with surgically induced complete heart block had a low 1-year survival rate of about 40%.[L1,L4]

Currently, the development of complete heart block, when properly managed, does not increase hospital mortality (e.g., see Chapter 43).

Sinus Node Dysfunction

The natural history of patients with this type of bradycardia has not been described clearly.

TECHNIQUE OF OPERATION

Pacing Modes

A number of different pacing modes are used (UAB). Discussion of these is facilitated by using the commonly employed abbreviations (Table 47-2).[P3]

VVI

Although the VVI mode is currently the most commonly used, technological advances may change this in the future. In the VVI mode, the ventricle is paced, sensing is from the ventricle, and the response to a sensed ventricular depolarization is inhibition of generation of the next electrical stimulus by the pulse generator.

With this pacing mode, the disadvantage is lack of atrial

Table 47-2 Pacemaker code describing the function of pulse generators. Usually, only the abbreviations for positions I–III are used (for example, VVI).

Position in Code	Description of Position	Alternatives and Their Abbreviations
I	Chamber(s) paced	V, ventricle A, atrium D, double
II	Chamber(s) sensed	V, ventricle A, atrium D, double 0, none
III	Mode of response(s)	T, trigger I, inhibit D, double 0, none R, reverse
IV	Programmable functions	P, programmable rate and/or output M, multiprogrammable 0, none
V	Special tachyarrhythmia functions	B, burst N, normal rate competition S, scanning E, external

contribution to ventricular filling. The advantage is simplicity of electrode placement and a relatively long life of the pulse generator.

AAI

The AAI mode requires normal AV conduction and some functioning atrial pathways to the AV node. In this mode, the atrium (nearly always the right atrium) is paced, sensing is from the atrium, and sensed atrial depolarization inhibits the next scheduled electrical impulse. This type of pacing mode was anticipated and pioneered by Lillehei and colleagues as early as 1963.[L1]

The AAI mode is used less than 5% of the time, primarily because many patients with sinus node dysfunction ultimately require ventricular pacing. The advantage of this mode is that the atrial contribution to ventricular filling is preserved.

VDD

The VDD mode, as well as the DVI and DDD modes, described below, require both an atrial and a ventricular electrode. The VDD mode also requires relatively normal sinus node function. The ventricle is paced, both the atrium and ventricle are sensed, and the response of the pulse generator may be either the triggering or the inhibition of the next electrical pulse. Generally, sensed atrial depolarization triggers a stimulating pulse to the ventricular electrode at a preset or variable PR interval. The ventricular stimulus is inhibited when spontaneous ventricular depolarization follows the atrial depolarization, within the set PR interval of the pulse generator. The pulse generator is so programmed that when the PP interval becomes excessively long, the pulse generator functions in the VVI mode.

The advantages of the VDD mode are that the atrial contribution to ventricular filling is preserved and that the ventricular rate follows the patient's own atrial rate and thus responds appropriately to stress and exercise. The disadvantages are the need for both atrial and ventricular electrodes and the possibility of the production of a reciprocating (loop) tachycardia by retrograde conduction.

DVI

Both atrium and ventricle are paced in the DVI mode, with an appropriate interval between the stimuli to each. Ventricular but not atrial depolarization is sensed. A sensed ventricular depolarization inhibits the next dual pacing stimulus in the noncommitted DVI mode; it does not in the committed DVI mode.

The advantages are that the atrial contribution to ventricular filling is maintained even when sinus node function fails. Raza and colleagues and Raichlen and colleagues, as well as others, have documented the hemodynamic advantages of this arrangement.[R2,R3] The disadvantage is that AV synchronization is lost when the atrial rate increases during exercise or emotion.

DDD

The DDD mode, or so-called *universal pacing mode,* can pace both atrium and ventricle, sense both atrial and ventricular depolarization, and either trigger or inhibit an electrical pacing pulse (Fig. 47-1).

Its advantage is the universality of its application. Its disadvantages are that dual stimulation reduces battery lifetime and that loop tachycardia may occur with variations in retrograde conduction from ventricles to atria. These disadvantages may be eliminated or reduced by reprogramming the pacemaker pulse generator characteristics when the patient's AV and ventriculoarterial (VA) conduction characteristics change.

Pulse Generators

Currently available pulse generators use lithium iodide batteries as a power source (UAB). Pulse generators are continuously improved by the manufacturers. While the pulse generators of choice are subject to change, the following have been in common use (UAB).

The Siemens-Elema 668 is a reliable single-chamber AAI or VVI pulse generator. It has the capability for measuring pacing thresholds noninvasively. It is relatively inexpensive, and the amplitude of the electrical pulse can be varied set at 2.5, 5, or 10 volts (v). The device is multiprogrammable. It has the special feature of allowing the pacing threshold to be checked by telephone (see "Special Features of Postoperative Care").

The Teletronics Optima MP has characteristics similar to those of the Siemens-Elema 668.

The Cordis 233F is the most commonly used dual-chamber pulse generator. It is a flexible device that can be reprogrammed with a small hand-held programmer with printing capabilities.

The Pacesetter 283 is a dual-chamber multiprogrammable pulse generator. In addition to its other features, it has nearly continuous variability of the amplitude of the electrical pulse. It generates a printed electrogram.

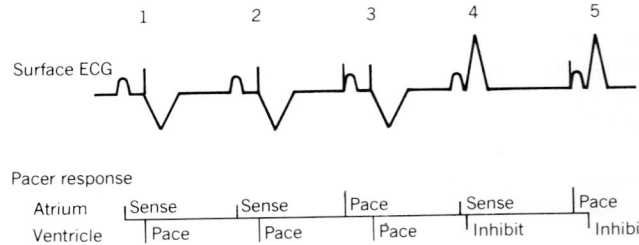

Figure 47-1 The possible responses to DDD pacing.
Reproduced with permission from Satler et al.[S5]

The Intermedics 283 is a dual-chamber pulse generator with an event counter that permits evaluation of the utilization of the pacing system.

Leads

For transvenous insertion and ventricular pacing, the Cordis 327-152 lead is most commonly used with the Cordis and the Siemens-Elema pulse generators (UAB); for atrial pacing, the Cordis 327–745 and the Medtronic 6990U leads are most commonly employed (UAB).

For insertion at open operation, the Medtronic 6917 screw-in and the Medtronic 5815 coiled-spring leads are most commonly placed for ventricular pacing (UAB). In infants and small children, the Medtronic coiled-spring lead with the coil bent back or the Medtronic 6917 screw-in lead (35 cm long, 2.5 turns) is used. When atrial pacing is to be used, the Medtronic 5815 coiled-spring electrode is modified by bending back the electrode and suturing the device to the atrial wall. For both ventricular and atrial pacing, the Medtronic 4951 stick-on epicardial lead has been used, but it has been found that its pacing threshold tends to be high.

Lead Testing

Each lead placed is tested at the time of insertion, but the *pacing threshold,* or the delivered voltage at which myocardial depolarization occurs, is tested first. For ventricular leads, a threshold of 0.3 (usually at 0.5 millisecond pulse duration) is optimal, but frequently the threshold is between 0.3 and 0.5 v. A threshold as high as 0.85 (UAB) to 1.0 (GLH) is acceptable; higher thresholds are undesirable, since they reduce the pulse generator life. For atrial leads, a stimulating threshold of 1.0 v is acceptable.

The lead is then tested for its sensing capabilities. For both endocardial and epicardial ventricular leads, a QRS complex in the electrogram greater than 5 millivolts (mv) with a satisfactory slew rate is desirable. For atrial leads, a P wave with peak-to-peak amplitude greater than 2 mv is acceptable.

Two additional criteria are particularly important in transvenously placed leads: the lead must not provoke ventricular tachycardia by its position, and its position must be mechanically stable.

In open chest insertion, it must be remembered that use of the electrocautery tends to increase the stimulating threshold.

Unipolar leads are generally used, and with them, the device itself is the indifferent electrode. Bipolar leads are

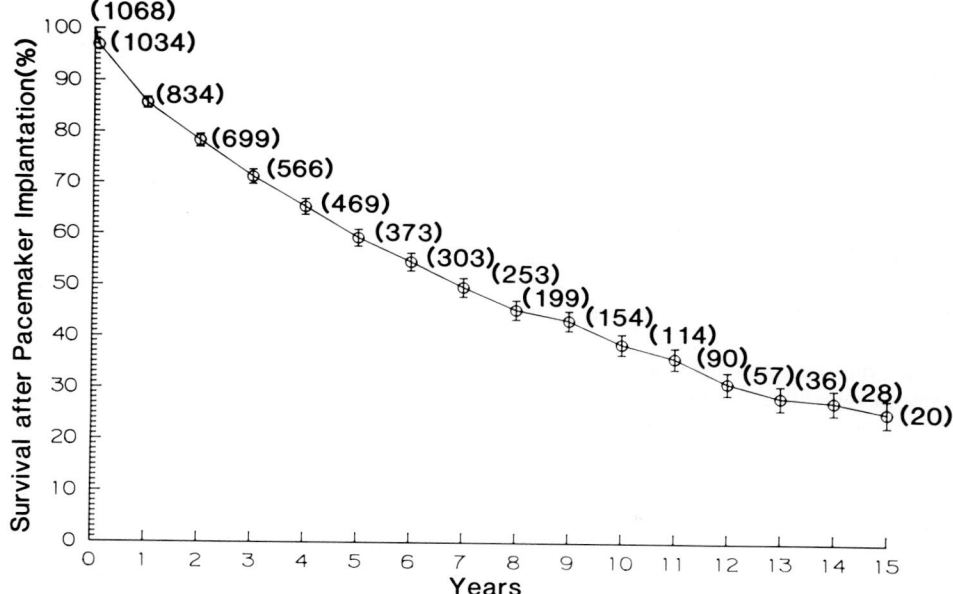

Figure 47-2 Actuarial survival of patients with permanent implantation of pulse generators (UAB; 1961–1984; *n* = 1,068; 502 deaths). Time zero is the end of surgery. The vertical lines encompass the standard error of the mean.

Reproduced with permission from Shepard and Pigott.[S6]

1984). The treatment is the insertion of an entirely new pacemaker system at a different site and complete removal of the old system, as has been emphasized by Beder and colleagues.[B3]

Excessive pressure of the pulse generator or wire against the overlying skin or subcutaneous tissue may cause necrosis and permit pacemaker or wire exposure, a problem said to occur in about 4% of cases.[S4] The true incidence of this condition is unknown, since it is often considered infection. Prevention of this problem is best achieved by the formation of the pulse generator pocket in the immediate prefascial space to permit as much tissue as possible to come between pulse generator and skin. In addition, the insertion of pulse generators in small pockets with skin closure under tension seems to increase the chance of skin necrosis. When the pulse generator and leads become exposed as a result of pressure necrosis, the treatment is the same as for an infected pacemaker.

Lead and Electrode Malfunction

Electrode Dislodgment
With or without right ventricular perforation, electrode dislodgment is the most common complication of the insertion of both ventricular and atrial endocardial leads. However, dislodgment occurs in less than 2% of cases.[F2,V1]

High Pacing Threshold
The threshold commonly increases within the first 6–8 days after implantation and becomes stable within 2–6 months. A high pacing threshold occurs in 3%–8% of patients.[F2] The incidence is higher (13%) in patients in whom the need for

pacing developed at the time of cardiac surgery and CPB (UAB). The incidence can be minimized by searching for the location with the lowest threshold at initial electrode placement and minimizing the use of the electrocautery at operation once the lead is in place (UAB).

The use of pacemakers that have high as well as normal output capabilities generally obviates the need for reoperation when a high pacing threshold develops. In intractable cases, placement of a new lead is necessary.

Undersensing
Most commonly, undersensing, or the lack of recognition of the heart's depolarization, is related to inadequate placement of the electrode; at times, it can be the result of later fibrosis at the electrode-myocardial junction. This complication leads to competitive pacing. Generally, undersensing can be treated by noninvasive programming to increase the sensitivity of the pulse generator.

Table 47-3 Survival by patient age after pacemaker implantation (UAB; 1961–August 1984; *n* = 1,068).

Age (yr)		5-Year Survival Rate
≤	<	
40 --- 50		83%
50 --- 60		66%
60 --- 70		67%
70 --- 80		62%
80 --- 90		51%

Lead Fracture

Currently, lead fracture, with its consequent loss of pacing, is an infrequent early complication of pacemaking but not uncommon years after implantation.

Pulse Generator Malfunction

Oversensing

One type of pulse generator malfunction, oversensing, consists of inappropriate inhibition of pacing by stimuli that do not originate from myocardial depolarization in the chamber being sensed. The most frequent cause of oversensing by an atrial circuit is skeletal muscle depolarization but may be the voltage of ventricular depolarization. This problem may be corrected by adjusting the sensitivity or in some instances prolonging the atrial refractory period in pulse generators in which this is possible. Oversensing by a ventricular circuit is usually the result of depolarization in skeletal muscle. The T wave may on occasions be sensed. This malfunction may be treated by altering the pulse generator sensitivity, changing the mode of pacing, or changing to bipolar pacing.

Pacemaker Arrhythmias

The introduction of dual-chamber pacing has been associated with a substantial increase in pacemaker-mediated rhythm disturbances. Retrograde conduction across the AV node and bundle of His (or across an accessory pathway; see Chapter 48) sets the stage for this type of rhythm disturbance. In such a setting, and when the pacemaker is in the VDD or DDD mode, ventricular depolarization is conducted retrograde to the atrium, where it stimulates atrial depolarization and a P wave. The pulse generator senses this as a P wave and stimulates another ventricular depolarization, which again is conducted retrograde to the atrium, and a reciprocating tachycardia is created. This persists until the retrograde loop is by chance stimulated during its refractory period or the pulse generator is reprogrammed.

The usual initial treatment is to reset the pulse generator to a simple VVI mode by external means, usually a magnet. Noninvasive reprogramming of the atrial refractory period can then usually prevent recurrence.

New Symptoms from Pacing

One of the most important new symptoms from pacing is syncope or near syncope, although it occurs in less than 10% of patients being paced in the VVI mode (Table 47-4). Arterial hypotension may also develop. These symptoms usually occur when ventriculoatrial conduction is intact and the indication for pacing has been sinus node dysfunction.[N1,N2] Their exact etiology is uncertain, but they may be caused by lack of atrial contribution to ventricular filling, secondary to atrioventricular asynchrony with or without atrial contraction against a closed AV valve. Also, AV valve incompetence may be caused by asynchronous contraction of atria and ventricles.[M3] The diagnosis is suspected from the situation and symptoms and is sometimes verified by a rise in blood pressure when pacing is stopped and a fall when pacing is begun. The treatment is a VDD or DDD mode of pacing.

Dizziness may be described as a symptom in about one-third of patients (Table 47-4). Since both dizziness and syncope are common in elderly patients in general, these symp-

Table 47-4 Symptoms during the follow-up period in patients with VVI pacing (GLH; 1981; n = 120; mean age, 72 years).

Symptoms	No.	%	CL
Neck flushing	1	1%	0.1%–3%
Postural hypotension	1	1%	0.1%–3%
Classic angina	10	10%	7%–14%
Atypical chest pain	27	26%	21%–31%
Muscle twitch[a]	22	21%	17%–26%
Syncope	7	7%	4%–10%
Dizziness	38	37%	31%–42%
Palpitations[b]	34	33%	28%–38%

KEY: CL, 70% confidence limits.

NOTE: Ten patients died over a 12-month period, one patient had the unit explanted, and 5 patients were lost to follow-up; thus, the follow-up data concern 104 patients.

[a] Transient in the vast majority of cases.

[b] In half of the cases, this was due to awareness of ventricular pacing.

toms may not be the result of the pacing itself in all instances. Palpitations are noted by about one-third of patients, sometimes due simply to awareness of ventricular pacing. Palpitations are noted frequently at night, when sinus slowing in patients with VVI units results in pacemaker activation. Such palpitations may be eliminated by AAI or DDD pacing or minimized by programming hysteresis into a VVI pacing system.

INDICATIONS FOR OPERATION

Indications for Pacing

The most common and noncontroversial indication for permanent cardiac pacing is symptomatic bradycardia. The symptomatic bradycardia may be intermittent or permanent and due to complete heart block, second-degree AV block, or sinus node dysfunction. The symptoms must be directly attributable to the bradycardia and may include syncope, dizziness, exercise intolerance, and congestive heart failure. Another noncontroversial indication is surgically induced complete heart block, because of the risk of an Adams-Stokes episode if a pacemaker is not placed.

Patients in sinus rhythm after the repair of congenital malformations but in whom complete heart block followed the repair and persisted for a number of days before the reversion to sinus rhythm are at increased risk of developing late symptomatic heart block. Such patients should be considered for prophylactic pacemaker implantation before hospital dismissal, particularly when subsidiary escape pacemakers have been absent or unreliable.

In some situations, permanent pacing may be indicated in patients with no symptoms.[F3] These situations include profound bradycardia (ventricular rate < 40), second-degree AV block at the infra-His level, advanced second-degree AV or complete heart block after myocardial infarction, and congenital heart block with a wide QRS escape rhythm. In such situations, permanent pacing is indicated because of the risk of an Adams-Stokes episode.

In asymptomatic patients, other rhythms can, under some circumstances, be an indication for pacing. Such circumstances include new bundle-branch block with transient second-degree AV block postmyocardial infarction,[H1] bifascicular bundle-branch block with intermittent type II second-degree AV block,[H1] sinus node dysfunction,[H1] and transient postsurgical AV block that reverts to bifascicular block in children.[F3] In addition, certain patients have major symptoms without documented bradycardia. Some of them require pacemakers after complete and thoughtful evaluation.

A special situation involves the patient after such extensive intra-atrial operations as the Senning or Mustard operation (see Chapter 39) or the Fontan type of operation with a complex atrial baffle (see Chapters 26 and 44). Late postoperatively, a junctional rhythm often develops, and the patient may be potentially subject to tachybradycardias and sudden death. Such a development is an indication for atrial pacing (AAI), the electrodes for which can be introduced through the subclavian vein (UAB).[M3]

Indications for Modes of Pacing

The indications for the various modes of pacing are still controversial, but some general guidelines are used (UAB). The single-chamber (AAI) mode (see Table 47-2) is recommended for patients with sinus node dysfunction and documented normal AV node and bundle of His function. The VVI mode, the most frequently used, is indicated for any symptomatic bradycardia except as otherwise noted. Dual-chamber pacing should be reserved for patients with the pacemaker syndrome or with a hemodynamic or symptomatic need for atrial contribution to cardiac output. If such an indication exists and the atrial rate is slow, DVI pacing is used; if the atrial rate is adequate, the VDD mode is used. If the hemodynamic state requires AV synchrony over a wide range of rates, the DDD mode is indicated, particularly in young patients.

REFERENCES

A

1. Alpert MA, Katti SK: Natural history of high-grade atrioventricular block following permanent pacemaker implantation. *J Chronic Dis* 35:341, 1982.

2. Alpert MA, Katti SK: Natural history of sinus node dysfunction after permanent pacemaker implantation. *South Med J* 75(10):1182, 1982.

B

1. Beyer J: Pacemaker implantation and sudden death, in C Meere (ed): *Cardiac Pacing. Proceedings of the VIth World Symposium on Cardiac Pacing.* Montreal: Laplante & Langevin, 1979.

2. Bigelow WG, Callaghan JC, Hopps JA: General hypothermia for experimental intracardiac surgery: The use of electrophrenic respirations, an artificial pacemaker for cardiac standstill, and radiofrequency rewarming in general hypothermia. *Ann Surg* 132:531, 1950.

3. Beder SD, Hanisch DG, Cohen MH, Van Heeckeren D, Ankenny JL, Riemenschneider TA: Cardiac pacing in children: A 15-year experience. *Am Heart J* 109:152, 1985.

C

1. Chardack WM, Gage AA, Greatbatch W: A transistorized, self-contained, implantable pacemaker for the long-term correction of complete heart block. *Surgery* 48:643, 1960.

D

1. Davies MJ, Anderson R, Becker A: *The Conduction System of the Heart.* London: Butterworth, 1983, p 207.

2. Davidson DM, Braall CA, Preston TA, Judge RD: Permanent ventricular pacing: Effect on long-term survival, congestive heart failure, and subsequent myocardial infarction and stroke. *Ann Intern Med* 77:345, 1972.

3. Dhingra RC, Palileo E, Strasberg B, Swiryn S, Bauerfeind RA, Wyndham CRC, Rosen KM: Significance of the HV interval in 517 patients with chronic bifasicular block. *Circulation* 64:1265, 1981.

E

1. Edhag O, Swahn A: Prognosis of patients with complete heart block or arrhythmic syncope who were not treated with artificial pacemakers. *Acta Med Scand* 200:457, 1976.

2. Esscher E, Michaelsson M: Assessment and management of complete heart block, in MJ Godman, RM Marquis (eds): *Pediatric Cardiology,* vol. 2. Edinburgh: Churchill Livingstone, 1979.

3. Elmquist R, Senning A: Implantable pacemaker for the heart, in CN Smyth (ed): *Medical Electronics: Proceedings of the Second International Conference on Medical Electronics, Paris, June 1959.* London: Iliffe & Sons, 1960.

F

1. Furman S, Pannizzo F: Output programmability and reduction of secondary intervention after pacemaker implantation. *J Thorac Cardiovasc Surg* 81:713, 1981.

2. Friedberg CK, Donoso E, Stein WG: Nonsurgical acquired heart block. *Ann NY Acad Sci* 111:835, 1964.

3. Frye RL, Collins JJ, DeSanctis RW, Dodge HT, Dreifus LS, Fisch C, Gettes LS, Gillette PC, Parsonnet V, Reeves TJ: Guidelines for permanent cardiac pacemaker implantation. *JACC* 4:434, 1984.

4. Furman S: Life expectancy of patients with implanted pacemakers. *PACE* 6:A28, 1983.

5. Furman S, Robinson G: The use of an intracardiac pacemaker in the correction of total heart block. *Surg Forum* 9:245, 1958.

H

1. Hindman MC, Wagner GS, JaRo M, Scheinman MM, DeSanctis RW, Hutter AH, Yeatman L, Rubenfire M, Pujura C, Rubin M, Morris JJ: The clinical significance of bundle branch block complicating acute myocardial infarction. II. Indications for temporary and permanent pacemaker insertion. *Circulation* 58(4):689, 1978.

2. Hauser RG, Jones J, Moss K, Edwards LM, Messer JV: Survival after pacemaker implantation, in K Steinbach, D Glogar, A Laszkovics, AW Scheibelhofer, H Weber (eds): *Cardiac Pacing: Proceedings of the VIIth World Symposium on Cardiac Pacing.* Vienna: Steinkopff-Verlag-Darmstadt, 1983.

3. Hyman AS: Resuscitation of the stopped heart by intracardial therapy. II. Experimental use of an artificial pacemaker. *Arch Intern Med* 50:283, 1932.

L

1. Lillehei CW, Sellers RD, Bonnabeau RC Jr, Elliot RS: Chronic postsurgical complete heart block: With particular reference to prognosis, management, and a new P-wave pacemaker. *J Thorac Cardiovasc Surg* 46:436, 1963.

2. Lev M: Pathogenesis of congenital atrioventricular block. *Prog Cardiovasc Dis* 15:145, 1972.

3. Lien WP, Lee YS, Chang FZ, Lee SY, Chen CM, Tsai HC: The sick sinus syndrome: Natural history of dysfunction of the sinoatrial node. *Chest* 72:628, 1977.

4. Lillehei CW, Levy MJ, Bonnabeau RC, et al: Direct wire electrical stimulation for acute postsurgical and postinfarction complete heart block. *Ann NY Acad Sci* 3:938, 1966.

M

1. Michaelsson M, Engle MA: Congenital complete heart block: An international study of the natural history. *Cardiovasc Clin* 4:86, 1972.

2. Mond HG: *The Cardiac Pacemaker: Function and Malfunction.* New York: Grune & Stratton, 1983, p 409.

3. McGoon MD, Maloney JD, McGoon DC, Danielson GK: Long-term endocardial atrial pacing in children with postoperative bradycardia-tachycardia syndrome and limited ventricular access. *Am J Cardiol* 49:1750, 1982.

4. Motte G, Coumel P, Abitol G, Dessertenne F, Slama R: Le syndrome QT long et syncopes par 'torsades de pointe.' *Arch Mal Coeur* 63:831, 1970.

N

1. Naclerio EA, Varriale P: Anterior axillary minithoracotomy: The optimal approach for left ventricular sutureless electrode implantation, in C Meere (ed): *Proceedings of the VIth World Symposium on Cardiac Pacing.* Montreal: Laplante & Langevin, 1979.

2. Nishimura RA, Gersh BJ, Holmes DR, Vlietstra RE, Broadbent JC: Outcome of dual-chamber pacing for the pacemaker syndrome. *Mayo Clin Proc* 58:452, 1983.

O

1. Otterstad JE, Selmer R, Strom O: Prognosis in cardiac pacing. *Acta Med Scand* 210:47, 1982.

P

1. Penton GB, Miller H, Levine SA: Some clinical features of complete heart block. *Circulation* 13(6):801, 1956.

2. Pinsky WW, Gillette PC, Garson A Jr, McNamara DG: Diagnosis, management and long-term results of patients with congenital complete atrioventricular block. *Pediatrics* 69(6):728, 1982.

3. Parsonnet V, Furman S, Smyth NP: A revised code for pacemaker identification: Pacemaker study group. *Circulation* 64:60A, 1981.

4. Phibbs B, Friedman HS, Graboys TB, Lown B, Marriott HJL, Nelson WP, Preston T: Indications for pacing in the treatment of bradycardias. Report of an independent study group. *JAMA* 252:1307, 1984.

R

1. Rokseth R, Hatle L: Prospective study on the occurrence and management of chronic sinoatrial disease, with follow-up. *Br Heart J* 36:582, 1974.

2. Raza ST, Lajos TZ, Bhayana JN, Lee AB Jr, Lewin AN, Gehring B, Schimert G: Improved cardiovascular hemodynamics with atrioventricular sequential pacing compared with ventricular demand pacing. *Ann Thorac Surg* 38:260, 1984.

3. Raichlen JS, Campbell FW, Edie RN, Josephson ME, Harken AE: The effect of the site of placement of temporary epicardial pacemakers on ventricular function in patients undergoing cardiac surgery. *Circulation* 70(suppl I):I-118, 1984.

S

1. Schechter DC: Background of clinical cardiac electrostimulation. *NY State J Med* 71:2575, 72:270, 1971, 1972.

2. Shaw DB, Holman RR, Gowers JI: Survival in sinoatrial disorder (sick-sinus syndrome). *Br Med J* 21:139, 1980.

3. Simon AB, Janz N: Symptomatic bradyarrhythmias in the adult: Natural history following ventricular pacemaker implantation. *PACE* 5:372, 1982.

4. Siddons H, Nowak K: Surgical complications of implanting pacemakers. *Br J Surg* 62:929, 1975.

5. Satler LE, Shepard RB: New trends in permanent cardiac pacing. *Ala J Med Sci* 20(2):192, 1983.

6. Shepard RB and Pigott J: (1984) Personal communication.

7. Scheinman MM, Peters RW, Modin G, Brennan M, Mies C, O'Young J: Prognostic valve of infranodal conduction time in patients with chronic bundle branch block. *Circulation* 56:240, 1977.

8. Shahar E, Feldman S, Shem-Tov A, Hegesh J, Barzilay Z, Neufeld HN: Permanent cardiac pacing in congenital heart disease: A follow-up study of 20 patients. *Europ Heart J* 5:829, 1984.

T

1. Thalen HJ, Meere CC: *Fundamentals of Cardiac Pacing.* London: Martinus Nijhoff, 1979, pp–1–22.

2. Thevenet R, Hodges PC, Lillehei CW: The use of a myocardial electrode inserted percutaneously for control of complete atrioventricular block by an artificial pacemaker. *Dis Chest* 34:1.

3. Thomas JE: Hyperactive carotid sinus reflex and carotid sinus syncope. *Mayo Clin Proc* 44:127, 1969.

4. Tonkin AM, Heddle WF: Electrophysiological testing of sinus node function. *PACE* 7:735, 1984.

V

1. Venditti J, Lajos TZ, Raza ST, Lewin AN, Bhayana JN, Lee AB Jr, Kohn R: 15 year experience with atrial electrodes and pacing, in K Steinbach, D Golgar, A Laszkovics, W Scheibelhofer, H Weber (eds): *Cardiac Pacing: Proceedings of the VIIth World Symposium on Cardiac Pacing.* Vienna: Steinkopff-Verlag-Darmstadt, 1983, p 401.

W

1. Weirich WL, Gott VL, Lillehei CW: Treatment of complete heart block by the combined use of a myocardial electrode and an artificial pacemaker. *Surgical Forum* 8:360, 1958.

Z

1. Zoll PM: Resuscitation of the heart in ventricular standstill by external electric stimulation. *N Engl J Med* 274:768, 1952.

48

TACHYCARDIAS

DEFINITION

Abnormal tachycardia is a rapid heartbeat out of proportion to the metabolic demands on the circulation. This chapter discusses the surgical aspects of symptomatic and life-threatening tachycardia.

Tachycardia may be supraventricular in origin, with accelerated antegrade and/or retrograde conduction through an atrioventricular (AV) bypass tract (Wolff-Parkinson-White syndrome); it may be an AV node reentrant tachycardia or an automatic or reentrant junctional tachycardia; or it may result from an intra-atrial automatic focus (ectopic atrial tachycardia). Tachycardia may also originate in atrial fibrillation or flutter. However, it may originate entirely within the ventricles and is then termed *ventricular tachycardia* or *ventricular fibrillation*.

SECTION 1

WOLFF-PARKINSON-WHITE SYNDROME

DEFINITION

As originally described, the Wolff-Parkinson-White syndrome (WPW) consisted of bundle-branch block with a short PR interval in healthy young people prone to paroxysmal tachycardia,[W1] but its definition now includes the presence of delta waves and a broad QRS complex in the electrocardiogram and accessory atrioventricular conduction pathways called *Kent bundles,* which conduct in at least an antegrade fashion. WPW is one of the *preexcitation syndromes,* a term that implies activation of a cardiac chamber partially or wholly by an impulse arising in another chamber and arriving earlier than would be expected if the impulse had proceeded over the normal conducting system.

HISTORICAL NOTE

Although Cohn in 1913[C1] and Wilson in 1915[W2] described what apparently was WPW, and Mines in 1914 described "circulating excitations" in the turtle heart,[M5] the specific electrocardiographic (ECG) syndrome of the WPW syndrome was not reported until 1930.[W1] The concept of an electrophysiologic bypass tract was first proposed in 1932 by Holtzmann and Scherf.[H1] In 1967, Durrer and Roos actually demonstrated by epicardial mapping that in patients with WPW, atrioventricular (AV) conduction occurs over an accessory AV conduction pathway, or bypass tract.[D1] This was confirmed in the same year by Burchell and colleagues, who also showed that ventricular preexcitation could be temporarily abolished by injecting procaine into the AV groove at the site of earliest ventricular activation.[B1]

In 1893, Kent had described muscular bridges connecting the right atrium to the right ventricle in several mammalian species,[K1] and Wood and colleagues supported those observations in 1943.[W6] Truex and colleagues in 1958 and in 1960 demonstrated the presence of muscular accessory pathways in human hearts,[T1,T2] and Lev and associates added further information on their morphology in the early 1960s.[L2,L3]

Further proof of the morphologic basis of the WPW syndrome came in 1968, when Cobb, Sealy and colleagues reported the division of the accessory pathway in a patient with the syndrome, in whom the PR interval and QRS complex became normal, the delta wave disappeared, and ventricular preexcitation and recurrent supraventricular tachycardia were eliminated.[C2] In that operation, an epicardial approach was used, and a transmural ventricular incision was made below the AV groove. Iwa and colleagues published a confirmatory report in 1970 and introduced the endocardial approach.[I3] Sealy then also adopted an endocardial approach from within the atria, which consisted of separating the atrium from the anulus after dissecting away the AV fat pad.[S5] Sealy and Gallagher also pioneered a successful surgical approach for patients whose accessory pathways were in the septal area[S2] and introduced cryosurgical ablation.[G6] This method has recently been combined with the epicardial approach with cardiopulmonary bypass (CPB) by Guiraudon and colleagues.[G5,K4]

These developments have led to an important place for surgical intervention in the treatment of many types of ventricular tachyarrhythmias.[C7]

MORPHOLOGY

Accessory atrioventricular (AV) conduction pathways (Kent bundles) mediating the WPW syndrome may occur at any point around the anulus of either AV valve, except along the aortic-mitral anulus.[B4] However, they are most commonly located (1) along the strong, well-formed mitral anulus, adjacent to the free wall of the left ventricle laterally or posteriorly (WPW type A); (2) at the less well-developed tricuspid valve anulus anterosuperiorly, adjacent to the right ventricular free wall (WPW type B); (3) along the tricuspid anulus, adjacent to the anterior aspect of the ventricular septum; (4) along the tricuspid or mitral anulus, adjacent to the posterior aspect of the ventricular septum, near the crux cordis. The accessory pathways adjacent to the posterior aspect of the ventricular septum lie in the potential space overlying the inlet portion of the ventricular septum[S2] and may be on either the right or the left ventricular aspect of the septum. Multiple functioning bundles are not uncommon (present in 10%–20% of selected cases) and considerably complicate the surgical problem.[I1,S6,U3]

The Kent bundles are said to have an average width of 1.8 mm.[S4] At least at times, they can actually be seen when the surgeon uses optical magnification.[B3]

From the standpoint of the cardiac surgeon, not only is the location of the accessory AV pathway important, but so are the normal location of the AV node and bundle of His (see Chapter 1, "Conduction System") and the details of the structures and spaces around the AV valve anuli and the fibrous skeleton of the heart. The *central fibrous body,* where the mitral, tricuspid, and aortic valves meet, is the most prominent part of the fibrous skeleton. The area of fibrous continuity between the aortic and the mitral valve, the *aortic-mitral anulus,* contributes to the fibrous skeleton. The leftward extension of this anulus is the *left fibrous trigone.* The *right fibrous trigone* is at the right-sided extremity of the mitral-aortic anulus and is part of the central fibrous body. It lies adjacent to the atrioventricular portion of the membranous septum, at the point where the tricuspid, mitral, and aortic anuli come together. Atrial muscle is not in juxtaposition with ventricular muscle in the area between the left and right fibrous trigones (along the aortic-mitral anulus), and thus accessory AV connections are not found in this area between the two trigones. As the surgeon views the mitral valve through the usual right-sided approach, the right fibrous trigone is just anterior to the medial commissure, and the left fibrous trigone is just lateral to the lateral commissure. As the surgeon views the tricuspid valve, the central fibrous body is in the region of the muscular portion of the atrioventricular septum (see Chapter 1).

The normal anatomy in the region of the crux cordis and contiguous posterior septal area is of critical importance in the surgery to ablate accessory AV conduction pathways in

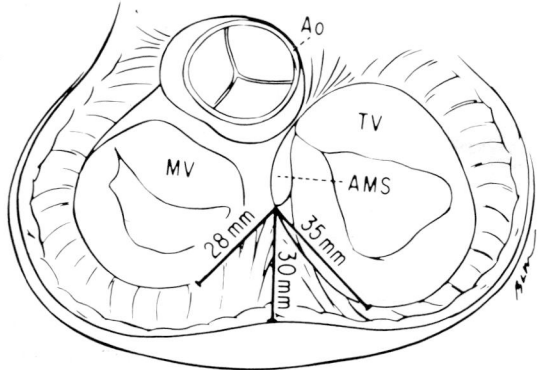

Figure 48-1 Schematic representation of the normal anatomy in the region of the crux cordis. Thirty millimeters is the distance from the crux cordis to the right fibrous trigone, which is essentially alongside the atrioventricular portion of the membranous septum which lies just on the atrial side of the anulus of the tricuspid valve. The distance from the most posterior aspect of the mitral valve to the right fibrous trigone is 28 mm, and that from the most posterior aspect of the tricuspid valve to the trigone is 35 mm. The latter is the area of Sealy's "toppled pyramid." Note the aorta, wedged into position between the mitral and tricuspid valves.

Ao, aorta; AMS, atrioventricular portion of the membranous septum; MV, mitral valve; TV, tricuspid valve.

Reproduced with permission from Sealy et al.[S7]

the region of the posterior aspect of the ventricular septum. This anatomy has been described by Sealy and colleagues as a "toppled pyramid enclosing a fat-filled space."[S2] The apex of the pyramid of space is the right fibrous trigone, described above, and the base is the epicardium over the crux. In adults, a distance of about 30 mm separates the base from the apex[S2] (Fig. 48-1). Two of the sides of the pyramid are the right and left atria, which fuse in the region of the right fibrous trigone to become the atrial septum. It is important to note that the mitral valve anulus lies a somewhat variable distance superior to the tricuspid anulus, which accounts for their being an atrioventricular septum (see Chapter 1, "Atrioventricular Septum"). Also, the interatrial groove, marking the posterior aspect of the atrial septum, lies somewhat to the left of the posterior aspect of the interventricular groove, and here the right atrium somewhat overlies or wraps around the interatrial groove (Fig. 48-2). The third side of the pyramid is the wall of the posterior superior process of the left ventricle and the muscular ventricular septum posteriorly. This pyramidal space contains fat, branches of the coronary artery, and the undersurface of the coronary sinus, with its branches from the right and left ventricles.

Most commonly in patients with the WPW syndrome, the heart is otherwise normal. However, in some patients the accessory muscle bundles coexist with Ebstein's anomaly,[S8] fossa ovalis type of atrial septal defect, atrioventricular discordant connection, and other anomalies.

CLINICAL FEATURES AND DIAGNOSTIC CRITERIA

Pathophysiology

Electrical impulses originate in the sinoatrial node and travel to the atrioventricular (AV) node through preferential path-

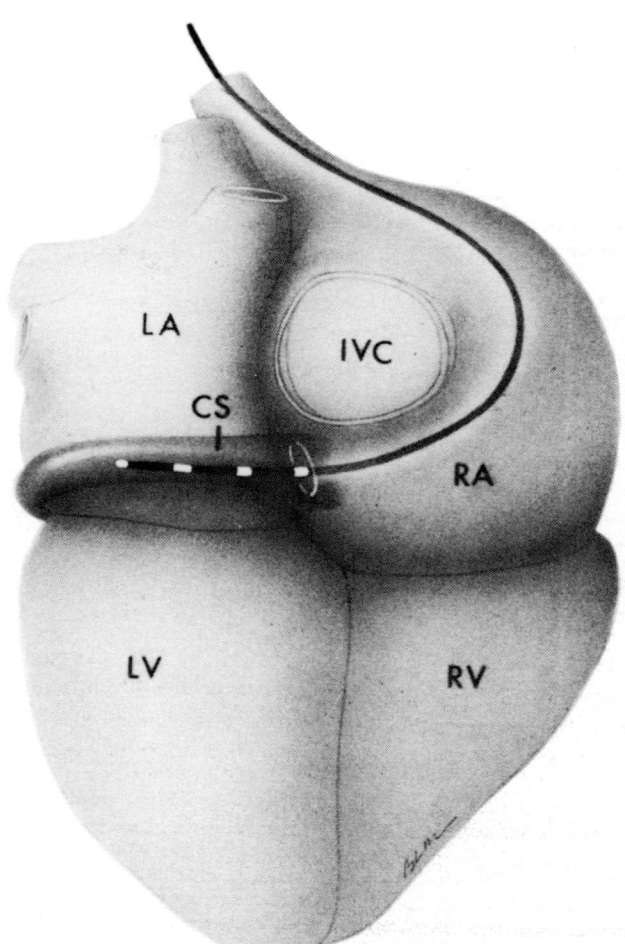

Figure 48-2 Schematic representation of the posterior surfaces of the heart. The interventricular groove between the right ventricle and left ventricle lies rightward of that between the right atrium and left atrium. The figure demonstrates well that electrophysiologic mapping from the coronary sinus reflects events in the left atrioventricular groove.

CS, coronary sinus; IVC, inferior vena cava; LA, left atrium; LV, left ventricle; RA, right atrium; RV, right ventricle.

Reproduced with permission from Sealy et al.[S7]

ways (see Chapter 1). Normally, the fibrous anuli of the mitral and tricuspid valves prevent the direct transmission of electrical impulses from atrium to ventricle (fibrous tissue, in contrast to muscle and specialized cells, does not conduct), and conduction occurs only via the AV node and bundle of His. At the AV node, a delay in AV conduction normally occurs before the impulse passes to the bundle of His and ultimately the Purkinje cells. This delay is reflected in the normal His bundle electrogram, in which an atrial electrogram is recorded at the time of the P wave in the standard electrocardiogram, a His bundle electrogram 60–100 milliseconds later, and ventricular electrical activity at the onset of the QRS complex (Fig. 48-3). In the WPW syndrome, with the Kent bundle offering an AV bypass tract, the electrical impulse travels antegrade down the normal pathway but also

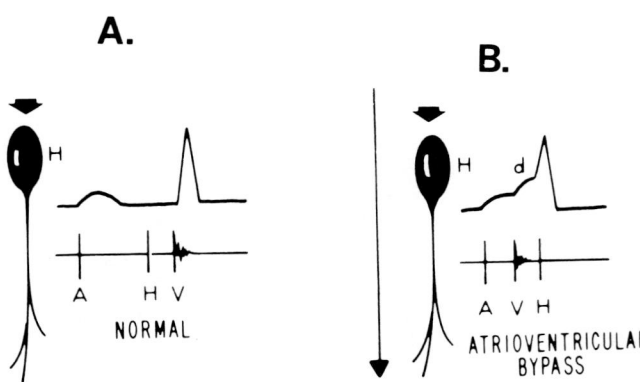

Figure 48-3 The electrocardiogram (top tracing), His bundle electrogram (bottom tracing), and a schematic diagram of the conduction pathways.
(a) Normal.
(b) WPW syndrome with complete AV bypass tract (accessory AV conduction pathway).
A, atrial electrogram; H, His bundle electrogram; V, ventricular electrogram. Reproduced with permission from Gallagher et al.[G1]

antegrade down the Kent bundle, where the delay normally imposed by the AV node is absent. This results in ventricular preexcitation at the insertion of the Kent bundle and the short PR interval, delta wave, and wide QRS complex characteristic of the WPW syndrome (see Fig. 48-3).

The normal AV conduction pathway and the accessory pathway constitute the basis for the reciprocating tachycardia sometimes seen in patients with the WPW syndrome. Most commonly, the circus movement uses the normal AV conduction system as the antegrade limb and the bypass tract as the retrograde limb of the reentrant circuit (so-called orthodromic circus movement tachycardia). Less commonly, the accessory pathway is used in an antegrade manner, and the normal AV conduction system in a retrograde manner (antidromic circus movement tachycardia).[K7]

When atrial fibrillation develops, rapid conduction via the accessory pathway may result in life-threatening ventricular responses, sometimes degenerating to ventricular fibrillation.

Symptoms

Patients with the WPW syndrome who present for treatment do so because of palpitations, with or without symptoms of acute cardiac failure. The palpitations and documented episodic tachycardias have often been present for 10–15 years and repeated hospitalizations may have been required.[H8] Over half the patients with paroxysmal tachycardia and the WPW syndrome give a history of syncope or near syncope.[H8] Rarely, they may present after resuscitation from an episode of sudden death.

Signs

The diagnosis is made from the characteristic ECG (see Fig. 48-3). Atrial fibrillation or flutter may coexist.

Preexcitation and the presence of accessory AV conduc-

tion pathways are confirmed preoperatively by electrophysiologic testing. For this, several multiple-electrode catheters are positioned in the right heart and in the coronary sinus, the latter for mapping in the left AV junction area. Multiple intracardiac and surface electrograms are recorded. With these, the presence and location of accessory pathways are determined by incremental atrial and ventricular pacing and extra stimulus techniques and recording of the sequence of retrograde atrial activation during ventricular pacing and orthodromic tachycardia. Supraventricular tachycardia is induced, and the participation of the accessory pathway in the reentrant circuit is confirmed. The antegrade and retrograde conduction characteristics of the accessory pathways and their refractory period are determined. In general, the shorter the refractory period, the faster the potential ventricular response during atrial fibrillation. Deliberate induction of atrial fibrillation during the study is therefore an important aspect of the electrophysiologic study. Multiple accessory pathways, enhanced AV nodal conduction, and dual AV nodal pathways are sought.

Associated electrophysiologic abnormalities are common in patients with WPW syndrome. About one-third have associated enhanced AV node conduction, and a few have dual AV nodal pathways.

NATURAL HISTORY

The electrocardiographic diagnosis of the preexcitation WPW syndrome is made in about 0.25% of healthy young people, with documented tachyarrhythmias occurring in about 2% of those with preexcitation.[D2] However, in other patient subsets of WPW, the prevalence of tachyarrhythmias is as high as 80%. Half the infants and children with supraventricular tachycardia difficult to control medically have WPW or concealed accessory muscle bundles (see Section 2).[G8]

Patients with WPW may present at any age, including the early month of life,[D6,W3] and the syndrome is more common in males.[D6] The majority of adults with WPW have otherwise normal hearts,[N1] although this syndrome may complicate a variety of acquired and congenital cardiac defects, including Ebstein's anomaly.[B2,S1] The patients with Ebstein's anomaly often have multiple right-sided accessory pathways, and preexcitation is said to be limited to the atrialized portion of the ventricle.[S1] Also, Rossi and Thiene have shown that a few other patients dying an arrhythmogenic death have accessory conduction pathways combined with very mild downward displacement of the tricuspid septal leaflet.[R2]

Eighty percent of patients with WPW and tachyarrhythmias have paroxysmal supraventricular tachycardias of a reciprocating type, 15% have atrial fibrillation, and 5% have atrial flutter. Sinus node dysfunction is said to be more common in patients with WPW than in those without it.[H2]

Patients with WPW, otherwise normal hearts, and no tachycardia have normal cardiac function and life expectancy. In patients with WPW and recurrent tachycardia, there is considerable morbidity, and sudden death occurs in a small proportion of patients. These sudden deaths are most likely the result of the combination of paroxysmal atrial fibrillation and fast antegrade conduction across the accessory AV pathways.[D5,K6] Some children and young adults with WPW and recurrent tachycardia lose the tendency toward developing tachyarrhythmias as they grow older. Also, preexcitation may be intermittent, and the delta wave may be intermittently lost, a situation suggesting a benign prognosis.[K5]

TECHNIQUE OF OPERATION

The object of the operative procedure is to isolate electrically the ventricles from the atria, except for the normal AV nodal pathway. The preparations for operation are those generally used (see Chapter 2, Section 3), in addition to preparations by a cardiologist competent in electrophysiologic techniques. After the median sternotomy incision is made, the pericardial stay sutures are placed, a left atrial monitoring line is inserted (UAB), and purse-string sutures are placed for cannulation. A pair of epicardial electrodes is sutured to the right atrium and another pair to the free wall of the right ventricle; similar pairs are sutured to the left atrium and left ventricle if left-sided accessory pathways are expected.

Electrophysiologic Mapping

A hand-held probe electrode is used to explore for the presence and location of accessory AV conduction pathways by recording epicardial electrograms and their timing at various locations using a standardized grid (Fig. 48-4). In the normal sequence of epicardial activation, the earliest epicardial breakthrough occurs low on the anterior surface of the right ventricle, 18–25 milliseconds after onset of the surface QRS complex (Fig. 48-5), with radial spread toward the apex and base. In patients with WPW, the identification of the location of the accessory pathway is easiest if the patient is in normal sinus rhythm with stable antegrade preexcitation. The map then identifies the site or sites of earliest ventricular activation, which in general establishes the ventricular insertion of the accessory pathway. Multiple areas of initial breakthrough may be noted.[G2] However, in the presence of a septal accessory pathway, the point of earliest epicardial excitation may be at a site remote from the actual location of the accessory AV tract; this site can be recognized as spurious by the fact that in this setting the earliest epicardial activation occurs after the onset of the delta wave in the surface electrocardiogram. Otherwise, it occurs about 15 seconds before or simultaneously with the delta wave. The identification of septal pathways frequently requires intracardiac mapping during cardiopulmonary bypass (CPB).

When stable antegrade preexcitation is not present in the operating room, atrial mapping is done during reciprocating tachycardia or ventricular pacing near the suspected site of the bypass tract.

Retrograde conduction over the accessory pathway is then sought during reentry tachycardia by mapping with the hand-held electrode to find possible sites of early atrial activation that identify the atrial insertion of the accessory bundles. If this is not possible, the mapping is done during ventricular pacing. In the presence of atrial fibrillation, the mapping can

LEFT ATRIUM   **RIGHT ATRIUM**

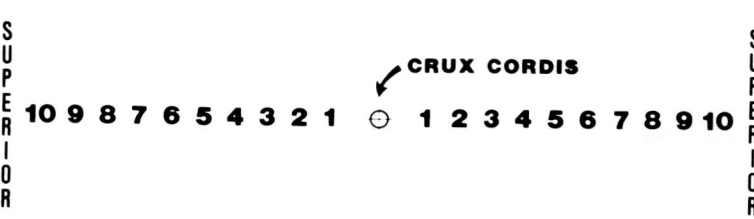

LEFT VENTRICLE   **RIGHT VENTRICLE**

Figure 48-4   Standardized grid for intraoperative epicardial mapping along the AV groove in the search of the location of accessory AV conduction pathways (Kent bundles) in patients with WPW syndrome or concealed retrograde conduction (UAB). The map is depicted with position 10 for both left atrium and right atrium being the most superior aspect of the atrioventricular groove. The orientation of the map is the same as that shown in Figure 48-2. The grid is useful in providing a standardized method of communication between the surgeon and cardiologist during surgery and a standardized method of record keeping for such patients.

ANTERIOR   **POSTERIOR**

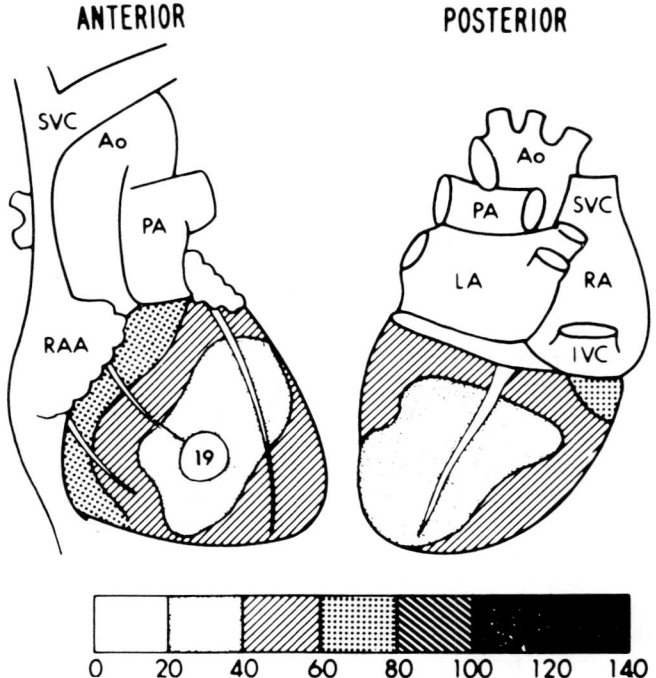

Figure 48-5   The normal sequence of anterior epicardial activation. Isochrones are drawn every 10 milliseconds and connect areas activating at the same time. All time intervals shown refer to the onset of the QRS complex.

Ao, aorta; IVC, inferior vena cava; LA, left atrium; PA, pulmonary artery; RA, right atrium; RAA, right atrial appendage; SVC, superior vena cava.

Reproduced with permission from Cox.[C3]

only be done ventricularly. A suture is placed to identify the site of earliest activation along the AV groove. After CPB is established at 37°C, endocardial mapping inside the right atrium is also performed during ventricular pacing if the precise location of the accessory pathway is uncertain. However, with the exception of patients with septal pathways, endocardial intracardial mapping is rarely necessary.

Division of Accessory Atrioventricular Conduction Pathways

After the epicardial mapping has been completed (it is often necessary to establish CPB to map the left atrioventricular groove), CPB is begun after direct cannulation of the superior and inferior vena cavae.

Right Atrioventricular Free Wall Pathways
The perfusate temperature is taken to 25°C, the right atrium is opened through the usual oblique incision (see Chapter 15, Fig. 15-12), the aorta is cross-clamped, and the cold cardioplegic solution is infused (see Chapter 3). An area of the tricuspid anulus is identified as corresponding to the area of preexcitation determined externally, and an incision is made through the atrial wall about 2 mm away from the hinge line of the tricuspid leaflets. The incision is extended about 1.5 cm on each side of the presumed location of the Kent bundles. The thin flap (2–3 mm thick) of atrial endocardium

between the incision and the tricuspid valve is then raised and the dissection carried down to the tricuspid anulus. The dissection is then extended until the underlying ventricular myocardium immediately adjacent to the tricuspid anulus is exposed. The fat pad containing the right coronary artery is dissected easily from the right ventricular wall. As the dissection is carried toward the epicardium, all the small bands and small vessels entering the ventricular myocardium are divided, so that the fibrous anulus becomes a nonconducting barrier to AV conduction except through the normal AV node and His bundle pathway. Because of the variable location of the accessory pathways, the underlying ventricular myocardium is cleared to a depth of 1 cm over the entire length of the endocardial incision.

The incision in the atrial wall is closed with continuous or interrupted 5-0 polypropylene sutures. The right atrium is closed. With strong suction on the aortic needle vent, the aortic clamp is released, rewarming of the patient by the perfusate having begun about 5 minutes earlier. The remainder of the period of CPB is completed as usual (see Chapter 2, Section 3). Electrophysiologic mapping is repeated and the electrocardiogram studied to determine whether preexcitation and the delta wave are absent. If they are still present, consideration is given to further mapping and efforts to find and interrupt the accessory conducting pathways.

Left Atrioventricular Free Wall Pathways
The mapping of left AV free wall pathways must usually be done on CPB at 37°C. The epicardial site of the accessory pathway is marked by a suture after mapping is completed. Cardiopulmonary bypass is established, using two venous cannulae and direct caval cannulation. The perfusate temperature is taken to 25°C, the aorta cross-clamped, and the cold cardioplegic infusion given. The left atrium is opened from the right side, as in other operations related to the mitral valve (see Chapter 11, Fig. 11-3). The point on the mitral anulus corresponding to the externally placed suture is marked with another suture. This point is in the periannular area between the area of the left fibrous trigone (a little anterior to the lateral commissure of the mitral valve) and counterclockwise nearly around to the area of the right fibrous trigone near the posteromedial commissure. A general incision is made in the left atrial wall over the region of the accessory AV connection 2–3 mm away from the hinge line of the mitral leaflet and extending 1.5–2.0 cm on each side of the anticipated location of the accessory pathway. Generally, the incision begins just behind the level of the left fibrous trigone and extends counterclockwise nearly to the termination of this area.[S9] The fat in the AV groove is separated from the superior aspect of the exposed ventricular myocardium, as in the approach to the right-sided free wall pathways. The tiny bands of connective tissue that bind the sulcus fat to the myocardium are divided, generally by blunt dissection. All superficial myocardial fibers that enter the mitral anulus fibrosus are interrupted. The left ventricular myocardium is exposed to a distance of about 1 cm in order to avoid missing any of the accessory pathways. Then the incision in the atrial wall is closed, the left atriotomy is closed, and with strong suction on the aortic needle, the aortic clamp is released. The remainder of the operation proceeds as usual, including the de-airing procedures (see Chap-

ter 2, Section 3). After CPB is discontinued, remapping is performed (see description under "Right Atrioventricular Free Wall Pathways").

Anterior Septal Pathways

As described for the interruption of right ventricular free wall accessory pathways, anterior septal pathways are approached through a right atriotomy on CPB. After the right atriotomy is made, an incision is begun in the right atrial wall about 2 mm away from the hinge line of the tricuspid leaflets, beginning just anterosuperior to the membranous septum, in the region of the right fibrous trigone and the commissure between septal and anterior tricuspid leaflets. This incision is carried anteriorly and superiorly in a clockwise fashion to the 12-o'clock position (as the surgeon views the tricuspid valve). The incision exposes the space on the superior aspect of the muscular ventricular septum, bounded also by the aortic root and the infundibulum of the right ventricle. The fat is cleared away from the right coronary artery. The fat and superficial muscle fibers are separated from the atrial septum and tricuspid anulus. As the dissection and separation of atrium and ventricle proceeds in this area, there is a small risk of injuring the bundle of His. After all connections between atrial and ventricular musculature have been interrupted, the incision in the atrial wall is closed with interrupted or continuous 5-0 polypropylene sutures. The right atriotomy is closed, and the remainder of the operation, including remapping, is carried out as described under "Right Atrioventricular Free Wall Pathways."

Posterior Septal Pathways

Lying in the region of the crux cordis, posterior septal pathways are the most difficult to locate electrophysiologically and to interrupt surgically.[S7] After CPB has begun, the right atrium has been opened, and cold cardioplegia has been established, an incision is made in the right atrial wall 2 mm from the hinge line of the tricuspid leaflets, just to the surgeon's right of the position of the AV node (see Chapter 1, Fig. 1-1). The incision is carried counterclockwise to the surgeon's right and anteriorly around the anulus for about 4 cm, about to the point overlying the right ventricular free wall rather than the septum. This exposes the fat pad, which contains the coronary vessels and lies above the posterior aspect of the ventricular septum below and the left atrial wall above. By dissecting the fat pad, coronary sinus, and AV node artery away from the entire inlet portion of the posterior ventricular septum, the surgeon can interrupt most of the posterior septal pathways without damaging the normal conduction system. The incision in the atrial wall is closed, the right atriotomy incision is closed, and the remainder of the operation is completed as described under "Right Atrioventricular Free Wall Pathways" and "Left Atrioventricular Free Wall Pathways."

When the posterior septal pathways are left-sided, after establishing CPB and cold cardioplegia, the usual right-sided left atriotomy incision is made. After the mitral valve is exposed, an incision is made 2 mm from the anulus about 1 cm anterior to the posteromedial commissure, in the region of the right fibrous trigone. The incision is carried clockwise around the anulus to the right and posteriorly to a point about 2 cm beyond the medial commissure. Again, the fat

pad and vessels are dissected away from the posterior aspect of the inlet portion of the ventricular septum. The incision in the atrial wall is closed, the left atrium is allowed to fill as the left atriotomy is closed, the tip of the left ventricle is aspirated for air, and with strong suction on the aortic needle vent, the aortic clamp is released. The remainder of the operation proceeds as described earlier, and in addition, two epicardial wires are attached on the atrial side and two on the ventricular side of the surgically interrupted bypass tracts to facilitate postoperative electrophysiologic study.

SPECIAL FEATURES OF POSTOPERATIVE CARE

The postoperative care is that generally given to patients after cardiac surgery (see Chapter 5). Electrophysiologic testing is repeated before the patient leaves the hospital to confirm the completeness of the division of the accessory pathways and to guide drug therapy if it is necessary. When appropriate epicardial wires have been left at operation, the electrophysiologic studies can be accomplished simply and without cardiac catheterization.

RESULTS

Hospital Mortality

Hospital mortality after operations for WPW is low but does not yet approach zero. Thus, 5 (2.5%, CL 1%–4%) of 200 consecutive patients undergoing surgery for WPW at Duke University died in hospital.[G3] None (0%, CL 0%–13%) among 14 patients undergoing such operations have died (UAB).

Termination of Wolff-Parkinson-White Syndrome

The operation for WPW is successful in terminating the syndrome in 80%–90% of patients. Among 14 patients, the results are not known in 4; among the other 10 patients, 8 (80%, CL 59%–93%) were asymptomatic, without delta waves, and with negative results of electrophysiologic studies postoperatively (UAB). Holmes and colleagues, of the Mayo Clinic, reported 20 (83%, CL 72%–81%) of 24 surgical patients to be without recurrence of their rhythm disturbance at a mean follow-up period of 16 months, although a few had return of delta waves in the ECG.[H8] Iwa and colleagues reported cure, with absence of delta waves, in 26 (93%, CL 84%–98%) of 28 recent patients.[12] Generally, the same results are obtained in pediatric patients, with Gillette and colleagues reporting 8 (80%, CL 59%–93%) among 10 patients as being cured.[G7] Ott and colleagues report a larger group of pediatric patients who have undergone surgical treatment for abnormal conduction pathways across the atrioventricular junction, among whom 47 (85%, CL 79%–90%) have a good long-term result over a follow-up period as long as 8 years.[O3]

According to the Duke experience, 39 (95%, CL 89%–98%) of 41 right free wall accessory AV conduction bundles were successfully divided, as were 93 (92%, CL 88%–95%) left free wall bundles, 17 (81%, CL 68%–90%) of 21 anterior septal bundles, and 42 (75%, CL 68%–81%) posterior septal bundles.[G3] Thus, the operation is more often successful when the AV accessory pathways are in the free wall than when they are in the ventricular septum.[B5]

Heart Block

Zero (0%, CL 0%–13%) of 14 patients developed complete heart block after operation (UAB). However, unintended division of the bundle of His and resultant complete heart block can occur. This was the case in 10 (5%, CL 3%–7%) of the 200 Duke patients.

In addition, in the Duke experience, complete heart block was intentionally produced by interruption of the bundle of His in 11 (5.5%, CL 3.8%–7.7%) of the 200 patients. This procedure effectively eliminates reciprocating tachycardia, but permanent pacemaking is of course required. Further, the procedure gives no protection to patients with atrial fibrillation and rapid antegrade conduction across the accessory pathway.

INDICATIONS FOR OPERATION

The presence of the WPW syndrome itself is not an indication for surgical treatment. Frequent or potentially life-threatening tachycardia, demonstrated to be related to the presence of the accessory AV conduction pathways, is generally an indication for preoperative and intraoperative electrophysiologic studies and surgical interruption of the accessory pathways, particularly in young patients in whom the long-term side effects of drug therapy are uncertain. In particular, operation is advisable in patients with very short antegrade refractory periods of the accessory pathways, in whom life-threatening tachycardia may result during atrial fibrillation.

When a cardiac operation is indicated (e.g., closure of an atrial septal defect, repair of Ebstein's anomaly, valvar repair or replacement, or coronary artery bypass grafting) in a patient asymptomatic from the WPW electrocardiographic syndrome, it is probably wise at operation to interrupt the accessory pathways, since serious postoperative tachycardias may result from their presence, and atrial fibrillation can be life-threatening.[K8] Such patients should undergo the usual preoperative and intraoperative electrophysiologic studies.

SPECIAL SITUATIONS AND CONTROVERSIES

Closed Techniques for Interruption of Atrioventricular Accessory Connections

An epicardial approach was used initially by Sealy and colleagues[C2] and has recently been again emphasized by Guiraudon and associates.[G5,K4] This approach can be considered somewhat hazardous to the coronary arteries and therefore less desirable than an open approach (UAB), but in certain circumstances its use may be considered.

When the accessory pathways are between the right atrium and the right ventricular free wall, an external dissection is made in the region of the pathway, generally during normothermic cardiopulmonary bypass. In this procedure,

the epicardium is incised at the junction of the right atrium and the fat pad, and a plane of dissection is established between them. The incision and dissection are carried about 1.5 cm beyond each side of the presumed location of the accessory AV connection. If this dissection can be made during sinus rhythm and stable antegrade preexcitation, the sudden disappearance of the delta wave in the surface electrocardiogram indicates that the accessory connection has been divided. In patients with Ebstein's anomaly, this dissection is often more difficult than usual because the atrioventricular junction may be folded over the fat pad and require division before the fat pad is reached. Once the pathway has been cut, cryosurgical ablation is performed with the application of a 1.5 cm cryoprobe at −60°C for 2 minutes.[G5] Cryosurgical ablation has been shown to be a useful technique for bundle of His ablation[H6] and in the surgery for ventricular tachycardia in ischemic heart disease (see Section 4) because it ablates myocardium, does not disrupt the collagenous structure of the heart, and results in a strong, discrete, fibrotic scar. However, coronary arteries can be damaged unless care is taken to keep them out of the surgical field;[M4] the coronary sinus has been shown to be relatively resistant to cryosurgical injury.[H9]

When the accessory AV connections are along the left ventricular free wall, CPB is established at 37°C using two venous cannulae and direct caval cannulation. The heart is lifted up and to the right, and an epicardial incision is made 4 cm in length and centered on the mapped location of the Kent bundle. Optical magnification is used. The left atrial branches of the circumflex artery are ligated and divided. This allows the fat pad and artery to be retracted away from the atrial wall as the dissection of the AV groove proceeds. Usually the preexcitation disappears during this dissection.[G5] Cryosurgery (see above) is then used to ablate that part of the atrial wall that received the atrial insertion of the Kent bundle.

Catheter Techniques for Interruption of Atrioventricular Accessory Pathways

As is the case in many other kinds of heart disease, the correction of the WPW syndrome by nonsurgical methods is undergoing trial. Ward and Camm report success in three patients by transvenous electrical ablation of the AV accessory pathway using an electrode lead and a conventional defibrillator.[W10] Further experience with such trials is required for their evaluation.

SECTION 2

PAROXYSMAL SUPRAVENTRICULAR TACHYCARDIA FROM CONCEALED ACCESSORY ATRIOVENTRICULAR CONDUCTION PATHWAYS

DEFINITION

Paroxysmal supraventricular tachycardia from concealed accessory atrioventricular (AV) pathways is a type of tachycardia, in which part of the reentry circuit is one or more accessory AV conduction pathways that conduct only in a retrograde direction and thus do not produce the electrocardiographic features of the WPW syndrome.

MORPHOLOGY

The morphologic bases for this type of supraventricular arrhythmia are accessory AV conduction pathways (Kent bundles), exactly as described for the WPW syndrome (see Section 1).

CLINICAL FEATURES AND DIAGNOSTIC CRITERIA

The patients present with a history of paroxysmal tachycardia, shown by ECG to be supraventricular in origin. Since there is no antegrade conduction over the accessory AV conduction pathway in this arrhythmia, none of the electrocardiographic features of WPW are present. The diagnosis is made by preoperative electrophysiologic studies that demonstrate retrograde conduction across an accessory pathway. The evidence for this diagnosis includes eccentric atrial activation during paroxysmal atrial tachycardia (PAT), with the earliest atrial activation site being other than the His bundle area and the proximal coronary sinus (free wall pathways). Also, during PAT, an initiated premature ventricular contraction (PVC) timed so as to occur during the refractory period of the bundle of His produces early atrial activation. Whether the stimulus for the PVC is given to the right or the left ventricle depends on the probable location of the accessory pathway.

NATURAL HISTORY

The natural history of patients with paroxysmal supraventricular tachycardia from concealed accessory AV conduction pathways is presumed to be similar to that for the WPW syndrome, except that the problem of a life-threatening ventricular rate in response to atrial fibrillation or flutter is not present.

TECHNIQUE OF OPERATION

The operation proceeds in general as does that for the WPW syndrome, but with the difference that only retrograde atrial mapping is relevant and is best carried out during paroxysmal atrial tachycardia, in which retrograde atrial activation occurs only via the accessory pathway. Once the site of atrial insertion of the retrograde conducting accessory AV conduction pathway has been identified, the pathway is divided as in the WPW syndrome.[S10]

SPECIAL FEATURES OF POSTOPERATIVE CARE

Usual care is given to the patients postoperatively (see Chapter 5). Electrophysiologic restudy is performed before hospital dismissal.

RESULTS

Less specific information is available concerning the results of surgical interruption of accessory conduction pathways with only retrograde conduction than of those with both retrograde and antegrade conduction, but in general they seem similar to those in the classical WPW syndrome.[S12] Among three patients in this category, all (100%, CL 53%–100%) were surgically cured (UAB).

INDICATIONS FOR OPERATION

The presence of a paroxysmal supraventricular tachycardia due to concealed accessory AV connections (Kent bundles) is an indication for operation when medical therapy is ineffective or contraindicated.

SECTION 3
OTHER SUPRAVENTRICULAR TACHYCARDIAS

Some paroxysmal supraventricular tachycardias are due to reentry phenomena confined to the region of the AV node. Such arrhythmias are most commonly related to dual AV nodal pathways but may be related to accessory AV node bypass tracts, which connect atrial muscle directly to the bundle of His. Others reflect the presence of Mahaim fibers connecting the AV node or bundle of His directly to the ventricular septal myocardium or right bundle branch. Atrial flutter and fibrillation can result in an excessively fast ventricular response when enhanced AV node conduction is present. The various types of such arrhythmias can usually be diagnosed by preoperative electrophysiologic studies.

At present, the only proven effective surgical therapy is surgical ablation of the bundle of His. The operation is done with the aid of electrophysiologic studies and provisions for atrial and ventricular pacing. After a median sternotomy incision is made and cardiopulmonary bypass established at 37°C, the right atrium is opened via the usual oblique incision, and stay sutures for exposure are placed. During atrial pacing, the area usually occupied by the bundle of His is explored with a hand-held exploring electrode. Once the characteristic His complex is identified, the exploring electrode is replaced with a hand-held cryoprobe with a 5-mm diameter tip. The temperature of the tip of the probe is reduced to 0°C, at which time AV conduction should cease; then the area is allowed to rewarm, and conduction should return. When this response has been confirmed, the temperature of the probe tip is reduced to −60°C for 2 minutes. A permanent cryoablation and heart block usually result. A permanent pacemaker is inserted.

The procedure is successful in controlling these refractory supraventricular tachycardias in about 90% of cases.[S3]

Closed chest methods of interrupting bundle of His conduction have now been developed and, while still incompletely evaluated, seem promising.[G9,S11] For example, Wood and colleagues reported three patients in whom the conduction was successfully interrupted by a DC electroversion stimulus through a catheter positioned against the bundle of His.[W7]

Other types of surgical procedures are currently under investigation and trial.[H7] These procedures are basically selective cryoablations of peri-AV nodal tissues, designed to ablate the electrophysiologic substrate required for AV nodal reentry tachycardia while preserving AV conduction.

SECTION 4
VENTRICULAR TACHYCARDIA IN ISCHEMIC HEART DISEASE

DEFINITION

Ventricular tachycardia is a form of tachycardia in which the abnormalities of impulse initiation or conduction arise in the ventricles. It is potentially fatal because of the usual association with important myocardial impairment and the tendency to degenerate into ventricular fibrillation.

HISTORICAL NOTE

In 1938, Parkinson and colleagues apparently first noticed the association between ventricular aneurysm and intractable ventricular tachycardia.[P2] However, the problem seemed to be known to Sir Thomas Lewis, who stated in 1909 the need for studying and understanding the condition by a controlled method of inducing tachycardia.[L1] This need was met in 1967 when Durrer and colleagues,[D3] in Holland, and Coumel and colleagues,[C4] in France, introduced the technique of programmed electrical stimulation of the human heart.

The first surgical approach to the treatment of the life-threatening ventricular tachycardia in patients with ischemic heart disease was reported in 1959 by Couch and colleagues, using simple aneurysmectomy.[C5] Fontaine, Frank, and Guiraudon reported surgical epicardial mapping as an adjunct to this kind of surgery in 1974,[F7] and Gallagher and colleagues reported the successful use of ventricular aneurysm resection guided by electrophysiologic mapping in 1975.[G11] In 1978, Guiraudon and colleagues introduced encircling endocardial ventriculotomy as a method of directly treating life-threatening ventricular tachycardia in patients with ischemic heart disease.[G4] Harken and colleagues reported electrophysiologically directed endocardial resection as a method of treatment in 1980.[H4]

MORPHOLOGY

Sustained ventricular tachycardia is an uncommon complication of ischemic heart disease in the absence of a previous myocardial infarction. It occurs most commonly in patients who have developed a large area of infarction and particularly in those with a left ventricular aneurysm. Thus, among 19 patients undergoing an operation for life-threatening ventricular tachycardia (UAB, 1977–1981) 13 (68%, CL 54%–80%) had also left ventricular resection for aneurysm.

Patients with ischemic heart disease who are subject to life-threatening ventricular tachycardia have, as a group, more left ventricular impairment than do patients with ischemic heart disease without this life-threatening complication. Thus, patients undergoing operations for ventricular tachycardia (UAB, 1977–1981) had a mean ejection fraction of 0.30, similar to that of patients undergoing surgical treatment for left ventricular aneurysm, whereas patients undergoing isolated coronary artery bypass grafting had one of 0.51 (P for difference = .0001).[K3] However, only a minority of patients with ischemic heart disease and left ventricular aneurysm with impaired left ventricular function develop life-threatening ventricular tachycardia. While the determinants of which patients are affected by ventricular tachycardia are not clear, septal involvement in the scarring does seem to be one of them.[C6]

The morphologic substrate for ventricular tachycardia in ischemic heart disease may reside for the most part in the subendocardium of the left ventricle and the left ventricular aspect of the ventricular septum, although this morphology is not completely established. Most commonly, this substrate is on the septum and near the border of an aneurysm or infarct. Virtually all hearts that have undergone a myocardial infarction have a mixture of myocardial cells and fibrous tissue in at least some areas of the left ventricle; such areas provide a basis for slow conduction and conduction block, two conditions necessary for ventricular reentry to occur.[W4] Thus, in areas of the subendocardium where ventricular tachycardia may begin, bundles of viable myocardial cells are imbedded in dense connective tissue.[F1,P1] These bundles may consist of Purkinje fibers, ventricular muscle fibers, or both. These generally parallel muscle bundles do not appear to connect to intramural fibers within the ventricular wall, and, indeed, regions where ventricular tachycardia seems to originate may have no surviving myocardial cells above the subendocardium. Thus, the surviving subendocardial muscle bundles are generally connected to the rest of the ventricle across the borders of the subendocardial portions of the scar.

This arrangement of parallel bundles of myocardial fibers separated by fibrous or connective tissue forms a nonuniform anisotropic (conducting in one direction) structure that could be considered an ideal substrate for reentrant circuits. Conduction between muscle bundles is probably slow, whereas conduction along the length of the muscle bundles is probably rapid. The fractionated character of electrograms recorded from such regions is also probably related to the nonuniform anisotropic anatomy. It can be hypothesized that the larger the proportion of the left ventricle involved with these morphologic characteristics, the greater the possibility that reentrant circuits will develop, activate contiguous subendocardium, and provoke ventricular tachycardia or ventricular fibrillation. The actual time and place of development of the electrical phenomenon responsible for the ventricular tachyarrhythmia (VT), according to current information, is determined by chance.

Even among individuals with life-threatening ventricular arrhythmias but without any other evidences of cardiac disease, a morphologic substrate likely to be responsible for the arrhythmia is usually found. Sugrue and colleagues report several different types of histopathologic abnormalities in such patients coming to autopsy, including myocardial cellular hypertrophy, interstitial fibrosis, myocardial degenerative changes, and acute myocarditis.[S18]

CLINICAL FEATURES AND DIAGNOSTIC CRITERIA

Pathophysiology

Many theories have been advanced as to the electrophysiologic basis of life-threatening ventricular arrhythmias in patients with ischemic heart disease, but it remains uncertain whether these arrhythmias arise as a result of macro- or micro-reentry circuits, normal or abnormal automaticity, or triggered activity. Most of the evidence favors the first two mechanisms. In any case, at least in many patients the abnormal impulse breaks through into the endocardial surface near its origin, resulting in the earliest ventricular electrical activation at this point during the tachycardia. Its breakthrough onto the epicardial surface may be some distance away.

Symptoms

In some patients, sudden death is the first manifestation of an important ventricular tachyarrhythmia. In others, premature ventricular contractions, ventricular tachycardia, or ventricular fibrillation cause the first symptoms during recovery from a myocardial infarction. In still other patients, frequent palpitations, sometimes accompanied by faintness or syncope, are the presenting complaint.

Signs

The diagnostic finding is a verified history of life-threatening ventricular tachycardia or fibrillation, or sustained ventricular tachycardia induced during electrophysiologic study.

Electrophysiologic Studies

The surgically important preoperative study is programmed electrical stimulation to induce sustained ventricular tachycardia and left ventricular endocardial mapping during the ventricular tachycardia. Up to 90% of patients with ischemic heart disease and clinically important sustained ventricular tachycardia or ventricular fibrillation develop sustained tachycardia when studied in this manner. The mapping electrode is introduced into the femoral artery and passed retrogradely up the aorta and into the left ventricular cavity. The catheter for programmed electrical stimulation is introduced transvenously and advanced to the apex of the right ventricle. Single, double, or triple extrastimuli at different basic cycle lengths and at different sites are used to induce sustained ventricular tachycardia. The earliest site of ventricular activation is sought. The mapping left ventricular catheter may record abnormal fractionated electrograms[K10] and slow conduction (one hallmark of the existence of reentry

circuits) or disorganized, asynchronous electrical activity. It may also demonstrate adjacent areas of systolic and diastolic activity,[H3] perhaps representing the latest areas of slow activation. Most important, an area of earliest endocardial activation during sustained ventricular tachycardia that precedes the onset of the QRS complex by 20–80 milliseconds is sought and is considered the most reliable indication of the location of a critical part of the reentry circuit responsible for the ventricular tachycardia (UAB).

Preoperative electrophysiologic studies are important because of the occasional inability to induce sustained ventricular tachycardia during operation, which precludes the direction of the endocardial resections or ablations by electrophysiologic study in the operating room.

NATURAL HISTORY

Patients may develop life-threatening ventricular tachyarrhythmias (VT) in the recovery phase of myocardial infarction or as a remote complication. Some patients present after resuscitation from sudden death. VT also may complicate other forms of heart disease and, rarely, may occur in the absence of demonstrable disease.

Sustained ventricular tachycardias and fibrillation may occur within the first 48 hours after an acute myocardial infarction but do not worsen prognosis; they are presumably ischemic in origin. Such arrhythmias later in the course of recovery are less common but more serious. The episodes are often multiple and in-hospital mortality as high as 60%.[G13,L4,W8] Such patients generally have inducible ventricular tachycardia when studied by programmed electrical stimulation and a poor long-term prognosis even with intense medical therapy. Marchlinski and colleagues reported only 20 (50%, CL 41%–59%) of 40 such patients alive after a mean follow-up period of 20 months, with over half the deaths occurring suddenly.[M8]

The natural history of individuals who have been retrieved from sudden death is highly variable, but in general is not a favorable one. Swerdlow and colleagues found that 34% of patients resuscitated from sudden death died suddenly within 3 years of their presentation.[S17] The most important risk factors for sudden death were advanced functional disability, as indicated by New York Heart Association (NYHA) functional class, and lack of response to therapy, as judged by programmed electrical stimulation. Depressed left ventricular function and the presence of ischemic heart disease seemed to be risk factors, although their risk was less certain than that of the major risk factors. As is the case in other patients with ischemic heart disease, the prognosis of medically treated patients with life-threatening ventricular tachyarrhythmias is adversely affected by the presence of severe proximal anterior descending coronary artery stenoses.[V2]

The ability of medical treatment to influence favorably the natural history of patients with life-threatening VT has been limited by the fact that an effective antiarrhythmic drug can be identified by electrophysiologic testing in less than 35% of cases.[S13,S14] Empirical therapy with high-dose amiodarone has been favorable in several large series.[H10,M11] However, an appreciable number of patients develop severe adverse reactions or aggravation of their arrhythmic symptoms with medical therapy.[F4,V1]

TECHNIQUE OF OPERATION

A variety of techniques of intraoperative electrophysiologic mapping and of surgical intervention have been used in recent years, with variable results. Here are described those currently in use (UAB).

The preliminary phases of the operation include the usual ones for open intracardiac operations (see Chapter 2, Section 3) in addition to the preparations and collaboration of a cardiologist competent in cardiac electrophysiology. A median sternotomy is made, pericardial stay sutures and purse-string sutures for cannulation are placed, and a left atrial pressure monitoring catheter is positioned (see Chapter 2). Electrodes are sutured onto the free wall of the right atrium and right ventricle. An epicardial electrophysiologic map of the left ventricle is then made in sinus rhythm. Ventricular tachycardia is induced, and epicardial mapping is repeated. If mapping disturbs cardiac function, it must be completed on cardiopulmonary bypass (Fig. 48-6).

Cardiopulmonary bypass (CPB) is begun at 37°C. The aorta is cross-clamped, and the left ventricle is opened through an infarct scar or the edge of a ventricular aneurysm, if one exists. The aorta is then declamped. When the aneurysm or scar is inferior, in the diaphragmatic portion of the left ventricle, the same procedure is followed. Occasionally, however, this approach results in inadequate exposure for endocardial mapping, necessitating enlargement of the incision. An initial endocardial electrophysiologic map is made during sinus rhythm, followed by mapping during sustained ventricular tachycardia (see Fig. 48-6). The purpose of the mapping is the identification of the point of earliest endocardial activation (see "Clinical Features and Diagnostic Criteria"). The CPB temperature may be increased to 38.5°C as an aid to sustaining VT. Once the mapping process is completed, the perfusate temperature is taken to 25°C, the aorta cross-clamped, and the cold cardioplegic infusion given. If a left ventricular aneurysm is present, it is excised (see Chapter 8).

Working through the left ventriculotomy, the previously identified area of earliest endocardial activation is electrically isolated from the rest of the ventricular mass by excision of the endocardial fibrosis as a wafer of endocardium and subendocardium about 2–3 mm thick and then creating around the area a full thickness scar that is fibrous and thus nonconducting. The latter is accomplished by a series of contiguous cryoablations of myocardium, with the cryoprobe tip placed against the endocardium, cooled to −60°C for 2 minutes, rewarmed, and then moved to the next position. (A cryolesion results in a homogeneous, nonarrhythmogenic, electrically inert scar with no disturbance of blood flow to adjacent tissues.[K2] Although in such a setting the lesions had been thought to be of full thickness, they have been shown not to extend to the outer layers of the myocardium.[M10]) Usually, the ventriculotomy is used as part of the perimeter of scar that is created.

The left ventricle is closed (see Chapter 8, "Technique of Operation"). The CABG procedure and the rest of the operation are performed in the usual fashion (see Chapter 7). In addition, six epicardial wires are left, two on the right atrium (as usual), two on the right ventricle, and two on the left ventricle, for use in the postoperative electrophysiologic study.

SPECIAL FEATURES OF POSTOPERATIVE CARE

The postoperative care is that usually given patients who have had surgery for ischemic heart disease (see Chapter 7).

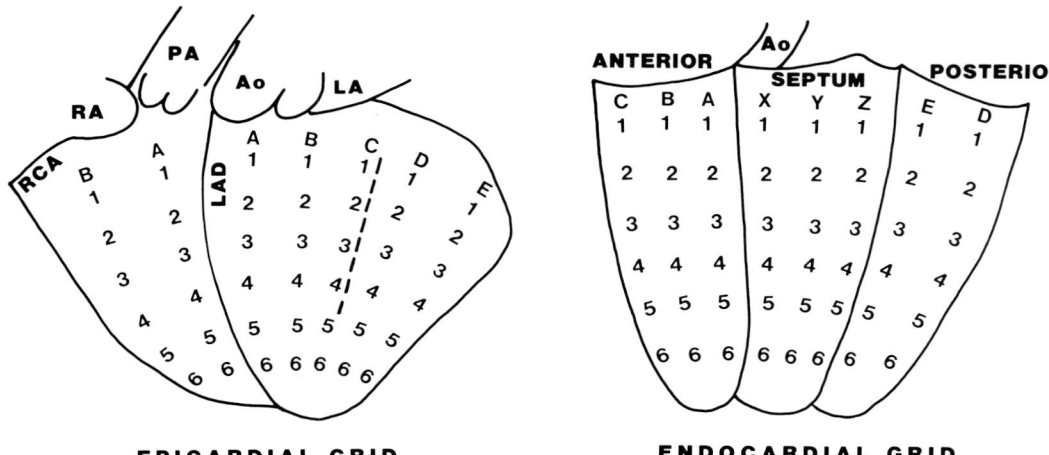

EPICARDIAL GRID   **ENDOCARDIAL GRID**

Figure 48-6 Grids for intraoperative epicardial and endocardial mapping during operations for life-threatening ventricular tachycardia (UAB). In the epicardial grid, the dashed line is the obtuse margin of the heart. The purposes of the grids are the same as those of the epicardial maps for the WPW syndrome (see Fig. 48-4).

Ao, aorta; LA, left atrium; LAD, left anterior descending coronary artery; PA, pulmonary artery; RA, right atrium; RCA, right coronary artery.

If ventricular electrical instability has been evident in the operating room after the operation, a continuous intravenous infusion of lidocaine is generally administered for at least 12 hours (see Chapter 5, Appendix 5E for details). Repeat electrophysiologic studies are performed before hospital dismissal. If six epicardial wires have been left at operation, this study can be done without cardiac catheterization.[P3] If inducible and sustained VT is still present, consideration is given to drug therapy or an implantable antiarrhythmic device (see "Special Situations and Controversies").

RESULTS

The results of surgery for patients with ischemic heart disease and life-threatening ventricular tachycardia are difficult to assess, and the success rates have varied widely. However, some general statements can be made based on past results, although these generalizations could be changed by improved diagnostic and therapeutic methods.

Survival

Less than 70% of surgically treated patients with ischemic heart disease and life-threatening ventricular tachycardia have survived 1 year after operation, and less than 50% have survived 5 years (UAB; Fig. 48-7). Most deaths occur within the first 3 months after operation, but there is a continuing later risk of death as well (Fig. 48-8). Similar results have been reported by others. Thus, Harken and Josephson re-

ported 60% (CL 52%–64%) actuarial survival at 4.5 years, with time zero being the time of operation and subendocardial resection the procedure used against ventricular tachycardia (Fig. 48-9).[H5,J1] Most of these deaths also occurred in the early months after operation. The mean ejection fraction of their patients was 28% (similar to that of UAB patients[K3]); 84 of their 90 patients had coronary artery disease; and 75 had concomitant left ventricular aneurysmectomy. Similar results were reported by Brodman and colleagues[B6] and Frank and colleagues.[F6]

Both early and late mortality appear to be at least in part related to the type of operation performed. Encircling endocardial myotomy probably carries a greater risk of death than does endocardial ablation (Table 48-1).[M2] This fact suggests that mortality rates may become lower with the more general adoption of safer operative procedures.

All these survival rates are lower than those for patients with ejection fractions of 0.3 undergoing only coronary artery bypass grafting (82%, CL 77%–83% at 4.5 years; see Chapter 7, Fig. 7-14) and those for patients without life-threatening VT undergoing left ventricular aneurysmectomy (76%, CL 72%–79% at 7.5 years; see Chapter 8, Fig. 8-7).

Modes of Death

Most commonly, patients undergoing operation for ventricular tachycardia in ischemic heart disease die in cardiac failure (Table 48-2). For example, among 40 deaths, the heart failure was acute and caused death within 48 hours of operation in 23% of the total deaths, was subacute and caused death 4–30 days after operation in 28%, and was chronic and caused death later in 13% (UAB).

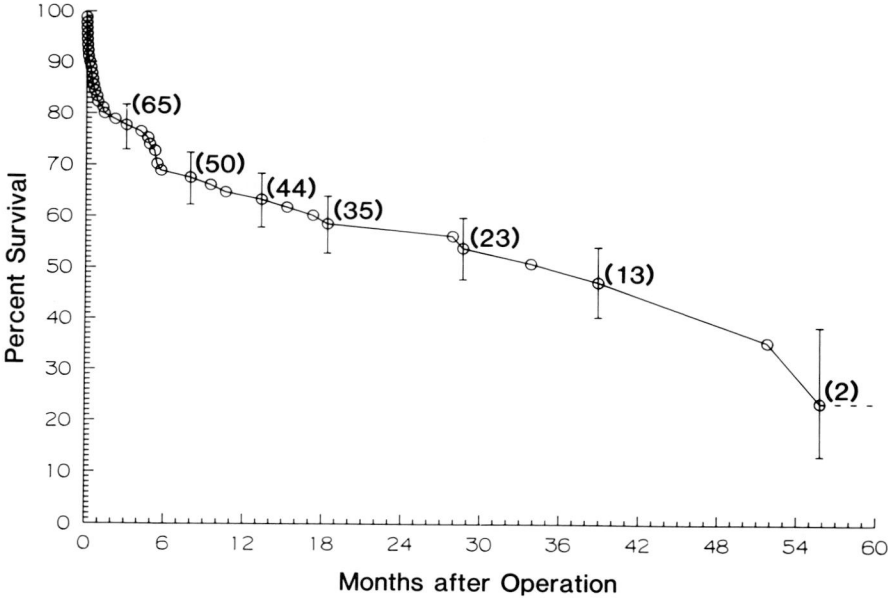

Figure 48-7 Actuarial survival of patients with ischemic heart disease after direct operations for life-threatening ventricular tachycardia (UAB; 1967–July 1984; *n* = 90; 40 deaths). Time zero is the end of cardiopulmonary bypass. Each circle represents a death. The vertical lines encompass the 70% confidence limits. The numbers in parentheses are patients traced to the times indicated. The dashed lines depict survival beyond the last event. The first operation was on May 16, 1978. Reproduced with permission from McGiffin et al.[M2]

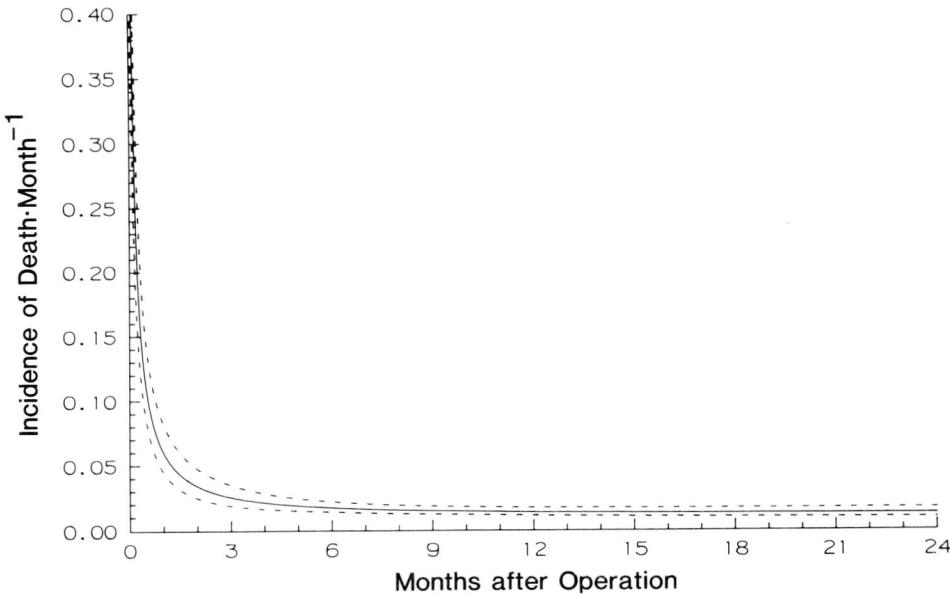

Figure 48-8   Hazard function (instantaneous risk of death) for death in patients with ischemic heart disease after direct operations for life-threatening ventricular tachycardia (UAB; 1967–July 1984; *n* = 90). The solid line is the point estimate, and the dashed lines enclose the 70% confidence limits. An early phase of risk begins with the end of operation and extends to about 3 months postoperatively, after which the late phase of risk is constant. For reference, the instantaneous risk (incidence) of death · month^{-1} of an age-, race-, and gender-matched general population is 0.001.
Reproduced with permission from McGiffin et al.[M2]

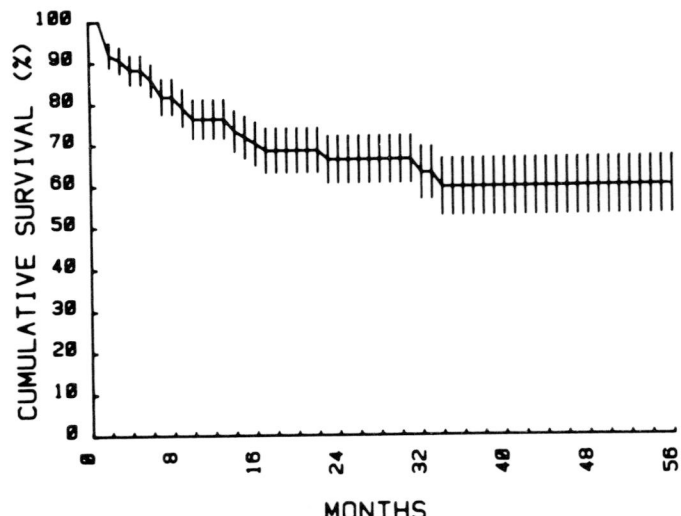

Figure 48-9   Actuarial survival curve of 90 patients after subendocardial resection with or without adjunctive procedures. Most of the deaths that occurred were early and included in a 9% operative mortality. The curve flattens after 2.5 years and ends in a 60% survival rate at 5 years.
Reproduced with permission from Harken et al.[H5]

A smaller proportion of patients die either suddenly or with documented ventricular tachyarrhythmias. Ninety-one percent of patients were free of these modes of death 1 year after operation (Fig. 48-10), but there was a constant hazard of such deaths occurring throughout the follow-up period (Fig. 48-11).

Relief of Life-threatening Ventricular Tachycardia

Freedom from Antiarrhythmic Drugs
Over half the patients surviving an electrophysiologic-guided direct operation for life-threatening ventricular tachycardia are without the need for antiarrhythmic drugs postoperatively and thus are surgical cures as regards their arrhythmia, at least currently (Table 48-3). Thus, among 50 such patients, 29 (58%, CL 50%–66%) are asymptomatic off drug therapy, a therapeutic plan believed indicated by the noninducibility of their VT at postoperative electrophysiologic study (UAB).

Freedom from Sustained Ventricular Tachycardia at Postoperative Study
Among 34 patients studied by epicardial programmed ventricular stimulation 7–30 days after operation, Page and colleagues were unable to induce sustained VT in 19 (56%, CL 46%–66%), and no arrhythmic events were observed in this group during a mean follow-up period of 19.5 months (UAB).[P3] Ventricular tachycardia was noninducible at study early postoperatively in 65 (79%, CL 74%–84%) of 82 patients reported by Harken and Josephson,[H5] in 25 (69%, CL 60%–78%) of 36 surviving patients reported by Kienzle and

Table 48-1 Hospital mortality after surgery for ischemic heart disease that included a procedure directed against life-threatening ventricular tachycardia (UAB; August 1978–July 1984; $n = 90$).[M2]

| Surgical Procedure | n | Early Hospital Deaths | | | | Late Deaths | | | Total Deaths | |
		No.	%	CL		No.	%	CL	No.	
LV resection	1		0%	0%–85%		1	100%	15%–100%	1	
More-or-less encircling endocardial myotomy	30	9	30%[a]	21%–41%		8	27%	18%–37%	17 }	$P(\chi^2) = .01$
Endocardial ablation[b]	32	4	12%[a]	6%–22%		4	12%	6%–22%	8 }	
Combined myotomy plus ablation	27	5	19%	11%–29%		9	33%	23%–45%	14	
Total	90	18	20%	15%–25%		22	24%	20%–30%	40	

KEY: CL, 70% confidence limits; LV, left ventricle.

[a] $P(\chi^2)$ for difference $= .09$.

[b] Subendocardial resection and/or cryoablation.

colleagues,[K9] in 30 (91%, CL 83%–96%) of 33 patients reported by Moran and colleagues,[M9] and in 27 (73%, CL 63%–81%) of 37 patients reported by Ostermeyer and colleagues. Current techniques, particularly the use of cryosurgery (see "Technique of Operation"), seem to bring more consistently good results.[P4] In patients with inducible sustained tachycardia at postoperative testing, the arrhythmia is often successfully suppressed by drug therapy, in contrast to the preoperative situation.[H5,M2]

Freedom from Spontaneous Ventricular Tachycardia or Sudden Death

Fifteen of the 34 patients studied by Page and colleagues postoperatively had inducible sustained VT, and 7 of those had ventricular tachycardia or sudden death during the follow-up period (*P* for difference from those with a negative postoperative study $= .0008$).[P3] Ventricular tachycardia may also recur later in patients without inducible VT at the early postoperative electrophysiologic study. This occurred in 2 (7%, CL 2%–16%) of 29 patients reported by Kienzle and colleagues.[K9] Harken and Josephson reported that, among 65 patients without inducible VT at postoperative electrophysiologic testing, 3 (5%, CL 2%–9%) had later recurrence of life-threatening ventricular tachycardia, and 3

others (5%, CL 2%–9%) died suddenly and unexpectedly late postoperatively.[H5]

Overall, over three-fourths of living patients are free of spontaneous sustained ventricular tachycardia 12 months after operation (Fig. 48-12).[M2] This is true for patients with inferior scars and aneurysms as well as for those with anterolateral ones.[14] When postoperative ventricular tachycardia does occur, it usually does so within the first week. Although the early risk phase persists only about 2 months after operation, there is a constant late risk of the development of spontaneous sustained ventricular tachycardia (Fig. 48-13). The early phase may be the result of persistent reentry circuits. The constant late phase may be the result of newly developed reentry circuits in areas of residual left ventricular or septal scarring.

If sudden death is also considered a ventricular arrhythmic event, then the actuarial freedom from a new ventricular arrhythmic event is about 72% at 12 months after operation (Fig. 48-14). The hazard function is similar to that just described for postoperative ventricular tachycardia and consists of an early and late phase (Fig. 48-15). Incremental risk factors for such events include a higher preoperative left ventricular end diastolic pressure and longer aortic cross-clamp time (Table 48-4). The former is a risk factor, in all probability, because of its reflection of the extent of left ventricular scarring; and longer aortic cross-clamp times generally result in more ventricular electrical instability postoperatively. In this regard, no surgical technique was clearly superior to others; the only two techniques that do not drop out in the analysis are more-or-less encircling myotomy and endocardial ablation by excision, and with neither is there a high degree of certainty that their inclusion is not by chance.

In addition, the majority of patients are found to have repetitive forms of ventricular arrhythmias postoperatively when studied by Holter monitoring, whether or not VT is inducible at electrophysiologic study early postoperatively.[K9] The significance of this finding is not certain at present.

Heart Block

Occasionally, patients come to operation with preexisting complete heart block. This was true in 2 of 90 patients at

Table 48-2 Mode of death in patients with ischemic heart disease after surgery directed against life-threatening ventricular tachycardia (UAB; 1967–July 1984; $n = 90$).[M2]

Mode of Death	n	% of 40	
Cardiac failure	26	65%	
Acute	9	23%	
Subacute	11	28%	
Chronic	6	15%	
Sudden	6	15% }	20%
Documented ventricular tachyarrhythmias	2	5% }	
Cancer	1	3%	
Subacute respiratory failure	1	3%	
Acute neurologic death	1	3%	
Alcoholic cirrhosis	1	3%	
Uncertain	2	5%	
Total	40	100%	

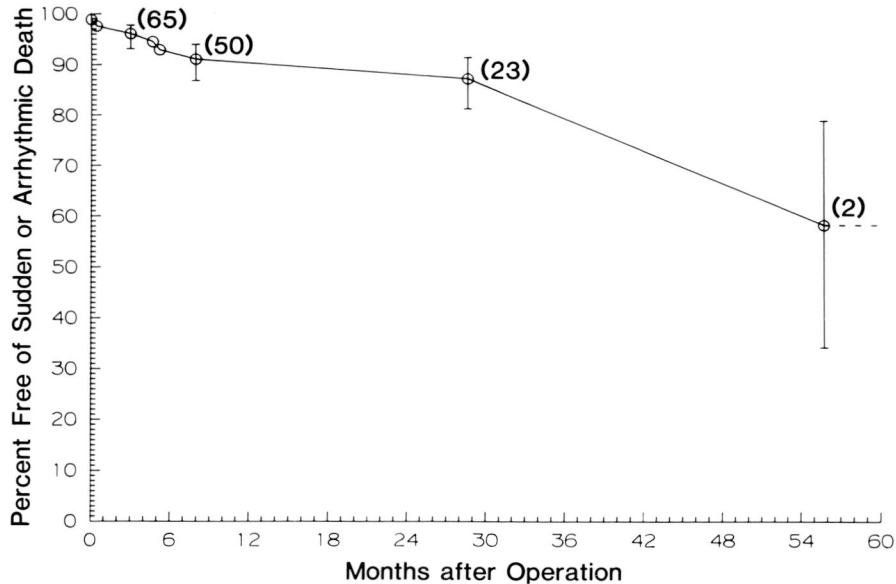

Figure 48-10 Actuarial depiction of freedom from death with documented sustained ventricular tachycardia and from sudden death in patients with ischemic heart disease after direct operations for life-threatening ventricular tachycardia (UAB; 1967–July 1984; *n* = 90; 9 events). Patients dying of other causes were censored at death.

Reproduced with permission from McGiffin et al.[M2]

UAB. A few patients develop complete heart block intraoperatively, probably related to trifascicular block. This occurred in 3 (3%, CL 1%–7%) of 88 patients at UAB. Heart block is managed by permanent pacing, preferably of the AV sequential type.

Rarely, patients require pacemaker insertion for severe sinus bradycardia.

Left Ventricular Function

Left ventricular function, as well as survival, appears to be affected by the specific type of surgical procedure used against the ventricular tachycardia. Ostermeyer and colleagues noted that 5 (45%, CL 27%–65%) of 11 patients treated by a complete encircling endocardial myotomy de-

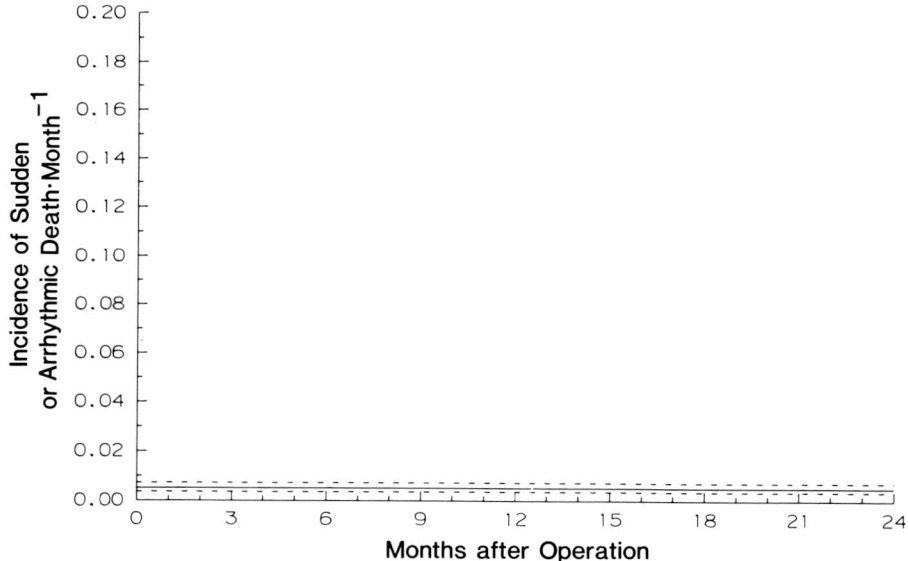

Figure 48-11 Hazard function (instantaneous risk of death with verified sustained ventricular tachycardia or suddenly) in patients with ischemic heart disease after direct operations for life-threatening ventricular tachycardia (UAB; 1967–July 1984; *n* = 90; 9 events). Patients dying of other causes were censored at death.

Reproduced with permission from McGiffin et al.[M2]

Table 48-3 Antiarrhythmic drug status among patients alive after surgery directed against life-threatening ventricular tachycardia (UAB; 1967–July 1984; n = 93).[M2]

Antiarrhythmic Drugs	Nonischemic		Ischemic	
	n	% of 2	n	% of 50
No	1	50%	29	58%
Yes	0	0%	20	40%
Not determined	1	50%	1	2%

NOTE: In some instances, the drugs have been indicated by atrial rather than ventricular arrhythmias. The n = 93 because of the inclusion of three patients (one death) with nonischemic VT.

veloped severe left ventricular dysfunction postoperatively, in contrast to 2 (8%, CL 3%–17%) of 26 in whom only a partial endocardial myotomy was performed.[O1]

Functional Status

Functional status separate from arrhythmic status is somewhat difficult to determine. However, most surviving patients are in NYHA functional class I or II late postoperatively (Table 48-5).[M2]

INDICATIONS FOR OPERATION

The indication for the direct operation for VT is the presence of life-threatening ventricular tachycardia and the preoperative demonstration of the focus for its development. Ventricular tachycardia in patients with ischemic heart disease is considered life-threatening when ventricular fibrillation has occurred outside the setting of acute ischemia; when documented symptomatic ventricular tachycardia has occurred while a patient is on optimal medical management; or when, in a patient with a suggestive history, sustained ventricular tachycardia can be induced by programmed electrical stimulation in spite of pharmacologic therapy. When necessary, surgical treatment can be performed without increased risk within the first few months after the acute myocardial infarction which has been responsible for the life-threatening arrhythmia.[M12]

The operation for the ventricular tachycardia is accompanied by appropriate procedures for the other aspects of ischemic heart disease that are present.

SPECIAL SITUATIONS AND CONTROVERSIES

Types of Indirect Operation

Coronary artery bypass grafting (CABG) has been proposed for the relief of life-threatening ventricular tachycardia. It may be efficacious in patients with severe coronary artery disease, no previous overt or silent myocardial infarction, and ventricular tachycardia or ventricular fibrillation induced by exercise or accompanying severe angina.[A1] However, CABG does not in general reliably reduce the risk of life-threatening ventricular arrhythmias in any other setting of ischemic heart disease (see Chapter 7, "Ventricular Arrhythmias" in section on Late Results).[S10]

Left ventricular aneurysmectomy with or without CABG is generally inadequate for the control of life-threatening

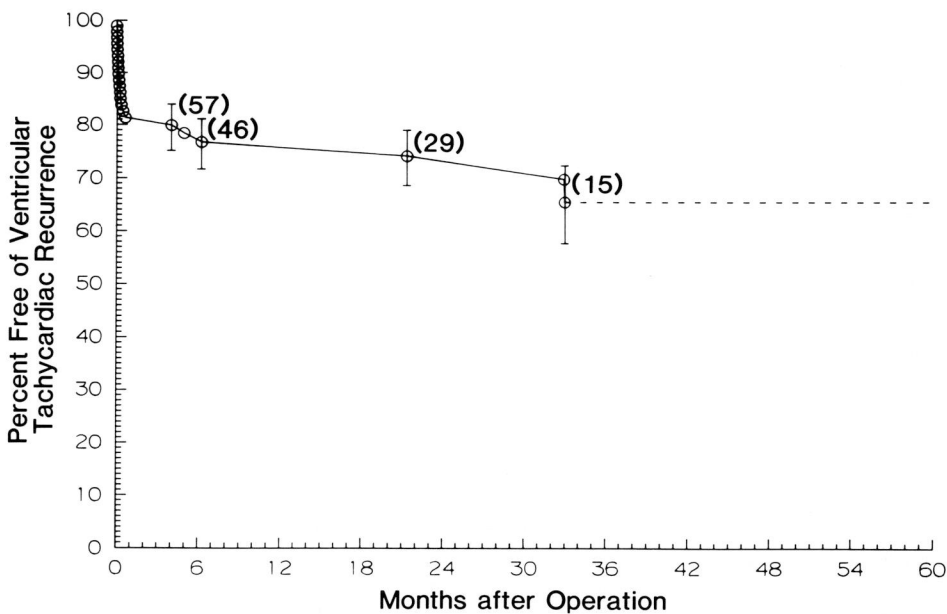

Figure 48-12 Actuarial depiction of freedom from recurrent spontaneous sustained ventricular tachycardia in patients with ischemic heart disease after direct operations for life-threatening ventricular tachycardia (UAB; 1967–July 1984; n = 90; 22 events). Patients dying of other causes were censored at death.

Reproduced with permission from McGiffin et al.[M2]

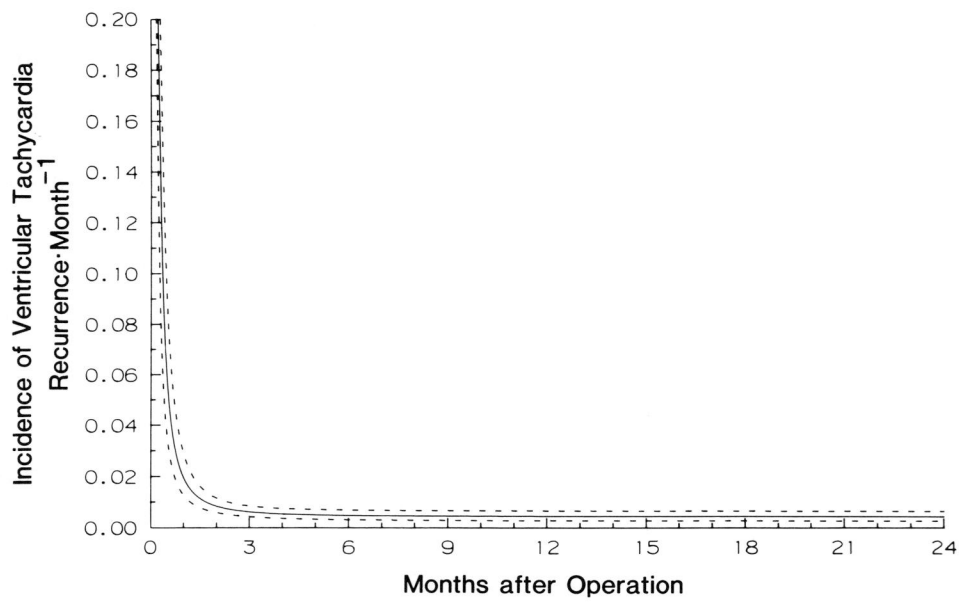

Figure 48-13 Hazard function for recurrence of spontaneous sustained ventricular tachycardia in patients with ischemic heart disease after direct operations for life-threatening ventricular tachycardia (UAB; 1967–July 1984; *n* = 90; 22 events). Patients dying of other causes were censored at death.

Reproduced with permission from McGiffin et al.[M2]

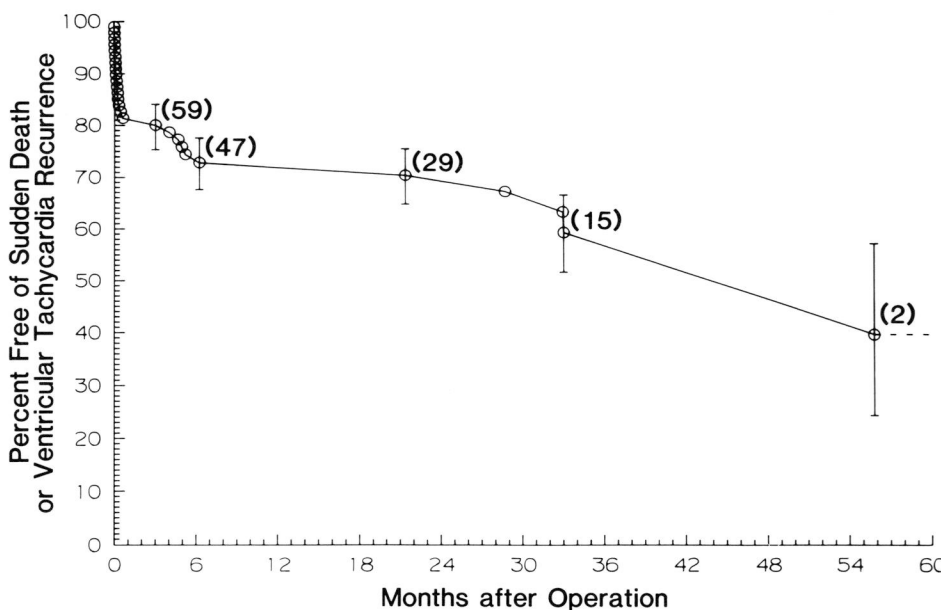

Figure 48-14 Actuarial depiction of freedom from sudden death or recurrence of spontaneous sustained ventricular tachycardia in patients with ischemic heart disease after direct operations for life-threatening ventricular tachycardia (UAB; 1967–July 1984; *n* = 90; 27 events). Patients dying of other causes were censored at death.

Reproduced with permission from McGiffin et al.[M2]

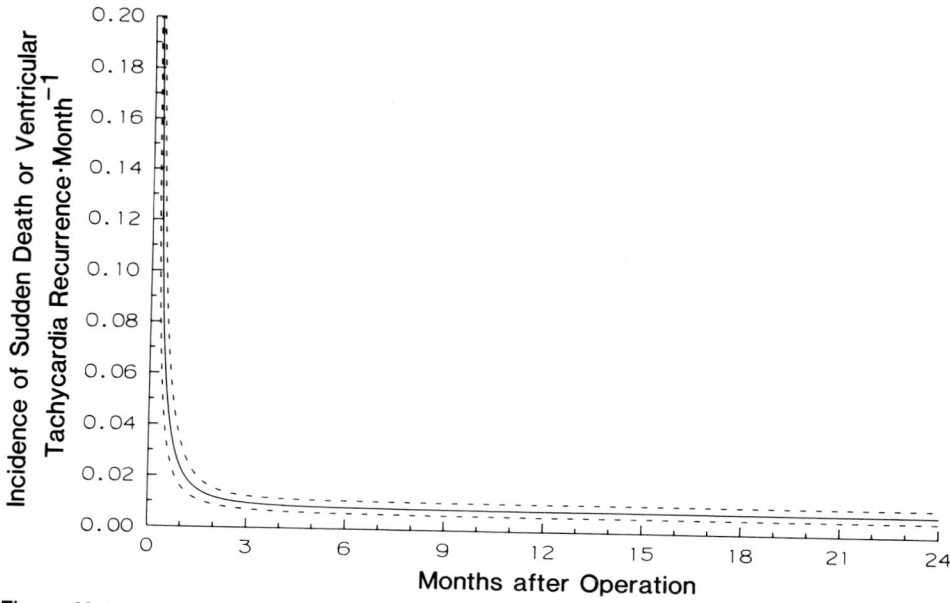

Figure 48-15 Hazard function for sudden death or the recurrence of spontaneous sustained ventricular tachycardia in patients with ischemic heart disease after direct operations for life-threatening ventricular tachycardia (UAB; 1967–July 1984; $n = 90$; 27 events). Patients dying of other causes were censored at death.

Reproduced with permission from McGiffin et al.[M2]

ventricular tachycardia.[M1] Thus, Mason and colleagues found a recurrence of the tachycardia within 1 month in 16 (50%, CL 39%–61%) of 32 patients treated in this manner, and in 32 (100%, CL 94%–100%) of 32 patients at 94 months.[M6] In a comparable group of 33 patients in which a direct operation guided by electrophysiologic mapping was also done, 4 (13%, CL 6%–21%) had a recurrence at 1 month and 10 (30%, CL 21%–41%) at 24 months.[M6] Similar findings have been reported by Harken and colleagues,[H4] by Ostermeyer and associates,[O2] and by Sami and colleagues,[S15] all of which strongly support the idea that left ventricular aneurysmectomy alone is an inadequate operation for the control

Table 48-4 Incremental risk factors for sudden death or recurrence of spontaneous sustained ventricular tachycardia in patients with ischemic heart disease after direct operations for life-threatening ventricular tachycardia (UAB; 1967–July 1984; $n = 90$; 27 events).

Incremental Risk Factor	Early Phase		Late Constant Phase	
	Coefficient ± SD	P value	Coefficient ± SD	P value
(Higher) preoperative left ventricular end diastolic pressure (mmHg)	0.12 ± 0.048	.01		
(Longer) aortic cross-clamp time (minutes)	0.032 ± 0.0135	.02		
More-or-less encircling endocardial myotomy with or without endocardial ablation	1.4 ± 0.82	.09		
Endocardial ablation by excision			1.0 ± 0.64	.11
Intercept	−7.4		−5.2	

NOTE: Patients were censored in the event of death from another cause. The risk factor analysis is in the parametric domain for time-related events (see Chapter 6). Variables analyzed were the usual demographic ones, preoperative left ventricular ejection fraction and end-diastolic pressure, preoperative NYHA functional class, previous surgery for ischemic heart disease, date of operation, the use of coronary artery bypass grafting (and, if used, the number of distal anastomoses) and aortic cross-clamp time. The analysis also evaluated the presence alone or in combination of more-or-less encircling endocardial myotomy, endocardial ablation, combined myotomy and ablation, and the individual procedures alone or in combination of left ventricular resection, myotomy, endocardial ablation by excision, and endocardial ablation by cryoablation.

Table 48-5 Functional status (NYHA class) of patients alive after surgery directed against life-threatening ventricular tachycardia (UAB; 1967–July 1984; n = 93).[M2]

NYHA Class	Nonischemic		Ischemic	
	n	% of 2	n	% of 50
I	0	0%	14	28%
II	1	50%	25	50%
III	0	0%	6	12%
IV	0	0%	1	2%
Unclassified	1	50%	4	8%

of life-threatening ventricular tachycardia (see Chapter 7, "Ventricular Arrhythmias," under "Special Situations and Controversies").

Types of Direct Operation

Subendocardial Resection
Currently, subendocardial resection can be considered the best direct operation for ventricular tachycardia. Its purpose is ablation of the origin of the ventricular tachycardia. It is a discreet approach, directed by pre- and intraoperative mapping. The procedure has not been reported to result in deterioration of left ventricular function. Its main disadvantage is that it cannot be carried out around the base of the papillary muscles. Also, it is not applicable to ventricular tachycardia arising within the septum or intramural myocardium.

Encircling Endocardial Ventriculotomy
The technique of encircling endocardial ventriculotomy was devised to isolate electrically all the scar tissue from which it is assumed the tachycardia arises. The procedure has been variably effective (Table 48-1).[G4,O1,O2] However, experimental studies by Ungerleider and colleagues have indicated that the procedure may have its favorable effect primarily through ablation of arrhythmogenic regions rather than their isolation.[U4] Both clinical experience[W5,O1,O2] and experimental studies have indicated that this procedure results in further myocardial ischemic damage and depression of ventricular function (see Chapter 8, "Ventricular Arrhythmias," under "Special Situations and Controversies").[U1,U5]

Automatic Implantable Defibrillation

Mirowski reported successful use of an implantable automatic defibrillator in patients with life-threatening ventricular arrhythmias.[M7] Watkins and colleagues combined endocardial resection controlled with intraoperative electrophysiologic studies and the implantation of the automatic defibrillator and reported two late deaths, neither related to arrhythmias among 12 patients surviving operation and traced 32 months.[W9] Although this technique is still in the early stages of development, it has already been demonstrated to be highly effective[E1] and is likely to play an important role in the management of refractory ventricular tachycardia and sudden death in the future.

Automatic Implantable Pacemakers

A further development is the testing of various fully implantable pacemakers that sense and interrupt tachycardias, that is, *tachycardia intervention pacemakers*.[N2] These sophisticated electronic devices sense the onset of tachycardia and operate in either scanning (delivery-coupled single or multiple extrastimuli) or overdrive (burst) modes. A small amount of experience[F8,R1] and theoretical considerations indicate that implantable devices can terminate ventricular tachycardia with critically timed single or double ventricular extrastimuli. Refinements of the devices and further experience may make this useful therapy in patients who are refractory to other methods.

SECTION 5
OTHER INTRACTABLE VENTRICULAR TACHYCARDIAS

About 25% of patients with ventricular tachycardia are without ischemic heart disease, and 10% have been said to be without any demonstrable morphologic cardiac disease.[F5] However, recent observations indicate that even in some patients who have been thought to be without morphologic cardiac disease, right ventricular morphologic abnormalities may be present.[S16] In surgical series, the cardiac pathology has most commonly been arrhythmogenic right ventricular dysplasia,[F2] an entity possibly comparable to Uhl's anomaly.[G12] Other less common morphologic bases include arrhythmogenic left ventricular dysplasia, idiopathic left ventricular aneurysms, congestive dilated cardiomyopathy, obstructive hypertrophic cardiomyopathy, and cardiac tumors.[F2,F5]

ARRHYTHMOGENIC RIGHT VENTRICULAR DYSPLASIA

The development of intractable ventricular tachycardia in childhood[D4] or adult life may be a manifestation of the rare arrhythmogenic right ventricular dysplasia.[M3] The right ventricular free wall has both thick and thin areas of pathologic development, and either may be arrhythmogenic. The basic pathologic process is said to be the progressive replacement of myocardial fibers in the subepicardium and midmyocardium by fatty tissue.[F3] The process does not occur in the subendocardium. It is believed that the strands of partially degenerated myofibrillar fascicles, which connect with normal myocardium, can provide a basis for slow conduction and reentry.[F2] Characteristically, on angiography the right ventricle is enlarged and deformed by bulging areas over the infundibulum, apex, and basal portion of the inferior wall.[G12]

In patients in whom the electrocardiographic findings and programmed electrical stimulation studies are diagnostic, operation with intraoperative mapping may be advised. A properly oriented simple ventriculotomy cutting across the arrhythmogenic focus is the recommended operation, although at times a localized resection has been done.[F2,F5,G12]

Some patients have had long-term remission of their ventricular tachycardia after the procedure.[F2] However, there is some evidence that this type of cardiomyopathy is progressive and that it may eventually involve the left ventricle as well.[H11]

In Uhl's anomaly, the free wall of the right ventricle is "like parchment," with only a few myocardial fibers between epicardium and endocardium.[U2] Occasionally, life-threatening ventricular tachycardia develops, and this may be controlled (one case at UAB) by pre- and intraoperative electrophysiologic studies and an appropriately placed ventriculotomy, as just described.

ARRHYTHMOGENIC LEFT VENTRICULAR DYSPLASIA

In arrhythmogenic left ventricular dysplasia, a rare cause of intractable ventricular tachycardia, the histopathologic state is the same as in arrhythmogenic right ventricular dysplasia but with more fibrosis.[F2] Preoperative and intraoperative electrophysiologic studies are said to identify the condition and encircling endocardial ventriculotomy to stop the arrhythmia.[F2]

IDIOPATHIC INTRACTABLE VENTRICULAR TACHYCARDIA

Idiopathic intractable ventricular tachycardia has also occasionally been treated surgically. In one report, the tachycardia seemed to originate in the left ventricular free wall in one of three cases and in the ventricular septum in the other two cases.[F2] However, the report of Sugrue and colleagues casts doubt on the idiopathic nature of such cases (see "Morphology").[S18]

REFERENCES

A

1. Anderson KP, Mason JW: Surgical management of ventricular tachyarrhythmias. *Clin Cardiol* 6:415, 1983.

B

1. Burchell HB, Frye RL, Anderson MW, McGoon DC: Atrioventricular and ventriculo-atrial excitation in Wolff-Parkinson-White syndrome (type B): Temporary ablation at surgery. *Circulation* 36:663, 1967.

2. Bharati S, Rosen K, Steinfield L, Miller RA, Lev M: The anatomic substrate for preexcitation in corrected transposition. *Circulation* 62:831, 1980.

3. Brodman R, Fisher J, Mitsudo S, Kim SG, Matos J: Kent pathways visualized in situ and removed at operation. *Am J Cardiol* 51:1457, 1983.

4. Becker AE, Anderson RH, Durrer D, Wellens JHH: The anatomical substrates of the Wolff-Parkinson-White syndrome: A clinicopathological correlation in seven patients. *Circulation* 57:870, 1978.

5. Burchell HB: The surgical treatment of re-entrant atrioventricular tachycardia (Wolff-Parkinson-White syndrome). *Mayo Clin Proc* 57:387, 1982.

6. Brodman R, Fisher JD, Johnston DR, Kim SG, Matos JA, Waspe LE, Scsavin GM, Furman S: Results of electrophysiologically guided operations for drug-resistant recurrent ventricular tachycardia and ventricular fibrillation due to coronary artery disease. *J Thorac Cardiovasc Surg* 87:431, 1984.

C

1. Cohn AE, Fraser FR: Paroxysmal tachycardia and the effect of stimulation of the vagus nerves by pressure. *Heart* 5:93, 1913.

2. Cobb FR, Blumenschein SD, Sealy WC, Boineau JP, Wagner GS, Wallace AG: Successful surgical interruption of the bundle of Kent in a patient with Wolff-Parkinson-white syndrome. *Circulation* 38:1018, 1968.

3. Cox JL: The surgical management of cardiac arrhythmias, in DC Sabiston, FC Spencer (eds): *Surgery of the Chest*, vol 2 (ed 4). Philadelphia: Saunders, 1983, p 1552.

4. Coumel P, Cabarol C, Fabiato A, Gourgon R, Slama R: Tachycardia permanente par rythme réciproque. *Arch Mal Coeur* 60:1830, 1967.

5. Couch OA Jr: Cardiac aneurysm with ventricular tachycardia and subsequent excision of aneurysm. *Circulation* 20:251, 1959.

6. Cohen M, Wiener I, Pichard A, Holt J, Smith H, Gorlin R: Determinants of ventricular tachycardia in patients with coronary artery disease and ventricular aneurysm. *Am J Cardiol* 51:61, 1983.

7. Cox JL: The status of surgery for cardiac arrhythmias. *Circulation* 71:413, 1985.

D

1. Durrer D, Roos JT: Epicardial excitation of the ventricles in a patient with Wolff-Parkinson-White syndrome. *Circulation* 38:1018, 1968.

2. Davidoff R, Schamroth CL, Myerberg DP: The Wolff-Parkinson-White pattern in healthy air crew. *Aviat Space Environ Med* 52:554, 1981.

3. Durrer D, Schoo L, Schuilenburg RM, Wellens HJJ: The role of premature beats in the initiation and the termination of supraventricular tachycardia in the Wolff-Parkinson-White syndrome. *Circulation* 36:644, 1967.

4. Dungan WT, Garson A, Gillette PC: Arrhythmogenic right ventricular dysplasia: A cause of ventricular tachycardia in children with apparently normal hearts. *Am Heart J* 102:745, 1981.

5. Dreifus LS, Haiat R, Watanabe Y, Arriaga J, Reitman NC: Ventricular fibrillation: A possible mechanism of sudden death in patients with the Wolff-Parkinson-White syndrome. *Circulation* 43:520, 1971.

6. Deal BJ, Keane JF, Gillette PC, Garson A Jr: Wolff-Parkinson-White syndrome and supraventricular tachycardia during infancy: Management and follow-up. *JACC* 5:130, 1985.

E

1. Echt DS, Armstrong K, Schmidt P, Oyer PE, Stinson EB, Winkle RA: Clinical experience, complications, and survival in 70 patients with the automatic implantable cardioverter/defibrillator. *Circulation* 71:289, 1985.

F

1. Fenoglio JJ Jr, Pham TD, Harken AH, Horowitz LN, Josephson ME, Wit AL: Recurrent sustained ventricular tachycardia: Structure and ultrastructure of subendocardial regions in which tachycardia originates. *Circulation* 68:518, 1983.

2. Fontaine G, Guiraudon G, Frank R, Tereau Y, Pavie A, Cabrol C, Chomette G, Grosgogeat Y: Surgical management of ventricular tachycardia not related to myocardial ischemia, in ME Josephson, HJJ Wellens (eds): *Tachycardias: Mechanism, Diagnosis, Treatment.* Philadelphia: Lea & Febiger, 1984.

3. Fontaine G, Guiraudon G, Frank R, Tereau Y, Fillette F, Marcus FI, Chomette G, Grosgogeat Y: Dysplasia ventriculaire droite arythmogene et maladie de Uhl. *Arch Mal Coeur* 75:361, 1982.

4. Fogoros RN, Anderson KP, Winkle RA, Swerdlow CD, Mason JW: Amiodarone: Clinical efficacy and toxicity in 96 patients with recurrent, drug refractory arrhythmias. *Circulation* 68:88, 1983.

5. Fontaine G, Guiraudon G, Frank R, Fillette F, Cabrol C, Grosgogeat Y: Surgical management of ventricular tachycardia unrelated to myocardial ischemia or infarction. *Am J Cardiol* 49:397, 1982.

6. Frank G, Klein H, Lichtlen P, Borst HG: Direct surgical therapy of ventricular arrhythmias in coronary heart disease. *Thorac Cardiovasc Surg* 29:315, 1981.

7. Fontaine G, Frank R, Guiraudon G: Surgical treatment of resistant re-entrant ventricular tachycardia by ventriculotomy: A new application of epicardial mapping. *Circulation* 50(suppl III):III-82, 1974 (abstr).

8. Fisher JD, Kim SG, Furman S, Matos JA: Role of implantable pacemakers in control of recurrent ventricular tachycardia. *Am J Cardiol* 49:194, 1982.

G

1. Gallagher JJ, Stevenson RH, Sealy WC, Wallace AG: The Wolff-Parkinson-White syndrome and the pre-excitation dysrhythmias: Medical and surgical management. *Med Clin North Am* 60:101, 1976.

2. Gallagher JJ, Kasell J, Sealy WC, Pritchett ELC, and Wallace AG: Epicardial mapping in the Wolff-Parkinson-White syndrome. *Circulation* 57:854, 1978.

3. Gallagher JJ, Sealy WC, Cox JL, Kasell JH: Results of surgery for pre-excitation in 200 cases. Fifty-fourth Scientific Sessions, American Heart Association, November 1981.

4. Guiraudon G, Fontaine G, Frank R, Escande G, Etievant P, Cabrol C: Encircling endocardial ventriculotomy: A new surgical treatment for life-threatening ventricular tachycardias resistant to medical treatment following myocardial infarction. *Ann Thorac Surg* 26:438, 1978.

5. Guiraudon GM, Klein GJ, Gulamhusein S, Jones DL, Yee R, Perkins DG, Jarvis E: Surgical repair of Wolff-Parkinson-White syndrome: A new closed-heart technique. *Ann Thorac Surg* 37:67, 1984.

6. Gallagher JJ, Sealy WC, Anderson RW, Kasell J, Millar R, Campbell RWF, Harrison L, Pritchett ELC, Wallace AG: Cryosurgical ablation of accessory atrioventricular connections: A

method for correction of the pre-excitation syndrome. *Circulation* 55:471, 1977.

7. Gillette PC, Garson A, Kugler JD, Cooley DA, Zinner A, McNamara DG: Surgical treatment of supraventricular tachycardia in infants and children. *Am J Cardiol* 46:281, 1980.

8. Gillette PC: Concealed anomalous cardiac conduction pathways: A frequent cause of supraventricular tachycardia. *Am J Cardiol* 40:848, 1977.

9. Gallagher JJ, Svenson RH, Kasell JH, German LD, Bardy GH, Broughton A, Critelli G: Catheter technique for closed-heart ablation of the atrioventricular conduction system: A therapeutic alternative for the treatment of refractory supraventricular tachycardia. *N Engl J Med* 306:194, 1982.

10. Garan H, Ruskin JN, Dimarco JP, Derkac WM, Akins CW, Daggett WM, Asten WG, Buckley MJ: Electrophysiologic studies before and after myocardial revascularization in patients with life-threatening ventricular arrhythmias. *Am J Cardiol* 51:519, 1983.

11. Gallagher JJ, Oldham HN, Wallace AG, Peter RH, Kasell J: Ventricular aneurysm with ventricular tachycardia. *Am J Cardiol* 35:696, 1975.

12. Guiraudon G, Fontaine G, Frank R, Leandri R, Barra J, Cabrol C: Surgical treatment of ventricular tachycardia guided by ventricular mapping in 23 patients without coronary artery disease. *Ann Thorac Surg* 32:439, 1981.

13. Goldberg R, Szkio M, Tonasdcia J, Kennedy HL: Length of time between hospital admission and ventricular fibrillation or cardiac arrest complicating acute myocardial infarction: Effect on prognosis. *Johns Hopkins Med J* 145:187, 1979.

H

1. Holzmann M, Scherf D: Über Elektrokardiogramme mit verkürzter Vorhof-Kammer-Distanz und positiven P-Zacken. *Z f klin Medizin* 121:404, 1932.

2. Hindman MC, Last JH, Rosen KM: Wolff-Parkinson-White syndrome observed by portable monitoring. *Ann Intern Med* 79:654, 1973.

3. Horowitz LN, Josephson ME, Harken AH: Epicardial and endocardial activation during sustained ventricular tachycardia in man. *Circulation* 61:1227, 1980.

4. Harken AH, Horowitz LN, Josephson ME: Comparison of standard aneurysmectomy and aneurysmectomy with directed endocardial resection for the treatment of recurrent sustained ventricular tachycardia. *J Thorac Cardiovasc Surg* 80:527, 1980.

5. Harken AH, Josephson ME: Surgical management of ventricular tachycardia, in ME Josephson, HJJ Wellens (eds): *Tachycardias: Mechanisms, Diagnosis, Treatment.* Chapter 24. Philadelphia: Lea & Febiger, 1984, p 495.

6. Harrison L, Gallagher JJ, Kasell J, Anderson RH, Mikat E, Hacket DB, Wallace AG: Cryosurgical ablation of the A-V node–His bundle: A new method for producing A-V block. *Circulation* 55:463, 1977.

7. Holman WL, Ikeshita M, Lease JG, Ferguson TB, Lofland GK, Cox JL: Alteration of antegrade atrioventricular conduction by cryoablation of peri-atrioventricular nodal tissue. *J Thorac Cardiovasc Surg* 88:67, 1984.

8. Holmes DR Jr, Osborn MJ, Gersh B, Maloney JD, Danielson GK: The Wolff-Parkinson-White syndrome: A surgical approach. *Mayo Clin Proc* 57:345, 1982.

9. Holman WL, Ikeshita M, Ungerleider RM, Smith PK, Ideker

RE, Cox JL: Cryosurgery for cardiac arrhythmias: Acute and chronic effects on coronary arteries. *Am J Cardiol* 51:149, 1983.

10. Heger JJ, Prystowsky EN, Zipes DP: Clinical efficacy of amiodarone in treatment of recurrent ventricular tachycardia and ventricular fibrillation. *Am Heart J* 106:887, 1983.

11. Higuchi S, Caglar NM, Shimada R, Yamada A, Takeshita A, Nakamura M: 16-year follow-up of arrhythmogenic right ventricular dysplasia. *Am Heart J* 108:1363, 1984.

I

1. Iwa T, Magara T, Watanabe Y, Kawasaji M, Misaki T: Interruption of multiple accessory conduction pathways in the Wolff-Parkinson-White syndrome. *Ann Thorac Surg* 30:313, 1980.

2. Iwa T, Kawasuji M, Misaka T, Iwase T, Magara T: Localization and interruption of accessory conduction pathway in the Wolff-Parkinson-White syndrome. *J Thorac Cardiovasc Surg* 80:271, 1980.

3. Iwa T, Kazui T, Sugii S, Wada J: Surgical treatment of Wolff-Parkinson-White syndrome. *Jpn J Thorac Surg* 23:513, 1970.

4. Ivey TD, Brady GH, Misbach GA, Greene HL: Surgical management of refractory ventricular arrhythmias in patients with prior inferior myocardial infarction. *J Thorac Cardiovasc Surg* 89:369, 1985.

J

1. Josephson ME, Harken AH, Horowitz LN: Long-term results of endocardial resection for sustained ventricular tachycardia in coronary disease patients. *Am Heart J* 104:51, 1982.

K

1. Kent AFS: Researches on structure and function of mammalian heart. *J Physiol* 14:233, 1893.

2. Klein GJ, Harrison L, Ideker RF, Smith WM, Kasell J, Wallace AG, Gallagher JJ: Reaction of the myocardium to cryosurgery: Electrophysiology and arrhythmogenic potential. *Circulation* 59:364, 1979.

3. Kirklin JW, Blackstone EH, Rogers WJ: The plights of the invasive treatment of ischemic heart disease. *JACC* 5:158, 1985.

4. Klein GJ, Guiraudon GM, Perkins DG, Jones DL, Yee R, Jarvis E: Surgical correction of the Wolff-Parkinson-White syndrome in the closed heart using cryosurgery: A simplified approach. *JACC* 3:405, 1984.

5. Klein GJ, Gulamhusein SS: Intermittent preexcitation in the Wolff-Parkinson-White syndrome. *Am J Cardiol* 52:292, 1983.

6. Klein GJ, Bashore TM, Sellers TD, Pritchett ELC, Smith WM, Gallagher JJ: Ventricular fibrillation in the Wolff-Parkinson-White syndrome. *N Engl J Med* 301:1080, 1979.

7. Kuck K, Brugada P, Wellens JHH: Observations on the antidromic type of circus movement tachycardia in the Wolff-Parkinson-White syndrome. *JACC* 2:1003, 1983.

8. Kugler JD, Gillette PC, Duff DF, Cooley DA, McNamara DG: Elective mapping and surgical division of the bundle of Kent in a patient with Ebstein's anomaly who required tricuspid valve replacement. *Am J Cardiol* 41:602, 1978.

9. Kienzle MG, Doherty JU, Roy D, Waxman HL, Harken AH, Josephson ME: Subendocardial resection for refractory ventricular tachycardia: Effects on ambulatory electrocardiogram, programmed stimulation and ejection fraction, and relation to outcome. *JACC* 2:853, 1983.

10. Klein H, Karp RB, Kouchoukos NT, Zorn GL, James TN, Waldo AL: Intraoperative electrophysiologic mapping of the ventricles during sinus rhythm in patients with a previous myocardial infarction. *Circulation* 66:847, 1982.

L

1. Lewis T: The experimental production of paroxysmal tachycardia and the effects of ligation of the coronary arteries. *Heart* 1:98, 1909.

2. Lev M, Sodi-Pallares D, Friedland C: A histopathologic study of the atrioventricular communication in a case of WPW with incomplete left bundle branch block. *Am Heart J* 66:399, 1963.

3. Lev M, Kennamer R, Prinzmetal M, de Mesquita QH: Histopathologic study of the atrioventricular communications in two hearts with the Wolff-Parkinson-White syndrome. *Circulation* 24:41, 1961.

4. Lie KI, Lim KL, Schuilenberg RM, David GK, Durrer D: Early identification of patients developing late in-hospital ventricular fibrillation after discharge from the coronary care unit. *Am J Cardiol* 41:674, 1978.

M

1. Mason JW, Stinson EB, Winkle RA, Oyler PE, Griffin JC, Ross DL: Relative efficacy of blind left ventricular aneurysm resection for the treatment of recurrent ventricular tachycardia. *Am J Cardiol* 49:241, 1982.

2. McGiffin DC, Kirklin JK, Blackstone EH, Plumb V, Waldo AL: (1984) Unpublished study.

3. Marcus FI, Fontaine GH, Guiraudon G, Frank R, Laurenceau J, Malergue C, Grosogeat Y: Right ventricular dysplasia: A report of 24 cases. *Circulation* 65:384, 1982.

4. Mikat EM, Hackel DB, Harrison L, Gallagher JJ, Wallace AG: Reaction of the myocardium and coronary arteries to cryosurgery. *Lab Invest* 37:632, 1977.

5. Mines GR: On circulating excitations in heart muscles and their possible relationship to tachycardia and fibrillation. Transactions of the Royal Society of Canada (third series) 8(section IV):43, 1914.

6. Mason JW, Stinson EB, Winkle RA, Griffin JC, Oyer PE, Ross DL, Derby G: Surgery for ventricular tachycardia: Efficacy of left ventricular aneurysm resection compared with operation guided by electrical activation mapping. *Circulation* 65:1148, 1982.

7. Mirowski M: Treatment of malignant ventricular tachyarrhythmias with the automatic implantable defibrillator. *Int J Cardiol* 2:409, 1983.

8. Marchlinski FE, Waxman HL, Buxton AE, Josephson ME: Sustained ventricular tachyarrhythmias during the early postinfarction period: Electrophysiologic findings and prognosis for survival. *JACC* 2:240, 1983.

9. Moran JM, Kehoe RF, Loeb JM, Lichtenthal PR, Sanders JH, Michaelis LL: Extended endocardial resection for the treatment of ventricular tachycardia and ventricular fibrillation. *Ann Thorac Surg* 34:538, 1982.

10. McGiffin D: (1984) Personal communication.

11. Morady F, Sauve MJ, Malone P, Shen EN, Schwartz AB, Bhandari A, Keung E, Sung RJ, Scheinman MM: Long-term efficacy and toxicity of high dose amiodarone therapy for ventricular tachycardia or ventricular fibrillation. *Am J Cardiol* 52:975, 1983.

12. Miller JM, Marchlinski FE, Harken AH, Hargrove WC, Josephson ME: Subendocardial resection for sustained ventricular tachycardia in the early period after acute myocardial infarction. *Am J Cardiol* 55:980, 1985.

N

1. Newman DJ, Donoso E, Friedbert CK: Arrhythmias in the Wolff-Parkinson-White syndrome. *Prog Cardiovasc Dis* 9:147, 1966.
2. Nathan A, Hellestrand K, Bexton R, Nappholz T, Spurrell R, Camm J: Clinical evaluation of an adaptive tachycardia intervention pacemaker with automatic cycle length adjustment. *PACE* 5:201, 1982.

O

1. Ostermeyer J, Breithardt G, Borggrefe M, Godehardt E, Seipel L, Bircks W: Surgical treatment of ventricular tachycardias. *J Thorac Cardiovasc Surg* 87:517, 1984.
2. Ostermeyer J, Breithardt G, Kolvenbach R, Borggrefe M, Seipel L, Schulte HD, Bircks W: The surgical treatment of ventricular tachycardias. *J Thorac Cardiovasc Surg* 84:704, 1982.
3. Ott DA, Gillette PC, Garson A Jr, Cooley DA, Reul GJ, McNamara DG: Surgical management of refractory supraventricular tachycardia in infants and children. *JACC* 5:124, 1985.

P

1. Pham TD, Fenoglio JJ Jr, Harken AH, Ursell PC, Josephson ME, Horowitz LN, Wit AL: Structural basis for recurrent sustained ventricular tachycardia. *Circulation* 64:IV-87, 1981.
2. Parkinson J, Bedford DE, Thompson WAR: Cardiac aneurysm. *Q J Med* 7:455, 1938.
3. Page PL, Arciniegas JG, Plumb VJ, Henthorn RW, Karp RB, Waldo AL: Value of early postoperative epicardial programmed ventricular stimulation studies after surgery for ventricular tachyarrhythmias. *JACC* 2:1046, 1983.
4. Plumb VJ, McGiffin DC, Kirklin JK, Henthorn RW, Epstein AE, Waldo AL: Cryosurgery for ventricular tachycardia. *JACC* 5:409, 1985 (abstr).

R

1. Reddy CP, Todd DP, Kuo CS, DeMaria AN: Treatment of ventricular tachycardia using an automatic scanning extrastimulus pacemaker. *JACC* 3:225, 1984.
2. Rossi L, Thiene G: Mild Ebstein's anomaly associated with supraventricular tachycardia and sudden death: Clinicomorphologic features in 3 patients. *Am J Cardiol* 53:332, 1984.

S

1. Smith WM, Gallagher JJ, Kerr CR, Sealy WC, Kasell JH, Benson DW Jr, Reiter MJ, Sterba R, Grant AO: The electrophysiologic basis and management of symptomatic recurrent tachycardia in patients with Ebstein's anomaly of the tricuspid valve. *Am J Cardiol* 49:1223, 1982.
2. Sealy WC and Gallagher JJ: The surgical approach to the septal area of the heart based on the experiences with 45 patients with Kent bundle. *J Thorac Cardiovasc Surg* 79:542, 1980.
3. Sealy WC, Gallagher JJ, and Kasell JH: His bundle interruption for control of inappropriate ventricular responses to atrial arrhythmias. *Ann Thorac Surg* 32:429, 1981.
4. Sealy WC, Gallagher JJ, Pritchett ELC: The surgical anatomy of Kent bundles based on electrophysiologic mapping and surgical exploration. *J Thorac Cardiovasc Surg* 76:804, 1978.
5. Sealy WC, Wallace AJ, Ramming KP, Gallagher JJ, Svenson RH: An improved operation for the definitive treatment of the Wolff-Parkinson-White syndrome. *Ann Thorac Surg* 17:107, 1974.

6. Sealy WC, Gallagher JJ: Surgical problems with multiple accessory pathways of atrioventricular conduction. *J Thorac Cardiovasc Surg* 81:707, 1981.
7. Sealy WC, Mikat EM: Anatomical problems with identification and interruption of posterior septal Kent bundles. *Ann Thorac Surg* 36:584, 1983.
8. Sealy WC, Gallagher JJ, Pritchett ELC, Wallace AG: Surgical treatment of tachyarrhythmias in patients with both an Ebstein anomaly and a Kent bundle. *J Thorac Cardiovasc Surg* 75:847, 1978.
9. Sealy WC, Gallagher JJ: Surgical treatment of left free wall accessory pathways of atrioventricular conduction of the Kent type. *J Thorac Cardiovasc Surg* 81:698, 1981.
10. Sealy WC: Surgical treatment of the two types of tachycardia caused by Kent bundles with only retrograde fashion. *J Thorac Cardiovasc Surg* 85:746, 1983.
11. Scheinman MM, Morady F, Hess DS, Gonzalez R: Catheter-induced ablation of the atrioventricular junction to control refractory supraventricular arrhythmias. *JAMA* 248:851, 1982.
12. Sealy WC, Anderson RW, Gallagher JJ: Surgical treatment of supraventricular tachyarrhythmias. *J Thorac Cardiovasc Surg* 73:511, 1977.
13. Spielman SR, Schwartz JS, McCarthy DM, Horowitz LN, Greenspan AM, Sadowski LM, Josephson ME, Waxman HL: Predictors of successor failure of medical therapy in patients with chronic recurrent sustained ventricular tachycardia: A discriminant analysis. *JACC* 1:401, 1983.
14. Swerdlow CD, Gong G, Echt DS, Winkle RA, Griffin JC, Ross DL, Mason JW: Clinical factors predicting successful electrophysiologic-pharmacologic study in patients with ventricular tachycardia. *JACC* 1:409, 1983.
15. Sami M, Chaitman BR, Bourassa MG, Carpin D, Chabot M: Long term follow-up of aneurysmectomy for recurrent ventricular tachycardia or fibrillation. *Am Heart J* 96:303, 1978.
16. Strain JE, Grose RM, Factor SM, Fisher JD: Results of endomyocardial biopsy in patients with spontaneous ventricular tachycardia but without apparent heart disease. *Circulation* 68:1171, 1983.
17. Swerdlow CD, Einkle RA, Mason JW: Determinants of survival in patients with ventricular tachyarrhythmias. *N Engl J Med* 308:1436, 1983.
18. Sugrue DD, Holmes DR Jr, Gersh BJ, Edwards WD, McLaran CJ, Wood DL, Osborn MJ, Hammill SC: Cardiac histologic findings in patients with life-threatening ventricular arrhythmias of unknown origin. *JACC* 4:952, 1984.

T

1. Truex RC, Bishof JK, Hoffman EL: Accessory atrial ventricular muscle bundles of developing human heart. *Anat Rec* 131:45, 1958.
2. Truex RC, Bishof JK, Downing DF: Accessory atrioventricular muscle bundles. II. Cardiac conduction system in a human specimen with Wolff-Parkinson-White syndrome. *Anat Rec* 137:417, 1960.

U

1. Ungerleider RM, Holman WL, Calacagno D, Williams JM, Lofland GK, Smith PK, Stanley TE, Quick G, Cox JL: Encircling endocardial ventriculotomy for refractory ischemic ventricular tachycardia. III. Effects on regional left ventricular function. *J Thorac Cardiovasc Surg* 83:857, 1982.
2. Uhl HS: A previously undescribed congenital malformation of

the heart: Almost total absence of the myocardium of the right ventricle. *Bull Johns Hopkins Hosp* 91:197, 1952.

3. Uther JB, Johnson DC, Baird DK, Richards DA, Denniss AR, Ross D, Leck BD: Surgical section of accessory atrioventricular electrical connections in 108 patients. *Am J Cardiol* 49:995, 1982.

4. Ungerleider RM, Holman WL, Stanley TE, Lofland GK, Williams JM, Ideker RE, Smith PK, Quick G, Cox JL: Encircling endocardial ventriculotomy for refractory ischemic ventricular tachycardia. I. Electrophysiological effects. *J Thorac Cardiovasc Surg* 83:840, 1982.

5. Ungerleider RM, Holman WL, Stanley TE, Lofland GK, Williams JM, Smith PK, Quick G, Cox JL: Encircling endocardial ventriculotomy for refractory ischemic ventricular tachycardia. II. Effects on regional myocardial blood flow. *J Thorac Cardiovasc Surg* 83:850, 1982.

V

1. Velebit V, Podrid P, Lown B, Cohen BH, Grayboys TB: Aggravation and provocation of ventricular arrhythmias by antiarrhythmic drugs. *Circulation* 65:886, 1982.

2. Vlay SC, Reid PR, Griffith LSC, Kallman CH: Relationship of specific coronary lesions and regional left ventricular dysfunction to prognosis in survivors of sudden cardiac death. *Am Heart J* 108:1212, 1984.

W

1. Wolff L, Parkinson J, White PD: Bundle branch block with short PR interval in healthy young people prone to paroxysmal tachycardia. *Am Heart J* 5:685, 1930.

2. Wilson FN: A case in which the vagus influenced the form of the ventricular complex of the electrocardiogram. *Arch Intern Med* 16:1008, 1915.

3. Wolff GS, Han J, Curran J: Wolff-Parkinson-White syndrome in the neonate. *Am J Cardiol* 41:559, 1978.

4. Wit AL, Cranefield PF: Reentrant excitation as a cause of cardiac arrhythmias. *Am J Physiol* 4:H1-17, 1978.

5. Waldo AL, Arciniegas JG, Klein H: Surgical treatment of life-threatening ventricular arrhythmias: The role of intraoperative mapping and consideration of presently available surgical techniques. *Prog Cardiovasc Dis* 23:247, 1981.

6. Wood FC, Wolferth CC, Geckeler GD: Histologic demonstration of accessory muscular connections between auricle and ventricle in a case of short PR interval and prolonged QRS complex. *Am Heart J* 25:454, 1943.

7. Wood DL, Hammill SC, Holmes DR, Osborn MJ, Gersh BJ: Catheter ablation of the atrioventricular conduction system in patients with supraventricular tachycardia. *Mayo Clin Proc* 58:791, 1983.

8. Wald RW, Waxman MB, Coney PN, Gunstensen J, Goldman BS: Management of intractable ventricular tachycardia after myocardial infarction. *Am J Cardiol* 44:329, 1979.

9. Watkins L, Platia EV, Mower MM, Griffith LSC, Mirowski M, Reid PR: The treatment of malignant ventricular arrhythmias with combined endocardial resection and implantation of the automatic defibrillator: Preliminary report. *Ann Thorac Surg* 37:60, 1984.

10. Ward DE, Camm AJ: Treatment of tachycardias associated with the Wolff-Parkinson-White syndrome by transvenous electrical ablation of accessory pathways. *Br Heart J* 53:64, 1985.

OTHER CARDIAC CONDITIONS

PART VI

49

CARDIAC TRAUMA

DEFINITION

Cardiac trauma is damage done to the heart by penetrating or nonpenetrating (closed or blunt) trauma.

Section 1
PENETRATING CARDIAC TRAUMA

HISTORICAL NOTE

Although homicide dates back to antiquity, apparently the suggestion that the resultant heart wounds could be sutured is a relatively recent one. It may be that Roberts in 1881 first suggested this in the surgical literature.[R1] In 1882 and again in 1895, studies of the experimental closure of cardiac wounds in animals were reported.[B1,D1] In an important paper in 1897, Rehn reported the first successful repair of a penetrating cardiac wound. It is said by Mead[M2] that Williams first successfully performed a heart operation in the United States when in 1889 at Providence Hospital in Chicago he repaired a stab wound of the heart.

The first published report of a successful heart operation in the United States was that of Hill, who repaired a stab wound of the heart in Montgomery, Alabama, in 1902.[H2] In his report, Hill not only described the successful suturing of the stab wound, but he also summarized 37 other cases reported by that time.

MORPHOLOGY

When a sharp long-bladed instrument, such as a knife, ice pick, stiletto, knitting needle, or screwdriver, is violently driven into the midportion of the thorax and penetrates the pericardium, a laceration of the heart or great arteries commonly results. In patients reaching a hospital after their traumatic episode, most commonly (35% of cases) the right ventricle alone is involved.[D2] The left ventricle alone is involved in about 25%, and very infrequently the right atrium alone. In nearly 30% of patients, more than one cardiac chamber is wounded.[S1] Also, coronary arteries can be transected and traumatic coronary arteriovenous fistulae produced.[L1]

When a missile penetrates the thorax and pericardium, a cardiac wound is frequently produced. Many high-velocity missiles produce massive through-and-through injuries of the heart. Occasionally, however, a missile may produce a tangential laceration of a ventricle or may penetrate a cardiac chamber and come to rest within it.

CLINICAL FEATURES AND DIAGNOSTIC CRITERIA

Pathophysiology

Most stab wounds of the heart result in acute pericardial tamponade, although occasionally rapidly exsanguinating hemorrhage may be the result. The patient thus usually presents with the symptoms and signs of acute cardiac tamponade complicated by acute blood loss. (For a discussion of cardiac tamponade, see Chapter 52, "Acute Cardiac Tamponade" in Section 1, Clinical Features and Diagnostic Criteria.)

Missile wounds usually result in acute hemorrhagic shock, which may be rapidly fatal. If not, the patient enters the hospital profoundly hypotensive and with tachycardia and collapsed veins.

Penetrating cardiac wounds are frequently accompanied by wounds involving the pleural space, internal mammary vessels, and lung and occasionally by wounds of the liver and other abdominal viscera.

Symptoms and Signs

The external evidences of a penetrating wound are usually apparent, although occasionally in the case of injury with a stiletto the external wound may initially escape discovery. The external wound and the evidence for either hemorrhagic shock or acute pericardial tamponade dominate the clinical presentation.

Special Studies

If the patient's condition allows it, a chest x-ray is made.

TECHNIQUE OF OPERATION

When a patient presents in the Emergency Room with a penetrating wound of the chest in a location and direction that could involve the heart, the assumption is made that a penetrating wound of the heart exists. Management protocols vary from hospital to hospital, depending on the ease of transfer of patients from the emergency room to the operating room, the facilities in the Emergency Room for performing thoracotomy, and the familiarity of the surgical service with cardiac operations. Since patients who have received penetrating wounds of the heart vary enormously in their condition on admission and in the number and type of coexisting wounds, rigid protocols are unwise.[T1] General guidelines used in a medical center whose staff is familiar with cardiac surgery can be given (UAB).

Stab Wounds

When a critically ill patient is admitted with the syndrome of acute cardiac tamponade from a stab wound of the heart, preparations are made for immediate transfer to the operating room. No more than 5 minutes need elapse between admission and the patient's transfer to the operating table. In the unlikely event that the stabbing device is still in place, it is not removed until preparations for operation are complete,

and ideally not until the pericardium has been opened. If during this brief interval for transportation the patient's condition worsens, a large-bore needle (13 F) is inserted into the pericardial space through the subxyphoid route. Because of the pathophysiology of acute cardiac tamponade (see Chapter 52), the removal of even 40–50 ml of blood usually improves the hemodynamic state at least temporarily.

The patient is rapidly anesthetized, prepared, and draped for operation. A large-bore needle is placed in an easily accessible large vein as these preparations are being made. The surgical draping should be wide so that the chest and abdomen are fully exposed. A median sternotomy incision is made and the pericardium opened. (In institutions where cardiac surgery is not a frequent occurrence, an anterolateral incision, usually left-sided, is made with the idea that this incision can be made the most rapidly and is the most generally useful. However, this is not true in a medical center where cardiac surgery is frequent.)

Blood is rapidly aspirated from the pericardial space with high-vacuum suckers. Ventricular wounds are best controlled immediately by digital compression. Atrial and caval wounds are generally not well controlled in this manner, and wide Allis clamps (so-called *Allis-Adair clamps*) serve ideally to establish hemostasis by opposing the wound edges. Only after digital or instrumental control of active bleeding has been accomplished should attention be turned to suturing the wounds. Ventricular wounds are best sutured with interrupted pledgetted mattress sutures of 2-0 or 3-0 Dacron or polypropylene. Occasionally a ventricular laceration is so extensive as to require cardiopulmonary bypass and patch grafting of the ventricular free wall. Wounds near a major coronary artery are similarly sutured, with pledgets on either side of the artery and the sutures passing beneath it. Atrial or caval wounds are closed by continuous 3-0 or 4-0 polypropylene sutures. Suturing is done beneath the clamp, and the clamp is removed only after the suture line is largely in place.

Unless there is near certainty that the pleural spaces have not been violated, both are opened widely through the median sternotomy. The internal mammary arteries, a potent source of hemorrhage, are examined and, if damaged, are suture-ligated. Damaged areas of lung are oversewn or stapled. The hilum of each lung is examined to ascertain whether there is injury to the pulmonary vessels.

Drainage catheters are placed in each pleural space, and one may be placed in the pericardial space as well. If hemostasis within the pericardium has been satisfactory, the pericardium is closed with widely spaced interrupted sutures. The sternotomy is closed in the usual manner (see Chapter 2, Section 3).

Missile Wounds

If shock and exsanguinating hemorrhage are the problem, as they usually are in missile wounds, a case can be made for immediate left anterolateral thoracotomy in the Emergency Room. If this is to be done, the patient is intubated and ventilated as the procedure is begun, and a large-bore needle is inserted into a vein. The incision curves beneath the breast, and the thorax is entered through the fifth or sixth interspace. An assistant spreads the wound with two hand-held retractors, or a self-retaining thoracotomy retractor is inserted. Digital control of the hemorrhage is obtained and the patient transported to the operating room. If digital control of the cardiac or great artery hemorrhage is not possible, the possibility of reclaiming the patient from death is unlikely.

Nearly always, the alternative plan of transporting the patient immediately to the operating room is followed (UAB). As noted earlier, only a few minutes are lost, and the ability to deal with the situation effectively is greatly enhanced. Once the operating room is reached, simultaneously a large-bore needle is inserted into a vein, the patient is intubated, and the surgical field is prepared and draped. If, in addition to the cardiac wound, there appears to be a major injury to the hilum of one of the lungs, an anterolateral incision is made on the affected side. (It may be necessary to carry this incision across the sternum if the cardiac wound is extensive.) Otherwise, a median sternotomy incision is rapidly made and the pericardium opened.

The principles of management are the same as described for penetrating wounds, but the result is less often successful.

SPECIAL FEATURES OF POSTOPERATIVE CARE

If a central venous line has not been inserted in the operating room, it is now placed. With this and the usual clinical criteria regarding the state of the circulation, the patient can be well managed. The principles of care are identical with those used in patients after other forms of cardiac surgery (see Chapter 5).

A special consideration is the possibility that a major coronary artery has been damaged by the trauma or at operation. Thus, in the first few postoperative hours, if the hemodynamic state is unexpectedly unsatisfactory, in spite of appropriate ventricular filling pressures, and particularly if the electrocardiogram suggests coronary injury, emergency coronary arteriography is performed. Should a major vessel be interrupted or importantly narrowed, emergency coronary artery bypass grafting is done.

During the early postoperative period, it also must be remembered that penetrating wounds may perforate a cardiac septum or damage an atrioventricular or, rarely, a semilunar valve.[S2] Should the findings suggest such an injury, appropriate studies are indicated. If the findings are positive, consideration is given to immediate, as opposed to delayed, repair. If the hemodynamic state is good, delay for 8–12 weeks allows a more secure repair to be made.

RESULTS

Prompt and effective therapy allows good results in most patients with stab wounds of the heart.[S3] The results in missile wounds are less good and depend on the extensiveness of the wound. Overall, about 75% of patients can be salvaged.[B3] The functional result in surviving patients is usually excellent, even when patch grafting of the left ventricular free wall is required.[S9]

INDICATIONS FOR OPERATION

The presence of a penetrating wound to the heart is an indication for immediate operation.[E1] A stab wound over the heart without bleeding or hypotension may not signify penetration of the heart and is therefore per se not an indication for operation.

SECTION 2
CLOSED CARDIAC TRAUMA

HISTORICAL NOTE

In earlier times, cardiac rupture was the only sequela of closed (or blunt) cardiac trauma to receive attention. Apparently, this catastrophic event was originally observed by Senac in 1778.[S4] Although rupture of the ventricular septum was described in 1847 by Hewett,[H1] Campbell and colleagues at the University of Minnesota first successfully repaired a ventricular septal defect produced by closed trauma in 1951.[C1] More recently, surgical attention has become focused on rupture of cardiac valves as a consequence of closed cardiac injuries, although in 1927 Adam described such injuries and the natural history of patients with valvar rupture secondary to trauma.[A1] Cardiac contusion has still more recently been recognized as one of the complications of closed cardiac trauma.[J1]

MORPHOLOGY

When the heart is compressed between two objects, such as the sternum and the vertebral column, or when there is sudden deceleration of the chest with the heart thrust forward against the sternum, intracardiac pressure suddenly becomes high, and the free cardiac wall, the ventricular septum, or the tensor apparatus of the atrioventricular valves may rupture. Rarely, a coronary artery fistula to a cardiac chamber develops after blunt chest trauma.[G10]

Less violent closed injuries may result simply in contusions of the myocardium. Such contusions may vary from small areas of subepicardial or subendocardial petechiae to contusions of the full thickness of the cardiac wall. Radionuclide angiography has shown that the anteriorly situated right ventricle is particularly susceptible to contusion in patients suffering closed chest injuries.[S8]

CLINICAL FEATURES AND DIAGNOSTIC CRITERIA
Cardiac Contusion

Patients with cardiac contusion may exhibit no symptoms, precordial pain, or symptoms indistinguishable from those of angina. Dysrhythmias of different types may develop.

Electrocardiographic abnormalities may be present shortly after the injury, or their onset may be delayed 12–24 hours. The abnormalities may be transient or longer lasting, depending on the extent of the myocardial damage.[J1] Actual

Q waves may develop similar to those seen in acute myocardial infarction. The level of the myocardial isoenzyme (MB) of creatine kinase (CK) may become elevated after injury and, if so, provides a near positive diagnosis of cardiac contusion.[K1] However, the electrocardiographic and isoenzymatic criteria are relatively insensitive and nonspecific indicators of cardiac contusion.[P1]

A relatively sensitive indicator is the radionuclide angiogram. The demonstration of decreased right ventricular or left ventricular ejection fraction in a previously healthy person and the demonstration of abnormalities of left ventricular segmental wall motion are sensitive methods of determining myocardial contusion in traumatized patients.[H3] These methods also allow sequential examination and indicate that considerable myocardial dysfunction can revert to normal within 3 weeks.

Cardiac Rupture

Patients with cardiac rupture usually develop immediate and severe acute cardiac tamponade. An exception is when there has been concomitant rupture of the pericardium, and then there is exsanguinating hemorrhage. Cardiac rupture may develop immediately upon injury, or the rupture may not occur for several days after the injury, and in the interim, there may be no suggestion of the impending catastrophe.

Ventricular Septal Rupture

When it occurs in a patient who has suffered closed chest trauma, rupture of the ventricular septum usually occurs at the time of injury. The characteristic murmur of a ventricular septal defect appears. When the septal rupture is small, the hemodynamic state remains good. When it is large, the patient exhibits the signs and symptoms of pulmonary venous hypertension, and cardiac output is likely to be low.

Atrioventricular Valve Rupture

When rupture of the tensor apparatus or the leaflet of an atrioventricular valve is a complication of closed trauma, its occurrence is usually immediate. Most commonly, it is the tricuspid valve that is ruptured. Thus, initially the clinical manifestations are minimal, and the diagnosis is not suggested until a number of weeks have passed, by which time the characteristic signs and symptoms are present (see Chapters 11, 14).[S6]

Less frequently, the tensor apparatus of the mitral valve is ruptured.[H4] With this injury, patients usually exhibit sudden pulmonary venous hypertension and rapidly developing symptoms, including frank pulmonary edema.[J2] Occasionally the severity of the mitral incompetence appears to increase and delayed operation is required one to two weeks after injury.[C2]

NATURAL HISTORY

Cardiac Contusion

Only fragmentary information is available concerning the natural history of patients with myocardial contusion, since no doubt this condition often goes undiagnosed. Probably the natural history is very similar to that of acute myocardial infarction. When the area involved is small, premature death is uncommon. When the area involved is of moderate size, and particularly when there is associated damage to the left anterior descending coronary artery, a typical large left ventricular aneurysm may develop.[S7] The natural history then is that of other large left ventricular aneurysms (see Chapter 8). When the area involved is very large, death may occur relatively early after injury, in the same modes as after acute myocardial infarction.

Pericarditis and hemopericardium may develop as complications of cardiac contusion. The natural history then becomes that of these conditions (see Chapter 52), with possible late development of chronic constrictive pericarditis.

Cardiac Rupture

Cardiac rupture is generally a rapidly fatal condition unless treated successfully by operation. However, if the rupture is small, and particularly if it involves the right ventricle, the hemopericardium that develops may tamponade the bleeding, and the hemodynamic state may remain reasonably good. Some patients survive such an episode, as evidenced by the very old finding of Cabriolanus (1604) of healed cardiac wounds in persons who had been thought to be well.[B2]

Ventricular Septal Rupture

As in naturally occurring ventricular septal defects, the natural history of ventricular septal rupture depends on the size of the hole (see Chapter 20). When it is small, the early posttraumatic hemodynamic state is good, as is the long-term outlook. When the hole is large, the hemodynamic state may not be good early after the injury and chronic congestive heart failure may ensue.

Atrioventricular Valve Rupture

In the same way that excision of the tricuspid valve is well tolerated (see Chapter 14), so is acute traumatic rupture of the tricuspid valve. Often the diagnosis is not made at the time of injury. Usually, within 2–3 months, the patient exhibits decreased exercise tolerance, and the signs of tricuspid valve incompetence become evident.

In mitral valve rupture, as in spontaneous rupture of chordi tendinae or postinfarction mitral incompetence, the patient often becomes acutely ill within a few hours of the injury.[S5] Perhaps because traumatic mitral valve rupture is associated with a variable amount of cardiac contusion and myocardial dysfunction, this condition often results in a rapidly progressing deterioration and death within 24 hours.[M1]

TECHNIQUE OF OPERATION

When the diagnosis is rupture of a cardiac free wall, immediate operation is undertaken, but preparations must be made for cardiopulmonary bypass (CPB). If the patient's condition allows it, the femoral artery is exposed and cannulated (after heparinization) before the median sternotomy.

After the median sternotomy, it may be seen that the rupture involves only a small area. In that case, digital control and the placement of pledgetted mattress sutures suffice. If digital control cannot be obtained, CPB is established; the blood is aspirated from the pericardium for venous return, and a reduced systemic blood flow rate is used. As soon as a single venous cannula can be inserted into the right atrium, CPB is converted to the usual techniques and flow rates. The repair of the free wall rupture is improvised but is generally similar to the repair of myocardial ruptures complicating acute myocardial infarction (see Chapter 8).

Posttraumatic ventricular septal defects and traumatic injuries of the tricuspid valve are managed in a manner similar to that for congenital ventricular septal defects[A2] and other kinds of tricuspid valve incompetence (see Chapters 20 and 14). In tricuspid valve rupture, the tensor apparatus is usually involved, and an attempt is made to reconstruct it, using pericardium.

SPECIAL FEATURES OF POSTOPERATIVE CARE

The care usually given to patients after cardiac surgery is used after repair of closed cardiac trauma (see Chapter 5).

RESULTS

Except in massive traumatic cardiac ruptures, the results of cardiac repair in the generally young and otherwise healthy individuals affected are good. Even in the face of cardiac rupture, aggressive therapy in an institution where cardiac surgery is frequent can salvage a number of patients. Five of 7 such patients survived after immediate operation and repair through a median sternotomy incision (UAB).

INDICATIONS FOR OPERATION

Cardiac Contusion

There is no indication for surgical treatment in patients with cardiac contusions. Close follow-up is indicated, however, in case delayed cardiac rupture or constrictive pericarditis develops.

Cardiac Rupture

When the patient survives the acute rupture long enough to reach a hospital, immediate operation is indicated.

Ventricular Septal Rupture

Unless the patient is asymptomatic and the ventricular septal rupture small, surgical closure is indicated. If the hemodynamic state remains good in the early posttraumatic period, the repair is deferred to 8–12 weeks after injury so that a more secure closure can be made.

Atrioventricular Valve Rupture

Since important valvular incompetence nearly always develops in cases of AV valve rupture, operation is advisable. When the tricuspid valve has been ruptured, operation is rarely urgently necessary and is often best delayed 8–12 weeks after the injury. In mitral valve rupture, operative repair is urgently indicated.

REFERENCES

A

1. Adam A: Über die traumatischen Veränderungen gesunder Klappen des Herzens. *Z Kreislaufforsch* 19:313, 1927.
2. Asfaw I, Thomas NW, Arbulu A: Interventricular septal defects from penetrating injuries of the heart: A report of 12 cases and review of the literature. *J Thorac Cardiovasc Surg* 69:450, 1975.

B

1. Block MH: Verhandlungen der deutschen Gesellschaft für Chirurgie, Part 1. Elften Congres, Berlin, 1882, p 108.
2. Ballance C: The surgery of the heart. *Lancet* 1:1, 73, 134, 1920.
3. Beall AC, Dietrich EB, Crawford HW, Cooley DA, De Bakey ME: Surgical management of penetrating cardiac injuries. *Am J Surg* 112:686, 1966.

C

1. Campbell GS, Vernier R, Varco RL, Lillehei CW: Traumatic ventricular septal defect. *J Thorac Surg* 37:496, 1959.
2. Caudros CL, Hutchinson JE, Mogtader AH: Laceration of a mitral papillary muscle and the aortic root as a result of blunt trauma to the chest. *J Thorac Cardiovasc Surg* 88:134, 1984.

D

1. Del Vecchio S: Suture of the heart. *Br Med J* 1:86, epitome 417, 1895.
2. Demetriades D: Cardiac penetrating injuries: Personal experience of 45 cases. *Br J Surg* 71:95, 1984.

E

1. Evans J, Gray LA Jr, Rayner A, Fulton RL: Principles for the management of penetrating cardiac wounds. *Ann Surg* 189:777, 1979.

H

1. Hewett P: Rupture of the septum ventriculorum. *London Medical Gazette* 4:870, 1847.
2. Hill LL: Report of a case of successful suturing of the heart, and table of 37 other cases of suturing by different operators and various terminations, and conclusions drawn. Medical Report #62, 29th Nov, p 846, 1902.
3. Harley DP, Mena I, Narahara KA, Miranda R, Nelson RJ: Traumatic myocardial dysfunction. *J Thorac Cardiovasc Surg* 87:386, 1984.

4. Harada M, Osawa M, Kosukegawa K: Isolated mitral valve injury from non-penetrating cardiac trauma. *J Cardiovasc Surg* 18:459, 1977.

J

1. Jones FL Jr: Transmural myocardial necrosis after nonpenetrating cardiac trauma. *Am J Cardiol* 26:419, 1970.
2. Jolly DT: Traumatic rupture of a papillary muscle of the mitral valve due to blunt thoracic trauma. *Can Fam Physician* 29:1960, 1983.

K

1. Kettunen P: Cardiac damage after blunt chest trauma, diagnosed using CK-MB enzyme and electrocardiogram. *International Journal of Cardiology* 6:355, 1984.

L

1. Lowe JE, Adams DH, Cummings RC, Wesly RLR, Phillips HR: The natural history and recommended management of patients with traumatic coronary artery fistulas. *Ann Thorac Surg* 36:295, 1983.

M

1. Munim A, Chodoff P: Traumatic acute mitral regurgitation secondary to blunt chest trauma. *Crit Care Med* 11:311, 1983.
2. Mead RH: *A History of Thoracic Surgery.* Springfield, Ill: Charles C Thomas, 1961.

P

1. Potkin RT, Werner JA, Trobaugh GB, Chestnutt CH III, Carrico CJ, Hallstrom A, Cobb LA: Evaluation of noninvasive tests of cardiac damage in suspected cardiac contusion. *Circulation* 66:627, 1982.

R

1. Roberts JB: The surgery of the pericardium. *Am Anat Surg* 4:247, 1881.
2. Rehn L: Über penetirende Herzwunden und Herznaht. *Arch Klin Chir* 55:315, 1897.

S

1. Symbas PN, Harlaftis N, Waldo WJ: Penetrating cardiac wounds: A comparison of different therapeutic methods. *Ann Surg* 183:377, 1976.
2. Symbas PN, Di Orio DA, Tyras DH: Penetrating cardiac wounds: Significant residual and delayed sequelae. *J Thorac Cardiovasc Surg* 66:526, 1973.
3. Sugg WL, Rea WJ, Ecker RR: Penetrating wounds of the heart: An analysis of 459 cases. *J Thorac Cardiovasc Surg* 56:531, 1968.
4. Senac JB: *Traité des Maladies du Coeur,* vol 1 (ed 2). Paris: Barbou, 1778.
5. Selmonosky CA, Ellison RG: Traumatic mitral valve incompetence: Case report. *J Trauma* 12:632, 1972.
6. Sheikhzadeh A, Langbehn F, Ghabusi P, Hakim C, Wendler G, Tarbiat S: Chronic traumatic tricuspid insufficiency. *Clin Cardiol* 7:299, 1984.
7. Stone DL, Fleming HA: Aneurysm of left ventricle and left coronary artery after non-penetrating chest trauma. *Br Heart J* 50:495, 1983.
8. Sutherland GR, Driedger AA, Holliday RL, Cheung HW, Sibbald WJ: Frequency of myocardial injury after blunt chest trauma as evaluated by radionuclide angiography. *Am J Cardiol* 52:1099, 1983.
9. Symbas PN, Lutz JF, Vlasis SE: Partial replacement of the left ventricular free wall with a Dacron graft: A 14 year follow-up. *J Thorac Cardiovasc Surg* 89:310, 1985.
10. Sareli P, Goldman AP, Pocock WA, Colsen P, Casari A, Barlow JB: Coronary artery-right ventricular fistula and organic tricuspid regurgitation due to blunt chest trauma. *Am J Cardiol* 54:697, 1984.

T

1. Tavares S, Hankins JR, Moulton AL, Attar S, Ali S, Lincoln S, Green DC, Sequeira A, McLaughlin JS: Management of penetrating cardiac injuries: The role of emergency room thoracotomy. *Ann Thorac Surg* 38:183, 1984.

W

1. Williams JB, Silver DG, Laws HL: Successful management of heart rupture from blunt trauma. *J Trauma* 21:534, 1981.

50

CARDIAC TUMORS

DEFINITION

Cardiac tumors include benign and malignant neoplasms arising within the cardiac chambers or in the myocardium. Metastatic neoplasms to the heart are not included.

HISTORICAL NOTE

The first recognition of a heart tumor is attributed to Columbus in 1559,[C1] followed by Malpighi, who in 1666 wrote a "dissertation de polypo cordis." Morgagni wrote of heart tumors in 1762.

The clinical diagnosis of a primary tumor, a sarcoma, was first recorded in 1934.[B1] The first antemortem diagnosis of a myxoma was made in 1951 using angiocardiography.[G1] A major diagnostic landmark occurred in 1968 with echocardiographic diagnosis of a left atrial myxoma, confirmed at operation and successfully treated.[S1]

By 1931, Yater had collected 75 cases of myxoma from the

literature, and advocacy for the removal of such tumors appeared as early as 1945.[Y1] In 1934, Beck partly removed an intrapericardial teratoma,[B2] and in 1951 Maurer successfully excised an intrapericardial lipoma.[M1] Among the earliest surgical approaches to myxomas was that of Bahnson and Newman, who in 1952 removed a myxoma from the right atrium via a right anterior thoracotomy using a short period of caval occlusion at normothermia. The patient died 24 days later from complications related to transfusion and electrolyte imbalance.[B3]

Using cardiopulmonary bypass (CPB), Crafoord in 1954 successfully excised a myxoma from the left atrium,[C2] as did Bigelow in 1955, using hypothermia and inflow occlusion.[B4] Successful excision of a right atrial myxoma was reported in 1957[H1] and in 1958.[C3] A left ventricular myxoma was excised in 1959 by Kay.[K1] The first successful excision of a right ventricular myxoma was undertaken in 1960.[B5] By 1964, only 60 cases of intracardiac myxoma had been successfully removed.[M2] Biatrial myxomas were removed in 1967.[Y2] In 1967, Gerbode described recurrence of a left atrial myxoma 4 years after initial excision.[G2]

TYPES OF CARDIAC TUMORS

Approximately 70% of cardiac tumors are benign, and 30% are malignant and potentially capable of invasion or metastasis (Table 50-1).

SECTION 1
MYXOMAS

DEFINITION

Cardiac myxomas are primary cardiac tumors that are generally pedunculated but may have a broad base. The cells are uniform, small, and polygonal, with round or oval nuclei and a moderate amount of cytoplasm. They lie in a myxomatous stroma in which other elements may be seen. One feature that distinguishes them from thrombi is that they are covered by endothelium and have endothelium-lined crevices and clefts.[W2]

MORPHOLOGY

Myxomas are intracavitary tumors occurring within any of the cardiac chambers, but they have a predilection for the atria (Table 50-2) and particularly the left atrium. They are usually 5–6 cm in diameter, with a range of 1–15 cm. Characteristically, they are polypoid and pedunculated, projecting into a cardiac chamber; rather gelatinous or mucoid, often with areas of hemorrhage; and either papillary or smooth or soft. Generally, they are not sessile but have a short, broad-based attachment. The papillary forms have a frondlike mass comprising the external surface of the neoplasm, which is friable and likely to produce embolisms.[M3]

Myxomas are composed of cells, primitive capillaries, and foci of extramedullary hematopoiesis within a myxoid matrix

Table 50-1 The incidence of neoplasms of the heart and pericardium.[M10]

Type	No.	%
Benign Tumors		
Myxoma	130	29.3%
Lipoma	45	10.1%
Papillary fibroelastoma	42	9.5%
Rhabdomyoma	36	8.1%
Fibroma	17	3.8%
Hemangioma	15	3.4%
Teratoma	14	3.2%
Mesothelioma of the AV node	12	2.7%
Granular cell tumor	3	0.7%
Neurofibroma	3	0.7%
Lymphangioma	2	0.5%
Subtotal	319	72%
Malignant Tumors		
Angiosarcoma	39	8.8%
Rhabdomyosarcoma	26	5.8%
Mesothelioma	19	4.2%
Fibrosarcoma	14	3.2%
Malignant lymphoma	7	1.6%
Extraskeletal osteosarcoma	5	1.1%
Neurogenic sarcoma	4	0.9%
Malignant teratoma	4	0.9%
Thymoma	4	0.9%
Leiomyosarcoma	1	0.2%
Liposarcoma	1	0.2%
Synovial sarcoma	1	0.2%
Subtotal	125	28%
Total	444	100%

KEY: AV, atrioventricular.

of acid mucopolysaccharide. The stroma contains variable numbers of reticulocytes and elastin fibers, smooth muscle cells, and collagen deposits. The matrix also contains polygonal cells with scant eosinophillic cytoplasm, either single and stellate, or multinuclear and in small nests. At the periphery of the tumor, the cells form a monolayer with clustering in the crevices, thereby stimulating primitive capillaries. The stalk has abundant large arteries and veins that communicate with the subendocardium, and at this interface, lymphocytes and plasma cells are prevalent. Microscopic foci of calcium and areas of metaplastic bone are found in 10% of myomas.[M3,M5]

Table 50-2 Types of cardiac tumors in surgical patients (UAB; 1967–July 1984, and GLH; 1958–October 1984).

Type of Tumor	No. of Patients
Atrial myxoma	38
Ventricular myxoma	1
Rhabdomyoma	6
Fibroma	2
Sarcoma	2
Right atrial extension of infradiaphragmatic tumor	4
Total	53

The nucleus of the polygonal cells is typically irregular and slightly hyperchromatic, but mitoses are not seen.[M5] The cells contain fine parallel filaments similar to those seen in glomangioma and fibromyxosarcoma. These filaments are believed to be the contractile components of smooth muscle cells. Immunologically identifiable smooth muscle–type filaments are recognized in endocardial cells, which have been noted to be more abundant in the left atrium, especially in the region of the fossa ovalis, than in other chambers.[M5]

Ferrans and Roberts[F1] think, however, that the organelle content of myxoma cells does not provide sufficient information to determine the cell of origin. They believe that although myxoma cells have a "vasoformative" tendency, the cytoarchitectural features of the variously differentiated blood vessel–like structures differ from those of normal blood vessels. Thus, myxomas are considered to arise from multipotential mesenchymal cells capable of differentiating into various types of cells, a view supported by the finding of bone and bone marrow tissue in myxomas. Histological examination of the atrial septum in 11 autopsied patients aged less than 4 months revealed myxomatous or myxofibrous tissue in the endocardium near the fossa ovalis, further supporting the concept that myxomas are derived from embryonal, undifferentiated mesenchyme.[F1]

The notion that myxomas are derived from thrombi appears to be thoroughly dispelled.[H3]

Increasing numbers of reports indicate the malignant potential of myxomas. Extensive local invasion has been noted.[H4] Death due to metastatic spread of an atrial myxoma has been reported once as a result of fatal brain-stem compression from an expanding cerebellar mass with histological features identical to those of a large, pedunculated left atrial myxoma also found at autopsy.[B6] There are now many reports of local recurrence[D2,G2,K2,R1,R2] and of distant metastases with invasion of vessel walls, aneurysmal change, and independent growth.[K3,P1,P2,R3,S4] Transgression beyond a blood vessel has also been noted by Price and associates.

In rare circumstances, atrial myxomas may become infected. Only 2 of 12 such cases have been diagnosed before death.[G3,J1] Central nervous system embolism has been a constant association.

Atrial Myxomas

The majority of atrial myxomas, whether left or right, arise from the atrial septum, usually from the region of the limbus of the fossa ovalis. About 10% of myxomas have other sites of origin, particularly the posterior and anterior atrial walls and the appendage (in order of frequency).[M3]

Eighty percent to 90% of myxomas are in the left atrium. Right atrial myxomas tend to be more solid and sessile than left atrial myxomas, with a wider attachment to the atrial wall or septum.[O1,S5] In one case, an atrial myxoma presenting in the right atrium arose from the inferior vena cava.[D1] Atrial myxomas may be multicentric (within a single chamber) or biatrial. The most common arrangement (75%) of biatrial tumors involves attachment of the two stalks to opposite sides of the same area of the septum.[I1]

Of 312 cases of right and left atrial myxomas reviewed by Newman and colleagues, only two were complicated by atrial septal defect;[N1] four additional cases have subsequently been reported.[N2] Such cases may have right-to-left shunts.

Ventricular Myxomas

Found mainly on the right ventricular free wall or ventricular septum, ventricular myxomas are sometimes described as infiltrating the ventricular myocardium. In about 15% of reported cases, right ventricular myxomas are associated with other cardiac myxomas. Left ventricular myxomas are rare, and little information about them is available.[M4]

Valvar Myxomas

The literature contains two reports of myxomas arising from the mitral valve[S3] and four reports of origin from the tricuspid valve.[S2] A cardiac myxoma originating from the pulmonary valve has also been reported.[C4]

CLINICAL FEATURES AND DIAGNOSTIC CRITERIA

Pathophysiology

Myxomas may produce symptoms of hemodynamic derangement from obstruction of flow within the cardiac chambers or from deformation of a cardiac valve, with resultant incompetence; they may produce symptoms by embolization; and, least commonly, they may produce so-called constitutional symptoms.[G4]

Hemodynamic Derangement

Myxomas may obstruct the pulmonary or systemic venous drainage or may impair flow across the atrioventricular valves, the likelihood of these events being greater with larger tumors. When such obstruction is intermittent, syncope, often related to postural change, or sudden death may occur. The obstruction is characteristically progressive.[G4] Intermittent obstruction causes syncope or sudden death in less than one-quarter of patients with left atrial myxomas,[G4,G1,M4] in one-third with right atrial or right ventricular myxomas,[H3,M4,M6,S9] and in one-half with left ventricular myxomas.[H3,M4]

Impairment of valve closure, either by obstruction or leaflet damage, may cause regurgitation.[P5] The valves may be structurally damaged by frequent tumor impingement, a sequence that also causes regurgitation. Although the regurgitation is the dominant abnormality in a few patients, as a rule, obstruction predominates.[H2] The symptoms are commonly of short duration, episodic, and associated with syncope.[G5]

Embolism

A major feature of cardiac myxomas is embolization. Emboli may arise from tumor fragmentation or detachment of the entire tumor, or from thrombi or infected foci on the neoplasm.[B8] Systemic emboli occur in 45% of patients with left atrial myxomas. They have been reported in every organ and may occlude coronary arteries.[E1,E2,F2,S11,S16] About 50% of emboli involve intra- or extracranial arteries to the central nervous system.[D3,S10,S11,T1] Cerebral emboli characteristically cause major permanent neurological deficits. On rare occasions, cerebral emboli are amenable to excision, with worthwhile results.[B6,B9,D3,N5,T1] Large emboli may obstruct the aortic bifurcation.[C10]

Although left ventricular myxomas are rare, the incidence of embolism from them is high (64%), apparently unrelated to tumor size, greater to the brain than elsewhere.[M4] Embolism from right-sided tumors occurs in about 10% of cases and may cause massive, fatal pulmonary obstruction.[G6] However, pulmonary arterial obstruction from this mechanism is much less common than is true thromboembolism to the pulmonary arteries in patients who have sustained systemic tumor emboli from a left atrial myxoma.[G4,G7] Multiple emboli from right-sided tumors may be a cause of pulmonary hypertension.[V2] Paradoxical embolism is rare.[N2,P4]

Constitutional Manifestations
A plethora of constitutional symptoms and certain laboratory findings may be the only manifestations of a cardiac myxoma. They include fever, weight loss, clubbing of the fingers and toes, Raynaud's phenomena, and myalgia and arthralgia.[B10,S12] In themselves, they are not pathognomonic of the diagnosis. Because the presence of antibodies to fresh heart muscle has been demonstrated preoperatively in some patients with myxomas, with appropriate postoperative diminution, it is speculated that patients may have an immune reaction to the neoplasm or to heart muscle mediated by the presence of neoplasm, which result in the constitutional symptoms.[C6] Total globulin levels are often elevated, and the electrophoretic patterns may reveal prominent alpha 2, beta 1, or heterogeneous gamma globulin peaks. Immunoelectrophoresis localizes the elevated globulins in either the IgM or IgA fractions. Elevated globulin levels are associated with a raised erythrocyte sedimentation rate and increased levels of C^+ reactive protein.[H5] Further nonspecific symptoms may be related to the seeding of multiple small emboli to muscle and joints, and hemorrhage or degeneration within the tumor.

Other unusual manifestations of cardiac myxomas include polycythemia with or without associated arterial hypoxia,[S9,W1] and clubbing (in both left and right atrial myxomas) associated with a right-to-left shunt at the atrial level through a patent foramen ovale or atrial septal defect.[G7,M8,W1] Hemolytic anemia occurs in about one-third of cases, particularly in association with a calcified myxoma; this and the thrombocytopenia which sometimes occurs, are probably due to mechanical destruction of formed blood elements. These features are reversible with tumor removal.[V1,W1]

Symptoms

Left atrial myxomas produce symptoms of hemodynamic origin which are entirely similar to those of mitral stenosis (see Chapter 11) in the majority of patients, with dyspnea and hemoptysis predominating.[B7,G2,L1,N4] The symptoms are commonly of short duration, episodic, and associated with syncope.[G5] They may rapidly become severe and intractable, and associated with congestive heart failure. *Right atrial myxomas* may also produce episodic symptoms, and the

symptoms may progress rapidly despite medical treatment. Abdominal protuberance from hepatomegaly and ascites, and peripheral edema are frequent presenting complaints in such settings.[M6] In the review by Morrisey and colleagues,[M6] all 18 patients had right heart failure, with a prominent *a* wave, raised venous pressure, hepatomegaly, ascites, and peripheral edema. Absence of orthopnea and of paroxysmal nocturnal dyspnea was notable.

Symptoms that result from embolization include various neurological deficits, coldness and pain in an extremity, occasionally angina from coronary embolization, and dyspnea from pulmonary embolization. Constitutional symptoms may be subtle or absent when the tumor is small,[H2] or they may uncommonly constitute the entire symptomotology.

Signs

The diagnosis of atrial myxoma is sometimes made immediately after admission by histologic examination of an embolus that has been removed from a peripheral artery;[K5] it must be recognized, however, that the absence of myxoma cells in the embolus does not deny the presence of myxoma, for thrombus forming on the neoplasm may be the cause of the embolism.

For *left atrial myxomas,* interpretation of the auscultatory findings has been aided by a combination of phonocardiographic and hemodynamic studies.[P5,P6] A loud first heart sound is prolonged by vibrations coinciding with the *c* wave of the left atrial pressure tracing and also with a characteristic notch in the left ventricular pressure curve; these vibrations occur after mitral valve closure when the tumor momentarily comes to rest in the left atrium.[P5] For mobile tumors moving from the left ventricle to the left atrium in early systole, a notch in the ascending limb of the left ventricular pressure tracing is considered to be due to a sudden increase in left atrial volume, which itself is manifested in the left atrial pressure pulse by a prominent *c* wave and subsequent dominant *v* wave. Accordingly, the first heart sound may be preceded by a loud ejection sound due to forceful ejection of the tumor from the left ventricle back into the left atrium.

When the tumor stays in the left atrium during the entire cardiac cycle, the diastolic murmur and the pressure tracings may be indistinguishable from those of mitral stenosis (i.e., there is no notch in the ventricular pressure wave, and the y descent is relatively slow).

The second heart sound is normally split, of low intensity, and followed by a third heart sound described as either an opening snap or a ventricular gallop. The opening snap occurs after the mitral valve opens and is thought to be due either to the tumor's striking the heart wall or to the diastolic sound of mitral regurgitation due to increased blood flow.

Systolic murmurs have also been recorded and have been attributed to associated mitral regurgitation.[P5,P6]

With *right atrial myxomas,* a loud, early systolic sound is heard, usually regarded as a widely split first heart sound, corresponding to expulsion of the tumor from the right ventricle.[H3] This sound is likely to correspond to a notch in the upstroke of the right ventricular pressure curve.[R4] A pulmonary ejection murmur with a delayed and accentuated pulmonic second sound and an early, late, or prolonged tricuspid diastolic murmur or rumble are heard.[S7] A systolic murmur is due to tricuspid regurgitation.

Ventricular myxomas are sufficiently rare that their auscultatory features are not fully known, but murmurs may suggest aortic or pulmonary stenosis.[B5] Occasionally, friction rubs are heard, presumably a result of physical contact of the tumor with the endocardium of one of the cardiac chambers.[H3]

Rarely, patients presenting with so-called constitutional manifestations exhibit cyanosis[S9,W1] and clubbing of the fingers and toes,[G7,M8,W1] or a gallop rhythm and sinus tachycardia.[H2]

Laboratory Studies

The results of laboratory studies are usually normal. In rare instances of presentation with so-called *constitutional manifestations,* some findings may be characteristic but not pathognomonic. Among such findings are anemia, thrombocytopenia, and findings associated with an immune response (see "Constitutional Manifestations").

Electrocardiogram

The changes in electrocardiographic findings associated with myxomas are not specific for such tumors but include arrhythmias and conduction disturbances, particularly atrial fibrillation, and bundle-branch block, and abnormal *P* waves.

Chest X-ray

The features on a plain chest x-ray are not specific for myxomas. Generalized cardiomegaly or specific chamber enlargement may be evident, particularly in the case of large left atrial myxomas causing obstruction. Septal lines, especially at the base and in the mid-zone, are fairly common findings because of coexisting pulmonary venous hypertension.[S13]

Echocardiogram

Two-dimensional echocardiography is now the most appropriate screening and diagnostic imaging modality for most cardiac tumors, particularly myxomas.[P8,V5] Valvular mitral stenosis can be excluded, and tumor prolapse through the atrioventricular valve may be demonstrated. Tumor prolapse is characteristically evident if echoes are seen behind the anterior cusp, particularly if those echoes are seen to move into the left ventricle during diastole.[B11] However, even large myxomas located within the body of the left atrium may not be apparent or may be underestimated in size with current two-dimensional or M-mode echocardiographic techniques, probably because the acoustic impedance characteristics of the tumor may be similar to those of blood.[C14]

Cardiac Catheterization and Angiocardiography

Unless other types of cardiac or coronary artery disease require assessment, catheterization and angiocardiography no longer constitute the investigative method of choice. If this invasive study is required for suspected left atrial tumors, a selective right heart study is performed, with injection of the radiopaque media into the pulmonary artery and filming as the dye passes through the left atrium. This method nearly always gives a clear demonstration of the lesion, whereas selective left ventricular cineangiography often fails to delineate it.

For right atrial myxomas, catheter placement into the right atrium is contraindicated, and the injection is made into one of the vena cavae.

NATURAL HISTORY

Myxomas occur in older adults and are two to three times more common in females than in males. They are very rare in children and have not been described in infancy.[A1,N3,S6,S7,S8] The literature contains six reports of familial myxoma (three with sibling restriction and three with a parent-child relationship)[C5,K6,K7,P4] and there is one additional example in the combined GLH-UAB series.

Myxomas are usually benign tumors, but rarely the tumor may metastasize.[N5,R1,R3] Such metastases have been reported in the brain[A2,B6,B9,R3] arteries,[N5] sternum, vertebral column,[R1,R3] pelvis,[R1] scapula,[S4] and soft tissues of the back.[R1] Metastasis can occur despite benign gross and microscopic appearances[R2] but is rare.

The course of surgically untreated patients with cardiac myxomas must be highly variable but cannot be clearly defined. However, once symptoms of dyspnea and hemoptysis develop, in the case of left atrial myxomas, or symptoms of abdominal protuberance from ascites or hepatomegaly develop, in the case of right atrial myxomas, there seems usually to be rapid progression to death within 1–2 years of onset. No information is available about the frequency of embolization in patients with myxomas or the tendency to repeated embolization if the cardiac myxoma is not removed. Likewise, there is no information concerning the course without treatment of patients presenting with constitutional symptoms only.

TECHNIQUE OF OPERATION

The preliminary steps are the usual ones for standard cardiopulmonary bypass (CPB). Direct caval cannulation is essential in the presence of a large right atrial myxoma but not otherwise, but it is routinely practiced for the removal of atrial myxomas as well as many other cardiac operations (UAB).

CPB is begun, and the patient is cooled to 25°C. A left atrial vent is not used. The aorta is cross-clamped and the cardioplegic solution infused through the aortic root in the usual fashion (see Chapter 3).

Left Atrial Myxomas

The usual vertical incision is made in the left atrium to the right of the interatrial groove (see Chapter 11, Fig. 11-6). Blood is removed from the left atrium with the high-vacuum sucker and discarded so that potential tumor emboli are not returned to the CPB circuit.[M7] The point of attachment of the tumor to the atrium is determined by inspection and the exploration of the tumor with the index finger. Assuming that it is attached to the atrial septum, which is usually the case, the tumor is not removed from the left atrial approach. Instead, a vertical right atriotomy is made and the interior of the right atrium examined in case a second tumor is present. As much as possible of the interior of the right ventricle is also inspected through the tricuspid valve. The atrial septum is then opened with a knife near the center of the fossa ovalis, and, with a finger in the left atrium as a guide to the attachment of the tumor, a sufficient amount of atrial septum is excised to include the tumor attachment and, if possible, uninvolved tissue 5 mm beyond it. The superior half of the fossa ovalis and the adjacent limbus are, if possible, included in the excision, since cells thought to be the precursor of myxoma are more abundant in this area. The tumor is then removed from the heart through the left or right atriotomy, whichever is the larger. Very large tumors may have to be removed piecemeal, although every attempt is made to keep the tumor intact and to avoid tumor embolization.[C9] After the tumor is removed, the interior of the left atrium is copiously irrigated with saline solution to evacuate any residual tumor fragments. The defect in the atrial septum is closed either by direct suture or, if too large for this, with a pericardial or knitted Dacron patch.

If the tumor is attached to the left atrial wall rather than the septum, the zone of attachment is excised, preferably with the full thickness of the adjacent wall but, if this is impracticable, with endocardium and some underlying muscle. Any wall defect created can generally be closed by direct suture.

The atria are closed. The usual precautions against air embolization are taken (see Chapter 2, Section 3) as the aortic clamp is released and rewarming begun. The rest of the procedure is completed in standard fashion.

Right Atrial Myxomas

Separate left and right atriotomies are not necessary unless there is preoperative evidence of an associated left atrial myxoma. Instead, the right atrium only is opened by the usual oblique incision (see Chapter 15, Fig. 15-12), and after the attachments of the tumor are defined, it is excised with the adjacent portion of atrial septum in the manner described under "Left Atrial Myomas." The left atrium is now carefully inspected via the surgically created atrial septal defect. Only if a tumor is seen in the left atrium is that chamber opened by a separate incision. The atrial septal defect is closed as described under "Left Atrial Myxomas," and the remainder of the procedure is also completed as described.

Other Myxomas

The removal of ventricular myxomas does not require excision of full-thickness ventricular wall, since such a procedure would increase risk and no recurrences have been recorded following less radical removal. Tumors in the left ventricular outflow tract are sometimes removed via an aortic approach.[G2] Otherwise the approach is through the right atrium for right ventricular tumors[B5,B16] and the left atrium for left ventricular tumors. The ventricle is opened directly only when the atrial approach is inadequate for the removal of the tumor. The procedure should include careful inspection of the interior of both right and left atria to exclude the presence of additional atrial tumors, which have been recorded in 15% of patients with right ventricular myxomas.[B5]

In those rare instances in which the tumor arises from an atrioventricular valve, the valve usually requires replacement. Also, valve replacement is occasionally required because of leaflet disruption from the "wrecking ball" action of the tumor. A markedly enlarged atrioventricular valve ring may require annuloplasty to correct residual valve incompetence. Such enlargement is particularly likely to occur in the tricuspid valve, since the tricuspid ring is more easily overstretched by a bulky tumor than is the mitral ring.

SPECIAL FEATURES OF POSTOPERATIVE CARE

Postoperative management is conducted in the usual fashion (see Chapter 5).

RESULTS

Survival

The hospital mortality after the removal of atrial myxomas is about 5% (Tables 50-3, 50-4). Virtually all of the deaths are in patients with advanced disability or old age, the mode of death being generally related, not to the atrial myxoma, but to coexisting cardiac or degenerative disease.

The early risks seem somewhat higher after the removal of myxomas from the ventricular cavities. Thus, among 32 patients undergoing the removal of right ventricular myxoma reported in the literature, there were three hospital deaths (9%, CL 4%–18%),[B5,L1,S14] and among 14 patients in whom a left ventricular myxoma was removed, there were three hospital deaths (21%, CL 10%–38%).[M4,S14,S15]

Death after hospital dismissal is uncommon, but recurrence of the myxoma (see "Recurrence") can lead to fatal complications (Fig. 50-1). Most of the other late deaths are from causes other than the cardiac tumor. Among 14 hospital survivors followed up to 96 months, two patients died (UAB; Fig. 50-1); and 23 patients followed up to 193 months, two patients also died (GLH).

Premature late death may occur more commonly when prosthetic valve replacement is necessary at the time of removal of the myxoma, for death can occur as a result of complications of the prosthesis.[R5,S5]

Recurrence

What has been classified as recurrence can be due theoretically to either tumor implantation (seeding at the time of removal), incomplete removal, or a growth from a new focus (multicentric origin). Two patients (5%, CL 2%–12%) of 37 hospital survivors in the combined UAB-GLH experience developed a recurrence, and both died as a result. In another combined series, there was one recurrence (4%, CL 0.5%–

Table 50-3 Hospital mortality after the removal of atrial myxomas (GLH; 1958–October 1984 and UAB; 1967–July 1984).

Cavity	UAB				GLH				Total			
	n	Hospital Deaths			n	Hospital Deaths			n	Hospital Deaths		
		No.	%	CL		No.	%	CL		No.	%	CL
LA	14	2[a]	14%	5%–31%	17		0%	0%–11%	31	2	6%	2%–15%
RA	2		0%	0%–61%	5		0%	0%–32%	7		0%	0%–24%
LV					1		0%	0%–85%	1		0%	0%–85%
Total	16	2	12%	4%–27%	23		0%	0%–8%	39	2	5%	2%–12%

KEY: CL, 70% confidence limits; LA, left atrium; LV, left ventricle; RA, right atrium.

[a] One patient aged 70 died suddenly 2 days after operation, and autopsy showed acute coronary occlusive disease; another, aged 74, died with subacute cardiac failure 10 days after operation.

12%) among 27 patients.[K2,R5] Among the 160 cases (Table 50-4) of excision of a left atrial myxoma reported in the literature, 10 (6%, CL 4%–9%) were reported to have had a recurrence, and 2 of the 10 suffered a second recurrence. In each instance, the recurrence was also in the left atrium. One patient had two reoperations for recurrences in the left atrium, the original tumor having been excised from the patient's left atrial wall, together with adjacent endocardium (UAB).

Recurrence following excision of a right atrial myxoma is very uncommon, and there have been no reports of recurrence of right or left ventricular myxomas. One patient is an example of recurrence in the left atrium following removal of a right atrial myxoma from the septum without septal excision (GLH). Dang and Hurley reported a case with a recurrence in the right ventricle following removal of a left atrial myxoma.[D2] These "recurrent" contralateral tumors may represent growth from a new focus.

Recurrences have been reported as early as 6 months following excision and at average about 30 months.[R1] They may be more rapidly growing than the parent tumor. Recurrence

figures may underestimate the incidence, since in reported series, follow-up has usually been incomplete and asymptomatic recurrences are seldom recognized. However, among the 15 long-term survivors reexamined with two-dimensional echocadiography, no unsuspected tumors have been seen (GLH).

Postoperative Arrhythmias

Atrial arrhythmias are common after the removal of atrial myxomas.[B14] Conduction disturbances are also reported and may be related to failure to limit the ressection to safe areas of the atrial septum or wall.

Functional Status

Living patients are generally in good health unless they have residual effects from a preoperative embolic event or have other disease processes.[H8] Thus, among 10 surviving patients, 5 were in New York Heart Association (NYHA) class I, 4 were in class II, and 1 was in class III (UAB).

Table 50-4 Results of operation for removal of cardiac myxomas using cardiopulmonary bypass as reported in the literature. Only series with five patients or more are analyzed.

Reference	LA	RA	Biatrial	RV	LV	Total
St. John Sutton et al.[S5a]	32 (1)	7	1			40
Larrieu et al.[L1]	12	2	0	1	0	15
Kabbani et al.[K2a]	15 (1)	2	0			17
Silverman[S15]	12	2	0	0	1	15
Donahoo et al.[D4a]	13	1	0			14
Collins et al.[C7]	4	3 (2)	0	0	1	8
Croxson et al.[C8a]	8	1	0			9
Desousa et al.[D3]	6 (2)	2	0	1	0	9
Gerbode et al.[G2]	7 (1)	0	0	0	1	8
Nasser et al.[N4a]	7	2	0			9
O'Neil et al.[O1]	4	1	0	0	0	5
Richardson et al.[R5a]	8	3	0			11
Melo et al.[M9]	14	4	0	0	0	18
Sasaki et al.[S14]	7	0	0	1	1	9
Kyllonen et al.[K4]	5	1	1 (1)	0	0	7
Hardin et al.[H6]	6 (1)	2 (1)	0	0	0	8
Total	160 (6)	33 (3)	2 (1)	3	4	202 (10)
% Hospital Mortality	4%	9%	50%	0%	0%	5%

KEY: LA, left atrium; LV, left ventricle; RA, right atrium; RV, right ventricle.

NOTE: The number of patients dying in hospital is in parentheses.

[a] Publication specifies atrial myxomas.

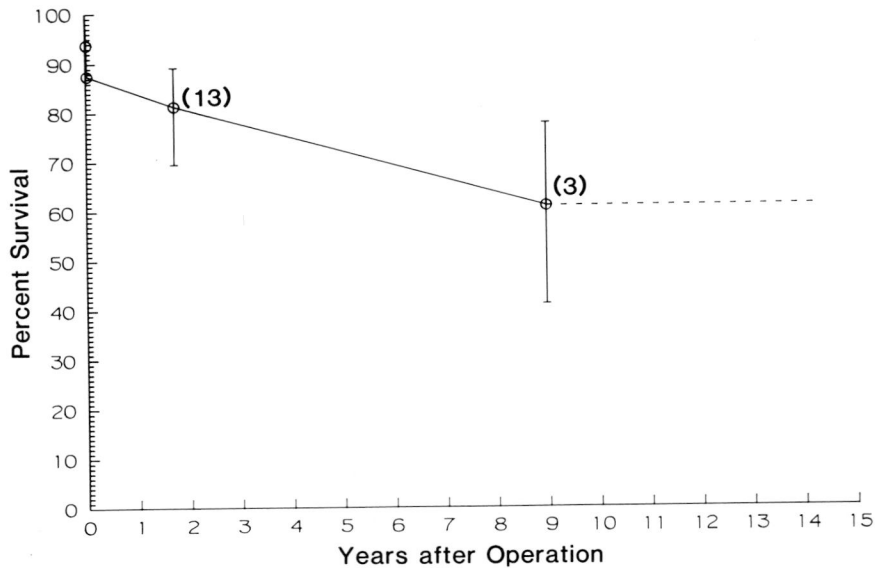

Figure 50-1 Actuarial survival, including hospital deaths, of patients undergoing surgical removal of atrial myxomas (UAB; 1967–July 1984; $n = 16$; two hospital deaths and two late deaths). All cases have been followed; follow-up date is September 1, 1984. The death 20 months after operation was in a patient who died at age 48 years after the second reoperation for recurrent left atrial myxoma. The patient dying 9 years postoperatively had metastatic carcinoma of the breast; that patient was 57 years old at operation.

INDICATIONS FOR OPERATION

Surgical removal is indicated whenever a diagnosis of cardiac myxoma is made. Generally it is considered a semiemergency procedure, particularly if the patient has a history of embolism or syncope since it has been noted that 8%–10% of patients die from embolic complications while waiting for operation.[N1,S10,T2]

SPECIAL SITUATIONS AND CONTROVERSIES

Extensiveness of the Operation

The surgical procedure described is recommended because of the possibility that the atrial myxoma is of multicentric origin from the atrial septum or atrial wall adjacent to the tumor base. However, at least six recurrences have been reported despite partial atrial septectomy,[D2] so there is little firm evidence on which to base these recommendations. Indeed, in the combined GLH-UAB series, some variability in this regard has been practiced (Table 50-5). Very radical operations that may increase the risk of hospital death are not indicated by the available information.

SECTION 2
RHABDOMYOMAS

DEFINITION

Cardiac rhabdomyomas are benign, yellow-gray tumors, the microscopic characteristic of which is the so-called *spider cell,* containing a central cytoplasmic mass suspended by fine, fibrillar processes radiating to the periphery.

MORPHOLOGY

Whether rhabdomyomas are true neoplasms or myocardial hamartomas is controversial, but the latter is generally considered the more likely situation.[B13,F4] Consistent with this view is the fact that at least half the patients have tuberous sclerosis with multiple hamartomatous lesions in the brain. Cardiac rhabdomyomas may be associated with hamartomas in other organs as well.[G8]

Rhabdomyomas invariably occur in the cardiac ventricles, with both sides equally involved. Very commonly, they are in multiple locations in the heart.

CLINICAL FEATURES AND DIAGNOSTIC CRITERIA

Cardiac rhabdomyomas are the most common primary tumors in children.[A1,B12,G9,M9] They may occur in siblings.[S18] The presentation is frequently at birth or in the first few days of life, with severe cardiac failure being the result of obstruction of cardiac pathways.[S17] Occasionally, the tumor is discovered somewhat later in a child known to have tuberous sclerosis, mental retardation, and, often, seizures.

The diagnosis can often be suspected on the basis of the clinical features and the results of two-dimensional echocardiography. Cardiac catheterization is usually carried out to determine whether inflow to or outflow from the ventricles is obstructed.

Table 50-5 The surgical procedure in the combined surgical series of cardiac myxomas (UAB; 1967–July 1984 and GLH; 1958–October 1984).

Procedures	UAB n	GLH n	Total n
Stalk excision only	9	6	15
Septum	5	6	
Atrial wall	4	0	
Septal resection	6[a]	17[b]	23
Wall excision	1	0	1
Total	16	23	39

NOTE: In addition, 1 patient had tricuspid annuloplasty, and one had coronary artery bypass grafting (GLH).

[a] In two operations, a Dacron patch was used for the repair; in four, closure was by direct suture.

[b] Closure by direct suture was used in all.

NATURAL HISTORY

Little documentation exists concerning the natural history of patients with cardiac rhabdomyomas. Even the incidence in infants with tuberous sclerosis has not been known until recently. Bass and colleagues determined by two-dimensional echocardiography that 8 (50%, CL 36%–64%) of 16 infants with tuberous sclerosis had also a cardiac rhabdomyoma.[B15] Presumably, death nearly always occurs in such patients in infancy or childhood, since older children and adults with such tumors are not seen.

TECHNIQUE OF OPERATION

Since rhabdomyomas usually protrude into the right or left ventricular cavity, their removal is done with the aid of cardiopulmonary bypass and/or profoundly hypothermic total circulatory arrest. The approach may need to be through the ventricular wall but at times may be done through the atrioventricular or semilunar valve.[K8] Excision is limited to the area of the tumor.

SPECIAL FEATURES OF POSTOPERATIVE CARE

The usual postoperative care is given (see Chapter 5). Catecholamine support may be necessary because of the extensive myocardial dissection.[C13]

RESULTS

The results of surgical treatment are generally unsatisfactory (Table 50-6). In some patients, the tumors are found at operation to be nonresectable. A few patients without tuberous sclerosis can obtain a good result.

INDICATIONS FOR OPERATION

In the presence of known tuberous sclerosis and severe mental retardation with seizures, operation may be contraindicated, especially if patient has multiple cardiac tumors and no cardiac symptoms. When the cardiac tumor is solitary and flow is obstructed, operation is indicated.

SECTION 3
FIBROMAS

DEFINITION

Cardiac fibromas are benign tumors, grossly resembling uterine leiomyomatas, with a whorled appearance on cut section. Microscopically, cardiac fibromas consist of elongated fibroblasts mixed with collagen and elastic fibers. Controversy exists as to whether fibromas should also be considered hamartomas.[C11,F3]

MORPHOLOGY

Fibromas occur almost exclusively within the ventricular myocardium and frequently in the ventricular septum.[H7] In

Table 50-6 Cardiac rhabdomyomas in the combined experience (UAB; 1967–July 1, 1984 and GLH; 1958–October 1984).

Age at Presentation	Size and Location	Surgery	Result	Tuberous Sclerosis
2 years	Large; RV outflow tract	Removal	NYHA class I 5 yr PO	No
5 days	Large multiple masses; all chambers	Exploration and biopsy	Alive 6 yr PO; cardiac status fair	Yes
12 days	Large; LV cavity	Subtotal removal	Alive 2 mo PO	Yes
Birth	Large multiple masses; ventricular septum and RV cavity	None[a]	Death 24 h after birth	
Birth	Large multiple masses; ventricular septum and free wall	None[a]	Death 18 h after birth	Yes; severe
2 years	Moderate sized; LV free wall and cavity	None[a]	Alive 12 mo later	Yes; severe

KEY: LV, left ventricular; NYHA, New York Heart Association; PO, postoperatively; RV, right ventricular.

[a] Operation considered, but condition deemed inoperable.

the two cases in the combined UAB-GLH series, one patient had a large tumor exclusively within the ventricular septum, and the other had a larger tumor mass within the ventricular septum extending beneath the left anterior coronary artery into the anterior and basal left ventricular free wall (UAB).

Patients with fibromas coming to surgical treatment tend to have large bulky tumors that are not infiltrating. In both cases in the combined series, the tumor was easily separated from the surrounding myocardium.

CLINICAL FEATURES AND DIAGNOSTIC CRITERIA

The presentation may be the result of the identification of a cardiac murmur in infancy and cardiomegaly on the chest x-ray. In both cases in this combined series, tumor calcification was seen on the chest x-ray, as it was in the cases reported by Geha and colleagues and by Reece and colleagues.[G10,R8] Many other and varied presentations are possible.[N5,V3]

Two-dimensional echocardiography identifies the solid mass and its location. Cardiac catheterization is indicated to determine encroachment upon ventricular cavities and any obstruction to flow.

NATURAL HISTORY

Fibromas are relatively rare tumors, two cases being seen in the entire UAB-GLH experience. Both presented at a young age (13 months and 28 months).

The natural history is unknown. In the two cases in this series, the presentation was because of incidental findings, as it was in the case of Lincoln and colleagues.[L2] Since most fibromas are diagnosed in infancy,[V3] and nearly all reported cases are in children less than 10 years of age, the presumption is that these tumors eventually cause death by obstructing ventricular inflow or outflow.

TECHNIQUE OF OPERATION

During cardiopulmonary bypass and cold cardioplegia, an incision is made through the epicardium and myocardium overlying the tumor. The tumor is enucleated by blunt and sharp dissection, which even when the tumor is large, is possible without entering a ventricular cavity to any extent. The ventricle is reconstructed by direct suture.

SPECIAL FEATURES OF POSTOPERATIVE CARE

The usual postoperative care is given (see Chapter 5).

RESULTS

Both patients survived, but considerable catecholamine support was required early postoperatively (UAB). At the most recent follow-up, both patients were alive, one 7 months and one 32 months after surgery, and both are in NYHA functional class I.

INDICATIONS FOR OPERATION

The diagnosis is an indication for operation, since all patients presenting probably have large fibromas.

SECTION **4**
LIPOMAS

DEFINITION

Cardiac lipomas are well encapsulated tumors typically composed of mature fat cells.

MORPHOLOGY

Cardiac lipomas seem most commonly to occur in the atrial septum, a condition termed *lipomatous hypertrophy of the interatrial septum*.[M10,P7,R6,R7] They are said also to occur in almost any location in the heart.

CLINICAL FEATURES AND DIAGNOSTIC CRITERIA

The one case of lipoma in the combined GLH-UAB series was discovered at operation in a 64-year-old woman in whom coronary artery bypass grafting was being done (UAB). The lipoma was bulky (3 × 4 cm) and in the atrial septum, impinging upon the superior vena caval orifice. It had produced no symptoms. Computed tomography can at least in some patients provide a specific preoperative diagnosis.[Z1]

NATURAL HISTORY

The natural history is unknown, since in most cases cardiac lipomas are incidental findings.

TECHNIQUE OF OPERATION

With cardiopulmonary bypass and cold cardioplegic myocardial protection, the lipoma is removed. If the tumor arises in the atrial septum, the septum may be excised and replaced with a Dacron patch.

SPECIAL FEATURES OF POSTOPERATIVE CARE

The usual postoperative care is given (see Chapter 5).

RESULTS

The prognosis is good. The patient in the combined series was well 6 months after operation.

INDICATIONS FOR OPERATION

The indications for operation are not known. If a large cardiac lipoma is encountered unexpectedly at operation, it should probably be removed if this can be done with little risk.

SECTION 5
SARCOMAS

DEFINITION

Sarcomas are malignant tumors of mesenchymal origin that display a wide variety of morphologic types.

MORPHOLOGY

Sarcomas may present as fibrosarcomas, angiosarcomas, rhabdomyosarcomas, or lymphosarcomas.[M3] In the combined series, one was an angiosarcoma (GLH), the other a fibrosarcoma (UAB). Any of the cardiac chambers may be involved. Sarcomas tend to metastasize widely. Sarcomas may arise from within the heart or ventricular epicardium. In the fibrosarcoma in the combined series, the origin was broad and from the posterior and inferior aspects of the left ventricle. In the angiosarcoma, the tumor involved the right ventricular wall, tricuspid anulus and leaflets, and epicardium.

CLINICAL FEATURES AND DIAGNOSTIC CRITERIA

The presentation was with cardiac tamponade in the two cases in the combined series. The patient with the angiosarcoma was 12 years old, the one with fibrosarcoma 22 months old. Cardiac sarcomas, however, may occur at any age and have variable presentations. Villasenor and colleagues describe a rhabdomyosarcoma producing subacute cardiac failure in an 82-year-old woman.[V4]

NATURAL HISTORY

The prognosis is poor for patients with cardiac sarcomas. Many of them have distant metastases when first seen.[W3]

TECHNIQUE OF OPERATION

The tumor is removed as completely as possible, usually during cardiopulmonary bypass. Additional therapy against the malignant disease may be indicated.

SPECIAL FEATURES OF POSTOPERATIVE CARE

The usual postoperative care is given (see Chapter 5).

RESULTS

Both patients in the combined series died within 6 months of operation.

INDICATIONS FOR OPERATION

Operation is indicated in order to secure a definitive histologic diagnosis. At the time of operation, as much of the tumor is removed as is possible.

SECTION 6
RIGHT ATRIAL EXTENSION OF INFRADIAPHRAGMATIC MALIGNANT TUMORS

DEFINITION

Infradiaphragmatic tumors extending into the right atrium and requiring cardiac surgical care are considered here.

MORPHOLOGY

In the combined UAB-GLH series, three patients with renal tumors and one with a recurrent uterine leiomyosarcoma were found to have tumor extension up the inferior vena cava and into the right atrium.[C12] In two adult patients, the renal tumors were adenocarcinomas; in one 43-month-old child, it was a Wilms' tumor. The tumor usually has some adherence to the endothelium of the inferior vena cava and the endocardium of the right atrium.

CLINICAL FEATURES AND DIAGNOSTIC CRITERIA

Usually infradiphragmatic tumors have no cardiac symptoms, and the extension of the tumor is found by two-dimensional echocardiography or venography.

NATURAL HISTORY

The natural history is not known with any degree of certainty, but presumably right atrial extension worsens the prognosis resulting in general from the primary tumor.

TECHNIQUE OF OPERATION

Operations for infradiaphragmatic tumors are best done as combined procedures, with simultaneous removal of the infradiaphragmatic tumor and its extension up the inferior vena cava and into the right atrium.

Typically, a median sternotomy incision is made and extended into the abdomen to the pubis as a midline incision. After the preparations for cardiopulmonary bypass (CPB), the abdominal tumor is appropriately mobilized, and preparations are made for its excision.

After the superior vena cava is directly cannulated, CPB is established, and the patient is cooled to 22°C. If venous return is insufficient, a sucker may be introduced through the right atrial appendage just into the right atrium without disturbing the tumor. At 22°C, the aorta is cross-clamped, the cold cardioplegic infusion given, the superior vena caval tape snugged down, and the right atrium opened. The flow is reduced to $0.5 \ 1 \cdot min^{-1} \cdot m^{-2}$, which can safely be continued for at least 20–30 minutes, or total circulatory arrest may be used. Blood returning into the right atrium is aspirated with a high-vacuum sucker and discarded to avoid tumor embolization.

The tumor is now dissected away from the endocardium and, if necessary, the tricuspid valve. It may be necessary to use a blunt dissector to separate the tumor gently from the endothelium of the inferior vena cava, to which it may adhere. If the concomitant operation is nephrectomy, the renal pedicle is controlled, and the kidney is removed, but the renal vein is not ligated until the tumor extension has been removed from the inferior vena cava and right atrium.

The right atrium is closed, a second venous cannula is inserted through the right atrial appendage into the inferior vena cava, CPB at full flow is reestablished, and rewarming of the patient is begun. The remainder of the operation is completed in the usual manner.

SPECIAL FEATURES OF POSTOPERATIVE CARE

The usual postoperative care is given (see Chapter 5).

RESULTS

The child with Wilms' tumor was alive, in NYHA class I, and continuing on chemotherapy 1 year after operation (UAB). The two adult patients with renal adenocarcinomata both died, one 8 months after operation and the other 13 months after operation (UAB). The 53-year-old woman with leiomyosarcoma is alive and in NYHA class II three years after operation (UAB).

INDICATIONS FOR OPERATION

If any extirpative surgery is to be done for malignant disease and there is known extension up the inferior vena cava and into the right atrium, the combined removal of the tumor and of the extension seems indicated.

REFERENCES

A

1. Arciniegas E, Hakimi M, Farooki Z, Truccone NJ, Green EW: Primary cardiac tumors in children. *J Thorac Cardiovasc Surg* 79:582, 1980.
2. Attar St, Lee Y-C, Singleton R, Scherlis R, David R, McLaughlin JS: Cardiac myxoma. *Ann Thorac Surg* 29:397, 1979.

B

1. Barnes AR, Beaver DC, Snell AM: Primary sarcoma of the heart: Report of a case with electrocardiographic and pathologic studies. *Am Heart J* 9:480, 1934.
2. Beck CS: Intrapericardial teratoma and a tumor of the heart: Both removed operatively. *Ann Surg* 116:161, 1942.
3. Bahnson HT, Newman EV: Diagnosis and surgical removal of intracavitary myxoma of the right atrium. *Bull Johns Hopkins Hosp* 93:150, 1953.
4. Bigelow WG, Dolan FG, Campbell FW: The effect of hypothermia and the risk of surgery. *Transact of the Soc Chir 16th Congress*, Copenhagen, 1955, p 631.
5. Bertolotti U, Mazzucco A, Valfre C, Valente M, Pennelli N, Gallucci V: Right ventricular myxoma: Review of the literature and report of two patients. *Ann Thorac Surg* 33:277, 1982.
6. Budzilovich G, Aleksie S, Greco A, Fernandez J, Harris J, Finegold M: Malignant cardiac myxoma with cerebral metastases. *Surg Neurol* 11:461, 1979.
7. Bulkley BH, Hutchins GM: Atrial myxomas: A fifty year review. *Am Heart J* 97:639, 1979.

8. Brewin TB: "Myxoma" of the heart: Report of a case in which death occurred as a result of detachment of the tumor from its pedicle. *Guy's Hospital Reports* 100:278, 1951.
9. Beran R, Hicks EP: The neurological aspects of atrial myxoma. *Clin Exp Neurol* 16:105, 1979.
10. Buchanan RRC, Cairns JA, Kraag G, Robinson JG: Left atrial myxoma mimicking vasculitis: Echocardiographic diagnosis. *Can Med Assoc J* 120:1540, 1979.
11. Bass NM, Sharratt GP: Left atrial myxoma diagnosed by echocardiography, with observations on tumor movement. *Br Heart J* 35:1332, 1973.
12. Bini RM, Westaby S, Bargeron LM Jr, Pacifico AD, Kirklin JW: Investigation and management of primary cardiac tumors in infants and children. *JACC* 2:351, 1983.
13. Bruni C, Prioleau PG, Ivey HH, Nolan SP: New fine structural features of cardiac rhabdomyoma: A case report. *Cancer* 46:2068, 1980.
14. Bateman TM, Gray RJ, Raymond MJ, Chaux A, Czer LSC, Matlof JM: Arrhythmias and conduction disturbances following cardiac operation for the removal of left atrial myxomas. *J Thorac Cardiovasc Surg* 86:601, 1983.
15. Bass JL, Breningstall GN, Swaiman KF: Echocardiographic incidence of cardiac rhabdomyoma in tuberous sclerosis. *Am J Cardiol* 55:1379, 1985.
16. Boulafendis D, Heine J, Samaan HA: Right ventricular myxoma. *Int J Cardiol* 5:216, 1984.

C

1. Columbus MR: *De Re Anatomica*, book XV, Venice: N Beui, 1559, p 269.

2. Crafoord C: Discussion on mitral stenosis and mitral insufficiency, in CR Lam (ed): *Proceedings of the International Symposium on Cardiovascular Surgery, Henry Ford Hospital, Detroit, Michigan, March 1955*. Philadelphia: Saunders, 1955, p 202.

3. Coates EO Jr, Drake EH: Myxoma of the right atrium with variable right-to-left shunt: Clinical and physiologic observations and report of a case with successful operative removal. *N Engl J Med* 259:165, 1958.

4. Catton RW, Guntheroth WG, Reichenbach DC: Myxoma of the pulmonary valve causing severe stenosis in infancy. *Am Heart J* 66:248, 1963.

5. Crawford FA, Selby JH, Watson D, Joransen J: Unusual aspects of atrial myxoma. *Ann Surg* 188:240, 1978.

6. Currey HFL, Matthews JA, Robinson J: Right atrial myxoma mimicking a rheumatic disorder. *Br Med J* 1:547, 1967.

7. Collins HA, Collins IS: Clinical experience with cardiac myxoma. *Ann Thorac Surg* 13:450, 1972.

8. Croxson RS, Jewitt D, Bentall HH, Cleland WP, Kristinsson A, Goodwin JF: Long-term followup of atrial myxoma. *Br Heart J* 34:1018, 1972.

9. Chamberlain SW, Carter JR, Richardson RL: Intraoperative coronary artery embolization from left atrial myxoma. *Anesthesiology* 47:301, 1977.

10. Carter AB, Lowe K, Hill I: Cardiac myxomata and aortic saddle embolism. *Br Heart J* 22:502, 1960.

11. Calhoun TR, Terry EE, Bet EB, Sunbury TR: Myocardial fibroma or fibrous hamartoma. *Ann Thorac Surg* 32:406, 1981.

12. Cleland DC, Westaby S, Karp RB: Treatment of intra-atrial cardiac tumors. *JAMA* 249:2799, 1983.

13. Corno A, de Simone G, Catena G, Marcelletti C: Cardiac rhabdomyoma: Surgical treatment in the neonate. *J Thorac Cardiovasc Surg* 87:725, 1984.

14. Come PC, Riley MF, Markis JE, Malagold M: Limitations of echocardiographic techniques in evaluation of left atrial masses. *Am J Cardiol* 48:947, 1981.

D

1. Devig PM, Clark TA, Aaron BL: Cardiac myxoma arising from the inferior vena cava. *Chest* 78:784, 1980.

2. Dang CR, Hurley EJ: Contralateral recurrent myxoma of the heart. *Ann Thorac Surg* 21:59, 1976.

3. Desousa AL, Muller J, Campbell R, Batnitzky S, Rankin L: Atrial myxoma: A review of the neurological complications, metastases, and recurrences. *J Neurol Neurosurg Psychiatry* 41:1119, 1978.

4. Donahoo JS, Weiss JL, Gardner TJ, Fortuin NJ, Brawley RK: Current management of atrial myxoma with emphasis on a new diagnostic technique. *Ann Surg* 189:763, 1979.

E

1. Edwards AT, Johnson W: A case of myxoma of the left atrium with peripheral arterial emboli. *Br J Surg* 46:391, 1959.

F

1. Ferrans VJ, Roberts WC: Structural features of cardiac myxomas: Histology, histochemistry and electron microscopy. *Hum Pathol* 4:111, 1973.

2. Franciosa JA, Lawrinson W: Coronary artery occlusion due to neoplasm: A rare cause of acute myocardial infarction. *Arch Intern Med* 128:797, 1971.

3. Feldman PS, Meyer MW: Fibroelastic hamartoma (fibroma) of the heart. *Cancer* 38:1976.

4. Fenoglio JJ, McAllister HA, Ferrans VJ: Cardiac rhabdomyoma: A clinicopathologic and electron microscopic study. *Am J Cardiol* 38:241, 1976.

G

1. Goldberg HP, Glenn F, Dotter CT: Myxoma of the left atrium: Diagnosis made during life with operative and postmortem findings. *Circulation* 6:762, 1952.

2. Gerbode F, Kerth WJ, Hill JD: Surgical management of tumors of the heart. *Surgery* 61:94, 1967.

3. Graham HV, von Hartitzsch B, Medina JR: Infected atrial myxoma. *Am J Cardiol* 38:658, 1976.

4. Greenwood WF: Profile of atrial myxoma. *Am J Cardiol* 21:367, 1968.

5. Goodwin JF: Symposium on cardiac tumors: The spectrum of cardiac tumors. *Am J Cardiol* 21:307, 1968.

6. Gonzalez A, Altieri PI, Marques E, Cox RA, Castillo M: Massive pulmonary embolism associated with a right ventricular myxoma. *Am J Med* 69:795, 1980.

7. Goodwin JF: Diagnosis of left atrial myxoma. *Lancet* 1:464, 1963.

8. Goyer RA and Bowden DH: Endocardial fibroelastosis associated with glycogen tumors of the heart and tuberous sclerosis. *Am Heart J* 64:539, 1962.

9. Golding R and Reed G: Rhabdomyoma of the heart. *N Engl J Med* 276:957, 1967.

10. Geha AS, Weidman WH, Soule EH, McGoon DC: Intramural ventricular cardiac fibroma: Successful removal in two cases and review of the literature. *Circulation* 36:427, 1967.

H

1. Hanlon CR: Discussion of Bahnson HT, Spencer FC, Andrus EC: Diagnosis and treatment of intracavity myxomas of the heart. *Ann Surg* 145:915, 1957.

2. Harvey WP: Clinical aspects of cardiac tumors. *Am J Cardiol* 21:328, 1968.

3. Hurst JW (ed): *The Heart, Arteries and Veins* (ed 5). New York: McGraw-Hill, 1982, p 1403.

4. Hannah H, Eisemann G, Hiszvzynskyj R, Winsky M, Cohen L: Invasive atrial myxoma: Documentation of malignant potential of cardiac myxomas. *Am Heart J* 104:881, 1982.

5. Hattler BG, Fuchs JCA, Cosson R, Sabiston JC: Atrial myxoma: An evaluation of clinical and laboratory manifestations. *Ann Thorac Surg* 10:65, 1970.

6. Hardin NJ, Wilson JM III, Gray GF, Gay WA: Experience with primary tumors of the heart: Clinical and pathological study of 17 cases. *Johns Hopkins Med J* 134:141, 1974.

7. Heath D: Pathology of cardiac tumors. *Am J Cardiol* 21:315, 1968.

8. Hanson EC, Gill CC, Razavi M, Loop TD: The surgical treatment of atrial myxomas. Clinical experience and late results in 33 patients. *J Thorac Cardiovasc Surg* 89:298, 1985.

I

1. Imperio J, Summers D, Krasnow N, Piccone VA: The distribution patterns of biatrial myxomas. *Ann Thorac Surg* 29:469, 1980.

J

1. Joseph P, Himmelstein DU, Mahowald JM, Stullman JS: Atrial myxoma infected with candida: First survival. *Chest* 78:340, 1980.

K

1. Kay JH, Anderson RM, Meihaus J, Lewis R, Magidsow O, Bernstein S, Griffith GC: Surgical removal of an intracavity left ventricular myxoma. *Circulation* 20:881, 1959.

2. Kabbani S, Cooley DA: Atrial myxoma: Surgical considerations. *J Thorac Cardiovasc Surg* 65:731, 1973.

3. Kimbrell DC, Kaasa LJ: Primary intraluminal aortic myxoma with involvement of several vertebrae. *JAMA* 226:459, 1973.

4. Kyllonen KEJ, Tala P, Merikallio E, Kala R: Cardiac myxoma: A report of 8 cases. *J Cardiovasc Surg* 17:392, 1976.

5. Koikkalainen K, Kostiainen S, Luosto R: Left atrial myxoma revealed by femoral embolectomy. *Scand J Thorac Cardiovasc Surg* 11:33, 1977.

6. Kleid JJ, Klugman J, Haas J, Battock D: Familiar atrial myxoma. *Am J Cardiol* 32:361, 1973.

7. Krause S, Adler LN, Reddy PS: Intracardiac myxoma in siblings. *Chest* 60:404, 171.

8. Kilman JW, Craenen J, Hosier DM; Replacement of entire right atrial wall in an infant with a cardiac rhabdomyoma. *J Pediatr Surg* 8:317, 1973.

L

1. Larrieu AJ, Jamieson WRE, Tyers GFO, Burr LH, Munro AI, Miyagishima RT, Gerein AN, Allen P: Primary cardiac tumors: Experience with 25 cases. *J Thorac Cardiovasc Surg* 83:339, 1982.

2. Lincoln JCR, Tynan MJ, Waterston DJ: Successful excision of an endocardial fibroma of the left ventricle in a 10-month-old infant. *J Thorac Cardiovasc Surg* 56:63, 1968.

M

1. Maurer ER: Successful removal of tumor of the heart. *J Thorac Cardiovasc Surg* 23:479, 1952.

2. Malm JR, Bowman FO Jr, Henry HB: Left atrial myxoma associated with an ASD. *J Thorac Cardiovasc Surg* 45:490, 1963.

3. McAllister HA: Primary tumors of the heart and pericardium. *Pathol Annu* 14:325, 1979.

4. Meller J, Teichholz LE, Pickard AD: Left ventricular myxoma: Echocardiographic diagnosis and review of the literature. *Am J Med* 63:816, 1977.

5. Merkow LP, Kooros MA, Macgovern G, Hayeslip DW, Weikers NJ, Pardo M, Fisher DL: Ultrastructure of a cardiac myxoma. *Arch Pathol* 88:390, 1969.

6. Morrisey JF, Campeti FL, Mahoney EB, Yu PN: Right atrial myxoma: Report of 2 cases and review of the literature. *Am Heart J* 66:4, 1963.

7. May IA, Kimball KG, Goldman PW, Dugan DJ: Left atrial myxoma: Diagnosis, treatment and pre- and postoperative physiological studies. *J Thorac Cardiovasc Surg* 53:805, 1967.

8. Meyers SN, Shapiro JE, Barresi V, De Boer AA, Pavel DI, Gracey DR, Suhre DE, Buehler JH: Right atrial myxoma with right to left shunting and mitral valve prolapse. *Am J Med* 62:308, 1977.

9. Melo J, Ahmad A, Chapman R, Wood J, Starr A: Primary tumors of the heart: A rewarding challenge. *Am Surg* 45:681, 1979.

10. McAllister HA, Fenoglio JJ: *Tumors of the Cardiovascular System, Atlas of Tumor Pathology,* series 2. Washington, DC: Armed Forces Institute of Pathology, 1978.

N

1. Newman HA, Cordell AR, Prichard RW: Intracardia myxomas: Review and report of 6 cases, one successfully treated. *Am Surg* 32:219, 1966.

2. Natarajan P, Vijayanagar RR, Eckstein PF: Right atrial myxoma with atrial septal defect: A case report and review of the literature. *Cathet Cardiovasc Diagn* 8:267, 1982.

3. Nadas AS, Ellison RC: Cardiac tumors in infancy. *Am J Cardiol* 21:363, 1968.

4. Nasser WK, Davis RH, Dillon JC, Tavel ME, Helman CH, Feigenbaum H, Fisch C: Atrial myxoma and pathologic features in 9 cases. *Am Heart J* 83:694, 1972.

5. Nicks R: Hamartoma of the right ventricle. *J Thorac Cardiovasc Surg* 47:762, 1967.

O

1. O'Neill MB, Grehl TM, Hurley EJ: Cardiac myxomas: A clinical diagnostic challenge. *Am J Surg* 138:68, 1979.

P

1. Pianov RP, Kanglova IN: Metastasizing cardiac myxoma. *Terpevticheskii Arkhiv* 44:107, 1972.

2. Pastakia B: Malignant atrial myxoma presenting as intracranial mass. *Chest* 75:531, 1979.

3. Price DL, Harris JL, New PF, Cantu RC: Cardiac myxoma: A clinicopathologic and angiographic study. *Arch Neurol* 23:558, 1970.

4. Powers JC, Falkoff M, Heinle RA: Familial cardiac myxoma: Emphasis on unusual clinical manifestations. *J Thorac Cardiovasc Surg* 77:782, 1979.

5. Penny JL, Gregory JJ, Ayres SM, Giannelli S, Rossi P: Calcified left atrial myxoma simulating mitral insufficiency: Hemodynamic and phonocardiographic effects of tumor movement. *Circulation* 36:417, 1967.

6. Pitt A, Pitt B, Schaefer J, Giley JM: Myxoma of the left atrium: Hemodynamic and phonocardiographic consequences of sudden tumor movement. *Circulation* 36:408, 1967.

7. Prior JT: Lipomatous hypertrophy of cardiac interatrial septum. *Arch Pathol* 78:11, 1964.

8. Poole GY, Breyer RH, Holliday RH, Hudspeth AS, Johnston FR, Cordell AR, Mills SA: Tumors of the heart: Surgical considerations. *J. Cardiovasc Surg* 25:5, 1984.

R

1. Read RC, White HJ, Murphy ML, Williams D, Sun CN, Flanagan WH: The malignant potentiality of left atrial myxoma. *J Thorac Cardiovasc Surg* 68:857, 1974.

2. Read RC: Cardiac myxoma and surgical history. *Ann Thorac Surg* 29:395, 1979.

3. Rankin LI, de Sousa AL: Metastatic atrial myxoma presenting as intracranial mass. *Chest* 74:451, 1978.

4. Roguin N, Amikam S, Riss E: Prolapsing right atrial myxoma: Clinical and hemodynamic considerations. *Br Heart J* 39:577, 1977.

5. Richardson JV, Brandt B III, Doty DB, Ehrenhaft JL: Surgical treatment of atrial myxomas: Early and late results of 11 opera-

tions and review of the literature. *Ann Thorac Surg* 28:354, 1979.

6. Reyes CV and Jablokow VR: Lipomatous hypertrophy of the cardiac interatrial septum. *Am J Clin Pathol* 72:785, 1979.

7. Reyes LH, Rubio PA, Korompai FL, Guinn GA: Lipoma of the heart. *Int Surg* 61:179, 1976.

8. Reece IJ, Cooley DA, Frazier OH, Hallman GL, Powers PL, Montero CG: Cardiac tumors. Clinical spectrum and prognosis of lesions other than classical benign myxoma in 20 patients. *J Thorac Cardiovasc Surg* 88:439, 1984.

S

1. Schattenberg TT: Echocardiographic diagnosis of left atrial myxoma. *Mayo Clin Proc* 43:620, 1968.

2. Suri RK, Pattankar VL, Singh H, Aikat BK, Gujral JS: Myxoma of the tricuspid valve. *Aust NZ J Surg* 48:429, 1978.

3. Sandrasago FA, Oliver WA, English TAH: Myxoma of the mitral valve. *Br Heart J* 42:221, 1979.

4. Seo S, Warner TFCS, Colyer RA, Winkler RF: Metastasizing atrial myxoma. *Am J Surg Pathol* 4:391, 1980.

5. St John Sutton MG, Mercier LA, Guiliani ER, Lie JT: Atrial myxomas: A review of clinical experience in 40 patients. *Mayo Clin Proc* 55:371, 1980.

6. Schmaltz AA, Apitz J: Primary heart tumors in infancy and childhood: Report of 4 cases and review of literature. *Cardiology* 67:12, 1981.

7. Snyder SN, Smith DC, Lau FYK, Turner AF: Diagnostic features of right ventricular myxoma. *Am Heart J* 91:240, 1976.

8. Steinke WE, Perry LW, Gold HR, McClenathan JE, Scott LP: Left atrial myxoma in a child. *Pediatrics* 49:580, 1972.

9. Sennerstedt R, Varnauskas E, Paulin S, Linder E, Ljunggren H, Werks L: Right atrial myxoma: Report of a case and review of the literature. *Am Heart J* 64:243, 1962.

10. Symbas PN, Hatcher CR Jr, Gravanis MB: Myxoma of the heart: Clinical and experimental observations. *Ann Surg* 183:470, 1976.

11. Silverman J, Olwin JS, Graehinger JS: Cardiac myxomas with systemic embolization: Review of the literature and report of a case. *Circulation* 26:99, 1962.

12. Skause B, Bava NO, Westfield TA: Atrial myxoma with Raynaud's phenomenon as the initial presenting symptom. *Acta Med Scand* 164:321, 1959.

13. Steiner RE: Radiologic aspects of cardiac tumors. *Am J Cardiol* 21:344, 1968.

14. Sasaki S, Lin YT, Redington JV: Primary intracavitory cardiac tumors: A review of 11 surgical cases. *J Cardiovasc Surg* 18:15, 1977.

15. Silverman NA: Primary cardiac tumors. *Ann Surg* 191:127, 1980.

16. Sybers HD, Booke WC: Coronary and retinal embolism from left atrial myxoma. *Arch Pathol* 91:179, 1971.

17. Shaher RM, Farina M, Alley R, Hansen P, Bishop M: Congenital subaortic stenosis in infancy caused by rhabdomyoma of the left ventricle. *J Thorac Cardiovasc Surg* 63:157, 1972.

18. Shaher RM, Mintzer J, Farina M, Alley R, Bishop M: Clinical presentation of rhabdomyoma of the heart in infancy and childhood. *Am J Cardiol* 30:95, 1972.

T

1. Tipton BK, Robertson JT, Robertson JH: Embolism to the central nervous system from cardiac myxoma: Report of 2 cases. *J Neurosurg* 47:937, 1977.

2. Thomas EK, Winchell CP, Varco RL: Diagnostic and surgical aspects of left atrial tumors. *J Thorac Cardiovasc Surg* 53:535, 1967.

V

1. Vuopia P, Nikkila EA: Hemolytic anemia and thrombocytopenia in a case of left atrial myxoma associated with mitral stenosis. *Am J Cardiol* 17:585, 1966.

2. Vidne B, Atsmon A, Aygen M, Levy MJ: Right atrial myxoma: Case report and review of the literature. *Isr J Med Sci* 7:1196, 1971.

3. Van der Hauwaert LG: Cardiac tumors in infancy and childhood. *Br Heart J* 33:125, 1971.

4. Villasenor HR, Fuentes F, Walker WE: Left atrial rhabdomyosarcoma mimicking mitral valve stenosis. *Tex Heart Inst J* 12:107, 1985.

5. Viswanathan B, Luber JM Jr, Bell-Thompson J: Right ventricular myxoma. *Ann Thorac Surg* 39:280, 1985.

W

1. Willman VL, Symbas PN, Mamiya RT, Cooper T, Hanlon CR: Unusual aspects of intracavity tumors of the heart. *Diseases of the Chest* 47:669, 1965.

2. Wold LE, Lie JT: Scanning electronmicroscopy of intracardiac myxoma. *Mayo Clin Proc* 56:198, 1981.

3. Whorton CM: Primary malignant tumor of the heart. *Cancer* 2:245, 1949.

Y

1. Yater WM: Tumors of the heart and pericardium: Pathology, symptomatology and report of 9 cases. *Arch Intern Med* 48:627, 1931.

2. Yipintsoi T, Donavanik L, Bhamarapravati N, Jumbala B, Prachaubmoh K: Bilateral atrial myxoma with successful removal. *Diseases of the Chest* 52:828, 1967.

Z

1. Zingas AP, Carrera JD, Murray CA, Kling GA: Case Report. Lipoma of the myocardium. *J Comput Assist Tomogr* 7:1098, 1983.

51

PRIMARY CARDIOMYOPATHIES AND CARDIAC TRANSPLANTATION

DEFINITION

Primary cardiomyopathies are those that are not the result of ventricular pressure or volume overload, hypoxia, or ischemia from coronary artery disease. Hypertrophic obstructive cardiomyopathy is considered separately, in Chapter 33.

HISTORICAL NOTE

Cardiomyopathies

Dilated and restrictive forms of cardiomyopathies have been recognized for a long time, but in the past 20 years considerable new knowledge has evolved concerning them. In contrast, the pathologic and clinical features of endomyocardial fibrosis began to be described only in the mid 1930s and 1940s.[B4,D2,L3,S4] Successful surgical treatment of endomyocardial fibrosis, by resection of the diseased endocardium and valve replacement, was first reported by Lepley and colleagues in 1974[L2] and then by Dubost in 1976.[D4]

Cardiac Transplantation

While knowledge about primary cardiomyopathies dates back many years, it was only with the advent of cardiac transplantation that definitive therapy became a possibility.

The development of this form of surgical treatment has not depended primarily on perfecting an operative technique but rather on developments in immunology and renal transplantation.

Regarding cardiac transplantation per se, Carrel and Guthrie first reported this procedure in 1905, with successful heterotopic cardiac transplantation procedures in dogs.[C4] For many years, little further was done, until in 1933 Mann and colleagues, at the Mayo Clinic, reported on successful transplantation of the heart into the neck of dogs.[M7] This work brought no clinical applications because of a lack of understanding of the immunologic features of organ transplantation.

A somewhat similar history has characterized the development of renal transplantation. Thus, Carrel in 1908, after earlier having perfected the method for blood vessel anastomoses, reported transplantation of the kidneys in experimental animals.[C10] Little was done in the years after these reports, and the next work on the subject was in two reports from Dederer, working in Mann's laboratory at the Mayo Clinic in 1918 and 1920.[D9,D10] His experiments were not very successful, but Williamson later commented that Dederer's short-term success in two members of the same litter of puppies "seems very suggestive that there are biologic phenomena which may be instrumental in the failures that have so frequently been attributed to mechanical difficulties."[W6] Williamson himself, in 1926, reported further studies on renal transplantation. He noted that autogenous kidney transplants functioned satisfactorily for months but that renal homografts functioned only for a period of days.[W7] Although Williamson described the histologic condition of the failed renal homograft as representing a form of glomerular nephritis, he also concluded that "the failure of homogenous kidney transplants seems attributable to a biologic incompatibility between the donor and recipient."[W7] He went on to state that "the value of kidney transplantation as a clinical measure is questionable with our present knowledge, although under proper conditions it might be worthy of serious consideration."[W7] Work continued in Mann's laboratory, but even by 1934, Wu and Mann had not increased the understanding of the failure of the transplanted kidney.[W8]

Twenty-two years then elapsed before the report of successful homotransplantation of the human kidney, and this was between identical twins.[M18,M20] In the interim, the work of Medawar had revolutionized the understanding of transplantation. Although antigens and antibodies were to some extent understood, at least as they were involved in various types of infectious disease, it was Medawar who first developed the concepts of immunology as applied to transplantation. His work was a result of the British government's research program early in World War II directed toward devising new methods of skin coverage for children extensively burned by the bombings of the Battle of Britain in 1939. His first paper, in 1944, described his classic experiments with skin transplants in rabbits.[M8] He found that the reaction of the rabbit to the transplantation of skin from another rabbit was very different from the benign reaction to transplantation of its own skin from one site to another, just as Williamson and others had found in the case of the kidney. Medawar determined that the skin transplant from an-

other rabbit developed a *cellular infiltrate* that destroyed the transplant in 7–10 days. Medawar termed this process *rejection*, and it is the analogue of the cellularly mediated acute rejection of cardiac transplantation as it occurs today (see "Results"). In the same paper, he also described *second set rejection*, which occurred when later a second transplant of skin was made to the same rabbit from the same donor rabbit. This second skin graft was destroyed in 5–6 days, more rapidly than in the *first set rejection*. Medawar deduced that preformed antibodies were responsible for the second set rejection, which is analogous to the humorally mediated *hyperacute rejection* that occurs rarely after cardiac transplantation.

In this and a second classic paper,[M14] Medawar developed a number of fundamental concepts. He confirmed his deduction that rejection under some circumstances was mediated by cells (lymphocytes) and in others by humoral antibodies. He recognized that the phenomena that he saw were the results of the enormous genetic diversity of individuals. He hypothesized that the phenomenon of second set rejection implied immunologic recollection of past events.

Methods for preventing rejection soon began to be discussed and studied, and Medawar himself in the early 1950s suggested that the recently discovered corticosteroids might help prevent rejection.[D11] However, techniques of immunosuppression developed slowly, and in the interim, at the Peter Bent Brigham Hospital in Boston in 1955, Merrill, Murray, Harrison, and Guild performed the first successful kidney transplantation in a human being; based on the immunologic concepts developed by Medawar, they chose identical twins for this procedure.[M18,M20] This successful case had been preceded at the Brigham Hospital by extensive investigations and some clinical renal homotransplantation between genetically diverse individuals with poor success. This work was summarized by Hume and colleagues in 1955.[H5] In 1960, Merrill and colleagues reported successful homotransplantation with mild immunosuppression between nonidentical twins.[M19] But it was not until 1962 that Murray, Merrill, and colleagues were able to report successful "kidney transplantation in modified recipients," and in this experience are reported the beginnings of modern immunosuppressive therapy.[M17] Calne had shown experimentally in 1961 that azathioprine (Imuran) prolonged the survival of kidney transplants.[C11,C12] Subsequently, intensive study has improved considerably the techniques of immunosuppression, with the development of cyclosporine being the latest reported advance (see "Special Situations and Controversies").

When Shumway in the late 1950s completed his training with Lillehei and Varco at the University of Minnesota in the early era of cardiac surgery, he went to Stanford University and began the development of an experimental program in cardiac transplantation. Lower and Shumway first reported successful experimental orthotopic cardiac transplantation in 1960,[L1] just at the time when renal transplantation was becoming established. This work was confirmed by Kondo and colleagues, who also obtained prolonged survivals.[K1] While laboratory work continued at Stanford and a few other institutions, Barnard (also a trainee at the University of Minnesota at the time of Shumway), in Cape Town, South Africa, unexpectedly performed the first successful cardiac transplantation in a human being in late 1966.[B1] In most but not all cardiac surgical centers around the world, clinical cardiac transplantation was then begun, but in that era few patients were more than short-term survivors. As a result, by the early 1970s cardiac transplantation had largely disappeared from clinical practice. An exception to this was the program at Stanford, where clinical and experimental transplantation continued at a steady pace. From the laboratory and clinical studies of the cardiac surgeons and their colleagues at Stanford, a continuous stream of new information emerged. As a result, in about 1980 cardiac transplantation began to reappear as a viable therapeutic modality. A major reason for its greater success at reappearance is the knowledge of immunosuppression that has come from research and from the experience with renal transplantation, with the most recent event being the discovery of cyclosporine. Another reason for the increased activity and improved success in cardiac transplantation in recent years has been the development of distant heart procurement programs. Watson and colleagues in 1977[W1] showed the feasibility of such programs, and Thomas and colleagues[T1] and later Watson and associates reported good clinical results using distant donors.[W2]

The historical note would be incomplete without emphasis on Medawar's concepts of acquired immunologic tolerance. This was the subject of his address upon receipt of the Nobel prize in 1961[M9] and was preceded by his work with Billingham (see below) and others. An observation that had early attracted Medawar's attention was that of Owen, who in 1945 observed that two genetically different calves sharing the same placenta (chimeras) can have transplants between themselves without rejection.[O3] Billingham, Brent, and Medawar then showed in 1953 that in mice the injection of a newborn with cells from another individual made that mouse tolerant of later transplants from the other individual.[B14] Subsequently, Lance and Medawar showed that under some circumstances long-term tolerance can be facilitated by injections of antilymphocyte serum.[L6] Other workers, particularly Monaco, have extended the knowledge of immunologic tolerance.[M21] While the techniques of inducing immunologic tolerance have not yet become clinically important in cardiac transplantation, it is the opinion of Diethelm[D11] and others experienced in the general field of transplantation that this may yet prove to be Medawar's most important contribution to the clinical success of cardiac and other organ transplantation.

MORPHOLOGY

Dilated Cardiomyopathy

The primary morphologic characteristic of the condition of dilated, or congestive cardiomyopathy is enlargement (increased volume) of the ventricles and, to a lesser extent, the atria. A variable degree of hypertrophy is often present.

Microscopic examination demonstrates extensive interstitial and perivascular fibrosis, occasionally with calcification, in the ventricular myocardium. Myocardial cell degeneration is usually seen.[S1] However, the specific diagnosis of dilated cardiomyopathy can usually not be made by endocardial biopsy.

Restrictive Cardiomyopathy

The uncommon form of cardiomyopathy known as *restrictive cardiomyopathy* is characterized morphologically by diffuse ventricular hypertrophy. The ventricular walls are excessively rigid. Microscopically, fibrosis and hypertrophy of myocytes are usually apparent.

Often there are no morphologic suggestions as to the primary process. However, this picture may be produced by amyloid infiltration of the myocardium as well as some other specific processes.

Endomyocardial Fibrosis

Characteristically, endomyocardial fibrosis also called obliterative cardiomyopathy, consists of fibrous endocardial lesions involving primarily the inflow portions of the right and left ventricles, along with the posterior wall and apex.[C3,D2] The atrioventricular (AV) valves are often involved and made incompetent. The outflow tract of the ventricle is usually spared.[C1] The heart may be more or less normal in size or somewhat enlarged, but massive cardiomegaly is rare,[C1,S2] as is ventricular hypertrophy. Both right and left ventricles are usually involved, but 40% of patients have purely left ventricular involvement and 10% purely right ventricular involvement.[S2] Metras and colleagues have described a more localized form of the disease that affects only the papillary muscles of the left ventricle and presents as isolated mitral regurgitation.[M2]

Microscopically, a thick layer of hyalinized fibrous tissue is usually seen.[D1] Calcification may be present, and thrombi may cover the inner portion of the involved ventricle. A characteristic feature of the disease is sparsity of elastic fibers, in contrast to the massive proliferation found in endocardial fibroelastosis. The myocardium is minimally affected. These changes may be associated with eosinophilia (Löffler's syndrome).[B15]

CLINICAL FEATURES AND DIAGNOSTIC CRITERIA

Etiology

Dilated cardiomyopathy frequently is of unknown etiology in the individual patient. However, there has been considerable speculation as to the possible progression of infective, particularly viral myocarditis to full-blown dilated cardiomyopathy. Such progression may be particularly frequent in children.[G6] Alcoholism, pregnancy, and systemic hypertension may provide a background for the development of dilated cardiomyopathy.

Restrictive cardiomyopathy may be secondary to amyloid infiltration and other processes, but in a number of cases the etiology is unknown.

Endomyocardial fibrosis is of unknown etiology. There has been speculation as to the possible role of a diet high in bananas, of malnutrition, and of various infections as well as consideration of this form of cardiomyopathy as an immunologic response.

Pathophysiology

Dilated cardiomyopathy is characterized pathophysiologically by impaired ventricular systolic function.[G1] However, particularly late in the disease, decreased left ventricular compliance may develop.[G2] As a consequence of these basic processes, both end-diastolic and end-systolic ventricular volumes are increased.

The primary physiologic abnormality in restrictive cardiomyopathy is severe impairment of ventricular compliance. Generally, ventricular systolic function is unimpaired. This condition simulates chronic constrictive pericarditis pathophysiologically to such an extent that the two conditions are separated hemodynamically with great difficulty.

Endomyocardial fibrosis is pathophysiologically complex. Early in this process, there are only scattered areas of fibrosis with little hemodynamic effect. As progressively increasing endomyocardial fibrosis develops, with consequent restriction of ventricular filling, ventricular end-diastolic pressures rise as do pulmonary or systemic venous pressures, depending on which ventricle is involved. The involvement of the AV valves then adds valvular incompetence to the already impaired hemodynamic state.[V1]

Symptoms and Signs

All forms of cardiomyopathy may have a prodromal phase, lasting weeks or months, that is nonspecific and suggests an infectious process. Then symptoms of left and/or right ventricular failure develop and progress to the stage of chronic congestive heart failure. The chest x-ray may be normal or may show cardiomegaly, which can be extreme in the case of dilated cardiomyopathy.

When endomyocardial fibrosis is present and involves both ventricles, right ventricular failure dominates the clinical picture, with liver enlargement, ascites, and peripheral edema in association with tricuspid incompetence. There are often pleural and pericardial effusions. With isolated left ventricular involvement, there are features of left ventricular failure and often mitral incompetence.[M22] There is usually a third heart sound. Right ventricular endomyocardial fibrosis is characterized by distinctive findings of right atrial enlargement, and hepatomegaly, ascites, and peripheral edema. The chest x-ray shows cardiomegaly, usually due to right atrial enlargement on pericardial effusion. Calcification may be seen diffusely within the myocardium.[C2]

Special Studies

Cardiac catheterization usually reveals the nonspecific findings to be expected from the pathophysiology of the disease. The right and/or left ventricular ejection fractions are reduced, and the diastolic pressure contour has the square root sign characterisic of pericardial constriction (see Chapter 52, ''Pathophysiology of Cardiac Compression'' in Section 1, Clinical Features and Diagnostic Criteria). Particu-

larly in restrictive cardiomyopathy, it may be impossible to exclude the diagnosis of chronic constrictive pericarditis on a hemodynamic basis. In some instances, thoracotomy is necessary for exclusion of the diagnosis of chronic constrictive pericarditis (see Chapter 52).[M1]

When endomyocardial fibrosis is present, angiocardiography often reveals obliteration of the apex of the ventricle involved. The left ventricle may show an apical diverticulum.

Endomyocardial biopsy may be useful in excluding other conditions in patients believed to have dilated cardiomyopathy. However, a positive diagnosis of dilated cardiomyopathy from biopsy is rarely possible.[O1] This is also true of restrictive cardiomyopathy. Myocardial biopsy may give a strong clue to the diagnosis of obliterative cardiomyopathy.

NATURAL HISTORY

Dilated Cardiomyopathy

Patients with dilated cadiomyopathy usually progressively deteriorate, and the majority die within 4 years of the onset of symptoms.[F1,G3] Eighty percent of patients are dead within 10 years of known onset (Fig. 51-1).[F2] The prognosis is particularly poor when marked cardiomegaly develops.[F2] Particularly relevant to cardiac transplantation is the fact that in some patients, only 12–24 months elapse between onset and death. Although death is usually in advanced cardiac failure, as in ischemic heart disease when left ventricular function is reduced, there is a high incidence of ventricular arrhythmia and sudden death.[M11]

The risk factors for early death (within 1 year) have been evaluated by Unverferth and colleagues,[U1] and their findings are useful in patients being considered for transplantation. The most powerful risk factors are left ventricular conduction delay, the presence of ventricular arrhythmias,[H6] and marked elevation of right atrial pressure.

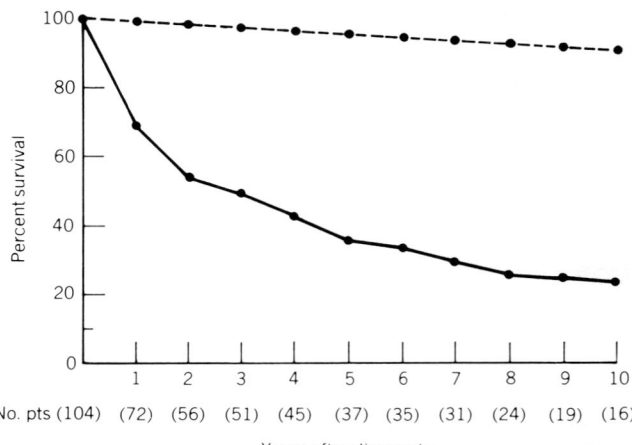

No. pts (104) (72) (56) (51) (45) (37) (35) (31) (24) (19) (16)

Years after diagnosis

Figure 51-1 Actuarial survival after diagnosis in patients with idiopathic dilated cardiomyopathy. The dashed line is the survival of an age- and sex-matched general population.

Reproduced with permission from Fuster et al.[F2]

Restrictive Cardiomyopathy

The natural history of patients with restrictive cardiomyopathy has not been well defined. Generally, the symptoms are of long duration, and death is delayed for 5–20 years after abnormalities of cardiac function become apparent.

Endomyocardial Fibrosis

The uncommon endomyocardial fibrosis (or obliterative cardiomyopathy) tends to affect children and young adults. It occurs primarily in Uganda, Nigeria, and India.[V1] However, cases have been sporadically reported in many countries of the world, including the United States.[L2] The natural history of patients with this type of cardiomyopathy is generally unfavorable, characterized by a slowly deteriorating course and death within 5–10 years,[C1] often within 1–2 years.[D3]

TECHNIQUE OF OPERATION: CARDIAC TRANSPLANTATION

Determination of Histocompatibility

For cardiac transplantation, the donor and recipient must have ABO (blood type) compatibility. Three procedures to study immunologic compatibility are also used: HLA typing, white blood cell antibody screen, and lymphocyte crossmatch (UAB).

HLA Typing

A lymphocyte preparation is made from the patient's peripheral blood, which is then added to a panel of approximately 180 wells containing different HLA-A, -B, and -C antisera (detecting antigens present on all lymphocytes) and a panel of 60 wells containing HLA-DR antisera (detecting antigens on B-lymphocytes), each in the presence of complement. If a cytotoxic antibody reacts with lymphocyte antigens, the cell membrane is damaged and lysis results, a process that can be detected by the passage of the trypan blue into the cell. In this way, the tissue antigen profile of the prospective recipient (patient)—and by the same process, that of the donor—is determined. However, currently HLA tissue typing is not part of the donor selection process, since no benefit from it has been demonstrated in cardiac transplantation.[S3] Some surgical groups have avoided performing transplantation in the setting of an HLA-A_2 or -A_3 mismatch because of possible predisposition to chronic graft rejection manifested by premature arteriosclerosis in the graft vessels.[P1] This, however, is not practiced currently (UAB).

White Blood Cell Antibody Screen

The lymphocyte cytotoxicity screen, or white blood cell antibody screen, is performed on prospective cardiac transplant recipients to detect the presence of preformed antibodies in the recipient reactive against a panel of HLA antigens. This is also a lymphocyte toxicity test, as is the HLA typing procedure, except that recipient *sera* are placed in 40–60 wells in a panel containing a wide range of HLA antigens. Any reactivity occurring in a well is regarded as a

positive reaction, and the result of the test is reported as the percentage of reactive antibody (PRA), which is the percentage of reactive wells in the panel. A prospective lymphocyte crossmarch is not performed if the antibody screen is negative (UAB).

Lymphocyte Crossmatch

If a recipient has reactive antibodies or positive results of screening for positive antibody, or if screening has not been done, a prospective crossmatch of recipient serum and a donor lymphocyte preparation is performed. This crossmatch is also a lymphocytotoxic test, a positive test being indicated by lymphocyte lysis. The probability of hyperacute rejection with a positive crossmatch is high, but rejection is not inevitable, since the antibodies may be directed against B cell antigens, which are thought not to result in graft destruction. In the setting of a positive crossmatch, the donor is rejected for the patient being tested.

Selection of the Recipient

Once the medical indications for transplantation have been identified (see ''Indications for Operation''), the recipient is reviewed to determine if there are any relative contraindications to cardiac transplantation.

The extremes of age are considered to contraindicate cardiac transplantation, although at the younger end of the scale there is no absolute contraindication, since Yacoub has performed cardiac transplantation in a neonate with hypoplastic left heart syndrome with at least early success.[Y1] An age below about 5 years is considered difficult for cardiac transplantation because of potential problems with repeated posttransplantation endomyocardial biopsies (UAB). Age older than about 55 years is a relative contraindication, since immunosuppressive complications tend to be more frequent and more severe in older patients.[G3]

Psychologic stability and likelihood of compliance with the treatment protocols are important considerations.[W4] If these factors are lacking, the important postoperative medical treatment may be knowingly or unknowingly aborted by the patient, with fatal consequences.

The patient must be free of infection. Insulin-dependent diabetes is a contraindication to cardiac transplantation, since this condition predisposes the patient to infection. In addition, many patients develop diabetes while on chronic steroid therapy, and preexisting diabetes may greatly increase the difficulty of its management. Active peptic ulcer disease is also a contraindication because of the propensity for its exacerbation in the presence of postoperative steroid therapy. A recent pulmonary embolus is an unfavorable finding, since patients with such a history are likely to develop fatal pulmonary infection at the infarct site during the necessary posttransplantation immunosuppression.[B2]

Pulmonary vascular disease is a contraindication to orthotopic cardiac transplantation, since the normal right ventricle usually fails when its afterload is increased by a pulmonary artery pressure of more than 60–79 mm Hg systolic. This means that a pulmonary vascular resistance greater than about 7 units $\cdot$ m^2 is not acceptable.

Preparation of the Recipient

The usual preparations for major cardiac surgery are made. In addition, when a donor has been identified, an event that makes transplantation within 6–12 hours almost certain, the patient is given 12–14 mg · kg^{-1} of cyclosporine orally.

If the recipient has a history of important renal dysfunction manifested by a serum creatinine level greater than 2.0 mg% at any time before cardiac transplantation, a modified pretransplant immunosuppressive regimen is utilized because of the increased incidence of acute renal failure using cyclosporine (see "Results"). A reduced dose of cyclosporine (1–5 mg · kg^{-1} orally) is combined with rabbit antithymocyte globulin (RATG; 2.5 mg · kg^{-1} intramuscularly) just before anesthetic induction.

The procurement of the donor heart and the preparations for placing the patient on cardiopulmonary bypass (CPB) are carefully synchronized. The patient is thus transferred to the operating room about 1½ hours before the estimated time of arrival of the donor heart at the patient's hospital (UAB).

Selection and Preparation of the Donor

The donor becomes available when brain death has occurred, and the criteria enumerated by the Ad Hoc Committee of the Harvard Medical School are generally used.[H1] The patient must be completely unreceptive and unresponsive, without reflexes or movements of breathing. Two flat electroencephalograms 24 hours apart are sometimes required.

Once a potential donor has been identified, other criteria apply. The donor should be less than 35 years of age. There should have been no episodes of profound hypotension at any time after injury because poor donor heart function after transplantation is likely to follow such an event.[G4] Any evidence of sepsis must be sought, and, if found, the donor is rejected. There should not be a great disparity between the size of the donor and recipient.

Findings upon physical examination relative to the heart must be normal. A 12-lead electrocardiogram is examined to exclude the possibility of the preexistence of Q wave abnormalities and conduction defects; nonspecific ST and T wave changes may be caused by head injury, hypothermia, and vasopressor agents and per se do not contraindicate use of the heart. If there has been any suggestion of hypotension or cardiac injury, serum cardiac enzymes, particularly the myocardial isoenzyme (MB fraction) of creatinine kinase (CK), are obtained and must be normal.

Once the donor has been screened and found acceptable, management of the donor becomes intense. Hypotension, hypothermia, and diabetes insipidus are frequent physiologic results of brain death and make careful attention to volume replacement, sometimes in large amounts, essential. Active warming may be required to counteract hypothermia.

The decision to use a specific donor must be based in part on the feasibility of keeping the cardiac ischemic time less than 180 minutes (UAB). This time limit is based on the demonstration of ultrastructural changes in hearts after 180 or more minutes of preservation.[B3] The cardiac ischemic time includes the time required to remove the heart from the donor after the aorta is cross-clamped, to transport the heart to the recipient's operating room (usually including air transport time, since most cardiac procurement is from distant sites), and to suture the donor heart into the recipient and release the recipient's aortic cross-clamp.

Procurement of the Donor Heart

The cardiac surgeon for the patient procures the heart (UAB). During cardiac procurement, consideration must be given to the fact that most donors are donating kidneys as well as hearts, and some the liver as well. The donor is prepared from the neck to the mid-thigh. Preferably, a central venous line and an arterial catheter are placed, since marked hypotension may occur during mobilization of the kidneys.

A long midline incison is made from the jugular notch to the pubis. Volume replacement continues actively, since considerable bleeding from the incisions is frequent due to the patient's vasodilated state. The usual median sternotomy is made and the self-retaining retractor inserted. While the donor nephrectomy team proceeds, the pericardium is opened, and the usual stay sutures are applied. The heart is examined for any evidence of cardiac injury, congenital anomalies, or acquired heart disease. The ascending aorta is dissected and mobilized as far as the takeoff of the innominate artery. The superior vena cava (SVC) is completely mobilized, including any pericardial reflection onto it. The inferior vena cava (IVC) is encircled with a heavy ligature. A purse-string suture is placed on the ascending aorta for the cardioplegic infusion.

When the donor nephrectomy surgeon is ready to clamp the renal pedicles, 200 units · kg^{-1} of heparin are given. While the surgeon waits for this to take full effect, the cardioplegia needle is inserted into the ascending aorta and secured. In this setting, the cardioplegic solution has only 10 mEq · l^{-1} of potassium and is in liter bags that have been in an ice cooler. The cardioplegic solution is infused by the anesthesiologist with a pressure bag.

If a central line is in place, it is withdrawn. The SVC is clamped as far distally as possible. The IVC is pulled up with the ligature, and a long straight clamp is placed across it as inferiorly as possible. The aorta is cross-clamped just proximal to the innominate artery. Infusion of the cardioplegic solution is begun, and the inferior vena cava and the right superior pulmonary vein are partially divided to allow the escape of warm blood from the heart. The cardioplegic infusion pressure is monitored digitally and kept appropriate (see Chapter 3), while at least 1,000 ml of solution are infused. Ice cold saline solution is poured into the pericardium.

After about 2 minutes (to allow cardiac cooling), the SVC is divided close to the clamp, the remainder of the IVC is divided, and the ascending aorta is divided just proximal to the cross-clamp. The apex of the heart is then elevated, and the left and right pulmonary veins are divided. The right and left pulmonary arteries are divided near the bifurcation, and after the pericardial reflections are cut, the heart is removed.

The heart is placed in a plastic bag containing ice cold saline solution, and the bag is then sealed with a tie gun. This bag is placed in a second heavy plastic bag, which is similarly sealed, and this package is placed in a stockinet slung inside a stainless steel canister, which is closed. The cannister is then placed in a heavy outer plastic bag, the last step taken under completely sterile conditions. The completed package is packed in ice in a commercial portable cooler, for transportation, usually by jet aircraft, to the recipient.

Initial Stages of the Operation

During procurement of the donor heart, the usual preparations for open cardiac operations (see Chapter 2, Section 3) are made for the patient by a colleague of the patient's surgeon. The right side of the neck is not used for any lines because inadvertent injury to the right internal jugular vein may compromise access for subsequent endomyocardial biopsy. A median sternotomy is made. The usual pursestring sutures are placed, except that the one for aortic can-

nulation is placed as high on the ascending aorta as possible (see Chapter 2, Section 3). The usual lines and attachments for cardiopulmonary bypass (CPB) are arranged. The hemodynamic state of the patient must be carefully protected during this stage of the operation.

Cardiac Transplantation

When the donor heart arrives in the operating room, it is prepared by the surgeon on a separate sterile table while preparation of the patient by the cardiac surgical colleague continues. The SVC of the donor heart is ligated and the right atrium is incised from the IVC upward toward the right atrial appendage to form a cuff of right atrium to match the right atrial cuff of the recipient (Fig. 51-2a). Similarly, the orifices of the pulmonary veins are connected, resulting in the formation of a left atrial cuff (Fig. 51-2b). The pulmonary artery and aorta are dissected free from the roof of the left atrium,

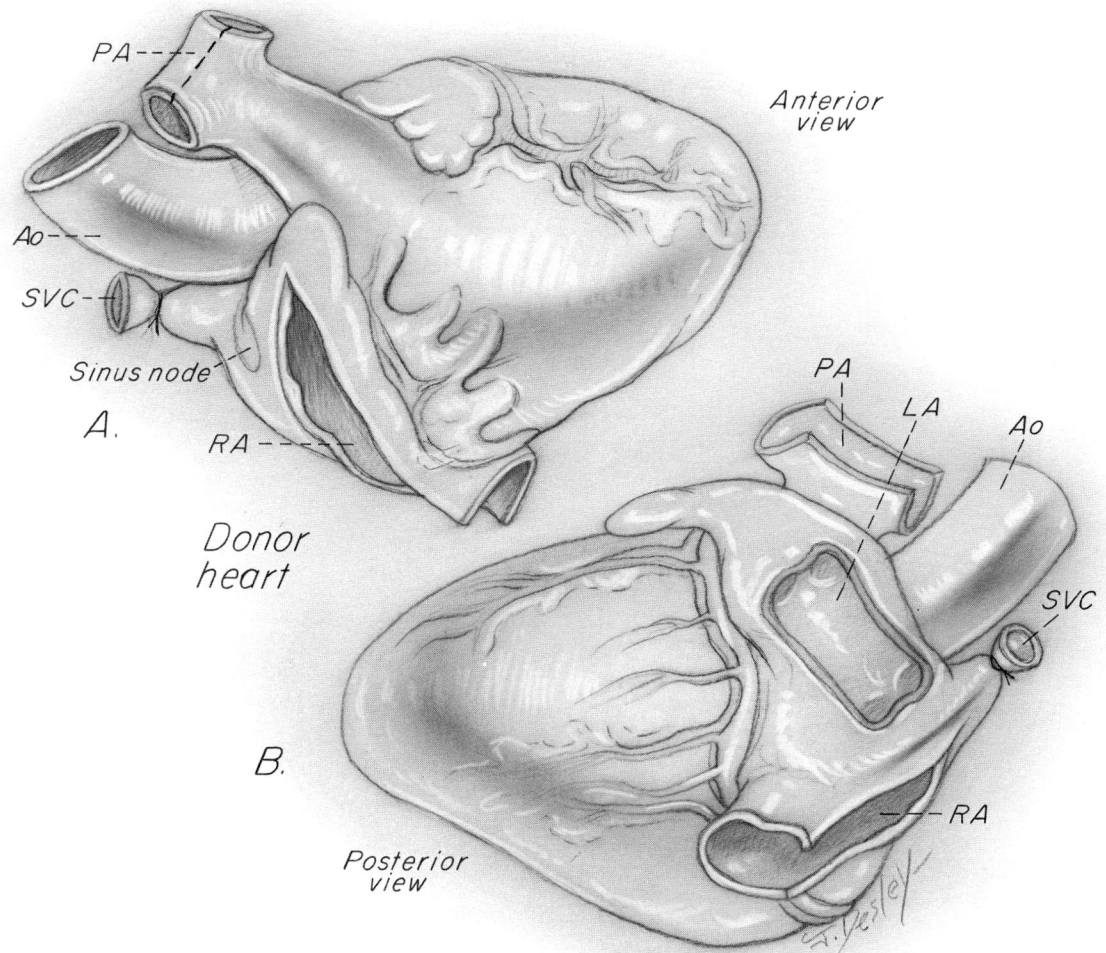

Figure 51-2 The cardiac transplantation operation.

(a) After being transported from the site of removal, the donor heart is prepared in the operating room in which the transplantation will be performed. An incision is made from the inferior vena caval orifice up the lateral wall of the right atrium. Care is taken to avoid damage to the sinus node.

(b) The orifices of the four pulmonary veins are connected, and the resultant square of posterior left atrial wall is removed. This creates the left atrial cuff. The pulmonary artery cuff is made.

Ao, aorta; CS, coronary sinus; LA, left atrium; MV, mitral valve; PA, pulmonary artery; RA, right atrium; SVC, superior vena cava; TV, tricuspid valve.

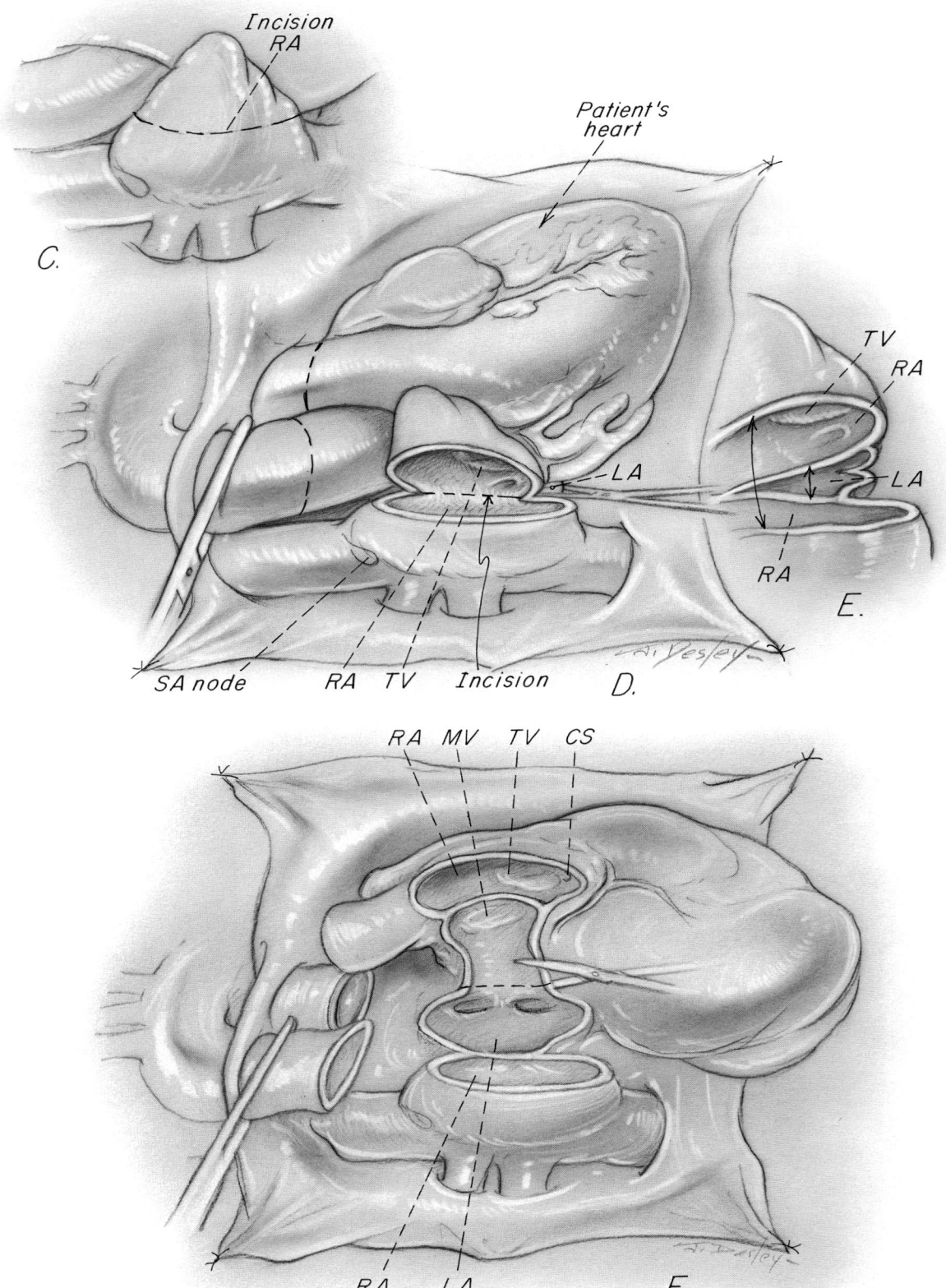

Figure 51-2 *(continued)*

(c) The cardiac transplantation operation in the patient begins with cardiectomy. For this, an initial right atriotomy is made lateral to the base of the atrial appendage.

(d) The right atriotomy is extended medially superiorly and inferiorly nearly to the AV groove, and then further above and below to cross the extremities of the atrial septum and enter the left atrium in both areas.

(e) The left atrium as well as the right atrium have been opened after step *d* has been completed.

(f) The aorta and then the pulmonary artery have been transected as proximally as possible. The left atrial incisions have been carried to the left, and in the drawing the inferior one is being extended superiorly at the base of the left atrial appendage to complete the cardiectomy.

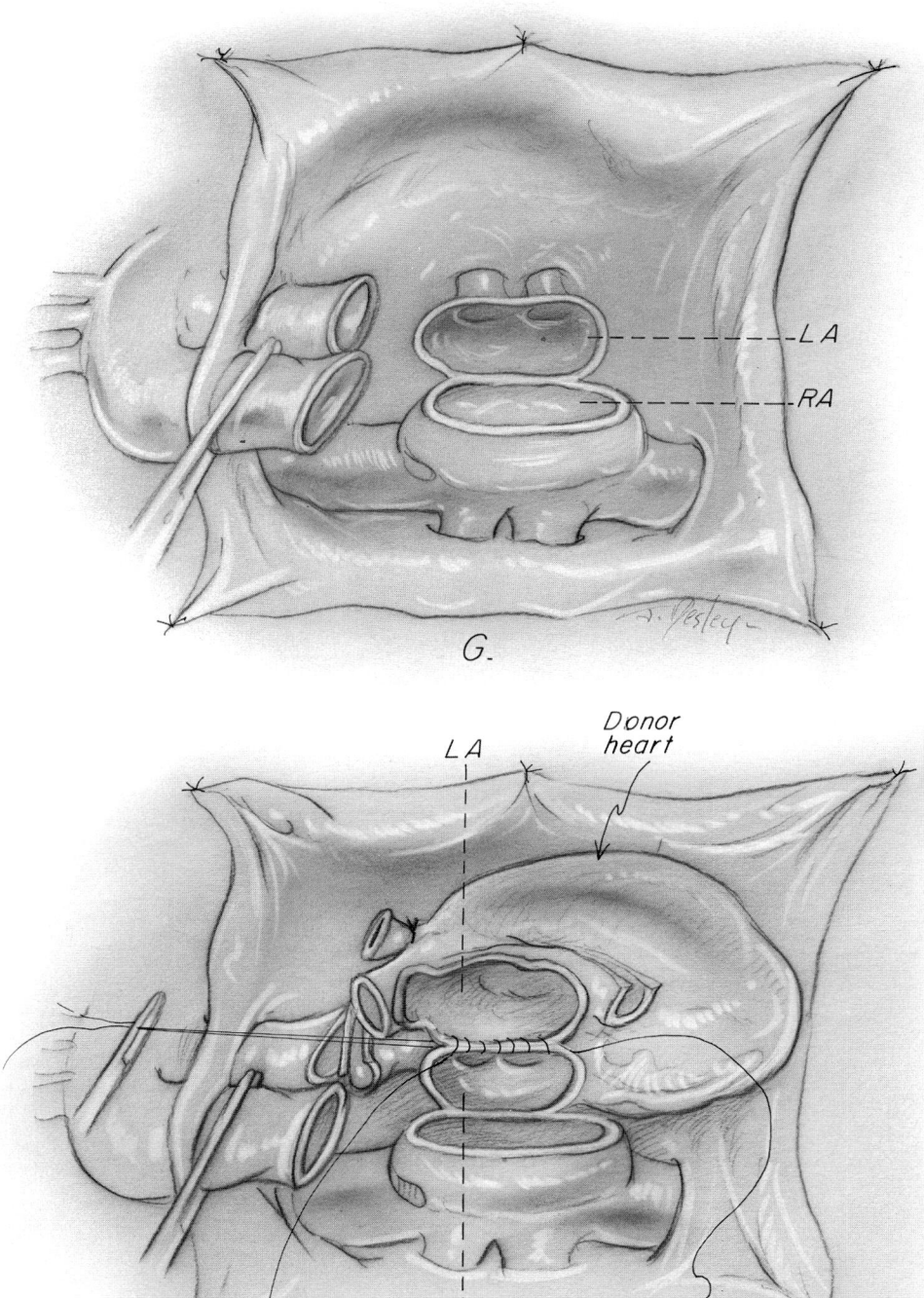

G.

Donor
heart

LA

LA

LA

H.

Figure 51-2 *(continued)*
(*g*) The appearance of the surgical field after the cardiectomy. The orifices of the right pulmonary veins are behind the posterior atrial septal remnant and are not visible.
(*h*) The insertion of the donor heart is the final step. For this, the donor heart is brought into the pericardium and allowed to fall off toward the patient's left side. A silk stay suture is placed superiorly, as shown. A double-armed 3-0 polypropylene suture is used to begin the suture line inferiorly and is continued from within as a whip stitch to join the left side of the atrial wall of the recipient and donor hearts. When this whip stitch reaches the superior stay suture, the stay suture is removed and the polypropylene suture held. With the other arm of the suture, the suture line is continued inferiorly and then to the right.

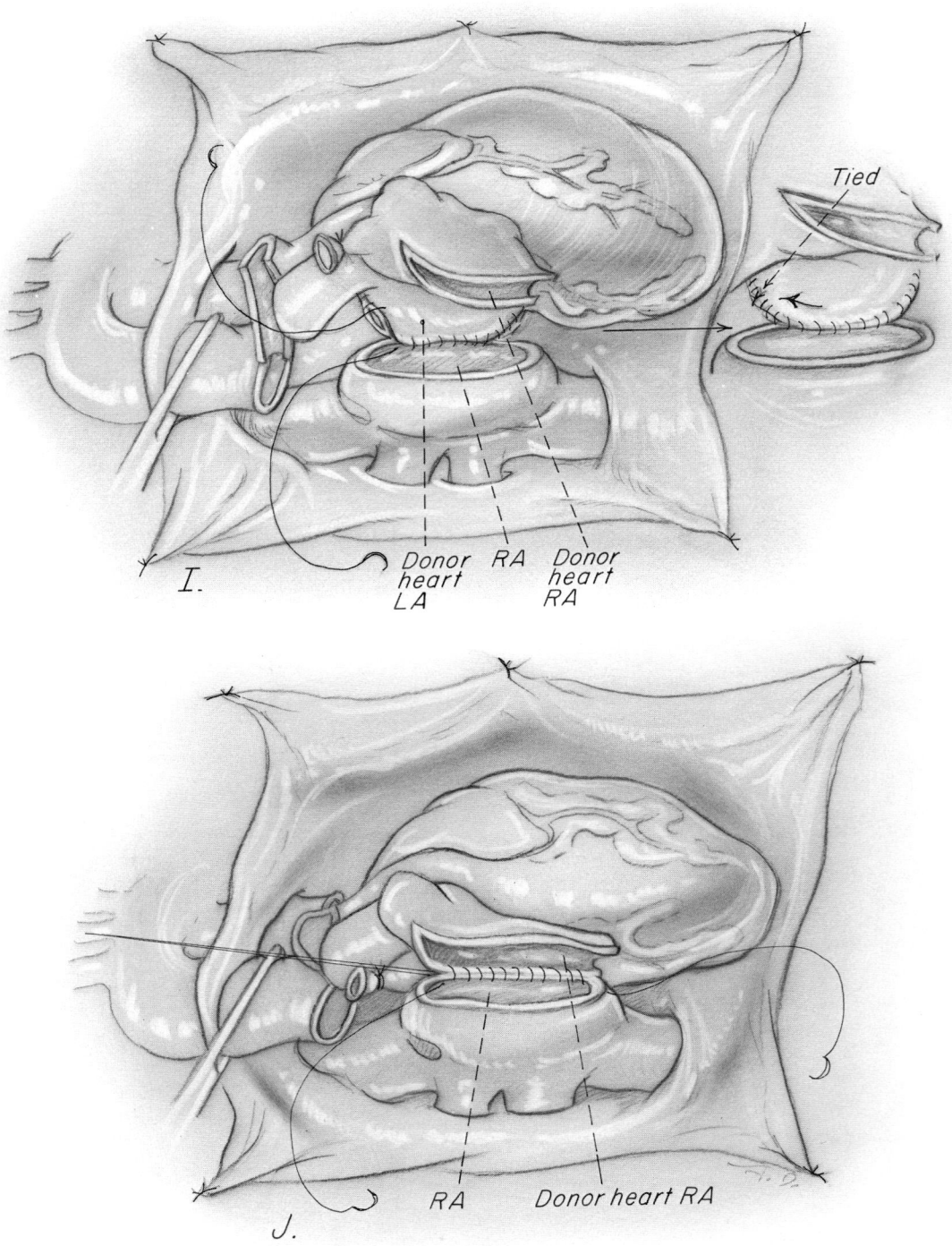

Figure 51-2 (*continued*)
(*i*) The suture line then extends superiorly to join the left atrial wall of the donor heart to the cut edge of the patient's atrial septum. The insert shows the suture line completed superiorly.

(*j*) The right atrium of the donor heart is now anastomosed to the remnant of the patient's right atrium. A stay suture is placed superiorly. A 3-0 polypropylene suture is used to begin the anastomosis inferiorly and is extended superiorly as a whip stitch. In the mid-portion of this suture line, the donor heart right atrium is joined to the suture line between the patient's atrial septum and the donor left atrium.

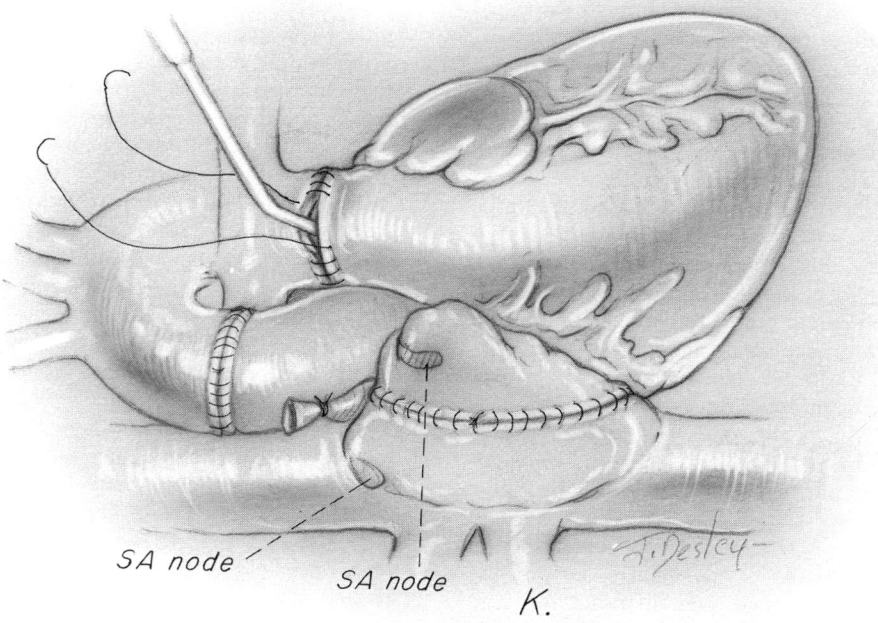

SA node   *SA node*   *K.*

Figure 51-2 *(continued)*
(k) The atrial anastomoses have been completed. An end-to-end anastomosis is made of the donor heart pulmonary artery to the patient's pulmonary artery, leaving the ends untied and a sucker in the pulmonary artery. The donor heart aorta is connected to the patient's aorta by a continuous whip stitch.

and the openings into the right and left pulmonary arteries are connected and then trimmed to provide a wide pulmonary artery orifice near the bifurcation (Figs. 51-2*a,b*).[M16]

As this is being done, the patient is placed on CPB using the usual direct caval cannulation (UAB). The aorta is cross-clamped, and the perfusate is lowered to 28–30°C. To begin the cardiectomy, a right atriotomy is made just lateral to the base of the appendage. As this incision is carried medially nearly to the atrioventricular groove and then superiorly, the roof of the left atrium is entered as the incision goes across the superior aspect of the atrial septum (Fig. 51-2*c*). The initial incision is then carried inferiorly around the right atrial appendage (to be removed with the heart) and then back nearly to the atrioventricular groove. As the incision is then carried inferiorly, the left atrium is entered adjacent to the coronary sinus in the same manner as superiorly (Fig. 51-2*d*). The superior and inferior incisions in the atrial septum are then connected (Fig. 51-2*e*). The aorta and main pulmonary artery are then transected as proximally as possible (Fig. 51-2*f*). Finally, the heart is allowed to roll off to the patient's left, and the left atrial incision is completed (removing the left atrial appendage with the specimen; Fig. 51-2*f*). The patient is now prepared for insertion of the donor heart (Fig. 51-2*g*).

The insertion of the donor heart is begun by connecting the left atrial cuff of the donor heart to the remnant of the patient's heart (Fig. 51-2*h*); the right side of the suture line connects the donor left atrial wall to the patient's atrial septum (Fig. 51-2*i*). The right atrial anastomosis is performed (Fig. 51-2*j*). The pulmonary artery anastomosis is then carried out in a standard end-to-end fashion with 4-0 polypropylene. The ends are tagged rather than tied for later de-airing

of the right ventricle (Fig. 51-2*k*). The end-to-end aortic anastomosis is then made (Fig. 51-2*k*).

The donor heart is at 4–6°C temperature on removal from the cannister in the operating room,[K2] and subsequent hypothermia is maintained during implantation by filling each atrial chamber with ice cold saline solution before securing the atrial suture line and by filling the pericardium with ice cold saline solution while each suture line is tied (UAB). Before the cross-clamp is removed, air is evacuated from the left ventricle by passage of a large-bore (13-g) needle from the right ventricle through the ventricular septum. A needle vent is placed in the ascending aorta in the previously placed purse-string suture, and with strong suction on this needle vent, the cross-clamp is removed. Air is evacuated from the right ventricle through the pulmonary artery anastomosis, and that suture is then tied.

The usual polyvinyl catheters and pacing wires are placed, as well as the usual drainage tubes. The incision is closed as usual.

Anatomic variations within the patient, such as persistent left superior vena cava or L-malposition of the aorta with congenitally corrected transposition of the great arteries, do not preclude transplantation but may require special techniques of insertion of the donor heart.[M13,R6]

TECHNIQUE OF OPERATION: ENDOMYOCARDIAL FIBROSIS

The operation for endomyocardial fibrosis is performed during cardiopulmonary bypass and cold cardioplegic myocardial protection. In left-sided disease, the mitral valve and interior of the left ventricle are exposed through the usual incision in the right side of the left atrium (see Chapter 11, Fig. 11-7). When exposure is unsatisfactory, an apical left ventriculotomy can be used.[G10,L2] The thickened and fibrotic endocardium in the inlet and apical portions of the left ventricle are excised. The endocardiectomy is made as extensive as needed, but no attempt is made to remove the fibrotic plaque in one block. The localization of the pathology to the inlet and apical portions in the ventricles facilitates the surgical procedure. Often the tensor apparatus of the mitral valve must be sacrificed as part of the excision, and, in any case, the valve is often incompetent preoperatively. Therefore, in most patients, mitral valve replacement is part of the procedure (see Chapter 11, "Mitral Valve Replacement" in section on Technique of Operation).

The approach is through the right atrium in cases of isolated right ventricular involvement. The procedure described above is carried out, usually associated with tricuspid valve replacement (see Chapter 14). However, a 5-mm strip of the endocardium is left on the ventricular septum along the anulus of the tricuspid valve, particularly in the region of the anteroseptal commissure, in order to avoid damage to the bundle of His.

SPECIAL FEATURES OF POSTOPERATIVE CARE: CARDIAC TRANSPLANTATION

General Measures

The usual care given to patients after cardiac surgery (see Chapter 5) is applied to patients who have received a cardiac transplant. Generally, the subsystems function normally, and little or no special therapy is required. Cardiac function early after transplantation is usually good, and inotropic agents are not required routinely (UAB). However, since the introduction of cyclosporine, and particularly in patients who have been in advanced heart failure with impaired renal function, transient renal failure may develop (see "Early Posttransplantation Renal Dysfunction with Cyclosporine").

Coumadin (sodium warfarin) administration is begun after 48 hours and continued for 14 days postoperatively as a prophylaxis against thromboembolism (see Chapter 5). Dipyrimadole administration is begun at the same time, in a dose of 100 mg every 6 hours, and is continued indefinitely to counteract, at least in part, the tendency of the donor heart to develop coronary arteriosclerosis.

Immunosuppressive Therapy

Current Protocol

Five hundred milligrams of methyl prednisolone are given in the operating room upon discontinuation of CPB. This drug is continued with a dose of 125 mg intravenously 4 hours later, and then every 8 hours for two more doses.

Cyclosporine is currently the main immunosuppressive agent.[M16] Experience has shown, however, that it must be supplemented with prednisone and under some circumstances with rabbit antithymocyte globulin (RATG).[G7] After the initial loading dose of cyclosporine before the transplantation, subsequent doses of this drug are generally 6–14 mg ·

kg^{-1} · day^{-1} in split doses orally, the exact dose depending on the cyclosporine levels, serum creatinine levels, and urinary output. An elevated bilirubin level dictates a lowering of cyclosporine dosage, since this drug is metabolized through the hepatic microsomal enzymes. The dosage of cyclosporine is adjusted by measurement of cyclosporine whole blood levels every other day in the early postoperative period. The therapeutic trough whole blood level is 250–1,000 ng · ml^{-1}. The drug is continued indefinitely.

Along with cyclosporine, prednisone is begun on the first postoperative day, in a dose of 0.5 mg · kg^{-1} twice daily. The dose is reduced by 0.1 mg · kg^{-1} each week until the permanent dose of 0.2 mg · kg^{-1} · day^{-1} is reached, by about the eighth postoperative week. This drug is continued indefinitely.

The regimen is altered when the probability that cyclosporine will induce acute renal failure is high. This side effect is likely to occur in recipients in whom severe heart failure has been associated with important creatinine elevation or medical measures have not returned renal function to a relatively normal level. In such patients (see "Preparation of the Recipient"), the reduction in cyclosporine dose instituted preoperatively is continued postoperatively, and generally the dose is 0.5–2 mg · kg^{-1} twice daily. Until the levels are therapeutic (cyclosporine blood levels exceeds 200 ng · ml^{-1}) and renal function has normalized, RATG is continued at a dose of 2.5 mg IgG · kg^{-1} · day^{-1} intravenously, administered over 4–6 hours.

Intravenous cyclosporine is used only when the oral route is contraindicated by abdominal distress. The intravenous dosage is one-third the oral dose and is given as a continuous infusion over 12 hours.

Azathioprine Protocol

The use of azathioprine as an immunosuppressive agent is currently not practiced (UAB). If it is used, 4 mg · kg^{-1} of azathioprine are administered orally 4–6 hours before transplantation. RATG is given upon induction of anesthesia (see "Preparation of the Patient"). The steroid administration is the same as with cyclosporine.

Postoperatively, azathioprine is begun on postoperative day 1 in a single oral dose of 2.5 mg · kg^{-1} · day^{-1}. Subsequent doses are adjusted so that the total white blood count is between 4,000–10,000 cells · cm^{-3}. RATG is given daily for 13 days in a dose of 2.5 mg IgG · kg^{-1} · day^{-1}.

Prednisone is begun on postoperative day 1 in a dose of 1.5 mg · kg^{-1} · day^{-1}, given as a split dose twice daily. The dose is reduced each day by 2.5 mg until a dose of 1 mg · kg^{-1} · day^{-1} is reached. Subsequent reductions are made when the patient is an outpatient to a minimum of 0.4 mg · kg^{-1} · day^{-1} by 6 months postoperatively.

Protection against Infection

Currently, the patient remains in the Cardiovascular Surgery Intensive Care Unit only 2–3 days unless complications develop (UAB). During this time, strict reverse isolation techniques are enforced. When the patient moves out of the Intensive Care Unit, the isolation techniques are relaxed, but hand washing and face masking by all staff and visitors coming into the patient's room are enforced. Whenever the patient leaves his or her room, the patient wears a mask, a practice that is continued until hospital dismissal, which is usually about 3 weeks postoperatively.

The usual pre-, intra- and postoperative antibiotic program is used (see Chapter 5), with cephamandol being given in a dose of 1 g every 6 hours intravenously until all intravascular lines are removed.

Sputum cultures are obtained at the time of removal of the endotracheal tube (usually 6–12 hours after operation) and urine cultures upon removal of the Foley catheter (usually 24–48 hours postoperatively). Sputum and urine cultures are obtained weekly while the patient is in the hospital. These special measures are used because of the vulnerability to infection imparted by the immunosuppressive regimen.

Identification of Rejection

The electrocardiogram is not helpful in identifying rejection in patients receiving cyclosporine. The most reliable method of identifying and following the course of rejection is endomyocardial biopsy. This procedure is performed every 7 days for the first 3 postoperative weeks and then every 2 weeks for approximately 6 weeks. Thereafter, biopsies are performed every 3–4 months (see "Cardiac Rejection," under "Special Situations and Controversies").

Treatment of Rejection

A 3-day course of methyl prednisolone (1,000 mg intravenously per day) is given. If the rejection is unresponsive, RATG is added in the doses previously described (see "Current Protocol" in section on Immunosuppressive Therapy).

When rejection is severe (or early graft function poor), retransplantation is necessary (three occurrences; UAB, July 1981–October 1984). The late results of retransplantation may be less good than those of the original cardiac transplant.[W5]

Treatment of Posttransplantation Renal Dysfunction

Renal dysfunction is common with the use of cyclosporine. In most patients, the first sign is a gradual rise in the blood urea and creatinine levels without oliguria under good hemodynamic conditions. Such renal dysfunction usually responds well to a temporary reduction in the cyclosporine dose.

Less commonly, acute renal failure develops with anuria, which generally lasts for 24–72 hours. Cyclosporine should be discontinued in such a setting and RATG substituted (2.5 mg $\cdot$ kg^{-1} $\cdot$ day^{-1}; UAB). Fluids are severely restricted until urine output returns.

In spite of such management, some patients develop left atrial hypertension and acute pulmonary edema. Treatment consists of hemofiltration (removal of only water) or hemodialysis for the several days required for the return of renal function.

When daily urine output has returned to at least 500 ml, cyclosporine administration is resumed at a low dose (.5–1 mg $\cdot$ kg twice daily) and gradually increased until therapeutic blood levels are reached, at which time RATG is discontinued.

Among the first 12 patients undergoing cardiac transplantation with cyclosporine, all patients received a preoperative cyclosporine dose of 12–14 mg $\cdot$ kg^{-1} (UAB). All 4 patients who had a recorded serum creatinine level greater than 2 mg $\cdot$ dl^{-1} at some time before transplantation developed acute renal failure requiring hemofiltration or hemodialysis. In contrast, none of the 8 patients without a preoperative serum creatinine level exceeding 2 mg $\cdot$ dl^{-1} required hemodialysis or hemofiltration (*P* for difference = .002).[K2] The current protocol for use of cyclosporine in patients with altered renal function has evolved as a result of this experience (UAB).

RESULTS: CARDIAC TRANSPLANTATION

Survival

Most patients survive the immediately postoperative period, but the instantaneous risk of death declines more slowly after this than it does after most cardiac operations. Thus, among 38 patients, 35 (92%, CL 86%–96%) survived for 1 week, 31 (87%, CL 80%–91%) for 1 month, 10 (68%, CL 59%–75%) for 1 year, and 3 (50%, CL 38%–63%) for 2 years (UAB; Fig. 51-3).[M2] This experience is similar to that of others in the current era (Fig. 51-4). Results are currently superior to those obtained in the late 1960s.[F3]

Hazard function analysis indicates that the greatest risk of dying is shortly after receipt of the heart transplant.[M2] The instantaneous risk of death falls after that and begins to level off after 3 months (Fig. 51-5). There is a relatively low constant risk of death thereafter, at least for the currently available periods of postoperative observation.

Modes of Death

Most deaths after cardiac transplantation are related to immunologic problems and efforts to prevent them (Table 51-1). Thus, rejection of the cardiac transplant is the commonest mode of death. Death with infection, no doubt related to the immunosuppressive therapy, is also frequent.[C5]

One patient with congenital heart disease (Table 51-2) died with acute right ventricular failure of the transplanted heart. He was known preoperatively to have a pulmonary vascular resistance of 9 units $\cdot$ m^2, but it was believed that reduction of his severely elevated left atrial pressure would result in acute reduction of the pulmonary vascular resistance. It did not. One patient died early postoperatively after receiving a heart that functioned poorly throughout.

The modes of death seem to be different in patients receiving conventional immunosuppression than in those receiving cyclosporine (Table 51-3). Thus, acute rejection has been less common in patients receiving cyclosporine (UAB), although the experience to date does not exclude the possibility that the difference is due to chance (overlapping 70% confidence limits).

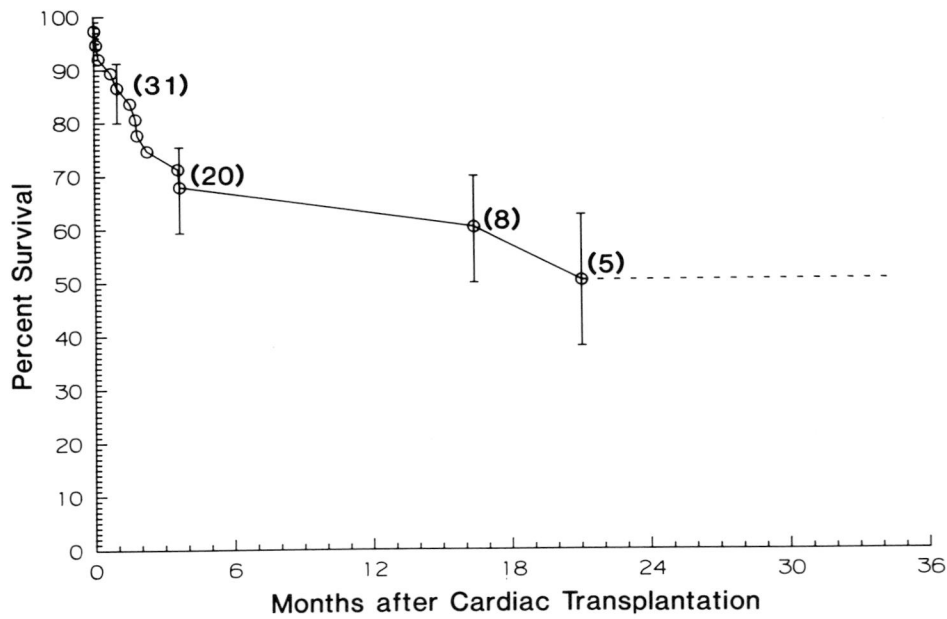

Figure 51-3 Actuarial survival, including hospital deaths, after cardiac transplantation (UAB; July 1981–October 1984; n = 38).

Reproduced with permission from McGiffin and Kirklin.[M2]

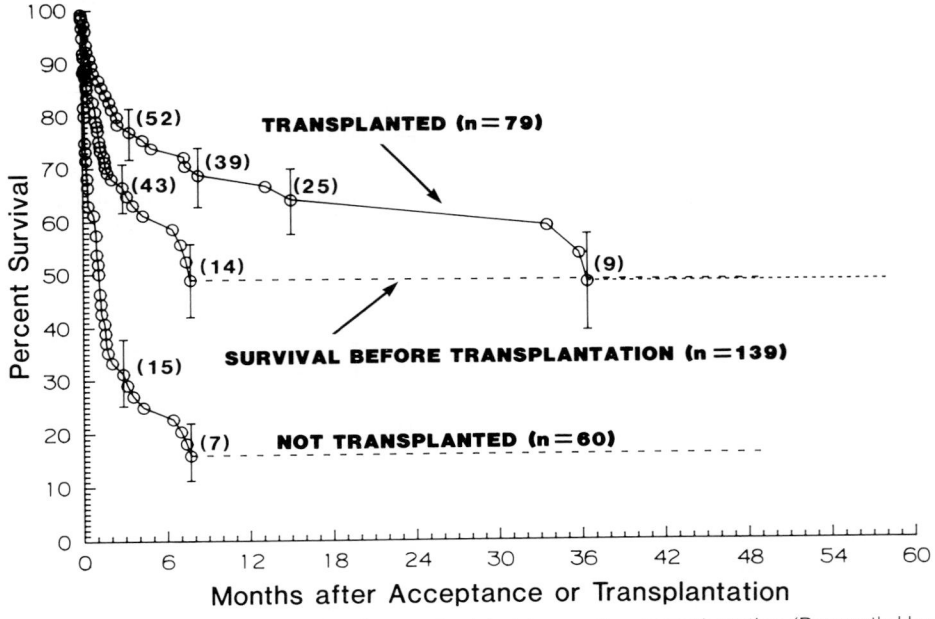

Figure 51-4 Actuarial survival of patients scheduled for cardiac transplantation (Papworth Hospital, Cambridge, England; December 1977–July 1984; follow-up as of July 1984). The survival is stratified into three curves. In the transplanted group, time zero is the time of cardiac transplantation. In the group entitled "survival before transplantation," time zero is the time of scheduling for transplantation; this group includes all patients scheduled, and they were censored at the time of transplantation. (See the text for discussion.) Time zero in the group entitled "not transplanted" is the time of scheduling; this group includes only patients who were never transplanted.

The data were supplied by Mr. Terence English, Papworth Hospital, Cambridge, England; analysis was by Blackstone and Naftel (UAB); the material is presented with the permission of Mr. English.

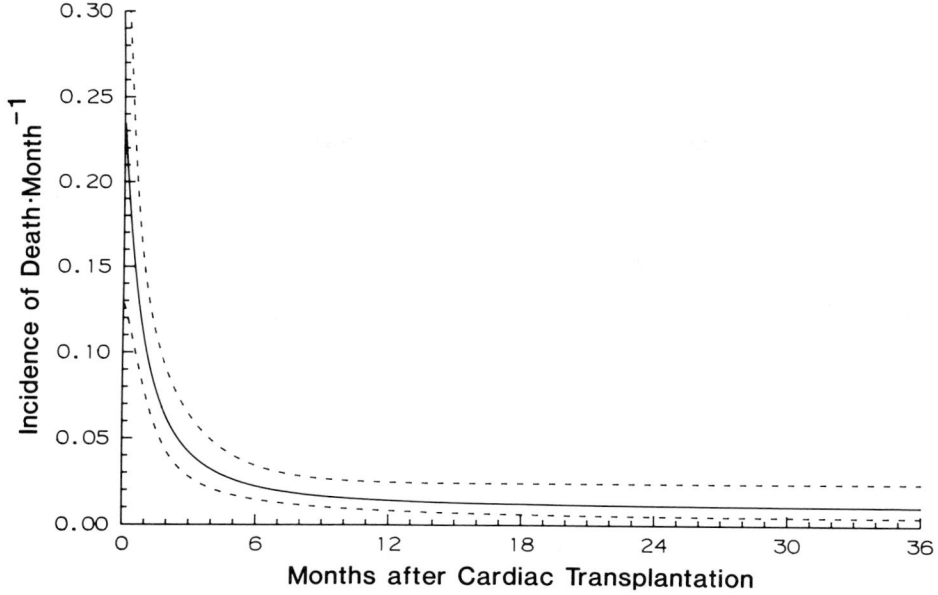

Figure 51-5 Hazard function for death (instantaneous risk per month) after cardiac transplantation (UAB; the data set is that depicted in Fig. 51-3). Time zero is the time of cardiac transplantation. There is an early phase and a later constant hazard phase.

Reproduced with permission from McGiffin and Kirklin.[M2]

Incremental Risk Factors for Premature Death

Absence of cyclosporine from the immunosuppressive regimen may in time be shown to be a risk factor for premature death, but the differences demonstrated to date could be due to chance (see above and Fig. 51-6). At least one death with infection was associated with a higher dosage of cyclosporine than is now considered advisable (UAB).

Recent results are improved not only because of cyclosporine but also because of general improvements in cardiac transplantation. Thus, at Stanford, the 1-year survival rate in 1968 was 22%, while in 1982 it was 88%.[J1]

Age at transplantation has had no demonstrable effect on survival (Table 51-4) or on the incidence of rejection episodes.

The patient's cardiac pathology has had no demonstrable effect on survival after transplantation (see Table 51-2). Noteworthy is the fact that in the patient with congenital

Table 51-1 Modes of premature (early and late) death after cardiac transplantation (UAB; July 1981–October 1984; n = 38).[M2]

Mode of Death	No. of Patients
Cardiac transplant rejection	6
Infection	4
Aspergillus	2
Cytomegalic virus	1
Brain abscess	1
Primary cardiac graft failure	1
Acute right ventricular failure (pulmonary vascular disease)	1
Pulmonary embolism	1
Total	13

heart disease and L-malposition of the aorta, no technical problems arose in the successful cardiac transplantation.

Functional Status

Little controversy exists as to the striking improvement in the functional status of many patients after cardiac transplantation, at least for a considerable period of time.[M3] Granting the difficulty of categorizing the post–cardiac transplant patient in a New York Heart Association (NYHA) functional class, 19 of 23 surviving and classifiable patients can be considered to be in NYHA functional class I and 4 in class II (UAB).[M2]

Cardiac Function

The transplanted donor heart appears to remain anatomically and functionally denervated indefinitely.[L4,S5] The patient's own sinus node is preserved with the atrial remnants but has a high incidence of dysfunction.[B6]

Gaudiani and colleagues found normal left ventricular ejection fractions both 1 year and 5 years after transplantation, with preservation of normal segmental wall motion as well.[G5] McGiffin and colleagues also found ejection fraction to be normal 6–21 months after transplantation, with an essentially normal increase during exercise (to an ejection fraction of 0.72 ± 0.08).[M10] Changes in ejection fraction were not found by them to predict rejection.

In other studies, the transplanted, chronically denervated, and nonrejecting heart has been found to have normal systolic function and contractile reserve.[B16] Left ventricular wall mass and end-diastolic wall thickness are greater in the chronically transplanted heart than in the normal heart.[B16] Some studies have indicated depression of left ventricular

Table 51-2 Relationship of the patient's cardiac pathologic condition to premature death after cardiac transplantation (UAB; July 1981–October, 1984; $n = 38$).

Cardiac Pathologic Condition	n	Deaths		
		No.	%	CL
Primary cardiomyopathy[a]	31	11	35%	26%–46%
Ischemic heart disease[b]	5	1	20%	3%–53%
Congenital heart disease[c]	2	1	50%	7%–93%
Total	38	13	34%	26%–44%
$P(\chi^2)$				.7

KEY: CL, 70% confidence limits.

[a] All patients but one (with endocardial fibroelastosis, aged 18, who died) had dilated cardiomyopathy; in two patients (one posttransplantation death), it was peripartum in origin, and in one (who is alive), it was believed rheumatic.

[b] All patients had advanced ischemic cardiomyopathy. All but one (who died) had previous coronary artery bypass grafting; all had had one to three previous myocardial infarctions.

[c] One patient, aged 22 at transplantation (who died), had repair of partial AV canal defect at age 3 years and residual severe left AV valve incompetence, followed by left AV valve replacement at age 21; he had severe secondary left ventricular cardiomyopathy and pulmonary hypertension (see the text). The other, aged 12 years, had situs solitus of the atria, AV discordant connection, double-outlet right ventricle, L-malposition of the aorta, straddling and overriding right AV valve, multiple ventricular septal defects, and pulmonary stenosis; there was severe secondary cardiomyopathy 11 years after a Waterston anastomosis.

function in the early days after transplantation.[C14,S9,S10] This and the subsequent increase in left ventricular mass may be related to the high systemic resistance in the recipient. Hypertension is common, and in some patients ejection fraction is decreased and left ventricular end-diastolic pressure increased.[G11] Left ventricular diastolic function after cardiac transplantation is decreased in some patients who are receiving cyclosporine.[H7]

A few patients develop accelerated coronary arteriosclerosis.[G5]

Complications

Nonlethal infectious complications occur mainly in the lungs and urinary tract and are primarily related to chronic immunosuppressive therapy.[M12,R1] Such infections include bacterial, fungal, and viral infections, particularly herpes simplex.[P2,W3] They usually respond to intensive medical treatment.

In addition, a member of noninfective complications occur that are also related primarily to immunosuppressive therapy (Table 51-5).

Comparison of Transplantation and Natural History

Assessing the overall efficacy of transplantation in prolonging life has been a difficult and complex task that has held the interest of physicians, surgeons, and statisticians.[A1] The depiction of the survival of patients receiving transplantation by the usual actuarial and parametric methods (see Chapter 6) is straightforward. The difficulty lies in assessing the probable survival of similar patients who did not undergo this surgical procedure. This dilemma may be forever difficult to resolve, since a randomized trial of cardiac transplantation is unlikely to be performed.

One method of assessing such natural history is by examining the survival of all patients scheduled for cardiac transplantation from a given moment on and censoring them at the time of transplantation, a method suggested by Turnbull and colleagues.[T2] Since the availability of a donor heart at a given time for a given patient is to a considerable extent a matter of chance, censoring of patients at transplantation can be considered appropriate. The resulting survival estimate, in which time zero is the time the patient is scheduled (so-called placed on the waiting list) can be used in comparison with a depiction of survival after transplantation, in which time zero is the moment of transplantation (see Figs. 51-4; and Figs. 51-7 and 51-8). This total group of patients is considered to give the best assessment available of the natural history without surgical treatment of patients submitted for cardiac transplantation (UAB).

Another reasonable method of assessment is the calculation of survival of all patients scheduled, and whether cardiac transplantation occurred is examined univariately or multivariately as a time-varying risk factor. In this analysis, assumptions are made as to the relative shape of the hazard function before and after transplantation.[C7]

Table 51-3 Modes of death in patients undergoing cardiac transplantation according to the type of immunosuppression used (UAB; July 1981–August 1984).[K2]

Mode of Death	Immunosuppression					
	Conventional (n = 17)			Cyclosporine (n = 17)		
	No.	% of 17	CL	No.	% of 17	CL
Acute rejection	5	29%	17%–45%	1	6%	0.8%–19%
Infection	3	18%	8%–32%	1	6%	0.8%–19%
Graft failure				1	6%	0.8%–19%
Pulmonary embolism	1	6%	0.8%–19%			
Right ventricular failure (pulmonary vascular disease)				1	6%	0.8%–19%
Total	9			4		

KEY: CL, 70% confidence limits.

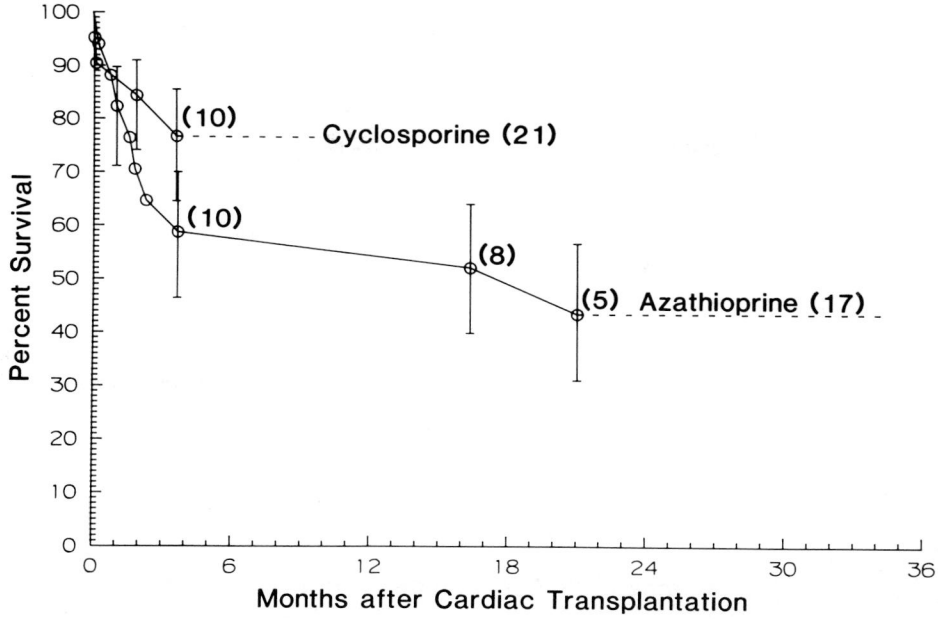

Figure 51-6 Stratified actuarial survival after cardiac transplantation (UAB; July 1981–October 1984). The azathioprine group, consisting of the first 17 patients, received no cyclosporine, and vice versa. *P* for difference (Wilcoxon) = .3.

Reproduced with permission from McGiffin and Kirklin.[M2]

Commonly, the survival of patients not receiving transplants at all has been used for the comparison, again with time zero as the time of placement on the waiting list.[C6] This group of patients is considered an inappropriate base for comparison, in view of the many variables that affect the appearance of a patient in the nontransplanted category rather than the transplanted one (UAB).

Several evaluations of the Stanford data, summarized by Aitkin and colleagues, find "insufficient evidence to support the conclusion that transplanted patients survive longer."[A1] However, examination of the hazard function of the two most appropriate groups for comparison (Fig. 51-7) suggests that the instantaneous risk of death is evidently (see Chapter 6) less in the transplanted group in the first month. This suggests the particular urgency of cardiac transplantation when it is inferred that the patient has a high probability of dying within 1 month without transplantation. Also, at least in the analysis of the Papworth series,[B13] survival for 3 years is appreciably better 57% (CL 52%–64%) in patients who have received transplants than in the "survival before transplantation" group (see Fig. 51-8), a situation reflected also in the hazard function analysis (see Fig. 51-7).

RESULTS: SURGERY FOR ENDOMYOCARDIAL FIBROSIS

One patient has received surgical treatment for endomyocardial fibrosis in the combined GLH-UAB experience, and the

Table 51-4 Relationship of age at cardiac transplantation to premature death (UAB; July 1981–October 1984; *n* = 38). The median age at transplantation is 36.5 years (range 12.0–57.5 years.)

Age at Transplantation (yr)				Deaths		
≤	<	n	No.	%	CL
	10				
10	20	9	3	33%	15%–56%
20	30	7	3	43%	20%–68%
30	40	8	4	50%	27%–73%
40	50	11	3	27%	12%–47%
50	60	3	0	6%	0%–47%
Total		38	13	34%	26%–44%
P(hazard domain)				.6	

KEY: CL, 70% confidence limits.

Table 51-5 Noninfective nonfatal complications of cardiac transplantation (UAB; July 1982–August 1984). The categories are not mutually exclusive.

Complication	No. of Patients
Hypertension with cyclosporine	9
Renal failure requiring dialysis or hemofiltration (early postoperatively)	4
Insulin-dependent diabetes	3
Acute myocardial infarction	2
Vertebral crush fracture	2
Pneumothorax following endocardial biopsy	2
Poor cardiac graft function or fibrosis requiring retransplantation	2
Avascular necrosis of femoral head requiring hip replacement	1
Ulnar neuropathy	1

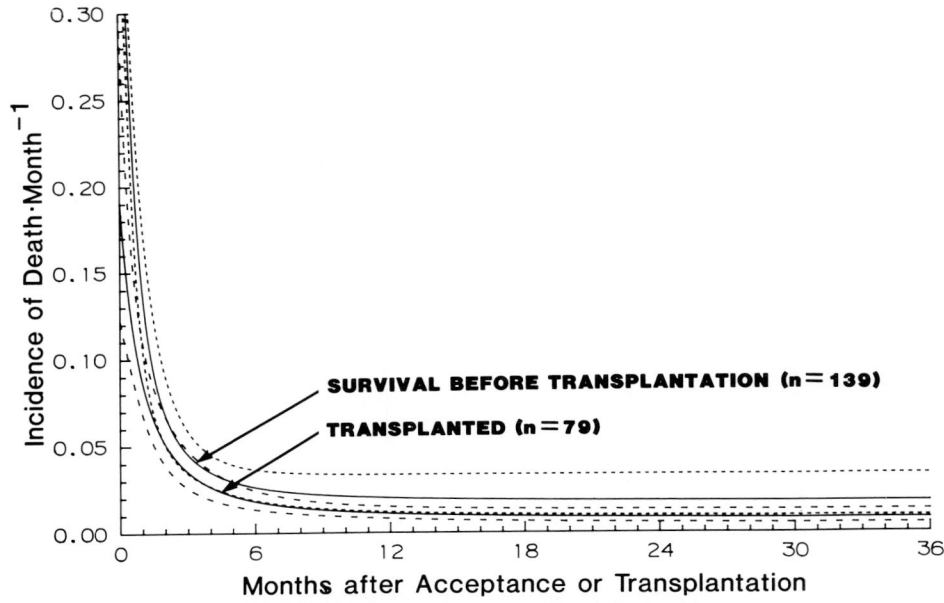

Figure 51-7   Hazard function for death (instantaneous risk per month) of the two groups represented in Figure 51-4. The dashed and dotted lines surround the 70% confidence limits. The groups are described in the legend of Figure 51-4.

The data were supplied by Mr. Terence English, Papworth Hospital, Cambridge, England; analysis was by Blackstone and Naftel (UAB); the material is presented with the permission of Mr. English.

result has been good (GLH). In general, the risk of operation has been 10%–20%, and higher in patients with biventricular disease. Thus, Metras and colleagues have reported 4 hospital deaths (20%, CL 10%–33%) among 20 patients operated on in the current era in the Ivory Coast.[M5]

The functional results of operation have been good.[D5,H2,M4,M6,V2] In most patients, the hemodynamic state of the left ventricle returns to normal after surgical treat-

ment of the left-sided form of the disease. However, in right ventricular endomyocardial fibrosis, despite clinical improvement, the hemodynamic status of the right ventricle usually remains abnormal.[M5] Right ventricular endocardiectomy may be complicated by complete heart block, but Metras and colleagues have avoided this in most cases by being conservative with the endocardial resection beneath the tricuspid valve.[M23]

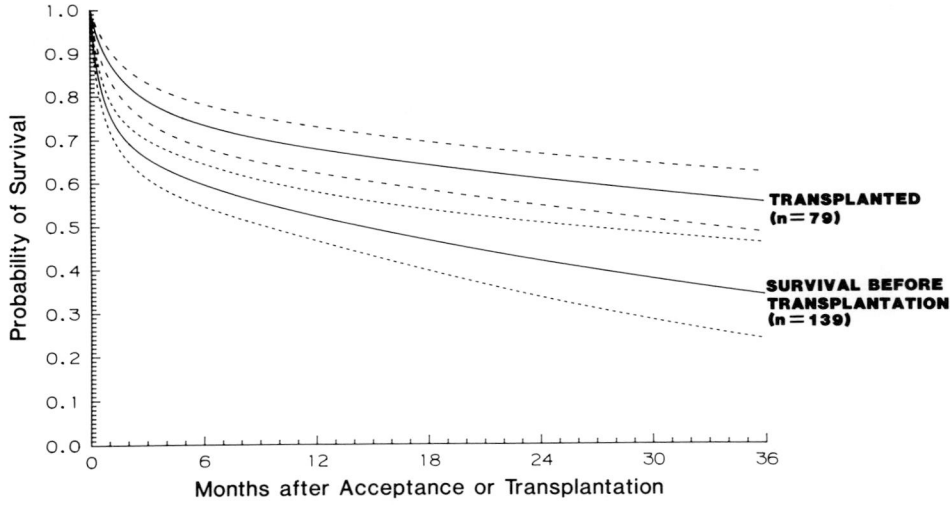

Figure 51-8   Parametric estimate of survival using the data displayed in Figure 51-4. The groups are described in the legend of Figure 51-4.

The data were supplied by Mr. Terence English, Papworth Hospital, Cambridge, England; analysis was by Blackstone and Naftel (UAB); the material is presented with the permission of Mr. English.

INDICATIONS FOR OPERATION

For most cardiomyopathies, cardiac replacement is the only effective surgical procedure. Cardiac replacement by homotransplantation is considered indicated in patients with cardiac disease (usually a severe cardiomyopathy which results from chronic volume or pressure overload, chronic hypoxia, or ischemia, or is idiopathic) in whom no other procedure or treatment can provide improved survival and functional status and in whom it is inferred that death will occur within 6 months, particularly if it is inferred that death will occur within 1–2 months (UAB). Consideration is also given to the possible contraindications presented by the patient (see ''Selection of the Recipient'' in section on Technique of Operation: Cardiac Transplantation).

A limitation to the use of cardiac transplantation is the limited supply of donor hearts. Investigations of the possible use of heterografts have begun,[B17] but a great deal of additional information is required to make this clinically successful. Insufficient information is available to assess the current usefulness of the artificial heart as a cardiac replacement device.

An exception to the need for cardiac replacement is endomyocardial fibrosis. With that condition, a corrective operation is indicated in patients whose disability has progressed and placed them in NYHA class III or IV.

SPECIAL SITUATIONS AND CONTROVERSIES

Cardiac Rejection

As in transplantation of any vascularized organ graft, the cardiac allograft is subject to rejection by the host immune system. The immune response consists of a humoral (antibody-mediated) response and a cellular response. The lymphocytes of the cellular response are categorized as T-lymphocytes and B-lymphocytes. The T-lymphocytes consist of cells with important effector functions, including cytotoxic T-cells, which lyse graft target cells; helper T-cells, which enhance both the humoral and cellular response; and suppressor T-cells, which can dampen the humoral and cellular response. Lymphocytes that are neither T-lymphocytes nor B-lymphocytes—are known as K, or killer cells. K cells depend on antibody for activity.

Hyperacute rejection is a humorally mediated phenomenon occurring within hours of transplantation resulting in death of the graft due to intense endothelial cell damage. No instance of this has been encountered (UAB). *Acute rejection*, usually occurring 7–90 days after transplantation, is mediated by the cellular immune response. It is characterized by cellular infiltration of the myocardium, particularly around blood vessels. If untreated, this process results in graft destruction. Rarely, an acute rejection can occur very early following transplantation (2–3 days), in which case it is called *accelerated acute rejection* but is still a predominantly cellular rejection. *Chronic rejection*, usually appearing more than 12 months after transplantation, is an antibody-mediated form of rejection manifested in cardiac transplantation as coronary atherosclerosis, presumably reflecting endothelial cell damage.

Currently, the only reliable method of detecting acute car-

Table 51-6 Histologic classification of severity of rejection (UAB).

Severity	Criteria
Mild	Few perivascular small lymphocytes
Moderate	More intense cellular infiltrate extending into interstitium
Severe	Heavy cellular infiltrate, focal or diffuse myonecrosis, vasculitis with hemorrhage

diac rejection is by use of percutaneous endomyocardial biopsy, introduced in 1973 by Caves and colleagues. The histologic appearance of the biopsied myocardium has been classified by Billingham,[B10] and a modification of this is employed (UAB; Table 51-6). However, the criteria were developed in an era of azathioprine treatment, and with cyclosporine, the amount of interstitial and myocardial edema is markedly reduced.[H4] Currently, in patients receiving cyclosporine, only the finding of myonecrosis on the biopsy is an indication for treatment. The inferences from endomyocardial biopsy from the right ventricle are limited by the probability that there is an irregular rather than uniform distribution of the morphologic features of rejection, and that these features may be more prominent in the right than in the left ventricle.[H8]

The summed electrocardiographic voltages are useful for the monitoring of rejection in patients treated with azathioprine, but this has not proved useful with cyclosporine therapy. Other subtle clinical signs of cardiac rejection are occasionally present, including the appearance of a third heart sound, diminution of peripheral pulses, and sudden normalization of blood pressure in a patient previously hypertensive on cyclosporine,[G8] and diffuse myalgias. The definitive diagnosis, however, currently relies on endocardial biopsy, although noninvasive studies may ultimately be useful. For example, Dawkins and colleagues have found echocardiographic evidences of changed ventricular diastolic function to correlate well with biopsy evidence of rejection.[D12]

Cyclosporine A

Cyclosporine A (usually termed simply *cyclosporine*) is a fungal metabolite that was first isolated from the fungus *Tolypocladium inflatum gams* in 1972.[B7,B9] The marked immunosuppressive properties of cyclosporine were discovered by Borel in 1972.[B7]

Cyclosporine has a specific and reversible effect on immunocompetent T cell lymphocytes by inhibiting the induction of cytotoxic effector and helper T cells without direct lymphocytotoxicity.[H3] A current hypothesis is that cyclosporine acts to inhibit the production and release of the lymphokines interleukin 1, from the activated macrophage, and interleukin 2 (T cell growth factor), from the activated T helper cells, thus preventing the formation of cytotoxic T-lymphocytes without affecting suppressor T-lymphocytes.[B8]

Animal studies suggest that cyclosporine may be most effective when given before the antigenic challenge, a situation perhaps related to the lower serum lymphokine concentration before the onset of rejection.

Cyclosporine is generally administered orally and is made more palatable by mixing the prescribed amount (drawn from the container using a pipette) with chocolate milk

(UAB). The absorption is somewhat variable, but peak blood levels are achieved at about 3.5 hours. The bioavailability of the oral solution at steady state is about 30%. Approximately 90% of circulating cyclosporine is protein bound, and the half-life is about 20 hours. Cyclosporine is eliminated primarily by the liver, with only about 6% of the dose eliminated by the kidneys.

Whole blood levels are monitored by radioimmunoassay[D6] and therapeutic trough levels range from 250–1,000 ng · ml^{-1}.[G10,O2]

The potential advantage of using cyclosporine in cardiac transplantation is related to its particularly specific immunosuppressive effects, compared to the global immunosuppressive actions of azathioprine.[N3] In addition, with cyclosporine, graft rejection can be prevented by lower doses of chronic steroid therapy. Although secure information is not yet available, current clinical experience with renal and heart transplantation[G7] suggests that the use of cyclosporine may be associated with less severe rejection episodes and less serious infections than is azathioprine. However, cyclosporine does appear to produce perimyocytic fibrosis in some transplanted hearts, the late functional significance of which is unknown, but there is a suggestion that left ventricular diastolic function may be impaired.[H7] This change does not occur in nontransplanted hearts.[K3]

The major toxicity of cyclosporine is renal toxicity, which in the acute phase is characterized by oliguria, a disproportionate elevation of blood urea level over creatinine level, and low urine sodium levels. The precise mechanism of the renal toxicity is unknown, but animal studies suggest that intense stimulation of the renin-angiotensin-aldosterone system occurs and is associated with arteriolar medial necrosis and tubular changes[S6] in the face of relatively well-preserved glomeruli.[D7] Even less is known about the effects of chronic cyclosporine therapy, but preliminary data from Stanford suggest that chronic elevation of serum creatinine levels is common, with renal biopsies in several patients showing extensive interstitial fibrosis, tubular atrophy, and focal glomerular sclerosis.[M15]

Less severe adverse side effects include reversible hepatotoxicity, fluid retention, hirsutism, gum hypertrophy, hypertension, tremor, and, rarely, late development of lymphoma (although this may be a result of overimmunosuppression with multiple agents).

Heterotopic Cardiac Transplantation

In 1975, Barnard and Losman introduced the technique of using the transplanted heart primarily as an assisting device, particularly for the left ventricle.[B5] Barnard and colleagues have continued to use this method and recently have reported good results in 46 patients.[N1] The method has advantages and deserves consideration in certain patients.

Heart-Lung Transplantation

Although heart-lung transplantation has not yet been undertaken clinically (UAB and GLH), it is considered an appropriate surgical approach in highly selected patients.

Historical Note

The first successful experimental heart and lung transplant was reported by Demikhov in the 1940s,[D8] but further attempts[G9] resulted in very limited survival, largely because of the problem of inadequate respiration following total pulmonary denervation in nonprimates.[N2] Castaneda and colleagues were the first to demonstrate the ability of primates to survive pulmonary denervation by using the technique of complete heart-lung autotransplantation.[C9] Reitz and colleagues, at Stanford, achieved long-term survival in primates following heart-lung transplantation with cyclosporine immunosuppression.[R2]

Early attempts at clinical heart-lung transplantation in three patients resulted in survival from hours to days.[B11,C8,L5] However, the results of single-lung transplantation were also poor,[V3] largely because of infection and impaired bronchial anastomotic healing. Later, a series of successful heart-lung transplants were performed at Stanford.[R3]

Technique of Operation

Potential recipients of heart-lung transplants are patients with primary cardiac disease with either secondary elevation of pulmonary arterial resistance or with developmental abnormalities of the pulmonary arteries. Possibly, patients with primary lung disease are potential recipients, the general criteria being the same as for cardiac transplantation.

One of the limiting factors in heart and lung transplantation is the availability of donors. Their lungs must remain free of tracheobronchial infection and meet the stringent requirements of normal peak inspiratory pressures and essentially normal gas exchange. A close match of thoracic dimensions is also required between both donor and recipient. Also, currently the donor is transported to the transplant center because of lack of satisfactory methods of lung presentation.[J2]

The donor and recipient procedures are performed in adjoining operating rooms and timed to keep the ischemic time of the transplanted heart-lung block to 1 hour or less. The donor heart-lung block is removed following standard cardioplegic infusion and administration of a cold crystalloid pulmonary artery flush. The recipient heart and lungs are removed through a median sternotomy on cardiopulmonary bypass with careful attention to preservation of both phrenic and vagus nerves. Separate removal of the heart and then the lungs probably minimizes mediastinal dissection, an important consideration in patients with extensive aortopulmonary collateral circulation. The donor heart-lung block is sutured in place with tracheal, right atrial, and aortic anastomoses.

Immunosuppression in these patients is similar to that for cardiac transplant recipients, except that (according to the Stanford protocol) after an initial four doses of methyl prednisolone in the immediate postoperative period, oral prednisone is not begun for 2 weeks, and azathioprine is temporarily used during this period, in addition to three doses of RATG. This regimen is adopted to promote healing of the tracheal anastomosis. Cyclosporine and prednisone are used for long-term maintenance immunosuppression.

Surveillance for rejection is by way of endomyocardial biopsy in the belief that rejection of the heart and lungs is concordant.[J3,R4] However, in the nonhuman primate, lethal pulmonary rejection has been demonstrated to occur in the absence of cardiac rejection.[S7] Rejection episodes are treated in a manner similar to that for rejection in cardiac transplant recipients.

A unique postoperative complication of heart-lung transplantation is a combination of impairment of gas exchange, pulmonary opacification as seen on the chest x-ray, and reduced lung compliance. This complication occurs in association with lung rejection, both in experimental and clinical single-lung and heart-lung transplants.[R2,R5,S8,V4] Such a reim-

plantation reponse is usually reversed within 3 weeks by vigorous diuresis and fluid restriction, but occasionally becomes severe and fatal. However, late death may occur from obliterative bronchiolitis.[D13]

In a series of 15 patients undergoing heart and lung transplantation at Stanford, 10 were alive between 3 and 30 months after operation.[B12] All surviving patients demonstrated normal gas exchange and normal spirometry. The long-term fate of the transplanted lung, however, remains unknown.

REFERENCES

A

1. Aitkin M, Laird N, Francis B: A re-analysis of the Stanford heart transplant data. *J Am Stat Assoc* 78:264, 1983.

B

1. Barnard CN: The operation. *S Afr Med J* 41:1271, 1967.
2. Baumgartner WA, Reitz BA, Oyer PE, Stinson EB, Shumway NE: Cardiac homotransplantation. *Curr Probl Surg* 16:1, 1979.
3. Billingham ME, Baumgartner WA, Watson DC, Reitz BA, Masek MA, Raney AA, Oyer PE, Stinson EB, Shumway NE: Distant heart procurement for human transplantation: Ultrastructural studies. *Circulation* 62(suppl 1):I-11, 1980.
4. Ball JD, Williams AW, Davies JNP: Endomyocardial fibrosis. *Lancet* 1:1049, 1954.
5. Barnard CN, Losman JG: Left Ventricular Bypass. *S Afr Med J* 49:303, 1975.
6. Bexton RS, Nathan AW, Hellestrand KJ, Cory-Pearce R, Spurrell RAJ, English TAH, Camm AJ: Sinoatrial function after cardiac transplantation. *JACC* 3:712, 1984.
7. Borel JF: The history of cyclosoprine A and its significance, in DJG White (ed): *Cyclosporine A: Proceedings of an International Conference on Cyclosporine A.* Amsterdam: Elsevier Biomedical, 1982, pp 5–17.
8. Bunjes D, Hardt C, Solbach W: Studies on the mechanism of action of cyclosporine A in the murine and human T-cell response in vitro, in DJG White (ed): *Cyclosporine A: Proceedings of an International Conference on Cyclosporine A.* Amsterdam: Elsevier Biomedical, 1982, pp 261–280.
9. Borel JF: Immunological properties of Cyclosporine A. *Heart Transplantation* 8:237, 1982.
10. Billingham ME: Diagnosis of autocardiac rejection. *Heart Transplantation* 1:25, 1982.
11. Barnard CN, Cooper DKC: Clinical transplantation of the heart: A review of 13 years' personal experience. *J R Soc Med* 74:670, 1981.
12. Baldwin JC, Jamieson JW, Stinson EB, Oyer PE, Shumway NE: Cardiopulmonary transplantation. *Cardiovascular Reviews and Reports* 5:148, 1984.
13. Blackstone EH, Naftel DC, English T: (1984) Personal communication.
14. Billingham RE, Brent L, Medawar PB: Actively acquired tolerance of foreign cells. *Nature* 172:603, 1953.
15. Brockington EF, Olsen EGJ: Loeffler's endocarditis and Davies' endocardial fibrosis. *Am Heart J* 85:308, 1973.

16. Borow KM, Neumann A, Arensman FW, Yacoub MH: Left ventricular contractility and contractile reserve in humans after cardiac transplantation. *Circulation* 71:866, 1985.
17. Bailey LL, Jang J, Johnson W, Jolley WB: Orthotopic cardiac xenografting in the newborn goat. *J Thorac Cardiovasc Surg* 89:242, 1985.

C

1. Cherian G, Vijayaraghavan G, Krishnaswami S, Sukumar IP, John W, Jairaj PS, Bhaktaviziam A: Endomyocardial fibrosis: Report on the hemodynamic data in 29 patients and review of the results of surgery. *Am Heart J* 105:659, 1983.
2. Cockshott WP, Saric S, Ikeme AC: Radiological findings in endomyocardial fibrosis. *Circulation* 35:913, 1967.
3. Connor DH, Somers K, Hutt MSR, Manion WC, D-Arbela PG: Endomyocardial fibrosis in Uganda: Part I. *Am Heart J* 74:687, 1967.
4. Carrel A, Guthrie CC: The transplantation of veins and organs. *Am J Med* 1:1101, 1905.
5. Cooper DKC, Lanza RP, Oliver S, Forder AA, Rose AG, Uys CJ, Novitzky D, Barnard DN: Infectious complications after heart transplantation. *Thorax* 38:822, 1983.
6. Clark DA, Stinson EB, Griepp RB, Schroeder JS, Shumway NE, Harrison DC: Cardiac transplantation in man. VI. Prognosis of patients selected for cardiac transplantation. *Ann Intern Med* 75:15, 1971.
7. Crowley J, Hu M: Covariance analysis of heart transplant survival data. *J Am Stat Assoc* 72:27, 1977.
8. Cooky PA, Bloodwell RD, Halloman GL, Hora JJ, Harrisen GM, Leachman RD: Organ transplantation for advanced cardiopulmonary disease. *Ann Thorac Surg* 8:30, 1969.
9. Castenada AR, Arnar O, Schmidt-Habelman P, Ollen JH, Zamora R: Cardiopulmonary autotransplantation in primates. *J Cardiovasc Surg* 37:523, 1972.
10. Carrel A: Transplantation in mass of the kidneys. *J Expl Med* 10:98, 1908.
11. Calne RY: Inhibition of the rejection of renal homografts in dogs by purine analogues. *Transplant Bull* 28:65, 1961.
12. Calne RY and Murray JE: Inhibition of the rejection of renal homografts in dogs by BW 57-322. *Surg Forum* 12:118, 1961.
13. Caves PK, Stinson EB, Billingham ME, Rider AK, Shumway NE: Diagnosis of human cardiac allograft rejection by serial cardiac biopsy. *J Thorac Cardiovasc Surg* 66:461, 1973.
14. Campeau L, Pospisil L, Grondin P, Dyrda I, Le Page G: Cardiac

catheterization findings at rest and after exercise in patients following cardiac transplantation. *Am J Cardiol* 25:523, 1970.

D

1. Davies JNP, Coles RM: Some considerations regarding obscure disease affecting the mural endocardium. *Am Heart J* 59:606, 1960.

2. Davies JNP, Ball JD: Pathology of endomyocardial fibrosis in Uganda. *Br Heart J* 17:337, 1955.

3. D'Arbela PG, Mutazindwa T, Patel AK, Somers K: Survival after first presentation with endomyocardial fibrosis. *Br Heart J* 34:403, 1972.

4. Dubost C, Maurice P, Gerbaux A, Bertrand E, Rulliere R, Vial F, Barrillon A, Prigent C, Carpentier A, Soyer R: The surgical treatment of constrictive fibrous echocarditis. *Ann Surg* 184:303, 1976.

5. Dubost C: Surgery for constrictive fibrous endocarditis. *Compr Ther* 5:28, 1979.

6. Donatsch P, Abisch E, Homerger M, Traber R, Trapp M, Voges R: A radioimmunoassay to measure cyclosporine A in plasma and serum samples. *J Immunoassay* 2:19, 1982.

7. Devineni R, McKenzie N, Duplan J, Keown P, Stiller C, Wallace AC: Renal effects of cyclosporine: Clinical and experimental observations, in BD Kuham (ed): *Cyclosporine, Biological Activity and Clinical Applications.* Orlando, FL: Grune & Stratton, 1984, p 503.

8. Denikhov VP: Some essential points of the techniques of transplantation of the heart, lungs and other organs. in B Haigh (trans): *Experimental Transplantation of Vital Organs.* Moscow: Medgiz State Press for Medical Literatures in Moscow, 1960, pp 29–48. New York: *Consultants Bureau*, 1962.

9. Dederrer C: Studies in the transplantation of whole organs. *J Amer Med Assoc* 70:6, 1918.

10. Dederrer C: Homotransplantation of the kidney and ovary. *Surg Gynec and Obstet* 31:47, 1920.

11. Diethelm AG: (1984) Personal communication.

12. Dawkins KD, Oldershaw, Billingham ME, Hunt SA, Oyer PE, Jamieson SW, Popp RL, Stinson EB, Shumway NE: Changes in disastolic function as a noninvasive marker of cardiac allograft rejection. *Heart Transplantation* III:286, 1984.

13. Dawkins KD, Jamieson SW, Hunt SA, Baldwin JC, Burke CM, Morris A, Billingham ME, Theodore J, Oyer PE, Stinson EB, Shumway NE: Long-term results, hemodynamics, and complications after combined heart and lung transplantation. *Circulation* 71:919, 1985.

F

1. Franciosa JA, Wilen M, Ziesche S, Cohn JN: Survival in men with severe chronic left ventricular failure due to either coronary heart disease or idiopathic dilated cardiomyopathy. *Am J Cardiol* 51:831, 1983.

2. Fuster V, Gersh BJ, Giuliani ER, Tajik AJ, Brandenburg RO, Frye RL: The natural history of idiopathic dilated cardiomyopathy. *Am J Cardiol* 47:525, 1981.

3. Frazier OH, Cooley DA, Painvin GA, Chandler LB, Okereke OUJ: Cardiac transplantation at the Texas Heart Institute: Comparative analysis of two groups of patients (1968–1969 and 1982–1983). *Ann Thorac Surg* 39:303, 1985.

G

1. Goodwin JF: Congestive and hypertrophic cardiomyopathies: A decade of study. *Lancet* 1:731, 1970.

2. Grossman W, McLaurin LP, Rolett EL: Alterations in left ventricular relaxation and diastolic compliance in congestive cardiomyopathy. *Cardiovasc Res* 13:514, 1979.

3. Griepp RB: A decade of human heart transplantation. *Transplant Proc* 11:285, 1979.

4. Griepp RB, Stinson EB, Clark DA, Dong E Jr, Shumway NE: The cardiac donor. *Surg Gynecol Obstet* 133:792, 1971.

5. Gaudiani VA, Stinson EB, Alderman E, Hunt SA, Schroeder JS, Perlroth MG, Bieber CP, Oyer PE, Reitz BA, Jamieson SW, Christopherson L, Shumway NE: Long-term survival and function after cardiac transplantation. *Ann Surg* 194:381, 1981.

6. Goldberg SJ, Valdes-Crux LM, Sahn DJ, Allen HD: Two-dimensional echocardiographic evaluation of dilated cardiomyopathy in children. *Am J Cardiol* 52:1244, 1983.

7. Griffith BP, Hardesty RL, Bahnson HT: Powerful but limited immunosuppression for cardiac transplantation with cyclosporine and low-dose steroid. *J Thorac Cardiovasc Surg* 87:35, 1984.

8. Griffith BP, Hardesty RL, Thompson ME, Dummer JS, Bahnson HT: Cardiac transplantation with cyclosporine: The Pittsburgh experience. *Heart Transplantation* 2:251, 1983.

9. Grinnan GB, Graham WH, Childs JW, Cowen RR: Cardiopulmonary transplantation. *J Thorac Cardiovasc Surg* 60:609, 1970.

10. Griffith BP, Hardesty RL, Trento A, Lee A, Bahnson HT: Targeted blood levels of cyclosporine for cardiac transplantation. *J Thorac Cardiovasc Surg* 88:952, 1984.

11. Greenburg ML, Uretsky BF, Reddy S, Bernstein RL, Griffith BP, Hardesty RL, Thompson ME, Bahnson HT: Long-term hemodynamic follow-up of cardiac transplant patients treated with cyclosporine and prednisone. *Circulation* 71:487, 1985.

H

1. Harvard Medical School: A definition of irreversible coma: Report of the Ad Hoc Committee of the Harvard Medical School to examine the definition of brain death. *JAMA* 205:337, 1968.

2. Hess OM, Turina M, Senning A, Goebel NH, Scholer Y, Krayenbuehl HP: Pre- and postoperative findings in patients with endomyocardial fibrosis. *Br Heart J* 40:406, 1978.

3. Hess Ad, Tutschka PJ: Effect of cyclosoprine A on human lymphocyte responses in vitro. *J Immunol* 124:2601, 1980.

4. Hunt SA: Complications of heart transplantation. *Heart Transplantation* 3:70, 1983.

5. Hume DM, Merrill JP, Miller BF, Thoran GW: Experiences with renal homotransplantation in the human: Report of nine cases. *J Clin Invest* XXXIV:327, 1955.

6. Holmes J, Kubo SH, Cody RJ, Klingfield P: Arrhythmias in ischemic and nonischemic dilated cardiomyopathy: Prediction of mortality by ambulatory electrocardiography. *Am J Cardiol* 55:146, 1985.

7. Humen DP, McKenzie FN, Kostuk WJ: Restricted myocardial compliance one year following cardiac transplantation. *Heart Transplantation* III:341, 1984.

8. Haverich A, Scott WC, Dawkins KD, Billingham ME, Jamieson SW: Asymmetric pattern of rejection following orthotopic cardiac transplantation in primates. *Heart Transplantation* III:280, 1984.

J

1. Jamieson SW, Oyer P, Baldwin J, Billingham M, Stinson E, Shumway N: Heart transplantation for end-stage ischemic heart

disease: The Stanford experience. *Heart Transplantation* III:224, 1984.

2. Jamieson SW, Stinson EB, Oyer PE, Baldwin JC, Shumway NE: Operative technique for heart-lung transplantation. *J Thorac Cardiovasc Surg* 87:930-935, 1984.

3. Jamieson SW, Stinson EB, Oyer PE, Reitz BA, Baldwin J, Modry D, Dawkins K, Theodore J, Hunt S, Shumway NE: Heart-lung transplantation for irreversible pulmonary hypertension. *Ann Thorac Surg* 38:554, 1984.

K

1. Kondo Y, Grodel F, Kantrowitz A: Heart transplantation in puppies: Long survival without immunosuppressive therapy. *Circulation* 31,32(suppl 1):181, 1965.

2. Kirklin JK: (1984) Personal communication.

3. Karch SB, Billingham ME: Cyclosporine induced myocardial fibrosis: A unique controlled case report. *Heart Transplantation* IV:210, 1985.

L

1. Lower RR, Shumway NE: Studies on orthotopic transplantation of the canine heart. *Surgical Forum* 11:18, 1960.

2. Lepley D, Aris A, Korns ME, Walker JA, D'Cunha RM: Endomyocardial fibrosis. *Ann Thorac Surg* 18:626, 1974.

3. Loeffler W: Endocarditis parietalis fibroplastica mit blunt Eosinophilia. *Schweiz Med Wochenschr* 66:817, 1936.

4. Leachman RD, Cokkinos DVP, Zamalloa O, Alvarez A: Electrocardiographic behavior of recipient and donor atria after human heart transplantation. *Am J Cardiol* 24:49, 1969.

5. Lillehei CW: discussion in CRH Wildevuun, JR Benfield: A series of 23 human lung transplantations by 20 surgeons. *Ann Thorac Surg* 9:515, 1970.

6. Lance EM, Medawar PB: quantitative studies on tissue transplantation immunity. IX. Induction of tolerance with antilymphocyte serum. *Proc R Soc Lond(Biol)* 173:447, 1969.

M

1. Meaney E, Shabetai R, Bhargana V, Shearer M, Weidner C, Mangiardi LM, Smalling R, Peterson K: Cardiac amyloidosis, constrictive pericarditis and restrictive cardiomyopathy. *Am J Cardiol* 38:547, 1976.

2. McGiffin DC, Kirklin JK, Naftel DC, Blackstone EH: (1984) Personal communication.

3. McGiffin DC, Karp RB, Whelchel JD, Diethelm AG: Cardiac transplantation: A review of the experience of the University of Alabama in Birmingham. *Ala J Med Sci* 20:425, 1983.

4. Moraes CR, Buffalo E, Victor E, Saravia L, Gomes JMP, Lira V, Lima R, Escobar M, Andrade JC: Endomyocardial fibrosis: Report of 6 patients and review of the surgical literature. *Ann Thorac Surg* 29:243, 1980.

5. Metras D, Coulibaly AO, Ouattara K, Chauvet J, Ekra A, Longechaud A, Bertrand E: Endomyocardial fibrosis. *J Thorac Cardiovasc Surg* 83:52, 1982.

6. Moraes CR, Buffalo E, Lima R, Victor E, Lira V, Escobar M, Rodrigues J, Saraiva L, Andrade JC: Surgical treatment of endomyocardial fibrosis. *J Thorac Cardiovasc Surg* 85:738, 1983.

7. Mann FC, Priestly JR, Markowitz J, Yates WM: Transplantation of the intact mammalian heart. *Arch Surg* 26:219, 1933.

8. Medawar PB: The behaviour and fate of skin autografts and skin homografts in rabbits. *J Anat* 78:176, 1944.

9. Medawar PB: Immunologic tolerance. *Nature* 189:14, 1961.

10. McGiffin DC, karp RB, Logic JR, Tauxe WN, Ceballos R: Results of radionuclide assessment of cardiac function following transplantation of the heart. *Ann Thorac Surg* 37:382, 1984.

11. Meinertz T, Hofmann T, Kasper W, Treese N, Bechtold H, Stienen U, Pop T, Leitner EV, Andresen D, Meyer J: Significance of ventricular arrhythmias in idiopathic dilated cardiomyopathy. *Am J Cardiol* 53:902, 1984.

12. Mason JW, Stinson EB, Hunt SA, Schroeder JS, Rider AK: Infections after cardiac transplantation: Relation to rejection therapy. *Ann Intern Med* 85:69, 1976.

13. McGiffin DC, Karp RB: Cardiac transplantation in a patient with a persistent left superior vena cava and an absent right superior vena cava. *Heart Transplantation* III:115, 1984.

14. Medawar PB: A second study of the behavior and fate of skin homografts in rabbits. *J Anat* 79:157, 1944.

15. Moran M, Newton L, Perlroth M, Myers B: Cyclosporine nephrotoxicity in man. *Proceedings of the American Society of Nephrology* 16:209A, 1983.

16. McGiffin DC, Kirklin JK: (1984) Personal communication.

17. Murray JE, Merrill JP, Dammin GJ, Dealy JB Jr, Alexandre GW, Harrison JH: Kidney transplantation in modified recipients. *Ann Surg* 156:337, 1962.

18. Merrill JP, Murray JE, Harrison JH: Successful homotransplantation of the human kidney between identical twins. *JAMA* 160:227, 1956.

19. Merrill JP, Murray JE, Harrison JH, Friedman EA, Dealy JB Jr, Dammin GJ: Successful homotransplantation of the kidney between nonidentical twins. *New Engl J Med* 262:1251, 1960.

20. Murray JE, Merrill JP, Harrison JH: Renal homotransplantation in identical twins. *Surg Forum* 6:432, 1955.

21. Monaco AP, Clark AW, Wood ML, Sahyoun AI, Codish SD, Brown RW: Possible active enhancement of a human cadaver renal allograft with antilymphocyte serum (ALS) and donor bone marrow: Case report of an initial attempt. *Surgery* 79:384, 1976.

22. Metras D, Quezzin-Coulibaly A, Quattara K, Bertrand E, Chauvet J: Endomyocardial fibrosis masquerading as rheumatic mitral incompetence. *J Thorac Cardiovasc Surg* 86:753, 1983.

23. Metras D, Coulibaly A, Ouattara K: The surgical treatment of endomyocardial fibrosis: results in 55 patients. *Circulation* 70(suppl II):II-329, 1984 (Abstr).

N

1. Novitzky D, Cooper DKC, Barnard CN: The surgical technique of heterotopic heart transplantation. *Ann Thorac Surg* 36:476, 1983.

2. Nakal S, Webb WR, Theolourides T, Sugg WL: Respiratory function following cardiopulmonary denervation in dog, cat and monkey. *Surg Gynecol Obstet* 125:1285, 1967.

3. Nelson PW: Cyclosporine. *Surg Gynecol Obstet* 159:297, 1984.

O

1. Olsen EGJ: Endomyocardial biopsy. *Br Heart J* 40:95, 1978.

2. Oyer PE, Stinson EB, Jamieson SW, Hunt S, Reitz BA, Bieber CP, Schroeder JS, Billingham M, Shumway NE: One year experience with cyclosporine A in clinical heart transplantation. *Heart Transplantation* 1:285, 1982.

3. Owen R: Immunogenetic consequences of vascular anastomoses between Bovine twins. *Science* 102:400, 1945.

P

1. Pennock JL, Oyer PE, Reitz BA, Jamieson SW, Bieber CP, Wallwork J, Stinson EB, Shumway NE: Cardiac transplantation in prospective for the future: Survival, complications, rehabilitation, and cost. *J Thorac Cardiovasc Surg* 83:168, 1982.
2. Pollard RB, Arvin AM, Gamberg P, Rand KH, Gallagher JG, Merigan TC: Specific cell-mediated immunity and infections with herpes viruses in cardiac transplant recipients. *Am J Med* 73:679, 1982.

R

1. Remington JS, Gaines JD, Griepp RB, Shumway NE: Further experience with infection after cardiac transplantation. *Transplant Proc* 4:699, 1972.
2. Reitz Ba, Burton NA, Jamieson SW, Bielson CP, Pennock JL, Stinson EB, Shumway NE: Heart and lung transplantation: Autotransplantation and allotransplantation in primates with extended survival. *J Thorac Cardiovasc Surg* 80:360, 1980.
3. Reitz BA, Wallwork JL, Hunt SA, Pennock JL, Billingham ME, Dyer PE, Stinson EB, Shumway NE: Heart-lung transplantation: Successful therapy for patients with pulmonary vascular disease. *N Engl J Med* 306:557, 1982.
4. Reitz BA, Gandiani VA, Hunt SA, Wallwork J, Billingham ME, Dyer PE, Baumgartner WA, Jamieson SW, Stinson EB, Shumway NE: Diagnosis and treatment of allograft rejection in heart-lung transplant recipients. *J Thorac Cardiovasc Surg* 85:354, 1983.
5. Reitz BA: Heart-lung transplantation: A review. *Heart Transplantation* 1:291, 1982.
6. Reitz BA, Jamieson SW, Gaudiani VA, Oyer PE, Stinson EB: Methol for cardiac transplantation in corrected transposition of the great arteries. *J Thorac Cardiovasc Surg* 23:293, 1982.

S

1. Schwarz F, Mall G, Zebe H, Blickle J, Derks H, Manthey J, Kubler W: Quantitative morphologic findings of the myocardium in idiopathic dilated cardiomyopathy. *Am J Cardiol* 51:501, 1983.
2. Shaper AG, Hutt MSR, Edington GM, Somers K, Fowler JM: Endomyocardial fibrosis. *Cardiologia* 52:20, 1968.
3. Stinson EB, Griepp RB, Payne R, Dong E Jr, Shumway NE: Correlation of histocompatibility matching with graft rejection and survival after cardiac transplantation in man. *Lancet* 11:459, 1971.
4. Samuel I, Anklesaria XJ: Endomyocardial fibrosis in South India. *Indian J Pathol Bacteriol* 3:157, 1960.
5. Stinson EB, Schroeder JS, Griepp RB, Shumway NE, Dong E: Observations on the behavior of recipient atria after cardiac transplantation in man. *Am J Cardiol* 30:615, 1972.
6. Siegl H, Ryffel B, Petric R, Shoemaker P, Muller A, Donatsch P, Mihatseh M: Cyclosoprine: The renin-angiotension-aldosterone system, and renal adverse reactions, in BD Kuhan (ed): *Cyclosporine: Biological Activity and Clinical Applications.* Orlando, FL: Grune & Stratton, 1984, p 503.
7. Scott WC, Hamerich A, Billingham ME, Dawkins KD, Jamieson SW: Lethal lung rejection without significant cardiac rejection in primate heart-lung allotransplants. *Heart Transplantation* IV:33, 1984 (abstr).
8. Siegelman SS, Siuha SBP, Veith FJ: Pulmonary reimplantation response. *Ann Surg* 177:30, 1971.

9. Stinson EB, Caves PK, Kriepp RB, Oyer PE, Rider AK, Shumway NE: Hemodynamic observations in the early period after human heart transplantation. *J Thorac Cardiovasc Surg* 69:264, 1975.
10. Schroeder JS: Hemodynamic performance of the human transplanted heart. *Transplant Proc* II:304, 1979.

T

1. Thomas FT, Szentpetery SS, Mammana RE, Wolfgang TC, Lower RR: Long-distance transportation of human hearts for transplantation. *Ann Thorac Surg* 26:346, 1978.
2. Turnbull BW, Brown BW, Hu M: Survivorship analysis of heart transplant data. *J Am Stat Assoc* 69:74, 1974.

U

1. Unverferth DV, Magorien RD, Moeschberger ML, Baker PB, Fetters JK, Leier CV: Factors influencing the one-year mortality of dilated cardiomyopathy. *Am J Cardiol* 54:147, 1984.

V

1. Vijayaraghavan G, Cherian G, Krishnaswami S, Sukumar IP: Left ventricular endomyocardial fibrosis in India. *Br Heart J* 39:563, 1977.
2. Valiathan MS, Sankarkumar R, Balakrishnan KG, Mohansingh MP: Surgical palliation for endomyocardial fibrosis: Early results. *Thorax* 38:421, 1983.
3. Veith FJ: Lung transplantation. *Surg Clin North Am* 58:357, 1978.
4. Veith FJ, Koerner SK, Siegelman SS, Torres M. Bardfeld PA, Attai LA, Boley JT, Takaro T, Gliedman M: Single lung transplantation in experimental and human emphysema. *Ann Surg* 178:463, 1973.

W

1. Watson DC Jr: Consistent survival after prolonged donor heart preservation. *Transplant Proc* 9:297, 1977.
2. Watson DC, Reitz BA, Baumgartner WA, Raney AA, Oyer PE, Stinson EB, Shumway NE: Distant heart procurement for transplantation. *Surgery* 86:56, 1979.
3. Whitley R, Barton N, Collins E, Whelchel J, Diethelm AG: Mucocutaneous herpes simplex virus infections in immunocompromised patients. *Am J Med* July:236, 1982.
4. Watts D, Freeman AM III, McGiffin DC, Kirklin JK, McVay R, Karp RB: Psychiatric aspects of cardiac transplantation. *Heart Transplantation* III:243, 1984.
5. Watson DC, Reitz BA, Oyer PE, Stinson EB, Shumway NE: Sequential orthotopic heart transplantation in man. *Transplantation* 30:401, 1980.
6. Williamson CS: Some observations of the length of survival and function of homogeneous kidney transplants. *J Urol* 10:275, 1923.
7. Williamson CS: Further studies of the transplantation of the kidney. *J Ucol* 16:231, 1926.
8. Wu PPT, Mann FC: Histologic studies of autogeneous and homogeneous transplants of the kidney. *Arch Surg* 28:889, 1934.

Y

1. Yacoub M: (1984) Personal communication.

52

PERICARDIAL DISEASE

SECTION 1
CHRONIC CONSTRICTIVE PERICARDITIS

DEFINITION

Chronic constrictive pericarditis is a chronic inflammatory process that involves both fibrous and serous layers of the pericardium and that leads to pericardial thickening and constriction of the ventricles. The resultant impairment in diastolic filling reduces cardiac function.

HISTORICAL NOTE

It is said that Galen in A.D. 160 described cicatricial thickening of the pericardium in an animal and surmised that the same condition might occur in humans. The first formal account of the condition in humans was apparently that of Lower, who described both acute and chronic constrictive pericarditis in 1669.[L1] Other early descriptions of the condition were those by Bonetus in 1679[B1] and Vieussens in 1715.[V1] Lancisi apparently understood the pathology of the condition, since in 1728 he described at autopsy a patient with a small heart encased by a thick adherent pericardium in association with marked swelling of the abdomen and jugular veins.[L2]

As a result of the observations of Morgagni in 1760[M1] and Lannec in 1819[L3] that pericardial adhesions were rarely associated with symptoms, little attention was paid to the possible clinical significance of chronic pericarditis for nearly 100 years because of ignorance of the difference between adhesive pericarditis and constrictive pericarditis. The literature contains only four largely ignored reports (Cheevers, 1842[C1]; Greisunger, 1856[G1]; Wilks, 1870[W1]; Kussmaul, 1873[K1]), all of which stressed that chronic constrictive pericarditis could be of clinical importance.

Interest was refocused on the condition by Pick's report in 1896 of three patients with chronic constrictive pericarditis whose clinical course had been thought in life to be due to cirrhosis of the liver.[P1] At about that time, surgeons were becoming more expert and aggressive, and Weill in 1895[W2] and Delorme in 1889[D1] suggested that pericardectomy be used as treatment for this condition. It is said that Brauer in 1902 suggested the removal of the bony precordium as a method of relief. Apparently the first operation directed against chronic constrictive pericarditis was carried out by Hallopeau.[H1] Both Rehn[R1] and Sauerbruck,[S1] in Germany, carried out a successful partial pericardectomy in 1913. Schmeiden and Fischer, in Germany, in 1926 reported a series of successful cases,[S2] as did Churchill in 1929, from Massachusetts General Hospital,[C4] and Beck in 1931, from Cleveland.[B2] The surgical experience was expanded by Harrington and Barnes, at the Mayo Clinic,[H2] and Heuer and Stewart, from New York Hospital.[H3] By 1941, Blalock and Burwell were able to report the surgical treatment of 28 patients.[B6]

An experimental approach began to clarify some of the perplexing problems that persisted in spite of the advent of surgical treatment. In 1929, Beck produced the syndrome of chronic constrictive pericarditis by injecting Dakin's solution into the pericardial cavity of dogs.[B3] He demonstrated that the obliteration of the pericardial cavity by adhesion did not produce the syndrome and that only a thick, dense scar around the heart would do so, thus solving the riddle of 100 years earlier.[B2] He then demonstrated in animals that the syndrome could be relieved by pericardectomy.[B4] He also demonstrated experimentally several efficient methods of controlling the hemorrhage that may develop from the heart during the dissection required in relieving chronic constrictive pericarditis.[B2] The pathogenesis was then further elucidated by the cardiac catheterization studies of Sawyer and colleagues[S4] and by the ingenious experiments of Isaacs and colleagues.[I1] These studies led directly to the development of better diagnostic and surgical methods.[B8]

MORPHOLOGY

The fibrous parietal pericardium and both layers of the visceral pericardium, the inner one of which (the epicardium) is intimately adherent to the myocardium, are all involved at least to some extent in patients with chronic constrictive pericarditis, but the details of the pathologic process vary. If the two layers of the visceral pericardium remain separate, the pericardial space contains variable amounts of fluid, often with extensive and sometimes hemorrhagic fibrinous deposits on both surfaces. This entire fibrous and fluid mass can be constricting to the heart. When the process has become far advanced, the two layers of the visceral pericardium thicken and fuse and, along with the fibrous pericardium, encase the heart in a thick, solid, fibrous, and often calcified envelope that is adherent to the myocardium.

In addition, cardiac muscle fiber atrophy occurs in many cases.[D2,R2] The atrophy may appear relatively early in the course of the disease.[D2] Myocardial fibrosis also complicates the late stages of chronic constrictive pericarditis.[L5]

CLINICAL FEATURES AND DIAGNOSTIC CRITERIA

Pathophysiology of Cardiac Compression

Cardiac compression occurs in chronic constrictive pericarditis but is also a feature of acute cardiac tamponade and effusive constrictive pericardial disease, a condition characterized by pericardial thickening and variable amounts of fluid in the pericardial space.

Normal
The pericardial pressure is subatmospheric and similar to intrapleural pressure. Both intrapericardial and intrapleural pressures become more negative during inspiration. There are very small fluctuations of intrapericardial pressure related to the cardiac cycle,[K4,S15] and the transpericardial pressure (pericardial minus pleural pressure) is highest at end diastole, the period of largest ventricular volume. Pericardial pressure does rise as ventricular volume is increased beyond normal limits by the rapid infusion of fluid. Under such circumstances, the effects of pericardial restraining are predominantly on the right ventricle.[T1]

The pressure-volume relationships and stress-strain characteristics of the normal pericardium are such that there is little rise in intrapericardial pressure when a small amount of fluid is placed intrapericardially. With the rapid addition of more fluid, the pressure slope rises progressively.[M6,R1] Finally, small further additions of fluid cause severe increases in intrapericardial pressure and, conversely, at this stage the removal of small amounts of intrapericardial fluid causes a relatively large decrease in intrapericardial pressure (the rationale of pericardiocentesis in acute pericardial tamponade). Further, because pericardial hysteresis exists,[M6] the intrapericardial pressure at a given volume during fluid removal is lower than during the addition of fluid.

Intrapericardial events, both normal and abnormal, have an effect on both cardiac filling and cardiac output. Such events are reflected in phasic and overall atrial and venous pressures. The effect on systemic venous pressure is of particular importance because it is easily observed in the jugular venous pressure. Normally, the inferior and superior vena caval pressures exceed atmospheric pressure by only a few millimeters of mercury. The jugular venous (and caval) pulse consists sequentially of three positive and upward waves and two downward movements. First is the *a* wave, generated by atrial systole. The *c* wave follows, caused by displacement of the tricuspid valvar apparatus toward the right atrium during isovolumic ventricular systole. A negative *x* descent is next, generated in part by the descent of the closed tricuspid valve apparatus at the beginning of ventricular ejection and in part by the decreased intrapericardial pressure resulting from the reduced ventricular volume as the ventricle ejects. A positive *v* wave is then generated by passive filling of the right atrium from the cavae and coronary sinus. Finally, a negative *y* descent occurs as blood rapidly flows from right atrium to right ventricle.

Acute Cardiac Tamponade

A rapid increase in intrapericardial fluid, usually blood, results in acute cardiac tamponade. In acute cardiac tamponade the intrapericardial pressure may rise as high as 20–30 mmHg. Such a pressure would be incompatible with life were it not for reflex venoconstriction, catecholamine release, and the immediate retention of sodium and water by the kidneys as part of the total bodily response to reduced cardiac output. As a result, the venous pressure rises to the level of intrapericardial pressure, and cardiac output is maintained, although usually at a reduced rate. This process has led to one definition of cardiac tamponade as a condition in which right atrial and systemic venous pressures are determined by the elevated intrapericardial pressure.[S11]

When the intrapericardial pressure rises, it exceeds left as well as right atrial pressure, and in patients who survive,[M8] both left and right atrial pressures rise in response to the neurohumeral compensatory mechanisms mentioned above. At this stage, right and left atrial pressures, right and left ventricular diastolic pressures, pulmonary artery diastolic pressure, and pulmonary artery wedge pressure are identical to intrapericardial pressure. Untreated, the patient dies when cardiac output continues to fall in spite of the compensatory mechanisms.

In this classic setting of acute cardiac tamponade, the heart is small and quiet, the venous pressure is elevated, and the systemic arterial blood pressure is depressed—a group of symptoms known as *Beck's triad*.[B10] The elevation of venous pressure may be mild, or it may reach 20 mmHg or more. The jugular venous pulse waves are altered, since the tamponade effect is least during ventricular ejection, when the ventricular volume is least. No cardiac filling occurs during diastole, and thus there is no *y* descent. All filling occurs during systole, and thus the *x* descent is preserved and exaggerated.

Unless hypotension is extreme, the condition is also characterized by *pulsus paradoxus,* an inspiratory decrease in arterial systolic blood pressure exceeding 10 mmHg during quiet respiration. The mechanism underlying pulsus paradoxus in acute cardiac tamponade is complex.[S11] During inspiration, caval flow into the right atrium increases, just as in the normal situation, and in fact, the percentage of increase is greater than normal. The resultant increase in right heart volume increases intrapericardial pressure still further, and pericardial transmural (intrapericardial versus intrapleural) pressure falls. Left ventricular volume is decreased as the ventricular septum is displaced leftward by the increased right ventricular volume.[S16] These phenomena result in a decreased left ventricular stroke volume and thus diminished arterial blood pressure. Another contributor to pulsus paradoxus is the delay in the passage of the increased caval flow of early inspiration to the left ventricle, so that by the time it has occurred respiration has generally shifted to the expiratory phase. Also, the inspiratory decrease in intrathoracic pressure tends to decrease aortic and arterial pressure; and inspiration tends directly to decrease left ventricular contraction.[M7]

Chronic Constrictive Pericarditis

The basic pathophysiology of chronic constrictive pericarditis has been debated for over half a century. By 1949, Holman and Willett had concluded that constriction of the caval orifices and atria was important in the pathogenesis of chronic constrictive pericarditis and adopted the median sternotomy approach for its surgical correction for this reason.[H4] In 1951, Burwell and colleagues had concluded, from cardiac catheterization study, that both right and left ventricular function was impaired and that constriction of caval orifices or atria played no role.[B9] In 1952, Isaacs and colleagues showed in dogs that a change in the volume-elasticity curves of the two ventricles resulted from experimentally produced constrictive pericarditis and that this was the fundamental pathophysiologic change associated with the disease (Fig. 52-1).[11] These investigators also demonstrated during the development of the constriction an increase in right and left ventricular diastolic pressure and a decrease in stroke volume. In their experimental animals, a small increase in volume resulted in a considerable increase in end-diastolic pressure. These studies indicated that lack of ventricular diastolic distensibility, and thus inability to generate an adequate preload (see Chapter 5, footnote 7), was a characteristic of hearts with chronic constrictive pericarditis. These considerations influenced Scannell and colleagues to adopt a left anterolateral thoracotomy as their surgical approach of choice by 1952.[S14]

A number of the features of clinical cases of chronic constrictive pericarditis derive from these basic abnormalities of diastolic function. Ventricular filling is impaired and ventricular stroke volume reduced as a result of the reduced com-

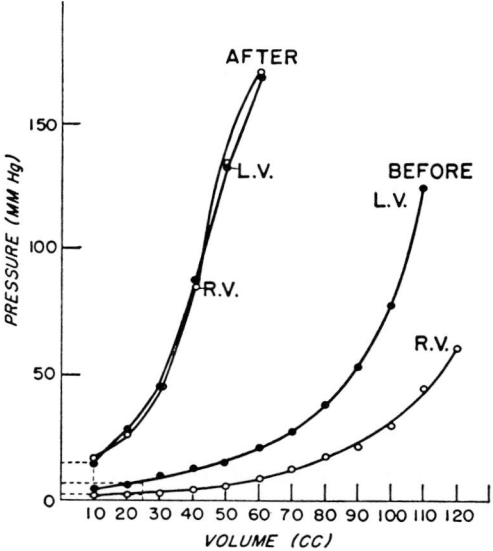

Figure 52-1 Pressure volume curves of left and right ventricles, made immediately after death by introducing 10-ml boluses of saline solution via the aorta or pulmonary artery into the closed ventricle. Note that in the normal dog's heart (labeled *before,* the compliance of the right ventricle is greater than that of the left. In the hearts of dogs with generalized pericardial constriction, the compliance is low and similar in both ventricles.

Reproduced with permission from Isaacs et al.[11]

pliance of the fused cardiac and pericardial mass. The phasic aspects of ventricular filling are also altered. For a brief period in early diastole, ventricular filling is rapid. However, the limit of ventricular distensibility is reached rapidly, and the right ventricular pressure pulse displays an early diastolic dip and then a high diastolic plateau (square root sign). There is nearly complete diastolic ventricular filling in the first 50 milliseconds of diastole.[G2]

Systemic venous pressures are correspondingly abnormal. The mean venous pressure is elevated. The *x* descent is steep and deep, corresponding to the beginning of ejection. The *y* descent is also steep and deep and corresponds to the early diastolic dip of right ventricular pressure. This is different from events during acute cardiac tamponade, where the *y* descent is absent. The normal inspiratory increase in vena caval flow and decrease in pressure is diminished and often absent.

Pulsus paradoxus is said to be infrequent in chronic constrictive pericarditis (it was observed in one-fourth of patients [GLH]), in contrast to the situation with acute cardiac tamponade. However, the frequency of its recognition is influenced by the cardiac rhythm; for it is usually present when there is sinus rhythm and impossible to detect when there is atrial fibrillation (a not uncommon accompaniment of chronic constrictive pericarditis).

The ventricular end-diastolic volumes are small in this disease, as are end-systolic volume and stroke index. The rate of rise of left ventricular systolic pressure and the ejection fraction are not altered.[L4] Thus, systolic left ventricular function under these circumstances is normal, but this does not necessarily indicate normal contractility.

Effusive Constrictive Pericardial Disease
Although it is seen in a number of settings, effusive congestive pericardial disease is common in nephrogenic pericarditis.[H5] In this condition, an increased volume of pericardial fluid produces the characteristic clinical picture of acute cardiac tamponade, with absence of a *y* descent and a preserved and prominent *x* descent in the jugular venous pulse. However, because of coexisting pericardial thickening, the aspiration of pericardial fluid does not return the situation to normal. Rather, the thickened pericardium begins to restrain the heart, but only after the rapid filling phase of the ventricles is over. Thus, the *y* descent is again present and is prominent, occurring during the time the right atrium is in free communication with the right ventricle through the open tricuspid valve and simultaneous with the early diastolic dip of ventricular pressure. In effusive constrictive pericardial disease, after the fluid is removed, there is no respiratory variation in the right atrial and venous pressures, just as in constrictive pericarditis.

Etiology

In most patients, the etiology of chronic constrictive pericarditis is not known. Thus, McCaughan and colleagues were able to identify a specific etiologic factor in only 27% of their patients,[M2] and Blake and colleagues in only 34%.[B5]

In about 10% of cases, documented acute pericarditis precedes the development of chronic constrictive pericarditis.

Less than 3% of patients in the recent era have evidence of tuberculous pericarditis, while before 1958, 13% had tuberculous pericarditis.[M2] Even in the very early report of 1948 from the Massachusetts General Hospital, in only 17% of the cases was tuberculosis proven as the etiology of the chronic constrictive pericarditis.[P2] Rarely, mediastinal irradiation appears to be a cause. Rheumatoid disease and sarcoidosis occasionally produce it. Trauma is another uncommon cause, with hemopericardium usually present as the precursor of the pericardial thickening and constriction.[M3,S5]

Previous cardiac surgery has also been implicated as a cause. However, McCaughan and colleagues present evidence that constrictive pericarditis is a rare complication of open heart surgery, occurring in less than 1% of cases, with open heart surgery being the cause of chronic constrictive pericarditis in only 4% of patients.[M2] Similar findings are reported by Kutcher and colleagues, who recognized only 11 instances (0.2%, CL 0.1%–0.3%) of chronic constrictive pericarditis among 5,207 adult patients undergoing open heart surgery.[K3] The interval between operation and the development of evidence of constriction tends to be surprisingly short, ranging between 14 and 186 days in the experience of Kutcher and colleagues.[K3]

Clinical Presentation

Classically, symptoms of chronic constrictive pericarditis are delayed for several years after the clinical or subclinical episode of acute pericarditis. The interval may, however, be as short as 2 weeks in those rare instances in which the pericarditis develops after cardiac surgery or 4–12 months after trauma or acute nonspecific pericarditis.

Initial symptoms may be only fatigue with or without modest effort breathlessness, and neck-vein distention may be noticed. Insidiously, however, hepatomegaly and ascites develop initially with or without peripheral edema. Even in the context of such evidence of significant fluid retention, breathlessness may occur only on exertion and not at rest; and although in very severe cases there may be orthopnea, paroxysmal nocturnal dyspnea is virtually unknown. Thus, among 27 surgical cases, 21 (78%) complained of abdominal distention, 17 (65%) complained of leg edema, and only 15 (56%) complained of dyspnea on exertion (UAB). The distribution of these symptoms was similar among the 231 cases reported by McCaughan and colleagues from the Mayo Clinic.[M2]

Clinical Findings

When constriction is not severe, the clinical findings may be limited to modest but persistent elevation of jugular venous pressure and slight liver enlargement with or without intermittent ankle edema. As constriction increases in severity, there is a progressive increase in venous pressure and hepatomegaly, with the eventual development of persistent peripheral edema, ascites, and pleural effusions. By this stage, pulsus paradoxus is to be expected if sinus rhythm persists, and there is often reduction in pulse pressure, as was the case in 8 (36%) of 22 patients in whom there was good information (UAB). The apex beat is usually not palpable, but there is often systolic retraction in the left parasternal region. This retraction may be followed by a visible and palpable forward thrust extending toward the expected site of the cardiac apex; and this impulse, which results from forceful ventricular filling with the onset of diastole, may be mistaken for the apex beat and taken to argue against the existence of pericardial constriction. Rapid ventricular filling in early diastole is associated also with an unusually early, often loud, third heart sound that is sometimes referred to as a *pericardial knock,* but usually there are no murmurs.

The chest x-ray may be unremarkable. However, pericardial calcification is evident in about 40% of cases. Radiologic evidence of restriction is present in about 60% of cases, and echocardiographic evidence in about 20%.[M2]

The electrocardiogram is usually abnormal, with nonspecific ST segment and T wave changes in 90% of cases; and in about 40% of patients with surgically verified chronic constrictive pericarditis, the QRS complexes have low voltage, and an atrial arrhythmia is present in 30%.[M2]

Computed tomography can be useful and demonstrates thickened pericardium in 80% of cases.[M2] However, pericardial thickening can be demonstrated by computed tomography in patients who are without cardiac compression or constriction.[S18]

Nuclear magnetic resonance may prove to be the most useful noninvasive method of diagnosing chronic constrictive pericarditis, when it is available. It allows measurement of pericardial thickness and also depicts the characteristic right atrial dilation and right ventricular narrowing.[S19]

Laboratory Investigation

A protein-losing enteropathy can be demonstrated in some patients with chronic constrictive pericarditis and ascites and hepatomegaly.[P4,P5,W3] The patient may have severe hypoproteinemia, with depression of albumin and gamma globulin, and an increased rate of leakage of plasma protein into the gastrointestinal tract. (This syndrome also develops after other conditions that chronically elevate inferior or superior vena caval pressure, such as the Fontan type of operation and atrial switch operations with inferior vena caval obstruction. See Chapter 26, "Protein-losing Enteropathy" in section on Late Results, and Chapter 39, "Superior Vena Caval Obstruction after Atrial Switch Procedure" and "Inferior Vena Caval Obstruction" in section on Special Situations and Controversies.)

Cardiac Catheterization

Characteristically, end-diastolic pressures are elevated to equal levels in the right atrium, pulmonary artery, and left atrium, and this is considered the hallmark of chronic constrictive pericardial disease.[B7,S3] Such findings were obtained in all the patients coming to catheterization, in the report by McCaughan and colleagues.[M2] The intraventricular pressure pulse contours characteristically demonstrate an early rapid fall in diastolic pressure in the right ventricle, followed by a rapid rise to an elevated diastolic plateau (square root sign).[H6,S3] The left ventricular pressure pulse usually has a similar contour.

Mean right atrial pressure fails to decrease normally during inspiration, or it may actually rise slightly. During inspiration, there is a transient increase in pulmonary blood volume and a slight reduction in right ventricular afterload, resulting in a fall in pulmonary artery and right ventricular systolic pressures and a decline in pulmonary venous pressure and left ventricular diastolic pressure as well.

When hemodynamic studies are equivocal, the rapid infusion (over 6–8 minutes) of 1,000 ml of normal saline solution produces diagnostic features of occult chronic constrictive pericardial disease.[B7] These features include not only striking elevations of filling pressures but also the development of typical pressure pulse morphologic characteristics of constriction, loss or reversal of the respiratory variation of right atrial pressure, and precise diastolic equilibration of cardiac pressures.

Minor Thoracotomy

The distinction between chronic constrictive pericarditis and restrictive cardiomyopathy can be difficult,[W5] and a minor thoracotomy may be useful in making that distinction in a few circumstances. A small anterior incision placed in the line of the formal anterolateral incision that would be used for pericardectomy (see Fig. 52-2) is made and the pericardium exposed through the interspace. A pericardial biopsy specimen is removed for study. If the surgical diagnosis is chronic constrictive pericarditis, the incision is extended and a formal pericardectomy performed. If no pericardial pathologic condition is found, the diagnosis is generally restrictive cardiomyopathy, and the operation is terminated as a minor procedure. If recurring pericardial effusion is found with a more or less normal pericardium, a wide removal of the pericardium can easily be accomplished with a less radical extension of the incision.

NATURAL HISTORY

Knowledge of the natural history of surgically untreated patients with chronic constrictive pericarditis is incomplete. The interval between an etiologic occurrence and the onset of clinical evidence of constriction varies between a few months and many years. But the factors determining the rate of progression of the disease and its symptomatology are unknown. Atrial fibrillation commonly occurs at some stage and results in a sudden deterioration in circulatory status.

Somerville has estimated that once the signs and symptoms of chronic constrictive pericarditis develop, only a semiinvalid life can be led over an interval of 5–15 more years.[S8] When the clinical syndrome includes ascites, progression is more rapid, particularly in children.[S9]

TECHNIQUE OF OPERATION

Since patients with chronic constrictive pericarditis coming to operation are often seriously ill, an arterial catheter is inserted in the radial artery for pressure recording, in addition to the usual preparations in the operating room. A cen-

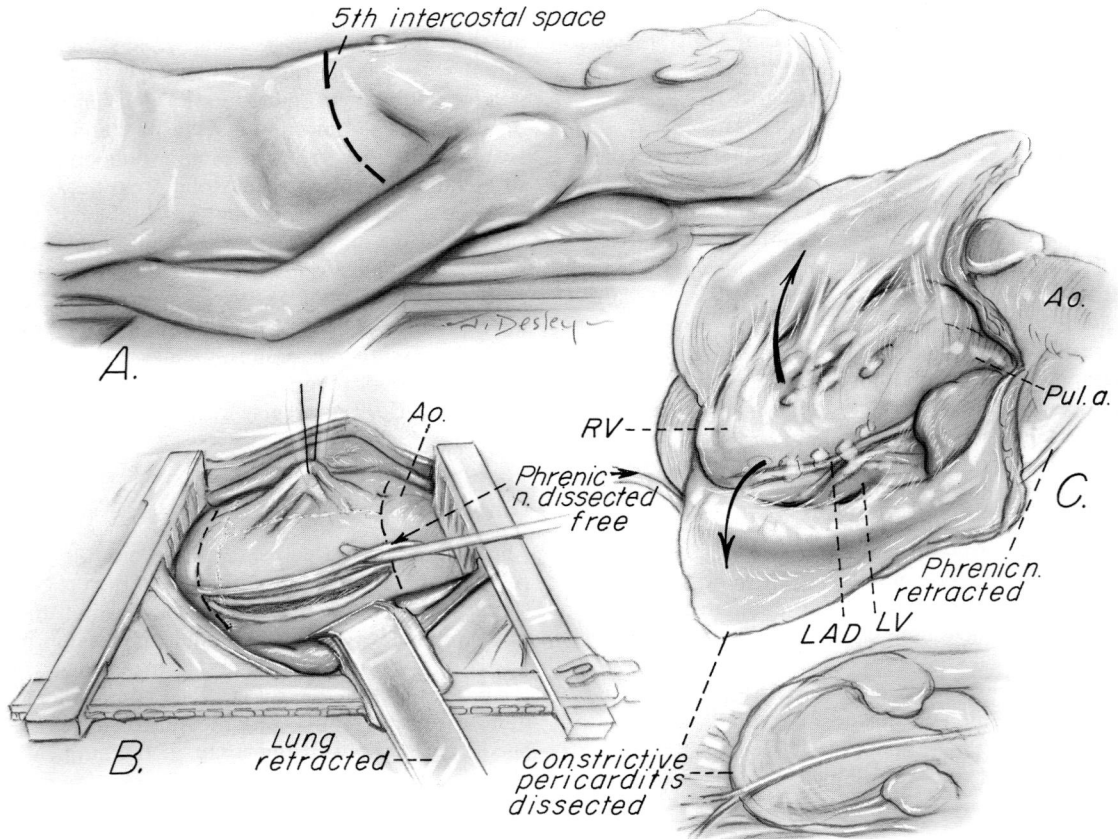

Figure 52-2 Pericardectomy for chronic constrictive pericarditis through a left anterolateral incision.

(a) Positioning of the patient and proposed incision.

(b) The phrenic nerve has been mobilized away from the pericardium. An initial longitudinal incision has been made in the thickened pericardium. The dashed lines illustrate the extensions of the incision first over the left ventricle and then over the right.

(c) The flaps have been dissected back, completely liberating both left ventricle and right ventricle, leaving where necessary small calcific plaques in situ. The first portion of the pulmonary artery has been completely unroofed. The final drawing shows the appearance at the end of the procedure. Note that the thickened pericardium has been removed from the diaphragm.

Ao, aorta; LAD, left anterior descending; LV, left ventricle; Pul. a., pulmonary artery; RV, right ventricle.

tral venous pressure line is also inserted, for right ventricular filling pressure must be prevented from rising excessively at the time the right ventricle is freed.

The approach may be through a left anterolateral thoracotomy (UAB) or a median sternotomy (GLH).

Left Anterolateral Thoracotomy Approach

The patient is positioned supine with a pillow beneath the left scapula. The patient's left hand is secured beneath the left buttocks, with the elbow hanging over the well-padded left side of the table (Fig. 52-2). A curving left anterolateral skin incision is made beneath the breast anteriorly and more laterally over the fifth interspace. The incision is carried through the pectoralis major muscle anteriorly, and the fifth interspace is opened. The interspace incision is carried well anteriorly, and usually the internal mammary vessels are ligated and divided and the fifth costal cartilage dis-

connected from the sternum. The rib spreader is inserted and the interspace incision laterally and posteriorly is extended with scissors as it is gradually opened (Fig. 52-2).

The left phrenic nerve is dissected away from the pericardium; as much fat and soft tissue should be left with the nerve as is possible, to minimize damage to it. The pericardium is incised through an area of minimal calcification, if possible posterolaterally over what is presumed to be left ventricle (see dashed line in Fig. 52-2). On occasions, this initial incision through the abnormal pericardium takes the dissection immediately onto the myocardium, and in other cases it enters a fluid-filled space (see "Morphology").

When a space is entered, the initial longitudinal incision is carried anteriorly and posteriorly from its superior and inferior extremities (Fig. 52-2). The anterior pericardial flap is dissected as far as the right side of the right atrioventricular groove, beneath the elevated thymus and prepericardial fat, and resected. The posterior flap is dissected far posteriorly and excised. The dissection must be carried superiorly onto the pulmonary trunk, since failure to relieve pericardial bands across the pulmonary trunk can result in postoperative gradients and severe right ventricular hypertension.[P3] The piece of pericardium left inferiorly is dissected off the diaphragm except in the area of the central fibrous tendon from which it cannot be removed. Now the fibrous plaques adherent to the epicardium are dissected off through the entire area of resection. If the epicardium is thin and relatively normal, it need not be disturbed. If it is thickened, it must be removed either in its entirety or in a sufficient number of areas to allow more normal diastolic filling of the two ventricles. Failure to do this will severely compromise the result of the operation.[W4]

If no pericardial space is found, the entire longitudinal incision and its anterior and posterior extensions are made only through the fibrous pericardium. Then the incision is deepened in an area that seems to be over myocardium rather than over the interventricular or atrioventricular groove. Slowly and carefully the posterior flap is dissected off the left ventricular myocardium. At first, this dissection is done only in areas in which it proceeds reasonably well, leaving the epicardium on the myocardium whenever it is thin and normal. When dissection in this plane is not possible, such as in an area of calcification or dense scarring, islands of calcification and scar may be left attached to the myocardium but separated from other areas. The dissection moves to the anterior pericardial flap whenever progress ceases posteriorly and vice versa. Particular care is exercised when the dissection passes across the interventricular groove containing the coronary vessels, and here, islands of calcific plaques may need to be left in place. The dissection is carried just across the atrioventricular groove and onto the atria. It is important to be certain that all constrictions in the atrioventricular groove are removed, since they can result in gradients between atrium and ventricle.[P2]

The anterior and posterior pericardial flaps are left long until the dissection is completed (Fig. 52-2) so they may be used temporarily to control any hemorrhage from the myocardium that occurs during the dissection. When the dissection has been completed, these pericardial flaps, as well as the diaphragmatic portion of the pericardium (see above), are excised.

A polyvinyl catheter is brought out from the left atrium via the appendage or left pulmonary veins, whenever possible, to assist in postoperative care. Two left pleural drainage tubes are placed, the tip of one being placed posteriorly and inferiorly and that of the other anteriorly and superiorly. The interspace incision is closed with heavy pericostal and perichondrial absorbable sutures, and the muscle layers are closed with continuous Dexon. The skin is closed with a continuous subcuticular suture.

Median Sternotomy Approach

The sternum is split in the usual manner (see Chapter 2, Section 3). The pericardium is opened vertically anteriorly. Often it is necessary to use a knife for this procedure, and particular care must be taken when the plane between the thickened (visceral) pericardium and the myocardium is

reached. The pericardial flaps are now dissected laterally superiorly and inferiorly, as already described. To the right, the dissection passes across the atrioventricular groove and proceeds across the anterior and lateral walls of the right atrium, provided the cleavage plane there is readily found. If it is not, this portion of thickened pericardium can be left in situ. In the former instance, the pericardial flap is excised about 2 cm anterior to the right phrenic nerve. To the left, the dissection proceeds across the front of the ventricles and then over the lateral left ventricular wall. This pericardial flap is excised about 1 cm in front of the left phrenic nerve. The dissection continues posterior to the phrenic nerve but in the plane between myocardium and epicardium until the entire left ventricle is freed (up to the atrioventricular groove posteriorly and over the diaphragm inferiorly). It is usually then possible to remove the thickened, often calcified outer pericardial layer, since there is usually a cleavage plane between this and the overlying, thickened pleura containing the phrenic nerve. The same is usually true of the thickened pericardial tissue inferiorly overlying the diaphragm. The operation is completed as described earlier.

SPECIAL FEATURES OF POSTOPERATIVE CARE

Low cardiac output may be associated with the development of marked cardiac dilatation during the pericardectomy, particularly dilatation of the right ventricle as it is freed from constriction in the context of a high venous pressure. Low cardiac output usually occurs in patients who have advanced disability, fluid retention, and ascites preoperatively.[M2] The low cardiac output may continue after operation, and maintenance of left atrial pressure at a relatively high level (15 mmHg or more) and the use of catecholamine infusions may be necessary for 12–48 hours.

Intra-aortic balloon pulsation is effective in these patients when cardiac output is low and unresponsive to other measures.[M2] Thus, when these conditions develop, the intra-aortic balloon pump should be introduced, preferably percutaneously (see Chapter 5, Appendix 5D).

EARLY RESULTS

Hospital Mortality

The hospital mortality after pericardectomy for chronic constrictive pericarditis does not approach zero, even in the current era, and remains at 5%–15%. In the Mayo Clinic experience during 1936–1983,[M2] which includes the cases reported by us in 1958,[C2] 32 (14%, CL 11%–17%) of 231 patients died in hospital, with improvement in mortality in the more recent eras. Two (7%, CL 2%–16%) of 29 patients operated on between 1967 and 1979 died (UAB), and 2 (4%, CL 1%–9%) of 52 patients operated on between 1960 and 1984 died (GLH, Table 52-1).

Mode of Death

The commonest mode of death is acute or subacute cardiac failure, accounting for about 75% of the hospital deaths;[M2]

Table 52-1 Hospital deaths according to surgical approach after pericardectomy for chronic constrictive pericarditis (GLH; 1960–1984).

Years	Surgical Approach	n	Hospital Deaths		
			No.	%	CL
1960–1971	Bilateral anterolateral thoracotomy	17	1	6%	8%–19%
1970–1977	Left anterolateral thoracotomy	11	1	9%	1%–28%
1975–1984	Median sternotomy	24	0	0%	0%–8%
	Total cases	52	2	4%	1%–9%

KEY: CL, 70% confidence limits.

this was the mode of death in one UAB and one GLH patient (see "Special Features of Postoperative Care"). Operative or early postoperative hemorrhage is the mode in 5%–10% of the deaths[M2]; this was the cause in the other UAB case. One GLH patient died 1 week postoperatively of respiratory failure (the operation was in 1966).

Incremental Risk Factors for Hospital Death

The preoperative functional status of the patient is the most important risk factor for hospital death.[M2] Thus, the risk approaches zero in patients preoperatively in New York Heart Association (NYHA) functional class I or II, is 10% (CL 8%–14%) for those in NYHA class III, and is 46% (CL 29%–64%) for those in NYHA class IV.[M2] Ascites and peripheral edema were also identified as risk factors in the recent Mayo Clinic study, as were higher intracardiac pressures and lower cardiac indexes preoperatively.[M2]

Noteworthy as not being a risk factor in the Mayo Clinic study was the surgical approach; median sternotomy was used in 61 patients, left anterolateral thoracotomy in 79, and cardiopulmonary bypass (CPB) in 5.[M2] The GLH experience (Table 52-1) and a comparison of it with the UAB experience indicate also that there is no difference in the results obtained with median sternotomy and those obtained with the left anterolateral thoracotomy. The presence of pericardial calcification, low-voltage QRS complexes, and atrial arrhythmias on the electrocardiogram were also not risk factors in the patients reported by McCaughan and colleagues.[M2]

LATE RESULTS

Survival

The survival of patients who have undergone surgical treatment of chronic constrictive pericarditis approaches that of an age-, sex-, and race-matched general population. The actuarial 5- and 15-year survival rates after pericardectomy, excluding hospital deaths, have been 83% and 59%, respectively; including hospital deaths, they have been 80% and 57%, respectively (GLH; Fig. 52-3). Similarly, in the report by McCaughan and colleagues, survival rates, excluding hospital deaths, are 84%, 71%, and 52% at 5, 15, and 30 years postoperatively, respectively (Fig. 52-4).[M2] One of 25

traced hospital survivors followed from 2.2–11.5 years (mean 7.5 years) died (UAB).

Modes of Premature Late Death

About 5% of patients remain in congestive heart failure after a satisfactory pericardectomy and die with this condition. Such patients are generally older and in NYHA class IV preoperatively (Table 52-2, Fig. 52-5).[M2] Most late deaths are unrelated to the constrictive pericarditis (Table 52-2) and may not be premature, as is suggested by the similarity between the actuarial survival of this subset and that of a matched general population.

Incremental Risk Factors for Premature Late Death

Poor preoperative functional status increases the risk of death in the early years after pericardectomy (Fig. 52-4). The type of surgical approach does not seem related to late survival (Fig. 52-6).

Reoperation

Proper use of either of the closed approaches to pericardectomy—median sternotomy or left anterolateral thoracotomy—results in a very low incidence (< 2%) of reoperation. Thus, no patient in the Mayo Clinic series, operated on after 1948 when one of these two incisions became near-routine, has required reoperation to date.[M2] No reoperations have been required in the UAB group (1967–1979), and one only (2%) in the GLH series of 50 hospital survivors.

Hemodynamic Results

Virtually all patients have normal resting hemodynamic characteristics after adequate surgical treatment of chronic constrictive pericarditis.[K2] During exercise, 10%–20% may show mild elevation of pulmonary artery pressure or failure to increase cardiac output. When considerable amounts of thickened pericardium are left over the ventricles, the hemodynamic improvement is less complete.[K2]

Functional Status

Most patients have a good long-term result from pericardectomy for chronic constrictive pericarditis, nearly all being in NYHA class I or II (Fig. 52-7, Table 52-3).

INDICATIONS FOR OPERATION

Almost without exception, the diagnosis of chronic constrictive pericarditis is an indication for operation. When the physiologic effects of the constriction are minimal and particularly when other serious disease is present, the operation may be delayed until more marked signs and symptoms are present.

Surgery for tuberculous pericarditis is best delayed until after at least a 6-week, and preferably a 3-month, course of antituberculous drug therapy. However, if there are clinical

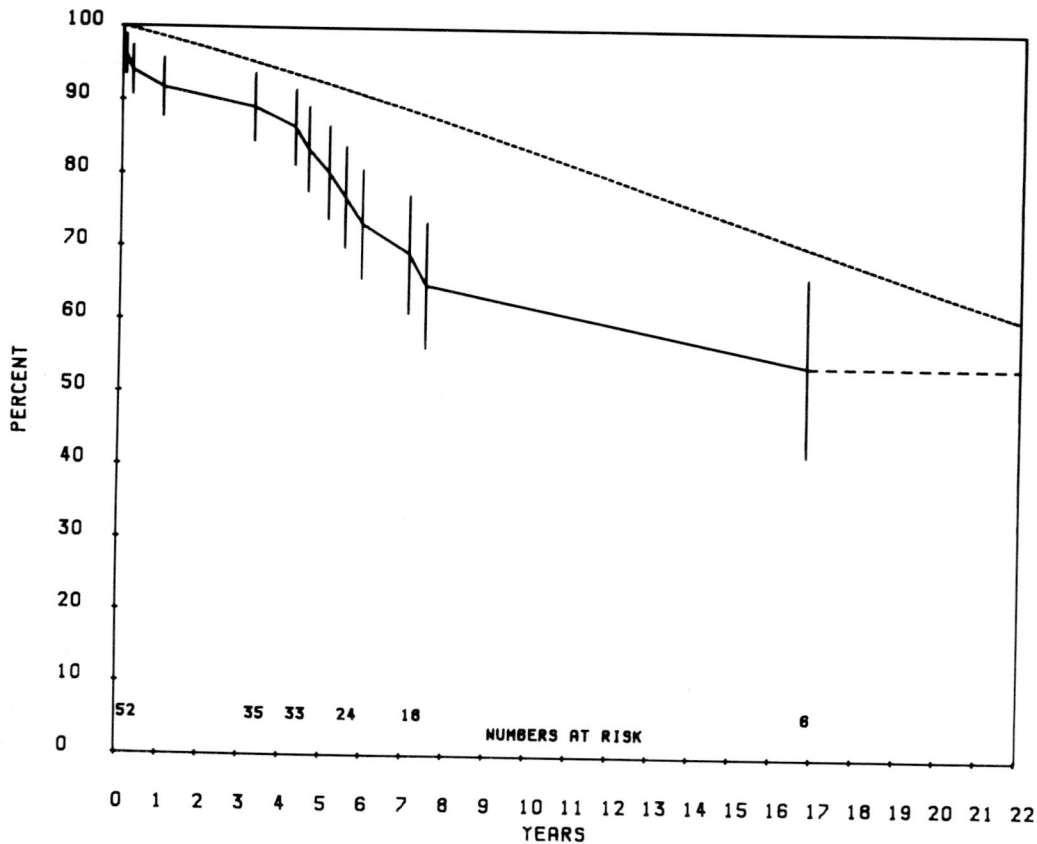

Figure 52-3 Actuarial survival, including hospital deaths, after pericardectomy for chronic constrictive pericarditis (solid line) compared with a matched general population (dashed line) (GLH; 1960–1984). The vertical bars enclose 1 standard error (essentially, the 70% confidence limits). The numbers at risk (the number of patients surviving at each time interval) are noted.

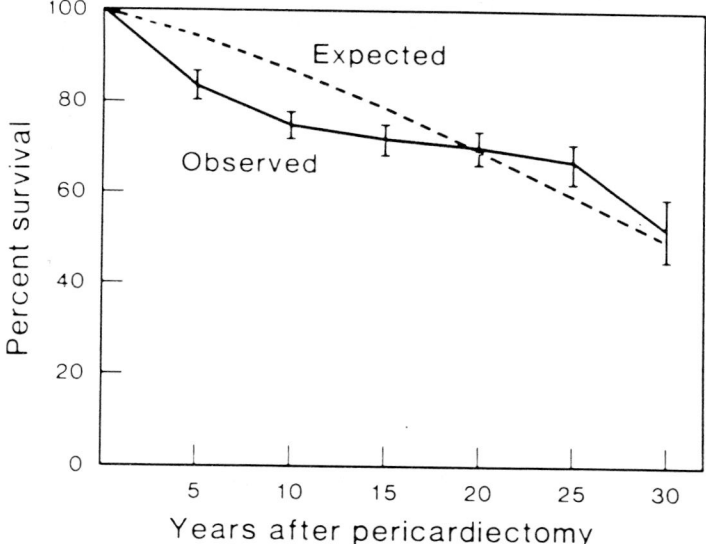

Figure 52-4 Actuarial survival, excluding hospital deaths, of patients after pericardectomy for chronic constrictive pericarditis (Mayo Clinic; 1936–1983; $n = 231$). The dashed line (*expected*) is the survival of an age- and sex-matched general population.

Reproduced with permission from McCaughan et al.[M2]

Table 52-2 Modes of late death among 46 hospital survivors of pericardectomy for constrictive pericarditis (GLH; 1960–1984).

Mode of Late Death	n	Age at Operation
Congestive heart failure	3	55, 67, 78
Coronary artery disease	2	64, 77
Reoperation for constrictive pericarditis	1	58
Carcinoma	4	44, 54, 67, 69
Gastric hemorrhage	1	65

NOTE: Follow-up was from 1 month to 22 years (mean 7.3 years). Four of 50 hospital survivors were lost to follow-up. Among the three patients dying with congestive heart failure, two were in NYHA class IV and one was in class III preoperatively; death occurred 44, 90, and 70 months postoperatively.

signs of progressive constriction, operation should not be delayed, despite the fact that active tuberculous granulation tissue may be encountered.

Occasional patients are seen with fatigue, dyspnea, and chest pain but without the characteristic clinical and laboratory features of chronic constrictive pericarditis. When the diagnosis of pericardial constriction is made by rapid volume expansion in the catheterization laboratory (see "Clinical Features and Diagnostic Criteria"), pericardectomy is indicated, since the symptomatic and long-term results are good.[B7]

SPECIAL SITUATIONS AND CONTROVERSIES

Techniques for Closed Operation

Controversy continues concerning the most appropriate technique of operation, although, clearly, any of several approaches is satisfactory. The more extensive bilateral anterior thoracotomy employed originally is, however, not necessary. The median sternotomy incision, originally advocated by Holman and Willett,[H4] gives good results,[S6] while the left anterolateral thoracotomy is equally satisfactory. It is more difficult to carry the dissection far to the left

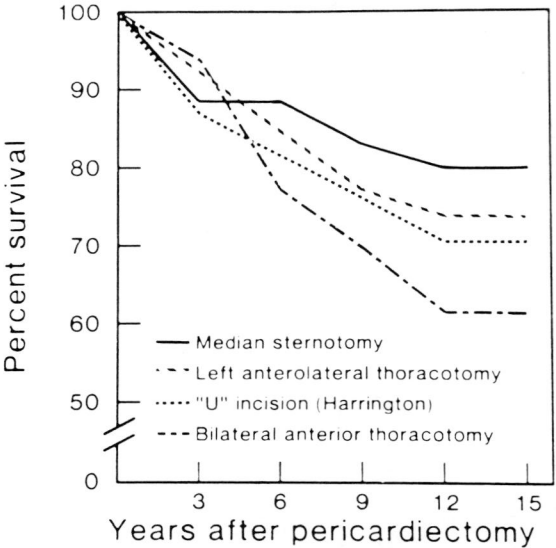

Figure 52-6 Actuarial survival, excluding hospital deaths, after pericardectomy according to the surgical approach. The data set is the same as in Figure 52-3.

Reproduced with permission from McCaughan et al.[M2]

with the median sternotomy and more difficult to carry it to the right anteriorly beyond the atrioventricular groove with a left anterolateral incision. An advantage of the median sternotomy approach is that, if difficulty occurs during the closed pericardectomy, including low cardiac output, arrhythmia, or bleeding, it is easy to institute cardiopulmonary bypass so that the operation can proceed under more controlled conditions. This is rarely necessary.

Median Sternotomy Approach with Cardiopulmonary Bypass

Copeland and colleagues,[C5] and more recently Culliford and colleagues,[C3] have advocated a more radical pericardectomy,

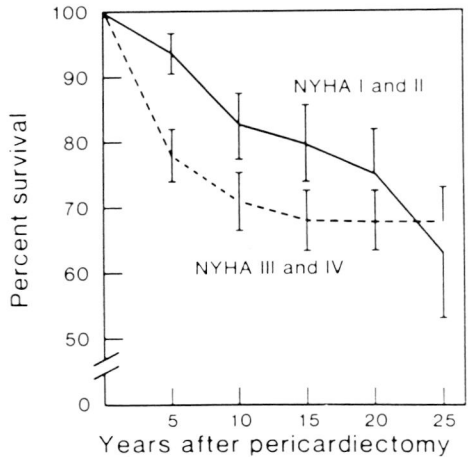

Figure 52-5 Actuarial survival, excluding hospital deaths, after pericardectomy according to preoperative functional status. The data set is the same as in Fig. 52-3.

Reproduced with permission from McCaughan et al.[M2]

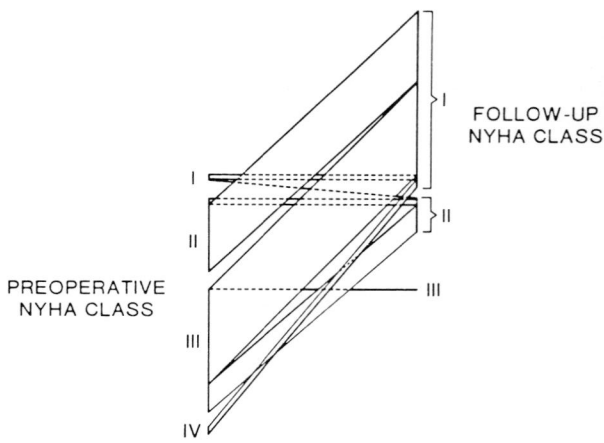

Figure 52-7 Preoperative and late postoperative functional class in 141 patients undergoing pericardectomy for chronic constrictive pericarditis.

Reproduced with permission from McCaughan et al.[M2]

Table 52-3 Preoperative and postoperative functional status among 52 patients undergoing pericardectomy for chronic constrictive pericarditis (GLH; 1960–1984). Follow-up is described in Table 52-2.

Preoperative NYHA Class	Postoperative NYHA Class			Dead	NFU
	I	II	III		
II	2	1			1
III	34	17	7		9	1
IV	16	7	2	1	4	2
Total	52	25	9	1	13	4

KEY: NFU, lost to follow-up; NYHA, New York Heart Association.

NOTE: One patient postoperatively in class II has been on chronic renal dialysis for 8 years; one required subsequent mitral and tricuspid valve replacement. The symptoms in the class III patient are the result of recurrent pulmonary tuberculosis.

with the aid of cardiopulmonary bypass. According to the combined data of their reports, 33 patients were operated on, with no deaths (0%, CL 0%–6%).[C3,C5] The difference between the hospital mortality associated with this method and that associated with closed methods (see "Early Results") could be due to chance (overlapping 70% confidence limits). Good long-term results for 12 years after operation have been reported by Culliford.[C3] However, a recent review of the Stanford experience by Seifert and colleagues shows no difference in early and late results between patients in whom CPB was used and those in whom it was not.[S17] CPB has been used in only 1 case each at UAB and GLH, in 2 of 26 cases reported from another large cardiac center by Miller and colleagues,[M4] in only 2 of 231 cases reported by McCaughan and colleagues,[M2] and rarely at another large referral center.[S6]

Proponents of the use of CPB indicate that it simplifies the surgical procedure, affords an opportunity for complete decortication of both ventricles, and allows complete liberation of the atrial and caval orifices. However, there is good evidence that liberation of the atria and cavae is unnecessary[K2] and that the closed techniques usually allow a complete operation. Although good results can be obtained using CPB, it is more expensive than the closed technique, and the evidence for its superiority overall remains incomplete. In highly selected cases—and these may include cases arising after open operations—CPB may be advantageous.

Section 2
NEPHROGENIC PERICARDITIS

DEFINITION

Pericarditis is usually nephrogenic when it occurs in patients with renal disease, especially those undergoing renal dialysis.

HISTORICAL NOTE

Until the introduction of hemodialysis, pericardial disease was generally considered a preterminal complication of uremia for which little could be done. It was assumed that the pericarditis was a response to chronically high levels of retained metabolic products, such as creatinine and urea, and part of a generalized hemorrhagic serositis. With the advent of dialysis, conceptual changes became necessary. It was observed that pericarditis may occur at any time during the course of hemodialysis and is not under such circumstances related to serum creatinine levels or the degree of nitrogen retention.[S10]

MORPHOLOGY

Nephrogenic pericarditis is usually of the so-called *bread and butter type,* with dense strands of fibrin bridging the space between the layers of the visceral pericardium. Both the visceral and parietal layers themselves may be thickened and adherent to one another, and the entire area may be hemorrhagic. There is likely to be considerable pericardial fluid, which may be loculated.

CLINICAL FEATURES AND DIAGNOSTIC CRITERIA
Pathophysiology

Rarely, acute cardiac tamponade develops in the nephrogenic pericarditis which occurs as a complication of hemodialysis. Pure chronic constrictive pericarditis occurs but is rare. Most commonly, there are the signs and symptoms of effusive constrictive pericardial disease.[H5] (See Section 1, "Pathophysiology of Cardiac Compression" for the pathophysiology of this and the other types of cardiac compression.)

Etiology

The precise cause of nephrogenic pericarditis, including that of pericarditis complicating dialysis, is unknown.[S11] In any event, the pericarditis complicating end-stage renal disease is no more likely to respond favorably to medical treatment including dialysis than is that developing during dialysis.[D3] Pericarditis occurs more frequently as a complication of hemodialysis than of peritoneal dialysis.[S11] It is more likely to develop in the young and in women,[M5] which suggests its possible relationship to the syndromes that develop after cardiopulmonary bypass (see Chapters 2, 5).

Inadequate dialysis has been suggested as a cause of nephrogenic pericarditis, but there is little support for this hypothesis. Infection has been blamed, but cultures of the pericardial fluid are nearly always negative.[R3]

Symptoms

The onset of the pericarditis may be heralded by chest pain that may be mild or excruciating and may be difficult or impossible to distinguish from angina. Some patients present with fever, leukocytosis, and a pericardial friction rub but have little pain. A few present with evidence of acute cardiac tamponade.

Signs

The most striking abnormality on physical examination is gross elevation of the jugular venous pulse. The characteristically absent y descent and preserved x descent are found in the jugular venous pulse wave. A pericardial friction rub may or may not be audible. The arterial blood pressure may be depressed, and pulsus paradoxus may be present.

Chest X-ray

An enlarging and globular cardiac silhouette on the chest x-ray supports the diagnosis.

Electrocardiogram

When nephrogenic pericarditis is acute, characteristically there is widespread ST segment elevation.[S12,S13] Later, the electrocardiogram may be normal, or if the disease becomes chronic, the typical electrocardiographic features of chronic constrictive pericarditis may evolve.

Echocardiogram

Variable amounts of fluid are demonstrated by echocardiography.

NATURAL HISTORY

About 15% of patients on chronic hemodialysis developed nephrogenic pericarditis (UAB). It has a tendency to occur early in the course of dialysis.[V2]

The natural history of this complication when no treatment is given is unknown. Presumably, some patients with a considerable effusion die with acute cardiac tamponade, and others develop chronic constrictive pericarditis and follow its natural history.

TECHNIQUE OF OPERATION

The treatment of nephrogenic pericarditis occurring during dialysis is controversial, and a number of different protocols are used.[F1]

Medical Treatment

Nonsurgical treatment may be used in mild cases or in debilitated patients. Such treatment includes intensification of the dialysis regimen, the use of nonsteroidal antiinflammatory agents, or the use of steroids systemically.[S11]

Pericardiocentesis

The cardiologist generally performs pericardiocentesis in the cardiac catheterization laboratory, under hemodynamic and electrocardiographic control, after localization of the fluid by echocardiography. Either the subxiphoid or the apical route is used, depending on the location of the fluid. The morbidity of this method is considerable, and currently it is rarely used (UAB). However, Callahan and colleagues have found pericardiocentesis directed by two-dimensional echocardiography to be a safe procedure.[C6]

Tube Drainage

In the operating room, the xiphoid process is removed through a small midline incision.[S7] As the sternum is elevated and the diaphragm depressed, fat is removed from over the pericardium, and the pericardium is opened under direct vision. The fluid is aspirated, and a sump type of drain[1] is inserted and placed on 10–20 mmHg suction. The wound is closed. Steroids may be placed in the pericardial cavity at intervals for 2–3 days; then the tube is removed.

Pericardectomy

As described in Section 1, pericardectomy is performed through a left anterolateral incision. An appropriate large piece of thickened pericardium can usually be easily removed.

RESULTS

After tube drainage and insertion of steroids, many patients are completely relieved of the signs and symptoms of pericarditis. In resistant cases, the results of pericardectomy are excellent, recurrence of acute tamponade or chronic constriction being rare.[R1]

INDICATIONS FOR OPERATION

When symptoms are significant and persist in spite of 7–10 days of intensive medical treatment or when acute pericardial tamponade develops, operation is indicated (UAB). Tube pericardial drainage with instillation of steroids is performed. When chronic constriction develops with or without pericardial fluid or when tube drainage fails to produce a satisfactory result, pericardectomy is indicated.[R3]

Section 3
OTHER TYPES OF PERICARDITIS

From a surgical viewpoint, other forms of pericarditis may (1) not require surgical treatment, because any pericardial fluid accumulates slowly and gradually stretches the fibrous pericardium so that it accommodates large amounts of fluid with little increase in transpericardial (pericardial minus pleural) pressure; (2) produce acute cardiac tamponade (see Chapter 49); (3) result in effusive constrictive pericardial disease (see Section 2); (4) result in chronic constrictive pericarditis (see Section 1); (5) present undrained purulent collections; and (6) cause recurrent chest pain of pericardial origin.

---

[1] Synder minihemovac flat silicone wound drainage device.

ACUTE PERICARDITIS

Acute, nonpurulent pericarditis may be a chronically recurring disease, and the disability from the recurrent chest pain may be sufficient to warrant subtotal pericardectomy. The pericardium is easily removed in this condition, through either a left anterolateral incision or a median sternotomy.

PERICARDIAL EFFUSION

Operation is rarely indicated for simple pericardial effusions, since the fluid accumulates slowly and rarely causes cardiac tamponade.

PURULENT PERICARDITIS

Intractable purulent pericarditis is uncommon in the current era. It is most commonly caused by *Staphylococcus aureus,* although *Hemophilus influenzae* may be etiologic. When it occurs and the pericardial abscess is not loculated, pericardiocentesis with two-dimensional echocardiographic control is usually the initial treatment.[B11] Unless the process subsides rapidly after one or two aspirations, more adequate drainage is required. This can be accomplished with a tube through the subxiphoid approach (see Section 2, "Technique of Operation").[A1] If a septic course continues of if loculations are present, evacuation and pericardectomy are indicated.

REFERENCES

A

1. Adebo OA: Purulent pericarditis in children. *J Thorac Cardiovasc Surg* 88:312, 1984 (Letter to the Editor).

B

1. Bonetus T: *De Ventric Tumore, Hydrope, Sepulchretum sive Anatomica Practica ex Cadaveribus Morbo Donatis,* book 3, section 21, observation 3, case 1. Geneva: L Chouët 1679.
2. Beck CS: The surgical treatment of pericardial scar. *J Am Med Assoc* 97:824, 1931.
3. Beck CS: The effect of surgical solution of chlorinated soda (Dakin's solution) in the pericardial cavity. *Arch Surg* 18:1659, 1929.
4. Beck CS, Griswold RA: Pericardiectomy in the treatment of the Pick syndrome: Experimental and clinical observations. *Arch Surg* 21:1064, 1930.
5. Blake S, Bonar S, O'Neill H, Hanly P, Drury I, Flanagan M, Garrett J: Aetiology of chronic constrictive pericarditis. *Br Heart J* 50:273, 1983.
6. Blalock A, Burwell CS: Chronic pericardial disease. *Surg Gynecol Obstet* 73:433, 1941.
7. Bush CA, Stang JM, Wooley CF, Kilman JW: Occult constrictive pericardial disease. *Circulation* 56:924, 1977.
8. Burwell CS: Constrictive pericarditis. *Circulation* 15:161, 1957.
9. Burwell CS: Some effects of pericardial disease on the pulmonary circulation. *Transactions of the Association of American Physicians* 64:74, 1951.
10. Beck CS: Two cardiac compressor triads. *JAMA* 104:714, 1935.
11. Björkhem G, Lundstrom N-R, Vitarelli A: Sequential study of echocardiographic changes in purulent pericarditis. *Pediatr Cardiol* 5:317, 1984.

C

1. Cheevers N: Observations on the diseases of the orifice and valves of the aorta. *Guy's Hospital Reports* VII:387, 1842.
2. Cooley JC, Clagett OT, Kirklin JW: Surgical aspects of chronic constrictive pericarditis: A review of 72 operative cases. *Ann Surg* 147:488, 1958.
3. Culliford AT, Lipton M, Spencer FC: Operation for chronic constrictive pericarditis: Do the surgical approach and degree of pericardial resection influence the outcome significantly? *Ann Thorac Surg* 29:146, 1980.

4. Churchill ED: Decortication of the heart (Delorme) for adhesive pericarditis. *Arch Surg* 19:1457, 1929.
5. Copeland JG, Stinson EB, Griepp RB, Shumway NE: Surgical treatment of chronic constrictive pericarditis using cardiopulmonary bypass. *J Thorac Cardiovasc Surg* 69:236, 1975.
6. Callahan JA, Seward JB, Tajik AJ: Cardiac tamponade: Pericardiocentesis directed by two-dimensional echocardiography. *Mayo Clin Proc* 60:344, 1985.

D

1. Delorme E: Sur un traitement chirurgical de la symphyse cardopericardique. *Bull et mém Soc de Chir de Paris* 24:918, 1889.
2. Dines DE, Edwards JE, Burchell HB: Myocardial atrophy in constrictive pericarditis. *Staff Meet Mayo Clin* 33:93, 1958.
3. De Pace NL, Nestico PF, Schwartz AB, Mintz GS, Schwartz JS, Kotler MN, Swartz C: Predicting success of intensive dialysis in the treatment of uremic pericarditis. *Am J Med* 76:38, 1984.

F

1. Frame JR, Lucas SK, Pederson JA, Elkins RC: Surgical treatment of pericarditis in the dialysis patient. *Am J Surg* 146:800, 1983.

G

1. Greisinger W: *Beitrag zur Diagnose der Mediastinitis.* Reported by Widenmann A, Tübingen, Germany, 1856.
2. Gaash WH, Peterson KL, Shabetai R: Left ventricular function in chronic constrictive pericarditis. *Am J Cardiol* 34:107, 1974.

H

1. Hallopeau MP: Un cas de cardiolyse. *Bull. et mem. Soc. de chir. de Paris* 47:1120, 1921.
2. Harrington SW, Barnes AR: Diagnosis and surgical treatment of chronic constrictive pericarditis. *The Southern Surgeon* 9:459, 1940.
3. Heuer GJ, Stewart HJ: The surgical treatment of chronic constrictive pericarditis. *Surg Gynecol Obstet* 68:979, 1939.
4. Holman E, Willett F: The surgical correction of constrictive pericarditis. *Surg Gynecol Obstet* 89:129, 1949.
5. Hancock EW: Subacute effusive-constrictive pericarditis. *Circulation* 43:183, 1972.

6. Hansen AT, Eskildsen P, Gotzsche H: Pressure curves from the right auricle and the right ventricle in chronic constrictive pericarditis. *Circulation* 3:881, 1951.

I

1. Isaacs JP, Carter BN II, Haller JA Jr: Experimental pericarditis: The pathologic physiology of constrictive pericarditis. *Bull Johns Hopkins Hosp* 90:259, 1952.

K

1. Kussmaul A: Uber schwielige Mediastine—Pericarditis und den paradoxen Puls. *Berliner Klinische Wochenschrift* 10:433, 445, 461, 1873.
2. Kloster FE, Crislip RL, Bristow JD, Herr RH, Ritzmann LW, Griswold HE: Hemodynamic studies following pericardiectomy for constrictive pericarditis. *Circulation* 32:415, 1965.
3. Kutcher MA, King SB III, Alimurung BN, Craver JM, Logue RB: Constrictive pericarditis as a complication of cardiac surgery: Recognition of an entity. *Am J Cardiol* 50:742, 1982.
4. Kenner HM, Wood EH: Intrapericardial, intrapleural, and intracardiac pressures during acute heart failure in dogs studied without thoracotomy. *Circ Res* 19:1071, 1966.

L

1. Lower R: *Tractatus de Corde item de motu, et colore sanguinis et chyli in eum transitu.* London: J. Allestry, 1669, pp 104–107.
2. Lancisi GM: *De Motu Cordis et Aneurysmatibus.* Rome: JM Salvioni, 1728, pp 38, 39.
3. Lannec RTH: *De l'auscultation médiate où traité du diagnostic des maladies des poumons et du coeur, fondé principalement sur ce nouveau moyen d'exploration.* Paris: 1819.
4. Lewis BS, Gotsman HS: Left ventricular function in systole and diastole in constrictive pericarditis. *Am Heart J* 86:23, 1973.
5. Levine HD: Myocardial fibrosis in constrictive pericarditis: Electrocardiographic and pathologic observation. *Circulation* 48:1268, 1963.

M

1. Morgagni GB: *De Sedibus et Causis Morborum.* Venice: Remondiniana, 1760, book ii, letters xxiii, xxiv.
2. McCaughan BC, Schaff HV, Piehler JM, Danielson GK, Orszulak TA, Puga FJ, Pluth JR, Connolly DC, McGoon DC: Early and late results of pericardiectomy for constrictive pericarditis. *J Thorac Cardiovasc Surg* 89:340, 1985.
3. McKusick VA, Kay JH, Isaacs JP: Constrictive pericarditis following traumatic hemopericardium. *Ann Surg* 142:97, 1955.
4. Miller JI, Mansour KA, Hatcher CR Jr: Pericardiectomy: Current indications, concepts, and results in a university center. *Ann Thorac Surg* 34:40, 1982.
5. Marini PD, Hull AR: Uremic pericarditis: A review of incidence and management. *Kidney Int* 7(suppl 2) S-163, 1975.
6. Morgan BC, Guntheroth WG, Dillard DH: Relationship of pericardial to pleural pressure during quiet respiration and cardiac tamponade. *Circ Res* 16:493, 1965.
7. McGreggor M: Current concepts: Pulsus paradoxus. *N Engl J Med* 301:480, 1979.
8. Metcalf J, Woodbury JW, Richards V, Burwell CS: Studies in experimental cardiac tamponade: Effects on intravascular pressures and cardiac output. *Circulation* 5:518, 1952.

P

1. Pick F: Über chronische unter dem Bilde dem Lebercirrhose verlaufende Perikarditis (perikardische Pseudolebercirrhose) nebst Bemerkungen über die Zuckergussleber (Curschmann). 29:385, 1896.
2. Paul O, Castleman B, White PD: Chronic constrictive pericarditis: A study of 53 cases. *Am J Med Sci* October:361, 1948.
3. Portal RW, Besterman EMM, Chambers RJ, Sellors TH, Somerville W: Prognosis after operation for constrictive pericarditis. *Br Med J* March:563, 1966.
4. Plauth WH, Waldmann TA, Wochner RD, Braunwald NS, Braunwald E: Protein-losing enteropathy secondary to constrictive pericarditis in childhood. *Pediatrics* 34:636, 1964.
5. Peterson VP, Hastrup J: Protein-losing enteropathy in constrictive pericarditis. *Acta Med Scand* 173:401, 1963.

R

1. Rehn L: Die perikardialen Verwachsungen im Kindesalter. *Arch f Klin Chir* 68:179, 1920.
2. Roberts JT, Beck CS: The effect of cardiac compression on the size of the heart muscle fibers. *Am Heart J* 22:314, 1941.
3. Rostand SG, Rutsky EA: Cardiac disease in dialysis patients, in D Gentile (ed): *Clinical Dialysis.* Englewood Cliffs, NJ: Appleton-Century-Crofts, 1983.

S

1. Sauerbruck F: *Die Chirurgie der Brustorgame,* vol 2. Berlin: Julius Springer 1925, p 1075.
2. Schmieden V, Fischer H: Die Herzbeutelentzunddung und ihre Folgezustande. *Ergebnisse des Chirurgie u Orthopädie* 19:98, 1926.
3. Shabetai R, Fowler NO, Guntheroth WG: The hemodynamics of cardiac tamponade and constrictive pericarditis. *Am J Cardiol* 26:480, 1970.
4. Sawyer CG, Burwell CS, Dexter L, Eppinger EC, Goodale WT, Gorlin R, Harken DE, Haynes FW: Chronic constrictive pericarditis: Further consideration of the pathologic physiology of the disease. *Am Heart J* 44:207, 1952.
5. Sbokos CG, Karayannocos PE, Kontaxis A, Kambylafkas J, Skalkeas GD: Traumatic hemopericardium and chronic constrictive pericarditis. *Ann Thorac Surg* 23:225, 1977.
6. Stewart RW: (1984) Personal communication.
7. Santos GH, Frater RWM: The subxiphoid approach in the treatment of pericardial effusion. *Ann Thorac Surg* 23:467, 1977.
8. Somerville W: Constrictive pericarditis with special reference to the change in natural history brought about by surgical intervention. *Circulation* 37,38(suppl V):V-102, 1968.
9. Stadler H, Stinger D: A case of Pick's syndrome as the basis for a study of hypoproteinemia. *J Pediatr* 18:84, 1941.
10. Silverberg S, Onepoulos DG, Wise D, Uden DE, Meindok H, Jones M, Rapaport A, De Veber G: Pericarditis in patients undergoing long-term hemodialysis and peritoneal dialysis. *Am J Med* 63:874, 1977.
11. Shabetai R, Rostand S: Nephrogenic pericardial disease, in RA O'Rourke, BM Brenner, JA Stein (eds): *Contemporary Issues in Nephrology,* vol 13, *The Heart and Renal Disease.* New York: Churchill Livingstone, 1984, pp 89–125.
12. Spodick DH: Pathogenesis and clinical correlations of the electrocardiographic abnormalities of pericardial disease. *Cardiovasc Clin* 8:201, 1977.

13. Surawicz BL, Lasseter KC: Electrocardiogram in pericarditis. *Am J Cardiol* 26:471, 1970.

14. Scannell JG, Myers GS, Friedlich AL: Significance of pulmonary hypertension in constrictive pericarditis. *Surgery* 32:184, 1952.

15. Stokland O, Miller MM, Lekvan J, Ilebekk A: The significance of the intact pericardium for cardiac performance in the dog. *Circ Res* 47:27, 1980.

16. Settle HP, Adolph RJ, Fowler NO, Engel P, Arguss NS, Levenson NI: Echocardiographic study of cardiac tamponade. *Circulation* 56:951, 1977.

17. Seifert FC, Miller DC, Oesterle SN, Stinson EB, Shumway NE: Results of surgery for constrictive pericarditis. *Circulation* 70(suppl II):II-327, 1984 (abstr).

18. Sutton FJ, Whitley NO, Applefeld MM: The role of echocardiography and computed tomography in the evaluation of constrictive pericarditis. *Am Heart J* 109:350, 1985.

19. Soulen RL, Stark DD, Higgins CB: Magnetic resonance imaging of constrictive pericardial disease. *Am J Cardiol* 55:480, 1985.

T

1. Tyson GS, Maier GW, Olsen CO, Davis JW, Rankin JS: Pericardial influences on ventricular filling in the conscious dog: An analysis based on pericardial pressure. *Circ Res* 54:173, 1984.

V

1. Vieussens R: *Traité nouveau de la structure et des causes du mouvement naturel du corier.* Toulouse: 1715, Chapter 1.

2. VanDevanter SH: discussion in JR Frame, SK Lucas, JA Pederson, RC Elkins: Surgical treatment of pericarditis in the dialysis patient. *Am J Surg* 146:800, 1983.

W

1. Wilks S: Adherent pericardium as a cause of cardiac disease. *Guy's Hospital Reports,* third series 16:196, 1870–1871.

2. Weill E: *Traité clinique des maladies du coeur chez les enfants.* Paris: 1895.

3. Wilkinson P, Pinto B, Senior JR: Reversible protein-losing enteropathy with intestinal lymphangiectasia secondary to chronic constrictive pericarditis. *New Engl J Med* 273:1178, 1965.

4. Walsh TJ, Baughman KL, Gardner TJ, Bulkley BH: Constrictive epicarditis as a cause of delayed or absent response to pericardiectomy. *J Thorac Cardiovasc Surg* 83:126, 1982.

5. Wood P: Chronic constrictive pericarditis. *Am J Cardiol* January:48, 1961.

THORACIC AORTIC DISEASE

PART VII

53

ACUTE TRAUMATIC AORTIC TRANSECTION

DEFINITION

Acute traumatic aortic transection is a dehiscence of all or part of the aortic wall, usually occurring as a result of intense deceleration of the body. Patients are considered to have acute transection when seen within 14 days of the accident. Chronic traumatic aortic transections and posttraumatic aneurysms are considered in Chapter 55.

HISTORICAL NOTE

Although the lethal nature of acute traumatic aortic transection had been recognized for centuries and was noted by Strassman in 1947,[S5] the data supporting the lethality of traumatic transection and the time relationships between the trauma and subsequent death were emphasized by Parmley and colleagues in 1958.[P2] The first report of successful repair of traumatic transection of the thoracic aorta was by Dshanelidze in 1923 (quoted in Clark and colleagues[C4]). In 1957, Gerbode and colleagues reported successful repair of such an injury,[G4] and Klassen and colleagues successfully repaired an acute traumatic aortic transection in 1958, as reported by Passaro and Pace[P3] and Vasko and colleagues.[V1]

MORPHOLOGY

Upper Descending Thoracic Aorta

Acute traumatic aortic transections occur most commonly in the upper descending thoracic aorta (71% of cases, according to Parmley and colleagues[P2]). With the abrupt deceleration of the thorax, such as occurs in a high-speed vehicular accident, with the body thrown violently against a near-stationary object, the ligamentum arteriosum and the intercostal arteries anchor the upper descending thoracic aorta to the thorax, as do the exits from the thorax of the brachiocephalic vessels, including the left subclavian artery. These portions decelerate with the thorax, but the distal end of the transvese aortic arch and the most proximal part of the descending thoracic aorta, heavily weighted with blood, continue to move forward until they, too, finally decelerate. An aortic transection tends to develop at the interface between these two parts, although the sum of the forces involved and the directions of their effects are complex. It has been calculated that in order to produce rupture, the forces generated by impact must be equivalent to an intravascular pressure of 2,500 mmHg.[Z1]

The transection is often complete, including the aortic adventitia and mediastinal pleura. If the forces have been less violent, the mediastinal pleura, and in some instances the adventitia, are spared. With still less violence, because of lesser initial velocity or less rapid decline to zero velocity, the mediastinal pleura, the adventitia, and parts of the aortic wall remain intact, while a fracture develops in a portion of the circumference of the aorta, usually posteriorly.

The location of the transection is variable. It usually occurs just proximal to the ligamentum arteriosum and about 1 cm distal to the origin of the left subclavian artery, but it may occasionally involve the aorta at the origin of the left subclavian artery. Uncommonly, the transection extends proximal to the left subclavian artery to involve the distal portion of the aortic arch.

When the patient survives the acute posttransection period, at least 14 days, the periaortic hematoma usually begins to liquify and is absorbed or evacuated back into the aorta and a false aneurysm (or so-called *pseudoaneurysm*) develops. The false aneurysm may remain stable for a long period and even calcify, but eventually it enlarges and ruptures.

Ascending Aorta

In patients reaching the hospital alive, the transection may be found in the ascending aorta (10% of Parmley's isolated cases of transection without other major visceral injuries[P2]), but this is uncommon. The mechanism of such a transection is similar to that of one in the upper descending thoracic aorta. Cammack and associates showed that vertical forces of deceleration lead to rupture of the ascending aorta and arch; horizontal forces lead to rupture of the descending aorta.[C9] The transection is most commonly in the distal portion of the ascending aorta, near the origin of the innominate artery. Less commonly, it is in the very proximal portion of the ascending aorta. As in the upper descending thoracic aorta, the transection may be complete or partial.

Other Sites

Rarely, traumatic aortic transections develop in the lower thoracic aorta (at times by direct violence in association with spine fractures) and in the abdominal aorta.

CLINICAL FEATURES AND DIAGNOSTIC CRITERIA

Pathophysiology

When a complete traumatic aortic transection develops and includes the investing mediastinal pleura and/or pericardium, hemorrhage is free and exsanguinating, and death occurs instantly or within a few minutes. When the tear involves all layers of the aortic wall but the mediastinal pleura remains intact, a large amount of blood suddenly escapes into the retropleural tissues, and the signs and symptoms of hemorrhagic shock appear. Usually under such circumstances some blood or plasma passes through the mediastinal pleura to produce a small left hemothorax or pleural fluid collection. When the adventitia of the aorta remains essentially intact, a smaller extravasation of blood occurs, and the mediastinal hematoma is less extensive. The aortic adventitia is more likely to remain intact when the tear does not involve the entire circumference of the aortic wall.

Usually the tear is complete (17 of 32 patients), but in many patients (15 of 32) it is partial (GLH).

Clinical Features

Patients with acute traumatic aortic transections frequently have other severe injuries, including liver and spleen lacerations with intra-abdominal hemorrhage, and head injuries. Such injuries have their own clinical features and diagnostic criteria and may affect management of the aortic rupture (see "Indications for Operation").

Patients who survive to reach the hospital may be in profound hemorrhagic shock if a large mediastinal extravasation has occurred or if there has been extensive intra-abdominal or extremity bleeding. Some patients, however, are hemodynamically stable after initial resuscitative measures, and a few show no signs of hemodynamic instability. In such patients, upper body hypertension is common.[F2,J2,R1]

Some patients in whom the overall trauma has not been great complain of severe interscapular back pain, but pain is generally not a major part of the presentation.

Evidence of impaired blood flow beyond the transection is uncommon. However, a small proportion of patients—5 (6%) of the 79 patients in the combined UAB-GLH experience—have paraplegia on hospital admission explainable only by the transection.[S4] Rarely, patients also have severe lower body and leg ischemia.

Chest X-ray

The chest x-ray is usually abnormal, but the abnormalities are variable. There may be opacification of the left hemothorax and shift of the mediastinum to the right due to a massive collection of fluid in the left pleural space. These features are not diagnostic of aortic transection, since bleeding after trauma may come from the intercostal or pulmonary vessels, cardiac and pericardial rupture, or from traumatic rupture of the left hemidiaphragm with intrathoracic splenic rupture.

Commonly, the film shows only diffuse upper mediastinal widening (Fig. 53-1), which, in the setting of a severe accident, strongly suggests acute traumatic upper descending

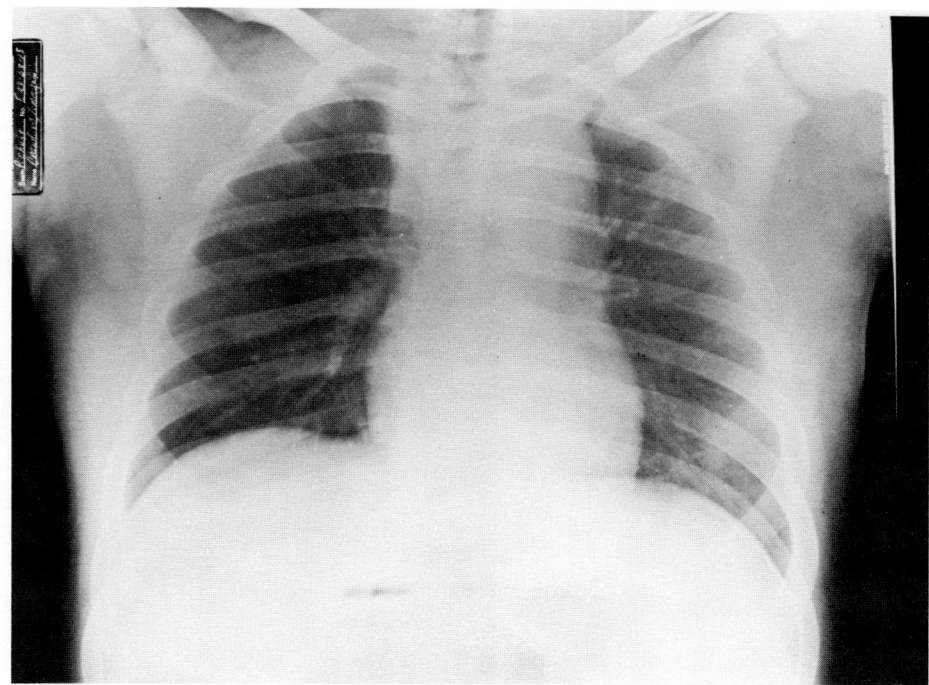

Figure 53-1 Chest x-ray of a patient 6 hours after a high-speed automobile accident (UAB). The upper mediastinal shadow is abnormally wide, and the outline of the distal aortic arch and upper descending thoracic aorta is blurred.

aortic transection. However, tracheal shift to the right, blurring of the normally sharp outline of the upper descending thoracic aorta, and opacification of the usually clear space between it and the pulmonary artery may be evident in the chest x-ray and all suggest aortic transection.[M2]

Aortogram

The diagnosis is made quickly and easily by thoracic aortography (Fig. 53-2), an examination urgently indicated whenever aortic transection is suspected. Subtraction aortography may prove to be the diagnostic method of choice in the future.

NATURAL HISTORY

The risk of death is greatest immediately after the accident, particularly in transections of the ascending aorta. As time passes after the injury, the hazard function (instantaneous risk of death) decreases, but the patient remains at great risk of death from hemorrhagic shock over the next several days (Fig. 53-3). The shock may be secondary either to the initial blood loss into a large mediastinal hematoma or to renewed bleeding into the adventitia and mediastinal pleura as the arterial blood pressure rises after the initial period of hypotension.[P2] About 40% of untreated patients are dead within 48 hours of hospital admission.

When death has not occurred by the seventh postinjury day, the risk of early death is less, and by 2 weeks after injury, it has fallen to relatively low levels (Fig. 53-3). How-

ever, a low but definite risk of death from hemorrhage persists because of the propensity of the false aneurysm (see "Morphology") to rupture even years later (Fig. 53-3).[C4] It has been estimated that, even after 10 years, 20% of patients with this kind of traumatic false aneurysm will die of rupture within the subsequent 5 years.[B1,G1]

TECHNIQUE OF OPERATION

Repair of Acute Traumatic Transection of Upper Descending Thoracic Aorta

An arterial catheter is inserted in the patient's right arm to monitor blood pressure; a nasopharyngeal thermistor is placed for temperature measurement; and, if it can be done expeditiously, a Swan-Ganz catheter is inserted for measurement of pulmonary artery wedge pressure (see Chapter 4). A double-lumen endotracheal tube is helpful and is inserted if the patient's condition is good and the intubation easy. A large-bore needle must be securely in position in a peripheral vein. The patient is placed in a right lateral decubitus position, but with the hips rolled back toward a more supine position so that the left femoral vessels are accessible. No attempt is made to warm the patient, since a body temperature of 32–33°C provides some spinal cord protection during the repair (see "Paraplegia" in section on Special Situations and Controversies). Since this operation is only rarely an urgent emergency (see "Indications for Operation"), there is usually time for the pump-oxygenator team to be assembled. Facilities for aspirating shed blood from the thorax in a

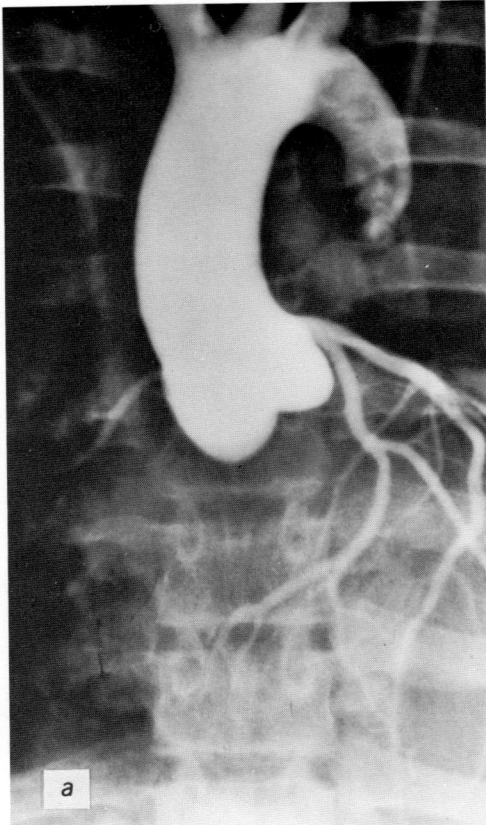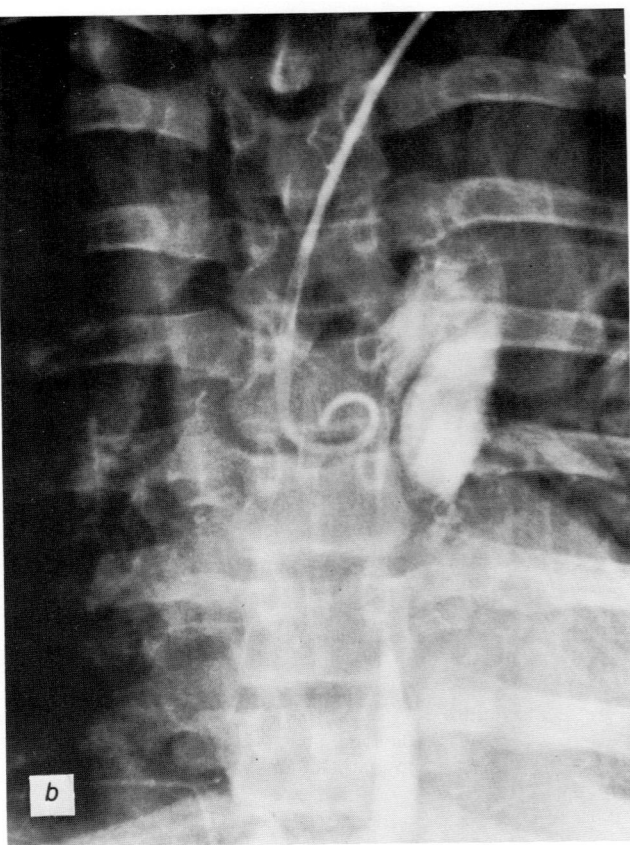

Figure 53-2   Aortogram, frontal view, in the same patient as in Figure 53-1, the catheter having been introduced through the left brachial artery (UAB).
(*a*) Early frame. The aorta seems to be obstructed at the site of a ragged mural laceration.
(*b*) Late frame. Extravasated contrast media is seen, which compresses the descending thoracic aorta.

sterile manner, washing and compacting the red blood cells, and rapidly returning them to the patient are organized.

A long left posterolateral incision is made, and the thorax is entered through the top of the bed of the nonresected fifth rib. The rib spreader is positioned and opened in stages over the next few minutes, and the opening into the thorax anteriorly and posteriorly is lengthened with scissors as this is done. As soon as the rib spreader has been partially opened, the surgeon (*not* the assistant) sucks the blood out of the thorax, taking great care not to provoke more bleeding by disturbing the mediastinal hematoma. Usually there is no active bleeding into the pleural space (patients with such bleeding have usually not reached the hospital alive), but if it is occurring, immediate control is obtained by digital compression.

Once the rib spreader has been well positioned, the lung is covered with a moist laparotomy pad and retracted anteriorly with a malleable retractor held by an assistant (the exposure is similar to that for repair of coarctation; see Chapter 34, Fig. 34-9). The mediastinal pleura is still undisturbed, and at this point a decision is made about the technique of spinal cord protection during aortic cross-clamping (see "Paraplegia" in section on Special Situations and Controversies). If the hematoma is small or of moderate size,

and if it does not engulf the distal portion of the transverse aortic arch and origin of the left subclavian artery, the transection is presumed to be in the usual location beyond the origin of the subclavian artery and repairable with simple aortic cross-clamping. This presumption should be based on the belief that the repair can very probably be accomplished within 30 minutes or less of aortic cross-clamping. If the patient's condition is stable and the temperature above 33°C, body temperature is reduced to that level by ice water lavage of the pleural space (see again "Paraplegia" in section on Special Situations and Controversies). If the hematoma extends over the origin of the left subclavian artery and distal aortic arch, its repair may take longer than 30 minutes, and provision is made for lower body and spinal cord blood flow during the period of aortic cross-clamping (see "Techniques of Minimizing the Incidence of Paraplegia after Aortic Cross-Clamping and Resection" in section on Special Situations and Controversies).

If the decision is made to proceed with simple aortic cross-clamping, a double-velour woven Dacron graft of appropriate size is selected and preclotted with blood, or a medium-porosity woven USCI Dacron graft preclotted with albumin (see "Grafts for Use in Thoracic and Thoracoabdominal Aortic Surgery," in section on Special Situations and Con-

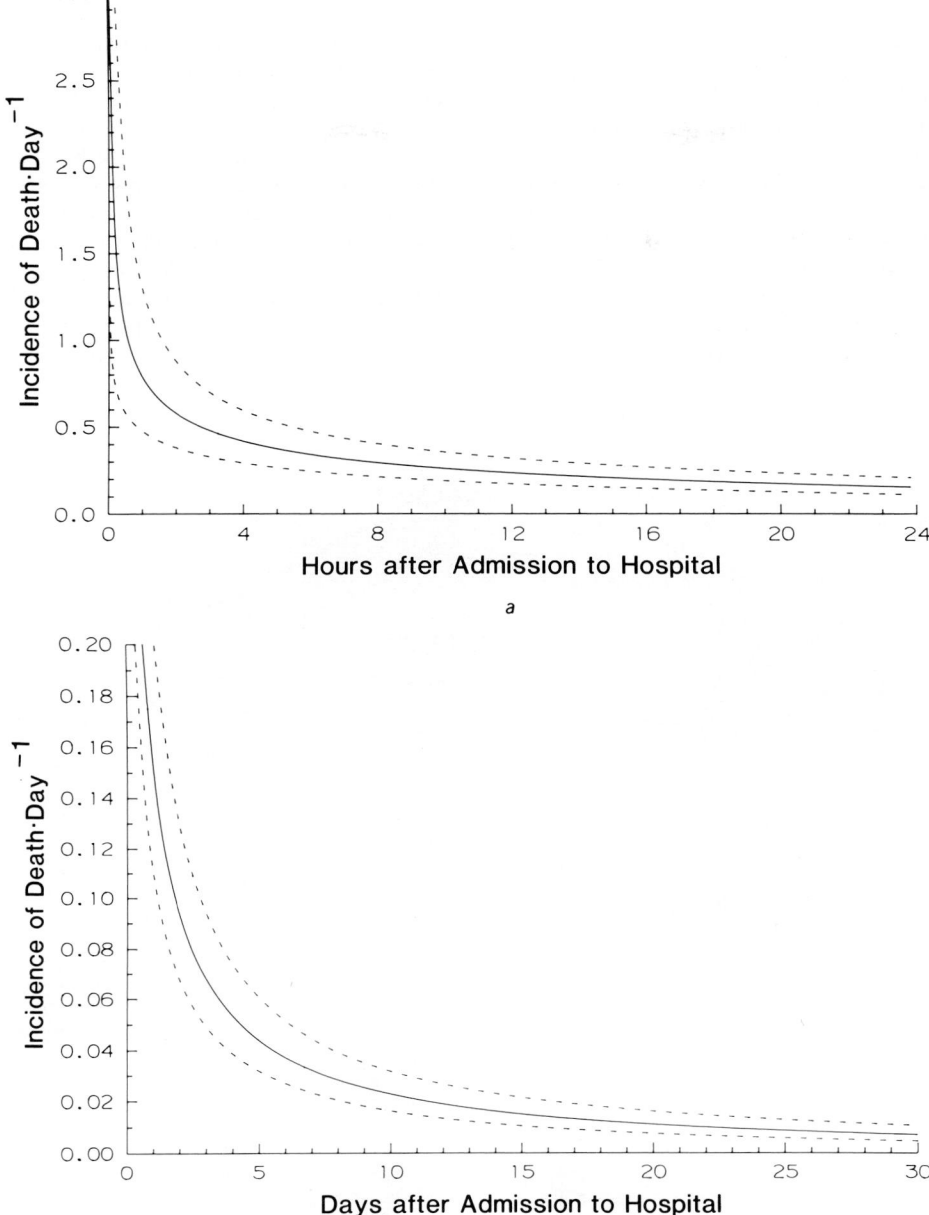

Figure 53-3 Hazard function, or instantaneous risk of death across time (see Chapter 6), after acute traumatic aortic transection. Time zero is admission to the hospital. The dashed lines enclose the 70% confidence limits. There is an early phase of rapidly falling risk and a constant late phase. (Analysis based on the 24 hospital admissions in the paper by Parmley and colleagues.[P2]) In (*a*) the horizontal axis encompasses only 24 hours (one day), and the vertical axis encompasses a large hazard. In (*b*) the horizontal axis encompasses 30 days and the vertical axis a smaller hazard. The relationships are such that the following are the probabilities of survival without treatment:

| Time after | Probability (%) of Survival for: | |
Hospital Admission	24 hours	7 days
0 hr	73%	50%
12 hr	85%	61%
24 hr	89%	66%
2 d	92%	73%
3 d	94%	77%
4 d	95%	80%
5 d	96%	82%

troversies for the details of graft selection and preclotting). The clamps for aortic control are selected. A few stay sutures are placed along the mediastinum behind the hilum of the lung and held anteriorly by clamps, which replace the cumbersome malleable retractor.

The mediastinal pleura is opened a short distance over the mid-thoracic aorta beyond the hematoma, over the transverse arch, and over the left subclavian artery beyond the hematoma (Fig. 53-4). Dissection is carried around the aorta and subclavian artery at these three points so that a cross-clamp can be placed. Tapes can be placed around the vessels, but they are not necessary and generally should be avoided. The dissection is now carried along the presenting surface of the aorta toward the hematoma from below and down the transverse arch and the subclavian artery from above.

When as much as seems safe has been accomplished in this manner, the cross-clamps are placed, one across the distal transverse arch, one across the subclavian artery, and one on the upper descending thoracic aorta (see Chapter 4 for discussion of anesthetic management during this phase of the operation). By this maneuver, reasonable control of bleeding can be established, but (1) there will be some bleeding retrogradely into the aorta via the intercostal arteries

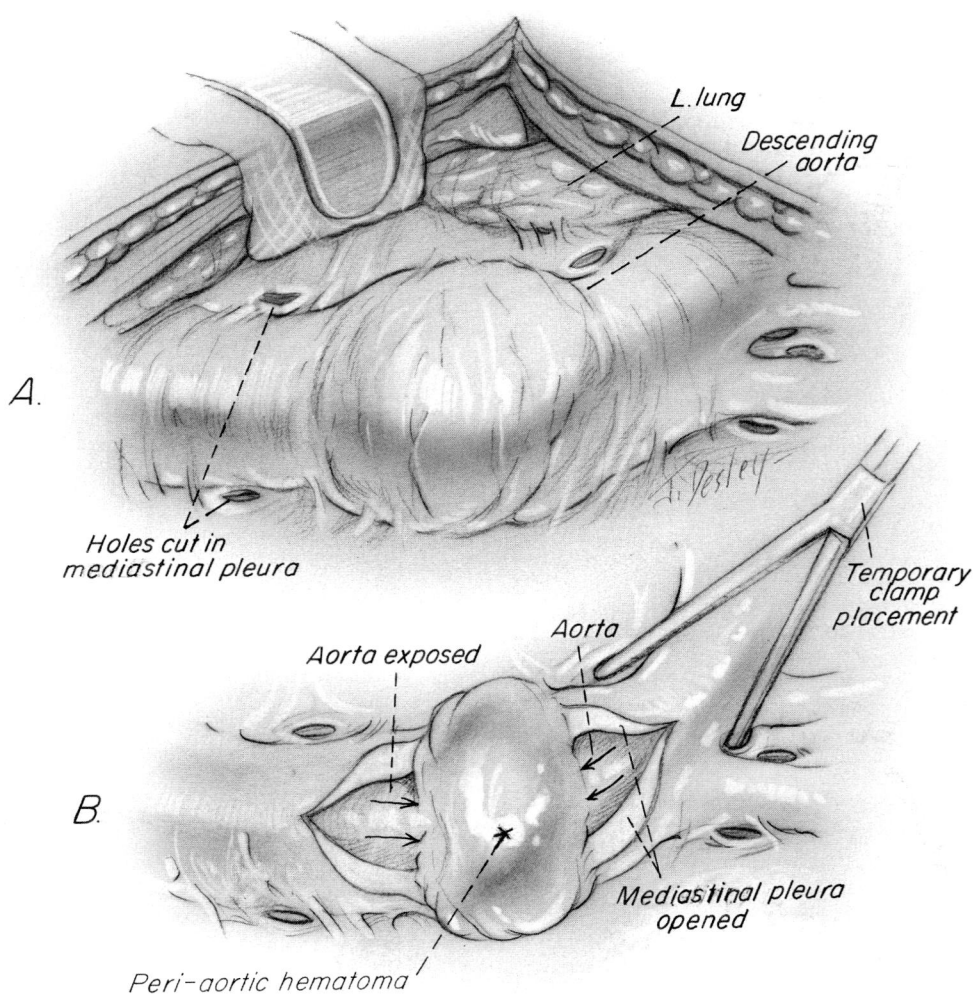

Figure 53-4 Repair of acute traumatic transection of the thoracic aorta.
(a) The appearance of the mediastinum at left thoracotomy. The subpleura hematoma around the aorta enlarges and distorts the area in the region of the ligamentum arteriosum. The initial step of making small cuts in the mediastinal pleura is shown.
(b) Initial stages of dissection. A temporary clamp has been placed on the aorta proximal to the origin of the left subclavian artery, but left open. The mediastinal pleura has been opened in a limited fashion and the dissection carried from above and below (indicated by arrows) toward the traumatic transection. The temporary proximal clamp is then closed, a temporary distal clamp is placed, and one is placed temporarily on the subclavian artery. The pleura over the mediastinal hematoma is opened, the hematoma largely removed, and the temporary clamps replaced with clamps just above and just below the area of transection.

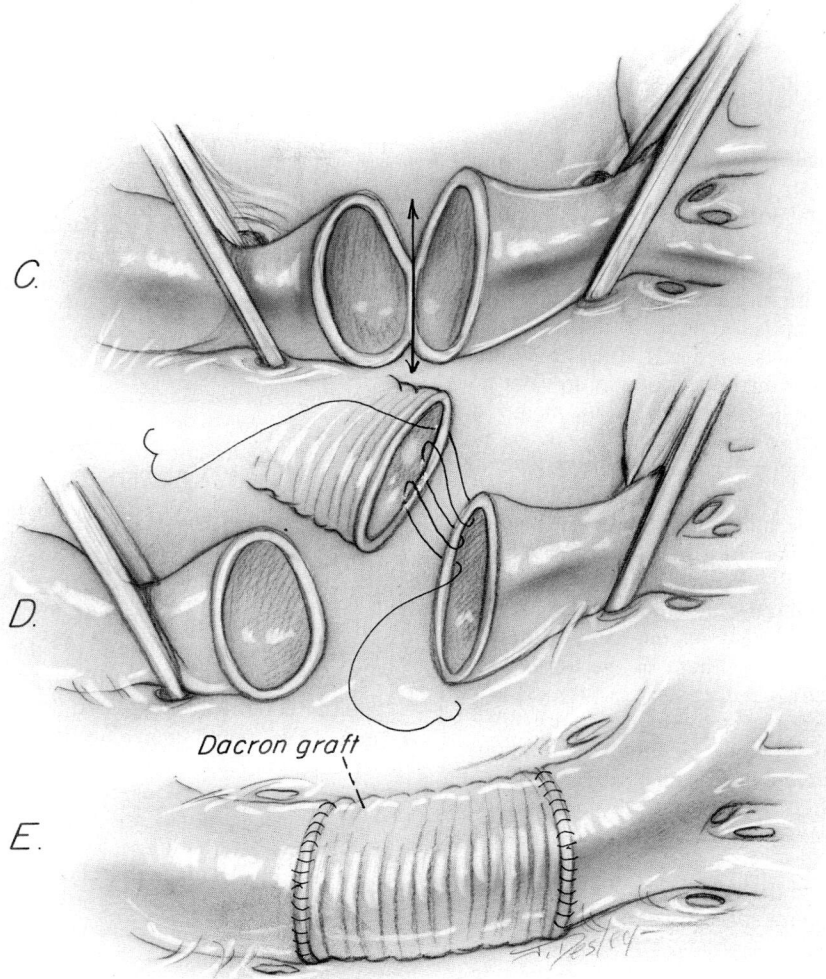

Figure 53-4 *(continued)*
(c) Rarely, end-to-end anastomosis can be made. Usually, the remaining bridge is cut and the field is prepared for graft insertion.
(d) A preclotted woven Dacron tube is sutured to the proximal aortic segment.
(e) The repair is complete.

above the distal cross-clamp, (2) absence of forward flow through these intercostal arteries puts the spinal cord at some risk of damage, and (3) cross-clamping the distal aortic arch rather than the aorta beyond the left subclavian artery causes a greater increase in left ventricular afterload and markedly decreases the collateral flow to the lower body via the left subclavian artery.

The dissection now continues expeditiously along the upper and lower aortic segments, adjacent to the transection, staying precisely in the periaortic tissue plane. At some point, the hematoma is entered, and the blood and clot are then evacuated rapidly. Usually there will be some bleeding into the field from the intercostal arteries between the transection and distal clamp. The two proximal clamps can now usually be replaced with a single clamp (sometimes a Satinsky or curved clamp) on the aorta just beyond the origin of the left subclavian artery, and the distal clamp can usually be replaced by one nearer the transection and above the

origin of most of the intercostal arteries. Blood coming into the field by retrograde flow through the intercostal arteries is aspirated through the system that returns blood to the patient. If possible, these arteries are not ligated or oversewn (see "Paraplegia" in section on Special Situations and Controversies), and the aorta is tailored to preserve their origins in the repair.

When the transection involves only a part of the circumference of the aorta, a direct repair can sometimes be made, with interrupted pledgetted everting mattress sutures of 4-0 polypropylene or a simple whip stitch. Although Fontan and colleagues report being always able to make a direct repair,[F1] this method is considered advisable only if the tissues seem of particularly good quality. Otherwise, a segment of the tube graft is interposed between the two ends (Fig. 53-4). After the proximal anastomosis is made, the proximal clamp is briefly released while the graft is occluded, and if there is any bleeding from the suture line, additional sutures are placed. Then the distal anastomosis is made, with aorta and graft tailored to preserve as many intercostal artery origins as possible. The distal clamp is released, any bleeding between sutures secured with fine interrupted sutures, and the proximal clamp slowly removed.

In cases in which a longer repair time may be anticipated (UAB) or routinely (GLH), provision is made to provide aortic flow beyond the distal aortic clamp. A Gott shunt may be inserted (see "Techniques of Minimizing the Incidence of Paraplegia after Aortic Cross-clamping and Resection" in the Section on Special Situations and Controversies), or, less often (when a Gott shunt is too difficult to position), left atrial-femoral artery bypass is used (GLH). The shunt is positioned before dissection of the site of rupture, but flow through it is not begun until just before the aortic clamps are placed. Alternatively, femoro-femoral bypass may be preferred when aortic flow must be maintained beyond the cross-clamp (UAB).

The availability of cardiopulmonary bypass (CPB) is also important[C6,C7] in circumstances in which it is recognized that the proximal cross-clamp will be very difficult to place safely or may need to be proximal to the left common carotid artery or when severe hemorrhage develops that can be controlled digitally but precludes safe placement of the aortic cross-clamps. Under such circumstances, the left femoral artery and vein are exposed (if necessary by the assistant while the surgeon digitally controls the bleeding), the patient heparinized, the vessels cannulated, and CPB begun at the greatest possible flow rate. The perfusate temperature is kept about 10°C below nasopharyngeal temperature (cooling is not rapidly induced, in an attempt to delay the onset of ventricular fibrillation), and the head of the operating table is gradually lowered (to minimize the chance of air's going to the brachiocephalic vessels). Cooling is continued until an inordinate amount of fluid needs to be added to the pump-oxygenator or cardiac dilation occurs, but the hope is to reduce nasopharyngeal temperature to about 22°C. Then CPB is discontinued, the proximal and distal aortic clamps are placed, and the head vessels are occluded with clamps if their origin is between the aortic clamps. The repair is then made, with the surgeon preserving as many intercostal arteries as possible. As CPB is again gradually begun, the distal clamp is released and any air allowed to escape between sutures or through a nick in the graft, the proximal clamp is released and any air massaged out the escape hole, and the brachiocephalic vessel or vessels are released. As rewarming by CPB proceeds, the heart may require defibrillation. Fresh-frozen plasma and platelet concentrates are given after discontinuing CPB.[1]

After the repair is completed, as much of the mediastinal pleura as possible is closed over the operative area. One intercostal drainage catheter is positioned posteroinferiorly in the gutter and another anterosuperiorly. The incision is closed after making certain that the lung has been reexpanded and the catheters are on suction.

---

[1]This special use of femoro-femoral bypass has been employed by Crawford[C7] but not at UAB or GLH.

Repair of Acute Traumatic Transection of Ascending Aorta

When a diagnosis of acute traumatic transection of the ascending aorta is made by aortography, preparations are made for a standard open heart operation with cardiopulmonary bypass (CPB) as the patient is being transferred to the operating room.

In the operating room, the usual peripheral devices are placed (see Chapter 2, Section 3). With the patient as well supported as possible by the anesthesiologist, one member of the surgical team makes a median sternotomy incision while the other exposes the left femoral artery in the groin. The pericardium is opened just enough to expose the right atrial appendage, every effort being made not to do any dissecting or disturb in any way the hematoma. If there is active bleeding, digital control is obtained.

The patient is heparinized, the femoral artery cannulated, a single right atrial venous cannula placed (see Chapter 2, Section 3), and CPB established with the perfusate temperature as low as possible so as to cool the patient rapidly. As this is being done, the thymus gland is divided, the pericardium opened more widely, and the pericardial reflection dissected off the hematoma over the distal portion of the ascending aorta. If massive hemorrhage is encountered during the dissection, the perfusate flow rate is reduced to $0.5 \text{ l} \cdot \text{min}^{-1} \cdot \text{m}^{-2}$ until enough of the aorta can be dissected to get an aortic cross-clamp beyond the transection. Usually this clamp can be placed just proximal to the origin of the innominate artery, although the clamp may have to be angled so that more of the undersurface of the aortic arch is exteriorized by it. Once this clamp is in position, full CPB flow may be resumed and the perfusate temperature stabilized at 25°C. After this clamp has been placed, a second more proximal clamp is placed in the mid-portion of the ascending aorta (the tear is usually between these two clamps), and the cold cardioplegic infusion is given directly into the proximal ascending aorta.

The area of the transection is dissected out. Usually there has been sufficient damage to the aorta that a securely preclotted tube graft is required for reconstruction of aortic continuity (see "Grafts for Use in Thoracic and Thoracoabdominal Aortic Surgery," in section on Special Situations and Controversies). The repair is made by the technique described for graft interposition for descending thoracic aortic transections. After the anastomosis is complete, the distal clamp is released, and while strong suction is maintained on the aortic needle vent placed for the cardioplegic infusion the proximal aortic clamp is similarly released. Rewarming has been started about 5 minutes previously.

After the patient has been rewarmed, CPB is discontinued, and the remainder of the operation is completed in the usual fashion (see Chapter 2, Section 3). Fresh-frozen plasma and concentrates rich in platelets are given after CPB has been discontinued and the protamine administered.

If the transection involves the innominate artery or aortic arch and digital control is possible, the CPB is continued until nasopharyngeal temperature reaches 20°C. Then total circulatory arrest is established, and the technique used in transverse arch resection is employed (see Chapter 55, "Repair of Transverse Arch Aneurysms'' in section on Technique of Operation).[A4]

SPECIAL FEATURES OF POSTOPERATIVE CARE

The postoperative care is that usually given after other major cardiovascular operations (see Chapter 5). Many of the patients have systemic hypertension early postoperatively, and particular care is taken in its control. Associated injuries are managed appropriately.

RESULTS

Survival

Unquestionably, many patients survive after repair of acute traumatic aortic transection who would otherwise have died, but the proportion surviving varies according to the circumstances. Associated severe injuries decrease the probability of survival. Paradoxically, rapid transport systems between the accident site and the hospital, while giving the individual patient a better chance to live, may decrease the proportion of surgical survivors because more severely injured patients reach the hospital while still alive.

The hospital mortality is generally about 25% (Table 53-1).[A3,A4,B5,T3] Results have improved in recent years (Table 53-2). Most deaths are the result of other injuries produced by the accident (Table 53-3). In general, older age decreases the probability of survival,[S6] although this is not necessarily the case (Table 53-4).

The long-term results are excellent.

Paraplegia

The proportion of patients developing paraplegia after surgical repair is variable but usually in the range of 5%–15% (Table 53-5; see ''Paraplegia'' in section on Special Situations and Controversies). The incidence may be lower in recent years because of better knowledge of appropriate techniques. Thus, among 31 patients undergoing repair in the current era (UAB and GLH from 1980 on), 25 of whom were known to be without prerepair paraplegia and who received adequate observation postrepair, only 2 (8%, CL 3%–18%) developed paraplegia or paraparesis. In one such patient (UAB), the hematoma extended 12 cm down the aorta from the level of the origin of the left subclavian artery, and the distal aortic clamp was left at that level during the 26 minutes

Table 53-2 Hospital deaths after surgical repair of acute traumatic transection of the aorta related to year of operation (GLH).

| Date of Operation | n | Hospital Deaths | | |
		No.	%	CL
1965–1980	15[a]	5	33%	22%–47%
1980–November 1984	17[b]	1	6%	2%–15%
Total	32	6	19%	11%–19%
$P(\chi^2)$			.04	

KEY: CL, 70% confidence limits.
[a] Twelve left atrial-femoral artery bypass, 1 femoro-femoral bypass, 1 full cardiopulmonary bypass, 1 simple aortic clamping.
[b] Sixteen Gott shunts, 1 left atrial-femoral artery bypass.

Table 53-3 Mode of death after repair of acute traumatic aortic transection (UAB; 1967–July 1984; $n = 47$, 13 deaths and GLH; 1965–November 1984; $n = 32$, 6 deaths).

Mode of Death	No. of Patients
Other subsystem trauma	13
Multiple	8
Head injury	3
Hemorrhagic shock during thoracotomy	2
Acute cardiac failure	4
Diffuse mediastinal and chest wall hemorrhage after repair	2
Total	19

Table 53-4 Hospital deaths according to age at operation (GLH; 1965–1984).

| Age (years) ≤ < | n | Hospital Deaths | | |
		No.	%	CL
20	12	3	25%	11%–44%
20 --- 30	12	2	17%	6%–35%
30 --- 40	5	0	0%	0%–32%
40 --- 50	1	0	0%	0%–85%
50 --- 60	0			
60 --- 70	2	1	50%	7%–93%
Total	32	6	19%	11%–29%
$P(\chi^2)$			.7	

KEY: CL, 70% confidence limits.

Table 53-1 Hospital deaths after surgical repair of acute traumatic transection of the aorta. (The UAB material concerns only patients operated on by the Division of Cardiothoracic Surgery.)

| Location of Transection | UAB, 1967–July 1984 | | | | GLH, 1965–November 1984 | | | | Total | | | |
| | | Hospital Deaths | | | | Hospital Deaths | | | | Hospital Deaths | | |
	n	No.	%	CL	n	No.	%	CL	n	No.	%	CL
Ascending aorta	2	0	0%	0%–61%					2		0%	0%–61%
Innominate artery					1	0	0%	0%–85%	1	0	0%	0%–85%
Upper descending aorta	45	13	29%	21%–37%	30	5	17%	9%–27%	75	18	24%	19%–30%
Lower descending aorta					1	1	100%	15%–100%	1	1	100%	15%–100%
Total	47	13	28%	20%–36%	32	6	19%	11%–29%	79	19	24%	19%–30%

KEY: CL, 70% confidence limits.

Table 53-5 Paraplegia or paraparesis developing after surgical treatment of acute traumatic aortic transection.

Location of Transection	UAB; 1967–July 1984					GLH; 1965–November 1984					Total			
	n	Corrected n	Spinal Cord Damage			n	Corrected n	Spinal Cord Damage			Corrected n	Spinal Cord Damage		
			No.	%	CL			No.	%	CL		No.	%	CL
Ascending aorta	2	2	0	0%	0%–61%						2	0	0%	0%–61%
Innominate artery						1	1	0	0%	0%–85%	1	0	0%	0%–85%
Upper descending aorta	45	37	6	16%	10%–25%	30	26	2[a]	8%	3%–17%	63	8	13%	8%–19%
Lower descending aorta						1					1	0	0%	0%–85%

KEY: CL, 70% confidence limits.

NOTE: Corrected *n* is the number of patients known to be without these events before surgery and with adequate observations after repair. The percent is percent of corrected *n*.

[a] One instance occurred after use of a Gott shunt, and one after simple aortic cross-clamping.

of aortic cross-clamping (no shunt). In the other (GLH), the Gott shunt was almost certainly not functioning (cross-clamp time 45 minutes).

INDICATIONS FOR OPERATION

When the diagnosis of acute traumatic aortic transection is made within 5 days of injury, prompt repair is indicated. The shorter the time between injury and diagnosis and the larger the mediastinal hematoma, the more urgent the operation. Thus, when the diagnosis is made within 12–24 hours of injury, the mediastinal hematoma is large, or there is considerable pleural fluid, emergency operation is advisable. Unless there is evidence of active and gross intra-abdominal bleeding, or of a head injury in urgent need of operation, the thoracic aortic injury takes precedence. If the hematoma is small or the interval between injury and operation is more than 24 hours, emergency repair is advisable, but essential and urgent intra-abdominal or neurologic surgery may take precedence.

When the diagnosis is made between about 24 hours and 5 days after injury, operation is advisable, but unless the hematoma is very large or there is evidence of active bleeding, the operation can be performed urgently but at a promptly scheduled time rather than as an emergency (see Fig. 53-3). In the interim, arterial hypertension is avoided by the use of sodium nitroprusside.[A3]

After about 14 days, the problem becomes similar to that of any thoracic aneurysm (see Chapter 55).

SPECIAL SITUATIONS AND CONTROVERSIES

Paraplegia

Paraplegia and paraparesis, and in some patients cord bladder, may complicate operations on the thoracic and thoracoabdominal aorta (Table 53-6). Although considerable information about this complication is available, it is not yet sufficient to eliminate it.

Tolerance of Normal Persons
to Thoracic Aortic Cross-clamping
When the thoracic aorta is cross-clamped just beyond the origin of the left subclavian artery, there is a risk of para-

plegia or paraparesis.[A1] In the study of Katz and associates, the incidence of paraplegia appeared to increase with longer aortic cross-clamp times (Fig. 53-5).[K1] In Crafoord's experience using aortic cross-clamping as part of the technique of repair of patent ductus arteriosus, paraplegia did not occur (0%, CL 0%–61%) when the cross-clamp time was less than 15 minutes but occurred in some patients with longer cross-clamp times (Fig. 53-6).[C2]

The Katz data must be interpreted with caution, since they were obtained from patients who had very recently suffered a severe whole body deceleration accident, which may itself have traumatized spinal cord blood supply and made the cord more susceptible to additional damage at operation. Indeed, paraplegia is occasionally present preoperatively in patients with acute aortic transection. Also, the body temperature of the patients and the exact number of intercostal arteries sacrificed at operation are not known. Nonetheless, the relationships derived by Katz and colleagues provide some quantitative information concerning the relationship in humans between cross-clamp time and the probability of paraplegia or paraparesis,[K1] and Crafoord's data[C2] are entirely compatible with these data (Fig. 53-6). Data from pigs[W1] are likewise compatible. Data derived from dogs by Pontius and associates[P4] and Beattie and colleagues[B8] appear to differ (Fig. 53-6), and species differences may well be the explanation.

The inference must be drawn that in normal humans the length of time the aorta may be cross-clamped just distal to the left subclavian artery without paraplegia or paraparesis resulting is limited. Since there is no better information than the probability curve supplied by Katz and associates concerning the interrelationship involved (Fig. 53-6), it represents the best guidelines for surgical procedures.

Source of Variability among Normal Persons
VERTEBRAL ORIGIN OF THE ANTERIOR SPINAL ARTERY. The data just discussed indicate that individuals do vary in their tolerance to thoracic aortic cross-clamping just beyond the origin of the left subclavian artery. This variation may depend in part on anatomic variability in the blood supply to the spinal cord. Usually the important but slim anterior spinal artery is formed at the level of the medulla by spinal artery branches from each of the vertebral arteries, which in turn are usually branches of the subclavian artery. As the

Table 53-6 Paraplegia or paraparesis developing after aortic surgery (UAB; 1967–July 1984).

Procedure	n	Spinal Cord Damage		
		No.	%	CL
Repair acute traumatic descending aortic transection	37	6	16%	10%–25%
Repair acute ascending aortic dissection	42	0	0%	0%–5%
Repair acute descending aortic dissection	12	1	8%	1%–26%
Repair descending arteriosclerotic or degenerative thoracic aneurysm	41	2	5%	2%–11%
Repair thoracoabdominal degenerative or arteriosclerotic aneurysm	6	0	0%	0%–27%
Repair chronic dissection of ascending aorta	18	0	0%	0%–10%
Repair chronic dissection of descending aorta	32	0	0%	0%–6%
Repair posttraumatic aneurysm of descending aorta	13	1	8%	1%–24%
Total	141	10	7%	5%–10%

KEY: CL, 70% confidence limits.

NOTE: The *n* in all instances is the number of patients for whom data are available as to the presence or absence of clinical evidence of spinal cord damage after operation. Excluded are patients whose preoperative status in this regard is not known or who were paraplegic. The *n* corresponds to the corrected *n* in Table 53-5. *P* for difference between incidence of postoperative paraplegia in acute lesions (6 in 37 patients) and in all others (3 in 110 patients) is .006, excluding those in ascending aorta.

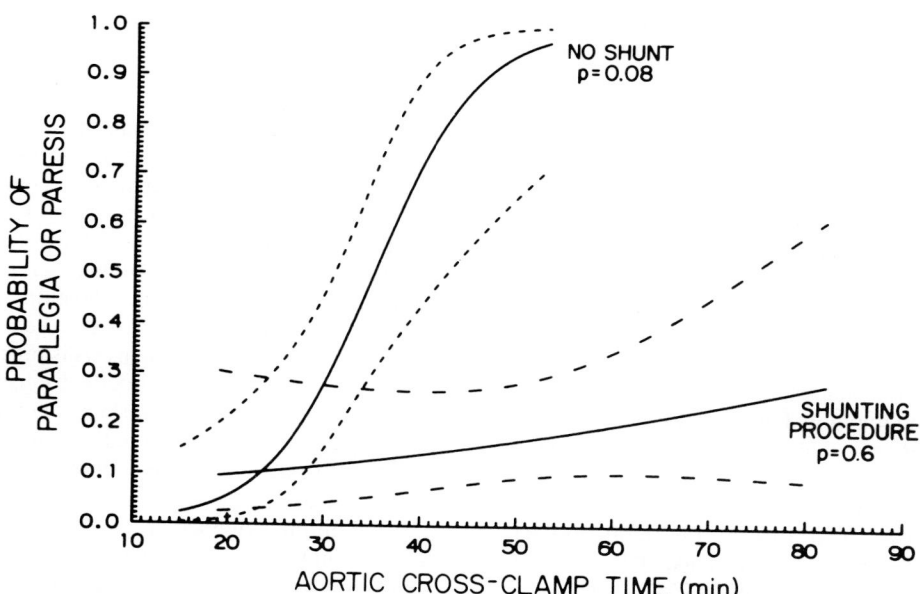

Figure 53-5 The risk of paraplegia according to the length of aortic cross-clamp time and the presence or absence of perfusion of the descending thoracic aorta. The data are from patients with acute aortic transection who were operated on with the aid of simple aortic cross-clamping just beyond the origin of the left subclavian artery (no shunt), or with an aorto-aortic bypass or some other form of perfusion of the aorta distal to the cross-clamping (shunting procedures).

Reproduced with permission from Katz et al.[K1]

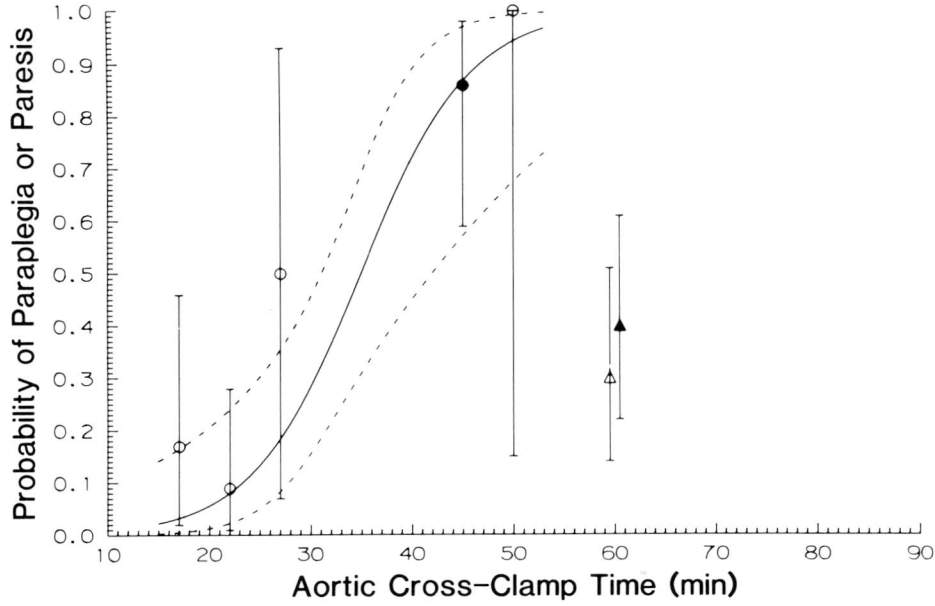

Figure 53-6 Composite presentation of data concerning the probability of paraplegia or paresis when the aorta is cross-clamped just distal to the left subclavian artery at more or less normothermia. The solid line, with the dashed lines enclosing the 70% confidence limits, is from the patients presented by Katz and colleagues (Fig. 53-5).[K1] The open circles with the vertical lines depicting the 70% confidence limits represent data from patients presented by Crafoord.[C2] The solid circle depicts data from pigs published by Wadouh and associates.[W1] The open triangle represents data in dogs published by Pontius and colleagues[P4] and the solid triangle data in dogs published by Beattie and colleagues.[B8]

anterior spinal artery passes down the spinal cord, it is contributed to by a variable number of radicular arteries, formed from spinal branches of the intercostal and lumbar arterial branches of the descending thoracic and abdominal aorta. Apparently the fewer the radicular arteries (and it is said that most commonly there are only five to eight in humans[D1,S1,W1]), the larger and more important is the anterior spinal artery and its origin from the two vertebral arteries (Kadyi,[K2] Piscol,[P1] Bartsch,[B3] quoted by Wadouh and colleagues[W1]). The more significant the vertebral origin of the anterior spinal artery, the longer is the safe descending thoracic aortic cross-clamp time likely to be.

ARTERY OF ADAMKIEWICZ. A particularly large radicular artery is present in most humans (the artery of Adamkiewicz,[A2] or the arteria radicularis magna anterior) that is vitally important to the functional integrity of the spinal cord inasmuch as its ligation usually results in paraplegia or paraparesis (in 5 of 7 pigs, 71%, CL 45%–90%).[W1] Among humans, this artery is said (Jellinger,[J1] Piscol,[P1] quoted by Wadouh and colleagues[W1]) to arise at T-9 (ninth thoracic vertebra level) to T-12 in 60% of individuals, at T-5 to T-8 in about 15%, and at L-1 or beyond in about 25%. Presumably, in normal persons the resection or exclusion of that part of the aorta from which this important artery arises entails a considerable probability of paraplegia, and methods of spinal cord protection cannot be relied on to minimize the incidence. The evidence for this inference is that paraplegia can result in some normal persons if the artery of Adamkiewicz[W1] or intercostal arteries that are important contributors to the anterior spinal artery are ligated.[S2] The inference is also supported by a report of paraplegia induced by the use of an intra-aortic balloon pump.[R2]

Effect of Level and Type of Aortic Cross-clamping

When the proximal one of a pair of cross-clamps is placed for 45–60 minutes on the abdominal aorta of a normal person beyond the origin of the renal arteries (at about the level of L-2), paraplegia or paraparesis occurs very rarely (in < 0.1% of cases),[C6] presumably because both clamps are beyond the origins of the artery of Adamkiewicz and consequently spinal cord ischemia does not develop. When the proximal aortic cross-clamp is at the level of the diaphragm for 45–60 minutes, paraplegia or paraparesis is presumed to develop in about 25% of persons. As already discussed, when the proximal cross-clamp is on the aorta just beyond the origin of the left subclavian artery for 45–60 minutes, 90% of persons are presumed to develop clinical evidence of permanent spinal cord damage.

In addition, evidence from the experimental studies of Spencer and colleagues[S2] indicates that clamping of the left subclavian artery along with the thoracic aorta increases the risk of paraplegia still further. This increase is understandable, since the anterior spinal artery originates from the vertebral artery, which originates from the subclavian artery.

The experiments of Pontius and colleagues[P4] suggest that as the distance between the two clamps on the thoracic aorta increases, so does the chance of paraplegia. This finding suggests that even the low pressure in the aorta distal to the cross-clamps provides some protective perfusion of the spinal cord, and that the absence of pressure in a long segment of aorta isolated between two clamps increases the risk of paraplegia.

Variability in Disease States

When the collateral circulation around that part of the aorta exteriorized by a pair of aortic cross-clamps is well developed, as in most patients undergoing the coarctation operation, the aorta can probably be cross-clamped at that level for many hours and perhaps indefinitely. Some patients with coarctation have an incomplete collateral circulation and a greater likelihood of developing paraplegia (a matter discussed in greater detail in Chapter 34).[B6]

Patients coming to operation for chronic arteriosclerotic or degenerative thoracic or thoracoabdominal aneurysm frequently have little or no flow through many or all of their intercostal arteries because of previous gradual thrombotic occlusion of their orifices. This process rarely if ever causes paraplegia, no doubt because it is slow and there is concomitant development of a collateral circulation. In these disease states, the collateral arteries are rarely large enough to be evident on examination. When well-developed, however, they may be sufficient in many patients with aneurysms to allow a 45–60-minute period of aortic cross-clamping without the development of paraplegia.

Mechanism of Paraplegia Development

The experimental studies of Wadouh and colleagues[W1,W3] and of Laschinger and colleagues[L1,L2] support firmly the hypothesis that paraplegia and paraparesis after descending thoracic aortic cross-clamping are due to spinal cord ischemia. However, ischemia may be increased by a concomitant increase in intracranial or intraspinal pressure developing during the cross-clamp period[B4,B7,M1] or by systemic arterial hypotension occurring before, during, or after the aortic repair.[C3]

Methods of Minimizing the Incidence of Paraplegia after Aortic Cross-clamping and Resection

PERFUSION OF THE DISTAL AORTA. When a pair of aortic cross-clamps is applied close together to the most proximal part of the descending thoracic aorta (such as in the operation for acute traumatic aortic transection), perfusion of the distal aorta by any one of a number of methods prevents spinal cord ischemia and the development of paraplegia.[L1,L2] This was demonstrated by Stranahan and colleagues as long ago as 1954.[S3] However, distal aortic perfusion prevents paraplegia only if the short segment of aorta exteriorized by the clamps does not give origin to the critical radicular blood supply to the spinal cord. If the critical arteries come off the exteriorized segment and the aortic clamps remain in position for a considerable period of time, perfusion of the distal aorta cannot be expected to afford protection to the spinal cord.

The Katz study supports the idea that perfusion of the distal aorta while a pair of aortic cross-clamps is on the upper descending thoracic aorta neutralizes the incremental risk of longer cross-clamp times (Fig. 53-5).[K1] Other studies

also support this concept by showing that distal aortic perfusion restores spinal cord blood flow, maintains spinal cord function, and restores the function temporarily lost by a brief period of inadequate perfusion of the distal aorta.[C5,L1,L2] The experimental study of Laschinger and colleagues suggests that the distal aortic pressure needs to be about 60 mmHg or more to ensure freedom from paraplegia.[L2]

HYPOTHERMIA. Hypothermia clearly prolongs the safe ischemic time for the spinal cord, just as it does for all other organs (see Chapter 2, Section 1). This was demonstrated about 40 years ago by Hufnagel and Gross[H1] and later by Beattie and colleagues,[B8] and reaffirmed by the elegant experimental study of Pontius and colleagues.[P4] These studies of Pontius and colleagues,[P4] as well as those of Beattie and colleagues[B8] and Parkins and colleagues,[P5] indicate that the spinal cord can recover normal function after ischemia of 60 minutes' duration at a whole body temperature of 30°C. The studies of Coles and colleagues indicate that profound cooling of the spinal cord itself imparts the same protection.[C8]

REATTACHMENT OF THE INTERCOSTAL AND LUMBAR ARTERIES. After resection of a segment of the thoracic or upper abdominal aorta, from which emerge arteries critical to spinal cord blood flow, reattachment of the intercostal and lumbar arteries to the graft would seem logical. Success of the method depends on preservation of spinal cord integrity during the period before the intercostal and lumbar arteries are reattached to the graft.

One way of accomplishing this reconstruction of spinal cord blood flow is tailoring the resection and the graft. Wakabayashi and Connolly suggested tailoring the resection of the descending thoracic aorta so that most of the posterior wall of the aneurysm with the origins of the intercostal arteries is preserved. The graft is then cut very obliquely on the distal end for an appropriate end-to-end anastomosis.[W2]

Another method is the use of the inclusion technique and the making of an oval opening in the graft, which is anastomosed to the aortic wall around the origin of the critical intercostal arteries. However, in the experience of Crawford, this method did not reduce the incidence of paraplegia and paraparesis.[C7] In that experience, 30%–40% of patients developed such complications after the resection of the entire descending thoracic and abdominal aorta.[C7]

Summary of Risk Factors for Paraplegia after Aortic Surgery

Minimizing the incidence of paraplegia after aortic surgery necessitates understanding as well as possible the incremental risk factors involved, even though they are incompletely elucidated. These risk factors include (1) the length of the aortic cross-clamp period, a factor now agreed to by Crawford[C7] and others; (2) the level of aortic cross-clamping; (3) the length of aorta exteriorized by the pair of clamps; (4) the inclusion of the subclavian artery in the cross-clamping; (5) the inclusion of intercostal arteries critical to spinal cord blood flow in the exteriorized segment of aorta; (6) the degree of development of the collateral circulation to the aorta distal to the clamp; (7) the degree of development of the collateral circulation to the spinal cord itself, which may have evolved as intercostal artery orifices in the diseased aortic segment were closed down by the disease process (see

P value in Table 53-6); (8) the body and spinal cord temperature during the period of aortic cross-clamping; (9) the total perfusion of the aorta distal to the cross-clamps, by collaterals and by a shunt or cardiopulmonary bypass; and (10) the completeness of spinal cord reperfusion after the removal of the cross-clamps.

Monitoring Spinal Cord Function during Operation

The technique of somatocortical evoked response (SEC) allows spinal cord function to be monitored during operations. In this technique, the posterior tibial nerve is stimulated and the response in the cerebral cortex recorded. Cunningham and colleagues have shown that this aspect of spinal cord function disappears 5–10 minutes after a pair of cross-clamps is applied to the thoracic or thoracoabdominal aorta.[C5] As noted earlier, they have also demonstrated reappearance of this function with distal aortic perfusion.

However, just as with brain function and the electroencephalogram, cessation of function does not indicate irreversible loss of function. However, the study of Laschinger and colleagues indicates that prolongation of spinal cord ischemia for 5–10 minutes after the onset of SEC quiescence is incompatible with functional recovery of the spinal cord after reperfusion.[L4]

Techniques of Minimizing the Incidence of Paraplegia after Aortic Cross-clamping and Resection

No one technique is always optimal for minimizing the incidence of paraplegia. The one best suited to the individual patient must be selected. With currently available information and techniques, it is not possible to eliminate the risk of paraplegia or paraparesis after descending thoracic and abdominal aortic operations. The prevalence of these complications can, however, be reduced to a minimum.

Whole Body Hypothermia

Hypothermia to a nasopharyngeal temperature of 32°C is achieved very simply. In neonates and infants, the operation is performed with the patient on a cooling blanket and with the operating room temperature cool (±60°F, or 16°C) during the making of the thoracotomy. If at the time for aortic cross-clamping the patient's temperature is not at 32–33°C, additional cooling is easily obtained by 5–10 minutes of ice water lavage of the left pleural space. Even in adults, such lavage is quite effective in dropping body temperature 2–3°C within 5 or 10 minutes. In neonates and small infants, rewarming after the clamps are removed is easily accomplished with the pad (now heating rather than cooling) and by warming the ambient temperature. The rewarming process is much slower in larger patients.

Cooling to 30°C requires formal surface cooling, which is cumbersome and time-consuming in large patients and generally inadvisable for thoracic and thoracoabdominal aortic operations.

Localized Cooling of the Spinal Cord

In a set of ingenious experiments, Coles and colleagues have shown in experimental animals that localized spinal cord cooling is protective against the paraplegia of aortic cross-

clamping.[C8] In these experiments, immediately after placing clamps across the upper descending thoracic aorta just beyond the left subclavian artery, across the left subclavian artery, and across the aorta at the level of the diaphragm, cold lactated Ringer's solution (50 ml · kg^{-1} at 5°C) was infused under pressure into the isolated aortic segment over a 3-minute period. Whereas all six animals subjected to 30 minutes of this type of aortic cross-clamping at normothermia developed paraplegia or paraparesis (100%, CL 73%–100%), none (0%, CL 0%–27%) developed permanent paraplegia or paraparesis when the spinal cord was cooled by this perfusion technique. This technique is applicable to some clinical situations.

Pharmacologic Intervention

Laschinger and colleagues have presented experimental evidence that methylprednisolone (30 mg per kilogram of body weight) given just before aortic cross-clamping and 4 hours later reduces the incidence of paraplegia.[L4] The mechanism of this apparent protection is unknown.

Perfusion of the Descending Thoracic and Abdominal Aorta

Since paraplegia is a rare complication of cardiopulmonary bypass (CPB), the nonpulsatile delivery of a reduced volume of blood flow into the thoracic aorta can be expected to nourish the spinal cord sufficiently to prevent paraplegia as long as intercostal arteries critical to spinal cord blood flow do not originate from the segment of aorta exteriorized by the cross-clamps. Assuming that during CPB about one-half of the blood flow goes into the descending aorta and beyond, during aortic cross-clamping at the level of the ligamentum arteriosum, a flow of about 1 l · min^{-1} · m^{-2} into the thoracic aorta and lower body at normothermia should be adequate to prevent paraplegia. Several methods of providing this perfusion are available.

AORTO-AORTIC SHUNT. The Gott shunt can be used to perfuse the descending thoracic and abdominal aorta (GLH),[G3] or a ¼-inch silastic tubing shunt can be made less expensively from components used for CPB (UAB; Fig. 53-7). Larger shunts are not necessary. The cannulae are introduced through purse-string sutures and secured in the same way as the aortic cannulae for CPB (see Chapter 2, Section 3). The proximal end of the shunt can be placed in the transverse arch, or in the ascending aorta after the pericardium has been opened, although the exposure for the latter can be difficult. The placement of a pack under the right side of the ascending aorta is helpful in improving exposure. The proximal end of the shunt may also be placed in the left subclavian artery, facing centrally, if the aortic cross-clamp is certain to be placed distal to the origin of the subclavian artery. The proximal end of the Gott shunt has also been placed at times in the left ventricle. The distal end of the shunt may be inserted directly into the lower descending thoracic aorta or into the left femoral artery, in which case the lower thoracic and abdominal aortas are perfused retrogradely.

With the silastic shunt, the patient is given one-half the usual dose of heparin (1.5 m · kg^{-1}) before the shunt is inserted. Generally, the heparin is not neutralized with prot-

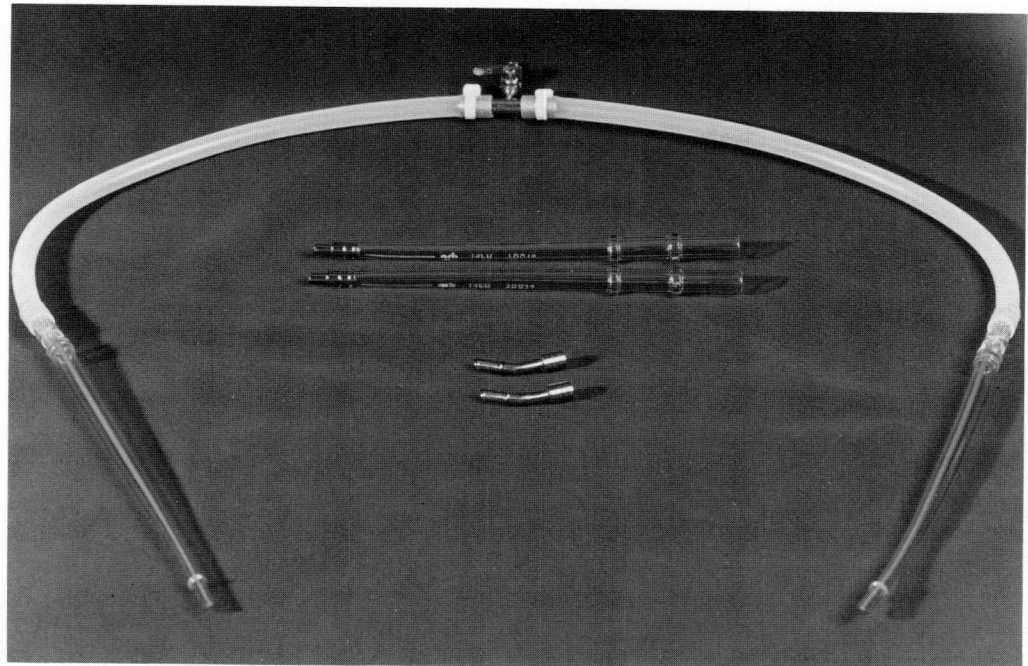

Figure 53-7 Shunt for aorto-aortic bypass (UAB). A standard aortic cannulation cannula has been affixed to each end of the ¼-inch silastic tubing. In the center are alternative cannulae for this purpose: the longer Pacifico arterial cannulae and the shorter, mildly angled cannulae. Usually clamps are placed on the tubing on both sides of the stopcock. For proximal cannula insertion, the proximal clamp is removed and the stopcock is open. The surgical nurse closes it as soon as blood appears in the silastic tubing. After the cannula is inserted and secured as is the aortic cannula for cardiopulmonary bypass, the surgeon opens the stopcock, fills the proximal tubing, and replaces the clamp proximal to the stopcock. The distal clamp is removed, the distal cannula is inserted, and again the nurse closes the stopcock when blood comes up into the silastic tubing. As soon as the aorta is cross-clamped, the clamp is removed from the proximal tubing, and the shunt is functioning.

amine at the end of the procedure. Because the Gott shunt is heparin coated, anticoagulation is not required, and intrathoracic bleeding and bleeding at other sites of injury is minimized.[A3]

FEMORO-FEMORAL BYPASS. For the procedure of femoro-femoral bypass, the femoral artery and vein are isolated through a small vertical incision in the groin, and tapes are placed around each vessel proximally. The patient is heparinized, clamps are placed proximally and distally on the femoral artery and vein, and transverse incisions are made in each. The arterial cannula is inserted, secured, attached to the arterial line of the pump-oxygenator, and de-aired. A long venous cannula (Fig. 53-8) is introduced into the femoral vein and advanced so that its tip lies in the inferior vena cava. The promontory of the sacrum is encountered as the cannula is introduced, and the cannula *must* be advanced about 3 cm beyond this point or venous drainage will be unsatisfactory. The tape is snugged around the venous cannula, and the cannula is attached to the venous line of the pump-oxygenator.

Femoro-femoral bypass is begun by starting the arterial pump at a flow rate of $0.5\ 1 \cdot min^{-1} \cdot m^{-2}$, with the perfusate temperature at 35°C, and then slowly opening the venous line. The level in the venous reservoir must not be allowed to rise over that present at the start, for this represents external

hemorrhage from the patient. To prevent this rise as venous return begins, the arterial flow is increased to the rate that keeps the reservoir level stable. A flow rate of $1.0–1.2\ 1 \cdot min^{-1} \cdot m^{-2}$ is satisfactory. If this flow rate cannot be obtained, fluid is added to the system. It may be necessary to accept a venous pressure of 12–15 mmHg.

When this technique is used, the anesthesiologist has generally placed a Swan-Ganz catheter after induction of anesthesia. During the perfusion, the anesthesiologist manipulates the cardiovascular subsystem with the aim of achieving a normal or mildly increased upper body arterial blood pressure while avoiding a left atrial (pulmonary artery diastolic) pressure above about 18 mmHg (see Chapter 4, ''Patients Undergoing Operations on the Descending Thoracic Aorta'' in Section 1).

At the end of the perfusion, decannulation is effected as usual, and the heparin reversed with protamine.

LEFT ATRIO-FEMORAL BYPASS. The use of an oxygenator is avoided with left atrio-femoral bypass, but this method is more difficult than the others to control. It may, however, be used in preference to femoro-femoral bypass in situations in which a Gott shunt is not appropriate (GLH). By its use, the occasional problems encountered with cannulation of the femoral vein and the risks of postoperative venous thrombosis can be avoided. The pericardium is opened in its upper

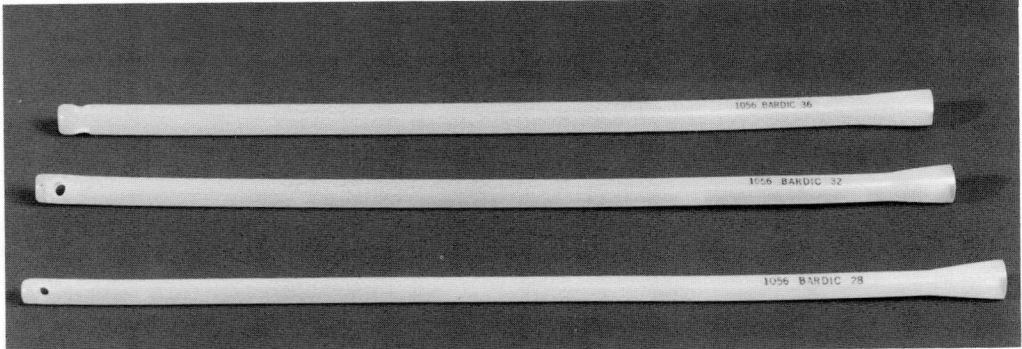

Figure 53-8   Long cannula for peripheral femoral vein cannulation for femoro-femoral bypass (UAB; venous catheters are of the Lillehei-Warden type; formerly Bardic 1056, currently USCI 007484–007296; USCI is Division of C. R. Bard, Inc.; Box 566, Billerica, MA 01821)

part in front of the phrenic nerve, and the left atrium is cannulated with a 7–8-mm cannula. Left atrial pressure is monitored by a pressure line incorporated in the cannula (see Chapter 2, Fig. 2-17). The arterial return catheter is inserted, usually into the femoral artery or into the external iliac artery (via a short transverse muscle-splitting iliac fossa incision and a retroperitoneal approach) with the tip pointing proximally. When appropriate it may be possible to insert it into the descending aorta above the diaphragm (with the tip pointing distally). The flow rate is set at approximately $1.5 \, 1 \cdot min^{-1} \cdot m^{-2}$ and left atrial pressure kept at approximately 5–8 mmHg. A disposable bubble oxygenator is incorporated in the circuit, but is used only as a reservoir unless the arterial blood becomes unsaturated.

Definition of Critical Length of Aortic Resection Using Somatosensory Evoked Potentials

When in the dog a single cross-clamp is placed just beyond the left subclavian artery, there is generally no immediate impairment of spinal cord blood flow or function or of somatosensory evoked potentials. The same is true when a second cross-clamp is placed a short distance beyond the first one. When the second cross-clamp is successively applied lower and lower on the thoracic aorta, most subjects finally exhibit immediate loss of somatosensory evoked potentials and a reduction in spinal cord blood flow. This usually occurs when the second cross-clamp is at the level of about the eighth thoracic vertebral body. Presumably, exclusion of that length of thoracic aorta between the clamps, if continued for a period of about 30 minutes, results in paraplegia, and exclusion of shorter segments does not result in paraplegia.[L3] If the longer segment of the aorta is excluded, shunting around the cross-clamp area would not help, and cooling of the body and spinal cord would seem to be the only useful protective technique.

Tailoring of the Aortic Resection and Graft

If intercostal arteries critical to spinal cord blood flow and function arise from the area of resection of a thoracic or thoracoabdominal aneurysm, the risk of paraplegia cannot be eliminated simply by techniques of spinal cord protection during the period of aortic cross-clamping. Complete protec-

tion under such circumstances also requires reestablishment of flow to the critical intercostal arteries after the period of aortic cross-clamping. Anastomosing the aortic wall around the intercostal arteries to an oval aperture in the graft is a logical way of accomplishing this, but it has not been demonstrated that this method reduces the incidence of paraplegia.[C7] Appropriate tailoring of the aneurysm resection and of the graft is another method that would seem likely to decrease the probability of postrepair paraplegia or paraparesis (see Chapter 55, Fig. 55-13).

Grafts for Use in Thoracic and Thoracoabdominal Aortic Surgery

Type of Graft
Through the years, both Teflon and Dacron grafts, knitted or woven and of various weaves, as well as homograft aorta processed in various ways, have been used as aortic replacements (see Chapter 55, "Historical Note"). Currently, Dacron grafts are used almost exclusively.

Knitted Dacron grafts have enjoyed favor in the past because of ease of handling and an allegedly thinner and more adherent neointima after insertion than with woven grafts. However, increasing numbers of operations on the aorta are being performed on heparinized patients, in whom knitted Dacron grafts allow massive hemorrhage through the graft; and newer types of woven Dacron grafts (particularly the double-velour woven Dacron graft[2]) are as soft and easy to handle and sew as are the knitted ones. Thus, currently, woven Dacron grafts have come to be the most commonly used grafts for aortic surgery, and they can be used exclusively (UAB).[C7] Woven Dacron grafts of low porosity are also available[3] and are useful in fully heparinized patients in whom even a small amount of bleeding through the graft is undesirable, but these grafts are very stiff.

---

[2] Meadox double-velour woven Dacron graft, manufactured by Meadox Medicals Incorporated, 103 Bauer Drive, Oakland, NJ 07436.

[3] Cooley low-porosity Veri-soft woven Dacron graft, manufactured by Meadox Medicals, Incorporated, 103 Bauer Drive, Oakland, NJ 07436.

Preclotting of Grafts

When using the woven double-velour graft in the thoracoabdominal or thoracic aorta in nonheparinized patients, after the proximal anastomosis is completed, the graft is clamped distally and the proximal aortic clamp released for 1–2 heartbeats and then reclosed. After a few minutes, the graft is well preclotted, the distal end is opened, and the clot and debris are removed with a sponge and sucker.

When this graft is used in heparinized patients, it is desirable to preclot it before patient heparinization by aspirating about 50 ml of the patient's blood from the heart or aorta, clamping one end of the graft and stretching it, and injecting the blood into the other end under as high a pressure as can be generated. As the blood exudes from the graft, it is collected in a small pan so that by the time the first injection is completed, the blood is reaspirated from the pan and again injected under high pressure. This process is continued until most of the blood has clotted. The graft is then set aside in a covered basin until ready for use. Before the graft is inserted, the clots are sucked or wiped out of the interior (not rinsed out with saline solution) and the device is ready for use.

It is alleged that the low-porosity graft (see footnote 3) can be used in heparinized patients without preclotting, but this is not totally reliable. Thus, this graft, too, is preclotted when used in patients who are to be heparinized, using either the simple whole blood preclotting technique just described or that of autoclaving the graft after preparing it by soaking in a 5% albumin solution or plasma (UAB), or blood (GLH).

The general technique of autoclaving as part of the preclotting process was suggested by Bethea and Reemtsma, who soaked the graft in heparinized blood before autoclaving.[B2] Cooley and associates recommend soaking the low-porosity Dacron graft (see footnote 3) in platelet-rich plasma (obtained by centrifuging heparinized blood removed from the patient) and then autoclaving the graft at 130°C for 5 minutes.[C1] Thurer and colleagues, again using the low-porosity Dacron graft, have found soaking of the graft with any albumin-containing solution (plasma or 5% albumin solution) before autoclaving to be satisfactory and more hemostatic than the traditional blood preclotting methods.[T1] Thurer has not found this technique satisfactory with other, higher-porosity woven Dacron grafts.[T2]

As an alternative to use of the rather stiff low-porosity graft, the medium-porosity woven USCI graft[4] may be employed after it is prepared by Crawford's method.[C7] This method consists of preparing the graft by stretching it over a long instrument, loosely filling it with gauze, and applying a generous coat of 5% albumin to the outside with a paintbrush or a strip of Teflon felt. The entire assembly is placed in the steam autoclave at 125°C for 3 minutes.

As could be expected, the various preclotting techniques also affect the inner surface thrombogenicity of the Dacron graft and the tendency toward thromboembolism. According to the experimental studies in dogs of Gloviezki and colleagues, with the low-porosity Dacron woven graft (see footnote 3), the area of desirable thrombus-free surface is greatest when the graft is not preclotted or when it is preclotted with blood in the standard manner.[G2] Among autoclaved grafts, those soaked with platelet-rich plasma rather than blood had the largest amount of thrombus-free surface, and this was correlated with the lowest incidence of thromboembolism. Albumin alone and platelet-free plasma were not tested.

---

[4] USCI DeBakey woven Dacron graft, catalog no. 0090. Manufactured by USCI, a division of C.R. Bard, Inc., Box 566, Billerica, MA 01821.

REFERENCES

A

1. Adams HD, Van Geertruyden HH: Neurologic complications of aortic surgery. *Ann Surg* 144:574, 1956.

2. Adamkiewicz A: Die Blutgefässe der menschlichen Rückenmarkes. *Sitsungsb d k Akad d Wissensch, Math-naturw* 85:101, 1882.

3. Akins CW, Buckley MJ, Daggett W, McIlduff JB, Austen WF: Acute traumatic disruption of the thoracic aorta: A ten-year experience. *Ann Thorac Surg* 31:305, 1981.

4. Appelbaum A, Karp RB, Kirklin JW: Surgical treatment for closed thoracic aortic injuries. *J Thorac Cardiovasc Surg* 71:458, 1976.

B

1. Bennett DE, Cherry JK: The natural history of traumatic aneurysms of the aorta. *Surgery* 61:516, 1967.

2. Bethea MC, Reemtsma K: Graft hemostasis: An alternative to preclotting. *Ann Thorac Surg* 27:374, 1979.

3. Bartsch W: *Die Durchblutung des Ruckenmarkes und ihre klinischen Storungen.* Würzburg: Hab Schrift, 1960, cited in Jellinger[35] and Piscol.[36]

4. Blaisdell FW, Cooley DA: The mechanism of paraplegia after temporary thoracic aortic occlusion and its relationship to spinal fluid pressure. *Surgery* 51:351, 1962.

5. Bodily K, Perry JF, Strate RG, Fischer RP: The salvageability of patients with post-traumatic rupture of the descending thoracic aorta in a primary trauma center. *J Trauma* 17:754, 1977.

6. Brewer LA III, Fosburg RG, Mulder GA, Verska JJ: Spinal cord complications following surgery for coarctation of the aorta: A study of 66 cases. *J Thorac Cardiovasc Surg* 64:368, 1972.

7. Berendes JN, Bredee JJ, Schipperheyn JJ, Mashhour YAS: Mechanisms of spinal cord injury after cross-clamping of the descending thoracic aorta. *Circulation* 66(suppl I):I-112, 1982.

8. Beattie EJ, Adovasio D, Keshishian JM, Blades B: Refrigeration in experimental surgery of the aorta. *Surg Gynecol Obstet* 96:711, 1953.

C

1. Cooley DA, Romagnoli A, Milan JD, Bossart MI: A method of preparing woven Dacron aortic grafts to prevent interstitial hemorrhage. *Cardiovasc Dis (Bull Tex Heart Inst)* 8:48, 1981.

2. Crafoord C: in G Ekstrom: The surgical treatment of patent ductus arteriosus: A clinical study of 290 cases. *Acta Chir Scand* 169(suppl):1, 1952.

3. Crawford ES, Rubio PA: Reappraisal of adjuncts to avoid ischemia in the treatment of aneurysms of descending thoracic aorta. *J Thorac Cardiovasc Surg* 66:693, 1973.

4. Clarke CP, Brandt PWT, Cole DS, Barratt-Boyes BG: Traumatic rupture of the thoracic aorta: Diagnosis and treatment. *Br J Surg* 54:353, 1967.

5. Cunningham JN Jr, Laschinger JC, Merkin HA, Nathan IM, Colvin S, Ransohoff J, Spencer FC: Measurement of spinal cord ischemia during operations upon the thoracic aorta: Initial clinical experience. *Ann Surg* 196:285, 1982.

6. Crawford ES, Crawford JL: *Diseases of the Aorta Including an Atlas of Angiographic Pathology and Surgical Technique.* Baltimore: Williams & Wilkins, 1984.

7. Crawford ES: (1984) Personal communication.

8. Coles JG, Wilson GJ, Sima AF, Klement P, Tait GA, Williams WC, Baird RJ: Intraoperative management of thoracic aortic aneurysm. *J Thorac Cardiovasc Surg* 85:292, 1983.

9. Cammack K, Rapport RL, Paul J, Baird WC: Deceleration injuries of the thoracic aorta. *Arch Surg* 79:244, 1959.

D

1. Djindjian R, Hurth M, Houdart M: Arterial supply of the spinal cord, in *Angiography of the Spinal Cord.* Baltimore: University Park Press, 1970, pp 3–13.

F

1. Fontan F, Chauve A, Deville Cl, Baudet E: Ruptures traumatiques de l'isthme aortique: Réparation chirurgicale. Résultats. *Chirurgie* 104:38, 1978.

2. Fleischaker RJ, Mazur JH, Baisch BF: Surgical treatment of acute traumatic rupture of the thoracic aorta. *J Thorac Cardiovasc Surg* 48:63, 1964.

G

1. Gundry SR, Burney RE, Mackenzie JR, Jafri SZ, Shirazi K, Cho KJ: Traumatic pseudoaneurysms of the thoracic aorta: Anatomic and radiologic correlations. *Arch Surg* 119:1055, 1984.

2. Gloviczki P, Hollier LH, Hoffman EA, Plate G, Trastek V, Kaye MP: The effect of preclotting on surface thrombogenicity and thromboembolic complications of Dacron grafts in the canine thoracic aorta. *J Thorac Cardiovasc Surg* 88:253, 1984.

3. Gott VL: Heparinized shunts for thoracic vascular operation. *Ann Thorac Surg* 14:219, 1972.

4. Gerbode F, Braimbridge M, Osborn JJ, Hood M, French S: Traumatic thoracic aneurysm: Treatment by resection and grafting with the use of an extracorporeal bypass. *Surgery* 42:975, 1957.

H

1. Hufnagel CA, Gross RE: Coarctation of the aorta: Experimental studies regarding its correction. *New Engl J Med* 233:287, 1945.

J

1. Jellinger K: *Zur Orthologie und Pathologie der Reckenmarksdurchblutung.* Vienna: Springer-Verlag, 1966, pp 8–41, 55–59.

2. Jahnke EJ, Fisher GW, Jones RC: Acute traumatic rupture of the thoracic aorta. *J Thorac Cardiovasc Surg* 48:63, 1964.

K

1. Katz NM, Blackstone EH, Kirklin JW, Karp RB: Incremental risk factors for spinal cord injury following operation for acute traumatic aortic transection. *J Thorac Cardiovasc Surg* 81:669, 1981.

2. Kadyi H: Über die Blutgefässe des menschlichen Rückenmarkes. Nach einer im 14, Bande der Denkschrift der Math Natur Classe der Akad der Wissenschaften in Krakau, erschienen in Monographie. *aus dem polnischen überzetzt vom Verfasser.* Gubrynowicz and Schmidt. Lemberg, 1889.

L

1. Laschinger JC, Cunningham JN Jr, Ctainella FP, Nathan IM, Knopp EA, Spencer FC: Detection and prevention of intraoperative spinal cord ischemia after cross-clamping of the thoracic aorta: Use of somatosensory evoked potentials. *Surgery* 92:1109, 1982.

2. Laschinger JC, Cunningham JN Jr, Nathan IM, Knopp EA, Cooper MM, Spencer FC: Experimental and clinical assessment of the adequacy of partial bypass in maintenance of spinal cord blood flow during operations on the thoracic aorta. *Ann Thorac Surg* 36:417, 1983.

3. Laschinger JC, Cunningham JN Jr, Isom OW, Nathan IM, Spencer FC: Definition of the safe lower limits of aortic resection during surgical procedures on the thoracoabdominal aorta: Use of somatosensory evoked potentials. *JACC* 2:959, 1983.

4. Laschinger JC, Cunningham JN Jr, Cooper MM, Kreiger K, Nathan IM, Spencer FC: Prevention of ischemic spinal cord injury following aortic cross-clamping: Use of corticosteroids. *Ann Thorac Surg* 38:500, 1984.

M

1. Miyamoto K, Keno A, Wada T, Kimoto S: A new and simple method of preventing spinal cord damage following temporary occlusion of the thoracic aorta by draining the cerebrospinal fluid. *J Thorac Cardiovasc Surg* 16:188, 1960.

2. Marsh DG, Sturm JT: Traumatic aortic rupture: Roentgenographic indications for angiography. *Ann Thorac Surg* 21:337, 1976.

P

1. Piscol K: *Die Blutversorgung des Ruckenmarkes und ihre klinische Relevanz.* Berlin: Springer-Verlag, 1972, pp 1–77.

2. Parmley LF, Mattingly TW, Manion WC, Jahnke EJ Jr: Nonpenetrating traumatic injury of the aorta. *Circulation* 17:1086, 1958.

3. Passaro E Jr, Pace WG: Traumatic rupture of the aorta. *Surgery* 46:787, 1959.

4. Pontius RG, Brockman HL, Hardy EG, Cooley DA, DeBakey ME: The use of hypothermia in the prevention of paraplegia following temporary aortic occlusion: Experimental observations. *Surgery* 36:33, 1954.

5. Parkins WM, Ben M, Vars HM: Tolerance of temporary occlusion of the thoracic aorta in normothermic and hypothermic dogs. *Surgery* 38:38, 1955.

R

1. Rice WG, Wittstruck KP: Acute hypertension and delayed traumatic rupture of the aorta. *JAMA* 147:915, 1951.

2. Rose DM, Jacobowitz IJ, Acinapura AJ, Cunningham JN Jr: Paraplegia following percutaneous insertion of an intra-aortic balloon. *J Thorac Cardiovasc Surg* 87:788, 1984.

S

1. Suh TH, Alexander L: Vascular system of human spinal cord. *Archives of Neurology and Psychiatry* 41:659, 1939.
2. Spencer FC, Zimmerman JM: The influence of ligation of intercostal arteries on paraplegia in dogs. *Surgical Forum* 9:340, 1958.
3. Stranahan A, Alley RD, Sewell WH, Kausel HW: Aortic arch resection and grafting for aneurysm employing an external shunt. *J Thorac Surg* 29:54, 1955.
4. Spencer FC, Guerin PF, Blake HA, Bahnson HT: A report of 15 patients with traumatic rupture of the thoracic aorta. *J Thorac Cardiovasc Surg* 41:1, 1961.
5. Strassman G: Traumatic rupture of the aorta. *Am Heart J* 33:508, 1947.
6. Sturm JT, Billiar TR, Dorsey JS, Luxenberg MG, Perry JF Jr: Risk factors for survival following surgical treatment of traumatic aortic rupture. *Ann Thorac Surg* 39:418, 1985.

T

1. Thurer RL, Hauer JM, Weintraub RM: A comparison of preclotting techniques for prosthetic aortic replacement. *Circulation* 66(suppl I):I-143, 1982.
2. Thurer RL: (1983) Personal communication.

V

1. Vasko JS, Raess DH, Williams TE Jr, Kakos GS, Kilman JW, Meckstroth CV, Cattanio SM, Klassen KP: Nonpenetrating trauma to the thoracic aorta. *Surgery* 82:400, 1977.

W

1. Wadouh F, Lindemann E-M, Arndt CF, Hetzer R, Borst HG: The arteria radicularis magna anterior as a decisive factor influencing spinal cord damage during aortic occlusion. *J Thorac Cardiovasc Surg* 88:1, 1984.
2. Wakabayashi A, Connolly JE: Prevention of paraplegia associated with resection of extensive thoracic aneurysms. *Arch Surg* 111:1186, 1976.
3. Wadouh F, Arndt C-F, Metzger H, Hartmann M, Wadouh R, Borst HG: Direct measurements of oxygen tension on the spinal cord surface of pigs after occlusion of the descending aorta. *J Thorac Cardiovasc Surg* 89:787, 1985.

Z

1. Zehnder MA: Delayed post-traumatic rupture of the aorta in a young healthy individual after closed injury: Mechanical-etiological considerations. *Angiology* 7:252, 1956.

3. Turney SZ, Attar S, Ayella R, Cowley RA, McLaughlin J: Traumatic rupture of the aorta: A five-year experience. *J Thorac Cardiovasc Surg* 72:727, 1976.

54

ACUTE AORTIC DISSECTION

DEFINITION

Acute aortic dissection is an event of sudden onset in which blood leaves the normal aortic channel through a usually discrete point of exit (the intimal tear) and rapidly dissects the inner from the outer layer of the media. Patients are considered to have an acute dissection when the process is less than 14 days old. (See Chapter 55 for a discussion of chronic dissection.)

HISTORICAL NOTE

Apparently, aortic dissection has been recognized since the sixteenth century,[D1] but knowledge concerning the entity has been incomplete, and through the centuries there has been confusion concerning many aspects of it. Laennec introduced the term *dissecting aneurysm* in 1826. A landmark in the development of knowledge of this entity came in 1934 with Shennan's treatise,[S3] which among other things documented that acute aortic dissection was a serious event.

Surgical approaches have been made only in the last 50 years. The early operations were indirect and consisted of the creation of a distal internal fenestration (reentry passage) or of an attempt to restore circulation directly to major branches sheared off by the dissection. Gurin and colleagues reported such procedures in 1935,[G1] as did Shaw in 1955.[S4] With the failure of these methods, the tendency toward acute rupture of the false lumen that results from acute dissection received surgical attention, and efforts were directed by Paullin and James in 1948 toward wrapping the area of dissection[P1] and by Johns in 1953 toward suturing the rupture.[J1]

The modern treatment of aortic dissection is a contribution of Michael DeBakey, who reported in 1955 the successful outcome of an operation, performed in 1954, in which the aneurysmal dilation of the false channel in the descending thoracic aorta was resected, the entry into the false channel distally oversewn, and end-to-end anastomosis performed.[D2] Subsequently, DeBakey devised the classification of aortic dissections most commonly used today (see "Morphology"). The first successful repair of chronic ascending aortic dissection with aortic incompetence was reported in 1962 by Spencer and Blake in a patient with chronic dissection,[S7] although the procedure was proposed by Bahnson and Spencer in 1960.[B1] Spencer and Blake carried out the operation used today, including suspension of the aortic valve commissure. The first successful repair of acute ascending aortic dissection with aortic incompetence was reported by Morris and colleagues in Houston in 1963.[M8] Moderate aortic incompetence persisted after the operation in that patient, and 15 years later the incompetence was severe, with moderate heart failure. Aortography showed the double lumen to persist and extend distally to the level of the aortic bifurcation. Aortic valve replacement was carried out in 1977.[L5] The patient remained well in 1985.[M10] Further successful surgical experiences with acute dissection of the ascending aorta were reported by DeBakey and colleagues in 1964.[D3]

The possibility of improving results in the management of acute aortic dissection by initial medical measures directed toward controlling arterial hypertension while maintaining adequate organ perfusion was demonstrated by Wheat and colleagues in 1965.[W1]

MORPHOLOGY

Morphologic Substrates

In many patients in whom an aortic dissection develops, the aortic wall shows only the changes that would be expected in a person of the patient's age.[D5,H1,L1,S5] Thus, it appears that, once blood is allowed to enter the aortic media, cleavage of the concentric elastic lamellar plates occurs in even an essentially normal aorta, and this event allows rapid and extensive dissection. The dissection usually proceeds distally, but it may extend proximally as well.

Medial degeneration (so-called *cystic medial necrosis*) of the aorta of a greater degree than is normal for age is present in about 20% of patients with acute aortic dissection[L1,S6] and predisposes patients to dissection. Rarely, aortitis may also be a predisposing factor.[H2]

Marfan's syndrome provides an important morphologic substrate for acute aortic dissection, with 20%–40% of patients with this syndrome developing acute dissection.[H2,R2,W2] In fact, aortic root dissection and rupture and chronic aortic regurgitation are the primary causes of reduced life expectancy in patients with Marfan's syndrome.[M9] However, many patients with Marfan's syndrome and aortic dissection exhibit no medial degeneration,[L1] and therefore this syndrome appears to be an independent risk factor for acute dissection.

A bicuspid aortic valve is associated with acute aortic dissection,[A2,E1,R3] and in the study of Larson and Edwards the process of acute dissection was found to occur nine times as frequently in patients with bicuspid as in those with tricuspid aortic valves.[L1] Possibly there is a higher incidence of congenital abnormalities of the aortic wall in persons with bicuspid than in those with tricuspid valves.[E1]

Atherosclerosis as a morphologic risk factor for the development of acute aortic dissection has been debated.[R1] Probably it is not a predisposing lesion,[L1] although rarely an intimal tear may develop in an ulcerated atheromatous plaque.

Aortic coarctation is associated with acute dissection in some patients, but probably this is because of the systemic arterial hypertension, which clearly is an important risk fac-

tor for the development of acute aortic dissection, and because of the congenital bicuspid aortic valve often present rather than the coarctation per se.[E2,R1] The role of pregnancy in the genesis of acute aortic dissection remains unresolved. Closed chest trauma may rarely result in a true aortic dissection,[R1,W2] as may aortic cannulation for cardiopulmonary bypass or a proximal coronary artery vein bypass graft anastomosis in older patients.

The Intimal Tear

Controversy exists as to whether an intimal tear is consistently present in acute aortic dissection and, thus, whether an intimal tear incites the dissection. One point of view is that rupture of aortic vasa vasorum is the inciting event and that it initiates an intramedial hemorrhage and subsequent dissection.[W2] However, Larson and Edwards found an intimal tear in each of 158 specimens personally examined,[L1] which supports the concept of the primacy of the intimal tear, a view held by Murray and Edwards[M3] and by Roberts.[R1]

The intimal tear develops commonly in the ascending aorta but also in the upper descending aorta just beyond the origin of the left subclavian artery.[B1] In the latter instance, the dissection usually proceeds only distally, but it may proceed proximally into the ascending aorta. Proximal disseciton occurred in 38% (CL 29%–47%) of autopsied cases studied by Larson and Edwards.[L1] Uncommonly, the intimal tear is in the transverse arch and, rarely, low in the descending thoracic aorta or in the abdominal aorta (Table 54-1).

The Dissection

In the few seconds in which the medial dissection occurs, the walls of any of the branches of the aorta may be involved with the dissection, may be sheared off from the lumen and be occluded by the dissection, may stay in communication with the aorta but only by the false channel, or may be

Table 54-1 Site of intimal tear in a surgical series of acute and chronic aortic dissection, based on findings on aortography and at operation (GLH; 1963–November 1984).

DeBakey Type	Site of Entry	n	%	CL
I	Ascending aorta	33	45%	38%–51%
	Proximal transverse arch	1	1%	0%–5%
II	Ascending aorta	5	7%	4%–11%
IIIa	Presumed adjacent to LSA (proximal dissection into ascending aorta)	5[a]	7%	4%–11%
IIIb	Adjacent LSA	22[b]	30%	24%–36%
	5–9 cm below LSA	6	8%	5%–13%
	Site uncertain	2	3%	1%–6%
Total		74	100%	

KEY: CL, 70% confidence limits. LSA, left subclavian artery.

[a]Surgery confined to ascending aorta.

[b]One inside aortic diverticulum (right arch with anomalous left subclavian artery), two associated with coarctation.

Table 54-2 Incidence of occlusion or significant narrowing of major branches after acute dissection involving the ascending aorta and beyond (GLH; 1963–November 1984; *n* = 39).

Major Vessel Involved	n	%	CL
To leg	10[a]	26%	18%–35%
To arm	9[b]	23%	16%–32%
Arch branch (stroke)	4	10%	5%–18%
Renal	1	3%	0%–8%
Mesenteric (infarction)	1	3%	0%–8%
Coronary (infarction)	3	8%	3%–15%

KEY: CL, 70% confidence limits.

[a]Left leg, five; right leg, three; both legs, two.

[b]Left arm, two; right arm, five; both arms, two.

uninvolved. Extension of the dissection into the branch wall is more common in the large arteries, such as the innominate, carotid, subclavian, or renal arteries, than in small ones (Table 54-2). The dissection more frequently involves the left, rather than the right, iliac artery. The extent and nature of the involvement of the branches, including the coronary and iliac arteries, is an important determinant of the clinical syndrome with which the patient presents.

A minority of patients have a discrete reentry tear at the distal end of the dissection, which puts the false channel in communication with the aortic lumen distally as well as proximally.

The False Channel

The false channel is in the outer half of the aortic media, and, as a consequence, its outer wall is thinner than the wall between the false and true channels.[R1] The false channel usually involves one-half to two-thirds of the circumference and rarely the entire wall. Although the false channel may be contained initially by the thin outer layer of media and the adventitia of the aorta, it often ruptures into the pericardium, the pleural space (usually the left), or, much less commonly, the abdomen. Even when initial rupture does not occur, blood from the false channel may extravasate through weak areas of media and adventitia to form a small or large mediastinal or pericardial hematoma. In any case, the false channel usually enlarges and produces marked increase in wall thickness and thus overall size of the involved portions of the aorta. In many instances, the aortic enlargement in the acute stage is diffuse and does not reach aneurysmal proportions. In the ensuing years, the thin outer wall of the false aneurysm tends to weaken, the channel tends to become aneurysmal, and eventually rupture may occur. Occasionally the false channel spontaneously becomes thrombosed.

Types of Aortic Dissection

DeBakey's classification of the anatomic location and extent of aortic dissections has won general acceptance (Fig. 54-1). An acceptable alternative is the Stanford classification into just two groups: dissections involving the ascending aorta (DeBakey types I and II) and those involving only the de-

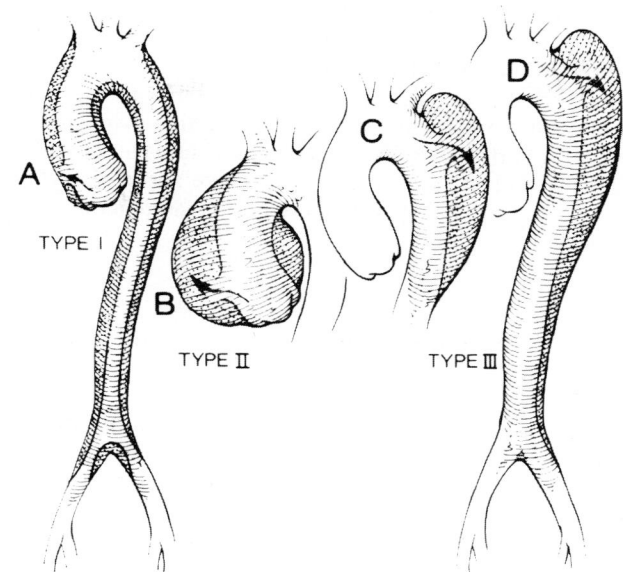

Figure 54-1 The DeBakey classification of aortic dissections (see the text for a description).

Reproduced with permission from DeBakey et al.[D1]

scending aorta with or without more distal extension (DeBakey type III).[D6] The Stanford classification, like DeBakey's, is not based on the site of the intimal tear, which may be difficult and at times impossible to identify, but rather on the portions of the aorta involved in the dissection. Both classifications take into account the fact that, although the dissection usually proceeds distally from the intimal tear, it may extend only proximally or in both directions.

In DeBakey's type I, not only is the ascending aorta involved but also the transverse arch and descending thoracic aorta. The intimal tear is usually in the anterior wall of the proximal portion of the ascending aorta. However, in a few patients with intimal tears distal to the left subclavian artery or in the transverse arch, the dissection extends proximally to involve the ascending aorta.[D1,L1] Patients with the intimal tear distal to the left subclavian artery comprise 10%–15% of those with an ascending aortic dissection.[M5] Aortic valvular incompetence and myocardial infarction may result from involvement of the proximal aorta in the dissection. In DeBakey type II dissection, only the ascending aorta is involved, and the dissection stops sharply just proximal to the innominate artery. This type of dissection may be found incidentally in operations for ascending aortic aneurysms. DeBakey's type III aortic dissection sometimes involves only the descending thoracic aorta (type IIIa) but most commonly extends into the abdominal aorta and occasionally the iliac arteries (type IIIb). In these types, the intimal tear is usually just beyond the left subclavian artery.

The proportion of patients with the various types of dissection depends on the nature of the series reported. In the large surgical series of DeBakey and colleagues containing both acute and chronic dissections (the latter is discussed in Chapter 55), type I and type II dissections constitute about 35% of the cases,[D1] while in the other surgical series of patients with dissection, they make up about 50% (GLH; table 54-1). In other clinical and autopsy series, acute dissections appear to involve the ascending aorta in 65%–85% of cases.[L1,L3] These differences may be related to the more rapid demise of patients with acute dissection involving the ascending aorta and to the promptness of surgical referral of the acute patient. Probably overall, acute aortic dissection involves the ascending aorta more often than other areas of the aorta.

CLINICAL FEATURES AND DIAGNOSTIC CRITERIA

Hemodynamic State

The presentation may be with sudden death, shortly after the onset of the dissection, the formation of the false channel, and free rupture through the thin outer wall into the pericardial, pleural, or peritoneal space. Sudden death can also follow the shearing off of the coronary arteries from their sinuses of Valsalva.

The presentation may be in hypovolemic shock of varying degrees. The shock may be the immediate result of the acute dissection when there has been loss of a moderate amount of blood from the false channel into periaortic tissues and spaces. Shock may also result from the development of acute aortic insufficiency when the dissection shears off the aortic attachment of the valve commissures, which occurs in 35%–60% of patients with acute dissection involving the ascending aorta.[L1,L4] Shock may also result from acute severe cardiac tamponade when the rupture into the pericardium temporarily seals off, as was the case in 10 (26%) of 39 patients (GLH). As time passes after the acute event, often with some lessening of the arterial hypotension, further extravasation of blood can occur from the false channel into periaortic tissues or spaces, leading to further hypovolemia and worsening of the hemodynamic state.

Aortic incompetence is usually present when the dissection involves the ascending aorta. Most often it is mild, as in 13, or 33%, of the 39 patients with acute ascending aortic dissection (GLH), but occasionally (23%) it is moderate or severe (26%).

In some patients, the hemodynamic state is reasonably good after the immediate event, and acute extravasation from the false channel or its rupture does not occur for some hours, days, or years after the acute dissection or may not occur at all. In still other patients, the acute dissection may result in no symptoms.

Symptoms and Signs

Although the dissection may be painless and at times even unknown to the patient, most patients experience sudden severe pain and a feeling of impending death. The pain is often interscapular, but it may be precordial and radiate into the neck or arms. Thus, it is at times difficult to distinguish from angina pectoris with or without acute myocardial infarction.

Once the acute dissection has occurred, there may be evidence of occlusion of a major vessel. Arch vessel occlusion causes stroke in about 10% of patients with a type I dissection coming to operation (Table 54-2). One leg (usually the left) may suddenly become numb, pale, and pulseless as the dissection occludes the iliac artery or the aortic bifurcation. Occasionally, the same process causes the pulses to disappear in an upper extremity. Uncommonly (in 2%–5% of patients[D1]), paraplegia suddenly develops as intercostal arteries are separated from the aortic lumen by the dissection (see Chapter 53, "Paraplegia," in the section on Special Situations and Controversies). Oliguria or anuria may appear with occlusion of the aortic origin of the renal arteries.

Historical Features

Many patients (80%–90%) presenting with the syndrome of acute aortic dissection are in the sixth decade of life or older and have a long history of arterial hypertension. Patients with acute dissection involving the ascending aorta tend to be younger than those with more distal dissections. The mean age of patients with ascending aortic dissections in the experience of Miller and associates was 55 ± 2 years (range 20–79 years), while that of patients with involvement of only the descending aorta and beyond was 63 ± 2 years (range 32–86 years).[M5]

Some patients have evidence of Marfan's syndrome, others develop their dissection during pregnancy, and a few have a history of coarctation or its repair (see "Morphology"). Occasionally, acute aortic dissection complicates both Turner's syndrome[S2] and Noonan's syndrome.[S1] It develops at a younger age, generally in the third or fourth decade of life, in this group of patients with specific predissection syndromes; and in them, and in younger persons in general, there is likely to be no history of hypertension, and the dissection usually originates in the ascending aorta.

Chest X-ray

In patients with acute aortic dissection, the chest x-ray frequently exhibits widening of the mediastinal shadow, particularly in its upper part and toward the left in types I and III. There may also be cardiomegaly secondary to a pericardial effusion or signs of pleural effusion, particularly in the left hemithorax. The aortic shadow is frequently prominent and unfolded.

Special Tests

Aortography is the conventional method of investigation in patients suspected of having acute aortic dissection and is usually performed whenever operation is considered. The false channel can be visualized, usually compressing the true channel, and at times, but not always, the intimal tear can be visualized (Fig. 54-2). The origin of the larger arteries from either the true or false lumen can usually be ascertained.

Examination by computed axial tomography has also been used for the diagnosis and delineation of acute aortic disease, as have two-dimensional and Doppler echocardiography.

Two-dimensional echocardiography is of particular value in identifying the intimal flap at the entry point into the false

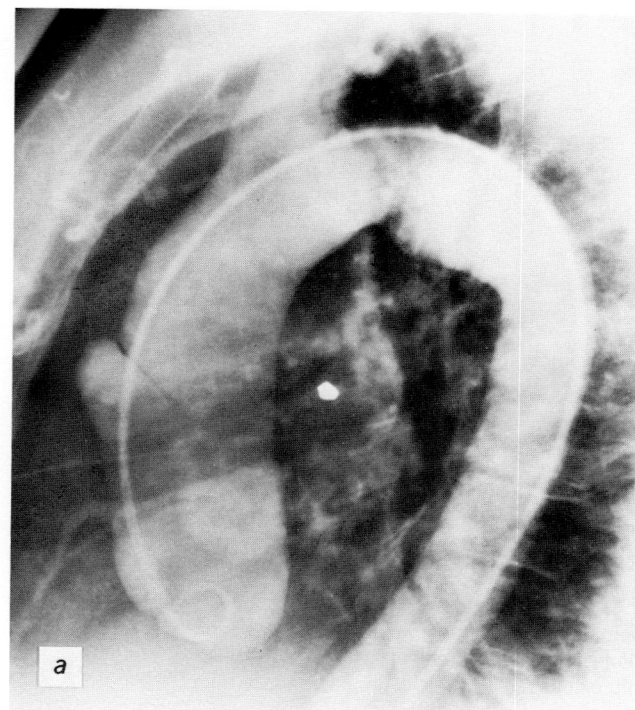

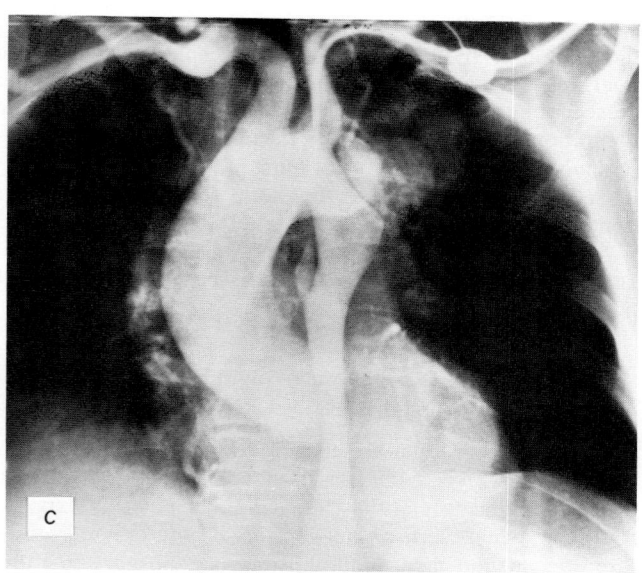

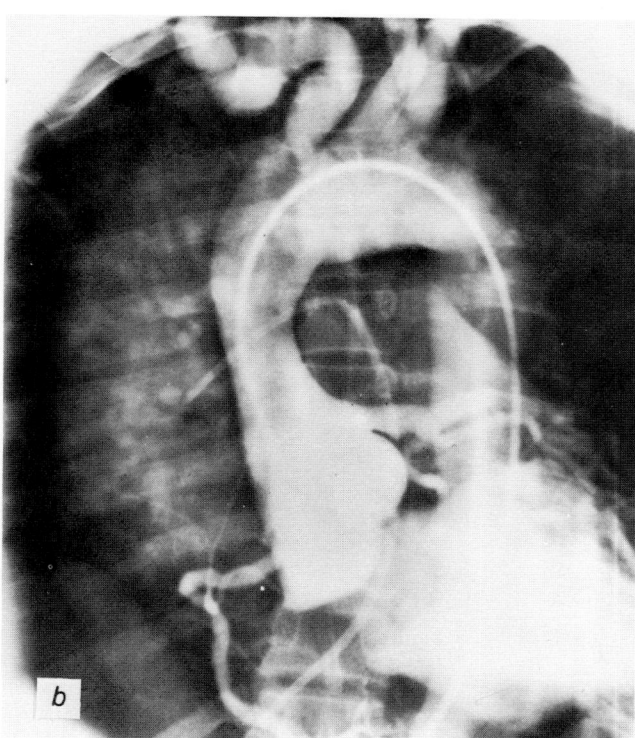

Figure 54-2 Aortography in acute aortic dissection (UAB).
(a) Aortogram (lateral view) in acute aortic dissection involving the ascending aorta. The intimal tear is evident in the anterior aspect of the ascending aorta.
(b) Acute aortic dissection involving only the ascending aorta. There is deformity of the noncoronary cusp, with aortic incompetence. The true lumen of the ascending aorta is compressed by the large false channel.
(c) Descending thoracic aortic dissection. The aortogram (frontal view) shows the true lumen compressed by the false channel, which begins just beyond the left subclavian artery and extends into the abdominal aorta.

channel, and thus in distinguishing aortic dissections from ordinary chronic aortic aneurysms.[11,M2] In fact, in patients with a classical history and an aortic diastolic murmur, operation may be undertaken without further tests when the two-dimensional echocardiographic findings identify an ascending aortic dissection.

NATURAL HISTORY

It is known that acute aortic dissection is a serious event, but a detailed portrayal of the natural history of the disease is

complicated by the great variability in the type and extent of the dissection and in the nature of the complications following it.

Survival

Overall, acute aortic dissection is highly lethal, with only about 40% of individuals surviving for 24 hours after the event.[S3] Survival for seven days occurs in only about 25% of patients, and for 90 days in only 10%.[A1,H2,S3]

Survival early after dissection is less likely in patients in whom the acute dissection involves the ascending aorta than in those in whom it is limited to the descending thoracic aorta and beyond. Thus, only about 8% of the former survive for 1 month or more after the acute dissection, compared with about 75% of the latter (Fig. 54-3).[L3]

Hypertension is an important risk factor in acute aortic dissection, in terms of both inciting the intimal tear and unfavorably affecting survival once dissection occurs.

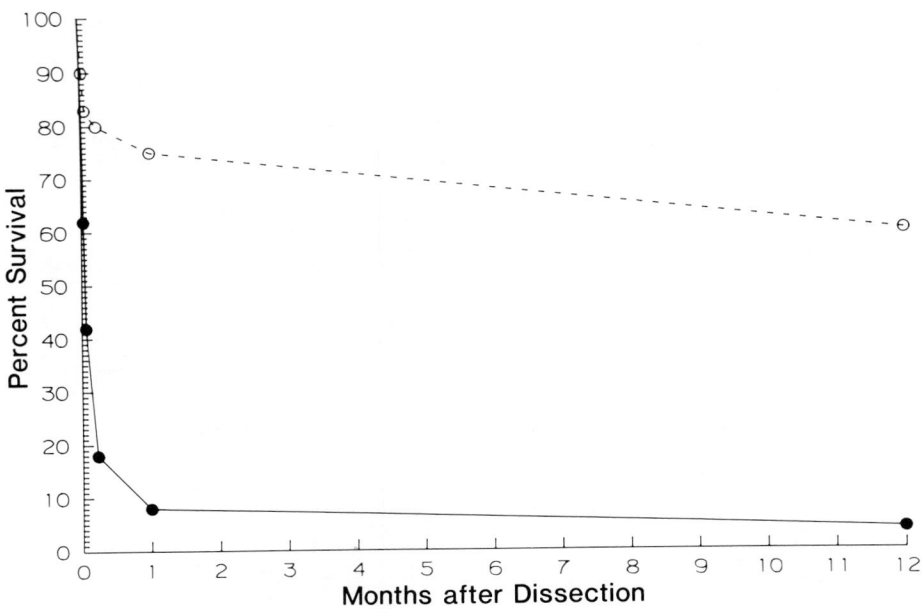

Figure 54-3 Freehand estimate of survival without surgical treatment after acute aortic dissection (solid circles, patients with ascending aortic involvement; open circles, patients with only descending aortic involvement with or without abdominal aortic extension). The estimate is based on data from the literature, primarily that of Lindsay and Hurst.[L1]

Modes of Death

Most patients who die acutely succumb from false channel rupture and consequent hemopericardium, hemomediastinum, or hemothorax. Deaths later in the early period after dissection may result from delayed rupture or organ dysfunction secondary to arterial occlusions.

Course after Survival from Acute Dissection

Persons who survive the acute dissecting episode continue to be at greater risk of dying than the general population. This is because the false channel generally persists (see "Morphology" and "Results") and usually gradually becomes aneurysmal and then ruptures months or years after the acute episode. Also, a new dissection (redissection) may occur in a previously uninvolved segment or portion of the wall of the aorta and present new risks to the patient.

TECHNIQUE OF OPERATION

Purpose of Surgical Treatment

The operation for acute aortic dissection is performed to prevent death of the patient from exsanguination and less frequently to reestablish blood flow in areas that have been occluded by the dissection. The operation must not isolate the false from the true lumen when important branches arise only from the false lumen. Areas of actual or impending rupture of the false channel need to be included in the resection, but no attempt is made to remove the entire distal false channel. Thus, the operation for acute aortic dissection does

not eliminate the disease process, except in patients with DeBakey type II dissections and those localized to the upper descending thoracic aorta (DeBakey type IIIa). Also, the operation should either remove the ascending aorta or, if it is uninvolved, isolate it from a more distal dissection, since false channels of the ascending aorta seem to have greater tendency to rupture than do those in the descending aorta.

The operative technique is based on the knowledge that after an acute dissection the aortic tissues are friable and of poor quality.

Repair of Acute Dissection Involving the Ascending Aorta

The usual preparations are made for operations in which cardiopulmonary bypass (CPB) is used (see Chapter 2, Section 3).

The femoral artery that has a normal pulse is exposed through a small vertical incision, or, if both femoral pulses are present, the right femoral artery is exposed, since it is more frequently spared from acute dissection. A median sternotomy is made, the pericardium is opened, and stay sutures are placed. The often hemorrhagic and distorted ascending aorta is not disturbed at this point. If easily done, a left atrial polyvinyl recording catheter is placed. A right atrial purse-string suture is placed for the single venous cannula (see Chapter 2, Section 3). An appropriately sized but not too large woven Dacron graft is selected and prepared (see Chapter 53, "Grafts for Use in Thoracic and Thoracoabdominal Aortic Surgery," in section on Special Situations and Controversies).

After heparinization, the femoral artery is cannulated. The femoral artery is used because it is difficult to be certain of getting a cannula into the true lumen of the distal ascending or transverse portion of the aortic arch in a patient with an acute dissection. A single venous cannula is inserted (see Chapter 2, Section 3), and CPB is established at 25°C. If severe aortic incompetence is present, a left atrial vent is often inserted and advanced into the ventricle (see Chapter 2, Section 3), although this is not necessary. A very limited dissection is made around the ascending aorta, just proximal to the origin of the innominate artery, and the aorta is cross-clamped at this point (Fig. 54-4). A longitudinal incision is made at a convenient site in the ascending aorta, and the

interior is examined. Often it becomes evident that the incision has been made into the false lumen (which is frequently anterior and to the right of the true lumen), in which case the true lumen is now opened. The cold cardioplegic solution is infused directly into the left and right coronary ostia (see Chapter 3), and this infusion is repeated about every 30 minutes. Stay sutures are applied to retract the aortic wall.

If one or more commissures of the aortic valve cusps have been separated from the outer aortic wall by the acute dissection, with consequent cusp prolapse, a pledgetted 4-0 polypropylene suture on a large needle is used to place a

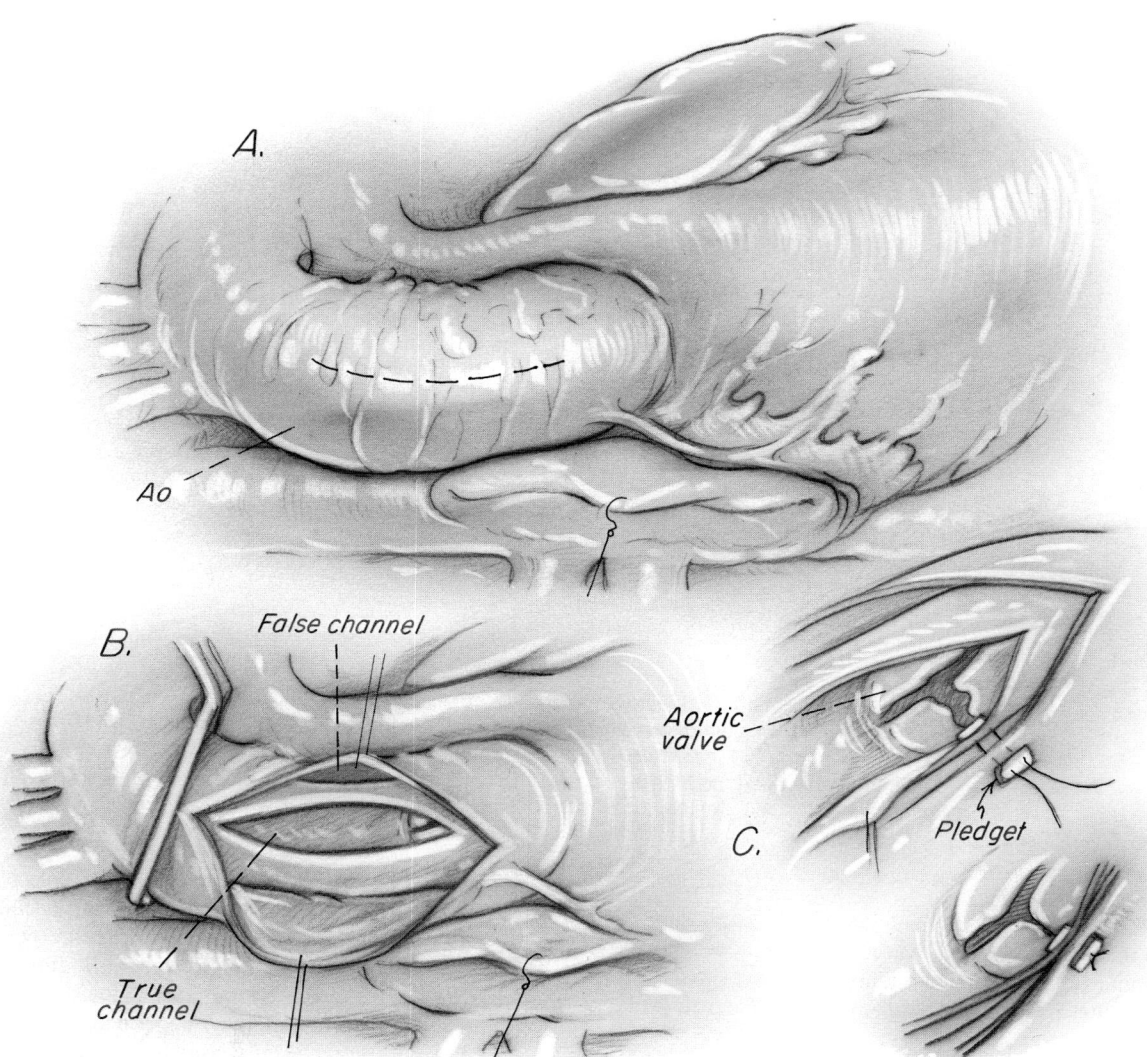

Figure 54-4 Repair of acute dissection of the ascending aorta with aortic incompetence by the interposition technique.

(a) The proposed line of incision into the enlarged and dissected ascending aorta.

(b) After cardiopulmonary bypass has been established, a clamp is placed across the aorta just proximal to the origin of the innominate artery. A longitudinal incision has been made into the ascending aorta and the cold cardioplegic infusion infused directly into the left and right coronary ostia. The true and false channels are visualized.

(c) A pledgetted mattress suture is used to bring the wall between the true and false lumen back against the outer aortic wall and thus to support the commissure between the right and noncoronary cusps.

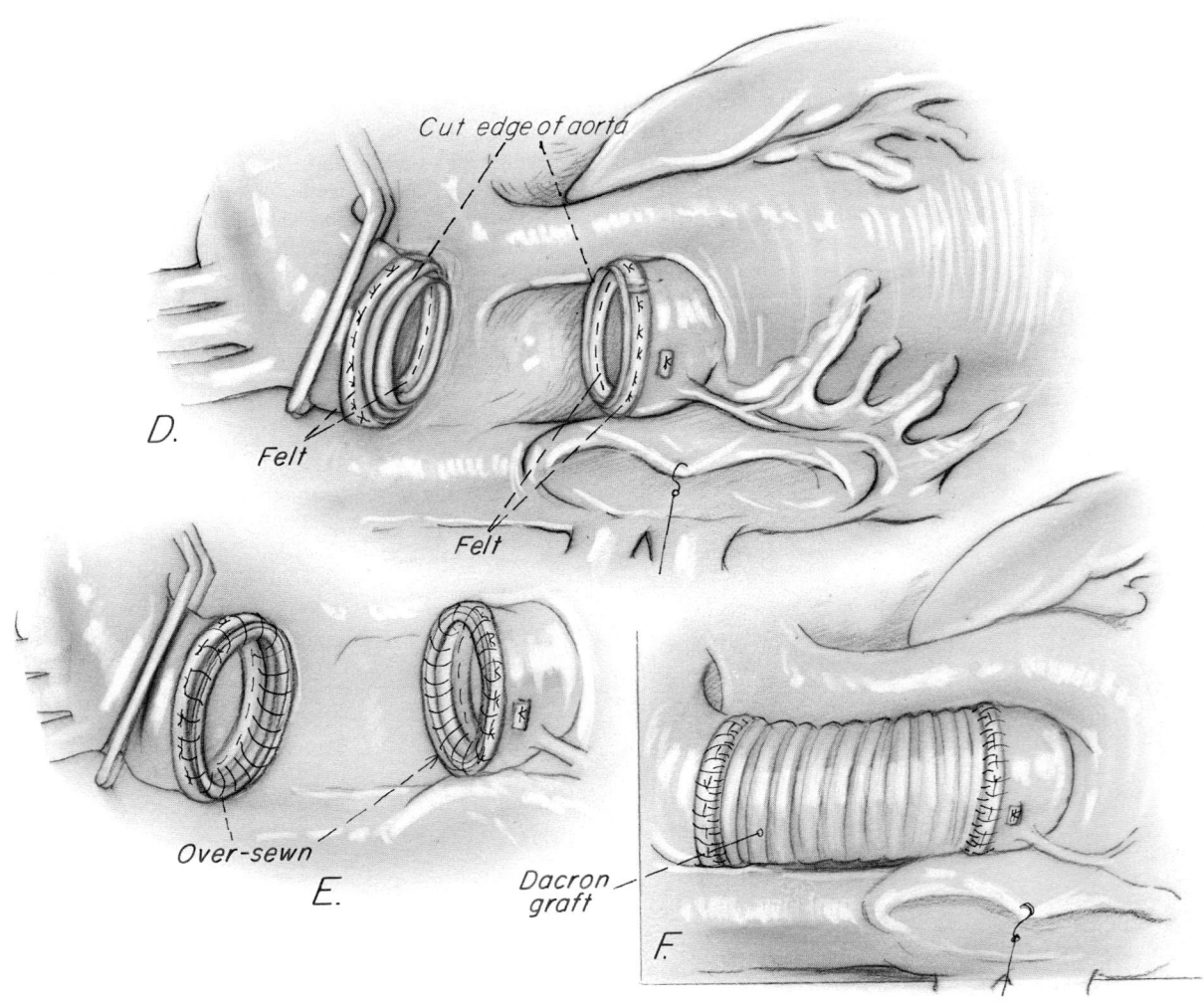

Figure 54-4   (continued)

(d) The aorta has been transected proximally and distally and each end treated by an inner and outer felt bolster sewn into place with interrupted mattress sutures. Note that the cut end of the aortic walls extends at least to the edge of the felt strips and preferably a little beyond.

(e) A whip stitch has been used to further prepare the proximal and distal end.

(f) A preclotted woven Dacron graft has been interposed between the two ends to reestablish aortic continuity.

Ao, aorta.

mattress suture across each affected commissure and through the aorta to be tied over a large felt pledget (Fig. 54-4). A similar repair is carried out around any coronary artery orifice that has been separated from the outer aortic wall by the dissection.

The aorta just proximal to the cross-clamp is examined. If the dissection ends before this point (DeBakey type II), the entire area of dissection is included in the repair. If, as is usual, the dissection extends distal to the cross-clamp, no effort is made to go further distally in the repair, except in a patient in whom the transverse arch has been shown to be a site of impending rupture, in which case the repair is extended to include this area (see Chapter 55, "Repair of Transverse Arch Aneurysms" in section on Technique of Operation).

The repair is effected by replacing the ascending aorta with a Dacron tube graft using either the interposition or the inclusion technique. With either method, after the proximal anastomosis is completed and part of the distal anastomosis is in place, the perfusion flow rate is reduced to $0.5 \, \text{l} \cdot \text{min}^{-1} \cdot \text{m}^{-2}$ and the aortic clamp momentarily released. If the flow is coming back through the true lumen, the clamp is replaced and the anastomosis completed. If the flow is coming back through the false lumen, action must be taken because completion of the suture line will not allow ascending aortic and coronary reperfusion with release of the cross-clamp or perfusion of any branches that may arise only from the false lumen after forward aortic flow is reestablished. Therefore, the cross-clamp is replaced; the perfusion is returned to full flow, still at 25°C; the patient is placed in Trendelenburg's position; the innominate and left common carotid arteries are identified and clamped (this step is probably not essential and may be omitted if difficult); CPB is virtually discontinued; and the cross-clamp is released.

At this point, two tested options are available. In one, a large V is excised from the septum between the true and false lumens to create a window to allow continued perfusion of both lumens after the repair. After the clamp is replaced, perfusion is recommenced, and the distal anastomosis is completed, with suturing only to the outer aortic wall in the area of excision. The disadvantage of this option is that the suture line is weakened at the site of the V excision, and continued free flow into the false channel is assured, with possible compression of the true lumen. The advantage is free flow into both channels after the repair, and this option may be advised as a routine in this situation (GLH). A second option is to complete the anastomosis, bring a $\frac{2}{16}$-inch Tygon tube as a side arm from the connector to the arterial cannula and attach to it a large-bore needle, and insert the needle into the graft (UAB). Without releasing the aortic cross-clamp, coronary perfusion is begun with perfusion into the graft through the needle. After the heart is beating well, the aortic clamp is gradually released as suction is placed on the aortic needle vent. The operation is completed in the usual manner. The disadvantage of this method is potential coronary and systemic air embolization, since the usual de-airing procedures are difficult, and possibly nonperfusion of branches that come solely from the false lumen. The advantages are good perfusion of the true lumen and security of the distal anastomosis, and the method may be advised as a routine in this situation (UAB).

After one of these maneuvers and the reestablishment of full flow, the patient is taken out of Trendelenburg's position. Rewarming with the perfusate is begun as the distal anastomosis is completed. The left atrial (or ventricular) vent, if present, has been turned off a few minutes previously and the left ventricle and graft allowed to fill with blood. A small slit is made in the graft, air is aspirated from the tip of the left ventricle, and the aortic clamp is gradually released while the graft is massaged to encourage air to exit through the slit. Since the aortic valve may still be mildly incompetent, the left ventricle is closely observed for distention; if distention develops, the vent is again placed on suction. The heart is defibrillated if necessary, and after a good cardiac action has been restored, the usual de-airing procedures are followed (see Chapter 2, Section 3).

The remainder of the operation is completed as usual. The circulation in the extremities, the presence of urine flow, and the integrity of the carotid pulses are verified before the patient leaves the operating table. If they are not satisfactory, aortographic studies are performed immediately, and, if necessary, remedial action is taken.

Interposition Method of Graft Insertion

First described by Austen and colleagues[A5] and currently used by Crawford[C1] and others, the interposition method of graft insertion is simple, and the anastomoses are usually completely hemostatic.[C1] This method requires a securely preclotted graft (see Chapter 53, "Grafts for Use in Thoracic

and Thoracoabdominal Aortic Surgery" in section on Special Situations and Controversies).[C1,C2] It is currently the method used routinely (UAB and GLH). After the ascending aorta and false lumen are opened, cardioplegia is administered, and the aortic commissures are resuspended if necessary and the aorta is transected about 1–2 cm distal to the level of the valve commissures, well beyond the coronary ostia. Dissection around the aorta before its transection is not necessary, and what little mobilization of the aortic wall is necessary proximal to the transection is more easily performed as the transection proceeds (see Fig. 54-4). Two Teflon felt strips are cut to a length a little longer than the circumference of the aorta at this point. One is placed outside the aorta and the other within the true lumen. Six to 8 pairs of interrupted mattress sutures are placed from without, passing through the external felt strip, the outer wall of false channel, the inner wall, and the inner felt strip and then returning to the outside. Each is tied and held in a clamp. The purpose of these interrupted sutures is to minimize any tendency of this preparation of the cut end of aorta to narrow the aortic lumen. As the sutures are placed, it is essential that all parts of the aortic wall protrude from between the strips (see Fig. 54-4). A whip stitch of 3-0 or 4-0 polypropylene suture is now placed around the circumference (see Fig. 54-4). The graft can be prepared and autoclaved while the proximal aorta is being prepared, and, if it is not yet ready, the distal aortic cuff is similarly prepared. The proximal anastomosis between the autoclaved graft and prepared aorta is made (Fig. 54-4). The aorta is now transected distally, if that has not yet been done, with the transection comfortably proximal to the cross-clamp. The distal end is prepared in the same fashion as was the proximal end. The graft is now trimmed to a proper length, and the distal anastomosis is made. The intervening aortic wall tissue does not need to be excised and can still be used to wrap the graft if bleeding through it is a problem. The remainder of the procedure is completed as described earlier.

Inclusion Technique of Graft Insertion

The inclusion technique (see Chapter 55, "Historical Note") has also been used for acute ascending aortic dissections (UAB). The proximal anastomosis is made first, fashioned so that the graft will lie within the true lumen of the ascending aorta. In preparation for this, a circumferential dissection is made around the aorta at this level. Sutures are placed from the outside through the outer wall of the false channel, through the inner wall between false channel and true lumen, and into the true lumen. These may be continuous mattress sutures of 2-0 or 3-0 polypropylene placed over a circumferential external felt strip and continuing as an everting mattress suture through the graft; or, if it seems easier, interrupted felt-pledgetted mattress sutures are placed from the outside in an entirely similar manner, to be tied from within. The suturing is usually begun to the left and posteriorly, and if interrupted sutures are used, four or five are placed before being tied.

If dissection and external placement of sutures through the aorta are not possible, the suturing is done from within with either a continuous mattress suture over a felt strip inside the

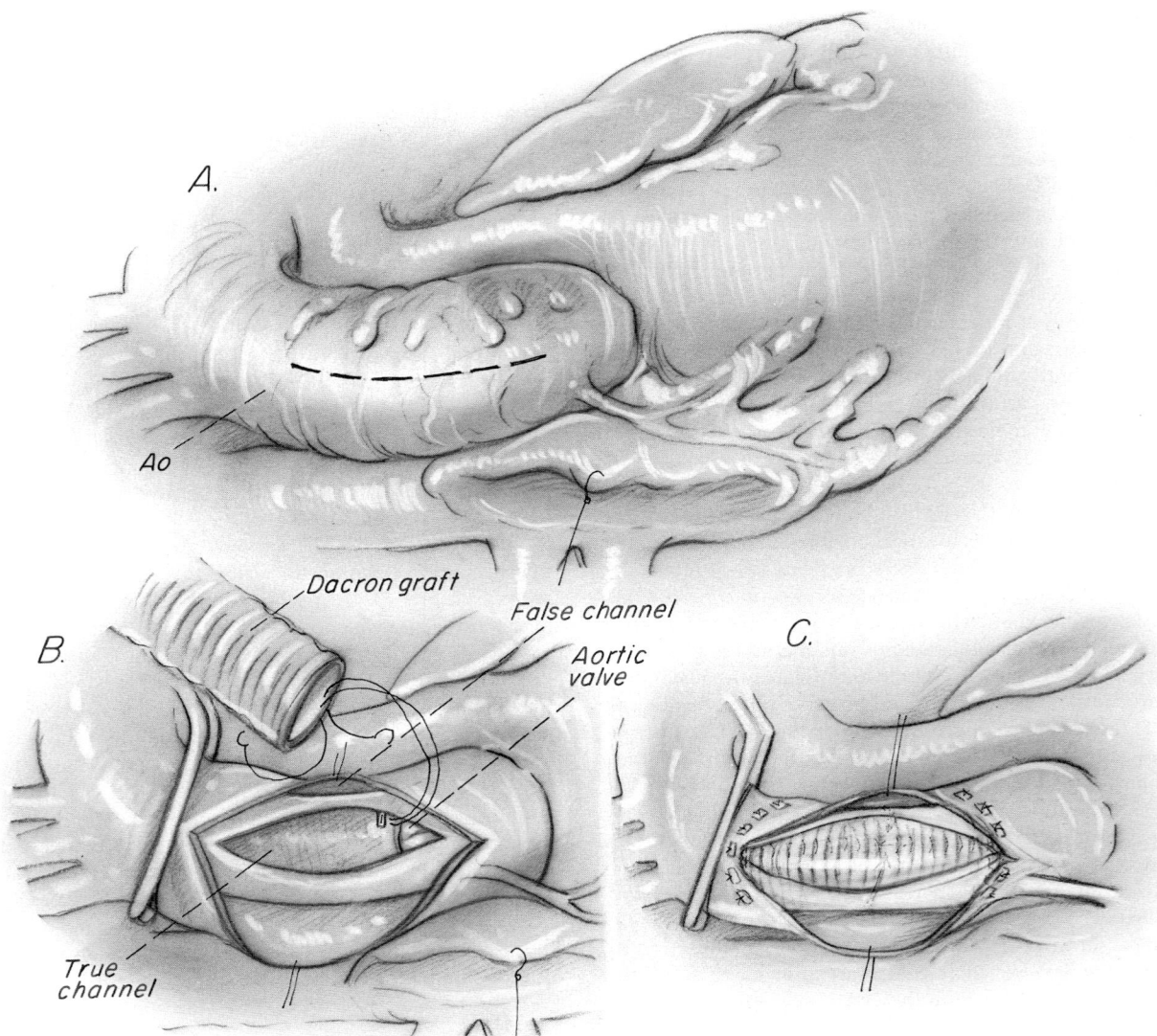

Figure 54-5 Alternative method of repair of acute ascending aortic aneurysms using the inclusion technique.
(a) The dashed line indicates the proposed longitudinal incision in the diffusely enlarged ascending aorta.
(b) Cardiopulmonary bypass is established, the aorta cross-clamped just proximal to the origin of the innominate artery, the longitudinal incision made, and the cold cardioplegic infusion given directly into the coronary ostia. A preclotted woven Dacron tube graft is sutured into place proximally (see the text for a description of the several methods for doing this).
(c) The method of placing sutures from within the true lumen. Posteriorly and laterally the sutures are placed from within the true lumen but grasping all layers. Anteriorly the pledgetted mattress sutures are placed from without. The distal anastomosis is made in a similar fashion. After the aortic cross-clamp is removed, the outer wall and that between the false and true channels are wrapped together around the graft and sutured together to complete hemostasis.
Ao, aorta.

aorta or interrupted felt-pledgetted mattress sutures (Fig. 54-5).

The graft is then cut to a proper length, and a similar distal anastomosis is made (Fig. 54-5). As described earlier, rewarming is begun, the aortic clamp is released, de-airing is accomplished, and the suture lines are inspected and made hemostatic. After CPB is discontinued, the aortic walls are

sutured around the graft to complete hemostasis. The operation is completed as described earlier.

Intraluminal Sutureless Prosthesis
Method of Graft Insertion
Some enthusiasm has developed for use of an intraluminal sutureless prosthesis in the treatment of both acute and

chronic dissection of both the ascending and descending aorta.[B2] Such prostheses were independently devised and used for this purpose by Dureau and colleagues,[D4] Ablaza[A3] and colleagues, and Lemole and associates.[L2]

A woven Dacron tube graft with a felt-covered metal spool at each end is manufactured for use with this technique. Nylon tapes are placed around the aorta just beyond each extremity of the proposed incision. After the aorta is clamped above and below, it is opened longitudinally. The device is slipped inside, and the tapes are tied down on the groove of the proximal and distal spool. The clamps are released.

The technique is basically that described by Carrel in 1912[C3] and used by Hufnagel in 1951 for his aortic valvular prosthesis placed in the upper descending thoracic aorta.[H3] Its disadvantages are that it cannot be used near coronary ostia or the orifice of large arterial branches of the aorta and that at times it can be extremely difficult to insert. It has the theoretical advantage that it shortens the length of the operation and avoids bleeding from graft suture lines. One of the seven patients so treated has required reoperation for severe recurrent aortic incompetence (this lesion was mild preoperatively) due to transection of the inner layer of the dissection at the proximal ligature (GLH). Another patient has important recurrent aortic incompetence and may require reoperation. This suggests that resuspension of the valve is less good with this technique, and the intraluminal sutureless prosthesis is no longer used when there is aortic valve incompetence.

Combined Ascending Aorta and Aortic Valve Replacement

Occasionally in patients with acute aortic dissection when resuspension of the aortic valve is inadequate (this is judged after the proximal graft suture line has been completed when the interposition technique is used) and particularly when the aortic anulus shows marked dilatation, combined ascending aorta and aortic valve replacement may be required. Also, the aortic valve may require replacement because it is structurally abnormal or diseased. Occasionally such replacement is accomplished by the Bentall method, and then the technique is similar to that described earlier (see Chapter 12, "Composite Graft Replacement of Aortic Valve and Ascending Aorta" in section on Technique of Operation, and Chapter 12, "Combined Aortic Incompetence and Ascending Aortic Aneurysm" in section on Special Situations and Controversies). However, since the distal anastomosis usually is made to a dissected aortic segment, the technique described in "Interposition Method of Graft Insertion" is often applicable. More commonly, in acute dissections the two parts of the operation are accomplished separately; the valve replacement is done first with the method used for isolated aortic valve replacement (see Chapter 12, "Technique of Operation"), and then the ascending aorta is replaced by the interposition method. One reason for preferring this approach in this situation is that the coronary anastomoses of the Bentall procedure can be difficult in patients with acute dissection, in whom the coronary ostia remain deep in the sinuses of Valsalva.

Repair of Acute Dissection Involving Only the Descending Thoracic Aorta and Beyond

The preparations for repair of acute dissection involving only the descending thoracic aorta and beyond are the same as those used for operations for acute aortic transection (see Chapter 53) and for aneurysm of the thoracic aorta (see Chapter 55 and Chapter 4), including organizing the method for retrieving aspirated blood and returning it as washed red blood cells to the patient. The room is cooled to about 60°F, and no attempt is made to keep the patient warm.

A long left posterolateral thoracic incision is made, and the thorax is entered through the top of the bed of the non-resected fifth rib. The rib spreader is inserted and opened gradually until a wide exposure is obtained. The lung is covered with a moist gauze and held forward with a malleable retractor. Often there is an extensive mediastinal hematoma, and the mediastinal pleura is opened only where the cross-clamps are to be placed.

From this point on, the operation is quite variable and depends on the individual situation as found at thoracotomy. When, as is usual, the operation is being done for a *complication* of acute aortic dissection, a 15-cm or longer segment of upper descending aorta, including areas of impending rupture, may need to be resected. However, every effort is made to limit the resection to as short a segment of the upper descending thoracic aorta as possible. The initial cross-clamps are placed across the distal transverse arch between left common carotid and left subclavian arteries, across the left subclavian artery, and across the descending aorta just beyond the proposed area of resection. After the aorta is opened, the clamps on the transverse arch and on the left subclavian artery are replaced, if possible, with a single aortic cross-clamp, placed just beyond the origin of the left subclavian artery (because of the disadvantages related to paraplegia of clamping the left subclavian artery).[1] The distal clamp should be placed as close to the proximal clamp as is consistent with removing areas of actual or impending rupture and good operating conditions, again with the purpose of minimizing the incidence of paraplegia.

Before the clamps are placed, and in the absence of the need for urgent aortic cross-clamping, the left chest is lavaged with ice cold saline solution for 5–10 minutes to reduce body temperature to about 33°C (UAB). Consideration is given to still further reducing spinal cord temperature by infusing under pressure into the aortic segment isolated by the cross-clamps about 2,000 ml of lactated Ringer's solution at 5°C over a 3-minute period (UAB). With these maneuvers for obtaining general and local spinal cord hypothermia, 45 minutes of aortic cross-clamping without paraplegia or paraparesis should be possible if arteries critical for the spinal cord are not sacrificed in the resection. If the need for a longer cross-clamp time is anticipated, femoro-femoral bypass is used (UAB).

---

[1] The details of paraplegia as a complication of the operation, and of the techniques used for minimizing its occurrence, as well as the details concerning selection of an appropriate type of graft and methods for preclotting it, are given in Chapter 53 in section on Special Situations and Controversies.

Alternatively, preparations are made routinely to provide flow beyond the distal aortic cross-clamp, based on the knowledge that in this group of patients the repair is frequently time-consuming (GLH). A left atrial-femoral artery bypass is positioned, or if cannulation of the transverse or even ascending aorta (from within the pericardium) is felt to be safe because a dissection at these levels is known not to be present, a Gott shunt is used.

After the aorta is opened longitudinally, the posterior aortic wall origin of the intercostal arteries is inspected. If this area is not involved in the dissection, it is not included in the resection, and the graft is appropriately contoured for the anastomosis (Fig. 54-6). Then the interposition technique of reconstruction is usually used. This technique is particularly advantageous since in the patients being operated on with a selective approach to surgery for acute dissection, the aorta is generally of very poor quality. Even though the patient is not heparinized, the graft is preclotted. If the proximal anastomosis is to undissected aorta, the inclusion technique of reconstruction rather than the interposition technique may be used (Fig. 54-7). The intraluminal sutureless prosthesis method of graft insertion may also be used in this location (see "Repair of Acute Dissection Involving the Ascending Aorta").

The technique of the operation may have to be modified according to the special circumstances of the pathologic condition encountered. Some of the maneuvers described for managing some of the problems in the repair of acute traumatic aortic dissection are applicable in this setting as well (see Chapter 53, "Technique of Operation").

When the dissection extends beyond the distal aortic clamp and major branches are known to arise from the false lumen, or if this information is not available, steps to ensure

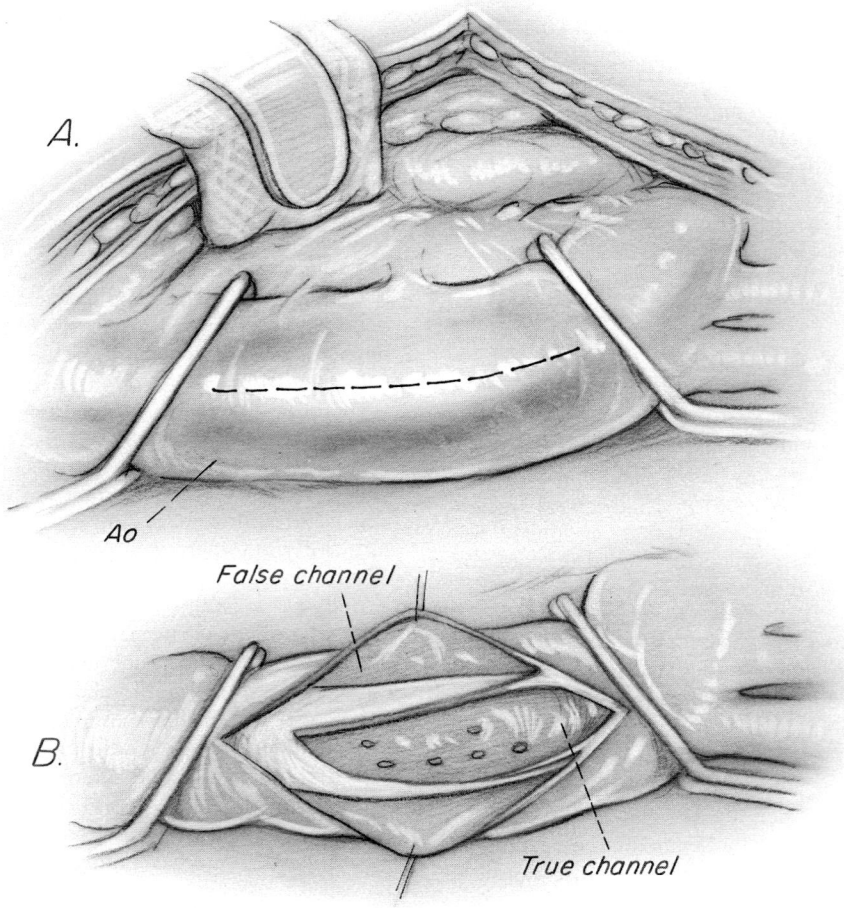

Figure 54-6 Repair of acute dissection of the descending thoracic aorta by the interposition technique.

(a) Through a left thoracotomy incision and after appropriate arrangements for protection of the spinal cord (see the text), the aorta is clamped just beyond the left subclavian artery at about the midportion of the descending thoracic aorta. The proposed longitudinal incision is indicated by the dashed line.

(b) The incision has been made with the electrocautery. Just beyond the proximal cross-clamp, the aortic wall is not dissected. More distally, the true channel is seen surrounded for the most part by a large false channel with a thin wall between it and the true channel. The external wall is also often very thin.

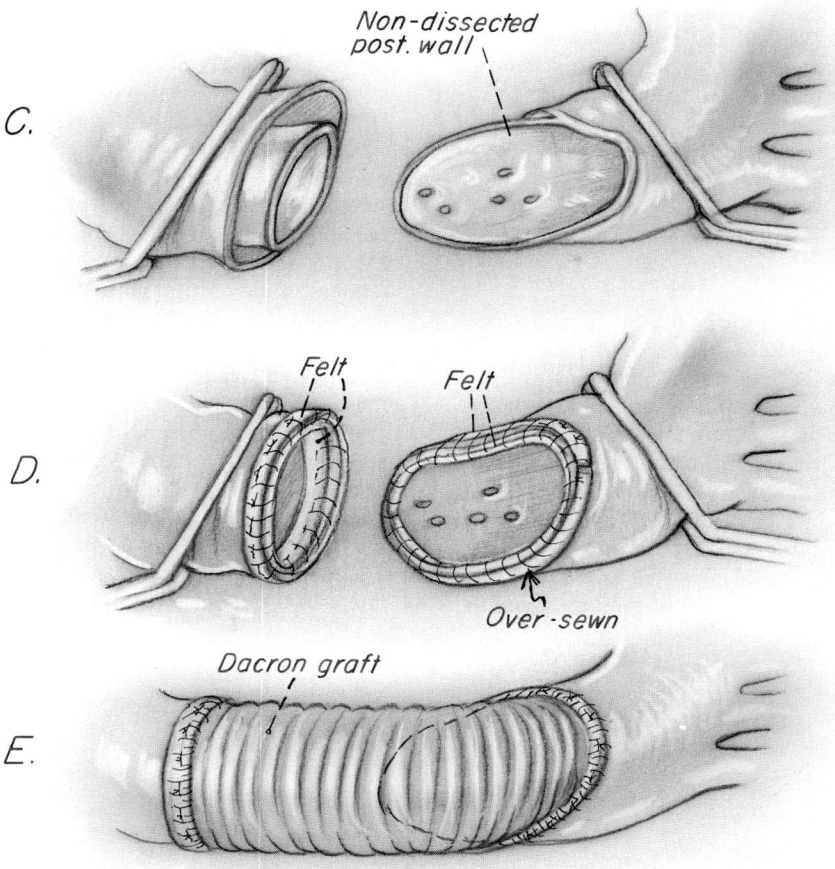

Figure 54-6 (continued)
(c) A segment of upper descending thoracic aorta about 10 cm in length has been resected. Whenever possible, a posterior tongue is left proximally in order to avoid sacrificing any more intercostal arteries than absolutely necessary.
(d) The proximal and distal ends are prepared with felt strips in the same manner as in the repair of acute dissection of the ascending aorta (see Fig. 54-4).
(e) Continuity is reestablished with a preclotted woven Dacron graft (see text for details).
Ao, aorta.

free communication between true and false lumens distal to the lower anastomosis are used (GLH; see "Repair of Acute Dissection Involving the Ascending Aorta").

It is to be noted that no emphasis is placed on removal of the site of the intimal tear, although this is done whenever convenient. Miller and colleagues have shown that the results are not affected by whether this area is included in the repair.[M1,M5] It is considered important to include the most *proximal* extent of the dissection in the repair so as to seal off the dissecting process from the ascending aorta, which seems particularly vulnerable to rupture when dissected.

After the anastomoses are completed by whatever technique is used, the distal clamp is removed and the suture lines are inspected for bleeding. The proximal clamp is then slowly removed while the anesthesiologist maintains the hemodynamic state of the patient in as good condition as possible. After time has passed and the wound is reasonably dry, the aortic shell is sutured around the graft.

Two catheters are left for temporary drainage, and the thoracotomy incision is closed in the usual manner.

SPECIAL FEATURES OF POSTOPERATIVE CARE

Early postoperatively, the care is that used after other types of major cardiovascular operations (see Chapter 5). Of particular importance is the prevention of arterial hypertension, since this predisposes the patient to early redissection or rupture of the retained false channel.

Long-term follow-up is mandatory for all patients who have experienced an acute aortic dissection, whether treated surgically or medically. One purpose is long-term pharmacologic control of arterial hypertension, since it has been shown that this prolongs survival, reduces the incidence of late aneurysm development in the false channel, and minimizes the incidence of new dissection (see "Results").

A second purpose of long-term follow-up of such patients is identification of enlarging aneurysms of the false channel so that they may be resected before they become unduly large and rupture. Thus, a chest x-ray, including a lateral film, is obtained at hospital dismissal in addition to examination by computed tomography to serve as a baseline for subsequent examinations, which are repeated every 3 months during the first postoperative year and every 6 months thereafter. Careful abdominal palpation and, if suspicion is aroused, ultrasound examination, will detect aneurysms developing below the diaphragm.

RESULTS

Hospital Mortality

The hospital mortality after the repair of acute aortic dissection generally does not approach zero even in the current era, indicating the seriousness of this condition.

In acute dissections involving the *ascending aorta,* hospital mortality has varied between about 20% and 40% (Tables 54-3, 54-4).[D1,M5] In the current era, the hospital mortality may be lower, being between 10% and 30% in reported series.[C1,C5,M5] Under proper circumstances and in the current era, the hospital mortality can now be very low, with 1 death (4%, CL 1%–13%) occurring in 24 patients (GLH-Table 54-4). In the case of involvement *limited to the de-scending aorta and beyond,* hospital mortality varies according to the indications for operation. When operation is performed as a routine in such cases, the mortality can be as low as 10%.[M1] When it is limited to those with complications of the acute dissection (GLH, UAB), mortality is 25% to 60% (Tables 54-3, 54-4).[C2]

Within the group of patients operated on acutely in earlier series, the risk of hospital death increased with a decrease in the interval between the dissection and the operation.[D1] Preoperative aortic rupture, loss of peripheral pulses, loss of renal or other visceral perfusion, older age, preoperative angina, congestive heart failure, and preoperative renal dysfunction have all been said to increase the risk of hospital death after repair of acute aortic dissection.[M1] However, these factors do not necessarily increase risk, as older age at operation has not been a risk factor in ascending aortic dissections (GLH; Table 54-5). Operation early after the dissection is, also, not necessarily a risk factor. Thus, the median interval between dissection and operation from 1980 to the present has been 18 hours in patients with ascending aortic dissection, and all patients operated on between 4 and 16 hours of the onset of rupture have survived (GLH).

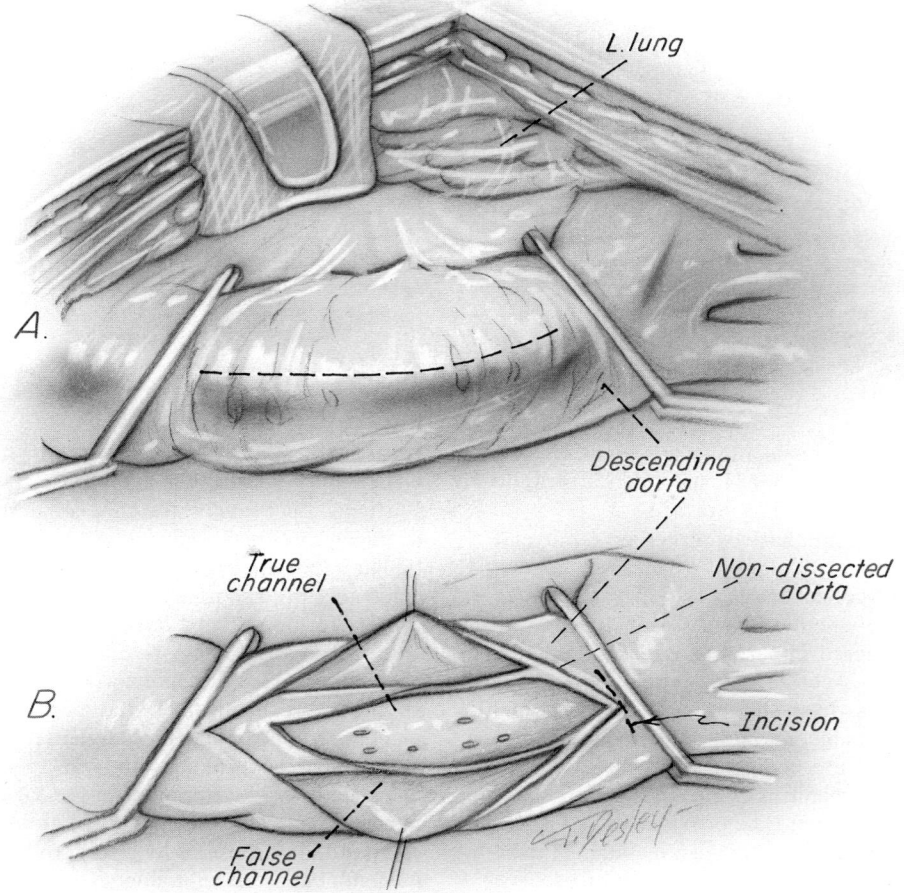

Figure 54-7   Repair of acute dissection of the descending thoracic aorta by the inclusion technique. (*a*) The diffusely enlarged and dissected thoracic aorta is shown with the proposed line of incision. (*b*) The segment of upper descending thoracic aorta has been opened longitudinally and a T extension is to be made at each angle. The proximal T extension is indicated by the dashed lines.

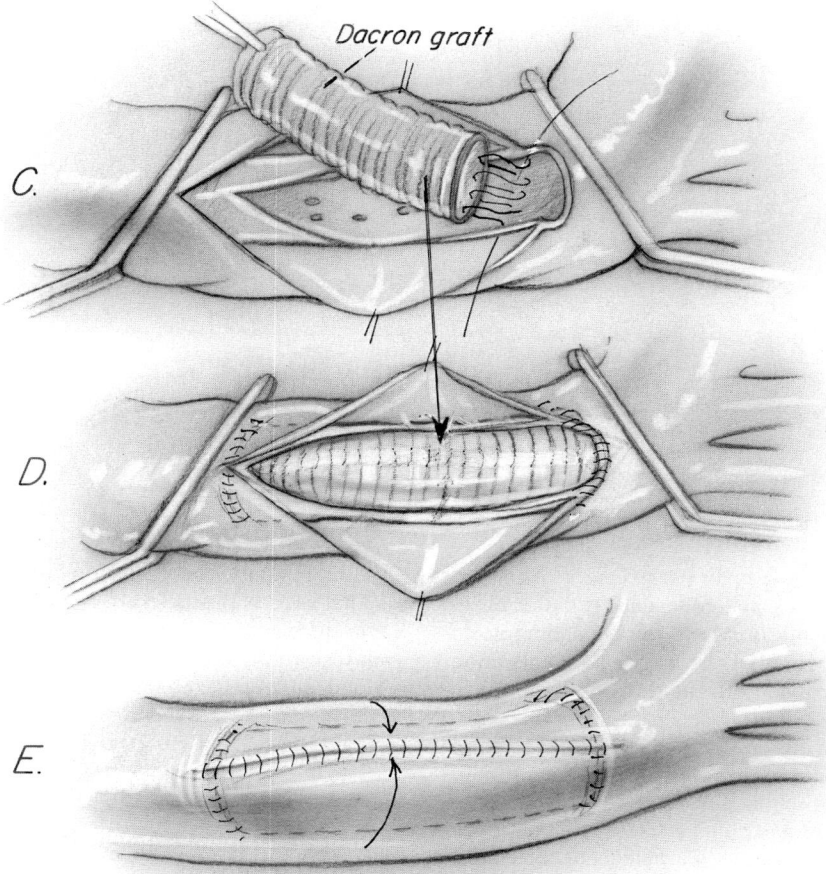

Figure 54-7 (*continued*)
(*c*) Since the aorta just beyond the proximal cross-clamp has not been dissected, the proximal anastomosis can be made with a simple whip stitch, as illustrated. The posterior one-third of the sutures are placed first, siting them all before pulling them up to be tight. The suturing is then continued anteriorly, first with one arm of the suture and then the other.
(*d*) The distal anastomosis has been completed by a similar method. Alternatively, interrupted pledgetted mattress sutures may be used (see Fig. 54-5).
(*e*) The walls of the descending thoracic aorta are brought together around the woven Dacron tube used for the reconstruction.

Modes of Death

In operations on the ascending aorta for acute aortic dissection, hemorrhage has been the most significant mode of death (Table 54-6) but is now largely avoidable using the interposition technique. Deaths related to occlusion or compression of major aortic branches are presumably lessened by very early operation, which in many instances restores flow through these vessels. In operations on the descending aorta, hospital death has been associated with either occlusion of abdominal aortic branches (with pancreatitis or renal failure) or abdominal rupture of the dissection (GLH).

Paraplegia after Repair

In addition to the 2%–3% of patients who have paraplegia or paraparesis with the onset of dissection, there is an additional risk of paraplegia developing at operation, no matter what technique is used for spinal cord protection and without any clear demonstration of the effect of the various tech-

Table 54-3 Hospital mortality after repair of acute aortic dissection (UAB; 1967–July 1984).

Site of Surgery	n	No.	%	CL
		\<Hospital Deaths\>		
Ascending	57	21	37%	30%–45%
Transverse arch	1	1	100%	15%–100%
Upper descending	16	8	50%	35%–65%
Total	74	30	41%	34%–47%

KEY: CL, 70% confidence limits.

NOTE: Excluded are patients with acute dissection in whom the aortic valve was also replaced, whose cases are included in Chapter 12. During 1975–July 1979, two deaths (22%, CL 8%–45%) occurred among nine patients in this category, and one death (33%, CL 4%–76%) occurred among three patients in whom coronary artery bypass grafting was also performed because of irreparable involvement of the coronary ostia in the dissection.

Table 54-4 Hospital mortality after repair of acute aortic dissection (GLH; 1963–November 1984).

	Site of Surgery											
	Ascending Aorta				Descending Aorta				All Cases			
		Hospital Deaths				Hospital Deaths				Hospital Deaths		
Years	n	No.	%	CL	n	No.	%	CL	n	No.	%	CL
1963–1975	8	3	38%	17%–62%	6	3	50%	24%–76%	14	6	43%	27%–60%
1975–1980	12	6	50%	32%–68%	2	1	50%	7%–93%	14	7	50%	33%–67%
1980–November 1984	24	1	4%	1%–13%	1	0	0%	0%–85%	25	1	4%	1%–13%
Total	44	10	23%	16%–31%	9	4	44%	24%–66%	53	14	26%	20%–34%
$P(\chi^2)$			.005				.6				.002	

KEY: CL, 70% confidence limits.

NOTE: Patients with the intimal tear in the region of the left subclavian artery and dissection proximally only are included in the group in which the site of surgery is the ascending aorta. Among the group with surgery to the ascending aorta and operated on from 1980–November 1984, the repair was with a Dacron graft in 12 patients, intraluminal prosthesis in 7, composite Dacron graft and prosthetic valve (Bentall's operation) in 4, and excision and direct suture in 1. In this group, 7 patients had severe preoperative cardiac tamponade, 4 had associated acute myocardial infarction and 1 an associated acute hemiparesis. The one death in this era was in a moribund patient with severe cardiac tamponade undergoing operation 24 hours after the acute dissection; the patient also had severe calcific aortic stenosis and underwent Bentall's operation.

niques on the incidence of postrepair paraplegia.[D1] Although in the experience of DeBakey and colleagues it did occur in 4% (CL 3%–7%) of patients in whom the ascending aorta was involved,[D1] it most commonly occurs as a complication of repair of dissections confined to the descending thoracic aorta and beyond. In the latter subset, paraplegia or neurogenic bladder occurred in 10% (CL 8%–12%) of the cases of DeBakey and colleagues,[D1] in most of which no perfusion of the distal aorta was performed, and in 17% (CL 9%–29%) of cases reported by Miller and colleagues, in most of which femoro-femoral bypass was used.[M1] Paraplegia occurred in 1 patient (11%, CL 1%–33%) among the 9 in this subset (GLH) and in 1 among 12 (UAB; Table 54-7).

Paraplegia may occur after repair of acute descending thoracic aortic aneurysms for several reasons. One reason is acute spinal cord ischemia secondary to temporary loss of flow through critical intercostal arteries coming off the segment of aorta isolated by the pair of cross-clamps. When the ischemia has been over a long enough period, paraplegia results even though reperfusion of the cord is adequate after removal of the clamps. Even though the aorta distal to the cross-clamp is perfused by some technique, if critical intercostal arteries come off the segment isolated by the clamps,

the perfusion will not be protective of the spinal cord. If the spinal cord is protected by some method such as hypothermia during the period of aortic cross-clamping, paraplegia may still result if intercostal arteries critical to spinal cord blood flow are excluded from the vascular reconstruction. (For a more detailed discussion see Chapter 53, "Paraplegia" in section on Special Situations and Controversies.)

Other In-Hospital Complications

The hospital stay after operation is considerably longer than that after most cardiac operations, averaging 18 days in the experience of Miller and colleagues.[M5] Pulmonary complications are frequent and are more common in operations through a left thoracotomy for repair of the descending aorta than after operations through a median sternotomy and directed at the ascending aorta.[M5] Postoperative moderate or severe renal dysfunction develops in about 25% of cases, in the experience of Miller and colleagues.[M5] Low cardiac output and its secondary complications also occur. Hemiplegia may delay convalescence. It is present preoperatively in about 10% of such patients and remains significant in about

Table 54-5 Hospital mortality after repair of acute ascending aortic dissection related to age and year of operation (GLH).

	Year of Operation							
	1963–1980				1980–November 1984			
		Hospital Deaths				Hospital Deaths		
Age (Yr)	n	No.	%	CL	n	No.	%	CL
≤ <								
20 --- 30	3	0	0%	0%–47%	1	0	0%	0%–85%
30 --- 40	0				2	0	0%	0%–61%
40 --- 50	6	3	50%	24%–76%	4	0	0%	0%–38%
50 --- 60	8	4	50%	27%–73%	7	0	0%	0%–24%
60 --- 70	3	2	67%	24%–96%	10	1	10%	1%–30%
Total	20	9	45%	32%–59%	24	1	4%	1%–13%
$P(\chi^2)$			.4				.8	

KEY: CL, 70% confidence limits.

Table 54-6 Mode of hospital death in patients operated on for acute dissection involving the ascending aorta (GLH; 1963–November 1984; n = 44.)

Mode of Death	n
Hemorrhage	5
Massive pulmonary embolism	1
Mesenteric infarction	1[a]
Stroke	1
Acute cardiac failure	2
Total	10

[a] Also stroke.

Table 54-7 Paraplegia or paraparesis developing after surgical treatment of acute aortic dissection (UAB; 1967–July 1984).

Most Proximal Aortic Involvement	n	Corrected n	Spinal Cord Damage		
			No.	%	CL
Ascending	57	42		0%	0%–5%
Transverse arch	1	0		0%	0%–85%
Upper descending	16	12	1	8%	1%–26%
Total	74	54	1	2%	0.2%–6%

KEY: CL, 70% confidence limits.

NOTE: Corrected n is the number of patients known to be without paraplegia or paraparesis before surgery and with adequate observations after repair. Among the corrected n of 12 patients with the most proximal extent of the disease in the upper descending thoracic aorta, 5 were repaired without shunting (1 paraplegia), 2 with aorto-aortic shunts, and 5 with femoro-femoral bypass.

half of them. A few additional patients develop it perioperatively.

Late Survival

Information concerning long-term survival after either medical or surgical treatment of acute dissection is difficult to interpret for a number of reasons. There is a certain degree of selection in all series of either medically or surgically treated patients. Reports of the results of both types of treatment often fail to distinguish between acute and chronic dissection. The disease is extremely variable, in both its location and its extent. The patient's associated medical conditions, such as hypertension and coronary artery disease, also have an important effect on survival. Therefore, any attempts to portray survival in patients with acute aortic dissection are limited.

The information available suggests that long-term survival is similar among patients with ascending aortic dissection, descending aortic dissection, and combinations of the two. Including a hospital mortality of 25%–45%, the survival rate appears to be about 50% at 5 years (Fig. 54-8, 54-9), although in some subsets of patients, such as those requiring operation for acute descending thoracic aortic dissection, the survival may be less good.[D7] Ten- and 20-year survival rates have been reported to be 32% and 5%, respectively.[D1] These data are compatible with the report of Haverich and colleagues of only 79% freedom from cardiovascular deaths at 5 years.[H5] Whether the false channel is eliminated by the operation or persists distally is the important determinant of long-term survival, rather than the point of origin of the dissection (see "Modes of Premature Late Death.")

Modes of Premature Late Death

Rupture of an aneurysm, usually of the false channel, is the commonest mode of late death after the surgical treatment of acute aortic dissection,[W4] this being the case in 30% of the late deaths reported by DeBakey and colleagues.[D1] Not unexpectedly, such rupture occurs in only 15% of cases in which the entire area of dissection is removed (DeBakey types II and IIIb) and in about 35% of cases in which it is not (DeBakey types I and IIIb).[D1] Patients with uncontrolled hypertension had a 46% incidence of false channel aneurysm development late postoperatively, whereas the incidence was 17% in those with controlled hypertension.

Acute myocardial infarction is associated with late death in 10% of cases, cerebrovascular complications in 10%, and congestive heart failure in 5%.[D1]

The False Channel after Repair

Although surgical treatment for acute aortic dissection is advised primarily to prevent early death of the patient, it had been hoped that it would also lead to gradual closure of the false channel distal to the operative area. This, however, is usually not the case, as demonstrated by the follow-up studies of Thomas and colleagues (seven of eight patients late postoperatively had persistence of the false channel),[T1] Cachera and colleagues,[C4] Turley and colleagues,[T2] and Guthaner and colleagues.[G2] In the latter study, 23 (85%, CL 75%–92%) of 27 patients had persistently patent false channels at restudy late postoperatively, with no demonstrable difference between those whose resections had been in the ascending as opposed to the descending aorta. Further, 6 patients (22%, CL 14%–33%) had aneurysms of the false channel, even though 3 of these had distal fenestrations (or reentry points). Thus, the operation, although useful, must be considered palliative.

Aortic Valve Competence after Commissural Resuspension

Successful resuspension, rather than valve replacement, does not increase the risk of operation in patients with acute aortic dissection and aortic incompetence.[A4,K1,M4,M5] Further, in most patients the aortic valve is competent or shows only mild leakage after this procedure. Thus, Koster and colleagues found five (71%, CL 45%–90%) of seven patients so treated to have no aortic valve incompetence and two to have mild incompetence,[K1] a finding almost identical to that of Appelbaum and colleagues (UAB).[A4] Late reoperation and valve replacement are usually not needed, Meng and colleagues reporting 55 (92%, CL 86%–95%) of 60 patients in a collected series[A4,K1,M4,M5] to be free of the need for valve replacement 2–10 years later.[M4]

A new dissection late postoperatively or late development of sinus of Valsalva aneurysm does of course predispose patients to the development of important aortic valve incompetence late postoperatively.

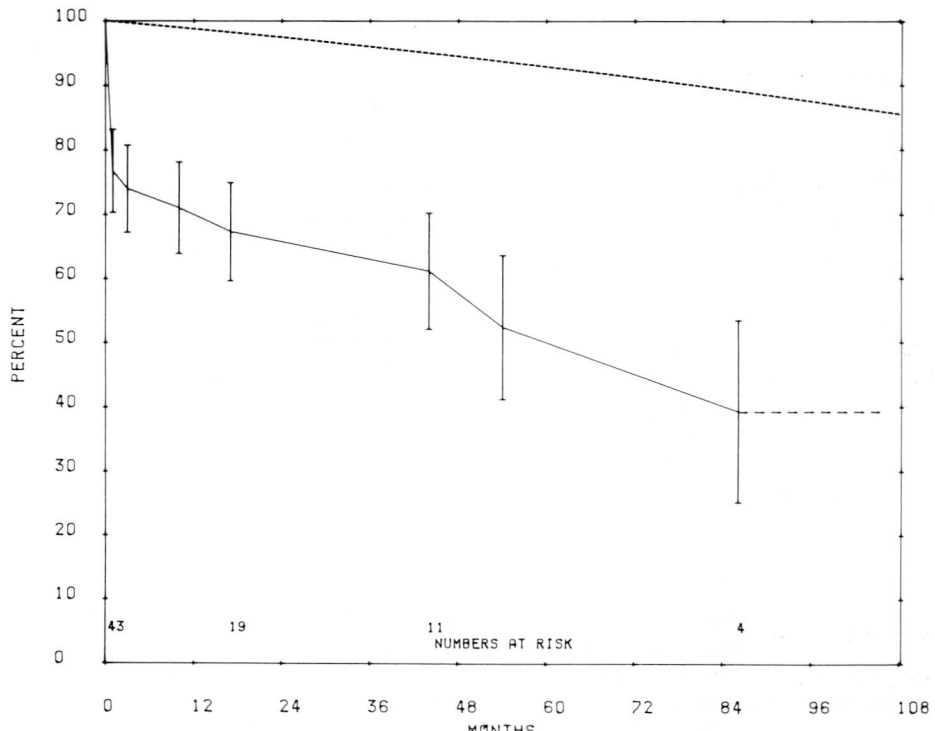

Figure 54-8 Actuarial survival after operation for acute dissection involving the ascending aorta (GLH; 1963–November 1984; *n* = 43; one patient lost to follow-up, 10 hospital deaths, 6 late deaths; follow-up 1–105 months, mean 36 months). The vertical lines indicate one standard error (70% confidence limits) and the interrupted line no further events. The upper dotted line is the survival curve for a matched general population.

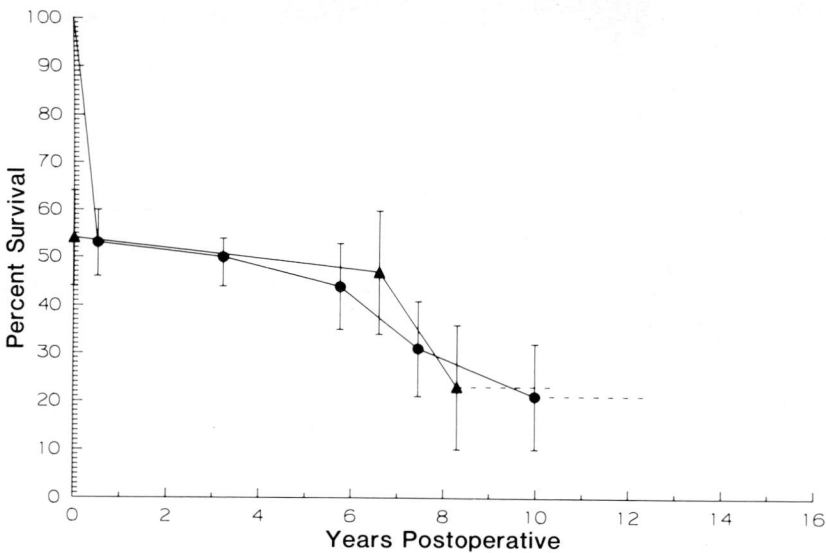

Figure 54-9 Actuarial survival after operation for acute aortic dissection involving the ascending aorta (solid circles) with or without more distal involvement (*n* = 53) and for acute dissection involving only the descending thoracic aorta and beyond (solid triangles; *n* = 20). Hospital deaths are included. The vertical lines enclose the 70% confidence limits (1 standard error of the mean).
Modified from Miller et al.[M5]

Redissection

Redissection (really a new aortic dissection in a different part of the aortic wall) sometimes develops years after the surgical or medical treatment of an acute aortic dissection. Redissection occurred in at least 6 (11%, CL 8%–21%) of 34 hospital survivors, all of whom required a second operation (UAB).

Reoperation

The need for later reoperation is relatively common, just as is operation after successful medical treatment. Reoperation is required most often for enlarging aneurysms of the false channel but occasionally for a new dissection. In the experience of Miller and colleagues, 6 (17%, CL 10%–26%) of 35 hospital survivors of resection of the ascending aorta required reoperation in a mean follow-up period of 4.4 years, as did 2 (18%, CL 6%–38%) of 11 survivors after descending aortic surgery.[M5]

INDICATIONS FOR OPERATION

When the acute aortic dissection is known to involve the ascending aorta or proximal portion of the transverse arch, immediate operation is indicated. This policy is the result of the informal comparison of natural history (see Fig. 54-3) with results of operation (Figs. 54-8, 54-9) and the belief that rupture is very likely to occur when acute aortic dissection involves the ascending aorta. The only contraindications are advanced age and frailty, associated severe incurable disease, paraplegia, and severe stroke.

When only the descending aorta is involved in an acute dissection, with or without involvement of the abdominal aorta and iliac vessels, and there have not been clinically evident complications of the acute dissection, medical treatment is indicated. This plan is supported by informal comparisons of results in such patients treated medically with those in patients treated surgically, which show no differences in comparable cases.[M7] With this protocol, 80% of selected patients survive at least 1 year after the acute dissection.[H4,W3] Medical treatment is directed toward maintaining normal (not elevated) arterial blood pressure with sodium nitroprusside, reducing the force of left ventricular ejection with β blockade[P2] and maintaining a good urine flow and good subsystem function. When initial medical treatment is accompanied by survival of the patient without important complications, close follow-up after hospital dismissal is essential. This need is emphasized by the experience of Wheat and colleagues[W3] and McFarland and colleagues[M6] that 50% of such patients die during the subsequent 3–5 years. The proper follow-up is precisely the same and is conducted for the same reasons as that required after surgical treatment (see "Special Features of Postoperative Care").

Complications in patients with acute aortic dissection involving only the descending thoracic and abdominal aorta indicate immediate surgical treatment by left thoracotomy and resection. Such complications include hemothorax, persisting pain, limb ischemia (operation is directed at the dissection, not the occluded iliac artery), evidence of acute renal failure, and paraparesis. Paraplegia per se is not an indication for operation, since recovery of function following repair of the acute dissection is not to be expected.

The Stanford group has proposed near-routine surgical treatment for acute aortic dissection limited to the descending thoracic aorta and beyond.[M1,M5] Although their results are good, it is not certain that in uncomplicated cases early survival rates are better than with medical therapy.

REFERENCES

A

1. Anagnostopoulos CE, Prabhakar MJS, Kittle CF: Aortic dissections and dissecting aneurysms. *Am J Cardiol* 30:263, 1972.
2. Abbott ME: Congenital cardiac disease, in T McCrae (ed): *Osler's Modern Medicine*, vol 4, (ed 3). Philadelphia: Lea & Febiger, 1927, p 744.
3. Ablaza SGG, Ghosh SC, Grana VP: Use of a ringed intraluminal graft in the surgical treatment of dissection aneurysms of the thoracic aorta. *J Thorac Cardiovasc Surg* 76:390, 1978.
4. Appelbaum A, Karp RB, Kirklin JW: Ascending vs. descending aortic dissections. *Ann Surg* 183:296, 1976.
5. Austen WG, Buckley MJ, McFarland J, DeSanctis RW, Sanders CA: Therapy of dissecting aneurysms. *Arch Surg* 95:835, 1967.

B

1. Bahnson HT, Spencer FC: Excision of aneurysm of ascending aorta with prosthetic replacement during cardiopulmonary bypass. *Ann Surg* 151:879, 1960.
2. Barner HB, Willman VL: Intraluminal graft for acute dissection of the ascending aorta. *Ann Thorac Surg* 17:58, 1974.

C

1. Crawford ES: (1984) Personal communication.
2. Crawford ES, Crawford JL: *Diseases of the Aorta including an Atlas of Angiographic Pathology and Surgical Technique*. Baltimore: Williams & Wilkins, 1984.
3. Carrel A: Results of the permanent intubation of the thoracic aorta. *Surg Gynecol Obstet* 15:245, 1912.
4. Cachera J-P, Vouhe PR, Loisance DY, Menu P, Poulain H, Bloch G, Vasile N, Aubry P, Galey J-J: Surgical management of acute dissections involving the ascending aorta: Early and late results in 38 patients. *J Thorac Cardiovasc Surg* 82:576, 1981.
5. Culliford AT, Ayvaliotis B, Shemin R, Colvin SB, Isom OW, Spencer FC: Aneurysms of the ascending aorta and transverse arch: Surgical experience in 80 patients. *J Thorac Cardiovasc Surg* 83:701, 1982.

D

1. DeBakey ME, McCollum CH, Crawford ES, Morris GC Jr, Howell J, Noon GP, Lawrie G: Dissection and dissecting aneurysms of the aorta: Twenty-year follow-up of five hundred twenty-seven patients treated surgically. *Surgery* 92:1118, 1982.

2. DeBakey ME, Cooley DA, Creech O Jr: Surgical considerations of dissecting aneurysm of the aorta. *Ann Surg* 142:586, 1955.

3. DeBakey ME, Henly WS, Cooley DA, Morris GC Jr, Crawford ES, Beall AC Jr: Surgical management of dissecting aneurysm involving the ascending aorta. *J Cardiovasc Surg* 5:200, 1964.

4. Dureau G, Villard J, George M, Deliry P, Froment JC, Clermont A: New surgical technique for the operative management of acute dissections of the ascending aorta: Report of two cases. *J Thorac Cardiovasc Surg* 76:385, 1978.

5. Dalen JE, Pape LA, Cohn LH, Koster JK Jr, Collins JJ Jr: Dissection of the aorta: Pathogenesis, diagnosis, and treatment. *Prog Cardiovasc Dis* 23:237, 1980.

6. Daily PO, Trueblood HW, Stinson EB, Wuerflein RD, Shumway NE: Management of acute aortic dissections. *Ann Thorac Surg* 10:237, 1970.

7. Doroghazi RM, Slater EE, DeSanctis RW, Buckley MJ, Austen WG, Rosenthal S: Long-term survival of patients with treated aortic dissection. *JACC* 3:1026, 1984.

E

1. Edwards WD, Leaf DS, Edwards JE: Dissecting aortic aneurysm with congenital bicuspid aortic valve. *Circulation* 57:1022, 1978.

2. Edwards JE: Aneurysms of the thoracic aorta complicating coarctation. *Circulation* 48:195, 1973.

G

1. Gurin D, Bulmer JW, Derby R: Dissecting aneurysm of the aorta: Diagnosis and operative relief of acute arterial obstruction due to this cause. *NY State J Med* 35:1200, 1935.

2. Guthaner DF, Miller DC, Silverman JF, Stinson EB, Wexler L: Fate of the false lumen following surgical repair of aortic dissections: An angiographic study. *Radiology* 133:1, 1979.

H

1. Hurley V: Dissecting aneurysm of the aorta: Histological appearances and an hypothesis of pathogenesis. *Australas Ann Med* 8:297, 1959.

2. Hirst AE Jr, Johns VJ Jr, Kime SW Jr: Dissecting aneurysm of the aorta: A review of 505 cases. *Medicine* 37:217, 1958.

3. Hufnagel CA: Aortic plastic valvular prosthesis. *Bull Georgetown Univ Med Ctr* 4:128, 1951.

4. Harris PD, Bowman FO Jr, Malm JR: The management of acute dissections of the thoracic aorta. *Am Heart J* 78:419, 1969.

5. Haverich A, Scott WC, Miller DC: Determinants of late survival and reoperation after aortic dissection repair. *Circulation* 70(suppl 2):2, 1984.

I

1. Iliceto S, Ettorre G, Francioso G, Antonelli G, Biasco G, Rizzon P: Diagnosis of aneurysm of the thoracic aorta: Comparison between two non invasive techniques: Two-dimensional echocardiography and computed tomography. *Eur Heart J* 5:545, 1984.

J

1. Johns TNP: Dissecting aneurysm of the abdominal aorta: Report of a case with repair of perforation. *Ann Surg* 137:232, 1953.

K

1. Koster JK Jr, Cohn LH, Mee RBB, Collins JJ Jr: Late results of operation for acute aortic dissection producing aortic insufficiency. *Ann Thorac Surg* 26:461, 1978.

L

1. Larson EW, Edwards WD: Risk factors for aortic dissection: A necropsy study of 161 cases. *Am J Cardiol* 53:849, 1984.

2. Lemole GM, Strong MD, Spagna PM, Karmilowicz NP: Improved results for dissecting aneurysms: Intraluminal sutureless prosthesis. *J Thorac Cardiovasc Surg* 83:249, 1982.

3. Lindsay J Jr, Hurst JW: Clinical features and prognosis in dissecting aneurysm of the aorta: A re-appraisal. *Circulation* 35:880, 1967.

4. Liotta D, Hallman GL, Milam JD, Cooley DA: Surgical treatment of acute dissecting aneurysm of the ascending aorta. *Ann Thorac Surg* 12:582, 1971.

5. Lawrie GM, Morris GC: Follow-up of dissecting aortic aneurysm. *JAMA* 239:724, 1978.

M

1. Miller DC, Mitchell RS, Oyer PE, Stinson EB, Jamieson SW, Shumway NE: Independent determinants of operative mortality for patients with aortic dissections. *Circulation* 70(suppl I)I-153, 1984.

2. Mathew T, Nanda NC: Two-dimensional and Doppler echocardiographic evaluation of aortic aneurysm and dissection. *Am J Cardiol* 54:379, 1984.

3. Murray CA, Edwards JE: Spontaneous laceration of ascending aorta. *Circulation* 47:848, 1973.

4. Meng RL, Najafi H, Javid H, Hunter JA, Goldin MD: Acute ascending aortic dissection: Surgical management. *Circulation* 64(suppl II), II-231, 1981.

5. Miller DC, Stinson EB, Oyer PE, Rossiter SJ, Reitz BA, Griepp RB, Shumway NE: Operative treatment of aortic dissections: Experience with 125 patients over a sixteen-year period. *J Thorac Cardiovasc Surg* 78:365, 1979.

6. McFarland J, Wirleson JT, Dinsmore RE, Austen WG, Buckley MJ, Sanders CA, DeSanctis EW: The medical treatment of dissecting aortic aneurysms. *N Engl J Med* 286:115, 1972.

7. Mills SE, Teja K, Crosby IK, Sturgill BC: Aortic dissection: Surgical and nonsurgical treatments compared, an analysis of seventy-four cases at the University of Virginia. *Am J Surg* 137:240, 1979.

8. Morris GC Jr, Henly WS, DeBakey ME: Correction of acute dissecting aneurysm of aorta with valvular insufficiency. *JAMA* 184:63, 1963.

9. McDonald GR, Schaff HV, Pyeritz RE, McKusick VA, Gott VL: Surgical management of patients with the Marfan syndrome and dilatation of the ascending aorta. *J Thorac Cardiovasc Surg* 81:180, 1981.

10. Morris GC Jr: (1985) Personal communication.

P

1. Paullin JE, James DF: Dissecting aneurysm of aorta. *Postgrad Med* 4:291, 1948.

2. Prokop EK, Palmer RF, Wheat MW Jr: Hydrodynamic forces in dissecting aneurysms: In-vitro studies in a tygon model and in dog aorta. *Circ Res* 27:121, 1970.

R

1. Roberts WC: Aortic dissection: Anatomy, consequences, and causes. *Am Heart J* 101:195, 1981.

2. Roberts WC, Honig HS: The spectrum of cardiovascular disease in the Marfan syndrome: A clinico-morphologic study of 18 necropsy patients and comparison to 151 previously reported necropsy patients. *Am Heart J* 104:115, 1982.

3. Roberts WC: The congenitally bicuspid aortic valve: A study of 85 autopsy cases. *Am J Cardiol* 26:72, 1970.

S

1. Shachter N, Perloff JK, Mulder DG: Aortic dissection in Noonan's Syndrome (46 XY Turner). *Am J Cardiol* 54:464, 1984.

2. Slater DN, Grundman MS, Mitchell L: Turner's syndrome associated with bicuspid aortic stenosis and dissecting aneurysm. *Postgrad Med J* 58:436, 1982.

3. Shennan T: *Dissecting Aneurysms.* Medical Research Clinical Special Report Series No. 193. London: His Majesty's Stationery Office, 1934.

4. Shaw RS: Acute dissecting aortic aneurysm: Treatment by fenestration of the internal wall of the aneurysm. *N Engl J Med* 253:331, 1955.

5. Stovin RGI: Dissecting the dissecting aneurysm. *Thorax* 33:273, 1978.

6. Schlatmann TJ, Becker AE: Pathogenesis of dissecting aneurysm of aorta: Comparative histopathologic study of significance of medial changes. *Am J Cardiol* 39:21, 1977.

7. Spencer FC, Blake H: A report of the successful surgical treatment of aortic regurgitation from a dissecting aortic aneurysm in a patient with the Marfan syndrome. *J Thorac Cardiovasc Surg* 44:238, 1962.

T

1. Thomas CS Jr, Alford WC Jr, Burrus GR, Frist RA, Stoney WS: The effectiveness of surgical treatment of acute aortic dissection. *Ann Thorac Surg* 26:42, 1978.

2. Turley K, Ullyot DJ, Godwin JD, Wilson JM, Lipton M, Carlsson E, Ebert PA: Repair of dissection of the thoracic aorta: Evaluation of false lumen utilizing computed tomography. *J Thorac Cardiovasc Surg* 81:61, 1981.

W

1. Wheat MW Jr, Palmer RF, Bartley TD, Seelman RC: Treatment of dissecting aneurysms of the aorta without surgery. *J Thorac Cardiovasc Surg* 50:364, 1965.

2. Wilson SK, Hutchins GM: Aortic dissecting aneurysms: Causative factors in 204 subjects. *Arch Pathol Lab Med* 206:175, 1982.

3. Wheat MW Jr, Harris PD, Malm JR, Kaiser G, Bowman FO Jr, Palmer RF: Acute dissecting aneurysms of the aorta: Treatment and results in 64 patients. *J Thorac Cardiovasc Surg* 58:344, 1969.

4. Wolfe GW, Oldham N, Rankin JS, Moran JF: Surgical treatment of acute ascending aortic dissection. *Ann Surg* 197:738, 1983.

55

CHRONIC THORACIC AND THORACOABDOMINAL AORTIC ANEURYSMS

DEFINITION

True aneurysms involving the ascending, transverse arch, descending thoracic, or thoracoabdominal portions of the aorta are localized enlargements contained by walls that, though attenuated, have all layers of the normal aortic wall. False aneurysms are localized enlargements of the aorta in which the wall consists of aortic adventitia and compressed periaortic fibrous tissue. This chapter excludes acute traumatic aneurysms (see Chapter 53) and acute dissecting aneurysms (see Chapter 54) in patients operated on within 14 days of onset.

HISTORICAL NOTE

An important contribution to modern aneurysm surgery was made by Rudolph Matas in New Orleans in 1902, when he described the basic maneuver of "getting inside the aneurysm" with minimal external dissection and after obtaining control of the artery above and below the aneurysm.[M1] Matas worked with both fusiform and sacciform aneurysms in the extremities. Interestingly, this basic maneuver was ignored as aortic aneurysm surgery began to develop, and in our early work with abdominal aortic aneurysms at the Mayo Clinic, we dissected out the aneurysm, often with a long and difficult operation and considerable hemorrhage from the lumbar arteries.[K2] DeBakey and Cooley described this same tedious method in their early classical paper of 1953.[D4] The publication of Javid and colleagues in 1962[J2] and Creech in 1966[C2] are generally credited with reintroducing the technique of working within the aneurysm. However, DeBakey and colleagues in Houston had reintroduced this concept into abdominal aortic aneurysm surgery by 1958,[C3] and we at the Mayo Clinic had learned it from them by about 1960. The inclusion technique of sewing the graft in place from within the aneurysm (see also Chapter 54, "Technique of Operation") is an embodiment of this concept (Fig. 55-1).[C1]

Throughout the first half of the twentieth century, sporadic attempts were made to treat abdominal aortic aneurysms by proximal partial or complete ligation of the aorta, but the results were generally unsatisfactory.[D3] Various other palliative procedures had also been used unsuccessfully. Then, in 1950, Estes, at the Mayo Clinic, published a classic paper that demonstrated the very poor prognosis of patients with abdominal aortic aneurysms, only 50% of whom survived 3 years after the diagnosis, with two-thirds of the deaths due to aneurysmal rupture.[E1] In response to that study, we at the Mayo Clinic began a surgical approach to this condition in 1951, and in 1953 reported the results of aneurysm reinforcement and of the tedious operation of aortoplasty and complete wrapping with fascia lata.[K2] In 1952, Shafer and Hardin, in Kansas City, reported resection and grafting with an aortic homograft (see below) of an abdominal aortic aneurysm, only to have the patient die 28 days after operation of numerous complications.[S2] Then Dubost and colleagues, working in Paris, reported in 1952 the first successful case of aortic resection for aneurysm and restoration of blood vessel continuity (in their case, an abdominal aortic aneurysm, which was approached retroperitoneally and replaced by a preserved aortic homograft).[D1] In 1953, reports of similar successes came from DeBakey and Cooley,[D4] in Houston, and us, at the Mayo Clinic.[H2,K2] Aortic homograft banks were promptly established in some centers to provide aortic replacement grafts.[M2]

The development of surgery for coarctation of the aorta (see Chapter 34) was antedated by a successful resection of a thoracic aortic aneurysm secondary to coarctation, although without restoration of aortic continuity, by Alexander and Byron in 1944.[A2] Aortic homografts were developed in 1948

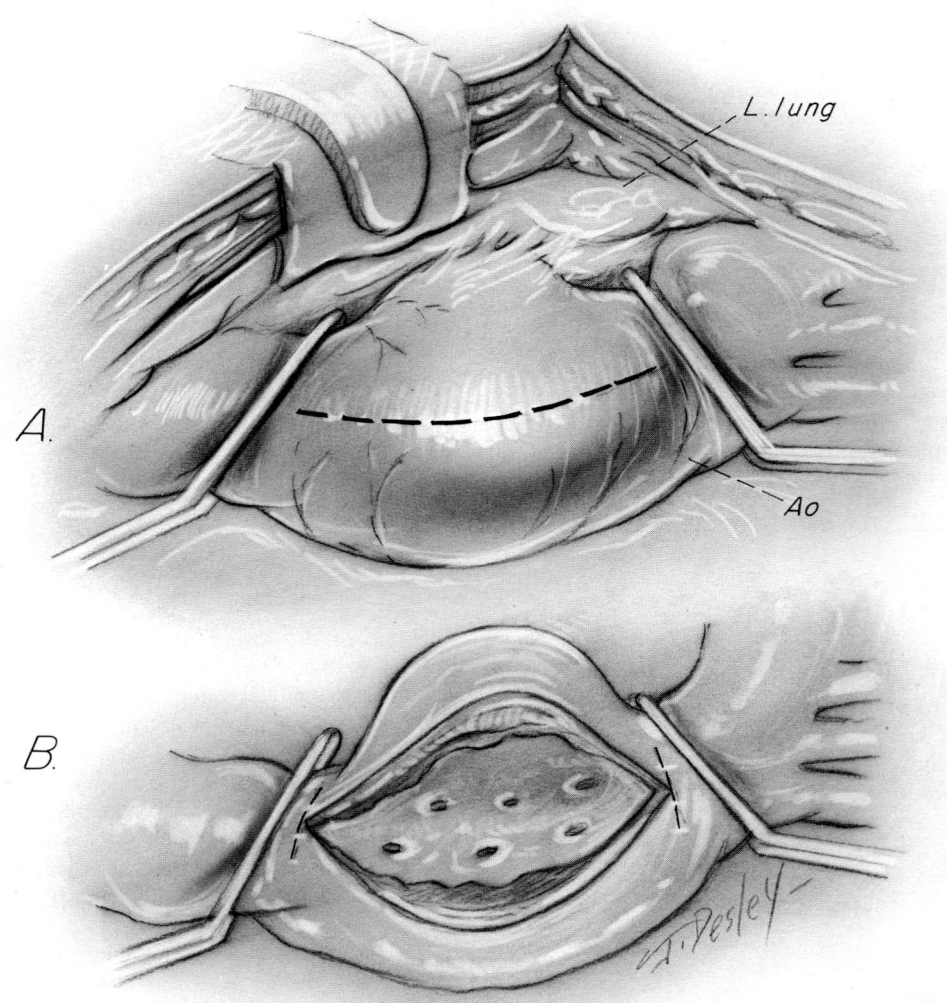

Figure 55-1 The inclusion technique of aortic grafting, in this instance a part of the repair of an upper descending thoracic aortic aneurysm.
(a) After appropriate maneuvers for protecting the spinal cord, cross-clamps are placed above and below the aneurysm. The dashed line indicates the proposed incision into the aneurysm.
(b) The aneurysm has been opened longitudinally with the electrocautery. T extensions will be made at the upper and lower ends to facilitate exposure for the anastomosis, as shown by the dashed lines. Thrombus usually partially fills the interior of these aneurysms. It has been removed in the area of the intercostal arteries.

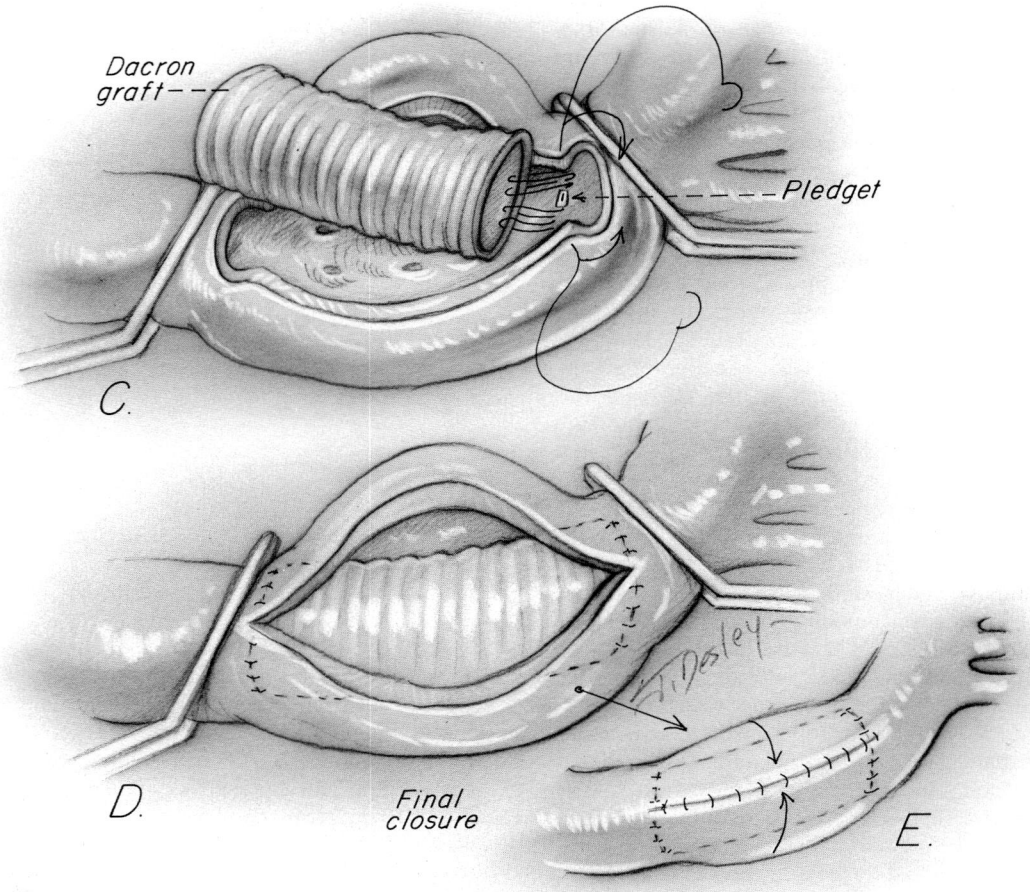

Figure 55-1 (*continued*)
(*c*) A predotted woven Dacron graft is being sutured into place proximally with a whip stitch, working entirely within the aneurysm. A pledgetted mattress suture was placed posteriorly as a beginning.
(*d*) Both proximal and distal anastomoses have been completed.
(*e*) Following this and the removal of the cross-clamps, and after any pulsatile bleeding has been controlled with additional sutures, the walls of the aneurysm are wrapped around the graft for final hemostasis.

Ao, aorta.

by Gross and colleagues, in Boston, to replace resected aortic segments.[G1,G3,P1] In 1950, Gross and colleagues reported successful clinical use of homografts for treating complex coarctations, including those with aneurysms,[G3] as did Swan in the same year.[S4] Lam and Aram, adopting this technique, reported in 1951 the resection and homograft replacement of a descending thoracic aortic aneurysm in an adult;[L2] prophetically, their patient developed paraparesis and died 6 weeks after operation from empyema. At about this time, Bahnson reported the successful management of a saccular aneurysm of the descending thoracic aorta by lateral resection and aortorrhaphy.[B2] In 1953, DeBakey and Cooley reported the first successful application of resection and grafting to a descending thoracic aortic aneurysm.[D7]

Ascending aortic aneurysms were also approached surgically before the advent of cardiopulmonary bypass (CPB). In 1952, Cooley and DeBakey reported the removal of sacciform ascending aortic aneurysms by lateral resection and aortorrhaphy,[C8] as did Bahnson[B2] and we, at the Mayo

Clinic,[J1] in 1953. Cooley and DeBakey, in 1956, reported the first successful modern operation for ascending aortic aneurysm, consisting of resection of the ascending aorta and grafting with an aortic homograft, with the aid of cardiopulmonary bypass;[C9] the operation was not quite modern, however, in that they separately perfused the right common carotid artery. Wheat and colleagues then reported the successful simultaneous but separate replacement of the ascending aorta and aortic valve with reimplantation of the coronary ostia into the graft.[W2] Bentall and de Bono in 1968[B5] and Edwards and Kerr (UAB) in 1970[E6] reported accomplishing this replacement with a composite valve and Dacron tube graft. Wheat and colleagues subsequently demonstrated the long-term patency of their anastomosis between the graft and the coronary ostia.[W1]

Transverse aortic arch aneurysms have presented a more difficult surgical challenge. Cooley and DeBakey had removed some sacciform aneurysms in this portion of the aorta by lateral resection by 1952,[C8] as had Bahnson by 1953.[B2]

Then DeBakey and Cooley published a paper in 1954 on "Successful Resection of Aneurysm of Distal Aortic Arch and Replacement by Graft,"[D6] but in fact the resection included only a short segment of the distal arch beyond the left subclavian artery for an aneurysm that had resulted from acute traumatic aortic transection (see Chapter 53). The case is of interest, however, in that the patient's temperature was reduced to 28°C by surface cooling before thoracotomy. The aorta was cross-clamped proximal to the left subclavian artery, which was also individually clamped, for 1 hour, and the patient did not develop paraplegia. (See Chapter 53, "Paraplegia" in section on Special Situations and Controversies for the significance of this.) Cooley, Mahaffey, and DeBakey reported the unsuccessful resection of an aneurysm of the entire transverse arch in 1955,[C12] using the very cumbersome method of temporary shunts without cardiopulmonary bypass, as did Stranahan and colleagues[S3] in a 15-hour operation in 1955 and Creech and colleagues in 1956.[C5] DeBakey and colleagues reported in 1957 the first successful and also modern type of repair, using homograft replacement of the transverse arch and CPB.[D5]

Thoracoabdominal aneurysms have also presented difficult surgical challenges, not only because of the magnitude of the operation but also because of the tendency of the patients to have renal and spinal cord dysfunction after the repair.[C3] During Bahnson's pioneering work with aneurysms of the aorta, he successfully repaired a saccular thoracoabdominal aneurysm in 1952 by lateral resection and aortorrhaphy.[B2] Ellis and colleagues, at the Mayo Clinic, first reported repair of such an aneurysm involving a visceral artery (in their case, the renal artery) by resection and grafting in 1955.[E3] Etheredge and colleagues reported successful repair of a more complex thoracoabdominal aneurysm including the coeliac axis and the superior mesenteric artery in that same year.[E4] Then DeBakey and colleagues in 1956 reported the successful repair of such an aneurysm involving all the visceral arteries (coeliac, superior mesenteric, and both renals).[D8] Subsequently, DeBakey, Crawford, and colleagues devised the technique of permanent Dacron aortic bypass and visceral arterial reattachment to appropriately located side-arm grafts, and in 1965 were able to report a 26% mortality rate among 42 patients operated on.[D9] Crawford modified and simplified the technique of the operation by applying the inclusion technique[C14] and thereby reduced the hospital mortality to 8% by 1978.[C3]

During this developmental phase, there was controversy about the lethality of thoracic aortic aneurysms, some reports indicating that the prognosis of patients with thoracic aneurysms was better than that of those with abdominal aneurysms.[L3] That this is not the case was established by Joyce and colleagues in 1964.[J3]

A series of technical improvements in the surgery of thoracic aneurysms evolved the techniques currently employed. Even after successful repair of aneurysms of the transverse arch had been accomplished using cardiopulmonary bypass, the methods remained complex, often with separate cannulation of the brachiocephalic vessels. In 1964, Borst and colleagues reported the repair of a traumatic aneurysm of the distal portion of the aortic arch via a left thoracotomy, using cardiopulmonary bypass to produce profound hypothermia

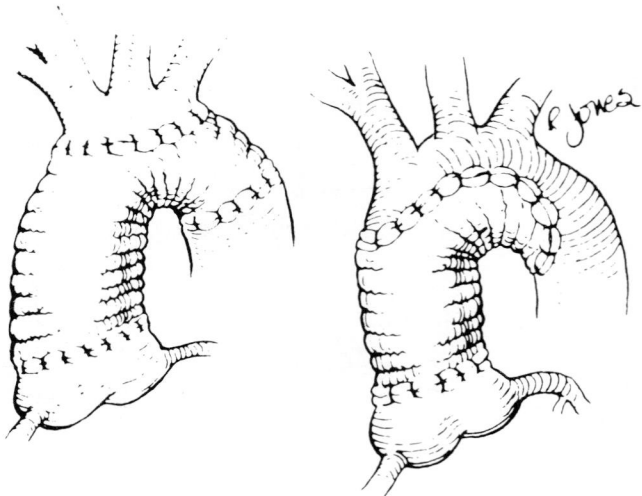

Figure 55-2 Methods of surgical repair of aneurysms of the transverse aortic arch. In both the methods, the resection and grafting are tailored to simplify the operation.

Reproduced with permission from Ott et al.,[O1] and the American Heart Association, Inc.

and performing the repair during total circulatory arrest.[B6] (For current application of a similar technique, see Chapter 53, "Repair of Acute Traumatic Transection of Upper Descending Thoracic Aorta" in Technique of Operation.) Much later, Griepp and colleagues established the value of profoundly hypothermic total circulatory arrest for the resection and grafting of more proximal and extensive aneurysms of the transverse portion of the aortic arch.[G2]

Among the technical improvements was the use of a single anastomosis between an oval opening in the graft and the aortic wall around all three head-vessel orifices in replacing transverse aortic arch aneurysms reported in 1968 by Bloodwell, Hallman, and Cooley and by Pearce and colleagues in the following year.[B3,P3] Later, Ott and colleagues[O1] reported tailoring the transverse arch resection and the graft so that a single distal anastomosis could be made (Fig. 55-2). Crawford and Saleh applied to transverse arch aneurysms the inclusion technique of working entirely within the aneurysm and wrapping the graft with aneurysm wall.[C10]

Technical improvements have also been made in the aortic replacement devices required in the modern treatment of aortic aneurysms and dissections. Those used by Dubost and others in the early surgical period were preserved aortic homografts. Soon the search for synthetic aortic substitutes was revived, Carrel's pioneering efforts in 1912[C6] and subsequent ones having been failures. The first satisfactory synthetic aortic substitute was a fabric tube made of Vinyon N cloth, and the first clinical application of this device was reported by Blakemore and Voorhees, in New York City, in 1954.[B1] Shumacker and colleagues in Indianapolis also used these fabric tubes in aortic replacement in the same year.[S1] For the next several years, surgeons, including us, at the Mayo Clinic and GLH, autoclaved and used in patients with aortic aneurysms fabric grafts made on the sewing machines of wives and friends, with generally good results! Intensive study of prosthetic grafts was quickly undertaken by several groups, and in 1955, Deterling and Bhonslay reported that Dacron was the best material then available for aortic replacement.[D2] Knitted and woven grafts of various types, mostly Dacron, have been widely used since then (see Chapter 53, ''Grafts for Use in Thoracic and Thoracoabdominal Aortic Surgery'' in section on Special Situations and Controversies).

MORPHOLOGY

Morphologic Substrates

Arteriosclerotic or Degenerative Aneurysms
Arteriosclerosis, or nonspecific aortic degenerative disease, is the commonest cause of thoracic and thoracoabdominal aneurysms, with approximately half these aneurysms in surgical series being in this category.[C20] The frequency of atherosclerosis as a cause has long been recognized, but only recently has credence been given to the idea that the thickened, degenerated, and aneurysmal thoracic aorta may be the site of a degenerative disease other than atherosclerosis.[C13]

Aortic Dissection with Persisting False Channel
When the false lumen persists after an acute aortic dissection (see Chapter 54, ''Morphology''), as it usually does, its thin outer wall (consisting only of the outer coat of the media and the adventitia) has a strong tendency gradually to weaken and enlarge. Because of the relationships expressed in Laplace's law, the wall stresses increase, and as this process proceeds, an aneurysm is formed and gradually enlarges. Chronic aortic dissection with persisting false channel is the second most common substrate for the development of chronic thoracic aneurysms.

Traumatic Aortic Transection
When neither death nor operation follows acute traumatic aortic transection, the disruption in at least part of the aortic circumference at the level of the ligamentum arteriosum allows an extravasation of blood into the periaortic area (see Chapter 53). This blood may remain in communication with the aorta and form a pulsating hematoma contained by aortic adventitia or the mediastinal tissues, or the hematoma may liquify and evacuate into the aorta. Because of the increased wall stress, the false aneurysm (or pulsating hematoma) begins to enlarge and form a typical thoracic aneurysm. Its life history is then similar to that of other thoracic aneurysms. About 10% of descending thoracic aortic aneurysms are in this category.

Annulo-Aortic Ectasia
The process of annulo-aortic ectasia in the ascending aorta is commonly encountered in patients with Marfan's syndrome and may be associated with cystic medial necrosis. When it leads to a true ascending aortic aneurysm, it is commonly associated with aortic valvular incompetence (see Chapter 12, ''Combined Aortic Incompetence and Ascending Aortic Aneurysm'' in section on Special Situations and Controversies, for discussion of this entity in patients with aortic valvular incompetence).

Aortitis
In the current era in developed countries, aortitis, either of the granulomatous type or secondary to syphilis, is an uncommon cause of thoracic aortic aneurysm. However, it was present in 8% of the unselected cases presented by Bickerstaff and colleagues.[B4] Granulomatous aortitis is an uncommon condition in which the microscopic appearance suggests an infectious etiology but bacteriologic studies are negative.[A3,Z1] It is said to be more common in adults and is sometimes associated with temporal arteritis, but several cases of aneurysm from granulomatous aortitis have been reported in children.[G5,Z1] A granulomatous arteritis may produce simultaneous aortic and pulmonary artery aneurysms.[D14]

When syphilis involves the aorta, it leads to the destruction of elastic fibers in the aortic media. Perhaps because of the relationships expressed in Laplace's law and the fact that the ascending aorta is generally the widest part of the aorta, syphilitic aortitis most commonly leads to aneurysm in that portion.

Location

The true anatomic distribution of thoracic aortic aneurysms is probably not known. However, the ascending aorta was involved in about 45% of the unselected cases reported by Bickerstaff and associates, the transverse arch in about 10%, the descending thoracic aorta in about 35%, and the thoracoabdominal aorta in about 10%.[B4]

CLINICAL FEATURES AND DIAGNOSTIC CRITERIA

Symptoms

At the time of presentation, many patients with thoracic aortic aneurysms are asymptomatic, although most give a history of hypertension.[B4] When symptoms are present, they often are sudden in onset and develop just before presentation coincident with sudden extension of the aneurysm.

Pain may, however, be chronic and of several months' duration. In ascending aortic aneurysms, it may be precordial in location, and particularly when the transverse part of the aortic arch is involved, it may radiate to the neck and jaw. Aneurysms of the descending thoracic aorta tend to produce back pain, usually between the scapulae, and those in the thoracoabdominal portion of the aorta, lower back pain.

Various symptoms may result from the aneurysm's compression of adjacent structures. Symptoms and signs of superior vena caval obstruction may be produced by the direct compression of the superior vena cava by an enlarging ascending aortic aneurysm. Aneurysms of the transverse arch or upper descending aorta may produce hoarseness by stretching the left vagus and recurrent laryngeal nerves.[J3]

Signs

Direct physical signs of the presence of a thoracic aortic aneurysm are uncommon. In earlier times, a pulsating mass anteriorly sometimes was the first evidence of the presence

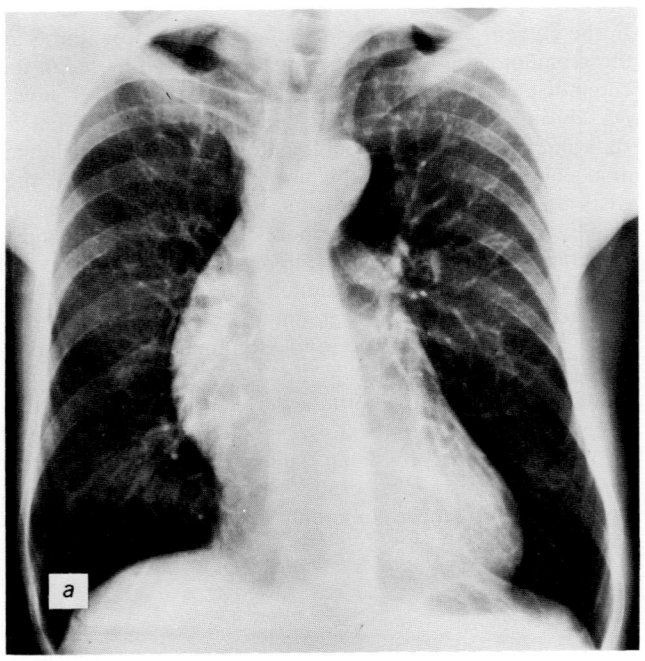

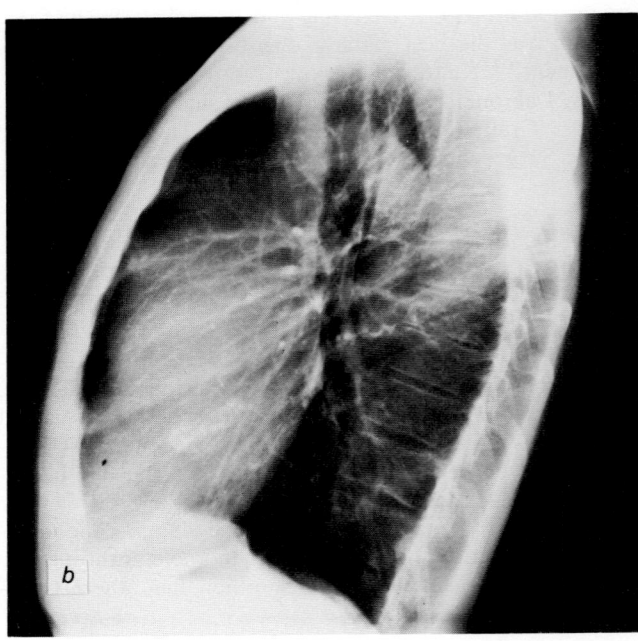

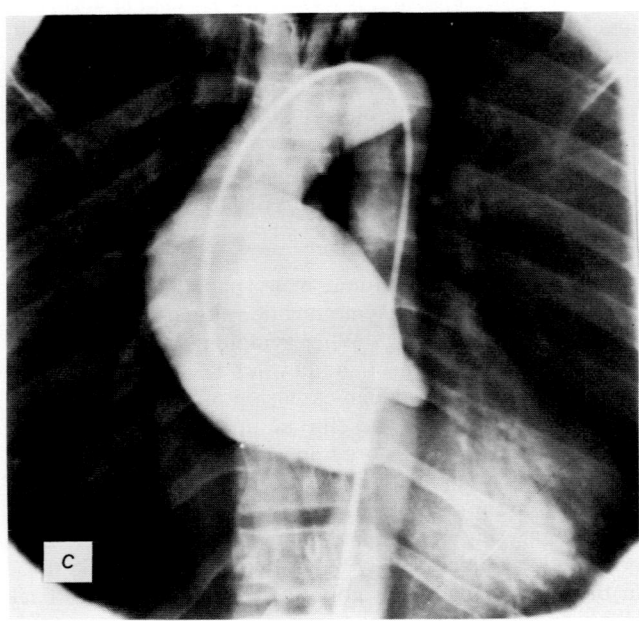

Figure 55-3 Chest x-rays and aortogram of a patient with aneurysm of the ascending aorta (UAB).
(a) The plain chest x-ray shows the typical convex deformity to the right in the frontal view.
(b) The x-ray shows increased contact of the ascending aorta with the anterior chest wall in the lateral view.
(c) The aortogram indicates that, as usual in this type of aneurysm, the sinuses of Valsalva are involved, and the aneurysm stops abruptly, before the takeoff of the innominate artery. Aortic incompetence is present.

Of particular surgical importance is the occasional presence in patients with thoracic aneurysm of ecchymosis and petechia. Such signs suggest disseminated intravascular coagulation. The occurrence of ecchymosis and petechia and their relationship to postoperative hemorrhage has been studied by Fisher and colleagues.[F1] Therefore, when this clinical sign is found, studies of the clotting mechanism are indicated. Rather than a contraindication to operation, these signs are an indication for surgery, but preparations should be made for administering large amounts of blood during the procedure and fresh-frozen plasma and platelet concentrate as soon as the aortic resection has been completed.[F1]

Chest X-ray

The chest x-ray can give a strong clue of the presence of a thoracic or thoracoabdominal aneurysm, and the aneurysm may be first discovered by a routine chest x-ray study. Ascending aortic aneurysms produce a convex shadow to the right of the cardiac silhouette (Fig. 55-3), those of the transverse arch an anterior and left-sided shadow (Figs. 55-4, 55-5, 55-6), and those of the descending aorta a shadow to the left and posteriorly (Fig. 55-7). The radiologic appearance of aneurysm is to be distinguished from that of elongation and

of a syphilitic aneurysm of the ascending aorta, and, rarely, such an aneurysm eroded the sternum and announced its presence by external rupture and exsanguinating hemorrhage.

Other stigmata of arteriosclerosis are frequently present in patients with thoracic aortic aneurysms. Joyce and colleagues found that 16% of their patients had evidence of coronary artery disease, 10% had evidence of peripheral vascular disease, 10% had evidence of cerebral vascular disease, and about 10% had an associated abdominal aortic aneurysm.[J3]

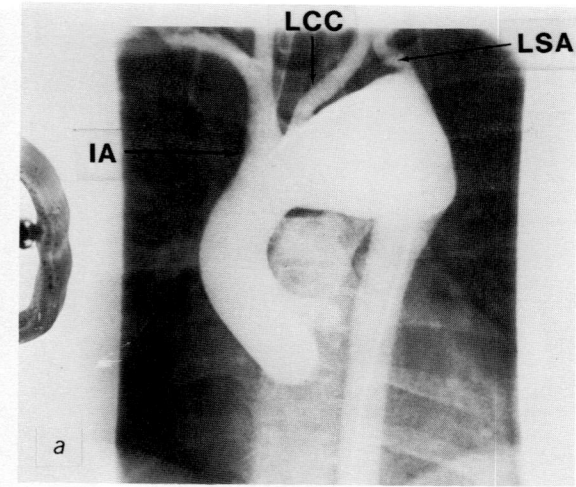

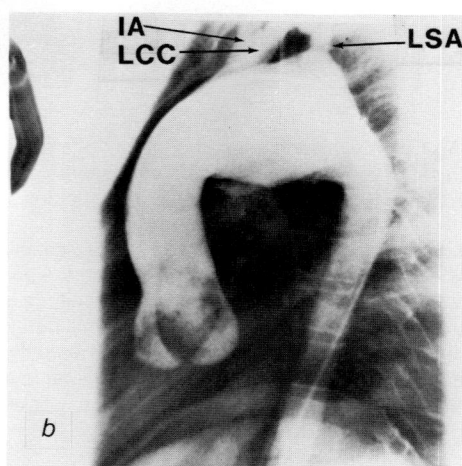

Figure 55-4   Thoracic aortograms of a patient with a moderately large fusiform transverse arch aortic aneurysm (UAB). The innominate artery originates just before the aneurysm, but the left common carotid artery and left subclavian arteries originate from the aneurysm. The aneurysm extends to the upper descending thoracic aorta.
(a) Frontal view.
(b) Lateral view.
IA, innominate artery; LCC, left common carotid artery; LSA, left subclavian artery.

tortuosity of the thoracic aorta without aneurysm formation (Fig. 55-8).

Thoracic Aortogram

Although not always necessary, thoracic aortography has been considered the definitive diagnostic procedure. Its most important contribution is the definition of the areas of relatively normal aorta proximal and distal to the aneurysm (Fig. 55-4), which at times requires visualization of the entire thoracic and abdominal aorta.[C7] Even large aneurysms may not be very dramatic in appearance at aortography, since luminal diameter may be near normal as a result of laminated thrombus within the aneurysm.

Computerized Axial Tomogram

With or without the use of contrast material, computerized axial tomography is a very useful method of evaluation of patients with thoracic aneurysms (Fig. 55-9). Currently, it is particularly useful for descending and thoracoabdominal aortic aneurysms.

NATURAL HISTORY

Aortic aneurysms gradually enlarge and eventually rupture no matter where they are located. Death may occur particularly early in patients with thoracic aortic aneurysms, compared with patients with abdominal ones (Fig. 55-10). Bickerstaff and colleagues found the 1-year survival rate of patients with thoracic aneurysms to be only 58% and the 5-year survival rate only 19%.[B4] Rupture of a thoracic aortic aneurysm occurred in 74% of the patients studied by Bickerstaff and colleagues[B4] and was the most common cause of death in the cases reported by Pressler and colleagues.[P2]

In particular, large aneurysms have a tendency to rupture,[M3] and recent increase in size usually precedes the catastrophic event. Likewise, the development of symptoms often precedes rupture, the symptoms resulting from prerupture expansion of the aneurysm. Once symptoms develop, the mean interval to rupture is 2 years.[B4]

The natural history may, however, depend in part on the etiology of the aneurysm. Patients whose chronic aneurysm is related to a previous acute aortic dissection may have a worse prognosis because of the possibility of redissection and sudden aneurysmal enlargement of other areas of the aorta. However, other than in patients with such a history, once a thoracic aneurysm forms, there is a strong tendency for its gradual enlargement and rupture, even in the case of chronic traumatic thoracic aneurysm.[F2,F3]

TECHNIQUE OF OPERATION

Preparations for Aneurysm Surgery

A thoracic or thoracoabdominal aortic aneurysm of any type is an extensive lesion, and a number of preparations for operation are required. An arterial pressure-recording catheter and adequate lines for intravenous therapy are placed after induction of anesthesia. Preferably, an internal jugular pressure-recording catheter is also placed. When the operation is performed through a median sternotomy, left atrial pressure is easily and inexpensively obtained by inserting the usual polyvinyl catheter into the left atrium (see Chapter 2, Section 3). When the operation is done through a left thoracotomy, a Swan-Ganz catheter can be placed to measure pulmonary artery wedge pressure.[K1] Also, when the operation is done through a left thoracotomy, a double-lumen endotracheal tube is used if it can be easily positioned. Facilities are made available for the rapid and sterile aspiration of blood from the surgical field, the washing and concentrating of red blood cells, and the rapid return of the packed red blood cells to the patient.

In operations on the descending thoracic and thoracoab-

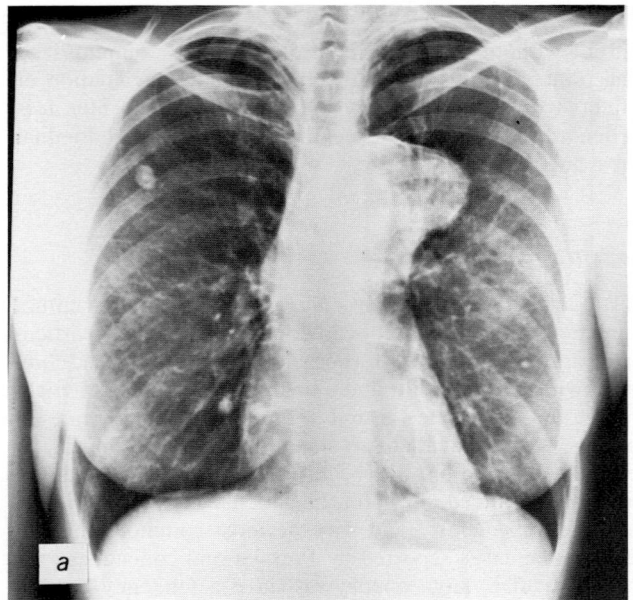

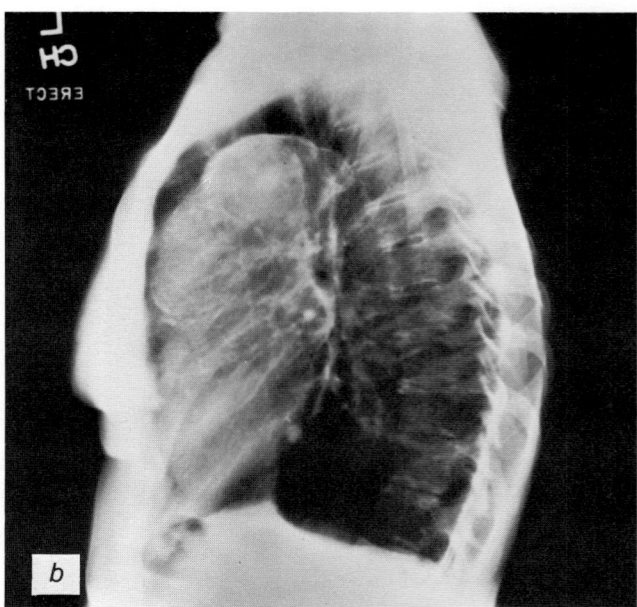

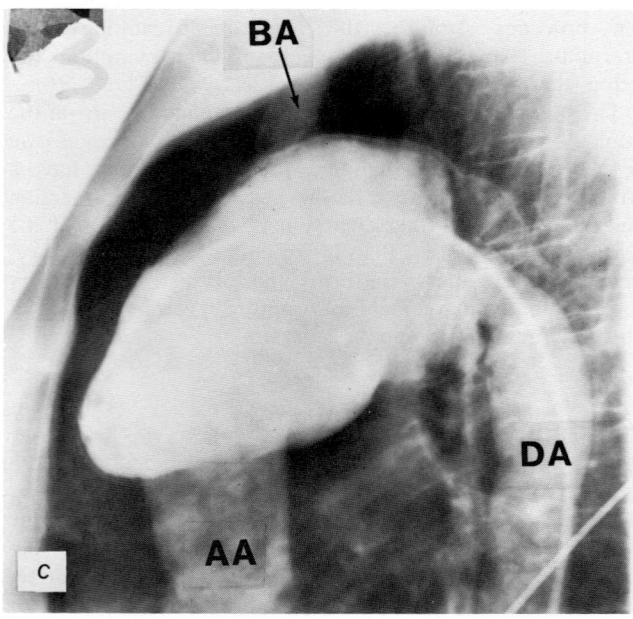

Figure 55-5   Chest x-ray and lateral aortogram of a patient with a large aneurysm of the transverse portion of the aortic arch (UAB). (*a*) In the frontal view, the chest x-ray shows the calcified aneurysm projecting to the left.
(*b*) In the lateral view, the position of the calcified aneurysm suggests that it originates in the transverse portion of the aortic arch.
(*c*) The lateral aortogram shows the somewhat sacciform aneurysm to involve the transverse portion of the aortic arch. It partly overlies the ascending aorta, obscuring the origin of the brachiocephalic arteries, and ends just short of the descending thoracic aorta.

AA, ascending aorta; BA, brachiocephalic arteries; DA, descending thoracic aorta.

dominal portions of the aorta, regulation of upper body arterial pressure requires care. Too high a pressure, with the resultant increase in left ventricular afterload, may increase left atrial pressure inordinately. This hemodynamic effect is further aggravated by the elevation in plasma epinephrine and norepinephrine levels that occurs after simple upper descending thoracic aortic cross-clamping.[S5] However, reducing upper body blood pressure with sodium nitroprusside carries the risk that the secondary reduction in aortic pressure beyond the cross-clamp will result in reduced renal blood flow and a tendency toward acute renal failure.[G6] Therefore, reduction of upper body arterial pressure must be done prudently during the period of aortic cross-clamping.

Particularly in operations on the descending and thoracoabdominal aorta, organ and subsystem function distally may be damaged not only during the ischemic period but also during the post–cross-clamping period. Thus, extensive bleeding from suture lines and hypotension after release of the cross-clamp increase the risk of renal failure or paraplegia. This period is often also characterized by metabolic acidosis secondary to the lower body ischemic period, and prompt treatment with sodium bicarbonate or other agents is important.[O2] Even with such treatment, renal blood flow may remain low for hours,[R1] and mannitol and Lasix (furosemide) are indicated if oliguria results.

Repair of Ascending Aortic Aneurysms

The preparations for operation, the median sternotomy, and the placement of stay sutures proceed as they do for most operations using cardiopulmonary bypass (see Chapter 2, Section 3). When the aneurysm extends nearly to the innominate artery or when the aneurysm is secondary to extensive chronic dissection, arterial cannulation through the femoral artery is elected. Otherwise, arterial cannulation may be into the distal portion of the ascending aorta or in the transverse arch if that is convenient.

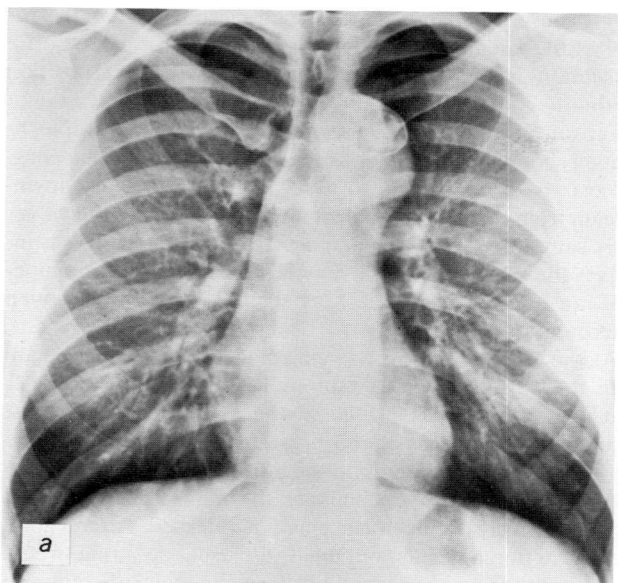

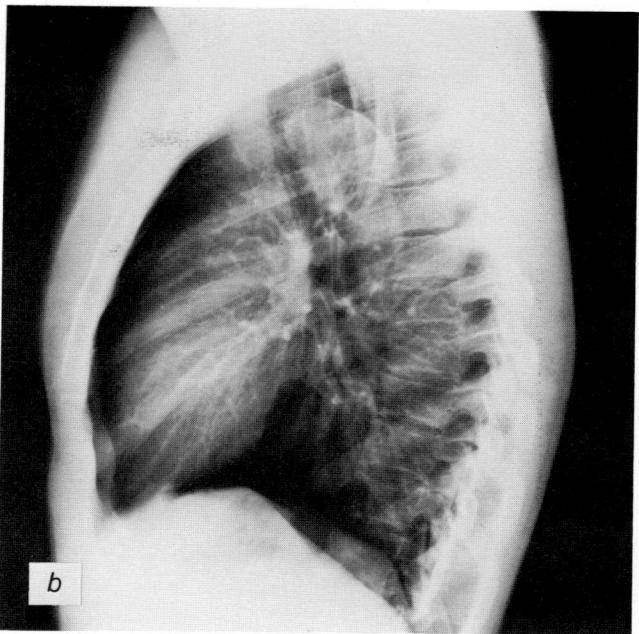

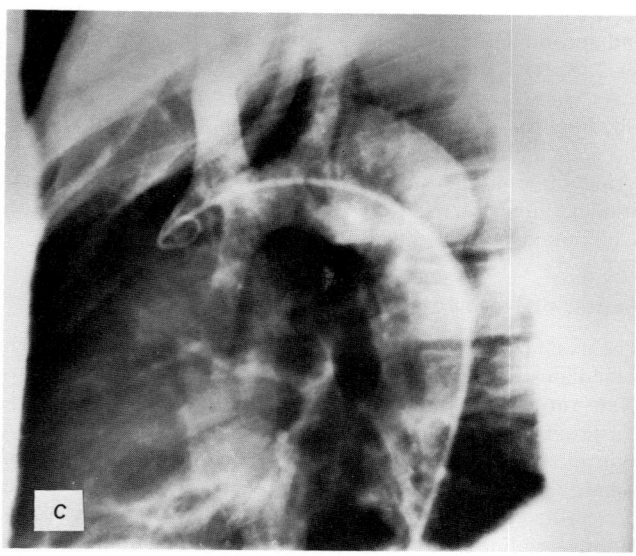

Figure 55-6 Small transverse aortic arch (UAB). Calcification can be seen within the wall of the aneurysm, which involves only that part of the arch beyond the origin of the left common carotid artery. (a) Frontal chest x-ray. (b) Lateral chest x-ray. (c) Aortogram.

Using a single venous cannula, cardiopulmonary bypass (CPB) is established in the usual manner at a perfusate temperature of 15°C. Generally a left atrial vent is not needed, but one may be inserted in the usual fashion (see Chapter 2, Section 3). After CPB has been established, minimal dissection of the aorta just beyond the aneurysm is accomplished so that if needed a felt strip may be passed behind this area. There must be room for the aortic cross-clamp to be placed distal to this area.

When *the aortic valve is to be replaced* because of important aortic valve incompetence, as well as the aneurysm of the ascending aorta resected, a composite graft and the inclusion technique are employed.[1] (For details of the compos-

ite graft technique, see Chapter 12 "Technique of Operation" and Fig. 12-5.) A modification of the technique described in Chapter 12 is used in patients with chronic dissection, in that the interposition technique of graft insertion is used at the distal anastomosis.[2] It is important to recognize that the composite graft technique is difficult and somewhat hazardous when the sinuses of Valsalva are not enlarged and thus the coronary arteries are not displaced distally from their normal location,[G4] and its advantage in such situations is minimal. Under such circumstances, it may be preferable separately to replace the aortic valve and graft the supra-annular portion of the aorta (see Chapter 54 "Combined Ascending Aorta and Aortic Valve Replacement" in section on Technique of Operation).

When *aortic valve replacement is not necessary* as a concomitant procedure, after CPB has been established the aortic cross-clamp is placed just proximal to the origin of the innominate artery. The cold cardioplegic solution is administered through a needle in the aneurysm itself. The aneurysm is opened longitudinally and its interior evaluated. If the aneurysm of the ascending aorta has resulted from a previous aortic dissection, generally the false channel extends beyond

---

[1]The inclusion technique of graft insertion *inside* the aneurysm is described in detail in Chapter 54, "Inclusion Technique of Graft

Insertion" in section on Technique of Operation, and in Figs. 54-5 and 54-7, as well as in Figs. 55-1, 55-12, and 55-14.

[2]The interposition technique of graft insertion by end-to-end anastomosis is described in Chapter 54, "Interposition Method of Graft Insertion" in section on Technique of Operation, and Figs. 54-4 and 54-6, as well as in Fig. 55-13.

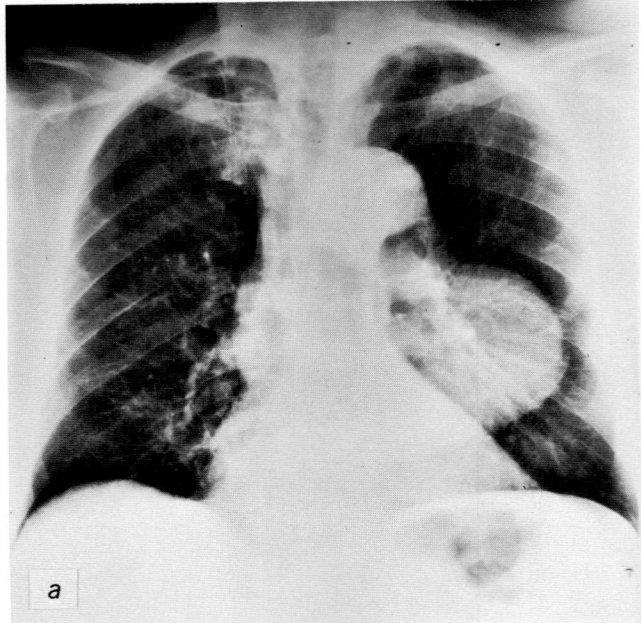

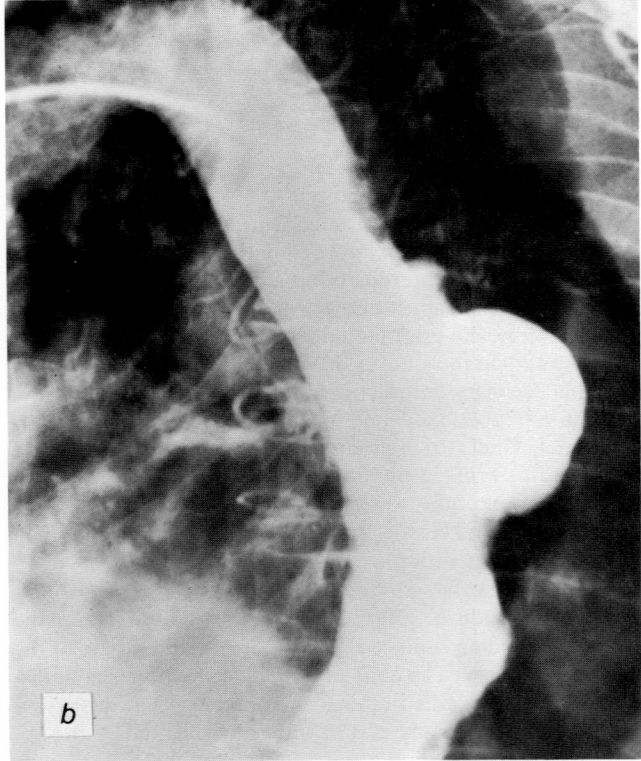

Figure 55-7 Aneurysms of the descending thoracic aorta (UAB). (a) Chest x-ray of a patient with a large but well-localized aneurysm of the mid descending thoracic aorta. (b) Thoracic aortogram, left anterior oblique view, of another patient with a localized aneurysm involving a short segment of the mid descending thoracic aorta.

the aortic cross-clamp. Under such circumstances, the repair of the aneurysm proceeds as described for acute aortic dissection, using either the inclusion or the interposition method (see footnotes 1 and 2). When the aneurysm is not the result of a previous acute dissection, the inclusion technique is commonly used (see footnote 1). The proximal anastomosis is usually made to a segment of aorta just downstream from the level of the commissures of the aortic valve. This same type of repair is made even if the aneurysm involves the sinuses of Valsalva or if the aortic valve is competent, an unusual occurrence. A securely preclotted woven Dacron graft is used.[3]

As the last anastomosis is being made, rewarming is begun with the perfusate, air is aspirated from the left ventricle, and a needle vent is placed in the segment of aorta just proximal to the cross-clamp or a small slit is made in the graft. With strong suction on the aortic needle vent, or with massage of the graft to facilitate the movement of air out from the small slit, the aortic clamp is released. After a good cardiac action has been obtained, the usual de-airing procedures are thoroughly carried out (see Chapter 2, Section 3). The suture lines are examined, and any pulsatile bleeding is secured by additional sutures. Then CPB is discontinued, and decannulation is effected in the usual manner (see Chapter 2, Section 3).

As soon as it is certain that there is no major pulsatile bleeding, the remnants of the aneurysm are sutured around the graft and suture lines (see footnote 1). The usual monitoring catheters and myocardial wires, as well as the usual drainage tubes, are placed, and the incision is closed in the usual manner.

Repair of Transverse Arch Aortic Aneurysms

The usual preparations are made for open operation through a median sternotomy (see Chapter 2, Section 3) and for aneurysm surgery. A femoral artery is exposed via a small vertical groin incision, the median sternotomy is made using a skin incision that extends 1–2 cm more into the neck than usual, and the pericardium is opened widely. The usual pericardial stay sutures are placed. A left atrial pressure-monitoring line is inserted (see Chapter 2, Section 3), and a right atrial purse-string stitch placed. An appropriate woven Dacron graft is securely preclotted (see footnote 3).

The patient is heparinized, the femoral artery is cannulated, a single venous cannula is inserted through the right atrial appendage, cardiopulmonary bypass (CPB) is established at the usual flow rate, cooling of the patient is begun (see Chapter 2, Section 4), and usually a left atrial vent is inserted and advanced into the ventricle (see Chapter 2, Section 3 for details). During cooling, the pericardial reflection is dissected off the distal portion of the ascending aorta, and the first portions of the innominate, left common carotid, and subclavian arteries are dissected. No attempt is made to dissect the aneurysm itself. Generally, the left pleural space is

---

[3]The types of graft and the methods of preclotting them are described in detail in Chapter 53, "Grafts for Thoracic and Thoracoabdominal Aortic Surgery" in section on Special Situations and Controversies.

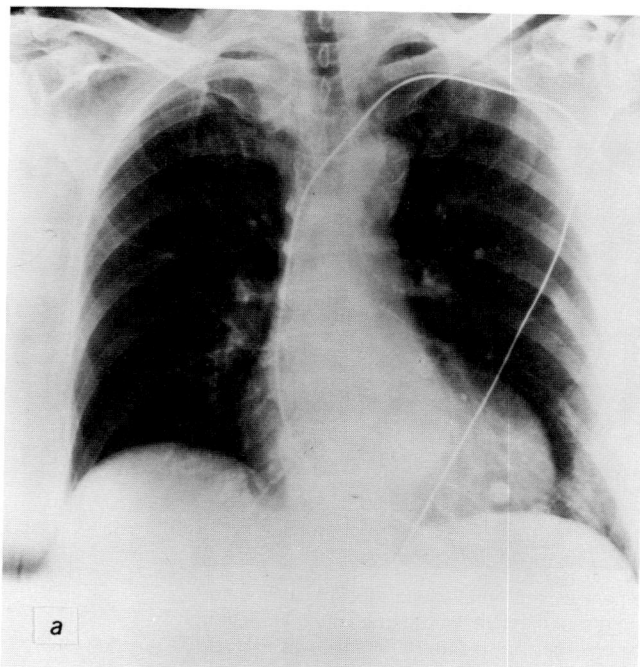

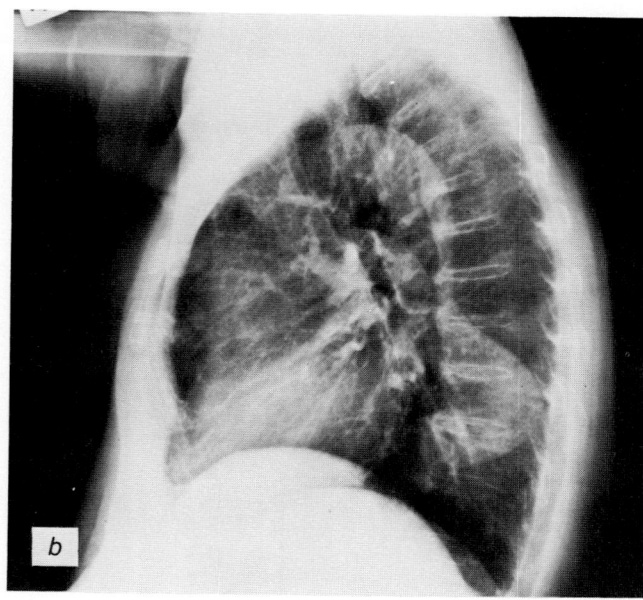

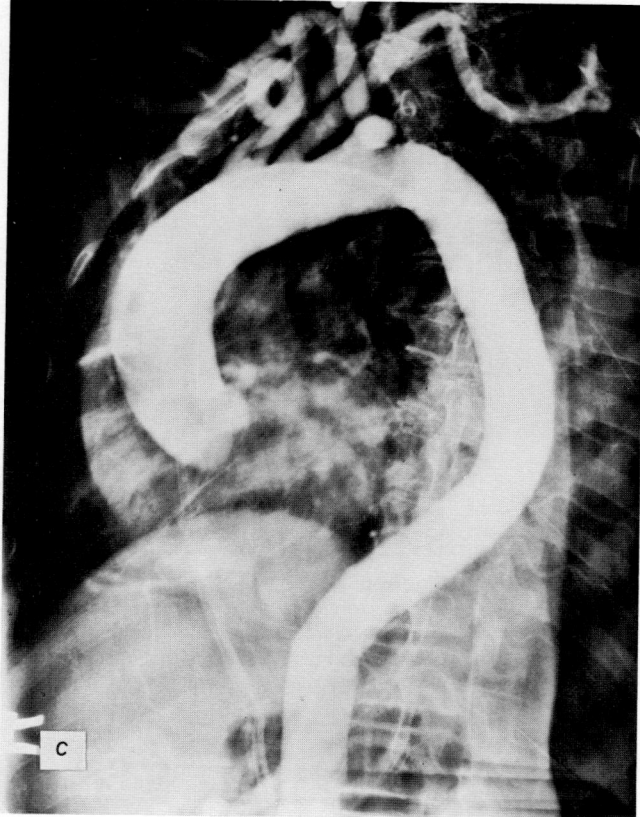

Figure 55-8 Frontal and lateral chest x-rays suggest aneurysm of the lower descending thoracic aorta (UAB). The aortogram indicates that aneurysm is not present but that the thoracic aorta has become tortuous and elongated by the aging process. Enhanced computerized tomography can also provide the correct diagnosis. (a) Frontal x-ray. (b) Lateral x-ray. (c) Aortogram.

entered in order to facilitate estimation of the distal extent of the aneurysm.

When the patient's nasopharyngeal temperature reaches 18–20°C, the three brachiocephalic vessels are clamped as near their origins as possible, and the ascending aorta is clamped well proximal to the aneurysm. The upper descending thoracic aorta is left unclamped. The cold cardioplegic solution is infused through the usual needle vent in the ascending aorta on the cardiac side of the proximal cross-clamp (see Chapter 3), total circulatory arrest is established, and the venous line is left open for about 10 seconds after arterial input to the patient is discontinued, so that the ve-

nous system is decompressed. Every effort is made to keep the total circulatory arrest time less than 45 minutes, although the risks of 60 minutes of arrest are accepted if this period is required for surgical treatment of this lesion (see Chapter 2, Sections 1, 4).

Because aneurysms of the transverse arch vary widely in size and extent, the actual techniques of repair are variable. In some circumstances, the aneurysm is localized, and the patient is treated by simple patch grafting of the defect in the wall between the transverse aorta and the aneurysm (Fig. 55-11). Occasionally, also, the aneurysm may involve only the proximal portion and undersurface of the transverse arch, and a relatively simple reconstruction by tailoring the resection and graft as described by Ott and colleagues (see Fig. 55-2) is possible.

Generally, however, the aneurysm diffusely involves the transverse arch, and a complete reconstruction is needed. Because of the difficulty of dissecting outside the aneurysm in this area and the need for the reinforcing wrap of the aneurysm walls around the graft at the completion of the operation, the inclusion technique is nearly always used (see

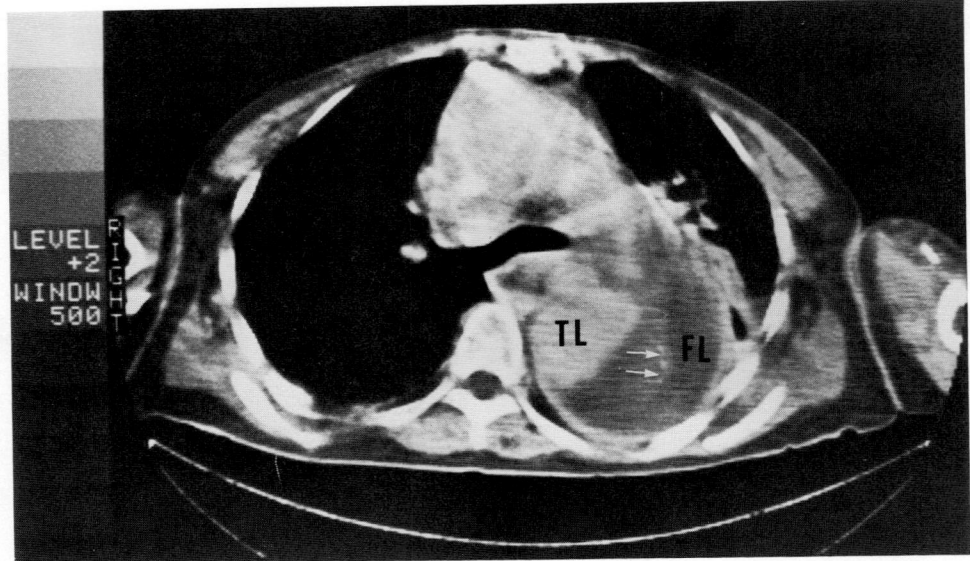

Figure 55-9 Computerized tomogram with enhancement by the intravenous ejection of a water-soluble contrast medium in a patient with chronic aortic dissection (UAB). The true lumen at the mid thoracic aorta level is deformed by the aneurysmally enlarged false lumen. The arrows indicate calcification within the aneurysm.

FL, false lumen; TL, true lumen.

footnote 1). A securely preclotted woven Dacron graft (see footnote 3) is prepared for the reconstruction.

The aneurysm is opened longitudinally in its mid-portion. The inside of the aneurysm is freed from any thrombotic debris, and care is taken not to lose any fragments down the unclamped descending thoracic aorta or in the orifices of the brachiocephalic vessels. The distal anastomosis is made first (Fig. 55-12). This often is the most difficult part of the operation. The exposure usually does not allow the placement of sutures from outside in, such as is often possible in the ascending aorta. Instead, the suturing is done entirely from within, with a stout needle and each bite taken deeply into the aortic wall. A 2-0 or 3-0 double-armed polypropylene suture is used, and the suturing is begun posteriorly where the exposure is most difficult. A simple continuous whip stitch may be used (GLH, UAB), a continuous everting mattress suture over felt strips (UAB), or interrupted everting mattress sutures over felt strips or with pledgets (UAB;

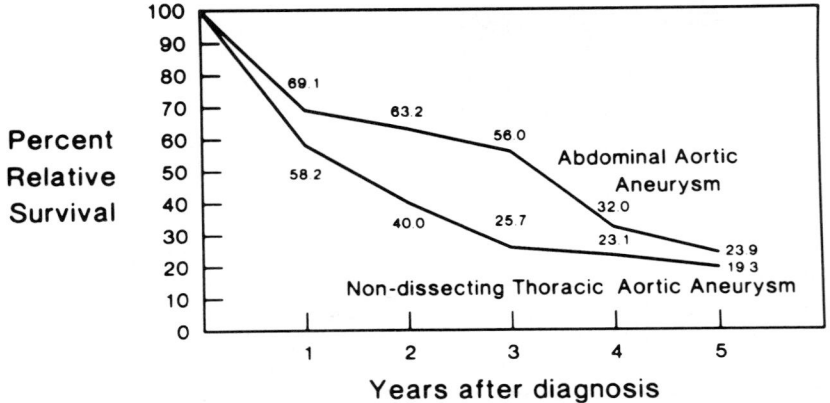

Figure 55-10 Actuarial survival of patients with chronic thoracic aortic aneurysm, nearly all of whom were without surgical treatment, compared to that of surgically untreated patients with abdominal aortic aneurysm, as reported earlier by Estes.[E1]

Reproduced with permission from Bickerstaff et al.[B4]

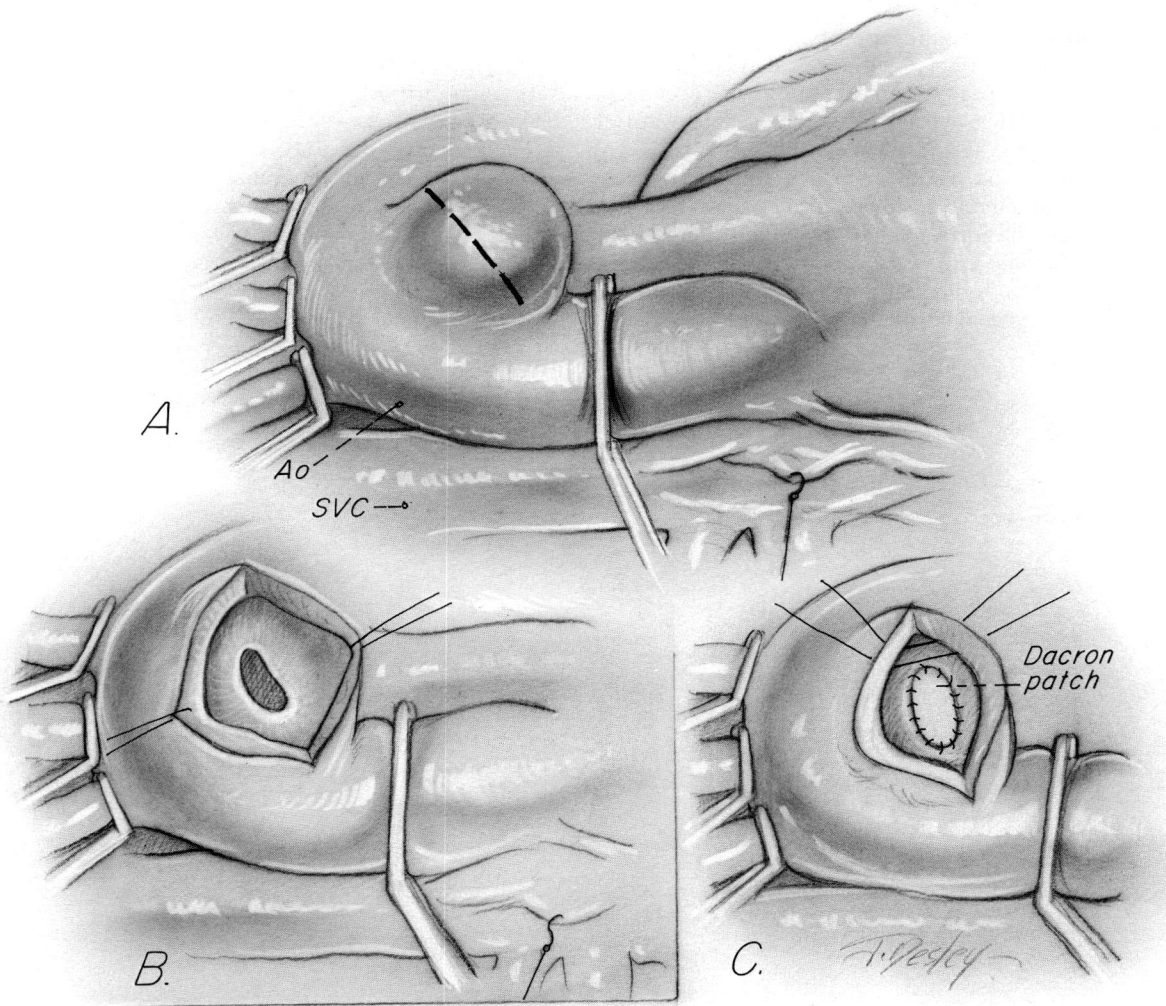

Figure 55-11   Repair of a saccular aneurysm arising from the undersurface of the transverse portion of the aortic arch.

(a) The innominate, left common carotid, and subclavian arteries have been dissected out, as has the proximal aspect of the transverse portion of the arch. Clamps have been placed on the aortic origin of the three brachiocephalic vessels, and on the mid-portion of the ascending aorta. The proposed incision into the saccular aneurysm is shown (alternatively, in some patients the opening may be made into the transverse portion of the aorta itself).

(b) After the aneurysm has been opened and the thrombotic material removed, a discrete opening between the transverse arch and the aneurysm is identified.

(c) This opening is closed with a preclotted woven Dacron patch. After cardiopulmonary bypass has been reestablished, all air removed, and the cross-clamps released, any important bleeding from the suture line is repaired. The aneurysm walls are brought together with interrupted sutures over the repair site.

Ao, aorta; SVC, superior vena cava.

see Fig. 55-12). It is better to take a little extra time to make a secure initial anastomosis than it is to have to attempt reinforcement of the anastomosis at a later time. In any case, the first four or five stitches are placed with the graft held at a distance, and then the graft is slid into position, and those sutures are snugged and tied if interrupted. With the interrupted suture technique, the last four or five sutures are held after placement and then tied when all are in place. The graft is clamped, and the arterial pump is turned on briskly, but for only about 5 seconds, to pressurize the descending aorta

and the suture line in order to check for suture line leaks. Whatever additional sutures are needed are now placed.

The graft is now contoured to lie nicely in place, and a properly located single oval aperture is made in its superior surface that is sufficiently large to give the graft access to the origins of the three brachiocephalic arteries (Fig. 55-12). The posterior suture line, between the edge of the graft aperture and the oval of aortic wall containing the three orifices, is made with a whip stitch of 3-0 polypropylene suture, again with deep bites of aortic wall taken (Fig. 55-12). A double-armed suture is used, and the sewing begins distally and progresses proximally toward the surgeon. After this suture line is carried around the right-sided angle, it is held. The other arm of the suture is used to carry the suture line around the left-sided angle and then anteriorly, worked again toward the surgeon to complete the anastomosis (Fig. 55-12).

The patient is placed in a rather steep Trendelenburg's position; the arterial pump is slowly turned until blood comes up the descending aorta and into the graft; the graft is massaged to dislodge any air, as are the orifices of the brachiocephalic arteries; and, when it is filled with blood, the graft is clamped at the place judged to be appropriate for the

anastomosis to the ascending aorta. CPB is then reestablished at 1.6 1 · min^{-1} · m^{-2} at 25°C, and the clamps are removed from the innominate, left common carotid, and left subclavian arteries. The suture line is examined, and any leaks are repaired with additional sutures.

The clamp on the graft is now moved more distally, the graft is cut, and the proximal anastomosis is made. This anastomosis may be made just as was the distal one, but preferably the sutures are placed from outside the aorta (UAB). The clamp is removed from the graft and the suture line examined for bleeding.

With strong suction on the aortic needle vent, the more

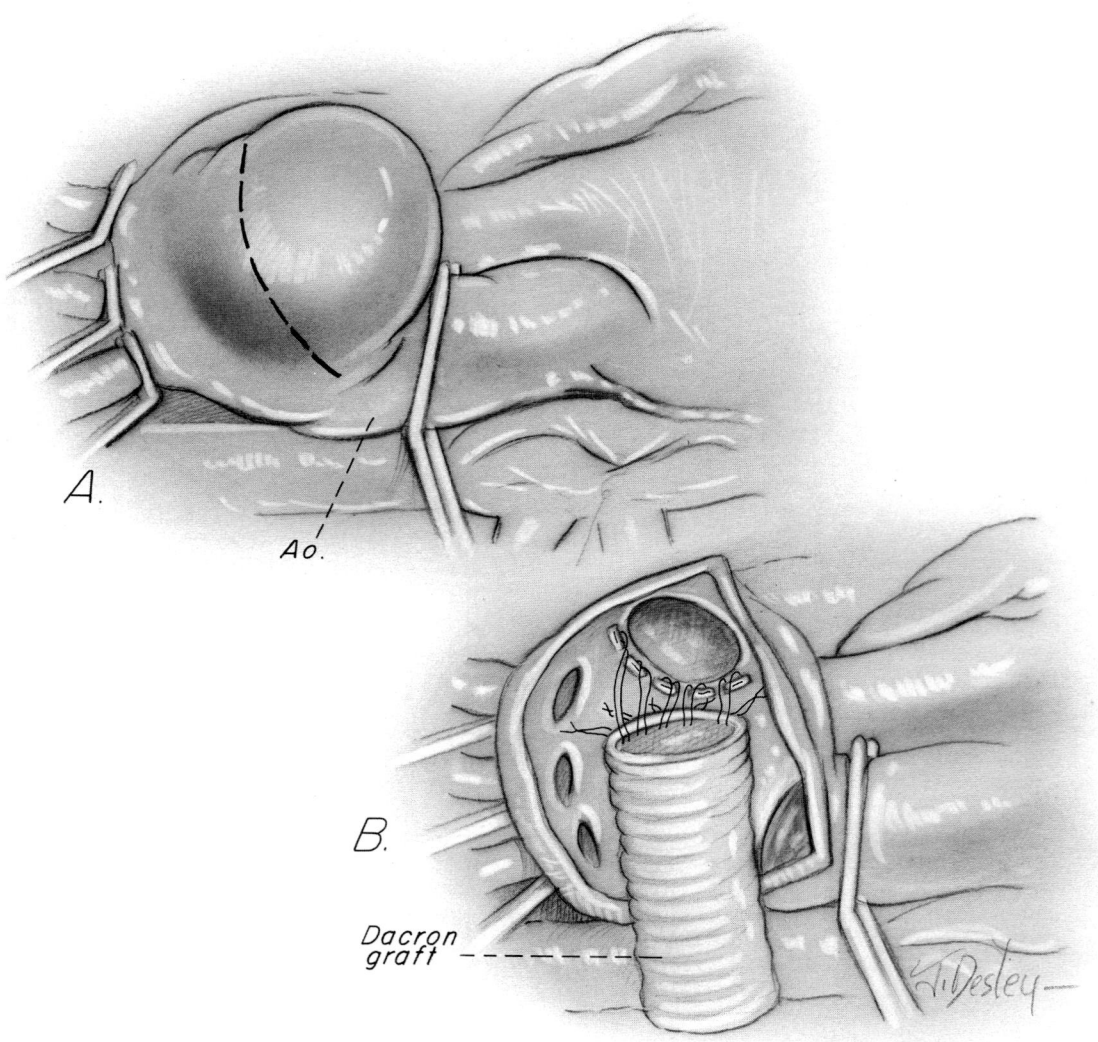

Figure 55-12   Repair of a large fusiform aneurysm of the transverse portion of the aortic arch using profound hypothermia and total circulatory arrest.
(a) After profound hypothermia has been induced, clamps are placed across the origin of the three brachiocephalic vessels, and on the mid-portion of the ascending aorta. The proposed incision into the aneurysm is shown with a dashed line.
(b) After total circulatory arrest is established, and without a distal aortic clamp, the aneurysm is opened widely. The securely preclotted woven Dacron tube graft is in this instance sutured into place distally with interrupted pledgetted mattress sutures. These sutures are placed mostly from within the aneurysm, and care is taken to take substantial, deep bites into the aortic wall with each stitch. A continuous whip stitch may be used.

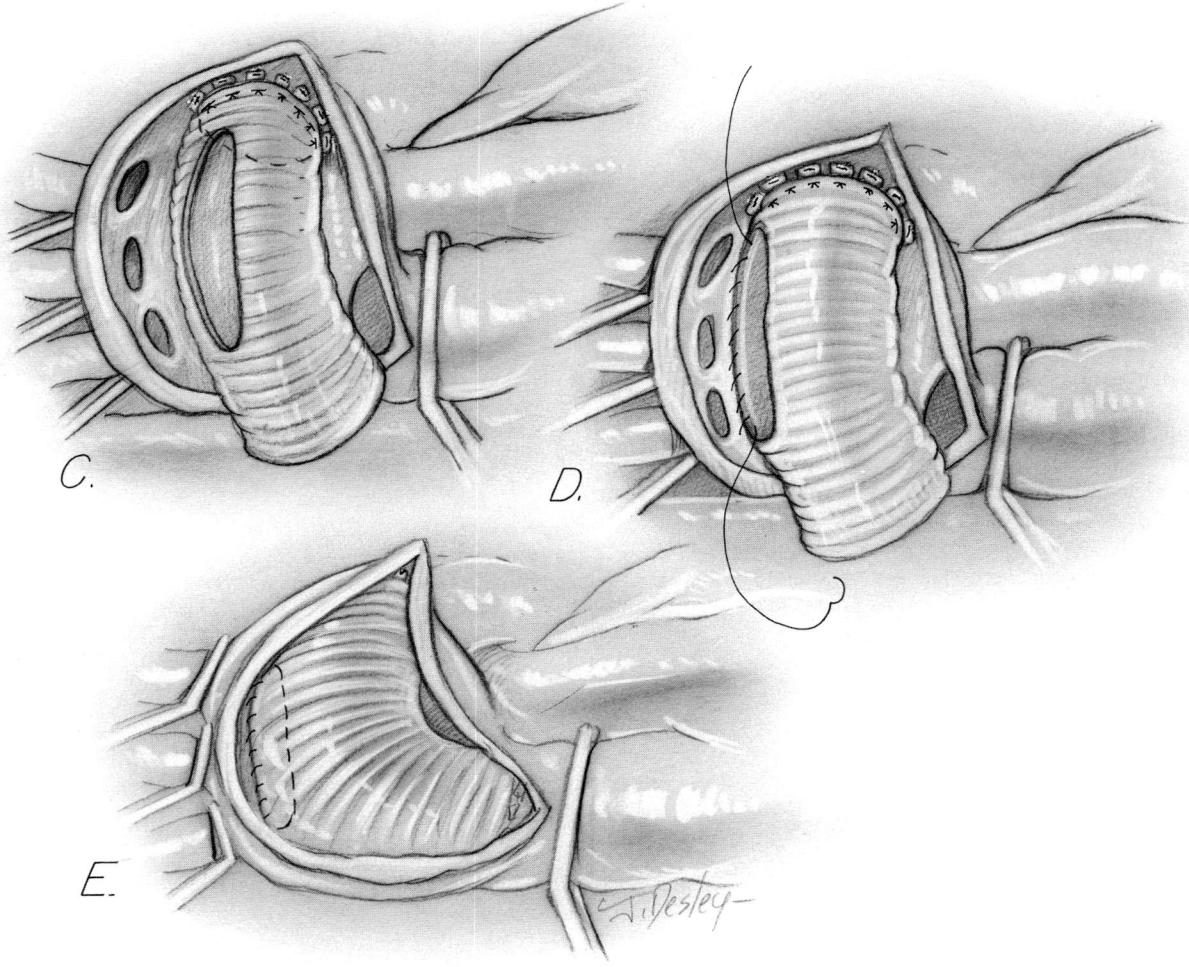

Figure 55-12   (continued)

(c) An oval segment has been removed from the superior surface of the graft to prepare for the single anastomosis around the origins of the brachiocephalic arteries.

(d) The posterior portion of the suture line is made from within, using a whip stitch.

(e) The anterior portion of the suture line around the origins of the brachiocephalic arteries has been completed. The proximal graft anastomosis is made as described in b for the distal anastomosis. After the clamps are removed and any important bleeding from the suture lines has been controlled, the walls of the aneurysm are brought together around the graft as in other inclusion techniques.

Ao, aorta.

proximal aortic clamp that was placed early in the procedure is released, rewarming having begun about 5 minutes before. When a strong cardiac action has returned, the usual de-airing procedures are followed. Again, all suture lines are examined for leaks, and any found are corrected. When rewarming is complete, CPB is discontinued and decannulation effected. After the heparin effect has been reversed with protamine sulfate, the aneurysm walls are wrapped snugly around the graft and held together with interrupted sutures. This wrap is not considered a substitute for a nonhemostatic suture line but, rather, a method of establishing final hemostasis in the face of oozing from suture lines or through the graft.

The remainder of the operation is completed in the usual manner (see Chapter 2, Section 3).

Repair of Descending Thoracic Aortic Aneurysms

The usual preparations for aneurysm surgery are made. Then the patient is placed in the right lateral decubitus position, with the left hip rolled back toward the surgeon so that the left femoral artery and vein are accessible if needed. A long posterolateral incision is made, and the thorax is entered through the top of the bed of the nonresected sixth rib. If the aneurysm is limited to the very upper portion of the descending thoracic aorta, the chest is entered through the top of the bed of the nonresected fifth rib. If the entire thoracic aorta is involved, a longer skin incision is made, curving inferiorly in its anterior portion, and the thorax is opened through the top of the bed of the nonresected fifth or sixth rib. For the distal clamp and anastomosis, a second entrance is made into the thorax through the top of the bed of the nonresected eighth rib. Interspace incisions may be preferred.

The procedure varies depending on the location and size of the descending thoracic aortic aneurysm, but the same general plan is followed for all. A limited dissection is made around the aorta just proximal to the aneurysm, liberating both sides of the aorta so that a cross-clamp can be placed. It is not necessary to dissect completely around the aneurysm. These aneurysms commonly have their proximal limit close to the left subclavian artery origin, in which case mobilization of the transverse arch between the left common carotid and subclavian arteries is required, the surgeon working between the phrenic and vagus nerves. Access to the aorta is often improved by opening the pericardium, particularly if a Gott shunt is to be inserted proximal to the cross-clamp site. A large vascular clamp is selected for placement at the appropriate point. The aneurysm is disturbed as little as possible as a similar dissection is made just beyond it, and a clamp is selected for placement there. The segment of aorta that is replaced is no longer than necessary, as prophylaxis against

unnecessarily interrupting intercostal arteries and increasing the risk of paraplegia.

The method of protecting the spinal cord during the period of cross-clamping is now selected and implemented.[4] A woven Dacron graft of the proper size is securely preclotted (see footnote 3). It is better that the graft is a little too small than too large in diameter. The proximal aortic clamp, and when necessary a left subclavian clamp, are placed, with the anesthesiologist maintaining an optimal hemodynamic state (see Chapter 4); the distal clamp is placed; and the aneurysm is opened longitudinally. The aortic origin of the intercostal arteries is studied. If possible, the aneurysmectomy is tailored so that an oblique anastomosis can be made of one end of the graft to the tailored aortic remnant and the maximum number of intercostal arteries preserved (see Chapter 54, Fig. 54-6). Otherwise, the aneurysmal portion of the aorta is simply replaced with the graft, using either the inclusion

---

[4]The risks of paraplegia after surgery on the descending thoracic and thoracoabdominal portions of the aorta, as well as methods of minimizing its occurrence, are discussed in Chapter 53, "Paraplegia" in section on Special Situations and Controversies.

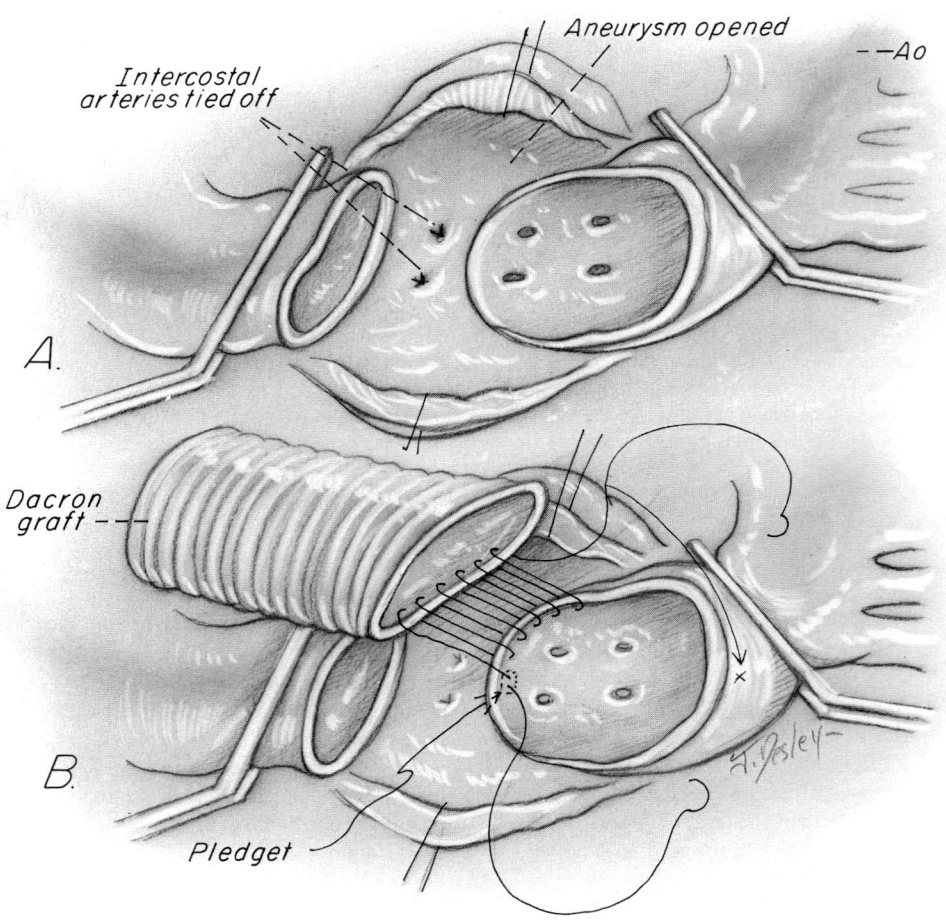

Figure 55-13 Interposition repair of a descending thoracic aortic aneurysm.
(a) The aortic resection and grafting are tailored to preserve intercostal arteries.
(b) The proximal anastomosis is made with a continuous whip stitch.

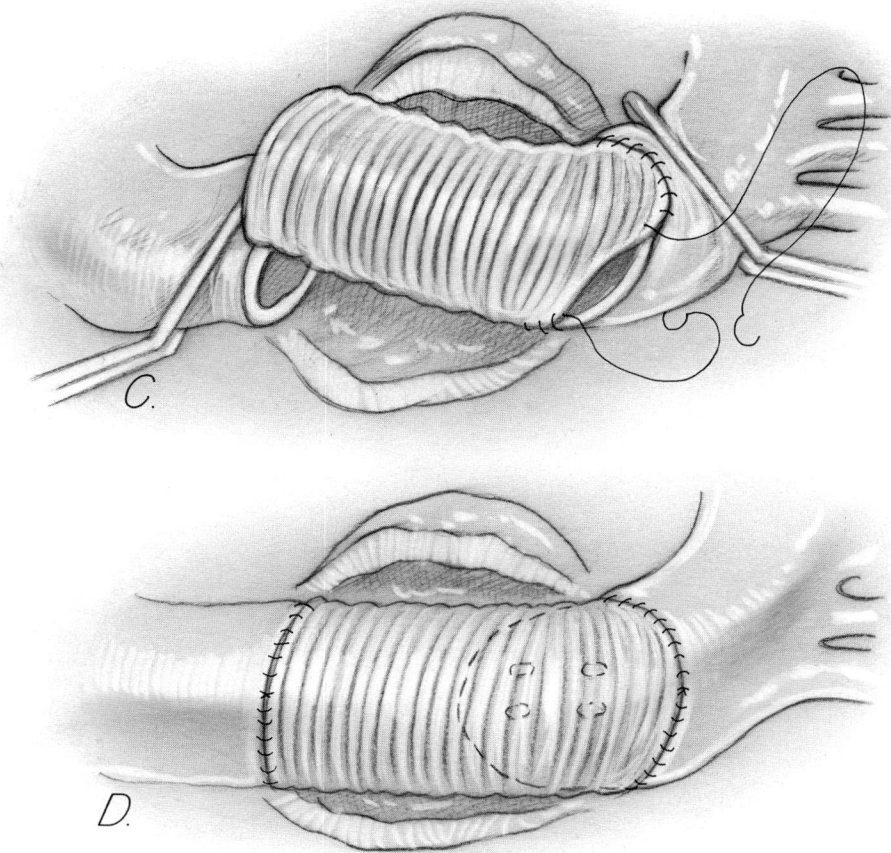

Figure 55-13 (continued)
(c) The proximal anastomosis is completed. The graft is trimmed to an appropriate length.
(d) The distal anastomosis is completed with a continuous whip stitch.
Ao, aorta.

technique (see Fig. 55-1) or the interposition method (Fig. 55-13; see footnotes 1 and 2). The interposition technique is always required when the aortic remnant is tailored to preserve intercostal arteries and an oblique anastomosis made (Fig. 53-13).

The utmost care is taken to make the suture lines entirely hemostatic. With either the inclusion or interposition technique, after the proximal anastomoses are made, the graft is clamped, the proximal clamp is opened for a few heartbeats to check for suture line leaks, and any leaks are repaired. After both anastomoses are completed, the distal clamp is released, and the proximal clamp is then gradually opened as the anesthesiologist monitors the hemodynamic state.[K1]

One intercostal drainage tube is brought out from the posterior gutter and one from the apex of the chest anteriorly. The incision is closed as usual.

Repair of Thoracoabdominal Aortic Aneurysms

The usual preparations for aneurysm surgery are made. The considerations with regard to paraplegia are particularly important because of the increased risk of this complication after repair of thoracoabdominal aneurysms (see footnote 4).

The patient is positioned in the same way as for descending aortic aneurysm surgery.

A thoracoabdominal incision is made,[H1] usually through the ninth intercostal space, and extended obliquely across the abdomen as an oblique incision or downward as a midline vertical abdominal incision (Fig. 55-14). A second intercostal incision, usually above the sixth rib, may be required when the aneurysm begins more proximally in the descending aorta. The diaphragm is opened by a peripheral incision. The peritoneum may not be opened, but, rather, the left side of the retroperitoneal space may be entered as the diaphragm is divided and the peritoneum and its contents as well as the left kidney are retracted forward and to the right. In many circumstances, it is easier to open the peritoneal cavity and reflect the spleen, descending colon, pancreas, and left kidney anteriorly and to the left.[C13]

Thoracoabdominal aneurysms vary greatly in location and extent, and these variations determine the details of the operative procedure. In most cases, an area just proximal to the aneurysm is selected for placement of the proximal clamp, and this area is prepared simply by clearing both sides of the aorta at this level. If the distal portion of the abdominal aorta is free of aneurysm, this is also prepared for

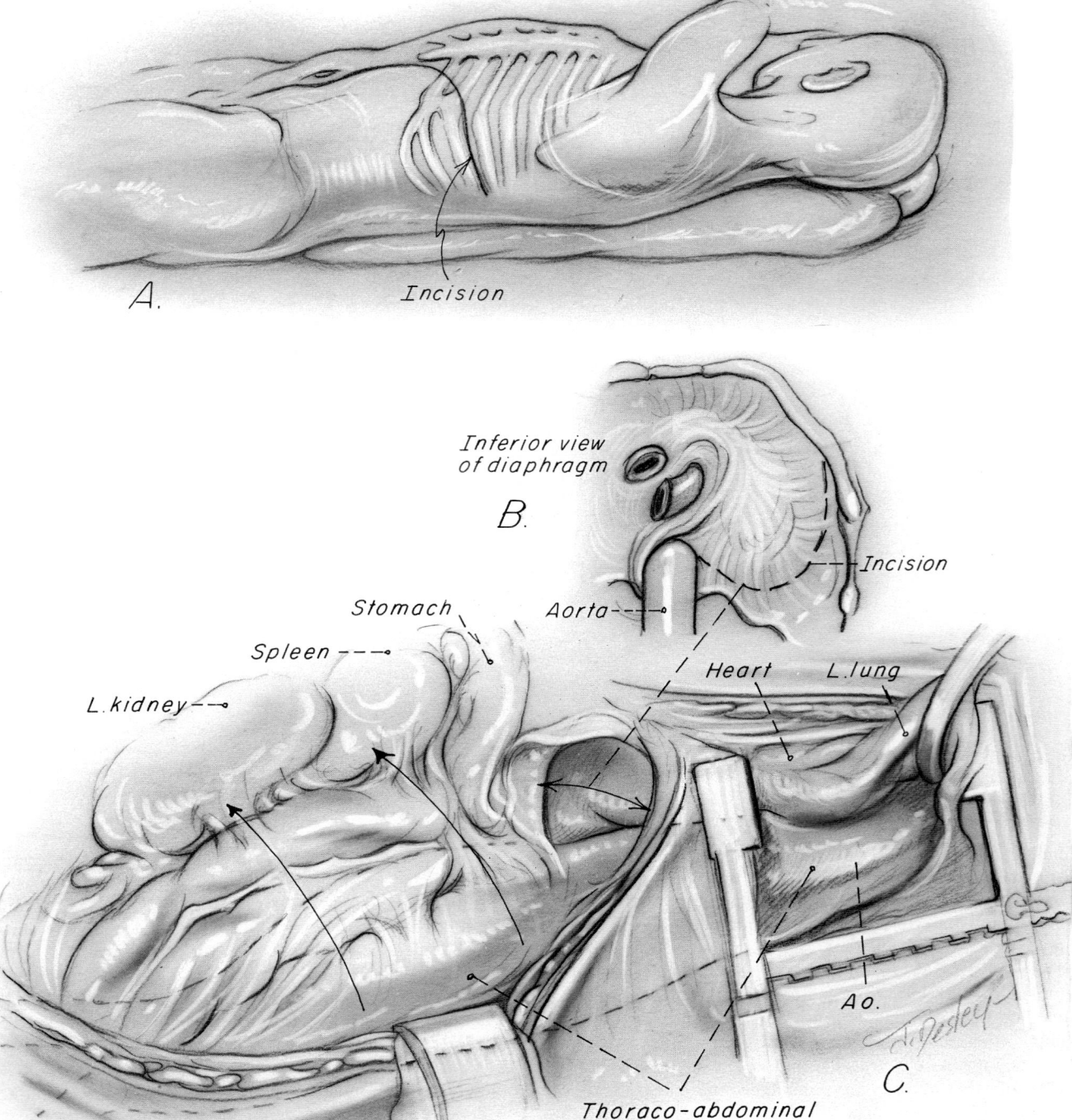

Figure 55-14 Repair of thoracoabdominal aneurysm

(a) The patient is placed in the right lateral decubitus position, with the hips rolled back so as to be in a 45° angled position. The thoracoabdominal incision is made as shown in the figure. For aneurysms extending to the mid-descending thoracic aorta, the incision is carried further posteriorly, and on occasions a second higher interspace incision is made.

(b) The diaphragm is opened with a peripheral radial incision that extends to the aorta.

(c) The abdominal viscera, including the left kidney, are reflected anteriorly and to the right.

Ao, aorta; Celiac a, celiac artery; Inf.mes.a, inferior mesenteric artery; L. renal a, left renal artery; Rt. renal a, right renal artery; sup.mes.a, superior mesenteric artery.

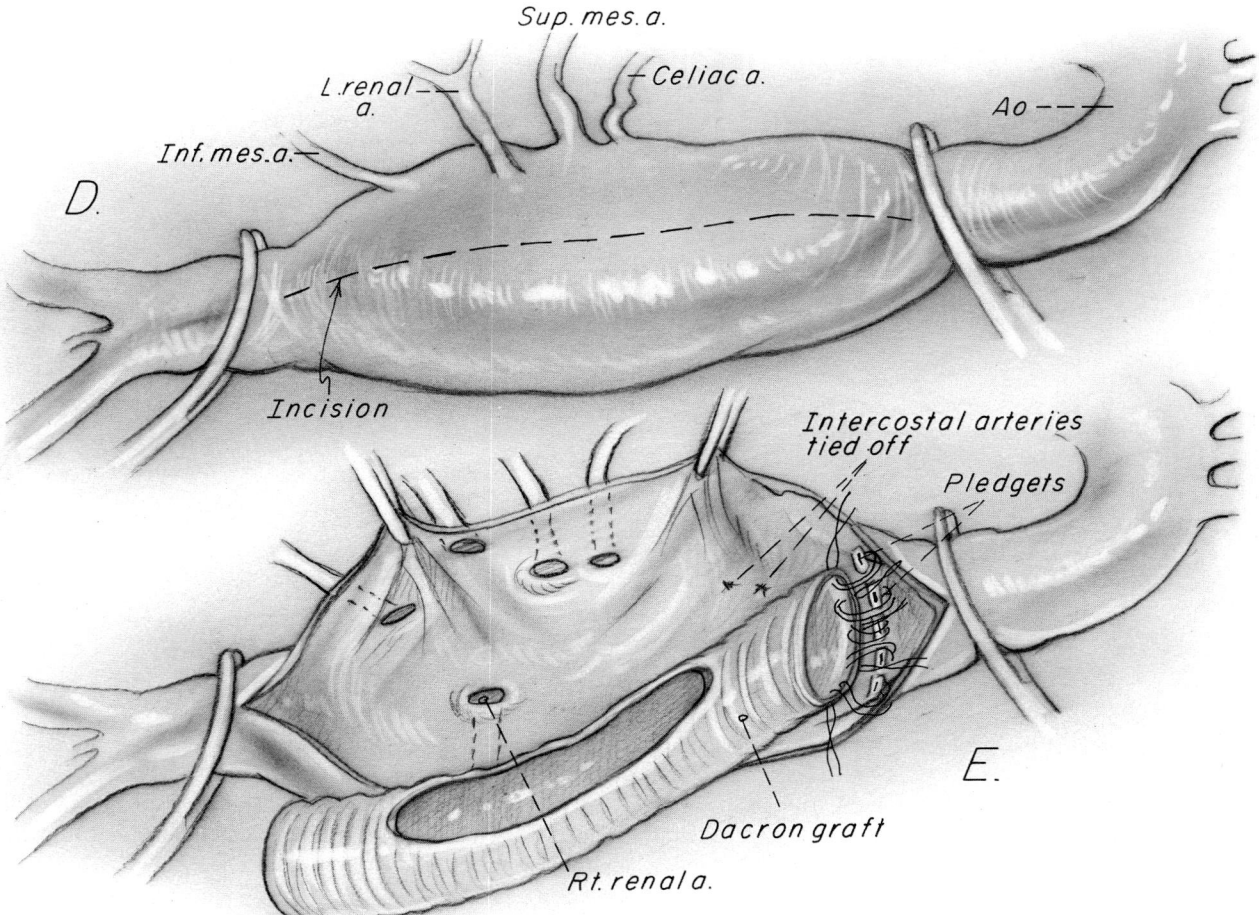

Figure 55-14 *(continued)*

(*d*) After the placement of appropriate occluding devices, the aneurysm is opened with a longitudinal incision. Retrograde bleeding from the visceral and intercostal arteries can be aspirated into a red blood cell–saving device for rapid return to the patient, or the arteries may be occluded from within by balloon-tipped catheters.

(*e*) The proximal anastomosis of a securely preclotted woven Dacron graft is made with continuous or interrupted pledgetted mattress sutures. A window is then cut in the graft through which blood will flow to the orifices of the visceral arteries.

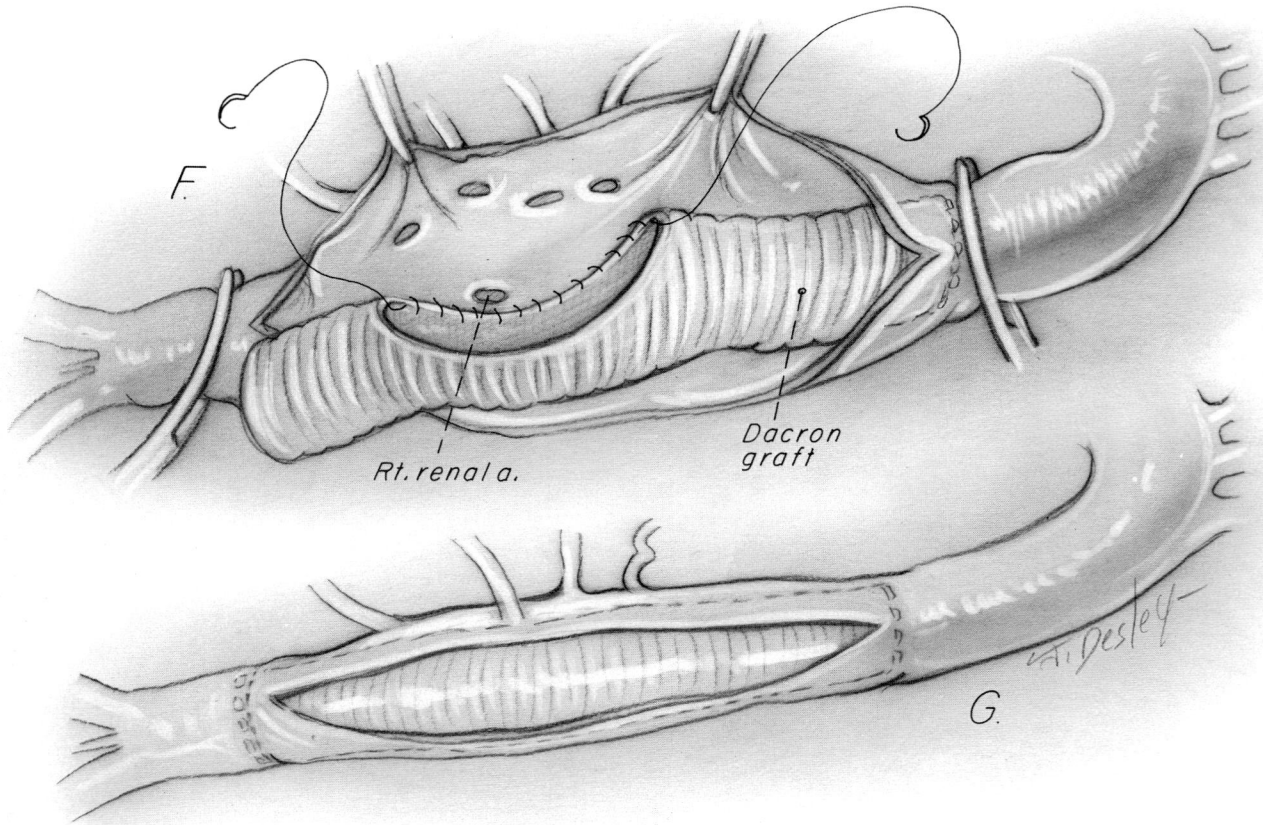

Figure 55-14 (*continued*)
(*f*) The edges around the window in the graft are sutured to the aortic wall around the cluster of visceral arterial orifices. After this is completed, the distal anastomosis will be made.
(*g*) The occluding devices are removed before closing the aneurysmal wall around the graft. The visceral arteries now receive blood flow through the window that has been made in the graft. The walls of the aneurysm are wrapped around the graft as a final step.

cross-clamping. If bleeding from the visceral arteries is considerable while the aneurysm is open, it can be controlled with Fogarty balloon catheters. Alternatively, both this and bleeding from the aorta beyond the aneurysm can be managed by simply aspirating the blood with the sterile system for processing and returning it to the patient.

After appropriate precautions against paraplegia are taken (see footnote 4) and an appropriately sized woven Dacron tube is securely preclotted (see footnote 3) the proximal aortic clamp is placed, the distal clamp is placed if it is to be used, and the aneurysm is opened longitudinally through its posterolateral surface. Before clamping, $1 \text{ mg} \cdot \text{kg}^{-1}$ of heparin is used and later reversed with a similar dose of protamine sulfate (GLH). The inclusion technique of graft insertion is employed (see footnote 1). After the proximal anastomosis is made and the proximal clamp is released briefly to allow checking for bleeding, an oval aperture is created in the graft opposite the area of the origin of the visceral arteries. The graft is then sewn to the aorta around these origins (Fig. 55-14). The proximal aortic clamp is again released briefly to allow checking for bleeding. The distal anastomosis is made, and both aortic clamps are released. When hemostasis has been obtained, the aneurysmal walls

are wrapped around the graft. The thoracoabdominal incisions are closed in the usual manner, and two intercostal drainage tubes are left in the left chest.

SPECIAL FEATURES OF POSTOPERATIVE CARE

Patients who have undergone repair of thoracic or thoracoabdominal aneurysm receive the same care given patients after major cardiac operations (see Chapter 5) except that intravenous (noncolloid) fluid administrations are more liberal to maintain a higher urinary output. Particular attention is paid to maintaining adequate ventricular preload by volume (colloid) infusions. The amount of chest drainage is closely observed, and the usual rules for reentry (see Chapter 5, Table 5-4) are enforced in these patients since major bleeding is one of the important risks.

When the repair has been made through a left thoracotomy, pulmonary complications are more apt to develop than after a median sternotomy. Thus, close attention to management of the pulmonary subsystem is mandatory (see Chapter 5 for details). Since renal blood flow is often reduced or absent for a time after the repair, evidence of acute renal dysfunction or failure is sought during the first few postoperative days, and, if present, appropriate treatment is promptly prescribed (see Chapter 5 for details).

RESULTS

Hospital Mortality

After repair of chronic thoracic and thoracoabdominal aortic aneurysm, hospital mortality is variable and depends, among other things, on the location and extent of the aneurysm. Also, older age at operation and the necessity that the operation be done as an emergency increase the risk of hospital death.[M5]

Ascending Aortic Aneurysms
The hospital mortality is low but does not yet approach zero for the repair of ascending aortic aneurysms.[D12] In a 15-year experience, the mortality was 6% in patients without concomitant aortic valve replacement and, in the 1975–1979 period, 5% when valve replacement is included (UAB; Table 55-1). Culliford and colleagues reported a similar mortality, with 3 deaths (9%, CL 4%–17%) among 35 patients,[C19] as did Grey, Ott, and Cooley, with 8 deaths (9%, CL 6%–13%) among 91 patients.[G4]

Transverse Arch Aortic Aneurysms
In the early era of thoracic aortic aneurysm surgery, hospital mortality following repair of transverse arch aneurysms was high, often greater than 50%, but in the recent era, several groups have reported hospital mortality rates of about 10% no matter what portion of the transverse arch was involved. Thus, Crawford and colleagues reported in 1979 only 1 hospital death (6%, CL 1%–19%) among 17 patients undergoing

repair of distal aortic arch aneurysms.[C11,C18] There has been 1 death (9%, CL 1%–28%) among 11 patients in whom the entire transverse arch was involved (GLH, Table 55-2), whereas comparable results have been obtained only in a recent era (UAB, Table 55-3). Crawford and Saleh have reported only 2 hospital deaths (12%, CL 4%–26%) among 17 patients in whom circulatory arrest techniques were used for extensive transverse aortic arch aneurysms.[C10]

The seriousness of the problem of transverse aortic arch aneurysms is evident, however, from the fact that several series report hospital mortality rates of about 25%. Culliford and colleagues have reported 2 deaths (25%, CL 9%–50%) among 8 patients treated by transverse arch resection and grafting under profoundly hypothermic total circulatory ar-

Table 55-1 Hospital mortality after resection of chronic aneurysms of the ascending aorta (UAB; 1967–July 1984).

Category of Aneurysm	n	Hospital Deaths		
		No.	%	CL
Arteriosclerotic or degenerative	8		0%	0%–21%
Chronic aortic dissection	18[a]	1	6%	1%–18%
Posttraumatic, closed	1		0%	0%–85%
Aortitis, including syphilis	2	1	50%	7%–93%
Postcardiovascular surgery	3[b]		0%	0%–47%
Total	32	2	6%	2%–14%

KEY: CL, 70% confidence limits.

NOTE: Patients in whom aortic valve replacement was also performed are not included; in the period 1975–July 1, 1979, 3 deaths (5%, CL 2%–9%) occurred among 63 patients in whom combined aortic valve replacement and resection of ascending aortic aneurysm were carried out (see Chapter 12, Table 12-6). Also excluded are patients with acute aortic dissection, who are included in Chapter 54, and those with acute traumatic transections, who are included in Chapter 53.

[a] Four patients (one death) had Marfan's syndrome.

[b] One late after aortic valve replacement; two late after coronary artery bypass grafting.

Table 55-2 Hospital mortality after resection of chronic ascending or transverse arch aortic aneurysms (GLH; 1963–1985).

Year of Operation	n	Hospital Deaths		
		No.	%	CL
1963–1972	7	2	29%	10%–55%
1972–1985	15	1	7%	0.9%–21%
Total	22	3	14%	6%–26%

KEY: CL, 70% confidence limits.

NOTE: Excluded is a 6-year-old patient with an acute mycotic aneurysm of the ascending and transverse arch, who died. Among the 22 patients, the aneurysm involved only the ascending aorta in 4 patients (no deaths), only the transverse arch in 3 (1 death), and both regions in 15 (2 deaths). The last category includes 4 patients (no deaths) undergoing concomitant aortic valve replacement (Bentall's procedure) and 1 patient who had a previous replacement of the descending aorta. In the 18 patients with transverse arch involvement, the entire arch was affected in 13 (1 death), only the proximal arch in 3 (1 death), and only the distal arch in 2 (1 death). Since 1980, only profoundly hypothermic circulatory arrest techniques have been used; before that, most patients had separate perfusion of the arch vessels during the aortic cross-clamp period. The one death in the 1972–1985 era occurred in a patient operated on in 1973.

Table 55-3 Hospital mortality after resection of chronic transverse arch aortic aneurysms (UAB; 1967–July 1984).

Category of Aneurysm	n	Hospital Deaths		
		No.	%	CL
Arteriosclerotic or degenerative	12	5	42%	25%–60%
Chronic aortic dissection	3	1[a]	33%	4%–76%
Marfan's syndrome, nondissecting	1	0	0%	0%–85%
Aortitis, including syphilis	1	1	100%	15%–100%
Postcardiovascular surgery	1	1[a]	100%	15%–100%
Total	18[b]	8	44%	30%–59%

KEY: CL, 70% confidence limits.

NOTE: Excluding the 2 patients who died during preparation, in 4 patients (0 death) the ascending aorta was also resected; in 6 patients (2 deaths) a portion of the descending aorta was also resected; in 2 patients (1 death) both the ascending and a portion of the descending thoracic aorta were also resected. No patient developed paraplegia.

[a] Died during preparations for cardiopulmonary bypass and repair.

[b] Excluding the 2 patients who died during preparations, in 1967–1980, there were 4 deaths (50%, CL 27%–73%) among 8 patients; in 1980–July 1984, there were 2 deaths (25%, CL 9%–50%) among 8 patients.

Table 55-4 Hospital mortality after resection of chronic aneurysms of the descending thoracic aorta (GLH; 1960–1985).

| Year of Operation | n | Hospital Deaths | | |
		No.	%	CL
1960–1972	22	6	27%	17%–40%
1972–1985	36	4	11%	6%–19%
Total	58	10	17%	12%–24%

KEY: CL, 70% confidence limits.

rest,[C19] Ergin and colleagues 3 deaths (21%, CL 10%–38%) among 14 such patients,[E5] and Columbi and colleagues a mortality of 23% (CL 10%–41%) among 13 such patients.[C16] However, the confidence limits of the mortality in these series overlaps with those in which the mortality is about 10%.

Hemorrhage and neurologic death are the most frequent modes of death in patients undergoing these extensive procedures.[A1,L1,M4]

Descending Thoracic Aortic Aneurysms
In the early era, hospital mortality was high. Thus, in 1958, we at the Mayo Clinic had experienced a hospital mortality of 33%,[E2] and in the 1960–1972 period, the mortality at GLH was 27% (Table 55-4). More recently, the results have improved (Tables 55-4, 55-5). Crawford and colleagues report 112 cases, with 10 (9%, CL 6%–13%) hospital deaths, and only 4 deaths (6%, CL 3%–10%) among 69 operated on between 1976 and 1980.[C4]

Hospital mortality is not related to the etiology of the aneurysm (Tables 55-5, 55-6) or to the age of the patient (Table 55-7), nor is there an effect of the technique of the repair on mortality. Thus, Donahoo and colleagues, using the Gott aorto-femoral or left ventricular-femoral shunt, experienced 3 deaths (15%, CL 7%–29%) among 20 patients undergoing repair of aneurysms of the descending aorta,[D11] whereas Crawford's patients have not had a shunt used. When repair is undertaken in the presence of acute rupture of the aneurysm, the mortality is higher.[L5,P4]

Thoracoabdominal Aortic Aneurysms
The repair of thoracoabdominal aneurysms has carried a hospital mortality of 30%–50% in many reported series (Table 55-8). Crawford and associates, however, have re-

Table 55-5 Hospital mortality after resection of chronic aneurysms of the descending thoracic aorta (UAB; 1967–July 1984).

| Category of Aneurysm | n | Hospital Deaths | | |
		No.	%	CL
Arteriosclerotic or degenerative	42	5	12%	7%–19%
Chronic aortic dissection	35	6	17%	10%–26%
Chronic posttraumatic	13	1	8%	1%–24%
Aortitis, including syphilis	1		0%	0%–85%
Postcardiovascular surgery	2		0%	0%–61%
Total	93	12	13%	9%–18%

KEY: CL, 70% confidence limits.

Table 55-6 Hospital mortality after resection of chronic descending thoracic aneurysms (GLH; 1960–1985; n = 58).

| Category of Aneurysm | n | Hospital Deaths | | |
		No.	%	CL
Arteriosclerotic or degenerative	20 (2)	6	30%	19%–44%
Chronic aortic dissection	26 (2)	3 (1)	12%	5%–22%
Chronic posttraumatic	11 (1)	1 (1)	9%	1%–28%
Postcardiovascular surgery	1	0	0%	0%–85%
Total	58 (5)	10 (2)	17%	12%–24%

KEY: CL, 70% confidence limits.
NOTE: The numbers in parentheses indicate the number of patients in the category who underwent an emergency operation for aortic rupture.

ported 4 (10%, CL 5%–17%) hospital deaths among 44 patients with thoracoabdominal aneurysms,[C3] and at GLH the mortality has also been low (Tables 55-9, 55-10).

Total Aortic Replacement
The feasibility of extensive aortic surgery is well illustrated by the experience of Crawford and colleagues, who report total aortic replacement, along with aortic valve replacement, in two stages, in two patients, both of whom survived.[C17] One developed paraparesis.

Paraplegia

It is rare for paraplegia or paraparesis to follow repair of ascending and transverse arch aortic aneurysms, but this complication does occur after the repair of descending and thoracoabdominal aortic aneurysms. It has occurred in 5% of patients undergoing the repair of descending thoracic aortic aneurysm in the combined UAB-GLH experience (Table 55-11), an incidence similar to that reported by others.[C15,N1] Paraplegia and paraparesis seem to occur most commonly after the repair of extensive thoracoabdominal aneurysms (Table 55-10), and in the experience of Crawford and colleagues, 5 (12%, CL 7%–19%) of 42 patients developed them.[C3] There is not a well-documented relationship between the methods used to minimize the incidence of paraplegia and the incidence of this complication.[C3,C4,C15,D11,N1] (See footnote 4.)

Renal Dysfunction and Failure

Renal dysfunction is a common complication of the repair of descending thoracic and thoracoabdominal aortic aneurysm, but it is uncommon that true renal failure develops. This latter complication occurred in 5% (CL 2%–9%) of the patients reported by Carlson and colleagues[C15] and in 3 (3%) of the 96 patients (GLH). Risk factors for renal dysfunction include older age, intraoperative hypotension, and, at least in the experience of Carlson and colleagues, failure to use some sort of shunting procedure.[C15]

Survival

The survival of patients with aneurysms of the aorta is similar, irrespective of the location of the aneurysm, except as

Table 55-7 Hospital mortality after resection of chronic thoracic and thoracoabdominal aortic aneurysms in all locations (GLH; 1960–1985; n = 96).

Age (years)		Descending Thoracic Aorta				Other Sites				Total			
			Hospital Deaths				Hospital Deaths				Hospital Deaths		
≤ <	n	No.	%	CL	n	No.	%	CL	n	No.	%	CL	
10 --- 20	4	0	0%	0%–38%	0				4	0	0%	0%–38%	
20 --- 30	5	0	0%	0%–32%	3	0	0%	0%–47%	8	0	0%	0%–21%	
30 --- 40	6	1	17%	2%–46%	1	0	0%	0%–85%	7	1	14%	2%–41%	
40 --- 50	7	3	43%	20%–68%	4	0	0%	0%–38%	11	3	27%	12%–47%	
50 --- 60	12	2	17%	6%–35%	12	2	17%	6%–35%	24	4	17%	9%–28%	
60 --- 70	17	2	12%	4%–26%	15	3	20%	9%–36%	32	5	16%	9%–25%	
70 --- 80	7	2	29%	10%–55%	3	0	0%	0%–47%	10	2	20%	7%–41%	
Total	58	10	17%	12%–24%	38	5	13%	7%–21%	96	15	16%	12%–20%	
$P(\chi^2)$		.4				.8				.7			

KEY: CL, 70% confidence limits.

Table 55-8 Hospital mortality after resection of chronic thoracoabdominal aortic aneurysms (UAB; 1967–July 1984).

		Hospital Deaths		
Category of Aneurysm	n	No.	%	CL
Arteriosclerotic or degenerative	10	5	50%	30%–70%
Chronic aortic dissection	3	2	67%	24%–96%
Total	13	7	54%	36%–71%

KEY: CL, 70% confidence limits.

Table 55-9 Hospital mortality after resection of chronic thoracoabdominal aortic aneurysms (GLH; 1969–1985).

		Hospital Deaths		
Category of Aneurysm	n	No.	%	CL
Arteriosclerotic or degenerative	14	2	14%	5%–31%
Chronic dissection	1	0	0%	0%–85%
Takayasu's arteritis	1	0	0%	0%–85%
Total	16	2[a]	12%	4%–27%

KEY: CL, 70% confidence limits.

[a] One death in 1971 using the old DeBakey technique[D9] and one from acute rupture during anesthetic induction (resection not performed).

dictated by differences in hospital mortality. Kitamura and colleagues reported a 5-year survival rate of 71% for combined aortic valve and ascending aortic aneurysm resection.[K3] Liddicoat and colleagues reported a similar 5-year survival rate among all patients in whom ascending aortic aneurysm have been resected and saw no difference when aortic valve replacement accompanied the aneurysm resection.[L4] The 5-year survival rate (including hospital mortality) was 60% after a Bentall-type procedure and similar (52%) when the operation was performed with separate valve and ascending aorta replacement (GLH; Fig. 55-15).

For patients who have undergone repair of transverse arch aortic aneurysms, the 5-year survival rate is 55% (GLH; Fig. 55-16). Crawford and colleagues reported a 5-year survival rate of 60% after the repair of descending thoracic aortic aneurysms (Fig. 55-17),[C4] comparable to that of DeBakey and colleagues (Fig. 55-18); and Carlson and colleagues a 5-year survival rate of 73% (UAB; Fig. 55-19).[C15] The 5-year actuarial survival rate after the repair of thoracoabdominal aortic aneurysm is 64% (GLH; Fig. 55-20); Crawford and colleagues have reported one of 62% (Fig. 55-21).[C3]

Survival is considerably better following repair of traumatic aneurysms of the descending thoracic aorta than

Table 55-10 Extent of aortic resection in thoracoabdominal aneurysms (excluding one patient with an aneurysm from the left subclavian artery to aortic bifurcation in whom resection was not performed) related to hospital mortality and incidence of spinal cord damage (GLH; 1969–1985).

Extent of Resection	n	Hospital Deaths	Paraplegia	Paraparesis
Left subclavian artery to inferior mesenteric artery or aortic bifurcation	2	0	1	1
Mid or lower thoracic aorta to inferior mesenteric artery or aortic bifurcation	11	1	0	1
Mid or lower thoracic aorta to superior mesenteric artery	2	0	0	0
Total	15	1 (7%)	1 (7%)	2 (14%)

NOTE: One patient has recovered completely from the paraparesis and the other almost completely.

Table 55-11 Incidence of paraplegia or paraparesis after repair of chronic descending thoracic aneurysms.

Category of Aneurysm	UAB; 1967–July 1984				GLH; 1960–1985				Total			
		Spinal Cord Damage				Spinal Cord Damage				Spinal Cord Damage		
	n	No.	%	CL	n	No.	%	CL	n	No.	%	CL
Arteriosclerotic or degenerative	41	2	5%	2%–11%	17	2	12%	4%–26%	58	4	7%	4%–12%
Chronic dissection	32	0	0%	0%–6%	24	2	8%	3%–19%	56	2	4%	1%–8%
Chronic posttraumatic	13	1	8%	1%–24%	11	0	0%	0%–16%	24	1	4%	0.5%–13%
Total	86	3	3.5%	1.5%–7%	52	4	8%	4%–14%	138	7	5%	3%–8%

KEY: CL, 70% confidence limits.

NOTE: The n in all instances is the number of patients in whom data on spinal cord injury are available. Those whose preoperative status in this regard is not known, those who were paraplegic, and those dying in the operating room are excluded.

when aneurysms in the same portion of the aorta are the result of arteriosclerosis or chronic dissection (Fig. 55-19), no doubt because the remainder of the aorta is more likely to be normal when the aneurysms are the result of trauma. This is evident also from the 5-year survival rate of 52% in Fig. 55-22, which excludes traumatic aneurysms.

Most late deaths in patients who have been surgically treated for atherosclerotic and dissecting aneurysms are due to rupture of new aneurysms that develop at other sites in the aorta, or occasionally to rupture of false aneurysms at graft suture lines. The next most common cause of late death is heart failure and rarely, renal failure.

Reoperation

In a significant number of patients, reoperation is necessary, particularly when there has been a previous aortic dissection. Thus, of 21 patients with adequate follow-up after repair of chronic descending aortic dissection, reoperation was required in 5 patients and an additional 4 died from aneurysm rupture, the latter being theoretically avoidable by reoperation (GLH). The actuarial incidence of new aneurysm formation (patient censored at the time of reoperation or late death from this cause) following surgery for both chronic and acute dissecting aneurysm is 32% at 5 years (Fig. 55-23). In the chronic atheromatous descending aortic aneurysm group, no patients had reoperation but 2 of 12 died from rupture of an associated aortic aneurysm. Thus, as in the case of acute aortic dissection (see Chapter 54), continued follow-up of all aneurysm patients is required and additional operations performed for aneurysms that develop or enlarge.

INDICATIONS FOR OPERATION

In asymptomatic patients, a moderately large or large aneurysm of the ascending or descending thoracic aorta is an indication for operation. Patients with small aneurysms may also be advised to have operation under these circumstances, but it is reasonable to follow them at 3-month intervals and advise prompt operation when enlargement occurs

or symptoms develop. A more pressing indication, such as large size or recent increase in size, may be required in patients with transverse arch or thoracoabdominal aneurysms because of the increased mortality and morbidity of resection of those areas.

Symptomatic aneurysms of any size and location, and those demonstrating an increase in size, are an indication for operation.

SPECIAL SITUATIONS AND CONTROVERSIES

Fibrin Glue

Most surgeons have experienced troublesome and at times exsanguinating hemorrhage from suture lines in friable aortic tissue. New technological advances, particularly fibrin glue, give promise of minimizing this problem in the future.[W3] Furthermore, highly porous grafts may be coated with the fibrin glue so that when in time the glue is absorbed, tissue ingrowth through the graft may anchor solidly into place a thin neointima.[W3]

Intraluminal Sutureless Prosthesis

An intraluminal sutureless prosthesis has been used in the treatment of acute aortic dissection and of chronic thoracic and thoracoabdominal aneurysms (for historical notes and technique of insertion see Chapter 54, ''Intraluminal Sutureless Prosthesis Method of Graft Insertion'' in section on Technique of Operation). Although uncommonly used (GLH and UAB), good results have been obtained by surgeons familiar with its use. Spagna and colleagues report 80 patients with thoracic and thoracoabdominal aneurysms in which the device has been used, with 9 (11%, CL 8%–16%) hospital deaths.[S6] The only complication of the device itself was one instance of dislodgement of the rings, necessitating reoperation early postoperatively. Even in experienced hands, in approximately 40% of patients it is necessary to remove one of the rings and make at that end of the graft a suture anastomosis.[S6]

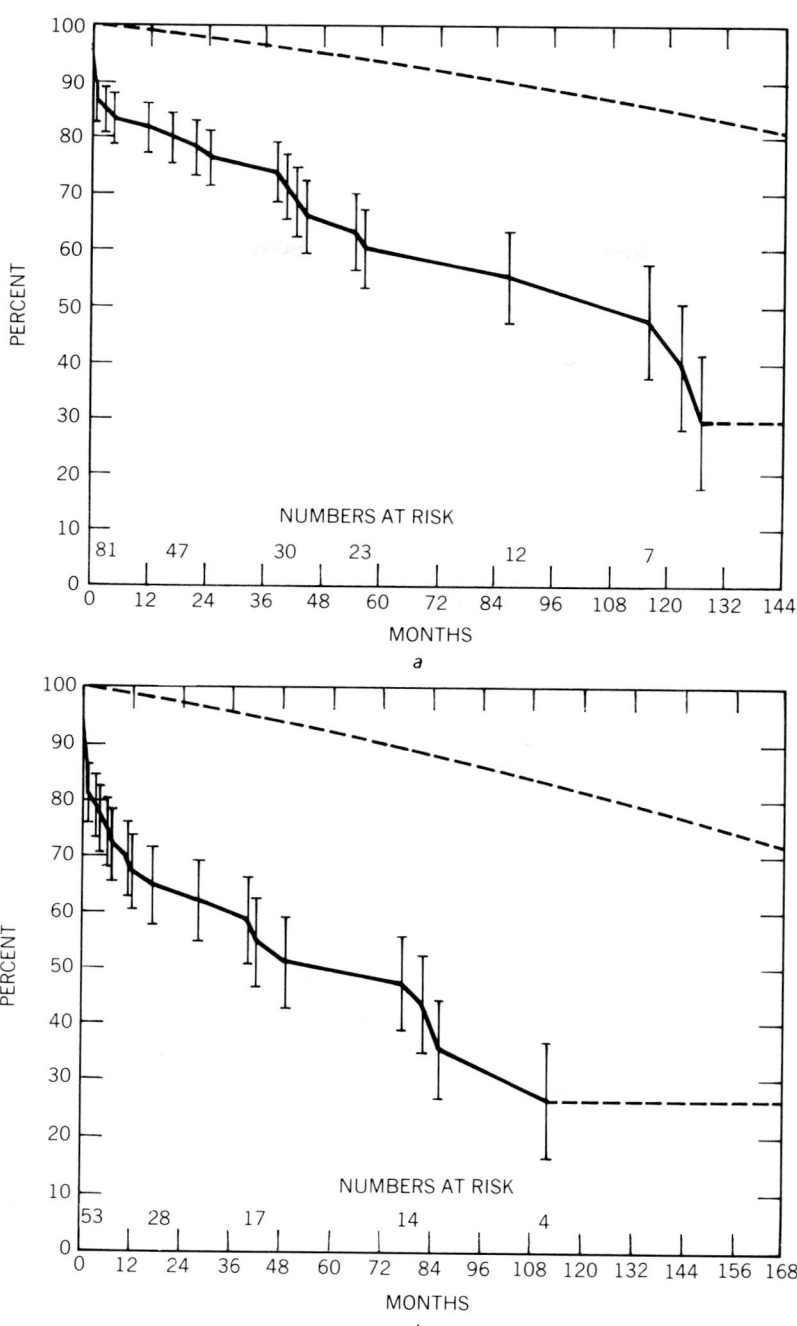

Figure 55-15 Actuarial survival after corrective surgery for ascending aortic arch aneurysm and aortic valve replacement (GLH; 1960–1985). The *n* includes both acute and chronic aneurysms and aneurysms that may have extended distal to the ascending aorta. The numbers at risk are shown. The bars indicate one standard error (equivalent to 70% confidence limits). The dashed line indicates survivors without additional events. The upper dashed line represents survival of a matched general population.
(*a*) Bentall-type procedure (*n* = 81, 11 hospital deaths, 16 late deaths).
(*b*) Non–Bentall-type procedure (*n* = 53, 10 hospital deaths, 16 late deaths).

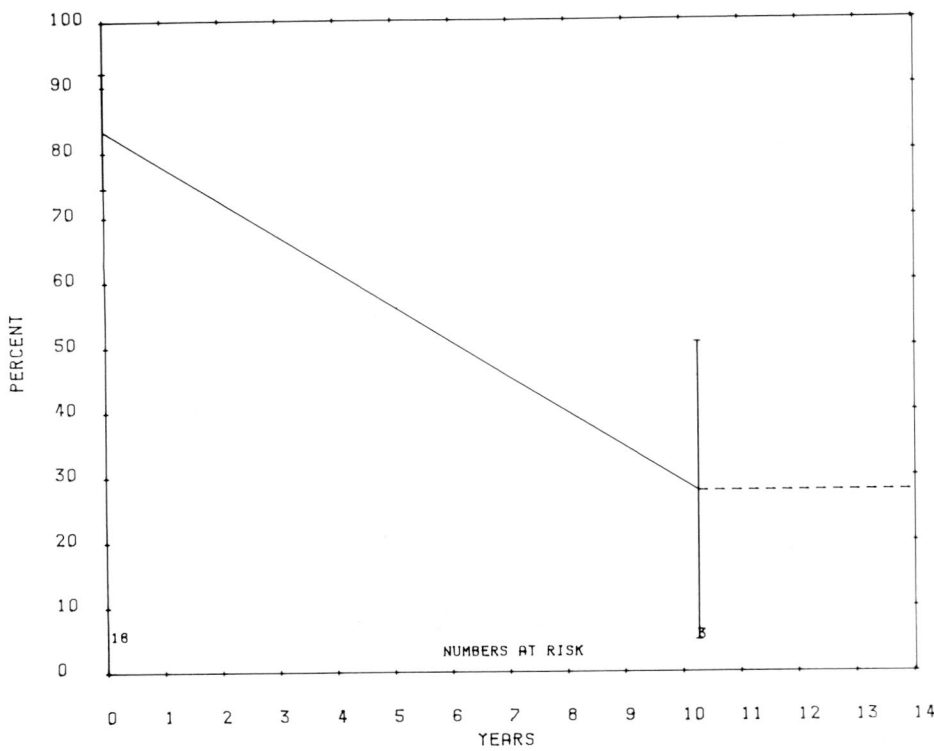

Figure 55-16 Actuarial survival after corrective surgery for chronic transverse aortic arch aneurysms (GLH; 1963–1985; *n* = 18). There were three hospital deaths and two late deaths, one due to ruptured suture line false aneurysm and one to heart failure. The presentation is as in Figure 55-15.

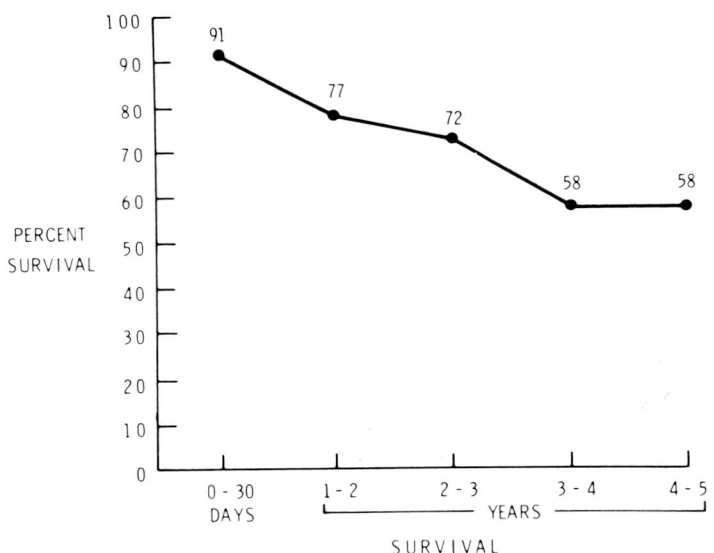

Figure 55-17 Actuarial survival, including hospital deaths, after resection of chronic aneurysms (including those from aortic dissection) of the descending thoracic aorta.

Reproduced with permission from Crawford et al.[C4]

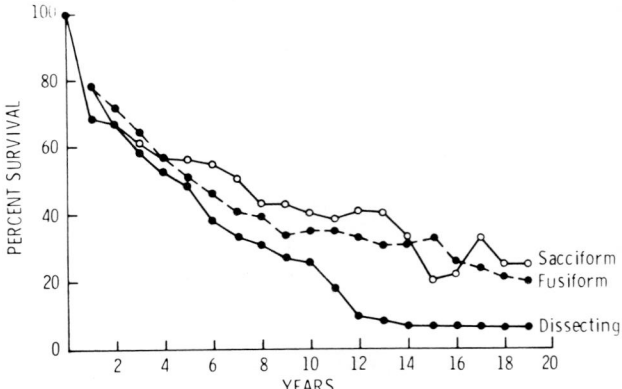

Figure 55-18 Actuarial survival, including an accounting of hospital deaths, after the repair of aneurysm of the descending thoracic aorta (*n* = 500).

Reproduced with permission from DeBakey et al.[D13]

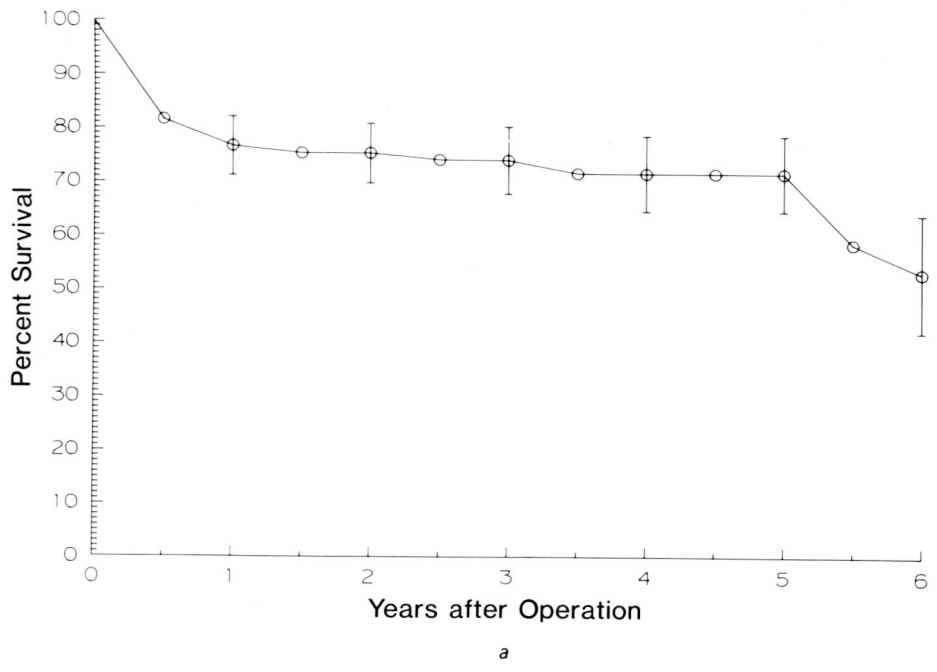

a

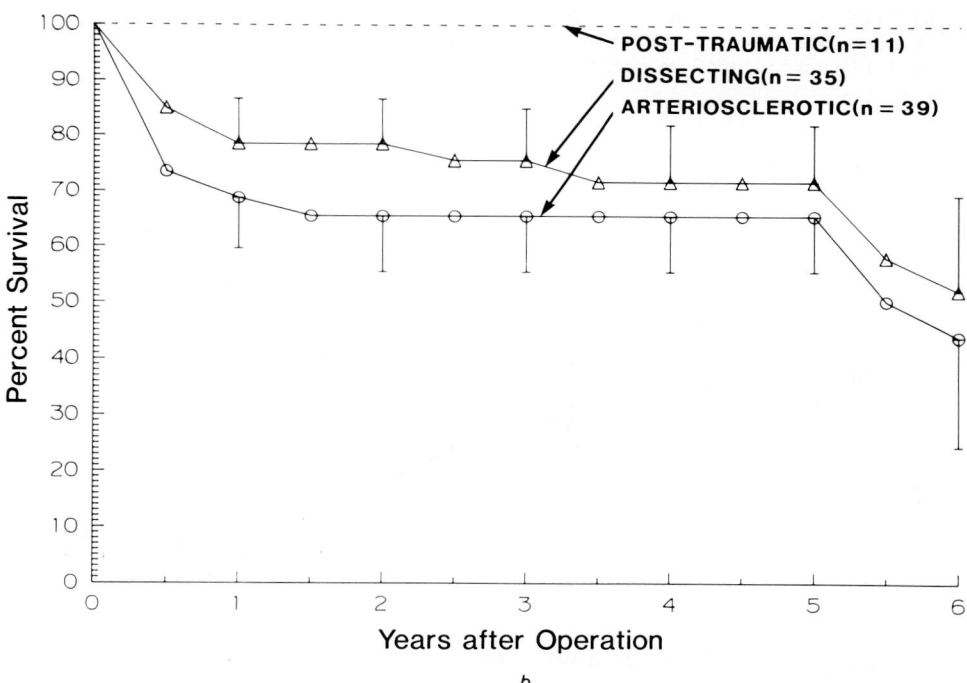

b

Figure 55-19 Actuarial survival, including an accounting of hospital deaths, after resection of aneurysm of the descending thoracic aorta (UAB; 1967–1980). The vertical bars indicate the 70% confidence limits.

(*a*) Survival of the entire group.

(*b*) Survival according to the type of aneurysm.

Modified from Carlson et al.[C15]

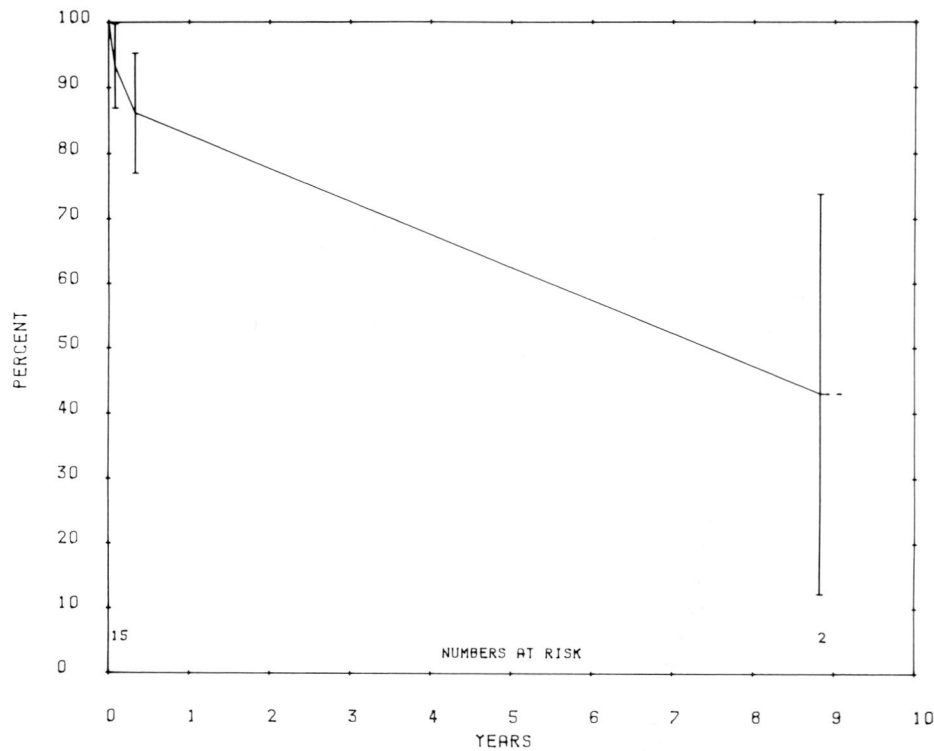

Figure 55-20 Actuarial survival after corrective surgery for chronic thoracoabdominal aortic aneurysms (GLH; 1969–1985; *n* = 15). There were one hospital death and two late deaths, one due to myocardial infarction and one to renal failure. The presentation is as in Figure 55-15.

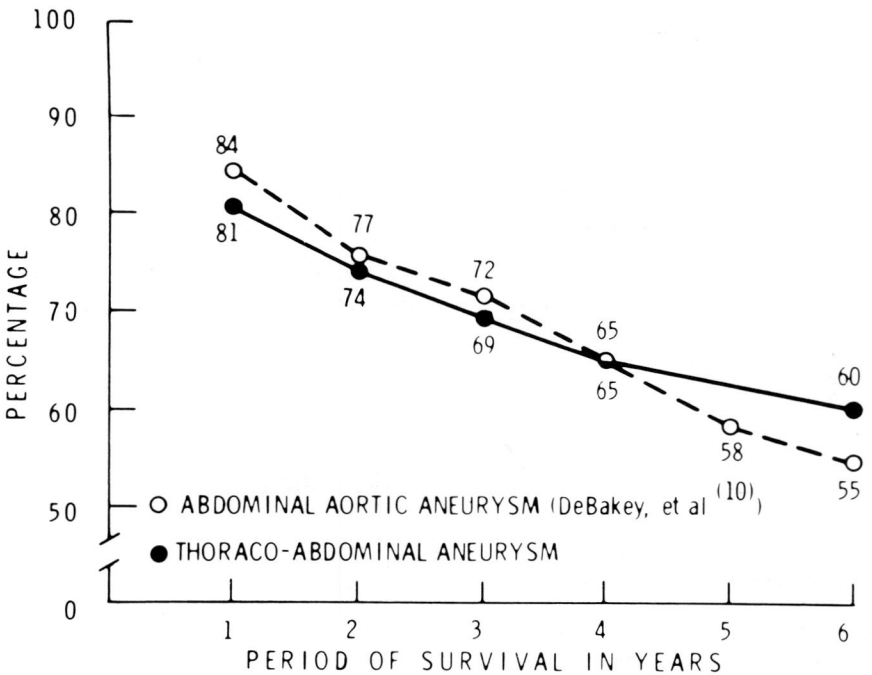

Figure 55-21 Actuarial survival after the repair of thoracoabdominal aortic aneurysms compared with that after resection of abdominal aortic aneurysms.

Reproduced with permission from Crawford et al.;[C3] the data concerning abdominal aortic aneurysms is from DeBakey et al.[D10]

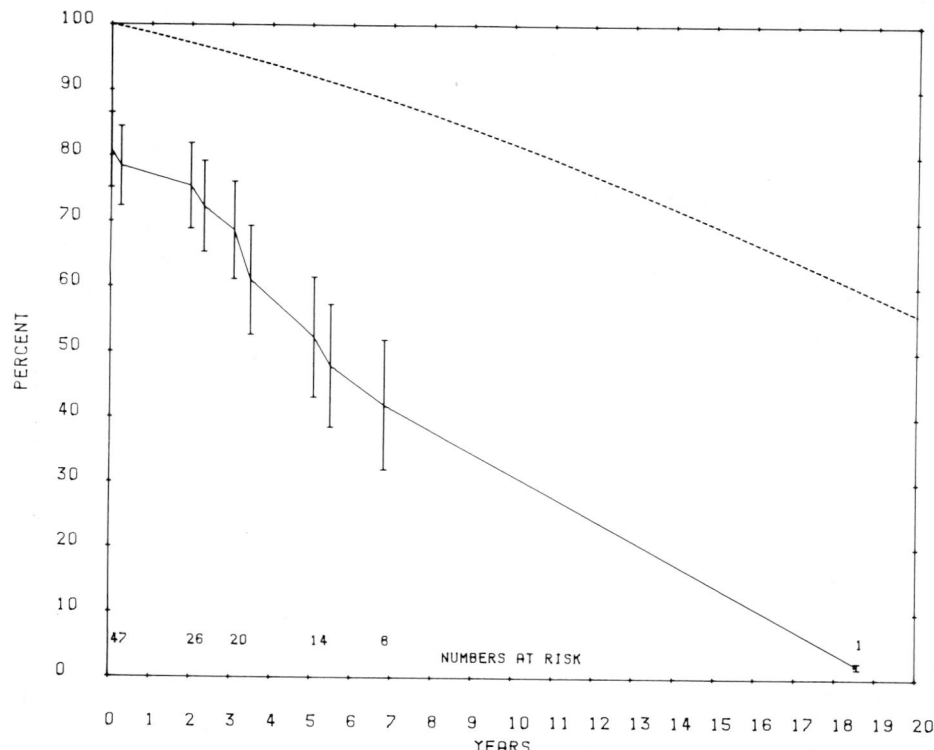

Figure 55-22 Actuarial survival after repair of chronic descending thoracic aortic aneurysm due to atherosclerosis or dissection, excluding traumatic aneurysms (GLH; 1960–1985; *n* = 47). There were 8 hospital deaths and 11 late deaths; 5 patients were lost to follow-up. Eight of the 11 late deaths were the result of further aneurysm formation. The presentation is as in Figure 55-15.

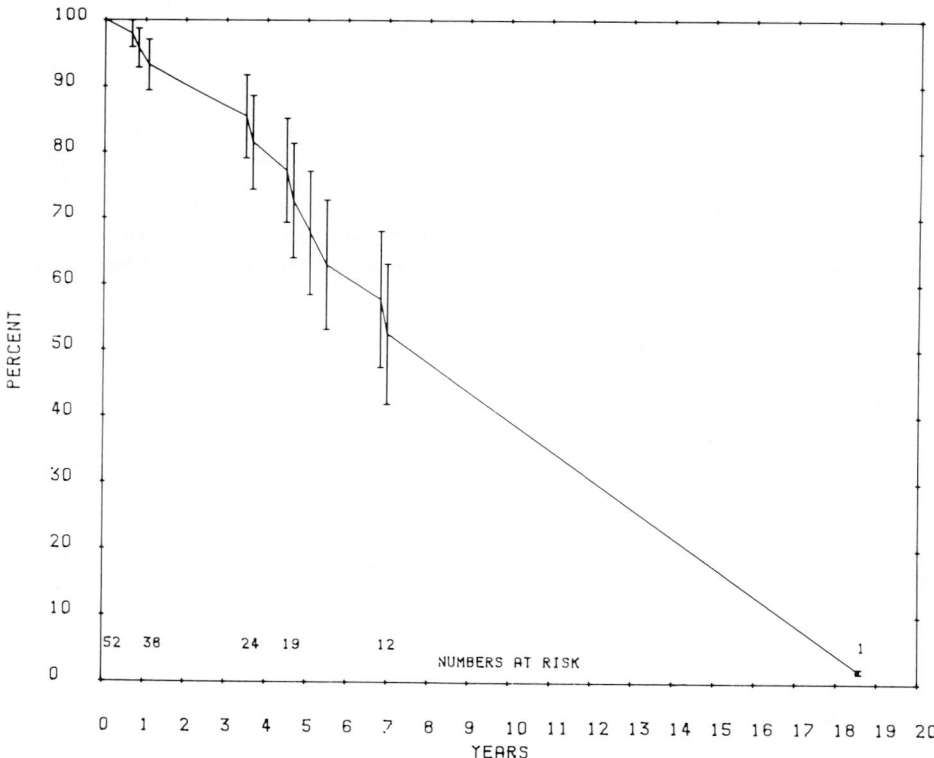

Figure 55-23 Actuarial incidence of patients free of new aneurysm formation requiring reoperation or causing late death after corrective surgery for acute or chronic aortic dissection (GLH; 1960–1985; *n* = 52; 13 events). The data include only hospital survivors and exclude 8 patients with no or an inadequate follow-up. The presentation is as in Figure 55-15.

REFERENCES

A

1. Antunes MJ, Colsen PR, Kinsley RH: Hypothermia and circulatory arrest for surgical resection of aortic arch aneurysms. *J Thorac Cardiovasc Surg* 86:576, 1983.
2. Alexander J, Byron FX: Aortectomy for thoracic aneurysm. *JAMA* 126:1139, 1944.
3. Austin WG, Bleunerhassett JB: Giant cell aortitis causing an aneurysm of the ascending aorta and aortic regurgitation. *N Engl J Med* 272:80, 1965.

B

1. Blakemore AH, Voorhees AB Jr: Aneurysm of the aorta: Review of 365 cases. *Angiology* 5:209, 1954.
2. Bahnson HT: Definitive treatment of saccular aneurysms of the aorta with excision of sac and aortic suture. *Surg Gynecol Obstet* 96:383, 1953.
3. Bloodwell RD, Hallman GL, Cooley DA: Total replacement of the aortic arch and the 'subclavian steal' phenomenon. *Ann Thorac Surg* 5:236, 1968.
4. Bickerstaff LK, Pairolero PC, Hollier LH, Melton LJ, Van Peenen JH, Cherry KJ, Joyce JW, Lie JT: Thoracic aortic aneurysms: A population-based study. *Surgery* 92:1103, 1982.
5. Bentall H, de Bono A: A technique for complete replacement of the ascending aorta. *Thorax* 23:338, 1968.
6. Borst HG, Schaudig A, Rudolph W: Arteriovenous fistula of the aortic arch: Repair during deep hypothermia and circulatory arrest. *J Thorac Cardiovasc Surg* 48:443, 1964.

C

1. Crawford ES, DeBakey ME, Morris GC Jr, Garrett HE, Howell JF: Aneurysm of the abdominal aorta. *Surg Clin North Am* 46:963, 1966.
2. Creech O Jr: Endo-aneurysmorrhaphy and treatment of aortic aneurysm. *Ann Surg* 164:935, 1966.
3. Crawford ES, Snyder DM, Cho GC, Roehm JOF Jr: Progress in treatment of thoraco-abdominal and abdominal aortic aneurysms involving celiac, superior mesenteric, and renal arteries. *Ann Surg* 188:404, 1978.
4. Crawford ES, Walker HSJ III, Saleh SA, Normann NA: Graft replacement of aneurysm in descending thoracic aorta: Results without bypass or shunting. *Surgery* 89:73, 1981.
5. Creech O Jr, DeBakey ME, Mahaffey DE: Total resection of the aortic arch. *Surgery* 40:817, 1956.
6. Carrel A: Permanent intubation of thoracic aorta. *J Exp Med* 16:17, 1912.
7. Crawford ES, Stowe CL, Crawford JL, Titus JL, Weilbaecher DG: Aortic arch aneurysm: A sentinel of extensive aortic disease requiring subtotal and total aortic replacement. *Ann Surg* 199:742, 1984.
8. Cooley DA, DeBakey ME: Surgical considerations of intrathoracic aneurysms of the aorta and great vessels. *Ann Surg* 135:660, 1952.
9. Cooley DA, DeBakey ME: Resection of entire ascending aorta in fusiform aneurysm using cardiac bypass. *JAMA* 162:1158, 1956.
10. Crawford ES, Saleh SA: Transverse aortic arch aneurysm: Improved results of treatment employing new modifications of aortic reconstruction and hypothermic cerebral circulatory arrest. *Ann Surg* 194:180, 1981.
11. Crawford ES, Saleh SA, Schuessler JS: Treatment of aneurysm of transverse aortic arch. *J Thorac Cardiovasc Surg* 78:383, 1979.
12. Cooley DA, Mahaffey DE, DeBakey ME: Total excision of the aortic arch for aneurysm. *Surg Gynecol Obstet* 101:667, 1955.
13. Crawford ES, Crawford JL: *Diseases of the Aorta including an Atlas of Angiographic Pathology and Surgical Technique.* Baltimore: Williams & Wilkins, 1984.
14. Crawford ES: Thoraco-abdominal and abdominal aortic aneurysms involving renal, superior mesenteric, and celiac arteries. *Ann Surg* 179:763, 1974.
15. Carlson DE, Karp RB, Kouchoukos NT: Surgical treatment of aneurysms of the descending thoracic aorta: An analysis of 85 patients. *Ann Thorac Surg* 35:58, 1983.
16. Columbi P, Rossi C, Porrini AM, Pellegrini A: Aneurysms involving the aortic arch: Report on thirteen surgically treated patients. *Thorac Cardiovasc Surg* 31:234, 1983.
17. Crawford ES, Crawford JL, Stowe CL, Safi HF: Total aortic replacement for chronic aortic dissection occurring in patients with and without Marfan's syndrome. *Ann Surg* 199:358, 1984.
18. Crawford ES, Snyder DM: Treatment of aneurysms of the aortic arch. *J Thorac Cardiovasc Surg* 85:237, 1983.
19. Culliford AT, Ayvaliotis B, Shemin R, Colvin SB, Isom OW, Spencer FC: Aneurysms of the ascending aorta and transverse arch. *J Thorac Cardiovasc Surg* 83:701, 1982.
20. Culliford AT, Ayvaliotis B, Shemin R, Colvin SB, Isom OW, Spencer FC: Aneurysms of the descending aorta. *J Thorac Cardiovasc Surg* 85:98, 1983.

D

1. Dubost C, Allary M, Oeconomos N: Resection of an aneurysm of the abdominal aorta: Reestablishment of the continuity by a preserved human arterial graft, with result after five months. *Arch Surg* 64:405, 1952.
2. Deterling RA Jr, Bhonslay SB: An evaluation of synthetic materials and fabrics suitable for blood vessel replacement. *Surgery* 38:71, 1955.
3. De Takats G, Reynolds JT: The surgical treatment of aneurysms of the abdominal aorta. *Surgery* 21:443, 1947.
4. DeBakey ME, Cooley DA: Surgical treatment of aneurysm of abdominal aorta by resection and restoration of continuity with homograft. *Surg Gynecol Obstet* 97:157, 1953.
5. DeBakey ME, Crawford ES, Cooley DA, Morris GC Jr: Successful resection of fusiform aneurysm of aortic arch with replacement by homograft. *Surg Gynecol Obstet* 105:657, 1957.
6. DeBakey ME, Cooley DA: Successful resection of aneurysm of distal aortic arch and replacement by graft. *JAMA* 155:1398, 1954.
7. DeBakey ME, Cooley DA: Successful resection of aneurysm of thoracic aorta and replacement by graft. *JAMA* 152:673, 1953.
8. DeBakey ME, Creech O Jr, Morris GC Jr: Aneurysm of thoraco-abdominal aorta involving the celiac, superior mesenteric, and renal arteries: Report of four cases treated by resection and homograft replacement. *Ann Surg* 144:549, 1956.
9. DeBakey ME, Crawford ES, Garrett HE: Surgical considerations in the treatment of aneurysms of the thoraco-abdominal aorta. *Ann Surg* 162:650, 1965.

10. DeBakey ME, Crawford ES, Cooley DA: Aneurysm of abdominal aorta: Analysis of results of graft replacement therapy one to eleven years after operation. *Ann Surg* 160:622, 1964.

11. Donahoo JS, Brawley RK, Gott VL: The heparin-coated vascular shunt for thoracic aortic and great vessel procedures: A ten-year experience. *Ann Thorac Surg* 23:507, 1977.

12. Donaldson RM, Ross DN: Composite graft replacement for the treatment of aneurysms of the ascending aorta associated with aortic valvular disease. *Circulation* 66(suppl I)I-116, 1982.

13. DeBakey ME, McCollum CH, Graham JM: Surgical treatment of aneurysms of the descending thoracic aorta: Long-term results in 500 patients. *J Cardiovasc Surg* 19:571, 1978.

14. Dennison AR, Watkins RM, Gunning AJ: Simultaneous aortic and pulmonary artery aneurysms due to giant cell arteritis. *Thorax* 40:156, 1985.

E

1. Estes JE Jr: Abdominal aortic aneurysm: A study of 102 cases. *Circulation* 2:258, 1950.

2. Ellis FH Jr, Kirklin JW, Bruwer AJ: Surgical experiences in the treatment of aneurysms of the thoracic aorta. *Surg Gynecol Obstet* 106:179, 1958.

3. Ellis FH Jr, Helden RA, Hines EA Jr: Aneurysm of the abdominal aorta involving the right renal artery: Report of case with preservation of renal function after resection and grafting. *Ann Surg* 142:992, 1955.

4. Etheredge SN, Yee J, Smith JV, Schonberger S, Goldman MJ: Successful resection of a large aneurysm of the upper abdominal aorta and replacement with homograft. *Surgery* 38:1071, 1955.

5. Ergin MA, O'Connor J, Guinto R, Griepp RB: Experience with profound hypothermia and circulatory arrest in the treatment of aneurysms of the aortic arch. *J Thorac Cardiovasc Surg* 84:649, 1982.

6. Edwards WS, Kerr AR: A safer technique for replacement of the entire ascending aorta and aortic valve. *J Thorac Cardiovasc Surg* 59:837, 1970.

F

1. Fisher DF, Yawn DH, Crawford ES: Preoperative disseminated intravascular coagulation associated with aortic aneurysms. *Arch Surg* 118:1252, 1983.

2. Finkelmeier BA, Mentzer RM Jr, Kaiser DL, Tegtmeyer CJ, Nolan ST: Chronic traumatic thoracic aneurysm. *J Thorac Cardiovasc Surg* 84:257, 1982.

3. Fleming AW, Green DC: Traumatic aneurysms of the thoracic aorta. *Ann Thorac Surg* 18:91, 1974.

G

1. Gross RE, Bill AH Jr, Peirce EC II: Methods for preservation and transplantation of arterial grafts: Observations on arterial grafts in dogs. Report of transplantation of preserved arterial grafts in nine human cases. *Surg Gynecol Obstet* 88:689, 1949.

2. Griepp RB, Stinson EB, Hollingsworth JF, Buehler D: Prosthetic replacement of the aortic arch. *J Thorac Cardiovasc Surg* 70:1051, 1975.

3. Gross RE, Hurwitt ES, Bill AH Jr, Peirce EC: Preliminary observations on the use of human arterial grafts in the treatment of certain cardiovascular defects. *New Engl J Med* 239:578, 1948.

4. Grey DP, Ott DA, Cooley DA: Surgical treatment of aneurysm of the ascending aorta with aortic insufficiency. *J Thorac Cardiovasc Surg* 86:864, 1983.

5. Gelfand M: Giant cell arteritis with aneurysmal formation in an infant. *Br Heart J* 17:264, 1955.

6. Gelman S, Reves JG, Fowler K, Samuelson PN, Lell WA, Smith LR: Regional blood flow during cross-clamping of the thoracic aorta and infusion of sodium nitroprusside. *J Thorac Cardiovasc Surg* 85:287, 1983.

H

1. Hood RT Jr, Kirklin JW: Usefulness of the abdominothoracic incision. *Surg Clin North Am* 33:1447, 1953.

2. Helden RA, Kirklin JW, Gifford RW Jr: The treatment of abdominal aortic aneurysms by excision and grafting. *Proc Staff Meet Mayo Clin* 28:707, 1953.

J

1. Johnston JB, Kirklin JW, Brandenburg RO: The treatment of saccular aneurysms of the thoracic aorta. *Proc Staff Meet Mayo Clin* 28:723, 1953.

2. Javid H, Julian OC, Dye WS, Hunter JA: Complications of abdominal aortic grafts. *Arch Surg* 85:142, 1962.

3. Joyce JW, Fairbairn JF, Kincaid OW, Juergens JL: Aneurysms of the thoracic aorta: A clinical study with special reference to prognosis. *Circulation* 29:176, 1964.

K

1. Kouchoukos NT, Lell WA, Karp RB, Samuelson PN: Hemodynamic effects of aortic clamping and decompression with a temporary shunt for resection of the descending thoracic aorta. *Surgery* 85:25, 1979.

2. Kirklin JW, Waugh JM, Grindlay JH, Openshaw CR, Allen EV: Surgical treatment of arteriosclerotic aneurysms of the abdominal aorta. *AMA Arch Surg* 67:632, 1953.

3. Kitamura S, Onishi K, Nakano S, Kawachi K, Kawashima Y: Early and late results of the Bentall operation for annulo-aortic ectasia. *J Cardiovasc Surg* 24:5, 1983.

L

1. Livesay JJ, Cooley DA, Reul GJ, Walker WE, Frazier H, Duncan JM, Ott DA: Resection of aortic arch aneurysms: A comparison of hypothermic techniques in 60 patients. *Ann Thorac Surg* 36:19, 1983.

2. Lam CR, Aram HH: Resection of the descending thoracic aorta for aneurysm: A report of the use of a homograft in a case and an experimental study. *Ann Surg* 134:743, 1951.

3. Lemann II: Aneurysms of the thoracic aorta: Its incidence, diagnosis, and prognosis: A statistical study. *Am J Med Sci* 152:210, 1916.

4. Liddicoat JE, Bekassy SM, Rubio PA, Noon GP, DeBakey ME: Ascending aortic aneurysms. *Circulation* 51,52(supp I):I-202, 1975.

5. Livesay JJ, Cooley DA, Ventemiglia RA, Montero CG, Warrian RK, Brown DM, Duncan JM: Surgical experience in descending thoracic aneurysmectomy with and without adjuncts to avoid ischemia. *Ann Thorac Surg* 39:37, 1985.

M

1. Matas RA: An operation for the radical cure of aneurysm based upon arteriorrhaphy: With the report of four cases successfully operated upon by the author. *Transactions of the American Surgical Association* 20:396, 1902.

2. Mortensen JD, Grindlay JH, Kirklin JW: The arterial homograft bank. *Proc Staff Meet Mayo Clin* 28:713, 1953.

3. McNamara JJ, Pressler VM: Natural history of arteriosclerotic thoracic aortic aneurysms. *Ann Thorac Surg* 26:468, 1978.

4. Mahfood S, Qasi A, Garcia J, Mispireta L, Corso P, Smyth N: Management of aortic arch aneurysm using profound hypothermia and circulatory arrest. *Ann Thorac Surg* 39:412, 1985.

5. Moreno-Cabral CE, Miller DC, Mitchell RS, Stinson EB, Oyer PE, Jamieson SW, Shumway NE: Degenerative and atherosclerotic aneurysms of the thoracic aorta. *J Thorac Cardiovasc Surg* 88:1020, 1984.

N

1. Najafi H, Dye WS, Javid H, Hunter JA, Goldin MD, Serry C: Aortic insufficiency secondary to aortic root aneurysm or dissection. *Arch Surg* 110:1401, 1975.

O

1. Ott DA, Frazier OH, Cooley DA: Resection of the aortic arch using deep hypothermia and temporary circulatory arrest. *Circulation* 58(suppl I):I-227, 1978.

2. Oyama M, McNamara J, Suehiro GT, Suehiro A, Sue-Ako K: The effects of thoracic aortic cross-clamping and declamping on visceral organ blood flow. *Ann Surg* 197:459, 1983.

P

1. Peirce EC II, Gross RE, Bill AH Jr, Merrill K Jr: Tissue-culture evaluation of the viability of blood vessels stored by refrigeration. *Ann Surg* 129:333, 1949.

2. Pressler V, McNamara JJ: Thoracic aortic aneurysm. *J Thorac Cardiovasc Surg* 79:489, 1980.

3. Pearce CW, Weichert RF III, del Real RE: Aneurysms of aortic arch. *J Thorac Cardiovasc Surg* 58:886, 1969.

4. Pressler V, McNamara JJ: Aneurysm of the thoracic aorta. Review of 260 cases. *J Thorac Cardiovasc Surg* 89:50, 1985.

R

1. Roberts AJ, Nora JD, Hughes WA, Quintanilla AP, Ganote CE, Sanders JH Jr, Moran JM, Michaelis LL: Cardiac and renal responses to cross-clamping of the descending thoracic aorta. *J Thorac Cardiovasc Surg* 86:732, 1983.

S

1. Shumacker HB Jr, King H: The use of pliable plastic tubes as aortic substitutes in man. *Surg Gynecol Obstet* 99:287, 1954.

2. Schafer PW, Hardin CA: The use of temporary polythene shunts to permit occlusion, resection and frozen homologous graft replacement of vital vessel segments: A laboratory and clinical study. *Surgery* 31:186, 1952.

3. Stranahan A, Alley RD, Sewell WH, Kausel HW: Aortic arch resection and grafting for aneurysm employing an external shunt. *J Thorac Surg* 29:54, 1955.

4. Swan H, Maaske C, Johnson M, Grover R: Arterial homografts. *Arch Surg* 61:732, 1950.

5. Symbas PN, Pfaender LM, Drucker MH, Lester JL, Gravanis MB, Zacharopoulos L: Cross-clamping of the descending aorta. *J Thorac Cardiovasc Surg* 85:300, 1983.

6. Spagna PM, Lemole GM, Strong M, Karmilowicz NP: Rigid intraluminal prosthesis for replacement of thoracic and abdominal aorta. *Ann Thorac Surg* 39:47, 1985.

W

1. Wheat MW, Boruchow IB, Ramsey HW: Surgical treatment of aneurysms of the aortic root. *Ann Thorac Surg* 12:593, 1971.

2. Wheat MW Jr, Wilson JR, Bartley TD: Successful replacement of the entire ascending aorta and aortic valve. *JAMA* 188:717, 1964.

3. Walterbusch G, Haverich A, Borst HG: Clinical experience with fibrin glue for local bleeding control and sealing of vascular prostheses. *Thorac Cardiovasc Surg* 30:234, 1982.

Z

1. Zumbro GL, Henley LB, Treasure RL: Saccular aneurysm of ascending aorta caused by granulomatous aortitis in a child. *J Thorac Cardiovasc Surg* 69:397, 1975.

INDEX

1525